THE LIPPINCOTT
MANUAL OF
Nursing
Practice

Sandra M. Nettina,
MSN, RN, CS, ANP

Nurse Practitioner,
Glenelg, Maryland

Adjunct Faculty
George Washington University
Washington, D.C.

George Mason University
Fairfax, Virginia

THE LIPPINCOTT

MANUAL OF
Nursing
Practice

SEVENTH EDITION

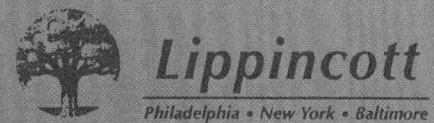

Lippincott

Philadelphia • New York • Baltimore

Acquisitions Editor: Lisa Stead
Managing Editor: Claudia Vaughn
Senior Project Editor: Tom Gibbons
Senior Production Manager: Helen Ewan
Production Coordinator: Michael Carcel
Art Director: Carolyn O'Brien
Interior Design: Holly Reid McGlaughlin
Indexer: Ellen Brennan

7th Edition

Library of Congress Cataloging in Publications Data

The Lippincott manual of nursing practice—7th ed. / [edited by Sandra M. Nettina].
    p. ; cm.
  Includes bibliographical references and index.
  ISBN 0-7817-2296-9 (cloth : alk. paper)
    1. Nursing—Handbooks, manuals, etc. I. Title: Manual of nursing practice. II. Title: Nursing practice. III. Nettina, Sandra M.
    [DNLM: 1. Nursing Care—Handbooks. WY 49 L765 2000]
  RT51.B78 2000
  610.73—dc21   00-034902

Care has been taken to confirm the accuracy of the information presented and to describe generally accepted practices. However, the authors, editors, and publisher are not responsible for errors or omissions or for any consequences from application of the information in this book and make no warranty, express or implied, with respect to the contents of the publication.

The authors, editors and publisher have exerted every effort to ensure that drug selection and dosage set forth in this text are in accordance with current recommendations and practice at the time of publication. However, in view of ongoing research, changes in government regulations, and the constant flow of information relating to drug therapy and drug reactions, the reader is urged to check the package insert for each drug for any change in indications and dosage and for added warnings and precautions. This is particularly important when the recommended agent is a new or infrequently employed drug.

Some drugs and medical devices presented in this publication have Food and Drug Administration (FDA) clearance for limited use in restricted research settings. It is the responsibility of the health care provider to ascertain the FDA status of each drug or device planned for use in their clinical practice.

9 8 7 6 5 4 3 2 1

Dedicated to the faculty, staff, and alumni of Sisters of Charity Hospital School of Nursing, Buffalo, New York. The doors closed in 1999 after 100 years of service, but the memories and culture of caring live on.

Also dedicated to Dan Nettina, my computer consultant, photographer, accountant, and messenger; and to Adam and Carol Nettina, who make everything worthwhile.

Contributors

Marg Brady, RN
Nephrology Clinic Nurse
The Hospital for Sick Children
Toronto, Canada

Chapter 49 Pediatric Renal and Genitourinary Disorders

Susan E. Brown, RN, MS
Clinical Coordinator, Transitional Care
Mercy Medical Center
Baltimore, Maryland

Chapter 16 Eye Disorders

Sarah Cameron, RN, BScN, Cneph
Clinical Nurse, Nephrology Department
The Hospital for Sick Children
Toronto, Canada

Chapter 49 Pediatric Renal and Genitourinary Disorders

Jeanette Campbell, RN, MSN, PNP
Quaker Medical Associates
Orchard Park, New York
PNP Preceptor, University of Buffalo
Buffalo, New York

Chapter 56 Developmental Disabilities

Jancintha Cauffield, PharmD, BCPS
Clinical Pharmacy Specialist
GeM Integrative Pharmacotherapy, Inc.
Jupiter, Florida

Appendix IV Herbal Preparations Used as Health Remedies

Joanne Coleman, RN, MS, ACNP, AOCN
Acute Care Nurse Practitioner
Gastrointestinal Surgery/Pancreas and Biliary
Department of Surgical Nursing
Johns Hopkins Hospital
Baltimore, Maryland

Chapter 19 Hepatic, Biliary, and Pancreatic Disorders

Carol De Clue, RN, MSN, CRNP
Nurse Practitioner, Breast Center
Johns Hopkins Hospital
Baltimore, Maryland

Chapter 8 Cancer Nursing

Lori DiMillo, RN, BSN
Quaker Medical Group
Orchard Park, New York
Student Pediatric Nurse Practitioner
University of Buffalo
Buffalo, New York

Chapter 48 Pediatric Gastrointestinal and Nutritional Disorders

Laureen Doloresco, MN, RN, CNAA
Assistant Chief of Nursing Services for Spinal Cord
    Injury/Rehabilitation
Nursing Services Department
James A. Haley Veteran's Hospital
Tampa, Florida

Chapter 15 Neurologic Disorders

Dale Drucker, MSN, CRNP
Nurse Practitioner, Adolescent Medicine
St. Christopher's Hospital for Children
Philadelphia, Pennsylvania

Chapter 55 Pediatric Integumentary Disorders

Carolyn Farrell, BS, MS, RN, CNP, CGC
Director, Clinical Genetics Service
Surgical Oncology
Rosewell Park Cancer Institute
Buffalo, New York

Chapter 4 Genetics and Health Applications

Marla Faust, MSN, FNP, PNP
Johns Hopkins School of Nursing
Baltimore, Maryland

Chapter 20 Nutritional Problems

Susan Dill Fishcera, RN, MSN
Family Nurse Practitioner
Southeastern Surgical Group
Tallahassee, Florida

Chapter 23 Breast Conditions

Cathy Flynn, RN, MSN, CPNP
Pediatric Nurse Practitioner
Pediatric Outpatient Services
University Medical Center
Las Vegas, Nevada

Chapter 50 Pediatric Metabolic and Endocrine Disorders

Catherine A. Freer, MS, RNC, CPNP
Pediatric Nurse Practitioner—Research Study Coordinator
Pediatric Hematology Department
Johns Hopkins University
Baltimore, Maryland

Chapter 52 Pediatric Hematologic Disorders

Christine Campion Fuller, RN
Clinical Nurse, Rheumatology Department
Royal Victoria Hospital
Montreal, Canada

Chapter 53 Pediatric Immunologic Disorders

Elizabeth Fuss, RN, MS, CIC
Infection Control Practitioner
Johns Hopkins Hospital
Baltimore, Maryland

Chapter 31 Infectious Diseases

Chris Garvey, RN, BSN, MPA
Coordinator, Pulmonary and Cardiac Rehabilitation
Seton Medical Center Dept. of Pulmonary Rehabilitation
Dale City, California

Chapter 10 Respiratory Function and Therapy
Chapter 11 Respiratory Disorders

Charles Gilkison, RN, MSP, FNP
Nurse Practitioner, Department of Endocrinology
Clinical Faculty
University of Texas School of Nursing at Galveston
Galveston, Texas

Chapter 24 Endocrine Disorders

Peggy Guin, PhD, ARNP, CNRN
Nursing Research, Quality Control
Nursing and Patient Services
Shands and the University of Florida
Gainesville, Florida

Chapter 15 Neurologic Disorders

Karen Hennessy, RN, MS, CPNP
Pediatric Nurse Practitioner
Johns Hopkins University
Baltimore, Maryland

Chapter 51 Pediatric Oncology

Ann Isaacs, RN, CS, MSN
Professor
Luzerne County Community College
Nanticoke, Pennsylvania

Chapter 57 Problems of Mental Health

Patricia L. Kane, RN, MSN, CS, CPNP
Nurse Practitioner—Pediatric Cardiology and Cardiac Surgery
Johns Hopkins Hospital
Baltimore, Maryland

Chapter 45 Pediatric Cardiovascular Disorders

Carol Kilmon, PhD, RN, CPNP
Pediatric Nurse Practitioner
General Pediatrics Department
The University of Texas Health Center at Tyler
Associate Professor, College of Nursing
The University of Texas at Tyler
Tyler, Texas

Chapter 47 Pediatric Eye and Ear Problems

Anna Komelasky, RN, MSN, CPNP
Pediatric Nurse Practitioner
Kaiser Permanente
Manassas, Virginia

Chapter 46 Pediatric Neurologic Disorders

Margaret Konefal, PhD, RN
Director of Women and Infant Services
Ben Taub Hospital
Houston, Texas

Chapter 43 Care of the Sick or Hospitalized Child

Debra Kosko, MN, FNP-C
Instructor, School of Nursing
Johns Hopkins Hospital
Baltimore, Maryland

Chapter 29 HIV Disease and AIDS

Adrianne Louloudes, MSN, RN
Pediatric Pulmonary Clinical Nurse Specialist
Chicago, Illinois

Chapter 44 Pediatric Respiratory Disorders

Ruth Manchester, RN, MA, OCN, CRNI
IV Therapist, IV Therapy Department
Holy Cross Hospital
Silver Spring, Maryland

Chapter 6 IV Therapy

Sally Matson, RN, BSN, MS, CWOCN
Private CWOCN Consultant
Orlando, Florida

Chapter 18 Gastrointestinal Disorders

Donna McCabe, RN, BSN, MSN, C.N.A. CEN
Nurse Manager
Emergency Department
Sisters of Charity Health Care System
Staten Island, New York

Chapter 35 Emergent Conditions

Cherly McGinnis, MA, MSN, ARNP
Nurse Practitioner/Clinical Coordinator
Pediatric Liver Transplant
University of Florida
Gainsville, Florida

Chapter 18 Gastrointestinal Disorders

Susan Miller, MSN, RN, CS
Advanced Practice Vascular Nurse
Cardiovascular/Transplant/Dialysis Nursing
Medical College of Virginia
Hospital of Virginia Commonwealth University
Richmond, Virginia

Chapter 14 Vascular Disorders

Nancy Mooney, MA, RN, ONC
Director of Nursing
NursingHands.com
New York, New York

Chapter 32 Musculoskeletal Disorders

Patricia Mosko, RN, MSN, CRNP
Adult Nurse Practitioner
General Medicine/Primary Care
Philadelphia Veterans Affairs Medical Center
Philadelphia, Pennsylvania

Chapter 30 Connective Tissue Disorders

Victoria Niederhauser, DrPH, APRN, PNP
Pediatric Nurse Practitioner
Kaiser Permanente
Honolulu, Hawaii
Adjunct Faculty
George Washington University
Washington, D.C.

Chapter 42 Pediatric Primary Care

Julia Olijnyk
Legal Nurse Consultant
Research Nurse Practitioner
George Washington University
Washington, D.C.

Chapter 2 Standards of Care, Ethical and Legal Issues

Lana Parson, MS, MA, ANRC
Burn Trauma Coordinator
Baltimore Regional Burn Center
Johns Hopkins Bayview Medical Center
Baltimore, Maryland

Chapter 34 Burns

Patricia Quigley, RhD, ARNP, CRRN
Rehabilitation Clinical Nurse Specialist
Nursing Services
James A. Haley Veterans' Hospital
Tampa, Florida

Chapter 15 Neurologic Disorders

Nancy Reilly, MSN, RN, CURN, NPC
Director, Clinical Services
Shore Continence Center, P. C.
Lakewood, New Jersey

Chapter 21 Renal and Urinary Disorders

Barbara Resnick, PhD, CRNP
Assistant Professor
Nursing Department
University of Maryland
Baltimore, Maryland

Chapter 9 Care of the Older Adult

Beth Rodgers, RN, BSN, CNOR
Advanced Clinical Nurse
Mercy Medical Center
Baltimore, Maryland

Chapter 7 Perioperative Nursing

Jane Shivnan, RN, MScN
Nurse Manager, Oncology Department
Johns Hopkins Hospital
Baltimore, Maryland

Chapter 26 Hematologic Disorders
Chapter 27 Transfusion Therapy and Blood and Marrow
Stem Cell Transplantation

Joan Bauman Skawski, RN, MA, CCRN
Nurse Case Manager
F. F. Thompson Hospital
Canandaigua, New York
President and Educator
Vinegar Hill, Ltd.

Chapter 12 Cardiovascular Function and Therapy
Chapter 13 Cardiac Disorders

Elizabeth Smith, RN, BSN, PNP
Quaker Medical Associates
Orchard Park, New York

Chapter 56 Developmental Disorders

Thomas Stuart, RN, BSN
Endocrine Specialty Representative
Humatrope Growth Hormone
Eli Lilly and Company
Phoenix, Arizona

Chapter 50 Pediatric Metabolic and Endocrine Disorders

Susan Thomason, MN, RN, CS, CETN
Coordinator, Spinal Cord Injuries/Disorders
Outpatient Center
Spinal Cord Injury/Disorder Services
James A. Haley Veterans' Hospital
Tampa, Florida

Chapter 15 Neurologic Disorders

Keiko Torgersen, RNC, BSN, MSM
Commander
82nd Aerospace Medicine Squadron
Air Education and Training Command Consultant for Perinatal
Nursing
Sheppard Air Force Base, Texas

Chapter 36 Maternal and Fetal Health
Chapter 37 Nursing Management During Labor and Delivery
Chapter 38 Care of the Mother and Newborn During the
Postpartum Period
Chapter 39 Complications of the Childbearing Experience

M. Claire Walsek, BSN, MS, CPNP
Pediatric Nurse Practitioner
National Institutes of Health
Bethesda, Maryland

Chapter 53 Pediatric Immunologic Disorders HIV and AIDS

Maria Zak, RN, BScN
Orthopedic Clinical Nurse Coordinator
The Hospital for Sick Children
Toronto, Canada

Chapter 54 Pediatric Orthopedic Problems

Clinical Consultants

Debbie Askin, MN, RNC
Neonatal Nurse Practitioner
Neonatal Intensive Care Unit
St. Boniface General Hospital
Winnipeg, Manitoba

Tom Bartol, MN, BSN
Family Nurse Practitioner
Health Reach
Richmond Area Health Center
Richmond, Maine

Bettina Braj, RN, MEd
Clinical Nurse Specialist and Nurse Practitioner
Dialysis Unit
The Hospital for Sick Children
Toronto, Ontario, Canada

Marie Scott Brown, RN, PNP, CNM, PhD
Professor of Family Nursing
Oregon Health Sciences University
Portland, Oregon

Marcia Gurber, MS, MSN, RN, CGRN
Administrative Director
Gastrointestinal Center
University of Texas, MD Anderson Cancer Center
Houston, Texas

Mary Lou Hayden, RN, MS, FNP
Virginia Allergy and Asthma, Inc.
Richmond, Virginia

Penny Hinkle, MSN, CRNP
Daycare Coordinator
Mental Health Treatment Program
Great Falls, Virginia

Mark F. Kern, PharmD
Assistant Clinical Professor
University of Maryland School of Pharmacy
Clinical Coordinator
Anticoagulation Services and Long Term Care Services
Mercy Medical Center
Baltimore, Maryland

Kathleen Loaffler, RN, MSN, CFNP
Family Nurse Practitioner
Primary Care Department
The Emory Clinic
Fayetteville, Georgia

Lily Luy, RN
Division of Rheumatology
The Hospital for Sick Children
Toronto, Ontario, Canada

Sheila O'Reilly, RN
Urology Clinic Nurse
The Hospital for Sick Children
Toronto, Ontario, Canada

Carol Palumbo, RN, BSN, OCN
Nurse Coordinator, Gynecology/Oncology
University of Virginia Cancer Center
Charlottesville, Virginia

Jay N. Parran, MD
Fellow, American Academy of Ophthalmology
Assistant Clinical Professor
University of Maryland School of Medicine
Private Practice in Ophthalmology
Mercy Medical Center
Baltimore, Maryland

Leslie Plauntz, RN, DNC
Clinical Nurse Specialist, Plastic Surgery
Sunnybrook and Women's College for Health Sciences Center
Toronto, Ontario, Canada

Rita Pool, RN
Clinical Coordinator, Renal Transplant Program
The Hospital for Sick Children
Toronto, Ontario, Canada

Susan Rudy, MSN, CRNP, CORLN
Research Otolaryngology Nurse Practitioner
Department of Otolaryngology Head and Neck Surgery
National Institute on Deafness and Other Communication
    Disorders
Silver Spring, Maryland

Diane B. Rush, CRNP
Nurse Practitioner, Division of Neurosurgery
Mercy Medical Center
Baltimore, Maryland

Carol Kay Scibetta, RN, BSN
1st Nurse
Head and Neck Center—Neurotology/Otolaryngology
    Department
State University of New York at Buffalo
Buffalo, New York

Laurie E. Scudder, RN,C, MS, PNP
Pediatric Nurse Practitioner
Vice President, Nurse Practitioner Education Associates, Ltd.
Columbia, Maryland

Karen A. Stawiasz, MS, RN, NP, OCN
Nurse Practitioner
Department of Oncology Services
Sisters Hospital, Head and Neck Center
Buffalo, New York

Maggie Whall, BSN, CRNP
Women's Health Nurse Practitioner
Columbia, Maryland

April Zarifian, MSN, RN, CNN, ARNP
Abdominal Transplant Department
Tulane University Medical Center
New Orleans, Louisiana

Reviewers

Barbara Bohanon, RNC
Director, Education Department
Huntsville Memorial Hospital
Joe G. Davis School of Nursing
Huntsville, Texas

Joy Britton, RN
Oncology Department
Monroe Medical Center
Highland, Indiana

Cori Burton, BSN, BS
Desert Regional Medical Center
Palm Springs, California

Barbara S. Cassidy, RN, MA
Director, Staff Development
Metrohealth Center for Skilled Nursing Care, East
Chicago, Illinois

Nancy Chess, BSN, MPA
Pro Start Nurse, Home Care IV Clinic
Bransan Hospital
Kalamazoo, Maine

Claudia Conroy, RN, MS, AOCN
Oncology Clinical Nurse Specialist
St. Alexius Medical Center
Hoffman Estates, Illinois

Jerilyn E. Hammon, RN, CPE
Director of Clinical Support Services
Nursing Administration
Sebring, Florida

Clair Homan, RN, BSN, PhN
Emergency Room
Fountain Valley Hospital
Fountain Valley, California

Janet K. Hunter, RN, MPA
Director of Patient Care Services
Patient Care Services
Dekalon Memorial Hospital
Dekalb, Indiana

Lori Komorowski, RN, MS
Clinical Nurse Specialist
Pediatrics
South Suburban Hospital
Lockport, Illinois

Doris Lugo, MSN
Instructor, Nursing Department
Eolegio Universitario De Humaccio
Humaccio, Puerto Rico

Donna Jo Mayo, RN, BSN
Research Nurse Coordinator
National Institutes of Health: Hematology/CPO
George Mason University
Fairfax, Virginia

Michelle Myers
Orthopedic Nurse
Loma Linda University Health Care
Loma Linda, California

Leah Olson, LPN
Hibbing Community College
Virginia, Minnesota

Anastasia M. Pietras, LPN
Cochise College
Sierra Vista, Arizona

Marci L. Robinson (AAS), RN
Director of Nursing Services
Carroll County Good Samaritan Center
Mt. Carroll, Illinois

Peggy Rochwood, RN
RN Manager
Eastern Idaho Regional Medical Center
Rigby, Idaho

Veach E. Rogers, RN, A.D.N.
Onslow Memorial Hospital
Jacksonville, North Carolina

Miriam Sapit, RN, BSN, OCN
Staff Nurse, Oncology Department
Montefiore Medical Center
Bronx, New York

Jean Shelton, BSN, MS
Director, Utilization Management
Business Operations/Beneficiary Support
Scott Air Force Base, 375th Medical Group
Scott Air Force Base, Illinois

Shyla Smith, BSN
State Surveyor, Long-Term Care Facilities
Facility Standards Department
Boise, Idaho

Elizabeth Tanner, A.D.N.
RN Case Manager—Home Health Care
Orem, Utah

Nicole A. Underdahl, RN
Intensive Care Unit
Trinity Medical Center
Munot, North Dakota

L. Dawn Welker, RN, AD
Collierville, Tennessee

G. Alan Young, MD
Chief Medical Resident
Internal Medicine Education Department
Baptist Health System Residency Training
Birmingham, Alabama

Preface

Looking back at past editions of the *Lippincott Manual of Nursing Practice*, I am reminded of the profound changes in nursing and health care over the years. As the book itself has grown in size and depth of information, the role of nurses has similarly expanded: the scope of nursing care has moved beyond the hospital, into homes and communities; nurses are now responsible for more comprehensive and advanced physical assessments of patients than ever before; procedures performed and assisted by nurses have become more technical; diagnostic tests for which nurses prepare patients are more numerous and far more enlightening; the number and types of medications administered by nurses is mind-boggling; and as we become increasingly knowledgeable about disease states, new treatment modalities are being developed continually.

At the same time, I am reassured by the fact that many things in nursing and health care remain the same. In fact, what seems like a change in nursing—the expanded practice to outpatient settings—is really a throwback to the past. Before the growth of large medical institutions and numerous community hospitals, much of health care was practiced in the home. The more comprehensive assessment now demanded from nurses actually finds its roots in the nursing process, which has been used since the 1960s as a systematic approach to identifying patients' problems and taking action to provide solutions. Finally, although the number of new medications is almost overwhelming, many patients are turning away from newer drugs to age-old herbal products and consulting older alternative health care practices.

So what does this mean for us as nurses in the 21st century? I think it is well explained by the title of a keynote lecture I recently attended: "The Past Informs the Future." We must take what we have learned from the past—the good and the bad, the successes and the failures—and build upon those lessons for the future. There are many health problems we have yet to fully understand; among these are addiction, many types of mental illness, the rapidly emerging antibiotic-resistant bacterias, new viral infections, autoimmune disease, and cancer. In the future, we as nurses will continue to meet the challenges of caring for people with these and other illnesses. We will not turn anyone away or quarantine, as we did in the past to people with illnesses such as leprosy and tuberculosis. And, going forward, we will meet our patients on their turf, whether it be in the home, a long-term care facility, the street, a clinic, or a hospital.

The *Lippincott Manual of Nursing Practice* has been updated to meet the needs of today's nurse as follows:

ORGANIZATION

The *Lippincott Manual of Nursing Practice* continues to follow a basic outline format for easy readability and access of information. The subheadings continue to follow both a medical model—Pathophysiology and Etiology, Clinical Manifestations, Diagnostic Evaluation, Management, and Complications—and a nursing process model—Nursing Assessment, Nursing Diagnoses, Nursing Interventions, Community and Home Care Considerations, Patient Education and Health Maintenance, and Outcome-Based Evaluation. Medical model information is presented because nurses need to understand the pathophysiology behind the patient's clinical manifestations as well as the rationale for diagnostic testing and treatment. In the nursing section, we have added the heading Community and Home Care Considerations to this edition because this information is a vital part of nursing care for many health problems. Although the whole book is written with care of the patient in any setting in mind, Community and Home Care Considerations offer additional interventions specific to the planning and implementation of care of the patient in the home.

The *Lippincott Manual of Nursing Practice* is divided into five parts to present a comprehensive reference for all types of nursing care. Part 1 discusses the role of the nurse in the health care delivery system. It comprises chapters on Nursing Practice and the Nursing Process, Standards of Care and Ethical and Legal Issues, Health Promotion and Preventive Care, and Genetics and Health Applications.

Part 2 encompasses medical-surgical nursing. General topics are presented in Unit 1, including Adult Physical Assessment, IV Therapy, Perioperative Nursing, Cancer Nursing, and Care of the Older Adult. Units 2 through 12 deal with body system function and dysfunction and the various disorders seen in adult medical and surgical nursing.

Part 3 is Maternity and Neonatal Nursing. Chapters include Maternal and Fetal Health, Nursing Management During Labor and Delivery, Care of the Mother and Newborn During the Postpartum Period, and Complications of the Childbearing Experience. Chapters reflect the routine childbearing experience as well as frequently encountered high-risk situations and problems that may arise for both the mother and baby.

Part 4 is Pediatric Nursing. Chapters are divided into two units. One unit covers General Practice Considerations comprising Pediatric Growth and Development, Pediatric Physical Assessment, Pediatric Primary Care, and Care of the Sick or Hospitalized Child. The remaining unit contains chapters based on body systems to describe the various disorders and corresponding nursing care seen in pediatric nursing.

Part 5 is on Psychiatric Nursing. Entries follow the Diagnostic and Statistical Manual (DSM) IV classification of mental illness. Treatments and nursing management for each are discussed.

NEW TO THIS EDITION

New and Expanded Material

Two new chapters have been added to this edition. Chapter 2, "Standards of Care, Ethical and Legal Issues," is included to raise the nurse's awareness of nursing care practiced in an environment in which outcomes are not always ideal. Ethical core concepts are presented and various ethical dilemmas frequently encountered are discussed. The bulk of the chapter presents legal aspects of nursing practice, such as accountability, advocacy, confidentiality, scope of practice, and standards of practice. Two important areas of liability, telephone triage and informed consent, are discussed. Telephone triage guidelines are given. Information is given to help the nurse provide and document care of the highest standard.

Also new is Chapter 4, "Genetics and Health Applications." The principles of genetics are reviewed, and the many applications to adult and pediatric health and illness are discussed. Information is given on the nurse's role in genetic counseling and other issues.

In addition to these new chapters is an expanded Chapter 38, "Care of the Mother and Newborn During the Postpartum Period." A new section has been added on Problems of Infants. This section covers common high-risk and problem situations in neonatal nursing such as prematurity, infant of the addicted mother, postmaturity, the septic infant, and others.

You will also find many new entries throughout the book. We have expanded the page length so as to include information on several new orthopedic, connective tissue, infectious, and dermatologic disorders.

Community and Home Care Considerations

Community and Home Care Considerations is a new heading that follows Nursing Interventions for many acute and chronic, adult and pediatric health problems. This information takes the place of Community-Based Nursing Tips in the last edition. This new section was created to ex-

pand coverage of skilled care provided to patients outside the hospital, in the home and other settings. This information is aimed at the home care nurse or case management nurse, or may even detail care that will be provided by a family member or caretaker once taught by a nurse. This section describes care that differs from that provided in the hospital due to the difference in setting.

Standards of Care Guidelines

Standards of Care Guidelines have been added to many chapters. They reflect the standard of care assessment and interventions for a particular health problem. They were designed as a quick guide to remind the nurse of the essential elements of care required when possible unexpected problems arise, such as chest pain or respiratory compromise. Some complex, chronic conditions are also represented. This information should serve as a general guideline only. Each patient situation presents a unique set of clinical factors and requires nursing judgment to guide care, which may include additional or alternative measures and approaches.

Patient Education Guidelines

This new feature offers many Patient Education tools that can be copied and given out to patients. They are written directly to the patient in language most patients can understand. These tools describe procedures, treatments, and self-monitoring techniques for many disorders.

Drug Alerts

Drug Alerts are also new to this edition. They are short, highlighted items that outline important drug information for a particular disorder, such as dangerous side effects, contraindications, interactions, dosage, or monitoring parameters. In addition to Drug Alerts, more drug tables and information on drugs have been added to the text wherever applicable.

Graphics

You will notice immediately that illustrations in the *Lippincott Manual of Nursing Practice* are now in color. We hope that this change will improve your understanding of various disorders and their treatment, as well as make the book more interesting to read. Tables and other graphics have been updated and enhanced as well.

It has been my pleasure preparing the seventh edition of the *Lippincott Manual of Nursing Practice* for you. I hope that it will not only meet your nursing reference needs, but also expand your horizons in providing quality nursing care.

Sandra M. Nettina, MSN, RN, CS, ANP

Acknowledgments

I would like to thank Kathleen Loeffler, MSN, FNP, and Cynthia Bumgarner, RN, MSN, for their editorial assistance. I would like to thank the following people for their assistance with photography: Florina Aquino, LPN, and Jessica Compos, RN, from The Mercy Villa, Baltimore, Maryland; Linda Scheguoe, Lucia Novak, Shelby Weaver, Kimberly Denner and their families; and Dan, Adam, and Carolyn Nettina.

I would like to thank the following people at Lippincott Williams & Wilkins for their contribution to the seventh edition: Mike Carcel, Production Coordinator; Helen Ewan, Senior Production Manager; Tom Gibbons, Senior Project Editor; Brett MacNaughton, Art Coordinator; Karin McAndrews, Editorial Assistant; Carolyn O'Brien, Art Director; Kamika Powell, Art Assistant; Barbara Ryalls, Managing Production Editor; Lisa Stead, Acquisitions Editor; and Claudia Vaughn, Managing Editor.

Contents

THE LIPPINCOTT

MANUAL OF
Nursing
Practice

Nursing Process
and Practice

Nursing Practice and the Nursing Process

NURSING PRACTICE

■ Basic Concepts in Nursing Practice

Understanding basic concepts in nursing practice, such as roles of nursing, theories of nursing, licensing, and legal issues, helps enhance performance.

Definition of Nursing
1. Nursing is an art and a science.
2. Earlier emphasis was on care of sick; now promotion of health is stressed.
3. American Nurses Association definition, 1980: Nursing is the diagnosis and treatment of human responses to actual and potential health problems.

Roles of Nursing
Whether in hospital-based or community health care setting, nurses assume three basic roles:
1. *Practitioner*—involves actions that directly meet the health care and nursing needs of patients, families, and significant others; includes staff nurses at all levels of the clinical ladder, advanced practice nurses, and community-based nurses.
2. *Leader*—involves actions such as deciding, relating, influencing, and facilitating that affect the actions of others and are directed toward goal determination and achievement; may be a formal nursing leadership role or an informal role periodically assumed by the nurse.
3. *Researcher*—involves actions taken to implement studies to determine the actual effects of nursing care to further the scientific base of nursing; can include all nurses, not just academicians, nurse scientists, and graduate nursing students.

History of Nursing
1. First nurses were trained by religious institutions to care for patients; no standards or educational basis.
2. In 1873, Florence Nightingale developed a model for independent nursing schools to teach critical thinking, attention to patient's individual needs, and respect for patient's rights.
3. During the early 1900s, hospitals used nursing students as cheap labor and most graduate nurses worked in private duty in homes.
4. After World War II, technological advancements brought more skilled and specialized care to hospitals, requiring more experienced nurses.
5. Development of intensive and coronary care units during the 1950s brought forth specialty nursing and advanced practice nurses.
   Greater interest in health promotion and disease prevention since the 1960s, along with a shortage of physicians serving rural areas, helped create the role of nurse practitioner.
   Whatever the role of the professional nurse or the practice setting, nurses must provide care in a culturally competent manner. The changing demographics of America brings a diverse array of individual needs to the health care marketplace. Nurses should be not only sensitive but must become knowledgeable about their patients' cultural identities.

Theories of Nursing
1. Nursing theories help define nursing as a scientific discipline of its own.
2. The elements of nursing theories are uniform—nursing, person, environment, and health; also known as the paradigm or model of nursing.
3. Nightingale was the first nursing theorist; she believed the purpose of nursing is to put the person in the best condition for nature to restore or preserve health.

4. More recent nursing theorists include:
   a. Levine—Nursing supports person's adaptation to change due to internal and external environmental stimuli.
   b. Orem—Nurses assist the person to meet universal, developmental, and health deviation self-care requisites.
   c. Roy—Nurses manipulate stimuli to promote adaptation in four modes—physiologic, self-concept, role function, and interdependence relations.
   d. Neuman—Nurses affect a person's response to stressors in the areas of physiologic, psychological, sociocultural, and developmental variables.
   e. King—Nurses exchange information with clients, who are open systems, to attain mutually set goals.
   f. Rogers—Nurses promote harmonious interaction between the person and environment to maximize health; both are four-dimensional energy fields.

Nursing in the Health Care Delivery System

1. Technology, education, society values, demographics, and health care financing all have an impact on where and how nursing is practiced.
   a. By the year 2030 the over-65 population will more than double to about 70 million.
   b. Almost 50% of the US population has one or more chronic conditions.
   c. The annual cost of medical care in the United States is greater than $900 billion and growing at a rate twice that of inflation.
2. Current trends to use health care dollars for primary care of many, rather than specialized care for a few, have shifted nursing care out of the acute care hospital and into the home and outpatient setting.
3. Inpatient staff nurses are now responsible for a greater number of patients who may be older, more acutely ill, and hospitalized for shorter stays.
   a. Diagnosis-related groups (DRGs), implemented in 1983, set rates for Medicare payment for inpatient services, fixing reimbursement based on diagnosis, not on actual charges. This set the standard for shorter hospital stays and other cost-cutting measures.
4. The concept of managed care has expanded for health maintenance organizations (HMOs) and preferred provider organizations (PPOs) to case management and reimbursement control for most insurance plans. Hence, more nurses are working in utilization management or for hospitals or insurance companies to determine the need for specialist consultations, costly procedures, surgeries, and hospitalizations.
5. More nurses are working for large outpatient centers run by hospitals or HMOs; responsibilities include less "hands on" care, but more assessment and health education for patients and their families.
6. The nursing role has expanded to meet health care challenges more efficiently with certification in a variety of specialties to provide direct care or support and educate other nurses in their roles (Table 1-1).

TABLE 1-1 American Nurses Association Credentialing Center Certification Programs

Generalist Examinations

Psychiatric and Mental Health Nurse
Medical-Surgical Nurse
Gerontologic Nurse
Nurse Administrator
Nurse Administrator, Advanced
College Health Nurse
Community Health Nurse
School Nurse
General Nursing Practice
Pediatric Nurse
Perinatal Nurse
Nursing Continuing Education/Staff Development
Home Health Nurse
Cardiac Rehabilitation Nurse

Clinical Nurse Specialist Examinations

Adult Psychiatric and Mental Health Nursing
Child and Adolescent Psychiatric Mental Health
Medical-Surgical Nursing
Gerontologic Nursing
Community Health Nursing
Home Health Nursing

Nurse Practitioner Examinations

Acute Care Nurse Practitioner
Adult Nurse Practitioner
Family Nurse Practitioner
Gerontologic Nurse Practitioner
School Nurse Practitioner
Pediatric Nurse Practitioner

Advanced Practice Nursing

1. Registered professional nurses with advanced training, education, and certification are allowed to practice in expanded scope.
2. This includes nurse practitioners, nurse midwives, nurse anesthetists, and clinical nurse specialists.
3. Scope of practice and legislation vary by state.
   a. Clinical nurse specialists are included in advanced practice nurse (APN) legislation in at least 25 states (some of these just include psychiatric/mental health clinical nurse specialists).
   b. Nurse practitioners have some type of prescriptive authority in all 50 states and the District of Columbia.
   c. Nurse practitioners are now eligible for Medicare reimbursement across the United States at 85% of the physician fee schedule in most cases and are eligible for Medicaid reimbursement in some states.
   d. Most states give authority to APNs through the Board of Nursing with some degree of physician collaboration/supervision required.
4. Master's degree preparation is becoming the requirement for most APN roles; however, many certificate programs have trained APNs in the past 30 years.

5. Regulation of Canadian APNs has been slower than in the United States, except for midwives, so practice of APNs has been restricted.

Licensing/Continuing Education

1. Every professional registered nurse must be licensed through the state Board of Nursing in the United States to practice in that state or the College of Nursing to practice in a Canadian province.
2. Continuing education requirements vary depending on state laws, institutional policies, and area of specialty practice. Continuing education units (CEUs) can be obtained through a variety of professional nursing organizations and commercial educational services.
3. Many professional nursing organizations exist to provide education, certification, support, and communication among nurses; for more information contact your state nurses' association, state Board of Nursing, or the American Nurses Association, 600 Maryland Avenue S.W., Suite 100, Washington, DC 20024-2571, 202-554-4444.

THE NURSING PROCESS

The nursing process is a deliberate, problem-solving approach to meeting the health care and nursing needs of patients. It involves assessment (data collection), nursing diagnosis, planning, implementation, and evaluation, with subsequent modifications used as feedback mechanisms that promote the resolution of the nursing diagnoses. The process as a whole is cyclical, the steps being interrelated, interdependent, and recurrent.

Steps in the Nursing Process

Assessment—systematic collection of data to determine the patient's health status and to identify any actual or potential health problems. (Analysis of data is included as part of the assessment. For those who wish to emphasize its importance, analysis may be identified as a separate step of the nursing process.)

Nursing diagnosis—identification of actual or potential health problems that are amenable to resolution by means of nursing actions.
Planning—development of goals and a plan of care designed to assist the patient in resolving the nursing diagnoses.
Implementation—actualization of the plan of care through nursing interventions or supervision of others to do the same.
Evaluation—determination of the patient's responses to the nursing interventions and of the extent to which the goals have been achieved.

Assessment

1. The nursing history
   a. Obtain subjective data through interviewing the patient, family members, or significant other and reviewing old records.
   b. Also provides the opportunity to convey interest, support, and understanding to the patient and to establish a rapport based on trust.
2. The physical examination
   a. Objective data obtained to determine the patient's physical alterations, limitations, and assets.
   b. Should be done in a private, comfortable environment with efficiency and respect.

Nursing Diagnosis

1. Organize, analyze, synthesize, and summarize the collected data.
2. Identify the patient's health problem(s), its (their) particular characteristic(s) and etiology(ies).
   State nursing diagnoses based on the North American Nursing Diagnosis Association (NANDA) list (Table 1-2). Nursing diagnoses continue to be developed and refined.
   Further work is being done through the University of Iowa College of Nursing to refine, extend, validate, and classify the NANDA taxonomy, called the Nursing Diagnosis and Extension Classification (NDEC) project.

TABLE 1-2 North American Nursing Diagnosis Association–Accepted Nursing Diagnoses	
Activity Intolerance	Breastfeeding, Interrupted
Activity Intolerance, Risk for	Breathing Pattern, Ineffective
Adaptive Capacity: Intracranial, Decreased	
Adjustment, Impaired	Cardiac Output, Decreased
Airway Clearance, Ineffective	Caregiver Role Strain
Anxiety	Caregiver Role Strain, Risk for
Aspiration, Risk for	Communication, Impaired Verbal
Autonomic Dysreflexia, Risk for	Community Coping, Ineffective
	Community Coping, Potential for Advanced
Body Image Disturbance	Confusion, Acute
Body Temperature, Risk for Altered	Confusion, Chronic
Breastfeeding, Effective	Constipation
Breastfeeding, Ineffective	Constipation, Colonic

(continued)

TABLE 1-2 North American Nursing Diagnosis Association–Accepted Nursing Diagnoses (Continued)

Constipation, Perceived
Constipation, Risk for
Coping, Defensive
Coping, Ineffective Individual

Death Anxiety
Decisional Conflict (Specify)
Denial, Ineffective
Dentition, Altered
Diarrhea
Disorganized Infant Behavior
Disorganized Infant Behavior, Risk for
Disuse Syndrome, Risk for
Diversional Activity Deficit
Dysreflexia

Energy Field Disturbance

Family Coping: Compromised, Ineffective
Family Coping: Disabling, Ineffective
Family Coping: Potential for Growth
Family Process: Alcoholism, Altered
Family Processes, Altered
Fatigue
Fear
Fluid Volume Deficit
Fluid Volume Deficit, Risk for
Fluid Volume Excess
Fluid Volume Imbalance, Risk for

Gas Exchange, Impaired
Grieving, Anticipatory
Grieving, Dysfunctional
Growth and Development, Altered

Health Maintenance, Altered
Health-Seeking Behaviors (Specify)
Home Maintenance Management, Impaired
Hopelessness
Hyperthermia
Hypothermia

Impaired Environmental Interpretation Syndrome
Incontinence, Bowel
Incontinence, Functional Urinary
Incontinence, Reflex Urinary
Incontinence, Stress
Incontinence, Total
Incontinence, Urge
Incontinence, Risk for Urinary Urge
Infant Feeding Pattern, Ineffective
Infection, Risk for
Injury, Risk for

Knowledge Deficit (Specify)

Latex Allergy Response
Latex Allergy, Risk for
Loneliness, Risk for

Memory, Impaired

Nausea
Noncompliance (Specify)
Nutrition, Altered: Less than Body Requirements
Nutrition, Altered: More than Body Requirements
Nutrition, Altered: Potential for More than Body Requirements

Oral Mucous Membrane, Altered
Organized Infant Behavior, Potential for Enhanced

Pain
Pain, Chronic
Parent/Infant/Child Attachment, Risk for Altered
Parental Role Conflict
Parenting, Altered
Parenting, Risk for Altered
Perioperative Positioning Injury, Risk for
Peripheral Neurovascular Dysfunction, Risk for
Personal Identity Disturbance
Physical Mobility, Impaired
Poisoning, Risk for
Post-Trauma Syndrome
Post-Trauma Syndrome, Risk for
Powerlessness
Protection, Altered

Rape Trauma Syndrome
Rape Trauma Syndrome: Compound Reaction
Rape Trauma Syndrome: Silent Reaction
Relocation Stress Syndrome
Role Performance, Altered

Self-Care Deficit
  Bathing/Hygiene
  Feeding
  Dressing/Grooming
  Toileting
Self-Esteem, Chronic Low
Self-Esteem, Situational Low
Self-Esteem, Disturbance
Self-Mutilation, Risk for
Sensory/Perceptual Alterations (Specify) (visual, auditory,
  kinesthetic, gustatory, tactile, olfactory)
Sexual Dysfunction
Sexuality Patterns, Altered
Skin Integrity, Risk for Impaired
Skin Integrity, Impaired
Sleep Pattern Disturbance
Social Interaction, Impaired
Social Isolation
Sorrow, Chronic
Spiritual Distress (Distress of the Human Spirit)
Spiritual Distress, Risk for
Spiritual Well-being, Potential for Enhanced
Suffocation, Risk for
Swallowing, Impaired

Therapeutic Regimen, Ineffective Management of
Therapeutic Regimen: Community, Ineffective Management of
Therapeutic Regimen: Families, Ineffective Management of
Therapeutic Regimen: Individual, Ineffective Management of
Thermoregulation, Ineffective
Thought Processes, Altered
Tissue Integrity, Impaired
Tissue Perfusion, Altered (Specify type) (renal, cerebral,
  cardiopulmonary, gastrointestinal, peripheral)
Trauma, Risk for

Unilateral Neglect
Urinary Elimination, Altered
Urinary Retention

Ventilation, Inability to Sustain Spontaneous
Ventilatory Weaning Response, Dysfunctional
Violence, Risk for: Self-Directed or Directed at Others

Planning

See Tables 1-3 and 1-4

1. Assign priorities to the nursing diagnoses. Highest priority is given to problems that are the most urgent and critical.
2. Establish goals or expected outcomes derived from the nursing diagnoses.
   a. Specify short-term, intermediate, and long-term goals as established by nurse and patient together.
   b. Goals should be specific, measurable, and patient focused and should include a time frame.
3. Identify nursing interventions as appropriate for goal attainment.
   a. Include independent nursing actions as well as medical orders.
   b. Should be detailed to provide continuity of care.
   c. Nursing Interventions Classification (NIC) is a language describing treatments that nurses from all settings and specialties perform. Over 400 NIC interventions have been developed through the University of Iowa College of Nursing. NIC interventions may serve a role in documentation, coding, and reimbursement for nursing care in the future.
4. Formulate the nursing care plan.
   a. Include nursing diagnoses, expected outcomes, interventions, and a space for evaluation.
   b. May use a standardized care plan—check off appropriate data and fill in target dates for expected outcomes and frequency and other specifics of interventions.
   c. May use a protocol that gives specific sequential instructions for treating patients with a particular problem, including who is responsible and what specific actions should be taken in terms of assessment, planning, interventions, teaching, recognition of complications, evaluation, and documentation.
   d. May use a care path or clinical pathway (also called care map or critical pathway) in which the nurse as case manager is responsible for outcomes, length of stay, and use of equipment during the patient's illness; includes the patient's medical diagnosis, length of stay allowed by DRG, expected outcomes, and key events that must occur for the patient to be discharged by that date. Key events are not as specific as nursing interventions but are categorized by day of stay and who is responsible—the nurse, physician, other health care team member, or patient or family.

Implementation

1. Coordinate the activities of the patient, the family, significant others, nursing team members, and other health team members.
2. Delegate specific nursing interventions to other members of the nursing team, as appropriate.
   a. Consider the capabilities and limitations of the members of the nursing team.
   b. Supervise the performance of the nursing interventions.
3. Record the patient's responses to the nursing interventions precisely and concisely.

Evaluation

Determines the success of nursing care and need to alter care plan.

1. Collect assessment data.
2. Compare the patient's behavioral outcomes to the expected outcomes to determine to what extent goals have been achieved.
3. Include the patient, family or significant others, nursing team members, and other health team members in the evaluation.
4. Identify alterations that need to be made in the goals and the nursing care plan.

Continuation of the Nursing Process

1. Continue all steps of the nursing process: assessment, nursing diagnosis, planning, implementation, and evaluation.
2. Continuous evaluation provides the means for maintaining the viability of the entire nursing process and for demonstrating accountability for the quality of nursing care rendered.

COMMUNITY AND HOME CARE NURSING

■ Home Health Concepts

The home care nurse functions in the home and community, outside the walls of a hospital or other health care facility. The role is more independent and the basic concepts of home health are different from hospital or outpatient nursing.

Roles and Duties of the Home Care Nurse

1. The home care nurse maintains a comprehensive knowledge base of the health of the client.
2. The home care nurse performs an extensive evaluation of the patient's medical history, physical condition, psychosocial well-being, living environment, and support systems.
3. The home care nurse functions independently, recommending to the primary or specialty health care provider what services are needed in the home.
4. The home care nurse coordinates the services of other disciplines such as physical therapy, occupational therapy, nutrition, and social work.
5. The home care nurse oversees the entire treatment plan and keeps the health care provider apprised of the patient's progress or lack of progress toward goals.
6. The home care nurse acts as a liaison between patient/family/caregivers and the primary health care provider and other members of the health care team.

(*text continues on page 12*)

TABLE 1-3 Example of a Nursing Care Plan

Mr. John Preston, a 52-year-old businessman, was admitted to the hospital with a diagnosis of angina pectoris. He stated that he had experienced substernal chest pain and weakness in his arms and hands after having lunch with a business associate. The pain had lessened by the time he arrived at the hospital. The nursing history revealed that he had been hospitalized 5 months previously with the same complaints and had been told by his physician to go to the emergency department if the pain ever recurred. He had been placed on a low-fat diet and had stopped smoking. Physical examination revealed that Mr. Preston's vital signs were within normal ranges and that his chest pain had been relieved with nitroglycerin. He stated that he had feared he was having a "heart attack" until his pain subsided and until he was told that his ECG was normal. He verbalized that he wanted to find out how he could prevent the attacks of pain in the future. The physician's requests on admission included activity as tolerated, low-cholesterol diet, and nitroglycerin 0.4 mg ($\frac{1}{150}$ gr) sublingually PRN.

NURSING DIAGNOSIS   Pain related to angina pectoris/rule out myocardial ischemia

GOALS

Short-term:	Relief of pain
Long-term:	Altered lifestyle to include measures that decrease myocardial oxygen demands
	Compliance with therapeutic regimen

Nursing Interventions	Expected Outcomes (Goals)	Critical Time*	Outcomes (Evaluation)
Continue assessment of cardiac function:			
Monitor blood pressure (BP), pulse (P), respirations (R) q4h.	BP, P, R will remain within normal limits.	24 h	BP: stable at 116–122/72–84 P: stable at 68–82 R: stable at 16–20
Assess frequency of chest pain and precipitating events.	Patient will remain free of chest pain.	24 h	Denies chest pain; able to walk length of hall, eat meals, and visit with family and friends without chest discomfort.
Encourage food and fluid intake that promotes normal nutrition, digestion, and elimination and that does not precipitate chest pain: light, regular meals; foods low in cholesterol; 1500–2000 mL fluid/d.	Will tolerate dietary regimen. Will not experience chest pain after meals. Will maintain normal bowel elimination. Will have intake of 1500–2000 mL fluid/d.	24 h	Denies chest pain after meals; no constipation or diarrhea; fluid intake 1700–2100 mL/d.
Request consultation with dietitian—for diet teaching.	Will identify foods low in cholesterol and those foods that are to be avoided. Will select well-balanced diet within prescribed restrictions.	48 h	Selects and eats a balanced diet consisting of foods low in cholesterol; dietitian reviewed diet restrictions with patient and wife; wife counseled in meal planning.
Encourage alterations in activities and exercise that are necessary to prevent episodes of anginal pain.	Will identify activities and exercises that could precipitate chest pain: those that require sudden bursts of activity and heavy effort. Will identify emotionally stressful situations; will explain the necessity for alternating periods of activity with periods of rest.	24 h	Patient and wife have identified activities and situations that should be avoided; patient and wife have studied their usual daily routine and have made plans to alter the routine to allow for rest periods; teenage son has volunteered to assist with strenuous home-maintenance chores.
Teach nitroglycerin regimen.	Will describe action, use, and correct administration of nitroglycerin.		Accurately stated action, use, and dosage of nitroglycerin; demonstrated correct administration.

*These times have not been standardized, but are individualized according to the patient's needs.

TABLE 1-4 Example of a Carepath: Free TRAM Breast Reconstruction

Locations/Phase	PTA/SDS/Prep	OR	PACU
Outcomes	1. Pt. verbalizes an understanding of expected limitations/restrictions post-discharge, positioning, ADL. 2. Pt. verbalizes tentative plan for support/caregiver post-discharge. 3. Pre-op exam & testing w/in accepted criteria. 4. Pt. verbalizes understanding of procedure, including indications. 5. Pt. verbalizes an understanding of expected hospital post-op course. 6. Pt. performs IS and volume documented. 7. Pt. verbalizes understanding of Advance Directives. 8. Pt. verbalizes understanding of pre-op teaching. • Pt./S.O. aware Pastoral Care is accessible. • Pt. received: – Reach to Recovery Hand in Hand referral (410-931-6856). – Comfort Pillow.	9. Pt. will experience minimal anxiety, per pt. report/assessment. 10. No apparent injury or trauma from physical, chemical, or electrical sources. 11. Follow OR standard for avoidance of pt. infection.	12. Temp. 95° or greater. 13. Aldrete score of 10. 14. Pain minimized per pt. report/assessment. 15. No evidence of surgical complication. • S.O. aware pt. in PACU. • Minimal nausea/vomiting. →
Discharge Planning	• Identify tentative D/C plan. • Identify primary caregiver post-discharge.		
Psychosocial	• Emotional support for pt./S.O. prn. →	→	↑
Safety Precautions		• Proper positioning. • Safety strap. • Pre-op count. • Post-op count.	• Per PACU protocol.
Consults/Referrals	• Social Work prn for discharge planning and/or psychosocial counseling. • Nursing education. • Anesthesia consult. • Occupational Therapy consult. • Pastoral Care for spiritual/ psychosocial counseling.	• Introduce pt. to OR environment and appropriate staff.	
Education	• IS, T, C, DB. • Pain management. • Med use pre-op. • Review procedure & indications. • Review expected post-op hospital course including drains, equipment, wound. • Review limitations post-discharge. • OR prep. • NPO. • Report time + location, day of surgery.		• IS, C, DB. → • Pain management. →

Assessments	• Post-op advancement of diet. • Advance Directives. • D/C smoking, alcohol, drugs. • Medical history and physical. • Nursing History. • Advance Directives obtained.	• Assessment per OR nursing standard. • Skin Assessment. • Flap checks, skin color, temperature & circulation.	• Assessments per PACU protocol. • Flap checks, skin color, temperature, capillary refill & circulation q1h × 12 h.
Medications/ IV Therapy		• IV fluids. → • Anesthesia. • Pre-op, prophylactic antibiotic.	→ Analgesia per surgeon + anesthesia order. • Antibiotics as ordered. → • PCA pump per protocol.
Type of I.V. access:			
Clinical Data	• Pre-op checklist.	• Verify room readiness.	• Pulse ox. • VS per PACU protocol.
Activities	• Verify informed consent obtained. • Vital signs	• Verify pre-op checklist information. • Verify functional OR table—able to flex.	• Bedrest. • HOB elevated 45–90° with knees flexed 45%.
Nutrition			• NPO.
Tests/Procedures	• CBC with diff. • SMA7. • Type and cross match. • 1 Auto unit (donated) (2 if bilateral)	• Tissue to pathology.	
Treatments		• Comfort measures. • Pt. prep per physician preference. • Athrombics per physician order. → • Foley. → • OR dressing. → • Follow OR nursing standard for avoidance of pt. infection. • JP drains—to axilla, abdomen and breast(s)—secure before moving pt.	• Use of IS, C+DB. → → → → • Empty JP drains q4h prn and record drainage. • JP dressings, change BID & prn.

Notify HO if:
T -
P -
R -
BP -

(continued)

TABLE 1-4 Example of a Carepath: Free TRAM Breast Reconstruction (Continued)

Locations/Phase	Day 1 (ICU/IMC) Eve. of Surg.	Day 2 (POD #1)	Day 3 (POD #2)	Day 4 (POD #3)
Outcomes	• Pt. verbalizes pain is at a level acceptable to the pt. • Pt. will demonstrate adequate lung expansion. → 16. VS WNL compared to baseline. 17. Tram flaps will reveal normal temp., pink coloration and no S+S of engorgement. → • U/O is > 30 cc/h. → • Pt. verbalizes an understanding of expected: discomfort, bruising, tightening and swelling. → 18. JP drainage will be within (written parameters). → 19. No S+S of wound infection. →	• Pt. pain is maintained at a level allowing mobility. → • Pt. is afebrile and VS WNL compared to baseline. → → → • Pt. identifies D/C plan and caregiver. → →	→ → → →	20. Pt. discharged to appropriate setting with appropriate resources. 21. Pt./S.O. verbalizes understanding of D/C instructions: – meds (pain, antibiotics) – diet – activity – S + Sx to call M.D. – f/u appt. – drain care – IS CDB – use of walker • Pt. activity/independence level appropriate for discharge setting and supports. • Discharge.
Discharge Planning		• Discuss tentative D/C plan. • Transfer to MS unit per Dr.'s orders.	↑ ↑ ↑	
Psychosocial	• Emotional support for pt./S.O. →			
Safety Precautions	• Side rails ↑ × 2 in PM and when on analgesia. → • Fall precautions. →	↑ ↑ ↑	↑ ↑ ↑	• D/C via wheelchair.
Consults/Referrals		• Occupational Therapy prn.		
Education	• IS, C, DB. → • Pain management. → • Orient to room and surroundings.	↑ • Initiate D/C teaching: – S + Sx of infection – wound care – drain care	• Reinforce teaching: → – drain care – meds (pain, antibiotics) – f/u appointment – S + Sx to notify M.D. – activity (HOB must remain elevated while in bed; OOB to chair; may ambulate) – limit operative arm ROM to 90° at shoulder	• No bra for 3 weeks. • No driving for 3 weeks. • No shower until drains removed—sponge bathe only.
Assessments	• Nursing Physical Assessment. → • Monitor OR drsg./site. → • TRAM flap circulation checks q1h × 12 h. – color – skin temp – capillary refill	↑ ↑ • TRAM flap circulation checks q2h until transfer to MS unit. • TRAM flap circulation checks q4h on MS unit. →	↑ ↑ ↑	↑ ↑ ↑

Medications/ IV Therapy	• IV fluids. → • Antibiotics as ordered. → • PCA per protocol. →	• D/C IV fluids. → • Convert to Med Lock after PCA and IV's discontinued. • Analgesia as ordered. → • D/C PCA when tolerating po analgesia.	• Med Lock. → →	
Type of I.V. access:				
Clinical Data	• VS q1h. • I&O q4h.	• VS q4h. • I&O q4h.	• VS q shift. → • I&O q shift. →	
Activities	• Bedrest. • HOB ↑ with knees flexed 45%. • OOB to chair in PM with assistance.	• HOB ↑ 45% when pt. in bed. • OOB with assistance to chair maintaining 45 to 90° waist flexion at all times. • Limit operative arm ROM to 90° at shoulder.	• HOB ↑ 45% when pt. in bed. • OOB ambulating with assistance. • No pressure to under-arm.	• Ambulating independently. • Do not raise arm above shoulder.
Nutrition	• NPO. • Clear liquid as tolerated when alert & stable.	• Advance as tolerated (once flap check done by physician in AM).	• Regular. →	
Tests/Procedures		• 6 AM CBC.		
Treatments	• Empty drains q4h & prn. → • IS, C, DB. → • Foley. • JP dressing changes BID & prn. → • Athrombics per Dr.'s order when in bed.	→ → • D/C Foley. • Athrombics when in bed. • D/C when ambulating. • OP site dressing changes by M.D. only.	→ → • PT/OT to begin. →	

Notify HO if:
T -
P -
R -
BP -

The Carepath is a guide. It can assist practitioners in making decisions about the treatment plan. None of the steps are mandatory or necessarily appropriate for every patient. Health care decisions are made by the patient with the advice of his or her physician. Medications, treatments, and procedures will only be done with a physician order.

Courtesy Mercy Medical Center, Baltimore, MD.

TRAM, transverse rectus abdominis myocutaneous; pt., patient; ADL, activities of daily living; HOB, head of bed; C + DB, cough and deep breathe; JP, Jackson-Pratt; IS, incentive spirometer; S.O., significant other; D/C, discontinue; prn, as needed; T, turn; C, cough; DB, deep breathe; OR, operating room; PTA, prior to admission; SDS, same day surgery; PACU, post anesthesia care unit; HO, house officer.

7. The home care nurse may function as supervisor of home health aides who provide direct daily care for the patient.
8. The home care nurse must honor patient rights as in the hospital (see p. 15).

Skills for Home Care Nursing

1. *Good rapport building*—to engage the patient, family, and caregivers in goal attainment.
2. *Clear communication*—to provide effective teaching to family and caregivers, to relate assessment information about the patient to the health care provider, and to share information with the home care team.
3. *Cultural competence*—knowledge and appreciation of the cultural norms being practiced in the home. Cultural practices may affect family structure, communication, and decision making in the home; health beliefs, nutrition, and alternative health practices; and spirituality and religious beliefs.
4. *Accurate documentation*—record keeping in home care is used for reimbursement of nursing services, accreditation and regulatory review, and communication among the home care team.

Reimbursement Issues

1. Home health care services are reimbursed by Medicare, Medicaid, and a variety of commercial insurances and managed care plans.
2. Some clients are willing to pay out of pocket for additional services not covered by insurance, because of the well-established value of home care services compared with more expensive hospital and nursing home services.
3. Services are reimbursed by Medicare if they meet the following criteria:
   a. Services are ordered by a physician (or, more recently, by a nurse practitioner).
   b. Services are intermittent or needed on a part-time basis.
   c. The client is homebound.
   d. The services required are skilled (need to be provided by a licensed nurse, physical therapist, or speech therapist, or by an occupational therapist, social worker, or home health aide along with the service of a nurse).
   e. The services requested are reasonable and medically necessary.
4. The home health nurse must evaluate the case and ensure that these criteria apply, and must document this so reimbursement will not be denied.

■ Home Health Practice

The nursing process is carried out in home care as it is in other nursing settings. Patient interactions are structured differently than in the hospital, however, because the nurse will interact with the patient for a limited time. Many procedures and nursing interventions are implemented in a similar manner as other nursing settings, as outlined in the rest of this book. Major concerns of the home care nurse are patient teaching, infection control, and maintenance of safety.

The Home Care Visit

1. The initial home care visit to a client should be preceded by information gathering and an introductory phone call.
2. Extensive assessment is carried out at the first visit, including complete medical and psychosocial history, physical examination, assessment of the home environment, nutritional assessment, medication review, and review of current treatment plan.
3. Once assessment (gathered from multiple sources) is complete, nursing diagnoses are formed.
4. Outcome planning (goal setting) is done with the patient, family, and caregivers involved.
5. The plan is implemented over a prescribed time period (the certified period of service). Interventions provided may be:
   a. *Cognitive interventions*—patient teaching
   b. *Psychosocial interventions*—reinforcing coping mechanisms, supporting caregivers, stress reduction
   c. *Technical interventions*—procedures such as wound care, catheter insertion
6. Evaluation is ongoing at every visit and by follow-up phone calls to adjust and refine the plan of care and frequency of service.
7. Recertification for continued service, discharge, or transfer (to a hospital or nursing home) ultimately occurs.

Patient Teaching

1. Patient teaching is directed toward the patient, family, caregivers, and involved significant others.
2. Patient teaching is usually considered skilled and is therefore reimbursable. Topics may include:
   a. Disease process/pathophysiology/signs and symptoms to monitor/treatment
   b. Administration of injectable medication or complex regimen of oral medications
   c. Diabetic management for a newly diagnosed diabetic
   d. Wound or ostomy care
   e. Catheterization
   f. Gastrostomy and enteral feedings
   g. Management of peripheral or central IV catheters
   h. Use of adaptive devices for carrying out activities of daily living and ambulation
   i. Transfer techniques and body alignment
   j. Preparation and maintenance of therapeutic diet
3. Barriers to learning should be evaluated and removed or compensated for.
   a. Environmental barriers such as noise, poor lighting, distractions
   b. Personal barriers such as sensory deficits, poor reading skills, drowsiness
4. The teaching plan should include the three domains of learning:

a. *Cognitive domain*—sharing facts and information

b. *Affective domain*—address patient's feelings about disease and treatment

c. *Psychomotor domain*—performance of desired behavior or steps in a procedure

5. Documentation of patient teaching should be specific and include the degree of patient competence of the procedure.

6. Patient teaching plans may take several sessions to implement successfully.

Infection Control

1. Nosocomial infection rates are much lower in home care, but patients are still at risk for infection due to weakened immune systems and the variability of a clean or sterile environment at home.

2. The nurse should assess and maintain a clean environment.

a. Ensure that clean or sterile supplies are readily available when needed.

b. Ensure that contaminated supplies are disposed of promptly and properly.

(i) Needles should be disposed of in sharps container (usually kept in the home), which can be disposed of through the home health agency or the patient's pharmacy.

(ii) Supplies such as dressings, gloves, catheters should be securely bagged and disposed of in small amounts through the regular trash collection at the patient's home. However, biohazardous waste disposal may be necessary in some cases.

3. The nurse should be aware of all methods of transmission of infection and implement and teach preventive practices.

NURSING ALERT

 Above all else, model and teach good handwashing practice to everyone in the home.

---

4. The nurse must perform ongoing assessment for signs and symptoms of infection, and teach patient, family, and caregivers what to look for.

5. The nurse should be aware of community-acquired infections that may be prevalent in certain populations such as tuberculosis, HIV disease, hepatitis, and sexually transmitted disease.

a. Teach preventive practices.

b. Encourage and institute screening programs.

c. Report infections according to the local public health department policy.

6. Encourage and provide vaccination for patient and household contacts for influenza, pneumococcal pneumonia, hepatitis B, and others as appropriate.

Ensuring Safety

1. Continually assess safety in the home, particularly if patient is very ill and a complex plan of care is being followed.

2. Assess for environmental safety issues such as cluttered spaces, stairs, use of throw rugs, slippery floors, poor lighting.

3. Assess for patient's personal safety issues such as sensory deficits, weakness, problems with eating or swallowing.

4. Assess safety for the patient using the bathroom—handrails, bathmat, raised toilet seat, water temperature.

5. Assess safety in the kitchen—proper refrigeration of food, ability to shop for and cook meals, oven safety.

6. Be alert for abuse and neglect, especially of children, dependent elders, and women.

7. Check equipment for electrical and fire safety and that it is being used properly.

8. Be continually cognizant of nurse's own safety—get directions, travel during daylight hours, wear seat belts, do not enter suspicious areas without escort, be alert to surroundings.

SELECTED REFERENCES

Andrew, M. A., & Boyle, J. S. (1999). *Transcultural concepts in nursing*. Philadelphia: Lippincott Williams & Wilkins.

Bozzo, J., & Minarik, P. (1999). Databases and nursing outcomes. *American Journal of Nursing, 99*(4), 22.

Carpenito, L. J. (1999). *Nursing care plans and documentation* (3rd ed.). Philadelphia: Lippincott Williams & Wilkins.

Carpenito, L. J. (1999). *Nursing diagnosis: Applications to clinical practice* (8th ed.). Philadelphia: Lippincott Williams & Wilkins.

Drevdahl, D. (1999). Sailing beyond: Nursing theory and the person. *Advances in Nursing Science, 21*(4), 1–13.

Green, K. (1998). *Home care survival guide*. Philadelphia: Lippincott Williams & Wilkins.

Haag-Heitman, B. H., & Kramer, A. (1998). Creating a clinical practice development model. *American Journal of Nursing, 98*(8), 39–43.

Haase, R., & Miller, K. (1999). Performance improvement in everyday clinical practice. *American Journal of Nursing, 99*(5), 52–54.

Hamric, A. B., Spross, J. A., & Hanson, C. M. (1996). *Advanced nursing practice: An integrative approach*. Philadelphia: W. B. Saunders.

Iowa Intervention Project. (1996). *Nursing interventions classification (NIC)* (2nd ed.). St. Louis: Mosby–Yearbook.

Lester, N. (1998). Cultural competency: A nursing dialog. *American Journal of Nursing, 98*(9), 26–33.

LeVasseur, J. J. (1999). Toward an understanding of art in nursing. *Advances in Nursing Science, 21*(4), 48–63.

Monti, E. J., & Tingen, M. S. (1999). Multiple paradigms of nursing science. *Advances in Nursing Science, 21*(4), 64–80.

North American Nursing Diagnosis Association. (1999). *NANDA nursing diagnoses: Definitions and classifications, 1999–2000*. Philadelphia: Author.

Pearson, L. J. (1999). Annual update of how each state stands on legislative issues affecting advanced nursing practice. *The Nurse Practitioner, 24*(1), 16–83.

Ryan, J. W. (1999). Collaboration of the nurse practitioner and physician in long term care. *Primary Care Practice, 3*(2), 127–134.

Wolfe, S. (2000). Hospitalists: Good or bad news for nurses? *RN, 63*(3), 31–33.

Zang, S., & Allender, J. A. (1999). *Home care of the elderly*. Philadelphia: Lippincott Williams & Wilkins.

Standards of Care, Ethical and Legal Issues

INTRODUCTION

Along with the privilege of providing professional health care services to consumers, the professional nurse has a commensurate degree of responsibility and accountability to follow ethical principles and standards of care integral to the profession. Ideally, such accountability should be promoted from within the profession by measures that are incorporated into daily practice. Such measures might include protocol implementation, preceptor performance review, peer review, continuing education, patient satisfaction surveys, and the implementation of risk management techniques. However, in certain instances, either despite or in the absence of such internal mechanisms, claims are made for an alleged injury or alleged malpractice liability. Although many claims may be without merit, many professional nurses, nonetheless, will come face to face with the unfamiliar legal system. A system of ethical principles and standards of care will be of benefit in such situations. Hence, it is preferable for the nursing profession to incorporate certain ethical and legal principles and protocols into practice to ensure that the patient consumer of nursing services receives only safe and appropriate care.

ETHICAL CORE CONCEPTS

Clinical ethics literature identifies four principles and values that are integral to the professional nurse's practice, namely, the nurse's ethical duty is to respect the patient's autonomy, and act with beneficence, nonmaleficence, and justice.

Respect for the Individual and His or Her Autonomy

1. Respect for the individual's autonomy incorporates principles of freedom of choice, self-determination, and privacy.
2. The professional nurse has the duty to view and treat each individual as an autonomous, self-determining person with the freedom to act in accordance with self-chosen, informed goals, as long as the action does not interfere or infringe on the autonomous action of another.
3. See the National League of Nursing Statement on Patients' Rights (Box 2-1).

Beneficence

The principle of beneficence affirms the inherent professional aspiration and duty to help promote the well-being of others, and often is the primary motivating factor for those who choose a career in the health care professions. Health care professionals aspire to help people achieve a better life through an improved state of health.

Nonmaleficence

1. The principle of nonmaleficence complements beneficence and obligates the professional nurse not to harm the patient directly or with intent.
2. In the health care profession, this principle is actualized only with the complementary principle of beneficence, because it is common for the nurse to cause pain or expose the patient to risk of harm when the harms or risks of harm are justified by the benefits of the procedures and/or treatments.
3. It is best to seek to promote balance of potential risk-induced harms with benefits, with the basic guideline being to strive to maximize expected benefits and min-

Nurses have a responsibility to uphold the following rights of patients:

To health care that is accessible and that meets professional standards, regardless of the setting.

To courteous and individualized health care that is equitable, humane, and given without discrimination as to race, color, creed, sex, national origin, source of payment, or ethical or political beliefs.

To information about their diagnosis, prognosis, and treatment—including alternatives to care and risks involved—in terms they and their families can readily understand, so that they can give their informed consent.

To informed participation in all decisions concerning their health care.

To information about the qualifications, names, and titles of personnel responsible for providing their health care.

To refuse observation by those not directly involved in their care.

To privacy during interview, examination, and treatment.

To privacy in communicating and visiting with persons of their choice.

To refuse treatment, medications, or participation in research and experimentation, without punitive action being taken against them.

To coordination and continuity of health care.

To appropriate instruction or education from health care personnel so that they can achieve an optimal level of wellness and an understanding of their basic health needs.

To confidentiality of all records (except as otherwise provided for by law or third party payer contracts) and all communications, written or oral, between patients and health care providers.

To access to all health records pertaining to them, and the right to challenge and correct their records for accuracy, and the right to transfer all such records in the case of continuing care.

To information on the charges for services, including the right to challenge these.

To be fully informed as to all their rights in all health care settings.

imize possible harms. Hence, nonmaleficence should be balanced with beneficence.

◼ Justice

1. Justice, or fairness, relates to the distribution of services and resources.
2. As the health care dollar becomes increasingly more scarce, justice seeks to allocate resources fairly and treat equals equally.
3. Dilemmas arise when resources are scarce and insufficient to meet the needs of everyone. How do we decide fairly who gets what in such situations?
4. One might consider whether it is just or fair for many people not to have funding or access to even the most

basic preventive care whereas others have insurance coverage for expensive and long-term hospitalizations.

5. Along with respect for people and their autonomy, the complex principle of justice is a culturally comfortable principle in countries such as the United States. Nonetheless, the application of justice is complex and often challenging.

ETHICAL DILEMMAS

◼ Conflicting Ethical Principles

1. Ethical dilemmas arise when two or more of the above-described ethical principles are in conflict.
2. Such dilemmas can best be addressed by applying the principles discussed above on a case-by-case basis once all available data are gathered and analyzed.
3. Clinicians should network with their colleagues and consider establishing multidisciplinary ethics committees to provide guidance.

Ethics Committees

1. Ethics committees identify, examine, and promote resolution of ethical issues and dilemmas by:
   a. Protecting the patient's rights
   b. Protecting the staff and the organization
   c. Reviewing decisions and standards of practice
   d. Improving the quality of care and services
   e. Serving as educational resources to staff
   f. Building a consensus on ethical issues with other professional organizations
2. Addressing and resolving ethical dilemmas is usually a shared burden.

◼ Examples of Ethical Dilemmas and Possible Responses

Unsafe Nurse-to-Patient Ratio

1. A pattern of unsafe nurse-to-patient ratio is apparent to the staff nurses due to sick calls or other staffing problems, be they temporary or longer term.
2. A series of actions to best resolve the problem includes the following:
   a. Address this unsafe situation verbally and document in letter form to the nurse unit charge nurse with copies to the nursing supervisor and director of nursing.
   b. This will likely prompt an appropriate action on the part of the hospital, such as creating a prn pool of nurses to call for such situations, hiring more staff, or, in the interim, securing contracts with outside nursing agencies and utilizing agency nursing personnel.
3. Tolerance by staff nurses employed under such circumstances will preclude appropriate resolution and will leave the nurse open to unsafe practice and unmet patient needs, and will increase the risk of liability.
4. The nurse will not be exonerated should a patient's care be compromised and an injury and legal claim ensue.

Nonresponse by Physician

1. A patient arrives to the rehabilitation unit at 9 PM with several positive criteria for falling, including poor short-term memory, daily use of a diuretic, daily use of a sleep aid, a history of a fall within the preceding 2 months, and a history of visual impairment.
   a. She is oriented to time, place, and person and is oriented to her new room, hospital bed, and call light equipment use.
   b. The nurse instructs the patient to summon her if she needs to void or otherwise get out of bed.
   c. Ten minutes later, upon returning to the patient's room, the nurse finds the patient out of bed, arranging her clothes in her closet, standing in a pool of urine on the floor.
   d. The nurse calls the physician to obtain an order for a posey vest and/or wrist restraints, but the doctor does not return her calls.
2. Again, a series of actions may resolve the problem or at least prevent injury to the patient. Address this situation with intermediate measures while waiting for the doctor's return call:
   a. Place side rails on the patient's bed.
   b. Move the patient to a room close to the nurse's station.
   c. Place a sign on the patient's room door and above the head of her bed identifying her as being at high risk for falling.
   d. Place a sign above the head of her bed instructing personnel to raise the bedside rails fully before leaving the patient's room.
   e. Check on the patient frequently during the initial 24 hours, reminding her of the call light and its use.
3. Call the patient's family, advising them of your concern about the patient's safety and discuss the issue of restraints with them. Discuss the high risk for falling, prevention of fall-induced injury versus the restriction of the patient's freedom of movement about the room.
4. Document assessment of potential problem, calls to the doctor, and discussion with family member.
5. Apply restraints per policy of rehabilitation unit until order is secured from doctor.
   a. Consider developing a standing order policy for restraint use to be utilized only in cases of special need.
   b. Secure order for restraints to be used prn from doctor.
6. Reassess patient's need for diuretic and sedative use. Discuss discontinuation of any unnecessary medications that increase patient's degree of confusion or risk for falling if possible.

Inappropriate Orders

1. Your 65-year-old patient with diagnosis of controlled congestive heart failure and presently in ICU is becoming increasingly anxious during your shift, but vital signs are stable and respiratory distress is absent. A house officer is summoned to evaluate this change in clinical status.
   a. The house officer, unfamiliar with the patient, spends 2 minutes reviewing the chart, examines the patient for 2 minutes, and orders a sedative to be administered stat and prn every 4 hours, as needed, thereafter.
   b. You ask the house officer if he heard decreased breath sounds in the left, lower lung, the possibility of him ordering some diagnostic tests such as a chest x-ray or arterial blood gases, and share your concern that administering the patient a sedative may mask the underlying cause of the anxiety, lead to respiratory compromise, and delay diagnosis and treatment of the underlying clinical problem.
   c. He leaves the unit. Do not give the sedative ordered by the house officer.
2. Although you cannot automatically follow an order you think is unsafe, you cannot just ignore a medical order, either.
   a. Document the scenario described above in the chart while you call the resident on call and notify your charge nurse.
   b. If assessment by the resident on call yields the same recommendation, call the attending physician, discuss your concerns with him/her, obtain appropriate stat orders, and notify the house officer and resident of the attending physician's orders and your actions taken.
   c. Notify all involved medical and nursing personnel of the patient's status.
   d. Document clearly, succinctly, and in a timely fashion.
3. Your actions reflect a concern about the best interest of the patient, and, although they may yield negative behaviors by the house officer and/or resident, it is more important to prevent potential injury to the patient.

LEGAL ASPECTS OF PROFESSIONAL NURSING PRACTICE

Accountability

1. Integral to the practice of any profession is the inherent need to be responsible for actions taken and for omissions.
2. The professional nurse must be proactive and take all appropriate measures to ensure that his/her own practice is not lacking, remiss, or deficient in any area or way.
3. Useful proactive measures include:
   a. Providing for self-audit
   b. Providing for peer review to assess reasonableness of care in a particular setting for a particular problem
   c. Working with local nursing organizations to make certain that local standards of practice are met
   d. Examining the quality (accuracy/completeness) of his/her documentation
   e. Establishing open working relationships with colleagues wherein honest constructive criticism is welcomed for the greater goal of quality patient care

4. Note that usually the local standards of practice are in step with those of nationally accepted standards.

■ Advocacy

The professional nurse has the duty to:
1. Promote what is best for the patient
2. Ensure that the patient's needs are met
3. Protect the client's rights

■ Confidentiality

1. The patient's privacy is consistent with the Hippocratic oath and with the law as part of the constitutional right to privacy.
2. Although the professional nurse should assure the patient of confidentiality, limits on this standard must be clarified and discussed with the patient at the earliest relevant opportunity.
3. It is imperative to understand clearly the process of informed consent and the legal standard for disclosure of confidential patient information to others.
4. The Medical Record Confidentiality Act of 1995, a federal statute, is the primary federal law governing the use of health treatment and payment records. Several practical guidelines include:
   a. Respect the individual's right to privacy when requesting or responding to a request for patient's medical records.
   b. Always require a signed medical authorization and consent form to release medical records and information to protect and respect patient–provider privilege statutes.
   c. Discuss confidentiality issues with patient and establish consent, aiming to elicit any concerns or special requests for information not to be disclosed.
5. The exceptions or limits to confidentiality include situations in which our society has judged that the need for information outweighs the principle of confidentiality. However, legal counsel should be consulted as these decisions are made on a case-by-case basis, and broad generalizations cannot be assumed.
6. It may be appropriate to breach confidentiality on a limited basis in situations such as the following:
   a. If a patient reveals an intent to harm someone, it is imperative to protect third parties from such harm.
   b. A clinician employed by a company, school, military unit, or court has split allegiances and the patient should be so advised at the appropriate time.
   c. Court orders, subpoenas, and summonses in some states may require the clinician to release records for review or testify in court with the appropriate information.
   d. Most insurance companies, health maintenance organizations, and governmental payors require participants to sign a release of their records to the payors.
   e. If a patient places his or her medical condition at issue, such as in personal injury cases, or in various other cases of patients claiming injuries for which they are seeking compensation.
   f. Many states have laws requiring clinicians to report the incidence of certain diseases, deaths, and other vital statistics.
   g. Criminal codes in many states require reporting gunshot wounds, incidents of rape, and incidents of child, spouse, or elder abuse if they have reasonable cause to suspect abuse.

■ Informed Consent

1. The doctrine of informed consent has become a fundamentally accepted principle governing the relationship between professional nurses and all other health care providers and patients.
2. Informed consent relates to the patient's right to accept or reject treatment by a nurse or any other health care provider and is a right of all legally competent adults or emancipated minors.
3. Emancipated minors are those individuals who are under 18 years of age and married, or are parents of their own children, or are self-sufficiently living away from the family domicile with parental consent.
4. In the case of a minor, informed consent would be obtained from the legal guardian.
5. In the case of individuals incapable of understanding medical treatment issues, informed consent must be obtained through a responsible person such as a guardian.
6. The professional nurse has the duty to verify with the patient that the physician or other health care provider has indeed explained each treatment or procedure in a language the patient (or the responsible person) can comprehend, warned him/her of any material risks, dangers, harms inherent in or collateral to the treatment, as well as advised him/her of the available alternatives, so as to enable the patient to make an intelligent and informed decision and choice about whether to undergo such treatment.
7. The informed consent should be obtained before rendering the treatment or performance of the procedure.
8. The professional nurse must document that the informed consent was obtained and that the patient understood the information.
9. The informed consent should be obtained in the presence of a witness.

NURSING ALERT

With the increasing cultural diversity of our client population, it is prudent to obtain an interpreter for the patient if there is a reasonable chance that the patient will not understand explanations in the English language.

■ Scope of Practice, Licensure, and Certification

1. The professional nurse's scope of practice is defined by the individual state regulations that govern practice.

2. The nurse should obtain a description of the RN's or LPN's scope of practice as outlined by the State Board of Nursing for the appropriate level of nursing.
3. Licensure is granted by an agency of state government and permits individuals accountable for the practice of professional nursing to engage in the practice of that profession, while prohibiting all others from doing so legally.
4. Licensure permits use of a particular title and protects the public by ensuring a minimum level of professional competence.
5. Certification is provided by a nongovernment association or agency and certifies that a person licensed to practice as a professional nurse has met certain predetermined standards described by that profession for specialty practice.
6. Additionally, certification assures the consumer that a person has mastered a body of knowledge and acquired the skills in a particular specialty.
7. The mechanisms for achieving certification vary by association and/or certifying body. Various types of criteria and national certification requirements are utilized.
8. The professional nurse with a specialty certification must meet certain conditions for certification maintenance or recertification, such as certain number of hours of clinical practice, continuing education, peer review, periodic self-assessment examination, and re-examination.
9. The American Nurses Association (ANA) may be contacted at 202-554-4444 for information related to specialty certification.
10. Credentialing is the process that protects the public by recognizing professional nurses who have successfully completed an approved course of study and achieved a level of specialized knowledge and skill to hold specialized positions.

Standards of Practice

General Principles

1. Like other professions, the practice of professional nursing has standards of practice setting minimum levels of acceptable performance for which its practitioners are accountable. These standards provide the patients with a means of measuring the quality of care they receive.
2. Standards of practice were first developed by the ANA in 1966 after an organizational revision of the ANA that resulted in the creation of five specialized divisions of practice.
3. Professional nurses are to be guided by the generic standards applicable to all nurses in all areas of practice as well as by specialty area standards.
4. A copy can be obtained from the ANA publications office, which can be reached at 1-800-637-0323.
5. The authority for the practice of nursing is based on a social contract that acknowledges rights and respon-

sibilities, along with mechanisms for public accountability.
6. Various specialty groups have developed their own additional standards, but addressing these exceeds the scope of this chapter. The professional nurse needs to be familiar with all standards applicable to his/her own practice areas.
7. Standards and parameters are a source of legal protection for the nurse practitioner.
8. They typically consist of a simple, realistic series of steps that will always apply to certain clinical scenarios.
9. Standards and parameters should outline only the minimum requirements for safe care and need to be updated as scientific knowledge changes.
10. A deviation from the protocol should be documented in the patient's chart with clear, concise statements of the nurse's decisions, actions, and reason(s) for the deviation. This is best done at the time the care is rendered because passage of time may lead to a less than accurate recollection of the specific events.
11. Informal or volunteer practice may afford the professional nurse some legal protection if it can be documented that the care rendered was the standard of practice within a community or state. Informal or volunteer care still needs to comply with the applicable standard of care.

The Standards of Professional Nursing Practice

1. The standards of professional nursing practice include standards of care and standards of professional performance (Box 2-2).
2. The standards of care for professional nursing include assessment, diagnosis, outcome identification, planning, implementation, and evaluation.
3. The standards of professional performance include quality of care, performance appraisal, education, collegiality and collaboration, ethics, resource utilization, and research.

BOX 2-2   Standards of Professional Nursing Practice

Standards of Care
Assessment
Diagnosis
Outcome Identification
Implementation
Evaluation

Standards of Professional Performance
Quality of Care
Performance Appraisal
Education
Collegiality
Ethics
Resource Utilization
Research

Common Departures from the Standards of Nursing Care

Claims most frequently made against professional nurses include failure to make appropriate assessments, follow physician orders, follow appropriate nursing measures, communicate information about the patient, follow institutional policy and procedures, and document appropriate information in the medical record (Box 2-3).

■ Quality Assurance

1. A quality assurance program allows for a systematic, deliberate, and ongoing mechanism for the evaluation and monitoring of professional nursing practice in terms of the quality of patient care and organizational management.
2. Such a proactive program promotes responsibility and accountability to deliver high-quality care, evaluates and improves patient care, and provides for an organized means of problem solving.
3. Consequently, use of a quality assurance program effectively reduces the professional nurse's exposure to liability, identifies educational needs, and improves the documentation of the care provided.
4. The components of quality assurance include:
   a. *Structure*—focuses on the organization of client care
   b. *Process*—focuses on tests ordered and procedures performed
   c. *Outcome*—focuses on the outcome achieved, such as improvement, absence of complications, timely discharge, patient satisfaction, or death
5. Mechanisms to incorporate in quality assurance programs may include:
   a. Patient satisfaction surveys to assess nurse interactions and maintain open lines of communication between provider and patient
   b. Peer review to recognize and reward care delivered, lead to higher standards of practice within a community, and discourage practice beyond the scope of legal authority
   c. Audit of clinical records to determine how well established criteria were met by the care rendered
   d. Utilization review to evaluate the extent to which services or resources were used as measured against a standard

■ Management of Liability

1. The sources of legal risk in a professional nurse's practice include patient care, procedures performed, and quality of documentation.
2. Liability can be minimized by the application of risk management systems and activities, which are designed to recognize and intervene to reduce the risk of injury to patients and subsequent claims against professional nurses.
3. Risk management systems and activities are based on the premise that many injuries to patients are preventable.

■ Malpractice

1. Nursing malpractice refers to a negligent act of a professional nurse engaged in the practice of that profession.
2. Although negligence embraces all negligent acts, malpractice is a specific term referring to negligent conduct in the rendering of professional services.
3. There is no guaranteed way to avoid a medical malpractice suit short of avoiding practicing as a professional nurse. Even the best nurses have been named as defendants.
4. A diligent and reflective nurse can reduce the risks of malpractice by consistently incorporating the following four elements into his/her practice:
   a. Excellent communication skills, with consistent efforts to elicit and address the expectations and requests of the patient

---

BOX 2-3 Common Legal Claims for Departure from Standards of Care

Failure to monitor or observe a patient's clinical status adequately

Failure to monitor or observe a change in a patient's clinical status

Failure to communicate and/or document a significant change in a patient's condition to appropriate professional

Failure to obtain a complete nursing history

Failure to formulate and/or follow the nursing care plan

Failure to perform a nursing treatment or procedure properly

Failure to provide a safe environment and to protect the patient from avoidable injury

Failure to implement a physician/NP/PA order properly and/or in a timely fashion

Failure to administer medications properly and in a timely fashion, and/or to report and administer omitted doses appropriately

Failure to observe a medication's action or adverse side effect

Failure to prevent infection

Failure to obtain help for a patient not receiving proper care from a physician or other health care provider

Failure to report that a patient is not receiving proper care from a physician or other health care provider

Failure to use equipment properly

Failure to evaluate and/or identify a patient at high risk for falling and/or to plan and implement a fall prevention program, appropriate to the individual patient

Failure to apply restraints when indicated and ordered

Failure to apply restraints in a proper manner

Utilizing equipment that is known to be defective

Failure to make prompt, accurate entries in a patient's medical record

Altering a medical record without noting it as a correction with signature, date, and time of change

Failure to adhere to hospital policy and/or procedural guidelines

b. Sincere compassion for each patient

c. Competent practice

d. Accurate and complete charting with notations of any deviations from the applicable standard of care with the specific reasons (eg, patient refused chest radiograph due to time constraint), and the patient's noncompliance

5. Generally, the professional nurse has the duty to:

a. Exercise that degree of diligence and skill that is ordinarily exercised by other professional nurses in the same state and specialty of practice

b. Apply such knowledge with reasonable care

c. Keep informed of approved standards of care in general use

d. Exercise his/her own best judgment in rendering care to the patient

6. Some states apply a geographic standard referred to as a locality rule, which asserts that providers in remote rural areas may have less access to continuing education and various equipment than their colleagues in urban areas. However, because communication and transportation continue to improve rapidly, the locality rule is becoming obsolete.

Burden of Proof for Malpractice

The plaintiff has the burden of proving four elements of malpractice, usually by means of expert testimony.

Duty

1. The plaintiff has a duty to prove that a patient–nurse relationship did, in fact, exist and, by virtue of that relationship, the nurse had the duty to exercise reasonable care when undertaking and providing treatment to the patient.

2. Limits and obligations of duty include:

a. This duty exists only when there is a patient–nurse relationship.

b. The professional nurse is not obligated to enter into a nurse–patient relationship with any individual.

c. Professional nurses generally have the right to decide to whom they will provide professional services and may request to be reassigned to another patient if the nurse–patient relationship is strained, difficult, or otherwise not comfortable.

d. Nurses have limits on their rights to decide, however, and may not refuse to treat a patient who has relied reasonably on the nurse's apparent willingness to treat all in need (eg, the emergency care department in a general hospital that advertises its emergency services) and may not abandon an established patient.

e. If a professional nurse wishes to terminate an established relationship with a patient, an available alternative with equivalent level nursing services must be made available to the patient in a timely fashion.

> **NURSING ALERT**
>
> The professional nurse must use caution when offering telephone advice for which there is no charge; there have been reported cases of patients suing providers successfully because they reasonably relied on the telephone advice of a nurse that caused them to delay seeking care and sustain permanent injuries as a result.

Breach of Duty

1. The plaintiff has the burden to establish that the professional nurse violated the applicable standard of care in treating the patient's condition.

2. The plaintiff must establish by way of expert professional nurse testimony that the "negligent" nurse failed to conform to the applicable standard of care, or rendered nursing care that fell below the level of care that would have been rendered by a prudent and diligent nurse under the same circumstances.

Proximate Cause

1. The plaintiff has the burden of establishing a causal relationship between the breach in the standard of care and the patient's injuries.

2. If a breach in standard of care did not cause the alleged injuries, then there is no proximate cause.

Damages

The plaintiff has the burden of establishing the existence of damages to the patient as a result of the malpractice.

Malpractice Insurance

1. Malpractice insurance will not protect the professional nurse from charges of practicing outside his/her scope of practice if he/she is practicing outside the legal scope of practice permitted within the state.

2. Hence, it is critical that he/she know the exact scope of practice permitted in his/her jurisdiction.

3. It is universally recommended that all professional nurses carry their own liability insurance coverage. This affords the nurse his/her own legal representation and an attorney who will be looking out solely for the nurse's best interests. Such coverage is recommended over and above the legal coverage and representation afforded by the employer's coverage.

The National Practitioner Databank

1. In 1986, The Health Care Quality Improvement Act established a databank to scrutinize members of the health care professions and list those physicians, nurses, and all other health care practitioners who have had a malpractice claim asserted against them.

2. At the time this databank was put into operation in 1991, it was limited to physicians and other health care providers in the hospital setting.

3. Recently, however, it has been expanded to include certain ambulatory care settings. Several more years of data

collection will be needed before meaningful numbers emerge.

4. At the present time, all hospitals must query the databank every 2 years regarding health care practitioners on their professional medical and nursing staffs, those to whom they have granted clinical privileges, or new appointments.
5. It is likely that continued health care industry evolution will yield statistics concerning health care practitioners' histories vis-à-vis malpractice claims.
   a. Exactly how these statistics will be utilized is not clear at the present time, but it would not be unanticipated for them to be used as one of several selection criteria for job applicant screening, for example.

▪ Telephone Triage, Advice, and Counseling

1. The use of telephone triage, advice, and counseling has become increasingly prevalent as health care providers have attempted to meet and satisfy the health care needs of their clients, increase access to care, and improve continuity of care, while limiting scheduled appointments to those truly requiring a patient–physician or other health care provider interaction.
2. However, those involved in the provision of such services must keep in mind that, even absent a face-to-face interaction, the professional nurse is nonetheless legally accountable for gathering of an accurate and complete history, application of appropriate protocols for diagnostic impressions, appropriate consultation with physicians and other health care providers, advice and counseling given, and facilitating timely and appropriate access to treatment facilities or referral to specialists to those in need.
3. A number of legal concepts of relevance to telephone triage are outlined in the next section.

Confidentiality
Just as in face-to-face interactions, all information exchanged during a telephone interaction is privileged and only to be used in the context of the advice being sought, with the sole purpose of providing the most appropriate and timely care needed by the client.

Implied Relationships
Even if the professional nurse rendering telephone advice never had or will have a face-to-face interaction with the client, the telephone interaction itself will establish a formal and legally binding patient–nurse relationship, for which the practitioner will be accountable legally.

Information Retrieval
1. The professional nurse has the duty to provide advice and counsel in the context of all medical data available to the practice from within the patient's medical record.

2. Therefore, a rapid method for retrieval of medical record data should be established and integrated into the telephone component of all practices.
3. Telephone advice must not be provided in a vacuum of knowledge about the patient's past history and so forth.
4. Because limited time will usually preclude gathering of all data available in the medical record already established, advice rendered without the benefit of all known medical history is more subject to error.

Respondeat Superior
1. Employers are held accountable, legally responsible, and liable for all inappropriate advice rendered by their employees, and all the damages that stem therefrom.
2. Therefore, employers must be responsible for educating and training the employees and updating protocols.

Vicarious Liability
1. Although similar to the concept of respondeat superior, vicarious liability is a broader concept in that a professional nurse rendering telephone advice or counseling may be viewed as a representative of the clinic physician, practice group, or clinic, thereby binding them legally for all acts of omission or commission, and damages that stem therefrom.
2. Thus, if telephone advice and counsel are rendered by an LPN, RN, or unlicensed personnel, the nurse and/or the health care facility and/or physicians in the practice may be viewed by a court as vicariously liable for inappropriate advice rendered and all resulting damages to the client.
3. This underscores the reasons for limiting this practice to well-trained nurses, physicians, and other health care providers and following carefully devised office protocols and standards.
4. The professional nurse must be encouraged to consult briefly with the in-office physician or other health care providers to reduce the possibility of advice that is not appropriate, oversights, and errors.

Negligent Supervisor
1. This concept relates to the failure of a supervising physician or other health care provider to provide the needed guidance and direction to the telephone advice nurse, despite a prevailing understanding, practice, or policy obligating this supervision.
2. Usually overlaps with respondeat superior or vicarious liability.

Negligence
1. Any telephone assessment and advice rendered must be in accordance with the generally accepted standards and protocols.
2. Violation of the applicable standards of practice/care is considered to be negligent.

3. Evidence of standards of care are established by:
   a. Publications on the topic
   b. Community practices
   c. Generally accepted guidelines or treatises on the topic

Abandonment

1. This concept becomes operational when a patient calls or comes in to report symptoms, seek advice, or request an on-site evaluation and/or treatment, and this communication is documented or otherwise established as fact, but the telephone advice nurse fails to follow through with the professional component of the interaction (advice).
2. Unless an undesirable outcome with serious and permanent damages occurred due to the absence of follow through by the telephone practitioner, however, it is doubtful that a legal claim could be brought successfully against the practitioner.

■ Electronic Communication and Telemedicine

1. In coming years, electronic communication is likely to become as prevalent as telephone advice, particularly for the 15% to 25% of Americans who reside in medically underserved or nonurban communities.
2. Although now communication is, for the most part, limited to the telephone or facsimile transmission, communication by high-tech computer systems that allow transmission of images (such as radiographs) and other data is likely to become just as prevalent in the near future.
3. Although legal accountability for such distance care is, as yet, unestablished, it is probable that the above-described principles will apply to those practices as well if a formal nurse–patient relationship is perceived to exist by the court.

■ Successful Telephone Practice

1. Policies aimed at minimizing the risk of an untoward outcome resulting from telephone advice, triage, and counseling should be established in every practice.
2. Policies should include protocol use, telephone practitioner training and education, use of established patient database, communication with physician or other health care providers, and appropriate documentation of interaction.
3. See Box 2-4 for components of a successful telephone advice practice.
4. The telephone advice nurse must gather and document certain fundamental information from the patient seeking health care advice or treatment. Although the following list is presented, it is not intended to limit inquiry or imply that the list is exhaustive. The inquiry and documentation must minimally include:
   a. Date and time of call
   b. Caller information including name of patient, relationship to the patient, telephone number with area code, when and where the caller may be reached for

---

> **BOX 2-4 Components of Successful Telephone Practice**
>
> - Apply standardized protocols and guidelines for the most frequently reported chief complaints.
> - Train nurses in proper history taking, protocol/guideline utilization, and documentation.
> - Apply a computer-based approach to manage the telephone encounters to complement existing protocols and guidelines to improve the process and documentation of the encounter.
> - Implement a quality assurance system to ensure a regular review of telephone logs.
> - Discuss problem cases with telephone advice nurses, and perform outcome surveys.
> - Maintain a constant availability of physicians and other health care providers to provide consultative assistance to the telephone advice nurse, as needed.
> - Ensure an ongoing review and revision of protocols and policies, to eliminate or improve on problematic policies and protocols.
> - Schedule patients with a possibly serious problem to be seen immediately.
> - Ask and confirm that the patient understands and feels comfortable with the plan at the end of the telephone interaction.
> - Invite the patient for an after-hours visit if he/she is uncomfortable with receiving home care instructions only, or with waiting until the next day to see the physician or other health care provider.
> - Encourage patients to call back if their condition worsens or if they have additional questions.
> - Advise patients to contact their health care provider the next day if the problem is not improving/resolving.
> - Document succinctly the components of telephone interaction, including the chief complaint, history of present illness, past medical history, allergies, home care or other instructions given, confirmation of patient's understanding and comfort with advice given, emergency precautions provided, and follow-up plans.

---

return calls, and alternative telephone numbers with area code, for backup
   c. Chief complaint
   d. History of present illness, with brief description of onset, symptoms, treatment used to date, effectiveness or lack of effectiveness of measures attempted, and aggravating or alleviating factors
   e. Whether the patient has had this problem before and, if so, when, diagnosis, and method of resolution
   f. If female, last menstrual period, method of birth control, and follow-up to rule out pregnancy
   g. Past medical history/other medical problems
   h. Allergies
   i. Likely differential diagnosis(es) based on the established protocols and guidelines being utilized by the organization or clinic
   j. Impact of the problem on the caller or patient

k. Accessibility of alternative sources of health care
l. Nurse's perception of the patient's vulnerability
m. Nurse's perception of the patient's understanding and comfort with the plan of care and follow-up plans

REFERENCES

Ahmed, D. S., & Hamrah, P. M. (1999). Med errors: Right drug, wrong dose. *American Journal of Nursing, 99*(1), 12.

American Nurses Association. (1999). *Standards of nursing practice* (2nd ed.). Washington, DC: American Nurses Publishing.

Awong, L. (1998). Asking patients about revising advance directives. *American Journal of Nursing, 98*(4), 71.

Bakzek, L., & Gross, L. (1999). Confidentiality and privacy: At the forefront for nurses. *American Journal of Nursing, 99*(6), 52.

Becker, J. H. (1997). Considerations in reporting elder abuse. *American Journal of Nursing, 97*(7), 22.

Beckman, J. P. (1995). *Nursing malpractice: Implications for clinical practice and nursing education.* Seattle: University of Washington Press.

Boucher, M. A. (1998). Delegation alert: how to delegate effectively while maintaining your nursing presence with patients. *American Journal of Nursing, 98*(2), 26–32.

Edwards, B. (1994). Telephone triage: How experienced nurses reach decisions. *Journal of Advanced Nursing, 19,* 717–724.

Eskreis-Nelson, T. R. (1997). Shedding some light on psychiatric care issues. *RN, 2,* 57–60.

Fiesta, J. (1998). Legal aspects of medication administration. *Nursing Management, 29,* 22–23.

Gobis, L. J. (1997). Can unlicensed staff relay verbal orders? *American Journal of Nursing, 97*(4), 20.

Haddad, A. (1997). Acute care decisions: Ethics in action. *RN, 1,* 21–24.

Kany, K. (1999). Workplace protections: Combating staffing problems. *American Journal of Nursing, 99*(4), 68.

Lewis, R. (1997). When a patient goes "AMA." *American Journal of Nursing, 97,* 13.

Lilley, L. L., & Guanci, R. (1999). Cross sensitivities: Medication errors waiting to happen. *American Journal of Nursing, 99*(2), 12.

Olijnyk, F. J. (2000). Legal and ethical issues. In P. V. Meredith & N. M. Horan (Eds.), *Adult primary care* (pp. 43–51). Philadelphia: W. B. Saunders.

Morgan, M. R. (1998). Falsifying an incident report. *American Journal of Nursing, 98*(1), 20–21.

Nguyen, B. Q. (1999). Workplace protections: When are you protected under the Americans with Disabilities Act? *American Journal of Nursing, 99*(6), 70.

Polston, M. D. (1999). Whistleblowing: Does the law protect you? *American Journal of Nursing, 99*(1), 26–32.

———. (1998). Reporting fraud. *American Journal of Nursing, 98,* 5, 70.

Poole, S. R. (1992). After-hours telephone coverage: The application of an area-wide telephone triage and advice system for pediatric practices. *Pediatrics, 92*(5), 670–679.

Ramsey, G. C. (1998). When long-term residents require emergent care. *American Journal of Nursing, 98*(9), 56.

Sheehan, J. P. (1997). Safeguard your license: The disciplinary process. *RN, 1,* 53–55.

Taylor, R. (1998). Forensic nursing: Standards for a new specialty. *American Journal of Nursing, 98*(2), 73.

The Virginia Law Foundation. (1998). Virginia lawyers practice handbook: Medical malpractice law in Virginia. *4,* 139–152.

Health Promotion and Preventive Care

CONCEPTS IN PROMOTION AND PREVENTION

■ Principles of Health Promotion

Health promotion is defined as the actions taken to develop a high level of wellness and is accomplished by influencing individual behavior and the environment in which people live.

Levels of Prevention
1. Disease prevention is aimed at avoidance of problems or minimizing problems once they occur.
   a. Primary prevention is the total prevention of a condition.
   b. Secondary prevention is the early recognition of a condition and measures taken to speed recovery.
   c. Tertiary prevention is the care given to minimize the effects of the condition and prevent long-term complications.
2. Preventive care should involve risk assessment to focus interventions at persons at risk for specific disorders.

Healthy People 2000 and 2010
1. Health promotion goes beyond prevention to help people manage their health and live longer and feel better.
2. Health promotion has become a priority since the US Department of Health and Human Services launched the Healthy People 2000 campaign in 1990 to focus public and health care worker attention on 21 health objectives, such as reducing tobacco use, reducing alcohol abuse, improving nutrition, improving environmental public health, preventing and controlling human immunodeficiency virus (HIV) infection and acquired immunodeficiency syndrome (AIDS), and improving maternal and infant health .

   Results of the Healthy People 2000 program have been generally good, with decreased infant mortality,

fewer deaths from car accidents and other violence, and decreased breast cancer deaths.
3. Negative results from the program have been an increase in asthma and asthma hospitalizations among young people, and an increase in obesity and inactivity in all ages.
4. A major goal for the Healthy People 2010 program is to reduce the disparity between races and ethnic groups on health issues. Hispanics and African Americans suffer higher rates of chronic disease such as diabetes and have poorer health outcomes in many areas. Another goal is to improve quality of life.
5. Healthy People 2010 is divided into four main categories:
   a. Promote healthy behaviors
   b. Promote healthy and safe communities
   c. Improve systems for personal and public health
   d. Prevent and reduce diseases and disorders

Nursing Role in Health Promotion
1. Nurses have played key roles in prevention in areas such as prenatal care, immunization programs, occupational health and safety, cardiac rehabilitation and education, and public health case finding and early intervention.
2. Nurses in all settings can meet health promotion needs of patients, whether practice is in the hospital, clinic, patient's home, health maintenance organization, private office, or community setting.
3. Health promotion is primarily accomplished through patient education, an independent function of nursing.
4. Health promotion should occur through the life cycle, with topics focused for infancy, childhood, adolescence, adulthood, and older age.
   a. For infancy, teach parents about the importance of prenatal care, basic care of infants, breast-feeding, nutrition, and infant safety.
   b. For childhood, stress the topics of immunizations; proper nutrition to enhance growth and development; and safety practices such as use of car seats and seat belts, fire prevention, and poison proofing the home.

c. For adolescence, focus topics on motor vehicle safety; avoidance of drug, alcohol, and tobacco use; sexual decision making and contraception; and prevention of suicide.

d. For adulthood, teach patients about nutrition, exercise, and stress management to help them feel better; also teach cancer screening techniques such as breast and testicular self-examination, and risk factor reduction for the leading causes of death—heart disease, stroke, and cancer.

e. For older age, stress the topics of nutrition and exercise to help them live longer and stay fit, safety measures to help them compensate for decreasing mobility and sensory function, and ways to stay active and independent.

Patient Teaching and Health Education

Health education is included in the American Nurses Association Standards of Care and is defined as an essential component of nursing care. It is directed toward promotion, maintenance, and restoration of health and toward adaptation to the residual effects of illness.

Learning Readiness

1. Assist the patient in physical readiness to learn by trying to alleviate any physical distress that may distract the patient's attention and prevent effective learning.
2. Assess and promote the patient's emotional readiness to learn.
   a. Motivation to learn depends on acceptance of the illness or that illness is a threat, recognition of the need to learn, values related to social and cultural background, and a therapeutic regimen comparable with the patient's lifestyle.
   b. Promote motivation to learn by creating a warm, accepting, positive atmosphere; encouraging the patient to participate in the establishment of acceptable, realistic, and attainable learning goals; and providing constructive feedback about progress.
3. Assess and promote the patient's experiential readiness to learn.
   a. Determine what past experiences the patient has had with health and illness, what success or failure the patient has had with learning, and what basic knowledge the patient has on related topics.
   b. Provide the patient with any prerequisite knowledge necessary to begin the learning process.

Teaching Strategies

1. Patient education can occur at any time and in any setting; however, you must consider how conducive the environment is to learning, how much time you are able to schedule, and what other family members or significant others can attend the teaching session.
2. Use a variety of techniques that are appropriate to meet the needs of each individual.
   a. Lecture or explanation should include discussion or a question and answer period.
   b. Group discussion is effective for individuals with similar needs; participants often gain support, assistance, and encouragement from other members.
   c. Demonstration and practice should be used when skills need to be learned; ample time should be allowed for practice and return demonstration.
   d. Teaching aids include books, pamphlets, pictures, slides, videos, tapes, and models and should be supplemental to verbal teaching. These can be obtained from government agencies such as the Department of Health and Human Services, the Centers for Disease Control and Prevention, and the National Institutes of Health; not-for-profit groups such as the American Heart Association or the March of Dimes; or pharmaceutical and insurance companies.
   e. Reinforcement and follow-up sessions offer time for evaluation and additional teaching if necessary and can greatly increase effectiveness of teaching.
3. Document patient teaching, including what was taught and how the patient responded; use standardized patient teaching checklists if available.

Selected Areas of Health Promotion

Counsel patients on the topics of proper nutrition, smoking cessation, exercise, relaxation, and sexual health to promote health.

Nutrition and Diet

1. It is projected that 35% of all cancer could be prevented with an improved diet recommended by the National Cancer Institute.
2. A low-fat, high-fiber diet is recommended.
   a. Fat should account for no more than 30% of calories.
   b. Fiber content should be 20 to 30 g daily.
   c. Five servings of fruits and vegetables should be included daily.
   d. Six servings of breads, cereals, and legumes should be included daily.
3. Dietary modifications are also necessary to treat and prevent disease such as hypertension, type II diabetes mellitus, coronary artery disease, and hyperlipidemia, as well as to promote optimal weight, energy, and well-being.
4. Educate patients about the five basic food groups and their placement on the food pyramid, optimum weight, calorie requirements, and ways to increase fiber and decrease fat in the diet.
   a. Total fat content can be reduced by cutting down on red and fatty cuts of meat; bacon and sausage; cooking oils; whole dairy products; eggs; baked goods; cookies and candy; and sauces, soups, and dressings made with cream, eggs, or oil. Also teach patients to save high-fat foods for a special treat, reduce portion

size, use fat substitutes, and prepare dishes at home using low-fat recipes.
  b. Teach patients to add fiber to the diet by choosing whole grain breads and cereals; raw or minimally cooked fruits and vegetables (especially citrus fruits, squash, cabbage, lettuce and other greens, beans); and any nuts, skins, and seeds. Fiber can also be increased by adding several teaspoons of whole bran to meals each day or taking an over-the-counter fiber supplement such as psyllium (Metamucil), as directed.
5. Encourage patients to keep diaries of their food intake and review them periodically to determine if other adjustments should be made.
6. If weight loss is desired, have the patient weigh in monthly, and review the diet and give praise or constructive criticism at this visit. Many people, especially women, respond to group therapy that focuses on education, support, and expression of feelings related to overeating.
7. Use and refer patients to resources such as:
   TOPS (Take Off Pounds Sensibly)
   P.O. Box 070360
   4575 South Fifth Street
   Milwaukee, WI 53207
   414-482-4620
   www.tops.org

Smoking Prevention and Cessation

1. It has been estimated that 30% of all cancer is linked to smoking and is preventable.
2. Studies show that 60% of all current smokers began by age 14 and that more than 3,000 children each day begin to use tobacco in the United States.
3. Smoking is a risk factor for hypertension, heart disease, peripheral vascular disease, chronic obstructive pulmonary disease (COPD), and cancer of the lung, colon, larynx, oral cavity, esophagus, bladder, pancreas, and kidney. It also worsens such conditions as respiratory infections, peptic ulcers, hiatal hernia, and gastroesophageal reflux.
4. Not smoking promotes health by increasing exercise tolerance; enhancing taste bud function; and avoiding facial wrinkles, bad breath, and odor on clothes.
5. Smoking prevention education should begin during childhood and stressed during adolescence, a time when peer modeling and confusion over self-image may lead to smoking.
6. Smoking cessation can be accomplished through an individualized, multidimensional program including:
   a. Information on the short- and long-term health effects of smoking.
   b. Practical behavior modification techniques to help break the habit—gum chewing, munching on carrot and celery sticks, sucking on mints and hard candy to provide oral stimulation; working modeling clay, knitting, or other ways to provide tactile stimulation; avoiding coffee shops, bars, or other situations that smokers frequent; incentive plans such as saving money for each cigarette not smoked and rewarding oneself when a goal is reached.
   c. Use of medications designed to reduce physical dependence and minimize withdrawal symptoms such as nicotine chewing gum, nasal spray or transdermal patches, as well as oral medication that acts on neurotransmitters in the central nervous system.
   d. Use of support groups, frequent reinforcement, and follow-up.
7. Use and refer patients to agencies such as:
   American Cancer Society
   19 West 56th Street
   New York, NY 10019
   212-586-8700
   www.acs.org

   American Lung Association
   1740 Broadway
   New York, NY 10019
   212-315-8700
   www.lungusa.org

Exercise and Fitness

1. Regular exercise as part of a fitness program helps achieve optimal weight, control blood pressure, increase high-density lipoprotein (HDL), lower risk of coronary artery disease, increase endurance, and improve the sense of well-being.
2. Long-term goals of regular exercise include decreased absenteeism from work, less disability, and reduced health care costs.
3. Studies have shown that both high-intensity exercise and low- to moderate-intensity exercise performed at least three times a week have positive effects.
   a. High-intensity exercise achieving 70% to 90% of maximum heart rate produces lactic acid in the muscles, which inhibits fat burning; however, calories will be burned at a high rate because carbohydrate is used for energy.
   b. Low- to moderate-intensity exercise achieving 50% to 70% of maximum heart rate begins to access fat stores for fuel after 30 minutes of exercise; with longer duration of exercise fewer calories but more fat will be burned.
4. Individual tolerance, time allotment, interests, and physical impairment must be figured into exercise planning.
5. Suggest walking, jogging, bicycling, swimming, water aerobics, and low-impact aerobic dancing as good low- to moderate-intensity exercise, performed three to five times a week for 45 minutes. Walking can be done safely and comfortably by most patients if the pace is adjusted to the individual's physical condition.
   a. Exercise programs should include 5- to 10-minute warm-up and cool-down periods with stretching activities to prevent injuries.
   b. Full intensity and duration of exercise should be worked up to gradually over a period of several weeks to months.

GERONTOLOGIC ALERT

Due to physiologic limitations of old age, maximum effective exercise for the elderly is 20 to 40 minutes at 50% to 60% of maximum heart rate.

6. Advise patients to stop if pain, shortness of breath, dizziness, palpitations, or excessive sweating is experienced.
7. Advise patients with cardiovascular, respiratory, and musculoskeletal disorders to check with their health care provider about specific guidelines or limitations for exercise.

NURSING ALERT

Severe cases of COPD, osteoarthritis, and coronary disease are contraindications for unsupervised exercise; check with the patient's health care provider to see if a physical therapy or occupational therapy referral would be helpful.

8. Use and refer patients to resources such as:
American Heart Association
772 Greenville Avenue
Dallas, TX 75231
214-373-6300
www.americanheart.org

Relaxation and Stress Management

1. *Stress* is a change in the environment that is perceived as a threat, challenge, or harm to the person's dynamic equilibrium. In times of stress, the sympathetic nervous system is activated to produce immediate changes of increased heart rate, peripheral vasoconstriction, and increased blood pressure. This response is prolonged by adrenal stimulation and secretion of epinephrine and norepinephrine, and is known as "the fight or flight" reaction.
2. A limited amount of stress can be a positive motivator to take action; however, excessive or prolonged stress can cause emotional discomfort, anxiety, possible panic, and illness.
3. Prolonged sympathetic-adrenal stimulation may lead to high blood pressure, arteriosclerotic changes, and cardiovascular disease; stress has also been implicated in acute asthma attack, peptic ulcer disease, irritable bowel syndrome, migraine headaches, and other illnesses.
4. Stress management can help control these illnesses as well as help individuals improve self-esteem, gain control over their lives, and enjoy life more fully.
5. Stress management involves identification of physiologic and psychosocial stressors through assessment of the patient's education, finances, job, family, habits, activities, personal and family health history, and responsibilities. Positive and negative coping methods should also be identified.
6. Relaxation therapy is one of the first steps in stress management; it can be used to reduce anxiety brought on by stress. Relaxation techniques include:

a. *Relaxation breathing*—the simplest technique that can be performed at any time. The patient breathes slowly and deeply until relaxation is achieved; however, it can lead to hyperventilation if done incorrectly.
b. *Progressive muscle relaxation*—relieves muscle tension related to stress. The patient alternately tenses, then relaxes muscle groups until the entire body feels relaxed.
c. *Autogenic training*—can help relieve pain and induce sleep. The patient replaces painful or unpleasant sensations with pleasant ones through self-suggestions; may require extensive coaching at first.
d. *Imagery*—uses imagination and concentration to take a "mental vacation." The patient imagines a peaceful, pleasant scene involving multiple senses. It can last as long as patient decides.
e. *Distraction*—uses patient's own interests and activities to divert attention from pain or anxiety and includes listening to music, watching television, reading a book, singing, knitting, doing crafts or projects, or physical activities.

7. To assist patients with relaxation therapy, follow these steps:
a. Review the techniques and encourage a trial with several techniques of the patient's choice.
b. Teach the chosen technique(s) and coach the patient until effective use of the technique is demonstrated.
c. Suggest that the patient practice relaxation techniques for 20 minutes a day to feel more relaxed and to be prepared to use them confidently when stress increases.
d. Encourage the patient to combine techniques such as relaxation breathing before and after imagery or progressive muscle relaxation along with autogenic training to achieve better results.

8. Additional steps in stress management include dealing with the stressors or problem areas and increasing coping behaviors.
a. Assist the patient to recognize specific stressors and determine if they can be altered. Then develop a plan for managing that stressor such as changing jobs, postponing taking an extra class, hiring a babysitter once a week, talking to the neighbor about his dog, or getting up an hour earlier to exercise.
b. Teach the patient to avoid negative coping behaviors such as smoking, drinking, using drugs, overeating, cursing, and using abusive behavior toward others. Teach positive coping mechanisms such as continued use of relaxation techniques, fostering of support systems—family, friends, church groups, social groups, or professional support groups.

Sexual Health

1. Because sexuality is inherent to every person and sexual functioning is a basic physiologic need of human beings, nurses must provide care in a way that is promotional to sexual health.

2. As a health educator and counselor in the area of sexual health, the nurse helps the patient gain knowledge, validate normalcy, prepare for changes in sexuality throughout the life cycle, and prevent harm gained through sexual activity.

3. Education about sexual activity should begin during school age, heighten during adolescence, and continue through adulthood.

4. Topics to cover include:

   a. Normal reproduction—the menstrual cycle, ovulation, fertilization (see p. 743).

   b. Unwanted pregnancy—approximately one million teen pregnancies occur in the United States each year.

   c. Contraception—ideally should begin before sexual activity is started, various methods, side effects, effectiveness, convenience (see p. 750).

   d. Sexually transmitted diseases (STDs)—mode of transmission, prevalence, signs and symptoms, methods of prevention (see p. 767).

      (i) Over 20 million people have genital herpes in the United States.

      (ii) Chlamydia is now the most common sexually transmitted pathogen and is often asymptomatic.

      (iii) Genital warts are highly recurrent and may lead to cervical dysplasia.

      (iv) Approximately 400,000 cases of AIDS were reported in the United States in 1993.

   e. Safer sex/abstinence—primarily adopted to prevent HIV transmission, but can also prevent other STDs and pregnancy.

      (i) Abstinence is the only 100% effective method for HIV prevention related to sexual transmission.

      (ii) Mutual monogamy can also be 100% effective if both partners enter the relationship HIV negative.

      (iii) Use of female or male latex condoms correctly and consistently is also highly effective.

      (iv) Use of spermicide containing nonoxynal-9 in addition to condoms provides additional protection.

      (v) For individuals infected with HIV, avoid vaginal, anal, and oral intercourse, deep kissing, and any practices that may injure tissues, if possible.

5. Other areas in which nurses can help promote healthy sexual functioning:

   a. Discuss with teenagers the value of delaying sexual activity—prevention of pregnancy and STDs, saving money on contraception, greater enjoyment of first sexual encounter when older, greater control of relationship and decision making if not sexually involved.

   b. Assist men to have greater respect for women, to allow women partnership in relationship, and to not equate sex with violence as often depicted in movies and television.

   c. Assist women to understand their sexuality needs, become comfortable with their bodies, communicate with sexual partners about their satisfaction, and seek medical help for gynecologic problems.

6. Use and refer patients to resources such as:

   American Social Health Association Herpes Hotline
   919-361-8488

   Centers for Disease Control and Prevention
   404-639-3534
   www.cdc.gov

   National AIDS Clearinghouse
   1-800-458-5231

PATIENT TEACHING AIDS

Copy and distribute the following patient teaching aids to enhance your counseling and promote health.

Stress is a common phenomenon among most individuals today, and can be related to job, relationship, financial, and other pressures. Known as the "fight or flight" reaction, the physiologic and emotional response to stress can lead to tension, anxiety, and a variety of health threats. Stress can be minimized by better coping with it and adapting to its causes. Follow this guide to better manage stress.

Recognize Stress

1. First, identify signs that you may be under stress (eg, irritability, tension, fatigue, insomnia, loss of interest in activities, feeling overwhelmed, or fighting with spouse and others).
2. Next, try to identify the true cause of stress. For example, you may snap at your children for playing the stereo too loudly, but what is the underlying cause of your irritability?
3. Examine areas of your job, family life, financial stability, and other roles and responsibilities that may be demanding or problematic.

Do Something About It

1. Try to manage stressful areas better—be assertive, negotiate, and say no if necessary. For example, confront the person with whom you are at odds and work out a mutual agreement, put the plan in writing, and try to stick to it.
2. Make more time for yourself and important relationships. Say no to responsibilities that you don't have time for and get help from a family member or friend, or hire a babysitter when necessary.

Relax

When you enter a stressful situation or you feel tension rising, practice the following relaxation techniques; you will be able to think more clearly and function more effectively.

RELAXATION BREATHING
Concentrate on breathing slowly and deeply with eyes closed (if possible) for several minutes when you need a quick tension reducer or before beginning one of the other methods.

1. Breathe in through your nose and mouth with face relaxed for a count of 1 and 2 and 3 and 4.
2. Hold your breath for 4 seconds, without straining.
3. Breathe out through your nose and pursed lips for a count of 6.
4. Repeat two or three times, breathe naturally for about 30 seconds, then repeat one or more sequences.
5. If you feel dizzy or tingling in your fingertips, you may be hyperventilating; slow down your breathing and don't take such deep breaths.

PROGRESSIVE MUSCLE RELAXATION
Because stress may cause you to subconsciously contract your muscles, in this exercise you will alternately tense and relax your muscle groups one by one, until your entire body is in a state of relaxation.

1. Assume a comfortable position, either sitting or reclining, and close your eyes.
2. Start with your forehead and tense the muscles so you feel tightness or strain; hold this position for 5 to 10 seconds.
3. Next, relax your forehead, noting the relief; concentrate on this for 10 to 15 seconds.
4. Progress from head to toe with each muscle group, including your jaw next, then shoulders, arms, hands, abdomen, buttocks, legs, and feet (you can do both sides simultaneously).
5. Note the feeling of total relaxation in your body once you have relieved tension from all your muscles.
6. Complete the exercise by opening your eyes, taking a few deep breaths, stretching, and arising slowly.

IMAGERY
Imagery allows you to take a mental vacation by using your imagination and diverting your attention from stressful thoughts.

1. Assume a comfortable position, breathe deeply, and close your eyes.
2. Count backward from 5 and begin to imagine a pleasant place such as a beach or garden.
3. Put yourself in that place by imagining it with all your senses (eg, hear the sound of waves washing up on the beach, feel the warm sun saturating your skin, or taste a tangy drink of lemonade).
4. Stay in that place for about 5 minutes, imagining different images.
5. Slowly let the images fade, breathe deeply, and count to 5 before opening your eyes.

DISTRACTION
You can use many methods of distraction to block your concentration from anxiety and stressful matters. Using your senses to listen to music, petting your dog, or reading can be relaxing.

1. Choose activities that you enjoy—reading, watching television, listening to music, taking a walk, playing an instrument, knitting, doing a craft, or drawing or painting.
2. Adjust the distraction method to your mood—if you are extremely tense, do not attempt a complex project or listen to loud, lively music. Rather, listen to quiet, soothing music or sketch a free-form design.
3. Use a variety of methods—some reserved for longer periods of time, and others that can be used on the spot when needed (eg, a portable tape player with headphones and your favorite music or a book of poetry).

PATIENT EDUCATION GUIDELINES Exercise Guidelines

Aerobic exercise provides a wide range of benefits including weight loss, muscle toning, endurance building, improved circulation, increased HDL (the "good" cholesterol), lowered risk of a heart attack, better controlled blood pressure, and a sense of reduced tension and feeling better. Aerobic exercise refers to any type of activity that uses oxygen to produce energy. The cardiovascular system is stimulated, and fat is burned. Most people can do aerobic exercise of some kind, adjusting the intensity as necessary. Follow these guidelines to develop your own exercise program.

1. Choose an activity that you enjoy, is convenient, and you are capable of; consider walking, bicycle riding, jogging, swimming, aerobics or step aerobics, sporting activities, or use of fitness equipment such as the rowing machine, stair stepper, or cross country ski machine.
2. Start out exercising 15 to 20 minutes at a time for the first week or two, then gradually increase the intensity and length of exercise time over several weeks to months.
3. Include 5- to 10-minute warm-up and cool-down periods with each exercise session, doing stretching of major muscles, deep breathing, and light calisthenics.
4. Exercise at least three times a week and be consistent.
5. Exercise at 50% to 70% of your maximum heart rate for moderate intensity or 70% to 90% for high intensity, as tolerated.

Calculating Target Heart Rate

To get the most out of exercise, calculate your heart rate. First, subtract your age from 220. This is your maximum heart rate; do not exceed this rate while exercising to avoid strain on your heart.

If you are 40 years old, your maximum heart rate is 220 minus 40, or 180. Your target heart rate is 40% to 50% of maximum for low-intensity exercise, 50% to 70% of maximum for moderate-intensity exercise, or 70% to 90% of max-

imum for high-intensity exercise. So, if you want to exercise at moderate intensity, 60% of 180 is 108 (180×0.6). Your target heart rate is 108. By taking your pulse several times during exercise, you can adjust your pace to stay close to your target heart rate and exercise optimally but safely.

Taking Your Pulse

First take your resting pulse before you begin exercise, counting for 30 seconds and multiplying by 2.

To take your pulse during exercise, slow down and find the carotid pulse point in your neck. Place two or three fingers on your trachea (windpipe) near the base of your neck and then move them over to the left or right about 2 to 3 inches until you feel the beating of your pulse. Press lightly so you do not cause an irregular heartbeat or interrupt circulation to your brain. Use a watch with a second hand to count the number of beats in 6 seconds. Now, multiply by 10 to get an estimate of your true 60-second pulse.

If you counted 10 beats in 6 seconds, your working heart rate is 100 (10×10). As you continue to exercise, you can work a little harder to reach your target rate. If your working heart rate is 10 beats or more greater than your target rate, slow down your pace and check your pulse again in 5 to 10 minutes.

When you complete your exercise, your pulse should be no more than 15 beats above your resting pulse; if it is, continue your cool-down activity.

When to Stop

You should usually never stop exercising abruptly; you must allow the heart to slow down and the blood to redistribute appropriately. You should slow down if you experience muscle cramps, shortness of breath, or fatigue. You should stop, however, if you experience chest pain, a cold sweat, dizziness, nausea or vomiting, heart palpitations, or fainting. Seek help and notify your health care provider immediately.

To help maintain optimal weight, feel better, and reduce the risk of heart disease, cancer, and a variety of health problems, the following dietary changes are recommended:

1. Increase fiber in diet to 20 to 30 g daily.
2. Reduce fat content to no more than 30% of total calories each day.
3. Eat five servings of fruits and vegetables each day. A serving consists of:
    a. One medium piece of fruit, ½ cup of cut-up fruit, or 6 oz of juice
    b. One half cup of cooked or raw vegetables, or 1 cup of leafy greens
4. Include six or more servings of cereal or bread per day.
5. Maintain moderate protein intake of fish, beans, nuts, or no more than 5 to 7 oz of lean meat per day.
6. Limit salt and alcohol consumption.

Reducing Fat

To determine how many grams of fat you should eat in your diet, first identify how many calories you should eat each day. This will vary depending on your body build and activity level, but approximately 2,100 calories is an average amount for an active medium-sized man or woman who is not trying to lose weight. Next, figure that 30% of 2,100 is 630 calories of fat. There are 9 calories per gram of fat, so 630 divided by 9 equals 70 g of fat. Now you are ready to read food labels to see how many grams of fat are in each serving of food you eat. Margarine, for example, contains 11 g of fat per tablespoon, and cheddar cheese contains about 8 g of fat per ounce. You will find that 70 g will add up quickly unless you include a variety of low-fat foods in your diet. *Note:* If you are trying to lose weight and are on a lower-calorie diet with a lower percentage of fat, this figure will be much lower.

Follow this guide to reduce fat:

BREADS, CEREALS, AND GRAINS

1. Eat whole grain (oat, bran, multigrain), light, wheat, or rye bread rather than pure white bread or other breads that list eggs as a major ingredient.
2. Eat pasta or rice rather than egg noodles, serve with light tomato sauce or vegetables as main dish, rather than meat.
3. Substitute angel food cake, low-fat cookies, crackers, and home-baked goods made with low-fat ingredients for higher-fat pies, cakes, cookies, doughnuts, biscuits, and muffins.

EGGS AND DAIRY PRODUCTS

1. Use only skim or 1% milk, no cream or half and half.
2. Use part skim and reduced-fat cheeses sparingly; substitute low-fat cottage cheese.
3. Use low-fat yogurt and frozen yogurt, pudding made from skim milk, and fat-free dessert items.

FATS AND OILS

1. Never use butter, lard, or coconut, palm, or palm kernel oil.
2. Use unsaturated vegetable oils sparingly (especially canola, safflower, sesame, soybean, sunflower, and olive).
3. Substitute margarine, especially diet or light margarine, for butter, but use sparingly.
4. Avoid egg yolks, chocolate, and bacon or beef fat for cooking; substitute two egg whites for one whole egg in recipes.
5. Use only low-fat mayonnaise and salad dressings.

MEATS, FISH, AND POULTRY

1. Use lean cuts of beef, lamb, and pork sparingly.
2. Eat white meat (chicken and turkey) with skin and fat removed before cooking, if possible.
3. Avoid organ meat, ribs, chicken wings, sausage, hot dogs, and bacon.
4. Use fillets of sole, salmon, mackerel, tuna, haddock, or canned tuna packed in water; avoid sardines, roe, and shrimp (high in cholesterol).
5. Eat small portions; bake or broil; blot with paper towel after cooking; and discard drained fat.

Increasing Fiber

Fiber is a plant cell wall component that is not broken down by the digestive system. It absorbs fluid and moves through the intestines in a bulky mass with the ability to absorb cholesterol and carcinogens. It decreases intestinal transit time, therefore decreasing constipation and related problems. Increase fiber in your diet gradually to prevent gas. Here are good sources of fiber:

1. Cereal containing 4 g or more of fiber per serving (read package label)
2. Whole grain breads and muffins
3. Fresh or frozen fruits and vegetables, not overcooked, with skin on
4. Nuts, seeds, and popcorn
5. Bran; add 1 teaspoon to food three times a day
6. Legumes (pods) such as peas or beans

PATIENT EDUCATION GUIDELINES   Smoking Cessation

Cigarette smoking is the single most preventable cause of death and disability today. Smoking is related to about 30% of all cancer deaths, is the leading risk factor for coronary artery disease and emphysema, and has many other effects on health and hygiene. People who smoke tend to have more dental problems, premature aging of the skin, increased acid in the stomach, decreased exercise tolerance, loss of taste bud function, problems with pregnancy and fetal growth, more frequent respiratory infections, and bad breath.

Smoking cessation, however, will reverse most of these risks and allow you to breathe more easily and feel better.

Plan to Quit

1. Make a list of all the positive things and all the negative things about smoking; consider the short- and long-term health risks on your list.
2. Talk to your health care provider about the use of nicotine chewing gum, nasal spray, or skin patch to aid your stop smoking program by reducing withdrawal symptoms and cravings for a cigarette. An oral medication that does not contain nicotine is also available by prescription.
3. Talk to family and friends and form a support network of people who have quit smoking.
4. Set the date to quit and don't make any excuses.
5. Stock up on low-calorie treats such as raw vegetables, sugarless gum, popcorn, and sugar-free soft drinks to enjoy when the urge to smoke hits.

6. Remove all ashtrays, cigarettes, matches, and lighters from your home, car, and office.

Stick With It

1. Avoid smoky environments such as bars and coffee shops and the smoking section of restaurants.
2. Restructure your routine to eliminate times you previously enjoyed a cigarette.
3. Anticipate feeling irritable for several days to several weeks while quitting, so avoid stressful situations.
4. Increase exercise, such as walking, biking, or sporting activities to relieve tension, fill free time, and concentrate on healthy activity.
5. Occupy your hands with modeling clay, knitting, doodling, or a craft project.
6. Brush your teeth often and enjoy fresher breath.
7. Reward yourself for not smoking.

Try, Try Again

1. If you start smoking again, don't be discouraged; many people are successful the second time around.
2. Review and revise your plan and pick a new quit date.
3. For more information on smoking cessation programs, contact:

    American Cancer Society 800-ACS-2345
    American Heart Association 214-373-6300
    American Lung Association 212-315-8700

SELECTED REFERENCES

Adatsi, G. (1999). Health going up in smoke. How can you prevent it? *American Journal of Nursing, 99*(3), 63–69.

Ammon, P. K. (1999). Individualizing the approach to treating obesity. *The Nurse Practitioner, 24*(2), 27–41.

Beech, B. M., Rice, R., Myers, L., Johnson, C., & Nicklas, T. A. (1999). Knowledge, attitudes, and practices related to fruit and vegetable consumption of high school students. *Journal of Adolescent Health, 24*(4), 244–250.

Bruccoliere, T. (2000). How to make patient teaching stick. *RN, 63*(2), 34–38.

Chlan, L., & Tracy, M. F. (1999). Music therapy in critical care: Indications and guidelines for intervention. *Critical Care Nurse, 19*(3), 35–41.

Ebomoyi, E. W., Bissonette, N. E., & Ukaga, O. M. (1998). Campus courtship behavior and fear of human immunodeficiency virus infection by university students. *Journal of the National Medical Association, 90*(7), 395–399.

Erikssen, G., Liestol, K., Bjornholt, J., Thaulow, E., Sandvik, L., & Erikssen, J. (1998). Changes in physical fitness and changes in mortality. *The Lancet, 352*(9130), 759–762.

Hernandez-Reif, M., Field, T., & Hart, S. (1999). Smoking cravings are reduced by self-massage. *Preventative Medicine, 28*(1), 28–32. Available at http://web.healthy.gov/healthypeople.

Lai, S. C., & Cohen, M. N. (1999). Promoting lifestyle changes. *American Journal of Nursing, 99*(4), 63–67.

Lyons, M. A. (1998). The phenomenon of compulsive overeating in a selected group of professional women. *Journal of Advanced Nursing, 27*(6), 1158–1164.

NHLBI Obesity Education Initiative Expert Panel on the Identification, Evaluation, and Treatment of Overweight and Obesity in Adults. (1998). *Clinical guidelines on the identification, evaluation, and treatment of overweight and obesity in adults. The evidence report.* Bethesda, MD: US Department of Health and Human Services.

Popkess-Vawter, S., Brandau, C., & Straub, J. (1998). Triggers of overeating and related intervention strategies for women who weight cycle. *Applied Nursing Research, 11*(2), 69–76.

Quesenberry, C. P., Caan, B., & Jacobson, A. (1998). Obesity, health services use, and health care costs among members of a health maintenance organization. *Archives of Internal Medicine, 158,* 466–472.

Royce, C. F. (1998). Condom use by Hispanic and African-American adolescent girls who use hormonal contraception. *Journal of Adolescent Health, 23*(4), 205–211.

Slatterly, L., Edwards, S. L., Boucher, K. M., Anderson, K., & Caan, B. J. (1999). Lifestyle and colon cancer: An assessment of factors associated with risk. *American Journal of Epidemiology, 150*(8), 869–877.

US Department of Health and Human Services. (1998). *Healthy people 2010 objectives, draft for public comments.* Washington, DC: US Department of Health and Human Services, Office of Public Health and Science.

———. (1997). *Healthy people 2000 review 1997.* Hyattsville, MD: US Department of Health and Human Services, Centers for Disease Control and Prevention, National Center for Health Statistics. DHHS Publication No. (PHS)98-1256.

———. (1990). *Healthy people 2000. National health promotion and disease prevention objectives.* Washington, DC: US Department of Health and Human Services. Public Health Service, 5, 416–417.

Wilson, L. M. (1999). Healthy people—a new millennium. *JONA's Healthcare, Law, Ethics, and Regulation, 1*(2), 29–32.

Genetics and Health Applications

HUMAN GENETICS

Human genetics is the study of the human condition as it is influenced by inherited factors that affect and determine growth and development and that can be transmitted from generation to generation. Furthermore, genetic factors extend beyond the limited view of solely distinct genetic syndromes to encompass influences on health, the occurrence of complex disorders, individual biologic responses to illness, potential treatment and medical management approaches, and strategies for prevention or cure.

This tremendous realization is readily apparent through the accomplishments of The Human Genome Project. This 15-year international collaborative effort, originally proposed for completion in 2005, has just been completed ahead of schedule in 2000. One significant goal is to identify the 50,000 to 100,000 human genes. These advances and the associated knowledge will continue to significantly impact the delivery of health care and nursing practice. Genetic evaluations, screening, testing, guided treatment, family counseling, and related legal, ethical, and psychosocial issues will become daily practice for nurses.

The impact of genetics on nursing is significant. In 1997, the American Nurses Association (ANA) officially recognized genetics as a nursing specialty. This effort was spearheaded by the International Society of Nurses in Genetics (ISONG). ANA and ISONG have collaborated in the establishment of Scope and Standards of Practice for nurses in genetics practice. The purpose of this chapter is to provide the nurse with practical information, resources, representative examples, and professional considerations critical to integration of genetics knowledge into nursing practice.

Underlying Principles
Biologic and Genetic Principles
Cell: The Basic Unit of Biology
1. Cytoplasm—contains functional structures important to cellular functioning, including mitochondria, which contain extranuclear deoxyribonucleic acid (DNA) important to mitochondrial functioning.
2. Nucleus—contains 46 chromosomes in each somatic (body) cell, or 23 chromosomes in each germ cell (egg or sperm) (Figure 4-1).

Chromosomes
1. Each somatic cell with a nucleus has 22 pairs of autosomes (the same in both sexes) and 1 pair of sex chromosomes.
2. Females have two X sex chromosomes; males have one Y sex chromosome and one X sex chromosome.
3. Normally, at conception, each individual receives one copy of each chromosome pair from the maternal egg cell and one copy of each chromosome pair from the paternal sperm cell, for a total of 46 chromosomes.
4. Karyotype is the term used to define the chromosomal complement of an individual, for example, 46, XY, as is determined by laboratory chromosome analysis.
5. Each chromosome contains about 2,000 genes.

Genes
1. The basic unit of inherited information.
2. Each human nucleated somatic cell has about 100,000 genes in the nucleus. Cells also have some non-nuclear genes located within the mitochondria within the cytoplasm.
3. Alternate forms of a gene are termed alleles.
4. For each gene, an individual receives one allele from each parent for the same trait, and thus has two alleles for

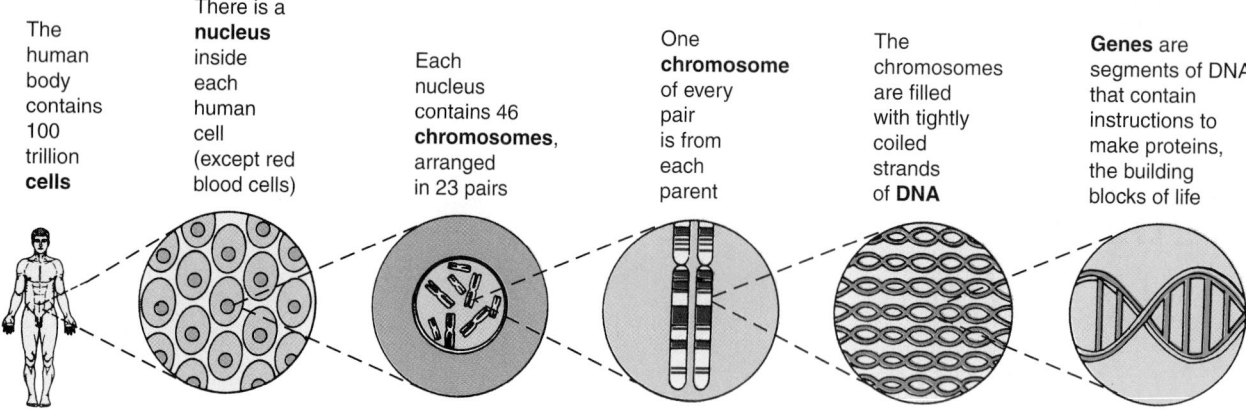

The human body contains 100 trillion **cells**

There is a **nucleus** inside each human cell (except red blood cells)

Each nucleus contains 46 **chromosomes**, arranged in 23 pairs

One **chromosome** of every pair is from each parent

The chromosomes are filled with tightly coiled strands of **DNA**

Genes are segments of DNA that contain instructions to make proteins, the building blocks of life

FIGURE 4-1 Cells, chromosomes, DNA, and genes.

each gene on the autosomes and also on the X chromosomes in females.

5. Males have only one X chromosome and therefore have only one allele for all genes on the X chromosome; they are hemizygous for all X-linked genes.

6. At any autosomal locus, or gene site, an individual can have two identical alleles and be termed homozygous for that trait or can have two different alleles at a particular locus, for example, for eye color, and be termed heterozygous.

7. Genotype refers to the gene constitution of an individual; for practical purposes it is commonly used to address a specific gene pair, for example, the gene for sickle cell disease, the gene for cystic fibrosis, or the gene for familial polyposis.

8. Phenotype refers to the physical or biochemical characteristics an individual manifests regarding expression of the presence of a particular feature, or set of features, associated with a particular gene.

9. Each gene is composed of a sequence of DNA bases.

DNA: Nuclear and Mitochondrial

1. Human DNA is a double-stranded helical structure comprising four different bases, the sequence of which codes for the assembly of amino acids to make a protein, or enzyme. These proteins are important for the following reasons:
   a. Body characteristics, such as eye color
   b. For biochemical processes, such as the gene for the digestion of phenylalanine
   c. For body structure, such as a collagen gene important to bone formation
   d. For cellular functioning, such as genes associated with the risk of cancer

2. The four DNA bases are adenine, guanine, cytosine, and thymine-A, G, C, and T

3. A change, or mutation, in the coding sequence, such as a duplicated or deleted region, or even a change in only one base, alters the production or functioning of the gene or gene product, thus affecting cellular processes, growth and development, etc.

4. DNA analysis can be done on almost any body tissue (blood, muscle, skin, etc.) using molecular techniques (not visible under a microscope) for mutation analysis of a specific gene with a known sequence or for DNA linkage of genetic markers associated with a particular gene.

Normal Cell Division

1. Mitosis occurs in all somatic cells, which under normal circumstances results in the formation of cells identical to the original cell, with the same 46 chromosomes.

2. Meiosis, or reduction division, occurs in the germ cell line, resulting in gametes (egg and sperm cells) with only 23 chromosomes, one representative of each chromosome pair.

3. During the process of meiosis, parental homologous chromosomes (from the same pair) pair and undergo exchanges of genetic material, resulting in recombinations of alleles on a chromosome and thus variation in individuals from generation to generation.

◼ Genetic Disorders

Presentations warranting genetic consideration include mental retardation, birth defects, biochemical or metabolic disorders, structural abnormalities, multiple miscarriages, and family history of the same or related disorder.

Disorders that result from abnormalities of chromosomes or genes or that are, at least in part, influenced by genetic factors are described in Table 4-1.

Classification of Genetic Alterations
Chromosomal

1. Entire chromosome or part of chromosome is affected. Usually associated with birth defects and mental retar-

(*text continues on page 40*)

TABLE 4-1 Selected Genetic Disorders

Disorder and Incidence	Characteristics	Etiology and Recurrence Risks	Considerations and Comments
Chromosomal Disorders			
Autosomal			
Down Syndrome (Trisomy 21) 1 in 700 newborns; incidence increases with advanced maternal age (eg, risk at maternal age 25 is 1 in 1,350; at age 35, 1 in 384; at age 45, 1 in 28)	Brachycephaly; oblique palpebral fissures; epicanthal folds; Brushfield spots; flat nasal bridge; protruding tongue; small, low-set ears; clinodactyly; simian crease; congenital heart defects; hypotonia; mental retardation; growth retardation; dry, scaly skin	Extra copy of number 21 chromosome (total of three copies): 94%—trisomy Down syndrome (karyotype 47, +21)—three distinct number 21 chromosomes due to nondisjunction (failure of chromosomal separation during meiosis); recurrence risk 1%, plus maternal age-related risk if over 35 4%—translocation Down syndrome—extra number 21 attached to another chromosome, usually a number 13 or number 14; half of these translocations are new occurrences, the other half are inherited from a parent. 2%—mosaic Down syndrome—affected has two different cell lines, one with the normal number of chromosomes and the other cell line trisomic for the number 21 chromosome; due to a postconception error in chromosomal division during mitosis.	• Recurrence risk for parents of affected are dependent on one or more of the following: chromosomal type of disorder, maternal age, parental karyotype, family history, and sex of transmitting parent and other chromosome involved (if translocation). • May demonstrate nuccal thickening prenatally on ultrasound examination. • Associated with moderate mental retardation. • No phenotypic differences between trisomy Down syndrome and translocation Down syndrome. • Chromosome analysis should be performed on all persons with Down syndrome.
Trisomy 13 (Patau Syndrome) 1 in 5,000 live births	Holoprosencephaly; cleft lip or palate, or both; abnormal helices; cardiac defects; rocker-bottom feet; overlapping positioning of fingers; seizures; severe mental retardation	Extra number 13 chromosome (total of three copies): Either trisomy form, due to nondisjunction, with less than a 1% recurrence risk; or translocation form, with recurrence risk less than that of translocation Down syndrome and dependent on other factors, including chromosomes involved.	• 44% die within the 1st month; 18% survive 1st year of life.
Trisomy 18 (Edwards Syndrome) 1 in 6,000 live births	Small for gestational age (may be detected prenatally); feeble fetal activity; weak cry; prominent occiput; low-set, malformed ears; short palpebral fissures; small oral opening; overlapping positioning of fingers (fifth digit over fourth, index over third); nail hypoplasia, short hallux; cardiac defects; inguinal or umbilical hernia; cryptorchidism in males; severe mental retardation	Extra number 18 chromosome (total of three copies): Majority due to trisomy with less than 1% recurrence risk.	• Most trisomy 18 conceptions miscarry; 90% of liveborn die within 1st year of life.

(continued)

TABLE 4-1 Selected Genetic Disorders (Continued)

Disorder and Incidence	Characteristics	Etiology and Recurrence Risks	Considerations and Comments
Sex Chromosome			
Klinefelter Syndrome 1 in 700 males; 47, XXY abnormality in 90%; other 10% have more than two X chromosomes in addition to the Y chromosome or have mosaicism (about 20%)	Body habitus may be tall, slim, and underweight; long limbs; gynecomastia; small testes; inadequate virilization; azoospermia or low sperm count; cognitive defects; behavioral problems	Due to nondisjunction during meiosis, except for cases of mosaicism, which are due to mitotic nondisjunction.	• No distinguishing features prenatally. • Diagnosis may not be suspected or pursued before puberty. • Diagnosis in childhood is beneficial in planning for testosterone replacement therapy, in addition to accurate understanding of learning or behavioral problems. • Tend to be delayed in onset of speech, have difficulty in expressive language; may be relatively immature; may have history of recurrent respiratory infections.
Turner Syndrome (45, X) 1 in 2,500 female births	Webbing of neck and short stature: lymphedema of hands and feet as newborn; congenital cardiac defects (especially coarctation of the aorta); low posterior hairline; cubitus valgus; widely spaced nipples; underdeveloped breasts; immature internal genitalia (eg, streak ovaries); primary amenorrhea; learning disabilities	About 50% due to a nondisjunctional error during meiosis (karyotype 45, X); 20% are mosaic due to nondisjunction during mitosis; 30% have two X chromosomes but one is functionally inadequate (eg, due to presence of abnormal gene); generally a sporadic occurrence.	• Webbing of neck and short stature may be detected prenatally by ultrasound. • Early diagnosis enhances optimal health care management, eg, planning for administration of growth hormone therapy, estrogen replacement. • Psychosocial implications associated with short stature, delayed onset of puberty. • Infertility associated with ovarian dysgenesis; adoption is generally the only option for having children.
Microdeletion/Microduplication			
Fragile X 1 in 1,200 males; 1 in 2,500 females	Motor delays; hypotonia; speech delay and language difficulty; hyperactivity; classic features including long face, prominent ears, and macroorchidism manifest around puberty; autism (about 7% of males); mental retardation in most males; learning disabilities in most affected females	Mutation in the fragile X mental retardation gene (FMR-1), represented as a large DNA expansion of a normally present trinucleotide. Carrier mother of an affected male has a 50% risk for future affected males and 50% risk to transmit the FMR-1 X chromosome to a daughter who would be a carrier, may be unaffected, or manifest features associated with the Fragile X syndrome and has a 50% risk to transmit that gene to future offspring.	• Both cytogenetic testing for expression of the fragile X site and DNA analysis for the expansion are available, but the latter is superior. • Phenotypic expression of this gene in males and females is variable; genetic mechanisms determining expression of this gene are very complicated. • Fragile X should be considered in the differential diagnosis of any mentally retarded male who is undiagnosed: it is the most common mental retardation in males.
Prader-Willi Syndrome Estimated incidence 1 in 25,000	Hypotonia and poor sucking ability in infancy; almond-shaped palpebral fissures; small stature; small, slow growth of hands and/or feet; small penis, cryptorchidism; insatiable appetite, behavioral problems onsetting in childhood; below-normal intelligence or mental retardation	Cytogenetic microdeletion in chromosome 15 q11–13 identified in 50–70% of cases; deletion associated with paternally inherited number 15 chromosome. Generally sporadic occurrence; empiric recurrence risk 1.6%.	• Consider diagnosis in infants presenting with hypotonia and sucking problems where etiology is unknown. • Associated with lack of a functioning paternal gene at this locus; presents clinical evidence for the necessity of two functioning genes, *both* a maternal and paternal contribution.

Mendelian Disorders—Single Gene

Autosomal Dominant

Achondroplasia
1 in 10,000 live births
Increased incidence associated with advanced paternal age (>40)

Megalocephaly; small foramen magnum and short cranial base with early spheno-occipital closure; prominent forehead; low nasal bridge; midfacial hypoplasia; small stature; short extremities; lumbar lordosis; short tubular bones; incomplete extension at the elbow; normal intelligence

Autosomal dominant inheritance; 80–90% are due to a new mutation. In those cases that are inherited, the affected parent has a 50% risk to transmit the gene to each child.

- Another distinct entity, termed Angelman syndrome, is associated with a deletion of the *maternal* contribution in this same cytogenetic region; it is also associated with mental deficiency, but with a different phenotypic presentation.
- Hydrocephalus can be a complication of achondroplasia and may be masked by megalocephaly.
- Risk for apnea secondary to cervical spinal cord and lower brain stem compression due to alterations in shape of cervical vertebral bodies; respiratory problems are also a risk because of the small chest and upper airway obstruction.
- Can be diagnosed prenatally by ultrasound.

Osteogenesis Imperfecta (Type 1)
1 in 15,000 live births

Blue sclerae; fractures (variable number); deafness may occur

Defect in the procollagen gene associated with decreased synthesis of a constituent chain important to collagen structure.
Can occur as a new mutation in that gene or can be inherited from a parent who has a 50% recurrence risk to transmit the gene; most severe cases represent a sporadic occurrence within a family.

- There are at least four general classifications of osteogenesis imperfecta, each with varying clinical severity, presentation, and pattern of genetic transmission.
- Treatment with calcitonin and fluoride may be beneficial in reducing the number of fractures.

Breast and Breast/Ovarian Cancer Syndrome
Accounts for 5–10% of breast cancer

Breast cancer (usually, but not exclusively, early age–onset, premenopausal)
Ovarian cancer

Mutation in the BRCA-1 or BRCA-2 gene; poses increased susceptibility (not certainty) for breast (56–87%) and/or ovarian (16–60%) cancer.

- Studies have also noted increased risk for prostate cancer, colon cancer in some families; also an association between male breast cancer and BRCA-2 mutations.

Familial Adenomatous Polyposis (FAP)
Accounts for about 1% of colon cancer

Associated with multiple adenomatous colorectal polyps (classic: > 100; atypical: < 100), desmoid tumors, other GI polyps, jaw cysts; family history of polyps and/or colorectal cancer; polyps progress to cancer; polyps can be present in childhood.

Mutations in the APC gene (a tumor suppressor gene). The majority of mutations result in a truncated protein.

- Genetic testing (protein truncation testing) is available. If mutation is identified in affected person, relatives can be tested for the same finding. Relatives at risk, whether by family history or by genetic testing, should start cancer screening by age 18, if not earlier, if there are symptoms or as a baseline. Screening includes colonoscopy, ophthalmologic examination.

(continued)

TABLE 4-1 Selected Genetic Disorders (Continued)

Disorder and Incidence	Characteristics	Etiology and Recurrence Risks	Considerations and Comments
Autosomal Recessive			
Sickle Cell Disease 1 in 400 live births of African American ancestry	Physically normal in appearance at birth; hemolytic anemia and the occurrence of acute exacerbations (crises), resulting in increased susceptibility to infection and vascular occlusive episodes	Point mutation in the sickle cell gene resulting in an altered gene product; red blood cells susceptible to sickling at times of low oxygen tension. Parents of an affected individual are both unaffected carriers of one abnormal copy of the sickle cell gene (sickle cell trait) and together have a 25% risk for recurrence in any offspring.	• 1 in 10 African Americans is a carrier of the sickle cell gene; population screening is indicated for these individuals. • Unaffected siblings of an affected individual have a 2/3, or 67%, risk to have the sickle cell trait and should be screened. • See p. 1541 for nursing care. • Prenatal testing is available through DNA analysis from specimen obtained during chorionic villus sampling or amniocentesis.
Cystic Fibrosis (CF) 1 in 2,000 live births (predominantly Caucasian)	Phenotypically normal at birth; may present with meconium ileus (10%) as neonate or later with persistent cough, recurrent respiratory problems, gastrointestinal complaints, abdominal pain, or infertility	Mutation in the cystic fibrosis transmembrane conduction regulator gene on chromosome 7 results in an abnormality of a protein integral to the cell membrane. Parents of an affected individual are both considered obligate carriers of one copy of the abnormal CF gene; thus, together they have a 25% recurrence risk with each conception.	• 1 in 20 whites is a carrier of a CF gene mutation. • Several different mutations have been identified within the CF gene, the most common of which is ΔF508, which accounts for about 70% of CF mutations. CF screening can identify about 85% of all CF mutations (95% in Jewish population); it is not yet being used for general population screening. • DNA analysis of the CF gene is advised for affected individuals and relatives of persons with CF. • See p. 1365 for nursing care.
Tay-Sachs Disease 1 in 3,600 Ashkenazic Jews	Normal at birth; progressive neurodegenerative manifestations, including loss of developmental milestones and lack of central nervous system (CNS) maturation; cherry-red spot on macula	Mutation in the gene for hexosaminidase A, an enzyme important to cellular metabolic processes, results in accumulation of metabolic by-products within the cell (especially brain), impairing functioning and causing the neurodegenerative effects. Parents of an affected individual are both considered unaffected obligate carriers of one copy of the Tay-Sachs disease gene; together they have a 25% risk of recurrence in their offspring.	• About 1 in 25 Ashkenazic Jews is a carrier of the Tay-Sachs gene; about 1 in 17 French Canadians is a carrier of an abnormal Tay-Sachs gene (different mutation from that of the Jewish ancestry); persons of these ancestries should be screened. • No treatment available; results in death in childhood. • Prenatal testing is available.
X-Linked Recessive			
Duchenne's Muscular Dystrophy (DMD) 1 in 3,500 males	Phenotypically normal at birth; dramatically elevated creatinine phosphokinase (CPK) level (detectable as early as 2 days of age); hypertrophy of the calves; history of tendency to trip and fall (at about 3 years of age); Gowers' sign (tendency to push off oneself when getting up from a sitting position)	DNA mutation, generally a deletion, detectable in 70% of affected males. Carrier females have a 25% risk with each pregnancy to have an affected male, a 25% risk to have a carrier female, a 25% chance to have a healthy male, and a 25% chance to have a healthy noncarrier female.	• 1 in 1,750 females is a carrier of the DMD gene. • In the case of an isolated affected male, the mother has a ⅔ statistical risk that she is a carrier of the DMD gene and a ⅓ chance that her affected son arose as the result of a new mutation in that gene (she is not a carrier).

Hemophilia A
1 in 7,000 males

Phenotypically normal at birth; bleeding tendency (ranging from frequent spontaneous bleeds associated with the severe form to bleeding only after trauma associated with the mild form)

Deficiency of Factor XIII (antihemophilic factor) due to abnormality in this gene located on the X chromosome.
Carrier females have a 25% risk with each pregnancy to have an affected son, a 25% risk for a carrier daughter, and a 25% chance each for a healthy unaffected daughter or son.

- DNA testing is recommended for affected males, and once type of gene mutation is known in that family, prenatal diagnosis and evaluation of potential female carriers can be carried out.
- DNA analysis may provide clues as to expected clinical severity.

Glucose 6-phosphate Dehydrogenase (G6PD)
10–14% of male live births of African American origin

Phenotypically normal at birth; many remain asymptomatic through life; may manifest acute hemolysis associated with exposure to outside factors, eg, certain medications

Abnormality of the G6PD gene on the X chromosome.
Carrier females have a 25% risk with each pregnancy to have an affected male and 25% risk to have a carrier female.

- Frequency of carrier females is about 1 in 3500.
- The severe form occurs in about 48% of cases.
- Moderate cases account for 31%
- The mild form accounts for 21% of cases.
- See p. 1549 for nursing care.
- Be aware of drugs, such as antimalarial drugs or sulfonamides; or chemicals, such as phenylhydrazine (used in silvering mirrors, photography, soldering) associated with hemolysis in G6PD-deficient individuals.

Multifactorial Disorders

Neural Tube Defects
1 in 1,000 live births

Abnormalities of neural tube closure, ranging from anencephaly to myelomeningocele to spina bifida occulta

Probably several genetic factors may predispose certain individuals, or families, to susceptibility, but certain environmental (eg, prolonged hyperthermia) and other unknown factors play an additive role in surpassing an arbitrary threshold, placing the developing fetus at risk.
Recurrence risk for isolated neural tube defects range between 1% and 5%.

- Recurrence risk for isolated neural tube defects is dependent on the severity of the defect, ie, a defect in the neurulation (the cranial end of the neural tube) versus cannulation (the development of the caudal end) and if there is a positive family history.
- Maternal screening can be performed prenatally (after 14 weeks' gestation) through alpha-fetoprotein levels in maternal serum.
- Can be associated with chromosomal or genetic disorders.

Cleft Lip and/or Cleft Palate
1 in 1,000 live births

Unilateral or bilateral; cleft lip and cleft palate may occur together or in isolation

Failure of migration and fusion of the maxillary processes during embryogenesis.
Recurrence risk for first-degree relatives of a person with an isolated cleft lip and/or cleft palate ranges between 2% and 6%.

- Clefting can occur as an isolated congenital abnormality or be one component of a syndrome, genetic defect, or chromosome abnormality, these latter three of which are associated with a recurrence risk specific to that disorder.
- Recurrence for isolated cleft lip and/or palate are dependent on the type of cleft, the sex of the affected individual, and the family history.

dation since there are extra or missing copies of all genes associated with the involved chromosome.

   a. Numerical—abnormal number of chromosomes due to nondisjunction (error in chromosomal separation during cell division). Examples are Down syndrome and Klinefelter syndrome.

   b. Structural—abnormality involving deletions, additions, or translocations (rearrangements) of parts of chromosomes. Examples are Prader-Willi syndrome and Angelman syndrome.

   c. Fragile sites—regions susceptible to chromosomal breakage, such as in fragile X syndrome.

2. May involve autosomes or sex chromosomes.

Single Gene or Pair of Genes

1. Manifestations are specific to cells, organs, or body systems affected by that gene.

2. *Autosomal dominant*—presence of a single copy of an abnormal gene results in phenotypic expression.

   a. These genes may involve proteins of a structural nature such as collagen. Affected individuals are usually of normal intelligence.

   b. Can be inherited from one parent, whose physical manifestations can vary, depending on specific disorder and the gene's penetrance and expressivity, for example, neurofibromatosis.

   c. Can arise as result of a new mutation in that gene in the affected individual.

   d. Individual with an autosomal dominant gene has a 50% risk of transmitting that gene to all offspring.

3. *Autosomal recessive*—requires that both alleles at a gene locus be abnormal for an individual to be affected.

   a. These genes are frequently important to biochemical functions, such as phenylalanine. Depending upon the gene and the nature of the mutation, affected individuals may be of normal intelligence or be mentally retarded.

   b. Generally, both parents are considered obligate carriers (unaffected) of one copy of the abnormal gene.

   c. Such a carrier couple has a 25% risk, with each pregnancy, to have an affected child, a 50% chance for the child to be an unaffected carrier, and a 25% chance for the child to be an unaffected noncarrier.

3. *X-linked recessive*—due to an abnormal gene, or genes, on the X chromosome.

   a. These genes may be important to structure or biochemical function. Depending upon the gene and the nature of the mutation, affected individuals may be of normal intelligence or be mentally retarded.

   b. Recessively inherited, in most cases, meaning that two abnormal genes are required to be affected. However, only one abnormal gene needs to be present for a male to be affected because males are hemizygous for all X-linked genes. An example is Duchenne muscular dystrophy.

   c. Females are typically only carriers of X-linked recessive disorders because the presence of a corresponding

normal gene on the other X chromosome in a female produces enough gene product for normal functioning; females can be affected to varying degrees in certain circumstances.

   d. A carrier female has a 25% risk, with each pregnancy, to have an affected son, a 25% risk to have a carrier daughter, a 25% chance to have an unaffected son, and a 25% chance to have an unaffected noncarrier daughter.

   e. A male with an abnormal X-linked gene who has children will transmit that gene to all of his daughters, who will be carriers of that gene (usually unaffected); none of his sons will inherit his abnormal X-linked gene, because they receive his Y chromosome.

4. *X-linked dominant*—relatively rare

   a. Mutations in these genes are usually lethal to male conceptions, as in Rett syndrome.

   b. Depending upon the gene and the nature of the mutation, affected females may be of normal intelligence or be mentally retarded. An example is incontinentia pigmenti.

5. *Mitochondrial*—genes whose DNA is within the mitochondria, which are located in the cytoplasm, not in the nucleus, and therefore do not follow mendelian laws of inheritance.

   a. Many of these genes are associated with respiratory functions within mitochondria and thus affect energy capacity of cells. Disorders may be manifested by diminished strength in the involved tissue, or myopathy.

   b. Essentially are maternally inherited, because the egg cell contains the cytoplasmic material that is involved in the zygote; the sperm cell contributes mainly only nuclear DNA.

   c. Varying phenotypes, depending on the number and distribution of abnormal mitochondrial genes.

   d. Can affect males or females, but males transmit few, if any, mitochondrial genes.

Multifactorial

1. Caused by several genetic factors in addition to other nongenetic influences (eg, environmental).

2. Because of the genetic components, affected individuals or close relatives are at an increased risk, compared with the general population, to have an affected child; that risk is generally 2% to 5%.

3. Elimination of known non-genetic risk factors or proactive treatment regimen, in some conditions, can reduce risk for occurrence (eg, diet modification to manage hypercholesterolemia, cessation of smoking to reduce risk of cancer, or weight control and exercise to prevent type II diabetes in susceptible individuals).

■ Genetic Counseling

Genetic counseling is a communication process that deals with human problems associated with the occurrence, or recurrence, of a genetic disorder in a family. There is a specific concern about risk associated with a certain problem or because of the relationship to someone who is affected, the proband. Several steps occur in the genetic evaluation, including obtaining and reviewing the medical history and records of the affected; eliciting the family history, with special attention to factors pertinent to the diagnosis in the proband; evaluating and examining the affected (if available and indicated); ordering appropriate tests and interpreting results; and then meeting with the person seeking the consultation and/or the proband.

Goals of Genetic Counseling
Assist the proband and/or consultant to:
1. Comprehend the medical facts, including the diagnosis, the possible course of the disorder, and the available management.
2. Understand the inheritance of the disorder and the risk of recurrence in specified relatives.
3. Understand the options for dealing with the risk of recurrence.
4. Choose the course of action that seems appropriate to the individuals involved, in view of their risk, family goals, and religious beliefs, and act in accordance with that decision.
5. Make the best possible adjustment to the disorder.

Identify Persons in Need of Genetic Assessment and Counseling
1. Parent(s) of a child with a birth defect(s), mental retardation, or known/possible genetic disorder
2. Any individual with a genetic or potentially genetic disorder
3. Persons with a family history of mental retardation, birth defect(s), genetic disorder, or condition that tends to run in the family
4. Pregnant women who will be 35 or older at the time of delivery
5. Couples of ethnic origin known to be at an increased risk for a specific genetic disorder
6. Couples who have experienced two or more miscarriages
7. Pregnant women who have an elevated or low maternal serum screening test result, such as alpha-fetoprotein
8. Women who have been exposed to drugs or infections during pregnancy
9. Couples who are related to each other
10. Persons who are concerned about the risk for a genetic disorder

Genetic Screening, Testing, and Research
Screening
1. Screening is the level of testing offered to large populations (eg, newborn) or to high-risk segments of the population (such as African Americans, Ashkenazi Jews, Mediterranean peoples) to identify individuals with a genetic disorder, increased risk for abnormality, or carriers of a genetic disorder.

2. Criteria include that the test itself must be reliable, appropriate to the designated population, and cost-effective and that the condition being tested for must be treatable or that early identification will enhance health.
3. Newborn screening varies among states, testing for disorders such as phenylketonuria (PKU), hypothyroidism, maple syrup urine disease (MSUD), and histidinemia.
4. Prenatal screening—maternal serum alpha-fetoprotein (AFP) or triple screen (includes measurement of maternal serum AFP, beta-human chorionic gonadotropin [bHCG], and estriol) or quad screen. After 14 weeks gestation can identify pregnancies at increased risk for neural tube defects (NTD), Down syndrome, and trisomy 18.

Testing
1. Biochemical testing is done on body tissue or fluid to measure enzyme levels and activity.
2. DNA testing is done on blood or tissue samples to look for a gene mutation or to study DNA linkage.
3. Chromosomal testing is done on nucleated cells (usually blood cells) or other tissue for detection of various conditions, such as extra, missing, deleted, duplicated, or rearranged chromosomes.

Prenatal Testing
1. Chorionic villus sampling (CVS)—for chromosomal, biochemical, and DNA testing; done at 9 to 12 weeks gestation.
2. Amniocentesis—for chromosomal, biochemical, and DNA testing at 13 weeks (early amniocentesis); AFP can be done at 14 to 18 weeks gestation.
3. Ultrasound—for dating pregnancy and assessing fetal structures, placenta, and amniotic fluid; done throughout pregnancy, but fetal structures are best visualized after 12 weeks.
4. Acetylcholinesterase (ACH) in amniotic fluid for suspected NTD.
5. Fetoscopy—for obtaining fetal blood samples or visualizing details of fetal structures; done during second trimester.
6. Percutaneous umbilical blood sampling (PUBS)—for obtaining fetal blood; done during second trimester.

Research
1. Testing done to further understand the genetics of a disorder or biochemical process.
2. *Not* clinical testing, and may have no clinical value to the patient's case.
   a. Some states, such as New York, mandate that genetic research specimens must be kept anonymous and that results not be provided to an individual for any clinical use.
3. There is ongoing and extensive research on cancer susceptibility genes.

Additional Genetic Testing Consideration
1. DNA banking—extraction and storage of one's DNA from blood through a qualified genetics laboratory; requires informed consent, proper collection, and prompt handling.

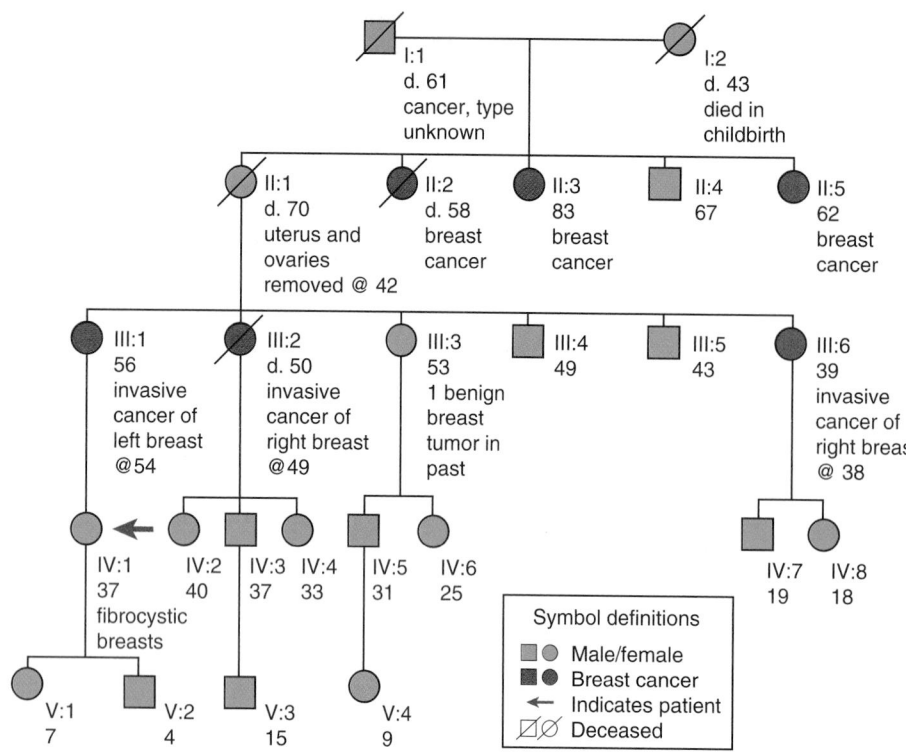

FIGURE 4-2 Genetic pedigree of a patient with breast cancer. Maternal side only is shown true to size; however, both maternal and paternal sides are assessed. Genetic risk may run through either side.

Nursing Roles and Responsibilities

1. Recognize or suspect genetic disorders by their physical characteristics and clinical manifestations.
2. Create a genetic pedigree (diagram of the family history), including cause of death and any genetically linked ailments (Figure 4-2).
3. Explain/review those aspects of diagnosis, prognosis, and treatment that affect the patient's growth and development and that parents or caretakers need to know to plan for the care of the patient.
4. Clear up misconceptions and allay feelings of guilt.
5. Assist with the diagnostic process by exploring medical and family history information, by using physical assessment skills, by obtaining blood samples, and/or by assisting with CVS or amniocentesis, as indicated.
6. Enhance and reinforce self-image and self-worth of parents and child.
7. Encourage interaction with family and friends; offer referrals, phone numbers of support groups.
8. Refer and prepare family for genetic counseling.
   a. Inform that prenatal testing does not mean termination of pregnancy (eg, it may confirm that the fetus is not affected, thus eliminating worry throughout pregnancy, although the determination of an abnormality is also a possibility).
   b. Encourage the parents to allow adequate time to deliberate on a course of action (eg, do not rush into a tubal ligation, because in a few years they may want more children).
   c. Remain nonjudgmental.
9. Check within state (for example, state health department) or with American Society of Human Genetics (301-571-1825) for information and resources regarding newborn testing required, state regulations on genetic testing and research, etc.
10. Recognize that there are many ethical, legal, psychosocial, and professional issues associated with obtaining, using, and storing genetic information.
    a. Be aware of associated professional responsibilities, including informed consent, documentation in medical records, medical releases, and individual privacy of information.
    b. Refer to federal legislation (Health Insurance Portability and Accountability Act, 1997) that deals with protection from genetic discrimination in medical insurance; individual state legislation; genetics professional societies (see below); and the World Health Organization document on ethical considerations in genetic testing and services.
11. Refer for further information and support to:
    March of Dimes Birth Defects Foundation, 1275 Mamaroneck Avenue, White Plains, New York 10605 (for educational materials and information on location of genetic services)

National Clearinghouse for Maternal and Child Health, 3520 Prospect Street NW, Suite 1, Washington, DC 20057 (for genetic and child health information and material)

International Society of Nurses in Genetics, 603-643-5706, **http://nursing.creighton.edu/isong/index.html** (genetics resource, network, and professional organization for nurses)

Genetic Alliance, 4301 Connecticut Avenue, NW, Suite 404, Washington, DC 20008, 800-336-GENE, **www.geneticalliance.org** (resource and advocate for national and local genetic support groups for lay persons and professionals)

Oncology Nursing Society, Genetics Special Interest Group, 610-520-2249

National Society of Genetic Counselors, **www.nsgc.org** (genetics resources, network and professional organization for genetic counselors)

SELECTED REFERENCES

Ad Hoc Committee on Genetic Counseling of the American Society of Human Genetics. (1975). Genetic counseling. *American Journal of Human Genetics, 27,* 240–242.

Diamond, E., Peters, J., & Jenkins, J. (1997). The genetic basis of cancer. *Cancer Nursing, 20,* 213–226.

Gelehrter, T., Collins, F., & Ginsburg, D. (1997). *Principles of medical genetics* (2nd ed.). Philadelphia: Lippincott-Raven.

Genetic susceptibility to breast and ovarian cancer: Assessment, counseling, and testing guidelines. Executive summary. (1999). American College of Medical Genetics Foundation (with support from New York State Department of Health).

Harper, P. S. (1998). *Practical genetic counseling* (5th ed.). Bristol: Wright.

International Society of Nurses in Genetics, Inc., and American Nurses Association. (1998). *Statement on the scope and standards of genetics clinical nursing practice.* Washington, D.C.: American Nurses Publishing.

King, R. C., & Stansfield, W. D. (1997). *A dictionary of genetics* (5th ed.). New York: Oxford University Press.

Lea, D. H., Jenkins, J. F., & Franconano, C. A. (1998). *Genetics in clinical practice: New directions for nursing and health care.* Boston: Jones and Bartlett.

McKusick, V. A. (1994). *Mendelian inheritance in man* (11th ed.). Baltimore: Johns Hopkins University Press.

Pillitteri, A. (1999). *Maternal and child health nursing* (3rd ed.). Philadelphia: Lippincott Williams & Wilkins.

Rimoin, D. L., Connor, J. M., & Pyeritz, R. E. (1997). *Emery and Rimoin's principles and practice of medical genetics* (3rd ed.). New York: Churchill Livingstone.

Scriver, C. R., Beaudet, A. L., Sly, W. S., et al. (1995). *Metabolic and molecular bases of inherited disease* (7th ed.). New York: McGraw-Hill Information Services.

Seideman, R., & Kleine, P. (1995). A theory of transformed parenting: Parenting a child with developmental delay/mental retardation. *Nursing Research, 44*(1), 38–44.

Wilcox-Honnold, P.M. (1998). Breast cancer and gene testing: Risk, rationale, and responsibilities of primary care providers. *Lippincott's Primary Care Practice, 2*(3), 271–283.

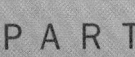

PART

2

Medical-Surgical Nursing

General Health Considerations

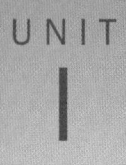

CHAPTER

5

Adult Physical Assessment

THE PATIENT HISTORY

▣ General Principles

1. The first step in caring for a patient and in soliciting active cooperation is to gather a careful and complete history.
   a. In all patient concerns and problems, an accurate history is the foundation on which data collection and the process of assessment are based.
   b. The comprehensiveness of the history elicited will depend on the information available in the patient's record.
2. Time spent early in the patient–nurse relationship gathering detailed information about what the patient knows, thinks, and feels about the problems will prevent time-consuming errors and misunderstandings later.
3. Skill in interviewing will affect both the accuracy of information elicited and the quality of the relationship established with the patient.

   This point cannot be overemphasized; the reader is encouraged to consult other sources for detailed discussion of techniques of health interviewing.

4. The purpose of the interview is to encourage an interchange of information between the patient and the nurse. The patient must feel that his or her words are understood and that concerns are being heard and dealt with sensitively.

▣ Interviewing Techniques

1. Provide privacy in as quiet a place as possible and see that the patient is comfortable.
2. Begin the interview with a courteous greeting and an introduction. Explain who you are and why you are there.
3. Be sure that facial expressions, body movements, and tone of voice are pleasant, unhurried, and nonevaluative, and that they convey the attitude of a sensitive listener, so the patient will feel free to express thoughts and feelings.
4. Avoid reassuring the patient prematurely (before you have adequate information about the problem). This only cuts off discussion; the patient may then be unwilling to bring up a problem causing concern.
5. At times, a patient gives cues or suggests information, but does not tell enough. It may be necessary to probe for

more information to obtain a thorough history; the patient must realize that this is done for his or her benefit.

6. Guide the interview so the necessary information is obtained, without cutting off discussion. Controlling the rambling patient is often difficult, but, with practice, it can be done skillfully, without jeopardizing the quality of the information gained.

Identifying Information

Purposes
1. To eliminate confusion about the patient's identity; to obtain the information required for contacting patient if the need arises
2. To provide an introduction to the patient and some indication of habits, lifestyle, and beliefs, which may be explored in greater depth in the personal and social history
3. To initiate a relationship based on recognition of the importance of the informant's role in sharing in the care of the patient (when this is the case)

Types of Information Needed
1. Date and time
2. Patient's name, address, telephone number, race, religion, birth date, and age
3. Name of referring practitioner
4. Insurance data
5. Name of informant—the patient may be the person giving this history; if not, record the name, address, telephone number, and relationship to the patient of the person giving the history.
6. Accuracy and reliability of informant—this is a judgment based on the consistency of responses to questions and on a comparison of information in the history with your own observations in the physical examination.

Method of Collecting Data
1. Careful interviewing of the patient or caregiver will provide most of the information.
2. The patient's hospital or clinic record may also be a valuable source.
3. Repeat information when necessary to verify accuracy (eg, to ensure that there has been no change in address or telephone number).
4. Assume a direct and courteous manner.
5. Explain the reasons why the information is needed—to help put the patient at ease.

Chief Complaint

Purposes
1. To allow the patient to describe his or her own problems and expectations with little or no direction from the interviewer
2. To identify the overriding problem for which the person is seeking help
   a. Adults with chronic conditions often have numerous complaints.

b. If possible, focus on a single problem or concern—the one most important to the patient.
3. To identify the patient's feelings about symptoms. The patient may show fear, guilt, or defensiveness in this first statement.

Types of Information Needed
The patient's primary problem(s) or concern in the patient's own words. A statement describing the duration of the complaint.

Method of Collecting Data
1. Ask the patient a direct question, for example, "How may I help you?" or "For what reason have you come to the hospital (clinic, etc.)?"
2. Avoid confusing questions, for example, "What brings you here?" ("The bus.") or "Why are you here?" ("That's what I came to find out.")
3. Ask how long the concern or problem has been present. If necessary, establish the time of onset precisely by offering such clues as "Did you feel this way a month (6 months or 2 years) ago?"
4. Let the patient speak freely without offering your opinion until he has had an opportunity to identify the problem as clearly as possible.
5. Write down what the patient says, using quotation marks to identify patient's words.

History of Present Illness

Purposes
1. To amplify the description of the chief complaint and to clarify its relationship to other symptoms and events
2. To carefully describe a symptom or problem that may be a clue to future diagnosis

Types of Information Needed
1. A detailed chronologic picture beginning with the time the patient was last well (or, in the case of a problem with an acute onset, the patient's condition just before the onset of the problem) and ending with a description of the patient's current condition.
2. If there is more than one important problem, each is described in a separate, chronologically organized paragraph in the written history of present illness.
3. The outline for reporting the present illness will vary with each case.

Method of Collecting Data
1. For each problem investigate the following:
   a. Quality (eg, sharp, dull, knifelike—referring to pain)
   b. Quantity (eg, ½ cup sputum)
   c. Location of symptoms, intensity, periodicity (eg, epigastric area; daily; after meals)
   d. Aggravating and alleviating factors (eg, medications, prescribed and over the counter; rest; diet)
   e. Associated phenomena (eg, shortness of breath)

2. Date the onset of the problem as accurately as possible because chronology is of the utmost importance (see section titled Chief Complaint).
3. Describe the character of the symptoms and state whether they have changed over time.
4. In the case of acute infections, inquire about possible exposure or an incubation period.
5. When the present illness has been characterized by attacks separated by free intervals, obtain the history of a typical attack: onset, duration, and associated symptoms—pain; fever; chills; relation to any activity, either physical or emotional, or to such factors as diet, medication, etc.
6. In both acute and chronic illnesses, note whether and when the patient stopped working or went to bed.
7. Get the patient's subjective appraisal of whether the symptom or problem is getting better or worse.
8. When a particular organ or system is disturbed, ask for a review of that system and related systems so important negative and positive information may be included in the written history. For instance, if a patient complains of chest pain, ask about both the respiratory and cardiac systems, as well as the musculoskeletal history of the chest.
9. Questioning may reveal that other systems must also be reviewed.
10. Ask about previous treatment, including medications, prescribing physician or practitioner, and place where treatment was obtained (name of hospital, clinic, etc.).
11. At the end, review the chronology and specifics and ask patient to affirm or correct the information.
12. Organize the information for recording or presentation.

Past Medical History
Purposes
1. To determine any change in the patient's normal patterns of living that may or may not be caused by illness
2. To identify clues that may aid in diagnosing the present illness
3. To participate in gathering and recording information that may be helpful in making a diagnosis, even though the nurse may not have the final responsibility for diagnosing the patient's particular problem

Types of Information Needed
1. General health and strength—sleeping patterns, appetite, stability of weight, usual activities
2. Acute infectious diseases—measles, mumps, whooping cough, chickenpox, pneumonia, pleurisy, tuberculosis, scarlet fever, acute rheumatic fever, rheumatic heart disease, tonsillitis, hepatitis, polio, sexually transmitted disease, tropical or parasitic diseases, any other acute infectious problem the patient describes
3. Immunization—polio, diphtheria, pertussis, tetanus, measles, mumps, rubella, hepatitis B, hepatitis A, pneu-

mococcal influenza, varicella, Lyme, and last PPD or other skin test, any abnormal or unusual reactions. Give date when possible.
4. Operation—indications, diagnosis, dates, hospital, surgeon, complications
5. Previous hospitalizations—physician, hospital data (year), diagnosis, treatment
6. Injuries—type; resulting disabilities
7. Major illnesses (any prolonged illnesses not requiring hospitalization)—dates, symptoms, course, treatment
8. Allergies (may appear in review of systems)—Asthma, hay fever, hives, food allergies, drug reactions, previous treatment with penicillin and any reactions
9. Obstetric history (may appear in review of systems)
   a. Pregnancies, miscarriages, abortions
   b. Describe course of pregnancy, labor, and delivery; date, place of delivery
10. Psychiatric history (may appear in review of systems)—treatment by a psychiatrist or psychologist, indications, date, place, medications for "nerves"

Method of Collecting Data
1. Begin by explaining the purpose and type of questions you will be asking; for example, "I am now going to ask you some questions about your past health."
2. Explain that these questions are important to obtain an accurate picture of all the events that affected or that did not affect the patient's health in the past.
3. Use direct questions; for example, "How would you describe your general health?" and then proceed with more specific queries, such as "Has your weight been stable over the past 5 years?"

Family History
Purposes
1. To present a picture of the patient's family health, including specifically that of grandparents, parents, brothers, sisters, aunts, and uncles. It also involves the health of close relatives because some diseases show a familial tendency or are hereditary.
2. To describe the health of the patient's spouse and children because this may give clues about possible communicable disease problems. It also will be important in determining what sort of condition a family is in and how this affects the patient.

Types of Information Needed
1. Age and health status of (or age at and cause of death of) parent, sibling
2. History, in immediate and close relatives, of heart disease, hypertension, stroke, diabetes, gout, kidney disease or stones, thyroid disease, asthma or allergies, blood problems, cancer (types), epilepsy, mental illness, arthritis, alcoholism, obesity

3. Hereditary diseases such as hemophilia or sickle cell disease
4. Age and health status of spouse and children

Method of Collecting Data

1. Begin with an explanation of what you are asking and why because the patient may not understand the purpose of your questions. For example:

   "I am going to ask now about the health of your immediate family and relatives. It is important to know if there are any conditions that tend to or could occur in your family, or in you as a member of the family."

2. Ask direct questions.
   a. Begin with the patient's siblings.
      "Do you have any brothers and sisters?"
      "How old are they and what is the state of their health?"
   b. List each sibling separately, giving age and state of health.

Review of Systems

Purpose

To obtain detailed information about the current state of the patient and any past symptoms, or lack of symptoms, patient may have experienced related to a particular body system.

Types of Information Needed

Subjective information about what the patient feels or sees with regard to the major systems of the body.

1. Skin—rash, itching, change in pigmentation or texture, sweating, hair growth and distribution, condition of nails
2. Skeletal—stiffness of joints, pain, deformity, restriction of motion, swelling, redness, heat. If there are problems, ask the patient to specify any activities of daily life that are difficult or impossible to perform.
3. Head—headaches, dizziness, syncope, head injuries
4. Eyes—vision, pain, diplopia, photophobia, blind spots, itching, burning, discharge, recent change in appearance or vision, glaucoma, cataracts, glasses/contact lenses worn, date of last refraction, infection
5. Ears—hearing acuity, earache, discharge, tinnitus, vertigo
6. Nose—sense of smell, frequency of colds, obstruction, epistaxis, postnasal discharge, sinus pain or therapy, use of nose drops or sprays (type and frequency)
7. Teeth—pain; bleeding, swollen or receding gums; recent abscesses, extractions; dentures; dental hygiene practices
8. Mouth and tongue—soreness of tongue or buccal mucosa, ulcers, swelling
9. Throat—sore throat, tonsillitis, hoarseness, dysphagia
10. Neck—pain, stiffness, swelling, enlarged glands or lymph nodes

11. Endocrine—goiter, thyroid tenderness, tremors, weakness, tolerance to heat and cold, changes in hat or glove size, changes in skin pigmentation, libido, bruisability, muscle cramps, polyuria, polydipsia, polyphagia, hormone therapy
12. Respiratory
    a. Pain in the chest and relationship to respirations
    b. Dyspnea, wheezing, cough, sputum (character, quantity), hemoptysis
    c. Night sweats (Does the patient have to change his bedding?)
    d. Last chest x-ray and result (indicate where obtained)
    e. Exposure to tuberculosis
13. Cardiac
    a. Presence of pain or distress and location (have patient point to location); radiation of pain; precipitating/aggravating causes; alleviating measures; timing and duration
    b. Palpitations, dyspnea, orthopnea (note number of pillows required for sleeping), edema, cyanosis
    c. Exercise tolerance (determine in relation to patient's regular activities—how much can he do before stopping to rest?)
    d. Blood pressure (if known): last electrocardiogram (ECG) and results (indicate where obtained)
14. Hematologic—anemia (if so, treatment received), tendency to bruise or bleed, thromboses, thrombophlebitis, any known abnormalities of blood cells
15. Lymph nodes—enlargement, tenderness, suppuration, duration and progress of abnormality
16. Gastrointestinal
    a. Appetite and digestion, intolerance to certain classes of foods
    b. Pain associated with hunger or eating, eructation, regurgitation, heartburn, nausea, vomiting, hematemesis
    c. Regularity of bowel movement (describe normal bowel habits and whether they have changed recently); diarrhea, flatulence, stools (color—brown, black, clay; tarry, fresh blood, mucus, etc.)
    d. Hemorrhoids, jaundice, dark urine, use of laxatives—type; frequency. (This should be included under past medical history with medications, but may be repeated here.)
    e. History of ulcer, gallstones, polyps, tumors
    f. Previous x-rays—where, when, results
17. Genitourinary—dysuria, pain, urgency, frequency, hematuria, nocturia, polydipsia, polyuria, oliguria, edema of the face, hesitancy, dribbling, loss in size or force of stream, passage of stones, stress incontinence, hernias, human immunodeficiency virus (HIV) status, history of sexually transmitted disease
    a. Males
       (1) Puberty—onset, voice change, erections, emissions
       (2) Libido—satisfaction with sexual relations

b. Females
   (1) Menses—onset, regularity, duration of flow, dysmenorrhea, last period, intermenstrual bleeding or discharge, dyspareunia
   (2) Libido—satisfaction with sexual relations
   (3) Pregnancies (see section titled Past Medical History)
   (4) Methods of contraception
   (5) Breasts—pain, tenderness, discharge, lumps, mammograms, breast self-examination—techniques and timing with regard to menstrual cycle

18. Neuromuscular
  a. Mental status—orientation to time, place, person, and distance. "How far is your home from the hospital?" (Interviewer must be able to verify the answer.)
  b. Memory
   (1) Distant memory shown by recalling past medical history
   (2) Recent memory shown by recalling what was eaten for breakfast
  c. Cognition, or ability of patient to conceptualize (very useful information in determining a health education plan for the patient)
  d. Patient's description of personality—how patient views self
  e. Presence of tics, twitching, weakness, paralysis, tremor, wasting of muscles, incoordination, fatigue, sensory loss with respect to pain, temperature, touch, muscle pain, cramps
  f. Psychiatric history may be entered here.

19. General constitutional symptoms—fever, chills, malaise, fatigability, recent loss or gain of weight

Method of Collecting Data

1. Begin by explaining to the patient—"I am going to ask you many questions about your body that will help in understanding your present problem."
2. Ask direct questions about each system, using terms that the patient understands.
3. Whenever the patient complains or suggests a symptom, ask the questions outlined under method of collecting data about the present illness (onset, duration, etc.).
4. Never assume that things are "OK" if the patient fails to mention something.
  a. Ask about every aspect of the function of a particular system and be sure to record the patient's responses.
  b. Often, the fact that a body system has been free of any symptoms is as important as any symptoms that have been experienced.
5. If necessary, memorize a list of questions for each system or use a list when interviewing the patient. Knowing what to ask about each system is based on knowledge of the function of each body system and of the way that normal function manifests itself.

Personal and Social History

Purposes

1. To describe the patient's life situation—may have bearing on the present condition or the patient's ability to cope with this problem
2. To develop a plan of care that "fits" the patient. Here the interviewer finds out the many personal and family resources an individual has to aid in coping with the situation—both long term and short term.
3. To have some idea of how the patient patterns his life
  a. Certain habits and patterns are more easily assimilated and changed, when necessary, than others.
  b. Knowing the patient's patterns is useful in helping to organize hospital routine in ways that will be least disruptive to the patient.
4. To help the patient develop a workable plan of care at home, based on knowledge of home conditions
5. To determine if the patient's occupation is directly or indirectly related to his condition
6. To determine if the patient's religious affiliation may affect therapy

Types of Information Needed

1. Personal status—birth place, education, armed service affiliation, position in the family, satisfaction with life situations (home and job), personal concerns
2. Habits/patterns
  a. Sleeping, activities/hobbies, nutrition/eating habits (diet for a typical day)
  b. Consumption of alcohol, coffee, tea, drugs (marijuana, over-the-counter medications)
  c. Tobacco (what form; how long)
  d. Sexual habits (can be part of genitourinary history)—relationships, frequency, satisfaction, HIV prevention
3. Home conditions
  a. Marital status, nature of family relationships
  b. Economic conditions—source of income; health insurance, Medicare, Medicaid
  c. Living arrangements and housing (owning/renting, heating, sewage, pets, etc.)
  d. Involvement with agencies (name, case worker, etc.)
4. Occupation
  a. Past and present employment and working conditions, including exposure to stress/tension, noise, pollution
  b. Working hours
  c. Job satisfaction
5. Religion—name, whether practicing or not, any stipulations with regard to health practices

Method of Collecting Data

1. Begin by explaining that you are now going to ask questions about the patient's life situation to gain a clearer perspective of the patient's condition and of how you might help.

2. Your manner should be matter-of-fact, yet concerned. If you are uncomfortable asking the questions, most likely the patient will sense that and be uneasy answering them.

3. A sensitive interviewer can ask most of the questions listed above in an initial interview without alienating the patient. For instance, ask "What has been your education?" instead of "How far have you gone in school?"

■ Ending the History

When you have completed the history, it is often helpful to say: "Is there anything else you would like to tell me?" or "What do you think is the matter with you?" This allows the patient to end the history by saying what is on his or her mind and what concerns the patient most.

PHYSICAL EXAMINATION

■ General Principles

1. A complete or partial physical examination is conducted following a careful comprehensive or problem-related history.
2. It is conducted in a quiet, well-lit room with consideration for patient privacy and comfort.

■ Approach to the Patient

1. When possible, begin with the patient in a sitting position, so both front and back can be examined.
2. Completely expose the part to be examined but drape the rest of the body appropriately.
3. Conduct the examination systematically from head to foot so as not to miss observing any system or body part.
4. While examining each region, consider the underlying anatomic structures, their function, and possible abnormalities.
5. Because the body is bilaterally symmetric for the most part, compare findings on one side with those on the other.
6. Explain all procedures to the patient while the examination is being conducted—to avoid alarming or worrying the patient and to encourage cooperation.

■ Techniques of Examination and Assessment

Use the following techniques of examination as appropriate for eliciting findings.

Inspection
1. Begins with first encounter with the patient and is the most important of all the techniques.
2. Is an organized scrutiny of the patient's behavior and body.
3. With knowledge and experience, the examiner can become highly sensitive to visual clues.
4. The examiner begins each phase of the examination by inspecting the particular part with the eyes.

Palpation
1. Involves touching the region or body part just observed and noting what the various structures feel like.
2. With experience comes the ability to distinguish variations of normal from abnormal.
3. Is performed in an organized manner from region to region.

Percussion
1. By setting underlying tissues in motion, percussion helps in determining whether the underlying tissue is air filled, fluid filled, or solid.
2. Audible sounds and palpable vibrations are produced, which can be distinguished by the examiner.

There are five basic notes produced by percussion, which can be distinguished by differences in the qualities of sound, pitch, duration, and intensity.

	Relative Intensity	Relative Pitch	Relative Duration	Example Location
Flatness	Soft	High	Short	Thigh
Dullness	Medium	Medium	Medium	Liver
Resonance	Loud	Low	Long	Normal lung
Hyperresonance	Very loud	Lower	Longer	Emphysematous lung
Tympany	Loud	*	*	Gastric air bubble or puffed out cheek

*Distinguished mainly by its musical timbre.
(From Bickley, L. S. [1999]. *Bates' guide to physical examination and history taking* [7th ed.]. Philadelphia: Lippincott Williams & Wilkins.)

3. The technique for percussion may be described as follows:

   a. Hyperextend the middle finger of your left hand, pressing the distal portion and joint firmly against the surface to be percussed.

   (1) Other fingers touching the surface will damp the sound.

   (2) Be consistent in the degree of firmness exerted by the hyperextended finger as you move it from area to area or the sound will vary.

   b. Cock the right hand at the wrist, flex the middle finger upward, and place the forearm close to the surface to be percussed. The right hand and forearm should be as relaxed as possible.

   c. With a quick, sharp, relaxed wrist motion, strike the extended left middle finger with the flexed right middle finger, using the tip of the finger, not the pad. (A very short fingernail is a must!) Aim at the end of the extended left middle finger (just behind the nail bed) where the greatest pressure is exerted on the surface to be percussed.

   d. Lift the right middle finger rapidly to avoid damping the vibrations.

   e. The movement is at the wrist, not at the finger, elbow, or shoulder; the examiner should use the lightest touch capable of producing a clear sound.

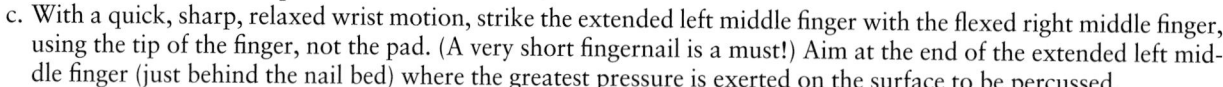

Auscultation

1. This method uses the stethoscope to augment the sense of hearing.

2. The stethoscope must be constructed well and must fit the user. Earpieces should be comfortable, the length of the tubing should be 25 to 38 cm (10–15 inches), and the head should have a diaphragm and a bell.

   a. The bell is used for low-pitched sounds such as certain heart murmurs.

   b. The diaphragm screens out low-pitched sounds and is good for hearing high-frequency sounds such as breath sounds.

   c. Extraneous sounds can be produced by clothing, hair, and movement of the head of the stethoscope.

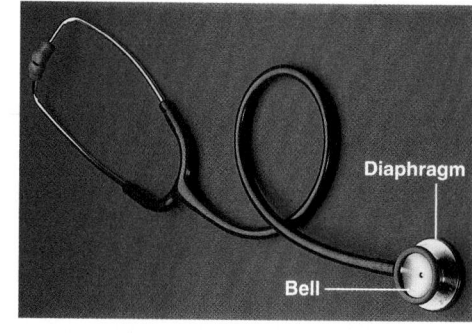

Diaphragm

Bell

◼ Equipment

Thermometer
Sphygmomanometer
Oto-ophthalmoscope
Flashlight
Tongue depressor

Cotton applicator stick
Stethoscope
Reflex hammer
Tuning fork
Safety pin

Additional items include disposable gloves and lubricant for rectal examination and a speculum for examination of female pelvis.

Technique	Findings

◼ Vital Signs

Importance—Many major therapeutic decisions are based on the vital signs; therefore, accuracy is essential.

Temperature

Routinely, where accuracy is not crucial, an oral temperature will suffice.

A rectal temperature is the most accurate.

Unless contraindicated (as in a patient with a severe cardiac arrhythmia), a rectal temperature is often preferred.

Temperature—may vary with the time of day.
  Oral: 37°C (98.6°F) is considered normal.
May vary from 35.8°C to 37.3°C (96.4°–99.1°F).
  Rectal: Higher than oral by 0.4°C to 0.5°C (0.7°–0.9°F).

Technique	Findings

Pulse

Palpate the radial pulse and count for at least 30 seconds.

If the pulse is irregular, count for a full minute and note the number of irregular beats/min.

Note whether the beat of the pulse against your finger is strong or weak, bounding or thready.

Pulse—Normal adult pulse is 60 to 80 beats/min; regular in rhythm. Elasticity of the arterial walls, blood volume, and mechanical action of the heart muscle are some of the factors that affect strength of the pulse wave, which normally is full and strong.

Respiration

Count the number of respirations taken in 15 seconds and multiply by 4.

Note rhythm and depth of breathing.

Respiration—Normally 16 to 20 respirations/min.

Blood Pressure

Measure the blood pressure in both arms.

Palpate the systolic pressure before using the stethoscope in order to detect an auscultatory gap.*

Apply cuff firmly; if too loose, it will give a falsely high reading.

Use cuff in appropriate size: a pediatric cuff for children; a leg cuff for obese people.

The cuff should be approximately 2.5 cm (1 inch) above the antecubital fossa.

Normal range
 Systolic—95–140 mm Hg
 Diastolic—60–90 mm Hg
A difference of 5 to 10 mm Hg between arms is common.
Systolic pressure in lower extremities is usually 10 mm Hg higher than reading in upper extremities.
Going from a recumbent to a standing position can cause the systolic pressure to fall 10 to 15 mm Hg and the diastolic pressure to rise slightly (by 5 mm Hg).

◼ Height and Weight

Determine the patient's height and weight. Use a measuring stick or tape rather than asking the patient's height.

◼ General Appearance

Begin observation on first contact with the patient (in the waiting room or while the patient is in bed); continue throughout the interview systematically—as the first step in the examination of each body part.

Inspection

Observe for: race, sex, general physical development, nutritional state, mental alertness, evidence of pain, restlessness, body position, clothes, apparent age, hygiene, grooming.

Careful observation of the general state of the individual provides many clues about a person's body image, how he behaves, and also some idea of how well or ill he is.

◼ Skin

1. Examination of the skin is correlated with the information obtained in the history and other parts of the physical examination.
2. Examine the skin as you proceed through each body system.

Auscultatory gap:
 1. *The first sound of blood in the artery is usually followed by continuous sound until nothing is audible with the stethoscope.*
 2. *Occasionally the sound is not continuous and there is a gap after the first sound, after which the sound of blood in the vessel is heard again.*
 3. *If one uses only the auscultatory method and pumps the cuff up until the sound is no longer heard, it is possible, when there is a gap in the sound or when the sound is not continuous, to get a falsely low systolic reading.*

Technique	Findings

Inspection

Observe for: skin color, pigmentation, lesions (distribution, type, configuration, size), jaundice, cyanosis, scars, superficial vascularity, moisture, edema, color of mucous membranes, hair distribution, nails.

"Normal" varies considerably depending on racial or ethnic background, exposure to sun, complexion, pigmentation tendencies (eg, freckles).

Palpation

Examine skin for temperature, texture, elasticity, turgor.

The skin is normally warm, slightly moist, and smooth and returns quickly to its original shape when picked up between two fingers and released. There is a characteristic hair distribution over the body associated with gender and normal physiologic function. Nails are present and smooth and cared for in some way.

Head

Inspection

Observe for: symmetry of face, configuration of skull, hair color and distribution, scalp.

Normally, the skull and face are symmetric, with distribution of hair varying from person to person. (However, determine by history if there has been any change.)

Palpation

Examine: hair texture, masses, swelling or tenderness of scalp, configuration of skull.

The scalp should be free of flaking, with no signs of nits (small, white louse eggs), lesions, deformities, or tenderness.

Eyes and Vision

Equipment
Ophthalmoscope

Anatomic Landmarks
Globes
Palpebral fissures
Lid margins
Conjunctivae
Sclerae
Pupils
Iris

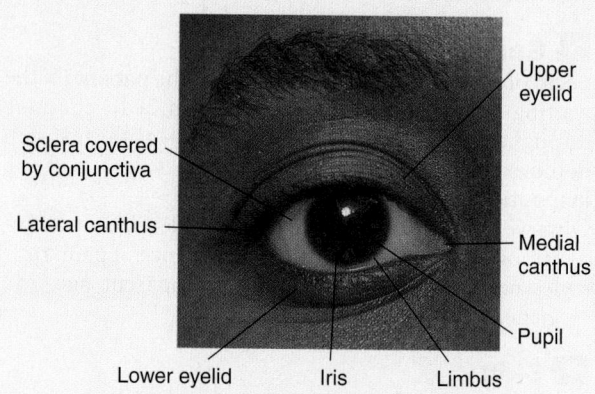

Inspection

1. *Globes*—for protrusion.
2. *Palpebral fissures* (longitudinal openings between the eyelids)—for width and symmetry.

2. *Palpebral fissures*—appear equal in size when the eyes are open.
   Upper lid—covers a small portion of the iris and cornea.
   Lower lid—margin is just below the junction of the cornea and sclera (limbus).
   Ptosis—drooping of eyelids.

3. *Lid margins*—for scaling, secretions, erythema, position of lashes.

3. *Lid margins*—are clear; the lacrimal duct openings (puncta) are evident at the nasal ends of the upper and lower lids.
   Eye lashes—normally are evenly distributed and turn outward.

Technique	Findings

4. *Bulbar and palpebral conjunctivae*—for congestion and color.
   Bulbar conjunctiva—membranous covering of the sclera (contains blood vessels).
   Palpebral conjunctiva—membranous covering of the inside of the upper and lower lids (contains blood vessels).

4. *Bulbar conjunctiva* (cover of sclera)—consists of transparent red blood vessels, which may become dilated and produce the characteristic "bloodshot" eye.
   Palpebral conjunctivae—are pink and clear.
   Conjunctivitis—inflammation of the conjunctival surfaces.

5. *Sclerae*—for color; *iris*—for color

5. *Sclerae*—should be white and clear.

6. *Pupils*—for size, shape, symmetry, reaction to light and accommodation (ability of the lens to adjust to objects at varying distances).

6. *Pupils*—normally constrict with increasing light and accommodation. Pupils are normally round and can range in size from very small ("pinpoint") to large (occupying the entire space of the iris).

7. *Eye movement*—extraocular movements, nystagmus, convergence.
   (Nystagmus: rapid, lateral, horizontal, or rotary movement of the eye.)
   (Convergence: ability of the eye to turn in and focus on a very close object.)
   (See neurologic examination, p. 83.)

7. *Extraocular movement*—movement of the eyes in conjugate fashion. (Six muscles control the movement of the eye.) Eyes normally move in conjugate fashion, except when converging on an object that is moving closer.
   Nystagmus—may be seen normally as a result of eye fatigue.
   Convergence—fails when double vision occurs, usually 10 to 15 cm (4–6 inches) from nose.

8. *Gross visual fields*—by confrontation. (See neurologic examination, p. 83.)

8. *Peripheral vision*—is full (medially and laterally, superiorly and inferiorly) in both eyes.

9. *Visual acuity*
   Check with a Snellen chart (with and without glasses).

9. *Normal vision*—20/20.
   Myopia—nearsightedness
   Hyperopia—farsightedness

Palpation

1. Determine strength of upper lids by attempting to open closed lids against resistance.
2. Palpate globes through closed lids for tenderness and tension.

1. The examiner should not be able to open the lids when the patient is squeezing them shut.
2. Globes normally are not tender when palpated.

Funduscopic Examination

1. *Red retinal reflex*—check the transparency of the anterior and posterior chambers.
2. *Cornea*—check for transparency.
3. *Lens*—check for transparency.
4. *Retina*—check for color, pigmentation, hemorrhages, and exudates.

1. *Red retinal reflex*—can be spotted by the examiner while standing 30 cm (12 inches) from the eye.
2. *Cornea*—should be transparent.
3. *Lens*—should be transparent (ie, retina can be seen).
4. *Retina*—color varies according to the amount of pigment present. There should be no hemorrhages or exudates.

5. *Optic disc*—check for color, distinction of margins, pigmentation, degree of elevation, cupping.

5. *Optic disc*—is circular and has a yellowish pink color. Although disc appearance may vary, the margins are normally distinct and regular, with varying amounts of pigment.

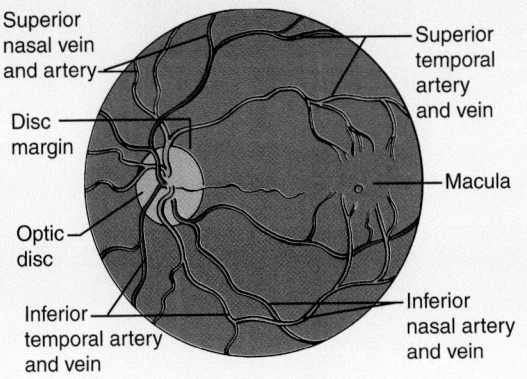

Superior nasal vein and artery
Disc margin
Optic disc
Inferior temporal artery and vein
Superior temporal artery and vein
Macula
Inferior nasal artery and vein

Technique

6. *Macula*—check for color. (Lies at a distance of 2 optic disc diameters laterally from the optic disc.)
7. *Blood vessels*—check for diameter, arteriovenous (A/V) ratio; origin and course; venous-arterial crossings. (Both arteries and veins are present and move outward from the disc nasally and temporally.)

Findings

6. *Macula*—because it is free of blood vessels, it is lighter in color than the rest of the retina.
7. *Retinal arteries and veins*—arteries are approximately ⅘ the size of the veins and lighter in color. Where arteries and veins cross, there is usually no disturbance in the course of either. Pulsations may occur in the vein near the optic disc.

Use of the Ophthalmoscope

1. Hold the instrument in your right hand and use your right eye to examine the patient's right eye.
   a. Reverse the procedure to examine the patient's left eye.
   b. This approach allows you to get close to the patient without bumping noses.
2. Hold the instrument so your last two fingers are straight, rather than curved around the handle. You can place these fingers against the patient's cheek to steady the instrument and to avoid hitting the patient with it.
3. Begin the funduscopic examination standing about 30 cm (a foot) from the patient. The room should be darkened.
4. Turn the dial on the head of the ophthalmoscope to +8 or +10 (black numbers).
5. Turn on the ophthalmoscope light and place the eyepiece up to your eye. If you wear glasses or contact lenses, it is best to wear them during the examination so you do not have to accommodate for your vision by turning the dial on the ophthalmoscope.
6. Aim the light at the pupil of the eye. You should see the red reflex immediately.
7. Slowly move in toward the patient, continuing to look through the eyepiece and keeping the light directed at the pupil, beyond which is the fundus.
8. With the index finger of the hand holding the ophthalmoscope, turn the dial toward zero as you move in.
   a. This allows you to focus on the various chambers of the eye.
   b. A way to find the eye and pupil is to put your hand on top of the patient's head and your thumb at the outer corner of the eye. If you lose the fundus, you can return to your thumb and get your bearings by moving medially from the thumb nail.
9. Once your hand is resting on the patient's cheek, continue to turn the dial until you can focus on the retina, and the blood vessels and the optic disc appear sharp.
10. Once you are focused on the optic disc, it is possible to follow the blood vessels out from the disc inferiorly and superiorly, medially and laterally. (See Chapter 16 [Eye Disorders] for visual fields, color vision tests, refraction, tonometry.)

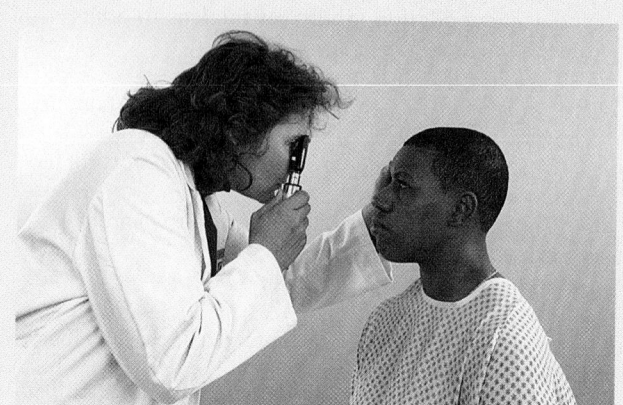

Technique   **Findings**

■ Ears and Hearing

Equipment
Tuning fork, otoscope

To Examine with Otoscope

1. Hold the helix of the ear and gently pull the pinna upward and back toward the occiput to straighten the external canal.
2. Gently insert the lighted otoscope, using an earpiece that is a comfortable size for the patient.
3. Once the otoscope is in place, put your eye up to the eyepiece and examine the external canal.

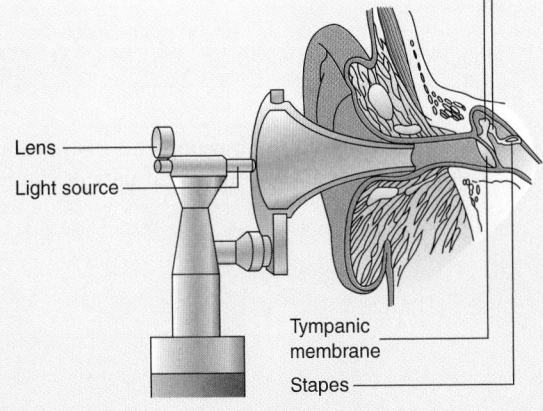

Techniques of Examination
Inspection

1. *Pinna*—examine for size, shape, color, lesions, masses.
2. *External canal*—examine with the otoscope for discharge, impacted cerumen, inflammation, masses, or foreign bodies.
3. *Tympanic membrane*—examine for color, luster, shape, position, transparency, integrity, and scarring.
4. *Landmarks*—note cone of light, umbo, handle and short process of the malleus, pars flaccida, and pars tensa.

   Gently move the otoscope to observe the entire drum.
   (Cerumen may obscure visualization of the drum.)

Palpation
Pinna—examine for tenderness, consistency of cartilage, swelling.

2. *External canal*—is normally clear with perhaps minimal cerumen.

3. *Tympanic membrane and landmarks.*

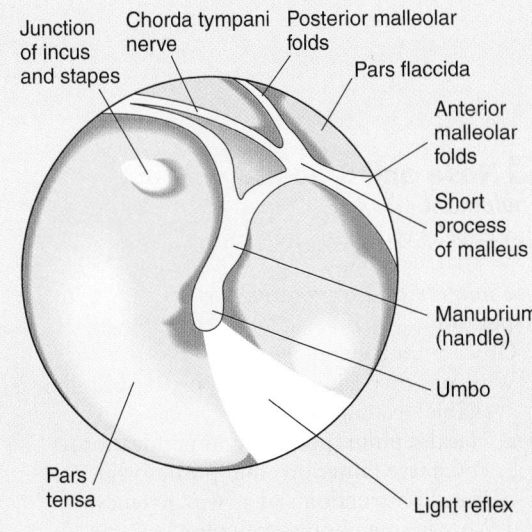

Right ear drum

Mechanical Tests

1. Test each ear for gross hearing acuity using whispered word or watch. Cover the ear not being tested.

1. A person with normal hearing can hear a whispered word from approximately 4.5 m (15 feet) and a watch from 30 cm (12 inches). The patient should hear the sound equally well in both ears, that is, there is no lateralization.

Technique	Findings

2. *Weber test*—test for lateralization of vibration. Place tuning fork in the center of the scalp near the forehead (*A*). (Also see Chapter 17 [Ear, Nose, and Throat Disorders]).

3. *Rinne test*—compares air and bone conduction.
   a. Place vibrating tuning fork on the mastoid process behind the ear and have the patient tell you when the vibration stops (*B*).
   b. Then quickly hold the buzzing end of the tuning fork *near* the ear canal and ask if patient can hear it (*C*).

2. Normally, sound is heard equally in both ears.

3. Normally, sound should be heard after vibration can no longer be felt, that is, air conduction is greater than bone conduction. Lateralization and conduction findings are altered by damage to the 8th cranial nerve and damage to the ossicles in the middle ear.

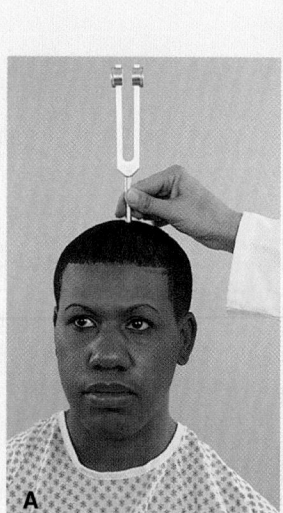
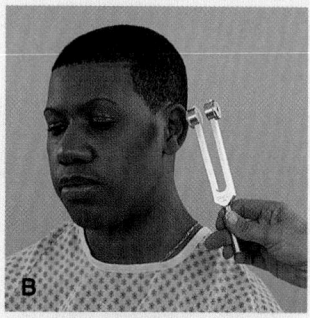
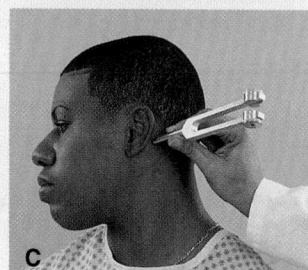

Nose and Sinuses

Equipment
Otoscope, nasal speculum

Techniques of Examination
Inspection
1. Observe for general deformity.
2. With nasal speculum (otoscope, if speculum is unavailable) examine for:
   a. Nasal septum (position and perforation)
   b. Discharge (anteriorly and posteriorly)
   c. Nasal obstruction and airway patency
   d. Mucous membranes for color
   e. Turbinates for color and swelling

Nasal septum—is normally straight and not perforated.
Discharge—none should be present.
Airways—are patent.
Mucous membranes—are normally pink.
Turbinates—three bony projections on each lateral wall of the nasal cavity covered with well-vascularized, mucous-secreting membranes. They warm the air going into the lungs and may become swollen and pale with colds and allergies.

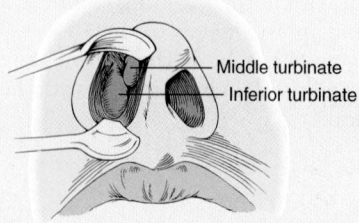

Technique	Findings

Palpation

Sinuses (frontal and maxillary)—for tenderness
   Frontal—direct manual pressure upward toward wall
      of sinus. Avoid pressure on eyes.
   Maxillary—with thumbs, direct pressure upward over
      lower edge of maxillary bones.

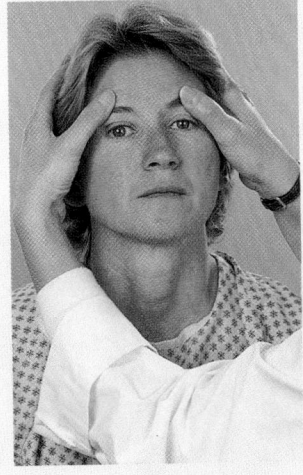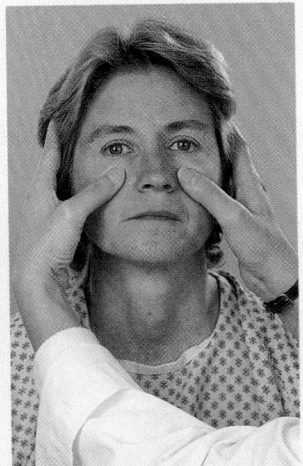

Tenderness of sinuses may indicate sinusitis.

◼ Mouth

Equipment
Flashlight, tongue depressor, gloves, gauze sponges

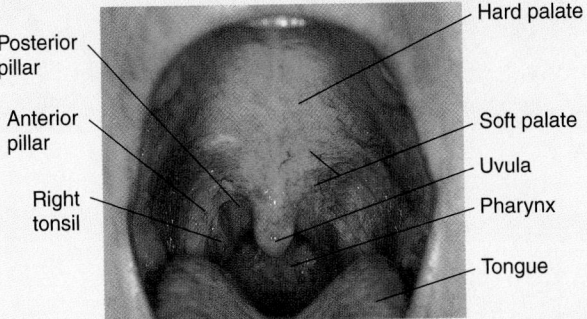

Techniques of Examination
Inspection
1. Observe lips for color, moisture, pigment, masses, ulcerations, fissures.
2. Use tongue depressor and penlight to examine:
   a. *Teeth*—number, arrangement, general condition
   b. *Gums*—for color, texture, discharge, swelling, or retraction
   c. *Buccal mucosa*—for discoloration, vesicles, ulcers, masses
   d. *Pharynx*—for inflammation, exudate, and masses
   e. *Tongue* (protruded)—for size, color, thickness, lesions, moisture, symmetry, deviations from midline, fasciculations
   f. *Salivary glands*—for patency
         Parotid glands

         Sublingual and submaxillary glands

   g. *Uvula*—for symmetry when patient says "ah"
   h. *Tonsils*—for size, ulceration, exudates, inflammation

Teeth—the adult normally has 32 teeth.
Gums—commonly recede in adults. Bleeding is fairly common and may result from trauma, gingival disease, or systemic problems (less common).

Tongue—is normally midline and covered with papillae, which vary in size from the tip of the tongue to the back. (The circumvallate papillae are large and posterior.)
Parotid glands—open in the buccal pouch at the level of the upper teeth halfway back.
Sublingual and submaxillary glands—open underneath the tongue.

Lingual tonsils—can often be seen on the posterior portion of the tongue.

Technique	Findings

    i. *Odor of breath*
    j. *Voice*—for hoarseness

Palpation

1. Examine oral cavity with gloved hand for masses and ulceration. Palpate beneath tongue and explore laterally the floor of the mouth (*A*).
2. Grasp tongue with gauze sponge to retract; inspect sides and undersurface of tongue and floor of mouth (*B*).

Odor of breath—may indicate dental caries.

1. Entire oral cavity should be pink and without ulcers, deep-red color, lesions, palpable masses, or swelling. An indurated mass raises the suspicion of malignancy.

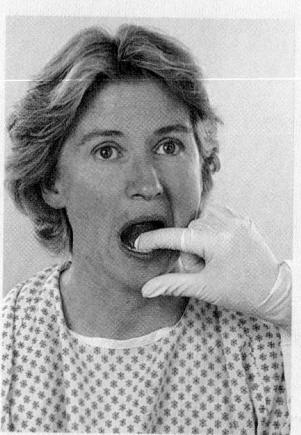
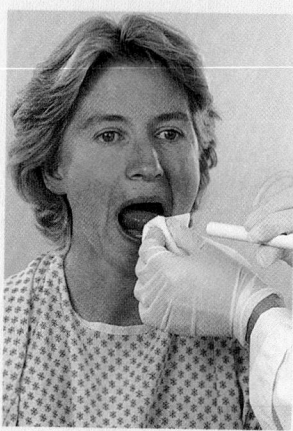

A   **B**

Neck

Equipment
Stethoscope

Techniques of Examination

1. Inspect all areas of the neck anteriorly and posteriorly for muscular symmetry, masses, unusual swelling or pulsations, and range of motion.

2. *Thyroid*—ask the patient to swallow and observe for movement of an enlarged thyroid gland at the suprasternal notch.

3. *Muscular strength*
    a. *Cervical muscles*—have patient turn the chin forcefully against your hand.
    b. *Trapezius muscles*—exert pressure on the patient's shoulders while he shrugs his shoulders.

4. *External jugular veins*—observe with patient sitting and then lying at 30° to 40° angle; patient's neck should not be flexed.

1. *Range of motion*—normally, the chin can touch the anterior chest, the head can be extended at least 45° from the vertical position and can be rotated 90° from midline to side.

2. *Thyroid*—is not usually visible, except in extremely thin persons.

3. *Strength*—see Findings, 11th cranial nerve.

4. *Jugular veins*—when the patient is lying with head elevated 30° to 40°, the jugular veins are approximately at the level of the right atrium, and pulsations that are transmitted from the right atrium can normally be seen with tangential lighting. Veins are not distended when the patient is sitting.

Technique	Findings

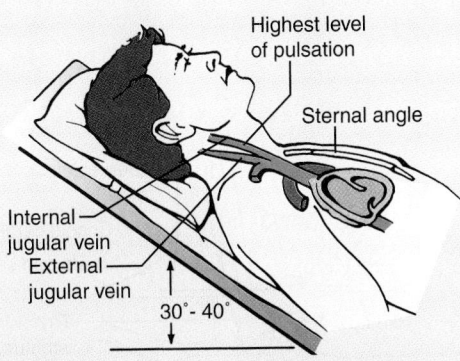

This serves as a fairly constant and therefore reliable landmark, when patient is supine or sitting, for estimating venous pressure, that is, the height in cm measured from level of distended internal jugular veins to level of sternal angle.

Note the sternal angle, the point on the surface anatomy that is approximately 5 to 7 cm (2–2.75 inches) above the right atrium.

Palpation

1. *Cervical nodes and salivary glands.*
2. *Trachea*—palpate at the sternal notch. Stand behind (or in front of) patient and allow the middle finger of each hand to glide off the head of the clavicle into the sternal notch.
   Palpate for deviation and tracheal tug.

1. *Cervical nodes*—in the adult, the cervical lymph nodes are not normally palpable unless the patient is very thin, in which case the nodes are felt as small, freely movable masses. Tender nodes suggest inflammation; hard, fixed nodes suggest malignancy.
2. *Trachea*—should be midline.
   Landmarks are easy to identify using this procedure. This is the downward pull synchronous with cardiac pulsation, usually the result of aneurysm of aorta.

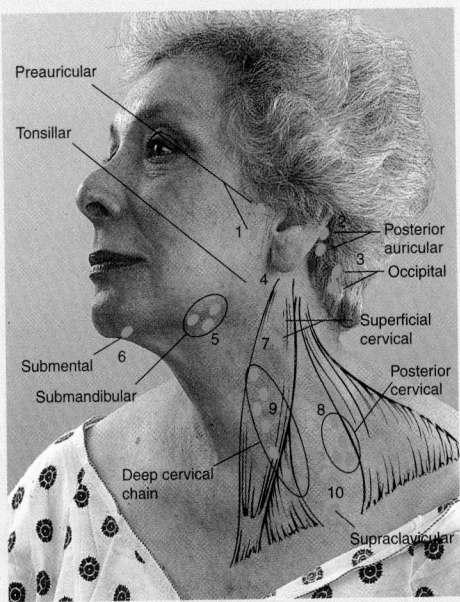

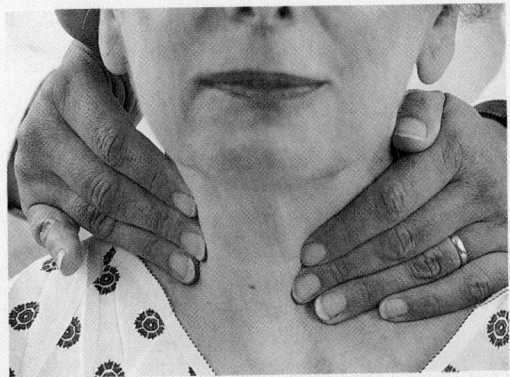

3. *Thyroid*
   a. Stand behind the patient and have him flex the neck to relax the cervical muscles.
   b. Place the fingertips of your left hand behind the left sternocleidomastoid muscle adjacent to the trachea just below larynx.
   c. Palpate the area over the trachea and to the left of the trachea to discern the outline of the isthmus of the left lobe of the thyroid gland.
   d. Note any enlargement, nodules, masses, consistency.

3. If the thyroid is palpable, it is normally smooth, without nodules, masses, or irregularities, or bruits (gushing sound produced by blood moving through a narrow vessel).

Technique   **Findings**

e. Reverse the procedure and examine the right lobe of the thyroid.

f. Because the thyroid gland moves upward on swallowing, have the patient swallow to facilitate examination.

4. *Carotid arteries*
   a. Palpate the carotids one side at a time.
   b. The carotids lie anterolaterally in the neck—avoid palpating the carotid sinuses at the level of the thyroid cartilage just below the angle of the jaw because this may cause slowing of heart rate.
   c. Note symmetry of pulsations, strength, and amplitude.

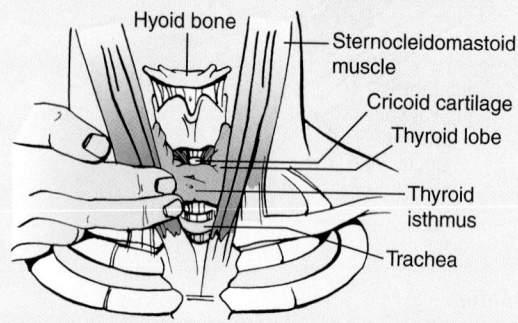

■ Lymph Nodes

1. It is important at some point in the examination to palpate all areas where lymphadenopathy might appear.
2. Often this is done as each region of the body is examined, for example, the cervical nodes are examined when the neck is examined.
3. However, in the record, the condition of the lymph nodes is described under a separate heading.

Techniques of Examination
Inspection
Note size, shape, mobility, consistency, tenderness, and inflammation.

Palpation
1. *Cervical, supra- and infraclavicular nodes.*

2. *Axillary nodes.*
   a. Examine while the patient is sitting.
   b. Place the patient's arm at his side and insert the examining fingers to the apex of the patient's axilla. (Use the fingers of your right hand to examine the left axilla and vice versa.)
   c. Rotate the examining hand so the fingers can palpate the anterior and posterior axillary fossae pressing against the chest wall. Press against the humerus bone in the axilla to examine the lateral fossa for nodes. Conclude the axillary examination by moving the fingers from the apex of the axilla downward in the midline along the chest wall.

Cervical nodes and supra- and infraclavicular nodes— not normally palpable. Enlargement may indicate a thoracic problem.

Axillary nodes—not normally palpable. Enlargement may occur with a breast or arm problem.

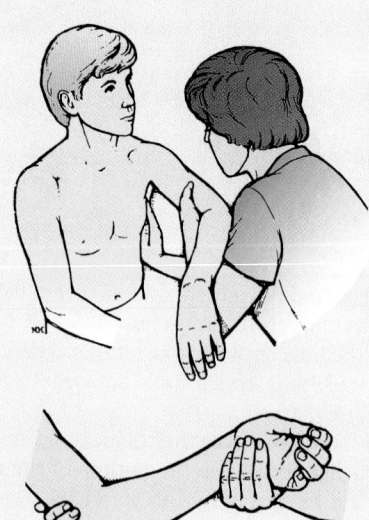

Technique	Findings

3. *Inguinal nodes*—are located in inguen and are usually examined when the abdomen is examined.

4. *Epitrochlear nodes*—are palpated just above the olecranon process.

Inguinal nodes—a few may be felt, but are small, movable, and nontender. Enlargement may indicate a genital or lower extremity problem.

Epitrochlear nodes—not usually palpable. Enlargement may indicate an arm or systemic problem.

■ Breasts (Male and Female)
Female Breast
Inspection
(With the patient sitting, arms relaxed at sides.)
1. Inspect the areolae and nipples for position, pigmentation, inversion, discharge, crusting, and masses. Extra, or supernumerary, nipples may occur normally, most commonly in the anterior axillary region or just below the normal breasts.
2. Examine the breast tissue for size, shape, color, symmetry, surface, contour, skin characteristics, and level of breasts. Note any retraction or dimpling of the skin.

3. Ask the patient to elevate her hands over her head; repeat the observation.

4. Have patient press her hands to her hips; repeat the observation.

Palpation
(This is best done with the patient recumbent.)
1. The patient with pendulous breasts should be given a pillow to place under the ipsilateral scapula of the breast being palpated so the tissue is distributed more evenly over the chest wall.

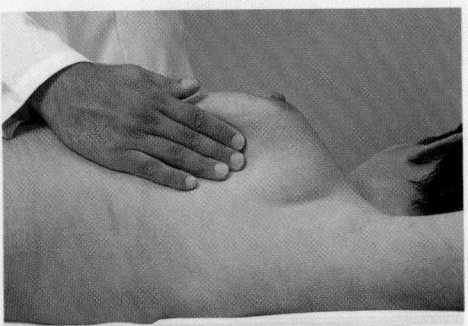

2. The arm on the side of the breast being palpated should be raised above the patient's head.
3. Palpate one breast at a time, beginning with the "asymptomatic" breast if the patient complains of symptoms.
4. To palpate, use the palmar aspects of the fingers in a rotating motion, compressing the breast tissue against the chest wall. (This is done quadrant by quadrant until the entire breast has been palpated—including

1. The *nipples* should be at the same level and protrude slightly. An *inverted nipple* (one that turns inward), if present since puberty, may be normal.
A *supernumerary nipple* usually consists of a nipple and a small areola and may be mistaken for a mole.
2. *Breast size*—in the female it is not uncommon to find a difference in the size of the two breasts. Normal asymmetry has usually been present since puberty and is not a recent phenomenon.
3. If there is a mass attached to the pectoral muscles, contracting the muscles will cause retraction of the breast tissue.

3. This allows the examiner to palpate the "normal" breast first and then compare the "symptomatic" breast to it.
4. *Breast texture*—varies according to the amount of subcutaneous tissue present.
   a. In young females, tissue is fairly soft and homogeneous; in postmenopausal women, tissue may feel nodular or stringy.

Technique	Findings

the "tail" of the breast tissue which extends into the axillary region in the upper outer quadrant of the breast.)

5. Note skin texture, moisture, temperature, or masses.

6. Gently squeeze the nipple and note any expressible discharge.
7. Repeat examination on the opposite breast and compare findings.

b. Consistency also varies with menstrual cycle, being more nodular and edematous just prior to menstruation.*

5. *Masses*—If a mass is palpated, its location, size, shape, consistency, mobility, and associated tenderness are reported.
6. *Discharge*—In the normal nonpregnant or nonlactating female, there is no nipple discharge.

Male Breast

Examination of the male breast can be brief and should never be omitted.

1. Observe the nipple and areola for ulceration, nodules, swelling, or discharge.
2. Palpate the areola for nodules and tenderness.

1. There should be no discharge.

Thorax and Lungs

General Information

1. Methodical inspection of the thorax requires reference to established "landmarks" to locate specific structures and to report significant findings.
2. The same structural landmarks are used in examining both the lung and the heart.
3. It is important to visualize the underlying structures and organs when examining the thorax.

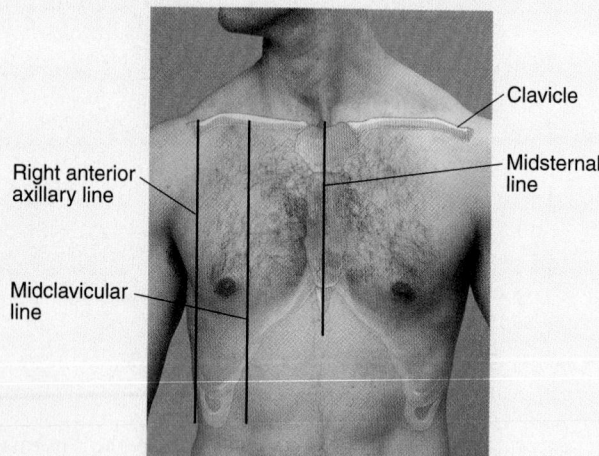

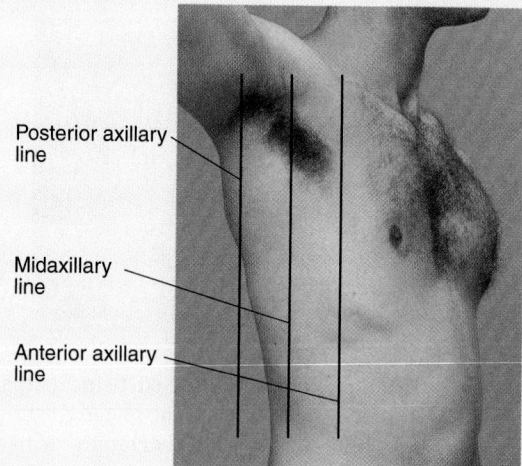

*In teaching women about breast self-examination, explain that the best time for performing the examination is a week after the menstrual period, when the breasts are least engorged and tender.

Technique	Findings

Techniques of Examination
Posterior Thorax and Lungs

Begin the examination with the patient seated; examine posterior chest and lungs.

Inspection

1. Inspect the spine for mobility and any structural deformity.
2. Observe the symmetry of the posterior chest and the posture and mobility of the thorax on respiration. Note any bulges or retractions of the costal interspaces on respiration or any impairment of respiratory movement.
3. Note the anteroposterior diameter in relation to the lateral diameter of the chest.

Palpation

1. Palpate the posterior chest with the patient sitting; identify areas of tenderness, masses, inflammation.
2. Palpate the ribs and costal margins for symmetry, mobility, and tenderness and the spine for tenderness and vertebral position.

3. To assess respiratory excursion—place the thumbs at the level of the 10th vertebra; with hands held parallel to the 10th ribs as they grasp the lateral rib cage, ask the patient to inhale deeply. Observe the movement of the thumbs while feeling the range, and observe the symmetry of the hands.

2. The thorax is normally symmetric; it moves easily and without impairment on respiration. There are no bulges or retractions of the intercostal spaces.

3. The anteroposterior (AP) diameter of the thorax in relation to the lateral diameter is approximately 1:2.

2. On palpation, there be no tenderness; chest movement should be symmetric and without lag or impairment. Tenderness may indicate musculoskeletal strain, fracture, or other problem.

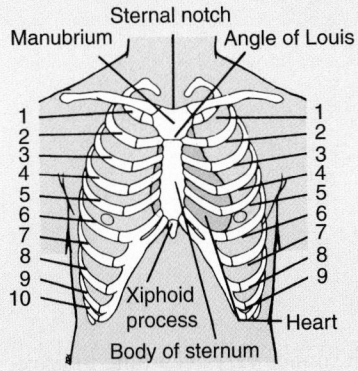

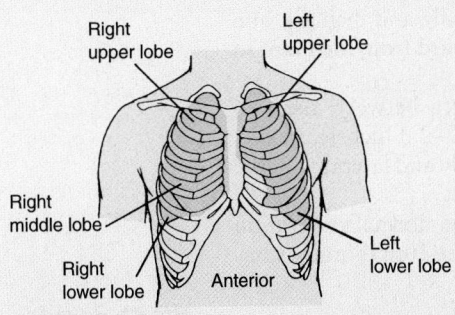

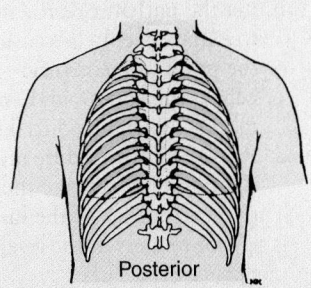

4. To elicit vocal and tactile *fremitus* (palpable vibrations transmitted through the bronchopulmonary system on speaking).
   a. Ask the patient to say "99"; palpate and compare symmetric areas of the lungs with the ball of one hand.

   b. Note any areas of increased or decreased fremitus.
   c. If fremitus is faint, ask the patient to speak louder and in a deeper voice.

4. Posteriorly, fremitus is generally equal throughout the lung fields.
It may be increased near the large bronchi.
   It may be decreased or absent anteriorly and posteriorly when vocal loudness is decreased, when posture is not erect, or when excessive tissue or underlying structures are present.

   One must distinguish the various normal causes of increased or decreased fremitus from the pathologic causes.

Technique

Findings

Percussion

As with palpation, the posterior chest is percussed with the patient sitting.

1. Percuss symmetric areas, comparing sides.
2. Begin across the top of each shoulder and proceed down between the scapulae and then under the scapulae, both medially and laterally in the axillary lines.
3. Note and localize any abnormal percussion sound.
4. For diaphragmatic excursion, percuss by placing the pleximeter (stationary) finger parallel to the approximate level of the diaphragm below the right scapula.
   a. Ask the patient to inhale deeply and hold his breath; percuss downward to the point of dullness. Mark this point.

Percussion normally reveals resonance over symmetric areas of the lung.

Percussion sound may be altered by poor posture and/or presence of excessive tissue.

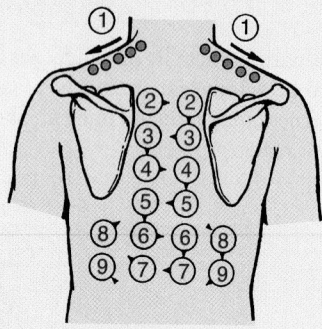

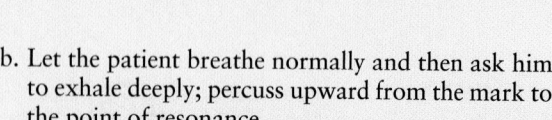

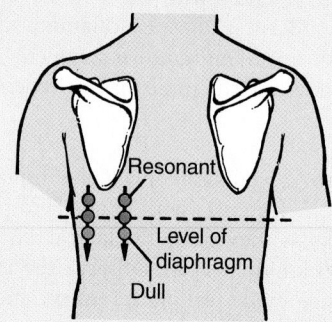

   b. Let the patient breathe normally and then ask him to exhale deeply; percuss upward from the mark to the point of resonance.
   c. Mark this point and measure between the two marks—normally 5 to 6 cm (2–2.3 inches).
   d. Repeat this procedure medially and laterally on the right and left sides of the chest.

The lower border of the lungs on normal respiration is approximately at the level of the 10th thoracic spinous process.

Auscultation

Aids in assessing air flow through the lungs, the presence of fluid or mucus, and the condition of the surrounding pleural space and lungs.

1. Have patient sit erect.*
2. With a stethoscope, listen to the lungs as the patient breathes somewhat more deeply than normally with mouth open. (Let the patient pause, as needed, to avoid hyperventilation.)

Note: If patient is unable to sit with or without assistance for examination of the posterior chest and lungs, position the patient first on one side and then on the other as you examine the lung fields.

Breath Sounds

On auscultation, breath sounds vary according to proximity of the large bronchi.

   a. They are louder and coarser near the large bronchi and over the anterior.
   b. They are softer and much finer (vesicular) at the periphery over the alveolae.

Breath sounds also vary in duration with inspiration and expiration.

Sounds may normally decrease in obese individuals.

Pathology will alter the normal bronchial, bronchovesicular, and vesicular breath sounds. (Abnormal breath sounds or adventitious sounds are to be noted and localized.)

Technique   **Findings**

3. Place the stethoscope in the same areas on the chest wall as those percussed, and listen to a complete inspiration and expiration in each area.
4. Compare symmetric areas methodically from the apex to the lung bases.
5. It should be possible to distinguish three types of normal breath sounds as indicated in the following table.

Breath Sounds	Duration of Inspiration and Expiration	Pitch of Expiration	Intensity of Expiration	Normal Location
Vesicular	Insp. > Exp.	Low	Soft	Most of lungs
Bronchovesicular	Insp. = Exp.	Medium	Medium	Near the main stem bronchi (ie, below the clavicles and between the scapulae, especially on the right).
Bronchial or tubular	Exp. > Insp.	High	Usually loud	Over the trachea

(From Bickley, L. S. [1999]. *Bates' guide to physical examination and history taking* [7th ed.]. Philadelphia: Lippincott Williams & Wilkins.)

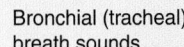
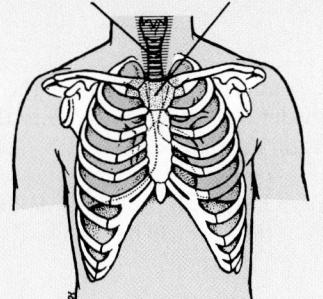

Bronchial (tracheal) breath sounds   Bronchovesicular breath sounds

Anterior Thorax and Lungs
The patient should be recumbent with arms at sides and slightly abducted.
Inspection
1. Inspect the chest for any structural deformity.
2. Note the width of the costal angle.

3. Observe rate and rhythm of breathing, any bulging or retraction of intercostal spaces on respiration, use of accessory muscles of respiration (sternocleidomastoid and trapezius on inspiration and abdominal muscles on expiration).
4. Note any asymmetry of chest wall movement on respiration.
Palpation
(Serves the same purposes in examining the anterior chest as in the posterior chest.)
1. To assess diaphragmatic excursion, place hands along the costal margins and note symmetry and degree of expansion as the patient inhales deeply.

2. The angle at the tip of the sternum is determined by the right and left rib margins at the xiphoid process. Normally, the angle is less than 90°.
3. The thorax is normally symmetric and moves easily without impairment on respiration. There are no bulges or retractions of the intercostal spaces.

Technique	Findings

2. Palpate for fremitus with the ball of the hand anteriorly and laterally.
   (Underlying structures [eg, heart, liver, etc.] may damp, or decrease, fremitus.)
3. Compare symmetric areas.
4. If necessary, displace the female breast gently.

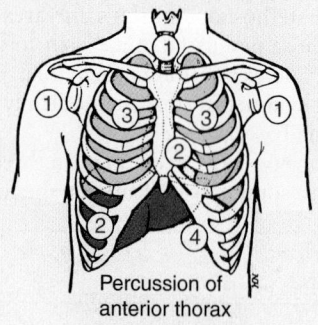

Percussion of
anterior thorax

① Flat   ③ Resonant
② Dull   ④ Tympanic

Percussion

1. With patient's arms resting comfortably at his sides, examiner percusses the anterior and lateral chest.
   Begin just below the clavicles and percuss downward from one interspace to the next, comparing the sound from the interspace on one side with that of the contra-lateral interspace.
2. Displace the female breast so breast tissue does not damp the vibration. Continue downward, noting the intercostal space where hepatic dullness is percussed on the right and cardiac dullness on the left.
3. Note effect of underlying structures.

2. A tympanic sound is produced over the gastric air bubble on the left somewhat lower than the point of liver dullness on the right.

3. Percussion over heart will produce a dull sound. The upper border of the liver will be percussed on the right side, producing a dull note.

Auscultation

Listen to the chest anteriorly and laterally for the distribution of resonance and any abnormal or adventitious sounds.

■ Heart

General Approach

1. The examiner must visualize the position of the heart under the sternum and the ribs and know certain landmarks for identification of specific structures and significant findings.
2. It is also important to identify those "areas" on the chest wall that will yield the most information initially about the function of the heart and its valves.
   a. In locating the intercostal spaces, begin by identifying the angle of Louis, which is felt as a slight ridge approximately 2.5 cm (1 inch) below the sternal notch, where the manubrium and the body of the sternum are joined.
   b. The 2nd ribs extend to the right and left of this angle.
   c. Once the 2nd rib is located, palpate downward and obliquely away from the sternum to identify the remaining ribs and intercostal spaces.

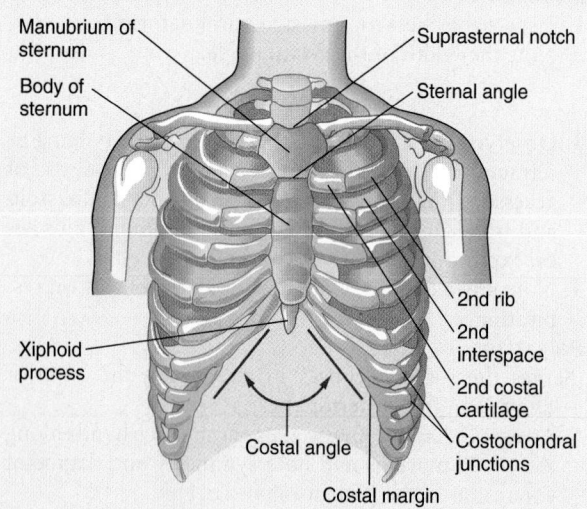

Manubrium of sternum
Body of sternum
Xiphoid process
Costal angle
Costal margin
Suprasternal notch
Sternal angle
2nd rib
2nd interspace
2nd costal cartilage
Costochondral junctions

Technique	Findings

Inspection

1. Inspect the precordium for any bulging, heaving, or thrusting.

2. Look for the apical impulse approximately in the 5th or 6th intercostal space at or just medial to the midclavicular line.

3. Note any other pulsations. Tangential lighting is most helpful in detecting pulsations.

1. Normally there are no bulges.

2. An apical impulse may or may not be observable.

3. There should be no other pulsations.

Palpation

1. Use the ball of the hand to detect vibrations, or "thrills," which may be caused by murmurs. (Use the fingertips or palmar surface to detect pulsations.)

1. There should be no thrills or other pulsations. (Thrills are vibrations caused by turbulence of blood moving through valves that are transmitted through the skin—feels similar to a purring cat.)

2. Proceed methodically through the examination so no area is omitted. Palpate for thrills and pulsations in each area (aortic, pulmonic, tricuspid, mitral).

a. Begin in the aortic area (2nd right intercostal space, close to the sternum) and proceed downward to the apex of the heart. (The mitral area is considered the apex of the heart.)

b. In the tricuspid area, use the palm of the hand to detect any heaving or thrusting of the precordium (tricuspid area—5th intercostal space next to the sternum).

Ordinarily, no heaving of the ventricle is felt, except, possibly, in the pregnant female.

c. In the mitral area (5th intercostal space, at or just medial to the midclavicular line) palpate for the apical beat; identify the point of maximal impulse (PMI) and note its size and force.

The apical pulse should be felt approximately in the 5th intercostal space, at or just medial to the midclavicular line. In the young, thin person, it is a sharp, quick impulse no larger than the intercostal space. In the older person, the impulse may be less sharp and quick.

Percussion

1. Outline the border of the heart or area of cardiac dullness.

a. The left border generally does not extend beyond 4, 7, and 10 cm left of the midsternal line in the 4th, 5th, and 6th intercostal spaces, respectively.

b. The right border usually lies under the sternum.

2. Percuss outward from the sternum with the stationary finger parallel to the intercostal space until dullness is no longer heard. Measure the distance from the midsternal line in centimeters.

Auscultation

1. Place the stethoscope in the pulmonic or aortic area.

2. Begin by identifying the 1st (S_1) and 2nd (S_2) heart sounds.

a. S_1 is caused by the closing of the tricuspid and mitral valves.

b. S_2 results from the closing of the aortic and pulmonary valves.

2. The two sounds are separated by a short systolic interval; each pair of sounds is separated from the next pair by a longer, diastolic interval. Normally, two sounds are heard—"lub," "dub."

a. In the aortic and pulmonic areas, S_2 is usually louder than S_1. In this way, each of the paired sounds can be distinguished from the other.

b. In the tricuspid area, S_1 and S_2 are of almost equal intensity, and, in the mitral area, S_1 is often slightly louder than S_2.

Technique   **Findings**

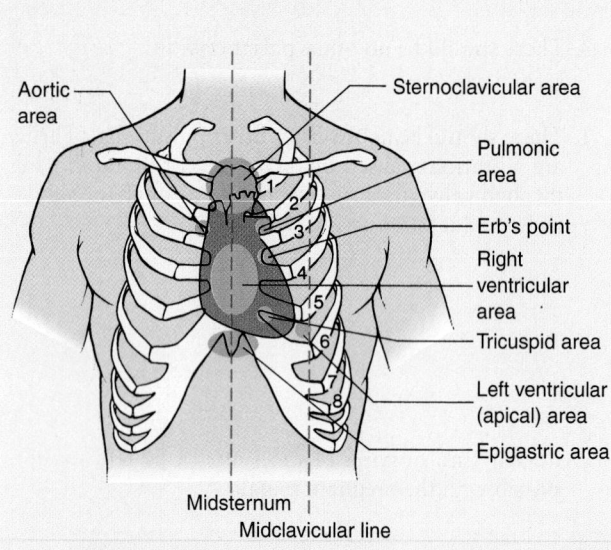

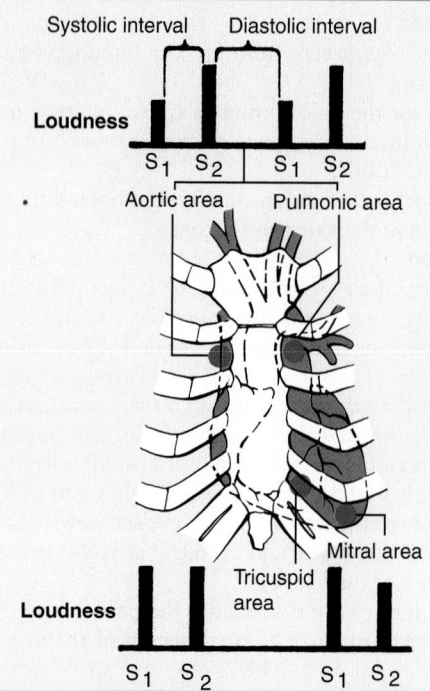

3. Once the heart sounds are identified, count the rate and note the rhythm as discussed under vital signs. If there is an irregularity, try to determine if there is any pattern to the irregularity in relation to the intervals, heart sounds, or respirations.

4. Once rate and rhythm are determined, listen in each of the four areas and at Erb's point (3rd left interspace, close to the sternum) systematically, first with the diaphragm (detects higher pitched sounds) and then with the bell (detects lower pitched sounds). In each area, listen to S_1 and then to S_2 for intensity and splitting.

3. Normally, the heart sounds are regular, with a rate of 60 to 80 beats/min (in the adult). In the athlete or jogger, the resting pulse may be between 40 and 60 beats/min.

4. An extra sound between S_1 and S_2 or S_2 and S_1 of longer duration indicates a systolic or diastolic murmur. Note the area of its greatest intensity (aortic, pulmonic, mitral, tricuspid). An extra sound of short duration usually indicates an S_3 or S_4 gallop.

Occasionally, there may be a splitting of S_2 in the pulmonary area. This is normal. Splitting of S_2 (two contiguous sounds are heard instead of one) is best heard at the end of inspiration, when right ventricular stroke volume is sufficiently increased to delay closure of the pulmonic valve *slightly* behind closure of the aortic valve.

▪ Peripheral Circulation

Jugular Veins

Evaluation of jugular venous distention is most useful in patients with suspected compromise of cardiac function.

Inspection

1. Inspect neck for internal jugular venous pulsations.

1. Jugular venous pulsations can be distinguished from carotid pulsations by the following chart:

Technique   Findings

Internal Jugular Pulsations	*Carotid Pulsations*
Rarely palpable	Palpable
Soft, undulating quality, usually with two or three outward components (a, c, and v waves)	A more vigorous thrust with a single outward component
Pulsation eliminated by light pressure on the vein just above the sternal end of the clavicle	Pulsation not eliminated
Level of pulsation usually descends with inspiration	Pulsation not affected by inspiration
Pulsations vary with position	Pulsations are unchanged by position

(From Bickley, L. S. [1999]. *Bates' guide to physical examination and history taking* [7th ed.]. Philadelphia: Lippincott Williams & Wilkins.)

2. Identify the highest point at which the pulsations can be seen and measure the vertical line between the point and the sternal angle.

    With the head raised to 45 degrees, the internal jugular venous pulsations should not be visible above 3 cm (1.18 inch).

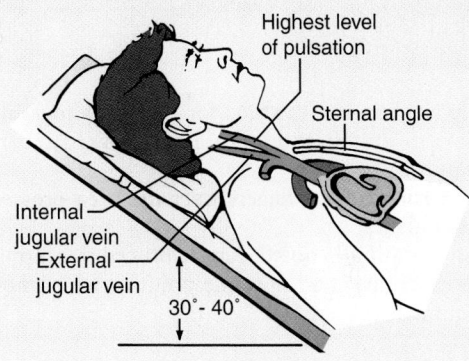

Extremities
Inspection
1. Observe skin over extremities for color, pallor, rubor, hair distribution.
2. Inspect for any superficial vessels.

1. Extremities should be symmetrically even in color, warmth, and moisture, without swelling.
    Swelling of feet may occur after prolonged standing or sitting, but will disappear readily when extremity is elevated.

Palpation
1. Note temperature of skin over extremities, comparing one side to the other.
2. Palpate pulses (radial, femoral, posterior tibial, dorsalis pedis), comparing symmetry from side to side.

2. There should be no arterial bruits.

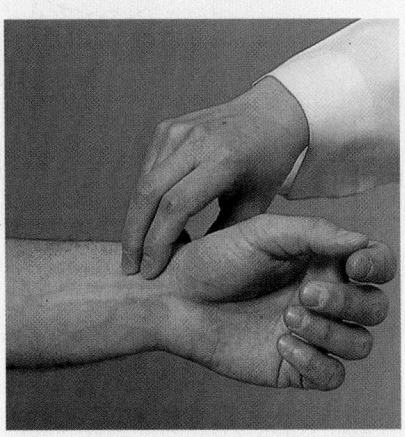
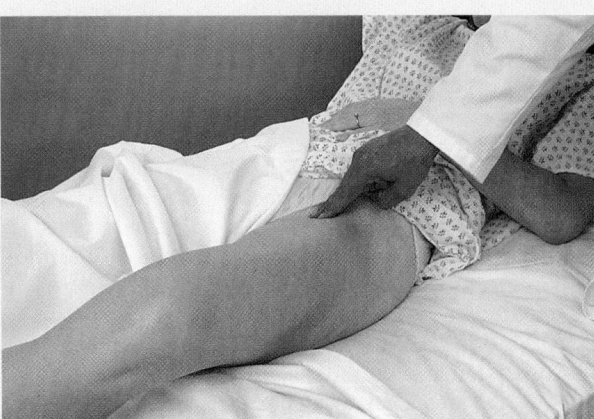

Palpating pulses.

Technique   **Findings**

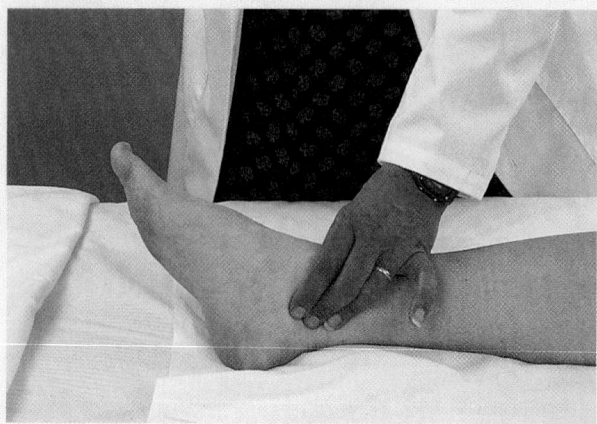 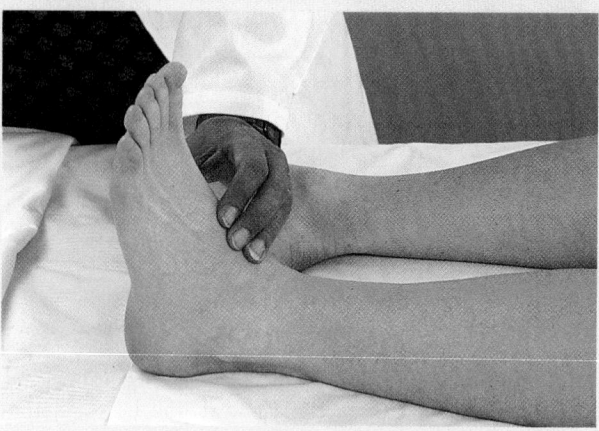

3. Palpate skin over the tibia for edema by pressing skin between thumb and index finger for 30 seconds to 1 minute.
   Then run pads of fingers over the area pressed and note indentation.
   If indentation is noted, repeat procedure, moving up the extremity, and note the point at which no more swelling is present.

3. Edema is usually graded from trace to 3+ or 4+ pitting (note scale used when recording data). Trace is a slight indentation that disappears in a short time. Grade 3+ or 4+, depending on the scale, is *deep* pitting that does not disappear readily. At best, these are subjective measurements, which are tried and confirmed through practice and comparison of findings with associates.

■ Abdomen
General Approach
1. Be sure the patient has an empty bladder.
2. The patient should be lying comfortably with arms at the side. Often, bending the knees slightly will help to relax the abdominal muscles and make palpation easier.
3. Expose the abdomen fully. Make sure your hands and the stethoscope diaphragm are warm.
4. Be methodical in visualizing the underlying organs as you inspect, auscultate, percuss, and palpate each quadrant or region of the abdomen.

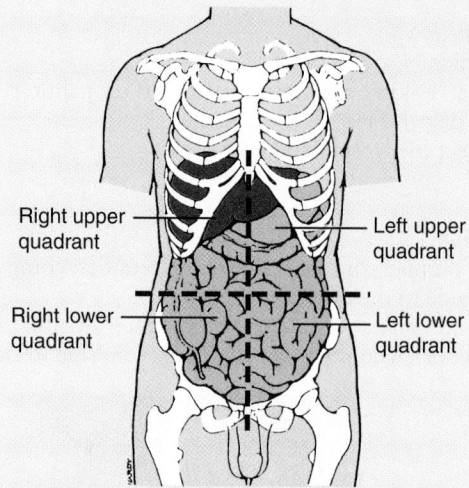

Inspection
1. Observe the general contour of the abdomen (flat, protuberant, scaphoid, or concave; local bulges). Also note symmetry, visible peristalsis, aortic pulsations.
2. Check the umbilicus for contour or hernia and the skin for rashes, striae, and scars.

1. The abdomen may or may not have any scars and should be flat or slightly rounded in the nonobese person.

Auscultation
1. This is done before percussion and palpation because palpation may alter the character of bowel sounds.
2. Note the frequency and character of bowel sounds (pitch, duration).
3. Listen over the aorta and renal arteries (either side of the umbilicus) for bruits.

2. Anywhere from 5 to 35 bowel sounds/minute. May have familiar sound of "growling."
3. There should be no bruits or rubs.

Technique	Findings

Percussion

1. Percussion provides a general orientation to the abdomen.
2. Proceed methodically from quadrant to quadrant, noting tympany and dullness.
3. In right upper quadrant (RUQ) in the midclavicular line, percuss the borders of the liver.

   a. Begin at a point of tympany in the midclavicular line of the right lower quadrant (RLQ) and percuss upward to the point of dullness (the lower liver border); mark the point.

   b. Percuss downward from the point of lung resonance above the RUQ to the point of dullness (the upper border of the liver); mark the point.

   c. Measure in centimeters the distance between the two marks in the midclavicular line (the liver span).

   d. Tympany of the gastric air bubble can be percussed in the left upper quadrant (LUQ) over the anterior lower border of the rib cage.

2. Tympany usually predominates, possibly with scattered areas of dullness due to fluid and feces.
3. Percussion of the liver should help guide subsequent palpation. The liver border in the midclavicular line should normally range from 6 to 12 cm (2.3–4.6 inches).

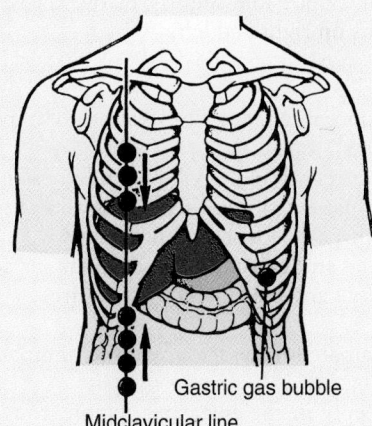

Gastric gas bubble

Midclavicular line

Palpation

1. Perform light palpation in an organized manner to detect any muscular resistance (guarding), tenderness, or superficial organs or masses.
2. Perform deep palpation to determine location, size, shape, consistency, tenderness, pulsations, and mobility of underlying organs and masses.
3. Move slowly and gently from one quadrant to the next to relax and reassure the patient.
4. Use two hands if the abdomen is obese or muscular, with one hand on top of the other. The upper hand exerts pressure downward while the lower hand feels the abdomen.

1. Tenderness and involuntary guarding indicate peritoneal inflammation.

2. Rebound tenderness (pain on quick withdrawal of the fingers following palpation) suggests peritoneal irritation, as in acute appendicitis.

Liver

1. Palpate the liver by placing the left hand under the patient's lower right rib cage and the right hand on the abdomen below the level of liver dullness. Press gently inward and upward with your fingertips while the patient takes a deep breath.

1. A normal liver edge may be palpable as a smooth, sharp, regular surface. An enlarged liver will be palpable and may be tender, hard, or irregular.

Spleen

1. Place your left hand around and under the patient's left lower rib cage and press your right hand below the left costal margin inward toward the spleen while the patient takes a deep breath.

2. Double check for an enlarged spleen by percussing in the lowest interspace in the left anterior axillary line as the patient takes a deep breath. An enlarged spleen will cause a change in percussion note from tympany to dullness.

1. A normal spleen is usually not palpable.

2. Be sure to start low enough so as not to miss the border of an enlarged spleen.

Technique	Findings

Kidney

1. Next palpate for the left and right kidneys.
2. Place the left hand under the patient's back between the rib cage and the iliac crest.
3. Support the patient while you palpate the abdomen with the right palmar surface of the fingers facing the left side of the body.
4. Palpate by bringing the left and right hands together as much as possible slightly below the level of the umbilicus on right and left.

4. The kidney is usually felt only in persons with very relaxed abdominal muscles (the very young, the aged, multiparous women). The right kidney is slightly lower than the left. The kidney is felt as a solid, firm, smooth elastic mass.

5. If the kidney is felt, describe its size and shape, and any tenderness.
6. Costal vertebral angle (CVA) tenderness is palpated with the patient sitting—usually during the examination of the posterior chest. Locate the CVA in the flank region and strike firmly with the ulnar surface of your hand. Note any tenderness over the area.

6. There should be no CVA tenderness.

Aorta

1. Next, palpate for the aorta with the thumb and index finger.
2. Press deeply in the epigastric region (roughly in the midline) and feel with the fingers for pulsations, as well as for the contour of the aorta.

1. The aorta is soft and pulsatile.

Other Findings

1. Palpation of the RLQ may reveal the part of the bowel called the cecum.
2. The sigmoid colon may be palpated in the LLQ.

1. The cecum will be soft.
2. The sigmoid colon is ropelike and vertical and, if filled with feces, may be quite firm.

3. The inguinal and femoral areas should be palpated bilaterally for lymph nodes.

3. Often small inguinal nodes are present; they are nontender, freely movable, and firm.

■ Male Genitalia and Hernias

This part of the examination, especially for hernias, is best done with the patient standing. (A *hernia* is the protrusion of a portion of the intestine through an abnormal opening.)

1. Drape the patient's chest and abdomen.
2. Expose the groin and genitalia.

Inspection

1. Inspect the pubic hair distribution and the skin of the penis.
2. Retract or have the patient retract the foreskin, if present.
3. Observe the glans penis and the urethral meatus. Note any ulcers, masses, or scars.
4. Note the location of the urethral meatus and any discharge.

2. The foreskin of the penis, if present, should be easily retractable.
3. The skin of the glans penis is smooth, without ulceration.
4. The urethral meatus normally is located ventrally on the end of the penis. Normally, there is no discharge from the urethra.

5. Observe the skin of the scrotum for ulcers, masses, redness, or swelling. Note size, contour, and symmetry. Lift the scrotum to inspect the posterior surface.

5. The scrotum descends approximately 4 cm (1.5 inches) in the adult; the left side is often larger than the right side.

Technique	Findings

6. Inspect the inguinal areas and groin for bulges (without and with the patient bearing down—as though having a bowel movement).

Palpation

Wear gloves.

1. Palpate any lesions, nodules, or masses, noting tenderness, contour, size, and induration. Palpate the shaft of the penis for any induration (firmness in relation to surrounding tissues).

2. Palpate each testis and epididymis separately between the thumb and first two fingers, noting size, shape, consistency, and undue tenderness (pressure on the testis normally produces pain).

   2. The testes are usually rubbery and of approximately equal size. The epididymis is located posterolaterally on each testis and is most easily palpable on the superior portion of the testis.

3. Also palpate the spermatic cord, including the vas deferens within the cord, from the testis to the inguinal ring. Note any nodules or tenderness.

4. Palpate for inguinal hernias, using the left hand to examine the patient's left side and the right hand to examine the patient's right side.

   4. Normally, there is no palpable herniating mass in the inguinal area.

   a. Insert the right index finger laterally, invaginating the scrotal sac to the external inguinal ring.

   b. If the external ring is large enough, insert the finger along the inguinal canal toward the internal ring and ask the patient to strain down, noting any mass that touches the finger.

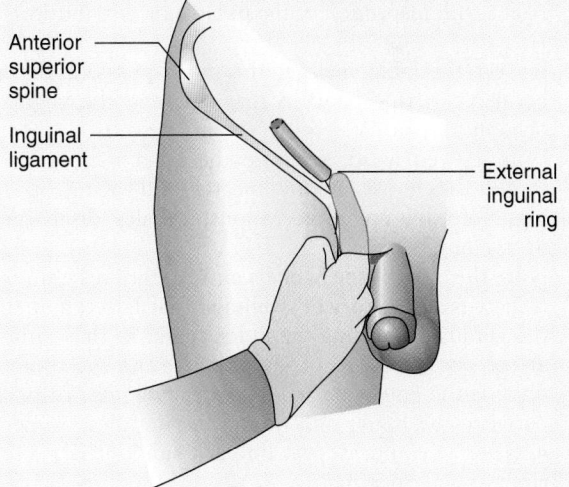

5. Also palpate the anterior thigh for a herniating mass in the femoral canal. Ask patient to strain down. (Femoral canal—not palpable, but is a potential opening in the anterior thigh, medial to the femoral artery below the inguinal ligament.)

   5. Ordinarily, there is no palpable mass in the femoral area.

■ Female Genitalia

Equipment

Disposable gloves, lubricant, speculum of appropriate size, excellent direct lighting, cervical scraper, glass slide, fluid for fixing Papanicolaou smear, cotton-tip applicator

Technique	Findings

General Approach

1. The patient's bladder should be empty.
2. The patient should lie in the lithotomy position with her buttocks extending slightly over the end of the examining table.
3. Her thighs are flexed and abducted; her feet are in the stirrups.
4. Her arms are at her side or crossed over her chest.
5. If a man is performing the examination, a female attendant must be present.
6. The examination will be most successful if the patient is relaxed. This can best be accomplished by draping the patient well so that the drape extends over the knees.
7. Explain each step of the procedure and avoid any quick, unexpected movements.
8. Be sure that your hands and the speculum are warm.

Inspection and Palpation

(These are performed almost simultaneously through the course of the examination.)

1. Begin with inspection of the pubic hair distribution.

2. Inspect the labia majora, the mons pubis, and the perineum (tissue between the anus and the vaginal opening).

3. With gloved hand, separate the labia majora and inspect the clitoris, urethral meatus, and vaginal opening. Note skin color, ulcerations, nodules, discharge, or swelling.

4. Note the area of the Skene's and Bartholin's glands. If there is any history of swelling of the latter, palpate the glands by placing the index finger in the vagina at the posterior end of the opening and the thumb outside the posterior portion of the vagina. Palpate between the finger and thumb for nodules, tenderness, or swelling. Repeat on each side of the posterior vaginal opening.

Speculum Examination

1. Have the appropriate size speculum available and lubricated with warm water. (Other lubricants may interfere with cytologic studies.)

2. Begin by inserting the first two fingers of the gloved hand into the vagina; locate the cervix, noting the angle of the fingers and the distance from the vaginal opening to the cervix.

3. Proceed by removing the two fingers to the edge of the vaginal opening. Press the two fingers downward against the perineum. Take the speculum in your other hand and, with the blades closed and held obliquely, guide the speculum past the two gloved fingers while exerting pressure downward. (This avoids putting painful pressure on the anterior urethral structures.) Avoid pinching the vagina with the speculum.

---

1. Normally, the pubic hair is distributed in an inverted triangle over the symphysis pubis.

2. In the virgin, the labia majora are full and rounded. They become thinner in older and multiparous women.

3. The labia minora and the prepuce around the clitoris are pinkish.

4. The hymen, or membranous fold that may partially occlude the vaginal opening, may or may not be present.

2. Normally, the uterus is positioned forward with the cervix at almost a right angle to the vagina.

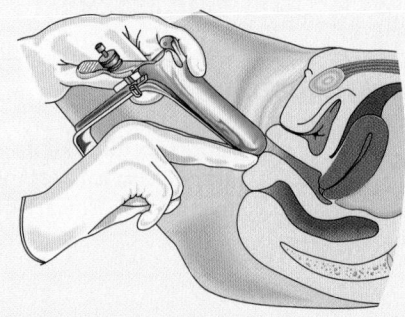

Technique   **Findings**

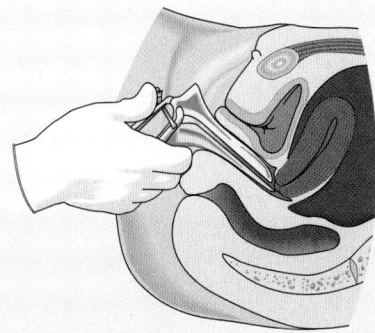
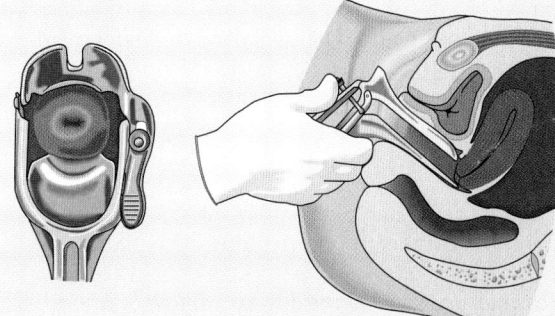

4. Once the speculum is inserted, remove the gloved fingers from the introitus (vaginal opening) and return the speculum blades to a horizontal position, maintaining pressure posteriorly.

5. Next, open the speculum blades and, with direct light, visualize the cervix. Maneuver the speculum so the cervix comes into full view. (The cervix lies within the *fornix,* or posterior portion of the vagina, dividing the fornix into the anterior, posterior, right, and left fornices.)

6. Inspect the cervix and its opening (os), noting position, color, and shape of the os, ulceration, nodules, bleeding, and discharge. (For Papanicolaou smear, see p. 747.)

6. The cervix of the nonpregnant woman is pink and smooth.

7. As you slowly pull the speculum out of the vagina, inspect the vaginal mucosa for color, inflammation, ulcers, masses, or discharge.

7. A small amount of clear lubricating mucus is normal in the vagina. Normally, there is no bleeding from the nonmenstruating female.

8. Close the blades before reaching the introitus, and remove the speculum without pinching the vaginal wall. (Also see Guidelines in Chapter 22, p. 744.)

Palpation (Bimanual Examination)

1. Lubricate the index and middle fingers of the gloved hand and insert them into the vagina, noting nodules, masses, or irregularities anteriorly and posteriorly.

2. Locate the cervix and fornices and note tenderness, shape, size, consistency, regularity, and mobility of the cervix.

2. The cervix of the nonpregnant women is smooth, firm, and slightly movable. It is nontender. The uterus is firm, smooth, and nontender.

3. Place the gloved finger in the posterior fornix and the ungloved hand on the abdomen approximately midway between the umbilicus and the symphysis pubis.

4. Press the two hands toward one another and palpate the uterus, noting its size, shape, regularity, consistency, mobility and tenderness, and any masses.

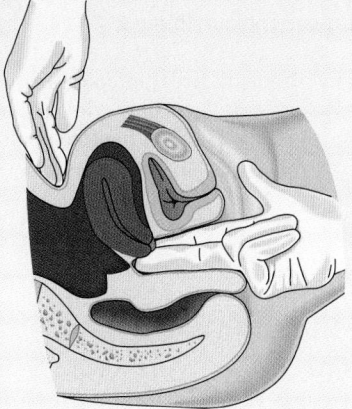

Technique	Findings
5. Next, place the gloved fingers in the right lateral fornix and the ungloved hand in the right lower quadrant. Palpate the ovaries, if possible, noting shapes, sizes, consistency, regularity, mobility, pain (the ovary is usually tender), or masses. Repeat the procedure on the left side.	5. The ovaries vary in size considerably, but average about $3.5 \times 2 \times 1.5$ cm ($1.4 \times 0.8 \times 0.6$ inches). The uterine (fallopian) tubes are generally not palpable.
6. Next, withdraw the gloved hand, leaving the index finger in the vagina and placing the middle finger in the rectum. Repeat the procedure of the bimanual examination.	6. Explain what you are doing because this is uncomfortable for the patient and may produce the sensation of wanting to defecate.
7. If possible, press the uterus downward toward the rectal finger so as much of the posterior surface of the uterus as possible can be examined.	
8. Proceed with the rectal examination (see below).	
9. On completing the examination, wipe genitalia and perineum with a tissue or offer the patient one so she may do it herself.	

▪ Rectum

Equipment
Glove, lubricant

Techniques of Examination
Male
General Approach
1. If the patient is ambulatory, have him stand and bend over the edge of the table.
2. It is also possible to examine the anus and rectum with the patient lying on his left side, knees drawn up and buttocks close to the edge of the table. (This is generally an uncomfortable position, and the patient should be told that he may feel as though he wants to move his bowels.)
3. The patient should be draped so only his buttocks are exposed.

Inspection
Spread the buttocks and inspect the anus, perianal region, and sacral region for inflammation, nodules, scars, lesions, ulcerations, or rashes. Ask the patient to bear down; note any bulges.

In males and females, the perianal and sacrococcygeal areas are dry, with varying amounts of hair covering them. In the sacrococcygeal region, it is not uncommon to find a small opening or sinus surrounded by a tuft of hair. This is a *pilonidal cyst*; it should be nontender and noninflamed.

Palpation
1. Palpate any abnormal area noted on inspection.
2. Lubricate the index finger of the gloved hand. Rest the finger over the anus as the patient bears down and, as the sphincter relaxes, insert finger slowly into the rectum.

Technique	Findings

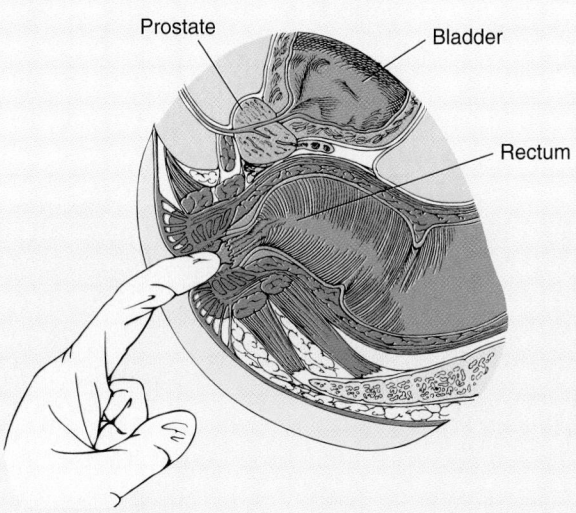

Prostate — Bladder — Rectum

3. Note sphincter tone, any nodules or masses, or tenderness.

4. Insert the finger further and palpate the walls of the rectum laterally and posteriorly while rotating your index finger. Note irregularities, masses, nodules, tenderness.

5. Anteriorly, palpate the two lateral lobes of the prostate gland and its median sulcus for irregularities, nodules, swelling, or tenderness.

6. If possible, palpate the superior portion of the lateral lobe, where the seminal vesicles are located. Note induration, swelling, or tenderness.

7. Just above the prostate anteriorly, the rectum lies adjacent to the peritoneal cavity. If possible, palpate this region for peritoneal masses and tenderness.

8. Continue to insert the finger as far as possible and have the patient bear down so more of the bowel can be palpated.

9. Gently withdraw your finger. Any fecal material on the glove should be tested for occult blood.

3. The anal canal is approximately 2.5 cm (1 inch) long; it is bordered by the external and internal anal sphincters, which are normally firm and smooth.

4. The wall of the rectum in males and females is smooth and moist.

5. The male prostate gland is approximately 2.5 cm (1 inch) long, smooth, regular, nonmovable, nontender, and rubbery.

6. The seminal vesicles are generally not palpable unless swollen.

9. There is normally no occult blood in the stools.

Female
General Approach

1. The examination is usually performed following the pelvic examination with the patient still in the lithotomy position.

2. If only the rectal examination is done, the patient may be positioned laterally, as for examination of the male. The lateral position permits better visualization of the sacral region.

3. The technique is basically the same for the female as for the male.

4. Anteriorly, the cervix, and perhaps a retroverted uterus, may be felt.

4. Anteriorly, the cervix is round and smooth.

Technique   Findings

Musculoskeletal System

General Approach

1. Examine the muscles and joints, keeping in mind the structure and functions of each.
2. This discussion will center on the technique for examining the patient who is asymptomatic and, therefore, will not present in detail the techniques for inspecting and palpating joints that are symptomatic or deformed.
3. It is important to ask in the history and to note in the examination whether the patient has difficulty performing activities of daily living:
   a. Bathing
   b. Dressing (buttoning, using zippers, tying shoelaces)
   c. Combing hair
   d. Brushing teeth
   e. Walking up and down stairs
   f. Bending
   g. Sitting
   h. Grasping and holding items without dropping them
   i. Standing from a sitting position, unaided
4. Once the above facts have been ascertained, the examination proceeds. Observe and palpate joints and muscles for symmetry and then examine each joint individually as indicated.
5. The examination is performed with the joints both at rest and in motion—moving through a full range of motion; joints and supporting muscles and tissues are noted.

Inspection

1. Inspect the upper and lower extremities for size, symmetry, and deformity, and muscle mass.

For the purpose of this text, it is sufficient to say that in the course of the history and examination, the examiner should not find any compromise or restriction of the patient's activities of daily living or any other normal activities. If any activity is restricted because of muscular or skeletal problems, the reader is referred to a more detailed text on physical examination.

2. Inspect the joints for range of motion (in degrees), enlargement, redness.
3. Note gait and posture; observe the spine for range of motion, lateral curvature, or any abnormal curvature.
4. Observe the patient for signs of pain during the examination.

Palpation

1. Palpate the joints of the upper and lower extremities and the neck for tenderness, swelling, temperature, and range of motion.
2. Hold the palm of the hand over the joint as it moves, or move the joint through the fullest range of motion and note any crepitation (crackling feeling within the joint).
3. Palpate the muscles for size, tone, strength, and tenderness.

Technique   **Findings**

4. Palpate the spine for bony deformities and crepitation. Gently tap the spine with the ulnar surface of your fist from the cervical to the lumbar region and note any pain or tenderness.

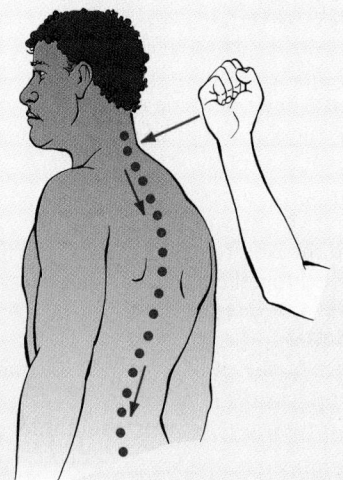

Neurologic System

Equipment
Safety pin, cotton, tuning fork, reflex hammer, flashlight, tongue blade, ophthalmoscope, vision screener, cloves, coffee, or other scented items

General Information
1. The examination described in this section is a screening neurologic examination.
   a. It is performed on individuals without specific neurologic complaints.
   b. A more detailed examination is used for patients with specific signs and symptoms.
   c. The student is referred to another text for the content and technique of a detailed neurologic examination.
2. The examination is performed with the patient in either the sitting or supine position.
3. Much of the neurologic examination can be performed as different regions of the body are being examined. This facilitates the flow of the entire examination.

   Example: The cranial nerves can be examined at the same time as the head and neck.

   A mental status evaluation can be done while the history is elicited and while the entire physical examination is performed.

Components of the Neurologic Examination
There are six components of the neurologic examination:
1. Mental status (cerebral function)
2. Cranial nerve function
3. Cerebellar function
4. Motor function
5. Sensory function
6. Deep tendon reflexes (DTRs)

The screening neurologic examination involves testing all of these components at least superficially. Learning these components in order will help in organizing the examination and in avoiding the omission of any part.

Technique	Findings

Basic Principles

1. Symmetry of function and findings on both sides of the body is important to note.

   Always compare one side of the body with the other side (eg, compare degree of motor strength of the right biceps with that of the left biceps).

2. Integrating the neurologic examination into the examination of the various body regions is advisable, although the results of the neurologic findings should be recorded together as an entity.

Carrying Out the Examination

Mental Status

Components of the mental status examination include the following:

- State of consciousness (alert, somnolent, stuporous, comatose)
- Memory (short-term, long-term, intermediate)
- Cognition (calculations, current events)
- Affect (mood)
- Ideational content (hallucinations)

In a screening examination, mental status is evaluated by observing the patient's affect during the history and the content of what he or she says.

1. While recording the history, ask the patient for identifying information (how to spell his name, where he lives), and ask what the date is. This tests orientation.

   1. Normally the individual is alert, knows who he is and where he lives, and can tell you the date.

2. The patient's ability to remember is also evaluated as the history is taken—by asking for his past medical history (long-term memory) and dietary habits: "What did you eat for breakfast?" (intermediate memory).

   2. The patient remembers recent and past events consistently, and willingly admits forgetting something. Elderly people often have much better long-term memory than recent memory.

3. Cognition and ideational content are evaluated throughout the history by what the patient says and by his articulateness, consistency, and reliability in reporting events.

4. Affect or mood is evaluated by observing the patient's verbal and nonverbal behavior in response to questions asked, to sudden noises, to interruptions—for example, does the patient laugh or smile when talking about normally sad events; is he easily startled by unexpected noises?

   4. Mood should be appropriate to the content of the conversation.

Cranial Nerve Function

First (Olfactory) Nerve

Is not usually tested unless the patient complains of a disturbance in sense of smell.

1. The airway must be patent.

2. Occlude one nostril; ask the patient to close his eyes and then present various substances to smell (eg, coffee, tobacco). Occlude the other nostril and repeat.

3. Use substances that do not have a lingering effect.

Second (Optic) Nerve

Includes tests of visual acuity and of gross visual fields and examination of the optic disc with a funduscope.

Technique	Findings

Visual Acuity

Is tested with the use of a Snellen chart (patient uses glasses if required).

1. Have the patient cover one eye at a time and read the smallest print possible on the chart from a distance of 6 m (20 feet).

1. Normal vision and corrected vision should be 20/20.

Visual Fields

1. Measure by having patient cover his right eye with his right hand. (You cover your left eye with your left hand.)

2. Stand approximately 60 cm (2 feet) from the patient and have him fix his gaze on your nose.

3. Bring two wagging fingers in from the periphery (in a plane equidistant from the patient and you) in all quadrants of the visual field and ask the patient to tell you when he sees your wagging fingers.

3. Assuming your visual fields are grossly normal, the patient and you should see the wagging fingers approximately simultaneously. (The patient's peripheral vision should approximate the examiner's, assuming that it is normal.)

Optic Disc

Is visualized as part of the funduscopic examination (see p. 56).

Third (Oculomotor), Fourth (Trochlear), and Sixth (Abducens) Nerves

Are tested together. These nerves control the movements of the extraocular muscles of the eye—the superior and inferior oblique and the medial and lateral rectus muscles. The oculomotor nerve also controls pupillary constriction.

1. Hold your index finger approximately 30 cm (1 foot) from the patient's nose. Ask the patient to hold his head steady.

2. Ask the patient to follow your finger with his eyes.

3. Move your finger to the right as far as the patient's eye moves. Before bringing your finger back to the center, move it up and then down, so that the patient glances up and peripherally and then down and peripherally.

4. Repeat the test, moving your finger to the left.

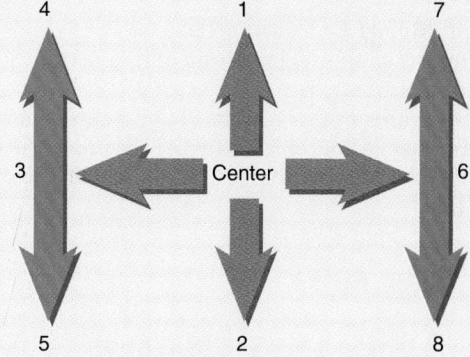

Fifth (Trigeminal) Nerve

Has motor component that controls muscles of mastication and a sensory component that controls sensations of the face.

Motor

1. Have the patient bite down on a tongue depressor with one side of his mouth while you try to pull the blade out.

2. Repeat the test on the other side of the mouth and compare muscle strength of the two sides.

1. Muscle strength in the face should be present and should be symmetric.

Sensory

Sensation to light touch.

1. Have the patient close his eyes.

1. Sensation should be present and symmetric. Always demonstrate to the patient how and with what you are testing sensation—to avoid startling the patient and to encourage cooperation.

2. Touch first one side of the patient's face and then the other (forehead, cheek, and chin), asking the patient if the sensation is present and feels the same on both sides.

3. Sensation to pain (pinprick) is tested similarly.

Technique	Findings

Seventh (Facial) Nerve

Motor function is tested by observing facial expression and symmetry of facial movement.

Ask the patient to frown, close his eyes, and smile.

The facial muscles should look symmetric when the patient frowns, closes his eyes, and smiles. Notice particularly the symmetry of the nasolabial folds.

Eighth (Acoustic) Nerve

Has two branches.

Cochlear (mediates hearing). (See ear examination, page 57.)

Vestibular (helps control equilibrium).

Romberg test: Have the patient stand erect with his eyes closed and feet close together.

Slight swaying may occur, but the patient should not fall. (Stand close to the patient so you can assist if he begins to fall.)

Ninth (Glossopharyngeal) and Tenth (Vagus) Nerves

Are tested together because both have a motor portion innervating the pharynx.

1. *Ninth:* Test the presence of the gag reflex.

2. *Tenth:* Ask the patient to say "ah" and observe the movement of the uvula and palate for deviation and asymmetry.

1. The gag reflex should be present, and there should be no difficulty in swallowing.
2. The palate and uvula should move symmetrically without deviation.

Eleventh (Spinal Accessory) Nerve

Mediates the sternocleidomastoid and upper portion of the trapezius muscles.

1. Ask the patient to turn his head to the side against resistance while your fingers apply pressure to the jaw.
2. Palpate the sternocleidomastoid muscle on the opposite side.

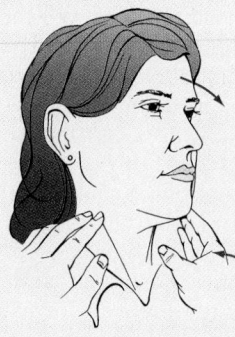

3. Then have the patient shrug his shoulders while you place your hands on his shoulders and apply slight pressure.

3. Neck and shoulder muscle strength should be symmetric.

Twelfth (Hypoglossal) Nerve

Innervates muscles of the tongue.

Test by noting articulation and by having the patient stick out his tongue, noting any deviation or asymmetry.

The tongue should be symmetric and should not deviate.

Cerebellar Function

Purpose: to screen for coordination.
1. Observe posture and gait.
2. Ask the patient to walk forward (and then backward) in a straight line.

3. To test for muscle coordination in the lower extremities, have the patient run his right heel down his left shin and vice versa.

2. The patient should be able to perform all the tests described with smooth, even movement and without losing balance.

Technique	Findings

4. To test coordination in upper extremities, have the patient close his eyes and touch his nose with his index finger (starting position: arms outstretched) first left, then right, in rapid succession.

4. The normal person can do this with rapid, smooth movements without undershooting or overshooting the target.

Motor Function

Tested in conjunction with the skeletal system because any bony deformity will affect motor function.

Evaluate muscle mass, tone, strength, and any abnormal movements (tics, fasciculations, twitching).

Muscle mass: Note symmetry between sides of the body and distribution distally and proximally.

Tone: Test by noting the resistance the muscle offers to movement on passive motion.

Muscle mass: Is usually considered in relation to sex and body build and to use of various muscle groups.

Tone: Generally there is slight resistance to passive movement of muscles as opposed to flaccidity (no resistance) or rigidity (increased muscle tone).

Strength: Will vary from person to person.

Strength

Lower extremity—have the patient do deep knee bends; walk on his toes and then his heels; hop on one foot and then the other.

Upper extremity—have the patient squeeze your fingers with both hands; compare sides of the body.

Also, apply resistance to the patient's outstretched arms and when the patient flexes the wrist and elbow; compare sides.

Unusual muscle movements: If present, are noted both when muscle is at rest and when it is moving.

Normally, tremors, tics, or fasciculations are not present either at rest or with movement.

Sensory Function

Should test sensitivity to light touch [cotton], pain [pinprick], vibration [tuning fork], and position. Compare both sides of body.

Light touch: Ask the patient to close his eyes. Brush his skin with a piece of cotton (on back of hands, forearms, upper arms, dorsal portion of foot laterally and medially; and along the tibia and thigh laterally and medially). Ask the patient to indicate when he feels the cotton and to compare the sensation bilaterally.

Pain: Use a safety pin; touch the skin as lightly as possible to elicit a sharp sensation.

Vibration sense: Test by placing a vibrating tuning fork on a bony prominence (wrist, medial and lateral malleoli). Ask the patient to tell you when he no longer feels vibration. Stop the vibration with your hand.

The patient should normally feel no vibration within a very short time.

Position Sense

1. Have the patient close his eyes.
2. Move the patient's digit (finger, great toe) up or down and ask the patient to say in what direction his finger or toe is pointing.
3. Place your thumb and index finger on either side of the digit being moved so the patient will not sense any pressure from your finger in the direction in which you are moving the digit.

2. Normally the patient can tell you without hesitation in what direction his digit is pointing.

Technique	Findings

Deep Tendon Reflexes

1. Have the patient relax; provide support for the extremity being tested.
2. Compare reflex amplitude of the same tendons on either side of the body.

2. Amplitude of the reflex may vary for different tendons.

Upper Extremities

Biceps

1. Place your right thumb on the patient's right biceps tendon (located in the antecubital fossa).
2. Rest the patient's forearm on your left hand and strike your thumb with the pointed end of the hammer head. Hold the hammer loosely so it pivots in your hand when it is moved with a wrist action.

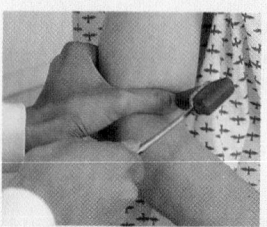

3. Strike your thumb with the least amount of pressure needed to elicit the reflex.

3. The forearm may move, and your thumb should feel the tendon jerk.

Triceps Tendon

1. Have the patient hang his arm freely, while you support it with your non-dominant hand
2. With the elbow flexed, strike the tendon directly, using the pointed end of the hammer.

2. The forearm should move slightly.

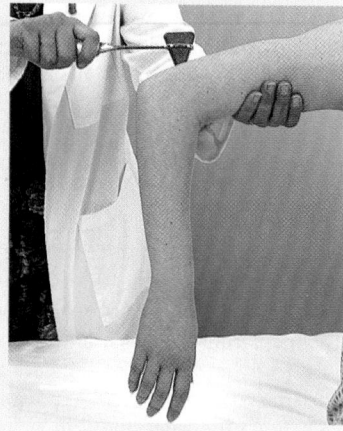

NURSING ALERT

If the reflexes are diminished symmetrically, have the patient grasp hands and contract arm muscles to check the lower extremities, and top feet to check the upper extremities.

Brachioradialis Tendon

1. Strike the forearm with the hammer about 2.5 cm (1 inch) above the wrist over the radius.
2. Be sure the forearm is supported and relaxed.

1. The thumb may be observed moving downward.

Technique	Findings

Lower Extremities

Quadriceps Reflex

1. Have the patient sitting with his legs hanging over the edge of the table or lying down while you support the legs at the knee (slightly bent).
2. Strike the tendon just below the patella.
3. If reflexes are difficult to elicit, have the patient interlace the fingers of both hands and then have patient try to pull his hands apart. While he is thus distracted, inhibition of the quadriceps reflex is diminished, and the reflex can be elicited more easily. If such a distraction is used to elicit the reflex, record this fact with the physical findings.

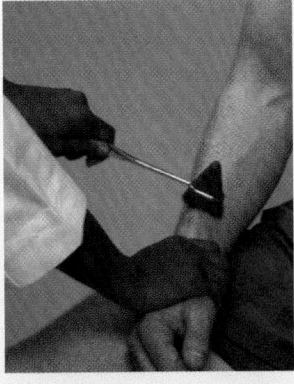

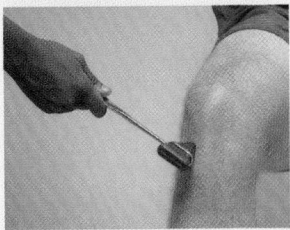

Achilles Reflex

1. Support the foot in dorsiflexed position.
2. Tap the Achilles tendon with the hammer head.

2. The foot should move downward into your hand.

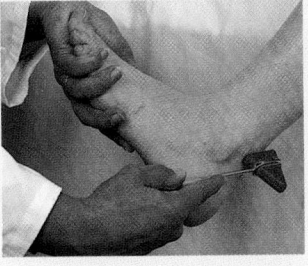

SELECTED REFERENCES

Bickley, L. S. (1999). *Bates' guide to physical examination and history taking* (7th ed.). Philadelphia: Lippincott Williams & Wilkins.

Fuller, J., & Schaller-Ayers, J. (1999). *Health assessment: A nursing approach* (3rd ed.). Philadelphia: Lippincott Williams & Wilkins.

Gallo, J. J., Fulmer, T., Paveza, G. J., & Reichel, W. (2000). *Geriatric assessment* (3rd ed.). Gaithersburg, MD: Aspen.

Gates, S. J., & Mooar, P. A. (1999). *Musculoskeletal primary care.* Philadelphia: Lippincott Williams & Wilkins.

Klingman, L. (1999). Assessing the female reproductive system. *American Journal of Nursing, 98*(8), 37–43.

———. (1999). Assessing the male genitalia. *American Journal of Nursing, 99*(7), 47–50.

O'Hanlon-Nichols, T. (1999). Neurologic assessment. *American Journal of Nursing, 99*(6), 44–50.

Orient, J. M. (2000). *Sapira's art and science of bedside diagnosis* (2nd ed.). Philadelphia: Lippincott Williams & Wilkins.

Warner, P. H., Rowe, T., & Whipple, B. (1999). Shedding light on the sexual history. *American Journal of Nursing, 99*(6), 34–40.

IV Therapy

GENERAL CONSIDERATIONS

Goals

The goals of intravenous (IV) therapy include:
1. Maintain or replace body stores of water, electrolytes, vitamins, proteins, fats, and calories in the patient who cannot maintain an adequate intake by mouth.
2. Restore acid–base balance.
3. Restore volume of blood components.
4. Administer safe and effective infusions of medications by using the appropriate vascular access.
5. Monitor central venous pressure (CVP).
6. Provide nutrition while resting the gastrointestinal tract.

Physiologic Assimilation of Infusion Solutions

Principles
1. Tissue cells (eg, epithelial cells, neurons) are surrounded by a semipermeable membrane.
2. Osmotic pressure is the "pulling" pressure demonstrated when water moves through the semipermeable membrane of tissue cells from an area of weaker concentration to stronger concentration of solute (eg, sodium ions, blood glucose). The end result is dilution and equilibration between the intracellular and extracellular compartments.
3. Extracellular compartment fluids primarily include plasma and interstitial fluid.

Types of Fluids
Isotonic
A solution that exerts the same osmotic pressure as that found in plasma.
1. Normal saline 0.9%
2. Lactated Ringer's
3. Blood components

a. Albumin 5%
b. Plasma
4. 5% dextrose in water (D5W)

Hypotonic
A solution that exerts less osmotic pressure than that of blood plasma. Administration of this fluid generally causes dilution of plasma solute concentration and forces water movement into cells to reestablish intracellular and extracellular equilibrium; cells will then expand or swell.
1. Half-strength normal saline, 0.45%
2. One-third sodium chloride, 0.3%

Hypertonic
A solution that exerts a higher osmotic pressure than that of blood plasma. Administration of this fluid increases the solute concentration of plasma, drawing water out of the cells and into the extracellular compartment to restore osmotic equilibrium; cells will then shrink.
1. Dextrose 5% in normal saline 0.9%
2. Dextrose 5% in half-strength normal saline (only slightly hypertonic because dextrose is rapidly metabolized and renders only temporary osmotic pressure)
3. Dextrose 10% in water
4. Dextrose 20% in water
5. Saline, 3% and 5%
6. Hyperalimentation solutions
7. Dextrose 5% in lactated Ringer's
8. Albumin 25%

Composition of Fluids
See Table 6-1.
1. Saline solutions—water and electrolytes (Na^+, Cl^-)
2. Dextrose solutions—water or saline and calories
3. Lactated Ringer's—water and electrolytes (Na^+, K^+, Cl^-, Ca^{++}, lactate)
4. Balanced isotonic—varies; water, some calories, electrolytes (Na^+, K^+, Mg^{++}, Cl^-, HCO^{-3}, gluconate)

TABLE 6-1 Composition of Selected IV Solutions

Solution	Tonicity	Na+	K+	Cl− (mEq/L)	Ca++	pH	mOsm/L	Calories
5% DW	Isotonic	—	—	—	—	5.0	253	170
10% DW	Hypertonic	—	—	—	—	4.6	561	340
0.9% NS	Isotonic	154	—	154	—	5.7	308	—
0.45% NS	Hypotonic	77	—	77	—	5.3	154	—
5% D and 0.9% NS*	Slightly hypertonic	154	—	154	—	4.2	561	170
5% and 0.45% NS	Slightly hypertonic	77	—	77	—	4.2	407	170
5% and 0.2% NS	Hypotonic	34	—	34	—	4.2	290	170
Lactated Ringer's†	Isotonic	148	4	156	4.5	6.7	309	9
5% D and lactated Ringer's	Slightly hypertonic	130	4	109	3.0	5.1	527	170
Normosol-R	Isotonic	140	5	96	—	6.4	295	—
Sodium lactate 1/6 molar	Slightly hypertonic	167	—	—	—	6.9	333	55
6% Dextran 75 and 0.9% NS	Isotonic	154	—	154	—	4.3	309	—

DW, dextrose in water; NS, normal saline

*5% Dextrose metabolizes rapidly in the blood and, in reality, produces minimal osmotic effects.

†Lactate converts to bicarbonate in the liver.

5. Whole blood and blood components
6. Plasma expanders—albumin, mannitol, dextran, plasma protein fraction 5% (Plasmanate), hetastarch (Hespan); exert increased oncotic pressure, pulling fluid from interstitium into the circulation and temporarily increasing blood volume
7. Parenteral hyperalimentation—fluid, electrolytes, amino acids, and calories

Uses and Precautions With Common Types of Infusions

See Table 6-2 for signs and symptoms of water excess or deficit, and Table 6-3 for signs and symptoms of isotonic fluid excess or deficit.

1. D5W
   a. Used to replace water (hypotonic fluid) losses, supply some caloric intake, or administer as carrying solution for numerous medications.
   b. Cautious use in patients with water intoxication (hyponatremia, syndrome of inappropriate antidiuretic hormone release). Should not be used as concurrent solution infusion with blood or blood components.

TABLE 6-2 Signs and Symptoms of Water Excess or Deficit

Site	Hyponatremia (Water Intoxication)	Hypernatremia (Water Deficit)
CNS	Muscle twitching Hyperactive tendon reflexes Convulsions Increased intracranial pressure, coma	Restlessness Weakness Delirium Coma
CV	Increased BP and pulse, if severe	Tachycardia Hypotension (if severe)
Tissues	Increased salivation, tears Watery diarrhea Fingerprinting of skin	Decreased saliva and tears Dry, sticky mucous membranes Red, swollen tongue Flushed skin
Renal	Oliguria	Oliguria
Other	None	Fever

TABLE 6-3 Signs and Symptoms of Isotonic Fluid Excess Deficit

Site	Deficit	Excess
CNS	Fatigue, apathy Anorexia Stupor, coma	Confusion (if severe)
CV	Orthostatic hypotension Flat neck veins Fast, thready pulse Hypotension Cool, clammy skin	Elevated venous pressure Distended neck veins Increased cardiac output Heart gallops Pulmonary edema
GI	Anorexia Thirst Silent ileus	Anorexia, nausea and vomiting Edema of stomach, colon, and mesentery
Tissues	Soft, small tongue with longitudinal wrinkling Sunken eyes Decreased skin turgor	Pitting edema Moist pulmonary crackles
Metabolism	Mild decrease in temperature	None

2. Normal saline
   a. Used to replace saline (isotonic fluid) losses, administer with blood components, or treat patients in hemodynamic shock.
   b. Cautious use in patients with isotonic volume excess (eg, heart failure, renal failure).
3. Lactated Ringer's
   a. Used to replace isotonic fluid losses, replenish specific electrolyte losses, and moderate metabolic acidosis

TYPES OF IV ADMINISTRATION

■ IV "Push"

Intravenous "push" (or "IV bolus") refers to the administration of a medication from a syringe directly into an ongoing IV infusion. It may also be given directly into a vein by way of saline or heparin lock.

Indications

1. For emergency administration of cardiopulmonary resuscitative procedures, allowing rapid concentration of a medication in the patient's bloodstream
2. When quicker response to the medication is required (eg, furosemide [Lasix], digoxin [Lanoxin])
3. To administer "loading" doses of a drug that will be continued by way of infusion (eg, heparin [Heparin])
4. To reduce patient discomfort by limiting need for intramuscular injections
5. To avoid incompatibility problems that may occur when several medications are mixed in one bottle
6. To deliver drugs to patients unable to take them orally (eg, coma) or intramuscularly (eg, coagulation disorder)
7. Cost-effective method—no need for extra tubing or syringe pump

Precautions and Recommendations

1. Before administration of the medication:
   a. Determine that the medication matches the order.
   b. Dilute the drug as indicated by pharmacy references. Many medications are irritating to veins and require sufficient dilution.
   c. Determine the correct (safest) rate of administration. Consult pharmacy or pharmaceutical text. Most medications are given slowly (rarely over less than 1 minute); sometimes as long as 30 minutes is required. Too rapid administration may result in serious side effects.
   d. If IV push is to be given with an ongoing IV infusion or to follow another IV push medication, check pharmacy for possible incompatibility. It is always wise to flush the IV tubing or cannula with saline before and after administration of a drug.
   e. Assess patient's condition and ability to tolerate the drug.
   f. Assess patency of IV line by presence of blood return.
      (i) Lower running IV bottle.
      (ii) Withdraw with syringe before injecting medication.

(iii) Pinch IV tubing gently.
   g. Ascertain dwell time of catheter. For infusion of vesicants (some chemotherapy agents), a catheter placement of 24 hours or less is advisable.
2. Watch patient's reaction to the drug.
   a. Be alert for major side effects, such as anaphylaxis, respiratory distress, tachycardia, bradycardia, or seizures. Notify the health care provider and institute emergency procedures as necessary.
   b. Assess for minor side effects such as nausea, flushing, skin rash, or confusion. Stop medication and consult health care provider.
3. Vesicants are always given through the side port of a running IV infusion.
4. Be familiar with hospital policies and guidelines regarding how, where, and by whom IV push medications can be given.

NURSING ALERT

Unusual dosages or unfamiliar drugs should always be confirmed with the health care provider and pharmacist before administration. The nurse is ultimately accountable for the drug that he or she administers.

■ Continuous or Intermittent Infusion Using Infusion Control Devices

Continuous or intermittent IV infusions may be given through traditionally hung bags of solution and tubing, with or without flow rate regulators. IV, intra-arterial, and intrathecal (spinal) infusion may be accomplished through the use of special external or implantable pumps. See Procedure Guidelines 6-1.

General Considerations

1. Advantages
   a. Ability to infuse large and small volumes of fluid with accuracy.
   b. An alarm warns of problem, such as air in line, high pressure required to infuse, or, ultimately, occlusion.
   c. Reduces nursing time in constantly readjusting flow rates.
2. Disadvantages
   a. Requires special tubing.
   b. There may be added cost to therapy.
   c. Infusion pumps will continue to infuse despite presence of infiltration.
3. Nursing responsibilities
   a. Remember that a mechanical infusion regulator is only as effective as the nurse operating it.
   b. Continue to check the patient regularly for complications, such as infiltration or infection.
   c. Follow the manufacturer's instruction carefully when inserting the tubing.
   d. Double-check the flow rate.
   e. Be sure to flush all air out of the tubing before connecting it to the patient's IV catheter.

f. Explain purpose of the device and the alarm system. Added machines in the room can evoke greater anxiety in the patient and family.

Types

1. Electronic flow rate regulators
   a. These devices deliver a prescribed fluid volume/hour.
   b. Often, pressure gradients may be adjusted so that high pressures are not used to deliver peripheral therapies.
   c. Use of an electronic flow-rate regulator is indicated for continuous infusions of:
      (i) Chemotherapy
      (ii) Infant and pediatric therapies
      (iii) Hyperalimentation
      (iv) Fluid and electrolytes on patients at risk for fluid overload
      (v) Most medications

2. Battery-powered ambulatory infusion pumps
   a. Example: CADD PLUS™ pump (Pharmacia Deltec, Inc.)
   b. These pumps deliver continuous or intermittent medications by way of IV, subcutaneous, or spinal routes.
   c. If used for pain control, patient may deliver a "bolus" injection if relief is not obtained from continuous, prescribed dose.
3. Freon-controlled spring pump (implanted)
   a. Example: Infusaid™ (Neuromed)
   b. This pump is placed subcutaneously, usually in the left lower quadrant of the abdomen.
   c. It will deliver continuous pain medication or chemotherapy by way of an artery, vein, or the spinal canal.
4. Computer-programmable pump (implanted)
   a. Example: synchromed pump™ (medtronics)
   b. Same actions as above

(text continues on page 94)

PROCEDURE GUIDELINES 6-1 **VENIPUNCTURE USING NEEDLE OR CATHETER**

EQUIPMENT

Rubber tourniquet
Disposable gloves
Antiseptic swab (alcohol, iodine, povidone-iodine)
If continuous infusion:
  IV solution
  IV Tubing
If saline heparin lock:
  Extension set or PRN adapter
  Heparin or normal saline solution (1–2 mL) in sterile syringe

Tape
Transparent IV dressing or other dressing supplies
Covered armboard (if necessary)
Desired cannula:
  Catheter (Teflon, Silastic polyurethane, or polyvinylchloride) in chosen bore size (gauges 14–25)
  Winged ("butterfly") needle

Note: Thorough handwashing is required before handling sterile supplies and initiating venipuncture.

PROCEDURE

Nursing Action	Rationale
PREPARATORY PHASE	
1. Explain procedure to patient. Have patient lie in bed. Ascertain whether patient is left- or right-handed.	1. Helps alleviate anxiety about the procedure. Determining "handedness" of patient suggests the infusion be started in opposite arm if possible.
2. Clear all IV tubing of air; winged needle tubing as well (may clear air with fluid from infusion tubing by attaching needle to it, or by irrigation needle with saline in sterile syringe).	2. To prevent infusion of air and potential air embolus.
3. Don gloves.	3. Complies with CDC requirements to minimize passing of blood-borne pathogens between the patient and nurse.
4. Select site for insertion (see discussion on site selection, p. 99).	
5. Apply tourniquet 5–10 cm (2–6 inches) above desired insertion site and ascertain satisfactory distention of the vein. Distal pulses should remain palpable.	5. The vein must be visible or palpable before venipuncture is attempted. The tourniquet should not be applied too tightly as to interfere with arterial blood flow.
6. Have patient open and close fist several times.	6. To increase blood supply in the area. Further techniques to aid in vein distention are discussed on p. 93. A tourniquet may not be necessary on greatly distended veins.
7. Remove tourniquet.	7. To prevent trauma to the arm from extended application of tourniquet. Can reapply later.
8. Cleanse the site: a. Clip hair if site is too obscured. b. Cleanse the skin with an alcohol swab.	8. To reduce number of skin microorganisms and minimize risk of infection.

PROCEDURE GUIDELINES 6-1 *CONTINUED*

Nursing Action	Rationale
c. Prepare skin with povidone-iodine (an iodophor) swab for 1 min, working from the center of proposed site to the periphery until a circle of 5–10 cm (2–4 inches) has been disinfected.	c. If a 1%–2% iodine solution is used, it should be used to prep the skin first (30–60 s), allowed to dry.
d. Allow area to air dry.	
9. Reapply tourniquet.	9. To facilitate catheter insertion.

PERFORMANCE PHASE: CATHETER INSERTION

Nursing Action	Rationale
1. Remove needle guard.	
2. Grasp patient's arm so the nurse's thumb is positioned approximately 5 cm (2 inches) from the site. Exert traction on skin in direction of hand.	2. To stabilize the vein and facilitate successful cannulation.
3. Insert the needle, bevel up, through the skin at an angle. Use a slow, continuous motion.	3. Bevel up position allows for the smallest and sharpest point of the needle to enter the vein first.
4. If the vessel rolls, it may be necessary to penetrate the skin first at a 20-degree angle and then apply a second thrust parallel to the skin.	4. Satisfactory penetration is evidenced by a sudden decrease in resistance and by appearance of blood coming back into catheter.
5. When the vein is entered, lower the catheter to skin level.	5. This will prevent puncturing through the vessel wall.
6. When inserting, always hold the catheter by the clear plastic flashback chamber and not by the colored hub.	
7. Advance the catheter approximately 0.6–1.3 cm. (¼–½ inch) into the vein.	7. To ensure entry into the vein.
8. Pull back on needle to separate needle from catheter 0.6 cm. (about ¼ inch) and advance catheter into vein.	8. Pulling back on needle prevents inadvertent puncture of vein and provides stability of catheter for insertion.
9. If resistance is met while attempting to thread catheter, stop, release tourniquet, and carefully remove both needle and catheter. Attempt another venipuncture with a *new* catheter.	9. The catheter may have become dislodged or encountered a turn or valve in the vein. It is better to start again than to cause further damage to vessel.

> ### NURSING ALERT
> **Never reinsert stylet back into catheter once it has been removed. You may puncture or sever catheter.**

Nursing Action	Rationale
a. Alternately, if catheter does not freely advance, attach IV tubing or heparin lock and flush, attempting to float catheter into vein.	a. Flow of flush solution may advance catheter.
10. Apply pressure on vein beyond catheter tip with the small or ring finger (see accompanying figure); release tourniquet and slowly remove needle while holding catheter hub in place.	10. This will reduce blood leakage while removing needle and connecting tubing to infusion set.

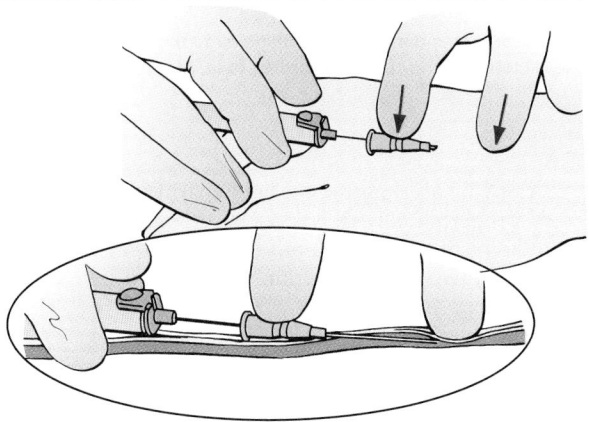

Finger palpation of dorsal venous arch.

continued

| PROCEDURE GUIDELINES 6-1 | VENIPUNCTURE USING NEEDLE OR CATHETER *CONTINUED* |

Nursing Action

Rationale

11. *If an IV,* attach the cleared administration set to the hub of the catheter and adjust the infusion flow at the prescribed rate.
12. *If a saline/heparin lock,* attach lock cap and extension set, taking care to maintain sterility of the set. Flush with 0.5 mL heparin or normal saline solution.
13. Apply transparent dressing to site or use dressing according to institutional protocol (see accompanying figure).
14. Loop tubing and tape to dressing or arm.

13. Transparent dressing secures IV catheter in place and prevents infection.
14. Prevents tension on IV catheter itself.

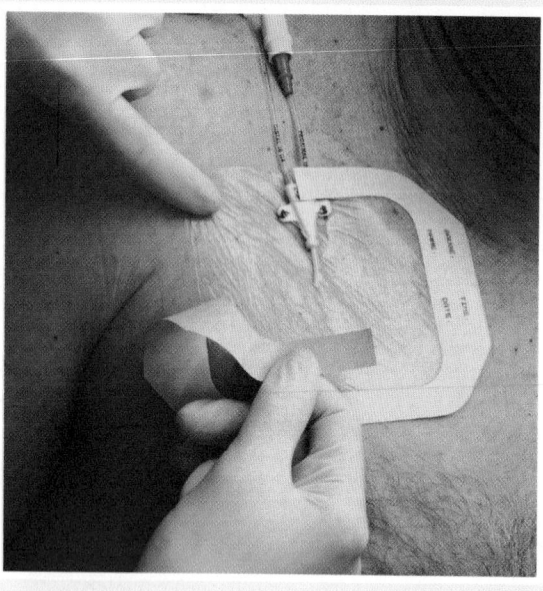

Transparent IV dressing. (Courtesy of 3M Health Care.)

15. Label strip of tape with an arrow indicating the path of the catheter, size of catheter, date, time of insertion and inserter's initials. Affix to dressing. Prepare similar label with each dressing change.

15. Labeling of dressing is dictated by hospital policy. Such a practice provides information useful in determining next dressing change and capability of needle to accommodate various types of infusion.

 NURSING ALERT

Standard dwell time for short peripheral catheter is 3 days. However, exceptions may be made due to patient's venous access, type of solution, and catheter material. If the catheter is not rotated according to institution policy, document reason.

Intermittent Infusions

Intermittent IV infusions may be given through a saline/heparin lock, "piggyback" to a continuous IV infusion, or for long-term therapy through a venous access device. See Procedure Guidelines 6-2, 6-3, and 6-4.

Saline/Heparin Lock

1. This intermittent infusion reservoir permits administration of periodic IV medications and solution without continuous fluid administration.

2. Many institutions do not use heparin solutions to keep short peripheral catheters open. A saline flush (2 mL) is administered and a clamp is tightened or the needle is withdrawn while injecting to create positive pressure and keep vein open.

"Piggyback" IV Administration

1. Means of administering medication by way of the fluid pathway of an established primary infusion line.
2. Drugs may be given on an intermittent basis through a primary infusion.

3. When a check valve is present on the primary tubing, it performs the following functions:
   a. Permits the primary infusion to flow after the medication has been administered.
   b. Prevents air from entering the system.
   c. Prevents secondary fluid from "running dry."
   d. Permits less mixing of primary fluid with secondary solution.
4. Use of an infusion pump or controller will permit rate changes between primary and secondary infusates.

Venous Access Devices

Indications
1. Long-term therapy—weeks, months, even years
2. Chemotherapy, medication, or blood product infusion; blood specimen collection
3. IV fluids in the home
4. Limited peripheral venous access due to extensive previous IV therapy, surgery, or previous tissue damage

Types
See Figure 6-1.
1. Central catheter—nontunneled; often called percutaneous
   a. Has one to four lumens
   b. Dwell time usually less than a month
   c. May be inserted in femoral, jugular, or subclavian veins

> **NURSING ALERT**
>
> An x-ray to determine placement of central catheter is necessary for all devices that deliver fluid into the subclavian vein or superior vena cava.

2. Central catheter—tunneled
   a. A tunneled catheter is inserted into a central vein (usually the subclavian, then the superior vena cava) and subcutaneously tunneled to an exit site approximately 10 cm from the insertion site.
   b. A Dacron cuff is located approximately 2 to 3 cm from the exit site, providing a barrier against microorganisms.
   c. Examples of the tunneled catheters in current use are Hickman™, Broviac™, and Groshong™.
3. Central implanted device
   a. A subcutaneous pocket is formed and a reservoir is placed; a catheter is attached to the reservoir and

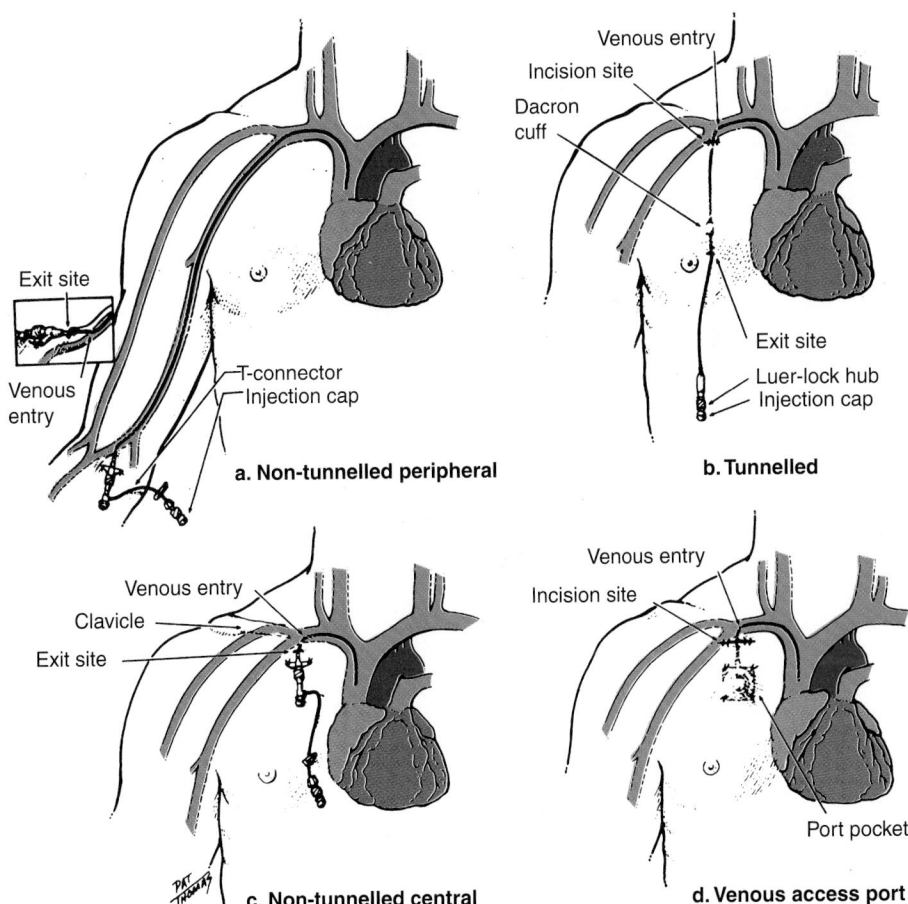

FIGURE 6-1 Common sites for long-term venous access devices. (Courtesy American Cancer Society.)

Exit site
Venous entry
T-connector
Injection cap
a. Non-tunnelled peripheral

Venous entry
Incision site
Dacron cuff
Exit site
Luer-lock hub
Injection cap
b. Tunnelled

Venous entry
Clavicle
Exit site
c. Non-tunnelled central

Venous entry
Incision site
Port pocket
d. Venous access port

tunneled subcutaneously and inserted into a central vein (usually the catheter tip is in the superior vena cava). This device cannot be visualized exteriorly.

  b. Examples of implanted devices in current use include the Port-A-Cath™, Medi-Port™, Infuse-A-Port™, and Groshong Port™.

4. Peripheral central—nontunneled

  a. Peripherally inserted central catheter (PICC); used in patients in acute, long-term, and home care settings.

    (i) Inserted in basilic, brachial, or cephalic veins.

    (ii) May be inserted by nurses with special training or interventional radiologists.

    (iii) PICC tip placement must be located in superior vena cava (verified by x-ray). Tip placement in subclavian or innominate vein contraindicated for hyperosmolar solutions (hyperalimentation).

    (iv) PICC insertion site and hub should be covered by a transparent dressing.

    (v) Extension tubing must be clamped when no solution infusing. Tape securely to arm.

    (vi) Positive pressure flushing will keep PICC from clotting (Table 6-4).

    (vii) PICCs placed in the medial cubital vein tend to follow the cephalic vein to central placement.

Observe carefully for pain and tenderness because cephalic vein is smaller than basilic.

  b. PAS Port™

    (i) Inserted in basilic vein

    (ii) Connected to a subcutaneously implanted port in the forearm

    (iii) Delivers fluid centrally into superior vena cava

NURSING ALERT

If central catheters are placed too deeply and extend into the right atrium, an irregular heartbeat may result. Monitor heart rhythm and notify health care provider immediately.

---

5. Midline catheters

  a. These catheters are inserted into the basilic or cephalic vein and extend 6 to 7 inches up the arm.

  b. They are inserted by specially trained nurses.

  c. Dwell time—for intermediate therapy of 2 to 6 weeks

  d. They are not appropriate for hyperosmolar solutions such as hyperalimentation and some antibiotics such as erythromycin (Ilotycin) and nafcillin (Unipen).

(*text continues on page 99*)

TABLE 6-4 IV Catheter Maintenance Guidelines

Catheter	Dressing Change	Flush (Maintenance)	Flush (After Blood Draw)
Short peripheral	3d when site changed	If used as a lock, 2 mL saline every shift or heparin 1:10 units/mL	N/A
Midline	q 3–5d	3 mL 1:10 units/mL heparin qd	5 mL normal saline 3 mL 1:100 units/mL heparin
PICC	3 times/wk postinsertion, weekly after that	2–3 mL 1:100 units/mL heparin qd	10 mL normal saline 3 mL 1:100 units/mL heparin
Groshong	q 1–2d postinsertion for a week postop, then q 3d until site fully healed, then every week. When site healed, no dressing. Secure catheter to chest with tape.	10 mL normal saline weekly	10–20 mL normal saline
Hickman/Broviac	Same as Groshong	3 mL 1:100 units qd if accessed q 8h or more frequently, no need for heparin between infusions	10 mL normal saline 3 mL 1:100 units/mL heparin
Implanted ports (including PAS Port)	Needle and dressing change every week when accessed	If accessed and locked: 5 mL normal saline and 5 mL 1:100 units/mL heparin after each infusion. Terminal flush: 5–7 mL 1:100 units/mL heparin and q 4wk thereafter	5 mL normal saline 5 mL 1:100 units/mL heparin
Percutaneous catheters (triple/double lumen)	q 2–3d	3 mL normal saline 2 mL 1:10 units heparin twice per day or after each infusion	3 mL normal saline 3 mL 1:10 units heparin
Quinton/Perm-A catheter (blue lumen, use only with order)	q 2–3d	2 mL 1000 units/mL heparin q 2–3d (always withdraw heparin first when using catheter)	10 mL normal saline 2 mL 1000 units/mL heparin

PROCEDURE GUIDELINES 6-2	SALINE/HEPARIN LOCK

Saline or heparin lock is an intermittent infusion reservoir that permits administration of periodic IV medications and solution without continuous fluid administration and aspiration of blood samples for laboratory analysis.

EQUIPMENT

Antiseptic swabs (usually alcohol)
Syringe with normal saline
Preflushed extension set with 2 mL sterile normal saline
 solution if converting IV line to existing cannula in vein.
Tape
Unsterile gloves

Optional:
 Syringe containing 1–2 mL heparin solution 1:10 units/mL

PROCEDURE

Nursing Action	Rationale
1. Wash hands.	
2. Explain procedure to patient.	2. To minimize patient anxiety.
3. Don gloves.	
4. Cleanse port of the heparin lock with alcohol. Insert normal saline syringe needle into port and aspirate slightly.	4. Use either a protected needle or a blunt-end syringe to access port. This equipment avoids accidental needle sticks. If small gauge catheter does not show a positive blood return, monitor site carefully.
5. Inject normal saline solution slowly to flush reservoir of saline or heparin solution and blood.	5. Not all institutions use heparin to maintain peripheral locks.
6. Check with patient to ensure no pain on flushing.	6. May indicate a clot or infiltration.
7. Check for swelling at needle site when flushing.	7. May indicate a clot or infiltration.
8. Insert medication tubing, administer drug, infuse at prescribed rate.	
9. After drug or solution administration, insert saline syringe and flush reservoir slowly. Remove syringe while still pushing plunger of syringe to ensure positive pressure.	9. To prevent blood clotting in the IV cannula. Central venous catheters require greater than 2.5 mL of solution to be effective.
10. Optional: Insert heparin solution into reservoir.	

FOLLOW-UP PHASE

1. Maintain patency of heparin lock by flushing it q8–12h, regardless of use.	1. If resistance is met, device should not be flushed. Attempt to remove occlusion via aspiration. If unable to restore patency, remove IV device.
2. IV administration set for intermittent therapy should be changed according to institutional policy. The tubing should only be used for the same medication.	2. It is recommended that the tubing be changed q24h because the tubing is not maintained as a closed system and therefore poses a risk for infection.

PROCEDURE GUIDELINES 6-3	SETTING UP AN AUTOMATIC INTRAVENOUS "PIGGYBACK"

EQUIPMENT

Sterile infusion set (primary)   Alcohol prep pad
Sterile infusion set (secondary)   Admixture

PROCEDURE

Follow procedure of particular manufacturer of "piggyback" infusion set.
In general, most procedures are similar to the following:

Nursing Action	Rationale
1. Wash hands thoroughly.	1. Minimizes possibility of infection.
2. Set up primary infusion set; this may have a check-valve (see A in accompanying figure).	2. The primary set should be functioning effectively before the secondary (piggyback) set can be attached. *continued*

PROCEDURE GUIDELINES 6-3   **SETTING UP AN AUTOMATIC INTRAVENOUS "PIGGYBACK"**
CONTINUED

Nursing Action	Rationale
3. Lower the primary flask on the IV pole; usually, an extension hook accompanies the set.	3. This will permit the check-valve to function.

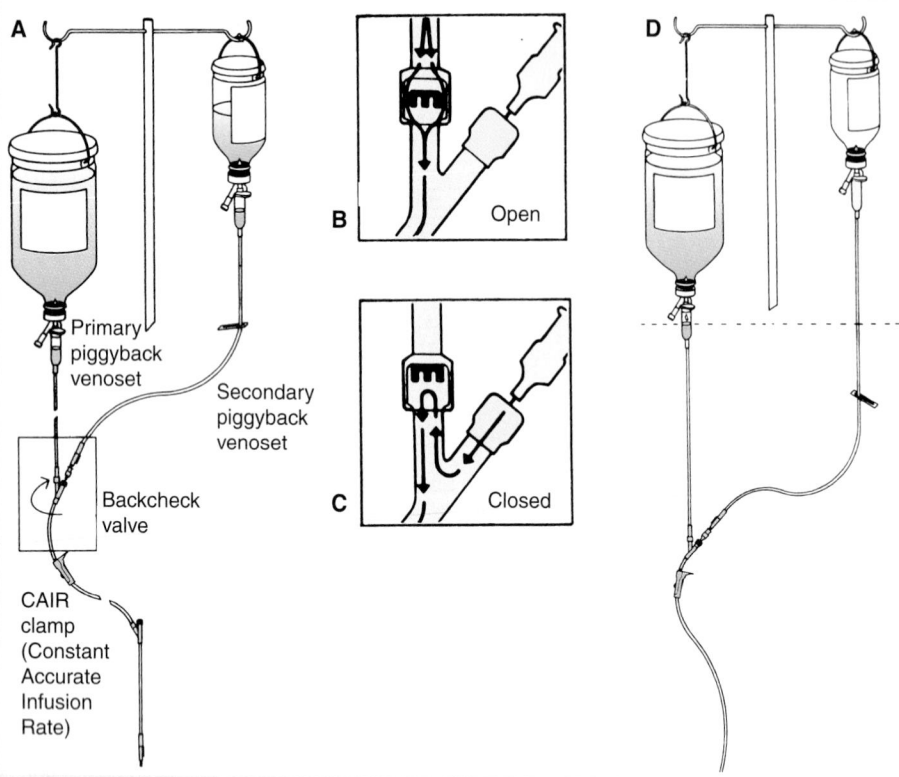

(A) "Piggyback" IV. On left is the primary infusion flask. Note use of extension hook (hanging from IV pole) to suspend primary flask. Backcheck valve is seen more clearly in B and C. Secondary "piggyback" source is seen on the right. (B) Open check-valve. Fluid from primary source flows down on either side of movable disc. Fluid from secondary source is closed off with clamp (not visible). (C) Closed check-valve. Note that fluid source from secondary flask (where pressure is greater because flask source is higher) is forcing movable disc upward, thereby closing off fluid from primary source. (D) When last of fluid from secondary source reaches the level of the fluid in the primary set drip chamber (as indicated by broken line), hydrostatic pressure between both sets will equalize. This releases check-valve; flow will shift from secondary to primary source. (Adapted from Abbott Laboratories)

4. Use alcohol swab to carefully cleanse injection site.	4. Usually this is a Y-connection on the primary site.
5. Attach secondary tubing to primary tubing—preferably with a protected needle—at entry port.	
6. Lower secondary bottle, open clamp, and allow infusate from primary bottle to prime secondary tubing. Close clamp.	6. This clears secondary tubing of air and prevents any loss of medication from secondary line.
7. Then hang secondary bottle higher than primary solution. Open roller clamp (see D in accompanying figure).	
8. Program pump or controller for rate of infusion for secondary medication.	8. To ensure medication administration over appropriate time period.

FOLLOW-UP PHASE

1. Change IV administration tubing according to your institutional guidelines.	
2. If possible, do not disattach secondary tubing from primary after infusion regimen started.	2. If using more than one secondary medication, the same tubing may be used. Back-flush tubing into old secondary bag or bottle. Dispose of bag or bottle. Hang new secondary medication to same tubing.

PROCEDURE GUIDELINES 6-4	ACCESSING AN IMPLANTED PORT

Implanted ports are becoming increasingly popular for patients with diseases such as cancer, sickle cell anemia, or cystic fibrosis to administer medications and continuous or intermittent IV fluids.

EQUIPMENT

5–10-mL syringes filled with normal saline
Noncoring Huber needle
Heparin flush solution 1:100 units/mL

Alcohol prep pads
3 povidone-iodine swab sticks
Sterile gloves

PROCEDURE

Nursing Action	Rationale
1. Wash hands thoroughly.	
2. Explain procedure to patient.	2. To minimize anxiety and facilitate learning.
3. Palpate port—feel septum.	3. To ensure placement and patency.
4. Select appropriate Huber needle—gauge and length.	
5. Flush Huber needle and extension with normal saline, leaving 5-mL syringe attached, being careful not to touch needle with unsterile gloves or fingers.	5. Priming of needle is essential to prevent infusion of air and ensure patency.
6. Don sterile gloves and cleanse site with alcohol and three povidone-iodine swabs. Allow to dry.	6. To prevent introduction of organisms into central line.
7. Grasp Huber needle with one hand and stabilize port with other hand—again locating septum.	
8. With a firm, steady motion, insert needle into port.	
9. Aspirate. If unable to aspirate, flush port with saline and try to aspirate blood again.	9. By aspirating first, you withdraw heparin solution that has been in port.
10. After aspirating blood, flush with 10 mL normal saline.	10. Presence of blood confirms correct needle placement in port.
11. If still no blood return, repeat port access or report findings to health care provider.	11. May order a radiologic study or urokinase declotting procedure.
12. When placement of needle confirmed, attach IV or "heparin lock" the port.	

FOLLOW-UP PHASE

1. Maintain patency by flushing according to your institutional guidelines. Change needle every 7 days.
2. Instruct patient to have port flushed monthly and notify health care provider of any problems.

NURSING ROLE IN IV THERAPY

◼ Initiating an IV

Nurses must be familiar with the procedure as well as the equipment involved in initiating an IV to provide effective therapy and prevent complications. See Standards of Care Guidelines.

Selecting a Vein

1. First verify the order for IV therapy unless it is an emergency situation.
2. Explain the procedure to the patient.
3. Select a vein suitable for venipuncture.
   a. Back of hand—metacarpal vein (Figure 6-2B). Avoid digital veins, if possible.
      (i) The advantage of this site is that it permits arm movement.
      (ii) If a vein problem develops later at this site, another vein higher up the arm may be used.
   b. Forearm—basilic or cephalic vein (see Figure 6-2A)
   c. Inner aspect of elbow, antecubital fossa—median basilic and median cephalic for relatively short-term infusion. However, use of these veins prevents bending of arm.

NURSING ALERT

The median basilic and cephalic veins are not recommended for chemotherapy administration due to potential for extravasation and poor healing resulting in impaired joint movement. In addition, these veins may be needed for intermediate or long-term indwelling catheters.

To prevent untoward effects of IV therapy, perform the following assessments and procedures:

- Before starting IV therapy, consider duration of therapy, type of infusion, condition of veins, and medical condition of the patient to assist in choosing IV site and type of catheter.
- Ensure that you are competent in initiating the type of IV therapy decided on and familiar with institutional policy and procedure before initiating therapy.
- After initiation of IV therapy, monitor the patient frequently for:

  Signs of infiltration or sluggish flow
  Signs of phlebitis or infection
  Correct solution, medication, volume, and rate
  Dwell time of catheter and need to be replaced
  Condition of catheter dressing and frequency of change
  Fluid and electrolyte balance
  Signs of fluid overload or dehydration
  Patient satisfaction with mode of therapy

This information should serve as a general guideline only. Each patient situation presents a unique set of clinical factors and requires nursing judgment to guide care, which may include additional or alternative measures and approaches.

d. Lower extremities
   (i) Foot—venous plexus of dorsum, dorsal venous arch, medial marginal vein
   (ii) Ankle—great saphenous vein

NURSING ALERT

Use lower extremities as a last resort. A patient with diabetes and peripheral vascular disease is not a suitable candidate. Obtain a health care provider order for the IV site and monitor lower extremity closely for signs of phlebitis and thrombosis.

4. Central veins are used:
   a. When medications and infusions are hypertonic or highly irritating, requiring rapid, high-volume dilution to prevent systemic reactions and local venous damage (eg, chemotherapy, hyperalimentation).
   b. When peripheral blood flow is diminished (eg, shock) or when peripheral vessels are not accessible (eg, obese patients).
   c. When CVP monitoring is desired.
   d. When moderate or long-term fluid therapy is expected.

Methods of Distending a Vein
1. Apply manual compression above site where cannula is to be inserted.

2. Have the patient periodically clench the fist (if arm is used).
3. Massage area in direction of venous flow.
4. Apply tourniquet (made of soft rubber tubing) at least 5 to 15 cm (2–6 inches) above planned insertion site, fastening it with a slip knot or hemostat.
5. An alternative is to apply blood pressure cuff (keep pressure just below systolic pressure).
6. Lightly tap vein site; this is to be done gently so the vein is not injured.
7. Allow extremity to be dependent (below heart level) for a few minutes.
8. Apply heat to a possible needle site by using a moist, warm towel.

Selecting Needle or Catheter
1. Use the smallest gauge catheter suitable for type and location of infusion.
2. If blood transfusion is to be given, use a larger-bore catheter, preferably a 20 gauge.
3. For very small veins and an infusion rate below 75 mL/h, a 24-gauge catheter may be appropriate.
4. Consider local anesthesia.
   a. If large-bore needle (greater than 18 gauge) is being inserted in an unusually sensitive patient, 0.1 mL 1% lidocaine (without epinephrine) may be ordered and infiltrated intradermally around the site to provide local anesthesia. Emla™ topical cream may also be applied 1 hour before vein cannulation.
   b. Local anesthesia is best avoided because it may cause collapse of desired veins, allergic reactions, and increased cost of the procedure.
5. For a short-term infusion of 1 hour or less, a steel needle may be used.
6. For longer-term therapy, choose a flexible catheter. These may be made of Teflon, Vialyon, and so forth.

NURSING ALERT

Needle sticks are a constant risk in IV therapy. Catheter companies manufacture many protective devices such as retractable stylets in IV catheters. Institutions are strongly encouraged to stock and use these safety devices to protect employees (Figure 6-3).

Cleansing the Infusion Site
1. If skin is unusually soiled, cleanse infusion site thoroughly with a good surgical soap and rinse.
2. Cleanse IV site with effective topical antiseptic (according to hospital protocol).
   a. Three alcohol swabs, used one at a time, in a circular movement from site outward and for ½ to 1 minute is an appropriate cleansing.
   b. Povidone-iodine, used for 1 minute and allowed to dry, is also appropriate, especially for the neutropenic patient.

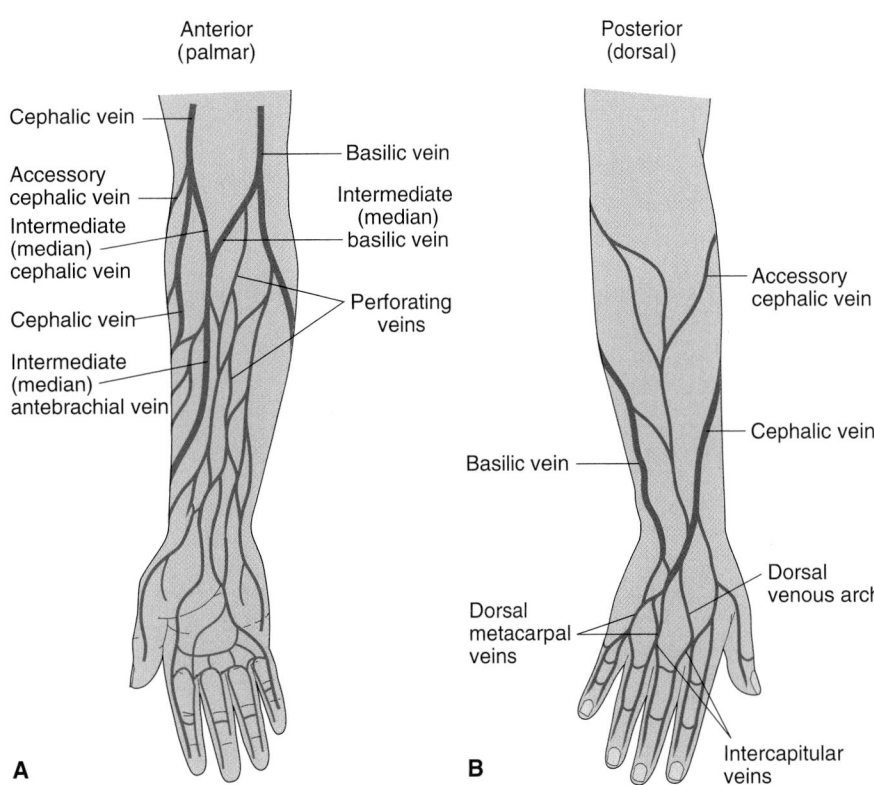

FIGURE 6-2 (**A**) Superficial veins, forearm. (**B**) Superficial veins, dorsal aspect of the hand.

Anterior
(palmar)

Cephalic vein

Accessory
cephalic vein

Intermediate
(median)
cephalic vein

Cephalic vein

Intermediate
(median)
antebrachial vein

Basilic vein

Intermediate
(median)
basilic vein

Perforating
veins

Posterior
(dorsal)

Accessory
cephalic vein

Cephalic vein

Basilic vein

Dorsal
venous arch

Dorsal
metacarpal
veins

Intercapitular
veins

A   B

 DRUG ALERT

Iodine solutions and iodophors (an iodine compound) may cause allergic reactions in some patients. Patient should be assessed for iodine allergies before IV insertion. Iodine and iodophor should dry to facilitate their antimicrobial properties.

Initiating the Venipuncture
Follow steps in Procedure Guidelines 6-1.

Infusion Tubing
1. Drip chambers
   a. A "microdrip" system delivers 60 drops/mL and is used when small volumes are being delivered (eg, less than 50 mL/h); this reduces the risk of clotting the IV line due to slow infusion rates.
   b. The "macrodrip" system delivers 10, 15, or 20 drops/mL and is used to deliver solution in large quantities or at fast rates.
2. Vents
   a. Vented tubing should be used with standard glass bottles; this permits air to enter the vacuum in the bottle and displace solution as it flows out.
   b. Nonvented tubing should be used for IV bags and glass bottles that have a built-in air vent.
3. Filters
   a. Filters help minimize the risk of contamination from certain microorganisms and particulate matter.
   b. Filters should be changed every 24 to 48 hours because bacteria may become trapped in the filter and release endotoxin, a small pyrogen capable of passing through the filter.
   c. Filters are found "in line" on conventional IV, blood, and hyperalimentation tubing. Check your institution's equipment and protocols to see if an additional filter is warranted. (An additional filter is needed for mannitol infusions.)
4. Special tubing
   a. Most mechanical infusion pumps and controllers require specialized tubing to fit their particular pumping chamber. Need for such a device should be determined before initiating infusion therapy.
   b. If added tubing length is required (especially for children and restless patients), extension tubing is available; this should be added at the time of IV setup.
   c. Secondary tubing is used for administration of intermittent "piggyback" medications that are connected to the port closest to the drip chamber.

Before activation

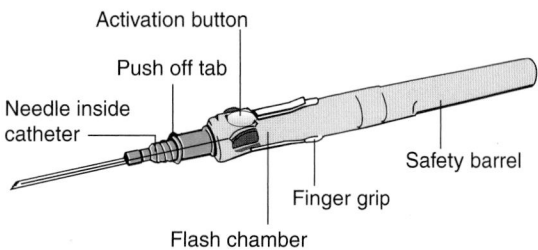

After activation

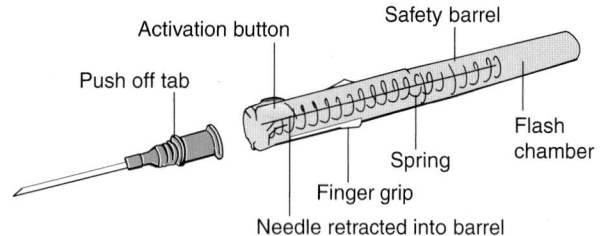

FIGURE 6-3 The activation button is pressed after the catheter is in the vein, so that the needle will retract into the safety barrel while the needle is still in the catheter. (Courtesy of Becton Dickinson)

d. Special coated tubing, designed to prevent leaching of polyvinyl chloride, is used for delivering medications such as nitroglycerin (Tridil), paclitaxel (Taxol), and cyclosporine (Sandimmune).

5. Tubing change
   a. Check your institutional protocol for time of tubing change. Standard is 48 to 72 hours.
   b. Label new tubing with date, time hung, and your initials.

6. Dressing changes and flushing of IV—vary depending on type of IV (see Table 6-4).

Adjusting Rate of Flow

The health care provider prescribes the flow rate. However, the nurse is responsible for regulating and maintaining the proper rate.

A. Patient—determining factors
   1. Surface area of the patient—the larger the patient, the more fluid may be required and tolerated.
   2. Patient condition—a patient in hypovolemic shock requires greater amounts of fluids, whereas the patient with heart or renal failure should receive fluids judiciously.
   3. Age of patient—fluids should be administered more slowly in the very young and elderly.

4. Tolerance to solutions—fluids containing medications causing potential allergic reactions or intense vascular irritation (eg, potassium chloride) should be well diluted or given slowly.
5. Prescribed fluid composition—efficacy of some drugs is based on speed of infusion (eg, antibiotics); other solutions are given at a rate titrated to the patient's response to them (eg, dopamine [Intropin], sodium nitroprusside [Nipride], heparin [Heparin]).

B. Factors affecting rate of flow
   1. Gauge of IV catheter
   2. Pressure gradient—the difference between two levels in a fluid system
   3. Friction—the interaction between fluid molecules and surfaces of inner wall of tubing
   4. Diameter and length of tubing
   5. Height of column of fluid
   6. Characteristics of fluid
      a. Viscosity
      b. Temperature—refrigerated fluids may cause diminished flow and vessel spasm; bring fluid to room temperature before infusion.
   7. Vein trauma, clots, plugging of vents, venous spasm, vasoconstriction, and so forth.
   8. Flow-control clamp derangement
      a. Some clamps may slip and loosen, resulting in a rapid, or "runaway," infusion. Many tubings now have safety clamps to prevent this rapid infusion.
      b. Plastic tubing may distort, causing "creep" or "cold flow"—the inside diameter of tubing will continue to change long after clamp is tightened or relaxed.
      c. Marked stretching of tubing may cause distortions of tubing and render clamp ineffective (may occur when patient turns over and pulls on a short tubing).
   9. If there is any question regarding rate of fluid administration, check with the health care provider.

GERONTOLOGIC ALERT

Be aware that veins are more likely to roll within the loose tissue beneath the skin, collapse, and become irritated in the elderly. In addition, fluid overload may be more pronounced, making IV therapy more difficult and potentially dangerous in the elderly.

C. Calculation of flow rate
   1. Most infusion rates are prescribed to be given at a certain volume per hour.
   2. The delivery of the prescribed volume is determined by calculating the necessary drops per minute to deliver the volume.
   3. Drops per milliliter will vary with commercial parenteral sets (eg, 10, 15, 20, or 60 drops/mL). Check directions on set.

4. Calculate infusion rate using the following formula:

$$\text{Drops/minute} = \frac{\text{total volume infused} \times \text{drops/mL}}{\text{total time for infusion in minutes}}$$

Example: Infuse 150 mL of D5W in 1 hour (set indicates 10 drops/mL)

$$\frac{150 \times 10}{60 \text{ minutes}} = 25 \text{ drops/minutes}$$

5. The nurse hanging a new IV solution should record date, time, and his or her initials on the container label.

NURSING ALERT

Never write directly on the IV bag to avoid leaks. Write on label or tape using a regular pen. Do not use magic markers because they are absorbed into the plastic bag and perhaps into the solution.

Complications of IV Therapy

Infiltration

Cause

1. Dislodgment of the IV cannula from the vein results in infusion of fluid into the surrounding tissues.

Clinical Manifestations

1. Swelling, blanching, and coolness of surrounding skin and tissues
2. Discomfort, depending on nature of solution
3. Fluid flowing more slowly or ceasing
4. Absence of blood backflow in IV catheter and tubing

Preventive Measures

1. Ensure that IV and distal tubing are secured sufficiently with tape to prevent movement.
2. Splint arm or hand as necessary.
3. Check IV site frequently for complications.

Nursing Interventions

1. Stop infusion immediately and remove IV needle or catheter.
2. Restart IV in the other arm.
3. If infiltration is moderate to severe, apply warm, moist compresses and elevate limb.
4. If a vasoconstrictor agent (eg, norepinephrine bitartrate [Levophed], dopamine [Intropin]) or a vesicant (various chemotherapy agents) has infiltrated, initiate emergency local treatment as directed. Serious tissue injury, necrosis, and sloughing may result if actions are not taken.
5. Document interventions and assessments.

Thrombophlebitis

Causes

1. Injury to vein during venipuncture, large-bore needle/catheter use, or prolonged needle/catheter use
2. Irritation to vein due to rapid infusions or irritating solutions (eg, hypertonic glucose solutions, cytotoxic agents,

strong acids or alkalis, potassium, and others). Smaller veins are more susceptible.
3. Clot formation at the end of the needle or catheter due to slow infusion rates
4. More often seen with synthetic catheters than steel needles

Clinical Manifestations

1. Tenderness at first, then pain along course of the vein
2. Swelling, warmth, and redness at infusion site; the vein may appear as a red streak above insertion site

Preventive Measures

1. Anchor needle or catheter securely at insertion site.
2. Change insertion site at least every 72 hours.
3. Use large veins for irritating fluid because of higher blood flow, which rapidly dilutes irritant.
4. Sufficiently dilute irritating agents before infusion.

Nursing Interventions

1. Apply cold compresses immediately to relieve pain and inflammation.
2. Later follow with moist, warm compresses to stimulate circulation and promote absorption.
3. Document interventions and assessments.

Bacteremia

Causes

1. Underlying phlebitis increases risk 18-fold.
2. Contaminated equipment or infused solutions (Figure 6-4)
3. Prolonged placement of an IV device (catheter/needle, tubing, solution container)
4. Nonaseptic IV insertion or dressing change
5. Cross-contamination by patient with other infected areas of body
6. The critically ill or immunosuppressed patient is at greatest risk of bacteremia.

Clinical Manifestations

1. Elevated temperature, chills
2. Nausea, vomiting
3. Elevated white blood cell count
4. Malaise, increased pulse
5. Backache, headache
6. May progress to septic shock with profound hypotension
7. Possible signs of local infection at IV insertion site (eg, redness, pain, foul drainage)

Preventive Measures

1. Follow same measures as outlined for thrombophlebitis.
2. Use strict asepsis when inserting IV or changing IV dressing.
3. Solutions should never hang longer than 24 hours.
4. Change insertion site at least every 48 to 72 hours.
5. Change IV administration set every 48 to 72 hours.
6. Change IV dressing every 48 to 72 hours.
7. Maintain integrity of infusion system.

Intrinsic
(present prior to use)

Extrinsic
(introduced during use)

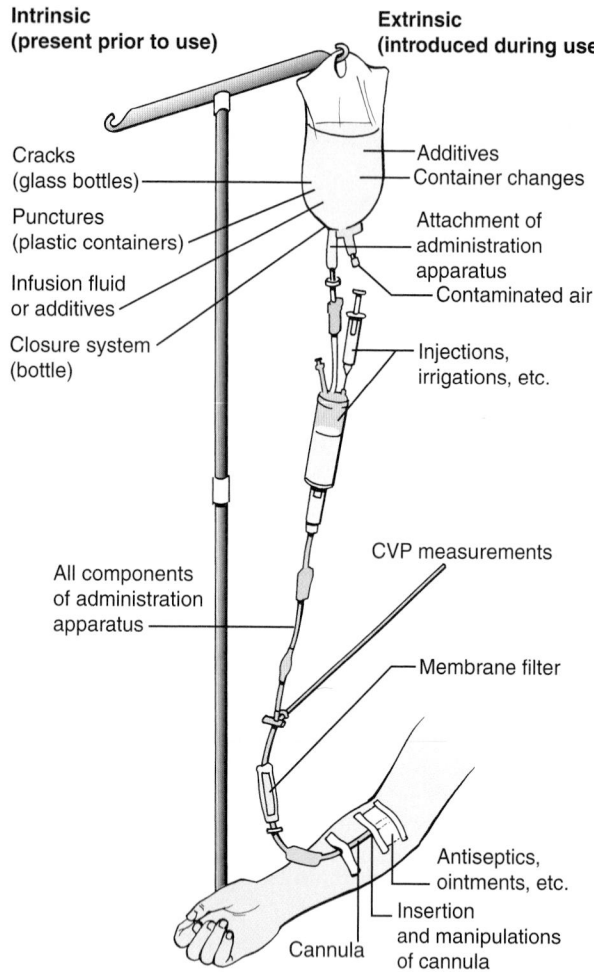

Cracks
(glass bottles)

Punctures
(plastic containers)

Infusion fluid
or additives

Closure system
(bottle)

All components
of administration
apparatus

Additives
Container changes

Attachment of
administration
apparatus
Contaminated air

Injections,
irrigations, etc.

CVP measurements

Membrane filter

Antiseptics,
ointments, etc.
Insertion
and manipulations
of cannula

Cannula

FIGURE 6-4 Potential mechanisms for contamination of IV in-fusion systems.

Nursing Interventions
1. Discontinue infusion and IV cannula.
2. IV device should be aseptically removed and the tip cut off with sterile scissors, placed in a dry sterile container, and immediately sent to the laboratory for analysis.
3. Check vital signs; reassure patient.
4. Obtain white blood cell count, as directed, and assess for other sites of infection (urine, sputum, wound).
5. Start appropriate antibiotic therapy immediately after receiving orders.
6. Document interventions and assessments.

Circulatory Overload
Cause
1. Delivery of excessive amounts of IV fluid (especially a risk for elderly patients, infants, or patients with cardiac or renal insufficiency).

Clinical Manifestations
1. Increased blood pressure and pulse
2. Increased CVP, venous distention (engorged neck veins)
3. Headache, anxiety
4. Shortness of breath, tachypnea, coughing
5. Pulmonary crackles
6. Chest pain (if history of coronary artery disease)

Preventive Measures
1. Know whether patient has existing heart or kidney con-dition. Be particularly vigilant in the high-risk patient.
2. Closely monitor infusion flow rate.
3. Splint arm or hand if IV flow rate fluctuates too widely with movement.

Nursing Interventions
1. Slow infusion to a "keep-open" rate and notify health care provider.
2. Monitor closely for worsening condition.
3. Raise patient's head to facilitate breathing.
4. Document interventions and assessments.

Air Embolism
Causes
1. A greater risk exists in central venous lines, when air en-ters catheter during tubing changes (air sucked in dur-ing inspiration due to negative intrathoracic pressure).
2. Air in tubing delivered by IV push or infused by infusion pump

Clinical Manifestations
1. Drop in blood pressure, elevated heart rate
2. Cyanosis, tachypnea
3. Rise in CVP
4. Changes in mentation, loss of consciousness

Preventive Measures
1. Clear all air from tubing before infusion to patient.
2. Change solution containers before they run dry.
3. Ensure that all connections are secure.
4. Use filter unless contraindicated.
5. Change IV tubing during expiration.

Nursing Interventions
1. Immediately turn patient on left side and lower head of bed; in this position, air will rise to right atrium.
2. Notify health care provider immediately.
3. Administer oxygen as needed.
4. Reassure patient.
5. Document interventions and assessments.

Mechanical Failure (Sluggish IV Flow)
Causes
1. Needle lying against the side of the vein, cutting off fluid flow
2. Clot at the end of the catheter or needle
3. Infiltration of IV cannula
4. Kinking of tubing or catheter

Clinical Manifestations

1. Sluggish IV flow
2. Alarm of flow regulator sounding
3. May be signs of local irritation—swelling, coolness of skin

Preventive Measures

1. Check IV often for patency, kinking, excessive movement by patient.
2. Secure IV well with tape and armboard, if necessary.

Nursing Interventions

1. Remove tape and check for kinking of tubing or catheter.
2. Pull back cannula because it may be lying against wall of vein, vein valve, or vein bifurcation.
3. Elevate or lower needle to prevent occlusion of bevel.
4. Move patient's arm to new position.
5. Lower solution container below level of patient's heart and observe for blood backflow.
6. If electronic flow-rate regulator is in use, check its integrity.
7. If none of the preceding steps produces the desired flow, remove needle or catheter and restart infusion.

Hemorrhage

Causes

1. Loose connection of tubing or injection port
2. Inadvertent or accidental removal of peripheral or central catheter
3. Anticoagulant therapy

Clinical Manifestations

1. Oozing or trickling of blood from IV site or catheter
2. Hematoma

Preventive Measures

1. Cap all central lines with PRN adapters and connect tubing to the cap—not directly to the line.
2. Tape all catheters securely—use transparent dressing when possible for peripheral and central catheters. Then tape the remaining catheter lumens and tubing in a loop so tension is not directly on the catheter.
3. Keep pressure on sites where catheters have been removed—a minimum of 10 minutes for an anticoagulated patient.

Venous Thrombosis

The vein in which the peripheral or central catheter lies becomes partially or fully occluded by a thrombus.

Causes

1. Infusion of irritating solutions
2. Infection along catheter may preclude this syndrome.
3. Fibrin sheath formation with eventual clot formation around catheter. This clot will eventually occlude vein.

Clinical Manifestations

1. Slowing of IV infusion or inability to draw blood from the central line
2. Swelling and pain in the area of catheter or in the extremity proximal to the IV line

Preventive Measures

1. Ensure proper dilution of irritating substances.
2. Ensure superior vena cava catheter tip placement for irritating solutions.

Nursing Interventions

1. Stop fluids immediately and notify health care provider.
2. Reassure patient and institute appropriate therapy:
   a. Anticoagulants
   b. Heat
   c. Elevation of affected extremity
   d. Antibiotics

SELECTED REFERENCES

Andris, D., & Krzywda, E. (1997, September/October). Catheter pinch-off syndrome: Recognition and management. *Journal of Intravenous Nursing, 20*, 233–237.

Bagnall-Reeb, H. (1998, September/October). Diagnosis of central venous access device occlusion: Implications for nursing practice. *Journal of Intravenous Nursing, 21*, S115–S121.

Camp-Sorrell, D. (Ed.) (1996). *Access device guidelines: Recommendations for nursing practice.* Pittsburgh: Oncology Nursing Society.

DeJong, M. (1998, December). Hyponatremia. *American Journal of Nursing, 98*, 36.

deMoissac, D., & Jensen, L. (1998, June). Changing IV administration sets: Is 48 versus 24 hours safe for neutropenic patients with cancer? *Oncology Nursing Forum, 25*, 907–913.

Dugger, B. (1997, November/December). Intravenous nursing competency: Why is it important? *Journal of Intravenous Nursing, 20*, 287–297.

Green, L., & Gerlach, C. J. (1994, May). Central lines have moved out. *RN, 57*, 26–31.

Hadaway, L. (1999, March/April). Developing an interactive intravenous education and training program. *Journal of Intravenous Nursing, 22*, 87–93.

Homer, L., & Holmes, K. (1998, September/October). Risks associated with 72- and 96-hour peripheral intravenous catheter dwell times. *Journal of Intravenous Nursing, 21*, 301–305.

Klotz, R. (1998, January/February). The effects of intravenous solutions of fluid and electrolyte balance. *Journal of Intravenous Nursing, 21*, 20–26.

Larovere, E. (1999). Accessing an implanted port. *Nursing 99, 29*(5), 56–58.

———. (1999). Deaccessing an implanted port. *Nursing 99, 29*(6), 60–61.

———. (2000). Placing a midline catheter. *Nursing 2000, 30*(3), 26.

Lawson, T. (1997, Winter). Infusion of medications via PICC and midline catheters in patients with AIDS. *Journal of Vascular Access Devices, 2*, 7–10.

Macklin, D. (1997, September). How to manage PICCs. *American Journal of Nursing, 97*, 26–33.

Mayo, D., Diamond, E., Kramer, W., & Horn, M. (1996, May). Discard volumes necessary for clinically useful coagulation studies from heparinized Hickman™ catheters. *Oncology Nursing Forum, 23*, 671–675.

Metheny, N. M. (2000). *Fluid and electrolyte balance* (4th ed.). Philadelphia: Lippincott Williams & Wilkins.

Miller, K., & Dietrick, C. (1997, May/June). Experience with PICC at a university medical center. *Journal of Intravenous Nursing, 20*, 141–147.

National Association of Vascular Access Networks Position Paper. (1998, Summer) Tip location of peripherally inserted central catheters. *Journal of Vascular Access Devices, 3*, 8–10.

Powers, F. (1999, July). Protecting elderly patients from IV complications. *Nursing 99, 29*, 54–55.

Pugliese, G. (1997, November/December). Reducing risks of infection during vascular access. *Journal of Intravenous Nursing, 20,* S11–S23.

Reed, T., & Phillips, S. (1996, November/December). Management of central venous catheter occlusions and repairs. *Journal of Intravenous Nursing, 19,* 289–302.

Richardson, D., & Brusso, P. (1993, January/February). Vascular access devices: Management of common complications. *Journal of Intravenous Nursing, 16,* 44–49.

Sansivero, G. (1998, September/October). Venous anatomy and physiology: Considerations for vascular access device placement and function. *Journal of Intravenous Nursing, 21,* S107–S114.

Schulmeister, L. (1998, September/October). A complication of vascular access device insertion: A case study and review of subsequent legal action. *Journal of Intravenous Nursing, 21,* 197–202.

Smith, J. (1998, March/April). Thrombotic complications in intravenous access. *Journal of Intravenous Nursing, 21,* 96–100.

Smith, M. (1998, May/June). Emergency access in pediatrics. *Journal of Intravenous Nursing, 21,* 149–152.

Terry, J., Baranowski, L., Lonsway, R., & Hedrick, C. (1995). *Intravenous therapy clinical principles and practice.* Philadelphia: W. B. Saunders.

Treston-Aurand, J., Olmsted, R., Allen-Bridson, K., & Craig, C. (1997, September/October). Impact of dressing materials on central venous catheter infection rates. *Journal of Intravenous Therapy, 20,* 201–206.

Weinstein, S. M. (1996). *Plumer's principles and practices of intravenous therapy* (6th ed.). Philadelphia: J. B. Lippincott.

Welk, T. (1999, January/February). Clinical and ethical considerations of fluid and electrolyte management in the terminally ill client. *Journal of Intravenous Nursing, 22,* 43–47.

Winters, V., Peters, B., Coila, S., & Jones, L. (1990). A trial with a new peripheral implanted vascular device. *Oncology Nursing Forum, 17,* 891–896.

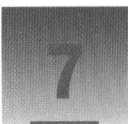
Perioperative Nursing

PERIOPERATIVE OVERVIEW

■ Introductory Information

Perioperative nursing is a term used to describe the nursing care provided in the total surgical experience of the patient: preoperative, intraoperative, and postoperative.

> *Preoperative phase*—from the time the decision is made for surgical intervention to the transfer of the patient to the operating room
>
> *Intraoperative phase*—from the time the patient is received in the operating room until admitted to the recovery room
>
> *Postoperative phase*—from the time of admission to the recovery room to the follow-up home/clinic evaluation

Types of Surgery

1. *Optional*—Surgery is scheduled completely at the preference of the patient (eg, cosmetic surgery).
2. *Elective*—The approximate time for surgery is at the convenience of the patient; failure to have surgery is not catastrophic (eg, superficial cyst).
3. *Required*—The condition requires surgery within a few weeks (eg, eye cataract).
4. *Urgent*—The surgical problem requires attention within 24 to 48 hours (eg, cancer).
5. *Emergency*—Situation requires immediate surgical attention without delay (eg, intestinal obstruction).

Common surgical incisions are pictured in Figure 7-1.

■ Ambulatory (Day) Surgery

Ambulatory surgery (same-day surgery, outpatient surgery) is a common occurrence for certain types of procedures. The office nurse is in a key position to assess patient status; plan perioperative experience; and monitor, instruct, and evaluate the patient.

Advantages

1. Reduced cost to patient, hospital, and insuring and governmental agencies
2. Reduced psychological stress to the patient
3. Less evidence of hospital-acquired infection
4. Less time lost from work by patient; minimal disruption of patient's activities and family life

Disadvantages

1. Less time to assess patient and perform preoperative teaching
2. Less time to establish rapport between patient and health personnel
3. Less opportunity to assess for late postoperative complications. This responsibility is primarily with the patient, although telephone and home care follow-up is possible.

Patient Selection

Criteria for selection include:
1. Surgery of short duration (varies by procedure and institution)
2. Noninfected conditions

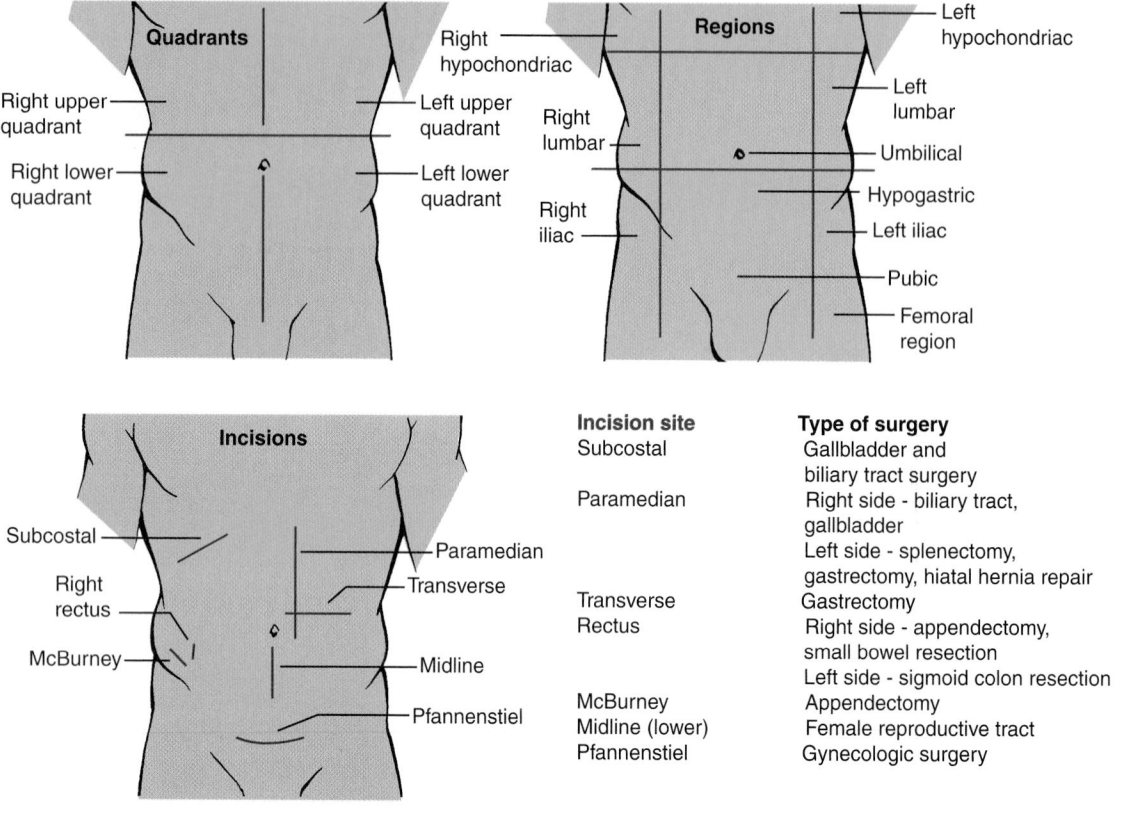

FIGURE 7-1   Regions and incisions of the abdomen.

3. Type of operation in which postoperative complications are predictably low
4. Age is usually not a factor, although too risky in a premature infant
5. Examples of frequently performed procedures:
   a. Ear-nose-throat (ENT; tonsillectomy, adenoidectomy)
   b. Gynecology (diagnostic laparoscopy, tubal ligation, dilatation and curettage)
   c. Orthopedics (arthroscopy, fracture or tendon repair)
   d. Oral surgery (wisdom teeth extraction, dental restorations)
   e. Urology (circumcision, cystoscopy, vasectomy)
   f. Ophthalmology (cataract)
   g. Plastic surgery (rhinoplasty, blepharoplasty, face lift)
   h. General surgery (laparoscopic hernia repair, lap-assisted cholecystectomy, biopsy, cyst removal)

Ambulatory Surgery Settings
Ambulatory surgery is performed in a variety of settings. A high percentage of outpatient surgery occurs in traditional hospital operating rooms in hospital-integrated facilities. Other ambulatory surgery settings may be hospital affiliated or independently owned and operated. Some types of outpatient surgeries can be performed safely in the health care provider's office.

Nursing Management
Initial Assessment
1. Develop a nursing history for the outpatient; this may be initiated in the health care provider's office.
2. Obtain a signed and witnessed informed consent form, which includes laterality of a limb if pertinent (eg, right arm, left leg, right eye).
3. Explain any additional laboratory studies needed and why.
4. Determine the following during initial assessment of the patient's physical and psychological status: Calm or agitated? Overweight? Disabilities or limitations? Allergies (be sure to include medication, food, and latex allergies)? Medications being taken (also include herbal medications because certain herbs, such as St. John's wort [a mild MAO inhibitor] and feverfew, can affect clotting)? Condition of teeth (dentures, caps, crowns)? Blood pressure problems? Major illnesses? Other surgeries? Seizures? Severe headaches? Smoker? Cardiac or respiratory problems?
5. Begin health education regimen. Instructions to patient:
   a. Notify health care provider and surgical unit immediately if you get a cold, have a fever, or have any illness before date of surgery.
   b. Arrive at specified time.

c. Do not ingest food or fluid from midnight previous to day of surgery.

d. Do not wear makeup or nail polish.

e. Wear comfortable, loose clothing and low-heeled shoes.

f. Leave valuables or jewelry at home.

g. Brush teeth in morning, rinse, but do not swallow liquid.

h. Shower the night before or day of surgery.

i. Have a responsible adult accompany you and drive you home—have person stay with you for 24 hours after surgery.

Preoperative Preparation

1. Administer preanesthetic medication; check vital signs.
2. Escort the patient to surgery after patient has urinated.
3. Review patient's chart for witnessed and informed consent, lab work, and pertinent medical history.

Postoperative Care

1. Check vital signs per protocol until stable.
2. Administer oxygen if necessary; check temperature.
3. Change patient's position and progress activity—head of bed elevated, dangling, ambulating. Watch for dizziness or nausea.
4. Ascertain, using the following criteria, that the patient has recovered adequately to be discharged:
   a. Vital signs stable for at least 1 hour
   b. Stands without dizziness and nausea; begins to walk
   c. Comfortable and free of excessive pain or bleeding
   d. Able to drink fluids and void
   e. Oriented as to time, place, person
   f. No evidence of respiratory depression (2 hours after extubation)

g. Has the services of a responsible adult who can escort patient home and remain at home

h. Understands postoperative instructions and takes instruction sheet home (Patient Education Guidelines)

Informed Consent (Operative Permit)

An *informed consent* (operative permit) is the process of informing the patient about the surgical procedure and obtaining consent from him or her. This is a legal requirement. Hospitals usually have a standard operative permit form approved by the hospital's legal department.

Purposes

1. To ensure that the patient understands the nature of the treatment, including potential complications
2. To indicate that the patient's decision was made without pressure
3. To protect the patient against unauthorized procedures, and to ensure that the procedure is performed on the correct body part
4. To protect the surgeon and hospital against legal action by a patient who claims that an unauthorized procedure was performed

Adolescent Patient and Informed Consent

1. An emancipated minor is usually recognized as one who is not subject to parental control:
   a. Married minor
   b. Those in military service
   c. College student under 18 but living away from home
   d. Minor who has a child

PATIENT EDUCATION GUIDELINES **Outpatient Postanesthesia and Postsurgery Instructions and Information**

1. Although you will be awake and alert in the Recovery Room, small amounts of anesthetic will remain in your body for at least 24 hours and you may feel tired and sleepy for the remainder of the day. Once you are home, take it easy and rest as much as possible. It is advisable to have someone with you at home for the remainder of the day.

2. Eat lightly for the first 12 to 24 hours, then resume a well-balanced, normal diet. Drink plenty of fluids. Alcoholic beverages are to be avoided for 24 hours after your anesthesia or intravenous sedation.

3. Nausea or vomiting may occur in the first 24 hours. Lie down on your side and breathe deeply. Prolonged nausea, vomiting, or pain should be reported to your surgeon.

4. Medications, unless prescribed by your physician, should be avoided for 24 hours. Check with your surgeon or anesthesiologist for specific instructions if you have been taking a daily medication.

5. Your surgeon will discuss your postsurgery instructions with you and prescribe medication for you as indicated. You will also receive additional instructions specific to your surgical procedure before leaving the hospital.

6. Your family will be waiting for you in the hospital's waiting room area near the Outpatient Surgery Department. Your surgeon will speak to them in this area before your discharge.

7. DO NOT OPERATE A MOTOR VEHICLE OR ANY MECHANICAL OR ELECTRICAL EQUIPMENT FOR *24 HOURS* AFTER YOUR ANESTHESIA.

8. DO NOT MAKE ANY IMPORTANT DECISIONS OR SIGN LEGAL DOCUMENTS FOR 24 HOURS AFTER YOUR ANESTHESIA.

(Courtesy of Doctor's Hospital of Prince George's County, Lanham, MD.)

2. Most states have statutes regarding treatment of minors.
3. Standards for informed consent are the same as for adults.

Procedures Requiring a Permit

1. Surgical procedures where scalpel, scissors, suture, hemostats, or electrocoagulation may be used
2. Entrance into a body cavity, such as paracentesis, bronchoscopy, cystoscopy, lumbar puncture
3. Radiologic procedure, particularly if contrast material is required (eg, myelogram, magnetic resonance imaging with contrast, angiography)
4. General anesthesia, local infiltration, and regional block

Obtaining Informed Consent

1. Before signing an informed consent, the patient should:
   a. Be told in clear and simple terms by the surgeon or other appropriate personnel (eg, anesthesiologist) what is to be done.
   b. Be aware of the risks, possible complications, disfigurement, and removal of body parts.
   c. Have a general idea of what to expect in the early and late postoperative periods.
   d. Have a general idea of the time frame involved from surgery to recovery.
   e. Have an opportunity to ask any questions.
   f. Sign a separate form for each procedure or operation.
2. Written permission is best and is legally acceptable.
3. Signature is obtained with the patient's complete understanding of what is to occur; it is obtained before the patient receives sedation and is secured without pressure or duress.
4. A witness is required—nurse, health care provider, or other authorized person.
5. In an emergency, witnessed permission by way of telephone or telegram is acceptable.
6. For a minor (or a patient who is unconscious or irresponsible), permission is required from a responsible member of the family—parent or legal guardian.
7. For married minor, permission from the husband or wife is acceptable.
8. If the patient is unable to write, an "X" to indicate his sign is acceptable if there is a signed witness to his mark.

■ Surgical Risk Factors and Preventive Strategies

Obesity

Danger

1. Increases difficulty involved in technical aspects of performing surgery (eg, sutures are difficult to tie because of fatty secretions); wound dehiscence is greater
2. Increases likelihood of infection because of lessened resistance

3. Increases potential for postoperative pneumonia and other pulmonary complications because greatly obese patients chronically hypoventilate
4. Increases demands on the heart, leading to cardiovascular compromise
5. Increases possibility of renal, biliary, hepatic, and endocrine disorders
6. Decreases ability to conserve heat due to radiant heat loss
7. Has altered response to many drugs and anesthetics
8. Decreases likelihood of early ambulation

Therapeutic Approach

1. Encourage weight reduction if time permits.
2. Anticipate postoperative obesity-related complications.
3. Be extremely vigilant for respiratory complications.
4. Carefully splint abdominal incisions when moving or coughing.
5. Be aware that some drugs should be dosed according to ideal body weight versus actual weight (owing to fat content), or an overdose may occur (eg, digoxin [Lanoxin], lidocaine [Xylocaine], aminoglycosides, and theophylline [Theo-Dur]).
6. Avoid intramuscular injections in morbidly obese individuals (intravenous [IV] or subcutaneous routes preferred).
7. Never attempt to move an impaired patient without assistance or without using proper body mechanics.
8. Obtain dietary consultation early in patient's postoperative course.

Poor Nutrition

Danger

1. Preoperative malnutrition (especially protein and calorie deficits and a negative nitrogen balance) greatly impairs wound healing.
2. Increases the risk of infection and shock.

Therapeutic Approach

1. Any recent (within 4–6 weeks) weight loss of 10% of patient's normal body weight should alert health care staff to poor nutritional status.
2. Attempt to improve nutritional status before and after surgery. Unless contraindicated, provide diet high in proteins, calories, and vitamins (especially vitamins C and A); this may require enteral and parenteral feeding. Reinforce that the postoperative period is not the appropriate time to diet.
3. Recommend repair of dental caries and proper mouth hygiene to prevent respiratory tract infection.

Fluid and Electrolyte Imbalance

Danger

Dehydration and electrolyte imbalances can have adverse effects in terms of general anesthesia and the anticipated volume losses associated with surgery, causing shock and cardiac dysrhythmias.

Therapeutic Approach

1. Assess patient's fluid and electrolyte status.
2. Rehydrate patient parenterally and orally as prescribed.
3. Monitor for evidence of electrolyte imbalance, especially Na^+, K^+, Mg^{++}, Ca^{++}.
4. Be aware of expected drainage amounts and composition; report excess and abnormalities.
5. Monitor the patient's intake and output; be sure to include all body fluid losses.

Aging
Danger

1. Potential for injury is greater in the aged.
2. Be aware that the cumulative effect of medications is greater in the older person.
3. Note that medications such as morphine and barbiturates in the usual dosages may cause confusion, disorientation, and respiratory depression.

Therapeutic Approach

1. Consider using lesser doses for desired effect.
2. Anticipate problems from chronic disorders such as anemia, obesity, diabetes, hypoproteinemia.
3. Adjust nutritional intake to conform to higher protein and vitamin needs.
4. When possible, cater to set patterns in older patients, such as sleeping and eating.

Presence of Cardiovascular Disease
Danger

Many surgical problems may be complicated in the presence of cardiovascular compromise.

Therapeutic Approach

1. Maintain diligence in nursing assessment.
2. Avoid fluid overload (oral, parenteral, blood products) because of possible myocardial infarction, angina, congestive failure, and pulmonary edema.
3. Prevent prolonged immobilization, which results in venous stasis. Monitor for potential deep vein thrombosis or pulmonary embolus.
4. Encourage change of position but avoid sudden exertion.
5. Use antiembolic hose or athrombic stockings intraoperatively and postoperatively.
6. Note evidence of hypoxia and initiate therapy.

Presence of Diabetes Mellitus
Danger

Hyperglycemia is potentiated by increased catecholamines and glucocorticoids due to surgical stress.

Therapeutic Approach

1. Recognize the signs and symptoms of ketoacidosis and glucosuria, which can threaten an otherwise uneventful surgical experience.
2. Monitor blood glucose and be prepared to administer insulin even though the patient may be NPO.
3. Reassure the diabetic patient that when the disease is controlled, the surgical risk may be no greater than it is for the nondiabetic person.

Presence of Alcoholism
Danger

Additional problem of malnutrition may be present in the presurgical patient with alcoholism. The patient may also have an increased tolerance to anesthetics.

Therapeutic Approach

1. Be prepared for rapid sequence induction to lessen the chance of vomiting and aspiration.
2. Note that the risk of surgery is greater for the person who has chronic alcoholism.
3. Anticipate the acute withdrawal syndrome (delirium tremens) within 72 hours of the last alcoholic drink.

Presence of Pulmonary and Upper Respiratory Disease
Danger

Chronic pulmonary illness may contribute to hypoventilation, leading to pneumonia and atelectasis. Surgery may be contraindicated in the patient who has an upper respiratory infection because it increases the likelihood of a more serious illness (eg, pneumonia).

Therapeutic Approach

1. Patients with chronic pulmonary problems such as emphysema or bronchiectasis should be treated for several days preoperatively with bronchodilators, aerosol medications, and conscientious mouth care, along with a reduction in weight and smoking, and methods to control secretions.
2. Chronic pulmonary disease increases the risk of atelectasis and pneumonia and potentiates respiratory depression from narcotics.

Concurrent or Prior Pharmacotherapy
Danger

Hazards exist when certain medications are given concomitantly with others (eg, interaction of some drugs with anesthetics can lead to hypotension and circulatory collapse). This also includes the use of many herbal substances. Although herbs are natural products, they can interact with other medications used in surgery.

Therapeutic Approach

1. An awareness of drug therapy is essential.
2. Notify health care provider and anesthesiologist if the patient is taking any of the following drugs:
   a. Certain antibiotics may interrupt nerve transmission when combined with a curariform muscle relaxant. This may cause respiratory paralysis and apnea.
   b. Antidepressants, particularly monoamine oxidase inhibitors (MAOs) and St. John's wort, an herbal product, increase hypotensive effects of anesthesia.
   c. Phenothiazines increase hypotensive action of anesthesia.
   d. Diuretics, particularly thiazides, may cause electrolyte imbalance and respiratory depression during anesthesia.
   e. Steroids inhibit wound healing.
   f. Anticoagulants such as warfarin or heparin; or medications or herbals that may affect coagulation such as aspirin, feverfew, ginkgo biloba, nonsteroidal anti-inflammatory drugs, ticlopidine (Ticlid), and clopidogrel (Plavix). Unexpected bleeding may result.

◆ DRUG ALERT

MAO inhibitors such as tranylcypromine (Parnate), phenelzine (Nardil), and selegeline (Eldepryl) must be discontinued before surgery or used with extreme caution due to danger of hypotension. St. John's wort must also be discontinued.

PREOPERATIVE CARE

Patient Education

Patient education is a vital component of the surgical experience. Preoperative patient education may be offered through conversation, discussion, the use of audiovisual aids, demonstrations, and return demonstrations. It is designed to help the patient understand the surgical experience to minimize anxiety and promote full recovery from surgery and anesthesia. The educational program may be initiated before hospitalization by the physician, nurse practitioner or office nurse, or other designated personnel. This is particularly important for patients who are admitted the day of surgery or undergo outpatient surgical procedures. The perioperative nurse can assess the patient's knowledge base and use this information in developing a plan for an uneventful perioperative course.

Teaching Strategies
Obtain a Database

1. Determine what the patient already knows or wants to know. This can be accomplished by reading the patient's chart, by interviewing the patient, and by communicating with the health care provider, family, and other members of the health team.
2. Ascertain patient's psychosocial adjustment to impending surgery.
3. Determine cultural or religious health beliefs and practices that may have an impact on the patient's surgical experience, such as refusal of blood transfusions, burial of amputated limbs within 24 hours, or special healing rituals.

Plan and Implement Teaching Program

1. Begin at the patient's level of understanding and proceed from there.
2. Plan a presentation, or series of presentations, for this individual patient or a group of patients.
3. Include family members and significant others in the teaching process.
4. Encourage active participation of patients in their care and recovery.
5. Demonstrate essential techniques; provide opportunity for patient practice and return demonstration.
6. Provide time for and encourage patient to ask questions and express concerns; make every effort to answer all questions truthfully and in basic agreement with the overall therapeutic plan.
7. Provide general information and assess the patient's level of interest in or reaction to it.
   a. Explain details of preoperative preparation and provide tour of area and view of equipment when possible.
   b. Offer general information on the surgery. Explain that the health care provider is the primary resource person.
   c. Tell when surgery is scheduled (if known) and approximately how long it will take; explain that afterward the patient will go to the recovery room. Emphasize that delays may be attributed to many factors other than a problem developing with this patient (eg, previous case in the operating room may have taken longer than expected or an emergency case has been given priority).
   d. Let patient know that family will be kept informed and that they will be told where to wait and when they can see patient; note visiting hours.
   e. Explain how a procedure or test may feel during or after.
   f. Describe the recovery room; what personnel and equipment the patient may expect to see and hear (specially trained personnel, monitoring equipment, tubing for various functions, and a moderate amount of activity by nurses and health care providers).
   g. Stress the importance of active participation in postoperative recovery.

8. Use other resource people: health care providers, therapists, chaplain, interpreters, and so forth.
9. Document what has been taught or discussed, as well as the patient's reaction and level of understanding.
10. Discuss with patient anticipated postoperative course (eg, length of stay, immediate postoperative activity, follow-up visit with the surgeon).

Use Audiovisual Aids If Available

1. Videotapes with sound or filmstrips with narration are effective in giving basic information to a single patient or group of patients. Many hospitals provide a television channel dedicated to patient instruction.
2. Booklets, brochures, and models, if available, are helpful.
3. Demonstrate any equipment that will be specific for the particular patient. Examples:
   a. Drains and drainage bags
   b. Monitoring equipment
   c. Side rails
   d. Incentive spirometer
   e. Ostomy bag

General Instructions

Preoperatively, the patient will be instructed in the following postoperative activities. This will allow a chance for practice and familiarity.

Diaphragmatic Breathing

This is a mode of breathing in which the dome of the diaphragm is flattened during inspiration, resulting in enlargement of the upper abdomen as air rushes into the chest. During expiration, abdominal muscles and the diaphragm relax. It is an effective relaxation technique.

Instruct the patient to:

1. Assume bed position similar to that most likely to be used postoperatively (semi-Fowler's).
2. Place both hands over lower rib cage; make a loose fist and rest the flat surface of the fingernails against the chest (to feel chest movement).
3. Exhale slowly and fully; ribs will sink downward and inward toward midline.
4. Inhale slowly and deeply through mouth and nose; permit abdomen to rise as lungs fill with air.
5. Hold this breath through a count of 5.
6. Exhale and let all air out through mouth and nose.
7. Repeat 15 times with a brief rest after each group of five.
8. Practice this twice each day preoperatively.

Incentive Spirometry

Preoperatively, the patient uses a spirometer to measure deep breaths (inspired air) while exerting maximum effort. The preoperative measurement becomes the goal to be achieved as soon as possible after the operation.

1. Postoperatively, the patient is encouraged to use the incentive spirometer about 10 to 12 times an hour.
2. Deep inhalations expand alveoli, which, in turn, prevents atelectasis and other pulmonary complications.

3. There is less pain with inspiratory concentration than with expiratory concentration, such as with coughing.

Coughing

Coughing promotes the removal of chest secretions. Instruct the patient to:

1. Interlace the fingers and place the hands over the proposed incision site; this will act as a splint during coughing and not harm the incision.
2. Lean forward slightly while sitting in bed.
3. Breathe, using the diaphragm as described under diaphragmatic breathing (see above).
4. Inhale fully with the mouth slightly open.
5. Let out three or four sharp "hacks."
6. Then, with mouth open, take in a deep breath and quickly give one or two strong coughs.
7. Secretions should be readily cleared from the chest to prevent respiratory complications (pneumonia, obstruction). *Note:* Certain position changes may be contraindicated after some surgeries (eg, craniotomy and eye or ear surgery).

Turning

Changing positions from back to side-lying (and vice versa) stimulates circulation, encourages deeper breathing, and relieves pressure areas.

1. Assist the patient to move onto side if assistance is needed.
2. Place the uppermost leg in a more flexed position than that of the lower leg and place a pillow comfortably between the legs.
3. Ensure that the patient is turned from one side to back and onto the other side every 2 hours.

Foot and Leg Exercises

Moving the legs improves circulation and muscle tone.

1. Have the patient lie on back; instruct patient to bend the knee and raise the foot—hold it a few seconds, extend the leg, and lower it to the bed.
2. Repeat above about five times with one leg and then with the other. Repeat the set five times every 3 to 5 hours.
3. Then have the patient lie on side; exercise the legs by pretending to pedal a bicycle.
4. Suggest the following foot exercise: Trace a complete circle with the great toe.

Evaluation of Teaching Program

1. Observe patient for correct demonstration of expected postoperative behaviors, such as foot and leg exercises and special breathing techniques.
2. Ask pertinent questions to determine patient's level of understanding.
3. Reinforce information when necessary.

▪ Preparation of the Operative Area

Skin

1. Human skin normally harbors transient and resident bacterial flora, some of which are pathogenic.

2. Skin cannot be sterilized without destroying skin cells.
3. Friction enhances the action of detergent antiseptics; however, friction should not be applied over a superficial malignancy (causes seeding of malignant cells) or areas of carotid plaque (causes plaque dislodgment and emboli).
4. It is ideal for the patient to bathe or shower, using a bacteriostatic soap (eg, Hibiclens), on the day of surgery. The surgical schedule may require that the shower be taken the night before.
5. The Centers for Disease Control and Prevention recommend that hair not be removed near the operative site unless it will interfere with surgery. Skin is easily injured during shaving and often results in a higher rate of postoperative wound infection.
6. If requested, shaving should be performed as close to the operative time as possible. The longer the interval between the shave and operation, the higher the incidence of postoperative wound infection.
   a. Use of electric clippers is preferable. Hair should be removed within 1 to 2 mm of the skin to avoid skin abrasion. Thorough cleaning of the clippers, after use, is essential.
   b. A sharp disposable razor, with a recessed blade, may be used as long as a "wet shave" is done. It is important that the shave be done in the direction of hair growth.
   c. Depilatory creams (hair-removing chemicals) offer the advantage of eliminating possible abrasions and cuts and producing clean, smooth, intact skin. Many patients even find this form of skin preparation relaxing. The depilatory creams may cause transient skin reactions in some patients, especially when used near the rectal and scrotal areas.
   d. Scissors may be used to remove hair greater than 3 mm in length.
7. For head surgery, obtain specific instructions from the surgeon concerning the extent of shaving.

Gastrointestinal Tract

1. Preparation of the bowel is imperative for intestinal surgery because escaping bacteria can invade adjacent tissues and cause sepsis.
   a. Cathartics and enemas remove gross collections of stool (eg, "Go Lightly").
   b. Oral antimicrobial agents (eg, neomycin, erythromycin) suppress the colon's potent microflora.
   c. Enemas "until clear" are prescribed the evening of elective surgery. No more than three enemas should be given because of negative effects on fluid and electrolyte balance. (It is also exhausting to the patient.) Notify the health care provider if the enemas never return clear.
2. Solid food is withheld from the patient for 6 hours before surgery. Patients having morning surgery are kept NPO overnight. Clear fluids (water) may be given up to 4 hours before surgery if ordered, to help the patient swallow medications.

Genitourinary Tract

A medicated douche may be prescribed preoperatively if the patient is to have a gynecologic (eg, hysterectomy) or urologic operation.

Preoperative Medication

With the increase of ambulatory surgery and same-day admissions, preanesthetic medications, skin preps, and douches are seldom ordered. However, medication may be prescribed preoperatively to facilitate the following goals:
1. To facilitate the administration of any anesthetic
2. To minimize respiratory tract secretions and changes in heart rate
3. To relax the patient and reduce anxiety

Types

1. *Opiates*—such as morphine (Roxanol) and meperidine (Demerol) are given to relax the patient and potentiate anesthesia.
2. *Anticholinergics*—such as atropine, scopolamine, and glycopyrrolate (Robinul) are given primarily to reduce respiratory tract secretions and to prevent severe reflex slowing of the heart during anesthesia. Typically given in conjunction with an opiate less than an hour before the patient's trip to the operating room.
3. *Barbiturates/tranquilizers*—such as pentobarbital (Nembutal) and other hypnotic agents are given the night before surgery to help ensure a restful night's sleep. It is important to note that reassurance from the nurse, anesthesiologist, and health care provider can do much to alleviate the patient's anxiety and insomnia.
4. *Prophylactic antibiotics*—are administered just before or during surgery when bacterial contamination is expected; ideally before skin incision is made.

Administering "On Call" Medications

> **NURSING ALERT**
>
> Preanesthetic medication, if ordered, should be given precisely at the time it is prescribed. If given too early, the maximum potency will have passed before it is needed; if given too late, the action will not have begun before anesthesia is started.

1. Have medication ready and administer as soon as call is received from the operating room.
2. Proceed with remaining preparation activities.
3. Indicate on the chart or preoperative checklist the time when medication was administered and by whom.

Admitting the Patient to Surgery
Final Checklist

The preoperative checklist is the last procedure before taking the patient to the operating room. Most facilities have a standard form for this check.

Identification and Verification

This includes verbal identification by the perioperative nurse while checking the identification band on the patient's wrist and written documentation (eg, chart) of the patient's identity, the procedure to be performed, the specific surgical site (includes right or left), the surgeon, and the type of anesthesia.

Review of Patient Record

Check for inclusion of the face sheet; allergies; history and physical; completed preoperative checklist; laboratory values, including most recent ones; electrocardiogram (ECG) and chest x-rays, if necessary; preoperative medications; and other preoperative orders by either the surgeon or anesthesiologist.

Consent Form

All nurses involved with patient care in the preoperative setting should be aware of the individual state laws regarding informed consent and the specific hospital policy. Obtaining informed consent is the responsibility of the surgeon performing the specific procedure. Consent forms should contain the stated procedure, the various risks, and alternatives to surgery, if any. It is a nursing responsibility to make sure the consent form has been obtained and is in the chart.

Patient Preparedness

1. NPO status
2. Proper attire (hospital gown)
3. Skin preparation, if ordered
4. IV started with correct gauge needle
5. Dentures or plates removed
6. Jewelry, contact lenses, glasses removed and secured in locked area or given to family member
7. Allow patient to void

Transporting Patient to the Operating Room

1. Adhere to the principle of maintaining the comfort and safety of the patient.
2. Accompany operating room attendants to the patient's bedside for introduction and proper identification.
3. Assist in transferring the patient from bed to stretcher (unless bed goes to operating room floor).
4. Complete chart and preoperative checklist; include laboratory reports and x-rays as required by hospital policy or health care provider's directive.
5. Recognize importance of coordinating team effort to ensure arrival of the patient in the operating room at the proper time.

The Patient's Family

1. Direct the patient's family to the proper waiting room where magazines, television, and coffee may be available.
2. Tell the family that the surgeon will probably contact them there immediately after surgery to inform them about the operation.
3. Acquaint the family with the fact that a long interval of waiting does not mean the patient is in the operating room all the while; anesthesia preparation and induction take time, and after surgery the patient is taken to the recovery room.
4. Tell the family what to expect postoperatively when they see the patient—tubes; monitoring equipment; and blood transfusion, suctioning, and oxygen equipment.

INTRAOPERATIVE CARE

Anesthesia and Related Complications

The goals of anesthesia are to provide analgesia, sedation, and muscle relaxation appropriate for the type of operative procedure, as well as to control the autonomic nervous system.

Common Anesthetic Techniques

Conscious Sedation
1. Patient remains conscious with some alteration of mood, drowsiness, and sometimes analgesia.
2. Protective reflexes remain intact.

Deep Sedation
1. Patient is asleep but easily arousable.
2. Protective reflexes are minimally depressed.

General Anesthesia
1. Complete loss of consciousness
2. A reversible state that provides analgesia, muscle relaxation, and sedation
3. Protective reflexes are lost
4. Produced by IV or inhaled anesthetics

Regional Anesthesia
1. Production of anesthesia in a specific body part
2. Achieved by injecting local anesthetics in close proximity (usually by injection) to appropriate nerves

Spinal Anesthesia
1. Local anesthetic is injected into lumbar intrathecal space.
2. Anesthetic blocks conduction in spinal nerve roots and dorsal ganglia; paralysis and analgesia occur below level of injection.

Epidural Anesthesia
1. Achieved by injecting local anesthetic into epidural space by way of a lumbar puncture
2. Results similar to spinal analgesia

Peripheral Nerve Blocks
Achieved by injecting local anesthetic to anesthetize the surgical site

Intraoperative Complications

1. Hypoventilation (hypoxemia, hypercarbia)—inadequate ventilatory support after paralysis of respiratory muscles and ensuing coma
2. Oral trauma (broken teeth, oropharyngeal, or laryngeal trauma)—due to difficult endotracheal intubation

3. Hypotension—due to preoperative hypovolemia or untoward reactions to anesthetic agents
4. Cardiac dysrhythmia—due to preexisting cardiovascular compromise, electrolyte imbalance, or untoward reactions to anesthetic agents
5. Hypothermia—due to exposure to cool ambient operating room environment and loss of normal thermoregulation capability from anesthetic agents
6. Peripheral nerve damage—due to improper positioning of patient (eg, full weight on an arm) or restraints
7. Malignant hyperthermia
   a. This is a rare reaction to anesthetic inhalants (notably enflurane, fluroxene, halothane, isoflurane) and muscle relaxants (eg, succinylcholine [Anectine]).
   b. Such drugs as theophylline (Theo-Dur), aminophylline (Aminophyllin), epinephrine (Adrenalin), and digoxin (Lanoxin) may also induce or intensify this reaction.
   c. This deadly complication is most likely to occur in younger people with an inherited muscle disorder (eg, forms of muscular dystrophy) or a history of subluxating joints, scoliosis.
   d. Malignant hyperthermia is due to abnormal and excessive intracellular accumulations of calcium with resulting hypermetabolism and increased muscle contraction.
   e. Clinical manifestations—tachycardia, pseudotetany, muscle rigidity, high fever, cyanosis, heart failure, and central nervous system damage
   f. Treatment—discontinue inhalent anesthetic; dantrolene sodium (Dantrium), oxygen, dextrose 50% (with extra insulin to enhance its utilization), diuretics, antiarrhythmics, sodium bicarbonate (for severe acidosis), and hypothermic measures (eg, cooling blanket, iced IV saline solutions, or iced saline lavages of stomach, bladder, or rectum)

POSTOPERATIVE CARE

Postanesthesia Care Unit (PACU)

To ensure continuity of care from the intraoperative phase to the immediate postoperative phase, the circulating nurse, anesthesiologist, or nurse anesthetist will give a thorough report to the PACU nurse. This should include the following:
1. Type of surgery performed and any intraoperative complications
2. Type of anesthesia (eg, general, local, sedation)
3. Drains and type of dressings
4. Presence of endotracheal (ET) tube or type of oxygen to be administered (eg, nasal cannula, T-piece)
5. Types of lines and locations (eg, peripheral IV, arterial line)
6. Catheters or tubes such as Foley, T-tube
7. Administration of blood, colloids, and fluid and electrolyte balance

8. Drug allergies
9. Preexisting medical conditions

Initial Nursing Assessment

Before receiving the patient, note proper functioning of monitoring and suctioning devices, oxygen therapy equipment, and all other equipment. The following initial assessment is made by the nurse in the PACU:
1. Verify the patient's identity, the operative procedure, and the surgeon who performed the procedure.
2. Evaluate the following signs and verify their level of stability with the anesthesiologist:
   a. Respiratory status
   b. Circulatory status
   c. Pulses
   d. Temperature
   e. Oxygen saturation level
   f. Hemodynamic values
3. Determine swallowing, gag reflexes, and level of consciousness, including patient's response to stimuli.
4. Evaluate any lines, tubes, or drains, estimated blood loss, condition of the wound (open, closed, packed), medications used, infusions, including transfusions, and output.
5. Evaluate the patient's level of comfort and safety by indicators such as pain and protective reflexes.
6. Perform safety checks to verify that side rails are in place and restraints properly applied, as needed, for infusions, transfusions, and so forth.
7. Evaluate activity status; movement of extremities.
8. Review health care provider's orders.

NURSING ALERT

It is important for the nurse to be able to communicate in the patient's language to provide an accurate assessment. Interpreters must be sought through the patient's family, hospital registry, Red Cross, or other agency.

Initial Nursing Diagnoses

- Ineffective Airway Clearance related to effects of anesthesia
- Impaired Gas Exchange related to ventilation–perfusion imbalance
- Altered Tissue Perfusion (Coronary) related to hypotension postoperatively
- Risk for Altered Body Temperature related to medications, sedation, and cool environment
- Risk for Fluid Volume Deficit related to blood loss, food and fluid deprivation, vomiting, and indwelling tubes
- Pain related to surgical incision and tissue trauma
- Impaired Skin Integrity related to invasive procedure, immobilization, and altered metabolic and circulatory state
- Risk for Injury related to sensory dysfunction and physical environment
- Sensory Alterations related to effects of medications and anesthesia

Initial Nursing Interventions
Maintaining a Patent Airway

1. Allow metal, rubber, or plastic airway to remain in place until the patient begins to waken and is trying to eject the airway.
   a. The airway keeps the passage open and prevents the tongue from falling backward and obstructing the air passages.
   b. Leaving the airway in after the pharyngeal reflex has returned may cause the patient to gag and vomit.

NURSING ALERT

Many seriously ill patients return from the operating room with an endotracheal tube in place; this may be left in place for hours or days and requires special management.

2. Aspirate excessive secretions when they are heard in the nasopharynx and oropharynx.

Maintaining Adequate Respiratory Function

1. Place patient in the lateral position with neck extended (if not contraindicated) and the upper arm supported on a pillow.
   a. This will promote chest expansion.
   b. Turn the patient every hour or two to facilitate breathing and ventilation.
2. Encourage patient to take deep breaths to aerate lungs fully and prevent hypostatic pneumonia; use incentive spirometer to aid in this function.
3. Assess lung fields frequently by auscultation.

STANDARDS OF CARE GUIDELINES
PACU Care

PACU or recovery room care is geared to recognizing the signs and anticipating and preventing postoperative difficulties. Carefully monitor the patient coming out of general anesthesia until:

1. Vital signs are stable for at least 30 minutes and are within normal range.
2. Patient is breathing easily.
3. Reflexes have returned to normal.
4. Patient is out of anesthesia, responsive, and oriented to time and place.

For the patient who had regional anesthesia, observe carefully until:

1. Sensation is restored and circulation is intact.
2. Reflexes have returned.
3. Vital signs have stabilized for at least 30 minutes.

This information should serve as a general guideline only. Each patient situation presents a unique set of clinical factors and requires nursing judgment to guide care, which may include additional or alternative measures and approaches.

4. Evaluate periodically the patient's orientation—response to name or command. *Note:* Alterations in cerebral function may suggest impaired oxygen delivery to tissues.
5. Administer humidified oxygen if required.
   a. Heat and moisture are normally lost during exhalation.
   b. Dehydrated patients may require oxygen and humidity because of higher incidence of irritated respiratory passages in these patients.
   c. Secretions can be kept moist to facilitate removal.
6. Use mechanical ventilation to maintain adequate pulmonary ventilation if required.

Assessing Status of Circulatory System

1. Take vital signs (blood pressure, pulse, and respiration) per protocol, as clinical condition indicates, until the patient is well stabilized. Then check every 4 hours thereafter or as ordered.
   a. Know the patient's preoperative blood pressure to make significant comparisons.
   b. Report immediately a falling systolic pressure and an increasing heart rate.
   c. Report variations in blood pressure, cardiac arrhythmias, and respirations over 30.
   d. Evaluate pulse pressure to determine status of perfusion. (A narrowing pulse pressure indicates impending shock.)
2. Monitor intake and output closely.
3. Recognize the variety of factors that may alter circulating blood volume.
   a. Reactions to anesthesia and medications
   b. Blood loss and organ manipulation during surgery
   c. Moving the patient from one position on the operating table to another on the stretcher
4. Recognize early symptoms of shock or hemorrhage.
   a. Cool extremities, decreased urine output (less than 30 mL/h), slow capillary refill (greater than 3 seconds), lowered blood pressure, narrowing of pulse pressure, and increased heart rate are often indicative of decreased cardiac output.
   b. Initiate oxygen therapy to increase oxygen availability from the circulating blood.
   c. Increase parenteral fluid infusion as prescribed.
   d. Place the patient in shock position with feet elevated (unless contraindicated).
   e. See Chapter 35 for more detailed consideration of shock.

Assessing Thermoregulatory Status

1. Monitor temperature hourly to be alert for malignant hyperthermia or to detect hypothermia.
2. A temperature over 37.7°C (100°F) or under 36.1°C (97°F) is reportable.
3. Monitor for postanesthesia shivering (PAS). It is most significant in hypothermic patients 30 to 45 minutes after admission to the PACU. It represents a heat-gain mechanism and relates to regaining thermal balance.

4. Provide a therapeutic environment with proper temperature and humidity; when cold, provide the patient with warm blankets.

Maintaining Adequate Fluid Volume

1. Administer IV solutions as ordered.
2. Monitor electrolytes and recognize evidence of imbalance, such as nausea and vomiting, weakness.
3. Evaluate mental status, skin color and turgor, and body temperature.
4. Recognize signs of fluid imbalance.
   a. Hypovolemia—decreased blood pressure and urine output, decreased central venous pressure (CVP), increased pulse
   b. Hypervolemia—increased blood pressure, changes in lung sounds such as crackles in the bases, and changes in heart sounds (eg, S_3 gallop), increased CVP
5. Monitor intake and output, including all drains. Observe for bladder distention.
6. Inspect skin and tissue surrounding maintenance lines to detect early infiltration. Restart lines immediately to maintain fluid volume.

Promoting Comfort

1. Assess pain by observing behavioral and physiologic manifestations.
2. Administer analgesics (change in vital signs may be a result of pain) and document efficacy.
3. Position the patient to maximize comfort.

Minimizing Complications
of Skin Impairment

1. Perform handwashing before and after contact with patient.
2. Inspect dressings routinely and reinforce if necessary.
3. Record amount and type of wound drainage (refer to Wound Care, p. 128).
4. Turn the patient frequently and maintain good body alignment.

Maintaining Safety

1. Keep side rails up until the patient is fully awake.
2. Protect the extremity into which IV fluids are running so the needle will not become accidentally dislodged.
3. Avoid nerve damage and muscle strain by properly supporting and padding pressure areas.
4. Recognize that the patient may not be able to complain of injury such as the pricking of an open safety pin or a clamp that is exerting pressure.
5. Check dressing for constriction.
6. Determine return of motor control following anesthesia—indicated by how the patient responds to a pinprick or a request to move a part.

Minimizing the Stress Factors
of Sensory Deficits

1. Know that the ability to hear returns more quickly than other senses as the patient emerges from anesthesia.
2. Avoid saying anything in the patient's presence that may be disturbing; patient may appear to be sleeping but still consciously hears what is being said.

3. Explain procedures and activities at the patient's level of understanding.
4. Minimize the patient's exposure to emergency treatment of nearby patients by drawing curtains and lowering voice and noise levels.
5. Treat the patient as a person who needs as much attention as the equipment and monitoring devices.
6. Respect the patient's feeling of sensory deprivation and overstimulation; make adjustments to minimize this fluctuation of stimuli.
7. Demonstrate concern for and understanding of the patient and anticipate needs and feelings.
8. Tell the patient repeatedly that the surgery is over and that he or she is in the recovery room.

Outcome-Based Evaluation

- Breathes easily
- Lung sounds clear to auscultation
- Vital signs stable
- Body temperature remains stable; minimal chills or shivering
- Intake and output are equal; no signs of volume imbalance
- Reports adequate pain control
- Wound edges intact without drainage
- Side rails up; positioned carefully
- Quiet, reassuring environment maintained

Transferring the Patient From the PACU
Transfer Criteria

Each facility may have an individual checklist or scoring guide used to determine a patient's readiness for transfer from the PACU based on the following:

1. Uncompromised cardiopulmonary status
2. Stable vital signs
3. Adequate urine output (at least 30 mL/h)
4. Orientation to person, place, events, and time
5. Satisfactory response to commands
6. Movement of extremities after regional anesthesia
7. Control of pain
8. Control or absence of vomiting

Transfer Responsibilities

1. Relay appropriate information to the unit nurse regarding condition; point out significant needs (eg, drainage, fluid therapy, incision and dressing requirements, intake needs, urinary output).
2. Physically assist in the transfer of the patient.
3. Orient patient to room, attending nurse, call light, and therapeutic devices.

■ Postoperative Discomforts

Most patients experience some discomforts postoperatively. These are usually related to the general anesthetic and the surgical procedure. The most common discomforts are nausea, vomiting, restlessness, sleeplessness, thirst, constipation, flatulence, and pain.

Nausea and Vomiting

Causes

1. Occurs in many postoperative patients
2. Most often related to inhalation anesthetics, which may irritate the stomach lining and stimulate the vomiting center in the brain
3. Results from an accumulation of fluid or food in the stomach before peristalsis returns
4. May occur as a result of abdominal distention, which follows manipulation of abdominal organs
5. Likely to occur if the patient believes preoperatively that vomiting will occur (psychological induction)
6. May be a side effect of narcotics

Preventive Measures

1. Insert nasogastric tube intraoperatively for operations on gastrointestinal tract to prevent abdominal distention, which triggers vomiting.
2. Determine whether patient is sensitive to morphine, meperidine (Demerol), or other narcotic because they may induce vomiting in some patients.
3. Be alert for any significant comment such as, "I just know I will vomit under anesthesia." Report such a comment to the anesthesiologist, who may prescribe an antiemetic drug and also talk to the patient before the operation.

Nursing Interventions

1. Encourage patient to breathe deeply to facilitate elimination of anesthetic.
2. Support the wound during retching and vomiting; turn patient's head to side to prevent aspiration.
3. Discard vomitus and refresh patient—mouthwash for mouth, clean linens for bed, and so forth.
4. Small sips of a carbonated beverage such as ginger ale, if tolerated or permitted.
5. Report excessive or prolonged vomiting so the cause may be investigated.
6. Maintain accurate intake and output record and replace fluids as ordered.
7. Detect presence of abdominal distention or hiccups, suggesting gastric retention.
8. Administer medications as ordered. Antiemetic medication such as prochlorperazine (Compazine), ondansetron HCl (Zofran), or promethazine (Phenergan) may be given; be aware that these drugs may potentiate the hypotensive effects of narcotics.
9. Consider accupressure as a nonpharmacologic method of relieving nausea. Wristbands that apply pressure 1 cm deep to the inner aspect of the wrists have been shown to reduce postoperative nausea by 10% over placebo.

◆ DRUG ALERT

Suspect idiosyncratic response to a drug if vomiting is worse when a medication is given (but diminishes thereafter).

Thirst

Causes

1. Inhibition of secretions by preoperative medication with atropine
2. Fluid lost by way of perspiration, blood loss, and dehydration due to preoperative fluid restriction

Preventive Measures

Unfortunately, postoperative thirst is a common and troublesome symptom that is often unavoidable due to anesthesia. The immediate implementation of nursing interventions is most helpful.

Nursing Interventions

1. Administer fluids by vein or by mouth if tolerated and permitted.
2. Offer sips of hot tea with lemon juice to dissolve mucus if diet orders allow.
3. Apply a moistened gauze square over lips occasionally to humidify inspired air.
4. Allow the patient to rinse mouth with mouthwash.
5. Obtain hard candies or chewing gum, if allowed, to help in stimulating saliva flow and in keeping the mouth moist.

Constipation and Gas Cramps

Causes

1. Trauma and manipulation of the bowel during surgery, as well as narcotic use, will retard peristalsis.
2. Local inflammation, peritonitis, or abscess
3. Long-standing bowel problem; this may lead to fecal impaction.

Preventive Measures

1. Encourage early ambulation to aid in promoting peristalsis.
2. Provide adequate fluid intake to promote soft stools and hydration.
3. Advocate proper diet to promote peristalsis.
4. Encourage early use of non-narcotic analgesia because many opiates increase chance of constipation.
5. Assess bowel sounds frequently.

Nursing Interventions

1. Ask patient about usual remedy for constipation and try it, if appropriate.
2. Insert gloved finger and break up the fecal impaction manually, if necessary.
3. Administer an oil retention enema (180–200 mL), if prescribed, to help soften the fecal mass and facilitate evacuation.
4. Administer a return-flow enema (if prescribed) or a rectal tube to decrease painful flatulence.
5. Administer gastrointestinal stimulants, laxatives, suppositories, and stool softeners, as prescribed.

■ Postoperative Pain

Pain is a subjective symptom in which the patient exhibits a feeling of distress. Stimulation of, or trauma to, certain nerve endings as a result of surgery causes pain.

General Principles

1. Pain is one of the earliest symptoms that the patient expresses on return to consciousness.
2. Maximal postoperative pain occurs between 12 and 36 hours after surgery and usually diminishes significantly by 48 hours.
3. Soluble anesthetic agents are slow to leave the body and therefore control pain for a longer time than insoluble agents; the latter produce rapid recovery, but the patient is more restless and complains more of pain.
4. Older people seem to have a higher tolerance for pain than younger or middle-aged people.
5. There is no documented proof that one sex tolerates pain better than the other.

Clinical Manifestations

1. Autonomic
   a. Elevation of blood pressure
   b. Increase in heart and pulse rate
   c. Rapid and irregular respiration
   d. Increase in perspiration
2. Skeletal muscle
   a. Increase in muscle tension or activity
3. Psychological
   a. Increase in irritability
   b. Increase in apprehension
   c. Increase in anxiety
   d. Attention focused on pain
   e. Complaints of pain
4. Patient's reaction depends on:
   a. Previous experience
   b. Anxiety or tension
   c. State of health
   d. Ability to concentrate away from the problem or be distracted
   e. Meaning that pain has for the patient

Preventive Measures

1. Reduce anxiety due to anticipation of pain.
2. Teach patient about pain management.
3. Review analgesics with patient and reassure that the pain relief will be available quickly.
4. Establish a trusting relationship and spend time with patient.

Nursing Interventions
Use Basic Comfort Measures

1. Provide therapeutic environment—proper temperature and humidity, ventilation, visitors.
2. Massage the patient's back and pressure points with soothing strokes—move patient easily and gently and with prewarning.
3. Offer diversional activities, soft radio music, or favorite quiet television program.
4. Provide for fluid needs by giving a cool drink; offer a bedpan.

5. Investigate possible causes of pain such as bandage or adhesive that is too tight, full bladder, cast that is too snug, or elevated temperature suggestive of inflammation or infection.
6. Instruct patient to splint wound when moving.
7. Keep bedding clean, dry, and free of wrinkles and debris.

Recognize the Power of Suggestion

1. Provide reassurance that the discomfort is temporary and that the medication will aid in pain reduction.
2. Clarify patient's fears regarding the perceived significance of pain.
3. Assist patient in maintaining a positive, hopeful attitude.

Assist in Relaxation Techniques

Imagery, meditation, controlled breathing, self-hypnosis/suggestion (autogenic training), and progressive relaxation

Apply Cutaneous Counterstimulation (Unless Contraindicated)

1. Vibration—a vigorous form of massage that is applied to a nonoperative site. It lessens patient's perception of pain. (Avoid applying this to calf, because doing so may dislodge an unheralded thrombus.)
2. Heat or cold—apply to operative or nonoperative site as prescribed. This works best for well-localized pain. Cold has more advantages than heat and fewer unwanted side effects (ie, burns). Heat works well with muscle spasm.

Give Analgesics as Prescribed in a Timely Manner

1. Instruct patient to request analgesic before the pain becomes severe.
2. If pain occurs consistently and predictably throughout a 24-hour period, analgesics should be given around the clock—avoiding the usual "demand cycle" of dosing that sets up eventual dependency and provides less adequate pain relief.
3. Administer prescribed medication to patient before anticipated activities and painful procedures (eg, dressing changes).
4. Monitor for possible side effects of analgesic therapy (eg, respiratory depression, hypotension, nausea, skin rash). Administer naloxone hydrochloride (Narcan) to relieve significant narcotic-induced respiratory depression.
5. Assess and document efficacy of analgesic therapy.

Pharmacologic Management
Oral and Parenteral Analgesia

1. Surgical patients are often prescribed a parenteral analgesic for 2 to 4 days or until incisional pain abates. At that time, an oral analgesic, narcotic or non-narcotic, will be prescribed.
2. Although the health care provider is responsible for prescribing the appropriate medication, it is the nurse's responsibility to ensure the drug is given safely and assessed for efficacy.

Patient-Controlled Analgesia (PCA)

1. Benefits
   a. Bypasses the delays inherent in traditional analgesic administration (the "demand cycle")
   b. Medication is administered by IV, producing more rapid pain relief and greater consistency in patient response.
   c. The patient retains control over pain relief (added placebo and relaxation effects).
   d. Decreased nursing time in frequent delivery of analgesics
2. Contraindications
   a. Patients under 10 to 11 years of age
   b. Patients with cognitive impairment (delirium, dementia, mental illness, hemodynamic or respiratory impairment)
3. A portable PCA device delivers a preset dosage of narcotic (usually morphine). An adjustable "lockout interval" controls the frequency of dose administration, preventing another dose from being delivered prematurely. An example of PCA settings might be a dose of 1 mg morphine with a lockout interval of 6 minutes (total possible dose is 10 mg/h).
4. Patient pushes a button to activate the device.
5. Instruction about PCA should occur preoperatively; some patients fear being overdosed by the machine and require reassurance.

Epidural Analgesia

1. Requires injections of narcotics into the epidural space by way of a catheter inserted by an anesthesiologist under aseptic conditions (Figure 7-2)
2. Benefits
   a. Produces effective analgesia without sensory, motor, or sympathetic changes
   b. Provides for longer periods of analgesia
3. Disadvantages
   a. The epidural catheter's proximity to the spinal nerves and spinal canal, along with its potential for catheter migration, make correct injection technique and close patient assessment imperative.
   b. Requires specific hospital protocol for injection and verification of nursing staff's injection technique
   c. Side effects include generalized pruritus (common), nausea, urinary retention, respiratory depression, hypotension, motor block, and sensory/sympathetic block. These side effects are related to the narcotic used (usually a preservative-free morphine [Duramorph] or fentanyl [Sublimaze]) and catheter position.
4. Strict asepsis is necessary when injecting the epidural catheter.
5. The catheter is initially aspirated gently; if blood or greater than 1 mL clear fluid is aspirated, hold injection and notify health care provider of possible catheter migration into spinal column.

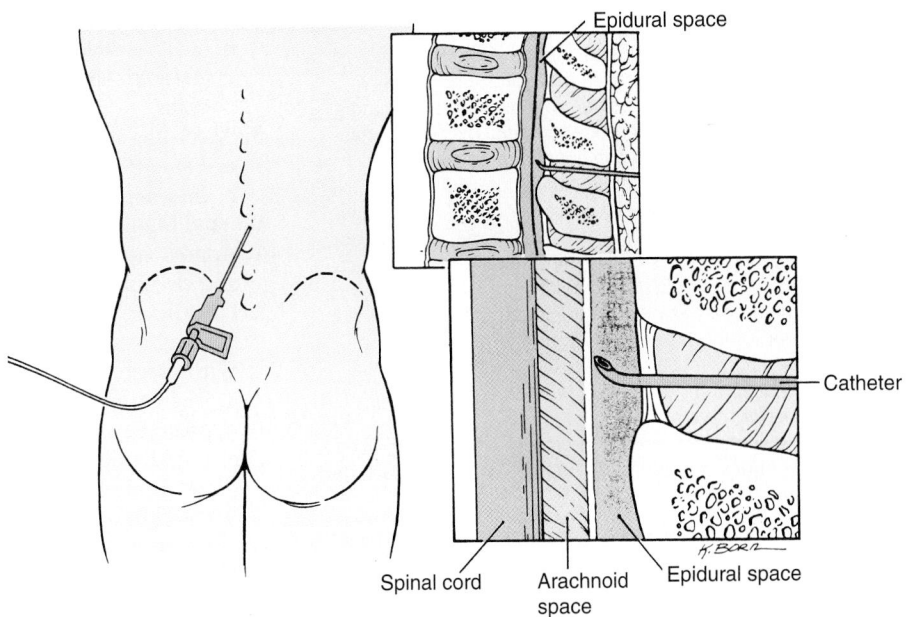

FIGURE 7-2 Epidural catheter placement.

6. Narcotic-related side effects are reversed with naloxone hydrochloride (Narcan).
7. The nurse ensures proper integrity of both the catheter and the dressing.
8. Occasionally, concurrent use of low-dose anesthetics such as bupivacaine (Marcaine) may be added to potentiate efficacy of epidural analgesia.

Postoperative Complications

Postoperative complications are a risk inherent in surgical procedures. They may interfere with the expected outcome of the surgery and may extend the patient's hospitalization and convalescence. The nurse plays a critical role in attempting to prevent complications and in recognizing their signs and symptoms immediately (see Standards of Care Guidelines). Implementing nursing interventions at an early stage of a complication is also of utmost importance.

STANDARDS OF CARE GUIDELINES
Preventing and Recognizing
Postoperative Complications

Care of the patient after surgery should include the following, until risk of complications has passed:

- Monitor vital signs (blood pressure, pulse, respirations, temperature, and level of consciousness) frequently until stable, and then periodically thereafter depending on the condition of the patient.
- Observe the wound site for drainage, odor, swelling, and redness, which could indicate infection.
- Observe the wound for intactness and stage of healing.
- Assess patient's pain level and monitor for unusual increase in pain (which may indicate infection or other problem) as well as oversedation related to narcotic administration.
- Monitor fluid status through vital signs, presence of edema, and intake and output measurements.
- Assess for presence of bowel sounds before resuming oral feedings, and monitor for abdominal distention, nausea, and vomiting, which could indicate paralytic ileus.
- Provide measures to enhance circulation of the lower extremities such as pneumatic compression, elastic wraps, range-of-motion exercises, and early ambulation, and assess for tenderness, swelling, and red streaking, which may indicate deep vein thrombosis.
- Assess pulmonary status including respiratory effort and rate; breath sounds; skin, mucous membrane, and nail bed color; and transcutaneous oxygen saturation.
- Ensure that patient is voiding regularly after surgery or after catheter removal.
- *Notify the surgeon if there is a significant deviation from the norm in any one of these parameters, or if a pattern of deviation is developing.*

This information should serve as a general guideline only. Each patient situation presents a unique set of clinical factors and requires nursing judgment to guide care, which may include additional or alternative measures and approaches.

Shock

Shock is a response of the body to a decrease in the circulating volume of blood; tissue perfusion is impaired culminating, eventually, in cellular hypoxia and death. (See p. 1076 for classification and emergency management of shock.)

Preventive Measures

1. Have blood available if there is any indication that it may be needed.
2. Measure accurately any blood loss and monitor all fluid intake and output.
3. Anticipate progression of symptoms on earliest manifestation.
4. Monitor vital signs per protocol until they are stable.
5. Assess vital sign deviations; evaluate blood pressure in relation to other physiologic parameters of shock and patient's premorbid values. Orthostatic pulse and blood pressure are important indicators of hypovolemic shock.
6. Prevent infection (eg, indwelling catheter care, wound care, pulmonary care) because this will minimize the risk of septic shock.

Hemorrhage

Hemorrhage is copious escape of blood from a blood vessel.

Classification

1. General
   a. *Primary*—occurs at the time of operation
   b. *Intermediary*—occurs within the first few hours after surgery. Blood pressure returns to normal and causes loosening of some ligated sutures and flushing out of weak clots from unligated vessels.
   c. *Secondary*—occurs some time after surgery due to ligature slip from blood vessel and erosion of blood vessel
2. According to blood vessels
   a. *Capillary*—slow general oozing from capillaries
   b. *Venous*—bleeding that is dark in color
   c. *Arterial*—bleeding that spurts and is bright red in color
3. According to location
   a. *Evident or external*—visible bleeding on the surface
   b. *Internal (concealed)*—bleeding that cannot be seen

Clinical Manifestations

1. Apprehension; restlessness; thirst; cold, moist, pale skin; and circumoral pallor
2. Pulse increases, respirations become rapid and deep ("air hunger"), temperature drops.
3. With progression of hemorrhage:
   a. Decrease in cardiac output and narrowed pulse pressure
   b. Rapidly decreasing blood pressure, as well as hematocrit and hemoglobin
   c. Patient grows weaker until death occurs.

Nursing Interventions and Management

1. Treat the patient as described for shock (see Chapter 35).
2. Inspect the wound as a possible site of bleeding. Apply pressure dressing over external bleeding site.

3. Increase IV fluid infusion rate and administer blood if necessary and as soon as possible.

Deep Vein Thrombosis

Deep vein thrombosis (DVT) occurs in pelvic veins or in deep veins of the lower extremities in postoperative patients. The incidence of DVT varies between 10% and 40% depending on the complexity of the surgery or the severity of the underlying illness. DVT is most common after hip surgery, followed by retropubic prostatectomy, and general thoracic or abdominal surgery. Venous thrombi located above the knee are considered the major source of pulmonary emboli.

Causes

1. Injury to intimal layer of the vein wall
2. Venous stasis
3. Hypercoagulopathy, polycythemia
4. High risks include obesity, prolonged immobility, cancer, smoking, estrogen use, advancing age, varicose veins, dehydration, splenectomy, and orthopedic procedures.

Clinical Manifestations

1. Majority of patients with DVT are asymptomatic.
2. Pain or cramp in the calf or thigh, progressing to painful swelling of entire leg
3. Slight fever, chills, perspiration
4. Marked tenderness over anteromedial surface of thigh
5. Intravascular clotting without marked inflammation may develop, leading to phlebothrombosis.
6. Circulation distal to the DVT may be compromised if sufficient swelling is present.

Nursing Interventions and Management

1. Hydrate the patient adequately postoperatively to prevent hemoconcentration.
2. Encourage leg exercises and ambulate the patient as soon as permitted by the surgeon.
3. Avoid any restricting devices such as tight straps that can constrict and impair circulation.
4. Avoid rubbing or massaging calves and thighs.
5. Instruct patient to avoid standing or sitting in one place for prolonged periods or crossing legs when seated.
6. Refrain from inserting IV catheters into legs or feet of adults.
7. Assess distal peripheral pulses, capillary refill, and sensation of lower extremities.
8. Check for positive Homans' sign—calf pain on dorsiflexion of the foot. This sign is present in nearly 30% of DVT patients.
9. Prevent the use of bed rolls or knee gatches in patients at risk because there is danger of constricting the vessels under the knee.
10. Initiate anticoagulant therapy either intravenously, subcutaneously, or orally, as prescribed.
11. Prevent swelling and stagnation of venous blood by applying appropriately fitting elastic stockings or wrapping the legs from the toes to the groin with elastic bandage.
12. Apply pneumatic stockings, intraoperatively, to patients at highest risk of DVT. Pneumatic stockings can reduce the risk of DVT by 30% to 50% (Figure 7-3).

Pulmonary Complications

Causes and Clinical Manifestations

1. Atelectasis
   a. Incomplete expansion of lung or portion of it occurring within 48 hours of surgery
   b. Attributed to absence of periodic deep breaths
   c. A mucous plug closes a bronchiole, causing alveoli distal to plug to collapse.
   d. Symptoms are often absent—may comprise mild to severe tachypnea, tachycardia, cough, fever, hypotension, and decreased breath sounds and chest expansion of affected side.
2. Aspiration
   a. Caused by inhalation of food, gastric contents, water, or blood into the tracheobronchial system.

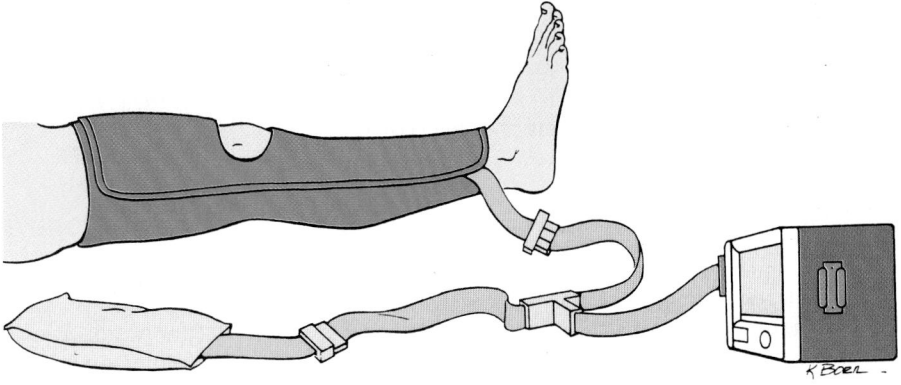

FIGURE 7-3 Pneumatic hose. Pressures of 35 mm Hg to 20 mm Hg are sequentially applied from ankle to thigh, producing an increase in blood flow velocity and improved venous clearing.

b. Anesthetic agents and narcotics depress the central nervous system, causing inhibition of gag or cough reflexes.

c. Nasogastric tube insertion renders both upper and lower esophageal sphincters partially incompetent.

d. Gross aspiration has a 50% mortality.

e. Symptoms depend on severity of aspiration; it may be silent. Usually evidence of atelectasis occurs within 2 minutes of aspiration. Other symptoms include tachypnea, dyspnea, cough, bronchospasm, wheezing, rhonchi, crackles, hypoxia, and frothy sputum.

3. Pneumonia

a. This is an inflammatory response in which cellular material replaces alveolar gas.

b. In postoperative patient, most often caused by gram-negative bacilli due to impaired oropharyngeal defense mechanisms.

c. Predisposing factors include atelectasis, upper respiratory infection, copious secretions, aspiration, dehydration, prolonged intubation or tracheostomy, history of smoking, impaired normal host defenses (cough reflex, mucociliary system, alveolar macrophage activity).

d. Symptoms include dyspnea, tachypnea, pleuritic chest pain, fever, chills, hemoptysis, cough (rusty or purulent sputum), and decreased breath sounds over involved area.

Preventive Measures

1. Report any evidence of upper respiratory infection to the surgeon.

2. Suction nasopharyngeal or bronchial secretions if patient is unable to clear own airway.

3. Prevent regurgitation and aspiration through proper patient positioning.

4. Recognize the predisposing causes of pulmonary complications:

a. Infections—mouth, nose, sinuses, throat

b. Aspiration of vomitus

c. History of heavy smoking, chronic pulmonary disease

d. Obesity

5. Avoid oversedation.

Nursing Interventions and Management

1. Monitor the patient's progress carefully on a daily basis to detect early signs and symptoms of respiratory difficulties.

a. Slight temperature, pulse, and respiration elevations

b. Apprehension and restlessness or a decreased level of consciousness

c. Complaints of chest pain, signs of dyspnea or cough

2. Promote full aeration of the lungs.

a. Turn the patient frequently.

b. Encourage the patient to take 10 deep breaths hourly, holding each breath to a count of 5 and exhaling.

c. Use a spirometer or any device that encourages the patient to ventilate more effectively.

d. Assist the patient in coughing in an effort to bring up mucous secretions. Have patient splint chest or abdominal wound to minimize discomfort associated with deep breathing and coughing.

e. Encourage and assist the patient to ambulate as early as the health care provider will allow.

3. Initiate specific measures for particular pulmonary problems.

a. Provide cool mist or heated nebulizer for the patient exhibiting signs of bronchitis or thick secretions.

b. Encourage patient to take fluids to help "liquefy" secretions and facilitate expectoration (in pneumonia).

c. Elevate the head of bed and ensure proper administration of prescribed oxygen.

d. Prevent abdominal distention—nasogastric tube insertion may be necessary.

e. Administer prescribed antibiotics for pulmonary infections.

Pulmonary Embolism
Causes

1. *Pulmonary embolism* (PE) is caused by the obstruction of one or more pulmonary arterioles by an embolus originating somewhere in the venous system or in the right side of the heart.

2. Postoperatively, the majority of emboli develop in the pelvic or iliofemoral veins before becoming dislodged and traveling to the lungs.

Clinical Manifestations

1. Sharp, stabbing pains in the chest

2. Anxiousness and cyanosis

3. Pupillary dilation, profuse perspiration

4. Rapid and irregular pulse becoming imperceptible—leads rapidly to death

5. Dyspnea, tachypnea, hypoxemia

6. Pleural friction rub (occasionally)

Nursing Interventions and Management

1. Administer oxygen with the patient in an upright sitting position (if possible).

2. Reassure and quiet the patient.

3. Monitor vital signs, ECG, and arterial blood gases.

4. Treat for shock or heart failure as needed.

5. Give analgesics or sedatives to control pain or apprehension.

6. Prepare for anticoagulation or thrombolytic therapy or surgical intervention. Management depends on the severity of the PE.

NURSING ALERT

Massive PE is life threatening and requires immediate interventions to maintain the patient's cardiorespiratory status.

Urinary Retention
Causes

1. Occurs postoperatively, especially after operations of the rectum, anus, vagina, or lower abdomen

2. Caused by spasm of bladder sphincter
3. More common in male patients owing to inherent increases in urethral resistance to urine flow
4. Can lead to urinary tract infection and possibly renal failure

Clinical Manifestations
1. Inability to void
2. Voiding small amounts at frequent intervals
3. Palpable bladder
4. Lower abdominal discomfort

Nursing Interventions and Management
1. Assist patient to sit or stand (if permissible) because many patients are unable to void while lying in bed.
2. Provide the patient with privacy.
3. Run the tap water—frequently, the sound or sight of running water relaxes spasm of the bladder sphincter.
4. Use warmth to relax sphincters (ie, sitz bath, warm compresses).
5. Notify physician if patient does not urinate regularly after surgery.
6. Administer bethanechol chloride (Urecholine) intramuscularly, if prescribed.
7. Catheterize only when all other measures are unsuccessful.

NURSING ALERT

Recognize that when a patient voids small amounts (30–60 mL every 15–30 minutes), this may be a sign of an overdistended bladder with "overflow" of urine.

Intestinal Obstruction
Bowel obstructions result in a partial or complete impairment to the forward flow of intestinal contents. Most obstructions occur in the small bowel, especially at its narrowest point—the ileum. (See p. 613 for full discussion of intestinal obstruction.)

Nursing Intervention and Management
1. Monitor for adequate bowel sound return after surgery. Assess bowel sounds and degree of abdominal distention (may need to measure abdominal girth); document these findings every shift.
2. Monitor and document characteristics of emesis and nasogastric drainage.
3. Relieve abdominal distention by passing a nasoenteric suction tube, as ordered.
4. Replace fluid and electrolytes.
5. Monitor fluid, electrolyte (especially potassium and sodium), and acid–base status.
6. Administer narcotics judiciously because these medications may further suppress peristalsis.
7. Prepare the patient for surgical intervention if obstruction continues unresolved.
8. Closely monitor patient for signs of shock.

9. Provide frequent reassurance to patient; use nontraditional methods to promote comfort (touch, relaxation, imagery).

Hiccups (Singultus)
Hiccups are intermittent spasms of the diaphragm causing the sound ("hic") that results from the vibration of closed vocal cords as air rushes suddenly into the lungs.

Causes
Irritation of the phrenic nerve between the spinal cord and terminal ramifications on undersurface of diaphragm
1. *Direct*—distended stomach, peritonitis, abdominal distention, pleurisy, tumors pressing on nerves
2. *Indirect*—toxemia, uremia
3. *Reflex*—exposure to cold, drinking very hot or very cold liquids, intestinal obstruction

Clinical Manifestations
1. Audible "hic"
2. Distress and fatigue
3. Vomiting
4. Wound dehiscence in severe cases

Nursing Interventions and Management
1. Remove the cause, if possible.
2. When removal of cause is not possible, remedies may include, if appropriate:
   a. Have patient swallow a large glass of water.
   b. Place tablespoon of coarse, granulated sugar on back of patient's tongue and have patient swallow it.
   c. Administer a phenothiazine drug such as prochlorperazine (Compazine) or chlorpromazine (Thorazine) as directed.
   d. Introduce a small catheter into the patient's pharynx (about 8–10 cm [3–4 inches]); rotate gently and jiggle back and forth.
   e. For rare, intractable hiccups, an extreme procedure is surgical alteration of the phrenic nerve.

Wound Infection
Wound infections are the second most common nosocomial infection. The infection may be limited to the surgical site (60%–80%) or may affect the patient systemically.

Causes
1. Drying tissues by long exposure, operations on contaminated structures, gross obesity, old age, chronic hypoxemia, and malnutrition are directly related to an increased infection rate.
2. The patient's own flora is most often implicated in wound infections (*Staphylococcus aureus*).
3. Other common culprits in wound infection include *Escherichia coli, Klebsiella, Enterobacter,* and *Proteus*.
4. Wound infections typically present 5 to 7 days postoperatively.
5. Factors affecting the extent of infection include:
   a. Kind, virulence, and quantity of contaminating microorganisms

b. Presence of foreign bodies or devitalized tissue

c. Location and nature of the wound

d. Amount of dead space or presence of hematoma

e. Immune response of the patient

f. Presence of adequate blood supply to wound

g. Presurgical condition of the patient (eg, elderly, alcoholism, diabetes, malnutrition)

Clinical Manifestations

1. Redness, excessive swelling, tenderness, warmth
2. Red streaks in the skin near the wound
3. Pus or other discharge from the wound
4. Tender, enlarged lymph nodes in axillary region or groin closest to wound
5. Foul smell from wound
6. Generalized body chills or fever
7. Elevated temperature and pulse
8. Increasing pain from incision site

GERONTOLOGIC ALERT

The elderly do not mount an inflammatory response to infection as readily, so may not present with fever, redness, and swelling. Increasing pain, fatigue, anorexia, and mental status changes are signs of infection in the elderly.

NURSING ALERT

Mild, transient fevers appear postoperatively due to tissue necrosis, hematoma, or cauterization. Higher sustained fevers arise with the following four most common postoperative complications: atelectasis (within the first 48 hours); wound infections (in 5–7 days); urinary infections (in 5–8 days); and thrombophlebitis (in 7–14 days).

Nursing Interventions and Management

1. Preoperative
   a. Encourage the patient to achieve an optimal nutritional level. Enteral or parenteral alimentation may be ordered preoperatively to reduce hypoproteinemia with weight loss.
   b. Reduce preoperative hospitalization to a minimum to avoid acquiring nosocomial infections.
2. Operative
   a. Follow strict asepsis throughout the operative procedure.
   b. When a wound has exudate, fibrin, desiccated fat, or nonviable skin, it is not approximated by primary closure but approximation is delayed (secondary closure).
3. Postoperative
   a. Keep dressings intact, reinforcing if necessary, until prescribed otherwise.
   b. Use strict asepsis when dressings are changed.
   c. Monitor and document amount, type, and location of drainage. Ensure that all drains are working properly. (See Table 7-1 for expected drainage amounts from common types of drains and tubes.)
4. Postoperative care of an infected wound

a. The surgeon removes one or more stitches, separates wound edges, and examines for infection using a hemostat as a probe.

b. A culture is taken and sent to the laboratory for bacterial analysis.

c. Wound irrigation may be done; have asepto syringe and saline available.

d. A drain may be inserted, or the wound may be packed with sterile gauze.

e. Antibiotics are prescribed.

f. Wet-to-dry dressings may be applied (see p. 129).

g. If deep infection is suspected, the patient may be taken back to the operating room.

Wound Dehiscence (Evisceration)

Causes

1. Commonly occurs between 5th and 8th day postoperatively when incision has weakest tensile strength; greatest strength is found between the 1st and 3rd postoperative day.
2. Chiefly associated with abdominal surgery.
3. This catastrophe is often related to the following:
   a. Inadequate sutures or excessively tight closures (the latter compromises blood supply)
   b. Hematomas; seromas
   c. Infections
   d. Excessive coughing, hiccups, retching, distention
   e. Poor nutrition; immunosuppression
   f. Uremia; diabetes mellitus
   g. Steroid use

Preventive Measures

1. Apply abdominal binder for heavy or elderly patients or those with weak or pendulous abdominal walls.
2. Encourage patient to splint incision while coughing.
3. Monitor for and relieve abdominal distention.

TABLE 7-1 Expected Drainage from Tubes and Catheters

Device	Substance	Daily Drainage
Foley catheter Ileal conduit Suprapubic catheter	Urine	500–700 mL/24 h first 48 h; then 1500–2500 mL/24 h
Gastrostomy tube	Gastric contents	Up to 1500 mL/24 h
Chest tube	Blood, pleural fluid, air	Varies: 500–1000 mL first 24 h
Ileostomy	Small bowel contents	Up to 4000 mL in first 24 h; then <500 mL/24 h
Miller-Abbott tube	Intestinal contents	Up to 3000 mL/24 h
Nasogastric tube	Gastric contents	Up to 1500 mL/24 h
T-tube	Bile	500 mL/24 h

4. Encourage proper nutrition with emphasis on adequate amounts of protein and vitamin C.

Clinical Manifestations

1. Dehiscence is heralded by sudden discharge of serosanguineous fluid from wound.
2. Patient complains that something suddenly "gave way" in the wound.
3. In an intestinal wound, the edges of the wound may part and the intestines may gradually push out. Observe for drainage of peritoneal fluid on dressing (clear or serosanguineous fluid).

Nursing Interventions and Management

1. Stay with the patient and have someone notify the surgeon immediately.
2. If intestines are exposed, cover with sterile moist saline dressings.
3. Monitor vital signs and watch for shock.
4. Keep the patient on absolute bed rest.
5. Instruct patient to bend knees, with head of bed elevated in semi-Fowler's position to relieve tension on abdomen.
6. Assure the patient that the wound will be properly cared for; attempt to keep patient quiet and relaxed.
7. Prepare the patient for surgery and repair of the wound.

Psychological Disturbances

Depression

1. Cause—perceived loss of health or stamina, pain, altered body image, various drugs, and anxiety about an uncertain future
2. Clinical manifestations—withdrawal, restlessness, insomnia, nonadherence to therapeutic regimens, tearfulness, and expressions of hopelessness
3. Nursing interventions and management
   a. Clarify misconceptions about surgery and its future implications.
   b. Listen to, reassure, and support patient.
   c. If appropriate, introduce patient to representatives of ostomy, mastectomy, or amputee support groups.
   d. Involve patient's partner and support people in care; psychiatric consultation is obtained for severe depression.

Delirium

1. Cause—prolonged anesthesia, cardiopulmonary bypass, drug reactions, sepsis, alcoholism (delirium tremens), electrolyte imbalances, and other metabolic disorders
2. Clinical manifestations—disorientation, hallucinations, perceptual distortions, paranoid delusions, reversed day–night pattern, agitation, insomnia; delirium tremens often appears within 72 hours of last alcoholic drink and may include autonomic overactivity—tachycardia, dilated pupils, diaphoresis, and fever.
3. Nursing interventions and management
   a. Assist with assessment and treatment of the underlying cause (restore fluid and electrolyte balance, discontinue offending drug, and so forth).
   b. Reorient to environment and time.
   c. Keep surroundings calm.
   d. Explain in detail every procedure done to patient.
   e. Sedate patient as ordered to reduce agitation, prevent exhaustion, and promote sleep. Assess for oversedation.
   f. Allow extended periods of uninterrupted sleep.
   g. Reassure family members with clear explanations of patient's aberrant behavior.
   h. Have contact with the patient as much as possible; apply restraints to patient only as last resort if safety is in question and if ordered by health care provider.

WOUND CARE

Wounds and Wound Healing

A *wound* is a disruption in the continuity and regulatory processes of tissue cells; *wound healing* is the restoration of that continuity. Wound healing, however, may or may not restore normal cellular function.

Wound Classification

Mechanism of Injury

1. *Incised wounds*—made by a clean cut of a sharp instrument, such as a surgical incision with a scalpel
2. *Contused wounds*—made by blunt force that typically does not break the skin but causes considerable tissue damage with bruising and swelling
3. *Lacerated wounds*—made by an object that tears tissues producing jagged, irregular edges; examples include glass, jagged wire, and blunt knife
4. *Puncture wounds*—made by a pointed instrument, such as an ice pick, bullet, and nail

Degree of Contamination

1. *Clean*—an aseptically made wound, as in surgery, that does not enter the alimentary, respiratory, or genitourinary tracts
2. *Clean-contaminated*—an aseptically made wound that enters the respiratory, alimentary, or genitourinary tracts. These wounds have slightly higher probability of wound infection than do clean wounds.
3. *Contaminated*—wounds exposed to excessive amounts of bacteria. These wounds may be open (avulsive) or accidentally made, or may be the result of surgical operations in which there are major breaks in aseptic techniques or gross spillage from the gastrointestinal tract.
4. *Infected*—a wound that retains devitalized tissue or involves preoperatively existing infection or perforated viscera. Such wounds are often left open to drain.

Physiology of Wound Healing

The phases of wound healing—inflammation, reconstruction (proliferation), and maturation—involve continuous and overlapping processes.

Inflammatory Phase (lasts 1–5 days)

1. Vascular and cellular responses are immediately initiated when tissue is cut or injured.
2. Transient vasoconstriction occurs immediately at the site of injury, lasting 5 to 10 minutes, along with deposition of a fibrinoplatelet clot to help control bleeding.
3. Subsequent dilation of small venules occurs; antibodies, plasma proteins, plasma fluids, leukocytes, and red blood cells leave the microcirculation to permeate the general area of injury, causing edema, redness, warmth, and pain.
4. Localized vasodilation is the result of direct action by histamine, serotonin, and prostaglandins.
5. Polymorphic leukocytes (neutrophils) and monocytes enter the wound to engage in destruction and ingestion of wound debris. Monocytes predominate during this phase.
6. Basal cells at the wound edges undergo mitosis; resultant daughter cells enlarge, flatten, and creep across the wound surface to eventually approximate the wound edges.

Proliferative Phase (lasts 2–20 days)

1. Fibroblasts (connective tissue cells) multiply and migrate along fibrin strands that are thought to serve as a matrix.
2. Endothelial budding occurs on nearby blood vessels, forming new capillaries that penetrate and nourish the injured tissue.
3. The combination of budding capillaries and proliferating fibroblasts is called *granulation tissue.*
4. Active collagen synthesis by fibroblasts begins by the 5th to 7th day, and the wound gains tensile strength.
5. By 3 weeks, skin obtains 30% of its preinjury tensile strength, the intestinal tissue about 65%, and fascia 20%.

Maturation Phase (21 days to months and even years)

1. Scar tissue is composed primarily of collagen and ground substance (mucopolysaccharide, glycoproteins, electrolytes, and water).
2. From the start of collagen synthesis, collagen fibers undergo a process of lysis and regeneration. The collagen fibers become more organized, aligning more closely to each other and increasing in tensile strength.
3. The overall bulk and form of the scar continue to change once maturation has started.
4. Typically, collagen production drops off; however, if collagen production greatly exceeds collagen lysis, keloid (greatly hypertrophied, deforming scar tissue) will form.
5. Normal maturation of the wound is clinically observed as an initial red, raised, hard immature scar that molds into a flat, soft, and pale mature scar.
6. The scar tissue will never achieve greater than 80% of its preinjury tensile strength.

Types of Wound Healing (Figure 7-4)

First Intention Healing (Primary Closure)

1. Wounds are made aseptic by minor débridement and irrigation, with a minimum of tissue damage and tissue reaction; wound edges are properly approximated with sutures.
2. Granulation tissue is not visible, and scar formation is typically minimal (keloid may still form in susceptible people).

Secondary Intention Healing (Granulation)

1. Wounds are left open to heal spontaneously or surgically closed at a later date; they need not be infected.
2. Examples in which wounds may heal by secondary intention include burns, traumatic injuries, ulcers, and suppurative infected wounds.
3. The cavity of the wound fills with a red, soft, sensitive tissue (granulation tissue), which bleeds easily. A scar (cicatrix) eventually forms.
4. In infected wounds, drainage may be accomplished by use of special dressings and drains. Healing is thus improved.
5. In wounds that are later resutured, two opposing granulation surfaces are brought together.
6. Secondary intention healing produces a deeper, wider scar.

◾ Wound Management

Many factors promote wound healing, such as adequate nutrition, cleanliness, rest, and position, along with the patient's underlying psychological and physiologic state. Of added importance is the application of appropriate dressings and drains. See Procedure Guidelines 7-1 and 7-2.

Dressings

Purpose of Dressings

1. To protect the wound from mechanical injury
2. To splint or immobilize the wound
3. To absorb drainage
4. To prevent contamination from bodily discharges (feces, urine)
5. To promote hemostasis, as in pressure dressings
6. To débride the wound by combining capillary action and the entwining of necrotic tissue within its mesh
7. To inhibit or kill microorganisms by using dressings with antiseptic or antimicrobial properties
8. To provide a physiologic environment conducive to healing
9. To provide mental and physical comfort for the patient

Advantages of Not Using Dressings

When the initial dressing on a clean, dry, and intact incision is removed, it is often not replaced. This may occur within 24 hours after surgery.

1. Permits better visualization of wound
2. Eliminates conditions necessary for growth of organisms (warmth, moisture, and darkness)

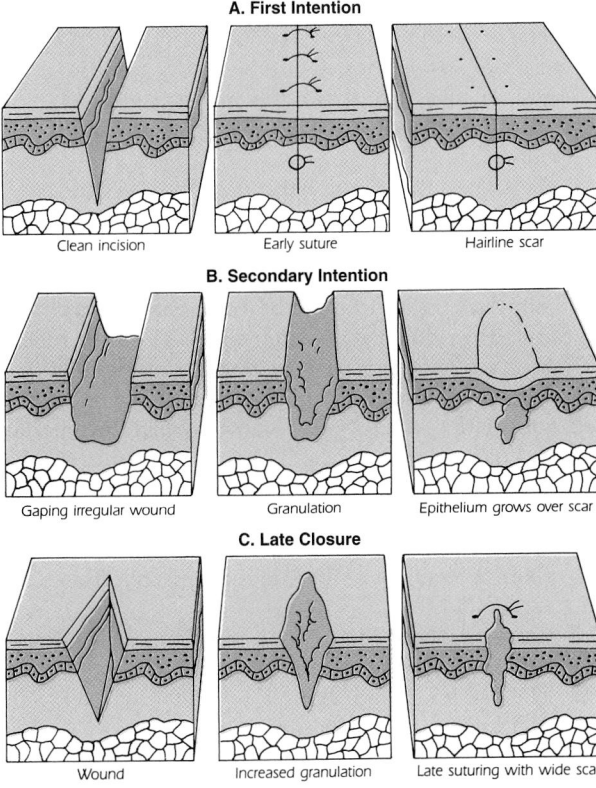

A. First Intention

Clean incision   Early suture   Hairline scar

B. Secondary Intention

Gaping irregular wound   Granulation   Epithelium grows over scar

C. Late Closure

Wound   Increased granulation   Late suturing with wide scar

FIGURE 7-4 Classification of wound healing. (**A**) First intention: A clean incision is made with primary closure; there is minimal scarring. (**B**) Second intention: The wound is left open so that granulation can occur; a large scar results. (**C**) Late closure: the wound is initially left open and later closed when there is no further evidence of infection.

3. Minimizes adhesive tape reaction
4. Is economical

Types of Dressings

1. Dry-to-dry dressings
   a. Used primarily for wounds closing by primary intention
   b. Offers good wound protection, absorption of drainage, and esthetics for the patient and provides pressure (if needed) for hemostasis
   c. Disadvantage—they adhere to the wound surface when drainage dries. Removal can cause pain and disruption of granulation tissue.
2. Wet-to-dry dressings
   a. These are particularly useful for untidy or infected wounds that must be débrided and closed by secondary intention.
   b. Gauze saturated with sterile saline (preferred) or an antimicrobial solution is packed into the wound, eliminating dead space.

c. The wet dressings are then covered by dry dressings (gauze sponges or absorbent pads).
   d. As drying occurs, wound debris and necrotic tissue are absorbed into the gauze dressing by capillary action.
   e. The dressing is changed when it becomes dry (or just before). If there is excessive necrotic debris on the dressing, more frequent dressing changes are required.
3. Wet-to-wet dressings
   a. Used on clean open wounds or on granulating surfaces. Sterile saline or an antimicrobial agent may be used to saturate the dressings.
   b. Provide a more physiologic environment (warmth, moisture), which can enhance the local healing processes as well as ensure greater patient comfort. Thick exudate is more easily removed.
   c. Disadvantage—surrounding tissues can become macerated, the risk of infection may rise, and bed linens become damp.

Types of Surgical Dressing Supplies

1. Hydrophobic occlusive (petrolatum gauze)
   a. This is an impermeable, nonadhering dressing that protects wounds from air- and moisture-borne contamination.
   b. It is used around chest tubes and any fistula or stoma that drains digestive juices.
   c. It is relatively nonabsorptive.
2. Hydrophilic permeable (oil-based gauze, Telfa pads)
   a. Allows drainage to penetrate dressing but remains somewhat nonadhering.
   b. For wounds with light to moderate exudate.
   c. Oil-based gauze used on abraded and open ulcerated or granulating wounds.
   d. May also be used to pack "caverns and sinuses" of large open wounds.
   e. Telfa pads are generally reserved for simple, closed, stable wounds.
3. Dressing sponges (Topper sponges or general-use gauze sponges)
   a. General-use gauze sponges come in various sizes (most commonly 2 × 2, 4 × 4 inches) and may be used for simple dry dressings, wet-to-dry dressings, or wet-to-wet dressings. Large-pore mesh allows for better absorption of drainage and necrotic wound debris.
   b. Topper sponges are primarily used over stable surgical incisions. Their smaller pore size and cotton filling make them less suitable for débriding activities.
4. All-absorbent combined dressing (Surgipad, ABD)
   a. Large (5 × 9 to 8 × 10 inches) cotton-filled dressing that is typically used as an "over-dressing," covering gauze or hydrophilic dressings for added wound protection, stabilization of dressings, and drainage absorption
   b. May also be used unaccompanied over intact surgical wounds

5. High-bulk gauze bandage ("fluffs")—primarily used for packing of large wounds undergoing healing by secondary intention
6. Drain sponge—similar to the Topper sponge except for the premade slit, which makes the dressing highly suitable for drain sites and tracheostomy sites
7. Transparent film dressing (Tegaderm, Op-Site)
   a. Highly elastic dressing, adjusts exceptionally well to body contours. It is permeable to oxygen and water vapor but generally impermeable to liquids and bacteria.
   b. Controversies surrounding its use (related to incidence of infection) have reduced its use.
   c. Most common indications include covering arterial and venous catheter sites as well as protecting vulnerable skin exposed to shearing forces.
   d. Is commonly used for surgical wounds over 4 × 4 dressing to replace tape.

Drains

Purpose of Drains

1. Drains are placed in wounds only when abnormal fluid collections are present or expected.
2. Drains are placed near the incision site:
   a. Usually in compartments (such as joints and pleural space) that are intolerant to fluid accumulation
   b. In areas with a large blood supply (such as the neck and kidney)
   c. In infected draining wounds
   d. In areas that have sustained large superficial tissue dissection (such as the breast)
3. Collection of body fluids in wounds can be harmful in the following ways:
   a. Provides culture media for bacterial growth
   b. Causes increased pressure at surgical site, interfering with blood flow to area
   c. Causes pressure on adjacent areas
   d. Causes local tissue irritation and necrosis (due to fluids such as bile, pus, pancreatic juice, and urine)

Wound Drainage

1. Drains are commonly made of Silastic and placed within either wounds or body cavities.
2. Drains placed within wounds are typically attached to portable (or, rarely, wall) suction with a collection container.
   a. Examples include the Hemovac, Jackson-Pratt, and Surgivac drainage systems.
3. Drains may also be used postoperatively to form hollow connections from internal organs to the outside to drain a body fluid, such as the T-tube (bile drainage), nephrostomy, gastrostomy, jejunostomy, and cecostomy tubes.
4. Drains act as foreign bodies; granulation tissue forms around them, walling them off rapidly.
5. Drains within wounds are removed when the amount of drainage decreases over a period of days or, rarely, weeks.
6. Fistula-forming tubes are often left in for longer periods of time.
   a. Careful handling of these drains and collection bags is essential.
   b. Accidental early removal may result in caustic drainage leaking within the tissues.
   c. The risk is reduced within 7 to 10 days when a wall of fibrous tissue has been formed.
7. The amount of drainage will vary with the procedure. Most common surgical procedures (eg, appendectomy, cholecystectomy, abdominal hysterectomy) have minimal wound drainage by the 3rd to 4th postoperative day. Drains are not commonly used after these operations.

NURSING ALERT

 The greatest amount of drainage is expected during the first 24 hours; closely monitor dressing and drains.

(text continues on page 134)

PROCEDURE GUIDELINES 7-1 **CHANGING SURGICAL DRESSINGS**

GENERAL CONSIDERATIONS

1. The procedure of changing dressings, then examining and cleansing the wound, uses principles of asepsis.

2. The initial dressing change is frequently done by the physician, especially for craniotomy, orthopedic, or thoracotomy procedures; subsequent dressing changes are the nurse's responsibility.

EQUIPMENT

STERILE

Gloves—disposable
Scissors, forceps (disposable packs available)
Appropriate dressing materials
Sterile saline

Cotton-tipped swabs
Culture tubes (if infection suspected)
For draining wound: add extra gauze and packing material, absorbent pads, and irrigation set

UNSTERILE

Gloves
Plastic bag for discarded dressings
Tape, proper size and type

Pads to protect patient's bed
Gown for nurse if wound is purulent/infected

PROCEDURE

PREPARATORY PHASE

1. Inform patient of dressing change. Explain procedure and have patient lie in bed.
2. Avoid changing dressings at mealtime.
3. Ensure privacy by drawing the curtains or closing the door; expose the dressing site.
4. Respect patient's modesty and prevent patient from being chilled.
5. Wash hands thoroughly.
6. Place dressing supplies on a clean, flat surface (overbed table).
7. If linen protection is needed, place clean towel or plastic bag under part of the body where wound is located.
8. Cut (or tear) off pieces of tape to be used in dressing change.
9. Place disposable bag nearby to collect soiled dressings.
10. Determine how many and what types of dressings are necessary. Open each dressing by peeling apart the edges of package (MAINTAIN STERILITY OF DRESSING). Leave each dressing within the open package.

Nursing Action	Rationale
REMOVING OLD DRESSING	
1. Don disposable gloves.	1. Unsterile gloves are sufficient if care is used not to touch wound.
2. Loosen all tape and gently pull tape ends toward the wound. It helps to hold skin taut with one hand while carefully peeling up an edge of the tape with the other hand. Wiping the back of tape with alcohol will hasten removal of "stuck" tape.	2. This process is less painful and less disturbing to the healing process (avoids pulling the wound edges apart and traumatizing sensitive skin).
3. Remove old dressings, one layer at a time, and place in disposable bag.	3. Hasty removal of dressings can cause trauma to wound and dislodge existing drains.
4. Removal of adherent dressings may be facilitated by moistening dressing with sterile saline.	4. This process is less painful and less traumatic to the delicate healing tissues.
OBTAINING A WOUND CULTURE	
1. Use aseptic technique.	1. To prevent contamination of a clean wound or culture media, or to prevent further contamination of a "dirty" wound.
2. Open sterile package of gloves; open package containing sterile syringe and needle; open package containing cotton-tipped culture swab. Keep all products within their sterile open packages until use.	2. Preparation for aseptic procedure.
3. Don sterile gloves.	
4. Aspirate generous amount of drainage liquid into syringe; inject into anaerobic tube. If liquid material is unobtainable, swab desired area with cotton-tipped culture swab, attempting to get maximum saturation.	4. It is important to collect culture specimen before wound is cleansed. The swab is the more common approach to wound cultures.
5. See that specimen is properly labeled and sent to laboratory for study.	
CLEANSING THE SIMPLE SURGICAL WOUND	
1. Use aseptic technique.	
2. Open package of sterile gloves; open sterile cleaning supplies (cotton-tipped applicators, sterile gauze sponges, sterile solution cup, sterile saline).	2. Preparation for aseptic procedure. Pour sterile cleansing solution (preferably saline) into the solution cup before donning sterile gloves.
3. Don sterile gloves.	
4. Clean along wound edges using a small circular motion from one end of the incision to the other; be sure to clean each side of the wound separately. Repeat the process using another moistened gauze or swab until the entire incision is cleansed. DO NOT SCRUB BACK AND FORTH ACROSS THE INCISION LINE.	4. To prevent contamination and mechanical trauma of wound.
5. Sterile saline is the cleansing agent of choice. Topical antiseptics (eg, povidone-iodine, hexachlorophene, alcohol, and boric acid) may be used on intact skin surrounding the wound but SHOULD NEVER BE USED WITHIN THE WOUND.	5. Most of the antiseptic agents are caustic to tissues and impair healing. The old saying "Never put anything in a wound that you couldn't put in your eye" is a truthful one.

continued

PROCEDURE GUIDELINES 7-1   CHANGING SURGICAL DRESSINGS *CONTINUED*

Nursing Action	Rationale
6. Repeat the same process with the drain site. Always clean the drain site separately from the primary incision site.	6. Reduces chance of cross-contamination.
7. Discard used cleaning supplies in the disposable bag.	7. This will be incinerated later.
8. Pat the incision site and drain site dry with a sterile dressing sponge.	8. To prepare wound for final dressing.

DRESSING THE WOUND

1. Maintain asepsis with use of sterile gloves.
2. After wound is dry, apply appropriate dressing, taking into consideration the nature of wound.
3. Tape dressing, using only the amount of tape required for secure attachment of dressing. Applying a "skin prep" on site to be taped can facilitate fixation and reduce irritation.

    3. Excessive use of tape can cause irritation and trauma to intact skin.

4. When *dressing the drain site:*
   a. Use premade drain sponge (can be prepared by making 5-cm [2-inch] slit, with sterile scissors, in 4 × 4-inch gauze sponge).

    a. The slit allows gauze to fit around the drainage tube.

   b. Gently slip sponge around drain; repeat process with second drain sponge, placing it at a right angle to the other sponge (see accompanying figure).

    b. Placement of the drain sponges in this manner allows for circumferential coverage of the drain site.

Dressing the drainage tube insertion site. Be sure that one sponge is placed at a right angle to the second sponge so the slits are going in different directions. If drainage is heavy, a sterile absorbent pad or extra gauze may be placed overall.

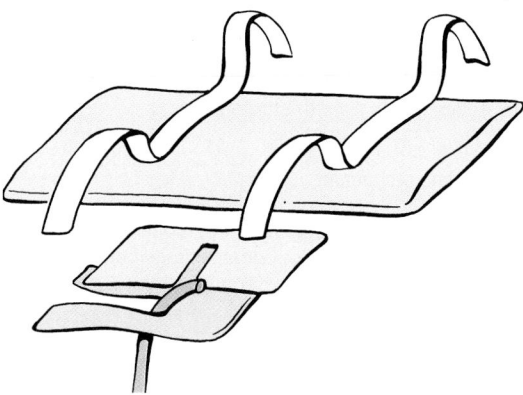

5. When *dressing an excessively draining wound:*
   a. Consider need for extra dressings and packing material.

    a. More dressing materials are needed to absorb excess fluid.

   b. Use Montgomery straps if frequent dressing changes are required (see accompanying figure).

    b. Frequent dressing changes can damage surrounding, intact skin owing to the frequent application and removal of tape. Montgomery straps alleviate the problem.

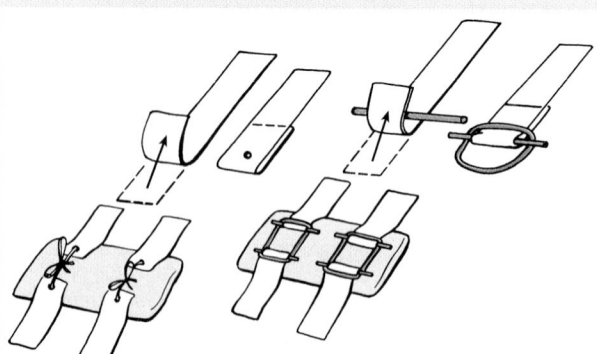

Montgomery straps; two styles are shown.

PROCEDURE GUIDELINES 7-1   *CONTINUED*

Nursing Action	Rationale
c. Excessively draining wounds may be "pouched," much like an ostomy bag.	c. To protect surrounding skin, save nursing time, and facilitate accurate assessment of drainage.
d. Protect skin surrounding wound from copious or irritating drainage (eg, gastrointestinal drainage) by applying some type of skin barrier.	d. Maintaining the cleanliness and integrity of surrounding tissue is essential for successful overall wound healing.

FOLLOW-UP CARE

1. Assess patient's tolerance to the procedure and help make patient more comfortable.	
2. Discard disposable items according to hospital protocol and clean equipment that is to be reused.	2. To prevent transmission of pathogenic organisms.
3. Wash hands.	
4. Record nature of procedure and condition of wound, as well as patient reaction.	

PROCEDURE GUIDELINES 7-2   **USING PORTABLE WOUND SUCTION**

EQUIPMENT

A calibrated collection container
Nonsterile gloves

Nursing Action	Rationale
1. When evacuator is full (200–800 mL—depending on size of evacuator), it is time to empty. A good rule is to empty every 8 h, or more frequently if necessary.	1. Negative pressure is dissipated as the evacuator fills.
2. Carefully remove plug, maintaining its sterility.	2. Minimizes risk of wound infection.
3. Empty contents of evacuator into calibrated container.	3. Measure drainage.
4. Place evacuator on flat surface.	4. To permit adequate compression.
5. Cleanse opening, as well as plug, with an alcohol sponge.	5. To maintain cleanliness of outlet.
6. Compress evacuator completely (see accompanying figure).	6. To remove air.

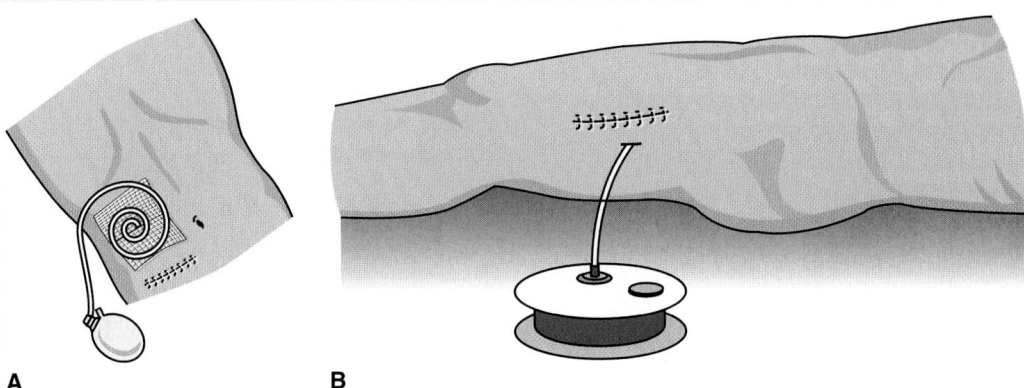

Types of surgical drains: (A) Jackson-Pratt, (B) Hemovac. Catheters drain the incision after surgery. Drainage is drawn into the portable wound-suction unit.

7. Replace plug while evacuator is compressed.	7. To reestablish negative pressure (suction).
8. As spring expands, a negative pressure of approximately 45 mm Hg is produced.	8. Any fluid and blood in tissues is sucked into evacuator. Negative pressure is not great enough to suck the soft tissues into the holes of the drainage catheter.

continued

PROCEDURE GUIDELINES 7-2   USING PORTABLE WOUND SUCTION *CONTINUED*

Nursing Action	Rationale
9. Check system for proper operation.	9. Look for fluid entering system; if none, look for disconnections.
10. Secure evacuator to patient's dressing; if patient is ambulatory, may fasten evacuator to clothing.	10. This permits patient to move without disturbing closed suction.
11. Ensure that the drainage catheters are positioned off of incisional site.	11. Minimizes trauma and contamination of wound.
12. Wash hands thoroughly.	12. To prevent cross-contamination with other patients and staff.
13. Record character and amount of drainage.	

■ Nursing Process Overview

Nursing Assessment

The wound should be assessed every 15 minutes while the patient is in the PACU. Thereafter, the frequency of wound assessment is determined by the nature of the wound, the degree of drainage, and the hospital protocol. Assessment and documentation of the wound's status should occur at least every shift until patient discharge.

Determine the following, which will affect wound healing:

1. What type of surgery did the patient have?
2. Was hemostasis in the operating room effective?
3. Has the patient received blood to sustain an adequate hematocrit (and promote perfusion to wound)?
4. What is the patient's age?
5. What is the nutritional status? What was it preoperatively?
   a. Is current intake of protein and vitamin C adequate?
   b. Is patient obese or cachectic?
6. What underlying medical conditions does patient have, and what medications is patient taking that could affect wound healing (eg, diabetes mellitus; steroids)?
7. How long has the patient been hospitalized preoperatively? (Longer preoperative hospital stays can increase complications.)
8. How is the wound held together?
   a. Staples, nylon sutures, adhesive strips, tension sutures?
   b. If the wound is left open, how is it being treated? Is granulation tissue present?
9. Are drains in place? What kind? How many?
   a. Is portable suction being used?
   b. Is the amount of drainage consistent with the nature of surgery?
10. What kinds of dressings are being used?
    a. Are they saturated?
    b. Is the amount and type of drainage consistent with nature of the surgery?
11. How does the wound appear?
    a. Is there evidence of edema, irritation, inflammation?
    b. Are the wound edges well approximated?
    c. Is the wound clean and dry?
12. How does the patient appear?
    a. Are there signs of wound pain or discomfort?
    b. Is fever or elevated white blood cell count present?
    c. Does patient express concern about the wound and potential disfigurement?
13. Does patient understand purpose of wound therapies, and can patient or significant other effectively carry out discharge instructions about wound care?

Nursing Diagnoses

- Risk for Infection related to surgical wound
- Impaired Tissue Integrity related to surgical wound
- Pain related to wound dressing procedures

Nursing Interventions

Preventing Infection

1. Ensure asepsis during dressing changes.
2. Reinforce or change dressings promptly when saturated with drainage.
3. Keep drainage tubing away from actual incision site.
4. Instruct patient to avoid touching incision to minimize wound contamination and injury.

Enhancing Tissue Integrity Through Healing

1. Assess patient's nutritional intake; consult with patient's health care provider if supplemental nutritional intake is required.
2. Minimize strain on incision site:
   a. Use appropriate tape, bandages, and binders.
   b. Have patient splint abdominal and chest incision when coughing.
   c. Instruct patient in proper way to get out of bed while minimizing incision strain (eg, for abdominal incision, turn on side and push self up with dependent elbow and opposite hand).
3. Assess and accurately document condition of incision site each shift.
4. Clarify patient's misconceptions of surgery and surgical incision.

5. Discuss the patient's feelings regarding the wound appearance and perceived disfigurement.

Relieving Pain

1. Give patient prescribed medication before painful dressing changes.
2. Continue to assess for pain from incision site.
3. Consider nonpharmacologic pain relief such as use of music therapy, relaxation exercises, and accupressure as indicated.

Patient Education

Before discharge, instruct patient and significant other on techniques and rationale for wound care.

1. Report immediately to health care provider if the following signs of infection occur:
   a. Redness, marked swelling (beyond ½ inch from incision site), tenderness, and increased warmth around wound
   b. Pus or unusual discharge, foul odor from wound
   c. Red streaks in skin near wound
   d. Chills or fever (over 37.7°C or 100°F)
2. Follow directives of the health care provider regarding activity allowances.
3. Keep suture line clean (may shower unless contraindicated by health care provider; avoid tub bathing until wound heals); never vigorously rub near suture line; pat dry.
4. Report to health care provider if after 2 months the incision site continues to be red, thick, and painful to pressure (probable beginning of keloid formation).

POSTOPERATIVE DISCHARGE INSTRUCTIONS

It is of primary importance that the nurse ensure that the patient has been given specific and individualized discharge instructions. These should be written by a provider and reinforced verbally by the nurse. A provider telephone contact should be included, as well as information regarding follow-up care and appointments. The instructions should be signed by the patient, provider, and nurse, and a copy becomes part of the patient's chart. Forms and procedures for discharge instructions may vary per facility.

■ Patient Education

Rest and Activity

1. It is common to feel tired and frustrated about not feeling able to do all the things you want; this is normal.
2. Plan regular naps and quiet activities, gradually increasing your exercise over the following weeks.
3. When you begin to exercise more, start by taking a short walk two or three times a day. Consult your health care provider if more specific exercises are required.

4. Climbing stairs in your home may be surprisingly tiring at first. If you have difficulty with this activity, try going upstairs backward ("scooching") on your "bottom" until your strength has returned.
5. Consult your health care provider to determine the appropriate time to return to work.

Eating

1. Follow dietary instructions provided at the hospital before your discharge.
2. It is not surprising to find that your appetite is limited at first or that you may feel bloated after meals; this should become less a problem as you become more active. (Some prescribed medications can cause this.) If symptoms persist, consult your health care provider.
3. Eat small, regular meals and make them as nourishing as possible to promote wound healing.

Sleeping

1. If sleeping is difficult because of wound discomfort, try taking your pain medication at bedtime.
2. Attempt to get sufficient sleep to aid in your recovery.

Wound Healing

1. Your wound will go through several stages of healing. After initial pain at the site, the wound may feel tingling, itchy, numb, or tight (a slight pulling sensation) as healing occurs.
2. Do not pull off any scabs because they protect the delicate new tissues underneath. They will fall off without any help when ready. Change the dressing according to surgeon's instructions.
3. Consult your health care provider if the amount of pain in your wound increases or if you notice increased redness, swelling, or discharge from wound.

Bowels

1. Irregular bowel habits can result from changes in activity and diet or the use of some drugs.
2. Avoid straining because it can intensify discomfort in some wounds; instead, use a rocking motion while trying to pass stool.
3. Drink plenty of fluids and increase the fiber in your diet through fruits, vegetables, and grains, as tolerated.
4. It may be helpful to take a mild laxative. Consult your health care provider if you have any questions.

Bathing, Showering

1. You may get your wound wet within 3 days of your operation if the initial dressing has already been changed (unless otherwise advised).
2. Showering is preferable because it allows for thorough rinsing of the wound.

3. If you are feeling too weak, place a plastic or metal chair in the shower so you may be seated during showering.
4. Be sure to dry your wound thoroughly with a clean towel and dress it as instructed before discharge.

Clothing

1. Avoid tight belts and underwear and other clothes with seams that may rub against the wound.
2. Wear loose clothing for comfort and to reduce mechanical trauma to wound.

Driving

It is important to ask your health care provider when you may resume driving. Safe driving may be affected by your pain medication. In addition, any violent jarring from an accident may disrupt your wound.

Bending and Lifting

1. How much bending, stretching, and lifting you are allowed depends on the location and nature of your surgery.
2. Typically, for most major surgeries, you should avoid lifting anything heavier than 5 lb for 4 to 8 weeks.
3. It is ideal to secure home assistance for the first 2 to 3 weeks after discharge.

SELECTED REFERENCES

American Society of PeriAnesthesia Nurses. (1999). *Standards of perianesthesia nursing practice.* Richmond, VA: Author.

Association of Perioperative Registered Nurses. (2000). *AORN standards and recommended practices for perioperative nursing.* Denver: Author.

Drain, C. B. (1994). *The post anesthesia care unit* (3rd ed.). Philadelphia: W. B. Saunders.

Erwin-Toth, P., & Hocevar, J. (1995). Wound care: Selecting the right dressing. *American Journal of Nursing, 95*(2), 46–51.

Fairchild, S. S. (1996). *Perioperative nursing, principles and practice.* Boston: Jones and Bartlett.

Ferrara-Love, R., Sekeres, L., & Bircher, N. C. (1998). Nonpharmacologic treatment of postoperative nausea. *Journal of Perianesthesia Nursing, 11*(6), 376–383.

Good, M., Stanton-Hicks, M., et al. (1999). Relief of postoperative pain with jaw relaxation, music, and their combination. *Pain, 81*(1–2), 163–172.

Kaiser, K. S. (1992). Assessment and management of pain in the critically ill trauma patient. *Critical Care Nursing Quarterly, 15*(2), 14–34.

Knoerl, D. V., Faut-Callahan, M., Paice, J., & Shott, S. (1999). Preoperative PCA teaching program to manage postoperative pain. *MEDSURG Nursing, 8*(1), 25–33, 36.

Litwick, K. (1994). *Core curriculum for post anesthesia nursing practice* (3rd ed.). Philadelphia: W. B. Saunders.

Meeker, M. H. (1995). *Alexander's care of the patient in surgery* (10th ed.). St. Louis: C. V. Mosby

Mimnaugh, L., Winegar, M., Mabrey Y., & Davis J. E. (1999). Sensations experienced during removal of tubes in acute postoperative patients. *Applied Nursing Research, 12*(2), 78–85.

Murphy, J. M. (1999). Preoperative consideration with herbal medicines. *AORN Journal, 69*(1), 173–183.

OR Manager. (1998). Campaign to end wrong-site surgery. *OR Manager, 14*(8), 7.

Pasero, C., Portenoy R. K., & McCaffery M. (1999). Using continuous infusion with PCA. *American Journal of Nursing, 99*(2), 22.

Pica-Furey, W. (1993). Ambulatory surgery—Hospital based versus freestanding. *AORN Journal, 57*(5), 1119–1127.

Roth, R. A. (1995). *Perioperative nursing core curriculum.* Philadelphia: W. B. Saunders.

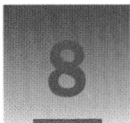

Cancer Nursing

GENERAL CONSIDERATIONS

Cancer is a disease of the cell in which the normal mechanisms of control of growth and proliferation are disturbed. This results in distinctive morphologic alterations of the cell and aberrations in tissue patterns.

The malignant cell is able to invade the surrounding tissue and regional lymph nodes. Primary cancer usually has a predictable natural history and pattern of spread.

Metastasis is the secondary growth of the primary cancer in another organ. The cancer cell migrates through a series of steps to another area of the body. This is the reason that cancer cannot always be cured by surgical removal alone. Most patients die as a result of metastases rather than progression of the primary cancer. Metastasis begins with local invasion followed by detachment of cancer cells that disseminate via the lymphatics and blood vessels and eventually establish a secondary tumor in another area of the body. Lymph nodes are often the first site of distant spread (Table 8-1).

■ Etiology, Detection, and Prevention

Epidemiology

1. In 1999, 1,2221,800 new cases of invasive cancer were reported and 563,100 deaths occurred. Although overall cancer incidence has decreased in the past 5 years, African Americans continue to have a higher incidence of cancer.
2. Age is the most outstanding risk factor for cancer.
   a. Cancer incidence increases progressively with age.
   b. Approximately 79% of persons diagnosed with cancer are over 55 years of age.
3. 80% of all cancers in America are related to lifestyle habits (i.e., smoking, alcohol consumption, diet) and environmental carcinogens.
   a. 90% of all cases of lung cancer are due to smoking.
   b. Excess alcohol intake is associated with cancers of the mouth, larynx, throat, esophagus, and liver, especially when combined with smoking.
   c. Exposure to carcinogens such as asbestos, benzene and radiation increases the risk of developing certain types of cancer.
   d. Solar ultraviolet radiation exposure is related to an increased risk of skin cancers.
4. There is a hereditary predisposition to specific forms of cancers that have been linked to certain events within a gene (i.e., BRCA1 and BRCA2 in breast cancer).
5. Infections and viruses are associated with an increased risk of certain forms of cancer.
   a. Human papilloma virus—cervical cancer
   b. Epstein-Barr virus—lymphoma
   c. Hepatitis B and C—hepatocellular cancer
   d. *Helicobacter pylori*—may be linked to gastric cancer
6. Five-year survival rates are increasing with improved therapy and earlier detection.
7. Ongoing genetic research is searching for the ability to correct and modify hereditary susceptibility.
8. Patterns of incidence and death rates vary with sex, age, race, and geographic location (Table 8-2).

Nutrition and Cancer

GERONTOLOGIC ALERT

 Elderly patients, especially those who live alone, may be malnourished before the initiation of therapy. Dietary consultation may be crucial before therapy.

1. Diet does influence the risk of cancer.
   a. High intake of fats may be associated with breast, colon, and prostate cancer.
   b. Low intake of fruit, vegetables, complex carbohydrates, and fiber is linked with cancer of the colon, larynx, esophagus, prostate, bladder, stomach, and lung.
   c. Salt-cured foods may influence cancers of the esophagus and stomach.

TABLE 8-1 Differences Between Malignant and Benign Tumors

Characteristic	Benign	Malignant
Growth	Slow, expansive	Invasive
Differentiation	Fully differentiated	Immature, poorly differentiated
Metastasis	Absent	Present

  d. Obesity is linked to cancers of the breast, colon, uterus, and gallbladder.
2. The role of heredity also is acknowledged.
3. The Unified Dietary Guidelines, established in July 1999, are a joint recommendation of the American Heart Association, the American Cancer Society (ACS), the American Dietetic Society, the American Academy of Pediatrics, and the National Institutes of Health. These guidelines closely follow the U.S. Department of Agriculture's Food Pyramid (Figure 8-1). Under the Unified Dietary Guidelines, a healthy diet would include:
  a. No more than 10% of total calories from saturated fat

TABLE 8-2 Leading Sites of Cancer Incidence and Death—1999 Estimates

Male	Female
Cancer Incidence by Site and Sex*	
Prostate 179,300	Breast 175,000
Lung 94,000	Lung 77,600
Colon 43,000	Colon 51,700
Bladder 39,100	Uterine 50,200
Lymphoma 36,400	Lymphoma 27,600
Melanoma 25,800	Ovarian 25,200
Oral 20,000	Melanoma 18,400
Rectal 19,400	Bladder 15,100
Kidney 17,800	Rectal 15,300
Leukemia 16,800	Pancreas 14,600
Pancreas 14,000	Thyroid 13,500
Stomach 13,700	Oral 9,800
All sites 623,800	*All sites 598,000*
Cancer Deaths by Site and Sex	
Lung 90,900	Lung 68,000
Prostate 37,000	Breast 43,300
Colon 23,000	Colon 24,900
Lymphoma 14,100	Pancreas 14,700
Pancreas 13,900	Ovarian 14,500
Leukemia 12,400	Lymphoma 12,900
Liver 8,400	Uterine 11,200
Bladder 8,100	Leukemia 9,700
Stomach 7,900	Brain 5,900
Brain 7,200	Multiple myeloma 5,600
Multiple myeloma 5,800	Kidney 4,700
Oral 5,400	Bladder 4,000
Rectal 4,800	Oral 2,700
All sites 291,100	*All sites 272,000*

*Excluding basal and squamous cell skin cancer and carcinoma in situ (American Cancer Society, 1999).

  b. No more than 30% of total calories from fat; 55% of total calories should come from complex carbohydrates, such as cereals, grains, fruits, and vegetables
  c. Dietary cholesterol should not exceed 300 mg/day
  d. Salt consumption should be limited to 6 g/day (one teaspoon)

Detection and Prevention
Primary prevention and secondary prevention are effective measures in decreasing mortality and morbidity of many cancers. Most cancers, however, are diagnosed after a reported symptom(s). The ACS recommends specific primary and secondary prevention measures to reduce an individual's risk of cancer (Table 8-3).

Primary Prevention
The assessment or reduction of risk factors before the disease occurs:
1. Make appropriate lifestyle changes.
2. Stop smoking.
3. Limit alcohol intake.
4. Eat a healthy diet: five or more servings of fruits and vegetables per day; eat other foods from plant sources: cereals, grains, rice, pasta or beans several times a day; limit fat foods, particularly animal sources.
5. Be physically active: maintain a healthy weight and participate in 20 to 30 minutes of exercise four to five days a week.
6. Avoid sun exposure, especially during the hours of 10 a.m. and 3 p.m.
7. Those at high risk for certain cancers should consider genetic counseling and testing.
8. Chemoprevention.
  a. Aspirin—low doses of ASA or NSAIDs (16 or more doses/month for at least 1 year) may protect against the development of colon cancer.
  b. Tamoxifen—can reduce the risk of breast cancer in women who are at high risk by nearly 50%.
  c. Finisteride—may prevent prostate cancer. This is currently under investigation.
  d. Certain other chemopreventive compounds are under investigation, i.e., selenium, vitamin E, and synthetic retinoids.

Secondary Prevention
Screening and early detection to improve overall outcome and survival:
1. Performing routine screening tests should be based on whether these tests are adequate to detect a potentially curable cancer in an otherwise asymptomatic person and are also cost effective.
2. Although all major authorities recommend routine screening for certain types of cancer, each has a different opinion on when screening should begin and how often.
3. Screening should be based on an individual's age, sex, family history of cancer, ethnic group or race, previous iatrogenic factors (prior radiation therapy or drugs such as DES), and history of exposure to environmental carcinogens.

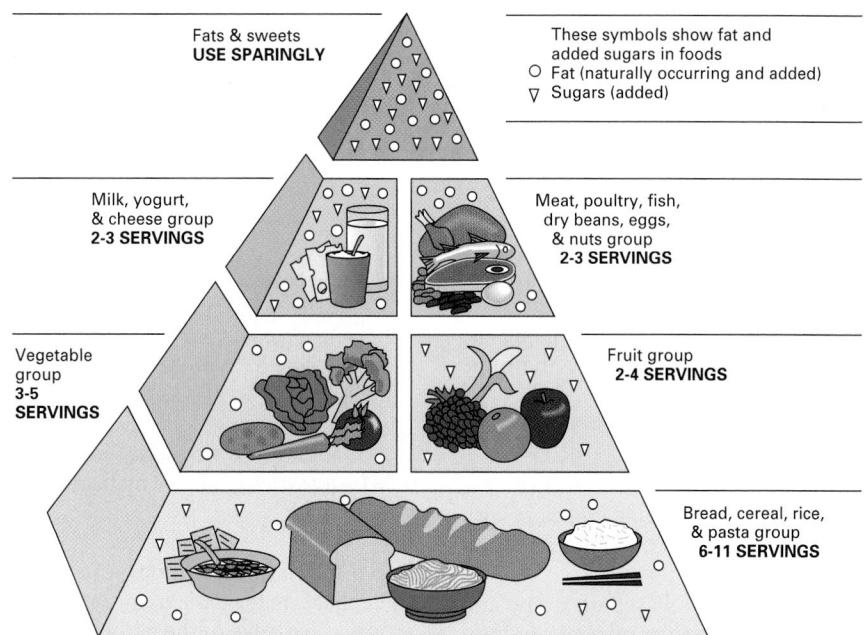

FIGURE 8-1 Dietary guidelines for cancer prevention. (U.S. Department of Agriculture/U.S. Department of Health and Services.)

a. Testicular cancer is the most common cancer of men between the ages of 15 and 34. Men with undescended testicles, Klinefelter syndrome, or exposure to diethylstilbestrol are at greatest risk. The American Urological Association (AUA) recommends annual screening beginning at age 15.

b. Prostate cancer occurs more commonly in men over age 60. With more widespread screening, younger men are being diagnosed in the early stages of the disease. The ACS and AUA recommend an annual PSA and digital rectal exam for men over age 50. The AUA also recommends annual testing for men aged

40 and over who are at high risk (African American, family history of prostate cancer).

c. Breast cancer is the most common type of cancer in women, and the incidence increases with age. The ACS recommends a clinical breast examination every 3 years from ages 20 to 39 and annually thereafter. Mammography should begin at age 40, but women with a first-degree relative with breast cancer should begin at age 35.

d. Colon cancer screening should begin with an annual digital rectal examination for all men and women over 40. Patients should be screened with sigmoidos-

TABLE 8-3 Recommendations for the Early Detection of Cancer in Asymptomatic Persons

Cancer Site	Test	Age	Frequency
Skin	Skin assessment	20–39	Every 3 years
		<40	Annually
Colon/rectal	Digital rectal exam/fecal occult test	40	Annually
	Sigmoidoscopy	50	Every 3 years
	Colonoscopy	50	Every 5 years
Cervix	Pelvic exam/Pap test	Onset of sexual activity or age 18	Yearly
Mouth	Oral exam	20–39	Every 3 years
		40	Annual
Prostate	Digital rectal exam/PSA	50	Annual
Breast	Self-breast exam	Any age	Monthly
	Clinical breast exam	Any age	Every 3 years
	Mammogram	35–39	Baseline
		40 and over	Annual
Testicular	Self-exam	Age 15–35	Annual

copy every 3 to 5 years beginning at age 50. Those at high risk should be screened with colonoscopy every 5 years.

  e. Lung cancer, although common in both men and women who have smoked, is not routinely screened for because there is no cost-effective method that would detect cancer early enough to make a difference in outcome.

Diagnostic Evaluation

1. Complete medical history and physical examination.
2. Biopsy of tumor site to determine pathologic diagnosis.
   a. The malignancy is classified according to anatomic extent and histopathologic analysis.
   b. Biopsy is obtained from the most accessible site (e.g., lymph node versus lung biopsy).
   c. All original slides should be reviewed with the pathologist. Clinical information should correlate with pathologic diagnosis. Be aware of possible errors and differences in interpretation.
   d. Classification of tumor type is based on tissue and cellular staining. Differences in cytoplasmic and nuclear staining distinguish one cell type from another and identify their stage of differentiation. The grade of the tumor (rating of 1 to 4) is based on how well differentiated the tissue or cells appear. For most tumors the higher grade, the less differentiated, which is associated with poorer prognosis.
   e. Flow cytometry testing of tumor tissue determines DNA content and indicates potential risk of recurrence.
   f. Estrogen/progesterone levels are obtained from breast tissue.
3. Laboratory tests including complete blood count (CBC) with differential, platelet count, and blood chemistries including liver function tests, blood urea nitrogen (BUN), and creatinine are done to determine baseline values.
   a. Further tests depend on cancer diagnosis.
   b. Blood markers (α-fetoprotein, β-human chorionic gonadotropin, CA15-3, CA125, etc.) may be appropriate to follow response to therapy.
4. Imaging procedures—chest x-ray, nuclear medicine scan, computed tomography (CT) scans, magnetic resonance imaging (MRI)—are used to determine evidence or extent of metastasis.

Staging

Staging is necessary at the time of diagnosis to determine the extent of disease (local versus metastatic), to determine prognosis, and to guide proper management.

1. The American Joint Committee of Cancer (AJCC) has developed a simple classification system (TNM) that can be applied to all tumor types. It is a numerical assessment of tumor size (T), presence or absence of regional lymph node involvement (N), and presence or absence of distant metastasis (Box 8-1).

BOX 8-1 AJCC Classification System of Tumors

T—primary tumor
Tx—primary tumor is unable to be assessed
T0—no evidence or primary tumor
Tis—carcinoma in situ
T1, T2, T3, T4—increasing size and/or local extent of primary tumor

N—presence or absence or regional lymph node involvement
Nx—regional lymph nodes are unable to be assessed
N0—no regional lymph node involvement
N1, N2, N3—increasing involvement of regional lymph nodes

M—absence or presence or distant metastasis
Mx—unable to assess
M0—absence of distant metastasis
M1—presence of distant metastasis

---

2. No standard evaluation exists for all cancers. Work-up depends on the patient, tumor type, symptoms, and medical knowledge of the natural history of that cancer.

MANAGEMENT

The method of treatment depends on the type of malignancy, the specific histologic cell type, stage, presence of metastasis, and condition of the patient. Cancer is treated by surgery, chemotherapy, radiation, or immunotherapy or by a combination of these modalities.

▣ Surgical Management

The principles of surgical management are based on a cooperative, multidisciplinary approach to various surgical resources. This is key to the management of the cancer patient. A surgical intervention usually provides the initial diagnosis; subsequent procedures may be needed for treatment.

Types of Surgical Procedures

1. Biopsy is surgical removal of a piece of tissue from the questionable area; the tissue sample is sent to the pathology laboratory for diagnostic verification.
2. Excisional biopsy is performed on small tumors to remove the entire mass and a small margin of normal tissues.
3. Reconstructive/rehabilitative surgery is the repair of defects from previous radical surgical resection; can be performed early (breast reconstruction) or delayed (head and neck surgery).
4. Palliative surgery is surgery that attempts to relieve the complications of cancer (e.g., obstruction of the gastrointestinal tract, pain produced by tumor extension into surrounding nerves).
5. Treatment of primary tumor is the removal of the primary site of malignancy. The goal of therapy is cure.

This depends on the biology of that particular cancer (e.g., basal cell carcinoma of the skin, early tumors of the rectum or colon).

6. Resection of metastases is used only in selected cases when a cure can be obtained or a reasonable prolongation of survival is possible. The primary cancer must be under control. The decision to proceed is influenced by the type of histology, number of lesions, their location, and whether they are bilateral.

7. Preventive/prophylactic surgery is the removal of lesions that, if left in the body, are at risk of developing into cancer. An example is polyps in the rectum.

8. Curative surgery is the removal of the primary site of malignancy and any lymph nodes to which the neoplasm has extended. Such surgery may be all that is required.

9. Debulking surgery is the removal of the bulk of the tumor; should be performed before the start of chemotherapy whenever possible.

▪ Chemotherapy for Cancer

Chemotherapy is the use of antineoplastic drugs to promote tumor cell destruction by interfering with cellular function and reproduction. It includes the use of various chemotherapeutic agents and hormones.

Principles of Chemotherapy Administration

1. The intent of chemotherapy is to destroy as many tumor cells as possible with minimal effect on healthy cells.

2. The goals of chemotherapy:
   a. Curative—complete response of the tumor.
   b. Control—to extend the life of the patient when a cure is not possible.
   c. Palliation—reduction of tumor burden to relieve symptoms such as pain and improve quality of life.

3. Chemotherapeutic agents can be effective on one of the four phases of the cell cycle or during any phase of the cell cycle. The cell cycle is divided into four stages:
   a. G1 (gap one) phase: RNA and protein synthesis (enzymes for DNA synthesis are manufactured)
   b. S (synthesis) phase: During a long time period the DNA component doubles for the chromosomes in preparation for cell division.
   c. G2 (gap two) phase: This is a short time period; protein and RNA synthesis occurs, and the mitotic spindle apparatus is formed.
   d. M (mitosis) phase: In an extremely short time period, the cell actually divides into two identical daughter cells.
   e. Cells not active in the cell cycle are designated as "resting" (G0). Cells in this phase are, for the most part, refractory to chemotherapy.

4. Therapeutic strategies:
   a. Adjuvant therapy is administered when no detectable disease is present. The goal is to decrease the rate of relapse and improve disease-free survival as well as maximize the potential for cure.
   b. Neoadjuvant therapy is the administration of several courses of chemotherapy before definitive surgical intervention (e.g., large breast masses). The goal of therapy is to decrease the amount of tissue that needs to be removed as well as to attempt to maximize cure potential.
   c. High dose/intensive therapy is the administration of high doses of chemotherapy, usually in association with growth factor support or before bone marrow transplant/stem cell rescue.
   d. Combination therapy is the use of multiple chemotherapeutic agents with different actions to provide maximal cell kill and minimize drug resistance. This is often more effective than single-agent chemotherapy.
   e. Malignant cells may exhibit resistance to some antineoplastic agents, thus limiting their usefulness. The tumor can be resistant to certain drugs from the start of therapy (natural resistance) or become resistant after therapy has begun (acquired resistance).

5. Routes of administration:
   a. Oral—capsule, tablet, or liquid
   b. Intravenous (IV)—push (bolus) or infusion over a specified time period
   c. Intramuscular
   d. Subcutaneous
   e. Intrathecal/intraventricular—given by injection through an Ommaya reservoir or by lumbar puncture
   f. Intra-arterial
   g. Intracavitary—such as peritoneal cavity
   h. Intravesical—into uterus or bladder
   i. Topical

6. Dosage is based on surface area (mg/m^2) in both adults and children.

7. Most chemotherapeutic agents have dose-limiting toxicities that require nursing interventions (Table 8-4). Chemotherapy predictably affects normal, rapidly growing cells (e.g., bone marrow, gastrointestinal tract lining, hair follicles). It is imperative that these toxicities be recognized early on by the nurse.

Safety Measures in Handling Chemotherapy

Cytotoxic drugs may be irritating to the skin, eyes, and mucous membranes (see Procedure Guidelines 8-1).

Personal Safety to Minimize Exposure via Inhalation

1. Chemotherapeutic agents should be prepared in a class II biologic safety cabinet (vertical laminar flow hood).

2. Vent vials with filter needle to equalize the internal pressure or use negative-pressure techniques.

3. Wrap gauze or alcohol pads around the neck of ampules when opening to decrease droplet contamination.

4. Wrap gauze or alcohol pads around injection sites when removing syringes or needles from IV injection ports.

(text continues on page 146)

TABLE 8-4 Frequently Used Chemotherapeutic Agents

Drug	Dose, Route, and Frequency	How Supplied	Major Side Effects			Other Side Effects or Comments
			Myelosuppression	Thrombocytopenia	Risk for Nausea and Vomiting	
Alkylators						
Cyclophosphamide (Cytoxan)	500–1500 mg/m² IV q3–4wk 100 mg/m² PO daily for 14 d	25 mg, 50 mg tablets 100 mg, 200 mg, 500 mg, 1 g, 2 g vials	Marked	Mild	Moderate	Hemorrhagic cystitis, alopecia Monitor liver function Drink 3 L fluids daily
Busulfan (Myleran)	2–8 mg PO, daily	2 mg tablets	Marked	Marked	Mild	Pulmonary fibrosis, skin pigmentation
BCNU (Carmustine)	75–100 mg/m² IV for 1–3 d q6wk	100 mg vial with 3 mL alcohol diluent	Marked delayed	Marked	Marked	Local pain during infusion, pulmonary fibrosis, crosses blood-brain barrier/irritant Requires reconstitution with supplied diluent
CBCDA (Carboplatin)	200–400 mg/m² IV q4wk	50 mg, 150 mg, 450 mg vials	Marked	Marked	Mild	Possible anaphylaxis, thrombocytopenia can be severe and prolonged
CCNU (Lomustine CeeNu)	130 mg/m² PO q6wk	10 mg, 40 mg, 100 mg capsules	Marked delayed	Marked	Moderate	Myelosuppression can be cumulative, Crosses blood-brain barrier. Take at bedtime on empty stomach
Chlorambucil (Leukeran)	0.1–0.2 mg/kg PO daily Usually 2 mg maintenance	2 mg tablet	Moderate	Moderate	Mild	Infertility. Leukopenia delayed up to 3 wk
Cisplatin (Platinol)	50–120 mg/m² IV q3–4wk 20 mg/m² IV daily for 5 d q3–4wk	10 mg, 50 mg vial	Moderate	Moderate	Severe	Nephrotoxicity/neurotoxicity, magnesium wasting, ototoxicity, anemia. Requires antiemetics before and after
Dacarbazine (DTIC)	150 mg/m² daily IV for 5 d q4wk 375 mg/m² on day 1 q15d	100 mg, 200 mg vial	Mild	Mild	Marked	Flulike syndrome, alopecia, facial flushing, parethesias, vesicant
Ifosfamide (Ifex)	1200 mg/m² IV for 5 d q3w	1 g, 2 g, 3 g	Moderate	Moderate	Mild	Neurotoxicity, hemorrhagic cystitis, alopecia, concomitant uroprotection with MESNA
Mesna	20 mg/kg 15 min before Ifex, repeated q3h for 4 doses	200 mg vial	None	None	None	Not an antineoplastic agent. Binds to reactive metabolite of Ifex or Cytoxan without affecting antitumor activity
MeCCNU (Semustine, Methyl CCNU)	130 mg/m² q6wk	10 mg, 40 mg, 100 mg capsules	Marked	Marked	Moderate	Delayed and cumulative myelosuppression, stomatitis, anorexia
Mechlorethamine hydrochloride (nitrogen mustard)	0.4 mg/kg intracavitary or 10 mg/m² q3–6wk	10 mg vials	Marked	Marked	Severe	Vesicant, stomatitis, alopecia, chemical thrombophlebitis

Drug	Dose	How Supplied				Toxicity
Melphalan (L-Pam, Alkeran)	6 mg orally, daily for 2–4 wk	2 mg tablet	Moderate	Moderate	Mild	Leukemia, second malignancies. Given on empty stomach.
Streptozocin (Zanosan)	500 mg/m² IV daily for 5 d q6wk	1 g vial	Mild	Mild	Moderate-marked	Irritant, renal failure, reactive hypoglycemia due to insulin release, diarrhea
Antibiotics						
Bleomycin (Blenoxane)	10–20 units/m² IV, IM, SQ weekly Total dose not to exceed 400 units 60–120 units in 100 mL normal saline for intracavitary therapy	15 unit vial	Rare	Rare	Mild	Skin reaction, pulmonary fibrosis, fever, allergic reaction, alopecia, stomatitis
Dactinomycin D (Actinomycin D, Cosmegen)	0.010–0.015 µg/kg IV for 5 d q3–4wk	0.5 mg vial	Marked	Marked	Moderate-severe	Alopecia, stomatitis, skin rash, hepatic dysfunction, vesicant, radiation recall
Daunorubicin (Cerubidine)	60 mg/m² IV for 3 d q3–4wk 550 mg/m² total IV dose	20 mg vial	Marked	Marked	Moderate-severe	Cardiomyopathy, alopecia, red urine, radiation recall, vesicant 450–550 mg/m² total dose with mediastinal radiation
Doxorubicin (Adriamycin)	60–75 mg/m² IV q3wk 30 mg/m² for 3 d q3–4 wk Total cumulative dose 550 mg/m²	10 mg, 20 mg, 50 mg vial	Marked	Marked	Moderate	Alopecia, cardiomyopathy, radiation recall, red urine, hepatic dysfunction, vesicant
Mitomycin (Mutamycin)	10–20 mg/m² IV q6–8wk	5 mg, 20 mg vial	Marked	Marked	Moderate	Renal and pulmonary dysfunction, alopecia, stomatitis, delayed myelosuppression, vesicant
Plant Alkaloids						
Vinblastine (Velban)	5 mg/m² IV q1–2wk	10 mg vial	Marked	Marked	Mild	Elevated uric acid, neurotoxicity, mucositis, alopecia, vesicant
Vincristine (Oncovin)	1–2 mg/m² IV maximum single dose 2 mg IV	1 mg/mL vial, 2 mg/mL vial	Mild	Mild	Mild	Distal neuropathy, constipation, vesicant
Vindesine (Eldisine)	2–4 mg/m² IV q1–2wk	10 mg ampule	Moderate	Mild	Mild	Neurotoxicity—can be cumulative if administered with other plant alkaloids, vesicant
Teniposide (VM 26)	50–100 mg/m² IV weekly for 4–6 wk	10 mg/mL ampule	Moderate	Mild	Mild	Distal neuropathy, can have cumulative neurotoxicity if administered with other plant alkaloids, alopecia, vesicant
Etoposide (VePesid) (VP-16)	45–75 mg/m²/d 3–5 d q3–5wk 125–140 mg/m² PO 3 times/wk q5wk	50 mg capsule, 100 mg/5 mL vial	Moderate	Mild	Mild-moderate	Distal neuropathy, alopecia, hypotension can occur following rapid infusion, headache, give over 30 minutes, irritant

(continued)

143

TABLE 8-4 Frequently Used Chemotherapeutic Agents (Continued)

Drug	Dose, Route, and Frequency	How Supplied	Myelosuppression	Thrombocytopenia	Risk for Nausea and Vomiting	Other Side Effects or Comments
			Major Side Effects			
Antimetabolites						
Azacytidine (5-azacytidine)	150 mg/m² IV for 5 d by continuous infusion 100 mg/m² continuous IV infusion q12h for 7 d	100 mg vial	Marked	Marked	Severe	Diarrhea, neurotoxicity, mucositis
Cytarabine (Cytosar, ARA-C)	50–100 mg in 100 mL saline for intrathecal	100 mg vial	Marked	Marked	Moderate	Stomatitis, headaches; anorexia, arachnoiditis with intrathecal. Cerebellar complications with high dose
5-Fluorouracil (5FU, Efudex)	300–500 mg/m² IV weekly or daily ×5	500 mg ampule cream, 1%, 5%	Moderate-marked	Mild	Mild	Stomatitis, diarrhea, alopecia, vein discoloration, photosensitivity, nail color changes
Capitabine (Xeloda)	110 mg/m²–2510 g/m² daily times 14 d, repeat every 21d	250 mg & 500 mg tablets	Moderate-marked	Mild	Moderate-high	Diarrhea, hand–foot syndrome, stomatitis
Hydroxyurea (Hydrea)	80 mg/kg PO daily	500 mg tablet	Marked	Marked	Mild	Alopecia, diarrhea, stomatitis. Crosses blood-brain barrier
6-Mercaptopurine (6 MP, Purinethol)	1.5–2.5 mg/kg PO	50 mg tablet	Moderate-marked	Moderate-marked	Mild	Stomatitis, hepatoxicity. Reduce dose if giving alopurinol concurrently
Methotrexate (Mexate)	2.5–5.0 mg PO daily; IV or IM dose varies 25–50 mg/m² intrathecal 5–10 mg/m² q3–7d	2.5 mg tablets 25 mg, 50 mg injection	Moderated-marked	Moderate-marked	Mild	Stomatitis, nephrotoxicity, diarrhea, crosses blood-brain barrier. Creatinine clearance must be >60 mL/min
Thioguanine (6 TG, Tabloid)	2 mg/kg daily PO	40 mg tablet	Moderate	Moderate	Mild	Cholestasis, stomatitis, diarrhea, hepatotoxicity

Taxanes

Drug	Dosage	Supplied				Nursing Considerations
Paclitaxel (Taxol)	175 mg/m² IV over 3 h q3wk, or 60–100 mg/m² weekly over 1 h	30 mg vial, 6 mg/mL with 5 mL	Marked	Mild	Mild	Peripheral neuropathy, myalgias, alopecia, fatigue, heart block, arrhythmia. Observe closely for hypersensitivity reaction; premedicate with Decadron 20 mg IV, Benadryl 150 mg IV and Zantac 50 mg IV. Requires non-PVC IV tubing
Docetaxel (Taxotere)	80–100 mg/m² IV over 1 h q3wk, or 40–80 mg/m² IV weekly	20 mg vial, 80 mg vial	Marked	Mild	Mild	Peripheral neuropathy, edema, alopecia, fatigue. Observe closely for hypersensitivity reaction; premedicate with Decadron 8 mg PO bid the day before, the day of, and the day after chemotherapy.

Miscellaneous Drugs

Drug	Dosage	Supplied				Nursing Considerations
Procarbazine (Matulane)	2–4 mg/kg daily PO	50 mg capsule	Moderate	Moderate	Mild	Sensitive to amines, neurotoxicity, crosses blood-brain barrier
Mitoxantrone (Novantrone)	12 mg/m² IV day 1–3	2 mg/mL in 10 mL, 12.5 mL, 15 mL vial	Moderate	Mild	Mild	Tachycardia, mucositis. Use extreme caution in preparation of drug
Gemcitabine (Gemzar)	1000 mg/m² IV over 30 min once a week for up to 7 wk or until signs of toxicity	200 mg/10 mL vial 1 g/50 mL vial	Moderate	Moderate	Mild	

5. Do not dispose of materials by clipping needles or removing needles from syringes.

6. Use puncture- and leak-proof containers for non-capped, non-clipped needles.

Personal Safety to Minimize Exposure via Skin Contact

1. Wear powder-free latex gloves with at least .007″ thickness at all times when preparing or working with chemotherapeutic agents. Individuals with latex allergies should use gloves made from nitrate or double glove with polyvinylchloride (PVC) gloves. Gloves manufactured of latex and nitrile material are now manufactured in greater thickness and offer more protection.

2. Wash hands before putting on and after removing gloves.

3. Change latex gloves after each use, tear, puncture, or medication spill or after every 30 minutes of wear.

4. Wear a long-sleeve, nonabsorbent gown with elastic at the wrists and back closure.

5. Eye and face shields should be worn if splashes are likely to occur.

6. Use syringes and IV tubing with Luer locks (which have a locking device to hold needle firmly in place).

7. Label all syringes and IV tubing containing chemotherapeutic agents as hazardous material.

8. Place an absorbent pad directly under the injection site to absorb any accidental spillage.

9. If any contact with the skin occurs, immediately wash the area thoroughly with soap and water.

10. If contact is made with the eye, immediately flush the eye with water and seek medical attention.

11. Spill kits should be available in all areas where chemotherapy is stored, prepared, and administered.

Personal Safety to Minimize Exposure via Ingestion

1. Do not eat, drink, chew gum, or smoke while preparing or handling chemotherapy.

2. Keep all food and drink away from preparation area.

3. Wash hands before and after handling chemotherapy.

4. Avoid hand-to-mouth or hand-to-eye contact while handling chemotherapeutic agents or body fluids of the person receiving chemotherapy.

Safe Disposal of Antineoplastic Agents, Body Fluids, and Excreta

1. Discard gloves and gown into a leak-proof container, which should be marked as contaminated or hazardous waste.

2. Use puncture- and leak-proof containers for needles and other sharp or breakable objects.

3. Linens contaminated with chemotherapy or excreta from patients who have received chemotherapy within 48 hours should be contained in specially marked hazardous waste bags.

4. Wear latex gloves for disposing of body excreta and handling soiled linens within 48 hours of chemotherapy administration.

5. In the home, wear gloves when handling bed linens or clothing contaminated with chemotherapy or patient excreta within 48 hours of chemotherapy administration. Place linens in a separate, washable pillow case. Wash separately in hot water and regular detergent.

Side Effects of Chemotherapy

Side effects of chemotherapy are graded on a scale from 0 to 4, with 0 being normal and 4 indicating life threatening. Scoring of side effects can determine a delay in therapy until the patient returns to normal, dose modification of drug(s), or cessation of therapy.

Alopecia

1. Most chemotherapeutic agents cause some degree of alopecia. This is dependent on the dose, half-life of drug, and duration of therapy.

2. Usually begins 2 weeks after administration of chemotherapy. Regrowth takes about 3 to 5 months.

3. The use of scalp hypothermia and tourniquets is highly controversial.

Anorexia

1. Chemotherapy changes the reproduction of taste buds.

2. Absent or altered taste can lead to a decreased food intake.

3. Concurrent renal or hepatic disease can increase anorexia.

Fatigue

The cause of fatigue is generally unknown but can be related to anemia, weight loss, altered sleep patterns, and coping.

Nausea and Vomiting

1. Caused by the stimulation of the vagus nerve by serotonin released by cells in the upper GI tract.

2. Incidence depends upon the particular chemotherapeutic agent.

3. Patterns of nausea and vomiting:
   a. Anticipatory: conditioned response from repeated association between therapy and vomiting.
   b. Acute: occurs 0 to 24 hours after chemotherapy administration.
   c. Delayed: can occur 1 to 4 days after chemotherapy administration.

Mucositis

1. Caused by the destruction of the oral mucosa, causing an inflammatory response.

2. Initially presents as a burning sensation with no changes in the mucosa and progresses to significant breakdown, erythema, and pain of the oral mucosa.

3. Consistent oral hygiene is important to avoid infection.

Anemia

1. Caused by suppression of the stem cell or interference with cell proliferation pathways.

2. May require red blood cell transfusion or injection of erythropoietin.

Neutropenia

1. Defined as an absolute neutrophil count (ANC) of 1500/mm^3 or less.

2. Risk of infection is greatest with an ANC less than 500/mm³.
3. Caused by suppression of the stem cell.
4. Usually occurs 7 to 14 days after administration of chemotherapy.
5. Can be prolonged.
6. Patients should be taught to avoid infection through proper hand washing, avoiding those with illness, proper hygiene, etc.
7. Patients need to be monitored and treated promptly for fever or other signs of infection.

Thrombocytopenia

1. Caused by suppression of megakaryocytes.
2. Incidence depends on the agent being used.
3. Risk of bleeding is present when platelet count falls below 50,000/mm³.
4. Risk is high when count falls below 20,000/mm³.
5. Risk is critical when count falls below 10,000/mm³.
6. Patient should be taught to avoid injury, e.g., no razors, avoid vaginal douches and rectal suppositories, and avoid dental floss during the period of thrombocytopenia.
7. May require platelet transfusions if count drops below 20,000/mm³.
8. Unexpected or adverse drug reaction should be reported to drug company or study chairperson.

Nursing Assessment

Integumentary System

1. Inspect for pain, swelling with inflammation or phlebitis, necrosis, or ulceration.
2. Inspect for skin rash, characteristics, whether pruritus, general or local.
3. Assess areas of erythema and associated tenderness or pruritus. Instruct patient to avoid irritation to skin, sun exposure, or irritating soaps.
4. Assess changes in skin pigmentation.
5. Note reports of photosensitivity, tearing of the eyes.
6. Assess condition of gums, teeth, buccal mucosa, and tongue.
   a. Determine whether any taste changes have occurred.
   b. Check for evidence of stomatitis, erythematous areas, ulceration, infection, or pain on swallowing.
   c. Determine whether the patient has any complaints of pain or burning of the oral mucosa or on swallowing.

Gastrointestinal System

1. Assess for frequency, timing of onset, duration, and severity of nausea and vomiting episodes before and after chemotherapy.
   a. Usually occurs from 1 to 24 hours after chemotherapy but may be delayed. Anticipatory vomiting may occur after first course of therapy. Can be initiated by various cues, including thoughts, smell, or even sight of the medical personnel.
2. Observe for alterations in hydration, electrolyte balance.
3. Assess for diarrhea or constipation.
   a. Ascertain any changes in bowel patterns.
   b. Discuss the consistency of stools.

c. Consider the frequency and duration of diarrhea (the number of stools each day for the number of days).
   d. Evaluate any dietary changes or use of medications such as narcotics that have had an impact on diarrhea or constipation.
4. Assess for anorexia.
   a. Discuss taste changes and changes in food preferences.
   b. Ask about daily food intake and normal eating patterns.
5. Assess for jaundice, right upper quadrant abdominal pain, changes in the stool or urine, and elevated liver function tests that indicate hepatotoxicity.

Hematopoietic System

NURSING ALERT

Fevers greater than 38.3°C (101°F) in a patient with an absolute neutrophil count less than 500/mm³ is an emergency requiring immediate administration of antibiotics.

1. Assess for neutropenia—absolute neutrophil count less than 500/mm³.
   a. Assess for any signs of infection (pulmonary, integumentary, central nervous system [CNS], gastrointestinal, and urinary).
   b. Auscultate lungs for adventitious breath sounds.
   c. Assess for productive cough or shortness of breath.
   d. Assess for urinary frequency, urgency, pain, or odor.
   e. Monitor for elevation of temperature above 38.3°C (101°F), chills.
2. Assess for thrombocytopenia—platelet count less than 50,000/mm³ (mild risk of bleeding); less than 20,000/mm³ (severe risk of bleeding).
   a. Assess skin and oral mucous membranes for petechiae, bruises on extremities.
   b. Assess for signs of bleeding (including nose, urinary, rectal, or hemoptysis).
   c. Assess for blood in stools, urine, or emesis.
   d. Assess for signs and symptoms of intracranial bleeding if platelet count is less than 20,00/mm³; monitor for changes in level of responsiveness, vital signs, and pupillary reaction.
3. Assess for anemia.
   a. Assess skin color, turgor, and capillary refill.
   b. Ascertain whether patient has experienced dyspnea on exertion, fatigue, weakness, palpitations, or vertigo. Advise rest periods as needed.

Respiratory and Cardiovascular Systems

1. Assess lung sounds.
2. Assess for pulmonary fibrosis, evidenced by a dry, nonproductive cough with increasing dyspnea. Patients at risk include those over 60 years old, smokers, those receiving or having had pulmonary radiation, those receiving cumulative dose of bleomycin (Blenoxane), or those with any preexisting lung disease.
3. Assess for signs and symptoms of congestive heart failure or irregular apical or radial pulses.

4. Verify baseline cardiac studies (e.g., electrocardiogram, multiple gated acquisition scan/ejection fraction) before administering doxorubicin (Adriamycin) or high-dose cyclophosphamide (Cytoxan).

Neuromuscular System

1. Ascertain whether patient is having difficulty with fine motor activities, such as zipping pants, tying shoes, or buttoning a shirt.
2. Determine the presence of paresthesia (tingling, numbness) of fingers or toes.
3. Evaluate deep tendon reflexes.
4. Evaluate patient for weakness, ataxia, or slapping gait.
5. Determine impact on activities of daily living and discuss changes.
6. Discuss symptoms of urinary retention or constipation.
7. Assess for ringing in ears or decreased hearing acuity.

Genitourinary System

1. Monitor urine output.
2. Assess for urinary frequency, urgency, or hesitancy.
3. Evaluate any changes in odor, color, or clarity of urine sample.
4. Assess for hematuria, oliguria, or anuria.
5. Monitor BUN, creatinine.

Nursing Diagnoses

- Risk for Infection related to neutropenia
- Risk for Bleeding related to thrombocytopenia
- Fatigue related to anemia
- Altered Nutrition: Less Than Body Requirements related to side effects of therapy
- Altered Oral Mucous Membranes related to stomatitis
- Altered Body Image related to alopecia and weight loss

Nursing Interventions

Preventing Infection

1. Monitor vital signs every 4 hours; report any occurrence of fever greater than 38.3°C (101.0°F) and chills.
2. Provide patient education
   a. Instruct patient to report signs and symptoms of infection, including:
      (i) Fever greater than 101.0°F and/or chills
      (ii) Mouth lesions, swelling, or redness
      (iii) Redness, pain, or tenderness at rectum
      (iv) Any change in bowel habits
      (v) Any areas of redness, swelling, induration, or pain on skin surface
      (vi) Any pain or burning when urinating or odor from urine
      (vii) Any cough or shortness of breath
   b. Reinforce good personal hygiene habits (routine bathing [preferably a shower], clean hair, nails, and mouth care).
   c. Avoid contact with persons who have a transmissible illness.
   d. Encourage deep-breathing and coughing to decrease pulmonary stasis.
3. Avoid performing invasive procedures—rectal temperatures, enemas, or insertion of indwelling urinary catheters.

4. Monitor white blood cell count (WBC) and differential.
5. Be aware that hematologic nadirs (lowest level) generally occur within 7 to 14 days after drug administration. Length of myelosuppression depends on specific drug. Institution of further therapy usually depends on an adequate WBC and absolute neutrophil count (ANC).
6. Calculate ANC to determine the number of neutrophils capable of fighting an infection by:

$$\text{Total WBC} \times (\% \text{ polys} + \% \text{ bands}) = \text{ANC}$$

Example: $700 \times (10\% + 5\%) = 105$

Interpretation: 105 of the 700 white blood cells are neutrophils and capable of fighting an infection (indicates severe neutropenia).

7. Administer prophylactic antibiotics as prescribed (if WBC is less than 500) and growth colony–stimulating factor with subsequent courses of chemotherapy to hasten neutrophil maturity.

Preventing Bleeding

1. Avoid invasive procedures when platelet count is less than 50,000 mm³, including intramuscular injections, suppositories, enemas, and insertion of indwelling urinary catheters.
2. Apply pressure on injection sites for 5 minutes.
3. Monitor platelet count; administer platelets as prescribed.
4. Monitor and test all urine, stools, and emesis for blood.
5. Provide patient education
   a. Instruct patient to avoid straight-edge razors, nail clippers, vaginal or rectal suppositories.
   b. Avoid intercourse when platelet count is less than 50,000/mm³.
   c. Encourage patient to blow his or her nose gently.
   d. Avoid dental work or other invasive procedures while thrombocytopenic.
   e. Avoid the use of NSAIDs, aspirin, and aspirin-containing products.

Minimizing Fatigue

1. Monitor blood counts (hemoglobin and hematocrit).
2. Administer blood products as prescribed.
3. Provide patient education
   a. Explain why fatigue and shortness of breath may occur.
   b. Caution the patient about physical overexertion; encourage rest frequently and warn patient to expect a tired feeling.
   c. Plan frequent rest periods between daily activities.
   d. Explain that blood transfusions, if given, are a part of therapy and not necessarily an indication of a setback.
   e. Observe skin color.
   f. Monitor nutritional status.

Promoting Nutrition

1. Administer antiemetics prior to chemotherapy and on a routine schedule (not prn).
2. Be aware that certain antiemetic combinations are more effective than single agents.

a. A 5Ht3 inhibitor (Zofran, Kytril), in combination with dexamethasone (Decadron)

b. Corticosteroids in combination with metoclopramide

3. For highly emetogenic chemotherapy regimens:

a. Premedicate with a 5Ht3 inhibitor (Zofran, Kytril) and dexamethasone (Decadron).

b. Include a prn antiemetic such as metoclopramide (Reglan), droperidol, prochlorperazine (Compazine), dexamethasone, or lorezapam (Ativan).

4. For moderately emetogenic regimens:

a. Premedicate with either droperidol or dexamethasone with metoclopramide plus diphenhydramine (Benadryl).

b. Include a prn antiemetic such as prochlorperazine (Compazine) or lorezapam (Ativan).

c. Failures may receive a 5Ht3 inhibitor (Zofran, Kytril).

5. For low emetogenic regimens: consider oral prochlorperazine (Compazine).

6. Extrapyramidal reactions occur frequently in patients under age 30 and over age 65. Treat dystonic reactions with diphenhydramine; treat restlessness with lorazepam.

7. If delayed nausea and vomiting begin 8 hours after acute prophylactic antiemetic therapy and continue for 24 to 36 hours, administer agents such as metoclopramide with dexamethasone plus diphenhydramine, haloperidol (Haldol), prochlorperazine, or lorezapam.

8. Consider alternative measures for relief of anticipatory nausea, such as relaxation therapy, imagery, and distraction.

9. Encourage small, frequent meals appealing to patient preferences.

10. Encourage patient to eat a diet high in calories and proteins. Provide high-protein supplement as needed.

11. Discourage smoking and alcoholic beverages, which may irritate mucous membranes.

12. Encourage fluid intake to prevent constipation.

13. Monitor intake and output, including emesis.

14. Consult dietitian concerning patient's food preferences, intolerances, and individual dietary interventions.

15. Recognize that the patient may have alterations in taste perception, such as a keener taste of bitterness and loss of ability to detect sweet tastes.

Minimizing Stomatitis

1. Report signs of infection—erythematous areas, white patches, ulcers.

2. Encourage the use of oral agents to promote cleansing, debridement, and comfort. Mouthwashes with more than 25% alcohol should be avoided.

3. Assess the need for antifungal, antibacterial, or antiviral therapy (each infection has a different appearance).

4. Administer local oral therapy such as combinations with viscous lidocaine (Xylocaine) for symptomatic control and maintenance of calorie intake.

Strengthening Coping With Altered Body Image

1. Reassure patient that hair will usually grow back. It may grow back a different texture or different color.

2. Suggest wearing a turban, wig, or headscarf, preferably purchased before hair loss occurs. Many insurance companies will pay for a wig with a prescription.

3. Encourage patient to stay on therapeutic program.

4. Be honest with the patient.

Patient Education and Health Maintenance

1. Ensure that patient uses good hygiene, knows symptoms of infection to report, and avoids crowds and persons with infection while neutropenic.

2. Advise patient to avoid using a razor blade to shave, contact sports, manipulation of sharp articles, use of hard bristle toothbrush, and passage of hard stool to prevent bleeding while thrombocytopenic.

3. Advise women to report symptoms of vaginal infection due to opportunistic fungal or viral infection.

4. Encourage patient participation in plan for chemotherapy and to set realistic goals for work and activities.

5. Assure patient that changes in menses, libido, and sexual function are usually temporary during therapy.

6. Obtain further information on chemotherapy at **http://cancernet.nci.nih.gov/peb/chemo_you**.

Outcome-Based Evaluation

- Afebrile, no signs of infection
- No bruising or bleeding noted; stool and urine heme test negative
- Denies shortness of breath or severe fatigue
- Tolerating small, frequent meals following antiemetic
- No oral lesions or pain on swallowing
- Maintaining proper hygiene

PROCEDURE GUIDELINES 8-1 **ADMINISTERING IV CHEMOTHERAPY**

EQUIPMENT

Supplies to start IV infusion or a running IV line	Alcohol swabs
Specific antidote for extravasation (if indicated)	Disposable plastic-backed absorbent liner
4 × 4 gauze pads	Medication to be administered

 NURSING ALERT

The handling and administration of chemotherapy requires specialized training and competency. Nurses without this training should not administer chemotherapy.

continued

PROCEDURE GUIDELINES 8-1   ADMINISTERING IV CHEMOTHERAPY *CONTINUED*

PROCEDURE

Nursing Action	Rationale

PREPARATORY PHASE

1. Patient education
   a. Review treatment goals.
   b. Review the treatment plan and side effects of chemotherapy.
   c. Review strategies to manage side effects.
   d. Instruct patient on reportable conditions, e.g., fever.
2. Compare written orders to drug protocol. If the drug is investigational, verify informed consent.
3. Check for appropriate dose and route of administration.
4. Calculate the dosage according to milligrams per kilogram (mg/kg) or milligrams per meter squared (mg/m²) by body surface area (BSA).
5. Check against the written order.
6. Check current lab values: CBC, differential, platelets, liver function tests, and creatinine.
7. Verify the patient's name and identification.
8. Identify a plan for antiemetic administration before, during, and after chemotherapy.
9. Review patient's medication history, including over-the-counter medications, for possible interactions.
10. Be aware of agents that cause anaphylactic reaction, such as asparaginase, paclitaxel, and docetaxel. Have emergency resuscitation equipment and drugs available.
11. Use a disposable, absorbent, plastic-backed pad under the work area.
12. Don protective gown, gloves, and eyewear if necessary.
13. If possible, prime all tubing prior to adding antineoplastics to the bag. If priming occurs at the administration site, the IV tubing should be primed with a non-drug fluid.

1. Patient education will prepare the patient for side effects, thus increasing tolerance of the drug.

3. Multiple ways to verify the drug and the dosage are necessary to prevent error.

6. Drug may be withheld in severe neutropenia, thrombocytopenia, or impaired liver or kidney function.

8. Antiemetics are more effective if given before administration and on a regular dosing schedule thereafter.

11. To absorb droplets of the drug that may inadvertently spill.

13. To prevent aeresolization/spillage of drug.

NURSING ALERT

If a small focal hematoma develops during insertion of the needle into the vein, do not use this site for chemotherapeutic administration because of the increased risk for extravasation and infiltration.

PERFORMANCE PHASE

1. Select venipuncture site free of sclerosis, thrombosis, or scar formation if at all possible. If the patient has an established IV, assess the site for erythema, pain, or tenderness.
2. Check for a blood return by aspirating at a y-site close to the IV catheter. Do not pinch the catheter tubing.
3. If any doubt exists regarding vein patency or safety of chemotherapy administration, discontinue the administration and treat as an extravasation if a vesicant chemotherapeutic agent has been used.
   a. Monitor for pain, which the patient may describe as localized to severe burning and radiating along the vein.
   b. Examine the site for erythema or swelling.
   c. If you suspect an extravasation, stop the infusion immediately and follow the procedure described below.
4. Drug administration:
   a. Monitor the patient, particularly during the first 15 minutes, for signs of hypersensitivity or anaphylaxis.
   b. Monitor the IV site throughout the infusion or IV push.

1. An optimal IV site reduces the risk of extravasation.

2. Pinching the catheter site may dislodge a small clot in a nonpatent IV.
3. A vesicant is a chemotherapeutic agent capable of causing blistering of tissues and possible tissue necrosis if it extravasates. Some agents are irritants, which cause pain along the vein wall with or without inflammation.

c. Tissue necrosis and sloughing may lead to permanent disability of an extremity.

a. Change in mentation or in vital signs may indicate hypersensitivity or anaphylactic reaction.

c. For IV push: use the y-site closest to the patient and check for blood return periodically throughout the procedure.
5. Dispose of syringes, IV tubing, protective clothing, etc., in hazardous waste bin.

5. Ensure universal precautions.

MANAGEMENT OF AN EXTRAVASATION
1. If an extravasation is suspected, stop the infusion of the chemotherapy.
2. Disconnect the IV tubing and attempt to aspirate all residual chemotherapy in the IV catheter using a syringe.
3. If an antidote is available, instill the appropriate amount through the existing IV and discontinue the IV.
4. Inject 5–6 mL of the antidote SQ in divided doses into the extravasated site with multiple injections. Repeat SQ dosing over several hours.
5. Apply warm or cold compress as indicated, depending on the chemotherapeutic agent that has extravasated.

2. To prevent release of medication as the IV is removed.

3. Antidote may prevent tissue necrosis.

5. To reduce extravasation and swelling.

TABLE 8-A Vesicants

Chemotherapeutic Agent	Antidote	Local Care
Adriamycin	None	Apply cold pack for 15–20 minutes at least 4 times a day.
Alkylating agents (nitrogen mustard, cisplatin)	Isotonic sodium thiosulfate	Prepare ⅙ molar solution and inject 1–4 mL into existing IV and SQ tissue. Heat or cold not proved effective.
Vinca alkaloids (vincristine, vinblastine)	Hyaluronidase	
Taxanes (paclitaxel, docetaxel)	Hyaluronidase	Mix 300 U with 3 cc of NS. Inject mL for mL infiltrated. Ice has been effective in reducing local tissue damage.
Antimetabolite (5-FU)	None—rare weak vesicant	

FOLLOW-UP PHASE
1. Document drug dosage, site, and any occurrence of extravasation, including estimated amount of drug extravasated and management. Photograph if possible.
2. Observe regularly after administration for pain, erythema, induration, and necrosis.

3. Monitor for other side effects of infusion.
   a. Patient may describe sensations of pain or pressure within the vessel, originating near the venipuncture site or extending 7.5–12.5 cm (3–5 inches) along the vein.
   b. Discoloration—red streak following the line of the vein (called a flare reaction) or darkening of the vein
   c. Itching, urticaria, muscle cramps, or pressure in the arm

1. To document extent of injury.

2. If only a small amount of drug extravasated and frank necrosis does not occur, phlebitis may still result, causing pain for several days or induration at the site that may last for weeks or months.
   a. Caused by irritation to the vein.

   b. Flare reaction common with doxorubicin (Adriamycin). Darkening of vein may occur with 5-fluorouracil (5-FU).
   c. Caused by irritation of surrounding subcutaneous tissue.

Radiation Therapy

Radiation therapy is the use of high-energy, ionizing beams to treat cancer and certain benign disorders. It causes molecular damage and biochemical changes and eventual cell death from disruption of the reproductive cycle.

General Considerations
Principles of Therapy
To deliver a precise dose of ionizing radiation without affecting healthy tissue.

1. Radiosensitivity is the degree and speed of response. This measure of susceptibility of cells to injury or death by radiation depends on cancer diagnosis and its inherent biologic activity. It is directly related to reproductive capability of the cell.
2. Role of oxygen: Oxygen must be present at the time of radiation's maximal killing effect. Poor circulation with resultant hypoxia can reduce cellular radiosensitivity. Giving multiple, daily doses allows reoxygenation and enhances radiosensitivity. The dose should allow for repair of normal tissues.

3. Cellular response can be modified by changing the dose rate, manipulating the process of cell repair, recruiting cells into replication cycle, and using hyperthermia (above 104°F).

4. Radioresistance is the lack of tumor response to radiation because of tumor characteristics (slow-growing tumor, less responsive), tumor cell proliferation, and circulation. Radiation is most effective during the mitotic stage of the cell cycle.

5. Radioresistant tumors: Many tumors are resistant to radiation, such as squamous cell, ovarian, soft tissue sarcoma, and gliomas. Many other tumors can become resistant after a period of time. Normal radioresistant tissues include mature bone, cartilage, liver, thyroid, muscle, brain, and spinal cord.

6. Beam energy and penetration: The majority of therapeutic radiation is administered using the cobalt 60 source or high-energy photons from linear accelerators. The radiation beam decreases in intensity with increasing depth. The penetration of the radiation into the body is directly proportional to the generating energy. Linear energy transfer (LET) is the rate at which energy is deposited per unit distance. High-energy electrons are used for tumors on or near the skin surface.

Types of Radiation Therapy

1. Teletherapy is external beam irradiation. Produces x-rays of varying energies. Administered by machines a distance from the body (80 to 100 cm).
   a. Types of machines: cobalt 60 teletherapy units and high-energy x-ray sources (linear accelerator, photons, megavoltage).
   b. Most common use of radiation is local therapy.
2. Brachytherapy is a high dose to a small tissue volume with less dose to adjacent normal tissue, using radioactive sources close to or within the tumor. Need direct access to the tumor.
   a. Interstitial therapy is implants with solid material such as seeds. May be temporary implants that are removed after several days or permanent. The permanent ones remain in place with gradual decay. Implant procedure is performed under local or general anesthesia. Used in breast and prostate disease.
   b. Intracavitary therapy is used in cancers of the uterine cervix.
   c. Surface radiation is used in choroid cancer.
   d. Systemic irradiation is parenteral or IV, oral ^{131}I for thyroid cancer, intraperitoneal.

Chemical and Thermal Modifiers of Radiation

1. Radiosensitization is the use of medications to enhance the sensitivity of the tumor cells.
2. Radioprotectors increase therapeutic ratio by promoting repair of normal tissues.
3. Hyperthermia is combined with radiation. Uses a variety of sources (ultrasound, microwaves) and produces a greater effect than radiation alone.

4. Intraoperative radiation therapy is surgically removing tumor followed by a single high dose to the tumor bed; usually prophylactic.

Units for Measuring Radiation Exposure or Absorption

1. Gray (Gy)—a unit to measure absorbed dose. One Gy equals 100 rads. (Rad—term used in the past to measure absorbed dose.) Joules/kg is also used to measure absorbed dose; 1 joule/kg = Gy.
2. Roentgen (R)—standard unit of exposure (usually applied to x-ray or gamma rays).
3. Radiation dose equivalent (rem)—unit of measure that relates to biologic effectiveness (roentgen equivalent in human beings). Standards were established by the International Committee on Radiation Protection (ICRP). The recommendation for maximum permissible dose (MPD) for radiation workers is 5 rems for persons over age 18; the maximum dose for women of reproductive capacity is 1.25 rems per quarter at an even rate.

Clinical Considerations
Nature and Indications for Use
Used alone or in combination with surgery or chemotherapy, depending on the stage of disease and goal of therapy.

1. Adjuvant radiation therapy—used when a high risk of local recurrence or large primary tumor exists.
2. Curative radiation therapy—used in anatomically limited tumors (retina, optic nerve, certain brain tumors, skin, oral cavity). Course is usually longer and the dose higher.
3. Palliative—for treatment of symptoms.
   a. Provides excellent pain control for bone metastases.
   b. Used to relieve obstruction.
   c. Relief of neurologic dysfunction for brain metastases.
   d. Given in short, intensive courses.

Treatment Planning
1. Accurate diagnosis is established by biopsy, and extent of disease is determined.
2. Goal of therapy is decided—cure versus palliation.
3. All patients undergo simulation and treatment planning.
   a. Target volume is identified by x-ray, scans, or physical examination.
   b. Treatment unit is selected.
   c. The design and pattern of delivery, total dose to be administered, time, and dose per day are determined.
   d. Usual schedule is Monday through Friday.
   e. Actual therapy lasts minutes. Most time is spent on positioning.
4. Computerized treatment plans are devised.
   a. Lead blocks are made to shape the beam and protect normal tissues.
   b. Immobilization devices (casts, head holders) are designed to ensure accurate positioning.
   c. Skin markings are applied to define the target and portal. These are replaced later by permanent tattoos.

Complications

Complications depend on the site of radiation therapy, type of radiation therapy (brachytherapy or teletherapy), total radiation dose, daily fractionated doses, and overall health of the patient. Side effects are predictable, depending on the normal organs and tissues involved in the field.

GERONTOLOGIC ALERT

Side effects may be prolonged due to decreased ability of the body to repair cellular damage.

Acute Side Effects

During treatment to 6 months after treatment:
1. Fatigue and malaise
2. Skin: erythema at the site, possible dry-to-wet desquamation
3. Gastrointestinal effects: nausea and vomiting, diarrhea, and esophagitis
4. Oral effects: changes in taste, mucositis, dryness, and xerostomia (dryness of mouth from lack of normal secretions)
5. Pulmonary effects: dyspnea, productive cough, pneumonitis
6. Renal and bladder effects: cystitis and urethritis
7. Cardiovascular: damage to vasculature of organs, thrombosis (heart is relatively radioresistant)
8. Recall reactions—acute skin and mucosal reactions when concurrent or past chemotherapy (doxorubicin [Adriamycin], dactinomycin [Actinomycin D])

Chronic Side Effects

After 6 months with a variability in time of expression:
1. Skin effects: fibrosis, telangiectasia, permanent darkening of the skin, and atrophy
2. Gastrointestinal effects: fibrosis, adhesions, obstruction, ulceration, and strictures
3. Oral effects: permanent xerostomia, permanent taste alterations, and dental caries
4. Pulmonary effects: fibrosis
5. Renal and bladder effects: radiation nephritis, fibrosis
6. Second primary cancer—patients who have received combined radiation and chemotherapy with alkylating agents have a 5% to 7% risk of acute leukemia

Nursing Assessment

1. Assess skin and mucous membranes for side effects of radiation.
2. Assess gastrointestinal, respiratory, and renal function for signs of side effects.
3. Assess patient's understanding of treatment and emotional status.

Nursing Diagnoses

- Risk for Impaired Skin Integrity related to radiation effects
- Altered Protection (for nurse and others) related to brachytherapy

Nursing Interventions
Maintaining Optimal Skin Care

1. Inform the patient that some skin reaction can be expected, but that it varies from patient to patient. Examples include dry erythema, dry desquamation, wet desquamation, epilation, and tanning.
2. Do not apply lotions, ointments, or cosmetics to the site of radiation unless prescribed. Cornstarch may be used when the skin is dry and itchy.
3. Discourage vigorous rubbing, friction, or scratching because this can destroy skin cells. Apply ointments as instructed by health professionals.
4. Avoid wearing tight-fitting clothing over the treatment field; prevent irritation by not using rough fabric such as wool and corduroy.
5. Take precautions against exposing the radiation field to sunlight and extremes in temperature.
6. Do not apply adhesive or other tape to the skin.
7. Avoid shaving the skin in the treatment field.
8. Use lukewarm water only and mild soap when bathing.

Ensuring Protection from Radiation

1. To avoid exposure to radiation while the patient is receiving therapy, consider the following:
   a. Time: exposure to radiation is directly proportional to the time spent within a specific distance to the source.
   b. Distance: amount of radiation reaching a given area decreases as resistance increases.
   c. Shield: sheet of absorbing material placed between the radiation source and the nurse decreases the amount of radiation exposure.
2. If exposed to penetrating radiation (x-ray or gamma rays), wear film badges on the front of the body.
3. Take appropriate measures associated with sealed sources of radiation implanted within a patient (sealed internal radiation).
   a. Follow directives on precaution sheet that is placed on the charts of all patients receiving radiotherapy.
   b. Do not remain within 1 meter (3 feet) of the patient any longer than required to give essential care.
4. Know that the casing material absorbs all alpha radiation and most beta radiation, but that a hazard concerning gamma radiation may exist.
5. Do not linger longer than necessary in giving patient care, even though all precautions are followed.
6. Be alert for implants that may have become loosened (those inserted in cavities that have access to the exterior); for example, check the emesis basin following mouth care for a patient with an oral implant.
7. Notify the radiation therapist of any implant that has moved out of position.
8. Use long-handled forceps or tongs and hold at arm's length when picking up any dislodged radium needle, seeds, or tubes. Never pick up a radioactive source with your hands.
9. Do not discard any dressings or linens unless you are sure that no radioactive source is present.

10. After the patient is discharged from the hospital, it is a good policy for the radiologist to check the room with a radiograph or survey meter to be certain that all radioactive materials have been removed.

11. Continue radiation precautions when a patient has a permanent implant, until the radiologist declares precautions unnecessary.

12. Obtain information at *http://cancernet.nci/gov/peb/radiation*.

Outcome-Based Evaluation
- Skin without breakdown or signs of infection
- Radiation precautions maintained

Cancer Immunotherapy

Cancer immunotherapy, or the use of biologic response modifiers (BRMs), is based on the hypothesis that the immune system can be manipulated to restore, augment, or modulate its own function. It is capable of altering the immune system with either stimulatory or suppressive effects. Cancer immunotherapy is rapidly becoming a fourth modality for cancer treatment.

Underlying Principles
Function
The primary function of the immune system is to detect and eliminate substances that are recognized as "non-self."
The Immune System
Two major components: nonspecific (innate) and specific (acquired).

1. Nonspecific or innate immunity is inherent in all individuals. The largest component of the nonspecific system is the skin. Other nonspecific defense mechanisms include mucous membranes, cilia, tears, sebaceous glands, and acidic urine.

2. Specific or acquired immunity has two primary features—specificity and memory. It is composed of three groups: cell-mediated immunity, humoral immunity, and null cells.
   a. Cell-mediated immunity is the T cells: T4 (helper/inducer cells) and T8 (cytotoxic and suppressor).
   b. Humoral immunity is the B cells, which ultimately secrete antibodies.
   c. Null cells are cells that are neither T nor B cells. Their principal function is still unknown. Natural killer (NK) cells and lymphokine-activated killer (LAK) cells are included in this group.

Types of Immunotherapy
1. Antibody therapy (serotherapy)
   a. Promotes targeting cells through antibody-antigen response.
   b. Monoclonal antibodies may be used alone or in combination with chemotherapy.
   c. Examples include rituximab (Rituxan) and trastuzumab (Herceptin).
   d. Rituximab is a murine/human chimeric monoclonal antibody specific for the CD20 surface marker on B cells. It is approved for the treatment of relapsed or refractory low-grade/follicular non-Hodgkin's lymphoma.
   e. Trastuzumab is a recombinant DNA–derived humanized monoclonal antibody that selectively binds with high affinity in a cell-based assay to the extracellular domain of the human epidermal growth factor receptor 2 protein, HER2. It is approved for the treatment of patients with metastatic breast cancer whose tumors overexpress the HER2 protein.

Cytokines
Cytokines are proteins produced by mononuclear cells of the immune system (usually the lymphocytes and monocytes) that have regulatory actions on other cells in the immune system.

1. Examples of cytokines include interleukins, interferons, colony-stimulating factors (CSFs), and tumor necrosis factor (TNF).
2. Many other biologic agents are currently under investigation.

Nursing Assessment
1. Review patient's chart to determine site of cancer, previous cancer therapies, current medications, and other medical conditions.
2. Assess patient's current cardiovascular and respiratory status.
3. Assess patient's understanding of immunotherapy and associated toxicities.

Nursing Diagnoses
- Hyperthermia as a side effect of immunotherapy
- Altered Tissue Perfusion (Cardiopulmonary) related to capillary permeability leak syndrome (third spacing of fluid) caused by immunotherapy

Nursing Interventions
Controlling Hyperthermia
1. Discuss the overall goal of immunotherapy, expected side effects, and the method of administration.
2. Instruct the patient to report any discomfort, including fever, chills, diarrhea, nausea and vomiting, itching, or weight gain.
3. Administer or advise self-administration of antipyretics such as acetaminophen (Tylenol) for fever.
4. Emphasize that side effects are temporary and will usually cease within 1 week after treatment ends.

Maintaining Tissue Perfusion
1. Monitor vital signs at least every 4 hours for hypotension, tachycardia, tachypnea, and fever.
   a. Instruct patient to remain in bed if blood pressure is low.
   b. Monitor apical heart rate.
2. Assess respirations for rate and depth, and auscultate breath sounds for evidence of pulmonary edema.

3. Assess for signs of restlessness, apprehension, discomfort, or cyanosis, which may indicate respiratory distress.
4. Administer oxygen as prescribed.
5. Maintain patent IV line and administer serum albumin as prescribed.
6. Check extremities for warmth, color, and capillary refill.

Outcome-Based Evaluation
- Relief of fever following medication
- Blood pressure stable; lungs clear

SPECIAL CONSIDERATIONS IN CANCER CARE

■ Pain Management
Pain related to cancer may be caused by direct tumor infiltration of bones, nerves, viscera, or soft tissue or by prior therapeutic measures (surgery, radiation).

Incidence
1. Pain is the most common symptom associated with cancer.
2. Approximately one-quarter of patients with newly diagnosed malignancies, one-third of patients undergoing treatment, and three-quarters of patients with advanced disease experience pain.

Causes
1. Pain induced by the disease, including pain secondary to direct tumor involvement of bone, nerves, viscera, or soft tissue.
2. Pain secondary to the treatment of cancer, such as surgery, chemotherapy, radiation, and immunotherapy.

Types of Pain
1. Somatic pain—caused by direct tumor involvement of sensory receptors in cutaneous and deep tissues.
   a. Usually described as dull, sharp, aching, and throbbing. It is usually constant and well localized.
   b. Most common somatic pain is bone pain caused by metastasis.
   c. Can usually be controlled with NSAIDs or oral opioids.
2. Neuropathic pain
   a. Results from nerve injury or compression.
   b. Neuropathic pain includes phantom pain and post-herpetic neuralgia.
   c. Described as burning, shooting, electric, and lancinating. It can be constant or sporadic.
   d. Usually is associated with abnormal sensations, such as paresthesias.
   e. Treatment usually includes adjuvant drugs such as tricyclic antidepressants and anticonvulsants in combination with opioids.

3. Visceral pain
   a. Usually described as a deep, dull, aching, squeezing, or pressure sensation. It can be vague or ill defined and can be referred to cutaneous sites, making it difficult to differentiate from somatic pain (e.g., right shoulder pain from liver metastases).
   b. Usually caused by the abnormal stretching of smooth muscle walls, ischemia of visceral muscle, and serosal irritation.
   c. Can be treated with surgery to remove the cause and oral opioids.

Other Clinical Manifestations
1. Fatigue from sleep disturbances; most patients may not have slept for extended periods of time.
2. Loss of appetite or weight loss; anxiety or depression.
3. Change in self-concept, change in quality of life.

Management
Pharmacologic Management
1. Use of NSAIDs
   a. Examples include aspirin, indomethacin (Indocin), and ibuprofen (Motrin)
   b. They produce analgesia by decreasing levels of inflammatory mediators at the site of tissue injury.
   c. There are newer NSAIDs called COX-2 inhibitors, such as celecoxib (Celebrex), with lower gastrointestinal bleeding rates. There are currently no data on these drugs specific to cancer.
   d. Used to treat mild to moderate pain.
2. Opioids
   a. Primary course of treatment for moderate to severe pain.
   b. Produce analgesia by binding to specific opiate receptors in the brain and spinal cord.
   c. Preparations:
      (i) Long acting—over 8 to 12 hours (MS Contin, Oromorph, OxyContin)
      (ii) Short acting—morphine sulfate, oxycodone, or hydromorphone (Dilaudid) may be used for breakthrough pain. Relief lasts 3 to 4 hours.
3. Should use oral route unless patient is unable to swallow or absorb medications through the GI tract.
4. Doses should be adjusted to achieve pain relief with an acceptable level of side effects.
5. Most important to administer on a schedule rather than prn.
6. Optimal treatment approach is to treat with long-acting drugs paired with short-acting drugs as needed for breakthrough pain.
7. Adjuvant drugs
   a. Used to enhance the effect of opioids.
   b. Commonly used drugs include:
      (i) Anticonvulsants, and antidepressants for neuropathic pain

(ii) Corticosteroids for tumor invasion of neural tissue, e.g., spinal cord compression

(iii) Muscle relaxants for musculoskeletal pain

Intraspinal Administration of Opiates

1. A catheter is placed into spinal epidural or subarachnoid (intrathecal) space for the management of acute or chronic pain.
2. Catheter may be placed percutaneously and sutured in site or tunneled subcutaneously to the abdominal wall and exteriorized, or the pump system may be implanted.
3. Catheter is positioned as near as possible to the spinal segment where the pain is projected.
4. Preservative-free sterile morphine or other analgesic/local anesthetic drug is injected into the system at specified intervals.
   a. May be delivered by patient-controlled analgesia (PCA) pump.
   b. May be continuous or bolus infusions.
5. Spinally administered local anesthetics produce their effects predominantly by action on axons of spinal nerve roots; produce long-lasting pain relief with relatively low doses with little or no blunting of patient's level of responsiveness.
6. Complications include respiratory depression, urinary retention, pruritus, infection, leakage, technical problems, and development of tolerance.
7. Patient education
   a. The patient and family are taught drug administration, pump instruction, catheter and exit site care, monitoring of respiration, and recognition of respiratory depression and its treatment.
   b. Arrange for home health care nurse to visit.

Nursing Assessment and Interventions

See Standards of Care Guidelines.

1. Screen for pain at each visit. Evaluate objectively the nature of the patient's pain: location, duration, quality, and impact on daily activities.
2. Use a pain intensity scale of 0 (no pain) to 10 (worst possible pain) or other pain scale as appropriate. Take careful history of prior and present medications, response, and side effects.
3. Assess relief from medications and duration of relief. (Use the same measuring scale every time.)
4. Base the initial analgesic choice on the patient's report of pain.
5. Administer drugs orally whenever possible; avoid intramuscular injection.
6. Administer analgesia "around the clock" rather than prn.
7. Convey the impression that the patient's pain is understood and that the pain can be controlled.
8. Take a careful pain history. Explore pain interventions that have been used and their effectiveness. Determine whether the intensity of the pain correlates with the prescribed analgesic.
9. Reevaluate the pain frequently. The requirement for analgesia should decrease if other treatment is given, including radiation or chemotherapy.
10. Use alternative measures to relieve pain such as guided imagery, relaxation, and biofeedback.
11. Provide ongoing support and open communication.
12. Consider referral to a pain specialist for intractable pain.
13. Provide education.
    a. A complete list of each medication prescribed with instructions on how to take each one.
    b. A list of potential side effects and how to manage them.
    c. Instruct patients that there is no benefit to suffering and that addiction is not a problem.
    d. Instruct patients that taking these medications now does not mean that they will not work later.
    e. Encourage patients to talk to their doctor or nurse about their pain and effectiveness of the treatment plan.
    f. Assure patients that there are other options if the medications prescribed do not work.
14. Take measures to prevent and treat side effects of opiates, such as constipation, nausea, and sedation.

■ Oncologic Emergencies

Septic Shock

Septic shock is a systemic disease associated with the presence and persistence of pathogenic microorganisms or their toxins in the blood.

Incidence and Mortality

The incidence of sepsis in cancer patients is estimated at 45%, with mortality rates exceeding 30%.

STANDARDS OF CARE GUIDELINES
Pain Management

To provide appropriate pain management for patients with cancer or other illnesses or injuries, consider the following:

- Assess pain repeatedly by questioning patient, looking for nonverbal signs of pain, and using appropriate pain rating scale.
- Administer analgesics on round-the-clock schedule as indicated with prn dosing for breakthrough pain.
- Utilize combination analgesic regimens and adjunct medications such as antiemetics, antidepressants, and antianxiety agents as needed for patient's comfort.
- Help the patient employ nonpharmacologic measures such as relaxation techniques, distraction, and massage.
- Assess for adverse reactions and patient's response to pain relief measures, and alter pain management plan as indicated.
- Communicate any significant adverse reactions or failure to provide adequate pain relief to health care provider.

This information should serve as a general guideline only. Each patient situation presents a unique set of clinical factors and requires nursing judgment to guide care, which may include additional or alternative measures and approaches.

Risk Factors

1. Neutropenia
2. Patients who are neutropenic greater than 7 days are most susceptible
3. Patients with HIV and concomitant neutropenia
4. Prolonged hospitalization
5. Elderly patients
6. Patients with co-morbid conditions such as diabetes and pulmonary diseases

Clinical Manifestations

1. Fever greater than 38.3°C
2. Warm, flushed, dry skin
3. Hypotension
4. Tachycardia
5. Tachypnea
6. Decreased level of consciousness
7. Decreased urine output

Diagnostic Evaluation

1. Vital signs
2. Culture—blood, urine, stool, sputum, central and peripheral IV lines, and any open wounds to determine source and type of infection
3. Chest x-ray—to detect underlying pneumonia
4. CT scans as necessary
5. Arterial blood gas evaluation—decreased pH reflects acidosis
6. BUN and creatinine—elevated due to decreased circulating blood volume
7. CBC with differential—elevated WBC with shift to left

Management

1. Antibiotics are started immediately; broad-spectrum antibiotics are given until organism is identified.
2. IV fluids and plasma expanders are used to restore circulating volume.
3. Colony-stimulating factors are administered to increase neutraphil count.
4. Vasopressors are administered to support blood pressure.
5. Oxygen is used to prevent tissue hypoxia.
6. Vital signs, respiratory status, urine output, and any signs of bleeding are monitored carefully.
7. Complications such as renal failure, respiratory failure, cardiac failure, metabolic acidosis, and disseminated intravascular coagulation are treated aggressively.

Spinal Cord Compression (SCC)

Metastatic epidural spinal cord compression is defined as compression on the spinal cord or cauda equina nerve roots from a lesion outside the spinal dura. Associated with vertebral metastases.

Incidence

1. 50% of diagnosed cases occur in patients with lung, breast, or colon cancer.
2. This is the second most common neurologic complication of cancer.

Clinical Manifestations

1. Clinical signs and symptoms relate to the site of the vertebral bony metastasis.
   a. Vertigo
   b. Cervical spine
      (i) Radicular pain in neck and back of head that is aggravated by neck flexion
      (ii) Upper extremity weakness
      (iii) Sensory loss in area of weakness, i.e., paresthesias, numbness
      (iv) Abnormal deep tendon reflexes
      (v) Gastric hypersecretion and paralytic ileus
   c. Thoracic spine
      (i) Local or radicular pain (or both)
      (ii) Lower extremity weakness
      (iii) Sensory loss below the level of the lesion
      (iv) Band of hyperesthesia at dermatome of tumor site
      (v) Impaired bladder and/or bowel control
   d. Lumbar spine
      (i) Local or radicular pain (or both)
      (ii) Lower extremity weakness, paralysis
      (iii) Atrophy of lower extremity muscles
      (iv) Sensory loss below level of the lesion
      (v) Urinary symptoms (hesitancy, retention), constipation, or bowel incontinence
2. Weakness and unsteadiness may be noted before changes in motor function. Progression is often rapid with foot drop and impaired ambulation. Urgent investigation and treatment are crucial to minimize the risk of paraplegia. The degree of weakness and ability to walk at presentation are important clinical predictors of outcome.
3. Changes in sensation—paresthesia, numbness, tingling. Severity usually mirrors the severity of motor weakness.

> **NURSING ALERT**
>
> Any abnormal neurologic symptoms in a patient with cancer should be considered an SCC until proved otherwise.

Diagnostic Evaluation

1. Neurologic examination—early diagnosis is important.
2. X-ray of the painful site—may or may not be abnormal. Can be used as an initial screen for complaints of back pain.
3. Bone scan—more sensitive to bony metastasis than x-ray to detect abnormal vertebral bodies.
4. MRI—most useful in detecting spinal cord lesions. The whole spine can be viewed. Immediately indicated if radiculopathy or myelopathy is present or x-rays are abnormal.
5. Myelogram with CT scan—no longer used unless MRI equipment is unavailable or patient is unable to tolerate MRI scanner.

Management

1. Treatment is usually palliative but may be curative in selected cases, such as metastatic seminoma.
2. Treatment goals are to relieve pain and restore function.
3. Corticosteroids—reduce inflammation and swelling at site, increase neurologic function, and relieve pain.
   a. A loading dose of decadron at 100 mg is often given prior to diagnostic procedures.
   b. Dose is then reduced to 16 to 24 mg/day during radiation therapy.
   c. Decadron must be tapered and not abruptly discontinued.
   d. Monitor patient's glucose levels while on decadron; it can cause hyperglycemia.
4. Radiation therapy to the tumor on spinal column.
   a. A common dose is 3000 cGy, delivered in 10 fractions over a period of 2.5 weeks.
5. Immediate decompressive surgery (laminectomy); not commonly used.

Complications

1. Respiratory impairment, including pneumonia and atelectasis
2. Mobility impairment, including immobility, foot drop, skin impairment, postural hypotension
3. Sensory losses creating safety concerns
4. Bladder or bowel dysfunction

Patient Education

1. Facilitate referral to home care services for nursing assessment, nursing intervention, and rehabilitation for residual deficits.
2. Facilitate referral to appropriate outpatient services, including physical therapy, occupational therapy, and psychosocial support.
3. Provide instruction regarding safety issues for residual sensory deficits (e.g., test bath water temperature, careful use of extreme hot or cold).

Hypercalcemia

Hypercalcemia is an elevated serum calcium level above 11.0 mg/dL. It results when bone resorption exceeds both bone formation and the ability of the kidneys to excrete extracellular calcium released from the bones.

Incidence

1. The most common life-threatening disorder associated with malignancy; occurs in 10% to 20% of patients with cancer.
2. Occurs most frequently in patients with carcinoma of the lung, breast, prostate, and multiple myeloma.
3. Can occur with or without skeletal metastasis, but more than 80% of patients do have bony disease.

Clinical Manifestations

1. Signs and symptoms may vary, depending on the severity of the hypercalcemia and the onset.
2. Symptoms may be nonspecific and insidious, such as nausea and vomiting, anorexia, weakness, constipation, polyuria, polydipsia, and change in mental status.

3. Neuromuscular changes such as muscle weakness may occur.
4. A very rapid and life-threatening increase in calcium may cause dehydration, renal failure, coma, and death.

Diagnostic Evaluation

1. Serum calcium level greater than 11.0 mg/dL in adults.
2. Electrolyte levels, BUN, and creatinine are obtained to determine hydration status and renal function.

Management

1. Management includes treating the primary malignancy with chemotherapy, surgery, or radiation.
2. Hydration with IV normal saline (0.9% NaCl) is the initial treatment for patients with acute hypercalcemia and clinical symptoms, to dilute the calcium and promote its renal excretion.
3. Pharmacotherapy
   a. Biphosphonates—administered IV (pamidronate [Aredia]) inhibit osteoclast resorption in the bone. Mainstay of drug therapy.
   b. Diuretics may be used to promote further diuresis and calcium excretion.
   c. Plicamycin—blocks PTH and may also inhibit bone resorption. Not readily used since the availability of biphosphonates.
   d. Calcitonin—used in combination with glucocorticoids, inhibits bone resorption. It has a rapid onset but a short duration of action. Used more often in patients with multiple myeloma.

Nursing Interventions

1. Prevent and detect hypercalcemia early.
   a. Recognize patients at risk and monitor for signs and symptoms, such as nausea and vomiting, constipation, lethargy, and anorexia.
   b. Emphasize importance of mobility to minimize bone demineralization and constipation.
   c. Instruct patient on the importance of adequate hydration.
2. Administer normal saline infusions as prescribed.
3. Administer medications as prescribed.
4. Maintain accurate intake and output; observe for oliguria or anuria.
5. Take vital signs every 4 hours, especially apical pulse and blood pressure.
6. Monitor electrolyte values and renal function.
7. Assess mental status.
8. Assess cardiorespiratory status for signs of fluid overload.

Superior Vena Cava Syndrome (SVCS)

Superior vena cava syndrome is obstruction and thrombosis of the superior vena cava by a tumor or an enlarged lymph node, resulting in impaired venous drainage of the head, neck, arms, and thorax.

Incidence

1. Approximately 3% to 4% of patients with cancer develop SVCS.
2. Occurs most often in men aged 50 to 70 who have tumors of the mediastinum (primary or metastatic).

3. The majority of cases arise from small cell lung cancers.
4. Other malignancies associated with SVCS include Hodgkin's and non-Hodgkin's lymphoma, thymoma, and breast cancer.

Clinical Manifestations

1. Signs and symptoms may vary, depending on the degree of obstruction and how rapidly the obstruction occurs.
2. SVCS that develops gradually results in subtle signs of edema and venous engorgement.
3. A rapid onset of SVCS is dramatic, potentially life threatening, and requires immediate intervention.
4. Dyspnea and "tight collar" syndrome (facial and neck swelling) occur for 2 to 4 weeks before diagnosis.
5. Chest pain, cough, and dysphagia are present.
6. Cyanosis and edema of the head and upper extremities may be apparent. Collateral circulation with dilated chest wall veins may be visible.
7. Progressive dyspnea, orthopnea, and neck vein distention occur.
8. CNS symptoms include headache, dizziness, irritability, lethargy, dysphagia, and visual disturbances.
9. Pleural effusion on chest x-ray may also be seen.

Diagnostic Evaluation

1. 60% of SVCS cases can be detected on plain chest x-ray.
2. CT scan may be necessary to make the diagnosis for some patients, but is usually used to determine the extent of tumor and obstruction.

Management

1. Radiation therapy is the gold standard of treatment for SVCS to reduce tumor size and relieve pressure. Most patients experience a relief of symptoms within the first 4 days of therapy.
2. Chemotherapy may be used in conjunction with radiation. Specific chemotherapeutic agents depend on the tumor type.
3. Surgery is rarely used due to the associated high morbidity and mortality risks.
4. Percutaneous stent placement may reopen occluded vessels.
5. Thrombolytic/anticoagulant therapy may be used if a thrombus is suspected or to prevent the formation of a thrombus; must be used within the first 7 days to be effective.
6. Oxygen is given for relief of dyspnea and maintenance of airway.
7. Analgesics and tranquilizers are used for discomfort and anxiety.

Nursing Interventions

1. Administer oxygen as prescribed to relieve hypoxia.
2. Place patient in Fowler's position—facilitates gravity drainage and reduces facial edema.
3. Limit the patient's activity and provide a quiet environment.
4. Reassure patient that cyanotic color and facial edema will subside with treatment.

Clinical Trials

A clinical trial is a scientific study designed to answer important clinical and biological questions. Trials provide a mechanism to tests the effectiveness of new drug and other therapies. Clinical trials are very important in the advancement of cancer treatment.

Phases of Clinical Trials

Phase I Trials

1. Phase 1 studies are offered to patients who have failed conventional therapy or for whom there is no treatment known to be superior.
2. Phase 1 trials are given to patients with various types of cancer to:
   a. Evaluate drug toxicities
   b. Establish the maximum tolerated dose of the drug
   c. Evaluate the pharmacokinetics of the drug

Phase II Trials

1. The goals of phase II studies are:
   a. Determine tumor activity in specific tumor types
   b. Design administration techniques
   c. Determine dose modifications

Phase III Trials

1. Designed to compare drug(s) with standard therapy
2. Evaluate response and duration of response

Phase IV Trials

1. Designed to determine new ways to use the drug
2. Determine effectiveness in the adjuvant setting

Nursing Interventions

1. Educate patients about the clinical trial process.
2. If involved in clinical trials, follow protocol and documentation as indicated.
3. Report all adverse events during the trial period.
4. Refer patients who are interested in clinical trials to CancerTrials at **http://cancertrials.nci.nih.gov**.

Psychosocial Components of Care

Nursing Assessment

1. Assess lifestyle prior to illness. How did patient solve other problems?
2. Assess for signs of anxiety and coexistence of depression: agitation/restlessness, sleep disturbances, excessive autonomic activity, weight gain or loss, mood changes.
3. What activities of daily living can the patient perform?
4. What changes in lifestyle have resulted from cancer and its treatment?
5. Ascertain the patient's perception of the disease and treatment.
6. Evaluate available social support; who is the most significant other?
7. Ask patient if any alternative modalities are being utilized for cancer treatment. Be aware that many patients seek herbal and other remedies despite lack of scientific evidence of any benefit. Encourage patient and family

TABLE 8-5 Alternative Therapies

In an effort to increase their chances of survival, bring a measure of control, and minimize side effects, a number of patients are turning to alternative therapies. Herbs are popular and have been used to treat cancer since 2838 BC. Many of these herbs, however, have not been adequately researched, so their impact on cancer is not known. Listed below are some common herbs and their advertised benefits. Neither the author nor the publisher makes any medical claims for any herbs listed.

Herb	Advertised Benefit	Precautions
Iscador	Derived from mistletoe—said to activate defense functions and help prevent metastatic spread after surgery	
Laetril	Derived from apricots and almonds—promoters say that enzymes in malignant neoplasms trigger the release of hydrogen cyanide from the drug. The cyanide is claimed to stop tumor respiration and kill the cancer cells	Has caused cyanide poisoning
Uritica	Derived from stinging nettle—used for prostate cancer in Germany	Can be irritating to the stomach
Essiac	Made from Indian rhubarb; thought to have anticancer activity	Studied in the 1980s—found to have no anti-tumor activity
Lily	Worldwide folk use for cancers	Can be toxic
Echinacea	Currently under investigation in liver and colon cancer for immune stimulation	Has cortisone-like activity
Hoxsey	Folk use in India; thought to have anticancer activity	Excessive use can cause headache, lethargy, heart failure, cardiac arrest
Pau D' arco	Anticancer activity noted, but studies were discontinued	Extremely toxic. Nausea, vomiting, potential for hemorrhage
Green tea	Chinese remedy; thought to have anticancer activity	Linked with high rates of esophageal cancer if consumed heavily
Ginseng	Old Chinese remedy; thought to stimulate immune system	Overdose may cause hemorrhage, vomiting, or death. Estrogen-like properties

to discuss alternative therapy use with health care provider to ensure safety (Table 8-5).

8. Try to gain a sense of emotional strengths and potential problem areas. Ask if patient and family have a plan for end of life care as appropriate.

Nursing Diagnoses
- Anxiety related to complex disease process, treatment options, and prognosis
- Ineffective Individual Coping related to life-altering disease process
- Fear of death and dying

Nursing Interventions
Reducing Anxiety
1. Establish and sustain an unhurried approach to give the patient time to organize fears, thoughts, and feelings.
2. Allow patient to share feelings about having cancer.
3. Reflect and amplify insights and judgments; try to reduce anxiety through reflection and reorientation.
4. Recognize feelings of losing control.
5. Discuss methods of stress reduction (imagery, relaxation, biofeedback).
6. Discuss the positive aspects of treatment.
7. Encourage expression of positive emotions—emphasis on living in the here and now, greater appreciation of life, etc.

8. Reinforce effective coping behaviors.
9. Encourage patient to join a support group. Refer to local chapter of the American Cancer Society or call 1-800-ACS-2345.
10. Remain available as problems arise. Give patient telephone numbers of persons to call when needed—creates a sense of security.
11. Initiate referrals for additional rehabilitation and psychosocial services as appropriate.

Promoting Effective Coping
1. Encourage patient and family members to enroll in cancer education program.
2. Encourage patient to learn everything about treatment plan, because this promotes a sense of control.
3. Provide expert physical care while teaching patient to take over care as able.
4. Assist patient in strengthening support system (family, friends, visitors, health care staff and volunteers, support groups)—strengthens self-esteem through the experience of feeling accepted and valued.
5. Help patient readjust expectations and goals to promote ongoing adjustment.
6. Support patient in coping mechanisms chosen.

Allaying Fear of Death and Dying
1. Educate patient and family about prognosis and end-of-life choices, as outlined by patient's health care provider.
2. Assess and respect the patient's beliefs.

3. Help the patient and family arrive at a consensus on treatment goals.
4. Facilitate emotional support for the patient.
5. Provide bereavement support to survivors.

Palliative Care

Palliative care, also known as comfort care, is primarily directed at providing relief to a terminally ill person through symptom management. The goal is not to cure but to provide comfort and maintain the highest possible quality of life for as long as possible. The focus of palliative care is not on death but on a compassionate, specialized care for the living. Palliative care is an integral part of oncology nursing. Most medical residents and nursing students do not get adequate training in palliative care. This is unfortunate since most will need to provide care for the terminally ill.

Management and Nursing Interventions

1. Discuss end-of-life issues early in patient's treatment plan.
   a. It is important for providers and nurses to have open and frank discussions with patients about their preferences regarding end-of-life care.
   b. This discussion should not occur during a life-threatening event when patients and families are stressed and feel rushed to make a decision.
2. Encourage patients to express their preferences about end of life in the form of a legal document.
   a. Advance Directives or a living will authorize a family member or friend to make decisions for the patient.
3. Educate about and provide hospice care.
   a. Hospice programs are not involved early enough for patients to fully benefit from the services available. This is largely due to the fact that providers wait to discuss hospice until very late in their care, and patients often have misconceptions about what hospice care can provide. Many patients resist hospice referral to pursue further treatment options.
   b. Hospice programs utilize a multidisciplinary approach to care for patients individually both at home or in a hospice facility.
4. Goals of hospice include:
   a. Symptom management
      (i) Pain control
      (ii) Air hunger
      (iii) Agitation
      (iv) Anxiety
      (v) GI discomfort
   b. Counseling
      (i) Pastoral care
      (ii) Bereavement counseling for families
      (iii) Facilitate emotional support for patients and families
   c. Respite care
      (i) Volunteers are available to help the family care for patients in the home.
      (ii) Patients can be transferred to an in-patient setting as necessary.

SELECTED REFERENCES

American Cancer Society@www.cancer.org

American Joint Committee on Cancer (1992). *Manual for staging of cancer* (4th ed.). Philadelphia: J. B. Lippincott.

Barnett, M.L. (1999). Hypercalcemia. *Seminars in Oncology Nursing, 15*(3), 190–20.

Bucholtz, J.D. (1999). Metastatic epidural spinal cord compression. *Seminars in Oncology Nursing, 15*(3), 150–159.

Byock, I. (2000). Completing the continuum of care: Integrating life prolongation and palliation. *CA: Cancer Journal for Clinicians, 50*, 123–132.

Cancer statistics. (1999). *Cancer Journal for Clinicians, 45*(1), 8–31.

Cancer Net @ cancernet.nci.nih.gov

Casciapo, D. (1995). *Manual of clinical oncology* (3rd ed.). Boston: Little, Brown.

Chang, H.M. (1999). Cancer pain management. *Medical Clinics of North America, 83*(3), 711–735.

Fauser, A.A., Fellhauer, M., Hoffman, M., Link, H., Schlimok, G., & Gralla, R.J. (1999). Guidelines for antiemetic therapy: Acute emesis. *European Journal of Cancer, 35*(3), 361–370.

Groenwald, S., Frogge, M., & Yarbro, C. (1992). *Cancer nursing: Principles and practice* (2nd ed.). Boston: James and Bartlett.

Grossman, S.A., Benededetti, C., Payne, R. & Syrjala, K. (1999). NCCN guidelines for cancer pain. *Oncology, 13*(11A), 33–34.

Haapoja, I.S., & Blendowski, C. (1999). Superior vena cava syndrome. *Seminars in Oncology Nursing, 83*(3), 183–189.

Harrison, R.A., & Waterbor, J.W. (1999). Understanding meta-analysis in cancer. Epidemiology: Dietary fat and breast cancer. *Cancer Detection and Prevention, 23*(2), 97–106:

Johnson, M.H., Moroney, C.E., & Gay, C.F. (1997). Relieving nausea and vomiting in patients with cancer: A treatment algorithm. *Oncology Nursing Forum, 24*(1), 51–56.

Kearney, N. (1999). New cancer strategies. *Oncology Nursing Forum, 22*(1), 28–33.

Labovich, T.M. (1999). Acute sensitivity reactions to chemotherapy. *Seminars in Oncology Nursing, 15*(3), 222–231.

Levy, M.H. (1999). Pain control in patients with cancer. *Oncology, 13*(Suppl. 2), 9–14.

Marcus, P.M., et al. (1999). Physical activity at age 12 and adult breast cancer risk. *Cancer Causes and Control, 10*, 293–302:

Montbraind, M.J. (1999). Past and present herbs used to treat cancer: Medicine, magic, or poison? *Oncology Nursing Forum, 26*(1), 49–60.

Mrozek, M.E., Frye, D.K., & Sanborn, H.M. (1999). Capecitabine: Nursing implications of a new oral chemotherapeutic agent. *Oncology Nursing Forum, 26*(4), 753–761.

Nielson, C. & Lang, R. (1999). Principles of screening. *Medical Clinics of North America, 83*(6), 1323–1337.

Oncology Nursing Society (1997). *Safe handling of cytotoxic drugs* (2nd ed.). Philadelphia: Oncology Nursing Press.

PDQ @ cancernet.nci.nih.gov/health.htm.

Portenoy, R.K. (1999). Managing cancer pain poorly responsive to systemic opioid therapy. *Oncology, 13*(Suppl. 2), 25–29.

Shelton, B. (1999). Sepsis. *Seminars in Oncology Nursing, 15*(3), 209–221.

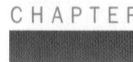
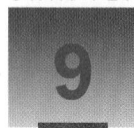

Care of the Older Adult

PHYSIOLOGY

Normal Changes of Aging

There are a number of normal age-related changes that occur in all major systems of the body. These may present at different times for different people. It is important to be able to differentiate between normal and abnormal changes in elderly people and to educate patients and families about these differences.

Vision
Characteristics
1. Decreased visual acuity
2. Decreased visual fields, and thus decreased peripheral vision
3. Decreased dark adaptation
4. Elevated minimal threshold of light perception
5. Presbyopia (farsightedness) due to decreased visual accommodation from loss of lens elasticity
6. Decreased color discrimination due to the yellowing of the lens; short wavelength colors, such as blues and greens are more difficult to see
7. Increased sensitivity to glare
8. Decreased depth perception
9. Decreased tears

Assessment Findings
1. Arcus senilis—deposits of lipid around the eye, seen as a white circle around the iris; causes no visual impairments
2. Cataracts—lens thickening and decreased permeability; noted on examination with the ophthalmoscope; results in fuzziness of vision
3. Smaller pupil size
4. Complaints of decreased ability to read, discomfort from light, changes in depth perception, falls, collisions, difficulty handling small objects, difficulty with activities of daily living (ADL), and tunnel vision
5. Glaucoma—increased intraocular pressure with tonometer testing
6. Dry, red eyes
7. Vitreous floaters, which are lightning flashes in the visual field

Nursing Considerations and Teaching Points
1. Make sure objects are in the patient's visual field, and do not move objects around.
2. Use large lettering to label medications and any distributed written information.
3. Allow the person more time to focus and adjust to the environment.
4. Avoid glare—may help to wear sunglasses.
5. Use nightlights to help with dark adaptation problems.
6. Use the colors red and yellow to stimulate vision.
7. Mark the edges of stairs and curbs to help with depth perception problems.
8. Use microspiral telescopes or magnifying glasses and high-intensity lighting.
9. Encourage yearly eye examination and/or refer for examination if visual changes persist (flashing lights in fields or "veil over the eye").
10. Encourage use of isotonic eyedrops as needed.
11. Refer patients to the following resource for visual impairments:
    American Foundation for the Blind
    11 Penn Plaza Suite 300
    New York, NY 10001
    212-502-7600
    www.AFB.org

Hearing
Characteristics
1. Approximately 30% to 50% of people older than 65 have significant hearing loss.
2. Three types of hearing disorders are common in the older population.

a. *Presbycusis*—progressive, irreversible bilateral loss of high-tone perception often associated with aging

b. *Central deafness*—occurs from nerve damage within the brain (considered a pathologic rather than normal change)

c. *Conduction deafness*—results from blockage or impairment of the mechanical movement in the outer or middle ear (also a pathologic condition)

3. Hearing loss in the elderly is often a combined problem. The majority of the loss is due to auditory nerve changes or deterioration of the structures of the ear. There may also be nerve damage beyond the ear. Presbycusis and central deafness can result in permanent hearing loss; conduction deafness is reversible.

4. Usual progression from high-tone or high-frequency loss to a general loss of both high and low tones.

5. Consonants (higher pitched sounds) not heard well.

6. Hearing loss increases with age and is greater in men.

7. Increase in the sound threshold (ie, greater sound needed to stimulate the older adult).

8. Decreased speech discrimination, especially with background noise.

9. Cerumen impaction, the most common cause of conductive hearing loss, is reversible.

Assessment Findings

1. Increased volume of patient's own speech
2. Turning of head toward speaker
3. Requests of a speaker to repeat
4. Inappropriate answers, but otherwise cognitively intact
5. The person may withdraw, demonstrate a short attention span, and become frustrated, angry, and depressed
6. Lack of response to a loud noise

Nursing Considerations and Teaching Points

1. Suggest hearing testing for further evaluation and consideration of an assistive device.
2. Face the person directly so he or she can lip read.
3. Use gestures and objects to help with verbal communication.
4. Touch the person to get his or her attention before talking.
5. Speak into the person's "good ear."
6. *Do not shout.* Shouting increases the tone of the voice, and elderly people are unable to hear these high tones.
7. Speak slowly and clearly.
8. Suggest amplifiers on telephones and alarms.
9. Allow the person more time to answer your questions.
10. Evaluate the person's ear canals regularly and assist with cerumen removal. Cerumen removal is facilitated by:
    a. Use of ceruminolytic agents such as Debrox, 10 drops in the affected ear twice a day for 5 days, followed by flushing the ear with warm water, or preferably an electronic irrigation device
    b. Careful use of an ear spoon to mechanically remove cerumen

11. Refer patients to the following organizations: American Association of Retired Persons—resource list for the deaf and hearing impaired (D14925) AARP Fulfillment (EE0569) P.O. Box 22796 Long Beach, CA 90801-5796

Self-Help Resources for Those Hard of Hearing 7910 Woodmont Ave, Suite 1200 Bethesda, MD 20814

Smell
Characteristics

1. Changes in smell are due to nasal sinus disease preventing odors from reaching smell receptors, a decrease in nerve fibers, chronic injury from infections, or bleeding.
2. Discrimination of fruity odors seems to persist the longest.
3. Generally, smells decrease in men more than in women.

Assessment Finding

1. Inability to notice unpleasant odors such as fires, body odor, or excessive perfume use
2. Decreased appetite

Nursing Considerations and Teaching Points

1. At mealtime, name food items and give the person time to think of the smell/taste of the food.
2. Suggest use of stronger spices and flavorings to stimulate smell.

Taste
Characteristics

1. Taste buds decrease with age, especially in men. People over 60 years of age have lost half of their taste buds. By age 80, only one sixth of the taste buds remain.
2. Taste buds are lost from the front to the back (ie, sweet and salty tastes are lost first, whereas bitter and sour tastes remain longer).

Assessment Findings

1. Complaints that food has no taste
2. Excessive use of sugar and salt
3. Inability to identify the foods
4. Decrease in appetite and weight loss
5. Decreased pleasure from food

Nursing Considerations and Teaching Points

1. Serve food attractively, and separate different types of foods.
2. Vary the texture of foods.
3. Encourage good oral hygiene.

Kinesthetic Sense
Characteristics

1. With age, the receptors in the joints and muscles that tell us where we are in space lose their ability to function. Therefore, there is a change in balance.

2. Walking with shorter step length, less leg lift, a wider base, and tendency to lean forward.
3. With age, less ability to stop a fall from occurring.

Assessment Findings
1. Alterations in posture, ability to transfer, and gait
2. Complaint of dizziness

Nursing Considerations and Teaching Points
1. Position items within reach.
2. Give person more time to move.

Cardiovascular
Characteristics
1. With age, the valves of the heart become thick and rigid as a result of sclerosis and fibrosis, compounding any cardiac disease already present.
2. Blood vessels also become thick and rigid, resulting in elevated blood pressure, which is present in half of the US population over the age of 65.
3. Maximum heart rate and aerobic capacity decrease with age.
4. Slower response to stress. Once the pulse rate is elevated, it takes longer to return to baseline.
5. Decline in maximum oxygen consumption.
6. About 50% of older adults have an abnormal resting ECG.
7. Subtle changes in artery walls result in a less flexible vasculature.

Assessment Findings
1. Elevated blood pressure up to 160/90 is considered normal over age 65 (goal BP 160/90)
2. Persistent tachycardia following stress

Nursing Considerations and Teaching Points
1. Encourage regular blood pressure evaluation.
2. Encourage longer cool-down period after exercise to return to baseline cardiac function.
3. Encourage regular aerobic exercise: walking, biking, or swimming for 20 minutes at least three times per week.

Pulmonary
Characteristics
1. With age, there is a weakening of the intercostal respiratory muscles, and the elastic recoil of the chest wall diminishes.
2. There is no change in total lung capacity, however residual volume and functional residual capacity increase.
3. PO_2 decreases with age due to ventilation–perfusion mismatches. However, elderly people are not hypoxic without coexistent disease.
4. There is a decrease in the mucous transport/ciliary system. Therefore, there is resulting decreased clearance of mucus and foreign bodies, including bacteria.

Assessment Findings
1. Prolonged cough, inability to raise secretions
2. Increased frequency of respiratory infections

Nursing Considerations and Teaching Points
1. Elderly people undergoing any surgical treatment need special attention paid to deep breathing exercises.
2. Teach measures to prevent pulmonary infections— avoid crowds during cold and flu season, wash hands frequently, report early signs of infection.

Immunologic
Characteristics
1. The function of T-cell lymphocytes, such as cell-mediated immunity, declines with age due to involution and atrophy of the thymus gland.
2. Decreased T-cell helper activity; increased T-cell suppressor activity.
3. Declining B-cell function as a result of T-cell changes.

Assessment Findings
1. More frequent infections
2. Increased incidence of many types of cancer

Nursing Considerations and Teaching Points
1. Teach people that they are at increased risk of infection, cancer, and autoimmune disease; therefore, routine follow-up and screening are essential.

Neurologic
Characteristics
1. There is gradual loss in the number of neurons with age, but no major change in neurotransmitter levels.
2. Some brain tissue atrophy is normal and does not relate to cognitive impairment.
3. Decreased muscle tone, motor speed, and nerve conduction velocity.
4. Decrease in gait speed of 1.6% per year after age 63, decreased step length, stride length, and arm swing.

Assessment Findings
1. Decreased position and vibration sense
2. Diminished reflexes, possible absent ankle jerks
3. Complaint of falls
4. Wide-based gait with decreased arm swing

Nursing Considerations and Teaching Points
1. Because of these changes in combination with sensory changes, fall prevention techniques are essential to teach to elderly people.
   a. Environmental safety techniques include nonslip surfaces, securely fastened handrails, sufficient light, glare-free lights, avoidance of low-lying objects, chairs of the proper height with armrests, skidproof strips or mats in the tub or shower, toilet and tub grab bars, elevated toilet seats.
   b. Home safety evaluations should be done on all community-dwelling elderly people to reduce the risk of falls. A home safety checklist can be obtained from:

National Safety Council
1025 Connecticut Avenue, NW
Washington, DC 20036
202-293-2270

Musculoskeletal
Characteristics
1. Declining muscle mass and endurance with age, although deconditioning may be an associated factor.
2. Decreased bone density, less so in men than in women.
3. Decreased thickness and resiliency of cartilage, with a resulting increase in the stiffness of joints.
4. Bone resorption exceeds bone formation, resulting in a decline in bone density.
5. Injuries to the cartilage accumulate with age.

Assessment Findings
1. Muscle atrophy
2. Increased incidence of fractures
3. Complaint of joint stiffness in absence of arthritis

Nursing Considerations and Teaching Points
Early intervention to encourage regular exercise in the elderly population is important to prevent exacerbation of these normal changes.

Community and Home Care Considerations
1. Encourage older adults to engage in 20 minutes of continuous aerobic exercise, including walking, biking, or swimming, at least three times per week.
2. For older adults who will be exercising at <80% of the maximum heart rate (220 – age), stress testing before starting an exercise program is not needed.
3. To help with adherence to the exercise program, older adults should be encouraged to exercise at a set time, to relieve pain before exercising, and to do an activity they enjoy. Provide positive reinforcement for those who do exercise, and continually reinforce the benefits of exercise (increased bone strength, cardiovascular fitness, decreased risks of falls, overall sense of well-being).

Endocrine
Characteristics
1. Decreased secretion of trophic hormones from the pituitary gland
2. Blunted growth hormone release during stress
3. Elevated vasopressin (antidiuretic hormone); exaggerated response to osmotic challenge
4. Elevated levels of follicle-stimulating hormone and luteinizing hormone because of reduced end-organ response
5. Normal insulin secretion at rest with an age-related decrease in secretion in response to a glucose load; this may be a function of weight or genetic factors

Assessment Findings
Usually asymptomatic

Nursing Considerations and Teaching Points
1. Encourage routine screening for elevated blood sugar.
2. Provide dietary education on well-balanced diet.

Reproductive
Characteristics
1. In women, menopause leads to decreases in the size of the ovaries and hormone production. This results in uterine involution, vaginal atrophy, and loss of breast mass.
2. In men, testosterone production and secretion decrease with age. However, serum levels may be in the low-normal range through age 80.

Assessment Findings
1. Vaginal dryness, painful intercourse
2. Atrophic vaginitis

Nursing Considerations and Teaching Points
1. Suggest the use of additional lubrication during sexual intercourse.
2. Advise sexually active older men that spermatogenesis may continue into advanced age.

Renal and Body Composition
Characteristics
1. Increased body fat and decreased lean muscle mass, even when weight remains stable.
2. Decreased renal function, measured by the glomerular filtration rate, or creatinine clearance.
3. Despite reduced total body creatinine due to decreased muscle mass in the older adult, serum creatinine often remains within normal range. This is because of decreased elimination of creatinine by the kidneys.
4. About 10% decline in creatinine clearance per decade after age 40; however, relatively unchanged serum creatinine.

Assessment Findings
1. Usually asymptomatic

Nursing Considerations and Teaching Points
1. Be aware that although creatinine level may be within normal range, creatinine clearance may be decreased. To obtain an accurate creatinine clearance in an elderly person, the following formula should be used: (140 – age)(weight [kg])/(72)(serum creatinine [mg per dL]).
2. Drugs that are cleared through the kidneys may be given in decreased dosage. Side effects and toxicity must be closely monitored.

Skin
Characteristics
1. Thinning of all three layers of the skin—epidermis, dermis, and subcutaneous tissue—leads to greater fragility

of the skin and decreased ability of the skin to function as a barrier to external factors.

2. Fewer melanocytes and decreased tanning.
3. Less efficient thermoregulation of heat because of fewer sweat glands.
4. Drier skin because the decreased number of sebaceous glands results in reduced oil production.
5. Other changes in aging skin include reduced sensory input, decreased elasticity, and impaired cell-related immune response.

Assessment Finding
1. Dry, irritated skin

Nursing Considerations and Teaching Points
1. Excessive use of soap, which can be drying to the skin, should be avoided.
2. Careful skin evaluation and lubrication are necessary to prevent fissures and breakdown.
3. Heat regulation needs to be controlled by proper clothing and avoidance of extreme temperatures.
4. Avoid direct application of extreme hot or cold to skin because damage may occur without feeling it.
5. **Encourage use of sunscreen during all outdoor activities.**

Community and Home Care Considerations
1. Xerosis is a common problem for older adults. Treatment should include:
   - Drinking 2000 mL of liquid daily
   - Total body immersion in warm water (90° to 105°) for 10 minutes
   - Use of nonperfumed soap without hexachlorophene
   - Application of emollient, particularly those with alpha-hydroxy acids (Lac-Hytrin), after bathing and at bedtime

Hematopoietic
Characteristics
1. Unchanged number of stem cells of all three cell lines; however, bone marrow cellularity is decreased by 33% during adult life.
2. Declining marrow activity, especially in response to stress, such as with blood loss or infection.

Assessment Finding
1. Asymptomatic

Nursing Considerations and Teaching Points
1. Anemia and granulocytopenia are not normal consequences of aging and should be investigated.
2. Teach patients that there is no need to take oral iron unless there is actually a documented loss in iron levels.
3. Dietary iron through green leafy vegetables, some red meat, and iron-fortified breads and cereals should be encouraged.

Altered Presentation of Disease
Characteristics
1. In part due to the physiologic changes that occur with aging, the manifestations of illness in the older patient are less dramatic than in younger patients.
2. Most elderly persons have at least one chronic condition. These coexisting conditions can complicate the evaluation of new symptoms.

Assessment Findings
1. The classic indicators of disease are often absent or disorders present atypically (Table 9-1).
2. Older people are less likely to complain of new symptoms but rather attribute them to aging or existing

TABLE 9-1 Atypical Presentation of Disorders in the Older Adult

Disorder	Atypical Presentation
Acute intestinal infection	1. Abdominal pain may be absent. 2. May present with acute confusional state, leukocytosis, and acidosis.
Appendicitis	1. Pain may be diffuse, not localized in right lower quadrant.
Biliary disease	1. Confusion, declining function, and other nonspecific symptoms. 2. Abnormal liver function tests may be only sign.
Congestive heart failure	1. Initially may have change in mental status and fatigue.
Hyperthyroidism	1. Apathy, palpitations, weight loss, weakness.
Hypothyroidism	1. Present with weight loss.
Myocardial infarction	1. Chest pain may be absent. 2. Syncope, dyspnea, vomiting, or confusion may be presenting symptoms.
Perforated ulcer	1. Rigidity may be absent until late.
Pneumonia	1. May present with confusion. 2. Fever and cough may be absent.
Pulmonary embolism	1. May present with change in mental status. 2. May not have fever, leukocytosis, or tachycardia.
Septicemia	1. May be afebrile.
Systemic lupus erythematosus	1. Pneumonitis, subcutaneous nodules, and discoid lesions are more common presentation. 2. Malar rash, Raynaud's phenomenon, and nephritis are less common.

conditions. Many elderly people minimize symptoms because of fears of hospitalization or health care costs.

Nursing Considerations and Teaching Points

1. Have a high index of suspicion for underlying illness if the older adult presents with an acute change in cognition, behavior, or function.

ASSESSMENT

Functional Assessment

Functional assessment is the measurement of a patient's ability to complete functional tasks and fulfill social roles, specifically addressing a person's ability to complete tasks ranging from simple self-care to higher-level activities.

Purpose

1. Functional assessment is essential in the care of the elderly because it:

a. Offers a systematic approach to assessing elderly people for deficits that often go undetected

b. Helps the nurse to identify problems and utilize appropriate resources

c. Provides a way to assess progress and decline over time

d. Helps the nurse evaluate the safety of the person's ability to live alone

2. Functional status includes the evaluation of sensory changes, ability to complete ADL, instrumental ADL, gait and balance problems, and elimination.

Instruments to Measure Functional Ability

1. Functional status may be assessed by several methods: self-report, direct observation, or family report. Direct observation is the method of choice, when possible.

2. The instrument chosen should be based on what is the specific goal or purpose for the evaluation. For example, if the focus is on basic self-care and mobility, the Barthel index should be used.

3. See Box 9-1 for scales measuring functional ability: Katz Index for Activities of Daily Living and Instrumental

---

BOX 9-1 Katz Index for Activities of Daily Living and Instrumental Activities of Daily Living

Activities of Daily Living

1. Bathing—Sponge bath, tub bath or shower
   0 = no assistance (gets in and out of tub by self)
   1 = uses a device to get in or out of tub but able to bathe self
   2 = requires partial assistance with bathing
   3 = full bath required (unable to bathe)

2. Dressing—includes getting clothes from closet and drawers (under and outer garments and able to use fasteners)
   0 = no assistance with getting clothes and dressing self
   1 = able to get clothes and get dressed, except for assistance with shoes
   2 = receives assistance with getting clothes or getting dressed
   3 = requires complete assistance or stays partly or completely undressed

3. Toileting—going to bathroom for bowel and urine elimination, self-cleaning and arranging clothes
   0 = requires no assistance
   1 = requires no assistance but uses device (cane, walker, wheelchair, bedpan at night, but able to empty in morning)
   2 = receives partial assistance with going to the bathroom or in cleansing or arranging clothing
   3 = receives full assistance or does not go to the bathroom

4. Transfer
   0 = moves well in and out of bed and/or chair without assistance
   1 = moves well in and out of bed and/or chair with device
   2 = moves in and out of bed and/or chair with assistance
   3 = requires full assistance

Instrumental Activities of Daily Living

1. Can you use the telephone?
   0 = without help, including looking up numbers and dialing
   2 = with some help (can answer phone or dial "O" in emergency, but need special help in getting the number or dialing)
   Why? _____
   3 = completely unable to use the telephone

2. Can you get to places out of walking distance?
   0 = without help (travels alone on buses, taxis, drives own car)
   1 = with some help in transferring on and off (device and/or person)
   2 = with help of someone while travelling
   3 = totally dependent on specialized arrangements for travel (ie, ambulance) or doesn't travel at all

3. Can you go shopping for groceries or clothing?
   0 = without help taking care of all shopping needs (assuming had own transportation)
   1 = able to take care of all shopping needs but requires companion to help
   2 = requires assistance in preparation of shopping list as well as a companion to help with shopping
   3 = totally dependent on another person for all shopping needs

4. Can you prepare your own meals?
   0 = without assistance (plan and cook full meals for yourself)
   2 = with some assistance (can prepare some things but unable to cook a full meal)
   Why? _____
   3 = totally unable to prepare meals

(continued)

BOX 9-1 Katz Index for Activities of Daily Living and Instrumental Activities of Daily Living (Continued)

Activities of Daily Living

5. Continence
   0 = controls urination and bowel movements completely by self
   1 = has occasional "accidents"
   2 = supervision helps keep bowel or urine control or is incontinent
   3 = catheter is used

6. Feeding
   0 = able to prepare foods, serve and feed self without assistance
   1 = requires help in preparation of food but is able to feed self
   2 = requires help in preparation of food, cutting of meat, buttering
   3 = receives full assistance or is fed partly or completely by tubes

   _____ SCORE
   Best score is 0, most independent; worst score is 18, most dependent.

Instrumental Activities of Daily Living

5. Can you do your housework?
   0 = without assistance (scrub floor, etc.)
   2 = able to do light housekeeping but needs help with heavy work
   ie _____
   3 = unable to do any housework

6. Can you take your own medicine?
   0 = without assistance (correct doses, correct time)
   1 = able if someone prepares it for you
   2 = able to if someone prepares it for you and reminds you to take it
   3 = require someone to prepare and give you your medication

7. Can you handle your own money?
   0 = without assistance (able to pay bills, write checks)
   2 = able to manage day-to-day buying but need help with managing check book and paying bills
   Why?_____
   How long has this been going on?
   3 = requires full assistance with money management

   _____ SCORE
   Best score is 0, most independent; worst score is 18, most dependent.

(Adapted from Katz, S., Ford, A. B., Moskowitz, R., et al. [1963]. Studies of illness in the aged, the index of ADL: A standardized measure of biologic and psychosocial function. *Journal of the American Medical Association, 185,* 914–919.)

Activities of Daily Living. Use these scales to determine how independent the older adult is, and repeat them periodically to compare level of functioning over time. See Selected References for reference to Barthel index.

Psychosocial Assessment

Altered Mental Status

1. Assessment of cognitive function to detect altered mental status involves examination of memory, perception, communication, orientation, calculation, comprehension, problem solving, thought processes, language, construction abilities, abstraction, attention, aphasia, and apraxia.
2. Assessment can be facilitated by use of the Folstein Mini-Mental State Examination (Box 9-2).
   a. This scale can help to follow the elderly person's mental status over time and assess for acute and or chronic changes.
   b. Although success on scales such as this has been associated with education and socioeconomic status, this scale continues to be used as an appropriate screening tool for abnormal cognitive function.
3. Assessment of altered mental status may elicit criteria that lead to a diagnosis of dementia. It is essential to differentiate dementia from delirium (which is treatable and reversible).

a. *Delirium* is abrupt in onset. Disorientation occurs early, and the behavior is variable hour to hour. There is a clouded, altered, or changing level of consciousness, short attention span, and disturbed sleep–wake cycle. Hallucinations are common.
b. *Dementia* has a gradual onset. Behavior is usually stable, and disorientation occurs late. Consciousness is not clouded, attention span generally is not reduced, day–night reversal of sleep–wake cycles can occur rather than hour-to-hour variation. Hallucinations do not occur until late.

Social Activities and Support

1. Important aspects of social function in geriatrics include social relationships (frequency, contacts, quality), activities, resources, and support. This information is important to help in making decisions about care.
2. Elicit information by asking questions such as:
   a. How often do you socialize with others?
   b. With whom do you socialize?
   c. What type of activities do you get involved in?
   d. Do you enjoy socializing?
   e. Who can you call for help?
   f. Do you know of any church or community groups you can call for help?

BOX 9-2 Folstein Mini-Mental State Examination

Maximum Score	Factor
	Orientation
5	What is the (year) (season) (date) (day) (month)?
5	Where are we (state) (county) (town) (hospital) (floor)?
	Registration
3	Name three objects; allow one second to say each. Then, ask the patient to repeat the three objects after you have said them. Give one point for each correct answer. Repeat until the patient learns all three. Count trials and record number.
	Attention and calculation
5	Ask the patient to begin with 100 and count backward by sevens (stop after five answers). Alternatively, spell "world" backward.
	Recall
3	Ask the patient to repeat the three objects that you previously asked him or her to remember.
	Language
2	Show the patient a pencil and a watch and ask him or her to name them.
1	Ask the patient to repeat the following: "No ifs, ands or buts."
3	Give the patient a three-stage command: "Take a paper in your right hand, fold it in half and put in on the floor."
1	Show the patient the written item "Close your eyes" and ask the patient to read and obey it.
1	Tell the patient to write a sentence.
1	Tell the patient to copy a design (complex polygon).
30	TOTAL SCORE POSSIBLE

Scoring: 24 to 30 correct—intact cognitive function
20 to 23 correct—mild cognitive impairment
16 to 19 correct—moderate cognitive impairment
15 or less correct—severe cognitive impairment

(Folstein, M. F., Folstein, S. E., & McHugh, P. R. [1975], "Mini-mental state." A practical method for grading the cognitive state of patients for the clinician. *Journal of Psychiatric Research, 12*[3], 189–198.)

Emotional/Affective Status
Characteristics
1. Depression may occur for the first time in older age and has been related to the many changes that occur with age:
   a. The independence of one's children
   b. The reality of retirement
   c. The loss of roles, income, spouse, friends, family, homes, pets, functional ability, health, and ability to participate in leisure activities such as reading
   d. Ageist messages from society supporting and encouraging the value of youth
2. Depression may also be caused by underlying illnesses such as Parkinson's disease and by drugs such as antihypertensives, antiarthritics, and antianxiety agents.
3. Depression is often difficult to identify in the elderly because the presentation is different than in younger people. Obtain the following information to assess for depression:
   a. Complaints of insomnia, weight loss, anorexia, and constipation (vegetative symptoms)
   b. Preoccupation with past life events
   c. Decrease in concentration, memory, and decision making (dementia syndrome)
   d. Other somatic complaints such as decreased appetite, musculoskeletal aches and pains, chest pain
   e. History of chronic illness or other health problems
   f. Current medications
4. Evaluate depression using the Brink Depression Scale as a screening tool (Box 9-3).
5. Suicide is sometimes associated with depression, with suicides being especially high in older white men. Assess for suicide risk.
6. Pain is underdetected and undertreated in the elderly and may be contributing to depression. Assess pain by asking and observing the patient, and provide appropriate measures to make the patient more comfortable.

Nursing and Patient Care Considerations
1. Treatment of depression should be given to older adults and includes drugs, psychotherapy, and, in some cases, electroconvulsive therapy.
2. Complement other therapeutic measures by providing opportunities to increase the person's self-esteem.
   a. Encourage participation in activities that are meaningful.

BOX 9-3 Geriatric Depression Scale (Short Form)

Choose the best answer for how you felt over the past week.

	YES	NO
1. Are you basically satisfied with your life?	☐	☐
2. Have you dropped many of your activities and interests?	☐	☐
3. Do you feel that your life is empty?	☐	☐
4. Do you often get bored?	☐	☐
5. Are you in good spirits most of the time?	☐	☐
6. Are you afraid that something bad is going to happen to you?	☐	☐
7. Do you feel happy most of the time?	☐	☐
8. Do you often feel helpless?	☐	☐
9. Do you prefer to stay at home rather than going out and doing new things?	☐	☐
10. Do you feel you have more problems with memory than most?	☐	☐
11. Do you think it is wonderful to be alive now?	☐	☐
12. Do you feel pretty worthless the way you are now?	☐	☐
13. Do you feel full of energy?	☐	☐
14. Do you feel that your situation is hopeless?	☐	☐
15. Do you think that most people are better off than you are?	☐	☐

TOTAL SCORE _____

The following answers count one point; scores 5 indicate probable depression.

1. NO	6. YES	11. NO
2. YES	7. NO	12. YES
3. YES	8. YES	13. NO
4. YES	9. YES	14. YES
5. NO	10. YES	15. YES

(Yesavage, J. A., & Brink, T. L. [1983]. Development and validation of a geriatric depression screening scale: A preliminary report. *Journal of Psychiatric Research, 17,* 37–49.)

   b. Compliment the person.
   c. Help the person develop a sense of mastery.
   d. Encourage reminiscence of meaningful past events.
3. Help the person identify and use social supports.

Motivation in the Elderly
Characteristics
1. Motivation is an important variable in the elderly person's ability to recover from any disabling event and the ability to maintain his or her highest level of wellness.
2. It is possible to evaluate a persons's motivation to comply with a given treatment plan and adopt interventions to help to improve the elderly person's motivation.
3. Factors that influence motivation in the elderly include:
   a. Needs, such as hunger
   b. Past experiences, specifically with health care providers
   c. Negative attitudes toward aging
   d. Self-efficacy expectations, or the belief in one's ability to perform a specific activity
   e. Outcome expectations, or the belief that if a specific activity is performed there will be an expected outcome
   f. The cost of performing a specific activity in terms of time, money, pain, fatigue, or fear

   g. Internal factors, such as sensory changes, cognitive status, and medication side effects
   h. External factors, such as social norms (particularly if those norms conflict with treatment) and the influence of social supports
4. Problems in motivation due to age-related differences include:
   a. A shift from achievement motivation to conservative motivation
   b. Increasing difficulty in the establishment of rewards for elderly people, due to their many losses
   c. A tendency to see a task as being more difficult than a younger person would
   d. A tendency to become easily discouraged; the older adult may not initiate behavior as readily
   e. Greater significance placed on the meaning of a task; it must be meaningful to the elderly person
   f. Evidence that elderly people do not do well on tasks if they are asked to do them rapidly, under a time limit, or in a stressful situation
   g. Increased importance placed on the cost of participating in an activity; fear of failing can be expressed either as increased anxiety or decreased willingness to take risks
   h. Increased need for elderly people to get approval for trying

5. The Motivation Wheel (Figure 9-1) can be used to evaluate motivation in the older adult.
   a. Motivation is influenced by personal expectations (self-efficacy and outcome expectations), spirituality, goals, self-determination, social support, individual care, and physical sensations.
   b. Motivation can be increased by strengthening self-efficacy and outcome expectations, spirituality, self-determination, by identifying appropriate goals, using social supports, individualized care, and decreasing any unpleasant sensations associated with an activity.

Nursing and Patient Care Considerations
1. Strategies to improve motivation include:
   a. Establish whose motives are being discussed—the patient's, the family's, or the health care provider's; involve the patient in setting the goals.
   b. Explore with the patient any indication of fear or other unpleasant sensation associated with the activity, such as pain or fatigue, and implement interventions to decrease these unpleasant sensations.
   c. Evaluate the spokes of the wheel to consider the many factors that influence motivation and implement interventions as appropriate.
   d. Encourage the patient to verbally express emotional factors associated with the activity.
   e. Examine the setting for the desired behavior to occur. Is the environment too stressful, too dark, or too noisy?

   f. Attempt to use role models. Elderly role models can change ageist attitudes and stimulate patients to perform the desired behavior.
   g. Set small goals to be met either daily or each shift. This provides frequent rewards.
   h. Do not be afraid to use yourself. Research has indicated that being nice, demonstrating caring, using humor, verbal encouragement and support can all help motivate the elderly person.
2. Educate the older adult about the benefits of the activity, whether these are physical or psychological.

HEALTH MAINTENANCE

■ Primary Prevention
Primary prevention is the prevention of disease before it occurs. Primary prevention can be broken down into counseling, immunizations, and chemoprophylaxis.

Counseling
1. Encourage smoking cessation.
   a. Approximately 20% of people between age 65 and 74 and 10% of those over age 75 still smoke cigarettes.
   b. Tobacco use has been linked to heart disease; peripheral vascular disease; cerebrovascular disease; chronic obstructive pulmonary disease; cancer such as lung, bladder, and esophageal malignancies; and numerous other health problems that decrease the quality of life or cause premature death.
   c. Although much damage has been done to the lungs and blood vessels by many years of smoking, elderly persons can still benefit from smoking cessation by increasing the quality of life.
2. Encourage physical activity.
   a. It has been stated that less than 10% of those over 65 are physically active and that almost 50% are sedentary.
   b. It has been recommended that elderly people participate in regular activity, especially aerobic activities that promote cardiovascular fitness, such as walking, cycling, or swimming.
   c. Refer to a physical, occupational, or rehabilitation therapist. An individualized exercise prescription should be developed and cleared with the health care provider.
3. Identify alcohol abuse in the elderly.
   a. The consequences of alcoholism include liver disease, gastrointestinal (GI) bleeding, and motor vehicle accidents.
   b. Question elderly people about drug or alcohol abuse. Although street drug use is rare, prescription drug abuse may be occurring.
   c. Recognize the signs and symptoms of alcohol abuse in the elderly (Box 9-4).
   d. Refer for counseling.

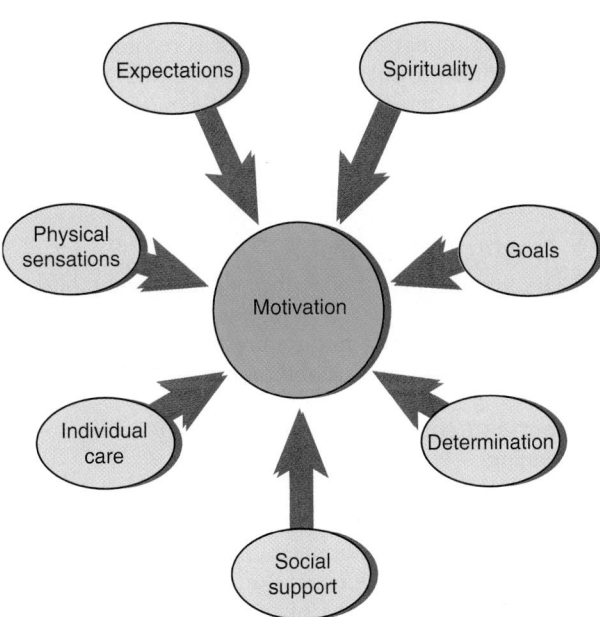

FIGURE 9-1 The wheel of motivation.

BOX 9-4 Signs of Alcohol Abuse in the Elderly

Difficulty with gait and balance
Acute change in cognition
Frequent falls or accidents
Change in drinking patterns
Poor nutritional intake
Poor hygiene and self-care
Lack of physical exercise
Social isolation

---

4. Evaluate and counsel on dental health.
   a. Dental problems in the elderly include missing teeth, ill-fitting dentures, periodontal disease, and decayed teeth.
   b. Dental problems often lead to poor eating habits, apathy, and fatigue.
   c. Regular dental health care should be encouraged to improve nutrition and the quality of life.

Immunizations
Pneumococcal Pneumonia and Influenza
1. Pneumococcal pneumonia and influenza are significant causes of mortality and morbidity in the elderly.
2. It is recommended that the pneumococcal vaccine be given at least once to all people over age 65. Individuals immunized before age 65 are candidates for revaccination, provided at least 6 or more years have passed since the last dose.
3. Two options are available for the prevention of influenza.
   a. Annual influenza vaccine for all people over 65.
   b. Amantadine (Symmetrel) or rimantadine (Flumadine) prophylaxis is only effective against influenza. These agents may be given for the entire flu season or initiated at the beginning of a flu outbreak; they are also effective in ameliorating symptoms if given within 48 hours of onset of illness.

Tetanus-Diphtheria
1. Tetanus-diphtheria immunization is an important but frequently forgotten component of health maintenance, especially in the elderly.
   a. The fatality rate of tetanus exceeds 50% in those over age 65.
   b. Combined tetanus-diphtheria boosters should be given every 10 years, but even a booster given after 25 to 30 years will be effective.
   c. For those with no history of immunization or unknown immunization status, a primary series should be initiated, consisting of two doses of tetanus-diphtheria vaccine at least 4 weeks apart, followed by a third dose 6 to 12 months later.

Chemoprophylaxis
1. It has been recommended that low-dose aspirin therapy be considered for people at risk for myocardial infarction or stroke.
   a. Contraindicated if patient is at risk for GI bleeding

2. Estrogen therapy is recommended in postmenopausal women who are at risk for coronary artery disease and osteoporosis. It is contraindicated if there is history of breast cancer, thrombophlebitis or undiagnosed genital bleeding.
3. Calcium, vitamin D, and other agents such as selective estrogen receptor modulators or biphosphonates may be considered for those at risk for osteoporosis.

Secondary Prevention
Secondary prevention is the detection of disease in an early stage, commonly for colorectal cancer, breast cancer, prostate cancer, uterine cancer, and tuberculosis screening.

Screening Recommendations
1. The recommendation for bowel cancer screening is for yearly stool specimens for occult blood and sigmoidoscopy every 3 years after age 50.
2. Monthly breast self-examination, yearly breast examination by a health care provider, and yearly mammography are suggested for breast cancer screening for women over age 50.
3. Yearly screening for tuberculosis via skin test is recommended for the older adult at increased risk, such as the institutionalized or those with medical risk factors such as diabetes or immunosuppression. A two-step test is indicated in those over age 55 because of waning immunogenicity. If the initial test is negative, a second test is given 1 to 2 weeks later.
4. Yearly rectal examinations and blood test for prostate specific antigen (PSA) are recommended in men over age 50 to screen for prostate disease.
5. Annual examination with Pap test is recommended in older women to rule out cervical or genital malignancies; after hysterectomy for noncancerous process, Pap test may be done every 3 to 5 years.
6. Yearly visual screening is important to assess for visual changes, glaucoma, and cataracts.

Tertiary Prevention
Tertiary prevention addresses the treatment of established disease to avoid complications and death. The major areas of focus for the older adult are preventing the complications of immobility and rehabilitation.

Preventing Complications of Immobility
Positioning
1. The goal of frequent position changes is to prevent contractures, stimulate circulation and prevent pressure sores, prevent thrombophlebitis and pulmonary embolism, promote lung expansion and prevent pneumonia, and decrease edema of the extremities. Changing position from lying to sitting several times a day can help prevent changes in the cardiovascular system known as deconditioning.

2. The recommendation is to change body position at least every 2 hours, and preferably more frequently in patients who have no spontaneous movement.

Proper Body Alignment

1. Dorsal or supine position
   a. The head is in line with the spine, both laterally and anteroposteriorly.
   b. The trunk is positioned so flexion of the hips is minimized to prevent hip contracture.
   c. The arms are flexed at the elbow with the hands resting against the lateral abdomen.
   d. The legs are extended in a neutral position with the toes pointed toward the ceiling.
   e. The heels are suspended in a space between the mattress and the footboard to prevent heel pressure.
   f. Trochanter rolls are placed under the greater trochanters in the hip joint areas.
2. Side-lying or lateral position
   a. The head is in line with the spine.
   b. The body is in alignment and is not twisted.
   c. The uppermost hip joint is slightly forward and supported by a pillow in a position of slight abduction.
   d. A pillow supports the arm, which is flexed at both the elbow and shoulder joints.
3. Prone position
   a. The head is turned laterally and is in alignment with the rest of the body.
   b. The arms are abducted and externally rotated at the shoulder joint; the elbows are flexed.
   c. A small, flat support is placed under the pelvis, extending from the level of the umbilicus to the upper third of the thigh.
   d. The lower extremities remain in a neutral position.
   e. The toes are suspended over the edge of the mattress.

Therapeutic Exercise

1. It has been reported that there is a daily loss of 1% to 1.5% of initial strength in an immobilized older adult.
2. The goals of therapeutic exercise are to develop and retrain deficient muscles, to restore as much normal movement as possible to prevent deformity, to stimulate the functions of various organs and body systems, to build strength and endurance, and to promote relaxation.
3. Perform passive range-of-motion exercise.
   a. Carried out without assistance from the patient.
   b. The purpose is to retain as much joint range of motion as possible, and to maintain circulation.
   c. Move the joint smoothly through its full range of motion (Box 9-5). Do not push beyond the point of pain.
4. Perform active assistive range of motion.
   a. Carried out by the patient with the assistance of the nurse.
   b. The purpose is to encourage normal muscle function.
   c. Support the distal part and encourage the patient to take the joint actively through its range of motion.
   d. Give only the amount of assistance necessary to accomplish the action.

5. Encourage active range of motion.
   a. Accomplished by the patient without assistance.
   b. The purpose is to increase muscle strength.
   c. When possible, active exercise should be done against gravity.
   d. Encourage the patient to move the joint through the full range of motion without assistance.
   e. Ensure that the patient does not substitute another joint movement for the one intended.
   f. Other active forms of exercise include turning from side to side, turning from back to abdomen, and moving up and down in bed.
6. Assist with resistive exercise.
   a. Carried out by the patient working against resistance produced by either manual or mechanical means.
   b. The purpose is to increase muscle strength.
   c. Encourage the patient to move the joint through its range of motion while you or someone else provides slight resistance at first and then progressively increases resistance.
   d. Weights may be used and are attached at the distal point of the involved joint.
   e. The movements should be done smoothly.
7. Teach isometric or muscle-setting exercise.
   a. Involve alternately contracting and relaxing a muscle while keeping the part in a fixed position; performed by the patient.
   b. The purpose is to maintain strength when a joint is immobilized.
   c. Teach the patient to contract or tighten the muscle as much as possible without moving the joint.
   d. The patient holds the position for several seconds, then relaxes.

Geriatric Rehabilitation and Restorative Care
Characteristics

1. The primary goal is restoring the older adult to maximum functional level.
2. Multidisciplinary service involving input from the primary care provider; nursing personnel; physical, occupational, speech, and recreational therapists; social worker; psychologist; and dietitian.
3. Rehabilitation/restorative nursing involves developing a rehabilitation philosophy of care.
   a. Patients are encouraged, and allowed sufficient time, to perform as much of their personal care as possible.
   b. Goals are set with the patient rather than for the patient.
   c. Prevention of further impairment is imperative.
   d. Focus on skin and wound care, regaining or maintaining bowel and bladder function, independent medication use, good nutritional status, psychosocial support, an appropriate activity/rest balance, and patient and family education.

(text continues on page 178)

BOX 9-5   Range of Motion

Shoulder   Flexion-Extension

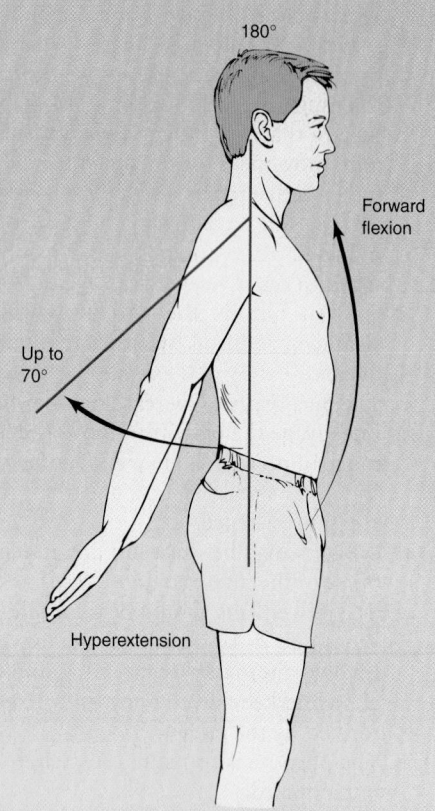

180°

Forward
flexion

Up to
70°

Hyperextension

Adduction-Abduction

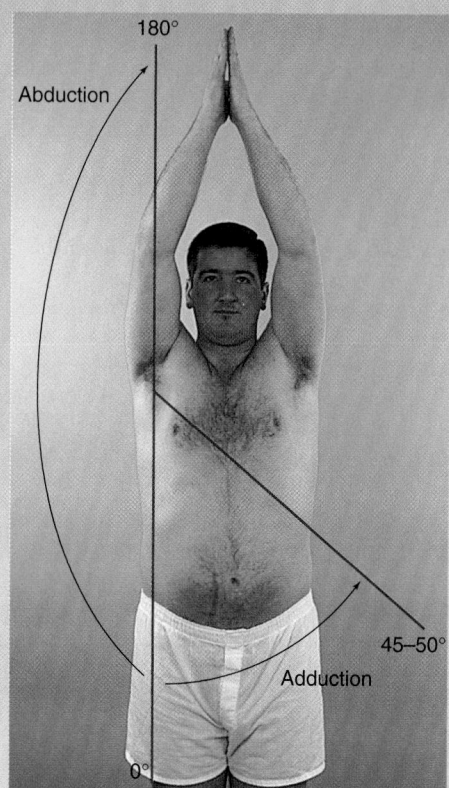

180°

Abduction

45–50°

Adduction

0°

Elbow   Flexion-Extension

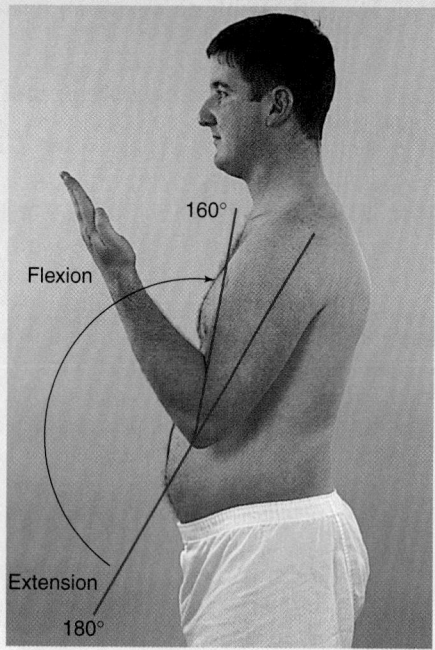

160°

Flexion

Extension

180°

Pronation-Supination

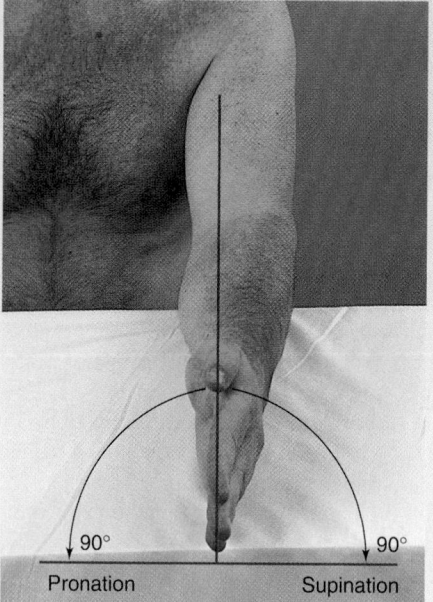

90°   90°
Pronation   Supination

BOX 9-5 Range of Motion (Continued)

Wrist
Dorsiflexion and Palmar Flexion

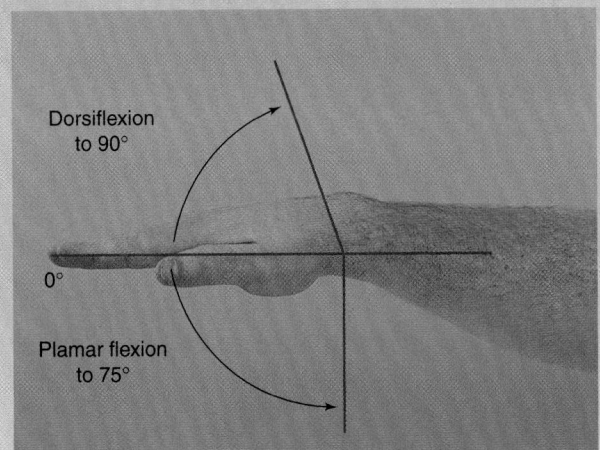

Dorsiflexion
to 90°

0°

Plamar flexion
to 75°

Ulnar-Radial Deviation

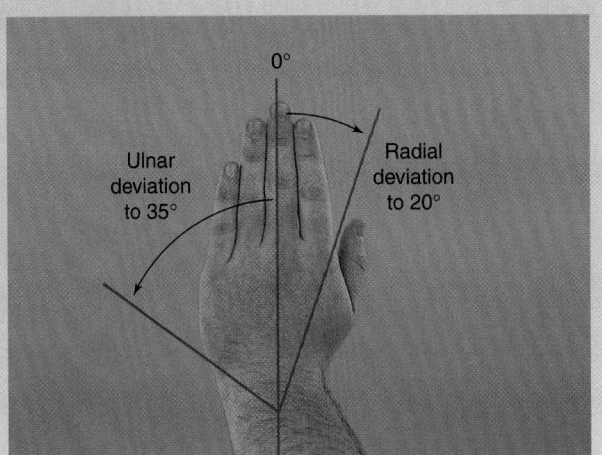

0°

Ulnar
deviation
to 35°

Radial
deviation
to 20°

Thumb   Adduction   Abduction   Opposition

 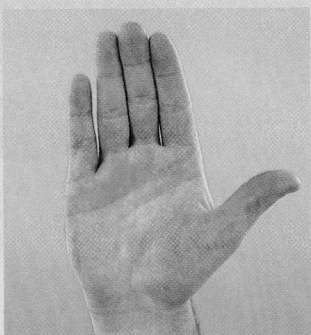 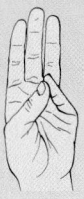

Fingers
  Adduction   Abduction   Flexion-Hyperextension

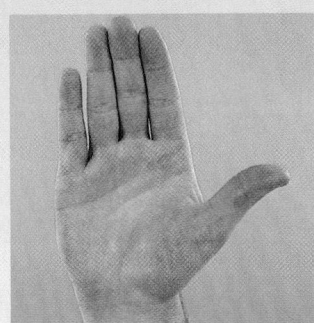 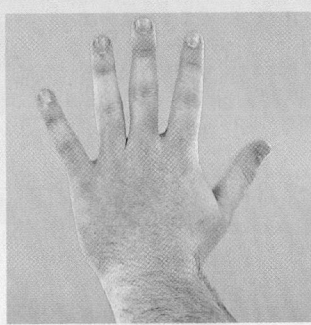 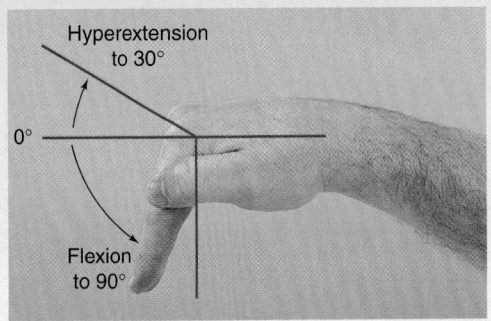

Hyperextension
to 30°

0°

Flexion
to 90°

(continued)

BOX 9-5 Range of Motion (Continued)

Ankle   Dorsiflexion-Plantar Flexion

Eversion-Inversion

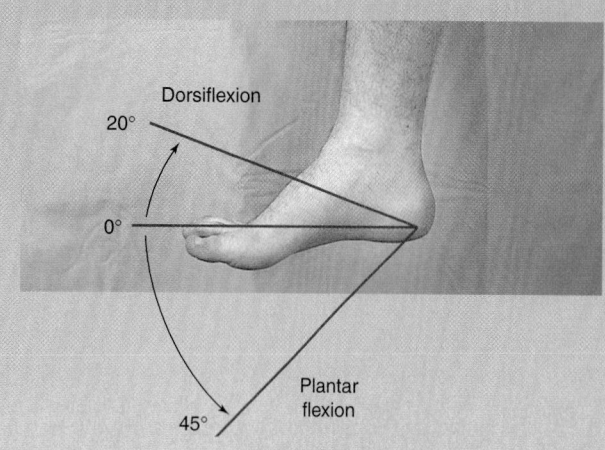

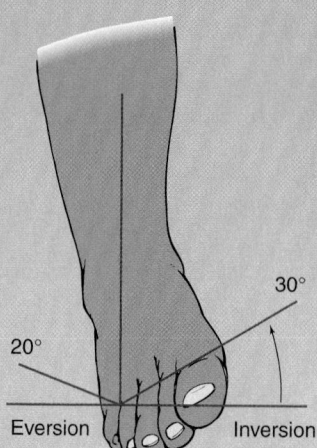

Toes   Flexion-Extension   Adduction-Abduction

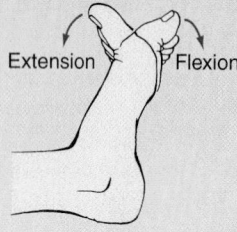

Hip   Adduction/Abduction   Internal Rotation/External Rotation

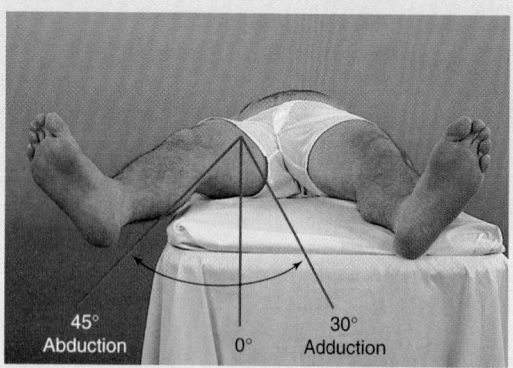

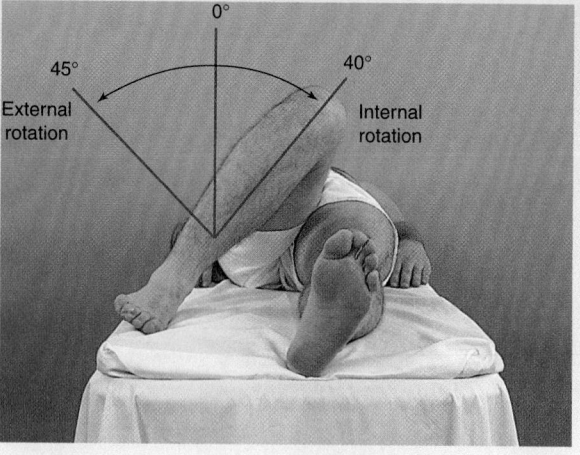

BOX 9-5 Range of Motion (Continued)

Knee   Flexion/Extension/Hyperextension

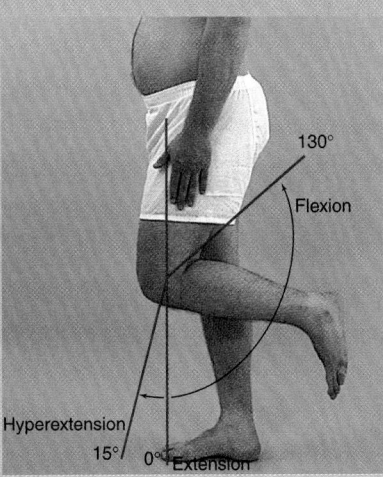

Cervical Spine   Flexion-Hyperextension   Rotation

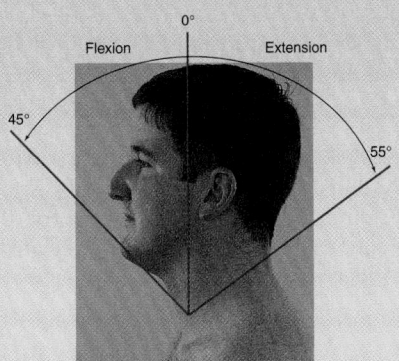   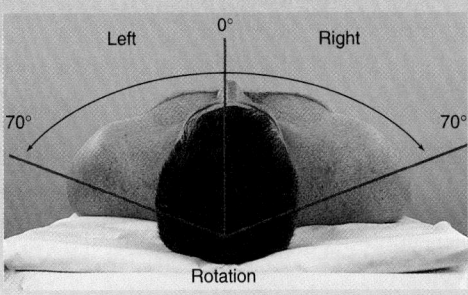

Lateral Bending

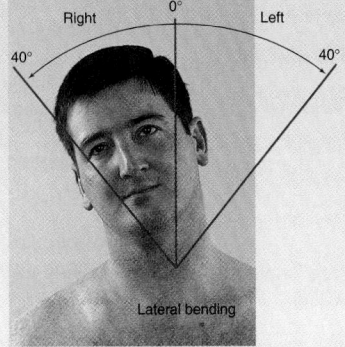

Nursing and Patient Care Considerations

1. Impaired cognitive function may have an impact on the quality of rehabilitation.
   a. Assess for physical problems that may exacerbate cognitive dysfunction (eg, infection, drug side effects, metabolic or circulatory problems, or fatigue).
   b. Provide innovative measures to encourage ambulation and increased function; provide frequent verbal cues and large print reminders; focus on basic self-care abilities.
   c. Implement appropriate safety measures such as bed side rails, proper lighting, appropriate staffing, and restraints if necessary.
2. Disability has a tremendous impact on the patient's body image and requires an adjustment by the patient. Be aware of the stages of psychological reaction the patient may undergo.
   a. Period of confusion, disorganization, and denial
   b. Period of depression and/or anxiety and grief
   c. Period of adaptation and adjustment
3. Interventions in rehabilitation nursing include:
   a. Provide an atmosphere of acceptance.
   b. Identify and encourage positive coping patterns.
   c. Encourage socialization and participation in group activities.
   d. Give positive reinforcement and feedback about progress.
   e. Involve families as much as possible.
4. Use interventions suggested above to motivate the older adult to engage in functional activities and exercise.

Community and Home Care Considerations

1. Family or significant other caring for the older adult at home can have a major impact on the rehabilitation process.
   a. Assist the family or significant other to face the reality of the patient's disability and to set appropriate goals.
   b. Involve the family or significant other in decision making and in the patient's care in order for them to develop and practice the skill necessary for the patient to reach rehabilitation goals.
   c. Help extend and enlarge the family's or significant other's skills by teaching problem solving, treatment needs of the patient, ways to communicate to health care providers, and the use of community resources.
   d. Assess the level of caregiver fatigue or burnout (Box 9-6).
2. For the older adult living independently:
   a. Encourage adherence to a regular exercise program to maintain optimal function.
   b. Exercise goals should be at least 20 minutes of continuous aerobic exercise (walking, biking, or swimming) three times a week.

SPECIAL HEALTH PROBLEMS OF THE OLDER ADULT

▪ Altered Response to Medication

Adults over age 65 consume 30% to 40% of all prescription drugs and an even higher proportion of the over-the-counter drugs consumed. Age-related changes predispose older adults to problems with medication side effects.

BOX 9-6 Caregiver Strain Index

Instructions given to the caregiver: I am going to read a list of things that other people have found to be difficult in caring for patients after they come home from the hospital. Would you tell me whether any of these apply to you? (Give the examples.)

Score one point for "yes" and zero for "no."

1. Sleep is disturbed (eg, because _____ is in and out of bed or wanders around at night).
2. It is inconvenient (eg, because helping takes so much time or it's a long drive over to help).
3. It is a physical strain (eg, because of lifting in and out of a chair).
4. It is confining (eg, because helping restricts free time or cannot visit).
5. There have been family adjustments (eg, because helping has disrupted routine or there has been no privacy).
6. There have been changes in personal plans (eg, had to turn down a job or could not go on vacation).
7. There have been other demands on my time (eg, from other family members).
8. There have been emotional adjustments (eg, because of severe arguments).
9. Some behavior is upsetting (eg, incontinence; _____ has trouble remembering things; _____ accuses others of taking things).
10. It is upsetting to find that _____ has changed so much from before (eg, _____ is a different person from before).
11. There have been work adjustments (eg, because of having to take time off).
12. It is a financial strain.
13. It has been completely overwhelming (eg, because of worry about _____ or concerns about how to continue to manage).

Scoring: Total score of 7 or more suggests a greater level of stress.

(Robinson, B. C. [1983]. Validation of a caregiver strain index. *Journal of Gerontology, 38*[3], 344–348. ©1983 The Gerontological Society of America.)

Pathophysiology and Etiology

1. Drug absorption is affected by the following age-related changes:
   a. Decreased gastric acid
   b. Decreased GI motility
   c. Decreased gastric blood flow
   d. Changes in GI villi
   e. Decreased blood flow and body temperature in rectum
2. Drug distribution is affected by:
   a. Decreased body size
   b. Decreased water content in the body
   c. Increased total body fat
   d. Drugs distributed in water have a higher concentration in the elderly (eg, gentamicin [Garamycin]).
   e. Drugs distributed in fat have a wider distribution and less intense but prolonged effect (eg, phenobarbital [Luminal]).
3. Drug metabolism in the older adult:
   a. Is altered by a decrease in liver size, blood flow, enzyme activity, and protein synthesis
   b. Requires more time than in younger adults. Therefore, there is increased drug activity time in drugs that are metabolized in the liver (eg, propranolol [Inderal], theophylline [Theo-Dur]).
4. Excretion of drugs is altered in older adults due to the following renal changes:
   a. Decreased renal tubular function and blood flow.
   b. This causes a decrease in renal filtration and an increase in blood levels of drugs that are excreted through the kidneys (eg, cimetidine [Tagamet]).

 DRUG ALERT

Drugs that may have severe adverse reactions in the elderly include anticholinergics (antihistamines, antidepressants), nonsteroidal anti-inflammatory drugs (NSAIDs), any drug with a long half-life, and drugs with action on the central nervous system.

Nursing Assessment

1. Drug toxicities are different than they are in younger people.
2. Fewer symptoms may be identified, and they may develop slower; however, the reactions may be more pronounced and further advanced once they do present.
3. Behavioral side effects are more common in elderly people because the blood–brain barrier becomes less effective; the first reaction to a drug is confusion.
4. Many potential drug side effects are not identified because they are attributed to old age; fatigue, confusion, anorexia, or indigestion as drug side effects may not be reported.
5. Allergic reactions to drugs increase with age due to a greater likelihood of earlier exposure.

Nursing and Patient Care Considerations

1. Maintain awareness that the older adult is at greater risk for adverse medication reactions.
   a. This risk increases from 6% when two drugs are taken to 50% when five different drugs are taken, and to 100% when eight or more medications are taken.
2. Assess the patient's ability to follow medication regimen by evaluation of:
   a. Cognition of the patient
   b. Ability to read drug labels
   c. Hand and muscle coordination
   d. Swallowing difficulty
   e. Lifestyle patterns, specifically smoking and alcohol use
   f. Cultural beliefs toward medication
   g. Ability to afford medication
   h. Caregiver involvement in medication administration; assess caregiver if indicated
3. Identify problems in the use of medications such as:
   a. Lack of knowledge about drugs
   b. Multiple medications and difficult administration techniques
   c. Caregiver misunderstanding of medication use
4. Appropriate interventions for safe drug use include:
   a. Obtain a complete drug history.
   b. Reinforce verbal instructions with written instructions using large print and simple wording. If necessary, use color coding rather than drug names.
   c. Write what the drug is used for and what the side effects can be.
   d. Make sure the patient or caregiver can open the medication container.
   e. Arrange medication schedules to coincide with regular activity, such as eating (if appropriate for that drug). Simplify the drug regimen as much as possible.
   f. If necessary, arrange a check-off system using a chart to ensure compliance.
   g. If possible, visibly evaluate all medications in the home, or ask patient to bring all medications for evaluation.
   h. Encourage patient to discard all old or unneeded medications, and to check expiration dates.
   i. Encourage patient to store medications in original containers and in a dry, dark place.
   j. Encourage patient to avoid over-the-counter medication without checking with the primary care provider before use.
   k. Encourage patient to report any drug side effects.
   l. Work with patient to maintain a drug regimen that follows the principles for geriatric drug use; start dosages low and go slow, use only necessary medications, titrate the dose to the patient response, simplify the regimen, and have frequent reevaluations done regarding the medication regimen.

Community and Home Care Considerations

1. Ask the patient or family to bring in all the patient's medications for clinic or office visits or whenever the patient goes to the hospital, in order to obtain an accurate medication history.
2. Ask the patient what vitamins, minerals, herbal supplements, and other over-the-counter products are being used. Many patients do not consider these medications and will not readily supply the information unless specifically asked.
3. Alert patients and family members that many "natural" products sold over the counter still may possess adverse reactions and toxicity, as well as interactions with other drugs.
4. Warn patients and families that many complementary and alternative therapies (CAM) do not have proven effectiveness despite advertisements of such. CAM should be used as an adjunct to conventional therapy, and the patient should notify all health care providers of supplements and therapies being used.

■ Altered Nutritional Status

Normal age-related changes, behavioral changes, and pathologic conditions may lead to malnutrition in the older adult.

Pathophysiology and Etiology

1. Changes in the oral cavity, including loss of teeth, diminished saliva production, and difficulty with mastication, may cause decreased food intake.
2. A decrease in gastric juice secretion with reduced pepsin hinders protein digestion, and iron, vitamin B_{12}, calcium, and folic acid absorption; there are no significant changes in the small or large bowel.
3. Sensory changes involving taste and smell cause anorexia.
4. Psychosocial factors including changes in living situation, widowhood, depression, loneliness, decreased choice of food for institutionalized elderly, need to adhere to special diets, economic status, and ability to obtain and prepare food all impact on what is eaten.
5. Alcohol use interferes with the absorption of the B-complex vitamins. Additionally, alcohol is high in calories and low in nutritional value.
6. Medications can alter nutrition by directly decreasing absorption and utilization of nutrients. Indirectly, medications can result in anorexia, serostomia, dysgeusia, and early satiety.
7. Dysphagia (difficulty swallowing), which commonly occurs after cerebral vascular accident, intubation, head and neck surgery, or related to Parkinson's disease and dementia, may cause decreased food intake.
8. With age, there is a decrease in energy needs because of a decrease in muscle mass (total caloric need decreases 30%).

Nursing Assessment

1. Patients with dysphagia may report difficulty swallowing and difficulty managing saliva. They cough after swallowing, they sound "wet" after eating, they may have pocketing of food, and they may have an absent or diminished gag reflex.
2. Protein-energy malnutrition can present with either a 10% weight loss over 6 months alone (marasmus) or weight loss with low serum albumin levels (kwashiorkor).
3. The single best predictor of a malnourished patient is a cholesterol level below 150 mg/dL.

Nursing and Patient Care Considerations

1. Educate older adult and family or significant other on basic nutritional requirements and on overcoming barriers that interfere with optimal nutrition.
   a. The Required Dietary Allowances (RDA) for healthy older adults are the same as that for younger adults, with three exceptions: decreased caloric intake, decreased protein intake (1 g/kg), and decreased iron requirements for postmenopausal women.
2. Encourage good mouth care.
3. Encourage patients to avoid alcohol if possible; refer for counseling if necessary and compensate for the nutritional consequences of alcohol abuse with liquid supplements, B vitamins.
4. Review all prescription and over-the-counter medications with patients, and evaluate the influence of these on nutritional status.
5. If food procurement, preparation, and enjoyment are a problem, identify community resources to offer assistance in obtaining food and community meals.
6. In institutional settings, environmental factors may influence food enjoyment. Encourage socialization when eating, and try to minimize the negative effects of disruptive people. Try to improve aesthetics.
7. To compensate for age-related changes in taste and smell, encourage use of low-sodium food additives.
8. Encourage proper body position (eg, sitting upright during mealtimes) and staying up for one half hour after eating to help with digestion.
9. If possible, encourage five to six small meals rather than three large meals.
10. If appropriate, encourage the family to bring in food favorites for the patient.
11. Position food on the plate so that if there is visual neglect, or impairment, the patient is best able to see the food served.
12. Identify patients with dysphagia and obtain a referral to a speech therapist.
    a. Work with the speech therapist and primary health care provider to determine what consistency of food is safe for the patient to swallow. If the patient is unable to swallow thin liquids, slushes, puddings, or applesauce should be given to ensure adequate hydration.

b. Use good compensatory techniques if indicated. These include sitting upright, tucking and turning the head, placing the food on the unaffected side of the tongue, swallowing twice to clear the pharyngeal tract, tucking the chin to the chest, and bringing the tongue up and back and holding the breath to swallow.

c. Write out swallowing instructions for patient and family, and educate family regarding the importance of maintaining these precautions.

Community and Home Care Considerations

1. To maintain an optimal nutritional state, the older adult at home should be encouraged to eat a well-balanced diet.
2. Take vitamin preparations with the fewest number of minerals and vitamins needed to prevent interactions, and avoid megadoses.
3. Take calcium, iron, and zinc at least 2 hours apart.
4. Take vitamins at the same time daily.
5. Take calcium and iron on an empty stomach.
6. Take fat-soluble vitamins (A, D, E, and K) with food.

Urinary Incontinence

Approximately 10 million Americans suffer from urinary incontinence, including 15% to 30% of community-dwelling elderly and 40% to 70% of institutionalized elderly. It is often not reported by elderly people because they consider it to be a normal age change, and there is a low expectation of benefit from treatment.

Pathophysiology and Etiology

1. There are four basic types of urinary incontinence:
   a. *Stress*—an involuntary loss of urine with increases in intra-abdominal pressure. Usually caused from weakness and laxity of pelvic floor musculature, or bladder outlet weakness.
   b. *Urge*—involves leakage of urine because of inability to delay voiding after sensation of bladder fullness is perceived. This is associated with detrusor hyperactivity, central nervous system disorders, or local genitourinary conditions.
   c. *Overflow*—due to a leakage of urine resulting from mechanical forces on an overdistended bladder. This results from mechanical obstruction or an acontractile bladder.
   d. *Functional*—involves urinary leakage associated with inability to get to the toilet because of cognitive and/or physical functioning.

Nursing Assessment

1. Identify reversible causes of incontinence using the DRIP acronym.
   a. **D**—Delirium, especially new onset delirium
   b. **R**—Restricted mobility, retention
   c. **I**—Infection (especially sudden onset cystitis), inflammation (such as atrophic vaginitis or urethritis), impaction (fecal)

d. **P**—Polyuria (from poorly controlled diabetes or diuretic treatment), pharmaceuticals (including psychotropics, anticholinergics, alpha agonists, beta agonists, calcium channel blockers, narcotics, alpha antagonists, and alcohol)

2. Evaluate lower urinary tract function.
   a. Stress maneuvers are evaluated by asking the patient, with a full bladder, to cough three times while standing. Observe for leakage of urine.
   b. Check for postvoid residual by inserting a 12 or 14 French straight catheter a few minutes after the patient voids.
   c. Evaluate bladder filling by leaving the straight catheter in place and using a 50-mL syringe to fill the bladder with sterile water. Hold the syringe approximately 15 cm above the pubic symphysis. Continue to fill the bladder in 25-mL increments until the patient feels the urge to void. Observe for involuntary bladder contractions. These contractions are detected by continuous upward movement of the column of fluid in the absence of abdominal straining.

Nursing and Patient Care Considerations

1. For stress or urge incontinence, teach Kegel (pelvic muscle) exercises.
   a. Tell the patient to first practice stopping stream of urine while voiding to identify proper contraction of the pubococcygeal muscle; contraction will result in stopping flow, and relaxation allows flow.
   b. Once proper contraction is verified, advise the patient to practice contraction for 5 to 10 seconds, then relaxation of the muscle for 5 to 10 seconds in sets of 10 three times a day.
   c. The exercise can be practiced anywhere at any time because it involves contraction of an internal muscle. The abdomen should be relaxed, and no movement should be visible by doing Kegel exercises.
2. Assist with biofeedback that involves the use of bladder, rectal, or vaginal pressure recordings to train patients to contract pelvic floor muscles and relax the bladder.
3. Institute a behavioral training program, using bladder records, biofeedback, and pelvic floor exercises for patients with stress or urge incontinence.
4. Other interventions include:
   a. Bladder retraining—progressive lengthening or shortening of voiding intervals to restore the normal pattern of voiding; this is useful after period of immobility or catheterization.
   b. Scheduled toileting—using a fixed toileting schedule to prevent wetting episodes for patients with urge or functional incontinence.
   c. Habit training—involves using a variable toileting schedule based on the patient's pattern of voiding; also incorporates positive reinforcement.
   d. Prompted voiding—includes regular prompts to void every 1 to 2 hours with positive reinforcement.

e. Appropriate use of incontinence aids such as pads/diapers.

f. Judicious use of medications to help control urge incontinence. These include oxybutinin (Ditropan and Ditropan XL) and tolterodine (Detrol). Contraindicated in urinary or gastric retention, myasthenia gravis, and uncontrolled glaucoma. Monitor carefully for anticholinergic effects—dry mouth, heat intolerance, urinary retention, constipation, drowsiness, dry eyes, blurred vision.

Urinary Retention

Urinary retention is a common problem in the older adult, often related to neurologic or other underlying condition.

Pathophysiology and Etiology

1. Frequently encountered in the acute care setting, post-catheterization, after stroke, in diabetics due to atonic neuropathic bladder, due to fecal impaction, and males with prostatic enlargement.
2. The patient with urinary retention may void small amounts or may be incontinent continuously due to overflow of urine.
3. Patients with urinary retention usually will have incontinence during the night.
4. Urinary retention may also be caused or aggravated by drugs with anticholinergic properties such as levodopa (Sinemet) or the tricyclic antidepressants, especially amitriptyline (Elavil).

> **NURSING ALERT**
>
> Urinary retention may cause urinary tract infection, which can lead to sepsis in the elderly.

Nursing Assessment

1. Take a complete history and perform physical examination to rule out causes of urinary retention.
2. Monitor for a distended bladder and perform postvoid catheterization; residual of greater than 300 mL of urine signals urinary retention.

Nursing and Patient Care Considerations

1. Remove fecal impaction to help patient regain bladder function.
2. If prostatic disease is suspected, appropriate referral is necessary.
3. Encourage male to use the standing position and female the sitting position to facilitate urinary flow; provide privacy.
4. Evaluate medication regimen and discuss the necessity or substitution of offending medication with health care provider.
5. If no underlying condition is suspected, attempt intermittent catheterizations every 8 hours, in combination with regular voiding attempts by patient. If there is no response in 2 weeks (ie, no decrease in postvoid residuals), referral to a urologist may be necessary for medical management of the urinary retention.

Fecal Incontinence

Fecal incontinence is an inability to voluntarily control the passage of gas or feces. Although not as common as urinary incontinence, fecal incontinence afflicts 13% to 47% of hospitalized elders and 10% to 30% of nursing home residents. It has been noted to affect 10.9 men and 13.3 women per 1,000 older adults living at home.

Pathophysiology and Etiology

1. Fecal continence depends on normal rectal and anal sensation, rectal reservoir capacity, and internal and external sphincter mechanisms.
2. In institutionalized elderly, fecal impaction is a primary cause of fecal incontinence due to stool leaking around a fecal mass.
3. In the noninstitutionalized elderly, fecal incontinence is often associated with dysfunction of one of the anorectal continence mechanisms such as impaired contractile strength of the sphincters, and lower rectal volume capacity. Stroke and spinal cord injuries cause loss of sensation in the rectal area.
4. Often, no cause can be determined for the fecal loss, and it is believed that the incontinence may be due to a degenerative injury to the pudendal nerve.

Nursing Assessment

1. Perform a rectal examination to check for impaction or decreased rectal sphincter tone.
2. If the fecal incontinence is diarrheal in nature, stool for leukocytes, culture and sensitivity, ova and parasites, and *Clostridium difficile* evaluation may be indicated.

Nursing and Patient Care Considerations

1. If there is no infection and no impaction, it may be helpful to increase dietary fiber in an attempt to add bulk to the stool to stimulate regular defecation.
2. Antidiarrheals, such as loperamide, may be effective in managing diarrhea.
3. Once an impaction is detected and removed, aggressive attempts should be made to set up a regular bowel pattern. This includes regular toileting times set preferably after breakfast, and increased fluid and fiber intake. Laxatives should be used only as a last resort.
4. In the bedbound patient, increased fiber in the diet is contraindicated. These patients may require a bisacodyl (Dulcolax) suppository or an enema to help with rectal evacuation two to three times per week.
5. Older adults with neurogenic fecal incontinence, such as patients with spinal cord injuries and post-CVA, should have treatment to induce fecal evacuation at regularly scheduled times.
6. A glycerin (Glycol) or bisacodyl (Dulcolax) suppository two to three times a week before breakfast (to use the normal gastrocolic reflex that starts after the first meal of the day) may help to induce a complete rectal evacuation and decrease stool incontinence.

Community and Home Care Considerations

1. Explain to patient and family that it is not necessary to have bowel movement every day.
2. Laxatives, which may induce diarrhea, should be avoided.
3. Fibrous foods that stimulate the bowel should be eaten daily, preferably at breakfast, such as stewed prunes, citrus fruit, bran cereals, etc. Help should be available to toilet the patient when the urge to defecate is felt.
4. One homeopathic remedy to maintain regular bowel movements is 3 tbsp applesauce, 2 tbsp bran, and 1 tbsp prune juice mixed, refrigerated, and given at least 1 tbsp each morning.

▣ Pressure Sores

Pressure sores (*decubitus ulcers*) are localized ulcerations of the skin or deeper structures. They most commonly result from prolonged periods of bed rest in acute or long-term care facilities (Figure 9-2).

Pathophysiology and Etiology
Factors in the Development of Pressure Sores

1. Pressure of 70 mm Hg applied for longer than 2 hours can produce tissue destruction; healing cannot occur without relieving the pressure.
2. Friction contributes to pressure sore development by causing abrasion of the stratum corneum.
3. Shearing force, produced by sliding of adjacent surfaces, is particularly important in the partial sitting position. This force ruptures capillaries over the sacrum.
4. Moisture on the skin results in maceration of the epithelium.

Risk Factors for Pressure Sores

1. Bowel or bladder incontinence
2. Malnourishment or significant weight loss
3. Edema, anemia, hypoxia, or hypotension
4. Neurologic impairment or immobility
5. Altered mental status, including delirium or dementia

Nursing Assessment

1. Assess for risk factors for pressure sore development and alter those factors, if possible.
2. Assess skin of the older adult frequently for the development of pressure sores.
3. Stage the ulcer so appropriate treatment can be started.
4. One commonly used staging system advocated by the National Pressure Ulcer Advisory Panel includes four levels (Figure 9-3):
   a. Stage one—nonblanching macule that may appear red or violet
   b. Stage two—skin breakdown as far as the dermis
   c. Stage three—skin breakdown into the subcutaneous tissue
   d. Stage four—penetrates bone, muscle, or joint

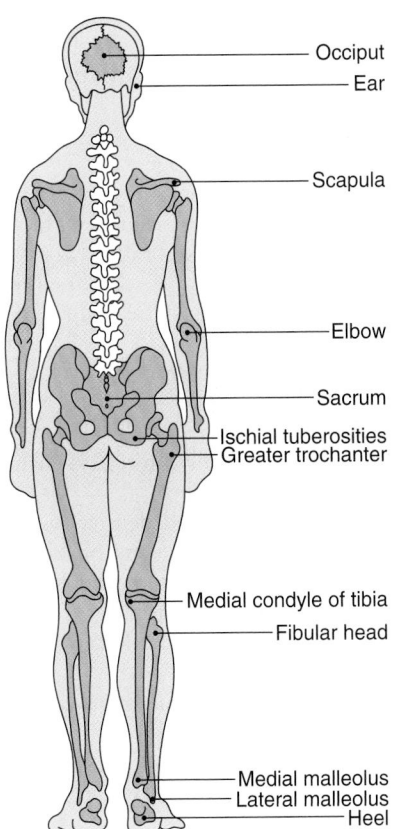

FIGURE 9-2 Areas susceptible to pressure sores.

Labels (top to bottom): Occiput; Ear; Scapula; Elbow; Sacrum; Ischial tuberosities; Greater trochanter; Medial condyle of tibia; Fibular head; Medial malleolus; Lateral malleolus; Heel

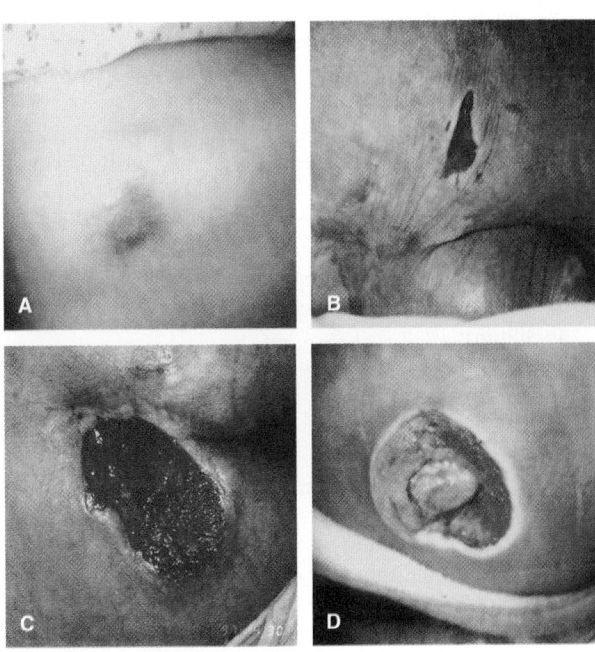

FIGURE 9-3 Pressure ulcer staging. (**A**) Stage I—erythema; (**B**) Stage II—breakdown of the dermis; (**C**) Stage III—full thickness skin breakdown; (**D**) Stage IV—bone, muscle, and supporting tissue involved.

Nursing and Patient Care Considerations
Prevent Pressure Sore Development
1. Provide meticulous care and positioning for immobilized patients.
   a. Inspect skin several times daily.
   b. Wash skin with mild soap, rinse, and blot dry with a soft towel.
   c. Lubricate skin with a bland lotion to keep skin soft and pliable.
   d. Avoid poorly ventilated mattress that is covered with plastic or impermeable material.
   e. Employ bowel and bladder programs to prevent incontinence.
   f. Encourage ambulation and exercise.
   g. Promote nutritious diet with optimal protein, vitamins, and iron.
2. Teach older adult and family or significant other the importance of good nutrition, hydration, activity, positioning, and avoidance of pressure, shearing, friction, and moisture.

Relieve the Pressure
1. Avoid elevation of head of bed greater than 30 degrees.
2. Reposition every 2 hours.
3. Use special devices to cushion specific areas, such as flotation rings, lamb's wool or fleece pads, egg-crate mattresses, booties, elbow pads.
4. Use an alternating-pressure mattress or air-fluidized bed for patients at high risk to prevent or treat pressure sores.
5. Provide for activity and ambulation as much as possible.
6. Advise frequent shifting of weight and occasional raising of bottom off chair while sitting.

Clean and Débride the Wound
1. Use normal saline for cleaning and disinfecting wounds.
2. Apply wet-to-dry dressings or enzyme ointments for débridement as directed; or assist with surgical débridement.

Treat Local Infection
1. Open wounds are always colonized with bacteria; hence, wound cultures are unnecessary unless there is evidence of systemic infection or progressive local infection such as cellulitis.
2. Apply topical antibiotics to locally infected pressure ulcer as prescribed.

Cover the Wound With a Protective Dressing
1. This minimizes disruption of migrating fibroblasts and epithelial cells and results in a moist, nutrient-rich environment for healing to occur.
   a. Polyurethane thin film dressings can be used for superficial low-exudate wounds. They are air and water permeable but do not absorb exudate.
   b. Hydrocolloids can provide padding to wounds but can lead to maceration; they are not oxygen permeable.
   c. Polyurethane foam/membrane dressings absorb exudate and are oxygen permeable.
   d. Hydrogel dressings are multilayered and include properties of both hydrocolloids and polyurethane. (See Table 9-2 for comparison of selected occlusive dressings.)

◼ Osteoporosis
Osteoporosis is a condition in which the bone matrix is lost, thereby weakening the bones and making them more susceptible to fracture. It is the most age-related metabolic bone disorder.

Pathophysiology and Etiology
1. The rate of bone resorption increases over the rate of bone formation, causing loss of bone mass.
2. Calcium and phosphate salts are lost, creating porous, brittle bones.
3. Occurs most frequently in postmenopausal women.
4. Other factors include:
   a. Age
   b. Inactivity
   c. Chronic illness
   d. Medications, such as corticosteroids, excessive thyroid replacement, cyclosporins
   e. Calcium and vitamin D deficiency
   f. Family history
   g. Smoking/alcohol use
   h. Diet—caffeine has been linked as a risk factor
   i. Race—whites and Asians have higher risk incidence
   j. Body type—small frame/short stature, low body fat

Clinical Manifestations
1. Asymptomatic until later stages.
2. Fracture after minor trauma may be first indication. Most frequent fractures associated with osteoporosis include fractures of the distal radius, vertebral bodies, proximal humerus, pelvis, and proximal femur (hip).
3. May have vague complaints related to aging process (stiffness, pain, weakness).
4. Estrogen deficiency may be noted.

Diagnostic Evaluation
1. X-rays show changes only after 30% to 60% loss of bone.
2. Studies that show decreased density of bone include computed tomography, dual photon absorptiometry, dual energy x-ray absorptiometry (DEXA).
3. Serum/urine calcium levels normal.
4. Serum bone GLA-protein (a marker for bone turnover) is elevated.
5. Bone biopsy shows thin, porous, otherwise normal bone.

Management
Management is primarily preventive.
1. Adequate intake of calcium—1 to 1.5 g—may be preventive.

TABLE 9-2 Comparison of Selected Occlusive Dressings

Dressing Type	Examples	Appropriate Use	Advantages	Disadvantages
Absorption	Debrisan Hydrophillic Beads	Stage II–IV ulcer with drainage	Absorbs drainage and deodorizes wound	Need to change dressing one to two times daily
Hydrocolloid	Duoderm	Stage I–II ulcer	Provides padding Easy to apply Water impermeable No skin excoriation	Poor absorptive capacity Poor oxygen exchange Messy residue Pressure areas possible
Polyurethane	Op-Site Tegaderm	Nondraining wounds	Transparent Self-adhesive Oxygen permeable	No absorptive capacity May cause excoriation Difficult to apply
Polyurethane membrane	Mitraflex	Skin tears Tape burns Blisters Stage II ulcers Low-moderate exudate wounds	Good absorptive ability Good oxygen exchange Water impermeable May débride	May cause excoriation
Polyurethane foam	Epi-Lock	Skin tears Tape burns Blisters Stage II ulcers Low-moderate exudate wounds	Good absorptive ability Good oxygen exchange Water impermeable May débride No skin excoriation	Nonadhesive
Hydrogel	Vigilon Biofilm	Stage I–III	No skin excoriation Transparent Some ability to absorb drainage Easy to apply	Difficult to apply Nonadherent
Débriding enzyme	Elase Travase	Stage III–IV	Acts against devitalized tissue Not appropriate for hard, dry eschar	May damage healthy tissue

2. Adequate intake of vitamin D (exposure to sunlight).
   a. Those receiving little sunlight exposure and limited dairy products should receive vitamin D supplement.
3. Weight-bearing exercise (walking) throughout life.
4. Use of estrogen replacement therapy for post-menopausal women, which is necessary in addition to calcium intake. Ideally, start within 5 years of menopause before osteoporosis is established, but may be of benefit in late stages as well.
5. Alternative to estrogen is an estrogen receptor agonist, raloxifene (Evista). Not as effective as estrogen, but does show some benefit in preserving bone density. No increase in risk of breast cancer.
6. Calcitonin (Miacalcin) administered by nasal spray preserves bone density. Side effect is nasal burning.
7. Risedronate (Actonel) and alendronate (Fosamax) bind to and inhibit osteoclast action, remain active on bone resorptive surfaces for 3 weeks, and do not impede normal bone formation.
   a. Associated with improved bone density and decreased fracture rate.
   b. They must be taken with fluid but not food, and patient must remain upright for 30 minutes after taking pill to prevent esophagitis.
8. Prevention of falls in the elderly to prevent fractures.

Complications
1. Fractures

Nursing Assessment
1. Obtain history of risk factors for osteoporosis, history of fractures, and other musculoskeletal disease.
2. Assess risk for falls and fractures—sensory or motor problems, improper footwear, lack of knowledge of safety precautions, and so forth.

Nursing Diagnosis
- Chronic Pain related to vertebral compression fractures in late stages of osteoporosis

Nursing Interventions
Reducing Pain
1. Administer narcotic analgesics as ordered for acute exacerbations of pain.

2. Encourage replacement with non-narcotic pain relievers as soon as possible to avoid addiction.

GERONTOLOGIC ALERT

Be alert for side effects of narcotics in the elderly, such as impairment of mental status; dizziness, which may contribute to falls and other accidents; and constipation.

---

3. Assist with putting on back brace and ensure proper fit. Encourage use as much as possible, especially while ambulatory.
4. Encourage compliance with physical therapy appointments and practicing exercises at home to increase muscle strength surrounding bones and to relieve pain.

Patient Education and Health Maintenance

1. Encourage exercise for all age groups. Teach the value of walking daily throughout life to provide stress required for strong bone remodeling.
2. Provide dietary education in relation to adequate daily intake of calcium 1,000 mg or more (1,500 mg if female is not on estrogen). Calcium can be obtained through milk and dairy products, vegetables, and supplements. Anyone with a history of urinary tract stones should consult with health care provider before increasing calcium intake.
3. Advise on vitamin D requirements, which can be obtained through sunlight exposure, drinking milk, and taking vitamin supplements. Vitamin D is required for calcium absorption, and requirements increase with age.
4. Encourage young women at risk to maximize bone mass through nutrition and exercise.
5. Suggest that perimenopausal women confer with the physician concerning need for calcium supplements and estrogen therapy.
6. Alert patients to resources, such as the National Osteoporosis Foundation (1-800-223-9994 or *www.nof.org*).

Community and Home Care Considerations

1. Identify women at high risk for osteoporotic fractures in the community—frail, elderly white or Asian women with poor dietary intake of dairy products and little exposure to sun—and provide education and safety measures to prevent falls and fracture.
2. Ensure that diet contains maximal calcium. Teach family and caregivers how to read labels, encourage dairy products, and add powdered milk to foods as possible. Use skim milk if cholesterol/fat intake is a consideration.
3. Ensure that supplements and other medications are being taken properly.
   a. Patient teaching is critical in dosing of alendronate sodium (Fosamax) to prevent esophagitis. Patient must take this upon waking with 6 to 8 oz of plain water, at least a half hour before first food, and must remain upright for 30 minutes after taking Fosamax. Risedronate may be better tolerated.
   b. Calcitonin nasal spray dose is one spray in one nostril once a day; alternate nostrils each day.
4. Teach strategies to prevent falls. Assess home for hazards (eg, scatter rugs, slippery floors, extension cords, adequate lighting).
5. Obtain physical and occupational therapy consults as needed to encourage use of walking aids when balance is poor and to improve muscle strength.

Outcome-Based Evaluation

• Pain tolerable with non-narcotic analgesics; no new fractures

Alzheimer's Disease

The most common form of dementia; characterized by progressive impairment in memory, cognitive function, language, judgment, and ADL. Ultimately, patients are unable to perform self-care activities and become dependent on caregivers.

Pathophysiology and Etiology

1. Gross pathophysiologic changes include cortical atrophy, enlarged ventricles, and basal ganglia wasting.
2. Microscopically, changes occur in the proteins of the nerve cells of the cerebral cortex and lead to accumulation of neurofibrillary tangles and neuritic plaques (deposits of protein and altered cell structures on the interneuronal junctions) and granulovascular degeneration. There is loss of cholinergic nerve cells, which are important in memory, function, and cognition.
3. Biochemically, neurotransmitter systems are impaired.
4. Cause unknown, but genetics and female gender are risk factors. Research is being conducted to locate specific genes involved in predisposition to Alzheimer's.
5. Viruses, environmental toxins, and previous head injury may also play a role.

Clinical Manifestations

1. Disease onset is subtle and insidious. Initially, a gradual decline of cognitive function from a previously higher level may be noticed. Short-term memory impairment is often the first characteristic in earliest stages of the disease. Patients are forgetful and have difficulty learning and retaining new information. In addition to memory impairment, at least one of the following functional deficits is present:
   a. Language disturbance (word-finding difficulty)
   b. Visual-processing difficulty
   c. Inability to perform skilled motor activities
   d. Poor abstract reasoning and concentration

2. Patients may have difficulty planning meals, managing finances, using a telephone, or driving without getting lost. Other classic signs include personality changes such as irritability and suspiciousness, personal neglect of appearance, and disorientation to time and space.
3. The following clinical manifestations are typical in the middle stage of Alzheimer's disease:
   a. Repetitive actions (perseveration)
   b. Nocturnal restlessness
   c. Apraxia (impaired ability to perform purposeful activity
   d. Aphasia (inability to speak)
   e. Agraphia (inability to write)
4. With disease progression, signs of frontal lobe dysfunction appear, including loss of social inhibitions and loss of spontaneity. Delusions, hallucinations, aggression, and wandering behavior often occur in the middle and late stages.
5. Patients in the advanced stage of Alzheimer's disease require total care. Symptoms may include:
   a. Urinary and fecal incontinence
   b. Emaciation
   c. Increased irritability
   d. Unresponsiveness or coma

Diagnostic Evaluation
1. Detailed patient history with corroboration by an informed source to determine cognitive and behavioral changes, their duration, and symptoms that may be indicative of other medical or psychiatric illnesses.
2. Noncontrast computed tomography (CT) to rule out other neurologic conditions. Magnetic resonance imaging (MRI) and single-photon emission computed tomography (SPECT) may be used.
3. Neuropsychological evaluation, including some form of mental status assessment, to identify specific areas of impaired mental functioning in contrast to areas of intact functioning.
4. Laboratory tests include complete blood count, sedimentation rate, chemistry panel, thyroid-stimulating hormone, test for syphilis, urinalysis, serum B_{12}, folate level, and test for human immunodeficiency virus (HIV) to rule out infectious or metabolic disorders.
5. Commercial assays for cerebrospinal fluid (CSF) tau protein and beta-amyloid are available, but their use is limited. Genetic testing is available, but its use is controversial. Three disease genes and one gene indicating susceptibility have been identified. In families with a history of Alzheimer's disease, tests are available to confirm Alzheimer's disease or to provide information to at-risk family members regarding their likelihood for development of Alzheimer's disease.

Management
1. Primary goals of treatment for Alzheimer's disease are to maximize functional abilities and improve quality of life by enhancing mood, cognition, and behavior. No curative treatment exists. Treatment includes pharmacologic and nonpharmacologic approaches.
2. Cholinesterase inhibitors are currently the only treatment for cognitive impairment of Alzheimer's disease. Tacrine (Cognex) and donepezil (Aricept) are two agents that may improve cognitive functioning by improving cholinergic neurotransmission.
3. Clinical trials of other agents to improve cognitive functioning are ongoing. They include estrogen, nonsteroidal anti-inflammatory drugs, and botanical agents, such as ginkgo biloba. It is hoped that a vaccine may be developed one day for use in genetically susceptible people.
4. Patients with depressive symptoms should be considered for antidepressant therapy.
5. Behavioral disturbances may require pharmacologic treatment with antipsychotics such as clozapine (Clozaril), risperidone (Risperdal), and olanzapine (Zyprexa).
6. Nonpharmacologic treatment used to improve cognition includes psychotherapeutic techniques such as reality orientation and memory retraining. Reminiscence therapy and stimulation-oriented treatment, such as art and other recreational therapies, are interventions that may improve mood and behavior.

 DRUG ALERT

Cholinesterase inhibitors are suggested for patients with mild or moderate Alzheimer's disease but have not been assessed for effectiveness for patients with severe Alzheimer's disease. Administration of tacrine for patients with mild to moderate Alzheimer's disease requires an introductory period and regular assessment of liver function. The starting dose for tacrine is 10 mg qid, which can be increased to a maximum of 40 mg qid. Patients should be observed for cholinergic adverse effects, most commonly gastrointestinal distress and elevations of serum transaminase levels.

Complications
1. Increased susceptibility to infections
2. Injury due to lack of insight, hallucinations, and confusion
3. Malnutrition due to inattention to mealtime and hunger or lack of ability to prepare meals

Nursing Assessment
1. Perform cognitive assessment for orientation, insight, abstract thinking, concentration, memory, and verbal ability.
2. Assess for changes in behavior and ability to perform ADL.
3. Evaluate nutrition and hydration; check weight, skin turgor, meal habits.

4. Assess motor ability, strength, muscle tone, and flexibility.

Nursing Diagnoses
- Altered Thought Processes related to physiologic changes
- Risk for Injury due to loss of cognitive abilities
- Sleep Pattern Disturbance secondary to disease process
- Caregiver Role Strain related to physical needs and behavioral manifestations of the disease process

Nursing Interventions
Improving Cognitive Response
1. Simplify the environment: decrease noise and social interaction to a level tolerable for the patient.
2. Maintain a strict routine, decrease the number of choices available to the patient, use pictures to identify activities. Use structured group activities.
3. Encourage participation in care as tolerated and provide positive feedback for tasks that are accomplished.
4. Provide rest periods between activities to reduce fatigue.
5. Post large calendar and clock in patient's view and orient frequently to time, person, and place (Figure 9-4).
6. Use lists and written instructions as reminders to daily activities.
7. Maintain consistency in interactions and introduce new people slowly.

Preventing Injury
1. Avoid restraints but maintain observation of the patient as necessary.
2. Provide for adequate lighting to avoid misinterpretation of the environment.
3. Remove unneeded furniture and equipment from the room.

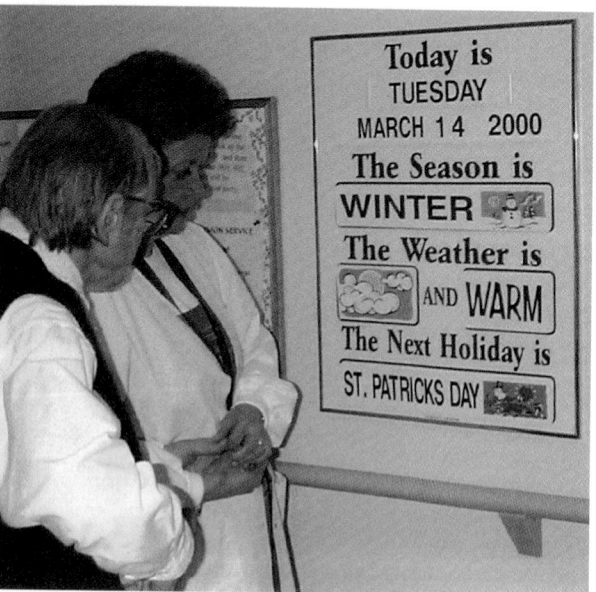

FIGURE 9-4 A large poster or calendar can be used to continually orient patient.

4. Provide identification tag and/or Medic-Alert bracelet.
5. Make sure patient has nonslip shoes or slippers that are easy to put on.
6. Encourage use of assistive safety devices such as handrails and shower chairs.
7. Ensure physical activity as tolerated and range-of-motion exercises to maintain mobility.

Ensuring Adequate Rest
1. Administer antipsychotics to manage agitation.
2. Provide periods of physical exercise to expend energy.
3. Support normal sleep habits and bedtime ritual.
   a. Keep regular bedtime.
   b. Have patient change into pajamas at bedtime.
   c. Allow desired bedtime activity, such as snack, warm noncaffeinated beverage, listening to music, or prayer.
4. Maintain quiet, relaxing environment to avoid confusion and agitation.

Supporting Caregiver
1. Encourage caregiver to discuss feelings.
2. Encourage caregiver to maintain own health and emotional well-being.
3. Stress the need for relaxation time or respite care.
4. Assist the caregiver in finding resources, such as community or church groups, social service programs, or hospital-based support groups.
5. Assess caregiver's stress and refer for counseling.
6. Support decision to place patient in a nursing facility.

Community and Home Care Considerations
1. Encourage regular medical checkups with attention to health maintenance every 3 to 6 months to provide ongoing medical surveillance of patient and stamina of caregivers. Include influenza vaccine and ensure that patient has had pneumococcal pneumonia vaccine.
2. Discuss advance directives for patients and discuss long-term placement options in anticipation of future needs, to help family members adjust and plan arrangements.
3. Encourage patients to be involved in social and intellectual activities as long as possible, such as family events, exercise and recreational activities, sharing the newspaper and other forms of media.
4. Assist caregivers to modify the home environment for safety, and advise families of safety hazards such as wandering and driving a car. Encourage use of door locks, electronic wander-alert guards, and registration with the "Safe Return" program through the Alzheimer's Association or local police department.
5. Remind family members of possible dangers around the house as patients becomes less responsible for behavior. Encourage caregivers to reduce the temperature of the hot water heater, remove dials from stove and other electrical appliances, remove matches and lighters, and safely store away tools and other potentially dangerous items.

Patient Education and Health Maintenance

1. Encourage activities that provide physical exercise and repetitive movement but that require little thought, such as dancing, painting, doing laundry, or vacuuming.
2. Teach patient and family to eliminate stimulants and maintain good nutrition.
3. Discuss with the family the need to organize finances and to make advanced directive decisions and guardianship arrangements before they are needed to allow the patient input into the process.
4. Over-the-counter products such as ginkgo biloba and vitamin E are gaining popularity; however, their clinical benefits are inconclusive at this time, so families should be encouraged to discuss their use with the health care provider and not abandon conventional treatment.
5. For additional information, refer families to:

   The Alzheimer's Association
   919 North Michigan Avenue, Suite 1100
   Chicago, IL 60611
   800-272-3900
   www.alz.org

Outcome-Based Evaluation

- Participates in ADL without confusion or agitation
- Remains free of injury
- Sleeps 6 to 8 hours at night with 1-hour rest period twice a day
- Caregiver reports using support systems and community resources

LEGAL AND ETHICAL CONSIDERATIONS

◼ Restraint Use

Since the Nursing Home Reform Act took effect in October 1990, long-term care facilities throughout the United States have been required to follow new guidelines emphasizing individualized, less restrictive care for residents. See Procedure Guidelines 9-1.

Guidelines

1. The following are the federal requirements for the use of restraints based on the 1987 Omnibus Budget Reconciliation Act.
2. These guidelines must be met in any long-term care facility that participates in Medicare or Medicaid. However, these guidelines are useful for health care providers working with elderly people in all settings.
   a. The resident has the right to be free from any physical restraints imposed or psychoactive drug administered for purposes of discipline or convenience and not required to treat the resident's medical symptoms.
   b. Physical restraints are any manual method of physical or mechanical device, material, or equipment attached or adjacent to the resident's body that the person cannot remove easily, which restricts freedom of movement or access to one's body (includes leg and arm restraints, hand mitts, soft ties or vest, wheelchair safety bars, and gerichairs).
   c. There must be a trial of less restrictive measures unless the physical restraint is necessary to provide lifesaving treatment.
   d. The resident or his or her legal representative must consent to the use of restraints.
   e. Residents who are restrained should be released, exercised, toileted, and checked for skin redness every 2 hours.
   f. The need for restraints should be reevaluated periodically.
   g. The specific institution will have to develop policies and procedures for the appropriate use of restraints and psychoactive drugs.
   h. Primary health care providers will have to write appropriate orders for restraints and/or psychoactive drugs.
3. The most frequently reported reason for nurses' use of restraints is to prevent patients from harming themselves or others. Specifically, they are used to prevent falls and prevent removal of catheters or intravenous lines.
4. Multiple studies have found that restraints actually increase the falls that occur, can result in patient strangulation, can increase patient confusion, can cause pressure ulcers and nosocomial infections, can decrease functional ability, and can result in social isolation.
5. In regard to the patient's personal and social integrity, restraints have resulted in emotional responses of anger, fear, resistance, humiliation, demoralization, discomfort, resignation, and denial.

Alternative Interventions Instead of Restraints

1. Evaluate those patients who are considered to be in need of a restraint. Evaluation should include physical function (see section titled Functional Assessment), cognitive status (see section titled Mental Status Testing), elimination history, history of falls, visual impairment, blood pressure (specifically evaluating for orthostatic hypotension), and medication use.
2. Attempt to correct any problems identified in the evaluation, such as visual impairment or unsafe gait.
3. Use the evaluation to determine patients at high risk of falling (ie, those with confusion, orthostatic hypotension, multiple medication regimens, and altered gait).
4. Alternatives to restraints for patients at high risk of falling when ambulating independently include:
   a. Use of beanbag chairs or specially designed chairs that make independent transfer difficult for the older adult

b. Tilting the front of a chair upward by inserting a small to medium folded blanket under the anterior portion of the cushion

c. Instituting increased exercise activities to help strengthen muscles and improve function

5. For the patient who interferes with treatment, it may be helpful to evaluate the need for the invasive treatments. When such treatments are essential, attempt the use of mittens or gloves rather than restraints.

6. For the patient who wanders, it may be helpful to provide an exercise program or establish a bounded environment in which the person can ambulate freely.

7. For aggressive and agitated patients, be aware that restraints may only make the behavior worse. Use of a low-stimulus environment, consistent caregivers, and appropriate medications may help control the agitation. Music therapy has also been shown to decrease aggressive behavior.

PROCEDURE GUIDELINES 9-1 — SAFETY GUIDELINES FOR RESTRAINT USE

EQUIPMENT

Restraint device
Full bed side rails
Side rail covers

PROCEDURE

Nursing Action	Rationale
PREPARATORY PHASE	
1. Select the least restrictive physical restraint.	1. Passive restraints such as geriatric chairs with trays are more desirable than active restraints (vests, leg, arm, wrist, hand restraints or seat belts).
2. Examine the restraint device to ensure that it is not torn or damaged, and that it works properly and is the proper size for the patient.	2. A damaged or improperly fitting restraint poses a significant safety risk because the patient could become suspended by the restraint, causing chest compression.

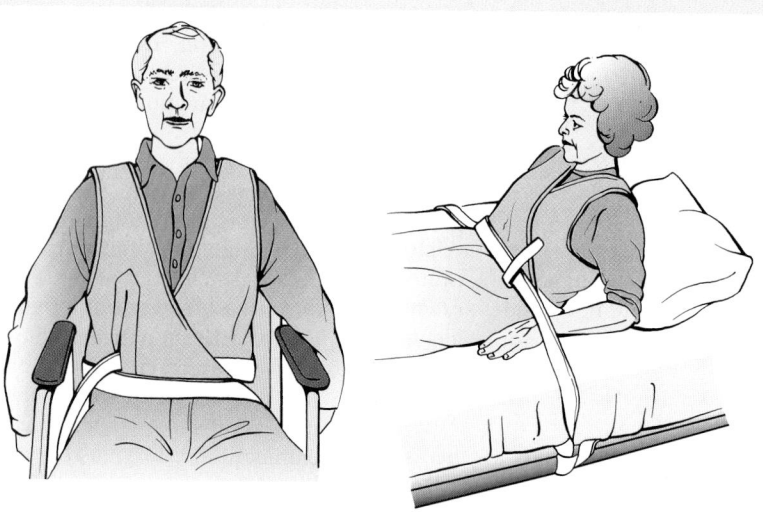

Proper position of patient restraint in wheelchair and bed. Straps of most vest-type restraints should cross in front of the patient. (Left) Safety vest. (Right) Budget vest.

Nursing Action	Rationale
3. If the restraint is being used in bed, make sure that full side rails can be placed in the up position. Obtain side rail covers if the patient's limbs could fit over, under, around, through, or between side rails.	3. Side rails that are only ½ or ¾ length of the bed may allow the patient to slip partially off the bed and to become suspended in the restraint.
4. Completely review manufacturer's instructions before applying the restraint.	4. Complete information can be obtained from Posey Co., 5635 Peck Rd., Arcadia, CA 91006, 800-44-POSEY.

PROCEDURE GUIDELINES 9-1   *CONTINUED*

Nursing Action	**Rationale**

PERFORMANCE PHASE

1. Apply the restraint with the patient positioned in the middle of the bed or sitting with hips well to the back of chair.

2. Make sure the front and back of restraint are positioned appropriately on the patient and that straps are crossed in the front, unless the vest is specifically designed with positioning slot in the back.

1. Proper positioning helps prevent injury or falls.

2. Crossing the straps in the back or applying a vest restraint backward may result in serious injury or death.

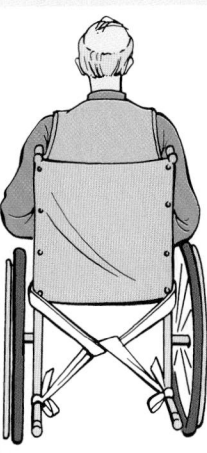

3. Secure straps out of patient's reach to the movable part of a spring bedframe or wheelchair kickspurs. Use quick-release knots.

3. Ensures that adjustment of bed position or siderails will not interfere with restraint. Quick-release knots allow timely intervention in emergency situations.

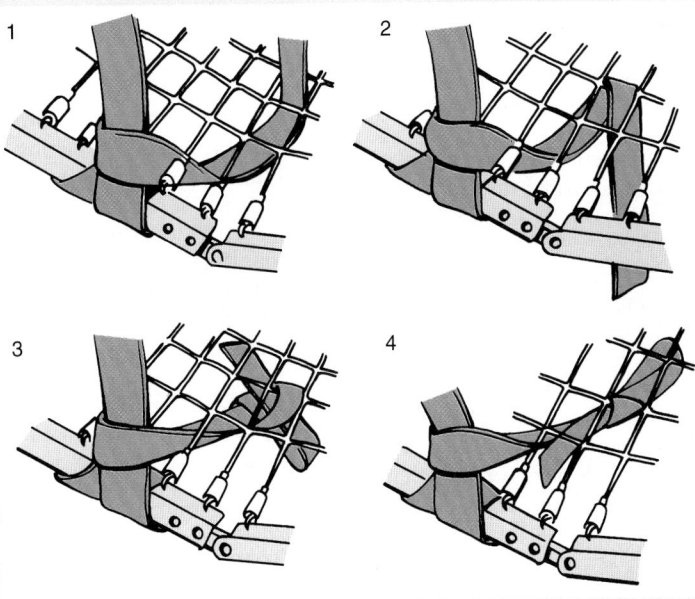

continued

PROCEDURE GUIDELINES 9-1	SAFETY GUIDELINES FOR RESTRAINT USE *CONTINUED*
Nursing Action	**Rationale**

FOLLOW-UP PHASE

1. Monitor the patient frequently once restraint is applied.

2. Use ancillary staff to sit with and try to calm agitated or restless patients whenever possible, even if restraint has been consented to.
3. Never use restraints on a toilet or commode or in a motor vehicle. Do not send restraint home with patient.

1. Will detect loosening, which may cause injury or restriction caused by the restraint.
2. Studies have shown that use of restraints only contributes to falls.

3. Restraints are specifically designed to be used with hospital beds, wheelchairs, and geriatric chairs, and by those trained in their proper use. Misuse may result in injury.

Advance Directives

The 1990 Patient Self-Determination Act, which requires that patients be asked about the existence of advanced directives at the time of enrollment into a health care facility, has increased awareness of older adults' rights to determine their own care. Based on the ethical principle of autonomy (a person's privilege of self-rule), advance directives provide a clear and detailed expression of a person's wishes for care.

Advance directives may be limited to a single situation, such as a "living will" for the terminally ill, or may address a multitude of different scenarios in detail.

Types of Advance Directives
Living Wills

1. Living Wills were the first and most widespread type of advance directive.
2. They were proposed as a mechanism for refusing "heroic" or unwanted medical intervention for the dying person.
3. They allow a person to state in writing that certain life-sustaining treatments should be withdrawn or withheld when that person is dying and unable to directly communicate his or her wishes.
4. Living Wills only allow for the refusal of further treatment. They are not precise in terms of directives and focus only on the patient who is clearly terminally ill.

**Durable Power of Attorney
for Health Care (DPOA-HC)**

1. This document appoints a person to act on behalf of another person, provides guidance for the proxy, and endures even when the maker is incapacitated.
2. The DPOA-HC is always a written document.
3. The document states the preferences and perhaps even the values of its maker: It outlines the types of decisions the person would want to have made on his or her behalf.
4. Because no DPOA-HC can cover all situations, the document should name a person who has the task of ensuring that the patient's wishes are honored. The proxy has the responsibility to interpret the DPOA-HC and extrapolate its contents to situations not specifically covered.

Nursing and Patient Care Considerations

1. Under the Patient Self-Determination Act, all patients who enter a Medicare- or Medicaid-certified hospital, nursing home or home health agency must:
   a. Be provided with information about the state's laws and the facility's policies regarding advance directive.
   b. Be asked if they have advance directives.
   c. Have their advance directives placed in their medical record.
2. Education of patients and families is essential in helping them to understand the difference between Living Wills or DPOA-HC and determining which document best suits their needs.
3. Patients and families need to be educated regarding what is involved in undergoing various life-sustaining procedures so they can make a decision regarding their future treatment.
4. Patients need to be informed that they can have more than one advance directive. That is, if a patient has a Living Will but is not terminally ill, he or she needs to be encouraged to obtain a DPOA-HC to ensure that health care wishes will be met in any situation.

Community and Home Care Considerations

1. Information on completing Advance Directives may be obtained by contacting Choice in Dying, 800-989-9455; *www.choices.org.*
2. Instruct older adults that the Medical Directive allows them to record their wishes regarding various types of medical treatment, and lets them appoint a proxy for if/when they are unable to make those decisions on their own.

SELECTED REFERENCES

Allen, L. A. (1999). Treating agitation without drugs. *American Journal of Nursing, 99*(4), 36–41.

Cassell, C., Cohen, H., Larson, E., Meier, D., Resnick, N., Ruenstein, L., & Sorensen, L. (Eds.). (1996). *Geriatric medicine.* New York: Springer.

Cavendish, R. (1999). Improving care for the elderly. *American Journal of Nursing, 99*(5), 88.

Clark, M. E., Lipe, A. W., & Bilbrey, M. (1998). Use of music to decrease aggressive behaviors in people with dementia. *Journal of Gerontological Nursing, 24*(7), 10–17.

Cowart, M., & Sutherland, M. (1998). Late-life drinking among women. *Geriatric Nursing, 19,* 214–219.

DeDeyn, P. P., Rabberu, K., Rasmussen, A., et al. (1999). A randomized trial of risperidone, placebo, and haloperidol for behavioral symptoms of dementia. *Neurology, 53,* 946.

Dunlap, R. (1997). Teaching advance directives: The why, when and how. *Journal of Gerontological Nursing, 23,* 11–16.

Ebersole, P., & Hess, P. (1998). *Toward healthy aging.* St. Louis: Mosby.

Ettinger, W. (1996). Physical activity and older people: A walk a day keeps the doctor away. *Journal of the American Geriatrics Society, 44,* 207–208.

Kessenich, C. R. (2000). Risedronate: A new biphosphonate for the treatment of osteoporosis. *The Nurse Practitioner, 23*(3), 106–108.

Loeb, J. L. (1999). Pain management in long-term care. *American Journal of Nursing, 99*(2), 48–52.

Mahoney, F., & Barthel, D. (1965). Functional evaluation: The Barthel Index. *Maryland State Medical Journal, 14,* 62–72.

Mayeaux, R., & Sano, M. (1999). Treatment of Alzheimer's disease. *New England Journal of Medicine, 341,* 1670.

Mosher, B., Cuddigan, J., Thomas, D., & Boudreau, D. (1999). Outcomes of 4 methods of debridement using a decision analysis methodology. *Advances in Wound Care, 12,* 81–89.

Ouslander, J., Osterweil, D., & Morley, J. (1997). *Medical care in the nursing home* (2nd ed.). New York: McGraw-Hill.

Resnick, B. (1999). Exercise for the older adult: The seven step approach to wellness. *Advance for Nurses, 20.*

———. (1998a). Health care practices of the old-old. *American Academy Journal of Nurse Practitioners, 10,* 147–155.

———. (1998b). Motivating the older adult to perform functional activities. *Journal of Gerontological Nursing, 24,* 23–31.

———. (1997). The presentation of acute illness in the older adult with dementia. *The Clinical Letter for Nurse Practitioners, 2,* 1–3.

———. (1996). Dermatological problems in the older adult. *Lippincott's Primary Care Practice, 1*(1), 14–23

———. (1993). Retraining the bladder after catheterization. *American Journal of Nursing, 93* (11), 46–50.

Ship, J., Pearson, J., Cruise, L., Brant, L., & Metter, E. (1996). Longitudinal changes in smell identification. *Journal of Gerontology, 51A,* A86.

Stolley, J. (1995). Freeing your patients from restraints. *RN, 95,* 26–30.

Tullman, D. F., & Dracup, K. (2000). Creating a healing environment for elders. *AACN Clinical Issues, 11*(1), 34–50.

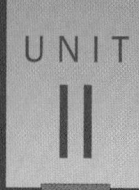

Respiratory Function and Therapy

GENERAL OVERVIEW

Respiratory Function

The major function of the pulmonary system (lungs and pulmonary circulation) is to deliver oxygen to cells and remove carbon dioxide from the cells (gas exchange). The adequacy of oxygenation and ventilation is measured by PaO_2 and $PaCO_2$. The pulmonary system also functions as a blood reservoir for the left ventricle when it is needed to boost cardiac output; as a protector for the systemic circulation by filtering debris/particles; as a fluid regulator so water can be kept away from alveoli; and as a provider of metabolic functions such as surfactant production and endocrine functions.

Terminology

1. *Alveolus*—air sac where gas exchange takes place
2. *Apex*—top portion of the upper lobes of lungs
3. *Base*—bottom portion of lower lobes, located just above the diaphragm
4. *Bronchoconstriction*—constriction of smooth muscle surrounding bronchioles
5. *Bronchus*—large airways; lung divides into right and left bronchi
6. *Carina*—location of division of the right and left main stem bronchi
7. *Cilia*—hairlike projections on the tracheobronchial surface lining, which aid in the movement of secretions and debris
8. *Compliance*—ability of the lungs to distend (eg, emphysema—lungs very compliant; fibrosis—lungs noncompliant or stiff)
9. *Dead space*—ventilation that does not participate in gas exchange; physiologic dead space occurs when there is adequate ventilation but no perfusion, as in pulmonary embolus
10. *Diaphragm*—dome-shaped muscle; the primary muscle used for respiration (located just below the lung bases)
11. *Diffusion* (of gas)—movement of gases from a higher to lower concentration
12. *Dyspnea*—subjective sensation associated with unpleasant, uncomfortable respiratory sensations, often caused by a dissociation between motor command and mechanical response of the respiratory system, eg:
    a. *Respiratory muscle abnormalities* (hyperinflation and airflow limitation from chronic obstructive pulmonary disease [COPD])
    b. *Abnormal ventilatory impedance* (narrowing airways and respiratory impedance from COPD or asthma)
    c. *Abnormal breathing patterns* (severe exercise, pulmonary congestion or edema, recurrent pulmonary emboli)
    d. *ABG abnormalities* (hypoxemia, hypercarbia)
13. *Hemoptysis*—bleeding from the lung; main symptom is coughing up blood
14. *Hypoxemia*—PaO_2 less than normal, which may or may not cause symptoms. Normal PaO_2 is 80 to 100 mm Hg on room air.
15. *Hypoxia*—insufficient oxygenation at the cellular level due to an imbalance in oxygen delivery and oxygen consumption. Usually causes symptoms reflecting decreased oxygen reaching the brain and heart.
16. *Mediastinum*—compartment between lungs containing lymph and vascular tissue that separates left from right lung
17. *Orthopnea*—shortness of breath when in reclining position
18. *Paroxysmal nocturnal dyspnea* (PND)—shortness of breath with sudden onset; occurs after going to sleep in recumbent position
19. *Perfusion*—blood flow, carrying oxygen and carbon dioxide, that passes by alveoli
20. *Pleura*—membrane that covers the outside of the lung (visceral pleura) and lines the thorax (parietal pleura) that creates a potential space
21. *Pulmonary circulation* (bronchial circulation)—circulatory system that supplies oxygenated blood to the respiratory system
22. *Respiration*—gas exchange from air to blood and blood to body cells
23. *Shunt*—adequate perfusion without ventilation, as in pulmonary edema, atelectasis, pneumonia, COPD
24. *Surfactant*—substance released by cells within the lung; maintains surface tension and keeps alveoli open allowing for better gas exchange
25. *Ventilation*—movement of air (gases) in and out of the lungs
26. *Ventilation–perfusion (V/Q) imbalance*—mismatch of ventilation and perfusion; a cause for hypoxemia. V/Q mismatch can be due to:
    a. Blood perfusing an area of the lung where ventilation is reduced or absent
    b. Excessive amount of blood flow for the amount of ventilation present

ASSESSMENT

Subjective Data

Explore the patient's symptoms through characterization and history taking to help anticipate needs and plan care.

Dyspnea

1. *Characteristics*—Is the dyspnea acute or chronic? Has it come about suddenly or gradually? Is more than one pillow required to sleep? Is the dyspnea progressive, recurrent, or paroxysmal? Walking how far leads to shortness of breath? How does it compare to the patient's baseline level of dyspnea? Are there any interventions that relieve the dyspnea? Ask patient to rate dyspnea on a scale of 1 to 10 scale with 1 being no dyspnea and 10 being the worst imaginable.

2. *Associated factors*—Is there a cough associated with the dyspnea and is it productive? What activities precipitate the shortness of breath? Does it seem to be worse when upset? Is it influenced by the time of day or seasons? Does it occur at rest or with exertion? Any fever, chills, night sweats? Any change in body weight?
3. *History*—Is there a patient history or family history of chronic lung disease, cardiac or neuromuscular disease? What is the smoking history?
4. *Significance*—Sudden dyspnea could indicate pulmonary embolus, pneumothorax, myocardial infarction, acute ventricular failure, or acute respiratory failure. In a postsurgical or postpartum patient, dyspnea may indicate pulmonary embolus or edema. Orthopnea can be indicative of heart disease or COPD. If dyspnea is associated with a wheeze, consider asthma or COPD.

Chest Pain
1. *Characteristics*—Is the pain sharp, dull, stabbing, or aching? Is it intermittent or persistent? Is the pain localized or does it radiate? If it radiates, where? How intense is the pain? Are there any interventions that relieve the pain?
2. *Associated factors*—What effect do inspiration and expiration have on the pain? What factors seem to precipitate the pain?
3. *History*—Is there a smoking history or environmental exposure? Has the pain ever been experienced before? What was the cause? Is there a preexisting pulmonary or cardiac diagnosis?
4. *Significance*—Chest pain related to pulmonary causes is usually felt on the side where pathology arises, but it can be referred. Dull persistent pain may indicate carcinoma of the lung, whereas sharp stabbing pain usually arises from the pleura.

Cough
1. *Characteristics*—Is the cough dry, hacking, or wheezy? Is it strong or weak?
2. *Associated factors*—Is the cough productive? If so, what is the consistency, odor, amount, and color of the sputum? How does sputum compare to the patient's baseline? Is there a particular time or event when coughing begins? Is the onset recent or gradual? Is it associated with food intake?
3. *History*—Has there been any environmental or occupational exposure to dust, fumes, or gases that could lead to cough? Is there a smoking history? Is the smoking current or in past? Are there past pulmonary diagnoses?
4. *Significance*—A dry, irritative cough may indicate viral respiratory tract infection. A cough at night should alert to potential left-sided heart failure or asthma. A morning cough with sputum might be bronchitis. A severe or changing cough should be evaluated for bronchogenic carcinoma. Consider bacterial pneumonia if sputum is rusty, and lung tumor if it is pink-tinged. A profuse pink frothy sputum could be indicative of pulmonary edema. A cough associated with food intake could indicate problems with aspiration.

Hemoptysis
1. *Characteristics*—Is the blood from the lungs? It could be from gastrointestinal system (hematemesis) or upper airway (epistaxis). Is it bright red and frothy? How much?
2. *Associated factors*—Is onset associated with certain circumstances or activities? Was the onset sudden and is it intermittent or continuous? Was there an initial sensation of tickling in the throat? Was there a salty taste, burning or bubbling sensation in the chest before bleeding?
3. *History*—Was there any recent chest trauma or respiratory treatment (chest percussion)?
4. *Significance*—Hemoptysis can be linked to pulmonary infection, lung carcinoma, abnormalities of the heart or blood vessels, pulmonary artery or vein abnormalities, or pulmonary emboli and infarction.

■ Physical Examination
Perform a physical examination of the chest using inspection, palpation, percussion, and auscultation to determine respiratory status and differentiate primary lung problems from cardiac problems.

Key Observations
1. What is the respiratory rate, depth, and pattern? Are accessory muscles being used?
2. Is there central cyanosis indicating possible hypoxemia or cardiac disease?
3. Are the jugular veins distended? Is there peripheral edema or other signs of cardiac dysfunction?
4. Does palpation of the chest cause pain? Is chest excursion symmetric?
5. Are the lung fields clear or are there rhonchi, wheezing, or crackles? Are breath sounds equal bilaterally?
6. Examine sputum or hemoptysis if available for amount, color, and consistency. Does it have an acidic pH (less than 7) indicating that it is from the stomach and not the lungs?
7. Is there an increase in the anterior to posterior chest diameter, suggesting air trapping? Is there clubbing of the fingers, suggesting polycythemia?

DIAGNOSTIC TESTS

■ Laboratory Studies
Arterial Blood Gas (ABG) Analysis
Description
1. A measurement of oxygen, carbon dioxide, as well as the pH of the blood that provides a means of assessing the adequacy of ventilation ($PaCO_2$), oxygenation (PaO_2).
2. Allows assessment of the acid–base (pH) status of the body—whether acidosis or alkalosis is present, whether

acidosis or alkalosis is respiratory or metabolic in origin and to what degree (compensated or uncompensated).

3. Allows evaluation of response to clinical interventions and/or diagnostic evaluation (oxygen therapy, exercise testing).

Nursing and Patient Care Considerations

1. Blood can be obtained from any artery but is most often drawn from the radial, brachial, or femoral site. It can be drawn directly by arterial puncture or accessed by way of indwelling arterial catheter (Procedure Guidelines 10-1). Determine hospital policy for qualifications for ABG sampling and site of arterial puncture.

2. If the radial artery is used, an Allen test must be performed before the puncture to determine if collateral circulation is present.

3. Arterial puncture should not be performed through a lesion, through or distal to a surgical shunt, or in area where peripheral vascular disease or infection is present.

4. Coagulopathy or medium- to high-dose anticoagulation therapy may be a relative contraindication for arterial puncture.

5. Interpret ABGs by looking at the following (normal values are listed):
   a. PaO_2—partial pressure of oxygen in arterial blood (80 to 100 mm Hg)
   b. $PaCO_2$—partial pressure of carbon dioxide in arterial blood (35 to 45 mm Hg)
   c. SaO_2—saturation of oxygen in arterial blood (greater than 95%)
   d. pH—hydrogen ion concentration, or degree of acid–base balance (7.35 to 7.45)

Sputum Examination

Description

1. Sputum is obtained for evaluation of gross appearance, microscopic examination, Gram's stain, culture, acid-fast bacillus, and cytology.
   a. The direct smear shows presence of white blood cells and intracellular (pathogenic) bacteria and extracellular (mostly nonpathogenic) bacteria.
   b. The sputum culture is used to make a diagnosis, determine drug sensitivity, and serve as a guide for drug treatment (ie, choice of antibiotic).
   c. Cytology (exfoliative cytology) is used to identify tumor cells.

Nursing and Patient Care Considerations

1. Patients receiving antibiotics, steroids, and immunosuppressive agents for prolonged time may have periodic sputum examinations, because these agents may give rise to opportunistic pulmonary infections.

2. It is important that the sputum be collected correctly and that the specimen be sent to a lab immediately. Allowing it to stand in a warm room will result in overgrowth of organisms, making identification of pathogen difficult; this also alters cell morphology.

3. Sputum can be obtained by various methods:
   a. Deep breathing and coughing
      (i) Obtain early morning specimen—yields best sample of deep pulmonary secretions from all lung fields.
      (ii) Have patient clear nose and throat and rinse mouth—to decrease sputum contamination.
      (iii) Instruct patient to take several deep breaths, exhale, and perform a series of short coughs.
      (iv) Have patient cough deeply and expectorate the sputum into a sterile container.
   b. Ultrasonic and/or hypertonic saline nebulization
      (i) Patient inhales through mouth slowly and deeply for 10 to 20 minutes.
      (ii) Nebulization increases the moisture content of air going to lower tract; particles will condense on tracheobronchial tree and aid in expectoration.
   c. Tracheal suction—aspiration of secretions through endotracheal or tracheostomy tube
   d. Bronchoscopic removal—provides sputum sampling by aspiration of secretions; brushing through a sterile catheter; bronchoalveolar lavage; and transbronchial biopsy
   e. Gastric aspiration (rarely necessary since advent of ultrasonic nebulizer)
      (i) Nasogastric tube is inserted into the stomach to siphon out swallowed pulmonary secretions.
      (ii) Useful only for culture of tubercle bacilli, but not for direct examination
   f. Transtracheal aspiration (Procedure Guidelines 10-2) involves passing a needle and then a catheter through a percutaneous puncture of the cricothyroid membrane. Transtracheal aspiration bypasses the oropharynx and avoids specimen contamination by mouth flora.

Pleural Fluid Analysis

Description

1. Pleural fluid is continuously produced and reabsorbed, with a thin layer of fluid normally in the pleural space. Abnormal accumulation of pleural fluid (effusion) occurs in diseases of the pleura, heart, or lymphatics. The pleural fluid is studied, along with other tests, to determine the underlying cause.

2. Obtained by aspiration (thoracentesis) or by tube thoracotomy (chest tube insertion; Procedure Guidelines 10-3).

3. The fluid is examined for cell count, differential, specific gravity, cytology, protein, glucose, pH, lactate dehydrogenase (LDH), and amylase. Pleural fluid is usually light straw colored.

Nursing and Patient Care Considerations

1. Observe and record total amount of fluid withdrawn, nature of fluid, and its color and viscosity.

2. Prepare sample of fluid and ensure transport to the laboratory.

(*text continues on page 203*)

PROCEDURE GUIDELINES 10-1	ASSISTING WITH ARTERIAL PUNCTURE FOR BLOOD GAS ANALYSIS

EQUIPMENT

Commercially available blood gas kit
or
2- or 3-mL syringe
23- or 25-gauge needle

0.5 mL sodium heparin (1:1,000)
Stopper or cap
Lidocaine

Sterile germicide
Cup or plastic bag with crushed ice
Gloves

PROCEDURE

Nursing Action	Rationale

PREPARATORY PHASE

1. Record patient's inspired oxygen concentration.

2. Take patient's temperature.

If not using a commercially available blood gas kit:
3. Heparinize the 2-mL syringe.
  a. Withdraw heparin into the syringe to wet the plunger and fill dead space in the needle.
  b. Hold syringe in an upright position and expel excess heparin and air bubbles.

1. Changes in inspired oxygen concentration alter the change in Pao_2. Degree of hypoxemia cannot be assessed without knowing the inspired oxygen concentration.
2. May be taken into consideration when results are evaluated. Hyperthermia and hypothermia influence oxygen release from hemoglobin.

3.
  a. This action coats the interior of the syringe with heparin to prevent blood from clotting.
  b. Air in the syringe may affect measurement of Pao_2 Heparin in the syringe may affect measurement of the pH.

PERFORMANCE PHASE (BY PHYSICIAN, NURSE, OR RESPIRATORY THERAPIST WITH SPECIAL INSTRUCTION)

1. Wash hands.
2. Don gloves.
3. Palpate the radial, brachial or femoral artery.

4. If puncturing the radial artery, perform the Allen test.

3. The radial artery is the preferred site of puncture. Arterial puncture is performed on areas where a good pulse is palpable.
4. The Allen test is a simple method for assessing collateral circulation in the hand. Ensures circulation if radial artery thrombosis occurs.

In the Conscious Patient:
  a. Obliterate the radial and ulnar pulses simultaneously by pressing on both blood vessels at the wrist.
  b. Ask patient to clench and unclench fist until blanching of the skin occurs.
  c. Release pressure on ulnar artery (while still compressing radial artery). Watch for return of skin color within 15 seconds.

  a. Impedes arterial blood flow into the hand.

  b. Forces blood from the hand.

  c. Documents that ulnar artery alone is capable of supplying blood to the hand, because radial artery is still occluded.

Note: If the ulnar does not have sufficient blood flow to supply the entire hand, the radial artery should not be used.

In the Unconscious Patient:
  a. Obliterate the radial and ulnar pulses simultaneously at the wrist.
  b. Elevate patient's hand above heart and squeeze or compress hand until blanching occurs.
  c. Lower patient's hand while still compressing the radial artery (release pressure on ulnar artery) and watch for return of skin color.
5. For the radial side, place a small towel roll under the patient's wrist.
6. Feel along the course of the radial artery and palpate for maximum pulsation with the middle and index fingers. Prepare the skin with germicide. The skin and subcutaneous tissues may be infiltrated with a local anesthetic agent (lidocaine).

5. To make the artery more accessible.

6. The wrist should be stabilized to allow for better control of the needle.

PROCEDURE GUIDELINES 10-1   *CONTINUED*

Nursing Action	Rationale
7. The needle is at a 45- to 60-degree angle to the skin surface (see accompanying figure) and is advanced into the artery. Once the artery is punctured, arterial pressure will push up the hub of the syringe and a pulsating flow of blood will fill the syringe.	7. The arterial pressure will cause the syringe to be filled within a few seconds.

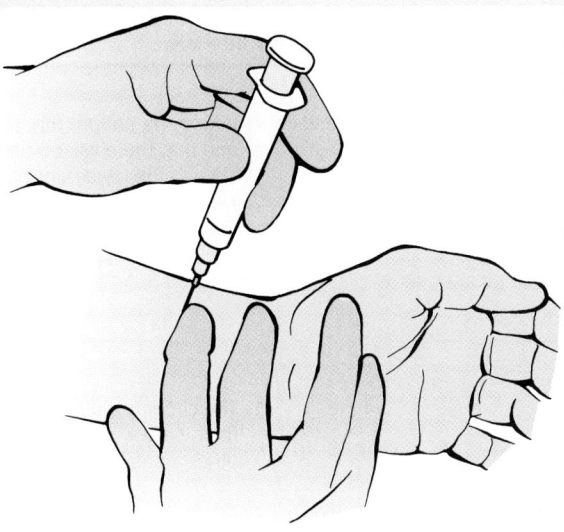

Technique of arterial puncture for blood gas analysis.

Nursing Action	Rationale
8. After blood is obtained, withdraw needle and apply firm pressure over the puncture with a dry sponge.	8. Significant bleeding can occur because of pressure in the artery.
9. Remove air bubbles from syringe and needle. Insert needle into rubber stopper.	9. Immediate capping of the needle prevents room air from mixing with the blood specimen.
10. Place the capped syringe in the container of ice.	10. Icing the syringe will prevent a clinically significant loss of O_2.
11. Maintain firm pressure on the puncture site for 5 minutes. If the patient is on anticoagulant medication, apply direct pressure over puncture site for 10 to 15 minutes and then apply a firm pressure dressing.	11. Firm pressure on the puncture site prevents further bleeding and hematoma formation.
12. For patients requiring serial monitoring of arterial blood, an arterial catheter (connected to a flush solution of heparinized saline) is inserted into the radial or femoral artery.	12. All connections must be tight to avoid disconnection and rapid blood loss. The arterial line also allows for direct blood pressure monitoring in the critically ill patient.

FOLLOW-UP PHASE

1. Send labeled, iced specimen to the laboratory immediately.	1. Blood gas analysis should be done as soon as possible because Pao_2 and pH can change rapidly.
2. Palpate the pulse (distal to the puncture site), inspect the puncture site, and assess for cold hand, numbness, tingling, or discoloration.	2. Hematoma and arterial thrombosis are complications following this procedure.
3. Change ventilator settings, inspired oxygen concentration or type and setting of respiratory therapy equipment if indicated by the results.	3. The Pao_2 results will determine whether to maintain, increase, or decrease the Fio_2. The Pao_2 and pH results will detect if any changes are needed in tidal volume of rate of patient's ventilator.

PROCEDURE GUIDELINES 10-2   ASSISTING WITH TRANSTRACHEAL ASPIRATION

EQUIPMENT

Sterile transtracheal set:

No. 14, No. 16, and No. 18 gauge needles	Local anesthetic	ECG monitoring equipment
Polyethylene catheter	Sterile gloves; mask	Endotracheal tube
Syringe	Specimen containers	Suction apparatus with catheters
Skin preparation solutions	Atropine	Cardiac resuscitation equipment

PROCEDURE

Nursing Action	Rationale
PREPARATORY PHASE	
1. Explain the procedure and give reassurance by skilled and empathic attention to the patient's needs. Instruct the patient to breathe quietly and to remain still.	1. Inform the patient that the procedure will cause coughing and that there will be an unpleasant sensation of a foreign body in the lower airway.
2. Administer supplemental oxygen, as directed, during the procedure if the patient's arterial oxygen tension is below normal while the patient is breathing room air.	2. This prevents worsening of hypoxemia.
3. Extend the patient's neck and place a pillow under shoulders.	3. This is the optimum position for cricothyroid puncture.
PERFORMANCE PHASE	
The cricothyroid membrane is identified by palpation.	
1. The skin over the cricothyroid area is cleansed, and the area is infiltrated with local anesthetic.	1. The cricothyroid membrane is less vascular and offers more safety in preventing posterior wall puncture than other areas.
2. A No. 14, 16, or 18 gauge needle is inserted through the cricothyroid membrane into the trachea, and a polyethylene catheter is threaded through the needle into the lower trachea. Caution the patient against swallowing or talking while the needle is introduced through the cricothyroid membrane.	
3. The needle is withdrawn, leaving the catheter in place.	3. The catheter's passage usually stimulates vigorous coughing.

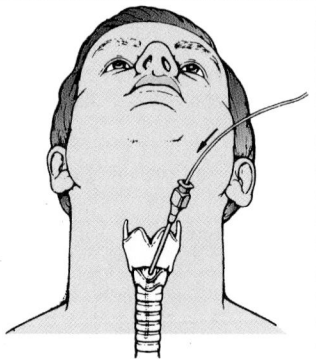

Transtracheal aspiration. After the catheter is positioned into the trachea, the needle is withdrawn, leaving the catheter in place.

4. A syringe is attached to the catheter, and secretions may be aspirated back into the syringe as the patient coughs. Request the patient to turn head while coughing.	4. Sterile saline (2 to 5 mL) may be injected into catheter to induce coughing, if necessary.

PROCEDURE GUIDELINES 10-2 · CONTINUED

Nursing Action	Rationale
5. Air is removed from the syringe, and the syringe is capped or the sample is injected into an anaerobic transfer vial. The specimen is sent to the laboratory for immediate processing.	5. This ensures anaerobic conditions. Cytologic, myco-bacterial, and other studies are carried out.
6. The catheter is withdrawn, and pressure is applied over the puncture site.	6. Gentle firm pressure over the site for about 5 minutes helps prevent bleeding and reduces subcutaneous emphysema.

FOLLOW-UP PHASE

1. Instruct the patient to rest quietly for about an hour.	
2. Observe for the following complications; local bleeding, puncture of posterior tracheal wall, subcutaneous emphysema, vasovagal reactions, cardiac dysrhythmias.	2. Assess for hoarseness after the procedure; this may be from a submucosal tracheal hematoma, which can cause suffocation. Inform the patient that minor blood streaking of sputum almost always occurs after this procedure.

PROCEDURE GUIDELINES 10-3 · ASSISTING THE PATIENT UNDERGOING THORACENTESIS

EQUIPMENT

Thoracentesis tray (if available)
or
Syringes: 5-, 20-, 50-mL
Needles: No. 22, No. 26, No. 16 (7.5 cm long)
Three-way stopcock and tubing
Hemostat
Biopsy needle

Germicide solution
Local anesthetic (eg, lidocaine 1%)
Sterile gauze sponges (4 × 4 and 2 × 2)
Sterile towels and drape
Sterile specimen containers
Sterile gloves

PROCEDURE

Nursing Action	Rationale
PREPARATORY PHASE	
1. Ascertain in advance if chest x-ray and/or other tests have been prescribed and completed. These should be available at the bedside.	1. Localization of pleural fluid is accomplished by physical examination, chest roentgenogram, ultrasound localization, or fluoroscopic localization.

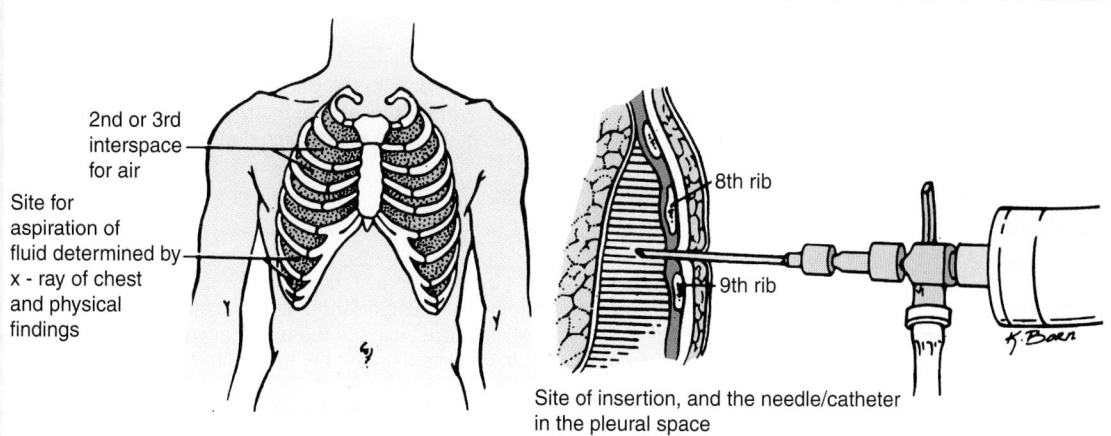

2nd or 3rd interspace for air

Site for aspiration of fluid determined by x-ray of chest and physical findings

8th rib

9th rib

Site of insertion, and the needle/catheter in the pleural space

Technique of thoracentesis.

continued

PROCEDURE GUIDELINES 10-3   ASSISTING THE PATIENT UNDERGOING THORACENTESIS
CONTINUED

Nursing Action	Rationale
2. See if consent form has been explained and signed.	
3. Determine if the patient is allergic to the local anesthetic agent to be used. Give sedation if prescribed.	

4. Inform the patient about the procedure and indicate how he or she can be helpful. Explain:
  a. The nature of the procedure.
  b. The importance of remaining immobile.
  c. Pressure sensations to be experienced.
  d. That no discomfort is anticipated after the procedure.
	4. An explanation helps orient the patient to the procedure, assists with coping, and provides an opportunity to ask questions and verbalize anxiety.

5. Assist patient to obtain comfortable position with adequate supports. If possible place upright (see accompanying figure) and help patient maintain position during procedure.	5. The upright position ensures that the diaphragm is most dependent and facilitates the removal of fluid that usually localizes at the base of the chest. A comfortable position helps the patient to relax.

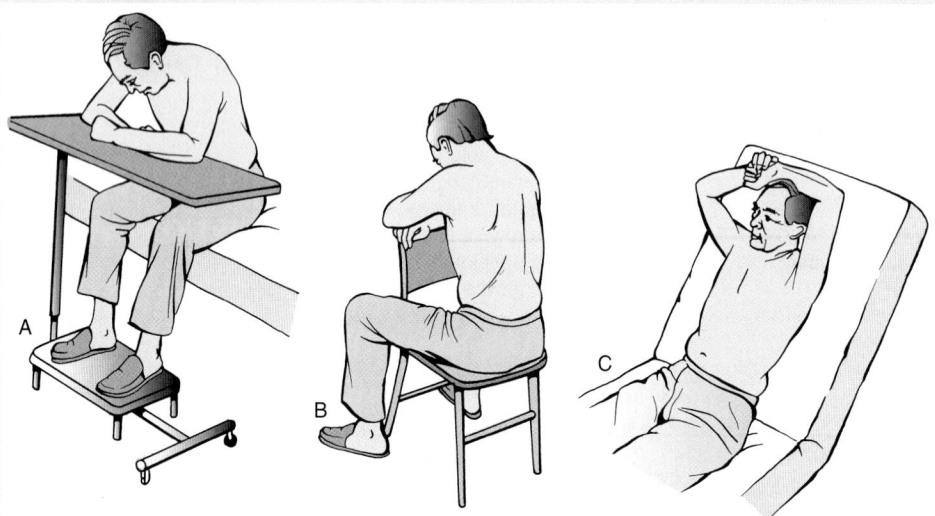

Positioning the patient for a thoracentesis. The nurse assists the patient to one of three positions, and offers comfort and support throughout the procedure. (A) Sitting on the edge of the bed with head and arms on and over the bed table. (B) Straddling a chair with arms and head resting on the back of the chair. (C) Lying on unaffected side with the bed elevated 30 to 45 degrees.

6. Support and reassure the patient during the procedure.
  a. Prepare the patient for sensations of cold from skin germicide and for pressure and sting from infiltration of local anesthetic agent.
  b. Encourage the patient to refrain from coughing.
  c. Be prepared to monitor patient's condition throughout the procedure.
	6. Sudden and unexpected movement by the patient can cause trauma to the visceral pleura with resultant trauma to the lung. A local anesthetic inhibits nerve conduction and is used to prevent pain during the procedure.

PERFORMANCE PHASE

1. The site for aspiration is determined from chest x-rays, by percussion, or by fluoroscopic or ultrasound localization. If fluid is in the pleural cavity, the thoracentesis site is determined by study of the chest x-ray and physical findings, with attention to the site of maximal dullness on percussion.	1. If air is in the pleural cavity, the thoracentesis site is usually in the 2nd or 3rd intercostal space in the midclavicular line. Air rises in the thorax because the density of air is much less than the density of liquid.
2. The procedure is done under aseptic conditions. After the skin is cleansed, the health care provider slowly injects a local anesthetic with a small-caliber needle into the intercostal space.	2. An intradermal wheal is raised slowly; rapid intradermal injection causes pain. The parietal pleura is very sensitive and should be well infiltrated with anesthetic before the thoracentesis needle is passed through it.

Nursing Action	Rationale
3. The thoracentesis needle is advanced with the syringe attached. When the pleural space is reached, suction may be applied with the syringe.	
a. A 20-mL or 50-mL syringe with a three-way adapter (stopcock) is attached to the needle. (One end of the adapter is attached to the needle and the other to the tubing leading to a receptacle that receives the fluid being aspirated.)	a. When a larger quantity of fluid is withdrawn, a three-way adapter serves to keep air from entering the pleural cavity. The amount of fluid removed depends on clinical status of the patient and absence of complications during the procedure.
b. If a considerable quantity of fluid is to be removed, the needle is held in place on the chest wall with a small hemostat.	b. The hemostat steadies the needle on the chest wall and prevents too deep a penetration of pleural space. Sudden pleuritic pain or shoulder pain may indicate that the visceral or diaphragmatic pleura are being irritated by the needle point.
c. A pleural biopsy may be performed.	
4. After the needle is withdrawn, pressure is applied over the puncture site and a small sterile dressing is fixed in place.	4. This is done to prevent air entry into pleural space.
FOLLOW-UP PHASE	
1. Place the patient on bed rest. A chest x-ray is usually obtained after thoracentesis.	1. Chest x-ray verifies that there is no pneumothorax.
2. Record vital signs every 15 minutes for 1 hour.	
3. Administer oxygen, as directed, if patient has cardio-respiratory disease.	3. Pulmonary gas exchange may worsen after thoracentesis in patients with cardiorespiratory disease.
4. Record the total amount of fluid withdrawn and the nature of the fluid, its color and viscosity. If prescribed, prepare samples of fluid for laboratory evaluation (usually bacteriology, cell count and differential, determinations of protein, glucose, LDH, specific gravity). A small amount of heparin may be needed for several of the specimen containers to prevent coagulation. A specimen container with preservative may be needed if a pleural biopsy is obtained.	4. The fluid may be clear, serous, bloody, or purulent.
5. Evaluate the patient at intervals for increasing respirations, faintness, vertigo, tightness in the chest, uncontrollable cough, blood-tinged mucus, and rapid pulse and signs of hypoxemia.	5. Pneumothorax, tension pneumothorax, hemothorax, subcutaneous emphysema, or pyogenic infection may result from a thoracentesis.

◾ Radiology and Imaging

Chest X-Ray (Roentgenogram)
Description
1. Normal pulmonary tissue is radiolucent and appears black on film. Thus, densities produced by tumors, foreign bodies, infiltrates, and so forth can be detected as lighter or white images.
2. This test shows the position of normal structures, displacement, and presence of abnormal shadows. It may reveal pathology in the lungs in the absence of symptoms.

Nursing and Patient Care Considerations
1. Should be taken upright if patient's condition permits. Assist technician at bedside in preparing patient for portable chest x-ray.
2. Encourage patient to take deep breath, hold breath, and remain still as x-ray is taken.
3. Ensure that all jewelry or metal objects in x-ray field are removed so as not to interfere with film.
4. Consider the contraindication of x-rays for pregnant patients.

Computerized Axial Tomography (CAT, CT)
Description
1. An imaging method in which the lungs are scanned in successive layers by a narrow x-ray beam. A computer printout is obtained of the absorption values of the tissues in the plane that is being scanned.
2. It may be used to define pulmonary nodules, pulmonary abnormalities, or to demonstrate mediastinal abnormalities and hilar adenopathy.

Nursing and Patient Care Considerations

1. Describe test to patient/family and ensure consent is obtained (if required by your institution). Test takes about 30 minutes.
2. Be alert to any allergies to iodine or other radiographic contrast media that might be used during testing.
3. Consider the contraindication of x-rays for the pregnant patient, especially for CT scans with contrast media.

Magnetic Resonance Imaging (MRI)
Description

1. A type of emission tomography based on magnetizing patient tissue, generating a weak electromagnetic signal, and mapping that signal for visualization.
2. Provides contrast between various soft tissues.
3. Traditional radiographic contrast media are not used but gadolinium injection may be necessary, depending on the patient's medical history.
4. It is helpful to synchronize the MRI image to the electrocardiogram in thoracic studies.
5. Consider the contraindication of x-rays for the pregnant patient.

Nursing and Patient Care Considerations

1. Explain procedure to patient and assess ability to remain still in a closed space; sedation may be necessary if the patient is claustrophobic.
2. Evaluate patient for magnetic implants such as pacemakers, prosthetic valves or joints, or metallic surgical clips, which preclude the use of MRI.
3. Check with MRI technician about the use of equipment such as ventilator or mechanical intravenous (IV) pump in MRI room.
4. Evaluate the patient for claustrophobia, and teach relaxation techniques to use during test. Sedation may be necessary.

Pulmonary Angiography
Description

1. An imaging method used to study the pulmonary vessels and the pulmonary circulation.
2. For visualization, radiopaque medium is injected by way of a catheter in the main pulmonary artery rapidly into the vasculature of the lungs. Films are then taken in rapid succession after injection.
3. It is considered the "gold standard" for diagnosis of pulmonary embolus, but spiral CT can also be effectively used.

Nursing and Patient Care Considerations

1. Determine whether the patient is allergic to radiographic contrast media (Standards of Care Guidelines).
2. Instruct patient that injection of dye may cause flushing, cough, and a warm sensation.
3. After the procedure, make sure pressure is maintained over access site and monitor pulse rate, blood pressure, and circulation distal to the injection site.

Ventilation–Perfusion (V/Q) Scan
Description

1. Radioisotope imaging of ventilation and blood flow to the lungs. The scintillation camera may be interfaced to a computer to record, collate, and refine data.
2. Perfusion scan is done after injection of a radioactive isotope.
   a. Measures blood perfusion through the lungs; evaluates lung function on a regional basis.
   b. Useful in perfusion (vascular) abnormalities such as pulmonary embolism.
3. Ventilation scan is done after inhalation of radioactive gas (xenon, krypton), which diffuses throughout the lungs.
   a. Useful in detecting ventilation abnormalities such as emphysema.

Nursing and Patient Care Considerations

Explain the procedure to the patient and encourage cooperation with inhalation and brief episodes of breath holding.

◼ Other Diagnostic Tests
Bronchoscopy
Description

1. The direct inspection and observation of the larynx, trachea, and bronchi through flexible or rigid bronchoscope.
   a. Flexible fiberoptic bronchoscope allows for more patient comfort and better visualization of smaller airways.
   b. Rigid bronchoscopy is preferred for small children and endobronchial tumor resection.
2. Has both diagnostic and therapeutic uses in pulmonary conditions. Diagnostic uses include:
   a. Collecting secretions for cytologic/bacteriologic studies.
   b. Determining location and extent of pathologic process and obtaining tissue or brush biopsy for cytologic examination or culture.
   c. Determining whether a tumor can be resected surgically.
   d. Diagnosing bleeding sites (source of hemoptysis).
3. Therapeutic uses include removal of foreign bodies or thickened secretions from tracheobronchial tree and the excision of lesions.

Nursing and Patient Care Considerations

1. See that an informed consent form has been signed and that risks and benefits have been explained to the patient. Review health care setting's policy and procedure for conscious sedation.

NURSING ALERT

 Determine if patient is allergic to radiographic dye before V/Q scan.

2. Administer prescribed medication to reduce secretions, block the vasovagal reflex, gag reflex, and relieve anxiety. Give encouragement and nursing support.
3. Restrict fluid and food for 6 to 12 hours before procedure (to reduce risk of aspiration when reflexes are blocked).
4. Remove dentures, contact lenses, and other prostheses.
5. After the procedure:
   a. Monitor cardiac rhythm and rate, blood pressure, and level of consciousness.
   b. Withhold cracked ice/fluids until patient demonstrates gag reflex.
   c. Monitor respiratory effort and rate.
   d. Monitor oximetry.
6. Promptly report cyanosis, hypoventilation, hypotension, tachycardia or dysrhythmia, hemoptysis, dyspnea, decreased breath sounds.

NURSING ALERT

 After bronchoscopy, be alert for complications: pneumothorax, dysrhythmias, and bronchospasm.

Lung Biopsy
Description
1. Procedures used for obtaining histologic material from the lung to aid in diagnosis. These include:
   a. *Transbronchoscopic biopsy*—biopsy forceps inserted through bronchoscope and specimen of lung tissue obtained.
   b. *Transthoracic needle aspiration biopsy*—specimen obtained through needle aspiration under fluoroscopic guidance.
   c. *Open lung biopsy*—specimen obtained through small anterior thoracotomy; used in making a diagnosis when other biopsy methods have not been effective or are not possible.

Nursing and Patient Care Considerations
1. Obtain permit for consent, if required.
2. Observe for possible complications including pneumothorax, hemorrhage (hemoptysis), and bacterial contamination of pleural space.
3. See bronchoscopy (above) or thoracic surgery (p. 259) for postprocedure care.

Pulmonary Function Tests (PFTs)
Description
1. Used to detect and measure abnormalities in respiratory function, and quantify severity of various lung diseases. Such tests include measurements of lung volumes, ventilatory function, diffusing capacity, gas exchange, lung compliance, airway resistance, and distribution of gases in the lung.
2. Ventilatory studies (spirometry) are the most common group of tests.
   a. Requires water spirometer, electronic spirometer, or wedge spirometer that plots volume against time (timed vital capacity).
   b. Patient is asked to take as deep a breath as possible and then to exhale into spirometer as completely and as forcefully as possible.
   c. Results are compared with normals for patient's age, height, and sex (Table 10-1).
   d. A reduction in the vital capacity, inspiratory capacity, and total lung capacity may indicate a restric-

TABLE 10-1 Pulmonary Function Tests

Term	Symbol	Description	Remarks
Vital capacity	VC	Maximum volume of air exhaled after a maximum inspiration	VC < 10–15 mL/kg suggests need for mechanical ventilation VC > 10–15 mL/kg suggests ability to wean
Forced vital capacity	FVC	Vital capacity performed with a maximally forced expiratory effort	Reduced in obstructive disease (COPD) due to air trapping Reflects airflow in large airways
Forced expiratory volume in 1 second	FEV_1	Volume of air exhaled in the first second of the performance of the FVC	Reduced in obstructive disease (COPD) due to air trapping Reflects airflow in larger airways
Ratio of FEV_1/FVC	FEV_1/FVC	FEV_1 expressed as a percentage of the FVC	Decreased in obstructive disease Normal in restrictive disease
Forced midexpiratory flow	$FEF_{25\%-75\%}$	Average flow during the middle half of the FVC	Reflects airflow in small airways Smokers may have change in this test before other symptoms develop
Peak expiratory flow rate	PEFR	Most rapid flow during a forced expiration after a maximum inspiration	Used to measure response to bronchodilators, airflow obstruction in patients with asthma
Maximal voluntary ventilation	MVV	Volume of air expired in a specified period (12 seconds) during repetitive maximal effort	An important factor in exercise tolerance

tive form of lung disease (disease due to increased lung stiffness).

e. An increase in functional reserve capacity, total lung capacity, and reduction in flow rates usually indicate an obstructive flow due to bronchial obstruction or loss of lung elastic recoil.

3. Lung volumes are determined by asking the patient to inhale a known concentration of inert gas such as helium or 100% oxygen and measuring concentration of inert gas or nitrogen in exhaled air (dilution method) or by plethysmography.

a. Yields thoracic volume (total lung capacity, plus any unventilated blebs or bullae).

b. An increased residual volume is found in air-trapping due to obstructive lung disease.

c. A reduction in several parameters usually indicates a restrictive form of lung disease or chest wall abnormality.

4. Diffusing capacity measures lung surface effective for the transfer of gas in the lung by having patient inhale gas containing known low concentration of carbon monoxide and measuring carbon monoxide concentration in exhaled air. Difference between inhaled and exhaled concentrations is related directly to uptake of carbon monoxide across alveolar-capillary membrane.

a. Is reduced in parenchymal lung disease, possibly in severe anemia, and in some forms of heart disease.

Nursing and Patient Care Considerations

1. Instruct patient in correct technique for completing PFTs; coach patient through test, if needed.

2. Instruct patient not to use oral or inhaled bronchodilator (such as albuterol), caffeine, or tobacco 4 hours before test.

Pulse Oximetry
Description

1. Provides an estimate of arterial oxyhemoglobin saturation by using selected wavelengths of light to noninvasively determine the saturation of oxyhemoglobin. Oximeters function by passing a light beam through a vascular bed, such as the finger or earlobe, to determine the amount of light absorbed by oxygenated (red) and deoxygenated (blue) blood.

2. Calculates the amount of arterial blood that is saturated with oxygen (SaO_2) and displays this as a digital value.

3. Indications include:

a. Monitor adequacy of oxygen saturation; quantify response to therapy.

b. Monitor unstable patient who may experience sudden changes in blood oxygen level.

c. Evaluation of need for home oxygen therapy.

d. Determine supplemental oxygen needs at rest and with exercise.

e. Need to follow the trend and need to decrease number of ABGs drawn.

4. The oxyhemoglobin dissociation curve allows for correlation between SaO_2 and PaO_2 (Figure 10-1).

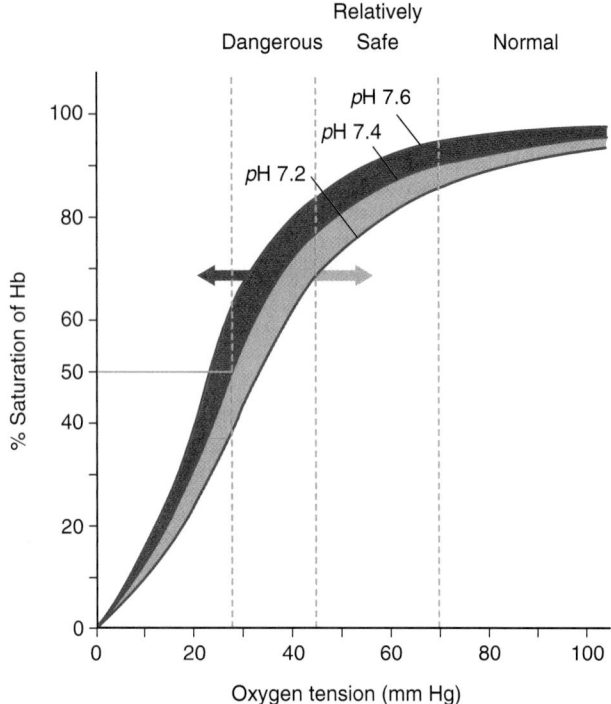

FIGURE 10-1   Oxygen-hemoglobin dissociation curve. The oxygen can attach to the hemoglobin more easily (higher SaO_2 per PO_2) but has more trouble coming off the hemoglobin at the tissues (less tissue oxygenation). Decreased oxygen affinity (shift to the right) means that it is more difficult for the oxygen to attach to the hemoglobin (lower SaO_2 per PO_2), but it can come off at the tissues more easily. P_{50} is normally 27 mmHg. A shift to the right gives a higher P_{50}, and a shift to the left gives a lower P_{50}.

a. Increased body temperature, acidosis, and increased 2,3 DPG cause a shift in the curve to the right, thus increasing the ability of hemoglobin to release oxygen to the tissues.

b. Decreased temperature, decreased 2,3 DPG, and alkalosis cause a shift to the left, causing hemoglobin to hold on to the oxygen, reducing the amount of oxygen being released to the tissues.

5. Increased bilirubin, increased carboxyhemoglobin, low perfusion or SaO_2 <80% may alter light absorption and interfere with results.

NURSING ALERT

If the SaO_2 drops below 80%, the reading displayed by the oximeter may vary by ±2% from the actual SaO_2. Oximeters rely on differences in light absorption to determine SaO_2. At lower saturations, oxygenated hemoglobin appears more blue in color and is less easily distinguished from deoxygenated hemoglobin. ABG should be used in this situation.

Nursing and Patient Care Considerations

1. Assess patient's hemoglobin. SaO_2 may not correlate well with PaO_2 if hemoglobin is not within normal limits.
2. Remove patient's nail polish because it can affect the ability of the sensor to correctly determine oxygen saturation.
3. Correlate oximetry with ABG and then use for single reading or trending of oxygenation (does not monitor $PaCO_2$).
4. Display heart rate should correlate with patient's heart rate.
5. To improve quality of signal, hold finger dependent and motionless (motion may alter results) and cover finger sensor to occlude ambient light.
6. Assess site of oximetry monitoring for perfusion on a regular basis, because pressure ulcer may occur from prolonged application of probe.
7. Device limitations: motion artifact, abnormal hemoglobins (carboxyhemoglobin and methemoglobin), IV dye, exposure of probe to ambient light, low perfusion states, skin pigmentation, nail polish or nail coverings, and nail deformities such as severe clubbing.
8. Document inspired oxygen or supplemental oxygen, type of oxygen delivery device.

Capnography

Description

1. Used to determine and monitor end-tidal CO_2 ($EtCO_2$)—the amount of carbon dioxide that is expired with each breath.
2. The $EtCO_2$ is displayed as a capnogram (a waveform and numeric reading).
3. Normally 3 to 8 torr less than $PaCO_2$, with the difference being greater in the presence of lung disease, or any increase in dead space.
4. Being increasingly used in the critical care setting, and as a pocket-sized model in the emergency department.

Nursing and Patient Care Considerations

1. Draw ABGs initially to correlate $EtCO_2$ with $PaCO_2$ and to establish the gradient between $PaCO_2$ and $EtCO_2$.
2. Does not evaluate pH or oxygenation.
3. Effective for confirming endotracheal tube placement and for monitoring CO_2 in patients who tend to retain CO_2 (COPD).

GENERAL PROCEDURES AND TREATMENT MODALITIES

Artificial Airway Management

Airway management may be indicated in patients with loss of consciousness, facial or oral trauma, copious respiratory secretions, respiratory distress, and the need for mechanical ventilation.

Types of Airways

1. Oropharyngeal airway—curved plastic device inserted through the mouth and positioned in the posterior pharynx to move tongue away from palate and open the airway
   a. Usually for short-term use in the unconscious patient, or may be used along with an oral endotracheal tube.
   b. Not used if recent oral trauma, surgery, or loose teeth are present.
   c. Does not protect against aspiration.

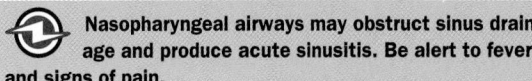

> **NURSING ALERT**
>
> Position patient on side and suction oral cavity frequently to prevent aspiration of oral secretions or vomitus when an oral airway is in place.

2. Nasopharyngeal airway (nasal trumpet)—soft rubber or plastic tube inserted through nose into posterior pharynx
   a. Facilitates frequent nasopharyngeal suctioning.
   b. Use extreme caution with patients on anticoagulants or bleeding disorders.
   c. Select size that is slightly smaller than diameter of nostril and slightly longer than distance from tip of nose to earlobe.
   d. Check nasal mucosa for irritation or ulceration, and clean airway with hydrogen peroxide and water.

> **NURSING ALERT**
>
> Nasopharyngeal airways may obstruct sinus drainage and produce acute sinusitis. Be alert to fever and signs of pain.

3. Endotracheal tube—flexible tube inserted through the mouth or nose and into the trachea beyond the vocal cords that acts as an artificial airway
   a. Allows for deep tracheal suction and removal of secretions.
   b. Permits mechanical ventilation.
   c. Inflated balloon seals off trachea so aspiration from the gastrointestinal (GI) tract cannot occur.
   d. Generally easy to insert in an emergency, but maintaining placement is more difficult so this is not for long-term use.
4. Tracheostomy tube—firm, curved artificial airway inserted directly into the trachea at the level of the second or third tracheal ring through a surgically made incision.
   a. Permits mechanical ventilation and facilitates secretion removal.
   b. Can be for long-term use.
   c. Bypasses upper airway defenses, increasing susceptibility to infection.

Endotracheal Tube Insertion

1. Orotracheal insertion is technically easier, because it is done under direct visualization (Procedure Guidelines 10-4). Disadvantages are increased oral secretions, de-

creased patient comfort, difficulty with tube stabilization, and inability of patient to use lip movement as a communication means.
2. Nasotracheal insertion may be more comfortable to the patient and is easier to stabilize.
   a. Disadvantages are that blind insertion is required; possible development of pressure necrosis of the nasal airway, sinusitis, and otitis media.
3. Tube types vary according to length and inner diameter, type of cuff, and number of lumens.
   a. Usual sizes for adults are 6.0, 7.0, 8.0, and 9.0 mm.
   b. Most cuffs are high volume, low pressure, with self-sealing inflation valves, or the cuff may be of foam rubber (Fome-Cuff).
   c. Most tubes have a single lumen; however, dual-lumen tubes may be used to ventilate each lung independently (Figure 10-2).
4. May be contraindicated when glottis is obscured by vomitus, bleeding, foreign body, or trauma, or cervical spine injury or deformity.

Tracheostomy Tube Insertion

1. Tube types vary according to presence of inner cannula and presence and type of cuff (Figure 10-3).
   a. Tubes with high-volume, low-pressure cuffs with self-sealing inflation valves; with or without inner cannula
   b. Fenestrated tube
   c. Foam-filled cuffs (Fome-Cuff)
   d. Speaking tracheostomy tube
   e. Tracheal button or Passy-Muir valve
   f. Silver tube (rarely used)

2. Vary according to length and inner diameter in millimeters. Usual sizes for an adult are 6.0, 7.0, 8.0, and 9.0 mm.
3. Tracheostomy is usually planned, either as an adjunct to therapy for respiratory dysfunction or for longer-term airway management when endotracheal intubation has been used for more than 14 days.
4. May be done at the bedside in an emergency when other means of creating an airway have failed (Procedure Guidelines 10-5).

Indications for Endotracheal Intubation or Tracheostomy

1. Acute respiratory failure, CNS depression, neuromuscular disease, pulmonary disease, chest wall injury
2. Upper airway obstruction (tumor, inflammation, foreign body, laryngeal spasm)
3. Anticipated upper airway obstruction from edema or soft tissue swelling due to head and neck trauma, some postoperative head and neck procedures involving the airway, facial or airway burns, decreased level of consciousness
4. Aspiration prophylaxis
5. Fracture of cervical vertebrae with spinal cord injury; requiring ventilatory assistance

Complications of Endotracheal or Tracheostomy Tubes

1. Laryngeal or tracheal injury
   a. Sore throat, hoarse voice
   b. Glottic edema
   c. Ulceration or necrosis of tracheal mucosa
   d. Vocal cord ulceration, granuloma, or polyps

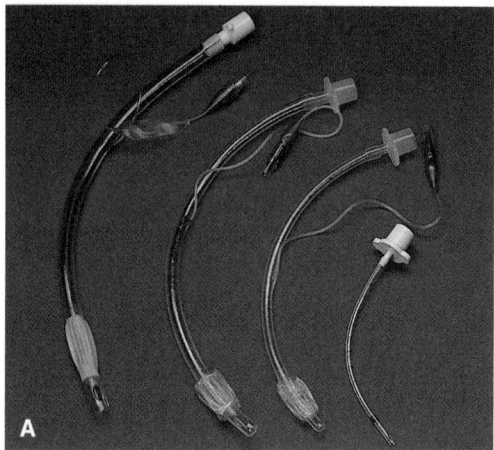
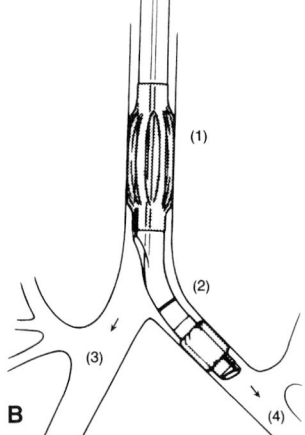

FIGURE 10-2 (**A**) Endotrachial tubes: single lumen and double lumen endotracheal tube. When the double lumen tube is used (**B**), two cuffs are inflated. One cuff (1) is positioned in the trachea and the second cuff (2) in the left mainstem bronchus. After inflation, air flows through an opening below the tracheal cuff (3) to the right lung and through an opening below the bronchial cuff (4) to the left lung. This permits differential ventilation of both lungs, lavage of one lung, or selective inflation of either lung during thoracic surgery. (Marshall, B. E., Longnecker, D. E., & Fairley, H. B. [Eds.]. [1988]. *Anesthesia for thoracic procedures* [p. 381]. Boston: Blackwell Scientific Publications. Used with permission.)

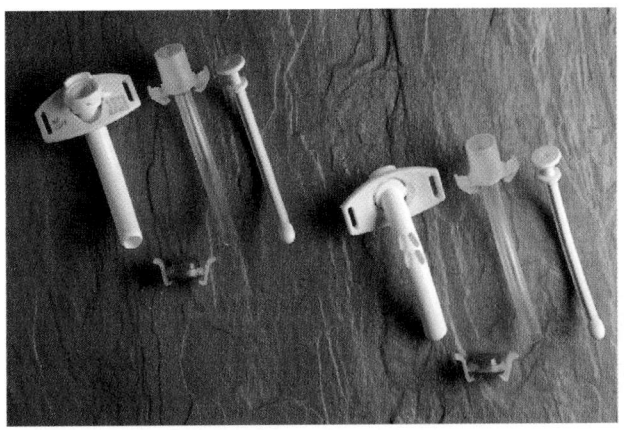

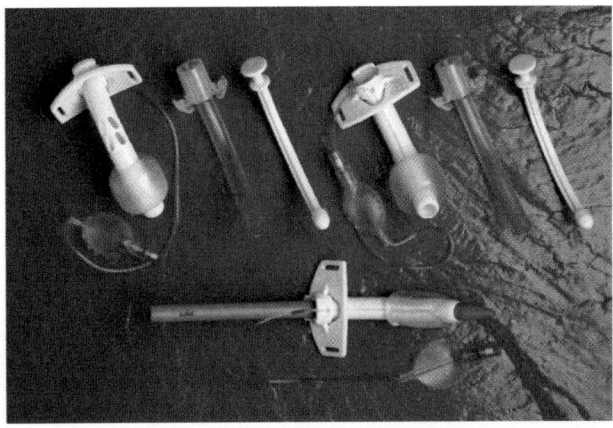

Cuffless: nonfenestrated (left) and fenestrated (right). Tracheostomy plug to allow breathing through upper airway also is shown.

Cuffed: fenestrated (left) and nonfenestrated (right) with inner cannula and obturator for insertion. Percutaneous tracheostomy inducer (bottom).

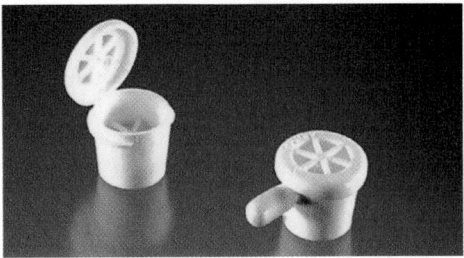

Speaking valve.

FIGURE 10-3 Types of tracheostomy tubes. (Courtesy of Mallinckrodt Medical, St. Louis, MO.)

e. Vocal cord paralysis
f. Postextubation tracheal stenosis
g. Tracheal dilation
h. Formation of tracheal-esophageal fistula
i. Formation of tracheal-arterial fistula
j. Innominate artery erosion
2. Pulmonary infection and sepsis
3. Dependence on artificial airway

Nursing Care for Patients With Artificial Airways
General Care Measures

1. Ensure adequate ventilation and oxygenation through the use of supplemental oxygen or mechanical ventilation as indicated.
2. Assess breath sounds every 2 hours. Note evidence of ineffective secretion clearance (rhonchi, crackles), which suggests need for suctioning.
3. Provide adequate humidity when the natural humidifying pathway of the oropharynx is bypassed.
4. Provide adequate suctioning of oral secretions to prevent aspiration and decrease oral microbial colonization.
5. Use clean technique when inserting an oral or nasopharyngeal airway, and take it out and clean it with hydrogen peroxide at least every 8 hours.
6. Perform frequent oral care with soft toothbrush or swabs and antiseptic mouthwash or hydrogen peroxide diluted with water.

7. Ensure that aseptic technique is maintained when inserting an endotracheal or tracheostomy tube. The artificial airway bypasses the upper airway, and the lower airways are sterile below the level of the vocal cords.
8. Elevate the patient to a semi-Fowler's or sitting position, when possible; these positions result in improved lung compliance. The patient's position, however, should be changed at least every 2 hours to ensure ventilation of all lung segments and prevent secretion stagnation and atelectasis. Position changes are also necessary to avoid skin breakdown.
9. If an oral or nasopharyngeal airway is used, turn the patient's head to the side to reduce the risk of aspiration (because there is no cuff to seal off the lower airway).

Nutritional Considerations

1. Consciousness is usually impaired in the patient with an oropharyngeal airway, so oral feeding is contraindicated.
2. To enhance comfort, remove a nasopharyngeal airway in the conscious patient during mealtime.
3. Recognize that an endotracheal tube holds the epiglottis open. Therefore, only the inflated cuff prevents the aspiration of oropharyngeal contents into the lungs. The patient must not receive oral feeding. Administer enteral tube feedings or parenteral feedings as ordered.
4. Administer oral feedings to a conscious patient with a tracheostomy, usually with the cuff inflated. The inflated

cuff prevents aspiration of food contents into the lungs, but causes the tracheal wall to bulge into the esophageal lumen, and may make swallowing more difficult. Patients who are not on mechanical ventilation and are awake, alert, and able to protect the airway are candidates for eating with the cuff deflated.

5. To assess ability to protect the airway, sit the patient upright and feed the patient colored gelatin or juice. If color from gelatin can be suctioned from the tracheostomy tube, aspiration is occurring, and the cuff must be inflated during feeding and for 1 hour afterward with head of bed elevated.

6. Patients should receive thickened rather than regular liquids; this will assist in effective swallowing.

> **NURSING ALERT**
>
> Consider the patient's nutritional needs early in process of intubation so nutritional status does not decline further. It is difficult to wean patients who have compromised nutritional status.

Cuff Maintenance

1. Endotracheal tube cuffs should be inflated continuously and deflated only during intubation, extubation, and tube repositioning.

2. Tracheostomy tube cuffs also should be inflated continuously in patients on mechanical ventilation or CPAP.

3. Tracheostomized patients who are breathing spontaneously may have the cuff inflated continuously (in the patient with decreased level of consciousness without ability to fully protect airway), deflated continuously, or inflated only for feeding if the patient is at risk of aspiration.

4. Monitor cuff pressure every 4 hours (Procedure Guidelines 10-6).

External Tube Site Care

1. Secure an endotracheal tube so it cannot be disrupted by the weight of ventilator or oxygen tubing or by patient movement.
   a. Use strips of adhesive tape or Velcro straps wrapped around the tube and secured to tape on the patient's cheeks or around the back of patient's head.
   b. Replace when soiled or insecure or when repositioning of tube is necessary.
   c. Position tubing so traction is not applied to endotracheal tube.

2. Perform tracheostomy site care at least every 8 hours using hydrogen peroxide and water, and change tracheostomy ties at least once a day (Procedure Guidelines 10-7).
   a. Make sure ventilator or oxygen tubing is supported so traction is not applied to the tracheostomy tube.

3. Have available at all times at the patient's bedside a resuscitation bag, oxygen source, and mask to ventilate the patient in the event of accidental tube removal. Anticipate your course of action in such an event.
   a. Endotracheal tube—know location and assembly of reintubation equipment including replacement endotracheal tube. Know how to contact someone immediately for reintubation.
   b. Tracheostomy—have extra tracheostomy tube, obturator, and hemostats at bedside. Be aware of reinsertion technique, if policy permits, or know how to contact someone immediately for reinserting the tube.

> **NURSING ALERT**
>
> In the event of accidental endotracheal or tracheostomy tube removal, use a bag/mask resuscitation device to ventilate the patient by mouth, while covering tracheostomy stoma. However, if the patient has complete upper airway obstruction, a gaping stoma, or a laryngectomy, mouth-to-stoma ventilation must be performed.

Psychological Considerations

1. Assist patient to deal with psychological aspects related to artificial airway.

2. Recognize that the patient is usually apprehensive, particularly about choking, inability to communicate verbally, inability to remove secretions, uncomfortable suctioning, difficulty in breathing, or mechanical failure.

3. Explain the function of the equipment carefully.

4. Inform the patient and family that speaking will not be possible while the tube is in place, unless using a tracheostomy tube with a deflated cuff, a fenestrated tube, a Passy-Muir speaking valve, or a speaking tracheostomy tube.

5. Develop with the patient the best method of communication (eg, sign language, lip movement, letter boards, paper and pencil, magic slate, or coded messages).
   a. Patients with tracheostomy tubes or nasal endotracheal tubes may effectively use orally operated electrolarynx devices.
   b. Devise a means for the patient to get the nurse's attention when someone is not immediately available at the bedside, such as call bell, hand-operated bell, rattle, and so forth.

6. Anticipate some of the patient's questions by discussing "Is it permanent?" "Will it hurt to breathe?" "Will someone be with me?"

7. Advise the patient that as condition improves a tracheostomy button may be used to plug the tracheostomy site. A tracheostomy button is a rigid, closed cannula that is placed into the tracheostomy stoma after removal of a cuffed or uncuffed tracheostomy tube. When in proper position, the button does not extend into the tracheal lumen. The outer edge of the button is at the skin surface and the inner edge is at the anterior tracheal wall (Procedure Guidelines 10-8).

> **NURSING ALERT**
>
> With the use of artificial airways, remember that although the patient may use a call bell, he or she will not be able to communicate verbally (unless device is used to allow speech).

Community and Home Care Considerations

1. Teach patient and/or caregiver procedure. Patient will need to use stationary mirror to visualize tracheostomy and perform procedure.
2. Suctioning patient in the home: whenever possible, patient and/or caregiver should be taught to perform procedure. Patient should use controlled cough and other secretion clearance techniques.
3. Preoxygenation and hyperinflation before suctioning may not be routinely indicated for all patients cared for in the home. Preoxygenation and hyperinflation are based on patient need and clinical status.
4. Normal saline should not be instilled unless clinically indicated (eg, to stimulate cough).

5. Clean technique and clean examination gloves are used. At the end of suctioning, the catheter or tonsil tip should be flushed by suctioning recently boiled or distilled water to rinse away mucus, followed by suctioning air through the apparatus. The outer surface may be wiped with alcohol or hydrogen peroxide. The catheter and tonsil tip should be air dried and stored in a clean, dry place. Generally, suction catheters should be discarded after 24 hours. Tonsil tips may be boiled and reused.
6. Care of tracheostomy stoma: clean with half-strength hydrogen peroxide (diluted with sterile water), and wipe with sterile water or sterile saline.

(*text continues on page 221*)

PROCEDURE GUIDELINES 10-4 ENDOTRACHEAL INTUBATION

EQUIPMENT

Laryngoscope with curved or straight blade and working light source (check batteries and bulb regularly)
Endotracheal tube with low-pressure cuff and adapter to connect tube to ventilator or resuscitation bag
Stylet to guide the endotracheal tube
Oral airway (assorted sizes) or bite block to keep patient from biting into and occluding the endotracheal tube
Adhesive tape or tube fixation system
Sterile anesthetic lubricant jelly (water-soluble)

10-mL syringe
Suction source
Suction catheter and tonsil suction
Resuscitation bag and mask connected to oxygen source
Sterile towel
Gloves
Face shield
End tidal CO_2 detector

PROCEDURE

Nursing Action	Rationale
PREPARATORY PHASE	
1. Assess the patient's heart rate, level of consciousness, and respiratory status.	1. Provides a baseline to estimate patient's tolerance of procedure.
PERFORMANCE PHASE	
1. Remove the patient's dental bridgework and plates.	1. May interfere with insertion. Will not be able to remove easily from patient once intubated.
2. Remove headboard of bed (optional).	
3. Prepare equipment.	3.
a. Ensure function of resuscitation bag with mask and suction.	a. Patient may require ventilatory assistance during procedure. Suction should be functional, because gagging and emesis may occur during procedure.
b. Assemble the laryngoscope. Make sure the light bulb is tightly attached and functional.	
c. Select an endotracheal tube of the appropriate size (6.0 to 9.0 mm for average adult).	
d. Place the endotracheal tube on a sterile towel.	d. Although the tube will pass through the contaminated mouth or nose, the airway below the vocal cords is sterile, and efforts must be made to prevent iatrogenic contamination of the distal end of the tube and cuff. The proximal end of the tube may be handled, because it will reside in the upper airway.
e. Inflate the cuff to make sure it assumes a symmetric shape and holds volume without leakage. Then deflate maximally.	e. Malfunction of the cuff must be ascertained before tube placement occurs.
f. Lubricate the distal end of the tube liberally with the sterile anesthetic water-soluble jelly.	f. Aids in insertion.
g. Insert the stylet into the tube (if oral intubation is planned). Nasal intubation does not employ use of the stylet.	g. Stiffens the soft tube, allowing it to be more easily directed into the trachea.

continued

PROCEDURE GUIDELINES 10-4   **ENDOTRACHEAL INTUBATION** *CONTINUED*

Nursing Action | **Rationale**

4. Aspirate stomach contents if nasogastric tube is in place.
5. If time allows, inform the patient of impending inability to talk and discuss alternative means of communication.
6. If the patient is confused, it may be necessary to apply soft wrist restraints.
7. Put on gloves and face shield.
8. During oral intubation if cervical spine is not injured, place patient's head in a "sniffing" position (ie, extended at the junction of the neck and thorax and flexed at the junction of the spine and skull).
9. Spray the back of the patient's throat with anesthetic spray if time is available.
10. Ventilate and oxygenate the patient with the resuscitation bag and mask before intubation.
11. Hold the handle of the laryngoscope in the left hand and hold the patient's mouth open with the right hand by placing crossed fingers on the teeth.
12. Insert the curved blade of the laryngoscope along the right side of the tongue, push the tongue to the left, and use right thumb and index finger to pull patient's lower lip away from lower teeth.
13. Lift laryngoscope forward (toward ceiling) to expose the epiglottis.
14. Lift laryngoscope upward and forward at a 45-degree angle to expose glottis and visualize vocal cords.
15. As the epiglottis is lifted forward (toward ceiling), the vertical opening of the larynx between the vocal cords will come into view (see accompanying figure).

6. Restraint of the confused patient may be necessary to promote patient safety and maintain sterile technique.
7. Prevents contact with patient's oral secretions.
8. Upper airway is open maximally in this position.

9. Will decrease gagging.

10. Preoxygenation decreases the likelihood of cardiac dysrhythmias or respiratory distress secondary to hypoxemia.
11. Leverage is improved by crossing the thumb and index fingers when opening the patient's mouth (scissor-twist technique).
12. Rolling the lip away from teeth prevents injury by being caught between teeth and blade.

13. Do not use teeth as a fulcrum; this could lead to dental damage.
14. This stretches the hypoepiglottis ligament, folding the epiglottis upward and exposing the glottis.
15. Do not use wrist. Use shoulder and arm to lift the epiglottis.

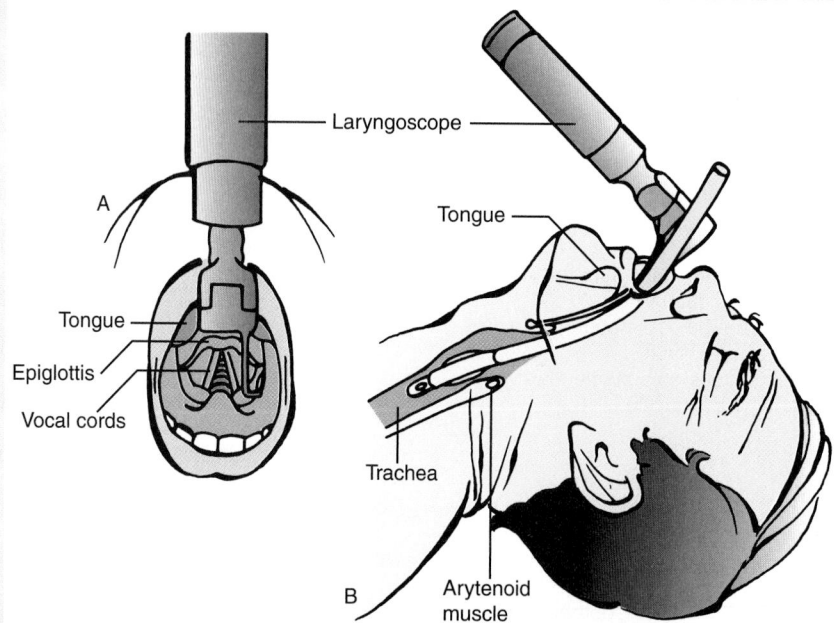

Endotracheal intubation. (A) *The primary glottic landmarks for tracheal intubation as visualized with proper placement of the laryngoscope.* (B) *Positioning the endotracheal tube.*

PROCEDURE GUIDELINES 10-4   *CONTINUED*

Nursing Action	Rationale
16. Once vocal cords are visualized, insert tube into the right corner of the mouth and pass the tube while keeping vocal cords in constant view.	16. Make sure you do not insert tube into esophagus; the esophageal mucosa is pink and the opening is horizontal rather than vertical.
17. Gently push the tube through the triangular space formed by the vocal cords and back wall of trachea.	17. If the vocal cords are in spasm (closed), wait a few seconds before passing tube.
18. Stop insertion just after the tube cuff has disappeared from view beyond the cords.	18. Advancing tube further may lead to its entry into a mainstem bronchus (usually the right bronchus) causing collapse of the unventilated lung.
19. Withdraw laryngoscope while holding endotracheal tube in place. Disassemble mask from resuscitation bag, attach bag to ET tube, and ventilate the patient.	
20. Inflate cuff with the minimal amount of air required to occlude the trachea.	20. Listen over the cuff area with a stethoscope. Occlusion occurs when no air leak is heard during ventilator inspiration or compression of the resuscitation bag.
21. Insert bite block if necessary.	21. This keeps patient from biting down on the tube and obstructing the airway.
22. Ascertain expansion of both sides of the chest by observation and auscultation of breath sounds.	22. Observation and auscultation help in determining that tube remains in position and has not slipped into the right mainstem bronchus.
23. Record distance from proximal end of tube to the point where the tube reaches the teeth.	23. This will allow for detection of any later change in tube position.
24. Secure tube to the patient's face with adhesive tape or apply a commercially available endotracheal tube stabilization device.	24. The tube must be fixed securely to ensure that it will not be dislodged. Dislodgement of a tube with an inflated cuff may result in damage to the vocal cords.
25. Obtain chest x-ray to verify tube position.	

FOLLOW-UP PHASE

1. Record tube type and size, cuff pressure, and patient tolerance of the procedure. Auscultate breath sounds every 2 hours or if signs and symptoms of respiratory distress occur. Assess ABGs after intubation if requested by the health care provider.	1. ABGs may be prescribed to ensure adequacy of ventilation and oxygenation. Tube displacement may result in extubation (cuff above vocal cords), tube touching carina (causing paroxysmal coughing), or intubation of a mainstem bronchus (resulting in collapse of the unventilated lung).
2. Measure cuff pressure with manometer; adjust pressure. Make adjustment in tube placement on the basis of the chest x-ray results.	2. The tube may be advanced or removed several centimeters for proper placement on the basis of the chest x-ray results.

PROCEDURE GUIDELINES 10-5   ASSISTING WITH TRACHEOSTOMY INSERTION

EQUIPMENT

Tracheostomy tube (sizes 6.0 to 9.0 mm. for most adults)
Sterile instruments: hemostat, scalpel and blade, forceps, suture material, scissors
Sterile gown and drapes, gloves
Cap and face shield
Antiseptic prep solution
Gauze sponges
Shave prep kit
Sedation
Local anesthetic and syringe
Resuscitation bag and mask with oxygen source
Suction source and catheters
Syringe for cuff inflation
Respiratory support available for post-tracheostomy (mechanical ventilation, tracheal oxygen mask, CPAP, T-piece)

continued

PROCEDURE GUIDELINES 10-5   ASSISTING WITH TRACHEOSTOMY INSERTION *CONTINUED*

PROCEDURE

Nursing Action	Rationale

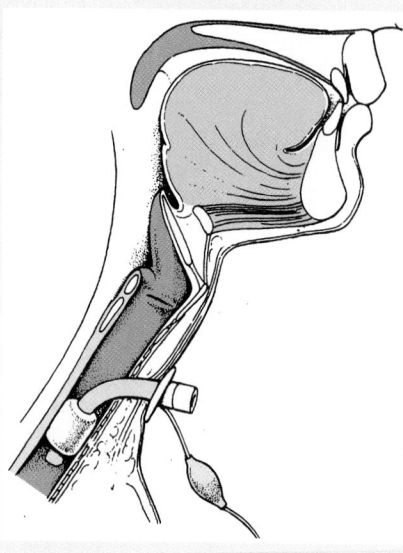

Tracheostomy tube placement.

PERFORMANCE PHASE

1. Explain the procedure to the patient. Discuss a communication system with the patient.
2. Obtain consent for operative procedure.
3. Shave neck region.

4. Assemble equipment. Using aseptic technique, inflate tracheostomy cuff and evaluate for symmetry and volume leakage. Deflate maximally.
5. Position the patient (supine with head extended, with a support under shoulders).
6. Obtain order for and apply soft wrist restraints if patient is confused.
7. Give medication if ordered.
8. Position light source.
9. Assist with antiseptic prep.
10. Assist with gowning and gloving.
11. Assist with sterile draping.
12. Put on face shield.

13. During procedure, monitor the patient's vital signs, suction as necessary, give medication as prescribed, and be prepared to administer emergency care.
14. Immediately after the tube is inserted, inflate the cuff. The chest should be auscultated for the presence of bilateral breath sounds.
15. Secure the tracheostomy tube with twill tapes or other securing device and apply dressing.
16. Apply appropriate respiratory assistive device (mechanical ventilation, tracheostomy, oxygen mask, CPAP, T-piece adapter).

1. Apprehension about inability to talk is usually a major concern of the tracheostomized patient.

3. Hair and beard may harbor microorganisms. If beard is to be removed, inform the patient or family.
4. Ensures that the cuff is functional before tube insertion.

5. This position brings the trachea forward.

6. Restraint of the confused patient may be necessary to ensure patient safety and preservation of aseptic technique.

12. Spraying of blood or airway secretions may occur during this procedure.
13. Bradycardia may result from vagal stimulation due to tracheal manipulation, or hypoxemia. Hypoxemia may also cause cardiac irritability.
14. Ensures ventilation of both lungs.

PROCEDURE GUIDELINES 10-5 *CONTINUED*

Nursing Action	Rationale
17. Check the tracheostomy tube cuff pressure.	17. Excessive cuff pressure may cause tracheal damage.
18. "Tie sutures" or "stay sutures" of 00 silk may have been placed through either side of the tracheal cartilage at the incision and brought out through the wound. Each is to be taped to the skin at a 45-degree angle laterally to the sternum.	18. Should the tracheostomy tube become dislodged, the stay sutures may be grasped and used to spread the tracheal cartilage apart, facilitating placement of the new tube.

FOLLOW-UP PHASE

Nursing Action	Rationale
1. Assess vital signs and ventilatory status; note tube size used, physician performing procedure, type, dose, and route of medications given.	1. Provides baseline.
2. Obtain chest x-ray.	2. Documents proper tube placement.

3. Assess and chart condition of stoma:
  a. Bleeding
	3.
	  a. Some bleeding around the stoma site is not unusual for the first few hours. Monitor and inform the physician of any increase in bleeding. Clean site aseptically when necessary. Do not change tracheostomy ties for first 24 hours, because accidental dislodgement of the tube could result when the ties are loose, and tube reinsertion through the as yet unformed stoma may be difficult or impossible to accomplish.

b. Swelling c. Subcutaneous air	c. When positive pressure respiratory assistive devices are used (mechanical ventilation, CPAP) before the wound is healed, air may be forced into the subcutaneous fat layer. This can be seen as enlargement of the neck and facial tissues and felt as crepitus or "cracking" when the skin is depressed. Report immediately.

4. An extra tube, obturator, and hemostat should be kept at the bedside. In the event of tube dislodgement, reinsertion of a new tube may be necessary. For emergency tube insertion:
  a. Spread the wound with a hemostat or stay sutures.
  b. Insert replacement tube (containing the obturator) at an angle.
  c. Point cannula downward and insert the tube maximally.
  d. Remove the obturator.
	4. The hemostat will open the airway and allow ventilation in the spontaneously breathing patient. Avoid inserting the tube horizontally, because the tube may be forced against the back wall of the trachea.

PROCEDURE GUIDELINES 10-6 ARTIFICIAL AIRWAY CUFF MAINTENANCE

EQUIPMENT

Suction catheter
Tonsil suction
Suction source
10-mL syringe

Pressure manometer (mercury or aneroid)
Manual resuscitation bag with reservoir, connected to 100% O_2 at 10 to 15 L/min
Face shield

PROCEDURE

Nursing Action	Rationale
PERFORMANCE PHASE	
1. Explain procedure to the patient.	1. Decreases the patient's anxiety and promotes cooperation.
2. Put on face shield.	2. Spraying of secretions may occur.

continued

PROCEDURE GUIDELINES 10-6 | **ARTIFICIAL AIRWAY CUFF MAINTENANCE** *CONTINUED*

PROCEDURE

Nursing Action	Rationale
DEFLATING THE CUFF	
1. Suction the trachea, then the oral and nasal pharynx. Then replace the catheter with a second sterile suction catheter.	1. Removes secretions collected above the cuff, which could be aspirated into the lungs when the cuff is deflated. Do not reenter the trachea with the same catheter used for suctioning the mouth.
2. Deflate the cuff slowly.	2. The small test balloon at the end of the tubing remains inflated as long as the cuff at the distal end of the tube is inflated. A vacuum within the syringe is sensed when no more air can be aspirated.
3. (Concomitant with step 2) Have the patient cough, or manually inflate the lungs with the resuscitation bag. Be ready to receive secretions in a tissue, or aspirate with tonsil suction.	3. Positive pressure in the airways may help force secretions upward and prevent aspiration of secretions.
4. Suction through the tracheostomy or endotracheal tube.	4. Secretions that may have been present above the inflated cuff and around the exterior tube have now seeped downward. Coughing reflex may be stimulated, helping to mobilize secretions.

5. Provide adequate ventilation while the cuff is deflated.
  a. If the patient does not require assisted ventilation, maintain humidified oxygen as directed.
  b. If the patient requires assisted ventilation, provide manual ventilation via a resuscitation bag. Leave cuff deflated for as long as the tube repositioning requires; then reinflate.
	5.
	
	  b. Monitor patient closely for tolerance. Loss of tidal volume or PEEP may promote hypoxemia and hypocarbia. Cuff should not be deflated for more than 30 to 45 seconds.

INFLATING A CUFF	

1. No leak technique.
  a. Attach air-filled syringe to cuff injection port.
  b. Slowly inject air until no air escapes from the patient's lungs around the cuff.
  c. Note amount of air injected to provide a seal.
	1. Air leakage will be heard when the intra-airway pressure is most positive (maximum peak airway pressure). For the spontaneously breathing patient, air leakage will be heard on exhalation. For the patient on positive pressure ventilation, air leakage will be heard at maximum ventilator inspiration.

2. Minimal leak technique (for mechanical ventilation):
 	
  a. Attach air-filled syringe to cuff injection port.
  b. Slowly inject air until no leak is heard at maximum peak airway pressure.
  c. Slowly remove air from cuff until a small air leak is heard at maximum peak airway pressure.
  d. Note amount of air injected.
	2. Inflates cuff at lowest possible pressure while still maintaining an adequate seal. Prevents tracheal necrosis from excessive or prolonged cuff pressure.
	
	  c. Adjustment in tidal volume setting may be necessary to compensate for the leak.

3. Measurement of minimal occluding volume (see accompanying figure).
  a. Inject sufficient air into the manometer tubing to raise the dial reading 1 cm H_2O above the zero reading.
  b. Insert male port of three-way stopcock into cuff injection port. One female port of stopcock holds the air-filled syringe, and one port holds the pressure manometer.
	
	  a. This "pressurizes" the tubing and prevents loss of air from the cuff to the tubing when the reading is taken.

PROCEDURE GUIDELINES 10-6   *CONTINUED*

Nursing Action   **Rationale**

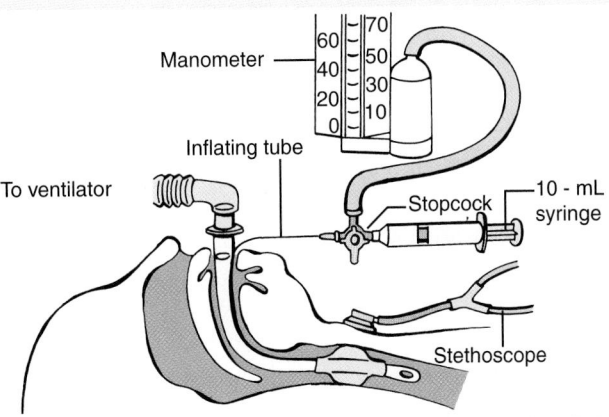

Determination of minimal occluding volume and cuff inflation pressure. A stopcock is inserted into the cuff injection port. When the stopcock is opened to the manometer, cuff pressure is registered on the manometer. An aneroid manometer can also be used. (Sills, J. [1986]. An emergency cuff inflation technique. Respiratory Care, 31[3], 201.)

c. Inject air into cuff until desired intracuff pressure is reached at maximum peak airway pressure.

    c. Aneroid manometer measures cuff pressure in cm H_2O: A pressure of 20 to 25 cm H_2O is desired. Mercury manometer pressure should be 15 to 20 mm Hg. Pressure greater than upper limit may cause compression of tracheal vessels, resulting in decreased blood flow to tissue. Pressure less than lower limit may allow aspiration of gastric or oral secretions.

d. Note amount of air needed to achieve the desired intracuff pressure.

e. Remove the stopcock from the injection port.

    e. Most injection ports have self-sealing valves. If not, a cap or closed stopcock may be left in the injection port (clamping of the inflation tubing is discouraged, because it may result in cracking or kinking of the line permanently).

MONITORING CUFF PRESSURE

1. While the cuff is inflated, monitor cuff pressure every 4 hours. Maintain cuff pressure between 15 and 20 mm Hg or 20 and 25 cm H_2O.
2. Document the amount of air required to maintain cuff pressure at this level.

    1. Excessive pressure will decrease blood flow to the tissue, resulting in tracheal necrosis. Insufficient cuff pressure predisposes to aspiration.
    2. Establishes a baseline for evaluation of change in pressure.

INABILITY TO MAINTAIN A SEAL

1. Assess the degree of leakage and length of time elapsed since cuff volume was replenished.

    1. If an inflated cuff leaks air within 10 minutes, assessment is necessary. Possibilities may be:
       a. Cuff positioned above the vocal cords (direct visualization necessary for repositioning).
       b. Incompetence of self-sealing valve on injection port.
       c. Tracheal dilatation (requiring larger size tube).
       d. Cuff may be ruptured, requiring a new tube.

continued

PROCEDURE GUIDELINES 10-6   ARTIFICIAL AIRWAY CUFF MAINTENANCE *CONTINUED*

Nursing Action	Rationale
2. Inflate the cuff to desired level.	
3. Disconnect syringe (and manometer if used).	
4. Assess for leakage.	
5. If leakage recurs, place three-way stopcock between syringe and injection port, inflate cuff, close stopcock. Remove syringe (and manometer if used) leaving closed stopcock in injection port.	5. Closed stopcock left in injection port acts as "plug" if self-sealing valve is incompetent.
6. If air leak persists, tube repositioning or replacement may be necessary. Consult with appropriate personnel.	

FOLLOW-UP PHASE

Nursing Action	Rationale
1. Note and record amount of air used for adequate seal, intracuff pressure, and inability to achieve seal. Document interventions necessary to reintubate, or change tracheostomy tube to obtain a desired seal.	
2. While the cuff is inflated, assess cuff pressure every 4 hours. The cuff pressure manometer is useful for this.	2. Leakage of air from the cuff or cuff injection port may occur. Assess the inflation status and adjust as needed.

PROCEDURE GUIDELINES 10-7   TRACHEOSTOMY CARE (ROUTINE)

EQUIPMENT

Assemble the following equipment or obtain a prepackaged tracheostomy care kit:
- Sterile towel
- Sterile gauze sponges (12)
- Track sparks (2)
- Sterile cotton swabs
- Sterile gloves

Hydrogen peroxide
Sterile water
Antiseptic solution and ointment (optional)
Tracheostomy tie tapes or commercially available tracheostomy securing device
Face shield

PROCEDURE

Nursing Action	Rationale
PREPARATORY PHASE	
1. Assess condition of stoma before tracheostomy care (redness, swelling, character of secretions, presence of purulence or bleeding).	1. The presence of skin breakdown or infection must be monitored. Culture of the site may be warranted by appearance of these signs.
2. Examine neck for subcutaneous emphysema.	2. Indicates air leak into subcutaneous tissue.
PERFORMANCE PHASE	
1. Suction the trachea and pharynx thoroughly before tracheostomy care.	1. Removal of secretions before tracheostomy care keeps the area clean longer.
2. Explain procedure to the patient.	
3. Wash hands thoroughly.	
4. Assemble equipment:	4.
a. Place sterile towel on patient's chest under tracheostomy site.	a. Provides sterile field.
b. Open 4 gauze sponges and pour hydrogen peroxide on them.	b. For removal of mucus and crust, which promotes bacterial growth.
c. Open 2 gauze sponges and pour antiseptic solution on them.	c. May be applied to fresh stoma or infected stoma. Not necessary for clean, healed stoma.
d. Open 2 gauze sponges; keep dry.	
e. Open 2 gauze sponges and pour sterile water on them.	
f. Place tracheostomy tube tapes on field.	

Nursing Action	Rationale
g. Put on face shield and sterile gloves.	g. Face shield prevents secretions from getting into the nurse's eyes. Sterile gloves prevent contamination of the wound by nurse's hands and also protect the nurse's hands from infection.
5. Clean the external end of the tracheostomy tube with 2 gauze sponges with hydrogen peroxide; discard sponges.	5. Designate the hand you clean with as contaminated and reserve the other hand as sterile for handling sterile equipment.
6. Clean the stoma area with 2 peroxide-soaked gauze sponges. Make only a single sweep with each gauze sponge before discarding.	6. Hydrogen peroxide may help loosen dry crusted secretions.
7. Loosen and remove crust with sterile cotton swabs.	
8. Repeat step 6 using the sterile water-soaked gauze sponges.	8. Ensures that all hydrogen peroxide is removed.
9. Repeat step 6 using dry sponges.	9. Ensures dryness of the area. Wetness promotes infection and irritation.
10. (Optional) An infected wound may be cleaned with gauze saturated with an antiseptic solution, then dried. A thin layer of antibiotic ointment may be applied to the stoma with a cotton swab.	10. May help clear wound infection.
11. Change a disposable inner cannula, touching only the external portion, and lock it securely into place. If inner cannula is reusable, remove it with your contaminated hand and clean it in hydrogen peroxide solution, using brush or pipe cleaners with your sterile hand. When clean, drop it into sterile saline solution and agitate it to rinse thoroughly with your sterile hand. Tap it gently to dry it and replace it with your sterile hand.	11. Because cannula is dirty when you remove it, use your contaminated hand. It is considered sterile once you clean it, so handle it with your sterile hand.
12. Change the tracheostomy tie tapes:	12.
a. Cut soiled tape while holding tube securely with other hand. Use care not to cut the pilot balloon tubing.	a. Stabilization of the tube helps prevent accidental dislodgement and keeps irritation and coughing due to tube manipulation at a minimum.
b. Remove old tapes carefully.	
c. Grasp slit end of clean tape and pull it through opening on side of the tracheostomy tube.	
d. Pull other end of tape securely through the slit end of the tape.	
e. Repeat on the other side.	
f. Tie the tapes at the side of the neck in a square knot. Alternate knot from side to side each time tapes are changed.	f. To prevent irritation and rotate pressure site.
g. Ties should be tight enough to keep tube securely in the stoma, but loose enough to permit two fingers to fit between the tapes and the neck.	g. Excessive tightness of tapes will compress jugular veins, decrease blood circulation to the skin under the tape, and result in discomfort for the patient.
13. Place a gauze pad between the stoma site and the tracheostomy tube to absorb secretions and prevent irritation of the stoma according to institution policy (see accompanying figure). Many clinicians believe that gauze should not be used around the stoma. In their opinion, the dressing keeps the area moist and dark, promoting stomal infection. They believe the stoma should be left open to the air and the surrounding area kept dry. A dressing is used only if secretions are draining onto subclavian or neck IV sites or chest incisions.	

Note: If only one clinician is available, the stoma is new (<2 weeks), or the patient's condition is unstable, follow steps c through f before removing old tapes. Two sets of ties will be in place at the same time. After completing step f, cut and remove the old tapes. Also, a tracheostomy-securing device can be used instead of the tracheostomy ties.

continued

PROCEDURE GUIDELINES 10-7   TRACHEOSTOMY CARE (ROUTINE) *CONTINUED*

Nursing Action	Rationale

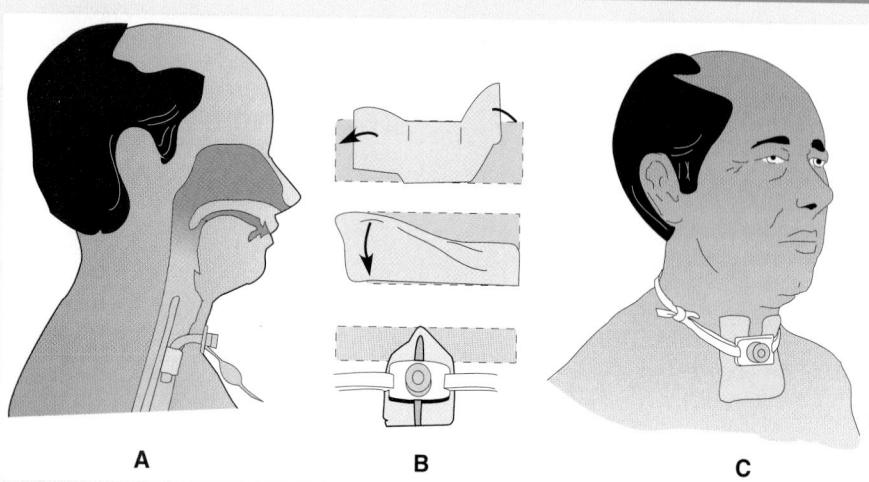

Placement of tracheostomy tube ties and elective gauze pad.

FOLLOW-UP PHASE

Nursing Action	Rationale
1. Document procedure performance, observations of stoma (irritation, redness, edema, subcutaneous air), and character of secretions (color, purulence). Report changes in stoma appearance or secretions.	1. Provides a baseline.
2. Cleaning of the fresh stoma should be performed every 8 hours, or more frequently if indicated by accumulation of secretions. Ties should be changed every 24 hours, or more frequently if soiled or wet.	2. The area must be kept clean and dry to prevent infection or irritation of tissues.

PROCEDURE GUIDELINES 10-8   INSERTION OF A TRACHEOSTOMY BUTTON

EQUIPMENT

Appropriate size tracheostomy button kit (includes cannula, solid closure plug, spacers, universal adapter)
Water-soluble lubricant
Syringe for deflation of tracheostomy cuff

Replacement tracheostomy tube
Flashlight
Gloves

PROCEDURE

Nursing Action	Rationale

PREPARATORY PHASE

Nursing Action	Rationale
1. Assess whether patient meets criteria for use of tracheostomy button. Criteria include: able to be adequately oxygenated with nasal cannula or face mask; able to swallow and protect the airway; able to cough up secretions; and a noninfected, nonirritated tracheal stoma.	1. If patient does not meet these criteria, use of tracheostomy tube as airway must be continued.
2. Determine vital signs, level of consciousness, SaO_2 or ABG.	2. Provides baseline for future assessment.

PROCEDURE GUIDELINES 10-8   CONTINUED

PROCEDURE

Nursing Action	Rationale
PERFORMANCE PHASE	
1. Elevate the head of the bed 45 degrees, suction the airway, deflate the tracheostomy tube cuff, and remove the tube.	1. Protects against aspiration.
2. Determine the distance from anterior tracheal wall to the outer edge of the stoma (skin surface) using a probe with a right angle bend (contained in the kit).	
3. Insert the angled end of the probe into the stoma, pull gently until the probe touches the anterior well, then mark the probe at the outer edge of the stoma (skin surface).	
4. Compare the length of the tracheostomy button cannula with this measurement. If the cannula is too long, it can be sized to fit by adding spacers included in the kit.	4. Spacer rings can be slipped over the cannula to size it for individualized patient requirements.
5. Coat the cannula with water-soluble lubricant. Ask the patient to relax and take several deep breaths. Insert the cannula into the stoma.	5. The cannula should pass easily into the stoma. If insertion is difficult, recheck cannula size. Several sizes are available.
6. Insert the closure plug into the cannula. Ties may be used to hold the button in place until the stoma closes around the button.	6. A slight snap will be heard as the plug enters the cannula. The plug causes the proximal end of the cannula to flare, holding it in place.
7. Remove button two times a week, clean with antibacterial soap, and replace it.	7. Periodic removal helps to keep tissue from granulating into the distal portion of the cannula.
FOLLOW-UP PHASE	
1. Observe immediate patient response and obtain Sao_2 or ABG after insertion. Report changes.	1. Use of the button increases dead space, which may increase work of breathing or cause a decrease in Sao_2.
2. Determine ability of patient to cough out secretions and swallow with button in place.	2. Confirms patient will not retain secretions or be at risk for aspiration with use of this device.

◾ Mobilization of Secretions

The goal of airway clearance techniques is to improve clearance of airway secretions, thereby decreasing obstruction of the airways. This serves to improve ventilation and gas exchange. Patients with respiratory disorders or other disorders such as loss of consciousness that may impair respiratory function often require help with mobilization and removal of secretions. Increased amount and viscosity of secretions and/or inability to clear secretions through the normal cough mechanism may lead to pooling of secretions in lower airways. Pooling of secretions leads to infection and inadequate gas exchange.

Secretions should be removed by coughing or, when necessary, by suctioning and can be mobilized through the chest physical therapy measures of postural drainage, percussion, vibration, directed cough, autogenic drainage, positive expiratory pressure, flutter mucus clearance device, and other secretion clearance measures. Breathing exercises are done with chest physical therapy to increase the efficiency of breathing.

Nasotracheal Suctioning

1. Intended to remove accumulated secretions or other materials that cannot be moved by the patient's spontaneous cough or less invasive procedures. Suctioning of the tracheobronchial tree in a patient without an artificial airway can be accomplished by inserting a sterile suction catheter lubricated with water-soluble jelly through the nares into the nasal passage, down through the oropharynx, past the glottis, and into the trachea (Procedure Guidelines 10-9).
2. Nasotracheal suction is a blind, high-risk procedure with uncertain outcome. Complications include mechanical trauma, hypoxia, dysrhythmias, bradycardia, increased blood pressure, vomiting, increased intracranial pressure, and misdirection of catheter.
3. Contraindications include:
   a. Bleeding disorders such as disseminated intravascular coagulation, thrombocytopenia, leukemia
   b. Laryngeal edema, laryngeal spasm
   c. Esophageal varices

d. Tracheal surgery

e. Gastric surgery with high anastomosis

f. Myocardial infarction

g. Occluded nasal passages or nasal bleeding

h. Epiglottitis

i. Head, facial, or neck injury

4. May cause trauma to the nasal passages.
   a. Do not attempt to force the catheter if resistance is met.
   b. Report if significant bleeding occurs.

5. Insert a nasal airway if repeated suctioning is necessary to protect the nasal passages from trauma.

6. Be alert for signs of laryngeal edema due to irritation and trauma. Stop if suctioning becomes difficult or if the patient develops new upper airway noise or obstruction.

   Duration of the suctioning should be limited to less than 15 seconds.

Suctioning Through an Endotracheal or Tracheostomy Tube

1. Ineffective coughing may cause secretion collection in the artificial airway or tracheobronchial tree, resulting in narrowing of the airway, respiratory insufficiency, and stasis of secretions.

2. Assess the need for suctioning at least every 2 hours through auscultation of the chest.
   a. Ventilation with a manual resuscitation bag will facilitate auscultation and may stimulate coughing, decreasing the need for suctioning.

3. Maintain sterile technique while suctioning (Procedure Guidelines 10-10).

4. Administer supplemental 100% oxygen through the mechanical ventilator or manual resuscitation bag before, after, and between suctioning passes to prevent hypoxemia.

5. Closed system suctioning may be done with the suction catheter contained in the mechanical ventilator tubing. Ventilator disconnection is not necessary so time is saved, sterility is maintained, and risk of exposure to body fluids is eliminated.

Community and Home Care Considerations

1. Teach caregivers to suction in the home situation using clean technique, rather than sterile. Wash hands well before suctioning.

2. Don fresh examination gloves for suctioning, and reuse catheter after rinsing it in warm water. Appropriate and aggressive airway clearance will assist in preventing pulmonary complications, thus lessening the need for hospitalization.

Chest Physical Therapy
Breathing Exercises

1. Techniques used to compensate for respiratory deficits and conserve energy by increasing efficiency of breathing (Procedure Guidelines 10-11).

2. The overall purposes for doing breathing exercises are:
   a. To relax muscles, relieve anxiety, and improve control of breathing.
   b. To eliminate useless uncoordinated patterns of respiratory muscle activity.
   c. To slow the respiratory rate.
   d. To decrease the work of breathing.
   e. To improve efficiency and strength of respiratory muscles.
   f. To improve ventilation and oxygen saturation during exercise.

3. Diaphragmatic breathing is used primarily to strengthen the diaphragm, which is the main muscle of respiration. It also aids in decreasing the use of accessory muscles and allows for better control over the breathing pattern, especially during stressful situations and increased physical demands.

4. Pursed-lip breathing is used primarily to slow the respiratory rate and assist in emptying the lungs of retained CO_2. This technique is always helpful to patients, but especially when they feel extreme dyspnea due to exertion.

5. Breathing exercises are most helpful to patients when practiced and used on a regular basis.

Percussion and Vibration

1. Postural drainage uses gravity and external manipulation of the thorax to improve mobilization of bronchial secretions, to enhance matching of ventilation and perfusion, and to normalize functional residual capacity.

2. Indicated for difficulty with secretion clearance, evidence of retained secretions, and lung conditions that cause increased production of secretions such as bronchiectasis, cystic fibrosis, chronic bronchitis, and emphysema.

3. Contraindicated in undrained lung abscess, lung tumors, pneumothorax, diseases of the chest wall, lung hemorrhage, painful chest conditions, tuberculosis, severe osteoporosis, and increased intracranial pressure.

4. Percussion is movement done by striking the chest wall in a rhythmic fashion with cupped hands or a mechanical device directly over the lung segment(s) to be drained. The wrists are alternately flexed and extended so the chest is cupped or clapped in a painless manner (Procedure Guidelines 10-12). A mechanical percussor may be used to prevent repetitive motion injury.

5. Vibration is the technique of applying manual compression, with oscillations or tremors to the chest wall during the exhalation phase of respiration.

Postural Drainage

1. Use of specific positions so the force of gravity can assist in the removal of bronchial secretions from affected lung segments to central airways by means of coughing or suctioning (Figure 10-4).

2. The patient is positioned so the diseased area(s) are in a near vertical position, and gravity is used to assist drainage of the specific segment(s).

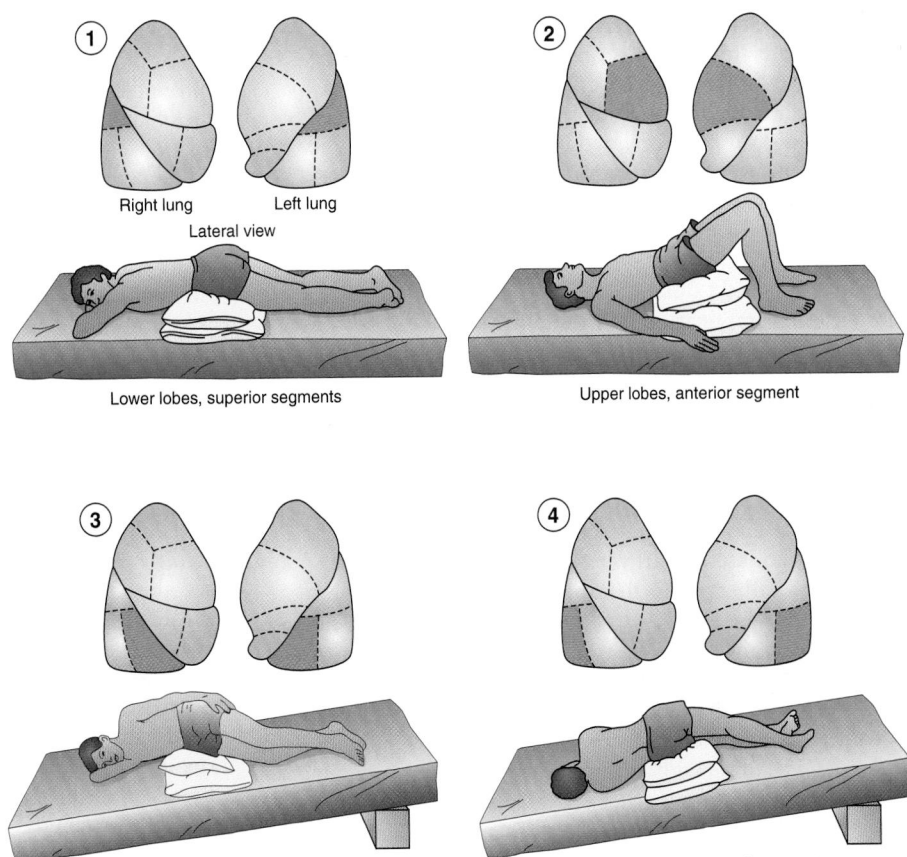

FIGURE 10-4 Postural drainage positions. Anatomic segments of the lung with four postural drainage positions. The numbers relate the position to the corresponding anatomic segment of the lung.

3. The positions assumed are determined by the location, severity, and duration of mucus obstruction.
4. The exercises are usually performed two to four times daily, before meals and at bedtime. Each position is held for 3 to 15 minutes.
5. The procedure should be discontinued if tachycardia, palpitations, dyspnea, or chest pain occur. These symptoms may indicate hypoxemia. Discontinue if hemoptysis occurs.
6. Contraindications: Increased intracranial pressure, unstable head or neck injury, active hemorrhage with hemodynamic instability, recent spinal surgery or injury, empyema, bronchopleural fistula, rib fracture, or flail chest.

NURSING ALERT

Postural drainage and chest percussion may result in hypoxia and should only be used if secretions are believed to be present.

7. Bronchodilators, mucolytic agents, water, or saline may be nebulized and inhaled, or bronchodilator metered-dose inhaler may be used before postural drainage and chest percussion to reduce bronchospasm, decrease thickness of mucus and sputum, and combat edema of the bronchial walls, thereby enhancing secretion removal (Procedure Guidelines 10–13).
8. Perform secretion clearance procedures before eating.
9. Ensure patient is comfortable before the procedure starts and as comfortable as possible while he or she assumes each position.
10. Auscultate the chest to determine the areas of needed drainage.
11. Encourage the patient to deep breathe and cough after spending the allotted time in each position (normally 3 to 15 minutes).
12. Encourage diaphragmatic breathing throughout postural drainage; this helps widen airways so secretions can be drained.

Directed Cough
1. Used to enhance effects of a spontaneous cough and compensate for physical limitations. Used for secretion clearance, atelectasis, prophylaxis against postoperative pulmonary complications, routine bronchial hygiene for cystic fibrosis, bronchiectasis, chronic bronchitis, and to obtain sputum specimen for diagnostic analysis.

2. Procedure includes a forced exhalation technique of one or two huffs (forced expirations), from mid- to low-lung volume, with glottis open, followed by a period of relaxed, controlled diaphragmatic breathing. The forced expiration can be augmented by brisk adduction of the upper arms to self-compress the thorax.
3. Contraindications include increased intracranial pressure or known intracranial aneurysm, as well as acute or unstable head, neck, or spinal injury.

Manually Assisted Cough
The external application of mechanical pressure to the epigastric region coordinated with forced exhalation.

Positive Expiratory Pressure (PEP)
1. Positive back pressure is created in the airways when the patient breathes in and out 5 to 20 times through a flow resistor.
2. During prolonged exhalation against positive pressure, peripheral airways are stabilized while air is pushed through collateral pathways (pores of Kohn and canals of Lambert) into distal lung units past retained secretions.
3. Expiratory airflow moves secretions to larger airways to be removed by coughing.
4. The pressure generated can be monitored and adjusted with a manometer (usually range from 10 to 20 cm H_2O).
5. Active exhalation with an inspiratory-to-expiratory ratio of 1:3 or 1:4 is suggested.
6. The cycle is repeated until secretions are expelled, usually within 20 minutes or less if patient tires.

Autogenic Drainage
1. Controlled breathing used at three lung volumes, beginning at low-lung volumes to unstick mucus, moving to mid-lung volume to collect mucus, and then to high-lung volume to expel mucus.
2. This method may be difficult for some patients to learn.

Flutter Mucus Clearance Device
1. Provides positive expiratory pressure (PEP) and high-frequency oscillations at the airway opening.
2. The flutter valve is a pipe-shaped device with an inner cone and bowl loosely supporting a steel ball. The bowl containing the steel ball is covered by a perforated cap.
3. Indications include atelectasis, bronchitis, bronchiectasis, cystic fibrosis, and other conditions producing retained secretions.
4. Mucus clearance is based on:
   a. Vibration of the airways, which loosens mucus from airway walls.
   b. Intermittent increase in endobronchial pressure that keeps airways open.
   c. Acceleration of expiratory airflow to facilitate upward movement of mucus.
5. Contraindications include pneumothorax and right-sided heart failure.
6. Directions:
   a. Patient should be seated upright with chin tilted slightly upward to further open airway.
   b. Instruct patient to inhale slowly.
   c. Place flutter in mouth with lips firmly sealed around stem or mouthpiece.
   d. Position flutter at horizontal level or raise bulb end up to 30 degrees for greater force.
   e. Instruct patient to hold breath for 2 to 3 seconds.
   f. Exhale through flutter at moderately fast rate, keeping cheeks stiff. Urge to cough should be suppressed.
   g. Repeat for 5 to 10 more breaths.
7. Have patient perform same technique with one to two forced exhalations to generate mucus elimination.
8. Generally used twice daily.
9. Clean flutter device every other day by disassembling and using a liquid soap and tap water. Disinfect regularly by soaking cleaned disassembled parts in one part alcohol to three parts tap water for 1 minute; rinse, wipe, reassemble, and store.

Intrapulmonary Percussive Ventilation (IPV)
Therapy is delivered by a percussionator, which delivers mini-bursts of air into the lungs at a rate of 100 to 300 per minute. Process includes delivery of a dense aerosol mist. The treatment lasts about 20 minutes.

The In-Exsufflator
Assists in secretion clearance by applying positive pressure to the airway, then rapidly shifting to negative pressure by way of a face mask, mouthpiece, endotracheal tube, or tracheostomy tube.

The ThAIRapy Vest
Enhances secretion clearance through high-frequency chest wall oscillation. High-frequency compression pulses are applied to the chest wall by way of an air pulse generator and inflatable vest.

Community and Home Care Considerations
1. Nebulizer tubing and mouthpiece can be reused at home repeatedly. Recommend thorough rinsing with hot water after each use.
2. Twice-weekly cleansing should include washing with liquid soap and hot water; followed by 30-minute soak in one part white vinegar and two parts tap water; and then rinsed with tap water, air dried, and stored in a clean, dry place.

(text continues on page 232)

PROCEDURE GUIDELINES 10-9   NASOTRACHEAL (NT) SUCTIONING

EQUIPMENT

Assemble the following equipment or obtain a prepackaged kit:
Disposable curved-tipped suction catheter
Sterile towel
Sterile disposable gloves
Sterile water

Anesthetic water-soluble lubricant jelly
Suction source at −80 to −120 mm Hg
Resuscitation bag with face mask. Connect 100% O_2
   source with flow of 10 L/min
Oximeter

PROCEDURE

Nursing Action	Rationale

PREPARATORY PHASE

1. Monitor heart rate, respiratory rate, color, ease of respirations. If the patient is on monitor, continue monitoring heart rate or arterial blood pressure. Discontinue the suctioning and apply oxygen if heart rate decreases by 20 beats per minute or increases by 40 beats per minute, if blood pressure increases, or if cardiac dysrhythmia is noted.

1. Suctioning may cause the occurrence of:
   a. Hypoxemia—Initially resulting in tachycardia and increased blood pressure, and later causing cardiac ectopy, bradycardia, hypotension, and cyanosis.
   b. Vagal stimulation resulting in bradycardia.

PERFORMANCE PHASE

1. Ascertain that the suction apparatus is functional. Place suction tubing within easy reach.

1. The procedure must be done aseptically, because the catheter will be entering the trachea below the level of the vocal cords, and introduction of bacteria is contraindicated.

2. Inform and instruct the patient regarding procedure.
   a. At a certain interval, the patient will be requested to cough to open the lung passage so the catheter will go into the lungs and not into the stomach. The patient will also be encouraged to try not to swallow, because this will also cause the catheter to enter the stomach.
   b. The postoperative patient can splint the wound to make the coughing produced by NT suctioning less painful.
3. Place the patient in a semi-Fowler's or sitting position if possible.

2. A thorough explanation will decrease patient anxiety and promote patient cooperation.

3. NT suctioning should follow chest physical therapy, postural drainage, and/or ultrasonic nebulization therapy. The patient should not be suctioned after eating or after a tube feeding is given (unless absolutely necessary) to decrease the possibility of emesis and aspiration.

4. Monitor oxygen saturation via oximetry and heart rate during suctioning.
5. Place sterile towel across the patient's chest. Squeeze small amount of sterile anesthetic water-soluble lubricant jelly onto the towel.
6. Open sterile pack containing curved-tipped suction catheter.
7. Aseptically glove both hands. Designate one hand (usually the dominant one) as "sterile" and the other hand as "contaminated."

7. The "contaminated" hand must also be gloved to ensure that organisms in the sputum do not come in contact with the nurse's hand, possibly resulting in infection of the nurse.

8. Grasp sterile catheter with sterile hand.
9. Lubricate catheter with the anesthetic jelly and pass the catheter into the nostril and back into the pharynx.
10. Pass the catheter into the trachea. To do this, ask the patient to cough or say "ahh." If the patient is incapable of either, try to advance the catheter on inspiration. Asking the patient to stick out tongue, or hold tongue extended with a gauze sponge, may also help to open the

9. If obstruction is met, do not force the catheter. Remove it and try the other nostril.
10. These maneuvers may aid in opening the glottis and allowing passage of the catheter into the trachea. To evaluate proper placement, listen at the catheter end for air, or feel for air movement against the cheek. An increase in intensity of breath sounds or more air movement

continued

PROCEDURE GUIDELINES 10-9   NASOTRACHEAL (NT) SUCTIONING *CONTINUED*

Nursing Action

Rationale

airway. If a protracted amount of time is needed to position the catheter in the trachea, stop and oxygenate the patient with face mask or the resuscitation bag-mask unit at intervals. If three attempts to place the catheter are unsuccessful, request assistance.

against cheek indicates nearness to the larynx. Gagging or sudden lessening of sound means the catheter is in the hypopharynx. Draw back and advance again. The presence of the catheter in the trachea is indicated by:
a. Sudden paroxysms of coughing.
b. Movement of air through the catheter.
c. Vigorous bubbling of air when the distal end of the suction catheter is placed in a cup of sterile water.
d. Inability of the patient to speak.

11. Specific positioning of catheter for deep bronchial suctioning:
    a. For left bronchial suctioning, turn the patient's head to the extreme right, chin up.
    b. For right bronchial suctioning, turn the patient's head to the extreme left, chin up.

11. Turning the patient's head to one side elevates the bronchial passage on the opposite side, making catheter insertion easier. Suctioning of a particular lung segment may be of value in patients with unilateral pneumonia, atelectasis, or collapse.

Note: The value of turning the head as an aid to entering the right or left mainstem bronchi is not accepted by all clinicians.

12. Never apply suction until catheter is in the trachea. Once correct position is ascertained, apply suction and gently rotate catheter while pulling it slightly upward. Do not remove catheter from the trachea.

12. Because entry into the trachea is often difficult, less change in arterial oxygen may be caused by leaving the catheter in the trachea than by repeated insertion attempts.

13. Disconnect the catheter from the suctioning source after 5 to 10 seconds. Apply oxygen by placing a face-mask over the patient's nose, mouth, and catheter, and instruct the patient to breathe deeply.

13. Be sure adequate time is allowed to reoxygenate the patient, as oxygen is removed, as well as secretions, during suctioning.

14. Reconnect suction source. Repeat as necessary.

14. No more than three to four suction passes should be made per suction episode.

15. During the last suction pass, remove the catheter completely while applying suction and rotating the catheter gently. Apply oxygen when catheter is removed.

15. Never leave the catheter in the trachea after the suction procedure is concluded, because the epiglottis is splinted open and aspiration may occur.

FOLLOW-UP PHASE
1. Dispose of disposable equipment
2. Measure heart rate, blood pressure, respiratory rate, and oxygen saturation. Record the patient's tolerance of procedure, type and amount of secretions removed, and complications.
3. Report any patient intolerance of procedure (changes in vital signs, bleeding, laryngospasm, upper airway noise).

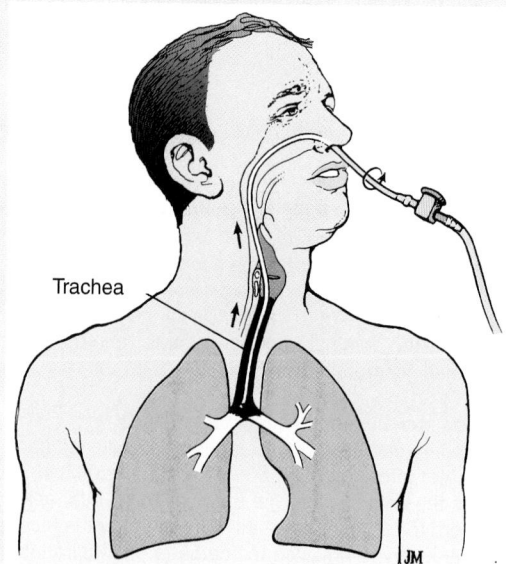

Trachea

Placement of nasotracheal tube for suctioning the tracheobronchial tree.

PROCEDURE GUIDELINES 10-10 — STERILE TRACHEOBRONCHIAL SUCTION BY WAY OF TRACHEOSTOMY OR ENDOTRACHEAL TUBE (SPONTANEOUS OR MECHANICAL VENTILATION)

EQUIPMENT

Assemble the following equipment or obtain a prepackaged suctioning kit:

Sterile suction catheters—No. 14 or 16 (adult), No. 8 or 10 (child). The outer diameter of the suction catheter should be no greater than one half the inner diameter of the artificial airway.

Two sterile gloves

Sterile towel

Suction source at 80 to 120 mm Hg

Sterile water

Resuscitation bag with a reservoir connected to 100% oxygen source (if patient is on positive end-expiratory pressure [PEEP] or continuous positive airway pressure [CPAP], add PEEP valve to exhalation valve on resuscitation bag in an amount equal to that on the ventilator or CPAP device)

Normal saline solution (in syringe or single-dose packet)

Sterile cup for water

Alcohol swabs

Sterile water-soluble lubricant jelly

Face shield

PROCEDURE

Nursing Action	Rationale
PREPARATORY PHASE	
1. Monitor heart rate and auscultate breath sounds. If the patient is monitored, continuously monitor heart rate and arterial blood pressure. If arterial blood gases are done routinely, know baseline values. It is important to establish a baseline because suctioning should be discontinued and oxygen applied or manual ventilation reinstituted if, during the suction procedure, the heart rate decreases by 20 beats per minute or increases by 40 beats per minute, blood pressure drops, or cardiac dysrhythmia is noted.	1. Suctioning may cause: a. Hypoxemia, initially resulting in tachycardia and increased blood pressure, progressing to cardiac ectopy, bradycardia, hypotension, and cyanosis. b. Vagal stimulation, which may result in bradycardia.
PERFORMANCE PHASE	
1. Instruct the patient how to "splint" surgical incision, because coughing will be induced during the procedure. Explain the importance of performing the suction procedure in an aseptic manner.	1. Thorough explanation lessens patient's anxiety and promotes cooperation.
2. Assemble equipment. Check function of suction and manual resuscitation bag connected to 100% O_2 source. Put on face shield.	2. Make sure that all equipment is functional before sterile technique is instituted to prevent interruption once the procedure is begun. Use of 100% O_2 will help to prevent hypoxemia.
3. Wash hands thoroughly.	
4. Open sterile towel. Place in a biblike fashion on patient's chest. Open alcohol wipes and place on corner of towel. Place small amount of sterile water-soluble jelly on towel.	
5. Open sterile gloves. Place on towel.	
6. Open suction catheter package.	
7. If the patient is on mechanical ventilation, test to make sure disconnection of ventilator attachment may be made with one hand.	
8. Don sterile gloves. Designate one hand as contaminated for disconnecting, bagging, and working the suction control. Usually the dominant hand is kept sterile and will be used to thread the suction catheter.	8. The hand designated as sterile must remain uncontaminated so organisms are not introduced into the lungs. The contaminated hand must also be gloved to prevent sputum from contacting the nurse's hand, possibly resulting in an infection of the nurse.
9. Use the sterile hand to remove carefully the suction catheter from the package, curling the catheter around the gloved fingers.	
10. Connect suction source to the suction fitting of the catheter with the contaminated hand.	

continued

PROCEDURE GUIDELINES 10-10	STERILE TRACHEOBRONCHIAL SUCTION BY WAY OF TRACHEOSTOMY OR ENDOTRACHEAL TUBE (SPONTANEOUS OR MECHANICAL VENTILATION) *CONTINUED*

Nursing Action	Rationale
11. Using the contaminated hand, disconnect the patient from the ventilator, CPAP device, or other oxygen source. (Place the ventilator connector on the sterile towel and flip a corner of the towel over the connection to prevent fluid from spraying into the area.)	11. Prevents contamination of the connection.
12. Ventilate and oxygenate the patient with the resuscitator bag, compressing firmly and as completely as possible approximately four to five times (try to approximate the patient's tidal volume). This procedure is called "bagging" the patient. In the spontaneously breathing patient, coordinate manual ventilations with the patient's own inspiratory effort.	12. Ventilation before suctioning helps prevent hypoxemia. When possible, two nurses or a nurse and a respiratory therapist work as a team to suction. Attempting to ventilate against the patient's own respiratory efforts may result in high airway pressures, predisposing the patient to barotrauma (lung injury due to pressure).
13. Gently insert suction catheter as far as possible into the artificial airway without applying suction. Most patients will cough when the catheter touches the carina.	13. Suctioning on insertion would unnecessarily decrease oxygen in the airway.
14. Withdraw catheter 2 to 3 cm and apply suction. Quickly rotate the catheter while it is being withdrawn.	14. Failure to withdraw and rotate catheter may result in damage to tracheal mucosa. Release suction if a pulling sensation is felt.
15. Limit suction time to no more than 10 seconds. Discontinue if heart rate decreases by 20 beats per minute or increases by 40 beats per minute, or if cardiac ectopy is observed.	15. Suctioning removes oxygen as well as secretions and may also cause vagal stimulation.
16. Bag patient between suction passes with approximately four to five manual ventilations.	16. The oxygen removed by suctioning must be replenished before suctioning is attempted again.
17. At this point, sterile normal saline may be instilled into the trachea by way of the artificial airway if secretions are tenacious.	17. Some clinicians believe secretion removal may be facilitated with saline instillation. Others believe saline does not mix with mucus and that suctioning of the saline just instilled is the only effect produced by performing this step. It is now thought that the greatest benefit of instilling sterile normal saline is to initiate a cough.
a. Open prepackaged container and instill 3 to 5 mL normal saline into the artificial airway during spontaneous inspiration.	a. Instillation of the saline during inspiration will prevent the saline from being blown back out of the tube.
b. Bag vigorously and then suction.	b. Bagging stimulates cough and distributes saline to loosen secretions.
18. Rinse catheter between suction passes by inserting tip in cup of sterile water and applying suction.	
19. Continue making suction passes, bagging the patient between passes, until the airways are clear of accumulated secretions. No more than four suction passes should be made per suctioning episode.	19. Repeated suctioning of a patient in a short time interval predisposes to hypoxemia, as well as being tiring and traumatic to the patient.
20. Give the patient four to five "sigh" breaths with the bag.	20. Sighing is accomplished by depressing the bag slowly and completely with two hands to deliver approximately $1\frac{1}{2}$ times the normal tidal volume to the patient, allowing for maximal lung expansion and prevention of atelectasis.
21. Return the patient to the ventilator or apply CPAP or other oxygen-delivery device.	
22. Suction oral secretions from the oropharynx above the artificial airway cuff.	
23. Clean elbow fitting of resuscitation bag with alcohol; cover with a sterile glove or 4×4.	

PROCEDURE GUIDELINES 10-10 *CONTINUED*

Nursing Action	Rationale
FOLLOW-UP PHASE	
1. Note any change in vital signs or patient's intolerance to the procedure. Record amount and consistency of secretions.	1. Evaluate the effectiveness of procedure and patient response.
2. Assess need for further suctioning at least every 2 hours, or more frequently if secretions are copious.	

Note: A closed system for suctioning may be in place in the ventilator circuit that allows suctioning without removal from the ventilator.

3. Teach caregivers to suction in the home situation using clean technique, rather than sterile. Wash hands well before suctioning and reuse catheter after rinsing it in warm water.	

PROCEDURE GUIDELINES 10-11 TEACHING THE PATIENT BREATHING EXERCISES

PROCEDURE

Nursing Action	Rationale
PREPARATORY PHASE	
1. Have patient clear the nasal passages before beginning exercises.	
PERFORMANCE PHASE	
Instruct the patient as follows:	
Diaphragmatic Breathing	
1. Place one hand on stomach just below the ribs and the other hand on the middle of the chest.	1. This helps the patient become aware of the diaphragm and its function in breathing.
2. Breathe in slowly and deeply through the nose, letting the abdomen protrude as far as it will. The abdomen enlarges during inspiration and decreases in size during expiration.	2. Slow inhalation provides ventilation and hyperinflation of the lungs.
3. Breathe out through pursed lips while contracting (tightening) the abdominal muscles. Press firmly inward and upward on the abdomen while breathing out. The ratio of inhalation to expiration should be 1:2. Inhale through the nose for the count of 2, exhale through pursed lips for the count of 4.	3. Contracting the abdominal muscles assists the diaphragm in rising to empty the lungs. The hand generates pressure on the abdomen to facilitate more complete expiration.
4. The chest should not move; attention is directed at the abdomen, not the chest.	4. Contraction of the abdominal muscles should take place during expiration.
5. Repeat for 1 minute (followed by a rest period of 2 minutes). Work up to 10 minutes, four times daily.	
6. Learn to do diaphragmatic breathing while lying, then sitting, and ultimately standing and walking.	6. Diaphragmatic breathing helps the patient breathe in a controlled manner during activities that produce dyspnea. If shortness of breath occurs, advise stopping the exercises until breathing pattern comes under control.

continued

PROCEDURE GUIDELINES 10-11 TEACHING THE PATIENT BREATHING EXERCISES *CONTINUED*

Nursing Action	Rationale
Pursed-Lip Breathing	
1. Inhale slowly and through the nose for a count of 2.	
2. Exhale slowly and evenly against pursed lips while contracting (tightening) the abdominal muscles. Avoid exhaling forcefully. Inhalation to exhalation rate is 1:2.	2. Pursing the lips increases intrabronchial pressure (helps maintain the bronchi in an open position) as well as intra-alveolar pressure. The pursed-lips maneuver also prolongs the expiratory phase of breathing, makes it easier to empty the air in the lungs, and promotes carbon dioxide elimination.
3. Sit in a chair. Fold arms across the abdomen. a. Inhale through the nose for a count of 2. b. Exhale slowly through pursed lips for a count of 4, contracting abdominal muscles. Bend over if necessary to contract abdominal muscles.	3. b. Leaning forward pushes the abdominal organs upward.
4. While walking. a. Inhale while walking two steps. b. Exhale through pursed lips while walking four steps.	4. Try any similar combinations according to breathing tolerance of patient.
5. While climbing stairs: a. Inhale through the nose while standing still. b. Exhale through pursed lips while climbing one to two steps. Repeat sequences. c. Stop and rest if short of breath.	

Lower Side Rib Breathing
1. Place hands on sides of lower ribs.
2. Inhale deeply and slowly while sides expand moving hands outward.
3. Exhale slowly through pursed lips and feel the hands and ribs move inward.
4. Rest.

Lower Back and Ribs Breathing
1. Sit in a chair. Place hands behind back; hold flat against lower ribs.
2. Inhale deeply and slowly while rib cage expands backward; the hands will move outward.
3. Keep hands in place. Blow out slowly; hands will move in.

Segmental Breathing
1. Place hands on sides of lower ribs.
2. Inhale deeply and slowly while concentrating on moving the right hand outward by expanding the right rib cage.
3. Ensure that the right hand moves outward more than the left hand.
4. Keeping hands in place, exhale slowly, and feel the right hand and ribs moving in.
5. Repeat, concentrating on expanding left side more than the right side.
6. Rest.

Patient Education
1. Instruct patient to always inhale through the nose. This permits filtration and humidification.
2. Tell patient to breathe slowly in a rhythmic and relaxed manner. This permits more complete exhalation and emptying of lungs; helps overcome anxiety associated with dyspnea and decreases oxygen requirement.
3. Advise patient to avoid sudden exertion.
4. Have patient practice breathing in several positions; air distribution and pulmonary circulation vary according to position of the chest. Practice for 10 breaths four times daily, before meals and at bedtime.
5. Educate patients about complementary therapies for breath control. Include yoga techniques and Qi Gong.
   a. Qi Gong is based on a 4000-year-old practice of breathing using a patient-centered approach from Taoist or Buddhist philosophy in which the individual is a microcosm of the universe.
   b. Qi (pronounced *chee*) is the vital force or energy, and Gong is the discipline, work, or skill. The study of Qi is roughly equivalent to bio-energy or electromagnetic energy, believed to control all functions and behavior. In other cultures, Qi or Chi is described as the soul or vital impulse.
   c. Breathing retraining is timed with movements. Inhaling brings the positive Qi and is usually accompanied with "opening" or "rising" movement. Exhaling releases the negative Qi and accompanies a "closing" or "sinking" movement.
   d. It is believed that respiration includes the skin as well as lungs. The back should be kept straight. The patient should stand firmly or sit so base of spine is aligned with top of head.

PROCEDURE GUIDELINES 10-12   PERCUSSION (CLAPPING) AND VIBRATION

EQUIPMENT

Pillows   Sputum cup
Tilt table   Paper tissues
Emesis basin

PROCEDURE

Nursing Action	Rationale

PERFORMANCE PHASE

1. Instruct the patient to use diaphragmatic breathing.

2. Position the patient in prescribed postural drainage position(s) (p. 222). The spine should be straight to promote rib cage expansion.

1. Diaphragmatic breathing helps the patient relax and helps widen airways.

2. The patient is positioned according to the area of the lung that is to be drained.

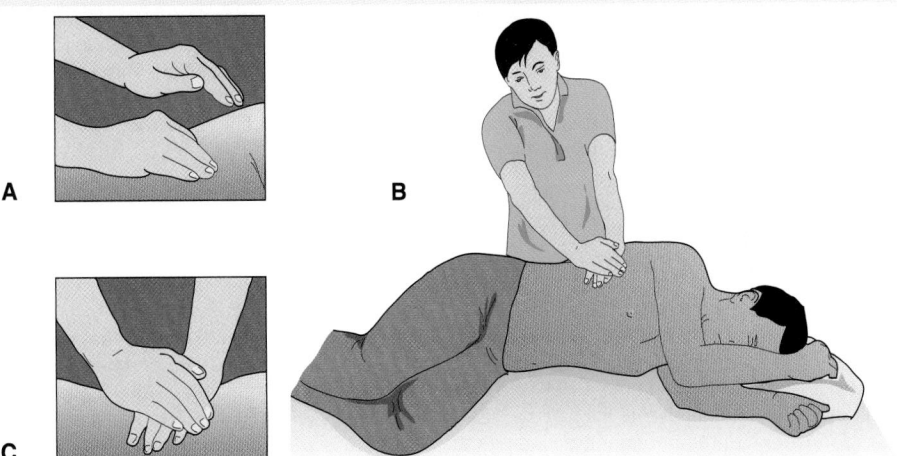

A **B** **C**

Percussion and vibration. (A) Proper hand positioning for percussion. (B) Proper technique for vibration. Note that the wrists and elbows are kept stiff and the vibrating motion is produced by the shoulder muscles. (C) Proper hand position for vibration.

3. Percuss (or clap) with cupped hands over the chest wall for 5 minutes over each segment for cystic fibrosis (or 1 to 2 minutes for other conditions). Work from:
   a. The lower ribs to shoulders in the back.
   b. The lower ribs to top of chest in the front.

4. Avoid clapping over the spine, liver, kidneys, spleen, breast, scapula, clavicle, or sternum.

5. Instruct the patient to inhale slowly and deeply. Vibrate the chest wall as the patient exhales slowly through pursed lips.
   a. Place one hand on top of the other over affected area or place one hand on each side of the rib cage.
   b. Tense the muscles of the hands and arms while applying moderate pressure downward and vibrate hands and arms.
   c. Relieve pressure on the thorax as the patient inhales.
   d. Encourage the patient to cough, using abdominal muscles, after three or four vibrations.

6. Allow the patient to rest several minutes.
7. Listen with a stethoscope for changes in breath sounds.

8. Repeat the percussion and vibration cycle according to the patient's tolerance and clinical response; usually 15 to 30 minutes.

3. This action helps dislodge mucous plugs and mobilize secretions toward the main bronchi and trachea. The air trapped between the operator's hand and chest wall will produce a characteristic hollow sound that resembles the sound of horses trotting.

4. Percussion over these areas may cause injuries to the spine or internal organs.

5. This sets up a vibration that carries through the chest wall and helps free the mucus.

b. This maneuver is performed in the direction in which the ribs move on expiration.

d. Contracting the abdominal muscles while coughing increases cough effectiveness. Coughing aids in the movement and expulsion of secretions.

7. The appearance of crackles and rhonchi indicates movement of air around mucus in the bronchi.

PROCEDURE GUIDELINES 10-13 — ADMINISTERING NEBULIZER THERAPY (SIDESTREAM JET NEBULIZER)

EQUIPMENT

Air compressor Nebulizer
Connection tubing Medication and saline solution

PROCEDURE

Nursing Action	Rationale
PREPARATORY PHASE	
1. Monitor the heart rate before and after the treatment for patients using bronchodilator drugs.	1. Bronchodilators may cause tachycardia, palpitations, dizziness, nausea, or nervousness.
PERFORMANCE PHASE	
1. Explain the procedure to the patient. This therapy depends on patient effort.	1. Proper explanation of the procedure helps to ensure the patient's cooperation and effectiveness of the treatment.
2. Place the patient in a comfortable sitting or a semi-Fowler's position.	2. Diaphragmatic excursion and lung compliance are greater in this position. This ensures maximal distribution and deposition of aerosolized particles to basilar areas of the lungs.
3. Add the prescribed amount of medication and saline to the nebulizer. Connect the tubing to the compressor and set the flow at 6 to 8 L/min.	3. A fine mist from the device should be visible.
4. Instruct the patient to exhale.	
5. Tell the patient to take in a deep breath from the mouthpiece, hold breath briefly, then exhale.	5. This encourages optimal dispersion of the medication.
6. Nose clips are sometimes used if the patient has difficulty breathing only through the mouth.	
7. Observe expansion of chest to ascertain that patient is taking deep breaths.	7. This will ensure that medication is deposited below the level of the oropharynx.
8. Instruct the patient to breathe slowly and deeply until all the medication is nebulized.	8. Medication will usually be nebulized within 15 minutes at a flow of 6 to 8 L/min.
9. On completion of the treatment, encourage the patient to cough after several deep breaths.	9. The medication may dilate airways, facilitating expectoration of secretions.
FOLLOW-UP PHASE	
1. Record medication used and description of secretions.	
2. Disassemble and clean nebulizer after each use. Keep this equipment in the patient's room. The equipment is changed every 24 hours.	
3. Each patient has own breathing circuit (nebulizer, tubing, and mouthpiece). Through proper cleaning, sterilization, and storage of equipment, organisms can be prevented from entering the lungs.	

Administering Oxygen Therapy

Oxygen is an odorless, tasteless, colorless, transparent gas that is slightly heavier than air. It is used to treat or prevent symptoms and manifestations of hypoxia. Oxygen can be dispensed from a cylinder, piped-in system, liquid oxygen reservoir, or oxygen concentrator. It may be administered by nasal cannula, transtracheal catheter, nasal cannula with reservoir devices, or various types of face masks. It may also be applied directly to the endotracheal or tracheal tube by way of a mechanical ventilator, T-piece, or manual resuscitation bag. The method selected depends on the required concentration of oxygen, desired variability in delivered oxygen concentration (none, minimal, moderate), and required ventilatory assistance (mechanical ventilator, spontaneous breathing).

Methods of Oxygen Administration

1. *Nasal cannula* (Procedure Guidelines 10–14)—nasal prongs that deliver low flow of oxygen.
   a. Requires nose breathing.
   b. Cannot deliver oxygen concentrations much higher than 40%.
2. *Simple face mask* (Procedure Guidelines 10–15)— mask that delivers moderate oxygen flow to nose and mouth. Delivers oxygen concentrations of 40% to 60%.

3. *Venturi mask* (Procedure Guidelines 10–16)—mask with device that mixes air and oxygen to deliver constant oxygen concentration.
    a. Total gas flow at the patient's face must meet or exceed peak inspiratory flow rate. When other mask outputs do not meet inspiratory flow rate of patient, room air (drawn through mask side holes) mixes with the gas mixture provided by the face mask, lowering the inspired oxygen concentration.
    b. Venturi mask mixes a fixed flow of oxygen with a high but variable flow of air to produce a constant oxygen concentration. Oxygen enters by way of a jet (restricted opening) at a high velocity. Room air also enters and mixes with oxygen at this site. The higher the velocity (smaller the opening), the more room air is drawn into the mask.
    c. Mask output ranges from approximately 97 L/min (24%) to approximately 33 L/min (50%).
    d. Virtually eliminates rebreathing of carbon dioxide. Excess gas leaves through openings in the mask, carrying with it the expired carbon dioxide.
4. *Partial rebreather mask* (Procedure Guidelines 10–17) has an inflatable bag that stores 100% oxygen.
    a. On inspiration, the patient inhales from the mask and bag; on expiration, the bag refills with oxygen and expired gases exit through perforations on both sides of the mask and some enters bag (Figure 10-5).
    b. High concentrations of oxygen (50% to 75%) can be delivered.
5. *Nonrebreathing mask* (Procedure Guidelines 10–17) has an inflatable bag to store 100% oxygen and a one-way valve between the bag and mask to prevent exhaled air from entering the bag.
    a. Has one-way valves covering one or both the exhalation ports to prevent entry of room air on inspiration.
    b. Has a flap or spring-loaded valves to permit entry of room air should the oxygen source fail or patient needs exceed the available oxygen flow.
    c. Optimally, all the patient's inspiratory volume will be provided by the mask/reservoir, allowing delivery of nearly 100% oxygen.
6. *Transtracheal catheter* (Procedure Guidelines 10–18)—accomplished by way of a small (8F) catheter inserted between the second and third tracheal cartilage.
    a. Does not interfere with talking, drinking, or eating and can be concealed under a shirt or blouse.
    b. Oxygen delivery is more efficient because all oxygen enters the lungs.
7. *Continuous positive airway pressure (CPAP) mask* (Procedure Guidelines 10–19) is used to provide expiratory and inspiratory positive airway pressure in a manner similar to positive end-expiratory pressure (PEEP) and without endotracheal intubation.
    a. Has an inflatable cushion and head strap designed to tightly seal the mask against the face.
    b. A PEEP valve is incorporated into the exhalation port to maintain positive pressure on exhalation.
    c. High inspiratory flow rates are needed to maintain positive pressure on inspiration.
8. *T-piece (Briggs) adapter* (Procedure Guidelines 10–20) is used to administer oxygen to patient with endotracheal or tracheostomy tube who is breathing spontaneously.
    a. High concentration of aerosol and oxygen delivered through wide bore tubing.
    b. Expired gases exit through open reservoir tubing.

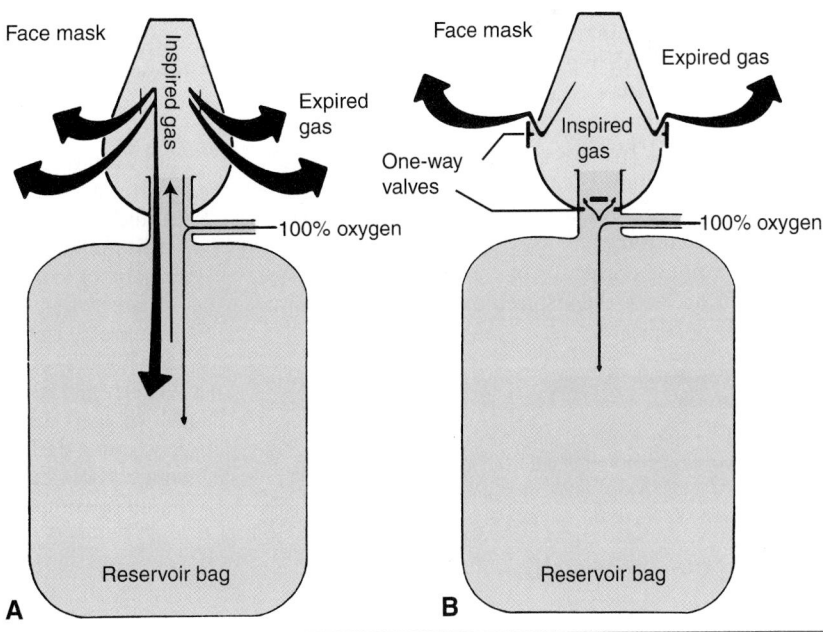

FIGURE 10-5 (A) Air flow diagram with partial rebreathing mask. (B) Air flow diagram with nonrebreathing mask. Arrows indicate direction of flow. (Burton, G. C., & Hodgkin, J. E. [Eds.], [1984]. *Respiratory care: A guide to practice* [2nd ed.]. Philadelphia: J.B. Lippincott.)

9. *Manual resuscitation bag* (Procedure Guidelines 10–21) delivers high concentration of oxygen to patient with insufficient inspiratory effort.
   a. With mask, uses upper airway by delivering oxygen to mouth and nose of patient.
   b. Without mask, adapter fits on endotracheal or tracheostomy tube.
   c. Usually used in cardiopulmonary arrest, hyperinflation during suctioning, or transport of ventilator-dependent patients.

Nursing Assessment and Interventions

1. Assess need for oxygen by observing for symptoms of hypoxia:
   a. Tachypnea
   b. Oxygen saturation <88%
   c. Tachycardia or dysrhythmias (premature ventricular contractions)
   d. A change in level of consciousness (symptoms of decreased cerebral oxygenation are irritability, confusion, lethargy, and coma, if untreated).
   e. Cyanosis occurs as a late sign (PaO_2 ≤45 mm Hg).
   f. Labored respirations indicate severe respiratory distress.
   g. Myocardial stress—increase in heart rate and stroke volume (cardiac output) is the primary mechanism for compensation for hypoxemia or hypoxia; pupils dilate with hypoxia.
2. Obtain ABGs and assess the patient's current oxygenation, ventilation, and acid–base status.
3. Administer oxygen in the appropriate concentration.
   a. Low concentration (24% to 28%)—appropriate for patients prone to retain carbon dioxide (COPD, drug overdose), who are dependent on hypoxemia (hypoxic drive) to maintain respiration. If hypoxemia is suddenly reversed, hypoxic drive may be lost and respiratory arrest may occur.
   b. High concentration (≥30%)—if hypoxemia is suddenly reversed, hypoxic drive may be lost and respiratory arrest may occur. High concentrations are appropriate in patients not predisposed to carbon dioxide retention.
4. Monitor response to therapy by oximetry and/or ABGs.
5. Increase or decrease the inspired oxygen concentration (FiO_2), as appropriate.

NURSING ALERT

All JCAHO-accredited hospitals must be smoke free; however, other health care facilities and homes where oxygen is used may allow smoking. Ensure that no smoking is conducted where oxygen is used.

Community and Home Care Considerations

1. Indications for supplemental oxygen based on Medicare reimbursement guidelines:
   a. Documented hypoxemia: In adults: PaO_2 ≤55 torr or SaO_2 ≤88% when breathing room air, or PaO_2 56 to 59 torr or SaO_2 ≤89% in association with cor pulmonale, CHF, or polycemia with hematocrit >56%.
   b. Some patients may not qualify for oxygen therapy at rest but will qualify for oxygen during ambulation, exercise, or sleep. Oxygen therapy is indicated during these specific activities when SaO_2 is demonstrated to fall to ≤88%.
   c. Determine oxygen prescription for rest, exercise, and sleep, and instruct patient and caregiver to follow these flow rates.
2. Precautions in the home
   a. In COPD with presence of CO_2 retention (generally due to chronic hypoxemia), oxygen administration at higher levels may lead to increased $PaCO_2$ level, and decreased respiratory drive.
   b. Fire hazard is increased in presence of higher than normal oxygen concentrations. Instruct patient and caregiver of home oxygen precautions:
      (i) Post NO SMOKING signs. Instruct in avoidance of cigarettes within 6 feet of oxygen.
      (ii) Avoid potential electrical sparks around oxygen (shave with blade razor instead of electric razor; keep away from heat sources).
      (iii) Keep oxygen at least 6 feet from any source of flame.
   c. Power failure may lead to inadequate oxygen supply when an oxygen concentrator is used without backup tank.
   d. Oxygen tanks must be secured in stand to prevent falling over.
   e. Improper use of liquid oxygen (touching liquid) may result in burns.
3. Oxygen delivered by way of tracheostomy collar or T-tube should be humidified.
4. Oxygen concentrators extract oxygen from ambient air and should deliver oxygen at concentrations of 85% or greater at up to 4 L/min.
5. Liquid oxygen is provided in large reservoir canisters with smaller portable units that can be transfilled by the patient or caregiver. Liquid oxygen evaporates from canister when not in use.
6. Compressed gas may be supplied in large cylinders (G or H cylinders) or smaller cylinders (D or E cylinders) with wheels for easier movement.
7. All oxygen delivery equipment should be checked at least once daily by the patient or caregiver, including function of equipment, prescribed flow rates, remaining liquid or compressed gas content, and backup supply.

(*text continues on page 248*)

PROCEDURE GUIDELINES 10-14	ADMINISTERING OXYGEN BY NASAL CANNULA

EQUIPMENT

Oxygen source
Plastic nasal cannula with connecting
   tubing (disposable)

Humidifier filled with distilled water
Flowmeter
NO SMOKING signs

PROCEDURE

Nursing Action	Rationale

PREPARATORY PHASE

1. Determine current vital signs, level of consciousness, and most recent ABG.

2. Assess risk of CO_2 retention with oxygen administration.

1. Provides a baseline for future assessment. Nasal cannula oxygen administration is often used for patients prone to CO_2 retention. Oxygen may depress the hypoxic drive of these patients (evidenced by a decreased respiratory rate, altered mental status, and further $Paco_2$ elevation).

2. If $Paco_2$ is decreased or normal, the patient is not experiencing CO_2 retention and can use oxygen without fear of the above consequences.

PERFORMANCE PHASE

1. Post NO SMOKING signs on the patient's door and in view of patient and visitors.
2. Show the nasal cannula to the patient and explain the procedure.
3. Make sure the humidifier is filled to the appropriate mark.

4. Attach the connecting tube from the nasal cannula to the humidifier outlet.
5. Set flow rate at prescribed liters/minute. Feel to determine if oxygen is flowing through the tips of the cannula.

3. Humidification may not be ordered if the flow rate is ≤4 L/min.

5. Because a nasal cannula is a low-flow system (patient's tidal volume supplies part of the inspired gas), oxygen concentration will vary, depending on the patient's respiratory rate and tidal volume. Approximate oxygen concentrations delivered are:
   1 L = 24% to 25%
   2 L = 27% to 29%
   3 L = 30% to 33%
   4 L = 33% to 37%
   5 L = 36% to 41%
   6 L = 39% to 45%

6. Place the tips of the cannula in the patient's nose and adjust straps around ears for snug, comfortable fit.

6. Inspect skin behind ears periodically for irritation or breakdown.

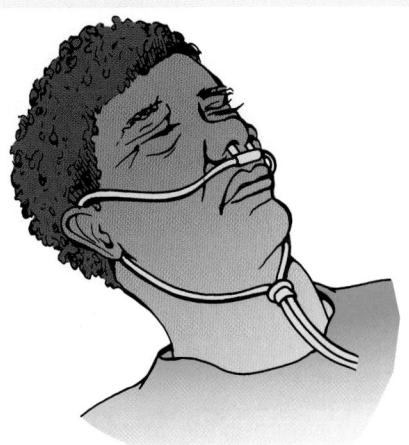

Administering oxygen by nasal cannula. Patient's inspiration consists of a mixture of supplemental oxygen supplied via the nasal cannula and room air. Oxygen concentration is variable and depends on patient's tidal volume and ventilatory pattern.

continued

PROCEDURE GUIDELINES 10-14   ADMINISTERING OXYGEN BY NASAL CANNULA *CONTINUED*

Nursing Action	Rationale
FOLLOW-UP PHASE	
1. Record flow rate used and immediate patient response.	1. Note the patient's tolerance of treatment. Report any intolerance noted.
2. Assess patient's condition, ABG or Sao_2 and the functioning of equipment at regular intervals.	2. Depression of hypoxic drive is most likely to occur within the first hours of oxygen use. Monitoring of Sao_2 with oximetry can be substituted for ABG if the patient is not retaining CO_2.
3. Determine patient comfort with oxygen use.	3. Flow rates in excess of 4 L/min may cause irritation to the nasal and pharyngeal mucosa.

 NURSING ALERT

Avoid use of petroleum jelly to lubricate nares, because it may clog openings of cannula.

PROCEDURE GUIDELINES 10-15   ADMINISTERING OXYGEN BY SIMPLE FACE MASK WITH/WITHOUT AEROSOL

EQUIPMENT

Oxygen source
Humidifier bottle with distilled water, if high humidity is desired

Plastic aerosol mask
Large-bore tubing (high humidity) or small-bore tubing
Flowmeter

NO SMOKING signs
For heated aerosol therapy:
    Humidifier heating element

PROCEDURE

Nursing Action	Rationale
PREPARATORY PHASE	
1. Determine current vital signs, level of consciousness, and Sao_2 or ABG, if patient is at risk for CO_2 retention.	1. Because the nebulizer face mask is a low-flow system (patient's tidal volume may supply part of inspired gas), oxygen concentration will vary depending on the patient's respiratory rate and rhythm. Oxygen delivery may be inadequate for tachypneic patients (flow does not meet peak inspiratory demand) or excessive for patients with slow respirations.
2. Assess viscosity and volume of sputum produced.	2. Aerosol is given to assist in mobilizing retained secretions.
PERFORMANCE PHASE	
1. Post NO SMOKING signs on patient's door and in view of the patient and visitors.	
2. Show the aerosol mask to the patient and explain the procedure.	
3. Make sure the humidifier is filled to the appropriate mark.	3. If the humidifier bottle is not sufficiently full, less moisture will be delivered.
4. Attach the large-bore tubing from the mask to the humidifier in the heating element, if used.	
5. Set desired oxygen concentration humidifier bottle and plug in the heating element, if used.	5. The inspired oxygen concentration is determined by the humidifier setting. Usual concentrations are 35% to 50%.
6. If the patient is tachypneic and concentration of 50% oxygen or greater is desired, two humidifiers and flowmeters should be yoked together.	6. The aerosol mask is a low-flow system. Yoking two humidifiers together doubles humidifier flow but does not change the inspired oxygen concentration.
7. Adjust the flow rate until the desired mist is produced (usually 10 to 12 L/min).	7. This ensures that the patient is receiving flow sufficient to meet inspiratory demand and maintains a constant accurate concentration of oxygen.

PROCEDURE GUIDELINES 10-15   *CONTINUED*

Nursing Action	Rationale

8. Apply the mask to the patient's face and adjust the straps so the mask fits securely.

9. Drain the tubing frequently by emptying condensate into a separate receptacle, not into the humidifier. If a heating element is used, the tubing will have to be drained more often.

    9. The tubing must be kept free of condensate. Condensate allowed to accumulate in the delivery tube will block flow and alter oxygen concentration. If condensate is emptied into the humidifier, bacteria may be aerosolized into the lungs.

10. If a heating element is used, check the temperature. The humidifier bottle should be warm, not hot, to touch.

    10. Excessive temperatures can cause airway burns; patients with elevated temperature should be humidified with an unheated device.

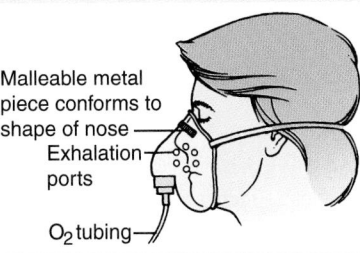

Malleable metal piece conforms to shape of nose
Exhalation ports
O_2 tubing

Simple face mask. Oxygen concentration varies with patient's tidal volume and respiratory rate.

FOLLOW-UP PHASE

1. Record Fio_2 and immediate patient response. Note the patient's tolerance of treatment. Notify the physician if intolerance occurs.

2. Assess the patient's condition and the functioning of equipment at regular intervals.

    2. Assess the patient for change in mental status, diaphoresis, changes in blood pressure, and increasing heart and respiratory rates.

3. If the patient's condition changes, assess Sao_2 or ABG.

    3. If the patient has a high V_E, flow from the mask may not be sufficient to meet inspiratory needs without pulling in room air. Room air will dilute the oxygen provided and lower the inspired oxygen concentration, resulting in hypoxemia. A change in mask or delivery system may be indicated.

4. Record changes in volume and tenacity of sputum produced.

    4. Indicates effectiveness of humidification.

PROCEDURE GUIDELINES 10-16   ADMINISTERING OXYGEN BY VENTURI MASK (HIGH AIR FLOW OXYGEN ENTRAINMENT [HAFOE] SYSTEM)

EQUIPMENT

Oxygen source
Flowmeter
Venturi mask for correct concentration (24%, 28%, 31%, 35%, 40%, 50%) or correct concentration adapter if interchangeable color-coded adapters are used

If high humidity desired:
  Compressed air source and flowmeter
  Humidifier with distilled water
  Large-bore tubing
NO SMOKING signs

PROCEDURE

Nursing Action	Rationale

PREPARATORY PHASE

1. Determine current vital signs, level of consciousness, and most recent ABG.

2. Assess risk of CO_2 retention with oxygen administration.

1. Provides a baseline for future assessment. Venturi masks are used for patients prone to CO_2 retention. Oxygen may depress the hypoxic drive of these patients (evidenced by a decreased respiratory rate, altered mental status, and further $Paco_2$ elevation).

2. Risk is greater if the patient is experiencing an exacerbation of illness.

PERFORMANCE PHASE

1. Post NO SMOKING signs on the door of the patient's room and in view of patient and visitors.
2. Show the Venturi mask to the patient and explain the procedure.
3. Connect the mask by lightweight tubing to the oxygen source.
4. Turn on the oxygen flowmeter and adjust to the prescribed rate (usually indicated on the mask). Check to see that oxygen is flowing out the vent holes in the mask.

5. Place Venturi mask over the patient's nose and mouth and under the chin. Adjust elastic strap.
6. Check to make sure holes for air entry are not obstructed by the patient's bedding.
7. If aerosol nebulizer used:
   a. Connect the humidifier to a compressed air source.
   b. Attach large-bore tubing to the humidifier and connect the tubing to the fitting for high humidity at the base of the Venturi mask.

4. To ensure the correct air/oxygen mix, oxygen must be set at the prescribed flow rate. Prescribed flow rates differ for different oxygen concentrations. Usually this information is printed on the mask or interchangeable color-coded source.

6. Proper mask function depends on mixing of sufficient amount of air and oxygen.
7. When a Venturi mask is used with aerosol, both an oxygen source and compressed air source are required. The compressed air source provides air for the air/oxygen mix. Excessive oxygen would be inspired if both tubings were connected to an oxygen source.

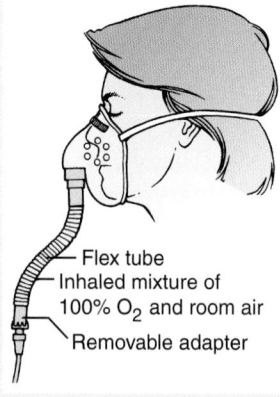

Flex tube
Inhaled mixture of
100% O_2 and room air
Removable adapter

Venturi mask. Constant high concentrations of oxygen can be delivered.

PROCEDURE GUIDELINES 10-16   *CONTINUED*

Nursing Action	Rationale
FOLLOW-UP PHASE	
1. Record flow rate used and immediate patient response. Note the patient's tolerance of treatment. Report if intolerance occurs.	1. Depression of hypoxic drive is most likely to occur within the first hours of oxygen use.
2. If CO_2 retention is present, assess ABG every 30 minutes for 1 to 2 hours or until the Pao_2 is >50 mm Hg and the $Paco_2$ is no longer increasing. Monitor pH. Report if the pH decreases below the initial assessment value.	2. A modest (5 to 10 mm Hg) increase in $Paco_2$ may occur after initiation therapy. A decreasing pH indicates failure of compensatory mechanisms. Mechanical ventilation may be required.
3. Determine patient comfort with oxygen use.	3. Venturi masks are best tolerated for relatively short periods because of their size and appearance. They also must be removed for eating and drinking. With improvement in patient condition, a nasal cannula may often be substituted.

PROCEDURE GUIDELINES 10-17   ADMINISTERING OXYGEN BY PARTIAL REBREATHING OR NONREBREATHING MASK

EQUIPMENT

Oxygen source
Plastic face mask with reservoir bag and tubing
Humidifier with distilled water

Flowmeter
NO SMOKING signs

PROCEDURE

Nursing Action	Rationale
PREPARATORY PHASE	
1. Determine current vital signs, level of consciousness.	1. Provides a baseline for evaluating patient response. Typically used for short-term support of patients who require a high inspired oxygen concentration.
2. Determine most recent Sao_2 or ABG.	2. Allows objective evaluation of patient response.
PERFORMANCE PHASE	
1. Post NO SMOKING signs on the patient's door and in view of the patient and visitors.	
2. Attach tubing to flowmeter.	
3. Show the mask to the patient and explain the procedure.	
4. Flush the reservoir bag with oxygen to inflate the bag and adjust flowmeter to 6 to 10 L/min.	4. Bag serves as a reservoir, holding oxygen for patient inspiration.
5. Place the mask on the patient's face.	5. Be sure the mask fits snugly, because there must be an airtight seal between the mask and the patient's face.
6. Adjust liter flow so the rebreathing bag will not collapse during the inspiratory cycle, even during deep inspiration.	6. With a well-fitting rebreathing bag adjusted so the patient's inhalation does not deflate the bag, inspired oxygen concentration of 60% to 90% can be achieved. Some patients may require flow rates higher than 10 L/min to ensure that the bag does not collapse on inspiration.

NURSING ALERT

1. Adjust the flow to prevent collapse of the bag, even during deep inspiration.
2. A partial rebreathing mask does not have a one-way valve between the mask and reservoir bag. If the bag is allowed to collapse on inspiration, more exhaled air can enter the reservoir and the patient can inhale high concentrations of CO_2.
3. A nonrebreathing mask will deliver a lower concentration of O_2 if the bag is allowed to collapse on inspiration. O_2 from the bag will be diluted by room air drawn in through the side holes of the mask.

continued

PROCEDURE GUIDELINES 10-17 | ADMINISTERING OXYGEN BY PARTIAL REBREATHING OR NONREBREATHING MASK *CONTINUED*

Nursing Action	Rationale
7. Stay with the patient for a time to make the patient comfortable and observe reactions.	
8. Remove mask periodically (if the patient's condition permits) to dry the face around the mask. Apply water-based lotion to skin and massage face around the mask.	8. These actions reduce moisture accumulation under the mask. Massage of the face stimulates circulation and reduces pressure over the area.

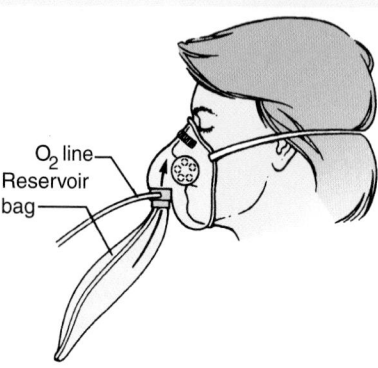

Partial rebreathing mask. 100% oxygen fills bag, but concentration delivered varies with respiration. Nonrebreathing mask is similar with the addition of a one-way valve that prevents expired air from entering bag and one-way flaps over exhalation ports.

FOLLOW-UP PHASE

1. Record flow rate and immediate patient response. Note the patient's tolerance of treatment. Report if intolerance occurs.	
2. Observe the patient for change of condition. Assess equipment for malfunctioning and low water level in humidifier.	2. Assess the patient for change in mental status, diaphoresis, change in blood pressure, and increasing heart and respiratory rates.

 NURSING ALERT

Monitor functioning of mask to ensure that side ports of mask do not get blocked. This could lead to patient inability to exhale and may lead to suffocation.

PROCEDURE GUIDELINES 10-18   ADMINISTERING OXYGEN BY TRANSTRACHEAL CATHETER

EQUIPMENT

Oxygen source
Transtracheal catheter with connecting tubing

Flowmeter
NO SMOKING signs

PROCEDURE

Nursing Action	Rationale
PREPARATORY PHASE	
1. Determine current vital signs, level of consciousness, and ABG, if patient is at risk for CO_2 retention.	1. Provides a baseline for future assessment.
2. Note evidence of infection (warmth, redness, swelling at insertion site) or temperature elevation.	2. The transtracheal catheter provides a direct communication between the skin and trachea. If the insertion site is not kept clean and dry, infection can develop.
3. Assess catheter patency. Obstruction is indicated by a decreased Sao_2, high pressure in the delivery tubing, or stimulation of a cough.	3. Mucus can form on the end of the catheter and restrict oxygen delivery. This increases pressure in the delivery tubing and humidifier. The mucus may touch the back of the trachea, stimulating a cough.
PERFORMANCE PHASE	
Stent Phase	
1. Post NO SMOKING signs on the patient's door and in view of the patient and visitors.	
2. Instruct the patient in purpose of stent.	2. The stent is used to maintain a patent tract during the first week after catheter insertion. It facilitates tract healing and allows gradual adjustment to use of the catheter. It is not used for oxygen delivery.
3. Teach that care of stent involves daily cleaning of the site with cotton-tipped applicators and observation for signs of infection. A 4×4 may be placed over the stent.	3. Until the tract heals, the patient is at increased risk for infection. Because the stent is open to the trachea, mucus may be coughed from the stent.
Immature Tract (Stent is Removed and Transtracheal Catheter Inserted)	
1. Instruct patient in cleaning and irrigation procedure. The patient should inject one half (1.5 mL) ampule of sterile normal saline into the catheter, insert and remove the cleaning rod three times, and inject the remaining sterile normal saline two to three times a day (morning, noon, evening).	1. The catheter cannot be removed from the tract for cleaning until the tract completely heals (about 2 months). Cleaning in place helps to prevent mucus from forming on the end of the catheter and obstructing oxygen delivery.
2. Teach the patient use of the staged cough technique (ie, sit with feet on floor, pillow over abdomen, inhale three to four times in through the nose and out through the mouth, on the last exhalation cough while bending forward with pillow against abdomen.)	2. Use of this cough technique helps to increase airflow during coughing. Higher airflows help to dislodge any mucus that has formed on the outside of the catheter and cannot be removed by the cleaning technique.
3. Instruct the patient to clean the insertion site daily with cotton-tipped applicators and report signs of infection.	3. Mucus may form at the insertion site. Keeping the tract clean and dry decreases infection risk. DO NOT use hydrogen peroxide because it can dry mucous membranes.
4. Teach the patient to place two small strips of transparent tape over the chain on either side of the catheter for the first 2 weeks of catheter use.	4. This helps to keep the catheter in place during the night when the patient is sleeping. Serves as a second security system to keep the catheter from being inadvertently pulled from the tract during the initial adjustment phase.
5. Instruct the patient to replace the nasal cannula and call for instruction if the catheter is displaced from the tract or if symptoms of subcutaneous emphysema develop (swelling at insertion site, tight chain, change in voice).	5. If the catheter comes out of the tract before it is mature, reinsertion may be difficult. If the tract is not completely healed, O_2 may enter the tissues around the insertion site. The patient may need to return to the clinic for assistance in replacing the catheter or delay using it until the tract is fully healed.

continued

PROCEDURE GUIDELINES 10-18 **ADMINISTERING OXYGEN BY TRANSTRACHEAL CATHETER**
CONTINUED

Nursing Action

Rationale

Mature Tract (Catheter is Removed for Cleaning)

1. Instruct the patient in steps involved in removing the tract for cleaning. Two catheters are used. The catheter in the tract is removed and replaced with a second catheter. The catheter removed from the tract is cleaned with antibacterial soap under warm running water. It then is air-dried and stored for reuse.
2. Instruct the patient to report immediately signs of infection and difficulty replacing the catheter.

1. The catheter should easily enter the tract. Practicing while looking in a mirror helps to develop skill in removing and reinserting the catheter. This step should be performed twice daily if a catheter with multiple side holes (SCOOP 2) is used. Removal daily, or less often, is necessary with a single end hole catheter (SCOOP 1).
2. These problems are less common with a mature tract, but can still occur.

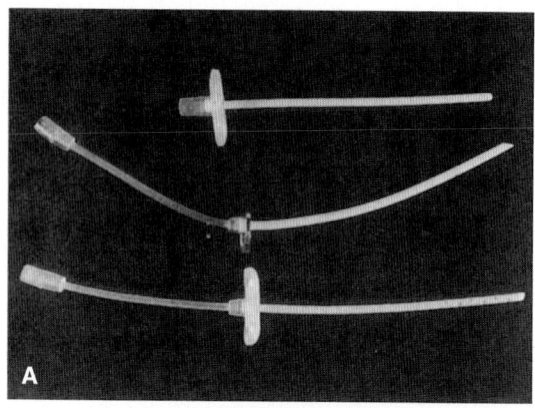
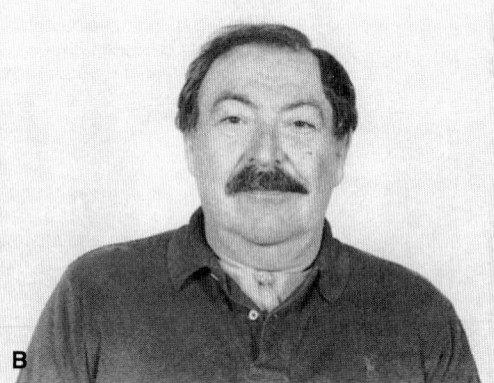
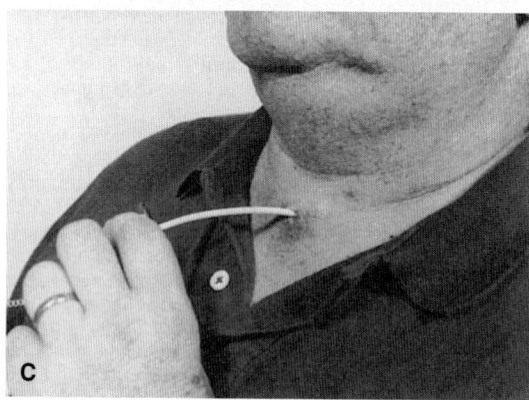
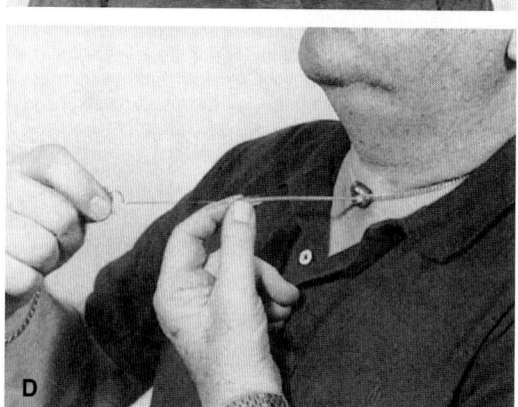

Administering oxygen by transtracheal catheter. *(A) Stent (upper), SCOOP 1 (middle), and SCOOP 2 (lower) catheter. (B) Transtracheal catheter in place. (C) While the tract is immature, the catheter is irrigated and cleaned two or three times a day with a cleaning rod. (D) When the tract is mature, the catheter can be removed from the tract for cleaning. (Courtesy of Medical Media Department, Veterans Administration Medical Center, Pittsburgh, PA.)*

FOLLOW-UP PHASE

1. Record flow rate of oxygen used and patient response.

2. Determine patient ability to perform care independently.

3. Ensure patient is able to demonstrate appropriate use of oxygen and attachment of oxygen to transtracheal catheter.
4. Discuss with patient signs and symptoms of oxygen toxicity and carbon dioxide retention.

1. Transtracheal oxygen delivery is more efficient. The same Sao_2 is typically maintained at one half of the former flow rate.
2. Repeat demonstration of care may be required before the patient masters self-care skills.

4. Too much carbon dioxide retention could lead to confusion, decreased level of consciousness or somnolence.

PROCEDURE GUIDELINES 10-19   **ADMINISTERING OXYGEN BY CONTINUOUS POSITIVE AIRWAY PRESSURE (CPAP) MASK**

EQUIPMENT

Oxygen blender
Flowmeter
CPAP mask
Valve for prescribed PEEP (2.5, 5, 7.5, 10 cm H_2O)
Nebulizer with distilled water

Large-bore tubing
Nasogastric tube (if ordered)
Sealing pad to accommodate nasogastric tube
NO SMOKING signs

PROCEDURE

Nursing Action	Rationale
PREPARATORY PHASE	
1. Assess the patient's level of consciousness and gag reflex.	1. CPAP mask may lead to aspiration unless the patient is breathing spontaneously and is able to protect the airway.
2. Determine current ABGs.	2. Document that patient meets criteria for use of this mask (normal or decreased $Paco_2$ and provides baseline to evaluate whether therapy results in CO_2 retention.

NURSING ALERT

1. CPAP is used when patients have not responded to attempts to increase Pao2 with other types of masks.
2. The patient will require frequent assessment to detect changes in respiratory status, cardiovascular status, and level of consciousness.
3. If the patient's level of consciousness decreases or ABGs deteriorate, intubation may be necessary.

PERFORMANCE PHASE	
1. Post NO SMOKING signs on the patient's door and in view of the patient and visitors.	
2. Show the mask to the patient and explain the procedure.	
3. Make sure nebulizer is filled to the appropriate mark.	
4. Insert nasogastric tube if ordered.	4. With CPAP, the patient may swallow air, causing gastric distention or emesis. Prophylactic nasogastric suction diminishes this risk.

Note: Some clinicians do not believe a nasogastric tube is needed.

5. Attach nasogastric tube adapter.	5. Use of adapter may decrease air leak around the mask.
6. Set desired concentration of oxygen blender and adjust flow rate so it is sufficient to meet the patient's inspiratory demand.	6. O_2 blenders are devices that mix air and O_2 using a proportioning valve. Concentrations of 21% to 100% may be delivered, depending on the model. Because the patient will be receiving all minute ventilation from this "closed system," it is essential that the flow rate be adequate to meet changes in the patient's breathing pattern.
7. Place the mask on the patient's face, adjust the head strap, and inflate the mask cushion to ensure a tight seal.	7. To maintain CPAP, an airtight seal is required. Head straps and the inflatable cushion help to ensure that difficult areas, such as the nose and chin, are sealed with greater comfort to the patient.
8. Organize care to remove the mask as infrequently as possible.	8. If mask is removed (for coughing, suctioning), CPAP is not maintained and inspired oxygen concentrations drop.

continued

PROCEDURE GUIDELINES 10-19   **ADMINISTERING OXYGEN BY CONTINUOUS POSITIVE AIRWAY PRESSURE (CPAP) MASK** *CONTINUED*

Nursing Action   **Rationale**

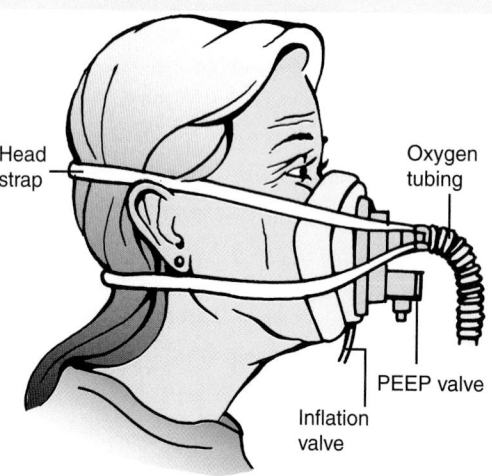

Administering oxygen by face mask with continuous positive airway pressure (CPAP).

FOLLOW-UP PHASE

1. Assess ABGs, hemodynamic status, and level of consciousness frequently.

2. Immediately report any increase in Paco$_2$.

3. Assess patency of nasogastric tube at frequent intervals.
4. Assess patient comfort and functioning of the equipment frequently.

5. Record patient response. With improvement, oxygen therapy without positive airway pressure can be substituted. With deterioration, intubation and mechanical ventilation may be required. Note the patient's tolerance of treatment. Report if intolerance occurs.

1. Provides objective documentation of patient response. CPAP may increase work of breathing, resulting in patient tiring and inability to maintain ventilation without intubation. CPAP may also decrease venous return (PEEP effect), resulting in decreased cardiac output.
2. An increase in Paco$_2$ suggests hypoventilation, resulting from tiring of the patient or inadequate alveolar ventilation. Need for intubation and mechanical ventilation should be evaluated.
3. May become obstructed, causing gastric distention.
4. Tight fit of the mask may predispose to skin breakdown. System may develop leaks, resulting in air escaping between the patient's face and mask.
5. Face mask CPAP is usually continued only for short periods (72 hours) because of patient tiring and the necessity to remove mask for suctioning and coughing.

Note: CPAP may be used as a therapy for sleep apnea only during nighttime hours.

PROCEDURE GUIDELINES 10-20	ADMINISTERING OXYGEN BY WAY OF ENDOTRACHEAL AND TRACHEOSTOMY TUBES WITH A T-PIECE (BRIGGS) ADAPTER

EQUIPMENT

Oxygen
Oxygen blender
Flowmeter

Humidifier with distilled water (heating element may be used as described in aerosol masks)
Large-bore tubing

T-piece and reservoir tubing
NO SMOKING signs

PROCEDURE

Nursing Action	Rationale

PREPARATORY PHASE

1. Assess patient's Sao$_2$, hemodynamic status, and level of consciousness frequently. If patient condition changes, assess ABGs.
2. Assess viscosity and volume of sputum produced.

1. Provides baseline to assess response.

2. Aerosol is given to assist in mobilizing retained secretions.

PERFORMANCE PHASE

1. Post NO SMOKING signs on the patient's door and in view of the patient and visitors.
2. Show the T-tube to the patient and explain the procedure.
3. Make sure the humidifier is filled to the appropriate mark.
4. Attach the large-bore tubing from the T-tube to the humidifier outlet.
5. Set desired oxygen concentration of O$_2$ blender or humidifier bottle and plug in heating element if used.

6. Adjust the flow rate until the desired mist is produced and meets the patient's inspiratory demand.

7. Drain the tubing frequently by emptying condensate into a separate receptacle, not into the humidifier. If a heating element is used, the tubing will have to be drained more often.

8. If a heating element is used, check the temperature. The humidifier bottle should be warm, not hot, to touch.

3. If humidifier is not sufficiently full, less aerosol will be delivered.

5. O$_2$ blenders are devices that mix air and O$_2$ using a proportioning valve. Concentrations of 21% to 100% may be delivered at flows of 2 to 100 L/min, depending on the model. Used when precise control is required.

6. The aerosol mist in the reservoir tubing attached to the T-tube should not be completely withdrawn on patient inspiration. If mist is withdrawn (does not extend from reservoir tubing) on inspiration, room air may be inspired and O$_2$ concentration decreased.

7. The tubing must be kept free of condensate. Condensate allowed to accumulate in the delivery tube will block flow and alter oxygen concentration. If condensate is emptied into the humidifier, bacteria may be aerosolized into the lungs.

8. Excessive temperatures can cause airway burns; patients with elevated temperatures will be better humidified with an unheated device.

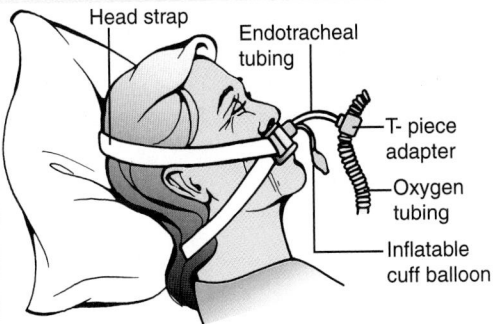

Administering oxygen via endotracheal tube with a T-piece adapter. A T-piece adapter is attached to the endotracheal tube and large-bore tubing, which serves as a source of oxygen and humidity.

continued

| PROCEDURE GUIDELINES 10-20 | ADMINISTERING OXYGEN BY WAY OF ENDOTRACHEAL AND TRACHEOSTOMY TUBES WITH A T-PIECE (BRIGGS) ADAPTER *CONTINUED* |

Nursing Action	Rationale

FOLLOW-UP PHASE

1. Record Fio_2 and immediate patient response. Note the patient's tolerance of treatment. Report if intolerance occurs.

2. Assess the patient's condition and the functioning of equipment at regular intervals.

2. Assess the patient for change in mental status, diaphoresis, perspiration, changes in blood pressure, and increasing heart and respiratory rates.

3. If the patient's condition changes, assess Sao_2 or ABGs and vital signs. Note changes suggesting increased work of breathing (diaphoresis, intercostal muscle retraction).

3. If the patient is being weaned, return to the ventilator if changes suggesting inability to tolerate spontaneous ventilation occur (see Weaning the Patient From Mechanical Ventilation, p. 255).

4. Record changes in volume and tenacity of sputum produced.

4. Indicates effectiveness of humidification therapy.

| PROCEDURE GUIDELINES 10-21 | ADMINISTERING OXYGEN BY MANUAL RESUSCITATION BAG |

EQUIPMENT

Oxygen source
Resuscitation bag and mask
Reservoir tubing or reservoir bag
O_2 connecting tubing

Nipple adapter to attach flowmeter to connecting tubing
Flowmeter
Gloves
Face shield

PROCEDURE

Nursing Action	Rationale

PREPARATORY PHASE

1. In cardiopulmonary arrest:
   a. Follow steps to establish that a cardiopulmonary arrest has occurred.

1.
   a. These steps are: establish unresponsiveness; call for help; position the patient on a firm, flat surface; open the mouth and remove vomitus or debris, if visible; assess presence of respirations with the airway open; if apneic, ventilate; palpate the carotid pulse; if absent, deliver chest compressions.

   b. Use caution not to injure or increase injury to the cervical spine when opening the airway.

   b. If cervical spine injury is a potential, the modified jaw thrust should be used. In other situations, the head-tilt/chin-lift method can be used. These maneuvers lift the tongue off the back of the throat and, in some situations, may be all that is needed to restore breathing.

2. In suctioning or transport situation, assess patient's heart rate, level of consciousness, and respiratory status.

2. Provides a baseline to stimulate patient's tolerance of procedure.

PERFORMANCE PHASE

1. Attach connecting tubing from flowmeter and nipple adapter to resuscitation bag.

1. A humidifier bottle is not used, because the high flow rates of oxygen required would force water into the tubing and clog it.

2. Turn flowmeter to "flush" position.

2. A high flow rate or "flush" position is necessary to meet the minute ventilation of the patient.

3. Attach reservoir tubing or reservoir bag to resuscitation bag.

3. A high inspired O_2 concentration is required. Without a reservoir, inspired O_2 concentration will be low (28% to 56%), because inspired gas will be air/O_2 mix. With a reservoir, manual resuscitation bags can achieve a Fio_2 of >96% at a flow rate of 15 L/min.

4. Put on face shield and gloves.

PROCEDURE GUIDELINES 10-21   *CONTINUED*

Nursing Action	Rationale

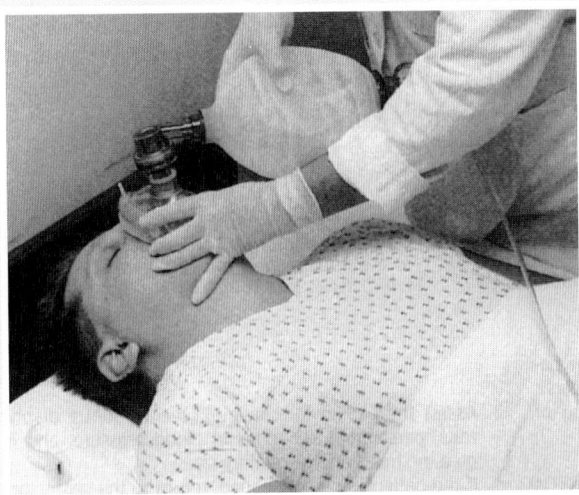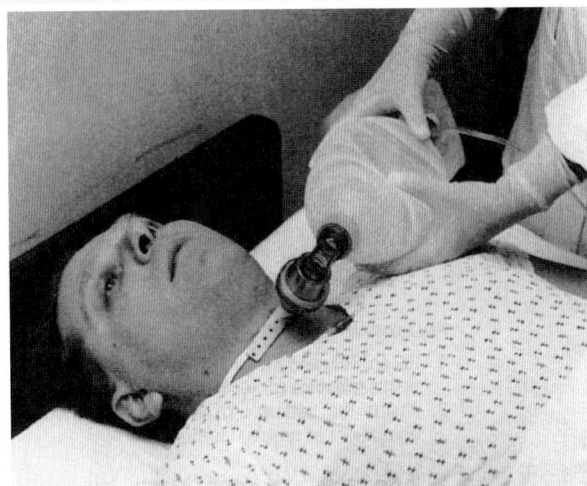

Using a manual resuscitation bag, with mask (left) or connected to an artificial airway (right).

 NURSING ALERT   Ensure that good seal is maintained between face and mask so volume delivered through compression of bag is not lost.

Cardiopulmonary Arrest

1. If respirations are absent after the airway is open, insert an oropharyngeal airway and ventilate twice with slow, full breaths of 1 to 1.5 seconds each. Allow 2 seconds between breaths.

1. The airway helps prevent obstruction from prolapse of the tongue in an unconscious patient. If ventilation is difficult, confirm that airway is unobstructed.

 NURSING ALERT   Airways are not appropriate in a conscious patient or patients with a gag reflex because stimulation of the oropharynx could cause vomiting and aspiration. Short nasal pumps can be used in conscious patients with a gag reflex.

2. Breaths will have to be quickly interposed between cardiac compressions. If the patient needs only respiratory assistance, watch for chest expansion and listen with the stethoscope to ensure adequate ventilation.

3. A rate of approximately 12 to 15 breaths per minute is used unless the patient is being given external cardiac compressions.

2. Squeeze resuscitation bag with sufficient force and at the rate necessary to maintain adequate minute ventilation.

3. Continue squeezing bag at appropriate interval until CPR is no longer required.

Preoxygenation and Suctioning

1. If hyperinflation is being used with suctioning, ventilate the patient before and after each suctioning pass (including after the last suction pass).

1. Hyperinflation before suctioning helps prevent hypoxemia. Hyperinflation after suctioning replaces O_2 removed during the procedure and helps to prevent atelectasis. The larger tidal volumes may also assist in mobilizing secretions and promote surfactant secretion.

continued

PROCEDURE GUIDELINES 10-21	ADMINISTERING OXYGEN BY MANUAL RESUSCITATION BAG *CONTINUED*

Nursing Action	Rationale
Transport	
1. If hyperinflation is used in transport, suction patient before disconnection for transport; monitor heart and respiratory rates and level of consciousness during procedure.	1. Establishes a patent airway before patient is moved. Provides information for assessing tolerance of transport.
2. Ventilate at rate of 12 to 15 breaths per minute.	
FOLLOW-UP PHASE	
1. In cardiopulmonary arrest, verify return of spontaneous pulse and respirations. Initiate further support as needed.	1. Establishes patient's need for definitive therapy (drugs, defibrillation, intensive care).
2. In suctioning or transport, return to previous support. Note patient tolerance of procedure.	2. Note Sao_2, heart rate, rate and ease of respirations, arterial blood pressure (if monitored), level of consciousness. Report if intolerance occurs.

Mechanical Ventilation

The mechanical ventilator device functions as a substitute for the bellows action of the thoracic cage and diaphragm. The mechanical ventilator can maintain ventilation automatically for prolonged periods. It is indicated when the patient is unable to maintain safe levels of oxygen or carbon dioxide by spontaneous breathing even with the assistance of other oxygen delivery devices.

Clinical Indications
Mechanical Failure of Ventilation
1. Neuromuscular disease
2. Central nervous system disease
3. Central nervous system depression (drug intoxication, respiratory depressants, cardiac arrest)
4. Musculoskeletal disease
5. Inefficiency of thoracic cage in generating pressure gradients necessary for ventilation (chest injury, thoracic malformation)

Disorders of Pulmonary Gas Exchange
1. Acute respiratory failure
2. Chronic respiratory failure
3. Left ventricular failure
4. Pulmonary diseases resulting in diffusion abnormality
5. Pulmonary diseases resulting in ventilation–perfusion mismatch

Underlying Principles
1. Variables that control ventilation and oxygenation include:
   a. Ventilator rate—adjusted by rate setting
   b. Tidal volume (VT)—adjusted by tidal volume setting; measured as inhaled volume
   c. Fraction inspired oxygen concentration (Fio_2)—set on ventilator or with an oxygen blender; measured with an oxygen analyzer
   d. Ventilator dead space—circuitry (tubing) common to inhalation and exhalation; tubing is calibrated
   e. PEEP—positive end-expiratory pressure; set within the ventilator or with the use of external PEEP devices; measured at the proximal airway
2. CO_2 elimination is controlled by tidal volume, rate, and dead space.
3. Oxygen tension is controlled by oxygen concentration and PEEP (also by rate and tidal volume).
4. In most cases, the duration of inspiration should not exceed exhalation.
   a. Rate, tidal volume, gas flow in liters per minute, and inspiratory pause all control inspiratory time.
   b. Inverse inspiration:exhalation (I:E) ratio results in "stacking" of breaths or buildup of pressure within the airway. Barotrauma and decreased cardiac output can result when inverse I:E ratio is used.
5. The inspired gas must be warmed and humidified to prevent thickening of secretions and decrease in body temperature. Sterile or distilled water is warmed and humidified by way of a heated humidifier.

Types of Ventilators
Negative Pressure Ventilators
1. Applies negative pressure around the chest wall. This causes intra-airway pressure to become negative, thus drawing air into the lungs through the patient's nose and mouth.
2. No artificial airway is necessary; patient must be able to control and protect own airway.
3. Indicated for selected patients with respiratory neuromuscular problems, or as adjunct to weaning from positive pressure ventilation.
4. Examples are the iron lung and cuirass ventilator.

Positive Pressure Ventilators
During mechanical inspiration, air is actively delivered to the patient's lungs under positive pressure. Exhalation is passive. Requires use of a cuffed artificial airway.
1. Pressure limited
   a. Terminates the inspiratory phase when a preselected airway pressure is achieved.

b. Volume delivered depends on lung compliance.

c. Use of volume-based alarms is recommended because any obstruction between the machine and lungs that allows a buildup of pressure in the ventilator circuitry will cause the ventilator to cycle, but the patient will receive no volume.

2. Volume limited

a. Terminates the inspiratory phase when a designated volume of gas is delivered into the ventilator circuit (10 to 15 mL/kg body weight—usual starting volume).

b. Delivers the predetermined volume regardless of changing lung compliance (although airway pressures will increase as compliance decreases). Airway pressures vary from patient to patient and from breath to breath.

c. Pressure-limiting valves, which prevent excessive pressure buildup within the patient-ventilator system, are used. Without this valve, pressure could increase indefinitely and pulmonary barotrauma could result. Usually equipped with a system that alarms when selected pressure limit is exceeded. Pressure-limited settings terminate inspiration when reached.

Modes of Operation

Controlled Ventilation (CV)

1. Cycles automatically at rate selected by operator.

2. Provides a fixed level of ventilation, but will not cycle or have gas available in circuitry to respond to patient's own inspiratory efforts. This typically increases work of breathing for patients attempting to breathe spontaneously.

3. Possibly indicated for patients whose respiratory drive is absent.

Assist/Control (A/C)

1. Inspiratory cycle of ventilator is activated by the patient's voluntary inspiratory effort and delivers preset volume or pressure.

2. Ventilator also cycles at a rate predetermined by the operator. Should the patient stop breathing, or breathe so weakly that the ventilator cannot function as an assistor, this mandatory baseline rate will prevent apnea. A minimum respiratory rate is provided.

3. Indicated for patients who are breathing spontaneously, but who have the potential to lose their respiratory drive or muscular control of ventilation. In this mode, the patient's work of breathing is greatly reduced.

Intermittent Mandatory Ventilation (IMV)

1. Allows patient to breathe spontaneously through ventilator circuitry.

2. Periodically, at preselected rate and volume or pressure, cycles to give a "mandated" ventilator breath. A minimum level of ventilation is provided.

3. Gas provided for spontaneous breaths usually flows continuously through the ventilator.

4. Indicated for patients who are breathing spontaneously, but at a tidal volume and/or rate less than adequate for their needs. Allows the patient to do some of the work of breathing.

Synchronized Intermittent Mandatory Ventilation (SIMV)

1. Allows patient to breathe spontaneously through the ventilator circuitry.

2. Periodically, at a preselected time, a mandatory breath is delivered. The patient may initiate the mandatory breath with own inspiratory effort, and the ventilator breath will be synchronized with the patient's efforts, or will be "assisted." If the patient does not provide inspiratory effort, the breath will still be delivered, or "controlled."

3. Gas provided for spontaneous breathing is usually delivered through a demand regulator, which is activated by the patient.

4. Indicated for patients who are breathing spontaneously, but at a tidal volume and/or rate less than adequate for their needs. Allows the patient to do some of the work of breathing.

Pressure Support

1. A positive pressure is set.

2. During spontaneous inspiration, ventilator circuitry is rapidly pressurized to the predetermined pressure and held at this pressure.

3. When the inspiratory flow rate decreases to a preset minimal level (20% to 25% or peak inspiratory flow), the positive pressure returns to baseline and the patient may exhale.

4. The patient ventilates spontaneously, establishing own rate, and inspiring the tidal volume that feels appropriate.

5. Pressure support may be used independently as a ventilatory mode or used in conjunction with CPAP or SIMV.

Special Positive Pressure Ventilation Techniques

Positive End-Expiratory Pressure (PEEP)

1. Maneuver by which pressure during mechanical ventilation is maintained above atmospheric at end of exhalation, resulting in an increased functional residual capacity. Airway pressure is therefore positive throughout the entire ventilatory cycle.

2. Purpose is to increase functional residual capacity (or the amount of air left in the lungs at the end of expiration). This aids in:

a. Increasing the surface area of gas exchange

b. Preventing collapse of alveolar units and development of atelectasis

c. Decreasing intrapulmonary shunt

3. Benefits

a. Because a greater surface area for diffusion is available and shunting is reduced, it is often possible to use a lower fraction of inspired oxygen concentration (FIO_2) than otherwise would be required to obtain adequate arterial oxygen levels. This reduces the risk of oxygen toxicity in conditions such as adult respiratory distress syndrome (ARDS).

b. Positive intra-airway pressure may be helpful in reducing the transudation of fluid from the pulmonary capillaries in situations where capillary pressure is increased (ie, left heart failure).

c. Increased lung compliance resulting in decreased work of breathing.

4. Hazards

a. Because the mean airway pressure is increased by PEEP, venous return is impeded. This may result in a decrease in cardiac output (especially noted in hypovolemic patients).

b. There is disagreement that the increased airway pressure may possibly result in alveolar rupture. The likelihood of damage is greater from peak airway pressure during mechanical ventilation than end-expiratory pressure. The likelihood is greater in patients with noncompliant lungs. This barotrauma may result in pneumothorax, tension pneumothorax, or development of subcutaneous emphysema.

c. The decreased venous return may cause antidiuretic hormone formation to be stimulated, resulting in decreased urine output.

5. Precautions

a. Monitor frequently for signs and symptoms of pneumothorax (increased pulmonary artery pressure, increased size of hemothorax, decreased lung movement, hyperresonant percussion, diminished breath sounds).

b. Monitor for signs of decreased venous return (decreased blood pressure, decreased cardiac output, decreased urine output, peripheral edema).

c. Abrupt discontinuance of PEEP is not recommended. The patient should not be without PEEP for longer than 15 seconds. The manual resuscitation bag used for ventilation during suction procedure or patient transport should be equipped with a PEEP device. In-line suctioning may also be used so PEEP can be maintained. Some clinicians believe that loss of PEEP for short periods is not detrimental in the lower ranges (less than 10 cm H_2O). An exception might be patients with increased intracranial pressure.

d. Intrapulmonary blood vessel pressure may increase with compression of the vessels by increased intra-airway pressure. Therefore, central venous pressure (CVP), pulmonary artery pressure (PAP), and pulmonary capillary wedge pressure (PCWP) may be increased. The clinician must bear this in mind when determining the clinical significance of these pressures.

Continuous Positive Airway Pressure (CPAP)

1. Also provides for positive airway pressure during all parts of a respiratory cycle, but refers to spontaneous ventilation rather than mechanical ventilation.

2. May be delivered through ventilator circuitry when ventilator rate is at "0" or may be delivered through a separate CPAP circuitry that does not require the ventilator.

3. Indicated for patients who are capable of maintaining an adequate tidal volume, but who have pathology preventing maintenance of adequate levels of tissue oxygenation or for sleep apnea.

4. CPAP has the same benefits, hazards, and precautions noted with PEEP. Mean airway pressures may be lower because of lack of mechanical ventilation breaths. This results in less risk of barotrauma and impedance of venous return.

Newer Modes of Ventilation
Inverse Ratio Ventilation (IRV)

1. I:E ratio is greater than 1 (normally, inspiration is shorter than expiration).

2. Potentially used in patients who are in acute severe hypoxemic respiratory failure. Oxygenation is thought to be improved.

3. Used with heavily sedated patients.

Noninvasive Positive Pressure Ventilation (NIPPV)

1. Uses a nasal mask, nasal pillow, oral mask, or mouthpiece attached to a standard ventilator. Delivers air through portable ventilator that is either volume cycled or flow cycled.

2. Used primarily in the past for patients with chronic respiratory failure associated with neuromuscular disease. Now, is being used successfully during acute exacerbations. Some patients are able to avoid invasive intubation. Other indications include weaning and post-extubation respiratory decompensation. Most successful with COPD.

3. Used easily in home setting. Equipment is portable and relatively easy to use.

4. May include BiPAP (bilevel positive airway pressure), which is essentially pressure support with CPAP. The system has a rate setting, as well as inspiratory and expiratory pressure setting.

High-Frequency Ventilation (HFV)

1. Uses very small tidal volumes (less than dead space volume) and high frequency (ratios greater than 100).

2. Gas exchange occurs through various mechanisms, not the same as conventional ventilation (convection).

3. Types
   a. High-frequency oscillatory ventilation (HFOV)
   b. High-frequency jet ventilation (HFJV)

4. Theory is that there is decreased barotrauma by having small tidal volumes and that oxygenation is improved by constant flow of gases.

5. Successful with IRDS (infant respiratory distress syndrome), much less successful with adult pulmonary complications.

Nursing Assessment and Interventions

1. Monitor for complications.

a. Airway obstruction (thickened secretions, mechanical problem with artificial airway or ventilator circuitry)
b. Tracheal damage
c. Pulmonary infection
d. Barotrauma (pneumothorax or tension pneumothorax)
e. Decreased cardiac output
f. Atelectasis
g. Alteration in GI function (dilation, bleeding)
h. Alteration in renal function
i. Alteration in cognitive-perceptual status
j. Respiratory acidosis or alkalosis
2. Suction the patient as indicated.
   a. When secretions can be seen or sounds resulting from secretions are heard with or without the use of a stethoscope
   b. After chest physiotherapy
   c. After bronchodilator treatments
   d. After a sudden rise or the "popping off" of the peak airway pressure in mechanically ventilated patients that is not due to the artificial airway or ventilator tube kinking, the patient biting the tube, the patient coughing or struggling against the ventilator, or a pneumothorax
3. Provide routine care for patient on mechanical ventilator (Procedure Guidelines 10-22).
4. Assist with the weaning process, when indicated (patient gradually assumes responsibility for regulating and performing own ventilations; Procedure Guidelines 10-23).
   a. Patient must have acceptable ABGs, no evidence of acute pulmonary pathology, and must be hemodynamically stable.
   b. Obtain serial ABGs and/or oximetry readings, as indicated.
   c. Monitor very closely for change in pulse and blood pressure, anxiety, and increased rate of respirations.
   d. The use of anxiolytics to assist with weaning the anxious patient is controversial; they may or may not be beneficial.
5. Once weaning is successful, extubate and provide alternate means of oxygen (Procedure Guidelines 10-24).
6. Extubation will be considered when the pulmonary function parameters of tidal volume (VT), vital capacity (VC), and negative inspiratory force (NIF) are adequate, indicating strong respiratory muscle function.

Community and Home Care Considerations

Patients may require mechanical ventilation at home to replace or assist normal breathing. Ventilator support in the home is used to keep the patient clinically stable and to maintain life.

1. Candidates for home ventilation are those patients who are unable to wean from mechanical ventilation, and/or have disease progression requiring ventilator support. Candidates for home mechanical ventilator support:

a. Require a tracheostomy tube.
b. No longer require intensive medical monitoring and services.
2. Patients may choose not to receive home ventilation. Examples of inappropriate candidates for home ventilation include patients who:
   a. Have FIO_2 requirement >0.40.
   b. PEEP >10 cm H_2O.
   c. Continuous invasive monitoring.
   d. Lack a mature tracheostomy.
   e. Lack able, willing, appropriate caregivers, and/or caregiver respite.
   f. Lack adequate financial resources for care in home.
   g. Lack adequate physical facilities:
      (i) Inadequate heat, electricity, sanitation
      (ii) Presence of fire, health, or safety hazards
3. For patients on mechanical ventilation in the home. a contract and relationship with a home medical equipment company must be developed to provide:
   a. Care of ventilator-dependent patient.
   b. Provision and maintenance of equipment.
   c. Timely provision of disposable supplies.
   d. Ongoing monitoring of patient and equipment.
   e. Training of patient, caregivers, and clinical staff on proper management of ventilated patient and use and troubleshooting of equipment.
4. Equipment required:
   a. Appropriate ventilator with alarms (disconnect and high pressure).
   b. Power source.
   c. Humidification system.
   d. Self-inflating resuscitation bag with tracheostomy adapter.
   e. Replacement tracheostomy tubes.
   f. Supplemental oxygen, as medically indicated.
   g. Communication method for patient.
   h. Backup charged battery to run ventilator during power failures.
5. Lay caregiver training and return demonstration must include:
   a. Proper setup, use, trouble shooting, maintenance, and cleaning of equipment and supplies.
   b. Appropriate patient assessment and management of abnormalities, including response to emergencies, power and equipment failure.
6. Potential complications include:
   a. Patient deterioration, need for emergency services.
   b. Equipment failure, malfunction.
   c. Psychosocial complications, including depression, anxiety, and/or loss of resources (caregiver, financial, detrimental change in family structure or coping capacity).
7. Communication is essential with local fire and utility companies from whom patient would need immediate and additional assistance in event of emergency (eg, power failure, fire).

(*text continues on page 259*)

PROCEDURE GUIDELINES 10-22	MANAGING THE PATIENT REQUIRING MECHANICAL VENTILATION

EQUIPMENT

Artificial airway
Mechanical ventilator
Ventilation circuitry

Humidifier
See manufacturer's directions for specific machine.

PROCEDURE

Nursing Action	Rationale

PREPARATORY PHASE

1. Obtain baseline samples for blood gas determinations (pH, Pao_2 $Paco_2$ HCO_3) and chest x-ray.

1. Baseline measurements serve as a guide in determining progress of therapy.

PERFORMANCE PHASE

1. Give a brief explanation to the patient.

2. Establish the airway by means of a cuffed endotracheal or tracheostomy tube (see p. 212).
3. Prepare the ventilator. (Respiratory therapist does this in many institutions.)
   a. Set up desired circuitry.
   b. Connect oxygen and compressed air source.
   c. Turn on power.
   d. Set tidal volume (usually 10 to 15 mL/kg body weight) or peak pressure.
   e. Set oxygen concentration.
   f. Set ventilator sensitivity.
   g. Set rate at 12 to 14 breaths per minute (variable).

   h. Adjust flow rate (velocity of gas flow during inspiration). Usually set at 40 to 60 L/min. Depends on rate and tidal volume. Set to avoid inverse inspiratory:expiratory (I:E) ratio. Usual I:E ratio is 1:2.

   i. Select mode of ventilation.
   j. Check machine function—measure tidal volume, rate, I:E ratio, analyze oxygen, check all alarms.
4. Couple the patient's airway to the ventilator.

5. Assess patient for adequate chest movement and rate. Note peak airway pressure and PEEP. Adjust gas flow if necessary to provide safe I:E ratio.
6. Set airway pressure alarms according to patient's baseline:
   a. High pressure alarm

1. Emphasize that mechanical ventilation is a temporary measure. The patient should be prepared psychologically for weaning at the time the ventilator is first used.
2. A closed system between the ventilator and patient lower airway is necessary for positive pressure ventilation.

   d. Adjusted according to pH and $Paco_2$.

   e. Adjusted according to Pao_2.

   g. This setting approximates normal ventilation. These machines' settings are subject to change according to the patient's condition and response, and the ventilator type being used.
   h. The slower the flow, the lower the peak airway pressure will result from set volume delivery. This results in lower intrathoracic pressure and less impedance of venous return. However, a flow that is too low for the rate selected may result in inverse inspiratory: expiratory ratios.

   j. Ensures safe function.
4. Be sure all connections are secure. Prevent ventilator tubing from "pulling" on artificial airway, possibly resulting in tube dislodgement or tracheal damage.
5. Ensures proper function of equipment.

6.

   a. High airway pressure or "pop off" pressure is set at about 20 cm H_2O above peak airway pressure. An alarm sounds if airway pressure selected is exceeded. Alarm activation indicates decreased lung compliance (worsening pulmonary disease); decreased lung volume (such as pneumothorax, tension pneumothorax, hemothorax, pleural effusion); increased airway resistance (secretions, coughing, breathing out of phase with the ventilator); loss of patency of airway (mucous plug, airway spasm, biting or kinking of tube).

Nursing Action	Rationale
b. Low pressure alarm	b. Low airway pressure alarm set at 5 to 10 cm H_2O below peak airway pressure. Alarm activation indicates inability to build up airway pressure because of disconnection or leak, or inability to build up airway pressure because of insufficient gas flow to meet patient's inspiratory needs.
7. Assess frequently for change in respiratory status by way of ABGs, pulse oximetry, spontaneous rate, use of accessory muscles, breath sounds, and vital signs. Other means of assessing are through the use of exhaled carbon dioxide (see sections titled Capnography, p. 207 or mixed venous oxygen saturation monitoring, p. 326). If change is noted, notify appropriate personnel.	
8. Monitor and troubleshoot alarm conditions. Ensure appropriate ventilation at all times.	8. Priority is ventilation and oxygenation of the patient. In alarm conditions that cannot be immediately corrected, disconnect the patient from mechanical ventilation and manually ventilate with resuscitation bag.
9. Positioning	9.
a. Turn patient from side to side every 2 hours, or more frequently if possible. Consider continuous lateral rotational therapy (CLRT) as early intervention to improve outcome.	a. For patients on long-term ventilation, this may result in sleep deprivation. Evolve a turning schedule best suited to a particular patient's condition.
b. Lateral turns are desirable; from right semiprone to left semiprone.	
c. Sit the patient upright at regular intervals if possible.	c. Upright posture increases lung compliance.
d. Consider prone positioning to improve oxygenation.	d. Proning has been shown to have some beneficial affects or the improvement of oxygenation in certain populations, such as patients with ARDS.

 NURSING ALERT **For patients in severe compromised respiratory state or who are unstable hemodynamically, consider use of specialty bed with rotational therapy. New versions may also have built-in vibration and percussion as adjunct therapy options.**

10. Carry out passive range-of-motion exercises of all extremities for patients unable to do so.	
11. Assess for need of suctioning at least every 2 hours.	11. Patients with artificial airways on mechanical ventilation are unable to clear secretions on their own. Suctioning may help to clear secretions and stimulate the cough reflex.
12. Assess breath sounds every 2 hours:	12.
a. Listen with stethoscope to the chest from bottom to top on both sides.	a. Auscultation of the chest is a means of assessing airway patency and ventilatory distribution. It also confirms the proper placement of the endotracheal or tracheostomy tube.
b. Determine whether breath sounds are present or absent, normal or abnormal, and whether a change has occurred.	
c. Observe the patient's diaphragmatic excursions and use of accessory muscles of respiration.	
13. Humidification	13.
a. Check the water level in the humidification reservoir to ensure that the patient is never ventilated with dry gas. Empty the water that condenses in the delivery and exhalation tubing into a separate receptacle, not	a. Water condensing in the inspiratory tubing may cause increased resistance to gas flow. This may result in increased peak airway pressures. Warm, moist tubing is a perfect breeding area for bacteria. If this water is

continued

PROCEDURE GUIDELINES 10-22   MANAGING THE PATIENT REQUIRING MECHANICAL VENTILATION *CONTINUED*

Nursing Action	Rationale
into the humidifier. Always wash hands after emptying fluid from ventilator circuitry. Humidification may also be achieved using a moisture enhancer.	allowed to enter the humidifier, bacteria may be aerosolized into the lungs. Emptying the tubing also prevents introduction of water into the patient's airways.
14. Assess airway pressures at frequent intervals.	14. Monitor for changes in compliance, or onset of conditions that may cause airway pressure to increase or decrease.
15. Measure delivered tidal volume and analyze oxygen concentration every 4 hours or more frequently if indicated.	

16. Monitor cardiovascular function. Assess for depression.
  a. Monitor pulse rate and arterial blood pressure; intra-arterial pressure monitoring may be carried out.
  b. Use pulmonary artery catheter to monitor pulmonary capillary wedge pressure (PCWP) mixed venous oxygen (SvO_2) and cardiac output (CO).
	16.
	  a. Arterial catheterization for intra-arterial pressure monitoring also provides access for ABG samples.
	  b. Intermittent and continuous positive pressure ventilation may increase the pulmonary artery pressures and decrease cardiac output.

17. Monitor for pulmonary infection.
  a. Aspirate tracheal secretions into a sterile container and send to laboratory for culture and sensitivity testing. This is done immediately after endotracheal intubation and in some instances on clinical assessment.
  b. Monitor for systemic signs and symptoms of pulmonary infection (pulmonary physical examination findings, increased heart rate, increased temperature, increased WBC count).
	17.
	  a. This technique allows for the earliest detection of infection or change in infecting organisms in the tracheobronchial tree.

18. Evaluate need for sedation or muscle relaxants.	18. Sedatives may be prescribed to decrease anxiety, or to relax the patient to prevent "competing" with the ventilator. At times, pharmacologically induced paralysis may be necessary to permit mechanical ventilation.

NURSING ALERT

Never administer paralyzing agents until the patient is intubated and on mechanical ventilation. Sedatives should be prescribed in conjunction with paralyzing agents, because the patient may not be able to move but can still have awareness of his surroundings and inability to move.

19. Report intake and output precisely and obtain an accurate daily weight to monitor fluid balance.	19. Positive fluid balance resulting in increase in body weight and interstitial pulmonary edema is a frequent problem in patients requiring mechanical ventilation. Prevention requires early recognition of fluid accumulation. An average adult who is dependent on parenteral nutrition can be expected to lose 0.25 kg (½ lb)/day; therefore, constant body weight indicates positive fluid balance.
20. Monitor nutritional status.	20. Patients on mechanical ventilation require inflation of artificial airway cuffs at all times. Patients with tracheostomy tubes may eat, if capable, or may require enteral feeding tubes or parenteral nourishment. Patients with endotracheal tubes are to be NPO (the tube splints the epiglottis open) and must be entirely tube fed or parenterally nourished.

21. Monitor GI function.
 	
  a. Test all stools and gastric drainage for occult blood.
 	
  b. Measure abdominal girth daily.
	21. Mechanically ventilated patients are at risk for development of stress ulcers.
	  a. Stress may cause some patients requiring mechanical ventilation to develop GI bleeding.
	  b. Abdominal distention occurs frequently with respiratory failure and further hinders respiration by elevation of the diaphragm. Measurement of abdominal girth provides objective assessment of the degree of distention.

PROCEDURE GUIDELINES 10-22	*CONTINUED*

Nursing Action	**Rationale**
22. Provide for care and communication needs of patient with an artificial airway.	
23. Provide psychological support.	23. Mechanical ventilation may result in sleep deprivation and loss of touch with surroundings and reality.
a. Assist with communication.	
b. Orient to environment and function of mechanical ventilator.	
c. Ensure that the patient has adequate rest and sleep.	

FOLLOW-UP PHASE

Nursing Action	**Rationale**
1. Maintain a flow sheet to record ventilation patterns, ABGs, venous chemical determinations, hemoglobin and hematocrit, status of fluid balance, weight, and assessment of the patient's condition. Notify appropriate personnel of changes in the patient's condition.	1. Establishes means of assessing effectiveness and progress of treatment.
2. Change ventilator circuitry every 24 hours; assess ventilator's function every 4 hours or more frequently if problem occurs.	2. Prevents contamination of lower airways.

PROCEDURE GUIDELINES 10-23	**WEANING THE PATIENT FROM MECHANICAL VENTILATION**

EQUIPMENT

Varies according to technique used
Briggs T-piece (see p. 245)

IMV or SIMV (set up in addition to ventilator or incorporated in ventilator and circuitry)
Pressure support

PROCEDURE

Nursing Action	**Rationale**

PREPARATORY PHASE

Nursing Action	**Rationale**
1. For weaning to be successful, the patient must be physiologically capable of maintaining spontaneous respirations. Assessments must ensure that:	1. Provides baseline; ensures that patient is capable of having adequate neuromuscular control to provide adequate ventilation.
a. The underlying disease process is significantly reversed, as evidenced by pulmonary examination, ABGs, chest x-ray.	
b. The patient can mechanically perform ventilation. Should be able to generate a negative inspiratory force (NIF) > -20 cm H_2O, have a vital capacity (VC) 10 to 15 mL/kg; have a resting minute ventilation (V_E) < 10 L/min; and be able to double this; have a spontaneous respiratory rate of <25 breaths per minute; without significant tachycardia; be normotensive; have optimal hemoglobin for condition; have adequate nutritional status.	
2. Assess for other factors that may cause respiratory insufficiency.	2. Weaning is difficult when these conditions are present.
a. Acid–base abnormality	
b. Nutritional depletion	
c. Electrolyte abnormality	
d. Fever	
e. Abnormal fluid balance	
f. Hyperglycemia	
g. Infection	

continued

PROCEDURE GUIDELINES 10-23 | WEANING THE PATIENT FROM MECHANICAL VENTILATION *CONTINUED*

Nursing Action	Rationale
h. Pain i. Sleep deprivation j. Decreased level of consciousness 3. Assess psychological readiness for weaning.	3. Patient must be physically and psychologically ready for weaning.

PERFORMANCE PHASE

Nursing Action	Rationale
1. Ensure psychological preparation. Explain procedure and that weaning is not always successful on the initial attempt. 2. Prepare appropriate equipment. 3. Position the patient in sitting or semi-Fowler's position. 4. Pick optimal time of day, preferably early morning. 5. Perform bronchial hygiene necessary to ensure that the patient is in best condition (postural drainage, suctioning) before weaning attempt.	1. Explaining procedure to patient will decrease patient anxiety and promote cooperation. The patient should not be discouraged if weaning is unsuccessful on the first attempt. 3. Increases lung compliance, decreases work of breathing. 4. The patient should be rested. 5. The patient should be in best pulmonary condition for weaning to be successful.

T-Piece

This system provides oxygen enrichment and humidity to a patient with an endotracheal or tracheostomy tube while allowing completely spontaneous respirations (for set-up and function see oxygen delivery section).

Nursing Action	Rationale

1. Discontinue mechanical ventilation and apply T-piece adapter.
2. Monitor the patient for factors indicating need for reinstitution of mechanical ventilation.
  a. Blood pressure increase or decrease greater than 20 mm Hg systolic or 10 mm Hg diastolic
  b. Heart rate increase of 20 beats/min or greater than 110
  c. Respiratory rate increase greater than 10 breaths/min or rate greater than 30
  d. Tidal volume less than 250 to 300 mL (in adults)
  e. Appearance of new cardiac ectopy or increase in baseline ectopy
  f. Pao_2 less than 60, $Paco_2$ greater than 55, or pH less than 7.35 (may accept lower Pao_2 and pH, and higher $Paco_2$ in patients with COPD)
3. Increase time off ventilator with each weaning attempt as the patient's condition indicates. Evaluate for toleration before moving to the next increment.
4. Institute other techniques helpful in encouraging weaning.
  a. Mental stimulation
  b. Biofeedback
  c. Participation in care
  d. Provision of rewards
  e. Contact with successfully weaned patients
5. When patient tolerates 40 to 60 min of continuous weaning, weaning increments can increase rapidly.
6. When the patient can maintain spontaneous ventilation throughout day, begin night weaning.
	1. Stay with the patient during weaning time to decrease patient anxiety and monitor for tolerance of procedure.
	2. Indicates intolerance of weaning procedure.
	
	3. The patient will progress as he or she becomes mentally and physically able to perform adequate spontaneous ventilation.
	4. Provides motivation and positive feedback.

CPAP Weaning

Nursing Action	Rationale
1. The principles and techniques for CPAP weaning are the same as for T-piece weaning. 2. The patient breathes with CPAP at low level (2.5 to 5 cm H_2O), rather than with the T-piece, for periods that increase in length.	1. This weaning technique is preferred for patients prone to atelectasis when placed on a T-piece.

IMV or SIMV Weaning

1. Set ventilator to IMV or SIMV mode.

PROCEDURE GUIDELINES 10-23   *CONTINUED*

Nursing Action	Rationale
2. Set rate interval.	2. This determines the time interval between machine-delivered breaths, during which the patient will breathe on own.
3. If the patient is on continuous flow IMV circuitry, observe reservoir bag to be sure that it remains mostly inflated during all phases of ventilation.	3. The gas flow rate into the bag must be adequate to prevent the bag from collapsing during inspiration. Flow rates of 6 to 10 L/min are usually adequate.
4. If gas for the patient's spontaneous breath is delivered via a demand valve regulator, ensure that machine sensitivity is at maximum setting.	4. Aids in decreasing work of breathing necessary to open demand valve.
5. Evaluate for tolerance of procedure. Monitor for factors indicating need for increase or decrease of mandatory respiratory rate (see step 3 of T-piece adapter section above). In rapid weaning, changes may be made approximately every 20 to 30 min.	5. If the patient does not tolerate the procedure, the $Paco_2$ will rise and pH will fall.
6. If $Paco_2$ and pH levels remain stable, then continue to decrease mandatory rate as patient tolerates.	6. May be done as frequently as every 20 to 30 min with ABG monitoring, pulse oximetry, documentation of successful weaning.

Pressure Support
1. May be beneficial adjunct to IMV or SIMV weaning.
2. The amount of pressure support (cm H_2O) provided to the airway is progressively decreased over time, allowing the patient to increase role in supporting own spontaneous ventilation.

FOLLOW-UP PHASE

1. Record at each weaning interval: heart rate, blood pressure, respiratory rate, Fio_2, ABG, pulse oximetry value, respiratory and ventilator rate (if IMV or SIMV), or length of time off ventilator (if T-piece weaning).	1. Provides record of procedure and assessment of progress.

Note: It is not within the scope of this manual to establish criteria for the use of one weaning modality as opposed to another.

PROCEDURE GUIDELINES 10-24   **EXTUBATION**

EQUIPMENT

Tonsil suction (surgical suction instrument)
10-mL syringe
Resuscitation bag and mask with oxygen flow
Face mask connected to large-bore tubing, humidifier, and oxygen source

Suction catheter
Suction source
Gloves
Face shield

PROCEDURE

Nursing Action	Rationale
PREPARATORY PHASE	
1. Monitor heart rate, lung expansion, and breath sounds before extubation. Record V_T, VC, NIF.	1. V_T, VC, and NIF are measured to assess respiratory muscle function and adequacy of ventilation.

2. Assess the patient for other signs of adequate muscle power.
  a. Instruct the patient to tightly squeeze the index and middle fingers of your hand. Resistance to removal of your fingers from the patient's grasp must be demonstrated.
  b. Ask the patient to lift head from the pillow and hold for 2 to 3 seconds.
	2. Adequate muscle strength is necessary to ensure maintenance of a patent airway.

continued

PROCEDURE GUIDELINES 10-24   EXTUBATION *CONTINUED*

Nursing Action	Rationale

 NURSING ALERT   Keep in mind that patient's underlying problems must be improved or resolved before extubation is considered. Patient should also be free from infection and malnutrition.

PERFORMANCE PHASE

1. Obtain orders for extubation and postextubation oxygen therapy.
2. Explain the procedure to the patient:
   a. Artificial airway will be removed.
   b. Suctioning will occur before extubation.
   c. Deep breath should be taken on command.
   d. Instruction will be given to cough after extubation.
3. Prepare necessary equipment. Have ready for use tonsil suction, suction catheter, 10-mL syringe, bag-mask unit, and oxygen by way of face mask.
4. Place patient in sitting or semi-Fowler's position (unless contraindicated).
5. Put on face shield.
6. Suction endotracheal tube.
7. Suction oropharyngeal airway above the endotracheal cuff as thoroughly as possible.
8. Put on gloves. Loosen tape or endotracheal tube-securing device.
9. Extubate the patient:
   a. Ask the patient to take as deep a breath as possible (if the patient is not following commands, give a deep breath with the resuscitation bag).
   b. At peak inspiration, deflate the cuff completely and pull the tube out in the direction of the curve (out and downward).
10. Once the tube is fully removed, ask the patient to cough or exhale forcefully to remove secretions. Then suction the back of the patient's airway with the tonsil suction.
11. Evaluate immediately for any signs of airway obstruction, stridor, or difficult breathing. If the patient develops any of the above problems, attempt to ventilate the patient with the resuscitation bag and mask and prepare for reintubation. (Nebulized treatments may be ordered to avoid having to reintubate patient.)
12. Oxygen therapy may be ordered.

1. Do not attempt extubation until postextubation oxygen therapy is available and functioning at the bedside.
2. Increases patient cooperation.

4. Increases lung compliance and decreases work of breathing. Facilitates coughing.
5. Spraying of airway secretions may occur.

7. Secretions not cleared from above the cuff will be aspirated when the cuff is deflated.

9.
   a. At peak inspiration, the trachea and vocal cords will dilate, allowing a less traumatic tube removal.

10. Frequently, old blood is seen in the secretions of newly extubated patients. Monitor for the appearance of bright red blood due to trauma occurring during extubation.
11. Immediate complications:
   a. Laryngospasm may develop, causing obstruction of the airway.
   b. Edema may develop at the cuff site. Signs of narrowing airway lumen are high-pitched crowing sounds, decreased air movement, and respiratory distress.

FOLLOW-UP PHASE

1. Note patient tolerance of procedure, upper and lower airway sounds postextubation, description of secretions.
2. Observe patient closely postextubation for any signs and symptoms of airway obstruction or respiratory insufficiency.
3. Observe character of voice and signs of blood in sputum.
4. Provide supplemental oxygen using face mask.

1. Establishes a baseline to assess improvement/development of complications.
2. Tracheal or laryngeal edema develops postextubation (a possibility for up to 24 hours). Signs and symptoms include high-pitched, crowing upper airway sounds and respiratory distress.
3. Hoarseness is a common postextubation complaint. Observe for worsening hoarseness or vocal cord paralysis.

Thoracic Surgeries

Thoracic surgeries (Table 10-2) are operative procedures performed to aid in the diagnosis and treatment of certain pulmonary conditions. Procedures include thoracotomy, lobectomy (Figure 10-6), pneumonectomy, segmental resection, and wedge resection. These procedures may or may not require chest drainage immediately after surgery.

NURSING ALERT

Meticulous attention must be given to the preoperative and postoperative care of patients undergoing thoracic surgery. These operations are wide in scope and represent a major stress on the cardiorespiratory system.

Preoperative Management

Goal is to maximize respiratory function to improve the outcome postoperatively and reduce risk of complications.

1. Encourage the patient to stop smoking to restore bronchial ciliary action and to reduce the amount of sputum and likelihood of postoperative atelectasis.
2. Teach an effective coughing technique.
   a. Sit upright with knees flexed and body bending slightly forward (or lie on side with hips and knees flexed if unable to sit up).
   b. Splint the incision with hands or folded towel.
   c. Take three short breaths, followed by a deep inspiration, inhaling slowly and evenly through the nose.
   d. Contract abdominal muscles and cough twice forcefully with mouth open and tongue out.
   e. Alternate technique—huffing and coughing—is less painful. Take a deep diaphragmatic breath and exhale forcefully against hand; exhale in a quick distinct pant, or "huff."
3. Humidify the air to loosen secretions.
4. Administer bronchodilators to reduce bronchospasm.
5. Administer antimicrobials for infection.
6. Encourage deep breathing with the use of incentive spirometer (Procedure Guidelines 10–25) to prevent atelectasis postoperatively.
7. Teach diaphragmatic breathing (see p. 229).
8. Carry out chest physical therapy and postural drainage to reduce pooling of lung secretions.
9. Evaluate cardiovascular status for risk and prevention of complication.
10. Encourage activity to improve exercise tolerance.
11. Administer medications and limit sodium and fluid to improve congestive heart failure, if indicated.
12. Correct anemia, dehydration, and hypoproteinemia with intravenous infusions, tube feedings, and blood transfusions as indicated.
13. Give prophylactic anticoagulant as prescribed to reduce perioperative incidence of deep vein thrombosis and pulmonary embolism.
14. Provide teaching and counseling.
    a. Orient the patient to events that will occur in the postoperative period—coughing and deep breath-

---

TABLE 10-2 Thoracic Surgery Types

Types	Descriptions	Indications
Exploratory thoracotomy	Internal view of lung • Usually posterolateral parascapular but could be anterior incision • Chest tubes after procedure	May be used to confirm carcinoma or for chest trauma (to detect source of bleeding)
Lobectomy	Lobe removal • Thoracotomy incision at site of lobe removal • Chest tubes after procedure	Used when pathology is limited to one area of lung: bronchogenic carcinoma, giant emphysematous blebs or bullae, benign tumors, metastatic malignant tumors, bronchiectasis and fungal infections
Pneumonectomy	Removal of an entire lung • Posterolateral or anterolateral thoracotomy incision • Sometimes there is a rib resection • No chest drains/tubes usually because fluid accumulation in empty space is desirable	Performed chiefly for carcinoma, but may be used for lung abscesses, bronchiectasis, or extensive tuberculosis *Note:* Right lung is more vascular than left; may cause more physiologic problems if removed
Segmentectomy (segmental resection)	Only certain segment of lung removed • Segments function as individual units	Used when pathology is very localized (ie, bronchiectasis) and when patient has preexisting cardiopulmonary compromise
Wedge resection	Small localized section of lung tissue removed—usually pie-shaped • Incision made without regard to segments • Chest tubes after procedure	Performed for random lung biopsy and small peripheral nodules

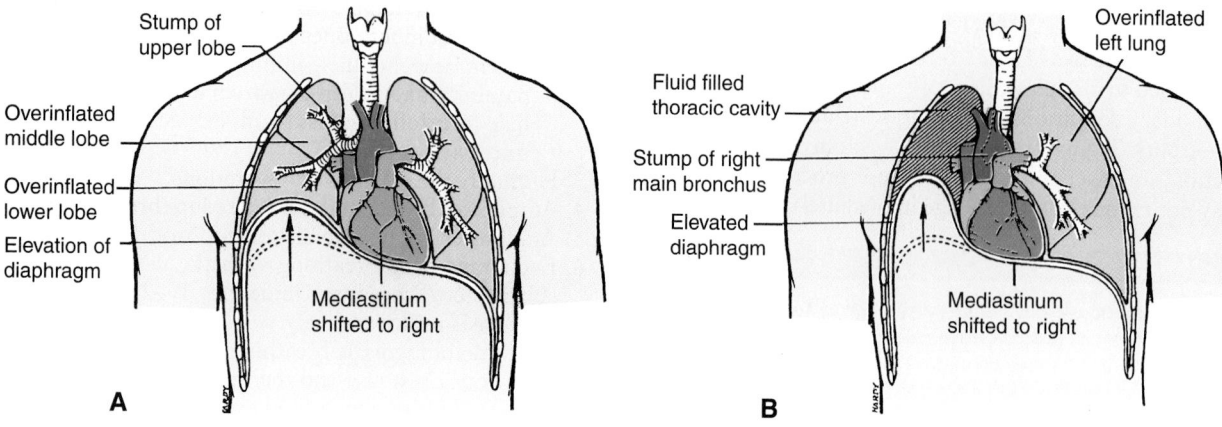

FIGURE 10-6   Operative procedures. (**A**) Lobectomy. (**B**) Pneumonectomy.

ing, suctioning, chest tube and drainage bottles, oxygen therapy, ventilator therapy, pain control, leg exercises and range-of-motion exercises for affected shoulder.

15. Ensure that patient fully understands surgery and is emotionally prepared for it; verify that informed consent has been obtained.

Postoperative Management

1. Use mechanical ventilator until respiratory function and cardiovascular status stabilize. Assist with weaning and extubation.
2. Auscultate chest, monitor vital signs, monitor electrocardiogram (ECG), and assess respiratory rate and depth frequently. Arterial line, CVP, and pulmonary artery catheter are usually used.
3. Monitor ABGs and/or SaO_2 frequently.
4. Monitor and manage chest drainage system to drain fluid, blood, clots, and air from the pleura after surgery (see p. 263). Chest drainage is usually not used after pneumonectomy, however, because it is desirable that the pleural space fill with an effusion, which eventually obliterates the space.

Complications

1. Hypoxia—watch for restlessness, tachycardia, tachypnea, and elevated blood pressure.
2. Postoperative bleeding—monitor for restlessness, anxiety, pallor, tachycardia, and hypotension.
3. Pneumonia; atelectasis.
4. Bronchopleural fistula from disruption of a bronchial suture or staple; bronchial stump leak.
   a. Observe for sudden onset of respiratory distress or cough productive of serosanguineous fluid.
   b. Position with the operative side down.
   c. Prepare for immediate chest tube insertion and/or surgical intervention.
5. Cardiac dysrhythmias (usually occurring third to fourth postoperative day); myocardial infarction or heart failure.

Nursing Diagnoses

- Ineffective Breathing Pattern related to wound closures
- Risk for Fluid Volume Deficit related to chest drainage and blood loss
- Pain related to wound closure and presence of drainage tubes in the chest
- Impaired Physical Mobility of affected shoulder and arm related to wound closure and the presence of drainage tubes in the chest

Nursing Interventions
Maintaining Adequate Breathing Pattern

1. Auscultate chest for adequacy of air movement to detect bronchospasm, consolidation.
2. Obtain ABGs and pulmonary function measurements as ordered.
3. Monitor level of consciousness and inspiratory effort closely to begin weaning from ventilator as soon as possible.
4. Suction frequently using meticulous aseptic technique.

> **NURSING ALERT**
>
> Tracheobronchial secretions are present in excessive amounts in postthoracotomy patients because of trauma to the tracheobronchial tree during operation, diminished lung ventilation, and diminished cough reflex.

> **NURSING ALERT**
>
> Look for changes in color and consistency of suctioned sputum. Colorless, fluid sputum is not unusual; opacification or coloring of sputum may mean dehydration or infection.

5. Elevate the head of the bed 30 to 40 degrees when patient is oriented and blood pressure is stabilized to improve movement of diaphragm.

6. Encourage coughing and deep-breathing exercises and use of an incentive spirometer to prevent bronchospasm, retained secretions, atelectasis, and pneumonia.

Stabilizing Hemodynamic Status

1. Take blood pressure, pulse, and respiration every 15 minutes or more frequently as indicated; extend the time intervals according to the patient's clinical status.
2. Monitor heart rate and rhythm by way of auscultation and ECG, because dysrhythmias are frequently seen after thoracic surgery.
3. Monitor the central venous pressure for prompt recognition of hypovolemia and for effectiveness of fluid replacement.
4. Monitor cardiac output and pulmonary artery systolic, diastolic, and wedge pressures. Watch for subtle changes, especially in the patient with underlying cardiovascular disease.
5. Assess chest tube drainage for amount and character of fluid.
   a. Chest drainage should progressively decrease after first 12 hours.
   b. Prepare for blood replacement and possible reoperation to achieve hemostasis if bleeding persists.
6. Maintain intake and output record, including chest tube drainage.
7. Monitor infusions of blood and parenteral fluids closely because patient is at risk for fluid overload if portion of pulmonary vascular system has been reduced.

Achieving Adequate Pain Control

1. Provide appropriate pain relief—pain limits chest excursions, thereby decreasing ventilation.
   Severity of pain varies with type of incision and with the patient's reaction to and ability to cope with pain. Usually a posterolateral incision is the most painful.

NURSING ALERT

Evaluate for signs of hypoxia thoroughly when anxiety, restlessness, and agitation of new onset are noted, before administering prn sedatives.

---

2. Give narcotics (usually by continuous IV infusion or by epidural catheter by way of patient-controlled analgesia (PCA) pump) for pain relief, as prescribed, to permit patient to breathe more deeply and cough more effectively. Avoid respiratory and CNS depression with too much narcotic; patient should be alert enough to cough.
3. Assist with intercostal nerve block or cryoanalgesia (intercostal nerve freezing) for pain control as ordered (see p. 288).
4. Position for comfort and optimal ventilation (head of bed elevated 15 to 30 degrees); this also helps residual air to rise in upper portion of pleural space, where it can be removed by the chest tube.
   a. Patients with limited respiratory reserve may not be able to turn on unoperated side, because this may limit ventilation of the operated side.

b. Vary the position from horizontal to semierect to prevent retention of secretions in the dependent portion of the lungs.
5. Encourage splinting of incision with pillow, folded towel, or hands, while turning.
6. Teach relaxation techniques such as progressive muscle relaxation and imagery to help reduce pain.

Increasing Mobility of Affected Shoulder

1. Begin range-of-motion exercise of arm and shoulder on affected side immediately to prevent ankylosis of the shoulder ("frozen" shoulder).
2. Perform exercises at time of maximal pain relief.
3. Encourage patient to actively perform exercises three to four times a day, taking care not to disrupt chest tube or IV lines.

Patient Education and Health Maintenance

1. Advise that there will be some intercostal pain for several weeks, which can be relieved by local heat and oral analgesia.
2. Advise that weakness and fatigability are common during the first 3 weeks after a thoracotomy, but exercise tolerance will improve with conditioning.
3. Suggest alternating walking and other activities with frequent short rest periods. Walk at a moderate pace and gradually extend walking time and distance.
4. Encourage continuing deep-breathing exercises for several weeks after surgery to attain full expansion of residual lung tissue.
5. Instruct on maintaining good body alignment to ensure full lung expansion.
6. Advise that chest muscles may be weaker than normal for 3 to 6 months after surgery, so patient must avoid lifting more than 20 lb until complete healing has taken place.
7. Warn that any activity that causes undue fatigue, increased shortness of breath, or chest pain should be stopped immediately.
8. Because all or part of one lung has been removed, warn to stay away from respiratory irritants (smoke, fumes, high level of air pollution).
   a. Avoid anything that may cause spasms of coughing.
   b. Sit in nonsmoking areas in public places.
9. Encourage to have an annual influenza injection and obtain a pneumococcal pneumonia vaccine.
10. Encourage to keep follow-up visits.
11. Prevent respiratory infections by frequent handwashing and avoiding others with respiratory infections.

Outcome-Based Evaluation

- Respirations 18–24, adequate depth; lungs clear; ABGs and SaO_2 within normal limits
- Blood pressure, CVP, and pulse stable
- Coughing and turning independently; reports relief of pain
- Performing active range of motion of affected arm and shoulder

PROCEDURE GUIDELINES 10-25   ASSISTING THE PATIENT USING AN INCENTIVE SPIROMETER

EQUIPMENT
According to the type of device used

PROCEDURE

Nursing Action	Rationale
PREPARATORY PHASE	
1. Measure the patient's normal tidal volume (V_T) and auscultate the chest.	1. The patient's baseline is established.
PERFORMANCE PHASE	
1. Explain the procedure and its purpose to the patient.	1. Optimal results are achieved when the patient is given pretreatment instruction. Preoperative instruction is also beneficial for the surgical patient.
2. Place the patient in a comfortable sitting or semi-Fowler's position.	2. Diaphragmatic excursion is greater in this position; however, if the patient is medically unable to be in this position, the exercise may be done in any position.
3. For the postoperative patient, try as much as possible to avoid discomfort with the treatment administration. Try to coordinate treatment with administration of pain-relief medications. Instruct and assist the patient with splinting of incision.	3. More likely to have best results in using incentive spirometry when patient has as little pain as possible.
4. Set the incentive spirometer V_T indicator at the desired goal the patient is to reach or exceed (500 mL is often used to start). The V_T is set according to the manufacturer's instructions.	4. The initial V_T may be prescribed, but the purpose of the device is to establish a baseline V_T and provide incentive to achieve greater volumes progressively.
5. Demonstrate the technique to the patient.	
6. Instruct the patient to exhale fully.	
7. Tell the patient to take in a slow, easy, deep breath from the mouthpiece.	7. Noseclips are sometimes used if the patient has difficulty breathing only through mouth. This will ensure full credit for each breath measured.
8. When the desired goal is reached (lungs fully inflated), ask the patient to continue the inspiratory effort for 3 seconds, even though the patient may not actually be drawing in more air.	8. Sustaining the inspiratory effort helps to open closed alveoli.
9. Instruct the patient to remove the mouthpiece, relax, and passively exhale; patient should take several normal breaths before attempting another one with the incentive spirometer.	9. Usually one incentive breath per minute minimizes patient fatigue. No more that four to five maneuvers should be performed per minute to minimize hypocarbia.
10. Continue to monitor the patient's spirometer breaths, periodically increasing the tidal volume as the patient tolerates.	
11. At the conclusion of the treatment, encourage the patient to cough after a deep breath.	11. The deep lung inflation may loosen secretions and enable the patient to expectorate them.
12. Instruct the patient to take 10 sustained maximal inspiratory maneuvers per hour and note the volume on the spirometer.	12. A total of 10 sustained maximal inspiratory maneuvers per hour during waking hours is a typical order. A counter on the incentive spirometer indicates the number of breaths the patient has taken.

Nursing Action	Rationale

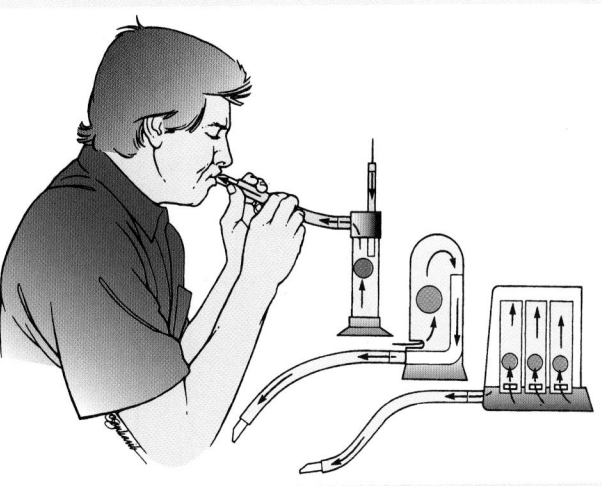

Flow incentive spirometer. Patients are instructed to inhale briskly to elevate the balls and to keep them floating as long as possible. The volume inhaled is estimated and variable.

FOLLOW-UP PHASE

1. Auscultate the chest. Chart any improvement or variation, the volume attained, effectiveness of cough, description of any secretions expectorated.

1. Note the effectiveness and patient tolerance of the treatment.

Chest Drainage

Chest drainage is the insertion of a tube into the pleural space to evacuate air or fluid, to help regain negative pressure. Whenever the chest is opened, from any cause, there is loss of negative pressure, which can result in collapse of the lung. The collection of air, fluid, or other substances in the chest can compromise cardiopulmonary function and even cause collapse of the lung, because these substances take up space.

It is necessary to keep the pleural space evacuated postoperatively and to maintain negative pressure within this potential space. Therefore, during or immediately after thoracic surgery, chest tubes/catheters are positioned strategically in the pleural space, sutured to the skin, and connected to some type of drainage apparatus to remove the residual air and drainage fluid from the pleural or mediastinal space. This assists in the reexpansion of remaining lung tissue.

Chest drainage can also be used to treat spontaneous pneumothorax, or hemothorax/pneumothorax caused by trauma. Sites for chest tube placement are:

1. For pneumothorax (air)—second or third interspace along midclavicular or anterior axillary line.
2. For hemothorax (fluid)—sixth or seventh lateral interspace in the midaxillary line.

Principles of Chest Drainage

1. Many types of commercial chest drainage systems are in use, most of which use the water-seal principle. The chest tube/catheter is attached to a bottle, using a one-way valve principle. Water acts as a seal and permits air and fluid to drain from the chest. However, air cannot reenter the submerged tip of the tube.
2. Chest drainage can be categorized into three types of mechanical systems (Figure 10-7).

Single-Bottle Water-Seal System

1. The end of the drainage tube from the patient's chest is covered by a layer of water, which permits drainage of air and fluid from the pleural space, but does not allow air to move back into the chest. Functionally, drainage depends on gravity, on the mechanics of respiration, and, if desired, on suction by the addition of controlled vacuum.

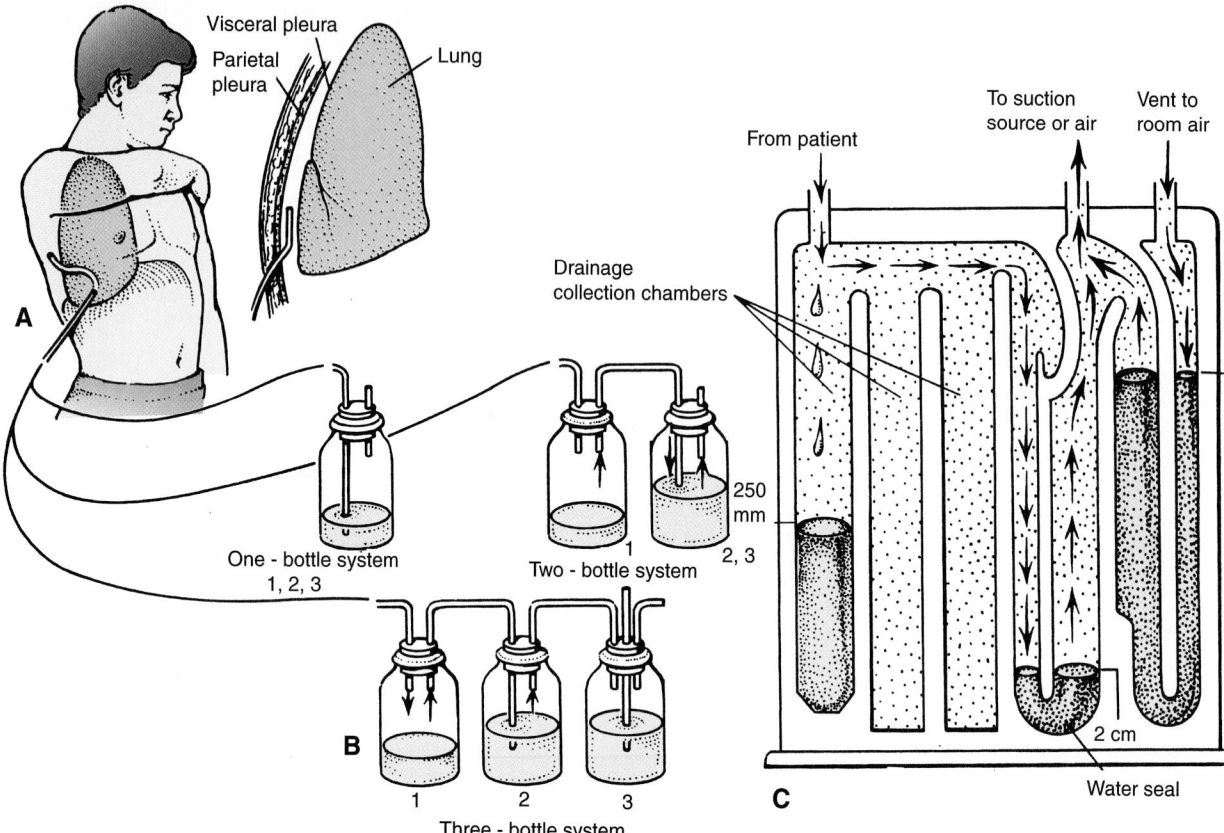

FIGURE 10-7 Chest drainage system. (**A**) Strategic placement of a chest catheter in the pleural space. (**B**) Three types of mechanical drainage systems. (**C**) A Pleur-Evac operating system: (1) the collection chamber, (2) the water seal chamber, and (3) the suction control chamber. The Pleur-Evac is a single unit with all three bottles identified as chambers.

2. The tube from the patient extends approximately 2.5 cm (1 inch) below the level of the water in the container. There is a vent for the escape of any air that may be leaking from the lung. The water level fluctuates as the patient breathes; it goes up when the patient inhales and down when the patient exhales.

3. At the end of the drainage tube, bubbling may or may not be visible. Bubbling can mean either persistent leakage of air from the lung or other tissues or a leak in the system.

Two-Bottle Water-Seal System

1. The two-bottle system consists of the same water-seal chamber, plus a fluid-collection bottle.

2. Drainage is similar to that of a single unit, except that when pleural fluid drains, the underwater-seal system is not affected by the volume of the drainage.

3. Effective drainage depends on gravity or on the amount of suction added to the system. When vacuum (suction) is added to the system from a vacuum source, such as wall suction, the connection is made at the vent stem of the underwater-seal bottle.

4. The amount of suction applied to the system is regulated by the wall gauge.

Three-Bottle Water-Seal System

1. The three-bottle system is similar in all respects to the two-bottle system, except for the addition of a third bottle to control the amount of suction applied.

2. The amount of suction is determined by the depth to which the tip of the venting glass tube is submerged in the water.

3. In the three-bottle system (as in the other two systems), drainage depends on gravity or the amount of suction

applied. The amount of suction in the three-bottle system is controlled by the manometer bottle. The mechanical suction motor or wall suction creates and maintains a negative pressure throughout the entire closed drainage system.

4. The manometer bottle regulates the amount of vacuum in the system. This bottle contains three tubes:
   a. A short tube above the water level comes from the water-seal bottle.
   b. Another short tube leads to the vacuum or suction motor, or to wall suction.
   c. The third tube is a long tube that extends below the water level in the bottle and opens to the atmosphere outside the bottle. This tube regulates the amount of vacuum in the system, depending on the depth to which the tube is submerged—the usual depth is 20 cm (7.6 inches).
5. When the vacuum in the system becomes greater than the depth to which the tube is submerged, outside air is sucked into the system. This results in constant bubbling in the manometer bottle, which indicates that the system is functioning properly.

> **NURSING ALERT**
>
> When the motor or the wall vacuum is turned off, the drainage system should be open to the atmosphere so intrapleural air can escape from the system. This can be done by detaching the tubing from the suction port to provide a vent.

6. In the commercially available systems, the three bottles are contained in one unit and identified as "chambers" (see Figure 10-7C). The principles remain the same for the commercially available products as they do for the glass bottle system.

Nursing and Patient Care Considerations

1. Assist with chest tube insertion (Procedure Guidelines 10–26).
2. Assess patient's pain at insertion site and give medication appropriately. If patient is in pain, chest excursion and lung inflation will be hampered.
3. Maintain chest tubes to provide drainage and enhance lung reinflation (Procedure Guidelines 10-27).

(*text continues on page 269*)

PROCEDURE GUIDELINES 10-26   ASSISTING WITH CHEST TUBE INSERTION

EQUIPMENT

Tube thoracostomy tray	Suture material
Syringes	Local anesthetic
Needles/trocar	Chest tube (appropriate size); connector
Basins/skin germicide	Chest drainage system—connecting tubes and tubing, collection bottles
Sponges	or commercial system, vacuum pump (if required)
Scalpel/sterile drape/gloves	Sterile water
Two large clamps	

PROCEDURE

Nursing Action	Rationale
PREPARATORY PHASE	
1. Assess patient for pneumothorax, hemothorax, presence of respiratory distress.	
2. Obtain a chest x-ray. Other means of localization of pleural fluid include ultrasound and/or fluoroscopic localization.	2. To evaluate extent of lung collapse or amount of bleeding in pleural space.
3. Assemble drainage system.	
4. Reassure the patient and explain the steps of the procedure. Tell the patient to expect a needle prick and a sensation of slight pressure during infiltration anesthesia.	4. The patient can cope by remaining immobile and doing relaxed breathing during tube insertion.
5. Position the patient as for an intercostal nerve block or according to physician preference.	5. The tube insertion site depends on the substance to be drained, the patient's mobility, and the presence/absence of coexisting conditions.
PERFORMANCE PHASE	
Needle or Intracath Technique	
1. The skin is prepared and anesthetized using local anesthetic with a short 25-gauge needle. A larger needle is used to infiltrate the subcutaneous tissue, intercostal muscles, and parietal pleura.	1. The area is anesthetized to make tube insertion and manipulation relatively painless.

continued

PROCEDURE GUIDELINES 10-26   **ASSISTING WITH CHEST TUBE INSERTION** *CONTINUED*

Nursing Action	Rationale
2. An exploratory needle is inserted.	2. To puncture the pleura and determine the presence of air/blood in the pleural cavity.
3. The IntraCath catheter is inserted through the needle into the pleural space. The needle is removed, and the catheter is pushed several centimeters into the pleural space.	
4. The catheter is taped to the skin.	4. To prevent it from being pushed out of the chest during patient movement or lung expansion.
5. The catheter is attached to a connector/tubing and attached to a drainage system (underwater-seal or commercial system).	

Trocar Technique for Chest Tube Insertion

A trocar catheter is used for the insertion of a large-bore tube for removal of a modest to large amount of air leak or for the evacuation of serous effusion.

1. A small incision is made over the prepared, anesthetized site. Blunt dissection (with a hemostat) through the muscle planes in the interspace to the parietal pleura is performed.	1. To admit the diameter of the chest tube.
2. The trocar is directed into the pleural space, the cannula is removed, and a chest tube is inserted into the pleural space and connected to a drainage system.	2. There is a trocar catheter available equipped with an indwelling pointed rod for ease of insertion.

Hemostat Technique Using a Large-Bore Chest Tube

A large bore chest tube is used to drain blood or thick effusions from the pleural space.

1. After skin preparation and anesthetic infiltration, an incision is made through the skin and subcutaneous tissue.	1. The skin incision is usually made one interspace below proposed site of penetration of the intercostal muscles and pleura.
2. A curved hemostat is inserted into the pleural cavity and the tissue is spread with the clamp.	2. To make a tissue tract for the chest tube.
3. The tract is explored with an examining finger.	3. Digital examination helps confirm the presence of the tract and penetration of the pleural cavity.
4. The tube is held by the hemostat and directed through the opening up over the ribs and into the pleural cavity.	
5. The clamp is withdrawn and the chest tube is connected to a chest drainage system.	5. The chest tube has multiple openings at the proximal end for drainage of air/blood.
6. The tube is sutured in place and covered with a sterile dressing.	

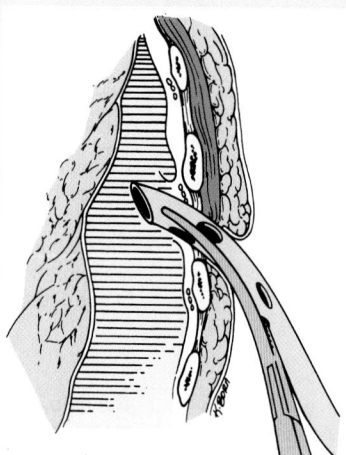

Chest tube (tube thoracostomy) inserted via hemostat technique.

PROCEDURE GUIDELINES 10-26 *CONTINUED*

Nursing Action	Rationale
FOLLOW-UP PHASE	
1. Observe the drainage system for blood/air. Observe for fluctuation in the tube on respiration. (See p. 268.)	1. If a hemothorax is draining through a thoracostomy tube into a bottle containing sterile normal saline, the blood is available for autotransfusion.
2. Secure a follow-up chest x-ray.	2. To confirm correct chest tube placement and reexpansion of the lung.
3. Assess for bleeding, infection, leakage of air and fluid around the tube.	

PROCEDURE GUIDELINES 10-27 **MANAGING THE PATIENT WITH WATER-SEAL CHEST DRAINAGE**

EQUIPMENT

Closed chest drainage system   Vacuum motor
Holder for drainage system (if needed)   Sterile connector for emergency use

PROCEDURE

Nursing Action	Rationale
PERFORMANCE PHASE	
1. Attach the drainage tube from the pleural space (the patient) to the tubing that leads to a long tube with end submerged in sterile normal saline.	1. Water-seal drainage provides for the escape of air and fluid into a drainage bottle. The water acts as a seal and keeps the air from being drawn back into the pleural space.
2. Check the tube connections periodically. Tape if necessary.	2. Tube connections are checked to ensure tight fit and patency of the tubes.
a. The tube should be approximately 2.5 cm (1 inch) below the water level.	a. If the tube is submerged too deep below the water level, a higher intrapleural pressure is required to expel air.
b. The short tube is left open to the atmosphere.	b. Venting the short glass tube lets air escape from the bottle.
3. Mark the original fluid level with tape on the outside of the drainage bottle. Mark hourly/daily increments (date and time) at the drainage level.	3. This marking will show the amount of fluid loss and how fast fluid is collecting in the drainage bottle. It serves as a basis for blood replacement, if the fluid is blood. Grossly bloody drainage will appear in the bottle in the immediate postoperative period and, if excessive, may necessitate reoperation. Drainage usually declines progressively after the first 24 hours.
4. Make sure the tubing does not loop or interfere with the movements of the patient.	4. Fluid collecting in the dependent segment of the tubing will decrease the negative pressure applied to the catheter. Kinking, looping, or pressure on the drainage tubing can produce back pressure, thus possibly forcing drainage back into the pleural space or impeding drainage from the pleural space.
5. Encourage the patient to assume a position of comfort. Encourage good body alignment. When the patient is in a lateral position, place a rolled towel under the tubing to protect it from the weight of the patient's body. Encourage the patient to change position frequently.	5. The patient's position should be changed frequently to promote drainage and body kept in good alignment to prevent postural deformity and contractures. Proper positioning helps breathing and promotes better air exchange. Pain medication may be indicated to enhance comfort and deep breathing.
6. Put the arm and shoulder of the affected side through range-of-motion exercises several times daily. Some pain medication may be necessary.	6. Exercise helps to avoid ankylosis of the shoulder and assist in lessening postoperative pain and discomfort.

continued

PROCEDURE GUIDELINES 10-27   MANAGING THE PATIENT WITH WATER-SEAL CHEST DRAINAGE
CONTINUED

Nursing Action	Rationale
7. "Milk" the tubing in the direction of the drainage bottle as often as ordered. (Many institutions do not advocate milking because of the increased intrapleural pressure it causes.)	7. "Milking" the tubing prevents it from becoming plugged with clots of fibrin. Constant attention to maintaining the patency of the tube will facilitate prompt expansion of the lung and minimize complications.
8. Make sure there is fluctuation ("tidaling") of the fluid level in the long glass tube.	8. Fluctuation of the water level in the tube shows that there is effective communication between the pleural space and the drainage bottle; provides a valuable indication of the patency of the drainage system, and is a gauge of intrapleural pressure.
9. Fluctuations of fluid in the tubing will stop when: a. The lung has reexpanded. b. The tubing is obstructed by blood clots or fibrin. c. A dependent loop develops (see step 4). d. Suction motor or wall suction is not operating properly.	
10. Watch for leaks of air in the drainage system as indicated by constant bubbling in the water-seal bottle. a. Report excessive bubbling in the water-seal change immediately. b. "Milking" of chest tubes in patients with air leaks should be done only if requested by surgeon.	10. Leaking and trapping of air in the pleural space can result in tension pneumothorax.
11. Observe and report immediately signs of rapid, shallow breathing, cyanosis, pressure in the chest, subcutaneous emphysema, or symptoms of hemorrhage.	11. Many clinical conditions may cause these signs and symptoms, including tension pneumothorax, mediastinal shift, hemorrhage, severe incisional pain, pulmonary embolus, and cardiac tamponade. Surgical intervention may be necessary.
12. Encourage the patient to breathe deeply and cough at frequent intervals. If there are signs of incisional pain, adequate pain medication is indicated.	12. Deep breathing and coughing help to raise the intrapleural pressure, which allows emptying of any accumulation in the pleural space and removes secretions from the tracheobronchial tree so the lung expands.
13. If the patient has to be transported to another area, place the drainage bottle below the chest level (as close to the floor as possible).	13. The drainage apparatus must be kept at a level lower than the patient's chest to prevent backflow of fluid into the pleural space.
14. If the tube becomes disconnected, cut off the contaminated tips of the chest tube and tubing, insert a sterile connector in the chest tube and tubing, and reattach to the drainage system. Otherwise, do not clamp the chest tube during transport.	
15. When assisting with removal of the tube: a. Administer pain medication 30 minutes before removal of chest tube. b. Instruct the patient to perform a gentle Valsalva maneuver or to breathe quietly. c. The chest tube is clamped and removed. d. Simultaneously, a small bandage is applied and made airtight with petroleum gauze covered by a 4 × 4-inch gauze and thoroughly covered and sealed with tape.	15. The chest tube is removed as directed when the lung is reexpanded (usually 24 hours to several days). During the tube removal, avoid a large sudden inspiratory effort, which may produce a pneumothorax.

FOLLOW-UP PHASE

1. Monitor patient's pulmonary status for signs and symptoms of decompensation.	1. Patient could have reformation of pneumothorax after removal.

SELECTED REFERENCES

American Association of Respiratory Care. (1995). Clinical practice guidelines: Long term mechanical ventilation in the home. *Respiratory Care, 40*(12), 1313–1320.

———. (1993a). Clinical practice guidelines: Directed cough. *Respiratory Care, 38*, 495–499.

———. (1993b). Clinical practice guidelines: Use of positive airway pressure adjuncts to bronchial hygiene therapy. *Respiratory Care, 38*, 516–521.

———. (1992a). Clinical practice guidelines: Nasotracheal suctioning. *Respiratory Care, 37*, 898–901.

———. (1992b). Clinical practice guidelines: Oxygen therapy in the home or extended care facility. *Respiratory Care, 37*, 918–922.

———. (1992c). Clinical practice guidelines: Sampling for arterial blood gas analysis. *Respiratory Care, 37*, 913–917.

———. (1991a). Clinical practice guidelines: Postural drainage therapy. *Respiratory Care, 36*, 1418–1426.

———. (1991b). Clinical practice guidelines: Pulse oximetry. *Respiratory Care, 36*, 1406–1409.

Baum, G., Celli, B., Crapo, J., & Karlinsky, J. (1998). *Textbook of pulmonary diseases* (6th ed.). Philadelphia: Lippincott-Raven.

Hardy, K. A. (1994, May). A review of airway clearance: New techniques, indications and recommendations. *Respiratory Care, 39*(5), 440–452.

Hess, D. (2000). Detection and monitoring of hypoxemia and oxygen therapy. *Respiratory Care, 45*(1), 65–80.

Kacmarek, R. (2000). Delivery systems for long-term oxygen therapy. *Respiratory Care, 45*(1), 84–92.

Langenderfer, B. (1998). Alternatives to percussion and postural drainage—A review of mucus clearance therapies: Percussion and postural drainage, autogenic drainage, positive expiratory pressure, flutter valve, intrapulmonary percussive ventilation, and high-frequency chest compression with the ThAIRapy vest. *Journal of Cardiopulmonary Rehabilitation, 18*, 283–298.

MacIntyre, N. (2000). Oxygen therapy and exercise response in lung disease. *Respiratory Care, 45*(2), 194–200.

Murray, J., & Nadal, J. (1994). *Respiratory medicine* (2nd ed.). Philadelphia: W. B. Saunders.

O'Donohue, W., & Bowman, T. (2000). Hypoxemia during sleep in patients with chronic obstructive lung disease: Significance, detection, and effects of therapy. *Respiratory Care, 45*(2), 188–191.

Perkins, L. A., & Shortall, S. P. (2000). Ventilation without intubation. *RN, 63*(1), 34–38.

Petty, T., & Bliss, P. (2000). Ambulatory oxygen therapy, exercise, and survival with advanced chronic obstructive pulmonary disease. *Respiratory Care, 45*(2), 204–211.

Pierson, D. (2000). Pathophysiology and clinical effects of chronic hypoxia. *Respiratory Care, 45*(1), 39–51.

Sabiston, D., & Spencer, F. (1995). *Surgery of the chest* (6th ed.). Philadelphia: W. B. Saunders.

Shapiro, B., Peruzzi, W., & Kozelowski-Templin, R. (1994). *Clinical application of blood gases* (5th ed.). St. Louis: Mosby.

Staff. (1999). Dyspnea: Mechanisms, assessment, and management: A consensus statement. *American Journal of Critical Care and Respiratory Medicine, 159*, 321–340.

Wong, F. W. (1999). A new approach to ABG interpretation. *American Journal of Nursing, 99*(8), 34–36.

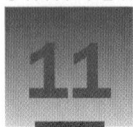
Respiratory Disorders

ACUTE DISORDERS

◼ Respiratory Failure

Respiratory failure is an alteration in the function of the respiratory system that causes the PaO_2 to fall below 50 mm Hg (hypoxemia) or the $PaCO_2$ to rise above 50 mm Hg (hypercapnia), as determined by arterial blood gas (ABG) analysis. Respiratory failure is classified as acute, chronic, or combined acute and chronic.

Classification
Acute Respiratory Failure
1. Characterized by hypoxemia (PaO_2 less than 50 mm Hg) or hypercapnia ($PaCO_2$ greater than 50 mm Hg) and acidemia (pH less than 7.35).
2. Occurs rapidly, usually in minutes to hours or days.
Chronic Respiratory Failure
1. Characterized by hypoxemia (decreased PaO_2) or hypercapnia (increased $PaCO_2$) with a normal pH (7.35 to 7.45).
2. Occurs over a period of months to years—allows for activation of compensatory mechanisms.
Acute and Chronic Respiratory Failure
1. Characterized by an abrupt increase in the degree of hypoxemia or hypercapnia in patients with preexisting chronic respiratory failure.
2. May occur after an acute upper respiratory infection or pneumonia, or without obvious cause.
3. Extent of deterioration is best assessed by comparing the patient's present ABG with previous ABG findings (patient "normals").

Pathophysiology and Etiology
Oxygenation Failure
Characterized by a decrease in PaO_2 and normal or decreased $PaCO_2$
1. Primary problem is inability to adequately oxygenate the blood, resulting in hypoxemia.
2. Hypoxemia occurs because damage to the alveolar-capillary membrane causes leakage of fluid into the interstitial space or into the alveoli and slows or prevents movement of oxygen from the alveoli to the pulmonary capillary blood.
   a. Typically, this damage is widespread, resulting in many areas of the lung being poorly ventilated or nonventilated.
   b. Consequences are severe ventilation–perfusion imbalance and shunt.
3. Hypocapnia results from hypoxemia and decreased pulmonary compliance. Fluid within the lungs makes the lung less compliant or stiffer.
   a. Change in compliance reflexively stimulates the increased ventilation.
   b. Ventilation is also increased as a response to hypoxemia.
   c. Ultimately, if treatment is unsuccessful, the $PaCO_2$ will increase, and the patient will experience both an increase in $PaCO_2$ and a decrease in PaO_2.
4. Etiology includes:
   a. Cardiogenic pulmonary edema (left ventricular failure; mitral stenosis)
   b. Adult respiratory distress syndrome (ARDS). Underlying causes of ARDS include shock of any etiology; infectious causes such as gram-negative sepsis, viral pneumonia, bacterial pneumonia; trauma such as fat emboli, head injury, lung contusion; aspiration

of gastric fluid, near drowning; inhaled toxins such as oxygen in high concentrations, smoke, corrosive chemicals; hematologic conditions such as massive transfusions, post-cardiopulmonary bypass; and metabolic disorders such as pancreatitis, uremia.

Ventilatory Failure With Normal Lungs

Characterized by a decrease in PaO_2, increase in $PaCO_2$, and a decrease in pH.

1. Primary problem is insufficient respiratory center stimulation or insufficient chest wall movement, resulting in alveolar hypoventilation.
2. Hypercapnia occurs because impaired neuromuscular function or chest wall expansion limits the amount of carbon dioxide removed from the lungs.
   a. Primary problem is not the lungs. The patient's minute ventilation (tidal volume times the number of breaths per minute) is insufficient to allow normal alveolar gas exchange.
3. The CO_2 not excreted by the lungs combines with H_2O to form carbonic acid (H_2CO_3). This predisposes to acidemia and a fall in pH.
4. Hypoxemia occurs as a consequence of hypercapnia. When the $PaCO_2$ rises, the PaO_2 must fall unless increased amounts of oxygen are added to the inspired air.
5. Etiology includes:
   a. Insufficient respiratory center activity (drug intoxication such as narcotic overdose, general anesthesia; vascular disorders such as cerebral vascular insufficiency, brain tumor; trauma such as head injury, increased intracranial pressure)
   b. Insufficient chest wall function (neuromuscular disease such as Guillain-Barré, myasthenia gravis, poliomyelitis; trauma to the chest wall resulting in multiple fractures; spinal cord trauma; kyphoscoliosis)

Ventilatory Failure With Intrinsic Lung Disease

Characterized by a decrease in PaO_2 and decreased pH

1. Primary problem is acute exacerbation or chronic progression of previously existing lung disease, resulting in CO_2 retention.
2. Hypercapnia occurs because damage to the lung parenchyma and/or airway obstruction limits the amount of carbon dioxide removed by the lungs.
   a. Primary problem is preexisting lung disease—usually chronic bronchitis, emphysema, or severe asthma. This limits CO_2 removal from the lungs.
3. The CO_2 not excreted by the lungs combines with H_2O to form carbonic acid (H_2CO_3). This predisposes to acidemia and a fall in pH.
4. Hypoxemia occurs as a consequence of hypercapnia. In addition, damage to the lung parenchyma and/or airway obstruction limits the amount of oxygen that enters the pulmonary capillary blood.
5. Etiology includes:
   a. Chronic obstructive pulmonary disease or COPD (chronic bronchitis, emphysema)
   b. Severe asthma
   c. Cystic fibrosis

Clinical Manifestations

1. Hypoxemia—restlessness, agitation, dyspnea, disorientation, confusion, delirium, loss of consciousness
2. Hypercapnia—headache, somnolence, dizziness, confusion
3. Tachypnea initially; then when no longer able to compensate, bradypnea
4. Accessory muscle use
5. Asynchronous respirations

NURSING ALERT

Obtain ABG whenever the history or signs and symptoms suggest the patient is at risk for developing respiratory failure. Initial and subsequent values should be recorded on a flow sheet or computer so comparisons can be made over time. Need for ABG can be decreased by using an oximeter to continuously monitor the SaO_2. Correlate oximeter values with ABG and then use oximeter for trending.

Diagnostic Evaluation

1. ABGs—show changes in PaO_2, $PaCO_2$, and pH from patient's normal; or PaO_2 less than 50 mm Hg, $PaCO_2$ greater than 50 mm Hg, pH less than 7.35.
2. Pulse oximetry—decreasing SaO_2.
3. End tidal CO_2 monitoring—elevated.
4. CBC, serum electrolytes, chest x-ray, urinalysis, electrocardiogram (ECG), blood and sputum cultures—to determine underlying cause and patient's condition.

Management

1. Oxygen therapy to correct the hypoxemia.
2. Chest physical therapy and hydration to mobilize secretions.
3. Bronchodilators and possibly corticosteroids to reduce bronchospasm and inflammation.
4. Diuretics for pulmonary congestion.
5. Mechanical ventilation as indicated. Noninvasive positive-pressure ventilation using a face mask has been tried in some patients.

NURSING ALERT

Avoid administration of oxygen at FIO_2 of 100% for COPD patients because you may eradicate the respiratory center drive. For COPD patients, the drive to breathe is hypoxemia.

Complications

1. Oxygen toxicity if prolonged high FIO_2 required
2. Barotrauma from mechanical ventilation intervention

Nursing Assessment

See Standards of Care Guidelines.

1. Note changes suggesting increased work of breathing (diaphoresis, intercostal muscle retraction) or pulmonary edema (fine, coarse crackles).
2. Assess breath sounds.
    a. Diminished or absent sounds indicate inability to ventilate the lungs sufficiently to prevent atelectasis.
    b. Crackles indicate ineffective airway clearance, fluid in the lungs.
    c. Wheezing indicates narrowed airways and bronchospasm.
    d. Rhonchi and crackles indicate ineffective secretion clearance.
3. Assess level of consciousness and ability to tolerate increased work of breathing.
    a. Confusion, rapid shallow breathing, abdominal paradox (inward movement of abdominal wall during inspiration), and intercostal retractions suggest inability to maintain adequate minute ventilation.
4. Assess for signs of hypoxemia and hypercapnia.
5. Determine vital capacity (VC), respiratory rate, minute ventilation (V_E), and negative inspiratory force (NIF) and compare with values indicating need for mechanical ventilation:
    a. VC <10 to 15 mL/kg
    b. Respiratory rate >35/min
    c. V_E >10 L/min
    d. NIF <−15 to −25 cm H_2O.
6. Analyze ABG and compare with previous values.

STANDARDS OF CARE GUIDELINES
Respiratory Compromise

When caring for patients at risk for respiratory compromise, consider the following assessments and interventions:

- Be aware of the status of the patient when assuming care so comparison can be made with subsequent assessments.
- Perform thorough systematic assessment, including mental status, vital signs, respiratory status, and cardiovascular status.
- Document patient's condition to provide a record for continuity of care.
- Evaluate for signs of hypoxia when anxiety, restlessness, confusion, or aggression of new onset are noted. Do not administer sedatives unless hypoxia has been ruled out by performing respiratory assessment.
- Notify appropriate health care provider of significant findings of hypoxia—cyanosis, circumoral pallor, rapid and shallow respirations, abnormal breath sounds, change in behavior or level of consciousness. Request assessment and intervention by health care provider as indicated.
- Use extreme caution in administering sedatives and narcotics to patients at risk for respiratory compromise.

This information should serve as a general guideline only. Each patient situation presents a unique set of clinical factors and requires nursing judgment to guide care, which may include additional or alternative measures and approaches.

a. If the patient cannot maintain a minute ventilation sufficient to prevent CO_2 retention, the pH will fall.
b. Mechanical ventilation or noninvasive ventilation may be needed if the pH falls to 7.30 or below.

7. Determine hemodynamic status (blood pressure, pulmonary wedge pressure, cardiac output, SvO_2) and compare with previous values. If patient is on mechanical ventilation and positive end-expiratory pressure (PEEP), venous return may be limited, resulting in decreased cardiac output.

Nursing Diagnoses

- Impaired Gas Exchange related to inadequate respiratory center activity or chest wall movement, airway obstruction, and/or fluid in lungs
- Ineffective Airway Clearance related to increased or tenacious secretions

Nursing Interventions
Improving Gas Exchange

1. Administer antibiotics, cardiac medications, and diuretics as ordered for underlying disorder.
2. Administer oxygen to maintain PaO_2 of 60 mm Hg or SaO_2 >90% using devices that provide increased oxygen concentrations (aerosol mask, partial rebreathing mask, nonrebreathing mask).
3. Monitor fluid balance by intake and output measurement, urine specific gravity, daily weight, and direct measurement of pulmonary capillary wedge pressure to detect presence of hypo/hypervolemia.
4. Provide measures to prevent atelectasis and promote chest expansion and secretion clearance, as ordered (incentive spirometer, nebulization, head of bed elevated 30 degrees, turn frequently, out of bed).
5. Monitor adequacy of alveolar ventilation by frequent measurement of respiratory rate, vital capacity, inspiratory force, and ABGs.
6. Compare monitored values with criteria indicating need for mechanical ventilation (see section titled Nursing Assessment). Report and prepare to assist with noninvasive ventilation or intubation and initiation of mechanical ventilation, if indicated.

Maintaining Airway Clearance

1. Administer medications to increase alveolar ventilation—bronchodilators to reduce bronchospasm, corticosteroids to reduce airway inflammation.
2. Perform chest physiotherapy to remove mucus. Teach slow, pursed-lip breathing to reduce airway obstruction.
3. Administer IV fluids and mucolytics to reduce sputum viscosity.
4. Suction patient as needed to assist with removal of secretions.
5. If the patient becomes increasingly lethargic, cannot cough or expectorate secretions, cannot cooperate with

therapy, or if pH falls below 7.30, despite use of the above therapy, report and prepare to assist with intubation and initiation of mechanical ventilation.

Patient Education and Health Maintenance

1. Instruct patient with preexisting pulmonary disease to seek early intervention for infections to prevent acute respiratory failure.
2. Teach patient about medication regimen.
3. Encourage patients at risk, especially the elderly and those with preexisting lung disease, to get yearly influenza and pneumococcal pneumonia (approximately once every 10 years) immunizations.

Outcome-Based Evaluation

- ABGs within patient's normal limits
- Decreased secretions; lungs clear

Adult Respiratory Distress Syndrome (ARDS)

ARDS is a clinical syndrome also called noncardiogenic pulmonary edema in which there is severe hypoxemia and decreased compliance of the lungs, which leads to both oxygenation and ventilatory failure. Mortality is 50% to 60% but is improved with early intervention.

Pathophysiology and Etiology

1. Pulmonary and/or nonpulmonary insult to the alveolar-capillary membrane causing fluid leakage into interstitial spaces.
2. Ventilation–perfusion (V/Q) mismatch caused by shunting of blood (Figure 11-1).
3. Etiologies are numerous and can be pulmonary or nonpulmonary. These include (but are not limited to):
   a. Pneumonia, sepsis, aspiration

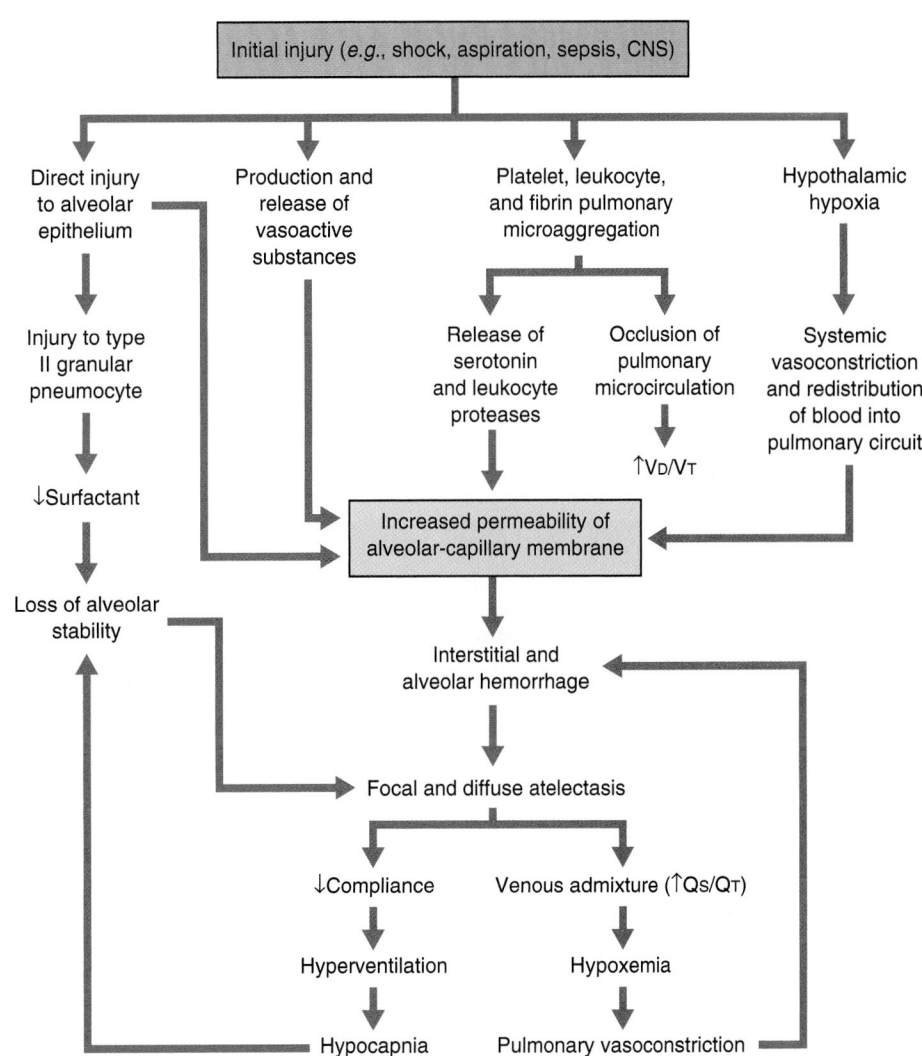

FIGURE 11-1 Pathogenesis of ARDS.

b. Shock (any cause), trauma
c. Metabolic, hematologic, and immunologic disorders
d. Inhaled agents—smoke, high concentration of oxygen, corrosive substances
e. Major surgery, fat or air embolism

Clinical Manifestations

1. Severe dyspnea, use of accessory muscles.
2. Increasing requirements of oxygen therapy. Hypoxemia refractory to supplemental oxygen therapy.
3. Severe crackles and rhonchi heard on auscultation.

Diagnostic Evaluation

1. The hallmark sign for ARDS is a shunt; hypoxemia remains despite increasing oxygen therapy.
2. Decreased lung compliance; increasing pressure required to ventilate patient on mechanical ventilation.
3. Chest x-ray exhibits bilateral infiltrates.
4. Pulmonary artery catheter readings: pulmonary artery wedge pressure >18 mm Hg.

Management

1. The underlying cause for ARDS must be determined so appropriate treatment can be initiated.
2. Ventilatory support with PEEP will be instituted. PEEP keeps the alveoli open, thereby improving gas exchange. Therefore, a lower oxygen concentration (FIO_2) can be used to maintain satisfactory oxygenation.
3. Fluid management must be maintained. The patient may be hypovolemic due to the movement of fluid into the interstitium of the lung. Pulmonary artery catheter monitoring and inotropic medication can be helpful.
4. Medications are aimed at treating the underlying cause. Corticosteroids are used infrequently due to the controversy regarding benefits of usage.
5. Adequate nutrition should be initiated early and maintained.

> **NURSING ALERT**
>
> The treatment for ARDS is aimed at symptom management, but the underlying cause must be treated or the ARDS will not resolve. Supportive measures will assist the patient while the underlying cause is being treated.

Complications

1. Infections such as pneumonia, sepsis.
2. Respiratory complications such as pulmonary emboli, barotrauma, oxygen toxicity, subcutaneous emphysema, or pulmonary fibrosis.
3. Gastrointestinal (GI) complications such as stress ulcer, ileus.
4. Cardiac complications such as decreased cardiac output and dysrhythmias.
5. Renal failure, disseminated intravascular coagulation (DIC).

Nursing Interventions

Care is similar to patient with respiratory failure (p. 270) and pulmonary edema (p. 385). Also see section titled Mechanical Ventilation, p. 248.

◼ Acute Bronchitis

Acute bronchitis is an infection of the lower respiratory tract that is generally an acute sequela to an upper respiratory tract infection.

Pathophysiology and Etiology

1. Primarily viral etiology, but may also arise from bacterial agents.
2. Airways become inflamed and irritated with increased mucous production.

Clinical Manifestations

1. Dyspnea, fever, tachypnea.
2. Productive cough, clear to purulent sputum.
3. Pleuritic chest pain, occasionally.
4. Diffuse rhonchi and crackles heard on auscultation.

Diagnostic Evaluation

Chest x-ray—no evidence of infiltrates or consolidation.

Management

1. Antibiotic therapy for 7 to 10 days may be indicated for patients with underlying respiratory problems or chronic illness.
2. Hydration and humidification.
3. Secretion clearance interventions (controlled cough, continuous positive airway pressure [PEP] valve therapy, chest physical therapy)
4. Bronchodilators for bronchospastic cough and bronchial irritation.
5. Symptom management for fever, cough.

Nursing Assessment

1. Obtain history of upper airway infection, course and length of symptoms.
2. Assess severity of cough and characteristics of sputum production.
3. Auscultate chest for diffuse rhonchi and crackles as opposed to localized crackles usually heard with pneumonia.

Nursing Diagnosis

- Ineffective Airway Clearance related to sputum production

Nursing Interventions

Establishing Effective Airway Clearance

1. Administer or teach self-administration of antibiotics as ordered.
2. Encourage mobilization of secretions, through hydration, chest physical therapy, and coughing. Educate patient that beverages with caffeine or alcohol do not promote hydration because of their diuretic effect.

3. If ordered, administer or teach self-administration of inhaled bronchodilators to reduce bronchospasm.
4. Caution patients on the use of over-the-counter cough suppressants, antihistamines, and decongestants that may cause drying and retention of secretions. Cough preparations containing the mucolytic guaifenesin may be appropriate.

Patient Education and Health Maintenance

1. Instruct patient about medication regimen, including the completion of the full course of antibiotics prescribed and the effects of meals on the absorption of the medications. If patient is not being treated with antibiotics, assure patient that the majority of people recover from bronchitis without antibiotic treatment.
2. Encourage patient to seek medical attention for shortness of breath and worsening condition.
3. Advise patient that a dry cough may persist after bronchitis due to irritation of the airways. A bedside humidifier and avoidance of dry environments may help.
4. Encourage patients to discuss alternative therapies with health care provider. Some people use garlic as an antimicrobial. It is believed to have antibacterial and antiviral activity due to the antiseptic oil, which is excreted through the lungs. It is believed to be useful in respiratory infections such as chronic bronchitis. It may be helpful as part of a broader approach to bronchitic asthma. Other herbs believed to have antimicrobial activity for bronchitis are echinacea, eucalyptus, and thyme. The antiseptic volatile oils contained in eucalyptus and thyme can also be used in the form of inhalations or baths.

Outcome-Based Evaluation

- Coughing up clear secretions effectively.

▣ Pneumonia

Pneumonia is an inflammatory process, involving the terminal airways and alveoli of the lung, caused by infectious agents (Table 11-1). It is classified according to its causative agent.

Pathophysiology and Etiology

1. The organism gains access to the lungs through aspiration of oropharyngeal contents, by inhalation of respiratory secretions from infected individuals, by way of the bloodstream, or from direct spread to the lungs as a result of surgery or trauma.
2. Patients with bacterial pneumonia may have an underlying disease that impairs host defense; pneumonia arises from endogenous flora of the person whose resistance has been altered, or from aspiration of oropharyngeal secretions.
   a. Immunocompromised patients include those receiving corticosteroids or immunosuppressants, those with cancer, those being treated with chemotherapy or radiotherapy, those undergoing organ transplantation, alcoholics, intravenous (IV) drug abusers, and those

with human immunodeficiency virus (HIV) disease and acquired immunodeficiency syndrome (AIDS).
   b. These people have an increased chance of developing overwhelming infection. Infectious agents include aerobic and anaerobic gram-negative bacilli, *Staphylococcus, Nocardia,* fungi, *Candida,* viruses such as cytomegalovirus (CMV), *Pneumocystis carinii,* reactivation of tuberculosis, and others.
3. When bacterial pneumonia occurs in a healthy person, there usually is a history of preceding viral illness.
4. Other predisposing factors include conditions interfering with normal drainage of the lung such as tumor, general anesthesia and postoperative immobility, depression of the central nervous system from drugs, neurologic disorders, or other conditions, and intubation or respiratory instrumentation.
5. Pneumonia may be divided into three groups:
   a. Community acquired, due to a number of organisms, including *Streptococcus pneumoniae*
   b. Hospital or nursing home acquired (nosocomial), due primarily to gram-negative bacilli and staphylococci
   c. Pneumonia in the immunocompromised person
6. Persons over 65 have a high mortality rate, even with appropriate antimicrobial therapy.

NURSING ALERT

Recurring pneumonia often indicates underlying disease such as cancer of the lung, multiple myeloma, or COPD.

Clinical Manifestations

For most common forms of bacterial pneumonia:
1. Sudden onset; shaking chill; rapidly rising fever of 39.5°C to 40.5°C (101°F to 105°F)
2. Cough productive of purulent sputum
3. Pleuritic chest pain aggravated by respiration/coughing
4. Dyspnea, tachypnea accompanied by respiratory grunting, nasal flaring, use of accessory muscles of respiration, fatigue.
5. Rapid, bounding pulse

Diagnostic Evaluation

1. Chest x-ray to show presence/extent of pulmonary disease.
2. Gram's stain, culture, and sensitivity studies of sputum— may indicate offending organism.
3. Blood culture to detect bacteremia (bloodstream invasion) occurring with bacterial pneumonia.
4. Immunologic test for detecting microbial antigens in serum, sputum, and urine.

Management

1. Antimicrobial therapy—depends on laboratory identification of causative organism and sensitivity to specific antimicrobials
2. Oxygen therapy if patient has inadequate gas exchange (*text continues on page 278*)

TABLE 11-1 Commonly Encountered Pneumonias

Type	Organism Responsible	Manifestations	Clinical Features	Treatment	Complications
Bacterial					
Streptococcal pneumonia (pneumococcal pneumonia)	*Streptococcus pneumoniae*	May be history of previous respiratory infection Sudden onset, with shaking and chills Rapidly rising fever; tachypnea Cough: with expectoration of rusty or green (purulent) sputum Pleuritic pain aggravated by cough Chest dull to percussion; crackles, bronchial breath sounds Confusion may be only presenting feature in elderly	Herpes simplex lesions often present on face or lips Usually involves one or more lobes	Cephalosporins; trimethoprim-sulfamethoxazole (Bactrim); amoxicillin clavulanate (Augmentin); macrolide antibiotics such as azithromycin (Zithromax) or clarithromycin (Biaxin)	Shock Pleural effusion Superinfections Pericarditis Otitis media
Staphylococcal pneumonia	*Staphylococcus aureus*	Often prior history of viral infection, especially influenza Insidious development of cough, with expectoration of yellow, blood-streaked mucus Onset may be sudden if patient is outside hospital Fever, pleuritic chest pain, progressive dyspnea Pulse varies; may be slow in proportion to temperature	Frequently seen in hospital setting; during influenza epidemics; in intravenous drug abuse These infections often lead to necrosis and destruction of lung tissue Treatment must be vigorous and prolonged owing to disease's tendency to destroy the lungs Organism may develop rapid drug resistance Prolonged convalescence usual	Cephalosporins; penicillinase-resistant extended-spectrum penicillins; vancomycin (Vancocin) for methicillin-resistant *S. aureus*	Effusion/pneumothorax Lung abscess Empyema Meningitis
Pneumonia due to gram-negative enteric bacilli	*Klebsiella* species: *Pseudomonas* organisms, *Escherichia coli*, *Serratia*, *Proteus* species	Sudden onset with fever, chills, dyspnea Pleuritic chest pain and production of purulent sputum	Usually infection occurs from aspiration of pharyngeal flora into bronchioles Seen in persons with severe illness; among the more common causes of hospital-acquired pneumonia	Usually multiple-drug regimens recommended: aminoglycosides; cephalosporins; and/or penicillinase-resistant extended-spectrum penicillin	Early necrosis of lung tissue with rapid abscess formation High mortality
Legionnaires' disease	*Legionella pneumophila*	High fever, chills, cough, chest pain, tachypnea Respiratory distress	Peak incidence in persons over 50 who are cigarette smokers and have underlying diseases that increase susceptibility to infection	Erythromycin (Eryc) or newer macrolide antibiotic such as clarithromycin (Biaxin)	Respiratory failure

	Organism	Signs and Symptoms	Notes	Treatment	Complications
Hemophilus influenza pneumonia	*Hemophilus influenzae*	Abrupt onset of coughing, fever, chills, chest pain	May affect healthy young adults	Erythromycin (Eryc), newer macrolide antibiotic, trimethoprim-sulfamethoxazole (Bactrim)	High mortality in patients with underlying disease (cancer; COPD) Pleural effusion common
Atypical and Non-bacterial Mycoplasma pneumonia or chlamydial pneumonia	*Mycoplasma pneumoniae*, *Chlamydia trachomatis*	Gradual onset; severe headache; irritating hacking cough producing scanty, mucoid sputum. Anorexia; malaise. Fever; nasal congestion; sore throat	Occurs most commonly in children and young adults, as well as in older adults in community or hospital setting. Rise in serum-complement-fixing antibodies to the organism	Erythromycin (Eryc); newer macrolide antibiotic; tetracycline (Tetracyn); doxycycline (Vibramycin)	Persisting cough, meningoencephalitis, polyneuritis, monoarticular arthritis, pericarditis, myocarditis
Viral pneumonia	Influenza viruses, Parainfluenza viruses, Respiratory syncytial viruses, Rhinoviruses, Adenovirus, Varicella, rubella, rubeola, herpes simplex, cytomegalovirus, Epstein-Barr virus	Cough. Constitutional symptoms may be pronounced (severe headache, anorexia, fever, and myalgia)	In majority of patients, influenza begins as an acute coryza; others have bronchitis and pleurisy, whereas still others develop gastrointestinal symptoms. Risk of developing influenza related to crowding and close contact with groups	Treat symptomatically. Amantadine (Symmetrel) relieves symptoms. Prophylactic vaccination recommended for high-risk persons (over 65; chronic cardiac or pulmonary disease, diabetes, and other metabolic disorders)	Persons with underlying disease have increased risk of complications; primary influenzal pneumonia; secondary bacterial pneumonia. Bacterial superinfection. Pericarditis. Endocarditis
Pneumocystis carinii pneumonia	*Pneumocystis carinii*	Insidious onset. Increasing dyspnea and nonproductive cough. Tachypnea; progresses rapidly to intercostal retraction, nasal flaring, and cyanosis. Lowering of arterial oxygen tension. Chest x-ray will reveal diffuse, bilateral interstitial pneumonia	Usually seen in host whose resistance is compromised; most common opportunistic infection in AIDS. Organism invades lungs of patients who have suppressed immune system (from cancer, AIDS, leukemia) or after immunosuppressive therapy for cancer, organ transplant, or collagen disease. Frequently associated with concurrent infection by viruses (cytomegalovirus), bacteria, and fungi	Trimethoprim-sulfamethoxazole (Bactrim); dapsone with trimethoprim (Trimpex); clindamycin (Cleocin) with primaquine. Pentamidine methanesulfonate	Patients are critically ill. Prognosis guarded, because it usually is a complication of a severe underlying disorder
Fungal pneumonia	*Aspergillus fumigatus*	Fever, productive cough, chest pain, hemoptysis. Chest x-ray reveals broad range of abnormalities from infiltration to consolidation, cavitation, and empyema	Neutropenic individual most susceptible. May develop *Aspergillus* as a superinfection	Amphotericin B (Fungizone); Itraconazole (Sporanox)	High fatality rate. Invades blood vessels and destroys lung tissue by direct invasion and vascular infarction

Complications

1. Pleural effusion.
2. Sustained hypotension and shock, especially in gram-negative bacterial disease, particularly in the elderly.
3. Superinfection: pericarditis, bacteremia, and meningitis.
4. Delirium—this is considered a medical emergency.
5. Atelectasis—due to mucous plugs.
6. Delayed resolution.

Nursing Assessment

1. Take a careful history to help establish etiologic diagnosis.
   a. History of recent respiratory illness? Mode of onset?
   b. Presence of fever, chills, chest pain, dyspnea?
   c. Any family illness?
   d. Medications? Alcohol, tobacco, or IV drug use?
2. Observe for anxious, flushed appearance, shallow respirations, splinting of affected side, confusion, and disorientation.
3. Auscultate for crackles overlying affected region, and for bronchial breath sounds when consolidation (filling of airspaces with exudate) is present.

Nursing Diagnoses

- Impaired Gas Exchange related to decreased ventilation secondary to inflammation and infection involving distal airspaces
- Ineffective Airway Clearance related to excessive tracheobronchial secretions
- Pain related to inflammatory process and dyspnea
- Risk for Injury related to resistant infection

Nursing Interventions

Improving Gas Exchange

1. Observe for cyanosis, dyspnea, hypoxia, and confusion, indicating worsening condition.
2. Follow ABGs/SaO_2 to determine oxygen need and response to oxygen therapy.
3. Administer oxygen at concentration to maintain PaO_2 at acceptable level. Hypoxemia may be encountered because of abnormal ventilation–perfusion ratios in affected lung segments.
4. Avoid high concentrations of oxygen in patients with COPD, particularly with evidence of CO_2 retention; use of high oxygen concentrations may worsen alveolar ventilation by removing the patient's only remaining ventilatory drive.
5. Place patient in an upright position to obtain greater lung expansion and improve aeration. Frequent turning and increased activity (up in chair, ambulate as tolerated) should be employed.

Enhancing Airway Clearance

1. Obtain freshly expectorated sputum for Gram's stain and culture, preferably early morning specimen, as directed. Instruct the patient as follows:
   a. Rinse mouth with water to minimize contamination by normal flora.
   b. Breathe deeply several times.
   c. Cough deeply and expectorate raised sputum into sterile container.
2. Encourage patient to cough. Retained secretions interfere with gas exchange. Suction as necessary.
3. Encourage increased fluid intake, unless contraindicated, to thin mucus and promote expectoration and replace fluid losses due to fever, diaphoresis, dehydration, and dyspnea.
4. Humidify air or oxygen therapy to loosen secretions and improve ventilation.
5. Employ chest wall percussion and postural drainage when appropriate to loosen and mobilize secretions.
6. Auscultate the chest for crackles and rhonchi.
7. Administer cough suppressants when coughing is nonproductive only if there is no evidence of retained secretions.
8. Mobilize patient to improve secretion clearance and reduce risk of atelectasis and worsening pneumonia.

Relieving Pleuritic Pain

1. Place in a comfortable position (semi-Fowler's) for resting and breathing; encourage frequent change of position to prevent pooling of secretions in lungs.
2. Demonstrate how to splint the chest while coughing.
3. Avoid suppressing a productive cough.
4. Administer prescribed analgesic agent to relieve pain. Avoid narcotics in patients with a history of COPD.

GERONTOLOGIC ALERT

Sedatives, narcotics, and cough suppressants should be used cautiously in the elderly, because of their tendency to suppress cough and gag reflexes and respiratory drive.

---

5. Apply heat and/or cold to chest as prescribed.
6. Assist with intercostal nerve block for pain relief.
7. Encourage modified bed rest during febrile period.
8. Watch for abdominal distention or ileus, which may be due to swallowing of air during intervals of severe dyspnea. Insert a nasogastric or rectal tube as directed.

Monitoring for Complications

1. Remember that fatal complications may develop during the early period of antimicrobial treatment.
2. Monitor temperature, pulse, respiration, blood pressure, and oximetry at regular intervals to assess the patient's response to therapy.
3. Auscultate lungs and heart. Heart murmurs or friction rub may indicate acute bacterial endocarditis, pericarditis, or myocarditis.
4. Employ special nursing surveillance for patients with the following conditions:
   a. Alcoholism, COPD, immunosuppression—these people, as well as elderly patients, may have little or no fever.

b. Chronic bronchitis—it is difficult to detect subtle changes in condition, because the patient may have seriously compromised pulmonary function.

c. Epilepsy—pneumonia may result from aspiration after a seizure.

d. Delirium—may be caused by hypoxia, meningitis, delirium tremens of alcoholism.

   (i) Prepare for lumbar puncture; meningitis may be lethal.

   (ii) Ensure adequate hydration and give mild sedation.

   (iii) Give oxygen to treat/prevent hypoxia.

   (iv) Delirium must be controlled to prevent exhaustion and cardiac failure.

5. Assess these patients for unusual behavior, alterations in mental status, stupor, and congestive heart failure.

6. Assess for resistant fever or return of fever, indicating bacterial resistance to antibiotics.

Patient Education and Health Maintenance

1. Advise patient that fatigue, weakness, and depression may be prolonged after pneumonia.

2. Encourage chair rest after fever subsides; gradually increase activities to bring energy level back to preillness stage.

3. Encourage breathing exercises to clear lungs and promote full expansion and function after the fever subsides.

4. Explain that a chest x-ray is taken 4 to 6 weeks after recovery to evaluate lungs for clearing and detect any tumor or underlying cause.

5. Advise smoking cessation. Cigarette smoking destroys tracheobronchial cilial action, which is the first line of defense of lungs; also irritates mucosa of bronchi and inhibits function of alveolar scavenger cells (macrophages).

6. Advise the patient to keep up natural resistance with good nutrition, adequate rest. One episode of pneumonia may make the person susceptible to recurring respiratory infections.

7. Instruct the patient to avoid fatigue, sudden extremes in temperature, and excessive alcohol intake, which lower resistance to pneumonia.

8. Encourage the yearly influenza immunization and immunization for *S. pneumoniae*, a major cause of bacterial pneumonia.

9. Advise avoidance of contact with people who have upper respiratory infections for several months after pneumonia resolves.

10. Practice frequent handwashing, especially after contact with others.

Outcome-Based Evaluation

- Cyanosis and dyspnea reduced; ABGs improved
- Coughing effectively; absence of crackles
- Appears more comfortable; free of pain
- Fever controlled, no signs of resistant infection

Aspiration Pneumonia

Aspiration is the inhalation of oropharyngeal secretions and/or stomach contents into the lungs. It may produce an acute form of pneumonia.

Pathophysiology and Etiology

1. Patients at risk and factors associated with risk:

a. Loss of protective airway reflexes (swallowing, laryngeal, cough) caused by altered state of consciousness, alcohol or drug overdose, during resuscitation procedures, seriously ill or debilitated patients, abnormalities of gag and swallowing reflexes

b. Nasogastric tube feedings

c. Obstetric patients—from general anesthesia, lithotomy position, delayed emptying of stomach from enlarged uterus, labor contractions

d. GI conditions—hiatal hernia, intestinal obstruction, abdominal distention

e. Prolonged endotracheal intubation/tracheostomy—can depress glottic and laryngeal reflexes from disuse

2. Effects of aspiration depend on volume and character of aspirated material

a. Particulate matter—mechanical blockage of airways and secondary infection

b. Anaerobic bacterial aspiration—from oropharyngeal secretions

c. Gastric juice—destructive to alveoli and capillaries; results in outpouring of protein-rich fluids into the interstitial and intra-alveolar spaces. Impairs exchange of oxygen and carbon dioxide, producing hypoxemia, respiratory insufficiency, and failure.

Clinical Manifestations

1. Tachycardia, fever
2. Dyspnea, cough, tachypnea
3. Cyanosis
4. Crackles, rhonchi, wheezing
5. Pink, frothy sputum (may simulate acute pulmonary edema)

Diagnostic Evaluation

1. Chest x-ray may be normal initially; with time, shows consolidation and other abnormalities

Management

Depends on the material aspirated.

1. Clearing the obstructed airway.

a. If foreign body becomes lodged in the patient's throat, remove object with forceps.

b. Place the patient in tilted head-down position on right side (right side more frequently affected if patient has aspirated solid particles).

c. Suction trachea/endotracheal tube—to remove any particulate matter.

2. Laryngoscopy/bronchoscopy if patient has been asphyxiated by solid material.

3. Fluid volume replacement for correction of hypotension.
4. Antimicrobial therapy if there is evidence of superimposed bacterial infection.
5. Correction of acidosis; respiratory acidosis and metabolic acidosis indicate a severe reaction due to aspiration of gastric contents.
6. Oxygen therapy and assisted ventilation if adequate blood gas values cannot be maintained.

Complications
1. Lung abscess; empyema
2. Necrotizing pneumonia

Nursing Assessment
1. Assess for airway obstruction.
2. Assess for risk factors for aspiration.
3. Assess for development of fever, foul-smelling sputum, and development of congestion.

Nursing Diagnoses
In addition to those for pneumonia, there is Risk for Aspiration.

Nursing Interventions
1. Be on guard constantly and monitor patients at risk as described above.
2. Elevate head of bed for debilitated patients, for those receiving tube feedings, and for those with motor diseases of the esophagus.
3. Place patients with impaired reflexes in a lateral position.
4. Be sure nasogastric tube is patent.
5. Give tube feedings slowly, with patient sitting up in bed.
   a. Check position of tube in stomach before feeding.
   b. Check seal of cuff of tracheostomy or endotracheal tube before feeding.
6. Keep the patient in a fasting state before anesthesia (at least 8 hours).
7. Feed patients with impaired swallowing slowly, and ensure that no food is retained in mouth after feeding.

> **NURSING ALERT**
>
> Morbidity and mortality rate of aspiration pneumonia remain high even with optimum treatment. Prevention is the key to the problem.

Pulmonary Embolism

Pulmonary embolism refers to the obstruction of one or more pulmonary arteries by a thrombus (or thrombi) originating usually in the deep veins of the legs, the right side of the heart, or, rarely, an upper extremity, which becomes dislodged and is carried to the pulmonary vasculature.

Pulmonary infarction refers to necrosis of lung tissue that can result from interference with blood supply.

Pathophysiology/Etiology
1. Obstruction, either partial or full, of pulmonary arteries, which causes decrease or absent blood flow; therefore, there is ventilation but no perfusion (ventilation–perfusion or V/Q mismatch).
2. Hemodynamic consequences:
   a. Increased pulmonary vascular resistance
   b. Increased pulmonary arterial pressure
   c. Increased right ventricular workload to maintain pulmonary blood flow
   d. Right ventricular failure
   e. Decreased cardiac output
   f. Decreased blood pressure
   g. Shock
3. Pulmonary emboli can vary in size and seriousness of consequences.
4. Predisposing factors include:
   a. Stasis, prolonged immobilization
   b. Concurrent phlebitis
   c. Previous heart (CHF, myocardial infarction) or lung disease
   d. Injury to vessel wall
   e. Coagulation disorders
   f. Metabolic, endocrine, vascular, or collagen disorders
   g. Malignancy
   h. Advancing age, estrogen therapy

> **NURSING ALERT**
>
> Be aware of high-risk patients for pulmonary embolism—immobilization, trauma to pelvis (especially surgical) and lower extremities (especially hip fracture), obesity, history of thromboembolic disease, varicose veins, pregnancy, CHF, myocardial infarction, malignant disease, postoperative patients, elderly.

Clinical Manifestations
1. Dyspnea, pleuritic pain, tachypnea, apprehension
2. Chest pain with apprehension and a sense of impending doom occurs when most of the pulmonary artery is obstructed.
3. Cyanosis, tachyarrhythmias, syncope, circulatory collapse, and possibly death encountered in patients with massive pulmonary embolism
4. Subtle deterioration in patient's condition with no explainable cause
5. Pleural friction rub

> **NURSING ALERT**
>
> Have a high index of suspicion for pulmonary embolus if there is a subtle deterioration in the patient's condition and unexplained cardiovascular and pulmonary findings.

Diagnostic Evaluation
1. ABGs—decreased PaO_2 is usually found, due to perfusion abnormality of the lung.

2. Chest x-ray—normal or possible wedge-shaped infiltrate.
3. Ventilation–perfusion (V/Q) lung scans—perfusion scan investigates regional blood flow to determine presence of perfusion defects; ventilation scan may be done in patient with large perfusion defects.
4. Pulmonary angiogram (most definitive)—emboli seen as "filling defects."

Management
Emergency Management
For massive pulmonary embolism, goal is to stabilize cardiorespiratory status

> **NURSING ALERT**
>
> Massive pulmonary embolism is a medical emergency; the patient's condition tends to deteriorate rapidly. There is a profound decrease in cardiac output, with an accompanying increase in right ventricular pressure.

1. Oxygen is administered to relieve hypoxemia, respiratory distress, and cyanosis.
2. An infusion is started to open an IV route for drugs/fluids.
3. Vasopressors, inotropic agents such as dopamine (Intropin) and/or antidysrhythmic agents may be indicated to support circulation if the patient is unstable.
4. The ECG is monitored continuously for right ventricular failure, which may have a rapid onset.
5. Small doses of IV morphine are given to relieve anxiety, to alleviate chest discomfort (which improves ventilation), and to ease adaptation to mechanical ventilator, if this is necessary.
6. Pulmonary angiography, hemodynamic measurements, ABG determinations, and other studies are carried out.

Subsequent Management—Anticoagulation and Thrombolysis
1. IV heparin (Heparin)—stops further thrombus formation and extends the clotting time of the blood; it is an anticoagulant and antithrombotic.
   a. IV loading dose usually followed by continuous pump or drip infusion or given intermittently every 4 to 6 hours.
   b. Dosage adjusted to maintain the activated partial thromboplastin time (PTT) at 1.5 to 2 times the pretreatment value (if the value was normal).
   c. Protamine sulfate may be given to neutralize heparin in event of severe bleeding.
2. Oral anticoagulation with warfarin (Coumadin) is usually used for follow-up anticoagulant therapy after heparin therapy has been established; interrupts the coagulation mechanism by interfering with the vitamin K-dependent synthesis of prothrombin and factors VII, IX, and X.
   a. Dosage is controlled by monitoring serial tests of prothrombin time; desired prothrombin time is 1.2 to 1.5 times control value.
   b. Reported as international normalized ratio (INR) of 1.2 to 1.5 by most laboratories.
   c. Anticoagulation is used to prevent new clot formation but does not dissolve previously formed clots. Thrombolytics are used to dissolve clots.

> **GERONTOLOGIC ALERT**
>
> Consider the patient's age in dosing of anticoagulation therapy. The elderly usually will need a decreased dosing regimen.

3. Thrombolytic agents such as streptokinase (Streptase) may be used in patients with massive pulmonary embolism; effective in lysing recently formed thrombi; improve circulatory and hemodynamic status. Administered IV in a loading dose followed by constant infusion.
4. Newer clot-specific thrombolytics (tissue plasminogen activator [t-PA], streptokinase activator complex, single-chain urokinase)—activate plasminogen only within thrombus itself rather than systematically; minimize occurrence of generalized fibrinolysis and subsequent bleeding.

Surgical Intervention
When anticoagulation is contraindicated or patient has recurrent embolization or develops serious complications from drug therapy.
1. Interruption of vena cava—reduces channel size to prevent lower extremity emboli from reaching lungs. Accomplished by:
   a. Ligation, plication, or clipping of the inferior vena cava.
   b. Placement of transvenously inserted intraluminal filter in inferior vena cava to prevent migration of emboli (Figure 11-2). Inserted through femoral or jugular vein by way of catheter.
2. Embolectomy (removal of pulmonary embolic obstruction).

Complications
1. Bleeding as a result of treatment
2. Respiratory failure

Nursing Assessment
1. Take nursing history with emphasis on onset and severity of dyspnea and nature of chest pain.
2. Examine the patient's legs carefully. Assess for swelling of leg, duskiness, pain on pressure over gastrocnemius muscle, pain on dorsiflexion of the foot (positive Homans's sign), which indicate thrombophlebitis as source.
3. Monitor respiratory rate—may be accelerated out of proportion to degree of fever and tachycardia.
   a. Observe rate of inspiration to expiration.
   b. Percuss for resonance, dullness, and flatness.
   c. Auscultate for friction rub, crackles, rhonchi, and wheezing.

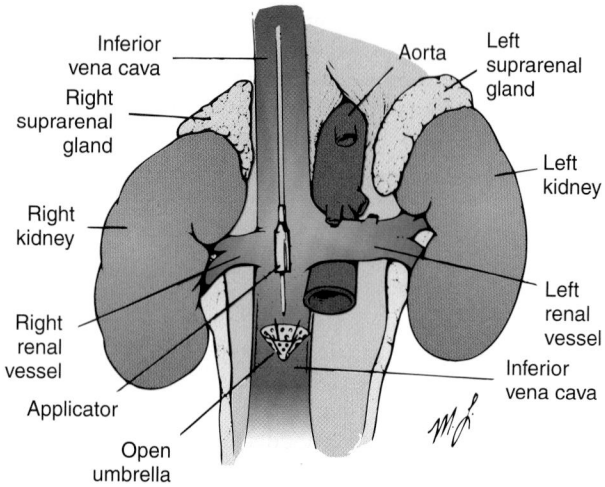

FIGURE 11-2 Insertion of umbrella filter in inferior vena cava to prevent pulmonary embolism. Filter (compressed within an applicator catheter) is inserted through an incision in the right internal jugular vein. The applicator is withdrawn when the filter fixes itself to the wall of the inferior vena cava after ejection from the applicator.

4. Auscultate heart; listen for splitting of second heart sound.
5. Evaluate results of PT/PTT tests for patients on anticoagulants and report results that are outside of therapeutic range; anticipate a dosage change.

Nursing Diagnoses

- Ineffective Breathing Pattern related to acute increase in alveolar dead airspace and possible changes in lung mechanics from embolism
- Altered Tissue Perfusion (pulmonary) related to decreased blood circulation
- Pain (pleuritic) related to congestion, possible pleural effusion, possible lung infarction
- Anxiety related to dyspnea, pain, and seriousness of condition
- Risk for Injury related to altered hemodynamic factors and anticoagulant therapy

Nursing Interventions
Correcting Breathing Pattern

1. Assess for hypoxia, headache, restlessness, apprehension, pallor, cyanosis, behavioral changes.
2. Monitor vital signs, ECG, oximetry, and ABG levels for adequacy of oxygenation.
3. Monitor patient's response to IV fluids/vasopressors.
4. Monitor oxygen therapy—used to relieve hypoxemia.
5. Prepare patient for assisted ventilation when hypoxemia is due to local areas of pneumoconstriction and abnormalities of ventilation–perfusion ratios.

Improving Tissue Perfusion

1. Closely monitor for shock—decreasing blood pressure, tachycardia, cool, clammy skin.
2. Monitor prescribed medications given to preserve right ventricular filling pressure and increase blood pressure.
3. Maintain patient on bed rest to reduce oxygen demands and risk of bleeding.
4. Monitor urinary output hourly, because there may be reduced renal perfusion and decreased glomerular filtration.

Relieving Pain

1. Watch patient for signs of discomfort and pain.
2. Ascertain if pain worsens with deep breathing and coughing; listen for friction rub.
3. Give prescribed morphine (Duramorph), and monitor for pain relief and signs of respiratory depression.
4. Position with head of bed slightly elevated (unless contraindicated by shock) and with chest splinted for deep breathing and coughing.
5. Evaluate patient for signs of hypoxia thoroughly when anxiety, restlessness, and agitation of new onset are noted, before administering prn sedatives. Consider physician evaluation when these signs are present, especially if accompanied by cyanotic nail beds, circumoral pallor, and increased respiratory rate.

Reducing Anxiety

1. Correct dyspnea and relieve physical discomfort.
2. Explain diagnostic procedures and the patient's role; correct any misconceptions.
3. Listen to the patient's concerns. Attentive listening relieves anxiety and reduces emotional distress.
4. Speak calmly and slowly.
5. Do everything possible to enhance the patient's sense of control.

Intervening for Complications

1. Shock—from low cardiac output secondary to resistance to right ventricular outflow or to myocardial dysfunction due to ischemia.
   a. Assess for skin color changes, particularly nail beds, lips, ear lobes, and mucous membranes.
   b. Monitor blood pressure.
   c. Measure urinary output.
   d. Monitor IV infusion of isoproterenol (Isuprel) or other prescribed agents.
2. Bleeding—related to anticoagulant or thrombolytic therapy.
   a. Assess patient for bleeding; major bleeding may occur from GI tract, brain, lungs, nose, and genitourinary (GU) tract.
   b. Perform stool guaiac test to detect occult blood loss.
   c. Monitor platelet count to detect heparin-induced thrombocytopenia.
   d. Minimize risk of bleeding by performing essential ABGs on upper extremities; apply digital compression at puncture site for 30 minutes; apply pressure

dressing to previously involved sites; check site for oozing.

e. Maintain patient on strict bed rest during thrombolytic therapy; avoid unnecessary handling.

f. Discontinue infusion in the event of uncontrolled bleeding.

g. Notify health care provider on call immediately for change in level of consciousness, ability to follow commands, sensation, ability to move limbs and respond to questions with clear articulation. Intracranial bleed may necessitate discontinuation of anticoagulation promptly to avert massive neurologic catastrophe.

Patient Education and Health Maintenance

1. Advise patient of the possible need to continue taking anticoagulant therapy for 6 weeks up to an indefinite period.

2. Teach about signs of bleeding, especially of gums, nose, bruising, blood in urine and stools.

3. For patients on anticoagulants, instruct to use soft toothbrush, avoid shaving with blade razor (use electric razor instead), and avoid aspirin-containing products. Notify health care provider of any bleeding or increased bruising.

4. Warn against taking medications unless approved by health care provider, because many drugs interact with anticoagulants.

5. Instruct patient to tell dentist about taking an anticoagulant.

6. Warn against inactivity for prolonged periods or sitting with legs crossed to prevent recurrence.

7. Warn against sports/activities that may cause injury to legs and predispose to a thrombus.

8. Encourage wearing a Medic-Alert bracelet identifying patient as anticoagulant user.

9. Instruct to lose weight if applicable; obesity is a risk factor for women.

10. Discuss contraceptive methods with patient if applicable; female patients are advised against taking oral contraceptives.

Outcome-Based Evaluation

- Verbalizes less shortness of breath
- Vital signs stable, adequate urinary output
- Reports freedom from pain
- Appears more relaxed; sleeping at long intervals
- Patient progressing without complications

Tuberculosis

Tuberculosis (TB) is an infectious disease caused by bacteria (*Mycobacterium tuberculosis*) that are usually spread from person to person through the air. It usually infects the lung but can occur at virtually any site in the body. HIV-infected patients are especially at risk. Drug-resistant TB is of particular concern in certain parts of the United States.

Pathophysiology and Etiology
Transmission

1. The term *mycobacterium* is descriptive of the organism, which is a bacterium that resembles a fungus. The organisms multiply slowly and are characterized as acid-fast aerobic organisms that can be killed by heat, sunshine, drying, and ultraviolet light.

2. TB is an airborne disease transmitted by droplet nuclei, usually from within the respiratory tract of an infected person who exhales them during coughing, talking, sneezing, or singing.

3. When an uninfected susceptible person inhales the droplet-containing air, the organism is carried into the lung to the pulmonary alveoli.

4. Most people who become infected do not develop clinical illness, because the body's immune system brings the infection under control.

Pathology

1. The bacilli of tuberculosis infect the lung, forming a tubercle (lesion).

2. The tubercle
   a. May heal, leaving scar tissue.
   b. May continue as a granuloma, then heal, or be reactivated.
   c. May eventually proceed to necrosis, liquefaction, sloughing, and cavitation.

3. The initial lesion may disseminate tubercle bacilli by extension to adjacent tissues, by way of the bloodstream, by way of the lymphatic system, or through the bronchi.

Clinical Manifestations

Patient may be asymptomatic or may have insidious symptoms that are ignored.

1. Constitutional symptoms
   a. Fatigue, anorexia, weight loss, low-grade fever, night sweats, indigestion.
   b. Some patients have acute febrile illness, chills, generalized influenzalike symptoms.

2. Pulmonary signs and symptoms
   a. Cough (insidious onset) progressing in frequency and producing mucoid or mucopurulent sputum.
   b. Hemoptysis; chest pain; dyspnea (indicates extensive involvement).

3. Extrapulmonary TB: *Mycobacterium* can infect any organ in the body, including pleurae, lymph nodes, genitourinary tract, bones/joints, peritoneum, central nervous system.

Diagnostic Evaluation

1. Sputum smear and culture—detection of acid-fast bacilli (AFB) in stained smears is the first bacteriologic clue of TB. Obtain first AM sputum on three consecutive days.

2. Sputum culture—a positive culture for *M. tuberculosis* confirms a diagnosis of TB.

3. Chest x-ray to determine presence and extent of disease.

4. Tuberculin skin test (PPD or Mantoux test)—inoculation of tubercle bacillus extract (tuberculin) into the intradermal layer of the inner aspect of the forearm (Procedure Guidelines 11-1). It is used to detect *M. tuberculosis* infection, either past or present, active or inactive.
5. Screening tests—multiple puncture tests such as tine test should not be used to determine if a person is infected.

Management

See Table 11-2.

1. A combination of drugs to which the organisms are susceptible is given to destroy viable bacilli as rapidly as possible and to protect against the emergence of drug-resistant organisms.
2. Current recommended regimen of uncomplicated pulmonary TB is 2 months of bactericidal drugs isoniazid (INH), rifampin (Rifadin; RIF), pyrazinamide (PZA), and ethambutol (EMB) (or streptomycin in children too young to be monitored for visual acuity). This regimen should be included until the results of drug susceptibility studies are available, unless there is little possibility of drug resistance. Follow with 4 months of isoniazid and rifampin.
3. Six months of therapy is usually effective for killing the three populations of bacilli: those rapidly dividing, those slowly dividing, and those only intermittently dividing.
4. Sputum smears may be obtained every 2 weeks until they are negative; sputum cultures do not become negative for 3 to 5 months.
5. Second-line drugs such as capreomycin (Capastat), kanamycin (Kantrex), ethionamide (Trecator-SC), para-aminosalicylic acid, and cycloserine (Seromycin) are used in patients with resistance, for retreatment, and in those with intolerance to other agents. Patients taking these drugs should be monitored by health providers experienced in their use.

 DRUG ALERT

Adverse reactions to anti-TB drugs may occur. Most common side effects are rash, GI intolerance, and liver toxicity. INH may produce peripheral neuropathy. Ethambutol may cause optic neuritis. Pyrazinamide may cause gout. Any anti-TB drug may cause rash. If rash occurs, hold all medications until rash subsides. Rechallenge drugs sequentially every 3 to 4 days to find cause. Usual sequence is INH, RIF, PZA, EMB, using the most important drug first. Liver toxicity is the most concerning adverse reaction. Toxic hepatitis may be caused by INH, RIF, and PZA. Instruct patients to seek immediate medical attention if symptoms or signs of hepatitis occur (nausea, emesis, anorexia, jaundice, and/or abdominal pain).

Complications

1. Pleural effusion
2. Tuberculosis pneumonia
3. Other organ involvement with tuberculosis

Nursing Assessment

1. Obtain history of exposure to tuberculosis.
2. Assess for symptoms of active disease—productive cough, night sweats, afternoon temperature elevation, weight loss, pleuritic chest pain.

TABLE 11-2   Recommended Drugs for the Initial Treatment of Tuberculosis in Adults

Drug	Dosage Forms	Daily Dose	Twice Weekly Dose	Thrice Weekly Dose	Major Adverse Reactions
Isoniazid (INH)	Tablets: 100 mg 300 mg Syrup: 50 mg/5 mL Vials: 1 g	5 mg/kg PO or IM	15 mg/kg Maximum 900 mg	15 mg/kg Maximum 900 mg	Hepatic enzyme elevation, peripheral neuropathy, hepatitis, hypersensitivity
Rifampin (Rifadin)	Capsules: 150 mg 300 mg Syrup: formulated from capsules, 10 mg/mL	10 mg/kg PO	10 mg/kg Maximum 600 mg	10 mg/kg Maximum 600 mg	Orange discoloration of secretions and urine; nausea, vomiting, hepatitis, febrile reaction, purpura (rare)
Pyrazinamide (PAZ)	Tablets: 500 mg	15–30 mg/kg PO	50–70 mg/kg	50–70 mg/kg Maximum 3 g	Hepatotoxicity, hyperuricemia, arthralgias, skin rash, gastrointestinal upset
Streptomycin	Vials: 1 g, 4 g	15 mg/kg IM	25–30 mg/kg	25–30 mg/kg Maximum 1.5 g	Ototoxicity, nephrotoxicity
Ethambutol (Myambutol)	Tablets: 100 mg 400 mg	15–25 mg/kg PO	50 mg/kg	25–30 mg/kg	Optic neuritis (decreased red-green color discrimination, decreased visual acuity), skin rash

3. Auscultate lungs for crackles.
4. If patient is on isoniazid, assess for liver dysfunction.
   a. Question the patient about loss of appetite, fatigue, joint pain, fever, and dark urine.
   b. Monitor for fever, right upper quadrant abdominal tenderness, nausea, vomiting, rash, persistent paresthesias of hands and feet.
   c. Monitor results of periodic liver function studies.

Nursing Diagnoses

- Ineffective Breathing Pattern related to decreased lung capacity
- Risk for Infection Transmission related to nature of the disease and patient's symptoms
- Altered Nutrition: Less Than Body Requirements related to poor appetite, fatigue, and productive cough
- Noncompliance related to lack of motivation and long-term treatment

Nursing Interventions

Improving Breathing Pattern

1. Administer and teach self-administration of medications as ordered.
2. Encourage rest and avoidance of exertion.
3. Monitor breath sounds, respiratory rate, sputum production, and dyspnea.
4. Provide supplemental oxygen as ordered.

Preventing Transmission of Infection

1. Be aware that TB is transmitted by respiratory droplets or secretions.
2. Provide care for hospitalized patient in a negative pressure room to prevent respiratory droplets from leaving room when door is opened.
3. Enforce that all staff and visitors use standard dust/mist/fume masks (Class C) for any contact with patient.
4. Use high-efficiency particulate masks such as HEPA filter masks for high-risk procedures such as suctioning, bronchoscopy, or pentamidine treatments.
5. Use Standard Precautions for additional protection: gowns and gloves for any direct contact with patient, linens or articles in room, meticulous handwashing, and so forth.
6. Educate the patient to control spread of infection through secretions.
   a. Cover mouth and nose with double-ply tissue when coughing or sneezing. Do not sneeze into bare hand.
   b. Wash hands after coughing or sneezing.
   c. Dispose of tissues promptly into closed plastic bag.

Improving Nutritional Status

1. Encourage and explain the importance of eating a nutritious diet to promote healing and improve defense against infection.
2. Provide small frequent meals and liquid supplements during symptomatic period.

3. Monitor weight.
4. Administer vitamin supplements, as ordered, particularly pyridoxine (vitamin B_6) to prevent peripheral neuropathy in patients taking isoniazid.

Avoiding Noncompliance

1. Educate the patient about the etiology, transmission, and effects of TB. Stress the importance of continuing to take medicine for the prescribed time because bacilli multiply very slowly and thus can only be eradicated over a long period of time.
2. Review the side effects of the drug therapy (see Table 11-2). Question the patient specifically about common toxicities of drugs being used, and emphasize immediate reporting should these occur.
3. Participate in observation of medication taking, weekly pill counts, or other programs designed to increase compliance with treatment for TB.

NURSING ALERT

Patient compliance remains a major problem in eradicating TB. Therefore, it may be helpful or necessary to have patient take medication in observed setting.

Community and Home Care Considerations

1. Improve ventilation in the home by opening windows in room of affected person, and keeping bedroom door closed as much as possible.
2. Instruct patient to cover mouth with fresh tissue when coughing or sneezing and to dispose of tissues promptly in plastic bags.
3. Discuss TB testing of persons residing with patient.
4. Investigate living conditions, availability of transportation, financial status, alcohol and drug abuse, and motivation, which may affect compliance with follow-up and treatment. Initiate referrals to a social worker for interventions in these areas.

Patient Education and Health Maintenance

1. Review possible complications: hemorrhage, pleurisy, symptoms of recurrence (persistent cough, fever, or hemoptysis).
2. Advise on avoidance of job-related exposure to excessive amounts of silicone (working in foundry, rock quarry, sand blasting), which increases chance of reactivation.
3. Encourage the patient to report at specified intervals for bacteriologic (smear) examination of sputum to monitor therapeutic response and compliance.
4. Instruct in basic hygiene practices and investigate living conditions. Crowded, poorly ventilated conditions contribute to development and spread of TB.
5. Encourage follow-up chest x-rays for rest of life to evaluate for recurrence.

6. Instruct on prophylaxis with isoniazid for persons infected with the tubercle bacillus without active disease to prevent disease from occurring, or to people at high risk of becoming infected.
7. Prophylaxis is recommended for the following groups:
   a. Household members and other close associates of potentially infectious TB cases
   b. Newly infected persons (positive skin test within 2 years)
   c. Persons with past TB who have not received adequate therapy
   d. Persons with significant reactions to tuberculin skin test and who are in special clinical situations (silicosis, diabetes, B-cell malignancies, end-stage renal disease, severe malnutrition, immunosuppression, HIV positive)
   e. Tuberculin skin reactors under age 35 years with none of the aforementioned risk factors

Outcome-Based Evaluation

- Afebrile; dyspnea relieved
- Standard precautions observed; patient disposing of respiratory secretions properly
- Maintains body weight
- Taking medications as prescribed

PROCEDURE GUIDELINES 11-1   TUBERCULIN SKIN TEST

EQUIPMENT

Purified protein derivative (PPD) tuberculin antigen; intermediate strength
Tuberculin syringe

Short 1.25 cm (½ inch) 26- or 27-gauge steel needle
Alcohol sponge
Gloves

PROCEDURE

Nursing Action	Rationale
PREPARATORY PHASE	
1. Determine if the patient has ever had BCG vaccine, recent viral disease, immunosuppression by disease, drugs, or steroids.	1. Any of these may cause false readings.
PERFORMANCE PHASE	
1. Draw up PPD-tuberculin into tuberculin syringe.	1. Follow the manufacturer's directions. Each 0.1-mL dose should contain 5 tuberculin units (TU of PPD-tuberculin). Use the antigen immediately to avoid absorption onto the plastic/glass syringe.
2. Don gloves.	2. Follow universal/standard infection control precaution.
3. Cleanse the skin of the inner aspect of forearm with alcohol. Allow to dry.	
4. Stretch the skin taut.	
5. Hold the tuberculin syringe close to the skin so the hub of the needle touches it as the needle is introduced, bevel up.	5. This reduces the needle angle at the skin surface and facilitates the injection of tuberculin just beneath the surface of the skin.
6. Inject the tuberculin into the superficial layer of the skin to form a wheal 6 mm to 10 mm in diameter.	6. If no wheal appears (because the injection was made too deep), inject again at another site at least 5 cm (2 inches) away.
7. Immediately place disposable needle and syringe into puncture-resistant sharps container.	
FOLLOW-UP PHASE	
To Read the Test	
1. Read the test within 48 to 72 hours when the induration is most evident.	1. Tuberculin skin tests are tests of *delayed hypersensitivity*.
2. Have a good light available. Flex the forearm slightly at the elbow.	
3. Inspect for the presence of induration; inspect from a side view against the light; inspect by direct light.	3. Induration refers to hardening or thickening of tissues.
4. Palpate: Lightly rub the finger across the injection site from the area of normal skin to the area of induration. Outline the diameter of induration.	4. Erythema (redness) without induration is generally considered to be of no significance.

PROCEDURE GUIDELINES 11-1   *CONTINUED*

Nursing Action	Rationale
5. Measure the maximum transverse diameter of induration (not erythema) in millimeters with a flexible ruler.	5. The extent of induration is measured in two diameters and recorded.

Interpretation

1. Induration of 5 mm or more in diameter	1. Considered positive in
	  a. People with known HIV or unknown HIV but with risk factors for HIV
	  b. People who have had recent contact with active tuberculosis
	  c. People who have fibrotic changes on chest x-ray, consistent with healed TB

2. Induration of 10 mm or more in diameter	2. Considered positive in:
	  a. People with certain medical conditions (diabetes mellitus, silicosis, head and neck cancer, leukemia, end-stage renal disease, gastrectomy, prolonged corticosteroid therapy)
	  b. Foreign-born people from areas of the world where TB is common (Asia, Africa, Latin America)
	  c. Medically underserved, low-income populations
	  d. Residents of long-term care facilities
	  e. Children less than 4 years of age
	  f. All people who do not meet above criteria but who have other risk factors for tuberculosis, such as homelessness, alcoholism, malnutrition, and health care work

3. Induration of 15 mm or more in diameter	3. Considered positive in people who do not meet the above criteria.

NURSING ALERT False-positive reaction may occur in people infected with mycobacteria other than *M. tuberculosis* and vaccination with bacille Calmette-Guérin (BCG).
False-negative reactions may occur in people with HIV infection, overwhelming miliary or pulmonary TB, severe or febrile illness, measles or other viral infections, Hodgkin's disease, sarcoidosis, live-virus vaccinations, and those receiving corticosteroids or immunosuppressive drugs.

Pleurisy

Pleurisy is a clinical term to describe *pleuritis* (inflammation of the pleura, both parietal and visceral).

Pathophysiology and Etiology

1. Inflammation of the pleura stimulates nerve endings, causing pain.
2. May occur in the course of many pulmonary diseases:
   a. Pneumonia (bacterial, viral)
   b. TB
   c. Pulmonary infarction, embolism
   d. Pulmonary abscess
   e. Upper respiratory tract infection
   f. Pulmonary neoplasm

Clinical Manifestations

1. Chest pain—becomes severe, sharp, and knifelike on inspiration (pleuritic pain)
   a. May become minimal or absent when breath is held
   b. May be localized or radiate to shoulder or abdomen
2. Intercostal tenderness

3. Pleural friction rub—grating or leathery sounds heard in both phases of respiration; heard low in the axilla or over the lung base posteriorly; may be heard for only a day or so
4. Evidence of infection; fever, malaise, increased white cell count

Diagnostic Evaluation

1. Chest x-ray may show pleural thickening.
2. Sputum examination may indicate infectious organism.
3. Examination of pleural fluid obtained by thoracentesis for smear and culture.
4. Pleural biopsy may be necessary to rule out other conditions.

Management

1. Treatment for the underlying primary disease (pneumonia, infarction, and so forth). Inflammation usually resolves when the primary disease subsides.
2. Pain relief, using both pharmacologic and nonpharmacologic methods.
3. Intercostal nerve block may be necessary when pain causes hypoventilation (Procedure Guidelines 11-2).

Complications
Severe pleural effusion.

Nursing Assessment
1. Assess patient's level of pain.
2. Observe for signs and symptoms of pleural effusion (dyspnea, pain, decreased local excursion of chest wall).
3. Auscultate lungs for pleural friction rub.

Nursing Diagnosis
- Ineffective Breathing Pattern related to stabbing chest pain

Nursing Interventions
Relieving Pain
1. Assist patient to find comfortable position that will promote aeration; lying on affected side decreases stretching of the pleura and, therefore, the pain decreases.
2. Instruct patient in splinting chest while taking a deep breath or coughing.
3. Administer or teach self-administration of pain medications as ordered.

4. Employ nonpharmacologic interventions for pain relief such as application of heat, muscle relaxation, and imagery.
5. Assist with intercostal nerve block if indicated.
6. Evaluate patient for signs of hypoxia thoroughly when anxiety, restlessness, and agitation of new onset are noted, before administering prn sedatives. Consider physician evaluation when these signs are present, especially if accompanied by cyanotic nail beds, circumoral pallor, and increased respiratory rate.

Patient Education and Health Maintenance
1. Instruct patient to seek early intervention for pulmonary diseases so pleurisy can be avoided.
2. Reassure and encourage patience because pain will subside.
3. Advise on reporting shortness of breath, which could indicate pleural effusion.

Outcome-Based Evaluation
- Respirations deep without pain.

PROCEDURE GUIDELINES 11-2   ASSISTING WITH AN INTERCOSTAL NERVE BLOCK

EQUIPMENT
Syringes, 10-mL Luer-Lok
Needles, No. 22 to 30 gauge

Anesthetic solution (lidocaine, bupivacaine, procaine)
Skin germicide; sterile gloves

PROCEDURE

Nursing Action	Rationale
PREPARATION PHASE	
1. Inform the patient that he or she will experience the prick of the needle and a slight sensation of pressure.	
2. Position the patient as directed:	
a. Have the patient sit up, bend forward, and hug a pillow, OR	a. This posture moves the scapulae forward and out of the way.
b. Place the patient prone with pillow under chest, OR	b. The prone position helps immobilize the patient.
c. Have the patient lie on unaffected side with upper arm hanging over the side of the table.	c. This pulls the scapula out of the way.
3. Ask the patient to identify the site of pain.	3. To determine which intercostal nerves are to be injected.
PERFORMANCE PHASE (BY THE PHYSICIAN)	
1. After the skin is prepared, the lower margin of the rib is palpated and a small skin wheal is raised, using a 25- to 30-gauge needle.	1. This is infiltration anesthesia.
2. Usually nerve blocks are done at the posterior angle of the ribs between the posterior axillary line and the spine.	2. The posterior angle is the most prominent and accessible, and an injection at this area produces a block of the entire distal nerve.
3. A fine needle is advanced through the wheal and directed downward so it slips under the edge of the rib into the upper portion of the interspace.	3. The intercostal nerve runs in a groove along the undersurface of the above rib.
4. The syringe (needle in place) is aspirated.	4. To ensure that the needle has not punctured the lung or that an intercostal vessel has been entered.
5. The local anesthetic (usually 3–5 mL) is injected into the area.	5. Usually the local anesthetic is injected above and below the painful rib to obtain complete relief of pain, as the sensory fields of intercostal nerves overlap.

PROCEDURE GUIDELINES 11-2   *CONTINUED*

Nursing Action	Rationale

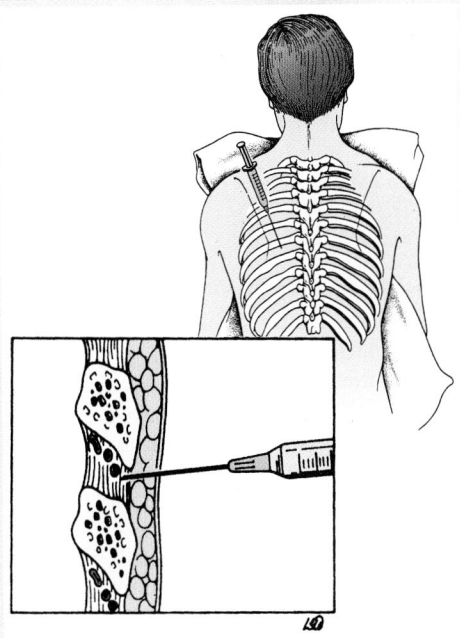

Intercostal nerve block

FOLLOW-UP PHASE

1. Assess for relief of pain and less painful coughing.
2. Obtain a chest x-ray.
3. Complications:
   a. Intravascular injection.
   b. Puncture of the lung with pneumothorax
   c. Hypotension

1. This is the expected outcome.
2. To ensure that a pneumothorax has not occurred.

▊ Pleural Effusion

Pleural effusion refers to a collection of fluid in the pleural space. It is almost always secondary to other diseases.

Pathophysiology and Etiology

1. May be either transudative or exudative.
2. Transudative effusions occur primarily in noninflammatory conditions; is an accumulation of low-protein, low cell count fluid.
3. Exudative effusions occur in an area of inflammation; is an accumulation of high-protein fluid.
4. Is a complication of:
   a. Disseminated cancer (particularly lung and breast), lymphoma.
   b. Pleuropulmonary infections (pneumonia).
   c. Congestive heart failure (CHF), cirrhosis, nephrosis.
   d. Other conditions—sarcoidosis, systemic lupus erythematosus (SLE), peritoneal dialysis, and so forth.

Clinical Manifestations

1. Dyspnea, pleuritic chest pain, cough
2. Dullness or flatness to percussion (over areas of fluid) with decreased or absent breath sounds

Diagnostic Evaluation

1. Chest x-ray or ultrasound to detect presence of fluid
2. Thoracentesis—biochemical, bacteriologic, and cytologic studies of pleural fluid to indicate cause

Management
General

1. Treatment is directed at underlying cause (heart disease, infection).
2. Thoracentesis is done to remove fluid, to collect a specimen, and to relieve dyspnea.

For Malignant Effusions

1. Chest tube drainage, radiation, chemotherapy, surgical pleurodectomy, pleuroperitoneal shunt, or pleurodesis.

2. In malignant conditions, thoracentesis may provide only transient benefits, because effusion may reaccumulate within a few days.
3. *Pleurodesis*—production of adhesions between the parietal and visceral pleura accomplished by tube thoracostomy, pleural space drainage, and intrapleural instillation of a sclerosing agent (tetracycline).
   a. Drug introduced through tube into pleural space; tube clamped.
   b. Patient is helped to assume varying positions for 3 to 5 minutes each to allow drug to spread to all surfaces of the pleura.
   c. Tube is unclamped as prescribed.
   d. Chest drainage continued for 24 hours or longer.
   e. Resulting pleural irritation, inflammation, and fibrosis cause adhesion of the visceral and parietal surfaces when they are brought together by the negative pressure caused by chest suction.

Complications
1. Large effusion could lead to respiratory failure.

Nursing Assessment
1. Obtain history of previous pulmonary condition.
2. Assess patient for dyspnea and tachypnea.
3. Auscultate and percuss lungs for abnormalities.

Nursing Diagnosis
- Ineffective Breathing Pattern related to collection of fluid in pleural space

Nursing Interventions
Maintaining Normal Breathing Pattern
1. Institute treatments to resolve the underlying cause, as ordered.
2. Assist with thoracentesis, if indicated (see p. 201).
3. Maintain chest drainage as needed (see p. 267).
4. Provide care after pleurodesis.
   a. Monitor for excessive pain from the sclerosing agent, which may cause hypoventilation.
   b. Administer prescribed analgesic.
   c. Assist patient undergoing instillation of intrapleural lidocaine if pain relief is not forthcoming.
   d. Administer oxygen as indicated by dyspnea and hypoxemia.
   e. Observe patient's breathing pattern, oxygen saturation, and other vital signs, for evidence of improvement or deterioration.

Patient Education and Health Maintenance
Instruct patient to seek early intervention for unusual shortness of breath, especially if patient has underlying chronic lung disease.

Outcome-Based Evaluation
- Reports absence of shortness of breath

Lung Abscess
A *lung abscess* is a localized, pus-containing, necrotic lesion in the lung characterized by cavity formation.

Pathophysiology and Etiology
1. Most often occurs due to aspiration of vomitus or infected material from upper respiratory tract.
2. Secondary causes include:
   a. Aspiration of foreign body into lung.
   b. Pulmonary embolus.
   c. Trauma.
   d. TB, necrotizing pneumonia.
   e. Bronchial obstruction (usually a tumor) causes obstruction to bronchus, leading to infection distal to the growth.
3. The right lung is involved more frequently than the left because of dependent position of the right bronchus, the less acute angle that the right main bronchus forms within the trachea, and its larger size.
4. In the initial stages, the cavity in the lung may or may not communicate with the bronchus.
5. Eventually, the cavity becomes surrounded or encapsulated by a wall of fibrous tissue, except at one or two points where the necrotic process extends until it reaches the lumen of some bronchus or pleural space and establishes a communication with the respiratory tract, the pleural cavity (bronchopleural fistula), or both.
6. The organisms most often seen are *Klebsiella pneumoniae* and *Staphylococcus aureus*.

Clinical Manifestations
1. Cough, fever, and malaise from segmental pneumonitis and atelectasis.
2. Headache, anemia, weight loss, dyspnea, weakness.
3. Pleuritic chest pain from extension of suppurative pneumonitis to pleural surface.
4. Production of mucopurulent sputum, often foul-smelling; blood streaking common; may become profuse after abscess ruptures into bronchial tree.
5. Chest may be dull to percussion, decreased or absent breath sounds, intermittent pleural friction rub.

Diagnostic Evaluation
1. X-ray of chest for diagnosis and location of lesion
2. Direct bronchoscopic visualization to exclude possibility of tumor or foreign body; bronchial washings and brush biopsy may be done for cytopathologic study
3. Sputum culture and sensitivity to determine causative organism(s) and antimicrobial sensitivity

Management
1. Administration of appropriate antimicrobial agent, usually by IV route, until clinical condition improves; then oral administration.
2. Chest physical therapy and postural drainage to drain cavity.
3. Bronchoscopy to drain abscess is controversial.

4. Surgical intervention only if patient fails to respond to medical management, sustains a hemorrhage, or has a suspected tumor.
5. Nutritional management usually is a high-calorie, high-protein diet.

Complications
1. Hemoptysis from erosion of a vessel
2. Empyema, bronchopleural fistula
3. Brain abscess

Nursing Assessment
1. Examine oral cavity, because poor condition of teeth and gums increases number of anaerobes in oral cavity and could be source for infection.
2. Perform chest examination for abnormalities.
3. Monitor for foul-smelling sputum, which may indicate an anaerobic pulmonary infection.
4. Review results of laboratory and x-ray findings for location of abscess and identification of causative organism.

Nursing Diagnoses
- Ineffective Breathing Pattern related to presence of suppurative lung disease
- Pain related to infection
- Altered Nutrition: Less Than Body Requirements related to catabolic state from chronic infection

Nursing Interventions
Minimizing Respiratory Dysfunction
1. Monitor patient's response to antimicrobial therapy; take temperature at prescribed intervals.
2. Carry out drainage procedures to hasten resolution.
   a. Postural drainage positions to be assumed depend on location of abscess.
   b. Carry out percussion, coughing, and breathing exercises.
   c. Measure and record the volume of sputum to follow patient's clinical course.
   d. Give adequate fluids to enhance liquefying of secretions.

Attaining Comfort
1. Use nursing measures to combat generalized discomfort; oral hygiene, positions of comfort, relaxing massage.
2. Take temperature, pulse, and respirations at regular intervals to determine type of fever and monitor the severity and duration of the infectious process.
3. Encourage rest and limitation of physical activity during febrile periods.
4. Monitor chest tube functioning.
5. Evaluate patient for signs of hypoxia thoroughly when anxiety, restlessness, and agitation of new onset are noted, before administering prn sedatives. Consider physician evaluation when these signs are present, especially if accompanied by cyanotic nail beds, circumoral pallor, increased respiratory rate, and so forth.

Improving Nutritional Status
1. Provide a high-protein and high-calorie diet.
2. Offer liquid supplements for additional nutritional support when anorexia limits patient's intake.
3. Monitor weight weekly.

Patient Education and Health Maintenance
1. Teach the patient that an extended course of antimicrobial therapy (4 to 8 weeks) is usually necessary; mixed infections are common and may require multiple antibiotics.
2. Encourage patient to have periodontal care, especially in presence of gingival lesions.
3. Stress importance of follow-up x-rays to monitor abscess cavity closure.
4. Remind family that patient may aspirate if weakness, confusion, alcoholism, seizures, and swallowing difficulties are present.
5. Encourage patient to assume responsibility for attaining/maintaining an optimal state of health through a planned program of nutrition, rest, and exercise.

Outcome-Based Evaluation
- Achieves improved respiratory function; temperature in normal range; less purulent sputum expectorated
- Appears more comfortable; verbalizes less pain
- Eating better; weight stable

▧ Cancer of the Lung (Bronchogenic Cancer)

Bronchogenic cancer refers to a malignant tumor of the lung arising within the wall or epithelial lining of the bronchus. The lung is also a common site of metastasis from cancer elsewhere in the body by way of venous circulation or lymphatic spread. Bronchogenic cancer is classified according to cell type:

Epidermoid (squamous cell)—most common
Adenocarcinoma
Small cell (oat cell) carcinoma
Large cell (undifferentiated) carcinoma

Pathophysiology and Etiology
Predisposing Factors
1. Cigarette smoking—amount, frequency, and duration of smoking have positive relationship to cancer of the lung.
2. Occupational exposure to asbestos, arsenic, chromium, nickel, iron, radioactive substances, isopropyl oil, coal tar products, petroleum oil mists alone or in combination with tobacco smoke.

NURSING ALERT

Suspect cancer of the lung in patients who belong to a susceptible, high-risk age group and who have repeated unresolved respiratory infections.

Staging

1. Refers to anatomic extent of tumor, lymph node involvement, and metastatic spread
2. Staging done by:
   a. Tissue diagnosis
   b. Lymph node biopsy
   c. Mediastinoscopy

Clinical Manifestations

Usually occur late and are related to size and location of tumor, extent of spread, and involvement of other structures

1. Cough, especially a new type or changing cough, results from bronchial irritation.
2. Dyspnea, wheezing (suggests partial bronchial obstruction)
3. Chest pain (poorly localized and aching)
4. Excessive sputum production, repeated upper respiratory infections
5. Hemoptysis
6. Malaise, fever, weight loss, fatigue, anorexia
7. Paraneoplastic syndrome—metabolic or neurologic disturbances related to the secretion of substances by the neoplasm
8. Symptoms of metastases—bone pain, abdominal discomfort, nausea and vomiting from liver involvement, pancytopenia from bone marrow involvement, headache from CNS metastasis
9. Usual sites of metastases—lymph nodes, bones, liver

Diagnostic Evaluation

1. X-ray of the chest, including fluoroscopy and tomography; lung cancers may be partly or completely hidden by other structures.
2. Cytologic examination of sputum/chest fluids for malignant cells.
3. Fiberoptic bronchoscopy for observation of location and extent of tumor; for biopsy.
4. CT—sensitive in detecting small nodules and metastatic lesions.
5. Lymph node biopsy; mediastinoscopy to establish lymphatic spread; to plan treatment.
6. Pulmonary function tests (PFTs) combined with split-function perfusion scan to determine if patient will have adequate pulmonary reserve to withstand surgical procedure.

Management

The treatment depends on the cell type, stage of disease, and the physiologic status of the patient. It includes a multidisciplinary approach that may be used separately or in combination, including:

1. Surgical resection
2. Radiotherapy
3. Chemotherapy
4. Immunotherapy

See Chapter 8 for more information on these methods.

Complications

1. Superior vena cava syndrome—oncologic complication caused by obstruction of major blood vessels draining the head, neck, and upper torso
2. Hypercalcemia—commonly from bone metastases
3. Syndrome of inappropriate antidiuretic hormone (SIADH) secretion with hyponatremia and abnormal water retention
4. Pleural effusion
5. Infectious complications, especially upper respiratory infections
6. Brain metastasis, spinal cord compression

Nursing Assessment

1. Determine onset and duration of coughing, sputum production, and the degree of dyspnea. Auscultate for breath sounds. Observe symmetry of chest during respirations.
2. Take anthropometric measurements; weigh patient; review laboratory biochemical tests; conduct appraisal of 24-hour food intake.
3. Ask about pain: location, intensity, factors influencing pain.

Nursing Diagnoses

- Ineffective Breathing Pattern related to obstructive and restrictive respiratory processes associated with lung cancer
- Altered Nutrition: Less Than Body Requirements related to hypermetabolic state, taste aversion, anorexia secondary to radiotherapy/chemotherapy
- Pain related to tumor effects, invasion of adjacent structures, toxicities associated with radiotherapy/chemotherapy
- Anxiety related to uncertain outcome and fear of recurrence

Nursing Interventions

See also Chapter 8.

Improving Breathing Patterns

1. Prepare patient physically, emotionally, and intellectually for prescribed therapeutic program.
2. Elevate head of bed to promote gravity drainage and prevent fluid collection in upper body (from superior vena cava syndrome).
3. Teach breathing retraining exercises to increase diaphragmatic excursion with resultant reduction in work of breathing.
4. Give prescribed treatment for productive cough (expectorant, antimicrobial agent) to prevent thickened secretions and subsequent dyspnea.
5. Augment the patient's ability to cough effectively.
   a. Splint chest manually with hands.
   b. Instruct patient to inspire fully and cough two to three times in one breath.
   c. Provide humidifier/vaporizer to provide moisture to loosen secretions.

6. Support patient undergoing removal of pleural fluid (by thoracentesis or tube thoracostomy) and instillation of sclerosing agent to obliterate pleural space and prevent fluid recurrence.

7. Administer oxygen by way of nasal cannula as prescribed.

8. Encourage energy conservation through decreasing activities.

9. Allow patient to sleep in a reclining chair if severely dyspneic.

10. Recognize the anxiety associated with dyspnea; teach relaxation techniques.

Improving Nutritional Status

1. Emphasize that nutrition is an important part of the treatment of lung cancer.
   a. Encourage small amounts of high-calorie and high-protein foods frequently, rather than three daily meals.
   b. Suggest eating major meal in the morning if rapidly becoming satiated and feeling full are problems.
   c. Ensure adequate protein intake—milk, eggs, chicken, fowl, fish, cheese, and oral nutritional supplements if patient cannot tolerate other meats.

2. Administer or encourage prescribed vitamin supplement to avoid deficiency states, glossitis, and cheilosis.

3. Change consistency of diet to soft or liquid if patient has esophagitis from radiation therapy.

4. Give enteral or total parenteral nutrition for malnourished patient who is unable or unwilling to eat.

Controlling Pain

1. Take a history of pain complaint; assess presence/absence of support system.

2. Administer prescribed drug, usually starting with nonsteroidal anti-inflammatory drugs (NSAID) and progressing to adjuvant analgesic and narcotic agents.
   a. Administer regularly to maintain pain at tolerable level.
   b. Titrate to achieve pain control.

3. Consider alternative methods, such as cognitive and behavioral training, biofeedback, relaxation, to increase patient's sense of control.

4. Evaluate problems of insomnia, depression, anxiety, and so forth that may be contributing to patient's pain.

5. Initiate bowel training program, because constipation is a side effect of some analgesic/narcotic agents.

6. Facilitate referral to pain clinic/specialist if pain becomes refractory (unyielding) to usual methods of control.

Minimizing Anxiety

1. Realize that shock, disbelief, denial, anger, and depression are all normal reactions to the diagnosis of lung cancer.

2. Try to have the patient express any concerns; share these concerns with health professionals.

3. Encourage the patient to communicate feelings to significant people in his or her life.

4. Expect some feelings of anxiety and depression to recur during illness.

5. Encourage the patient to keep active and remain in the mainstream. Continue with usual activities (work, recreation, sexual) as much as possible.

Patient Education and Health Maintenance

1. Teach patient to use NSAID or other prescribed medication as necessary for pain without being overly concerned about addiction.

2. Help the patient realize that not every ache and pain is due to the results of lung cancer; some patients do not even experience pain.

3. Tell the patient that radiation therapy may be used for pain control if tumor has spread to bone.

4. Advise the patient to report any new or persistent pain; it may be due to some other cause, such as arthritis.

5. Suggest talking to a social worker about financial assistance, or other services that may be needed.

6. For additional information, call American Cancer Society. Call local unit or 1-800-ACS-2345; *www.cancer.org*.

Outcome-Based Evaluation

- Able to perform self-care without dyspnea
- Eating small meals four to five times a day; weight stable
- Reports pain decreased from level 6 to level 2 with medication
- Verbalizing anger; practicing relaxation techniques

CHRONIC DISORDERS

Bronchiectasis

Bronchiectasis is a chronic dilatation of the bronchi and bronchioles due to inflammation and destruction of their walls.

Pathophysiology and Etiology

1. There is damage to the bronchial wall, which leads to the buildup of thick sputum, causing obstruction.

2. Severe coughing results in the permanent dilation of the bronchial walls.

3. Usually involves the lower lobes.

4. As the process progresses, there is atelectasis and fibrosis, which lead to respiratory insufficiency.

5. Pulmonary infections, obstruction of bronchi, aspiration of foreign bodies, vomitus, or material from upper respiratory tract, and immunodeficiency are common causes.

Clinical Manifestations

1. Persistent cough with production of copious amounts of purulent sputum

2. Intermittent hemoptysis; breathlessness

3. Recurrent fever and bouts of pulmonary infection

4. Crackles and rhonchi heard over involved lobes

5. Finger clubbing

Diagnostic Evaluation

1. Chest x-ray may reveal areas of atelectasis with widespread dilatation of bronchi.
2. Sputum examination may detect offending pathogens.
3. High-resolution computed tomography (CT) scan useful in diagnosis of bronchiectasis.

Management

Goal: prevent progression of disease.
1. Infection controlled by:
   a. Smoking cessation
   b. Prompt antimicrobial treatment of exacerbations of infection
   c. Immunization against potential pulmonary pathogens (influenza and pneumococcal vaccine)
2. Secretion clearance techniques such as postural drainage, percussion, vibration, PEP valve, flutter valve, and so forth.
3. Bronchodilators for bronchodilatation and improved secretion clearance.
4. Surgical resection (segmental resection) when conservative management fails.

Complications

1. Progressive suppuration
2. Hemoptysis, major pulmonary hemorrhage
3. COPD, emphysema, chronic respiratory insufficiency

Nursing Assessment

1. Obtain history regarding amount and characteristics of sputum produced, including hemoptysis.
2. Auscultate lungs for diffuse rhonchi and crackles.

Nursing Diagnosis

- Ineffective Airway Clearance related to tenacious and copious secretions

Nursing Interventions

Maintaining Airway Clearance

1. Encourage use of chest physical therapy techniques to empty the bronchi of their accumulated secretions.
   a. Assist with postural drainage positioning for involved lung segment(s) to drain the bronchiectatic areas by gravity, thus reducing degree of infection and symptoms.
   b. Employ percussion and vibration to assist in mobilizing secretions.
   c. Encourage productive coughing to help clear secretions.
   d. Consider PEP valve or flutter valve for enhanced secretion clearance
2. Encourage increased intake of fluids to reduce viscosity of sputum and make expectoration easier.
3. Consider vaporizer to provide humidification and keep secretions thin.

Patient Education and Health Maintenance

1. Instruct the patient to avoid noxious fumes, dusts, smoke and other pulmonary irritants.
2. Teach the patient to monitor sputum. Report if change in quantity (increase/decrease) or character occurs.
3. Instruct the patient and family about importance of pulmonary drainage.
   a. Teach drainage exercises and chest physical therapy techniques.
   b. Encourage postural drainage before rising in the morning, because sputum accumulates during night.
   c. Encourage patient to engage in physical activity throughout day to help mobilize mucus.
4. Encourage regular dental care because copious sputum production may affect dentition.
5. Emphasize the importance of influenza and pneumococcal immunizations and prompt treatment of all respiratory infections.

Outcome-Based Evaluation

- Decreased sputum; lungs clear after chest physical therapy

Chronic Obstructive Pulmonary Disease (COPD)

COPD is a term that refers to a group of conditions characterized by continued increased resistance to expiratory airflow. COPD includes chronic bronchitis and pulmonary emphysema. Some clinicians consider asthma as part of COPD, but due to its reversibility, it is considered by most to be a separate entity (see section titled Bronchial Asthma, Chapter 28).

Chronic bronchitis is a chronic inflammation of the lower respiratory tract characterized by excessive mucous secretion, cough, and dyspnea associated with recurring infections of the lower respiratory tract.

Pulmonary emphysema is a complex lung disease characterized by destruction of the alveoli, enlargement of distal airspaces, and a breakdown of alveolar walls. There is a slowly progressive deterioration of lung function for many years before the development of illness.

Pathophysiology and Etiology

1. The person with COPD may have (Figure 11-3):
   a. Excessive secretion of mucus and chronic infection within the airways (bronchitis)—infection, irritation, hypersensitivity → local hyperemia → hypertrophy of mucous glands → increase in size and number of mucus-producing elements in bronchi (mucous glands and goblet cells) → inflammation and edema → narrowing and obstruction of airflow.
   b. Increase in size of airspaces distal to the terminal bronchioles, with loss of alveolar walls and elastic recoil of the lungs (emphysema).
   c. There may be an overlap of these conditions.
2. As a result of these conditions, there is a subsequent derangement of airway dynamics (eg, obstruction to airflow).
3. The etiology of COPD includes:
   a. Cigarette smoking
   b. Air pollution, occupational exposure

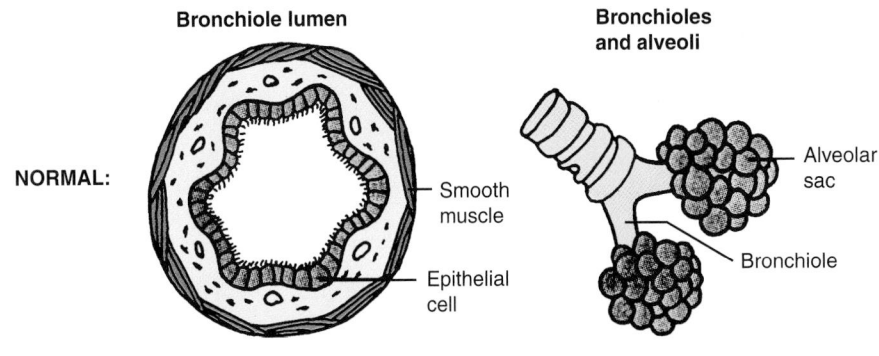

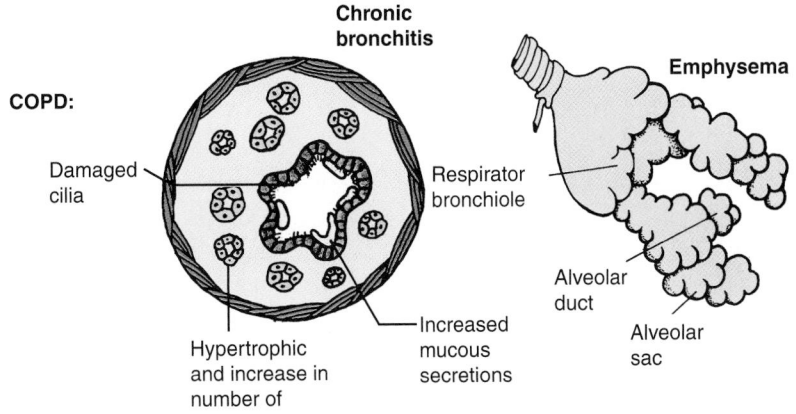

FIGURE 11-3 Airway changes in COPD compared with normal.

c. Allergy, autoimmunity

d. Infection

e. Genetic predisposition, aging

4. Alpha$_1$-antitrypsin deficiency is a genetically determined cause of emphysema and occasionally liver disease. Alpha$_1$-antitrypsin serves primarily as an inhibitor of neutrophil elastase, an elastin-degrading protease released by neutrophils. When alveolar structures are left unprotected from exposure to elastase, progressive destruction of elastin tissues results in the development of emphysema.

Clinical Manifestations

Chronic Bronchitis

Usually insidious, developing over a period of years

1. Presence of a productive cough lasting at least 3 months a year for 2 successive years

2. Production of thick, gelatinous sputum; greater amounts produced during superimposed infections

3. Wheezing and dyspnea as disease progresses

Emphysema

Gradual in onset and steadily progressive

1. Dyspnea, decreased exercise tolerance.

2. Cough may be minimal, except with respiratory infection.

3. Sputum expectoration—mild.

4. Increased anteroposterior diameter of chest (barrel chest) due to air trapping with diaphragmatic flattening.

Diagnostic Evaluation

1. PFTs demonstrate airflow obstruction—reduced FEV$_1$, FEV$_1$ to FVC ratio; increased residual volume to total lung capacity (TLC) ratio, possibly increased TLC (see p. 205)

2. ABGs—decreased PaO$_2$, pH, and increased CO$_2$

3. Chest x-ray—in late stages, hyperinflation, flattened diaphragm, increased retrosternal space, decreased vascular markings, possible bullae

4. Alpha$_1$-antitrypsin assay useful in identifying genetically determined deficiency in emphysema

Management

Goal: reverse airflow obstruction.

1. Smoking cessation.

2. Bronchodilators, of which there are two main categories (Table 11-3):

a. Anticholinergics: ipratropium (Atrovent) and beta agonists such as albuterol (Proventil, Ventolin)—given to reduce and protect against bronchospasm.

(1) Aerosol formulations provide optimum therapy, because drug is applied directly to receptors in airways.

(*text continues on page 299*)

TABLE 11-3 Commonly Used Pulmonary Drugs

Drugs/Administration	Pharmacologic Effects	Indications	Undesired Effects	Nursing Implications
Bronchodilators				
Aminophylline (Amoline) (intravenous injection)	Methylxanthine compound—relaxes smooth muscle by increasing level of cyclic adenosine monophosphate	Acute exacerbation of asthma or bronchitis	CNS—irritability, restlessness, insomnia CV—palpitations, tachycardia, hypotension GI—nausea, vomiting, diarrhea	Too rapid administration can cause hypotension, extra systoles, muscle tremors. Administer at prescribed rate with an intravenous infusion pump.
Theophylline preparations (Theo-Dur) (oral)	Methylxanthine compound—relaxes muscle by increasing cyclic adenosine monophosphate	Mild bronchodilator, maintenance therapy for bronchospasm	CNS—irritability, restlessness, insomnia, seizures in toxic ranges CV—palpitations, tachycardia, hypotension GI—nausea, vomiting, diarrhea	Teach patients to take at equal intervals throughout the day. To decrease GI irritation, take with milk or crackers. Monitor theophylline blood level q 6–12 mo to ensure therapeutic range, prevent toxicity.
Albuterol (Proventil, Ventolin) (oral, metered-dose inhaler [MDI], nebulized liquid)	Sympathomimetic (beta₂-agonist) with highly selective beta₂ activity	*Oral:* Maintenance therapy for bronchospasm, works within 30 minutes MDI, nebulized liquid: rapid relief of bronchospasm, dyspnea—works within 3–5 min	Nervousness, tachycardia, headache, nausea, tremors Continuous nebulization may cause hypokalemia.	Observe inhalation by patient to be certain that correct technique is used. Caution patient not to exceed prescribed dose. Side effects often associated with excessive use. Does not reduce inflammation.
Terbutaline (Brethine) (oral, MDI, subcutaneous injection)	Sympathomimetic with selective beta₂ activity	Acute exacerbation of asthma or bronchitis (subcutaneous preparation) Maintenance therapy for bronchospasm (inhaled and oral preparation)	Nervousness, tachycardia, headache, nausea (subcutaneous preparation) Hand tremors (subcutaneous and oral preparations)	Caution patients that hand tremors may occur. Tremors decrease with prolonged oral use. Observe inhalation by patient to be certain that correct technique is used.
Metaproterenol (Alupent) (oral, MDI, inhalant solution	Sympathomimetic with selective beta₂ activity	Maintenance therapy for bronchospasm MDI onset of action 5–30 min	Nervousness, tachycardia, headache, nausea	Observe inhalation by patient to be certain that correct technique is used.
Pirbuterol acetate (Maxair) (MDI)	Sympathomimetic with selective beta₂ activity	Maintenance therapy for bronchospasm	Nervousness, tachycardia, headache, nausea	Observe inhalation by patient to be certain that correct technique is used.
Salmeterol xinafoate (Serevent) (MDI)	Sympathomimetic with selective beta₂ activity	Maintenance therapy for bronchospasm, long-acting (12 h)	Nervousness, tachycardia, headache, nausea	Observe inhalation by patient to be certain that correct technique is used. Instruct patient that not for immediate relief of bronchospasm, dyspnea. Maximum dose two puffs every 12 h

Drug	Action	Use	Side Effects	Nursing Considerations
Ipratropium bromide (Atrovent) (MDI, nebulized liquid)	Anticholinergic	Maintenance therapy for bronchospasm Acts within 15 minutes	Rare: Can cause blurring of vision if sprayed into the eyes (atropine derivative) Voice hoarseness	Instruct patient to use spacer device with MDI or close lips around inhaler mouthpiece, close eyes during inhalation.
Combivent (albuterol with ipratropium combination MDI)	Sympathomimetic with selective beta₂ and anticholinergic activity	Fast acting and maintenance therapy for bronchospasm	See albuterol and ipratropium	See albuterol and ipratropium One puff of Combivent equals one puff of albuterol and one puff of ipratropium

Corticosteroids

Drug	Action	Use	Side Effects	Nursing Considerations
Hydrocortisone/prednisone (Deltasone) (intravenous injection, oral preparation)	Potent anti-inflammatory activity	Acute exacerbation of asthma or bronchitis (IV preparation) Acute exacerbation or maintenance therapy (oral preparation)	CNS—depression, euphoria, mood changes GI—gastric irritation, peptic ulcer Metabolic—hypernatremia, hypokalemia, hyperglycemia, water retention and weight gain Long term, high dose: adrenal insufficiency, osteoporosis, muscle weakness, cataracts, glaucoma, fragile and easily bruised skin, immunosuppression	Long-term use: Do not stop abruptly due to adrenal suppression Take oral form with food. Usually given as taper from higher dose to lowest possible dose that achieves desired effect
Beclomethasone (Vanceril, Beclovent) (MDI)	Synthetic corticosteroid with potent anti-inflammatory activity; effective only by inhalation Not effective in acute attack; must be used for 2 to 4 weeks to show effectiveness	Asthma (alternative to use of oral steroids) COPD	Oral candidiasis Systemic side effects associated with oral steroids do not occur May experience skin bruising in high doses	Inhaled as a aerosol. May precipitate bronchospasm in acute exacerbation. Not used with status asthmaticus or acute asthma episodes. Use a spacer device with MDI, and use water gargle, rinse and spit after use to prevent oral candidiasis
Triamcinolone acetonide (Azmacort) (MDI)	Anti-inflammatory steroid; effective only by inhalation Not effective in acute attack; must be used for 2 to 4 weeks to show effectiveness	Asthma COPD	Oral candidiasis Systemic side effects associated with oral steroids do not occur May experience skin bruising in high doses	Packaged with a spacer. Decreases oral deposition and oral candidiasis. Use water gargle, rinse and spit after use to prevent oral yeast growth
Flunisolide (AeroBid) (MDI)	Anti-inflammatory steroid; effective only by inhalation Not effective in acute attack; must be used for 2 to 4 weeks to show effectiveness	Asthma COPD	Oral candidiasis Systemic side effects associated with oral steroids do not occur May experience skin bruising in high doses	Longer acting. May be prescribed twice a day, rather than four times a day. Use a spacer device with MDI, and use water gargle, rinse and spit after use to prevent oral candidiasis
Fluticasone (Flovent)	Anti-inflammatory steroid; effective only by inhalation Not effective in acute attack; must be used for 2 to 4 weeks to show effectiveness	Asthma COPD	Oral candidiasis Systemic side effects associated with oral steroids do not occur May experience skin bruising in high doses	Longer acting. May be prescribed twice a day, rather than four times a day. Use a spacer device with MDI, and use water gargle, rinse and spit after use to prevent oral candidiasis

(continued)

TABLE 11-3 Commonly Used Pulmonary Drugs (Continued)

Drugs/Administration	Pharmacologic Effects	Indications	Undesired Effects	Nursing Implications
Pulmocort (Budesonide Dry Powder Inhaler)	Anti-inflammatory steroid; effective only by inhalation Not effective in acute attack; must be used for 2 to 4 weeks to show effectiveness	Asthma COPD	Oral candidiasis Systemic side effects associated with oral steroids do not occur May experience skin bruising in high doses	Longer acting. May be prescribed twice a day, rather than four times a day. Use water gargle, rinse and spit after use to prevent oral candidiasis
Miscellaneous				
Cromolyn sodium (Intal) (solution for inhalation, powder used with special inhaler)	Inhibits activation of a variety of inflammatory cells associated with asthma, *prevents* bronchospasm Not effective in acute attack; must be used for 2 to 4 weeks to show effectiveness	Maintenance therapy for asthma	Cough, bronchospasm	Should not be used with status asthmaticus or acute asthma episodes. May be given in combination with bronchodilator or if administration causes bronchospasm.
Nedocromil (Tilade) (MDI)	Inhibits activation of a variety of inflammatory cells associated with asthma, *prevents* bronchospasm Not effective in acute attack; must be used for 2 to 4 weeks to show effectiveness	Maintenance therapy for asthma	Cough, bronchospasm GI: nausea, vomiting	Should not be used with status asthmaticus or acute asthma episodes. May be given in combination with bronchodilator or if administration causes bronchospasm.
Zafirlukast (Accolate)	Blocks leukotriene receptors	Prophylaxis and chronic treatment of mild to moderate asthma for persons older than 12 years	Potential drug interactions, particularly warfarin	Will not reverse acute bronchospasm
Zileuton (Zyflo)	Blocks leukotriene receptors	Prophylaxis and chronic treatment of mild to moderate asthma for persons older than 12 years	Potential drug interactions	Will not reverse acute bronchospasm
Montelukast (Singulair)	Blocks leukotriene receptors	Prophylaxis and chronic treatment of mild to moderate asthma for persons older than 5 years	Potential drug interactions, particularly phenobarbitol	Will not reverse acute bronchospasm

(2) Bronchodilating aerosols delivered by metered-dose inhalers (MDI) or hand-held or pump-driven devices.

    b. Methylxanthines such as theophylline (Theodur) given orally as sustained-release formulation for chronic maintenance therapy.

3. Antimicrobial agents for episodes of respiratory infection.
4. Corticosteroids used in acute exacerbations for anti-inflammatory effect can be given by mouth, IV, or inhaler.
5. Chest physical therapy, including postural drainage for secretion clearance, breathing retraining for improved ventilation and control of dyspnea.
6. Supplemental oxygen therapy for patient with hypoxemia. CO_2 must be monitored to determine increased CO_2 retention.
7. Pulmonary rehabilitation to improve function, strength, symptom control, disease self-management techniques, independence, and quality of life.
8. Lung volume reduction surgery is under investigation for treatment of heterogeneous emphysema
9. Treatment for alpha$_1$-antitrypsin deficiency:
    a. Regular IV infusions (every 1 to 2 weeks) of human alpha$_1$-antitrypsin (Prolastin) replacement therapy can effectively correct the antiprotease imbalance in the lungs.
    b. Prevent damage to lungs by quitting smoking.
    c. Lung transplantation may be considered for persons with severely disabling alpha$_1$-antitrypsin disease.

 DRUG ALERT

Theophylline is not in favor as much as it was in the past due to systemic side effects, need for regular blood level monitoring, and blood level changes from multiple other drugs. More emphasis is now placed on the use of inhaled bronchodilators.

Complications
1. Respiratory failure
2. Pneumonia, overwhelming respiratory infection
3. Right heart failure, dysrhythmias
4. Depression
5. Skeletal muscle dysfunction

Nursing Assessment
1. Determine smoking history, exposure history, positive family history of respiratory disease, onset of dyspnea.
2. Note amount, color, and consistency of sputum.
3. Inspect for use of accessory muscles of respiration and use of abdominal muscles during expiration; note increase of anteroposterior diameter of chest.
4. Auscultate for decreased/absent breath sounds, crackles, decreased heart sounds.
5. Determine level of dyspnea, how it compares to patient's baseline.
6. Determine oxygen saturation at rest and with activity.

Nursing Diagnoses
- Ineffective Airway Clearance related to bronchoconstriction, increased mucous production, ineffective cough, possible bronchopulmonary infection
- Ineffective Breathing Pattern related to chronic airflow limitation
- Risk for Infection related to compromised pulmonary function and defense mechanisms
- Impaired Gas Exchange related to chronic pulmonary obstruction, ventilation–perfusion abnormalities due to destruction of alveolar capillary membrane
- Altered Nutrition: Less Than Body Requirements related to increased work of breathing, air swallowing, medication effects with resultant wasting of respiratory and skeletal muscles
- Activity Intolerance related to compromised pulmonary function, resulting in shortness of breath and fatigue
- Sleep Pattern Disturbance related to hypoxemia and hypercapnia
- Impaired Individual Coping related to the stress of living with chronic disease, loss of independence

NURSING ALERT

 Early in the patient's course, issues of a living will, advanced directives, and resuscitation status need to be addressed. It is better to have these discussions with the patient before crisis situations.

Nursing Interventions
Improving Airway Clearance
1. Eliminate all pulmonary irritants, particularly cigarette smoking.
    a. Cessation of smoking usually results in less pulmonary irritation, sputum production, and cough.
    b. Keep patient's room as dust-free as possible.
    c. Add moisture (humidifier, vaporizer) to indoor environment, if appropriate.
2. Administer bronchodilators to control bronchospasm and assist with raising sputum.
    a. Assess for side effects—tremulousness, tachycardia, cardiac dysrhythmias, central nervous system stimulation, hypertension.
    b. Auscultate the chest after administration of aerosol bronchodilators to assess for improvement of aeration and reduction of adventitious breath sounds.
    c. Observe if patient has reduction in dyspnea.
    d. Monitor serum theophylline level, as ordered, to ensure therapeutic level and prevent toxicity.
3. Use postural drainage positions to aid in clearance of secretions, if mucopurulent secretions are responsible for airway obstruction (see p. 222).
4. Use controlled coughing (see p. 223).
5. Keep secretions liquid.
    a. Encourage high level of fluid intake (8 to 10 glasses; 2 to 2.5 L daily) within level of cardiac reserve.

b. Give inhalations of nebulized water to humidify bronchial tree and liquefy sputum if appropriate.

c. Avoid dairy products if these increase sputum production.

Improving Breathing Pattern

1. Teach and supervise breathing retraining exercises to strengthen diaphragm and muscles of expiration to decrease work of breathing (see p. 229).

   a. Teach diaphragmatic, lower costal, and abdominal breathing, using a slow and relaxed breathing pattern to reduce respiratory rate and decrease energy cost of breathing.

   b. Use pursed-lip breathing at intervals and during periods of dyspnea to control rate and depth of respiration and improve respiratory muscle coordination. Diaphragmatic and pursed-lip breathing should be practiced for 10 breaths four times daily before meals and before sleep. Inspiratory to expiratory ratio should be 1:2.

2. Discuss and demonstrate relaxation exercises to reduce stress, tension, and anxiety.

3. Encourage patient to assume position of comfort to decrease dyspnea. Positions might include leaning trunk forward with arms supported on a fixed object.

Controlling Infection

1. Recognize early manifestations of respiratory infection—increased dyspnea, fatigue; change in color, amount, and character of sputum; nervousness; irritability; low-grade fever.

2. Obtain sputum for smear and culture.

3. Administer prescribed antimicrobials to control secondary bacterial infections in the bronchial tree, thus clearing the airways.

Improving Gas Exchange

1. Watch for and report excessive somnolence, restlessness, aggressiveness, anxiety, or confusion; central cyanosis; and shortness of breath at rest, which frequently is caused by acute respiratory insufficiency and may signal respiratory failure.

2. Review ABGs; record values on a flow sheet so comparisons can be made over time.

3. Monitor oxygen saturation and give supplemental oxygen as ordered to correct hypoxemia in a controlled manner. Monitor and minimize CO_2 retention. Patients that experience CO_2 retention may need lower oxygen flow rates.

NURSING ALERT

Normally, CO_2 levels in the blood provide a stimulus for respiration. However, in patients with COPD, chronically elevated CO_2 impairs this mechanism and low oxygen levels act as stimulus for respiration. Giving a high concentration of supplemental oxygen to persons who retain CO_2 may suppress the hypoxic drive, leading to increased hypoventilation, respiratory decompensation, and the development of a worsening respiratory acidosis.

---

4. Be prepared to assist with noninvasive ventilation *or* intubation and mechanical ventilation if acute respiratory failure and rapid CO_2 retention occur.

Improving Nutrition

1. Take nutritional history, weight, and anthropometric measurements.

2. Encourage frequent small meals if patient is dyspneic; even a small increase in abdominal contents may press on diaphragm and impede breathing. Encourage snacking on high-calorie, high-protein snacks such as cheese, nuts, and so forth.

3. Offer liquid nutritional supplements to improve caloric intake and counteract weight loss.

4. Avoid foods producing gas and abdominal discomfort.

5. Employ good oral hygiene before meals to sharpen taste sensations.

6. Encourage pursed-lip breathing between bites if patient is very short of breath; rest after meals.

7. Give supplemental oxygen while patient is eating to relieve dyspnea, as directed.

8. Monitor body weight.

Increasing Activity Tolerance

1. Reemphasize the importance of graded exercise and physical conditioning programs (enhances delivery of oxygen to tissues; allows a higher level of functioning with greater comfort). This may be part of a formalized pulmonary rehabilitation program or a referral to physical or occupational therapy.

   a. Discuss walking, stationary bicycling, swimming.

   b. Encourage use of portable oxygen system for ambulation for patients with hypoxemia and marked disability.

2. Encourage patient to carry out regular exercise program 3 to 7 days per week to increase physical endurance.

3. Train patient in energy conservation techniques.

Improving Sleep Patterns

1. Maintain a balanced schedule of activity and rest.

2. Use nocturnal oxygen therapy when appropriate.

3. Avoid use of sedatives that may cause respiratory depression.

Enhancing Coping

1. Understand that the constant shortness of breath and fatigue make the patient irritable, apprehensive, anxious, and depressed, with feelings of helplessness/hopelessness.

2. Assess the patient for reactive behaviors (anger, depression, and acceptance).

3. Demonstrate a positive and interested approach to the patient.

   a. Be a good listener and show that you care.

   b. Be sensitive to patient's fears, anxiety, and depression; may provide emotional relief and insight.

   c. Provide patient with control of as many aspects of his or her care as possible.

4. Strengthen the patient's self-image.
5. Allow the patient to express feelings. Be aware that (within a controlled degree) the mechanisms of denial and repression may be useful defense mechanisms.
6. Be aware that sexual dysfunction is common in patients with COPD. Encourage discussion of concerns, and clarify misunderstandings. Encourage patient to use a bronchodilator and secretion clearance techniques before sexual activity, plan for sexual relations at time of day when patient has highest level of energy, use supplemental oxygen if needed, and consider alternative displays of affection to loved one.
7. Support spouse/family members. Refer to local or national support groups (American Lung Association 1-800-LUNGUSA; Well Spouse Foundation 1-800-838-0879).

Community and Home Care Considerations

1. Encourage patient to live within the limitations that emphysema imposes.
2. Help to relax and work at a slower pace. Obtain occupational therapy consult to help employ work simplification techniques such as sitting for tasks, pacing activities, using dressing aids (grabber, sock aid, long-handled shoe horn), shower bench, and hand-held shower head.
3. Encourage enrollment in a pulmonary rehabilitation program where available and Better Breathers club or other support group. Resources include American Lung Association 1-800-LUNGUSA. Pulmonary rehabilitation programs are offered in most communities. Components include breathing retraining techniques, proper use of medications and inhalers, secretion clearance techniques, prevention and management of respiratory infection, panic control, controlling dyspnea with activities of daily living (ADLs) and stair climbing, control of pulmonary irritants, monitored and supervised exercise, and group support.
4. Studies on pulmonary rehabilitation demonstrate increased strength, function and independence, ADL management, improved symptom control, coping, well-being, and quality of life as well as decreased hospital admissions and decreased length of stay. Studies have not shown to improve lung function or survival, however.
5. Suggest vocational counseling to secure a sedentary job if presently in a demanding manual job.
6. Warn to avoid overfatigue, which is a factor in producing respiratory distress.
7. Advise to adjust activities according to individual fatigue patterns.
8. Advise to try to cope with emotional stress as positively as possible. Such stress triggers attacks of dyspnea. Teach coping strategies such as relaxation techniques, meditation, guided imagery, and so forth.

9. Stress that progression of worsening lung function may be slowed through health supervision for rest of life.

Patient Education and Health Maintenance
General Education

1. Give the patient a clear explanation of the disease, what to expect, how to treat and live with it. Reinforce by frequent explanations, reading material, demonstrations, and question and answer sessions (see Patient Education).
2. Review with the patient the objectives of treatment and nursing management.
3. Work with the patient to set goals (eg, stair climbing, return to work, and so forth).
4. Encourage patient involvement in disease self-management techniques, such as identification and prompt reporting of respiratory infection or respiratory deterioration. Encourage patient to have open communication and partnership with primary care physician.

Avoid Exposure to Respiratory Irritants

1. Advise patient to stop smoking and avoid exposure to second-hand smoke.
2. Advise patient to avoid sweeping, dusting, and exposure to paint, aerosols, bleaches, ammonia, and other respiratory irritants.
3. Advise patient to keep entire house well ventilated.
4. Warn patient to stay out of extremely hot/cold weather to avoid aggravating bronchial obstruction and sputum production.
   a. Keep a warm mask or scarf over nose and mouth, and drink a warm beverage to warm inspired air in cold weather.
   b. Stay indoors with air conditioning when air pollution level is high.
   c. Try to avoid abrupt environmental changes.
   d. Shower in warm (not too hot or too cold) water.
5. Instruct patient to humidify indoor air in winter; maintain 30% to 50% humidity for optimal mucociliary function.
6. Suggest the use of an HEPA air cleanser to remove dust, pollen, and other particulates. This is controversial as to the benefit to the patient.

Prevent and Treat Respiratory Infections

1. Warn against exposure to persons with respiratory infections; a respiratory infection makes symptoms worse and can produce further irreversible damage.
2. Advise patient to avoid crowds and areas with poor ventilation.
3. Stress the importance of obtaining influenza vaccine (annual) and pneumococcal vaccine to decrease likelihood of developing these infections.
4. Teach how to recognize and report evidence of respiratory infection promptly—changes in character of sputum (amount, color, or consistency), increasing cough/wheezing, increasing shortness of breath, increasing difficulty in raising sputum, chest pain.

PATIENT EDUCATION GUIDELINES   Chronic Obstructive Pulmonary Disease (COPD)

There are two types of COPD, chronic bronchitis and emphysema, which may occur together or separately. Chronic bronchitis is diagnosed when there is a chronic cough with phlegm (sputum) for at least 3 months over a period of 2 years. With emphysema, there is a loss of elasticity of the lung tissue. Both result in inflammation and blockage of the airways. Smoking is the leading cause.

Controlling Symptoms

TO CONTROL COUGH AND PHLEGM:

1. Drink plenty of water (8–10 glasses a day) to keep phlegm thin.
2. Use inhalers on a regular basis as prescribed:
   a. Bronchodilators such as Proventil to open up the airways.
   b. Atrovent to decrease cough and mucous production.
   c. Corticosteroids to reduced swelling.
3. Avoid irritants to the lungs such as cigarette smoke, dust, smog, perfume, cold air, and very hot air.
4. Report any change in color, amount, or thickness of phlegm that could indicate an infection.
5. Try to avoid respiratory infections by limiting contact with people during cold and flu season. Get the flu and pneumonia vaccines and wash hands frequently.

TO CONTROL SHORTNESS OF BREATH:

1. Practice "pursed-lip breathing" by breathing in through the nose and out through pursed lips (like you are whistling), with a long, slow expiration.
2. Position yourself for better breathing by leaning forward while sitting with elbows on table or resting on knees.
3. Use relaxation techniques such as listening to soft music, imagining you are in a quiet peaceful place, or having someone give you a massage.

4. If prescribed, use oxygen as directed, especially while performing activities such as bathing, dressing, eating, and walking.

TO CONTROL FATIGUE:

1. Do not stop doing physical activity; instead, learn how to manage by planning activities to conserve energy.
2. Start with an exercise program that is easy, and progress slowly to increase your activity.
3. Talk to your health care provider about joining a pulmonary rehabilitation program.
4. Eat a well-balanced diet.
5. Sleep with head elevated using several pillows or in a reclining chair to reduce shortness of breath and increase rest.
6. If awakened by cough, sit up, sip fluid, and use inhaler to try to clear lungs of phlegm.
7. Avoid overuse of inhalers, which may cause shakiness and insomnia.

TO COMPENSATE FOR POOR APPETITE:

1. Eat six or more small meals and snacks a day rather than two or three larger meals.
2. Eat slowly; plan at least 30 minutes per meal. Sit forward with elbows propped on table.
3. Unless otherwise directed, try a high-protein, moderate-fat, and lower-carbohydrate diet of sufficient calories to cover the increased work of breathing.
4. Consider a high-calorie, high-protein drink if you do not feel like eating.

Adapted from Wright, L. (1998). Learning to cope with chronic obstructive pulmonary disease. *Lippincott's Primary Care Practice, 2*(6), 647–649.

---

5. Instruct patient to discuss with physician taking prescribed antimicrobial at first sign of infection.
   a. Have a current prescription available.
   b. Have periodic sputum cultures when receiving long-term antimicrobial therapy; this may be a controversial practice.
   c. Discuss with physician use of corticosteroids for respiratory infections.

Reduce Bronchial Secretions

1. Advise to maintain an adequate fluid intake (8 to 10 glasses daily); mark down the amount of liquid consumed daily.
2. Encourage use of bronchodilators as directed.
3. Teach postural drainage exercises as prescribed.
   a. Stay in each position 5 to 15 minutes as tolerated.
   b. Use controlled cough after each position.

4. Use other secretion clearance techniques, such as chest percussion, PEP valve, flutter valve, huff cough, if needed for enhanced secretion clearance.

Improve Airflow

1. Teach use of MDI properly to maximize aerosol deposition in the bronchial tree.
   a. Use spacer device, breathe out normally; place MDI (attached to spacer device) in mouth, make tight seal around mouthpiece (if not using spacer device: place inhaler 1 inch in front of open mouth).
   b. Actuate cartridge to release spray and inhale slowly over 5 seconds.
   c. Pause, holding breath for about 10 seconds; exhale slowly.
2. Encourage routine use of a spacer device to allow easier inhalation of bronchodilator medication and enhanced medication deposition.

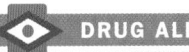
Breathing Exercises

1. Explain that goal is to strengthen and coordinate muscles of breathing to lessen work of breathing and help lung empty more completely.
2. Stress the importance of controlled breathing.
3. Teach diaphragmatic breathing and pursed-lip breathing for episodes of dyspnea and stress.
4. Encourage muscle toning by regular exercise.

General Health

1. Teach good habits of well-balanced, nutritious intake.
2. Encourage high-protein diet with adequate mineral, vitamin, and fluid intake.
3. Advise against excessive hot or cold fluids/foods, which may provoke an irritating cough.
4. Advise to avoid hard-to-chew foods (causes tiring) and gas-forming foods, which cause distention and restrict diaphragmatic movement.
5. Encourage five to six small meals daily to ease shortness of breath during and after meals.
6. Suggest rest periods before and after meals if eating produces shortness of breath.
7. Advise against eating when upset or angry.
8. Warn against potassium depletion. Patients with COPD tend to have low potassium levels; also patient may be taking diuretics.
   a. Watch for weakness, numbness, tingling of fingers, leg cramps.
   b. Foods high in potassium include bananas, dried fruits, dates, figs, orange juice, grape juice, milk, peaches, potatoes, tomatoes.
9. Advise on restricting sodium, as directed.
10. Limit carbohydrates if CO_2 is retained by patient, because they increase CO_2.
11. Use community resources (Meals on Wheels) if energy level is low.

Outcome-Based Evaluation

- Coughing up secretions easily; decreased wheezing and crackles
- Reports less dyspnea; effectively using pursed-lip breathing
- No signs of superimposed respiratory infection
- ABGs and/or SpO_2 improved on low-flow oxygen
- Tolerating small, frequent meals; weight stable
- Reports walking longer distances without tiring
- Reports better sleep; using low-flow oxygen at night
- Demonstrates more effective coping; expresses feelings; seeking support group

Pulmonary Heart Disease (Cor Pulmonale)

Pulmonary heart disease is an alteration in the structure or function of the right ventricle resulting from disease affecting lung structure or function or its vasculature (except when this alteration results from disease of the left side of the heart or from congenital heart disease). Cor pulmonale refers to heart disease caused by lung disease.

Pathophysiology and Etiology

1. Condition that deprives lungs of oxygen: hypoxemia → hypercapnia → acidosis → circulatory complications → pulmonary hypertension → right heart enlargement → right heart failure.
2. Etiology includes:
   a. Pulmonary vascular disease
   b. Pulmonary embolism
   c. COPD

Clinical Manifestations

1. Increasing dyspnea and fatigue; progressive dyspnea (orthopnea, paroxysmal nocturnal dyspnea), chronic cough
2. Distended neck veins, peripheral edema, hepatomegaly
3. Bibasilar crackles and split second heart sound on auscultation of chest
4. Manifestations of carbon dioxide narcosis—headache, confusion, somnolence, coma

Diagnostic Evaluation

1. ABGs—decreased PaO_2 and pH, increased $PaCO_2$.
2. PFTs may show airway obstruction.
3. Electrocardiogram changes are consistent with right ventricular hypertrophy.
4. Chest x-ray shows right heart enlargement.
5. Echocardiogram shows right heart enlargement.

Management

Goal: treatment of underlying lung disease and management of heart disease.

1. Long-term, low-flow oxygen to improve oxygen delivery to peripheral tissues, thus decreasing cardiac work and lessening sympathetic vasoconstriction. Liter flow individualized during activities, rest, and sleep.
2. Diuretics to lower pulmonary artery pressure (PAP) by reducing total blood volume and excess fluid in lungs.
3. Pulmonary vasodilators such as nitroprusside (Nitropress); hydralazine (Apresoline); calcium channel blockers to dilate pulmonary vascular bed and reduce pulmonary vascular resistance. Use is controversial.
4. Bronchodilators to improve lung function.
5. Mechanical ventilation, if patient in respiratory failure.
6. Sodium restriction to reduce edema.

Complications

1. Respiratory failure
2. Dysrhythmias

Nursing Assessment

1. Determine if patient has longstanding history of lung disease.
2. Assess degree of dyspnea, fatigue, hypoxemia.
3. Inspect for jugular venous distention and peripheral edema.

Nursing Diagnoses

- Impaired Gas Exchange related to excess fluid in lungs; increased pulmonary vascular resistance
- Fluid Volume Excess related to right heart failure

Nursing Interventions

Improving Gas Exchange

1. Monitor ABG values and/or oxygen saturation as a guide in assessing adequacy of ventilation.
2. Use continuous low-flow oxygen as directed to reduce PAP.
3. Avoid central nervous system depressants (narcotics, hypnotics). They have depressant action on respiratory centers and mask symptoms of hypercapnia.
4. Monitor for signs of respiratory infection, because infection causes carbon dioxide retention and hypoxemia.

Attaining Fluid Balance

1. Watch alterations in electrolyte levels, especially potassium, which can lead to disturbances of cardiac rhythm.
2. Employ ECG monitoring when necessary, and monitor closely for dysrhythmias.
3. Limit physical activity until improvement is seen.
4. Restrict sodium intake based on evidence of fluid retention.

Patient Education and Health Maintenance

1. Emphasize the importance of stopping cigarette smoking; cigarette smoking is a major cause of pulmonary heart disease.
   a. Query the patient about smoking habits.
   b. Inform the patient of risks of smoking and benefits to be gained when smoking is stopped.
2. Teach the patient to recognize and treat infections immediately.
3. Inform the patient of interrelationship among infection, air pollution, and cardiopulmonary disease.
4. Explain to the patient/family that restlessness, depression, and poor sleeping, as well as irritable and angry behavior, may be characteristic; patient should improve with rise in O_2 and fall in CO_2 levels in ABG values.
5. Treat hypoxemia with supplemental oxygen, which will reduce further work load on the right heart.
6. Explain that if the patient has chronic lung disease, it may be necessary to have continuous low-flow oxygen therapy at home.

Outcome-Based Evaluation

- Less dyspneic; ABGs improved, oxygen saturation ≥90%
- Edema reduced; no dysrhythmias

Interstitial Lung Disease (Pulmonary Fibrosis)

Pulmonary fibrosis is a general term that refers to a variety of chronic lung disorders, such as *asbestosis, silicosis, coal worker's pneumoconiosis,* and *sarcoidosis*. There are estimated to be 130 types of interstitial lung disease, only about a third have known causes. Causes include occupational exposure, environmental exposure, drugs and poisons, radiation, infections as well as connective tissue disease. Pulmonary fibrosis may also be idiopathic.

Pathophysiology and Etiology

1. May be related to occupational exposure:
   a. Asbestosis (increased risk for lung cancer)
   b. Silicosis
   c. Coal worker's pneumoconiosis
2. May be related to environmental exposure:
   a. Hard metal disease (cobalt, tungsten, carbide)
   b. Gas, fumes, vapors, aerosols
   c. Drug and poison exposure
   d. Cancer drugs (nitrofurantoin, methotrexate, busulfan, bleomycin)
   e. Anti-inflammatory drugs (aspirin, gold, penicillamine)
   f. Heart drugs (amiodarone)
   g. Abused substances: heroin, methadone, Darvon, talc used in IV drug abuse
   h. Exposure to radiation
   i. Exposure to infections
   j. Connective tissue disease
3. Chronic changes include lung tissue damage, inflammation of alveoli with scarring, and fibrosis and stiffening of the interstitium (tissue between the alveoli).
4. The damage limits oxygen transport through scarred alveolar capillary membrane into bloodstream.

Clinical Manifestations

1. The most prevalent symptom is dyspnea, particularly with exercise.
2. Dry cough.
3. Symptoms may vary in severity, and the course of the disease may be unpredictable.

Idiopathic Pulmonary Fibrosis

Incidence and Etiology

1. Idiopathic pulmonary fibrosis has no identifiable cause.
2. Incidence is approximately five cases per 100,000 people.
3. It is generally diagnosed at 40 to 70 years of age.

Clinical Manifestations

1. Slow onset of dyspnea and dry cough are present.
2. Hypoxia with exercise.
3. Rarely, patients may have weight loss, fever, myalgias.
4. Breath sounds often include crackles.
5. Clubbing of fingertips is common.

Diagnostic Evaluation
1. Pulmonary function test shows decreased total lung capacity and vital capacity, with decreased diffusion capacity.
2. ABGs show low arterial oxygen level
3. Chest x-ray may demonstrate patchy, nonuniform infiltrates, ground glass pattern, reticular nodular pattern, honeycomb pattern, and small lung volumes.
4. Exercise test shows hypoxia with exercise.

Management
1. Corticosteroids: About one third of patients respond to corticosteroids within 4 to 6 weeks. Patients may be started on 60 to 100 mg/day for 6 weeks then tapered over 3 months to a maintenance dose of 20 mg/day.
2. Azathioprine (Imuran) 1 to 3 mg/kg/day.
3. Cyclophosphamide (Cytoxan) 2 mg/kg/day; may have toxic side effects
4. Lung transplantation may offer improved symptoms, function, and survival for some.
5. Oxygen for hypoxemia.

 DRUG ALERT

Long-term use of oral steroids may cause osteoporosis, decreased immune function, muscle wasting, glaucoma, cataracts, friable skin, mood changes, weight gain, hyperglycemia, gastric upset, and ulcers. Side effects are often related to higher doses of steroids used over an extended period of time. Review the potential side effects with the patient when therapy is begun. Instruct the patient not to abruptly cease therapy. If unable to continue oral steroids, patient should notify the health care provider immediately.

Sarcoidosis and Other Connective Tissue Diseases

Causes
1. Rheumatoid arthritis (RA): Twenty percent of patients with rheumatoid arthritis develop interstitial lung disease due to pleural inflammation by age 50 to 60 years. Pulmonary involvement is most common in females.
2. Systemic lupus erythematosus (SLE)
3. Scleroderma: CREST syndrome (*c*alcinosis, *R*aynaud's syndrome, *e*sophageal dysmotility, *s*clerodactyly, *t*elangiectasia)
4. Ankylosing spondylitis
5. Sarcoidosis
   a. Granulomatous disease in which clumps of inflammatory epithelial cells occur in many organs, primarily in lungs.
   b. Lymph node enlargement seen on chest x-ray.
   c. Sarcoidosis usually occurs from 20 to 40 years of age.

Management
Comprehensive management of the inflammatory process and multisystem effects. (See Chapter 30.)

Occupational Lung Diseases

Types
1. *Asbestosis* is a diffuse interstitial fibrosis of the lung caused by inhalation of asbestos dust and particles.
   a. Found in workers involved in manufacture, cutting, and demolition of asbestos-containing materials; there are over 4,000 known sources of asbestos fiber (asbestos mining and manufacturing, construction, roofing, demolition work, brake linings, floor tiles, paints, plastics, shipyards, insulation).
   b. Asbestos fibers are inhaled and enter alveoli, which, in time, are obliterated by fibrous tissue that surrounds the asbestos particles.
   c. Fibrous pleural thickening and pleural plaque formation produce restrictive lung disease, decrease in lung volume, diminished gas transfer, and hypoxemia with subsequent development of cor pulmonale.
2. *Silicosis* is a chronic pulmonary fibrosis caused by inhalation of silica dust.
   a. Exposure to silica dust is encountered in almost any form of mining because the earth's crust is composed of silica and silicates (gold, coal, tin, copper mining); also stone cutting, quarrying, manufacture of abrasives, ceramics, pottery, and foundry work.
   b. When silica particles (which have fibrogenic properties) are inhaled, nodular lesions are produced throughout the lungs. These nodules undergo fibrosis, enlarge, and fuse.
   c. Dense masses form in the upper portion of the lungs; restrictive and obstructive lung disease results.
3. *Coal worker's pneumoconiosis* (CWP; "black lung") is a variety of respiratory disease found in coal workers in which there is an accumulation of coal dust in the lungs, causing a tissue reaction in its presence.
   a. Dusts (coal, kaolin, mica, silica) are inhaled and deposited in the alveoli and respiratory bronchioles.
   b. There is an increase of macrophages that engulf the particles and transport them to terminal bronchioles.
   c. When normal clearance mechanisms no longer can handle the excessive dust load, the respiratory bronchioles and alveoli become clogged with coal dust, dying macrophages, and fibroblasts, which lead to the formation of the coal macule, the primary lesion of CWP.
   d. As macules enlarge, there is dilation of the weakening bronchiole, with subsequent development of focal or centrilobular emphysema.

Pathophysiology
1. Effects of inhaling organic dust (moldy hay, mushroom compost, malt, moldy maple bark, pigeon or parrot droppings, feathers, or contaminated grain), noxious particles, gases, or fumes. Development of disease depends on composition of inhaled substance, its antigenic (precipitating an immune response) or irritating properties, the dose inhaled, the length of time inhaled, and the host's response.

2. Exposure to inorganic dusts stimulates pulmonary interstitial fibroblasts, resulting in pulmonary interstitial fibrosis.

3. Acute symptoms of fever, cough, and chills may occur 4 to 12 hours after exposure and reoccur with repeated exposure. Chronic disease develops years later.

4. Noxious fumes may cause acute injury to alveolar wall with increasing capillary permeability and pulmonary edema.

5. Occupational lung diseases usually develop slowly (over 20 to 30 years) and are usually asymptomatic in the early stages.

NURSING ALERT

Asbestosis is strongly associated with bronchogenic cancer and mesotheliomas of the pleura and peritoneal surfaces. Smoking increases the risk of lung cancer 50 to 100 times.

Clinical Manifestations

1. Chronic cough; productive in silicosis and CWP
2. Dyspnea on exertion; progressive and irreversible in asbestosis and CWP
3. Susceptibility to lower respiratory tract infections
4. Bibasilar crackles in asbestosis
5. Expectoration of varying amounts of black fluid in CWP

Diagnostic Evaluation

1. Chest x-ray—nodules of upper lobes in silicosis and CWP; diffuse parenchymal fibrosis, especially of lower lobes, in asbestosis.
2. PFTs primarily show restrictive pattern.
3. Bronchoscopy with lavage to identify specific exposure.
4. CT, sputum examination, and lung biopsy may be needed to rule out other disorders.

Management

1. There is no specific treatment; exposure is eliminated, and the patient is treated symptomatically.
2. Give prophylactic isoniazid (INH) to patient with positive tuberculin test, because silicosis is associated with high risk of TB.
3. Persuade people who have been exposed to asbestos fibers to stop smoking to decrease risk of lung cancer.
4. Keep asbestos worker under cancer surveillance; watch for changing cough, hemoptysis, weight loss, melena, and so forth.
5. Bronchodilators may be of some benefit if any degree of airway obstruction is present.

Complications

1. Respiratory failure
2. Lung cancer

Nursing Assessment

1. Obtain occupational and environmental exposure history. Determine length and degree of exposure.

2. Obtain full medical history and family history for connective tissue disorders.
3. Obtain medication history.
4. Obtain history of smoking, respiratory infections, and other chronic lung disease.
5. Evaluate symptoms, functional capacity, and auscultate lungs for crackles.

Nursing Diagnoses

- Ineffective Breathing Pattern related to fibrotic lung tissue causing restriction
- Impaired Gas Exchange related to fibrotic lung tissue and secretions

Nursing Interventions

Improving Breathing Pattern

1. Administer oxygen therapy as required.
2. Administer or teach self-administration of bronchodilators, as ordered.
3. Encourage smoking cessation.

Promoting Gas Exchange

1. Encourage mobilization of secretions through hydration and breathing and coughing exercises.
2. Advise on pacing activities to prevent fatigue.

Patient Education and Health Maintenance

1. Provide information regarding the importance of smoking cessation as well as methods of smoking cessation.
2. Instruct patient in methods of health maintenance, such as adequate nutrition and exercise, so additional medical problems can be avoided.
3. Advise patient that compensation may be obtained for impairment related to occupational lung disease through the Worker's Compensation Act.
4. Provide information to healthy workers on prevention of occupational lung disease.
   a. Enclose toxic substances to reduce their concentration in the air.
   b. Employ engineering controls to reduce exposure.
   c. Monitor air samples.
   d. Ventilate the environment properly to reduce dust content of work atmosphere.
   e. Use protective devices such as face masks, respirators, hoods, and so forth.

Outcome-Based Evaluation

- Reports less dyspnea
- Effectively mobilizes secretions

TRAUMATIC DISORDERS

Pneumothorax

Air in the pleural space occurring spontaneously or from trauma (Figure 11-4). In patients with chest trauma, it is usually the result of a laceration to the lung parenchyma,

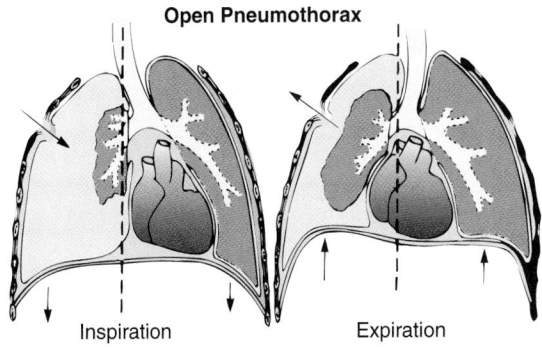

Open Pneumothorax

Inspiration   Expiration

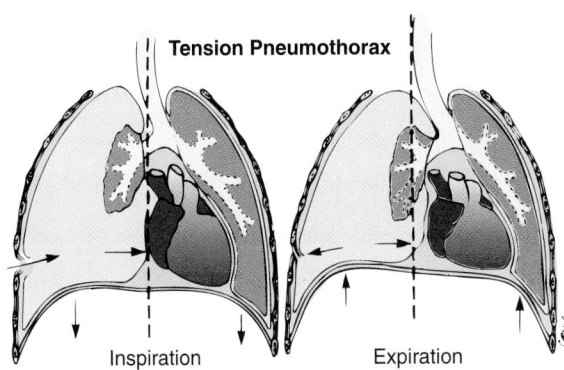

Tension Pneumothorax

Inspiration   Expiration

FIGURE 11-4 Open pneumothorax and tension pneumothorax. In open pneumothorax, air enters the chest during inspiration and exits during expiration. There may be slight inflation of the affected lung due to a decrease in pressure as air moves out of the chest. In tension pneumothorax, air can enter but not leave the chest. As the pressure in the chest increases, the heart and great vessels are compressed and the mediastinal structures are shifted toward the opposite side of the chest. The trachea is pushed from its normal midline position toward the opposite side of the chest, and the unaffected lung is compressed.

tracheobronchial tree, or esophagus. The patient's clinical status depends on the rate of air leakage and size of wound. Pneumothorax is classified as:

Spontaneous pneumothorax—sudden onset of air in the pleural space with deflation of the affected lung in the absence of trauma.

Open pneumothorax (sucking wound of chest)—implies an opening in the chest wall large enough to allow air to pass freely in and out of thoracic cavity with each attempted respiration.

Tension pneumothorax—buildup of air under pressure in the pleural space resulting in interference with filling of both the heart and lungs.

Pathophysiology and Etiology

1. When there is a large open hole in the chest wall, the patient will have a "steal" in ventilation of other lung.

2. A portion of the tidal volume will move back and forth through the hole in the chest wall, rather than the trachea as it normally does.

3. Spontaneous pneumothorax is usually due to rupture of a subpleural bleb.
   a. May occur secondary to chronic respiratory diseases or idiopathically.
   b. May occur in healthy people, particularly in thin, white males and those with family history of pneumothorax.

Clinical Manifestations

1. Hyperresonance; diminished breath sounds.
2. Reduced mobility of affected half of thorax.
3. Tracheal deviation away from affected side in tension pneumothorax.
4. Clinical picture of open or tension pneumothorax is one of air hunger, agitation, hypotension, and cyanosis.
5. Mild to moderate dyspnea and chest discomfort may be present with spontaneous pneumothorax.

Diagnostic Evaluation

1. Chest x-ray to confirm presence of air in pleural space

Management
Spontaneous Pneumothorax

1. Treatment is generally nonoperative if pneumothorax is not too extensive.
   a. Observe and allow for spontaneous resolution for less than 50% pneumothorax in otherwise healthy person.
   b. Needle aspiration or chest tube drainage may be necessary to achieve reexpansion of collapsed lung if greater than 50% pneumothorax.
2. Surgical intervention by pleurodesis (see p. 259) or thoracotomy with resection of apical blebs is advised for patients with recurrent spontaneous pneumothorax.

Tension Pneumothorax

1. Immediate decompression to prevent cardiovascular collapse by thoracentesis or chest tube insertion to let air escape
2. Chest tube drainage with underwater-seal suction to allow for full lung expansion and healing

Open Pneumothorax

1. Close the chest wound immediately to restore adequate ventilation and respiration.
   a. Patient is instructed to inhale and exhale gently against a closed glottis (Valsalva maneuver) as a pressure dressing (petroleum gauze secured with elastic adhesive) is applied. This maneuver helps to expand collapsed lung.
2. Chest tube is inserted and water-seal drainage set up to permit evacuation of fluid/air and produce reexpansion of the lung.
3. Surgical intervention may be necessary to repair trauma.

Complications
1. Acute respiratory failure
2. Cardiovascular collapse with tension pneumothorax

Nursing Assessment
1. Obtain history for chronic respiratory disease, trauma, and onset of symptoms.
2. Inspect chest for reduced mobility and tracheal deviation.
3. Auscultate chest for diminished breath sounds and percuss for hyperresonance.

Nursing Diagnoses
- Ineffective Breathing Pattern related to air in the pleural space
- Impaired Gas Exchange related to atelectasis and collapse of lung

Nursing Interventions
Achieving Effective Breathing Pattern
1. Provide emergency care as indicated.
    a. Apply petroleum gauze to sucking chest wound (see section titled Management, above)
    b. Assist with emergency thoracentesis or thoracostomy.
    c. Be prepared to perform cardiopulmonary resuscitation (CPR) or administer medications if cardiovascular collapse occurs.
2. Maintain patent airway; suction as needed.
3. Position upright if condition permits to allow greater chest expansion.
4. Maintain patency of chest tubes.
5. Assist patient to splint chest while turning or coughing and administer pain medications as needed.

Resolving Impaired Gas Exchange
1. Encourage patient in the use of inspiratory spirometer.
2. Monitor oximetry and ABGs to determine oxygenation.
3. Provide oxygen as needed.

Patient Education and Health Maintenance
1. Instruct patient to continue use of the inspiratory spirometer at home.
2. For patients with spontaneous pneumothorax, there is an increased chance of repeat occurrence; therefore, encourage these patients to report sudden dyspnea immediately.

Outcome-Based Evaluation
- Breath sounds equal bilaterally; less dyspneic
- ABGs improved

▪ Chest Injuries

Chest injuries are potentially life-threatening because of (1) immediate disturbances of cardiorespiratory physiology and hemorrhage and (2) later developments of infection, damaged lung, and thoracic cage. Traumatic chest injuries include *rib fracture, hemothorax, flail chest, pulmonary contusion,* and *cardiac tamponade.* Patients with chest trauma may have injuries to multiple organ systems. The patient should be examined for intra-abdominal injuries, which must be treated aggressively.

Pathophysiology and Clinical Manifestations
Rib Fracture
1. Most common chest injury
2. May interfere with ventilation and may lacerate underlying lung
3. Causes pain at fracture site; painful, shallow respirations; localized tenderness and crepitus (crackling) over fracture site

Hemothorax
1. Blood in pleural space as a result of penetrating or blunt chest trauma.
2. Accompanies a high percentage of chest injuries.
3. Can result in hidden blood loss.
4. Patient may be asymptomatic, dyspneic, apprehensive, or in shock.

Flail Chest
1. Loss of stability of chest wall as a result of multiple rib fractures, or combined rib and sternum fractures.
2. When this occurs, one portion of the chest has lost its bony connection to the rest of the rib cage.
3. During respiration, the detached part of the chest will be pulled in on inspiration and blown out on expiration (paradoxical movement).
4. Normal mechanics of breathing are impaired to a degree that seriously jeopardizes ventilation, causing dyspnea and cyanosis.
5. Generally associated with other serious chest injuries; lung contusion, lung laceration, diffuse alveolar damage.

Pulmonary Contusion
1. Bruise of the lung parenchyma that results in leakage of blood and edema fluid into the alveolar and interstitial spaces of the lung
2. May not be fully developed for 24 to 72 hours
3. Signs and symptoms include:
    a. Tachypnea, tachycardia
    b. Crackles on auscultation
    c. Pleuritic chest pain
    d. Copious secretions
    e. Cough—constant, loose, rattling

Cardiac Tamponade
1. Compression of the heart as a result of accumulation of fluid within the pericardial space
2. Caused by penetrating injuries
3. Signs and symptoms include:
    a. Falling blood pressure
    b. Distended neck veins, elevated central venous pressure (CVP)
    c. Muffled heart sounds

d. Pulsus paradoxus (systolic blood pressure drops and fluctuates with respiration)
e. Dyspnea, cyanosis, shock

NURSING ALERT

A rapidly developing tamponade interferes with ventricular filling and causes impairment of circulation. Thus, there is a reduced cardiac output and poor venous return to the heart. Cardiac collapse can result. In the patient with hypovolemia due to associated injuries, the CVP may not rise, thus masking the signs of cardiac tamponade.

Management and Nursing Interventions

The goal is to restore normal cardiorespiratory function as quickly a possible. This is accomplished by performing effective resuscitation while simultaneously assessing the patient, restoring chest wall integrity, and reexpanding the lung. The order of priority is determined by the clinical status of the patient.

Rib Fracture

1. Give analgesics (usually non-narcotic) to assist in effective coughing and deep breathing.
2. Encourage deep breathing with strong inspiration; give local support to injured area by splinting with hands.
3. Assist with intercostal nerve block (see Procedure Guideline 11-2) to relieve pain so coughing and deep breathing may be accomplished. An intercostal nerve block is the injection of a local anesthetic into the area surrounding the intercostal nerves to relieve pain temporarily after rib fracture(s), chest wall injury, or thoracotomy.
4. For multiple rib fractures, epidural anesthesia may be used.

Hemothorax

1. Assist with thoracentesis to aspirate blood from pleural space, if being done before a chest tube insertion.
2. Assist with chest tube insertion and set up drainage system to accomplish complete and continuous removal of blood and air.
   a. Auscultate lungs and monitor for relief of dyspnea.
   b. Monitor amount of blood loss in drainage.
3. Replace volume with IV fluids or blood products.

Flail Chest

1. Stabilize the flail portion of the chest with hands; apply a pressure dressing and turn the patient on injured side, or place 10-lb sandbag at site of flail.
2. Thoracic epidural analgesia may be used for some patients to relieve pain and improve ventilation.
3. If respiratory failure is present, prepare for immediate endotracheal intubation and mechanical ventilation—treats underlying pulmonary contusion and serves to stabilize the thoracic cage for healing of fractures, improves alveolar ventilation, and restores thoracic cage stability and intrathoracic volume by decreasing work of breathing.

4. Prepare for operative stabilization of chest wall in select patients.

Pulmonary Contusion

For moderate lung contusion
1. Employ mechanical ventilation to keep lungs inflated.
2. Administer diuretics to reduce edema.
3. Correct metabolic acidosis with IV sodium bicarbonate.
4. Use pulmonary artery pressure monitoring.
5. Monitor for development of pneumonia.

Cardiac Tamponade

For penetrating injuries
1. Assist with pericardiocentesis (see p. 343) to provide emergency relief and improve hemodynamic function until operation can be undertaken.
2. Prepare for emergency thoracotomy to control bleeding and to repair cardiac injury.

Additional Responsibilities

1. Suction as indicated through nose or mouth or endotracheal tube.
2. Prepare for tracheostomy, if indicated.
   a. Tracheostomy helps to clear tracheobronchial tree, helps the patient breathe with less effort, decreases the amount of dead airspace in the respiratory tree, and helps reduce paradoxical motion.
   b. When used with mechanical ventilation, provides a closed system and stabilizes the chest.
3. Secure one or more IV lines for fluid replacement, and obtain blood for baseline studies such as hemoglobin and hematocrit.
4. Monitor serial CVP readings to prevent hypovolemia and circulatory overload.
5. Monitor ABG/SpO$_2$ results to determine need for supplemental oxygen, mechanical ventilation.
6. Obtain urinary output hourly to evaluate tissue perfusion.
7. Continue to monitor thoracic drainage to provide information about rate of blood loss, whether bleeding has stopped, whether surgical intervention is necessary.
8. Institute ECG monitoring for early detection and treatment of cardiac dysrhythmias (dysrhythmias are a frequent cause of death in chest trauma).
9. Maintain ongoing surveillance for complications:
   a. Aspiration
   b. Atelectasis
   c. Pneumonia
   d. Mediastinal/subcutaneous emphysema
   e. Respiratory failure

Patient Education and Health Maintenance

1. Instruct patient in splinting techniques.
2. Ensure that patient is aware of importance of automobile seat belt use.
3. Teach patient to report signs of complications—increasing dyspnea, fever, cough.

SELECTED REFERENCES

American Association for Cardiovascular and Pulmonary Rehabilitation. (1998). *Guidelines for pulmonary rehabilitation programs* (2nd ed.). Champaign, IL: Human Kinetics.

American Thoracic Society (2000). Idiopathic pulmonary fibrosis: Diagnosis and treatment. *American Journal of Respiratory Care Medicine, 161,* 646–664.

American Thoracic Society and Centers for Disease Control. (1994). Treatment of tuberculosis and tuberculosis infection in adults and children. *American Journal of Respiratory Critical Care Medicine, 149,* 1359–1374.

Antonelli, M., et al. (1998). A comparison of noninvasive positive-pressure ventilation and conventional mechanical ventilation in patients with acute respiratory failure. *New England Journal of Medicine, 339,* 429–435.

Baum, G., Celli, B., Crapo, J., & Karlinsky, J. (1998). *Textbook of pulmonary diseases* (6th ed.). Philadelphia: Lippincott-Raven.

Cadek, J. (1996, December). Alpha$_1$-antitrypsin: A world view. *Cest, 110*(6) [Suppl.].

Casaburi, R., & Petty, T. (1993). *Principles and practice of pulmonary rehabilitation.* Philadelphia: W. B. Saunders.

Christie, F. (1998). Pulmonary embolism. *American Journal of Nursing, 98*(11), 36–37.

Garvey, C. (1998). COPD and exercise. *Lippincott's Primary Care Practice, 2*(6), 589–598.

Gordin, F., et al. (2000). Rifampin and pyrazinamide vs. isoniazid for prevention of tuberculosis in HIV-infected persons. *Journal of the American Medical Association, 283,* 1445–1450.

Kwiatkowski, M., & Jain, M. (1998). Current trends and treatments in chronic obstructive pulmonary disease. *Lippincott's Primary Care Practice, 2*(6), 545–558.

Mackin, L. (1998). Screening for tuberculosis in the primary care setting. *Lippincott's Primary Care Practice, 2*(6), 599–610.

Murray, J., & Nadal, J. (1994). *Respiratory medicine* (2nd ed.). Philadelphia: W. B. Saunders.

Nuorti, J.P., et al. (2000). Cigarette smoking and invasive pneumococcal disease. *New England Journal of Medicine, 342,* 681–689.

Sabiston, D., & Spencer, F. (1995). *Surgery of the chest* (6th ed.). Philadelphia: W. B. Saunders.

Sause, W., et al. (2000). Final results of phase III trials in regionally advanced unresectable non–small cell lung cancer. *Chest, 117*(2), 358–364.

US Department of Health and Human Services. (1994). *Core curriculum on tuberculosis: What the clinician should know* (3rd ed.). Atlanta: US Department of Health and Human Services.

Williams, R. M. (1998). Pneumococcal vaccination. *Lippincott's Primary Care Practice, 2*(6), 625–633.

Wintermeyer, S. F. (1998). Occupational asthma. *Lippincott's Primary Care Practice, 2*(6), 614–624.

Wright, L. (1998). Learning to cope with chronic obstructive pulmonary disease. *Lippincott's Primary Care Practice, 2*(6), 647–649.

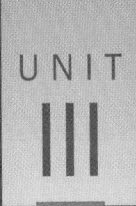

UNIT

III

Cardiovascular Health

CHAPTER

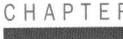
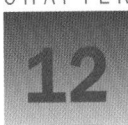

*Cardiovascular
Function
and Therapy*

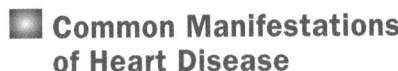

Common Manifestations of Heart Disease

Chest pain is the most common manifestation among patients with cardiac disease. Other complaints include shortness of breath, palpitations, weakness or fatigue, and dizziness or syncope.

Chest Pain
Characterization
1. Nature and intensity

a. Ask patient to describe in own words what the pain is like—dull, sharp, crushing, burning, heaviness, ache, pressure?
b. Ask patient to rate pain relative to pain experienced in the past, using a scale of 1 to 10 (10 being the most severe pain and 1 the least).
2. Onset and duration
a. When did the pain start?
b. How long did the pain episode last?
3. Location and radiation
a. Ask patient to point to area where it hurts most. (Positive Levine's sign: Clenched fist brought to patient's chest; indicative of diffuse visceral pain associated with unstable cardiac disease.)

b. Ask the patient if the pain seems to travel (most commonly radiates to left arm, jaw, back, and abdominal region).
4. Precipitating and relieving factors
   a. What activity was patient doing just before pain (rapid walking, exposure to cold, eating a spicy meal, sitting quietly, awakened from sleep)?
   b. What relieves the pain (rest, medications, change of position)?
5. Associated signs/symptoms: observe for nausea, diaphoresis, dyspnea, fatigue, palpitations, disorientation.

Significance
1. Ischemia caused by an increase in demand for coronary blood flow and oxygen delivery, which exceeds available blood supply; due to coronary artery disease, or a decreased supply without an increased demand due to coronary artery spasm or thrombus.
2. Excruciating "shearing" pain radiating to back and flanks may indicate acute dissecting aneurysm of the aorta.
3. Sharp precordial pain (over heart area) radiating to left shoulder and upper back, aggravated by respirations—indicates acute pericarditis.

Shortness of Breath (Dyspnea)
Characterization
1. What precipitates or relieves dyspnea?
2. How many pillows does patient sleep with at night? (Using several pillows is indicative of advanced heart failure.)
3. How far can patient walk or how many flights of stairs can patient climb before becoming dyspneic?
4. Determine the type of dyspnea.
   a. *Exertional*—breathlessness on moderate exertion that is relieved by rest.
   b. *Paroxysmal nocturnal*—sudden dyspnea at night; awakens patient with feeling of suffocation; sitting up relieves breathlessness.
   c. *Orthopnea*—shortness of breath when lying down. Patient must keep head elevated with more than one pillow to minimize dyspnea.

Significance
1. It may be a sign of left ventricular failure or transient congestive heart failure.

Palpitations
Characterization
1. Do you ever feel your heart pound, beat too fast, or skip beats?
2. Do you feel dizzy or faint when you experience these sensations?
3. What brings on this sensation?
4. How long does it last?
5. What do you do to relieve these sensations?

Significance
1. Pounding, jumping sensations in chest usually due to tachydysrhythmias
2. Skipped beats usually due to premature atrial or ventricular beats

Weakness and Fatigue
Characterization
1. What activities can you perform without becoming tired?
2. What activities cause you to become tired?
3. Is the fatigue relieved by rest?
4. Is leg weakness accompanied by pain or swelling?

Significance
1. Fatigue is produced by low cardiac output. The heart is unable to provide sufficient blood to meet the increased metabolic needs of cells.
2. As heart disease advances, fatigue is precipitated by less effort.
3. Weakness or tiring of the legs may be caused by peripheral arterial or venous disease.

Dizziness and Syncope
Characterization
1. How many episodes of syncope/near syncope have been experienced?
2. Did a hot room, hunger, sudden position change, or pressure on your neck precipitate the episode (rules out incidents that may cause a vasovagal response)?
3. How long does dizziness last?
4. What relieves dizziness?

Significance
1. Syncope is a transient loss of consciousness due to a fall in cardiac output with resulting cerebral ischemia. Near syncope refers to lightheadedness, dizziness, temporary confusion.
2. Dysrhythmias related to cardiac disease may cause syncope.

■ Nursing History
History of Present Illness
1. What other symptoms has the patient noticed?
2. How long has the patient been ill? What has the course of the illness been?
3. Obtain a review of systems.

Past Medical History
Medical and Surgical History
1. Hypertension, diabetes mellitus, hyperlipidemia, or other chronic illnesses which cause or aggravate cardiovascular disease.
2. Past illnesses/hospitalizations: trauma to chest (possible myocardial contusion); sore throat/dental extractions

(possible endocarditis); rheumatic fever (valvular dysfunction, endocarditis); thromboembolism (MI, pulmonary embolism)

3. Medications—many cardiac drugs must be tapered off to prevent a "rebound effect"; many drugs affect heart rate and may cause orthostatic hypotension; estrogen preparations may lead to thromboembolism.

Family History
1. Ask if patient's family members (patients, grandparents, siblings, blood relatives) were diagnosed with coronary artery disease, hypertension, hyperlipidemia, diabetes.

Lifestyle
1. Assess for risk factors to cardiovascular disease such as smoking, obesity, pattern of recurrent weight gain after dieting, sedentary lifestyle, stress, alcohol consumption.

■ Physical Examination
Vital Signs
Determine Heart Rate
1. Time for 1 full minute; note regularity.
2. Compare apical and radial heart rate (pulse deficit).

Monitor Blood Pressure
1. Take pressure in both arms and note differences (5- to 10-mm Hg difference is normal). Difference >10 may indicate subclavian steal syndrome or dissecting aortic aneurysm.
2. Determine pulse pressure (systolic pressure minus diastolic pressure) to evaluate cardiac output (30 to 40 mm Hg normal; less than 30 mm Hg indicates decreased cardiac output).
3. Note presence of pulsus alternans—loud sounds alternate with soft sounds with each auscultatory beat (hallmark of left ventricular failure).
4. Note presence of pulsus paradoxus—abnormal fall in blood pressure during inspirations (cardinal sign of cardiac tamponade).

Assess for Postural or Orthostatic Hypotension
1. Autonomic compensatory factors for upright posture are inadequate due to volume depletion, bed rest, drugs such as beta- or alpha-adrenergic blockers, or neurologic disease; prompt hypotension occurs with assumption of the upright position.
2. Note changes in heart rate and blood pressure in at least two of three positions: lying, standing, sitting; allow at least 3 minutes between position changes before obtaining rate and pressure.
3. Orthostatic changes evident if blood pressure decreases by 15 mm Hg (systolic) or 5 mm Hg diastolic and/or heart rate increases 15 beats with position changes. Keep in mind that patients on beta blockers may not exhibit a compensatory increase in heart rate.

Skin and Extremities
Palpate for Temperature and Evidence of Diaphoresis
1. Warm/dry skin indicates adequate cardiac output.
2. Cool, clammy skin indicates compensatory vasoconstriction due to low cardiac output.

Observe for Cyanosis, Jaundice, and Fatty Skin Deposits (Xanthomas)
1. Cyanosis—bluish discoloration of the skin and mucous membranes.
   a. *Central cyanosis*—low oxygen saturation of arterial blood. Noted on tongue, buccal mucosa, and lips. Indicative of cardiorespiratory disease; may be evident in heart failure or pulmonary edema.
   b. *Peripheral cyanosis*—reduced blood flow through extremities due to vasoconstriction. Noted on distal aspects of extremities, tip of nose, and ear lobes; due to cold exposure or obstructive peripheral vascular disease.
2. Jaundice—yellow discoloration of sclera of eyes and/or skin; may be sign of right-sided heart failure or chronic hemolysis from prosthetic heart valve.
3. Yellow plaque (fatty deposits) evident on skin; associated with hyperlipidemia and coronary artery disease.

Inspect Nail Beds for Splinter Hemorrhages and Clubbing
1. Thin brown lines in nail bed are associated with endocarditis.
2. Clubbing (swollen nail base and loss of normal angle) is associated with congenital heart disease and cor pulmonale.

Inspect and Palpate for Edema
1. Edema is an abnormal accumulation of serous fluid in soft tissue.
2. Location of edema is influenced by gravity—fluid collects bilaterally in lower parts of the body: sacral area (bedridden patients), ankles, and feet (ambulatory patients), and "pits" with pressure (dependent-pitting edema).
3. Weight gain occurs before clinical evidence of edema. Edema is a late sign of heart failure.
4. Describe degree of edema in terms of depth of pitting that occurs with slight pressure; mild—0 to ¼ inch, moderate—½ inch, severe—¾ to 1 inch.

Palpate Arterial Pulses
1. Examine the pulses bilaterally; peripheral pulses should be equal.
   a. Note amplitude (fullness), which depends on pulse pressure (difference between systolic and diastolic pressures); this gives an estimate of stroke volume.
   b. Small volume pulse may be from low stroke volume and peripheral vasoconstriction (MI, shock, constrictive pericarditis, vasoconstrictive drugs).

c. Large volume pulse produced by large stroke volume (aortic regurgitation, pregnancy, thyrotoxicosis, bradycardia, patent ductus arteriosus).

d. Palpate carotid artery—reveals character of pulse in the proximal aorta and provides indication of any abnormality causing disease of left ventricle.

Chest and Neck
General Assessment
1. Palpate the precordial area with palmar base of hand.
2. Note pulsation in apical area (fifth intercostal space—midclavicular line).
3. Pulsation (apical impulse) should be approximately 2 cm in diameter; lateral displacement of greater than 7 to 9 cm from sternal border indicates left ventricular hypertrophy.

Respiration
1. Note rate, depth, and respiratory pattern, use of accessory muscles.

Jugular Venous Pulse
1. Venous pulsation can be more easily seen than felt.
2. Identification of venous pulse permits assessment of height of venous pressure.
3. See page 71 for technique.

Heart Auscultation
1. Four main areas of auscultation: aortic area, pulmonary area, mitral area, and the tricuspid area.
2. Listen with diaphragm for rate and regularity of rhythm.
   a. Determine if an irregularity is related to respiratory movements.
   b. Evaluate the sequence in which an irregularity occurs.
3. During auscultation, feel the pulsation of the right carotid artery and the radial artery to assess for pulse deficit.
4. Auscultate with bell of stethoscope for an S_3 gallop (may indicate ventricular failure), an S_4 gallop (may be present in left ventricular hypertrophy, pulmonary or aortic stenosis, and hypertension), murmurs (indicate incompetent or stenotic valves), or pericardial friction rub (pericarditis).

DIAGNOSTIC TESTS

Cardiovascular function and disease are evaluated by a variety of blood tests, ultrasound techniques, fluoroscopy and nuclear imaging studies, and electrocardiography. The ECG and its application in exercise stress testing are invaluable in the evaluation of chest pain and cardiac dysfunction.

■ Laboratory Studies
Enzyme and Isoenzyme Tests
Description
1. When myocardial tissue is damaged (myocardial infarction; MI), certain cardiac enzymes are released into the bloodstream and result in elevated peripheral blood enzyme levels:
   a. Creatine kinase (CK)
   b. Lactic dehydrogenase (LDH)
   c. Aspartate aminotransferase (AST, formerly SGOT). However, these enzymes may be widely distributed in tissues and elevated in conditions not associated with MI such as damage to skeletal muscles, liver, brain, kidneys, and other organs.
2. Isoenzymes of CK and LDH can be identified by laboratory methods to reveal the specific tissue that is damaged.
3. Cardiac troponins—cardiac troponins T and I begin to rise 3 to 5 hours after myocardial injury occurs.
4. Myoglobin levels—levels usually peak within 6 hours of acute MI; not as specific as CK-MB.

Nursing and Patient Care Considerations
1. Ensure that enzymes are drawn in a serial pattern, usually on admission and every 6 to 24 hours until three samples are obtained; enzyme activity then is correlated to the extent of heart muscle damage.
2. Normal values, rise, and peak of enzymes following MI include:
   a. CK—rise in 12 hours; peak in 36 to 72 hours; normalize (35 to 232 IU) in 3 to 5 days.
   b. LDH—rise in 12 hours; peak in 12 to 24 hours; normalize (100 to 190 IU) in 10 days.
   c. AST—rise in 8 to 12 hours; peak in 18 to 36 hours; normalize in 3 to 4 days.
   d. CK-MB—rise in 4 to 8 hours, peak in 24 hours, normalize (less than 5 IU) in 72 hours.
   e. LDH_1 and LDH_2—LDH_2 is normally greater than LDH_1, except when the heart muscle is damaged a reversal occurs; a "flipped" pattern results, with LDH_1 exceeding the value of LDH_2, usually within 12 to 24 hours.
   f. Cardiac troponin T—rise 3 to 5 hours, remain elevated for 14 to 21 days.
   g. Cardiac troponin I—rise 3 hours, peak at 14 to 18 hours, and remain elevated for 5 to 7 days.
   h. Myoglobin—detected as early as 2 hours, peak in 3 to 15 hours.

NURSING ALERT

The greater the peak in enzyme activity and the length of time an enzyme remains at peak level correlate with serious damage of the heart muscle and a poorer prognosis for the patient.

■ Radiology and Imaging
Chest X-Ray
Description
Shows heart size, contour, and position; reveals cardiac and pericardial calcifications and demonstrates physiologic alterations in pulmonary circulation

Nursing and Patient Care Considerations

1. Advise patient to remove all metal jewelry before having x-ray.
2. If portable chest x-ray is being done on bedridden or critically ill patient, assist with high Fowler's position during x-ray and ensure that all tubes, IV lines, and monitoring remain in place.

Myocardial Imaging
Description

With the use of radionuclides and scintillation cameras, radionuclide angiograms can be used to assess left ventricular performance.

1. "Hot spot" or positive imaging using technetium 99m stannous pyrophosphate is used when diagnosis of MI is unclear.
2. "Cold spot" imaging using thallium 201 can be used to rule out MI if negative. However, if positive, it cannot differentiate between old and new infarction and areas of ischemia versus infarction.
3. Radionuclide ventriculogram using technetium 99m provides measurements of right and left ventricular ejection fraction, distinguishes regional from global ventricular wall motion, and allows for subjective analysis of cardiac anatomy to detect intracardiac shunts or valvular or congenital abnormalities.

Nursing and Patient Care Considerations

Advise patient that a radionuclide will be injected through a central venous, Swan-Ganz, or IV catheter or antecubital vein. Reassure the patient that the radionuclide will not cause radiation injury or affect heart function.

Angiography
Description

1. Injection of contrast medium into the vascular system (to outline the heart and blood vessels) accompanied by cineangiograms (rapidly changing films or movies on an intensified fluoroscopic screen), which record the passage of contrast medium through the vascular tree.
2. Useful for providing information regarding coronary anatomy, structural abnormalities (occlusions, defects, fistulae), or abnormal heart valve function.
3. Types of angiography include:
   a. *Selective angiocardiography*—contrast medium is injected through a catheter directly into one of the heart chambers, coronary arteries, or greater vessel.
   b. *Aortography*—a form of angiography that outlines the lumen of the aorta and major arteries arising from it.
   c. *Coronary arteriography* (most common form of selective angiocardiography)—used as an evaluation tool before coronary artery surgery or myocardial revascularization and after surgery to evaluate graft patency. (See section titled Cardiac Catheterization, p. 319.)
   d. *Peripheral arteriography*—to determine arterial patency of extremities.

Nursing and Patient Care Considerations

1. Before angiogram, keep the patient in a fasting state—to minimize danger of pulmonary aspiration should emesis occur.
2. After angiogram:
   a. Record vital signs every 15 minutes × 4 (or more often as patient's condition indicates until vital signs are stable).
   b. Check for bleeding at puncture or cutdown site.
   c. Check distal extremity for normal color and intact pulses.
   d. The patient may complain of mild headache and/or discomfort in the groin or other site depending on route by which contrast medium was administered.
   e. Check for bed rest and special fluid instructions.

Echocardiography (Ultrasound Cardiography)
Description

1. A record of high-frequency sound vibrations that have been sent into the heart through the chest wall. The cardiac structures return the echoes derived from the ultrasound. The motions of the echoes are traced on an oscilloscope and recorded on film.
2. Clinical usefulness includes: demonstration of valvular and other structural deformities, detection of pericardial effusion, evaluation of prosthetic valve function, diagnosis of cardiac tumors of asymmetric thickening of interventricular septum, diagnosis of cardiomegaly (heart enlargement).
3. Types include two-dimensional and M mode. The methods are complementary and are often used in conjunction.
   a. *Two-dimensional echocardiography*—provides a wider view of the heart and its structures because it involves a planar ultrasound beam
   b. *M-mode*—utilizes a single ultrasound beam and provides a narrow segmental view
4. Transesophageal echocardiography
   a. The ultrasound transmitter is located at the end of a catheter, which is passed through the esophagus; allows for a more clear and accurate diagnostic evaluation.
   b. This is an invasive procedure; the patient will require mild sedation and must be kept NPO for a specified time, usually 4 to 6 hours, before the procedure.

Nursing and Patient Care Considerations

Advise the patient that traditional echocardiography is noninvasive and that no preparation is necessary. Position the patient on the left side, if tolerated, to bring the heart closer to the chest wall. Assist patient to cleanse chest of transducer gel after the test.

Doppler Ultrasound

1. Noninvasive method of evaluating peripheral venous patency and valvular competence and arterial patency.
2. The entire test takes about 5 to 10 minutes, and no special preparation is necessary.

3. Tell the patient that a cuff is applied to the leg to detect arterial patency, and will be inflated and deflated similar to blood pressure measurement.

Plethysmography (Pulse Volume Recording [PVR])

1. A noninvasive measurement of changes in calf volume corresponding to changes in blood volume brought about by temporary venous occlusion with a high pneumatic cuff.
2. Ocular pneumoplethysmography (OPG)—measures indirectly carotid artery blood flow; this is done by the application of pneumatic pressure on the eye to measure ophthalmic artery pressure.
3. Advise the patient that cuff inflation may cause brief discomfort, but not pain.

Oscillometry

1. Degree of arterial occlusion may be measured by an oscillometer, which measures pulse volume. One extremity may be compared with the other to evaluate arterial patency.
2. An inflatable cuff is wrapped around the extremity, and the oscillometric index is determined by inflating the cuff and reading the dial.
3. Advise patient to remain still while cuff is inflated and deflated to prevent interference with pressure readings.

Phlebography (Venography)
Description
An x-ray visualization of the vascular tree after the injection of a contrast medium (Renografin) to detect venous occlusion
Nursing and Patient Care Considerations
1. Inform the patient that he or she may experience an intense burning sensation in the vessel where the solution is injected. This will last for only a few seconds.
2. Note any evidence of allergic reaction to the contrast medium; this may occur as soon as the contrast medium is injected, or it may occur after the test.
   a. Perspiring, dyspnea, nausea, vomiting
   b. Rapid heart rate, numbness of extremities
   c. Hives
3. Advise the patient to notify the health care provider of any signs of allergic reaction.
4. Observe injection site for signs of redness, swelling, bleeding, thrombosis.

Digital Subtraction Angiography (DSA) or Digital Intravenous Angiography
Description
Radiologic technique that uses computer subtraction to display an enhanced image of the arterial system. Contrast medium is injected by way of a catheter inserted into the brachial vein, and a guidewire is threaded into the superior vena cava.

Nursing and Patient Care Considerations
1. Advise on no food intake within 2 hours of the test to prevent vomiting if there is a reaction to the contrast medium.
2. Make sure the patient will be able to hold breath and lie very still when directed.
3. Instruct the patient to increase fluid intake over next 24 hours (1,500 to 2,000 mL) to aid in excretion of contrast medium.

Other Diagnostic Tests
The Electrocardiogram (ECG)
Basic Principles
1. Electrical activity is generated by the cells of the heart as ions are exchanged across cell membranes.
2. Electrodes that are capable of conducting electrical activity from the heart to the ECG machine are placed at strategic positions on the extremities and chest precordium (Figure 12-1).

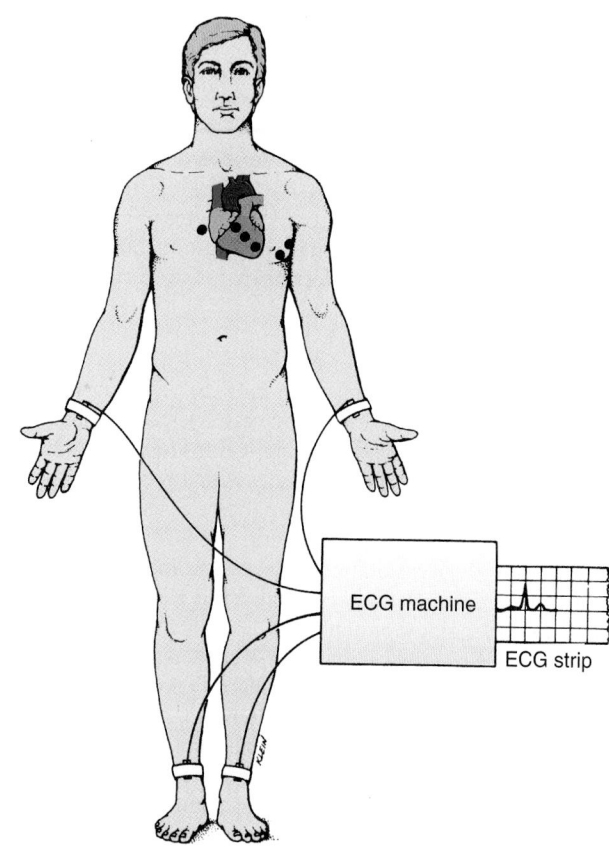

ECG machine

ECG strip

FIGURE 12-1 Transmission of heart's impulse to a graphic display by ECG machine. The electrodes that are capable of conducting electrical activity from the heart to the ECG machine are placed at strategic positions on the extremities and chest precordium.

3. The electrical energy sensed is then converted to a graphic display by the ECG machine. This display is referred to as the *electrocardiogram.*

4. A heart contraction is represented by wave forms on the ECG graph paper, which are designated P, Q, R, S, and T waves.

5. Wave forms are referred to as deflections relative to an isoelectric line (a line that expresses no energy). The isoelectric line can be determined by looking at the T–P interval.

   a. The P wave is the first positive deflection and represents atrial depolarization.

   b. The Q wave is the first negative deflection after the P wave; the R wave is the first positive deflection after the P wave.

   c. The S wave is the negative deflection after the R wave.

   d. The QRS wave form is generally regarded as a unit and represents ventricular depolarization.

   e. The T wave follows the S wave and is joined to the QRS complex by the S–T segment. The T wave represents the return of ions to the appropriate side of the cell membrane. This signifies relaxation of the muscle fibers and is referred to as *repolarization* of the ventricles.

   f. The Q–T interval is the time between the Q wave and the T wave.

Indications

The ECG is a useful tool in the diagnosis of those conditions that may cause aberrations in the electrical activity of the heart. Examples of these conditions are as follows:

1. MI and other types of coronary artery diseases, such as angina
2. Cardiac dysrhythmias
3. Cardiac enlargement
4. Electrolyte disturbances, especially of calcium and potassium levels
5. Inflammatory diseases of the heart
6. Effects on the heart by drugs such as digoxin (Lanoxin) and tricyclic antidepressants

ECG Leads and Normal Wave Form Interpretation (Figure 12-2)

1. The standard ECG consists of 12 leads (I, II, III, AVR, AVL, AVF, V_1, V_2, V_3, V_4, V_5, V_6).

   a. Each lead records the heart's electrical activity from a different anatomic position.

   b. Identification of specific myocardial changes on certain leads assists in defining pathologic conditions.

2. The normal amplitude of the P wave is 3 mm or less; the normal duration of the P wave is 0.04 to 0.11 second. P waves that exceed these measurements are considered to be a deviation from normal.

3. The P–R interval is measured from the upstroke of the P wave to the Q–R junction and is normally between 0.12 and 0.20 second.

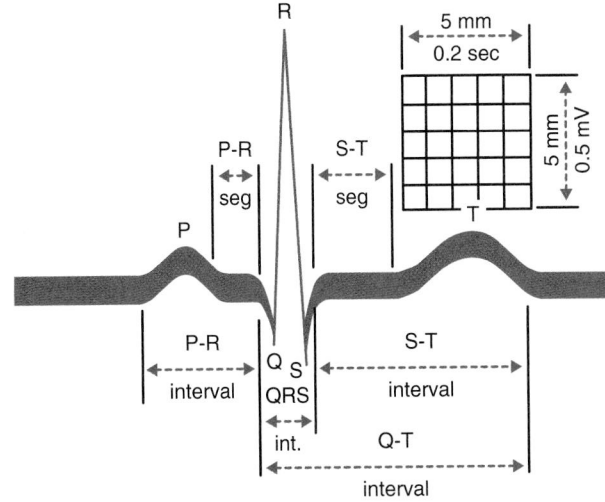

FIGURE 12-2 Wave form analysis.

   a. The P–R interval represents the time of impulse transmission from the sinoatrial (SA) node to the atrioventricular (AV) node.

   b. There is a built-in delay in time at the AV node to allow for adequate ventricular filling to maintain normal stroke volume (the amount of blood ejected with each contraction).

4. The QRS complex contains separate waves and segments, which should be evaluated separately. Normal QRS complex should be between 0.06 and 0.10 second.

   a. The Q wave, or first downward stroke after the P wave, is usually less than 3 mm in depth. A Q wave of significant deflection is not normally present in the healthy heart. A pathologic Q wave usually indicates a completed MI.

   b. The R wave is the first positive deflection after the P wave, normally 5 to 10 mm in height. Increases and decreases in amplitude become significant in certain disease states. Ventricular hypertrophy produces very high R waves because the hypertrophied muscle requires a stronger electrical current to depolarize.

5. The S–T segment begins at the end of the S wave, the first negative deflection after the R wave, and terminates at the upstroke of the T wave.

6. The T wave represents the repolarization of myocardial fibers or provides the resting state of myocardial work; the T wave should always be present.

   a. Normally, the T wave should not exceed a 5-mm amplitude in all leads except the precordial (V_1 to V_6) leads, where it may be as high as 10 mm.

Nursing and Patient Care Considerations

1. Perform ECG or begin continuous ECG monitoring as indicated.

a. Provide privacy, and ask the patient to undress, exposing chest, wrists, and ankles. Assist with draping as appropriate.

b. Place leads on chest and extremities as labeled, using self-adhesive electrodes or water-soluble gel or other conductive material.

c. Instruct patient to lie still, avoiding movement, coughing, or talking while ECG is recording to avoid artifact.

d. Make sure ECG machine is plugged in and grounded, and operate according to manufacturer's directions.

e. If continuous cardiac monitoring is being done, advise patient on the parameters of mobility as movement may trigger alarms and false readings.

2. Interpret ECG (Figure 12-3). Develop a systematic approach to assist in accurate interpretation for dysrhythmias, myocardial damage, or other changes.

a. Determine the rate. Is it fast, slow, or normal?

(i) A gross determination of rate can be accomplished by counting the number of QRS complexes within a 6-second time interval (use the superior margin of ECG paper) and multiplying the complexes by a factor of 10.

Note: One must be cautioned that this method is accurate only for rhythms that are occurring at normal intervals and should not be used for determining rate in irregular rhythms. Irregular rhythms are always counted for 1 full minute for accuracy.

(ii) Another means of obtaining rate is to divide the number of large five-square blocks between each two QRS complexes into 300. Three hundred large blocks represent 1 minute on the ECG paper.

Example: In Figure 12-3, the number of large square blocks between complexes #5 and #6 equals 5, or a rate of 60.

b. Next, determine the rhythm. Is it regular, irregular, regularly irregular, or irregularly irregular? Use calipers or count blocks between QRS complexes to determine regularity.

c. Finally, examine each wave and segment for abnormality.

(i) Find the P waves. Is one present for each QRS complex? Are they absent as in junctional rhythm? Are they replaced by other wave forms? What is the configuration like? Are they identical, well-formed, or do they change shape as in atrial fibrillation or paroxysmal atrial tachycardia?

(ii) Measure the P–R interval. Prolonged P–R interval may be a precursor to a variety of heart blocks due to drug therapy or myocardial disease.

(iii) Look for pathologic Q waves, or one that is greater than 0.04 second in time and greater than 3 mm in depth or greater than one third the height of the R wave.

(iv) Measure the QRS complex. Are they identical in configuration? Do they fall early? Does the configuration vary? Are any wide and bizarre, representing a premature ventricular contraction?

(v) Examine the S–T segments. Elevation of the S–T segment heralds a pattern of injury and usually occurs as an initial change in acute MI. S–T depression occurs in ischemic states. Calcium and potassium changes also affect the S–T segment.

(vi) Look at the T wave. Is it positively or negatively deflected? Is it peaked? Inverted T waves may indicate ischemia.

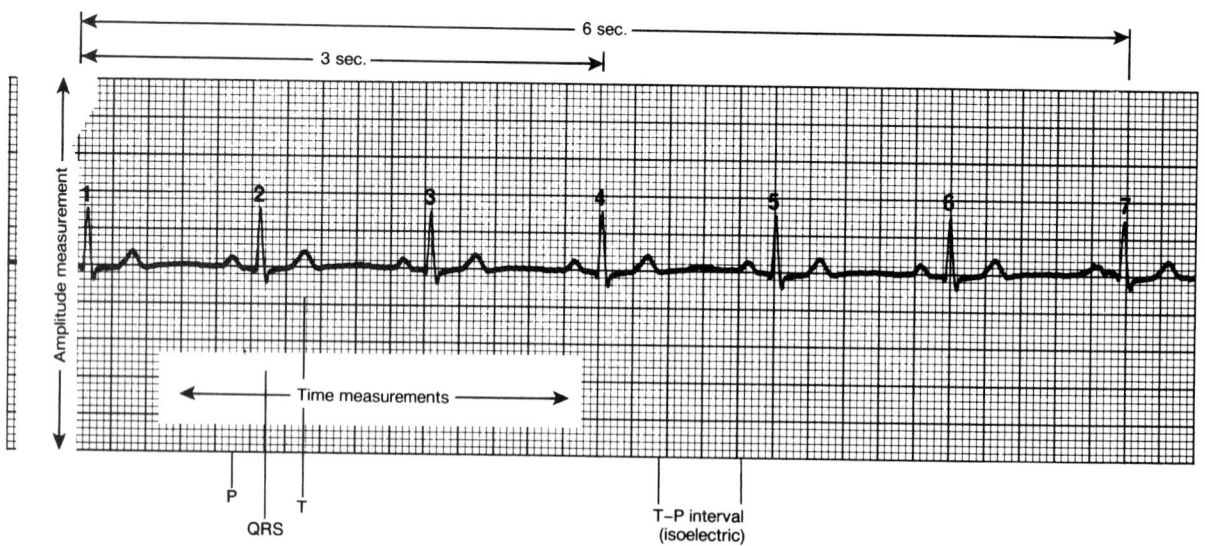

FIGURE 12-3 Lead II normal sinus rhythm and ECG paper.

(vii) Measure the Q–T interval. The normal Q–T interval should be less than one half the R–R interval. Prolonged Q—T interval may indicate digitalis toxicity, long-term quinidine (Quinaglute) or procainamide (Pronestyl) therapy, or hypomagnesemia.

Cardiac Catheterization

Description

1. Cardiac catheterization is a diagnostic procedure in which a catheter(s) is (are) introduced into the heart and blood vessels to (1) measure oxygen concentration, saturation, tension, and pressure in the various heart chambers; (2) detect shunts; (3) provide blood samples for analysis; and (4) determine cardiac output and pulmonary blood flow.
2. Right-heart catheterization—a radiopaque catheter is passed from an antecubital or femoral vein into the right atrium, right ventricle, and pulmonary vasculature under direct visualization with a fluoroscope.
   a. Right atrium and right ventricle pressures are measured; blood samples are taken for hematocrit and oxygen saturation.
   b. After entering the right atrium, the catheter is then passed through the tricuspid valve, and similar tests are performed on blood within the right ventricle.
   c. Finally, the catheter is passed through the pulmonic valve and as far as possible beyond that point; capillary samples are obtained, capillary wedge pressure is recorded, and cardiac output can be determined.
   d. Complications—cardiac dysrhythmias, venous spasm, thrombophlebitis, infection of cutdown site, cardiac perforation, and cardiac tamponade.
3. Left-heart catheterization—usually done by retrograde catheterization of the left ventricle or by transseptal catheterization of the left atrium.
   a. Retrograde approach—catheter may be introduced percutaneously by puncture of the femoral artery and advanced under fluoroscopic control into the ascending aorta and into the left ventricle, or catheter is inserted under direct vision into the right brachial artery.
   b. Transseptal approach—catheter is passed from the right femoral vein (percutaneously or by saphenous vein cutdown) into right atrium. A long needle is passed up through the catheter and is used to puncture the septum separating the right and left atria; needle is withdrawn, and the catheter is advanced under fluoroscopic control into left ventricle.
   c. The catheter tip is placed at the coronary sinus, and contrast medium is injected directly into one or both of the coronary arteries to evaluate patency.
   d. Gives hemodynamic data—permits flow and pressure measurements of left heart.
   e. Most often performed to evaluate the function of the left ventricular muscle and mitral and aortic valves, or the patency of coronary arteries.
   f. Used to evaluate patients before and after cardiac surgery.
   g. Complications of left-heart catheterization and implications for nursing assessment are
      (i) Dysrhythmias (ventricular fibrillation), syncope, vasospasm.
      (ii) Pericardial tamponade, MI, pulmonary edema.
      (iii) Allergic reaction to contrast medium.
      (iv) Perforation of great vessels of heart; systemic embolization (stroke, MI).
      (v) Loss of pulse distal to arteriotomy and possible ischemia of lower arm and hand.
4. Angiography is usually combined with heart catheterization for coronary artery visualization.

Nursing and Patient Care Considerations

Preprocedure:

1. Know which approach is to be used in order to anticipate possible complications.
2. Withhold food and fluid 6 hours before procedure to prevent vomiting and aspiration.
3. Ascertain history of previous allergies.
4. Mark distal pulses for easy reference after catheterization.
5. Explain that patient will be lying on an examining table for a prolonged period and that certain sensations may be experienced:
   a. Occasional thudding sensations in the chest—from extrasystoles, particularly when the catheter is manipulated in ventricular chambers.
   b. Strong desire to cough may occur during contrast medium injection into right heart during angiography.
   c. Transient feeling of heat, particularly in the head, from injection of contrast medium.
6. Remove dentures; give prescribed medication.

Postprocedure:

1. Record the blood pressure and apical pulse every 15 minutes (or more frequently) until vital signs are stable after the procedure to discern dysrhythmias.
2. Check peripheral pulses in affected extremity (dorsalis pedis, posterior tibial pulse in the lower extremity, and radial pulse in upper extremity); evaluate extremity temperature, color, and complaints of pain, numbness, or tingling sensation to determine signs of arterial insufficiency.
3. Watch puncture (cutdown) sites for hematoma formation. Question patient about increase in pain/tenderness at site.
4. Assess for complaints of chest pain and report occurrence immediately. MI may occur and is a serious complication of cardiac catheterization.
5. Enforce activity restrictions, which are based on coagulation status and whether avascular closure method was employed (2–24 hours).
6. Evaluate complaints of back pain, thigh or groin pain (may indicate retroperitoneal bleeding).
7. Be alert for signs/symptoms of vagal reaction (nausea, diaphoresis, hypotension, bradycardia); treat as directed with atropine and fluids.

GENERAL PROCEDURE AND TREATMENT MODALITIES

Hemodynamic Monitoring

Hemodynamic monitoring is the assessment of the patient's circulatory status; it includes measurements of heart rate, intra-arterial pressure, pulmonary artery and pulmonary capillary wedge pressures (PCWP), central venous pressure (CVP), cardiac output, and blood volume. See Procedure Guidelines 12-1, 12-2, and 12-3.

Central Venous Pressure (CVP) Monitoring

1. Refers to the measurement of right atrial pressure or the pressure of the great veins within the thorax.
   a. Right-sided cardiac function is assessed through the evaluation of the CVP.
   b. Left-sided heart function is less accurately reflected by the evaluation of CVP but may be useful in assessing chronic right and left heart failure and/or differentiating right and left ventricular infarctions.
2. Requires the threading of a catheter into a large central vein (subclavian, internal/external jugular, median basilic, or femoral). The catheter tip then is positioned in the right atrium, upper portion of the superior vena cava, or the inferior vena cava (femoral approach only).
3. Purposes of CVP monitoring include:
   a. To serve as a guide for fluid replacement.
   b. To monitor pressures in the right atrium and central veins.
   c. To administer blood products, total parenteral nutrition, and drug therapy contraindicated for peripheral infusion.
   d. To obtain venous access when peripheral vein sites are inadequate.
   e. To insert a temporary pacemaker.
   f. To obtain central venous blood samples.

Pulmonary Artery Pressure (PAP) Monitoring

Purposes
1. To monitor pressures in the right atrium (CVP), right ventricle, pulmonary artery, and distal branches of the pulmonary artery (PCWP). The latter reflects the level of the pressure in the left atrium (or filling pressure in the left ventricle); thus, pressures on the left side of the heart are inferred from pressure measurement obtained on the right side of the circulation.
2. To measure cardiac output through thermodilution.
3. To obtain blood for central venous oxygen saturation.
4. To continuously monitor mixed venous oxygen saturation (SvO_2); available on special catheters
5. To provide for temporary atrial/ventricular pacing and intra-atrial electrocardiography (available only on special catheters)

Underlying Considerations
1. Left atrial pressure is closely related to left ventricular end diastolic pressure (LVEDP—filling pressure of the

left ventricle) and is therefore an indicator of left ventricular function.
2. The pulmonary artery diastolic pressure (PADP) reflects the LVEDP in patients with normal lungs and mitral valve. The PADP can be continuously monitored as an approximation of LVEDP (limits excessive balloon inflation to obtain a PCWP and subsequent risk of balloon rupture or damage to the pulmonary artery).
3. The SvO_2 is affected by four factors: cardiac output, hemoglobin, arterial oxygen saturation (SaO_2), and tissue oxygen consumption.
4. Changes in SvO_2 alert the clinician to changes in these factors. More rapid detection of change facilitates interventions to correct problems before significant deterioration in patient's condition occurs.
5. If the amount of oxygen supplied to the tissues is inadequate to meet demands, more oxygen will be extracted from venous blood and the SvO_2 will decrease. If oxygen supply exceeds demand, the SvO_2 will increase.

Methods
1. The Swan-Ganz catheter is a flow-directed, balloon-tipped, four- to five-lumen catheter that is percutaneously inserted at the bedside and allows for continuous PAP monitoring as well as periodic measurement of PCWP and other parameters.
2. The catheter is 110 cm long, marked at increments of 10 cm, and is available in varying diameters.
3. Most catheters in use incorporate thermodilution for determination of cardiac output.
4. If monitoring of SvO_2 is desired, a pulmonary artery catheter incorporating fiberoptics is used.
5. If temporary cardiac pacing capability is desired, a catheter with a lumen for a pacing wire may be used.
6. Catheter may be inserted under fluoroscopy or at the bedside using the hemodynamic wave form as a guide to correct position.

Cardiac Output

Cardiac output is the amount (volume) of blood ejected by the left ventricle into the aorta in 1 minute. The normal cardiac output is 4 to 8 L/min.

Underlying Concepts
1. Cardiac output is determined by stroke volume (SV) and heart rate (HR).
   a. HR = number of cardiac contractions per minute. The integrity of the conduction system and nervous system innervation of the heart influence functioning of this determinant.
   b. SV = amount of blood ejected from ventricle per beat. The amount of blood returning to the heart (preload), venous tone, resistance imposed on the ventricle before ejection (afterload), and the integrity of the cardiac muscle (contractility) influence the functioning of this determinant.
2. The body alters cardiac output by increases/decreases in one of both of these parameters. Cardiac output is main-

tained if the HR fails by an increase in SV. Likewise, a decrease in SV produces a compensatory rise in HR to keep the cardiac output normal.

3. Cardiac output will decrease if either of the determinants cannot inversely compensate for the other.

4. Cardiac output measurements are adjusted to patient size by calculating the cardiac index (CI). CI = cardiac output divided by body surface area (BSA); BSA is determined through standard charts based on individual height and weight. Normal CI is 2.5 to 4.0 L/min/m^2.

Assessment of Cardiac Output

Low cardiac output may be detected by:

1. Changes in mental status
2. An increase in heart rate
3. Shortness of breath
4. Cyanosis or duskiness of buccal mucosa, nail beds, and ear lobes
5. Falling blood pressure
6. Low urine output
7. Cool, moist skin

Methods

1. Cardiac output is measured by a variety of techniques. In the clinical setting, it is usually measured by the thermodilution technique used in conjunction with a flow-directed balloon catheter (Swan-Ganz catheter).

2. The Swan-Ganz catheter is positioned in its final position in a branch of the pulmonary artery; it has a thermistor (external sensing device) situated 4 cm from the tip of the catheter, which measures the temperature of the blood that flows by it (see p. 328).

(*text continues on page 329*)

PROCEDURE GUIDELINES 12-1	CENTRAL VENOUS PRESSURE (CVP) MONITORING

EQUIPMENT

Venous pressure tray	Arm board (for antecubital insertion)
Cutdown tray	Sterile dressing/tape
Infusion solution/infusion set with CVP manometer	Gowns, masks, caps, and sterile gloves
Heparin flush system/pressure bag (if transducer to be used)	ECG monitor
IV pole	Carpenter's level (for establishing zero point)

 NURSING ALERT

A CVP line is a potential source of septicemia.

PROCEDURE

Nursing Action	Rationale
PREPARATORY PHASE (BY NURSE)	
1. Assemble equipment according to manufacturer's directions. Evaluate patient's PT, PTT, CBC.	1. To assess for coagulopathies or anemia.
2. Explain the procedure to the patient and obtain informed consent.	2. Procedure is similar to an IV, and the patient may move in bed as desired after passage of catheter.
a. Explain to patient how to perform the Valsalva maneuver.	a. The Valsalva maneuver performed during catheter insertion and removal decreases chance of air emboli.
b. NPO 6 hours before insertion.	
3. Position patient appropriately.	3. Provides for maximum visibility of veins.
a. Place in supine position.	
(i) Arm vein—extend arm and secure on armboard.	
(ii) Neck veins—place patient in Trendelenburg's position. Place a small rolled towel under shoulders (subclavian approach).	(ii) Trendelenburg's position prevents chance of air emboli. Anatomic access and clinical status of the patient are considered in site selection.
4. Flush IV infusion set and manometer (measuring device) *or* prepare heparin flush for use with transducer. Secure all connections to prevent air emboli and bleeding.	4.
a. Attach manometer to IV pole. The zero point of the manometer should be on a level with the patient's right atrium.	a. The level of the right atrium is at the fourth intercostal space midaxillary line.
b. Calibrate/zero transducer and level port with patient's right atrium.	b. Mark midaxillary line with indelible ink for subsequent readings to ensure consistency of the zero level.
5. Place patient on ECG monitor.	5. Dysrhythmias may be noted during insertion as catheter is advanced.

continued

PROCEDURE GUIDELINES 12-1   **CENTRAL VENOUS PRESSURE (CVP) MONITORING** *CONTINUED*

Nursing Action	Rationale
INSERTION PHASE (BY PHYSICIAN)	
1. Physician dons gown, cap, and mask.	1. CVP insertion is a sterile procedure.
2. The CVP site is surgically cleansed. The physician introduces the CVP catheter percutaneously or by direct venous cutdown.	2. Patient may be asked to perform Valsalva maneuver to protect against chance of air embolus.
3. Assist patient to remain motionless during insertion.	
4. Monitor for dysrhythmias as catheter is threaded to great vein or right atrium.	
5. Connect primed IV tubing/heparin flush system to catheter and allow IV solution to flow at a minimum rate to keep vein open (25 mL maximum).	5. Catheter placement must be verified before hypertonic or blood products can be administered.
6. The catheter should be sutured in place.	6. Prevents inadvertent catheter advancement or dislodgement.
7. Place a sterile occlusive dressing over site.	
8. Obtain a chest x-ray.	8. Verify correct catheter position.
TO MEASURE THE CVP	
1. Place the patient in a position of comfort.	1. This is the baseline position used for subsequent readings.
2. Position the zero point of the manometer at the level of the right atrium (see accompanying figure).	

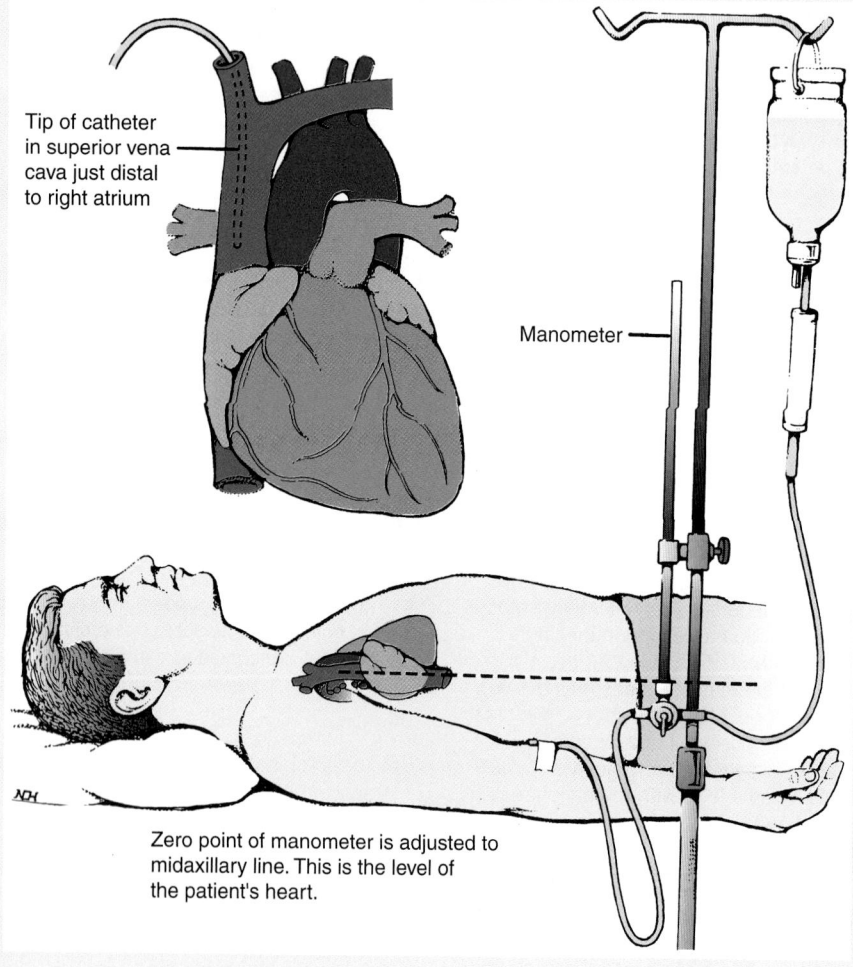

Tip of catheter in superior vena cava just distal to right atrium

Manometer

Zero point of manometer is adjusted to midaxillary line. This is the level of the patient's heart.

Nursing Action	Rationale

3. Turn the stopcock so the IV solution flows into the manometer, filling to about the 20- to 25-cm level. Then turn stopcock so solution in manometer flows into patient.

4. Observe the fall in the height of the column of fluid in manometer. Record the level at which the solution stabilizes or stops moving downward. This is the central venous pressure. Record CVP and the position of the patient.

4. The column of fluid will fall until it meets an equal pressure (ie, the patient's central venous pressure). The CVP reading is reflected by the height of a column of fluid in the manometer when there is open communication between the catheter and the manometer. The fluid in the manometer will fluctuate slightly with the patient's respirations. This confirms that the CVP line is not obstructed by clotted blood.

5. The CVP catheter may be connected to a transducer and an electrical monitor with either digital or calibrated CVP wave readout.

6. The CVP may range from 5 to 12 cm H_2O (absolute numeric values have not been agreed on) or 2 to 6 mm Hg.

6. The change in CVP is a more useful indication of adequacy of venous blood volume and alterations of cardiovascular function. The management of the patient is not based on one reading, but on repeated serial readings in correlation with patient's clinical status.

7. Assess the patient's clinical condition. Frequent changes in measurements (interpreted within the context of the clinical situation) will serve as a guide to detect whether the heart can handle its fluid load and whether hypovolemia or hypervolemia is present.

7. CVP is interpreted by considering the patient's entire clinical picture; hourly urine output, heart rate, blood pressure, cardiac output measurements.
   a. A CVP near zero indicates that the patient is hypovolemic (verified if rapid IV infusion causes patient to improve).
   b. A CVP above 15 to 20 cm H_2O may be due to either hypervolemia or poor cardiac contractility.

8. Turn the stopcock again to allow IV solution to flow from solution bottle into the patient's veins.

8. When readings are not being made, flow is from a very slow microdrip to the catheter, bypassing the manometer.

FOLLOW-UP PHASE

1. Observe for complications.

1. Patient's complaints of new or different pain or shortness of breath must be assessed closely; may indicate development of complications.

   a. *From catheter insertion:* Pneumothorax, hemothorax, air embolism, hematoma, and cardiac tamponade

   a. Signs/symptoms of air embolism include severe shortness of breath, hypotension, hypoxia, rumbling murmur, cardiac arrest.

   b. *From indwelling catheter:* Infection, air embolism
   c. If air embolism is suspected, immediately place patient in left lateral Trendelenburg's position and administer oxygen. Air bubbles will be prevented from moving into the lungs and will be absorbed in 10 to 15 minutes in the right ventricular outflow tract.

2. Carry out ongoing nursing surveillance of the insertion site and maintain aseptic technique.
   a. Inspect entry site twice daily for signs of local inflammation/phlebitis. Remove immediately if there are any signs of infection.
   b. Change dressings as prescribed.
   c. Label to show date/time of change.
   d. Send the catheter tip for bacteriologic culture when it is removed.

PROCEDURE GUIDELINES 12-2 — MEASURING PULMONARY ARTERY PRESSURE (PAP) BY FLOW-DIRECTED BALLOON-TIPPED CATHETER (SWAN-GANZ CATHETER)

EQUIPMENT

Swan-Ganz catheter set
ECG, monitor and display unit with paper recorder
For Svo₂ monitoring, fiberoptic PA catheter, optical module, and microprocessor unit
Defibrillator
Pressure transducer (disposable/reusable)
Cutdown tray
Sterile saline solution

Pressurized bag
Heparin infusion in plastic bag
Continuous flush device
Local anesthetic
Skin antiseptic
Transparent/gauze dressing
Tape

PROCEDURE

Nursing Action	Rationale

PREPARATORY PHASE (BY NURSE)

1. Explain procedure to the patient and family/significant other. Obtain informed consent.
2. Check vital signs and apply ECG electrodes.
3. Place patient in a position of comfort; this is the baseline position.

1. Explain that patient may feel the catheter moving through veins, and this is normal.

3. Note the angle of elevation if patient cannot lie flat, because subsequent pressure readings are taken from this baseline position to ensure consistency. Patient may need to be in Trendelenburg's position briefly if the jugular or subclavian vein is used.

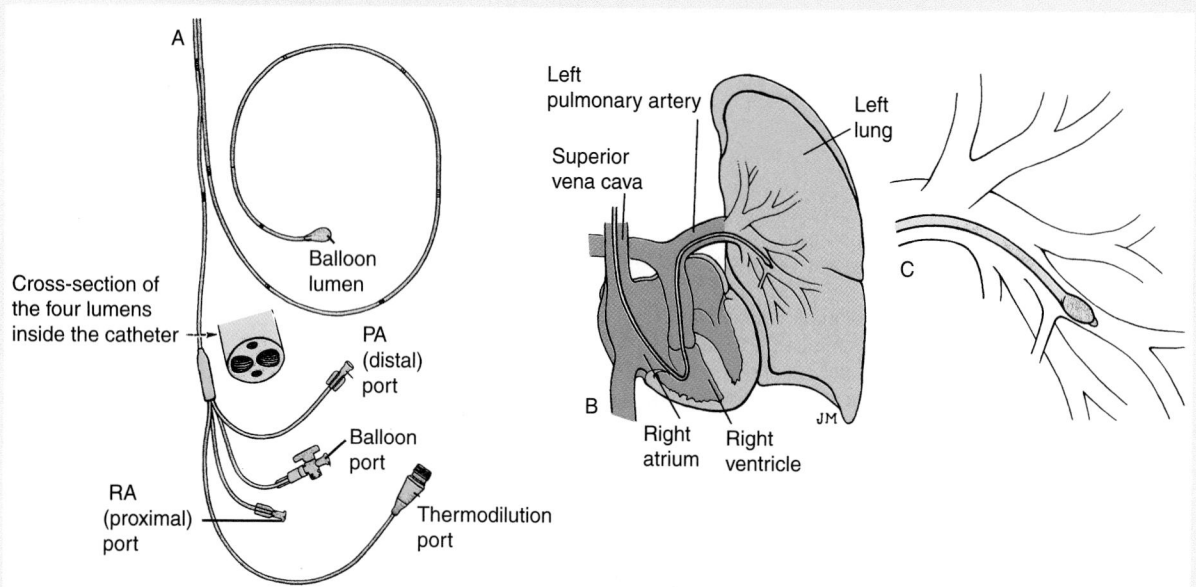

(A) Swan-Ganz catheter. (B) Location of the Swan-Ganz catheter within the heart. The catheter enters the right atrium via the superior vena cava. The balloon is then inflated, allowing the catheter to follow the blood flow through the tricuspid valve, through the right ventricle, through the pulmonic valve, and into the main pulmonary artery. Waveform and pressure readings are noted during insertion to identify location of the catheter within the heart. The balloon is deflated once the catheter is in the pulmonary artery and properly secured. (C) Pulmonary capillary wedge pressure (PCWP). The catheter floats into a distal branch of the pulmonary artery when the balloon is inflated and becomes "wedged." The wedged catheter occludes blood flow from behind, and the tip of the lumen records pressures in front of the catheter. The balloon is then deflated, allowing the catheter to float back into the main pulmonary artery.

PROCEDURE GUIDELINES 12-2   *CONTINUED*

Nursing Action	Rationale
4. Set up equipment according to manufacturer's directives: a. The pulmonary artery catheter requires a transducer and recording, amplifying, and flush systems. b. Flush system according to manufacturer's directions.	4. a. Monitoring systems may vary greatly. The complexity of equipment requires an understanding of the equipment in use. A constant microdrip of heparin flush solution is maintained to ensure catheter patency. b. Flushing of the catheter system ensures patency and eliminates air bubbles.
5. Adjust transducer to level of patient's right atrium (phlebostatic axis fourth intercostal space, midaxillary line).	5. Differences between the level of the right atrium and the transducer will result in incorrect pressure readings; the phlebostatic axis is at the level of the right atrium.
6. Calibrate pressure equipment (especially important when reusable transducers are employed).	6. A known quantity of pressure is applied to the transducer (usually by mercury manometer) to ensure accurate monitoring of pressure readings.
7. Clip excess hair. Prepare skin over insertion site.	7. The catheter is inserted percutaneously under sterile conditions.

PERFORMANCE PHASE (BY PHYSICIAN)

1. Physician dons sterile gown and gloves, and places sterile drapes over patient.	1. Sterile field is established to prevent chance of infection.
2. The balloon is inflated with air under sterile water or saline to test for leakage (bubbles). The catheter may be flushed with saline at this time.	2. To ensure that the balloon is intact and to remove air from catheter.
3. The Swan-Ganz catheter is inserted through the internal jugular, subclavian, or any easily accessible vein by either percutaneous puncture or venotomy.	3. The internal jugular vein establishes a short route into the central venous system.
4. The catheter is advanced to the superior vena cava. Oscillations of the pressure waveforms will indicate when the tip of the catheter is within the thoracic cavity. The patient may be asked to cough.	4. Catheter placement may be determined by characteristic waveforms and changes. Coughing will produce deflections in the pressure tracing when the catheter tip is in the thorax.
5. The catheter is then advanced gently into the right atrium and the balloon is inflated with air.	5. The amount of air to be used is indicated on the catheter.
6. The inflated balloon at the tip of the catheter will be guided by the flowing stream of blood through the right atrium and tricuspid valve into the right ventricle. From this position, it finds its way into the main pulmonary artery. The catheter tip pressures are recorded continuously by specific pressure waveforms as the catheter advances through the various chambers of the heart.	6. Watch ECG monitor for signs of ventricular irritability as catheter enters the right ventricle. Report any signs of dysrhythmia to the physician.
7. The flowing blood will continue to direct the catheter more distally into the pulmonary tree. When the catheter reaches a pulmonary vessel that is approximately the same size or slightly smaller in diameter than the inflated balloon, it cannot be advanced any further. This is the wedge position, called pulmonary capillary wedge pressure (PCWP) or pulmonary artery wedge pressure (PAWP).	7. With the catheter in the wedge position, the balloon blocks the flow of blood from the right side of the heart toward the lungs. The sensor at the tip of the balloon detects pressures distally, which results in the sensing of retrograde left atrial pressures. The PCWP is thus equal to left atrial pressures. a. Normal PCWP is 8 to 12 mm Hg. Optimal LV function appears to be at a wedge between 14 and 18 mm Hg. b. Wedge pressure is a valuable parameter of cardiac function. Filling pressures less than 8 to 10 mm Hg may indicate hypovolemia and in an acutely injured heart are often associated with reduction in cardiac output, hypotension, and tachycardia. Filling pressures greater than 20 mm Hg are associated with left ventricular failure, pulmonary congestion, and hypervolemia.

continued

PROCEDURE GUIDELINES 12-2   **MEASURING PULMONARY ARTERY PRESSURE (PAP) BY FLOW-DIRECTED BALLOON-TIPPED CATHETER (SWAN-GANZ CATHETER)** *CONTINUED*

Nursing Action	Rationale
8. The balloon is deflated, causing the catheter to retract spontaneously into a larger pulmonary artery. This gives a continuous pulmonary artery systolic, diastolic, and mean pressure.	8. The normal systolic pulmonary pressure ranges are 20 to 30 mm Hg, and the diastolic pulmonary pressure ranges are 8 to 12 mm Hg. The normal mean pulmonary artery pressure (average pressure in pulmonary artery throughout the entire cardiac cycle) is 15 to 20 mm Hg.
9. The catheter is then attached to a continuous heparin flush and transducer.	9. A low-flow continuous irrigation ensures that the catheter remains patent. The transducer converts the pressure wave into an electronic wave that is displayed on the oscilloscope.
10. The catheter is sutured in place and covered with a sterile dressing.	
11. A chest x-ray is obtained after Swan-Ganz insertion if fluoroscopy was not used to guide insertion.	11. To confirm catheter position and to provide a baseline for future reference.

TO OBTAIN WEDGE PRESSURE READING

Nursing Action	Rationale
1. Note amount of air to be injected into balloon, usually 1 mL. Do not introduce more air into balloon than specified.	
2. Inflate the balloon slowly until the contour of the pulmonary arterial pressure changes to that of pulmonary wedge pressure. As soon as a wedge pattern is observed, no more air is introduced.	2. The transducer converts the pressure wave into an electronic wave that is displayed on a screen.
a. Note the digital pressure recordings on the monitor (an average of pressure waves is displayed, but these waves are not taken at end expiration).	a. PCWP should be determined at end expiration because respiratory variation of the waveform occurs due to changes in intrathoracic pressures.
b. Obtain a strip of the pressure tracing.	b. A calibrated oscilloscope or graph paper is needed to read pressures at end expiration.
c. Determine PCWP from strip at end expiration.	
3. Deflate the balloon as soon as the pressure reading is obtained. Do not draw back with force on the syringe because too forceful a deflation may damage the balloon.	3. Segmental lung infarction may occur if the catheter balloon is left inflated for long periods. PCWP is only measured intermittently. Do not allow catheter to remain in wedge position when patient is unattended or when not directly making the measurement.
4. Record PCWP reading and amount of air needed to obtain wedge reading. Document recorded waveform by placing a strip of the waveform in patient's chart showing wedge tracing reverting to pulmonary artery waveform.	4. Overinflation of the balloon may cause a "superwedge" waveform, and data obtained will be inaccurate. Overinflation of balloon may cause balloon to lose elastic properties and rupture. The strip provides documentation that catheter was not left in wedge position.

TO OBTAIN Svo₂ READING

Nursing Action	Rationale
1. Before insertion, perform a preinsertion calibration of the catheter.	1. This calibrates the catheter to light intensity in the environment.
2. After insertion, perform a calibration for light intensity and an in vivo calibration every 8 hours.	2. The in vivo calibration ensures that there is minimal difference, or "drift" between the actual Svo_2 value and the value displayed on the monitor. The light calibration adjusts for changes in light in the environment.

 NURSING ALERT

Also perform in vivo calibration if the optical module is disconnected at the catheter junction, if calibration data are lost, or if the Svo_2 is ±4% of the Svo_2 value calculated from mixed venous values obtained from the pulmonary artery catheter.

Nursing Action	Rationale

3. Monitor SvO_2 at frequent intervals. Values of 60% to 80% are normal.	3.
	  a. Causes of an SvO_2 < 60% include:
	    (i) Decrease in cardiac output
	    (ii) Decrease in SaO_2
	    (iii) Decrease in hemoglobin
	    (iv) Increase in O_2 consumption
	  b. Causes of an SvO_2 > 80% include:
	    (i) Increase in SaO_2
	    (ii) Decrease in O_2 consumption

4. If the SvO_2 changes ±10% from the prior value, confirm that the change reflects a change in patient condition.	4. The value displayed may not be accurate if fibrin or a clot is obstructing the catheter tip (low-intensity signal), if the catheter is touching the vessel wall or in a wedged position (high-intensity signal), or if the catheter is no longer calibrated accurately.
5. If the catheter is not functioning properly, initiate steps to resolve the problem.	5. These steps may include aspiration to determine if a clot is obstructing the catheter or notifying the physician of the need to reposition the catheter.
6. If no catheter malfunction is identified, report changes to the physician, initiate therapy based on standard of care.	6. Prompt intervention can restore normal tissue oxygen delivery before untoward effects occur.

FOLLOW-UP PHASE

Nursing Action	Rationale
1. Inspect the insertion site daily. Look for signs of infection, swelling, and bleeding.	1. A foreign body (catheter) in the vascular system increases the risk of sepsis.
2. Record date and time of dressing change and IV tubing change.	
3. Assess contour of waveform frequently and compare with previously documented waveforms.	3. Catheter may move forward and become lodged in wedge position or drift back into right ventricle. Turn patient to left side and ask him to cough (may dislodge catheter from wedge position). If not dislodged, notify physician.
4. Assess for complications: pulmonary embolism, dysrhythmias, heart block, damage to tricuspid valve, intracardiac knotting of catheter, thrombophlebitis, infection, balloon rupture, rupture of pulmonary artery.	4. Blood coming back into syringe indicates balloon rupture. Notify physician immediately.
5. When indicated, the catheter is removed without excessive force of traction; pressure dressing is applied over the site. The site should be checked periodically for bleeding.	

PROCEDURE GUIDELINES 12-3 — MEASUREMENT OF CARDIAC OUTPUT BY THERMODILUTION METHOD

EQUIPMENT

Flow-directed thermodilution catheter in place
CO set, which includes IV tubing
10-mL syringe and three-way stopcock
Normal saline or D5W solution bag
Cardiac monitor with CO computation capability or stand-alone CO computer
Temperature sensor cable

PROCEDURE

Nursing Action	Rationale
1. Explain procedure to patient.	1. Allays anxiety.
2. Connect IV solution bag and CO set maintaining aseptic technique.	2. Solution will be injected directly into the heart and must be sterile.
3. If you do not have a prepackaged CO set, attach IV solution bag to IV tubing, connect a three-way stopcock to the end of the tubing; connect a 10-mL syringe to the middle part of the three-way stopcock.	
4. Attach the three-way stopcock to the proximal injectate port of the thermodilution catheter. This port should be reserved solely for determination of CO. No medications.	4. The proximal injectate port should have its distal end in the right atrium. If medications are infusing in this port, they will be flushed through in bolus form when CO measurements are taken.
5. Another three-way stopcock may be used to allow for IV solution to run at a keep-open rate.	5. Once the CO set is connected, the system should remain closed.
6. Connect temperature sensor cable to the thermistor port of the thermodilution catheter.	6. When solution is injected through catheter, it mixes with the blood in the right side of the heart and flows to the pulmonary artery where blood temperature is detected by the thermistor.
7. Set cardiac monitor to CO computation format. If using a stand-alone CO computer, enter the temperature of the injectable solution and the code number for the size of thermodilution catheter in use (code will be located on the thermodilution catheter packaging).	7. The injectate solution should be 15° to 20° cooler than the patient's body temperature. Room temperature injectate is usually adequate.
8. Fill 10-mL syringe with injectate solution by turning stopcock off to patient and open to syringe and solution.	
9. Turn off IV keep-open solution if present.	9. Need closed system from syringe to catheter.
10. Turn stopcock off to inject solution and open to patient and syringe.	
11. Press "inject" button on the CO computer or monitor and inject 10 mL rapidly (within 4 seconds) and smoothly into the proximal port.	11. Delay will interfere with results.
12. Wait for computation to be complete. Repeat the procedure two or three times to obtain an average.	12. Some monitors display a waveform for the injectate dispersal to evaluate the adequacy of dispersal and temperature sensing.
13. Turn stopcock off to the syringe and injectate and allow keep-open IV fluid to infuse through the proximal port.	

PROCEDURE GUIDELINES 12-3   *CONTINUED*

Nursing Action	Rationale

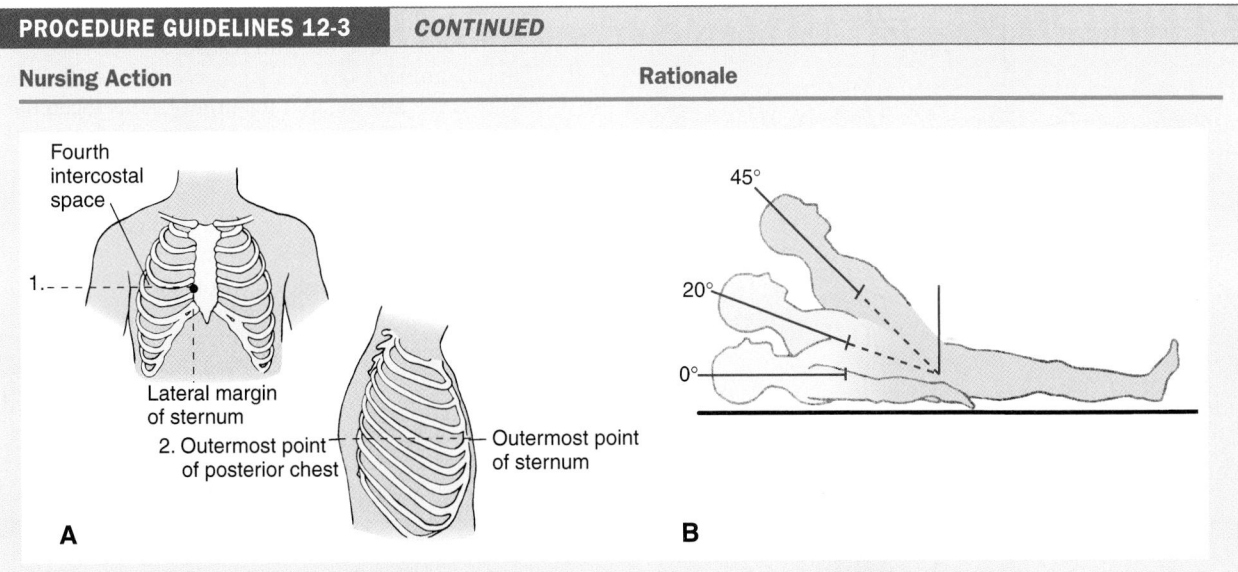

The phlebostatic axis and the phlebostatic level. (A) The phlebostatic axis is the crossing of two reference lines: (1) a line from the fourth intercostal space at the point where it joins the sternum, drawn out to the side of the body beneath the axilla; (2) a line midpoint between the anterior and posterior surfaces of the chest. (B) The phlebostatic level is a horizontal line through the phlebostatic axis. The transducer or the zero mark on the manometer must be level with this axis for accurate measurements. As the patient moves from the flat to erect positions, the chest moves and therefore the reference level; the phlebostatic level stays horizontal through the same reference point. (After Shinn, J., et al: Heart and Lung, 8[2], 324.)

Cardiac Pacing

A cardiac pacemaker is an electronic device that delivers direct stimulation to the heart. The purpose of the pacemaker is to initiate and maintain the heart rate when the heart's natural pacemaker is unable to do so. Pacing may be accomplished through a permanent implantable system; a temporary system with an external pulse generator and percutaneously threaded leads; or a transcutaneous external system with electrode pads placed over the chest. See Procedure Guidelines 12-4.

Pacemaker Design
Pulse Generator

Contains the circuitry and batteries to generate the electrical signal
1. Pulse generators may be temporary (external) or permanently implanted (internal).
   a. Pulse generators are outside the body in temporary pacing systems and subcutaneously implanted in permanent systems.
   b. Temporary pacing systems are for short-term therapy; permanent pacing systems provide for long-term therapy.

c. Temporary external (transcutaneous) pacemakers are used frequently during emergency situations requiring immediate cardiac pacing.
2. The pulse generator in a permanent pacing system is encapsulated in a metal can, which protects the generator from electromagnetic interferences.
3. A temporary pacing system generator is contained in a small box with dials for programming (Figure 12-4). The external box is attached to the patient with Velcro straps.
   a. Transcutaneous external pacing systems house the generator in a piece of equipment similar to an ECG portable monitor. Dials for programming the unit and ECG monitoring are contained in the device.
   b. Electromechanical interference is more likely to occur with temporary systems.
   c. Temporary pacing systems use batteries, which need replacement based on use of device. The transcutaneous system has rechargeable battery circuitry.
4. Permanent pacing systems use reliable power sources such as lithium or nuclear batteries. Lithium batteries have a projected life span of 8 to 12 years, whereas nuclear power sources, although used infrequently, offer a 20-year projected life span.

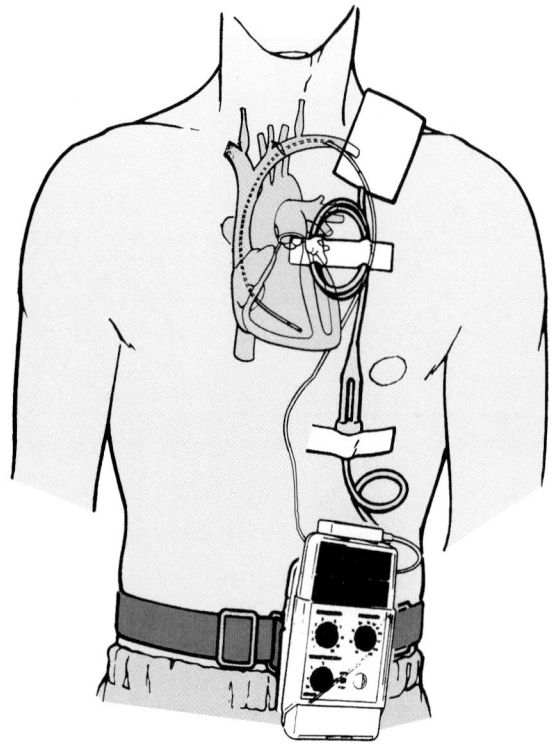

FIGURE 12-4 Temporary transvenous pacer wire with external pulse generator. (Courtesy of MEDTRONIC, Inc.)

Pacemaker Lead

Transmits the electrical signal from the pulse generator to the heart

1. One or two leads may be placed in the heart.
   a. A "single-chamber" pacemaker has one lead in either the atrial or ventricular chamber. The sensing and pacing capabilities of the pacemaker are confined to the chamber where the lead is placed.
   b. "Dual-chamber" pacemakers have two leads. One lead is in the atrium, and the other lead is located in the ventricle. Pacing and sensing can occur in both heart chambers, closely "mimicking" normal heart function (physiologic pacing).
   c. Pacemaker leads may be threaded through a vein into the right atrium and/or right ventricle (endocardial/transvenous approach) or introduced by direct penetration of the chest wall and attached to the left ventricle or right atrium (Figure 12-5).
   d. Fixation devices located at the end of the pacemaker lead allow for secure attachment of the lead to the heart, reducing the possibility of lead dislodgement.
   e. Temporary lead(s) protrude from the incision and are connected to the external pulse generator. Permanent lead(s) are connected to the pulse generator implanted underneath the skin (epicardial/transthoracic approach).
2. One (unipolar) or two (bipolar) electrodes are contained on the tip of the pacemaker lead in contact with the heart.
   a. A unipolar system better senses intrinsic cardiac signals, but the bipolar system is less affected by electromechanical interference.
   b. Unipolar leads produce a large spike on the ECG; bipolar leads produce a small, almost invisible spike.
3. Transcutaneous external pacing system noninvasively delivers electrical stimuli to the heart.
   a. The transcutaneous lead system consists of large pads containing electrodes.
   b. The pads or "leads" are applied to the anterior chest (V_2, V_3, or V_5 position) and a second pad on the back

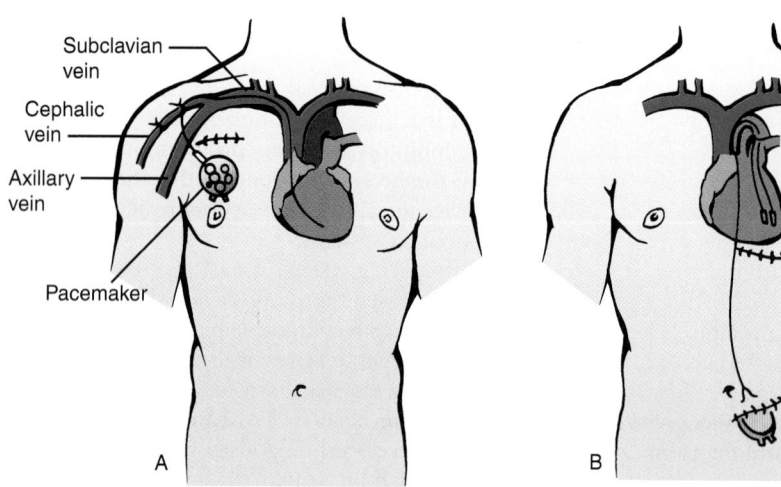

FIGURE 12-5 (**A**) The catheter is unipolar and is threaded to the apical area of the right ventricle via a major vein. (**B**) The catheter is bipolar and is passed through an opening in the chest wall and is sutured to the external surface of the left ventricle.

(between the spine and left scapula at heart level). Leads must be placed so the current travels through most of the myocardium.

c. The lead system then is connected to the external console.

Pacemaker Function

Cardiac pacing refers to the ability of the pacemaker to stimulate either the atrium, the ventricle, or both heart chambers in sequence and initiate electrical depolarization and cardiac contraction. Cardiac pacing is evidenced on the ECG by the presence of a "spike" or "pacing artifact."

Pacing Functions

1. *Atrial pacing*—direct stimulation of the right atrium producing a "spike" on the ECG preceding a P wave.
2. *Ventricular pacing*—direct stimulation of the right or left ventricle producing a "spike" on the ECG preceding a QRS complex.
3. *Atrioventricular pacing*—direct stimulation of the right atrium and either ventricle in sequence; mimics normal cardiac conduction, allowing the atria to contract before the ventricles. ("Atrial kick" received by the ventricles allows for an increase in cardiac output.)

Sensing Functions

Cardiac pacemakers have the ability to "see" intrinsic cardiac activity when it occurs (sensing).

1. *Demand*—ability to "sense" intrinsic cardiac activity and deliver a pacing stimulus only if the heart rate falls below a preset rate limit.
2. *Fixed*—no ability to "sense" intrinsic cardiac activity; the pacemaker is unable to "synchronize" with the heart's natural activity and consistently delivers a pacing stimulus at a preset rate.
3. *Triggered*—ability to deliver pacing stimuli in response to "sensing" a cardiac event.
   a. "Sees" atrial activity (P waves) and delivers a pacing spike to the ventricle after an appropriate delay (usually 0.16 second, similar to P–R interval).
   b. Maintains atrioventricular synchrony and increases heart rate based on increases in the body demands that occur with exercise or during stress.
   c. "Physiologic" sensors are being developed as alternatives to "trigger" a ventricular response, because many patients have atrial dysfunction.
   d. "Sensor-driven" rate-responsive pacemakers do not sense atrial activity; a triggered ventricular beat occurs when the pacemaker senses either increases in muscle activity, temperature, oxygen utilization, or changes in blood pH.

Capture Function

1. The pacemaker's ability to generate a response from the heart (contraction) after electrical stimulation is referred to as *capture*.
   a. "Electrical" capture is indicated by a P wave or QRS following and corresponding to a pacemaker spike.
   b. "Mechanical" capture of the ventricles is determined by a palpable pulse corresponding to the electrical event.

Pacemaker Codes

The Intersociety Commission for Heart Disease (ICHD) has established a five-letter code (1984) to describe the normal functioning of today's sophisticated pacemakers.

1. Letters 1, 2, 3
   a. The first letter of the code refers to the chamber paced.
   b. The second letter refers to the chamber sensed.
   c. The third letter refers to the response to sensing.
2. Letters 4 and 5
   a. The fourth and fifth letters refer to special functions of today's pacemakers.
   b. The fourth letter refers to the programmability of the pacemaker.
   c. The fifth letter refers to the various modes of operation for antitachycardic pacemakers. These pacemakers are used to control tachydysrhythmias in patients who have failed conventional drug therapy.

Clinical Indications

1. Symptomatic bradydysrhythmias
2. Symptomatic heart block
   a. Mobitz II second-degree heart block
   b. Complete heart block
   c. Bifascicular and trifascicular bundle branch blocks
3. Prophylaxis
   a. After acute MI: dysrhythmia and conduction defects
   b. Before or after cardiac surgery
   c. During diagnostic testing:
      (i) Cardiac catheterization
      (ii) Electrophysiology studies
      (iii) Percutaneous transluminal coronary angioplasty (PTCA)
      (iv) Stress testing
      (v) Before permanent pacing
4. Tachydysrhythmias; to break rapid rhythm disturbances
   a. Supraventricular
   b. Ventricular

Nursing Assessment

Assess patient's knowledge level of procedure: nothing by mouth (NPO) before procedure; IV line insertion; performed in operating or special procedures room with fluoroscope and continuous ECG monitoring; local anesthetic to minimize discomfort; sedation.

Nursing Diagnoses

- Decreased Cardiac Output related to potential pacemaker malfunction and dysrhythmias
- Risk for Injury related to pneumothorax, hemothorax, bleeding, microshock, and accidental malfunction
- Risk for Infection related to surgical implantation of pacemaker generator and/or leads

- Anxiety related to pacemaker insertion, fear of death, lack of knowledge, and role change
- Impaired Physical Mobility related to imposed restrictions of arm movement and bed rest
- Pain related to surgical incision and transcutaneous external pacing stimuli
- Disturbance in Body Image, related to pacemaker implantation

Nursing Interventions

Maintaining Adequate Cardiac Output

1. Record the following information after insertion of the pacemaker:
   a. Pacemaker manufacturer, model, and lead type
   b. Operating mode (based on ICHD code)
   c. Programmed settings: lower rate limit; upper rate limit; AV delay; pacing thresholds
   d. Patient's underlying rhythm
   e. Patient's response to procedure
2. Attach ECG electrodes for continuous monitoring of heart rate and rhythm.
   a. Set alarm limits 5 beats below lower rate limit and 5 to 10 beats above upper rate limits (ensures immediate detection of pacemaker malfunction or failure).
   b. Keep alarms on at all times.
   c. Analyze ECG strip every 4 hours.
      (i) Identify presence/absence of pacing artifact.
      (ii) Differentiate paced P waves and paced QRS complexes from spontaneous beats.
      (iii) Measure AV delay (if pacemaker has dual chamber functions).
      (iv) Determine the paced rate.
      (v) Analyze the paced rhythm for presence and consistency of capture (every pacing spike is followed by atrial and/or ventricular depolarization).
      (vi) Analyze the rhythm for presence and consistency of proper sensing. (After a spontaneous beat, the pacemaker should not fire unless the interval between the spontaneous beat and the paced beat equals the lower pacing rate and/or the paced beat follows the programmed AV delay).
3. Monitor vital signs every 15 minutes until stable; then as directed.
4. Monitor urine output and level of consciousness—ensures adequate cardiac output achieved with paced rhythm.
5. Observe for the presence of dysrhythmias (ventricular ectopic activity can occur because of irritation of ventricular wall by lead wire).
   a. Monitor for competitive rhythms such as runs of atrial fibrillation or flutter, accelerated junctional or idioventricular or ventricular tachycardia.

b. Report all dysrhythmias.
   c. Administer antidysrhythmic therapy as directed.
6. Obtain 12-lead ECG daily as directed.

NURSING ALERT

Transport patient to other parts of hospital with portable ECG monitoring and nurse. Patients with temporary pacemakers should never be placed in unmonitored areas.

Avoiding Injury

1. Note that a postinsertion chest x-ray has been taken to ensure correct lead wire position and that no fluid is in lungs.
2. Monitor for signs/symptoms of hemothorax or pneumothorax:
   a. *Hemothorax*—inadvertent puncture of the subclavian vein or artery; can cause fatal hemorrhage; observe for diaphoresis, hypotension, and restlessness; immediate surgical intervention may be necessary.
   b. *Pneumothorax*—inadvertent puncture of the lung; observe for acute onset of dyspnea, cyanosis, chest pain, absent breath sounds over involved lung, acute anxiety, hypotension. Prepare for chest tube insertion.
3. Evaluate continually for evidence of bleeding.
   a. Check incision site frequently for bleeding.
      (i) Apply manual pressure and pressure dressing to control bleeding.
      (ii) Palpate for pulses distal to insertion site. (Swelling of tissues from bleeding may impede arterial flow.)
4. Monitor for evidence of lead migration and perforation of heart.
   a. Observe for muscle twitching and/or hiccups (may indicate chest wall or diaphragmatic pacing).
   b. Evaluate patient's complaints of chest pain (may indicate perforation of pericardial sac).
   c. Auscultate for pericardial friction rub.
   d. Observe for signs/symptoms of cardiac tamponade: distant heart sounds, distended neck veins, pulsus paradoxus.
5. Provide an electrically safe environment for patient. Stray electrical current can enter the heart through temporary pacemaker lead system and induce dysrhythmias.
   a. Protect exposed parts of electrode lead terminal in temporary pacing systems with a rubber glove. (Newer external generators have the lead terminals enclosed in a case; a rubber glove is not necessary.)
   b. Wear rubber gloves whenever touching temporary pacing leads. (Static electricity from your hands can enter the patient's body through the lead system.)

c. Make sure all equipment is grounded with three-prong plugs inserted into a proper outlet; biomedical engineer should routinely check room to ensure safe environment.

d. Temporary epicardial pacing wires (most common after cardiac surgery) should have the terminal needles protected by a plastic tube; place tube in rubber glove to protect it from fluids or electrical current.

6. Be aware of hazards in the hospital environment that can interfere with pacemaker function or cause pacemaker failure and/or permanent pacemaker damage.

a. Avoid use of electric razors.

b. Avoid direct placement of defibrillator paddles over pacemaker generator; anterior placement of paddles should be 4 to 5 inches away from pacemaker; always evaluate pacemaker function after defibrillation.

c. Electrocautery devices and transcutaneous nerve stimulators (TENS units) pose a risk.

d. Patients with permanent pacemakers should never be exposed to magnetic resonance imaging (MRI) because the strength of the magnetic field may alter or erase pacemaker program memory.

e. Caution must be used if patient is to receive radiation therapy; the pacemaker should be repositioned if unit lies directly in the radiation field.

7. Prevent possible accidental pacemaker malfunctions.

a. Use clear plastic covering over external temporary generators at all times (eliminates potential manipulation of programmed settings).

b. Secure temporary pacemaker generator to patient's chest or waist; never hang on IV pole.

c. Transfer of patient from bed to stretcher should only be attempted with an adequate number of personnel, so that patient can remain passive; caution personnel to avoid underarm lifts.

d. Place a sign over patient's bed alerting personnel to presence of temporary pacemaker.

e. Evaluate transcutaneous pacing electrodes every 2 hours for secure contact to chest wall; change electrode pads as directed or if patient is diaphoretic.
   Note: Transcutaneous pacing should not be employed continuously for longer than 2 hours.

8. Monitor for electrolyte imbalances, hypoxia, and myocardial ischemia. (The amount of energy the pacemaker needs to stimulate depolarization may need adjustment if any of these are present.)

Preventing Infection

1. Take temperature every 4 hours; report elevations. (Suspect pacemaker system for infection source if elevation occurs.)

2. Observe incision site for signs/symptoms of local infection: redness, purulent drainage, warmth, soreness.

3. Be alert to manifestations of bacteremia. (Patients with endocardial leads are susceptible to endocarditis; see p. 372.)

4. Clean incision site as directed, using sterile technique.

5. Monitor vein through which the pacing lead wire was placed for evidence of phlebitis.

6. Evaluate patient's complaints of increasing tenderness and discomfort at incision site.

7. Administer antibiotic therapy as prescribed.

Relieving Anxiety

1. Offer careful explanations regarding anticipated procedures and treatments, and answer the patient's questions with concise explanations.

2. Encourage the patient to use coping mechanisms to overcome anxieties—talking, crying, walking.

3. Encourage the patient to accept responsibility for care.

a. Review plan of care with the patient.

b. Encourage the patient to make decisions regarding a daily schedule of self-care activities.

c. Engage the patient in goal setting. Establish with the patient priorities of care and time frames to accomplish goals up until discharge.

4. Monitor for unwarranted fears expressed by the patient (commonly, pacemaker failure), and provide explanations to alleviate fear. Explain to the patient life expectancy of batteries and the measures taken to check for failure (see section titled Patient Education, below).

Minimizing the Effects of Immobility

1. Explain the purpose for bed rest (24 to 48 hours) and immobilization of extremity nearest to permanent or temporary pacemaker lead implant (allows for stabilization of lead in heart and prevents lead dislodgement).

2. Encourage patient to take deep breaths frequently each hour—promotes pulmonary function; caution against vigorous coughing (lead dislodgement may occur).

3. Instruct patient in dorsiflexion exercises of ankles and tightening of calf muscles. This promotes venous return and prevents venous stasis. Exercises should be done hourly.

4. Restrict movement of affected extremity.

a. Place arm nearest to permanent pacemaker implant in sling as directed; extremity with temporary pacing wire should be immobilized and kept straight as prescribed.

b. Instruct patient to gradually resume range of motion of extremity as directed (usually 24 hours for permanent implants); avoid over-the-head motions for approximately 5 days.

c. Evaluate patient's arm movements to ensure normal range-of-motion progression; assist patient with passive range of motion of extremity as necessary

(prevents development of shoulder stiffness caused by prolonged joint immobility); consult physical therapy as directed if stiffness and pain occur.
5. Assist patients with activities of daily living (ADLs) as appropriate.

Relieving Pain

1. Prepare patient for discomfort that may be experienced after pacemaker implant or initiation of transcutaneous pacing.
   a. Explain to patient that incisional pain will occur after procedure; pain will subside after the first week, but some soreness will be experienced for up to 3 to 4 weeks.
   b. Explain to patient the potential for discomfort during transcutaneous pacing; ensure patient that the lowest energy possible will be used and analgesics will be given.
2. Administer analgesics as directed; attempt to coincide peak analgesic effect with performance of range-of-motion exercises and ADLs.
3. Offer back rubs to promote relaxation.
4. Provide patient with diversional activities.
5. Evaluate effectiveness of pain-relieving modalities.

Maintaining a Positive Body Image

1. Encourage the patient to express concerns regarding self-image and pacer implant.
2. Reassure the patient that sexual activity and modes of dressing will not be altered by pacemaker implantation.
3. Offer the patient the opportunity to talk to others who have had a pacemaker implantation.
4. Encourage spouse of patient or significant other to discuss concerns of self-image with the patient.

Patient Education and Health Maintenance
Anatomy and Physiology of the Heart

Use diagrams to identify heart structure, conduction system, area where pacemaker is inserted, and why the pacemaker is needed.

Pacemaker Function

1. Give the patient the manufacturer's instructions (for particular pacemaker), and help familiarize patient with pacemaker.
2. If available, give the patient a pacemaker to hold, and identify unique features of patient's pacemaker; or show patient picture of pacemaker.
3. Explain to patient the purpose and function of the component parts of the pacemaker: generator and lead system.

Activity

1. Reassure patient that normal activities will be able to be resumed.
2. Explain to patient that it takes about 2 months to develop full range of motion of arm (fibrosis occurs around the lead and stabilizes it in heart).

3. Specific instructions include:
   a. Instruct patient not to lift items over 3 lb or perform difficult arm maneuvers.
   b. Caution patient against excessive stretching or bending exercises.
   c. Avoid contact sports, tennis, golfing, bowling, and yardwork until resumption of these activities is permitted by physician.
   d. Caution patient not to fire rifle with it resting over pacemaker implant.
   e. Sexual activity may be resumed when desired.
4. Instruct patient to gauge activities according to sensations of moderate pain in arm or site of implant and stretching sensation in and around implant site.

Pacemaker Failure

1. Teach the patient to check own pulse rate at least every week for 1 full minute at rest to be certain that preset rate remains constant. (Patients may check pulse daily to ensure all is well and promote a sense of control.)
2. Teach the patient to:
   a. Report immediately any slowing of pulse greater than 4 to 5 beats per minute, or any increase in pulse rate.
   b. Report signs and symptom of dizziness, fainting, palpitation, prolonged hiccups, and chest pain to health care provider immediately. These signs are indicative of pacemaker failure.
   c. Take pulse while these feelings are being experienced.
3. Encourage the patient to wear identification bracelet and carry pacemaker identification card that lists pacemaker type, rate, health care provider's name, and the hospital where the pacemaker was inserted; encourage significant other to keep a card with patient's pacemaker information so someone else will have it.

Electromagnetic Interference

Advise the patient that improvements in pacemaker design have reduced problems of electromagnetic interference (EMI).

1. High-energy radar, television and radio transmitters, industrial arc welders, electrocautery equipment, TENS, large motors (cars, boats), oversized magnets (MRI equipment found at hospitals, junkyards where magnets lift cars), ultrasonic dental cleaning equipment, electric razors.
   a. Avoid direct contact and close proximity with these devices because they may affect the functioning of the pacemaker. (In many cases, no damage to the generator will occur; devices may confuse the pacemaker and readjust the settings.)
   b. Teach the patient, if dizziness or sensations of a fast heart rate occur, to move 4 to 6 feet away from source and check pulse. Pulse should return to normal.

2. Antitheft devices and airport security alarms will not affect pacemaker function, although the metal may trigger the alarm. Instruct patient to show ID card.

3. Household and kitchen appliances will not affect pacemaker function. Microwave ovens are no longer a threat to pacemaker operation (old warning signs may still be near microwave ovens).

Care of Pacemaker Site

1. Advise patient to wear loose-fitting clothing around the area of pacemaker implantation until healing has taken place.

2. Watch for signs and symptoms of infection around generator and leads—fever, heat, pain, skin breakdown at implant site.

3. Advise patient to keep incision clean and dry. Encourage tub baths for the first 10 days after pacemaker implant rather than showers.
   a. Instruct patient not to scrub incision site or clean site with bath water.
   b. Teach patient to clean incision site with antiseptic as directed.

4. Explain to patient that healing will take approximately 3 months.
   a. Instruct patient to maintain a well-balanced diet to promote healing.

GERONTOLOGIC ALERT

Elderly patients may experience delayed wound healing because of poor nutritional status. Evaluate nutritional intake carefully, and offer a balanced diet to ensure proper healing.

---

5. Instruct patient to inform dentist of pacemaker so antibiotic prophylaxis can be administered before extractions or vigorous dental cleaning (prevents development of endocarditis).

Follow-Up

1. See that the patient has a copy of ECG tracing (according to agency policy) for future comparisons. Encourage patient to have regular pacemaker checkup for monitoring function and integrity of pacemaker.

2. Transtelephonic evaluation of implanted cardiac pacemakers for battery and electrode failure is available.

3. Review medications with the patient before discharge.

4. Inform the patient that the pulse generator will have to be surgically removed for a variety of reasons (eg, battery depletion) and replaced; improved power sources and circuitry make reoperation less frequent.
   a. Relatively simple procedure performed under local anesthesia.

Outcome-Based Evaluation

- Vital signs stable; pacing spikes rated on ECG tracing
- Breath sounds noted throughout; respirations unlabored
- Incision without drainage
- Asking questions and participating in care
- Exercising in bed; arm remains immobilized
- Reports relief of pain
- Verbalizes acceptance of pacemaker

PROCEDURE GUIDELINES 12-4   **TRANSCUTANEOUS CARDIAC PACING**

EQUIPMENT

Disposable electrode pads
External pacing module
Resuscitative equipment

PROCEDURE

Nursing Action	Rationale
PREPARATORY PHASE	
1. Explain procedure to patient.	
2. Explain sensation of discomfort with external pacing	2. Discomfort is felt with each firing, but can be relieved with analgesics.

continued

PROCEDURE

Nursing Action	Rationale
PERFORMANCE PHASE	
1. Place electrodes as follows: a. Anterior/posterior: The negative electrode is placed on the anterior chest at the V_3–V_1 position; the positive electrode is placed on the back to the left of the spine. b. Anterior/anterior: The negative electrode is placed under the right clavicle; the positive electrode is placed at the V_6 position.	1. Electrodes must be placed so the current passes through as much of the myocardium as possible with the least distance between the pads.
2. Ensure that pacing module is off or on standby and that milliamp output is set at the minimal level before connecting electrodes to external module.	2. Prevents accidental shock on connection.
3. Connect pacing electrodes to external module.	
4. Determine rate setting according to instructions and/or patient condition. If patient heart is consistently too low to maintain adequate cardiac output, set rate at 70 to 80. If the patient's rate falls only intermittently and the pacemaker will be used in the demand mode, set rate at 60.	4. Can be set at a fixed rate or on demand, to pace only if heart rate falls below 60 (or other rate).
5. Gradually increase milliamp output until a pacing spike and corresponding QRS complex are seen. Palpate pulse to ensure adequate response to electrical event.	5. If using the demand mode, set the rate higher than the patient's rate to establish the correct output and capture, then return the rate to 60.
6. Check pad placement frequently.	6. Patient perspiration may cause pads to loosen or slip.
FOLLOW-UP PHASE	
1. Check vital signs at least every 15 minutes while continuous pacing is employed.	1. To determine if cardiac output is adequate.
2. Monitor ECG continuously for pacer functioning.	2. To detect malfunction (may occur due to electrode loosening).
3. Assure patient that treatment is temporary.	3. Should only be used continuously for 2 hours.
4. Prepare patient for transvenous or permanent pacemaker insertion as indicated.	

◼ Defibrillation and Cardioversion

Electrical cardioversion (or counter shock) is the passing of an electrical shock of short duration through the heart to terminate tachydysrhythmia (eg, ventricular fibrillation or ventricular tachycardia without pulse). A defibrillator is an instrument that delivers an electric shock to the heart to convert the dysrhythmia to normal sinus rhythm. (Defibrillators are not used to convert other abnormal and rapid cardiac rhythms.) See Procedure Guidelines 12-5.

An automatic external defibrillator (AED) may be used inside the hospital or out in the community to deliver electric shock to the heart before trained personnel can arrive with a manual defibrillator. See Procedure Guidelines 12-6.

Synchronized cardioversion is the term used to describe a timed delivery of electric current to the heart for the purpose of terminating certain dysrhythmias. It is timed not to hit the T wave during the cardiac cycle, because an electric discharge during this phase may cause ventricular fibrillation. See Procedure Guidelines 12-7.

Indications
Defibrillation
1. Ventricular fibrillation
2. Ventricular tachycardia without a pulse
Synchronized Cardioversion
1. Atrial fibrillation
2. Atrial flutter
3. Supraventricular tachycardia
4. Ventricular tachycardia with a pulse

> **NURSING ALERT**
> Synchronized cardioversion is generally contraindicated when a patient has been taking a significant amount of digoxin (Lanoxin), because more lethal dysrhythmias may ensue after electric discharge.

PROCEDURE GUIDELINES 12-5	DIRECT CURRENT DEFIBRILLATION FOR VENTRICULAR FIBRILLATION

EQUIPMENT

DC defibrillator with paddles
Interface material (disposable conductive gel pads, electrode gels and pastes)
Resuscitative equipment

PROCEDURE

Nursing Action	Rationale

PERFORMANCE PHASE

Monitored Patient

1. If ventricular fibrillation recognized within 2 minutes, give precordial thump, assess rhythm and carotid pulse, and expose anterior chest.
2. If within 2 minutes of detection of ventricular fibrillation, defibrillate before initiating cardiopulmonary resuscitation. Beyond 2 minutes, START RESUSCITATION EFFORTS IMMEDIATELY.

1. This procedure should be carried out immediately after ventricular fibrillation is detected to minimize cerebral and circulatory deterioration.
2. Cardiopulmonary resuscitation is essential before and after defibrillation to ensure blood supply to the cerebral and coronary arteries.

Unmonitored Patient

1. Expose anterior chest.
2. START CARDIOPULMONARY RESUSCITATION IMMEDIATELY.
3. Apply interface material to the patient (gel pads) or to the paddles (gel, paste). The electrode paddles should be in firm contact with the patient's skin.

3. The interface material helps provide better conduction and prevents skin burns. Do not allow any paste on the skin between the electrodes. If the paste areas touch, the current may short circuit (severely burning the patient) and may not penetrate the heart. Saline pads are not recommended because the saline can easily drip, forming a path for the current.

4. Remove oxygen from immediate area.
5. A second person should turn on the defibrillator to the prescribed setting. The American Heart Association recommends that initial defibrillation should be 200 to 300 watt-seconds of *delivered* energy. A second attempt at same level should be given if first attempt is unsuccessful. A third attempt with an increase of energy level to 360 watt-seconds should be attempted. Allow only approximately 5 seconds between the successive attempts to assess rhythm and pulse.

4. Prevents danger of fire or explosion.
5. The shock is measured in joules or watt-seconds (the dose is 2 joules/kg in pediatric patients based on estimated body weight). Less time between successive shocks enhances effectiveness.

6. Apply one electrode just to the right of the upper sternum below the clavicle and the other electrode just to the left of the cardiac apex or left nipple (see accompanying figure). About 20 to 25 lb of pressure are applied to paddles to ensure good contact with the patient's skin.

6. The paddles are placed so the electrical discharge flows through as much myocardial mass as possible. If anteroposterior paddles are used, the anterior paddle is held with pressure on the middle sternum while the patient lies on the posterior paddle under the left infrascapular region. In this method, the countershock more directly traverses the heart.

continued

PROCEDURE GUIDELINES 12-5	DIRECT CURRENT DEFIBRILLATION FOR VENTRICULAR FIBRILLATION *CONTINUED*

Nursing Action   **Rationale**

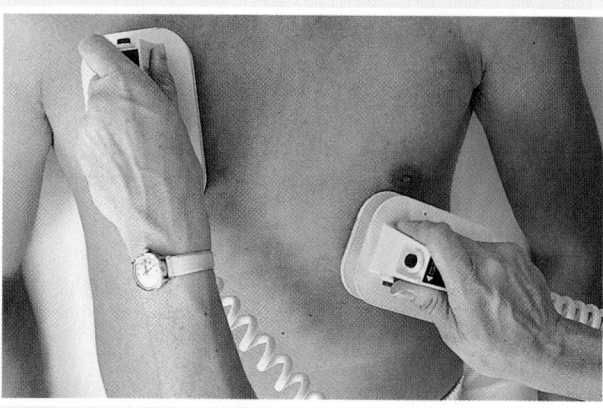

Paddle placement in ventricular defibrillation.

7. Grasp the paddles only by the insulated handles.

8. Charge the paddles. Once paddles are charged, GIVE THE COMMAND FOR PERSONNEL TO STAND CLEAR OF THE PATIENT AND THE BED. Look quickly to make sure all are away from the patient and bed.

8. If a person touches the bed, he or she may act as a ground for the current and receive a shock, especially if there are electrolyte solutions on the floor.

9. Push the discharge buttons in both paddles simultaneously.

10. Remove the paddles from the patient *immediately* after the shock is administered (unless paddles are being used as monitor leads).

11. Resume cardiopulmonary resuscitation efforts until stable rhythm, spontaneous respirations, pulse, and blood pressure return.

11. After the third attempt to countershock, CPR efforts should be resumed; total delay should be no more than 5 seconds to oxygenate the patient and restore circulation.

12. Look at the ECG monitor to determine the specific therapy for the resultant electrical mechanism. Further high-energy countershocks may be necessary.

FOLLOW-UP PHASE

1. After the patient is defibrillated and rhythm is restored, lidocaine is usually given to prevent recurrent episodes.

1. Any resultant dysrhythmia may require appropriate drug intervention.

2. Continue with intensive monitoring/care.

PROCEDURE GUIDELINES 12-6	SYNCHRONIZED CARDIOVERSION

EQUIPMENT

Cardioverter and ECG machine
Conduction jelly or gel pads and cardiac medications
Resuscitative equipment

PROCEDURE

Nursing Action   **Rationale**

1. If the procedure is elective, it is advisable to have the patient NPO 12 hours before the cardioversion.

1. During sedation or the procedure, the patient may vomit and aspirate if the stomach is full.

PROCEDURE GUIDELINES 12-6 **CONTINUED**

Nursing Action	Rationale
a. Reassure the patient and see that informed consent has been obtained. b. Make sure the patient has not been taking digitalis and that the serum potassium is normal. 2. Make sure IV line is secure. 3. Obtain a 12-lead ECG before and after cardioversion with the ECG machine. The ECG machine wires are best left on the patient, because the ECG printout is of much better quality than that of the monitor. This fact is especially important when one is trying to dissect complicated dysrhythmias. 4. a. Allow the patient to receive oxygen before and after cardioversion. b. Remove oxygen from the immediate area during delivery of the shock. 5. Place the paddles in one of the following two positions: a. Anterior-posterior position One paddle—left infrascapular area Other paddle—upper sternum at third interspace b. Anterior position One paddle—just to right of sternum at second interspace Other paddle—just under left nipple 6. Determine if the machine's synchronization mechanism is working before applying the paddles. a. The discharge should hit near the peak of the R wave. b. The R wave usually must be of substantial height; if it is not, adjust the gain (sensitivity) or change the lead. On many machines, the R wave must be upright before there is synchronization. 7. If using paste, apply to all of the paddle surface, but make sure there is no excess around the edges of the paddles. a. The paste should be rubbed into the skin very thoroughly; this allows more electricity to penetrate the body surface. b. Make sure paddles are clean because surface material will interfere with the flow of electricity. c. Apply firm pressure to the paddle. 8. If using gel pads, place pads where paddles are to be positioned. 9. Set dial for lowest level of electrical energy that can be expected to convert the dysrhythmia. Some dysrhythmias (such as atrial flutter) can be converted with very low energies, such as 25 watt-seconds (joules). 10. A short-acting sedative such as midazolam (Versed) should be given if the patient is conscious. 11. After the patient is in a light sleep from the IV medication and when no one is touching the bed or patient, discharge the cardioverter. If cardioversion does not occur, proceed to a higher energy level. 12. Monitor the ECG after conversion occurs. Blood pressures should be recorded about every 15 minutes until the preshock blood pressure is reached.	a. Do not use word "shock" because this will increase the patient's apprehension. b. Low potassium may precipitate postshock dysrhythmias. 2. An IV line may be necessary for administration of emergency medications. 3. An ECG is taken to ensure that the patient has not had a recent myocardial infarction (either just before or after the cardioversion). 4. a. Oxygen will help prevent unwanted dysrhythmias after cardioversion b. An explosion could occur if a spark from the paddles should ignite the oxygen during the procedure. 6. a. If the electrical discharge hits the T wave, ventricular fibrillation may occur. b. Synchronization is not used for ventricular fibrillation. (The machine will not work for defibrillation if the synchronization mode is on.) 7. If there is excess paste around the paddles, the discharge may run onto the skin, causing a burn. If there is not firm contact between the paddle and skin, a burn may occur; also, electricity is lost from the heart. 8. Excessive energies may cause unnecessary discomfort to the patient and create unnecessary electrical hazards. 10. This helps produce amnesia concerning the cardioversion. 12. The patient may revert to previous dysrhythmias after conversion.

PROCEDURE GUIDELINES 12-7 | AUTOMATED EXTERNAL DEFIBRILLATOR

EQUIPMENT

Automated external defibrillator (AED) unit
Electrodes

PROCEDURE

Nursing Action	Rationale
1. Ascertain unconsciousness and pulselessness.	
2. Position patient in the supine position.	
3. Start CPR while AED is being applied.	3. Early restoration of oxygenation and perfusion is imperative in enhancing the resuscitative effort.
4. Place electrodes on the patient's anterior chest, just below the right clavicle and lateral and below the left nipple (apex of the heart). See paddle placement for Defibrillation, p. 339.	4. Appropriate electrode position ensures passage of current through the majority of the myocardium. Anterior placement is preferred because attempting anterior-posterior electrode placement may delay treatment.
5. Turn AED on.	
6. Follow audio and/or visual instructions from the AED.	6. The AED will analyze the rhythm in 5 to 15 seconds and determine the need for defibrillation based on that analysis. It will then let the operator know how to proceed.
7. Suspend CPR or any movement of the patient during the analysis.	7. External movement will impair the AED's accuracy in analyzing the rhythm.
8. If after analyzing the rhythm a shock is advised, the AED will instruct the operator to prepare for a shock. It will charge the unit, give warning to "stand clear," and then deliver the shock.	
9. After the first shock, do not restart CPR. Allow the AED to reanalyze the rhythm. If a second shock is indicated, the AED will proceed as above. Most AEDs will deliver three successive shocks as in the American Heart Association guidelines for defibrillation.	9. Delivering the shocks in rapid succession or "stacking" the shocks decreases resistance and enhances the effectiveness of defibrillation.
10. After the third shock is delivered, if there is no pulse, continue CPR for 1 minute, then begin the analysis procedure again.	10. The patient will have been pulseless for this time. Oxygenation and circulation must be restored or the patient's chances of survival decrease markedly.
11. Continue the sequence of allowing the AED to complete its program, then CPR for 1 to 2 minutes, then allowing the AED to run through its program again until the resuscitation team arrives.	
12. If *no* shock is indicated, continue CPR for 1 minute, then allow the AED to analyze the rhythm. Proceed as above if a shock is now indicated. If no shock is indicated again, continue CPR and recheck pulse and rhythm (with the AED) every 1 to 2 minutes. The patient's rhythm may change to a "shockable" rhythm during the course of the resuscitative effort.	
13. If the patient regains a pulse, continue to support ventilations. Keep AED electrodes attached and the unit on in case the patient again loses consciousness.	

■ Automatic Implantable Defibrillator

The automatic implantable defibrillator is a device that delivers electric shocks directly to the heart muscle (defibrillation) in order to terminate lethal dysrhythmias: ventricular fibrillation and ventricular tachycardia (Figure 12-6). The automatic implantable defibrillator is surgically placed by one of four approaches: lateral thoracotomy, median sternotomy (in conjunction with cardiac surgery), subxiphoid, or subintercostal.

Design

The implantable defibrillator is slightly larger than a pacemaker and consists of two component parts:

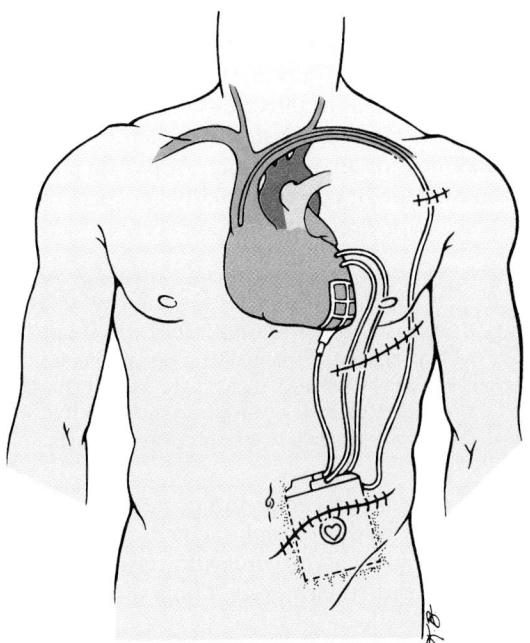

FIGURE 12-6 Automatic implantable defibrillator.

1. *Pulse generator*—contains the circuitry and battery to detect dysrhythmias and generate the electric shock. The generator is placed in a subcutaneous pocket in the upper abdominal quadrant.
   a. Battery life depends on usage. Longevity is estimated at 12 to 24 months or 100 shocks.
   b. The direct current electric shock delivered is 25 to 32 joules.
2. *Lead system*—two sets of leads are used and can be placed in various positions on or in the heart.
   a. One set of lead electrodes senses lethal dysrhythmias in the heart.
   b. The other set of lead electrodes transmits the electric shock from the pulse generator to the heart.
3. The implantable defibrillator is noninvasively turned on and off by a doughnut-shaped magnet.

Function

Four electric shocks are delivered in a programmed sequence:
1. The device allows 10 to 35 seconds to detect a lethal dysrhythmia, charge, and "defibrillate" the heart. The lethal dysrhythmia must meet two programmed criteria (rate and amount of time spent from the isoelectric line) to trigger the device to emit an initial electric shock. The amount of joules necessary to convert each patient is determined during insertion and testing of the device, usually 15 to 25 joules.

2. Nontermination of the lethal dysrhythmia by the initial shock triggers the device to continue the sequence (detect, charge, and defibrillate) until a total of four or five shocks have been delivered (number of shocks depends on device model implanted).
   a. Subsequent shocks are slightly higher, at 30 to 32 joules.
   b. The total sequence lasts approximately 2 minutes.
3. Nontermination of the lethal dysrhythmia after the shock sequence signals the device to revert to the "detection" mode of operation and not to reinitiate the shocking sequence. The device will reinitiate the shocking sequence only if a rhythm other than the lethal dysrhythmia is detected and maintained for at least 35 seconds. If this criterion is met and another lethal dysrhythmia is detected, the device will cycle through the shocking sequence again.
4. Termination of a lethal dysrhythmia at any time during the shocking sequence signals the device to interrupt the sequence, return to a detection mode and reinitiate the shocking sequence if another lethal dysrhythmia is detected.

Indications

1. Failure of maximal conventional medical therapy to control ventricular fibrillation and/or ventricular tachycardia (as determined by electrophysiology studies)
2. Survival of one episode of sudden cardiac death not associated with acute MI

Complications

1. Infection
2. Bleeding
3. Device failure
4. Pacemaker interaction
5. Constrictive pericarditis

Nursing Diagnoses

- Anxiety related to invasive procedure and fear of death
- Risk for Infection related to invasive procedure and implanted device
- Decreased Cardiac Output related to surgical procedure and/or dysrhythmias
- Ineffective Breathing Pattern related to surgical procedure and discomfort

Nursing Interventions
Reducing Anxiety

1. Explain to patient and family reason for implant, surgical procedure, and pre- and postprocedure management:
   a. Performed in the operating room; anesthesia required
   b. Incision location
   c. Endotracheal intubation; chest tubes
   d. Intravenous (IV) line; continuous ECG monitoring
   e. Early mobilization after procedure

f. Cough and deep breathing exercises

g. Management of incisional pain

h. Turning on the device (usually 48 to 72 hours after implantation)

2. Provide emotional support to patient and family.

a. Encourage patient and family to verbalize fears and/or expectations of hospitalization, lifestyle adjustments, self-concept, body image, and device malfunction (misfiring/failure to fire).

b. Reinforce to patient that daily activities will not increase the risk of the device misfiring.

c. Explain the sensation that might be felt if the device fires and the patient is conscious. (Many patients will become unconscious before the device fires and therefore feel no sensations.) Sensations experienced in conscious patients vary, but are often described as a severe chest blow.

3. Allow patient to participate in care as much as possible.

a. Encourage patient to dress in street clothes during hospitalization. (Loose-fitting clothes are recommended to prevent chafing/irritation at implant site.)

b. Allow patient to look at incision site.

c. Offer patient instructional booklets on the device.

Preventing Infection

1. Check temperature every 4 hours; report elevations. (Suspect defibrillator system as infection source if elevation occurs; infections commonly occur within 5 to 10 days.) Early postoperative fever may also be due to atelectasis; auscultate lungs.

2. Evaluate incision site every 4 hours; note redness, swelling, purulent/serous drainage; palpate around incision site for tenderness, warmth, and/or drainage.

3. Culture all drainage from incision.

4. Evaluate incision for tissue erosion.

5. Monitor white blood cell (WBC) count and differential.

6. Cleanse incision and change dressing as directed, using aseptic technique.

7. Encourage a high-calorie/high-protein diet to promote wound healing and decrease chance of postoperative complications.

> **GERONTOLOGIC ALERT**
>
> Elderly patients may not demonstrate abnormal temperature elevations with infections and experience prolonged wound healing.

Maintaining Adequate Cardiac Output

1. Monitor vital signs frequently until stable.

2. Evaluate incision site for evidence of bleeding and/or hematoma.

3. Monitor chest tube drainage for excessive amount and note color.

4. Evaluate urine output.

5. Be alert to potential for dysrhythmias postoperatively. (Manipulation of heart and swelling may induce dysrhythmias 24 to 48 hours after implant.)

6. Treat dysrhythmias as directed—antidysrhythmic therapy and/or electric countershock (standard anterior paddle placement or anterior/posterior paddle placement is recommended); correct underlying causes such as hypoxia and/or electrolyte disturbances.

> **NURSING ALERT**
>
> CPR should be started immediately on any patient with an implantable defibrillator who becomes unconscious and has no pulse. A slight "buzz" sensation will be felt if the implanted device delivers a shock, but it is not harmful. Gloves may be worn to minimize the sensation.

7. Evaluate carefully all complaints of chest pain (noncardiac pain may be due to lead fracture or dislodgement; pain may be noted along wire pathways).

8. Auscultate heart sounds every 4 hours for presence of friction rub.

Promoting Effective Breathing Pattern

1. Ask patient to take several deep breaths every hour to expand lung fields.

2. Encourage cough and deep breathing exercises frequently; medicate with analgesics before exercises and provide a pillow for splinting.

3. Monitor use of incentive spirometer.

4. Elevate head of bed to promote adequate ventilation.

5. Auscultate lung fields every 4 hours.

6. Assist with position changes every 2 hours while on bed rest.

7. Encourage early ambulation.

8. Administer analgesics as ordered.

Patient Education and Health Maintenance
Introduction to Implantable Defibrillator

1. Review anatomy of the heart with emphasis on the conduction system, using a diagram of the heart.

2. Give accurate explanations, using correct medical terminology (allows patient to interact with the health care team more effectively), regarding reason for device implantation, component parts of system, function of device.

a. Use manufacturer's instructional booklet and video presentation about the device.

b. Encourage family members to participate in education process.

Living With the Implantable Defibrillator

1. Instruct patient and family on actions to be taken should the device fire.

a. Explain signs/symptoms that may be experienced if a lethal dysrhythmia occurs: palpitations, dizziness, shortness of breath, chest pain.

b. If signs/symptoms are experienced, lie down and try to call "911" for help if alone.

c. Family members should check for a pulse if patient becomes unconscious. CPR should be started immediately if no pulse is present and "911" has been called.

d. Reinforce that shocks emitted from device are not harmful, and CPR should never be delayed to wait for device to complete the shocking sequence.

e. If patient remains conscious and/or is unconscious with a pulse, family members should monitor patient during episode, continually assessing for a pulse during shocking sequence. After the episode, follow instructions as directed by health care provider.

f. Keep a diary of all episodes and shocks received from device. Include date, time, and associated symptoms.

2. Explore with patient/family fears regarding failure of device, sensation associated with a shock, and injury to others if a shock occurs.

a. Sensations experienced vary but are most commonly described as a severe blow to the chest.

b. No injury will occur to others if in contact with patient during a shock; a slight shock may be felt by your partner if the device fires during sexual intercourse.

c. Battery life depends on frequency of use. The device is evaluated every 2 months for 1 year and every month thereafter.

3. Review sources of electromechanical interference that should be avoided (see p. 334).

a. The device will usually not become damaged but may be turned off due to interference.

b. A "beeping" sound may be audible if device is turned off by interferences.

c. Airport security devices and hand-held airport security devices may affect device function. These devices must be avoided. Carry Medic-Alert card and show to security personnel.

d. Areas/diagnostic tests using large magnets must be avoided.

e. Notify health care provider if contact with sources of potential interference has occurred.

4. Notify dentist of implanted device because prophylaxis with antibiotics may be necessary before dental care.

5. Review with health care provider resumption of activities such as driving and sports.

Other Instructions

1. Review care of incision site (see p. 335).

2. Loose-fitting clothing should be worn until healing takes place.

3. Provide Medic-Alert card; encourage carrying card at all times and obtaining a corresponding Medic-Alert bracelet.

4. Reinforce how to keep diary of episodes and date of 2-month follow-up appointment.

5. Provide information to family members regarding CPR training courses.

Outcome-Based Evaluation

- Verbalizes understanding of device and surgical procedure
- Afebrile; incision without drainage
- Vital signs stable; no dysrhythmias
- Respirations unlabored, lungs clear

Pericardiocentesis

Pericardiocentesis is the puncturing of the pericardial sac to aspirate fluid. Excessive fluid within the pericardial sac can cause compression of the heart chambers, resulting in an acute decrease in cardiac output (cardiac tamponade). Fluid accumulation (pericardial effusion) can occur rapidly (acute) or slowly (stable).

Acute—a rapid increase of fluid into pericardial space (as little as 200 mL) causes a marked rise in intrapericardial pressure. Emergency intervention is required to prevent severe circulatory compromise.

Stable—slow accumulation of fluid into pericardial sac over weeks or months, causing pericardium to stretch and accommodate up to 2 L of fluid without severe increases in intrapericardial pressure. See Procedure Guidelines 12-8.

Purposes

1. To remove fluid from the pericardial sac caused by:
   a. Infection
   b. Malignant neoplasm or lymphoma
   c. Trauma
      (i) Accidental—blunt or penetrating wounds
      (ii) Iatrogenic—cardiac surgery; cardiopulmonary resuscitation; perforation of heart by catheter or transvenous pacemaker
   d. Drug reactions
   e. Radiation
   f. MI
2. To obtain fluid for diagnosis
3. To instill certain therapeutic drugs

Sites for Pericardiocentesis

1. Subxiphoid—needle inserted in the angle between left costal margin and xiphoid
2. Near cardiac apex, 2 cm (0.8 inch) inside left border of cardiac dullness
3. To the left of the fifth or sixth interspace at the sternal margin
4. Right side of fourth intercostal space just inside border of dullness

PROCEDURE GUIDELINES 12-8   ASSISTING THE PATIENT UNDERGOING PERICARDIOCENTESIS

EQUIPMENT

Pericardiocentesis tray
Intracath set
Skin antiseptic
1% to 2% lidocaine
Sterile gloves

ECG for monitoring purposes
Sterile ground wire—to be connected between pericardial
   needle and V lead of ECG (use alligator clip type connectors)
Equipment for cardiopulmonary resuscitation

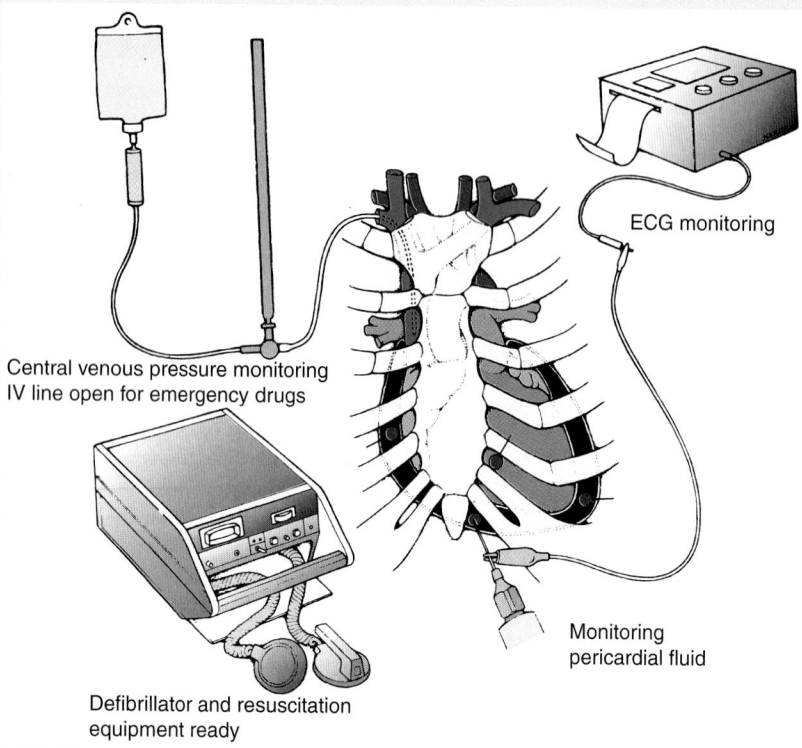

ECG monitoring

Central venous pressure monitoring
IV line open for emergency drugs

Monitoring
pericardial fluid

Defibrillator and resuscitation
equipment ready

Nursing support of the patient undergoing pericarditis. (Small circles indicate sites for pericardial aspiration.)

PROCEDURE

Nursing Action	Rationale

PREPARATORY PHASE

1. Medicate the patient as prescribed.
2. Establish venous access.

2. This preserves a route for intravenous therapy in the event of an emergency.

3. Place the patient in a comfortable position with the head of the bed or treatment table raised to a 45-degree angle.
4. Apply the limb leads of the ECG to the patient.
5. Have defibrillator available for immediate use.
6. Have pacemaker available.
7. Open the tray using aseptic technique.

3. This position makes it easier to insert needle into pericardial sac.
4. The patient is monitored during the procedure by ECG.
5. In case the procedure has severe adverse effect.

PERFORMANCE PHASE (BY PHYSICIAN)

1. The site is prepared with skin antiseptic; the area is draped with sterile towels and injected with anesthetic.

Nursing Action	Rationale
2. The pericardial aspiration needle is attached to a 50-mL syringe by a three-way stopcock. The V lead (precordial lead wire) of the ECG is attached to the hub of the aspirating needle by a sterile wire and alligator clips or clamp.	2. There is danger of laceration of myocardium/coronary artery and of cardiac dysrhythmias.
3. The needle is advanced slowly until fluid is obtained.	3. Fluid is generally aspirated at a depth of 2.5 to 4 cm (1 to 1½ inches).
4. When the pericardial sac has been entered, a hemostat is clamped to the needle at the chest wall just where it penetrates the skin. Pericardial fluid is aspirated slowly.	4. This prevents movement of the needle and further penetration while fluid is being removed. Aspirated fluid may be cloudy, clear, or bloody.
5. Monitor the patient's ECG, blood pressure, and venous pressure constantly.	5. a. The S–T segment rises if the point of the needle contacts the ventricle; there may be ventricular ectopic beats.
	b. The P–R segment is elevated when the needle touches the atrium.
	c. Large, erratic QRS complexes indicate penetration of the myocardium.
6. If a large amount of fluid is present, a polyethylene catheter may be inserted through a needle (an intracath) and left in the pericardial sac.	6. An indwelling catheter left in the pericardial space permits further slow drainage of fluid and prevents recurrence of cardiac tamponade.
7. Watch for presence of bloody fluid. If blood accumulates rapidly, an immediate thoracotomy and cardiorrhaphy (suturing of heart muscle) may be indicated.	7. Bloody pericardial fluid may be due to trauma. Bloody pericardial effusion fluid does not clot readily, whereas blood obtained from inadvertent puncture of one of the heart chambers does clot.
FOLLOW-UP PHASE	
1. Monitor patient closely.	1. After pericardiocentesis, careful monitoring of blood pressure, venous pressure, and heart sounds will be necessary to indicate possible recurrence of tamponade; repeated aspiration is then necessary.
a. Watch for rising venous pressure and falling arterial pressure.	
b. Auscultate the area over the heart.	2. In the presence of these signs, the patient is probably experiencing cardiac tamponade.
2. Prepare for surgical drainage of pericardium if:	
a. Pericardial fluid repeatedly accumulates, or	
b. The aspiration is unsuccessful, or	
c. Complications develop	
3. Listen for decrease in intensity of heart sounds indicating recurring cardiac tamponade.	
4. Assess for complications:	
Inadvertent puncture of heart chamber	
Dysrhythmias	
Puncture of lung, stomach, or liver	
Laceration of coronary artery or myocardium	

Percutaneous Transluminal Coronary Angioplasty (PTCA)

Percutaneous transluminal coronary angioplasty is a technique used for the treatment of coronary artery disease (CAD). A balloon-tipped catheter is introduced through a guidewire into a coronary vessel with a non-calcified atheromatous lesion. The balloon of the catheter is then inflated, causing disruption of the intima and changes in the atheroma. The result is an increase in the diameter of the lumen of the coronary vessel (as judged by angiographic criteria) and improvement of blood flow below the lesion. Balloon inflation/deflation may be repeated until satisfactory results are achieved (Figure 12-7).

Indications

Patients meeting these criteria are generally acceptable candidates for PTCA:

1. Stable angina (less than 1 year) or unstable angina (less than 6 months), despite optimal medical therapy.
2. Single-vessel or multivessel disease (balloon dilatation of the most severe "culprit" lesion is initially attempted to determine if successful angioplasty can be achieved); surgery to bypass the lesion may be recommended if PTCA is unsuccessful.

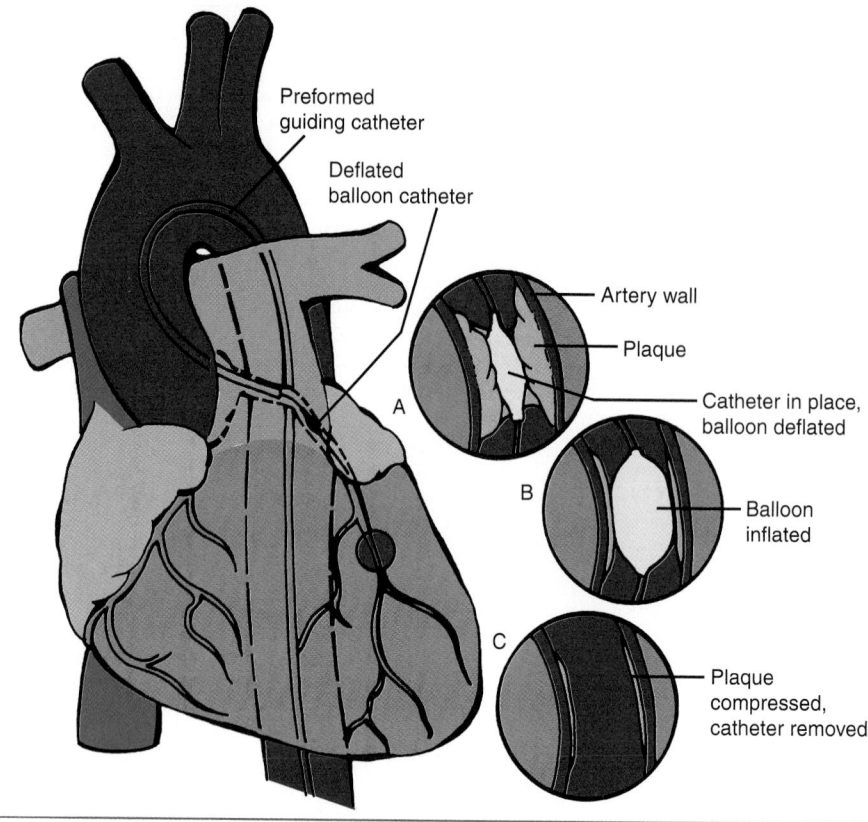

FIGURE 12-7 Percutaneous transluminal coronary angioplasty. (**A**) The balloon-tipped catheter is passed into the affected coronary artery. (**B**) The balloon is then rapidly inflated and deflated with controlled pressure. (**C**) The balloon disrupts the intima and causes changes in the atheroma, resulting in an increase in the diameter of the lumen of the vessel and improvement of blood flow. (Redrawn after Purcell, J. A., & Giffin, P. A. [1981]. Percutaneous transluminal coronary angioplasty. *American Journal of Nursing 9*, 1620–1626.)

3. Proximal, accessible noncalcified lesions; midvessel lesions may also be attempted with success.
4. Suitable candidate for heart surgery and has consented to heart surgery as an alternative treatment.
5. Evolving MI (may be in combination with thrombolytic therapy) and obstructed coronary bypass grafts.

Contraindications
1. Patients with left main coronary artery disease
2. Patients with severe left ventricular dysfunction

Complications
1. Coronary occlusion, coronary dissection, MI, coronary artery spasm, and prolonged angina may necessitate immediate coronary artery bypass graft surgery. A cardiac surgical team must be on standby during all PTCA procedures.
2. PTCA is associated with a restenosis rate of 30% to 40%. Restenosis may occur acutely (within 24 hours) or within 6 months. A second angioplasty may be performed with improved long-term results.

Other Procedures
1. Laser-assisted balloon angioplasty
   a. A laser light is directed by a percutaneously inserted flexible fiberoptic catheter and is able to "vaporize" atheromatous lesions in the coronary vessels.
   b. Balloon angioplasty of the vessel may then be performed.

   c. This new technique may minimize damage to the intimal lining, open diseased vessels more effectively, prevent early and long-term restenosis, and expand the use to calcified, unusual lesions and total occlusions.
2. Atherectomy
   a. A burr-tipped, high-speed, rotating catheter is inserted percutaneously into a coronary vessel and "drills" through the atheromatous lesion, changing it to microscopic debris.
   b. This technique may open diseased vessels more effectively, especially in patients who have coronary lesions not amenable to standard angioplasty.
3. Intracoronary stenting
   a. A tiny coil or diamond mesh tubular device (stent) is placed in the coronary artery immediately after successful balloon angioplasty.
   b. The stent remains in the vessel to prevent restenosis.

Nursing Diagnoses
- Anxiety related to impending invasive procedure
- Decreased Cardiac Output related to dysrhythmias, vessel restenosis, or spasm
- Risk for Injury (bleeding) related to femoral catheter and effect of anticoagulant and/or thrombolytic therapy
- Pain related to invasive procedure or myocardial ischemia

Nursing Interventions
Reducing Anxiety
1. Reinforce the reasons for the procedure.
   a. Describe the location of the coronary vessels using a diagram of the heart.
   b. Describe/draw the location of the patient's lesion using heart diagram.
2. Explain the events that will occur before, during, and after the procedure. Preparation minimizes anxiety and increases compliance with care regimen.
   a. Performed in the cardiac catheterization laboratory; similar to the cardiac catheterization procedure. Review auditory and tactile stimuli.
   b. Mild sedation given; patient remains awake throughout procedure to report any chest pain (indicates myocardial ischemia) and to cough when instructed (enhances catheter placement).
   c. Medication (nitroglycerin) will be given prophylactically to prevent and relieve episodes of chest pain.
3. Prepare patient for complications of procedure. Provide preoperative teaching to patient and family regarding heart surgery (see p. 350).
4. Explain the necessity of the IV, ECG monitoring, frequent vital sign and groin checks, and remaining NPO before the procedure.

Maintaining Adequate Cardiac Output
1. Check vital signs every 15 minutes for 1 hour, then every half hour for 2 hours, and subsequently every 1 to 2 hours.
2. Continually evaluate for signs/symptoms of restenosis.
   a. Emphasize importance of reporting any chest discomfort or jaw, back, arm pain and/or nausea, abdominal distress.
   b. Take ECG for all complaints suspicious of possible myocardial ischemia.
   c. Administer oxygen and vasodilator therapy for pain as directed.
   d. Obtain CK and isoenzymes as directed.
   e. Keep patient NPO if prolonged chest pain occurs (patient may return to catheterization laboratory).
3. Administer medications to maintain vessel patency.
   a. Antiplatelet agents may be given after procedure to prevent reocclusion (eg, abciximab [ReoPro]).
   b. Low-dose heparin or low-molecular-weight heparin (enoxaparin [Lovenox]) may also be used.
   c. Many patients are then maintained on ticlopidine (Ticlid) or clopidogrel (Plavix).
4. Evaluate fluid and electrolyte balance.
   a. Record intake and output.
   b. Encourage fluid intake to prevent dehydration. Contrast medium used during procedure causes diuresis.
   c. Observe for dysrhythmias possibly related to potassium imbalance. Excessive diuresis causes potassium depletion.
   d. Administer potassium supplement as prescribed.
5. Be alert to potential of vasovagal reaction during removal of groin catheter.
   a. Observe for bradycardia, hypotension, diaphoresis, nausea.
   b. Administer IV atropine as directed.
   c. Place patient in Trendelenburg's position to promote blood return to the heart and improve hypotension.
   d. Give fluid challenge as directed.

Preventing Bleeding
1. Maintain bed rest with affected extremity immobilized and head of bed elevated no more than 30 degrees 12 to 24 hours after procedure to prevent catheter dislodgement, bleeding, and prolonged healing of vessel lining; less restriction if an intra-arterial suture was used.
2. Mark peripheral pulses before procedure with indelible ink.
3. Check peripheral pulse of affected extremity and insertion site after each vital sign check.
4. Observe color, temperature, and sensation of affected extremity with each vital sign check.
   a. Catheter remains in the groin 4 to 6 hours after procedure to avoid bleeding complications (patient remains anticoagulated after procedure).
5. Report if extremities become cool and pale, and pulses become significantly diminished or absent.
6. Look for presence of hematoma, and mark hematoma to note change in size. Report if hematoma continues to enlarge.
7. Note petechiae, hematuria, and complaints of flank pain (vessel patency is maintained by not reversing intraprocedure heparinization; chance of bleeding is increased).
8. Hold direct pressure over insertion site if bleeding is observed, and report immediately.
9. Check bed linen under patient frequently for blood.
10. Ask patient to report any sensation of warmth at groin area.

Relieving Pain
1. Administer analgesics/anxiolytic medication as directed.
2. Ensure a restful environment.
   a. Provide back rubs for muscle relaxation.
   b. Minimize noise and interruptions.
   c. Offer sleep medication as indicated.
3. Progress patient's diet as tolerated (clear liquids/full liquid diet until catheters removed); assist patient with meals.

Patient Education and Health Maintenance
Instruct patient as follows:
1. Modification of cardiac risk factors as means of controlling progression of coronary artery disease.
2. Name of medications, action, dosage, and side effects.
   a. Common medications to prevent clot formation include aspirin, dipyridamole (Persantine), clopidogrel (Plavix)
   b. Medications to increase blood flow to heart such as isosorbide dinitrate (Isordil)
   c. Medications to slow heart rate/decrease chest pain such as metoprolol (Lopressor) or propranolol (Inderal)

d. Medications to increase blood flow and prevent coronary artery spasm, calcium channel blockers such as diltiazem (Cardizem), nifedipine (Procardia)

3. Dates and importance of follow-up tests—exercise ECG, thallium 201 perfusion imaging.

4. Symptoms for which patient should seek medical attention—side effects of medications, chest pain, or weight increases greater than 5 lb.

5. Chest pain unrelieved with nitroglycerin and persisting longer than 15 minutes after rest is significant.

6. Stenosis can recur within 6 months. Second angioplasty is usually successful for more than 1 year.

Outcome-Based Evaluation

• Verbalizes understanding of procedure
• Vital signs stable; urine output adequate
• No bleeding or hematoma at insertion site
• Verbalizes relief of pain

■ Intra-aortic Balloon Pump (IABP) Counterpulsation

Counterpulsation is a method of assisting the failing heart and circulation by mechanical support. The mechanism of counterpulsation therapy is opposite to the normal pumping action of the heart; counterpulsation devices pump while the heart muscle relaxes (diastole) and relax when the heart muscle contracts (systole).

Function

Intra-aortic Balloon Pump (Figure 12-8)

A balloon catheter is introduced into the femoral artery percutaneously or surgically, threaded to the descending

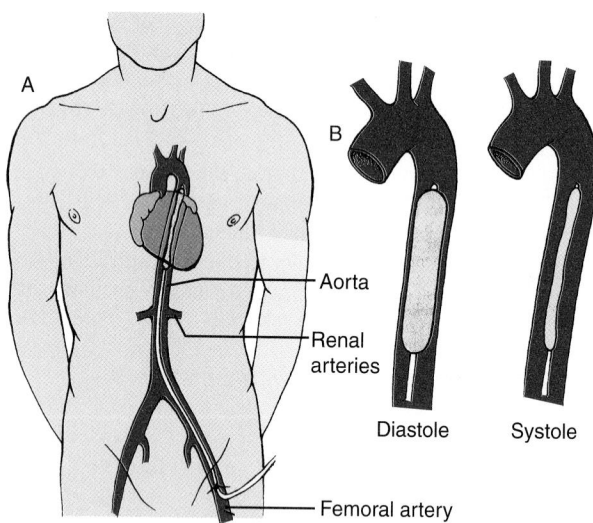

Aorta

Renal arteries

Diastole   Systole

Femoral artery

FIGURE 12-8 Counterpulsation. (**A**) Introduction of the intra-aortic balloon catheter via the femoral artery. (**B**) The intra-aortic balloon pump augments diastole, resulting in increased perfusion of the coronary arteries and myocardium and a decrease in the left ventricular work load.

thoracic aorta, and positioned distal to the subclavian artery.

1. The balloon catheter is attached to an external console, allowing for inflation/deflation of the balloon with gas such as carbon dioxide.

2. The external console integrates the inflation/deflation sequence with the mechanical events of the cardiac cycle (systole/diastole) by "triggering" gas delivery in synchronization with the patient's ECG and "timing" the duration of inflation and point of deflation in conjunction with the patient's arterial pressure waveform.

Counterpulsation With IABP

1. Eases the workload of a damaged heart by increasing coronary blood flow (diastolic augmentation) and decreasing the resistance in the arterial tree against which the heart must pump (afterload reduction).

2. This results in an increase in cardiac output and a reduction in myocardial oxygen requirements.

3. The balloon is inflated at the onset of diastole; this results in an increase in diastolic pressure (diastolic augmentation), which increases blood flow through the coronary arteries.

4. The balloon is deflated just before the onset of systole, facilitating the emptying of blood from the left ventricle.

5. Clinical uses
   a. Treatment of cardiogenic shock after MI
   b. Low cardiac output states—after open heart surgery; life-threatening dysrhythmias
   c. High cardiac output states—sepsis, hemorrhage
   d. Myocardial ischemia unresponsive to medical therapy and external counterpulsation pressure

Contraindications

1. Aortic valve insufficiency
2. Aortic aneurysm and/or dissection
3. Severe aortoiliac disease

Complications

1. Ischemia of limb distal to insertion site
2. Impairment of cerebral circulation due to balloon migration occluding the subclavian artery or by embolus
3. Impairment of renal circulation due to balloon malposition or embolus
4. Dissection of the aorta
5. Thrombocytopenia
6. Septicemia
7. Infection at insertion site
8. Hemorrhage due to anticoagulation

Nursing Diagnoses

• Anxiety related to invasive procedure, critical illness, and environment
• Decreased Cardiac Output related to myocardial ischemia and/or mechanical intervention
• Altered Tissue Perfusion related to foreign body in aorta
• Impaired Skin Integrity related to decreased mobility

Nursing Interventions
Relieving Anxiety

1. Explain IABP therapy to patient and family geared to their level of understanding.
   a. Review purpose of therapy and how the IABP functions.
   b. Reinforce mobility restrictions: supine with head of bed elevated 15 to 30 degrees, no movement or flexing of leg with IABP catheter.
   c. Explain need for frequent monitoring of vital signs, rhythm, affected extremity, and pulses.
   d. Discuss the sounds associated with functioning external console: balloon inflation/deflation and alarms.
2. Encourage family members to participate in care of patient.
   a. Allow family to visit patient frequently.
   b. Solicit family members' assistance in reinforcing mobility restrictions to patient and notifying nursing staff of patient comfort needs.
3. Allow patient to verbalize fears regarding therapy and illness.
4. Ensure that informed consent is obtained.
5. Administer anxiolytic medications as prescribed and indicated.

Maintaining Adequate Cardiac Output

1. Assist during insertion of IABP catheter.
   a. Offer patient reassurance and comfort measures (patient is only mildly sedated).
   b. Ensure strict aseptic environment during insertion.
   c. Establish ECG monitoring, choosing the lead with the largest R wave (external console senses R wave of ECG to trigger gas delivery) and without artifact (integration of the patient's cardiac cycle with the inflation/deflation balloon sequence depends on a continuous clear ECG tracing).
   d. Record date, time, and the patient's tolerance to procedure.
2. Start IABP immediately after insertion, as directed; review manufacturer's manual for IABP equipment in use.
   a. Adjust the duration of balloon inflation/deflation by the arterial waveform; inflation is "timed" to begin at the dicrotic notch of the arterial waveform, and deflation occurs before the next systole.
   b. Compare the patient's arterial pressure waveform with/without balloon augmentation to evaluate effectiveness of therapy. Note difference in patient's end diastolic pressure and balloon-assisted end diastolic pressure (the balloon-assisted end diastolic pressure should be lower, indicating a reduction in afterload).
   c. Monitor hemodynamic parameters with Swan-Ganz catheter (see p. 324). Record mean arterial pressure, CVP, PAP, PCWP, and cardiac output to evaluate overall effectiveness of therapy. Perform hemodynamic calculations to evaluate SVR and left ventricular stroke work (LVSW).

3. Monitor vital signs every 15 to 30 minutes for 4 to 9 hours then hourly, if stable.
4. Monitor neurologic status at least every 2 hours.
5. Monitor urine output from indwelling catheter every hour.
6. Maintain accurate intake/output.
7. Report chest pain immediately.
8. Treat dysrhythmias as directed.
9. Check for blood oozing around IABP catheter every hour for 8 hours, then every 4 hours (anticoagulation therapy is used to prevent thrombus formation); apply direct pressure and report bleeding.

Maintaining Adequate Tissue Perfusion

1. Evaluate for ischemia of extremity with IABP catheter.
   a. Mark pulses with indelible ink to facilitate checks.
   b. Monitor peripheral pulses (dorsalis pedis, posterior tibial, popliteal, and left radial) for rhythm, character, and pulse quality every 15 minutes for 1 hour, then every 30 minutes for 1 hour, and then hourly.
   c. Use Doppler device for pulses difficult to palpate and to auscultate for bruits/hums.
   d. Observe skin temperature, color, sensation, and movement of affected extremity. Dusky, cool, mottled, painful, numb/tingling extremity indicates ischemia.
2. Observe for possible indications of thromboemboli.
   a. Note decreases in urine output after initiation of therapy—may indicate renal artery emboli.
   b. Perform neurologic checks every hour to evaluate for cerebral emboli.
   c. Auscultate bowel sounds to detect evidence of ischemia.
3. Recognize early signs/symptoms of compartment syndrome. Increased pressure in tissue reduces blood flow.
   a. Note complaints of pain, pressure, and numbness of affected extremity induced by passive stretching.
   b. Palpate affected extremity for swelling and tension.
   c. Monitor CK values. Highly elevated CKs may indicate compartment syndrome.
4. Keep head of bed elevated 15 to 30 degrees if tolerated to prevent upward migration of catheter.

Maintaining Skin Integrity

1. Assess skin frequently for signs of redness or breakdown.
2. Place patient on specialty mattress or bed designed to prevent pressure sores (preferably before balloon insertion).
3. Pad bony prominences.
4. Implement passive range-of-motion exercises with exception of extremity with IABP catheter.
5. Turn patient from side to side as a unit every 2 hours. Patients are usually debilitated and prone to pressure sores.

Outcome-Based Evaluation

- Patient states activity restrictions and rationale
- BP and cardiac output readings improved

- Peripheral pulses strong; extremities warm and nail beds pink
- No skin redness or breakdown

Heart Surgery

Open heart surgery is most commonly performed for coronary artery disease, valvular dysfunction, and congenital heart defects. The procedure requires temporary cardiopulmonary bypass (blood is diverted from the heart and the lungs and mechanically oxygenated and circulated) to provide a dry, bloodless field during the operation.

Newer and less invasive procedures include *minimally invasive direct coronary artery bypass (MIDCAB)* and *port access procedures.*

Types of Procedures

1. Traditional coronary artery bypass surgery
   a. A graft (leg and arm veins) is anastomosed to the aorta, and the other end of the graft is secured to a distal portion of a coronary vessel.
   b. The graft "bypasses" the obstructive lesion in the vessel, and adequate blood flow is restored to the heart muscle supplied by the artery.
   c. Multiple grafts can be placed to bypass lesions, and the internal mammary artery may also be used for grafts.
   d. Traditional procedure is done through sternotomy. The heart is stopped, and the cardiopulmonary bypass machine is used.
2. Valvular surgery
   a. Prosthetic or biologic valves are placed in the heart as definitive therapy for incompetent heart valves.
   b. Valve replacement can be done in conjunction with coronary artery bypass surgery.
   c. Usually done as open heart procedure through sternotomy incision.
3. Congenital heart surgery
   a. Defects of the heart can be surgically repaired and reconstructed.
   b. Temporary cardiopulmonary bypass is not always required.
4. MIDCAB procedure is done through small thoracotomy incision, and cardiopulmonary bypass is not needed because the heart remains beating.
   a. Limited to single-vessel disease.
   b. Graft may be taken from the internal thoracic artery.
   c. The heart may be slowed during anastomosis of the graft.
   d. Cuts postoperative length of stay to 2 to 4 days.
   e. Cannot be done following an acute MI, in the severely obese, or in someone needing the intra-aortic balloon pump.
5. Postaccess procedures are performed through a small anterior thoracotomy incision and a few 1-cm lateral port incisions that allow direct access to the heart and good visualization through a thoracoscope.
   a. Multiple vessel bypass can be performed as well as mitral valve surgery and repair of atrial septal defect.
   b. The heart is stopped, and cardiopulmonary bypass is used.
   c. Cuts postoperative length of stay to 1 to 3 days.
   d. Contraindicated in patients with occlusion in posterior arteries, severe atherosclerosis, and aortic aneurysms.

Preoperative Management

1. Review of patient's condition to determine status of pulmonary, renal, hepatic, hematologic, and metabolic systems.
   a. Cardiac history; history of cardiac dysrhythmias.
   b. Pulmonary health. Patients with COPD may require prolonged postoperative respiratory support.
   c. Depression—can produce a serious postoperative depressive state and can affect postoperative morbidity and mortality.
   d. Present alcohol intake; smoking history.
2. Preoperative laboratory studies.
   a. Complete blood count; serum electrolytes; lipid profile; and nose, throat, sputum, and urine cultures.
   b. Antibody screen.
   c. Preoperative coagulation survey (platelet count, prothrombin time, partial thromboplastin time)—Extracorporeal circulation will affect certain coagulation factors.
   d. Renal and hepatic function tests.
3. Evaluation of medication regimen. These patients are usually on multiple drugs.
   a. Digitalis—may be receiving large doses to improve myocardial contractility; may be stopped several days before surgery to avoid digitoxic dysrhythmias from cardiopulmonary bypass.
   b. Diuretics—assess for potassium depletion and volume depletion; give potassium supplement to replenish body stores. May be omitted several days preoperatively to avoid electrolyte imbalance and consequent dysrhythmias postoperatively.
   c. Beta-adrenergic blockers (propranolol [Inderal])—usually continued.
   d. Psychotropic drugs (diazepam [Valium]; chlordiazepoxide [Librium])—postoperative withdrawal may cause extreme agitation.
   e. Antihypertensives (reserpine [Serapsil])—omitted as far in advance of procedure as possible to allow norepinephrine repletion.
   f. Alcohol—sudden withdrawal may produce delirium.
   g. Anticoagulant drugs—discontinued several days before operation to allow coagulation mechanism to return to normal.
   h. Corticosteroids—if taken within the year before surgery, may be given supplemental doses to cover stress of surgery.
   i. Prophylactic antibiotics may be given preoperatively.
   j. Drug sensitivities or allergies are noted.

4. Improvement of underlying pulmonary disease and respiratory function to reduce risk of complications.
   a. Encourage patient to stop smoking.
   b. Treat infection and pulmonary vascular congestion.

GERONTOLOGIC ALERT

Elderly and debilitated patients are at greater risk for postoperative respiratory complications.

5. Preparation for events in the postoperative period.
   a. Take the patient and family on tour of ICU. This lessens anxiety about being in ICU.
      (i) Introduce the patient to staff personnel who will be caring for him or her.
      (ii) Give family a schedule of visiting hours and times for phone contact.
   b. Teach chest physical therapy procedures to optimize pulmonary function.
      (i) Have the patient practice with incentive spirometer.
      (ii) Show and practice diaphragmatic breathing techniques.
      (iii) Have the patient practice effective coughing, leg exercises.
   c. Prepare patient for presence of monitors, chest tubes, IVs, blood transfusion, endotracheal tube, nasogastric tube, pacing wires, arterial line, indwelling catheter.
      (i) Explain to the patient that two chest tubes will be inserted below incision into chest cavity for drainage and maintenance of negative pressure.
      (ii) Explain to the patient that endotracheal tube will prevent speaking, but communication will be possible through writing until tube is removed (usually within 24 hours).
      (iii) Explain to the patient that diet will consist of liquids until 24 hours after surgery.
      (iv) Explain to the patient that monitoring equipment and IV lines will restrict movement, and nursing staff will position the patient comfortably every 2 hours and as necessary.
   d. Discuss with the patient the need to monitor vital signs frequently and the likelihood of frequent disturbances of the patient's rest.
   e. Discuss pain management with the patient; assure the patient that analgesics will be administered as necessary to control pain.
   f. Tell the patient that both hands may be loosely restrained for a number of hours after surgery to eliminate possibility of pulling out tubes and IV lines inadvertently.
6. Evaluation of emotional state to reduce anxieties. Patients undergoing heart surgery are more anxious and fearful than other surgical patients. (Moderate anxiety assists patient to cope with stresses of surgery. Low anxiety level may indicate that the patient is in denial. High anxiety may impair the patient's ability to learn and listen.)
   a. Offer support and help patient and family mobilize positive coping mechanisms.
   b. Answer questions and allay fears and misconceptions.
7. Surgical preparation:
   a. Shave anterior and lateral surfaces of trunk and neck; shave entire body down to ankles (for coronary bypass).
   b. Shower/bathe with Betadine soap.
   c. Give sedative before going to the operating room.

Potential Complications

1. Cardiac dysrhythmias frequently occur after heart surgery.
   a. Premature ventricular contractions occur most frequently after aortic valve replacement and coronary bypass surgery. May be treated with pacing, lidocaine (Xylocaine), potassium.
   b. Atrial arrhythmias also occur after valvular surgery.
   c. Dysrhythmias also apt to occur with ischemia, hypoxia, alterations in serum potassium, edema, bleeding, acid–base or electrolyte disturbances, digitalis toxicity, myocardial failure.
2. Cardiac tamponade results from bleeding into the pericardial sac or accumulation of fluids in the sac, which compresses the heart and prevents adequate filling of the ventricles.
3. MI.
4. Cardiac failure (low output syndrome).
5. Persistent bleeding from cardiac incision, tissue fragility, trauma to tissues, clotting defects; blood clotting disturbances usually transitory after cardiopulmonary bypass; however, a significant platelet deficiency may be present.
6. Hypovolemia.
7. Renal insufficiency or failure. Renal injury may be caused by deficient perfusion, hemolysis, low cardiac output before and after open-heart surgery; use of vasopressor agents to increase blood pressure.
8. Hypotension may be caused by inadequate cardiac contractility and reduction in blood volume or by mechanical ventilation (when the patient "fights" the ventilator, or PEEP is used), all of which can produce a reduction in cardiac output.
9. Embolization may result from injury to the intima of the blood vessels, dislodgement of a clot from a damaged valve, venous stasis aggravated by certain dysrhythmias, loosening of mural thrombi, and coagulation problems.
   a. Common embolic sites are lungs, coronary arteries, mesentery, extremities, kidneys, spleen, and brain.
10. Postpericardiotomy syndrome—a group of symptoms occurring after cardiac and pericardial trauma and MI.
    a. Cause is not certain; may be from anticardiac antibodies, viral etiology, or other cause.
    b. Manifestations—fever, malaise, arthralgias, dyspnea, pericardial effusion, pleural effusion, friction rub.

11. Postperfusion syndrome—diffuse syndrome characterized by fever, splenomegaly, lymphocytosis.
12. Febrile complications—probably from body's reaction to tissue trauma or accumulation of blood and serum in pleural and pericardial spaces.
13. Hepatitis.

Postoperative Management

1. Adequate oxygenation is ensured; respiratory insufficiency is common after open heart surgery.
    a. Assisted or controlled ventilation is employed. Respiratory support is used during first 24 hours to provide airway in the event of cardiac arrest, to decrease the work of the heart, and to maintain effective ventilation.
    b. Chest x-ray taken immediately after surgery and daily thereafter to evaluate state of lung expansion and to detect atelectasis; to demonstrate heart size and contour, confirm placement of central line, endotracheal tube, and chest drains.
2. Hemodynamic monitoring during the immediate postoperative period for cardiovascular and respiratory status and fluid and electrolyte balance to prevent or recognize complications.
3. Drainage of mediastinal and pleural chest tubes is monitored.
4. Fluid and electrolyte balance is monitored closely.
5. Hypokalemia may be caused by inadequate intake, diuretics, vomiting, excessive nasogastric drainage, stress from surgery.
    a. Hyperkalemia may be caused by increased intake, red cell breakdown from the pump, acidosis, renal insufficiency, tissue necrosis, and adrenal cortical insufficiency.
    b. Hyponatremia may be due to reduction of total body sodium or to an increased water intake, causing a dilution of body sodium.
    c. Hypocalcemia may be due to alkalosis (which reduces the amount of calcium in the extracellular fluid) and multiple blood transfusions.
    d. Hypercalcemia may cause dysrhythmias imitating those caused by digitalis toxicity.
6. Postoperative medications include:
    a. Aspirin daily as MI prophylaxis.
    b. Analgesics.
    c. Antihypertensives or antiarrhythmics if needed.
7. Monitoring for complications.
8. Cardiac pacing, if indicated, by way of temporary pacing wires from the incision.

Nursing Diagnoses

- Anxiety related to fear of unknown, fear of death, and fear of pain
- Impaired Gas Exchange related to alveolar capillary membrane changes, immobility, altered blood flow
- Decreased Cardiac Output, related to mechanical factors: decreased preload and impaired contractility
- Risk for Fluid Volume Deficit and Electrolyte Imbalance related to physiologic effects of heart–lung machine
- Pain related to sternotomy and leg incisions
- Sensory/Perceptual Alterations related to intensive care environment, sleep deprivation, inability to speak, and immobility

Nursing Interventions
Minimizing Anxiety

1. Orient the patient to surroundings as soon as awakens from surgical procedure. Tell the patient that operation is over, location, the time of day, and your name.
2. Allow family members to visit the patient as soon as condition stabilizes. Encourage family members to talk to and touch the patient. (Family members may be overwhelmed by critical care environment.)
3. As the patient becomes more alert, explain purpose of all the equipment in environment. Continually orient the patient to time and place.
4. Administer anxiolytics as directed.

Promoting Adequate Gas Exchange

1. Frequently check function of mechanical ventilator, patient's respiratory effort, and ABGs.
2. Check endotracheal tube placement.
3. Auscultate chest for breath sounds. Crackles indicate pulmonary congestion; decreased or absent breath sounds indicate pneumothorax.
4. Sedate patient adequately to help tolerate endotracheal tube and cope with ventilatory sensations.
5. Use chest physiotherapy for patients with lung congestion to prevent retention of secretions and atelectasis.
6. Promote coughing, deep breathing, and turning to keep airway patent, prevent atelectasis, and facilitate lung expansion.
7. Suction tracheobronchial secretions carefully. Prolonged suctioning leads to hypoxia and possible cardiac arrest.
8. Restrict fluids (per request) for first few days. There is danger of pulmonary congestion from excessive fluid intake.
9. Assist with weaning process and extubation (see p. 255) when indicated.

Maintaining Adequate Cardiac Output

1. Monitor cardiovascular status to determine effectiveness of cardiac output. Serial readings of blood pressure by way of intra-arterial line, heart rate, CVP, left atrial or PAP, and PCWP from monitor modules are observed, correlated with the patient's condition, and recorded.
    a. Monitoring is continuous.
2. Check urine output every $\frac{1}{2}$ to 1 hour (from indwelling catheter).
3. Observe buccal mucosa, nail beds, lips, ear lobes and extremities for duskiness, cyanosis—signs of low cardiac output.

4. Feel the skin; cool, moist skin reveals lowered cardiac output. Note temperature and color of extremities.
5. Monitor neurologic status.
   a. Observe for symptoms of hypoxia—restlessness, headache, confusion, dyspnea, hypotension, and cyanosis.
   b. Note the patient's neurologic status hourly in terms of level of responsiveness, response to verbal commands and painful stimuli, pupillary size and reaction to light, and movement of extremities, hand-grasp ability.
   c. Monitor for and treat postoperative convulsive seizures.

Maintaining Adequate Fluid Volume

1. Administer IV fluids as ordered, but limit if signs of fluid overloading occur.
2. Keep intake and output flow sheets as a method of determining positive or negative fluid balance, and the patient's fluid requirements.
   a. IV fluids (including flush solutions through arterial and venous lines) are considered intake.
   b. Measure postoperative chest drainage—should not exceed 200 mL/h for first 4 to 6 hours.
3. Be alert to changes in serum electrolytes.
   a. Hypokalemia may cause dysrhythmias, digitalis toxicity, metabolic alkalosis, weakened myocardium, cardiac arrest.
      (i) Watch for specific ECG changes.
      (ii) Give IV potassium replacements as directed.
   b. Hyperkalemia may cause mental confusion, restlessness, nausea, weakness, and paresthesia of extremities. Be prepared to administer an ion-exchange resin, sodium polystyrene sulfonate (Kayexalate), which binds the potassium.
   c. Hyponatremia may cause weakness, fatigue, confusion, convulsions, and coma.
   d. Hypocalcemia may cause numbness and tingling in the fingertips, toes, ears, and nose; carpopedal spasm, muscle cramps, and tetany. Give replacement therapy as needed.
   e. Hypercalcemia may cause digitalis toxicity. Institute treatment as directed. This condition may lead to asystole and death.

Relieving Pain

1. Examine sternotomy incision and leg dressing.
2. Record nature, type, location, and duration of pain.
3. Differentiate between incisional pain and anginal pain.
4. Report restlessness and apprehension not corrected by analgesics—may be from hypoxia or a low-output state.
5. Administer medications as often as prescribed, or monitor constant infusion to reduce amount of pain and to aid the patient in performing deep breathing and coughing exercises more effectively.
6. Assist patient to position of comfort.
7. Encourage early mobilization.

Promoting Perceptual and Physical Orientation

1. Watch for symptoms of postcardiotomy delirium (may appear after brief lucid period).
   a. Signs and symptoms include delirium (impairment of orientation, memory, intellectual function, judgment), transient perceptual distortions, visual and auditory hallucinations, disorientation, and paranoid delusions.
   b. Symptoms may be related to sleep deprivation, increased sensory output, disorientation to night and day, prolonged inability to speak because of endotracheal intubation, age, and preoperative cardiac status.
2. Keep the patient oriented to time and place; notify the patient of procedures and expectations of cooperation.
3. Encourage family to come in at regular times—helps patient regain sense of reality.
4. Plan care to allow rest periods, day–night pattern, and uninterrupted sleep.
5. Encourage mobility as soon as possible. Keep environment as free as possible of excessive auditory and sensory input. Prevent bodily injury.
6. Reassure the patient and the family that psychiatric disorders after cardiac surgery are usually transient.
7. Remove patient from the ICU as soon as possible. Allow patient to talk about psychotic episode—helps deal with and assimilate experience.

Other Nursing Responsibilities:
Avoiding Complications

1. Dysrhythmias
   a. Monitor ECG continuously.
   b. Treat dysrhythmias immediately because they may lead to decreased cardiac output.
   c. Evaluate cause of dysrhythmias—inadequate oxygenation, electrolyte imbalance, MI, mechanical irritation (eg, pacing wires, invasive lines, chest tubes).
2. Cardiac tamponade
   a. Assess for signs of tamponade—arterial hypotension; rising CVP; rising left atrial pressure; muffled heart sounds; weak, thready pulse; neck vein distention; falling urinary output.
   b. Check for diminished amount of drainage in the chest-collection bottle; may indicate that fluid is accumulating elsewhere.
   c. Prepare for pericardiocentesis.
3. MI
   a. Check cardiac enzymes daily. Elevations may indicate MI.
   b. Symptoms may be masked by the usual postoperative discomfort.
      (i) Watch for decreased cardiac output in the presence of normal circulating volume and filling pressure.
      (ii) Obtain serial ECGs and isoenzymes to determine extent of myocardial injury.
      (iii) Assess pain to differentiate myocardial pain from incisional pain.
   c. Treatment is individualized. Postoperative activity level may be reduced to allow heart adequate time for healing.

4. Embolization
   a. Initiate preventive measures such as antiembolic stockings; omit pressure on popliteal space (leg crossing, raising knee gatch); start passive and active exercises.
   b. Assess respiratory and mental status as described above.
   c. Maintain integrity of all invasive lines.
5. Bleeding
   a. Watch for steady and continuous drainage of blood.
   b. Assess for arterial hypotension, low CVP, increasing pulse rate, and low left atrial and pulmonary artery wedge pressures.
   c. Prepare to administer blood products, IV solutions, or protamine sulfate or vitamin K (AquaMEPHYTON)
   d. Prepare for potential return to surgery for bleeding persisting (over 300 mL/h) for 2 hours.
6. Fever/infection
   a. Control higher degrees of fever by use of hypothermia mattress.
   b. Evaluate for atelectasis, pleural effusion, or pneumonia if fever persists. (The most common cause of early postoperative fever [within 24 hours] is atelectasis.)
   c. Evaluate for urinary tract infection/wound infection.
   d. Bear in mind the possibility of infective endocarditis if fever persists.
   e. Draw blood for culture to rule out endocarditis.
7. Renal insufficiency
   a. Measure urine volume; less than 20 mL/h can indicate decreased renal function.
   b. Carry out specific gravity tests to determine kidneys' ability to concentrate urine in renal tubules.
   c. Watch BUN and serum creatinine levels, as well as urine and serum electrolyte levels.
   d. Give rapid-acting diuretics and/or inotropic drugs (dopamine [Intropin], dobutamine [Dobutrex]) to increase cardiac output and renal blood flow.
   e. Prepare the patient for peritoneal dialysis or hemodialysis if indicated. (Renal insufficiency may produce serious cardiac dysrhythmias.)

Community and Home Care Considerations

Preparing the patient with cardiovascular disease or after cardiac surgery for the return home and/or optimizing the patient's health status in the home are important nursing functions. The key areas on which to focus include assessment, education, and evaluating responses.

Assessment

1. Optimally, the discharge plan begins at hospital admission. The patient's physical condition will determine to some extent his or her needs at home (ie, ability to care for self). But the available support systems will allow the nurse to individualize the plan of care.
2. Assess the patient's functional abilities. Patients with cardiovascular disorders may need to conserve their energy and/or rest often at least temporarily.

3. Assess the patient's available support systems, family, friends, neighbors.
   a. Will the patient have someone to facilitate care? If so, that person should be included in the treatment planning.
   b. Does the patient have other avenues of support (eg, neighbors, friends)?
   c. Does the patient have access to transportation for physician visits?
   d. Will the patient or someone else be able to provide meals, shopping?
   e. Will the patient need assistance with ADLs and personal care?
4. Assess the patient's home for safety hazards (eg, stairs, narrow walkways, unsafe electric systems, poor sanitation).

Plan for Home Care

1. Based on the above assessment, determine the patient's need for supportive services.
2. Coordinate services such as home health aides.
3. Refer patients to area meal delivery service as appropriate. These services provide special diets in most cases (eg, low sodium or low cholesterol).
4. Coordinate outpatient cardiac rehabilitation services as appropriate.
5. Establish outpatient or home-based physical and occupational therapy as appropriate for graduated exercise and energy conservation techniques.

Patient Education

1. Include caregivers in the educational sessions, especially if they will be directly involved in the patient's care.
2. Assess knowledge of disease, complications, and medications.
3. Begin with teaching about the disease process and the patient's particular manifestations and complications.
4. Outline the potential complications and how to avoid them and when to contact the health care provider.
5. Review current medications: Name (brand and generic), regimen, purpose, rationale, adverse/side effects, dosage and administration.
6. Provide written materials on the above for the patient's reference.

Patient Education and Health Maintenance

Note: Specific guidelines will vary slightly among institutions and health care providers. Check hospital policy and orders.

1. Instruct about activities.
   a. Increase activities gradually within limits. Avoid strenuous activities until after exercise stress testing.
   b. Take short rest periods.
   c. Avoid lifting more than 20 lb.
   d. Participate in activities that do not cause pain or discomfort.
   e. Increase walking time and distance each day.

f. Stairs (one to two times daily) the first week; increase as tolerated.

g. Avoid large crowds at first.

h. Avoid driving until after first postoperative checkup. At this time, check with health care provider.

i. Resumption of sexual relations parallels ability to participate in other activities. Usually may resume sexual activities 2 weeks after surgery. Avoid if tired or after heavy meal. Consult health care provider if chest discomfort, difficult breathing, or palpitations occur and last longer than 15 minutes after intercourse.

j. Return to work after first postoperative checkup, as advised by health care provider.

k. Expect some chest discomfort.

2. Advise about diet.

a. Some patients are placed on minimum salt restriction (eg, no salt added at table); cholesterol may be limited.

b. Weigh daily and report weight gain of more than 5 lb per week.

3. Teach about medications.

a. Label all medications; give purposes and side effects.

b. Patients with prosthetic valves may continue warfarin (Coumadin) regimen indefinitely. Explain bleeding precautions.

4. Advise patients with prosthetic valves:

a. Pregnancy is usually discouraged.

b. Need for antibiotic coverage before dental and surgical procedures.

c. Patients on anticoagulants should watch for bleeding and should avoid use of aspirin (and many other drugs)—interferes with action of warfarin.

5. Advise the patient to carry an identification card stating cardiac condition and medications being taken.

6. Encourage compliance with rehabilitation and exercise program after exercise stress testing.

7. Inform the patient whom to contact (and how) in case of an emergency.

8. See also section on patient education after MI, page 368, and patient education about infective endocarditis, page 375.

9. Explore community support groups such as: American Heart Association, *www.americanheart.org.*

Outcome-Based Evaluation

- Verbalizes understanding of surgical procedure, reduction in fear
- Extubated 24 hours postoperative; spontaneous unlabored respirations 14 to 18 per minute
- Blood pressure and heart rate stable; adequate urine output
- Serum electrolytes within normal range
- Verbalizes reduced pain
- Oriented to time and place; no hallucinations
- No bleeding noted; afebrile; ECG shows normal sinus rhythm

SELECTED REFERENCES

American Heart Association. (1997). *Textbook for advanced cardiac life support.* Dallas: Author.

Brown, L. M., & Brown, A. S. (1994). Transesophageal echocardiography: Implications for the critical care nurse. *Critical Care Nurse, 14*(3), 55–59.

Corona, G. G. (1999). Pacemakers: Keeping the beat today. *RN, 62*(12), 50–54.

Darling, E. (1994). Overview of electrophysiologic testing. *Critical Care Nursing Clinics of North America, 6*(1), 1–14.

Edgar, W. F., & Ebersole, N. (1999). MIDCAB. *American Journal of Nursing, 99*(7), 40–45.

Futterman, L. G., & Lemberg, L. (1999). Low-molecular-weight heparin: An antithrombotic agent whose time has come. *American Journal of Critical Care, 8*(1), 520–523.

Gaw-Ens, B. (1994). Informational support for families immediately after CABG surgery. *Critical Care Nurse, 14*(1), 41–50.

Gawlinski, A. (2000). Measuring cardiac output: Intermittent bolus thermodilution method. *Critical Care Nurse, 20*(2), 118–122.

Gibbar-Clements, T., Shirrell, D., Dooley, R., & Smiley, B. (2000). The challenge of warfarin therapy. *American Journal of Nursing, 100*(3), 38–40.

Harrison, H. (1999). Troponin I. *American Journal of Nursing, 99*(5), 24 TT.

Hodgins, C., & Sorenson, G. (1994). Directional coronary athrectomy: A new treatment for coronary artery disease. *Critical Care Nurse, 14*(1), 61–66.

Hudak, C. M., & Gallo, M. (1997). *Critical care nursing: A holistic approach* (7th ed.). Philadelphia: J. B. Lippincott.

Kimura, B. J., et al. (2000). Accuracy and cost effectiveness of single-view echocardiographic screening for suspected mitral valve prolapse. *American Journal of Medicine, 108*(3) 331–333.

Kline-Rogers, E., Martin, J. S., & Smith, D. D. (1999). New era of reperfusion in acute myocardial infarction. *Critical Care Nurse, 19*(1), 21–31.

Livorsi-Moore, J., Gulanick, M., & Rosko, P. (1999). Port access. Another advance in cardiovascular surgery. *American Journal of Nursing, 99*(7), 52–55.

Mancini, M. E., & Kaye, W. (1999). AEDs: Changing the way you respond to cardiac arrest. *American Journal of Nursing, 99*(5), 26–30.

Meyer, N. (1999). Using physiologic and pharmacologic stress testing in the evaluation of coronary artery disease. *The Nurse Practitioner, 24*(4), 70–82.

Morse, D., Campbell, R., & Riddle, M. (1998). Transmyocardial revascularization: A case study. *American Journal of Critical Care, 7*(6), 426–428.

Murphy, M. J., & Berding, C. B. (1999). Use of measurement of myoglobin and cardiac troponins in the diagnosis of acute myocardial infarction. *Critical Care Nurse, 19*(1), 58–65.

Pelter, M. M., Adams, M. G., Wung, S., Paul, S. M., & Drew, B. J. (1998). Peak time occurrence of myocardial ischemia in the coronary care unit. *American Journal of Critical Care, 7*(6), 411–417.

Pettney, L., & Leflar-Dileva, K. (1994). Preparing for cardiomyoplasty: A new horizon in cardiac surgery. *Dimensions of Critical Care Nursing, 13*(5), 226–236.

Ryan, D. (2000). A lab primer. *RN, 63*(1), 26–30.

Thorbs, N., Barbiere, C., Wayland, R., & Morgan, P. (2000). Coronary rotational atherectomy: A nursing perspective. *Critical Care Nurse, 20*(2), 77–84.

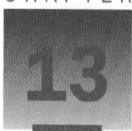

Cardiac Disorders

CARDIAC DISORDERS

▨ Coronary Artery Disease

Coronary artery disease (CAD) is characterized by the accumulation of fatty deposits along the innermost layer of the coronary arteries. The fatty deposits may develop in childhood and progressively enlarge and thicken throughout the life span. The enlarged lesion (atheroma/plaque) can cause a critical narrowing (75% occlusion) of the coronary artery lumen, resulting in a decrease in coronary blood flow and an inadequate supply of oxygen to the heart muscle.

Pathophysiology and Etiology

1. The most widely accepted cause of CAD is the accumulation of lipids (mainly cholesterol) and fibrous materials (smooth muscle cells) within the coronary artery lumen.
   a. Increased blood levels of low-density lipoprotein (LDL—known as the "bad" cholesterol because it transports cholesterol to body tissues) irritate and damage the inner layer of the coronary vessels.
   b. LDL enters the vessel after damaging the protective barrier, accumulates, and forms fatty streaks.
      (i) Fatty streaks are yellow, flat, and cause no significant coronary artery obstruction.
      (ii) These lesions develop frequently between the ages of 8 and 18 years.
   c. Smooth muscle cells (from the middle layer of the coronary artery) move to the inner layer to engulf the fatty substance, produce fibrous tissue, and stimulate calcium deposition.
2. This cycle continues, resulting in the transformation of the fatty streak into a fibrous plaque, and eventually a "complicated" CAD lesion evolves.
   a. A complicated lesion develops as small blood vessels grow into the fibrous plaque and the core of the lesion enlarges and calcifies.
   b. The complicated lesion can cause significant coronary obstruction by hemorrhage and ulceration of the plaque.
3. Risk factors
   a. The three major risk factors include high blood cholesterol levels, hypertension, and cigarette smoking.
   b. Unmodifiable risk factors include age, male sex, race, and family history of CAD.
   c. Other risk factors include diabetes mellitus, obesity, sedentary lifestyle, and stress.
4. Research is being conducted to explain the association of other factors such as chlamydial infection, increased homocysteine levels, hypothyroidism, and lipoprotein (a) in the pathogenesis of atherosclerosis and CAD.

Clinical Manifestations

See Standards of Care Guidelines.

Stable (Effort) Angina Pectoris

Chest pain precipitated by physical exertion or emotional stress; increased oxygen demands are placed on the heart muscle, but the ability of the coronary artery to deliver blood to the muscle is impaired because of obstruction by a significant coronary lesion (75% narrowing of the vessel). Rest and nitroglycerin relieve the pain.

1. *Character*—substernal chest pain, pressure, heaviness, or discomfort. Other sensations include a squeezing, aching, burning, choking, strangling, and/or cramping pain.
   a. Pain may be mild or severe and typically presents with a gradual buildup of discomfort and subsequent gradual fading away.
   b. May produce numbness or weakness in arms, wrists, or hands.
   c. Associated symptoms include diaphoresis, nausea, indigestion, dyspnea, tachycardia, and increase in blood pressure.
2. *Location*—behind middle or upper third of sternum; the patient generally will make a fist over the site of the pain

- Thoroughly evaluate any complaint of chest pain.
- Be alert to those at highest risk for myocardial infarction—smokers, those with hypertension, those with hyperlipidemia—but do not discount that MI may occur in those without risk factors.
- Be alert to common alternative presentation of coronary artery disease and MI in women, diabetics, and the elderly (nausea, indigestion, fatigue).
- Notify health care provider and obtain ECG for any complaint of chest pain.
- For chest pain not relieved by rest, assist/advise patient to go to emergency facility immediately.

This information should serve as a general guideline only. Each patient situation presents a unique set of clinical factors and requires nursing judgment to guide care, which may include additional or alternative measures and approaches.

(positive Levine sign; indicates diffuse deep visceral pain) rather than point to it with his or her finger.

3. *Radiation*—usually radiates to neck, jaw, shoulders, arms, hands, and posterior intrascapular area. Pain occurs more commonly on the left side than the right.
4. *Duration*—usually lasts 1 to 5 minutes after stopping activity; nitroglycerin relieves pain within 1 minute.
5. *Other precipitating factors*—exposure to hot or cold weather, eating a heavy meal, and sexual intercourse increase the workload of the heart and, therefore, increase oxygen demand.

Unstable (Preinfarction) Angina Pectoris

Chest pain occurring at rest; no increase in oxygen demand is placed on the heart muscle, but an acute lack of blood flow to the muscle occurs because of coronary artery spasm aggravated by the presence of an enlarged plaque or hemorrhage/ulceration of a complicated lesion. Critical narrowing of the vessel lumen occurs abruptly in either instance.

1. A change in frequency, duration, and intensity of stable angina symptoms is indicative of progression to unstable angina.
2. Unstable angina pain lasts longer than 10 minutes, is unrelieved by rest or sublingual nitroglycerin, and mimics signs and symptoms of impending myocardial infarction (see section titled MI, p. 360).

NURSING ALERT

Unstable angina can cause sudden death or result in a myocardial infarction. Early recognition and treatment are imperative to prevent complications.

Silent Ischemia

The absence of chest pain with documented evidence of an imbalance between myocardial oxygen supply and demand (S–T depression of 1 mm or more) as determined by ECG, exercise stress test, or ambulatory (Holter) ECG monitoring

1. Silent ischemia most commonly occurs in the early morning hours (6AM to 12PM).

2. Arousal causes an increase in sympathetic stimulation and blood viscosity, and coronary vessel tone increase in the morning, causing silent ischemic episodes.

Diagnostic Evaluation

1. *Characteristic chest pain* and clinical history
2. *Nitroglycerin test*—relief of pain with nitroglycerin
3. *ECG stress testing*—progressive increases of speed and elevation of walking on a treadmill increase the workload of the heart. ST and T wave changes occur if myocardial ischemia is induced.
4. *Radionuclide imaging*—a radioisotope, thallium 201, injected during exercise is imaged by camera. Low uptake of the isotope by heart muscle indicates regions of ischemia induced by exercise. Images taken during rest show a reversal of ischemia in those regions affected.
5. *Radionuclide ventriculography* (gated blood pool scanning)—red blood cells tagged with a radioisotope are imaged by camera during exercise and at rest. Wall motion abnormalities of the heart can be detected and ejection fraction estimated.
6. *Cardiac catheterization*—coronary angiography performed during the procedure determines the presence, location, and extent of coronary lesions.
7. *Positron emission tomography (PET)*—cardiac perfusion imaging with high resolution to detect very small perfusion differences due to stenotic arteries. Not available in all settings.

Management
Drug Therapy

Antianginal medications (nitrates, beta blockers, calcium channel blockers) are used to maintain a balance between oxygen supply and demand. Reduction of the workload of the heart decreases oxygen demand and consumption. Coronary vessel relaxation promotes blood flow to the heart muscle, thereby increasing oxygen supply.

1. *Nitrates*—cause generalized vasodilation throughout the body.
   a. Nitrates can be administered orally, sublingually, transdermally, or IV and provide short- or long-lasting effects.
   b. Short-acting nitrates provide immediate relief of acute anginal attacks or prophylaxis if taken before activity.
   c. Long-acting nitrates prevent anginal episodes and/or reduce severity and frequency of attacks.
2. *Beta blockers*—inhibit sympathetic stimulation of receptors that are located in the conduction system of the heart and in heart muscle.
   a. Some beta blockers inhibit sympathetic stimulation of receptors in the lungs as well as the heart ("nonselective" beta blockers); vasoconstriction of the large airways in the lung occurs; generally contraindicated for patients with chronic obstructive lung disease.
   b. "Cardioselective" beta blockers (in recommended drug ranges) affect only the heart and can be used safely in patients with lung disease.

3. *Calcium channel blockers*—inhibit movement of calcium within the heart muscle and coronary vessels; promote vasodilation and prevent/control coronary artery spasm.

4. *Antilipid agents*—decrease cholesterol and triglyceride.

Percutaneous Transluminal Angioplasty

1. A balloon-tipped catheter is placed in a coronary vessel narrowed by plaque.
2. The balloon is inflated and deflated to stretch the vessel wall and flatten the lesion (see section titled Percutaneous Transluminal Coronary Angioplasty (PTCA), p. 345).
3. Blood flows freely through the unclogged vessel to the heart.

Intracoronary Atherectomy

1. A blade-tipped catheter is guided into a coronary vessel to the site of the plaque.
2. Depending on the type of blade, the plaque is either cut, shaved, or pulverized, and then removed.
3. Requires a larger catheter introduction sheath so its use is limited to larger vessels.

Intracoronary Stent

1. A diamond mesh tubular device is placed in the coronary vessel.
2. Prevents restenosis by providing a "skeletal" support.

Coronary Artery Bypass Surgery

1. A graft is surgically attached to the aorta, and the other end of the graft is attached to a distal portion of a coronary vessel.
2. Bypasses obstructive lesions in the vessel and returns adequate blood flow to the heart muscle supplied by the artery (see section titled Heart Surgery, p. 350).

Transmyocardial Revascularization

By means of a laser beam, small channels are formed in the myocardium to encourage new blood flow.

Lifestyle Modification

1. Cessation of smoking
2. Control of high blood pressure
3. Lowering of blood cholesterol level
4. Dietary modifications
5. Folate and B-complex vitamins for hyperhomocystinemia

Complications

1. Sudden death due to lethal dysrhythmias
2. Congestive heart failure (CHF)
3. MI

Nursing Assessment

1. Ask patient to describe anginal attacks.
   a. When do attacks tend to occur? After a meal? After engaging in certain activities? After physical activities in general? After visits of family/others?
   b. Where is the pain located? Does it radiate?
   c. Was the onset of pain sudden? Gradual?
   d. How long did it last—seconds? minutes? hours?
   e. Was the pain steady and unwavering in quality?
   f. Is the discomfort accompanied by other symptoms? Sweating? Lightheadedness? Nausea? Palpitations? Shortness of breath?
   g. How is the pain relieved? How long does it take for pain relief?
2. Obtain a baseline 12-lead ECG.
3. Assess patient's and family's knowledge of disease.
4. Identify patient's and family's level of anxiety and use of appropriate coping mechanisms.
5. Gather information regarding the patient's cardiac risk factors.
6. Evaluate patient's medical history for conditions that may influence choice of drug therapy (diabetes, heart failure, previous myocardial infarction, obstructive lung disease).
7. Identify factors that may contribute to noncompliance with prescribed drug therapy.
8. Review renal/hepatic studies and complete blood count.
9. Discuss with patient current activity levels. (Effectiveness of antianginal drug therapy is evaluated by patient's ability to attain higher activity levels.)
10. Discuss patient beliefs regarding modification of risk factors and willingness to change.

Nursing Diagnoses

- Pain related to an imbalance in oxygen supply and demand
- Decreased Cardiac Output related to reduced preload, afterload, contractility, and heart rate secondary to hemodynamic effects of drug therapy
- Anxiety related to chest pain, uncertain prognosis, and threatening environment

Nursing Interventions

Relieving Pain

1. Determine intensity of patient's angina.
   a. Ask patient to compare the pain with other pain experienced in the past and, on a scale of 1 (lowest) to 10 (highest), rate current pain.
   b. Observe for other signs and symptoms: diaphoresis, shortness of breath, protective body posture, dusky facial color, and/or changes in level of consciousness.
2. Place patient in comfortable position.
3. Administer oxygen if prescribed.
4. Obtain blood pressure, apical heart rate, and respiratory rate.
5. Obtain a 12-lead ECG as directed.
6. Administer antianginal medication as prescribed.
7. Report findings to health care providers.
8. Monitor for relief of pain, and note duration of anginal episode.
9. Take vital signs every 5 to 10 minutes until angina pain subsides.
10. Monitor for progression of stable angina to unstable angina: increase in frequency and intensity of pain, pain occurring at rest or at low levels of exertion, pain lasting longer than 15 minutes.

11. Determine level of activity that precipitated anginal episode.
12. Identify specific activities patient may engage in that are below the level at which anginal pain occurs.
13. Reinforce the importance of notifying nursing staff whenever angina pain is experienced.

Maintaining Cardiac Output

1. Monitor carefully the patient's response to drug therapy.
   a. Take blood pressure and heart rate in a sitting and lying position on initiation of long-term therapy (provides baseline data to evaluate for orthostatic hypotension that may occur with drug therapy).
   b. Recheck vital signs as indicated by onset of action of drug and at time of drug's peak effect.
   c. Note changes in blood pressure of more than 10 mm Hg and changes in heart rate of more than 10 beats.
   d. Note patient complaints of headache (especially with use of nitrates) and dizziness.
      (i) Administer or teach self-administration of analgesics as directed for headache.
      (ii) Encourage supine position for dizziness (usually associated with a decrease in blood pressure; preload is enhanced by this mechanism, thereby increasing blood pressure).
   e. Institute continuous ECG monitoring or obtain 12-lead ECG as directed. Interpret rhythm strip every 4 hours for patients on continuous monitoring (beta blockers and calcium channel blockers can cause significant bradycardia and various degrees of heart block).
   f. Evaluate for development of heart failure (beta blockers and some calcium channel blockers decrease contractility, thus increasing the likelihood of heart failure).
      (i) Obtain serial weights.
      (ii) Auscultate lung fields for crackles.
      (iii) Monitor for the presence of edema.
2. Be sure to remove previous nitrate patch or paste before applying new paste or pad (prevents hypotension).
3. Be alert to adverse reaction related to abrupt discontinuation of beta blocker and calcium channel blocker therapy. These drugs must be tapered to prevent a "rebound phenomenon": tachycardia, increase in chest pain, hypertension.
4. Report all untoward drug effects to health care provider.

Decreasing Anxiety

1. Rule out physiologic etiologies for increasing or new onset of anxiety before administering prn sedatives. Physiologic causes must be identified and treated in a timely fashion to prevent irreversible adverse or even fatal outcomes; sedatives may mask symptoms delaying timely identification/diagnosis and treatment.
2. Assess patient for signs of hypoperfusion, auscultate heart and lung sounds, obtain a rhythm strip and administer oxygen as prescribed. Notify the health care provider immediately.

3. Document all assessment findings, health care provider notification and response, and interventions and response.
4. Explain to the patient and family reasons for hospitalization, diagnostic tests, and therapies administered.
5. Encourage the patient to verbalize fears and concerns regarding illness through frequent conversations—conveys to the patient a willingness to listen.
6. Answer the patient's questions with concise explanations.
7. Administer medications to relieve patient anxiety as directed. *Sedatives and tranquilizers* may be used to prevent attacks precipitated by aggravation, excitement, or tension.
8. Explain to the patient the importance of anxiety reduction to assist in control of angina. (Anxiety and fear put an increased stress on the heart, requiring the heart to use more oxygen.) Teach relaxation techniques.
9. Discuss measures to be taken when an anginal episode occurs. (Preparing patient decreases anxiety and allows patient to accurately describe angina.)
   a. Review the questions that will be asked during anginal episodes.
   b. Review the interventions that will be employed to relieve anginal attacks.

Patient Education and Health Maintenance
Instruct Patient and Family About CAD

1. Review the chambers of the heart and the coronary artery system, using a diagram of the heart.
2. Show patient a diagram of a clogged artery; explain how the blockage occurs; point out on the diagram the location of the patient's lesions.
3. Explain what angina is (a warning sign from the heart that there is not enough blood and oxygen because of the blocked artery or spasm).
4. Review specific risk factors that affect CAD development and progression; highlight those risk factors that can be modified and controlled to reduce risk.
5. Discuss the signs and symptoms of angina, precipitating factors, and treatment for attacks. Stress to patient the importance of treating angina symptoms at once.
6. Distinguish for patient the different signs and symptoms associated with stable angina versus preinfarction angina.

Identify Suitable Activity Level to Prevent Angina

Advise the patient on the following:

1. Participate in a normal daily program of activities that do not produce chest discomfort, shortness of breath, and undue fatigue. Begin regular exercise regimen as directed by health care provider.
2. Avoid activities known to cause anginal pain—sudden exertion, walking against the wind, extremes of temperature, high altitude, emotionally stressful situations; these may accelerate heart rate, raise blood pressure, and increase cardiac work.

3. Refrain from engaging in physical activity for 2 hours after meals. Rest after each meal if possible.
4. Do not undertake activities requiring heavy effort (eg, carrying heavy objects).
5. Try to avoid cold weather if possible; dress warmly and walk more slowly. Wear scarf over nose and mouth when in cold air.
6. Reduce weight, if necessary, to reduce cardiac load.

Instruct About Appropriate Use of Medications and Side Effects

1. Carry nitroglycerin at all times.
   a. Nitroglycerin is volatile and is inactivated by heat, moisture, air, light, and time.
   b. Keep nitroglycerin in original dark glass container, tightly closed to prevent absorption of drug by other pills or pillbox.
   c. Nitroglycerin should cause a slight burning or stinging sensation under the tongue when it is potent.
2. Place nitroglycerin under tongue at first sign of chest discomfort.
   a. Stop all effort or activity; sit, and take nitroglycerin tablet—relief should be obtained in a few minutes.
   b. Bite the tablet between front teeth and slip under tongue to dissolve if quick action is desired.
   c. Repeat dosage in a few minutes for total of 3 tablets if relief is not obtained.
   d. Keep a record of number of tablets taken to evaluate any change in anginal pattern.
   e. Take nitroglycerin prophylactically to avoid pain known to occur with certain activities.

NURSING ALERT

Instruct patient to go to the nearest health facility if chest pain persists more than 15 minutes, is unrelieved by 3 nitroglycerin tablets, or is more intense and widespread than the usual angina episodes. (Patient should not drive self.)

3. Demonstrate for patient how to administer nitroglycerin paste correctly.
   a. Place paste on calibrated strip.
   b. Remove previous paste on skin by wiping gently with tissue.
   c. Rotate site of administration to avoid skin irritation.
   d. Apply paste to skin; use plastic wrap to protect clothing if not provided on strip.
   e. Have patient return demonstration.
4. Instruct patient on administration of transdermal nitroglycerin patches.
   a. Remove previous patch; wipe area with tissue to remove any residual medication.
   b. Apply patch to a clean, dry, nonhairy area of body.
   c. Rotate administration sites.
   d. Instruct patient not to remove patch for swimming or bathing.

5. Teach about side effects of other medications.
   a. Constipation—verapamil (Calan)
   b. Ankle edema—nifedipine (Procardia)
   c. Heart failure (shortness of breath, weight gain, edema)—beta or calcium channel blockers
   d. Dizziness—vasodilators, antihypertensives
6. Ensure that patient has enough medication until next follow-up appointment or trip to the pharmacy. Warn against abrupt withdrawal of beta or calcium channel blockers to prevent rebound effect.

Counsel on Risk Factors and Lifestyle Changes

1. Inform patient of methods of stress reduction such as biofeedback and relaxation techniques.
2. Review low-fat/low-cholesterol diet. Suggest available cookbooks (American Heart Association) that may assist in planning and preparing foods. Have dietitian visit patient to design a menu plan.
3. Inform patient of available cardiac rehabilitation programs that offer structured classes on exercise, smoking cessation, and weight control.
4. Avoid excessive caffeine intake (coffee, cola drinks), which can increase the heart rate and produce angina.
5. Do not use "diet pills," nasal decongestants, or any over-the-counter medications that can increase the heart rate or stimulate high blood pressure.
6. Avoid the use of alcohol or drink only in moderation (alcohol can increase hypotensive side effects of drugs).
7. Encourage follow-up visits for control of diabetes and hypertension.
8. Have patient discuss adjunctive vitamin therapy (ie, vitamins E and C) with health care provider.

Outcome-Based Evaluation

- Verbalizes relief of pain
- Blood pressure and heart rate stable
- Verbalizes lessening anxiety, ability to cope

Myocardial Infarction

Myocardial infarction (MI) refers to a dynamic process by which one or more regions of the heart muscle experience a severe and prolonged decrease in oxygen supply because of insufficient coronary blood flow; subsequently, necrosis or "death" to the myocardial tissue occurs. The onset of the myocardial infarction process may be sudden or gradual, and the progression of the event to completion takes approximately 3 to 6 hours.

Pathophysiology and Etiology

1. Acute coronary thrombosis (partial or total)—associated with 90% of MIs.
   a. Severe coronary artery disease (greater than 70% narrowing of the artery) precipitates thrombus formation.
   b. Intramural hemorrhage into atheromatous plaques causes the lesion to enlarge and occlude the vessel; dissecting hemorrhage can also occur.

c. The plaque ruptures into the vessel lumen, and a thrombus forms on top of the ulcerated lesion, with resultant vessel occlusion.
2. Other etiologic factors include coronary artery spasm, coronary artery embolism, infectious diseases causing arterial inflammation, hypoxia, anemia, and severe exertion or stress on the heart in the presence of significant coronary artery disease (ie, surgical procedures or shoveling snow).
3. Different degrees of damage occur to the heart muscle (Figure 13-1):
   a. *Zone of necrosis*—death to the heart muscle caused by extensive and complete oxygen deprivation; irreversible damage
   b. *Zone of injury*—region of the heart muscle surrounding the area of necrosis; inflamed and injured, but still viable if adequate oxygenation can be restored
   c. *Zone of ischemia*—region of the heart muscle surrounding the area of injury, which is ischemic and viable; not endangered unless extension of the infarction occurs
4. According to the layers of the heart muscle involved, MIs can be classified as:
   a. Transmural (Q wave) infarction—area of necrosis occurs throughout the entire thickness of the heart muscle.
   b. Subendocardial (nontransmural/non-Q) infarction—area of necrosis is confined to the innermost layer of the heart lining the chambers.

NURSING ALERT

Patients with subendocardial infarctions should be considered as having an uncompleted MI; monitor carefully for signs and symptoms of extension of heart muscle damage.

---

5. Location of MI is identified as the location of the damaged heart muscle within the left ventricle: inferior, anterior, lateral, and posterior or right ventricle.
   a. Left ventricle is the most common and dangerous location for an MI, because it is the main pumping chamber of the heart.
   b. Right ventricular infarctions commonly occur in conjunction with damage to the inferior and/or posterior wall of the left ventricle.
6. Region of the heart muscle that becomes damaged— determined by the coronary artery that becomes obstructed (Figure 13-2).
7. The amount of heart muscle damage and the location of the MI—determine prognosis.

Clinical Manifestations

1. Chest pain
   a. Severe, diffuse steady substernal pain of a crushing and squeezing nature
   b. Not relieved by rest or sublingual vasodilator therapy, but requires narcotics
   c. May radiate to the arms (commonly the left), shoulders, neck, back, and/or jaw
   d. Continues for more than 15 minutes
   e. May produce anxiety and fear, resulting in an increase in heart rate, blood pressure, and respiratory rate
2. Diaphoresis, cool clammy skin, facial pallor
3. Hypertension or hypotension
4. Bradycardia or tachycardia

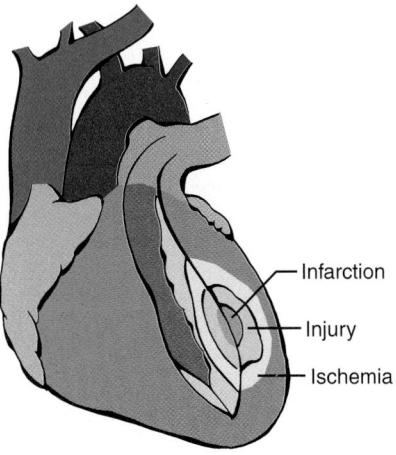

FIGURE 13-1 Different degrees of damage occur to the heart muscle after a myocardial infarction. The diagram shows the zones of necrosis, injury, and ischemia.

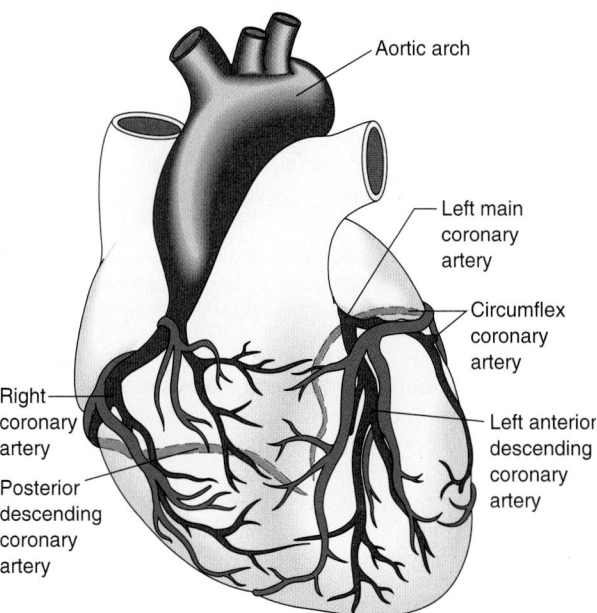

FIGURE 13-2 Diagram of the coronary arteries arising from the aorta and encircling the heart. Some of the coronary veins also are shown. (Chaffee, E. E., & Greisheimer, E. M. *Basic physiology and anatomy*. Philadelphia: J.B. Lippincott.)

5. Premature ventricular and/or atrial beats
6. Palpitations, severe anxiety, dyspnea
7. Disorientation, confusion, restlessness
8. Fainting, marked weakness
9. Nausea, vomiting, hiccups
10. Atypical symptoms: epigastric or abdominal distress, dull aching or tingling sensations, shortness of breath, extreme fatigue

> **NURSING ALERT**
>
> Many patients do not have symptoms; these are "silent myocardial infarctions." Nevertheless, there still is resultant damage to the heart. Women often present with atypical and/or vague complaints (eg, epigastric pain, "gas," feeling tired).

> **GERONTOLOGIC ALERT**
>
> Elderly patients are more likely to experience silent MIs or have atypical symptoms: hypotension, low body temperature, vague complaints of discomfort, mild perspiration, strokelike symptoms, dizziness, change in sensorium.

Diagnostic Evaluation

ECG Changes
1. Generally occur within 2 to 12 hours, but may take 72 to 96 hours.
2. Necrotic, injured, and ischemic tissue alters ventricular depolarization and repolarization.
   a. S–T segment depression and T wave inversion indicate a pattern of ischemia.
   b. S–T elevation indicates an injury pattern.
   c. Q waves (Figure 13-3) indicate tissue necrosis and are permanent. A pathologic Q wave is one that is greater than 3 mm in depth or greater than one third the height of the R wave.

> **NURSING ALERT**
>
> A normal ECG does not rule out the possibility of infarction, as ECG changes can be subtle and obscured by underlying conditions (bundle branch blocks, electrolyte disturbances).

Elevation of Serum Enzymes and Isoenzymes
1. Enzymes are drawn in a serial pattern, usually on admission and every 6 to 24 hours until three samples are obtained; enzyme activity then is correlated to the extent of heart muscle damage (see p. 314).
2. Enzymes commonly evaluated include creatinine kinase (CK), lactic dehydrogenase (LDH), and aspartate aminotransferase (AST).
3. CK and LDH can be broken down further into isoenzymes, which are more organ specific.
   a. CK-MB is specific to heart muscle and thus the most sensitive enzyme for determining heart muscle damage.

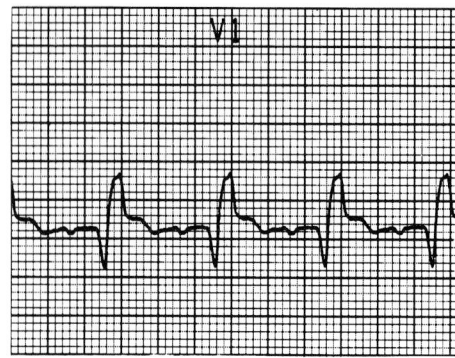

FIGURE 13-3 Abnormal Q wave.

   b. LDH_1 and LDH_2 are specific to heart muscle and thus elevated.

Other Findings
1. Elevated cardiac troponins
2. Elevated myoglonins
3. White blood cell count and sedimentation rate elevate due to inflammatory process associated with the damaged heart muscle.
4. Radionuclide imaging allows recognition of areas of decreased perfusion.
5. PET determines the presence of reversible heart muscle injury and irreversible or necrotic tissue; extent to which the injured heart muscle has responded to treatment also can be determined.
6. Cardiac muscle dysfunction noted on echocardiography.

Management

Therapy is aimed at the protection of ischemic and injured heart tissue to preserve muscle function, reduce the infarct size, and prevent death. Innovative modalities provide early restoration of coronary blood flow, and the use of pharmacologic agents improves oxygen supply and demand, reduces and/or prevents dysrhythmias, and inhibits the progression of coronary artery disease.

Oxygen Therapy
Improves oxygenation to ischemic heart muscle.

Pain Control
Endogenous catecholamine release during pain imposes an increased workload on the heart muscle, thus causing an increase in oxygen demand.
1. Opiate analgesic therapy
   a. Morphine is used to relieve pain, to improve cardiac hemodynamics by reducing preload and afterload, and to provide anxiety relief.
   b. Meperidine (Demerol) is useful for pain management in those patients allergic to morphine or sensitive to respiratory depression.
2. Vasodilator therapy
   a. Nitroglycerin (sublingual, IV, paste) promotes venous (low-dose) and arterial (high-dose) relaxation

as well as relaxation of coronary vessels and prevention of coronary spasm.
   b. Myocardial oxygen demand is reduced with subsequent pain relief.
   c. Persistent chest pain requires prompt action (IV nitroglycerin.)
3. Anxiolytic therapy
   a. Benzodiazepines are used with analgesics when anxiety complicates chest pain and its relief.

Pharmacologic Therapy

1. Thrombolytic agents, such as tissue plasminogen activator (Activase), streptokinase (Streptase), and reteplase (Retavase), reestablish blood flow in coronary vessels by dissolving obstructing thrombus.
   a. No effect on the underlying stenosis that precipitated the thrombus to form.
   b. Administered IV or intracoronary.
2. Adjunctive therapy aimed at preventing fibrinogen from adhering to activated platelets may include administration of eptifibatide (Integrilin) or abciximab (ReoPro), or, to prevent platelet activation, aspirin.
3. Anticoagulation therapy is useful as an adjunct to thrombolytic therapy. Also used in situations of prolonged bed rest, pulmonary embolism, deep vein thrombosis, mural thrombi, cardiogenic shock, and patients with atrial fibrillation.
4. Beta-adrenergic blocking agents improve oxygen supply and demand, decrease sympathetic stimulation to the heart, promote blood flow in the small vessels of the heart, and have antidysrhythmic effects.
   a. Appears to lower mortality and decrease chance of reinfarction and sudden death post-MI.
5. Antidysrhythmic therapy—lidocaine (Xylocaine) decreases ventricular irritability, which commonly occurs after MI.
6. Calcium channel blockers improve the balance between oxygen supply and demand by decreasing heart rate, blood pressure, and dilating coronary vessels.
   a. Diltiazem has been shown to decrease the incidence of reinfarction in patients with non-Q-wave MIs and is currently the only calcium blocker proven to be beneficial.

Percutaneous Transluminal Coronary Angioplasty (PTCA)

1. Mechanical opening of the coronary vessel can be performed during an evolving infarction.
2. PTCA can be used as an adjunct to thrombolytic therapy (see section titled PTCA, p. 345).

Surgical Revascularization

1. Emergency coronary artery bypass surgery can be performed within 6 hours of evolving infarction.
2. Definite treatment of the stenosis and less scar formation on the heart are the benefits of this therapy.

Complications

1. Rhythm disturbances
2. Cardiac failure
   a. Infarct expansion (thinning and dilation of the necrotic zone)
   b. Infarct extension (additional heart muscle necrosis occurring after 24 hours of acute infarction)
   c. CHF (with 20% to 35% left ventricle damage)
   d. Cardiogenic shock (see p. 370)
   f. Reinfarction
   g. Ischemic cardiomyopathy
3. Cardiac rupture
4. Papillary muscle rupture
5. Ventricular mural thrombus
6. Thromboemboli
7. Ventricular aneurysm
8. Cardiac tamponade
9. Pericarditis (2 to 3 days after MI)
10. Psychiatric problems—depression, personality changes

Nursing Assessment

1. Gather information regarding the patient's chest pain:
   a. Nature and intensity—describe the pain in patient's own words and compare it with pain experienced in the past.
   b. Onset and duration—exact time pain occurred, as well as the time pain relieved or diminished (if applicable).
   c. Location and radiation—point to the area where the pain is located and to other areas where the pain seems to travel.
   d. Precipitating and aggravating factors—describe the activity performed just before the onset of pain and if any maneuvers and/or medications alleviated the pain.
2. Question patient about other symptoms experienced associated with the pain. Observe patient for diaphoresis, facial pallor, dyspnea, guarding behaviors, rigid body posture, extreme weakness, confusion.
3. Evaluate cognitive, behavioral, and emotional status.
4. Question patient regarding prior health status with emphasis on current medications, allergies (opiate analgesics, iodine, shellfish), recent trauma or surgery, aspirin ingestion, peptic ulcers, fainting spells, drug and alcohol use.
5. Analyze information for contraindications for thrombolytic therapy and/or PTCA.
6. Gather information on presence or absence of cardiac risk factors.
7. Identify patient's social support system and potential caregiver(s).
8. Identify significant other's reaction to the crisis situation.

Nursing Diagnoses

Also see Nursing Care Plan 13-1.
- Pain related to an imbalance in oxygen supply and demand

NURSING CARE PLAN 13-1   Caring for a Patient With Acute MI

Mr. M. is a 60-year-old male admitted to your unit with a diagnosis of an acute inferior wall MI. From your assessment and knowledge of acute MI, you develop your plan of care.

Subjective data: Mr. M. is complaining of severe crushing chest pain unrelieved by rest, which has lasted for 2 hours. The pain is substernal and does not radiate. He tells you that he smokes two packs of cigarettes per day, is a manager at an electronics firm, and that his father died at age 59 from a heart attack.

Objective data: Vital signs: pulse 110 and irregular, BP 90/68, respirations 28. His cardiac monitor shows sinus tachycardia with frequent PVCs and his 12-lead ECG shows ST elevation in leads II, III, and AVF. He has no significant Q waves at this time. His heart sounds are normal except for the irregularity, and his lungs are clear. He is pale, diaphoretic, and holding his chest.

NURSING DIAGNOSIS   **Pain related to an imbalance in oxygen supply and demand**

GOAL (EXPECTED OUTCOME)   **Pain will be reduced.**

Nursing Interventions	Rationale	Outcomes (Evaluation)
1. Position Mr. M. in bed in semi-Fowler's position.	1. This allows for rest and adequate chest excursion, to increase available oxygen, and to decrease cardiac work.	1. Resting in semi-Fowler's position.
2. Administer oxygen by way of nasal cannula at 4 L/min.	2. To increase oxygen supply. May decrease pain and PVCs.	2. Color improved and verbalizes decreased pain.
3. Administer nitroglycerin and morphine based on vital signs and pain relief.	3. Both medications will help to alleviate pain by decreasing venous return to the heart, thereby decreasing cardiac work. Morphine will also help to decrease the patient's sensation of pain.	3. Verbalizes decreased pain.
4. Monitor BP closely by way of non-invasive BP monitor.	4. Both of the above medications may decrease the BP because both will decrease venous return. Intra-arterial blood pressure monitoring may be used if condition warrants.	4. BP remains stable.
5. Attach electrodes for continuous bedside cardiac monitor. Monitor heart rate and rhythm frequently.	5. Increases in heart rate may indicate heart blocks. Dysrhythmias are common during the initial stages of an acute MI.	5. Heart rate within normal limits.
6. Administer and monitor thrombolytic therapy.	6. May help to relieve the coronary occlusion.	6. Blood flow restored as evidenced by decreased pain and no further ECG changes.
7. Monitor for signs of bleeding; avoid unnecessary venous or arterial punctures.	7. Thrombolytics cause clot lysis, may cause bleeding.	7. No signs of bleeding.

NURSING DIAGNOSIS   **Decreased Cardiac Output related to decreased cardiac contractility and dysrhythmias**

GOAL (EXPECTED OUTCOME)   **Cardiac output will improve.**

Nursing Interventions	Rationale	Outcomes (Evaluation)
1. Administer IV fluids as ordered.	1. IV fluid may be necessary to compensate for the decreased venous return caused by nitrates and morphine.	1. BP improved.
2. Monitor closely for signs of developing left ventricular failure (ie, auscultate lung sounds for crackles and heart sounds for S_3).	2. Left ventricular failure may develop as a result of the decreased myocardial contractility and/or the administration of excess IV fluids.	2. Lungs clear and heart sounds normal.
3. Monitor urine output hourly.	3. A decrease in urine output may indicate a decrease in renal blood flow.	3. Urine output greater than 30 mL/h.
4. Monitor mental status.	4. A change in mental status may indicate a decrease in cardiac output.	4. Remains alert and oriented.

(continued)

NURSING CARE PLAN 13-1 Caring for a Patient With Acute MI (Continued)

Nursing Interventions	Rationale	Outcomes (Evaluation)
5. Employ hemodynamic monitoring: CVP and pulmonary artery pressures by way of a pulmonary artery catheter; calculate cardiac index and systemic vascular resistance.	5. These parameters will help to guide fluid volume administration, vasoactive drug administration, and assess cardiac performance.	5. CVP, PAP, PCWP, CI, and SVR remain within normal limits.
6. Interpret rhythm strip at least every 4 hours, more frequently as condition warrants. Administer antiarrhythmics, if indicated.	6. Dysrhythmias such as PVCs result in a decreased stroke volume and less coronary artery filling time. Frequent monitoring, especially during the first few hours of an acute MI and during thrombolytic therapy administration, is necessary to prevent/treat lethal dysrhythmias.	6. PVCs decreasing in frequency.
7. Administer vasopressors; titrate to BP response.	7. Administration of vasopressors in the setting of acute MI is controversial in that they may cause an increase in systemic vascular resistance, which increases cardiac work.	7. BP improved without worsening chest pain or ECG changes.

NURSING DIAGNOSIS   Anxiety related to chest pain, fear of death, threatening environment, invasive therapies, and uncertain prognosis

GOAL (EXPECTED OUTCOME)   Anxiety will be alleviated.

Nursing Interventions	Rationale	Outcomes (Evaluation)
1. Explain equipment, procedures, and need for frequent assessment to Mr. M. and his family. Discuss visiting hours and the need to allow for rest.	1. Aids in decreasing anxiety due to threatening environment.	1. Mr. M. and family verbalize understanding of plan of care. Plan for visiting established.
2. Observe for autonomic signs/symptoms of anxiety (eg, increased heart rate, BP, and respiratory rate).	2. Anxiety is associated with an increase in sympathetic activity, which increases cardiac work.	2. No autonomic signs of anxiety.
3. Administer diazepam (Valium).	3. May aid in limiting Mr. M.'s anxiety.	3. Verbalizes decrease in anxiety after medication.
4. Offer back massage.	4. Touch and massage may promote relaxation.	4. Verbalizes decrease in tension after massage.
5. Maintain continuity of care.	5. Consistency of routine and staff promotes trust and confidence.	5. Cooperative with care and talkative with staff.

- Anxiety related to chest pain, fear of death, threatening environment
- Decreased Cardiac Output related to impaired contractility
- Activity Intolerance related to insufficient oxygenation to perform activities of daily living (ADL), deconditioning effects of bed rest
- Risk for Injury (bleeding) related to dissolution of protective clots
- Altered Tissue Perfusion (myocardial) related to coronary restenosis, extension of infarction
- Ineffective Individual Coping related to threats to self-esteem, disruption of sleep–rest pattern, lack of significant support system, and loss of control

Nursing Interventions
Reducing Pain

1. Handle patient carefully while providing initial care, starting IV infusion, obtaining baseline vital signs, and attaching electrodes for continuous ECG monitoring.
2. Administer oxygen by nasal cannula if prescribed, and encourage patient to take deep breaths—may decrease incidence of dysrhythmias by allowing the heart to be less ischemic and less irritable; may reduce infarct size, decrease anxiety, and resolve chest pain.
3. Offer support and reassurance to patient that relief of pain is a priority.
4. Administer sublingual nitroglycerin as directed; recheck blood pressure (BP), heart rate (HR), and respiratory rate

before administering nitrate therapy and 10 to 15 minutes after dose.

5. Administer narcotics as prescribed (morphine [Duramorph] or meperidine [Demerol])—decreases sympathetic activity and reduces heart rate, respirations, blood pressure, muscle tension, and anxiety.
   a. Use caution in administering narcotics to patients with chronic obstructive pulmonary disease, hypotension, dehydration, and to the elderly.
   b. Be alert that meperidine can have a vagolytic effect and cause tachycardia, thus increasing myocardial oxygen demands.

GERONTOLOGIC ALERT

Elderly patients are extremely susceptible to respiratory depression in response to narcotics. Analgesic agents with less profound effects on the respiratory center should be used. Anxiolytic agents also should be used with caution.

6. Obtain baseline vital signs before giving agents and 10 to 15 minutes after each dose. Place patient in a supine position during administration to minimize hypotension.

7. Give IV nitroglycerin as prescribed. Monitor BP continuously with automatic blood pressure machine or intra-arterially or every 5 minutes with auscultatory method while titrating for pain relief.

NURSING ALERT

Intravenous (IV) administration is the preferred route for analgesic medication, because intramuscular injections can cause elevations in serum enzymes, resulting in an incorrect diagnosis of myocardial infarction.

8. Review with patient frequently the importance of reporting any chest pain, discomfort, and/or epigastric distress without delay.

Alleviating Anxiety

1. Rule out physiologic etiologies for increasing or new onset of anxiety before administering prn sedatives. Physiologic causes must be identified and treated in a timely fashion to prevent irreversible adverse or even fatal outcomes; sedatives may mask symptoms, delaying timely identification/diagnosis and treatment.

2. Assess patient for signs of hypoperfusion, auscultate heart and lung sounds, obtain a rhythm strip, and administer oxygen as prescribed. Notify the health care provider immediately.

3. Document all assessment findings, health care provider notification and response, and interventions and response.

4. Explain to the patient and family reasons for hospitalization, diagnostic tests, and therapies administered.

5. Explain equipment, procedures, and need for frequent assessment to patient and significant others.

6. Discuss with patient and family member the anticipated nursing and medical regimen.
   a. Explain visiting hours and need to limit number of visitors at one time.
   b. Offer family members preferred times to phone unit to check on patient's status.

7. Observe for autonomic signs of anxiety such as increases in heart rate, BP, respiratory rate, tremulousness.

8. Administer antianxiety agents as prescribed.
   a. Explain to patient the reason for sedation: undue anxiety can make the heart more irritable and require more oxygen.
   b. Assure patient that the goal of sedation is to promote comfort and, therefore, should be requested if anxious, excitable, or "jittery" feelings occur.
   c. Observe for adverse effects of sedation such as lethargy, confusion, and/or increased agitation.

9. Maintain consistency of care with one or two nurses regularly assisting patient, especially if severe anxiety is present.

10. Offer back massage to promote relaxation, decrease muscle tension, and improve skin integrity.

11. Use techniques such as guided imagery to relieve tension and anxiety.

Maintaining Hemodynamic Stability

1. Monitor BP every 2 hours or as directed—hypertension increases afterload of the heart, elevating oxygen demand; hypotension causes reduced coronary and tissue perfusion.

2. Monitor respirations and lung fields every 2 to 4 hours or as prescribed.
   a. Auscultate for normal and abnormal breath sounds (crackles may indicate left ventricular failure; diffuse crackles indicate pulmonary edema).

NURSING ALERT

Auscultation of clear lungs in the presence of cool, clammy skin, jugular venous distention, and hypotension may indicate right ventricular infarction.

   b. Observe for dyspnea, tachypnea, frothy pink sputum, orthopnea—may indicate left ventricular failure, pulmonary embolus, pulmonary edema.

3. Evaluate heart rate and heart sounds every 2 to 4 hours or as directed.
   a. Compare apical heart rate with radial pulse rate, and determine the pulse deficit.
   b. Auscultate heart for the presence of a third heart sound (failing ventricle), fourth heart sound (stiffening ventricular muscle due to MI), friction rub (pericarditis), murmurs (valvular and papillary muscle dysfunction, intraventricular septal rupture).

4. Note presence of jugular venous distention and liver engorgement.

a. Estimate right atrial pressure by determining jugular venous pressure.

b. Observe for hepatojugular reflux.

5. Evaluate the major arterial pulses (weak pulse and/or presence of pulsus alternans indicates decreased cardiac output; irregularity results from dysrhythmias).

6. Take body temperature every 4 hours or as directed (most patients develop an increase in temperature within 24 to 48 hours due to tissue necrosis).

7. Observe for presence of edema.

8. Monitor skin color and temperature (cool, clammy skin and pallor associated with vasoconstriction secondary to decreased cardiac output).

9. Be alert to change in mental status, such as confusion, restlessness, disorientation.

10. Employ hemodynamic monitoring as indicated.

11. Evaluate urine output (30 mL/h)—decrease in volume reflects a decrease in renal blood flow.

12. Monitor for life-threatening dysrhythmias (common within 24 hours following infarctions).

a. Be vigilant for occurrence of any type of premature ventricular beats—may predict ventricular fibrillation or ventricular tachycardia.

b. Anticipate possibility of reperfusion dysrhythmias after thrombolytic therapy.

c. Correct dysrhythmias immediately as directed. Lidocaine (Xylocaine) may be given prophylactically to protect against ventricular fibrillation and ventricular tachycardia.

Increasing Activity Tolerance

1. Promote rest with early gradual increase in mobilization—prevents deconditioning, which occurs with bed rest.

a. Minimize environmental noise.

b. Provide a comfortable environmental temperature.

c. Avoid unnecessary interruptions and procedures.

d. Structure routine care measures to include rest periods after activity.

e. Discuss with patient and family members the purpose of limited activity and visitors—to help the heart heal by lowering heart rate and blood pressure to maintain cardiac workload at lowest level and decrease oxygen consumption.

f. Promote restful diversional activities for patient (reading, listening to music, drawing, crossword puzzles, crafts).

g. Encourage frequent position changes while in bed.

2. Assist patient with prescribed activities.

a. Assist patient to rise slowly from a supine position to minimize orthostatic hypotension.

b. Encourage passive and active range-of-motion exercise as directed while on bed rest.

c. Measure the length and width of the unit so patients can gradually increase their activity levels with specific guidelines (walk one width [150 ft] of the unit).

d. Elevate patient's feet when out of bed in chair to promote venous return.

e. Implement a step-by-step program for progressive activity as directed.

Preventing Bleeding

1. Take vital signs every 15 minutes during infusion of thrombolytic agent and then hourly.

2. Observe for presence of hematomas or skin breakdown, especially in potential pressure areas such as the sacrum, back, elbows, ankles.

3. Be alert to verbal complaints of back pain indicative of possible retroperitoneal bleeding.

4. Observe all puncture sites every 15 minutes during infusion of thrombolytic therapy and then hourly for bleeding.

5. Apply manual pressure to venous or arterial sites if bleeding occurs. Use pressure dressings for coverage of all access sites.

6. Observe for blood in stool, emesis, urine, and sputum.

7. Minimize venipunctures and arterial punctures; use heparin lock for blood sampling and medication administration.

8. Avoid intramuscular injections.

9. Caution patient about vigorous tooth brushing, hair combing, or shaving.

10. Avoid trauma to patient by minimizing frequent handling of patient.

11. Monitor lab work: prothrombin time (PT), partial thromboplastin time (PTT), hematocrit (Hct), and hemoglobin (Hgb).

12. Check for current blood type and crossmatch.

13. Administer antacids as directed to prevent stress ulcers.

14. Implement emergency interventions as directed in the event of bleeding: fluid, volume expanders, blood products.

15. Monitor for changes in mental status and headache.

16. Avoid vigorous oral suctioning.

17. Avoid use of automatic BP device above puncture sites or hematoma. Use care in taking BP; use arm not being used for thrombolytic therapy.

Maintaining Tissue Perfusion

1. Observe for persistent and/or recurrence of signs and symptoms of ischemia: chest pain, diaphoresis, hypotension—may indicate extension of MI and/or reocclusion of coronary vessel.

2. Report immediately.

3. Administer oxygen as directed.

4. Record a 12-lead ECG.

5. Prepare patient for possible emergency procedure(s): cardiac catheterization, bypass surgery, PTCA, thrombolytic therapy.

Strengthening Coping Abilities

1. Listen carefully to patient and family members to ascertain their cognitive appraisals of stressors and threats.

2. Assist patient to establish a positive attitude toward illness and progress adaptively through the grieving process.
3. Manipulate environment to promote restful sleep by maintaining patient's usual sleep patterns.
4. Be alert to signs and symptoms of sleep deprivation—irritability, disorientation, hallucinations, diminished pain tolerance, aggressiveness.
5. Minimize possible adverse emotional response to transfer from the intensive care unit to the intermediate care unit:
   a. Introduce the admitting nurse from the intermediate care unit to the patient before transfer.
   b. Plan for the intermediate care nurse to answer questions the patient may have and to inform patient what to expect relative to physical layout of unit, nursing routines, and visiting hours.

Patient Education and Health Maintenance

Goals are to restore patient to optimal physiologic, psychological, social, and work level; aid in restoring confidence and self-esteem; develop patient's self-monitoring skills, and assist in managing cardiac problems; modify risk factors.

1. Inform the patient and family member about what has happened to heart.
   a. Explain basic cardiac anatomy and physiology
   b. Identify the difference between angina and MI.
   c. Describe how the heart heals and that healing is not complete for 6 to 8 weeks after attack.
   d. Discuss what the patient can do to assist in the recovery process and reduce the chance of future heart attacks.
2. Instruct patient on how to judge the body's response to activity.
   a. Introduce the concept that different activities require varied expenditures of oxygen.
   b. Emphasize the importance of rest and relaxation alternating with activity.
   c. Instruct patient how to take pulse before and after activity, as well as guidelines for the acceptable increases in heart rate that should occur.
   d. Review signs and symptoms indicative of a poor response to increased activity levels: chest pain, extreme fatigue, shortness of breath.
3. Design an individualized activity progression program for patient as directed.
   a. Determine activity levels appropriate for patient as prescribed and by predischarge low-level exercise stress test.
   b. Encourage patient and family member to list activities they enjoy and would like to resume.
   c. Establish the energy expenditure of each activity (ie, which are most demanding on the heart), and rank activities from lowest to highest.
   d. Instruct patient to move from one activity to another after the heart has been able to manage the previous workload as determined by signs and symptoms and pulse rate.
4. Give patient specific activity guidelines, and explain that activity guidelines will be reevaluated after heart heals:
   a. Walk daily, gradually increasing distance and time as prescribed.
   b. Avoid activities that tense muscles, such as weight lifting, lifting heavy objects, isometric exercises, pushing and/or pulling heavy loads.
   c. Avoid working with arms overhead.
   d. Gradually return to work.
   e. Avoid extremes in temperature.
   f. Do not rush; avoid tension.
   g. Advise getting at least 7 hours of sleep each night and take 20- to 30-minute rest periods twice a day.
   h. Advise limiting visitors to three to four daily for 15 to 30 minutes and shorten phone conversations.
5. Tell patient that sexual relations may be resumed on advice of health care provider, usually after exercise tolerance is assessed.
   a. If patient can walk briskly or climb two flights of stairs, he or she can usually resume sexual activity with familiar partner; resumption of sexual activity parallels resumption of usual activities.
   b. Sexual activity should be avoided after eating a heavy meal, after drinking alcohol, or when tired.
6. Advise eating three to four small meals per day rather than large, heavy meals. Rest 1 hour after meals.
7. Advise limiting caffeine and alcohol intake.
8. Driving a car must be cleared with health care provider at a follow-up visit.
9. Teach patient about medication regimen and side effects.
10. Instruct the patient to notify the health care provider when the following symptoms appear:
    a. Chest pressure or pain not relieved in 15 minutes by nitroglycerin or rest
    b. Shortness of breath
    c. Unusual fatigue
    d. Swelling of feet and ankles
    e. Fainting, dizziness
    f. Very slow or rapid heart beat
11. Assist patient to reduce risk of another MI by risk factor modification.
    a. Explain to patient the major risk factors that can increase chances for having another MI: smoking, high blood cholesterol levels, and hypertension. Related risk factors include obesity, family history, diabetes, stress, and lack of exercise.
    b. Instruct patient in strategies to modify risk factors.
12. For additional information and support refer to:
    The American Heart, Lung, and Blood Institute
    Public Inquiries and Reports Office
    Building 31
    Bethesda, MD 20205

Outcome-Based Evaluation

- Patient pain free; easily arousable
- No signs of anxiety or agitation
- Vital signs stable, lung fields clear, urine output adequate
- Activity slowly progressing and tolerated well
- No signs of bleeding
- No recurrent chest pain
- Sleeping well; emotionally stable

▣ Hyperlipidemia

Hyperlipidemia is a group of metabolic abnormalities resulting in combinations of elevated serum total cholesterol (hypercholesterolemia), elevated low-density lipoprotein, elevated triglycerides (hypertriglyceridemia), and decreased high-density lipoprotein. Up to 50% of Americans may have elevated cholesterol. These abnormalities are the primary risk factor for atherosclerosis and coronary artery disease.

Pathophysiology and Etiology

Primary Hyperlipidemias

1. Genetic metabolic abnormalities resulting in the overproduction or underproduction of specific lipoproteins or enzymes. They are rare but tend to run in families.
2. Primary hyperlipidemias include hypercholesterolemia, defective apolipoproteinemia, hypertriglyceridemia, combined hyperlipidemia, dysbetalipoproteinemia, polygenic hypercholesterolemia, lipoprotein lipase deficiency, apoprotein C-II deficiency, lethicin cholesterol acetyltransferase deficiency.

Secondary Hyperlipidemias

1. Very common and are multifactorial.
2. Etiologic factors include chronic diseases such as diabetes, hypothyroidism, nephrotic syndrome, liver disease obesity, dietary intake, conditions such as pregnancy and alcoholism, medications such as beta blockers and diuretics.

Consequences

1. Atherosclerotic plaque formation in blood vessels.
2. Causes narrowing, possible ischemia, and may lead to thromboembolus formation.
3. Result in cardiovascular, cerebrovascular, and peripheral vascular disease.

Clinical Manifestations

1. Usually asymptomatic until significant target organ damage is done
2. May be metabolic signs such as corneal arcus, xanthoma, xanthelasma, pancreatitis
3. Chest pain, myocardial infarction
4. Transient ischemic attacks, stroke
5. Intermittent claudication, arterial occlusion of lower extremities

Diagnostic Evaluation

1. Screening cholesterol and HDL may be done on non-fasting basis.
2. Total cholesterol (TC) and high-density lipoproteins (HDL)
   a. If TC <200 mg/dL and HDL >35 mg/dL, screening is repeated in 5 years.
   b. If TC <200 mg/dL and HDL <35, do fasting lipoprotein analysis.
   c. If TC 200 to 239 mg/dL and HDL ≥35 mg/dL and patient has less than two risk factors, repeat screening in 1 to 2 years.
   d. If TC 200 to 239 mg/dL and HDL <35 mg/dL or patient has two or more risk factors, do lipoprotein analysis.
3. Base treatment and follow-up on lipoprotein analysis.
   a. If LDL is <130 mg/dL, repeat in 5 years.
   b. If LDL is 130 to 159 mg/dL and patient has less than two risk factors, repeat in 1 year.
   c. If LDL is >160 mg/dL or patient has two or more risk factors, initiate therapy and repeat in 1 year.
4. If patient already has established coronary artery disease:
   a. And LDL <100 mg/dL, no therapy but repeat in 1 year.
   b. And LDL >100 mg/dL, start therapy and repeat as needed.

Management

National Cholesterol Education Program (NCEP) Guidelines

1. Correction or control of secondary disorders such as diabetes, alcoholism, hypothyroidism.
2. Multidimensional approach including diet, exercise, weight loss, and drug treatment.
3. Lifestyle modification is indicated for all with TC >200 mg/dL—decreased fat intake, increased exercise, and risk factor awareness and reduction.
4. Step 1 diet allows no more than 30% of total required calories from fat, including no more than 8% to 10% saturated fat calories, and less than 300 mg daily cholesterol intake.
5. Step 2 diet allows no more than 7% of calories from saturated fat and <200 mg cholesterol.
6. Those with TC >239 mg/dL, or cholesterol >200 and HDL <35 or LDL >160 should follow heart healthy diet with no more than 30% of calories coming from fat, including no more than 8% to 10% of calories coming from saturated fat, and less than 300 mg cholesterol per day.
7. Drug therapy should be considered if LDL >190 mg/dL with less than two risk factors, or LDL >160 and two or more risk factors.
8. If patient already has coronary artery disease, diet and exercise therapy should be instituted for LDL >100 mg/dL; drug therapy should be instituted for LDL >130.

Drug Therapy Options

1. Bile acid sequestrants such cholestyramine (Questran) or colestipol (Colestid). Main side effects are gastro-intestinal (GI) related—bloating, flatus, interaction with other medications taken orally.
2. Nicotonic acid. Main side effect is severe flushing; taking aspirin 325 mg before may help.
3. Fibrinic acid derivatives such as gemfibrozil (Lopid)—may cause myopathy.
4. HMG CoA reductase inhibitors ("statins") such as pravastatin (Pravachol) and atorvastatin (Lipitor).
   a. Most expensive agents but best tolerated
   b. Require liver function monitoring because can elevate transaminases
   c. Also may cause myopathy

Complications

1. Disability from myocardial infarction, stroke, and lower extremity ischemia.

Nursing Assessment

1. Obtain history of chronic diseases; medications; and cardiovascular risk factors such as smoking, family history of premature CAD, postmenopausal, and so forth.
2. Obtain diet history.
3. Inspect for xanthomas (cholesterol deposits on skin), xanthalasmas (cholesterol deposits on eyelids), and corneal arcus (ring around cornea, significant in patients under 50).
4. Examine for signs of peripheral vascular disease—decreased pulses; cool, pale extremities; loss of hair; and shiny skin.
5. Examine for carotid bruit.
6. Obtain ECG for ischemic changes.

Nursing Interventions and Patient Education

1. Teach diet basics and obtain nutritional consult.
2. Teach patient to engage in exercise, approximately 30 minutes a day, including walking, stationary bicycle riding, and so forth. Tell patients that studies have shown significant decreased mortality from walking 2 miles a day.
3. Engage the patient in smoking cessation program.
4. Tell patients that 1% decrease in cholesterol results in 2% reduced risk of coronary artery disease.
5. Explain goal LDL numbers (<130 if no CAD, <100 if CAD present) for patients on drug therapy, and have patient keep log of lipid results.
6. Encourage follow-up laboratory work—repeat lipoprotein analysis and liver function test monitoring every 3 months for those on HMG CoA reductase inhibitors.
7. Teach patient on bile acid sequestrants not to take other medications for 1 hour before or 2 hours afterward, because it prevents absorption of many medications.

Cardiogenic Shock

Cardiogenic shock occurs when the heart muscle loses its contractile power. Extensive damage of the left ventricle (40% or greater) due to myocardial infarction commonly initiates a perpetuating "shock cycle."

Pathophysiology and Etiology

1. Impaired contractility causes a marked reduction in cardiac output.
2. Decreased cardiac output results in a lack of blood and oxygen to the heart as well as other vital organs (brain and kidneys).
3. Lack of blood and oxygen to the heart muscle results in continued damage to the muscle, a further decline in contractile power, and a continued inability of the heart to provide blood and oxygen to vital organs.
4. End-stage cardiomyopathy, severe valvular dysfunction, and ventricular aneurysm also can precipitate cardiogenic shock.

Clinical Manifestations

1. Confusion, restlessness, mental lethargy (due to poor perfusion of brain)
2. Low systolic pressure (80 mm Hg or 30 mm Hg less than previous levels)
3. Oliguria—urine output less than 30 mL/h for at least 2 hours—due to decreased perfusion of kidneys
4. Cold, clammy skin (blood is shunted from the peripheral circulation to perfuse vital organs)
5. Weak, thready peripheral pulses, fatigue, hypotension—due to inadequate cardiac output
6. Dyspnea, tachypnea, cyanosis (increased left ventricular pressures result in elevation of left atrial and pulmonary pressures, causing pulmonary congestion)
7. Dysrhythmias (due to lack of oxygen to heart muscle) and sinus tachycardia (as a compensatory mechanism for a decreased cardiac output)
8. Chest pain (due to lack of oxygen and blood to heart muscle)

Diagnostic Evaluation

1. Altered hemodynamic parameters (PCWP 18 mm Hg or greater, cardiac index less than 2.2, systemic vascular resistance elevation, decreased SvO_2)
2. Chest x-ray—pulmonary vascular congestion
3. Abnormal laboratory values—elevated blood urea nitrogen (BUN) and creatinine, elevated liver enzymes, elevated serum lactate

Management
Pharmacologic Therapy

1. Cardiac glycosides (digoxin, [Lanoxin]) and positive inotropic drugs (dopamine [Intropin], dobutamine [Dobutrex], amrinone [Inocor], milrinone [Primacor]) stim-

ulate cardiac contractility. Use dobutamine, amrinone, and milrinone with caution because they may lower the blood pressure.

NURSING ALERT

 Use vasoactive drugs with extreme caution in the presence of cardiogenic shock. They require constant vigilance and astute observation to maintain an adequate perfusion pressure while achieving afterload reduction.

---

2. Vasodilator therapy
   a. Decreases the workload of the heart by reducing venous return and lessening the resistance against which the heart pumps (preload and afterload reduction).
   b. Cardiac output improves, left ventricular pressures and pulmonary congestion decrease, and myocardial oxygen consumption is reduced.
3. Vasopressor therapy is controversial because it may increase systemic vascular resistance.
4. Diuretic therapy
   a. Decreases total body fluid volume
   b. Relieves systemic and pulmonary congestion

Counterpulsation Therapy (see p. 348)
1. Improves blood flow to the heart muscle and reduces myocardial oxygen needs
2. Results in improved cardiac output and preservation of viable heart tissue

Cardiopulmonary Bypass
Left Ventricular Assist Device (LVAD)
1. Involves cannulation of the left atrium and aorta to shunt blood to an external pump and return it to the central circulation, thereby assisting the left ventricle in its work.
2. May only be performed in areas where immediate access to emergency cardiac surgery is available.

Emergency Cardiac Surgery (see p. 350)
1. Bypass graft
2. Heart transplantation

Complications
1. Neurologic impairment
2. Acute respiratory distress syndrome (ARDS)
3. Renal failure
4. Multiorgan dysfunction syndrome
5. Death

Nursing Assessment
1. Identify patients at risk for development of cardiogenic shock.
2. Assess for early signs and symptoms indicative of shock:
   a. Restlessness, confusion, or change in mental status
   b. Increasing heart rate
   c. Decreasing pulse pressure (indicates impaired cardiac output)

   d. Presence of pulsus alternans (indicates left heart failure)
   e. Decreasing urine output, weakness, fatigue
3. Observe for presence of central and peripheral cyanosis.
4. Observe for development of edema.
5. Identify signs and symptoms indicative of extension of myocardial infarction—recurrence of chest pain, diaphoresis.
6. Identify patient's and significant other's reaction to crisis situation.

NURSING ALERT

 Cardiogenic shock carries an extremely high mortality rate. Astute assessments and immediate actions are essential in preventing death.

Nursing Diagnoses
- Decreased Cardiac Output related to impaired contractility due to extensive heart muscle damage
- Impaired Gas Exchange related to pulmonary congestion due to elevated left ventricular pressures
- Altered Tissue Perfusion (renal, cerebral, cardiopulmonary, GI, and peripheral) related to decreased blood flow
- Anxiety related to intensive care environment and threat of death

Nursing Interventions
Improving Cardiac Output
1. Establish continuous ECG monitoring to detect dysrhythmias, which increase myocardial oxygen consumption.
2. Monitor hemodynamic parameters continually with Swan-Ganz catheter (see p. 320) to evaluate effectiveness of implemented therapy.
   a. Obtain PAP, PCWP, and CO readings as indicated.
   b. Calculate the cardiac index (CI; cardiac output relative to body size) and systemic vascular resistance (SVR; measurement of afterload).
   c. Cautiously titrate vasoactive drug therapy according to hemodynamic parameters.
      (i) Be alert to adverse responses to drug therapy; dopamine (Intropin) may cause increase in heart rate; vasodilators nitroglycerin (Tridil) and nitroprusside (Nipride) may worsen hypotension; digoxin (Lanoxin) may result in dysrhythmias from toxicity; diuretics may cause hyponatremia, hypokalemia, and hypovolemia.
      (ii) Administer vasoactive drug therapy through central venous access (peripheral tissue necrosis can occur if peripheral IV access infiltrates, and peripheral drug distribution may be lessened from vasoconstriction).
3. Monitor blood pressure and mean arterial pressure (MAP) with intra-arterial line (cuff pressures are diffi-

cult to ascertain and may be inaccurate) every 30 minutes and every 5 minutes during active titration of vasoactive drug therapy.

4. Maintain MAP greater than 60 mm Hg (blood flow through coronary vessels is inadequate with a MAP less than 60 mm Hg).

5. Measure and record urine output every hour from indwelling catheter and fluid intake.

6. Obtain daily weights.

7. Evaluate serum electrolytes for hyponatremia and hypokalemia.

8. Be alert to incidence of chest pain (indicates myocardial ischemia and may further extend heart damage).
   a. Report immediately.
   b. Obtain a 12-lead ECG recording.
   c. Anticipate use of counterpulsation therapy.

Improving Oxygenation

1. Monitor rate and rhythm of respirations every hour.

2. Auscultate lung fields for abnormal sounds (coarse crackles indicate severe pulmonary congestion) every hour; notify health care provider.

3. Evaluate arterial blood gases (ABGs).

4. Administer oxygen therapy to increase oxygen tension and improve hypoxia.

5. Elevate head of bed 20 to 30 degrees as tolerated (may worsen hypotension) to facilitate lung expansion.

6. Reposition patient frequently to promote ventilation and maintain skin integrity.

7. Observe for frothy pink-tinged sputum and cough (may indicate pulmonary edema); report immediately.

Maintaining Tissue Perfusion

1. Perform a neurologic check every hour, using the Glasgow Coma Scale.

2. Report changes immediately.

3. Obtain BUN and creatinine blood levels to evaluate renal function.

4. Auscultate for bowel sounds every 2 hours.

5. Evaluate character, rate, rhythm, and quality of arterial pulses every 2 hours.

6. Monitor temperature every 2 to 4 hours.

7. Employ sheepskin foot and elbow protectors to prevent skin breakdown.

Relieving Anxiety

1. As with the above, always evaluate signs of increasing anxiety and/or new onset anxiety for a physiologic cause before treating with anxiolytics.

2. Explain equipment and rationale for therapy to patient and family. Increasing knowledge assists in alleviating fear and anxiety.

3. Encourage patient to verbalize fears concerning diagnosis and prognosis.

4. Explain sensations patient will experience before procedures and routine care measures.

5. Offer reassurance and encouragement.

6. Provide for periods of uninterrupted rest and sleep.

7. Assist patient to maintain as much control as possible over environment and care.
   a. Develop a schedule for routine care measures and rest periods with patient.
   b. Ensure that a calendar and clock are in view of patient.

Patient Education and Health Maintenance

1. Teach patients on digoxin (Lanoxin) the importance of taking their medication as prescribed, taking pulse before daily dose, and reporting for periodic blood levels.

2. Teach signs of impending heart failure—increasing edema, shortness of breath, decreasing urine output, decreasing blood pressure, increasing pulse—and tell patient to notify health care provider immediately.

3. See specific measures for myocardial infarction (see p. 360), cardiomyopathy (see p. 380), and valvular disease (see p. 387).

Outcome-Based Evaluation

- CO greater than 4 L/min; CI greater than 2.2, PCWP less than 18 mm Hg
- Respirations unlabored and regular; normal breath sounds throughout lung fields
- Normal sensorium; urine output adequate; skin warm and dry
- Verbalizes lessened anxiety and fear

◼ Infective Endocarditis

Infective endocarditis (IE; bacterial endocarditis) is an infection of the inner lining of the heart caused by direct invasion of bacteria or other organisms leading to deformity of the valve leaflets.

Pathophysiology and Etiology

1. When the inner lining of the heart (endocardium) becomes inflamed, a fibrin clot (vegetation) forms.

2. The fibrin clot may become colonized by pathogens during transient episodes of bacteremia resulting from invasive procedures (venous/arterial cannulation, dental work causing gingival bleeding, GI tract surgery, liver biopsy, sigmoidoscopy, and so forth), indwelling catheters, urinary tract infections, and wound/skin infections.

3. Platelets and fibrin surround the invading microorganisms, forming a protective covering and causing the infected vegetation to enlarge.
   a. The enlarged vegetation (the basic lesion of endocarditis) can deform, thicken, stiffen, and scar the free margins of valve leaflets, as well as the fibrous ring (annulus) supporting the valve.
   b. The vegetation(s) may also travel to various organs/tissues (spleen, kidney, coronary artery, brain, and lungs) and obstruct blood flow.
   c. The "protective covering" surrounding the vegetation makes it difficult for white blood cells and anti-

microbial agents to infiltrate and destroy the infected lesion.

4. Causal organisms include:
   a. Bacteria
      (i) *Streptococcus viridans*—bacteremia occurs after dental work or upper respiratory infection.
      (ii) *Staphylococcus aureus*—bacteremia occurs after cardiac surgery or parenteral drug abuse.
      (iii) Enterococci (penicillin-resistant group D streptococci)—bacteremia usually occurs in elderly patients (over age 60) with genitourinary tract infection.
   b. Fungi (*Candida albicans, Aspergillus*)
   c. Rickettsieae

5. Infective endocarditis may develop on a heart valve already injured by rheumatic fever, congenital defects, on abnormally vascularized valves, normal heart valves, and mechanical/biologic heart valves.

6. Infective endocarditis may be acute or subacute, depending on the microorganisms involved. Acute IE manifests rapidly with danger of intractable heart failure and occurs more commonly on normal heart valves.

7. Subacute IE manifests a prolonged chronic course with a lesser chance of complications and occurs more commonly on damaged or defective valves.

8. Infective endocarditis may follow cardiac surgery, especially when prosthetic heart valves are used. Foreign bodies such as pacemakers, patches, grafts, and dialysis shunts predispose to infection.

9. High incidence among drug abusers, in whom the disease mainly affects normal valves, usually the tricuspid.

10. Hospitalized patients with indwelling catheters, those on prolonged IV therapy or prolonged antibiotic therapy, and those on immunosuppressive drugs or steroids may develop fungal endocarditis.

11. Relapse due to metastatic infection is possible, usually within the first 2 months after completion of antibiotic regimen.

Clinical Manifestations

Severity of manifestations depends on invading microorganism.

General Manifestations

1. Fever, chills, sweats (fever may be absent in elderly or in patients with uremia)
2. Anorexia, weight loss, weakness
3. Cough, back and joint pain (especially in patients over age 60)
4. Splenomegaly

Skin and Nail Manifestations

1. Petechiae—conjunctiva, mucous membranes.
2. Splinter hemorrhages in nail beds.
3. Osler's nodes—painful red nodes on pads of fingers and toes; usually late sign of infection and found with a subacute infection.

4. Janeway's lesions—light pink macules on palms or soles, nontender, may change to light tan within several days, fade in 1 to 2 weeks. Usually an early sign of endocardial infection.

Heart Manifestations

1. New pathologic or changing murmur—no murmur with other signs and symptoms may indicate right heart infection.
2. Tachycardia—related to decreased cardiac output.

Central Nervous System Manifestations

1. Localized headaches
2. Transient cerebral ischemia
3. Altered mental status, aphasia
4. Hemiplegia
5. Cortical sensory loss
6. Roth's spots on fundi

Pulmonary Manifestations

1. Usually occur with right-sided heart involvement
2. Pneumonitis, pleuritis, pulmonary edema, pulmonary infiltrates

Embolic Phenomena

1. Lung—hemoptysis, chest pain, shortness of breath
2. Kidney—hematuria
3. Spleen—pain in upper left quadrant of abdomen radiating to left shoulder
4. Heart—myocardial infarction
5. Brain—sudden blindness, paralysis, brain abscess, meningitis
6. Blood vessels—mycotic aneurysms
7. Abdomen—melena, acute pain

Diagnostic Evaluation

Varied clinical manifestations and similarities to other diseases make early diagnosis of IE difficult.

1. Blood cultures—at least two positive serial blood cultures isolating bacteria or fungi
2. Elevated sedimentation rate, tests indicative of anemia, mild leukocytosis, urine abnormalities indicating nephrosis
3. ECG—usually normal
4. Echocardiography—identification of vegetations and assessment of location and size of lesions

Management

1. Antimicrobial therapy based on sensitivity of causative agent: penicillin G (Megacillin), nafcillin (Unipen), vancomycin (Vancocin), gentamicin (Garamycin), clindamycin (Cleocin), rifampin alone or in combination for 4 to 6 weeks. Bactericidal serum levels of selected antibiotics are monitored by titering it against the causative organism; if serum lacks adequate bactericidal activity, more antibiotic or a different antibiotic is given.
   a. Note that missed doses of antibiotics due to the patient's unavailability while off the unit for diagnostic tests are given after return to the unit.

b. Missed antibiotic doses may have irreversible deleterious consequences.

c. Notify health care provider if doses will be missed to ensure that appropriate alternative measures are taken.

2. Audiogram obtained before antibiotic regimen initiated

3. Urine cultures obtained after 48 hours to assess efficacy of drug therapy

4. Repeat blood cultures obtained after 48 hours to assess efficacy of drug therapy

5. Close follow-up by cardiologist

6. Supplemental nutrition

7. Surgical intervention for:
   a. Acute destructive valvular lesion—excision of infected valves or removal of prosthetic valve
   b. Hemodynamic impairment
   c. Recurrent emboli
   d. Infection that cannot be eliminated with antimicrobial therapy
   e. Drainage of abscess or empyema—for patient with localized abscess or empyema
   f. Repair of peripheral or cerebral mycotic aneurysm

Complications

1. Severe heart failure due to valvular insufficiency

2. Uncontrolled/refractory infection

3. Embolic episodes (ischemia or necrosis of extremities and organs)

4. Conduction disturbances

Nursing Assessment

1. Identify factors that may predispose to endocarditis, such as rheumatic heart disease, congenital heart defects, idiopathic hypertrophic subaortic stenosis (IHSS), IV drug abuse, prosthetic heart valves, aortic or mitral stenosis, previous history of endocarditis.

2. Determine onset of signs and symptoms of endocarditis (early treatment of infection improves prognosis).

3. Identify potential incidents that may have precipitated a transient bacteremia capable of causing endocarditis.

4. Obtain blood cultures, complete blood count, renal and hepatic studies, and a baseline 12-lead ECG.

5. Assess patient for allergies, with special emphasis on untoward reactions to antibiotic therapy.

6. Note if patient is currently on antibiotic therapy (may affect blood culture results).

7. Identify patient's and family's level of anxiety and use of appropriate coping mechanisms.

Nursing Diagnoses

- Decreased Cardiac Output related to structural factors (incompetent valves)

- Altered Tissue Perfusion (renal, cerebral, cardiopulmonary, GI, and peripheral) related to interruption of blood flow

- Hyperthermia related to illness, potential dehydration, and aggressive antibiotic therapy

- Altered Nutrition: Less Than Body Requirements related to anorexia

- Anxiety related to acute illness and hospitalization

Nursing Interventions

Maintaining Adequate Cardiac Output

1. Auscultate heart to detect new murmur or change in existing murmur; presence of gallop.

2. Monitor blood pressure and pulse.
   a. Note presence of pulsus alternans (indicative of left heart failure).
   b. Evaluate pulse pressure (30 to 40 mm Hg normal; indicates adequate cardiac output).

3. Evaluate jugular venous distention.

4. Record intake and output.

5. Record daily weight.

6. Auscultate lung fields for evidence of crackles (rales).

Maintaining Tissue Perfusion

1. Observe the patient for altered mentation, hemoptysis, hematuria, aphasia, loss of muscle strength, complaints of pain.

2. Observe for splinter hemorrhages of nail beds, Osler's nodes, and Janeway's lesions.

3. Notify health care provider of observed changes in the patient's status.

4. Position patient frequently to prevent skin breakdown and pulmonary complications associated with bed rest.

Maintaining Normothermia

1. Observe basic principles of asepsis, good handwashing techniques, and continuity of patient care by primary nurse.

2. Employ meticulous IV care for long-term antibiotic therapy.
   a. Note the date of needle or cannula insertion on nursing care plan.
   b. If a peripheral site is used, rotate the site every 72 hours or if site becomes tender, reddened, infiltrated, or has purulent drainage.
   c. Change gauze or transparent dressing every 24 hours to prevent infection.
   d. If a continuous venous access device (CVAD) is used, follow nursing policy for site care and dressing changes and flushing procedures.

3. Administer parenteral antibiotic therapy as directed.
   a. Develop chart for rotation of sites for intramuscular administration of antibiotic therapy.
   b. Observe for untoward reaction to antibiotic therapy (severe respiratory distress, rash, itching, fever).
   c. Observe for side effects of long-term antibiotic therapy—ototoxicity, renal failure.

4. Monitor temperature every 2 to 4 hours.
   a. Document results on graph.
   b. Note increases in heart rate and/or respirations with elevated temperatures.

c. Provide blankets and temperature-controlled comfortable environment if patient has shaking chills; change bed linens as necessary.

d. Administer analgesic medications as directed.

5. Observe patient for a general "sense of well-being" within 5 to 7 days after initiation of therapy.

6. Monitor laboratory values—hematocrit, BUN, creatinine, WBC, antibiotic levels, blood cultures.

7. Promote adequate hydration, because diaphoresis and increased metabolic rate may cause dehydration.

a. Encourage oral fluid intake.

b. Administer IV fluids as directed.

c. Observe skin turgor and mucous membranes.

Improving Nutritional Status

1. Assess the patient's daily caloric intake.

2. Discuss food preferences with the patient.

3. Consult with a dietitian regarding nutritional needs of patient and food preferences.

4. Encourage small meals and snacks throughout the day.

5. Record daily caloric intake and weight.

6. Educate family members about the patient's caloric needs.

7. Encourage family members to assist the patient with meals and bring in the patient's favorite foods.

Reducing Anxiety

1. Rule out physiologic etiologies for increasing or new onset of anxiety before administering prn sedatives. Physiologic causes must be identified and treated in a timely fashion to prevent irreversible adverse or even fatal outcomes; sedatives may mask symptoms, delaying timely identification/diagnosis and treatment.

2. Assess patient for signs of hypoperfusion, auscultate heart and lung sounds, obtain a rhythm strip and administer oxygen as prescribed. Notify the health care provider immediately.

3. Document all assessment findings, health care provider notification and response, and interventions and response.

4. Explain to the patient and family reasons for hospitalization, diagnostic tests, and therapies administered.

5. Encourage the patient to verbalize fears regarding illness and hospitalization.

6. Explain all procedures to patient before initiation.

7. Offer the patient literature, if available, about his or her disease.

8. Encourage diversional activities for the patient such as television, reading, and interaction with other patients.

9. Encourage family members to interact with the patient as frequently as possible.

Patient Education and Health Maintenance
For Patients at Risk for Infective Endocarditis

1. Discuss anatomy of heart and changes that occur during endocarditis, using diagrams of the heart.

2. Give the patient written literature on early signs and symptoms of disease; review these with the patient.

3. Discuss with individual the mode of entry of infection.

4. Indicate that antibiotic prophylaxis is recommended for persons with:

a. Congenital heart defects, prosthetic/biologic heart valves, IHSS

b. Past history of endocarditis

c. Mitral valve prolapse with insufficiency

d. Rheumatic heart disease and valvular dysfunction

e. Undergoing procedures most likely to cause bacteremia (dental procedures causing gingival bleeding, surgery on or instrumentation of GI tract, certain genitourinary procedures, and so forth)

5. Identify individual steps necessary to prevent infection.

a. Practice good oral hygiene, regular tooth brushing, and flossing.

b. Notify health care personnel of any history of congenital heart disease or valvular disease.

c. Discuss importance of carrying emergency identification with information of medical history at all times.

d. Take temperature if infection is suspected, and notify health care provider of elevation.

e. Educate persons at risk to look for and treat signs and symptoms of illness indicating bacteremia—injuries, sore throats, furuncles, and so forth.

6. Provide patient with American Heart Association Bacterial Endocarditis wallet card outlining recommended antibiotic prophylaxis for procedures (obtain at local American Heart Association chapter).

7. Encourage susceptible individuals to receive pneumococcal and influenza vaccines.

a. Teach that vaccines reduce the risk of severe infections that could precipitate heart failure.

8. Teach women in childbearing years the risks of using intrauterine devices (IUDs) for birth control (source of infection) and that antibiotic therapy is not necessary for individuals having normal deliveries.

For Individuals Who Have Had Endocarditis
Regarding Possible Relapse

1. Discuss importance of keeping follow-up appointments after hospital discharge (infection can recur in 1 to 2 months).

2. Review the tests that will be performed after hospital discharge—blood cultures, physical examination.

3. Teach individual to inspect soles of feet for Janeway's lesions (indicative of possible relapse).

4. Contact social worker to assist the patient with financial planning and home discharge arrangements if applicable.

Outcome-Based Evaluation

- Blood pressure stable; no change in murmur; no gallop noted

- No change in level of consciousness (LOC), strength, or neurologic function

- Normal temperature; negative blood cultures; normal WBC count, BUN, and creatinine; no hearing impairments
- Increased daily caloric intake tolerated well
- Verbalizes decrease in anxiety

◼ Rheumatic Endocarditis (Rheumatic Heart Disease)

Rheumatic endocarditis is damage done to the heart, particularly the valves, resulting in valve leakage (regurgitation) and/or obstruction (narrowing or stenosis). There are associated compensatory changes in the size of the heart's chambers and the thickness of chamber walls.

Pathophysiology and Etiology
1. *Rheumatic fever* is a sequela to group A streptococcal infection. It is a preventable disease through the detection and adequate treatment of streptococcal pharyngitis.
2. Symptoms of streptococcal pharyngitis
   a. Sudden onset of sore throat; throat reddened with exudate
   b. Swollen, tender lymph nodes at angle of jaw
   c. Headache and fever 38.9° to 40°C (101° to 104°F)
   d. Abdominal pain (children)
3. Some cases of streptococcal throat infection are relatively asymptomatic.

Clinical Manifestations
1. Polyarthritis; warm and swollen joints
2. Carditis
3. Chorea (irregular, jerky, involuntary, unpredictable muscular movements)
4. Erythema marginatum (wavy, thin red-line rash on trunk and extremities)
5. Subcutaneous nodules
6. Fever
7. Prolonged P–R interval demonstrated by ECG
8. Heart murmurs; pleural and pericardial rubs

Diagnostic Evaluation
1. Throat culture—to determine presence of streptococcal organisms
2. Increased sedimentation rate, WBC count and differential, and C-reactive protein—increase during acute phase of infection
3. Elevated antistreptolysin titer

Management
1. Antimicrobial therapy
   a. Note that missed doses of antibiotics due to the patient's unavailability while off the unit for diagnostic tests are given after return to the unit.
   b. Missed antibiotic doses may have irreversible deleterious consequences.
   c. Notify health care provider if doses will be missed to ensure that appropriate alternative measures are taken.
2. Rest—to maintain optimal cardiac function
3. Salicylates—to control fever and pain
4. Prevention of recurrent episodes

Complications
1. Valvular heart disease
2. Cardiomyopathy
3. CHF

Nursing Assessment
1. Ask patient about symptoms of fever or throat or joint pain.
2. Ask patient about chest pain, dyspnea, fatigue.
3. Observe for skin lesions or rash on trunk and extremities.
4. Palpate for firm, nontender movable nodules near tendons or joints.
5. Auscultate heart sounds for murmurs and/or rubs.

Nursing Diagnoses
- Hyperthermia related to disease process
- Decreased Cardiac Output related to decreased cardiac contractility
- Activity Intolerance related to joint pain and easy fatigability

Nursing Interventions
Reducing Fever
1. Administer penicillin therapy as prescribed to eradicate hemolytic streptococcus; an erythromycin preparation may be used if the patient is allergic to penicillin.
2. Give salicylates as prescribed to suppress rheumatic activity by controlling toxic manifestations, to reduce fever, and to relieve joint pain.
3. Assess for effectiveness of drug therapy.
   a. Take and record temperature every 3 hours.
   b. Evaluate the patient's comfort level every 3 hours.

Maintaining Adequate Cardiac Output
1. Assess for signs and symptoms of acute rheumatic carditis.
   a. Be alert to the patient's complaints of chest pain, palpitations, and/or precordial "tightness."
   b. Monitor for tachycardia (usually persistent when the patient sleeps) or bradycardia.
   c. Be alert to development of second-degree heart block or Wenckebach's disease (acute rheumatic carditis causes P–R interval prolongation).
2. Auscultate heart sounds every 4 hours.
   a. Document presence of murmur or pericardial friction rub.
   b. Document extra heart sounds (S_3 gallop, S_4 gallop).
3. See discussion on rheumatic fever in children, Chapter 45.

4. Monitor for development of chronic rheumatic endocarditis, which may include valvular disease and CHF.

Maintaining Activity

1. Maintain bed rest for duration of fever or if signs of active carditis are present.
2. Provide range-of-motion exercise program.
3. Provide diversional activities that prevent exertion.
4. Discuss need for tutorial services with parents to help child keep up with school work.

Patient Education and Health Maintenance

Preventing Recurrence

1. Counsel the patient to maintain good nutrition.
2. Counsel the patient on hygienic practices.
   a. Discuss proper handwashing, disposal of tissues, laundering of handkerchiefs (decrease chance of exposure to microbes).
   b. Discuss importance of using patient's own toothbrush, soap, and washcloths when living in group situations.
3. Counsel the patient on importance of receiving adequate rest.
4. Counsel the patient to seek treatment immediately should sore throat occur.
   a. Explore with patient his or her ability to pay for medical treatment. If appropriate, contact social services for the patient. (Financial difficulties may inhibit the patient from seeking early treatment of symptoms.)

Other Points

1. Instruct the patient to use prophylactic penicillin therapy before undergoing surgery of genitourinary tract, lower GI tract, and respiratory tract.
2. See section titled Patient Education, Endocarditis, page 375.

Outcome-Based Evaluation

- Afebrile
- Denies chest pain; normal sinus rhythm
- Bed rest maintained while febrile

■ Myocarditis

Myocarditis is an inflammatory process involving the myocardium.

Pathophysiology and Etiology

1. Focal or diffuse inflammation of the myocardium; may be acute or chronic.
2. May follow infectious process—viral (particularly coxsackie group B, and may develop after influenza A or B, herpes simplex), bacterial, mycotic, parasitic, protozoal, rickettsial, and spirochetal infections.
3. May be associated with chemotherapy (especially doxorubicin [Adriamycin]) or immunosuppressive therapy.
4. Conditions such as sarcoidosis and collagen diseases may lead to myocarditis.

Clinical Manifestations

1. Symptoms depend on type of infection, degree of myocardial damage, capacity of myocardium to recover, and host resistance. Can be acute or chronic and can occur at any age. Symptoms may be minor and go unnoticed.
   a. Fatigue and dyspnea
   b. Palpitations
   c. Occasional precordial discomfort
2. Cardiac enlargement.
3. Abnormal heart sounds: murmur, S_3 or S_4, or friction rubs.
4. Signs of CHF (eg, pulsus alternans, dyspnea, crackles).
5. Fever with tachycardia.

Diagnostic Evaluation

1. Transient ECG changes—S–T segment flattened, T wave inversion, conduction defects, extrasystoles, supraventricular and ventricular ectopic beats
2. Elevated WBC count and sedimentation rate
3. Chest x-ray—may show heart enlargement and lung congestion
4. Elevated antibody titers (antistreptolysin-O [ASO titer] as in rheumatic fever)
5. Stool and throat cultures isolating bacteria or a virus
6. Endomyocardial biopsy for definitive diagnosis

Management

Treatment objectives are targeted toward management of complications.

1. Diuretic and digoxin (Lanoxin) therapy for CHF and atrial fibrillation
2. Antidysrhythmic therapy (usually quinidine [Quinaglute] or procainamide [Pronestyl])
3. Strict bed rest to promote healing of damaged myocardium
4. Antimicrobial therapy if causative bacteria is isolated

Complications

1. CHF
2. Cardiomyopathy

Nursing Assessment

1. Assess for fatigue, palpitations, fever, dyspnea, and chest pain.
2. Auscultate heart sounds.
3. Evaluate history for precipitating factors.

Nursing Diagnoses

- Hyperthermia related to inflammatory/infectious process
- Decreased Cardiac Output related to decreased cardiac contractility and dysrhythmias
- Activity Intolerance related to impaired cardiac performance and febrile illness

Nursing Interventions
Reducing Fever
1. Administer antipyretics as directed.
2. Check temperature every 4 hours.
3. Administer antibiotics as directed.

Maintaining Cardiac Output
1. Evaluate for clinical evidence that disease is subsiding—monitor pulse, auscultate for abnormal heart sounds (murmur or change in existing murmur), check temperature, auscultate lung fields, monitor respirations.
2. Record daily intake and output.
3. Record weight daily.
4. Check for peripheral edema.
5. Elevate head of bed, if necessary, to enhance respiration.
6. Treat the symptoms of CHF as prescribed (see p. 382).

 DRUG ALERT

Patients with myocarditis may be sensitive to digitalis. Assess for toxic signs and symptoms such as anorexia, nausea, fatigue, weakness, yellow-green halos around visual images, prolonged P–R interval.

7. Evaluate the patient's pulse and apical rate for signs of tachycardia and gallop rhythm—indications that CHF is recurring.
8. Evaluate for evidence of dysrhythmias—patients with myocarditis are prone to develop dysrhythmias.
   a. Institute continuous cardiac monitoring if evidence of a dysrhythmia develops.
   b. Have equipment for resuscitation, cardiac defibrillation, and cardiac pacing available in the event of life-threatening dysrhythmia.

Reducing Fatigue
1. Ensure bed rest to reduce heart rate, stroke volume, blood pressure, and heart contractility; also helps to decrease residual damage and complications of myocarditis, and promotes healing.
   a. Prolonged bed rest may be required until there is reduction in heart size and improvement of function.
2. Provide diversional activities for patient.
3. Allow the patient to use bedside commode rather than bedpan (reduces cardiovascular workload).
4. Discuss with the patient activities that can be continued after discharge.
   a. Discuss the need to modify activities in the immediate future.
   b. Explore with the patient lifestyle modifications and discuss adequacy of self-concept.

Patient Education and Health Maintenance
Instruct the patient as follows:
1. There is usually some residual heart enlargement; physical activity may be slowly increased; begin with chair rest for increasing periods; follow with walking in the room and then outdoors.
2. Report any symptom involving rapidly beating heart.
3. Avoid competitive sports, alcohol, and other myocardial toxins (doxorubicin [Adriamycin]).
4. Pregnancy is not advisable for women with cardiomyopathies associated with myocarditis.
5. Prevent infectious diseases with appropriate immunizations.
6. Encourage family members to support the patient and learn about the illness.

Outcome-Based Evaluation
- Afebrile
- BP and heart rate stable; no dysrhythmias noted
- Bed rest maintained

Pericarditis
Pericarditis is an inflammation of the pericardium, the membranous sac enveloping the heart. It is often a manifestation of a more generalized disease.

Pericardial effusion is an outpouring of fluid into the pericardial cavity seen in pericarditis.

Constrictive pericarditis is a condition in which a chronic inflammatory thickening of the pericardium compresses the heart so it is unable to fill normally during diastole.

Pathophysiology and Etiology
1. Acute idiopathic pericarditis is the most common and typical form; etiology unknown
2. Other causes include:
   a. Infection
      (i) Viral (influenza, coxsackievirus)
      (ii) Bacterial—*Staphylococcus*, meningococcus, Streptococcus, pneumococcus, gonococcus, *Mycobacterium tuberculosis*
      (iii) Fungal
      (iv) Parasitic
   b. Connective tissue disorders (lupus erythematosus, periarteritis nodosa)
   c. Myocardial infarction; early, 24 to 72 hours; or late, 1 week to 2 years after MI (Dressler's syndrome)
   d. Malignant disease; thoracic irradiation
   e. Chest trauma, heart surgery, including pacemaker implantation
   f. Drug induced (procainamide [Pronestyl]; phenytoin [Dilantin])

Clinical Manifestations
1. Pain in anterior chest, aggravated by thoracic motion—may vary from mild to sharp and severe; located in precordial area (may be felt beneath clavicle, neck, scapular region)—may be relieved by leaning forward
2. Pericardial friction rub—scratchy, grating, or creaking sound occurring in the presence of pericardial inflammation

3. Dyspnea—from compression of heart and surrounding thoracic structures
4. Fever, sweating, chills—due to inflammation of pericardium
5. Dysrhythmias

Diagnostic Evaluation
1. Echocardiogram—most sensitive method for detecting pericardial effusion
2. Chest x-ray—may show heart enlargement
3. ECG—to evaluate for myocardial infarction
4. WBC and differential elevations indicating infection
5. Antinuclear antibody serologic tests elevated in lupus erythematosus
6. PPD test positive in tuberculosis; ASO titers—elevated if rheumatic fever is present
7. Pericardiocentesis—for examination of pericardial fluid for etiologic diagnosis
8. BUN—to evaluate for uremia

Management
The objectives of treatment are targeted toward determining the etiology of the problem; administering pharmacologic therapy for specified etiology, when known; and being alert to the possible complication of cardiac tamponade.
1. Bacterial pericarditis—penicillin or other antimicrobial agents
2. Rheumatic fever—penicillin G and other antimicrobial agents (see p. 373)
3. Tuberculosis—antituberculosis chemotherapy (see p. 284)
4. Fungal pericarditis—amphotericin B and fluconazole
5. Systemic lupus erythematosus—steroids
6. Renal pericarditis—dialysis, indomethacin (Indocin), biochemical control of end-stage renal disease
7. Neoplastic pericarditis—intrapericardial instillation of chemotherapy; radiotherapy
8. Postmyocardial infarction syndrome—bed rest, aspirin, prednisone
9. Postpericardiotomy syndrome (after open-heart surgery)—treat symptomatically
10. Emergency pericardiocentesis if cardiac tamponade develops
11. Partial pericardiectomy (pericardial "window") or total pericardiectomy for recurrent constrictive pericarditis

Complications
1. Cardiac tamponade
2. CHF
3. Hemopericardium (especially patients post-MI receiving anticoagulants)

Nursing Assessment
1. Evaluate complaint of chest pain.
   a. Ask the patient if pain is aggravated by breathing, turning in bed, twisting body, coughing, yawning, or swallowing.
   b. Elevate head of bed; position pillow on over-the-bed table so the patient can lean on it.
   c. Assess if above intervention relieves the patient's chest pain (associated pleuritic pain of pericarditis is usually relieved by sitting up and/or leaning forward).
   d. Be alert to the patient's medical diagnoses when assessing pain. Postmyocardial infarction patients may experience a dull, crushing pain radiating to neck, arm, and shoulders, mimicking an extension of infarction.
2. Auscultate heart sounds.
   a. Listen for friction rub by asking patient to hold breath briefly.
   b. Listen to the heart with patient in different positions.
3. Evaluate history for precipitating factors.

Nursing Diagnoses
- Chest Pain related to pericardial inflammation
- Decreased Cardiac Output related to impaired ventricular expansion

Nursing Interventions
Reducing Discomfort
1. Give prescribed drug regimen for pain and symptomatic relief.
   a. Nonsteroidal anti-inflammatory drugs (NSAIDs) suppress inflammatory symptoms of acute pericarditis
   b. Corticosteroids—for more severe symptoms
2. Relieve anxiety of the patient and family by explaining the difference between pain of pericarditis and pain of recurrent myocardial infarction. (Patients may fear extension of myocardial tissue damage.)
3. Explain to the patient and family that pericarditis does not indicate further heart damage.
4. Encourage the patient to remain on bed rest when chest pain, fever, and friction rub occur.
5. Assist patient to position of comfort.

Maintaining Cardiac Output

> **NURSING ALERT**
>
> Normal pericardial sac contains less than 25 to 30 mL of fluid; pericardial fluid may accumulate slowly without noticeable symptoms. However, a rapidly developing effusion can produce serious hemodynamic alterations.

1. Assess heart rate, rhythm, BP, respirations at least hourly in the acute phase.
2. Assess for signs of cardiac tamponade—increased heart rate, decreased BP, presence of paradoxical pulse, distended neck veins, restlessness, muffled heart sounds.
3. Prepare for emergency pericardiocentesis or surgery. Keep pericardiocentesis tray at bedside (see p. 344).
4. Assess for signs of CHF (see p. 382).
5. Monitor closely for the development of dysrhythmias.

Patient Education and Health Maintenance

1. Teach patient the etiology of pericarditis.
2. Instruct patient about signs and symptoms of pericarditis and the need for long-term medication therapy to help relieve symptoms.
3. Review all medications with the patient—purpose, side effects, dosage, and special precautions.

Outcome-Based Evaluation

- Patient verbalizes relief of pain
- BP and heart rate stable, no dysrhythmias, no friction rub

Cardiomyopathy

Cardiomyopathy refers to any disease of the heart muscle. In primary cardiomyopathy, the cause of the disorder is unknown; in secondary cardiomyopathy, the cause of the disorder is known or suspected (coronary artery disease can cause ischemic cardiomyopathy).

The cardiomyopathies are categorized into three major groups (dilated, hypertrophic, restrictive) to delineate the variations in structural and functional abnormalities that can occur.

Pathophysiology and Etiology

Dilated Cardiomyopathy

1. Both the right and left ventricle enlarge (dilate) significantly, causing a decrease in the ability of the heart to pump blood efficiently to the body.
2. Blood remaining in the ventricles after contraction causes increases in ventricular, atrial, and pulmonary pressures.
3. The increased pressures continue to diminish the ability of the heart to pump blood to the body, and heart failure occurs.
4. Alcohol abuse, chemotherapy, chemical agents, pregnancy (third trimester, postpartum), and infections can cause dilated cardiomyopathy.

Hypertrophic Cardiomyopathy (HCM)

1. HCM is primarily due to the abnormal thickening of the ventricular septum of the heart.
2. The thickening of the heart muscle commonly occurs asymmetrically (septum is proportionately thicker than the other ventricular walls), but also may occur symmetrically (septum and the ventricular free wall both become equally thickened).
3. The ultrastructure of the heart is also disrupted by patches of myocardial fibrosis, disorganization of myocardial fibers, and abnormalities of the coronary microvasculature.
4. The thickened heart muscle and ultrastructure disruption change the shape, size, and distensibility of the ventricular cavity and alter the normal thickness and functioning of the mitral valve; as a result, the heart's ability to relax and contract normally is impaired.
    a. Muscle stiffness impairs the filling of the ventricle with blood during relaxation.
    b. Forceful contractions eject blood from the heart too rapidly, causing abnormal pressure gradients; mechanical narrowing of the passage by which the blood leaves the heart also may occur, acutely obstructing blood flow to the body.
5. HCM is a genetically transmitted disorder.

Restrictive Cardiomyopathy

1. The heart muscle becomes infiltrated by various substances, resulting in severe fibrosis.
2. The heart muscle becomes stiff and nondistensible, impairing the ability of the ventricle to fill with blood adequately.
3. Amyloidosis and hemochromatosis (excess iron deposition) may cause restrictive cardiomyopathy.

Clinical Manifestations

1. Exertional dyspnea
2. Chest pain
3. Signs of CHF (see p. 382)
4. Pulmonary edema (see p. 385)
5. Dysrhythmias (frequent atrial/ventricular ectopic beats; sinus, atrial, and ventricular tachycardia)
6. Pericardial effusions (with restrictive cardiomyopathy)

Diagnostic Evaluation

1. Chest x-ray (cardiomegaly).
2. ECG—may show dysrhythmia.
3. Echocardiogram detects abnormalities of heart wall movements.
4. 24-hour Holter monitoring to detect dysrhythmias.
5. Radionuclide imaging to assess ventricular function.
6. Cardiac catheterization may help determine cause (ischemic or nonischemic).

Management

The goal of therapy is to maximize ventricular function and prevent complications.

Dilated Cardiomyopathy

1. Effective management of heart failure by conventional therapy (see p. 383).
2. Oral anticoagulants may be instituted to prevent thrombus and pulmonary embolus.
3. Heart transplantation must be considered in the terminal disease phase.

 DRUG ALERT

Patients with dilated cardiomyopathy are susceptible to digoxin toxicity. Monitor patient carefully for evidence of nausea, vomiting, yellow vision, and dysrhythmias.

Hypertrophic Cardiomyopathy

1. *Beta-adrenergic blockers*—reduce the force of the heart muscle's contraction, diminish obstructive pressure gra-

dients, and decrease oxygen requirements. Metoprolol [Lopressor] is the agent of choice.

2. *Calcium channel blockers*—decrease heart rate and contractility and vasodilate, thereby providing symptom relief. Verapamil (Calan) and diltiazem (Cardizem) are agents of preference and are usually implemented after failure of beta-adrenergic agents to control symptoms.

3. *Antidysrhythmic therapy*—amiodarone (Cordarone) is the agent of choice to prophylactically prevent lethal dysrhythmias.

4. *Myotomy and myectomy*—surgical resection of a portion of the septum to reduce muscle thickness and provide symptom relief.

5. *Device implantation*—pacemakers and automatic internal defibrillators may be implanted to treat severe bradycardias and lethal tachycardias.

NURSING ALERT

Chest pain experienced by HCM patients is managed by rest and elevation of the feet (improves venous return to the heart). Vasodilator therapy (nitroglycerin) may worsen chest pain by decreasing venous return to the heart and further increasing obstruction of blood flow from the heart; agents that increase contractility of the heart muscle (dopamine, dobutamine) should also be avoided or used with extreme caution.

Restrictive Cardiomyopathy

1. Therapy is palliative unless specific underlying process is established.
2. Heart failure can be controlled with fluid restriction and diuretic therapy.
3. Digoxin (Lanoxin) is beneficial for controlling atrial fibrillation.
4. Oral anticoagulants are instituted to prevent emboli.

Complications

1. Mural thrombus (due to blood stasis in ventricles with dilated cardiomyopathy)
2. Severe heart failure
3. Sudden cardiac death
4. Pulmonary embolism

Nursing Assessment

1. Evaluate the patient's chief complaint, which may include fever, syncope, general aches, fatigue, palpitations, dyspnea.
2. Evaluate etiologic factors such as alcohol abuse, pregnancy, recent infection, or history of endocrine disorders.
3. Assess for positive family history.
4. Auscultate lung sounds for crackles (pulmonary edema) or decreased sounds (pleural effusion).
5. Assess heart size, and auscultate for abnormal sounds.
6. Evaluate cardiac rhythm and ECG for evidence of atrial or ventricular enlargement and infarction.

Nursing Diagnoses

- Decreased Cardiac Output related to decreased ventricular function and/or dysrhythmias
- Anxiety related to fear of death and hospitalization
- Fatigue related to disease process

Nursing Interventions

Improving Cardiac Output

1. Monitor heart rate, rhythm, temperature, and respiratory rate at least every 4 hours.
2. Evaluate CVP, pulmonary artery and pulmonary capillary wedge pressures by way of a pulmonary artery catheter to assess progress and effect of drug therapy.
3. Calculate cardiac output, cardiac index, and systemic vascular resistance.
4. Observe for changes in cardiac output, such as decreased BP, change in mental status, decreased urine output.
5. Administer pharmacologic support as directed, and observe for changes in hemodynamic and clinical status.
6. Administer medications to control or eradicate dysrhythmias as directed.
7. Administer anticoagulants as directed, especially for patients in atrial fibrillation.
   a. Monitor coagulation studies.
   b. Observe for evidence of bleeding.

Relieving Anxiety

1. As above, always evaluate increasing and/or new onset anxiety for a physiologic cause, and report to the health care provider before administration of anxiolytics.
2. Explain all procedures and treatments.
3. Inform patient and visitors of visiting hours and policy and whom to contact for information.
4. Orient patient to unit, purpose of equipment, and plan of care.
5. Encourage questions and voicing of fears and concerns.

Reducing Fatigue

1. Ensure that patient and visitors understand the importance of rest.
2. Assist patient in identifying stressors and reducing their effect (especially important for patients with HCM because stress worsens the outflow obstruction).
3. Provide uninterrupted periods, and assist with ambulation as ordered.
4. Teach the use of diversional activities and relaxation techniques to relieve tension.

Patient Education and Health Maintenance

1. Teach about medications such as digoxin (Lanoxin).
   a. Take daily only after taking pulse; notify health care provider if pulse is below 60 (or other specified rate).
   b. Report signs of digitalis toxicity—anorexia, nausea, vomiting, yellow vision.
   c. Follow-up for periodic blood levels.
2. Advise about low-sodium diet. Teach how to read labels.

3. Advise reporting signs of heart failure—weight gain, edema, shortness of breath, increased fatigue.
4. Ensure that family members know cardiopulmonary resuscitation (CPR) because sudden cardiac arrest is possible.

Outcome-Based Evaluation

- BP and hemodynamic parameters stable; urine output adequate; alert
- Asking questions and cooperating with care
- Resting at intervals

Heart Failure

Heart failure, also called *congestive heart failure (CHF)*, is a clinical syndrome that results from the heart's inability to pump the amount of oxygenated blood necessary to meet the metabolic requirements of the body.

Pathophysiology and Etiology

1. Cardiac compensatory mechanisms (increases in heart rate, vasoconstriction, heart enlargement) occur to assist the failing heart.
   a. These mechanisms are able to "compensate" for the heart's inability to pump effectively and maintain sufficient blood flow to organs and tissue at rest.
   b. Physiologic stressors that increase the workload of the heart (exercise, infection) may cause these mechanisms to fail and precipitate the "clinical syndrome" associated with a failing heart (elevated ventricular/atrial pressures, sodium and water retention, decreased cardiac output, circulatory and pulmonary congestion).
   c. The compensatory mechanisms may hasten the onset of failure because they increase afterload and cardiac work.
2. Caused by disorders of heart muscle resulting in decreased contractile properties of the heart; coronary heart disease leading to myocardial infarction; hypertension; valvular heart disease; congenital heart disease; cardiomyopathies; dysrhythmias.
3. Other causes include:
   a. Pulmonary embolism; chronic lung disease
   b. Hemorrhage and anemia
   c. Anesthesia and surgery
   d. Transfusions or infusions
   e. Increased body demands (fever, infection, pregnancy, arteriovenous fistula)
   f. Drug-induced
   g. Physical and emotional stress
   h. Excessive sodium intake

Clinical Manifestations

Initially, there may be isolated left ventricular failure, but in time the right ventricle fails because of the additional workload. Combined left and right ventricular failure is common.

Left-Sided Heart Failure (Forward Failure)

1. Congestion occurs mainly in the lungs from backing up of blood into pulmonary veins and capillaries.
   a. Shortness of breath, dyspnea on exertion, paroxysmal nocturnal dyspnea (due to reabsorption of dependent edema that has developed during day), orthopnea, pulmonary edema
   b. Cough—may be dry, unproductive; often occurs at night
2. Fatigability—from low cardiac output, nocturia, insomnia, dyspnea, catabolic effect of chronic failure.
3. Insomnia, restlessness.
4. Tachycardia—S_3 ventricular gallop.

Right-Sided Heart Failure (Backward Failure)

Signs and symptoms of elevated pressures and congestion in systemic veins and capillaries:

1. Edema of ankles; unexplained weight gain (pitting edema is obvious only after retention of at least 4.5 kg [10 lb] of fluid)
2. Liver congestion—may produce upper abdominal pain
3. Distended neck veins
4. Abnormal fluid in body cavities (pleural space, abdominal cavity)
5. Anorexia and nausea—from hepatic and visceral engorgement
6. Nocturia—diuresis occurs at night with rest and improved cardiac output
7. Weakness

Cardiovascular Findings in Both Types

1. Cardiomegaly (enlargement of the heart)—detected by physical examination and chest x-ray
2. Ventricular gallop—evident on auscultation; ECG
3. Rapid heart rate
4. Development of pulsus alternans (alternation in strength of beat)

Diagnostic Evaluation

1. ECG may show ventricular hypertrophy and strain.
2. Echocardiography may show ventricular hypertrophy, dilation of chambers, and abnormal wall motion.
3. Chest x-ray may show cardiomegaly, pleural effusion, and vascular congestion.
4. ABG studies may show hypoxemia due to pulmonary vascular congestion.
5. Liver function studies may be altered because of hepatic congestion.

Management

Treatment is directed at eliminating excessive accumulation of body water, increasing the force and efficiency of myocardial contraction, and reducing the workload of the heart. These goals are achieved through promoting rest and administering pharmacologic agents.

Diuretics

1. Eliminate excess body water and decrease ventricular pressures.
2. A low-sodium diet and fluid restriction complement this therapy.
3. Some diuretics may have slight venodilator properties.

Positive Inotropic Agents

1. Increase the heart's ability to pump more effectively by improving the contractile force of the muscle.
2. Digoxin (Lanoxin) may only be effective in severe cases of failure.
3. Dopamine (Intropin) also improves renal blood flow in low dose range.
4. Dobutamine (Dobutrex).
5. Milrinone (Primacor) and amrinone (Inocor) are potent vasodilators.

Vasodilator Therapy

1. Decreases the workload of the heart by dilating peripheral vessels.
2. By relaxing capacitance vessels (veins and venules), vasodilators reduce ventricular filling pressures (preload) and volumes.
3. By relaxing resistance vessels (arterioles), vasodilators can reduce impedance to left ventricular ejection and improve stroke volume.
4. Vasodilators used in CHF:
   a. Nitrates such as nitroglycerin (Tridil), isosorbide dinitrate (Isordil), nitroglycerin ointment (Nitrobid)—predominantly dilate systemic veins
   b. Hydralazine (Apresoline)—predominantly affects arterioles; reduces arteriolar tone
   c. Prazosin (Minipress)—balanced effects on both arterial and venous circulation
   d. Sodium nitroprusside (Nipride)—predominantly affects arterioles
   e. Morphine sulfate (Duramorph)—decreases venous return, decreases pain and anxiety and thus cardiac work

Angiotensin-Converting Enzyme Inhibitors (ACE Inhibitors)

1. Inhibit the adverse effects of angiotensin II (potent vasoconstrictor).
2. Decreases left ventricular afterload with a subsequent decrease in heart rate associated with heart failure, thereby reducing the workload of the heart and increasing cardiac output.
3. Captopril (Capoten) and enalapril (Vasotec) are commonly used.

Beta-adrenergic Blocking Agents

1. Decrease myocardial workload and protect against fatal dysrhythmias by blocking norepinephrine effects of the sympathetic nervous system.
2. Metoprolol (Lopressor) or metoprolol CR or XL (Toprol XL) are commonly used.
3. Carvedilol is a nonselective beta and alpha blocking agent. Patients may actually experience increase in general malaise for a 2- to 3-week period while they adjust to the medication.

Diet

1. Restricted sodium
2. Restricted fluids

 NURSING ALERT

High serum sodium levels are the most common finding in patients readmitted with a diagnosis of CHF.

Heart Transplantation

Used in advanced heart failure

Complications

1. Intractable or refractory heart failure—patient becomes progressively refractory to therapy (does not yield to treatment).
2. Cardiac dysrhythmias.
3. Myocardial failure.
4. Digitalis toxicity—from decreased renal function, potassium depletion, and so forth.
5. Pulmonary infarction; pneumonia; emboli.

Nursing Assessment

1. Obtain history of symptoms, limits of activity, and response to rest.
2. Assess peripheral arterial pulses; note quality, character; assess heart and blood pressure rhythm and rate.
3. Inspect/palpate precordium for lateral displacement of point of maximum impulse.
4. Identify sleeping patterns and sleep aids commonly used by patient.

Nursing Diagnoses

- Decreased Cardiac Output related to impaired contractility and increased preload/afterload
- Impaired Gas Exchange related to alveolar edema due to elevated ventricular pressures
- Fluid Volume Excess related to sodium and water retention
- Activity Intolerance related to oxygen supply and demand imbalance

Nursing Interventions

Maintaining Adequate Cardiac Output

1. Place patient at physical and emotional rest to reduce work of heart.
   a. Provide rest in semirecumbent position or in armchair in air-conditioned environment—reduces work of heart, increases heart reserve, reduces blood pressure, decreases work of respiratory muscles and oxygen utilization, improves efficiency of heart contraction; recumbency promotes diuresis by improving renal perfusion.

b. Provide bedside commode—to reduce work of getting to bathroom and for defecation.

c. Provide for psychological rest—emotional stress produces vasoconstriction, elevates arterial pressure, and speeds the heart.
  (i) Promote physical comfort.
  (ii) Avoid situations that tend to promote anxiety/agitation.
  (iii) Offer careful explanations and answers to the patient's questions.

2. Evaluate frequently for progression of left ventricular failure. Take frequent blood pressure readings.
  a. Observe for lowering of systolic pressure.
  b. Note narrowing of pulse pressure.
  c. Note alternations in strong and weak pulsations (pulsus alternans).

3. Auscultate heart sounds frequently.
  a. Note presence of S_3 or S_4 gallop (S_3 gallop is a significant indicator of CHF).
  b. Monitor for premature ventricular beats.

4. Observe for signs and symptoms of reduced peripheral tissue perfusion: cool temperature of skin, facial pallor, poor capillary refill of nail beds.

5. Administer pharmacotherapy as directed.

6. Monitor clinical response of patient with respect to relief of symptoms (lessening dyspnea and orthopnea, decrease in crackles, relief of peripheral edema).

NURSING ALERT

Watch for sudden unexpected hypotension, which can cause myocardial ischemia and decrease perfusion to vital organs.

Improving Oxygenation

1. Raise head of bed 20 to 30 cm (8 to 10 inches)—reduces venous return to heart and lungs; alleviates pulmonary congestion.
  a. Support lower arms with pillows—to eliminate pull of their weight on shoulder muscles.
  b. Sit orthopneic patient on side of bed with feet supported by a chair, head and arms resting on an over-the-bed table, and lumbosacral area supported with pillows.

2. Auscultate lung fields every 4 hours for crackles and wheezes in dependent lung fields (fluid accumulates in areas affected by gravity).
  a. Mark with water-soluble ink the level on the patient's back where adventitious breath sounds are heard.
  b. Use markings for comparative assessment during changes in tours of duty with other nursing personnel.

3. Observe for increased rate of respirations (could be indicative of falling arterial pH).

4. Observe for Cheyne-Stokes respirations (may occur in elderly because of a decrease in cerebral perfusion stimulating a neurogenic response).

5. Position the patient every 2 hours (or encourage the patient to change position frequently)—to help prevent atelectasis and pneumonia.

6. Encourage deep-breathing exercises every 1 to 2 hours—to avoid atelectasis.

7. Offer small, frequent feedings—to avoid excessive gastric filling and abdominal distention with subsequent elevation of diaphragm that causes decrease in lung capacity.

8. Administer oxygen as directed.

Restoring Fluid Balance

1. Administer prescribed diuretic as ordered.

2. Give diuretic early in the morning—nighttime diuresis disturbs sleep.

3. Keep input and output record—the patient may lose large volume of fluid after a single dose of diuretic.

4. Weigh the patient daily—to determine if edema is being controlled: weight loss should not exceed 0.45 to 0.9 kg (1 to 2 lb/day).

5. Assess for weakness, malaise, muscle cramps—diuretic therapy may produce hypovolemia and electrolyte depletion, namely hypokalemia. Hypokalemia may cause weakening of cardiac contractions and may precipitate digitalis toxicity in the form of dysrhythmias.

6. Give oral potassium as prescribed.

7. Watch for problems associated with diuretic therapy including disorders of hyperuricemia, volume depletion, hyponatremia, magnesium depletion, hyperglycemia, and diabetes mellitus.

8. Watch for signs of bladder distention in the elderly male with prostatic hyperplasia.

9. Observe for symptoms of electrolyte depletion—lassitude, apathy, mental confusion, anorexia, decreasing urinary output, azotemia.

10. Limit IV fluid administration through use of heparin lock (allows for periodic drug administration without increasing excessive fluid intake).

11. Monitor for pitting edema of lower extremities and sacral area. Use "egg crate" mattress and sheepskin to prevent pressure sores (poor blood flow and edema increase susceptibility).

12. Observe for the complications of bed rest—pressure sores (especially in edematous patients), phlebothrombosis, pulmonary embolism.

13. Be alert to complaints of right upper quadrant abdominal pain, poor appetite, nausea, and abdominal distention (may indicate hepatic and visceral engorgement).

14. Monitor the patient's diet. Diet may be limited in sodium—to prevent, control, or eliminate edema; may also be limited in calories.

15. Caution patients to avoid added salt in food and foods with high sodium content.

Improving Activity Tolerance

1. Increase the patient's activities gradually. Alter or modify the patient's activities—to keep within the limits of his cardiac reserve.

a. Assist the patient with self-care activities early in the day (fatigue sets in as day progresses).

b. Be alert to complaints of chest pain or skeletal pain during or after activities.

2. Observe the pulse, symptoms, and behavioral response to increased activity.

a. Monitor the patient's heart rate during self-care activities.

b. Allow heart rate to decrease to preactivity level before initiating a new activity.

   (i) Note time lapse between cessation of activity and decrease in heart rate (decreased stroke volume causes immediate rise in heart rate).

   (ii) Document time lapse and revise patient care plan as appropriate (progressive increase in time lapse may be indicative of increased left ventricular failure).

3. Relieve nighttime anxiety and provide for rest and sleep—Patients with CHF have a tendency to be restless at night because of cerebral hypoxia with superimposed nitrogen retention. Give appropriate sedation—to relieve insomnia and restlessness.

Patient Education and Health Maintenance

1. Explain the disease process to the patient; the term *failure* may have terrifying implications.

a. Explain the pumping action of the heart—"to move blood through the body to provide nutrients and aid in the removal of waste material."

b. Explain the difference between heart attack and CHF.

2. Teach the signs and symptoms of recurrence. Watch for:

a. Gain in weight—report weight gain of more than 2 to 3 lb (0.9 to 1.4 kg) in a few days. Weigh at same time daily to detect any tendency toward fluid retention.

b. Swelling of ankles, feet, or abdomen.

c. Persistent cough.

d. Tiredness, loss of appetite.

e. Frequent urination at night.

3. Review medication regimen.

a. Label all medications.

b. Give written instructions.

c. Make sure the patient has a check-off system that will show that he or she has taken medications.

d. Teach the patient to take and record pulse rate and blood pressure.

e. Inform the patient of adverse drug effects.

f. If the patient is taking oral potassium solution, it may be diluted with juice and taken after a meal.

g. Tell the patient to weigh self daily and log weight if on diuretic therapy.

h. Ask whether patient is taking Coenzyme Q10 or other supplements; should discuss with health care provider.

4. Review activity program. Instruct the patient as follows:

a. Increase walking and other activities gradually, provided they do not cause fatigue and dyspnea.

b. In general, continue at whatever activity level can be maintained without the appearance of symptoms.

c. Avoid excesses in eating and drinking.

d. Undertake a weight reduction program until optimal weight is reached.

e. Avoid extremes in heat and cold, which increase the work of the heart; air conditioning may be essential in a hot, humid environment.

f. Keep *regular* appointment with health care provider or clinic.

5. Restrict sodium as directed.

a. Give patient a booklet containing sodium content of common foods from local chapter of American Heart Association.

b. Give patient a written diet plan with lists of permitted and restricted foods.

c. Advise patient to look at all labels to ascertain sodium content (antacids, laxatives, cough remedies, and so forth).

d. Teach the patient to rinse the mouth well after using tooth cleansers and mouthwashes—some of these contain large amounts of sodium. Water softeners are to be avoided.

e. Teach the patient that sodium is present in alkalizers, cough remedies, laxatives, pain relievers, estrogens, and other drugs.

f. Encourage use of flavorings, spices, herbs, and lemon juice.

g. Avoid salt substitutes in the presence of renal disease.

Outcome-Based Evaluation

- Normal blood pressure and heart rate
- Respiratory rate 16 to 20, ABGs within normal limits, no signs of crackles or wheezes in lung fields
- Weight decrease of 1 kg (2.2 lb) daily, no pitting edema of lower extremities and sacral area
- Heart rate within normal limits, rests between activities

Acute Pulmonary Edema

Acute pulmonary edema refers to the presence of excess fluid in the lung, either in the interstitial spaces or in the alveoli.

Pathophysiology and Etiology

1. The presence of fluid in the alveoli impedes gas exchange, especially oxygen movement into pulmonary capillaries.

2. May be caused by:

a. Heart disease—acute left ventricular failure, myocardial infarction, aortic stenosis, severe mitral valve disease, hypertension, CHF

b. Circulatory overload—transfusions and infusions

c. Drug hypersensitivity, allergy, poisoning

d. Lung injuries—smoke inhalation, shock lung, pulmonary embolism, or infarct

e. Central nervous system injuries—stroke, head trauma

f. Infection and fever—infectious pneumonia (viral, bacterial, parasitic)

g. Postcardioversion, postanesthesia, postcardiopulmonary bypass

h. Narcotic overdose

Clinical Manifestations

1. Coughing and restlessness during sleep (premonitory symptoms).
2. Extreme dyspnea and orthopnea—patient usually uses accessory muscles of respiration with retraction of intercostal spaces and supraclavicular areas.
3. Cough with varying amounts of white- or pink-tinged frothy sputum.
4. Extreme anxiety and panic.
5. Noisy breathing—inspiratory and expiratory wheezing and bubbling sounds.
6. Cyanosis with profuse perspiration.
7. Distended neck veins.
8. Tachycardia.
9. Precordial pain (if pulmonary edema secondary to myocardial infarction).

Diagnostic Evaluation

1. Chest x-ray—shows interstitial edema
2. Echocardiogram to detect valvular disease
3. Measurement of pulmonary artery wedge pressure by Swan-Ganz catheter (differentiates etiology of pulmonary edema—cardiogenic or altered alveolar-capillary membrane)
4. Blood cultures in suspected infection—may be positive
5. Cardiac enzymes in suspected myocardial infarction—may be elevated

Management

1. The immediate objective of treatment is to improve oxygenation and reduce pulmonary congestion.
2. Identification and correction of precipitating factors and underlying conditions are then necessary to prevent recurrence.
3. Increasing oxygen tension (oxygen therapy), reducing fluid volume (diuretics, vasodilators), improving the heart's ability to pump effectively (glycosides, beta agonists), and decreasing anxiety guide therapeutic interventions.
4. *Oxygen therapy*—high concentrations of oxygen are used to combat hypoxemia. Intubation and ventilatory support may be necessary to improve hypoxemia and prevent hypercarbia.
5. *Morphine sulfate (Duramorph)*—reduces anxiety, promotes venous pooling of blood in the periphery, and reduces resistance against which the heart must pump.
6. *Vasodilator therapy* (nitroglycerin [Tridil] and nitroprusside [Nipride])—reduces the amount of blood returning to the heart and resistance against which the heart must pump.
7. *Diuretic therapy* (furosemide [Lasix], ethacrynic acid [Edecrin])—reduces blood volume and pulmonary congestion by producing prompt diuresis.

8. *Contractility enhancement therapy* (digoxin [Lanoxin], dopamine [Intropin], dobutamine [Dobutrex].
   a. Improves the ability of the heart muscle to pump more effectively, allowing for complete emptying of blood from the ventricle and a subsequent decrease in fluid backing up into the lungs.
   b. Aminophylline may prevent bronchospasm associated with pulmonary congestion. Use with caution because it may also increase heart rate and induce tachydysrhythmias.

Complications

1. Dysrhythmias
2. Respiratory failure

Nursing Assessment

1. Be alert to development of a new nonproductive cough.
2. Assess for signs and symptoms of hypoxia—restlessness, confusion, headache.
3. Auscultate lung fields frequently.
   a. Note inspiratory and expiratory wheezes, rhonchi, moist fine crackles appearing initially in lung bases and extending upward.
4. Auscultate for extra heart sounds.
   a. Note presence of third heart sound (may be difficult to hear because of respiratory sounds).
5. Identify precipitating factors that place patient at risk for development of pulmonary edema.

NURSING ALERT

 Acute pulmonary edema is a true medical emergency; it is a life-threatening condition.

Nursing Diagnoses

- Impaired Gas Exchange related to excess fluid in the lungs
- Anxiety related to sensation of suffocation and fear

Nursing Interventions
Improving Oxygenation

1. Give oxygen in high concentration—to relieve hypoxia and dyspnea.
2. Take steps to reduce venous return to the heart.
   a. Place patient in upright position; head and shoulders up, feet and legs hanging down—to favor pooling of blood in dependent portions of body by gravitational forces; to decrease venous return.
3. Give morphine in small titrated intermittent doses (IV) as directed.
   a. Morphine usually is not given if pulmonary edema is caused by stroke or occurs in the presence of chronic pulmonary disease or cardiogenic shock.
   b. Watch for excessive respiratory depression.
   c. Monitor blood pressure because morphine may intensify hypotension.

d. Have morphine antagonist available—naloxone hydrochloride (Narcan).
4. Give injections of diuretic IV.
   a. Insert an indwelling catheter—large urinary volume will accumulate rapidly.
   b. Watch for falling blood pressure, increasing heart rate, and decreasing urinary output—indications that the total circulation is not tolerating diuresis and that hypovolemia may develop.
   c. Check electrolyte levels because potassium loss may be significant.
   d. Watch for signs of urinary obstruction in men with prostatic hyperplasia.
5. Administer vasodilator if patient fails to respond to therapy.
   a. Monitor by measuring pulmonary artery pressure and cardiac output.
6. Administer aminophylline (Amoline) if ordered.
   a. Monitor blood levels of drug.
   b. Evaluate for side effects of drug—ventricular dysrhythmias, hypotension, headache.
7. Administer cardiac glycosides as ordered.
8. Assist with cardioversion if indicated (pulmonary edema may precipitate tachycardias).
9. Give appropriate drugs for severe, sustained hypertension.
10. Continually evaluate the patient's response to therapy. Reevaluate lung fields and cardiac status (see section titled Nursing Assessment).

Decreasing Anxiety
1. Stay with the patient and display a confident attitude—the presence of another person is therapeutic, because the acute anxiety of the patient may tend to intensify the severity of patient's condition. (Arterial vasoconstriction diminishes as anxiety is relieved.)
2. Explain to the patient in a calm manner all therapies administered and the reason for their use.
   a. Give brief explanations related to goal of therapies (eg, "Morphine will help you relax and ease the work of breathing").
   b. Explain to the patient importance of wearing oxygen mask. Assure the patient that mask will not increase sensation of suffocation.
3. Inform the patient and family of progress toward resolution of pulmonary edema.
4. Allow time for the patient and family to voice concerns and fears.

Patient Education and Health Maintenance
During convalescence, instruct the patient as follows to prevent recurrences of pulmonary edema:
1. Remind patient of early symptoms before onset of acute pulmonary edema; these should be reported promptly.
2. If coughing develops (a wet cough), sit with legs dangling over side of bed.
3. See section titled Patient Education, Heart Failure, page 385.

Outcome-Based Evaluation
- Unlabored respirations at 14 to 18 times per minute, lungs clear on auscultation
- Appears calm; rests comfortably

Acquired Valvular Disease of the Heart
The function of normal heart valves is to maintain the forward flow of blood from the atria to the ventricles and from the ventricles to the great vessels.

Valvular damage may interfere with valvular function by stenosis or by impaired closure that allows backward leakage of blood (valvular insufficiency, regurgitation, or incompetence).

Pathophysiology and Etiology
Mitral Stenosis
1. *Mitral stenosis* is the progressive thickening and contracture of valve cusps with narrowing of the orifice and progressive obstruction to blood flow.
2. Acute rheumatic valvulitis has "glued" the mitral valve flaps (commissures) together, thus shortening the chordae tendineae, so that the flap edges are pulled down, greatly narrowing the mitral orifice.
3. The left atrium has difficulty in emptying itself through the narrow orifice into the left ventricle; therefore, it dilates and hypertrophies. Pulmonary circulation becomes congested.
4. As a result of the abnormally high pulmonary arterial pressure that must be maintained, the right ventricle is subjected to a pressure overload and may eventually fail.

Mitral Insufficiency
1. Mitral insufficiency (regurgitation) is incomplete closure of the mitral valve during systole, allowing blood to flow back into the left atrium.
2. Left atrial pressures increase.
3. Left ventricular hypertrophy may develop due to inefficient emptying.
4. May be due to valve distortion or shortening or damage to chordae tendineae or papillary muscles caused by mitral valve prolapse, chronic rheumatic heart disease, postinfarction mitral regurgitation, infective endocarditis, and penetrating and nonpenetrating trauma.

Aortic Stenosis
1. Aortic stenosis is a narrowing of the orifice between the left ventricle and the aorta.
2. The obstruction to the aortic outflow places a pressure load on the left ventricle that results in hypertrophy and failure.
3. Left atrial pressure increases.
4. Pulmonary vascular pressure increases, which may eventually lead to right ventricular failure.
5. May be caused by congenital anomalies, calcification, or rheumatic fever.

Aortic Insufficiency

1. Valve flaps fail to completely seal the aortic orifice during diastole and thus permit backflow of blood from the aorta into the left ventricle.
2. The left ventricle increases the force of contraction to maintain an adequate cardiac output, often resulting in hypertrophy.
3. The low aortic diastolic pressures result in decreased coronary artery perfusion.
4. May be caused by rheumatic endocarditis, infective endocarditis, or congenital malformation, Marfan's syndrome, Ehler-Danlos syndrome, systemic lupus erythematosus, or by diseases that cause dilation or tearing of the ascending aorta (syphilitic disease, rheumatoid spondylitis, dissecting aneurysm).

Tricuspid Stenosis

1. Tricuspid stenosis is restriction of the tricuspid valve orifice due to commissural fusion and fibrosis.
2. Usually follows rheumatic fever and is commonly associated with diseases of the mitral valve.

Tricuspid Insufficiency (Regurgitation)

1. Tricuspid insufficiency allows the regurgitation of blood from the right ventricle into the right atrium during ventricular systole.
2. Common cause is dilation of right ventricle or rheumatic fever.

Clinical Manifestations

1. Fatigue, weakness
2. Dyspnea, cough, orthopnea, nocturnal dyspnea
3. Murmur
   a. Mitral stenosis—increased first heart sound, opening snap, and low-pitched rumbling diastolic murmur heard at the apex
   b. Mitral insufficiency—soft first heart sound and a blowing pansystolic murmur heard at the apex and transmitted to the axilla (characteristic of mild regurgitation due to papillary muscle dysfunction of mitral prolapse)
   c. Aortic stenosis—loud, rough systolic murmur over aortic area; often associated with a palpable thrill
   d. Aortic insufficiency—high-pitched blowing decrescendo diastolic murmur audible along the left sternal edge
   e. Tricuspid stenosis—similar to those of rheumatic mitral disease; blowing diastolic murmur along left sternal border
   f. Tricuspid insufficiency—pansystolic murmur in tricuspid area
4. Dysrhythmias, palpitations
5. Hemoptysis (from pulmonary hypertension) and hoarseness (from compression of left recurrent laryngeal nerve) in mitral stenosis
6. Low blood pressure, dizziness, syncope, angina, and symptoms of CHF in aortic stenosis
7. Arterial pulsations visible and palpable over precordium and visible in neck; widened pulse pressure; and water-hammer (Corrigan's) pulse (pulse strikes palpating finger with a quick, sharp stroke and then suddenly collapses) in aortic insufficiency
8. Symptoms of right-sided heart failure—edema, ascites, hepatomegaly—in tricuspid stenosis and insufficiency

Diagnostic Evaluation

1. ECG may show dysrhythmias.
2. Echocardiography may show abnormalities of valve structure and function and chamber size and thickness.
3. Chest x-ray may show cardiomegaly and pulmonary vascular congestion.
4. Cardiac catheterization and angiocardiography—to confirm diagnosis and determine severity.

Management

Medical Therapy

1. Antibiotic prophylaxis for endocarditis before invasive procedures—indicated in most cases
2. Treatment of heart failure—diuretics, sodium restriction, vasodilators, cardiac glycosides, and so forth as indicated

Surgical Intervention

See page 350 for care of the patient undergoing heart surgery.

1. For mitral stenosis:
   a. Closed mitral valvotomy—introduction of a dilator through the mitral valve to split its commissures.
   b. Open mitral valvotomy—direct incision of the commissures.
   c. Mitral valve replacement.
   d. Balloon valvuloplasty—a balloon-tipped catheter is percutaneously inserted, threaded to the affected valve, and positioned across the narrowed orifice. The balloon is inflated/deflated, causing a "cracking" of the calcified commissures and enlargement of the valve orifice.
2. For mitral insufficiency—mitral valve replacement or annuloplasty (retailoring of the valve ring)
3. For aortic stenosis or insufficiency:
   a. Replacement of aortic valve with prosthetic or tissue valves.
   b. Balloon valvuloplasty (aortic stenosis).
4. For tricuspid stenosis or insufficiency—valvuloplasty or replacement may be done at time of surgical intervention for associated rheumatic mitral or aortic disease.

Complications

1. CHF
2. Possible right-sided heart failure
3. Dysrhythmias

Nursing Assessment

Mitral Stenosis

1. Auscultate for accentuated first heart sound, usually accompanied with an "opening snap" (due to sudden

tensing of valve leaflets) at apex with diaphragm of stethoscope.

2. Place the patient in left lateral recumbent position. With bell of stethoscope at apex, auscultate for a low-pitched diastolic murmur (rumbling murmur). Note duration of murmur (long duration is indicative of significant stenosis).

Mitral Insufficiency

1. Auscultate for diminished first heart sound.
2. Auscultate for systolic murmur (prominent finding), commencing immediately after first heart sound at apex, and note radiation of sound to axilla and left intrascapular area.
3. Mild insufficiency may produce a pansystolic murmur (little connection between severity of mitral insufficiency and intensity of murmur auscultated).

Aortic Stenosis

1. Auscultate for prominent fourth heart sound and possible paradoxical splitting of second heart sound (suggestive of associated left ventricular dysfunction). First heart sound is normal.
2. Auscultate for a midsystolic murmur at the base of the heart (heard best) and at the apex of heart. Note harsh and rasping quality at base of heart and a higher pitch at apex of heart.

Aortic Insufficiency

1. Auscultate for soft first heart sound.
2. Place the patient in sitting position leaning forward.
3. Place diaphragm of stethoscope along left sternal border at the third and fourth intercostal space and then along the right sternal border. Auscultate for a high-pitched diastolic murmur. To increase audibility of murmur, ask the patient to hold breath at end of deep expiration. Reauscultate for murmur.

Tricuspid Stenosis

Auscultate for a blowing diastolic murmur at the lower left sternal border (increases with inspiration).

Tricuspid Insufficiency

1. Auscultate for a third heart sound (may be accentuated by inspiration).
2. Auscultate for a pansystolic murmur in the parasternal region at the fourth intercostal space. Murmur is usually high pitched.

Nursing Diagnoses

- Decreased Cardiac Output related to altered preload, afterload, or contractility
- Activity Intolerance related to reduced oxygen supply
- Ineffective Individual Coping related to acute/chronic illness

Nursing Interventions

Maintaining Adequate Cardiac Output

1. Assess frequently for change in existing murmur or new murmur.

2. Assess for signs of left and/or right ventricular failure.
3. Monitor and treat dysrhythmias as ordered.
4. Prepare the patient for surgical intervention (see p. 350).

Improving Tolerance

1. Maintain bed rest while symptoms of CHF are present.
2. Allow patient to rest between interventions.
3. Begin activities gradually (eg, chair sitting for brief periods).
4. Assist or perform hygiene needs for patient to reserve strength for ambulation.

Strengthening Coping Abilities

1. Instruct the patient regarding specific valvular dysfunction, possible etiology, and therapies implemented to relieve symptoms.
   a. Include family members in discussions with the patient.
   b. Stress the importance of adapting lifestyle to cope with illness.
2. Discuss with the patient surgical intervention as the treatment modality, if applicable.
3. Assess the patient's use of appropriate coping mechanisms to deal with illness.
4. Refer the patient to appropriate counseling services, if indicated (vocational, social work, cardiac rehabilitation).

Patient Education and Health Maintenance

1. Review activity restriction/schedule with patient and family.
2. Instruct patient to report signs of impending or worsening heart failure—dyspnea, cough, increased fatigue, ankle swelling.
3. Review sodium and/or fluid restrictions.
4. Review medications—purpose, action, schedule and side effects.
5. See sections titled Patient Education, Heart Failure, page 387; Infective Endocarditis, page 375; and Rheumatic Endocarditis, page 377.

Outcome-Based Evaluation

- Blood pressure and heart rate within normal limits
- Tolerating chair sitting for 15 minutes every 2 hours
- Discussing ways to cope with lifestyle/activity changes

Cardiac Dysrhythmias

Cardiac dysrhythmias are disturbances in regular heart rate and/or rhythm due to change in electrical conduction or automaticity. Dysrhythmias may arise from the SA node (sinus bradycardia or tachycardia) or anywhere within the atria or ventricles (known as ectopy or ectopic beats). Some may be benign and asymptomatic, whereas other dysrhythmias are life-threatening.

Dysrhythmias may be detected by change in pulse, abnormality on auscultation of heart rate, or ECG abnormality. Continuous cardiac monitoring is indicated for potentially life-threatening dysrhythmias.

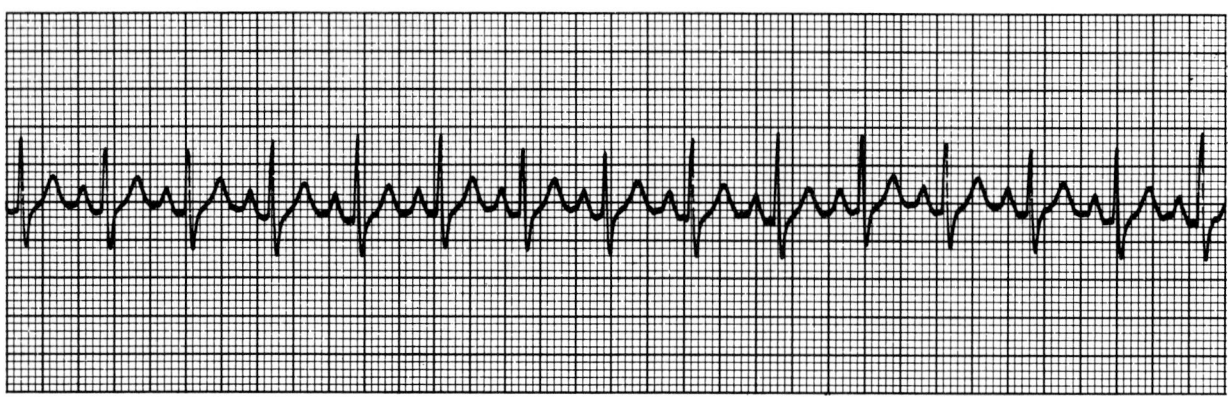

FIGURE 13-4   Sinus tachycardia.

Sinus Tachycardia (Figure 13-4)
Etiology
1. Sympathetic nerve fibers, which act to speed up excitation of the SA node, are stimulated by underlying causes such as anxiety, exercise, fever, shock, drugs, altered metabolic states (such as hyperthyroidism), or electrolyte disturbances.
2. The wave of impulse is transmitted through the normal conduction pathways; the rate of sinus stimulation is simply greater than normal (rate exceeds 100 beats per minute).

Analysis
Rate: 130
Rhythm: R–R intervals are regular

P wave: present for each QRS complex, normal configuration, and each P wave is identical
P–R interval: falls between 0.12 and 02.0, or 0.16 second
QRS complex: normal in appearance, one follows each P wave
QRS interval: 0.06 second
T wave: follows each QRS complex and is positively conducted

Management
1. Treatment is directed toward elimination of the cause, rather than the dysrhythmia.
2. Urgency is dependent on the effect of rapid heart rate on coronary artery filling time to prevent cardiac ischemia.

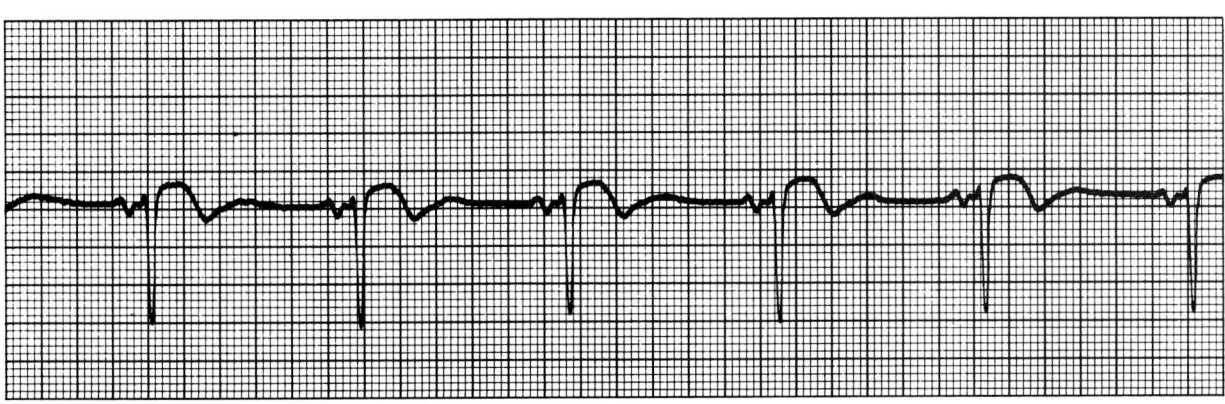

FIGURE 13-5 Sinus bradycardia.

Sinus Bradycardia (Figure 13-5)
Etiology
1. The parasympathetic fibers (vagal tone) are stimulated and cause the sinus node to slow.
2. Underlying causes
   a. Can be expected in the well-trained athlete
   b. Drugs
   c. Altered metabolic states, such as hypothyroidism
   d. The process of aging, which causes increasing fibrotic tissue and scarring of the SA node
   e. Certain cardiac diseases, such as acute MI (especially inferior wall MI)
3. The wave of impulse is transmitted through the normal conduction pathways; the rate of sinus stimulation is simply less than normal (less than 60 beats per minute).

Analysis
Rate: 55
Rhythm: R–R interval is regular
P wave: present for each QRS complex, normal configuration, and each P wave is identical
P–R interval: falls between 0.12 and 0.18 second
QRS complex: normal in appearance, one follows each P wave
QRS interval: 0.04–0.08 second
T wave: follows each QRS and is positively conducted

Management
1. The urgency of treatment depends on the effect of the slow rate on maintenance of cardiac output.
2. Atropine 0.5 mg IV push blocks vagal stimulation to the SA node and therefore accelerates heart rate.
3. If the bradycardia persists, a pacemaker may be required.

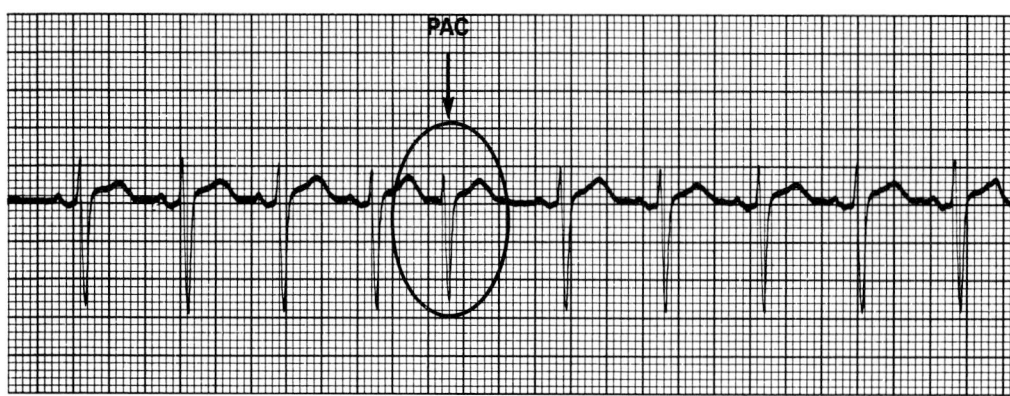

FIGURE 13-6   Normal sinus rhythm with premature atrial contraction.

Premature Atrial Contraction (PAC; Figure 13-6)
Etiology

1. May occur in the healthy or diseased heart. Is of no particular significance in the healthy heart. In the diseased heart, it may represent ischemia and a resultant irritability in the atria.
2. The PAC may increase in frequency and be the precursor of more serious dysrhythmias in the diseased heart.
3. The wave of impulse of the PAC originates within the atria and outside the sinus node.
4. Because the impulse originates within the atria, the P wave will be present, but it will be different in appearance as compared with those beats originating within the sinus node.
5. The impulse traverses the remainder of the conduction system in a normal pattern; thus, the QRS complex is identical in configuration to the normal sinus beats.

Analysis

Rate: may be slow or fast.

Rhythm: will be irregular; this is caused by the early occurrence of the PAC.

P wave: will be present for each normal QRS complex; the P wave of the premature contraction will be distorted in shape.

P–R interval: may be normal but can also be shortened, depending on where in the atria the impulse originated. The closer the site of atrial impulse formation to the AV node, the shorter the P–R interval will be.

QRS complex: within normal limits because all conduction below the atria is normal.

T wave: normally conducted.

Management

1. Generally requires no treatment.
2. PACs should be monitored for increasing frequency.

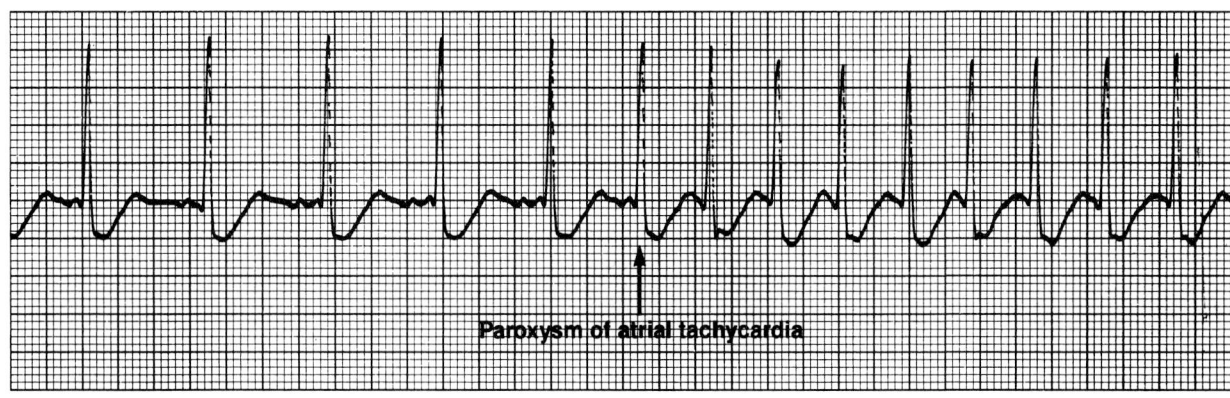

FIGURE 13-7 Paroxysmal atrial tachycardia.

Paroxysmal Atrial Tachycardia (PAT; Figure 13-7)
Etiology
1. Causes include:
   a. Syndromes of accelerated pathways (eg, Wolff-Parkinson-White syndrome)
   b. Syndrome of mitral valve prolapse
   c. Ischemic coronary artery diseases
   d. Excessive use of alcohol, cigarettes, caffeine
   e. Drugs—digoxin (Lanoxin) is a frequent cause
2. An ectopic atrial focus captures the rhythm of the heart and is stimulated at a very rapid rate; the impulse is conducted normally through the conduction system so the QRS complex usually appears within normal limits.
3. The rate is often so rapid that P waves are not obvious but may be "buried" in the preceding T wave.

Analysis
Rate: between 150 and 250 beats per minute
Rhythm: regular
P waves: present before each QRS complex; however, the faster the rate, the more difficult it becomes to visualize P waves. The P waves can frequently be measured with calipers by observing the varying configuration of the preceding T waves
P–R interval: usually not measurable
QRS complex: will appear normal in configuration and within 0.06 to 0.10 second
T waves: will be distorted in appearance as a result of P waves being buried in them

Management
1. Treatment is directed first to slowing the rate and, second, to reverting the dysrhythmia to a normal sinus rhythm.
2. Reducing the rate may be accomplished by having the patient perform a Valsalva maneuver. This stimulates the vagus nerve to slow the heart.
   a. A Valsalva maneuver may be done by having the patient gag or "bear down" as though attempting to have a bowel movement.
   b. The health care provider may choose to perform carotid massage.
3. Adenosine (Adenocard) is the drug of choice for PAT associated with hypotension, chest pain, or shortness of breath.
   a. The initial dose is 6 mg rapid IV push followed by 12 mg. If no response in 1 to 2 minutes, a third bolus of 12 mg may be needed.
   b. Has a very short half-life and is therefore eliminated quickly.
4. Beta-adrenergic blockers such as esmolol (Brevibloc) may be used.
5. The calcium channel blocking agents (eg, verapamil [Calan]) are effective in reverting this dysrhythmia. Beware of hypotension especially in the volume-depleted patient.
6. If drug therapy is ineffective, elective cardioversion can be used.

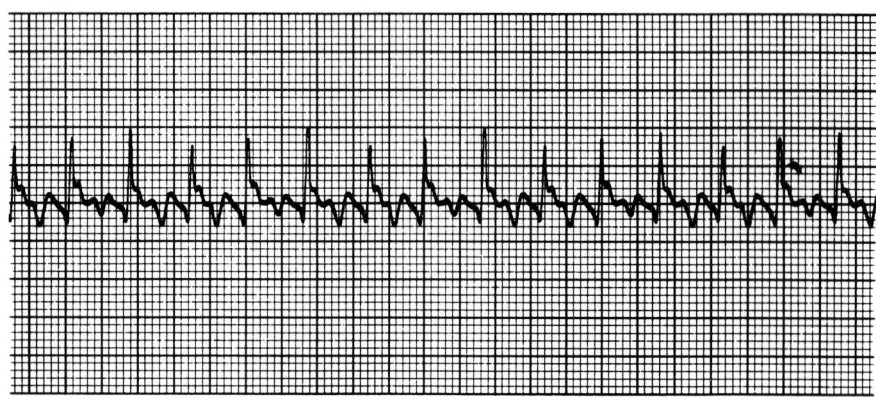

FIGURE 13-8   Atrial flutter.

Atrial Flutter (Figure 13-8)
Etiology
1. Occurs with atrial stretching or enlargement (as atrioventricular valvular disease), myocardial infarction, and congestive heart failure.
2. An ectopic atrial focus captures the rhythm in atrial flutter and fires at an extremely rapid rate (200 to 400) with regularity.
3. Conduction of the impulse through the conduction system is normal; thus, the QRS complex is unaffected.
4. An important feature of this dysrhythmia is that the AV node sets up a therapeutic block, which disallows some impulse transmission.
   a. This can produce a varying block or a fixed block (ie, sometimes the AV node will transmit every second flutter wave, producing a 2:1 block, or the rhythm can be 3:1 or 4:1).
   b. If the AV node conducted 1:1, then the outcome would be a ventricular rate of about 300/min. This would rapidly deteriorate.

Analysis
Rate: atrial rate between 250 and 400 beats per minute; ventricular rate will depend on degree of block.
Rhythm: regular or irregular, depending on kind of block (eg, 2:1, 3:1, or a combination).

P wave: not present; instead, it is replaced by a sawtoothed pattern that is produced by the rapid firing of the atrial focus. These waves are also referred to as "F" waves.
P–R interval: not measurable.
QRS complex: normal configuration and normal conduction time.
T wave: present but may be obscured by flutter waves.

Management
1. The urgency of treatment depends on the ventricular response rate and resultant symptoms. Too rapid or slow a rate will decrease cardiac output.
2. A calcium channel blocker such as diltiazem (Cardizem) may be used to slow AV nodal conduction. Use with caution in the patient with CHF, hypotension, or concomitant beta-blocker therapy.
3. Digitalis and quinidine preparations may be used.
4. A beta-adrenergic blocking drug such as esmolol (Brevibloc) may also be used.
5. If drug therapy is unsuccessful, atrial flutter will often respond to cardioversion. Small doses of electrical current are often successful.
6. Electrophysiologic studies and subsequent ablation therapy are highly effective because the ectopic focus is usually readily identified.

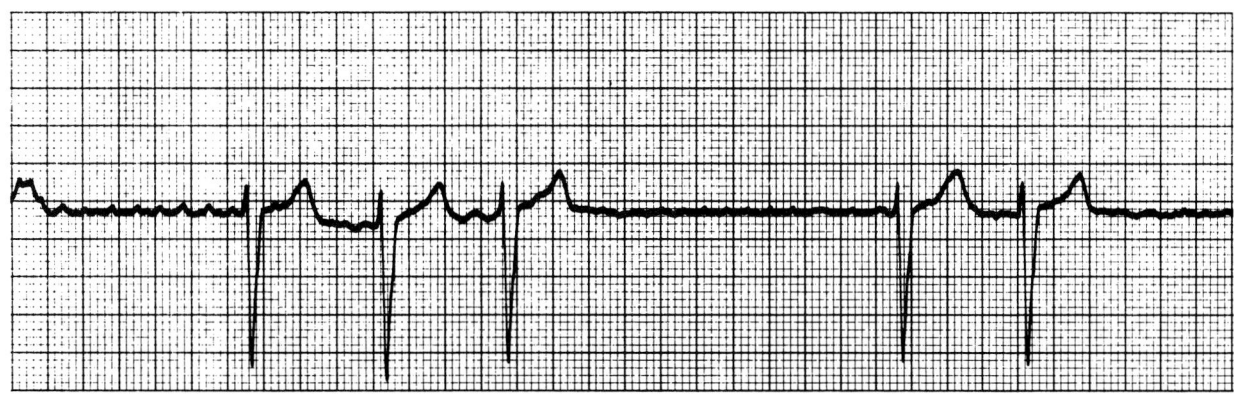

FIGURE 13-9 Atrial fibrillation with slow ventricular response (controlled).

Atrial Fibrillation (Figure 13-9)
Etiology
1. Fibrotic changes associated with the aging process, acute MI, valvular diseases, and digitalis preparations may cause atrial fibrillation.
2. Multiple atrial foci fire impulses at rapid and disorganized rates.
3. The atria are not depolarized effectively; hence, there are no well-formed P waves.
4. Instead, the baseline between QRS complexes is filled with a "wiggly" line that is described as fine or coarse.
5. If the atrial rate is rapid enough, the line will appear almost flat. The atria are said to be firing at rates of between 300 and 500 times per minute.
6. The conduction of a QRS complex is so random that the rhythm is extremely irregular.
7. Atrial fibrillation may be described as controlled if the ventricular response is 100 beats per minute or less; the dysrhythmia is uncontrolled if the rate is above 150 beats per minute.

Analysis
Rate: atrial fibrillation is usually immeasurable because fibrillatory waves replace P waves; ventricular rate may vary from bradycardia to tachycardia.
Rhythm: classically described as an "irregular irregularity."

P wave: replaced by fibrillatory waves, sometimes called "little f" waves.
P–R interval: not measurable.
QRS complex: a normally conducted complex.
T wave: normally conducted.

Management
1. Controlled atrial fibrillation of long-standing duration requires no treatment as long as the patient is experiencing no untoward effects. Most cardiologists agree that reversion of long-standing atrial fibrillation is hazardous because of the potential for a thrombus to be dislodged from the atria at the time of reversion.
2. Uncontrolled atrial fibrillation (ventricular responses of 100 beats per minute or greater) is treated with digitalis preparations. If the atrial fibrillation is of recent onset, the cardiologist may choose to revert the rhythm to a sinus rhythm.
3. Atrial fibrillation is treated with electrical cardioversion if the patient is unstable.
4. The beta-adrenergic blocking drugs or calcium ion antagonists may also be used if digitalis and quinidine prove ineffective.
5. Adenosine (Adenocard) may be used to assist in diagnosing the rhythm.

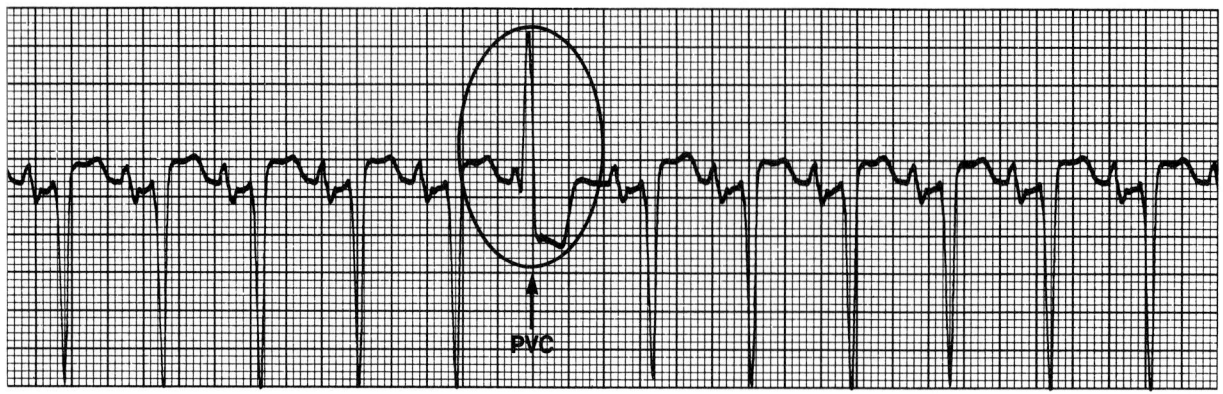

FIGURE 13-10 Normal sinus rhythm with premature ventricular contraction.

Premature Ventricular Contraction
(PVC; Figure 13-10)
Etiology
1. May be caused by acute MI, other forms of heart disease, pulmonary diseases, electrolyte disturbances, metabolic instability, and drug abuse.
2. The wave of impulse originates from an ectopic focus (foci) within the ventricles at a rate faster than the next normally occurring beat.
3. Because the normal conduction pathway is bypassed, the configuration of the PVC is wider than normal and is distorted in appearance.
4. PVCs may occur in regular sequence with normal rhythm—every other beat (bigeminy), every third beat (trigeminy), and so forth (Figure 13-11).

Analysis
  Rate: may be slow or fast.
  Rhythm: will be irregular because of the premature firing of the ventricular ectopic focus.
  P wave: will be absent, because the impulse originates in the ventricle, bypassing the atria and AV node.
  P–R interval: not measurable.

QRS complex: will be widened greater than 0.12 second, bizarre in appearance when compared with normal QRS complex. The QRS of a PVC is often referred to as having a "sore thumb" appearance.
T wave: the T wave of the PVC is usually deflected opposite to the QRS.

Management
1. PVCs are usually the precursors of more serious ventricular dysrhythmias. The following conditions involving PVCs require prompt and vigorous treatment:
   a. PVCs occurring at a rate exceeding six per minute
   b. Occur as two or more consecutively
   c. PVCs fall on the peak or down slope of the T wave (period of vulnerability)
   d. Are of varying configurations, indicating a multiplicity of foci
2. The standard treatment of PVCs is with lidocaine hydrochloride (Xylocaine) by IV push.
   a. For effective treatment of PVCs, it is important to raise the serum level of lidocaine as rapidly as possible without causing toxic effects.
   b. An initial bolus of 1 to 1.5 mg/kg may be administered.

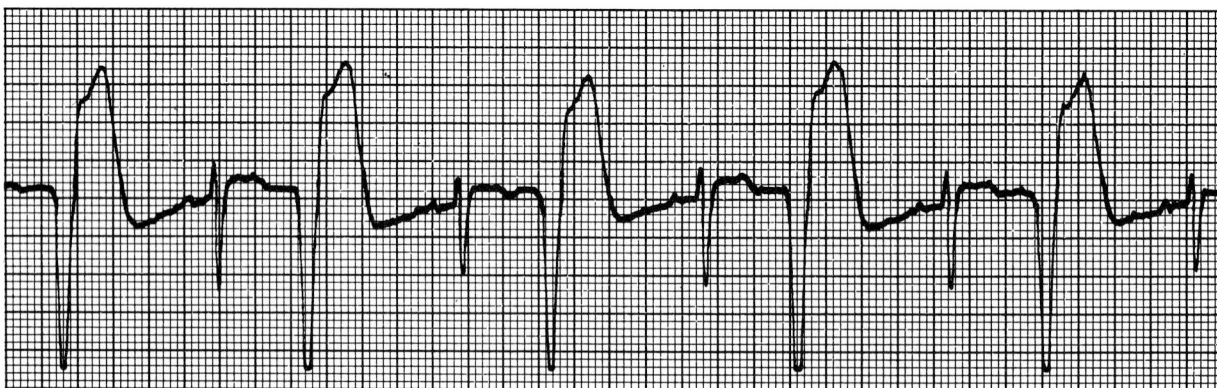

FIGURE 13-11 Ventricular bigeminy.

c. If the dysrhythmia continues to "break through," another 1 mg/kg bolus may be given within 15 minutes.

d. The bolus should be followed by a continuous IV infusion of lidocaine 2 g/500 mL D5W at 1 to 4 mg/min.

3. Be alert to the development of confusion, slurring of speech, and diminished mentation, because lidocaine toxicity affects the central nervous system. Should these symptoms appear, slowing the lidocaine may cause them to abate.

 DRUG ALERT

Lidocaine (Xylocaine) must be used with extreme caution in patients with liver disease and in the elderly.

4. If ventricular ectopy occurs concomitantly with a bradycardia, use lidocaine with caution, if at all. The ectopy may be compensation for the bradycardia. If lidocaine abolishes compensatory beats, the cardiac output may be seriously compromised, to the patient's detriment.

5. If ventricular premature beats occur in conjunction with a bradydysrhythmia, atropine may be chosen to accelerate the heart rate and eliminate the need for ectopic beats.

6. Atropine should be used with caution in the acute MI. The injured myocardium may not be able to tolerate the accelerated rate.

7. If lidocaine proves to be ineffective in controlling PVCs, procainamide (Pronestyl) may be given (IV push), followed by a continuous drip. The average bolus dose is 300 mg. Procainamide may cause hypotension.

8. If lidocaine and procainamide prove ineffective, either alone or in combination therapy, bretylium tosylate (Bretylol) may be used. Bretylium is administered in a continuous infusion.

9. Magnesium sulfate may be used, especially in patients with acute MI. It may be given as 1 g IV over 5 minutes to 24 hours depending on the urgency of the situation.

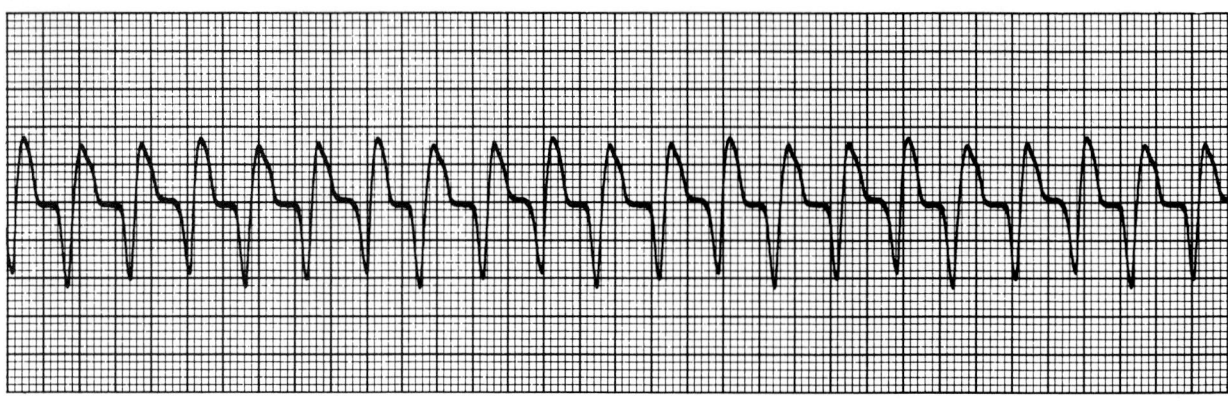

FIGURE 13-12   Ventricular tachycardia.

Ventricular Tachycardia (Figure 13-12)

Etiology

1. Occurs in:
   a. Acute MI
   b. Syndromes of accelerated rhythm that deteriorate (eg, Wolff-Parkinson-White syndrome)
   c. Metabolic acidosis, especially lactic acidosis
   d. Electrolyte disturbances
   e. Toxicity to certain drugs, such as digoxin (Lanoxin) or isoproterenol (Isuprel)
2. A life-threatening dysrhythmia that originates from an irritable focus within the ventricle at a rapid rate.
3. Because the ventricles are capable of an inherent rate of 40 beats per minute or less, a ventricular rhythm at a rate of 100 beats per minute may be considered tachycardia.

Analysis

Rate: usually between 140 and 220 beats per minute
Rhythm: usually regular but may be irregular
P wave: not present
P–R interval: not measurable
QRS complex: broad, bizarre in configuration, widened greater than 0.12 second
T wave: usually deflected opposite to the QRS complex

Management

1. If the patient is alert and not hemodynamically decompensating, lidocaine hydrochloride (Xylocaine) is administered as a bolus. This is followed by a continuous lidocaine infusion.
2. If the event is witnessed and the patient is unconscious, administer a precordial blow.
3. If the patient loses consciousness and pulse, immediate defibrillation is indicated.

NURSING ALERT

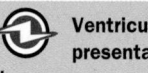 Ventricular tachycardia is life-threatening, and its presentation calls for immediate intervention by the nurse.

4. If the patient remains alert and drug therapy is not working, then synchronized cardioversion is applied. The purpose of cardioversion is to abolish all cardiac rhythm and allow the normal pacemaker the opportunity to capture the rhythm.
5. In some cases, ventricular tachycardia may be refractory to drug therapy. Nonpharmacologic treatments such as endocardial resection, aneurysmectomy, antitachycardia pacemakers, cryoablation, automatic internal defibrillators, and catheter ablation are alternative treatment modalities.
6. An atypical form of ventricular tachycardia, referred to as polymorphous ventricular tachycardia or torsades de pointes, can result as a consequence of drug therapy (eg, quinidine [Quinaglute] therapy) or electrolyte imbalance such as hypomagnesemia. It is important to differentiate this atypical form because its therapy differs from that of the more typical ventricular tachycardia.
   a. Torsades de pointes is characterized by a Q–T interval prolonged to greater than 0.60 second, varying R–R intervals, and polymorphous QRS complexes.
   b. The treatment of choice is administration of magnesium sulfate 1 g IV over 5 to 60 minutes.
   c. If the patient loses consciousness and pulse, defibrillate.
   d. Ventricular pacing to override the ventricular rate and, hence, capture the rhythm is also an acceptable treatment.
   e. Procainamide (Pronestyl) is avoided, because its effect is to prolong the Q–T interval.

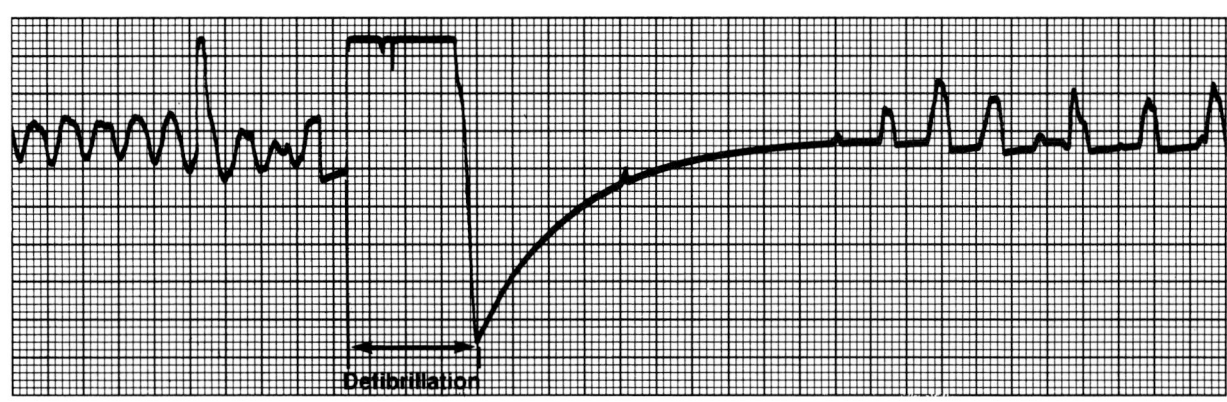

FIGURE 13-13 Ventricular fibrillation with defibrillation.

Ventricular Fibrillation (Figure 13-13)
Etiology
1. Occurs in acute MI, acidosis, electrolyte disturbances, and other deteriorating ventricular rhythms.
2. The ventricles are firing chaotically at rates that exceed 300 beats per minute and so do not allow for effective impulse conduction.
3. Cardiac output ceases, and the patient loses pulse, blood pressure, and consciousness.
4. Clinical death occurs and must be reversed immediately, or the patient will succumb.

Analysis
Rate: not measurable because of absence of well-formed QRS complexes
Rhythm: chaotic
P wave: not present
QRS complex: bizarre, chaotic, no definite contour
T wave: not apparent

Management
1. The only treatment for ventricular fibrillation is immediate defibrillation. Defibrillate at 200 watts/sec, then 200 to 300, then 360; pause only to check rhythm and pulse quickly between these defibrillations. Epinephrine may make the fibrillation more vulnerable to defibrillation.
2. If the third shock is unsuccessful, begin CPR and administer epinephrine (Adrenalin) 1 mg IV push.
3. Unsuccessful defibrillation may be a result of lactic acidosis.
4. Check adequacy of CPR.

Atrioventricular (AV) Block
Etiology
1. May be caused by ischemia or inferior wall MI, digitalis toxicity, hypothyroidism, or Stokes-Adams syndrome.
2. Impaired tissue at the level of the AV node prevents the timely passage of the wave of impulse through the conduction system.
3. In first-degree AV block, the impulse is transmitted normally, but it is delayed longer at the level of the AV node. The P–R interval exceeds 0.20 second.
4. In second-degree AV block, there is no relationship between the atrial activity recorded on the monitor and the ventricular activity. Both chambers are discharging impulses, but activity of the atria and activity of the ventricles bear no relationship to each other.

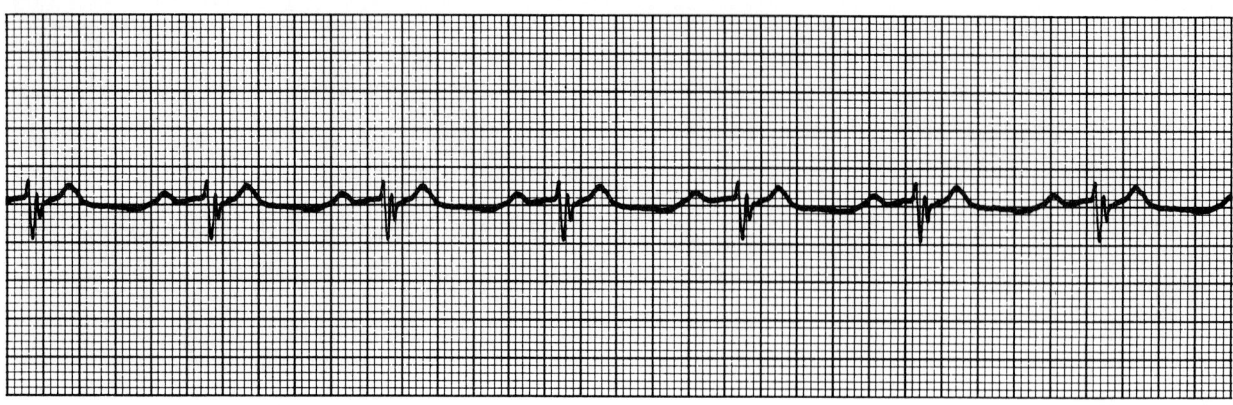

FIGURE 13-14   First-degree AV block.

Analysis

1. First-degree AV block (Figure 13-14)
   Rate: usually normal but may be slow
   Rhythm: regular
   P wave: present for each QRS complex, identical in configuration
   P–R interval: prolonged to greater than 0.20 second
   QRS complex: normal in appearance and between 0.06 and 0.10 second
   T wave: normally conducted
2. Second-degree AV block (Figure 13-15)
   Rate: usually normal.
   Rhythm: may be regular or irregular.
   P wave: present but some may not be followed by a QRS complex. A ratio of two, three, or four P waves to one QRS complex may exist.
   P–R interval: varies in Mobitz I (Wenckebach), usually lengthens until one is nonconducted; constant in Mobitz II, but not all Ps conducted.
3. Third-degree AV block (complete heart block) (Figure 13-16)
   Rate: atrial rate is measured independently of the ventricular rate. The ventricular rate is usually very slow.
   Rhythm: each independent rhythm will be regular, but they will bear no relationship to each other.
   P wave: present but no consistent relationship with the QRS.
   P–R interval: not really measurable.
   QRS complex: depends on the escape mechanism (ie, AV nodal will have normal QRS, ventricular will be wide and the rate will be slower).

Management

Like that of other dysrhythmias, the treatment of heart blocks depends on the effect the rate is having on cardiac output.

1. First-degree AV block usually requires no treatment.
2. Second-degree AV block may require treatment if the ventricular rate falls too low to maintain effective cardiac output.

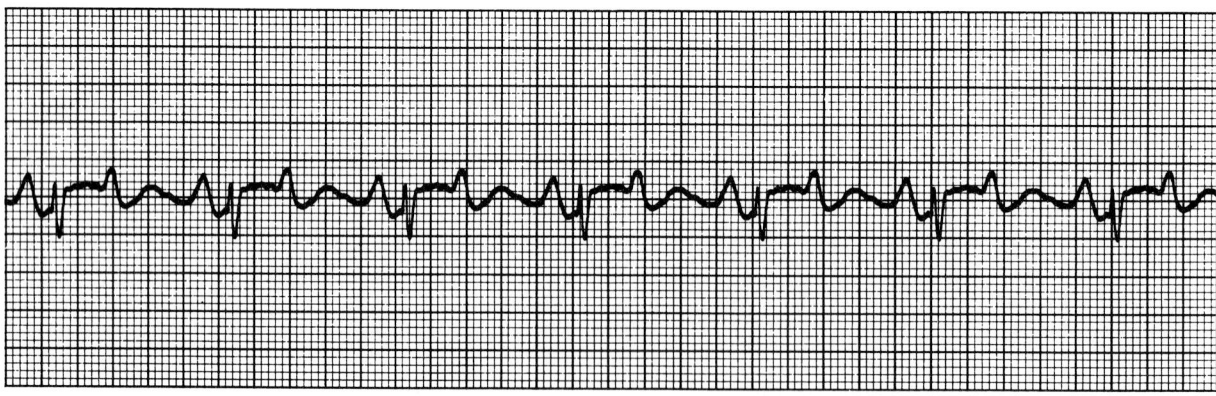

FIGURE 13-15   Second-degree AV block (Mobitz I).

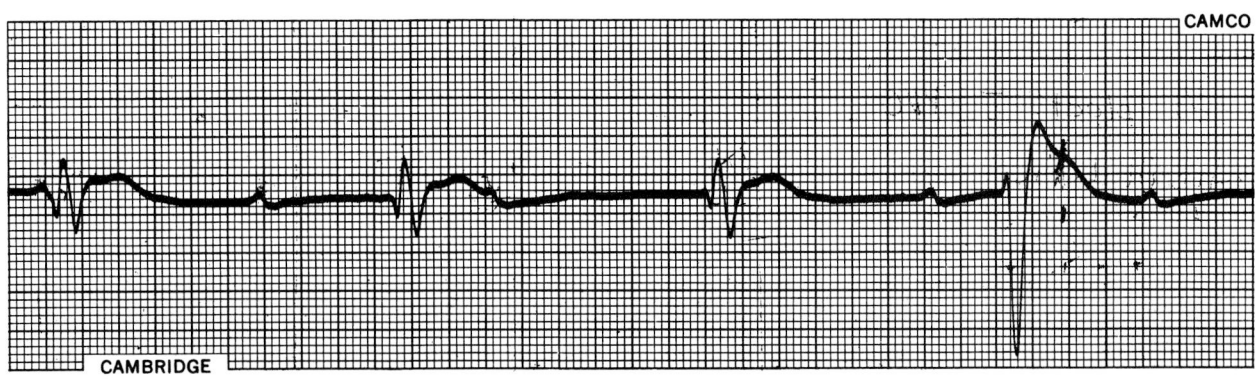

FIGURE 13-16 Third-degree AV block.

3. Third-degree AV block may require treatment of choice when intervention is called for.
4. Transcutaneous pacing should be employed in the emergent situation.
5. Atropine may be given while awaiting the pacemaker, but it must be remembered that the effect of atropine is to block vagal tone, and the vagus acts on the sinus node. Because the AV node is the culprit in heart block, atropine may not be helpful.

SELECTED REFERENCES

Andersen, R. E., Wadden, T. A., Bartlett, S. J., et al. (1999). Effects of lifestyle activity vs. structured aerobic exercise in obese women: A randomized trial. *Journal of the American Medical Association, 281,* 335.

Branum, K. (1999). Using beta-blockers in the treatment of heart failure. *Nurse Practitioner, 24*(7), 75–83.

Cantin, B., Gagnon, F., Moorjani, S., et al. (1998). Is lipoprotein (a) an independent risk factor for ischemic heart disease in men? The Quebec Cardiovascular Study. *Journal of the American College of Cardiology, 31,* 519–525.

Chyun, D. (1997). Nursing management of coronary heart disease in women: Using research findings. *Critical Care Nurse, 17*(2), 10–14.

Deckelbaum, R. J., Fisher, E. A., Winston, M., et al. (1999). Summary of a scientific conference on preventative nutrition: Pediatric to geriatric. *Circulation, 94,* 1795.

Freed, L. A., Levy, D., Levine, R. A., et al. (1999). Prevalence and clinical outcome of mitral valve prolapse. *New England Journal of Medicine, 34*(1), 1–7.

Grundy, S., Balady, G., Criqui, M., et al. (1997). Guide to primary prevention of cardiovascular diseases. A statement for healthcare professionals from the task force on risk reduction. *Circulation, 95,* 2329–2331.

Hak, A. E., Pols, H. A., Visser, T. J., et al. (2000). Subclinical hypothyroidism is an independent risk factor for atherosclerosis and myocardial infarction in elderly women: The Rotterdam study. *Annals of Internal Medicine, 132*(4), 270–278.

Halm, M. A., & Penque, S. (1999). Heart disease in women. *American Journal of Nursing, 99*(4), 26–31.

Hjalmarson, A., et al. (2000). Effects of controlled release metoprolol on total mortality, hospitalizations, and well-being in patients with heart failure: The Metoprolol CR/XL Randomized Intervention Trial in Congestive Heart Failure (MERIT-HF). *Journal of the American Medical Association, 283*(6), 1295–1302.

Leighton, C. (1998). A change of heart. *American Journal of Nursing, 98*(10), 33–37.

Malinow, M., Bostom, A., et al. (1999). Homocysteine, diet, and cardiovascular diseases. A statement for healthcare professionals from the nutrition committee, American Heart Association. *Circulation, 99*(1), 178.

McCarthy, R. E., et al. (2000). Long-term outcomes of fulminant myocarditis as compared with acute (nonfulminant) myocarditis. *New England Journal of Medicine, 342*(6), 690–695.

Metules, T. (1999). Cardiac tamponade. *RN, 62*(12), 26–30.

Milner, K. A., Funk, M., Richard, S., et al. (1999). Gender differences in symptom presentation associated with coronary heart disease. *American Journal of Cardiology, 84,* 396–399.

National Institutes of Health. (1993). *Second report of the expert panel on detection, evaluation and treatment of high blood cholesterol in adults: Adult treatment panel II.* Washington, DC: National Institutes of Health (Publication NIH 93-3095).

Pfister, S. M. (1999). Using clopidogrel bisulfate: A new antiplatelet drug. *Nurse Practitioner, 24*(9), 100–110.

Vaughn, C. J., Gotto, A. M., & Basson, C.T. (2000). The evolving role of statins in the management of atherosclerosis. *Journal of the American College of Cardiology, 35*(1), 1–10.

Wannamethee, S. G., Sharper, A. G., & Walker, M. (1998). Changes in physical activity, mortality, and incidence of coronary heart disease in older men. *Lancet, 351,* 1603.

Yug, B. S. (1999). Would you look for this CAD risk factor? *RN, 62*(11), 41–42.

Yusuf, S., Dagenais, G., Pogue, J., et al. (2000). Vitamin E supplementation and cardiovascular events in high-risk patients: The Heart Outcomes Prevention Evaluation Study Investigators. *New England Journal of Medicine, 342,* 154–160.

Yusuf, S., Sleight, P., Pogue, J., et al. (2000). Effects of an angiotensin-converting enzyme inhibitor, ramipril, on cardiovascular events in high-risk patients: The Heart Outcomes Prevention Evaluation Study Investigators. *New England Journal of Medicine, 342,* 145–153.

Vascular Disorders

MANAGEMENT OF VASCULAR DISORDERS

Anticoagulant Therapy

Anticoagulant therapy is the administration of medications to achieve the following:

- Disrupt the blood's natural clotting mechanism.
- Prevent formation of a thrombus in immobile and/or postoperative patients.
- Intercept the extension of a thrombus once it has formed.

Types of anticoagulants include coumarin derivatives such as warfarin sodium (Coumadin) given orally, and heparin sodium (Heparin) given parenterally. A new low-molecular-weight heparin, enoxaparin (Lovenox), is being given prophylactically following some orthopedic surgical procedures, such as total hip replacement. The benefits are its more steady bioavailability, longer half-life, and less platelet inhibition than standard heparin. Anticoagulants may be contraindicated or used with extreme caution in conditions that may lead to bleeding, in patients who may have poor follow-up, and in patients with hepatic and renal insufficiency (Procedure Guidelines 14-1).

◆ DRUG ALERT

Oral anticoagulants should be discontinued preoperatively to reduce the risk of hemorrhage in the intraoperative phase. IV anticoagulants may be prescribed preoperatively as their half-life is short; thus, the anticoagulant effects are reversed within 30 minutes to 1 hour after discontinuation.

Nursing Interventions

Administering Heparin

1. Weigh patient prior to initiating therapy as dose is calculated on the basis of weight.
2. For subcutaneous administration, see p. 405.
3. For intravenous administration, begin continuous infusion.
   a. Use continuous infusion pump.
   b. Assess frequently to ensure the pump is functioning properly, there are no kinks or leaks in IV tubing, and IV site is without signs/symptoms of infiltration.
4. Double-check concentration and dose of heparin, especially when giving high dosages.
5. Be aware that heparin may be continued for 4 to 5 days after oral anticoagulant is initiated due to the delayed onset of therapeutic effectiveness with oral anticoagulants.

Administering Coumadin

1. Give orally at the same time every day.
2. Usually given in the afternoon at dinnertime.

Administering Low-Molecular-Weight Heparin

1. Administered subcutaneously.
2. Dosage of enoxaparin is 30 mg every 12 hours.
3. Usually begun 12 to 24 hours after surgery and limited to 7 to 10 days.

NURSING ALERT

Obtain baseline coagulation and hematologic studies before initiating any anticoagulation therapy to ensure that the patient does not have an underlying bleeding/clotting disorder.

Monitoring Clotting Profiles

1. Activated partial thromboplastin time (APTT or PTT) is the coagulation test used to monitor the anticoagulation effects of heparin.
   a. The patient's PTT should be 2 to 2.5 times the control.
   b. Obtain PTT levels daily or as ordered. Heparin dose will be adjusted to achieve the desired level of anticoagulation.
2. Other lab studies to monitor as ordered and/or if bleeding is suspected:
   a. Platelet count
   b. Hemoglobin and hematocrit
   c. Fibrinogen
3. Prothrombin time (PT) and international normalized ratio (INR) are the coagulation tests used to monitor the anticoagulation effects of Coumadin.
   a. The patient's INR should be 2 to 3.5 times the control. *Note:* The desired levels of INR are determined by the health care provider.
   b. Obtain PT/INR levels daily or as ordered. Coumadin dose will be adjusted to achieve the desired level of anticoagulation.
4. Other lab studies to monitor as ordered and/or if bleeding is suspected while patient is on Coumadin:
   a. Platelet count
   b. Hemoglobin and hematocrit
5. Be aware of drug–drug (including over the counter and herbal supplements) and food–drug interactions that may alter the effects of Coumadin. This occurs because of alterations in the clearance of the drug or the rate of intestinal absorption. The following is a partial list of drugs/food that alter the metabolism of Coumadin. Please consult a pharmacist and/or medication reference book for a complete list.
   a. Decreases INR:
      (i) Barbiturates
      (ii) Antacids
      (iii) Oral contraceptives
      (iv) Estrogen
      (v) Adrenal corticosteroids
      (vi) Quinidine
      (vii) Tamoxifen
      (vii) Rifampin
      (viii) Vitamin K–rich foods (green leafy vegetables)
   b. Increases INR:
      (i) Aspirin
      (ii) Heparin
      (iii) Nonsteroidal anti-inflammatories (NSAIDs)
      (iv) Cimetidine
      (v) Antibiotics—high-dose penicillins, "mycins," cephalosporins
      (vi) Fluconazole
      (vii) Ticlodipine
      (viii) Thyroxine
      (ix) Indomethacin
      (x) Sulfa compounds
      (xi) Alcohol
      (xii) Gingko biloba
      (xiii) Ginseng
      (xiv) Garlic
6. No monitoring of PTT or other coagulation tests is required for low-molecular-weight heparin except in patients with renal disease and patients weighing <50kg or >80kg.

DRUG ALERT

Drug and food interactions can alter the effect of anticoagulants. Review the effect of other medications and herbal supplements the patient may be taking during anticoagulant therapy.

Preventing Bleeding

1. Follow precautions to prevent bleeding.
   a. Handle patient carefully while turning and positioning.
   b. Maintain pressure on IV and venipuncture sites for at least 5 minutes. Apply ice if patient is prone to bleeding.
   c. Assist with ambulation and keep walkways/hallways free from clutter to prevent falls.
2. Observe carefully for any possible signs of bleeding and report immediately so that anticoagulant dosage may be reviewed and altered if necessary:
   a. Hematuria—frank blood in urine or microhematuria as detected on test strip.
   b. Melena—assess for dark/tarry stools, use test cards for occult blood.
   c. Hemoptysis—assess for frank blood in emesis, use test cards for occult blood.
   d. Bleeding gums—note any pink saliva or frank bleeding with dental hygiene.
   e. Epistaxis—frequent/persistent nosebleeds.
   f. Inspect skin carefully for any bruising/hematomas.
3. Have on hand the antidotes to reverse anticoagulants being used:
   a. Heparin—protamine sulfate
   b. Warfarin—phytonadione (vitamin K_1, Aquamephyton)

NURSING ALERT

There is a risk of bleeding in any patient receiving anticoagulants.

Patient Education and Health Maintenance

1. Instruct patient about taking anticoagulant.
   a. Follow instructions carefully and take medications exactly as prescribed.
   b. Notify all health care providers, including dentist, that you are taking anticoagulants.
   c. Avoid foods that may alter the effects of anticoagulation medication or that if used, should be used in

the same quantity every day: green leafy vegetables, fish, liver, green tea, tomatoes.

d. Take medications at the same time each day and do not stop taking them even if symptoms of thrombus/embolus are not present.

e. Wear a bracelet or carry a card indicating that anticoagulants are being taken; include name, address, and telephone number of health care provider.

2. Advise the patient to notify the health care provider of any of the following:

a. All medications both prescribed and over the counter (including vitamins and herbal supplements) that he or she is currently taking.

b. Accidents, infections, excessive diarrhea, and other significant illnesses that may affect blood clotting.

c. Scheduled invasive procedures by other health care providers, including routine dental exams and other dental procedures, cardiac catheterizations, etc. If surgical care by another health care provider or dentist is needed, inform other provider that anticoagulants are being taken.

d. Missed doses—if anticoagulation dose is forgotten, do not take extra pills to make up for a skipped dose.

3. Advise the patient to avoid:

a. Taking any other medications without first checking with health care provider, particularly:

(i) Vitamins
(ii) Herbal supplements
(iii) Aspirin
(iv) Mineral oil
(v) Cold medicines
(vi) Antibiotics
(vii) Phenylbutazone (Butazolidin)

b. Excessive use of alcohol because alcohol may affect clotting ability; check on acceptable limits for social drinking.

c. Participation in activities in which there is high risk of injury.

d. Foods that may cause diarrhea or upset stomach.

4. Instruct the patient to be alert for these warning signs:

a. Excessive bleeding that does not stop quickly (such as following shaving, a small cut, toothbrushing with gum injury, nosebleed)

b. Excessive menstrual bleeding

c. Skin discoloration or bruises that appear suddenly

d. Black or bloody bowel movements; for questionable stool discoloration, test for occult blood

e. Blood in urine

f. Faintness, dizziness, or unusual weakness

5. Stress the importance of close follow-up and compliance with periodic laboratory work for blood clotting profiles. Notify health care provider if you are unable to keep scheduled appointments.

| PROCEDURE GUIDELINES 14-1 | SUBCUTANEOUS INJECTION OF HEPARIN |

PURPOSE

When prolonged therapy is indicated, heparin may be given subcutaneously into fatty tissues. Low-dose subcutaneous heparin may be given postoperatively to prevent deep vein thrombosis.

EQUIPMENT

1- or 2-mL syringe or disposable tuberculin syringe
Fine sharp needle, no. 27, 1.6-cm (⅝ in.) long (or premeasured Tubex cartridge-needle unit)
Skin antiseptic

CONSIDERATIONS

1. Most convenient sites are along lower abdominal fat pad—to avoid inadvertent intramuscular injection and hematoma formation.

a. A common location site is the fatty area anterior to either iliac crest.

b. Avoid injection sites within 5 cm (2 in.) of the umbilicus because of possibility of entering a larger blood vessel.

2. Areas where subcutaneous layer is thin should be avoided.

GERONTOLOGIC ALERT

The aging individual begins to lose subcutaneous fat padding. Examine patient for best site for subcutaneous administration of heparin.

continued

PROCEDURE GUIDELINES 14-1   SUBCUTANEOUS INJECTION OF HEPARIN *CONTINUED*

Nursing Action	Rationale
PERFORMANCE PHASE	
1. Sponge the area gently with alcohol. Do not rub!	1. Rubbing or pinching skin might initiate damage to the tissue; heparin would aggravate any bleeding.
2. Attempt to stretch skin out, using palm of left hand. Some prefer to (gently) pick up a well-defined fold of skin.	2. Try to empty blood vessels in local area to lessen likelihood of their being pierced by needle—with subsequent hematoma formation.
3. Holding the shaft of the syringe in dart fashion, insert needle directly through the skin at a right angle just into the subcutaneous fatty layer.	
4. Move right hand into position to direct plunger. a. Do not move needle tip once it is inserted. b. Do not pull back plunger for testing.	4. Aspiration in a forcible manner can damage small blood vessels and frequently lead to bleeding and hematoma formation, especially in the presence of high local concentration of heparin.
5. Firmly push plunger down as far as it will go.	5. This ensures administration of total dose of heparin.
6. When injection has been made, withdraw needle gently at the same angle at which it entered, releasing skin roll on withdrawal of needle.	6. To minimize tissue damage.
7. Press an alcohol sponge to the site for a few seconds.	7. To minimize oozing or bleeding.
FOLLOW-UP CARE	
1. *Do not rub the area. Instruct patient not to rub area.*	1. Rubbing would increase the likelihood of bleeding.
2. *Site of injection* a. Change site of injection each time heparin is administered. b. A chart can be marked with time, date, and measured dosage so that rotation of sites can be ensured.	

Note: Low-dose heparin may be used to prevent deep vein thrombosis postoperatively.

Thrombolytic Therapy

Thrombolytic therapy is administration of thrombolytic agents to dissolve any formed thrombus and inhibit the body's hemostatic function. Thrombolytic agents are available for parenteral use only. Commonly used thrombolytics include streptokinase (Streptase) and tissue plasminogen activator (tPA, Activase).

Thrombolytic therapy is contraindicated in conditions that may lead to bleeding and should only be given in a controlled setting such as a cardiac catheterization laboratory or an intensive care unit. Thrombolytic therapy for deep vein thrombosis, however, may be given on step-down units or medical/surgical floors.

Clinical Indications

1. Acute MI from coronary thrombosis
2. Pulmonary embolus
3. Acute occlusion of peripheral arteries/prosthetic grafts
4. Deep vein thrombosis

Nursing Interventions

1. Monitor clotting profiles; these are essential before the initiation of treatment to disclose any bleeding tendencies and to serve as a baseline for assessment of drug efficacy.

2. Observe for signs of bleeding and report immediately.
   a. Have typed and cross-matched blood on hold in case bleeding is severe.
   b. Have aminocaproic acid (Amicar) on hand to treat bleeding.
3. Monitor for allergic reaction. A small number of patients (fewer than 5%) may experience an allergic reaction.
   a. Observe the patient for the onset of a new rash, fever, and chills.
   b. Report any suspected allergic reaction immediately.
   c. Administer corticosteroids, if ordered, to treat reaction.
4. Monitor electrocardiogram (ECG) for arrhythmias after reperfusion if thrombolytic therapy is being used for coronary thrombus.
5. Frequently assess color, warmth, and sensation of extremity if therapy is being used for peripheral arterial occlusion.

Care of the Patient Undergoing Vascular Surgery

Vascular surgery may involve operations of the arteries, veins, or lymphatic system. Surgery may be performed on an urgent basis, as in *embolectomy* for acute arterial embolism, or electively for *vein ligation and stripping* for varicose veins after conservative management fails. Other vascular procedures include *thrombectomy* and *vena caval filter insertion* for venous problems and *arterial bypass grafting* (aortoiliac, aortofemoral, femoropopliteal, and femoral-distal), *endarterectomy, endovascular grafting,* and *percutaneous transluminal angioplasty (PTA)* for arterial problems with or without placement of an intraluminal stent.

Preoperative Management

1. Additional health conditions such as heart disease, hypertension, diabetes mellitus, and chronic lung disease are fully evaluated, and management is adjusted to decrease operative risks.
2. Chronic skin and tissue changes are assessed preoperatively, and impairment is minimized through protection of the affected part(s), treatment with antibiotics, and proper positioning to enhance circulation (elevated for venous and lymphatic problems, level or slightly dependent for arterial problems).
3. Nutritional status is assessed and improved preoperatively to aid in wound healing postoperatively.
4. Risk factors for vascular disease, such as smoking, obesity, and sedentary lifestyle, are reviewed and patient teaching is begun to prevent recurrence/progression of vascular disorder.
5. The patient is prepared emotionally and physically for surgery, with teaching focusing on positioning in bed, exercises and activity expected to be followed postoperatively, frequently checking of circulation and wound, and preventing complications such as bleeding, infection, and neurovascular compromise.

Postoperative Management

1. Bed rest may be maintained for 24 hours to reduce swelling and the risk of bleeding.
2. If surgery involved revascularization, peripheral pulses are assessed distal from operative site to ensure adequate tissue perfusion.
3. If surgery involved use of bypass graft(s), the graft site(s) are protected and assessed for patency as well.
4. Extremity(s) is positioned with the popliteal space supported to prevent trauma and promote circulation.
5. Anticoagulation may be continued, but it increases chance of bleeding following surgery.
6. Hydration, nutrition, and oxygenation are promoted to ensure wound healing.
7. Surgical incisions are assessed for redness, drainage, and approximation and may be covered with dry dressings.
8. Breathing exercises using incentive spirometer are done every 2 hours while awake to prevent postoperative pulmonary complications.

Nursing Diagnoses

• Altered Tissue Perfusion (peripheral) related to underlying vascular disorder, postoperative swelling

• Risk for Infection related to surgical incision and impaired circulation
• Pain related to surgical incision and swelling
• Impaired Physical Mobility related to pain and imposed restrictions

Nursing Interventions

Promoting Tissue Perfusion

1. Maintain dressing or compression bandages as directed.
2. Monitor for bleeding through dressing—reinforce and notify surgeon as indicated.
3. Monitor for hematoma formation beneath skin—increased pain and swelling. Apply pressure and notify surgeon.
4. Measure vital signs frequently for tachycardia and hypotension, which may indicate hemorrhage.
5. Perform frequent neurovascular checks to involved extremity. Check warmth, color, capillary refill, sensation, movement, and pulses; compare with other side.
6. Position as directed—usually legs elevated and fully supported.

Preventing Infection

1. Maintain IV infusion or heparin lock for antibiotic administration as ordered and assess daily for signs of infiltration/infection.
2. Check incision site for drainage, warmth, and erythema, which indicate infection.
3. Change incision dressing(s) as ordered and prn for drainage/soiling.
4. Monitor temperature for elevation.
5. Monitor hematologic profiles for elevation in white blood cell count (WBC).

Relieving Pain

1. Assess pain level and administer analgesic as ordered.
2. If patient-controlled anesthesia (PCA) is being used, instruct patient on use and ensure proper functioning of pump.
3. Position for comfort, using pillows for support.
4. Watch for side effects of narcotics such as hypotension, respiratory depression, nausea and vomiting, and constipation.
5. Time pain medication before activity.
6. Instruct patient in alternative coping methods such as visualization.

Minimizing Immobility

1. Encourage isometric and range-of-motion exercises while on bed rest.
   a. Exercise affected extremity by pushing foot into footboard, making a fist, or simply contracting muscles without movement if approved by surgeon.
   b. Perform full range of motion of other extremities.
2. Encourage ambulation as soon as allowed.
   a. Avoid dangling legs because of possible compression against the back of bed or chair.
   b. Avoid long periods of sitting or standing.
   c. Encourage short periods of walking every 2 hours.

Patient Teaching and Health Maintenance

1. Instruct patient/significant other in care of incision and/or wound at home. Ensure that patient has proper resources available.
2. Instruct on wearing of elastic stockings as ordered.
3. Instruct patient/significant other in signs of infection, graft failure, or worsening circulatory problem that should be reported.
4. Refer patient to vascular rehabilitation, physical therapy, and occupational therapy as indicated.
5. Refer for additional support for risk factor modification, such as supervised weight loss programs, nutritional counseling, smoking cessation.
6. Instruct patient to avoid restrictive clothing (including socks, hose, shoes, etc.), especially over areas of revascularization.
7. Instruct patient to inspect feet, including plantar aspect and between toes, daily and to inspect shoes for foreign objects, such as small stones, prior to putting them on.
8. Instruct patient to wear thick socks and well-fitting shoes with wide toebox to avoid development of breakdown/ulceration on pressure points.
9. Review any medications, especially anticoagulants (see p. 403).
10. Ensure that the patient knows when and where to follow up.

Outcome-Based Evaluation

- Affected extremity(s) with good color, capillary refill, and pulses; warm and sensitive to touch; moving adequately
- Incision site(s) are well approximated and without signs and symptoms of infection
- Patient reports adequate pain control on current regimen
- Patient is ambulating for 10 minutes every 2 hours without difficulty or shows signs of progressing independence with the assistance of physical/occupational therapy

CONDITIONS OF VEINS

See Table 14-1.

Venous Thrombus

Phlebitis is an inflammation in the wall of a vein. The term is used clinically to indicate a superficial and localized condition that can be treated with application of heat.

Superficial thrombophlebitis is a condition in which a clot forms in a vein secondary to phlebitis or because of partial obstruction of the vein. More commonly seen in the greater or lesser saphenous veins of the lower extremities.

Phlebothrombosis is the formation of a thrombus or thrombi in a vein; in general, the clotting is related to (1) stasis, (2) abnormality of the walls of the vein(s), and (3) abnormality of the clotting mechanism. Deep veins of the lower extremities are most commonly involved.

TABLE 14-1   Comparison of Arterial and Venous Obstruction

Factor	Arterial Obstruction	Venous Obstruction
Onset	May be sudden	Gradual
Color	Pale	Slightly cyanotic
	Later—mottled, cyanotic	Rubescent
Skin temperature	Cold	Warm
Leg size	May be reduced	Enlarged
Leg hair and nails	Decreased hair; thick, brittle nails	No change
Edema	None to mild	Typically calf to foot
Sensation	Sensory changes	Normal sensation
Arterial pulses	Pulse deficit	Normal
Effect of elevating leg	Condition worsens	Slight improvement

Deep vein thrombosis (DVT) is thrombosis of deep rather than superficial veins. Two serious complications are pulmonary embolism and postphlebitic syndrome.

Note: While the terms do not necessarily represent identical pathologies, for clinical purposes they are used interchangeably when discussing the same process.

Pathophysiology and Etiology
General Points

1. Three antecedent factors are believed to play a significant role in the development of venous thromboses: (1) stasis of blood, (2) injury to the vessel wall, and (3) altered blood coagulation (Virchow's triad).
2. Usually two of the three factors occur before thrombosis develops.

Thrombosis-Related Situations

1. Venous stasis—following operations, childbirth, or bed rest for any prolonged illness.
2. Prolonged sitting or as a complication of varicose veins.
3. Injury (bruise) to a vein; may result from direct trauma or internal trauma as from IV catheters, infusion of medications, and/or infiltration of medications.
4. Extension of an infection of tissues surrounding the vessel.
5. Continuous pressure of a tumor, aneurysm, or excessive weight gain in pregnancy.
6. Unusual activity in a person who has been sedentary.
7. Hypercoagulability associated with malignant disease, blood dyscrasias.

High-Risk Factors

1. Malignancy
2. Previous venous insufficiency
3. Conditions causing prolonged bed rest—MI, congestive heart failure (CHF), sepsis, traction, end-stage cancer, HIV/AIDS
4. Leg trauma—fractures, cast, joint replacements
5. General surgery—over 40 years of age
6. Obesity, smoking

Clinical Manifestations

Clinical features vary with site and length of affected vein.

1. DVT may occur asymptomatically or may produce severe pain, fevers, chills, malaise, and swelling and cyanosis of affected arm or leg.
2. Superficial thrombophlebitis produces visible and palpable signs such as heat, pain, swelling, erythema, tenderness, and induration along the length of the affected vein.
3. Extensive vein involvement may cause lymphadenitis.

Diagnostic Evaluation

1. Venous duplex/color duplex ultrasound is commonly done. This noninvasive test allows for visualization of the thrombus, including any free-floating or unstable thrombi that may cause emboli. Most effective in the detection of thrombus in the lower extremities.
2. Impedance plethysmography (IPG): a noninvasive measurement of changes in calf volume corresponding to changes in blood volume brought about by temporary venous occlusion with a high-pneumatic cuff. Electrodes measure electrical impedance as cuff is deflated. Slow decrease in impedance indicates diminished blood flow associated with thrombus.
3. RF testing: radioactive fibrinogen (fibrinogen I^{125}) is administered intravenously. Images are taken through nuclear scanning at 12 to 24 hours; the radioactive fibrinogen will be concentrated at the area of clot formation.
4. Venography: intravenous injection of a radio-contrast agent. The vascular tree is visualized and obstruction is identified.
5. Coagulation profiles: APTT, PT/INR, circulating fibrin, monomer complexes, fibrinopeptide A, serum fibrin, protein C & S, antithrombin III levels. Detect intravascular coagulation.

Management

Goals: To prevent propagation of the thrombus, prevent recurrent thrombus formation, prevent pulmonary emboli, and limit venous valvular damage.

Anticoagulation

For documented cases of DVT to prevent embolization.

1. Heparin is given IV initially, followed by 3 to 6 months of oral anticoagulant therapy (see p. 403).
2. Heparin and enoxaparin may also be given subcutaneously as prophylaxis for the prevention of DVT, especially in postoperative and/or immobile patients.

Thrombolytic Therapy

May be used in life- or limb-threatening situations.

Most effective in dissolving existing clots within the first 24 hours of thrombolic event.

Nonpharmacologic Therapies

For superficial thrombophlebitis and as an adjunct to anticoagulation with DVT.

1. Bed rest: usually recommended for 5 days. Prevents muscle contraction with walking, which may dislodge clot.
2. Elevation of effected extremity: at least 10 to 20 degrees above the level of the heart to enhance venous return and decrease swelling.
   a. Pillows should be used to support the popliteal space.
   b. If the upper extremity is effected, a sling or stockingette attached to an IV pole may be used.
3. Compression: promotes venous return and reduces swelling.
   a. Electrically or pneumatically controlled stockings, boots, or sleeve
   b. Elastic stockings/garments
4. Dry heat
   a. Warm water bottles
   b. Ultrasound (acoustic vibration with frequencies beyond human ear perception)
5. Moist heat
   a. Hydrotherapy
   b. Whirlpool bath
   c. Warm compresses

Surgery

1. Placement of a filter into the inferior vena cava to prevent pulmonary embolism in a patient who cannot tolerate prolonged anticoagulant therapy.
2. Thrombectomy may be necessary for severely compromised venous drainage of the extremity.
3. See page 406 for surgical care.

Complications

1. Pulmonary embolism
2. Postphlebitic syndrome

Nursing Assessment

1. Obtain history of risk factors for thrombophlebitis.
2. Note symmetry or asymmetry of legs. Measure and record leg circumferences daily (Procedure Guidelines 14-2).
3. Observe for evidence of venous distention or edema, puffiness, stretched skin, hardness to touch.
4. Examine for signs of obstruction due to occluding thrombus—swelling, particularly in loose connective tissue or popliteal space, ankle, or suprapubic area.
5. Hand-test extremities for temperature variations—use dorsum (back) of same hand; first compare ankles, then move to the calf and up to the knee.
6. Assess for calf pain, which may be aggravated when foot is dorsiflexed with the knee flexed (Homans' sign) (Figure 14-1). Unfortunately, this sign is nonspecific and has a low sensitivity for detecting thrombophlebitis.
7. Assess all IV catheter insertion sites for signs and symptoms of infection and infiltration. Rotate peripheral IV sites every 72 hours or prn.

Nursing Diagnoses

- Pain related to decreased venous blood flow
- Risk for Injury (bleeding) related to anticoagulant therapy
- Impaired Physical Mobility related to pain and imposed treatment

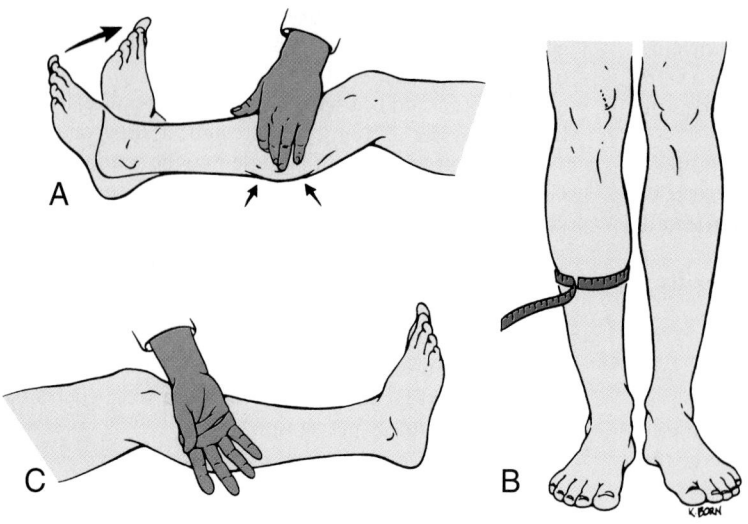

FIGURE 14-1 Nursing assessment for deep vein thrombosis. (**A**) Pain and tenderness in the calf of the affected extremity, especially on dorsiflexion of the foot (Homans' sign). (**B**) The affected extremity may have a larger circumference than the unaffected extremity, caused by edema. (**C**) The affected extremity will be warm to touch compared to the unaffected extremity.

Nursing Interventions
Relieving Pain

1. Elevate legs as directed to promote venous drainage and reduce swelling.
2. Apply warm compresses or heating pad as directed to promote circulation and reduce pain.
   a. Ensure that water temperature is not too hot.
   b. Cover plastic water bottle or heating pad with towel before applying to skin.
3. Administer acetaminophen (Tylenol), codeine, or other analgesic as prescribed and as needed. Avoid the use of aspirin (or aspirin-containing drugs) and nonsteroidal anti-inflammatory drugs (NSAIDs) during anticoagulant therapy to prevent further risk of bleeding.

NURSING ALERT

Avoid massaging or rubbing calf because of the danger of breaking up the clot, which can then circulate as an embolus.

Preventing Bleeding

See page 403 for nursing interventions for patients on anticoagulant therapy.

Preventing Other Hazards of Immobility

1. Prevent venous stasis by proper positioning in bed.
   a. Support full length of legs when they are to be elevated (Figure 14-2).
   b. Prevent pressure ulcers that may occur over bony prominences such as sacrum, hips, knees, and heels.

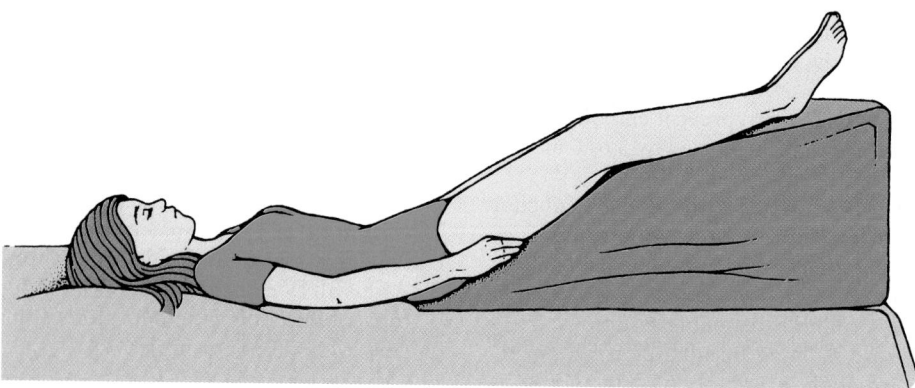

FIGURE 14-2 This leg elevator is of foam construction with a removable cotton cover that may be machine washed. It is clamped to the lower end of the mattress. This position is anatomically correct and provides adequate support to all parts of the leg. Edema and stasis of the lower extremities can be controlled. (Courtesy of Jobst.)

Be aware of bony prominence of one leg pressing on soft tissue of other leg (in side-lying position, place a soft pillow between legs).

   c. Avoid hyperflexion at knee as in jackknife position (head up, knees up, pelvis and legs down); this promotes stasis in pelvis and extremities.

2. Initiate active exercises unless contraindicated, in which case use passive exercises.
   a. If the patient is on bed rest:
     (i) Simulate walking if lying on back—5 minutes every 2 hours.
     (ii) Simulate bicycle pedaling if lying on side—5 minutes every 2 hours.
   b. If contraindicated, resort to passive exercises—5 minutes every 2 hours.

3. Encourage adequate fluid intake, frequent changes of position, and effective coughing and deep-breathing exercises.

4. Be alert for signs of pulmonary embolism—chest pain, dyspnea, anxiety, and apprehension—and report immediately.

5. After the acute phase (5-7 days), apply elastic stockings as directed (Figure 14-3). Remove twice daily and check for skin changes, pressure points, and calf tenderness.

6. Encourage ambulation when allowed (usually after 5-7 days, when clot has fully adhered to vessel wall).
   a. If permissible, have the patient sit up and move to side of bed in sitting position. Provide a foot support (stool or chair)—dangling of feet is not desirable because pressure may be exerted against popliteal vessels and may obstruct blood flow.
   b. If the patient is permitted out of bed, encourage walking 10 minutes each hour.
   c. Discourage crossing of legs and long periods of sitting because compression of vessels can restrict blood flow.

Community and Home Care Considerations

Practice preventive measures for bedridden patients who are prone to develop thrombosis:

1. Have the patient lie in bed in the slightly reversed Trendelenburg position because it is better for the veins to be full of blood than empty.

2. Place a footboard across the foot of the bed.

3. Instruct the patient to press the balls of the feet against the footboard, as if rising up on toes.
   a. Then have the patient relax the foot.
   b. Request that the patient do this 5 to 10 times each hour.

Patient Education and Health Maintenance

1. Teach patient signs of recurrent thrombophlebitis and pulmonary embolism to report immediately.

2. Provide thorough instructions about anticoagulant therapy (see p. 404).

3. Teach patient to promote circulation and prevent stasis by applying elastic hose at home.

Put on supports early in the morning, before swelling occurs.

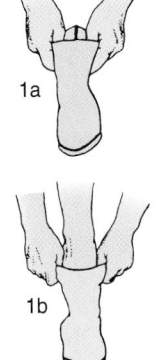

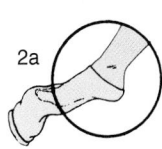

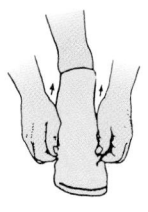

Always begin with supports "inside out"....as they are when you receive them.

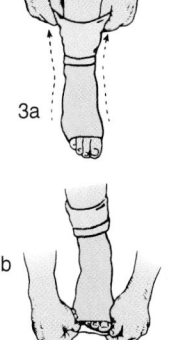

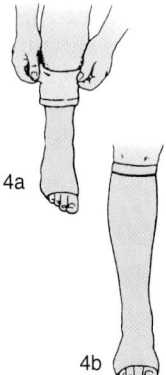

Sit with feet in easy reach. Support must be "inside out," with its foot inverted back to heel. Seam faces own (sketch 1a). Grasp each side firmly and pull onto foot (sketch 1b).

Pull past midpoint of heel (skech 2a), so support will not slip back. Then, reach just beyond toes and grasp fabric between fingers and start pulling over foot. Pull from sides... never by seams.

Pull all the way up past ankle (sketch 3a). Seat heel in place. Pull foot portion of support out toward tips of toes (sketch 3b) to set fabric evenly on foot. Allow to settle back normally.

Using short (2 inches at a time) snappy pulls (sketch 4a) pull support up to point it was measured to end (sketch 4b). Smooth evenly down leg. Never allow top to roll or turn down.

FIGURE 14-3 Method of applying supporting hose. (Courtesy of Jobst.)

4. Advise against straining or any maneuver that increases venous pressure in the leg. Eliminate the necessity to strain at stool by increasing fiber and fluids in the diet.

5. Warn patient of hazards of smoking and obesity: nicotine constricts veins, decreasing venous blood flow. Extra pounds increase pressure on leg veins. Make appropriate referrals to nutritionist, smoking-cessation classes, etc., as needed.

6. Advise patient to avoid prolonged periods of sitting or standing. If necessary, perform exercises to encourage venous return.

Outcome-Based Evaluation

- Patient verbalizes reduced pain
- No bleeding is observed
- Normal respiratory status is maintained

Chronic Venous Insufficiency

Chronic venous insufficiency, also called *postphlebitic syndrome,* is a form of chronic venous stasis; it may be a residual effect of phlebitis. It results from chronic occlusion of the veins or destruction of the valves.

Pathophysiology and Etiology

1. Smaller vessels have dilated because main channel for returning blood from the leg to the heart was blocked by a thrombus.

2. Valves of diseased veins can no longer prevent backflow, thereby → chronic venous stasis → swelling and edema → superficial varicose veins.

3. Lower leg becomes discolored because of venous stasis and pigmentation ulceration (postphlebitis).

4. Most commonly involves iliac and femoral veins and occasionally saphenous vein.

Clinical Manifestations

1. Chronic edema; worse while legs dependent.

2. Intractable induration, discoloration, pain, ulceration; area surrounding medial malleolus is the most common site.

Diagnostic Evaluation and Management

1. Doppler, plethysmography—noninvasive screening that shows obstruction and valve incompetency.

2. Best treatment is prevention of phlebitis and constant use of compression if phlebitis has occurred.

3. After this syndrome has developed, only palliative and symptomatic treatment is possible because the damage is irreparable.

Complications

1. Stasis ulcers
2. Cellulitis
3. Recurrent thrombosis

Nursing Interventions and Patient Education

Instruct the patient as follows:

1. Wear elastic stockings to prevent edema.

2. Avoid sitting or standing for long periods of time or sitting with legs crossed.

3. Elevate legs on a chair for 5 minutes every 2 hours.

4. Elevate legs above level of head by lying down two to three times daily.

5. Raise foot of bed 15 to 20 cm (6–8 in.) at night to allow venous drainage by gravity.

6. Apply bland, oily lotions to prevent scaling and dryness of skin.

7. Avoid constricting bandages.

8. Prevent injury, bruising, scratching, or other trauma to skin of leg and foot.

9. Be alert for signs of ulceration, drainage, warmth, erythema, and pain, indicating infection.

PROCEDURE GUIDELINES 14-2   **OBTAINING LEG MEASUREMENTS TO DETECT EARLY SWELLING**

PURPOSE

To obtain leg measurements for detection and monitoring of thrombophlebitis

EQUIPMENT

Flexible tape measure in centimeters/inches
Black felt-tip pen

PROCEDURE

Nursing Action	Rationale

PREPARATORY PHASE

1. Instruct patient to lie in dorsal recumbent position.

PROCEDURE GUIDELINES 14-2   **CONTINUED**

Nursing Action	Rationale
PERFORMANCE PHASE	
1. On admission of the patient, measure the circumference of the ankle, calf, and thigh.	1. This will provide baseline data.
2. Obtain measurements at the widest part of the ankle, calf, and thigh.	2. To provide a consistent anatomic place of measurement, some clinics have a predetermined starting point, such as 15 or 20 cm from the knee cap.
3. Mark the leg with a black felt-tip pen where measurement taken.	3. To promote accuracy of measurements
4. Thereafter, when measuring, place the measuring tape on the marked line.	
5. Repeat measurements taken on admission the next morning before any patient activity.	5. Otherwise, later measurements may give a false reading because of gravitational edema.
6. Thereafter, obtain measurements at the same time of day weekly unless there is evidence of swelling, in which case it is done daily.	6. Weekly—to detect swelling Daily— to monitor swelling and its response to treatment

7. Record measurements:
   Leg Measurements
   Date:
   Time:
	7. To evaluate trends

	Right				Left	
Ankle _____		cm/in.	Ankle _____			cm/in.
Calf _____		cm/in.	Calf _____			cm/in.
Thigh _____		cm./in.	Thigh _____			cm./in.

8. Compare measurements:

   a. Check one leg with the other.

   b. Check each leg with baseline data.

Significant Findings:
1.5 cm (males) difference between legs or compared with baseline
1.2 cm (females) difference between legs or compared with baseline

Stasis Ulcers

Stasis ulcer is an excavation of the skin surface produced by sloughing of inflammatory necrotic tissue, usually caused by vascular insufficiency in the lower extremity.

Pathophysiology and Etiology
1. Stasis ulcer results from inadequate oxygen and other nutrients to the tissues because of edema and decreased circulation.
2. Secondary bacterial infection occurs because of decreased circulation that limits the body's response to infection.
3. Postphlebitic syndrome and stasis are responsible for most leg ulcers.

Clinical Manifestations
Severity of symptoms depends on the extent and duration of vascular insufficiency.
1. Open sore that is inflamed (Figure 14-4)
2. Drainage may be present or the area may be covered by a dark crust.
3. Patient may complain of swelling, heaviness, aching, and fatigue.
4. Edema and pigmentation around ulcer.

GERONTOLOGIC ALERT

 The occurrence of stasis ulcers is increasing, especially in the aging population.

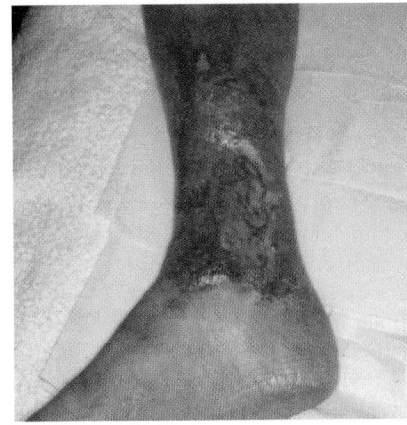

FIGURE 14-4 Venous ulcer.

Diagnostic Evaluation

1. Noninvasive tests such as plethysmography and venous Doppler may show impeded blood flow and incompetent valves.
2. Wound cultures will identify microorganisms if infected.

Management

Removing Devitalized Tissue

1. Necrotic material is flushed out with cleansing agents to dissolve slough. These agents are chemically or naturally derived enzymes that are proteolytic or fibrinolytic.
2. Surgical excision of slough—if necrotic tissue is loose, this procedure can be done without anesthesia; if the tissue is adherent, anesthesia will be required.

Stimulating Formation of Granulation Tissue

1. Dressing of choice
   a. Nonadherent so that removal is painless and does not damage newly forming tissue
   b. Highly absorbent
   c. Safe, nontoxic
   d. Sterile, accessible, and inexpensive
2. Application of compression over dressings, generally through the use of bandages or elastic stockings. In some circumstances, inflatable pneumatic leggings may be appropriate.
3. Unna's boot, an effective treatment of choice, is an example of a combined dressing and compression bandage.
4. Bed rest with leg elevation
5. Systemic drug therapy
   a. No single agent affects ulcer healing.
   b. Diuretic therapy for edema reduction may improve capillary circulation.
6. Application of skin grafts
   a. Skin grafts are used for ulcers that will not heal.
   b. They are not recommended for first-line treatment.

Preventing Recurrence

1. Ligation of the saphenofemoral or saphenopopliteal vessels with stripping
2. Ligation of the lower leg communicating veins
3. Deep vein bypass or reconstruction
4. Injection compression sclerotherapy
5. See page 406 for surgical care

Complications

1. Infection
2. Sepsis

Nursing Assessment

1. Observe appearance and temperature of the skin.
2. Note location and appearance of ulcer.
3. Determine presence and quality of all peripheral pulses. Use Doppler if needed.
4. Observe for drainage and signs of infection.

Nursing Diagnoses

- Impaired Tissue Integrity related to stasis ulcer
- Pain related to stasis ulcer

Nursing Interventions

Restoring Tissue Integrity

1. Elevate affected extremity to decrease edema.
2. Place cotton between toes to prevent pressure on a toe.
3. Provide overbed cradle to protect leg from pressure of bed linens.
4. Consider air-fluidized bed to provide pressure relief.
5. Administer prescribed antibiotics.
6. Apply wet to dry dressings, chemical beads or ointments, and topical antibiotics as ordered.
7. Apply Unna's boot to lower extremity as ordered.
8. Ensure adequate nutritional intake to enhance wound healing.

Reducing Pain

1. Administer prescribed analgesics, such as NSAIDs, to reduce pain and inflammation.
2. Medicate 30 to 45 minutes before a dressing change.
3. Encourage short periods of ambulation after pain medication is given.

Community and Home Care Considerations

1. Ensure that all supplies are obtained for home care. Utilize social services and other resources to help with financial arrangements as needed.
2. Assess the patient's ability to perform dressing changes at home. Include other persons in teaching to assist patient.
3. Make home visits several times a week to assess healing of ulcer, assess for infection, and assist family in carrying out dressing changes and other measures.

Patient Education and Health Maintenance

1. Stress the importance of following explicitly the recommendations of the health care provider.
2. Explain the hazards of trying other remedies without professional advice.
3. Indicate that the treatment may be long but that patience is an important aspect.
4. Encourage maintenance of healthy tissue when the ulcer is healed by continuing with the safeguards practiced before because breakdown of healthy tissue frequently occurs.
5. Encourage participation in physical therapy and a regular exercise program.
6. Encourage weight control and proper dietary intake to ensure adequate amounts of protein and vitamins and a reduced sodium intake.
7. Teach patient the correct method of dressing changes.
8. Instruct patient on injury prevention, including keeping hallways and walkways clear of obstacles, using a night light to avoid injury if awakened at night, etc.

Outcome-Based Evaluation

- Skin is of normal color and temperature, nontender and nonswollen, and demonstrates new epithelium
- Patient verbalizes only minimal discomfort with dressing changes

Varicose Veins

Primary varicose veins—bilateral dilatation and elongation of saphenous veins; deeper veins are normal. As the condition progresses, because of hydrostatic pressure and vein weakness, the vein walls become distended, with asymmetric dilatation, and some of the valves become incompetent. The process is irreversible. *Secondary varicose veins* result from obstruction of deep veins.

Telangectasias (spider veins) are dilated superficial capillaries, arterioles, and venules. They may be cosmetically unattractive but do not pose a threat to circulation.

Pathophysiology and Etiology

1. Dilatation of the vein prevents the valve cusps from meeting; this results in increased back-up pressure, which is passed into the next lower segment of the vein. The combination of vein dilatation and valve incompetence produces the varicosity (Figure 14-5).
2. Varicosities may occur elsewhere in the body (esophageal and hemorrhoidal veins) when flow or pressure is abnormally high.
3. Predisposing factors:
   a. Hereditary weakness of vein wall or valves
   b. Long-standing distention of veins brought about by pregnancy, obesity, or prolonged standing
   c. Old age—loss of tissue elasticity

Clinical Manifestations

1. Disfigurement due to large, discolored, tortuous leg veins
2. Easy leg fatigue, cramps in leg, heavy feeling, increased pain during menstruation, nocturnal muscle cramps

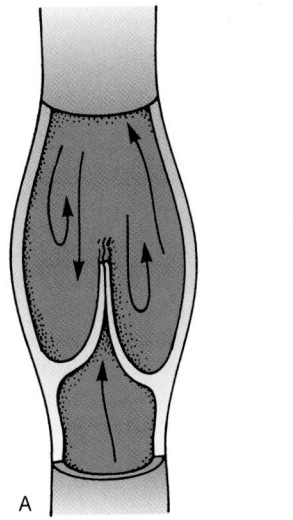 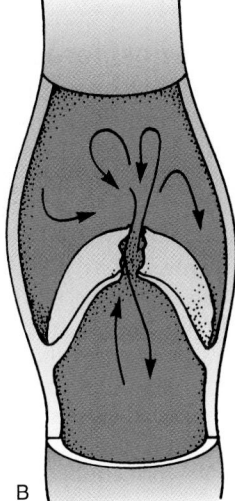

A   B

FIGURE 14-5 Valve incompetence develops as dilatation of a vessel prevents effective approximation of valve cusps. **(A)** Closed venous valve. **(B)** Incompetent venous valve.

Diagnostic Evaluation

1. Walking tourniquet test—to demonstrate presence or absence of valvular incompetence of communicating veins.
   a. A tourniquet is snugly fastened around the lower extremity just above the highest noted varicosities.
   b. The patient is directed to walk briskly for 2 minutes.
   c. Failure of varicosities to empty suggests valvular incompetence of communicating veins distal to tourniquet.
2. Photoplethysmography—a noninvasive technique to observe venous flow hemodynamics by noting changes in the blood content of the skin; used to detect incompetence in valves located inside the vein.
3. Doppler ultrasound—can detect accurately and rapidly the presence or absence of venous reflux in deep or superficial vessels.
4. Venous outflow and reflux plethysmography—able to detect deep venous occlusion.
5. Ascending and descending venography—an invasive technique that can also demonstrate venous occlusion and patterns of collateral flow. This test is expensive; it may not be required if a careful history, physical examination, and laboratory testing are done.

Management

1. Conservative therapies such as encouraging weight loss if appropriate and avoiding activities that cause venous stasis by obstructing venous flow.
2. Surgery may be considered for ulceration, bleeding, and cosmetic purposes in selected patients, if patency of deep veins is ensured.
3. Surgical procedures—a single method or combination of methods is tailored to meet the needs of the individual:
   a. Sclerosing injection—may be combined with ligation or limited to treatment of isolated varicosities. The affected vessel may be sclerosed by injecting sodium tetradecyl sulfate or similar sclerosing agent. Compression bandage is then applied without interruption for 6 weeks; inflamed endothelial surfaces adhere by direct contact.
   b. Multiple vein ligation
   c. Ligation and stripping of the greater and lesser saphenous systems. This is the most effective procedure.
   d. Venous reconstruction or venous valvular transplant
   e. Laser therapy

Complications

1. Hemorrhage due to weakening of the vein wall and pressure on it
2. Skin infection and breakdown, producing ulcers (rare in primary varices)

Nursing Assessment

1. Inspect for dilated, tortuous vessel.
2. Perform the manual compression test to determine severity of varicose vein.

a. With the fingertips of one hand, feel the dilated vein.

b. With your other hand, compress firmly at least 20 cm (8 in) higher on the leg.

c. Feel for an impulse transmitted toward your lower hand.

d. Competent saphenous valves should block the impulse. If you feel the impulse, the patient has varicose veins with incompetent valves.

3. Assess for any ulceration, chronic venous insufficiency, or signs of infection.

Nursing Diagnoses

- Impaired Tissue Integrity related to chronic changes and postoperative inflammation
- Pain related to surgical incisions, inflammation

Nursing Interventions

Promoting Tissue Integrity Postoperatively

1. Maintain elastic compression bandages from toes to groin. Monitor neurovascular status of feet (color, warmth, capillary refill, sensation, pulses) to prevent compromise from swelling.

2. Elevate legs about 30 degrees, providing support for the entire leg. Ensure that knee gatch is positioned for straight incline.

3. Monitor for signs of bleeding, especially in the first 24 hours.

a. Blood soaked through bandages

b. Increased pain, hematoma formation

c. Hypotension and tachycardia

4. If incisional bleeding occurs, elevate the leg above the level of the heart, apply pressure over the site, and notify the surgeon.

5. Be alert for complaints of pain over bony prominences of the foot and ankle; if the elastic bandage is too tight, loosen it—later, have it reapplied.

6. Maintain IV infusion for fluids and antibiotics as ordered.

7. After removal of compression bandages (about 7 days postoperatively), observe or teach patient to observe for signs of cellulitis or incisional infection.

8. Encourage use of elastic stockings for several weeks to months following surgery.

Relieving Pain

1. Administer analgesics as prescribed.

2. Encourage mostly bed rest the first day with legs elevated. The second day, encourage ambulation for 5 to 10 minutes every 2 hours.

3. Advise, when ambulatory, to avoid prolonged standing, sitting, or crossing or dangling legs to prevent obstruction.

Patient Education and Health Maintenance

Postoperative Instructions

Instruct the patient to:

1. Wear pressure bandages or elastic stockings as prescribed—usually 3 to 4 weeks after surgery.

2. Elevate legs about 30 degrees and provide adequate support for entire leg.

3. Take analgesics for pain as ordered.

4. Report signs such as sensory loss, calf pain, or fever to the health care provider.

5. Avoid dangling of legs.

6. Walk as able.

7. Note that complaints of patchy numbness can be expected but should disappear in less than a year.

8. Follow conservative management instructions (below) to prevent recurrence.

Conservative Management

Instruct the patient to:

1. Avoid activities that cause venous stasis by obstructing venous flow:

a. Wearing tight garters, tight girdle

b. Sitting or standing for prolonged periods of time

c. Crossing the legs at knees for prolonged periods while sitting (reduces circulation by 15%)

2. Control excessive weight gain.

3. Wear firm elastic support as prescribed, from toe to thigh when in upright position.

a. Put elastic stockings on in bed before getting up.

b. Waist-high elastic support hose are available and may be useful.

4. Elevate foot of bed 15 to 20 cm (6–8 in) for night sleeping.

5. Avoid injuring legs.

Outcome-Based Evaluation

- Skin is of normal color and temperature, nontender and nonswollen, and intact
- Patient is actively moving extremity; verbalizes reduced pain

CONDITIONS OF THE ARTERIES

Arteriosclerosis and Atherosclerosis

Arteriosclerosis is an arterial disease manifested by a loss of elasticity and a hardening of the vessel wall. More commonly known as "hardening of the arteries," it is a normal part of the aging process and generally occurs uniformly throughout the arterial system.

Atherosclerosis is the most common type of arteriosclerosis, manifested by the formation of atheromas (patchy lipoidal degeneration of the intima). Lesions, or plaques, form throughout the arterial wall, reducing the size of the vessel and limiting the flow of blood. Over time, atherosclerotic lesions can completely occlude the lumen by buildup of the plaque material and may contribute to thrombus formation.

Pathophysiology and Etiology

1. Etiology thought to be a reaction to injury:

a. Endothelial cell injury causes increased platelet and monocyte aggregation to site of injury.

b. Smooth muscle cells migrate and proliferate.

c. Matrix of collagen and elastic fibers forms.

2. Atherosclerotic lesions are two types: fatty streaks and fibrous plaques (Figure 14-6).

3. Risk factors include heredity, increasing age, male gender, cigarette smoking, hypertension, elevated blood cholesterol levels, diabetes mellitus, obesity, physical inactivity, and stress.

Clinical Manifestations

1. May affect entire vascular system or one segment of the vascular tree.

2. Symptoms are based on area affected.

a. Brain (cerebroarteriosclerosis)—transient ischemic attacks (TIA); stroke or cerebrovascular accident (CVA); visual disturbances such as amaurosis fugax, which is described by patients as a shade over a portion of the eye. See Chapter 15.

b. Heart (coronary artery disease, CAD)—angina, myocardial infarction (MI), congestive heart failure (CHF). See Chapter 13.

c. Gastrointestinal tract (aortic occlusive disease, aortic aneurysm, and mesenteric ischemia)—abdominal pain, unintentional weight loss, lower back pain.

d. Kidneys (renal artery stenosis)—renal insufficiency, poorly controlled hypertension.

e. Extremities (lower extremity arterial occlusive disease)—intermittent claudication (pain in legs associated with exercise), rest pain, tissue loss (with or without presence of infection and/or gangrene), embolic events.

3. Decreased or absent pulses; bruits.

GERONTOLOGIC ALERT

Atherosclerotic cardiovascular disease afflicts 80% of the population over age 65 and is the most common condition of the arterial system in the elderly.

Diagnostic Evaluation

Specific to body system affected:

1. Arteriography of involved area may show stenosis and increased collateral circulation.

2. CT scan

3. MRI/MRA

4. Noninvasive testing of the vascular system:

a. Duplex studies

b. Sequential Doppler studies

c. Pulse volume resistance

d. Ankle-brachial index (ABI) (Figure 14-7)

5. ECG, echocardiogram, Holter monitoring, exercise stress testing, myocardial imaging, and cardiac catheterization may be done to evaluate coronary artery disease.

Management

Medical Management

1. Modification of risk factors

2. Prescriptive management—anticoagulants, antiplatelet therapy (Table 14-2), lipid-lowering agents, antihypertensives

3. Specific treatment for end-organ dysfunction—see cerebrovascular insufficiency (p. 457), angina (p. 356), occlusive arterial disease (p. 419).

4. Vascular rehabilitation/exercise

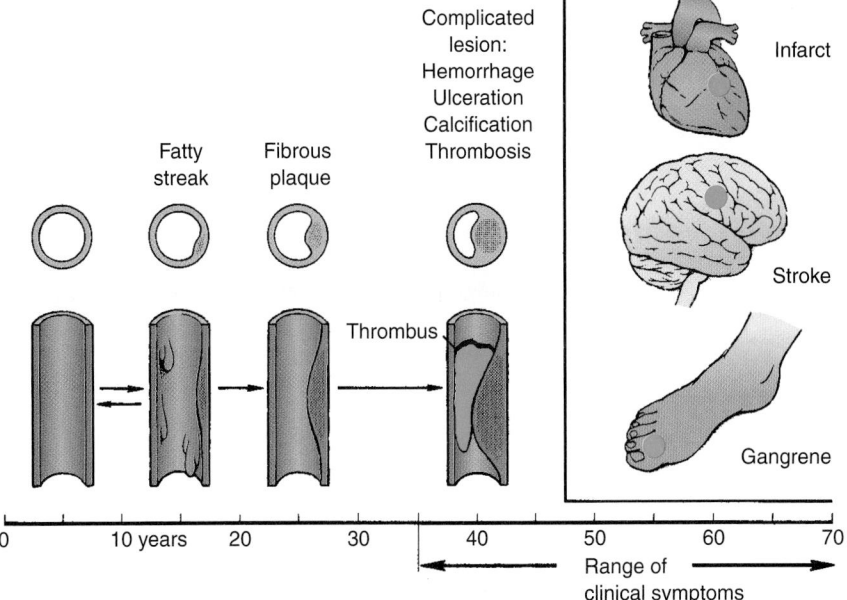

FIGURE 14-6 Schematic concept of the progression of atherosclerosis. Fatty streaks constitute one of the earliest lesions of atherosclerosis. Many fatty streaks regress, whereas other progress to fibrous plaques and eventually to atheroma, which may be complicated by hemorrhage, ulceration, calcification, or thrombosis and may produce myocardial infarction, stroke, or gangrene.

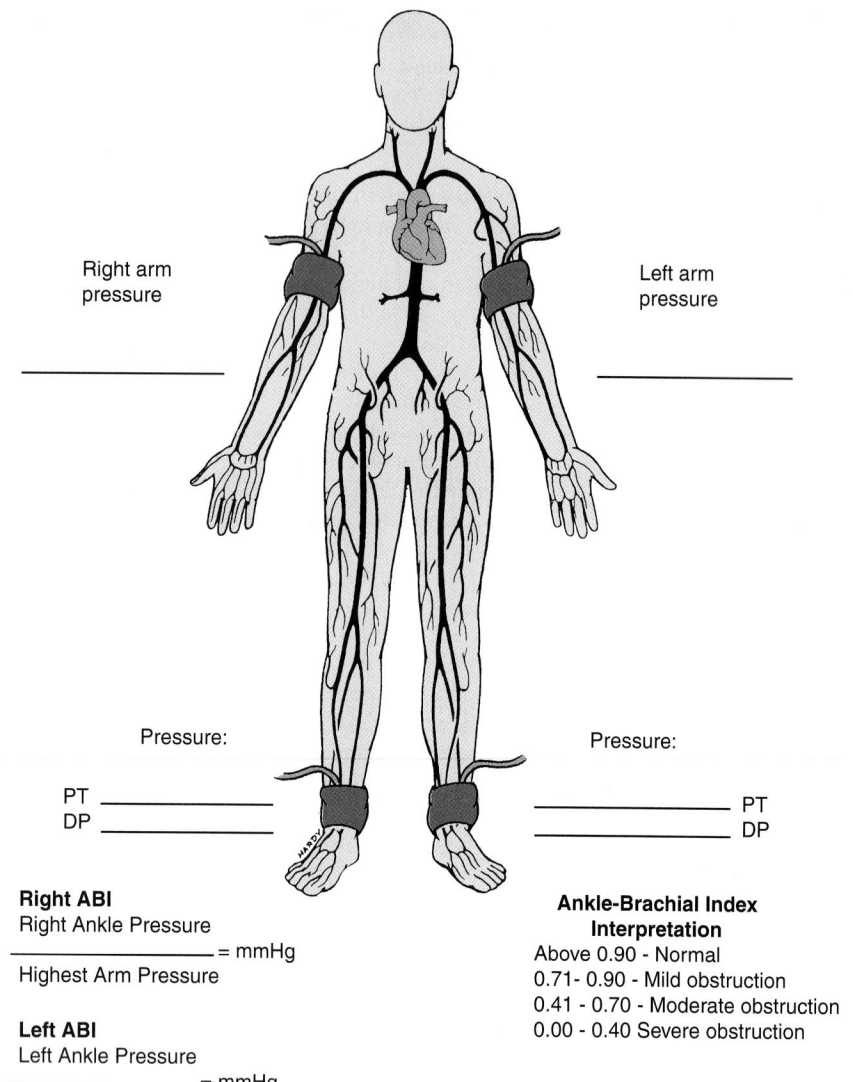

Right arm pressure

Left arm pressure

_____

_____

Pressure:

Pressure:

PT _____
DP _____

_____ PT
_____ DP

Right ABI
Right Ankle Pressure
_____ = mmHg
Highest Arm Pressure

Left ABI
Left Ankle Pressure
_____ = mmHg
Highest Arm Pressure

**Ankle-Brachial Index
Interpretation**
Above 0.90 - Normal
0.71- 0.90 - Mild obstruction
0.41 - 0.70 - Moderate obstruction
0.00 - 0.40 Severe obstruction

FIGURE 14-7 Determining ankle-brachial index (ABI).

Surgical Management

1. Endovascular procedures:
   a. Percutaneous transluminal angioplasty (PTA) with or without placement of intralumenal stent—to relieve arterial stenosis when lesions are accessible, as in superficial femoral and iliac arteries, through the use of special inflatable balloon catheters and metal stents.
   b. Endovascular grafting—placement of prosthetic graft via a transluminal approach. Graft material covers a metallic stent. The stent is placed via femoral artery and is deployed.
   c. Rotational atherectomy—high-speed rotary cutter that removes lesions by abrading plaque. Benefits of this therapy are minimal damage to the normal endothelium and low incidence of complications.
   d. Laser angioplasty—amplified light waves are transmitted by fiberoptic catheters. Laser beam heats the tip of a percutaneous catheter and vaporizes the atherosclerotic plaque.
2. Surgical revascularization of the affected vessels, including:
   a. Embolectomy—removal of blood clot from the artery
   b. Thrombectomy—removal of thrombus from the artery
   c. Endarterectomy—removal of atherosclerotic plaque from the artery
   d. Bypass—use of a graft, either vein graft or prosthetic material, to route blood flow around blocked area.

TABLE 14-2 Antiplatelet Therapy

Antiplatelet therapy is used to prevent platelet aggregation and thrombus formation. It is used in the treatment of cerebrovascular disease, coronary artery disease, and intermittent claudication. The table lists some common antiplatelet medications, their indications, and potential side effects.

Medication	Use	Contraindications
Aspirin	Prevention of myocardial infarction (MI), transient ischemic attacks (TIAs), cerebrovascular accidents (CVA)	Allergy to acetylsalicylic acid (ASA) Active gastric ulcers
Ticlopidine (Ticlid)	Prevention of TIA, CVA	Sensitivity to drug Renal impairment Liver impairment Other risk factors for bleeding
Pentoxifylline (Trental)	Treatment of intermittent claudication	Sensitivity to drug Recent cerebral or retinal hemorrhage Caffeine or theophylline intolerance
Clopidogrel (Plavix)	Prevention of CVA, TIA	Sensitivity to drug Active pathologic bleeding, eg, peptic ulcer, intracranial hemorrhage Severe hepatic disease
Cilostazol (Pletal)	Treatment of intermittent claudication—has antiplatelet, vasodilatory, and antithrombotic effects	Sensitivity to drug CHF Liver impairment See drug–drug interactions
Dipyridamole 200 mg, aspirin 25 mg (Aggrenox)	Prevention of stroke	Allergy to ASA Active ulcer disease Renal and hepatic impairment Bleeding disorders

Complications

Long-term complications of atherosclerosis are related to the specific body system affected.

1. Brain—long- and short-term disabilities associated with stroke
2. Heart—stable/unstable angina, myocardial infarction (MI), congestive heart failure (CHF)
3. Aorta—ischemic bowel, aneurysms, impotence, renal failure, nephrectomy
4. Lower extremities—intermittent claudication, non-healing ulcers, infections/gangrene, amputation

Nursing Interventions and Patient Education

Attention is directed to reducing risk factors by smoking cessation (p. 26), stress reduction (p. 27), weight reduction (p. 26), adequate control of diabetes (p. 848) and/or hypertension (p. 426), and adjusting diet to reduce cholesterol intake (p. 25). Encourage active lifestyle to promote cardiovascular health.

■ Peripheral Arterial Occlusive Disease (Aorta and Distal Arteries)

Peripheral arterial occlusive disease is a form of arteriosclerosis in which the peripheral arteries become blocked. Chronic occlusive arterial disease occurs much more frequently than does acute (which is the sudden and complete blocking of a vessel by a thrombus or embolus).

Pathophysiology and Etiology
Arteriosclerosis Obliterans

1. Most commonly caused by atherosclerosis with contributing factors as discussed in previous section.
2. May involve the following vessels in isolation or combination:
   a. Aortoiliac system
   b. Femoral arteries—superficial femoral (SFA), profunda femoris
   c. Popliteal artery
   d. Trifurcating vessels—anterior tibial (AT), posterior tibial (PT), and peroneal arteries
   e. Dorsalis pedis artery (DP)
   f. Pedal arch
3. Lesions tend to form at areas of bifurcation of the vessels.
4. Pattern of disease differs in non-diabetics and diabetics:
   a. Non-diabetics—disease usually involves the macrocirculation (larger vessels, eg, aorta, iliac, femoral arteries) and is more common in isolated segments.
   b. Diabetics—disease usually involves the microcirculation (smaller vessels, eg, popliteal, tibial, peroneal, and small vessels in the foot/digits) and occurs in more diffuse segments.

Thromboangiitis Obliterans (Buerger's Disease)

Inflammatory process of arterial wall, which is followed by thrombosis. Also affects adjacent veins and nerves. Associated with heavy cigarette smoking.

Clinical Manifestations

Symptoms appear gradually and are specific to the area affected:

Aortoiliac

1. Mesenteric ischemia, pain after eating
2. Unintentional weight loss
3. Renal insufficiency
4. Poorly controlled hypertension
5. Impotence
6. Intermittent claudication

Femoral, Popliteal, and Distal Arteries

1. Intermittent claudication
2. Rest pain—associated with severe arterial ischemia. Severe pain in feet aggravated by elevation of lower extremity. Pain is relieved by placing foot in dependent position.
3. Dependent rubor—dusky purple color of extremity when in dependent position; changes to pallor when elevated.
4. Numbness/tingling of feet/toes.
5. Trophic changes associated with tissue malnutrition:
   a. Hair loss
   b. Thick toenails
   c. Thin, shiny skin
   d. Cool temperature of extremity
6. Tissue loss/nonhealing ulcers, which may develop wet or dry gangrene (Figure 14-8).

Diagnostic Evaluation

Noninvasive

1. Vascular physical examination
2. Ankle-brachial index—comparison of systolic blood pressure in arm with that of ankle. May be done before and after exercise. Normally, the systolic pressures are equal. In presence of atherosclerotic disease, the pressure below an occluded area is less than the arm pressure (see Figure 14-7).
3. Doppler ultrasound—increased velocity of flow through a stenotic vessel, or no flow with total occlusion

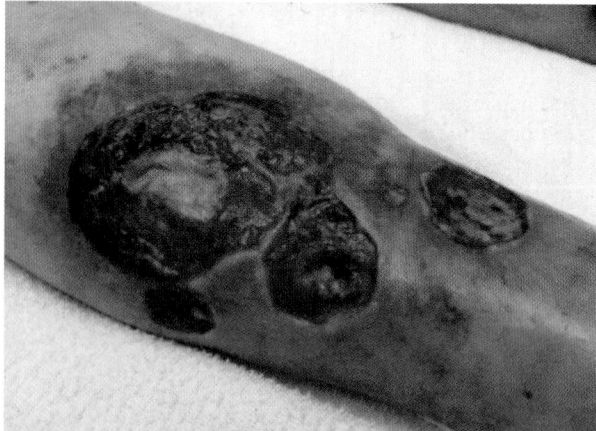

FIGURE 14-8 Arterial ulcer.

4. Segmental plethysmography—decreased pressure distal to region of occlusion

Invasive

Angiography—to confirm occlusion

Management

1. Goals
   a. Reestablish blood flow to areas of critical ischemia.
   b. Preserve the extremity.
   c. Relieve pain associated with intermittent claudication or rest pain.
   d. Provide sufficient blood flow for wound healing.
2. Conservative treatment includes modification of risk factors: walking, weight reduction, smoking cessation, and control of other conditions such as hypertension and diabetes mellitus.
3. Pharmacologic treatment with antiplatelet agents or anticoagulants to improve blood flow by increasing erythrocyte flexibility and lowering blood viscosity.
4. When conservative measures clearly are not enough, revascularization surgery (endarterectomy, arterial bypass grafting, or a combination) may be required.
5. Endovascular procedures such as PTA may be used alone or with revascularization surgery for dilatation of localized noncalcified segments of narrowed arteries with or without intralumenal stenting.
6. Amputation of affected extremity in cases of severe infection/gangrene, failed attempts at revascularization, or when revascularization is not considered a viable option.
7. See page 406 for surgical care.

Complications

1. Ulceration with slow healing
2. Gangrene, sepsis
3. Severe occlusion may necessitate limb or partial limb amputation

Nursing Assessment

1. Auscultate abdomen and listen for presence of bruits.
2. Observe lower extremities for color, sensation, and temperature. Compare bilaterally for differences.
3. Palpate pulses (Figure 14-9) and record. If pulses are nonpalpable, attempt to locate pulse with a handheld Doppler.
4. Inspect nails for thickening and opacity; inspect skin for shiny, atrophic, hairless, and dry appearance—reflect chronic changes.
5. Assess for pain:
   a. Severe abdominal pain after eating
   b. Pain in legs with exercise
   c. Pain in legs at rest
6. Assess for ulcers of toes and feet.

Nursing Diagnoses

• Altered Tissue Perfusion (peripheral) related to decreased arterial blood flow

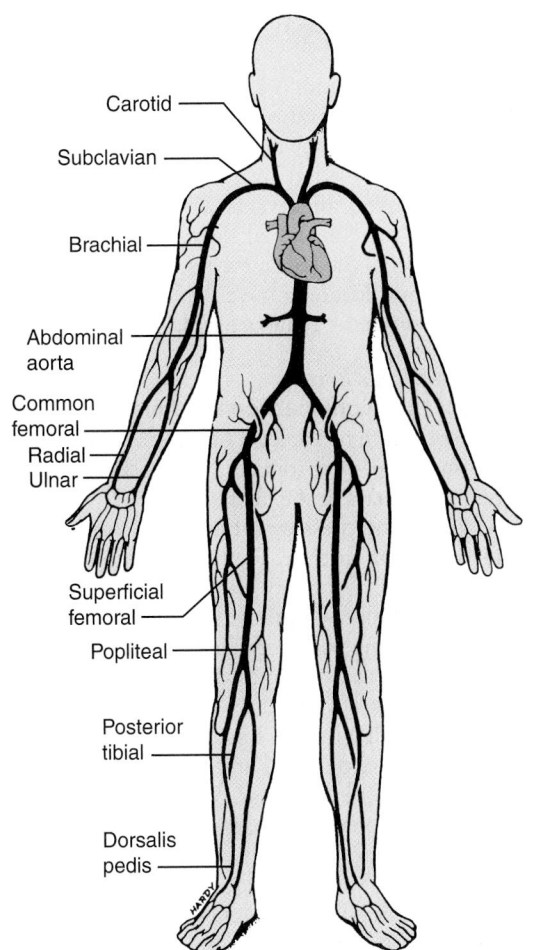

Carotid
Subclavian
Brachial
Abdominal aorta
Common femoral
Radial
Ulnar
Superficial femoral
Popliteal
Posterior tibial
Dorsalis pedis

FIGURE 14-9 Salient points in evaluating peripheral arterial insufficiency. Reduced or absent femoral pulses indicate aortoiliac disease. Absent popliteal pulses indicate superficial femoral occlusion. Pulse deficits in one extremity, with normal pulses in the contralateral extremity, suggest acute arterial embolus. Absent pedal pulses indicate tibioperoneal artery involvement.

- Sensory/Perceptual Alteration (tactile) of lower extremities
- Risk for Infection related to decreased arterial flow

Nursing Interventions
Promoting Tissue Perfusion
1. Perform frequent neurovascular checks of affected extremity.
2. Inspect lower extremity/feet for new areas of ulceration or extension of existing ulceration.
3. Provide and encourage well-balanced diet to enhance wound healing.
4. Encourage walking or performance of range-of-motion exercises to increase blood flow, which will increase collateral circulation.
5. Administer or teach self-administration of pain medication to achieve comfort level conducive to ambulation.

Protecting Lower Extremities
1. Encourage patient to wear protective footwear such as rubber-soled slippers or shoes with closed, wide toebox when out of bed.
2. Instruct patient/family to keep hallways and walkways free of clutter to avoid injury.
3. Avoid tight-fitting socks/shoes.
4. Instruct patient to avoid sitting with legs crossed.
5. Avoid using adhesive tape and harsh soaps on affected skin.
6. Instruct patient to check temperature of bath water with forearm before entering tub.
7. Perform and teach foot care, including washing and carefully drying and inspecting feet daily.

Preventing Infection
1. Apply lanolin or petrolatum to intact skin of lower extremities to prevent drying and cracking of skin.
2. Encourage patient to wear clean hose/socks daily: woolen socks for winter, cotton for summer.
3. Teach patient to:
   a. Trim toenails straight across after soaking the feet in warm water.
   b. Place wisps of cotton under corner of great toenail if there is a tendency toward ingrown toenails.
   c. Have a podiatrist cut corns and calluses; do not use corn pads or strong medications.
4. Teach patient signs to report:
   a. Redness, swelling, irritation, blistering, foul odor
   b. Itching, burning; rashes
   c. Bruises, cuts, unusual appearance of skin
   d. New areas of ulceration
5. Instruct patient to check with physician before using any over-the-counter or topical lotions or creams to wound.
6. For patients post-operative revascularization in which prosthetic graft material was used, instruct patient on the need for prophylactic antibiotics before any invasive procedure, including routine dental examinations and other surgical procedures.

Patient Education and Health Maintenance
1. Instruct patient on the importance of walking to improve circulation.
2. Instruct patient not to sit or stand in one position for long periods of time.
3. Instruct patient, when sitting, to keep knees below the level of the hips to avoid hip flexion.
4. Instruct patient to avoid tight-fitting clothing, eg, elastic-topped socks or clothing made out of Lycra/Spandex, especially over area of graft placement.
5. Instruct patient not to cross legs when sitting or lying down.
6. Instruct patient on methods to promote vasodilatation by keeping extremity warm, ceasing smoking, and stopping use of other vasoconstricting substances such as caffeine.
7. Instruct patient on the importance of daily foot care.

Outcome-Based Evaluation
- No new ulcer formation
- Verbalizes importance of wearing protective shoes and washing and inspecting feet daily
- No signs of infection of lower extremities

Aneurysm

An aneurysm is a distention of an artery brought about by a weakening/destruction of the arterial wall. They are lined with intralumenal debris such as plaque and thrombi. Because of the high pressure in the arterial system, aneurysms can enlarge, producing complications by compressing surrounding structures; left untreated, they may rupture, causing a fatal hemorrhage. A dissection occurs when the layers of the artery become separated. Blood flows between the layers, causing further disruption of the arterial wall. Additionally, the intralumenal thrombus may totally occlude the artery, leading to acute ischemia to all arteries distal to the area of thrombosis, or they may embolize clot and/or plaque to the arteries distal to the aneurysm.

The *aorta* is the most common site for aneurysms; however, they may form in any vessel. Peripheral vessel aneurysms may involve the renal artery, subclavian artery, popliteal artery (knee), or any major artery. These produce a pulsating mass and may cause pain or pressure on surrounding structures.

Pathophysiology and Etiology
1. Aneurysms may form as the result of:
   a. Atherosclerosis
   b. Trauma
   c. Infection
   d. Heredity
   e. Immunologic conditions
2. False aneurysms (pseudoaneurysm) are associated with trauma to the arterial wall, as in blunt trauma or trauma associated with arterial punctures for angiography and/or cardiac catheterization.
3. The ascending aorta and the aortic arch are the sites of greatest hemodynamic stress and also are the most common sites of arterial dissection.
4. Contributing factors include:
   a. Hypertension
   b. Arteriosclerosis
   c. Local infection, pyogenic or fungal (mycotic aneurysm)
   d. Congenital weakness of vessels
   e. Syphilis
   f. Trauma

> **GERONTOLOGIC ALERT**
>
> Because of vascular changes that occur as a natural process of aging, all patients over age 65 are assessed for the potential for aneurysms.

5. Morphologically, aneurysms may be classified as follows:

   a. Saccular—distention of a vessel projecting from one side
   b. Fusiform—distention of the whole artery (ie, entire circumference is involved)
   c. Dissecting—hemorrhagic or intramural hematoma, separating the medial layers of the aortic wall
6. Abdominal aortic aneurysms are described as infrarenal, when the "neck" of the aneurysm is located below the level of the renal arteries, or suprarenal, when the aneurysm is located above the level of the renal arteries or involves the renal arteries.

Clinical Manifestations
Aneurysm of the Thoracoabdominal Aorta
From the aortic arch to the level of the diaphragm. At first no symptoms; later symptoms may come from CHF or a pulsating tumor mass in the chest.
1. Pulse and blood pressure difference in upper extremities if aneurysm interferes with circulation in left subclavian artery
2. Pain and pressure symptoms
3. Constant, boring pain because of pressure
4. Intermittent and neuralgic pain because of impingement on nerves
5. Dyspnea, causing pressure against trachea
6. Cough, often paroxysmal and brassy in sound
7. Hoarseness, voice weakness, or complete aphonia, resulting from pressure against recurrent laryngeal nerve
8. Dysphagia due to impingement on esophagus
9. Edema of chest wall—infrequent
10. Dilated superficial veins on chest
11. Cyanosis because of vein compression of chest vessels
12. Ipsilateral dilatation of pupils due to pressure against cervical sympathetic chain
13. Abnormal pulsation apparent on chest wall, due to erosion of aneurysm through rib cage—in syphilis

Abdominal Aneurysm
1. Many of these patients are asymptomatic.
2. Abdominal pain is most common, either persistent or intermittent—often localized in middle or lower abdomen to the left of midline
3. Low back pain
4. Feeling of an abdominal pulsating mass, palpated as a thrill, auscultated as a bruit
5. Hypertension
6. Distal variability of blood pressure, pressure in arm greater than thigh
7. If rupture, will present with hypotension and/or hypovolemic shock

> **GERONTOLOGIC ALERT**
>
> Most abdominal aneurysms occur between the ages of 60 and 90. Rupture of the aneurysm is likely if there is coexistent hypertension or if the aneurysm is larger than 6 cm.

Diagnostic Evaluation

1. Abdominal or chest x-ray may show calcification that outlines aneurysm.
2. Computed tomography (CT) scanning and ultrasonography are used to detect and monitor size of aneurysm.
3. MRI/MRA.
4. Arteriography allows visualization of aneurysm and vessel.

Management

1. May follow small aneurysms (4 cm or less) with CT scanning or ultrasound every 6 months and aggressively control blood pressure.
2. The prognosis is poor for untreated patients as aneurysm enlarges.
3. Surgery:
   a. Resection of the aneurysm via abdominal incision and placement of a prosthetic graft to restore vascular continuity.
   b. Endovascular grafting—repair of aneurysm using a stent graft, which is deployed via the femoral artery.
   c. Thoracic aneurysms are the most difficult to treat and require use of atrial-femoral circulatory bypass intraoperatively.

Complications

1. Fatal hemorrhage
2. Myocardial ischemia
3. Stroke
4. Paraplegia due to interruption of anterior spinal artery
5. Abdominal ischemia
6. Ileus
7. Graft occlusion
8. Graft infections
9. Acute renal failure
10. Impotence
11. Lower extremity ischemia
12. "Trash toes"—results from distal emobolization of plaque and/or blood clots

Nursing Assessment

1. In patient with thoracoabdominal aortic aneurysm, be alert for sudden onset of sharp, ripping, or tearing pain located in anterior chest, epigastric area, shoulders, or back, indicating acute dissection or rupture.
2. In patients with abdominal aortic aneurysm, assess for pain and intense low back pain caused by rapid expansion. Be alert for syncope, tachycardia, and hypotension, which may be followed by fatal hemorrhage due to rupture.

Nursing Diagnoses

- Altered Tissue Perfusion (vital organs) related to aneurysm or aneurysm rupture and/or dissection
- Risk for Infection related to surgery
- Pain related to pressure of aneurysm on nerves and postoperatively

Nursing Interventions

Maintaining Perfusion of Vital Organs

Preoperatively:
1. Assess for chest pain and abdominal pain.
2. Prepare patient for diagnostic studies or surgery as indicated.
3. Monitor for signs and symptoms of hypovolemic shock.
4. Perform neurovascular checks to distal extremities.

Postoperatively:
1. Monitor vital signs frequently.
2. Assess for signs and symptoms of bleeding:
   a. Hypotension
   b. Tachycardia
   c. Tachypnea
   d. Diaphoresis
3. Monitor lab values as ordered.
4. Monitor urinary output hourly.
5. Assess abdomen for bowel sounds and distention.
6. Perform neurovascular checks to distal extremities.
7. Assess feet for signs and symptoms of embolization:
   a. Cold feet
   b. Cyanotic toes
   c. Pain in feet
8. Maintain IV infusion to administer medications to control blood pressure and provide fluids postoperatively.
9. Position patient to avoid hip flexion, keeping knees below the level of the hips when sitting in chair.
10. If thoracoabdominal aneurysm repair has been performed, monitor for signs and symptoms of spinal cord ischemia:
    a. Pain
    b. Numbness
    c. Parasthesia
    d. Weakness

Preventing Infection

1. Monitor temperature.
2. Monitor changes in WBC count.
3. Monitor incision for signs of infection.
4. Administer antibiotics, if ordered.

Relieving Pain

1. Administer pain medication as ordered or monitor patient-controlled analgesia.
2. Keep head of bed elevated no more than 45 degrees for the first 3 days postoperatively to prevent pressure on incision site.
3. Administer nasogastric decompression for ileus following surgery, until bowel sounds return.
4. Assess abdomen for bowel sounds and distention.

Patient Education and Health Maintenance

1. Instruct patient about medications to control blood pressure and the importance of taking them.
2. Discuss disease process and signs and symptoms of expanding aneurysm or impending rupture, or rupture, to be reported.

3. For postsurgical patients, discuss warning signs of post-operative complications (fever, inflammation of operative site, bleeding, and swelling).
4. Encourage adequate balanced intake for wound healing.
5. Encourage patient to maintain an exercise schedule postoperatively.
6. Instruct patient that due to use of a prosthetic graft to repair the aneurysm, he or she will require prophylactic antibiotic use for invasive procedures, including routine dental examinations and dental cleaning.

Outcome-Based Evaluation
- Tissue color, sensation, and temperature normal; non-tender, nonswollen, and intact
- Afebrile, no signs of infection
- Reports control of pain with medication

Acute Arterial Occlusion
Acute arterial occlusion is the sudden interruption of blood flow, which may cause complete or partial obstruction of the artery. Critical ischemia of the extremity develops and may result in loss of affected extremity and/or death.

Pathophysiology and Etiology
1. Embolization is the most common cause of acute arterial occlusion.
2. Emboli may consist of thrombus, atheromatous debris, or tumor.
3. Emboli most commonly originate in the heart as a result of atrial fibrillation, MI, or CHF (about 85%), but can also occur after invasive procedures such as cardiac catheterization, angiography, and surgery.
4. Arteriosclerosis may cause roughening or ulceration of atheromatous plaques, which can lead to emboli.
5. May also be associated with immobility, anemia, and dehydration.
6. Emboli tend to lodge at bifurcations and atherosclerotic narrowings.
7. Other causes of acute occlusion include:
   a. Trauma
   b. Thrombus
   c. Venous outflow obstruction, which includes compartment syndrome

Clinical Manifestations
1. The patient may experience acute pain and loss of sensory and motor function due to emboli blocking the artery and associated vasomotor reflex.
   a. Paralysis of part
   b. Anesthesia of part
   c. Pallor and coldness
   d. Edema
   e. Rigidity of extremity

Diagnostic Evaluation
1. Neurovascular assessment of affected area.
2. Doppler ultrasonography, segmental limb pressure, and pulse volume recordings—may indicate decreased flow.

3. Radionuclide scan—may identify clot.
4. Arteriography—confirms diagnosis.
5. Digital subtraction angiography and MRI may be done for cerebral emobolization.

Management
1. Drug therapy—anticoagulants (see p. 403), thrombolytics (see p. 406)
2. Surgery:
   a. Embolectomy (Figure 14-10) must be performed within 6 to 10 hours to prevent muscle necrosis and loss of extremity.
   b. Fasciotomy—incisions made over leg compartments to aid expansion of edematous tissue and relief of pressure on the arterial system.
   c. Amputation of affected limb if revascularization is inappropriate due to metabolic complications.
3. Treatment of shock
4. Bed rest

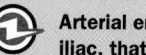

> **NURSING ALERT**
>
> Arterial embolization of a large artery, such as the iliac, that has major systemic effects is life threatening and requires emergency operative intervention.

Complications
1. Irreversible ischemia and loss of extremity
2. Metabolic complications:
   a. Acidosis
   b. Hyperkalemia
   c. Renal failure
3. Shock

Nursing Assessment
1. Assess for acute, severe pain.
2. Assess for gradual or acute loss of sensory and motor function.
3. Check for aggravation of pain by movement of and pressure on the extremity.
4. Palpate for loss of distal pulses.
5. Inspect for pale, mottled, and numb extremity.
6. Inspect for collapse of superficial veins due to decreased blood flow to the extremity.
7. Inspect for sharp line of color and temperature demarcation. This may occur distal to the site of occlusion as a result of ischemia.
8. Assess for edema.

Nursing Diagnoses
- Sensory/Perceptual Alteration (tactile) related to impaired blood supply
- Altered Tissue Perfusion (peripheral) related to lack of blood flow by clot
- Risk for Infection related to surgery

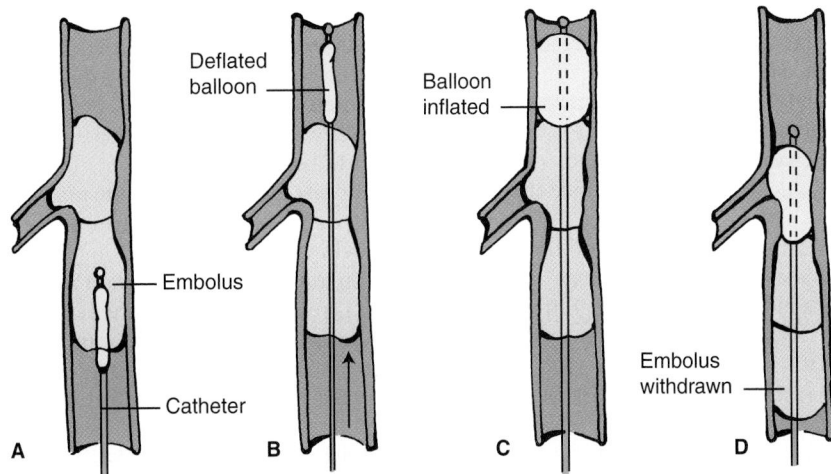

FIGURE 14-10 Extracting an embolus from a vessel can be done with the use of a Fogarty embolectomy catheter. The catheter, with a soft, deflated balloon near the tip, is threaded through the artery via an arteriotomy. (**A, B**) It is passed through the embolus and its thrombus; (**C**) it is then inflated. (**D**) A steady pull downward withdraws the embolus along with the catheter.

Nursing Interventions
Protecting the Extremity
1. Protect extremity by keeping it at or below the body's horizontal plane.
2. Protect leg from hard surfaces, tight or heavy surfaces, and tight or heavy overlying bed linens.
3. Handle extremity gently and prevent pressure or friction while repositioning.
4. Administer pain medications as ordered.

Promoting Tissue Perfusion
1. Administer heparin IV to reduce tendency of emboli to form or expand (useful in smaller arteries).
2. Monitor thrombolytic therapy IV to dissolve clot as ordered.
3. Monitor patient for signs of bleeding (gums, urine, stool).
4. Monitor coagulation, hematology, and electrolyte studies.
5. Prepare the patient for surgery (see p. 406).
6. Postoperatively, promote movement of extremity to stimulate circulation and prevent stasis.

Preventing Infection
1. Postoperatively, check surgical wound for bleeding, swelling, erythema, and discharge.
2. Maintain IV infusion or venous access device to administer IV antibiotics if indicated.
3. Continue to monitor the patient for tachycardia, fever, pain, erythema, warmth, swelling, and drainage at incision site.

Patient Education and Health Maintenance
1. Teach prevention techniques such as daily aerobic activity, observation for skin breakdown, and prevention of injury.
2. Teach patient the medical regimen and importance of taking prescribed medications such as oral anticoagulants to prevent reembolization (see p. 403).
3. Encourage patient to report symptoms of arterial occlusion: paralysis, numbness, tingling, pallor, and coldness of extremity.

Outcome-Based Evaluation
- Extremity without injury
- Limb has normal color, sensation, movement, and temperature
- No signs of infection

▨ Vasospastic Disorder (Raynaud's Phenomenon)
Raynaud's phenomenon or syndrome is a vasospastic disorder that is brought on by an unusual sensitivity to cold or to emotional stress.

Pathophysiology and Etiology
1. The condition is a form of intermittent arteriolar vasoconstriction that results in coldness, pain, and pallor of fingertips, toes, or tip of the nose.
2. The cause is unknown, although it may be secondary to connective tissue and other immunologic disorders.
3. Episodes may be triggered by emotional factors or by unusual sensitivity to cold.
4. Most common in women between ages 16 and 40 and seen much more frequently in cold climates and during the winter months.

Clinical Manifestations

1. Intermittent arteriolar vasoconstriction resulting in coldness, pain, pallor.
2. Involvement of the fingers appears to be asymmetric; thumbs are less often involved.
3. Characteristic color changes: white-blue-red
   a. White—blanching, dead-white appearance if spasm is severe
   b. Blue—cyanotic, relatively stagnant blood flow
   c. Red—a reactive hyperemia on rewarming
4. Occasionally, there is ulceration of the fingertips.

Diagnostic Evaluation

1. Clinical symptoms must last at least 2 years to confirm the diagnosis.
2. Tests may be done to rule out secondary disease processes such as chronic arterial occlusive or connective tissue disease.

Management

1. Avoidance of trigger and aggravating factors.
2. Calcium channel blockers are frequently used to prevent or reduce vasospasm.
3. Nitroglycerin or sympatholytics such as reserpine (Serpasil), guanethidine (Ismelin), or prasozin (Minipress) may be helpful for some. Side effects such as headache, dizziness, and orthostatic hypotension may be prohibitive.
4. Antiplatelet agents such as aspirin or dipyridamole (Persantine) may be given to prevent total occlusion.
5. Sympathectomy—removal of the sympathetic ganglia or division of their branches may offer some improvement.

Complications

1. Chronic disease may cause atrophy of skin and muscles.
2. Ulceration and gangrene (rare).

Nursing Assessment

1. Perform thorough history and review of systems for clues to underlying disorder.
2. Assess for blanching of digits when exposed to cold. Color turns cyanotic, then red with normal temperature.
3. Note whether warmth brings about symptom relief.

Nursing Diagnoses

- Sensory/Perceptual Alteration (tactile) related to vasospastic process
- Pain related to hyperemic stage

Nursing Interventions

Minimizing Sensory Alteration

1. Assist patient in avoiding exposure to cold; for example, use gloves to handle cold items (water pitcher, refrigerated items).
2. Encourage patient to stop smoking.
3. Help patient to understand the need to avoid stressful situations.

4. Offer patient options for stress management.
5. Administer and teach patient about drug therapy.
6. Need to take drugs every day to prevent or minimize symptoms.
7. Follow orthostatic hypotension precaution if on sympatholytics.
8. Advise patient that episode may be terminated by placing hands (or feet) in warm water.

Relieving Pain

1. Explain to patient that pain may be experienced when spasm is relieved—hyperemic phase.
2. Administer or teach self-administration of analgesics.
3. Reassure patient that pain is temporary; persistent pain, ulceration, or signs of infection should be reported.

Patient Education and Health Maintenance

1. Avoid whatever provokes vasoconstriction of vessels of hands.
2. Prevent injury to hands, which can aggravate vasoconstriction and lead to ulceration.
3. Minimize exposure to cold because this precipitates a reaction.
4. Wear warm clothing—boots, gloves, and hooded jackets—when going out in cold weather.
   a. Turn heat on in automobile during travel.
   b. Shop in heated stores; avoid unheated buildings.
   c. Avoid getting wet.
5. Avoid placing hands in cold water, the freezer, or the refrigerator unless protective gloves are worn.
6. Use extra precautions to avoid injuries to fingers and hands from needle sticks and knife cuts.

Outcome-Based Evaluation

- Wears gloves while handling cold items; follows medication regimen
- Reports decreased length of painful phase with episodes

HYPERTENSIVE DISORDERS

◼ Hypertension

Hypertension (high blood pressure) is a disease of vascular regulation in which the mechanisms that control arterial pressure within the normal range are altered. Predominant mechanisms of control are the central nervous system (CNS), the renal pressor system (renin-angiotensin-aldosterone system), and extracellular fluid volume. Why these mechanisms fail is not known. The basic explanation is that blood pressure is elevated when there is increased cardiac output plus increased peripheral vascular resistance. There are an estimated 50 million Americans with hypertension, and this number is expected to increase due to the aging of the population. Only a fraction of these people are aware of their hypertension and are treated for it, and even fewer have gained adequate control of their blood pressure.

Pathophysiology and Etiology

Primary or Essential Hypertension

(Approximately 95% of patients with hypertension)

1. When the diastolic pressure is 90 mm Hg or higher and other causes of hypertension are absent, the condition is said to be primary hypertension. More specifically, an individual is considered hypertensive when the average of three or more blood pressure readings taken at rest several days apart exceeds the upper limits shown in Table 14-3.
2. Cause of essential hypertension is unknown; however, there are several areas of investigation:
   a. Hyperactivity of sympathetic vasoconstricting nerves
   b. Presence of vasoactive substance released from the arterial endothelial cells that acts on smooth muscle, sensitizing it to vasoconstriction
   c. Increased cardiac output, followed by arteriole constriction
   d. Excessive dietary sodium intake, sodium retention, insulin resistance, and hyperinsulinemia play roles that are not clear
   e. Familial (genetic) tendency
3. Systolic blood pressure elevation in the absence of elevated diastolic blood pressure is termed isolated systolic hypertension and is treated in the same manner.

Secondary Hypertension

1. Occurs in approximately 5% of patients with hypertension secondary to other pathology
2. Renal pathology
   a. Congenital anomalies, pyelonephritis, renal artery obstruction, acute and chronic glomerulonephritis
   b. Reduced blood flow to kidney causes release of renin. Renin reacts with serum protein in liver (α2-globulin) $\rightarrow$ angiotensin I; this plus angiotensin-converting enzyme (ACE) $\rightarrow$ angiotensin II $\rightarrow$ leads to increased blood pressure.
3. Coarctation of aorta (stenosis of aorta)—blood flow to upper extremities is greater than flow to lower extremities—hypertension of upper part of body.
4. Endocrine disturbances
   a. Pheochromocytoma—a tumor of the adrenal gland that causes release of epinephrine and norepinephrine and a rise in blood pressure.
   b. Adrenal cortex tumors lead to an increase in aldosterone secretion (hyperaldosteronism) and an elevated blood pressure.
   c. Cushing's syndrome leads to an increase in adrenocortical steroids (causing sodium and fluid retention) and hypertension.
   d. Hyperthyroidism—causes increased cardiac output.
5. Medications such as estrogens, sympathomimetics, NSAIDs, steroids, antidepressants.

Consequences of Hypertension

1. Prolonged hypertension damages blood vessels in the brain, eyes, heart, and kidneys and increases the risk of stroke, angina, myocardial infarction, blindness, and heart and kidney failure.
2. Blood vessel damage occurs through arteriosclerosis in which smooth muscle cell proliferation, lipid infiltration, and calcium accumulation occur in the vascular epithelium.
3. Damage to heart, brain, eyes, and kidneys is termed target organ disease; this is the major object of prevention in patients with high blood pressure.

Prevalence and Risk Factors

1. Hypertension is one of the most prevalent chronic diseases for which treatment is available; however, most patients with hypertension are untreated.
2. There are no symptoms; thus, it is termed "the silent killer."
3. Increase in incidence is associated with the following risk factors:
   a. Age—between 30 and 70
   b. Race—African American
   c. Overweight, sleep apnea
   d. Family history
   e. Smoking
   f. Sedentary lifestyle
   g. Diabetes mellitus
4. Prevalence in African Americans is 32.4%; in non-Hispanic whites, 23.3%; and in Mexican Americans, 22.6%.
5. In addition to higher prevalence, hypertension occurs earlier and is more severe in African Americans.
6. Recent data have shown that only 68% of adults with hypertension are aware of it, 53% receive treatment, and only 27% reach good blood pressure control.

TABLE 14-3 Classification of Blood Pressure for Adults Age 18 and Older[a]

Category	Blood Pressure (mm Hg)		
	Systolic		Diastolic
Optimal[b]	<120	and	<80
Normal	<130	and	<85
High-normal	130–139	or	85–89
Hypertension[c]			
Stage 1	140–159	or	90–99
Stage 2	160–179	or	100–109
Stage 3	≥180	or	≥110

[a] Not taking antihypertensive drugs and not acutely ill.
[b] Optimal blood pressure with respect to cardiovascular risk is below 120/80 mm Hg; unusually low readings should be evaluated for clinical significance.
[c] Based on the average of two or more readings taken at each of two or more visits after initial screening visit.
(From Joint National Committee on Prevention, Detection, Evaluation, and Treatment of High Blood Pressure. [1997]. The sixth report of the Joint National Committee on Prevention, Detection, Evaluation, and Treatment of High Blood Pressure. [JNC VI]. *Archives of Internal Medicine, 157*, 2413–2446.)

Clinical Manifestations

1. Usually asymptomatic
2. May cause headache, dizziness, blurred vision when greatly elevated
3. Blood pressure readings as shown in Table 14-3

Diagnostic Evaluation

1. ECG—to determine effects of hypertension on the heart (left ventricular hypertrophy, ischemia) or presence of underlying heart disease
2. Chest x-ray—may show cardiomegaly
3. Proteinuria, elevated serum blood urea nitrogen (BUN), and creatinine levels—indicate kidney disease as a cause or effect of hypertension; first voided urine micro-albumin is the earliest sign
4. Serum potassium—decreased in primary hyperaldosteronism; elevated in Cushing's syndrome, both causes of secondary hypertension
5. Urine (24 hour) for catecholamines—increased in pheochromocytoma
6. Renal scan to detect renal vascular diseases; may include ingestion of captopril, an ACE inhibitor, to detect its effect on renal blood flow

Management
Lifestyle Modifications

1. Lose weight if body mass index (BMI) is greater than or equal to 27.
2. Limit alcohol—no more than 1 oz ethanol daily for men, 0.5 oz for women
3. Get regular aerobic exercise equivalent to 30 to 45 minutes of brisk walking most days.
4. Cut sodium intake to 2.4 g or less per day.
5. Include recommended daily allowances of potassium, calcium, and magnesium in diet. This can be accomplished through following the DASH diet (Dietary Approaches to Stop Hypertension)—rich in fruits, vegetables, low-fat dairy products, and fiber and low in saturated and total fat (see Patient Education Guidelines).
6. Stop smoking.
7. Reduce dietary saturated fat and cholesterol.
8. Consider reducing coffee intake (five cups per day has been shown to increase blood pressure in hypertensive men).
9. If, despite lifestyle changes, the blood pressure remains at or above 140/90 mm Hg (or is not at optimal level in the presence of other cardiovascular risk factors) over 3 to 6 months, drug therapy should be initiated.

Drug Therapy
See Table 14-4.
1. Considerations in selecting therapy include:
   a. Race—African Americans respond well to diuretic therapy; Caucasians respond well to ACE inhibitors.
   b. Age—some side effects may not be tolerated well by elderly persons.
   c. Concomitant diseases and therapies—some agents also treat migraines, benign prostatic hyperplasia, CHF; have beneficial effects on conditions such as renal insufficiency; or have adverse effects on conditions such as diabetes or asthma.
   d. Quality of life impact—tolerance of side effects.
   e. Economic considerations—newer agents very expensive.
   f. Doses per day—may be compliance problem.
2. Agents include:
   a. Diuretics—lower blood pressure by promoting urinary excretion of water and sodium to lower blood volume
   b. β Blockers—beta-adrenergic inhibitors that lower blood pressure by slowing the heart and reducing cardiac output as well as release of renin from the kidneys
   c. α-Receptor blockers—alpha-adrenergic inhibitors that lower blood pressure by dilating peripheral blood vessels and lowering peripheral vascular resistance
   d. Central alpha agonists—lower blood pressure by diminishing sympathetic outflow from the brain, thereby lowering peripheral resistance
   e. Peripheral adrenergic agents—inhibit peripheral adrenergic release of vasoconstricting catecholamines, such as norepinephrine
   f. Combined alpha and beta blockers—adrenergic inhibitors that work through both alpha and beta receptors
   g. Angiotensin converting enzyme (ACE) inhibitors—lower blood pressure by blocking the enzyme that converts angiotensin I to the potent vasoconstrictor angiotensin II. These drugs also raise the level of bradykinin, a potent vasodilator, and lower aldosterone levels.
   h. Angiotensin II antagonists—similar action to ACE inhibitors
   i. Calcium antagonists (calcium channel blockers)—stop the movement of calcium into the cells; relax smooth muscle, which causes vasodilation; and inhibit reabsorption of sodium in the renal tubules
   j. Direct vasodilators—direct smooth muscle relaxants that primarily dilate arteries and arterioles
3. If hypertension is not controlled with the first drug within 1 to 3 months, three options can be considered:
   a. If the patient has faithfully taken the drug and not developed any side effects, the dose of the drug may be increased.
   b. If the patient has had adverse effects, another class of drugs can be substituted.
   c. A second drug from another class could be added. If adding the second agent lowers the pressure, the first agent can be slowly withdrawn or, if necessary, combination therapy will be continued.
4. The best management of hypertension is to use the fewest drugs at the lowest doses while encouraging the patient

PATIENT EDUCATION GUIDELINES **The Dietary Approaches to Stop Hypertension (DASH) Diet**

This diet is rich in fruits, vegetables, and low-fat dairy products and low in saturated and total fat. It has been shown to reduce blood pressure. The following eating plan is based on a 2000-calorie-a-day diet. Depending on calorie needs, the number of daily servings in a food group may vary from those listed. Further information about the DASH diet is available online at **http://dash.bwh.harvard.edu.**

Food Group	Daily Serving	Serving Sizes	Examples and Notes
Grains and grain products	7–8	1 slice bread ½ cup dry cereal ½ cup cooked rice, pasta, or cereal	Whole wheat bread, English muffin, pita bread, bagel, cereals, grits, oatmeal
Vegetables	4–5	1 cup raw leafy vegetable ½ cup cooked vegetable 6 oz vegetable juice	Tomatoes, potatoes, carrots, peas, squash, broccoli, turnip greens, collards, kale, spinach, artichokes, beans, sweet potatoes
Fruits	4–5	6 oz fruit juice 1 medium fruit ¼ cup dried fruit ½ cup fresh, frozen, or canned fruit	Apricots, bananas, dates, grapes, oranges, orange juice, grapefruit, grapefruit juice, mangoes, melons, peaches, pineapples, prunes, raisins, strawberries, tangerines
Low-fat or nonfat dairy	2–3	8 oz milk 1 cup yogurt 1.5 oz cheese	Skim or 1% milk, skim or low-fat buttermilk, non-fat or low-fat yogurt, part-skim mozzarella cheese, non-fat cheese
Meats, poultry, fish	2 or less	3 oz cooked meats, poultry, or fish	Select only lean meats; trim away visible fats; broil, roast, or boil instead of frying; remove skin from poultry
Nuts, seeds, and legumes	4–5/ week	1.5 oz or ⅓ cup nuts ½ oz or 2 tbsp seeds ½ cup cooked legumes	Almonds, filberts, mixed nuts, peanuts, walnuts, sunflowers, kidney beans, lentils

(From Joint National Committee on Prevention, Detection, Evaluation, and Treatment of High Blood Pressure. [1997]. The sixth report of the Joint National Committee on Prevention, Detection, Evaluation, and Treatment of High Blood Pressure [JNC VI]. *Archives of Internal Medicine, 157*, 2413–2446.)

TABLE 14-4 Oral Antihypertensive Drugs

Drug	Trade Name	Usual Dose Range in Total mg/Day[a] (Frequency per Day)	Selected Adverse Effects[b]
Diuretics (partial list)			
Chlorthalidone (G)[c]	Hygroton	12.5–50 (1)	Short term: increases cholesterol and glucose levels
Hydrochlorothiazide (G)	HydroDIURIL, Microzide, Esidrix	12.5–50 (1)	Biochemical abnormalities: decreases potassium, sodium, and magnesium levels, increases uric acid and calcium levels
Indapamide	Lozol	1.25–5 (1)	
Metolazone	Mykrox	0.5–1.0 (1)	Rare: blood dyscrasias, photosensitivity, pancreatitis, hyponatremia
	Zaroxolyn	2.5–10 (1)	
Loop Diuretics			
Bumetanide (G)	Bumex	0.5–4 (2–3)	(Short duration of action, no hypercalcemia)
Ethacrynic acid	Edecrin	25–100 (2–3)	(Only nonsulfonamide diuretic, ototoxicity)
Furosemide (G)	Lasix	40–240 (2–3)	(Short duration of action, no hypercalcemia)
Torsemide	Demadex	5–100 (1–2)	
Potassium-Sparing Agents			
Amiloride HCl (G)	Midamor	5–10 (1)	Potassium-sparing agents only: hyperkalemia
Spironolactone (G)	Aldactone	25–100 (1)	(Gynecomastia)
Triamterene (G)	Dyrenium	25–100 (1)	
Adrenergic Inhibitors			
Peripheral Agents			
Guanadrel	Hylorel	10–75 (2)	(Postural hypotension, diarrhea)
Guanethidine monosulfate	Ismelin	10–150 (1)	(Postural hypotension, diarrhea)
Reserpine[d] (G)	Serpasil	0.05–0.25 (1)	(Nasal congestion, sedation, depression, activation of peptic ulcer)

(*continued*)

TABLE 14-4 Oral Antihypertensive Drugs (Continued)

Drug	Trade Name	Usual Dose Range in Total mg/Day[a] (Frequency per Day)	Selected Adverse Effects[b]
Central α-Agonists			
Clonidine HCl (G)	Catapres	0.2–1.2 (2–3)	Sedation, dry mouth, bradycardia, withdrawal hyper-
Guanabenz acetate (G)	Wytensin	8–32 (2)	tension (more with clonidine, less with guanfacine)
Guanfacine HCl (G)	Tenex	1–3 (1)	(Hepatic and "autoimmune" disorders)
Methyldopa (G)	Aldomet	500–3000 (2)	
α-Blockers			
Doxazosin mesylate	Cardura	1–16 (1)	Postural hypotension
Prazosin HCl (G)	Minipress	2–30 (2–3)	
Terazosin HCl	Hytrin	1–20 (1)	
β-Blockers			
Acebutolol[e,f]	Sectral	200–800 (1)	Bronchospasm, bradycardia, heart failure, may
Atenolol (G)[e]	Tenormin	25–100 (1–2)	mask insulin-induced hypoglycemia; less serious:
Betaxolol[e]	Kerlone	5–20 (1)	impaired peripheral circulation, insomnia, fatigue,
Bisoprolol fumarate[e]	Zebeta	2.5–10 (1)	decreased exercise tolerance, hypertriglyceridemia
Carteolol HCl[f]	Cartrol	2.5–10 (1)	(except agents with intrinsic sympathomimetic
Metoprolol tartrate (G)[e]	Lopressor	50–300 (2)	activity)
Metoprolol succinate[e]	Toprol-XL	50–300 (1)	
Nadolol (G)	Corgard	40–320 (1)	
Penbutolol sulfate[f]	Levatol	10–20 (1)	
Pindolol (G)[f]	Visken	10–60 (2)	
Propranolol HCl (G)	Inderal	40–480 (2)	
	Inderal LA	40–480 (1)	
Timolol maleate (G)	Blocadren	20–60 (2)	
Combined α- and β-Blockers			
Carvedilol	Coreg	12.5–50 (2)	Postural hypotension, bronchospasm
Labetalol HCl (G)	Normodyne, Trandate	200–1200 (2)	
Direct Vasodilators			
Hydralazine HCl (G)	Apresoline	50–300 (2)	Headaches, fluid retention, tachycardia (lupus syn-
Minoxidil (G)	Loniten	5–100 (1)	drome with hydralazine, hirsutism with minoxidil)
Calcium Antagonists			
Nondihydropyridines[g]			
Diltiazem HCl	Cardizem SR	120–360 (2)	Conduction defects, worsening of systolic dysfunc-
	Cardizem CD, Dilacor XR, Tiazac	120–360 (1)	tion, gingival hyperplasia (nausea and headache with diltiazem, constipation with verapamil)
Verapamil HCl	Isoptin SR, Calan SR	90–480 (2)	
	Verelan, Covera HS	120–480 (1)	
Dihydropyridines			
Amlodipine besylate	Norvasc	2.5–10 (1)	Ankle edema, flushing, headache, gingival hypertrophy
Felodipine	Plendil	2.5–20 (1)	
Isradipine	DynaCirc	5–20 (2)	
	DynaCirc CR	5–20 (1)	
Nicardipine	Cardene SR	60–90 (2)	
Nifedipine	Procardia XL, Adalat CC	30–120 (1)	
Nisoldipine	Sular	20–60 (1)	
Angiotenrin-Converting Enzyme Inhibitors			
Benazepril HCl	Lotensin	5–40 (1–2)	Common: cough; rare: angioedema, hyperkalemia,
Captopril (G)	Capoten	25–150 (2–3)	rash, loss of taste, leukopenia
Enalapril maleate	Vasotec	5–40 (1–2)	
Fosinopril sodium	Monopril	10–40 (1–2)	
Lisinopril	Prinivil, Zestril	5–40 (1)	
Moexipril	Univasc	7.5–15 (2)	
Quinapril HCl	Accupril	5–80 (1–2)	
Ramipril	Altace	1.25–20 (1–2)	
Trandolapril	Mavik	1–4 (1)	

(continued)

TABLE 14-4 Oral Antihypertensive Drugs (Continued)

Drug	Trade Name	Usual Dose Range in Total mg/Day[a] (Frequency per Day)	Selected Adverse Effects[b]
Angiotensin II Receptor Blockers			
Candesartan cilexetil[h]	Atacand	8–32 (1–2)	Angioedema (very rare), hyperkalemia
Irbesartan	Avapro	150–300 (1)	
Losartan potassium	Cozaar	25–100 (1–2)	
Valsartan	Diovan	80–320 (1)	
HCl = hydrochloride			

[a] These dosages may vary from those listed in the *Physicians' Desk Reference* (51st edition), which may be consulted for additional information.
[b] Adverse effects are for the class of drugs except where noted for individual drugs (in parentheses); refer to the individual package inserts for drug-specific information.
[c] (G) indicates generic available.
[d] Also acts centrally.
[e] Cardioselective.
[f] Has intrinsic sympathomimetic activity.
[g] Mibefradil (Posicor) was withdrawn from the market in June 1998.
[h] This drug was not approved at the time JNC VI was released.
(From Joint National Committee on Prevention, Detention, Evaluation, and Treatment of High Blood Pressure [1997]. The sixth report of the Joint National Committee on Prevention, Detection, Evaluation, and Treatment of High Blood Pressure [JNC VI]. *Archives of Internal Medicine*, 157, 2413–2446.)

to maintain lifestyle changes. After blood pressure has been under control for at least a year, a slow, progressive decline in drug therapy can be attempted.

5. If the desired blood pressure is still not achieved with the addition of a second drug, a third agent or a diuretic or both (if not already prescribed) could be added.

Complications
See Figure 14-11.
1. Angina pectoris or MI due to decreased coronary perfusion
2. Left ventricular hypertrophy and CHF due to consistently elevated aortic pressure

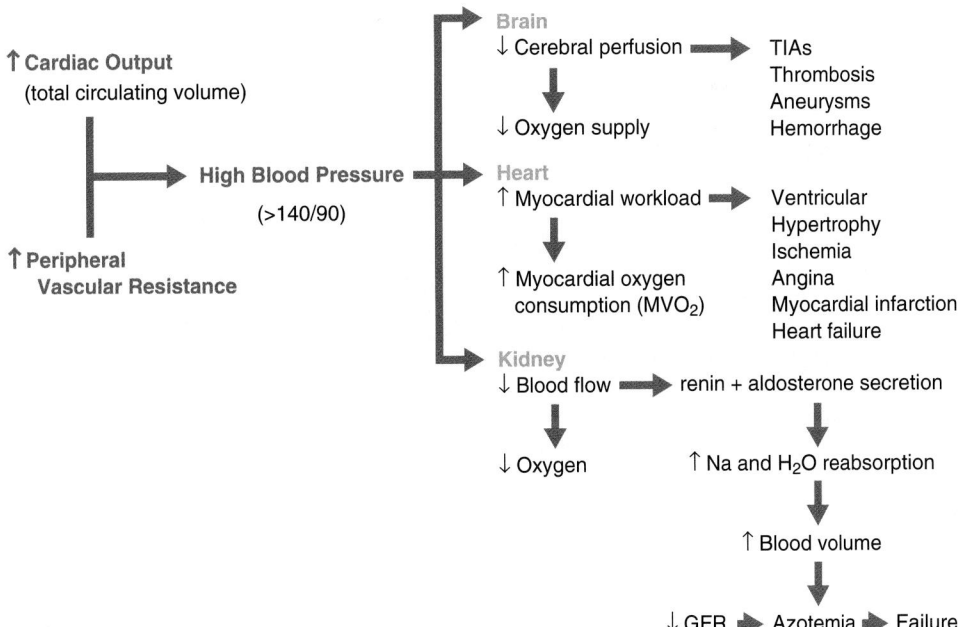

FIGURE 14-11 Determinants and clinical effects of high blood pressure. GFR, glomerular filtration rate; TIA, transient ischemic attack.

3. Renal failure due to thickening of renal vessels and diminished perfusion to the glomerulus
4. Transient ischemic attacks (TIAs), stroke, or cerebral hemorrhage due to cerebral ischemia and arteriosclerosis
5. Retinopathy
6. Accelerated hypertension (see p. 433)

Nursing Assessment
Nursing History
Query the patient with regard to the following:
1. Family history of high blood pressure
2. Previous episodes of high blood pressure
3. Dietary habits and salt intake
4. Target organ disease or other disease processes that may place the patient in a high-risk group—diabetes, coronary artery disease, kidney disease
5. Cigarette smoking
6. Episodes of headache, weakness, muscle cramp, tingling, palpitations, sweating, visual disturbances
7. Medication that could elevate blood pressure:
    a. Oral contraceptives, steroids
    b. NSAIDs
    c. Nasal decongestants, appetite suppressants, tricyclic antidepressants
8. Other disease processes, such as gout, migraines, asthma, heart failure, and benign prostatic hypertrophy, that may be helped or worsened by particular hypertension drugs.

Physical Examination
1. Auscultate heart rate and palpate peripheral pulses; determine respirations.
2. If skilled in doing so, perform funduscopic examination of the eyes for the purpose of noting vascular changes. Look for edema, spasm, and hemorrhage of the eye vessels.
3. Examine the heart for a shift of the point of maximal impulse to the left, which occurs in heart enlargement.
4. Auscultate for bruits over peripheral arteries to determine the presence of atherosclerosis, which may be manifested as obstructed blood flow.
5. Determine mentation status by asking patient about memory, ability to concentrate, and ability to perform simple mathematical calculations.

Blood Pressure Determination
1. Measure the blood pressure of the patient under the same conditions each time.
2. Avoid taking blood pressure readings immediately after stressful or taxing situations. Wait 30 minutes after patient has smoked.
3. Place the patient in a position of comfort and have him or her remain silent.
4. Support the bared arm; avoid constriction of arm by a rolled sleeve.
5. Use a blood pressure cuff of the correct size.
    a. The bladder within the cuff should encircle at least 80% of the patient's arm.
    b. Many adults will require a large cuff.

c. Two or more readings separated by 2 minutes should be averaged.
6. Be aware that falsely elevated blood pressures may be obtained with a cuff that is too narrow; falsely low readings may be obtained with a cuff that is too wide.
7. Auscultate and record precisely the systolic and diastolic pressures based on Korotkoff sounds.
    a. Systolic—the pressure within the cuff indicated by the level of the mercury column at the moment when the first clear, rhythmic pulsatile sound is heard (phase 1).
    b. First diastolic—the pressure within the cuff indicated by the level of the mercury column at the moment when the sound becomes muffled (phase 4).
    c. Second diastolic—the pressure within the cuff at the moment the sound disappears, ie, the onset of silence (phase 5).
    d. Phases 2 and 3 are less distinct sounds produced between systolic and first diastolic and are not identified clinically or recorded.

NURSING ALERT

The finding of an isolated elevated blood pressure does not necessarily indicate hypertension. However, the patient should be regarded as at risk for high blood pressure until further assessment through history taking, repeat blood pressure measurements, and diagnostic testing either confirms or denies the diagnosis.

Nursing Diagnoses
- Knowledge Deficit regarding the relationship between the treatment regimen and control of the disease process
- Ineffective Management of Therapeutic Regimen related to medication side effects and difficult lifestyle adjustments

Nursing Interventions
Providing Basic Education
1. Explain the meaning of high blood pressure, risk factors, and their influences on the cardiovascular, cerebral, and renal systems.
2. Stress that there can never be total cure, only control, of essential hypertension; emphasize the consequences of uncontrolled hypertension.
3. Stress the fact that there may be no correlation between high blood pressure and symptoms; the patient cannot tell by the way he or she feels whether blood pressure is normal or elevated.
4. Have the patient recognize that hypertension is chronic and requires persistent therapy and periodic evaluation. Effective treatment improves life expectancy; therefore, follow-up health care visits are mandatory.
5. Present a coordinated and complementary plan of guidance.
    a. Inform the patient of the meaning of the various diagnostic and therapeutic activities to minimize anxiety and to obtain cooperation.

b. Solicit the assistance of the patient's spouse/family/friend—provide information regarding the total treatment plan.

c. Be aware of the dietary plan developed for this particular patient.

6. Explain the pharmacologic control of hypertension.

a. Explain that the drugs used for effective control of elevated blood pressure will likely produce side effects.

b. Warn the patient of the possibility that orthostatic hypotension may occur initially with some drug therapy.

(i) Instruct the patient to get up slowly to offset the feeling of dizziness.

(ii) Encourage the patient to sit or lie down immediately if he or she feels faint.

c. Alert the patient to expect initial effects such as anorexia, light-headedness, and fatigue with many medications.

d. Inform the patient that the goal of treatment is to control blood pressure, reduce the possibility of complications, and use the minimum number of drugs with the lowest dosage necessary to accomplish this.

7. Educate the patient to be aware of serious side effects and report them immediately so that adjustments can be made in individual pharmacotherapy.

8. Note that dosages are individualized; therefore, they may need to be adjusted because it is often impossible to predict reactions.

9. Warn the patient on vasodilating drugs to use caution in certain circumstances that produce vasodilation—a hot bath, hot weather, febrile illness, consumption of alcohol—which may exacerbate blood pressure reduction.

10. Warn patients that blood pressure is often decreased when circulating blood volume is reduced—as in dehydration, diarrhea, hemorrhage—so blood pressure should be monitored closely and treatment adjusted.

GERONTOLOGIC ALERT

Polypharmacy, cognitive changes, and sensory deficits in the elderly may make dosage adjustment and control of blood pressure difficult. Work with the patient, family, and home care nurse to devise a simple method for the patient to take the proper medications. Elderly patients are also more sensitive to therapeutic levels of drugs and may demonstrate side effects while on an otherwise average dosage. Monitor closely for safety and efficacy of therapy. They may be more sensitive to postural hypotension and should be cautioned to change positions with great care.

Encouraging Self-Management

1. Enlist the patient's cooperation in redirecting lifestyle in keeping with the guidelines of therapy, acknowledge the difficulty, and provide support and encouragement.

2. Develop a plan of instruction for medication self-management.

a. Plan the patient's medication schedule so that the many medications are given at proper and convenient times; set up a daily checklist on which the patient can record the medication taken.

b. Be sure the patient knows the generic and brand names for all medications and throws away old medications and dosages so they will not be mixed up with current medications.

3. Instruct the patient regarding proper method of taking blood pressure at home and at work if health care provider so desires. Inform patient of desired range and the readings that are to be reported.

4. Determine recommended dietary plans and provide dietary education as appropriate.

a. Most patients have a basic knowledge of nutrients and minerals such as fats and sodium and can be taught to read labels.

b. Some patients may require consultation with a dietician to understand how diet may affect blood pressure and health.

Outcome-Based Evaluation

- Demonstrates increased knowledge about high blood pressure, medication effects, and prescribed therapeutic activities
- Takes medications, keeps follow-up appointments

Accelerated Hypertension

Accelerated hypertension, also called malignant hypertension, occurs when the blood pressure elevates extremely rapidly, threatening one or more of the target organs: brain, kidney, heart.

Pathophysiology

1. Elevated diastolic pressure → strain on arterial wall → thickening and calcification of arterial media (sclerosis) → narrowed blood vessel lumen.

2. Sclerosis of vessels →increased wall permeability → deposits placed on intima and media of vessels → cerebral, myocardial, or renal ischemia.

Clinical Manifestations

1. Brain effects:
   a. Encephalopathy
   b. Stroke
   c. Progressive headache, stupor, seizures

2. Kidney effects:
   a. Decreased blood flow, vasoconstriction
   b. BUN elevated
   c. Plasma renin activity increased
   d. Urine specific gravity lowered
   e. Proteinuria

3. Heart effects:
   a. Left ventricular failure
   b. Acute MI
   c. Heart failure

Management

Goal is to lower blood pressure to reduce the probability of permanent damage to a target organ: brain, heart, kidney.

1. If diastolic blood pressure exceeds 115 to 130 mm Hg, clinical condition is assessed very carefully.
2. Immediate hospitalization and treatment if the following are present:
   a. Seizures
   b. Abnormal neurologic signs
   c. Severe occipital headache
   d. Pulmonary edema
3. The patient is hemodynamically monitored in the intensive care unit.
4. Antihypertensive agents are administered parenterally. Agents include:
   a. Vasodilators such as sodium nitroprusside (Nipride), nitroglycerin (Tridil), diazoxide (Hyperstat), or hydralazine (Apresoline)
   b. Adrenergic inhibitors such as phentolamine (Regitine), labetalol (Normodyne), and methyldopa (Aldomet)
   c. The short-acting calcium antagonist nifedipine is rarely used at present due to the danger of precipitating an ischemic event.
5. Diuretics may be administered to maintain a sodium diuresis when the arterial pressure falls.
6. Vasopressor agents should be available if the blood pressure responds too vigorously to antihypertensive agents.

Nursing Interventions

1. Record blood pressure frequently or monitor blood pressure via an intra-arterial line or electronically controlled cuff. Some drugs necessitate the taking of blood pressure readings every 5 minutes or more frequently while titrating drug therapies.

NURSING ALERT

The blood pressure should be reduced gradually and wide pressure variations avoided because lowered blood pressure may not be adequate to perfuse vital organs.

2. Monitor for side effects of medications—headache, tachycardia, orthostatic hypotension.
3. Measure urine output accurately.
4. Observe for hypokalemia, especially if patient is placed on diuretic therapy. Monitor for ventricular dysrhythmias.
5. Observe for CNS complications.
   a. Note signs of confusion, irritability, lethargy, and disorientation.
   b. Listen for complaints of headache, difficulty with vision.
   c. Check for evidence of nausea or vomiting.
   d. Be alert for signs of seizure activity. Provide a safe environment—padded side rails. Keep bed in lowest position.

6. Reduce activity and provide quiet environment.
7. Monitor ECG continuously.
8. Maintain constant vigilance until blood pressure is decreased and stable, then begin a hypertension teaching program.

LYMPHATIC DISORDERS

The lymphatic system is a network of vessels and nodes that are interrelated with the circulatory system. It removes tissue fluid from intercellular spaces and protects the body from bacterial invasion. Lymph nodes are located along the course of the lymphatic vessels and filter lymph before it is returned to the bloodstream.

Lymphedema and Lymphangitis

Lymphedema is a swelling of the tissues (particularly in the dependent position) produced by an obstruction to the lymph flow in an extremity.

Lymphangitis is an acute inflammation of lymphatic channels, which most commonly arises from a focus of infection in an extremity.

Pathophysiology and Etiology

Lymphedema

1. Classified as primary (congenital malformations) or secondary (acquired obstruction).
2. Swelling in the extremities occurs due to an increased quantity of lymph fluid that results from an obstruction of lymphatics.
3. Obstruction may be in both the lymph nodes and the lymphatic vessels.
4. It may be associated with radical mastectomy, varicose veins, chronic phlebitis, and elephantiasis.

Lymphangitis

1. Arises most commonly from infection in an extremity.
2. The characteristic red streak extending up an arm or leg from the infected wound outlines the course of the lymphatics as they drain.
3. Recurrent lymphangitis is often associated with lymphedema.

Clinical Manifestations

1. Edema may be massive and is often firm in lymphedema.
2. Lymphangitis:
   a. Displays characteristic red streaks that extend up an arm or leg from an infection that is not localized and that can lead to septicemia
   b. Produces general symptoms—high fever, chills
   c. Produces local symptoms—local pain, tenderness, swelling along involved lymphatics
   d. Produces local lymph node symptoms—enlarged, red, tender (acute lymphadenitis)
   e. Produces an abscess—necrotic, pus-producing (suppurative lymphadenitis)

Diagnostic Evaluation
1. Lymphangiography—outlines lymphatic system
2. Lymphoscintigraphy—reliable alternative to lymphangiography using radioactive colloid material; detects obstruction or inflammation
3. CT
4. MRI

Management
Lymphedema
1. Bed rest with leg elevation
2. Active and passive exercises
3. External compression devices
4. Elastic stockings (when ambulatory)
5. Diuretics (controversial)
6. Surgery
   a. Excision of affected subcutaneous tissue and fascia with skin grafting
   b. Transfer of superficial lymphatics to deep lymphatic system by buried dermal flap
   c. Complications include flap necrosis, hematoma, abscess under flap, cellulitis

Lymphangitis
1. Administer antibiotic agents because causative organisms usually are streptococci and staphylococci.
2. Treat affected part by rest, elevation, and the application of hot, moist dressings.
3. Incise and drain if necrosis and abscess formation occur.

Complications
1. Abscess formation (rare with lymphangitis)
2. Firm, nonpitting lymphedema unresponsive to treatment (congenital lymphedema, called lymphedema praecox)
3. Elephantiasis secondary to parasite (filaria)—chronic fibrosis of subcutaneous tissue and chronic swelling of the extremity
4. Septicemia

Nursing Assessment
1. Assess extremity for edema and inflammation.
   a. Palpate edema to evaluate its quality (soft and pitting or firm and nonpitting).
   b. Note any areas of abscess formation (suppurative lymphadenitis).
2. Watch for signs of fever and chills.

Nursing Diagnoses
- Risk for Impaired Skin Integrity related to edema and/or inflammation
- Pain related to incision and/or surgery

Nursing Interventions
Maintaining Skin Integrity
1. Apply elastic bandages or stockings (after acute attack with lymphangitis).
2. Advise the patient to rest frequently with affected part elevated—each joint higher than the preceding one.

3. Administer diuretics as prescribed to control excess fluid.
4. Give antibiotics as prescribed.
5. Recommend isometric exercises with extremity elevated.
6. Suggest moderate sodium restriction in diet.
7. Observe postoperatively for signs of infection.

Relieving Pain Postoperatively
1. Encourage comfortable positioning and immobilization of affected area.
2. Administer or teach patient to administer analgesics as prescribed; monitor for side effects.
3. Use bed cradle to relieve pressure from bed covers.

Patient Education and Health Maintenance
1. Instruct patient on proper application of support stockings and/or compression device.
2. Encourage use of elastic bandage or stocking. May need for several months to prevent long-term edema.
3. Advise patient to avoid trauma to extremity.
4. Instruct patient to use lotions that are free of perfumes that may irritate skin.
5. Advise patient to practice good hygiene to avoid superimposed infections.
6. Instruct patient about the signs and symptoms of infection to report to health care providers.
7. Instruct patient to inspect feet and legs daily for evidence of skin breakdown.

Outcome-Based Evaluation
- Skin is normal color and temperature, nontender, nonswollen, and intact
- Patient verbalizes no pain on actively moving extremity

SELECTED REFERENCES
Albers, G.W., Easton, J.D., Sacco, R.L. et al. (1998). Antithrombotic and thrombolytic therapy for ischemic stroke. *Chest, 114*, 683S–698S.
Appel, L.J., Moore, T.J., Obarzanek, E., et al., for the DASH Cooperative Research Group (1997). A clinical trial of the effects of dietary patterns on blood pressure. *New England Journal of Medicine, 336*, 1117–1124.
Breen, P. (2000). DVT: What every nurse should know. *RN, 63*(4), 58–62.
Bryant, J.L. & Turkoski, B.B. (1999). Relieving intermittent claudication: A nursing approach. *Journal of Vascular Nursing 17*(4), 81–85.
Burt, V.L., Cutler, J.A., Higgins, M., et al. (1995). Trends in the prevalence, awareness, treatment, and control of hypertension in the adult US population: Data from the health examination surveys, 1960 to 1991. *Hypertension, 26*, 60–69.
Cairns, J.A. Theroux, P., Lewis, H.D., et al. (1998). Antithrombotic agents in coronary artery disease. *Chest, 114*, 611S–633S.
Dyken, M.L. (1998). Antiplatelet agents and stroke prevention. *Seminars in Neurology, 18*, 441–450.
Fahey, V.A. (1999). *Vascular nursing* (3rd ed.). Philadelphia: W.B. Saunders.
Fink, H.A., et al. (2000). The accuracy of physical examination to detect abdominal aortic aneurysm. *Archives of Internal Medicine, 160*(6), 833–836.
Gibbar-Clements, T., Shirrell, D., Dooley, R., & Smiley, B. (2000). The challenge of warfarin therapy. *American Journal of Medicine, 100*(3), 38–40.

Gress, T.W., et al. (2000). Hypertension and antihypertensive therapy as risk factors for type 2 diabetes mellitus. *New England Journal of Medicine, 342*(6), 905–912.

Hansson, L. Zanchetti, A., Carruthers, S.G., et al. (1998). Effects of intensive blood-pressure lowering and low-dose aspirin in patients with hypertension: Principal results of the hypertension optimal treatment (HOT) randomized trial. *Lancet, 351*, 1755–1762.

Hirsh, J. Anderson, D.R., Bussey, H., et al. (1998). Oral anticoagulants: Mechanism of action, clinical effectiveness, and optimal therapeutic range. *Chest, 114*, 445S–469S.

Hirsh, J. & Poller, L. (1994). The international normalized ratio: A guide to understanding and correcting its problems. *Archives of Internal Medicine, 152*, 278–288.

Jackson, R.R. & Clagett, G.P. (1998). Antithrombotic therapy in peripheral artery occlusive disease. *Chest, 114*, 666S–682S.

Joint National Committee on Prevention, Detection, Evaluation, and Treatment of High Blood Pressure. (1997). The sixth report of the Joint National Committee on Prevention, Detection, Evaluation, and Treatment of High Blood Pressure. *Archives of Internal Medicine, 157*, 2413–2446.

Kozen, V., Fortner, N., & Hölzenbein, T. (1998). An empirical study of nursing in patients undergoing two different procedures for abdominal aneurysm repair. *Journal of Vascular Nursing, 16*(1), 1–5.

Kupecz, D. (2000). Intermittent claudication treatment. *Nurse Practitioner, 25*(5), 112–116.

Lavine, P., et al. (2000). Obstructive sleep apnea syndrome as a risk factor for hypertension: Population study. *British Medical Journal, 320*(4), 479–482.

Meissner, I., Whisnant, J.Pl, Sheps, S.G., et al. (1999). Detection and control of high blood pressure in the community: Do we need a wake-up call? *Hypertension, 34*, 466–471.

MacVittie, B.A. (1998). *Vascular surgery*. St. Louis: Mosby.

Moser, M. & Black, H.R. (1998). The role of combination therapy in the treatment of hypertension. *American Journal of Hypertension, 11*, 73S–78S.

National Heart, Lung, and Blood Institute. (1997). *Fact book fiscal year 1996*. Bethesda, MD: National Institutes of Health.

Patrono, C. Coller, B. Dalen, J.E., et al. (1998). Platelet-active drugs. The relationships among dose, effectiveness, and side effects. *Chest, 114*, 470S–488S.

Perez-Stable, E.J., et al. (2000). The effects of propranolol on cognitive function and quality of life: A randomized trial among patients with diastolic hypertension. *American Journal of Medicine, 108*(7), 359–365.

Prisant, L.M. & Doll, N.C. (1997). Hypertension: The rediscovery of combination therapy. *Geriatrics, 52*(11), 28–30, 33–38.

Rakic, V., Burke, V., & Beilin, L.J. (1999). Effects of coffee on ambulatory blood pressure in older men and women. *Hypertension, 33*(3), 869–873.

Sharis, P.J., Cannon, C.P., & Loscalzo, J. (1998). The antiplatelet effects of ticlopidine and clopidogrel. *Annals of Internal Medicine, 129*, 394–405.

Society for Vascular Medicine and Biology and Society for Vascular Nursing (1998). *Peripheral vascular disease: Marker for cardiovascular risk*. Society for Vascular Medicine and Biology/Society for Vascular Nursing.

Stop Hypertension in the Elderly Cooperative Research Group. (1991). Prevention of strokes by antihypertensive drug treatment in older persons with isolated systolic hypertension. Final results of the Systolic Hypertension in the Elderly Program (SHEP). *Journal of the American Medical Association, 265*, 3255–3264.

Treadway, K.T. (1995). Screening for hypertension. In Goroll, A.H., May, L.A., & Mulley, A.G. (1995). *Primary Care Medicine*. Philadelphia: J. B. Lippincott.

U.S. Department of Health and Human Services. (1994). *Clinician's handbook of preventative services*. Washington, D.C.: U.S. Government Printing Office.

U.S. Renal Data System. (1997). *USRDS 1997 annual report*. Bethesda, MD: National Institute of Diabetes, Digestive and Kidney Disease.

Veterans Administration Cooperative Study Group on Antihypertensive Agents. (1967). Effects of treatment on morbidity in hypertension I: Results in patients with diastolic blood pressures averaging 115 through 129 mm Hg. *Journal of the American Medical Association, 202*, 1028.

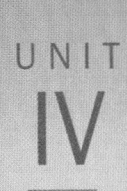

CHAPTER

15

*Neurologic
Disorders*

ASSESSMENT

Common manifestations of neurologic dysfunction include motor, sensory, autonomic, and cognitive deficits. By exploring these symptoms, obtaining a pertinent history, and performing a thorough neurologic examination, you will gain an understanding of the underlying disorder and become skilled in planning care for patients with neurologic disorders. See Chapter 5 for neurologic examination techniques.

DIAGNOSTIC TESTS

 Radiology and Imaging

Recent developments in anatomical and physiologic imaging techniques have facilitated the rapid detection and evaluation of neurologic disorders. Anatomic imaging reveals information about the structure of the nervous system, including the brain and spinal cord. Physiologic imaging focuses on the function of the brain and biochemical and metabolic processes in brain cells.

Computed Tomography (CT) Scan
Description
1. An anatomic imaging study that uses a computer-based x-ray to provide a cross-sectional image of the brain. Intravenous (IV) contrast dye may be used to examine the integrity of the blood–brain barrier.
2. Spinal CT scan may be used to evaluate low back pain due to herniated intervertebral disk or other spinal lesions.
3. *Advantages of CT:* Widespread availability, short imaging time, excellent visualization of skull and vertebrae, and sensitivity for detection of calcification and acute hemorrhage.
4. *Disadvantages of CT:* Does not provide information about function of tissues; exposes the patient to ionizing radiation.
5. Preferred procedure for detection of subarachnoid hemorrhage (SAH) and other rapidly evolving neurologic disorders. When magnetic resonance imaging (MRI) is contraindicated, CT is often the scan of choice.

Nursing and Patient Care Considerations
1. Instruct the patient to remove metal objects, such as earrings, eyeglasses, and hair clips.
2. Ask if the patient has an allergy to iodine or history of previous allergy to IV dye, to determine if premedication is indicated for prevention of allergic reaction to the contrast agent.
3. Tell the patient to expect a sensation of feeling flushed if contrast dye is injected through the IV catheter.
4. Inform the patient the procedure normally takes 10 to 30 minutes.
5. Request that the patient remain as immobile as possible during the examination.
6. Tell the patient to resume usual activities after the procedure.
7. Encourage increased fluid intake for the rest of the day to assist in expelling the contrast dye.

Magnetic Resonance Imaging (MRI)
Description
1. Anatomic imaging technique that uses a powerful magnetic field and radio frequency waves to create an image. When tissue is placed in a strong magnetic field, hydrogen atoms in the tissue line up within the field. In MRI, pulsating radio frequency waves are applied to the magnetic field to alter the tissue magnetization, creating a clear image of the tissue.
2. The imaging procedure of choice for most neurologic diseases (eg, detection of demyelinating diseases, nonacute hemorrhage, and cerebral infarction).
3. *Advantages of MRI:* Absence of ionizing radiation, sensitivity to blood flow, imaging in several planes, and superior visualization of soft tissues. An important advantage is its ability to distinguish water, iron, fat, and blood.
4. Sensitive to detection of white matter changes and valuable in detecting changes associated with Alzheimer's disease and multiple sclerosis.
5. Contraindicated for patients with pacemakers, aneurysm clips, or other implanted objects that could be dislodged by the magnetic field. Dental amalgam, gold, and stainless steel are generally considered safe, but may distort the image.
6. MRI scanner has the appearance of a tunnel-like chamber, and its constricted opening prevents its use for extremely obese people. Because of its narrow dimensions, MRI may induce claustrophobic and anxiety reactions and is not recommended for people with these tendencies.

Nursing and Patient Care Considerations
1. Encourage the patient to use the bathroom before the procedure, because it may take from 40 to 90 minutes.
2. Instruct the patient to remove any metal items, including eyeglasses, jewelry, hair clips, hearing aids, dentures, and clothing with zippers, buckles, or metal buttons.
3. Encourage the patient to remain as still as possible during the procedure. Sedate patient, as directed.
4. Describe the tunnel-like narrow chamber of the MRI scanner, and inform the patient it sometimes causes feelings of anxiety or claustrophobia.
5. Inform the patient the scanner will make a dull, thumping noise throughout the procedure.
6. Tell the patient to resume usual activities after the procedure.

Positron Emission Tomography (PET) Scan
Description
1. A computer-based physiologic imaging technique that permits study of the brain's metabolism and chemical function. PET measures emissions of particles of injected radioisotopes, called positrons, and converts them to an image of the brain.
2. PET scanners are not frequently used or widely available due to their high cost ($2 million to $3 million). PET requires sophisticated equipment to produce its radioisotopes, or positron emitters.
3. A glucose-like solution and mildly radioactive tracers are combined for injection or inhalation. After injection or inhalation of this radioactive compound, pairs of gamma rays are emitted into adjacent tissue during radioactive decay. The PET scanner measures the gamma rays to determine how quickly tissues absorb the radioactive isotopes. A computer processes the data into an image that shows where radioactive material is located, corresponding to cellular metabolism.
4. Provides information on patterns of glucose utilization that reflect neuronal metabolism. Areas of decreased metabolism indicate dysfunction.
5. Useful in early detection of dementia, tumors, seizures, head trauma, Parkinson's disease, amyotrophic lateral sclerosis, and multiple sclerosis.

Nursing and Patient Care Considerations

1. Inform the patient that this procedure requires injection or inhalation of a radioactive substance that emits positively charged particles. Explain that the image is created when the negative particles found in the body combine with the positive particles of the imaging substance.
2. Explain that, after injection of the radioisotope, the patient will be asked to rest quietly on a stretcher for about 45 minutes to allow the substance to circulate to the brain.
3. Reassure the patient that radiation exposure is minimal.
4. Encourage the patient to void before the test, because the scan and associated procedures may take several hours.
5. Advise the patient to increase fluid intake after the procedure to flush out the radioisotope, and resume meals.
6. Tell the patient that it may take a few days to get results of the PET scan, because it requires processing before it is available for interpretation.

Single Photon Emission Computed Tomography (SPECT)
Description
1. A noninvasive physiologic imaging technique that measures blood perfusion in the brain, in contrast to the neuronal uptake of glucose in PET. It uses principles similar to PET, but the radioactive tracer decays to emit only a single photon.
2. Uses a rotating camera to track the single photons emitted from radioactive decay, collecting information from multiple views. Radioactive tracers reveal cerebral blood flow in various regions of the brain.
3. The radioactive tracer compounds used in SPECT are commercially prepared and do not require the specialized equipment used in PET scanning. SPECT scanning does not require an IV line.
4. Used to evaluate cerebral blood flow of patients with ischemic stroke, SAH, migraine, Alzheimer's disease, epilepsy, and other degenerative diseases.

Nursing and Patient Care Considerations
1. Inform the patient that this is a noninvasive procedure that should cause minimal discomfort.
2. Tell the patient that results of the scan are typically available for interpretation by a specialist immediately after the procedure.

Cerebral Angiography
Description
1. An invasive x-ray study in which a radiopaque dye is injected into the brachial or femoral artery to assess cerebral circulation. Serial x-rays are taken after contrast dye illuminates each common carotid artery and each vertebral artery. The structure and patency of cerebral arteries are examined.
2. Useful in detection of stenosis or occlusion, aneurysms, and vessel displacement due to pathologic processes (eg, tumor, abscess, hematoma).
3. Potential complications: temporary or permanent neurologic deficit, anaphylaxis, bleeding or hematoma at the IV site, and impaired circulation in the extremity distal to the injection site.

Nursing and Patient Care Considerations
1. Omit the meal before the test, although clear liquids may be taken.
2. Ask patient about allergies and specifically rule out presence of iodine allergy, which requires pretest preparation. Often, patients with allergy to iodine also have allergies to radiopaque contrast media that may cause severe reaction.
3. Options for pretest preparation include:
   a. Administration of IV steroid 24 hours in advance of procedure and diphenhydramine 50 mg PO 1 hour before procedure *or*
   b. 50 mg Benadryl PO 1 hour before the procedure *or*
   c. Intramuscular (IM) injection of steroid, in the event the test is emergent, followed by Benadryl 50 mg PO
4. Mark pedal peripheral pulses.
5. Explain that a local anesthetic will be used to insert a catheter into the femoral artery (brachial artery may be used) and threaded into the required cerebral vessel.
6. Tell the patient to expect some discomfort when the catheter is inserted into the artery. Additionally, the sensation of a warm, flushed feeling and metallic taste should be expected when the dye is injected.
7. Caution the patient to lie still during the procedure.
8. After the angiography:
   a. Maintain bed rest, as ordered, and monitor vital signs.
   b. Apply an ice pack or sandbag to the IV site, as ordered, to prevent hematoma. Remove the sandbag frequently to observe for bleeding, swelling, or redness.
   c. Check the patient frequently for neurologic symptoms, such as motor or sensory alterations, reduced level of consciousness (LOC), speech disturbances, dysrhythmias, or blood pressure fluctuations.
   d. Monitor for adverse reaction to contrast medium (eg, restlessness, respiratory distress, tachycardia, facial flushing, nausea and vomiting).
   e. Assess skin color, temperature, and peripheral pulses of the extremity distal to the IV site—change may indicate impaired circulation due to occlusion.

Digital Subtraction Angiography (DSA)
Description
1. A variation of cerebral angiography. First, an x-ray is taken of the patient's skull and stored by a computer. Next, contrast material is administered IV, and serial x-rays are taken of the area. The computer digitally

subtracts the original image from subsequent images, producing a clear image of the highlighted arterial vessels.

2. There is less potential for bleeding than in cerebral angiography because the injection of dye is IV rather than arterial.
3. Used to evaluate extracranial circulation. Size of vessels, patency, stenosis, or displacement can be determined.
4. May be done on an outpatient basis.

Nursing and Patient Care Considerations

1. Tell the patient to restrict food 4 hours before the test.
2. Ask patient about allergies and specifically rule out presence of iodine allergy, which requires pretest preparation. Often, patients with allergy to iodine also have allergies to radiopaque contrast media, which may cause severe reaction. Options for pretest preparation include:
   a. Administration of IV steroid 24 hours in advance of procedure and Benadryl 50 mg PO 1 hour before procedure *or*
   b. IM injection of steroid, in the event the test is emergent, followed by Benadryl 50 mg PO
3. Explain that a contrast dye will be administered through an IV catheter, and injection of the dye may cause a warm, flushed feeling and metallic taste.
4. Instruct the patient to remain absolutely motionless during the procedure.
5. After the IV is removed, instruct the patient to resume usual activities.
6. Encourage increased fluids for the rest of the day to help flush out the contrast medium.

Myelography
Description

1. A lumbar puncture is performed to inject a contrast dye or air into the subarachnoid space. After injection of a local anesthetic into the lumbar area, a hollow needle is inserted through which a dye or air is injected into the subarachnoid space surrounding the spinal cord. Fluoroscopy, x-rays, or CT scans are used to view selected areas.
2. The patient is secured on an x-ray table, which is tilted in various directions while spinal films are taken.
3. Observation of the subarachnoid space reveals obstructions due to bone displacement, spinal cord compression, herniated intervertebral disks, or other lesions.

Nursing and Patient Care Considerations

1. Omit the meal before the procedure.
2. Administer sedative before the procedure as prescribed.
3. Explain that the patient will likely experience some discomfort. The contrast medium often results in a headache due to central nervous system (CNS) irritation by the chemical. Back pain may be exacerbated by the lumbar puncture and dye injection.
4. Explain the patient will be strapped to a table that will tilt up or down during the procedure while x-rays are taken.
5. Ask patient about allergies, and specifically rule out presence of iodine allergy, which requires pretest prepa-

ration. Often, patients with allergy to iodine also have allergies to radiopaque contrast media, which may cause severe reaction. Options for pretest preparation include:
   a. IV steroid 24 hours in advance of procedure and diphenhydramine 50 mg PO 1 hour before *or*
   b. IM injection of steroid, in the event the test is emergent, followed by diphenhydramine 50 mg PO
6. Postprocedure care is determined by the type of contrast dye used:
   a. If the patient has received Metazamide (a water-based contrast medium), elevate the head of the bed 15 to 30 degrees for 8 hours to reduce upward dispersion of the medium.
      (i) Keep patient quiet for first several hours.
      (ii) Avoid administration of phenothiazines.
   b. If Pantopaque (an oil-based contrast medium) is used, instruct the patient to lie flat in bed for 12 to 24 hours to reduce cerebrospinal fluid (CSF) leakage and decrease headache.
      (i) Encourage the patient to force fluids for rehydration and replacement of CSF.
      (ii) Observe the patient for signs and symptoms of meningeal irritation (eg, headache, fever, stiff neck, back spasms, nausea and vomiting, seizures).
7. Check patient's ability to void.

Brain Scan
Description

1. A scanner measures the brain's uptake of a radioactive isotope that is administered IV. Radioactive uptake is increased at the site of damaged brain tissue, probably due to abnormal permeability of the blood–brain barrier.
2. Shows location and size of cerebral lesions, but does not specify the source of the lesion (eg, abscess, tumor, cerebral infarction).

Nursing and Patient Care Considerations

1. Withhold medications, as ordered, 24 hours before the test (eg, antihypertensives, vasoconstrictors, vasodilators).
2. Explain that, after injection of the dye, the patient will be asked to change positions while the scanner takes pictures of various views of the brain.
3. Assure the patient that no discomfort will be felt during this procedure.

Magnetic Source Imaging (MSI)
Description

1. Provides information about electric function of the brain without injection of isotopes, attachment of electrodes, or other types of invasive procedures.
2. Currents in the neurons of the brain produce magnetic fields outside the body.

   Using detectors placed near the head, MSI measures external magnetic fields to evaluate the flow of electric currents within the brain.

3. May be used in surgery for intractable epilepsy to locate an epileptic focus.

Nursing and Patient Care Considerations

1. Remove all metal from patient; report any metal implants.
2. Change patient into clothing without metal clasps, buttons, and so forth.
3. Explain that dental work may need to be demagnetized.
4. Tell the patient washable markings will be penned on his or her head as reference points.

Cerebral Blood Flow Studies
Description

1. Injection or inhalation of a radioisotope or nitrous oxide, which is absorbed by the brain. The information is read by 16 to 32 probes placed on the head and analyzed by a computer.
2. Provides regional or overall data regarding cerebral blood flow. Normal blood flow is 50 to 55 mL flow/100 g of cerebral tissue/minute.

Nursing and Patient Care Considerations

1. Reassure the patient that this is a relatively noninvasive procedure and requires cooperation only during the inhalation or injection process.

Transcranial Doppler Studies
Description

1. Noninvasive tests that measure the velocity of blood flow through cerebral arteries, providing information about the circulation to the brain.

   A technician applies a gel to skin at temporal, transorbital, or foramen magnum areas of the skull. A probe is applied to transmit a signal to the cerebral artery being studied. Detected velocities are recorded.

Nursing and Patient Care Considerations

1. Explain the study will be done with the patient in a reclining position.
2. Inform the patient the test normally takes less than 1 hour, depending on the number of arteries that will be studied.

Intracarotid Amobarbital Procedure (Wada Test)
Description

1. A technique used to assess language dominance and memory function before ablative surgery for epilepsy.
2. The patient undergoes cerebral angiography to visualize the cerebral vasculature, and a catheter is placed into the internal carotid artery. Once the catheter is positioned, a short-acting barbiturate is injected (sodium amobarbital [Amytal]) to anesthetize the cerebral hemisphere to mimic the proposed surgery.
3. Electroencephalogram (EEG) and clinical symptoms are used to determine effectiveness. The patient is then tested for language and memory. Drug effects wear off in 2 to 12 minutes.

Nursing and Patient Care Considerations

1. Prepare patient as for a cerebral angiography.
2. Instruct the patient to be NPO after 8 PM the night before the test.
3. Reassure the patient that any speech alterations will be temporary.

Other Diagnostic Tests

Other diagnostic tests include lumbar puncture, which provides information about the CNS through direct contact with the CSF; a variety of tests that measure electrical impulses in portions of the nervous system; and neuropsychological evaluation.

Lumbar Puncture
Description

1. A needle is inserted into lumbar subarachnoid space, usually between the third and fourth lumbar vertebrae, and CSF is withdrawn for diagnostic and therapeutic purposes.
2. Purposes include:
   a. Obtaining CSF for examination (microbiologic, serologic, cytologic, or chemical analysis).
   b. Measuring cerebrospinal pressure and assisting in detection of obstruction of CSF circulation.
   c. Determining the presence or absence of blood in the spinal fluid.
   d. Aiding in the diagnosis of viral or bacterial meningitis, subarachnoid or intracranial hemorrhage, tumors, and brain abscesses.
   e. Administering antibiotics and cancer chemotherapy intrathecally in certain cases.
   f. Determining levels of tau protein and beta-amyloid in the CSF, a new test that may be used to assist the diagnosis of Alzheimer's disease. Elevated tau and decreased levels of beta-amyloid are associated with Alzheimer's disease.

Nursing and Patient Care Considerations

See Procedure Guidelines 15-1.

Electroencephalography (EEG)
Description

1. Electrodes are attached to the scalp to provide a recording of electrical activity that is generated in the cerebral cortex. Electrical impulses are transmitted to an electroencephalograph, which magnifies them and records them as brain waves on a strip of paper.
2. Usually performed in a room designed to eliminate electrical interference; however, may be performed at bedside using a portable unit.
3. Provides physiologic assessment of cerebral activity for diagnosis of epilepsy, coma, organic brain syndrome, sleep disorders, and confirmation of brain death.
4. Restlessness and fatigue can alter brain wave patterns.
5. For a baseline recording, the patient is instructed to lie still and relax with eyes closed. After a baseline record-

ing in a resting phase, the patient may be tested in various stress situations (eg, asked to hyperventilate for 3 minutes, look at a flashing strobe light) to elicit abnormal electrical patterns.

Nursing and Patient Care Considerations

1. For routine EEG, tranquilizers, anticonvulsants, sedatives, and stimulants should be held for 24 to 48 hours before the study.
2. Thoroughly wash and dry the patient's hair to remove hair sprays, creams, or oils.
3. Explain that electrodes will be attached to the patient's skull with a special paste.
4. Assure patient that electrodes will not cause any shock, and encourage the patient to relax during the procedure, because anxiety can affect brain wave patterns.
5. Meals should be taken as usual to avoid sudden changes in blood glucose levels.

Magnetoencephalogram (MEG)
Description

A magnetoencephalogram uses a magnetometer to measure the location, depth, orientation, and polarity of spike field strength. Used in determination of epileptogenic focus.

Nursing and Patient Care Considerations

1. Remove all metal.
2. Demagnetize dental work.
3. Assure the patient that the procedure will cause no discomfort.

Evoked Potential Studies
Description

1. These tests measure evoked potentials, or the brain's electrical responses to visual, auditory, or sensory stimuli. Three types of responses are measured: visual, somatosensory, and auditory.
   a. Visual evoked potentials are produced by asking the patient to look at rapidly reversing checkerboard patterns. They assist in evaluating multiple sclerosis and traumatic injury. EEG electrodes are placed over the occiput and record the transmission time from the retina to the occiput.
   b. Somatosensory evoked potentials are generated by stimulating a peripheral sensory nerve and are useful in diagnosing peripheral nerve disease. They measure transmission time up the spinal cord to the sensory cortex.
   c. Auditory evoked potentials are produced by applying sound such as clicks to help locate auditory lesions and evaluate integrity of the brain stem. The transmission time up the brain stem into the cortex is measured.

Nursing and Patient Care Considerations

1. Explain that electrodes will be attached to the patient to measure the electrical activity of the nervous system. Placement of the electrodes will depend on the type of evoked potentials being measured.
2. Ask patient to remove all jewelry.

3. Assure the patient the procedure is not painful and does not cause any electric shock.
4. Inform the patient the test normally takes from 45 to 60 minutes.

Electromyography (EMG)
Description

1. EMG is a recording of a muscle's electrical impulses at rest and during contraction. A needle is attached to an electrode and inserted into a muscle. A mild electric charge is delivered to stimulate the muscle at rest and during voluntary contraction. The response of the muscle is measured on an oscilloscope screen.
2. Useful in distinguishing lower motor neuron disorders from muscle disorders (eg, ALS from muscular dystrophy).
3. Nerve conduction time (NCT), another diagnostic test, is often measured simultaneously.

Nursing and Patient Care Considerations

1. Explain that this test measures the electrical activity of muscles.
2. Inform the patient the procedure normally takes 1 hour.
3. Advise the patient a needle will be inserted into selected muscles, and to expect some degree of discomfort from needle insertion.

Tensilon Test
Description

1. The patient is administered an IV injection of Tensilon (edrophonium), a short-acting anticholinesterase, which improves muscle strength by increasing muscle response to nerve impulses. After the injection of Tensilon, the patient is asked to perform repetitive muscle movements (eg, open and close eyes, cross and uncross legs) to evaluate the muscle response.
2. Useful in the diagnosis of myasthenia gravis. If the patient has myasthenia gravis, muscle strength should improve as soon as Tensilon is injected. EMG may supplement Tensilon test findings to confirm this disease.
3. Contraindicated in patients with hypotension, bradycardia, apnea, or obstruction of the urinary or intestinal tract.

Nursing and Patient Care Considerations

1. Check the patient's history for use of medications that may affect muscle function, anticholinesterase therapy, medication hypersensitivities, and respiratory disease. Hold medications as ordered.
2. Explain that this test helps to determine the cause of muscle weakness.
3. Inform patient the test normally takes 15 to 30 minutes.
4. Do not describe the exact response that is expected because this may influence test results.
5. Explain that, after administration of an IV medication, the patient will be instructed to make specific repetitive muscle movements. Explain the test may be repeated several times to ensure accuracy.
6. Inform the patient there may be some unpleasant side effects felt after injection of medication, but the reaction should disappear quickly.

7. Assure the patient that someone will be available at all times.
8. Observe the patient closely during the test to monitor for adverse reactions to Tensilon.
9. Keep resuscitation equipment nearby, in case of respiratory distress.

Nerve Conduction Studies
Description
1. A peripheral nerve is stimulated electrically through the skin and underlying tissues. A recording electrode detects the response from the stimulated nerve. The time between the stimulation of the nerve and the response is measured on an oscilloscope, and speed of conduction along the nerve is calculated.
2. In peripheral nerve injuries and disease, nerve conduction time is delayed.

Nursing and Patient Care Considerations
1. Inform the patient some discomfort may be experienced from the external stimulation and uncontrolled muscle activity.

Neuropsychological Testing
Description
A series of tests that evaluate effects of neurologic disorders on cognitive functioning and behavior. A neuropsychologist selects appropriate tests to determine the extent and type of functional deficits. Paper and pencil tests, puzzles, word and recall games are commonly used. Testing may assess the following:
1. Intelligence, attention span, memory, judgment
2. Motor, speech, and sensory function
3. Affect, coping, and adaptation
4. Language quality, abstraction, distractibility
5. Ability to sequence learned behaviors
6. Used in diagnosis of organic brain dysfunction and dementia
7. Valuable in determining vocational rehabilitation training needs

Nursing and Patient Care Considerations
1. Assure the patient that these tests are not intended to evaluate mental illness.
2. Explain that testing evaluates the ability to remember, calculate numbers, and perform abstract reasoning.
3. The patient should be well rested, because testing is mentally tiring and lengthy. A complete examination is a 4- to 6-hour process, depending on the patient's ability to concentrate.
4. Anticipate fatigue and frustration after the examination.

Stereotaxis
Description
1. In conjunction with CT scan monitoring, stereotactic biopsy of brain lesions is performed when deep lesions are inaccessible to surgical resection, or when preoperative neurologic symptoms are absent and risks of craniotomy outweigh benefits.
2. Allows for precise targeting of deep brain lesions for biopsy or surgery. Minimizes tissue trauma to surrounding cerebral areas. Can also be used for aspiration of intracranial hematomas, abscesses, and cystic lesion.

Nursing and Patient Care Considerations
1. Explain to the patient that, although the stereotactic surgery penetrates the skull, it does not penetrate the brain.
2. Tell the patient that a CT scan will help pinpoint the exact surgical site and that the position of the electrode or microinstrument will be checked by x-ray or CT scan before the procedure begins.
3. Keep patient NPO before the procedure.
4. Administer analgesics for headaches as ordered.

Polysomnography (PSG)
Description
1. PSG is a noninvasive, all-night sleep study that measures character of sleep, simultaneously monitoring EEG, cardiac and respiratory function, and movements during sleep. It is used to confirm fragmented sleep patterns in narcolepsy and sleep-related epilepsy.
2. Testing is time consuming and labor intensive. Procedures typically include multiple physiologic measures such as EEG, EMG, electrocardiogram (ECG), heart rate, respiratory effort, air flow, and oxygen saturation.

Nursing and Patient Care Considerations
1. Explain that the electrodes placed on the scalp, chest, extremities, and face will be uncomfortable but do not deliver electrical current.
2. Reassure the patient that a technician will be in the next room.
3. Advise the patient to wear comfortable nightwear.

Multisleep Latency Test (MSLT)
Description
1. MSLT is a sleep study performed during the day. It is the most widely objective assessment of daytime sleepiness and is commonly used to confirm a diagnosis of narcolepsy.
2. Testing consists of four "napping" periods of 20 to 35 minutes, during which time the patient lies down on a bed in a darkened room and is allowed to fall asleep. The multiple short sleep periods during the MSLT increase the observation of rapid eye movement (REM) periods.

Nursing and Patient Care Considerations
1. Explain the time and duration of the naps.
2. Reassure the patient that he or she will be free to move about between naps.
3. Tell the patient to wear comfortable clothing and to bring reading or other materials for use between naps.

PROCEDURE GUIDELINES 15-1 — ASSISTING THE PATIENT UNDERGOING LUMBAR PUNCTURE

EQUIPMENT

Sterile lumbar puncture set   Skin antiseptic
Sterile gloves   Band-Aid
Xylocaine 1%–2%

PROCEDURE

Nursing Action	Rationale
PREPARATORY PHASE	
1. Before procedure, the patient should empty bladder and bowel.	1. To enhance comfort.
2. Give a step-by-step summary of the procedure. For lying position, see accompanying figure.	2. Reassures the patient and gains cooperation.

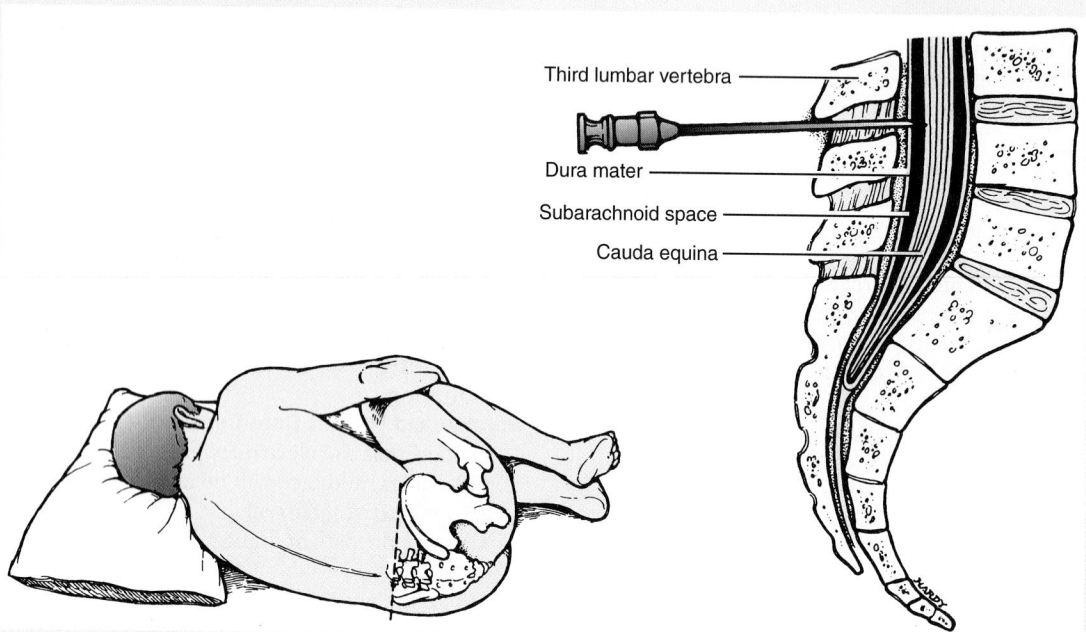

Third lumbar vertebra
Dura mater
Subarachnoid space
Cauda equina

Technique of lumbar puncture.

3. If patient has signs of increased intracranial pressure, a CT scan should be done to rule out mass effect before a lumbar puncture.	3. Removal of CSF in the presence of mass effect may precipitate brain herniation.
4. Position the patient on side with a small pillow under head and a pillow between legs. Patient should be lying on a firm surface.	4. The spine is maintained in a horizontal position. The pillow between the legs prevents the upper leg from rolling forward.
5. Instruct the patient to arch the lumbar segment of back and draw knees up to abdomen, chin to chest, clasping knees with hands.	5. This posture offers maximal widening of the interspinous spaces and affords easier entry into the subarachnoid space.
6. Assist the patient in maintaining this position by supporting behind the knees and neck. Assist the patient to maintain the posture throughout the examination.	6. Supporting the patient helps prevent sudden movements, which can produce a traumatic (bloody) tap and thus impede correct diagnosis.
7. Alternately, for sitting position, have the patient straddle a straight-back chair (facing the back) and rest head against arms, which are folded on the back of the chair.	7. In obese patients and those who have difficulty in assuming an arched side-lying position, this posture may allow more accurate identification of the spinous processes and interspaces.

PROCEDURE GUIDELINES 15-1   CONTINUED

Nursing Action	Rationale
PERFORMANCE PHASE (BY THE PHYSICIAN)	
1. The skin is prepared with antiseptic solution, and the skin and subcutaneous spaces are infiltrated with local anesthetic agent.	1. To reduce risk of contamination; to decrease pain.
2. A spinal puncture needle is introduced at the L3–L4 interspace. The needle is advanced until the "give" of the ligamentum flavum is felt and the needle enters the subarachnoid space. The manometer is attached to the spinal puncture needle.	2. L3–L4 interspace is *below* the level of the spinal cord.
3. After the needle enters the subarachnoid space, help the patient to slowly straighten legs.	3. This maneuver prevents a false increase in intraspinal pressure. Muscle tension and compression of the abdomen give falsely high pressures.
4. Instruct the patient to breathe quietly (not to hold breath or strain) and not to talk.	4. Hyperventilation may lower a truly elevated pressure. Talking can elevate CSF pressure.
5. The initial pressure reading (opening pressure) is obtained by measuring the level of the fluid column after it comes to rest.	5. With respiration, there is normally some fluctuation of spinal fluid in the manometer. Normal range of spinal fluid pressure with the patient in the lateral recumbent position is 70–200 mm H_2O. Opening pressure exceeds normal range when hydrocephalus or increased ICP is present.
6. About 2–3 mL of spinal fluid is placed in each of three test tubes for observation, comparison, and laboratory analysis. Spinal fluid should be clear and colorless.	6. Bloody spinal fluid may indicate subarachnoid hemorrhage or a traumatic tap. If traumatic tap, blood should gradually clear with subsequent specimens.
7. Closing pressure is the pressure on the manometer after the CSF specimen is collected and/or excess CSF removed.	7. Closing pressure should be within normal CSF pressure range.
FOLLOW-UP PHASE	
1. After the procedure, the patient is asked to remain flat for about 2 hours.	1. This reduces pressure on tissue surfaces along the needle track to prevent CSF leakage.
2. Ensure adequate hydration with oral or parenteral fluids.	2. This facilitates replacement of CSF and prevents spinal headache.
3. Monitor for spinal headache, and observe for CSF leak.	3. CSF leaks from lumbar punctures are characterized by intractable spinal headache.

GENERAL PROCEDURES AND TREATMENT MODALITIES

Nursing Management of the Patient With an Altered State of Consciousness

Unconsciousness is a condition in which there is a depression of cerebral function ranging from stupor to coma. Coma results from an impairment in both the arousal and the awareness of consciousness. The arousal of consciousness is mediated by the reticular activating substance (RAS) in the brain stem. The awareness component of consciousness is mediated by the cortical activity within the cerebral hemispheres.

Both arousal and awareness are assessed when using the Glasgow Coma Scale (GCS) as a measure of LOC. When using the GCS, *coma* may be defined as no eye opening on stimulation, absence of comprehensible speech, and failure to obey commands.

An altered state of consciousness may be caused by many factors including hypoxemia, trauma, vascular disorders, neoplasms, degenerative and infectious disorders as well as a variety of metabolic disorders and structural neurologic lesions. Diagnostic evaluation and management depend on the underlying cause, overall intracranial dynamics, age, comorbidities, and general state of health.

Nursing Assessment
1. Assess the patient's level of responsiveness (arousal and awareness).
2. Assess patient's response to command or painful stimulation (if patient does not obey commands, press pen against proximal portion of patient's nail bed, near cuticle, for stimulation).

a. Avoid stimulation techniques likely to result in tissue trauma.
b. Assess eye opening.
c. Assess verbal responses.
d. Assess motor responses.

3. Record the patient's best response. Use the GCS for documentation (Table 15-1).

4. Assess motor function of upper and lower extremities for strength and symmetry, assessing for pronator drift proximally and grip strength distally in upper extremities; leg lifts proximally and dorsi/plantar flexion distally in lower extremities.

5. Test cranial nerve reflexes to assess for brain stem dysfunction.
   a. Assess pupil size, symmetry, and reaction to light.
   b. Assess extraocular movements (CN 3, 4, 6) and reflex eye movements elicited by head turning (oculocephalic response). The oculovestibular (caloric) response (CN 3, 4, 6, 8) is tested by medical staff when the patient is comatose and the oculovestibular response is absent, as a determination of brain death.
   c. Assess CN 5, 7 together to evaluate facial pain, blink, eye closure, and grimace.
   d. Assess CN 9, 10, 12 to evaluate gag, swallowing reflex, tongue protrusion, and patient's ability to handle own secretions.

6. Assess respiratory rate and pattern (normal, Kussmaul, Cheyne-Stokes, apneic).

7. Assess deep tendon reflexes; evaluate for paratonia or flexor/extensor posturing.

8. Examine head for signs of trauma, and mouth, nose, and ears for evidence of edema, blood, and CSF (may indicate basilar skull fracture).

9. Monitor any change in neurologic status over time, and report changes to health care provider as indicated.

TABLE 15-1   The Glasgow Coma Scale (GCS)

Parameter	Finding	Score
Eye opening	Spontaneously	4
	To speech	3
	To pain	2
	Do not open	1
Best verbal response	Oriented	5
	Confused	4
	Inappropriate speech	3
	Unintelligible speech	2
	No verbalization	1
Best motor response	Obeys command	6
	Localizes pain	5
	Withdraws from pain	4
	Abnormal flexion	3
	Abnormal extension	2
	No motor response	1

Interpretation: best score = 15; worst score = 3; 7 or less generally indicates coma; changes from baseline are most important.

> **NURSING ALERT**
>
> A change in GCS of two or more points may be significant and requires investigation. If patient demonstrates deterioration as evidenced by a change in neurologic checks, notify physician without delay, and reevaluate neurologic status more often than required by orders, based on nursing judgment.

Nursing Diagnoses
- High Risk for Secondary Brain Injury
- Ineffective Airway Clearance related to upper airway obstruction by tongue and soft tissues; inability to clear respiratory secretions
- Risk for Fluid Volume Deficit related to inability to ingest fluids, dehydration from osmotic therapy (when used to reduce intracranial pressure)
- Altered Oral Mucous Membranes related to mouth breathing, absence of pharyngeal reflex, inability to ingest fluid
- Risk for Impaired Skin Integrity related to immobility or restlessness
- Impaired Tissue Integrity of cornea related to diminished/absent corneal reflex
- Hyperthermia related to infectious process; damage to hypothalamic center
- Altered Urinary Elimination (Incontinence or Retention) related to unconscious state
- Bowel Incontinence related to unconscious state

Nursing Interventions
Minimizing Secondary Brain Injury

1. Monitor for change in neurologic status, decreased LOC, onset of cranial nerve deficits.

2. Identify emerging trends in neurologic function, and communicate findings to medical staff.

3. Monitor response to pharmacologic therapy including drug levels.

4. Monitor laboratory data, CSF cultures, and Gram's stain, if applicable, and communicate findings to medical staff.

5. Assess neurologic drains/dressings for patency, security, and characteristics for drainage.

6. Institute measures to minimize risk for increased intracranial pressure (IICP), cerebral edema, seizures, or neurovascular compromise.

7. Adjust care to reduce risk of increasing intracranial pressure (ICP): body positioning without flexing head, reduce hip flexion, distribute care throughout 24-hour period sufficiently for ICP to return to baseline.

Maintaining an Effective Airway

1. Position patient to prevent tongue from obstructing the airway, encourage drainage of respiratory secretions, and promote adequate exchange of oxygen and carbon dioxide.

2. Keep the airway free of secretions with suctioning. In the absence of cough and swallowing reflexes, secre-

tions rapidly accumulate in the posterior pharynx and upper trachea and can lead to respiratory complications (eg, aspiration).

a. Insert oral airway if tongue is paralyzed or is obstructing the airway. An obstructed airway increases ICP. This is considered a short-term measure.

b. Prepare for insertion of cuffed endotracheal tube to protect the airway from aspiration and to allow efficient removal of tracheobronchial secretions.

c. See page 225 for technique of tracheal suctioning.

d. Use oxygen therapy as prescribed to deliver oxygenated blood to the CNS.

Attaining and Maintaining Fluid and Electrolyte Balance

1. Monitor prescribed IV fluids carefully, minimizing large volumes of "free water," which may aggravate cerebral edema.

2. Maintain hydration and enhance nutritional status with use of enteral or parenteral fluids.

3. Measure urinary output and specific gravity.

4. Evaluate pulses (radial, carotid, apical, and pedal); measure blood pressure; these parameters are a measure of circulatory adequacy/inadequacy.

5. Maintain circulation; support the blood pressure and treat life-threatening cardiac dysrhythmias.

Maintaining Healthy Oral Mucous Membranes

1. Remove dentures. Inspect patient's mouth for dryness, inflammation, and the presence of crusting.

2. Provide mouth care by brushing teeth and cleansing the mouth with appropriate solution every 2 to 4 hours to prevent parotitis (inflammation of parotid gland).

3. Apply lip emollient to maintain hydration and prevent dryness.

Maintaining Skin Integrity

1. Keep the skin clean, dry, and free of pressure because comatose patients are susceptible to the formation of pressure ulcers.

2. Turn the patient from side to side on a regular schedule to relieve pressure areas and help clear lungs by mobilizing secretions; turning also provides kinesthetic (sensation of movement), proprioceptive (awareness of position), and vestibular (equilibrium) stimulation.

3. Reposition carefully after turning to prevent ischemic and shearing over pressure areas.

4. Position extremities in functional position, and monitor skin underneath splints/orthoses to prevent skin breakdown and pressure neuropathies.

5. Perform range-of-motion exercises of extremities at least four times daily; contracture deformities develop early in unconscious patients.

Maintaining Corneal Integrity

1. Protect the eyes from corneal irritation as the cornea functions as a shield. If the eyes remain open for long periods, corneal drying, irritation, and ulceration are likely to result.

a. Make sure the patient's eye is not rubbing against bedding if blinking and corneal reflexes are absent.

b. Inspect the condition of the eyes with a flashlight.

c. Remove contact lenses, if worn.

d. Irrigate eyes with sterile saline or prescribed solution to remove discharge and debris.

e. Instill prescribed ophthalmic ointment in each eye to prevent glazing and corneal ulceration.

f. Instill artificial tears as prescribed.

g. Apply eye patches, when indicated, ensuring that eyes remain closed under patch.

2. Prepare for temporary tarsorrhaphy (suturing of eyelids in closed position) if unconscious state is prolonged.

Reducing Fever

1. Look for possible sites of infections (respiratory, CNS, urinary tract, wound) when fever is present in an unconscious patient.

2. Monitor temperature frequently or continuously.

3. Control persistent elevations of temperature. Fever increases metabolic demands of brain, decreases circulation and oxygenation, resulting in cerebral deterioration.

a. Maintain cool ambient temperature. Anticipate potential for overcooling and make environmental adjustments accordingly (eg, operating room environment).

b. Minimize excess covering on bed.

c. Administer prescribed antipyretics.

d. Use cool-water sponging and an electric fan blowing over the patient to increase surface cooling for hyperthermia resistant to antipyretics.

e. Consider use of hypothermia blanket if hyperthermia is of neurogenic origin.

f. Monitor core temperature continuously, and avoid rapid overcooling.

Promoting Urinary Elimination

1. Palpate over the patient's bladder at intervals to detect urinary retention and an overdistended bladder.

2. Insert an indwelling urethral catheter for short-term management.

3. Use intermittent bladder catheterization for distention as soon as possible to minimize risk of infection.

4. Monitor for fever and cloudy urine.

5. Initiate a bladder training program as soon as consciousness is regained.

Promoting Bowel Function

1. Observe for constipation due to immobility and lack of dietary fiber. Stool softener or laxative may be prescribed to promote bowel elimination.

2. Monitor for diarrhea resulting from infection, antibiotics, hyperosmolar fluids, and fecal impaction.

a. Patients on tube feedings may develop diarrhea.

b. Perform a rectal examination if fecal impaction is suspected.

c. Use fecal collection bags, and provide meticulous skin care if patient has fecal incontinence.

3. Auscultate for bowel sounds; palpate lower abdomen for distention.

Family Education and Support

1. Develop a supportive and trusting relationship with the family or significant other(s).
2. Provide information and frequent updates on patient's condition and progress.
3. Involve them in routine care, and teach procedures that they can perform at home.
4. Demonstrate and teach methods of sensory stimulation to be used frequently.
   a. Use physical touch and reassuring voice.
   b. Talk in meaningful way even when patient does not seem to respond.
   c. Orient patient periodically to person, time, and place.
5. Encourage adequate room lighting to prevent hallucinations.
6. Teach family to recognize and report unusual restlessness, which could indicate cerebral hypoxia or metabolic imbalance.
7. Enlist help of social worker, home health agency, or other resources to assist family with such issues as financial concerns, need for medical equipment in home, and respite care.

Outcome-Based Evaluation

- Neurologic status remains at baseline or improved
- Maintains clear airway; coughs up secretions
- Absence of signs of dehydration
- Intact, pink mucous membranes
- No skin breakdown or erythema
- Absence of trauma to cornea
- Core temperature within normal limits
- Catheterized at intervals for clear urine
- Bowel movement on regular basis in response to bowel regimen

◼ Nursing Management of the Patient With Increased Intracranial Pressure

ICP is the pressure exerted by the contents inside the cranial vault—the brain tissue (gray and white matter), CSF, and the blood volume. These three components exist in the following volume ratio: brain tissue, 80%; CSF, 10%; blood volume, 10%. The pressure relationship of these elements constantly adjusts to achieve an acceptable steady state or equilibrium between the components of the intracranial system.

Increased ICP is defined as CSF pressure greater than 15 mm Hg.

Factors that influence the ability of the body to achieve this steady state include systemic blood pressure, ventilation and oxygenation, metabolic rate and oxygen consumption (fever, shivering, activity), regional cerebral vasospasm, and oxygen saturation/hematocrit. Inability to maintain a steady state, resulting in increased ICP, can result from head injury, cerebral edema, abscess and infection, lesions, intracranial surgery, and radiation therapy. Increased ICP constitutes an emergency and requires prompt treatment.

ICP can be monitored by means of an intraventricular catheter, a subarachnoid screw or bolt, or an epidural pressure-recording device. However, noninvasive assessment of continuous ICP curves are being researched. Certain parameters called transcranial Doppler (TCD) are being calculated with arterial blood pressure (ABP) and cerebral blood flow velocity (FV), as a promising method to monitor ICP with noninvasive techniques.

Pathophysiology and Etiology

The Monro-Kellie doctrine states that when brain, blood, and CSF exist in the above ratio, the intracranial compartment is filled to capacity. The brain contents must be kept in equilibrium, and the ratio between volume and pressure must remain constant. Any increase in the volume of one component must be accompanied by a reciprocal decrease in one of the other components. When this volume–pressure relationship becomes unbalanced, ICP increases. The brain attempts to compensate for rises in ICP by:

1. Displacement/shunting of CSF from the intracranial compartment to the lumbar subarachnoid space (SAS). Normally, about 500 mL of CSF are produced and absorbed in 24 hours. About 125 to 150 mL circulate throughout the ventricular system and the SAS in the following ratio: 25 mL in the ventricles, 90 mL in the lumbar SAS, 35 mL in the cisterns and surrounding SAS.
2. Increased CSF absorption.
3. Decreased cerebral blood volume by displacement of cerebral venous blood into the venous sinuses. Compensatory measures are finite. Increased ICP will ultimately occur if the volume of the intracranial mass exceeds the volume compensated for.
4. Intracranial compliance ("tightness" of the brain). Compliance is the relationship between intracranial volume and ICP. It is a nonlinear relationship; as ICP increases, compliance decreases. With functional compensatory mechanisms, an increase in volume causes a small, transient increase in ICP. As compliance decreases, small increases in volume result in moderate increases in pressure. When compensatory mechanisms are exhausted, very slight increases in volume will produce large increases in pressure. The patient's response to changes in ICP will depend on where the patient is on the volume–pressure curve.

Nursing Assessment
Change in Level of Consciousness
Caused by increased cerebral pressure. Assess for:
1. Falling score on the GCS (GCS ≤7)
2. Early behavioral changes: restlessness, irritability, drowsiness, confusion, apathy
3. Change in orientation: disorientation to time, place, or person
4. Difficulty/inability to follow commands
5. Difficulty/inability in verbalization or in responsiveness to auditory stimuli
6. Change in response to painful stimuli (eg, purposeful to inappropriate/absent responses)
7. Posturing (abnormal flexion/extension)

Changes in Vital Signs
Caused by pressure on brain stem. Assess for:
1. Rising blood pressure or widening pulse pressure (the difference between systolic and diastolic blood pressure)
2. Pulse changes with bradycardia changing to tachycardia as ICP rises
3. Respiratory irregularities; tachypnea (early sign of increased ICP); slowing of rate with lengthening periods of apnea; Cheyne-Stokes or Kussmaul breathing, central neurogenic hyperventilation, apneustic, ataxic breathing
4. Moderately elevated temperature

Pupillary Changes
1. Caused by increased pressure on optic and oculomotor nerves.
2. Inspect the pupils with a flashlight to evaluate size, configuration, and reaction to light.
3. Compare both eyes for similarities, differences.
   a. Uncal herniation
      (i) Unilaterally dilating pupil ipsilateral to lesion.
      (ii) Anisocoria with sluggish light reaction in dilated pupil.
      (iii) If treatment is delayed or unsuccessful, contralateral pupil becomes dilated and fixed to light.
      (iv) Ultimately, both pupils assume midposition and remain fixed to light.
   b. Central transtentorial herniation
      (i) Pupils are small bilaterally (1 to 3 mm).
      (ii) Reaction to light is brisk but with small range of constriction.
      (iii) Treatment is delayed or unsuccessful; small pupils dilate moderately (3 to 5 mm) to fix irregularly at midposition.
      (iv) Ultimately, both pupils dilate widely.
4. Inspect the retina and optic nerve for hemorrhage and papilledema.

Extraocular Movements
1. Evaluate gaze to determine if it is conjugate (paired, working together) or if eye movements are abnormal.
2. Evaluate ability of eyes to abduct and adduct.

   a. Alteration in vision (eg, blurred vision, diplopia, field cut)
   b. Spontaneous roving, random eye movements
   c. Deviation of one or both eyes
   d. Nystagmus on horizontal/vertical gaze
3. Oculocephalic reflex (doll's eyes): brisk turning of the head left, right, up, or down with observation of eye movements in response to the stimulus. Tests brain stem pathways between cranial nerves III, IV, VI, and VIII.
4. Oculovestibular reflex (ice water calorics): 30 to 60 mL of ice water instilled into the ear with the head of the bed elevated to 30 degrees.
5. Tests brain stem pathways between cranial nerves III, IV, VI, and VIII. Response preserved longer than the doll's eyes maneuver.

Other Changes
1. Be alert for: Headache increasing in intensity; aggravated by movement/straining
2. Vomiting recurrent with little or no nausea; especially in early morning; may be projectile
3. Papilledema from optic nerve compression
4. Subtle changes such as restlessness, headache, forced breathing, purposeless movements, and mental cloudiness
5. Motor and sensory dysfunctions (proximal muscle weakness, presence of pronator drift)
6. Contralateral hemiparesis progressing to complete hemiplegia
7. Speech impairment when dominant hemisphere involved
8. Seizure activity: focal or generalized
9. Decreased brain stem reflexes (cranial nerve deficits; eg, corneal, gag, and swallow)
10. Pathologic reflexes: Babinski, grasp, chewing, sucking

Nursing Diagnosis
• Decreased Adaptive Capacity: Intracranial

Nursing Interventions
Decreasing Intracranial Pressure

> **NURSING ALERT**
>
> Increased ICP is a true life-threatening medical emergency that requires immediate recognition AND prompt therapeutic intervention.

1. Establish and maintain airway, breathing, and circulation.
2. Assist with hyperventilation with a volume ventilator. P_{CO_2} is a potent cerebral vasodilator. Hyperventilation causes cerebral vasoconstriction and decreases cerebral blood volume and results in reduced ICP.
3. Avoid hypoxia. Decreased P_{O_2} (less than 60) also causes cerebral vasodilation, thus increasing ICP. A high level of continuous positive airway pressure (CPAP) causes

decreased venous return secondary to increased intra-thoracic pressure and increased ICP.

4. Maintain adequate cerebral perfusion pressure (CPP). CPP is determined by subtracting the ICP from the mean arterial pressure (MAP): CPP = MAP − ICP.

5. Administer osmotic diuretics such as mannitol (Osmitrol) or urea (Ureaphil), as ordered, to remove water and fluid from areas of brain with an intact blood–brain barrier, thus dehydrating brain tissue. Osmotic diuretics act by establishing an osmotic gradient across the blood–brain barrier that depletes the intracellular and extracellular fluid volume within the brain and throughout the body.

6. Insert an indwelling urinary catheter for management of diuresis.

7. Administer corticosteroids such as dexamethasone (Decadron), as ordered, to reduce edema surrounding brain tumor, if present. Corticosteroids are used to reduce inflammation and to decrease cerebral edema although the use in trauma is controversial.

8. Maintain balanced fluids and electrolytes. Diabetes insipidus (DI) results from the absence of antidiuretic hormone (ADH). The syndrome of inappropriate antidiuretic hormone secretion (SIADH) results from the secretion of ADH in the absence of changes in serum osmolality. Either extreme may occur with ICP.

9. Monitor effects of neuromuscular paralyzing agents, such as pancuronium (Pavulon), which may be given along with mechanical ventilation to prevent sudden changes in ICP due to coughing, straining, or fighting the ventilator.

10. Treat fever aggressively, because fever increases cerebral blood flow and cerebral blood volume; acute increases in ICP occur with fever spikes. Also, infection is a common complication of ICP.

11. Administer high-dose barbiturates and other anesthetic agents, as ordered, to induce comatose state and suppress brain metabolism, which, in turn, reduces cerebral blood flow and ICP.
    a. Be alert to the high level of nursing support required. All responses to environmental and noxious stimuli (suctioning, turning) are abolished as well as all protective reflexes.
    b. Barbiturate coma requires complete supportive care of a comatose, mechanically ventilated patient. With no cough or gag reflex to protect the airway, the patient is very susceptible to pneumonia.
    c. Monitor ICP, EEG, arterial pressure, and serum barbiturate levels as indicated.
    d. Monitor temperature because barbiturate coma causes hypothermia.

12. Avoid positions or activities that may increase ICP. Keep head in alignment with torso; neck flexion or rotation increases ICP by impeding venous return.
    a. Minimize suctioning or other stimuli that precipitously increase ICP.
    b. Keep head of bed elevated 30 degrees to reduce jugular venous pressure and decrease ICP.

13. Use ICP monitoring when ordered for sustained increased ICP (above 20 mm Hg persisting 15 minutes or more or if there is a significant shift in pressure).

14. Avoid taking pressure readings immediately after a procedure. Allow patient to rest for approximately 5 minutes.

15. Record ICP readings every hour, and correlate with significant clinical events or treatments (suctioning, turning).

Outcome-Based Evaluation
- ICP and vital signs stable; alert and responsive

Continuous Intracranial Pressure Monitoring
ICP monitoring is a technology that assists the nurse to assess, plan, intervene, and evaluate patient responses to care. See Procedure Guidelines 15-2.

Monitoring Systems
1. Intraventricular catheter inserted into lateral ventricle using a drill or burr hole opening; connected to fluid-filled transducer, which converts mechanical pressure to electrical impulses and waveform; allows for ventricular drainage.
2. Subarachnoid (bolt) hollow screw inserted into SAS beneath skull and dura through drill hole; also connected to pressure transducer system.
3. Epidural sensor inserted beneath skull but not through dura, so does not measure pressure directly; fiberoptic cable is connected directly to monitor.

Waveforms
1. ICP fluctuates, creating three distinct waveforms.
2. Plateau or A waves are characterized by rapid increases and decreases of pressure with recurring elevations of 15 to 50 mm Hg or higher and may last 2 to 15 minutes.
   a. A waves are clinically significant.
   b. May be accompanied by transient symptoms of headache, nausea, decreased consciousness.
3. B waves are of shorter duration and smaller amplitude than A waves and are not clinically significant unless they occur frequently; then they may precede A waves.
4. C waves are small, rhythmic oscillations that are not clinically significant but fluctuate with changes in blood pressure.

Nursing Interventions
1. Note the pattern of waveforms and any sustained elevation of pressure above 15 mm Hg.
2. Note what stimuli cause increased pressure, such as bathing, suctioning, repositioning.
3. Watch for developing or increasing frequency of plateau waves. Report these, and begin measures to lower increased ICP as described above.

PROCEDURE GUIDELINES 15-2 — INTRACRANIAL PRESSURE (ICP) MONITORING

EQUIPMENT

Sterile gloves
Airway
Ambu Bag
ICP monitoring system (intraventricular, subarachnoid, epidural)
IV pole or standard on which to mount the system

IV solutions as ordered
IV high-pressure tubing
Burr hole tray for insertion or as needed
Topical anesthetic
Vital sign records

PROCEDURE

Nursing Action	Rationale
PREPARATORY PHASE	
1. Explain the need for extensive, continuous assessment and appropriate nursing intervention to the family and patient.	1. Explanations will decrease anxiety, allow patient and family a sense of control, and encourage compliance with procedure.
2. Gather and assemble equipment. Flush lines with ordered solution according to manufacturer's directions.	2. Availability of equipment will enhance success of procedure.
3. Calibrate equipment according to directions.	3. Accurate interpretation of ICP values and wave patterns will depend on appropriate baseline function.
4. Perform neurologic assessment.	4. Patient baseline must be established to determine changes and guide therapy.
5. Administer light sedation/analgesia if patient is agitated.	5. Procedure is invasive, and injury may result with excessive patient movement.
PERFORMANCE PHASE	
1. Establish head of bed at 30 degrees.	1. Head elevation is a conventional nursing intervention used to control elevated intracranial pressure and avoid complications in patients with neurotrauma. 　a. Head elevation facilitates venous drainage, decreasing intracranial volume, and prevents collapse of the ventricles if ventricular placement. 　b. However, elevating the head of the bed may decrease cerebral perfusion pressure, creating ischemia.
2. Shave and cleanse the operative site.	2. Removes bacteria from the site, reducing the risk of infection.
3. Establish the sterile field.	3. A sterile field reduces the risk of infection.
4. Assist with burr hole and placement of intracranial monitoring system.	4. Direct monitoring of intracranial pressure allows for early detection of decompensation and management of complications.
5. Connect monitoring catheter to transducer/monitoring equipment according to directions.	5. Allows for conduction of intracranial and cerebral perfusion pressures to the interpretive component of the system.
6. Observe numeric readings and wave patterns. Adjust characteristics to obtain optimal visual reading.	6. Changes in baseline readings indicate alterations in intracranial pressure or problems with the mechanics of the monitoring system.

continued

PROCEDURE GUIDELINES 15-2   INTRACRANIAL PRESSURE (ICP) MONITORING *CONTINUED*

Nursing Action   **Rationale**

A.   Normal ICP waveform

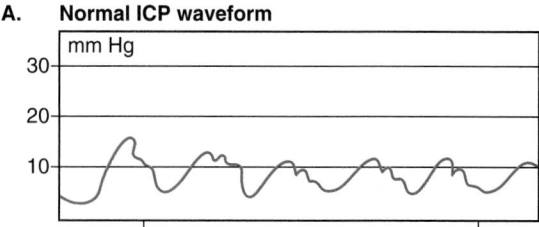

B.   A waves (plateau waves)

B waves

C waves

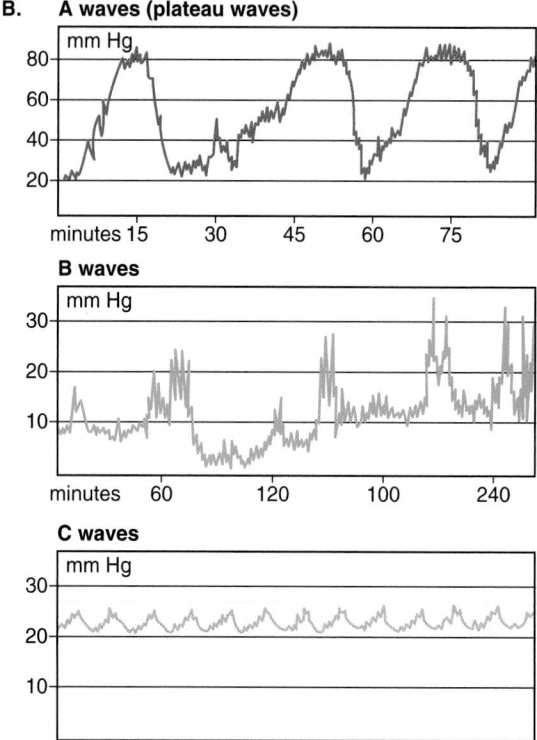

(A) Normal waveform. (B) A waves (plateau waves), B waves, and C waves.

7. Cover the catheter insertion site with a sterile dressing. Observe for possible CSF drainage depending on the placement of the catheter.

8. Adjust alarm system according to ordered parameters.

7. The skull and meninges have been penetrated, leaving the patient at risk for infection.

8. Alarms should be on at all times to alert the nurse away from the bedside of ongoing adverse changes.

FOLLOW-UP PHASE

1. Frequently assess the patient and the system to ascertain neurologic status, assessing ICP and cerebral perfusion pressure (CPP), and patency of the system.

2. Irrigate the system using sterile technique according to policy or prn as indicated to maintain patency.

3. Report dampened wave forms, and have 1 cc of normal saline available for irrigation if indicated.

4. Assess head dressing for CSF drainage. Change dressing according to policy.

5. Adjust the height of the transducer of the system to the level of the patient's ventricles (inner canthus of eye and tip of ear) with every position change for accurate readings.

1. Manipulation of the system may inadvertently close the system, leaving the patient without benefit of monitoring.

2. Irrigation helps maintain the patency of the system.

3. The tip of the catheter may have migrated against the ventricular wall or cerebral tissue depending on location, or ventricular collapse may be imminent. Irrigation is done by the health care provider in this case.

4. Because of its high glucose content, CSF is an excellent medium for bacterial growth.

5. Position of the transducer in relation to the ventricles will influence the accuracy of the readings because of fluid gradient pressures.

Nursing Management of the Patient Undergoing Intracranial Surgery

Craniotomy is the surgical opening of the skull to gain access to intracranial structures to remove a tumor, relieve IICP, evacuate a blood clot, stop hemorrhage, or remove epileptogenic tissue (Figure 15-1). Surgical approach may be supratentorial (above the tentorium or dural covering that divides the cerebrum from cerebellum) or infratentorial (below the tentorium, including the brain stem). Craniotomy may be performed by means of burr holes (made with a drill or hand tools) or by making a bony flap.

Craniectomy is excision of a portion of the skull. *Cranioplasty* is repair of a cranial defect by means of a plastic or metal plate. *Transsphenoidal surgery* is an approach that gains access to the pituitary gland through the nasal cavity and sphenoidal sinus (discussed in Chapter 24, Endocrine Disorders, p. 818).

Preoperative Management

1. Diagnostic findings, surgical procedure, and expectations are reviewed with the patient.
2. Presurgical shampoo with an antimicrobial agent may be ordered. Shave and prep often do not occur until patient is in the OR.
3. Corticosteroids are ordered to reduce cerebral edema.
4. Anticonvulsants are ordered to reduce risk of seizures.

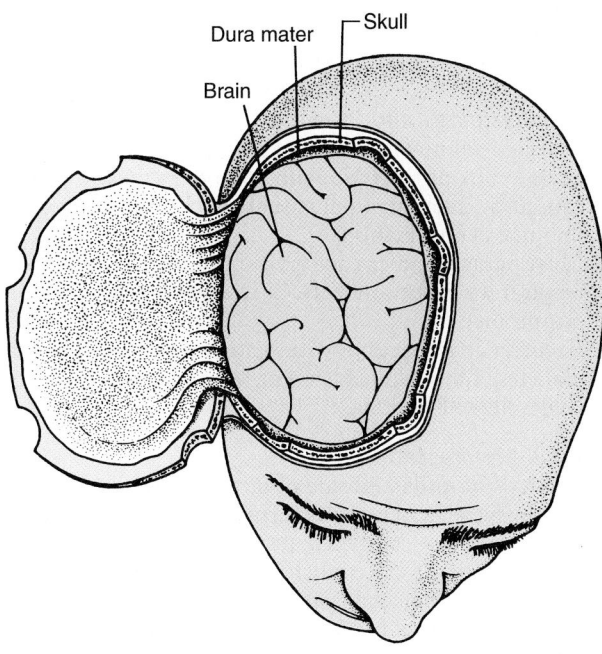

Dura mater — Skull

Brain

FIGURE 15-1 Craniotomy.

5. The patient is prepared for the use of intraoperative antibiotics to reduce risk of infection and urinary catheterization to assess urinary volume during operative period.
6. A hyperosmolar agent (mannitol [Osmitrol]) and a diuretic (furosemide [Lasix]) may be administered immediately preoperatively if needed to reduce cerebral edema.
7. Neurologic assessment is performed to evaluate and record the patient's neurologic baseline and vital signs for postoperative comparison.
8. Family and patient are made aware of the immediate postoperative care and where the physician will contact the family after surgery.
9. Supportive care is given as needed for neurologic deficits.

Postoperative Management

1. Respiratory status is assessed by monitoring rate, depth, and pattern of respirations. A patent airway is maintained.
2. Vital signs and neurologic status are monitored, using GCS (see p. 446); findings are documented.
3. Arterial and central venous pressure (CVP) are monitored, possibly with Swan-Ganz line for accurate manipulation of blood pressure and fluid status.
4. Pharmacologic agents are prescribed to control ICP according to procedure for increased ICP.
5. Incisional and headache pain are controlled with mild analgesic such as codeine and acetaminophen, as prescribed.
6. Patient undergoing supratentorial craniotomy is given anticonvulsants and placed on back or unoperative side.
7. After an infratentorial operation, patient is kept on side and off back with only a small, firm pillow under patient's head.
8. CT of the brain is performed if patient's status deteriorates.
9. Oral fluids are provided after swallow reflex and bowel sounds have returned. Intake and output are monitored.
10. Signs of infection are monitored by checking craniotomy site, ventricular drainage, nuchal rigidity, or presence of CSF.
11. Periorbital edema is controlled by such measures as cold compresses or moist tea bags.
12. Changes in CPP are observed with raising the head of the bed to lower ICP.

Potential Complications

1. Intracranial hemorrhage/hematoma
2. Cerebral edema
3. Infections (eg, postoperative meningitis, pulmonary, wound)
4. Seizures
5. Cranial nerve dysfunction
6. Decreased CPP causing cerebral ischemia

Nursing Diagnoses
- Impaired Cerebral Tissue Perfusion due to increased ICP
- Potential for Cerebral Ischemia secondary to decreased CPP
- Risk for Aspiration related to decreased swallow reflex and postsurgical positioning
- Risk for Infection related to invasive procedure
- Pain related to physiologic changes produced due to invasive procedure
- Constipation related to use of narcotic medication and immobility

Nursing Interventions
Maintaining ICP Within Normal Range (<15 mm Hg) and CPP (>53 mm Hg)
1. Closely monitor LOC, vital signs, pupillary response, and ICP, if indicated.
2. Teach patient to avoid activities that can raise ICP, such as excessive flexion or rotation of the head and Valsalva maneuver (coughing, straining at stool).
3. Administer corticosteroids and other medications as prescribed to reduce ICP.
4. Avoid noxious tactile stimuli (suctioning).

Preventing Aspiration
1. Offer fluids only when patient is alert and swallow reflex has returned.
2. Have suction equipment available at bedside. Suction only if necessary and do so carefully to prevent rise in ICP.
3. Elevate head of bed to maximum of order and patient comfort.

Preventing Nosocomial Infections
1. Use sterile technique for dressing changes, catheter care, and ventricular drain management.
2. Be aware of patients at higher risk of infection—those undergoing lengthy operations, those with ventricular drains left in longer than 72 hours, and those with operations of the third ventricle.
3. Assess surgical site for redness, tenderness, and drainage.
4. Watch for leakage of CSF, which increases the danger of meningitis.
   a. Watch for sudden discharge of fluid from wound; massive leak requires surgical repair.
   b. Warn against coughing, sneezing, or nose blowing, which may aggravate CSF leakage.
   c. Assess for moderate elevation of temperature and neck rigidity.
   d. Note patency of ventricular catheter system.
5. Institute measures to prevent respiratory or urinary tract infection postoperatively (see p. 124).

Relieving Pain
1. Medicate patient according to assessment findings.
2. Elevate head of bed per procedure protocol to relieve headache.
3. Provide distractive measures for pain management.
4. Darken room if patient is photophobic.

Avoiding Constipation
1. Encourage fluids when patient is able to manage liquids.
2. Ambulate as soon as possible.
3. Change to non-narcotic agents for pain control as soon as possible.
4. Avoid Valsalva-like maneuvers.

Family Education and Support
1. Keep patient and family aware of progress and plans to transfer to step-down unit, general nursing unit, subacute care, or rehabilitation facility.
2. Encourage frequent visiting and interaction of family for stimulation of patient as care allows.
3. Begin discharge planning early, and obtain referral of home care nursing, social work, physical and occupational therapy as needed.

Outcome-Based Evaluation
- Decrease ICP and maintain CPP (>53 mm Hg).
- Easily arousable to verbal stimulation, vital signs stable, ICP and CPP within normal limits, pupils equal and reactive, no vomiting
- Gag reflex present; breath sounds clear
- Afebrile without signs of infection
- Verbalization of decreased pain
- Passed soft stool

CRANIAL NERVE DISORDERS

Bell's Palsy
Idiopathic Bell's palsy is an acute peripheral facial paralysis of the infratemporal portion of the seventh cranial nerve (facial) unilaterally. It is typically a self-limiting process that usually improves in 4 to 6 months.

Pathophysiology and Etiology
1. Cause is unknown. Possible etiologies include sensory ganglionitis of the CNS with secondary muscle palsy, caused by inflammation, vascular ischemia, and autoimmune demyelination.
2. Most patients experience a viral prodrome (eg, upper respiratory infection 1 to 3 weeks before onset of symptoms).
3. Recurrence in patients with history of Bell's palsy or diabetes, although incidence of recurrence is <10%.
4. Generally self-limiting.

Clinical Manifestations
1. Paralysis of ipsilateral side of face from vertex of scalp to chin; facial muscles weak throughout forehead, cheek, and chin; can affect speech, distort face
2. Involvement of all branches of facial nerve: facial weakness, diminished taste from anterior two thirds of tongue, decreased blink reflex, decreased lacrimation, inability to close eye, painful eye sensations; photophobia

3. Hyperacusis on the affected side
4. Distorted body image due to change in facial appearance

Diagnostic Evaluation
1. History to determine sequelae of onset
2. Physical examination for evaluation of seventh cranial nerve function and corneal sensation
3. Exclusion of lesions that mimic Bell's palsy such as tumor, infection, trauma, or stroke
4. Electrophysiologic testing, specifically action potentials and EMGs and NCVs to evaluate nerve function.

Management
1. Corticosteroid therapy initiated early to decrease inflammation (eg, prednisone 1 mg/kg/day for 10 to 14 days, followed by a tapering dose).
2. Eye care to maintain lubrication and moisture if unable to close. May need to be patched during sleep.
3. Physical therapy, electrical stimulation to maintain muscle tone.
4. Biofeedback (controversial).
5. Surgery to anastomose facial nerve to other cranial nerve (CNVII–XI or CNVII–XII; controversial due to natural history); surgical closure of eyelid to protect cornea (tarsorrhaphy).
6. Nonsteroidal anti-inflammatory drugs to relieve pain.

Complications
1. Corneal ulceration
2. Impairment of vision
3. Body image disturbance related to facial nerve paralysis

NURSING ALERT
Keratitis (inflammation of the cornea), ulceration, and vision loss are major threats to a patient with Bell's palsy. Protect the cornea if eye does not close.

Nursing Assessment
1. Test motor components of facial nerve by assessing patient's smile, ability to whistle, purse lips, wrinkle forehead, and close eyes. Observe for facial asymmetry.
2. Observe patient's ability to handle secretions, food, fluids; observe for drooling.
3. Assess patient's ability to blink and speak clearly.
4. Assess effect of altered appearance on body image.

Nursing Diagnoses
- Impaired Tissue Integrity related to loss of protective eye closure
- Pain related to physiologic alterations of disorder
- Body Image Disturbance related to facial nerve paralysis

Nursing Interventions
Protecting Corneal Integrity
1. Administer or teach patient to administer artificial tears and ophthalmic ointment as prescribed.
2. Patch eye to keep shut at night as directed.
3. Inspect eye for redness or discharge.
4. Advise patient to report eye pain immediately.

Relieving Pain
1. Administer or teach patient to administer corticosteroids to reduce inflammation and non-narcotic analgesics to relieve pain.
2. Teach patient to apply moist heat to face.
3. Perform or teach patient to perform facial massage to alleviate feelings of stiffness.

Enhancing Body Image
1. Encourage patient to express feelings related to body image disturbance.
2. Assist patient to use mirror as means to obtain feedback about actual versus perceived appearance and identify factors that impede or enhance.

Patient Education and Health Maintenance
1. Instruct the patient to wear wrap-around sunglasses to decrease normal evaporation from the eye from sun and wind, to avoid eye irritants, and to increase environmental humidity.
2. Instruct the patient in use of ophthalmic drops and ointment, proper methods of lid closure, and patching of the eye.
3. Demonstrate facial exercises (eg, raise eyebrows, squeeze eyes shut, purse lips) and stress their importance to prevent muscle atrophy.

Outcome-Based Evaluation
- Cornea without redness, pain, or discharge
- Patient reports adequate pain control
- Patient verbalizes adjustment to body image disturbance

Trigeminal Neuralgia (Tic Douloureux)
Trigeminal neuralgia (tic douloureux) is an intensely painful neurologic condition that affects one or more branches of the fifth cranial (trigeminal) nerve. Patients experience sudden paroxysms of "lancinating" or electric shock–like facial pain (Figure 15-2) localized to one or more branches of the nerve. The pain is often precipitated by trigger points that "fire" when the patient talks, shaves, eats, touches the face, brushes the teeth, or is exposed to cold wind.

Trigeminal Nerve Branches
1. V_1: ophthalmic branch; pain involves the eye and forehead
2. V_2: maxillary branch; pain involves the cheek, upper teeth, upper gums, and nose
3. V_3: mandibular branch; pain involves the lower jaw, side of tongue, lower teeth, lower gum, extends to ear

Pathophysiology and Etiology
1. Unknown cause
2. Degenerative or viral causes suspected
3. Compression from artery adjacent to the nerve strips myelin from nerve when it pulsates. Loss of myelin acts

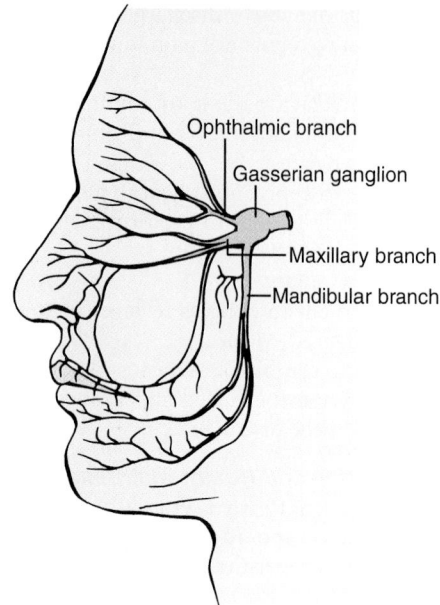

FIGURE 15-2 The main divisions of the trigeminal nerve are the ophthalmic, maxillary, and mandibular. Sensory root fibers arise in the gasserian ganglion.

like an uninsulated wire that "fires" abnormally in response to stimuli.

> **GERONTOLOGIC ALERT**
>
> Trigeminal neuralgia is often seen in the elderly population. Pain often appears to be localized to one or more teeth. Patients may seek dental care for pain relief, resulting in one or more tooth extractions without alleviation of pain.

Clinical Manifestations

1. Sudden, severe episodes of intense facial pain localized to one or more of the branches of the nerve, lasting less than 30 to 60 seconds and ending abruptly.
2. Pain is precipitated by activation of trigger points, such as touching the face, talking, chewing, yawning, and brushing the teeth, that place pressure on the terminal end of the branch affected.
3. Pain is always unilateral and does not cross the midline. Bilateral pain is sometimes seen in patients with multiple sclerosis.
4. Some patients experience numbness, particularly around corner of mouth.

Diagnostic Evaluation

1. History of characteristic symptoms and pattern
2. CT, MRI, skull x-rays to rule out other disorders
3. Initial response to pharmacologic treatment in the majority of cases

Management
Pharmacologic

1. Use of carbamazepine (Tegretol) is first and most effective medication used to treat condition. Other drugs such as imipramine (Tofranil), phenytoin (Dilantin), baclofen (Lioresal), divalproex (Depakote), or gabapentin (Neurontin) may be added or substituted over time.
2. Although pain generally responds to pharmacologic intervention, it gradually becomes refractory over time or patients suffer undesirable side effects.

Surgical

1. Alcohol or phenol block for pain may last several months after injection.
2. Percutaneous radiofrequency trigeminal gangliolysis low-voltage stimulation of nerve by electrode inserted through foramen ovale; sensory function destroyed but attempt to preserve motor function; may cause decreased corneal sensation if V_1 affected; paresthesias, jaw weakness, undesirable, painful numbness (anesthesia dolorosa). Pain may recur as nerve regenerates, necessitating repeat procedure.
3. Rhizotomy (transection of nerve root at gasserian ganglion) causes complete loss of sensation; other complications include burning, stinging, discomfort in and around eye, herpetic lesions of face, keratitis, and corneal ulceration.
4. Microvascular decompression of trigeminal nerve intracranial procedure (see p. 453 for nursing care). Most effective form of therapy, with 75% to 80% of patients pain free without need for medication long term after procedure. Treatment of choice for younger patients willing to accept craniotomy.

Complications

1. Anorexia and weight loss
2. Dehydration
3. Anxiety/fear
4. Depression/social isolation/suicidal ideations in extreme cases

Nursing Assessment

1. Take history of the pain, including duration, severity, and aggravating factors.
2. Assess nutritional status and hydration.
3. Assess for anxiety and depression, including problems with sleep, social interaction, coping ability.

Nursing Diagnoses

- Pain related to physiologic changes of the disorder
- Altered Nutrition: Less Than Body Requirements due to fear of eating
- Anxiety/Depression related to lack of control over painful episodes

Nursing Interventions
Relieving Pain

1. To minimize painful episodes, review with the patient potential trigger factors, and develop individualized methods of coping with identified triggers.

2. Encourage the patient to take medication regularly, including "rescue" medication for breakthrough periods.
3. Help patient maintain a method of communication without causing pain from talking.

Maintaining Adequate Nutrition

1. To maximize nutritional intake, instruct the patient to take foods and fluids at room temperature and to chew on the unaffected side.
2. Have the patient consult with the dietitian for appropriate meal texture and composition.
3. Encourage small, frequent meals to avoid fatigue and pain.
4. Advise nutritional supplements if indicated.

Reducing Anxiety

1. Support patient through treatment trials.
2. Teach relaxation exercises, such as relaxation breathing, progressive muscle relaxation, and imagery to relieve tension.
3. Encourage participation in support groups (eg, Trigeminal Neuralgia Association), and facilitate therapeutic relationship with health care provider.

Patient Education and Health Maintenance

1. Educate the surgical patient regarding self-care after denervation procedures.
2. Instruct patient to look at eye in mirror three to four times/day if corneal sensation is impaired.
3. Instill eyedrops every 4 hours for loss of corneal sensation.
4. Instruct patient to avoid drinking hot liquids through a straw.
5. Instruct patient to chew on unaffected side to avoid biting tongue, lips, and inside of mouth.
6. Instruct patient who wears dentures that jaw muscle will regenerate over time; avoid having dentures refitted.
7. Instruct patient to maintain regular dental checkups, because pain will not be felt with caries.
8. Ask patient if face is numb, and instruct patient to report any change in sensation.
9. Refer patient to the Trigeminal Neuralgesia Association for education and support network: 609-361-6250; *www.tna.support.org*.

Outcome-Based Evaluation

- Patient verbalizes reduced pain
- Weight maintained
- Patient verbalizes decreased anxiety/depression

CEREBROVASCULAR DISEASE

■ Cerebrovascular Insufficiency

Cerebrovascular insufficiency is an interruption or inadequate blood flow to a focal area of the brain resulting in transient or permanent neurologic dysfunction. *Transient ischemic attack (TIA)* lasts less than 24 hours. *Ischemic stroke* is similar to myocardial infarction, in that the pathogenesis is loss of blood supply to the tissue, which can result in irreversible damage if blood flow is not restored quickly.

> **NURSING ALERT**
>
> The professional nurse is often the first health care provider to assess the patient during entry into the emergency care system. Critical assessment by the nurse can determine if the patient is a candidate for emergency medications within the first 2 to 3 hours of symptoms. Thus, the nurse's role in assessment is critical during this therapeutic window for treatment.

Pathophysiology and Etiology

1. Cerebrovascular insufficiency is caused by atherosclerotic plaque or thrombosis, increased PCO_2, decreased PO_2, decreased blood viscosity, hyperthermia/hypothermia, increased ICP.
2. Carotid arteries, major intracranial vessels, or microcirculation may be affected.
3. Cardiac causes of emboli include atrial fibrillation, mitral valve prolapse, infectious endocarditis, and prosthetic heart valve.
4. Event may be classified as transient ischemic attack (TIA)—transient episode of cerebral dysfunction with associated clinical manifestations lasting usually minutes to an hour, possibly up to 24 hours.
5. Symptoms persisting longer than 24 hours are classified as stroke.

Clinical Manifestations of Transient Ischemic Attacks

1. History of intermittent neurologic deficit, sudden in onset, with maximal deficit within 5 minutes and lasting less than 24 hours.
2. Carotid system involvement: amaurosis fugax, homonymous hemianopsia, unilateral weakness, unilateral numbness/paresthesias, aphasia, dysarthria.
3. Vertebrobasilar system involvement: vertigo, bilateral homonymous hemianopsia, diplopia, weakness that is bilateral or alternates sides, dysarthria, dysphagia, ataxia, perioral numbness.
4. Carotid bruit.
5. History of headaches of duration of days before ischemia.

Diagnostic Evaluation

1. Cerebral angiography, carotid angiography, oculoplethysmography, Doppler ultrasound—all provide information about carotid and intracranial circulation.
2. Prothrombin time if anticoagulation is considered.
3. Diffusion-weighted MRI may be done to rule out stroke.
4. Transesophageal echocardiography to rule out emboli from heart.

Management

1. Platelet aggregation inhibitors, such as aspirin and ticlopidine (Ticlid), to reduce risk of stroke.
2. Surgical intervention to increase blood flow to brain—carotid endarterectomy, extracranial/intracranial anastomosis, or angioplasty.

3. Reduction of other risk factors to prevent stroke, such as control of blood pressure, diabetes, and hyperlipidemia and smoking cessation.

4. Anticoagulation/thrombolytic agents for patients who continue to have symptoms despite antiplatelet therapy and those with major source of cardiac emboli. Thrombolytic agents include streptokinase or recombinant tissue plasminogen activator (rt-PA) 3 to 5 hours after onset.

Complications
Complete ischemic stroke

Nursing Assessment
1. Obtain history of possible TIA; hypertensive and diabetic control; hyperlipidemia; cardiovascular disease, such as atrial fibrillation; smoking.
2. Perform physical examination, including neurologic, cardiac, and circulatory systems; be sure to listen for carotid bruit.
3. Assess patient for history of headache and, if positive, for duration of headache.

Nursing Diagnoses
• Altered Cerebral Tissue Perfusion related to underlying atherosclerosis
• Risk for Injury: stroke

Nursing Interventions
Improving Cerebral Perfusion
1. Teach patient signs and symptoms of TIA and need to notify health care provider immediately.
2. Administer or teach self-administration of anticoagulants, antihypertensives, and other medication, monitoring for side effects and therapeutic effect.
3. Prepare patient for surgical intervention as indicated (carotid endarterectomy or extracranial-intracranial anastomosis).

Providing Care and Preventing Complications
After Carotid Endarterectomy
For postoperative extracranial-intracranial care, see Nursing Management of the Patient Undergoing Intracranial Surgery, page 453.
1. After surgery, closely monitor vital signs and administer medication as prescribed to avoid hypotension (which can cause cerebral ischemia) or hypertension (which may precipitate cerebral hemorrhage).
2. Perform frequent neurologic checks, including pupil size, equality, and reaction; handgrip and plantar flexion strength; sensation; mental status; and speech. Notify the health care provider of any deficits immediately.
3. Monitor for hoarseness, impaired gag reflex, or difficulty swallowing and facial weakness, which indicate cranial nerve injury.
4. Keep head in neutral position to relieve stress on surgical site; monitor drainage.

5. Keep tracheostomy tube at bedside and assess for stridor; hematoma formation can cause airway obstruction.
6. Observe operative area closely for swelling; mild swelling is expected, but if hematoma formation is suspected, prepare patient for immediate surgery.
7. Medicate for pain, and avoid agitation or sudden changes in position, which could affect blood pressure.
8. Elevate head of bed when vital signs are stable.

NURSING ALERT

Extracranial-intracranial anastomosis is used for focal areas of ischemia. Pressure over the anastomosis of the superior temporal artery (extracranial) and the middle cerebral artery (intracranial) can result in rupture or ischemia of the site. If the patient wears glasses, remove the bow on the operative side to avoid this possible pressure point.

Patient Education and Health Maintenance
1. Encourage patient receiving anticoagulants to comply with follow-up monitoring of prothrombin time and/or partial thromboplastin time and to report any signs of bleeding.
2. Encourage the use of electric razors and toothbrushes.
3. Provide information on smoking cessation, low-fat/low-cholesterol diet, birth control alternatives, and exercise, and stress the need to change lifestyle to halt cerebrovascular disease and prevent stroke.
4. Provide patient with community-based support groups for community resources.
5. Reinforce with patient and family importance of accessing the medical system, by calling 911, when symptoms first occur.

Outcome-Based Evaluation
• Patient is alert without neurologic deficits
• Respirations unlabored, vital signs stable, no swelling of neck; reports relief of pain
• Patient able to discuss risk factors to prevent stroke: obesity, hypertension, smoking

■ Cerebrovascular Accident (Stroke)
Stroke or cerebrovascular accident is the onset and persistence of neurologic dysfunction lasting longer than 24 hours and resulting from disruption of blood supply to the brain and indicates infarction rather than ischemia. Strokes are classified as ischemic or hemorrhagic. Stroke is the third leading cause of death in the US, affecting 400,000 persons annually.

Pathophysiology and Etiology
1. Partial or complete occlusion of a cerebral blood vessel resulting from cerebral thrombosis (due to arteriosclerosis) or embolism.

2. Ischemia related to decreased blood flow to an area of the brain secondary to systemic disease, such as cardiac or metabolic disease.

3. Hemorrhage occurring outside the dura (extradural), beneath the dura mater (subdural), in the SAS (subarachnoid), or within the brain substance (intracerebral).

4. Risk factors include hypertension, TIA, heart disease, elevated cholesterol, diabetes mellitus, obesity, carotid stenosis, polycythemia, cigarette smoking.

5. Cardiac causes of stroke account for approximately 20% of strokes occurring in the United States.

Clinical Manifestations

1. Clinical manifestations vary depending on the vessel affected and the cerebral territories it perfuses. Symptoms are usually multiple. Headache may be a sign of impending SAH and cerebral infarction.

2. Sudden, severe headache due to spontaneous SAH is usually the result of rupture of an intracranial saccular aneurysm or arteriovenous malformation; it is cataclysmic, heralded by severe headache, meningeal signs and neurologic dysfunction.

3. Numbness (paresthesia), weakness (paresis), or loss of motor ability (plegia) on one side of the body.

4. Difficulty in swallowing (dysphagia).

5. Aphasia (expressive, receptive, global).

6. Visual difficulties of inattention and neglect, including loss of half of a visual field, double vision.

7. Altered cognitive abilities and psychological affect.

8. Self-care deficits.

Diagnostic Evaluation

1. Carotid ultrasound—to detect carotid stenosis.

2. CT—to determine cause and location of stroke.

3. Cerebral angiography—to determine extent of cerebrovascular insufficiency.

4. PET, MRI may be done to localize ischemic damage.

Management

Acute Treatment

1. Support of vital functions—maintain airway, breathing, oxygenation, circulation.

2. Reperfusion and hemodilution with volume expanders (dextran or pentastarch); thrombolytic therapy with tissue plasminogen activator (t-PA, Activase); vasodilation with nimodipine (Nimotop).

3. Management of increased ICP (see p. 448).

4. Diuretic treatment to reduce cerebral edema, which peaks 3 to 5 days after infarction.

5. Calcium channel blockers to reduce blood pressure and prevent cerebral vasospasm.

Subsequent Treatment

1. Anticoagulation after hemorrhage is ruled out.

2. Antiplatelet agents such as ticlopidine (Ticlid) or aspirin.

3. Antispasmodic agents for spastic paralysis.

4. A rehabilitation program, including physical therapy, occupational therapy, and speech therapy as needed.

5. Treatment of poststroke depression with antidepressants, such as selective serotonin reuptake inhibitor citalopram.

Complications

1. Aspiration pneumonia

2. Dysphagia in 25% to 50% of patients after stroke

3. Spasticity, contractures

4. Deep-vein thrombosis, pulmonary embolism

5. Brain stem herniation

6. Poststroke depression

Nursing Assessment

1. Maintain neurologic flow sheet during acute phase.

2. Assess for voluntary or involuntary movements, tone of muscles, presence of deep tendon reflexes (reflex return signals end of flaccid period and return of muscle tone).

3. Also assess mental status, cranial nerve function, sensation/proprioception, bladder control.

4. Monitor bowel and bladder function.

5. Monitor effectiveness of anticoagulation therapy.

6. Frequently assess level of function and psychosocial response to condition.

 DRUG ALERT

Prothrombin time levels are reported in international normalized ratios (INR). Anticoagulants are adjusted to maintain an INR at 2.0 to prevent stroke and the associated complication of intracranial and subdural hemorrhage. Report INRs that are elevated to reduce the risk of bleeding or decreased levels to adjust therapy to be more effective.

Nursing Diagnoses

- Risk for Injury related to neurologic deficits
- Impaired Physical Mobility related to motor deficits
- Altered Thought Processes related to brain damage
- Impaired Verbal Communication related to brain injury
- Self-Care Deficit (bathing, dressing, toileting) related to hemiparesis/paralysis
- Altered Nutrition: Less Than Body Requirements, related to impaired self-feeding, chewing, swallowing
- Altered Urinary Elimination related to motor/sensory deficits
- Altered Family Process related to catastrophic illness, cognitive and behavioral sequelae of stroke, and caregiving burden

NURSING ALERT

Use of clinical pathways maximizes stroke patient outcomes. Case management models of care foster interdisciplinary utilization, timeliness of referrals, patient education, patient satisfaction, and efficient use of health care resources. The specific role of the nurse in stroke recovery integrates therapeutic aspects of coordinating, maintaining, and training.

Nursing Interventions
Preventing Falls and Other Injuries
1. Maintain bed rest during acute phase (24 to 48 hours after onset of stroke) with head of bed slightly elevated and side rails in place.
2. Administer oxygen as ordered during acute phase to maximize cerebral oxygenation.
3. Frequently assess respiratory status, vital signs, heart rate and rhythm, and urinary output to maintain and support vital functions.
4. When patient becomes more alert after acute phase, maintain frequent vigilance and interactions aimed at orienting, assessing, and meeting the needs of the patient.
5. Try to allay confusion and agitation with calm reassurance and presence.
6. Assess patient for risk for fall status.

Preventing Complications of Immobility
(Figure 15-3)
Interventions to improve functional recovery require active participation of the patient and repetitive training. Functional demand and intensive training are believed to trigger CNS reorganization—responsible for late functional recovery after stroke.
1. Use a foot board during flaccid period after stroke to keep foot dorsiflexed; avoid its use after spasticity develops.

2. Avoid excessive pressure on ball of foot after spasticity develops.
3. Do not allow top bedding to pull affected foot into plantar flexion.
4. Maintain functional position of all extremities.
   a. Apply splints and braces as needed—Volar splint to support functional position of wrist, sling to prevent shoulder subluxation of flaccid arm, high-top sneaker for ankle and foot support. Splints support flaccid extremities and can also be used on spastic extremities to decrease stretch stimulation and reduce spasticity.
   b. Apply a trochanter roll from the crest of the ilium to the midthigh to prevent external rotation of the hip.
   c. Place a pillow in the axilla of the affected side when there is limited external rotation to keep arm away from chest and prevent adduction of the affected shoulder.
   d. Place the affected upper extremity slightly flexed on pillow supports with each joint positioned higher than the preceding one to prevent edema and resultant fibrosis; alternate elbow extension.
   e. Place the hand in slight supination with fingers slightly flexed.
   f. Place the patient in a prone position for 15 to 30 minutes daily, and avoid sitting up in chair for long periods to prevent knee and hip flexion contractures.

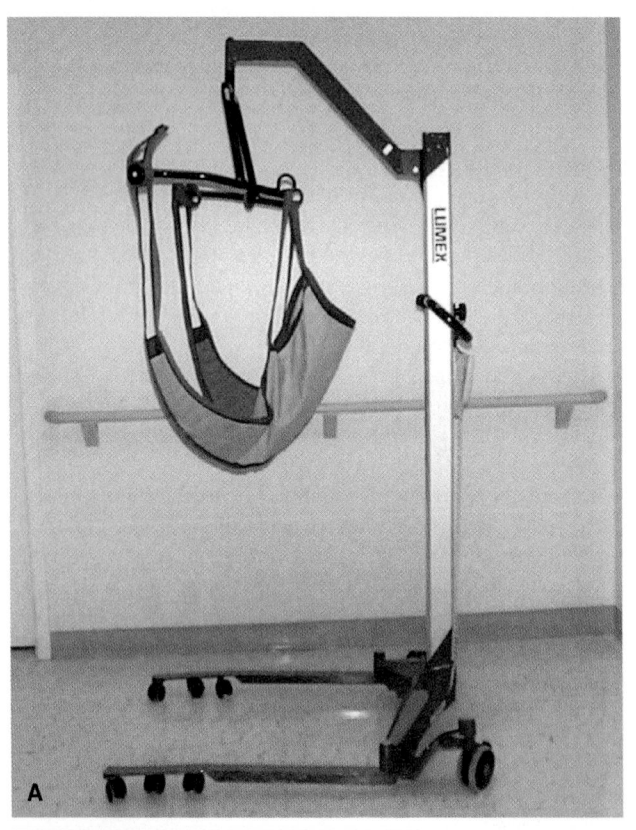

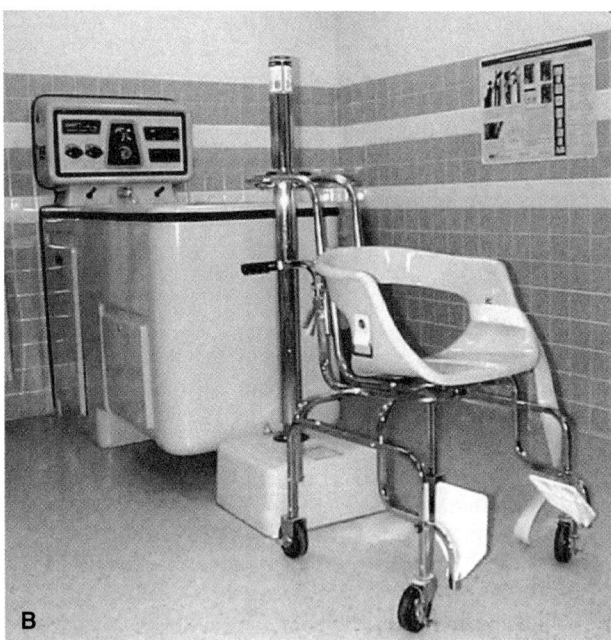

FIGURE 15-3 Preventing complications of immobility: (**A**) electronic chair for transferring patients out of bed; (**B**) whirlpool tub with chair for immersing patients for bathing or treatment.

g. Place patient in reflex positioning to foster functional recovery.

h. "Forced use" is an experimental treatment designed to overcome nonuse of the hemiparetic upper extremity in regaining functional use of the affected arm with selected chronic hemiparetic patients.

i. "Constraint-induced (CI) movement therapy" restricts the contralateral upper extremity in effort to force use of the affected arm.

5. Exercise the affected extremities passively through range of motion four to five times daily to maintain joint mobility and enhance circulation; encourage active range-of-motion exercise as able (see p. 174).

6. Teach patient to use unaffected extremity to move affected one.

7. Reflex-inhibiting positions are therapeutic and will enhance functional recovery.

8. Prepare for ambulation cautiously.

a. Check for orthostatic hypotension.

b. Graduate the patient from a reclining position to head elevated, and dangle legs at the bedside before transferring out of bed or ambulating; assess sitting balance in bed.

c. Assess the patient for excessive exertion.

d. Have patient wear walking shoes.

e. Assess standing balance, and have patient practice standing.

f. Help patient begin walking as soon as standing balance is achieved; ensure safety with a patient waist belt.

Optimizing Cognitive Abilities

1. Be aware of the patient's cognitive alterations, and adjust interaction and environment accordingly.

2. Participate in cognitive retraining program—reality orientation, visual imagery, cueing procedures—as outlined by rehabilitation nurse and/or therapist.

3. Use pictures of family members, clock, calendar; post schedule of daily activities where patient can see.

4. Focus on patient's strengths, and give positive feedback.

Facilitating Communication

1. Speak slowly, using visual cues and gestures; be consistent, and repeat as necessary.

2. Speak directly to the patient while facing him or her.

3. Give plenty of time for response, and reinforce attempts as well as correct responses.

4. Minimize distractions.

5. Use alternative methods of communication other than verbal, such as written words, gestures, or pictures.

Fostering Independence

1. Teach patient to use nonaffected side for activities of daily living (ADLs) but not to neglect affected side.

2. Adjust the environment (eg, call light, tray) to side of awareness if spatial neglect or visual field cuts are present; approach patient from uninvolved side.

3. Teach the patient to scan environment if visual deficits are present.

4. Encourage family to provide clothing that is a size larger than the patient wears, with front closures, Velcro, and stretch fabric; teach patient to dress while sitting to maintain balance.

5. Ensure that personal care items, urinal, commode, and so forth are nearby and that patient obtains assistance with transfers and other activities as needed.

6. ADLs require both anticipatory and reactive postural adjustments.

7. Patients often have clear goals in relation to functional abilities, against which all success and forward progress will be measured.

Promoting Adequate Oral Intake

1. Help patient relearn swallowing sequence using compensatory techniques.

a. Place ice on tongue, and encourage sucking.

b. Progress to popsicle and soft foods.

c. Make sure mechanical soft or pureed diet is provided, based on ability to chew.

2. Encourage small, frequent meals, and allow plenty of time to chew and swallow.

3. Remind patient to chew on unaffected side.

4. Encourage patient to drink small sips from a straw with chin tucked to the chest, strengthening effort to swallow while chin is tucked down.

5. Inspect mouth for food collection and pocketing before entry of each new bolus of food, and teach patient compensatory techniques for safe swallowing.

6. Inspect oral buccosa for injury from biting tongue or cheek.

7. Encourage frequent oral hygiene.

8. Teach the family how to assist the patient with meals to facilitate chewing and swallowing.

a. Reduce environmental distractions to improve patient concentration.

b. Provide oral care before eating to improve aesthetics and afterward to remove food debris.

c. Position the patient so he or she is sitting with 90 degrees of flexion at the hips and 45 degrees of flexion at the neck. Use pillows behind the back and along the weak side to achieve correct position.

d. Maintain position for 30 to 45 minutes after meals to prevent regurgitation and aspiration.

Attaining Bladder Control

1. Perform intermittent catheterization if needed after positive bladder scan results.

2. Perform indwelling bladder catheterization during acute stage, only if intermittent catheterization is contraindicated.

3. Establish regular schedule of voiding—every 2 to 3 hours, correlated with fluid intake—once bladder tone returns.

4. Assist with standing or sitting to void (especially males).

5. See page 181 for bladder retraining program details.

Strengthening Family Coping

1. Encourage the family to maintain outside interests.

2. Teach stress management techniques, such as relaxation exercises, use of community and church support networks.

3. Encourage participation in support group for family of stroke victim and respite program or other available resources in area.
4. Involve as many family and friends in care as possible.
5. Provide information about stroke and expected outcome.
6. Teach family that stroke survivors do show depression in the first 3 months of recovery.

Community and Home Care Considerations

1. Hemiplegic complications resulting from stroke commonly include "frozen" shoulder; adduction and internal rotation of arm with flexion of elbow, wrist, and fingers; external rotation of the hip with flexion of the knee and plantar flexion of the ankle.
2. Perform range-of-motion exercises, and instruct the patient and family on these as well as proper positioning.
3. Reinforce that these muscle and ligament deformities resulting from stroke can be prevented with daily stretching and strengthening exercises.
4. Depression after stroke is a major problem because it can increase the morbidity.
5. Monitor for signs of depression such as difficulty sleeping, frequent crying, anorexia, feelings of guilt or sadness.
6. Notify health care provider for possible medication therapy.
7. Continue to support family who may be caring for a hemiplegic or aphasic person at home or in long-term

care for a long time. Six months after stroke, around 9% to 21% of survivors are severely disabled, fully dependent in self-care tasks, and live in institutions.

Patient Education and Health Maintenance

1. Teach the patient and family to adapt home environment for safety and ease of use.
2. Instruct patient in need for rest periods throughout day.
3. Reassure the family that it is common for poststroke patients to experience emotional lability and depression; treatment can be given.
4. Encourage consistency in the environment without distraction.
5. Assist family to obtain self-help aids for the patient.
6. Instruct the family in management of aphasia (Box 15-1).
7. Refer the patient/family for more information and support to such agencies as:

> The National Stroke Association
> 9707 East Easter Lane
> Englewood, CO 80112
> 303-649-9299
> *www.stroke.org*

Outcome-Based Evaluation

- No falls, vital signs stable
- Body alignment maintained, no contractures
- Oriented to person, place, and time
- Communicates appropriately

BOX 15-1 Aphasia

Aphasia is an acquired disorder of communication resulting from brain damage due to stroke, head injury, brain tumors, or brain cysts. It may involve impairment of the ability to speak, to understand the speech of others, to read, write, calculate, and understand gestures. The majority of aphasic individuals have difficulty with expression and comprehension to varying degrees. Fatigue will have adverse effect on speech.

To enhance your communication with the aphasic patient, keep the environment simple and relaxed, minimize distractions, and use multiple sensory channels.

Refer the family to:

American Speech-Language-Hearing Association
10801 Rockville Pike
Rockville, MD 20852
301-897-5700
www.asha.org

Aphasia Syndromes

1. Fluent aphasia: Patient retains verbal fluency but may have difficulty in understanding speech.
2. Wernicke's aphasia, receptive aphasia: Patient speaks readily but speech lacks clear content, information, and direction; jargon frequently used.
3. Broca's aphasia, expressive aphasia: Broken and dysarthric speech patterns.
4. Anomic or amnesiac aphasia: Speech is almost normal, but marred by word-finding difficulty.

5. Conduction aphasia: Comprehension of language is good but has difficulty repeating spoken material.

Nursing Interventions

1. Speak at your normal rate and volume: The patient is not hard of hearing.
2. Allow plenty of time to answer.
3. Do not ask questions that require complex answers.
4. Rote phrases can be spontaneous.
5. Provide pad and pen if the patient prefers and is able to write.
6. Avoid forcing speech.
7. Watch the patient for clues and gestures if his or her speech is jargon; make neutral statements.
8. Nonfluent aphasia: Speech is sparse and produced slowly and with effort and poor articulation; usually has a relative preservation of auditory comprehension.
9. Allow plenty of time for response.
10. Ask for minimal word response.
11. Encourage patient to speak slowly.
12. Expect frustration and anger at inability to communicate.
13. Global aphasia; severe disruption of all aspects of communication (verbal speech, written, reading, understanding).
14. Keep environment simple.
15. Use gestures as well as language.
16. Allow patient to manipulate objects for additional sensory input.

- Brushing teeth, putting on shirt and pants independently
- Feeds self two thirds of meal
- Voiding on commode at 2-hour intervals
- Family seeking help and assistance from others

■ Rupture of Intracranial Aneurysm or Arteriovenous Malformation (AVM)

An *intracranial aneurysm* is an abnormal localized dilatation of the wall of a cerebral artery due to congenital absence of the muscle layer of the vessel. Consistent blood flow against the weakened area results in growth of the aneurysm and thinning of the vessel wall. Aneurysms usually occur in an artery or major branches of the circle of Willis. They may be of congenital, traumatic, arteriosclerotic, or infectious origin. Most are saccular and asymptomatic until rupture. When aneurysms rupture, sudden bleeding occurs in the SAS between the arachnoid and the pia (*SAH*), which produces symptoms of a hemorrhagic stroke. They also may obstruct CSF flow and/or prevent reabsorption, decrease blood flow, and/or irritate the hypothalamus.

An *AVM* is a system of dilated arteries and veins in which the normal capillary bed is absent. AVMs are described as a tangled mass of discolored vessels that have the appearance of a cluster of grapes. Because of back flow of pressure, a fistula develops, resulting in vascular dilatation and chronic hypoperfusion. Approximately 50% of patients with AVMs present with hemorrhage. Other signs of AVM rupture include seizures and signs of mass effect.

The Hunt-Hess grading scale is used to determine prognosis and timing of surgical intervention for both aneurysm and AVM rupture. Studies show surgery is more effective if done before vasospasm occurs. Cerebral vasospasm only rarely occurs in AVMs due to their superficial rather than deep location within the brain.

Grading of Aneurysms (Hunt-Hess Scale)

0 Unruptured; asymptomatic discovery
I Asymptomatic or minimal headache with slight nuchal rigidity
II Moderate to severe headache, nuchal rigidity; no neurologic deficit other than cranial nerve deficit
III Drowsiness, confusion, or mild focal deficit (eg, hemiparesis), or combination of these findings
IV Stupor, moderate to severe deficit, possibly early decerebrate rigidity and vegetative disturbances
V Deep coma, decerebrate rigidity, moribund appearance

Etiology and Pathophysiology

1. Cause unknown or related to atherosclerosis, intracranial AVM, hypertensive vascular disease, head trauma.
2. May become symptomatic due to pressure of enlarging aneurysm on nearby cranial nerves or brain tissue.
3. Rupture and hemorrhage into SAS may cause increased ICP and ischemia.
4. Vasospasm may occur 4 to 12 days after rupture, causing ischemia and infarction.
5. Rebleeding may occur due to lysis of clot.

Clinical Manifestations

1. Sudden onset of severe headache, often accompanied by nausea, vomiting, but no neurologic deficits; may be a warning bleed caused by leaking of aneurysm or rupture of the AVM.
2. May present with loss of consciousness and severe deficits if massive bleed. Focal signs or deficits dependent on the location of the bleed and compression of adjacent brain structures (visual disturbances, cranial nerve deficits, hemiparesis, and so forth).
3. Other signs and symptoms include visual disturbances, dizziness, nuchal rigidity, photophobia, papilledema.

Diagnostic Evaluation

1. History and physical examination
2. CT scan—to determine presence of blood in SAS, rule out other lesions.
   Increased density if blood present, may also show increased ICP or mass effect.
3. Lumbar puncture (if no mass effect on CT): grossly bloody CSF with >25,000 RBCs, CSF will not clear with subsequent taps as a traumatic tap would.
4. Cerebral angiogram—only definitive diagnosis of aneurysmal etiology: documents presence, location, and configuration. Will also indicate vasospasm.

Management

1. Intracranial aneurysm precautions to minimize the risk of rebleeding and control BP.
2. Management of increased ICP with osmotic diuretics such as mannitol (Osmitrol).
3. Antifibrinolytic therapy with aminocaproic acid (Amicar) to inhibit clot lysis and prevent additional bleeding (controversial).
4. Management of systemic hypertension with nitroprusside (Nipride) and close monitoring to prevent precipitous drop in blood pressure, aggravating ischemia.
   a. Prevention of vasospasm with calcium channel blockers such as nimodipine (Nimotop) and plasma expanders and hypervolemia to increase cerebral perfusion.
   b. Nimodipine has cerebral specificity to block the influx of calcium at the intracellular space. It is the only drug approved by the FDA for treatment of vasospasm.
   c. Nimodipine is administered at a dose of 60 mg PO q4h (for 21 consecutive days from the time of SAH. For optimal effect, the nimodipine should be started within 96 hours of SAH.
5. Prophylactic seizure management with phenytoin (Dilantin) and phenobarbital (Luminal).

6. Surgical/endovascular interventions to prevent further bleeding.
   a. Craniotomy for clipping/ligation of aneurysm/AVM, evacuation of clot.
   b. Strengthening the wall by wrapping if inaccessible to clipping or ligation.
   c. Endovascular management with detachable coils or balloon angioplasty (aneurysm).
   d. Embolization with particles or balloon occlusion (AVM).
   e. Radiosurgery procedures with gamma knife or LINAC scalpel (AVMs).
   f. See page 453 for care of craniotomy patient.
7. Surgical treatment of hydrocephalus with ventriculostomy and/or shunt.

Complications
1. The greatest risk for rebleeding is in the first 7 to 14 days after initial bleed.
2. Hydrocephalus; obstructive initially requiring ventriculostomy, nonobstructive long term, may require shunt.
3. Cerebral vasospasm: arterial constriction that occurs 4 to 12 days after SAH, which produces decreased blood flow, ischemia, and potential infarction.
4. Seizures.

Nursing Assessment
1. Perform and document neurologic assessment with vital signs and as patient condition warrants.
2. Monitor for changes in or decreasing LOC, cranial nerve function, pupillary function, and motor function with drift.
3. Assess for increasing headache, which could signal rebleeding.
4. Monitor for focal neurologic deficits, which may indicate vasospasm.
5. Assess vital signs and pupillary changes frequently for development of increased ICP.

Nursing Diagnoses
- High Risk for Secondary Brain Injury related to potential rebleeding, vasospasm, hydrocephalus, and seizures
- Altered Cerebral Perfusion related to disease process and vasospasm
- Pain secondary to cerebral hemorrhage, meningeal irritation, surgical procedure
- Anxiety of patient/family related to treatment, intracranial surgery, uncertainty of patient outcome

Nursing Interventions
Modifying Activity to Prevent Complications
1. Institute aneurysm/SAH precautions to reduce environmental stimuli, limit stress, and decrease the risk of rebleed and/or increased ICP:
   a. Maintain complete bed rest with head elevated 30 degrees to reduce cerebral edema.
   b. Maintain quiet environment with low lighting, no noise, and no unnecessary activity to prevent photophobia, agitation, and pain. Limit use of TV and telephone.
   c. Restrict visitors to only immediate family or significant other who has been counseled to ensure quiet environment.
   d. Encourage the awake patient to avoid activities that increase blood pressure or ICP: straining, sneezing, acute flexion/rotation of the neck, cigarette smoking; assist patient with position changes.
   e. Teach the awake patient to exhale through mouth during defecation, avoiding Valsalva maneuver to reduce strain; administer stool softeners as ordered; avoid rectal temperature, enemas, and suppositories.
   f. Avoid caffeinated beverages and extremes of temperatures.
   g. Provide physical care, such as bathing and feeding, as needed.
2. Medicate patient as ordered during periods of extreme agitation.
3. Institute seizure precautions by providing padded side rails, suction equipment, and oral airway at the bedside.
4. Perform and document neurologic assessment with vital signs and as patient condition warrants; to include LOC, cranial nerve function, pupillary function, and motor function with drift.
5. Assess for signs of increased ICP, including bradycardia and widening pulse pressure, changes in respiratory pattern (Cheynes-Stokes pattern, apneustic, ataxic, and so forth).
6. Implement nursing interventions to minimize ICP and cerebral swelling (ie, elevate head of bed 30 degrees, maintain proper head and neck alignment to avoid jugular vein compression, avoid prolonged suctioning procedures, keep procedure less than 15 seconds, collaborate with physicians to use lidocaine presuctioning if intubated).
7. Monitor arterial blood gas (ABG) values for hypoxia and hypercapnia, which aggravate ICP.
8. Monitor ventriculostomy, if present, for patency, amount and character of drainage, and correct height level every 4 hours.
9. Recognize need for maintenance of BP parameters based on status of clipped vs unclipped aneurysm: (ie, clipped: sBP 160 to 180; unclipped: sBP 120 to 140).
10. Evaluate effectiveness of antihypertensive or vasopressor therapy.
11. Perform ongoing physical assessment including respiratory, cardiac, gastrointestinal (GI), genitourinary (GU) function to detect potential complications.
12. Maintain safety factors (eg, prevent sensory overload, physical injury related to vision, hearing, body awareness deficits).

Maintaining Cerebral Perfusion

1. Frequently monitor neurologic status based on condition, including LOC, pupillary reaction, motor and sensory function, cranial nerve function, speech, presence of headache.
2. Administer hypervolemia/hypertensive therapy with colloid and crystalloid to increase cerebral perfusion.
3. Monitor fluid and electrolytes; monitor hematocrit and hemoglobin throughout hydrotherapy.
4. Evaluate adequacy of hypervolemic therapy regimen by assessment of BP, hemodynamic monitoring, neurologic status, and input and output status at least every 2 hours, while in the ICU.
5. Assess for subjective neurologic complaints specific to decreased perfusion (eg, diplopia, headache, blurred vision), and recognize peak time for vasospasm occurrence is 4 to 12 days after bleed.
6. Assess for signs and symptoms of vasospasm: insidious onset of confusion, disorientation, and decreased LOC, or focal deficit associated with area of bleed.
7. Document findings and report changes; subtle change in LOC, such as drowsiness and speech slurring, or onset of pronator drift, may be first sign of deterioration.
8. See page 445 for care of patients with altered state of consciousness.

Reducing Pain

1. Assess level of pain and pain relief; report any increase in headache.
2. Administer analgesics as prescribed; if narcotic being given with sedative, monitor for CNS depression, decreased respirations, decreased blood pressure.
3. Encourage distraction and relaxation techniques that will promote calming effect.
4. Explain to patient/significant other limited use of narcotics secondary to need to assess patient's LOC at all times.
5. Encourage elevated head of bed to minimize cerebral swelling.
6. Provide cool compresses to head.
7. Provide quiet, dark environment.
8. If patient experiences unrelieved or increased pain, assess for any changes in neurologic signs, nuchal rigidity, photophobia, and/or changes in vision, which could signal hemorrhage, hydrocephalus, or meningeal irritation.

Reducing Anxiety

1. Provide ongoing assessment of psychosocial issues (sexuality, anxiety, fear, depression, frustration, emotional lability).
2. Be attuned to verbal and nonverbal cues from the patient/family that signal problems with coping.
3. Inform the patient regarding all treatment modalities.
4. Encourage discussion of risks/benefits with the surgeon.
5. Use reassurance and therapeutic conversation to relieve fear and anxiety.
6. Provide support to the patient/family in dealing with the stress and uncertainty of hospitalization.

7. Consult Social Services for assistance with patient/family support and long-term care decisions as needed.
8. Prepare patient and family for surgery (see p. 453).

Community and Home Care Considerations

1. Assess level of knowledge and ability of patient/significant other to retain information.
2. Assess ongoing home care needs.
3. Assess need for nursing home placement or rehab center, and obtain social service referral to help with planning.
4. Provide teaching to family and caregivers, and act as liaison between health care team and family.
5. Teach patient and family how to deal with permanent neurologic deficits, and ensure that they obtain needed supplies and services.

Patient Education and Health Maintenance

1. Instruct patient/family on purpose and frequency of neurologic radiologic procedures.
2. Explain what an aneurysm is, signs/symptoms of rupture, and possible threats of rupture.
3. Educate the patient to the risk of rebleed, which is highest within first 2 weeks of rupture, but may remain for rest of life if not definitively treated.
4. Educate the patient to activities to avoid to prevent sudden increased pressure, such as heavy lifting and straining.
5. Encourage lifelong medical follow-up and immediate attention if severe headache develops.
   Instruct patient/family on need for and use of invasive monitoring and drainage systems.
6. Reinforce the need for head of bed not to be adjusted.
7. Explain aneurysm precautions and rationale.
8. Provide educational material for procedures.
9. Set mutual goals for discharge, and communicate discharge preparations with other disciplines (registered nurse, physician, physical therapist, discharge coordinator).
10. Explain medications to patient/significant other and potential side effects. Explain importance of continued nimodipine therapy and correct usage.
11. Have patient verbalize discharge instructions regarding wound care, activity restrictions, medications, and reportable signs/symptoms.

Outcome-Based Evaluation

- No signs of rebleeding, IICP, decreased cerebral perfusion, or seizures; quiet environment maintained; vital signs stable; neurologic parameters stable
- Patient verbalizes decreased pain or control of pain to an intensity that is acceptable
- Patient and family able to state reason for surgery, possible risks
- Decrease in anxiety sufficient to allow the completion of necessary procedures and to promote recovery

INFECTIOUS DISORDERS

Meningitis

Meningitis is the inflammation of the meninges, the membranes lining the brain and spinal cord. Pathogenic organisms cross the blood–brain barrier, invade the SAS, and cause an inflammatory response.

Pathophysiology and Etiology

1. In the United States, the incidence of acute, bacterial meningitis is approximately 3 cases/100,000 a year. The organisms causing these infections seem to vary depending on the age and immune status of the patient. These organisms may have epidemic potential.
2. There has been a decrease in the incidence of *Haemophilus influenzae* meningitis due to the hemophilus b conjugate vaccine, and an increase in the incidence of *Streptococcus pneumoniae* meningitis.
3. Other common organisms causing adult meningitis include *Neisseria meningitidis* and *Listeria monocytogenes*. In neonates, *L. monocytogenes, Escherichia coli,* and group B streptococci are most common.
4. In patients who are elderly, are debilitated, or have immunosuppression, *L. monocytogenes,* gram-negative bacilli such as *E. coli,* and pneumococcus may be responsible. Viral meningitis is uncommon in older adults.
5. Cryptococcal and candidal meningitis are opportunistic infections that occur in patients with acquired immunodeficiency syndrome (AIDS) and other immunosuppressive conditions. Cryptococcal infections may be related to exposure to pigeon droppings.
6. Hospital-acquired meningitis, frequently associated with neurosurgical procedures, is of growing concern.
7. Patients at high risk for sinusitis, otitis media, and pneumonia have a greater risk for developing meningitis.

Other factors predisposing to meningitis include alcoholism, cirrhosis, sickle cell disease, splenectomy, and very young and old patients.
8. Organism colonization frequently precedes community-acquired meningitis, most frequently caused by *S. pneumoniae, H. influenzae* type B, and *N. meningitidis.*

Clinical Manifestations

1. Headache.
2. Fever.
3. Altered mental status; confusion in older patients.
4. Petechial or purpuric rash, especially with *N. meningitidis.*
5. Photophobia.
6. Nuchal rigidity, or a bulging fontanelle in infants.
7. Positive Brudzinski's and Kernig's signs (Figure 15-4).
8. Poor feeding, altered breathing patterns, or listlessness in neonates.
9. Onset may be over several hours or several days and vary depending on the infectious agent, the patient's age, immune status, comorbidities, and other variables.

Diagnostic Evaluation

1. Complete blood count with differential is indicated to detect an elevated leukocyte count in bacterial and viral meningitis, with a greater percentage of polymorphonuclear leukocytes (90%) in bacterial and (<50%) in viral meningitis (normal 0 to 15%).
2. Blood cultures are obtained to indicate the organism.
3. Lumbar puncture with CSF examination reveals leukocytosis, culture to organism, low glucose levels, high protein levels, and positive gram stain frequently seen with meningitis. A polymerase chain reaction test for DNA is performed to rule out bacterial meningitis.
4. MRI/CT with and without contrast rules out other disorders.

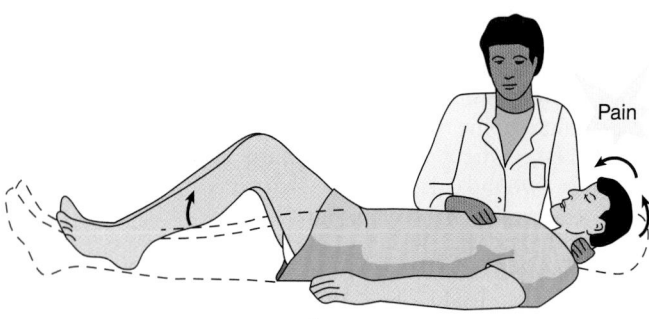
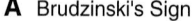
A Brudzinski's Sign

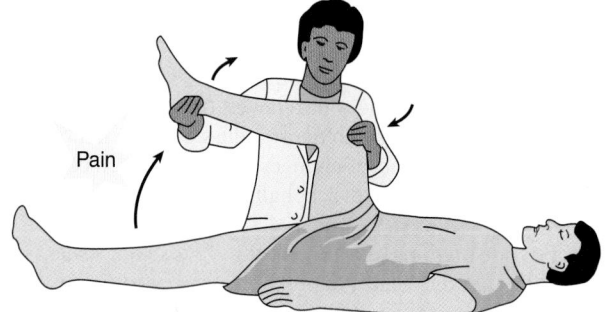
B Kernig's Sign

FIGURE 15-4 Signs of meningeal irritation include nuchal rigidity and positive Brudzinski's and Kernig's signs. (**A**) To elicit Brudzinski's sign, place the patient supine and flex the head upward. Resulting flexion of both hips, knees, and ankles with neck flexion indicates meningeal irritation. (**B**) To test for Kernig's sign, once again place the patient supine. Keeping one leg straight, flex the other hip and knee to a bent knee to form a 90-degree angle. Slowly extend the lower leg. This places a stretch on the meninges, resulting in pain and spasm of the hamstring muscle. Resistance to further extension can be felt.

5. Low CD-4 counts in patients indicate immunosuppression in HIV+ patients and other patients with immunosuppressive disorders.
6. Latex agglutination may be positive for antigens in meningitis.

Management
1. Acute bacterial meningitis must be differentiated from acute viral meningitis.
2. If there is a greater percentage of polymorphonuclear leukocytes (neutrophils), the patient should be placed on antibiotic therapy for bacterial meningitis.
3. Pharmacotherapy for bacterial meningitis, initiated immediately after taking blood cultures, is directed at treating the usual causative agents.
4. If meningitis is suspected after neurosurgical procedures, potential IV line bacteremia, CSF leak, or immunosuppression, therapy is also indicated for *Staphylococcus aureus* and gram-negative bacilli.
5. Antifungal agents, such as amphotericin B and the triazoles, fluconazole and itraconazole, are indicated for cryptococcal meningitis. Relapse is common if the patient does not have chronic suppressive therapy with fluconazole or another antifungal agent (20% to 60% relapse).
6. Large doses of IV antibiotics allow adequate amounts to cross the blood–brain barrier. Typical antibiotics include penicillin G, ampicillin, ceftriazone, cefotaxime, rifampin, trimethoprim/sulfamethoxazole, vancomycin, and chloramphenicol. Antibiotics may be given in combination or singularly.

NURSING ALERT
Be aware that increasing bacterial resistance to antibiotics has been developing, making this life-threatening illness very difficult to treat in some instances.

7. Pharmacotherapy ranges from 4 days of penicillin therapy with meningococcal meningitis to 21 days in immunosuppressed patients with *Listeria*.
8. Tuberculosis meningitis may present with cranial nerve deficits. Because cultures for *Mycobacterium tuberculosis* take approximately 4 weeks, empiric antituberculosis drugs must be initiated.
9. Adjunctive therapies to minimize inflammation include corticosteroids (dexamethasone) and hyperosmolar agents (mannitol, glycerol).

Complications
1. Bacterial meningitis, particularly in children, may result in deafness, learning difficulties, spasticity, paresis, or cranial nerve disorders.
2. Increased ICP in AIDS patients with cryptococcal meningitis has resulted in severe visual losses.
3. Seizures occur in 20% to 30% of patients.
4. Increased ICP may result in cerebral edema, decreased perfusion, and tissue damage.
5. Severe brain edema may result in herniation or compression of the brain stem.
6. Purpura may be associated with disseminated intravascular coagulation.

Nursing Assessment
1. Obtain a history of recent infections, such as upper respiratory infection.
2. Assess neurologic status and vital signs.
3. Evaluate for signs of meningeal irritation.

Nursing Diagnoses
- Hyperthermia related to the infectious process and cerebral edema
- Risk for Fluid Volume Deficit related to fever and decreased intake
- Altered Cerebral Tissue Perfusion related to infectious process and cerebral edema
- Pain related to meningeal irritation
- Impaired Physical Mobility related to prolonged bed rest

Nursing Interventions
Reducing Fever
1. Administer antibiotics on time to maintain optimal blood levels.
2. Monitor temperature frequently or continuously, and administer antipyretics as ordered.
3. Institute other cooling measures, such as a hypothermia blanket, as indicated.

Maintaining Fluid Balance
1. Prevent IV fluid overload, which may worsen cerebral edema.
2. Monitor intake and output closely.
3. Monitor CVP frequently.

Enhancing Cerebral Perfusion
1. Assess LOC, vital signs, and neurologic parameters frequently.
2. Maintain a quiet, calm environment to prevent agitation, which may cause an increased ICP.
3. Prepare patient for a lumbar puncture for CSF evaluation, and repeat spinal tap, if indicated. Lumbar puncture typically precedes neuroimaging.
4. Notify the health care provider of signs of deterioration: increasing temperature, decreasing LOC, seizure activity, or altered respirations.

Reducing Pain
1. Administer analgesics as ordered; monitor for response and adverse reactions. Avoid narcotics, which may mask a decreasing LOC.
2. Darken the room if photophobia is present.
3. Assist with position of comfort for neck stiffness, and turn patient slowly and carefully with head and neck in alignment.

Promoting Return to Optimal Level of Functioning
1. Implement rehabilitation interventions after admission (eg, turning, positioning).
2. Progress from passive to active exercises based on the patient's neurologic status.

NURSING ALERT

Note and report any missed doses of antibiotics, osmotic diuretics, and steroids; administer prn doses as soon as possible to avert deleterious consequences due to missed doses.

Community and Home Care Considerations

1. Prevent bacterial meningitis by eliminating colonization and infection with the offending organism.
   a. Administer vaccines against *H. influenzae* type B for children, *N. meningitidis* serogroups A,C,Y, and W135 for patients at high risk, and *S. pneumoniae* for patients with chronic illnesses and the elderly.
   b. Administer vaccines for travelers to countries with a high incidence of meningococcal disease and household contacts of someone who has had meningitis.
   c. Chemoprophylaxis for meningococcal disease, most commonly with rifampin, may be necessary for health care workers, household contacts in the community, day care centers, and other highly susceptible populations.
2. If maintenance antifungal prophylaxis is initiated for patients with low CD-4 counts, as seen in some patients with AIDS, the patient must understand the importance of long-term pharmacologic therapy.

Patient Education and Health Maintenance

1. Advise close contacts of the patient with meningitis that prophylactic treatment may be indicated; they should check with their health care providers or the local public health department.
2. Encourage the patient to follow medication regimen as directed to fully eradicate the infectious agent.
3. Encourage follow-up and prompt attention to infections in future.

Outcome-Based Evaluation

- Afebrile
- Adequate urine output; CVP in normal range
- Alert LOC; normal vital signs
- Pain controlled
- Optimal level of functioning after resolution

■ Encephalitis

Encephalitis is an inflammation of cerebral tissue, typically accompanied by meningeal inflammation, that is caused by a viral infection. It presents as either *acute viral encephalitis* or *postinfectious encephalomyelitis*.

Pathophysiology and Etiology

1. Acute viral encephalitis, accounting for the vast majority of cases, is caused by a direct infection of the gray matter containing neural cells.
   a. Results in perivascular inflammation and neuronal destruction.
   b. More common in children, and is most commonly caused by the herpes simplex virus and, to a lesser degree, by the arboviruses.
   c. Herpes simplex type 1 is responsible for almost all cases of herpes simplex encephalitis in children and adults. Herpes simplex type 2 is more common in neonates who are born to mothers with this infection during pregnancy.
2. Postinfectious encephalomyelitis follows a viral or bacterial infectious process, but organisms do not directly affect the neural tissue in the white matter; however, perivascular inflammation and demyelination do occur in the cerebral tissue.
   a. The incidence of postinfectious encephalomyelitis has decreased considerably with immunization against measles, mumps, and rubella and the infrequent administration of vaccines due to the eradication of smallpox. Rare in infancy.
   b. The most common cause is respiratory or GI infection 1 to 3 weeks before the acute onset of encephalomyelitis symptoms.
   c. May be caused by specific species of mosquitoes and ticks (arthropods), which may be seasonal and geographic hosts (eg, *California encephalitis, St. Louis equine encephalitis*).
3. *Herpes simplex encephalitis* may result from reactivation of the virus that has been dormant in the cranial and other ganglia, or to reinfection. Direct spread to the brain by the olfactory or trigeminal nerve is suspected with herpes simplex virus type 1.
4. *Cytomegalovirus encephalitis* should be considered in patients who have advanced HIV infection, have evidence of the cytomegalovirus in other sites, and have progressive neurologic deterioration.
5. *Toxoplasma* encephalitis is the most common cause of intracranial mass lesions in patients with AIDS.

Clinical Manifestations

1. ICP may result in alteration in consciousness, nausea, and vomiting.
2. Seizures may be present.
3. Motor weakness, such as hemiparesis, may be detected.
4. Increased deep tendon reflexes and extensor plantar response are noted.
5. Fever may be present.
6. Headache may indicate signs of meningeal irritation.
7. Bizarre behavior and personality changes may present at onset.
8. Hypothalamic-pituitary involvement may result in hypothermia, diabetes insipidus, SIADH.
9. Neurologic symptoms may include superior quadrant visual field defects, aphasia, dysphagia, ataxia, syndrome of inappropriate antidiuretic hormone (SIADH), and paresthesias.

Diagnostic Evaluation

1. Lumbar puncture with evaluation of CSF is performed to detect leukocytosis, increased mononuclear cell pleocytosis, increased proteins, and normal or slightly lowered glucose.
2. Polymerase chain reaction (PCR) analysis of the virus' DNA and the detection of intrathecally produced viral antibodies are essential in diagnosing the specific virus (eg, herpes simplex virus, cytomegalovirus). Arbovirus-specific IgM in CSF and a fourfold change in specific IgG antibody are diagnostic for arboviral encephalitis.
3. EEG may demonstrate slow brain wave complexes in encephalitis.
4. Gadolinium-enhanced MRI differentiates postinfectious encephalomyelitis from acute viral encephalitis.
   a. Enhanced multifocal white matter lesions are seen in encephalomyelitis, which may remain for months after clinical recovery.
   b. Herpes simplex virus encephalitis typically has medial-temporal and orbital-frontal lobe inflammation and necrosis; there may be low-density abnormalities in the temporal lobes.
   c. Cytomegalovirus, seen in patients who have advanced HIV disease, may have enhanced periventricular areas.
5. Brain tissue biopsy indicates presence of infectious organisms.

Management

1. Differentiate acute viral encephalitis from noninfectious diseases such as sarcoidosis, vasculitis, systemic lupus erythematosis, and others.
2. In patients who are immunosuppressed, such as HIV+ patients, differentiate acute viral encephalitis from cytomegalovirus encephalitis, toxoplasmic encephalitis, and fungal infections.
   a. Patients with cytomegalovirus may be treated with ganciclovir (Cytovene) and foscarnet (Foscavir), commonly used to treat cytomegalovirus retinitis in HIV+ patients.
   b. Pyrimethamine (Daraprim) and sulfadoxine (Fansidar) are commonly used to treat *Toxoplasma* encephalitis.
   c. When encephalomyelitis develops, supportive care is indicated because there is no known treatment; corticosteroids may be used.
3. IV acyclovir over 10 days to 3 weeks duration is indicated for herpes simplex virus. Mothers who have genital herpes simplex may be treated with acyclovir during the third trimester to avoid shedding the virus to their babies.
4. Anticonvulsants manage seizures.

 DRUG ALERT

Acyclovir, indicated for acute viral encephalitis caused by herpes simplex type 1, inhibits replication of the virus DNA. Acyclovir should be infused over 1 hour, because crystalluria and renal failure may result if administration is too rapid.

Complications

1. Sequelae of the herpes simplex virus may cause temporal lobe swelling, which can result in compression of the brain stem. This virus may also cause aphasia, major motor and sensory deficits, and Korsakoff's psychosis (amnestic syndrome).
2. Relapse of encephalitis may be seen after initial improvement and completion of antiviral therapy.
3. Mortality and morbidity rates depend on the infectious agent, host status, and other considerations. With herpes simplex, the mortality rate is approximately 30%.

Nursing Assessment

1. Obtain patient history of recent infection, animal exposure, tick or mosquito bite, recent travel, exposure to ill contacts.
2. Before delivery, women should be questioned regarding a history of congenital herpes simplex virus and examined for evidence of this virus; a cesarean section should be explored with the physician.
3. Strict universal (standard) precautions should be adhered to in order to contain drainage from herpetic lesions.
4. Vesicular lesions or rashes on neonates should be reported immediately, because these could indicate active herpes simplex infection.
5. Perform a complete clinical assessment.

Nursing Diagnoses

- Risk for Injury related to seizures and cerebral edema
- Altered Cerebral Tissue Perfusion related to disease process
- Hyperthermia related to infectious process
- Alteration in Thought Processes due to personality changes
- Risk of Infection Transmittal

Nursing Interventions

Preventing Injury

1. Maintain quiet environment and provide care gently, avoiding overactivity and agitation, which may cause increased ICP.
2. Maintain seizure precautions with side rails padded, airway and suction equipment at bedside.
3. Administer medications as ordered; monitor response and adverse reactions.

Promoting Cerebral Perfusion

1. Monitor neurologic status closely. Observe for subtle changes, such as behavior or personality changes, weakness, or cranial nerve involvement. Notify health care provider.
2. In arbovirus encephalitis, restrict fluids to passively dehydrate the brain.
3. Reorient patient frequently.
4. Provide supportive care if coma develops; may last several weeks.

5. Encourage significant others to interact with patient, and participate in the patient's rehabilitation, even while the patient is in a coma.

Relieving Fever
1. Monitor temperature and vital signs frequently.
2. Administer antipyretics and other cooling measures as indicated.
3. Monitor fluid intake and output, and provide fluid replacement through IV lines as needed. Be alert to signs of other coexisting infections, such as urinary tract infection or pneumonia, and notify health care provider so cultures can be obtained and treatment started.

Managing Aberrations in Thought Processes
1. Orient to person, place, time.
2. Maintain memory book, and provide cues to perform required activities.

Avoiding Infectious Disease Transmission
1. Maintain strict universal (standard) precautions.
2. Initiate and maintain isolation per facility policy.

Community and Home Care Considerations
1. Promote vaccination of patient/family/significant others for measles, mumps, and rubella.
2. Pregnant women who have a history of genital herpes simplex, or their partners, should inform their physician of this history.
3. Contacts of rabies-infected patients should be offered rabies prophylaxis.

Patient Education and Health Maintenance
1. Explain the effects of the disease process and the rationale for care.
2. Reassure significant others based on patient's prognosis.
3. Encourage follow-up for evaluation of deficits and rehabilitation progress.
4. Educate others about the signs and symptoms of encephalitis if epidemic is suspected.

Outcome-Based Evaluation
- No seizures or signs of IICP
- Alert with no neurologic deficits
- Afebrile
- Oriented, memory intact
- No transmission of infection

◼ Brain and Spinal Abscesses
A brain abscess is a free or encapsulated collection of infectious material of brain parenchyma, between the dura and the arachnoid linings (*subdural empyema*) or between the dura and the skull (*cranial epidural abscess*). Spinal abscesses typically occur in the epidural, subdural, and intermedullary regions.

Etiology and Pathophysiology
1. A brain abscess is usually a result of direct inoculation of organisms, as from the paranasal sinuses, middle ear, teeth, penetrating brain injury, cranial surgery, or bacteremias from extracranial sources (eg, intracardiac lesions).
   a. *S. aureus* is the etiologic agent in 60% of spinal epidural abscesses.
   b. Intermedullary abscesses are more common in the pediatric population, and are associated with lumbosacral dermal sinuses. Approximately 20% to 30% are "cryptic" abscesses with no apparent source of infectious seeding.
2. In the initial inoculation period, organisms invade the brain parenchyma resulting in local inflammation and edema. The resulting cerebritis develops into a necrotic lesion and then becomes encapsulated.
3. Fungal brain abscess is commonly seen in HIV+ patients and other populations who are immunosuppressed. Diffuse microabscesses may occur with infections caused by *Candida* species.
4. *M. tuberculosis* may cause abscesses of pus containing acid-fast bacilli (AFB) surrounded by a dense capsule. These abscesses are also found in patients who are HIV+ or have other immunosuppressive diseases.

Clinical Manifestations
1. Headache is poorly localized with a dull ache.
2. Increased ICP may result in nausea, vomiting, decreased LOC.
3. Fever is found in less than 50% of cases.
4. Neurologic findings such as hemisensory and paresis deficits, aphasia, ataxia may be present.
5. Seizures are frequently present.
6. Dental abscess, sinusitis, and otitis media may be present.
7. Backache is the presenting symptom in 94% of patients with spinal epidural abscesses and is a common finding with spinal subdural abscesses.

Diagnostic Evaluation
1. CT, MRI with contrast locate the site(s) of abscess, follow evolution and resolution of suppurative process.
   a. On CT scan, early cerebritis presents as hypodensity, and progressive encapsulation is represented by a hypodense ring around the lesion.
   b. There may be decreased ring enhancement with patients who are immunosuppressed, which may be due to a lack of inflammatory response.
   c. Microabscesses may not be detected by the CT scan or MRI.
2. Blood cultures are obtained to identify organism, positive Gram's stain, leukocytosis, and elevated erythrocyte sedimentation rate (ESR).
3. Cultures are obtained from the suspected source of infection, using stereotaxic needle aspiration or brain surgery, to identify the organism and sensitivity to antimicrobials.
4. A metastatic brain abscess may be differentiated from a metastatic tumor by CT scan or MRI. Abscesses have hypodense centers with a smooth surrounding capsule, whereas tumors may have irregular borders and diffuse enhancement
5. EEG detects seizure disorders.

Management

1. Closed stereotaxic needle biopsy, under CT guidance, may be used for drainage evacuation instead of craniotomy.
2. Radical surgical débridement, especially with fungal infections, may be indicated with antimicrobial therapy.
3. Initiation of empiric antimicrobial therapy is based on Gram's stain and the suspected site of origin.
   a. Because brain abscesses are frequently caused by multiple organisms, antimicrobial therapy is directed toward the most common etiologic agents: streptococci, anaerobic bacteria (eg, *Bacteroides* species).
   b. *S. aureus* may be suspected if surgical procedures have been performed.
   c. Gram-negative bacteria (eg, *Clostridium* species) should be suspected if a cranial wound has been contaminated with soil.
   d. Penicillin G, metronidazole, and third-generation cephalosporins are common therapeutic agents.
   e. A 6- to 8-week course of parenteral antibiotics is typical, followed by a 2- to 3-month course of oral antimicrobial therapy.
4. Antifungal therapy, such as amphotericin B, is initiated for candidiasis and other fungal infections.
5. Antituberculosis pharmacotherapy, such as rifampin, isoniazid, and pyrazinamide, should be used to treat abscesses containing AFB.
6. Adjunctive therapy includes corticosteroids and osmotic diuretics to reduce cerebral edema, and anticonvulsants to manage seizures.

Complications

1. The brain abscess can rupture into the ventricular space, causing a sudden increase in the severity of the patient's headache. This complication is often fatal.
2. Papilledema may occur <25% of cases, indicating intracranial hypertension.
3. Lumbar puncture may be dangerous due to the possibility of a brain stem herniation.
4. Permanent neurologic deficits, such as seizure disorders, visual defects, hemiparesis, and cranial nerve palsies, may be present.
5. There is greater mortality if the patient has symptoms of short duration, has severe mental status changes, and has rapid progression of neurologic impairment.

Nursing Assessment

1. Obtain history of previous infection, immunosuppression, headache, and related symptoms.
2. Perform neurologic assessment, including cranial nerve evaluation, motor, and cognitive status.

Nursing Diagnoses

- Pain related to cerebral mass
- Altered Thought Processes related to disease process
- Risk for Injury related to neurologic deficits
- Anxiety related to surgery, prognosis, and relapse

Nursing Interventions

Relieving Pain

1. Administer pain medications as ordered.
2. Provide comfort measures, such as quiet environment, positioning with head slightly elevated, and assistance with hygiene needs.
3. Provide passive relaxation techniques, such as soft music and backrubs.

Promoting Thought Processes

1. Frequently monitor vital signs, LOC, orientation, and seizure activity.
2. Report changes to health care provider; changes could signal increased ICP.
3. Administer medications as ordered, noting response and adverse reactions.
4. Prepare patient for repeated diagnostic tests to evaluate response to therapy and surgery.

Minimizing Neurologic Deficits

1. Maintain a safe environment with side rails up, call light within reach, and frequent observation.
2. Evaluate other cranial nerve function, and report changes.
3. Refer to occupational therapy, speech therapist, or other rehabilitation specialist to provide adjunct to nursing rehabilitation.

Reducing Anxiety

1. Prepare patient and family for surgery when indicated. Encourage discussion with surgeon to understand risks, benefits of the procedure.
2. Explain nursing care (see care related to craniotomy, p. 453).

Community and Home Care Considerations

1. Patient follow-up is essential for sinusitis, otitis media, respiratory infections, and other infectious processes that may result in a brain abscess.
2. Continue with rehabilitation to regain or compensate for neurologic deficits.
3. Continue with pharmacologic regimen in community setting.
4. Observe for recurrence of brain and spinal abscesses.

Patient Education and Health Maintenance

1. Maintain wellness with vaccinations, immunizations, and overall health.
2. Reinforce need for dental procedure prophylaxis to avoid dental abscesses.
3. Instruct in need for immediate assessment of head wounds.

Outcome-Based Evaluation

- Patient verbalizes reduced pain
- Patient oriented to person, place, and time; following simple commands
- No injury related to neurologic deficits
- Reduced anxiety regarding disease process and procedures

DEGENERATIVE DISORDERS

■ Parkinson's Disease

Parkinson's disease is a chronic, progressive neurologic disease affecting the brain centers responsible for control and regulation of movement. It is characterized by tremor, bradykinesia, rigidity, and postural abnormalities. Parkinson's can complicate the diagnosis, clinical course, and recovery from other illness. Approximately 1% of the total US population older than 60 is affected by idiopathic Parkinson's disease, and it less commonly affects people of younger age. It is the second most common neurodegenerative disease.

Pathophysiology and Etiology

1. A deficiency of dopamine in the substantia nigra of the brain is thought to be responsible for the symptoms of parkinsonism.
2. Underlying etiology may be related to a virus, genetic susceptibility, toxicity, or other unknown cause.
3. The clinical diagnosis of Parkinson's disease may be difficult because elderly patients may have other causes of rigidity, bradykinesia, and tremor.

Clinical Manifestations

1. Bradykinesia (slowness of movement), loss of spontaneous movement.
2. Resting tremor of 4 to 5 Hz.
3. Rigidity in performance of all movements.
4. Autonomic disorders—sleeplessness, salivation, sweating, orthostatic hypotension.
5. Depression, dementia.
6. Masklike facies.
7. Verbal fluency may be impaired.
8. Finger tapping responses are slowed.

Diagnostic Evaluation

1. Observation of clinical symptoms; may do imaging studies to rule out other disorders.
2. Physical examination of upper extremity elbow flexion/extension reveals rigidity on extension.
3. Sensorimotor assessment of grip reveals abnormally high grip forces and longer than normal to complete object lift, particularly with lighter loads.
4. Favorable response to a single dose of levadopa helps confirm the diagnosis.

Management
Pharmacologic

1. Anticholinergics to reduce transmission of cholinergic pathways, which are thought to be overactive when dopamine is deficient.
2. Amantadine (Symmetrel), which is thought to increase release of dopamine in the brain.
3. Levodopa, a dopamine precursor, combined with carbidopa, a decarboxylase inhibitor, to inhibit destruction

of L-dopa in the bloodstream, making more available to the brain. The combination of levodopa-carbidopa (Sinemet) usually is used.
4. Bromocriptine (Parlodel), a dopaminergic agonist that activates dopamine receptors in the brain.
5. Use of the monoamine oxidase inhibitor selegiline (Eldepryl) to delay the onset of disability and need for levodopa therapy.
6. Tolcapone (Tasmar) is in a new drug class (COMT inhibitors) for adjunct treatment.

GERONTOLOGIC ALERT

Elderly patients may have reduced tolerance to anti-parkinsonism drugs and may require smaller doses. Watch for and report psychiatric reactions, such as anxiety and confusion; cardiac effects, such as orthostatic hypotension and pulse irregularity; and blepharospasm (twitching of the eyelid), an early sign of toxicity.

Surgery

1. New surgical treatments for Parkinson's disease and essential tremor are promising.
2. Medical pallidotomy often improves longstanding symptoms such as dyskinesia, akinesia, rigidity, and tremor.
3. Chronic deep brain stimulation of the thalamus decreases tremor unresponsiveness to medication.

Complications

1. Dementia
2. Aspiration
3. Injury from falls

Nursing Assessment

1. Obtain history of symptoms and their effect on functioning.
2. Assess cranial nerves, cerebellar function (coordination), motor function.
3. Observe gait and performance of activities.
4. Assess speech for clarity and pace.
5. Assess for signs of depression.
6. Assess family dynamics, support systems, and access to social services.

Nursing Diagnoses

- Impaired Physical Mobility related to bradykinesia, rigidity, and tremor
- Altered Nutritional Status: Less Than Body Requirements related to motor difficulties with feeding, chewing, and swallowing
- Impaired Verbal Communication related to decreased speech volume and facial muscle involvement
- Constipation related to diminished motor function and inactivity
- Ineffective Individual Coping related to physical limitations and loss of independence

Nursing Interventions
Improving Mobility
1. Encourage the patient in daily exercise, such as walking, riding a stationary bike, swimming, or gardening.
2. Advise the patient to do stretching and postural exercises as outlined by physical therapist.
3. Encourage the patient to take warm baths and receive massages to help relax muscles.
4. Instruct the patient to take frequent rest periods to overcome fatigue and frustration.
5. Teach postural exercises and walking techniques to offset shuffling gait and tendency to lean forward.
   a. Instruct patient to use a broad-based gait.
   b. Have patient make a conscious effort to swing arms, raise the feet while walking, use a heel–toe gait, and increase the width of stride.
   c. Tell patient to practice walking to marching music or sound of ticking metronome—provides sensory reinforcement.

Optimizing Nutritional Status
1. Teach patient to think through the sequence of swallowing—close lips with teeth together; lift tongue up with food on it; then move tongue back and swallow while tilting head forward.
2. Instruct patient to chew deliberately and slowly, using both sides of mouth.
3. Tell patient to make conscious effort to control accumulation of saliva by holding head upright and swallowing periodically.
4. Have patient use secure, stabilized dishes and eating utensils.
5. Suggest smaller meals and additional snacks.
6. Monitor weight.

Maximizing Communication Ability
1. Encourage compliance with medication regimen.
2. Suggest referral to speech therapist.
3. Teach patient facial exercises and breathing methods to obtain appropriate pronunciation, volume, and intonation.
   a. Take a deep breath before speaking to increase the volume of sound and number of words spoken with each breath.
   b. Exaggerate pronunciation and speak in short sentences; read aloud in front of a mirror or into a tape recorder to monitor progress.
   c. Exercise facial muscles by smiling, frowning, grimacing, and puckering.

Preventing Constipation
1. Encourage foods with moderate fiber content—whole grains, fruits, and vegetables.
2. Increase water intake.
3. Obtain a raised toilet seat to encourage normal position.
4. Encourage patient to follow regular bowel routine.

Strengthening Coping Ability
1. Help the patient establish realistic goals and outline ways to achieve goals.
2. Provide emotional support and encouragement.
3. Encourage use of all resources, such as therapists, primary care provider, social worker, social support network.
4. Encourage open communication, discussion of feelings, and exchange of information about Parkinson's disease.
5. Have patient take active role in activity planning and evaluation of treatment plan.
6. Observe for changes in depression to determine if the patient is responding to antidepressants.

Community and Home Care Considerations
1. Recommend interdisciplinary home health care program. Requires skilled assessment of needs of patient, professional nursing and therapeutic services, patient and family education, and case management to optimize patient outcomes.
2. Encourage use of soothing music to reduce pain and depression.
3. Assess safety in environment to reduce risk of falls.
4. Utilize physical therapy services to encourage safe ambulation and reduce fear of falls.
5. Encourage use of social services, respite care and health visitors, mental health counselors, and support groups to prevent caregiver strain.
6. Use occupational therapy aids to ensure mobility and safety, such as grab rails in the tub or shower, raised toilet seat, hand rails on both sides of the stairway, rope secured to foot of bed to achieve sitting position, and straight-backed wooden chairs with armrests.

Patient Education and Health Maintenance
1. Instruct the patient to avoid sedatives, unless specifically prescribed, which have additive effect with other medications, and to avoid vitamin B preparations, and vitamin-fortified foods, which can reverse effects of medication.
2. Instruct the patient in medication regimen and adverse reactions, such as orthostatic hypotension, dry mouth, dystonia, muscle twitching, urinary retention, impaired glucose tolerance, anemia, and elevated liver function tests.
3. Encourage follow-up and monitoring for diabetes, glaucoma, hepatotoxicity, and anemia while undergoing drug therapy.
4. Teach patient ambulation cues to avoid "freezing" in place and possibly avoid falls by doing one of the following:
   a. Raise head, raise toes, then rock from one foot to another while bending knees slightly.
   b. Raise arms in a sudden short motion.
   c. Take a small step backward, then start forward.
   d. Step sideways, then start forward.
5. Instruct the family not to pull patient during episodes of "freezing," which increases the problem and may cause falling.

6. Refer the patient/family for more information and support to such agencies as:

National Parkinson's Foundation
www.parkinson.org
National Institute of Neurological Disorders and Stroke
www.ninds.nih.gov

Outcome-Based Evaluation

* Attending physical therapy sessions, doing facial exercises 10 minutes twice a day
* Eating three small meals and two snacks, no weight loss
* Enunciation clear, speaking in four to five words per breath
* Passing soft stool every day
* Asking questions about Parkinson's, obtaining help from son or daughter

■ Multiple Sclerosis

Multiple sclerosis (MS) is a chronic, frequently progressive neurologic disease of the CNS of unknown etiology and uncertain trajectory. MS is characterized by the occurrence of small patches of demyelination of the white matter of the optic nerve, brain, and spinal cord. MS is the most common CNS disease among young adults and the third leading cause of disability in the United States. It is estimated that 400,000 Americans have this disorder of the brain and spinal cord, causing disruption of electrical messages from the brain to the peripheral nervous system.

Pathophysiology and Etiology

1. *Demyelination* refers to the destruction of the myelin, the fatty and protein material that covers certain nerve fibers in the brain and spinal cord.
2. Demyelination results in disordered transmission of nerve impulses.
3. Inflammatory changes lead to scarring of the affected nerve fibers.
4. Cause unknown but possibly related to autoimmune dysfunction, genetic susceptibility, or an infectious process.
5. More prevalent in the northern latitudes and among Caucasians.

Clinical Manifestations

Lesions can occur anywhere within the white matter of the CNS. Symptoms reflect the location of the area of demyelination.
1. Fatigue and weakness.
2. Abnormal reflexes—absent or exaggerated.
3. Visual disturbances—impaired and double vision, nystagmus.
4. Motor dysfunction—weakness, tremor, incoordination.
5. Sensory disturbances—paresthesias, impaired deep sensation, impaired vibratory and position sense.
6. Impaired speech—slurring, scanning (dysarthria).
7. Urinary dysfunction—hesitancy, frequency, urgency, retention, incontinence; upper urinary tract infection. Urinary dysfunction affects about 90% of patients with MS and may exacerbate relapse of MS.
8. Neurobehavioral syndromes—depression, cognitive impairment, emotional lability.

Diagnostic Evaluation

1. Establishing a definitive diagnosis is often difficult, with much uncertainty concerning prognosis once the diagnosis is made.
2. Serial brain MRI studies have proven to be useful for diagnosing and monitoring patients with MS—show small plaques scattered throughout white matter of CNS.
3. A new technique, magnetic resonance spectroscopy, is now being used in vivo to monitor specific pathophysiology of evolving MS plaques.
4. Electrophoresis study of CSF shows abnormal IgG antibody.
5. Visual, auditory, and somatosensory evoked potentials—slowed conduction is evidence of demyelination.

Management

MS treatment is dynamic and rapidly evolving, covering two main areas: direct treatment of MS, and treatment of the effects or symptoms resulting from MS. Treatment is aimed at relieving symptoms and helping the patient function. However, a therapeutic relationship between the patient and nurse creates a critical and strong bond that is essential across the long trajectory of the illness.

Acute Attacks

1. Corticosteroids or adrenocorticotropic hormone are used to decrease inflammation, shorten duration of relapse or exacerbation.
2. Immunosuppressive agents may stabilize the course.
3. Beta-interferon (Betaseron, Avonex) is being used for treatment of rapidly progressing symptoms in some persons.
4. Copolymer-1, a mixture of synthetic polypeptides composed of four amino acids, has been effective in reducing relapse rates and disability in patients with relapsing-remitting MS.
5. Glatiramer acetate (Copaxone), an immunomodulator, is used in relapsing-remitting disease.

Chronic Symptom Management

1. Treatment of spasticity with agents such as baclofen (Lioresal), dantrolene (Dantrium), diazepam (Valium); physical therapy; nerve blocks and surgical intervention
2. Control of fatigue with amantadine (Symmetrel)
3. Treatment of depression with antidepressant drugs and counseling
4. Bladder management with anticholinergics, intermittent catheterization for drainage, prophylactic antibiotic
5. Bowel management with stool softeners, bulk laxative, suppositories
6. Multidisciplinary rehabilitation management with physical therapy, occupational therapy, and so forth
7. Control dystonia with carbamazepine (Tegretol)

8. Management of pain syndromes with carbamazepine (Tegretol), phenytoin (Dilantin), perphenazine/amitriptyline (Triavil)

Complications
1. Respiratory dysfunction
2. Infections: bladder, respiratory, sepsis
3. Complications from immobility
4. Speech, voice, and language disorders, such as dysarthria

Nursing Assessment
1. Observe motor strength, coordination, and gait.
2. Perform cranial nerve assessment.
3. Evaluate elimination function.
4. Explore coping, effect on activity and sexual function, emotional adjustment.
5. Assess patient and family coping, support systems, available resources.

Nursing Diagnoses
- Impaired Physical Mobility related to muscle weakness, spasticity, and incoordination
- Fatigue related to disease process and stress of coping
- Sensory-Perceptual Alteration (Tactile, Kinesthetic, Visual) related to disease process
- Altered Urinary Elimination related to disease process
- Altered Family Processes related to inability to fulfill expected roles
- Sexual Dysfunction related to disease process

Nursing Interventions
Promoting Motor Function
1. Perform muscle stretching and strengthening exercises daily, or teach patient or family to perform, using stretch–hold–relax routine to minimize spasticity and prevent contractures.
2. Apply ice packs before stretching to reduce spasticity.
3. Tell patient to avoid muscle fatigue by stopping activity just short of fatigue and take frequent rest periods.
4. Encourage ambulation and activity, and teach patient how to use such devices as braces, canes, and walkers when necessary.
5. Inform the patient to avoid sudden changes in position, which may cause fall due to loss of position sense, and to walk with a wide-based gait.
6. Encourage frequent change in position while immobilized to prevent contractures; sleeping prone will minimize flexor spasm of hips and knees.

Minimizing Fatigue
1. Help patient and family understand that fatigue is an integral part of multiple sclerosis.
2. Plan ahead, and prioritize activities. Take brief rest periods throughout the day.
3. Avoid overheating, overexertion, and infection.
4. Encourage energy conservation techniques, such as sitting to perform activity, limiting trips up and down stairs, pulling or pushing rather than lifting.

5. Help patient develop healthy lifestyle with balanced diet, rest, exercise, and relaxation.

Optimizing Sensory Function
1. Suggest use of an eyepatch or frosted lens (alternate eyes) for patients with double vision.
2. Encourage ophthalmologic consultation to maximize vision.
3. Provide a safe environment for patient with any sensory alteration.
   a. Orient patient to the environment, and keep arrangement of furniture and personal articles constant.
   b. Make sure floor is free of obstacles, loose rugs, or slippery areas.
   c. Teach the use of all senses to maintain awareness of environment.

Maintaining Urinary Elimination
1. Ensure adequate fluid intake to help prevent infection and stone formation.
2. Assess for urinary retention, and catheterize for residual urine as indicated.
3. Teach patient to report signs of urinary tract infection immediately.
4. Set up bladder training program to reduce incontinence.
   a. Encourage fluids every 2 hours.
   b. Follow regular schedule of voiding, every 1 to 2 hours, lengthening as tolerated.
   c. Restrict fluid volume and salty foods 1 to 2 hours before bedtime.
5. See pages 181 and 182 for more information on urinary retention and incontinence.

Normalizing Family Processes
1. Encourage verbalization of feelings of each family member.
2. Encourage counseling and use of church or community resources.
3. Suggest dividing up household duties, child care responsibilities to prevent strain on one person.
4. Explore adaptation of some roles so patient can still function in family unit.
5. Expand treatment efforts to include the whole family.
6. Support mothers with MS who often face fatigue and episodic exacerbations during their child-rearing years.

Promoting Sexual Function
1. Encourage open communication between partners.
2. Discuss birth control options, if appropriate.
3. Suggest sexual activity when patient is most rested.
4. Suggest consultation with sexual therapist to help obtain greater sexual satisfaction.

Community and Home Care Considerations
1. The nurse case manager functions as care provider, facilitator, advocate, educator, counselor, and innovator aimed at intervention in a wide variety of settings to improve patient function and mobility.
2. Teach the patient and family to use their own judgment, knowledge, and ingenuity to control MS symptoms.

3. Teach patient and family how to conduct periodic self-assessment of daily functioning, so home care team can continue to make modifications in treatment plan.

Patient Education and Health Maintenance

1. Encourage the patient to maintain previous activities, although at a lowered level of intensity.
2. Teach the patient to respect fatigue and avoid physical overexertion and emotional stress; remind patient that activity tolerance may vary from day to day.
3. Advise the patient to avoid exposure to heat and cold or infectious agents.
4. Encourage nutritious diet that is high in fiber to promote health and good bowel elimination.
5. Advise the patient that some medications may accentuate weakness such as some antibiotics, muscle relaxants, antiarrhythmics and antihypertensives, antipsychotics, oral contraceptives, and antihistamines; check with health care provider before taking any new medications.
6. Teach the patient receiving beta-interferon (Betaseron) to expect side effects of flulike symptoms, fever, asthenia, chills, myalgias, sweating, and local reaction at the injection site. Liver function test elevation and neutropenia may also occur. Side effects may persist for up to 6 months of treatment before subsiding.
7. Instruct the patient receiving Betaseron in self-injection technique.
8. Try to include children in the education of MS and the relationship of fatigue and functional status.
9. Refer the patient/family for more information and support to such agencies as:

   The National Multiple Sclerosis Society
   733 Third Avenue
   New York, NY 10017
   212-986-3240
   www.nmss.org

Outcome-Based Evaluation

- Performing exercises correctly without spasm
- Resting at intervals, tolerating activity well
- Moving about in environment without injury
- Voiding every 2 hours, two episodes incontinence
- Family sharing care, discussing feelings
- Patient reports satisfaction with sexual activity

◼ Amyotrophic Lateral Sclerosis (ALS)

Amyotrophic lateral sclerosis, also known as Lou Gehrig's disease, is an incapacitating disease that results in progressive weakness accompanied by other lower motor neuron signs, such as atrophy or fasciculations.

Pathophysiology and Etiology

1. Degeneration of upper motor neurons (nerves leading from the brain to medulla or spinal cord) and lower motor neurons (nerves leading from the spinal cord to the muscles of the body).
2. Results in progressive loss of voluntary muscle contraction and functional capacity.
3. Cause is unknown.
4. Usually affects men in the fifth or sixth decade of life.

Clinical Manifestations

1. Progressive weakness and wasting of muscles of arms, trunk, and legs
2. Fasciculations and signs of spasticity
3. Progressive difficulty swallowing (drooling, regurgitation of liquids through nose), speaking (nasal and unintelligible), and, ultimately, breathing

Diagnostic Evaluation

1. Electromyography to evaluate denervation and muscle atrophy
2. Nerve conduction study to evaluate nerve pathways
3. Pulmonary function tests to evaluate respiratory function
4. Barium swallow to evaluate ability to achieve various phases of swallow
5. MRI, CT to rule out other disorders
6. Laboratory tests: creatine kinase, heavy metal screen, thyroid function tests, CSF evaluation to rule out other causes of muscle weakness

Management

No specific treatment available to arrest or alter course of the disease. Treatment is palliative and symptomatic.

1. Baclofen (Lioresal) to control spasticity.
2. Diazepam (Valium) to control fasciculations.
3. Antidepressants, sleep medications.
4. Feeding gastrostomy.
5. Mechanical ventilation eventually becomes necessary.

Complications

1. Respiratory failure
2. Aspiration pneumonia
3. Cardiopulmonary arrest

Nursing Assessment

1. Evaluate respiratory function: rate, depth, tidal volume.
2. Perform cranial nerve assessment, particularly gag reflex and swallowing.
3. Assess voluntary motor function and strength.

Nursing Diagnoses

- Ineffective Breathing Pattern related to respiratory muscle weakness
- Impaired Physical Mobility related to disease process
- Altered Nutrition: Less Than Body Requirements related to inability to swallow
- Fatigue related to denervation of muscles
- Social Isolation related to fatigability and decreased communication skills
- Risk for Infection related to inability to clear airway

Nursing Interventions
Maintaining Respiration
1. Monitor vital capacity frequently. Document pattern, and report any decrease below patient's baseline.
2. Position patient upright, suction upper airway, and perform chest physical therapy to enhance respiratory function.
3. Encourage use of incentive spirometer to exercise respiratory muscles.
4. Assess for signs of hypoxia, such as tachypnea, hypopnea, restlessness, poor sleep, and excessive fatigue.
5. Obtain ABGs as ordered.
6. Establish the wishes of the patient in terms of life-support measures; obtain copy of living will for chart, if applicable.
7. Assist with intubation, tracheostomy, and mechanical ventilation when indicated (see Chapter 10).
8. Provide suctioning and routine care of a patient with artificial airway and mechanical ventilation.

Optimizing Mobility
1. Encourage the patient to continue usual activities as long as possible, but modify exertion to avoid fatigue.
2. Encourage physical therapy exercises to strengthen unaffected muscles, and perform range-of-motion exercises to prevent contractures.
3. Encourage energy-conservation techniques.
4. Obtain assistive devices as needed to help patient maintain independence, such as special feeding devices, remote controls, and a motorized wheelchair.

Meeting Nutritional Requirements
1. Provide high-calorie, small, frequent feedings.
2. Provide meals that are of a texture the patient can handle; semisolid food is usually easiest to swallow.
   a. Avoid easily aspirated, pureed, and mucus-producing foods (eg, milk).
   b. Try warm or cold foods that stimulate temperature receptors in mouth and may help in swallowing.
   c. Do not wash down solids with fluids—may cause choking and aspiration.
3. Allow patient to make own food selection.
4. Provide assistive devices for self-feeding when possible.
5. Make mealtime a pleasant experience in a bright room, with quiet company so the patient may concentrate on eating and avoid undue embarrassment.
6. Examine oral cavity for food debris before and after meals, and assess swallowing function and buildup of saliva.
7. Encourage rest periods before meals to alleviate muscle fatigue.
8. Place patient upright for meals with neck flexed to partially protect the airway.
9. Instruct patient to take a breath before swallowing, hold breath to swallow, exhale or cough after swallow, and swallow again.
10. Tell patient to avoid talking while eating.
11. Prepare patient for gastrostomy or other alternate feeding methods when appropriate.

Minimizing Fatigue
1. Encourage activity alternating with frequent naps.
2. Encourage patient to accomplish most important activities early in day.
3. Consult with occupational therapist about energy-conservation techniques in performing ADLs.

Maintaining Social Interaction
1. Use mechanical speech aids or communication board.
2. Use an environmental control board.
3. Eye movements/blinks may be the last voluntary movement; develop a code system to serve as a communication method.
4. Because standard call lights cannot be activated by the severely debilitated ALS patient, provide some type of constant monitoring and surveillance to meet patient's needs.
5. Allow patient to select which social activities are meaningful.
6. Refer to counselor or psychologist for coping with communication barriers and inevitability of losses.

Preventing Aspiration and Infection
1. Consult with speech therapist for techniques and devices to assist swallowing.
2. Discourage bed rest to prevent pulmonary stasis.
3. Perform chest physiotherapy as tolerated.
4. Monitor for fever and tachycardia, and obtain sputum, urine, and other cultures as indicated.

Community and Home Care Considerations
1. Teach caregivers how to perform suctioning, tracheostomy care, and ventilator care in the home as indicated. Clean technique will be used rather than sterile.
2. Teach caregivers how to perform gastrostomy feedings and care of tube.
3. Assess for adequate supplies for care and ability of caregivers to carry out procedures.
4. Encourage cleanliness in home environment and avoidance of contact with anyone with respiratory infection. Give influenza and pneumonia vaccines as indicated.

Patient Education and Health Maintenance
1. Stress the importance of maintaining physical exercise.
2. Review with the patient and family proper eating mechanics to avoid fatigue and aspiration.
3. Inform the patient of right to make decisions regarding a living will if he or she decides against artificial ventilation.
4. Encourage the family to seek support and respite care.
5. Remind the family that the patient with ALS maintains full alertness, sensory function, and intelligence. Encourage them to maintain interaction, socialization, and stimulation.
6. Refer the patient/family for more information and support to such agencies as:
   The Amyotrophic Lateral Sclerosis Association
   1021 Ventura Boulevard, Suite 321
   Woodland Hills, CA 91364
   800-782-4747
   www.alsa.org

Outcome-Based Evaluation

- Respirations 28, shallow, unlabored at rest
- Feeding self with assistive utensils
- Tolerating small, frequent feedings without aspiration
- Napping twice a day for 1 to 2 hours
- Communicating needs effectively to staff and family
- No signs of respiratory or urinary infection

NEUROMUSCULAR DISORDERS

Guillain-Barré Syndrome (Polyradiculoneuritis)

Guillain-Barré syndrome (GBS) is an acute, rapidly progressing, inflammatory demyelinating polyneuropathy of the peripheral sensory and motor nerves and nerve roots. GBS is most often, but not always, characterized by muscular weakness and mild distal sensory loss. GBS is the most frequently acquired demyelinating neuropathy. It affects one in 100,000 people and must be identified quickly to initiate treatment and decrease life-threatening complications. Mortality rate is about 5% despite intensive medical care.

Pathophysiology and Etiology

1. Believed to be an autoimmune disorder that causes acute neuromuscular paralysis.
2. Viral infection, immunization, or other event may trigger the autoimmune response.
3. About 30% to 40% of cases are preceded by *Campylobacter* infection, an acute infectious diarrheal illness.
4. Cell-mediated immune reaction is aimed at peripheral nerves, causing demyelination and possibly axonal degeneration.

Clinical Manifestations

1. Paresthesias.
2. Acute onset of symmetric progressive muscle weakness; most often beginning in the legs and ascending to involve the trunk, upper extremities, and facial muscles. Paralysis may develop.
3. Difficulty with swallowing, speech, and chewing due to cranial nerve involvement.
4. Decreased or absent deep tendon reflexes, position and vibratory perception.
5. Autonomic dysfunction (increased heart rate and postural hypotension).
6. Decreased vital capacity, depth of respirations, and breath sounds.
7. Occasionally spasm and fasciculations of muscles.
8. May be dysthesias and muscle spasms.

Diagnostic Evaluation

1. CSF examination—low blood cell count, high protein.
2. Electrophysiologic studies—NCT shows decreased conduction velocity of peripheral nerves.

Management

1. Plasmapheresis produces temporary reduction of circulating antibodies.
2. Electrocardiography monitoring and treatment of cardiac dysrhythmias.
3. Analgesics and muscle relaxants as needed.
4. Intubation and mechanical ventilation if respiratory paralysis develops.

Complications

1. Respiratory failure
2. Cardiac dysrhythmias
3. Complications of immobility and paralysis
4. Anxiety and depression

Nursing Assessment

1. Assess pain level due to muscle spasms and paresthesias.
2. Assess cardiac function including orthostatic blood pressures.
3. Assess respiratory status closely to determine hypoventilation due to weakness.
4. Perform cranial nerve assessment, especially ninth cranial nerve for gag reflex.
5. Assess motor strength.

Nursing Diagnoses

- Ineffective Breathing Pattern related to weakness/paralysis of respiratory muscles
- Impaired Physical Mobility related to paralysis
- Altered Nutrition: Less Than Body Requirements, related to cranial nerve dysfunction
- Impaired Verbal Communication related to intubation, cranial nerve dysfunction
- Pain related to disease pathology
- Anxiety related to communication difficulties and deteriorating physical condition

Nursing Interventions

Maintaining Respiration

1. Monitor respiratory status through vital capacity measurements, rate and depth of respirations, breath sounds.
2. Monitor level of weakness as it ascends toward respiratory muscles.
3. Watch for breathlessness while talking, a sign of respiratory fatigue.
4. Maintain calm environment, and position patient with head of bed elevated to provide for maximum chest excursion.
5. Avoid narcotics and sedatives, which may depress respirations.
6. Monitor the patient for signs of impending respiratory failure; heart rate above 120 or below 70 beats/minute; respiratory rate above 30/minute; prepare to intubate.

Avoiding Complications of Immobility

1. Position patient correctly, and provide range-of-motion exercises (see p. 174).

2. Encourage physical and occupational therapy exercises to regain strength during rehabilitative period.

3. Assess for complications, such as contractures, pressure sores, edema of lower extremities, and constipation.

4. Provide assistive devices as needed, such as cane or wheelchair, for patient to take home.

5. Recommend referral to rehabilitation services or physical therapy for evaluation and treatment.

Promoting Adequate Nutrition

1. Auscultate for bowel sounds; hold enteral feedings if bowel sounds are absent to prevent gastric distention.

2. Assess chewing and swallowing ability by testing fifth and ninth cranial nerves; if function is inadequate, provide alternate feeding.

3. During rehabilitation period, encourage a well-balanced, nutritious diet in small, frequent feedings with vitamin supplement if indicated.

4. Recommend referral to dietitian for evaluation and proper diet therapy.

Maintaining Communication

1. Develop a communication system with patient who cannot speak.

2. Have frequent contact with patient, and provide explanation and reassurance, remembering that patient is fully conscious.

3. Provide some type of patient call system.

4. Recommend referral to speech therapy for evaluation and treatment.

Relieving Pain

1. Administer analgesics as required; monitor for adverse reactions, such as hypotension, nausea and vomiting, and respiratory depression.

2. Provide adjunct pain management therapies, such as therapeutic touch, massage, diversion, imagery.

3. Provide explanations to relieve anxiety, which augments pain.

4. Turn the patient frequently to relieve painful pressure areas.

Reducing Anxiety

1. Get to know the patient, and build a trusting relationship.

2. Discuss fears and concerns while verbal communication is possible.

3. Reassure patient that recovery is probable.

4. Use relaxation techniques, such as listening to soft music.

5. Provide choices in care, and give patient a sense of control.

6. Enlist the support of significant others.

Community and Home Care Considerations

1. Be aware that GBS is a significant cause of new long-term disability for at least 1,000 persons per year in the United States, necessitating long-term rehabilitation and community reintegration. Outcome can range from mild paresthesia to death. The chance of recovery is significantly affected by age, antecedent gastroenteritis, disability, electrophysiologic signs of axonal degeneration, latency to nadir, and duration of active disease.

2. Given the young age at which GBS sometimes occurs, the patient and family care must be treated as an integral unit, assessing family communication, knowledge, adjustment, and use of support systems.

3. Include in caregiver training strategies the need for exercise, positioning, and activity to prevent secondary complications such as contractures, deep vein thrombosis, hypercalcemia, and pressure ulcers.

Patient Education and Health Maintenance

1. Advise patient and family that acute phase lasts 1 to 4 weeks, then patient stabilizes and rehabilitation can begin; however, convalescence may be lengthy, from 3 months to 2 years.

2. Instruct patient in breathing exercises or use of incentive spirometer to reestablish normal patterns.

3. Teach patient to wear good supportive and protective shoes while out of bed to prevent injuries due to weakness and paresthesias.

4. Instruct patient to check feet routinely for injuries, because trauma may go unnoticed due to sensory changes.

5. Reinforce maintenance of normal weight; additional weight will further stress the motor abilities.

6. Encourage the use of scheduled rest periods to avoid overfatigue.

7. Refer the patient/family for more information and support to such agencies as:
   The Guillain-Barré Syndrome Foundation International
   PO Box 262
   Wynnewood, PA 19096
   610-667-0131
   www.webmast.com

Outcome-Based Evaluation

- Respirations—24, deep, unlabored
- Providing assistive range-of-motion exercises every 2 hours; no pressure sores or edema present
- Gag reflex present, eating small meals without aspiration
- Using short phrases and head nodding to communicate effectively
- Patient verbalizes decreased pain
- Patient verbalizes reduced anxiety

Myasthenia Gravis

Myasthenia gravis is a chronic autoimmune disorder affecting the neuromuscular transmission of impulses in the voluntary muscles of the body. It is due to an antibody-mediated attack against acetylcholine receptors at the neuromuscular junction. Cardinal features are muscle weakness and fatigue.

Pathophysiology and Etiology

1. Depletion of acetylcholine receptors at neuromuscular junctions brought about by an autoimmune attack. The origin of this autoimmune response is unknown.

2. The reduced number of acetylcholine receptors results in diminished amplitude of end-plate potentials. Failed

transmission of nerve impulses to skeletal muscle at the myoneuronal junction results in decreased muscle power, clinically manifested as extreme fatigue and weakness.
3. About 80% to 90% of patients with myasthenia gravis have serum antibodies to acetylcholine.
4. Thyroid gland abnormalities are present in 80% of patients.
5. An acute *myasthenic crisis* may result from natural deterioration, emotional upset, upper respiratory infection, surgery, trauma, or adrenocorticotropic hormone therapy.
6. *Cholinergic crisis* can result from overmedication with anticholinergic drugs, which release too much acetylcholine at the neuromuscular junction.
7. *Brittle crisis* occurs when the receptors at the neuromuscular junction become insensitive to anticholinesterase medication.
8. Women are three times more susceptible to developing myasthenia gravis.

Clinical Manifestations
1. Extreme muscular weakness and easy fatigability
2. Visual disturbances—diplopia and ptosis from ocular weakness
3. Masklike facial expression from involvement of facial muscles
4. Dysarthria and dysphagia from weakness of laryngeal and pharyngeal muscles
5. Impending crisis:
   a. Sudden respiratory distress
   b. Signs of dysphagia, dysarthria, ptosis, and diplopia
   c. Tachycardia, anxiety
   d. Rapidly increasing weakness of extremities and trunk

Diagnostic Evaluation
1. Serum test for acetylcholine receptor antibodies—positive in up to 90% of patients.
2. Edrophonium (Tensilon) test—IV injection relieves symptoms temporarily. After injection, a marked but temporary improvement in muscle strength suggests myasthenia gravis. Also differentiates myasthenic crisis from cholinergic crisis.
3. Electrophysiologic (electromyogram [EMG]) testing—reveals decremental response to repetitive nerve stimulation.
4. CT scan to assess enlargement of thymus gland

Management
1. With treatment, most patients can lead fairly normal lives.
2. Anticholinesterase drugs such as neostigmine (Prostigmin) and pyridostigmine (Mestinon, Regonol) to enhance neuromuscular transmission.
3. Immunosuppressive drugs such as prednisone (Orasone) and azathioprine (Imuran) when weakness is not adequately controlled by anticholinergic medication. Immunosuppressant treatment is often permanent.
4. Plasmapheresis removes antibodies from the blood and is used for patients in myasthenic crisis or for short-term treatment of patients undergoing thymectomy.
5. Thymectomy for those people with tumor or hyperplasia of the thymus gland.
6. Interventions for crisis:
   a. Immediate hospitalization
   b. Edrophonium (Tensilon) to differentiate crisis and treat myasthenic crisis; temporarily worsens cholinergic crisis; unpredictable results with brittle crisis
   c. Aggressive respiratory support—tracheostomy, ventilator, vigorous suctioning
   d. Plasmapheresis
   e. Neostigmine (Prostigmin) IV for myasthenic crisis
   f. Discontinue anticholinergic medications until respiratory function improves; give atropine to reduce excessive secretions for cholinergic crisis

Complications
1. Aspiration
2. Complications of decreased physical mobility
3. Respiratory failure

Nursing Assessment
1. Assess cranial nerve function, motor fatigability with repetitive activity, and speech. Observe eye muscles (often affected first) for ptosis, ocular palsy, diplopia.
2. Assess respiratory status—breathlessness, respiratory weakness, tidal volume, and vital capacity measurements.

Nursing Diagnoses
- Fatigue related to disease process
- Risk of Aspiration related to muscle weakness of face and tongue
- Social Isolation related to diminished speech capabilities and increased secretions

Nursing Interventions
Minimizing Fatigue
1. Plan exercise, meals, and other ADLs during energy peaks. Time administration of medications 30 minutes before meals to facilitate chewing and swallowing.
2. Assist the patient in developing realistic activity schedule.
3. Provide an eyepatch, and alternate eyes for the patient with diplopia to allow safe participation in activity.
4. Allow for rest periods throughout the day.
5. Obtain assistive devices to help patient perform ADLs.

◆ **DRUG ALERT**

Many medications can accentuate the weakness experienced by the patient with myasthenia, including some antibiotics, antiarrhythmics, local and general anesthetics, muscle relaxants, and analgesics. Assess function after administering any new drug, and report deterioration in condition.

Preventing Aspiration

1. Assess patient's oral motor strength before each meal.
2. Teach patient to position head in a slightly flexed position to protect airway during eating.
3. Modify diet as needed to minimize risk of aspiration; for instance, soft, solid foods instead of liquid.
4. Have suction available that patient can operate.
5. Administer IV fluids and nasogastric tube feedings to patient in crisis or with impaired swallowing; elevate head of bed after feeding.
6. Suction the patient frequently if on a mechanical ventilator; assess breath sounds, and check chest x-ray reports, because aspiration is a common problem.

Maintaining Social Interactions

1. Encourage patient to use an alternate communication method, such as flash cards or a letter board, if speech is affected.
2. Instruct patient to speak in a slow manner to avoid voice strain; refer to speech therapy as needed.
3. Show the patient how to cup chin in hands during speech to support lower jaw and assist with speech.
4. Teach patient to tilt head, and to carry a handkerchief to manage secretions in public.
5. Encourage family participation in care.

Community and Home Care Considerations

1. Assess home environment for physical and emotional stressors, such as uncomfortable temperature, draft, loud noises, and encourage avoidance of such.
2. Emphasize continued follow-up and compliance with treatment regimen.
3. Make referrals to community agencies as indicated, such as home respiratory care, physical therapy, nutritional services.
4. Assess patient frequently for fluctuation in condition, and inform caregivers that this is common.
5. Teach patient and family how to use home suction in case of aspiration. Make sure everyone in household knows Heimlich maneuver.

Patient Education and Health Maintenance

1. Instruct the patient and family regarding the symptoms of crisis.
2. Review the peak times of medications and how to schedule activity for best results. For patients on anticholinesterase therapy:
   a. Stress accurate dosage and times.
   b. Tell patient not to skip medication
   c. Instruct patient to avoid taking medication with fruit, coffee, tomato juice, or other medications.
   d. Inform patient of adverse side effects such as GI distress.
3. Stress the importance of scheduled rest periods before fatigue develops.
4. Teach the patient ways to prevent crisis and aggravation of symptoms.

   a. Avoid exposure to colds and other infections.
   b. Avoid excessive heat and cold.
   c. Inform the dentist of condition, because use of procaine (Novocain) is not well tolerated.
   d. Avoid emotional upset.
5. Encourage patient to wear a Medic-Alert bracelet.
6. Stress importance of adequate nutrition; instruct to chew food thoroughly and eat slowly.
7. Advise patient to avoid alcohol, tonic water.
8. Refer patient/family for more information and support to such agencies as:
   The Myasthenia Gravis Foundation, Inc.
   61 Gramercy Park North, Room 605
   New York, NY 10010
   212-533-7005
   www.myasthenia.org

Outcome-Based Evaluation

- Demonstrates optimal self-care in bathing, eating, toileting, and dressing without fatigue
- Breathes effectively, cough is effective, suctioning own secretions, lungs clear
- Visits with friends, participates in social activities, using alternative method of communications

TRAUMA

Head Injury

Head injury, also known as traumatic brain injury (TBI), is the disruption of normal brain function due to trauma-related injury resulting in compromised neurologic function resulting in focal or diffuse symptoms. TBI is classified as mild (GCS 13 to 15 with loss of consciousness to 15 minutes), moderate (GCS 9 to 12 with loss of consciousness for up to 6 hours), or severe (GCS 3 to 8 with loss of consciousness greater than 6 hours). Studies have shown that mild TBI with positive CT scan is more indicative of moderate injury resulting in a more pronounced neurobehavioral presentation and extended neurologic recovery time frame, beyond the typical 3 months. (Also see Chapter 35, p. 1070, for emergency management of head injury.)

Pathophysiology and Etiology

1. Types of brain injuries include concussion, cerebral contusion, brain stem contusion, epidural hematoma, subdural hematoma, and skull fracture.
2. Caused by blunt or penetrating injury.
3. Neurologic deficits result from shearing of white matter, ischemia and mass effect from hemorrhage, and cerebral edema of surrounding brain tissue.

Clinical Manifestations

1. Disturbances in consciousness: confusion to coma
2. Headache, vertigo
3. Agitation, restlessness

4. Respiratory irregularities
5. Cognitive deficits
6. Pupillary abnormalities
7. Sudden onset of neurologic deficit
8. Coma and coma syndromes; persistent vegetative state

Diagnostic Evaluation
1. CT scan to identify and localize lesions, edema, bleeding
2. Skull and cervical spine films to identify fracture, displacement
3. Neuropsychological tests during rehabilitation phase to determine cognitive deficits

Management
1. Management of increased ICP
2. Antibiotics to prevent infection with open skull fractures or penetrating wounds
3. Surgery for evacuation of intracranial hematomas, débridement of penetrating wounds, elevation of skull fractures, or repair of CSF leaks

Complications
1. Infections: systemic (respiratory, urinary), neurologic (meningitis, ventriculitis)
2. Increased ICP, hydrocephalus
3. Posttraumatic seizure disorder
4. Permanent neurologic deficits: cognitive, motor, sensory, speech
5. Neurobehavioral alterations: impulsivity, uninhibited aggression, emotional lability

Nursing Assessment
1. Monitor for signs of increased ICP—altered LOC, abnormal pupil responses, vomiting, increased pulse pressure, bradycardia, hyperthermia.
2. Observe for CSF leakage.
3. Note contusions about eyes and ears.
4. Perform cranial nerve, motor, sensory, and reflex assessment.
5. Assess for behavior that warrants potential for injury to self or others

---

NURSING ALERT

Regard every patient who has a brain injury as having a potential spinal cord injury. A significant number of patients are under the influence of alcohol at the time of injury, which may mask the nature and severity of the injury.

Nursing Diagnoses
- Altered Cerebral Tissue Perfusion related to increased ICP
- Ineffective Breathing Pattern related to increased ICP or brain stem injury
- Altered Nutrition: Less Than Body Requirements related to compromised neurologic function and stress of injury
- Altered Thought Processes related to physiology of injury
- Risk for Injury related to altered thought processes
- Ineffective Family Coping related to unpredictability of outcome

Nursing Interventions
Maintaining Adequate Cerebral Perfusion
1. Maintain a patent airway.
2. Monitor ICP (see p. 448).
3. Monitor for changes in neurologic status, decreased LOC, and onset of cranial nerve deficits.
4. Identify emerging trends in neurologic function, and communicate findings to medical staff.
5. Monitor response to pharmacologic therapy including drug levels.
6. Monitor laboratory data, CSF cultures and Gram's stain, if applicable, and communicate findings to medical staff.
7. Monitor results of serial serum and urine electrolyte and osmolality studies to maintain the level of dehydration ordered to reduce cerebral edema.
8. Assess dressings and drainage tubes after surgery for patency, security, and characteristics of drainage.
9. Institute measures to minimize IICP, cerebral edema, seizures, or neurovascular compromise such as careful positioning to avoid flexing head, reducing hip flexion, and spreading out care evenly over 24-hour period.

Maintaining Respiration
1. Monitor respiratory rate, depth, and pattern of respirations; report any abnormal pattern, such as Cheyne-Stokes respirations or periods of apnea.
2. Assist with intubation and ventilatory assistance, if needed.
3. Turn patient every 2 hours, and assist with coughing and deep breathing.
4. Suction patient as needed; however, hyperventilate the patient before suctioning to prevent hypoxia.

Meeting Nutritional Needs
1. Provide nasogastric feedings once bowel sounds have returned if patient is unable to swallow; elevate the head of the bed after feedings, and check residuals to prevent aspiration. Feed the patient as soon as possible after a head injury and administer H_2-blocking agents to prevent gastric ulceration and hemorrhage from gastric acid hypersecretion.
2. Consult with dietitian to provide the increased calories and nitrogen requirement resulting from the metabolic changes of brain injury.

NURSING ALERT

Caloric needs of the head-injured patient are similar to those of a patient with 30% body burns. Consult your dietitian to institute hyperalimentation within the first 2 to 3 days after injury to support the recovery process.

---

3. Administer IV hyperalimentation as ordered.
4. During rehabilitation, recognize the dysphagic patient and encourage oral feeding of soft or pureed foods in an

unhurried manner. Refer to speech or physical therapist as indicated for feeding difficulties.

Promoting Cognitive Function

1. Periodically, assess patient's LOC, and compare to baseline.
2. Be aware of patient's cognitive alteration, and adjust interaction and environment accordingly.
3. Provide meaningful stimulation using all senses—visual, olfactory, gustatory, acoustic, and tactile.
4. Observe patient for fatigue or restlessness from over-stimulation.
5. Involve family in sensory stimulation program.
6. Decrease environmental stimuli when patient is in agitated state.
7. Reorient to surroundings using repetition, verbal and visual cues, and memory aids; routinely orient patient after awakening.
8. Use pictures of family members, clock, calendar as outlined by occupational therapist.
9. Encourage family to provide items from home to increase sense of identity and security.
10. Anticipate need for additional help with toileting, eating, performing ADLs due to cognitive impairment.
11. Break down ADLs into simple steps that patient can progressively take part in.
12. Structure the environment and care activities to minimize distraction and provide consistency.
13. Identify and maintain usual patterns of behavior—sleep, medication use, elimination, food intake, and self-care routine.
14. Refer patient for cognitive retraining, if appropriate.

Preventing Injury

1. Instruct the family regarding the behavioral phases of recovery from brain injury, such as restlessness and combativeness.
2. Investigate for physical sources of restlessness, such as uncomfortable position, signs of urinary tract infection, or pressure ulcer development.
3. Reassure patient and family during periods of agitation and irrational behavior.
4. Pad side rails, and wrap hands in mitts if patient is agitated. Maintain constant vigilance, and avoid restraints if possible.
5. Keep environmental stimuli to a minimum.
6. Provide adequate light if patient is hallucinating.
7. Perform passive range-of-motion exercises to release muscle tension from inactivity.
8. Avoid sedatives to avoid medication-induced confusion and altered states of cognition.

Strengthening Family Coping

1. Refer family to community support services, such as respite care.
2. Assist the family members to establish stress management techniques that can be integrated into their lifestyle, such as ventilation of feelings, use of respite care, relaxation techniques.
3. Consult with social worker or psychologist to assist the family in adjusting to patient's permanent neurologic deficits.
4. Help the family assist the patient to recognize current progress and not focus on limitations.

Community and Home Care Considerations

1. Observe for signs of postconcussion syndrome (PCS), which include headache, decreased concentration, irritability, dizziness, insomnia, restlessness, diminished memory, anxiety, easy fatigability, and alcohol intolerance.
2. Be aware that persistence of these symptoms can interfere with relationships and employability of the patient.
3. Encourage the patient and family to report these symptoms and obtain additional support and counseling as needed. PCS may persist as long as 2 years.
4. Act as liaison to coordinate all the home care services the patient will need, while keeping in touch with the patient's primary care provider, neurologist, and neurosurgeon.
5. Provide the necessary education to caregivers in tube feedings, positioning, range-of-motion exercises, and so forth.

Patient Education and Health Maintenance

1. Review with the family the signs of increased ICP.
2. Reinforce the lability of cognitive, language, and physical functioning of the person with brain injury and the lengthy recovery period.
3. Teach the family therapeutic use of touch, massage, and music to calm the agitated patient.
4. Refer the patient/family for more information and support to such agencies as:

    Brain Injury Association
    105 North Alfred Street
    Alexandria, VA 22314
    703-236-6000

Outcome-Based Evaluation

- ICP stable
- Respirations—24, regular
- Tube feedings tolerated well without residual
- Oriented to person, place, and time
- Less agitated; side rails maintained
- Family reports using respite care

▌ Spinal Cord Injury

Spinal cord injury (SCI) is a traumatic injury to the spinal cord that may vary from a mild cord concussion with transient numbness to immediate and complete tetraplegia. The most common sites are the cervical areas C5, C6, and C7 and the junction of the thoracic and lumbar vertebrae, T12, L1. Injury to the spinal cord may result in loss of function below the level of cord injury. Approximately 200,000 persons with SCI are living in the United States and are typically young, white males (median age 26). (Also see Chapter 35, p. 1071, for emergency management of SCI.)

Pathophysiology and Etiology

1. SCI may result from trauma, vascular disorders, infectious conditions, tumor, and other insults.
2. The most common etiologies are motor vehicle accidents (MVA), falls, sports injuries, and violence.
3. Patients who have SCI later in life are more likely to have incomplete cervical injuries.

GERONTOLOGIC ALERT

Older patients are more likely to have comorbidities such as hypertension, myocardial infarction, and chronic obstructive pulmonary disease.

Clinical Manifestations

1. Clinical manifestations vary and depend on the location and severity of cord damage. In general, complete transection causes all loss of function below the level of the lesion (Figure 15-5), and incomplete cord damage results in a partial loss of movement and sensation (Table 15-2).
   a. Patients with injuries T1 and above have *tetraplegia* (formerly called quadriplegia), and injuries T2 and below have *paraplegia*.
   b. The neurologic level of injury is the lowest neural level with normal sensation and movement.
2. Classification is typically based on an impairment scale set forth by the American Spinal Injury Association (ASIA). This scale is based on whether injury is complete (no sensory or motor function) or incomplete (some motor and/or sensory function).
3. Various syndromes (incomplete injuries) may characterize the clinical presentation.
   a. *Central cord syndrome*—cervical injury with predominant weakness of the upper limbs; tetraplegia but able to ambulate
   b. *Brown-Séquard syndrome*—motor and proprioceptor loss of the ipsilateral side, and pain and temperature loss on the contralateral side
4. Most recovery occurs within 6 months of injury; patients with incomplete injuries have greater recovery than patients with complete injuries.

Diagnostic Evaluation

1. X-ray of spinal column to include open mouth studies for adequate visualization of C1 and C2.
2. MRI of spine—to detect soft tissue injury, hemorrhage, edema, bony injury. Syringomyelia may present as more pronounced cord compression, syrinx at the fracture site, and kyphosis at the fracture site.
3. Electrophysiologic monitoring to determine function of neural pathways.

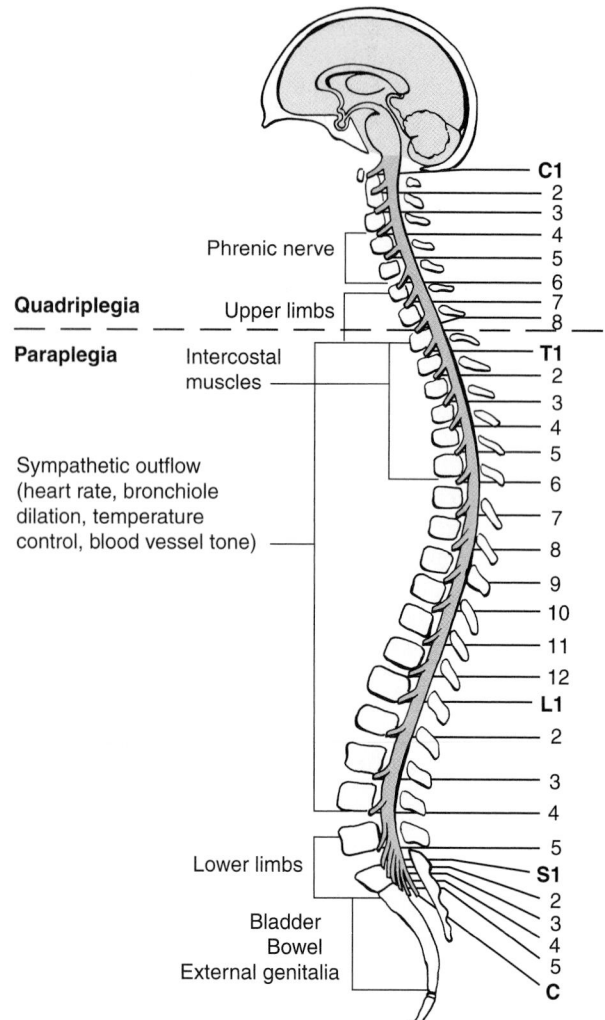

FIGURE 15-5 Levels of spinal cord innervation.

4. Urodynamic studies may include uroflow to detect bladder outlet obstruction and/or impaired bladder contractility; cystometrogram (CMG) to determine bladder sensation, compliance, and capacity; sphincter EMG and other studies. The gold standard in urodynamics is to measure both bladder and urethral pressure under fluoroscopy monitoring.
5. If deep vein thrombosis or pulmonary emboli are suspected, an ultrasound of the lower extremity or ventilation/perfusion scan is performed.
6. Heterotopic ossification may be diagnosed in the inflammatory stages using ultrasound. Alkaline phosphatase and ESR are typically elevated.
7. Nutritional status should be assessed using nutritional history, anthropometric measurements, prealbumin (half-life 12 to 36 hours) and transferrin (half-life 6 to 10 days). Total lymphocyte count and creatinine height index are also used to establish nutritional risk.

TABLE 15-2 Incomplete Cord Syndromes

Lesion	Mechanism of Injury	Preserved	Impaired
Anterior cord syndrome (dorsal columns of the spinal cord are spared)	Flexion	Light touch Vibratory sensation Proprioception	Motor function Pain and temperature sensation
Posterior cord syndrome (anterior columns of the cord are spared)	Extension	Motor function Pain and temperature sensation	Light touch Vibratory sensation Proprioception
Central cord syndrome (central gray matter of the cord is injured)	Flexion or extension	Motor function of lower extremities	Motor function of upper extremities
Brown-Séquard syndrome (hemisection of the cord)	Penetrating trauma	Contralateral—pain and temperature sensation Ipsilateral—movement, light touch, proprioception	Contralateral—movement, light touch, proprioception Ipsilateral—pain and temperature

From Neff, J., & Kidd, P. (1993). *Trauma nursing: The art and science.* Chicago: Mosby.

Management

1. Requires a multidisciplinary approach because of multiple systems involvement and the psychosocial aspects of catastrophic injuries.

Immediately After Trauma (Less Than 1 Hour)

1. Immobilization with rigid cervical collar, sandbags, and rigid spine board to transport from the field to acute care facility.
2. Methylprednisolone (Solu-Medrol) IV given within 8 hours of injury to decrease the extent of injury. Contraindicated in systemic fungal infection, hypersensitivity, and pregnancy.

Acute Phase (1 to 24 Hours)

1. Maintenance of pulmonary and cardiovascular stability.
   a. Intubation and mechanical ventilation, if needed.
   b. Vasopressors to maintain adequate perfusion.
   c. Medical stabilization before spinal stabilization and decompression.
2. Spinal cord immobilization.
   a. Traction to reduce cervical spine injuries.
   b. Kinetic turning bed such as RotoRest to immobilize patients with thoracic and lumbar injuries.
3. Management of neurogenic bladder—insert Foley catheter to drain bladder and monitor kidney perfusion.
4. Pressure ulcer prevention.
   a. Pressure reduction mattress or kinetic turning frame.
   b. When spine is stable, patient is turned every 2 hours and heels are suspended to avoid pressure.

Subacute Phase (Within 1 Week)

1. Stabilize vertebral column and ligamentous injuries through traction or surgical intervention (Figure 15-6).
2. GM-1 ganglioside sodium salt IV, begun within 72 hours after injury, and continued for 18 to 32 days.
3. H_2-receptor blockers to prevent gastric irritation and hemorrhage.
4. Early mobilization and passive exercise as soon as patient is surgically and medically stable.
5. Hyperalimentation to retard negative nitrogen balance.
6. Small doses of heparin to reduce risk of thrombophlebitis and pulmonary emboli within 72 hours of SCI, unless there is active bleeding, coagulopathy, or head injury.
7. Possible vena cava filter to prevent thromboembolism in patients who have failed anticoagulant prophylaxis, or in whom anticoagulants are contraindicated.
8. Neurogenic bowel program.

Chronic Phase (Beyond 1 Week)

1. Anticoagulants are continued until discharge with incomplete injuries; for 8 weeks with uncomplicated motor injury; and for 12 weeks (or discharge from rehabilitation) for complete motor injury and other complications.
2. Management of complications may include treatment of infections with antibiotics; treatment of respiratory compromise with phrenic nerve pacing, mechanical ventilation, and other methods; pressure ulcer treatment; management of heterotopic ossification with calcium chelators and anti-inflammatory agents; drainage of syringomyelia; management of spasticity with oral or intrathecal antispasmodics, surgical procedure, or spinal cord stimulation; and management of central neuropathic pain with anticonvulsants, minor sedatives, antidepressants, nerve block, or surgical procedure.
3. Rehabilitation includes medical and psychosocial support, physical therapy, urologic evaluation, occupational therapy, and multiple other interventions to facilitate an increased level of function and community participation.

Complications

1. Spinal shock lasting a few hours to a few weeks noted by loss of all reflex, motor, sensory, and autonomic activity below the level of the lesion.
2. Respiratory arrest, pneumonia, atelectasis; mechanical ventilation often required with cervical injury.
3. Cardiac arrest may result from initial trauma, worsening of initial injury from edema, concomitant injuries, and other illnesses.

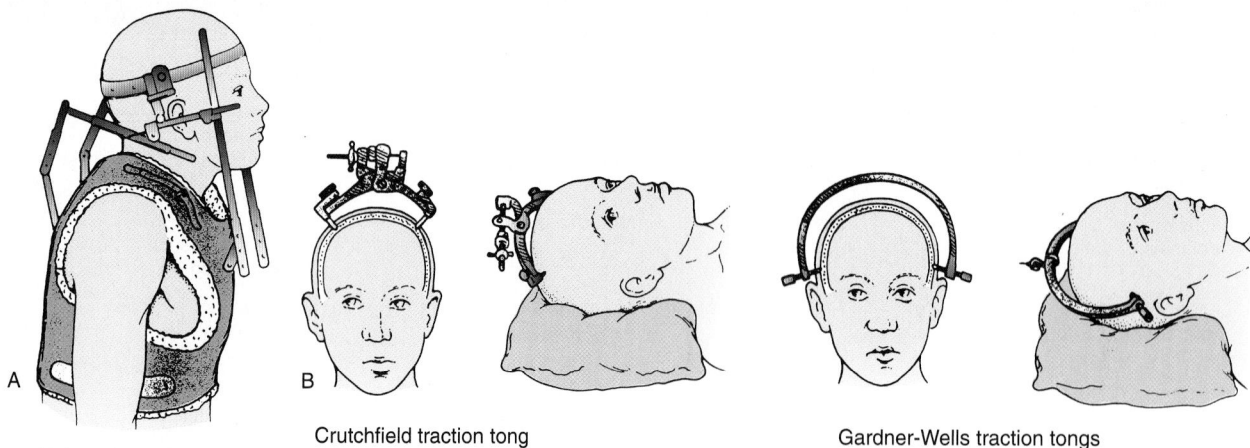

A
Halo vest traction

B
Crutchfield traction tong

Gardner-Wells traction tongs

FIGURE 15-6 Cervical traction. Cervical spine injuries are managed with immediate immobilization, early reduction, and stabilization of the vertebral column. Cervical traction with either skeletal tongs or a halo device accomplishes these goals.
(**A**) Halo-vest device.
(1) A halo ring is fixed to the skull by four pins and connected to a removable vest by a metal frame. (2) The halo ring may initially be connected to bed traction or may be applied after tongs are removed; the vest is used to attain mobility. (3) To care for a patient in a vest, inspect skin under the vest; encourage position changes frequently, including the prone position to relieve pressure; wash and dry skin well through slide openings; avoid using powder under vest, which causes friction and possibly pressure ulcers; turn the patient and vest as a unit; and make sure a vest wrench is taped to the front of the vest for quick release if CPR is required. (4) To provide halo care, cleanse pin sites daily and observe for redness, drainage, and tenderness; observe for loosening of pins and stabilize the patient's head while notifying surgeon if pin becomes detached; provide assistance with activities, because the patient is top-heavy and cannot scan the environment easily; provide emotional support to help the patient adjust to his or her bizarre appearance. *Do not turn the patient by grasping the halo apparatus.*
(**B**) Skeletal tongs.
(1) Crutchfield and Vinke tongs require predrilled holes in the skull under local anesthesia; Gardner-Wells and Heifitz tongs do not. (2) Weight is added to traction gradually to accomplish reduction of vertebral fracture, then enough weight is kept to maintain vertebral alignment. (3) Make sure that tongs are several inches from the head of the bed and weights hang freely. (4) To care for a patient in skeletal tongs, inspect tong sites for signs of infection; shave hair around sites as needed; cleanse the sites with providone-iodine (Betadine) solution or other antiseptic; and check back of head for signs of pressure and massage the head periodically without moving the neck.

4. Thromboembolic complications—in 15% of patients.
5. Infections—respiratory, urinary, pressure sores, sepsis.
6. Autonomic dysreflexia—exaggerated autonomic response to stimuli below the level of the lesion in patients with lesions at or above T6 is a medical emergency and can result in dangerous elevation of blood pressure.
7. Autonomic dysfunction resulting in orthostatic hypotension, thermodysregulation, and vasomotor abnormalities.
8. Neurogenic bladder—bladder storage pressure >35 to 40 cm may result in renal deterioration.
9. Paralytic ileus—common in subacute and acute stage.
10. Heterotopic ossification—bony overgrowth that occurs below the level of injury any time after SCI.
11. Syringomyelia—cystic formation in the spinal cord may occur any time after SCI.
12. Depression—occurs in 25% of men and 47% of women with SCI.
13. Pressure ulcers may occur in up to 35% of persons with SCI.
14. Spasticity may result in contractures.
15. Amenorrhea occurs in 60% of women with SCI, usually temporary.
16. Neuropathic pain occurs in 34% to 94% of patients with SCI.

Nursing Assessment

1. Assess cardiopulmonary status and vital signs to help determine degree of autonomic dysfunction, especially in patients with tetraplegia.
2. Determine LOC and cognitive indicating involvement of TBI and other factors.
3. Perform frequent motor and sensory assessment of trunk and extremities—extent of deficits may increase due to edema and hemorrhage. Later, increasing neurologic deficits and pain may indicate development of syringomyelia.
4. Note signs and symptoms of spinal shock such as flaccid paralysis, urinary retention, absent reflexes.
5. Assess bowel and bladder function.
6. Assess quality, location, severity of pain.
7. Perform psychosocial assessment to evaluate motivation, support network, financial or other problems.
8. Assess for indicators of powerlessness, including verbal expression of no control over situation, depression, nonparticipation, dependence on others, passivity.

Nursing Diagnoses

- Ineffective Breathing Pattern related to paralysis of respiratory muscles or diaphragm
- Impaired Physical Mobility related to motor dysfunction
- Risk for Impaired Skin Integrity related to immobility
- Urinary Retention related to neurogenic bladder
- Constipation related to neurogenic bowel
- Risk for Injury: autonomic dysreflexia and orthostatic hypotension
- Powerlessness related to loss of function, long rehabilitation, depression
- Sexual Dysfunction related to erectile dysfunction and fertility changes

Nursing Interventions

Attaining an Adequate Breathing Pattern

1. For patients with high-level lesions, continuously monitor respirations and maintain a patent airway. Be prepared to intubate if respiratory fatigue or arrest occurs.
2. Frequently assess cough and vital capacity. Teach effective coughing, if patient is able (Box 15-2).
3. Provide adequate fluids and humidification of inspired air to loosen secretions.
4. Suction as needed; observe vagal response (bradycardia—should be temporary).
5. When appropriate, implement chest physiotherapy regimen to assist pulmonary drainage and prevent infection.
6. Monitor results of ABGs, chest x-ray, and sputum cultures.
7. Tape wrench to body jacket or halo traction in the event the jacket must be removed for basic or advanced life support.

Promoting Mobility

1. Place patient on firm kinetic turning bed until spinal cord stabilization. After stabilization, turn every 2 hours on a pressure reduction surface, ensuring good alignment.

BOX 15-2   Assisted Coughing

Many patients with tetraplegia have an impairment of the diaphragmatic and intercostal muscles. The result is a weak or ineffective cough. To increase the mechanical effectiveness of the patient's cough, perform or teach the assisted cough technique.

1. Place the patient in supine, low semi-Fowler's position.
2. Place the heels of your hands on the costophrenic angle of the patient's rib cage.
3. With the patient's head turned away, ask the patient to hyperventilate and exhale once or twice. Allow your hands to move with the patient.
4. During the next breath, ask the patient to take a deep breath and cough while exhaling.
5. As patient coughs, thrust your hands down and in (inferiorly and medially) to add power to the diaphragm during exhalation.
6. Allow one or two normal breaths, and repeat the procedure.

 NURSING ALERT

Incorrect hand placement may cause injury to the internal organs, ribs, and xyphoid process.

---

2. Log roll patient with unstable SCI.
3. Perform range-of-motion exercises to prevent contractures and maintain rehabilitation potential.
4. Monitor blood pressure with position change in the patient with lesions above midthoracic area to prevent orthostatic hypotension.
5. Encourage physical therapy and practicing of exercises as tolerated.
6. Encourage weight-bearing activity to prevent osteoporosis and risk of kidney stones.
7. Apply pneumatic compression device or compression hose to legs for the first 2 weeks after SCI to avoid thromboembolic complications.

Protecting Skin Integrity

1. Pay special attention to pressure points when repositioning patient.
2. Obtain pressure relief mattress and appropriate wheelchair with cushion for patient.
3. Inspect for pressure ulcer development daily over bony prominences, including the back of head, ears, trunk, heels, and elbows. Observe under stabilization devices for pressure areas, particularly on the scapulae. Use a risk assessment tool to determine risk of developing pressure ulcer.
4. Keep skin clean, dry, and well lubricated.
5. Turn a minimum of every 2 hours, and instruct patient to perform wheelchair weight shifts every 15 minutes. Place patient in prone position at intervals, unless contraindicated.
6. Institute treatment for pressure ulcers immediately, and relieve pressure to promote healing.

Promoting Urinary Elimination

1. Consider use of intermittent catheterization as an alternative to an indwelling catheter, typically beginning every 4 hours.
2. If patient has an upper motor neuron lesion (above L1) and no indwelling catheter, promote reflex voiding by tapping the bladder, gently pulling the patient's pubic hair, or stroking the patient's inner thigh.
3. If the patient has a lower motor neuron lesion (L1 or below) and no indwelling catheter, promote voiding by using a bladder Crede's method by gently compressing the suprapubic area to promote voiding.
4. Encourage fluid intake of 3,000 to 4,000 mL of fluid a day (2,000 mL per day if intermittent catheterization is used) to prevent infection and urinary calculi. Space fluids out over 24-hour period to avoid bladder overdistention.
5. Monitor for urinary retention by percussing the suprapubic area for dullness or catheterizing for residual urine after voiding.
6. Monitor intake and output as indicated.

Promoting Bowel Activity

1. Assess bowel sounds, and note abdominal distention. Paralytic ileus is common immediately after injury.
2. Encourage intake of high-calorie, high-protein, and high-fiber (15 g) diet when bowel sounds return and food is tolerated.
3. Assess for loose stool oozing from rectum, and perform rectal examination to check for fecal impaction; remove fecal matter if necessary.
4. Institute a bowel program as early as possible.
   a. Schedule bowel care at the same time of day to develop a predictable outcome.
   b. Stimulate the gastrocolic reflex 30 minutes before bowel care with food or liquid intake.
   c. Perform bowel care with patient in bowel chair or in left side-lying position, confine procedure to 2 hours.
   d. Use abdominal massage, deep breathing, warm fluids, and leaning forward in the chair to enhance success.
5. For patients with upper motor neuron lesions, perform reflexic bowel care.
   a. Insert a glycerin or bisacodyl suppository or mini-enema (4 mL).
   b. Alternatively, use digital stimulation with gloved, lubricated finger—perform a semicircular motion against rectal wall. Repeat every 5 to 10 minutes until evacuation is complete.
6. For patients with lower motor neuron lesions, perform areflexic bowel care.
   a. Perform manual stool elimination.
7. Have patient perform Valsalva maneuver (after urinary elimination to prevent vesicoureteral reflux of urine).

STANDARDS OF CARE GUIDELINES
Autonomic Dysreflexia

Risk for autonomic dysreflexia occurs after spinal cord injury at the level of T6 or above and may result in dangerously elevated blood pressure. Follow these assessment and treatment measures to protect the patient:

Be aware of and try to prevent common causes of autonomic dysreflexia whenever possible:
- Bladder distention, urinary tract infection, bladder or kidney stones
- Cystoscopy, detrusor sphincter dysynergia, urodynamic testing
- Bowel distention, bowel impaction
- Constrictive clothing, shoes, or apparatus
- Noxious stimuli such as pain, strong smells, pressure

Be alert for signs and symptoms of autonomic dysreflexia:
- Sudden and significant increase in systolic and diastolic blood pressure above patient's baseline. (Normal systolic BP for a person with tetraplegia is 90–110 mm Hg.)
- Pounding headache
- Profuse sweating, piloerection, and flushing above the level of the lesion
- Blurred vision and spots in visual field
- Nasal congestion
- Apprehension and anxiety
- Cardiac irregularity in rhythm and rate

Take the following actions if autonomic dysreflexia does occur:

- Check blood pressure; if elevated, call health care provider immediately.
- Immediately sit the patient up.
- Loosen clothing and other constrictive apparatus.
- Monitor BP every 2–5 minutes.
- Check the urinary system—catheterize patient; if catheter in place, check for kinks in tubing obstructing drainage; if catheter blockage suspected, gently irrigate with small amount normal saline; replace catheter if not draining adequately.
- Check the rectum for stool, and gently remove if present. Topical anesthetic such as 2% lidocaine jelly is usually used before rectal examination or catheter insertion.
- If BP remains elevated, administer immediate release nifedipine 10 mg (bite and swallow) or nitroglycerin ointment 2% 1 inch above the level of injury, as directed.

After the episode of autonomic dysreflexia, do the following:
- Monitor BP for at least 2 hours for recurrent hypertension or symptomatic hypotension. Notify health care provider as indicated.
- Provide patient teaching for prevention and treatment of complication.
- Be sure all caregivers understand autonomic dysreflexia and the patient carries an identification card.

This information should serve as a general guideline only. Each patient situation presents a unique set of clinical factors and requires nursing judgment to guide care, which may include additional or alternative measures and approaches.

8. For chronic constipation without relief from more conservative approaches, consider a bulk-forming agent or laxative 8 hours before bowel care.

Preventing Autonomic Dysfunction and Orthostatic Hypotension

Also see Standards of Care Guidelines.

1. Protect the patient from possible stimuli causing autonomic dysreflexia.
   a. Bowel or bladder distention caused by fecal impaction, urinary retention, or a kinked indwelling catheter
   b. Abnormal skin stimulation, such as lying on wrinkled sheets, hot or cold stimulation, or pain from constricting clothing
   c. Distention or contraction of visceral organs such as gastric distention or emptying an overdistended bladder too fast
   d. Infection, especially of the urinary tract
2. Be alert to signs of autonomic dysreflexia, such as pounding headache, profuse sweating, nasal congestion, piloerection (goosebumps), bradycardia, and severe hypertension.
3. If autonomic dysreflexia does occur, immediately place the patient in a sitting position to help lower the blood pressure and diminish ICP and initiate treatment.
   a. Remove possible causative stimuli.
   b. Administer antihypertensive medication as ordered.
   c. Monitor blood pressure every 2 to 5 minutes until return to normal.
4. Be alert for, prevent, and manage orthostatic hypotension, especially in patients with cervical SCI.
5. Use tilt table as ordered to gradually increase the patient's ability to tolerate sitting after acute SCI.
6. Other conservative strategies consist of use of embolic hose, abdominal binder, and high-salt diet.
7. Administer a sympathomimetic such as ephedrine or pseudoephedrine, as ordered, before patient is transferred to wheelchair.

Empowering Patient

1. Explain all procedures to the patient. Answer any questions.
2. Ensure that patient plays an integral part in decision making regarding plan of care. Allow patient to make modifications to treatment plan when possible.
3. Schedule procedures and planning sessions when patient is rested and experiencing decreased anxiety.
4. Praise patient for incremental gains in function or participation.
5. Discuss stress management techniques, such as relaxation therapy, counseling, and problem solving.
6. Identify motivating factors and priorities with the patient.
7. Use peer counseling for patient to gain support from other people with SCI.
8. Be alert for signs of depression (problems with sleep, loss of interest, guilt, loss of energy, lack of concentration, change in appetite, feeling sad) or risk for suicide, and refer to mental health counselor.
9. Administer antidepressant medications as directed.

 DRUG ALERT

Caution should be exercised for persons with spinal cord injuries who are taking tricyclic antidepressants because of autonomic dysfunction. SCI patients are more vulnerable to anticholinergic side effects and orthostatic hypotension. There are also numerous potential drug reactions associated with monoamine oxidase (MAO) inhibitors and SCI.

Minimizing Alteration in Sexuality and Fertility

1. Encourage patient to discuss alternate expression of feelings with partner.
2. Advise bowel care and urinary elimination before intercourse.
3. Advise women that 90% regain regular menstrual cycles by 1 year. Pregnancy can occur, and delivery occurs in 40% before 37 weeks gestation. Autonomic dysreflexia may occur as a complication of delivery.

Community and Home Care Considerations

1. Alert caregivers that autonomic dysreflexia is a complication that may occur up to several years after SCI involving T6 and above. Teach patient and caregivers preventive and emergency treatment measures.
2. Coordinate continued rehabilitation effort to ensure social support, ongoing pharmacologic treatment, and monitoring for long-term complications such as depression, vocational training, and adaptation to the home and work environment. Use Functional Independence Measure (FIM) or other instrument to set and achieve goals with the patient in ADLs, transferring, locomotion, and other functional aspects.
3. Teach bowel care and urinary elimination procedures to patient and all caregivers to ensure continuity.
4. Teach care of traction and immobilization devices including daily cleansing with soap and water of pin sites for skeletal traction.
5. Enlist help of occupational therapist, physical therapist, vocational therapist, recreational therapist, and others as needed.

Patient Education and Health Maintenance

1. Teach patient and family about the physiology of nerve transmission and how spinal injury has affected normal function, including mobility, sensation, bowel and bladder function.
2. Reinforce that rehabilitation is lengthy and involves compliance with therapy to increase function.
3. Explain that spasticity may develop 2 weeks to 3 months after injury and may interfere with routine care and ADLs. Spasticity should be managed by:
   a. Maintaining calm, stress-free environment.
   b. Allowing plenty of time for activities such as positioning and transferring.
   c. Performing joint range-of-motion exercises with slow, smooth movements.

d. Avoiding temperature extremes.

e. Administering muscle relaxants such as baclofen (Lioresal), diazepam (Valium), and dantrolene (Dantrium) as prescribed.

4. Teach patient to protect skin from pressure ulcer development by frequent repositioning while in bed, weight-shifting and lift-offs every 15 minutes while in a wheelchair, and avoiding shear forces and friction.

5. Teach inspection of skin daily for development of pressure sores, using a mirror if necessary.

6. Encourage sexual counseling, if indicated, to promote satisfaction in personal relationships.

a. Women with spinal cord injuries experience little sensation during sexual intercourse, but fertility and ability to bear children are usually not affected.

b. Men with spinal cord injuries may consider implantation of a penile prosthesis to obtain an erection.

7. Teach all people the importance of seat belts.

Outcome-Based Evaluation

- Respirations adequate, ABGs within normal limits
- Repositioning hourly, no orthostatic changes
- No evidence of pressure ulcers
- Reflex (or areflexic) voiding without retention
- Bowel evacuation controlled
- No episodes of autonomic dysreflexia
- Patient verbalizes feeling of control over condition
- Patient and partner exploring sexuality and sexual options

◼ Peripheral Nerve Injury

Peripheral nerve injury (PNI) is an injury to nerves in the upper extremity (radial, ulnar, median) or lower extremity (peroneal, sciatic, femoral, tibial). PNI may include damage to major nerves, the nerve root, plexus (brachial or lumbar), and other peripheral sites.

Pathophysiology and Etiology

1. The incidence of PNI is approximately 2% to 3% in populations with multiple injuries. Males have higher incidence than females.

2. The most frequently injured site is the upper extremity, specifically the upper arm. Childhood PNIs occur predominantly in the lower extremities.

3. Traumatic head and skeletal injuries are frequently associated with PNI.

4. PNI may result from penetration, laceration, contusion, stretch, missile, or crushing. MVA account for the majority of PNI; other mechanisms of injury include industrial accidents, stab and gunshot wounds, and motorcycle accidents.

5. Nerve injuries are classified according to the Sunderland system, which establishes grades of nerve function on which to base recovery and need for surgery. Grade I indicates neuropraxia in which the patient recovers in days to weeks and no surgery is required; Grade V indicates complete laceration of the nerve with guarded prognosis.

6. Within hours of injury, the regeneration process begins with axons sprouting "growth cones" with a proliferation of Schwann cells. These specialized cells guide regenerating fibers into the muscle and facilitate axonal growth.

7. With the exception of neuropraxia, in which nerve damage is minimal, the rate of axon regeneration is approximately 1 to 2 mm/day.

Clinical Manifestations

1. Flaccid paralysis

2. Absence of deep tendon reflexes

3. Atonic/hypotonic muscles

4. Progressive muscle atrophy

5. Fasciculations peak 2 to 3 weeks after injury

6. Trophic changes: skin is warm and dry 3 weeks after injury, then becomes cold and cyanotic with loss of hair, brittle fingernails, and ulceration development

7. Causalgia (chronic pain syndrome)

8. Specifics to area affected:

a. Radial nerve injury—weakness in extension, possible wrist drop, inability to grasp objects/make a fist, impaired sensation over posterior forearm and dorsum of the hand

b. Brachial plexus—difficulty in abduction of shoulder, weakness with supination and flexion of the forearm (upper trunk) or extension of the forearm (middle trunk) or paralysis and atrophy of small muscles of the hand (lower trunk)

c. Median and ulnar nerve injuries—sensory (median nerve) and motor (ulnar) loss of function in the hand (pronation, opposition of thumb, paralysis of finer flexor muscles)

d. Femoral—weakness of knee and hip extension, atrophy of quadriceps, absence of knee jerk, loss of sensation of anterior aspect of the thigh

e. Common peroneal—footdrop, sensory loss on dorsum of foot, difficulty with eversion

f. Sciatic—footdrop, pain across gluteus and thigh, loss of knee flexion, weakness/paralysis of muscles below knee.

Diagnostic Evaluation

1. Muscle ultrasonography to evaluate extent of muscle involvement and assess acute nerve injuries.

2. MRI and electrophysiologic studies such as ENG and EMG—to detect site and degree of nerve injury.

3. Muscle imaging may detect atrophy and mesenchymal alteration of skeletal muscles.

4. Tinel's sign (tapping the axons of the regenerating nerve produces a paresthesia in the normal distribution of the nerve) to determine rate of axonal regeneration.

Management

1. Microsurgical repair with tension-free coaptation using technology such as CO_2 laser welding, fibrin gluing, and ring coupling. Autogenous nerve grafts are the gold standard.
2. Small segments of nerve grafts may be placed to create a bridge to facilitate axonal and Schwann cell growth. Nerve "conduits," connectors of nerve sites, may be comprised of bone, vein, artery, silicone, or other material.
3. Tissue expansion is used to compensate for tissue deficit.
4. Insulinlike growth factor (IGF) and acidic fibroblast growth factor (aFGF) have enhanced regeneration when administered systematically or topically and other factors are being investigated.
5. Corticosteroids may be used to decrease edema.
6. Splinting or casting may be indicated for reducing tension on the PNI site to facilitate healing.

Complications

1. Infection, if injury is penetrating and site becomes contaminated
2. Compartment syndrome due to edema or positioning
3. Muscle atrophy/flaccid paralysis
4. Sensory deficit

Nursing Assessment

1. Perform frequent neurovascular checks of the affected extremity (pressure, vibration, and two-point discrimination sensation; motor function, strength; pulses, temperature, capillary refill, degree of swelling).
2. Assess degree of pain on 0 to 10 scale.
3. Test reflexes of affected extremity.
4. Observe for signs of infection if there is an open wound.
5. Assess for concomitant injuries such as head or skeletal trauma.

Nursing Diagnoses

- Sensory/Perceptual Alteration (Tactile) related to injury
- Pain related to injury
- Risk for Infection secondary to tissue disruption

Nursing Interventions

Optimizing Sensory and Motor Function

1. Administer corticosteroids and diuretics as ordered to decrease swelling and development of compartment syndrome.
2. Keep extremity elevated to promote venous drainage.
3. Perform neurovascular check to evaluate status of injury.
   a. Incorporate Tinel's sign into assessment.
   b. Report any changes in condition.
4. Postoperatively assist rehabilitation team in reeducating nerves and muscles to achieve function.
5. Observe for paresthesias, pain, or altered skin integrity in areas of splinting and casting.

Promoting Comfort

1. Administer and teach self-administration of analgesics as ordered.
2. Elevate extremity.
3. Avoid exposure of denervated areas to temperature extremes.
4. Apply such devices as splints and slings as ordered.
5. Maintain mobility with range-of-motion exercises. Perform gently and after administration of analgesics.

Preventing Infection

1. Assess wound and dressing frequently for erythema, warmth, swelling, odor, and drainage.
2. Monitor temperature with vital signs for hyperthermia and tachycardia indicating infection.
3. Encourage deep-breathing exercises and ambulation to prevent pulmonary complications.

Patient Education and Health Maintenance

1. Teach management of wound and dressing.
2. Review analgesia schedule and need for elevation of injured area.
3. Teach exercises for involved area.
4. Suggest assistive devices to promote independence.
5. Stress the importance of complying with long-term rehabilitation, physical therapy, and follow-up evaluations.
6. Support a community accident prevention program including seat belts, industrial regulations, and sports and recreational safety measures.

Outcome-Based Evaluation

- Stable neurovascular status; functional use of extremity.
- Patient reports adequate relief of pain.
- Wound/surgical site is free of erythema, drainage, odor.

CENTRAL NERVOUS SYSTEM TUMORS

Brain Tumors

Primary intracranial neoplasms are the result of proliferation of normal cells within the CNS. These include tumors of the brain itself, the skull or meninges, the pituitary gland, and the blood vessels. CNS tumors may also consist of metastatic tumors that spread from systemic organs. Primary CNS tumors only rarely metastasize outside the CNS.

Pathophysiology and Etiology

1. May originate in the CNS or metastasize from tumors elsewhere in the body.
2. May be benign or malignant; all produce effects of space-occupying lesion (edema, increased ICP). Malignancy may be related not to cell type or invasiveness, but rather to location and inoperability.

3. May arise from any tissue of the CNS. 40% to 50% of intracranial neoplasms are gliomas.
   a. Astrocytoma—arising from connective tissue of the brain (astrocytes); highly invasive, poorly marginated; grades 1 and 2
   b. Glioblastoma—Grade 3 and 4 astrocytomas; highly invasive, infiltrative, poorly marginated
   c. Oligodendrogliomas—arise from the frontal and temporal lobes of the cerebrum
   d. Ependymoma
   e. Medulloblastoma
   f. Colloid cysts—develop within lateral or third ventricles
   g. Meningioma—arising from linings of the brain
   h. Acoustic neuroma—develops in or on the eighth cranial nerve
   i. Metastatic lesions—commonly from lung and breast cancer, usually multiple and unresectable
   j. Developmental tumors (dermoid and epidermoid cysts, craniopharyngioma, pituitary or pineal, teratoma)
   k. Hemangioma—angioma from blood vessels of the brain
4. Malignant tumors (chondrosarcoma, osteogenetic sarcoma, fibrosarcoma, chordoma) account for 2% of all cancer deaths each year; second most common malignancy in children.

Clinical Manifestations

Depend on tumor location and biologic nature of the tumor. If the tumor is in a noneloquent area of the brain or slow growing, specific symptoms may not develop until the late stages of the process. Instead, the tumor may produce generalized symptoms related to the increasing size of the tumor and the expanding area of cerebral edema surrounding the margins of the tumor. This is referred to as the "mass" effect of the tumor.

1. Generalized symptoms (due to increased ICP)—headache (especially in the morning), vomiting, papilledema, malaise, altered cognition and consciousness.
2. Focal neurologic deficits (related to region of tumor):
   a. Parietal area—sensory alterations, speech and memory disturbances, neglect, visuospatial deficits, right–left confusion, depression
   b. Frontal lobe—personality, behavior, and memory changes; contralateral motor weakness; Broca's aphasia
   c. Temporal area—memory disturbances, auditory hallucinations, Wernicke's aphasia, complex partial seizures, visual field deficits
   d. Occipital area—visual agnosia and visual field deficits
   e. Cerebellar area—coordination, gait, and balance disturbances, dysarthria
   f. Brain stem—dysphagia, incontinence, cardiovascular instability, respiratory depression, coma, cranial nerve dysfunction
   g. Hypothalamus—loss of temperature control, diabetes insipidus, SIADH
   h. Pituitary/sella turcica—visual field deficits, amenorrhea, galactorrhea, impotence, cushingoid symptoms, elevated growth hormone, panhypopituitarism
3. Referred symptoms (related to the vasogenic edema of the tumor presence)—usually present symptoms of ischemia of region distal to the actual lesion.
4. Seizures.

Diagnostic Evaluation

1. Skull radiographs—to determine bone involvement, identify pineal shift, helpful in children
2. CT—with and without contrast to visualize tumor, hemorrhage, shift of midline, cerebral edema
3. EEG—to detect locus of irritability
4. Lumbar puncture for elevated CSF protein, cytology; risk of herniation if IICP
5. Angiogram—to detect vascular tumor
6. Cerebral blood flow studies—to follow progression of tumor
7. MRI—to visualize tumor; more useful than CT in posterior fossa evaluation
8. Stereotactic biopsy/surgery—needed for definitive diagnosis, cell type

Management

Effectiveness of treatment depends on tumor type and location, capsulation, or infiltrative status. Tumors in vital areas, such as the brain stem, or nonencapsulated and infiltrating tumors may not be surgically accessible, and treatment may produce severe neurologic deficits (blindness, paralysis, mental impairment). Treatment is usually multimodal.

1. Surgery—removal/debulking by way of craniotomy, laser resection, or ultrasonic aspiration.
   a. Craniotomy is treatment of choice for most tumors, although about 10% are inoperable.
   b. Laser resection or ultrasonic aspiration may augment surgical resection.
2. Radiation therapy—external radiation to tumor bed with 2-cm border.
   a. Conventional therapy daily for 6 weeks; shorter to brain stem.
   b. Prophylactic radiation to brain stem for other brain tumors with high risk of metastasis.
   c. Brachytherapy—can use radioisotopes implanted through interstitial catheters to permit high doses for high-grade malignant tumors.
3. Radiosurgery—stereotactic radiosurgery by way of LINAC scalpel or gamma knife delivers a single, high dose of radiation to a precisely targeted tumor area. Destroys only abnormal tissue, limiting damage to surrounding brain tissue.
4. Chemotherapy with single or combination drug therapy; may require autologous bone marrow transplantation

(aspirated before chemotherapy and reinfused afterward to treat bone marrow depression).

   a. As adjunct to surgery and radiation.

   b. Many agents do not cross blood–brain barrier.

5. Shunting procedure—to manage hydrocephalus, which may be obstructive or nonobstructive depending on location, tumor type, degree of necrosis, and associated edema and inflammation.

6. Supportive therapy and medications.

   a. Antiepileptic drug (AED) therapy.

   b. Dexamethasone (Decadron) to reduce swelling and reduce radiation edema; also given during end stage to enhance quality of life.

Complications

1. Increased ICP and brain herniation
2. Neurologic deficits from expanding tumor or treatment

Nursing Assessment

1. Assess vital signs and signs of increased ICP (see p. 449).
2. Assess cranial nerves, LOC, mental status, affect, and behavior.
3. Monitor for seizures.
4. Assess level of pain using visual analogue scale (0 to 10) or face scale as indicated.
5. Assess level of anxiety.
6. Assess patient and family patterns of coping, support systems, and resources.

Nursing Diagnoses

- Pain related to brain mass, surgical intervention
- Risk for Injury related to altered LOC, possible seizures, IICP, and sensory and motor deficits
- Anxiety related to diagnosis, surgery, radiation, and/or chemotherapy
- Altered Nutrition: Less Than Body Requirements related to compromised neurologic function and stress of injury
- Altered Family Processes related to changes in role

Nursing Interventions

Relieving Pain

1. Provide analgesics around the clock at regular intervals, that will not mask neurologic changes.
2. Maintain the head of the bed at 15 to 30 degrees to reduce cerebral venous congestion.
3. Provide a darkened room or sunglasses if the patient is photophobic.
4. Maintain a quiet environment to increase patient's pain tolerance.
5. Provide scheduled rest periods to help patient recuperate from stress of pain.
6. Instruct the patient to lie with the operative side up.
7. Alter diet as tolerated if patient has pain on chewing.
8. Collaborate with patient on alternative ways to reduce pain, such as use of music therapy.

Preventing Injury

1. Report any signs of increased ICP or worsening neurologic condition immediately.
2. Adjust care to reduce risk of IICP; body positioning without flexion of head, reduce hip flexion, distribute care throughout the 24-hour period to allow ICP to return to baseline.
3. Monitor laboratory data, CSF cultures, and Gram's stain, and communicate results to medical staff.
4. Monitor results of serial serum and urine electrolyte and osmolality studies to maintain the level of dehydration ordered to reduce cerebral edema.
5. Monitor response to pharmacologic therapy including drug levels.
6. Initiate seizure precautions; pad the side rails of the bed to prevent injury if seizures occur; have suction equipment available.
7. Maintain availability of medications for management of status epilepticus (see p. 497).
8. Initiate fall precautions; side rails up at all times, call light within reach at bedside, assist with toileting on a regular basis.
9. Gradually progress patient to ambulation with assistance as tolerated, enlist help from physical therapist, occupational therapist early as indicated to prevent falls.
10. If the patient is dysphagic or unconscious, initiate aspiration precautions; elevate the head of the bed 30 degrees and position patient's head to the side to prevent aspiration.
11. If dysphagic, position the patient upright and instruct in sequenced swallowing to maintain feeding function.
12. Maintain oxygen and suction at the bedside in case of aspiration.
13. For the patient with visual field deficits, place materials in visual field.
14. Provide appropriate care and teaching for patient receiving chemotherapy (see p. 146).
15. Provide appropriate care and teaching for the patient receiving radiation (see p. 153).
16. Provide routine postoperative care for the patient undergoing craniotomy (see p. 453).

Minimizing Anxiety

1. Provide a safe environment in which the patient may verbalize anxieties.
2. Help patient to express feelings related to fear and anxiety.
3. Answer questions and provide written information.
4. Include the patient/family in all treatment options and scheduling.
5. Introduce stress management techniques.
6. Provide consistency in care, and continually provide emotional support.
7. Assess the patient's usual coping behaviors, and provide support in these areas.
8. Consult with social worker for community resources.

Optimizing Nutrition

1. Medicate for nausea before position changes, radiation, or chemotherapy, and as needed.
2. Maintain adequate hydration within guidelines for cerebral edema.
3. Offer small, frequent meals as tolerated.
4. Consult with dietitian to evaluate food choices and provide adequate caloric needs through enteral or parenteral nourishment if unable to take oral nutrition.
5. Alter consistency of diet as necessary to enhance intake.

Strengthening Family Coping

1. Recognize stages of grief.
2. Foster a trusting relationship.
3. Provide clear, consistent explanations of procedures and treatments.
4. Encourage family involvement in care from the beginning.
5. Establish a means of communication for family with patient when verbal responses are not possible.
6. Consult with social worker and mental health provider when family needs assistance in adjusting to neurologic deficits.
7. Assist family to use stress management techniques and community resources such as respite care.
8. Encourage discussion with health care provider about prognosis and functional outcome.

Patient Education and Health Maintenance

1. Explain the side effects of treatment.
2. Encourage close follow-up after diagnosis and treatment.
3. Explain the importance of continuing corticosteroids and how to manage side effects, such as weight gain and hyperglycemia.
4. Encourage the use of community resources for physical and psychological support, such as transportation to medical appointments, financial assistance, respite care.
5. Refer the patient/family for more information and support to such agencies as:
   National Institute of Neurologic Disorders and Stroke
   www.ninds.nih.gov
   American Cancer Society
   800-ACS-2345

Outcome-Based Evaluation

- Patient reports satisfactory comfort level
- No new neurologic deficits, seizures, falls, or other injuries
- Patient expresses decreased anxiety
- Nutritional intake meeting metabolic demands
- Patient and family verbalize understanding of treatment and available resources

Tumors of the Spinal Cord and Canal

Tumors of the spinal cord and canal may be extradural (existing outside the dural membranes), including chordoma and osteoblastoma; intradural-extramedullary (within the SAS), including meningiomas, neurofibromas, and schwannomas; or intramedullary (within the spinal cord), including astrocytomas, ependymomas, and neurofibromatosis "dumbbell tumors."

Pathophysiology and Etiology

1. Cause for abnormal cell growth is unknown.
2. Extradural tumors spread to the vertebral bodies.
3. Spinal cord and/or nerve compression results.
4. Approximately 5% to 10% of patients with primary tumors of the breast, lung, and prostate present with malignant spinal cord compression.
5. Spinal cord tumors comprise approximately 10% of childhood tumors; the majority of these tumors are extradural.

Clinical Manifestations

Depends on location and type of tumor and extent of spinal cord compression.

1. Back pain that is localized or radiates; may be absent in over 50% of patients
2. Weakness of extremity with abnormal reflexes
3. Sensory changes
4. Bladder, bowel, or sexual dysfunction

Diagnostic Evaluation

1. A plain x-ray or CT scan can detect a pathologic fracture, collapse, or destruction resulting from a mass.
2. MRI is sensitive to tumor detection.
3. CT myelography with lumbar puncture is sensitive to tumor detection but may be uncomfortable and result in complications from lumbar puncture.

Management

1. Surgical interventions include vertebral body resection with stabilization, laminectomy, or bony decompression.
   a. Surgery may provide better outcome in terms of ambulation for patients with paresis or plegia before treatment.
   b. Outcome is the same given surgery or radiation therapy for those who were ambulatory before treatment.
2. Radiation therapy may be used over 2 to 4 weeks; dosing protocols vary.
3. Corticosteroids such as dexamethasone and prednisone in moderate to high doses are indicated for use before radiation therapy to improve the ambulation rate in the paretic patient.
   a. Corticosteroids are not typically used in nonparetic ambulatory patients.
   b. They are tapered over 2 weeks before discontinuing.

Complications

1. Spinal cord infarction secondary to compression
2. Malignant spinal cord compression
3. Nerve or spinal compression from tumor expansion

Nursing Assessment

1. Perform motor and sensory components of the neurologic examination.

2. Assess pain using 0 to 10 scale as indicated.

3. Assess autonomic nervous system relative to level of lesion—pupillary responses, vital signs, bowel and bladder function.

4. Assess for spinal or nerve compression—progressive increase in pain, paralysis or paresis, sensory loss, loss of rectal sphincter tone, and sexual dysfunction.

Nursing Diagnoses

- Anxiety related to surgery and outcome
- Pain related to nerve compression
- Sensory/Perceptual Alteration (Tactile, Kinesthetic) related to nerve compression
- Altered Urinary Elimination related to spinal cord compression
- Risk for Injury related to surgery

Nursing Interventions

Relieving Anxiety

1. Provide a safe environment for patient to verbalize anxieties.

2. Provide explanations regarding all procedures. Answer questions or refer patient to someone who can answer questions.

3. Refer to cancer and spinal cord lesion support groups as needed.

4. Provide the patient/family with written information regarding disease process and medical interventions.

5. Reduce environmental stimulation.

6. Promote periods of rest to enhance coping skills.

7. Involve the family in distraction techniques.

8. Provide options in care when possible.

Relieving Pain

1. Administer analgesics as indicated and evaluate for pain control.

2. Instruct the patient in the use of patient control analgesia, if available.

3. Instruct the patient in relaxation techniques, such as deep breathing, distraction, imagery.

4. Position patient off surgical site postoperatively.

Compensating for Sensory Alterations

1. Reassure patient that degree of sensory/motor impairment may decrease during the postoperative recovery period as the amount of surgical edema decreases.

2. Instruct the patient with sensory loss to visually scan the extremity during use to avoid injury related to lack of tactile input.

3. Instruct the patient with painful paresthesias in appropriate use of ice, exercise, or rest.

4. Assess the patient with sensory and motor alterations, and refer to physical therapy for assistance with ADLs, ambulation.

Achieving Urinary Continence

1. Assess the urinary elimination pattern of the patient.

2. Instruct the patient in the therapeutic intake of fluid volume and relationship to elimination.

3. Instruct the patient in an appropriate means of urinary elimination and bowel management (see p. 488).

Providing Additional Postoperative Care

1. Provide routine postoperative care to prevent complications.

2. Monitor surgical site for bleeding, CSF drainage, signs of infection.

3. Keep surgical dressing clean and dry.

4. Cleanse surgical site as ordered.

5. Pad the bed rails and chair if the patient experiences numbness or paresthesias, to prevent injury.

6. Support the weak/paralytic extremity in a functional position.

Patient Education and Health Maintenance

1. Encourage the patient with motor impairment to use adaptive devices.

2. Demonstrate proper positioning and transfer techniques.

3. Instruct the patient with sensory losses about dangers of extreme temperatures and the need for adequate foot protection at all times.

4. If the patient has suspected or confirmed neurofibromatosis, suggest referral to genetic counselor. Also encourage follow-up for MRI every 12 months to monitor disease progression.

5. Refer to cancer and SCI support groups as needed.

Outcome-Based Evaluation

- Anxiety managed
- Reports that pain is relieved
- Compensates for sensory deficits; ambulatory postoperatively
- Voiding at intervals without residual
- Incision healing, skin intact

OTHER DISORDERS

Seizure Disorders

Seizures (also known as epileptic seizures and, if recurrent, epilepsy) are defined as a sudden alteration in normal brain activity that causes distinct changes in behavior and body function. Seizures are thought to result from disturbances in the cells of the brain that cause them to give off abnormal, recurrent, uncontrolled electrical discharges.

Pathophysiology and Etiology

Altered Physiology

1. The pathophysiology of seizures is unknown. It is known, however, that the brain has certain metabolic needs for oxygen and glucose. Neurons also have certain permeability gradients and voltage gradients that are affected by changes in the chemical and humoral environment.

2. Factors that change the permeability of the cell population (ischemia, hemorrhage) and ion concentration (Na^+, K^+) can produce neurons that are hyperexcitable and demonstrate hypersynchrony, producing an abnormal discharge.

Classification

Seizures are classified by the origin of the seizure activity and associated clinical manifestations.

1. Anything the brain can do as a normal function, it can do as seizure behavior.
2. *Simple partial seizures* can have motor, somatosensory, psychic, or autonomic symptoms *without impairment* of consciousness.
3. *Complex partial seizures* have an *impairment* (but not a loss) of consciousness with simple partial features, automatisms, or impairment of consciousness only.
4. *Generalized seizures* have a loss of consciousness with convulsive or nonconvulsive behaviors.
5. Simple partial seizures can progress to complex partial seizures, and complex partial seizures can secondarily become generalized.
6. Nonepileptogenic behaviors can emulate seizures but have a psychogenic rather than organic origin.

Cause

The cause may be unknown or due to one of the following:

1. Trauma to head or brain resulting in scar tissue or cerebral atrophy
2. Tumors
3. Cranial surgery
4. Metabolic disorders (hypocalcemia, hypoglycemia/hyperglycemia, hyponatremia, anoxia)
5. Drug toxicity, such as theophylline (Theo-dur), lidocaine (Xylocaine), penicillin
6. CNS infection
7. Circulatory disorders
8. Drug withdrawal states (alcohol, barbiturates)
9. Congenital neurodegenerative disorders

Clinical Manifestations

Related to area of the brain involved in the seizure activity. May range from single abnormal sensations, aberrant motor activity, altered consciousness/personality to loss of consciousness and convulsive movements.

1. Impaired consciousness
2. Disturbed muscle tone or movement
3. Disturbances of behavior, mood, sensation, or perception
4. Disturbances of autonomic functions

Diagnostic Evaluation

1. EEG with or without video monitoring—locates epileptic focus, spread, intensity, and duration; helps classify seizure type
2. MRI, CT scan—to identify lesion that may be cause of seizure
3. SPECT or PET scan or MSI—additional tests to identify seizure foci
4. Neuropsychological studies—to evaluate for behavioral disturbances

Management

1. Pharmacotherapy—drug selected according to seizure type (Table 15-3)
2. Biofeedback—useful in the patient with reliable auras

3. Surgery—resective and palliative operations (temporal lobectomy, extratemporal resection, corpus callosotomy, hemispherectomy)
4. Vagal nerve stimulation

Complications

1. Status epilepticus
2. Injuries due to falls

Nursing Assessment

1. Obtain seizure history, including prodromal signs and symptoms, seizure behavior, postictal state, history of status epilepticus.
2. Document the following about seizure activity:
   a. Circumstances before attack, such as visual, auditory, olfactory, or tactile stimuli; emotional or psychological disturbances; sleep; hyperventilation
   b. Description of movement, including where movement or stiffness started; type of movement and parts involved; progression of movement; whether beginning of seizure was witnessed
   c. Position of the eyes and head; size of pupils
   d. Presence of automatisms, such as lip smacking or repeated swallowing
   e. Incontinence of urine or feces
   f. Duration of each phase of the attack
   g. Presence of unconsciousness and its duration
   h. Behavior after attack, including inability to speak, any weakness or paralysis, sleep
3. Psychosocial effect of seizures.
4. History of drug or alcohol abuse.
5. Compliance and medication-taking strategies.

 DRUG ALERT

Nonadherence to medication regimen as well as toxicity of antiepileptic medications can increase seizure frequency. Obtain drug levels before implementing medication changes.

Nursing Diagnoses

- Altered Cerebral Tissue Perfusion related to seizure activity
- Risk for Injury related to seizure activity
- Ineffective Individual Coping related to psychosocial and economic consequences of epilepsy

Nursing Interventions

Maintaining Cerebral Tissue Perfusion

1. Maintain a patent airway until patient is fully awake after a seizure.
2. Provide oxygen during the seizure if color change occurs.
3. Stress the importance of taking medications regularly.
4. Monitor serum levels for therapeutic range of medications.
5. Monitor patient for toxic side effects of medications.
6. Monitor platelet and liver functions for toxicity due to medications.

TABLE 15-3 Antiepileptic Medications

Drug/Dosage/Indications	Adverse Reactions	Patient Teaching
Clonazepam (Klonopin): Generalized seizures such as absence, atonic, myoclonic; PO up to 20 mg/day, increase 0.5 mg over 3-day period	Dose-related: Visual disturbances, ataxia, cognitive impairment. Idiosyncratic: Rash, hirsutism, vivid dreams.	Take with meals. Avoid driving. Avoid alcohol ingestion.
Carbamazepine (Tegretol): Partial and generalized seizures; give PO up to 1,600 mg/day in divided doses or to clinical toxicity	Dose-related: Blurred vision, dizziness, visual disturbances, ataxia, lethargy. Idiosyncratic: Skin rash, hepatic dysfunction (bleeding, dark urine), leukopenia, aplastic anemia.	Dose-related effects may diminish. Take PO with food. Must comply with ordered lab studies. Available in chewable tablets, if preferred. Drug induces own metabolizing enzymes, effectiveness of dose may decrease within 3–6 weeks.
Ethosuxamide (Zarontin): Generalized seizures initially 1,000 mg/day in divided doses; increase by 250 mg every 4–7 days to 1.5 g	Dose-related: GI upset, sedation, unsteadiness. Idiosyncratic: Skin rash, psychotic behaviors.	Take with food, milk to decrease GI upset. Use hard candy, gum to prevent dry mouth.
Felbamate (Felbatol): Partial and generalized seizures: 2,400–3,600 mg/day in divided doses	Dose-related: Decreased appetite, weight loss, GI upset. Idiosyncratic: Sleep disturbances.	Take with food, milk.
Gabapentin (Neurontin): For partial and generalized seizures: PO 900–1,800 mg/day in divided doses	Dose-related: Somnolence, dizziness, fatigue, and nystagmus. Idiosyncratic: Hypotension, rash, hematuria.	Avoid working around machinery or driving if somnolence is experienced
Phenytoin (Dilantin): Partial and generalized seizures, IV 900 mg–1.5 g run at 50 mg/min, if previously on phenytoin 100–300 mg same rate. PO 300 mg/day in divided doses	Dose-related: Nystagmus, ataxia, visual changes, seizure exacerbation, slurred speech. Idiosyncratic: Aplastic anemia, rash, Steven-Johnson syndrome.	Urine may turn pink. Good oral hygiene is necessary (brushing and flossing) to prevent gingival hyperplasia.
Primidone (Mysoline): Partial seizures, PO 250 mg/day up to 2 g/day in divided doses	Dose-related: Visual disturbances, sedation. Idiosyncratic: Thrombocytopenia, lymphadenopathy, hallucinations.	Do not withdraw medication without first consulting health care provider.
Valproic acid (Depakene, Depakote): Partial and generalized seizures, PO initially 15 mg/kg/day, add 5–10 mg/kg/day, up to 60 mg/kg/day in divided doses	Dose-related: GI upset, tremor, increased liver enzymes, hyperammonemia, somnolence, thrombocytopenia. Idiosyncratic: Hepatic failure, pancreatitis.	Do not dilute elixir with carbonated beverages. Avoid driving. Take with food.

Preventing Injury

1. Provide a safe environment by padding side rails and removing clutter.
2. Place the bed in a low position.
3. Do not restrain the patient during a seizure.
4. Do not put anything in the patient's mouth during a seizure.
5. Place the patient on side during a seizure to prevent aspiration.
6. Protect the patient's head during a seizure.
7. Stay with the patient who is ambulating or who is in a confused state during seizure.
8. Provide a helmet to the patient who falls during seizure.
9. Manage the patient in status epilepticus (Box 15-3).

Strengthening Coping

1. Consult with social worker for community resources for vocational rehabilitation, counselors, support groups.
2. Teach stress reduction techniques that will fit into patient's lifestyle.
3. Initiate appropriate consultation for management of behaviors related to personality disorders, brain damage secondary to chronic epilepsy.
4. Answer questions related to use of computerized video EEG monitoring and surgery for epilepsy management.

Community and Home Care Considerations

1. Counsel patients with uncontrolled seizures about driving or operating dangerous equipment.

BOX 15-3 Emergency Management of Status Epilepticus

Status epilepticus (acute, prolonged, repetitive seizure activity) is a series of generalized seizures without return to consciousness between attacks. The term has been broadened to include continuous clinical and/or electrical seizures lasting at least 5 minutes, even without impairment of consciousness. Status epilepticus is considered a serious neurologic emergency. It has a high mortality and morbidity rate (permanent brain damage, severe neurologic deficits). Factors that precipitate status epilepticus include medication withdrawal, fever, metabolic or environmental stresses, alcohol withdrawal, sleep deprivation, and so forth in patient with preexisting seizure disorder.

Nursing Interventions
1. Establish an airway, and maintain blood pressure.
2. Obtain blood studies for glucose, blood urea nitrogen, electrolytes, and anticonvulsant drug levels to determine metabolic abnormalities and serve as a guide for maintenance of biochemical homeostasis.
3. Administer oxygen—there is some respiratory arrest at height of each seizure, which may produce venous congestion and hypoxia of brain.
4. Establish IV lines, and keep open for blood sampling, drug administration, and infusion of fluids.
5. Administer IV anticonvulsant (lorazepam [Ativan], phenytoin [Dilantin]) *slowly* to ensure effective brain tissue and serum concentrations.
   a. Additional anticonvulsants given as directed—effects of lorazepam are of short duration.
   b. Anticonvulsant drug levels monitored regularly.
6. Monitor the patient continuously; depression of respiration and blood pressure induced by drug therapy may be delayed.
7. Use mechanical ventilation as needed.
8. If initial treatment is unsuccessful, general anesthesia may be required.
9. Assist with search for precipitating factors.
   a. Monitor vital and neurologic signs on a continuing basis.
   b. Use electroencephalographic monitoring to determine nature and abolition (after diazepam administration) of epileptic activity.
   c. Determine (from family member) if there is a history of epilepsy, alcohol/drug use, trauma, recent infection.

2. Be familiar with state laws.
3. Assess home environment for safety hazards in case the patient falls, such as crowded furniture arrangement, sharp edges on tables, glass. Soft flooring and furniture and padded surfaces may be necessary.
4. Support patient in discussion about seizures with employer, school, and so forth.

Patient Education and Health Maintenance
1. Encourage the patient to determine existence of trigger factors for seizures (eg, skipped meals, lack of sleep, emotional stress).

2. Remind the patient of the importance of following medication regimen.
3. Tell the patient to avoid alcohol, because it interferes with metabolism of antiepileptic medications.
4. Encourage the patient and family to discuss feelings and attitudes about epilepsy.
5. Encourage patient to carry/wear a Medic-Alert card or bracelet.
6. Encourage a moderate lifestyle that includes exercise, mental activity, and nutritional diet.
7. For the surgical candidate, reinforce instructions related to surgical outcome of the specific surgical approach (temporal lobectomy, corpus callosotomy, hemispherectomy, and extratemporal resection).
8. Refer the patient/family for more information and support to such agencies as:
   The Epilepsy Foundation of America
   300 East Joppa Road
   Suite 1103
   Towson, MD 21286
   800-492-2523

Outcome-Based Evaluation
- Taking medication as ordered, drug level within normal range
- No injuries observed
- Reports using support services and stress management techniques

◼ Narcolepsy

Narcolepsy is a neurologic disorder characterized by abnormalities of rapid eye movement (REM) sleep, some abnormalities of non-REM (NREM) sleep, and excessive daytime somnolence.

Pathophysiology and Etiology
1. Pathology associated with neurotransmitters in REM sleep. Increased frequency of sleep-onset, rapid eye movement periods (SOREMP).
2. Genetic susceptibility—associated with class II human leukocyte antigens (HLAs).
3. Although considered a hypersomnia disorder, the person does not experience excessive amounts of sleep in a 24-hour period.
4. Onset is usually between ages 15 and 25.

Clinical Manifestations
1. Four classic symptoms (all symptoms not present in all patients):
   a. Excessive daytime sleepiness (usually first symptom)
   b. Cataplexy (abrupt loss of muscle tone after emotional stimulation such as laughter, anger)
   c. Sleep paralysis (powerless to move limbs, speak, open eyes, or breathe deeply while fully aware of condition)
   d. Hypnagogic hallucinations associated with drowsiness before sleep, usually visual or auditory
2. Symptoms enhanced by high temperature, indoor activity, and idleness.

3. Clinical manifestations may abate, but never phase out completely.
4. Patient may complain of inability to focus vision or thought process rather than have a feeling of sleepiness.
5. Nocturnal sleep disturbance—occurs 2½ to 3 hours after falling asleep.
   a. After being awake for 45 to 60 minutes, the patient will fall back to sleep for another 2½ to 3 hours and then awaken again.
   b. This is believed to be the source of the daytime somnolence.

Diagnostic Evaluation
1. Polysomnograph to assess nighttime sleep—indicates the underlying cause for the complaint of sleepiness
2. Multisleep latency test (MSLT) to assess daytime sleepiness—indicates severity of the problem

Management
1. Mutual goal setting, because not everyone derives benefit from treatment. Even with medication, patients may never attain normal levels of alertness.
2. Nonpharmacologic therapy: support groups, short naps (10 to 20 minutes, three times daily), caffeinated beverages, exercise, and avoidance of heavy meals.
3. Stimulants: pemoline (Cylert), methylphenidate (Ritalin), dextroamphetamine (Dexedrine), methamphetamine (Desoxyn)
4. Antidepressants for cataplexy; protriptyline (Vivactil), desipramine (Norpramin), fluoxetine (Prozac).

Complications
1. Injury related to falling asleep
2. Psychosocial problems such as disturbed relationships, loss of employment, depression

Nursing Assessment
1. Obtain history of sleep and activity pattern.
2. Assess emotional status and social interactions.
3. Assess response to medication and lifestyle treatment.

Nursing Diagnoses
- Sleep Pattern Disturbance related to disease process
- Fatigue related to disrupted nighttime sleep
- Ineffective Individual Coping related to interference with activity

Nursing Interventions
Promoting Normal Sleep–Wake Cycle
1. Review daily schedule to determine periods of sleep and cataplexy.
2. Help patient establish nondrug therapies (exercise, diet) that will fit into lifestyle.
3. Administer or teach self-administration of prescribed medications.
   a. Advise of side effects of amphetamines, such as nervousness, irritability, tremors, and GI upset.
   b. Warn patient to take only as prescribed and to not increase dosage because of tolerance and drug dependence.

Reducing Fatigue
1. Schedule 10- to 20-minute rest periods two to three times/day.
   a. Help patient incorporate naps into lifestyle.
2. Encourage patient to incorporate small amounts of caffeinated beverages at intervals, and smaller, more frequent meals rather than large, heavy meals during the day to maintain energy.
3. Plan diversional activities and relaxation during fatigued periods.

Strengthening Coping
1. Encourage active participation in selection of treatment modalities.
2. Assist patient in identifying trigger factors of worsening symptoms.
3. Teach problem-solving strategy to promote sense of control over activities and symptoms during the day.
4. Review patient coping mechanisms, and reinforce positive ones.
5. Encourage use of support groups and community resources.

Patient Education and Health Maintenance
1. Review the normal sleep cycle and the pathophysiology of narcolepsy.
2. Stress the importance of nonpharmacologic measures as an adjunct to treatment.
3. Inform the patient of rights of employment conditions under the Americans with Disabilities Act.
4. Advise caution with using alcohol, working with machinery, or using dangerous equipment to prevent injury to self or others during sleepiness or cataplexy.
5. If patient drives, advise using caution and avoiding lengthy trips.
6. Encourage patient to wear a Medic-Alert bracelet.
7. Encourage follow-up with health care provider, specialist, and mental health counselor as needed.

Outcome-Based Evaluation
- Patient complying with medication regimen
- Reports working without undue fatigue
- Identifying trigger factors

Headache Syndromes

Headaches are one of the most common complaints of people seeking health care. Pain in the head is a symptom of underlying pathology. Most chronic headaches are *tension/muscle contraction headaches, migraine headaches,* or *cluster headaches.* Acute severe headaches may be a symptom of serious neurologic disease. Identifying the etiology of headaches requires an understanding of the characteristics of each type of headache.

Pathophysiology and Etiology

1. Tension/muscle contraction
   a. Due to irritation of sensitive nerve endings in the head, jaw, and neck from prolonged muscle contraction in the face, head, and neck.
   b. Precipitating factors include fatigue, stress, poor posture.
   c. Characterized by hatband distribution.
2. Migraine headache
   a. Hyperactivity to the neurotransmitter serotonin.
   b. Familial predisposition.
   c. Consists of initial vasospasm, then dilation of intracranial and extracranial arteries.
   d. Migraine attack may consist of any of five phases: prodrome, aura, headache, resolution, and postdrome.
   e. Migraines are labeled with or without aura (usually visual); aura is due to reduced cortical neuronal activity.
   f. Migraines occur in 10% of Americans.
3. Cluster headaches
   a. Usually unilateral, recurring.
   b. Occur mostly in men.
   c. Release of increased histamine results in vasodilation.
4. Other headaches
   a. Traction-inflammation—due to infection such as meningitis, encephalitis, increased or decreased ICP, lesions.
   b. Temporal arteritis—attributed to autoimmune disorder; inflammation of arterial wall; may result in vision loss due to involvement of the ophthalmic nerve. Usually occurs in persons over age 50.
   c. Sinus headache—results from inflammation of one or more of the paranasal sinuses.

Clinical Manifestations

1. Tension/muscle contraction: dull, bandlike, constricting, persistent pain and pressure in the back of the head and neck, across forehead, bitemporal areas; may be tender points of head or neck.
2. Migraine: sensory, motor, or mood alterations precede headache; gradual onset of severe unilateral, throbbing headache, may become bilateral.
   a. With classic migraine, characteristic aura may include scintillating scotoma (area of decreased vision surrounded by area of less abnormal or normal vision with zigzag appearance), hemianopia (loss of half of field of vision) and paresthesias; usually lasts less than a day.
   b. Headache follows aura in less than an hour.
   c. With common migraine, nausea, vomiting, and photophobia may accompany headache; may last 4 to 72 hours and leave the person with limited food tolerance.
   d. May be triggered in women by hormonal fluctuations (menses, pregnancy).
3. Cluster headache: pain is sudden, sharp, burning, excruciating, unilateral, always involving facial area from neck to temple, and often occurs during the evening or night.
   a. Occurs in clusters of 2 to 8 weeks followed by headache-free periods.
   b. Associated with unilateral excessive tearing, redness of the eye, stuffiness of nostril on affected side, facial swelling, flushing, and sweating.
   c. Attacks last several minutes to several hours. Multiple attacks may occur in 1 day.
4. Temporal arteritis: unilateral or bilateral pain, particularly severe at night, with tender temporal arteries.
5. Sinus headache: pain is usually felt over sinus areas, above eyes, along the side of the nose, and behind ears or may be referred to points on the head.
   a. May or may not be accompanied by varying degrees of congestion, nasal drainage, postnasal drip, and other symptoms.

Diagnostic Evaluation

1. Skull/sinus films to rule out lesions, sinusitis
2. CT/MRI scan to rule out lesions, hemorrhage, chronic sinusitis
3. Erythrocyte sedimentation rate (ESR) and other blood studies to help determine inflammatory process with temporal arteritis

Management

Pharmacologic Treatment

Medications are intended to reduce the frequency, severity, and duration of the headache. Effectiveness of medication is individualized. Some persons may need a combination of medications.

1. Aspirin, acetaminophen, and nonsteroidal anti-inflammatory drugs for mild to moderate pain of tension, sinus, or mild vascular headaches.
2. Some drugs may abort vascular headaches if taken at the onset, including methysergide (Sansert), a serotonin antagonist; ergotamine (Ergostat), a vasoconstrictor; or sumatriptan (Imitrex), a 5HT agonist.
3. Sumatriptan is available in subcutaneous injection as well as oral form.
4. Other oral 5HT agonists include zolmitriptan (Zomig), naratriptan (Amerge), and rizatriptan (Maxalt).

> ◆ **DRUG ALERT**
>
> **Vasoconstrictors and 5HT agonists used to abort vascular headaches are contraindicated in patients with uncontrolled hypertension, coronary artery disease, and peripheral vascular disease.**

5. Inhalation of 100% oxygen may abort a cluster headache.
6. Some drugs may be used continuously as prophylactic treatment for recurrent migraines, including beta blockers, calcium channel blockers, and tricyclic antidepressants.

7. Antihistamines and decongestants may be effective for sinus headaches.

8. Corticosteroids may be used for temporal arteritis.

9. Occasionally, narcotic analgesics, muscle relaxants, and antianxiety agents may be needed for severe pain.

Nonpharmacologic Management

1. Relaxation techniques, guided imagery, paced breathing.

2. Biofeedback, cognitive therapy.

3. Trigger identification and control of such factors as intake of alcohol (red wine), skipped meals, over- or undersleeping.

4. To prevent migraine: avoidance of monosodium glutamate (MSG), mixed spices such as "seasoned salt," nitrates and nitrites commonly contained in bacon, hot dogs, or deli meats.

5. Rest in a quiet, dark room at onset of headache.

6. If caffeine user, spread caffeine intake evenly over the day.

7. Routine exercise program.

Complications

1. Usually none.

Nursing Assessment

1. Obtain a history of related symptoms, triggering factors, degree of pain, and medications used.

2. Perform a complete neurologic examination to detect any focal deficits or signs of increased ICP that indicate tumor or hemorrhage.

3. Assess coping mechanisms and emotional status.

Nursing Diagnoses

- Pain related to headache
- Ineffective Individual Coping related to chronic and/or disabling pain

Nursing Interventions

Controlling Pain

1. Reduce environmental stimuli: light, noise, movement.

2. Suggest light massage to tight muscles in neck, scalp, back for tension headaches.

3. Apply warm, moist heat to areas of muscle tension.

4. Encourage patient to lie down and attempt to sleep.

5. Teach progressive muscle relaxation to treat and prevent tension headaches.
   a. Alternately tense and relax each group of muscles for a count of 5, starting with the forehead and working downward to the feet.
   b. Try to maintain state of relaxation of each muscle group until whole body feels relaxed.
   c. Relaxation of just head and neck may also be helpful if time is limited.

6. Teach patient the cause of headache and proper use of medication.

7. Encourage adequate rest once headache is relieved to recover from fatigue of the pain.

Promoting Positive Coping

1. Encourage patient to become aware of triggering factors and early symptoms of headache, so headache can be prevented or promptly treated.

2. Encourage adequate nutrition, rest and relaxation, and avoidance of stress and overexertion to better cope with headaches.

3. Implement problem solving to help patient manage problems that arise in social or work situations related to headaches.

4. Review coping mechanisms, and strengthen positive ones.

Patient Education and Health Maintenance

1. Teach proper administration of medication.
   a. Self-injection of sumatriptan (Imitrex) given subcutaneously with autoinjector.
   b. Inhalation of ergotamine (Ergostat) through metered-dose inhaler.

2. Teach side effects of medications.
   a. GI upset, gastritis, and possible ulcer formation with nonsteroidal anti-inflammatory drugs—take with food.
   b. Numbness, coldness, paresthesias, and pain of extremities with ergot derivatives—report to health care provider.
   c. Chest pain, wheezing, flushing with sumatriptan (Imitrex)—report to health care provider.
   d. Hypotension with beta blockers and calcium channel blockers—arise slowly, do not exceed prescribed dosage, do not discontinue beta blockers abruptly.

3. Advise avoidance of alcohol, which can worsen headaches.

4. Teach about foods that are high in tyramine that may trigger migraines—aged cheese, red wine, liver.

Outcome-Based Evaluation

- Patient reports fewer, less severe headaches
- Describes use of positive coping mechanisms

■ Herniated Intervertebral Disk (Ruptured Disk)

Herniation of the intervertebral disk is a protrusion of the nucleus of the disk into the annulus (fibrous ring around the disk) with subsequent nerve compression. The herniation may occur in any portion of the vertebral column (Figure 15-7).

Pathophysiology and Etiology

1. The intervertebral disk is a cartilaginous plate made up of gelatinous material in the center, known as the nucleus pulposus, and is encapsulated in the fibrous annulus.

2. Risk factors for herniation include:
   a. Degeneration (aging), trauma, and congenital predisposition
   b. Biomechanical factors, such as twisting and repetitive motions in occupational settings

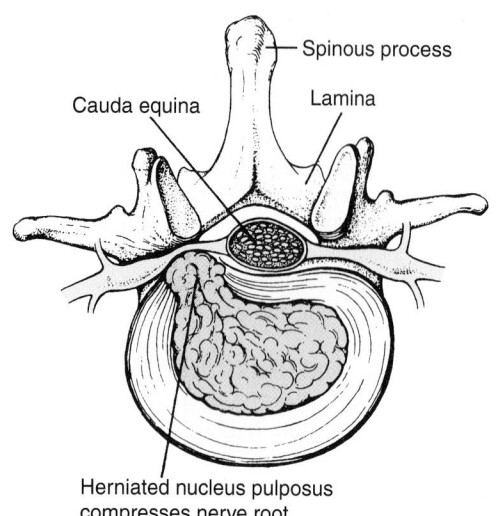

FIGURE 15-7 Ruptured vertebral disk. (Chaffee, E.E. & Greisheimer, E.M. *Basic physiology and anatomy* [3rd ed.]. Philadelphia: J.B. Lippincott.)

c. Sedentary occupations
d. Obesity
e. Smoking
3. The herniation compresses the spinal nerve root on one side and, with further degeneration of the disk, may eventually produce pressure on the spinal cord.
4. This sequence may take months to years, producing acute and chronic symptoms.

Clinical Manifestations
General Considerations
1. An intervertebral disk may herniate without causing symptoms.
2. Symptoms depend on location, size, rate of development, and effect on surrounding structures.
3. Most symptomatic disk herniations result in pain, sensory changes, loss of reflex, and muscle weakness that resolve without surgery.

Cervical
1. Pain and stiffness in the neck, top of shoulders, and region of the scapula
2. Pain in upper extremities and head
3. Paresthesias and numbness of upper extremities
4. Weakness of upper extremities

Lumbar
1. Low back pain with varying degrees of sensory and motor dysfunction.
2. Pain radiating from the low back into the buttocks and down the leg.
3. Postural deformity of the lumbar spine.
4. Positive straight-leg raise test: pain occurs in leg below the knee when leg raised from a supine position.

5. Weakness and asymmetric reflexes.
6. Sensory loss.

NURSING ALERT

Cauda equina syndrome is an emergency caused by compression of the cauda equina area of the spinal cord. Symptoms include bowel, bladder, or sexual dysfunction or saddle area numbness. It must be recognized early, and compression must be relieved to prevent permanent loss of these functions.

Diagnostic Evaluation
1. Myelogram—demonstrates herniation and pressure on spinal cord or nerve roots
2. CT or MRI—demonstrates herniation; MRI has greater sensitivity
3. Electromyography—localizes specific spinal nerve involvement

Management
Supportive Measures
1. Conservative treatment 4 to 6 weeks, if no progressive neurologic deficit.
2. Bed rest on a firm mattress (2 days usually sufficient).
3. Heat or ice massage to affected area.
4. Cervical collar or possibly cervical traction are widely used, although efficacy is not proven.
5. Physical therapy.

Pharmacotherapy
1. Anti-inflammatory drugs, such as ibuprofen (Motrin) or prednisone (Orasone).
2. Muscle relaxants, such as diazepam (Valium) or cyclobenzaprine (Flexeril).
3. Analgesics, narcotics may be necessary during acute phase.

Surgical Intervention
1. May be done if there is progression of neurologic deficit or failure to improve with conservative management.
2. Surgical procedures include diskectomy (decompression of nerve root), laminectomy, spinal fusion, microdiskectomy, and percutaneous diskectomy.

Chemonucleolysis
1. Less common invasive treatment for lumbar disk herniation
2. Injection of chymopapain (Chymodiactin) into herniated disk that produces loss of water and proteoglycans from the disk, reducing the size of the disk and subsequent pressure on the nerve root
3. May cause severe complications such as transverse myelitis, allergic reactions, persistent muscle spasm

Alternative and Complementary Measures
1. Acupuncture
2. Manipulative therapy
3. Massage therapy for adjunct pain relief
4. Homeopathic remedies
5. Various nutritional supplements

Complications

1. Permanent neurologic dysfunction (weakness, numbness)
2. Chronic pain with associated psychosocial issues
3. Cauda equina syndrome

Nursing Assessment

1. Perform repeated assessments of motor function, sensation, and reflexes to determine progression of condition.
2. Assess level at which straight-leg raise test is positive; generally, radiation of pain below knee at 45 degrees of elevation is considered positive for nerve root involvement; positive at lesser elevation may indicate worsening condition.
3. Assess pain level on scale of 1 to 10.

Nursing Diagnoses

- Pain related to area of compression
- Impaired Physical Mobility related to pain and disease physiology

Nursing Interventions

Minimizing Pain

1. Administer or teach self-administration of anti-inflammatory drugs as prescribed and with food or antacid to prevent GI upset.
2. Administer or teach self-administration of prescribed muscle relaxant; observe safety, because drowsiness may result.
3. Administer or teach self-administration of analgesics as prescribed; be prepared for sedation.
4. Use bedboards under mattress and maintain bed rest except for short trips to bathroom; maintain supine or low-Fowler's position or side-lying position with slight knee flexion and pillow between knees.
5. Apply moist heat to affected area of back as desired.
6. Encourage relaxation techniques, such as imagery and progressive muscle relaxation.

Maintaining Mobility

1. Encourage range-of-motion exercises while in bed.
2. Properly fit and use a cervical collar (if appropriate to level of injury).
3. Apply a back brace or cervical skin traction, if ordered.
4. Inspect skin several times a day, especially under stabilization devices, for redness and evidence of pressure sore development.
5. Provide massage and good skin care to pressure-prone areas.
6. Assist patient with activities at bedside, and discourage lifting or straining of any kind.
7. Encourage compliance with physical therapy treatments and activity restrictions as ordered.

Community and Home Care Considerations

1. Encourage lifestyle changes if needed—smoking cessation, weight reduction.
2. Demonstrate and encourage aerobic exercise, back strengthening, and endurance exercises.
3. Ensure that patient avoids heavy lifting and uses proper body mechanics around the house.
4. Discourage prolonged bed rest and inactivity.
5. Refer for vocational counseling, if indicated.
6. If cervical skin traction is ordered for home use, teach the patient how to apply the chin strap and head halter. The weight should hang freely over the back of a chair or doorknob near the head of the bed. Make sure the patient maintains proper alignment of the neck and removes traction before moving the head.

Care of the Patient Having Disk Surgery

Preparing the Patient for Surgery

1. Educate patient about surgical procedure.
   a. Procedure is generally short.
   b. Small incision will be made on back of neck; second incision will be on hip if bone graft is taken from iliac crest for spinal fusion.
   c. Routine postoperative care will include frequent assessment of vital signs and neurologic function, frequent turning and deep breathing, pain control, and ambulation on the first postoperative day.
2. Document baseline neurologic assessment to compare with after surgery.
3. Explain your actions to patient as you shave operative area, administer preoperative medications, and perform any other preoperative order.

Preventing Complications Postoperatively

1. Monitor vital signs and surgical dressing frequently, because hemorrhage is a possible complication.
2. Assess movement and sensation of extremities, report any new deficit.
3. Administer analgesics and steroid medications to control pain from incision and swelling around nerve roots and spinal cord due to surgery.
4. Maintain cervical collar if ordered.
5. Log-roll patient to reposition frequently and encourage coughing and deep breathing.
6. Position for comfort with small pillow under head (but avoid extreme neck flexion) and pillow under knees to take pressure off lower back.
7. Provide fluids as soon as gag reflex and bowel sounds are noted.
8. Assess for hoarseness, indicating that cervical surgery has resulted in recurrent laryngeal nerve injury; may cause ineffective cough.
9. Watch for dysphagia due to edema of the esophagus, and provide blenderized diet.
10. Ensure that patient voids after surgery; report urinary retention.
11. Encourage ambulation as soon as possible by having patient lie on side close to edge of bed and push up with arms while swinging legs toward floor in one motion; alternate walking with bed rest, discourage sitting.
12. Report any sudden reappearance of radicular pain (may indicate nerve root compression from slipping of

bone graft or collapsing of disk space) or burning back pain radiating to buttocks (may indicate arachnoiditis).

Patient Education and Health Maintenance

1. Educate patient regarding lifestyle changes—smoking cessation, increased activity, loss of weight.
2. Provide instructions regarding back anatomy and back care to reduce symptoms.
3. Teach patient the importance of complying with bed rest, use of cervical collar, and other conservative measures to try to reduce inflammation and heal disk herniation.
4. Tell patient who has had a cervical disk herniation to avoid extreme flexion, extension, or rotation of the neck and to keep the head in neutral position during sleep.
5. Encourage the patient with a lumbar disk herniation to remain on bed rest at home with ambulation to the bathroom only until inflammation and pain are sufficiently reduced; then ambulation can be increased, but lifting and sitting are discouraged.
6. Encourage patient to do stretching and strengthening exercises of extremities and abdomen after acute symptoms have subsided. The back can be gently stretched by lying on the back and bringing the knees up toward the chest.
7. Teach the patient about proper body mechanics and the use of leg and abdominal muscles rather than the back. Knees should be bent on lifting, and load should carried close to midtrunk.
8. Encourage follow-up with physical therapy as indicated for reconditioning and work hardening.
9. Tell patient to avoid the prone position, long car rides, and sitting in a soft chair.
10. Instruct the patient to report any changes in neurologic function or recurrence of radicular pain.
11. Encourage good nutrition, avoidance of obesity, and proper rest to reduce risk of recurrence.

Outcome-Based Evaluation

- Patient verbalizes reduced pain
- Maintains mobility with active lifestyle

SELECTED REFERENCES

Albers, G. W., et al. (2000). Intravenous tissue-type plasminogen activator for treatment of acute stroke: The Standard Treatment with Alteplase to Reverse Stroke (STARS) study. *Journal of the American Medical Association, 283*(5), 1145–1150.

Aldrich, M. (1998). Diagnostic aspects of narcolepsy. *Neurology, 50*(Suppl. 1), S2–S7.

American Association of Neuroscience Nurses. (1996). *Core curriculum for neuroscience nursing* (3rd ed.). Chicago: AANN.

Barker, F., & Janetta, P. (1996). The long-term outcome of microvascular decompression for trigeminal neuralgia. *New England Journal of Medicine, 334*(17), 1077–1083.

Barnett, H. J. M., et al. (2000). Causes and severity of ischemic stroke in patients with internal carotid artery stenosis. *Journal of the American Medical Association, 283*(6), 1429–1436.

Barnwell, A., & Kavanagh, D. (1997). Prediction of psychological adjustment to multiple sclerosis. *Social Science & Medicine, 45*(3), 411–418.

Bergman, S. B., Yarkoney, G. M., & Stiens, S. A. (1997). Spinal cord injury rehabilitation. Medical complications. *Archives of Physical Medical Rehabilitation, 78*(Suppl.), S53–S58.

Bisnaire, D. (1998). Nursing research in stroke: A review. *Axone, 20*(1), 10–13.

Bisnaire, D., & Robinson, L. (1997). Accuracy of leveling intraventricular collection drainage systems. *Journal of Neuroscience Nursing, 29*(4), 261–268.

Brimioulle, S., Moraine, J., Norrenberg, D., & Kahn, R. (1997). Effects of positioning and exercise on intracranial pressure in a neurosurgical intensive care unit. *Physical Therapy, 77*(12), 1682–1689.

Bryant, G. (2000). When spinal cord injury affects the bowel. *RN, 63*(2), 26–29.

Campbell, P., & Edwards, S. (1997). Hyperdynamic therapy: The nurse's role in the treatment of cerebral vasospasm. *Journal of Neuroscience Nursing, 29*(5), 318–324.

Caplan, L. (1997). New therapies for stroke. *Archives of Neurology, 54*(10), 1222–1224.

Cawley, M., Marburger, R., & Earl, G. (1998). Investigational neuroprotective drugs in traumatic brain injury. *Journal of Neuroscience Nursing, 30*(6), 369–374.

Choo, K., & Guilleminault, C. (1998). Narcolepsy and idiopathic hypersomnolence. *Clinics in Chest Medicine, 19*(1), 169–181.

Chotikul, L. (2000). Spinal implants. *RN, 63*(5), 26–31.

Chow, T., & Cummings, L. (1998). Treatment of depression in the patient with Parkinson's disease. *Clinical Geriatrics, 6*(11), 34–35, 39–41, 45–46.

Collice, M. (1999). Multidisciplinary (surgical and endovascular) approach to intracranial aneurysms. *Journal of Neurosurgical Sciences, 42*(Suppl. 1), 131–140.

Consortium for Spinal Cord Medicine. (1998). *Depression following spinal cord injury: A clinical practice guideline for primary care physicians.* Washington, DC: Paralyzed Veterans of America.

———. (1998). *Neurogenic bowel management in adults with spinal cord injury. Clinical practice guidelines.* Washington, DC: Paralyzed Veterans of America.

———. (1997). *Acute management of autonomic dysreflexia: Adults with spinal cord injury presenting to health-care facilities. Clinical practice guidelines.* Washington, DC: Paralyzed Veterans of America.

———. (1997). *Prevention of thromboembolism in spinal cord injury. Clinical practice guidelines.* Washington, DC: Paralyzed Veterans of America.

Cunning, S. (2000). When the Dx is myasthenia gravis. *RN, 63*(4), 26–30.

DiFabio, R., Soderberg, J., Choi, T., Hansen, C., & Schapiro, R. (1998). Extended outpatient rehabilitation: Its influence on symptom frequency, fatigue, and functional status for persons with progressive multiple sclerosis. *Archives of Physical Medicine & Rehabilitation 79*(2), 141–146.

Dorsher, P. (1997). Evaluation and treatment of low back pain. *Journal of Florida Medical Association, 84*(1), 24–27.

Dubowitz, V. (1989). *Color atlas of muscle disorders in childhood.* Chicago: Year Book Medical Publishers.

Duff, D., & Wells, D. (1997). Postcomatose unawareness/vegetative state following severe brain injury: A content methodology. *Journal of Neuroscience Nursing, 29*(5), 305–317.

Duncan, B., & Siegal, A. (1998). Early diagnosis and management of Alzheimer's disease. *Journal of Clinical Psychiatry, 59*(Suppl. 9), 15–21.

Eide, P. K. (1998). Pathophysiological mechanisms of central neuropathic pain after spinal cord injury. *Spinal Cord, 36*, 601–612.

Faerber, E. N., & Roman, N. V. (1997). Central nervous system tumors of childhood. *Pediatric Oncology Imaging, 35*(6), 1301–1328.

Formal, C. S., Cawley, M. F., & Steins, S. A. (1997). Spinal cord injury rehabilitation. Functional outcomes. *Archives of Physical Medicine and Rehabilitation, 78*(Suppl.), S59–S64.

Fox, S. (1999). Neuralgic mechanisms in traumatic brain injury. *Journal of Neuroscience Nursing, 31*(2), 87–96.

———. (1998). The use of a quality of life instrument to improve assessment of brain tumor patients in an outpatient setting, *Journal of Neuroscience Nursing, 30*(5), 322–325.

Frymoyer, J. (1988). Back pain and sciatica. *New England Journal of Medicine, 318*(5), 291–300.

Geldmacher, D., & Whitehouse, P. (1997). Differential diagnosis of Alzheimer's disease. *Neurology, 48*(Suppl. 6), S2–S9.

Geraci, E., & Geraci, T. (1996). A look at recent hyperventilation studies: Outcomes and recommendations for early use in head-injured patient. *Journal of Neuroscience Nursing, 28*(4), 222–224, 229–233.

Gilman, S. (1998). Imaging the brain. *New England Journal of Medicine, 338*(12), 812–820.

Goldsmith, C. (1998). Continuing education. Advances in treatment for Parkinson's disease. *Nurseweek, 11*(4), 12–3, 19.

Gordon, S., & Morrison, C. (1998). Fibromyalgia and its primary care complications. *MEDSURG Nursing, 7*(4), 207–213, 216.

Gulick, E. (1998). Symptom and activities of daily living trajectory in multiple sclerosis: A 10-year study. *Nursing Research, 47*(3), 137–146.

———. (1997). Correlates of quality of life among persons with multiple sclerosis. *Nursing Research, 46*(6), 305–311.

Gutierrez, K. M., & Prober, C. G. (1998). Encephalitis: Identifying the specific cause is key to effective management. *Postgraduate Medicine, 103*(3), 123–143.

Gutmann, D. H., Aylsworth, A., Carey, J. C., Korf, B., Marks, J., Pyeritz, R. E., Rubenstein, A., & Viskochil, D. (1997). The diagnostic evaluation and multidisciplinary management of neurofibromatosis 1 and neurofibromatosis 2. *Journal of the American Medical Association, 278*(1), 51–57.

Hart, R. G., et al. (2000). Aspirin for the primary prevention of stroke and other major vascular events: Meat-analysis and hypotheses. *Archives of Neurology, 57*(3), 326–332.

Heath, D. (1999). Secondary mechanisms in traumatic brain injury: A nurse's perspective. *Journal of Neuroscience Nursing, 31*(2), 97–103.

Heye, M. L. (1997). Pain assessment in elders: Practical tips. *Nurse Practitioner Forum, 8*(4), 133–139.

Hickey, J. V. (1993). *The clinical practice of neurological and neurosurgical nursing.* Philadelphia: J. B. Lippincott,

Hodgson, T. (1998). Proximal aneurysms in association with arteriovenous malformations: Do they resolve following obliteration of the malformation with stereotactic radiosurgery? *British Journal of Neurosurgery, 12*(5), 434–437.

Hudak, C., & Gallo, B. (1997). Quick review of neurodiagnostic testing. *American Journal of Nursing, 97*(7), 16CC–16FF.

Indications for Polysomnography Task Force, American Sleep Disorders Association Standards of Practice Committee. (1997). Practice parameters for the indications for polysomnography and related procedures. *Sleep, 20*(6), 406–422.

Koller, W., & Montgomery, E. (1997). Issues in the early diagnosis of Parkinson's disease. *Neurology, 49*(1), S10–S25.

Kuether, T. (1999). Clinical and angiographic outcomes, with treatment data, for patients with cerebral aneurysms treated with Guglielmi detachable coils: A single center experience. *Neurosurgery, 43*(5), 1016–1025.

Levitz, R. E. (1998). Herpes simplex encephalitis: A review. *Heart & Lung, 27*(3), 209–212.

Lightner, D. J. (1998). Contemporary urologic management of patients with spinal cord injury. *Mayo Clinic Proceedings, 73*(5), 434–438.

Loblaw, D. A., & Laperriere, N. J. (1998). Emergency treatment of malignant extradural spinal cord compression: An evidence-based guideline. *Journal of Clinical Oncology, 16*(4), 1613–1624.

Loeb, J. L. (1999). Pain management in long-term care. *American Journal of Nursing, 99*(2), 48–52.

Mathisen, G. E., & Johnson, J. P. (1997). Brain abscess. *Clinical Infectious Diseases, 25,* 763–781.

McGuinness, S., & Peters, S. (1999). The diagnosis of multiple sclerosis: Peplau's Interpersonal Relations Model in practice. *Rehabilitation Nursing, 24*(1), 30–33.

McMahon-Parkes, K., & Cormock, M. (1997). Guillain-Barré syndrome: Biological basis, treatment, and care. *Intensive & Critical Care Nursing, 13*(1), 42–48.

Meythaler, J. (1997). Rehabilitation of Guillain-Barré syndrome. *Archives of Physical Medicine and Rehabilitation, 78*(8), 872–879.

Morgenlander, J. C. (1997). Recognizing peripheral neuropathy: How to read the clues to an underlying cause. *Postgraduate Medicine, 102*(3), 71–80.

Morrison, S. (1997). Guglielmi detachable coils: An alternative therapy for surgically high risk aneurysms. *Journal of Neuroscience Nursing, 29*(4), 232–237.

Multiple Sclerosis Council. (1998). *Fatigue and multiple sclerosis. Evidence-based management strategies for fatigue in multiple sclerosis. Clinical practice guidelines.* Washington, DC: Paralyzed Veterans of America.

Nikas, D. L. (1995). Commentary on cerebral perfusion pressure: Management protocol and clinical results. *AACN Nursing Scan in Critical Care, 16*(3), 13.

Noble, J., Munro, C. A., Prasad, V. S. S. V., & Midha, R. (1998). Analysis of upper and lower extremity peripheral nerve injuries in a population of patients with multiple injuries. *The Journal of Trauma: Injury, Infection, and Critical Care, 45*(1), 116–122.

Nowotny, M. (1999). My hourly journey with amyotrophic lateral sclerosis. *Journal of Neuroscience Nursing, 30*(1), 68–70.

Ozuna, J. (1997). Pharmacologic management of epilepsy: An update. *Journal of Neuroscience Nursing, 29*(5), 330–337.

Phillips, E. J., & Simor, A. E. (1998). Bacterial meningitis in children and adults. *Postgraduate Medicine, 103*(3), 102–117.

Reddy, M., & Reddy, V. (1997). Stroke rehabilitation. *American Family Physician, 55*(5), 1742–1748.

Richards, K. C., Gibson, R., & Overton-McCoy, A. L. (2000). Effects of massage in acute and critical care. *AACN Clinical Issues, 11*(1), 77–96.

Rosenblum, D., & Saffir, M. (1998). The natural history of multiple sclerosis and its diagnosis. *Physical Medicine and Rehabilitation Clinics of North America , 9*(3), 537–549.

Sackley, C., & Gladman, J. (1998). The evidence for rehabilitation after severely disabling stroke. *Physical Therapy Review, 3*(1), 19–29.

Schurch, B., Wichmann, W., & Rossier, A. B. (1996). Post-traumatic syringomyelia (cystic myelopathy): A prospective study of 449 patients with spinal cord injury. *Journal of Neurology, Neurosurgery and Psychiatry, 60*(1), 61–67.

Sementilli, M. (1999, July/August). Targeting the beast: Meeting the challenge of treating those with MTBI. *Continuing Care,* 30–35.

Siddall, P. J., Taylor, D. A., & Cousins, M. J. (1997). Classification of pain following spinal cord injury. *Spinal Cord, 35,* 69–75.

Simmon, J. M. (1996). Chronic pain syndrome: Nursing assessment and intervention. *Rehabilitation Nursing, 21*(1), 13–37.

Simmons, B. J. (1997). Management of intracranial hemodynamics in the adult: A research analysis of head positioning and recommendations for clinical practice and future research. *Journal of Neuroscience Nursing, 29*(1), 44–49.

Small, G., & Leiter, F. (1998). Neuroimaging for diagnosis of dementia. *Journal of Clinical Psychiatry, 59*(Suppl. 11), 4–7.

Souder, E., & Alavi, A. (1995). A comparison of neuroimaging modalities for diagnosing dementia. *Nurse Practitioner, 20*(1), 66–74.

Stewart-Amidei, C. (1998). The 1998 neuro-oncology symposium: New horizons, new hope. *Journal of Neuroscience Nursing, 30*(6), 361–368.

Stewart-Amidei, C. (1996). Epilepsy: Abstracts from the 1996 neuroscience nursing clinical symposium. *Journal of Neuroscience Nursing, 28*(6), 388–398.

Tapper, V. (1997). Pathophysiology, assessment and treatment of Parkinson's disease. *The Nurse Practitioner, 22*(7), 76, 78, 80.

Toyota, B. (1999). The efficacy of an abbreviated course of nimodipine in patients with good-grade aneurysmal subarachnoid hemorrhage. *Journal of Neurosurgery, 90*(2), 203–206.

Vickers, L., & O'Neill, C. (1998). An interdisciplinary home healthcare program for patients with Parkinson's disease. *Rehabilitation Nursing, 23*(6), 236–239.

Wantanabe, T. (1996). Urodynamics of spinal cord injury. *Urologic Clinics of North America, 23*(3), 459–473.

Ward-Smith, P. (1997). Stereotactic radiosurgery for malignant brain tumors: The patient's perspective. *Journal of Neuroscience Nursing, 29*(2), 117–122.

Watchmaker, G. P., & Mackinnon, S. E. (1997). Advances in peripheral nerve repair. *Hand Surgery Update II, 24*(1), 63–73.

Whetten-Goldstein, K., Sloan, F., Kulas, E., Cutson, T., & Schenkman, M. (1997). The burden of Parkinson's disease on society, family, and the individual. *Journal of the American Geriatrics Society, 45*(7), 844–849.

Winkelman, C. (1999). A review of pharmacodynamics and pharmacokinetics in seizure management. *Journal of Neuroscience Nursing, 31*(1), 50–53.

Worsham, T. L. (2000). Easing the course of Guillian-Barré syndrome. *RN, 63*(3), 46–50.

Yamashita, T., Ishii, S., & Usui, M. (1998). Pain relief after nerve resection for post-traumatic neuralgia. *Journal of Bone and Joint Surgery (Br), 80*(3), 499–503.

Yarkony, G. M., Formal, C. S., & Cawley, M. F. (1997). Spinal cord injury rehabilitation: Assessment and management during acute care. *Archives of Physical Medicine Rehabilitation, 78*, S48–S52.

INTRODUCTORY INFORMATION

◼ Definition of Terms

1. *Vision:* Passage of rays of light from an object through the cornea, aqueous humor, lens, and vitreous humor to the retina, and its appreciation in the cerebral cortex.
2. *Emmetropia:* Normal vision: rays of light coming from an object at a distance of 6 m (20 ft) or more are brought to focus on the retina by the lens (Figure 16-1).
3. *Ametropia:* Abnormal vision.
   a. *Myopia:* Nearsightedness: rays of light coming from an object at a distance of 6 m (20 ft) or more are brought to a focus in front of the retina (see Figure 16-1).
   b. *Hyperopia:* Farsightedness: rays of light coming from an object at a distance of 6 m (20 ft) or more are brought to a focus in back of the retina (see Figure 16-1).
4. *Accommodation:* Focusing apparatus of the eye adjusts to objects at different distances by means of increasing the convexity of the lens (brought about by contraction of the ciliary muscles).
5. *Presbyopia:* The elasticity of the lens decreases with increasing age; an emmetropic person with presbyopia will read the paper at arm's length and will require prescription lenses to correct the problem.
6. *Astigmatism:* Uneven curvature of the cornea causing the patient to be unable to focus horizontal and vertical rays of light on the retina at the same time.

◼ Common Abbreviations

OD (oculus dexter) or RE—right eye
OS (oculus sinister) or LE—left eye
OU (oculus unitas)—both eyes
IOP—intraocular pressure
IOL—intraocular lens
EOL—extraocular lens

◼ Eye Care Specialists

Ophthalmologist

Medical doctor specializing in diagnosis and treatment of the eye. Ophthalmology specialists may focus their practice to a specific part of the eye or disorder, such as a cornea specialist or glaucoma specialist.

Optometrist

Doctor of optometry who can examine, diagnose, and manage visual problems and diseases of the eye, but does not do surgery.

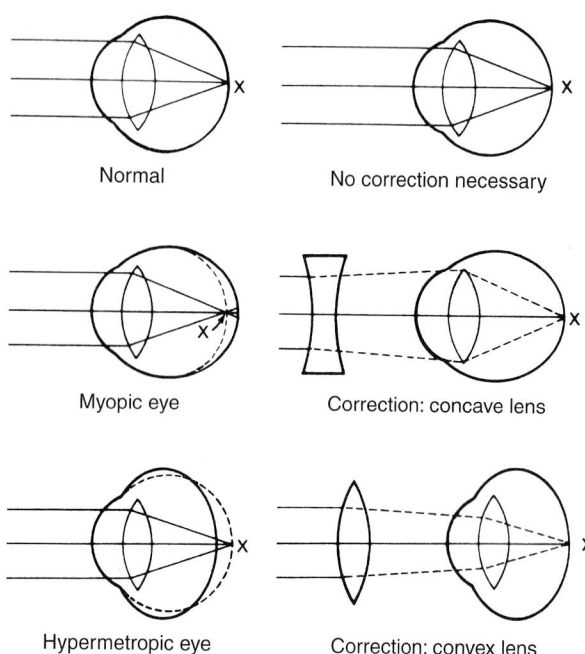

Normal

No correction necessary

Myopic eye

Correction: concave lens

Hypermetropic eye

Correction: convex lens

FIGURE 16-1 Normal vision and refractory errors.

Optician
Fits, adjusts, and gives eyeglasses or other devices on the written prescription of an ophthalmologist or optometrist.

Ocularist
Technician who makes ophthalmic prostheses.

ASSESSMENT

Subjective Data
Subjective data for eye assessment include complaints of altered vision or other symptoms, associated lifestyle and other factors, and recent and past health history.

Presenting Symptoms
1. Any blurred vision, double vision, loss of vision or a portion of the visual field?
2. Is there pain, headache, foreign body sensation (scratchy, something in the eye), photophobia, redness, itchiness, lacrimation, or drainage?
3. Is there difficulty in functioning such as driving or reading due to visual problem?

> **GERONTOLOGIC ALERT**
>
> Question older patients about driving. Change in driving pattern such as avoidance of night driving and less rush hour driving may indicate visual dysfunction as well as impaired reflexes and ability to concentrate in complex situations.

Associated Factors
1. Does the patient wear contact lenses or glasses?
2. What is the patient's occupation and common sports activities?
3. How long have there been symptoms?
4. What treatments has the patient tried?

History
1. Eye injury or accident
2. Recent infection, such as an upper respiratory infection
3. Ocular history, such as previous injury, surgery, or use of medication
4. Medical history, such as diabetes, hypertension, arthritis, or allergies

Ocular Examination (Figure 16-2)

> **NURSING ALERT**
>
> Every patient who seeks medical attention for an eye complaint should have his or her visual acuity tested.

External Examination
Includes examination of the eye and accessory organs without the aid of special apparatus.

Visual Acuity (Snellen Chart and other methods)
1. Each eye is tested separately, with and without glasses.
2. Letters and objects are of a size that can be seen by the normal eye at a distance of 6 m (20 ft) from the chart.
3. Letters appear in rows and are arranged so the normal eye can see them at distances of 9, 12, 15 m (30, 40, 50 ft), and so forth.
4. A person who can identify letters of the size 6 at 6 m (20 at 20 feet) is said to have 6/6 (20/20) vision.
5. Additionally, if vision is less than 6/60 (20/200), tests may be recorded as follows:
   a. Counting fingers (CF) at—meters (feet)
   b. Hand motion (HM)—ability to detect hand movement at a certain distance
   c. Light perception and projection (LP & P)
   d. Light perception only (LP)
   e. No light perception (NLP)

Visual Fields
To determine function of optic pathways.
1. Equipment—light source and test objects. Can be done manually or as new automated visual fields.
2. Peripheral field—useful in detecting decreased peripheral vision in one or both eyes.
   a. Patient is seated 18 to 24 inches in front of the examiner.
   b. The left eye is covered while the patient focuses with the right eye on a spot about 1 ft from the eye.
   c. A test object is brought in from the side at 15-degree intervals, through complete 360 degrees.

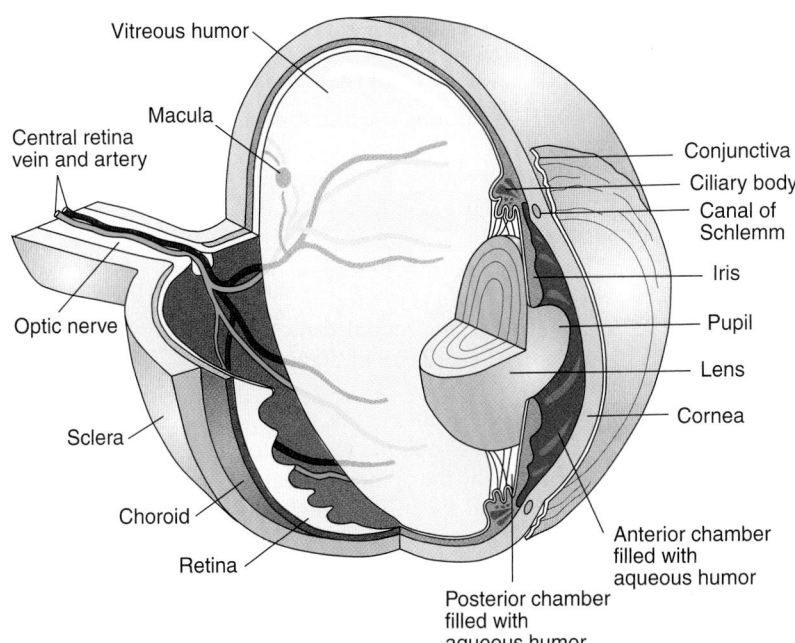

FIGURE 16-2 Three-dimensional cross-section of the eye.

d. The patient signals when he or she sees the test object and again when the object disappears through the 360 degrees.

Color Vision Tests

These tests are done to determine the person's ability to perceive primary colors and shades of colors; it is particularly significant for people whose occupation requires discerning colors, such as artists, interior decorators, transportation workers, surgeons, and nurses. (Useful in diagnosing diffuse retinal dysfunction and various types of optic neuropathies.)

1. Equipment
   a. Polychromatic plates—these are dots of primary colors printed on a background of similar dots in a confusion of colors.
   b. Individual colored disks—each disk is matched to its next closest color.
2. Procedure
   a. Various polychromatic plates are presented to the patient under specified illumination.
   b. The patterns may be letters or numbers that the normal eye can perceive instantly, but that are confusing to the person with a perception defect.
3. Outcome
   a. Color-blindness—person is unable to perceive the figures.
   b. Red–green blindness—8% of males, 0.4% of females
   c. Blue–yellow blindness—rare

Refraction

Refraction is a clinical measurement of the error of focus in an eye.

1. Refraction and internal examination may be accomplished by instilling a medication with cycloplegic and mydriatic properties into the conjunctiva of the eye. Tropicamide (Mydriacyl) or cyclopentolate (Cyclogyl) are two such medicines that cause ciliary muscle relaxation, pupil dilation (mydriasis), and lowered accommodative power (cycloplegia).
2. In older children and adults, refraction without the use of drugs is preferred.
3. The use of a multiple pinhole can help screen for refractive causes of decreased vision versus decreased vision secondary to organic disease.
4. The refractive state of the eye can be determined as follows:
   a. Objectively—through retinoscopy or by automatic refraction (special instrument that measures, computes, and prints out refraction errors of each eye)
   b. Subjectively—trial of lenses to arrive at the best visual image

Internal Examination

Ophthalmoscopic Examination

1. Direct ophthalmoscopy—uses a strong light reflected into the interior of the eye through an instrument called an ophthalmoscope.
2. Indirect ophthalmoscopy—allows the examiner to obtain a stereoscopic view of the retina. Light source is from a head-mounted light. The examiner views the retina through a convex lens held in front of the eye and a viewing device on the head mount. The image appears inverted. This method of examination allows the examiner

to use binocular vision with depth perception and wider viewing field.

3. Clinical significance
   a. Detection of cataracts, vitreous opacities, corneal scars
   b. Close examination for the pathologic changes in retinal blood vessels that may occur with diabetes or hypertension
   c. Examination of the choroid for tumors or inflammation
   d. Examination of the retina for retinal detachment, scars, or exudates and hemorrhages of diabetes

Slit-Lamp Examination

1. Special equipment that magnifies the cornea, sclera, and anterior chamber, and provides oblique views into the trabeculum for examination by the ophthalmologist.
2. The patient sits with chin and forehead resting against equipment supports.
3. The room is generally darkened, and the pupils are dilated.
4. Helps detect disorders of the anterior portion of the eye.

Tonometry

1. Schiotz's tonometry
   a. After instillation of topical anesthesia, the Schiotz's tonometer is gently rested on the eyeball (Figure 16-3).
   b. The indicator measures the ocular tension in millimeters of mercury (mm Hg).
   c. Normal tension is approximately 11 to 22 mm Hg.
2. Applanation tonometry
   a. This is the most effective measuring method for determining intraocular pressure; however, it requires a biomicroscope and a trained interpreter. May be part of the slit-lamp examination.
   b. After instillation of topical anesthesia, the cornea is flattened by a known amount (3.14 mm).
   c. The pressure necessary to produce this flattening is equal to the intraocular pressure, counterbalancing the tonometer.
3. Air applanation tonometry—this requires no topical anesthesia and measures tension by sensing deformation of the cornea in reaction to a puff of pressurized air.
4. Clinical significance: measurement of intraocular tension or pressure (elevated in glaucoma).

DIAGNOSTIC TESTS

◼ Radiology and Imaging

Several imaging studies beyond the basic eye examination may be done to further evaluate eye disease.

Fluorescein Angiography
Description

1. Introduction of sodium fluoresce intravenously (IV) over several minutes, usually through a brachial vein.

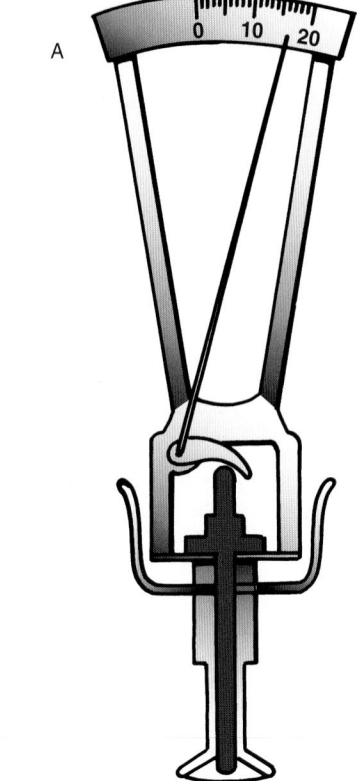
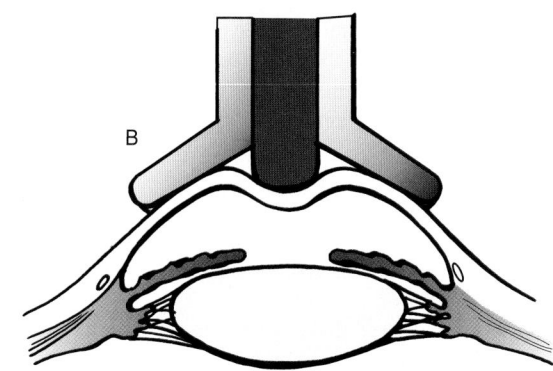

FIGURE 16-3 (**A**) Schiotz's tonometer in which the plunger, in black, measures the ease of indentation of cornea. (**B**) Indentation of the anesthetized cornea by the plunger of the tonometer in order to measure ocular tension. (Newell, F. W. *Ophthalmology: Principles and concepts.* [4th ed.]. St. Louis: CV Mosby)

2. Indirect ophthalmoscopy using a blue filter may be done, and photographs of the ocular fundus are obtained.
3. Provides information concerning vascular obstructions, microaneurysms, abnormal capillary permeability, and defects in retinal pigment permeability.

Nursing and Patient Care Considerations

1. Advise the patient that a series of eyedrops will be given to dilate the pupil for better visualization of the retina. The patient will be positioned in a special chair with head immobilized.
2. Dye will be injected into the arm over several minutes. Photographs will be taken during injection and up to 1 hour after injection.
3. Side effects include nausea due to dye injection, burning in eye from eyedrop instillation, blurred vision and photophobia for 4–8 hours due to pupil dilation, and possible yellow skin and urine discoloration for up to 48 hours after dye injection.

Eye and Orbit Sonography
Description
Sound waves are used in the diagnosis of intraocular and orbital lesions. Two types of ultrasonography are used in ophthalmoscopy:

1. A-scan—uses stationary transducers to measure the distance between changes in acoustic density. This is used to differentiate benign and malignant tumors and to measure the length of the eye to determine the power of an intraocular lens.
2. B-scan—moves linearly across the eye; increases in acoustic density are shown as an intensification on the line of the scan that presents a picture of the eye and the orbit.
3. Abnormal patterns are seen in alkali burns, detached retina, keratoprosthesis, thyroid ophthalmopathy, foreign bodies, vascular malformations, benign and malignant tumors, and a variety of other conditions.

Nursing and Patient Care Considerations
1. Advise the patient that topical anesthetic drops are applied to the eye before the procedure so the patient will not feel the transducer contacting the eye.

2. The procedure may take as little as 8–10 minutes or 30 minutes or longer, if a lesion is detected, in order to locate the lesion.
3. Warn patient not to rub eyes until the anesthetic has worn off to avoid trauma to the eye.

Electroretinography (ERG)
Description
Used to evaluate hereditary and acquired disorders of the retina; an electrode is placed over the eye to evaluate the electrical response to light.

Nursing and Patient Care Considerations
1. Advise the patient that the eyes are propped open and he or she will be positioned lying or sitting down.
2. Topical anesthetic drops are instilled.
3. A cotton wick electrode saturated in saline is applied to the cornea.
4. Various intensities of light are produced, and the electrical potential is measured.
5. Caution the patient not to rub eyes for up to 1 hour after procedure to avoid trauma while eyes are anesthetized.

GENERAL PROCEDURES AND TREATMENT MODALITIES

■ Instillation of Medications
See Procedure Guidelines 16-1.

Ophthalmic medications may be used for diagnostic and therapeutic purposes:

1. To dilate or contract the pupil
2. To relieve pain, discomfort, itching, and inflammation
3. To act as an antiseptic in cleansing the eye
4. To combat infection

See Table 16-1 for ophthalmic pharmacologic agents.

PROCEDURE GUIDELINES 16-1   INSTILLATION OF EYE MEDICATIONS

EQUIPMENT
Sterile solution or medication (most medications have accompanying dropper or are in squeeze bottle or tube)
Small gauze squares or cotton balls

PROCEDURE

Nursing Action	Rationale
PREPARATORY PHASE	
1. Inform the patient of the need and reason for instilling drops or ointment.	
2. Allow the patient to sit with head tilted backward or to lie in a supine position.	

continued

PROCEDURE GUIDELINES 16-1   INSTILLATION OF EYE MEDICATIONS *CONTINUED*

Nursing Action	Rationale
PERFORMANCE PHASE	
1. Check the patient's name.	1. For proper patient identification.
2. Check written prescription and bottle, vial, or tube for correct medication.	2. To avoid medication error.

3. Check prescription designating eye requiring drops and confirm with patient.
    OD (oculus dexter)—right eye
    OS (oculus sinister)—left eye
    OU (oculus uterque)—both eyes	

4. Wash hands before instilling medication.	4. To prevent transfer of microorganisms to patient.
5. Remove cap from container and place on clean surface.	5. To prevent contamination of lid.
6. If eyedropper is used, fill eyedropper with medication by squeezing bulb. Do not tip eyedropper upside down so medication can flow back into bulb end.	6. Loose particles of rubber from bulb end may slip into medication.
7. Using forefinger, pull lower lid down gently.	7. To expose inner surface of lid and cul-de-sac.
8. Instruct patient to look upward.	8. Prevents medication from hitting sensitive cornea.
9. Drop medication amount prescribed into center of lower lid (cul-de-sac) (see Fig. *A*).	9. Prevents medication from hitting sensitive cornea.

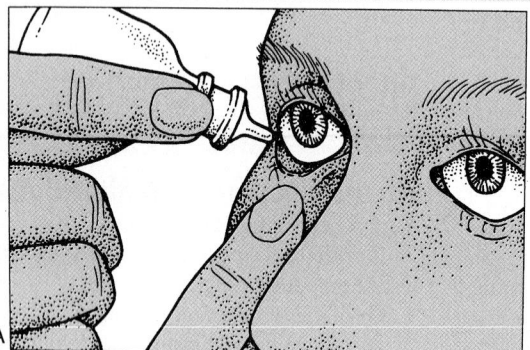 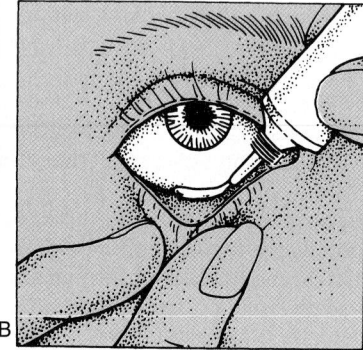

10. If ointment is to be instilled, squeeze out a ribbon of medication from the tube into the lower lid without touching the eye with the end of the tube (see Fig. *B*).	10. To prevent contamination of the tube.
11. Instruct patient to close eyes slowly but not to squeeze or rub them. Open eye.	11. Squeezing or rubbing would express medication from eye; closing allows medication to be distributed evenly over eye.
12. Wipe off excess solution with gauze or cotton balls.	12. Prevents possible skin irritation.
13. Wash hands after instilling medication.	13. Prevents transfer of microorganisms to self or other patients.
14. If additional eyedrops are ordered, wait 5 minutes between each medication.	14. To allow time for absorption of medication.

FOLLOW-UP PHASE

Record time, type, strength, and amount of medication and the eye into which medication was instilled.

Irrigation of the Eye

See Procedure Guidelines 16-2.

Ocular irrigation is often necessary for the following:
1. To irrigate chemicals or foreign bodies from the eyes
2. To remove secretions from the conjunctival sac
3. To treat infections
4. To relieve itching
5. To provide moisture on the surface of the eyes of an unconscious patient

(*text continues on page 515*)

TABLE 16-1 Ophthalmic Pharmacologic Agents*

Pharmacology/Action	Products
1. *Sympathomimetics.* Given topically for the treatment of glaucoma. Immediate effect is decrease in production of aqueous humor. Long-term effect is an increase in outflow facility. May be used in combination with miotics, beta blockers, carbonic anhydrase inhibitors, or hyperosmotic agents.	Epinephrine (Epifrin, Glaucon, Epitrate, Propine)
2. *Miotics, direct-acting.* Cholinergic agents given topically that affect the muscarinic receptors of the eye; results include miosis and contraction of the ciliary muscle. In narrow-angle glaucoma, miosis opens the angle to improve aqueous outflow. Contraction of the ciliary muscle enhances the outflow of aqueous humor by indirect action of the trabecular network—the exact mechanism is unknown. Primary use of miotics is in glaucoma but can be used to counter the effects of cycloplegics/mydriatics.	Acetylcholine (Miochol) Carbachol (Isocarbachol, Niostat) Pilocarpine (Pilocar, Isopto Carpine)
3. *Miotics, cholinesterase inhibitors.* Topical agents that inhibit the enzyme cholinesterase, causing an increase in the activity of the acetylcholine already present in the body. Causes intense miosis and contraction of the ciliary muscle. Decrease in intraocular pressure that is seen is a result of increased outflow of aqueous humor. Used for treatment of open-angle glaucoma, conditions where the outflow of aqueous is obstructed; postiridectomy problems; and accommodative esotropia (inward deviation of one eye).	Demecarin bromide (Humorsol) Isoflurophate (Floropryl) Physostigmine (IsoptoEserine)
4. *Beta-adrenergic-blocking agents.* Act on the beta receptors of the adrenergic nervous system. Two types of beta sites: B_1 and B_2. B_1 site primarily the myocardium resulting in decreased heart rate and cardiac output. B_2 primarily bronchial and vascular smooth muscle resulting in bronchoconstriction, decreased blood pressure. There are two types of ophthalmic beta blockers: cardioselective blocker (betaxolol) acts only on B_1 sites and may on rare occasions cause cardiac effects if absorbed systemically. All other nonselective blockers act on B_1 and B_2 sites and cause significant cardiac and pulmonary effects if absorbed systemically. Used for treatment of increased intraocular pressure by decreasing the formation of aqueous humor and causing a slight increase in the outflow facility.	Betaxolol (Betoptic) Levubunolol (Betagan) Timolol (Timoptic) Carteolol (Ocupress)
5. *Carbonic anhydrase inhibitors.* Oral agents that act to inhibit the action of carbonic anhydrase. Suppression of this enzyme results in a decreased production of aqueous humor. Used in combination regimen to treat glaucoma and postoperative rise in IOP.	Acetazolamide (Diamox) Methazolamide (Neptazane)
6. *Osmotic diuretics.* Osmotic agents given intravenously used for reduction of IOP in acute attack of glaucoma or before ocular surgery where preoperative reduction of IOP is indicated.	Mannitol (Osmitrol) Glycerin (Glycerol)
7. *Prostaglandin analogues.* Newer agents used in the lowering of IOP presumably by increasing transuveal flow or filtration of aqueous. Used in open-angle glaucoma resistant to other agents.	Latanoprost (Xalatan)
8. *Mydriatics.* Topical agents that result in dilation of the pupil, vasoconstriction, and an increase in the outflow of aqueous humor. Used for pupillary dilatation for surgery and examination.	Phenylephrine (Ak-Dilate, Mydfrin)
9. *Cycloplegic mydriatics.* Topical agents that block the reaction of the sphincter muscle of the iris and the muscle of the cilliary body to cholinergic stimulation resulting in dilatation of the pupil (mydriasis) and paralysis of accommodation (cycloplegia). Used in conditions requiring pupil to be dilated and kept from accommodation.	Atropine Homatropine (Ak-Homatropine) Scopolamine (Isopto-Hyoscine) Cyclopentolate (Cyclogel) Tropicamide (Mydriacyl)
10. *Ophthalmic anti-infectives.* Topical agents used for treatment of ophthalmic infections. Commercial products are intended for treatment of superficial ocular problems, such as conjunctivitis and blepharitis. Extemporaneous (compounded) drops are used for more serious topical infections (ie, corneal ulcer, endophthalmitis [intraocular infection]).	*Antibiotics:* Bacitracin (Ak-Tracin) Chloramphenicol (Chloroptic) Ciprofloxacin (Ciloxan) Erythromycin (Ilosone) Gentamycin (Garamycin, Genoptic) Neomycin/polymixin/bacitracin (Neosporin) Norfloxacin (Chibroxin) Sulfacetamide (Sulamyd, Bleph-10) Tobramycin (Tobramycin, Tobrex) *Antifungal:* Amphotericin B (Fungizone) Fluconazole Natamycin (Natcyn) *Antiviral:* Trifluridine (Viroptic) Vidarabine (Vira A)
11. *Local anesthetics.* Block the transmission of nerve impulses. Used topically to provide local anesthetic for tests, such as tonometry and for procedures of short duration. Injections used in ophthalmology for retrobulbar blocks.	*Topical:* Proparacaine (Ophthaine) Tetracaine (Pontocain) *Injection:* Lidocaine

(continued)

TABLE 16-1 Ophthalmic Pharmacologic Agents* (Continued)

Pharmacology/Action	Products
12. *Ophthalmic steroid anti-inflammatories.* Mostly corticosteroids. Used topically to relieve pain, photophobia, as well as suppress other inflammatory processes of the conjunctiva, cornea, lid, and interior segment of the globe.	Dexamethasone (Maxidrex, Decadron) Flurometholone (FML, Flarex) Loteprednol (Alrex, Lotemax) Prednisolone acetate (PredForte, Econopred Plus)
13. *Nonsteroidal anti-inflammatory drugs* (NSAIDs). Act by inhibiting an enzyme involved in the synthesis of prostaglandins, which are key in the body's response to inflammation. These drugs, given topically, are analgesics and anti-inflammatories.	Diclofenac sodium (Voltaren) Flurbiprofen (Ocufen) Ketorolac (Acular) Suprofen (Profenal)
14. *Anti-allergy medications.* There are a number of different types of drugs, given topically, in this category, including antihistamine, mast cell stabilizers, NSAID anesthetic, and astringents (some in combination).	*Antihistamines:* Emedastine (Emadine) Levocabastine ((Livostin) Olopatadine (Patanol) Pheniramine (Naphcon A) *Mast cell stabilizer:* Cromolyn (Opticrom, Crolom) Lodoxamide (Alomide) *Astringent:* Zinc sulfate
15. *Vasoconstrictors.* Topical agents that contract local blood vessels resulting in less redness and irritation.	Naphazoline (Vasocon)

*All pharmacologic agents should be reviewed from a drug handbook before administration for contraindications, adverse reactions, and cautions. IOP: intraocular pressure.

PROCEDURE GUIDELINES 16-2 — IRRIGATING THE EYE (CONJUNCTIVAL IRRIGATION)

STERILE EQUIPMENT

An eyedropper, asepto bulb syringe, or plastic bottle with prescribed solution depending on the extent of irrigation needed. For copious use (ie, chemical burns), sterile normal saline or prescribed solution and IV set-up with attached tubing.

PROCEDURE

Nursing Action	Rationale
PREPARATORY PHASE	
1. Verify the eye to be irrigated and the solution and amount of irrigant.	
2. The patient may sit with head tilted back or lie in a supine position.	
3. Instruct the patient to tilt head toward the side of the affected eye.	3. To prevent fluid from draining into unaffected eye.
PERFORMANCE PHASE	
1. Wash eyelashes and lids with prescribed solution at room temperature; a curved basin should be placed on the affected side of the face to catch the outflow.	1. Any materials on the lids and lashes should be washed off before exposing conjunctiva.
2. Evert the lower conjunctival sac. (If feasible, have the patient pull down lower lid with index finger.)	2. Exposes inner surfaces of lower lid and conjunctival sac (involves the patient and gives a sense of control).
3. Instruct the patient to look up; avoid touching eye with equipment.	3. Prevents injury to the sensitive cornea.
4. Allow irrigating fluid to flow from the inner canthus to the outer canthus along the conjunctival sac.	4. Prevents solution from flowing toward the lacimal sac, duct, and nose, possibly transmitting infection.
5. Use only enough force to flush secretions from conjunctiva. (Allow patient to hold curved basin near the eye to catch fluid.)	5. Prevents eye injury (involves the patient in the treatment).
6. Occasionally, have patient close eyes.	6. Allows upper lid to meet lower lid with the possibility of dislodging additional particles.

PROCEDURE GUIDELINES 16-2 | *CONTINUED*

Nursing Action	Rationale
FOLLOW-UP PHASE	
1. Pat eye dry and dry the patient's face with a soft cloth.	1. Provides comfort.
2. Record kind and amount of fluid used as well as its effectiveness.	2. Provides documentation of nursing actions.

◼ Application of Dressing or Patch

See Procedure Guidelines 16-3.

One or both eyes may need shielding for the following:
1. To keep an eye at rest, thereby promoting healing
2. To prevent the patient from touching eye
3. To absorb secretions
4. To protect the eye
5. To control or lessen edema

PROCEDURE GUIDELINES 16-3 | **APPLICATION OF AN EYE PATCH, EYE SHIELD, AND PRESSURE DRESSING TO THE EYE**

EQUIPMENT

Eye covering to be used — Scissors
Transparent or adhesive tape — Water
Rubber glove

PROCEDURE

Nursing Action	Rationale
EYE PATCH	
1. Instruct patient to close both eyes.	1. It is difficult to close only the affected eye.
2. Place patch over the affected eye.	
3. Secure the patch with three or more strips of transparent tape diagonally from midforehead to below the ear.	3. Transparent tape is easy to remove—use hypoallergenic tape if patient has allergies to tape.
4. For unconscious patient, close eyelid and moisten the eye patch.	4. Dry patch can irritate cornea if eyelid opens.
EYE SHIELD (PLASTIC OR METAL)	
1. Apply over dressings or directly over the undressed eye, fastening with two strips of transparent tape.	1. Used primarily to protect the eye. Place tape on outer edges of shield so as not to obstruct vision through holes in shield.
2. For metal eye shields, a guard can be placed around flanged edges before use.	2. Protects skin from metal. Ensure that patient is not allergic to latex.
a. Cut 1.2–2.5-cm (½–1-in.) wide strip from a rubber glove finger.	a. Covers metal edges of shield or guard.
b. Stretch it around perimeter of shield.	b. Two such pieces add cushioning and provide comfort.
PRESSURE DRESSINGS	
1. Prepare 8–10 adhesive strips by cutting 2.5-cm (1-in.) adhesive tape in 35-cm (9-in.) lengths. Stretch tape (3M) may also be used.	1. Ensure that skin is dry so tape will adhere.
2. Apply two eye patches to the affected eye.	2. Provides pressure dressing bulk.
3. Apply strips from forehead above unpatched eye across dressings to the cheek bone (maxillary prominence).	3. To secure dressing and apply pressure while permitting freedom of movement of the head.

 NURSING ALERT

Prolonged use of pressure dressings may cause increased temperature in the interior of the covered eye because they act as a moisture chamber. Pressure dressings also may need to be removed periodically for a short time so air can freely circulate over cornea.

Removing a Particle From the Eye

See Procedure Guidelines 16-4.
1. Typically, removing a foreign body from the eye is an uncomplicated first-aid measure.
2. However, if the object appears to be embedded, medical intervention is required, that is, local anesthetic, antibiotic therapy, and clinical expertise in using other instruments.
3. The cornea should be evaluated for abrasion from the foreign body by use of fluorescein staining, even if a foreign body cannot be found.

PROCEDURE GUIDELINES 16-4   **REMOVING A PARTICLE FROM THE EYE AND FLUORESCEIN STAINING**

EQUIPMENT

Local anesthesia	Cotton applicator sticks or tongue blades
Hand lens	Irrigating saline
Sterile fluorescein strips and illumination source	Antibiotic solution

PROCEDURE

Nursing Action   **Rationale**

PREPARATORY PHASE

> **NURSING ALERT**
>
> It is very important to take a patient history to determine the nature of the foreign body. If the particle is metal or entered the eye with projectile force, trauma to the eye could result. It may be necessary for the ophthalmologist to remove the foreign body immediately without attempting this method, to prevent further injury.

1. Instill anesthetic eyedrops as directed.

1. To facilitate comfort.

PERFORMANCE PHASE

Removal of Particle

1. As patient looks upward, evert lower lid to expose the conjunctival sac.

1. Particles are often washed downward by the upper lid.

2. With small cotton applicator dipped in saline, gently remove particle.

2. Wipe gently across lid—inner to outer aspect. Use hand magnifying lens if necessary.

3. If offending particle is not found, proceed to examine upper lid.
   a. Have the patient look downward while you stand in front of patient.
   b. Encourage the patient to relax; move slowly and reassure patient that you will not hurt him or her.

   c. Place cotton applicator stick or tongue blade horizontally on outer surface of upper lid. Apply pressure about 1 cm above lid margin (see Fig. *A*).
   d. Grasp upper eyelashes with fingers of other hand and pull the upper lid outward and upward over cotton applicator (see Fig. *B*). Remove particle if present.

   a. Moves sensitive cornea down and away from area of activity.
   b. Relaxation prevents squeezing the lids shut, a maneuver that contracts the obicularis muscle, making eversion of lid impossible.
   c. Because the upper tarsal plate extends 10–12 mm above the lid margin, pressure must be applied at least 1 cm above the lid margin for easy eversion of lid.
   d. Because particles may be washed under the lid, visual exposure assists in detection. Eyelid will remain everted by itself during inspection and removal.

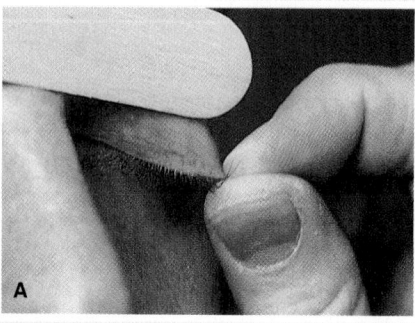

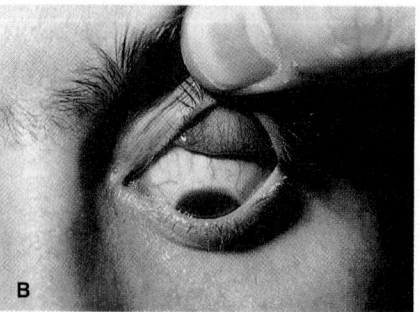

PROCEDURE GUIDELINES 16-4	*CONTINUED*

Nursing Action	Rationale

Fluorescein Staining

1. Use fluorescein strip to detect corneal abrasion.	1. Green stain will indicate if abrasion is present.
2. After telling patient what you are going to do, pull the lower eyelid down and gently touch the tip of a sterile fluorescein strip to the inner aspect of the eyelid.	2. The strip will moisten with patient's own tears to activate the dye.
3. Ask the patient to blink several times to distribute the dye.	3. Green dye will be dispersed over the conjunctive and cornea, and concentrate at an area of abrasion or ulceration.
4. Cornea is viewed through a slit lamp, Woods lamp, or other green light to best illuminate area of concentrated dye.	4. Because cornea reflects a dark pupil, viewing with naked eye may not detect abrasion.

FOLLOW-UP PHASE

1. Apply antibiotic ointment as directed.	1. To prevent potential serious infection from break in cornea.
2. Apply patch as directed.	2. To rest eye and protect cornea for healing.

Removing Contact Lenses

Because contact lenses need regular cleaning and changing, if a person is injured and incapacitated because of an accident, sickness, or other cause, the lenses should be removed. See Procedure Guidelines 16-5.

1. If a person is injured or unconscious and unable to remove lenses, the eyes should be thoroughly examined for injury and the contact lenses removed. An optometrist or ophthalmologist may need to be called.
2. Determine the type of lens from the patient or family.

a. Soft corneal lenses are widely used. The diameter covers the cornea plus a portion of the sclera of the eye. Extended- and daily-wear soft lenses are available.
b. Rigid or gas-permeable lenses are usually smaller than the cornea of the eye, although some are made to extend beyond the cornea onto the sclera of the eye. These lenses need to be removed promptly.
3. Do not remove lenses if the iris is not visible on opening the eyelids; await the arrival of an ophthalmologist. If patient is to be transported, note that contacts are in the eyes. (Write out the message and tape it to the patient or send with transporter.)

PROCEDURE GUIDELINES 16-5	REMOVING CONTACT LENSES

EQUIPMENT

Containers	Normal saline
Marker	Eye suction cup
Labels	

PROCEDURE

Nursing Action	Rationale

PREPARATORY PHASE

1. Because the patient will undoubtedly be in the recumbent position, it is acceptable to remove the lens while he or she is in this position.	
2. Wash your hands thoroughly.	2. To prevent contamination from hands to eyes.

PERFORMANCE PHASE

Hard Type Lenses

1. If an eye suction cup is available (as in Emergency Department), simply separate eyelids to expose lens fully; then, place cup over lens and apply slight pressure to cup.	1. The suction produced will permit cup to lift contact lens from cornea.
2. If a suction cup is not available, follow this procedure. For right eye, stand on right side of patient.	2. Hands will have easier access to eye.
3. Lightly place left thumb on upper eyelid and right thumb on lower eyelid close to the edge and parallel with lids.	3. Thumbs are placed in a leverage position on the eyelids.

continued

PROCEDURE GUIDELINES 16-5   REMOVING CONTACT LENSES *CONTINUED*

Nursing Action	Rationale
4. Gently pull lids apart and observe if contact lens is visible. If contact lens is not visible, wait for an experienced practitioner.	
5. If contact lens is visible, it should slide with the movement of the eyelids while thumbs are still kept at the edges of the eyelids.	
6. Gently open the lids wide beyond the edge of the lens and maintain this position (see Fig. *A*).	
7. Press gently downward with right thumb on eyeball (see Fig. *B*).	7. This should cause the contact lens to tip up on the edge.
8. Gently slide the eyelids and thumbs together (see Fig. *C*).	8. This should allow the contact lens to slide out between the lids where it can be taken off.

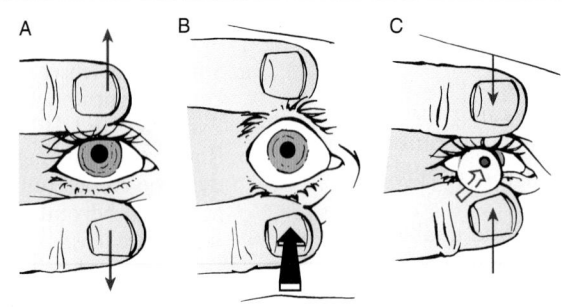

9. FORCE SHOULD NOT BE USED.	9. Cornea may be irreparably damaged.
10. If contact lens can be seen but cannot be removed, gently slide it to the white sclera.	10. This moves it away from the sensitive cornea.
11. For left eye, move to left side of patient and repeat procedure.	

Soft Contact Lenses

May be removed by gently grasping and pinching contact lens between thumb and forefinger. If a contact lens cannot be removed with relative ease, discontinue efforts and wait for the ophthalmologist to remove it.

> **⊘ NURSING ALERT**
>
> **Extended-wear contacts or disposable contacts worn for more than 1 week may precipitate corneal damage.**

DISPOSITION OF LENSES

1. When lenses are found and removed, place in a case or bottle; label "right" and "left."	1. Because right and left lenses are often different, storing them with proper labels will be appreciated.
2. Store in normal saline solution.	2. This prevents drying because soft lenses must be kept moist.

◼ Ocular Surgery

Follow this nursing process overview for any patient having ocular surgery. Specific nursing interventions are listed in the next section for particular types of surgical procedures.

Nursing Assessment

1. Collect subjective and objective data about patient's general state of health.
2. Ascertain what symptoms the patient has been having (eye pain, visual loss, drainage, history of trauma) and how that has impacted usual activity.

3. Assess patient's mobility and self-care ability.
4. Assess visual and other sensory impairments.
5. Gather data regarding usual support systems used by patient. Is family near? Do friends visit regularly?
6. Review patient's daily schedule.
7. Record pertinent data in patient's record.

Nursing Diagnoses
- Knowledge Deficit of postoperative expectations and continuing care
- Risk for Injury related to altered vision
- Sensory/Perceptual Alterations (Visual) related to disease, trauma, or postoperative eye condition
- Fear of blindness related to invasive procedure to eye(s)
- Self-Care Deficits related to reduced or altered vision

Nursing Interventions
Preparing for Surgery
1. Explain to the patient preoperative orders as well as postoperative expectations. (These will be specific for each type of surgery and particular health care provider.)
   a. Postoperatively, a specific position in bed may be maintained for a few hours, for example, patient may lie on unoperated side.
   b. Postoperatively, a small pillow may be used while patient is in supine position.
2. Instruct patient to wash hair the evening before surgery; long hair of female patients should be arranged so it is off the face.
3. Check agency surgical policy regarding skin preparation. Patients may be requested to shower with antibacterial soap the evening before or morning of surgery.
4. Check that operative permit is correct and signed with specified eye having surgery noted.
5. Remove dentures, contact lenses, or artificial eye and any metal before patient goes to the operating room. (Wedding band can usually be taped in place.)
6. Inform patient if any eye bandages are necessary postoperatively.
7. Administer any preoperative medications, including eyedrops as prescribed.
8. Position side rails (up) after administering any medications and place call bell next to patient.
9. Be available to answer any questions the patient may have relating to the surgery or postoperative period.

> **NURSING ALERT**
>
> For patients requiring bed rest (ie, after keratoplasty, injury, retinal detachment surgery), measures should be taken to prevent pulmonary and/or circulatory complications. This may include passive range-of-motion exercises, antiembolism stockings, and special positioning.

Preventing Injury Postsurgery
1. Position the patient as permitted for specific surgery.
2. Position side rails (up) to offer patient a sense of security.

3. Place call bell next to patient; have patient call the nurse rather than risk increased intraocular pressure from the stress and strain of attempting to be self-sufficient.
4. Advise patient to avoid bending over or straining that may cause increase in intraocular pressure.
5. Instruct caregivers to tell the patient when they enter and leave the room.
6. Avoid activities such as combing hair that will disturb the patient's head or cause tension on sutures or operative site.

Compensating for Altered Vision
1. Orient patient to any new environment—room arrangement and/or people.
2. Encourage self-care within the patient's limits.
3. Supervise attempts of patient to feed himself or herself and in other self-care activities.

> **GERONTOLOGIC ALERT**
>
> Be aware that older people may have additional sensory/perceptual alterations such as hearing loss and decreased position sense, which increases their risk of falls and feeling of isolation.

Reducing Fear
1. Recognize that dependence on sight is exaggerated when one faces diminishment or loss of sight.
2. Recognize that patients' concern of surgical outcome may be manifested differently, for example, fear, depression, tension, resentment, anger, or rejection.
3. Encourage the patient to express feelings.
4. Demonstrate interest and understanding.
5. Reassure the patient that rehabilitative programs and personnel are available.

Increasing Self-Care Activities
1. Provide diversional and occupational therapy to keep the patient occupied mentally within the limits of decreased vision.
2. Provide rest periods as necessary.
3. Provide adequate diet and fluids to promote proper elimination and decreased straining.
4. Discourage patient from smoking, reading, and self-shaving for safety reasons.
5. Caution the patient against rubbing eyes or wiping them with soiled tissues.
6. Instruct patient to wear dark glasses if eyes are light-sensitive.
7. Maintain safe environment—doors should be completely open or closed, floors kept clear of articles.

Patient Education and Health Maintenance
1. Advise patient to consult ophthalmologist before undertaking diversional or recreational therapy that may be fatiguing to the eyes—no reading; television in moderation.
2. Emphasize that lights should not be too bright or glaring.
3. Inform the patient before he or she leaves the hospital regarding medications, eyeglasses, follow-up visits.

4. Instruct the patient and family on instillation of eye medications and proper cleansing of eyes.
   a. Instillation of eyedrops
   b. Application of an eye shield or patch
5. Inform the patient of talking books, records, tapes, and machines available from most public libraries without charge.
6. Confirm the following with patient/family before discharge:
   a. Is a return appointment date with health care provider confirmed?
   b. Are patient's medications properly identified and labeled? Do the patient and family member know how to use the prescribed medications?
   c. Does the patient understand the restrictions placed on him/her and the reasons for them?
   d. Does patient/family know what signs/symptoms must be reported to health care provider between appointments (ie, pain, temperature above 101°F, discharge)?

Outcome-Based Evaluation

- Compliant with preoperative routine; asks appropriate questions
- Describes precautions that must be taken as safety measures, carries cane to prevent possible falls
- Demonstrates improved vision in accordance with expectations of the surgery
- Appears relaxed and positive concerning outcome of surgery
- Manages self-care with minimal assistance

Corneal Transplantation (Keratoplasty)
Description

The transplantation of a donor cornea, usually obtained at autopsy, to repair a corneal scar, burn, deformity, or dystrophy.

1. Types of grafts
   a. Full-thickness (6.5–8 mm)—most common
   b. Partial-thickness-lamellar
2. Fresh cornea is the preferred tissue; it is removed from the donor within 12 hours after death and used within 24 hours.
3. Special solutions for storage of fresh cornea are available, which may extend storage up to 3 days.
4. *Cryopreservation* is the care and handling of a corneal graft by freezing to retain its transparency.

Preoperative Management and Nursing Care

1. Discuss psychological, cultural, and spiritual concerns with patient and health care personnel.
2. Advise patient that the surgery is usually performed under local anesthesia and that he or she will be awake and must remain still during procedure.
3. Cleanse the face thoroughly with antibacterial solution as ordered.
4. Administer preoperative medications as ordered.

Postoperative Management and Nursing Care

1. Assess for:
   a. Anxiety—healing may be slow.
   b. Security of the eye patch—patch helps protect the eye from disruption of sutures or injury due to increased inflammmation.
   c. Level of discomfort—pain may be symptomatic of complication.
   d. Bowel and bladder habits—to prevent straining which may raise intraocular pressure, or urinary retention which may result in urinary tract infection
   e. Activity—avoid activities that increase intraocular pressure (sneezing, coughing, quick movement of the head).
2. Administer medications as prescribed (ie, pain medication, steroid eyedrops).
3. Prevent infection—use aseptic technique with medication administration and dressing change.
4. Instruct patient to avoid touching dressing and eyes.

Complications

1. Hemorrhage
2. Graft dislocation
3. Infection
4. Postoperative glaucoma
5. Graft rejection—may occur 10 to 14 days postoperatively
   a. Signs and symptoms include decreased vision, ocular irritation, corneal edema, red sclera

Patient Education and Health Maintenance

1. Teach patient signs of graft rejection occurring about 10 to 14 days postoperatively.
2. Instruct patient to monitor eye daily for graft rejection. Recommend assessment be done at the same time daily for comparison.
3. Teach patient that vision varies and that functional vision does not return until sutures are removed.
4. Emphasize the importance of follow-up visits.

Refractive Surgery
Types of Procedures

1. Radial keratotomy (RK)
   a. Procedure designed to provide correction of myopia (nearsightedness).
   b. The cornea is anesthetized topically, and, under a microscope, the surgeon marks the visual axis.
   c. Eight to 16 radial incisions are made into the corneal surface to flatten it. This permits images to fall on the retina instead of in front of it.
   d. Time to optimal correction is about 3 months. (Procedure is being performed less frequently now with the development of laser surgery for refraction.)
2. Excimer photorefractive keratectomy (PRK)
   a. Limited to correcting myopia and some astigmatism.
   b. The front surface of the corneal epithelium is removed (by laser, manual scraping, or both).

c. The laser is then used to change the corneal curvature by vaporizing the tissue (reshaping or sculpting the cornea).

d. Optimal visual recovery about 6 months.

3. Laser-assisted in-situ keratomileusis (LASIK); also laser-automated lamellar keratoplasty (Laser ALK)

a. Procedure is designed to treat a wider range of prescriptions than the other refractive procedures.

b. Microsurgical instrument (microkeratome) is used to create a corneal flap.

c. A cool laser beam (using an excimer laser) reshapes the cornea, and the flap is then closed.

d. The excimer laser can remove corneal tissue with an accuracy of up to 0.25 microns (0.00004 inch).

e. Only about 50 microns of tissue are removed to achieve the desired correction.

f. Refractive recovery about 3 months.

4. Holmium laser thermokeratoplasty (Holmium LTK)

a. Tissue is heated, not vaporized.

b. Cornea is marked to pinpoint where to aim the laser.

c. The laser heats only selected portions of the cornea to shrink collagen fibers around the cornea edges.

Patient Education and Nursing Care

1. Procedure performed in physician's office or clinic

2. Specific procedures used to correct nearsightedness, farsightedness, astigmatism

3. May or may not eliminate need for glasses especially with aging

4. No guarantee of desired effects

5. May not be appropriate for patients with corneal disease, retinal disease, glaucoma, severe diabetes, uncontrolled vascular disease, autoimmune diseases, pregnancy

6. Elective procedure may be costly

7. Frequent concerns:

a. Pain—generally no pain with most procedures

b. Length of procedure—laser itself 15–40 seconds; entire procedure as little as 30 minutes

c. Activity—minor restriction, resume full activity in 1–3 days

d. Postoperative instructions—differ with physician and procedure; include antibiotic drops, anti-inflammatory drops, eye protection

Note: Many new procedures are being developed that have not yet received FDA approval including new lasers and implanted contact lenses.

Vitrectomy
Description

1. This procedure is performed for conditions such as unresolved hemorrhage with diabetic retinopathy, intraocular foreign body, and vitroretinal adhesions.

2. It involves the removal of all or part of the vitreous humor, the transparent, gelatinlike substance behind the lens.

3. As the vitreous is removed, saline is infused to replace the vitreous. At the end of the procedure, gas, air, or silicone oil may be introduced into the eye to keep the retina in place.

Preoperative Management and Nursing Care

1. Provide explanations of procedure and answer any questions the patient may have.

2. Assess patient's baseline visual acuity and level of function.

3. Give preoperative medication as ordered.

4. Advise patient that if gas is used he or she may be restricted to prone position for 1–6 days.

Postoperative Management and Nursing Care

1. Place pressure patch on one or both eyes after surgical closure.

2. Assist with activities to ensure patient safety.

3. Apply cold compresses to control edema and associated discomfort.

4. Restrict activity to bed rest with bathroom privileges.

5. Medicate for pain, nausea, and vomiting, as indicated.

6. Monitor vital signs and patient's underlying medical condition, such as a diabetic's glucose levels.

7. Monitor for activities that increase intraocular pressure (eg, sneezing, coughing, straining, bending).

8. Instill eye medications as ordered.

9. Properly position patient—if the eye was injected with air during surgery, he or she will remain face down to keep the air/gas bubble over the retina. If not, a semi-Fowler's position is appropriate to keep the visual axis clear.

10. Evaluate drainage—a moderate amount is to be expected for about 2 postoperative days. Unusual amounts of color should be reported immediately.

11. Encourage patience, because the patient will be anxious to witness immediate improvement in vision.

Enucleation
Description

1. Complete removal of the eyeball, usually performed due to trauma, infection, tumor such as melanoma, or prevention of sympathetic ophthalmia.

2. At surgery, the eye is removed by opening the conjunctiva and extraocular muscles, severing the optic nerve, and removing the eyeball.

3. A ball implant is then covered by the muscles and maintains the contour of the eye. The conjunctiva is then closed, and a plastic conformer is placed to maintain the integrity of the eyelid.

4. An individualized prosthesis can be fitted 4–6 weeks later, and a second procedure may be done to improve ocular motility.

Preoperative Management and Nursing Care

1. Review the procedure with patient and family members.

2. Describe postoperative expectations in detail.

3. Begin teaching preoperatively in care of enucleated eye socket and prosthesis.

a. Inspecting eye and lid

b. Instilling medication

c. Irrigating site to remove mucus

d. Removing the prosthesis

e. Using aseptic technique when performing procedures

4. Assess fear and anxiety associated with loss of body part.

5. Advise patient and family of support systems available, and make appropriate referrals.

6. Prepare the patient for surgery, and give preoperative medications as ordered.

Postoperative Management and Nursing Care

1. Instill medications, usually antibiotic and steroid ointments, to prevent infection.

2. Apply pressure/ice dressings as ordered to reduce swelling.

3. Irrigate conformer area to reduce mucus.

4. Cleanse eyelid to reduce chance of infection.

5. Assist patient in adjusting to body image change.

6. Assist patient in adjusting to monocular vision—especially with loss of peripheral vision and depth perception.

7. Review that in 4 to 6 weeks after surgery, the patient will receive an ocular prosthesis (artificial eye).

Complications

1. Hemorrhage

2. Infection

3. Implant extrusion

COMMON EYE DISORDERS

▪ Conditions of the Conjunctiva and Eyelids

The eyelids are the outermost defense mechanisms of the eyes, functioning as a physical barrier as well as to maintain moisture and dispersement of tears. The palpebral conjunctiva lines the upper and lower lids, and the bulbar conjunctiva forms a protective coating over the sclera. The conjunctiva responds to infections, inflammatory disorders, and environmental irritants. Blood vessels in the conjunctiva dilate readily causing redness, and pain receptors respond to inflammatory changes. Inflammatory disorders are outlined in Table 16-2. Structural disorders that may be amenable to surgery include:

• Entropion—inward turning of the eyelid margin

• Ectropion—outward turning of the eyelid margin

• Ptosis—drooping of the upper eyelid

• Lagophthalmos—inadequate closure of the eyelids

▪ Disorders of the Cornea and Uveal Tract

The cornea is the outermost tissue that functions in vision. It must remain clear and smooth to admit light to the retina. Blood vessels are contained in the limbus (periphery). Epithelial layers of the cornea repair rapidly, but if they are penetrated, infection can rapidly spread inward and vision may be lost.

The uveal tract is made up of the iris, which controls pupil size; ciliary body, which secretes aqueous humor and controls accommodation; and choroid layer, which provides vasculature to the anterior uveal tract. Disorders of the uveal tract may cause pupil changes, problems with accommodation, clouding of the anterior chamber or vitreous, and more serious problems due to adhesions (Table 16-3).

▪ Cataract

Clouding or opacity of the crystalline lens that impairs vision.

Pathophysiology and Etiology

1. Senile cataract—commonly occurs with aging

2. Congenital cataract—occurs at birth

3. Traumatic cataract—occurs after injury

4. Aphakia—absence of crystalline lens

5. Additional risk factors for cataract formation include diabetes; ultraviolet light exposure; high-dose radiation; and drugs such as corticosteroids, phenothiazines, and some chemotherapy agents.

Clinical Manifestations

1. Blurred or distorted vision.

2. Glare from bright lights.

3. Gradual and painless loss of vision.

4. Previously dark pupil may appear milky or white.

Diagnostic Evaluation

1. Slit-lamp examination—to provide magnification and visualize opacity of lens

2. Tonometry—to determine IOP and rule out other conditions

3. Direct and indirect ophthalmoscopy to rule out retinal disease

4. Perimetry—to determine the scope of the visual field (normal with cataract)

Management
General

1. Surgical removal of the lens is indicated.

a. A patient with one cataract can usually manage without surgery.

b. If cataract occurs in both eyes, surgery is recommended when vision in the better eye causes problems in daily activities. Surgery is done on only one eye at a time.

2. Cataract surgery is usually done under local anesthesia. Preoperative eyedrops produce decreased response to pain and lessened motor activity (neuroleptanalgesia). Oral medications may be given to reduce intraocular pressure.

3. Intraocular lens (IOL) implants are usually implanted at the time of cataract extraction, replacing thick glasses that may provide suboptimal refraction.

TABLE 16-2 Conditions of the Eyelids and Conjunctiva

Condition	Treatment and Nursing Considerations
Blepharitis An inflammatory reaction of the eyelid margin caused by bacteria (usually *S aureus*) or seborrheic skin condition, resulting in flaking, redness, irritation, and possibly recurrent styes of the upper or lower lid, or both.	Diagnostic culture usually not necessary. Mild cases treated with eyelid margin scrub at least once daily (baby shampoo may be used). If *S aureus* likely, antibiotic ointment is prescribed 1 to 4 times a day to eyelid margin. Teach patient to scrub eyelid margin(s) with cotton swab to remove flaking and then apply ointment with cotton swab as directed.
Hordeolum (stye)/Chalazion The term *stye* refers to an inflammation or infection of the glands and follicles of the eyelid margin. *External hordeolum* involves the hair follicles of the eyelashes; *chalazion* is a granulomatous (chronic) infection of the meibomian glands. Bacteria, usually staphylococcus, and seborrhea are the causes. Pain, redness, foreign body sensation, and a pustule may be present.	Treatment usually consists of warm soaks to help promote drainage, good handwashing and eyelid hygiene, and possible application of antibiotic ointment. In some cases, incision and drainage in the office with local anesthetic may be necessary. Teach patient how to clean eyelid margins and not to squeeze the stye.
Conjunctivitis Inflammation or infection of the bulbar (covering the sclera and cornea) or palpebral (covering inside lids) conjunctiva. May be *allergic, bacterial (S aureus, Streptococcus pneumoniae, Hemophilus influenzae,* and others), *gonococcal, viral* (adenovirus, herpes simplex, coxsackievirus, and others), or *irritative* (topical medication, chemicals, wind, smoke, contact lenses, ultraviolet light) causes. *Trachoma* is caused by *Chlamydia trachomatis* and is a major cause of blindness worldwide, but is rare in North America. Symptoms of conjunctivitis vary from mild pruritus and tearing to severe drainage, burning, hyperemia, and chemosis (edema). Term "*pink eye*" usually refers to infectious conjunctivitis.	Fluorescein staining may be done to rule out ulceration or keratitis (involvement of cornea). Culture if purulent exudate; special culture for *Neisseria gonorrhoeae*. Warm soaks (10 min four times a day) used when crusting and drainage present; cold compresses helpful for allergic and irritative causes. If topical antibiotic ordered, teach patient instillation technique. Urge good handwashing to prevent spread. Allergic conjunctivitis treated with topical or oral antihistamines, vasoconstrictors, and mast cell stabilizers.

TABLE 16-3 Conditions of the Cornea and Uveal Tract

Condition	Treatment and Nursing Considerations
Corneal Abrasion and Ulceration (Keratitis) Loss of epithelial layers of cornea due to some type of trauma—contact with fingernail, tree branch, spark or other projectile, or overwearing contact lens. May lead to corneal ulceration and secondary infection into cornea (keratitis), which may lead to blindness. Symptoms are pain, redness, foreign body sensation, photophobia, increased tearing, and difficulty opening eye.	Treatment is urgent. Fluorescein staining and examination with Woods lamp or slit lamp to identify the abrasion or ulceration. Antibiotic ointment may be instilled and eye patched for 24 h. Cycloplegic drops may also be used in large abrasions or ulcers. Abrasion heals in 24–48 h. Ulceration should be followed by an ophthalmologist. Ensure that patch is secure enough so patient cannot open eyelid, but not so tight that patient "sees stars." Teach patient to use topical antibiotic (or antiviral in cases of herpes simplex dendritic keratitis) after patch is removed, and follow-up as directed. Review safety practices such as wearing protective eye shields, not rubbing eyes, using contact lenses properly, and washing hands frequently.
Iritis/Uveitis Uveitis is an inflammation of the intraocular structures. It is classified by involved structures (1) *anterior uveitis*—iris (iritis) or iris and ciliary body (iridocyclitis), (2) *intermediate uveitis*—structures posterior to the lens (pars plantis or peripheral uveitis), and (3) *posterior uveitis*—choroid (choroiditis), retina (retinitis), or vitreous near the optic nerve and macula. Anterior uveitis is most common and is usually unilateral. Posterior uveitis is usually bilateral. Causes of uveitis are infections; immune-mediated disorders such as ankylosing spondylitis, Crohn's disease, Reiter's syndrome, lupus; trauma; or it may be idiopathic. Onset is acute with deep eye pain, photophobia, conjunctival redness, small pupil that does not react briskly, ciliary flush (redness around limus), and decreased visual acuity.	Urgent ophthalmology evaluation is needed. Inflammation is treated with a topical corticosteroid and a cycloplegic agent. Teach patient how to instill medications and adhere to dosing schedule to prevent permanent eye damage. Suggest sunglasses to decrease pain from photophobia. Encourage follow-up for IOP measurements because corticosteroids can increase IOP.

4. If intraocular lens implant is not used, the patient will be fitted with appropriate eyeglasses or a contact lens to correct refraction after the healing process.

Surgical Procedures

Two types of extractions:

1. Intracapsular extraction—the lens as well as the capsule are removed through a small incision.
2. Extracapsular extraction—the lens capsule is incised, and the nucleus, cortex, and anterior capsule are extracted.
   a. The posterior capsule is left in place and is usually the base to which an IOL is implanted.
   b. A conservative procedure of choice, simple to perform, is usually done under local anesthesia.

Two types of procedures for extraction are:

1. Cryosurgery—a special technique in which a pencil-like instrument with a metal tip is supercooled (−35°C), then is touched to the exposed lens, freezing to it so the lens is easily lifted out.
2. Phacoemulsification—the mechanical breaking up (emulsifying) of the lens by a hollow needle vibrating at ultrasonic speed. This action is coupled with irrigation and aspiration of the emulsified particles from the anterior chamber.

Intraocular Lens Implantation

1. The implantation of a synthetic lens (intraocular lens) is designed for distance vision; the patient may wear prescription glasses for reading and near vision.
   a. Intraocular lens implant restores binocular vision.
   b. Sophisticated calculations are required to determine the prescription for the lens.
2. Numerous types of intraocular lenses are available. Designs and materials change as new developments occur.
3. Advantages of intraocular lens include the following:
   a. Provides an alternative for the person who cannot wear contact lenses
   b. Cannot be lost or misplaced like conventional glasses
   c. Provides superior vision correction and depth perception than glasses
4. Complications (specific to implantation):
   a. Pain from inflammation of various eye structures—usually controlled by nonsteroidal anti-inflammatory drugs, but systemic antibiotics and immunosuppression may be required.
   b. Rosy vision (glare) due to keeping pupil from full constriction; excessive light enters pupil, causing a dazzling of macula (minute corneal opacity).
   c. Degeneration of the cornea.
   d. Malpositioning or dislocation of lens.
5. Implants may not be advisable for patients with severe myopia, history of chronic iritis, retinal detachment, diabetic retinopathy, glaucoma, and complications during surgery.

Contact Lens

Extended-wear contact lens is an option for those who do not receive intraocular lens implants. They restore binocular vision and result in magnification of images in the range of 7% to 10%.

The patient will need to take the lens out for cleaning periodically, or, if patient is elderly or debilitated, he or she will need to follow up at intervals for cleaning at the ophthalmologist's office.

Complications

1. Blindness

Nursing Assessment

Preoperative

1. Assess knowledge level regarding procedure.
2. Assess level of fear and anxiety.
3. Determine visual limitations.

Postoperative

1. Assess pain level.
   a. Sudden onset—may be due to ruptured vessel or suture and may lead to hemorrhage.
   b. Severe pain—accompanied by nausea and vomiting; may be caused by increased intraocular pressure and may require immediate treatment.
2. Assess visual acuity in unoperated eye.
3. Assess for signs of infection—fever, inflammation, pain, drainage.
4. Assess patient's level of independence.

Nursing Diagnoses

• Knowledge Deficit regarding operative course
• Pain related to surgical complications

Nursing Interventions

Preparing the Patient for Surgery

1. Orient patient and explain procedures and plan of care to decrease anxiety.
2. Instruct patient not to touch eyes to decrease contamination.
3. Obtain conjunctival cultures, if requested, using aseptic technique.
4. Administer preoperative eyedrops—antibiotic, mydriatic-cycloplegic, and other medications—mannitol solution IV, sedative, antiemetic, and narcotic as directed.

Preventing Complications Postoperatively

1. Medicate for pain as prescribed to promote comfort.
2. Administer medication to prevent nausea and vomiting as needed.
3. Notify health care provider of sudden pain associated with restlessness and increased pulse, which may indicate increased IOP, or fever, which may indicate infection.
4. Caution patient against coughing or sneezing to prevent increased IOP.
5. Advise patient against rapid movement or bending from the waist to minimize IOP. Patient may be more comfortable with head elevated 30 degrees and lying on the unaffected side.
6. Allow patient to ambulate as soon as possible and to resume independent activities.
7. Assist patient in maneuvering through environment with the use of one eye while eye patch is on (1–2 days).

8. Encourage patient to wear shield at night to protect operated eye from injury while sleeping.

Patient Education and Health Maintenance
Promoting Independence
1. Advise patient to increase activities as tolerated unless given restrictions by the surgeon.
2. Caution against activities that cause patient to strain (eg, lifting heavy objects, straining at defecation, and strenuous activity) for up to 6 weeks as directed.
3. Instruct patient and family in proper eyedrop or ointment instillation.
4. Advise patient to bring all medications to follow-up visits to permit dosage adjustments by ophthalmologist. Discontinued medications can then be discarded to prevent confusion.

Adjusting to Visual Change
1. Inform the patient receiving corrective lenses that fitting for temporary corrective lenses for the first 6 weeks will occur several days after surgery.
   a. Prescription for permanent lenses will be determined 6 to 12 weeks after surgery.
   b. Prescription for a permanent contact lens will be determined about 3 to 6 weeks after surgery.
2. Encourage patient to use dark glasses after eye dressings are removed to provide comfort from photophobia due to lack of pupil constriction from mydriatic-cycloplegic drops.

Adjusting to the Eyeglasses
1. Stress the importance of patience in the coming weeks of adjustment—it is easy to become frustrated.
2. Tell patient that if glasses are to be worn, they will cause the perceived image to be about one third larger than normal. Glasses cannot restore binocular vision as an intraocular lens implant or contact lens will because of the discrepancy of image size between the treated eye and untreated eye.
3. If glass is used in the prescription, it is heavier and thicker than the more expensive plastic cataract eyeglass lenses.
4. Instruct the patient to look through the center of the corrective glasses and to turn head when looking to the side, because peripheral vision is markedly distorted.
5. It is necessary to relearn space judgment—walking, using stairs, reaching for articles on the table (such as a cup of coffee), pouring liquids—due to loss of binocular vision and peripheral distortion.
6. Advise patients to use handrails while walking and doing steps, and to reach out slowly for objects to be picked up.

Becoming Familiar With Contact Lenses
Teach the patient that:
1. With contact lenses, magnification is only about 7% to 10%; peripheral vision is not distorted so binocular vision is achieved and spatial distortion is usually not an issue.
2. Patients do need to learn how to remove daily-wear and extended-wear lenses or return to the ophthalmology office for replacement of extended-wear lens periodically.

Becoming Familiar With Intraocular Lens
1. Teach patient that with an intraocular lens, magnification problems are negligible. Both the operated eye and the unoperated eye can work together after cataract surgery with lens implantation, and the preoperative glasses can usually be worn in the recuperative period.
2. Advise that no eyeglasses may be required for distance but may be needed for reading and writing.
3. Caution against straining of any type. Bend knees only if necessary to reach for something on the floor.
4. Recommend sponge bathing. Avoid getting soap in the eyes.
5. Advise avoidance of tilting head forward when washing hair; tilt head slightly backward. Vigorous shaking of the head is to be avoided.

Outcome-Based Evaluation
- Vision maximized and distortions or limitations in vision described by patient
- Independent activities demonstrated, and patient denies discomfort

■ Acute (Angle-Closure) Glaucoma
A condition in which an obstruction occurs at the access to the trabecular meshwork and the canal of Schlemm. Intraocular pressure is normal when the anterior chamber angle is open, and glaucoma occurs when a significant portion of that angle is closed. Glaucoma is associated with progressive visual field loss and eventual blindness if allowed to progress. This is most often an acute painful condition not to be confused with chronic open-angle glaucoma.

Pathophysiology and Etiology
1. Mechanical blockage of anterior chamber angle results in accumulation of aqueous humor (fluid).
2. Anterior chamber is anatomically shallow in most cases.
3. The shallow chamber with narrow anterior angles is more prone to physiologic events that result in closure.
4. Angle closure occurs because of pupillary dilation or forward displacement of the iris.
5. Angle closure can occur in subacute, acute, or chronic forms.
6. Episodes of subacute closure may precede an acute attack and cause transient blurred vision and pain but no increased IOP.
7. Acute angle closure causes a dramatic response with sudden elevation of IOP and permanent eye damage within several hours if not treated.
8. Within several days, scar tissue forms between the iris and cornea, closing the angle. The iris and ciliary body begin to atrophy, the cornea degenerates because of edema, and the optic nerve begins to atrophy.

Clinical Manifestations
1. Pain in and around eyes due to increased ocular pressure; may be transitory attacks.
2. Rainbow of color (halos) around lights.

3. Vision becomes cloudy and blurred.
4. Pupil mid-dilated and fixed
5. Nausea and vomiting may occur.
6. Hazy-appearing cornea due to corneal edema.
7. Although onset may have initial subclinical symptoms, severity of symptoms may progress to cause acute symptoms of increased intraocular pressure—nausea and vomiting, sudden onset of blurred vision, severe pain, profuse lacrimation, and ciliary injection.

> **NURSING ALERT**
>
> This type of glaucoma is a medical emergency and requires immediate treatment. Untreated, it can result in blindness in less than a week.

Diagnostic Evaluation

1. Tonometry—elevated IOP, usually greater than 50 mm Hg.
2. Ocular examination may reveal a pale optic disk.
3. Gonioscopy (using special instrument called gonioscope) to study the angle of the anterior chamber of the eye.

> **DRUG ALERT**
>
> Dilatation of pupils is avoided if the anterior chamber is shallow. This is determined by oblique illumination of the anterior segment of the eye. A flashlight is shined across the iris from the temporal side. If the iris is bulging (with a shallow anterior chamber), a crescent shadow appears on the nasal side of the iris.

Management
Pharmacology

1. Emergency pharmacotherapy is initiated to decrease eye pressure before surgery.
2. Medications are prescribed at the discretion of the ophthalmologist according to the patient's condition and needs.
3. Medication classifications prescribed include:
   a. Parasympathomimetic drugs used as miotic drugs—pupil contracts; iris is drawn away from cornea; aqueous humor may drain through lymph spaces (meshwork) into canal of Schlemm.
   b. Carbonic anhydrase inhibitor—restricts action of enzyme that is necessary to produce aqueous humor.
   c. Beta blockers—nonselective—may reduce production of aqueous humor or may facilitate outflow of aqueous humor.
   d. Hyperosmotic agents—to reduce intraocular pressure by promoting diuresis.

Surgery

1. Surgery is indicated if:
   a. Intraocular pressure is not maintained within normal limits by medical regimen.
   b. There is progressive visual field loss with optic nerve damage.

2. Types of surgery include:
   a. Peripheral iridectomy—excision of a small portion of the iris whereby aqueous humor can bypass pupil; treatment of choice. Most often a laser procedure.
   b. Trabeculectomy—partial-thickness scleral resection with small part of trabecular meshwork removed and iridectomy. Necessary if peripheral anterior adhesions (synechiae) have developed due to repeated glaucoma attacks.
   c. Laser iridotomy—multiple tiny laser incisions to iris to create openings for aqueous flow; may be repeated.
3. Other eye is usually operated on eventually as a preventive measure.

Complications

Uncontrolled intraocular pressure that can lead to optic atrophy and total blindness.

Nursing Assessment

1. Evaluate patient for severe pain, nausea and vomiting, signs of increased intraocular pressure.
2. Assess visual symptoms.
3. Establish history of onset of attack and previous attacks.
4. Assess patient's level of anxiety and knowledge base.

Nursing Diagnoses

- Pain related to increased IOP
- Fear related to pain and potential loss of vision

Nursing Interventions
Relieving Pain

1. Notify health care provider immediately of patient's condition.
2. Administer narcotics and other medications as directed. Medications that may produce nausea and vomiting are avoided. Patient may be medicated with antiemetic if nausea occurs.
3. Explain to patient that the goal of treatment is to reduce IOP as quickly as possible.
4. Explain procedures to patient.
5. Reassure patient that, with reduction in IOP, pain and other signs and symptoms should subside.
6. Explain side effects of medications:
   a. Mannitol (Osmitrol) (IV)—transient blurred vision, rhinitis, thirst, nausea, transient circulatory overload, headache
   b. Acetazolamide (Diamox) or methazolamide (Neptazane) (oral)—drowsiness, anorexia, paresthesia, stomach upset, tinnitus, fluid and electrolyte imbalance, rare kidney or liver dysfunction
   c. Pilocarpine (Pilocar, Isopto carpine, Ocupress) (topical)—burning and redness of eye, headache, constricted pupil, poor vision in dim light, retinal detachment, rare lens opacity

Relieving Fear

1. Provide reassurance and calm presence to reduce anxiety and fear.

2. Prepare patient for surgery, if necessary.
3. Describe procedure to patient; surgery will likely be done on outpatient basis.
   a. Patch will be worn for several hours, and sunglasses may help with photophobia.
   b. Vision will be blurred for first few days after the procedure.
   c. Frequent initial follow-up will be necessary for tonometry to ensure control of intraocular pressure.

Patient Education and Health Maintenance

1. Instruct patient in use of medications. Stress the importance of long-term medication use to control this chronic disease. Patients often forget that eyedrops are medications and that glaucoma is a chronic illness.
2. Remind patient to keep follow-up appointments.
3. Instruct patient to seek immediate medical attention if signs and symptoms of increased intraocular pressure return—severe eye pain, photophobia, excessive lacrimation.
4. Advise patient to notify all health care providers of condition and medications and to avoid use of medications that may increase IOP such as corticosteroids and anticholinergics (such as antihistamines) unless the benefit outweighs the risk.

Outcome-Based Evaluation

- Patient states that pain is decreased
- Patient describes treatment regimen and verbalizes reduced fear

Chronic (Open-Angle) Glaucoma

Glaucoma is characterized as a disorder of increased intraocular pressure, degeneration of the optic nerve, and visual field loss. Open-angle glaucoma makes up 90% of primary glaucoma cases (angle-closure glaucoma makes up the other 10%), and its incidence increases with age. Incidence with chronic open-angle glaucoma—2% at age 40, 7% at age 70, 8% at age 80.

Pathophysiology and Etiology

Degenerative changes occur in the trabecular meshwork and canal of Schlemm, causing microscopic obstruction. Aqueous fluid cannot be emptied from the anterior chamber, increasing IOP.

IOP varies with activity, and some people tolerate elevated IOP without optic damage (ocular hypertension), whereas others exhibit visual field defects and optic damage with minimal or transient IOP elevation. The risk of eye damage increases with age, family history of glaucoma, diabetes, and hypertension.

Clinical Manifestations

1. Mild, bilateral discomfort (tired feeling in eyes, foggy vision).
2. Slowly developing impairment of peripheral vision—central vision unimpaired.
3. Progressive loss of visual field.
4. Halos may be present around lights with increased ocular pressure.

Diagnostic Evaluation

1. Tonometry—IOP usually greater than 24 mm Hg but may be within normal limits
2. Ocular examination—to check for clipping and atrophy of the optic disk
3. Visual fields testing for deficits

> **NURSING ALERT**
>
> Because of the relative ease of developing chronic glaucoma asymptomatically, encourage people of all ages to have an eye examination that includes measurement of eye pressure (tonometry) periodically to facilitate early detection and treatment to prevent loss of eyesight.

Management

1. Often treated with a combination of topical miotic agents (increase the outflow of aqueous humor by enlarging the area around trabecular meshwork) and oral carbonic anhydrase inhibitors and beta blockers (decrease aqueous production).
2. Remission may occur; however, there is no cure. The patient should continue to see health care provider at 3- to 6-month intervals for control of IOP.
3. If medical treatment is not successful, surgery may be required, but is delayed as long as possible.
4. Types of surgery include:
   a. Laser trabeculoplasty
      (i) An outpatient procedure, treatment of choice if increased ocular pressure unresponsive to medical regimen only.
      (ii) As many as 100 superficial surface burns are placed evenly at junction of pigmented and nonpigmented trabeculum meshwork for 360 degrees in anesthetized eye, which allows increased outflow of aqueous humor.
      (iii) Maximum decrease in IOP is achieved in 2 to 3 months, but IOP may rise again in 1 to 2 years.
   b. Iridencleisis—an opening is created between anterior chamber and space beneath the conjunctiva; this bypasses the blocked meshwork, and aqueous humor is absorbed into conjunctival tissues.
   c. Cyclodiathermy or cyclocryotherapy—the ciliary body's function of secreting aqueous humor is decreased by damaging the body with high-frequency electrical current or supercooled probe applied to the surface of the eye over the ciliary body.
   d. Corneoscleral trephine (rarely done)—a permanent opening at the junction of the cornea and sclera is made through the anterior chamber so aqueous humor can drain.

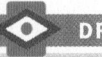
DRUG ALERT

Using beta blocker eyedrops in the treatment of glaucoma can cause an adverse reaction in patients on beta blockers for cardiovascular disease. Potential for bradycardia exists. Monitor vital signs.

Nursing Assessment

1. Assess frequency, duration, and severity of visual symptoms.
2. Assess patient's knowledge of disease process and anxiety about the diagnosis.
3. Assess patient's motivation to participate in long-term treatment.

Nursing Diagnoses

- Knowledge Deficit of glaucoma and surgical procedure

Nursing Interventions

Providing Information About Glaucoma

1. Review the normal anatomy and physiology of the eye as well as the changes that occur in the drainage of aqueous humor with glaucoma.
2. Be sure that the patient understands that, although he or she may be asymptomatic, intraocular pressure could still be elevated, and damage to the eye could be occurring. Therefore, ongoing use of medication and follow-up are essential.
3. Teach patient the action, dosage, and side effects of all medications. Ensure adequate administration of eyedrops by watching return demonstration.
   a. Timolol maleate (Timoptic) and betaxolol (Betoptic)—side effects include headache, eye irritation, decreased corneal sensitivity, blurred vision, bradycardia, palpitations, bronchospasm, hypotension, and heart failure
   b. Pilocarpine (Pilocar, Isopto Carpine)—side effects include eye irritation, blurring, and redness; headache; pupil constriction; poor vision in dim light; possible hypertension and tachycardia; and rare retinal detachment and lens opacity
   c. Acetazolamide (Diamox) and methazolamide (Neptazane)—side effects include drowsiness, anorexia, paresthesia, stomach upset, tinnitus, fluid and electrolyte imbalance, and rare kidney and liver dysfunction
4. Discuss visual defects with patient and ways to compensate. Vision loss is permanent, and treatment is aimed at stopping the process.
5. Inform patient that surgery is done on outpatient basis and recovery is quick. Prolonged restrictions are not required.
   a. After surgery, elevation of head 30 degrees will promote aqueous humor drainage after a trabeculectomy.
   b. Additional medications after surgery will include topical steroids and cycloplegics to decrease inflammation and to dilate the pupil.

Patient Education and Health Maintenance

1. The patient must remember that glaucoma cannot be cured, but it can be controlled.
2. Remind the patient that periodic eye checkups are essential, because pressure changes may occur.
3. Alert patient to avoid, if possible, circumstances that may increase IOP:
   a. Upper respiratory infections
   b. Emotional upsets—worry, fear, anger
   c. Exertion, such as snow shoveling, pushing, heavy lifting
4. Recommend the following:
   a. Continuous daily use of eye medications as prescribed
   b. Moderate use of the eyes
   c. Exercise in moderation to maintain general well-being
   d. Unrestricted fluid intake: alcohol and coffee may be permitted unless they are noted to cause increased intraocular pressure in the particular patient
   e. Maintenance of regular bowel habits to decrease straining
   f. Wearing a medical identification tag indicating the patient has glaucoma

Outcome-Based Evaluation

- Verbalizes understanding of glaucoma as a chronic disease; demonstrates proper instillation of ophthalmic medications

Retinal Detachment

Detachment of the sensory area of the retina (rods and cones) from the pigmented epithelium of the retina. A break in the continuity of the retina may first occur from small degenerative holes and tears, which may lead to detachment.

Pathophysiology and Etiology

1. Spontaneous detachment may occur due to degenerative changes in the retina or vitreous.
2. Trauma, inflammation, or tumor causes detachment by forming a mass that mechanically separates the retinal layers.
3. Diabetic retinopathy often leads to retinal degeneration and tears disrupting the integrity of the retina.
4. Myopia and loss of a lens from a cataract (aphakia) also predisposes to retinal tears and detachment because the posterior chamber is enlarged leading to vitreous pull.
5. Once detachment occurs, that portion of the retina is unable to perceive light because the blood and oxygen supply is cut off; hence, part of visual field will be lost.
6. Detachment occurs most commonly in patients older than age 40.

Clinical Manifestations

1. Retinal detachment may occur slowly or rapidly, but without pain.
2. The patient complains of flashes of light or blurred, "sooty" vision due to stimulation of the retina by vitreous pull.

3. The patient notes sensation of particles moving in line of vision (more so than usual—"floaters" that a person can see floating across field of vision when looking at a light background).

4. Delineated areas of vision may be blank.

5. A sensation of a veil-like coating coming down, coming up, or coming sideways in front of the eye may be present if detachment develops rapidly.
   a. This veil-like coating, or shadow, is often misinterpreted as a drooping eyelid or elevated cheek.
   b. Straight-ahead vision may remain good in early stages.

6. Unless the retinal holes are sealed, the retina will progressively detach; ultimately there will be a loss of central vision as well as peripheral vision, leading to legal blindness.

Diagnostic Evaluation

Indirect ophthalmoscopy shows gray or opaque retina. The retina is normally transparent. Slit-lamp examination and three-mirror gonioscopy magnify the lesion.

Management

General

1. Sedation, bed rest, and eye patch may be used to restrict eye movements.

2. Surgical intervention may be indicated.

3. Return of visual acuity with a reattached retina depends on:
   a. Amount of retina detached before surgery
   b. Whether the macula (area of central vision) was detached
   c. Length of time the retina was detached
   d. Amount of external distortion caused by the scleral buckle
   e. Possible macular damage as a result of diathermy of cryocoagulation

4. Surgical reattachment is successful approximately 90% to 95% of the time. If retina remains attached 2 months postoperatively, condition likely to be corrected and unlikely to reoccur.

Surgical Procedures

1. Photocoagulation—a light beam (either laser or xenon arc) is passed through the pupil, causing a small burn and producing an exudate between the pigment epithelium and retina.

2. Electrodiathermy—an electrode needle is passed through the sclera to allow subretinal fluid to escape. An exudate forms from the pigment epithelium and adheres to the retina.

3. Cryosurgery or retinal cryopexy—a supercooled probe is touched to the sclera, causing minimal damage; as a result of scarring, the pigment epithelium adheres to the retina.

4. Scleral buckling—a technique whereby the sclera is shortened to allow a buckling to occur, which forces the pigment epithelium closer to the retina (often accompanied by vitrectomy).

Complications

1. Glaucoma
2. Infection

Nursing Assessment

Preoperative

1. Assess for history of trauma or other risk factors.

2. Assess level of anxiety and knowledge level regarding procedures.

3. Determine visual limitations and obtain visual description from patient to determine assistance needed.

Postoperative

1. Assess pain level.

2. Assess visual acuity if unoperated eye not patched.

3. Determine patient's ability to ambulate and assume independent activities as tolerated.

Nursing Diagnoses

- Fear related to visual deficit and surgical outcome
- Risk for Injury related to eye surgery

Nursing Interventions

Preparing the Patient for Surgery

1. Instruct patient to remain quiet in prescribed position. (Detached area of retina remains in dependent position.) Assist with all activities and offer frequent reassurance.

2. Patch both eyes. Ensure that patient is oriented to surroundings and can call for assistance.

3. Describe preoperative procedures before carrying them out.

4. Wash face with antibacterial solution.

5. Administer preoperative medications as ordered.

6. Instruct patient not to touch eyes.

Preventing Complications Postoperatively

1. Caution patient to avoid bumping head.

2. Encourage patient not to cough or sneeze or to perform activities that will increase IOP.

3. Assist patient with activities as needed.

4. Encourage ambulation and independence.

5. Administer medications for pain, nausea, and vomiting as prescribed.

6. Provide sedate, diversional activities such as radio, audio books.

Patient Education and Health Maintenance

1. Encourage self-care at discharge, if done in an unhurried manner. (Avoid falls, jerks, bumps, or accidental injury.)

2. Instruct patient in following:
   a. Rapid eye movements should be avoided for several weeks.
   b. Driving is restricted.
   c. Within 3 weeks, light activities may be pursued.
   d. Within 6 weeks, heavier activities and athletics are possible. Define such activities for the patient.
   e. Avoid straining and bending head below the waist.

f. Use meticulous cleanliness when instilling eye medications.

g. Apply a clean, warm, moist washcloth to eyes and eyelids several times a day for 10 minutes to provide soothing and relaxing comfort.

h. Symptoms that indicate a recurrence of the detachment: floating spots, flashing light, progressive shadows. Recommend that the patient contact health care provider if they occur.

3. Advise patient to follow up. The first follow-up visit to the ophthalmologist should occur in 2 weeks, with other visits scheduled thereafter.

Outcome-Based Evaluation

• Patient verbalizes understanding of treatment
• Patient following activity restrictions

◼ Other Problems of the Retina and Vitreous

The retina is a multilayered structure that receives images and transmits them to the brain. It is nourished by retinal arteries and veins. Problems result from inflammation, trauma, vascular changes, congenital defects, and aging. Central lesions affect the macula, impairing central vision, near vision, and color discrimination. Peripheral lesions impair peripheral vision causing blind spots, night blindness, and eventual tunnel vision. See Table 16-4 for treatment of individual disorders.

Nursing Assessment

1. Take history of eye problems, general health, and family history of eye disease.

TABLE 16-4 Other Conditions of the Retina and Vitreous

Condition	Treatment and Nursing Considerations
Vitreous Hemorrhage Bleeding into the vitreous may occur due to trauma, sickle cell disease, hypertension, diabetic retinopathy, retinal tear or detachment, intraocular lens displacement, and clotting abnormalities. It causes decrease or loss of vision in affected eye.	The underlying cause is treated and surgery to repair the retina may include photocoagulation, cryotherapy, scleral buckle, or vitrectomy. See section titled Retinal Detachment. Assist the patient with visual deficit and activity and position restrictions before surgery. Maintain eye patches, activity restriction, and medication administration after surgery.
Central Retinal Artery Occlusion Sudden occlusion of the central retinal artery causes painless loss of vision in one eye with loss of light perception. It may have been preceded by episodes of transient blindness (amaurosis fugax) for 10 to 15 min. It is caused by an embolus, usually from the ipsilateral carotid artery.	Medical emergency! Vision may be salvaged if occlusion occurred within 24 h. Treatment consists of massaging the globe in an attempt to break up the embolus or get it to move distally, inhalation of a mixture of 95% oxygen and 5% CO_2 to get the retinal vessels to dilate, and IV infusion of acetazolamide to lower IOP. Position the patient in Trendelenburg's position and monitor vital signs as directed. Offer reassurance and assist with additional testing and treatment as indicated.
Central Retinal Vein Occlusion Occlusion of the central retinal vein or a branch causes sudden (over several hours), painless decrease in visual acuity. Usually occurs in people with hypertension or other vascular disorders.	Urgent ophthalmologic evaluation is needed. Photocoagulation may be used to prevent local hemorrhage and promote neovascularization. Corticosteroids are used to treat retinal edema, and an aspirin or anticoagulant may be used to prevent further occlusive disease. Encourage regular screening for glaucoma in follow-up as a complication from scar tissue formation after photocoagulation.
Macular Degeneration Age-related changes in the choroid deprive the fovea centralis of blood supply causing a dry (atrophic) form (onset over several years) or wet (exudative) form (onset over several days to weeks with neovascularization and hemorrhaging). Central and near vision are affected, but some peripheral vision remains; bilateral.	Support patient and family. Be realistic about prognosis—there is no treatment, and condition is progressive. Refer patient to local chapter of The Lions Club or other agency to help with adaptive devices for low vision.
Retinitis Inflammation of the retina, usually caused by cytomegalovirus (CMV) as a complication of HIV disease (see p. 930).	
Diabetic Retinopathy A vascular disorder of the retina that leads to diminished vision as a complication of diabetes mellitus (see p. 850).	

2. Obtain functional history of how eye problem may be impairing work, recreation, and other activities.
3. Assess bilateral visual acuity, peripheral vision, and color discrimination.
4. Assist with pupil dilation and ophthalmoscopy as directed.

Nursing Diagnoses
- Sensory/Perceptual Alteration (Visual) related to sudden visual loss
- Sensory/Perceptual Alteration (Visual) related to gradual visual loss
- Risk for Injury related to visual impairment
- Anxiety related to fear of further visual loss

Nursing Interventions
Compensating for Sudden Loss of Vision
1. Orient to unit/clinic and explain all procedures.
2. Assist with self-care activities.
3. Have personal articles placed nearby.

Compensating for Gradual Loss of Vision
1. Discuss strategies/modifications to carry out usual activities.
2. Engage support people in assistance with patient activity.
3. Refer patients with vision less than 20/70 to the Blind Association or other resource for assistive devices.
4. Advise patient to memorize environment while some vision is intact, then do not rearrange furniture or change environment.

Ensuring Safe Activities
1. Help patient understand visual weaknesses such as where blind spots are and how to compensate by turning head to scan environment, using magnifying glass, having environment brightly lit.
2. Discourage use of throw rugs, furniture placed in the middle of room or in cramped spaces.
3. Encourage arranging of frequently used items (kitchen wares, clothing, personal care items) in accessible areas.
4. Use side rails as needed, and ensure that patient can call for help if needed.
5. Assist patient on stairs, ensure good footwear, and obtain order for assistive devices as needed.

Relieving Anxiety
1. Keep patient informed during the diagnostic process.
2. Educate about resources.
3. Encourage participation in support groups.

Patient Education and Health Maintenance
1. Encourage frequent follow up with ophthalmologist.
2. Advise patient to use corrective lenses as directed, keep lens prescription up to date, and to have a spare pair of glasses available.
3. Warn patient against straining eyes by excessive exposure to the sun, reading, or computer work.

4. Rest eyes as needed.
5. Report sudden deterioration in vision or other changes: sudden loss of vision, increase in floaters, flashes of light, sharp pain.

Outcome-Based Evaluation
- Patient bathing and dressing with assistance
- Patient performing self-care activities independently
- No falls or other injuries
- Patient reports understanding of disease and acceptance of treatment plan

Eye Trauma

Trauma to the eye may be caused by blunt or sharp injury, chemical or thermal burns. The eyelids, protective layers, surrounding soft tissue, or the globe itself may be injured. Vision may be impaired by direct injury or latent scarring. See Table 16-5 for specific conditions.

Nursing Assessment
1. Obtain history of mechanism of injury as well as extent of other injuries.
2. Assess level of pain and visual symptoms.
3. Perform neurologic assessment, and assess vital signs.
4. Assess visual acuity.

Nursing Diagnoses
- Pain from tissue trauma
- Sensory Perceptual Alteration (Visual) related to swelling and disruption of tissue
- Fear related to loss of vision

Nursing Interventions
Relieving Pain
1. Medicate for pain as directed; however, monitor for respiratory depression, hypotension, and decreased level of consciousness if narcotic analgesic is used. *Note:* Medications that depress the central nervous system may be contraindicated if head injury is suspected.
2. Provide ice and cool compresses to relieve swelling and pain.
3. Provide additional comfort measures such as positioning, dimmed lights, and quiet environment.
4. Irrigate and patch eye as directed.
5. Monitor vital signs and neurologic status as indicated.
6. Watch for and report signs of infection such as fever, drainage, increased pain, warmth, and redness.

Compensating for Visual Impairment
1. Maintain bed rest.
2. Assist with all activity and care.
3. Maintain safe environment.

Reducing Fear
1. Provide psychological support.
2. Describe all procedures and treatments to patient and family.
3. Prepare patient for surgery as indicated.

TABLE 16-5 Eye Trauma

Condition	Signs and Symptoms	Medical Management
Blunt Contusion—bruising of periorbital soft tissue	Swelling and discoloration of the tissue Bleeding into the tissue and structures of the eye Pain *Dx:* Tests must determine if injury to parts of eye and systemic trauma	*Rx:* To reduce swelling Pain management dependent on structures involved *Note:* If there is any possibility of a ruptured globe, a loose patch and shield should be placed and ocular manipulation discouraged until ophthalmologist assessment completed.
Hyphema—presence of blood in the anterior chamber	Pain Blood in anterior chamber Increased intraocular pressure	*Rx:* Usually spontaneous recovery If severe, bed rest or chair rest with bathroom privileges, eye shield, interior chamber paracentesis, topical steroids, and cycloplegics
Orbital Fracture—fracture and dislocation of walls of the orbit, orbital margins, or both	May be accompanied by other signs of head injury Rhinorrhea Contusion Diplopia *Dx:* X-ray, CT	*Rx:* May heal on own if no displacement or infringement on other structures Surgery (repair the orbital floor with plate freeing entrapped orbital tissue)
Foreign body—on cornea (25% all ocular injuries), conjunctiva Intraocular particles penetrate sclera, cornea, globe	Severe pain Lacrimation Foreign body sensation Photophobia Redness Swelling *Wood and plant foreign body may cause severe infection within hours	*Rx:* MEDICAL EMERGENCY Removal of foreign body through irrigation, cotton-tipped applicator, or magnet Treatment of intraocular foreign body depends on size, magnetic properties, tissue reaction, location Surgical removal
Laceration/perforation—cutting or penetration of soft tissue or globe	Pain Bleeding Lacrimation Photophobia	*Rx:* MEDICAL EMERGENCY Surgical repair—method of repair depends on severity of injury Antibiotics—topically and systemically

Ruptured globe—concussive injury to globe with tears in the ocular coats, usually the sclera	Pain
	Altered intraocular pressure
	Limitation of gaze in field of rupture
	Hyphema
	Hemorrhage (poor prognostic sign)
	Dx: CT, ultrasound
		Rx: MEDICAL EMERGENCY
		Surgical repair
		  Vitrectomy
		  Scleral buckle
		Antibiotics
		Steroids
		Enucleation

Burns (determine causative agent) Burns, chemical—caused by alkali or acid agent	Pain Burning Lacrimation Photophobia	*Rx:* MEDICAL EMERGENCY Copious irrigation until pH is 7 Severe scarring may require keratoplasty Antibiotics
Burns, thermal—usually burn to eyelids—may be first-, second-, or third-degree	Pain Burned skin Blisters	*Rx:* First aid—apply sterile dressings Pain control Leave fluid blebs intact Suture eyelids together to protect eye—if perforation a possibility Skin grafting with severe second- and third-degree burns
Burns, ultraviolet—excessive exposure to sunlight, sunlamp, snow blindness, welding	Pain—delayed several hours after exposure Foreign body sensation Lacrimation Photophobia *Symptoms occur some time after exposure	*Rx:* Pain relief Condition self-limiting Bilateral patching with antibiotic ointment and cycloplegics

Patient Education and Health Maintenance

1. Teach patient how to administer medications such as topical antibiotics.
2. Instruct on use of patch or shield.
3. Advise patient to report increase in pain, decrease in vision, redness, fever.
4. Teach safety measures with decreased visual acuity.
5. Advise use of corrective lenses as prescribed.
6. Stress follow-up care.
7. Attempt to prevent future trauma with protective eyewear.

Outcome-Based Evaluation

- Patient resting comfortably, reports less pain
- No fall or injury reported
- Patient cooperating with procedures

RESOURCES

For further information regarding eye disorders and resources, contact:

American Council for the Blind
1155 15th Street, N.W., Suite 1004
Washington, D.C. 20005
202-467-5081
www.acb.org

Association for Macular Diseases, Inc.
210 East 64th Street
New York, NY 10021
212-605-3719
www.macular.org

Wilmer Eye Institute at Johns Hopkins Hospital
600 North Wolfe Street
Baltimore, MD 21287-9255

SELECTED REFERENCES

Albert, D. M., & Jakobiec, F. A. (1994). *Principles and practices of ophthalmology*. Philadelphia: W. B. Saunders.

American Academy of Ophthalmology, EyeNet. (1997). *Refractive eye surgery. www.eyenet.org/public/ref_surg/ref_surg.html*

American Society of Cataract and Refractive Surgery. (1999). *Refractive surgery, new options in vision correction. www.ascr.org/eye/refract.html*

Atwood, J. D. (Ed.) (1998). What's new in contact lenses. *Review of Ophthalmology, 5*(5), 115–116.

Blecher, M. H. (Ed.) (1998). What's new in cataract surgery. *Review of Ophthalmology, 5*(5), 62–65.

Boyd-Monk, H., & Steinmetz, C. G. III. (1987). *Nursing care of the eye*. Norwalk, CT: Appleton & Lange.

Cassel, G., Billig, M., & Randall, H. (1998). *The eye book, a complete guide to eye disorders and health*. Baltimore: Johns Hopkins University Press.

Cioffi, L. A. (1997). *The Devers manual: Ophthalmology for the health care professional*. Philadelphia: Lippincott Williams & Wilkins.

Dambro, M. R. (2000). *Griffith's 5 minute clinical consult*. Philadelphia: Lippincott Williams & Wilkins.

Goldberg, S. (1993). *Ophthalmology made ridiculously simple*. Miami: Med Masters.

Heffner, D. (1997). Protocol: Allergic conjunctivitis. *Primary Care Practice, 1*(2), 217–219.

Jampel, H. (1998). Laser trabeculoplasty is the treatment of choice for chronic open-angle glaucoma. *Archives of Ophthalmology, 116*, 240–241.

Lakhanpol, R., Robin, A., Gabelt, B. T., & Kaufman, P. (1998). A global guide to glaucoma medications. *Review of Ophthalmology, 5*(5), 42–47.

Lewis, C. (1998, July-August). Laser surgery: Is it worth looking into? *FDA Consumer Magazine.*

Newell, F. W. (1992). *Ophthalmology principles and concepts* (7th ed.). St. Louis: Mosby.

Regillo, C. (Ed.) (1998). What's new in the retina. *Review of Ophthalmology, 5*(5), 77–82.

Rhee, D. J., & Deramo, V. A. (1998). *The Wills Eye drug guide*. Philadelphia: Lippincott Williams & Wilkins.

Rhee, D. J., & Pyfer, M. F. (1999). *Office and emergency room diagnosis and treatment of eye disease*. Philadelphia: Lippincott Williams & Wilkins.

Roizen, M. F. (2000). More preoperative assessment by physicians and less by laboratory tests. *New England Journal of Medicine, 342*(2), 204–205.

Schein, O. D., et al. (2000). The value of routine preoperative medical testing before cataract surgery. *New England Journal of Medicine, 342*(2), 168–175.

Szucs, P. A., et al. (2000). Safety and efficacy of diclofenac ophthalmic solution in the treatment of corneal abrasions. *Annals of Emergency Medicine, 35*(2), 131–137.

Thompson, J. M., McFarland, G. K., Hirsch, J. E., & Tucker, S. M. (1997). *Mosby's clinical nursing*. St. Louis: Mosby.

Ear, Nose, and Throat Disorders

ASSESSMENT

History

Obtaining a history, including the patient's signs and symptoms, current health patterns, and previous illnesses, will help in identifying ear, nose, and throat (ENT) problems and an appropriate plan of care.

Key Signs and Symptoms

1. Epistaxis
   a. Is the bleeding an anterior trickling or a posterior gushing?
   b. Unilateral or bilateral?
2. Headache
   a. Exactly what parts of the head or face hurt? Is it pain or a pressure sensation?
   b. Is it associated with nasal congestion and postnasal drip? Visual changes?
3. Sore throat
   a. Is it accompanied by swollen glands, high fever, nasal congestion, and postnasal drip?
   b. Is it acute or chronic? Was there any exposure to others with throat infection?
4. Nasal congestion
   a. Is it acute or chronic? Accompanied by fever and purulent drainage?
   b. Accompanied by itching and paroxysmal sneezing and/or wheezing? Seasonal or perennial?

5. Hoarseness
   a. Is it related to infection, voice abuse, dietary habits, tobacco use, or alcohol abuse?
   b. Is it acute (<2 weeks), recurrent, or chronic (>2 weeks)?
   c. Is there any dysphagia, odynophagia, globus sensation, sore throat, weight loss, or neck lump?
6. Earache
   a. Is it worsened by manipulation of the auricle or is it a deep throbbing pain? Is there any otorrhea?
   b. Were there preceding upper respiratory infection (URI) symptoms?
7. Hearing loss
   a. Was it sudden or gradual in onset?
   b. Unilateral or bilateral?
8. Dizziness
   a. Is the patient lightheaded or experiencing vertigo (as if the room or self is spinning)?
   b. Is the dizziness associated with any change in head or body position?

Current Health Patterns

1. Inquire about nutrition, dental care, normal mouth care habits, dental caries, use of partial or full dentures, stress-related grinding, clenching or clamping of teeth.
2. Ask about consumption of alcohol, smoking, use of a pipe, and smokeless tobacco.
3. Determine personal hygiene in regard to ears. Are cotton swabs or other objects used for cleaning?

4. Is there any loud noise exposure?
5. Does the patient frequently strain voice through talking, singing, or shouting?
6. What medications is the patient taking? Have antibiotics been used? For how long?

Previous Illnesses

1. Is there a history of allergies?
2. Is there any immunosuppressive illness, such as diabetes mellitus, cancer, human immunodeficiency virus (HIV) infection?
3. Has there been any trauma?
4. Is there a history of rhinitis, sinusitis, or ear infections?
5. Is there a family history of any ENT problems or cancer?

▌ Physical Examination

Assessment of the Mouth and Oropharynx

1. Remove dentures, if present.
2. Inspect mouth.
   a. Observe the lips for color, moisture, ulcers, lumps, localized discoloration, and cracking.
   b. Inspect the tongue for smoothness, moisture, condition of papillae, and color; note the presence of redness, swelling, lesions, or cracks (a thin white coat is normal). Note any deviation or tremor when the tongue is moved (cranial nerve XII).
   c. Observe the hard and soft palates and note any redness, fissures, cracks, abnormal coloring, or nodules. Note the position and relative length of the uvula.
   d. Observe the buccal and labial mucosa for moisture, discoloration, lesions.
   e. Inspect the gums and number of teeth; note any missing, cracked, or discolored teeth; note obvious caries and local irritations; observe the gingiva for color, retraction, evidence of bleeding, or edema.
   f. Observe toothbrushing and flossing technique, if possible.
   g. With a tongue blade, depress the tongue and note the position of the uvula (cranial nerve X) when the soft palate rises as the patient says "ah"; note discoloration, enlargement, exudate, ulceration of the posterior oropharyngeal wall. Observe the tonsils for size, symmetry, inflammation, exudate, and collection of food debris in crypts. Note any halitosis.
   h. Test the gag reflex (cranial nerve IX).
3. Palpate.
   a. Wearing gloves, palpate the outer lips, the gingiva, the buccal mucosa, and the floor of the mouth for lesions, masses, or tenderness.
   b. Palpate the temporomandibular joint (TMJ) while patient opens and closes mouth, then moves the jaw from side to side. Note crepitus, tenderness, or spasm. Note maximum oral opening (patient should be able

to place three fingers of nondominant hand stacked vertically between the central incisors).

Assessment of Nose and Sinuses

1. Inspect external nose for swelling, discoloration, deformity, and skin lesions. (Look from the front, side, and with patient's head tilted back.)
2. Have patient tilt head backward and use flashlight or otoscope with aural speculum to assess position of septum, edema of nasal mucosa, drainage, and patency of nasal passages.
3. Inspect, palpate, and percuss the frontal and maxillary sinuses for tenderness or inflammation.
4. Observe oropharynx for evidence of postnasal drip.
5. Test sense of smell (cranial nerve I) by having patient close eyes and sniff samples of coffee, vanilla, or other common scents.

Assessment of the Ears

1. Examine unaffected ear first in patient with ear pain. If gentleness is demonstrated during examination of good ear, patient is more likely to submit to examination of painful ear.
2. Inspect and palpate pinna for deformity, swelling, warmth, and tenderness on manipulation of auricle or tragus.
3. Perform otoscopic examination for presence of foreign body, inflammation, drainage, or tympanic membrane abnormalities, as indicated.
4. Assess hearing (cranial nerve VIII) through the use of a tuning fork. Tuning fork tests (Weber's and Rinne tests) are used only for screening purposes (Table 17-1).
   a. Weber's (lateralization) test—place base of lightly vibrating tuning fork on top of patient's head or in middle of forehead; ask where patient hears it, one or both sides.
   b. Rinne test—place base of lightly vibrating tuning fork on mastoid process until patient can no longer hear it; then quickly place vibrating fork near the ear canal and ask if patient can still hear it.

TABLE 17-1 Tuning Fork Tests

Ear Condition	Weber's Test	Rinne Test
Normal, no hearing loss	No shifting of sounds laterally	Sound perceived longer by *air* conduction
Conductive loss	Shifting of sounds to poorer ear	Sound perceived as long or longer by *bone* conduction
Sensorineural loss	Shifting of sounds to better ear	Sound perceived longer by *air* conduction

DIAGNOSTIC TESTS

Audiometry

Description

1. Audiometry is a battery of tests to measure hearing and ear function. These tests are usually done by an audiologist to confirm and define hearing loss.
2. Pure-tone audiometry consists of a pure (musical) tone of increasing loudness.
3. Speech audiometry consists of the spoken word to determine the ability to hear and discriminate sounds.
4. The stimulus may be applied directly over the ear canal to determine air conduction (conductive hearing loss), or over the mastoid to determine nerve conduction (sensorineural hearing loss). Mixed hearing loss can also be evaluated.
5. Results are plotted on a graph known as an audiogram.
6. Tympanography (impedance audiometry) is a separate procedure in which air pressure is manipulated in a sealed ear canal. This measures middle ear muscle reflex to sound stimulation, as well as compliance of the tympanic membrane.
   a. Function problems such as middle ear effusion, scarring of the tympanic membrane, and eustachian tube dysfunction can be evaluated.

Nursing and Patient Care Considerations

1. The patient wears earphones and signals upon hearing a tone.
2. A soundproof room is used to increase accuracy.
3. No special patient preparation or participation is necessary for tympanography.

Electronystagmography (ENG)

Description

1. ENG is the measurement of changes in electrical potentials created by eye movement during spontaneous, positional, and calorically evoked nystagmus.
2. It is used to evaluate the oculomotor and vestibular systems to differentiate the cause of vertigo, tinnitus, and hearing loss of unknown origin.
3. The test takes place in a darkened room. It lasts about 1 hour.
4. Electrodes are taped to the patient's face, and the patient is asked to look in different directions and change positions.
5. Air is gently blown into the external ear canal.
6. Water may be used to irrigate the external ear canal.

Nursing and Patient Care Considerations

1. Patient preparation includes avoiding a heavy meal before the procedure and avoiding caffeine and alcohol for 48 hours before the procedure.
2. Medications that may affect the vestibular system, such as sedatives, antianxiety agents, antihistamines, and medications ordered for dizziness, may be held for up to 5 days before the procedure.

GENERAL PROCEDURES AND TREATMENT MODALITIES

Nasal Surgery

Indications

Facial Trauma and Nasal Fractures

Reduction of nasal fractures may be done by a closed manipulation with external casting in the office or by open surgical technique in the operating room. Repair and stabilization of other maxillofacial fractures usually require an operating room procedure for wiring or plating.

Nasal Septal Surgery

1. Submucous resection of the septum is an operation in which cartilaginous and/or osseous portions of the septum that lie between the flaps of the mucous membrane and perichondrium are removed or straightened to establish a midline partition between the right and left nasal cavities to provide a clear nasal airway.
2. Nasal septal reconstruction involves resection or removal of cartilaginous (or bony) septum followed by reconstruction of all parts of the septum that may produce nasal airway obstruction.

Rhinoplasty

1. Involves changing the nose's external appearance. Grafted cartilage or bone harvested from other parts of the body may be used.
2. A septorhinoplasty may be done when there are both external and internal nasal deformities.

Sinus Surgery

1. Functional endoscopic sinus surgery (FESS) is done with rigid endoscopes and long-handled forceps working through the nose to widen the natural sinus ostia and to facilitate the natural sinus drainage patterns.
2. Polyps and other small intranasal growths can be removed endoscopically.
3. The packing used after FESS is very small, filling only the area adjacent to the sinus ostia, so is not visible except for a retrieval string extending outside the nasal ala.
4. Other traditional approaches to the sinuses such as the Caldwell-Luc procedure (opening under lip to enter maxillary sinus and strip out diseased mucosa), a nasoantral window (creating an opening between the maxillary sinus and the anterior inferior nose), and external or internal ethmoidectomies, with their historically extensive postoperative nasal and sinus packing, are now used only in selected complicated cases.

Preoperative Management

1. If a fracture or trauma has occurred, head of bed should be raised to promote drainage, lessen edema, and make patient more comfortable.

2. Intermittent cold compresses and pain medications should be utilized as ordered.
3. Antibiotics may be used to reduce bacterial colonization of nose and sinuses.
4. The patient should be advised that a sensation of pressure may be felt in the nasal area during surgery if done under local anesthetic.
5. The patient should be told about the use of nasal packing to effect hemostasis and the appearance of facial or periorbital ecchymosis (bruising) that may be present and will subside over a course of weeks.
6. The patient should avoid use of aspirin, nonsteroidal anti-inflammatory agents, and drugs that may affect platelet function before surgery.

Complications
1. Hematoma/hemorrhage
2. Local infection—contaminated nasal packing is an excellent culture medium for pathogens
3. Aspiration
4. Pressure necrosis (from packing)
5. Blindness from orbital hematoma or unintended orbital involvement in endoscopic sinus surgery
6. Cerebrospinal fluid rhinorrhea from unintended or traumatic violation of the cribiform plate
7. Pulmonary decompensation

Nursing Diagnoses
- Ineffective Breathing Pattern (nasal airway clearance) related to nasal packing and swelling
- Risk for Aspiration related to bleeding, inability to blow nose
- Knowledge Deficit related to performance of nasal hygiene
- Potential for Altered Oral Mucous Membranes related to mouth breathing
- High Risk for Infection related to alterations in nasal/sinus mucous membranes and drainage patterns

Nursing Interventions
Facilitating Breathing and Comfort
1. Keep head elevated (three to four pillows) day and night to keep swelling down.
2. Apply cold compresses or ice packs intermittently for 24 hours to lessen edema and discoloration and to promote comfort. (Use great caution and only with approval of surgeon after rhinoplasty.)
3. Advise patient that packing will be removed within 1 week of placement.
4. Encourage the use of a humidifier to relieve crusting of nasal mucosa and prevent irritation from dryness in nose and throat.
5. Encourage relaxation techniques and deep-breathing exercises for anxiety associated with nasal passages being blocked.

6. Be alert for worsening pulmonary conditions such as asthma, chronic obstructive pulmonary disease (COPD), and sleep apnea when the nose is congested or packed.
7. Encourage use of analgesics but caution overuse, which may cause respiratory depression.

Preventing Bleeding and Aspiration
1. Monitor closely for bleeding; check for increased swallowing, blood dripping down back of throat (use flashlight and tongue blade).
2. Change the gauze pad under the nose as it becomes soaked with blood; bleeding should gradually decrease.
3. Check other external dressings for saturation.
4. Notify surgeon if bleeding increases. Expect a temporary minor increase in bleeding with vomiting, sneezing, ambulation, or crying in the first 48 hours.
5. Reassure the patient about the sucking sound that will be experienced on swallowing; the nasal packing prevents air from moving through the nose, and a partial vacuum is created in the throat during swallowing.
6. Instruct the patient not to blow nose but to blot secretions with tissue.
7. Regularly observe and document visible packing retrieval strings external to nose, taped to cheek if present.

Ensuring Proper Nasal Hygiene
1. Encourage patient to use a vaporizer to help relieve crusting of nasal mucosa from dryness.
2. Remind patient that sneezing, straining, and nose blowing increase venous pressure and can result in bleeding/hematoma.
3. Advise patient to keep the mouth open while sneezing if unable to control sneezing.
4. Teach patient an appropriate effective method of nasal hygiene as approved by surgeon. After FESS, the patient will need regular appointments for professional nasal cleaning by the surgeon and will also need to flush the nose regularly to control nasal crusting and to facilitate healing (see Patient Education, p. 548).
5. In general, patient may gently clean nasal ala area with saline and/or peroxide for comfort, but large crusts should be removed by surgeon or allowed to work themselves free.
6. Instruct to avoid environmental irritants, especially smoke.

Protecting Oral Mucous Membranes
1. Administer frequent mouth care, because the patient is forced to breathe through the mouth.
2. Use flexible straw to sip mouthwash for rinsing purposes.
3. Encourage fluid intake and use of lip protectant.

Preventing Infection
1. Advise the patient to notify surgeon for uncontrolled postoperative pain, fever, foul odor or taste in mouth, or unusual drainage.
2. Prophylactic antibiotics should be taken on time if ordered.
3. Patient must keep follow-up appointment for packing removal.

Patient Education and Health Maintenance

1. Tell patient to notify surgeon immediately for uncontrolled postoperative pain, any visual change postoperatively, fever, unilateral clear nasal discharge with leaning the head forward, uncontrolled excessive nasal bleeding, dyspnea, blanching or necrosis of the external nasal tissues or the palate while packing is in place.
2. After Caldwell-Luc procedure or rhinoplasty, advise patient that numbness in operative area may be present for several weeks to months.
3. Instruct patient to avoid strenuous activity, lifting, and trauma to nose; the motion of bony fragments (after fracture) within soft tissue will produce laceration and bleeding.
4. After rhinoplasty, even the pressure of wearing eyeglasses or pulling on a tight shirt over the head can disrupt the intended cosmetic result.
5. Sun exposure should also be avoided after rhinoplasty due to a tendency for hyperpigmentation.
6. If a nasal splint is present, tell patient to avoid getting it wet; do not attempt to remove it.
7. Advise patient that postoperative follow-up may need to continue for 6 to 12 months to monitor for excess scar formation or cosmetic deformity.

Outcome-Based Evaluation

- Mouth breathing without difficulty
- Patient protecting airway without aspiration
- Nasal and palatal tissues without blanching or darkening
- Oral mucous membranes dry, but pink and intact
- Afebrile

■ Ear Surgery

Ear surgery may involve the tympanic membrane, the middle ear cavity, the mastoid, or the inner ear. It may be done for perforation of the eardrum, to facilitate drainage and remove diseased tissue in cases of infection, to relieve vertigo, or to treat hearing loss.

Types of Surgery

1. Myringotomy—creating a surgical opening into tympanic membrane (with knife or laser) for possible drainage tube insertion
2. Tympanoplasty—reconstruction of diseased or deformed middle ear components (Table 17-2)
   a. Type I (myringoplasty)—purpose is to close perforation by placing a graft over it in order to create a closed middle ear to improve hearing and decrease risk of infection and cholesteatoma. Perforation is closed using one of the following:
      (i) Fascia from temporalis muscle
      (ii) Vein grafts from hand or forearm
      (iii) Epithelium from auditory canal (eustachian tube)
   b. Type II–V—suitable replacement (polyethylene, stainless steel wire, bone, cartilage) is used to maintain continuity of conduction sound pathway. The necessity of a two-stage procedure is determined.
      (i) First stage—eradication of all diseased tissues; area is cleaned out to achieve a dry, healed middle ear.
      (ii) Second stage—performed 2 to 3 months after first stage; reconstruction, using grafts.
3. Mastoidectomy—removal of mastoid process of temporal bone
   a. Simple—performed through the ear with a tympanoplasty (closed approach)
   b. Modified or radical—wide excision of the mastoid and diseased middle ear contents through an occipital incision (open)
4. Stapedectomy—removal of footplate of stapes and insertion of a graft or prosthesis
5. Labyrinthectomy—destruction of the labyrinth (inner ear) through the middle ear and aspiration of the endolabyrinth

TABLE 17-2 Types of Tympanoplasty

Type	Middle Ear Damage		Repair Process
	Tympanic Membrane	Ossicles	
I	Perforated	Normal	Close perforation—myringoplasty
II	Perforated	Erosion of malleus and/or incus	Close perforation; graft against incus or whatever remains of malleus
III	Tympanic membrane destroyed or widely perforated	Rest of ossicular chain destroyed but stapes are intact and mobile	Grafts implanted to contact the normal stapes Tympanostapedopexy
IV	Tympanic membrane destroyed or widely perforated	Ossicular chain destroyed. Head, neck, and crura of stapes destroyed. Stapes footplate mobile	Expose mobile stapes footplate—graft implanted. Air pocket between graft and round window provides protection The cavum minor operation
V	Tympanic membrane destroyed or widely perforated	Ossicular chain destroyed. Head, neck, and crura of stapes destroyed. Stapes footplate fixed	Make opening in horizontal semicircular canal; graft seals off middle ear to give sound protection for round window Tympanoplasty and fenestration of lateral semicircular canal

6. Endolymphatic decompression and shunt—release of pressure on the endolymphatic system in the labyrinth and creation of a shunt for fluid to the subarachnoid space or the mastoid
7. Cochlear implant—implantation of electronic device that bypasses cochlea and stimulates auditory nerve

Preoperative Management

1. Hearing function is fully evaluated.
2. Antibiotics are given to treat infection.
3. The patient is prepared emotionally for the effects of surgery.
4. Careful assessment for signs of acute infection is performed, which may delay surgery.

Postoperative Management

1. Antibiotics may be continued to prevent local and central nervous system (CNS) infection.
2. Bed rest may be maintained for the first 24 hours or longer to decrease symptoms of nausea and vertigo (if the inner ear was disturbed) or to prevent disruption of prosthesis.
3. Analgesics, antiemetics, and antihistamines are given as needed.
4. The patient is positioned to promote drainage but maintain some immobility.
5. Packing may be removed up to 6 days postoperatively if prosthesis or graft procedure was performed.
6. Hearing will be reevaluated after edema has subsided and healing has occurred.

Complications

1. Infection: local, CNS (meningitis, brain abscess)
2. Hearing loss
3. Facial nerve paralysis

Nursing Diagnoses

- Pain related to surgical incision and swelling
- Risk for Infection related to local CNS infection
- Risk for Injury related to vertigo

Nursing Interventions

Relieving Pain

1. Administer or teach self-administration of analgesic as indicated postoperatively.
2. Tell patient to expect pain to subside within first few hours with simple procedures or within first day or two with major procedures.
3. Position for comfort following the instructions from the surgeon.
   a. On side with surgical ear upward to maintain graft position and immobility
   b. Lying on side with surgical ear down to promote drainage from ear canal
   c. Position of patient preference
4. Elevate head of bed to reduce swelling and pressure.

5. Advise patient to avoid sudden movement. Use pillows for support.

Preventing Infection

1. Reinforce external dressings as needed until after first changed by surgeon, then change when saturated to prevent bacterial growth in damp dressings.
2. Loosely pack cotton or gauze in ear canal as indicated, without causing increased pressure.
3. Do not probe or insert anything into ear canal.
4. Administer or teach self-administration of antibiotics as prescribed. Do not use eardrops unless specifically ordered postoperatively.
5. Wash hands before any ear care, and instruct patient not to touch ear.
6. Take care not to get dressing or ear wet.
7. Advise patient not to blow nose, which could cause nasopharyngeal secretions to be forced up eustachian tube into middle ear.
8. Report and teach patient to report any increased pain, fever, ear inflammation, or drainage, indicating local infection.
9. Be alert for headache, fever, stiff neck, or altered level of consciousness, which may indicate CNS infection.

Ensuring Safety

1. Be aware that dizziness or vertigo may occur for the first several days postoperatively.
2. Maintain side rails up while patient is in bed.
3. Assist patient on ambulating for the first time after surgery and as needed thereafter.
4. Encourage the patient to move slowly, because sudden movements may exacerbate vertigo.
5. Administer or teach self-administration of antiemetics and antihistamines as ordered and as needed; watch for sedation.
6. Instruct the patient not to blow nose, cough, lean forward, or perform Valsalva maneuver to prevent disrupting graft or prosthesis, aggravating vertigo, or forcing bacteria up the eustachian tube. If coughing or blowing nose is necessary, do so with open mouth to relieve pressure.

Patient Education and Health Maintenance

1. Advise the patient that there may be a temporary hearing loss for a few weeks after surgery because of tissue edema, packing, and so forth. The effects of a hearing restoring operation will not be known for several weeks, and additional rehabilitation may be necessary to optimize results.
2. Advise patient to protect ear, perform dressing changes, or place loose cotton in outer ear as indicated. Replace cotton twice daily or sooner if saturated by drainage.
3. Encourage follow-up for packing removal as directed.
4. Instruct the patient to avoid sudden pressure changes in the ear.
   a. Do not blow nose.
   b. Do not fly in a small plane.
   c. Do not dive.

5. Advise against smoking.
6. Tell patient to protect ears when going outdoors for the first week.
7. Tell patient to avoid getting ear wet until completely healed.
8. Tell patient to avoid crowds or exposure to colds so upper respiratory infection is prevented.
9. Instruct patient about signs and symptoms of complications to report.
   a. Return of tinnitus
   b. Vertigo
   c. Fluctuations of hearing ability
   d. Fever, headache, ear inflammation, increased pain, stiff neck
   e. Facial drooping or numbness
10. Advise patient that facial nerve paralysis may be temporary and to increase fluid intake through a straw during this time.

Outcome-Based Evaluation

- Verbalizes relief of pain
- No signs of infection
- Ambulating without difficulty

CONDITIONS OF THE MOUTH AND JAW

Candidiasis

Candidiasis is a fungal infection commonly caused by *Candida albicans,* usually occurring in the mouth and pharynx, but it also occurs in the esophagus and can become a source of systemic dissemination, particularly in high-risk persons.

Pathophysiology and Etiology

1. More common with immunosuppression from disease states or treatment regimens (eg, HIV infection, chemotherapy, corticosteroids).
2. Altered oral environment from loss of epithelial layer, antibiotic therapy, preexisting infections, poor oral hygiene or nutritional status, wearing dentures.

Clinical Manifestations

1. Oral discomfort, burning, altered taste, erythema
2. White, raised, painless plaques, loosely adherent
3. Possible spread to the esophagus with pain on swallowing and chest pain

Diagnostic Evaluation

1. Microscopic smear of plaques shows characteristic hyphae.
2. Fungal culture positive for *C. albicans.*
3. Occasionally, biopsy of lesions may be necessary to rule out leukoplakia (premalignant plaques).

Management

1. Topical antifungal agents in oral rinses, troches, or creams such as clotrimazole (Mycelex) or nystatin.
2. Systemic treatment is indicated if topical agents fail or for esophageal cases with fluconazole (Diflucan), ketoconazole (Nizoral), or amphotericin B (Fungizone)
3. Analgesics for pain.
4. Oral prostheses are also treated to avoid harboring and reintroducing infection.

Complications

1. Candidal infection throughout the gastrointestinal tract
2. Candidal sepsis

Nursing Assessment

1. Assess extent of lesions and inflammation in mouth as well as any chest discomfort indicating spread to esophagus.
2. Assess level of pain.
3. Assess nutritional status and effect of pain on oral intake.
4. Obtain history for risk factors for candidal infection.

Nursing Diagnoses

- Altered Nutrition: Less Than Body Requirements related to oral discomfort
- Knowledge Deficit related to antifungal therapy

Nursing Interventions

Attaining Adequate Nutrition

1. Administer analgesics as prescribed ½ to 1 hour before meals.
2. Provide soft foods, soothing liquids; avoid temperature extremes.
3. Encourage saline rinses with lukewarm water or loosen crusts with dilute hydrogen peroxide mouth rinses, followed by water rinses, as prescribed.
4. Provide gentle suctioning if pain becomes so severe that patient cannot handle secretions, and provide intravenous (IV) fluids.

Ensuring Adequate Therapy

1. Administer antifungal agents as prescribed. Observe patient for proper use of topical preparation.
   a. Ensure that mouth is clean and free of food debris before administering drug.
   b. For swish-and-swallow preparations, tell patient to swish and hold in mouth for at least 5 minutes (preferably 20 minutes) before swallowing.
   c. For troches, have patient suck until dissolved, over 20 minutes.
2. Observe for signs and symptoms of systemic drug side effects: nausea; vomiting; diarrhea; renal, bone marrow, cardiovascular, hepatic, or neurologic toxicities.
3. Explain the importance of continuing therapy for duration prescribed, usually at least 3 weeks.

Patient Education and Health Maintenance

1. Instruct high-risk patients on daily oral examination and signs and symptoms to observe.
2. Teach patient to avoid highly seasoned foods, extremes in temperature, alcoholic beverages, and smoking, all of which irritate the oral mucosa.
3. Encourage good oral hygiene.
4. Oral prosthesis should be soaked in antifungal solution each night during treatment. May need to refrain from wearing denture due to oral discomfort.
5. Encourage patient on long-term systemic antifungal therapy to follow up for liver function test monitoring as directed.

Outcome-Based Evaluation

- Adequate intake of liquids and soft foods as evidenced by stable body weight, and lack of orthostasis
- Swishes oral suspension for 10 minutes before spitting or swallowing

Herpes Simplex Infection (Type 1)

Also known as *cold sores* or *fever blisters,* herpes simplex virus (HSV; usually type 1) is often associated with lip and oral lesions.

Pathophysiology and Etiology

1. After a primary infection, it is thought that the herpes virus remains latent in the neural ganglia and is activated by some stimulus that triggers the migration of the virus to the epithelium.
2. Recurrent herpes labialis or oral or pharyngeal herpes may by precipitated by sun exposure, fever, oral trauma, fatigue, emotional upset, hormonal changes, and other factors.
3. Spread is through contact with oral secretions.
4. Herpes simplex virus type 2 is associated with genital lesions and is sexually transmitted.

Clinical Manifestations

1. Prodromal period—tingling, soreness, burning in area where lesion will develop.
2. Small vesicles appear on erythematous, edematous base, frequently near the mucocutaneous junction of the lips and adjacent skin.
3. May also occur in oral mucosa, especially in immunocompromised persons.
4. Vesicles rupture, causing ulcerations.
5. Lesions heal spontaneously in 7 to 14 days.

Management

1. No diagnostic tests are necessary. Clinical appearance forms diagnosis.
2. Treatment may not be necessary if cases are mild and usually short-lived.
3. Comfort measures such as mild oral or topical analgesic, or drying agent (zinc oxide).
4. Good hygiene to prevent spread to self and others.
5. Antiviral agents are available to decrease the duration of symptoms.
6. Penciclovir (Denavir) 1% cream applied every 2 hours while awake at earliest sign.
7. Acyclovir (Zovirax) topical, oral, or IV—often used for immunocompromised patients with severe cases.

Nursing Interventions and Patient Education

1. Advise adequate rest and nutrition and avoidance of identified triggers.
2. Advise that virus is transmitted through close contact such as kissing and sharing food and cups, so to avoid these from prodromal period until well healed.
3. Recommend good handwashing and hygiene.
4. Tell patient and significant others that many people have been exposed to HSV type 1 but have not developed lesions because they are not susceptible.

Temporomandibular Disorders (TMD)

Temporomandibular disorders are conditions affecting the jaw joint that consist of one or more of the following:

1. Myofascial pain—pain in the muscles serving the jaw (temporalis, masseter, medial and lateral pterygoids), neck, and shoulder
2. Internal derangement of the jaw joint (dislocated or displaced joint disk or injured condyle)
3. Degenerative joint disease (eg, arthritis)

Pathophysiology and Etiology

1. Causes include rheumatoid or osteoarthritis; scleroderma; ankylosing spondylitis; trauma; teeth clenching or bruxism (teeth grinding); neoplasms; acute infections such as parotitis, dental infections, and peritonsillar abscess; congenital anomalies; and tetanus.
2. Any mental and physical stresses can induce or exacerbate symptoms.
3. Above factors result in inflammation and muscle spasm of temporomandibular joint (TMJ).

Clinical Manifestations

1. Pain at the joint, temples, mandible, or masticatory muscles worsens with jaw movement. Referred muscle spasm of the neck, trapezius, and sternocleidomastoid muscle causes discomfort.
2. Clicking or crepitus from grating or popping of the joint.
3. Limitation of movement, dislocation, or jaw locking.
4. Headaches, earaches, or tinnitus; even dizziness and hearing problems.
5. Change in the bite (upper and lower teeth do not match in the normal comfortable way).
6. May experience deteriorating oral hygiene/halitosis from limited oral opening (trismus), making dental hygiene difficult.

7. May experience difficulty chewing due to limited jaw excursion, resulting in altered diet and weight loss.
8. Jaw clicking alone is common and requires no workup or intervention if asymptomatic. It probably represents a displaced joint disk.

Diagnostic Evaluation

1. Diagnosis can usually be achieved by history and physical examination without extensive testing.
2. Dental and TMJ x-rays may or may not be helpful.
3. Occlusal analysis evaluates for malocclusion of the jaw and teeth in a bite position.
4. Computed tomography (CT) and magnetic resonance imaging (MRI) are usually normal unless there is underlying degenerative changes, fracture, or neoplasm of jaw or cervical spine.
5. Arthrography (joint x-rays using dye).
6. Arthroscopy (endoscopic invasive joint examination).

Management

1. Initial management employs jaw rest (soft, no-chew diet for 2 weeks, plus avoiding extreme jaw movements such as wide yawning, and gum chewing).
2. Anti-inflammatory/analgesic medications such as ibuprofen (Motrin).
3. Application of warm, moist heat or ice packs.
4. Muscle relaxants may be prescribed.
5. Therapeutic nightguard or splint—to realign malocclusion or joint disk and to optimize muscle relaxation.
6. Physical therapy for gentle stretching and relaxing exercises with or without ultrasound (deep-heat) therapy—to enhance analgesia and muscle relaxation and to promote local tissue metabolism.
7. Transcutaneous electrical nerve stimulation (TENS) reduces muscle spasm of head, neck, and back and reduces pain.
8. In general, conservative reversible measures above are employed as long as possible before progressing to invasive/surgical management.
   a. Arthroscopy—investigational procedure to visualize joint, reposition disk, lyse adhesions, or débride joint
      (i) Reserved for conditions not improved by medical management.
      (ii) Complications include cranial nerve VII damage with facial paralysis and paresis, perforation of the external auditory canal, piercing of the middle cranial fossa.
   b. Surgery—to remove the disk or reshape bony prominences
9. Complications include malocclusion, cranial nerve VII damage, infection.

Nursing Interventions and Patient Education

1. Assess the character, frequency, location, and duration of pain. Evaluate what triggers and relieves the pain. Determine how effective previous treatments have been.
2. Explore the effect of the disorder on the patient's lifestyle, especially eating habits. Assist patient to alter methods of oral hygiene and eating if severe trismus is present.
3. Instruct the patient on the indications, dosages, and side effects of analgesics and anti-inflammatory medications.
4. Teach the patient proper use of heat therapies. Cold applications may be preferred by some patients to reduce pain and spasm.
5. Encourage the patient to perform active mouth opening, protrusion, and lateral movement exercises of the jaw for 5 minutes, four to five times per day, as prescribed to stretch muscles and reduce spasm.
6. Encourage the use of soft food and liquid supplements during times of acute pain exacerbated by eating. Advise reduction of foods that require excessive chewing, such as raw vegetables, tough meat, nuts. Discourage gum chewing.
7. Explore tension-reducing modalities with the patient, especially progressive muscle relaxation to reduce muscle tension and spasm.
8. Encourage follow-up with dentist, oral surgeon, ENT specialist, or other caregiver as indicated.
9. Encourage proper use of the night guard or dental splint including periodic appointments to assess fit.
10. May need Medic-Alert bracelet and preoperative anesthesia consultation for elective surgeries if maximum jaw opening is less than 30 mm, limiting access for airway intubation.

▉ Maxillofacial and Mandibular Fractures

Fractures of the maxillofacial bones or mandible may occur as the result of industrial, athletic, and vehicular accidents; violent acts; and falls.

Pathophysiology and Etiology

1. Mandibular fractures frequently occur due to blow to the chin.
2. Maxillofacial fractures usually occur due to blow to the cheek or face.
3. May be nondisplaced or displaced, usually closed, and includes soft tissue injury.
4. May also occur as part of planned surgical reconstruction for jaw problems.
5. Injuries sustained in altercations or motor vehicle accidents may be associated with alcohol intoxication or recreational drug use.

Clinical Manifestations

1. Malocclusion, asymmetry, abnormal mobility, crepitus (grating sound with movement), pain, or tenderness
2. Tissue injury: swelling, ecchymosis, bleeding, pain

Diagnostic Evaluation

1. X-rays (posterioanterior, oblique, occlusal, panorex)—to show fracture and possible displacement
2. CT scan—to evaluate extent of complicated injuries

Management

1. Maintenance of adequate respiratory functioning—may include oxygen support, endotracheal intubation, or tracheostomy. See Chapter 35, Emergent Conditions.
2. Control of bleeding—usually accomplished with direct pressure.
3. Reduction of the fracture—usually closed reduction.
4. Immobilization—depends on location, type, and severity of the fracture.
   a. Barton's bandage with a Kling or stockinette bandage
   b. Interdental fixation with rubberbands or wiring
   c. Intermaxillary fixation with rubberbands or wiring
   d. Interosseous fixation with open reduction
5. Maintenance of adequate nutritional intake with liquid or soft diet—to maintain immobilization of fracture site.
6. Pain control—to promote comfort.
7. Prevention of infection with antibiotics in the presence of positive cultures.

Complications

1. Airway obstruction, aspiration
2. Hemorrhage, infection
3. Disfigurement
4. Extraocular muscle entrapment/orbital globe displacement with resultant visual disturbance
5. Acute drug/alcohol withdrawal

Nursing Assessment

1. Obtain description of injury and review chart and diagnostic tests for extent of injury.
2. Continually assess respiratory status.
3. Assess level of pain.
4. Assess visual acuity and extraocular movement.
5. Assess for tremors, delirium/hallucinations, anxiety, seizure activity related to alcohol or drug withdrawal.

Nursing Diagnoses

- Risk for Aspiration related to immobilization of jaw
- Altered Nutrition: Less Than Body Requirements related to pain, injury, and immobilization
- Pain related to injury and surgical intervention
- Body Image Disturbance related to disfigurement of injury or surgical repair
- Risk for Injury related to complications of surgery

Nursing Interventions

Preventing Aspiration

1. Maintain effective airway.
   a. Elevate head of bed 30 to 45 degrees, or position leaning over a bedside stand to reduce edema and improve handling of secretions.
   b. Ensure readily accessible suctioning equipment; teach patient oral and nasal suctioning; position on side or upright during suctioning.
   c. Administer antiemetics as prescribed for nausea and vomiting to prevent aspiration.
   d. Make sure wire cutters or scissors are present for immediate removal of the wires or rubberbands if the airway becomes obstructed. (Vertical rubber bands or wires should be cut.)
   e. Ensure that a method for calling the nurse (call bell) is within easy access for the patient at all times in case of emergency.
2. Monitor blood pressure, pulse, respirations, and temperature to note early onset of infection or aspiration.

Maintaining Nutritional Status

1. Administer liquid diet as prescribed; place straw against teeth or through any gaps in the teeth. Teeth may initially be sensitive to hot and cold.
2. Position in upright position before, during, and for 45 to 60 minutes after all feedings.
3. Evaluate ongoing nutritional and hydration status; weight; intake, output, and specific gravity; laboratory values—24-hour urea nitrogen, transferrin level, electrolytes, and albumin.
4. Advance to blenderized diet as tolerated.
5. Make environment as pleasant as possible to enhance appetite—remove all sources of odor, decrease interruptions, position comfortably.

Increasing Comfort

1. Administer liquid or a suspension of analgesics as prescribed—avoid narcotics on an empty stomach, which may cause nausea and vomiting.
2. Administer diazepam (Valium) as prescribed to reduce anxiety and control reflex muscle spasm.
3. Apply paraffin wax to the ends of wire fixation devices to decrease irritation to the gums and oral mucosa.
4. Apply petroleum jelly to the lips to decrease dryness and prevent cracking.

Strengthening Body Image

1. Provide firm reassurance regarding progress to reduce anxiety and allay fears.
2. Avoid unrealistic promises in relation to scars or disfigurement.
3. Allow the patient to choose the first time for looking in the mirror.
4. Provide privacy as requested. The patient may be sensitive to appearance.

Preventing Complications

1. Provide mouth care every 2 hours while awake for the first several days, then four to six times per day.
2. Initially, provide mouth care with warm normal saline mouth swishes.
3. As diet is progressed, remove collected debris with a pressurized water stream cleaner (Water Pik) and encourage the patient to brush teeth with a soft, child-sized toothbrush.
4. Observe facial injuries for swelling, erythema, pain, or warmth to detect onset of infection.

5. Change facial dressings as needed to prevent soiling with secretions, food, or drainage, which may promote bacterial growth.
6. Provide alternative form of communication such as magic slate or picture board because maxillomandibular fixation limits articulating ability, making speech difficult to understand.

Patient Education and Health Maintenance

1. Encourage adequate nutrition—inform the patient and family that foods can be blenderized and thinned with juices or broths to a consistency that can be taken through a straw.
2. Explore with the patient options for maintaining proper oral care; encourage the patient to practice the options of choice.
3. Discuss the use of antiemetic medications to prevent nausea and vomiting, stressing the complications this could cause.
4. Make sure the patient has wire cutters or scissors at all times and knows how to use them should airway obstruction occur.
5. Encourage follow-up health care visits, including counseling for alcohol or drug abuse.

Outcome-Based Evaluation

- No evidence of aspiration.
- Tolerating fluids through straw. Maintains adequate body weight.
- Expresses relief of pain.
- Views self in mirror; notices improvement in appearance.
- No signs of infection; oral hygiene maintained.

PROBLEMS OF THE NOSE, THROAT, AND SINUSES

Rhinopathies

Rhinopathies are disorders of the nose that interrupt its normal functions of olfaction, and warming, filtering, and humidifying inspired air. These include *allergic rhinitis, non-allergic rhinitis, vasomotor rhinitis,* and other conditions.

Pathophysiology and Etiology

1. Allergic rhinitis—IgE-mediated response causing release of vasoactive substances from mast cells (see p. 916)
2. Nonallergic rhinitis
3. Infectious—viral (common cold) and bacterial (purulent)
4. Drug-induced (rebound rhinitis; rhinitis medicamentosa)—caused by excessive use of topical nasal decongestants
5. Vasomotor rhinitis—unexplained autonomic nasal dysfunction as a result of overactivity of the parasympathetic nerve supply to the mucous membranes of the nose and paranasal sinuses

6. Rhinitis of pregnancy—nasal congestion resulting from estrogen-mediated mucosal engorgement (may occur with oral contraceptive use also)

Clinical Manifestations

1. Hypersecretion—wet, running/dripping nose or postnasal drip
2. Nasal obstruction symptoms—nasal congestion, pressure, or stuffiness (Figure 17-1)
3. Headache

Management

1. Treatment of underlying cause
   a. Allergy—antihistamines (see Chapter 28)
   b. Infection—supportive care for viral; antibiotics for bacterial
2. Topical decongestants (for short-term use); systemic decongestants

> ◆ **DRUG ALERT**
>
> Severe rebound nasal obstruction may occur with overuse of topical decongestants. Stress the importance of only using for 2 to 3 days as directed.

3. Intranasal corticosteroids—preferred treatment in vasomotor rhinitis; may also be used in other types

Nursing Interventions and Patient Education

1. Avoid irritating inhalants, especially smoke, aerosols, noxious fumes.
2. Do not overuse topical nasal sprays/drops.
3. Do not blow nose too frequently or too hard; doing so may cause infection to spread, sinuses to become infected, and an eardrum to be perforated.
4. Blow through both nostrils at the same time to equalize pressure.
5. Side effect of systemic decongestants is stimulation of sympathetic nervous system—insomnia, nervousness, palpitations.
6. Intranasal corticosteroids do not cause significant systemic absorption in usual doses, but occasionally may cause pharyngeal fungal infections and rarely cause nasal septal perforation.
7. Be aware that many people use a variety of herbal products to prevent and treat nasal and sinus infections. Echinacea, zinc, and vitamin C are generally safe, but should not be taken in greater amounts than recommended. All products should be reported to the patient's health care provider.

▪ Epistaxis

Epistaxis refers to nosebleed or hemorrhage from the nose. It most commonly originates in the anterior portion of the nasal cavity. Posterior nasal bleeding usually originates from the turbinates or lateral nasal wall.

A. Rhinitis

B. Sinusitis

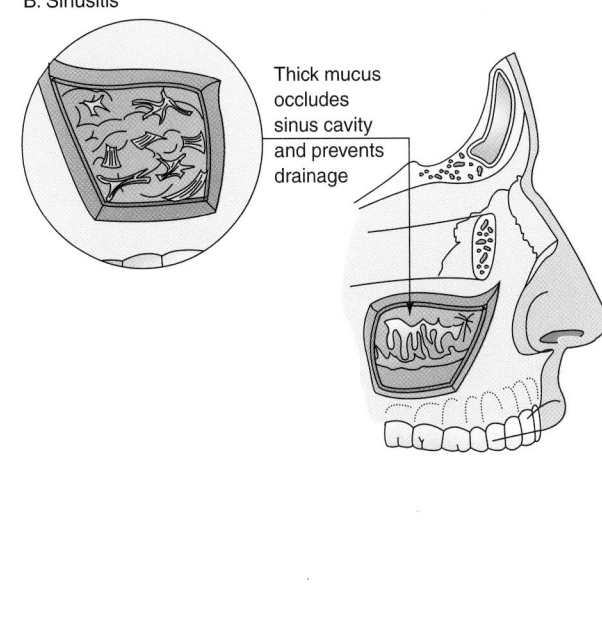

Edematous conchae; polyps may develop

Thick mucus occludes sinus cavity and prevents drainage

Occluded sinus openings

Enlarged nasal mucosa

Discharging mucus

FIGURE 17-1 Rhinitis and sinusitis. (**A**) The mucous membranes lining the nasal passages become inflamed, congested, and edematous, blocking sinus openings and obstructing air passage. (**B**) The sinus cavity mucous membranes are also marked by inflammation and congestion, with thickened mucous secretions filling the sinus cavities and further occluding the openings.

Pathophysiology and Etiology

1. Local causes:
   a. Dryness leading to crust formation—bleeding occurs with removal of crusts by nose picking, rubbing, or blowing.
   b. Trauma—direct blows.
2. Systemic causes are less common—hypertension, arteriosclerosis, renal disease, bleeding disorders (most common systemic cause).
3. Majority of nosebleeds are anterior; posterior bleeds are more difficult to control.

Diagnostic Evaluation

1. Inspection with nasal speculum to determine site of bleeding. Important to determine which side bled first.
2. Laboratory evaluation to exclude blood dyscrasias.

Management

Depends on severity and source of bleeding in nasal cavity.
1. Patient is placed in an upright posture, leaning forward to reduce venous pressure, and instructed to breathe gently through the mouth to prevent swallowing of blood.
2. With anterior bleeds, patient is instructed to compress the soft part of nose with index finger and thumb for 5 to 10 minutes to maintain pressure on the nasal septum.
3. A cotton pledget soaked with a vasoconstricting agent may be inserted into each nostril, and pressure is applied if bleeding is not controlled by compression alone. After

5 to 10 minutes, the cotton is removed, and the site of bleeding is identified.
4. The blood vessel may be cauterized.
5. If bleeding continues or posterior bleeding is initially identified, packing may be layered into nasal cavity and nasopharynx or balloon tamponade may be required to apply pressure over a larger area.

NURSING ALERT

 Monitor the patient for a vasovagal episode during insertion of nasal packing.

---

6. Surgical ligation of vessels may be required.

Complications

1. Rhinitis, maxillary and frontal sinusitis
2. Hemotympanum, otitis media

Nursing Interventions and Patient Education

1. Monitor vital signs and assist with control of bleeding.
2. Be aware that packing is uncomfortable and painful and may be in place for 2 to 5 days.
3. Monitor patient with posterior packing for hypoxia (from aspiration of blood, sedation, and preexisting pulmonary dysfunction).
4. Monitor for respiratory difficulty or obstruction—secondary to slippage of packing or balloon, swelling of palate, relaxation of tongue.

5. Instruct the patient as follows for self-management of minor bleeding episodes:
   a. Sit up and lean forward while compressing the soft part (lower half) of nose between index finger and thumb.
   b. If bleeding continues, moisten a small piece of cotton with vasoconstricting nosedrops (phenylephrine hydrochloride [Neo-Synephrine] or oxymetazoline hydrochloride [Afrin]) and place inside nose. Press against bleeding site 5 to 10 minutes.
6. Instruct patient to avoid blowing or picking nose after a nosebleed.
7. Advise patients prone to nosebleeds to:
   a. Apply a lubricant to nasal septum twice daily to reduce dryness.
   b. Use a humidifier if environmental air is dry.

Sinusitis

Sinusitis is an inflammation of the mucous membranes of one or more paranasal sinuses. It is usually precipitated by congestion from viral upper respiratory infection and/or nasal allergy. Obstruction of the sinus ostia (resulting from mucosal swelling and/or mechanical obstruction) leads to retention of secretions and is the usual precursor to sinusitis.

Chronic sinusitis is a suppurative inflammation of the sinuses with chronic irreversible change in the mucosa and sinus bony area.

Clinical Manifestations
Acute Sinusitis
1. Pain—stabbing or aching, over the infected sinus and referred to face and head (Figure 17-2)
2. Nasal congestion and discharge; may or may not be present
3. Anosmia (lack of smell): inspired or expired air cannot reach the olfactory groove
4. Red and edematous nasal mucosa
5. May have fever
Chronic Sinusitis
1. Persistent nasal obstruction; chronic nasal discharge, clear or purulent when infected

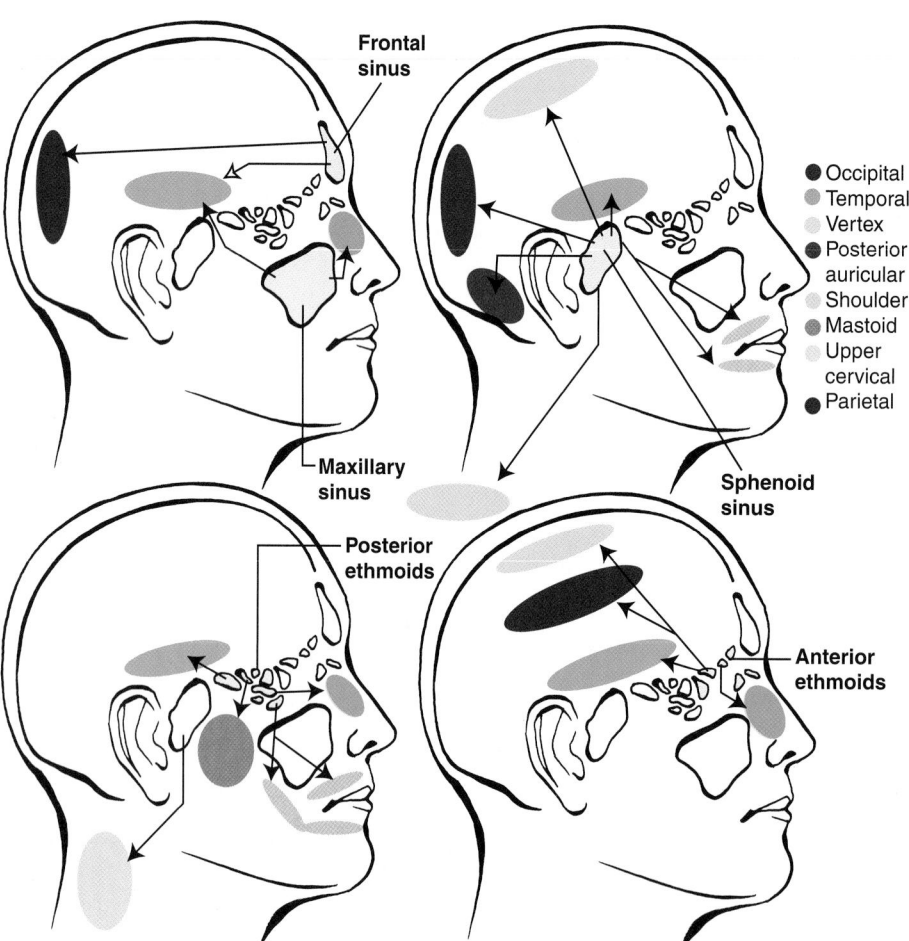

FIGURE 17-2 Paranasal sinuses. (Galen, B. [1997]. Chronic recurrent sinusitis: Recognition and treatment. *Lippincott's Primary Care Practice, 1* [2], 183–197.)

2. Cough—produced by constant dripping of discharge back into nasopharynx
3. Feeling of facial fullness/pressure
4. Headache—may be vague or in same pattern as acute sinusitis, more noticeable in the morning; fatigue

Diagnostic Evaluation

1. Sinus x-rays and CT scan show air–fluid level in acute sinusitis; thickening of sinus mucous membranes, opacification, and anatomic obstruction patterns in chronic sinusitis.
2. Antral puncture and lavage—provides culture material to identify infectious organism; also a therapeutic modality to clear sinus of bacteria, fluid, and inflammatory cells.
3. Nasal and sinus endoscopy (the sinuses can be easily accessed after the patient has had an antrostomy).

Management

1. Topical decongestant spray or drops or systemic decongestants for mucosal shrinkage to encourage drainage from sinus. Topical therapy should be limited to no more than three successive days of use.
2. Topical nasal corticosteroids are frequently used in chronic sinusitis, and may be used in acute cases.
3. Antibiotic, usually trimethoprim–sulfamethoxazole (Bactrim), penicillinase-resistant penicillins, cephalosporins, or macrolide antibiotics.
4. Usually 10- to 14-day course for acute sinusitis
5. Prolonged therapy for chronic sinusitis (up to several months).
6. Analgesics—pain may be significant.
7. Warm compresses; cool vapor humidity for comfort and to promote drainage.
8. Surgical interventions (for chronic sinusitis when conservative treatment is unsuccessful).
   a. Endoscopic sinus surgery—endoscopic removal of diseased tissue from affected sinus; used to treat chronic sinusitis of maxillary, ethmoid, and frontal sinuses.
   b. Nasal antrostomy (nasal–antral window)—surgical placement of an opening under inferior turbinate to provide aeration of the antrum and to permit exit for purulent materials.
   c. For nursing care, see page 537.

Complications

Depend on anatomic location of sinus involved.
1. Extension of infection to the orbital contents and eyelids.

NURSING ALERT

Watch for lid edema, edema of ocular conjunctiva, drooping lid, limitation of extraocular motion, visual loss. May indicate orbital cellulitis, which necessitates immediate treatment.

---

2. Bone infection (osteomyelitis) may spread by direct extension or through blood vessels. Frontal bone commonly affected.
3. CNS complications include meningitis, subdural and epidural purulent drainage, brain abscess, cavernous sinus thrombosis (acute thrombophlebitis originating from an infection in an area having venous drainage to cavernous sinus).

Nursing Interventions and Patient Education

1. Advise patient to promptly seek medical attention for acute sinus infection to prevent chronic sinus disease.
2. Discourage swimming/diving while patient has upper respiratory infection, which may cause contaminated water to be forced into a sinus, usually the frontal sinus.
3. Stress the importance of complying with antibiotic therapy for complete duration, and following up for recurrence.
4. Advise patient with asthma that sinusitis has been associated with exacerbation of asthma symptoms; patient should be alert for increased wheezing, chest tightness, or cough, and seek treatment.
5. Teach patient with recurrent sinusitis how to irrigate nasal passages with saline to remove crusted mucus near the sinus openings and enhance drainage. (See Patient Education, p. 548.)

Pharyngitis

Pharyngitis is an inflammation of the pharynx, including palate, tonsils, and posterior wall of the pharynx, most commonly caused by acute infection, usually transmitted through respiratory secretions. Streptococcal pharyngitis (*strep throat*) and rhinoviruses (the common cold) are frequent causes.

Pathophysiology and Etiology

1. Acute bacterial pharyngitis is usually caused by group A beta-hemolytic streptococci (streptococcal pharyngitis/"strep throat"). Peak age group for streptococcal pharyngitis is 5 to 18, but it may occur in all age groups.
2. Other bacterial causes include *Haemophilus influenzae, Moraxella catarrhalis, Corynebacterium diphtheriae* (diphtheria), *Neisseria gonorrhoeae* (gonorrhea), and other groups of streptococcus. Transmission of *N. gonorrhoeae* is through oral contact with genital secretions; it is a sexually transmitted disease.
3. Viral pharyngitis is common and causes include rhinovirus, adenovirus parainfluenza virus, coxsackievirus, coronavirus, and others.
4. More chronic causes are irritation from postnasal drip of allergic rhinitis and chronic sinusitis, chemical irritation, and systemic diseases.

Clinical Manifestations

1. For acute bacterial infections, abrupt onset of sore throat and fever (usually above 38.2°C [101°F] in streptococcal pharyngitis).

PATIENT EDUCATION GUIDELINES   Nasal Saline Irrigation

This procedure will help clear your nasal passages of crusted drainage that may be blocking the sinus opening. Perform this once or twice a day to feel less nasal congestion and to help your sinuses drain.

1. Prepare saline solution right before irrigation.
2. Mix ½ tsp table salt and ¼ tsp baking soda with 8 oz warm tap water until well dissolved.
3. Lean forward from the waist over a sink.
4. Fill a bulb syringe (1 oz baby ear or nasal bulb) with the saline solution by squeezing it in the solution and letting it fill by suction.
5. Insert the tip of the filled syringe into one nostril, aimed toward the eye, away from the nasal septum.
6. Squeeze the syringe gently and feel the solution run backward in the nose and out the other nostril and possibly down the back of the throat and out of the mouth.
7. Once you are comfortable with this procedure, you may be able to rotate your head forward, backward, and from side to side to irrigate the sinuses as well as the nose.

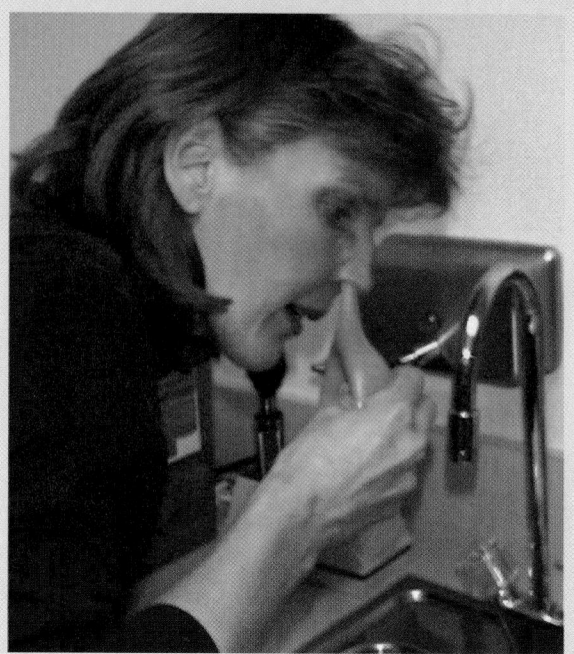

Nose irrigation with bulb syringe.

a. Throat pain is aggravated by swallowing.
b. Pharynx appears reddened with edema of uvula; tonsils enlarged and reddened; pharynx and tonsils may be covered with exudate (Figure 17-3).
2. Varying degrees of sore throat, nasal congestion, fatigue, and fever with other bacterial and viral causes.
3. Swollen, palpable, and tender cervical lymph nodes in most cases.

Diagnostic Evaluation

1. Throat culture or rapid streptococcal antigen detection test to rule out streptococci. Rapid strep tests provide results within 5 minutes; false-negative rate is higher than with culture method.
2. Throat culture on Thayer-Martin medium or gonococcal antigen detection test to rule out gonococcal pharyngitis if genital gonococcal infection or positive sexual contact is suspected.
3. Viral testing is not practical, and viral causes are self-limiting.

Management

1. For streptococcal pharyngitis, penicillin V (Pen-Vee-K) 250 mg qid orally for 10 days or penicillin G benzathine (Bicillin) in a single intramuscular dose of 2.4 million units appears to shorten duration of symptoms and prevents rheumatic fever.

2. Erythromycin for patient who is allergic to penicillin.
3. Other penicillins, macrolides, and cephalosporins are also used.

Complications

1. Acute rheumatic fever
2. Peritonsillar abscess/cellulitis
3. Acute glomerulonephritis
4. Scarlet fever
5. Sinusitis, otitis media, mastoiditis

NURSING ALERT

Acute rheumatic fever, a complication of streptococcal pharyngitis, can be prevented if patient is treated adequately with penicillin, and possibly another antibiotic. Unfortunately, there is no evidence that antibiotic therapy will prevent acute glomerulonephritis.

Nursing Interventions and Patient Education

1. Advise patient to have any sore throat with fever evaluated, especially in the absence of cold symptoms.
2. Encourage compliance with full course of antibiotic therapy, despite feeling better in several days, to prevent complications.
3. Advise lukewarm saline gargles and use of antipyretic/analgesics as directed to promote comfort.

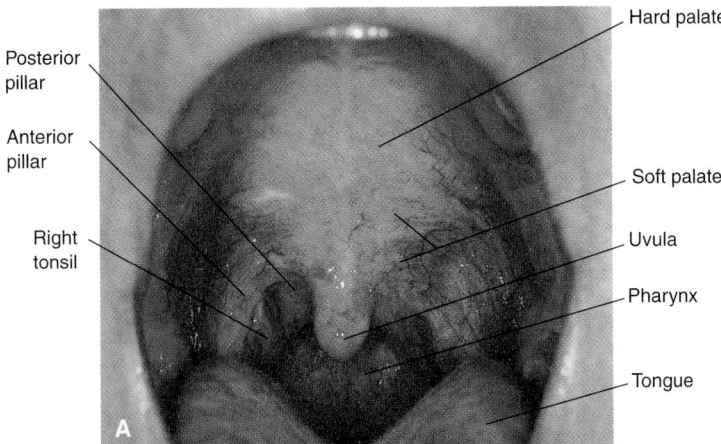
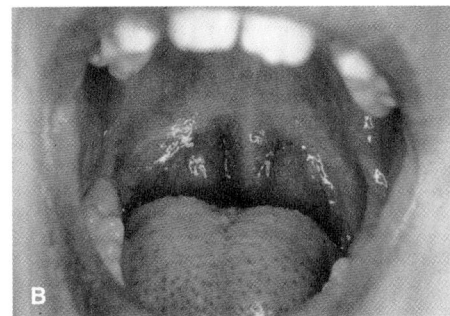
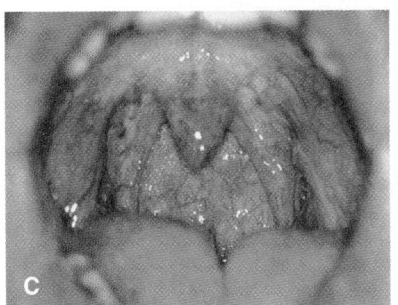
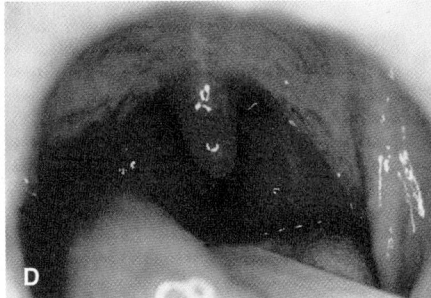
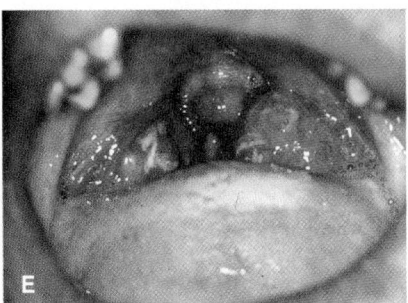

FIGURE 17-3 Assessment of pharyngitis. (**A**) Normal throat. (**B**) Normal large tonsils without redness. (**C**) Mild redness without exudate. (**D**) Intense redness without exudate. (**E**) Redness with exudate on tonsils (probably indicates group A streptococcal infection).

4. Encourage bed rest with increased fluid intake during fever.

EAR DISORDERS

◼ Hearing Loss

Hearing loss ranks high as a health disability. There are multiple causes, and the range of hearing loss varies from mild high-frequency loss to severe loss with complete inability to understand the spoken word. Two major types of hearing loss are conductive and sensorineural. There are 20 million Americans with hearing loss.

Classification of Hearing Loss

1. Conductive loss—hearing loss due to an impairment of the external or middle ear or both. If causative problem cannot be corrected, a hearing aid may help.
2. Sensorineural (perceptive) loss—hearing loss due to disease of the inner ear or nerve pathways; sensitivity to and discrimination of sounds are impaired. Hearing aids usually are helpful.
3. Combined hearing loss—combination of the above.

4. Psychogenic hearing loss—usually a manifestation of an emotional disturbance and unrelated to evident structural changes in the hearing mechanisms. Loss is often total, but without physical basis; thus, the patient may suddenly recover.

Presbycusis

A progressive, bilaterally perceptive hearing loss of older people, usually involving high frequencies, that occurs with the aging process.

1. All other possibly treatable hearing disorders should be ruled out before this diagnosis. There is no effective medical or surgical treatment.
2. The patient should be counseled by an otologist (physician who specializes in the ear) in collaboration with an audiologist (nonphysician provider who can suggest nonmedical treatment).
3. Helpful aids should be considered, such as a telephone amplifier, radio and television earphone attachments, buzzers instead of doorbell.
4. Understanding and help from family members are important.

Otosclerosis

Otosclerosis is a pathologic condition in which there is formation of new spongy bone in the labyrinth, fixation of the stapes, and prevention of sound transmission through the ossicles to the inner fluids, resulting in deafness.

The cause is unknown, but there is a familial tendency and more women are affected than men.

Clinical Manifestations

1. Young adult presents with a history of slow, progressive hearing loss of soft, spoken tones, with no middle ear infection.
2. A frequent complaint is tinnitus; both ears may be affected equally.
3. History reveals gradual hearing loss.
4. Audiometry findings substantiate conductive or mixed hearing loss.
5. Bone conduction is much better than air conduction.

Management

1. No known medical treatment exists for this form of deafness, but amplification with a hearing aid may be helpful.
2. Surgery—stapedectomy.
   a. The removal of otosclerotic lesions at the footplate of stapes or complete removal of the stapes and the creation of a tissue implant with prosthesis to maintain suitable conduction.
   b. To perform such delicate surgery, the otologic binocular microscope is used.

Cochlear Implant

A cochlear implant is a device that emits auditory signals for profoundly deaf people (Figure 17-4). The single-electrode system bypasses the damaged cochlear system and stimulates the remaining auditory nerve fibers. This results in the perception of sound.

Description

1. Purpose is for patient to detect louder environmental sounds, but will not restore normal hearing.
2. The microphone and sound processor are positioned externally; the electrode is implanted internally and inserts into the cochlea.
3. Electrical stimuli converted from the sound processor are sent inside the body to the implanted electrode. These electrical signals stimulate the auditory nerve fibers, which are interpreted by the brain.
4. Success rate is highly variable, which has made the cochlear implant controversial.
   About 25,000 cochlear implants have been inserted worldwide.

Patient Criteria

There are no standardized criteria for patient selection. Some data that are considered include:

1. Severe to profound sensorineural hearing loss in both ears.
2. Little to no benefit with hearing aids.
3. No medical contraindications.
4. Physically healthy adult or child as young as 18 months.

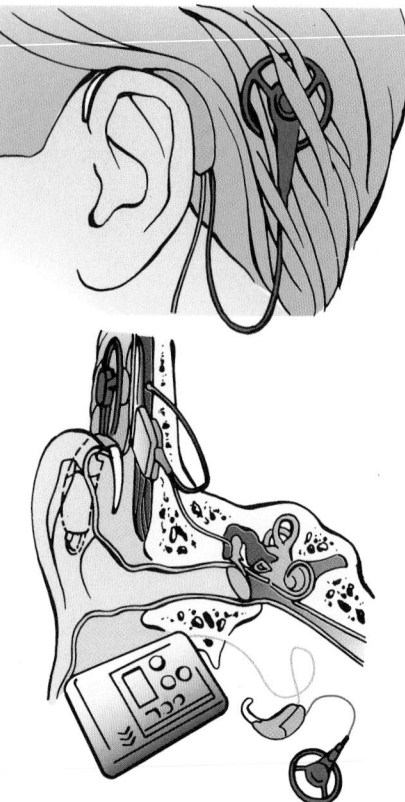

FIGURE 17-4 Nucleus 24 cochlear implant system. Sounds are picked up by the small, directional microphone located in the headset at the ear. A thin cord carries the sound from the microphone to the speech processor, a powerful miniaturized computer. The speech processor filters, analyzes, and digitizes the sound into coded signals that are sent from the speech processor to the transmitting coil. The transmitting coil sends the coded signals as FM radio signals to the cochlear implant under the skin. The cochlear implant delivers the appropriate electrical energy to the array of electrodes, which have been inserted into the cochlea. The electrodes along the array stimulate the remaining auditory nerve fibers in the cochlea. The resulting electrical sound information is sent through the auditory system to the brain for interpretation. The entire process takes microseconds.

5. No evidence of brain impairment, psychoses, or mental retardation.
6. Reasonable expectations and optimism. Motivation must be present.

Nursing Interventions

1. Encourage the prospective patient to visit with someone who is currently using an implant to learn the positive and negative results of a cochlear implant.
2. Explain the rehabilitation process: usually begins 2 months after surgery. Included are:

a. Adjustment of controls.

b. Operation and maintenance of stimulator unit.

c. Listening critically and learning lip reading.

d. Learning discrimination of sounds through cochlear implant. Understanding speech through cochlear implant is not possible with this device alone.

e. Many people trained with such an implant can lip read more easily and can distinguish voices and environmental sounds.

3. For care after surgery, see page 539.

Other Implantable Devices

1. Bone conduction devices transmit sound from an external device, worn above the ear, through the skin and into the skull to the inner ear. This device is indicated in those with conductive hearing loss when a hearing aid is contraindicated, such as chronic ear infection.

2. Semi-implantable hearing aids are being tested for conductive and mixed hearing loss.

Maximizing Communication With the Person Who is Hearing Impaired

When hearing loss is permanent or not amenable to medical or surgical intervention, aural rehabilitation is necessary for the patient to maintain communication and prevent isolation. Aural rehabilitation is a multifaceted process that includes auditory training (listening skills), speech reading (formerly called lip reading), and the use of hearing aids. Nurses strive to maintain effective communication with patients. These suggestions promote better communication.

When the Person Is Hearing Impaired and Able to Lip Read

1. Face the person as directly as possible when speaking.

2. Place yourself in good light so he or she can see your mouth.

3. Do not chew, smoke, or have anything in your mouth when speaking.

4. Speak slowly and enunciate distinctly.

5. Provide contextual clues that will assist the person in following your speech. For example, point to a tray if you are talking about the food on it.

6. To verify that patient understands your message, write it for him or her to read (ie, if you doubt that patient is understanding you).

When the Person Is Hearing Impaired and Difficult to Understand

1. Pay attention when the person speaks; facial and physical gestures may help you understand what person is saying.

2. Exchange conversation with person when it is possible to anticipate replies. This is particularly helpful in your initial contact with person and may help you become familiar with speech peculiarities.

3. Anticipate context of speech to assist in interpreting what the person is saying.

4. If unable to understand person, resort to writing or include in your conversation someone who does understand; request that person repeat that which is not understood.

Organizations That Help the Hearing Impaired

Alexander Graham Bell Association for the Deaf
3417 Volta Place NW
Washington, DC 20007
202-337-5220

American Speech-Language-Hearing Association
10801 Rockville Pike
Rockville, MD 20852
301-897-5700
www.asha.org

National Association of the Deaf
814 Thayer Avenue
Silver Springs, MD 20910
301-587-1788
www.nad.org

Community and Home Care Considerations

1. Prevention of hearing loss should be discussed in the community—in schools, the workplace, and community gatherings.

2. Preventable hearing loss includes:

a. Noise-induced hearing loss—long periods of exposure to loud noise from machinery or engines.

b. Acoustic trauma—single exposure to intense noise such as an explosion or amplified music.

3. Prevention involves avoidance of both types of noise, generally any noise above 85 or 90 decibels.

4. Teach people to be aware of their surroundings and avoid noisy places or turn off sources of noise in the environment whenever possible.

5. Teach proper use of ear protection including earplugs and headsets both in the workplace and elsewhere.

6. Advise people that the Occupational Safety and Health Administration (OSHA) requires ear protection when noise exposure is above the legal limits, so workers have a right to this.

Otitis Externa

Otitis externa is an inflammation of the external ear canal, usually caused by acute infection.

Pathophysiology and Etiology

1. Bacterial causes, usually *Pseudomonas, Proteus vulgaris,* streptococci, and *Staphylococcus aureus.*

2. Fungal infection with *Aspergillus niger, C. albicans.*

3. Dermatologic conditions such as seborrhea, eczema, and contact dermatitis.

4. Trauma to the ear canal, frequently from cleaning the canal.

5. Stagnant water in ear canal after swimming.

6. Necrotizing malignant otitis externa is a serious infection into deeper tissue adjacent to the ear canal, including cellulitis and osteomyelitis. It is frequently caused by *Pseudomonas* and may be seen in diabetics, the elderly, or debilitated people.

Clinical Manifestations
1. Pain, increased by manipulation of auricle or tragus; itching
2. Fever; periauricular lymphadenopathy
3. Foul-smelling white to purulent drainage
4. Red, swollen ear canal with discharge on otoscopic examination

Management
1. Instillation of isopropyl alcohol drops (dries moisture), acetic acid (Vosol) solution (restores acidity), or topical antibiotics (curb infection). A combination of these treatments may be used.
   a. Prophylactic use of alcohol drops or acetic acid solution by swimmers or those prone to otitis externa may be indicated.
   b. Antibiotic drops include combination products containing polymyxin, neomycin, and hydrocortisone (Cortisporin, Pediotic); ciprofloxacin (Cipro HC Otic); and ofloxacin (Floxin Otic).
   c. A 10-day course of treatment is usually indicated.
   d. Parenteral antibiotics will be used for necrotizing otitis externa.
2. If canal is swollen and tender, an antibiotic solution containing a corticosteroid is chosen to decrease inflammation and swelling. If acute inflammation and closure of the ear canal prevent drops from saturating canal, a wick may need to be inserted by an ENT specialist so drops will gain access to walls of entire ear canal.
3. Burow's solution (aluminum acetate solution) or topical corticosteroid cream or lotion is used in otitis externa caused by dermatitis.
4. Fungal infection may be treated with a topical antifungal such as nystatin.
5. In chronic otitis externa, debris from ear canal may need to be removed through irrigation or suction, after pain and swelling have subsided.
6. Warm compresses and analgesics may be needed.

Nursing Interventions and Patient Education
1. Demonstrate proper application of eardrops.
   a. Lie or sit with head tilted to side and affected ear up.
   b. Pull auricle upward and outward and instill four drops or amount prescribed.
   c. Maintain position for 5 minutes to ensure proper saturation.
   d. Do not put cotton in ear because it will soak up drops and impair contact with canal.
2. Advise that otitis externa can be prevented or minimized by thoroughly drying the ear canal after coming into contact with water or moist environment.
3. Teach patient to use prophylactic eardrops after swimming to assist in preventing swimmer's ear, as directed by health care provider.
4. Advise the use of properly fitting earplugs for recurrent cases.

5. Teach proper ear hygiene: clean auricle and outer canal with washcloth only; do not insert anything smaller than finger wrapped in washcloth in ear canal.

NURSING ALERT

 Use of cotton-tipped applicators to dry the canal or remove earwax should be avoided because:

1. Cerumen may be forced against the tympanic membrane.
2. The canal lining may be abraded, making it more susceptible to infection.
3. Cerumen that coats and protects the canal may be removed.

■ Impacted Cerumen and Foreign Bodies

Accumulated cerumen (earwax) may become impacted due to use of cotton swabs to clean ears and may be a problem for some people. Cerumen becomes drier in the elderly, making impaction more likely. Foreign bodies may be lodged in ear canal intentionally or accidentally by patient or other person (usually in children), or patient may be completely unaware, as in insect obstruction.

Etiology and Clinical Manifestations
1. Cerumen usually builds up over period of time, causing slightly decreased hearing acuity and feeling that ear(s) is plugged.
   a. May be underlying seborrhea or other dermatologic condition that causes flaking of skin that mixes with cerumen and becomes obstructive.
   b. Cerumen may be pushed back over tympanic membrane by action of cotton swab.
   c. Patient may instill cerumenolytic, which actually makes condition worse by softening cerumen and causing it to coalesce into larger clump.
2. Insect may fly or crawl into ear, causing initial low rumbling sound; later, feeling that ear is plugged and decreased hearing acuity.
3. Pain, fever, and drainage may occur as otitis externa develops.

Management
1. Accumulated cerumen (earwax) does not have to be removed unless it becomes impacted and interferes with hearing; may be removed by irrigating ear canal (Figure 17-5). See Procedure Guidelines 17-1.
2. Foreign bodies may be removed by instrumentation or irrigation.
   a. Insects—treat by instilling oil drops to smother insect, which then can be removed with ear spatula or irrigation.
   b. Vegetable foreign bodies (eg, peas)—irrigation is contraindicated because vegetable matter absorbs water, which would further wedge it in the canal.

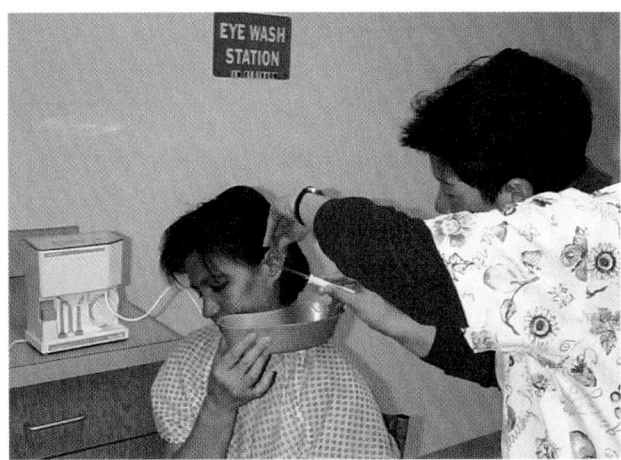

FIGURE 17-5 Using a dental irrigation device to irrigate the external auditory cavity.

c. Only a skilled person should attempt to remove foreign body to prevent tympanic membrane perforation and trauma to canal.

d. General anesthesia may be required for young children.

NURSING ALERT

 Do not attempt to irrigate ear or instill anything into external canal if eardrum may be perforated; otoscopic examination should be done to rule out tympanic membrane rupture. Some antibiotic eardrops are contraindicated if the tympanic membrane is not intact.

Nursing Interventions and Patient Education

1. Teach proper ear hygiene, especially not putting anything in ears.

2. Explain the normal protective function of cerumen.

3. If patient has problem with cerumen buildup and has been advised by health care provider to use a cerumenolytic periodically, ensure that patient is getting cerumen out of ear before more medication is instilled. A bulb syringe may be used by the patient at home to help remove softened cerumen.

4. Advise patient to report persistent fever, pain, drainage, or hearing impairment.

PROCEDURE GUIDELINES 17-1 | **IRRIGATING THE EXTERNAL AUDITORY CANAL**

PURPOSES

1. To remove discharge from the canal.
2. To facilitate removal of cerumen or foreign body.

NURSING ALERT

Ask if patient has a history of draining ears or has ever had a perforation or other complications from a previous ear irrigation. If the reply is "yes," check with the health care provider before proceeding with the irrigation.

EQUIPMENT AND SOLUTIONS

Kind and amount of solution desired (usually warm water)
Ear syringe or irrigating container with tubing, clamp,
  and catheter
Protective towels

Cotton balls and cotton-tipped applicators
Solution bowl and emesis basin
Bag for disposable items

PREPARATORY PHASE

1. After explaining procedure to the patient, place in a position of sitting or lying with head tilted forward and toward affected ear.
2. Position protective towels.

continued

PROCEDURE GUIDELINES 17-1   IRRIGATING THE EXTERNAL AUDITORY CANAL *CONTINUED*

Nursing Action	Rationale

PERFORMANCE PHASE

1. Use a cotton applicator to remove any discharge on outer ear.
2. Place basin close to the patient's head and under the ear.
3. Test temperature of solution. It should be comfortable to the inner aspect of wrist area.

1. To prevent carrying discharge deeper into canal.
2. To provide a receptacle to receive irrigating solution.
3. Solutions that are hot or cold are most uncomfortable and may initiate a feeling of dizziness.

 GERONTOLOGIC ALERT

Take special care not to irrigate an older adult's ear with cool water, because dizziness may be pronounced.

4. Ascertain whether impaction is due to a foreign hydroscopic (attracts or absorbs moisture) body before proceeding.
5. Gently pull the outer ear upward and backward (adult) or downward and outward (child).
6. Place tip of syringe or irrigating catheter at opening of ear; gently direct stream of fluid against sides of canal.
7. If an irrigating container is used, elevate only high enough to remove secretions or no more than 15 cm (6 in.) above patient's ear.
8. Observe for signs of pain or dizziness.
9. If irrigating does not dislodge the wax, instill several drops of prescribed glycerin, carbamide peroxide (Debrox), or other solutions as directed two or three times daily for 2 to 3 days.

4. If water contacts such a substance, it may cause it to swell and produce intense pain.
5. To straighten the ear canal (see accompanying figure)
6. To decrease direct force of irrigation against eardrum and possibility of rupturing it.
7. To provide safe and effective pressure of fluid; if height is more than 15 cm (6 inches), pressure will be too great and may damage tissue.
8. Discontinue treatment if they occur.
9. To soften and loosen impaction.

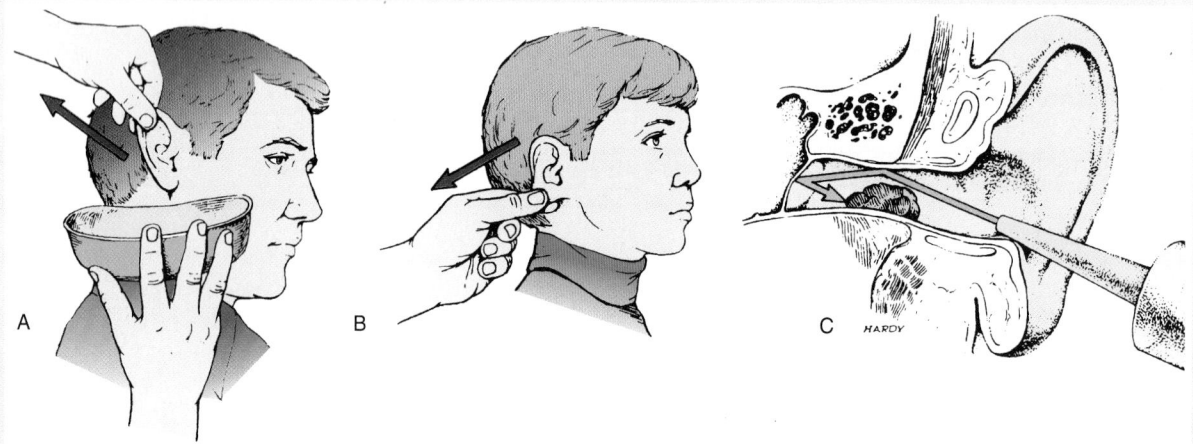

Ear irrigation. (A) The external auditory canal in the adult can best be exposed by pulling the earlobe upward and backward. (B) The same exposure can be achieved in the child by gently pulling the auricle of the ear downward, outward, and backward. (C) An enlarged diagram showing the direction of irrigating fluid against the side of the canal. Note: *This is more effective in dislodging cerumen than if the flow of solution were directed straight into the canal.*

FOLLOW-UP PHASE

1. Dry external ear.
2. Remove soiled equipment and make the patient comfortable.
3. Patient should lie on irrigated (affected) side for a few minutes after procedure to allow any remaining solution to drain out.
4. Record time of irrigation, kind and amount of solution, nature of return flow, and effect of treatment.

Acute Otitis Media

Acute otitis media is an inflammation/infection of the middle ear caused by the entrance of pathogenic organisms, with rapid onset of signs and symptoms. It is a major problem in children but may occur at any age.

Pathophysiology and Etiology

1. Pathogenic organisms gain entry into the normally sterile middle ear, usually through a dysfunctional eustachian tube (suppurative otitis media).
2. Organisms include *Streptococcus pneumoniae, H. influenzae, M. catarrhalis,* and *S. aureus.*
3. In serous (secretory) otitis media, no purulent infection occurs, but blockage of the eustachian tube causes negative pressure and transudation of fluid from blood vessels and development of effusion in the middle ear.

Clinical Manifestations

1. Pain is usually the first symptom.
2. Fever may rise to 40 to 40.6°C (104 to 105°F).
3. Purulent drainage (otorrhea) is present if tympanic membrane is perforated.
4. Irritability may be noted in the young person.
5. Headache, hearing loss, anorexia, nausea, and vomiting may be present.
6. Purulent effusion may be visible behind tympanic membrane, or tympanic membrane may be reddened on otoscopic examination.
7. History may reveal prior upper respiratory infection, allergic rhinitis, or smoking in household and sibling otitis media in children.

Diagnostic Evaluation

1. Pneumatic otoscopy shows a tympanic membrane that is full, bulging, and opaque with impaired mobility (or retracted with impaired mobility).
2. Cultures of discharge through ruptured tympanic membrane may suggest causative organism.

Management

1. Antibiotic treatment—amoxicillin (Amoxil) is first-line treatment; cephalosporins, macrolides, or trimethroprim–sulfamethoxazole (Bactrim) may be used in penicillin allergy.
2. Amoxicillin/clavulanic acid (Augmentin) and cephalosporins are used for treatment failure due to increasing rate of beta-lactamase–producing bacteria that inactivate penicillin and other antibiotics.
3. Usual treatment course is 10 days.
4. Follow-up is indicated to determine effectiveness of therapy.
5. Nasal or topical decongestants and antihistamines have a very limited role to promote eustachian tube drainage.
6. Surgery—myringotomy.

a. An incision is made into the posterior inferior aspect of the tympanic membrane for relief of persistent effusion.
b. Performed on selected patients to prevent recurrent episodes.
c. May be done because of failure of patient to respond to antimicrobial therapy; for severe, persistent pain; and for persistent conductive hearing loss.

Complications

1. Perforation of tympanic membrane
2. Chronic otitis media and mastoiditis
3. Conductive hearing loss
4. Meningitis, brain abscess

Nursing Assessment

1. Obtain history of upper respiratory infection, previous ear infections, allergies, and progression of symptoms.
2. Assess fever and level of pain.
3. Obtain baseline hearing evaluation, if indicated.

Nursing Diagnosis

• Pain related to inflammation and increased middle ear pressure

Nursing Interventions

Relieving Pain

1. Administer or teach self-administration of aspirin and other analgesics as prescribed. (Sedation is usually avoided because it may interfere with early detection of intracranial complications.)
2. Administer or teach self-administration of antibiotics, as prescribed.
3. Encourage the use of local warm compresses or heating pad to promote comfort and help resolve infectious process.
4. Be alert for such symptoms as headache, slow pulse, vomiting, and vertigo, which may be significant for sequelae that involve the mastoid or even the brain.

Patient Education and Health Maintenance

1. Encourage follow-up after treatment to ensure resolution.
2. Advise patient that sudden relief of pain may indicate tympanic membrane rupture. Do not instill anything in ear, and call health care provider.
3. Instruct patient to follow up for any recurrence of symptoms such as pain, fever, ear congestion.

Outcome-Based Evaluation

• Patient verbalizes relief of pain at follow-up visit.

Chronic Otitis Media

Chronic otitis media is a chronic inflammation of the middle ear with tissue damage, usually caused by repeated episodes of acute otitis media. It may be caused by an antibiotic-resistant organism or a particularly virulent strain of organism.

Pathophysiology and Etiology

1. The accumulation of pus inflammatory exudate under pressure in the middle ear cavity may result in necrosis of tissue, with damage to the tympanic membrane and possibly the ossicles.
   a. The most common organisms are group A beta-hemolytic streptococcus, *S. pneumoniae*, and *H. influenzae*.
   b. Other organisms may be present, such as *Pseudomonas*, *Proteus*, and *Bacteroides* species.
2. Persistent rupture of the tympanic membrane and damage to the ossicles lead to conductive hearing loss.
3. Extension of infection may occur into the mastoid cells (mastoiditis).
4. Cholesteatoma may form (mass of squamous epithelium and desquamated debris in the middle ear).
5. Chronic systemic disease and immunosuppression are risk factors.

Clinical Manifestations

1. Painless or dull ache and tenderness of mastoid.
2. Otorrhea may be odorless or foul smelling.
3. Vertigo and pain may be present if CNS complications have occurred.
4. History will indicate several episodes of acute otitis media, possible rupture of tympanic membrane.
5. Fever and postauricular erythema and edema.

Diagnostic Evaluation

1. Air conductive hearing loss is present through audiometric tests.
2. X-rays may note mastoid pathology, for example, cholesteatoma or haziness of mastoid cells.
3. Culture of exudate from middle ear (through ruptured tympanic membrane or at time of surgery).

Management

Note: If advanced chronic ear disease is left untreated, inner ear and life-threatening CNS complications may develop because of erosion of surrounding structures.

Medical Therapy

1. Antibiotic and steroid eardrops may control middle ear infection and inflammation, but once mastoiditis develops, parenteral antibiotic therapy is necessary.
2. Eardrops containing neomycin, garamycin, tobramycin, and quinolones such as Ciprofoxacin (Cipro) are instilled into the middle ear when the tympanic membrane is ruptured.
3. IV antibiotics must cover beta-lactamase–producing organisms—ampicillin–sulbactam (Unasyn), cefuroxime (Ceftin).
4. Frequent removal of epithelial debris and purulent drainage may protect tissue from damage.

Surgical Interventions

1. Indicated when cholesteatoma is present.
2. Indicated when there is pain, profound deafness, dizziness, sudden facial paralysis, or stiff neck (may lead to meningitis or brain abscess).
3. Types of procedures
   a. *Simple mastoidectomy*—removal of diseased bone and insertion of a drain; indicated when there is persistent infection and signs of intracranial complications.
   b. *Radical mastoidectomy*—removal of posterior wall of ear canal, remnants of the tympanic membrane, and the malleous and incus.
   c. *Posteroanterior mastoidectomy*—combines simple mastoidectomy with tympanoplasty (reconstruction of middle ear structures).

Complications

1. Acute and chronic mastoiditis
2. Cholesteatoma
3. CNS infection (meningitis, intracranial abscess)
4. Postoperatively—facial nerve paralysis, bleeding, vertigo

Nursing Assessment

1. Assess for history of ear infection and treatment compliance. Identify factors that may prevent compliance with treatment in future—lack of money/prescription coverage, lack of transportation, lack of knowledge on severity of infection, and so forth.
2. Assess for ear drainage, patency of tympanic membrane.
3. Assess for hearing loss.
4. Palpate for mastoid tenderness.

For nursing process related to patients undergoing surgical treatment, see care related to Ear Surgery, page 539.

Patient Education and Health Maintenance

1. Teach patient to keep ear dry—avoid showers, washing hair, swimming—to prevent any water from gaining access to middle ear.
2. Encourage patient to follow up for frequent ear cleaning.
3. Stress the importance of adhering to antibiotic schedule (usually home IV therapy) and to notify home care nurse or health care provider if there is any problem with venous access or a dose is missed for any reason.
4. Advise of complications and to report headache, change in mental status or arousal, or increased ear pain.
5. Stress the importance of follow-up hearing evaluations and early intervention for any signs of ear infection in the future.

■ Meniere's Disease

Meniere's disease (endolymphatic hydrops) is a chronic disease that involves the inner ear and causes a triad of symptoms—vertigo, hearing loss, and tinnitus.

Pathophysiology and Etiology

1. Cause is unknown.
2. Fluid distention of the endolymphatic spaces of the labyrinth destroys cochlear hair cells.
3. Usually unilateral, later may become bilateral.
4. Occurs most frequently between age 30 and 60.
5. Severity of attacks may diminish over the years, but hearing loss increases.

Clinical Manifestations

1. Sudden attacks occur, in which patient feels that the room is spinning (vertigo); may last 10 minutes to several hours.
2. Dizziness, tinnitus, and reduced hearing occur on involved side.
3. Headache, nausea, vomiting, and incoordination are present.
4. Sudden motion of the head may precipitate vomiting.
5. History often reveals ear trouble, vasomotor rhinitis, and allergies.
6. The most comfortable position for the patient is lying down.
7. Irritability; other personality changes.
8. After multiple attacks, tinnitus and impaired hearing may be continuous.

Diagnostic Evaluation

1. Caloric test/ENG to differentiate Meniere's disease from intracranial lesion.
   a. Fluid, above or below body temperature, is instilled into the auditory canal.
   b. Will precipitate an attack in patients with Meniere's disease.
   c. Normal patient complains of dizziness; patient with acoustic neuroma has no reaction.
2. Audiogram shows sensorineural hearing loss.
3. CT, MRI to rule out acoustic neuroma.

Management

Medical

1. Patient can be asked to keep a diary noting presence of aural symptoms (eg, tinnitus, distorted hearing) when episodes of vertigo occur. This may help diagnose which ear is involved and whether surgery will be needed.
2. Administration of the vestibular suppressant to control symptoms.
   a. Meclizine (Antivert, Bonine) up to 25 mg qid
   b. Diphenhydramine (Benadryl) 25 to 50 mg tid to qid
   c. Diazepam (Valium) 2 mg tid or 5 to 10 mg IM or IV (addictive potential)
3. Streptomycin (IM) or gentamycin (transtympanic injection) may be given to selectively destroy vestibular apparatus if vertigo is uncontrollable.
4. Additional antiemetic such as promethazine (Phenergan) may be needed to reduce nausea, vomiting, and resistant vertigo.

Surgical

1. Conservative—simple endolymphatic sac decompression or endolymphatic subarachnoid or mastoid shunt to relieve symptoms without destroying function.
2. Destructive surgery:
   a. Labyrinthectomy—recommended if the patient experiences progressive hearing loss and severe vertigo attacks so normal tasks cannot be performed; results in total deafness of affected ear.
   b. Vestibular nerve section—neurosurgical suboccipital approach to the cerebellopontine angle for intracranial vestibular nerve neurectomy.

Complications

1. Irreversible hearing loss
2. Disability and social isolation due to vertigo and hearing loss
3. Injury due to falls

Nursing Assessment

1. Assess for frequency and severity of attacks.
2. Provide screening hearing tests.
3. Evaluate effect on patient's activities, potential for fall or injury.

Nursing Diagnoses

- Risk for Injury related to sudden attacks of vertigo
- Social Isolation related to fear of attack and hearing loss

Nursing Interventions

For care related to labyrinth surgery, see page 539.

Ensuring Safety

1. Help patient recognize aura so patient has time to prepare for an attack.
2. Encourage patient to lie down during attack, in safe place, and lie still.
3. Put side rails up on bed if in hospital.
4. Have patient close eyes if this lessens symptoms.
5. Inform patient that the dizziness may last for varying lengths of time. Maintain safety precautions until attack is complete.

Minimizing Feelings of Isolation

1. Provide encouragement and understanding. Show the patient that you understand the seriousness of this disorder, even though there is little that can be done to ease the discomfort:
2. Assist patient to identify specific triggers to control attacks.
   a. Remind the patient to move slowly, because jerking or making sudden movements may precipitate an attack.
   b. Avoid noises and glaring, bright lights, which may initiate an attack.
   c. Control environmental factors and personal habits that may cause stress or fatigue.
   d. If there is a tendency to allergic reactions to foods, eliminate those foods from the diet.

3. Avoid oversedation of the patient through polypharmacy with sedatives, anticholinergics, and narcotics that may increase risk of falling if attack occurs.
4. Teach patient to be aware of other sensory cues from the environment, visual, olfactory, and tactile, if hearing is affected.

Patient Education and Health Maintenance
1. Teach about medication therapy, including side effects of vestibular suppressants—drowsiness, dry mouth.
2. Advise sodium restriction as adjunct to vestibular suppressant therapy.
3. Advise patient to keep a log of attacks, triggers, and severity of symptoms.
4. Encourage follow-up hearing evaluations and provide information about surgical care if planned.
5. Teach patient hearing conservation methods—avoid loud noises, wear earplugs if necessary, avoid smoking, avoid use of ototoxic drugs such as aspirin, quinine, and some antibiotics.

Outcome-Based Evaluation
- Patient lying down with side rails up and eyes closed during attack; resolved without injury
- Identified caffeine, bright lights, and stress as triggering factors; verbalizes desire to eliminate these factors

Labyrinthitis

Labyrinthitis is an inflammation of the inner ear vestibular labyrinth system. It may be due to a viral or bacterial infection, occur as a symptom of a tumor or other pathology in the nervous system, or occur due to a physiologic response from external stimuli. The hallmark is vertigo.

Pathophysiology and Etiology
1. Bacterial labyrinthitis is rare and usually a complication of bacterial meningitis, although it may rarely be seen with otitis media or cholesteatoma.
2. Viral labyrinthitis is more common, but poorly understood. It may be caused by a common upper respiratory virus or occur with mumps, rubella, rubeola, and influenza.
3. Conflicting visual, vestibular, and somatosensory signals may be caused by stimuli such as a roller coaster ride, a sudden stop, or a quick change in position. The elderly and those with cerebrovascular disease are at risk.
4. Both hearing and balance may be affected by infectious or pathologic causes.

Clinical Manifestations
1. Sudden onset of incapacitating vertigo, with varying degrees of nausea and vomiting, hearing loss, and tinnitus.
2. The first attack is most severe; repeated attacks occur over a week to several months with infectious labyrinthitis.
3. Symptoms may remain steady or gradually increase with CNS pathology.

Diagnostic Evaluation
1. Characteristic infectious labyrinthitis may be monitored for improvement without diagnostic testing.
2. ENG with caloric and doll's eye testing to differentiate cause.
3. CT or MRI for suspected tumors of cranial nerve VIII.
4. Forced hyperventilation for 1 to 3 minutes to mimic symptoms—differentiates physiologic cause.

Management
1. The rare cases of bacterial labyrinthitis are treated with antibiotics, as with the suspected predisposing infection.
2. Viral and physiologic causes are treated with symptomatic support.
3. Prevention and management of attacks.
4. Vestibular suppressant and antiemetic medication as with Meniere's disease (meclizine, diazepam, promethazine).
5. Presumed pathologic causes are worked up, and the cause is treated with neurosurgery or another measure.

Complications
1. Permanent hearing loss
2. Injury from fall

Nursing Assessment
1. Assess frequency and severity of attacks and how patient handles them.
2. Assess for fever related to bacterial infection.
3. Assess for additional neurologic symptoms—visual changes, change in mental status, sensory and motor deficits, and so forth—that may indicate CNS pathology.
4. Assess for effectiveness of vestibular stimulants and antiemetics.
5. If fall occurs, assess for injury.

Nursing Diagnoses
- High Risk for Injury related to gait disturbance secondary to vertigo
- Anxiety related to sudden onset of symptoms
- Risk for Fluid Volume Deficit related to vomiting and impaired intake
- Self-Care Deficit (bathing, dressing, feeding, toileting) related to vertigo

Nursing Interventions
Preventing Injury
1. At onset of attack, have patient lie still in darkened room with eyes closed or fixed on stationary object, until the vertigo passes.
2. Ensure that patient can obtain help at all times through use of call system, close proximity to staff, or companion.
3. Remove any obstacles in patient's environment.
4. Ensure that sensory aids are available—glasses, hearing aid, proper lighting.
5. Use side rails while patient is in bed.
6. Administer medications as directed; assess for and avoid oversedation.

Minimizing Anxiety

1. Explain the physiology behind vertigo and the possible triggers.
2. Support patient and family through the diagnostic process.
3. Assist patient to adjust activities to minimize the impact.
4. Teach stress reduction techniques such as deep breathing, talking and asking questions, and distraction.

Ensuring Adequate Fluid

1. Keep diet light while vertigo is present.
2. Administer antiemetics as directed.
3. Assess intake and output as indicated.
4. Encourage fluids and small feedings while patient is feeling better.

Encouraging Safe Self-Care

1. Encourage activity while vertigo is minimal; rest during attacks.
2. Set up environment for patient's safety and convenience—chair near sink, walker to hold on to while walking if necessary, and so forth.
3. Assist patient with hygiene and other care as needed.

Patient Education and Health Maintenance

1. Teach patients with viral labyrinthitis that attacks are self-limiting, will become less severe, and should leave no permanent disability.
2. Teach safety measures during vertigo attacks.
3. Tell patient that vertigo is best tolerated while lying flat in bed in a darkened room, with eyes closed or looking at stable object.
4. Teach patients how to take medications, and to avoid other CNS depressants such as alcohol.
5. Encourage follow-up.

Outcome-Based Evaluation

- Resting in bed during attack with side rails up
- Patient verbalizing feelings and questions about treatment
- Taking fluids, light diet every 4 hours, after medication administration
- Performing appropriate hygiene and dressing by self at bedside

MALIGNANT DISORDERS

Cancer of the Oral Cavity

Cancer of the oral cavity may arise from the lips, buccal mucosa, gums, hard palate, floor of the mouth, salivary glands, and anterior two thirds of the tongue.

Pathophysiology and Etiology

1. Most prevalent in men ages 50 to 70 years; approximately 90% are squamous cell carcinoma.
2. High-risk factors: use of tobacco and alcohol (particularly in combination), use of smokeless tobacco (snuff), pipe smoking, and chronic sun exposure.
3. Overall 5-year survival rate is 30% to 40%, depending on the stage of disease at diagnosis.

Clinical Manifestations

1. Often asymptomatic in early stages.
2. Mucosal erythroplasia—red inflammatory or erythroplastic mucosal changes; appears smooth, granular, and minimally elevated, with or without a white component (leukoplakia); persisting longer than 14 days.
3. Cancer of the lip—presence of a lesion that fails to heal.
4. Cancer of the tongue—swelling, ulceration, areas of tenderness or bleeding, abnormal texture, or limited movement of the tongue.
5. Floor-of-the-mouth cancer—red, slightly elevated, mucosal lesion with ill-defined borders, leukoplakia, indurated, ulceration, or wartlike growth.
6. More advanced stages characterized by ulceration, bleeding, pain, induration, and/or cervical lymphadenopathy.

Diagnostic Evaluation

1. Careful inspection of the oral cavity with indirect mirror examination of pharynx.
2. Staining of the oral lesion with toluidine blue—the lesion stains dark blue after rinsing with acetic acid (normal tissue does not absorb stain).
3. Excisional biopsy of suspected tissue.
4. Radiologic studies: chest x-ray, CT, and MRI to determine local invasiveness and metastasis.

Management

Selection of treatment depends on the size and site of lesion and how extensively surrounding tissues are involved.

1. Small lesions can be removed by wide excision or treated with radiotherapy or interstitial irradiation.
2. Large lesions may be excised widely or treated by radical neck dissection for extensive lymphatic involvement, followed by external irradiation to decrease recurrence rate but maintain appearance.
3. Radiation therapy can be palliative, providing it has not been given previously.
4. Chemotherapy of previously untreated patients with locally advanced tumors has shown high response rates in clinical trials.

Complications

1. Second primary cancers of the larynx, hypopharynx, esophagus, and lungs
2. Secondary to treatment:
   a. Surgery: transient salivary outflow obstruction, infection, voice changes, fistula formation, loss of swallowing, cosmetic defects
   b. Radiation: temporary loss of taste, xerostomia, radiation caries, osteoradionecrosis

Nursing Assessment

1. Obtain complete history, noting risk factors such as smoking and alcohol use.
2. Question the patient regarding changes in swallowing, smell or taste, salivation, discomfort when eating, sore throat, foul breath odor.
3. Note the quality of voice patterns and odor of breath.
4. Inspect the oral cavity: erythema, red velvety areas; white patches; bleeding; swelling; record the size, location, and description.
5. Palpate the cervical lymph nodes for size, firmness, or tenderness.

Nursing Diagnoses

- Pain related to malignant infiltration, lesion(s), difficulty swallowing, surgery, radiation therapy
- Altered Nutrition: Less Than Body Requirements related to pain, difficulty in chewing or swallowing, history of alcohol abuse
- Body Image Disturbance related to changes in facial contour, cosmetic defect from surgery

Nursing Interventions

Also see page 561 if radical neck dissection has been performed.

Achieving an Acceptable Level of Comfort

1. Provide systemic analgesics or analgesic gargles as prescribed.
2. If the patient can tolerate it, provide mouth care with soft toothbrush and flossing between teeth.
3. If patient cannot tolerate brushing and flossing:
   a. Gently lavage oral cavity with a catheter inserted between the patient's cheek and gums with warm water or mouthwash.
   b. Use power water spray to clean inaccessible areas if patient's comfort allows.
4. Encourage use of mouthwashes that do not contain alcohol, which may irritate the gums.
5. Provide management of excessive salivation and mouth odors.
   a. Insert a gauze wick in corner of mouth; place basin conveniently to catch drooling; replace frequently to absorb and direct excess saliva.
   b. Suction secretions with a soft rubber catheter as needed; instruct patient on suctioning methods.
6. Provide management of decreased salivation, if necessary.
   a. Encourage intake of fluids, if not contraindicated.
   b. Instruct the patient to avoid dry, bulky, and irritating foods.
   c. Offer lemon lozenges or chewing gum to stimulate salivation.
7. Maintain a clean and odor-free environment by removing soiled dressings, tissues, and gauzes, and providing room deodorants.

Improving Nutritional Status

1. Handle feeding problems in one or a combination of the following ways, as ordered:
   a. Intravenously
   b. Nasogastric tube feedings or gastrostomy tube feedings
   c. Orally—serve meals high in protein and vitamin content, low in acidity and salt
2. Provide mouth care before and after eating.
3. Allow the patient to have meals in privacy, if desired.
4. Offer easily chewed foods; mash or blenderize, if necessary.
5. Add herbs or sweeteners to enhance flavor.
6. If swallowing difficulties persist, see Procedure Guidelines 18-8, page 600, or consult the occupational or speech therapist.
7. Monitor weight, intake and output, and laboratory tests, such as blood urea nitrogen, creatinine, albumin, and total proteins.

Strengthening Body Image

1. Assess the patient's reaction to condition.
   a. Evaluate the patient's apprehension, and offer emotional support.
   b. Correct any misinformation.
   c. Determine therapeutic plan of care for the patient's rehabilitation.
2. Recognize that face and neck surgery can be disfiguring and the patient often is embarrassed, withdrawn, and depressed.
3. Assist the patient in caring for personal appearance.
4. Observe closely for indications of the patient's needs, which may be communicated in other ways, such as acting out or withdrawn behavior.
5. Allow verbalization of fears, anger, distaste with body changes in a nondefensive manner.
6. Communicate acceptance of appearance in an honest manner.
7. Encourage the patient's family and friends to visit so patient is aware that others care about him or her.
8. Provide diversional activities.

Community and Home Care Considerations

1. Teach mouth care procedure and dressing care to maintain cleanliness and prevent odor.
2. Emphasize adequate nutrition—proper consistency, proper seasoning, and right temperature. Show family how to prepare food in blender or food processor as necessary.
3. If suctioning is required, instruct as to method, use and care of equipment, and obtain supplies for family.
4. Provide detailed instructions and demonstration to the patient and caregiver on incisional care.
5. Assess for signs of obstruction, hemorrhage, infection, and depression, and teach caregivers what to do about them if they occur.

Patient Education and Health Maintenance

1. Encourage follow-up with speech-language pathologist, if indicated.
2. Encourage cessation of high-risk behaviors to all—smoking, alcohol consumption, use of smokeless tobacco, pipe smoking.
3. Emphasize the need for routine follow-up examinations.

Outcome-Based Evaluation

- Reports adequate comfort levels, is pain free, handles secretions adequately
- Achieves adequate nutritional status, able to eat prescribed diet
- Verbalizes acceptance of body image, demonstrates behaviors that reflect self-esteem (eg, shaves, dresses, applies makeup)

Radical Neck Dissection for Head and Neck Malignancy

Radical neck dissection, which may be indicated for head and neck cancer, refers to a group of malignant tumors that may occur at one or more anatomic locations in the upper respiratory and digestive tract. Specific sites include ear, nasopharynx, nose and paranasal sinuses, palate, oral cavity, larynx, hypopharynx, and thyroid gland. Most are squamous cell carcinomas. Local extension to adjacent muscle, bone, and vital structures often occurs before detection, and metastasis to cervical lymph nodes is common.

Surgical Procedures

1. Resection of lesion is the primary intervention.
2. Radical neck dissection—removal of all tissue under the skin from the ramus of the jaw down to the clavicle, from midline back to the angle of the jaw. This includes sternocleidomastoid muscle, other smaller muscles, jugular vein in the neck.
3. Modified (functional) radical neck dissection—removal of lymph nodes only.
4. Concomitant hemilaryngectomy or total laryngectomy may be necessary.
5. Often followed by postoperative radiation therapy. In some instances where resection is impossible, radical radiation therapy is the sole treatment for head and neck malignancy.
6. Surgical reconstruction may be performed with a rotational flap, skin graft, or free flap to promote healing and improve aesthetics.

Preoperative Management

1. Interventions to improve nutritional status preoperatively include nutritional supplements, hyperalimentation, alcohol withdrawal, and counseling.
2. Patient's general health status is evaluated, and underlying conditions, such as cirrhosis and obstructive pulmonary or cardiovascular disease, are identified and treated, if possible.
3. Patient is evaluated for level of understanding of disease process, treatment regimen, and follow-up care.
4. Emotional preparation for major surgery, long rehabilitation, and change in body image is provided.

Postoperative Management

1. A major goal of postoperative management is protection of the airway. After the patient has fully recovered from anesthesia, the endotracheal tube is removed (unless respiratory compromise occurs).
2. The patient is closely monitored for hemorrhage. Wound drainage through portable suction should not exceed 120 mL on the first postoperative day, then decreases.
3. Prophylactic antibiotics are given to prevent infection because of extensive incision, lymph node resection, and close proximity to oral secretions.
4. Oral nutritional supplements, enteral feedings, or hyperalimentation is provided until oral intake is adequate and nutritional status is improved.

Complications

1. Surgery—salivary incontinence, malocclusion, unintelligible speech, difficulty eating or swallowing, unacceptable deformity
2. Radiation
   a. Early—radiation mucositis, erythema, desquamation, dysphagia, secondary infection, oral pain
   b. Long-term—atrophy, fibrosis, salivary dryness, hoarseness, difficulty swallowing, bone pain, osteonecrosis, pathologic fractures, limitation of movement

Nursing Diagnoses

- Ineffective Breathing Pattern related to laryngeal edema, secretions, presence of a tracheostomy
- Risk for Infection related to surgery, proximity of secretions to suture line, postoperative radiation
- Altered Nutrition: Less Than Body Requirements related to anorexia, inability to swallow, pain on swallowing
- Impaired Verbal Communication related to laryngeal edema, laryngectomy, tracheostomy
- Body Image Disturbance related to surgical therapy, radiation changes

Nursing Interventions
Maintaining Effective Breathing Pattern

1. Place the patient in Fowler's position.
2. Observe for signs of respiratory embarrassment, such as dyspnea, cyanosis, edema, hoarseness, or dysphagia.
3. Provide supplemental oxygen by face mask, if necessary; if tracheostomy is present, provide oxygen by collar or T-piece, providing adequate humidification.
4. Auscultate for decreased breath sounds, crackles, wheezes; auscultate over the trachea in the immediate postoperative period to assess for stridor indicative of edema.
5. Encourage deep breathing and coughing.

6. Assist the patient in assuming a sitting position to bring up secretions (support the patient's neck with the nurse's hands).
7. Suction secretions orally or aseptically through a tracheostomy if patient is unable to cough them up.

Preventing Infection
1. Assess vital signs for indication of infection—increased heart rate, elevation of temperature.
2. Inspect wound for hemorrhage, drainage, or tracheal constriction; reinforce dressings as needed.
3. Inspect incision for signs of infection—redness, warmth, swelling, drainage.
4. If portable suction is used, expect approximately 80 to 120 mL of serosanguineous secretions to be drawn off during the first postoperative day; this diminishes with each day.
5. Aseptically cleanse skin area around drain exit, using saline or prescribed solution.
6. Ensure that the incision site remains clean and dry; cleanse away any secretions immediately.

Improving Nutritional Status
1. Postoperatively provide IV fluids and hyperalimentation, tube feedings through nasogastric tube or gastrostomy tube, or oral feedings as soon as swallowing is established.
2. Provide mouth care before and after meals.
3. Assess for excessive or decreased salivation, which may impair swallowing.
4. Ensure that emergency suctioning and airway equipment is available at the bedside during meals in the event of choking or aspiration.
5. Position patient in an upright position, supporting shoulders and neck with pillows, if necessary.
6. Inquire whether the patient would prefer privacy during meals.
7. Provide an environment that is clean and free of interruptions and odor.
8. Assist with oral intake, providing easily chewed foods. Mash or blenderize meals, if necessary.

Improving Ability to Communicate
1. If tracheostomy or laryngectomy has been performed, provide alternative methods of communication (letter board, chalk and slate, paper and pencil). If writing is a problem, it may be due to denervation of the trapezius muscle.
2. Allow adequate time for patient to communicate.
3. Place call bell and other articles that patient may need within easy access.
4. Recognize that patient may have difficulty nodding "yes" or "no" because of neck dissection.
5. Provide support and encouragement during communication attempts, recognizing that this patient often is depressed and frustrated even during limited communication.
6. Refer patient to speech-language pathologist, if indicated.

Strengthening Body Image
1. Respect the patient's desire for privacy during treatments, dressing changes, and feedings.
2. Inform visitors of appearance before they see patient so their expressions do not upset patient.
3. Provide frequent aeration of the room, and use deodorants to prevent unpleasant odors.
4. Observe for lower facial paralysis; this may indicate facial nerve injury.
5. Watch for shoulder dysfunction, which may follow resection of spinal accessory nerves.
   a. Use postoperative muscle exercises and muscle re-education.
   b. Work with the patient to obtain good functional range of motion.
6. Talk with the surgeon and patient about decisions on future cosmetic surgery or in the use of a prosthetic device.
7. Encourage the patient to verbalize concerns and feelings.
   a. Consult the health care provider to determine the nature and extent of explanation and prognosis that has been given to the patient.
   b. Encourage the patient to seek confirmation of personal philosophy and religious beliefs, because this may provide answers.
   c. Accentuate the positive.
   d. Encourage the patient to participate in the plan of care.
   e. Recognize that a great effort has to be made in behavior modification to change a lifestyle that included alcohol consumption and cigarette smoking. It is difficult to do.

Community and Home Care Considerations
If patient has a permanent tracheostomy or laryngectomy, instruct the patient and family regarding:
1. Need for increased humidification in home environment
2. Protective stoma cover to help filter air
3. Avoiding activities that may cause aspiration (eg, swimming)
4. Referral for speech-language pathologist, social worker to meet ongoing communication needs

Patient Education and Health Maintenance
Exercises
Instruct the patient and family regarding exercises to prevent limited range of motion and discomfort (Figure 17-6).
1. Perform exercises morning and evening. Initially, exercises are done only once; the number is increased by one each day until each exercise is done 10 times.
2. After each exercise, the patient is instructed to relax.
3. For neck:
   a. Gently rotate head to each side as far as possible.
   b. Tilt head to the right side as far as possible; repeat for left side.
   c. Drop chin to chest, and then raise chin as high as possible.

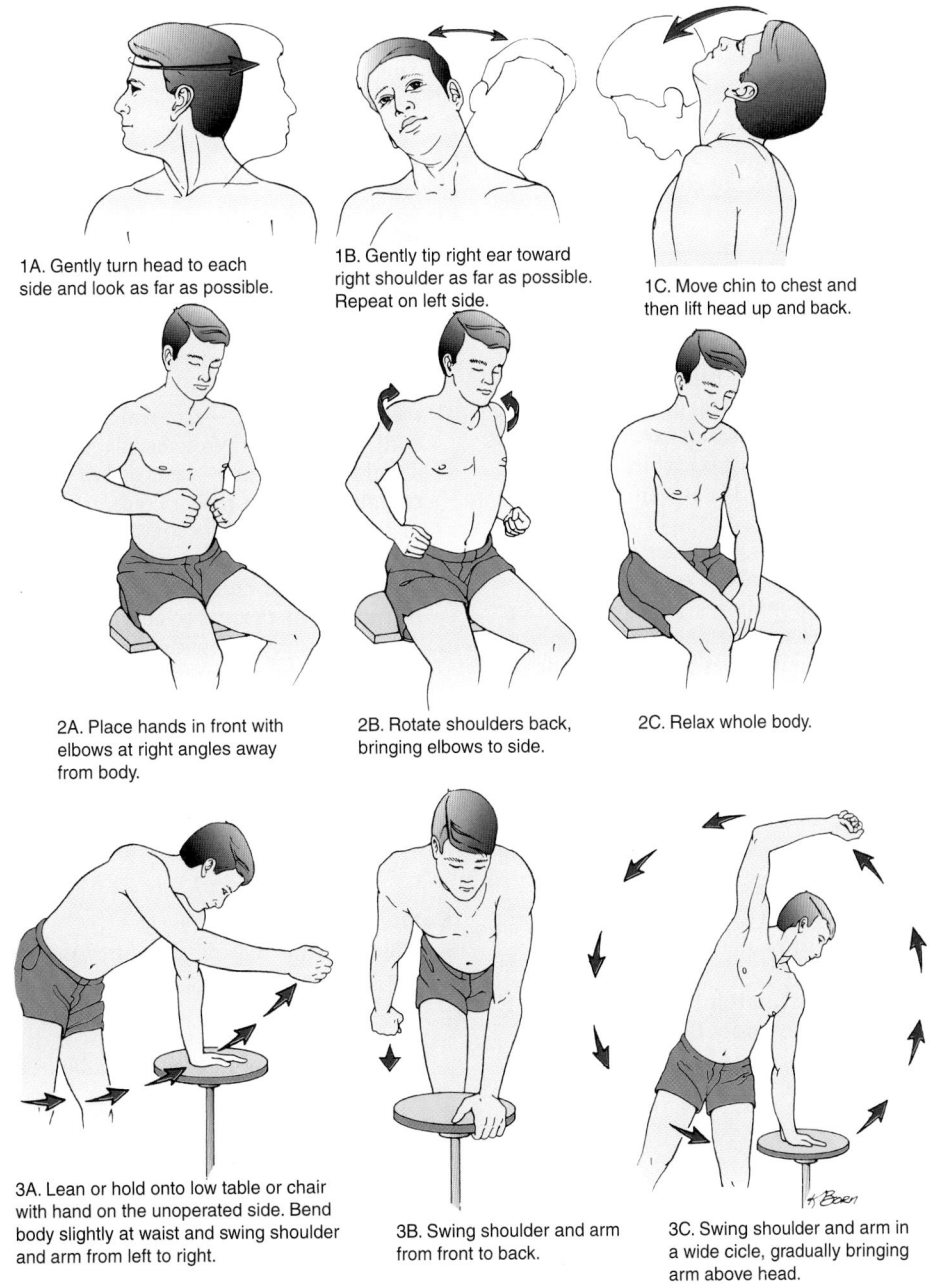

1A. Gently turn head to each side and look as far as possible.

1B. Gently tip right ear toward right shoulder as far as possible. Repeat on left side.

1C. Move chin to chest and then lift head up and back.

2A. Place hands in front with elbows at right angles away from body.

2B. Rotate shoulders back, bringing elbows to side.

2C. Relax whole body.

3A. Lean or hold onto low table or chair with hand on the unoperated side. Bend body slightly at waist and swing shoulder and arm from left to right.

3B. Swing shoulder and arm from front to back.

3C. Swing shoulder and arm in a wide cicle, gradually bringing arm above head.

FIGURE 17-6 Rehabilitation exercises after head and neck surgery to regain maximum shoulder function and neck motion.

4. For shoulder:
   a. Standing beside bed, place hand from unoperated side on bed for support.
   b. Gradually swing arm on operated side up and back as far as is comfortable for the patient.
   c. Each day, work toward finishing a complete circle.

Follow-Up Visits

Emphasize the need for frequent follow-up visits and completion of radiation therapy, if prescribed.

Outcome-Based Evaluation

- Maintains adequate breathing pattern; absence of dyspnea, shortness of breath; is able to handle secretions
- Is free of signs and symptoms of infection; vital signs stable; incision is clean, dry, without redness or drainage
- Is adequately hydrated, maintains stable nutritional status, is able to tolerate diet without choking or aspiration
- Able to communicate and make needs known

- Discusses concerns regarding condition, verbalizes positive aspects of self

Cancer of the Larynx

Cancer of the larynx is a malignant growth of the vocal cords (intrinsic) or any portion of the larynx (extrinsic). When treated early, the likelihood of cure is great.

Pathophysiology and Etiology

1. Occurs predominantly in men older than 60.
2. Most patients have a history of smoking; those with supraglottic laryngeal cancer frequently have a history of smoking and a high alcohol intake. Other risk factors include vocal straining, chronic laryngitis, industrial exposure, nutritional deficiency, and family predisposition.
3. In North America, about two thirds of carcinomas of the larynx arise in the glottis, almost one third arise in the supraglottic region, and about 3% arise in the subglottic region of the larynx.
4. When limited to the vocal cords (intrinsic), spread is slow because of lessened blood supply.
5. When cancer involves the epiglottis (extrinsic), cancer spreads more rapidly because of abundant supply of blood and lymph and soon involves the lymph nodes of the neck.

Clinical Manifestations

Depend on tumor location; sequence in appearance related to pattern and extent of tumor growth.

Supraglottic Cancer

1. Tickling sensation in throat
2. Dryness and fullness (lump) in throat
3. Painful swallowing (odynophagia) associated with invasion of extralaryngeal musculature
4. Coughing on swallowing
5. Pain radiating to ear (late symptom)

Glottic Cancer (Cancer of the Vocal Cord)

1. Most common cancer of the larynx
2. Hoarseness or voice change
3. Aphonia (loss of voice)
4. Dyspnea
5. Pain (in later stages)

Subglottic Cancer (Uncommon)

1. Coughing
2. Short periods of difficulty in breathing
3. Hemoptysis; fetid odor, which results from ulceration and disintegration of tumor

Diagnostic Evaluation

1. Indirect mirror examination of larynx may indicate lesion.
2. Direct laryngoscopy and biopsy to identify lesion.
3. CT scan and other special radiologic tests to detect tumor.
4. Laryngography—contrast study of larynx to define blood vessels and lymph nodes.

Management

Depends on sites and stages of cancer.

Endoscopic Removal of Early Malignancy

Radiation

1. Singly or in combination with surgery.
2. Complications of radiation—edema of larynx, soft tissue and cartilage necrosis, chondritis (inflammation of cartilage).

Surgery

1. Carbon dioxide laser for early-stage disease.
2. Partial laryngectomy—removal of small lesion on true cord, along with a substantial margin of healthy tissue.
3. Supraglottic laryngectomy—removal of hyoid bone, epiglottis, and false vocal cords; tracheostomy may be done to maintain adequate airway; radical neck dissection may be done.
4. Hemilaryngectomy—removal of one true vocal cord, false cord, one half of thyroid cartilage, arytenoid cartilage.
5. Total laryngectomy—removal of entire larynx (epiglottis, false or true cords, cricoid cartilage, hyoid bone; two or three tracheal rings are usually removed when there is extrinsic cancer of the larynx [extension beyond the vocal cords]). A radical neck dissection may also be done because of metastasis to cervical lymph nodes.
6. Total laryngectomy with laryngoplasty—voice rehabilitation may be attempted through the Asai operation.
   a. A dermal tube is made from the upper end of the trachea into the hypopharynx.
   b. The tracheostomy opening is closed off with a finger.
   c. The patient expires air up the dermal tube into the pharyngeal cavity.
   d. The sound produced is transformed into almost normal speech.

Complications

1. Salivary fistula may develop after any surgical procedure that involves entering the pharynx or esophagus.
   a. Monitor for saliva collecting beneath the skin flaps or leaking through suture line or drain site.
   b. Management—nasogastric tube feeding, meticulous local wound care with frequent dressing changes, promotion of drainage.
2. Hemorrhage (carotid artery rupture) or hematoma formation.
   a. A major postoperative complication such as skin necrosis or salivary fistula usually precedes carotid artery rupture.
   b. Management—immediate wound exploration in operating room.
3. Stomal stenosis.
4. Aspiration.
5. Long-term complications:
   a. Chest infections (from repeated aspiration)
   b. Recurrence of cancer in stoma

Preoperative Management
Preparing for Total Laryngectomy

1. Collaborate with the surgeon in preparing the patient; interpret and amplify what surgeon and speech-language pathologist have explained.

2. Patient is informed that breathing will occur through an opening (tracheostoma) in the neck.

3. Patient is made aware of the fact that speech will be altered by surgery.

   a. Expect reactions of anxiety and depression, because the psychosocial effects of voice loss are substantial.

   b. Practice a means of communication (pad and pencil, sign language, pictures, word cards, artificial larynx) that can be used until speech therapy begins.

   c. Arrange for patient to be visited by laryngectomee (one who has had larynx removed) for hope and encouragement.

   d. Inform patient of available community services.

4. Information about alternative modes of communication is provided.

   a. Artificial larynx, using either neck or intraoral placement. Electrolarynx provides communication assistance in early postoperative period or later to those unable to learn alternative method.

   b. Tracheoesophageal puncture with voice prosthesis. A puncture is made between posterior wall of tracheostoma and underlying esophagus; a one-way valved voice prosthesis is inserted through tracheoesophageal puncture that allows patient to shunt pulmonary air into esophagus for voice production (Figure 17-7).

   c. Esophageal speech is accomplished by training patient to force air down the esophagus and release it in a controlled manner.

   d. Surgical reconstructive procedures to restore voice.

Nursing Assessment

1. Ask about smoking history, alcohol intake, drug history, chronic illnesses.

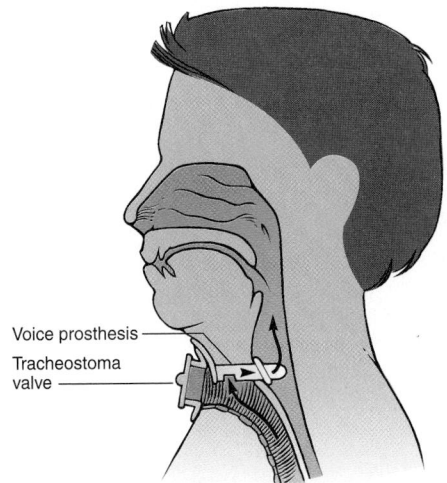

FIGURE 17-7 Schematic representation of tracheoesophageal puncture speech. Air travels from the lungs through a voice prosthesis, which enters a puncture in the posterior wall of the trachea. Air travels into the esophagus and out the mouth.

2. Take a nutrition history and 24-hour food intake recall. Review results of laboratory test. Weigh the patient.

3. Observe ability to swallow.

4. Review recommendations of speech-language pathologist and social worker.

5. Assess for independence, self-assuredness, and willingness to try new things; these are strengths on which to build.

6. Assess reality of patient's expectations.

7. Find out about patient's social support system.

Nursing Diagnoses

- Ineffective Breathing Pattern related to presence of artificial airway, accumulation of secretions, inability to cough secondary to surgical procedure
- Altered Nutrition: Less Than Body Requirements related to impaired swallowing secondary to surgical alteration of pharynx and larynx; laryngeal edema and pain; radiation-induced mucositis
- Impaired Verbal Communication related to surgery/absence of larynx; presence of artificial airway
- Knowledge Deficit related to stoma care and living with effects of laryngectomy

Nursing Interventions
Improving Breathing Pattern

1. Monitor for signs of difficult breathing—suprasternal and intercostal retractions, tachypnea, dyspnea, tachycardia, changes in sensorium.

2. Auscultate trachea/chest for evidence of stridor, wheezing, and absence of breath sounds.

3. Be sure that the patient uses a specific signal to indicate need for suctioning; enter on nursing care plan.

4. Suction secretions as they accumulate to clean and protect the airway and prevent subsequent aspiration.

   a. Suction nasal secretions also, because patient is unable to blow nose.

   b. Remove crusts from nares and apply ointment.

5. Use chest physical therapy as necessary to remove secretions.

6. Remember that postoperative patient is unable to cough.

   a. Teach to bend forward until stoma is below lung level and to exhale rapidly. This aids in secretion removal from lungs.

   b. Teach to wipe resultant secretions away from tracheostoma with a handkerchief.

7. Encourage breathing exercises, because most patients have been heavy smokers.

8. Supply constant humidification to moisten tracheostoma and avoid viscous secretions; tracheal air will require additional warmth and moisture.

9. Keep calm and maintain sense of security.

   a. Reassure patient that someone is always near to assist.

   b. Have call bell within reach.

10. In the event of clogging or obstruction of the stoma, follow Procedure Guidelines 17-2.

PROCEDURE GUIDELINES 17-2   EMERGENCY FIRST AID FOR THE LARYNGECTOMEE

EQUIPMENT (IF AVAILABLE)

Suction equipment	Sterile gloves
Sterile disposable catheter	Sterile saline
#14–16 F (adult)	Portable mask and bag
#8–10 F (child)	

PROCEDURE FOR TOTAL NECK BREATHER

One who breathes ONLY through the neck opening:
1. There is no connection between lungs and nose or mouth.
2. A tracheostomy or laryngectomy tube may or may not be in the neck opening.

NURSING ALERT

No air can get through to lungs of a total laryngectomee when stoma is clogged.

Nursing Action	Rationale
1. PLACE PATIENT ON BACK, on a firm surface, head straight, chin up. Bare the neck down to the sternum.	1. Access to the laryngeal stoma and observation of thoracic movement are facilitated.
2. Position a blanket or any article of clothing under the shoulders.	2. This promotes extension of the neck area, permitting access.
3. Make a rapid assessment of the situation:	3.
a. Is victim wearing a tracheostomy or laryngectomy tube?	a. In a laryngectomee, tube removal cannot cause immediate danger.
b. Has patient been operated on recently?	b. If so, tracheostomy tube cannot be removed.
c. Check for tracheal obstruction. Clean stomal opening of mucus and encrusted matter.	c. Mucus and so forth may account for obstruction. Use a clean cloth or handkerchief—never tissue.
4. START MOUTH-TO-NECK BREATHING PROMPTLY: Position yourself at side of victim. Place your mouth and lips tightly over neck opening or around the tracheal tube if the person is wearing one.	4. SECONDS COUNT. Do not remove the tube.
5. If suction equipment is available, insert a soft rubber tube 7.5–12.5 cm (3–5 inches) into opening for a few seconds.	5. A partially open airway transporting air to the victim is infinitely better than a clean airway that does not supply air at this crucial time.
6. Blow in a sufficient amount of air to see chest rise; then release and allow chest to fall.	
7. For the first 5 seconds, repeat every 1–2 seconds; then slow down to a steady pace of every 4–5 seconds (12–20 times per minute).	
8. Continue until spontaneous breathing returns.	

FOLLOW-UP PHASE

1. When spontaneous breathing occurs, provide oxygen from a portable supply.	1. To relieve hypoxemia.
2. If breathing fails again, resume mouth-to-neck breathing.	
3. You can also use a manual resuscitation bag with an infant-size mask.	3. Attach baby-sized mask; be sure there is a tight seal against neck opening. Because a tight seal is difficult to maintain and because pressure of the mask on the major blood vessels of the neck may interfere with blood supply to the brain, mouth-to-neck breathing is safer and better.
4. Watch the chest rise.	4. This is the easiest way to detect spontaneous breathing.
5. Observe the patient constantly.	

PROCEDURE FOR PARTIAL NECK BREATHER

One who breathes MAINLY through the neck opening:
1. A connection between the lungs and the nose and mouth still exists.
2. The larynx may or may not be present.
3. A tracheostomy or laryngectomy tube may or may not be in the neck opening.

PROCEDURE GUIDELINES 17-2	CONTINUED

Nursing Action   **Rationale**

 NURSING ALERT

With mouth-to-neck breathing, **FAILURE OF THE CHEST TO RISE** is reliable proof that the patient is a partial neck breather. The rescuer may hear or feel air escaping from the victim's nose or mouth, but it is not getting into the lungs.

1. a. Immediately place the palm of your hand (the one nearest to the patient's head) over the lips and mouth.
   b. Pinch the nose shut between your third and fourth fingers.
   c. Place your thumb in the soft space under the chin and firmly press upward and backward.
	1. This will close the area between the trachea and throat and at the same time raise the base of the tongue against the palate and pharynx.

2. Remove the patient's dentures.	2. To ensure better lip closure and effective underchin thumb closure.
3. Begin mouth-to-neck breathing as described above.	3. Now mouth-to-neck breathing will fill the lungs and the chest will rise.

Facilitating Adequate Nutrition

1. Monitor IV fluids during first few postoperative days.
2. Administer fluids and nutrients by nasogastric or esophagostomy tube.
   a. Tube feedings started after bowel sounds are heard and continued until sufficient healing of pharynx has occurred (10 to 12 days) and patient is ready to resume oral feedings.
   b. Avoid manipulating nasogastric tube as it is resting on/near suture line.
   c. Cleanse nostrils and lubricate with water-soluble lubricant.
   d. Cleanse crust on outside of tube.
   e. Pay attention to oral hygiene, with regular toothbrushing and prescribed antiseptic mouthwashes.
3. Encourage patient to relearn swallowing.
   a. Ensure quiet environment, because relearning how to swallow causes frustration and requires concentration. Have standby suction available.
   b. Place patient in sitting position, leaning slightly forward. This allows larynx to move forward and hypopharynx to partially open.
   c. Explain that the epiglottis normally prevents fluid/food from entering larynx during swallowing.
4. Teach technique for swallowing.
   a. Inhale before swallowing, swallow, cough gently while exhaling, and reswallow.
   b. This ensures adequate air in lungs to cough out any food that has passed into the unguarded laryngeal region, thus preventing aspiration.

Providing Alternative Communication

1. Advise patient to communicate by writing until voice work can begin with speech-language pathologist.
2. Discourage forced whispering, which increases pharyngeal tension.

3. Reassure that speech therapy will begin as soon as patient can swallow comfortably.
4. Encourage patient to join local laryngectomy support group (Lost Chord Club, New Voice Club), which gives opportunity to practice new speech and serves as a bridge between therapy and return to social life.

Providing Information About Laryngectomy

1. Inform patient that a laryngectomy or tracheostomy tube is usually worn until stoma heals (1 to 2 months); patient then starts gradual process of leaving tube out 1 hour at a time.
2. Demonstrate procedure for cleaning and changing tube.
   a. See page 218 for tracheostomy tube care.
   b. Place gauze dressing under tube to absorb secretions as prescribed. Change when it becomes soiled to prevent skin irritation and odor.
   c. Encourage patient to practice changing tracheostomy tie tapes.
3. Tracheostoma care—teach patient to:
   a. Wash hands before touching stoma to prevent infection.
   b. Wet washcloth with warm water; wring dry and gently wipe stoma. Do not use soap, tissues, or cotton balls, because these may enter airway.
   c. Apply petroleum around exterior of stoma to prevent skin irritation.
   d. Report excessive redness, swelling, purulent secretions, or bleeding.
4. Stoma cover
   a. Stoma cover is necessary to filter air and increase humidity of air; also necessary for hygienic purposes.
   b. Stoma cover can be crocheted or made of cotton cloth.
   c. For men: ascot or turtleneck sweaters may be worn. When a regular shirt is worn, the second button

from the top can be sewed over the buttonhole as though it were fastened. This leaves a wide opening through which a handkerchief can be inserted when coughing.

d. For women: a variety of fashionable scarves, jewelry, high-neck dresses, and turtleneck sweaters can be worn.

5. Bowel care: discuss high-fiber diet and use of stool softener, because patient with tracheostoma is usually not able to hold breath to "bear down" for bowel movement.

Community and Home Care Considerations

1. Provide humidification in the home; use pans of water in the rooms, a humidifier, or cool-mist vaporizer, especially in bedroom and when dry heat is used.
2. Tell patient to avoid cold air; cover tracheostoma with thin layer of foam rubber or other cover to warm and humidify air.
3. Encourage patient to drink fluids liberally (2 to 3 L) to help liquefy secretions.
4. Have patient always keep stoma covered for hygienic management of secretions and to keep dust/foreign matter from entering trachea.
5. Place a protective shield over stoma before bathing, showering, or shampooing hair and while getting a haircut or shaving. Use an electric razor instead of blade, because shaving cream can irritate.
6. Swimming is not recommended.

Patient Education and Health Maintenance

1. Tell the patient to expect some loss of smell and impairment of taste sensation.
2. Advise the patient to check with health care provider before taking any medication, because many drugs (such as antihistamines and cold products) tend to dry the mucous membranes of the stoma.
3. Warn the patient to seek immediate attention for the following: pain, difficulty in breathing or swallowing, appearance of pus or blood-streaked sputum.

Outcome-Based Evaluation

- Breathing quietly; no evidence of noisy secretions
- Swallowing soft foods; maintaining weight
- Able to make needs known; speech therapy has started
- Able to manage tracheostomal care; has made provisions for home humidification and tracheostomal supplies

SELECTED REFERENCES

Abaza, M.M., Spiegel, J.R., & Sataloff, R.T. (1999). Managing uncommon causes of pharyngitis. *Hospital Medicine*, 35(1), 12–19.

American Academy of Allergy, Asthma and Immunology/American College of Allergy, Asthma and Immunology/Joint Council of Allergy, Asthma and Immunology. (1998). *Diagnosis and management of rhinitis.* Accessed at **www.guidelines.gov**.

———. (1998). *Parameters for diagnosis and management of sinusitis.* Accessed at **www.guidelines.gov**.

American Academy of Neurology. (1996). *Assessment: Electronystagmography.* Accessed at **www.guidelines.gov**.

Cavendish, R. (1998). Adult hearing loss. *American Journal of Nursing*, 98(8), 50–51.

Centers for Disease Control and Prevention. (1999). *Acute otitis media: Management and surveillance in an era of pneumococcal resistance.* Accessed at **www.guidelines.gov**.

Dowell, S., Butler, J., Giebink, S. & the Drug-Resistant *Streptococcus pneumoniae* Therapeutic Working Group. (1999). Acute otitis media: Management and surveillance in an era of pneumococcal resistance—A report from the Drug-Resistant *Streptococcus pneumoniae* Therapeutic Working Group. *Pediatric Infectious Disease Journal*, 18(1), 1–9.

Galen, B. (1997). Chronic recurrent sinusitis: Recognition and treatment. *Primary Care Practice*, 1(2), 183–197.

Harris, L. L., & Huntoon, M. B. (Eds.) (1998). *Core curriculum for otorhinolaryngology and head and neck nursing.* New Smyrna Beach, FL: Society of Otolaryngology and Head and Neck Nursing.

Harrison, L. B., Sessions, R. B., Hong, W. K., & Wenig, B. M. (1998). *Head and neck cancer.* Philadelphia: Lippincott Williams & Wilkins.

Infectious Diseases Society of America. (1997 [Reviewed 1999]). *Diagnosis and management of group A streptococcal pharyngitis: A practice guideline.* Accessed at **www.guidelines.gov**.

Kupecz, D. (1999). Managing allergic rhinitis. *The Nurse Practitioner*, 24(5), 107–120.

Leiner, S. (2000). Acute pharyngitis with lifelong implications. *The Nurse Practitioner*, 25(4), 119–122.

Lucente, F. E. (Ed.) (1999). *Essentials of otolaryngology* (4th ed.). Philadelphia: Lippincott Williams & Wilkins.

Office of Medical Applications of Research. (1995). *Cochlear implants in adults and children.* Accessed at **www.guidelines.gov**.

Rontal, M., Bernstein, J.M., Rontal, E., & Anon, J. (1999). Bacteriologic findings from the nose, ethmoid and bloodstream during endoscopic surgery for chronic rhiosinusitis: Implications for antibiotic therapy. *American Journal of Rhinology*, 13(2), 91–96.

Shellenbarger, T. (2000). Nosebleeds: Not just kids' stuff. *RN*, 63(2), 50–54.

Tigges, B.B. (2000). Acute otitis media and pneumococcal resistance: Making judicious management decisions. *The Nurse Practitioner*, 25(1), 69, 73–80, 85.

Tupper, S. Z. (1999). When the inner ear is out of balance. *RN*, 62(11), 36–39.

United States Preventive Services Task Force. (1996). *Screening for hearing impairment.* Accessed at **www.guidelines.gov**.

Weaver, E.M., Czibulka, A., & Sasaki, C.T. (1999). Acute epistaxis: A step-by-step guide to controlling hemorrhage. *Consultant*, 40(3), 901.

Zwart, S., et al. (2000). Penicillin for acute sore throat: Randomized double blind trial of seven days versus three days treatment or placebo in adults. *British Medical Journal*, 320(2), 150–154.

UNIT V

Gastrointestinal and Nutritional Health

CHAPTER

18

Gastrointestinal Disorders

GENERAL OVERVIEW

The gastrointestinal (GI) system comprises the alimentary canal and its accessory organs, beginning at the mouth; extending through the pharynx, esophagus, stomach, small intestine, colon, rectum, and anal canal; and ending at the anus.

The GI system is responsible for the following essential bodily functions: ingestion and propulsion of food, mechanical and chemical digestion of food, absorption of nutrients into the bloodstream, and the storage and elimination of waste products from the body through feces.

ASSESSMENT

See Standards of Care Guidelines.

Subjective Data

A comprehensive health history should be obtained to elicit subjective data related to major manifestations of GI problems. Common manifestations include nutritional problems, abdominal pain, indigestion, nausea and vomiting, diarrhea, constipation, and dysphagia.

Nutritional Problems

1. Characteristics: What is your normal 24-hour food intake? What is your usual weight? Has there been a recent weight gain or loss? If a recent weight change, how many pounds? How is your appetite?
2. Associated factors: Explore other factors that may influence weight changes—food preferences; family/individual routines associated with eating; cultural and religious values; psychological factors, such as depres-

---

STANDARDS OF CARE GUIDELINES
Gastrointestinal Dysfunction

When caring for a patient after abdominal surgery or with any type of gastrointestinal disorder:

- Ensure that adequate bowel sounds are present before allowing anything by mouth. Reassess for bowel sounds, any bloating, and abdominal tenderness periodically.
- Monitor food intake and fluid intake and output as indicated.
- Periodically monitor weight, and watch for trend in weight loss or weight gain.
- Assess stools for frequency, consistency, color, and amount.
- Report increase in pain, fever, nausea and vomiting, bloating, change in stools, sign of wound infection to health care provider promptly.

This information should serve as a general guideline only. Each patient situation presents a unique set of clinical factors and requires nursing judgment to guide care, which may include additional or alternative measures and approaches.

---

sion, anxiety, stress; physical factors, such as activity level, health status, dental problems, allergies; access/transportation to grocery stores; eating habits, self-imposed dietary restrictions; body image; nutritional knowledge.
3. History: Any history of eating disorders? Any family history of ulcer disease, GI cancer, inflammatory bowel disease, obesity?

Abdominal Pain

1. Characteristics: Can you describe the pain (sharp, dull, superficial, or deep)? Is the pain intermittent or continuous? Can you point to where the pain is located? What makes the pain better, worse?
2. Associated factors: Are there other symptoms associated with the pain—fever, nausea, vomiting, diarrhea, constipation, anorexia, weight loss, dyspepsia?
3. History: Any family history of GI cancer, ulcer disease, inflammatory bowel disease? Any previous history of tumors, malignancy, or ulcers?

Indigestion (Dyspepsia)

1. Characteristics: Have you experienced any of the following symptoms—a feeling of fullness, heartburn, excessive belching, flatus, nausea, a bad taste, mild or severe pain? How is your appetite? If pain or tenderness, where is it located? Does the pain radiate to any other areas? What precipitating factors are associated with the pain? What makes the symptoms better, worse? Are the symptoms associated with food intake? If associated with food, the amount and type?
2. Associated factors: Is there nausea, vomiting, or diarrhea? Is there a history of alcohol or aspirin use?
3. History: Any family history of cancer, inflammatory bowel disease? Any history of bowel obstruction? Any previous abdominal surgeries?

Nausea and Vomiting

1. Characteristics: Is the nausea or vomiting associated with certain stimuli, such as specific foods, odors, activity, or a certain time of day? Does it occur before or after food intake? How many times a day does vomiting occur? What specific fluids/foods can be tolerated when vomiting occurs? What is the amount, color, odor, and consistency of the vomitus (Table 18-1)?
2. Associated factors: Is there fever, headache, dizziness, weakness, diarrhea? Any weight loss?
3. History: Any history of gallbladder disease? Ulcer disease? GI cancer?

Diarrhea

1. Characteristics: How long has the diarrhea been present? Determine the frequency, consistency, color, quantity, and odor of stools. Is there blood, mucus, pus, or food particles in the stools? Does this represent a change in bowel habits? Any nocturnal diarrhea? What makes the diarrhea worse, better? Any associated weight loss (see Box 18-1)?

TABLE 18-1   Nature of Vomitus

Color/Taste/Consistency	Possible Source
Yellowish or greenish	May contain bile Medication—senna
Bright red (arterial)	Hemorrhage, peptic ulcer
Dark red (venous)	Hemorrhage, esophageal or gastric varices
"Coffee grounds"	Digested blood from slowly bleeding gastric or duodenal ulcer
Undigested food	Gastric tumor Ulcer, obstruction
"Bitter" taste	Bile
"Sour" or "acid"	Gastric contents
Fecal components	Intestinal obstruction

2. Associated factors: Any fever, nausea, vomiting, abdominal pain, abdominal distention, flatus, cramping, urgency with straining? Is the patient taking antibiotics? Has there been any recent travel to foreign countries? (Mexico, South America, Africa, and Asia are countries with the highest risk of traveler's diarrhea.) Is the patient experiencing emotional stress or anxiety?
3. History: Is there a history of colon cancer, ulcerative colitis, Crohn's disease, malabsorption syndrome?

BOX 18-1   Causes of Diarrhea and Constipation

Causes of Diarrhea
Infectious agents (*E coli*, *Salmonella*, *Shigella*, *Campylobacter*, *Giardia*, Amoeba, *Clostridium difficile*, *Cyclospora*, *Cryptosporidium*, Rotavirus)
Food poisoning
Drugs (antibiotics, magnesium)
Fecal impaction
Bowel disease (irritable bowel syndrome, ulcerative colitis, Crohn's disease)
Malabsorption syndromes (lactose intolerance, celiac sprue, fat malabsorption)
Short bowel syndrome
Malignant syndromes (Zollinger-Ellison syndrome, carcinoid syndrome)

Causes of Constipation
Inadequate fluid intake
Psychological factors
Electrolyte imbalances
Hormonal abnormalities
Mechanical bowel obstruction, ileus
Drugs (laxative abuse, anticholinergic agents, opiates)
Loss of innervation (Hirschsprung's disease)
Neuromuscular (paralysis, spinal cord injury or sacral lesion, multiple sclerosis)
Anorectal disorders (hemorrhoids, fecal impaction, cancer, abscess, fissures)

DRUG ALERT

Obtain history of any over-the-counter (OTC), herbal, or "natural" products the patient may be taking. Ginger is often used as an antiemetic, is generally safe, but can cause heartburn. Licorice root is used for upset stomach and to soothe ulcers but can cause sodium and fluid retention and loss of potassium. Goldenseal is used as an antidiarrheal but can cause a number of adverse reactions including skin and mucous membrane irritation, interference with anticoagulation, cardiac and nervous system excitability. Many herbs can impair absorption of other medicines. Remind patients that herbal products are not found naturally in the body or in significant amounts in the daily diet, so should be treated like drugs.

Constipation

1. Characteristics: What is the frequency, consistency, color of the stools? Is this a change in bowel habits? If a change, has this been gradual or sudden? What is the size of the stools? Have there been dietary changes? Is there blood or mucus in the stools?
2. Associated factors: Are there periods of diarrhea? Is there abdominal pain or distention? Is the patient experiencing stress? Is there a change in activity level? Does the patient have a regular time for defecation? Does the patient use antacids containing calcium or an anticholinergic?
3. History: Any family history of colorectal cancer? Any history of depression or metabolic disorders, such as hypothyroidism or hypercalcemia?

Dysphagia

1. Characteristics: Is the onset acute or gradual? Is the problem with swallowing intermittent or continuous? Is this associated with solid foods, liquids, or both?
2. Associated factors: Is there any regurgitation, heartburn, chest or back pain, weight loss? Any hoarseness, voice change, or sore throat?
3. History: Is there a family history of esophageal cancer? Is there a history of stroke, palsy, or any other neurologic conditions? Is there a history of alcohol or tobacco intake?

Physical Examination

When performing a physical examination of the abdomen, include the following: inspection of the abdomen, auscultation of all four abdominal quadrants, percussion for tympany or dullness, light and deep palpation.

NURSING ALERT

Auscultation should be performed before percussion and palpation, which may stimulate bowel sounds. Deep palpation in noted areas of tenderness or pain should be performed last.

Key Findings

1. Tenting of the skin when skin is rolled between thumb and index finger. Tenting may indicate dehydration.
2. Mouth lesions, missing teeth, swollen or bleeding gums may contribute to weight loss and nutritional deficiencies.
3. Body weight may indicate obesity or such problems as anorexia nervosa or malignancy.
4. Palpable mass may indicate an enlarged organ, inflammation, malignancy, hernia.
5. Rebound tenderness, guarding, and rigidity may indicate appendicitis, cholecystitis, peritonitis, pancreatitis, duodenal ulcer.
6. Protuberant or bulging abdomen or flanks can indicate ascites. Two physical assessment skills that may help to confirm the presence of ascites are testing for shifting dullness and testing for a fluid wave.
7. Distention and absence of bowel sounds may indicate intestinal obstruction.

Characteristics of Stool

1. The appearance of blood in stool may be characteristic of its source.
   a. Upper GI bleeding—tarry black (melena)
   b. Lower GI bleeding—bright red blood
   c. Lower rectal or anal bleeding—blood streaking on surface of stool or on toilet paper
2. Other characteristics of stool may indicate a particular GI problem.
   a. Bulky, greasy, foamy, foul smelling, gray with silvery sheen—steatorrhea (fatty stool)
   b. Light gray "clay-colored" (due to absence of bile pigments, acholic)—biliary obstruction
   c. Mucus or pus visible—chronic ulcerative colitis, shigellosis
   d. Small, dry, rocky-hard masses—constipation, obstruction
   e. Marble-sized stool pellets—spastic colon syndrome

DIAGNOSTIC TESTS

Laboratory Tests

Laboratory tests for GI disorders include stool testing for blood (Hemoccult), other stool tests, and a variety of blood tests, such as hematocrit and hemoglobin for monitoring GI bleeding.

Hemoccult Guaiac Tests (Hemoquant, Hemoccult II)
Description

Commercially available guaiac-impregnated slides or wipes present a simple, inexpensive, and aesthetically acceptable method of testing feces for blood.

Nursing and Patient Care Considerations

Advise patient as to the test preparation procedure. Common practices are listed below. For 3 days before the test and during the stool collection period:

1. Diet should have a high fiber content.
2. Avoid red meat in the diet.
3. Avoid foods with a high peroxidase content, such as turnips, cauliflower, broccoli, horseradish, and melon.
4. Avoid iron preparations, iodides, bromides, aspirin, nonsteroid anti-inflammatory drugs (NSAIDs), or vitamin C supplements greater than 250 mg/day.
5. Avoid enemas or laxatives before the stool specimen collection.

NURSING ALERT

Certain protocols may specify to avoid aspirin and NSAIDs for at least a week before Hemoccult testing to prevent bleeding. Vitamin C (ascorbic acid) can cause a false-negative reading.

Procedure

1. A wooden applicator is used to apply a stool specimen to the slide, or a special wipe is used and placed in the packet. Three stool samples are taken because of the possibility of intermittent bleeding and false-negative results.
2. Slides (or wipes) applied inside a packet can be brought or mailed to the health care provider or laboratory.
3. When hydrogen peroxide (denatured alcohol-stabilizing mixture) is added to samples, any blood cells present liberate their hemoglobin, and a bluish ring appears on the electrophoretic paper. Read precisely at 30 seconds.
4. A single positive test is an indication for further diagnostic evaluation for GI lesions. False-positive results occur in about 10% of tests. Test may become false-negative in 10% of specimens tested 4 or more days after streaking on paper.

Community and Home Care Considerations

1. Nonadherence to the diet/medication restrictions can cause false-positive or false-negative readings.
2. The stool must not be contaminated with urine or toilet tissue.
3. The stool guaiac specimen packets do not require refrigeration.
4. Stool specimen packets should be submitted for laboratory testing within 6 days.

Stool Specimen
Description

The stool is examined for its amount, consistency, and color. Normal color varies from light to dark brown, but various foods and medications may affect stool color. Special tests may be made for fecal urobilinogen, fat nitrogen, food residue, and other substances. Fecal leukocytes are tested by Wright's stain, and stool cultures are obtained to identify bacteria, virus, or ova and parasites.

Nursing and Patient Care Considerations

1. Use a tongue blade to place a small amount of stool in a disposable waxed container.
2. Save a sample of fecal material if unusual in appearance, contains worms or blood, blood streaked, unusual color, or excess mucus; show to health care provider.
3. Specimens for parasitology must be collected in vials containing special preservatives. For accurate specimen results, the vials must be sent to the laboratory as soon as possible. The vials should be refrigerated if unable to submit quickly to the laboratory.
4. Send specimens to be examined for parasites to the laboratory immediately so the parasites may be observed under microscope while viable, fresh, and warm.
5. Test for occult blood or to confirm grossly visible melena or blood—Hemoccult guaiac test.
6. Consider that barium, bismuth, mineral oil, and antibiotics may alter the results.

Hydrogen Breath Test
Description

1. The hydrogen breath test is used to evaluate carbohydrate absorption.
2. A radioactive substance is ingested, and, after a certain time period, exhaled gases are measured.
3. The test measures the amount of hydrogen produced in the colon, absorbed in the blood, and then exhaled in the breath.
4. This test is used as a diagnostic test for short bowel syndrome, lactose intolerance, and bacterial overgrowth of the intestine (blind loop syndrome, Crohn's disease, distal ileal disease).

Nursing and Patient Care Considerations

1. The patient should be NPO 12 hours before the procedure.
2. The patient should not smoke after midnight before the test.
3. Antibiotics and laxative/enemas should not be used for 1 week before the test. These products may alter the laboratory results.
4. Appropriate diet instructions should be given before discharge if the test is positive.

Helicobacter pylori (H. pylori) Testing
Description

1. Laboratory tests for *H. pylori* include a serum IgG antibody test and an *H. pylori* breath test.
2. A positive antibody test may not differentiate between active and inactive disease.
3. A negative test can be interpreted to mean no antibodies or antibodies present at a lower level than detectable.

Nursing and Patient Care Considerations

1. Symptomatic patients and patients with an active or past history of ulcer disease should be tested for *H. pylori*. Endoscopy may be necessary for patients with symptoms of weight loss, anemia, occult blood loss, and patients older than 50 years.
2. It is recommended that negative *H. pylori* test results in a patient with ulcer-related complications be confirmed by a second test.
3. Contact laboratory for the type of serologic test being performed for *H. pylori* and the appropriate tube for blood.
4. Due to the potential for false-negative *H. pylori* breath test, preparation includes stopping treatment 2 weeks before testing.
5. False-positive results from *H. pylori* breath testing may be caused by achlorhydria or urease production associated with other GI disorders.

■ Radiology and Imaging Studies
Upper Gastrointestinal Series and Small-Bowel Series
Description

1. Upper GI series and small-bowel series are fluoroscopic x-ray examinations of the esophagus, stomach, and small intestine after the patient ingests barium sulfate.
2. As the barium passes through the GI tract, fluoroscopy outlines the GI mucosa and organs.
3. Spot films record significant findings.
4. Double-contrast studies administer barium first followed by a radiolucent substance, such as air, to produce a thin layer of barium to coat the mucosa. This allows for better visualization of any type of lesion.

Nursing and Patient Care Considerations

1. Explain procedure to patient.
2. Instruct patient to maintain low-residue diet for 2 to 3 days before test and a clear liquid dinner the night before the procedure.
3. Emphasize NPO after midnight before the test.
4. Encourage patient to avoid smoking before the test.
5. Explain that the health care provider may prescribe all narcotics and anticholinergics to be held 24 hours before the test because they interfere with small intestine motility. Other medications may be taken with sips of water, if ordered.
6. Tell the patient that he or she will be instructed at various times throughout the procedure to drink the barium (480 to 600 mL).
7. Explain that a cathartic will be prescribed after the procedure to facilitate expulsion of barium.
8. Instruct the patient that stool will be light in color for the next 2 to 3 days from the barium.
9. Instruct patient to notify health care provider if he or she has not passed the barium in 2 to 3 days, because retention of the barium may cause obstruction or fecal impaction.
10. Note that water-soluble iodinated contrast agent (such as Gastrografin) may be used for a patient with a suspected perforation or colonic obstruction. Barium is toxic to the body if it leaks into the peritoneum

with perforation. It can also worsen an obstruction, thus is not used if an obstruction is suspected.

Barium Enema
Description
1. Fluoroscopic x-ray examination visualizing the entire large intestine is administered after the patient is given an enema of barium sulfate.
2. Can visualize structural changes, such as tumors, polyps, diverticula, fistulas, obstructions, and ulcerative colitis.
3. Air may be introduced after the barium to provide a double-contrast study.

Nursing and Patient Care Considerations
1. Explain to the patient:
   a. What the x-ray procedure involves.
   b. That proper preparation provides a more accurate view of the tract and that preparations may vary.
   c. That it is important to retain the barium so all surfaces of the tract are coated with opaque solution.
2. Instruct the patient on the objective of having the large intestine as clear of fecal material as possible:
   a. The patient may be given a low-fiber, low-fat diet, 1 to 3 days before the examination.
   b. The day before examination, intake may be limited to clear liquids (no drinks with red dye).
   c. The day before the examination, a oral laxative, suppository, and/or cleansing enema may be prescribed.
3. The patient will be NPO after midnight the day of procedure.
4. An enema or cathartic may be ordered after the barium enema to cleanse bowel of barium and prevent impaction.
5. Inform the patient that barium may cause light-colored stools for several days after the procedure.

NURSING ALERT

If barium enema and upper GI series are both ordered, the upper GI series is done last so barium traveling down the digestive tract does not interfere with the results of the barium enema.

Ultrasonography (Ultrasound)
Description
1. A noninvasive test focuses high-frequency sound waves over an abdominal organ to obtain an image of the structure.
2. Ultrasound can detect small abdominal masses, fluid-filled cysts, gallstones, dilated bile ducts, ascites, and vascular abnormalities.
3. Ultrasound with Doppler may be ordered for vascular assessment.

Nursing and Patient Care Considerations
1. If indicated, prepare the patient before the procedure with a special diet, laxative, or other medication to cleanse the bowel and decrease gas.

2. Abdominal ultrasound usually requires the patient to be NPO for at least 6 hours before the procedure.
3. Change position of patient, as indicated, for better visualization of certain organs.

Computed Tomography (CT) Scan
Description
1. This is a x-ray technique that provides excellent anatomic definition and is used to detect tumors, cysts, and abscesses.
2. The CT can also detect dilated bile ducts, pancreatic inflammation, and some gallstones.
3. It identifies changes in intestinal wall thickness and mesenteric abnormalities.
4. Ultrasound and CT can be used to perform guided needle aspiration of fluid or cells from lesions anywhere in the abdomen. The fluid or cells are then sent for laboratory tests (such as cytology or culture).
5. A newer technique of focused appendiceal CT can be used to diagnose appendicitis.
   a. Rectal contrast media is given so the colon is opacified quickly without waiting for oral contrast to reach the appendix.
   b. The right lower quadrant is focused on to visualize the appendix, so the procedure is quick.

Nursing and Patient Care Considerations
1. Instruct the patient that fasting for 4 hours before the procedure and an enema or cathartic may be necessary. This is to cleanse the bowel for better visualization.
2. Ask the patient if she is pregnant. If yes, do not proceed with scan and notify health care provider.
3. Ask if there are known allergies to iodine or contrast media. A contrast medium may be given intravenously (IV) to provide better visualization of body parts. If allergic, notify the technician and health care provider immediately.
4. Instruct the patient to report symptoms of itching or shortness of breath if receiving contrast media, and observe patient closely.

◼ Endoscopic Procedures

Endoscopy is the use of a flexible tube (the fiberoptic endoscope) to visualize the GI tract and to perform certain diagnostic and therapeutic procedures. Images are produced through a video screen or telescopic eyepiece. The tip of the endoscope moves in four directions, allowing for wide-angle visualization. The endoscope can be inserted through the rectum or mouth, depending on which portion of the GI tract is to be viewed.

Endoscopes contain multipurpose channels that allow for air insufflation, irrigation, fluid aspiration, and the passage of special instruments. These instruments include biopsy forceps, cytology brushes, needles, wire baskets, laser probes, and electrocautery snares.

Endoscopic functions other than visualization include biopsy or cytology of lesions, removal of foreign objects or polyps, control of internal bleeding, and opening of strictures.

Esophagogastroduodenoscopy (EGD)

Description

1. This allows for visualization of the esophagus, stomach, and duodenum.
2. EGD can be used to diagnose acute or chronic upper GI bleeding, esophageal or gastric varices, polyps, malignancy, ulcers, gastritis, esophagitis, esophageal stenosis, and gastroesophageal reflux.
3. Instruments passed through the scope can be used to perform a biopsy or cytologic study, remove polyps or foreign bodies, control bleeding, or open strictures.

Nursing and Patient Care Considerations

1. Explain the following to the patient:
   a. The type of procedure to be performed on the patient. As an outpatient, advise that someone must accompany the patient to drive home due to the patient being sedated.
   b. NPO for 8 to 12 hours before the procedure to prevent aspiration and allow for complete visualization of the stomach.
   c. Remove dentures and partial plates to facilitate passing the scope and preventing injury.
2. Inform the health care provider of any known allergies and current medications. Medications may be held until after the test is completed.
3. Obtain prior x-rays, and send with the patient.
4. Describe what will occur during and after the procedure:
   a. The throat will be anesthetized with a spray or gargle.
   b. An IV sedative will be administered.
   c. The patient will be positioned on the left side with a towel or basin at the mouth to catch secretions.
   d. A plastic mouthpiece will be used to help relax the jaw and protect the endoscope. Emphasize that this will not interfere with breathing.
   e. The patient may be asked to swallow once while the endoscope is being advanced. Then the patient should not swallow, talk, or move tongue. Secretions should drain from the side of the mouth, and the mouth may be suctioned.
   f. Air is inserted during the procedure to permit better visualization of the GI tract. Most of the air is removed at the end of the procedure. The patient may feel bloated, burp, or pass flatus from remaining air.
   g. Keep patient NPO according to protocol until patient is alert and gag reflex has returned.
   h. May resume regular diet after gag reflex returns and tolerating fluids.
   i. May experience a sore throat for 24 to 36 hours after the procedure. When the gag reflex has returned, throat lozenges or warm saline gargles may be prescribed for comfort.
5. Monitor vital signs every 30 minutes for 3 to 4 hours, and keep the side rails up until the patient is fully alert.

6. Monitor the patient for abdominal or chest pain, cervical pain, dyspnea, fever, hematemesis, melena, dysphagia, lightheadedness, or a firm distended abdomen. These may indicate complications.
7. Instruct the patient on the above listed signs and symptoms, and advise to report immediately should any occur, even after discharge.
8. Possible complications include perforation of the esophagus or stomach, pulmonary aspiration, hemorrhage, respiratory depression or arrest, infection, cardiac arrhythmias or arrest.

NURSING ALERT

Perforation of the GI tract is a complication of endoscopy. Assess for abdominal or chest pain, dyspnea, fever, tachycardia, lightheadedness, and distended abdomen. Report immediately.

Proctosigmoidoscopy and Colonoscopy

1. Proctosigmoidoscopy (rectosigmoidoscopy) is the visualization of the anal canal, rectum, and sigmoid colon through a fiberoptic sigmoidoscope. See Procedure Guidelines 18-1: Assisting With a Proctosigmoidoscopy.
2. Colonoscopy is the visualization of the entire large intestine, sigmoid colon, rectum, and anal canal.
3. Sigmoidoscopy or colonoscopy can be used to diagnose malignancy, polyps, inflammation, or strictures.
4. Colonoscopy is used for surveillance in patients with a history of chronic ulcerative colitis, previous colon cancer, or colon polyps.
5. Lower GI endoscopy can be used to perform biopsy, remove foreign objects, or obtain specimen for culture or cytology.
6. Colonoscopy, a more extensive procedure than proctosigmoidoscopy, requires several days of bowel preparation and use of conscious sedation during the procedure. The bowel preparation includes approximately 1 gallon or less iso-osmolar electrolyte solution to consume over a 3- to 4-hour period the day before the procedure, clear liquid diet the day before the procedure, and an oral laxative the night before the procedure. Protocols may vary.

Endoscopic Ultrasound (EUS)

Description

1. This procedure is a combination of endoscopy and ultrasonography to visualize the GI tract.
2. An ultrasonic transducer is built into the distal end of the endoscope.
3. This procedure allows for high-quality resolution and imaging of the walls of the esophagus, stomach, duodenum, small intestines, and colon. Adjacent abdominal structures can also studied.
4. Endoscopic ultrasound is also indicated to evaluate and stage lesions of the GI tract.

Nursing and Patient Care Considerations

1. Verify the patient's compliance with the pretest bowel preparation the day before the procedure, usually an oral laxative (such as magnesium citrate) and a clear liquid diet.
2. The patient must be NPO after midnight.
3. Explain to the patient that a feeling of fullness will occur when water is introduced into the GI tract. This eliminates air space and provides for high resolution.
4. If an upper endoscopic ultrasound is performed, maintain the NPO status until the gag reflex returns. A lower endoscopic ultrasound can be performed using a rectal approach.
5. Observe the patient for a change in vital signs, bleeding, pain, vomiting, abdominal distention or rigidity.
6. Ensure that patients who have had endoscopic procedures requiring sedation have a caregiver to drive home after the procedure.

PROCEDURE GUIDELINES 18-1	ASSISTING WITH A PROCTOSIGMOIDOSCOPY

EQUIPMENT

Fleet-type enema—used at least 1 hour before the sigmoidoscopy
Water-soluble lubricant
Sigmoidoscope
Biopsy forceps
Culture swab
Long applicator sticks (cotton)
Drapes or sheets
Specimen bottles containing 10% formalin

Culture tubes
4 × 4 gauze sponges
Cytology brush
Glass eyepiece to fit on scope during insufflation of air
Disposable gloves for preliminary digital examination
Suction machine
Microscopic slides with fixative or 95% ethyl alcohol
Specimen labels

NURSING ALERT

Need to have emergency resuscitation equipment available in case a vagal reaction occurs with signs and symptoms of pallor, diaphoresis, dizziness, weakness, unconsciousness, decrease in blood pressure and pulse rate, sometimes causing vital signs to be unobtainable.

PROCEDURE

Nursing Action	Rationale

PREPARATORY PHASE

Inform the health care provider of any known allergies and current medications. Certain medications, such as anticoagulants, may be held before the test.

Obtain prior x-rays and results of blood or radiologic studies, and send with the patient.

Nursing Action	Rationale
1. Record baseline vital signs. Leave the blood pressure cuff in place. An automatic blood pressure machine may be used; however, a manual cuff is preferred in the event the patient has a vagal reaction (see Nursing Alert above).	1. Monitoring of the blood pressure and pulse throughout the procedure will be necessary.

2. Have the patient assume the knee–chest or Sims' lateral position.
  a. Knee–chest position
    (i) Knees are spread comfortably apart.
    (ii) Thighs are perpendicular to table.
    (iii) Feet are extended over the edge.
    (iv) Head is turned sideways to right (head shares pillow with chest).
    (v) Left arm is flexed to side of chest.
    (vi) Right arm may rest above head.
  b. Sims' lateral position
    (i) Place patient on left side with left leg partially flexed at hip and knees; right leg should be fully flexed.
    (ii) Pelvis to be perpendicular to table
	2. The position used depends on physician preference, patient condition, and nature of examining table (or bed).
	  a. This position permits the sigmoid to hang forward, diminishing the angle at the rectosigmoid junction.
	
	  b. Used for elderly, ill, or arthritic patients or those who are reluctant to assume the knee–chest position.

3. Drape the patient so only perineum is visible.	3. A disposable large sheet with a circular opening is practical. This will minimize embarrassment.

Nursing Action	Rationale
4. Explain to the patient to take slow, deep breaths as the physician examines the rectum by digital examination.	4. The physician is examining for tenderness, mucus, blood fistula, inflammation, ulceration, and feces. The digital examination also indicates the direction of the anal canal, its patency, and the presence of any abnormality; it promotes anal relaxation and helps to lubricate the orifice.
5. Warm sigmoidoscope in tap water or sterilizer to slightly above body temperature; lubricate tip of scope.	5. A cold scope would cause discomfort and promote contraction rather than relaxation of perianal muscles. Water-soluble lubricant permits easier passage of scope. It also minimizes the urge to defecate at tube insertion.
6. Physician spreads buttocks and anal margins with left hand and inserts instrument with right hand (or vice versa). Have the patient breathe deeply.	6. Keep instrument out of view of patient. Breathing slowly and deeply will help relax abdominal muscles and minimize cramping.
7. Nurse encourages relaxation and explains each step in advance.	7. Reassuring the patient promotes relaxation.
8. Physician may use a glass eyepiece over viewing end of scope; an insufflation bulb and tubing are attached. A small quantity of air may be pumped into the bowel. Tell patient as the air moves down the bowel he may experience flatulence. This is normal.	8. The purpose of inflating lower bowel with air is to expand the area viewed so vision is not obstructed by mucosal folds and to facilitate passage into the sigmoid colon.
9. Examination of the sigmoid, rectum, and mucosa are done while the scope is being removed. If a rigid scope is used, passage of a large cotton swab through the scope may be done to remove blood, mucus, and feces. If a flexible scope is used, only suction is necessary to clear the field. Turn suction to lowest setting initially.	9. This clears the field of vision.
10. Passage of biopsy forceps, cytology brush, or culture swab through the scope is done to collect specimens.	10. Specimens will be placed in 10% formalin and labeled. A specimen for cytology is placed in a container of 95% ethyl alcohol or affixed to a microscopic slide with slide fixative. Specimens for cultures will be sent in specimen tubes.
11. Relay to the physician any expressions or complaints of pain by the patient.	11. Tenderness and pain may be experienced by the patient with a history of abdominal surgery; procedure may have to be terminated in order not to risk perforation.

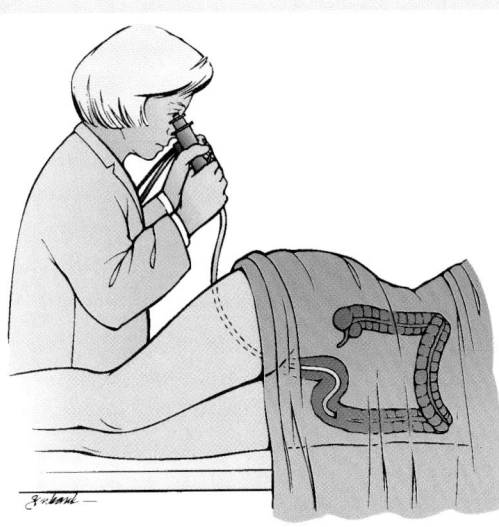

Proper positioning and draping for sigmoidoscopy.

continued

PROCEDURE GUIDELINES 18-1	ASSISTING WITH A PROCTOSIGMOIDOSCOPY *CONTINUED*

Nursing Action	Rationale

FOLLOW-UP PHASE

1. On withdrawal of scope, assist patient into gradually assuming a relaxed position.
2. Wipe perianal area.
3. If disposable scope is used, rinse and discard in proper receptacle. Reusable scopes are properly cleaned with solution and water, per protocol. Sterilizable parts are sterilized before scope is stored.
4. Record the procedure, preparation of the patient, reaction of the patient, and patient's vital signs.
5. Label all specimens immediately and send to the laboratory.
6. Observe the patient for complications: hemorrhage (increased pulse, decreased blood pressure, weakness, pallor, rectal bleeding, and possible abdominal pain), perforation (sudden, severe abdominal pain, fever, malaise, changes in vital signs, bloody or mucoid rectal drainage, and possible abdominal distention).
7. Instruct the patient on these signs and symptoms, and advise to notify health care provider immediately should they occur, even after discharge.

1. To promote comfort.
2. Prevent soilage of garments.
3. Prevents contamination and infection.

5. Minimizes error; allows fresh samples for evaluation.
6. Early identification allows immediate action and better outcome.

7. A slow leak from hemorrhage or perforation may not show up for several hours.

GENERAL PROCEDURES AND TREATMENT MODALITIES

Relieving Constipation and Fecal Impaction

A common procedure to relieve constipation or evacuate the lower bowel is an enema, the installation of a solution into the rectum and sigmoid colon. See Procedure Guidelines 18-2.

Fecal impaction may cause constipation or small amounts of diarrhea or liquid fecal seepage around the obstructing impaction. Impaction may be removed manually to promote bowel elimination (Figure 18-1).

Purposes of Enema Administration

1. Bowel preparation for diagnostic tests or surgery to empty the bowel of fecal content
2. Delivery of medication into the colon (such as enemas containing neomycin to decrease the bowel's bacteria count or a kayexalate enema to decrease the serum potassium level)
3. To soften the stool (oil-retention enemas)
4. To relieve gas (tidal, milk and molasses, or Fleet's enemas)
5. Promote defecation and evacuate feces from the colon for patients with constipation or an impaction

Indications and Contraindications of Fecal Impaction Removal

1. Consider manual removal of fecal impaction in the following patients at risk:

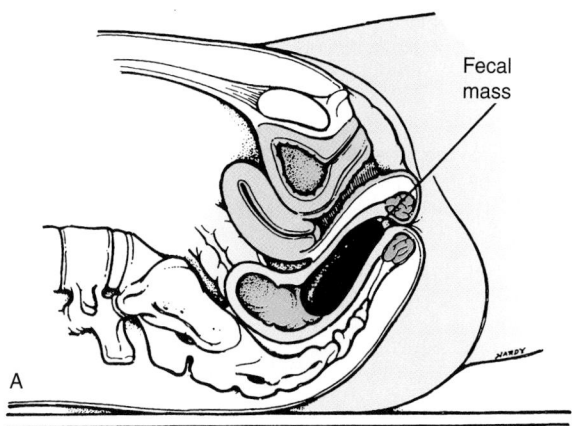
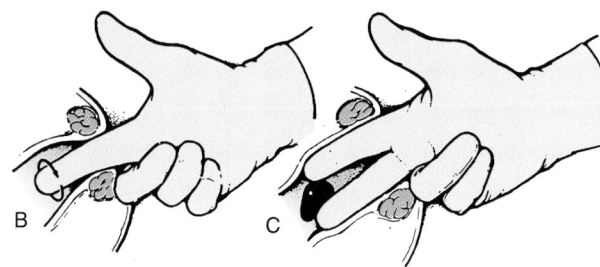

FIGURE 18-1 Fecal impaction. (**A**) Note shaded area inside rectal sphincter—this indicates fecal impaction. (**B**) By gently stimulating the rectal wall with a gloved index finger and using a circular motion, it is possible to loosen fecal material. (**C**) It may be necessary to gently insert two fingers in an attempt to crush the fecal mass. A scissor-like motion is used.

a. Elderly persons with chronic constipation or insufficient hydration, or who are inactive

b. Orthopedic patients who have been in traction or in body casts

c. Patients who have just undergone rectal surgery or when barium has not been adequately removed after radiologic examination

d. Patients with neurologic or psychotic disorders

2. Fecal impaction can occur with a descending/sigmoid colostomy. The fingers may be used to break up feces through the stoma, followed by cleansing irrigation.

3. Manual removal of fecal impaction can stimulate the vagus nerve and cause syncope and tachycardia. It is contraindicated in the following conditions:

a. Pregnancy

b. After genitourinary, rectal, perineal, abdominal, or gynecologic surgery

c. Myocardial infarction, coronary insufficiency, pulmonary embolus, congestive heart failure, heart block

d. GI or vaginal bleeding

e. Blood dyscrasias, bleeding disorders

f. Hemorrhoids, fissures, and rectal polyps

PROCEDURE GUIDELINES 18-2	ADMINISTERING AN ENEMA

EQUIPMENT

Prepackaged enema or enema container	Waterproof pad	Washcloth and towel
Disposable gloves	Bath blanket	Basin
Water-soluble jelly	Bedpan or commode	Toilet tissue

PROCEDURE

Nursing Action	Rationale

PREPARATORY PHASE

Nursing Action	Rationale
1. Assess the patient's bowel habits (last BM, laxative usage, bowel patterns) and physical condition (hemorrhoids, mobility, external sphincter control).	1. Enema should not be given if there is a suspicion of appendicitis or bowel obstruction.
2. Provide for privacy, and explain procedure to patient.	2. Provides comfort.

PERFORMANCE PHASE

Nursing Action	Rationale
1. Wash hands.	1. Promotes hygiene.
2. Place patient on left side with right knee flexed (Sims' position). Place waterproof pad underneath patient, and cover with bath blanket.	2. Allows for enema solution to flow by gravity along the natural curve of the sigmoid colon and rectum.
3. Place bedpan or bedside commode in position for patients who cannot ambulate to the toilet or who may have difficulty with sphincter control.	3. Allows for easy accessibility.
4. Remove plastic cover over tubing, and lubricate tip of enema tubing 3–4 inches (7.5–10 cm) unless prepackaged (tip is already lubricated). Even prepackaged enema may need more lubricant.	4. Prevents trauma and eases application.
5. Apply disposable gloves.	
6. Separate buttocks, and locate rectum.	
7. Instruct patient that you will be inserting tubing and to take slow, deep breaths.	7. Allows for patient relaxation and readiness.
8. Insert tubing 3–4 inches for adult patients.	8. Prevents tissue trauma of rectum.
9. Slowly instill the solution using a clamp and the height of the container to adjust flow rate if using an enema bag and tubing. For high enemas, raise enema container 12–18 inches above anus; for low enemas, 12 inches. If using a prepackaged enema, slowly squeeze the container until all solution is instilled.	9. Rapid infusion can cause colon distention and cramping. Container elevated past 12–18 inches and controller on tubing not regulated contribute to rapid infusion.
10. Lower container or clamp tubing if patient complains of cramping.	
11. Withdraw rectal tubing after all enema solution has been instilled or until clear (usually not more than three enemas).	11. "Until clear" means until results do not contain fecal matter and are clear.
12. Instruct patient to hold solution as long as possible and that a feeling of distention may be felt.	12. Promotes better results.
13. Discard supplies in the appropriate trash receptacle.	13. Maintains hygiene, minimizes patient embarrassment.

continued

PROCEDURE GUIDELINES 18-2 | ADMINISTERING AN ENEMA *CONTINUED*

Nursing Action	Rationale
14. Assist patient on the bedpan or to the bedside commode or toilet when urge to defecate occurs.	14. Prompt action will prevent soiling.
15. Observe enema return for amount, fecal content. Instruct patient not to flush toilet until the nurse has seen the results.	15. If enema has not had sufficient time to absorb, result may be mostly clear with little fecal material.

> **NURSING ALERT** Enemas should not be given routinely to treat constipation, because they disrupt normal defecation reflexes and the patient becomes dependent.

FOLLOW-UP PHASE

1. Document the type of enema given, volume, and results on the appropriate chart forms.	
2. Assess and document presence or absence of abdominal distention after enema was given.	2. Relief of abdominal distention indicates success of gas relief.
3. Assist the patient with washing perineum and rectal area, if indicated; may also need a clean gown or linen change.	3. Fecal soiling may result, especially in bedridden patients.

Nasogastric and Nasointestinal Intubation

Nasogastric (NG) intubation refers to the insertion of a tube through the nasopharynx into the stomach. See Procedure Guidelines 18-3: Nasogastric Intubation and Procedure Guidelines 18-4: Nasogastric Tube Removal.

Nasointestinal intubation is performed by inserting a small-bore, weighted tube that is carried by way of peristalsis into the duodenum or jejunum. It is primarily used for administering feedings and maintaining nutritional intake. See Procedure Guidelines 18-5: Nasointestinal Intubation.

Purposes of Nasogastric Intubation

1. Remove fluids and gas from stomach (decompression)
2. Prevent or relieve nausea and vomiting after surgery or traumatic events by decompressing the stomach
3. Determine the amount of pressure and motor activity in the GI tract (diagnostic studies)
4. Irrigate the stomach (lavage) for active bleeding or poisoning
5. Treat mechanical obstruction
6. Administer medications and feeding (gavage) directly into the GI tract
7. Obtain a specimen of gastric contents for laboratory studies when pyloric or intestinal obstruction is suspected

Nursing and Patient Care Considerations

1. If the patient is unconscious, advance the tube between respirations to make sure it does not enter the trachea.
   a. You will need to stroke the unconscious patient's neck to facilitate passage of the tube down the esophagus.
   b. Watch for cyanosis while passing the tube in an unconscious patient. Cyanosis indicates the tube has entered the trachea.

2. If the patient has a nasal condition that prevents insertion through the nose, the tube is passed through the mouth.
   a. Remove dentures, slide the distal end of the tube over the tongue, and proceed the same way as a nasal intubation.
   b. Make sure to coil the end of the tube and direct it downward at the pharynx.
3. Pain or vomiting after the tube is inserted indicates tube obstruction or incorrect placement.
4. If the NG tube is not draining, the nurse should reposition tube by advancing or withdrawing it slightly (with a physician's order). After repositioning, always check for placement.
5. Recognize the complications when the tube is in for prolonged periods: nasal erosion, sinusitis, esophagitis, esophagotracheal fistula, gastric ulceration, and pulmonary and oral infections.
6. Extended-use NG tubes are made of flexible, soft, plastic material with manufacturer's recommendations that may include leaving the tube in place for up to 30 days before changing the tube.
7. Assess the color, consistency, and odor of gastric contents. Coffee ground–like contents may indicate GI bleeding. Report findings immediately.
8. The tube should be irrigated before and after medication administration through the tube.
   a. Medications should be given in liquid form, if possible.
   b. Clamp the tube for 30 to 45 minutes to ensure medication absorption before reconnecting to suction, if ordered.
9. Check GI function by auscultating for bowel sounds on a regular basis after the tube has been clamped for 30 minutes.

(*text continues on page 585*)

PROCEDURE GUIDELINES 18-3   NASOGASTRIC INTUBATION

EQUIPMENT

Nasogastric tube—usually single-lumen
  Levin or double-lumen Salem sump tube
Water-soluble lubricant
Suction equipment if ordered
Clamp for tubing
Towel, tissues, and emesis basin
Glass of water and straw
Tincture of benzoin
Hypoallergenic tape: ½ inch and 1 inch

Bio-occlusive transparent dressing
Irrigating set with 20-mL syringe or
  a 50-mL catheter-tip syringe
Stethoscope
Tongue blade
Penlight
Disposable gloves
Normal saline

PROCEDURE

Nursing Action	Rationale

PREPARATORY PHASE

1. Ask the patient if he or she has ever had nasal surgery, trauma, a deviated septum, or bleeding disorder.

2. Explain procedure to the patient, and tell how mouth breathing, panting, and swallowing will help in passing the tube.

3. Place the patient in a sitting or high-Fowler's position; place a towel across chest.

4. Determine with the patient what sign he or she might use, such as raising the index finger, to indicate "wait a few moments" because of gagging or discomfort.

5. Remove dentures; place emesis basin and tissues within the patient's reach.

6. Inspect the tube for defects; look for partially closed holes or rough edges.

7. Place rubber tubing in ice-chilled water for a few minutes to make the tube firmer. Plastic tubing may already be firm enough; if too stiff, dip in warm water.

8. Determine the length of the tube needed to reach the stomach (see accompanying figure).

9. Have the patient blow nose to clear nostrils.

10. Inspect the nostrils with a penlight, observing for any obstruction. Occlude each nostril, and have the patient breathe. This will help determine which nostril is more patent.

11. Wash your hands. Put on disposable gloves.

12. Measure the patient's NEX (nose, earlobe, xiphoid), and mark the tube appropriately. Some tubes may be pre-marked to indicate length, but this may not correlate exactly with the measurement obtained.
    a. The distance from the nose to the earlobe is the first mark on the tube. This measurement represents the distance to the nasal pharynx.
    b. When the tube reaches the xiphoid process (tip of the breast bone) a second mark is made on the tube. This measurement represents the length required to reach the stomach.

---

1. Nasogastric tubes may be contraindicated in patients with nasopharyngeal or esophageal obstruction, severe uncontrolled coagulopathy, or severe maxillofacial trauma.

2. Improves comfort and compliance.

3. Facilitates passage of tube into esophagus.

4. Provides a method of communication, which is reassuring to the patient.

5. Dentures may become loose and interfere with tube insertion.

6. Irrigation and suction may be affected by defective tube.

7. A firm tube that is not too rigid will pass easiest, without causing trauma.

8. To prevent coiling of tube in stomach or tube ending in esophagus.

11. To protect nurse from patient's secretions.

continued

PROCEDURE GUIDELINES 18-3   NASOGASTRIC INTUBATION *CONTINUED*

Nursing Action   **Rationale**

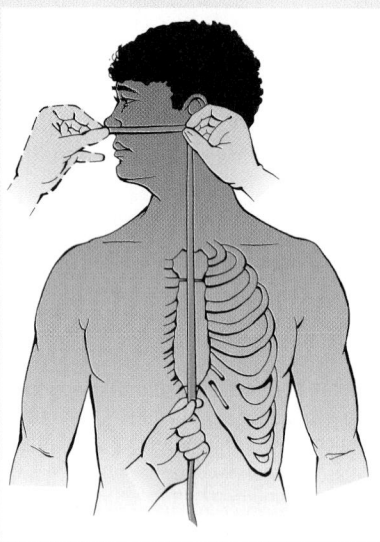

Obtaining the NEX measurement.

PERFORMANCE PHASE

1. Coil the first 7–10 cm (3–4 inches) of the tube around your fingers.
2. Lubricate the coiled portion of the tube with water-soluble lubricant. Avoid occluding the tube's holes with lubricant.

3. Tilt back the patient's head before inserting tube into nostril, and gently pass tube into the posterior nasopharynx, directing downward and backward toward the ear.

4. When tube reaches the pharynx, the patient may gag; allow patient to rest for a few moments.
5. Have the patient tilt head slightly forward. Offer several sips of water through a straw, or permit patient to suck on ice chips, unless contraindicated. Advance tube as patient swallows.

6. Gently rotate the tube 180 degrees to redirect the curve.
7. Continue to advance tube gently each time the patient swallows.
8. If obstruction appears to prevent tube from passing, do not use force. Rotating tube gently may help. If unsuccessful, remove tube and try other nostril.
9. If there are signs of distress such as gasping, coughing, or cyanosis, immediately remove tube.
10. Continue to advance the tube when the patient swallows, until the tape mark reaches the patient's nostril.
11. To check whether the tube is in the stomach:
    a. Ask the patient to talk.

    b. Use the tongue blade and penlight to examine the patient's mouth—especially an unconscious patient.

1. This curves tubing and facilitates tube passage.
2. Lubrication reduces friction between the mucous membranes and tube and prevents injury to the nasal passages. Using a water-soluble lubricant prevents oil aspiration pneumonia if the tube accidentally slips into trachea.
3. The passage of the tube is facilitated by following the natural contours of the body. The slower the advancement of the tube at this point, the less likelihood of putting pressure on the turbinates, which could cause pain and bleeding.
4. Gag reflex is triggered by the presence of the tube.
5. Flexed head position partially occludes the airway, and the tube is less likely to enter trachea. Swallowing closes the epiglottis over the trachea and facilitates passage of tube into the esophagus. Actually, once the tube passes the cricopharyngeal sphincter into the esophagus, it can be slowly and steadily advanced even if the patient does not swallow.
6. This prevents the tube from entering the patient's mouth.

8. Avoid discomfort and trauma to patient.

9. May have entered the trachea.

10. This is the reference point where the tube was measured.
11.
    a. If the patient cannot talk, the tube may be coiled in throat or passed through vocal cords.
    b. If the patient is choking or has difficulty breathing, the tube has probably entered the trachea.

PROCEDURE GUIDELINES 18-3   *CONTINUED*

Nursing Action	Rationale
c. Attach a syringe to the end of the NG tube. Place a stethoscope over the left upper quadrant of the abdomen, and inject 10–20 cc of air while auscultating the abdomen.	c. Air can be detected by a "whooshing" sound entering stomach rather than the bronchus. If belching occurs, the tube is probably in the esophagus.
d. Aspirate contents of stomach with a 50-mL catheter tip syringe. If stomach contents cannot be aspirated, place the patient on left side and advance the tube 2.5–5 cm (1–2 inches) and try again.	d. Aspirated stomach contents indicate that the tube is in the stomach.
e. X-rays may be done to confirm tube placement.	

> **NURSING ALERT**
>
> **Never place the end of the tube in water while checking placement. If the tube is in the trachea, the patient could aspirate.**

Nursing Action	Rationale
12. After tube is passed and the correct placement is confirmed, attach the tube to suction or clamp the tube.	12. Clamping can be done using a clamp, plastic plug, or folding the tube over and slipping the bend into the tube end.
13. Apply tincture of benzoin to the area where the tape is placed.	13. This helps make the tube adhere, especially with diaphoretic patients.
14. Anchor tube with: a. Hypoallergenic tape; split lengthwise and only halfway, attach unsplit end of tape to nose, and cross split ends around tubing. Apply another piece of tape to bridge of nose. b. Bio-occlusive transparent dressing where it exits the nose.	14. Prevents the patient's vision from being disturbed; prevents tubing from rubbing against nasal mucosa. This will ensure tape being secure. Do not tape to forehead, this could cause necrosis of the nostril.
15. Anchor the tubing to the patient's gown. Use a rubber band to make a slip-knot to anchor the tubing to the patient's gown. Secure the rubber band to the patient's gown using a safety pin.	15. To permit mobility of patient. This prevents tugging on the tube when the patient moves.
16. Clamp the tube until the purpose for inserting the tube takes place.	16. See #12.
17. Attach the larger lumen of the Salem sump tube to suction equipment if ordered. Low continuous suction or high intermittent suction may be used with the Salem sump tube. If the Levin tube is used, low intermittent suction is recommended.	17. To prevent gastric mucosal damage, if a vacuum forms and the tube adheres to the gastric wall.

FOLLOW-UP PHASE

Nursing Action	Rationale
1. Assure the patient that most discomfort he or she feels will lessen as he or she gets used to the tube.	
2. Irrigate the tube at regular intervals (every 2 hours unless otherwise indicated) with small volumes of prescribed fluid to ensure the tube patency. a. If the tube is a Salem sump, it will require periodic placing of 10–20 mL of air through the vent port (blue port or smaller lumen). Do not instill water into the vent, and, if the vent is draining fluid, instill air to clear it. b. Check the Salem sump tube patency by placing the vent port next to your ear.	2. b. A soft hissing sound is heard if the tube is patent. If the port hangs downward and the tube backs up, stomach contents will spill over the patient.
3. Cleanse nares and provide mouth care every shift.	3. Promotes patient comfort and decreases risk of infection.
4. Apply petrolatum to nostrils as needed, and assess for skin irritation or breakdown.	4. To keep tissue soft and prevent crusting and skin breakdown.
5. Keep head of bed elevated at least 30 degrees.	5. To minimize gastroesophageal reflux.
6. Record the time, type, and size of tube inserted. Document placement checks after each assessment, along with amount, color, consistency of drainage.	6. To ensure proper tube and placement at all times, and assist in evaluation of tube effectiveness.

PROCEDURE GUIDELINES 18-4   NASOGASTRIC TUBE REMOVAL

EQUIPMENT

Towel   Lip pomade
Disposable gloves   Mouth hygiene materials

PROCEDURE

Nursing Action	Rationale
PREPARATORY PHASE	
1. Be certain that gastric or small bowel drainage is not excessive in volume.	1–3. Tube may not be discontinued unless drainage is minimal, bowel sounds are present, and patient is passing flatus.
2. Ensure, by auscultation, that audible peristalsis is present.	
3. Determine whether the patient is passing flatus; this indicates peristalsis.	
4. There is a health care provider's order for removal.	
PERFORMANCE PHASE	
1. Place a towel across the patient's chest, and inform him or her that the tube is to be withdrawn.	1. No doubt, the patient will be happy to have progressed to this stage.
2. Apply disposable gloves.	2. Provides protection from contaminated body fluids.
3. Turn off suction; disconnect and clamp tube.	3. Prevents fluids from leaking from tube.
4. Remove the tape from the patient's nose.	
5. Instruct the patient to take a deep breath and hold it.	5. This maneuver closes the epiglottis.
6. Slowly, but evenly, withdraw tubing and cover it with a towel as it emerges. (As the tube reaches the nasopharynx, you can pull quickly.)	6. Covering the tubing helps dispel patient's nausea.
7. Provide the patient with materials for oral care and lubricant for nasal dryness.	7. Mouthwash and a nasal lubricant will be appreciated by the patient.
8. Dispose of equipment in appropriate receptacle.	
9. Document time of tube removal and the patient's reaction.	
10. Document tube removal and color, consistency, and amount of drainage in suction canister.	
11. Continue to monitor the patient for signs of GI difficulties.	11. Recurrence of nausea or vomiting may require reinsertion of nasogastric tubing. Changes in vital signs may suggest infection.

PROCEDURE GUIDELINES 18-5   NASOINTESTINAL INTUBATION (SMALL-BORE FREEDING TUBES)

EQUIPMENT

Type of tube ordered by health care provider   Tape, rubber band, clamp, safety pin
30-mL or 60-mL luer-lock or tip syringe   Glass of water
Water-soluble lubricant   Stethoscope

 NURSING ALERT

Intestinal feeding tubes are longer, measuring up to 120 cm as compared to approximately 76 cm for gastric feeding tubes. Some tubes are weighted at the distal end of the tube. All tubes should be routinely pretested for patency and function before passage.

PROCEDURE

Nursing Action	Rationale
PREPARATORY AND PERFORMANCE PHASES (BY HEALTHCARE PROVIDER—NURSE ASSISTED)	
1. Tube Preparation:	
a. Do not ice plastic tubes.	a. Become too stiff to work with.
b. Inject 10 mL of water into the tube.	b. Aids in insertion.

Nursing Action	Rationale
c. Insert guidewire or stylet into tube, making sure it is positioned snugly against tube.	c. Prevents trauma.
d. Dip weighted tip into glass of water.	d. Activates lubricant.
2. Similar to passing a short nasogastric tube and taping to patient (see Procedure Guidelines 18-3).	
3. After the tube enters the stomach, it passes by peristalsis and gravity into the small intestine. Change patient's position from Fowler's to a position in which the patient is leaning forward.	3. This will assist in advancing the tubing to and through the pylorus; tilting to the right is helpful.
4. Obtain an x-ray of the abdomen after tube insertion.	4. Confirms placement.
5. Stylet should remain in place until position is confirmed.	

NURSING/PATIENT CARE CONSIDERATIONS

1. Be aware of risk of aspiration in an unconscious patient.
2. Instruct patient on complications associated with tube feedings, such as nausea, vomiting, diarrhea.
3. A continuous drip infusion delivered with an infusion pump may lessen the risk of aspiration, abdominal distention, and/or diarrhea.
4. If abdominal distention, vomiting, or diarrhea occurs, notify the health care provider; the rate of infusion may need to be adjusted.

■ Caring for the Patient Undergoing Gastrointestinal Surgery

Types of Procedures

Gastric Surgeries

1. Total gastrectomy—complete excision of the stomach with esophageal-jejunal anastomosis
2. Subtotal or partial gastrectomy—a portion of the stomach excised:
   a. Billroth I procedure—gastric remnant anastomosed to the duodenum
   b. Billroth II procedure—gastric remnant anastomosed to the jejunum
3. Gastrostomy (Janeway or Spivak)—rectangular stomach flap created into abdominal stoma, used for intermittent tube feedings

Hernia Surgeries

1. Herniorrhaphy—surgical repair of a hernia with suturing of the abdominal wall
2. Hernioplasty—reconstructive hernia repair with mesh sewn over the defect for reinforcement

Bowel Surgeries

1. Appendectomy—excision of the vermiform appendix
2. Bowel resection—segmental excision of small and/or large bowels with varied approaches:
   a. Anastomosis of proximal and distal ends of bowel
   b. Anastomosis of proximal and distal ends of bowel with temporary diverting loop ostomy
   c. Both ends of bowel exteriorized to the abdominal wall with proximal ostomy and distal mucous fistula
   d. Hartmann's procedure—proximal large bowel as ostomy; distal end of large bowel oversewn inside abdomen as Hartmann's pouch
3. Low-anterior resection—subtotal resection of the rectum with colorectal or coloanal anastomosis
4. Abdominoperineal resection—a combined abdominal and perineal approach for removal of the rectum and anus with permanent colostomy
5. Subtotal colectomy—partial removal of the large bowel or colon
6. Total colectomy—complete removal of the large bowel or colon with varied approaches:
   a. Ileorectal anastomosis—colon removal with ileum anastomosed to rectum
   b. Proctocolectomy—colon removal including the rectum and anus with permanent ileostomy
   c. Ileal reservoir—anal anastomosis. Colon removal, subtotal proctectomy, possible distal rectal mucosectomy, creation of pelvic reservoir from two, three, or four loops of ileum with anastomosis at anal canal. Usually a temporary loop ileostomy is performed as fecal diversion to protect the reservoir and the ileal-anal anastomosis. After takedown of temporary loop ileostomy (2 to 3 months postoperatively), the reservoir stores feces and patient eliminates under voluntary control through the anus.
   d. Kock or Barnett continent internal reservoir (BCIR) procedures—proctocolectomy, creation of a continent small bowel reservoir with nipple valve abdominal stoma used for stool removal through routine

intubation. Continence is provided through the nipple valve.

7. Roux-en-Y jejunostomy—jejunum severed with distal end exteriorized as permanent stoma for intermittent tube feedings; proximal end reanastomosed to GI tract distal to stoma to reestablish pathway

Laparoscopic Surgery

1. GI surgical procedures are increasingly being assisted by the use of a laparoscope, either partially or totally. The laparoscope is usually inserted through a 1-cm umbilical incision with additional trocars used for visualization and assistance. Dissection is performed with endocautery, scissors, or laser.
2. Advantages may include reduction in postoperative pain, shorter hospital and recuperative periods, cost effectiveness, and improved cosmetic outcome.
3. Contraindications may include obesity, internal adhesions, and bowel obstruction with distention.
4. Cholecystectomies and appendectomies are routinely done through laparoscopy; other GI surgeries, including ostomies and bowel resections, are increasingly being done through this surgical approach.

Preoperative Management

1. All diagnostic tests and procedures are explained to promote cooperation and relaxation.
2. The patient is prepared for the type of surgical procedure as well as postoperative care (ie, IV, patient-controlled analgesia pump, NG tube, surgical drains, incision care, possibility of ostomy).
3. Measures to prevent postoperative complications are taught, including coughing, turning, and deep breathing; using the incentive spirometer; and splinting the incision.
4. IV fluids or total parenteral nutrition (TPN) before surgery may be ordered to improve fluid and electrolyte balance and nutritional status.
5. Intake and output is monitored.
6. Preoperative laboratory studies are obtained.
7. Bowel cleansing will be initiated 1 to 2 days before surgery for better visualization. Preparation may include diet modifications, such as liquid or low residue, oral laxatives, suppositories, enemas, or polyethylene glycoelectrolyte solution (CoLyte, GoLYTELY).
8. Antibiotics are ordered to decrease the bacterial growth in the colon.
9. An ostomy specialty nurse is consulted if patient is scheduled for an ostomy to initiate early understanding and management of postoperative care.
10. Patient may not have anything by mouth after midnight the night before surgery. Medications may be withheld, if ordered. This will keep the GI tract clear.

Postoperative Management and Nursing Care
See Table 18-2.

1. Physical assessment is completed at least once per shift, or more frequently, as indicated.
   a. Monitor vital signs for signs of infection and shock—fever, hypotension, tachycardia.
   b. Monitor intake and output for signs of imbalance, dehydration, and shock. Include all drains in evaluating intake and output.
   c. Assess abdomen for increased pain, distention, rigidity, and rebound tenderness, because these may indicate postoperative complications. Report abnormal findings.
   d. Expect diminished or absent bowel sounds in the immediate postoperative phase.
   e. Evaluate dressing and incision. Check for purulent or bloody drainage, odor, and unusual tenderness or redness at incision site, which may indicate bleeding or infection.
   f. Evaluate for passing of flatus or feces.
   g. Monitor for nausea and vomiting. Note the presence of fecal smell or material in vomitus, because it may indicate an obstruction.
   h. Check NG aspirate, vomitus, and stools for signs of bleeding. Record and report findings if present.
2. Laboratory values are monitored and patient is evaluated for signs and symptoms of electrolyte imbalance.
3. Wound drains, IVs, and all other catheters are monitored and evaluated for signs of infection or infiltration.
4. To maintain patency of NG tube, the tube may be irrigated with 30 mL of normal saline solution (NSS) every 2 hours and as needed. If there are large amounts of NG output, IV replacement may be necessary.

NURSING ALERT

Due to the type of abdominal surgery and location of the suture line, the health care provider may order not to irrigate or manipulate the NG tube.

---

5. Subcutaneous heparin may also be ordered to prevent embolus. Antiembolism stockings may be used.
6. Turning, coughing, deep breathing, and incentive spirometry are performed every 2 hours. Dangling at bedside is encouraged the night of surgery and an attempt at ambulation the first postoperative day is made, unless ordered otherwise.
7. Patient-controlled analgesia for pain control or other analgesics, as ordered, are administered to promote comfort.
8. Wound dressing is changed every day or as needed, maintaining aseptic technique.
9. Diet is advanced as ordered, after presence of bowel sounds indicates GI tract has regained motility. After 1 to 2 days of NPO postoperatively, the usual diet progression is ice chips, sips of water, clear liquids, full liquids, soft or regular diet.

TABLE 18-2 Critical Pathway* for Elective Small- and Large-Bowel Surgery (Courtesy of St. Luke's Hospital, Jacksonville, Florida)

	Pre-Admission	Pre-Op	Post-Op	Level 1	Level 2	Level 3	Level 4	Level 5
Laboratory	CBC UA Chem 7 (opt) UCG/Beta HCG			CBC (opt) Chem 7 (opt)				Complete Staging Form
Radiology	CXR							
Diagnostic Cardiology	ECG (Case Specific)							
Respiratory			Incentive Spirometer Q1 Hour WA Aerosal (opt) →					
Medication/IVs		IV Hydration PO Antibiotics → Home Medication Evaluation	Perioperative ATB Sub Q Heparin (if at risk) PCA/Epidural or other analgesia →	TPN (opt) Reglan (opt) Antiemetics (opt)		IV to Hep Lock PO Pain Meds D/C PCA		
Treatment	Pre-op Evaluations with special attention to: Contact risk Medication Diabetes Steroid Aspirin Anticoagulants	Bowel Prep/Enemas → Enterostomal Therapy Consult (opt) →	Maintain drains Maintain NG (opt) Maintain Foley Antiembolism stockings (PAS) I & O Daily Weights	Enterostomal Consult Wound Care		D/C Drains Clamp NG D/C Foley D/C PAS: Change to TEDS	D/C NG	Independent Stomal Care
Activity	MOS SP 36 Survey†	Assess Ambulation →	Dangle Feet at Bedside	Sit in chair Ambulate with assistance →	Phy. Therapy (opt) Ambulate × 4	Ambulate × 6	Ambulate independently	
Nutrition	Nutrition Screen Calorie/Protein Supplements (if indicated) →	NPO after MN	Nutrition screening within 48 h NPO →	NPO/Ice Chips	Nutrition (opt) Assessment	Clear Liquids →	Advance Diet Consult for Food Preferences (opt)	

Level 5 (Medication/IVs): Oncology consult if needed

(continued)

TABLE 18-2 Critical Pathway* for Elective Small- and Large-Bowel Surgery (Courtesy of St. Luke's Hospital, Jacksonville, Florida) (Continued)

	Pre-Admission	Pre-Op	Post-Op	Level 1	Level 2	Level 3	Level 4	Level 5
Elimination								
Education/Teaching	Ostomy teaching (opt)			Ostomy Teaching (opt) →				
	Incentive Spirometer		Incentive Spirometer →					
	PCA use—other pain management		Pain Management →					
	Activity expectations			Walking Schedule →				
	Dietary Schedule				Dietary Schedule →			
	Splinting/coughing: leg exercises		Splinting/coughing: leg exercises →					
Discharge Planning		Social Service evaluation Assess home situation, need for referral		Assess discharge needs			Referral needs assessed Medical equipment needs Discharge Meds ECF Transfer Form	

ATB: antibiotic; CBC: complete blood count; CXR: chest x-ray; ECF: extended care facility; ECG: electrocardiogram; HCG: human chorionic gonadotropins; Hep: heparin; I&O: intake and output; IV: intravenous; MN: midnight; NG: nasogastric; Opt: optional; PAS: passive antiembolism stockings; PCA: patient-controlled analgesic; PO: by mouth; PT: prothrombin time; PTT: partial thromboplastin time; Q1: hourly; SF: short form functional status; SubQ: subcutaneous; TPN: total parenteral nutrition; UA: urinalysis; UCG: urinary chorionic gonadotropins; WA: while awake

The Clinical Pathway established for this procedure does not replace the exercise of independent clinical judgment on the part of the physician treating the individual patient.

NOTE: THIS IS NOT A PHYSICIAN ORDER

MOS SF 36 Survey—standard form used to assess functional ability. © 1992 with permission by Medical Outcomes Trust Inc., Boston, MA.

10. Dietary education includes fiber, avoiding gas-producing foods, and maintaining adequate fluid intake.
11. Reinforcement of teaching and assistance with ostomy care.
12. Administration of medications, as ordered, which may include a stool softener or laxative when bowel function has returned.

Potential Complications
1. Paralytic ileus or obstruction
2. Peritonitis or sepsis
3. Anastomotic leakage, which may result in peritonitis

Nursing Diagnoses
- Pain related to surgical incision
- Altered Nutrition: Less Than Body Requirements, related to dietary modifications after surgery
- Impaired Skin Integrity related to surgical incision
- Constipation related to surgery
- Risk for Infection related to surgical incision
- Fluid Volume Deficit related to surgical procedure
- Knowledge Deficit of surgical procedure and postoperative care

Nursing Interventions
Promoting Comfort
1. Assess pain location, intensity, and characteristics, and ensure they are appropriate for postoperative stage.
2. Administer prescribed pain medications, and provide instructions if using a patient-controlled analgesia pump, to keep patient comfortable.
3. Assess the effectiveness of the pain medications. If ordered, promethazine (Phenergan) can potentiate the effectiveness of pain medication.
4. Encourage the patient to change positions frequently and to splint incision when turning, coughing, or deep breathing to minimize discomfort.

Improving Nutritional Status
1. Monitor intake and output every 8 hours, or more frequently if indicated, to maintain fluid balance.
2. Advance diet as tolerated.
3. Weigh patient daily to ensure adequate calorie intake.
4. Provide snacks or high-protein, high-calorie supplements, and assist in menu selection, if needed.
5. Instruct patient to avoid gas-producing foods, and encourage ambulation.

Improving Skin Integrity
1. Assess wound for signs of erythema, swelling, and purulent drainage, which may indicate infection.
2. Change surgical dressing every 24 hours and as needed to protect skin from drainage and decrease risk of infection.
3. Apply gauze on skin to protect against leaking from drains or stomas.
4. Turn patient frequently or encourage position changes to prevent skin breakdown at pressure areas.

Promoting Bowel Elimination
1. Assess for presence of bowel sounds to evaluate return of bowel function.
2. Ask the patient if passing flatus rectally—also indicative of return of bowel function.
3. Evaluate for abdominal distention, nausea, or vomiting, which may indicate obstruction.
4. Monitor stool for frequency, amount, and consistency.
5. Administer stool softener or laxative, as ordered, to promote comfort with elimination.
6. Encourage diet with adequate fiber and fluid content for natural laxative effect.
7. Encourage and assist with ambulation to promote peristalsis.

Preventing Infection
1. Monitor temperature every shift or as ordered, and review previous readings to recognize early increases.
2. Change surgical dressings every 24 hours or more frequently, as indicated. Maintain aseptic technique to avoid contamination.
3. Monitor wound for signs and symptoms of infection, such as redness, swelling, purulent drainage, odor, and pain.
4. Obtain a wound culture, as ordered.
5. Monitor patient with a Foley catheter for signs and symptoms of urinary tract infection, such as concentrated, cloudy urine; hematuria; fever. If Foley discontinued, monitor for the above plus complaints of burning and frequency.
6. Assist patient in washing perineum daily and as needed if incontinence is present, for increased comfort and hygiene.
7. Assess breath sounds, and monitor for crackles.
8. Instruct patient to turn, cough, deep-breathe, and use incentive spirometer every 2 hours to minimize complications.
9. Encourage early ambulation to initiate bowel function and reduce risk of embolus.
10. Administer antibiotics, as ordered, to maintain constant blood level.

Maintaining Fluid Volume
1. Monitor intake and output every 8 hours, or more frequently, if ordered, to assess recent status. Include amount of wound drainage from dressing changes and drains that may be in place.
2. Assess patient for signs of dehydration—flushed, dry skin; tenting of skin; oliguria; tachycardia, hypotension, and rapid respirations; increase in hematocrit, blood urea nitrogen, electrolytes; fever; weight loss.
3. Monitor laboratory results, and report abnormal findings.
4. Assess patient for signs of electrolyte imbalance—nausea, vomiting; cardiac dysrhythmia, tremor, seizures, anorexia, malaise, weakness, irregular pulse; changes in behavior, mental status.
5. Weigh daily to ensure adequate caloric intake.

6. Administer parenteral fluids, enteral feedings, and blood products as ordered to maintain volume during period of decreased oral intake.

Community and Home Care Considerations

1. Reinforce discharge instructions and the importance of postsurgical regimen to include health provider follow-up appointments, laboratory and other scheduled tests or therapies.
2. A person who has undergone a total gastrectomy needs lifelong parenteral administration of vitamin B_{12} to prevent pernicious anemia. This may also apply to persons with the terminal ileum removed, and sometimes for those with ileostomies.
3. Change dressing, and reinforce ostomy care as directed by health care provider. Report any signs of infection—unusual drainage, redness, warmth, increased pain, swelling.
4. Instruct to gradually increase activities of daily living. No heavy lifting (more than 10 lb), pushing, pulling, or driving for 6 to 8 weeks postoperatively.
5. Referral to additional community resources if applicable (support groups, meal programs, social services).

Patient Education and Health Maintenance

1. Review signs and symptoms of wound infection so early intervention may be instituted.
2. Explain signs and symptoms of other postoperative complications to report—elevated temperature, nausea or vomiting, abdominal distention, changes in bowel function and stool consistency or color.
3. Instruct patient to report promptly blood in the stool or the coughing up of blood.
4. Teach patient regarding wound and/or ostomy care, if applicable, to promote healing and self-confidence.
5. Encourage patient to turn, cough, deep-breathe; use of incentive spirometer; and ambulation. Discuss the importance of these functions during the recovery period.
6. Review dietary changes, such as increased fiber content and fluid intake, and their importance in improving bowel function.
7. Review actions and side effects of prescribed medications to encourage compliance and understanding of management.
8. Assess the need for home health follow-up, and initiate appropriate referrals if indicated.

Outcome-Based Evaluation

- Verbalizes increased comfort (using a 0 to 10 pain scale with 0 being no pain and 10 being the highest score to measure pain)
- Consumes 50% to 75% of each meal; no weight loss
- Incisional flaps approximated and healing ridge present
- Passing flatus and stool
- No signs and symptoms of infection
- Vital signs stable, fluid and electrolytes in balance
- Verbalizes and/or demonstrates increased knowledge regarding surgical and postoperative care

■ Caring for the Patient Undergoing Ostomy Surgery

See Standards of Care Guidelines.

Types of Fecal Ostomies
Colostomy
See Figure 18-2.

1. A surgically created opening between the colon and the abdominal wall to allow fecal elimination. It may be a temporary or permanent diversion.
2. A colostomy may be placed in any segment of the large intestine (colon), which will influence the nature of fecal discharge. The more right-sided the colostomy, the looser the stool. Transverse and descending/sigmoid colostomies are the most common types.
3. A colostomy may be performed as part of an abdominoperineal resection for rectal cancer; a fecal diversion for unresectable cancer; a temporary measure to protect an anastomosis; surgical treatment for inflammatory bowel diseases, trauma, ischemic bowel, and congenital conditions.

STANDARDS OF CARE GUIDELINES
Care of the Patient With an Ostomy

- Prepare patient preoperatively by explaining the surgical procedure, stoma characteristics, and ostomy management with a pouching system.
- If possible preoperatively, have ostomy nurse mark an optimal stoma site.
- Postoperatively, monitor the stoma color and amount and color of stomal output every shift; document, and report any abnormalities.
- Periodically change a properly fitting pouching system over the ostomy to avoid leakage and protect the peristomal skin. Use this time as an opportunity for teaching.
- Assess peristomal skin with each pouching system change, document findings, and treat any abnormalities (skin breakdown due to leakage, allergy, or infection) as indicated.
- Teach the patient and/or caregiver self-care skills of routine pouch emptying, cleansing skin and stoma, and changing of the pouching system until independence is achieved.
- Instruct the patient and family in lifestyle adjustments regarding gas and odor control; procurement of ostomy supplies; and bathing, clothing, and travel tips.
- Encourage patient to verbalize feelings regarding the ostomy, body image changes, and sexual issues.
- Inform patient of community resources such as United Ostomy Association, local ostomy supply dealers, ostomy nurse specialists, American Cancer Society, and Crohn's & Colitis Foundation.

This information should serve as a general guideline only. Each patient situation presents a unique set of clinical factors and requires nursing judgment to guide care, which may include additional or alternative measures and approaches.

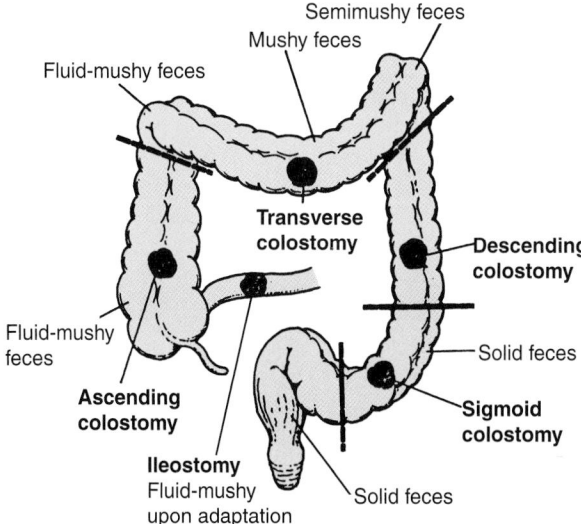

FIGURE 18-2 A diagrammatic representation of the placement of fecal ostomies and nature of discharge at these sites.

Ileostomy

1. A surgically created opening between the ileum of the small intestine and the abdominal wall to allow elimination of small bowel effluent.
2. An ileostomy is usually formed at the terminal ileum of the small bowel and is usually placed in the right lower quadrant of the abdomen. Stool from an ileostomy drains frequently (average four to five times per day) and contains proteolytic enzymes, which can be harmful to skin.
3. Diagnoses that may require a temporary or permanent ileostomy include ulcerative colitis, Crohn's disease, familial polyposis, congenital defects, and trauma.

Characteristics of Stomas

1. A stoma is that part of the intestine (small or large) that is brought above the abdominal wall and that becomes the outlet for discharge of intestinal contents. It is often used interchangeably with the word "ostomy."
2. Normal stomal characteristics: pink-red, moist, bleeds slightly when rubbed, no feeling to touch, stool functions involuntary, and postoperative swelling gradually decreases over several months.
3. Stoma classifications:
   a. *End stoma:* After bowel is divided, the proximal bowel is exteriorized to abdominal wall, everted (which exposes mucosal lining), and sutured to dermis or subcutaneous tissue. There is only one opening that drains stool. The distal bowel is either surgically removed or sutured closed within abdominal cavity.
   b. *Double-barrel stoma:* After bowel is divided, the proximal and distal ends of bowel are exteriorized to abdominal wall, everted, and sutured to the dermis or subcutaneous tissue. If the stomas are brought up

next to each other requiring them to be pouched together, they are referred to as a double-barrel stoma; if the stomas are apart to be pouched separately, they may be referred to as an end stoma (proximal), which drains stool, and a mucous fistula (distal), which drains mucus. This type of stoma is usually temporary.
   c. *Loop stoma:* A bowel loop is brought to the abdominal wall through an incision and stabilized temporarily with a rod, catheter, or a skin or fascial bridge. The anterior wall of bowel is opened surgically or by electrocautery to expose the proximal and distal openings. The posterior wall of bowel remains intact and separates the functioning proximal opening and the nonfunctioning distal opening. This type of stoma is usually temporary.
4. Ostomy specialty nurse
   a. An ostomy specialty nurse has the title of certified ostomy nurse (CON) or certified wound, ostomy and continence nurse (CWOCN), known previously as a certified enterostomal therapy nurse (CETN). These nurses play a vital role in the rehabilitation of patients with ostomies and related problems.
   b. The Wound Ostomy and Continence Nurses Society (WOCN), 2755 Bristol Street #110, Costa Mesa, CA 92626 has an official publication called the *Journal of Wound, Ostomy, and Continence Nursing,* published monthly by Mosby, 11830 Westline Industrial Drive, St. Louis, MO 63146-3318, *www.wocn.org.*

Preoperative Management and Nursing Care

1. Prepare the patient for general abdominal surgery (see p. 585).
2. Administer replacement fluid as ordered before surgery due to possible increased output during the postoperative phase.
3. Provide low-residue diet before NPO status.
4. Explain that the abdomen will be marked by the ostomy specialty nurse or surgeon to ensure proper positioning of the stoma.
      Note: The abdominal location of the stoma is usually determined by anatomical location of bowel segment (eg, a sigmoid colostomy is ideally located in left lower abdominal quadrant).
5. Other considerations when selecting a stoma include:
   a. Positioning within rectus muscle.
   b. Avoidance of bony prominences, such as iliac crest and costal margin.
   c. Clearance from umbilicus, scars, and deep creases, observed in lying, sitting, and standing positions.
   d. Positioning on a flat pouching surface.
   e. Avoidance of beltline when possible.
   f. Positioning within patient's visibility to optimize independent ostomy care.
6. Support the patient and family with the many psychosocial considerations of ostomy surgery.

Postoperative Management and Nursing Care

1. Administer general abdominal surgery care (see p. 260).
2. Assess stoma every shift for color and record findings:
   a. Normal color: pink-red
   b. Dusky: dark red; purplish hue (ischemic sign)
   c. Necrotic: brown or black; may be dry (notify health care provider to determine extent of necrosis)
3. Apply pouching system with ⅛-inch clearance to prevent stomal constriction, which contributes to edema (Box 18-2).
4. Check for abdominal distention, which reduces blood flow to stoma through mesenteric tension.
5. Evaluate and empty drains and ostomy pouch frequently to promote patency and maintain seal.

BOX 18-2 Fecal Ostomy Pouching Systems

1. Pouching systems are varied according to manufacturer and patient needs. Systems are classified as one-piece or two-piece and disposable or reusable. A disposable, one-piece pouch is commonly used with backing as adhesive tape, skin barrier, or both. A disposable two-piece system consists of a skin barrier wafer with or without a tape border and a pouch. Disposable systems are popular and are discarded after one use. Reusable systems are declining in use and are made of heavier material, allowing use for weeks to months. They require the use of double-backed adhesive disks, cement, and/or belt to provide a seal.
2. Pouching systems are available in precut sizes and cut-to-fit options as well as with a flat backing versus degrees of convexity. Convex pouching systems are used with flush or retracted stomas to increase stomal protrusion and reduce undermining of feces.
3. Fecal pouches are available in closed-end and drainable styles. Drainable pouches require the use of a tail closure and may be used more than once. Closed-end pouches may contain a built-in filter to release gas and require no tail closure. A closed-end pouch is discarded after one use. Pouch selection depends on the patient's preference or ability to manipulate the volume and frequency of fecal output.
4. Many accessory products are available to assist in the management of a fecal ostomy. They include skin sealants, skin barrier powders, pastes, washers, adhesive removers, tapes, belts, pouch covers, and deodorants.
5. The goal is to change a pouching system on a routine basis to prevent leakage. Usually, this is every 3–7 days and will vary per individual needs. Routine changes allow for examination of the peristomal skin for breakdown. Schedule the change when the bowel is least active, usually early morning before breakfast, 2–4 hours after a meal, or before bedtime. At times, the pouching system may need to be changed immediately if leakage is imminent, itching or burning of peristomal skin is present, odor is detected with a closed system, or the wafer is dissolving.

---

6. Monitor intake and output with extreme accuracy, because output may remain high during early postoperative period.
7. Suction and irrigate NG tube frequently, as ordered, to relieve pressure and decrease gastric contents.
8. Offer continued support to patient and family.

Complications

1. Mucocutaneous separation (between skin and stoma)
2. Stomal ischemia
3. Stomal stricture or stenosis (usually long-term complication)
4. Stomal prolapse
5. Peristomal hernia
6. Peristomal skin breakdown from exposure to fecal output, allergic reaction to products, or infection, such as candidiasis

Nursing Diagnoses

- Knowledge Deficit related to surgical procedures and ostomy management
- Body Image Disturbance related to change in structure, function, and appearance
- Anxiety related to loss of bowel control and autonomy
- Impaired Skin Integrity related to irritation of peristomal skin by drainage and equipment
- Altered Nutrition: Less Than Body Requirements, related to increased output and inadequate intake
- Sexual Dysfunction related to altered body structure

Nursing Interventions

Educating the Patient

1. Review the surgical procedure with patient, and discuss the information that the surgeon and other providers have given. Clarify any misunderstandings.
2. Avoid overwhelming the patient with information.
3. Include family in discussions, when appropriate.
4. Use available educational materials, including pictures and drawings, if patient is receptive.
5. Involve the ostomy specialty nurse (CWOCN) in ostomy teaching, and reinforce information, including lifestyle modifications.
6. Use a team approach; the need for information may come from many disciplines.
7. Assess patient's response to teaching. If patient not interested, provide alternative times for teaching and review.
8. Consider the psychosocial issues of the patient and their effect on learning.

Promoting a Positive Self-Image

1. Encourage the patient to verbalize feelings about the surgical outcome.
2. Provide support during initial viewing of the stoma, and encourage patient to touch the area.
3. Encourage spouse or significant other to view the stoma.

4. Arrange a visit by a United Ostomy Association ostomy visitor if the patient desires. This is preferably done pre-operatively.
5. Offer counseling, as necessary, and encourage patient to use normal support systems, such as family, church, community groups.

Reducing Anxiety

1. Provide information regarding expected outcomes, such as the type and consistency of bowel function.
2. Introduce gradual steps toward achieving independent ostomy management. Have the patient:
   a. First observe stoma, pouch change, and emptying procedure. See Procedure Guidelines 18-6: Changing a Two-Piece Drainable Fecal Pouching System.
   b. Learn tail closure application and removal.
   c. Empty pouch by cuffing tail and using tail closure.
   d. Assist with pouching system change until independent.
      Note: Some patients may have decreased vision or dexterity and may require additional assistance and encouragement.
3. Teach colostomy irrigation procedure, if appropriate. See Procedure Guidelines 18-7: Irrigating a Colostomy.
   a. Review that irrigating involves inserting an enema into a descending or sigmoid colostomy.
   b. Reinforce its purposes of cleansing the colon and stimulating the colon to move at a desired time regularly to regain control of fecal elimination.
   c. It is a patient preference whether colostomy irrigations are attempted for control. Irrigation may occur every day or every other day depending on bowel pattern. It usually takes 1 to 2 months to establish control. Patients with a preoperative history of regular, formed bowel movements are more likely to realize success.
   d. Disadvantages to the colostomy irrigation include that it is time-consuming and requires consistency, and that bowel dependency to irrigation may occur.
   e. Only a patient with a descending or sigmoid colostomy is an irrigation candidate for fecal control. A colostomy more proximal than descending has too liquid and higher volume of fecal output to be managed through irrigation.
   f. If a patient discontinues colostomy irrigations after months or years of performance, due to illness, hospitalization, or preference, a bulk laxative or other stimulant may be routinely necessary to maintain regular bowel function.
4. Acknowledge that it is normal to have negative feelings toward ostomy surgery; empathize with patient.
5. Describe behaviors to attain a sense of control, such as resuming activities of daily living.

Maintaining Skin Integrity

1. Select pouching system based on type of ostomy and condition of stoma and skin (see Box 18-2).
2. Empty pouch when one third to one half full to avoid overfilling, which interferes with pouch seal.
   a. Remove tail closure from pouch tail.
   b. Cuff bottom of pouch tail.
   c. Drain stool from pouch.
   d. Clean pouch tail with toilet tissue or wipe (may rinse pouch if desired).
   e. Uncuff pouch, and reapply tail closure.
3. Treat peristomal skin breakdown as needed.
   a. Dust skin breakdown with skin barrier powder (such as Stomahesive powder).
   b. Seal powder with water or skin sealant (such as Skin Prep).
   c. Allow skin to dry before applying pouching system.

NURSING ALERT

When peristomal skin is exposed to excess moisture, candidiasis can occur. It presents as an erythematous rash, which may include papules, pustules, or white patches. Patients may complain of pruritus. The treatment procedure is the same as treating skin breakdown, using a prescribed antifungal powder (Mycostatin) in place of the skin barrier powder. The antifungal powder should be used at each pouching system change and continued 2 weeks after the condition has cleared. Positive identification of *Candida albicans* can be done through a culture or scraping. Treatment is usually initiated without culture or scraping if the signs and symptoms are classic.

Maximizing Nutritional Intake

1. Review dietary habits with patient to determine patterns, preferences, and bowel irritants.
2. Advise the patient to avoid foods that stimulate elimination, such as nuts, seeds, and certain fruits.
3. Recommend consistency in dietary habits as well as moderation.
4. Coordinate consult with nutritionist, as needed.
5. Weigh daily; monitor vital signs and electrolytes to determine patient's nutritional status.

Achieving Sexual Well-Being

1. Encourage patient and significant other to express feelings about the ostomy.
2. Discuss ways to conceal pouch during intimacy, if desired: pouch covers, special ostomy underwear. May briefly use small-capacity pouch (minipouch or cap).
3. Recommend different positions for sexual activity to decrease stoma friction and skin irritation.
4. Review, when appropriate, that an ostomy in a woman does not prevent a successful pregnancy.
5. Recommend counseling as needed.

Patient Education and Health Maintenance
Skin Care

1. Instruct patient to inspect peristomal skin with each pouching system change.
2. Review techniques for treating peristomal skin problems.
3. Recommend alternative products if patient develops allergic reaction to a ostomy product.

4. Teach patient to notify health care provider when skin care problems do not resolve by usual methods.

Odor Control

1. Encourage pouch hygiene through rinsing, keeping pouch tail free of stool, airing of reusable pouches, discarding odor-impregnated pouches.
2. Recommend the use of pouch deodorants, room deodorizers, and oral deodorizers, such as bismuth subgallate (Devrom) or parsley.
3. Avoid use of pinholes in pouch.

Gas Control

1. Suggest avoidance of straws, excessive talking while eating, chewing gum, and smoking to reduce swallowed air.
2. Instruct about gas-forming foods, such as beans and cabbage, and eliminate when appropriate. It takes about 6 hours for gas to travel from mouth to colostomy.
3. Recommend using arm over stoma to muffle gas sounds when appropriate.

Activities of Daily Living

Educate the patient about the following:

1. Resumption of normal bathing habits (tub or shower) with or without pouching system.
2. Picture framing the edges of the pouching system with waterproof tape, if needed for bathing or swimming.
3. Clothing modifications usually minimal. Girdles without stays and pantyhose acceptable.

4. Carrying an ostomy supply kit during work or travel in case of an emergency.
5. Participating in sports as desired. Caution must be exercised with contact sports. During vigorous activities, a belt or binder may provide extra security.
6. The United Ostomy Association, a self-help group for ostomates and other interested persons. The national headquarters is located at 19772 MacArthur Blvd., Suite 200, Irvine, CA 92612-2405, 800-826-0826; *www.uoa.org/*. The official membership publication is the *Ostomy Quarterly*. Encourage ostomy patients to participate in a local chapter. Chapters usually publish a local newsletter, conduct monthly meetings, and provide trained ostomy visitors on request by health care providers.
7. Ostomy manufacturers offer literature covering a wide variety of ostomy-related topics.
8. Encourage patient to maintain contact with health care providers.

Outcome-Based Evaluation

- Verbalizes knowledge regarding ostomy surgery
- Demonstrates skills for care of the ostomy
- Incorporates ostomy management into activities of daily living
- Verbalizes acceptance of body image changes and resumption of sexual activities

---

PROCEDURE GUIDELINES 18-6   **CHANGING A TWO-PIECE DRAINABLE FECAL POUCHING SYSTEM**

EQUIPMENT

Duplicate wafer and pouch	Washcloth and towel	Accessory products
Tail closure	Mild nonoily soap (optional)	prescribed for patient

PROCEDURE

Nursing Action	Rationale
PREPARATORY PHASE	
1. Have patient assume a relaxed position and provide privacy. The best position may be sitting, reclining, or standing.	1. Patient must see stoma site to learn care.
PERFORMANCE PHASE	
1. To remove pouching system:	
a. Wear nonsterile gloves.	a. Maintains universal precautions.
b. Push down gently on skin while lifting up on the wafer (ostomy adhesive remover may be used).	b. Minimizes skin trauma.
c. Discard soiled pouch and wafer in odorproof plastic bag. Save tail closure for reuse.	c. Removes room odor and maintains universal precautions.
2. To cleanse skin:	
a. Use toilet tissue to remove feces from stoma and skin if needed.	a. Stoma may function during the change.
b. Cleanse stoma and peristomal skin with soft cloth and water, soap optional. The patient may shower with or without pouching system in place. Clip or shave peristomal hair if appropriate.	b. Minimizes skin breakdown and promotes hygiene.

PROCEDURE GUIDELINES 18-6   *CONTINUED*

Nursing Action	Rationale
c. Rinse and dry skin thoroughly after cleansing. It is normal for the stoma to bleed slightly during cleansing and drying.	c. Removes residue, which may interfere with adhesion of wafer.
3. To apply wafer:	
a. Use measuring guide or pattern to determine stoma size.	a. This step is omitted when stomal shrinkage is complete, about 2 months postop.
b. Trace correct size onto back of wafer and cut to stoma size. It is acceptable to cut $\frac{1}{16}$–$\frac{1}{8}$ inch larger than stoma.	b. Avoids wafer rubbing stoma; omit this step if the wafer is precut.
c. Apply a line of skin barrier paste around stoma or on lip of wafer opening. Allow to set according to manufacturer's instructions. (Other barrier may be used in place of paste, such as strips or washer. Some may find the paste too difficult to see or have developed an allergy to the alcohol within the paste.)	c. Extra skin protection is imperative for ileostomy and right-sided colostomy. A left-sided colostomy may not need a secondary barrier because formed stool is less harmful to skin. Paste acts as "caulking" to prevent undermining of feces.
d. Remove paper backing(s) from the wafer, center opening over stoma, and press wafer down onto peristomal skin.	d. Ensures adherence.
4. Snap pouch onto the flange of the wafer according to manufacturer's directions (see accompanying figure).	4. If attached properly, there will be no leakage or odor.
5. Apply tail closure to pouch tail.	5. Proper closure controls odor.

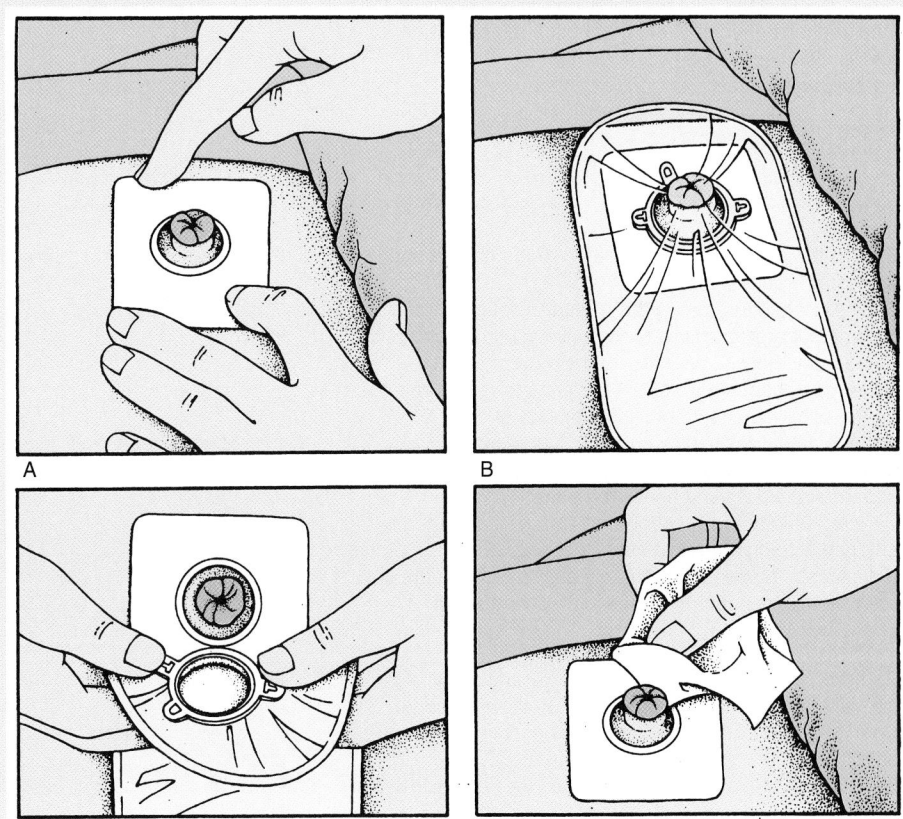

A

B

C

D

(A) A wafer with flange (1$\frac{1}{2}$", 1$\frac{3}{4}$", 2$\frac{1}{4}$", 2$\frac{3}{4}$", 4") is applied after cleaning and drying of peristomal skin. (B) A transparent or opaque drainable pouch is positioned over stoma at desired angle. (C) Pouch may be removed without removal of wafer. (D) Stoma may be assessed without removing wafer. (Adapted by permission from Convatec, A Bristol-Myers, Squibb Company.)

continued

PROCEDURE GUIDELINES 18-6	CHANGING A TWO-PIECE DRAINABLE FECAL POUCHING SYSTEM *CONTINUED*

Nursing Action	Rationale
FOLLOW-UP PHASE	
1. Dispose of plastic bag with waste materials.	1. Complies with universal precautions.
2. Clean drainable pouch with soap and water, if appropriate. Drainable pouches may be reused several times.	2. Controls odor; reduces cost.
3. A commercial deodorant can be placed in the pouch to reduce odor.	
4. Gas can be released from the pouch by releasing the tail closure or by snapping off an area on the pouch flange. Never make a pinhole in the pouch to release gas.	4. Destroys the odorproof seal.

PROCEDURE GUIDELINES 18-7	IRRIGATING A COLOSTOMY

EQUIPMENT

Reservoir for irrigating fluids; irrigator bag or enema bag if irrigator bag not available

Irrigating fluid: 500–1,500 mL lukewarm water or other solution prescribed by health care provider (Volume is titrated based on patient tolerance and results; average amount is 1,000 mL.)

Irrigating tip: Cone tip or soft rubber catheter #22 or #24 with shield to prevent backflow of irrigating solution (Use only if cone not available. The cone is the preferred method to avoid possibility of bowel perforation.)

Irrigation sleeve (long, large-capacity bag with opening at top to insert cone or catheter into stoma); available in different styles: Snap-on, self-adhering to skin, or held in place by belt

Large tail closure

Water-soluble lubricant

PROCEDURE

Nursing Action	Rationale
PREPARATORY PHASE	
1. Explain the details of the procedure to the patient and answer any questions.	1. Relieves anxiety and promotes compliance.
2. Select a consistent time, free from distractions. If the patient is learning to irrigate for bowel control, choose the time of day that will best fit into the patient's lifestyle.	2. Establishes regularity.
3. Have the patient sit in front of the commode on chair or on the commode itself, providing privacy and comfort.	
4. Hang irrigating reservoir with prescribed solution so the bottom of the reservoir is approximately at the level of the patient's shoulder and above the stoma. *Note:* Colostomy irrigation may also be performed to empty the colon of its contents (feces, gas, mucus) before a diagnostic procedure or surgery and to cleanse the colon after fecal impaction removal or with constipation.	4. Height of irrigation bag regulates pressure of irrigant.
PERFORMANCE PHASE	
1. Remove pouch or covering from stoma, and apply irrigation sleeve, directing the open tail into the commode.	1. Allows water and feces to flow directly into commode.
2. Open tubing clamp on the irrigating reservoir to release a small amount of solution into the commode.	2. Removes air from the setup; avoids air from being introduced into the colon, which can cause crampy pain.
3. Lubricate the tip of the cone/catheter, and gently insert into the stoma. Insert catheter no more than 3 inches. Hold cone/shield gently, but firmly, against stoma to prevent backflow of water.	3. Prevents intestinal perforation and irritation of mucous membranes.
4. If catheter does not advance easily, allow water to flow slowly while advancing catheter. NEVER FORCE CATHETER.	4. Slow rate relaxes bowel to facilitate passage of catheter.

PROCEDURE GUIDELINES 18-7   *CONTINUED*

Nursing Action	Rationale
Dilating the stoma with lubricated, gloved pinky finger may be necessary to direct cone/catheter properly.	
5. Allow water to enter colon slowly over a 5- to 10-minute period. If cramping occurs, slow flow rate or clamp tubing to allow cramping to subside. If cramping does not subside, remove cone/catheter to release contents.	5. Cramping may occur from too rapid flow, cold water, excess solution, or colon ready to function.
6. Hold cone/shield in place 10 seconds after water is instilled, then gently remove cone/catheter from stoma.	6. Discourages premature evacuation of fluid.
7. As feces and water flow down sleeve, periodically rinse sleeve with water. Allow 10–15 minutes for most of the returns, then dry sleeve tail and apply tail closure.	
8. Leave sleeve in place for approximately 20 more minutes while patient gets up and moves around.	8. Ambulation stimulates peristalsis and completion of irrigation return.
9. When returns are complete, clean stomal area with mild soap and water; pat dry; reapply pouch or covering over stoma.	9. Cleanliness and dryness promote comfort.
FOLLOW-UP PHASE	
1. Clean equipment with soap and water; dry and store in well-ventilated area.	1. This will control odor and mildew, prolonging the life of equipment.
2. If applicable, the patient should use a pouch until the colostomy is sufficiently controlled.	2. It may take several months to establish control. The patient can then use minipouch, stoma cap, or gauze covering as desired.

ESOPHAGEAL DISORDERS

Esophageal varices are covered in Chapter 19.

Gastroesophageal Reflux Disease (GERD) and Esophagitis

Gastric contents flow back into the esophagus in GERD due to incompetent lower esophageal sphincter (LES). Esophagitiis, or inflammation of the esophageal mucosa, may result.

Pathophysiology and Etiology

1. Gastroesophageal reflux associated with an incompetent LES—gastric contents reflux (flow backward) through the LES into the esophagus.
2. Can be the result of impaired gastric emptying from gastroparesis or partial gastric outlet obstruction.
3. The acidity of gastric content and amount of time in contact with esophageal mucosa are related to the degree of mucosal damage.
4. Inflammation and ulceration of the esophagus may result, causing esophagitis.
5. May be caused by motility disorders—achalasia, scleroderma, esophageal spasm.

Clinical Manifestations
GERD

1. The most common symptom is heartburn (pyrosis), often occurring 30 to 60 minutes after meals and with reclining positions. Complaints of spontaneous reflux (regurgitation) of sour or bitter gastric contents into the mouth.
2. Dysphagia is a less common symptom.
3. Other symptoms include atypical chest pain, hoarseness, chronic cough, bronchospasm (asthma/wheezing), and odynophagia (sharp substernal pain on swallowing).
4. Symptoms that may suggest other disease etiologies need further evaluation: atypical chest pain (rule out possible cardiac causes), dysphagia, odynophagia, or weight loss (rule out cancer or esophageal stricture).

Esophagitis

1. Esophagitis is an acute or chronic inflammation of the esophagus. Severity of symptoms may be unrelated to the degree of esophageal tissue damage.
2. Symptoms vary according to etiology of esophagitis. Symptoms include dysphagia, odynophagia, severe burning, chest pain.
3. Causes of esophagitis other than GERD
   a. Infectious—*Candida,* herpes, HIV, cytomegalovirus
   b. Chemical—alkali or acid
   c. Medication-induced—may include doxycycline, ascorbic acid, quinidine, potassium chloride, bisphosphonates

Diagnostic Evaluation

1. Endoscopy can visualize inflammation, lesions, or erosions. Biopsy can confirm diagnosis.
2. Esophageal manometry measures LES pressure and determines if esophageal peristalsis is adequate. This study should be used before patients undergo surgical treatment for reflux.
3. Acid perfusion (Bernstein test)—onset of symptoms after ingestion of dilute hydrochloric acid and saline is

considered positive. This test differentiates between cardiac and noncardiac chest pain.
4. Ambulatory 24-hour pH monitoring is frequently performed for diagnostics. It determines the amount of gastroesophageal acid reflux.
5. Barium esophagography—use of barium with radiographic studies to diagnose mechanical and motility disorders.

Management

Management is divided into a five-phase approach:

Phase I: Lifestyle Changes
1. Head of bed raised 15 to 20 cm (6 to 8 inches).
2. Do not lie down for 3 hours after eating—time frame for greatest reflux.
3. Bland diet—avoid garlic, onion, peppermint, fatty foods, chocolate, coffee (even decaffeinated), citrus juices, colas, and tomato products.
4. Avoid overeating—causes LES relaxation.
5. No tight-fitting clothes.
6. Weight control.
7. Smoking cessation.
8. Reduce alcohol.

Phase II: First-Line Drug Therapy
1. Antacids—reduce gastric acidity. Use on an as-needed basis. Provide symptomatic relief but do not heal esophageal lesions.
2. Histamine-(H_2) receptor blockers, such as ranitidine (Zantac), cimetidine (Tagamet), famotidine (Pepcid)—decrease gastric acid secretions. Provide symptomatic relief. May require lifelong therapy.

> **◆ DRUG ALERT**
>
> OTC H_2 receptor blockers include Axid AR, Pepcid AC, Tagamet HB, and Zantac 75. These OTC medications are half the strength of the same medications through prescription.

Phase III: Second-Line Drug Therapy
1. Use of high-dose H_2 blocker
2. Addition of a prokinetic agent, metoclopramide (Reglan), to promote gastric emptying
3. Addition of a proton pump inhibitor, such as omeprazole (Prilosec) or lansoprazole (Prevacid), to block gastric acid secretion

Phase IV: Drug Maintenance Therapy
1. May be needed depending on the severity of disease and recurrence of symptoms after initial drug therapy is stopped.
2. Use the lowest effective drug dose of H_2 receptor blocker or proton pump inhibitor.

Phase V: Surgery
1. May be indicated for patients who do not respond to other approaches or who cannot adhere to strict lifestyle and pharmacologic management. Common procedure is Nissen fundoplication.

a. Upper portion of the stomach is wrapped around the distal esophagus and sutured, creating a tight LES.
b. This procedure can be performed laparoscopically.
c. Combined with vagotomy-pyloroplasty if associated with gastroduodenal ulcer.

Complications
1. Esophageal stricture formation
2. Ulceration of the esophagus, with or without fistula formation
3. Aspiration, may be complicated by pneumonia
4. Development of Barrett's esophagus—presence of columnar epithelium above the gastroesophageal junction associated with adenocarcinoma of the esophagus

Nursing Interventions and Patient Education
1. Teach the patient about prescribed medications, side effects, and when to notify the health care provider.
2. Inform the patient regarding medications that may exacerbate symptoms.
3. Advise the patient to sit or stand when taking any solid medication (pills, capsules): emphasize the need to follow the drug with at least 100 mL of liquid.
4. Emphasize to the patient and family what foods and activities to avoid: fatty foods, garlic, onions, alcohol, coffee, and chocolate; straining, bending over, tight-fitting clothes, smoking.
5. Encourage the patient to sleep with the head of the bed elevated (not pillow elevation).
6. Encourage a weight-reduction program if the patient is overweight—to decrease intra-abdominal pressure.

> **◆ DRUG ALERT**
>
> Anticholinergics may further impair functioning of the LES, allowing reflux; antihistamines, antidepressants, antihypertensives, antispasmodics, and some neuroleptics and antiparkinsonian drugs decrease saliva production, which may decrease acid clearance from the esophagus.

Hiatal Hernia

A hiatal hernia is a protrusion of a portion of the stomach through the hiatus of the diaphragm and into the thoracic cavity.

Pathophysiology and Etiology
1. There are two types of hiatal hernias:
   a. *Sliding hernia:* Stomach and gastroesophageal junction slip up into the chest (most common)
   b. *Paraesophageal hernia (rolling hernia):* Part of the greater curvature of the stomach rolls through the diaphragmatic defect
2. Caused by muscle weakening due to aging or other conditions, such as esophageal carcinoma or trauma, or following certain surgical procedures

Clinical Manifestations

1. May be asymptomatic
2. Heartburn (with or without regurgitation of gastric contents into the mouth)
3. Dysphagia, chest pain

Diagnostic Evaluation

1. Barium study of the esophagus outlines hernia.
2. Endoscopic examination visualizes defect.

Management

1. Elevation of head of bed (15 to 20 cm [6 to 8 inches]) to reduce nighttime reflux.
2. Antacid therapy—to neutralize gastric acid.
3. H_2 receptor antagonist (cimetidine, ranitidine) if patient has esophagitis.
4. Surgical repair of hernia if symptoms are severe.

Complications

Incarceration of the portion of the stomach in the chest—constricts the blood supply

Nursing Interventions and Patient Education

1. Instruct patient on the prevention of reflux of gastric contents into esophagus by:
   a. Eating smaller meals.
   b. Avoiding stimulation of gastric secretions by omitting caffeine and alcohol.
   c. Refraining from smoking.
   d. Avoiding fatty foods: promote reflux and delay gastric emptying.
   e. Refraining from lying down for at least 1 hour after meals.
   f. Losing weight, if obese.
   g. Avoiding bending from the waist and/or wearing tight-fitting clothes.
2. Advise patient to report to health care facility immediately for the onset of acute chest pain, which may indicate incarceration of a large paraesophageal hernia.

▣ Esophageal Trauma and Perforations

Esophageal trauma or perforations are injuries to the esophagus caused by external or internal insult.

Pathophysiology and Etiology

1. *External:* stab or bullet wounds, crush injuries, blunt trauma.
2. *Internal*
   a. Swallowed foreign objects (coins, pins, bones, dental appliances, caustic poisons).
   b. Spontaneous or postemetic rupture—usually in the presence of underlying esophageal disease (reflux, hiatal hernia).
   c. Mallory-Weiss syndrome—nonpenetrating mucosal tear at the gastroesophageal junction. Caused by an increase in transabdominal pressure from lifting, vomiting, or retching. A predisposing condition is alcoholism.

Clinical Manifestations

1. Pain at the site of injury or impaction, aggravated by swallowing; chest pain, may be severe
2. Dysphagia or odynophagia
3. Persistent foreign object sensation
4. Subcutaneous emphysema and crepitus of face, neck, or upper thorax—noted in cervical, thoracic, and esophageal perforations
5. Temperature elevation occurring within 24 hours of trauma
6. Blood-stained saliva or excessive salivation
7. Hematemesis; previous history of vomiting or retching—Mallory-Weiss syndrome
8. Respiratory difficulty if there is pressure on the tracheobronchial tree from injury or edema

Diagnostic Evaluation

1. History of recent esophageal trauma
2. Chest x-ray to look for foreign body
3. Esophagogram to outline trauma
4. Endoscopy to directly visualize trauma

Management

1. Maintenance of adequate respiratory functioning; may require oxygen support or endotracheal intubation—to ensure an open airway in the presence of edema of the neck.
2. Replacement of fluids. May need blood transfusion. Bleeding may stop spontaneously; if not, endoscopic hemostatic therapy or surgery is indicated.
3. Restoration of the continuity of the esophagus by removing the cause.
4. For external wound injury, emergency first-aid wound care and surgical repair may be indicated.
5. For swallowed foreign bodies:
   a. Barium swallow determines location of foreign body; usually removed through endoscopy.
   b. Some patients with a history of food impaction may be treated with a spasmolytic, such as IV glucagon.
6. For chemical ingestion:
   a. If lye or other caustic or organic solvent was swallowed, do NOT try to induce vomiting.
   b. Treat with IV fluids and analgesics.
   c. A gastrostomy may be performed, either as a temporary or a permanent means of feeding the patient.
   d. Resulting strictures may be relieved by dilating the narrow esophagus.
   e. Reconstructive surgery may be necessary to create a new passageway for food between pharynx and stomach.

Complications

1. Airway occlusion
2. Shock
3. Perforation with mediastinitis or pleural effusion
4. Stricture formation
5. Abscess or fistula formation

Nursing Assessment

1. Assess the following to determine status of patient:
   a. Vital signs
   b. Respiratory status
   c. Intake and output
   d. Bleeding
   e. Ability to swallow—choking, gagging
2. Monitor the patient for hypovolemic shock.

Nursing Diagnoses

- Fluid Volume Deficit related to blood loss from injury
- Altered Nutrition: Less Than Body Requirements, related to esophageal injury
- Ineffective Breathing Pattern related to pain and trauma
- Pain related to injury

Nursing Interventions

Maintaining Fluid Volume

1. Administer IV fluids and blood transfusion for volume replacement, if indicated.
2. Monitor intake and output. Urine output should be greater than 30 mL/h.
3. Monitor laboratory results (electrolytes, hemoglobin, and hematocrit), and report abnormal findings.

Maintaining Nutritional Status

1. Monitor daily weights and skin turgor.
2. Administer parenteral hyperalimentation as prescribed—to prevent gastric reflux into the esophagus, which may occur with enteral feedings.
3. Encourage progression of diet through NG, esophagostomy, or oral feedings once esophagoscopy or esophagogram reveals healing of the esophagus.
4. Continue to monitor intake and output.

Maintaining Respiratory Function

1. Auscultate the lungs and trachea for stridor, crackles, or wheezes. Assess respiratory rate, depth, use of accessory muscles, and skin color.
2. Position patient in semi-Fowler's position to facilitate breathing and reduce neck edema.
3. Monitor vital signs frequently for signs and symptoms of shock and infection.
4. Administer oxygen as prescribed.
5. Have emergency airway equipment at bedside.

Reducing Pain

1. Administer analgesics as prescribed—IV analgesia may be required to control pain and allow the esophagus to rest.
2. Provide reassurance and support.
3. Assess and record pain relief.
4. Evaluate for symptoms that may indicate spillage of digestive contents into the mediastinum, pleura, or abdominal cavity—sudden onset of acute pain.

Patient Education and Health Maintenance

1. Instruct the patient on the indications and side effects of analgesics.
2. Inform the patient on the signs and symptoms to report on possible complications: increase in severity or nature of pain; difficulty breathing or swallowing.
3. See Procedures Guidelines 18-8: Teaching the Patient With Dysphagia How to Swallow. This assists the patient who has difficulty swallowing after injury or surgical correction of the oropharynx or upper esophagus (also helpful with neurologic deficit or stroke).
4. Teach the patient about tests or surgical procedures that may be performed.

Outcome-Based Evaluation

- Fluid volume is maintained; hypovolemic shock is prevented/treated
- Nutritional status is maintained; intake sufficient; diet progressing, if possible
- Respiratory function is maintained; vital signs stable; lungs clear
- Demonstrates increased comfort

PROCEDURE GUIDELINES 18-8	TEACHING THE PATIENT WITH DYSPHAGIA HOW TO SWALLOW

EQUIPMENT

Suction	Face mask	Glass with straw
Oxygen	Selected foods	

PROCEDURE

Nursing Action	Rationale
PREPARATION	
1. Explain to the patient that you plan to work with him or her in developing an effective swallow.	1. The patient's cooperation, concentration, and directed participation are essential to the success of this learning experience.

PROCEDURE GUIDELINES 18-8   *CONTINUED*

Nursing Action	Rationale
2. Ensure that emergency equipment is available at the bedside—suction, oxygen, face mask.	2. For use in the event that the patient chokes, vomits, or aspirates.
3. Place the patient in an upright sitting position in a chair or support with pillows in high-Fowler's position if unable to get out of bed—for about 20 minutes before and 45–60 minutes after meals.	3. This will allow time to adjust and relax in this position before meals; allows gravity to assist the swallowing procedure during meals; helps prevent reflux or regurgitation after meals.
4. Provide mouth care before meals. Suction the patient if secretions are present. If the patient's mouth is dry, provide a lemon wedge or pickle to suck on.	4. This will increase patient's ability to taste and enjoy the sensation of eating.
5. Prepare an environment that is pleasant, peaceful, and without interruptions. Remove distracters, such as TV, radio.	5. Patient must be able to concentrate on the process of swallowing in a relaxed manner.

FOOD AND FLUID SELECTION

Nursing Action	Rationale
6. Foods should be chosen that hold some shape; moist enough to prevent crumbling but dry enough to hold a bolus shape—casseroles, custards, scrambled eggs.	6. Foods that crumble may be aspirated when they fall apart; foods that are too moist may be drooled through the lips.
7. Mugs and glasses with spouts or a straw should be used for liquids.	7. These utensils help prevent liquids from leaking out of corners of patient's mouth.
8. Avoid sticky foods—peanut butter, chocolate, milk, ice cream.	8. These foods stimulate thick mucus and will make swallowing more difficult.
9. Dry foods can be moistened with margarine, gravy, or broths. If liquids are a problem, juices can be thickened with sherbets.	9. Foods need to be of a consistency that will hold a bolus form until swallowed.
10. Avoid tepid or room-temperature foods.	10. Hot and cold foods are thought to maximally stimulate receptors that activate swallowing mechanism.

INSTRUCTIONS DURING MEALS

Nursing Action	Rationale
11. Have patient position head in the midline and forward, chin pointed toward chest.	11. Improves ability to consciously swallow without food falling down the posterior pharynx. Support patient's forehead with a hand if the patient lacks neck control.
12. Instruct the patient to smell the food before each bite; hold each bite for a few seconds; hold lips together firmly; concentrate on swallowing; then swallow.	12. Concentrating on each step before swallowing will increase the effectiveness of the swallow.
13. If the patient has an increase in saliva during the meal, instruct the patient to collect the saliva with the tongue and consciously swallow it between bites throughout the meal.	13. This will help prevent aspiration of saliva between mouthfuls.
14. If the patient complains of a dry mouth during meals, instruct the patient to move the tongue in a circular fashion against the insides of the cheeks.	14. This will help stimulate salivation.
15. Caution the patient against talking during the meal or with the mouth full of food.	15. Talking or laughing during eating is a common cause of airway obstruction.

FEEDING THE PATIENT WITH AN AFFECTED SIDE OF THE MOUTH (FACIAL PARALYSIS, HEMIPLEGIA)

Nursing Action	Rationale
1. Turn the patient to the unaffected side.	1. This helps prevent food from falling down the weaker/paralyzed part of the oral cavity, a possible cause of aspiration.
2. Place food on the unaffected side of mouth rather than in the middle of the mouth.	2. Permits food to be managed more effectively.
3. Encourage the patient to form a bolus by moving the food around the mouth with the tongue.	3. This assists in placing food in a proper position for swallowing, rather than permitting food to collect near the cheek.

FOLLOW-UP CARE

Nursing Action	Rationale
1. Provide mouth care after meals.	1. Food particles may collect in the mouth or cheeks.
2. Record the amount of intake, the patient's taste and food preferences, progress, and any special tactics that were effective in helping the swallowing process.	2. Progress notes will assist in moving toward self-care.
3. Encourage family members to participate in the patient's feeding program.	3. This will help provide continuity on discharge.

▓ Motility Disorders of the Esophagus

Primary motility disorders include achalasia, diffuse esophageal spasm, and those of nonspecific origin. Secondary motility disorders may be caused by neuromuscular, GI, endocrine, or connective tissue disorders.

Pathophysiology and Etiology

Primary Motility Disorders

1. Achalasia refers to excessive resting tone of the LES, incomplete relaxation of the LES with swallowing, and failure of normal peristalsis in the lower two thirds of the esophagus. The pathology is related to defective innervation of the myenteric plexus innervating the involuntary muscles of the esophagus.
2. Diffuse esophageal spasm is a motor disorder in which high-amplitude, nonpropulsive, nonperistaltic tertiary contractions (a form of aperistalsis) are present. LES functioning is frequently normal.

Secondary Motility Disorders

1. Neuromuscular dysfunction includes myasthenia gravis, Parkinson's disease, muscular dystrophy, amyotrophic lateral sclerosis, and cerebral palsy.
2. Connective tissue disorders include scleroderma.
3. GI causes include GERD.
4. Other secondary causes include the autonomic neuropathy of diabetes mellitus.

Clinical Manifestations

Achalasia

1. Gradual onset of dysphagia with solids and liquids
2. Substernal discomfort or a feeling of fullness
3. Regurgitation of undigested food during a meal or within several hours after a meal
4. Weight loss

Diffuse Esophageal Spasm

1. Intermittent dysphagia for solids or liquids—does not progress to continuous dysphagia.
2. Stress large volume of food and hot or cold liquids may aggravate symptoms.
3. Anterior chest pain.

Secondary Motility Disorders

Symptoms of esophagitis from gastroesophageal reflux.

Diagnostic Evaluations

Achalasia

1. Chest x-ray, which may show an enlarged, fluid-filled esophagus
2. Barium esophagography showing dilation, decreased or absence of peristalsis, decreased emptying, and a "bird beak" narrowing of the distal esophagus
3. Esophageal manometry to confirm the diagnoses suspected
4. Endoscopic ultrasound or a chest CT for suspected tumor

Diffuse Esophageal Spasm

1. Barium esophagography showing simultaneous contractions of the esophagus having a "corkscrew" or "rosary bead" appearance
2. Esophageal manometry showing intermittent contractions with episodes of normal peristalsis

Secondary Motility Disorders

Diagnostic workup may include barium esophagography or manometry.

Management

Achalasia

1. Drug therapy using calcium channel blockers, such as nifedipine (Procardia), to reduce the LES pressure. This type of treatment is usually best for patients presenting with mild symptoms and a nondilated esophagus or patients who are medically unstable to undergo invasive therapies.
2. Esophageal dilation using a balloon-tipped catheter is the preferred treatment for most patients.
3. Surgical therapy (Heller's myotomy of the LES) may be used on patients who do not respond to balloon dilation. This surgery requires a laparotomy or thoracotomy or may be done through a thoracoscope.

Diffuse Esophageal Spasm

1. Drug therapy using nitrates and calcium channel blockers is the primary treatment.
2. Dilation may provide some symptom relief.
3. Surgical myotomy is used rarely for patients with a debilitating disorder who are able to withstand a surgical procedure.

Other Motility Disorders

1. Treatment of the gastroesophageal reflux.
2. Dilation may be required for peptic stricture.

Complications

1. Malnutrition
2. Pneumonia, lung abscess, bronchiectasis from nocturnal regurgitation causing aspiration
3. Esophagitis, esophageal diverticula
4. Perforation from dilation procedure
5. Peptic stricture or Barrett's esophagus from severe erosive esophagitis

Nursing Assessment

1. Assess for difficulty with swallowing, vomiting, weight loss, chest pain associated with eating.
2. Inquire as to what facilitates passage of food, such as position changes, use of liquids.

Nursing Diagnoses

- Altered Nutrition: Less Than Body Requirements, related to dysphagia
- Pain related to heartburn or surgical procedure

Nursing Interventions
Improving Nutritional Status
1. Direct patient to eat sitting in an upright position; eat slowly and chew food thoroughly.
2. Avoid food and beverages that precipitate symptoms.
3. Suggest that the patient sleep with head elevated to avoid reflux or aspiration.
4. Provide a bland diet, and tell the patient to avoid alcohol as well as spicy, very hot, and very cold foods, to minimize symptoms.
5. Eliminate sources of tension as a precipitating factor producing stress during mealtime.
6. Administer pharmacologic agents as prescribed.

Promoting Comfort
1. Assess patient for discomfort, chest pain, regurgitation, and cough. If surgical procedure was performed, assess for incisional pain.
2. Provide appropriate postoperative care. Incisional approach determines nature of postoperative care (eg, an incision through chest implies nursing care similar to that given to a patient with a thoracotomy [see p. 259]).
3. Administer analgesics as ordered.
4. Assess for effectiveness of pain medication.

Patient Education and Health Maintenance
1. Encourage lifestyle activity changes similar to those for patients with reflux (see p. 598).
2. See Procedure Guidelines 18-8: Teaching the Patient With Dysphagia How to Swallow (see p. 600).
3. Advise patients to avoid medications with anticholinergic properties (such as antihistamines), which increase LES pressure and cause dysphagia.
4. Provide information on all diagnostic procedures or surgery performed.

Outcome-Based Evaluation
- Demonstrates proper positioning for eating; describes dietary habits that minimize symptoms; compliant with medications regimen
- Demonstrates improved comfort
- Verbalizes how to take medications and potential side effects

Esophageal Diverticulum

An esophageal diverticulum is an outpouching of the esophageal wall, usually in the cervical posterior side, secondary to an obstructive or inflammatory process.

Pathophysiology and Etiology
1. Zenker's diverticulum—protrusion of pharyngeal mucosa at the pharyngoesophageal junction between the interior pharyngeal constrictor and cricopharyngeal muscle.
2. Mid or distal esophageal diverticula may develop above strictures or may be secondary to motility disorders.

Clinical Manifestations
Zenker's Diverticulum
1. Difficulty in swallowing, fullness in neck, throat discomfort, a feeling that food stops before it reaches the stomach, and regurgitation of undigested food
2. Belching, gurgling, or nocturnal coughing brought about by diverticulum becoming filled with food or liquid, which is regurgitated and may irritate the trachea
3. Halitosis and foul taste in mouth caused by food decomposing in a pouch (diverticulum)
4. Weight loss due to nutritional depletion

GERONTOLOGIC ALERT

Hoarseness, asthma, and pneumonitis may be the only signs of esophageal diverticula in the very elderly.

Mid or Distal Esophageal Diverticula
Generally no symptoms.

Diagnostic Evaluation
1. Barium esophagogram outlines diverticulum.
2. Endoscopy is not indicated and may be dangerous due to the possibility of rupture.

Management
Zenker's Diverticulum
1. Small diverticula may not be treated, but the underlying cause is treated with dilatation or myotomy.
2. A transverse cervical diverticulectomy or diverticuloplexy with suspension and cricopharyngeal myotomy may be done.
   a. Caution is taken to avoid injury to common carotid artery and internal jugular vein.
   b. Sac is dissected free and then excised flush with esophageal wall.

Mid or Distal Esophageal Diverticula
Underlying primary condition must be treated.

Complications
1. Aspiration pneumonia
2. Malnutrition
3. Lung abscess

Nursing Assessment
1. Obtain history of dysphagia, coughing, throat discomfort, choking, regurgitation of food.
2. Evaluate for halitosis.
3. Determine what measures assist the patient with food intake; what foods/fluids the patient is able to tolerate.
4. Evaluate weight loss and dietary habits.

Nursing Diagnoses
- Altered Nutrition: Less Than Body Requirements, related to dysphagia
- Pain related to symptoms and surgical procedure

Nursing Interventions

Improving Nutritional Status

1. Provide frequent, small meals, which are better tolerated.
2. Elevate head of bed for 2 hours after eating.
3. Monitor intake and output.
4. Weigh daily.

Maintaining Comfort and Preventing Complications

1. Preoperatively, or if the condition is nonoperative, implement nursing interventions similar to those for esophagitis.
2. Postoperatively, wound care is similar to that of other surgical incisions of the same anatomical position (eg, thoracotomy [see p. 561] or neck surgery).
3. Administer appropriate pain medications, and assess effectiveness.
4. Patient may need oral suctioning to control drooling.
5. Maintain NG tube if in place.
   a. Irrigate tube as ordered.
   b. Do not manipulate NG tube due to location of tube and suture line.

Patient Education and Health Maintenance

1. Instruct patient regarding treatment of esophagitis caused by gastroesophageal reflux (see p. 598).
2. Instruct patient on importance of good oral hygiene.

Outcome-Based Evaluation

- Tolerates oral feedings; maintains weight or shows gradual increase
- Demonstrates improved comfort

■ Cancer of the Esophagus

Malignant lesions of the esophagus occur in four types worldwide: squamous cell, adenocarcinoma, carcinosarcoma, and sarcoma.

Pathophysiology and Etiology

Incidence

1. Incidence of adenocarcinoma of the distal and middle third of the esophagus appears to be increasing in the Western world.
2. Squamous cell carcinoma, most often originating in the upper half of the esophagus, appears to have an equal incidence to adenocarcinoma.
3. Highest rate in the United States occurs in men, who are usually older than age of 60; more common in nonwhite males.

Associated Factors

Cause is unknown but has been associated with:
1. Barrett's esophagus.
2. Achalasia.
3. Chronic use of alcohol and tobacco (squamous cell carcinoma).
4. Genetic predisposition—nonwhite male population.

5. Ingestion of caustic substances (such as lye), which cause esophageal strictures.
6. Other head and neck cancers.

Clinical Manifestations

1. Dysphagia is the usual presenting symptom, although it is a late sign, by which time there often is regional or systemic involvement.
2. Mild, atypical chest pain associated with eating precedes dysphagia but is rarely significant enough for the patient to seek health care.
3. Pain on swallowing (odynophagia).
4. Progressive weight loss.
5. Hoarseness (if laryngeal involvement).
6. Lymphadenopathy (supraclavicular or cervical) or hepatomegaly with metastatic involvement.
7. Later symptoms—hiccups, respiratory difficulty, foul breath, regurgitation of food and saliva.

Diagnostic Evaluation

1. Chest x-ray may show adenopathy; mediastinal, widening, metastasis; or a tracheoesophageal fistula.
2. Endoscopy with cytology and biopsy.
3. Barium esophagram may show polypoid, infiltrative, or ulcerative lesion requiring biopsy.
4. CT may be helpful in delineating the extent of the tumor as well as in identifying presence of adjacent tissue invasion and metastases.

Management

1. The goal of treatment may be cure or palliation, depending on the staging of the tumor and the patient's overall condition in relation to nutritional, cardiovascular, pulmonary, and functional status.
2. The wide variability in treatment reflects the overall poor results from any one approach.
3. Surgery.
   a. Lesions of the middle and lower esophagus are excised with use of the thoracotomy approach with esophagogastrectomy or colon interposition (section of colon is used to replace the excised portion of the esophagus).
   b. Lesions of the cervical esophagus are excised with a bilateral neck dissection and esophagogastrectomy; laryngectomy and thyroidectomy may be necessary.
   c. A two-step approach may be selected when resection with a cervical esophagostomy and feeding gastrostomy are performed initially; subsequent reconstructive surgery is performed.
4. Radiation, chemotherapy, or their combination; combination therapy appears to have better results.
5. Palliative treatment of dysphagia through dilation done by endoscopy or laser therapy.
6. The goal of palliative treatment is to reduce the complications of the tumor to improve quality of life. Any one or a combination of the aforementioned therapies can be used for palliative treatment.

Complications

1. *Preoperatively:* malnutrition, aspiration pneumonitis; hemorrhage; sepsis; tracheoesophageal fistula
2. *Postoperatively:* dumping syndrome, nutritional deficiencies, reflux esophagitis, anastomosis leakage

Nursing Assessment

1. Obtain history of symptoms, such as dysphagia, pain, cough, hoarseness.
2. Evaluate for weight loss and dietary changes.
3. Assess support system and personal coping mechanisms.

Nursing Diagnoses

- Altered Nutrition: Less Than Body Requirements, related to disease process and treatment
- Risk for Infection related to chronic disease, invasive procedures and treatment
- Ineffective Individual Coping

Nursing Interventions

Improving Nutritional and Fluid Status

1. Provide the preoperative patient with a high-protein, high-calorie diet. Nutritional supplements may be indicated. TPN may be ordered if unable to take foods/fluids orally.
2. Postoperatively, administer IV fluids as prescribed. Initially, the patient may require large volumes if extensive excision of lymph nodes was performed. TPN may be ordered.
3. Assess for bowel sounds; administer fluids per NG tube, as prescribed.
4. Encourage patient in advancing diet from liquids to soft foods.
5. Remind patient to remain in upright position for approximately 2 hours after eating to promote digestion.
6. Provide mouth care for patient comfort and hygiene.

Monitoring for Complications

1. Monitor blood pressure, pulse, respiration, and temperature to note early onset of hemorrhage, infection, dysrhythmias, aspiration, or anastomosis leakage.
2. Observe drainage from incision and/or chest tube for bleeding or purulence.
3. Administer oxygen as prescribed to facilitate tissue oxygenation.

Strengthening Individual Coping

1. Encourage patient to utilize support system during treatment and recovery process.
2. Provide information about laryngectomy, gastrostomy, and other procedures related to surgery, as indicated.
3. Provide training in relaxation techniques and diversional therapy for anxiety and pain control after surgery.

Patient Education and Health Maintenance

1. Encourage the patient to avoid overeating, take small bites, chew food well; avoid chunks of meat and stringy raw vegetables and fruit.
2. Depending on type of surgery, frequent small meals may be better tolerated.
3. Encourage rest postoperatively and advancing activities as tolerated.
4. Instruct patient regarding signs and symptoms of complications to report: nausea, vomiting, elevated temperature, cough, difficulty swallowing.

Outcome-Based Evaluation

- Maintains nutritional status: weight gain; good skin turgor; eating small, frequent meals if possible
- No evidence of complications
- Performing self-care with help of support persons

GASTRODUODENAL DISORDERS

▨ Gastrointestinal Bleeding

GI bleeding is not just a gastroduodenal disorder but may occur anywhere along the alimentary tract. Bleeding is a symptom of an upper or lower GI disorder. It may be obvious in emesis or stool, or it may be occult (hidden).

Pathophysiology and Etiology

1. Trauma anywhere along the GI tract
2. Erosions or ulcers
3. Rupture of an enlarged vein, such as a varicosity (esophageal or gastric varices)
4. Inflammation, such as esophagitis (caused by acid or bile), gastritis, inflammatory bowel disease (chronic ulcerative colitis, Crohn's disease), and bacterial infection
5. Alcohol and drugs (aspirin-containing compounds, NSAIDs, anticoagulants, corticosteroids)
6. Diverticular disease
7. Cancers
8. Vascular lesions or disorders, such as bowel ischemia, aortoenteric fistula
9. Mallory-Weiss tear
10. Anal disorders, such as hemorrhoids or fissure

Clinical Manifestations

Characteristics of Blood

1. Bright red: vomited from high in esophagus (hematemesis): from rectum or distal colon (coating stool)
2. Mixed with dark red: higher up in colon and small intestine: mixed with stool
3. Shades of black ("coffee ground"): esophagus, stomach, and duodenum; vomitus from these areas
4. Tarry stool (melena): occurs in patient who accumulates excessive blood in the stomach

Signs and Symptoms of Bleeding

1. Massive bleeding
   a. Acute, bright red hematemesis or large amount of melena with clots in the stool
   b. Rapid pulse, drop in blood pressure, hypovolemia, and shock

2. Subacute bleeding
    a. Intermittent melena or coffee-ground emesis
    b. Hypotension
    c. Weakness, dizziness
3. Chronic bleeding
    a. Intermittent appearance of blood
    b. Increased weakness, paleness, or shortness of breath
    c. Occult blood

Diagnostic Evaluation

1. It is not difficult to diagnose bleeding, but it may be difficult to locate the source of bleeding.
2. History: change in bowel pattern, presence of pain or tenderness, recent intake of food and what kind (eg, red beets?), alcohol consumption, drugs such as aspirin or steroids.
3. Complete blood count (hemoglobin, hematocrit, platelets) and coagulation studies (PTT, PT with INR) may show abnormalities.
4. Endoscopy: identifies source of bleeding, determines risk of rebleeding, and provides endoscopic therapy if needed.
5. Imaging may detect etiology of bleeding.
6. Test of stool for occult blood.

Management
Based on Etiology

1. If aspirin or NSAIDs are the cause, discontinue medication and treat bleeding.
2. If ulcer is the cause, medications, dietary and lifestyle modifications.
3. Therapeutic endoscopic procedure (cautery, injection).
4. Surgery may be indicated for cancers, inflammatory diseases, and vascular disorders.

Emergency Intervention

1. Patient remains on NPO status.
2. IV lines and oxygen therapy initiated.
3. If life-threatening bleeding occurs, treat shock, administer blood replacement, intra-arterial vasopressin or embolization.
4. Surgical therapy, if indicated.

Nasogastric Intubation

1. An NG tube should be in place for most patients with acute or upper GI bleeding.
2. If the aspirate continues to be bloody after 2 to 3 L of tap water lavage, the patient may have an active bleed requiring more emergent intervention or endoscopic therapy.

Other Measures

1. Electrocoagulation using a heater probe.
2. Injection of sclerosant or epinephrine.

> **NURSING ALERT**
>
> Because of the action of topical thrombin, it is used only on the surface of bleeding tissue and never is injected into the blood vessels, where intravascular clotting could occur.

3. Endoscopy used in conjunction with management measures as well as in diagnostic evaluation.
4. Pharmacotherapy depends on cause; can include histamine blockers as either continuous IV (preferred) or bolus infusion to block the acid-secreting action of histamine. Intra-arterial vasopressin can be used to slow or stop active bleeding from diverticulum or vascular ectasia.
5. Surgery is indicated when more conservative measures fail.

Complications

1. Hemorrhage
2. Shock
3. Death

Nursing Assessment

1. Obtain history regarding:
    a. Change in bowel patterns or hemorrhoids.
    b. Change in color of stools (dark black, red, or streaked with blood).
    c. Alcohol consumption.
    d. Medications, such as aspirin, NSAIDs, antibiotics, anticoagulants, corticosteroids.
    e. Hematemesis.
    f. Other medical conditions.
2. Evaluate for presence of abdominal pain or tenderness.
3. Monitor vital signs and laboratory tests for changes that indicate bleeding (hemoglobin, hematocrit, platelet count, coagulation studies).
4. Test for occult blood, if indicated.

Nursing Diagnoses

- Fluid Volume Deficit related to blood loss
- Altered Nutrition: Less Than Body Requirements, related to nausea, vomiting, diarrhea

Nursing Interventions
Attaining Normal Fluid Volume

1. Maintain NG tube and NPO status to rest GI tract and evaluate bleeding.
2. Monitor intake and output as ordered to evaluate fluid status.
3. Monitor vital signs as ordered.
4. Observe for changes indicating shock, such as tachycardia, hypotension, increased respirations, decreased urine output, change in mental status.
5. Administer IV fluids and blood products as ordered to maintain volume.

Attaining Balanced Nutritional Status

1. Weigh daily to monitor caloric status.
2. Administer IV fluids, TPN if ordered to promote hydration and nutrition while on PO restrictions.
3. Begin liquids when patient is no longer NPO. Advance diet as tolerated. Diet should be high calorie, high protein. Frequent, small feedings may be indicated.
4. Offer snacks; high-protein supplements.

Patient Education and Health Maintenance

1. Discuss the cause and treatment of GI bleeding with patient.
2. Instruct patient regarding signs and symptoms of GI bleeding: melena, emesis that is bright red or "coffee ground" color, rectal bleeding, weakness, fatigue, shortness of breath.
3. Instruct patient on how to test stool or emesis for occult blood, if applicable.

Outcome-Based Evaluation

- Fluid volume is maintained; hypovolemic shock is prevented
- Nutritional status is maintained; body weight is maintained or increased

◼ Peptic Ulcer Disease

Peptic ulcer disease refers to ulcerations in the mucosa of the lower esophagus, stomach, or duodenum (Figure 18-3).

Pathophysiology and Etiology

1. Etiology of peptic ulcers disease is multifactorial.
   a. *H. pylori* infection—present in most patients with peptic ulcer disease
   b. Ulcerogenic drugs such as NSAIDs
   c. Zollinger-Ellison syndrome and other hypersecretory syndromes
2. Risk factors may include drugs (NSAIDs, prolonged high-dose corticosteroids), family history, Zollinger-Ellison syndrome, cigarettes, stress, blood group O, lower socioeconomic status.
3. Recent studies have shown that alcohol is poorly associated with peptic ulcer disease. There are conflicting results on the role of caffeine in peptic ulcer disease.

Clinical Manifestations

1. Gnawing or burning epigastric pain occurring 1 to 3 hours after a meal
2. Nocturnal epigastric, abdominal pain or burning
3. Early satiety, anorexia, weight loss, heartburn, belching (may indicate reflux disease)
4. Dizziness, syncope, hematemesis, or melena (may indicate hemorrhage)
5. Anemia

> **NURSING ALERT**
>
> Sudden, intense midepigastric pain radiating to the right shoulder may indicate ulcer perforation.

Diagnostic Evaluation

1. Upper GI endoscopy with possible biopsy and cytology—more accurate detection
2. Upper GI radiographic examination (barium study)
3. Serial stool specimens to detect occult blood
4. Gastric secretory studies (gastric acid secretion test and serum gastric level test)—elevated in Zollinger-Ellison syndrome
5. Serology to test for *H. pylori* antibodies
6. C-urea breath test to diagnose *H. pylori*

Management

General Measures

1. Eliminate use of NSAIDs or other causative drugs.
2. Eliminate cigarette smoking.
3. Well-balanced diet with meals at regular intervals. Avoid dietary irritants.

Drug Therapy

1. Multiple drug regimens are used to treat *H. pylori* (Table 18-3)

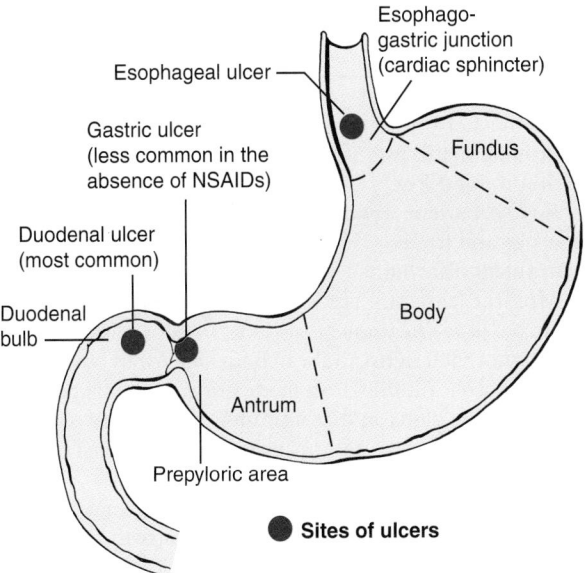

FIGURE 18-3 Esophageal, gastric, and duodenal ulcer sites.

TABLE 18-3 Drug Regimens for Eradication of *Helicobacter pylori*

Drug	Dosage	Duration
Omeprazole (Prilosec)	20 mg PO bid	14 days
Amoxicillin or	1000 mg PO bid or	
Metronidazole (Flagyl)	500 mg PO bid	
Clarithromycin (Biaxin)	500 mg PO bid	
Bismuth subsalicylate	2 tabs PO qid	14 days
(Pepto-Bismol)		
Metronidazole (Flagyl)	250 mg PO qid	
Tetracycline	500 mg PO qid	
BMT regimen	Above	7 days
(above) along with		
Omeprazole (Prilosec)	20 mg PO bid	
Ranidine (Zantac)	400 mg PO bid	28 days
Clarithromycin (Biaxin)	500 mg PO tid	14 days

Surgery

1. Surgical interventions may be indicated for hemorrhage, obstruction, perforation, and acid reduction (Figure 18-4). Surgery may also be indicated with ulcer disease of long duration or severity or difficulty with medical regimen compliance.
2. Gastroduodenostomy (Billroth I).
   a. Partial gastrectomy with removal of antrum and pylorus of stomach.
   b. The gastric stump is anatomosed with the duodenum.
3. Gastrojejunostomy (Billroth II)
   a. Partial gastrectomy with removal of antrum and pylorus of stomach.
   b. The gastric stump is anatomosed with the jejunum.
4. Antrectomy
   a. Gastric resection includes a small cuff of duodenum, the pylorus, and the antrum (lower half of stomach).
   b. The duodenal stump is closed, and the jejunum is anastomosed to the stomach.
5. Total gastrectomy
   a. Also called an esophagojejunostomy
   b. Removal of the stomach with attachment of the esophagus to the jejunum or duodenum.
6. Pyloroplasty
   a. A longitudinal incision is made in the pylorus, and it is closed transversely to permit the muscle to relax and to establish an enlarged outlet.
   b. Often, a vagotomy is performed at the same time.
7. Vagotomy
   a. The surgical division of the vagus nerve to eliminate the impulses that stimulate HCL secretion.
   b. There are three types: *selective vagotomy,* which severs only the branches that interrupt acid secretion; *truncal vagotomy,* which severs both the anterior and posterior trunks to decrease acid secretion and gastric motility; and *parietal vagotomy,* which severs only the part of vagus that innervates the parietal acid-secreting cells.

Complications

1. GI hemorrhage
2. Ulcer perforation
3. Gastric outlet obstruction

Nursing Assessment

1. Determine location, character, radiation of pain, factors aggravating or relieving pain, how long it lasts, when it occurs.
2. Ask about eating patterns, regularity, types of food, eating circumstances.
3. Ask about medications (especially aspirin, anti-inflammatory drugs, or steroids).
4. History of illnesses including previous GI bleeds.
5. Obtain psychosocial history.
6. Physical assessment with documentation of positive abdominal findings.
7. Take vital signs, including lying, standing, and sitting blood pressures and pulses, to determine if orthostasis is present due to bleeding.

Nursing Diagnoses

- Fluid Volume Deficit related to hemorrhage
- Pain related to epigastric distress secondary to hypersecretion of acid, mucosal erosion, or perforation
- Diarrhea related to GI bleeding
- Altered Nutrition: Less Than Body Requirements, related to the disease process
- Knowledge Deficit related to physical, dietary, and pharmacologic treatment of disease

Nursing Interventions

Avoiding Fluid Volume Deficit

1. Monitor intake and output continuously to determine fluid volume status.
2. Monitor stools for blood and emesis.
3. Monitor hemoglobin and hematocrit and electrolytes.
4. Administer prescribed IV fluids and blood replacement, as prescribed.
5. Insert NG tube as prescribed, and monitor the tube drainage for signs of visible and occult blood.
6. Administer medications through the NG tube to neutralize acidity, as prescribed.
7. Prepare patient for saline lavage, as ordered.
8. Observe patient for an increase in pulse and a decrease in blood pressure (signs of shock).
9. Prepare patient for diagnostic procedure or surgery to determine or stop the source of bleeding.

Achieving Pain Relief

1. Administer prescribed medication.
2. Provide small, frequent meals to prevent gastric distention if not NPO.
3. Advise patient about the irritating effects of certain drugs and foods.

Decreasing Diarrhea

1. Monitor patient's elimination patterns to determine effects of medications.
2. Monitor vital signs, and watch for signs of hypovolemia.
3. Administer antidiarrheal medication as prescribed.
4. Watch for signs and symptoms of impaired skin integrity (erythema, pain, pruritus) around anus to promote comfort and decrease risk of infection.

Achieving Adequate Nutrition

1. Eliminate foods that cause pain or distress; otherwise, the diet is usually not restricted.
2. Provide small, frequent meals that neutralize gastric secretions and may be better tolerated.

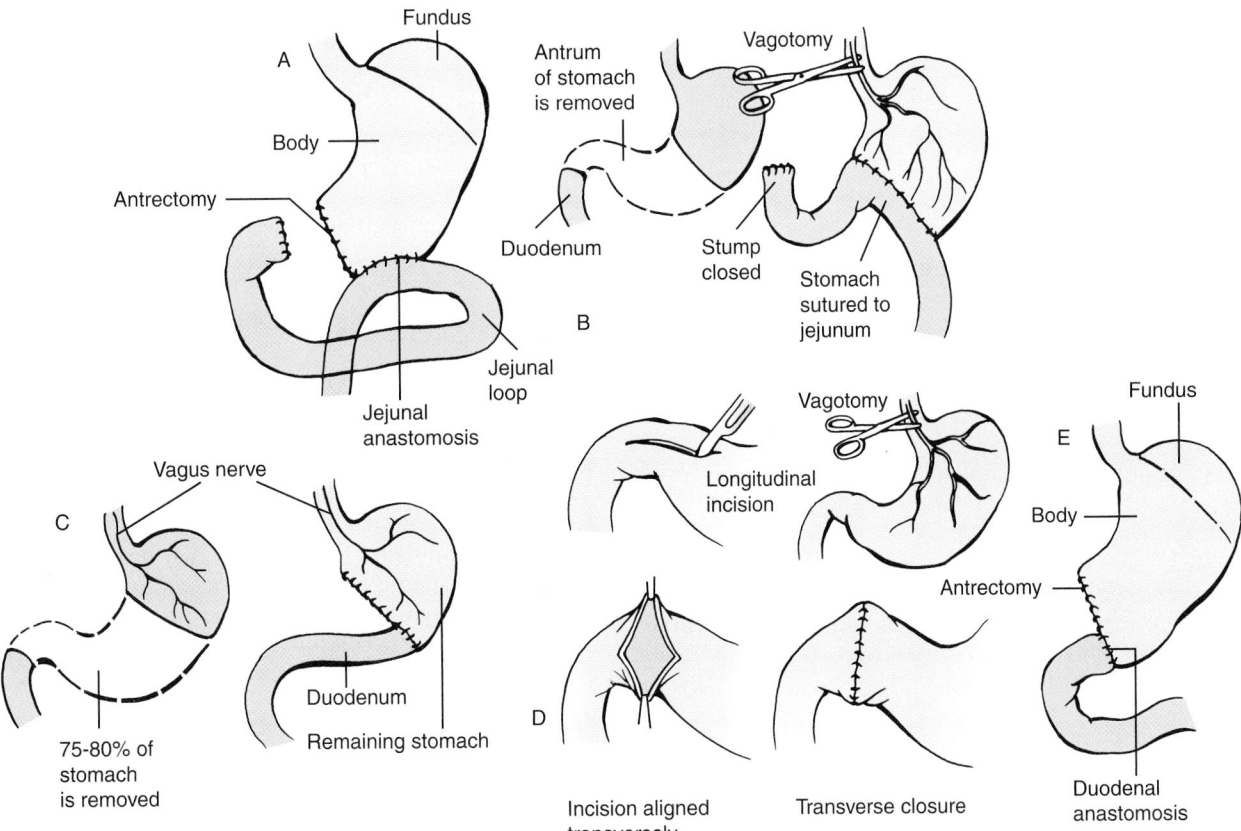

FIGURE 18-4 Surgical procedures for peptic ulcer. (**A**) Gastrojejunostomy (Billroth II). The jejunum is anastomosed to the gastric stump after a partial gastrectomy (removal of antrum and pylorus). (**B**) Antrectomy and vagotomy. The resected portion includes a small cuff of duodenum, the pylorus, and the antrum (about one half of the stomach). The stump of the duodenum is closed by suture, and the side of the jejunum is anastomosed to the cut end of the stomach. (**C**) Subtotal gastrectomy. The resected portion includes a small cuff of the duodenum, the pylorus, and from two thirds to three quarters of the stomach. The duodenum or side of the jejunum is anastomosed to the remaining portion of the stomach. (**D**) Vagotomy and pyloroplasty. A longitudinal incision is made in the pylorus, and it is closed transversely to permit the muscle to relax and to establish an enlarged outlet. This compensates for the impaired gastric emptying produced by vagotomy. (**E**) Gastroduodenostomy (Billroth I). The duodenum is anastomosed to the gastric stump after removal of the antrum and pylorus (partial gastrectomy).

3. Provide high-calorie, high-protein diet with nutritional supplements as ordered.
4. Administer parenteral nutrition as ordered if bleeding is prolonged and patient is malnourished.

Educating About the Treatment Regimen

1. Explain all tests and procedures to increase knowledge and cooperation; minimize anxiety.
2. Review the health care provider's recommendations for diet, activity, medication, and treatment. Allow time for questions, and clarify any misunderstandings.

3. Give the patient a chart listing medications, dosages, times of administration, and desired effects to promote compliance.
4. Teach patient signs and symptoms of bleeding and when to notify the health care provider.

Patient Education and Health Maintenance

1. Teach patient signs and symptoms of bleeding and when to notify the health care provider.

2. Promote healthy lifestyle changes to include adequate nutrition, cessation of smoking, decreased alcohol consumption, stress reduction strategies.
3. Teach purpose, dosage, and side effects of each medication prescribed.

Outcome-Based Evaluation

- Vital signs stable; fluid volume maintained
- Pain free
- No more than two to three loose stools per day
- Eating frequent small meals each day; reports no loss of weight
- Can describe peptic ulcer disease, its treatment, and complications; complies with treatment regimen

Gastric Cancer

Malignant tumor of the stomach.

Pathophysiology and Etiology

1. Risk factors include:
   a. Chronic atrophic gastritis with intestinal metaplasia.
   b. Pernicious anemia or having had gastric resections (greater than 15 years).
   c. Adenomatous polyps.
2. Related factors:
   a. More common in men and blacks.
   b. Incidence increases with age.

Clinical Manifestations

Early Manifestations

Most often, patient presents with same symptoms as gastric ulcer; later, on evaluation, the lesion is found to be malignant.
1. Progressive loss of appetite
2. Noticeable change in, or appearance of GI symptoms—gastric fullness (early satiety), dyspepsia lasting more than 4 weeks
3. Blood (usually occult) in the stools
4. Vomiting
   a. May indicate pyloric obstruction or cardiac-orifice obstruction.
   b. Occasionally, vomiting has a coffee-ground appearance because of slow leaks of blood from ulceration of the cancer.

Later Manifestations

1. Pain, often induced by eating and relieved by vomiting
2. Weight loss, loss of strength, anemia, metastasis (usually to liver), hemorrhage, obstruction
3. Abdominal or epigastric mass

Diagnostic Evaluation

1. History—weight loss and fatigue over several months
2. Upper GI radiography and endoscopy—afford visualization and provide means for obtaining tissue samples for histologic and cytologic review
3. Imaging, such as bone or liver scan—may determine extent of disease

Management

1. The only successful treatment of gastric cancer is surgical removal. Gastric resection is surgical removal of part of the stomach.
2. If tumor has spread beyond the area that can be excised surgically, cure cannot be accomplished.
   a. Palliative surgery such as subtotal gastrectomy with or without gastroenterostomy may be performed to maintain continuity of the GI tract.
   b. Surgery may be combined with chemotherapy to provide palliation and prolong life.

Complications

1. If surgery is performed, there may be a risk of hemorrhage or infection.
2. Metastasis and death.

Nursing Assessment

1. Assess for anorexia, weight loss, GI symptoms (gastric fullness, dyspepsia, vomiting).
2. Evaluate for pain, noting characteristics/location.
3. Check stool for occult blood.
4. Monitor complete blood count to assess for anemia.

Nursing Diagnoses

- Pain related to disease process or surgery
- Risk for Injury, shock and other complications related to surgery and impaired gastric tissue function
- Altered Nutrition: Less Than Body Requirements, related to malignancy and treatment

Nursing Interventions

Promoting Comfort and Wound Healing

1. Turning, coughing, deep breathing every 2 hours to prevent vascular and pulmonary complications and promote comfort.
2. Institute NG suction, if ordered, to remove fluids and gas in the stomach and prevent painful distention.
3. Administer parenteral antibiotics, as ordered, to prevent infection.
4. Administer analgesics, as ordered.

Preventing Shock and Other Complications

1. Shock and hemorrhage.
   a. Monitor changes in blood pressure, pulse, and respiration.
   b. Observe the patient for evidence of changes in mental status, pallor, clammy skin, dizziness.
   c. Check the dressings and suction canister frequently for evidence of bleeding.
   d. Administer IV infusions and blood replacement as prescribed.
2. Cardiopulmonary complications.
   a. Encourage the patient to cough and take deep breaths to promote ventilatory exchange and enhance circulation.

b. Assist the patient to turn and move, thereby mobilizing secretions.

c. Promote ambulation, as prescribed, to increase respiratory exchange.

3. Thrombosis and embolism.

a. Initiate a plan of self-care activities to promote circulation.

b. Encourage early ambulation to stimulate circulation.

c. Prevent venous stasis by use of elastic stockings, if indicated.

d. Check for tight dressings or binder that might restrict circulation.

4. Dumping syndrome—a complex reaction that may occur because of excessively rapid emptying of gastric contents. Manifestations include nausea, weakness, perspiration, palpitation, some syncope, and possibly diarrhea. Instruct the patient as follows:

a. Eat small, frequent meals rather than three large meals.

b. Suggest a diet high in protein and fat and low in carbohydrates, and avoid meals high in sugars, milk, chocolate, salt.

c. Reduce fluids with meals, but take them between meals.

d. Take anticholinergic medication before meals (if prescribed) to lessen GI activity.

e. Relax when eating; eat slowly and regularly.

f. Take a rest after meals.

5. Phytobezoar formation (formation of gastric concretion composed of vegetable matter).

a. Can be seen with partial gastrectomy and vagotomy.

b. Avoid fibrous foods, such as citrus fruits (skins and seeds), because they tend to form phytobezoars.

(i) After a gastric resection, the remaining gastric tissue is not able to disintegrate and digest fibrous foods.

(ii) This undigested fiber congeals to form masses that become coated by mucus secretions of the stomach.

(iii) Stress the importance of adequate chewing.

Attaining Adequate Nutritional Status

1. Administer parenteral nutrition, if ordered.

2. Follow prescribed diet progressions.

a. Give fluids by mouth when audible bowel signs are present.

b. Increase fluids according to the patient's tolerance.

c. Offer a diet with vitamin supplements when the patient's condition permits.

d. Avoid high-carbohydrate foods, such as milk, which may trigger dumping syndrome.

e. Offer diet as prescribed—usually high in protein and calories to promote wound healing.

Patient Education and Health Maintenance

1. Emphasize the importance of coping with stressful situations. Provide information about support groups.

2. Review nutritional requirements with the patient.

3. Stress the importance of vitamin B_{12} supplements after gastrectomy to prevent surgically induced pernicious anemia.

4. Encourage follow-up visits with the health care provider.

5. Recommend annual blood studies and medical checkups for any evidence of pernicious anemia or other problems.

6. Instruct on measures to prevent dumping syndrome.

Outcome-Based Evaluation

- Verbalizes increased comfort (using a 0 to 10 point pain scale with 0 being no pain and 10 being the highest score to measure pain)
- Vital signs stable; no evidence of complications
- Body weight is maintained or increased

INTESTINAL CONDITIONS

Abdominal Hernias

A hernia is a protrusion of an organ, tissue, or structure through the wall of the cavity in which it is normally contained. It is often called a "rupture."

Pathophysiology and Etiology

Causes

1. Results from congenital or acquired weakness (traumatic injury, aging) of the abdominal wall.

2. May result from increased intra-abdominal pressure due to heavy lifting, obesity, pregnancy, straining, coughing, or proximity to tumor.

Classification by Site

1. *Inguinal*—hernia into the inguinal canal (more common in males).

a. *Indirect inguinal hernia*—due to a weakness of the abdominal wall at the point through which the spermatic cord emerges in the male and the round ligament in the female. Through this opening, the hernia extends down the inguinal canal and often into scrotum or labia.

b. *Direct inguinal*—passes through the posterior inguinal wall; more difficult to repair than indirect inguinal hernia.

2. *Femoral*—hernia into the femoral canal, appearing below the inguinal ligament (Poupart's ligament; ie, below the groin).

3. *Umbilical*—intestinal protrusion at the umbilicus due to failure of umbilical orifice to close. Occurs most often in obese women, children, and in patients with increased intra-abdominal pressure from cirrhosis and ascites.

4. *Ventral* or *incisional*—intestinal protrusion due to weakness at the abdominal wall; may occur after impaired incisional healing due to infection, drainage, and so forth.

5. *Parastomal*—hernia through the fascial defect around a stoma and into the subcutaneous tissue.

Classification by Severity

1. *Reducible*—the protruding mass can be placed back into abdominal cavity.
2. *Irreducible*—the protruding mass cannot be moved back into the abdomen.
3. *Incarcerated*—an irreducible hernia in which the intestinal flow is completely obstructed.
4. *Strangulated*—an irreducible hernia in which the blood and intestinal flow are completely obstructed; develops when the loop of intestine in the sac becomes twisted or swollen and a constriction is produced at the neck of the sac.

Clinical Manifestations

1. Bulging over herniated area appears when patient stands or strains, and disappears when supine.
2. Hernia tends to increase in size and recurs with intra-abdominal pressure.
3. Strangulated hernia presents with pain, vomiting, swelling of hernial sac, lower abdominal signs of peritoneal irritation, fever.

Diagnostic Evaluation

Based on clinical manifestations:

1. Abdominal x-rays—reveal abnormally high levels of gas in the bowel.
2. Laboratory studies (complete blood count, electrolytes)—may show hemoconcentration (increased hematocrit), dehydration (increased or decreased sodium), and elevated WBC, if incarcerated.

Management

1. Mechanical (reducible hernia only).
   a. A truss is an appliance with a pad and belt that is held snugly over a hernia to prevent abdominal contents from entering the hernial sac. A truss provides external compression over the defect and should be removed at night and reapplied in the morning before patient arises. This nonsurgical approach may be used only when a patient is not a surgical candidate.
   b. Parastomal hernia is often managed with a hernia support belt with Velcro, which is placed around an ostomy pouching system (similar to a truss).
   c. Conservative measures—no heavy lifting, straining at stool, or other measures that would increase intra-abdominal pressure.
2. Surgical—recommended to correct hernia before strangulation occurs, which then becomes an emergency situation.
   a. Herniorrhaphy—removal of hernial sac; contents replaced into the abdomen; layers of muscle and fascia sutured. Laparoscopic herniorrhaphy is a possibility and often performed as outpatient procedure.
   b. Hernioplasty involves reinforcement of suturing (often with mesh) for extensive hernia repair.
   c. Strangulated hernia requires resection of ischemic bowel in addition to repair of hernia.

Complications

1. Bowel obstruction
2. Recurrence of hernia

Nursing Assessment

1. Ask patient if hernia is enlarging and uncomfortable.
2. Determine if patient is exhibiting signs and symptoms of strangulation, such as distention, fever, nausea, and vomiting.

Nursing Diagnoses

- Pain related to bulging hernia (mechanical)
- Pain related to surgical procedure
- Risk for Infection related to emergency procedure for strangulated or incarcerated hernia

Nursing Interventions

Achieving Comfort

1. Fit patient with truss or belt when hernia is reduced, if ordered.
2. Trendelenburg's position may reduce pressure on hernia, when appropriate.
3. Emphasize to patient to wear truss under clothing and to apply before getting out of bed when hernia is reduced.
4. Evaluate for signs and symptoms of hernial incarceration or strangulation.
5. Insert NG tube, if ordered, to relieve intra-abdominal pressure on herniated sac.
6. Give stool softeners as directed.

Relieving Pain Postoperatively

1. Have the patient splint the incision site with hand or pillow when coughing to lessen pain and protect site from increased intra-abdominal pressure.
2. Administer analgesics, as ordered.
3. Teach about bed rest, intermittent ice packs, and scrotal elevation as measures used to reduce scrotal edema or swelling after repair of an inguinal hernia.
4. Encourage ambulation as soon as permitted.
5. Advise patient that difficulty in urinating is common after surgery; promote elimination to avoid discomfort, and catheterize if necessary.

Preventing Infection

1. Check dressing for drainage and incision for redness and swelling.
2. Monitor for other signs/symptoms of infection: fever, chills, malaise, diaphoresis.
3. Administer antibiotics, if appropriate.

Patient Education and Health Maintenance

1. Advise that pain and scrotal swelling may be present for 24 to 48 hours after repair of an inguinal hernia.
   a. Apply ice intermittently.
   b. Elevate scrotum, and use scrotal support.
   c. Take medication prescribed to relieve discomfort.

2. Teach to monitor self for signs of infection: Pain, drainage from incision, temperature elevation. Also report continued difficulty in voiding.
3. Inform that heavy lifting should be avoided for 4 to 6 weeks. Athletics and extremes of exertion are to be avoided for 8 to 12 weeks postoperatively, per provider instructions.

Outcome-Based Evaluation
- Hernia effectively reduced with truss or belt; patient comfortable
- Pain controlled postoperatively
- No swelling present; no signs/symptoms of infection

Intestinal Obstruction

Intestinal obstruction is an interruption in the normal flow of intestinal contents along the intestinal tract. The block may occur in the small or large intestine, may be complete or incomplete, may be mechanical or paralytic, and may or may not compromise the vascular supply. Obstruction most frequently occurs in the young and the old.

Pathophysiology and Etiology
Types and Causes
1. *Mechanical obstruction*—a physical block to passage of intestinal contents without disturbing blood supply of bowel. High small-bowel (jejunal) or low small-bowel (ileal) obstruction occurs four times more frequently than colonic obstruction (Figure 18-5). Causes include:
   a. Extrinsic—adhesions from surgery, hernia, wound dehiscence, masses, volvulus (twisted loop of intestine).
   b. Intrinsic—hematoma, tumor, intussusception (telescoping of intestinal wall into itself), stricture or stenosis, congenital (atresia, imperforate anus), trauma, inflammatory diseases (Crohn's, diverticulitis, ulcerative colitis)
   c. Intraluminal—foreign body, fecal or barium impaction, polyp, gallstones, meconium in infants
   d. In postoperative patients, approximately 90% of mechanical obstructions are due to adhesions. In nonsurgical patients, hernia (most often inguinal) is the most common cause of mechanical obstruction.
2. *Paralytic (adynamic, neurogenic) ileus*
   a. Peristalsis is ineffective (diminished motor activity perhaps because of toxic or traumatic disturbance of the autonomic nervous system).
   b. There is no physical obstruction and no interrupted blood supply.
   c. Disappears spontaneously after 2 to 3 days.
   d. Causes include:
      (i) Spinal cord injuries; vertebral fractures.
      (ii) Postoperatively after any abdominal surgery.
      (iii) Peritonitis, pneumonia.
      (iv) Wound dehiscence (breakdown).
      (v) GI tract surgery.
3. *Strangulation*—obstruction compromises blood supply, leading to gangrene of the intestinal wall. Caused by prolonged mechanical obstruction.

Altered Physiology
1. Increased peristalsis, distention by fluid and gas, and increased bacterial growth proximal to obstruction. The intestine empties distally.
2. Increased secretions into the intestine are associated with diminution in the bowel's absorptive capacity.
3. The accumulation of gases, secretions, and oral intake above the obstruction causes increasing intraluminal pressure.

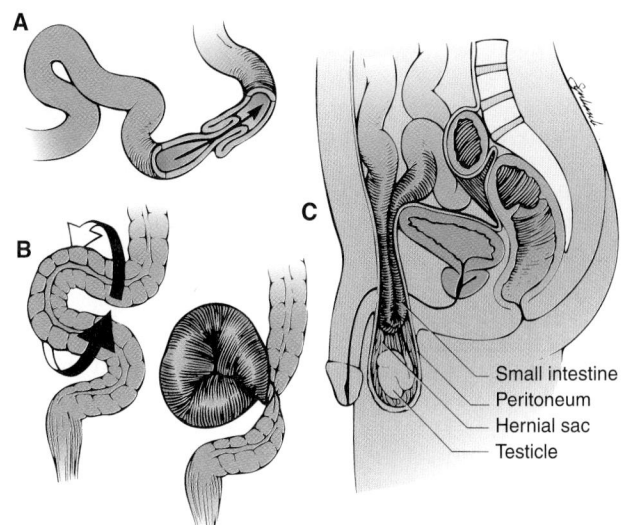

FIGURE 18-5 Three causes of intestinal obstruction. (**A**) Intussusception. Note shortening of the colon by the movement of one segment of bowel into another. (**B**) Volvulus of the sigmoid colon. The twist is counterclockwise in most cases of sigmoid volvulus. (**C**) Hernia (inguinal). Note that the sac of the hernia is a continuation of the peritoneum of the abdomen and that the hernial contents are intestine, omentum, or other abdominal contents that pass through the hernial opening into the hernial sac.

Small intestine
Peritoneum
Hernial sac
Testicle

4. Venous pressure in the affected area increases, and circulatory stasis and edema result.

5. Bowel necrosis may occur because of anoxia and compression of the terminal branches of the mesenteric artery.

6. Bacteria and toxins pass across the intestinal membranes into the abdominal cavity, thereby leading to peritonitis.

7. "Closed-loop" obstruction is a condition in which the intestinal segment is occluded at both ends, preventing either the downward passage or the regurgitation of intestinal contents.

Clinical Manifestations

Fever, peritoneal irritation, increased white blood cell count, toxicity, and shock may develop with all types of intestinal obstruction.

1. Simple mechanical—high small-bowel: colic (cramps), mid- to upper abdomen, some distention, early bilious vomiting, increased bowel sounds (high-pitched tinkling heard at brief intervals), minimal diffuse tenderness

2. Simple mechanical—low small-bowel: significant colic (cramps), midabdominal, considerable distention, vomiting slight or absent, later feculent, increased bowel sounds and "hush" sounds, minimal diffuse tenderness

3. Simple mechanical—colon: cramps (mid- to lower abdomen), later-appearing distention, then vomiting may develop (feculent), increase in bowel sounds, minimal diffuse tenderness.

4. Partial chronic mechanical obstruction—may occur with granulomatous bowel in Crohn's disease. Symptoms are cramping, abdominal pain, mild distention, and diarrhea.

5. Strangulation symptoms are initially those of mechanical obstruction, but later progress rapidly—pain is severe, continuous, and localized. There is moderate distention, persistent vomiting, usually decreased bowel sounds and marked localized tenderness. Stools or vomitus become melenous or bloody or contain occult blood.

Diagnostic Evaluation

1. Abdominal and chest x-rays
   a. May show presence and location of small or large intestinal distention, gas or fluid.
   b. "Bird beak" lesion in colonic volvulus.
   c. Foreign body visualization.
2. Contrast studies
   a. Barium enema may diagnose colon obstruction or intussusception.
   b. Ileus may be identified by oral barium or Gastrografin.
3. Laboratory tests
   a. May show decreased sodium, potassium, and chloride levels due to vomiting.
   b. Elevated WBC counts with necrosis, strangulation, or peritonitis.
   c. Serum amylase may be elevated from irritation of the pancreas by the bowel loop.
4. Rigid proctoscopy/flexible sigmoidoscopy

Management

Nonsurgical Management

1. Correction of fluid and electrolyte imbalances with normal saline or Ringer's solution with potassium as required.
2. NG suction to decompress bowel.
3. Treatment of shock and peritonitis.
4. TPN may be necessary to correct protein deficiency from chronic obstruction, paralytic ileus, or infection.
5. Analgesics and sedatives, avoiding opiates due to GI motility inhibition.
6. Antibiotics for peritonitis.

Surgery

Consists of relieving obstruction. Options include:

1. Closed bowel procedures: lysis of adhesions, reduction of volvulus, intussusception, or incarcerated hernia.
2. Enterotomy for removal of foreign bodies, bezoars, and so forth.
3. Resection of bowel for obstructing lesions, or strangulated bowel with end-to-end anastomosis.
4. Intestinal bypass around obstruction.
5. Temporary ostomy may be indicated (see Caring for Patient Undergoing Ostomy Surgery, p. 590).

Complications

1. Dehydration due to loss of water, sodium, and chloride
2. Peritonitis
3. Shock due to loss of electrolytes and dehydration
4. Death due to shock

Nursing Assessment

1. Assess the nature and location of the patient's pain, the presence or absence of distention, flatus, defecation, emesis, obstipation.
2. Listen for high-pitched bowel sounds, peristaltic rushes.

GERONTOLOGIC ALERT

Watch for air–fluid lock syndrome in elderly, who often remain in the recumbent position for extended periods.
1. Fluid collects in dependent bowel loops.
2. Peristalsis is too weak to push fluid "uphill."
3. Obstruction primarily occurs in the large bowel.

3. Conduct frequent checks of the patient's level of responsiveness; decreasing responsiveness may offer a clue to an increasing electrolyte imbalance or impending shock.

Nursing Diagnoses

• Pain related to obstruction, distention, and strangulation
• Risk for Fluid Volume Deficit related to impaired fluid intake, vomiting, and diarrhea from intestinal obstruction
• Diarrhea related to obstruction

- Ineffective Breathing Pattern related to abdominal distention, interfering with normal lung expansion
- Anxiety related to complications and severity of illness
- Fear of death related to life-threatening symptoms of intestinal obstruction

Nursing Interventions

Achieving Pain Relief

1. Administer prescribed analgesics.
2. Provide supportive care during NG intubation to assist with discomfort.
3. To relieve air–fluid lock syndrome, turn the patient from supine to prone position every 10 minutes until enough flatus is passed to decompress the abdomen. A rectal tube may be indicated.

Maintaining Electrolyte and Fluid Balance

1. Measure and record all intake and output.
2. Administer IV fluids and parenteral nutrition as prescribed.
3. Monitor electrolytes, urinalysis, hemoglobin, and blood cell counts, and report any abnormalities.
4. Monitor urinary output to assess renal function and to detect urinary retention due to bladder compressions by the distended intestine.
5. Monitor vital signs; a drop in blood pressure may indicate decreased circulatory volume due to blood loss from strangulated hernia.

Maintaining Normal Bowel Elimination

1. Collect stool samples to test for occult blood if ordered.
2. Maintain adequate fluid balance.
3. Record amount and consistency of stools.
4. Maintain NG tube as prescribed to decompress bowel.

Maintaining Proper Lung Ventilation

1. Keep the patient in Fowler's position to promote ventilation and relieve abdominal distention.
2. Monitor arterial blood gases for oxygenation levels if ordered.

Reducing Anxiety and Preventing Complications

1. Prevent infarction by carefully assessing the patient's status; pain that increases in intensity or becomes localized or continuous may herald strangulation.
2. Detect early signs of peritonitis, such as rigidity and tenderness, in an effort to minimize this complication.
3. Avoid enemas, which may distort an x-ray or make a partial obstruction worse.
4. Observe for signs of shock—pallor, tachycardia, hypotension.
5. Watch for signs of:
   a. Metabolic alkalosis (slow, shallow respirations; changes in sensorium; tetany).
   b. Metabolic acidosis (disorientation; deep, rapid breathing; weakness; and shortness of breath on exertion).

Relieving Fears

1. Recognize the patient's concerns, and initiate measures to provide emotional support.
2. Encourage presence of support person.

Patient Education and Health Maintenance

1. Explain the rationale for NG suction, NPO status, and IV fluids initially. Advise patient to progress diet slowly as tolerated once home.
2. Advise plenty of rest and slow progression of activity as directed by surgeon or other health care provider.
3. Teach wound care if indicated.
4. Encourage patient to follow up as directed and to call surgeon or health care provider for increasing abdominal pain, vomiting, or fever in meantime.

Outcome-Based Evaluation

- Experiences minimal pain
- Urine output adequate; vital signs stable
- Demonstrates relief of bowel obstruction—passes flatus, has first bowel movement
- Demonstrates improved breathing ability
- Exhibits no signs of complications
- Appears relaxed and reports feeling better

▪ Appendicitis

Appendicitis is inflammation of the vermiform appendix caused by an obstruction of the intestinal lumen from infection, stricture, fecal mass, foreign body, or tumor.

Pathophysiology and Etiology

1. Obstruction is followed by edema, infection, and ischemia.
2. As intraluminal tension develops, necrosis and perforation usually occur.
3. Appendicitis can affect any age group, but is most common in males 10 to 30 years old.

Clinical Manifestations

1. Generalized or localized abdominal pain in the epigastric or periumbilical areas and upper right abdomen. Within 2 to 12 hours, the pain localizes in the right lower quadrant and intensity increases.
2. Anorexia, moderate malaise, mild fever, nausea and vomiting.
3. Usually constipation occurs; occasionally diarrhea.
4. Rebound tenderness, involuntary guarding, generalized abdominal rigidity.

Diagnostic Evaluation

1. Physical examination consistent with clinical manifestations.
2. White blood cell (WBC) count reveals moderate leukocytosis (10,000 to 16,000/mm) with shift to the left (increased neutrophils).
3. Urinalysis to rule out urinary disorders.
4. Abdominal x-ray may visualize shadow consistent with fecalith in appendix; perforation will reveal free air.
5. Abdominal ultrasound or CT scan can visualize appendix and rule out other conditions, such as diverticulitis and Crohn's disease. Focused appendiceal CT can now be done to more quickly evaluate for appendicitis.

GERONTOLOGIC ALERT

In older adults, be aware of vague symptoms: milder pain, less pronounced fever, and leukocytosis with shift to the left on differential.

Management

1. Surgery (appendectomy) is indicated.
   a. Simple appendectomy or laparoscopic appendectomy in absence of rupture or peritonitis.
   b. An incisional drain may be placed if an abscess or rupture occurs.
2. Preoperatively maintain bed rest, NPO status, IV hydration, possible antibiotic prophylaxis, and analgesia.

Complications

1. Perforation (in 95% of cases)
2. Abscess
3. Peritonitis

Nursing Assessment

1. Obtain history for location and extent of pain.
2. Auscultate for presence of bowel sounds; peristalsis may be absent or diminished.
3. On palpation of the abdomen, assess for tenderness anywhere in the right lower quadrant, but often localized over McBurney's point (point just below midpoint of line between umbilicus and iliac crest on the right side). Assess for rebound tenderness in the right lower quadrant as well as referred rebound when palpating the left lower quadrant.
4. Assess for positive psoas sign by having the patient attempt to raise the right thigh against the pressure of your hand placed over the right knee. Inflammation of the psoas muscle in acute appendicitis will increase abdominal pain with this maneuver.
5. Assess for positive obturator sign by flexing the patient's right hip and knee and rotating the leg internally. Hypogastric pain with this maneuver indicates inflammation of the obturator muscle.

Nursing Diagnoses

- Pain related to inflamed appendix
- Risk for Infection related to perforation

Nursing Interventions

Preoperative nursing care is listed; for postoperative care, see Caring for the Patient Undergoing Gastrointestinal Surgery, page 585.

Relieving Pain

1. Monitor pain level, including location, intensity, pattern.
2. Assist patient to comfortable positions, such as semi-Fowler's and knees up.
3. Restrict activity that may aggravate pain, such as coughing and ambulation.
4. Apply ice bag to abdomen for comfort.

5. Give analgesics only as ordered after diagnosis is determined.
6. Avoid indiscriminate palpation of the abdomen to avoid increasing the patient's discomfort.

NURSING ALERT

Do not give analgesics/antipyretics to mask fever, and do not administer cathartics, because they may cause rupture.

Preventing Infection

1. Monitor frequently for signs and symptoms of worsening condition indicating perforation, abscess, or peritonitis: increasing severity of pain, tenderness, rigidity, distention, ileus, fever, malaise, tachycardia.
2. Administer antibiotics as ordered.
3. Promptly prepare patient for surgery.

Patient Education and Health Maintenance

1. Instruct patient to avoid heavy lifting for 4 to 6 weeks after surgery.
2. Instruct patient to report symptoms of anorexia, nausea, vomiting, fever, abdominal pain, incisional redness or drainage postoperatively.

Outcome-Based Evaluation

- Verbalizes increased comfort with positioning and analgesics
- Afebrile; no rigidity or distention

◼ Diverticular Disease

Diverticular disease consists of prediverticular disease, diverticulosis, and diverticulitis. A *diverticulum* is a pouch or saccular dilatation of the colon wall. *Diverticulosis* is a condition exhibiting multiple diverticula. *Diverticulitis* is an inflammation of one or more diverticula.

Pathophysiology and Etiology

Prediverticular Disease

1. Characterized as a weakening and degeneration of the colonic musculature. The muscle thickening narrows the bowel lumen, thereby increasing intraluminal pressure results.
2. No diverticula are yet formed.

Diverticulosis

1. Marks the formation of diverticula, which are herniations of the mucosal and submucosal layers of the colon developing at weak points where nutrient blood vessels penetrate the colon wall (Figure 18-6).
2. Causes for diverticular disease are unclear, but data suggest excessive intraluminal pressure plays a key role. A contributing factor may be a low-residue diet, which reduces fecal residue, narrows the bowel lumen, and leads to higher pressure intra-abdominally during defecation.
3. Diverticulosis occurs most often in persons older than age 60.

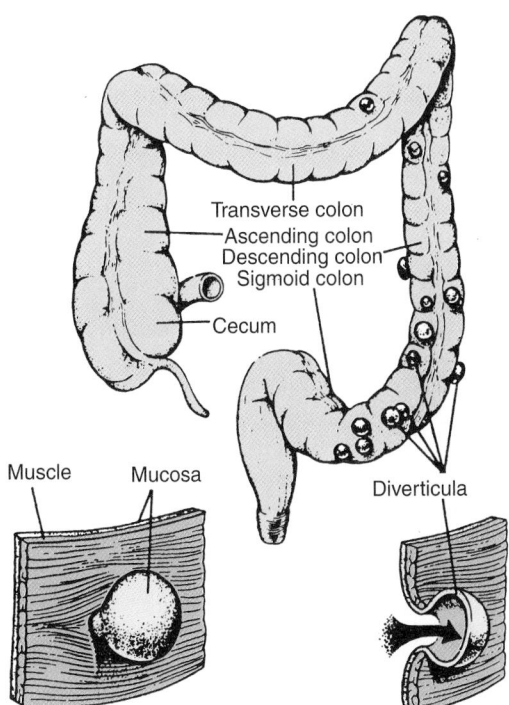

FIGURE 18-6 Diverticula are most common in the sigmoid colon; they diminish in number and size as the colon approaches the cecum. Diverticula are rarely found in the rectum.

Diverticulitis

1. Results when one or more diverticula become inflamed and usually perforate the thin diverticular wall, which consists of mucosal and serosal layers. The inflammation may be caused by a combination of a fecalith plug and accumulating bacteria.
2. If diverticulum perforates, local abscess or peritonitis may occur.
3. Uninflamed or minimally inflamed diverticula may erode adjacent arterial branches causing acute massive rectal bleeding.
4. It is estimated that some persons with diverticulosis will develop diverticulitis.

Clinical Manifestations
Prediverticular Disease
1. May be asymptomatic.
2. Intermittent or chronic abdominal pain; worsening after eating or before bowel movements.
3. Constipation and/or diarrhea.
Diverticulosis
1. May be asymptomatic.
2. Crampy abdominal pain.
3. Bowel irregularity—constipation and/or diarrhea.
4. Periodic abdominal distention.
5. Sudden massive hemorrhage may be first symptom.

Diverticulitis
1. Mild.
   a. Bouts of soreness, mild lower abdominal cramps.
   b. Bowel irregularity, constipation, and diarrhea.
   c. Mild nausea, gas, low-grade fever, and leukocytosis.
2. Severe acute diverticulitis.
   a. Crampy pain in lower left quadrant of abdomen.
   b. Low-grade fever, chills, leukocytosis.
   c. Ruptured diverticula produce abscesses or peritonitis with abdominal rigidity; signs of shock and sepsis (hypotension, chills, high fever). Near a blood vessel, a rupture may cause massive hemorrhage.
   d. Sometimes, fistulae form with the bladder, the adjacent small bowel, the vagina, and the perianal area or skin.
   e. Sepsis may spread through portal vein to liver, causing liver abscesses.
   f. Chronic diverticulitis may cause adhesions that narrow the bowel's opening and can cause partial or complete bowel obstruction.
3. Urinary frequency and dysuria are associated with bladder involvement in the inflammatory process.

Diagnostic Evaluation
1. Laboratory studies: WBC may show leukocytosis with shift to the left; hemoglobin/hematocrit may be low with chronic or acute bleeding.
2. Flat film of abdomen, ultrasonography/CT scan—free air under diaphragm with perforation into the abdominal cavity. Computed tomography is recommended for complicated cases.
3. Sigmoidoscopy; colonoscopy—to rule out carcinoma and confirm diagnosis.
4. Barium enema (after infection subsides)—may visualize diverticular sacs, narrowing of colonic lumen, partial or complete obstruction or fistulae.

NURSING ALERT

 In patients with acute diverticulitis, a barium enema may rupture the bowel.

Management
Prediverticular Disease
1. High-fiber diet.
2. Bran therapy or psyllium hydrophilic mucilloid (Metamucil) prescribed to counteract tendency toward constipation.
Diverticulosis
1. High-fiber diet with possible avoidance of large seeds or nuts, which may clog diverticular sac.
2. Bran therapy, psyllium preparation, or stool softeners, such as docusate sodium (Colace), to avoid constipation.
3. Intestinal diverticulosis with pain usually responds to a liquid or low-residue diet and stool softeners to relieve symptoms, minimize irritation, and reduce progression to diverticulitis.

Diverticulitis

1. Medical management
   a. Bed rest, liquid or low-residue diet, stool softeners.
   b. Broad-spectrum antibiotic.
   c. Medications to control pain and muscle spasms.
   d. Blood transfusions may be needed during massive bleeding episodes. Vasopressin (Pitressin) may be used to control bleeding.
   e. NPO, IV therapy, NG placement if signs/symptoms of peritonitis or massive bleed.
2. Surgical management—if there is little response to medical treatment or if complications such as hemorrhage, obstruction, or perforation occur, surgery is necessary.
   a. Segment of intestine involved with diverticula is resected; two ends reanastomosed to maintain continuity.
   b. Temporary colostomy is sometimes performed to divert fecal stream with continuity restored in later second-stage procedure (Hartmann pouch procedure).
3. Primary laparoscopic sigmoid resection with anastomosis is a common surgical option for peridiverticulitis, stenosis, or recurrent attacks of inflammation (uncomplicated cases).

Complications

1. Hemorrhage from colonic diverticula, usually in the right colon
2. Bowel obstruction
3. Fistula formation
4. Septicemia

Nursing Assessment

1. Have patient describe amount of fiber and fluid intake per day and past and present bowel patterns. Any constipation, diarrhea, or alternating of both?
2. Ask if experiencing abdominal cramping or pain, bloody stools, or stool/gas passage from vagina or in urine.
3. Watch for signs and symptoms of peritonitis: increasing abdominal pain, guarding, rebound tenderness, abdominal distention, nausea/vomiting.
4. Monitor vital signs: temperature may be elevated; tachycardia and hypotension may indicate peritonitis/massive bleed.

Nursing Diagnoses

- Pain related to intestinal discomfort, diarrhea, and/or constipation
- Altered Nutrition: Less Than Body Requirements, related to diarrhea, fluid and electrolyte loss, nausea, and vomiting
- Constipation or Diarrhea, related to the disease process
- Knowledge Deficit of the relationship between diet and diverticular disease

Nursing Interventions
Achieving Pain Relief

1. Observe for signs and location of pain, type, and severity, and intervene when appropriate.
   a. Administer nonopiate analgesics as prescribed (opiates may mask signs of perforation).
   b. Administer anticholinergics as prescribed to decrease colon spasm.
2. Auscultate bowel sounds to monitor bowel motility.
3. Palpate abdomen to determine rigidity or tenderness due to perforation or peritonitis.

Maintaining Adequate Nutrition

1. Follow prescribed diet that is high in soft residue and low in sugar.
   a. Provide lists of these foods to enhance familiarity with proper dietary control.
   b. Emphasize that proper food intake influences how well the intestinal tract functions.
2. Inform patient that bran products will add bulk to the stool and can be taken with milk or sprinkled over cereal.
3. Monitor intake and output and weight daily to determine caloric status.

Promoting Normal Bowel Elimination

1. Advise patient to establish regular bowel habits to promote regular and complete evacuation.
2. Observe and record color, consistency, and frequency of stools.
3. Encourage fluids if constipated to promote bowel stimulation.
4. Provide high-residue diet to provide bulk and more consistency to the stool.

Increasing Understanding of Disease

1. Explain the disease process to the patient and its relationship to diet.
2. Have the patient continue periodic medical supervision and follow-up; report problems and untoward symptoms.
3. Refer to nutritionist, as needed.

Patient Education

1. Instruct on high-residue diet choices.
2. Emphasize the importance of establishing regular bowel habits.
3. Advise patient to report left lower quadrant pain, generalized abdominal tenderness, and fever.

Outcome-Based Evaluation

- Expresses relief of pain and has a decrease in symptoms
- Consumes a prescribed diet and can relate what foods to include or avoid
- Reports near-normal bowel function; no diarrhea or constipation
- Delineates the general nature of diverticulosis and can list dietary regimen that helps or aggravates the condition

Peritonitis

Peritonitis is a generalized or localized inflammation of the peritoneum, the membrane lining the abdominal cavity and covering visceral organs.

Pathophysiology and Etiology
Primary Peritonitis
Acute, spontaneous condition; relatively rare
1. Persons with nephrosis or cirrhosis; the offending organism is most often *Escherichia coli.*
2. May occur in young females; introduced through uterine tubes or blood due to pathogenic bacteria such as streptococci, pneumococci, or gonococci.

Secondary Peritonitis
Contamination of peritoneal cavity by GI fluid and microorganisms.
1. Complication of appendicitis, diverticulitis, peptic ulceration, biliary tract disease, colon inflammation, volvulus, strangulated obstruction, perforation, abdominal cancers.
2. May occur after abdominal trauma: gunshot wound, stab wound, or blunt trauma from motor vehicle accident.
3. May occur as postoperative complication.
   a. May occur after intraoperative intestinal spillage.
   b. Compromised patients are vulnerable (those with diabetes, malignancy, malnutrition, or steroids.
4. May result from continuous ambulatory peritoneal dialysis.

Clinical Manifestations
1. Initially, local type of abdominal pain tends to become constant, diffuse, and more intense.
2. Abdomen becomes extremely tender and muscles become rigid; rebound tenderness and ileus may be present; patient lies very still, usually with legs drawn up.
3. Percussion: resonance and tympany due to paralytic ileus; loss of liver dullness may indicate free air in abdomen.
4. Auscultation: decreased bowel sounds.
5. Nausea and vomiting often occur; peristalsis diminishes; anorexia is present.
6. Elevation of temperature and pulse as well as leukocytosis.
7. Fever; thirst; oliguria; dry, swollen tongue; signs of dehydration.
8. Weakness, pallor, diaphoresis, and cold skin are a result of the loss of fluid, electrolytes, and protein into the abdomen.
9. Hypotension, tachycardia, and hypokalemia may occur.
10. Shallow respirations may result from abdominal distention and upward displacement of the diaphragm.
   Note: With generalized peritonitis, large volumes of fluid may be lost into abdominal cavity (can account for losses to 5 L/day).
11. Ascites

Diagnostic Evaluation
1. WBC to show leukocytosis (leukopenia if severe).
2. Arterial blood gases may show metabolic acidosis with respiratory compensation.

3. Urinalysis may indicate urinary tract problems as primary source.
4. Peritoneal aspiration (paracentesis) to demonstrate blood, pus, bile, bacteria (Gram's stain), amylase.
5. Abdominal x-rays may show free air in peritoneal cavity, gas and fluid collection in small and large intestines, generalized bowel dilatation, intestinal wall edema.
6. CT of abdomen or sonography may reveal intra-abdominal mass, abscess, ascites.
7. Chest x-ray may show elevated diaphragm.
8. Laparotomy to identify the underlying cause.

Management
1. Treatment of inflammatory conditions preoperatively and postoperatively with antibiotic therapy may prevent peritonitis. Broad-spectrum antibiotic therapy to cover aerobic and anaerobic organisms is initial treatment, followed by specific antibiotic therapy after culture and sensitivity results.
2. Bed rest, NPO status, respiratory support if needed.
3. IV fluids and electrolytes, possibly TPN.
4. Analgesics for pain; antiemetics for nausea and vomiting.
5. NG intubation to decompress the bowel.
6. Possibly rectal tube to facilitate passage of gas.
7. Operative procedures to close perforations, remove infection source (ie, inflamed organ, neurotic tissue), drain abscesses, and lavage peritoneal cavity.
8. Abdominal paracentesis may be done to remove accumulating fluid.
9. Blood transfusions, if appropriate.
10. Oral feedings after return of bowel sounds and passage of gas and/or feces.

Complications
1. Intra-abdominal abscess formation (ie, pelvic subphrenic space)
2. Septicemia
3. Hypovolemic problems
4. Renal or liver failure
5. Respiratory insufficiency

Nursing Assessment
1. Assess for abdominal distention and tenderness, guarding, rebound, hypoactive or absent bowel sounds to determine bowel function.
2. Observe for signs of shock—tachycardia and hypotension.
3. Monitor vital signs, arterial blood gases, complete blood count, electrolytes, and central venous pressure to monitor hemodynamic status and assess for complications.

Nursing Diagnoses
- Pain related to peritoneal inflammation
- Fluid Volume Deficit related to vomiting and interstitial fluid shift
- Altered Nutrition: Less Than Body Requirements, related to GI symptomatology

Nursing Interventions
Achieving Pain Relief
1. Place the patient in semi-Fowler's position before surgery to enable less painful breathing.
2. After surgery, place the patient in Fowler's position to promote drainage by gravity.
3. Provide analgesics as prescribed.

Maintaining Fluid and Electrolyte Volume
1. Keep patient NPO to reduce peristalsis.
2. Provide IV fluids to establish adequate fluid intake and to promote adequate urinary output, as prescribed.
3. Record accurately intake and output, including the measurement of vomitus and NG drainage.
4. Minimize nausea, vomiting, and distention by use of NG suction, antiemetics.
5. Monitor for signs of hypovolemia: dry mucous membranes, oliguria, postural hypotension, tachycardia, diminished skin turgor.

Achieving Adequate Nutrition
1. Administer TPN, as ordered, to maintain positive nitrogen balance until patient can resume oral diet.
2. Reduce parenteral fluids and give oral food and fluids per order, when the following occur:
   a. Temperature and pulse return to normal.
   b. Abdomen becomes soft.
   c. Peristaltic sounds return (determined by abdominal auscultation).
   d. Flatus is passed, and patient has bowel movements.

Patient Education and Health Maintenance
1. Teach patient and family how to care for open wounds and drain sites, if appropriate.
2. Assess the need for home care nursing to assist with wound care and assess healing; refer as necessary.

Outcome-Based Evaluation
- Minimal analgesics needed; abdomen soft, nontender, and no distention
- Balanced intake and output, no evidence of dehydration or electrolyte imbalances
- Bowel sounds present; tolerating soft diet

◼ Ulcerative Colitis

Ulcerative colitis is a chronic idiopathic inflammatory disease of the mucosa and, less frequently, the submucosa of the colon and rectum. If only the rectum is involved, it may be called ulcerative proctitis.

Pathophysiology and Etiology
1. The exact cause of ulcerative colitis is unknown. Possible theories include:
   a. Genetic predisposition.
   b. Environmental factors may trigger disease (viral or bacterial pathogens, dietary).
   c. Immunologic imbalance or disturbances.
   d. Defect in intestinal barrier causing hypersensitive mucosa and increased permeability.
   e. Defect in repair of mucosal injury, which may develop into a chronic condition.
2. Multiple crypt abscesses develop in intestinal mucosa that may become necrotic and lead to ulceration.
3. Most common in young adulthood and middle life, peak incidence at 20 to 40 years of age.
4. Incidence greatest in Caucasians of Jewish descent.

Clinical Manifestations
1. Diarrhea—may be bloody or contain pus and mucus.
2. Tenesmus (painful straining), sense of urgency, and frequency.
3. Increased bowel sounds; abdomen may appear flat, but, as condition continues, abdomen may appear distended.
4. There often is weight loss, fever, dehydration, hypokalemia, anorexia, nausea and vomiting, iron-deficiency anemia, and cachexia (general lack of nutrition and wasting with chronic disease).
5. Crampy abdominal pain.
6. The disease usually begins in the rectum and sigmoid and spreads proximally, at times, involving the entire colon. Anal area may be irritated and reddened; left lower abdomen may be tender on palpation.
7. There is a tendency for the patient to experience remissions and exacerbations.
8. Increased risk of developing colorectal cancer.
9. May inhibit extracolonic manifestations of eye, joint, and skin complaints.

Diagnostic Evaluation
Diagnosis is based on a combination of laboratory, radiologic, endoscopic, and histologic findings.

Laboratory Tests
1. Stool examination to rule out enteral pathogens; fecal analysis positive for blood during active disease.
2. Complete blood count—hemoglobin and hematocrit may be low due to bleeding; WBC may be increased.
3. Increased prothrombin time possible.
4. Elevated erythrocyte sedimentation rate (ESR).
5. Decreased serum levels of potassium, magnesium, and albumin may be present.

Other Diagnostic Tests
1. Barium enema to assess extent of disease and detect pseudopolyps, carcinoma, and strictures. May show absence of haustral markings; narrow, lead-pipe appearance; superficial ulcerations.
2. Flexible proctosigmoidoscopy/colonoscopy findings reveal mucosal erythema and edema, ulcers, inflammation that begins distally in the rectum and spreads proximally for variable distances. Pseudopolyps and friable tissue may be present.
3. Changes in crypt height, loss of crypts, crypt abscess with neutrophils infiltrates on biopsy.

Management

General Measures

1. Bed rest, IV fluid replacement, clear liquid diet.
2. For patients with severe dehydration and excessive diarrhea, TPN may be recommended to rest the intestinal tract and restore nitrogen balance.
3. Treatment of anemia—iron supplements for chronic bleeding, blood replacement for massive bleeding.

Drug Therapy

1. 5-aminosalicylic acid—sulfasalazine (Azulfidine)—mainstay drug for acute and maintenance therapy. Dose-related side effects include vomiting, anorexia, headache, skin discoloration, dyspepsia, and lowered sperm count.
2. Oral salicylates, such as mesalamine (Pentasa), olsalazine (Dipentum)—appear to be as effective as sulfasalazine and are used when patients are allergic to sulfa.
   a. Nephrotoxicity can occur with mesalamine; diarrhea with olsalazine.
3. Mesalamine enema available for proctosigmoiditis; suppository for proctitis.
4. Corticosteroids—primary agent used in the management of inflammatory disease. Should be treated concomitantly with 5-aminosalicylic acid preparations to benefit from their potential steroid-sparing effects. Corticosteroids must be tapered slowly over a 6- to 8-week period:
   a. Prednisolone (Delta-Cortef)—IV, to induce remission of acute severe disease.
   b. Prednisone (Orasone)—orally, for moderate to severe disease.
   c. Hydrocortisone (Cortef)—enema used for proctitis and left-sided colitis.
5. Immunosuppressive drugs—purine analogues, 6-mercaptopurine, azathioprine may be indicated when patient is refractory or dependent on corticosteroids.
6. Antidiarrheal medications may be prescribed to control diarrhea, rectal urgency and cramping, abdominal pain; not routinely ordered—treat with caution.

Surgical Measures

1. Surgery is recommended when patients fail to respond to medical therapy, if clinical status is worsening, for uncontrollable side effects of medications, severe hemorrhage, perforation, toxic megacolon, dysplasia, or cancer.
2. Surgical procedures include:
   a. Noncurative approaches—possible curative, reconstructive procedure at later date
      (i) Temporary loop colostomy for decompression if toxic megacolon present without perforation
      (ii) Subtotal colectomy, ileostomy, and Hartmann's pouch
      (iii) Colectomy with ileorectal anastomosis
   b. Reconstructive procedures—curative
      (i) Total proctocolectomy with permanent end-ileostomy
      (ii) Total proctocolectomy with continent ileostomy (Kock or BCIR)
      (iii) Total colectomy with ileal reservoir—anal (or ileal reservoir–distal rectal) anastomosis—procedure of choice (Figure 18-7)
      (iv) The ultimate surgical goal is to remove the entire colon and rectum to cure patient of ulcerative colitis.

Complications

1. Perforation, hemorrhage
2. Toxic megacolon—fever, tachycardia, abdominal distention, peritonitis, leukocytosis, dilated colon on abdominal x-ray—life-threatening
3. Abscess formation, stricture, anal fistula
4. Malnutrition, anemia, electrolyte imbalance
5. Skin lesions (erythema nodosum, pyoderma gangrenosum)
6. Arthritis, ankylosing spondylitis
7. Colon malignancy
8. Liver disease
9. Eye lesions (uveitis, conjunctivitis)
10. Growth retardation in prepubertal children
11. Possible infertility in females

Nursing Assessment

1. Review nursing history for patterns of fatigue and overwork, tension, family problems that may exacerbate symptoms.

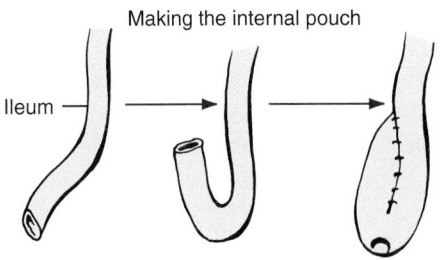

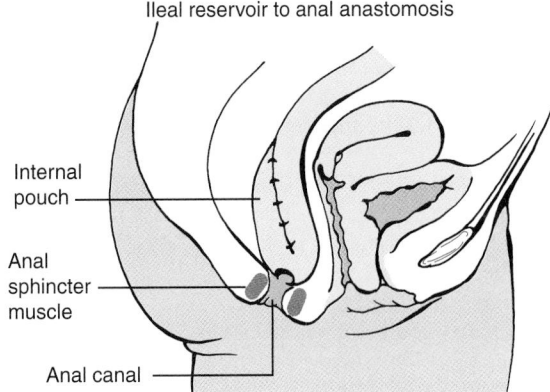

FIGURE 18-7 Ileal reservoir–anal anastomosis. This reservoir is constructed of two loops of small intestine forming a J configuration (J pouch).

2. Assess food habits and use of any dietary or herbal supplements used as alternative therapies that may have a bearing on triggering symptoms (milk intake may be a problem). Many patients use vitamins, herbs, and homeopathic remedies without realizing the effect on bowel function.
3. Determine number and consistency of bowel movements, any rectal bleeding present.
4. Listen for hyperactive bowel sounds; assess weight.

Nursing Diagnoses
- Pain related to disease process
- Altered Nutrition: Less Than Body Requirements, related to diarrhea, nausea, and vomiting
- Fluid Volume Deficit related to diarrhea and loss of fluid and electrolytes
- Risk for Infection related to disease process, surgical procedures
- Ineffective Individual Coping related to fatigue, feeling of helplessness, and lack of support system

Nursing Interventions
Promoting Comfort
1. Follow prescribed treatment of reducing or eliminating food and fluid and instituting parenteral feeding or low-residue diets to rest the intestinal tract.
2. Give sedatives and tranquilizers, as prescribed, not only to provide general rest, but also to slow peristalsis.
3. Be aware of skin breakdown around anus.
   a. Cleanse the skin gently after each bowel movement.
   b. Apply a protective emollient, such as petroleum jelly, skin sealant, or moisture-barrier ointment.
4. Relieve painful rectal spasms (produced by frequent diarrheal stools) with anodyne suppositories, as prescribed.
5. Report any evidence of sudden abdominal distention—may indicate toxic megacolon.
6. Reduce physical activity to a minimum, or provide frequent rest periods.
7. Provide commode or bathroom next to bed, because urgency of movements may be a problem.

Achieving Nutritional Requirements
1. Maintain acutely ill patient on parenteral replacement of vitamins, fluids, and electrolytes (potassium), as prescribed.
2. When resuming oral fluids and foods, select those that are nonirritating to the mucosa (mechanically, thermally, and chemically). If this fails, an elemental diet may be prescribed to provide low residue to rest the lower intestinal tract.
3. Avoid dairy products if patient is lactose intolerant.
4. Provide a well-balanced, low-residue, high-protein diet to correct malnutrition.
5. Determine which foods the patient can tolerate, and modify diet plan accordingly.
6. Bolster with supplemental vitamin therapy, including vitamins C, B complex, and K, as prescribed.

7. Possibly avoid cold fluids, which may increase intestinal motility.
8. Administer prescribed medications for symptomatic relief of diarrhea.

Maintaining Fluid Balance
1. Maintain accurate intake and output records.
2. Weigh daily; rapid increase or decrease may relate to fluid imbalance.
3. Monitor serum electrolytes, and report any abnormalities.
4. Observe for decreased skin turgor, dry skin, oliguria, decreased temperature, weakness, increased hemoglobin, hematocrit, blood urea nitrogen, and specific gravity, which all are signs of fluid loss leading to dehydration.

Minimizing Infection and Complications
1. Give antibacterial drugs as prescribed.
2. Administer corticosteroids as prescribed.
3. Provide conscientious skin care after severe diarrhea.
4. For severe proctitis, instill rectal steroids as prescribed to produce a remission of symptoms.
5. Administer prescribed therapy to correct existing anemia.
6. Observe for signs of colonic perforation and hemorrhage—abdominal rigidity, distention, hypotension, tachycardia.

Providing Supportive Care
1. Recognize psychological needs of the patient.
   a. Fear, anxiety, and discouragement.
   b. Hypersensitivity may be evident.
2. Acknowledge patient's complaints.
3. Encourage the patient to talk; listen and offer psychological support.
4. Answer questions about the permanent or temporary ostomy, if appropriate.
5. Initiate patient education about living with chronic disease.
6. For up-to-date information and education, contact Crohn's & Colitis Foundation of America, Inc., 386 Park Avenue Soth, New York NY 10016, 212-685-3440; *www.ccfa.org/*.
7. Include the patient as part of the health care team to provide continuity of care, communication, and periodic evaluation.
8. Offer educational and emotional support to family members.
9. Refer for psychological counseling, as needed.

Community and Home Care Considerations
Pouchitis
1. Patients undergoing one of the continent restorative procedures (Kock, BCIR, or ileal reservoir–anal anastomosis) must be alert for a common late postoperative complication called pouchitis.
2. The symptoms include increased stool output, cramps, and malaise.
3. It is thought to be related to stasis within the pouch/reservoir and usually responds to metronidazole (Flagyl).
4. Assess for these symptoms and notify health care provider.

Food Blockage

1. Patients with a temporary or permanent ileostomy must be alert for signs and symptoms of a food blockage.
   a. This is a mechanical blockage of undigested food-stuffs at the level of the fascia.
   b. It is most likely to occur in the first 6 weeks postoperatively when the bowel is edematous; however, patients with an ileostomy must be aware that it can occur at any time if precautions are not taken.
2. Symptoms may include spurty, watery stool with strong odor, decreased or no stool output, abdominal discomfort, cramping or bloating, and stomal swelling. Nausea and vomiting is a late symptom and requires immediate attention.
3. Treatment includes:
   a. Avoiding solid foods and drinking clear liquids when symptoms occur. Patients with ileostomies must never take laxatives.
   b. A larger opening in the pouching system to allow for stomal swelling.
   c. Gently massaging the abdomen around the stoma and/or pulling the knees to chest and rocking the body back and forth.
   d. A warm shower or bath may help with relaxation.
   e. If the blockage lasts for more than 2 to 3 hours or if nausea/vomiting occurs, seek medical attention immediately. Usually, an ileostomy lavage is done to relieve the blockage by the health care provider or ostomy specialty nurse.
4. It is best to instruct the patient how to prevent a food blockage by limiting certain foods the first few months after surgery—Chinese vegetables, skins and seeds, fatty meats, bean hulls, popcorn, and other foods that do not digest well.
5. Instruct the patient to avoid problem foods, chew food well, drink plenty of fluids while eating, eat possible problem foods in small amounts, and reintroduce problem foods slowly into the diet.
6. Some persons may need to avoid problem foods permanently.

Patient Education and Health Maintenance

1. Teach patient about chronic aspects of ulcerative colitis and each component of care prescribed.
2. Encourage self-care in monitoring symptoms, seeking annual checkup, and maintaining health.
3. Alert patient to possible postoperative problems with skin care, aesthetic difficulties, and surgical revisions.
4. Inform patients that early indications of relapse, such as bleeding or increased diarrhea, should be reported immediately so treatment may be initiated.
5. If the patient has an ileostomy, provide information about the local chapter of the United Ostomy Association.
6. Encourage patient to share experiences with others undergoing similar procedures.

Outcome-Based Evaluation

- Reports lessening of pain; functions well with minimal analgesics
- Demonstrates improved food and fluid intake; avoids roughage intake
- Diarrhea is controlled; fluid and electrolyte balance is maintained
- Absence of complications
- Shows improved psychological outlook; participates in counseling, if desired; uses support systems

Crohn's Disease

Crohn's disease is a chronic idiopathic inflammatory disease that can affect any part of the GI tract, usually the small and large intestines. It is predominantly a transmural disease of the bowel wall. Other names for this disease include *regional enteritis, granulomatous colitis, transmural colitis, ileitis,* and *ileocolitis.*

Pathophysiology and Etiology

1. Exact etiology is unknown for this disease. It is thought to be multifactorial with the following theories:
   a. Genetic predisposition.
   b. Environmental agents may trigger the disease such as infections (viral or bacterial overload) or dietary factors.
   c. Immunologic imbalance or disturbances.
   d. Defect in the intestinal barrier that increases the permeability of the bowel.
   e. Defect in the repair of mucosal injury leading to chronic condition.
   f. Cigarette smoking is a risk factor in developing disease and increases exacerbations. In contrast, cigarette smoking seems to have a protective effect with ulcerative colitis.
2. Intestinal tissue is thickened and edematous; ulcers enlarge, deepen, and form transverse and longitudinal linear ulcers that intersect, resembling cobblestone appearance. The deep penetration of these ulcers may form fissures, abscesses, and fistulae. The healing and fibrosis of these lesions may lead to stricture.
3. The rectum is typically spared from disease, and "skip lesions" are discontinuous areas of diseased bowel.
4. Transmural inflammation is a characteristic finding of this disease as well as granulomas.
5. Involvement of the upper GI (mouth, esophagus, stomach, and duodenum) is rare, and, if present, there is usually disease elsewhere.
6. May occur at any age, but occurs mostly in those between 15 and 35 years of age.
7. Highest incidence with Caucasians of Jewish descent.
8. The clinical presentation can be divided into three patterns:
   a. Inflammatory
   b. Fibrostenotic (stricturing)
   c. Perforating (fistulizing)

9. Recurrences tend to fall into the same pattern for each individual patient and may provide an approach to treatment.

Clinical Manifestations

These are characterized by exacerbations and remissions—may be abrupt or insidious.

1. Crampy pain usually in the right lower quadrant.
2. Chronic diarrhea—usual consistency is soft or semi-liquid. Bloody stools or steatorrhea (due to malabsorption) may occur.
3. Fever may indicate infectious complication, such as abscess.
4. Fecal urgency and tenesmus.
5. Palpable right lower quadrant fullness or mass may be palpated, which corresponds to adherent loops of bowel or abscess.
6. Rectal examination may reveal a perirectal abscess, fistula, fissure, or skin tags, which represent healed perianal lesions.
7. The *inflammatory pattern* may display malabsorption, weight loss, and less abdominal pain; *fibrostenotic pattern* may display a partial small bowel obstruction, diffuse abdominal pain, nausea, vomiting, and bloating; *perforating pattern* may display a sudden profuse diarrhea due to enteroenteric fistula, fever, and localized tenderness due to abscess, or other fistulizing symptoms such as pneumaturia and recurrent urinary tract infections.

Diagnostic Evaluation

1. The diagnosis is based on a combination of laboratory, radiologic, endoscopic, and histologic findings.
2. CBC may show mild leukocytosis, thrombocytosis, anemia.
3. Elevated ESR, hypoalbuminemia.
4. Stool analysis may reveal leukocytes but no enteric pathogens.
5. Upper GI and SB follow-through barium studies may show the classic "string sign" at the terminal ileum, which suggests a constriction of an intestinal segment.
6. A barium enema may permit visualization of lesions in the large intestine and terminal ileum.
7. CT of the abdomen and pelvis are helpful with diagnosis but more often used to evaluate complications such as abscess or fistulae.
8. Colonoscopy is the procedure of choice. Typical findings include presence of skip lesions, cobblestoning, ulcerations, and rectal sparing.
9. Biopsy may reveal granulomas, infiltration of lymphocytes, and monocytes.

Management
Medical Management

1. The goals of medical management include managing symptoms, reducing complications, inducing remissions, improving nutrition, and avoiding surgical interventions when possible.
2. 80% of patients experience weight loss; water and electrolyte imbalances; iron, vitamin, mineral, and protein deficiencies.
3. During acute episodes, bowel rest is usually required.
4. Nutritional replacements may include an elemental diet (Vivonex) administered orally or through an NG tube.
5. TPN may be ordered.
6. For milder cases, a low-residue diet may be indicated and avoidance of untolerated foods. Nutritional supplements may be ordered to provide additional nutrients and calories.

Drug Therapy

1. There is no known cure for this disease; it is primarily treated with medications. The disease severity and the area of the GI tract influence drug therapy.
2. 5-Aminosalicylic acid (5-ASA; Asacol, Pentasa, Dipentum)—first-line drug to induce and maintain remission. Has anti-inflammatory effect and is used in patients allergic to sulfa. Asacol releases mesalamine in the terminal ileum and colon. Pentasa releases mesalamine throughout the GI tract.
3. Topical 5-ASA (Rowasa suppositories or enemas) is used for distal colitis.
4. Sulfasalazine (Azulfidine)—first-line agent with unfavorable side effects: nausea, vomiting, headache, rash, fever. Less common side effects may include anemia, pancreatitis, pulmonary fibrosis, and sperm motility disorder.
5. Antibiotics (Flagyl, Cipro)—may be used in conjunction with 5-ASA or sulfasalazine to induce remission.
6. Corticosteroids—to reduce inflammation; given PO (prednisone, budesonide), IV (Solu-Medrol), or by suppository (Anusol-HC), retention enema (Cortenema), or foam (Proctofoam-HC) depending on the severity of disease.
   a. Long-term use of corticosteroids has severe side effects: cushingoid appearance, osteoporosis, hypertension, diabetes, psychosis, neuropathy, and myopathy.
   b. Steroids should be tapered off whenever possible.
7. Immunomodulators (6-mercaptopurine, azathioprine, methotrexate, Purinethol) used in patients who are steroid dependent or steroid refractory. May allow for decrease or elimination of steroid use.
   a. Assists with fistula improvement or healing.
   b. Side effects include marrow suppression, pancreatitis, hepatitis, and infections.
8. Antidiarrheals (Imodium, Lomotil, paregoric, codeine) decrease stool frequency in mild to moderate disease; use with caution.
9. Fish oil—may be used in maintaining remission. The side effects (diarrhea, flatulence, halitosis, heartburn) may limit patient use.

10. Miscellaneous drugs may include antispasmodics (Bentyl), bulking agents (Citrucel, Metamucil), or tricyclic antidepressants (Elavil, Pamelor) for treatment of abdominal pain.
11. Infliximab (Remicade)—new drug used in the treatment of this disease; a monoclonal antibody that blocks the activity of the inflammatory agent, tumor necrosis factor (TNF).
    a. It is indicated for moderate to severe disease not responding to traditional therapies or those with draining fistulae.
    b. Side effects may include infusion reactions (fever, chills, pruritus, or urticaria), cardiopulmonary reactions (chest pain, hypotension or hypertension, dyspnea), and infections (pneumonia, cellulitis, sepsis).

Surgery

Indicated only for the complications of Crohn's disease. Approximately 70% of Crohn's disease patients will eventually require one or more operations for relieving obstruction, closing fistulae, draining abscesses, repairing perforations, managing hemorrhage, or widening strictures. Depending on the individual patient, surgical options include:

1. Segmental bowel resection with anastomosis
2. Subtotal colectomy with ileorectal anastomosis
3. Total colectomy with ileostomy for severe disease in colon and rectum (see p. 590 for care of the ostomy patient).
4. Kock pouch and ileal reservoir–anal anastomosis are contraindicated in Crohn's patients. These procedures require the use of the small intestine in which Crohn's disease may develop.

Complications

1. Abscess (occurs in 20%), and fistulae (occur in 40%)
2. Strictures—may result from inflammation, edema, abscess, adhesions, but usually from fibrostenosis
3. Hemorrhage, bowel perforation, intestinal obstruction
4. Nutritional deficiencies: poor caloric intake due to food avoidance, malabsorption of bile salts and fat, vitamin B_{12} deficiency with ileal disease, short-gut syndrome after extensive surgical resections
5. Dehydration and electrolyte disturbances
6. Peritonitis and sepsis
7. Believed to have increased risk of small bowel and colorectal cancers

Nursing Assessment

1. Assess frequency and consistency of stools to evaluate volume losses and effectiveness of therapy.
2. Have the patient describe the location, severity, and onset of abdominal cramping or pain.
3. Ask the patient about weight loss and anorexia. Weigh daily to monitor changes.
4. Have the patient describe foods eaten to elicit dietary exacerbations
5. Determine if the patient smokes, including duration and amount.
6. Ask about family history of GI diseases.

Nursing Diagnoses

- Altered Nutrition: Less Than Body Requirements, related to pain, nausea
- Fluid Volume Deficit related to diarrhea
- Pain related to the inflammatory disease of the small intestine
- Ineffective Individual Coping related to feelings of rejection and embarrassment

Nursing Interventions
Achieving Adequate Nutritional Balance

1. Encourage diet that is low in residue, fiber, and fat and high in calories, protein, and carbohydrates, with vitamin and mineral supplements.
2. Monitor weight daily.
3. Provide small, frequent feedings to prevent distention.
4. Have patient participate in meal planning to encourage compliance and increase knowledge.
5. Prepare patient for elemental diet or TPN if the patient is debilitated.

Maintaining Fluid and Electrolyte Balance

1. Monitor intake and output.
2. Provide fluids as prescribed to maintain hydration (1,000 mL/24 hours is minimum intake to meet body fluid needs).
3. Monitor stool frequency and consistency.
4. Monitor electrolytes (especially potassium) and acid–base balance, because diarrhea can lead to metabolic acidosis.
5. Watch for cardiac dysrhythmias and muscle weakness due to loss of electrolytes.

Controlling Pain

1. Administer medications for control of inflammatory process, as prescribed.
2. Observe and record changes in pain—frequency, location, characteristics, precipitating events, and duration.
3. Monitor for distention, increased temperature, hypotension, and rectal bleeding—all signs of obstruction due to the inflammation.
4. Clean rectal area, and apply ointments as necessary to decrease discomfort from skin breakdown.
5. Prepare patient for surgery if response to medical and drug therapy is unsatisfactory.
6. Surgery is determined specifically for each patient.
7. Recurrence of the disease is possible after surgery.

Providing Psychosocial Support

1. Offer understanding, concern, and encouragement—this person is often embarrassed about frequent and malodorous stools and often is fearful of eating.
2. Facilitate supportive psychological counseling, if appropriate.

3. Encourage patient's usual support persons to be involved in management of the disease and seek additional support groups as needed.
4. Encourage health-promoting behavior.

Patient Education and Health Maintenance

1. Provide comprehensive education about anatomy and physiology of the GI system, the chronic disease process, drug therapy, potential complications, and potential surgery.
2. Instruct patient about all prescribed medications, including the purpose, dosage, and side effects, as well as to discuss use of any over-the-counter drugs with health care provider.
3. Encourage regular follow-up and to report signs of complications: increasing abdominal distention, cramping pain, diarrhea, malaise, anorexia, fever, and passing stool through urethra or vagina.
4. Explain the importance of adequate hydration and nutrition (based on individual tolerance) and monitoring weight.
5. Encourage patient to participate in stress-reducing activities such as exercise, relaxation techniques, music therapy.
6. For further information, have patient contact Crohn's & Colitis Foundation, 386 Park Avenue South, New York, NY 10016, 212-685-3440, *www.ccfa.org*.

Outcome-Based Evaluation

- Improved nutritional intake; weight stable
- Adequate fluid intake; no evidence of dehydration; electrolyte levels within normal limits
- Demonstrates relief of pain and symptoms manageable
- Verbalizes improved attitude toward ways to live with the disease

Colorectal Cancer

Colorectal cancer refers to malignancies of the colon and rectum. This type is the second most common visceral cancer in the United States. Colorectal tumors are nearly all adenocarcinomas. Lymphoma, carcinoid, melanoma, and sarcomas account for only 5% of colorectal lesions.

Pathophysiology and Etiology

1. Risk factors include:
   a. Age: risk increases sharply after age 40 with 90% of cases occurring in persons over age 50.
   b. Previous history of resected colorectal cancer.
   c. Family history of colorectal cancer is present in 25% of persons with colon cancer.
   d. Polyposis syndromes:
      (i) Villous polyps, adenomatous polyps carry malignant potential (especially if multiple or greater than 1 cm in size) and are routinely removed during colonoscopy. Persons with polyps need periodic colonoscopic surveillance.
      (ii) Familial adenomatous polyposis (FAP; also a variant called Gardner's syndrome) is an inherited condition characterized by multiple adenomatous polyps of the colon, in which cancer will inevitably develop in all affected individuals. This only accounts for less than 1% of colon cancer.
      (iii) Turcot syndrome—an inherited condition characterized by adenomatous polyps and the coexistence of a central nervous system malignant tumor, such as glioblastoma.
   e. Hereditary nonpolyposis colorectal cancer (HNPCC)—hereditary condition with a markedly increased risk of developing colorectal cancer as well as other cancers, such as endometrial, ovarian, renal, pancreatic, gastric, and small intestinal. There are few or no adenomatous polyps, and the bowel may undergo rapid change from normal tissue to polyp to cancer. Tends to develop at an average age of 44 years, and 70% arise most often in the right colon. Accounts for about 3% to 6% of all colorectal cancers. A thorough family history is essential for assessment of suspected HNPCC.
   f. Chronic ulcerative colitis—increasing risk after 10-year history.
   g. Incidence is higher in industrialized countries and lower in underdeveloped countries. Reason unclear but may be related to diet.
   h. Immunodeficiency disease.
2. Colorectal lesions occur most frequently in the rectum and sigmoid areas; however, it appears there is a trend toward increasing frequency of right-sided lesions.
3. Most adenocarcinomas are ulcerative in appearance. A left-sided lesion tends to be annular and scarlike; a right-sided lesion tends to be a cauliflowerlike mass that protrudes into the bowel lumen.
4. A lesion starts in the mucosal layers of the colonic wall and eventually penetrates the wall and invades surrounding structures and organs (bladder, prostate, ureters, vagina). Cancer spreads by direct invasion, lymphatic spread, and through the bloodstream. The liver and lungs are the most common metastatic sites.

Clinical Manifestations

Colorectal cancer is often asymptomatic. If present, symptomatology varies according to the location of the lesion and the extent of involvement.

1. Right-sided lesions—change in bowel habits, usually diarrhea; vague abdominal discomfort; black, tarry stools; anemia; weakness; weight loss; palpable mass in right lower quadrant.
2. Left-sided lesions—change in bowel habits, often increasing constipation with bouts of diarrhea due to partial obstruction; bright, streaked, red blood in stool; cramping pain; weight loss; anemia; palpable mass.
3. Rectal lesions—change in bowel habits with possibly urgent need to defecate, alternating constipation and di-

arrhea, and narrowed caliber of stool; bright red blood in stool; feeling of incomplete evacuation; rectal fullness progressing to dull constant ache.

Diagnostic Evaluation

1. Stool examination for blood (Hemoccult)—often reveals evidence of carcinoma when the patient is otherwise asymptomatic.
2. Colonoscopy with biopsy—diagnostic procedure of choice after strong suspicious clinical history or abnormal barium enema.
3. Pelvic MRI and endorectal ultrasonography provide information about cancer penetration and pararectal lymph nodes.
4. Carcinoembryonic antigen (CEA)—70% of patients have elevated CEA levels. The CEA level monitors possible recurrence or metastasis.
5. CT scan of abdomen, liver, lung, and brain may reveal metastatic disease.

Management

Blood Replacement

Administration of whole blood or packed red blood cells if severe anemia exists.

Surgical Resection

Treatment of choice for those with resectable lesions. Regional lymph node dissection determines staging and guides decisions regarding adjuvant therapy. Surgical options include:

1. Laparotomy with wide segmental bowel resection of tumor, including regional lymph nodes and blood vessels (right hemicolectomy, transverse colectomy, left hemicolectomy, or sigmoid resection).
2. Transanal excision—selected persons with tumors less than 3 cm and well differentiated less than 7.5 cm from the anal verge, and localized to the rectal wall may avoid laparotomy.
3. Low anterior resection for upper rectal lesions—may include temporary loop colostomy to protect anastomosis with second procedure for takedown of colostomy.
4. Abdominoperineal resection with permanent end colostomy for lower rectal lesions when adequate margins cannot be obtained, or there is involvement of anal sphincters. Due to improved stapling devices used deep in the pelvis, abdominoperineal resection accounts for fewer than 5% of most colorectal resections.
5. Temporary loop colostomy to decompress bowel and divert fecal stream, followed by later bowel resection, anastomosis, and takedown of colostomy.
6. More extensive surgery involving the removal of other organs if cancer has spread, such as liver wedge, bladder, uterus, and/or small intestine may be performed.
7. Unresectable colorectal cancer—diverting colostomy or ileostomy as palliation for obstructing tumor, laser fulguration, or the placement of an expandable wire stent.
8. Total proctocolectomy or ileal reservoir–anal anastomosis procedure for patients with FAP and chronic ulcerative colitis before colorectal cancer develops.

Radiation Therapy

1. May be used preoperatively to improve resectability of the tumor
2. May be used postoperatively as adjuvant therapy to treat residual disease

Chemotherapy

1. May be used as adjuvant therapy to improve survival time.
2. May be used for residual disease, recurrence of disease, unresectable tumors, and metastatic disease.
3. Drug combinations may include 5-fluorouracil plus levamisole or 5-fluorouracil plus leucovorin (Wellcovorin).

Complications

1. Obstruction
2. Hemorrhage
3. Anemia

Nursing Assessment

1. Interview patient regarding dietary habits and family and medical history to identify risk factors.
2. Question the patient regarding symptomatology of colorectal cancer, changes in bowel habits, rectal bleeding, tarry stools, abdominal discomfort, weight loss, weakness, and anemia.
3. Palpate abdomen for tenderness (usually not tender), presence of mass.
4. Test stool for occult blood.

Nursing Diagnoses

- Altered Nutrition: Less Than Body Requirements, related to malignancy effects and weight loss
- Constipation and/or Diarrhea related to change in bowel lumen
- Pain related to malignancy, inflammation, and possible intestinal obstruction
- Fatigue related to anemia, radiation, chemotherapy, and metastatic disease
- Fear related to diagnosis, prognosis, potential for complications

Nursing Interventions

Achieving Adequate Nutrition

1. Meet the patient's nutritional needs by serving a high-calorie, low-residue diet for several days before surgery, if condition permits.
2. Observe and record fluid losses, such as may be sustained by vomiting and diarrhea.
3. Maintain hydration through IV therapy, and record urinary output. Metabolic tissue needs are increased, and more fluids are needed to eliminate waste products.
4. Serve smaller meals spaced throughout the day to maintain adequate calorie and protein intake if not NPO.

5. Encourage patient to participate in meal planning to promote compliance.

6. Adjust diet before and after treatments, such as chemotherapy or radiation. Serve clear liquids, bland diet, or NPO, as prescribed.

7. Instruct patient to take prescribed antiemetic as needed, especially if receiving chemotherapy.

Relieving Constipation or Diarrhea

1. Monitor amount, consistency, frequency, and color of stool.

2. For constipation, use laxatives or enemas as needed, and encourage exercise and adequate fluid/fiber intake to promote bowel motility.

3. For diarrhea, encourage adequate fluid intake to prevent fluid volume deficit and electrolyte imbalance.

4. For diarrhea related to radiation or chemotherapy, administer antidiarrheal medications and discuss foods that may slow transit time of bowel, such as bananas, rice, peanut butter, and pasta.

NURSING ALERT

Antidiarrheal medications and foods to control diarrhea are contraindicated for the patient with an obstructing lesion. Use these measures only postoperatively after lesion resection for control of diarrhea related to cancer therapy.

Relieving Pain

1. Assess type and severity of pain, and administer analgesics as needed for pain.

2. Evaluate effectiveness of analgesic regimen.

3. Investigate different approaches, such as relaxation techniques, repositioning, imaging, laughter, music, reading, and touch for control or relief of pain.

Maintaining Energy Level

1. Institute an individualized activity plan after assessing patient's activity level and tolerance, noting shortness of breath or tachycardia.

2. Allow for frequent rest periods to regain energy.

3. Administer blood products, as ordered, if fatigue is related to severe anemia.

Minimizing Fear

1. Encourage patient and family to express feelings and fears together and separately.

2. Acknowledge that it is normal to have negative feelings toward cancer, surgery, colostomy, and treatment options.

3. Provide information and answer questions regarding disease process, treatment modalities, and complications. Offer diverse educational materials, such as brochures, videotapes.

4. Refer patient and family to the American Cancer Society (1-800-ACS-2345) for information about cancer support groups and classes.

5. Refer for counseling, if desired.

Community and Home Care Considerations

1. Colorectal cancer screening is recommended for all persons aged 50 or older with annual fecal occult blood testing (Hemoccult II) or flexible sigmoidoscopy or both.

2. Persons with positive fecal occult blood tests usually undergo colonoscopy with removal of polyps, if present.

3. Genetic testing can confirm a hereditary diagnosis such as FAP or HNPCC.

Patient Education and Health Maintenance

1. Provide detailed information or resources about treatment modalities of radiation and chemotherapy.

2. Teach and demonstrate to patient and/or family the skills necessary for colostomy management, which may include colostomy irrigation. The ostomy specialty nurse can provide formal education in this area.

3. Initiate a home care nursing referral to assist with wound care, to manage treatment side effects, and to continue teaching colostomy care.

Outcome-Based Evaluation

- Exhibits weight gain and improves nutritional status by adequate dietary intake
- Has regular soft bowel movements
- Minimal pain, controlled with analgesics or other techniques
- Able to perform activities of daily living with adequate amounts of energy; no shortness of breath on exertion
- Sleeping well; able to discuss feelings and fears related to surgery, prognosis, and treatment options

ANORECTAL CONDITIONS

Hemorrhoids

Hemorrhoids are vascular masses in the lower rectum or anus that have become loosened from connective tissue as a result of congestion in the veins of the hemorrhoidal plexus; external hemorrhoids appear outside the external sphincter, whereas internal hemorrhoids appear above the internal sphincter (Figure 18-8). When blood within the hemorrhoids becomes clotted due to obstruction, the hemorrhoids are referred to as thrombosed.

Pathophysiology and Etiology

1. Predisposing factors include:
   a. Pregnancy, prolonged sitting/standing
   b. Straining at stool, chronic constipation/diarrhea
   c. Anal infection, rectal surgery, or episiotomy
   d. Hereditary factor, alcoholism
   e. Portal hypertension (cirrhosis)
   f. Coughing, sneezing, vomiting
   g. Loss of muscle tone due to old age
   h. Anal intercourse

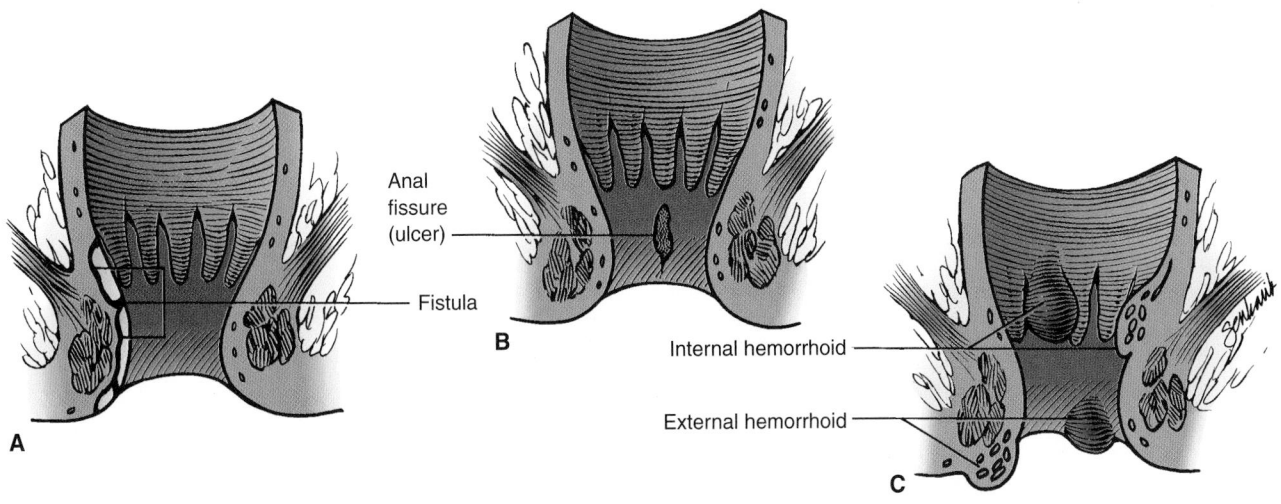

FIGURE 18-8 Various types of anal lesions. (**A**) Fistula. (**B**) Fissure. (**C**) External and internal hemorrhoids.

2. Increased intra-abdominal pressure causes engorgement in the vascular tissue lining the anal canal.
3. Loosening of vessels from surrounding connective tissue occurs with protrusion or prolapse into anal canal.

Clinical Manifestations
1. Sensation of incomplete fecal evacuation
2. Visible (if external) and palpable mass
3. Constipation, anal itching
4. Bleeding during defecation, bright red blood on stool due to injury of mucosa covering hemorrhoid
5. Infection or ulceration, mucus discharge
6. Pain noted more in external hemorrhoids
7. Sudden rectal pain due to thrombosis in external hemorrhoids

Diagnostic Evaluation
1. History and visualization by external examination and the use of an anoscope or proctoscope
2. Barium enema or sigmoidoscopy, to rule out more serious colonic lesions causing rectal bleeding

Management
Asymptomatic hemorrhoids require no treatment.
Medical
1. Bowel habits should be regulated with nonirritating stool softeners and high-fiber diet to keep stools soft.
2. Frequent, warm sitz baths to ease pain and combat swelling.
3. Insertion of soothing anal suppository two to three times daily.
4. Application of witch hazel compresses for comfort.
5. Control of itching by improved anal hygiene measures and control of moisture.

6. Do not use topical anesthetics chronically on hemorrhoids or fissures, because they often produce hypersensitive (allergic) perianal skin rashes with severe itching.
7. Manual reduction of external hemorrhoids if prolapsed.
8. Injection of sclerosing solutions to produce scar tissue and decrease prolapse.
9. Cryodestruction—freezing of hemorrhoids.
   a. Reported to be less painful.
   b. Some patients have a foul-smelling discharge for about a week to 10 days after cryosurgery.

Surgical
1. Surgery may be indicated when the following conditions exist:
   a. Prolonged bleeding
   b. Disabling pain
   c. Intolerable itching
   d. General unrelieved discomfort
2. Ligation with a rubber band is treatment of choice.
   a. A large anoscope is used; the apex of the internal hemorrhoid is grasped and drawn through a double-sleeved cylinder.
   b. An elastic band is loaded on the inner cylinder and released by a trigger device so the band encircles the base of the hemorrhoid.
   c. After a period of time, the hemorrhoid sloughs away.
3. Dilatation of the anal canal and lower rectum under general anesthesia is another treatment.
   a. This procedure is not advocated for patients whose main complaints are prolapse or incontinence.
   b. It also is not recommended for aging patients with weak sphincters.
4. Incision and removal of clot from acutely thrombosed hemorrhoid.
5. Hemorrhoidectomy—excision of internal/external hemorrhoids.

TABLE 18-4 Anorectal Disorders

Condition	Etiology	Clinical Manifestations	Management	Nursing Considerations
Fissure: Linear laceration of anal epithelium; typically located in the posterior midline.	1. Constipated stools may tear anal lining 2. Perineum strain during childbirth 3. Tuberculosis, syphilis, Crohn's disease may be cause	Tearing acute pain during and after bowel movement; spotting of bright red blood with stool; possibly spasm of anal canal; burning/discomfort may continue for several hours after bowel movement	1. Promotion of regular, soft bowel movements through bran, psyllium, stool softeners, suppositories 2. Fissurectomy 3. Lateral internal sphincterotomy	1. Assist with warm sitz baths and local application of anesthetic ointment to reduce pain 2. Instruct to eat high-fiber foods and drink fluids to prevent constipation
Abscess: Localized area of pus from inflammation of anorectal tissue	1. Infection develops from abrasion from foreign object, such as enema tip or fishbone 2. Acute phase of anal fistula, suspect Crohn's disease 3. Tuberculosis or actinomycosis	Painful, reddened bulge or swelling near anus; pain increases with sitting; moderate to severe pain; pus may drain	1. Incision and drainage of purulent exudate 2. Placement of drainage catheter for 7–10 days; possible packing dressing 3. Warm sitz baths	1. Wound assessment 2. Pain medications as needed 3. Alert for passage of bowel movements, postoperatively
Fistula: Abnormal tubelike passage from skin near anus into anal canal	1. Often preceded by anal abscess 2. May be associated with inflammatory bowel disease, cancer, or foreign body 3. Hidradenitis suppurativa	Purulent drainage from opening; itching and pain	1. Fistulotomy 2. Fistulectomy 3. Bowel rest to allow fistula to heal; possible fecal diversion temporarily	1. Wound assessment 2. Pain medications as needed 3. Alert for passage of bowel movement postoperatively
Anal Condylomas (venereal warts)	1. Infectious cauliflower-like papillomas; probably sexually transmitted papillomavirus 2. Differentiate from syphilitic warts, hemorrhoids, and anal/skin cancers	1. Thrive in moist, macerated surfaces, as with purulent drainage 2. Often recur 3. Rarely invade urethra, bladder, or rectum	1. Application of podophyllum resin (may be painful) 2. Electrofulguration 3. Alpha-interferon injections/ synergistic with podophyllum resin 4. Fluorouracil	1. Encourage good anal hygiene and frequent use of talc dusting powder 2. Schedule follow-up visits to assess area periodically for recurrence
Proctitis: Acute or chronic inflammation of rectal mucosa	1. Common infecting organisms are *Neisseria gonorrhoeae*, *Chlamydia*, herpes simplex virus, *Treponema pallidum*	1. Anorectal pain; purulent or bloody discharge; constipation; tenesmus 2. Often seen in homosexual men	Treatment specific to isolated organism	Explain rectal procedures and assist with examination and treatment
Stricture: Narrowing of the anorectal lumen, preventing dilation of sphincter	1. Usually results from scarring after anorectal surgery (hemorrhoidectomy) or inflammation 2. Status postradiation to pelvic area	1. Constipation, ribbon stools, pain with passage of bowel movements; may not completely evacuate stools; itching	1. Treatment of inflammatory cause 2. Dilation by digital, instrumentation, or balloon methods 3. If stenosis severe, may need plastic surgery to anal canal	1. Prevention of stenosis after anal surgery facilitated by anal hygiene, warm sitz baths, and dilation 2. Postoperative care includes stool softeners, warm sitz baths, and wound care
Rectal prolapse: Mucosal membrane protrudes through anus	1. The support structures are weakened (sphincters and muscles) leading to rectal intussusception 2. Conditions may include neurologic disorders, chronic diseases, aging	1. Associated with constipation and straining; rectal fullness; bloody diarrhea; rectal ulcer secondary to intussusception	1. Treatment depends on underlying cause 2. Sclerosing agent injection may fix rectum in place 3. Surgery may include sphincter repair or resection of prolapsed tissue	1. Diet/fluid instructions to avoid constipation 2. Teach perineum-strengthening exercises

Complications
1. Hemorrhage, anemia
2. Incontinence
3. Prolapse and strangulation

Nursing Interventions and Patient Education
1. After thrombosis or surgery, assist with frequent positioning, using pillow support for comfort.
2. Provide analgesics, warm sitz baths, or warm compresses to reduce pain and inflammation.
3. Apply witch hazel dressing to perianal area or anal creams or suppositories, if ordered, to relieve discomfort.
4. Observe anal area postoperatively for drainage and bleeding; report if excessive.
5. Administer stool softener/laxative to assist with bowel movements soon after surgery, to reduce risk of stricture.
6. Encourage regular exercise, high-fiber diet, and adequate fluid intake (8 to 10 glasses/day) to avoid straining and constipation.
7. Discourage regular use of laxatives—firm, soft stools dilate the anal canal, decreasing stricture formation.
8. Determine patient's normal bowel habits, and identify predisposing factors in order to educate patient about changes necessary to prevent recurrence of symptoms.

■ Other Conditions of the Anorectum
See Table 18-4.

SELECTED REFERENCES
Breitfeller, J. M. (1999). Peritonitis. *American Journal of Nursing, 99* (4), 33.

Brenner, H., Rothenbacher, D., Bode, G., & Adler, G. (1997). Relation of smoking and alcohol and coffee consumption to active *Helicobacter pylori* infection: Cross sectional study. *British Medical Journal, 315* (7121), 1489–1492.

Cavalieri, J., & Franklin, B. (1998). Hereditary nonpolyposis colon cancer. *American Journal of Nursing, 98* (10), 42–43.

Claussen, J. (1999). Gastroesophageal reflux disease: A rational approach to management. *Clinician Reviews, 9* (6), 69–82.

Cupp, M. (1999). Herbal remedies: Adverse effects and drug interactions. *American Family Physician, 59* (5), 239.

Dambro, M., & Griffith, J. (1999). *Griffith's 5 minute clinical consult* (7th ed.). Baltimore: Williams & Wilkins.

Goldsmith, C. (1998). Gastroesophageal reflux disease. *American Journal of Nursing, 98* (9), 44–45.

Gondzur, N., Morse, T., & Schlossberg, N. (1998). *Gastroenterology nursing.* St. Louis: Mosby, Inc.

Gruber, M., & Lance, P. (1998). Colorectal cancer detection and screening. *Primary Care Practice, 2* (4), 369–376.

Hilsden, R. J., Scott, C. M., & Verhoef, M. J. (1998). Complimentary medicine use by patients with inflammatory bowel disease. *American Journal of Gastroenterology, 93,* 697.

Hull, T. L., & Erwin-Toth, P. (1996). The pelvic pouch procedure and continent ostomies: Overview and controversies. *WOCNJ, 23* (3), 156–170.

Hyman, N. H. (1997). Anorectal disease: How to relieve pain and improve other symptoms. *Geriatrics, 52* (4), 75–77.

Kim, E. C., & Dundon, M. (1998). Medical and psychological aspects of irritable bowel syndrome. *Primary Care Practice, 2* (4), 329–340.

Laine, L., Estrada, R., Trujillo, M., et al. (1998). Effect of proton-pump inhibitor therapy on diagnostic testing for *Helicobacter pylori. Annals of Internal Medicine, 129,* 547–550.

Margolin, D. A., & Beck, D. E. (1997). Surgical therapy for ulcerative colitis. *Ostomy Quarterly, 34* (1), 36–40:

McQuaid, K. (1999). *Current medical diagnosis & treatment* (38th ed.). Los Altos, CA: Lange.

Ng, E. K. W, et al. (2000). Eradication of *Helicobacter pylori* prevents recurrence of ulcer after simple closure of duodenal ulcer perforation: Randomized control trial. *Annals of Surgery, 231*(2), 153–158.

Norton, B. (1998). Crohn's disease. *Advance for Nurse Practitioners, 6* (9), 42–50 .

O'Hara, M., Kiefer, W., Farrell, K., & Kemper, K. (1998). A review of 12 commonly used medicinal herbs. *Archives of Family Medicine, 7* (3), 536.

Pramik, M. J. (1999). Gutting IBD. *Drug Topics, 143* (2), 43–51.

Present, D. H., Rutgeerts, P., Targan, S., et al. (1999). Infliximab for the treatment of fistulas in patients with Crohn's disease. *New England Journal of Medicine, 337,* 1029.

Salcedo, J., & Al-Kawas, F. (1998). Treatment of *Helicobacter pylori* infection. *Archives of Internal Medicine, 158,* 842–851.

Schatzkin, A., et al. (2000). Lack of effect of low-fat, high-fiber diet on the recurrence of colorectal adenomas. *New England Journal of Medicine, 342*(8), 1149–1155.

Schmeller, E. (1998). Traveler's diarrhea. *Clinician Reviews, 8* (6), 71–83.

Schoenfeld, P. S. (1998). Acid peptic diseases in the era of *Helicobacter pylori. Primary Care Practice, 2* (4), 358–368.

Slattery, M. L., Edwards, S. L., Boucher, K. M., Anderson, K., & Caan, B. J. (1999). Lifestyle and colon cancer: An assessment of factors associated with risk. *American Journal of Epidemiology, 150*(8), 869–877.

Sonnenberg, A., Schwartz, S., Cutter, A., Vakil, N., & Bloom, B. (1998). Cost savings in duodenal ulcer therapy through *Helicobacter pylori* eradication compared with conventional therapies. *Archives of Internal Medicine, 158,* 852–860.

Swearingen, P., & Ross, D. (1999). *Manual of medical-surgical nursing care.* St. Louis: Mosby.

Tierney, L., McPhee, S., & Papadaris, M. (1997). *Current medical diagnosis & treatment* (36th ed.). Englewood Cliffs, NJ: Appleton & Lange.

Timby, B. (1996). *Fundamental skills and concepts in patient care* (6th ed.). Philadelphia: J. B. Lippincott.

Tobillo, E., & Schwartz, S. (1998). Acute diarrhea. *Advance for Nurse Practitioners, 6* (10), 39–44.

Tucker, K., & Schumann, L. (1999). Gastroesophageal reflux disease. *The Clinical Advisor, 52*–58.

Winslow, L., & Kroll, D. (1998). Herbs as medicines. *Archives of Internal Medicine, 158,* 2192–2199.

Hepatic, Biliary, and Pancreatic Disorders

ASSESSMENT

◼ Assessment of Accessory Organ Dysfunction

The liver, the gallbladder and its bile ducts, and the pancreas are called accessory glands in the gastrointestinal (GI) system. Their function is to aid digestion through the delivery of enzymes to the small intestine. The liver plays additional roles in detoxification of chemicals and synthesis and storage of important nutrients. The pancreas also functions as an endocrine gland, as discussed in Chapter 25.

Major liver, biliary, and pancreatic problems can be differentiated by characterization of manifestations and through history taking and physical examination.

Common Manifestations
1. Jaundice—any yellow color of sclerae and skin, pruritus, dark tea-colored urine, light gray or clay-colored (acholic) stools?
2. Any dyspepsia, anorexia, nausea, vomiting, right upper quadrant or epigastric pain, or pain radiating to the back or shoulder blade? What is the relationship of pain to eating or to position?
3. Has there been fatigue, malaise, loss of vigor and strength, easy bruising, or weight loss?
4. Any fever, chills, headache, myalgias, arthralgias, photophobia?
5. Any steatorrhea—stools that are loose, greasy, foamy, foul in odor, and that float?

History
1. Have there been recent blood transfusions? Are there known blood disorders? Gastrointestinal bleeding?
2. Has there been contact with a person who has an infection, such as hepatitis? Any unprotected sexual activity or ingestion of potentially contaminated food?
3. Has there been drug or chemical toxicity, such as carbon tetrachloride, chloroform, phosphorus, arsenicals, ethanol, halothane (Fluothane), isoniazid (INH), or acetaminophen (Tylenol)? Have Amanita mushrooms been ingested recently? Are certain medications being taken, such as phenothiazine derivatives, sulfonamides, antidiabetic drugs, propylthiouracil (PTU), monoamine oxidase inhibitors, methyldopa (Aldomet), Imuran, corticosteroids, thiazide diuretics, estrogens, valproic acid, or didanosine (DDI), a nucleoside reverse transcriptase inhibitor to treat HIV infection?
4. Is there a history of nonsterile needle puncture?
5. Does medical history include gallstone(s), hepatitis, pancreatitis, Wilson's disease, Budd-Chiari syndrome, liver surgery, or transplantation?
6. Any family history of gallstones, pancreatitis, gallbladder or pancreatic cancer?
7. How much alcohol, if any, is or has been ingested during the years?

Physical Examination Findings
1. Skin—yellow sclerae or skin? Rashes or scratches on body from severe scratching because of pruritus? Any signs of bruising or petechiae on body, palmar erythema, or overt bleeding?
2. Abdomen—any tenderness or liver enlargement in the right upper quadrant? Any ascites? Any palpable masses in the abdomen?
3. Peripheral vascular—any edema, anasarca or telangiectasia?

4. Neurologic—what is the level of consciousness? Any asterixis (flapping tremor elicited when the arms are extended and wrists dorsiflexed)?

DIAGNOSTIC TESTS

Laboratory Tests
See Table 19-1, Liver Diagnostic Studies.

CA 19-9
Description
A tumor antigen found in serum; used as a marker for pancreatic cancer
Nursing and Patient Care Considerations
1. Tell patient a blood test will be taken and the results will be ready in 1 to 3 days.

2. Not a screening test for pancreatic cancer, this is an adjunct with other tests to provide support for a diagnosis of pancreatic cancer and to better measure the recurrence of pancreatic cancer after treatment.
3. Acute pancreatitis also causes elevated levels of the antigen.

Radiology and Imaging
Hepatobiliary Scan
Description
A noninvasive nuclear medicine study (also referred to as a HIDA scan based on isotope used) using radioactive materials to aid in the diagnoses of hepatobiliary disorders, such as common bile duct obstruction, acute and chronic cholecystitis, bile leaks, biliary dyskinesia, biliary atresia, and liver transplant function.

TABLE 19-1 Liver Diagnostic Studies

Test and Purpose	Normal	Clinical and Nursing Significance
Bile Formation and Secretion		
1. *Serum bilirubin (van den Bergh's reaction)* Measures bilirubin in the blood; this determines the ability of the liver to take up, conjugate, and excrete bilirubin. Bilirubin is a product of the breakdown of hemoglobin.		
Direct (conjugated)—soluble in water	0–5.1 µmol/L	Abnormal in biliary and liver disease, causing jaundice clinically.
Indirect (unconjugated)—insoluble in water	0–14 µmol/L	Abnormal in hemolysis and in functional disorders of uptake or conjugation.
Total serum bilirubin	1.7–20.5 µmol/L	
2. *Urine bilirubin* Not normally found in urine, but if direct serum bilirubin is elevated, some spills into urine.	None (0)	Mahogany-colored urine; when specimen is shaken, yellow-tinted foam can be observed. Confirm with Ictotest tablet or dipstick. If phenazopyridine (Pyridium) is being taken, there may be a false-positive bilirubin result. (Mark laboratory slip if this medication is being taken.)
3. *Urobilinogen* Formed in small intestine by action of bacteria on bilirubin. Related to amount of bilirubin excreted into bile.	Urine urobilinogen up to 0.09–4.23 µmol/24 hr. Fecal urobilinogen 0.068–0.34 mmol/24 hr	Urine specimen is collected over 2-h period after lunch. Place specimen in dark brown container and send it to laboratory immediately to prevent decomposition. If the patient is receiving antimicrobials, mark laboratory slip to this effect, as production of urobilinogen can be falsely reduced.
Protein Studies		
1. *Albumin and globulin measurement* Is of greater significance than total protein measurement		As one increases, the other decreases; hence,
Albumin—produced by liver cells	35–55 g/L	Albumin ↓ cirrhosis chronic hepatitis
Globulin—produced in lymph nodes, spleen, and bone marrow and Kupffer's cells of liver	15–30 g/L	Globulin ↑ cirrhosis chronic obstructive jaundice viral hepatitis
Total serum protein	60–80 g/L	
2. *Prothrombin time (PT)* Prothrombin and other clotting factors are manufactured in the liver; its rate is influenced by the supply of vitamin K.	100% of control	Prothrombin time may be prolonged in liver disease, in which case it will not return to normal with vitamin K. It may also be prolonged in malabsorption of fat and fat-soluble vitamins, in which case it will return to normal with vitamin K.

(continued)

TABLE 19-1 Liver Diagnostic Studies (Continued)

Test and Purpose	Normal	Clinical and Nursing Significance
Fat Metabolism		
1. *Cholesterol* It is possible to measure lipid metabolism by determining serum cholesterol levels.	3.90–6.50 mmol/L Esters = 60% of total	Serum cholesterol level is decreased in parenchymal liver disease. Serum lipid level is increased in biliary obstruction.
Liver Detoxification		
1. *Serum alkaline phosphatase* Because bile disposes this enzyme, any impairment of liver cell excretory function will cause an elevation. In cholestasis or obstruction, increased synthesis of enzyme causes very high levels in blood.	20–90 U/L at 30°C	*Abnormalities:* The level is elevated to more than 3 times normal in obstructive jaundice, intrahepatic cholestasis, liver metastasis, or granulomas. Also elevated in osteoblastic diseases, Paget's disease, and hyperparathyroidism.
Enzyme Production		
1. Aspartate aminotransferase or AST (formerly SGOT)	4.8–19 U/L	An elevation in these enzymes indicates liver cell damage.
2. Alanine aminotransferase or ALT (formerly SGPT)	2.4–7 U/L	**Note:** Opiates may also cause a rise in AST and ALT.
3. Lactic dehydrogenase (LDH)	80–192 U/L	Aspirin may cause an increase or decrease in AST and ALT.
4. Gamma glutamyl transpeptidase (GGT)	0–30 U/L at 30°C	Enzyme found in liver, kidney, heart, pancreas, spleen, brain. An elevation confirms hepatic involvement in elevated alkaline phosphatase.
5. Ammonia (serum)	11.1–67.0 μmol/L	Ammonia levels rise when the liver is unable to convert them to urea.
6. Bile acids radioimmunoassay (after cholecystokinin stimulation) Total Chenodeoxycholic acid Cholic acid Deoxycholic acid Lithocholic acid	35.0–148.0 mmol/L 10.0–61.4 mmol/L 6.8–81.0 mmol/L 2.0–18.0 mmol/L 0.8–2.0 mmol/L	Elevated serum bile acids are seen in hepatic diseases.

SGOT: serum glutamic oxaloacetic transaminase; SGPT: serum glutamic pyruvic transaminase.

Nursing and Patient Care Considerations

1. The patient should have nothing by mouth (NPO) at least 4 hours before the procedure.
2. If possible, no opiates should be administered for at least 4 hours before the procedure.
3. Tell the patient that scan time may be up to 4 hours, and that additional images may need to be taken up to 24 hours later.

Oral Cholecystography
Description

Oral iodide-containing contrast medium excreted by the liver and concentrated in the gallbladder is administered to assist in the radiographic examination of the gallbladder to detect gallstones and to assess the ability of the gallbladder to fill, concentrate its contents, contract, and empty.

Nursing and Patient Care Considerations

1. Assess for any allergies to iodine, seafood, or contrast media.
2. Administer or teach self-administration of contrast medium 10 to 12 hours before the x-ray study, usually the evening before.
3. Instruct patient to remain NPO after taking the contrast medium to prevent contraction and emptying of the gallbladder.
4. Explain that a repeat study may be necessary if the gallbladder is not visualized on the first attempt.
5. Should not be performed on jaundiced patients, because the liver cannot excrete the dye into the gallbladder.

Endoscopic Retrograde Cholangiopancreatography (ERCP)
Description

1. Endoscopic visualization of the common bile, pancreatic, and hepatic ducts with a flexible fiberoptic endoscope inserted into the esophagus, passed through the stomach and into the duodenum.
2. The common bile duct and the pancreatic duct are cannulated and contrast medium is injected into the ducts, permitting visualization and radiographic evaluation.
3. Done to detect extrahepatic biliary obstruction, such as stones, tumors of the bile duct, strictures or injuries to the bile duct; intrahepatic biliary obstruction caused by stones or tumor; and pancreatic disease, such as chronic pancreatitis, pseudocyst, or tumor.

4. May be combined with a therapeutic biliary or pancreatic procedure, such as endoscopic sphincterotomy, placement of biliary or pancreatic stents, tissue biopsy or fluid cytology, or retrieval of retained gallstones.

Nursing and Patient Care Considerations

Preprocedure

1. Assess for any allergies to iodine, seafood, or contrast media.
2. The patient must be NPO at least 4 hours before the procedure.
3. Ensure that dentures are removed; instruct patient to gargle and swallow topical anesthetic to decrease gag reflex, as ordered.
4. Verify that patient has a signed informed consent before sedation is given.
5. Establish baseline vital signs.
6. Establish intravenous (IV) access.
7. Administer antibiotic prophylaxis as ordered.

Postprocedure

1. Monitor and document vital signs.
2. Observe for and report abdominal distention and signs of perforation, gastrointestinal bleeding or possible pancreatitis, including chills, fever, pain, vomiting, tachycardia. Notify the physician immediately.
3. Maintain NPO status until gag reflex returns. Check for gag reflex by applying gentle pressure on a tongue depressor placed on the back of the tongue.

Endoscopic Ultrasound (EUS)

Description

A high-frequency ultrasound probe is placed at the tip of an endoscope to assess the pancreas through the gastrointestinal lumen. This helps to provide images of the pancreas and adjacent organs. It is useful in staging pancreatic tumors; establishing the size of the tumor, its extension into adjacent structures, local and regional nodal involvement, and any blood vessels that may be involved. Tissue may also be obtained by fine needle aspiration through EUS-guidance to confirm the diagnosis of a pancreatic malignancy.

Nursing and Patient Care Considerations

Preprocedure

1. The same as for ERCP.
2. Instruct the patient that tissue may be obtained for analysis.
3. Verify the patient has a signed informed consent for the procedure and tissue aspiration before sedation is given.

Postprocedure

The same as for ERCP.

Magnetic Resonance Cholangiopancreatography (MRCP)

Description

A noninvasive radiologic technique that produces images of the pancreatic ducts and biliary tree that are similar in appearance to those obtained from an ERCP. MRCP does not require the administration of any contrast material and provides ideal imaging for patients with allergies to iodine-based contrast materials.

Nursing and Patient Care Considerations

Preprocedure

1. Confirm that the patient does not have a pacemaker because the magnetic field could cause pacer malfunction.
2. Confirm that the patient does not have any metal hardware in or on the body, such as artificial joint replacements or steel sutures, because this will cause artifact and a distorted picture from the magnetic pull by the metal.
3. Remove all metal attachments from the patient, such as watch, rings, IV poles, and infusion devices.
4. The patient must be NPO at least 4 hours before the procedure.
5. Inform the patient that the test takes about 10 to 30 minutes.

Postprocedure

Patient may resume usual activities.

Percutaneous Transhepatic Cholangiography (PTC)

Description

1. Fluoroscopic examination of the intrahepatic and extrahepatic biliary ducts after injection of contrast medium into the biliary tree through percutaneous needle injection.
2. Helps to distinguish obstructive jaundice caused by liver disease from jaundice caused by biliary obstruction, such as from a tumor, injury to the common bile duct, stones within the bile ducts, or sclerosing cholangitis.
3. A biliary catheter may be placed during the procedure to drain the biliary tree, called percutaneous transhepatic biliary drainage (PTBD). This relieves jaundice, decreases pruritus, improves nutritional status, allows easy access into the biliary tree for further procedures, and can be used as an anatomic landmark and stent at the time of surgery.

Nursing and Patient Care Considerations

Preprocedure

1. Assess for allergies to iodine, seafood, or contrast media to determine need to be premedicated with antihistamines and steroids to prevent reaction.
2. The patient must be NPO at least 4 hours before the procedure.
3. Verify that patient has a signed informed consent before sedatives are given.
4. Establish baseline hemoglobin and hematocrit.
5. Ensure prothrombin time is within normal limits
6. Establish baseline vital signs
7. Establish IV line.
8. Administer antibiotic prophylaxis as ordered.

Postprocedure

1. Monitor and document vital signs and assess puncture site for bleeding, hematoma, or bile leakage.
2. Check for and report signs of peritonitis from bile leaking into the abdomen: fever, chills, diffuse abdominal

pain, tenderness, distention, or cholangitis (infection in the biliary tree) from bacteria in the bile being released into the GI tract and then into the blood stream.

3. Continue antibiotic prophylaxis per protocol.
4. If the patient has a PTBD, monitor catheter exit site for bleeding or bile drainage and monitor drainage in bile bag for color, amount, and consistency. The drainage initially may have some blood mixed with bile but should clear within a few hours. Remember the liver makes 700–1000 ml of bile in 24 hours and there should be adequate drainage when bile is draining into a bile bag (called external drainage).
   a. Report frank blood and/or blood clots that appear in the bile bag.
   b. Large amounts of bile drainage may require fluid replacement.
   c. Maintain patency and security of biliary catheter; perform routine care and dressing at catheter exit site.
   d. Perform routine flushing of biliary catheter per order.

NURSING ALERT

Do not aspirate from a PTBD catheter, because this draws bacteria from the bowel back through the liver and may cause cholangitis. Gently push solution into the PTBD catheter to prevent increased pressure within the biliary tree.

---

   e. Cap off end of biliary catheter to allow internal drainage of bile, if indicated. Teach patient the care and flushing of biliary catheter and signs of complications, if indicated.
5. Signs of complications include fever, chills, jaundice, inability to flush the catheter, bleeding from the catheter, leakage around the exit site of the catheter, dislodgment of the catheter.

Other Diagnostic Tests

Liver Biopsy

Description

Sampling of liver tissue through needle aspiration to establish a diagnosis of liver disease through histologic study.

Nursing and Patient Care Considerations

Preprocedure

1. Establish baseline hemoglobin and hematocrit.
2. Ensure that prothrombin time is within normal limits.
3. Verify informed consent.
4. Establish baseline vital signs.
5. Tell patient that cooperation in holding breath for about 10 seconds during the procedure is important to obtain biopsy without damaging the diaphragm.

Postprocedure

1. Position patient on right side with pillow supporting lower rib cage for several hours.
2. Check vital signs and observe biopsy site frequently for bleeding or drainage.
3. Report increasing pulse, decreasing blood pressure, increasing pain, and apprehension, which may indicate hemorrhage.

GENERAL PROCEDURES AND TREATMENT MODALITIES

Cholecystectomy

Cholecystectomy is surgical removal of the gallbladder for acute and chronic cholecystitis. It is one of the most frequent surgical procedures, with more than 600,000 performed each year in the United States.

Procedure

1. Open laparotomy—gallbladder removed after making an abdominal incision.
2. Laparoscopy—gallbladder removed from a small opening just above the umbilicus by the use of a laparoscope for viewing.
3. Three other small punctures are made in the abdomen to place other special instruments used to assist in the manipulation and removal of the gallbladder.
4. The organs in the abdomen can be viewed through the laparoscope and via a television monitor through a camera attached to the laparoscope.
5. If the patient is scheduled for a laparoscopic cholecystectomy, consent is also obtained for a traditional open cholecystectomy in case the gallbladder is not accessible through the laparoscopic technique.
6. After cholecystectomy, bile ducts will eventually dilate to accommodate the volume of bile once held by the gallbladder to aid in the digestion of fats.

Preoperative Management

1. IV fluids are given before surgery to improve hydration status if the patient has been vomiting.
2. Antibiotics are ordered for acute cholecystitis.
3. The patient is educated about the procedure and what to expect postoperatively.
4. Patient must remain NPO from midnight the night before surgery and must void before surgery.

Postoperative Management

1. Postoperatively, the patient is evaluated for:
   a. Vital signs, level of consciousness.
   b. Level of pain.
   c. Wound appearance: wound drain or T-tube patency, security and drainage (if present).
   d. Intake and output.
2. Early ambulation is encouraged to prevent thromboembolus, to facilitate voiding, and to stimulate peristalsis.
3. Complications to assess for include incisional infection, hemorrhage, and bile duct injury (persistent pain, fever, abdominal distention, nausea, anorexia, or jaundice).

Nursing Diagnoses

- Pain Related to surgical procedure
- Risk for Infection related to surgical procedure
- Impaired Skin Integrity related to surgical procedure
- Altered Nutrition: Less Than Body Requirements related to surgical procedure, wound pain, or T-tube drainage

Nursing Interventions
Relieving Pain
1. Assess pain location, level, and characteristics.
2. Administer prescribed pain medications or monitor patient-controlled analgesia.
3. Encourage splinting of incision when moving.
4. Encourage ambulation as soon as prescribed to decrease flatus and abdominal distention and to promote bowel motility.
5. Instruct patient that usual activities can usually be resumed within 5 to 7 days after laparoscopic cholecystectomy or within 4 to 6 weeks of open cholecystectomy.
   a. Sexual activity may be resumed when pain has abated.
   b. Obtain specific instructions for wound care, activity such as heavy lifting, strenuous activity, showers and tub baths, and driving per surgeon's protocol.

Preventing Infection
1. Assess wound dressings for any increased or purulent drainage.
2. Assess wound drain or T-tube site for any drainage, and note amount, color, and odor.
3. Assess bile drainage from T-tube into bile bag:
   a. Report any decrease in drainage.
   b. Maintain T-tube patency and security.
4. Report right upper quadrant pain, abdominal distention, fever, chills, or jaundice because this may indicate a bile duct injury.
5. Administer antibiotics as prescribed.
6. Encourage use of incentive spirometer, coughing and deep breathing, and ambulation to decrease risk of pulmonary infection.

Maintaining Skin Integrity
1. Assess wounds for healing.
2. Perform wound care as prescribed.
3. Assess for adequate hydration.
4. Tell the patient to keep the incision or wound sites dry for 5 to 7 days and to report any signs of redness, pain, or drainage.

Providing Adequate Nutrition
1. Assess for nausea and vomiting and administer antiemetics as prescribed.
2. Encourage fluid intake and advance to regular diet as tolerated.
3. Administer replacement fluids for bile drainage from T-tube if indicated.
4. Clamp T-tube when indicated and assess tolerance of food and color of stools.

Patient Education and Health Maintenance
1. Teach patient and family that rapid postoperative recovery should be expected.
2. Advise patient and family to notify the surgeon immediately of any subtle change in a patient's postoperative course or persistent symptoms. A bile duct injury should always be suspected after a laparoscopic cholecystectomy in patients who do not show the expected recovery during the early postoperative period.

3. Advise patient to advance diet as tolerated. Fats can be taken as tolerated, because the bile ducts dilate to accommodate storage of bile as needed.

Outcome-Based Evaluation
- Verbalizes decreased pain
- No fever or no signs of infection
- Wound healing without drainage
- Tolerating fluids and small solid feedings

HEPATIC DISORDERS

Functions of the liver include:
- Storage of vitamins A, B, D; iron; and copper.
- Synthesis of plasma proteins, including albumin and globulins.
- Synthesis of the clotting factors vitamin K and prothrombin.
- Storage of glycogen and synthesis of glucose from other nutrients (gluconeogenesis).
- Breakdown of fatty acids for energy.
- Production of bile.
- Detoxification and excretion of waste products.

▪ Hepatitis
Hepatitis is a viral infection of the liver associated with a broad spectrum of clinical manifestations from asymptomatic infection through icteric hepatitis to hepatic necrosis. Five types of hepatitis virus have been identified.

Pathophysiology and Etiology
Type A Hepatitis (HAV)
1. Hepatitis A is caused by an RNA virus of the enterovirus family.
2. Mode of transmission is primarily fecal-oral, usually through the ingestion of food or liquids contaminated with the virus.
   a. Prevalent in underdeveloped countries or in instances of overcrowding and poor sanitation.
   b. Infected food handler can spread the disease, and people can contract it by consuming water or shellfish from contaminated waters.
   c. Commonly spread by person-to-person contact and rarely by blood transfusion.
3. Incubation period is 3 to 5 weeks, with the average being 4 weeks.
4. Occurrence is worldwide, usually among children and young adults.
5. Mortality is 0% to 1%, with recovery the rule.

Type B Hepatitis (HBV)
1. Hepatitis B is a double-shelled particle containing DNA. This particle is composed of the following:
   a. HBcAg—hepatitis B core antigen (antigenic material in an inner core).
   b. HBsAg—hepatitis B surface antigen (antigenic material in an outer coat).

c. HBeAg—an independent protein circulating in the blood.

2. Each antigen elicits a specific antibody:
   a. Anti-HBc—persists during the acute phase of illness; may indicate continuing hepatitis B virus in the liver.
   b. Anti-HBs—detected during late convalescence; usually indicates recovery and development of immunity.
   c. Anti-HBe—usually signifies reduced infectiousness.

3. Significance:
   a. HBcAg—found only in liver cells, not serum.
   b. HBsAg—usually detected transiently in blood of 80% to 90% of infected persons; may be noted in blood for months or years, indicating that the patient has acute or chronic hepatitis B or is a carrier.
   c. HBeAg—if absent, the patient is an asymptomatic carrier. If present, it indicates highly infectious period of acute, active hepatitis. If it persists, indicates progression to chronic state.

4. Mode of transmission is primarily through blood (percutaneous and permucosal route).
   a. Oral route through saliva or through breast-feeding.
   b. Sexual activity through blood, semen, saliva, or vaginal secretions.
   c. Gay men are at high risk.

5. Incubation period is 2 to 5 months.

6. Occurrence is for all ages, but mostly affects young adults worldwide.

7. Mortality can be as high as 10%, with another 10% of patients progressing to carrier status or developing chronic hepatitis. It is the main cause of cirrhosis and hepatocellular carcinoma worldwide.

Type C Hepatitis (HCV)

1. Formerly called non-A, non-B hepatitis; an RNA virus.

2. Mode of transmission in most cases is through blood or blood product transfusion, usually from commercial or paid blood donors.
   a. Found among IV drug users and renal dialysis patients and personnel.
   b. Can be transmitted through sexual intercourse.
   c. Can be transmitted through contaminated piercing and tatooing tools.

3. Incubation period varies from 1 week to several months.

4. Occurs in all age groups.
   a. Most common form of posttransfusion hepatitis.
   b. May be seen sporadically or in epidemic proportions.

Type D Hepatitis (HDV, Delta Hepatitis)

1. Hepatitis D virus is a defective RNA agent that appears to replicate only with the hepatitis B virus. It requires HBsAg to replicate.
   a. Occurs along with HBV or may superinfect a chronic HBV carrier.
   b. Cannot outlast a hepatitis B infection.
   c. May be acute or chronic.

2. Mode of transmission and incubation are the same as for HBV.

3. Occurrence in the United States is primarily among IV drug abusers or multiply-transfused patients. The highest incidence exists in the Mediterranean, Middle East, and South America.

4. Mortality—causes about 50% of fulminant hepatitis, which has an extremely high mortality rate.

Type E Hepatitis (HEV)

1. A recently identified nonenveloped single-strand RNA virus.

2. Mode of transmission is fecal-oral, but because this virus is inconsistently shed in feces, detection is difficult.

3. Incubation is the same as for HAV.

4. Occurrence is primarily in India, Africa, Asia, and Central America, but may be found in recent travelers to these areas and is more common in young adults and more severe in pregnant women.

Clinical Manifestations

Type A Hepatitis

1. May have no symptoms.

2. Prodromal symptoms: fatigue, anorexia, malaise, headache, low-grade fever, nausea, and vomiting.

3. Highly contagious during this period, usually 2 weeks before the onset of jaundice.

4. Icteric phase: jaundice, tea-colored urine, clay-colored stools, and right upper quadrant tenderness.

5. Symptoms may be mild in children; adults are more likely to have severe symptoms and a prolonged course of disease.

Type B Hepatitis

1. Symptom onset usually more insidious and prolonged compared with HAV.

2. May be asymptomatic.

3. One week to 2 months of prodromal symptoms: fatigue, anorexia, transient fever, abdominal discomfort, nausea and vomiting, headache.

4. Extrahepatic manifestations may include myalgias, photophobia, arthritis, angioedema, urticaria, maculopapular eruptions, skin rashes, vasculitis.

5. Jaundice in icteric phase.

6. May in rare cases progress to fulminant hepatic failure, also called fulminant hepatitis.

7. May become chronic active or chronic persistent (asymptomatic) hepatitis.

Type C Hepatitis

1. Similar to those associated with HBV but often less severe.

2. Symptoms usually occur 6 to 7 weeks after transfusion.

3. Approximately 50% develop chronic liver disease and at least 20% progress to cirrhosis.

Type D Hepatitis

1. Similar to HBV but more severe.

2. With superinfection of chronic HBV carriers, causes sudden worsening of condition and rapid progression of cirrhosis.

Diagnostic Evaluation

1. Elevated serum transferase levels (aspartate transaminase [AST], alanine transaminase [ALT]) for all forms of hepatitis.

2. Radioimmunoassays that reveal IgM antibodies to hepatitis virus in the acute phase of HAV.
3. Radioimmunoassays to include HBsAg, anti-HBc, anti-HBsAg detected in various stages of HBV (Figure 19-1).
4. Hepatitis C antibody—may not be detected for 3 to 6 months after onset of HCV illness; antigen tests for HCV are being developed that will confirm diagnosis sooner.
5. Antidelta antibodies of HBsAg for HDV or the detection of IgM in acute disease and IgG in chronic disease.
6. Hepatitis E antigen (with HCV ruled out).
7. Liver biopsy to detect chronic active disease, progression, and response to therapy.

Management
All Types of Hepatitis
1. Rest according to patient's level of fatigue.
2. Therapeutic measures to control dyspeptic symptoms and malaise.
3. Hospitalization for protracted nausea and vomiting or life-threatening complications.
4. Small, frequent feedings of a high-caloric, low-fat diet; proteins are restricted when the liver cannot metabolize protein by-products, as demonstrated by symptoms.
5. Vitamin K injected subcutaneously if prothrombin time is prolonged.
6. Intravenous fluid and electrolyte replacement as indicated.
7. Administration of antiemetic for nausea.
8. After jaundice has cleared, gradual increase in physical activity. This may require many months.

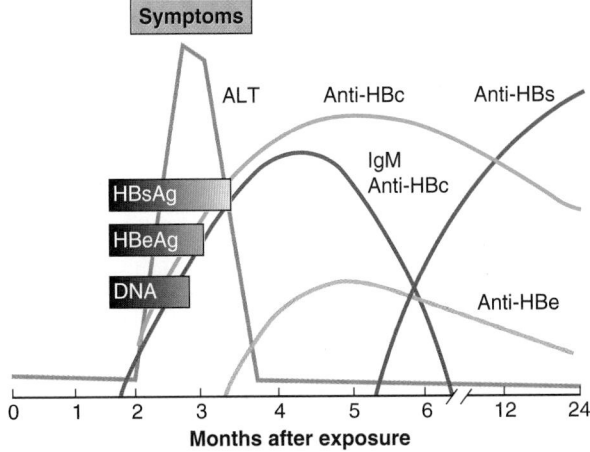

FIGURE 19-1 Time course for clinical, laboratory, and virologic features of acute hepatitis B infection. ALT: alanine aminotransferase; anti-HBc: antibody to hepatitis B core antigen; anti-HBe: antibody to hepatitis Be antigen; anti-HBs: antibody to hepatitis B surface antigen; HBeAg: hepatitis Be antigen; HBsAg: hepatitis B surface antigen. (Perrillo, R.P., & Regenstein, F.G. [1996]. Viral and immune hepatitis. In Kelley, W.N. [Ed.]. *Textbook of internal medicine.* [3rd ed.]. Philadelphia: J.B. Lippincott.)

For HCV patients
1. Long-term interferon (Betaseron) therapy may produce at least temporary remission.
2. Combination interferon and ribaviron (AZT) treatment.

Complications
1. Dehydration, hypokalemia.
2. Chronic "carrier" hepatitis or chronic active hepatitis.
3. Cholestatic hepatitis.
4. Fulminant hepatitis (liver transplantation may be necessary).
5. HBV and HCV carriers have a higher risk of developing hepatocellular carcinoma.

Nursing Assessment
1. Assess for systemic and liver-related symptoms.
2. Obtain history, such as IV drug use, sexual activity, travel, and ingestion of possible contaminated food or water to assess for any mode of transmission of the virus.
3. Assess size and shape of liver to detect enlargement or characteristics of cirrhosis.
4. Obtain vital signs, including temperature.

Nursing Diagnoses
For all patients:
- Altered Nutrition: Less Than Body Requirements related to effects of liver dysfunction
- Fluid Volume Deficit related to nausea and/or vomiting
- Activity Intolerance related to anorexia and liver dysfunction
- Risk for Infection Transmission related to communicable disease

For HBV patients:
- Risk for Injury related to coagulopathy because of impaired liver function
- Altered Thought Processes related to encephalopathy because of impaired liver function

Nursing Interventions
Maintaining Adequate Nutrition
1. Encourage frequent small feedings of high-calorie, low-fat diet. Avoid large quantities of protein during acute phase of illness.
2. Encourage eating meals in a sitting position to decrease pressure on the liver.
3. Encourage taking pleasing meals in an environment with minimal noxious stimuli (odors, noise, interruptions).
4. Administer or teach self-administration of antiemetics as prescribed. Avoid phenothiazines, such as chlorpromazine (Thorazine), which have a cholestatic effect and may cause or worsen jaundice.

Maintaining Adequate Fluid Intake
1. Provide frequent oral fluids as tolerated.
2. Administer IV fluids for patients with inability to maintain oral fluids.
3. Monitor intake and output.

Maintaining Adequate Rest and Activity

1. Promote periods of rest during symptomatic phase, according to level of fatigue.
2. Promote comfort by administering or teaching self-administration of analgesics as prescribed.
3. Provide emotional support and diversional activities when recovery and convalescence are prolonged.
4. Encourage gradual resumption of activities and mild exercise during convalescent period.

Ensuring Prevention of Disease Transmission

1. Educate patient about disease and about disease transmission.
2. Emphasize the self-limiting nature of most forms of hepatitis and the need for follow-up of liver function tests.
3. Stress importance of proper public and home sanitation and of proper preparation and dispensation of foods.
4. Encourage specific protection for close contacts.
   a. Immune globulin (Gammar) as soon as possible to household contacts of HAV patients.
   b. Hepatitis B immune globulin as soon as possible to blood or body fluid contacts of HBV patients, followed by HBV vaccine series.
5. Explain precautions to patient and family about transmission and prevention of transmission to others.
   a. Good handwashing and hygiene after using bathroom.
   b. Avoidance of sexual activity (especially for HBV) until free of HBsAg.
   c. Avoidance of sharing needles, eating utensils, and toothbrushes to prevent blood or body fluid contact (especially for HBV).
6. Report all cases of hepatitis to public health officials.

Preventing and Controlling Bleeding

1. Monitor and teach patient to monitor and report any signs of bleeding.
2. Monitor prothrombin time and administer vitamin K as ordered.
3. Avoid trauma that may cause bruising, limit invasive procedures, if possible, and maintain adequate pressure on needle stick sites.

Monitoring Thought Processes

1. Monitor for signs of encephalopathy—lethargy and somnolence with mild confusion and personality changes, such as excessive sexual or aggressive activity, loss of usual inhibitions. Lethargy may alternate with excitability, euphoria, or unruly behavior.
2. Monitor for worsening of condition, from stupor to coma; assess for asterixis, the irregular flapping of the forcibly dorsiflexed outstretched hands.
3. Maintain calm, quiet environment and reorient patient as needed.

Patient Education and Health Maintenance

1. Identify persons or groups at high risk, such as IV drug abusers or their sexual contacts and those living in crowded conditions with potentially poor hygiene or sanitation, and teach them proper hygiene, waste disposal, food preparation, use of condoms, proper use of needles, and other preventive measures.
2. Educate adolescents about the risk of piercing and tattooing in transmission of hepatitis C.
3. Encourage vaccination for HBV with series of three shots (at 0, 1, and 6 months) for high-risk patients, such as health care workers or institutionalized persons, as well as vaccination of all children from birth or at adolescence.
4. Instruct all patients who have received a blood transfusion to refrain from donating blood for 6 months (the incubation period of HBV). After hepatitis infection, blood should never be given if patient is a hepatitis B carrier or was infected with hepatitis C.
5. Stress the need to follow precautions with blood and secretions until the patient is deemed free of HBsAg.
6. Explain to HBV carriers that their blood and secretions will remain infectious.

Outcome-Based Evaluation

- Tolerating small carbohydrate feedings
- No vomiting, tolerating fluids
- Maintaining self-care and light ambulation
- Family members seeking active immunization
- No signs of bleeding
- Lethargic but oriented, no tremor

■ Hepatic Cirrhosis

Cirrhosis of the liver is characterized by scarring. It is a chronic disease in which there has been diffuse destruction and fibrotic regeneration of hepatic cells. As necrotic tissue is replaced by fibrotic tissue, normal liver structure and vasculature is altered, impairing blood and lymph flow, resulting in hepatic insufficiency and portal hypertension.

Pathophysiology and Etiology

1. Laennec's cirrhosis (macronodular)
   a. Fibrosis—mainly around central veins and portal areas.
   b. Cirrhosis most common because of chronic alcoholism and malnutrition.
2. Postnecrotic cirrhosis (micronodular)
   a. Broad bands of scar tissue.
   b. Because of previous acute viral hepatitis or drug-induced massive hepatic necrosis.
3. Biliary cirrhosis
   a. Scarring around bile ducts and lobes of the liver.
   b. Results from chronic biliary obstruction and infection (cholangitis).
   c. Much rarer than Laennec's and postnecrotic cirrhosis.

Clinical Manifestations

1. Onset is insidious; may take years to develop.
2. Early complaints include fatigue, anorexia, edema of the ankles in the evening, epistaxis and bleeding gums, and weight loss.
3. Later complaints because of chronic failure of the liver and obstruction of portal circulation.

a. Chronic dyspepsia, constipation, or diarrhea.

b. Esophageal varices, dilated cutaneous veins around the umbilicus (caput medusa), internal hemorrhoids, ascites, splenomegaly, and pancytopenia.

c. Plasma albumin is reduced, leading to edema and contributing to ascites.

d. Anemia and poor nutrition lead to fatigue and weakness, wasting, and depression.

e. Deterioration of mental function from lethargy to delirium to coma and eventual death.

f. Estrogen-androgen imbalance cause spider angiomata and palmar erythema; menstrual irregularities in females; testicular and prostatic atrophy, gynecomastia, loss of libido, and impotence in males.

4. Bleeding tendencies, such as nosebleeds, easy bruising, hematemesis, or profuse hemorrhage from stomach and esophageal varices.

Diagnostic Evaluation

1. Liver biopsy detects destruction and fibrosis of hepatic tissue.

2. Liver scan shows abnormal thickening and a liver mass.

3. Computed tomography (CT) scan determines the size of the liver and its irregular nodular surface.

4. Esophagoscopy to determine esophageal varices.

5. Paracentesis to examine ascitic fluid for cell, protein, and bacterial counts.

6. PTC differentiates extrahepatic from intrahepatic obstructive jaundice.

7. Laparoscopy and liver biopsy permit direct visualization of the liver.

8. Serum liver function test results are elevated.

Management

1. Minimize further deterioration of liver function through the withdrawal of toxic substances, alcohol, and drugs.

2. Correction of nutritional deficiencies with vitamins and nutritional supplements and a high-calorie and moderate-to high-protein diet.

3. Treatment of ascites and fluid and electrolyte imbalances.

a. Restrict sodium and water intake, depending on amount of fluid retention.

b. bed rest to aid in diuresis.

c. Diuretic therapy, frequently with spironolactone (Aldactone), a potassium-sparing diuretic that inhibits the action of aldosterone on the kidneys.

d. Abdominal paracentesis to remove fluid and relieve symptoms (see Procedure Guidelines 19-1); ascitic fluid may be ultrafiltrated and reinfused through a central venous access.

e. Administration of albumin to maintain osmotic pressure.

4. Peritoneovenous shunt may be performed in patients whose ascites are resistant to other forms of treatment.

a. Complications include bacterial infections, shunt obstruction, and intravascular coagulopathies.

5. Symptomatic relief measures, such as pain medication and antiemetics.

6. Treatment of other problems associated with liver failure. Administration of lactulose (Cephulac), neomycin (Myciguent) for hepatic encephalopathy.

7. Orthotopic liver transplantation may be necessary.

Complications

1. Hyponatremia and water retention.

2. Bleeding esophageal varices.

3. Coagulopathies.

4. Spontaneous bacterial peritonitis.

5. Hepatic encephalopathy, which may be precipitated by the use of sedatives, high-protein diet, sepsis, or electrolyte imbalance.

Nursing Assessment

1. Obtain history of any precipitating factors, such as alcohol abuse, hepatitis, or biliary disease. Establish present pattern of alcohol intake.

2. Assess mental status through interview and interaction with the patient.

3. Perform abdominal examination, assessing for ascites (Figure 19-2).

4. Observe for any bleeding.

5. Assess daily weight and abdominal girth measurements.

Nursing Diagnoses

• Activity Intolerance related to fatigue, general debility, and discomfort

• Altered Nutrition: Less Than Body Requirements related to anorexia and GI disturbances

• Impaired Skin Integrity related to edema, jaundice, and compromised immunologic status

• Risk for Injury related to altered clotting mechanisms

• Altered Thought Processes related to deterioration of liver function and increased serum ammonia level

Nursing Interventions
Promoting Activity Tolerance

1. Encourage alternating periods of rest and ambulation.

2. Maintain some periods of bed rest with legs elevated to mobilize edema and ascites.

3. Encourage and assist with gradually increasing periods of exercise.

Improving Nutritional Status

1. Encourage patient to eat high-calorie, moderate-protein meals and to have supplementary feedings.

2. Suggest small, frequent feedings and attractive meals in an aesthetically pleasing setting at mealtime.

3. Encourage oral hygiene before meals.

4. Administer or teach self-administration of medication for nausea, vomiting, diarrhea, or constipation.

Protecting Skin Integrity

1. Note and record degree of jaundice of skin and sclerae and scratches on the body.

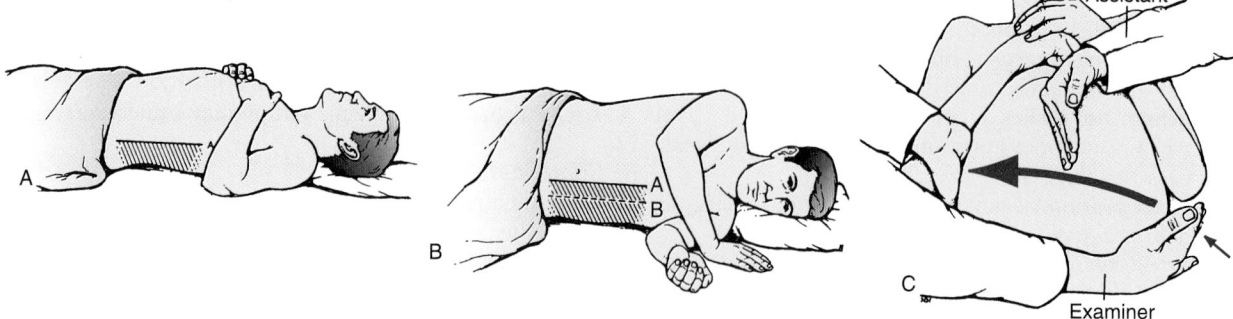

FIGURE 19-2 Assessing for ascites. (**A**) To percuss for shifting dullness, each flank is percussed with the patient in a supine position. If fluid is present, dullness is noted at each flank. The most medial limits of the dullness should be marked as indicated in *A*. The patient should then be shifted to the side. (**B**) Note what happens to the area of dullness if fluid is present. (**C**) To detect the presence of a fluid wave, the examiner places one hand alongside each flank. A second person then places a hand, ulnar side down, along the patient's midline and applies light pressure. The examiner then strikes one flank sharply with one hand, while the other hand remains in place to detect any signs of a fluid impulse. The assistant's hand dampens any wave impulses traveling through the abdominal wall.

2. Encourage frequent skin care, bathing without soap, and massage with emollient lotions.
3. Advise patient to keep fingernails short.

Preventing Injury Through Bleeding
1. Observe stools and emesis for color, consistency, and amount; test each one for occult blood.
2. Be alert for symptoms of anxiety, epigastric fullness, weakness, and restlessness, which may indicate GI bleeding.
3. Observe for external bleeding: ecchymosis, leaking needle stick sites, epistaxis, petechiae, and bleeding gums.
4. Keep patient quiet and limit activity if signs of bleeding exhibited.
5. Administer vitamin K (AquaMEPHYTON) as prescribed.
6. Stay in constant attendance during episodes of bleeding.
7. Institute and teach measures to prevent trauma:
   a. Maintain safe environment.
   b. Gentle blowing of nose.
   c. Use of soft toothbrush.
8. Encourage intake of foods with high vitamin C content.
9. Use small-gauge needles for injections, and maintain pressure over site until bleeding stops.

Promoting Improved Thought Processes
1. Restrict high-protein loads while serum ammonia is high to prevent hepatic encephalopathy. Monitor ammonia levels.
2. Protect from sepsis through good handwashing and prompt recognition and management of infection.
3. Monitor fluid intake and output and serum electrolyte levels to prevent dehydration and hypokalemia (may occur with the use of diuretics), which may precipitate hepatic coma.
4. Keep environment warm and limit visitors.

5. Pad the side rails of the bed and provide careful nursing surveillance to ensure patient's safety.
6. Assess level of consciousness and frequently reorient as needed.

 DRUG ALERT

Narcotics, sedatives, and barbiturates are used cautiously in the restless patient with cirrhosis to prevent precipitation of hepatic coma.

7. Administer lactulose (Cephulac) or neomycin (Myciguent) through a retention enema or nasogastric tube, as ordered, for elevated ammonia levels and decreasing level of consciousness.

Patient Education and Health Maintenance
1. Stress the necessity of giving up alcohol completely.
2. Urge acceptance of assistance from a substance abuse program.
3. Provide written dietary instructions.
4. Encourage daily weighing for self-monitoring of fluid retention or depletion.
5. Discuss side effects of diuretic therapy.
6. Emphasize the importance of rest, a sensible lifestyle, and an adequate, well-balanced diet.
7. Involve the person closest to the patient, because recovery often is not easy and relapses are common.
8. Stress the importance of continued follow-up for laboratory tests and evaluation by a health care provider.

Outcome-Based Evaluation
• Ambulating for 10 minutes each hour
• Tolerating small, frequent feedings
• Skin without breakdown or scratches

- No bleeding or bruising; results of stool tests are negative for occult blood
- Patient drowsy but easily aroused and oriented

Bleeding Esophageal Varices

Esophageal varices are dilated tortuous veins usually found in the submucosa of the lower esophagus; however, they may develop higher in the esophagus or extend into the stomach.

Pathophysiology and Etiology

1. Nearly always because of portal hypertension, which may result from obstruction of the portal venous circulation and cirrhosis of the liver.
   a. Because of increased obstruction of the portal vein, venous blood from the intestinal tract and spleen seeks an outlet through collateral circulation, which creates new pathways of return to the right atrium and causes an increased strain on the vessels in the submucosal layer of the lower esophagus and upper part of the stomach.
   b. These collateral vessels are tortuous and fragile and bleed easily.
2. Other causes of varices are abnormalities of the circulation in the splenic vein or superior vena cava and hepatic venothrombosis.
3. Mortality rate is high because of further deterioration of liver function to hepatic coma and complications, such as aspiration pneumonia, sepsis, and renal failure.

Clinical Manifestations

1. Hematemesis—vomiting of bright red blood
2. Melena—passage of black, tarry stools
3. Bright red rectal bleeding from hypermotility of the bowel or rectal varicies
4. Blood loss may be sudden and massive, causing shock

Diagnostic Evaluation

1. Upper GI endoscopy to identify the cause and site of bleeding.
2. Serum liver function tests, including ammonia level—elevated.

Management

Emergency Treatment

1. Restoration of circulation blood volume with blood and IV fluids.
2. Vasopressin (Pitressin) IV may be used to reduce portal pressure by decreasing splanchnic blood flow and to increase clotting and hemostasis, although its efficacy is not proven. Complications include hypertension, bradycardia, esophageal ulceration or perforation, aspiration pneumonitis, worsening variceal hemorrhage, water intoxication, cardiac ischemia in patients with preexisting cardiac disease.
3. Gastric lavage to remove blood from the GI tract, and to enhance visualization for endoscopic examination.

4. Esophageal balloon tamponade, whereby balloons are inflated in the distal esophagus and the proximal stomach to collapse the varices and induce hemostasis (see Procedure Guidelines 19-2).
   a. Complications include esophageal necrosis, perforation, aspiration, asphyxiation, and stricture.
   b. This procedure should be reserved for patients who are known, without a doubt, to be bleeding from esophageal varices and in whom all forms of conservative therapy have failed.
5. Endoscopic sclerotherapy.
   a. A sclerosing agent is injected directly into the varix with a flexible fiberoptic endoscope to promote thrombosis and sclerosis of bleeding sites.
   b. To control bleeding and reduce the frequency of subsequent variceal hemorrhages, but repeated treatments may be required.
   c. Complications include esophageal ulceration, stricture, and perforation.
6. Endoscopic esophageal ligation (variceal banding) may be urgent or nonurgent.

Nonurgent Treatment

1. Administration of parenteral feedings to allow the esophagus to rest.
2. Surgical ligation of varices to tie off blood vessels at the site of bleeding.
3. Esophageal transection and devascularization that separate bleeding site from portal system.
4. Surgical interventions to lower portal pressure by shunting blood around the liver—care is similar to abdominal surgery (see p. 259) complicated by severe cirrhotic liver (see p. 314).
   a. Portal-systemic (portacaval) shunt: portal vein is anastomosed to the inferior vena cava to reduce variceal blood flow and pressure.
   b. Splenorenal shunt: a shunt is made between the splenic vein and the left renal vein after splenectomy; this is done when the portal vein cannot be used because of thrombosis or for other reasons.
   c. Interposition mesocaval shunt: superior mesenteric vein is grafted to the inferior vena cava.
5. Transjugular intrahepatic portosystemic shunting (TIPS)—a nonsurgical approach.

Complications

1. Exsanguination or recurrent hemorrhage
2. Portal systemic encephalopathy

Nursing Assessment

1. Monitor vital signs and respiratory function.
2. Assess level of consciousness and impending signs of liver failure.

Nursing Diagnoses

- Altered Tissue Perfusion related to GI bleeding
- Risk for Aspiration related to GI bleeding and intubation
- Anxiety related to fear of unknown procedures and consequences of GI bleeding

Nursing Interventions
Maintaining Adequate Tissue Perfusion
1. Assess blood pressure, heart rate, skin condition, and urine output for signs of hypovolemia and shock.
2. Monitor patient frequently having vasopressin infusion for complications: hypertension, bradycardia, abdominal cramps, chest pain, or water intoxication.
3. Observe patient for straining, gagging, or vomiting; these increase pressure in the portal system and increase risk of further bleeding.
4. Check all GI secretions and feces for occult and frank blood.
5. Monitor infusion of blood products.
6. Administer vitamin K (AquaMEPHYTON) as prescribed.

Preventing Aspiration
1. Assess respirations and monitor oxygen saturation of blood.
2. Note and report occurrence of signs of obstructed airway or ruptured esophagus from the esophageal balloon: changes in skin color, respirations, breath sounds, level of consciousness, or vital signs; chest pain.
3. Check location and inflation of esophageal balloon; maintain traction on tubes if applicable.
4. Have scissors readily available. Cut tubing and remove esophageal balloon immediately if the patient develops acute respiratory distress.
5. Keep head of bed elevated to avoid gastric regurgitation and aspiration of gastric contents.
6. When using the Sengstaken-Blakemore esophageal balloon tube, ensure removal of secretions above the esophageal balloon: position nasogastric tube in the esophagus for suctioning purposes; provide intermittent oropharyngeal suctioning.
7. Inspect nares for skin irritation; cleanse and lubricate frequently to prevent bleeding.

Reducing Anxiety and Fear
1. Provide care in a concerned, nonjudgmental manner.
2. Explain all procedures to the patient.
3. Remain with the patient or maintain close observation and place call bell within patient's reach.
4. Work swiftly and confidently, not hurriedly and anxiously.
5. Provide alternate means of communication if tubes or other equipment interfere with the patient's ability to talk.
6. Use touch and other tactile stimuli to provide reassurance to the patient.
7. Use protective restraints to prevent dislodging of tubes in confused, combative patient.

Patient Education and Health Maintenance
1. Discuss signs and symptoms of recurrent bleeding and the need to seek emergency medical treatment if these occur.
2. Instruct the patient to avoid behaviors that increase portal system pressure: straining, gagging, Valsalva's maneuver.
3. Instruct the patient in the effects of high-protein diets and alcohol consumption in causing further complications.

4. Encourage the patient to abstain from alcohol consumption; discuss support organizations, such as Alcoholic Anonymous.

Outcome-Based Evaluation
• Blood pressure stable, urine output adequate
• Airway maintained without aspiration
• Patient cooperative and indicates understanding of treatment

■ Liver Cancer

Cancer of the liver, or *hepatocellular carcinoma*, is a primary cancer of the liver and is relatively uncommon in the United States. It is, however, one of the most common malignancies in the world, particularly in Africa and Asia. *Cholangiocarcinoma* is a primary malignant tumor of the bile ducts, which can be intrahepatic or extrahepatic. This type of cancer is uncommon in the United States but is more frequently seen in Asia. These two types of cancer are often combined for reporting purposes and make the incidence data harder to interpret.

Liver metastasis may occur from a primary site, which is found in about one-half of all late cancer cases.

Pathophysiology and Etiology
1. Incidence of primary cancer of the liver is increasing in the United States in the younger population and in females.
2. Cirrhosis, hepatitis B virus, and hepatitis C virus have been implicated in its etiology.
3. Rarer associated causes are hemachromatosis; alpha 1-antitrypsin deficiency; aflatoxins; chemical toxins, such as vinyl chloride and Thorotrast; carcinogens in herbal medicines; nitrosamines; and ingestion of hormones, as in oral contraceptives.
4. Arises in normal tissue as a discrete tumor or in end-stage cirrhosis in a multinodular pattern.
5. Liver metastasis reaches the liver by way of the portal system or the lymphatic channels or by direct extension from an abdominal tumor.

Clinical Manifestations
1. Depends on the state of the liver in which it arises; without cirrhosis and with good liver function, carcinoma of the liver may grow to huge proportions before becoming symptomatic, but in a cirrhotic patient, the lack of hepatic reserve usually leads to a more rapid course.
2. Most common presenting symptom is right upper quadrant abdominal pain, usually dull or aching, and may radiate to the right shoulder.
3. A right upper quadrant mass, weight loss, abdominal distention with ascites, fatigue, anorexia, malaise, and unexplained fever.
4. Jaundice is present only in a minority of patients at diagnosis in primary cancer of the liver. In cholangiocarcinoma, the presenting symptom is usually obstructive jaundice.

5. With portal vein obstruction, ascites and esophageal varices occurs.

Diagnostic Evaluation
1. Increased levels of serum bilirubin, alkaline phosphatase, and liver enzymes
2. Alpha-fetoprotein (AFP) is the principal tumor marker for hepatocellular carcinoma and is elevated in 70% to 95% of patients with the disease.
3. Ultrasonography and CT along with magnetic resonance imaging (MRI) are the most useful noninvasive tests to detect liver cancer and assess if the tumor can be surgically removed.
4. Arteriography is necessary to determine the resectability of any tumor of the liver.
5. Percutaneous needle biopsy or biopsy assisted by ultrasonography may be done.
6. Laparoscopy with liver biopsy may be performed.

Management
Nonsurgical Treatment
Varying degrees of success with chemotherapy and radiation. These therapies may prolong survival and improve the patient's quality of life by reducing pain, but the overall effect is palliative.
1. Liver cancer is radiosensitive, but treatment is restricted by the limited radiation tolerance of the normal liver.
2. Radiation therapy can help reduce pain and discomfort.
3. Chemotherapy is used as an adjuvant therapy after surgical resection of liver cancer.
   a. Systemic chemotherapy is the only treatment applicable once the cancer has spread outside the liver.
   b. Regional infusion chemotherapy by implantable pump has been used to deliver a high concentration of chemotherapy directly to the liver through the hepatic artery.
4. Hyperthermia has been used to treat hepatic metastases.
5. Hepatic artery occlusion and embolization with the use of chemotherapeutic agents is another possible method.
6. Immunotherapy is under investigation.
7. PTBD is used to drain obstructed biliary ducts in patients with inoperable tumors or in patients considered poor surgical risks.
8. Percutaneous or endoscopic placement of internal stents may also palliate a patient with obstructed bile ducts with a terminal diagnosis.

Surgical Treatment
Surgery is the best treatment but is only feasible in 25% of cases.
1. Surgery is an option only after the extent of tumor and hepatic reserve have been considered.
2. Surgical resection may be along anatomic divisions of the liver or nonanatomic resections.
3. Freezing hepatic tumors by cryosurgery is a new modality that preserves normal liver.
4. Liver transplantation has been performed to treat liver tumors, but results have been poor because of the high rate of recurrent primary liver malignancy. It is now recommended that the patient be treated before and after transplantation with chemotherapy and radiation therapy.
5. Care of the patient after liver surgery is similar to general abdominal surgery (see p. 259).

Complications
1. Malnutrition, biliary obstruction with jaundice.
2. Sepsis, liver abscesses.
3. Fulminant liver failure, metastasis.

Nursing Assessment
1. Obtain history of hepatitis, alcoholic liver disease and cirrhosis, exposure to toxins, or other potential causes.
2. Assess for signs and symptoms of malnutrition, including recent weight loss, loss of strength, anorexia, and anemia.
3. Assess for abdominal pain, any right shoulder pain, and enlargement of the liver.
4. Assess for fever, jaundice, ascites, or bleeding.
5. Note any change in mental status as precipitating hepatic encephalopathy.

Nursing Diagnoses
- Pain related to growth of tumor
- Altered Nutrition: Less Than Body Requirements related to anorexia
- Fluid Volume Excess related to ascites and edema formation

Nursing Interventions
Controlling Pain
1. Administer pharmacologic agents as ordered to control pain, considering metabolism through a liver with decreased function.
   a. Use caution not to administer doses more frequently than prescribed.
   b. Monitor for signs of drug toxicity.
2. Provide nonpharmacologic methods of pain relief, such as massage and guided imagery.
3. Position patient for comfort, usually in semi-Fowler's position.
4. Assess patient's response to pain control measures.

Improving Nutritional Status
1. Encourage patient to eat small meals and to take supplementary feedings, such as Ensure.
2. Assess and report changes in factors affecting nutritional needs: increased body temperature, pain, signs of infection, stress level. Encourage additional calories as tolerated.
3. Monitor daily weight changes.

Relieving Excess Fluid Volume
1. Monitor vital signs and record accurate intake and output of fluid.
2. Restrict sodium and fluid intake as prescribed.
3. Administer diuretics and replacement potassium as prescribed.

4. Administer albumin and protein supplements as prescribed to draw fluid from interstitial to intravascular space.
5. Measure and record abdominal girth daily.
6. Weigh daily, watching for increases that indicate more fluid retention.
7. Monitor laboratory values pertinent to liver function.

Patient Education and Health Maintenance

1. Instruct patient and family on preparation for surgery, reinforce and clarify surgical procedure proposed, and review postoperative instructions.

2. Instruct patient and family on nonsurgical treatment, if appropriate.
3. Explore options for pain management.
4. Inform patient of signs and symptoms of complications.
5. Instruct patient in continued surveillance for recurrence.
6. Instruct patient and family in care of any tubes or drains.

Outcome-Based Evaluation

- Verbalizes reduced pain
- Tolerates small feedings; no weight loss
- Abdominal girth decreased; urine output greater than intake

---

PROCEDURE GUIDELINES 19-1   ASSISTING WITH ABDOMINAL PARACENTESIS

EQUIPMENT

Sterile paracentesis tray and gloves	Drape or cotton blankets	Skin preparation tray with antiseptic
Local anesthetic	Collection bottle (vacuum bottle)	Specimen bottles and laboratory forms

PROCEDURE

Nursing Action	Rationale
PREPARATORY PHASE	
1. Explain procedure to the patient.	1. This may reduce the patient's fear and anxiety.
2. Record the patient's vital signs.	2. Provides baseline values for later comparison.
3. Have the patient void before treatment is begun. See that consent form has been signed.	3. This will lessen the danger of accidentally piercing the bladder with the needle or trocar.
4. Position the patient in Fowler's position with back, arms, and feet supported (sitting on the side of the bed is a frequently used position).	4. The patient is more comfortable, and a steady position can be maintained.
5. Drape the patient with sheet exposing abdomen.	5. Minimizes exposure of patient and keeps patient warm.
PERFORMANCE PHASE	
1. Assist in preparing skin with antiseptic solution.	1. This is considered a minor surgical procedure that requires aseptic precautions.
2. Open sterile tray and package of sterile gloves; provide anesthetic solution.	
3. Have collection bottle and tubing available.	
4. Assess pulse and respiratory status frequently during procedure; watch for pallor, cyanosis, or syncope (faintness).	4. Watch preliminary indications of shock. Keep emergency drugs available.
5. Physician administers local anesthesia and introduces needle or trocar.	
6. Needle or trocar is connected to tubing and vacuum bottle or syringe; fluid is slowly drained from peritoneal cavity.	6. Drainage is usually limited to 1–2 L to relieve acute symptoms and minimize risk of hypovolemia and shock.
7. Apply dressing when needle is withdrawn.	7. Elasticized adhesive patch is effective, serving as waterproof adhering dressing.
FOLLOW-UP PHASE	
1. Assist the patient to a comfortable position after treatment.	
2. Record amount and characteristics of fluid removed, number of specimens sent to laboratory, the patient's condition during treatment.	
3. Check blood pressure and vital signs every ½ h for 2 h, every hour for 4 h, and every 4 h for 24 hr.	3. Close observation will detect poor circulatory adjustment and possible development of shock.
4. Usually, a dressing is sufficient; however, if the trocar wound appears large, the physician may close the incision with sutures.	
5. Watch for leakage or scrotal edema after paracentesis.	5. If seen, report at once.

PROCEDURE GUIDELINES 19-2	USING BALLOON TAMPONADE TO CONTROL ESOPHAGEAL BLEEDING (SENGSTAKEN-BLAKEMORE TUBE METHOD, MINNESOTA TUBE METHOD)

EQUIPMENT

Esophageal balloon
  (Sengstaken-Blakemore or Minnesota)
Basin with cracked ice
Clamps for tubing

Water-soluble lubricant
Syringe (50 mL with catheter tip)
Towel and emesis basin
Glass of water and straw

Adhesive tape
Device to apply traction (eg, football helmet)
Large scissors (for emergency deflation)
Manometer (to measure balloon pressure)

PROCEDURE

Nursing Action   **Rationale**

PREPARATORY PHASE

1. Provide support and reassure the patient that this procedure will help to control bleeding.
2. Explain procedure to the patient and explain how breathing through the mouth and swallowing can help in passing the tube. (See accompanying figure.)
3. Elevate head of bed slightly, unless the patient is in shock.

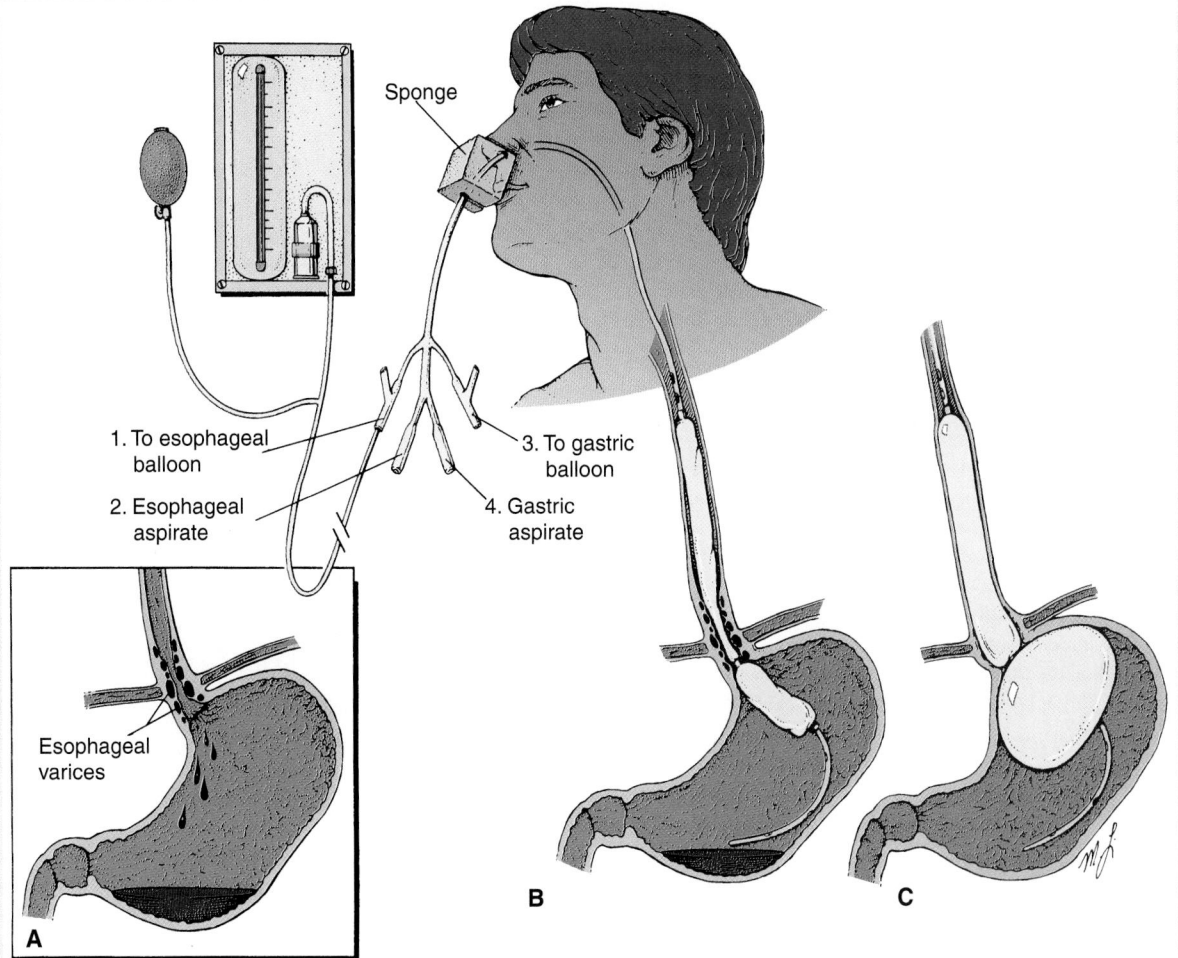

Sponge

1. To esophageal balloon
2. Esophageal aspirate
3. To gastric balloon
4. Gastric aspirate

Esophageal varices

A   B   C

Esophageal varices and their treatment by a compressing balloon tube (Sengstaken-Blakemore). (A) Dilated veins of the lower esophagus. (B) The tube is in place in the stomach and the lower esophagus but is not inflated. (C) Inflation of the tube causing compression of the veins. It may be necessary to pass an additional tube through the other nostril to aspirate. Note: The Minnesota four-lumen esophagogastric tamponade tube has an additional outlet for aspiration of the esophagus.

continued

PROCEDURE GUIDELINES 19-2	USING BALLOON TAMPONADE TO CONTROL ESOPHAGEAL BLEEDING (SENGSTAKEN-BLAKEMORE TUBE METHOD, MINNESOTA TUBE METHOD) *CONTINUED*

Nursing Action	**Rationale**

PERFORMANCE PHASE

Nursing Action	Rationale
1. Check balloons by trial inflation to detect leaks.	1. This is best done under water because it is easier to see escaping air bubbles.
2. Chill the tube, then lubricate it before the physician passes it via mouth or nose (preferable).	2. Chilling makes the tube more firm and lubrication lessens friction.
3. Provide the patient with a few sips of water.	3. This will help pass the tube more easily.
4. After the tube has entered the stomach, verify its placement by irrigating the gastric tube with air while auscultating over the stomach.	4. It is imperative that the tube is in the stomach so that the gastric tube is not inflated in the esophagus.
5. After obtaining an x-ray film of the lower chest and upper abdomen to verify placement in the stomach, inflate gastric balloon (200–250 mL) with air and gently pull tube back to seat balloon against gastroesophageal junction.	5. This is to exert force against the cardia.
6. Clamp gastric balloon; mark tube location at nares.	6. This prevents air leakage and tube migration. The mark on the tube allows easy visualization of movement of the tube.
7. Apply gentle traction to the balloon tube and secure it with a foam rubber cube at the nares or tape it to the faceguard of a football helmet.	7. This prevents the tube from migrating with peristalsis and assists in exerting proper pressure.
8. Attach Y connector to esophageal balloon opening. Attach syringe to one arm of the Y connector and manometer to the other. Inflate esophageal balloon to 25–35 mm Hg. Clamp esophageal balloon.	8. Maintains enough pressure to tamponade bleeding while preventing esophageal necrosis.
9. Apply suction to gastric aspiration opening. Irrigate at least hourly.	9. Suctioning and irrigating the tube can remove old blood from the stomach and prevent hepatic encephalopathy; allows monitoring of bleeding status.
10. **[If using Sengstaken-Blakemore tube]** Insert a nasogastric tube, positioning it above the esophageal balloon and attach to suction.	10. Suctions saliva accumulated above the esophageal balloon, which may be aspirated, and checks for bleeding above the esophageal balloon.
11. **[If using a Minnesota tube]** Attach fourth port, esophageal suction port, to suction. a. Label each port. b. Tape scissors to head of bed.	a. Prevents accidental deflation or irrigation. b. Airway occlusion may occur if the esophageal balloon is pulled into the hypopharynx. If this occurs, the esophageal balloon tube must be cut and removed immediately.

NURSING RESPONSIBILITIES

1. Maintain *constant* vigilance while balloons are inflated in the patient.
2. Keep balloon pressures at required level to control bleeding. (Clamps help to maintain pressure.)
3. Observe and record vital signs; monitor color and amount of nasogastric lavage fluid (subtracting lavage input) for evidence of bleeding.
4. Be alert for chest pain—may indicate injury or rupture of esophagus.
5. Irrigate suction tube as prescribed; observe and record nature and color of aspirated material.
6. Keep head of bed elevated to avoid gastric regurgitation and to diminish nausea and a sensation of gagging.
7. Maintain nutritional and electrolyte levels parenterally.
8. Maintain nasogastric suction or suction to esophageal suction port to aspirate any collected saliva.
9. Note nature of breathing; if counterweight pulls the tube into oropharynx, the patient may be asphyxiated.

NURSING ALERT

Keep a pair of scissors taped to the head of the bed. In the event of *acute respiratory distress*, use the scissors to cut across tubing (to deflate both balloons) and remove tubing.

Note: This procedure should be reserved for patients who are known, without a doubt, to be bleeding from esophageal varices and in whom all forms of conservative therapy have failed.

Fulminant Liver Failure

Fulminant liver failure is acute necrosis of the liver cells without preexisting liver disease, resulting in the inability of the liver to perform its many functions.

Pathophysiology and Etiology

1. Viral hepatitis is the most common cause.
2. Poisons, chemicals, and drugs such as acetaminophen (Tylenol), tetracycline (Tetracyn), isoniazid (INH), halogenated anesthetics, monoamine oxidase inhibitors, valproate (Depakene), amiodarone (Cordarone), methyldopa (Aldomet), and Amanita mushrooms may cause liver toxicity.
3. Ischemia and hypoxia because of hepatic vascular occlusion, hypovolemic shock, acute circulatory failure, septic shock, heat stroke may be causes.
4. Miscellaneous causes include hepatic vein obstruction, Budd-Chiari syndrome, acute fatty liver of pregnancy, partial hepatectomy, complication of liver transplantation.
5. Progression of hepatocellular injury and necrosis is rapid, with development of hepatic encephalopathy within 8 weeks of onset of disease.
6. Mortality rate is high, 60% to 85%, despite intensive treatment.

Clinical Manifestations

1. Malaise, anorexia, nausea, vomiting, fatigue.
2. Jaundice, especially mucous membranes.
3. Urine is tea-colored and frothy when shaken.
4. Pruritus caused by bile salts deposited on skin.
5. Steatorrhea and diarrhea because of decreased fat absorption.
6. Peripheral edema as the fluid moves from the intravascular to the interstitial spaces, secondary to hypoproteinemia.
7. Ascites from hypoproteinemia and/or portal hypertension.
8. Easy bruising, petechiae, overt bleeding because of clotting deficiency.
9. Altered levels of consciousness, ranging from irritability and confusion to stupor, somnolence, and coma.
10. Change in deep tendon reflexes—initially hyperactive, become flaccid, asterixis (tremor)
11. Fetor hepaticus—breath odor of acetone.
12. Portal systemic encephalopathy, also known as hepatic coma or hepatic encephalopathy, can occur in conjunction with cerebral edema.
13. Cerebral edema is often the cause of death because of brain stem herniation or because of respiratory arrest.

Diagnostic Evaluation

1. Prolonged prothrombin time, decreased platelet count.
2. Elevated ammonia, amino acid, and mercaptan levels.
3. Hypoglycemia or hyperglycemia.
4. Dilutional hyponatremia or hypernatremia, hypokalemia, hypocalcemia, and hypomagnesemia,

Management

1. Oral or rectal administration of lactulose (Cephulac) to minimize formation of ammonia and other nitrogenous by-products in the bowel.
2. Rectal administration of neomycin (Myciguent) to suppress urea-splitting enteric bacteria in the bowel and decrease ammonia formation.
3. Low-molecular-weight dextran or albumin followed by a potassium-sparing diuretic (spironolactone) to enhance fluid shift from interstitial back to intravascular spaces.
4. Pancreatic enzymes, if diarrhea and steatorrhea are present, to permit better tolerance of diet.
5. Mannitol (Osmitrol) IV for management of cerebral edema when indicated.
6. Cholestyramine (Questran) to promote fecal excretion of bile salts to decrease itching.
7. Antacids and histamine-2 (H_2) antagonists to reduce the risk of bleeding from stress ulcers.
8. Restriction of dietary protein and sodium while maintaining adequate caloric intake with diet or hypertonic dextrose solutions.
9. Supplemental vitamins (A, B complex, C, and K) and folate.
10. Infusion of fresh-frozen plasma to maintain prothrombin time; cryoprecipitate as needed.
11. Additional medical interventions, depending on the patient's condition, may include hemodialysis, hemofiltration, hemoperfusion, or plasmapheresis.
12. Liver transplantation has become the treatment of choice.

Complications

1. Acute respiratory failure.
2. Infections and sepsis.
3. Cardiac dysfunction, hypotension.
4. Hepatorenal failure.
5. Hemorrhage.

Nursing Assessment

1. Obtain history of exposure to drugs, chemicals, or toxins; exposure to infectious hepatitis; and course of illness.
2. Assess respiratory status, breath, level of consciousness, and vital signs.
3. Assess for ascites, edema, jaundice, bleeding, asterixis, presence or absence of reflexes.
4. Assess results of arterial blood gas evaluations, electrolytes, prothrombin time, and hemoglobin and hematocrit determinations.

Nursing Diagnoses

- Fluid Volume Deficit related to hypoproteinemia, peripheral edema, ascites
- Ineffective Breathing Pattern related to anemia and decreased lung expansion from ascites

- Altered Nutrition: Less Than Body Requirements related to GI side effects and decreased absorption, storage, and metabolism of nutrients
- Risk for Impaired Skin Integrity related to malnutrition, deposition of bile salts, peripheral edema, decreased activity
- Risk for Infection related to altered immune response
- Risk for Injury related to encephalopathy

Nursing Interventions

Maintaining Adequate Fluid Volume
1. Monitor vital signs frequently.
2. Weigh patient daily and keep an accurate intake and output record; record frequency and characteristics of stool.
3. Measure and record abdominal girth daily.
4. Assess and record peripheral edema.
5. Restrict sodium and fluids; replace electrolytes as directed.
6. Administer low-molecular-weight dextran or albumin and diuretics as prescribed.
7. Assess for any signs and symptoms of hemorrhage or bleeding.

Improving Respiratory Status
1. Monitor respiratory rate, depth, use of accessory muscles, nasal flaring, and breath sounds.
2. Evaluate results of arterial blood gases and hemoglobin and hematocrit evaluations.
3. Elevate head of the bed to lower diaphragm and decrease respiratory effort.
4. Turn frequently to prevent stasis of secretions.
5. Administer oxygen therapy as directed.

Improving Nutritional Status
1. Enlist a nutrition specialist to help evaluate nutritional status and needs.
2. Encourage the patient to eat in a sitting position to decrease abdominal tenderness and feeling of fullness.
3. Provide small, frequent meals or dietary supplements to conserve the patient's energy.
4. Provide mouth care if the patient has bleeding gums or fetor hepaticus.
5. Restrict sodium intake and protein based on ammonia levels and symptoms of encephalopathy.
6. Provide enteral and parenteral feedings as needed.

Maintaining Skin Integrity
1. Inspect skin for any alteration in integrity.
2. Provide good skin care.
3. Bathe without soap and apply soothing lotions.
4. Keep the patient's fingernails short to prevent scratching from pruritus.
5. Administer medications as prescribed for pruritus.
6. Assess for signs of bleeding from broken areas on the skin.
7. Turn the patient frequently to prevent pressure sores.
8. Avoid trauma and friction to the skin.

Preventing Infection
1. Be alert for signs of infection, such as fever, cloudy urine, abnormal breath sounds.
2. Use good handwashing and aseptic technique when caring for any break in the skin or mucous membranes.
3. Restrict visits with anyone who may have an infection.
4. Encourage the patient to try and not scratch itching skin.

Preventing Injury
1. Maintain close observation, side rails, and nurse call system.
2. Assist with ambulation as needed and avoid obstructions to prevent falls.
3. Have well-lit room and frequently reorient patient.
4. Observe for subtle changes in behavior (such as unkempt appearance), worsening of sample of handwriting, and change in sleeping pattern to detect worsening encephalopathy.

Patient Education and Health Maintenance
1. Teach patient and family to notify health care provider of increased abdominal discomfort, bleeding, increased edema or ascites, hallucinations, or lapses in consciousness.
2. Instruct to avoid activities that increase the risk of bleeding: scratching, falling, forceful nose blowing, aggressive tooth brushing, use of straight-edged razor.
3. Advise limiting activities when fatigued and encourage use of frequent rest periods.
4. Maintain close follow-up for laboratory testing and evaluation by health care provider.

Outcome-Based Evaluation
- Blood pressure stable, urine output adequate
- Respirations unlabored
- Tolerating three to four small feedings a day
- Skin intact without abrasions
- No fever or signs of infection
- No falls

BILIARY DISORDERS

The gallbladder stores and concentrates bile produced by the liver. The hormone cholecystokinin, secreted by the small intestine, stimulates contraction of the gallbladder and relaxation of the sphincter of Oddi for delivery of bile into the small intestine.

Bile assists in the emulsification (breakdown) of fat; absorption of fatty acids, cholesterol, and other lipids from the small intestine; and excretion of conjugated bilirubin from the liver.

Cholelithiasis, Cholecystitis, Choledocholithiasis

Cholelithiasis is stones in the gallbladder. Cholecystitis, inflammation of the gallbladder, may be acute or chronic. Choledocholithiasis is stones in the common bile duct.

Pathophysiology and Etiology

Cholelithiasis

1. Stones occur when cholesterol supersaturates the bile in the gallbladder and precipitates out of the bile. The cholesterol-saturated bile predisposes to the formation of gallstones and acts as an irritant, producing inflammatory changes in the gallbladder.
   a. Cholesterol stones are the most common type of gallstones found in the United States.
   b. Four times more women than men develop cholesterol stones.
   c. Women are usually older than 40 years of age, multiparous, and obese.
   d. Stone formation increases in users of contraceptives, estrogens, and cholesterol-lowering drugs, which are known to increase biliary cholesterol saturation.
   e. Bile acid malabsorption, genetic predisposition, and rapid weight loss are also risk factors for cholesterol gallstones.
2. Pigment stones occur when free bilirubin combines with calcium.
   a. Found in patients with cirrhosis, hemolysis, and infections in the biliary tree.
   b. These stones cannot be dissolved.
3. An estimated 25 million people in the United States have gallstones, with 1 million new cases discovered each year.
   a. Incidence of stone formation increases with age because of increased hepatic secretion of cholesterol and decreased bile acid synthesis.
   b. Increased risk in patients with malabsorption of bile salts with GI disease, bile fistula, gallstone ileus, carcinoma of the gallbladder, or in those who have had ileal resection or bypass.

Cholecystitis

1. Acute cholecystitis, an acute inflammation of the gallbladder, is most commonly caused by gallstone obstruction.
   a. Secondary bacterial infection may occur and progress to empyema (purulent effusion of the gallbladder).
2. Acalculous cholecystitis is acute gallbladder inflammation without obstruction by gallstones.
3. Occurs after major surgical procedures, severe trauma, or burns.
4. Chronic cholecystitis occurs when the gallbladder becomes thickened, rigid, and fibrotic and functions poorly. Results from repeated attacks of cholecystitis, calculi, or chronic irritation.

Choledocholithiasis

1. Small gallstones can pass from the gallbladder into the common bile duct and proceed to the duodenum. More often they remain in the common bile duct and can cause obstruction, resulting in jaundice and pruritis.
2. Common duct stones are frequently associated with infected bile and can lead to cholangitis (inflammation/infection of a bile duct).
3. A typical clinical picture includes biliary pain in the upper abdomen, jaundice, chills and fever, mild hepatomegaly, abdominal tenderness, and occasionally, rebound tenderness.

Clinical Manifestations

1. Gallstones that remain in the gallbladder are usually asymptomatic.
2. Biliary colic can be caused by gallstones.
   a. Steady, severe, aching pain or sensation of pressure in the epigastrium or right upper quadrant, which may radiate to the right scapular area or right shoulder.
   b. Begins suddenly and persists for 1 to 3 hours until the stone falls back into the gallbladder or is passed through the cystic duct.
3. Acute cholecystitis causes biliary colic pain that persists more than 4 hours and increases with movement, including respirations.
   a. Also causes nausea and vomiting, low-grade fever, and jaundice (with stones or inflammation in the common bile duct).
   b. Right upper quadrant guarding and Murphy's sign (inability to take a deep inspiration when examiner's fingers are pressed below the hepatic margin) are present.
4. Chronic cholecystitis causes heartburn, flatulence, and indigestion. Repeated attacks of symptoms may occur resembling acute cholecystitis.

Diagnostic Evaluation

1. Oral cholecystography, ultrasonography, and hepatobiliary (HIDA) scan may visualize stones or inflammation.
2. ERCP or PTC to visualize location of stones and obstruction.
3. Elevated conjugated bilirubin because of obstruction.

Management

1. Supportive management may include IV fluids, nasogastric suction, pain management, and antibiotics (with a positive culture).
2. Surgical management:
   a. Cholecystectomy, open or laparoscopic (see p. 310).
   b. Intraoperative cholangiography and choledochoscopy for common bile duct exploration.
   c. Placement of a T-tube in the common bile duct to decompress the biliary tree and allow access into the biliary tree postoperatively.
3. Oral therapy with chenodeoxycholic acid (CDCA), ursodeoxycholic acid (Actigall), or a combination of both to decrease the size of existing cholesterol stones or to dissolve small ones.
   a. Indicated for patients at high risk for surgery because of comorbid conditions.
   b. Major side effects include diarrhea, abnormal liver function tests, increases in serum cholesterol.

4. Direct contact therapy by which a local cholelitholytic agent is infused by a catheter directly into the gallbladder or through a percutaneous transhepatic biliary catheter.
   a. Indicated for symptomatic, high-risk patients whose gallbladder can be visualized by a radiographic study.
   b. Side effects include pain from the catheter, nausea, transient elevations of liver function tests and white blood count.
5. After cholecystectomy, intracorporeal lithotripsy may be used to fragment retained stones in the common bile duct by pulsed laser, or hydraulic lithotripsy applied through an endoscope directly to the stones. The stone fragments are removed by irrigation or aspiration. Retained stones may also be removed by basket retrieval through the endoscopic or percutaneous transhepatic biliary approach.

Complications

1. Cholangitis.
2. Necrosis, empyema, or perforation of the gallbladder.
3. Biliary fistula through the duodenum.
4. Gallstone ileus.
5. Adenocarcinoma of the gallbladder.

Nursing Assessment

1. Obtain history and demographic data that may indicate risk factors for biliary disease.
2. Assess patient's pain for location, description, intensity, relieving and exacerbating factors.
3. Assess for signs of dehydration: dry mucous membranes, poor skin turgor, low urine output with elevated specific gravity.
4. Assess sclera and skin for jaundice.
5. Monitor temperature and white blood count for indications of infection.

Nursing Diagnoses

- Pain related to biliary colic or stone obstruction
- Fluid Volume Deficit related to nausea and vomiting and decreased intake

Nursing Interventions
Relieving Pain
1. Assess pain location, severity, and characteristics.
2. Administer medications or monitor patient-controlled analgesia to control pain.
3. Assist in attaining position of comfort.
Restoring Normal Fluid Volume
1. Administer IV fluids and electrolytes as prescribed.
2. Administer antiemetics as prescribed to decrease nausea and vomiting.
3. Maintain nasogastric decompression, if needed.
4. Begin food and fluids as tolerated, after acute symptoms subside or postoperatively.
5. Observe and record amount of biliary tube drainage, if applicable.

Patient Education and Health Maintenance

1. Instruct patient in care of any tubes or catheters that may be in place at discharge.
   a. Observe for bleeding or drainage around insertion site.
   b. Replace dressing per protocol.
   c. Report any change in drainage.
2. Review discharge instructions for activity, diet, medications, and postoperative follow-up.
3. Emphasize symptoms of complications to be reported, such as increased or persistent pain, fever, abdominal distention, nausea, anorexia, jaundice, unusual drainage.
4. Encourage follow-up as indicated.

Outcome-Based Evaluation

- Patient verbalizes reduced pain level
- Tolerates oral fluids and solid food; adequate urine output

PANCREATIC DISORDERS

The pancreas secretes pancreatic enzymes, including amylase and lipase, through the pancreatic duct when stimulated by cholecystokinin and secretin to aid in digestion of carbohydrates and fat in the small intestine. The pancreas also secretes hormones, such as insulin and glucagon, that help to regulate and maintain normal serum glucose.

■ Acute Pancreatitis

Acute pancreatitis is an inflammation of the pancreas, ranging from mild edema to extensive hemorrhage, resulting from various insults to the pancreas. It is defined by a discrete episode of abdominal pain and serum enzymes elevations. The structure and function of the pancreas usually return to normal after an acute attack.

Pathophysiology and Etiology

1. Excessive alcohol consumption is the most common cause in the United States.
2. Also commonly caused by biliary tract disease, such as cholelithiasis, acute and chronic cholecystitis.
3. Less common causes are bacterial or viral infection, blunt abdominal trauma, peptic ulcer disease, ischemic vascular disease, hyperlipidemia, hypercalcemia; the use of corticosteroids, thiazide diuretics, and oral contraceptives; surgery on or near the pancreas or after instrumentation of the pancreatic duct; tumors of the pancreas or ampulla; and a small incidence of congenital pancreatitis.
4. Mortality is high (10%) because of shock, anoxia, hypotension, or multiple organ dysfunction.
5. Attacks may resolve in complete recovery, may recur without permanent damage, or may progress to chronic pancreatitis.
6. Autodigestion of all or part of the pancreas is involved, but the exact mechanism is not completely understood.

Clinical Manifestations

(Depend on severity of pancreatic damage.)

1. Abdominal pain, usually constant, midepigastric or periumbilical, radiating to the back or flank. Patient assumes a fetal position or leans forward while sitting to relieve pressure of the inflamed pancreas on celiac plexus nerves. Pain can be mild to incapacitating.
2. Nausea and vomiting.
3. Fever.
4. Involuntary abdominal guarding, epigastric tenderness to deep palpation, and reduced or absent bowel sounds.
5. Dry mucous membranes; hypotension; cold, clammy skin; cyanosis; and tachycardia, which may reflect mild to moderate dehydration from vomiting or capillary leak syndrome (third space loss).
6. Shock may be the presenting manifestation in severe episodes, with respiratory distress and acute renal failure.
7. Purplish discoloration of the flanks (Grey Turner's sign) or of the periumbilical area (Cullen's sign) occurs in extensive hemorrhagic necrosis of the pancreas.

Diagnostic Evaluation

1. Serum amylase, lipase, glucose, bilirubin, alkaline phosphatase, lactic dehydrogenase (LDH), AST, ALT, potassium, and cholesterol may be elevated.
2. Serum albumin, calcium, sodium, magnesium, and possibly potassium may be low because of dehydration, vomiting, and the binding of calcium in areas of fat necrosis.
3. Abdominal x-ray to detect an ileus or isolated loop of small bowel overlying the pancreas. Pancreatic calcifications or gallstones may suggest an alcohol or biliary etiology.
4. CT scan is the most definitive for determining pancreatic changes.
5. Chest x-ray for detection of pulmonary complications. Pleural effusions are common, especially on the left, but may be bilateral.

Management

Depending on severity of episode, the management focuses on alleviation of symptoms and support of the patient to prevent complications.

1. Restoration of circulating blood volume with IV crystalloid or colloid solutions or blood products.
2. Maintenance of adequate oxygenation reduced by pain, anxiety, acidosis, abdominal pressure, or pleural effusions.
3. Pain control to alleviate pain and anxiety, which increases pancreatic secretions.
4. Rest of the GI tract.
   a. Withhold oral feedings to decrease pancreatic secretions.
   b. Nasogastric intubation and suction to relieve gastric stasis, distention, and ileus, if needed.
5. Maintenance of alkaline gastric pH with H_2 antagonists and antacids to suppress acid drive of pancreatic secretions and to prevent stress ulcer complications of acute illness.
6. Nutrition provided or treatment of malnutrition with parenteral feedings, as needed.
7. Pharmacotherapy
   a. Electrolyte replacements as needed.
   b. Sodium bicarbonate to reverse metabolic acidosis.
   c. Regular insulin to treat hyperglycemia.
   d. Antibiotic therapy for infection or sepsis.
8. Surgical intervention if complications occur.
   a. Incision and drainage of infection and pseudocysts.
   b. Debridement or pancreatectomy to remove necrotic pancreatic tissue.
   c. Cholecystectomy for gallstone pancreatitis.

Complications

1. Pancreatic ascites, abscess or pseudocyst.
2. Pulmonary infiltrates, pleural effusion, adult respiratory distress syndrome.
3. Hemorrhage with hypovolemic shock.
4. Acute renal failure.
5. Sepsis and multiple organ dysfunction syndrome.

Nursing Assessment

1. Obtain history of gallbladder disease, alcohol use, or any precipitating factors.
2. Assess GI distress, including nausea and vomiting, diarrhea, and passage of stools containing fat.
3. Assess characteristics of abdominal pain.
4. Assess nutritional and fluid status.
5. Assess respiratory rate and pattern and breath sounds.

GERONTOLOGIC ALERT

 The incidence of severe, systemic complications of pancreatitis increases with age. Assess for any changes in mental status in an older person with pancreatitis as an indicator of an underlying complication. Acute pancreatitis in an older person may indicate an underlying pancreatic tumor obstructing the pancreatic duct.

Nursing Diagnoses

- Pain related to disease process
- Fluid Volume Deficit related to vomiting, self-restricted intake, fever, and fluid shifts
- Ineffective Breathing Pattern related to severe pain and pulmonary complications

Nursing Interventions

Controlling Pain

1. Administer narcotic analgesics as ordered to control pain.
2. Assist patient to a comfortable position.
3. Maintain NPO status to decrease pancreatic enzyme secretion.
4. Maintain patency of nasogastric suction to remove gastric secretions and to relieve abdominal distention, if indicated.

5. Provide frequent oral hygiene and care.
6. Administer antacids as prescribed.
7. Report increase in severity of pain, which may indicate hemorrhage of the pancreas, rupture of a pseudocyst, or inadequate dosage of the analgesic.

Restoring Adequate Fluid Balance

1. Monitor and record vital signs, skin color, and temperature.
2. Monitor intake and output and weigh daily.
3. Evaluate laboratory data for hemoglobin, hematocrit, albumin, calcium, potassium, sodium, and magnesium levels and administer replacements as prescribed.
4. Observe and measure abdominal girth if pancreatic ascites is suspected.
5. Report any trend in decreasing blood pressure or urine output or rising pulse, because this may indicate hypovolemia and shock or renal failure.

Improving Respiratory Function

1. Assess respiratory rate and rhythm, effort, oxygen saturation, and breath sounds frequently.
2. Position in upright or semi-Fowler's position to enhance diaphragmatic excursion.
3. Administer oxygen supplementation as prescribed to maintain adequate oxygen levels.
4. Report signs of respiratory distress immediately.
5. Instruct patient in coughing and deep breathing to improve respiratory function.

Patient Education and Health Maintenance

1. Instruct patient to gradually resume a low-fat diet.
2. Instruct patient to increase activity gradually, providing for daily rest periods.
3. Reinforce information about disease process and precipitating factors. Stress that subsequent bouts of acute pancreatitis may destroy the pancreas, cause additional complications, and lead to chronic pancreatitis.
4. If pancreatitis is a result of alcohol abuse, the patient needs to be reminded of the importance of eliminating all alcohol; advise about Alcoholics Anonymous or other substance abuse counseling.

Outcome-Based Evaluation

- Verbalizes reduced pain level
- Blood pressure stable; urine output adequate
- Respirations unlabored; breath sounds clear

▪ Chronic Pancreatitis

Chronic pancreatitis is defined as the persistence of pancreatic cellular damage after acute inflammation and decreased pancreatic endocrine and exocrine function.

Pathophysiology and Etiology

1. Alcohol abuse is the most common cause; less common causes are hyperparathyroidism, hereditary pancreatitis, malnutrition, and trauma to the pancreas.
2. With chronic inflammation, destruction of the secreting cells of the pancreas causes maldigestion and malabsorption of protein and fat and possibly diabetes mellitus if islet cells of the pancreas have been affected.
3. As cells are replaced by fibrous tissue, obstruction of the pancreatic and common bile ducts and duodenum may result.

Clinical Manifestations

1. Pain is usually located in the epigastrium or left upper quadrant, often radiating to the back; similar to that observed in acute pancreatitis, but more constant and occurring at unpredictable intervals. As the disease progresses, recurring attacks of pain will be more severe, more frequent, and of longer duration.
2. Weight loss, nausea, vomiting, anorexia.
3. Malabsorption and steatorrhea occur late in the course of the disease.
4. Diabetes mellitus.

Diagnostic Evaluation

1. Serum amylase and lipase may be normal to low because of decreased pancreatic exocrine function.
2. Bilirubin and alkaline phosphatase may be elevated if biliary obstruction occurs.
   a. Secretin and cholecystokinin stimulatory test results—abnormal.
   b. Fecal fat analysis determines need for pancreatic enzyme replacement.
3. Plain abdominal x-ray to determine diffuse calcification of the pancreas.
4. CT scan identifies pancreatic structural changes, such as calcifications, masses, ductal irregularities, enlargement, and pseudocysts.
5. ERCP defines ductal anatomy and localizes complications, such as pancreatic pseudocysts and ductal disruptions.

Management

1. Pain management.
2. Correction of nutritional deficiencies.
3. Pancreatic enzyme replacement.
4. Treatment of diabetes mellitus.
5. Endoscopic placement of pancreatic stent allowing free flow of pancreatic juices through distorted and irregular/narrowed pancreatic duct.
6. Surgical interventions to reduce pain, restore drainage of pancreatic secretions, correct structural abnormalities, and manage complications. Care is similar to the patient undergoing abdominal surgery (see p. 259).
   a. Pancreaticojejunostomy—side-to-side anastomosis of pancreatic duct to jejunum to drain pancreatic secretions into jejunum.
   b. Revision of sphincter of ampulla of Vater—sphincteroplasty.

c. Drainage of pancreatic pseudocyst into nearby structures or by external drain.
d. Resection of part of pancreas (Whipple, distal pancreatectomy) or removal of entire pancreas (total pancreatectomy).
e. Autotransplantation of islet cells.

Complications
1. Pancreatic pseudocyst.
2. Pancreatic ascites and pleural effusions.
3. Gastrointestinal hemorrhage.
4. Biliary tract obstruction.
5. Pancreatic fistula.

Nursing Assessment
1. Assess level of abdominal pain.
2. Assess nutritional status.
3. Assess for steatorrhea and malabsorption.
4. Assess for signs and symptoms of diabetes mellitus.
5. Assess current level of alcohol intake and motivation and resources available to abstain from drinking.

Nursing Diagnoses
- Pain related to chronic insult to pancreas
- Altered Nutrition: Less Than Body Requirements related to fear of eating, malabsorption, and glucose intolerance
- Anxiety related to surgical intervention

Nursing Interventions
Controlling Pain
1. Assess and record the character, location, frequency, and duration of pain.
2. Determine precipitating and alleviating factors of the patient's pain.
3. Explore the effect of pain on the patient's lifestyle and eating habits.
4. Administer or teach self-administration of analgesics (narcotics) as ordered to control pain.
5. Use nonpharmacologic methods and pain medications to promote relaxation, such as distraction, imagery, and progressive muscle relaxation.
6. Assess response to pain control measures, and refer to chronic pain management clinic, if indicated.

Improving Nutritional Status
1. Assess nutritional status, history of weight loss, and dietary habits, including alcohol intake.
2. Administer pancreatic enzyme replacement with meals, as prescribed.
3. Administer antacids and/or H_2 receptor antagonists to prevent neutralization of enzyme supplements, as indicated.
4. Monitor intake and output and daily weight.
5. Assess for GI discomfort with meals and character of stools.

6. Monitor blood glucose levels and teach balanced, low concentrated carbohydrate diet and insulin therapy as indicated.

NURSING ALERT

Warn patient that dangerous hypoglycemic reaction may result from use of insulin while drinking alcohol and skipping meals.

7. Identify foods that aggravate symptoms and teach low-fat diet.

Relieving Anxiety About Surgical Intervention
1. Describe planned surgical intervention and the expected results.
   a. Decreased pain.
   b. Ability to eat better and improve general condition.
2. Prepare patient for side effects/complications of surgery.
   a. Total pancreatectomy will cause permanent diabetes mellitus, dependence on insulin, severe malabsorption, and the need for lifelong pancreatic enzyme replacement.
   b. Malnutrition and debility increase patient's risk for poor healing and complications of surgery.
3. Assist patient to prepare for surgery by encouraging abstinence of alcohol and intake of nutritional and vitamin supplements.
4. Encourage patient to enlist help of support network and strengthen appropriate coping mechanisms.
5. After surgery, provide meticulous care to prevent infection, promote wound healing, and prevent routine complications of surgery (see p. 263).

Patient Education and Health Maintenance
1. Instruct the patient regarding correct use of analgesics.
2. Instruct in proper administration of pancreatic enzyme replacement.
   a. Take just before or during meals.
   b. May be enteric coated. Do not crush or chew tablets; powder may be obtained if difficulty swallowing tablets.
   c. Take with antacid or take H_2 antagonist as directed to prevent pancreatic enzyme from being destroyed by gastric acid secretions.
3. Advise patient to monitor number and characteristics of stools; report increased stools or food intolerance.
4. Diabetic teaching with follow-up to monitor progression of condition, if applicable.
5. Stress that no treatment will be effective if alcohol consumption is continued.

Outcome-Based Evaluation
- Verbalizes reduced pain level
- Weight stabilized or weight gain noted
- Verbalizes understanding of effects of surgical procedure

Pancreatic Cancer

Cancer of the pancreas may arise in the head (70%) or body and tail (30%) of the pancreas. Adenocarcinoma of the cells that line the ducts of the pancreas is the most common (80%) type. Pancreatic cancer is the fourth leading cause of cancer deaths in the United States, because 90% of tumors are unresectable at the time of diagnosis.

Pathophysiology and Etiology

1. Incidence is increasing.
2. Usually occurs between the ages of 60 and 80, but can be found in younger patients.
3. Smoking, prolonged exposure to industrial chemicals, high-fat diet, diabetes mellitus, and chronic pancreatitis are considered risk factors. Small percentage of pancreatic cancer is inherited.
4. Obstruction of bile flow may occur with tumors in the head of the pancreas because of compression of the distal common bile duct.
5. Obstruction of pancreatic duct produces pain and exocrine dysfunction.

Clinical Manifestations

1. Symptoms are often vague and nonspecific, preventing early detection.
2. Weight loss, abdominal pain, anorexia, nausea, vomiting, and weakness occur.
3. Pain usually occurs in the upper abdomen and is gnawing or boring and may radiate to the back.
   a. Pain is often worse at night, and patients tend to lie with legs drawn up in the fetal position or may lean forward when seated (proning).
   b. Pain becomes more localized, severe, and unremitting as the disease progresses.
4. Early satiety and a feeling of bloating after eating may occur.
5. Biliary obstruction produces jaundice, dark tea-colored urine, clay-colored stools, and pruritus.
6. Depression and lethargy may be present.

Diagnostic Evaluation

1. Ultrasonography and CT scan—detect tumors larger than 1 cm.
2. ERCP and EUS—defines anatomy and allows biopsy or fine needle aspiration for cytology to confirm diagnosis.
3. MRCP—defines anatomy without the use of contrast dye.
4. Liver function tests elevated; coagulation studies may be prolonged.
5. Carcinoembryonic antigen (CEA) and CA 19-9—may be elevated.
6. Percutaneous needle aspiration or biopsy through ultrasonography or CT scan guidance to determine malignancy.
7. Endoscopic ultrasonography for preoperative staging.

Management

The goal of treatment may be cure or palliation, depending on the staging of the tumor. Most cases are usually too far advanced for cure. Longer palliation is now being achieved.

Surgery

1. Whipple procedure (pancreaticoduodenectomy) is the removal of the head of the pancreas, distal portion of the common bile duct including the gallbladder, duodenum, and the distal stomach with anastomosis of the remaining pancreas, stomach, and common bile duct to the jejunum (Figure 19-3). If the gallbladder is present it is removed also.
   a. Stomach and pylorus may be preserved—pyloruspreserving Whipple procedure.
   b. Done for carcinoma of the head of the pancreas, periampullary area, chronic pancreatitis of the head of the pancreas, and trauma.
2. Total pancreatectomy, including a splenectomy, may be performed for diffuse tumor throughout the pancreas.

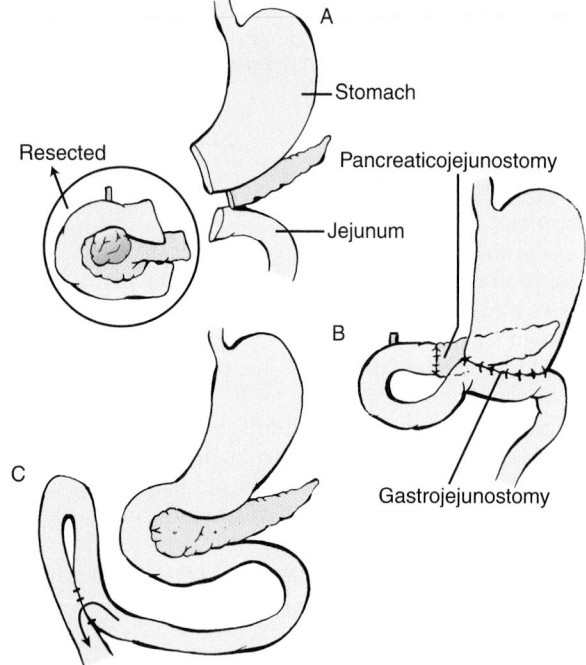

FIGURE 19-3 Pancreaticoduodenectomy (Whipple procedure or resection). (**A**) End result of resection of the carcinoma of the head of the pancreas or the ampulla of Vater. The common duct is sutured to the end of the jejunum, and the remaining portion of the pancreas and the end of the stomach are sutured to the side of the jejunum. (**B**) Lines indicate removal of the head of the pancreas, duodenum, adjacent stomach, and distal segment of common bile duct.

3. Distal pancreatectomy is the removal of the distal pancreas and spleen for tumors localized in the body and tail.
4. Palliative bypass of the bile duct (choledochojejunostomy or cholecystojejunostomy) and/or stomach (gastrojejunostomy) for unresectable tumors of the pancreas.
5. Care is similar to that of patient undergoing abdominal surgery (see p. 259).

Other Measures

1. Chemotherapy may be used in combination with radiation therapy before surgery to shrink tumors.
   a. Chemotherapy combined with radiation therapy may be given for resectable tumors after surgery for microscopic or undetectable disease left behind.
   b. Chemotherapy and radiation therapy may be given for tumors deemed unresectable at the time of surgery and after palliative bowel bypass surgery.
2. Chemotherapy may be given alone for treatment of unresectable or metastatic disease.
3. Radiation therapy may be used alone.
   a. External beam irradiation for local control, reduction of pain, and to palliate obstruction.
   b. Intraoperative radiation therapy has also been used in some centers.
4. Endoscopic or percutaneous stent placement for relief of biliary obstruction (usually for patients near end of life).
5. Endoscopic or percutaneous stent for relief of duodenal obstruction (usually for patients near end of life).
6. Chemical splanchnicectomy, injection of alcohol into the celiac axis nerves, numbs the nerves in the area of the pancreas for pain relief.
   a. May be performed intraoperatively by the surgeon or percutaneously under CT guidance as an outpatient procedure by an anesthesia pain service.
   b. Provides temporary pain relief and can be repeated.
7. Novel therapies, including immunotherapy and gene and vaccine therapies, are being investigated.
8. Clinical investigations combining various treatments are aimed at improving the prognosis of pancreatic cancer.

Complications

1. Biliary, gastric, and duodenal obstruction.
2. Metastases and liver failure secondary to metastasis.
3. Portal hypertension because of encasement of major blood vessels in the area of the pancreas.

Nursing Assessment

1. Obtain history for risk factors, pain, and symptoms of pancreatic dysfunction.
2. Assess nutritional status, including diet history, anorexia, weight loss, nausea and vomiting, steatorrhea, skin turgor.
3. Evaluate laboratory results for alterations in glucose, pancreatic enzymes, liver function, and coagulation studies.
4. Assess psychosocial status to determine depression, usual coping strategies, support systems, and experience with past serious illness.

5. Assess use of alternative therapies or any over-the-counter medications.

NURSING ALERT

The efficacy of herbal medications to treat or cure pancreatic cancer has not been proved. Little information is known about the interaction of herbal medications with conventional medications or treatments. Herbal medications may interact with chemotherapy drugs and compromise treatment. If a patient is using any alternative treatments or herbal medications, this must be known to all health care providers. Alternative therapies, other than those that are ingested, may be of benefit to a patient with pancreatic cancer if used adjunctly; however, much research is needed.

Nursing Diagnoses

- Pain related to pancreatic tumor or surgical incision
- Altered Nutrition: Less Than Body Requirements related to disease process and/or surgical intervention
- Fluid Volume Deficit related to proteinemia, surgical alterations
- Impaired Tissue Integrity related to malnutrition, surgical incisions, and altered pancreatic or bile drainage

Nursing Interventions

Controlling Pain

1. Administer narcotics as ordered or monitor patient-controlled analgesia.
2. Teach relaxation techniques, such as relaxation breathing, progressive muscle relaxation, and imagery, as adjuncts for pain relief.
3. Assist with frequent turning and comfortable positioning.
4. Administer adjuvant medications, such as antidepressants, as prescribed.
5. Assess patient's response to pain and symptom control measures.
6. Consider hospice services for symptom management if patient no longer benefits from therapy.

Improving Nutritional Status

1. Administer parenteral nutrition as prescribed preoperatively and postoperatively.
2. Monitor serum glucose level for hyperglycemia or hypoglycemia.
3. Progress diet slowly when oral intake is tolerated; observe for nausea, vomiting, and gastric distention.
4. Administer high-protein, high-carbohydrate diet with vitamin supplements and pancreatic enzymes as prescribed.
5. Encourage use of spices to stimulate taste buds, provide cool foods to decrease odor, use plastic utensils if patient complains of metallic taste from treatments, offer small, frequent meals.
6. Provide appetite stimulant, such as megestrol acetate (Megace) or cannabinoids, as needed.
7. Monitor serum albumin.

8. Weigh daily.

9. Assess for fat and protein malabsorption.

Attaining Adequate Fluid Volume

1. Monitor vital signs and record accurate intake and output.

2. Monitor any wound drain output.

3. Evaluate laboratory values for hypoalbuminemia, hyponatremia, hypochloremia, and metabolic alkalosis; replace electrolytes as prescribed.

4. Administer fluid replacement as indicated.

5. Report change in vital signs or increased pain, which may indicate hemorrhage or leak from anastomosis.

Maintaining Tissue Integrity

1. Observe skin for jaundice, breakdown, irritation, or excoriation.

2. Administer antipruritics, provide frequent skin care without soap and with thorough rinsing, apply emollient lotions, keep fingernails short to prevent scratching.

3. Inspect skin around drains for irritation and protect skin from leakage of fluids from any drains or tubes.

4. Inspect surgical dressings and incision for bleeding, drainage, or signs of infection.

5. Prevent tension on anastomoses by monitoring for abdominal distention and maintaining patency of surgically placed tubes and drains.

6. Maintain aseptic technique in handling wound dressings and drainage of all secretions.

Community and Home Care Considerations

1. Educate patient and family about course of disease and support them through the process.

2. Provide assistive devices and direct care to help with energy conservation. Patients who die from pancreatic cancer usually have progressive weight loss from anorexia leading to severe cachexia, fatigue, and muscle wasting, which is refractory to any intervention.

3. Assess for bowel obstruction, which may also deplete energy and lower nutritional status. Notify health care provider of reduced bowel activity, increased pain.

4. Emphasize to the patient and family that pain can always be managed and patients need not die in pain. The plan for pain management should be aggressive and should provide the patient an optimal quality of life.

Patient Education and Health Maintenance

1. Instruct patient and family on self-care measures for pancreatic insufficiency.
   a. Glucose monitoring, insulin administration, signs and symptoms of hypoglycemia and hyperglycemia.
   b. Pancreatic enzyme replacement, high-protein, high-carbohydrate diet.

2. Teach wound and drain care, as needed:

3. Explore options for pain management.

4. Coordinate referral for home care for any wound or drain care, new diabetic management, new medications, change in diet, or referral for hospice care.

Outcome-Based Evaluation

- Verbalizes reduced pain
- Weight stable
- Vital signs stable; urine output adequate
- Incision intact without drainage or bleeding

SELECTED REFERENCES

Apte, M.V., Keogh, G.W., & Wilson, J.S. (1999). Chronic pancreatitis: Complications and management. *Journal of Clinical Gastroenterology, 29*(3), 225–240.

Barish, M.A., Yucel, E.K., & Ferrucci, J.T. (1999). Magnetic resonance cholangiopancreatography. *New England Journal of Medicine, 341*(4), 258–264.

Berger, A.M., Portenoy, R.K., & Weissman, D.E. (Eds.). (1998). *Principles and practice of supportive oncology.* Philadelphia: Lippincott-Raven.

Bhutani, M.S. (1999). Endoscopic ultrasound in pancreatic diseases. Indications, limitations, and the future. *Gastroenterology Clinics of North America, 28*(3), 747–770.

Bodner, W.R., Hilaris, B.S., & Mastoras, D.A. (2000). Radiation therapy in pancreatic cancer: Current practice and future trends. *Journal of Clinical Gastroenterology, 30*(3), 230–233.

Caletti, G., & Fusaroli, P. (1999). Endoscopic ultrasonography. *Endoscopy, 31*(1), 95–102.

Dervenis, C., & Bassi, C. (2000). Evidence-based assessment of severity and management of acute pancreatitis. *British Journal of Surgery, 87*(3), 257–258.

Coleman, J. (1999). Bile duct injuries in laparoscopic cholecystectomy: Nursing perspective. *AACN Clinical Issues, 10*(4), 442–454.

Fletcher, L.L., & Thomas, D. J. (1999). The challenge of diagnosing the cause of jaundice. *The Nurse Practitioner, 24*(10), 98–102.

Freeny, P.C. (1999). Pancreatic imaging. New modalities. *Gastroenterology Clinics of North America, 28*(3), 723–746.

Greenfield, L.J., Mulholland, M., Oldham, K.T., Zelenock, G.B., & Lillemoe, K.D. (Eds.). (1997). *Surgery: Scientific principles and practice* (2nd ed.). Philadelphia: Lippincott-Raven.

Kavanagh, P.V., van Sonnenberg, E., Wittich, G.R., Goodacre, B.W., & Walser, E.M. (1997). Interventional radiology of the biliary tract. *Endoscopy, 29*(6), 570–576.

Lillemoe, K.D., & Yeo, C.J. (1998). Management of complications of pancreatitis. *Current Problems in Surgery, 35*(1), 1–98.

Ponchon, T. (2000). Diagnostic endoscopic retrograde cholangiopancreatography. *Endoscopy, 32*(3), 200–208.

Rosenthal, R.J., Rossi, R.L., & Martin, R.F. (1998). Options and strategies for the management of choledocholithiasis. *World Journal of Surgery, 22*(11), 1125–1132.

Sauter, P.K., & Coleman, J. (1999). Pancreatic cancer: A continuum of care. *Seminars in Oncology Nursing, 15*(1), 36–47.

Schaffner, M. (1994). *Manual of gastrointestinal procedures* (3rd ed.). Baltimore: Williams & Wilkins.

Seef, L.B., et al. (2000). 45-year follow-up of hepatitis C virus infection in healthy young adults. *Annals of Internal Medicine, 132*(2), 105–111.

Shovein, J.T., Damazo, R.J., & Hyams, I. (2000). Hepatitis A—How benign is it? *American Journal of Nursing, 100*(3), 43–47.

Strasberg, S.M. (1997). Cholelithiasis and acute cholecystitis. *Baillieres Clinical Gastroenterology, 11*(4), 643–661.

Yeo, C.J., & Cameron, J.L. (1999). Pancreatic cancer. *Current Problems in Surgery, 36*(2), 57–152.

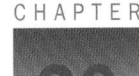
Nutritional Problems

GENERAL CONSIDERATIONS

Nutrition Overview

Knowledge of nutrients and the basic principles of nutrition is important in the role of patient teaching for disease prevention and health promotion. The four basic food groups and their placement on a pyramid serves as a guide to basic, healthy nutrition.

Key Principles

1. Nutrients, including carbohydrates, fats, proteins, vitamins, and minerals have specific functions within the body. They work together to provide energy, regulate metabolic processes, and synthesize tissues.
2. Nutrition influences all body systems both favorably and unfavorably. Examples of unfavorable effects include the link between cholesterol and heart disease or salt intake and high blood pressure. Favorable effects are many, such as the association of fiber intake with improved gastrointestinal (GI) function and the role of antioxidant vitamins A, C, and E, in preventing cancer.
3. Nutritional needs vary in response to metabolic changes, age, sex, growth periods, stress (trauma, disease, pregnancy, lactation), and physical condition.
4. Dietary and vitamin supplements may be needed depending on disease states, dietary intake, and other factors.
5. The types of foods eaten and eating patterns are developed during a lifetime and are determined by psychosocial, cultural, religious, and economic influences.
6. The nurse works with the dietitian or nutritionist to promote optimum nutrition for each patient.

Basic Food Groups and Food Pyramid

1. Developed in 1958, the four basic food groups are grains, vegetables and fruits, meat, and milk. A fifth group is considered when looking at fat in the diet. A well-balanced diet consists of foods from each group.

2. In response to growing scientific knowledge regarding the linkage of diet and disease, the U. S. Department of Agriculture developed the Food Guide Pyramid (Figure 20-1). It reflects an increased emphasis on carbohydrates in the form of grains, fruits, and vegetables as primary food sources, with a decreased emphasis on meats, dairy products, and fats.
3. In addition, seven basic dietary guidelines have been developed to promote sound eating habits and optimal health. They are:
   a. Eat a variety of foods.
   b. Maintain a healthy weight.
   c. Choose a diet low in fat, especially saturated fat and cholesterol.
   d. Choose a diet with plenty of vegetables, fruits, and grains.
   e. Use sugar in moderation.
   f. Use salt and sodium in moderation.
   g. Drink alcoholic beverages in moderation.
4. Nurses are often called upon to teach and explain these guidelines.

Nutritional Assessment

There are many methods to assess the type and amount of food consumed, including a 24-hour recall of foods eaten, a food diary kept by the patient for several days, and a food frequency questionnaire that reflects food intake patterns.

In addition to these specific tools, the following information is useful to determine nutritional patterns and status.

Key History Points

1. General background information—name, age, sex, family composition, socioeconomic status, occupation.
2. General health status and any chronic conditions, including diabetes and associated dietary restrictions.
3. Cultural/religious factors influencing dietary patterns.
4. Family history of diseases, including diabetes and obesity.

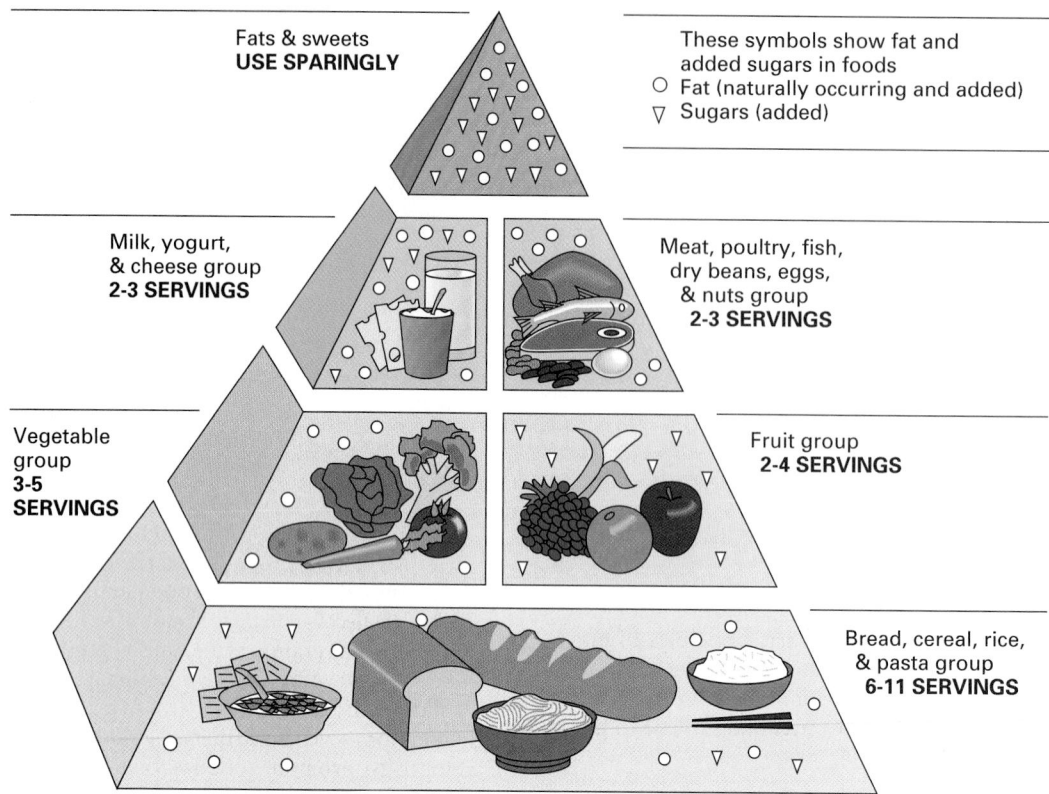

FIGURE 20-1   The Food Guide Pyramid. (Source: U.S. Department of Agriculture, April 1992.)

5. Current medications.
6. Food habits.
   a. Typical daily intake, including meal frequency, meal timing, meal location.
   b. Snacking patterns.
   c. Food intolerance or dislikes.
   d. Nutritional supplements, including vitamins, drinks, and food.
   e. Alcohol consumption.
   f. Use of specific diets/dietary restrictions.
7. Food purchase and preparation.
   a. Who purchases and prepares food and where food is purchased.
   b. Facilities for food storage and preparation.
   c. Factors influencing the types of food purchased.
8. Nutritionally related problems
   a. General well-being, energy level.
   b. Weight change during the past 6 months.
   c. Difficulty chewing or swallowing, use of dentures.
   d. Change in sense of taste or smell.
   e. Eructation, flatulence, nausea, vomiting, diarrhea, constipation, or abdominal pain or swelling, and relation to food intake.
   f. Bowel habits.

Physical Examination and Anthropometrics
1. Perform a systematic physical examination, observing for a wide variety of physical findings associated with nutritional status.
   a. Listlessness, apathy.
   b. Poor muscle tone.
   c. Dull, brittle hair; hair may be thin or sparse, easily plucked.
   d. Rough, dry, and scaly skin.
   e. Cheilosis (fissures at angles of mouth).
   f. Stomatitis (inflammation of mouth).
   g. Inflammation and easy bleeding of gums.
   h. Glossitis (inflammation of tongue).
   i. Dental caries and poor dentition.
   j. Spoon-shaped, brittle, ridged nails.
   k. Skeletal deformities, such as bowlegs.
2. Perform anthropometry as indicated. (Anthropometry comes from the word anthropology and is the science that studies the size, weight, and proportions of the human body to determine body fat mass and nutritional status.)
3. Types of anthropometric measurements include height and weight, skin-fold thickness, and circumferential tests.

4. Height and weight are determined on patient admission and are later used as a baseline for comparisons in nutritional status.
   a. Height is the distance from the patient's feet to the top of the head.
   b. Weight is the measure of total body energy stores.
   c. Weight should be measured using a consistent and reliable scale and at a consistent time.
   d. Weight loss of more than 10% of body weight during 6 months is considered clinically significant and may be associated with physiologic abnormalities and increased mortality.
5. Body mass index is the ratio of weight in kilograms and height in meters. It consists of the weight divided by the height squared (Table 20-1).
   a. BMI of <18.5 is classified as underweight.
   b. BMI of 18.5 to 24.9 is classified as normal.
   c. BMI of 25 to 29.9 is classified as overweight.
   d. BMI of 30 to 39.9 is classified as obesity.
   e. BMI ≥40 is classified as extreme obesity.
6. Metabolism is faster in younger people. For this reason, babies and children need 50 kcal per kg per day and adults need 28 kcal per kg per day. More exact measurement of caloric requirements for infants can be obtained by using charts; these estimate the body surface area by height and weight and the standard basal metabolic rate for a given weight (See Appendix).

TABLE 20-1 Body Mass Index (BMI)*

Weight	Height					
	5′	5′3″	5′6″	5′9″	6′	6′3″
140	27	25	23	21	19	18
150	29	27	24	22	20	19
160	31	28	26	24	22	20
170	33	30	28	25	23	21
180	35	32	29	27	25	23
190	37	34	31	28	26	24
200	39	36	32	30	27	25
210	41	37	34	31	29	26
220	43	39	36	33	30	28
230	45	41	37	34	31	29
240	47	43	39	36	33	30
250	49	44	40	37	34	31

* Body mass index = weight (kg)/height (m²).

7. Skin-fold thickness provides an estimate of body fat based on the amount of fat in subcutaneous tissue (Figure 20-2).
   a. Triceps skin-fold thickness:
      (i) At the midpoint of the nondominant upper arm, grasp skin and subcutaneous fat, pulling it away from the underlying muscle, and place the caliper jaws over the skin-fold flap.

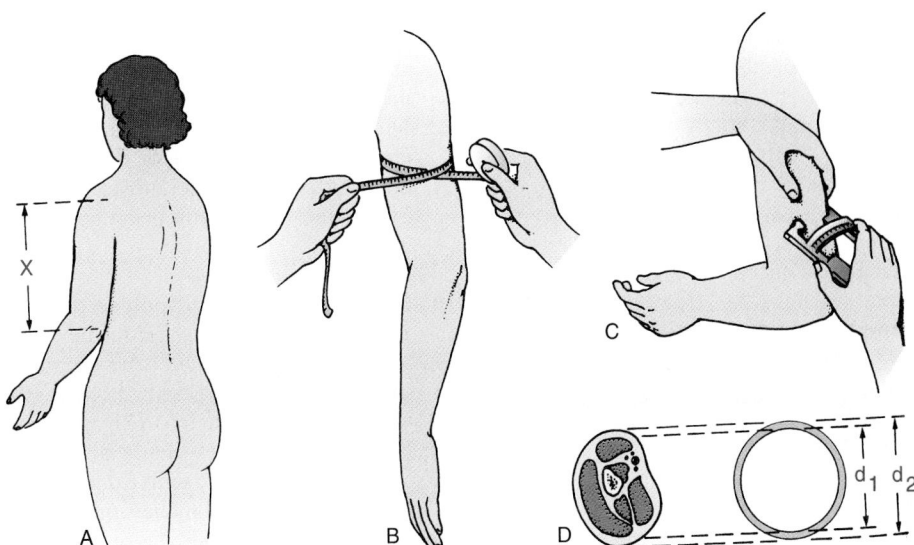

FIGURE 20-2 Anthropometric measurements. Proper positioning of the patient is required: (**A**) for measuring the mid-upper arm, (**B**) to determine mid-upper arm circumference (MAC); this position is also used to measure (**C**) the triceps skinfold (TSF) thickness, which is measured with a caliper; (**D**) shows the relation between d1 (MAMC)—mid-upper arm muscle circumference—and d2 (MAC—mid-upper arm circumference). Mid-upper arm muscle circumference is a significant measurement in determining protein-calorie malnutrition. Formula for calculation: MAMC = MAC − (0.314 × TSF). (Adapted from Blackburn, G.L., & Harvey, K.B. [1982]. Nutritional assessment as a routine in clinical medicine. *Postgraduate Medicine, 71* [5], 51.)

(ii) Take the reading within 2 to 3 seconds and without using excessive pressure.

(iii) Repeat the reading twice and take an average of the three readings to increase accuracy.

b. Subscapular skin-fold thickness: Grasp the skin and subcutaneous tissue just below the inferior boarder of the left scapula and measure with calipers as noted.

8. Circumferential tests provide information on the amount of skeletal muscle and adipose tissue. Mid-upper arm circumference—an indirect estimate of the body's muscle mass:

a. Place a tape measure around the midpoint of the nondominant upper arm and secure it snugly.

b. To calculate, multiply the triceps skin fold by 3.14 and subtract the product from the mid-upper arm circumference.

c. Adult standards are 16.5 mm for women and 12.5 mm for men.

Diagnostic Tests

1. Serum albumin—albumin is responsible for maintaining blood volume and serum and electrolyte balance. A decrease in nutritional status may result in a drop in albumin synthesis. Albumin levels reflect nutritional status during the past 30 days. Prealbumin is a more sensitive but expensive test that measures more recent nutritional status.

2. Hemoglobin—decreased amounts are related to iron deficiency anemia or other defect in hemoglobin synthesis.

3. Serum transferrin—responsible for binding iron to plasma and transporting it to the bone marrow. Reduced levels are found in catabolic states and some chronic diseases.

4. Twenty-four hour urine creatinine—an increase in this measure indicates increased tissue breakdown.

5. Twenty-four hour urea nitrogen—this test can be used to determine nitrogen balance.

GENERAL PROCEDURES AND TREATMENT MODALITIES

■ Enteral Feeding

See Procedure Guidelines 20-1.

Administration of nutrients directly into the stomach, duodenum, or jejunum through a tube is more physiologically beneficial and cost-effective than parenteral feeding. Enteral feeding carries less risk of infection than parenteral feeding and maintains a functional GI tract by preventing mucosal atrophy and biliary and pancreatic dysfunction. Enteral therapy is appropriate for patients with at least a minimally functional GI tract who cannot take nutrition by mouth.

Enteral therapy has become increasingly used as more commercially available enteral formula have been developed and long-term enteral feeding tubes have become safer and more easily inserted.

Clinical Indications

1. Increased metabolic needs—trauma, burns, cancer.
2. Coma.
3. Head/neck surgery.
4. Malabsorption.
5. Obstruction of esophagus or oropharynx.
6. Severe anorexia nervosa.
7. Recurrent aspiration.

Sites of Tube Insertion
Short-Term Nutritional Support

1. Nasogastric tube passed through the nose or mouth (orogastric) into the stomach and secured in place.
2. Tube placement must be verified before use by x-ray, aspiration of contents for pH and bilirubin concentration, or auscultation of air infected through tube.
3. If there is any question about tube placement in the respiratory tract, an x-ray should be taken and the tube should be removed.
4. Nasoduodenal or nasojejunal—tube passed through the nose into duodenum or jejunum and secured in place. X-ray is usually needed to verify correct tube placement.

Long-Term Nutritional Support

1. Gastrostomy—insertion of a tube either surgically or through a percutaneous endoscopic procedure into the stomach.
2. Gastrostomy button—small device inserted through gastrostomy stoma to allow for long-term feeding with minimal effect on body image.
3. Jejunostomy—insertion of a tube directly into the jejunum either surgically or through a percutaneous endoscopic procedure. Jejunostomy feedings are generally by continuous infusion using a volume control infuser.

Types of Tubes

1. Large-bore nasogastric polyurethane Levine tube—size 12 to 18F, used very short-term.
2. Small-bore nasogastric tube—made of polyurethane, silicone, or polyvinyl chloride with a tungsten-weighted tip at distal end, size 6 to 12F and 30 to 36 inches long.
3. Nasointestinal tube—made of silicone, polyurethane, or polyvinyl chloride with tungsten-weighted tip, size 6 to 12F and 40 to 60 inches long.
4. Gastrostomy tube—Foley or mushroom catheter type made of silicone, polyurethane, polyvinyl chloride, or latex; a balloon on the distal end to stabilize tube may be used and ranges from 5 to 30 mL capacity.
5. Gastrostomy button—silicone; ranging from 18 to 28F and 1 in. long; useful for person wanting minimal alteration in body image.
6. Jejunostomy tube—size ranging from 5 to 14F with or without a balloon (a balloon may obstruct lumen of jejunum).

Delivery Systems for Feeding Solution

1. Intermittent or continuous infusion of feeding solution by gravity is accomplished by hanging container of feeding solution from an intravenous (IV) pole and adjusting delivery rate by flow regulator.
2. Continuous feeding by controller feeding pump allows uniform flow, particularly of viscous solutions.
3. Bolus feeding involves enteral formula poured into barrel of a large (60 mL) syringe attached to a feeding tube and allowed to infuse by gravity.

NURSING ALERT

Bolus feeding may precipitate dumping syndrome, particularly if given into the small intestine. Dumping syndrome occurs when the GI system is overworked and the body is forced to decrease certain metabolic processes to provide excess energy to the GI system. People with dumping syndrome may feel dizzy or lightheaded, nervous, and nauseated.

Community and Home Care Considerations

Teach patient and family:

1. Technique for administration of tube feeding outlined in Procedure Guidelines 20-1.
2. Signs and symptoms of potential complications.
3. Need to assess tube placement and residual before each feeding.
4. Principles of medical asepsis, including careful handwashing, refrigeration of formula, cleaning of equipment with soap and water and thorough drying between feedings.
5. When the gastrostomy or jejunostomy tube insertion site is well healed, surrounding skin can be cleaned with soap and water.
6. Gauze dressing can be applied as needed.
7. Leakage around tube or signs of peristomal skin irritation should be reported.

Complications

See Table 20-2.

(text continues on page 666)

TABLE 20-2 Complications of Enteral Feeding and Treatment

Complications	Causes	Interventions
Tube displacement	Tube migration into esophagus	Observe for eructation of air when injecting air to test for tube placement in stomach. Aspirate gastric contents; if none is obtained, suspect esophageal placement. Advance tube and auscultate for "whooshing" sound of air entering stomach and aspiration of gastric contents.
	Tube placement into respiratory tract	Observe for gagging, dyspnea, inability to speak, coughing when tube insertion attempted. Aspirate gastric contents; if pH greater than 6, suspect respiratory tract placement. Obtain chest x-ray.* Withdraw tube and attempt reinsertion with patient's head flexed forward.*
Tube obstruction	Tube kinking Tube clogging	Obtain chest x-ray to confirm and withdraw and reinsert new tube.* Flush tube every 4 hrs with 30 cc of water and after administration of intermittent feeding and medication administration. Administer medications in liquid form if possible. Crush medications finely.
Vomiting	Tube migration into esophagus	See interventions for tube displacement above.
	Decreased absorption	Auscultate for decreased bowel sounds, observe for abdominal distention. Consider decreasing amount of tube feeding, change type of feeding to one requiring less digestive effort and a lower fat content.* Consider administration on a continuous basis.* Consider placement of a small bore, weighted-tip nasointestinal tube.*
	Rapid rate of infusion	Administer no faster than 200–300 cc during 10–20 min. Consider administration on a continuous basis.*
	Excessive infusion of air	If giving a bolus feeding, pinch tubing off when refilling syringe with formula. If giving continuous feeding, make certain bag does not empty before closing off tubing.
	Patient position	Maintain patient at 30°–45° angle of head elevation during and 30–60 min after feeding. If administering continuous feeding, maintain head elevation at all times.
Diarrhea	Drug therapy	Evaluate drug regimen for possible causes of drug-induced diarrhea from antibiotics, elixirs with high osmolarity, H_2 blockers, magnesium-containing antacids.
	Hypoalbuminemia	Check serum albumin levels. Administer formula requiring less digestion.*
	High osmolarity of formula	Begin administration of formula at slow rate.* Consider continuous feeding rather than intermittent.* Consider diluting formula with water and gradually increasing concentration.*
	Lactose intolerance	Administer lactose-free formula.*
	Bacterial contamination of formula	Change administration set daily or per agency protocol. Maintain strict medical asepsis, including careful hand washing before administration of formula. Allow formula to hang no longer than 8 h.
	Rapid infusion rate	Administer slowly; consider continuous rather than intermittent infusion.*

(continued)

TABLE 20-2   Complications of Enteral Feeding and Treatment (Continued)

Complications	Causes	Interventions
Constipation	Lack of fiber Decreased fluid intake Drug therapy	Administer formula with fiber.* Increase intake of water.* Evaluate drug regimen for possible cause, including aluminum-containing antacids.
Hyperglycemia	High caloric density formula (1.5–2 kcal/mL)	Monitor serum glucose, assess for dehydration caused by hyperosmotic diuresis; observe for symptoms of hyperglycemia, including polyuria, polydipsia. Change formula to lower calorie content.* Administer insulin.* Observe for hypercapnea (increased respirations, elevated P_{CO_2}).
Electrolyte imbalance Hypernatremia	Dehydration	Assess for signs and symptoms of dehydration (I&O, daily weights, skin turgor, blood urea nitrogen, central venous pressure, tachycardia, hypotension). Rehydrate with D5W and/or hypotonic saline solutions.*
Hyponatremia	Overhydration	Observe for signs and symptoms of hypervolemia (shortness of breath, rales, I&O, daily weight, peripheral edema, elevated CVP). Observe for signs and symptoms of hyponatremia (lethargy, headaches, mental status change, nausea, vomiting, abdominal cramping). Replace sodium, administer diuretics, restrict fluids.*
Hyperkalemia	Metabolic acidosis/renal insufficiency	Observe for signs and symptoms of hyperkalemia (dysrhythmias, nausea, diarrhea, muscle weakness). Treat underlying cause. Administer exchange resin, glucose, and insulin.*
Hypokalemia	Diarrhea	See interventions for diarrhea. If severe, replace potassium.*

H_2: histamine; I&O: intake and output; CVP: central venous pressure.
* Obtain orders from health care provider.

PROCEDURE GUIDELINES 20-1

ADMINISTRATION OF ENTERAL (TUBE) FEEDINGS: INTERMITTENT OR CONTINUOUS

EQUIPMENT

Tube feeding formula
Graduated containers
30–60 mL catheter-tipped syringe
Water
Stethoscope

pH strip
Gavage feeding bag (optional)
For continuous tube feeding:
Tube feeding bag and tubing and volume control infuser

PROCEDURE

Nursing Action	Rationale
PREPARATORY PHASE	
1. Remove formula from refrigerator and allow to come to room temperature.	1. Use prepared dietary formulas within 24 h.
2. Explain procedure to patient.	
3. Wash hands.	3. Prevent bacterial contamination of formula.
4. Protect patient from spillage.	
5. Shake formula container.	5. Shaking prevents separation of formula.
6. Elevate head of bed 30°–45°.	6. Prevents aspiration.
7. Using the catheter-tipped syringe, inject 20 cc–30 cc of air while listening with a stethoscope positioned at the epigastric area (for nasogastric tubes). For nasointestinal tubes, 20 cc of air may be injected, but auscultation site may be displaced laterally and inferiorly.	7. Auscultation of a "whooshing" or bubbling sound assists in confirmation of proper tube placement. Should the patient burp immediately after injection of air, suspect esophageal placement of tube.

PROCEDURE GUIDELINES 20-1   *CONTINUED*

Nursing Action	Rationale
8. Aspirate stomach contents.	8. If residual gastric contents exceed 100 cc for intermittent tube feedings or greater than 1.5 times the hourly rate for continuous tube feeding, hold feeding and notify health care provider. No residual will be obtained with intestinal placement.
9. Measure pH of residual.	9. pH of gastric contents should be between 1 and 6. Intestinal pH may be greater than 6. Respiratory tract secretions usually measure greater than 6. Measurement of bilirubin by test strip may also be done; bilirubin over 5 predicts lung placement.
10. If residual is within normal limits, and stomach or intestinal placement has been confirmed, return gastric contents to stomach through syringe using gravity to assist flow. If there is a question about the tube placement, notify the provider and obtain an order for an x-ray.	10. Returning gastric contents to stomach prevents acid-base and electrolyte imbalance.

PERFORMANCE PHASE

1. For intermittent tube feeding, attach barrel of catheter-tipped syringe to pinched-off feeding tube.	1. Pinching off the feeding tube prevents air from entering the stomach and causing distention.
2. Fill catheter-tipped syringe with formula and allow fluid to flow in by gravity.	2. The rate of flow is regulated by raising or lowering the syringe.
3. Pour additional formula into barrel of syringe when it is three-quarters empty.	3. Prevents air from entering stomach.
4. After administering the prescribed amount of formula, flush tubing with at least 30 cc of water.	4. Prevents clogging of feeding tube.
5. If using a gavage bag for intermittent feeding, fill bag with prescribed amount of feeding, purge feeding bag tubing of air, attach distal end to feeding tube, and regulate to run over at least 10–20 min.	
6. For continuous tube feeding, fill bag with 4 h of tube feeding, flush tubing, attach to volume control infuser according to manufacturer's instructions, attach distal end to feeding tube, and start. Flush with 30–60 cc of water every 4 hours after first checking residual.	6. Prevents bacterial contamination. Maintains tube patency.
7. After intermittent feeding is completed, cover end of feeding tube with plug or clamp.	7. Prevents leakage.

FOLLOW-UP PHASE

1. Rinse equipment with warm water, and dry. Replace every 24 h or per agency policy.	1. Limits bacterial contamination.
2. Maintain head of bed elevation for 30–60 min. after feeding is completed. If continuous feeding, maintain head elevation continuously.	2. Prevents aspiration.
3. Document type and amount of feeding, amount of water given, and patient tolerance of procedure.	
4. Monitor breath sounds, bowel sounds, gastric distention, diarrhea or constipation, intake and output, daily weight, and serum chemistry results.	4. Evaluates for aspiration, effect on gastrointestinal system, and therapeutic effect of feedings.

PATIENT EDUCATION

1. Instruct patient to notify nurse if experiencing sensation of fullness, nausea, or vomiting.	1. May indicate intolerance of feeding.

GASTROSTOMY OR JEJUNOSTOMY CARE

1. Special care of ostomy tube insertion site should include:
   a. Cleaning around tube with prescribed cleansing solution every shift and as needed.
   b. Applying sterile 4 × 4 gauze pad and taping in place.
   c. Applying skin barrier should peristomal skin become excoriated.
   d. Taping of tube to skin or skin barrier with hypoallergenic tape.

▪ Parenteral Nutrition

See Procedure Guidelines 20-2.

Parenteral nutrition is the introduction of nutrients, including amino acids, lipids, carbohydrates, vitamins, minerals, and water, through a venous access device (VAD) directly into the intravascular fluid to provide nutrients required for metabolic functioning of the body.

Clinical Indications
1. Patient cannot tolerate enteral nutrition because of:
   a. Paralytic ileus.
   b. Intestinal obstruction.
   c. Acute pancreatitis.
   d. Malabsorption.
   e. Persistent vomiting.
   f. Severe diarrhea.
   g. Fistula.
   h. Inflammatory bowel disease.
2. Hypermetabolic states for which enteral therapy is either not possible or inadequate.
   a. Burns.
   b. Trauma.
   c. Sepsis.
3. In these situations additional components are added to the enteral therapy or individualized solutions are developed to meet the nutritional needs of the patient.

Methods of Parenteral Nutrition
Total Nutrient Admixture (TNA)
1. Given through a central vein, often into the superior vena cava, this parenteral formula combines carbohydrates in the form of a concentrated (20% to 70%) dextrose solution; proteins in the form of amino acids; lipids in the form of an emulsion (10% to 20%), including triglycerides, egg phospholipids, glycerol, and water; and vitamins and minerals.
2. Central TNA is indicted for patients requiring parenteral feeding for 7 or more days.

Peripheral Parenteral Nutrition (PPN)
1. Given through a peripheral vein, this parenteral formula combines a lesser concentrated glucose solution with amino acids, vitamins, minerals, and lipids.

2. Unlike TNA given centrally, peripheral parenteral nutrition provides fewer calories, and generally a larger percentage of calories is supplied by lipids rather than by carbohydrates.
3. Indicated for patients requiring parenteral nutrition for fewer than 7 days.

Total Parenteral Nutrition (TPN)
1. Combines glucose, amino acids, vitamins, and minerals and is given through a central IV line.
2. If lipids are needed, they are given intermittently or mixed in with the TPN solution, through a central IV.

Fat Emulsion (Lipids)
1. Ten percent or 20% emulsion composed of triglycerides, egg phospholipids, glycerol, and water.
2. May be given centrally or peripherally.

Delivery Systems for Parenteral Nutrition
1. Central venous access devices:
   a. Insertion of long-term VADs, such as Hickman, Broviac, or Groshung catheters.
   b. Peripherally inserted central catheters (PICC lines) may be used.
   c. If multilumen, these VADs can allow concomitant administration of TNA and other solutions, including medications or blood, each running through a separate lumen.
2. Peripheral IV access:
   a. Insertion of an angiocatheter into a vein in the arm or leg.
   b. Midline catheters of longer length and with the ability to remain in place for more than 3 days.
3. Delivery of parenteral nutrition should be controlled by a volume control infuser.
4. Filters should be used whenever possible.
   a. A 0.22-micron filter may be used for TPN (without added fat emulsion).
   b. A 1.2-micron filter may be used for TNA or fat emulsion.

Complications
See Table 20-3.

TABLE 20-3 Complications of Administration of Total Nutrient Admixture (TNA) and Treatment

Complications	Causes	Interventions
Sepsis	High glucose content of fluid Venous access device contamination	Monitor temperature, WBC count, insertion site for signs and symptoms of infection. Maintain strict surgical asepsis when changing dressing and tubing. Consider decreasing glucose content of fluid.* Consider removal of venous access device with replacement in alternate site.* If blood cultures positive, consider institution of antibiotic therapy.*
Electrolyte imbalance	Iatrogenic Effect of underlying diseases, ie, fistula, diarrhea, vomiting	Monitor electrolyte levels at least every 2–3 days. Monitor signs and symptoms of electrolyte imbalance. Treat underlying cause.* Change concentration of electrolytes in TNA as necessary to address blood levels.*

(continued)

TABLE 20-3 Complications of Administration of Total Nutrient Admixture (TNA) and Treatment (Continued)

Complications	Causes	Interventions
Hyperglycemia	High glucose content of fluid Insufficient insulin secretion	Monitor blood glucose frequently. Decrease glucose content of fluid if possible.* Administer exogenous insulin per addition to TNA, subcutaneously or through a separate intravenous drip.*
Hypoglycemia	Abrupt discontinuation of TNA administered through a central vessel	After discontinuation of centrally administered TNA, start $D_{10}W$ at the same rate.*
Hypervolemia	Iatrogenic Underlying disease, ie, CHF, renal failure	Monitor intake and output, daily weights, CVP, breath sounds, peripheral edema. Consider administering more concentrated TNA solution.*
Hyperosmolar diuresis	High osmolarity of TNA	Monitor intake and output, daily weights, CVP. Consider decreasing concentration or amount of fluid administered.*
Hepatic dysfunction	High concentration of carbohydrates and/or fats relative to protein in TNA	Monitor liver function tests, triglyceride levels, presence of jaundice. Consider alteration in formula content.*
Hypercapnea	High carbohydrate content of fluid	Consider changing formula to increase the proportion of fat relative to carbohydrate.
Lipid intolerance	Low birth weight or premature infant History of liver disease History of elevated triglycerides	Monitor for bleeding (check stools for occult blood, coagulation studies, platelet levels). Monitor O_2 levels for impaired oxygenation. Monitor for fat overload syndrome: monitor triglyceride levels and liver function tests, hepatosplenomegaly, decreased coagulation, cyanosis, dyspnea. Monitor allergic reaction: nausea, vomiting, headache, chest pain, back pain, fever. Administer lipid-containing solutions slowly, initially, while observing for symptoms.
Lipid particulate aggregation	Unstable mixture of dextrose solution with lipid emulsion	Observe for cracking or creaming of fluid, and avoid use of fluid with these characteristics.

WBC: white blood cell; CHF: congestive heart failure; CVP: central venous pressure.
* Obtain orders from health care provider.

PROCEDURE GUIDELINES 20-2

ADMINISTRATION OF TOTAL NUTRIENT ADMIXTURE (TNA) (SIMILAR PROCEDURE FOR TOTAL PARENTERAL NUTRITION [TPN] AND OTHER COMPONENTS)

EQUIPMENT

Volume control infuser
Bag of TNA
Administration tubing with luer-lock connections
1.2-μm filter
Hypoallergenic tape, 1 in
Face mask (optional)

Clean gloves
Sterile dressing kit to include:
  Alcohol swab sticks (3)
  Povidone-iodine sticks (3)
  Sterile gloves
  Transparent dressing

PROCEDURE

Nursing Action	Rationale

To change bag and bottle:

PREPARATORY PHASE

1. Remove TNA from refrigerator at least 1 h before hanging.	1. Decreases incidence of hypothermia, pain, and venospasm.
2. Inspect fluid for presence of cracking or creaming.	2. Indicates fluid separation, do not use. If infusing TPN, solution should be clear without clouding.
3. Wash hands.	3. Prevents bacterial contamination.

continued

PROCEDURE GUIDELINES 20-2 | **ADMINISTRATION OF TOTAL NUTRIENT ADMIXTURE (TNA) (SIMILAR PROCEDURE FOR TOTAL PARENTERAL NUTRITION [TPN] AND OTHER COMPONENTS)** *CONTINUED*

Nursing Action	Rationale

PERFORMANCE PHASE

1. Using strict sterile technique, attach tubing (with filter) to TNA bag and purge of air.

1. Prevent air embolus.
   * Tubing should be changed on a regular basis (every 2–3 d). Filter will be different for TPN, because lipids are not included.

2. Close all clamps on new tubing. Insert tubing into volume control infuser.
3. If venous access device (VAD) has a clamp at proximal end, clamp tubing.

3. Prevents air embolus if VAD is inserted in a central vein.

4. If no clamp is available on central VAD, instruct patient to Valsalva maneuver (bear down and hold breath) while new tubing is connected.

4. Valsalva's maneuver creates positive pressure, preventing air from getting sucked into tubing.

5. Sterilely connect tubing to hub of VAD, making certain the connection is securely fastened using luer-lock connections.

5. Prevents disconnection of tubing.

6. Open all clamps and regulate flow through volume control infuser.

FOLLOW-UP PHASE

1. Monitor administration hourly, assessing for integrity of fluid and administration system and patient tolerance and complications.

1. See Table 20-3 for complications of TNA.

2. Document tubing change and fluid administration, observations, presence of complications, and any treatment given.

PATIENT EDUCATION

1. Teach patient signs and symptoms of complications, including sepsis, phlebitis, extravasation, and to report any changes to nursing personnel.

1. Patient can assist nursing personnel in monitoring therapy and in detecting complications.

2. If patient is to be discharged to home with TNA, begin instruction regarding proper storage, handling, and administration of TNA. Include family members as appropriate.

2. Long-term therapy may be indicated in burns, emaciation due to cancer treatment, and other conditions. Home care nurses will reinforce your teaching.

To change central venous catheter dressing:

PREPARATORY PHASE

1. Obtain equipment.
2. Explain procedure to patient.
3. Place patient in a comfortable supine position and turn head away from site.

3. Turning patient's head away from site will decrease possible microbial contamination of site.

4. Wash hands.

4. All precautions are taken to prevent bacterial contamination.

5. Don mask (optional).

PERFORMANCE PHASE

1. Don clean gloves and carefully remove old dressing.
2. Inspect insertion site for complications.

2. Observe for edema, erythema, tenderness, and leakage of fluid.

3. Clean insertion site with each alcohol swab beginning at insertion site and moving outward in a circular pattern.

3. Moves potential contaminants away from insertion site.

4. Repeat using each povidone-iodine swab.

4. Removes bacteria from insertion site.

5. Allow to dry.

5. Drying allows adhesive dressing to adhere securely.

6. Remove adhesive backing of transparent dressing. Center dressing over site.

6. Application of transparent dressing provides a bacterial barrier while allowing full visualization of insertion site.

7. Loop and tape tubing to skin using 1-in tape. Do not tape over dressing.

7. Prevent dislodgement of tubing.

PROCEDURE GUIDELINES 20-2   *CONTINUED*

Nursing Action	Rationale
FOLLOW-UP PHASE	
1. Document dressing change and observation of insertion site.	
2. Observe insertion site frequently for signs of complications.	2. Observe for edema, erythema, tenderness, and leakage of fluid.
PATIENT EDUCATION	
1. Teach patient signs and symptoms of infection, phlebitis, and fluid extravasation and to report any changes to nursing personnel.	1. Patient may be first to notice complications.
2. If patient is to be discharged to home with TNA, begin instruction regarding sterile dressing change. Include family members as appropriate.	2. Because risk of sepsis is so great, sterile technique is still required for home dressing changes.

NUTRITIONAL DISORDERS

Obesity

Obesity is an overabundance of body fat resulting in body weight of 20% or more than the average weight for the person's age, height, sex, and body frame. Increasingly, obesity is being diagnosed using the Body Mass Index (to account for body build) and/or Body Surface Area and Basal Metabolic Rates (to account for metabolic activity of the person). A BMI greater than 30 is considered obese. About 18% of Americans are obese (up from 12% in 1991) and 63% of men and 55% of women are overweight.

Pathophysiology and Etiology

1. Increasing evidence reveals that heredity plays a part in the development of obesity. Identical twins raised apart are more likely to have similar amounts of body fat than fraternal twins raised separately.
2. Environment plays a role.
   a. Some evidence shows that children reared by obese parents have an increased tendency toward obesity.
   b. In addition, social class may influence weight; that is, higher social class may be associated with more weight-conscious behavior.
3. A variety of psychological factors may contribute to weight gain, including depression and anxiety.
4. Physiologic factors.
   a. Endocrine abnormalities (rare causes of obesity)—Cushing's syndrome, hypothyroidism, hypogonadism, or hypothalamic lesions.
   b. Age—advancing age may be associated with obesity often because of changes in activity level or in women, because of hormonal changes; early childhood and the start of puberty may also be associated with obesity.
      (i) Overeating after puberty may increase the total number of fat cells.

(ii) Despite dieting, these extra fat cells can never be eliminated; they only decrease in size.

Clinical Manifestations

1. Body weight greater than 20% of acceptable weight for height or BMI >30.
2. Increased weight is correlated with increased incidence of:
   a. Cardiovascular disease.
   b. Diabetes mellitus.

Diagnostic Evaluation

1. Nutritional assessment—to evaluate dietary habits.
2. Anthropometric and physical assessment—to evaluate increased body fat and effects of obesity on body.
3. Selected hormonal studies (thyroid, adrenal)—to look for underlying cause.

Management
Conservative Measures

1. Diet therapy—has been controversial, but a well-balanced diet containing all the major food groups is still advised.
   a. One thousand calories per day must be eliminated from a diet to lose 1 kg (2.2 lb) of body weight per week.
   b. A 1,200-calorie diet for women and a 1,500-calorie diet for men with variations depending on patient size and activity level are basic to diet management. Fats should compose no more than 30% of all calories, proteins approximately 15 to 20%, and carbohydrates should constitute the remaining portion.
   c. A balance of food groups is essential to maintain vitamin and nutrient balance. Nutrient supplements may be necessary (iron, B_6, zinc, and folate).
   d. Food preparation should include seasoning with herbs, onion, garlic, and pepper, and foods should be baked, broiled, steamed, or sautéed using minimal polyunsaturated oil.

e. Food attractively arranged on smaller plates, using whole rather than processed foods and eaten slowly, will assist the overall process.

f. Eliminating entire food groups from the diet, such as carbohydrates (in many popular protein and fat-based diets), will eventually result in craving of those foods eliminated, disruption of normal metabolic processes, and quick weight gain when the food is added to the diet.

2. Exercise—a daily exercise program may include walking or other aerobic activities for approximately 180 minutes per week, or 1 hour at least three times a week, however daily exercise is optimal.

3. Behavior modification is a cornerstone of any successful diet.

a. Identify and eliminate situations or cues leading to overeating or high-calorie foods with use of a food diary.

b. Provide positive reinforcement of proper dietary habits.

c. Should a lapse in diet habits occur, focus on a prompt and positive return to appropriate dietary habits.

d. Stress reduction techniques, such as visual imagery or progressive relaxation; peer support may be helpful.

Pharmacotherapy

1. Anorexia medications, such as amphetamines and norepinephrine-releasing agents or reuptake inhibitors, reduce appetite and stimulate weight loss initially.

2. However, tolerance develops within 2 to 4 weeks and weight is rapidly regained when the drugs are discontinued.

3. Numerous long-term studies have failed to show long-term success with these agents.

4. Phentermine (Ionamin, Fastin) is one of the most widely prescribed agents; however, it causes stimulating effects and should not be used in uncontrolled hypertension, advanced heart disease, history of drug abuse, and with MAO inhibitors.

5. Sibutramine (Meridia) is a mixed neurotransmitter reuptake inhibitor that acts on the central nervous system to reduce appetite.

a. The long-term risks of this medication are not known, but it must be used cautiously with hypertension, coronary artery disease, heart failure, arrhythmia, renal and hepatic impairment, narrow angle glaucoma, and seizure disorders.

b. Multiple drug interactions include monamine oxidase inhibitors, other serotonergic drugs (selective serotonin reuptake inhibitors [SSRIs] antidepressants, sumatriptan and other migraine agents), lithium, dextromethorphan, and possibly erythromycin and ketoconazole.

c. Side effects include dry mouth, constipation, dizziness, nervousness, insomnia. Has not been shown to be addictive.

6. Recently, scientists have found success in weight loss with the use of orlistat (Xenical), a gastrointestinal lipase inhibitor, which blocks the breakdown of fat in the GI system. About 30% of dietary fat is eliminated.

a. Side effects include oily or fatty stools, flatulence, and GI distress.

b. Long-term safety of the drug has not been determined, but addition of a fat-soluble vitamin supplement (vitamin A, D, E, K and beta carotene) taken 1 hour before or 2 hours after orlistat is taken will prevent a theoretical vitamin deficiency.

c. Should not be used in cases of cholestasis or malabsorption.

d. These medications are only adjunct to diet and exercise therapy.

Surgical Interventions

Numerous surgical procedures have been used. However, gastroplasty is the current procedure of choice. These therapies are generally reserved for morbidly obese patients who cannot lose weight through the above therapies.

1. Gastroplasty—most common procedure is vertical banding involving creation of a 30-mL pouch along the lesser gastric curvature with a small outlet created with the use of a ring of plastic at the distal end to prevent dilation (Figure 20-3).

2. Gastric bypass—a Roux-en-Y gastroenterostomy is constructed by first creating a 50-mL pouch in the proximal stomach by stapling horizontally and completely separating the smaller proximal stomach pouch from the larger distal stomach pouch. To this proximal pouch, the distal jejunum is attached, thus bypassing the distal stomach pouch. The transected proximal portion of the jejunum is anastomosed to the distal jejunum.

Complications

1. Obesity is a risk factor for diabetes, gallbladder disease, osteoarthritis of weight-bearing joints, high blood pressure, and coronary artery disease.

2. Vitamin and mineral deficiencies because of surgical intervention and/or severely restricted diet.

a. A moderate, well-balanced weight reduction diet will generally not cause deficiencies, although a multiple vitamin/mineral supplement may be used.

b. A low-calorie diet (fewer than 800 to 1,000 calories/day) will require careful monitoring and vitamin/mineral supplements.

Nursing Assessment

1. Obtain a complete nutritional assessment (may be in collaboration with a nutritionist).

2. Assess behavioral/emotional components of eating, coping mechanisms, and past successes/failures with dieting.

Nursing Diagnoses

• Altered Nutrition: More Than Body Requirements related to high-calorie, high-fat diet, and limited exercise

• Fluid Volume Deficit related to gastroplasty or gastric bypass surgery

• Self-Esteem Disturbance related to weight

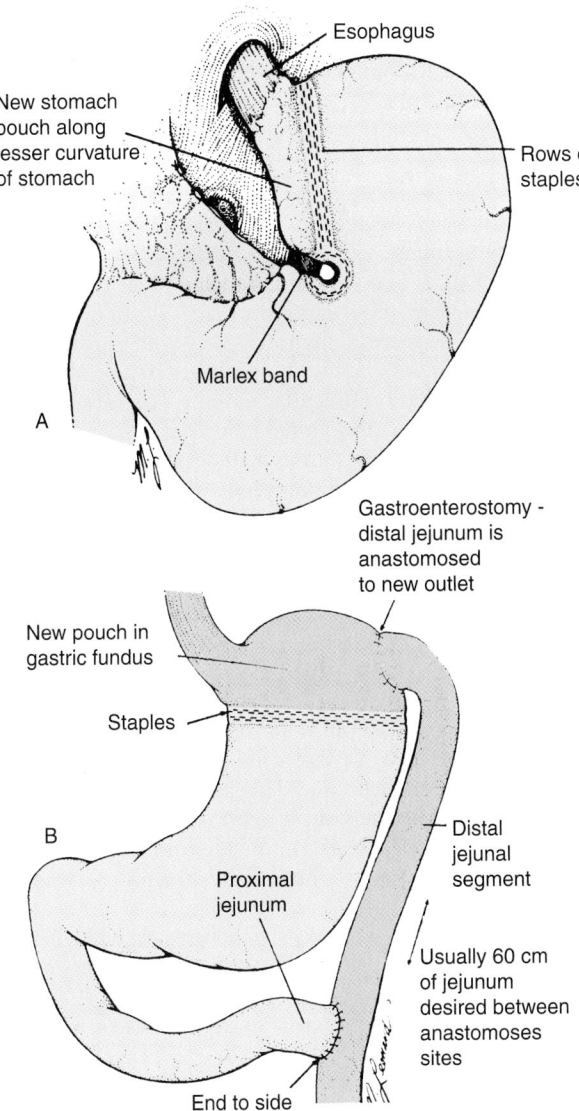

Esophagus

New stomach pouch along lesser curvature of stomach

Rows of staples

Marlex band

A

Gastroenterostomy - distal jejunum is anastomosed to new outlet

New pouch in gastric fundus

Staples

B

Proximal jejunum

Distal jejunal segment

Usually 60 cm of jejunum desired between anastomoses sites

End to side anastomosis

FIGURE 20-3 (**A**) Gastroplasty with vertical banding. (**B**) Gastric bypass with Roux-en-Y anastomosis.

Nursing Interventions
Modifying Nutritional Intake

1. Assist patient in assessing current dietary habits and identifying poor dietary habits.
2. Assist patient in developing appropriate diet plan based on likes and dislikes, activity level, and lifestyle.
3. Suggest behavior modification strategies, such as shortening lunch break, preventing access to quick snacks, eating only at mealtimes at the table.
4. Provide emotional support to patient during weight-reduction efforts through positive reinforcement and creative problem solving.

5. Provide patient with alternative coping mechanisms, including stress reduction techniques, such as progressive relaxation and guided imagery.
6. Assess patient's ability to tolerate exercise through measurement of vital signs before, during, and after exercise and ask about symptoms of shortness of breath and chest pain.

Preventing Complications Postoperatively

1. Provide initial postoperative care as for gastric resection (see p. 586).
2. Administer IV fluids as directed. Record intake and output.
3. When bowel sounds return, give oral fluids to prevent dehydration.
4. If fluids are tolerated, begin six small feedings for a total of 600 to 800 calories.
5. Observe for and report increased pain and distention, which may indicate leakage at staple sites or obstruction.
6. Monitor vital signs and wound for signs of wound infection and dehiscence.
7. Watch for and report signs of dehydration (thirst, oliguria, dry mucous membranes) and hypokalemia (muscle weakness, anorexia, nausea, decreased bowel sounds, and dysrhythmias).
8. Warn patient that overeating will cause vomiting and painful esophageal distention.
9. Stress the importance of good dietary habits and behavior modification to lose weight, because gastroplasty is only an adjunct to treatment.
10. Encourage close, long-term follow-up for monitoring of weight loss and nutritional status. Additional long-term complications include esophagitis and malnutrition.

Strengthening Self-Esteem

1. Direct patient education and conversation in a nonjudgmental manner.
2. Get to know the patient and point out the positive aspects of patient's health and well-being.
3. Encourage patient to make change in weight for the positive health aspects, not just for cosmetic reasons.
4. Be a good role model—show a healthy attitude toward sensible eating, exercise, and other healthy practices.

Patient Education and Health Maintenance

1. Discuss fat, carbohydrate, and protein, their inclusion in common foods, and their calories per gram.
2. Describe the five basic food groups and their placement on the food pyramid.
3. Explain the purpose of a balanced diet and the need for vitamins and minerals.
4. Review the health hazards of obesity and recent evidence that repeated losing and regaining of weight carries a greater risk of heart disease.

5. Advise patient of plateau period that may occur without weight loss for some time, but advise patient not to get discouraged.
6. Tell patient to keep a food diary to show to nutritionist and to weigh self no more than once a week.
7. If patient is interested in liquid diets or herbal supplements to lose weight, encourage discussion with his or her health care provider. Some preparations may contain ephedra, a powerful stimulant that may cause increased blood pressure, significant side effects, and many drug interactions.
8. Refer to agencies such as American Dietetic Association, 216 West Jackson Boulevard, Chicago, IL 60606-6995, 800-366-1655; and TOPS (Take Pounds Off Sensibly), P.O. Box 070360, 4575 South Fifth Street, Milwaukee, WI 53207, 414-482-4620; *www.tops.org*.

Outcome-Based Evaluation
- Five-pound weight loss during first month
- No abdominal distention, nausea or vomiting, or wound infection
- Patient verbalizes feeling good about self secondary to change in diet and exercise habits

Anorexia Nervosa

Anorexia nervosa is an eating disorder characterized by self-induced weight loss greater than 15% of minimally normal weight for age and height and associated with psychological and endocrine abnormalities. Periods of starvation may be mixed with gorging and purging.

Pathophysiology and Etiology
1. A semistarvation state with glucose and protein sparing, fat utilization, endocrine changes, and fluid and electrolyte disturbances is induced.
   a. Loss of fat stores.
   b. Decreased protein synthesis.
   c. Hypothalamic/pituitary dysfunction—decrease in follicle stimulating hormone (FSH), luteinizing hormone (LH), and estrogen.
   d. Decrease in thyroid hormone.
   e. Decrease in catecholamines.
2. The biopsychosocial etiologic components of this disease interact differently in each patient.
   a. Biologic/genetic predisposition remains unclear.
   b. Psychological components include:
      (i) Distorted body image.
      (ii) Fear of gaining weight.
      (iii) Self-esteem dependent on body image.
      (iv) Ability to achieve weight loss viewed as a sign of self-control.
      (v) Denial of problem.
   c. Social influences
      (i) Most patients are between the age of 14 and 24, and 90% are female.
      (ii) Seen most often in the middle and upper class social strata.
      (iii) Patients may relate high family expectations.
      (iv) Frequent peer/social pressure to strive toward an esthetic of thinness.

Clinical Manifestations
1. Symptoms vary widely and often are dependent on the severity of illness.
2. Physical signs and symptoms include loss of adipose tissue and weight loss of greater than 15% of ideal body weight, bradycardia, hypotension, cold intolerance, hypothermia, dry skin, thinning scalp hair, lanugo, amenorrhea for 3 consecutive months, decreased libido, constipation, and abdominal pain.
3. Psychological manifestations include perfectionistic and/or obsessive-compulsive behavior with high performance expectations, anxiety, increased exercise activity, inhibited or destructive social interactions, sleep disturbance, depression, and diminished sexual interest.

Diagnostic Evaluation
1. Serum chemistry may show electrolyte imbalance that may be life-threatening (decreased chloride, potassium, phosphate, magnesium, zinc levels); increased blood urea nitrogen (BUN), creatinine, liver function tests, bicarbonate, amylase; and decreased albumin levels.
2. Hormone studies may show decreased LH, FSH, estrogen, testosterone (in men), and thyroid hormone and decreased response to luteinizing hormone-releasing hormone.
3. Complete blood count may show decreased white blood cells and hematocrit, indicating starvation's effect on immunity and anemia.
4. Electrocardiogram to detect dysrhythmias or signs of electrolyte imbalance.
5. Urinalysis may show ketonuria.

Management
1. Dietary modification to achieve gradual weight gain and normal eating habits.
2. Enteral/parenteral feeding may be necessary if prescribed diet cannot be maintained by patient and physical status warrants.
3. Individual counseling focuses on patient's need to control weight, alteration in body image, and associated diagnoses, including depression and suicidal ideation.
4. Antidepressants and other pharmacologic agents for associated psychiatric problems may be tried.

Complications
1. Severe electrolyte disturbances, especially hypokalemia; dehydration; and anemia.
2. Cardiac dysrhythmias, hypotension, cardiac arrest.
3. Amenorrhea and other endocrine dysfunctions.

4. Comorbid psychiatric conditions such as depression, anxiety disorders, and high risk for suicide.

Nursing Assessment

1. Obtain detailed dietary history and complete review of systems, including psychological, gynecologic, endocrine, GI systems, activities of daily living, and exercise history.
2. Perform physical examination, including vital signs, height and weight, heart rate and rhythm, bowel sounds, and observation for hematemesis and dental caries (which may indicate self-induced vomiting).

Nursing Diagnoses

- Altered Nutrition: Less Than Body Requirements related to self-restricted intake
- Body Image Disturbance related to weight
- High Risk for Suicide related to psychological distress

Nursing Interventions

Promoting Weight Gain

1. Monitor daily intake and output and weight (before breakfast).
2. Assess bowel function. Promote fluids and activity to prevent constipation if the patient cannot tolerate food high in fiber.
3. Encourage small, frequent meals or snacks of high calorie foods and beverages. Liquid nutritional supplements may be best tolerated.
4. Provide positive reinforcement for improved intake and weight gain.

Fostering a Healthy Body Image

1. Establish a trusting relationship and provide for patient's safety and security needs.
2. Be alert for lying and manipulation that the patient may display to preserve control.
3. Involve patient in the treatment plan, offering choices to increase patient's sense of control.
4. Encourage patient to verbalize feelings about body image, self-concept, fears, and frustrations.
5. Emphasize the importance of counseling, stress management, assertiveness training, and other therapies.

Preventing Suicide

1. Assess level of risk by obtaining history of past suicide attempts, recent suicidal thoughts, and current ideation, plan, and possible method.
2. Maintain level of observance called for by situation.
3. Ensure that access to sharp objects is prohibited.
4. Ensure that a crisis intervention team is on call if needed.

Patient Education and Health Maintenance

1. Teach principles of nutrition and healthful diet and eating habits. Discuss food matter-of-factly to avoid reinforcing the patient's preoccupation with food.
2. Teach the effect of starvation on both physiologic and psychological functioning.

3. Involve the patient's family and significant others in the treatment plan, as appropriate.
4. Describe the dangers of using laxatives and diuretics in weight control, such as electrolyte imbalances, dehydration, and bowel atony.
5. Refer to agencies such as American Anorexia-Bulimia Association, 212-575-6200.

Outcome-Based Evaluation

- One-pound weight gain during 1 week
- Verbalizes satisfaction with body image and weight
- Patient denies suicidal thoughts

▨ Bulimia Nervosa

Bulimia is recurrent episodes of binge eating and a feeling of lack of control over eating behavior during these episodes, with associated inappropriate methods to prevent weight gain, including self-induced vomiting, excessive use of laxatives, diuretics, fasting, or excessive exercise. These episodes occur at least twice a week for 3 months. Self-image is significantly influenced by body weight and shape.

Pathophysiology and Etiology

1. Onset of illness often occurs in late adolescence or early 20s and is approximately 10 times more common in young women than in young men.
2. Bulimia is associated with a personal or family history of obesity, substance abuse, depression, anxiety, or mood disorders.
3. Self-induced vomiting may result in electrolyte imbalance (hypokalemia, hyponatremia, hypochloremia, elevated bicarbonate) or esophageal tears or gastric rupture.
4. Starvation and its physiologic effects may or may not be as evident as they are in anorexia nervosa.

Clinical Manifestations

1. The course of the disease may be chronic or intermittent during many years.
2. Weight is often maintained within normal range or may be significantly elevated or decreased.
3. Binge eating may be followed by inappropriate compensatory mechanisms, including self-induced vomiting, self-induced diarrhea through the use of laxatives or cathartics, the use of diuretics, excessive fasting, and excessive exercise.
4. Physical signs may include callouses or skin changes on hands and fingers, loss of dental enamel, swollen lymph nodes, and bad breath or mouthwash smell on breath because of self-induced vomiting.
5. Endocrine changes, such as amenorrhea, may be present.

Diagnostic Evaluation

1. Serum chemistry for electrolytes, blood urea nitrogen, and creatinine, and bicarbonate—may be abnormal, indicating fluid and electrolyte imbalances.

2. Additional tests may include thyroid function tests, luteinizing hormone, follicle stimulating hormone, estrogen, and electrocardiogram to determine effects of bulimia on body.

Management

1. Nutritional plan to accomplish weight goal (gain or loss).
   a. Balanced diet with incremental inclusion of foods previously perceived by patient as "fattening."
   b. Exercise.
2. Psychological counseling and support.
   a. Assist patient to develop insight into behavior and a more realistic body image.
   b. Assist patient to develop effective coping strategies and problem-solving mechanisms.

Complications

1. Fluid and electrolyte disturbances, particularly hypokalemia, metabolic alkalosis, and associated cardiac dysrhythmias.
2. Obesity or anorexia nervosa.
3. Dental erosion.
4. Esophageal tear or gastric rupture.

Nursing Assessment

1. Perform complete nutritional assessment.
2. Evaluate fluid and electrolyte status and manifestations of associated problems.
3. Assess for signs and symptoms of depression, anxiety, personality disorder, and associated eating behaviors and history of family dysfunction.

Nursing Diagnoses

- Altered Nutrition: More/Less than Body Requirements related to binge/purge behavior
- Ineffective Individual Coping related to lack of control over eating habits

Nursing Interventions

Attaining Appropriate Weight

1. Assist patient to select well-balanced diet and maintain appropriate eating habits.
   a. Educate patient to choose low-fat foods in small portions to gain control of caloric intake.
   b. Encourage patient to keep a food log and to eat only at mealtime.
2. Provide positive reinforcement for appropriate eating behaviors.
3. Teach patient the risks associated with abnormal eating behavior and the benefits of maintaining healthful nutritional and exercise habits.
4. Assess daily weight, intake and output, urine for ketones, and serum electrolytes to determine physical response to nutritional interventions.

Improving Coping

1. Encourage patient to set realistic goals for weight and appearance.
2. Assist patient to identify and implement alternative coping strategies in times of stress, including expression and exploration of feelings, problem solving, appropriate use of exercise, and relaxation techniques.
3. Include family in counseling and teaching sessions, as appropriate.
4. Set limits so patient will feel in control of self.

Patient Education and Health Maintenance

1. Stress the importance of maintaining follow-up visits and counseling.
2. Refer to agencies such as American Anorexia-Bulimia Association, 212-575-6200; and Eating Disorder Information Center, 200 Elizabeth Street, CW1211, Toronto, Ontario, Canada M5G 2C4, 416-340-4156; *www.nedic.on.ca.*

Outcome-Based Evaluation

- Well-balanced dietary intake without evidence of vomiting
- Verbalizing correct problem-solving approach

Malabsorption Syndrome

Malabsorption syndrome is a group of symptoms and physical signs that occur because of poor nutrient absorption in the small intestine, particularly fat absorption, with a resultant decrease in absorption of fat-soluble vitamins A, D, E, and K. Poor absorption of other nutrients, including carbohydrates, minerals, and proteins may also occur. *Celiac sprue* and *lactase deficiency* are common types.

Pathophysiology and Etiology

Malabsorption has multiple etiologies, including gallbladder or pancreatic disease, lymphatic obstruction, vascular impairment, and bowel resection. Outlined below are two common causes.

1. Celiac sprue—malabsorption of fat resulting from atrophy of villi and microvilli of the small intestine because of an intolerance to gluten found in common grains, such as wheat, rye, oats, and barley.
2. Lactase deficiency—often of genetic origin, this digestive enzyme deficiency prevents the digestion of lactose found in milk, causing osmosis of water into the lumen of the intestine.

Clinical Manifestations

1. Steatorrhea.
2. Abdominal distention and pain.
3. Flatulence.
4. Anorexia, fatigue, weight loss, edema.
5. Vitamin deficiency—fat soluble (A, D, E, K).
6. Protein deficiency and negative nitrogen balance.

Diagnostic Evaluation

1. Fecal fat analysis—72-hour stool collection; may be increased.
2. Serum measurement of vitamin levels, total protein, and albumin may be decreased.
3. Prothrombin time may be prolonged because of vitamin K deficiency.

Management

1. Treatment of the underlying cause, if possible, by eliminating causative agents, such as grains or milk.
2. Promotion of adequate nutritional intake through a carefully designed diet that substitutes alternatives to the offending agent and that ensures replacement of deficient nutrients through oral, enteral, or parenteral therapy.

Complications

1. Dehydration.
2. Electrolyte imbalance with possible cardiac dysrhythmias.
3. Protein deficiency with muscle atrophy and edema.
4. Vitamin deficiency with tetany, bleeding, and anemia.
5. Skin breakdown.

Nursing Assessment

1. Assess fluid and electrolyte status through careful monitoring of intake and output, daily weight, serum electrolytes, vital signs, and other signs and symptoms of dehydration and electrolyte imbalance.
2. Assess GI function through observation of frequency and characteristics of stool, bowel sounds, and distention, pain, and other associated symptoms.
3. Assess nutritional status.

Nursing Diagnoses

- Altered Nutrition: Less Than Body Requirements related to malabsorption of nutrients
- Fluid Volume Deficit related to loss of fluid through stool
- Pain related to abdominal distention and cramps
- Risk for Impaired Skin Integrity related to irritation of anal area by stool

Nursing Interventions

Improving Nutritional Status

1. Ensure that diet is free of causative agent(s), such as milk or wheat products.
2. Provide diet high in missing nutrients, including proteins, carbohydrates, fats, vitamins, and minerals.
3. Teach patient to use substitute products for causative agents, such as gluten-free flour, corn, soybean, milk substitutes.
4. Monitor weight and characteristics of stool closely.

Restoring Fluid Balance

1. Monitor intake and output and urine-specific gravity.
   a. Include watery stool in output.
   b. Be aware that edema is because of low serum proteins, not because of fluid overload.
2. Monitor vital signs frequently, based on condition.
3. Be alert for dehydration—orthostatic hypotension, tachycardia, decreased skin turgor, dry mucous membranes, thirst, oliguria.
4. Observe for signs and symptoms of potential electrolyte disturbances—nausea, vomiting, dysrhythmias, tremors, seizures, anorexia, weakness—and report abnormal results of serum electrolytes.
5. Administer IV fluids or parenteral or enteral nutrition as ordered.

Relieving Pain

1. Assess timing, frequency, and character of pain and its relationship to food.
2. Encourage Fowler's position and frequent change in position for comfort.
3. Administer analgesics, antidiarrheals, and antiflatulents as ordered.

Maintaining Tissue Integrity

1. Provide meticulous perineal care after each stool with application of hydrophobic ointments if necessary to prevent skin breakdown.
2. Give careful attention to general skin condition, assessing for redness, breakdown, and poor turgor, and maintain general skin integrity through cleanliness, lubrication, padding of bony prominences, frequent turning, and adequate hydration and nutrition.

Patient Education and Health Maintenance

1. Provide nutritional counseling for patient and/or family, particularly if symptoms are secondary to food intolerance; stress which foods to avoid and the importance of carefully reading all food labels, recommend appropriate food substitutions, and necessary nutritional supplements.
2. Advise regarding signs and symptoms that indicate worsening of disease—increased frequency of stool, diarrhea or steatorrhea, increased pain.

Outcome-Based Evaluation

- Weight maintained
- Vital signs stable; urinary output adequate
- Verbalizes decreased pain after meals
- No skin breakdown noted

■ Vitamin and Mineral Deficiencies

Vitamins are organic compounds found in natural foods and are needed for growth, reproduction, good health, and resistance to infection. Minerals are inorganic compounds found in nature and serve a variety of physiologic functions. Specific requirements depend on age, activity, metabolic rate (increased fever), and special processes, such as pregnancy, lactation, and disease processes.

See Table 20-4 for management of vitamin and mineral imbalances.

(text continues on page 681)

TABLE 20-4 Vitamin and Mineral Requirements and Imbalances

Vitamin, RDA Requirements	Function	Clinical Manifestations of Imbalance	Diagnostic Evaluation	Management
Vitamin A (Retinol) RDA: 4,000–5,000 IU Fat soluble	Tissue maintenance via antioxidant ability. Skeletal and soft tissue growth and development. Visual adaptation to light and dark. Supports reproductive function.	Deficiency: Night blindness, xerophthalmia, keratinization, generalized mucosa dryness/damage, vomiting, diarrhea, weight loss, urinary and vaginal infections, tooth decay, follicular hyperkeratosis. Toxicity: Yellow-orange skin coloring, hair loss, joint pain, dry skin, mouth soreness, anorexia, vomiting, cirrhosis.	Deficiency: History and physical findings are helpful in diagnosis of most vitamin imbalances. Serum level less than 35 mg/dL suggests vitamin deficiency.	Deficiency: Replacement therapy of 30,000 IU to treat night blindness Good dietary sources of vitamin A are green and yellow fruits and vegetables and liver. In patients with malabsorption of fat soluble vitamins and patients with low dietary intake of vitamin A, IV supplements are required.
Vitamin B_1 (Thiamine) RDA: 1.0–1.5 mg Water soluble	Carbohydrate metabolism. Necessary for neurologic, gastric, cardiac, and musculoskeletal function.	Deficiency: Appetite loss, constipation, dyspnea, fatigue, irritability, nervousness, memory loss, paresthesias, muscle pain. Toxicity: Large doses may be given generally without difficulty, although anaphylaxis has been reported.	Deficiency: Erythrocyte transketolase activity less than 15–20%.	Deficiency: Treat underlying cause. High protein diet with supplemental B complex vitamins. Food sources rich in thiamine are brewer's yeast, meat, wheat germ, and enriched grains and beans. Parenteral therapy with 50–100 mg/d followed by 5–10 mg/d PO.
B_2 (Riboflavin) RDA: 0.6 mg/ 1,000 kcal Water soluble	Carbohydrate metabolism. Promotes growth, red blood cell formation, and healthy eyes and skin.	Deficiency: Sore throat, cheilosis, dermatitis, burning and itching of eyes, tearing and vascularization of corneas; late-stage symptoms include neuropathy and growth retardation. Toxicity: Flushing, gastric irritation, liver enzyme elevation.	Deficiency: Erythrocyte glutathione activity greater than 1.2–1.3. Decreased urinary riboflavin levels.	Deficiency: Good dietary sources of B_2 are dairy products, vegetables, enriched grains, eggs, nuts, and liver. Oral supplements of 5–15 mg/d. Toxicity: Supportive measures.
B_6 (Pyridoxine) RDA: 1.6–2 mg Water soluble	Promotes protein metabolism. Maintains neurologic function and RBC production.	Deficiency: Anemia, weakness, glossitis, cheilosis, irritability, seizures. Toxicity: Neuromuscular damage.	Deficiency: Pyridoxal phosphate levels less than 50 ng/mL	Deficiency: Oral supplementation— 10–20 mg. Good dietary sources of B_6 are bananas, brewer's yeast, fish, meat, whole grains, and liver. Individuals taking oral contraceptives or isoniazid may need to supplement their diets with pyridoxine. Pregnancy also increases need.

(continued)

TABLE 20-4 Vitamin and Mineral Requirements and Imbalances (Continued)

Vitamin, RDA Requirements	Function	Clinical Manifestations of Imbalance	Diagnostic Evaluation	Management
B₁₂ (Cobalamin) RDA: 2 mcg Water soluble	Maintains neurologic function and RBC development via hemoglobin synthesis.	Deficiency: Megaloblastic anemia, memory impairment, confusion, depression, fatigue, nervousness, decreased reflex response, balance impairment, speech difficulties, demyelination of the large fibers of the spinal cord, anorexia, vomiting, weight loss, yellowing of skin, abdominal pain, dyspnea, diarrhea, glossitis.	Deficiency: Serum levels of less than 100 pg/mL. Decreased hematocrit with elevation of MCV. Schilling test also measures absorption of radioactive B₁₂.	Deficiency: B₁₂ 200 mcg/d IM for 1 wk, then every mo for life if deficiency is due to pernicious anemia. Oral vitamin B₁₂ may be necessary for strict vegetarians. Good dietary sources of B₁₂ are eggs, fish, organ meats, lean meat, dairy products.
Biotin RDA: 30–100 mcg Water soluble	Metabolism of proteins, fats, and carbohydrates.	Deficiency: Dry skin, fatigue, grayish skin discoloration, muscle pain, depression, insomnia and anorexia.		Deficiency: Good sources of biotin are egg yolks, vegetables, yeast, milk, grains.
Folate (folic acid) RDA: 180–200 mcg Water soluble	RBC formation. DNA and RNA synthesis and support of cell growth and reproduction. Prevention of birth defects.	Deficiency: Glossitis, diarrhea, megaloblastic anemia, digestive problems.	Deficiency: Serum level less than 3 ng/mL.	Deficiency: Nutritional supplementation—1 mg/d PO Avoid alcohol. Good sources of folate are citrus fruits, eggs, milk, green leafy vegetables, dairy products, organ meats, seafood, whole grains, and yeast.
Niacin RDA: 13–19 mg Water soluble	Metabolism of carbohydrates, fats and proteins. Works with thiamine and riboflavin for the production of cellular energy. Promotes skin, neurologic, and gastrointestinal function.	Deficiency: Apathy, fatigue, appetite loss, headaches, indigestion, muscle weakness, nausea, insomnia, dermatitis, diarrhea, confusion, disorientation, memory impairment, glossitis, and stomatitis.	Deficiency: Serum levels less than 30 mcg/100 mL. Diminished or absent metabolites in urine.	Deficiency: Good sources of niacin are eggs, lean meats, organ meats, poultry, seafood, fish, dairy products, nuts, whole and enriched grains, brewer's yeast. Nutritional supplementation: 10–150 mg. Supplemental niacin may also be necessary when taking oral contraceptives.
Pantothenic acid RDA: 4–7 mg Water soluble	Vital for overall metabolism. Aids in formation of carbohydrates, proteins, and fats. Aids in cortisone production, ATP production, stress tolerance, vitamin utilization, hemoglobin synthesis.	Deficiency: Diarrhea, hair loss; respiratory infections, nervousness, muscle cramps, premature aging, intestinal disorders, eczema, kidney disorders.		Deficiency: This vitamin is widely available in foods, especially organ meats, legumes, vegetables, and fruits.

(continued)

TABLE 20-4 Vitamin and Mineral Requirements and Imbalances (Continued)

Vitamin, RDA Requirements	Function	Clinical Manifestations of Imbalance	Diagnostic Evaluation	Management
Vitamin C RDA: 50–60 mg Water soluble	Antioxidant action decreases cellular dysfunction. Promotes wound healing. Aids in connective tissue, bone, tooth, and cartilage formation. Promotes capillary integrity. Promotes nonheme iron absorption.	Deficiency: Bleeding gums, tooth decay, nosebleeds, low infection resistance, bruising, anemia, delayed wound healing, anorexia, joint pain, lethargy. Toxicity: Gastrointestinal distress.	Deficiency: Serum levels less than 0.1 mg/100 dL.	Deficiency: Nutritional supplementation: 100–1,000 mg/d of vitamin C. Good sources of vitamin C are citrus fruits, green leafy vegetables, broccoli, tomatoes, peppers, potatoes, strawberries. Avoid smoking.
Vitamin D RDA: 200–400 IU Fat soluble	Regulates calcium and phosphate absorption and metabolism and bone formation. Aids in renal phosphate clearance, myocardial function, nervous system maintenance and normal blood clotting.	Deficiency: Rickets, osteomalacia. Toxicity: Hypercalcemia, bone pain, weakness.	Deficiency: Low levels of vitamin D and calcium (calcium less than 8.5 mg/100 mL). Radiographic bone deformities. Abnormal bone densitometry.	Deficiency: Nutritional supplementation: Ergocalciferol, 25 mcg/d PO Good sources of vitamin D are egg yolks, yeast, enriched milk, fish liver oils. Exposure to sunlight.
Vitamin E (Tocopherol) RDA: 8–10 mg Fat soluble	Antioxidant action decreases cellular dysfunction. Aids in RBC formation.	Deficiency: Neuromuscular disturbances, including decreased reflexes, vibratory and position sense, and ataxia.	Deficiency: Serum levels less than 0.5 mg/dL.	Deficiency: Nutritional supplementation: 100–400 IU/d PO. Parenteral therapy may be necessary to treat neurologic symptoms. Good sources of vitamin E are vegetable oils, milk, eggs, meat, fish, green leafy vegetables.
Vitamin K RDA: 65–80 mcg Fat soluble	Promotes coagulation through the formation of prothrombin and other clotting factors.	Deficiency: Abnormal bleeding times, hemorrhage, epistaxis, hemetemesis and bleeding at any orifice or puncture site is possible.	Deficiency: Prothrombin time extended longer than PTT.	Deficiency: Administration of vitamin K 15 mg subcutaneously. Good sources of vitamin K are green leafy vegetables, liver, wheat germ, cheese, egg yolk, soy bean oil.
Minerals Calcium RDA: 800–1,200 mg	Aids in: Bone and tooth formation. Muscle contraction. Blood coagulation. Nerve impulse transmission. Cardiac function. Cell membrane permeability. Enzyme activation.	Deficiency: Tooth decay, muscle cramps, tetany, nervousness and delusion, cardiac palpitations, congestive heart failure, and paresthesias. Toxicity: Muscle weakness, diminished deep tendon reflexes, anorexia, nausea, vomiting, personality changes, decreased memory, renal disturbances.	Deficiency: Serum level less than 8.5 mg/dL. Toxicity: Serum level greater than 10.5 mg/dL.	Deficiency: Oral supplements of 1–2 g/d of elemental calcium. In severe hypocalcemia, 10 mL of 10% calcium gluconate IV administered no faster than 2 mL/min. Good sources of calcium are milk products, green leafy vegetables, whole grains, and egg yolks. Toxicity: Force fluids, diuretics, and limit dietary *(continued)*

TABLE 20-4 Vitamin and Mineral Requirements and Imbalances (Continued)

Vitamin, RDA Requirements	Function	Clinical Manifestations of Imbalance	Diagnostic Evaluation	Management
				intake. Administration of phosphate salts and glucocorticoids may also be necessary.
Chromium RDA: 0.29 mg.	Maintains serum glucose levels. Maintains fat metabolism.	Deficiency: Glucose intolerance, vertigo, abdominal pain, shock, convulsions, anuria, dermatitis.	Deficiency: Serum levels less than 0.3 mg/mL.	Deficiency: Nutritional supplements: 50–200 mg/d. Good sources of chromium are brewer's yeast, whole grains, cereals.
Copper RDA: 1.5–3 mg	Hemoglobin synthesis. Maintenance of hemostasis. Energy production.	Deficiency: Hypochromic anemia, bone disease, weakness, skin lesions, altered respiratory status. Toxicity: Nausea, vomiting, diarrhea, abdominal pain, malaise.	Deficiency: In addition to diminished serum levels, 24-hour urine samples showing levels of urinary excretion of copper below 15–60 mcg/24 h.	Deficiency: Nutritional supplementation: 0.1 mg/kg/d PO. IV supplementation— 1–2 mg/d. Good sources of copper are nuts, seeds, organ meats and seafood.
Iodine RDA: 150 mcg	Thyroid hormone synthesis.	Deficiency: Hypothyroidism/goiter, nervousness, irritability, obesity, cold hands and feet, chills, brittle hair, fatigue, bradycardia, decreased cardiac output, thick tongue, hoarseness, poor memory, hearing loss, anorexia.	Deficiency: Low T_3 and T_4 levels. Thyroid scan.	Deficiency: Nutritional supplementation: 50–100 mg daily PO Good sources of iodine are iodized salt, seafood.
Iron RDA: 10–15 mg	Hemoglobin synthesis. Cellular oxidation. Transportation of oxygen.	Deficiency: Iron deficiency anemia, fatigue, tachycardia, palpitations, dyspnea, susceptibility to infection, brittle nails, cheilosis, glossitis.	Deficiency: Decreased hemoglobin, hematocrit, iron, and ferritin levels and increased total iron-binding capacity.	Deficiency: Nutritional supplementation: 325 mg PO TID; Imferon 250 mg/d IM for each gram of hemoglobin below normal. IV supplementation: 1.5–2 g over 4–6 h. Good sources of iron are eggs, fish, organ meats, wheat germ, beans, lentils, beef, potatoes, and peas.
Magnesium RDA: 280–350 mg	Parathyroid hormone regulation. Acid-base balance. Enzyme activation. Smooth muscle regulation. Metabolism of carbohydrates and protein. Cell growth and reproduction.	Deficiency: Tetany, tremors, confusion, depression, tachycardia, dysrhythmias, seizures. Toxicity: Nausea, vomiting, drowsiness, muscle weakness, decreased deep tendon reflexes, hypotension, respiratory depression.	Deficiency: Serum levels less than 1.3 mEq/L. Toxicity: Serum levels greater than 2.1 mEq/L.	Deficiency: Nutritional supplementation: 1–2 g IV during 15 min. Good sources of magnesium are nuts, meat, grain, green vegetables, seafood, dairy products. Toxicity: Supportive measures.
Phosphorus				

(continued)

TABLE 20-4 Vitamin and Mineral Requirements and Imbalances (Continued)

Vitamin, RDA Requirements	Function	Clinical Manifestations of Imbalance	Diagnostic Evaluation	Management
RDA: 800–1200 mg	Nerve and muscle activity. Vitamin utilization. Kidney function. Metabolism of carbohydrates, proteins and fats. Cell growth and repair. Myocardial contraction. Energy production. Bone and tooth formation. Acid-base balance. Red blood cell function.	Deficiency: Anorexia, weakness, tremor, paresthesias, anemia, mental status change, hypoxia, osteomalacia. Toxicity: Tetany, soft tissue calcification, seizures, renal damage.	Deficiency: Serum levels less than 2.5 mg/dL. Toxicity: Serum levels greater than 4.5 mg/dL.	Deficiency: Nutritional supplementation: PO or IV phosphate. Good sources of phosphate are dairy products, eggs, fish, grains, meat, poultry, yellow cheeses, almonds, beans, cocoa, chocolate, liver, milk, peas, peanuts, walnuts, whole wheat, and rye. Toxicity: Administration of phosphate-binding agents (Amphojel). Hemodialysis or peritoneal dialysis.
Potassium RDA: 2,000–3,500 mg	Muscle contraction. Cardiac function. Protein synthesis. Nerve impulse transmission. Carbohydrate metabolism. Acid-base balance. Major intracellular cation.	Deficiency: Muscle weakness, fatigue, malaise, flaccidity, mental confusion, irritability, depression, dysrhythmias, hypotension, nausea, vomiting, anorexia, decreased GI motility, muscle cramps, paresthesias, hyperglycemia, polyuria, metabolic alkalosis. Toxicity: Muscle weakness, paralysis, paresthesias, nausea, vomiting, diarrhea, metabolic acidosis, prolonged cardiac conduction, ventricular dysrhythmias.	Deficiency: Serum levels less than 3.5 mEq/L. Toxicity: Serum levels greater than 5 mEq/L.	Deficiency: Nutritional supplementation: PO or IV, IV replacement generally at a rate of 10 mEq/h with careful cardiac monitoring and frequent measurements of serum potassium levels. Good sources of potassium are bananas, oranges, beef, prunes, beans, seafood, raisins. Toxicity: Infuse calcium gluconate 10% (10 mL). Sodium bicarbonate infusion. Insulin and glucose infusion. Oral or rectal exchange resins. Hemodialysis or peritoneal dialysis.
Sodium RDA: 500 mg	Maintains fluid balance. Cell membrane permeability and absorption of glucose. Bioelectric potential of tissues. Cardiac function. Acid-base balance. Regulation of neuromuscular function.	Deficiency: Muscle weakness, irritability, headache, seizures, nausea, vomiting, malaise, abdominal cramping, hypotension, tachycardia. Toxicity: Flushed skin, oliguria, agitation, thirst, dry mucous membranes, seizures.	Deficiency: Serum levels less than 135 mEq/L. Toxicity: Serum levels greater than 145 mEq/L.	Deficiency: Restrict free water intake. Infuse 0.9% saline solution if patient is hypovolemic. Infuse 3% saline and administer diuretic if sodium levels significantly low. Demeclocycline may be used to block ADH in the renal tubules to promote water excretion.

(continued)

TABLE 20-4 Vitamin and Mineral Requirements and Imbalances (Continued)

Vitamin, RDA Requirements	Function	Clinical Manifestations of Imbalance	Diagnostic Evaluation	Management
				Toxicity: Administer salt-free solutions such as D_5W followed by 0.45% saline solution. Low sodium diet. Administer vasopressin if diminished ADH is the cause.
Zinc RDA: 12–15 mg	Cellular metabolism. Maintenance of taste and smell. Burn and wound healing. Gonadal function. Maintenance of serum vitamin A concentration. Acid-base balance. Protein digestion. Promotion of growth.	Deficiency: Fatigue, hair loss, poor wound healing, impaired growth, bone deformities, loss of taste, anorexia, iron deficiency anemia, hypogonadism, hyperpigmentation. Toxicity: Diminished deep tendon reflexes, malaise, decreased level of consciousness, diarrhea, leukopenia.	Deficiency: Serum levels less than 75 mcg/dL.	Deficiency: Nutritional supplementation: zinc sulfate 200 mg TID PO. Good sources of zinc are liver, seafood, beans, lentils, oatmeal, wheat bran, eggs, peas, pasta, chicken, and milk. Toxicity: Supportive measures.

IV: intravenous; PO: by mouth; RBC: red blood cell; MCV: mean corpuscular volume; IM: intramuscular; ATP; adenosine triphosphate; PTT: partial thromboplastin time; TID: three times a day; GI: gastrointestinal; ADH: antidiuretic hormone.

SELECTED REFERENCES

Andersen, R.E., Wadden, T.A., Bartlett, S.J., et al. (1999). Effects of lifestyle activity vs. structured aerobic exercise in obese women: A randomized trial. *Journal of the American Medical Association, 281,* 335–340.

Aronne, L.J. (1998). Modern medical management of obesity: The role of pharmaceutical intervention. *Journal of the American Dietetic Association, 98*(suppl 2), S23–26.

Blecker, V., & Mehta, D.I. (2000). Nutritional problems in patients who have chronic disease. *Pediatric Review, 21*(1), 29–31.

Bliss, D.Z. & Lehmann, S. (1999). Tube feeding: Immune boosting formula. *RN, 62*(8), 26–28.

Bliss, D.Z. & Lehmann, S. (1999). Tube feeding: Administration tips. *RN, 62*(8), 29–31.

Galica, L.A. (1997). Parenteral nutrition. *Nursing Clinics of North America, 32*(4), 705–717.

Gianino, S., et al. (1996). The ABC's of TPN. *RN, 59*(2), 42–47.

Loranskaia, T. (1998) Current approaches to diet therapy of malabsorption. *Medical Clinics of Russia, 76*(1), 50–53.

Metheney, N.A., et al. (1999). pH and concentration of bilirubin in feeding tube aspirates as predictors of tube placement. *Nursing Research, 48*(4), 189.

Miller, D. & Miller, H. (1995). Giving meds through the tube. *RN, 58*(1), 44–47.

Muscari, M. (1996). Primary care of adolescents with bulimia nervosa. *Journal of Pediatric Health Care, 10*(1), 17–25.

Nelson, K., et al. (1998) Hunger in an adult patient population. *Journal of the American Medical Association, 279*(15), 1211–1214.

Reilly, H. (1998). Parenteral nutrition: An overview of current practice. *British Journal of Nursing, 7*(8), 461–467.

Pendelton, V.R., et al. (1998). The predictive validity of the diet readiness test in a clinical population. *International Journal of Eating Disorders, 24*(40), 363–369.

Shick, S.M., et al. (1998). Persons successful at long term weight loss and maintenance continue to consume a low energy , low fat diet. *Journal of the American Dietetic Association, 98*(4), 408–413.

Subar, A.F., et al. (1998). Dietary sources of nutrients among US children. *Pediatrics, 102*(1 of 4), 913–923.

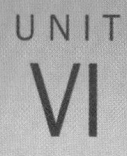

CHAPTER

21

*Renal and
Urinary Disorders*

ASSESSMENT

■ Subjective Data

Subjective data include characterization of symptoms, history of present illness, past medical and surgical history, demographic data, and lifestyle factors. Signs and symptoms involving the urinary tract may be due to disorders of the kidneys, ureters, or bladder, surrounding structures, or disorders of other body systems. See Standards of Care Guidelines.

Changes in Micturition (Voiding)
Changes in Amount or Color of Urine

1. *Hematuria*—blood in the urine.
   a. Considered a serious sign and requires evaluation.
   b. Color of bloody urine depends on several factors including the amount of blood present and the anatomical source of the bleeding.
      (i) Dark, rusty urine indicates bleeding from the upper urinary tract.
      (ii) Bright red bloody urine indicates lower urinary tract bleeding.
   c. Microscopic hematuria is the presence of red blood cells in urine, which can only be seen under a microscope; urine appears normal.

STANDARDS OF CARE GUIDELINES
Renal Impairment

- Be aware that urinary output reflects urinary and renal status of the patient. Notify health care provider of decreased urine output.
- Patients at risk for renal impairment include those with cardiovascular disease, diabetes, and hypertension; postoperative patients; hypotensive patients; and those with prostate and other diseases of the urinary tract.
- Thorough assessment of the urinary tract includes:
  —Hourly intake and output measurement
  —Assessment of color, clarity, and specific gravity of the urine
  —Palpation of the abdomen for suprapubic tenderness
  —Percussion of the flanks for costovertebral angle tenderness
  —Prostate examination
  —Subjective assessment for symptoms such as urgency, frequency, nocturia, hesitancy, dribbling, decreased force of stream, hematuria, and incontinence
- Be alert to drugs that may impair urinary and renal function such as nonsteroidal anti-inflammatory drugs, anticholinergics, sympathomimetics, aminoglycoside antibiotics.
- Report abnormal urinalysis, urine culture, and renal function test results to health care provider promptly.

This information should serve as a general guideline only. Each patient situation presents a unique set of clinical factors and requires nursing judgment to guide care, which may include additional or alternative measures and approaches.

---

   d. Hematuria may be due to systemic cause such as blood dyscrasias, anticoagulant therapy, neoplasms, trauma, extreme exercise.
   e. Painless hematuria may indicate neoplasm in the urinary tract.
   f. Hematuria is common in patients with urinary tract stone disease and may also be seen in renal tuberculosis, polycystic disease of kidneys, acute pyelonephritis, thrombosis and embolism involving renal artery or vein.
2. *Polyuria*—large volume of urine voided in given time.
   a. Volume is out of proportion to usual voiding pattern and fluid intake.
   b. Demonstrated in diabetes mellitus, diabetes insipidus, chronic renal disease, use of diuretics.
3. *Oliguria*—small volume of urine.
   a. Output between 100 and 500 mL/24 h.
   b. May result from acute renal failure, shock, dehydration, fluid–electrolyte imbalance.
4. *Anuria*—absence of urine output.
   a. Output less than 50 mL/24 h.
   b. Indicates serious renal dysfunction requiring immediate medical intervention.
5. *Pneumaturia*—passage of gas in urine during voiding. Caused by fistulous connection between bowel and bladder, rectosigmoid cancer, regional ileitis, sigmoid diverticulitis (most common), and gas-forming urinary tract infections.

Symptoms Related to Irritation of the Lower Urinary Tract

1. *Dysuria*—pain or difficult urination.
   a. Burning sensation seen in wide variety of inflammatory and infectious urinary tract conditions.
2. *Frequency*—voiding occurs more often than usual when compared with the patient's usual pattern or with a generally accepted norm of once every 3 to 6 hours.
   a. Determine if habits governing fluid intake have been altered—it is essential to know normal voiding pattern to evaluate frequency.
   b. Increasing frequency can result from a variety of conditions, such as infection and diseases of urinary tract, metabolic disease, hypertension, medications (diuretics).
3. *Urgency*—strong desire to urinate that is difficult to postpone.
   a. Due to inflammatory conditions of the bladder, prostate, or urethra, acute or chronic bacterial infections, neurogenic voiding dysfunctions, chronic prostatitis or bladder outlet obstruction in men, and urogenital atrophy in postmenopausal women.
4. *Nocturia*—excessive urination at night, which interrupts sleep.
   a. Causes include urologic conditions affecting bladder function, poor bladder emptying, bladder outlet obstruction, or overactive bladder.

b. Metabolic causes include decreased renal concentrating ability or heart failure, diabetes mellitus, and the increased urine production at rest that occurs with aging.

5. *Strangury*—slow and painful urination; only small amounts of urine voided.

a. Blood staining may be noted.

b. Seen in severe cystitis and interstitial cystitis.

Symptoms Related to Obstruction of the Lower Urinary Tract

1. *Weak stream*—decreased force of stream when compared to usual stream of urine when voiding.

2. *Hesitancy*—undue delay and difficulty in initiating voiding.

a. May indicate compression of urethra, outlet obstruction, neurogenic bladder.

3. *Terminal dribbling*—prolonged dribbling or urine from the meatus after urination is complete. May be caused by bladder outlet obstruction.

4. *Incomplete emptying*—feeling that the bladder is still full even after urination. Indicates either urinary retention or a condition that prevents the bladder from emptying well; leads to infection.

Types of Urinary Incontinence

Urinary incontinence is the involuntary loss of urine; may be due to pathologic, anatomical, or physiologic factors affecting the urinary tract.

1. *Stress incontinence*—intermittent leakage of urine due to increased abdominal pressure, such as coughing, sneezing, or straining.

a. Indicates weakness of pelvic floor and sphincter muscles in women, and damage to the internal sphincter mechanism (usually from prostatic surgery) in men.

2. *Urge incontinence*—sensation of the need to urinate followed by sudden, involuntary loss of urine.

a. May be related to neurologic disease affecting the bladder, acute or chronic irritation of the bladder wall, and the effects of prolonged bladder outlet obstruction.

b. Idiopathic causes include changes in the bladder and urethra with aging, urogenital atrophy in women.

3. *Overflow incontinence*—loss of urine caused by overdistention of the bladder. Associated with complete urinary retention.

4. *Total incontinence*—continuous leakage of urine from the bladder. Occurs with injury to the sphincteric mechanisms, bladder neck, and urethra.

5. *Functional incontinence*—loss of urine due to functional impairment that causes difficulty in ambulation or dexterity in getting to the bathroom and positioned to void.

6. *Mixed incontinence*—combination of two or more types of incontinence.

7. *Enuresis*—involuntary voiding during sleep. May be physiologic during early childhood; thereafter, may be functional or symptomatic of obstructive or neurogenic disease (usually of lower urinary tract) or dysfunctional voiding.

Urinary Tract Pain

1. Genitourinary pain is not always present in renal disease, but is generally seen in the more acute conditions of the urinary tract.

2. Kidney pain—may be felt as a dull ache in costovertebral angle; or may be a sharp, colicky pain felt in the flank area that radiates to the groin or testicle. Due to distention of the renal capsule; severity related to how quickly it develops.

3. Ureteral pain—felt in the back and radiates to the groin or scrotum if the upper ureter is the source, to the suprapubic area, penis, and urethra if the lower ureter is the source.

4. Bladder pain (lower abdominal pain or pain over suprapubic area)—may be due to bladder infection or overdistended bladder.

5. Urethral pain from irritation of bladder neck, from foreign body in canal, or from urethritis due to infection or trauma; pain increases when voiding.

6. Pain in scrotal area due to inflammatory swelling of epididymis or testicle, or torsion of the testicle.

7. Testicular pain due to injury, mumps orchitis, torsion of spermatic cord.

8. Perineal or rectal discomfort due to acute prostatitis, prostatic abscess.

9. Back and leg pain due to cancer of prostate with metastases to bone.

10. Pain in glans penis is usually from prostatitis; penile shaft pain is from urethral problems.

Related Symptoms

1. Gastrointestinal (GI) symptoms related to urologic conditions include nausea, vomiting, diarrhea, abdominal discomfort, paralytic ileus, and GI hemorrhage with uremia.

2. Occur with urologic conditions because the GI and urinary tracts have common autonomic and sensory innervation and because of renointestinal reflexes.

3. Fever and chills may also occur with infectious processes.

History

Seek the following historical data related to urinary and renal function:

1. What is (are) the patient's present and past occupation(s)? Look for occupational hazards related to the urinary tract—contact with chemicals, plastics, tar, rubber, also truck or school bus drivers.

2. What is the patient's smoking history?

3. What is the past medical and surgical history, especially in relation to urinary problems?

4. Is there any family history of renal disease?

5. What childhood diseases did the patient have?

6. Is there a history of urinary tract infections? Did any occur before the age of 12?

7. Did enuresis continue beyond the age when most children gain control?

8. Any history of genital lesions or sexually transmitted diseases (STDs)?

9. For the female patient: Number of children? Their ages? Any forceps deliveries? When? Any signs of vaginal discharge? Vaginal/vulvar itch or irritation? Family history of pelvic organ prolapse ("dropped" bladder or uterus) or urinary incontinence?
10. Does the patient have diabetes mellitus? Hypertension? Allergies? Neurologic disease or dysfunction?
11. Has the patient ever been hospitalized for a urinary tract infection? What diagnostic tests were performed? Cystoscopy? Urodynamics? Kidney x-ray procedures? Was the patient catheterized for a period of time? Were antibiotics given, either intravenously (IV) or orally?
12. Has the patient ever had surgery for bladder or prostate problems or any traumatic injuries involving the pelvis?
13. Is the patient taking any prescription or over-the-counter drugs or herbal preparations that may affect renal or urinary function? Have any drugs been prescribed for renal or urinary problems?
14. Is the patient at risk for urinary tract infection?

■ Objective Data

Objective data should focus on physical examination of the abdomen and the genitalia. Complete body system assessment may be indicated in some conditions, such as renal failure.

Examination of the Abdomen

1. Inspect the abdomen for any visible masses or bulges; auscultate for the presence of bowel sounds.
2. Percussion may reveal a distended bladder when dullness is found above the symphysis pubis.
3. Light palpation may detect tenderness or resistance; deep palpation can be used to assess the kidneys although this is difficult in most patients.
4. With the patient in a sitting position, tenderness of the costovertebral angle can be detected by placing the palm of your right hand over the costovertebral angle and striking your right hand with the fist of your left hand. Tenderness here indicates infection.

NURSING ALERT

In the patient who complains of back pain or who is in obvious discomfort, percussion over the costovertebral angle may be adequate to elicit tenderness, without causing undue pain.

Examination of the Female Genitalia

1. Inspection of the female external genitalia may reveal inflammation, ulcerations, nodules, or lesions. Inspect the skin of the labia into the groins for rashes or irritation. Note any vaginal discharge present; its color, consistency, and odor (if present).
2. With the labia spread, ask the patient to bear down; a cystocele, urethrocele, or rectocele may be visible.
3. With two fingers in the vagina, ask the patient to contract her muscles around your fingers as long as possible; this allows for assessment of pelvic floor muscle strength.
4. Inspect the vaginal tissue for vascularity and evidence of urogenital atrophy in which the tissue is smooth, pale, and dry.

Examination of the Male Genitalia

1. Inspect the urethral meatus for discharge.
2. Retract the foreskin, and assess for hygiene and the presence of smegma.
3. Inspect the shaft of the penis, the glans, and prepuce for lesions or indurated areas.
4. Palpate the testis and the epididymis for evidence of inflammation, tenderness, or masses; palpate the scrotal contents for hydrocele or varicocele.
5. Inspect the inguinal and femoral areas for bulges or hernias; ask the patient to bear down or cough during this portion of the examination.
6. Perform a rectal examination in men over age 40; assess for size and consistency of the prostate as well as anal sphincter tone.

General Examination

1. Assess the patient's cardiac and respiratory status, including presence of adventitious lung sounds, cardiac arrhythmias, or evidence of congestive heart failure.
   a. Examination for jugular venous pressure, bulging neck vessels, and peripheral edema is important in patients suspected of having renal disease.
   b. Measure blood pressure, which may be elevated in renal disease.
2. Palpate inguinal lymph nodes for enlargement—important in patients suspected of having genitourinary cancer or STD.
3. Assess skin color and changes that may occur in chronic renal failure.

DIAGNOSTIC TESTS

■ Laboratory Studies

Common laboratory studies pertaining to renal and urologic disorders include blood and urinary excretion tests for renal function, prostate-specific antigen (PSA), and urinalysis.

Tests of Renal Function
Description

1. Renal function tests are used to determine effectiveness of the kidneys' excretory functioning, to evaluate the severity of kidney disease, and to follow the patient's progress.
2. There is no single test of renal function; best results are obtained by combining a number of clinical tests.
3. Renal function is variable from time to time.

Nursing and Patient Care Considerations

Renal function may be within normal limits until about 50% of renal function has been lost. See Table 21-1.

TABLE 21-1 Tests of Renal Function

There is no single test of renal function; renal function is variable from time to time. The rate of change of renal function is more important than the result of a single test.

Test	Purpose/Rationale	Test Protocol

Renal concentration test
  Specific gravity
  Osmolality of urine
	Tests the ability to concentrate solutes in the urine. Concentration ability is lost early in kidney disease; hence, this test detects early defects in renal function.	Fluids may be withheld 12–24 h to evaluate the concentrating ability of the tubules under controlled conditions. Specific gravity measurements of urine are taken at specific times to determine urine concentration.

Creatinine clearance	Provides a reasonable approximation of rate of glomerular filtration. Measures volume of blood cleared of creatinine in 1 min. Most sensitive indication of early renal disease. Useful to follow progress of the patient's renal status.	Collect all urine over 24-h period. Draw one sample of blood within the period.
Serum creatinine	A test of renal function reflecting the balance between production and filtration by renal glomerulus. Most sensitive test of renal function.	Obtain sample of blood serum.
Serum urea nitrogen (blood urea nitrogen [BUN])	Serves as index of renal excretory capacity. Serum urea nitrogen depends on the body's urea production and on urine flow. (Urea is the nitrogenous end-product of protein metabolism.) Affected by protein intake, tissue breakdown.	Obtain sample of blood serum.
Protein	Random specimen may be affected by dietary protein intake. Proteinuria >150 mg/24 h may indicate renal disease.	Collect all urine over 24-h period.
Urine casts	Mucoproteins and other substances present in renal inflammation; help to identify type of renal disease (eg, red cell casts present in glomerulonephritis, fatty casts in nephrotic syndrome, white cell casts in pyelonephritis).	Collect random urine specimen.

Prostate-Specific Antigen (PSA)

Description

1. This amino acid glycoprotein is measured in the serum by a simple blood test.
2. An elevated PSA indicates the presence of prostate disease, but is not exclusive to prostate cancer.
3. Level rises continuously in the presence of prostate cancer.
4. Normal serum PSA level is less than 4.0 ng/mL. Levels less than 10.0 ng/mL may be indicative of benign prostatic hyperplasia (BPH) and not necessarily prostate cancer.
5. Patients who have undergone treatment for prostate cancer are monitored periodically with PSA levels for recurrence.

Nursing and Patient Care Considerations

1. No patient preparation is necessary.
2. Some clinicians prefer not to perform digital rectal examinations of the prostate at the same time that a PSA is drawn, to prevent artificial elevation of PSA level, although this association has not been proven.
3. Clinical laboratories may differ slightly in methods used for determining PSA; patients having serial PSA should be sent to the same lab.

Urinalysis

Description

Involves examination of the urine for overall characteristics, such as appearance, pH, specific gravity, and osmolality, as well as microscopic evaluation for the presence of normal and abnormal cells.

1. *Appearance*—normal urine is clear.
   a. Cloudy urine (phosphaturia) is not always pathologic, related only to the precipitation of phosphates in alkaline urine. Normal urine may also develop cloudiness on refrigeration or from standing at room temperature.
   b. Abnormally cloudy urine (pyuria or chyluria)—due to pus, blood, epithelial cells, bacteria, fat, colloidal particles, phosphate, or lymph fluid.
2. *Odor*—normal urine has a faint aromatic odor.
   a. Characteristic odors produced by ingestion of asparagus, thymol.
   b. Cloudy urine with ammonia odor—urea-splitting bacteria such as *Proteus,* causing urinary tract infections.
   c. Offensive odor—may be due to bacterial action in presence of pus.
3. *Color* shows degree of concentration and depends on amount voided.

a. Normal urine is clear yellow or amber because of the pigment urochrome.

b. Dilute urine is straw-colored.

c. Concentrated urine is highly colored; a sign of insufficient fluid intake.

d. Cloudy or smoky colored—may be from hematuria, spermatozoa, prostatic fluid, fat droplets, chyle.

e. Red or red-brown—due to blood pigments, porphyria, transfusion reaction, bleeding lesions in urogenital tract, some drugs and food (beets).

f. Yellow-brown or green-brown—may reveal obstructive lesion of bile duct system or obstructive jaundice.

g. Dark brown or black—due to malignant melanoma, leukemia.

4. pH of urine reflects the ability of kidney to maintain normal hydrogen ion concentration in plasma and extracellular fluid; indicates *acidity* or *alkalinity* of urine.

a. pH should be measured in fresh urine because the breakdown of urine to ammonia causes urine to become alkaline.

b. Normal pH is around 6 (acid); may normally vary from 4.6 to 7.5.

c. Urine acidity or alkalinity has relatively little clinical significance unless the patient is on special diet or therapeutic program or is being treated for renal calculous disease.

5. *Specific gravity* reflects the kidney's ability to concentrate or dilute urine; may reflect degree of hydration or dehydration.

a. Normal specific gravity ranges from 1.005 to 1.025.

b. Specific gravity is fixed at 1.010 in chronic renal failure.

c. In a person eating a normal diet, inability to concentrate or dilute urine indicates disease.

6. *Osmolality* is an indication of the amount of osmotically active particles in urine (specifically, it is the number of particles per unit volume of *water*). It is similar to specific gravity, but is considered a more precise test; it is also easy to do—only 1 to 2 mL of urine are required. Average value is 300 to 1,090 mOsm/kg for female patients; 390 to 1090 mOsm/kg for male patients.

Nursing and Patient Care Considerations

1. Freshly voided urine provides the best results for routine urinalysis; some tests may require first morning specimen.

2. Obtain sample of about 30 mL.

3. Urine culture and sensitivities are often performed using the same specimen obtained for urinalysis; therefore, use clean-catch (Procedure Guidelines 21-1) or catheterization techniques.

4. Patients with urinary diversions, especially ileal conduit diversions, require special techniques to obtain urine that is not contaminated with bacteria from the intestinal diversion.

PROCEDURE GUIDELINES 21-1	TECHNIQUE FOR OBTAINING CLEAN-CATCH MIDSTREAM VOIDED SPECIMEN

A *clean-catch midstream specimen* is the best clinically effective method of securing a voided specimen for urinalysis. It is not a simple procedure and requires patient education and active assistance of the female patient.

EQUIPMENT

Antiseptic solution or liquid soap solution
Sterile water
4 × 4-inch sponges

Disposable gloves for nurse assisting female patient
Sterile specimen container

PROCEDURE

Nursing Action	Rationale
MALE PATIENT	
1. Instruct the patient to expose glans and cleanse area around meatus. Wash area with mild antiseptic solution or liquid soap. *Rinse thoroughly.*	1. The urethral orifice is colonized by bacteria. Urine readily becomes contaminated during voiding. Rinse antiseptic solution or soap solution thoroughly because these agents can inhibit bacterial growth in a urine culture.
2. Allow the initial urinary flow to escape.	2. The first portion of urine washes out the urethra and contains debris.
3. Collect the midstream urine specimen in a sterile container.	3. The midstream sample reflects the status of the bladder.
4. Avoid collecting the last few drops of urine.	4. Prostatic secretions may be introduced into urine at the end of the urinary stream.

continued

PROCEDURE GUIDELINES 21-1	TECHNIQUE FOR OBTAINING CLEAN-CATCH MIDSTREAM VOIDED SPECIMEN *CONTINUED*

Nursing Action	Rationale

FEMALE PATIENT

1. Ask the patient to separate her labia to expose the urethral orifice.

   If no one is available to assist the patient, she may sit backwards on the toilet seat facing the water tank or sit on (straddle) the wide part of the bedpan.
2. Cleanse the area around the urinary meatus with sponges soaked with antiseptic/soap solution. Rinse thoroughly.
   a. Wipe the perineum from the front to the back.
   b. Do not use sponges more than once.
3. While the patient keeps the labia separated (see accompanying figure), instruct her to void forcibly.

1. Keeping the labia separated prevents labial or vaginal contamination of the urine specimen. By straddling the toilet seat/bedpan, the patient's labia are spread apart for cleansing.

2. The urethral orifice is colonized by bacteria. Urine readily becomes contaminated during voiding.

3. This helps wash away urethral contaminants.

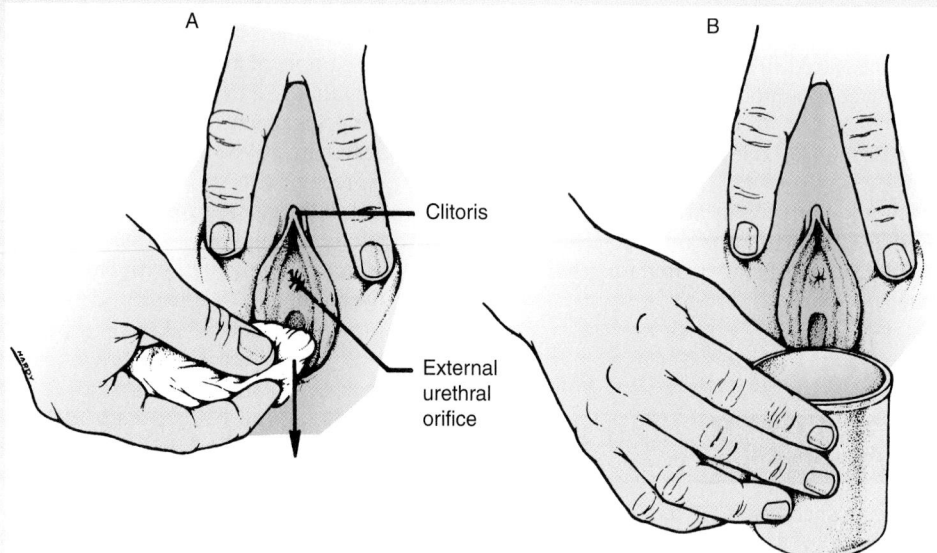

Obtaining a clean-catch midstream urine specimen in the female patient. *(A)* instruct the patient to hold the labia apart and wash from high up front toward the back with gauze soaked in soap. *(B)* The collection cup is held so that it does not touch the body, and the sample is obtained only while the patient is voiding with the labia held apart.

4. Allow initial urinary flow to drain into bedpan (toilet) and then catch the midstream specimen in a sterile container, making sure that the container does not come in contact with the genitalia.

4. The first portion of urine washes out the urethra. Have the patient remove the container from the stream while she is still voiding.

FOLLOW-UP PHASE

1. Send specimen to laboratory immediately.

1. A culture should be performed as soon as possible to avoid multiplication of urinary bacteria and lysis of cells.

■ Radiology and Imaging

These tests include simple x-rays, x-rays with the use of contrast media, ultrasound, nuclear scans, and imaging through computed tomography (CT) and magnetic resonance imaging (MRI).

X-ray of Kidneys, Ureters, and Bladder (KUB)
Description
1. Consists of plain film of the abdomen
2. Delineates size, shape, and position of kidneys
3. Reveals any deviations, such as calcifications (stones), hydronephrosis, cysts, tumors, or kidney displacement

Nursing and Patient Care Considerations
1. No preparation is needed.
2. Often done before other testing.

Intravenous Pyelogram
(IVP; Intravenous Urogram [IVU])
Description
1. IV introduction of a radiopaque contrast medium that concentrates in the urine and thus facilitates visualization of the kidneys, ureter, and bladder.
2. The contrast medium is cleared from the bloodstream by renal excretion.

Nursing and Patient Care Considerations
1. Contraindicated in patients with renal failure, uncontrolled diabetes, or multiple myeloma.
2. Contraindicated in patients receiving drug therapy for chronic bronchitis. emphysema, or asthma and in patients taking metformin HCL (Glucophage).
3. Patients with known iodine/contrast material allergy must have steroid/antihistamine preparation; in some cases, an anesthesiologist must be available.
4. Bowel preparation is necessary:
    a. Clear liquids only the day before the examination.
    b. Cathartics/laxatives are given the evening before the examination.
    c. NPO after midnight the day of the examination (if scheduled for afternoon, clear liquids only in the morning).

Retrograde Pyelography
Description
1. Injection of opaque material through ureteral catheters, which have been passed up ureters into renal pelvis by means of cystoscopic manipulation. The opaque solution is introduced by gravity or syringe injection.
2. May be done when IVP is contraindicated or if IVP provides inadequate visualization of the collecting system.

Nursing and Patient Care Considerations
Contraindicated in patients with urinary tract infection, or with suspected perforation of the ureter or bladder; allergic reactions to contrast material are rare in this examination.

Cystourethrogram
Description
1. Visualization of urethra and bladder by x-ray after retrograde instillation of contrast material through a catheter. An examination of only the bladder is a *cystogram*; of only the urethra is a *urethrogram*.
2. Used to identify injuries, tumors, or structural abnormalities of the urethra or bladder; or to evaluate emptying problems or incontinence (voiding cystourethrogram).

Nursing and Patient Care Considerations
1. Carries risk of infection due to instrumentation.
2. Allergy to contrast material is not a contraindication.
3. Additional x-rays may be taken after catheter is removed and patient voids (voiding cystourethrogram).
4. Provide reassurance to allay patient's embarrassment.

Renal Angiography
Description
1. IV catheter is threaded through the femoral and iliac arteries into the aorta or renal artery.
2. Contrast material is injected to visualize the renal arterial supply.
3. Evaluates blood flow dynamics, demonstrates abnormal vasculature, and differentiates renal cysts from renal tumors.
4. May be done to embolize a kidney before nephrectomy for renal tumor.

Nursing and Patient Care Considerations
1. Clear liquids only after midnight before the examination; adequate hydration is essential.
2. Continue oral medications (special orders needed for diabetic patients).
3. IV required.
4. May not be done on the same day as other studies requiring barium or contrast material.
5. Maintain bed rest for 8 hours after the examination, with the leg kept straight on the side used for groin access.
6. Observe frequently for hematoma or bleeding at access site. Keep sandbag at bedside for use if bleeding occurs.

Renal Scans
Description
1. Radiopharmaceuticals (also called radiotracers or isotopes) are injected IV.
    a. Tc-DTPA or Tc99m-DMSA is used for anatomical visualization and evaluation of glomerular filtration.
    b. Other radiopharmaceuticals may also be used depending on the purpose of the scan.
2. Evaluates renal size, shape, position, and function or blood flow to the kidneys.
3. Studies are obtained with a scintillation camera placed posterior to the kidney with the patient in a supine, prone, or sitting position.

Nursing and Patient Care Considerations
1. The patient should be well hydrated. Give several glasses of water or IV fluids as ordered before scan.

2. Furosemide (Lasix) or captopril (Capoten) may be administered in conjunction with the scan to determine their effects.

Ultrasound
Description
1. Uses high-frequency sound waves passed into the body and reflected back in varying frequencies based on the composition of soft tissues. Organs in the urinary system create characteristic ultrasonic images that are electronically processed and displayed as an image.
2. Abnormalities such as masses, malformations, or obstructions can be identified; useful in differentiating between solid and fluid-filled masses.
3. A noninvasive technique.

Nursing and Patient Care Considerations
1. Ultrasound examination of the prostate is performed using a rectal probe. A Fleet's enema may be ordered just within hours of the examination.
2. Ultrasound examination of the bladder requires that the bladder be full.
3. Patient should not have had any studies using barium for 2 days before ultrasound of the kidney or bladder.

Computed Tomography and Magnetic Resonance Imaging
See descriptions, page 438.

Other Tests
Other tests that may be done to evaluate disorders of the renal and urologic systems include cystoscopy, urodynamic testing, and needle biopsy of the kidney.

Cystoscopy
Description
1. Cystoscopy is a method of direct visualization of the urethra and bladder by means of a cystoscope that is inserted through the urethra into the bladder. It has a self-contained optical lens system that provides a magnified, illuminated view of the bladder.
2. Uses include:
   a. To inspect bladder wall directly for tumor, stone, or ulcer and to inspect urethra for abnormalities or to assess degree of prostatic obstruction.
   b. To allow insertion of ureteral catheters for radiographic studies, or before abdominal or genitourinary surgery.
   c. To see configuration and position of ureteral orifices.
   d. To remove calculi from urethra, bladder, and ureter.
   e. To diagnose and treat lesions of bladder, urethra, and prostate.

Nursing and Patient Care Considerations
1. Simple cystoscopy is often performed in an office setting. More complicated cystoscopy involving resections or ureteral catheter insertions are done in the operating room cystoscopy suite, where IV sedation or general anesthesia may be used.
2. The patient's genitalia are cleaned with an antiseptic solution just before the examination. A local topical anesthetic (Xylocaine gel) is instilled into the urethra before insertion of cystoscope.
3. Because fluid flows continuously through the cystoscope, the patient may feel an urge to urinate during the examination.
4. Contraindicated in patients with known urinary tract infection.
5. Nursing interventions after cystoscopic examination:
   a. Monitor for complications: urinary retention, urinary tract hemorrhage, infection within prostate or bladder.
   b. Expect the patient to have some burning on voiding, blood-tinged urine, and urinary frequency from trauma to mucous membrane of the urethra.
   c. Administer or teach self-administration of antibiotics prophylactically as ordered to prevent urinary tract infection.
   d. Advise warm sitz baths or analgesics such as ibuprofen or acetaminophen to relieve discomfort after cystoscopy.
   e. Provide routine catheter care if urinary retention persists and an indwelling catheter is ordered.

Urodynamics
Description
Urodynamics is a term that refers to any of the following tests that provide physiologic and functional information about the lower urinary tract. They measure the ability of the bladder to store and empty urine. Most urodynamic equipment uses computer technology with results visible in real time on a monitor.
1. Uroflowmetry (flow rate)—a record of the volume of urine passing through the urethra per unit of time (mL/s). It is shown on graph paper and gives information about the rate and flow pattern of urination.
2. Cystometrogram—recording of the pressures exerted during filling and emptying of the urinary bladder to assess its function. Data about the ability of the bladder to store urine at low pressure and the ability of the bladder to contract appropriately to empty urine are obtained.
   a. One or more small catheters are placed through the urethra (or suprapubic area) into bladder. The residual volume is measured if the patient recently voided, and the catheters are left in place.
   b. The catheters are connected to urodynamic equipment designed to measure pressure at the distal end of the catheter.
   c. Water, saline, or contrast material is infused at a slow rate into the bladder.
   d. When the bladder feels full, the patient is asked to "void." A normal detrusor contraction of the bladder appears as a sharp rise in bladder pressure on the

graph. If the patient is unable to void, the test may be considered normal because it is difficult to void normally with catheters in place.

3. Sphincter electromyelography (EMG) measures the activity of the pelvic floor muscles during bladder filling and emptying. EMG activity may be measured using surface (patch) electrodes placed around the anus or with percutaneous wire or needle electrodes.

4. Pressure-flow studies involve all of the above components, along with the simultaneous measurement of intra-abdominal pressure by way of a small tube with a fluid-filled balloon that is placed in the rectum. This permits better interpretation of actual bladder pressures without the influence of intra-abdominal pressure.

5. Video urodynamics use all of the above components. The fluid used to fill the bladder is contrast material, and the entire study is performed under fluoroscopy, providing radiographic pictures in combination with the recording of bladder and intra-abdominal pressures. Video urodynamics are reserved for patients with complicated voiding dysfunction.

Nursing and Patient Care Considerations

1. Contraindicated in patients with urinary tract infection.
2. Frequently performed by nurses; essential to provide information and support throughout the test to ensure clinically significant results.
3. Patients will have burning on urination afterward (due to instrumentation); encourage the patient to force fluids.
4. Short-term antibiotics are often given to prevent infection.

Needle Biopsy of Kidney
Description

Performed by percutaneous needle biopsy through renal tissue with ultrasound guidance or by open biopsy through a small flank incision; useful in securing specimens for electron and immunofluorescent microscopy to determine the diagnosis, treatment, and prognosis of renal disease.

Nursing and Patient Care Considerations

1. Prebiopsy nursing management
   a. Ensure that coagulation studies are carried out to identify the patient at risk for postbiopsy bleeding and that serum creatinine, urinalysis, and urine culture are done.
   b. Ensure that patient fasts for several hours before the procedure, as ordered.
   c. Establish an IV line, as ordered.
   d. Describe the procedure to the patient, including holding breath (to stop movement of the kidney) during insertion of the biopsy needle.

2. Postbiopsy nursing management
   a. Place the patient in a prone position immediately after biopsy and on bed rest for 8 to 24 hours to minimize bleeding.
   b. Take vital signs every 5 to 15 minutes for first hour and then with decreasing frequency if stable to assess for hemorrhage, which is a major complication.
   c. Watch for rise or fall in blood pressure, anorexia, vomiting, or development of a dull, aching discomfort in abdomen.
   d. Assess for flank pain (usually represents bleeding into the muscle) or colicky pain (clot in the ureter).
   e. Assess for backache, shoulder pain, or dysuria.
   f. Persistent bleeding may be suspected when an enlarging hematoma is palpable through the abdomen.
   g. If perirenal bleeding develops, avoid palpating or manipulating the abdomen after the first examination has determined that a hematoma exists.
   h. Collect serial urine specimens to evaluate for hematuria.
   i. Assess for any patient complaints, especially frequency and urgency on urination.
   j. Keep fluid intake at 3,000 mL daily if tolerated, unless the patient has renal insufficiency.
   k. Check results of hematocrit and hemoglobin (done the following morning) to assess for anemia, unless the vital signs change before then.
   l. Prepare for transfusion and surgical intervention for control of hemorrhage, which may necessitate surgical drainage or nephrectomy.

3. Instruct the patient on the following after biopsy:
   a. Avoid strenuous activity, strenuous sports, and heavy lifting for at least 2 weeks.
   b. Notify health care provider if any of the following occur: flank pain, hematuria, lightheadedness and fainting, rapid pulse, or any other signs and symptoms of bleeding.
   c. Report for follow-up 1 to 2 months after biopsy; will be checked for hypertension, and the biopsy area is auscultated for a bruit.

GENERAL PROCEDURES AND TREATMENT MODALITIES

■ Catheterization

Catheterization may be done to relieve acute or chronic urinary retention, to drain urine preoperatively and postoperatively, to determine the amount of residual urine after voiding, or to determine accurate measurement of urinary drainage in critically ill patients. See Procedure Guidelines 21-2 and 21-3.

Suprapubic catheterization establishes drainage from the bladder by introducing a catheter percutaneously or by an incision through the anterior abdominal wall into the bladder. It may be done for acute urinary retention when urethral catheterization is not possible; for urethral trauma, stricture, or fistula to divert flow of urine from the urethra; or for obtaining an uncontaminated urine specimen for culture. See Procedure Guidelines 21-4.

(*text continues on page 697*)

PROCEDURE GUIDELINES 21-2   CATHETERIZATION OF THE URINARY BLADDER

EQUIPMENT

Sterile gloves
Disposable sterile catheter set with
    single-use packet of lubricant
Antiseptic solution for periurethral
    cleansing (sterile)

Gloves, drape, sponges
Sterile container for culture
Bath blanket/sheet for draping
Standing lamp (preferred) or flashlight

SELECTION OF CATHETER SIZE

Use the smallest catheter capable of providing adequate drainage.

PROCEDURE

Nursing Action	Rationale

FEMALE PATIENT

Preparatory Phase

1. Put the patient at ease.

2. Open catheter tray using aseptic technique. Place waste receptacle in accessible place.

3. Place the patient in a supine position with knees bent, hips flexed, and feet resting on bed about 0.6 m (2 feet) apart. Drape the patient.
4. Direct light for visualization of genital area.
5. Position moisture-proof pad under the patient's buttocks.
6. Wash hands. Put on sterile gloves.

Performance Phase

1. Separate labia minora so urethral meatus is visualized; one hand is to maintain separation of the labia until catheterization is finished.

1. The patient will feel reassured if the procedure is explained and if she is handled gently and considerately.
2. Catheterization requires the same aseptic precautions as a surgical procedure.
     The principal danger of catheterization is urinary tract infection, which is associated with increased morbidity and longer, more costly hospitalization.

5. To absorb urine if necessary.
6. To prevent bacterial contamination.

1. This maneuver helps prevent labial contamination of the catheter (see accompanying figure).

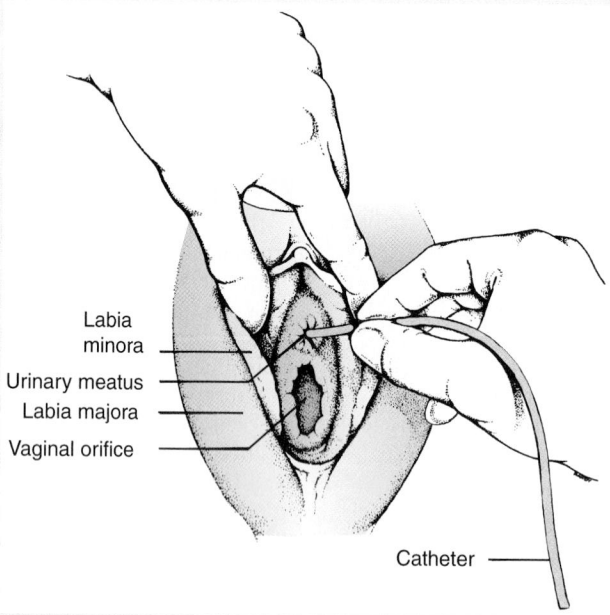

Labia minora
Urinary meatus
Labia majora
Vaginal orifice

Catheter

Catheterization of urinary bladder in the female patient.

PROCEDURE GUIDELINES 21-2   *CONTINUED*

Nursing Action	Rationale
2. Cleanse around the urethral meatus with a povidone-iodine solution.	2. Bacteria that normally colonize the distal urethra may be introduced into the bladder during or immediately after catheter insertion. Inadequate preparation of the urethral meatus is a major cause of infection.

a. Manipulate cleansing sponges with forceps, cleansing with downward strokes from anterior to posterior.
  b. Dispose of cotton sponge after each use.
  c. If the patient is sensitive to iodine, benzalkonium chloride or other cleansing agent is used.	

3. Introduce well-lubricated catheter 5–7 cm (2–3 inches) into urethral meatus using strict aseptic technique.	3. A well-lubricated catheter reduces friction and trauma to the meatus. The female urethra is a relatively short canal, measuring 3–4 cm in length.
a. Avoid contaminating surface of catheter. b. Ensure that catheter is not too large or too tight at urethral meatus.	b. Too large a catheter may cause painful distention of the meatus and cause damage to the uroepithelium.
4. Allow some bladder urine to flow through catheter before collecting a specimen.	4. To obtain representative bladder sample.

MALE PATIENT

Nursing Action	Rationale
1. Lubricate the catheter well with lubricant or prescribed topical anesthetic.	1. A well-lubricated catheter prevents urethral trauma (decreasing the opportunity for bacterial invasion).
2. Wash off glans penis around urinary meatus with an iodophor solution (Betadine) using forceps to hold cleansing sponges. Keep the foreskin retraction. Maintain sterility of dominant hand.	2. Cleanse urethral meatus from tip to foreskin with downward stroke on one side. Discard sponge. Repeat as required.
3. Grasp shaft of penis (with nondominant hand) and elevate it. Apply gentle traction to penis while catheter is passed.	3. This maneuver straightens the penile urethra and facilitates catheterization. Maintaining a grasp of the penis prevents contamination and retraction of penis.
4. Using sterile gloves, insert catheter into the urethra; advance catheter 15–25 cm (6–10 inches) until urine flows.	4. The male urethra is a canal extending from the bladder to the end of the glans penis. The length varies within wide limits; the average length is about 21 cm.
5. If resistance is felt at the external sphincter, slightly increase the traction on the penis and apply steady, gentle pressure on the catheter. Ask patient to strain gently (as if passing urine) to help relax sphincter.	5. Some resistance may be due to spasm of external sphincter. Inability to pass the catheter may mean that a urethral stricture or other forms of urethral pathology exist. The urethra may have to be dilated with a sound by a urologist.
6. When urine begins to flow, advance the catheter another 2.5 cm (1 inch).	6. Advancing the catheter ensures its position in the bladder.
7. Replace (or reposition) the foreskin.	7. Paraphimosis (retraction and constriction of the foreskin behind the glans penis), secondary to catheterization, may occur if the foreskin is not replaced.

FOLLOW-UP PHASE

Nursing Action	Rationale
1. Pinch off catheter and remove gently when urine ceases to flow.	1. Pinching off the catheter prevents air from entering the bladder as the catheter is removed.
2. Dry area; make patient comfortable.	
3. Send specimen to laboratory as indicated.	
4. Record time, procedure, amount, and appearance of urine.	

COMMUNITY AND HOME CARE CONSIDERATIONS

- Caregiver or patient can catheterize using clean technique.
- Assemble catheter (usually flexible, red rubber catheter; clear plastic, firmer catheter may be used by men), lubricant and liquid soap.
- Cleanse area around urethral meatus with liquid soap, if desired.
- Wash hands; wear unsterile gloves if desired.
- Catheterize; remove catheter when drainage ceases.
- Wash catheter with soap and water; rinse and dry well with paper towel.
- Store in new zip-lock type plastic bag.
- Nurse catheterizing patient in home usually maintains sterile technique.
- Replace catheters as often as possible, at least once a month.

PROCEDURE GUIDELINES 21-3   MANAGEMENT OF THE PATIENT WITH AN INDWELLING (SELF-RETAINING) CATHETER AND CLOSED DRAINAGE SYSTEM

EQUIPMENT

Catheter tray with closed system of urinary drainage
Antibacterial solution for cleansing

Gauze squares
Single-use packet of lubricant

PROCEDURE

Nursing Action

Rationale

GENERAL CONSIDERATIONS

1. Catheterize the patient (p. 692), using a catheter that is preconnected to a closed drainage system.
   a. Advance catheter almost to its bifurcation (for male patient).
   b. Inflate the balloon according to manufacturer's directions. Be sure catheter is draining properly before inflating balloon, then withdraw catheter slightly.
2. Secure the indwelling catheter.
   a. Female: Tape the catheter and drainage tubing to the thigh.
      Male: Tape the catheter to the patient's thigh.
   b. Allow some slack of the tubing to accommodate the patient's movements.
   c. Keep the tubing over the patient's leg.

1. A closed drainage system is one that is closed to outside air.
   a. This prevents the balloon from becoming trapped in the urethra.
   b. Inadvertent inflation of the balloon within the urethra is painful and causes urethral trauma.
2. Properly securing the catheter prevents catheter movement and traction on the urethra.

   c. This tubing position helps prevent kinking or forming loops of stagnant urine.

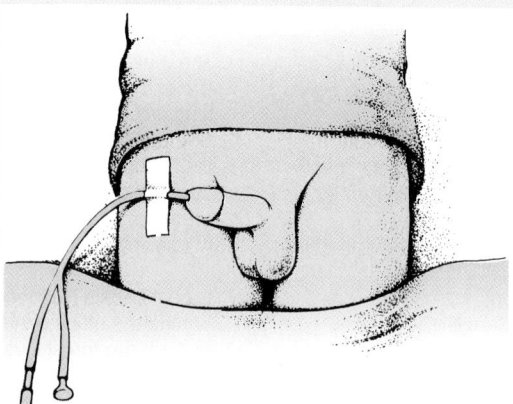

In the male patient, the indwelling catheter is taped to the thigh to straighten the angulation of the penoscrotal junction, thus reducing pressure on the urethra exerted by the catheter.

CARE OF THE INDWELLING CATHETER

1. Cleanse around the area where catheter enters urethral meatus (meatal–catheter junction) with soap and water during the daily bath to remove debris.

2. Avoid using powders and sprays on the perineal area.
3. Avoid pulling on the catheter during cleansing.

1. Suppurative drainage and encrustation occur at the exit of any tube. Infectious organisms can migrate to the bladder along the outside of any indwelling catheter; however, excessive manipulation of the catheter may promote migration of bacteria.
2. Powder can encrust and cause soreness and infection.
3. Pulling on the catheter may be painful. Backward and forward displacement of the catheter introduces contaminants into the urinary tract.

Nursing Action	Rationale

TO OBTAIN URINE FOR CULTURE

1. Clamp the drainage tubing below the aspiration (sampling) port for a *few minutes* to allow urine to collect.
2. Cleanse the aspiration port with povidone-iodine or 70% alcohol.
3. Insert a sterile No. 21-gauge needle (attached to a sterile syringe) into the aspiration port of the catheter tubing.
4. Aspirate a small volume of urine for culture.
5. Remove needle from syringe and release urine carefully into sterile specimen container.
6. *Unclamp the drainage tube.*
7. Send specimen to laboratory immediately.

1. Avoid separating catheter and connecting tube. Disconnection of the catheter and tubing is a major cause of urinary tract infection.

3. Avoid inserting needle into the shaft of the catheter because this may cause balloon deflation.

6. To prevent retention of urine and potential infection.
7. The specimen should be marked as a "catheterized specimen" because the presence of any number of colonies of an organism indicates a urinary tract infection.

TO IRRIGATE THE CATHETER

Note: This is not done unless obstruction is anticipated (bleeding after bladder/prostate surgery).

1. Wash hands. Don gloves.
2. Using aseptic technique, pour sterile irrigating solution into sterile container.
3. Cleanse around catheter/drainage tubing connection with sterile gauze pads soaked in povidone-iodine solution.

4. Disconnect catheter from drainage tubing. Cover tubing with a sterile cap.
5. Place a sterile drainage basin under the catheter.

6. Connect a large-volume syringe to the catheter and irrigate catheter using prescribed amount of sterile irrigant.

7. Remove syringe and place end of catheter over drainage basin, allowing returning fluid to drain into basin.
8. Repeat irrigation procedure until fluid is clear or according to physician's directives.
9. Disinfect the distal end of the catheter and end of drainage tubing; reconnect the catheter and tubing. Remove gloves. Wash hands.
10. Document type and amount of irrigating solution, color and character of returning fluid, presence of sediment/blood clots, and patient's reaction.

3. If frequent irrigations are necessary to keep the catheter open, change the catheter because the catheter itself is probably contributing to the problem.

5. You are opening the closed system and must maintain sterility.
6. Instill about 30 mL irrigating solution at a time. Avoid instilling the solution forcibly to prevent bladder irritation and spasms.
7. This provides gravitational flow.

8. After prostatic surgery, the goal of irrigation is to clear bloody fluid that may clot.
9. Use irrigating equipment one time and then discard.

CHANGING THE CATHETER

Change catheter according to the needs of the patient.

An indwelling catheter should *not* be changed at arbitrarily fixed intervals.

MAINTAINING A CLOSED DRAINAGE SYSTEM

1. Wash hands immediately before and after handling any part of the system. Wear clean, disposable gloves when handling the drainage system.
2. Maintain unobstructed urine flow.
   a. Keep the drainage bag in a dependent position, below the level of the bladder.
   b. Urine should not be allowed to collect in the tubing, because a free flow of urine must be maintained to prevent infection.
   c. Keep the bag off the floor.

1. Hands are the major route of transmission of gram-negative bacteria.

2. Urine flow must be downhill.
   a. Raising the bag will cause reflux of contaminated urine from the bag into the patient's bladder.
   b. Improper drainage occurs when the tubing is kinked or twisted, allowing pools of drainage to collect in the loops of tubing.
   c. To prevent bacterial contamination.

continued

PROCEDURE GUIDELINES 21-3   **MANAGEMENT OF THE PATIENT WITH AN INDWELLING (SELF-RETAINING) CATHETER AND CLOSED DRAINAGE SYSTEM** *CONTINUED*

Nursing Action	Rationale
3. To empty the drainage bag. a. Wash hands; don gloves.	a. Empty the bag at regular intervals, taking care to see that the drainage valve/spout is not contaminated.
b. Disinfect spigot. Empty the bag in a separate collecting receptacle for each patient. Disinfect spigot again.	b. Each patient should have his or her own collecting receptacle that is labeled and kept in the bathroom, not on the floor—to prevent cross-contamination.
c. Avoid letting the drainage bag touch the floor. d. Change the drainage bag if contamination occurs, if the urine flow becomes obstructed, or if the connecting junctions start to leak.	

PREVENTING CROSS-CONTAMINATION

Nursing Action	Rationale
1. Wash hands before and after handling the catheter/drainage system and between patients.	1. Many urinary tract infections are due to extrinsically acquired organisms transmitted by cross-contamination.
2. Assign only one patient with an indwelling catheter to a room. If this is not possible, separate the infected patient with an indwelling catheter from an uninfected patient.	2. There appears to be a greater risk of microbial transmission between catheterized patients.
3. Know the patients at risk.	3. Female, elderly, debilitated, and critically ill patients, those in the postpartum state, and patients with obstructed neurologically impaired bladders are at risk for infection.

COMMUNITY AND HOME CARE CONSIDERATIONS

For care of catheter at home, instruct patient to:
- Wash hands before and after handling the catheter.
- Wash around urinary opening daily, taking care to avoid pulling on the catheter during cleansing.
- Drink 8–12 glasses of fluids daily; increase fluid intake if urine becomes dark and concentrated.
- Wipe all connecting junctions with alcohol before changing from leg-bag drainage to overnight drainage bag.
- Keep the drainage bag at a lower level than the bladder; do not place the bag on your chair.
- Avoid letting the bag lay on its side because urine may flow back into the drainage tube.
- Usually the catheter is not changed except when obstruction or malfunction occurs.
- Inspect the catheter after removal for evidence of encrustation; if there are no signs of encrustation and blocking of lumen, the interval between catheter changes may be increased.
- Call health care provider if fever and/or cloudy, bloody, or odoriferous urine develops.

PROCEDURE GUIDELINES 21-4   **ASSISTING THE PATIENT UNDERGOING SUPRAPUBIC BLADDER DRAINAGE (CYSTOSTOMY)**

Suprapubic bladder drainage is a method of establishing drainage from the bladder by introducing a catheter percutaneously or by an incision through the anterior abdominal wall into the bladder.

EQUIPMENT

Sterile suprapubic drainage system package (disposable)	Skin germicide for suprapubic skin preparation; sterile gloves Local anesthetic agent if needed

PROCEDURE

Nursing Action	Rationale

PREPARATORY PHASE

Nursing Action	Rationale
1. Place the patient in a supine position with one pillow under head.	1. Allows access to suprapubic area but reduces muscle tension.
2. Expose the abdomen.	

PROCEDURE GUIDELINES 21-4 CONTINUED

Nursing Action	Rationale

PERFORMANCE PHASE (BY PHYSICIAN)

1. The bladder is distended with 300–500 mL sterile saline in a urethral catheter, which is removed, or the patient is given fluids (PO or IV) before the procedure.
2. The suprapubic area is surgically prepared. After the skin is dried, the needle entry point is located.
3. The skin and subcutaneous tissues are infiltrated with local anesthesia.
4. A small stab wound (incision) may be made.
5. The catheter* is introduced via a guidewire, needle, or cannula through the incision and advanced in a slightly caudal direction.
6. The catheter is advanced until the flange is against the skin where it is secured with tape, a body seal system, or sutures.
7. The catheter is connected to a sterile drainage system.
8. Secure drainage tubing to lateral abdomen with tape.
9. If the catheter is not draining properly, withdraw the catheter 2.5 cm (1 inch) at a time until urine begins to flow. Do not dislodge catheter from bladder.
10. The drainage is maintained continuously for several days.
11. If a "trial of voiding" is requested, the catheter is clamped for 4 h.
    a. Have the patient attempt to void while the catheter is clamped.
    b. After the patient voids, unclamp the catheter and measure residual urine.
    c. Usually, if the amount of residual urine is less than 100 mL on two separate occasions (AM and PM), the catheter may be removed.
    d. If the patient complains of pain or discomfort, or if the residual urine is over the prescribed amount, the catheter is usually left open.
12. When the catheter is removed, a sterile dressing is placed over the site. Usually the tract will close within 48 h.
13. Monitor for complications.

1. Distention of the bladder makes the bladder easier to locate by the suprapubic route.
2. The needle entry point is in the midline, 2–3 cm above the symphysis pubis and directly over the palpable bladder.
3. An adequate level of local anesthesia is achieved to facilitate catheter introduction.

5. Entrance into the bladder is usually felt and can be verified by free flow of urine.

6. Another method is to advance a long needle into the bladder until urine flow verifies the needle is in the bladder.

7. Aseptic technique is used in the area around the cystostomy tube.
8. Prevents undue tension on the catheter.

11. Usually, patients will void earlier after surgery with suprapubic drainage than with indwelling catheters.

12. Suprapubic drainage is considered more comfortable than an indwelling urethral catheter. It allows greater patient mobility, and there is less risk of bladder infection.
13. Complications of this procedure: Inadvertent peritoneal and bowel damage, leakage around catheter, kinking of catheter, hematuria, abdominal wall abscess.

* It is necessary to become familiar with the manufacturer's directions for the system being used.

◼ Dialysis

Dialysis refers to the diffusion of solute molecules through a semipermeable membrane, passing from the side of higher concentration to that of lower concentration. The purpose of dialysis is to maintain the life and well-being of the patient. It is a substitute for some kidney excretory functions but does not replace the kidneys' endocrine and metabolic functions. Methods of dialysis include:

1. Peritoneal dialysis.
    a. Intermittent peritoneal dialysis (acute or chronic)— see Procedure Guidelines 21-5
    b. Continuous ambulatory peritoneal dialysis
    c. Continuous cycling peritoneal dialysis—uses automated peritoneal dialysis machine overnight with prolonged dwell time during day
2. Hemodialysis (see p. 698).
3. Continuous renal replacement therapy (CRRT)—this includes special procedures such as continuous arteriovenous hemofiltration (CAVH), continuous venovenous hemodialysis (CVVHD), continuous arteriovenous ultrafiltration (CAVU), and slow continuous ultrafiltration (SCUF). These use extracorporeal blood circulation through a small-volume, low-resistance filter to provide continuous removal of solutes and fluid in the intensive care setting.

Continuous Ambulatory Peritoneal Dialysis (Figure 21-1)

Continuous ambulatory peritoneal dialysis (CAPD) is a form of intracorporeal dialysis that uses the peritoneum for the semipermeable membrane.

Procedure

1. A permanent indwelling catheter is implanted into the peritoneum; the internal cuff of the catheter becomes embedded by fibrous ingrowth, which stabilizes it and minimizes leakage.
2. A connecting tube is attached to the external end of the peritoneal catheter, and the distal end of the tube is inserted into a sterile plastic bag of dialysate solution.
3. The dialysate bag is raised to shoulder level and infused by gravity into the peritoneal cavity (approximately 10 minutes for a 2-L volume).
4. The typical dwell time is 4 to 6 hours.
5. At the end of the dwell time, the dialysate fluid is drained from the peritoneal cavity by gravity. Drainage of 2 L plus ultrafiltration takes about 10 to 20 minutes if the catheter is functioning optimally.
6. After the dialysate is drained, a fresh bag of dialysate solution is infused using aseptic technique, and the procedure is repeated.
7. The patient performs four to five exchanges daily, 7 days a week, with an overnight dwell time allowing uninterrupted sleep; most patients become unaware of fluid in the peritoneal cavity.

Advantages Over Hemodialysis

1. Physical and psychological freedom and independence

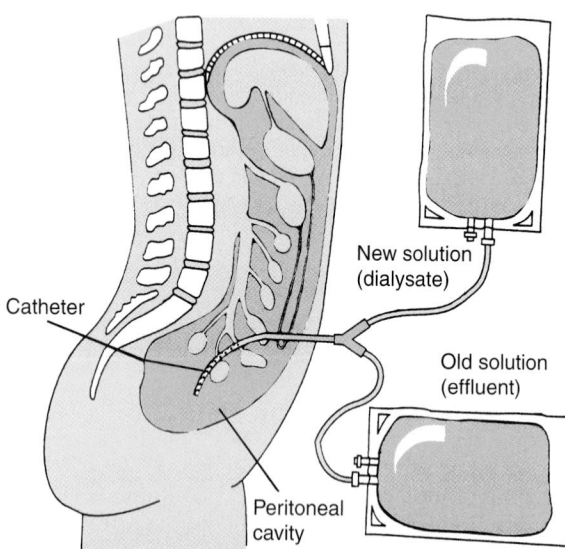

FIGURE 21-1 Continuous ambulatory peritoneal dialysis. The peritoneal catheter is implanted through the abdominal wall. Fluid infuses into the peritoneal cavity and drains after a prescribed time.

2. More liberal diet and fluid intake
3. Relatively simple and easy to use
4. Satisfactory biochemical control of uremia

Complications

1. Infectious peritonitis, exit-site and tunnel infections.
2. Noninfectious catheter malfunction, obstruction, dialysate leak.
3. Peritoneal–pleural communication, hernia formation.
4. GI bloating, distention, nausea.
5. Hypervolemia, hypovolemia.
6. Bleeding at catheter site.
7. Bloody effluent secondary to internal bleeding. In female patients, this may occur during menstruation.
8. Obstruction may occur if omentum becomes wrapped around the catheter or the catheter becomes caught in a loop of bowel.

Patient Education

1. The use of CAPD as a long-term treatment depends on prevention of recurring peritonitis.
   a. Use strict aseptic technique when performing bag exchanges.
   b. Perform bag exchanges in clean, closed-off area without pets and other activities.
   c. Wash hands before touching bag.
   d. Inspect bag, tubing for defects and leaks.
2. Do not omit bag changes—this will cause inadequate control of renal failure.
3. Some weight gain may accompany CAPD—the dialysate fluid contains a significant amount of dextrose, which adds calories to daily intake.
4. Report signs and symptoms of peritonitis—cloudy peritoneal fluid, abdominal pain or tenderness, malaise, fever.

Hemodialysis

Hemodialysis is a process of cleansing the blood of accumulated waste products. It is used for patients with end-stage renal failure or for acutely ill patients who require short-term dialysis.

Procedure

1. The patient's access is prepared and cannulated.
2. Heparin is administered (unless contraindicated).
3. Heparinized blood flows through a semipermeable dialyzer in one direction, and dialysis solution surrounds the membranes and flows in the opposite direction.
4. Dialysis solution consists of highly purified water to which sodium, potassium, calcium, magnesium, chloride, and dextrose have been added. Bicarbonate or acetate is also added to achieve the proper pH balance.
5. Through the process of diffusion, solute in the form of electrolytes, metabolic waste products, and acid–base components can be removed or added to the blood.
6. Excess water is removed from the blood (ultrafiltration).
7. The blood is then returned to the body through the patient's access.

Requirements for Hemodialysis

1. Access to the patient's circulation
2. Dialysis machine and dialyzer with semipermeable membrane

3. Appropriate dialysate bath
4. Time—approximately 4 hours, three times weekly
5. Place—dialysis center or home (if feasible)

Methods of Circulatory Access

1. Arteriovenous fistula (AVF)—creation of a vascular communication by suturing a vein directly to an artery.
   a. Usually, radial artery and cephalic vein are anastomosed in nondominant arm; vessels in the upper arm may also be used.
   b. After the procedure, the superficial venous system of the arm dilates.
   c. By means of two large-bore needles inserted into the dilated venous system, blood may be obtained and passed through the dialyzer. The arterial end is used for arterial flow and the distal end for reinfusion of dialyzed blood.
   d. Healing of AVF requires several weeks; a central vein catheter is used in the interim.
2. Arteriovenous graft—arteriovenous connection consisting of a tube graft made from autologous saphenous vein or from polytetrafluoroethylene (PTFE). Ready to use in 2 to 3 weeks.
3. Central vein catheters (CVC)—direct cannulation of veins (subclavian, internal jugular, or femoral); may be used as temporary or permanent dialysis access.

Complications of Vascular Access

1. Infection
2. Catheter clotting
3. Central vein thrombosis or stricture
4. Stenosis or thrombosis
5. Ischemia of the hand (steal syndrome)
6. Aneurysm or pseudoaneurysm

Monitoring During Hemodialysis

1. Involves constant monitoring of hemodynamic status, electrolyte, and acid–base balance, as well as maintenance of sterility and a closed system.
2. Usually performed by a specially trained nurse who is very familiar with the protocol and equipment being used.

Lifestyle Management for Chronic Hemodialysis

1. Dietary management involves restriction or adjustment of protein, sodium, potassium, or fluid intake.
2. Ongoing health care monitoring includes careful adjustment of medications that are normally excreted by the kidney or are dialyzable.
3. Surveillance for complications.
   a. Arteriosclerotic cardiovascular disease, congestive heart failure, disturbance of lipid metabolism (hypertriglyceridemia), coronary heart disease, stroke
   b. Intercurrent infection
   c. Anemia and fatigue
   d. Gastric ulcers and other problems
   e. Bone problems (renal osteodystrophy, aseptic necrosis of hip)—from disturbed calcium metabolism
   f. Hypertension
   g. Psychosocial problems: depression, suicide, sexual dysfunction
4. Supportive agencies: American Association of Kidney Patients, 100 South Ashley Drive, Suite 200, Tampa, FL 33602, 1-800-749-AAKP, *www.aakp.org*; National Kidney Foundation, 30 E. 33rd St., New York, NY 10016, 212-889-2210, *www.kidney.org*; National Kidney and Urologic Diseases Information Clearing House, Information Way, Bethesda, MD 20892, 301-654-4415 *www.niddk.nih.gov.*

(*text continues on page 702*)

PROCEDURE GUIDELINES 21-5 **ASSISTING THE PATIENT UNDERGOING (ACUTE) PERITONEAL DIALYSIS***

Peritoneal dialysis is a substitute for kidney function during renal failure. The peritoneum acts as a dialyzing membrane, and dialysate is delivered into the peritoneal cavity.

EQUIPMENT

Dialysis administration set (disposable, closed system)	Local anesthesia	Suture set
Peritoneal dialysis solution as requested	Central venous pressure monitoring equipment	Sterile gloves
Supplemental drugs as requested		Skin antiseptic

PROCEDURE

Nursing Action	Rationale
PREPARATORY PHASE	
1. Prepare the patient emotionally and physically for the procedure.	1. Nursing support is offered by explaining procedure mechanics, providing opportunities for the patient to ask questions, allowing verbalization of feelings, and giving expert physical care.

continued

PROCEDURE GUIDELINES 21-5   **ASSISTING THE PATIENT UNDERGOING (ACUTE) PERITONEAL DIALYSIS*** *CONTINUED*

Nursing Action	Rationale
2. See that the consent form has been signed.	
3. Weigh the patient before dialysis and every 24 h thereafter, preferably on an in-bed scale.	3. The weight at the beginning of the procedure serves as a baseline of information. Daily weight confirms ultrafiltration results and evaluates volume status.
4. Take temperature, pulse, respiration, and blood pressure readings before dialysis.	4. Measurement of vital signs at the beginning of dialysis is necessary for comparing subsequent changes in vital signs.
5. Have the patient empty bladder.	5. If the bladder is empty, there is less likelihood of perforating it when the trocar is introduced into the peritoneum.
6. Flush the tubing with dialysis solution.	6. The tubing is flushed to prevent air from entering the peritoneal cavity. Air causes abdominal discomfort and drainage difficulties.
7. Make the patient comfortable in a supine position. Have the patient and health care personnel wear masks.	7. This helps protect the patient from airborne contamination.

PERFORMANCE PHASE (BY THE PHYSICIAN)

The following is a brief summary of the method of insertion of a temporary peritoneal catheter (*done under strict asepsis*).

1. The abdomen is prepared surgically, and the skin and subcutaneous tissues are infiltrated with a local anesthetic.	1. Surgical preparation of the skin minimizes or eliminates surface bacteria and decreases the possibility of wound contamination and infection.
2. A small midline stab wound is made 3–5 cm below the umbilicus.	
3. The trocar is inserted through the incision with the stylet in place, or a thin stylet cannula may be inserted percutaneously.	
4. The patient is requested to raise head from the pillow after the trocar is introduced.	4. This maneuver tightens the abdominal muscles and permits easier penetration of the trocar without danger of injury to the intra-abdominal organs.
5. When the peritoneum is punctured, the trocar is directed toward the left side of the pelvis. The stylet is removed, and the catheter is inserted through the trocar and maneuvered into position.	
a. Dialysis fluid is allowed to run through the catheter while it is being positioned.	a. This prevents the omentum from adhering to the catheter, impeding its advancement or occluding its opening.
6. After the trocar is removed, the skin may be closed with a purse-string suture. (This is not always done.) A sterile dressing is placed around the catheter.	6. The catheter is attached to the skin to prevent loss of the catheter in the abdomen.
7. Attach the catheter connector to the administration set, which has been previously connected to the container of dialysis solution (warmed to body temperature, 37°C.)	7. The solution is warmed to body temperature for patient comfort and to prevent abdominal pain. Heating also causes dilatation of the peritoneal vessels and increases urea clearance.
8. Drugs (heparin, potassium, antibiotic) are added in advance.	8. The addition of heparin prevents fibrin clots from occluding the catheter. Potassium chloride may be added on request unless patient has hyperkalemia. Antibiotics are added for the treatment of peritonitis.
9. Permit the dialyzing solution to flow unrestricted into the peritoneal cavity (usually takes 5–10 min for completion). If the patient experiences pain, slow down the infusion.	9. The inflow solution should flow in a steady stream. If the fluid flows in too slowly, the catheter may need to be repositioned, because its tip may be buried in the omentum, or it may be occluded by a blood clot. Flushing may help.
10. Allow the fluid to remain in the peritoneal cavity for the prescribed time period (20–30 min). Prepare the next exchange while the fluid is in the peritoneal cavity.	10. For potassium, urea, and other waste materials to be removed, the solution must remain in the peritoneal cavity for the prescribed time (dwell or equilibration time). The maximum concentration gradient takes place in the first 5–10 min for small molecules, such as urea and creatinine.

Nursing Action	Rationale
11. Unclamp the outflow tube. Drainage should take approximately 20–30 min, although the time varies with each patient.	11. The abdomen is drained by a siphon effect through the closed system. Gravity drainage should occur fairly rapidly, and steady streams of fluid should be observed entering the drainage container. The drainage is usually straw-colored.
12. Check outflow for cloudy appearance, blood, and/or fibrin.	12. May be an early sign of peritonitis.
13. If the fluid is not draining properly, move the patient from side to side to facilitate the removal of peritoneal drainage. The head of the bed may also be elevated.	13. If the drainage stops, or starts to drip before the dialyzing fluid has run out, the catheter tip may be buried in the omentum. Rotating the patient may be helpful (or it may be necessary for the physician to reposition the catheter).
14. Ascertain if the catheter is patent. Check for closed clamp, kinked tubing, or air lock. *Never push the catheter in.*	14. Pushing in the catheter introduces bacteria into the peritoneal cavity.
15. When the outflow drainage ceases to run, clamp off the drainage tube and infuse the next exchange, using strict aseptic technique.	
16. Take blood pressure and pulse q15min during the first exchange and every hour thereafter. Monitor the heart rate for signs of dysrhythmia.	16. A drop in blood pressure may indicate excessive fluid loss from glucose concentrations of the dialyzing solutions. Changes in the vital signs may indicate impending shock or overhydration.
17. Take the patient's temperature q4h (especially after catheter removal).	17. An infection is more apt to become evident after dialysis has been discontinued.
18. The procedure is repeated until the blood chemistry levels improve. The usual duration for short-term dialysis is 48–72 h. Depending on the patient's condition, 48–72 exchanges will be necessary.	18. The duration of dialysis depends on the severity of the condition and on the size and weight of the patient.
19. Keep an exact record of patient's fluid balance during the treatment. a. Know the status of the patient's loss or gain of fluid at the end of each exchange. Check dressing for leakage and weight on gram scale if significant. b. The fluid balance should be about even or should show slight fluid loss or gain, depending on the patient's fluid status.	19. Complications (circulatory collapse, hypotension, shock, and death) may occur if the patient loses too much fluid through peritoneal drainage. Large fluid losses around the catheter may not be noted unless the dressings are checked carefully.
20. Promote patient comfort during dialysis.	20. The dialysis period is lengthy, and the patient becomes fatigued.
a. Provide frequent back care and massage pressure areas. b. Have the patient turn from side to side. c. Elevate head of bed at intervals. d. Allow the patient to sit in chair for brief periods if condition permits (only with surgically implanted catheter; with trocar, patient is usually on bed rest).	
21. Observe for the following: a. Abdominal pain—note the time of discomfort during exchange cycle and duration of symptoms.	a. Pain may be caused by the dialyzing solution's not being at body temperature, incomplete drainage of the solution, chemical irritation, pressure by the catheter, peritonitis, or air pressing on the diaphragm, causing referred shoulder pain.
b. Dialysate leakage—change the dressings frequently, being careful not to dislodge the catheter; use sterile plastic drapes to prevent contamination.	b. Leakage around the catheter predisposes the patient to infection at the exit site and peritonitis. Dialysis may need to be terminated if leakage persists.
c. Place the patient in a more upright position and use smaller fluid volumes to try to relieve pain and leakage.	
22. Keep accurate records. a. Exact time of beginning and end of each exchange: starting and finishing time of drainage b. Amount of solution infused and recovered	

continued

PROCEDURE GUIDELINES 21-5   **ASSISTING THE PATIENT UNDERGOING (ACUTE) PERITONEAL DIALYSIS* CONTINUED**

c. Fluid balance

d. Number of exchanges

e. Medications added to dialyzing solution

f. Pre- and postdialysis weight, plus daily weight

g. Level of responsiveness at beginning, throughout, and at end of treatment

h. Assessment of vital signs and patient's condition

COMPLICATIONS

1. Peritonitis
   a. Watch for nausea and vomiting, anorexia, abdominal pain, tenderness, rigidity, and cloudy dialysate drainage.
   b. Send specimen of dialysate for white cell count and full set of cultures.
2. Bleeding
   a. A hematocrit of the drainage fluid may be taken to determine the amount of bleeding.

1. Peritonitis is the most common complication. Antibiotics may be added to dialysate and also given systemically.

2. A small amount of bleeding around the catheter is not significant if it does not persist. During the first few exchanges, blood-tinged fluid from subcutaneous bleeding is not uncommon. Small amounts of heparin may be added to inflow solution to prevent the catheter from becoming clogged.

* Automated closed-system peritoneal cycling machines are available.

Kidney Surgery

Kidney surgery may include *nephrectomy* (removal of the kidney), *kidney transplantation* for end-stage renal disease (ESRD), procedures to remove stones or tumors, and procedures to insert drainage tubes (*nephrostomy*). Incisional approaches vary but may involve the flank, thoracic, and abdominal regions. Nephrectomy is most often performed for malignant tumors of the kidney but may also be indicated for trauma and kidneys that no longer function due to obstructive disorders and other renal disease. The absence of one kidney does not result in impaired renal function when the remaining kidney is normal.

Many surgical procedures were previously performed as "open" procedures, but are now being done with laparoscopic "keyhole" surgeries. An endoscope is introduced, and the abdomen is inflated with CO_2. Instruments are passed through other sites, or a sleeve may be used, which allows a hand to be introduced at the operative site. Advantages are decreased postoperative pain, decreased blood loss, and decreased length of stay (3 to 4 days for nephrectomy patients).

Preoperative Management

1. The patient is prepared for surgery, and consent is witnessed. Preoperative antibiotics and bowel cleansing regimen are prescribed.
2. Risk factors for thromboembolism are identified (smoking, oral contraceptive use, varicosities of lower extremities), and antiembolism stockings may be applied. Leg exercises are taught, and the patient is prepared for pneumatic/sequential compression stockings that will be used postoperatively.
3. Pulmonary status is assessed (presence of dyspnea, productive cough, other related cardiac symptoms), and deep-breathing exercises, effective coughing, and use of incentive spirometer are taught.
4. If embolization of the renal artery is being done preoperatively for patients with renal cell carcinoma, the following symptoms of postinfarction syndrome are observed for (may last up to 3 days):
   a. Flank pain
   b. Fever
   c. Leukocytosis
   d. Hypertension

Postoperative Management

1. Vital signs are monitored, and incisional area is assessed for evidence of bleeding or hemorrhage.

NURSING ALERT

 Use frequent and close observation of blood pressure, pulse, and respiration to recognize hemorrhage (and shock)—chief danger after renal surgery. Watch for pain, sanguineous drainage from drain site(s), or expanding pulsatile flank mass. Prepare for rapid blood and fluid replacement and reoperation.

2. Pulmonary complications of atelectasis, pneumonia, and pneumothorax are observed for. Pulmonary toilet through deep breathing, percussion, and vibration is maintained. Chest tube drainage may be used (the prox-

imity of the thoracic cavity to the operative area may result in the need for chest tube drainage postoperatively).

3. Patency of urinary drainage tubes is maintained (nephrostomy, suprapubic, or urethral catheter). Ureteral stents may be used.

4. Respiratory status and lower extremities are assessed for thromboembolic complications.

5. Bowel sounds, abdominal distention, and pain are monitored, which may indicate paralytic ileus and need for nasogastric decompression.

6. For kidney transplantation patients, immunosuppressant drugs (corticosteroids in combination with azathioprine [Imuran] or similar agent) are ordered. Early signs of rejection include temperature greater than 100.4°F (38.5°C), decreased urine output, weight gain of 3 lb or more overnight, pain or tenderness over the graft site, hypertension, increased serum creatinine.

Nursing Diagnoses
- Pain related to surgical incision
- Altered Urinary Elimination related to urinary drainage tubes or catheter(s)
- Risk for Infection related to incision, potential pulmonary complications, and possibly immunosuppression
- Risk for Fluid Volume Deficit or Excess related to fluid replacement needs and transplanted/remaining kidney function

Nursing Interventions
Relieving Pain
1. Assess pain location, level, and characteristics. Transient renal coliclike pain may be caused by passage of blood clots down the ureter; however, report any persistent increasing or unrelievable pain, which may indicate obstruction of urinary drainage or hemorrhage.

2. Administer pain medications; evaluate effectiveness of patient-controlled analgesia (PCA).

3. Encourage patient to ambulate, splint incision to move or cough.

Promoting Urinary Elimination
1. Maintain patency of urinary drainage tubes and catheter(s) while in place. Prevent kinking or pulling.

2. Use handwashing and asepsis when providing care and handling urinary drainage system (especially important for the patient taking immunosuppressants).

3. Make sure indwelling catheter is dependent and draining.
   a. Report any decrease in output or excessive clots.
   b. Be alert for signs of urinary infection such as cloudy urine, fever, or bladder or flank ache.

4. Intervene to encourage removal of catheter when patient becomes ambulatory.

5. Maintain adequate fluid intake, IV or oral when allowed.

Preventing Infection
1. Monitor for fever, elevated leukocyte count, abnormal breath sounds.

2. Administer antibiotics as prescribed.

3. Assist patient with use of incentive spirometer, coughing and deep breathing, and ambulation to decrease risk of pulmonary infection. Provide meticulous care to chest tube sites.

4. Change dressings promptly if drainage is present—drainage is an excellent culture medium for bacteria.

5. Obtain specimens for bacteriologic testing of urine, wounds, sputum, and discontinued catheters, drains, and IV lines as indicated. Before removing catheters or urinary drains, disinfect skin around entry site, then remove. Using aseptic technique, cut off tip of catheter or drain and place in sterile container for laboratory culture.

6. Monitor vascular access to hemodialysis to ensure patency and watch for evidence of infection.

7. For kidney transplantation patients, give oral antifungal to prevent mucosal candidiasis, which often occurs due to immunosuppression.

8. Provide regular skin care, and assist with hygiene.

Maintaining Fluid Balance
1. Closely monitor intake and output, especially after kidney transplantation.
   a. Expect normal urine output to be 30 to 100 mL/h.
   b. Report oliguria with less than 30 mL/h or polyuria of 100 to 500 mL/h.

2. Monitor serum electrolyte results and electrocardiogram (ECG) for changes associated with electrolyte imbalance.
   a. Report arrhythmias or other cardiac symptoms immediately.

3. Monitor blood pressure and heart rate, central venous pressure, and pulmonary artery pressure (if indicated) to anticipate adjustment of fluid replacement.

4. Avoid using dialysis access extremity for IV lines, intra-arterial monitoring, or restraints.

5. Prepare for hemodialysis in postoperative period until transplanted kidney is functioning well.

Patient Education and Health Maintenance
After Nephrectomy
1. Provide information about continued recovery from surgery; regular exercise, refraining from heavy lifting or strenuous activities, resumption of normal dietary intake.

2. Advise wearing a Medic-Alert bracelet, and inform all health care providers of solitary kidney status.

3. Encourage close follow-up and need to seek medical attention for any signs of urinary infection or urinary tract disease if only one kidney present to prevent damage to that kidney.

After Kidney Transplantation
1. Explain and reinforce symptoms of rejection—fever, chills, sweating, lassitude, hypertension, weight gain, peripheral edema, decrease in urine output. Acute rejection is common and usually reversible; often occurs in first 2 months after transplantation.

2. Prepare patient for possible need for maintenance dialysis when rejection occurs. If the transplanted kidney is rejected, it may be removed in the initial postoperative period. For chronic rejection, the kidney is not commonly removed.
3. Explain continued protection of vascular access graft, which may still be enlarged, tender to palpation, associated with edema of overlying tissues.
4. Encourage compliance with laboratory tests (serum blood urea nitrogen [BUN] and creatinine, serum chemistry, hematology, bacteriology, cyclosporine, or tacrolimus levels) to monitor recipient's immune status and detect early signs of rejection.
5. Instruct patient and family about prescribed immunosuppressants and complications of therapy—infection or incomplete control of rejection.
   a. Review immunosuppressive medications in detail, including color identification of pills, dose schedules, side effects, and the necessity for taking the medication.
   b. Review other medications such as histamine₂ blockers to prevent stress ulcers and prophylaxis for *Candida* and community-acquired infections.
6. Review in detail postoperative self-care regimen (may be inpatient or outpatient), including adequate fluid intake, daily weight, measurement of urine, stool test for occult blood, prevention of infection, exercise.
7. Instruct to report immediately:
   a. Decrease in urinary output
   b. Weight gain, edema
   c. Malaise, fever
   d. Graft swelling and tenderness (visible and palpable below the skin)
   e. Changes in blood pressure readings
   f. Respiratory distress
   g. Anxiety, depression, change in appetite or sleep
8. Advise avoidance of contact sports for life to prevent trauma to the transplanted kidney.
9. Stress that follow-up care after transplantation is a lifelong necessity.
10. For additional support and information, refer to American Association of Kidney Patients, 100 South Ashley Drive, Suite 200, Tampa, FL 33602, 1-800-749-AAKP; *www.aakp.org*.

Outcome-Based Evaluation
- Verbalizes relief of pain
- Urinary drainage clear without clots
- Absence of fever or signs of infection
- Vital signs stable; urine output 50 mL/h

Urinary Diversion

Urinary diversion refers to diverting the urinary stream from the bladder so that it exits by way of a new avenue. A number of operative procedures may be performed to achieve this (Figure 21-2). Methods of urinary diversion include:

1. *Ileal conduit* (or "Bricker's loop")—most common; transplants the ureters into an isolated section of the terminal ileum, bringing one end through the abdominal wall to create a stoma. Urine flows from the kidney into the ureters, then through the ileal conduit, and exits through urinary stoma. The ureters may also be transplanted into a segment of the transverse colon (colon conduit).
2. *Nephrostomy*—insertion of a catheter into the renal pelvis by way of an incision into the flank or by percutaneous catheter placement into the kidney. They are rarely placed for long periods of time; they are a short-term method of diverting urine away from an obstruction or lesion below the level of the renal pelvis.
3. *Continent urinary diversion* procedures—create a urinary reservoir from an intestinal segment that is either brought to the skin using a valve mechanism that permits catheterization, or is anastomosed directly to the proximal urethra.
   a. *Continent urinary reservoir* (Kock pouch, Indiana pouch, Mainz pouch, and others)—transplants the ureters into a pouch created from small bowel or large and small bowel. Mechanisms to discourage ureteral reflux are used to implant the ureters into the pouch, including an intussuscepted nipple valve or tunneling the ureters through the taeniae of the bowel. The existing ileocecal valve, or a surgically created intussuscepted nipple valve, provides the continence mechanism. Patient does not have to wear an external appliance, but the procedure does require intermittent self-catheterization of the pouch.
   b. *Orthotopic bladder replacement* (Hemi-Kock pouch, Neobladder, and others)—pouch created from small or large and small bowel is anastomosed to urethral stump; voiding is through the urethra. Patient usually has nocturnal incontinence; not all patients are candidates for this procedure.

Preoperative Management
1. Functional assessment should be performed including degree of manual dexterity and visual acuity—essential for stoma care or self-catheterization postoperatively.
2. The patient's psychosocial resources are evaluated, including available support persons, education, occupation, and economic resources (including insurance coverage of ostomy supplies if needed), coping strengths, attitudes toward urinary diversion.
3. Bowel preparation is performed to prevent fecal contamination during surgery and the potential complication of infection.
   a. Clear liquids only and prescribed laxatives for mechanical cleansing of the bowel.
   b. Antibiotics as prescribed (nonabsorbable; active against enteric organisms) to reduce bacterial count in the bowel lumen.

Types of Cutaneous Diversions

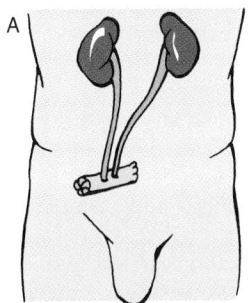

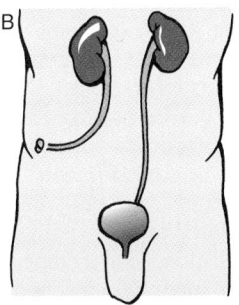

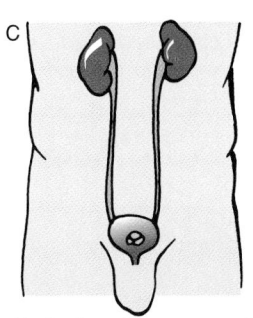

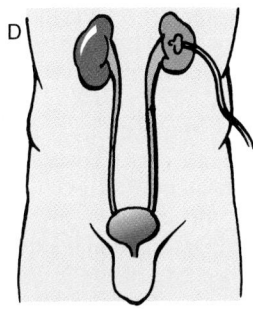

A Conventional ileal conduit. The surgeon transplants the ureters to an isolated section of the terminal ileum (ileal conduit), bringing one end to the abdominal wall. The ureter may also be transplanted into the transverse sigmoid colon (colon conduit) or proximal jejunum (jejunal conduit).

B Cutaneous ureterostomy. The surgeon brings the detached ureter through the abdominal wall and attaches it to an opening in the skin.

C Vesicostomy. The surgeon sutures the bladder to the abdominal wall and creates an opening (stoma) through the abdominal and bladder walls for urinary drainage.

D Nephrostomy. The surgeon inserts a catheter into the renal pelvis via an incision into the flank or by percutaneous catheter placement, into the kidney.

Types of Continent Urinary Diversions

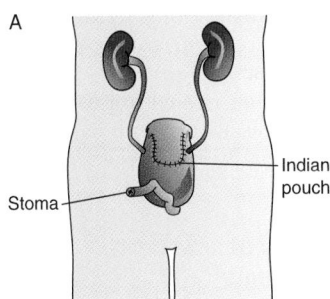

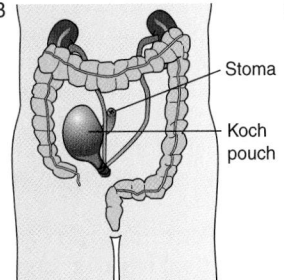

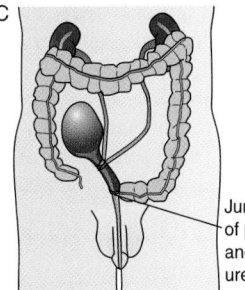

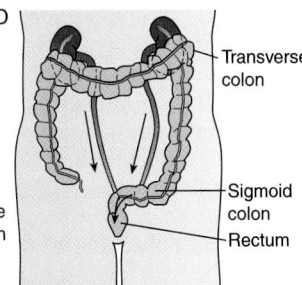

A Indiana pouch. The surgeon introduces the ureters into a segment of ileum and cecum. Urine is drained periodically by inserting a catheter into the stoma.

B Continent ileal urinary diversions (Koch pouch). The surgeon transplants the ureters to an isolated segment of small bowel, ascending colon, or ileocolonic segment and develops an effective continence mechanism or valve. Urine is drained by inserting a catheter into the stoma.

C In male patients, the Koch pouch can be modified by attaching one end of the pouch to the urethra, allowing more normal voiding. The female urethra is too short for this modification.

D Ureterosigmoidostomy. The surgeon introduces the ureters into the sigmoid, thereby allowing urine to flow through the colon and out of the rectum.

FIGURE 21-2 Methods of urinary diversion.

4. Adequate hydration is ensured, including IV infusions, to ensure urine flow during surgery and to prevent hypovolemia.
5. The procedure is explained by the surgeon and the enterostomal therapist before surgery.
   a. For ileal or colon conduit, the stoma site is planned preoperatively with the patient standing, sitting, and lying—to place the stoma away from bony prominences, skin creases, and scars, and where the patient can see it.
   b. Stoma site may also be marked even though continent urinary diversion procedure is planned, in case findings during surgery prevent continent procedure and standard ileal or colon conduit is necessary.

Postoperative Management
1. The patient is assessed for immediate postoperative complications; wound or urinary tract infection, urinary or fecal anastomotic leakage, small bowel obstruction, paralytic ileus, pelvic thrombophlebitis, pulmonary embolism, and necrosis of stoma.
2. Intake and output are monitored including amount of urinary output, patency of drainage catheter(s), and degree of hematuria.
3. Pelvic gravity or suction drains are evaluated—sudden increase in drainage suggests an anastomotic leak; send specimen of drainage for BUN and creatinine, if ordered. (Presence of measurable BUN and creatinine in the drainage indicates urine in drainage, confirming a urine leak.)

4. Ureteral stents are used to protect ureterointestinal anastomoses; stents will emerge from stoma or through separate wound (stents are not visible in orthotopic bladder replacement patients). They are removed in 3 weeks.

Nursing Diagnoses
- Altered Urinary Elimination related to urinary diversion
- Pain related to surgery
- Body Image Disturbance related to urinary diversion
- Sexual Dysfunction related to reconstructive surgery and impotence (in men)

Nursing Interventions
Achieving Urinary Elimination
For ileal or colon conduit patients:
1. Maintain a transparent urostomy pouch over the stoma postoperatively to allow for easy assessment.
2. Inspect the stoma for color and size; whether it is flush, nippled, or retracted; and the condition of the skin around the stoma. Document baseline information for subsequent comparison.
   a. Stoma should be red, wet with mucus, soft, and slightly rubbery to the touch (stoma lacks nerve ending, so feeling in stoma is absent).
   b. Cyanotic stoma indicates poor circulation.
   c. Necrotic stoma is blue-black or tan-brown.
3. Report any bleeding, necrosis, sloughing, suture separation.
4. Check patency of ureteral stents.
5. Keep the pouch on at all times, and observe normal urine (but not fecal) drainage at all times.
   a. Connect pouches to drainage bag when patient is in bed, and record urine volume hourly.
   b. Initial urostomy pouch remains in place for several days postoperatively; it is changed every 3 to 5 days when patient teaching begins.

For continent urinary diversion patients:
1. Maintain patency of drainage catheters placed into internal urinary pouch during surgery; irrigate with 30 mL saline every 2 to 4 hours to prevent obstruction from mucous accumulation.
2. Assess stoma—should be very small and flush.
3. Record urine output and character of urine.
4. Monitor output of pelvic drain (on gentle suction or gravity drainage) every 8 hours.
5. Advise patient that approximately 3 weeks after surgery the drainage catheter is removed from the pouch after a radiographic study ("pouch-o-gram") confirms healing of all anastomoses.

Controlling Pain
1. Administer analgesic medications, or teach use of and monitor PCA (IV or epidural).
2. Assess response to pain control.
3. Provide positioning for comfort, alternating with ambulation, as able.

Resolving Body Image Issues
1. Assess patient's reaction to looking at new urinary stoma, if applicable; provide reassurance and support.

2. Accept the patient's depression, which may be manifested in irritability or lack of motivation to learn.
   a. Give extra support until the patient can cope.
   b. Reinforce the concept that the stoma will be manageable.
   c. Acknowledge feelings of fear and anxiety as normal.
3. Encourage patient to gradually participate in care of stoma or catheters.
4. Encourage verbalization of feelings and concerns related to urinary diversion.
5. If possible, arrange for patient to speak with another patient who has undergone the same surgery; this provides realistic expectations and support for a positive outcome.
6. Help patient/family to gain independence through learning to manage the ostomy. Provide for demonstrations, supervised practice, written instructions, and return demonstrations until patient is independent in self-care.

Coping With Sexual Dysfunction
1. Be aware that most men experience impotence as a result of surgery; provide information or referrals about options including medications, pharmacologic erection programs, and penile prostheses.
2. Allow patient to express feelings related to loss of sexual function, and encourage discussion with partner.
3. Tell women that they may usually resume sexual activity after healing is complete.

Patient Education and Health Maintenance
For Ileal or Colon Conduit Patients
1. Obtain and familiarize the patient with the appropriate equipment. Most urostomy pouching systems are disposable. The choice of pouch is determined by location of stoma, patient activity, body build, and economic status.
   a. Two-piece pouches consist of a skin barrier (or wafer) that fits around the stoma and adheres to the skin, and a pouch that snaps onto the skin barrier.
   b. One-piece pouches may be precut for the correct stoma size and include the adhesive; the pouch is applied directly to the peristomal skin.
2. Assist the patient to determine stoma size (for ordering correct appliance). The stoma will shrink considerably as edema subsides, and the size is recalibrated several times during the first 3 to 6 weeks postoperatively.
   a. Measuring guides are included with most urostomy pouches.
   b. The inside diameter of the skin barrier should not be more than $\frac{1}{16}$ to $\frac{1}{8}$ inch larger than the diameter of the stoma.
3. Teach how to change the pouch.
   a. Change pouch early in morning before taking fluids or before evening meal—urine output is lower at these times.
   b. Prepare the new pouching system according to manufacturer's directions.

c. Wash the peristomal skin with noncream-based soap and water. Rinse and pat dry. *The skin must be dry or appliance will not adhere.*

d. A gauze or tissue wick may be applied over the stoma to absorb urine while the appliance is being changed. Keep the skin free from direct contact with urine. Suggest the use of tampons to soak up urine from stoma while changing pouch at home if desired.

e. Center the skin barrier directly over the stoma, and apply it carefully. Apply gentle pressure around appliance for secure adherence.

f. Apply a belt to keep pouch in place if desired; it is especially useful in patients with soft abdomens.

4. Advise that additional adhesives, such as pastes or cements, are not usually necessary with a well-fitting pouch.

5. Tell patient that frequency of pouch changes depends on the type of pouch used—generally pouches should be changed every 3 days (for one-piece pouches) to every 4 to 7 days (for two-piece pouches).

6. Advise emptying the pouch when it is a third to half full to prevent weight of urine from loosening adhesive seal—open drain valve (spigot) for periodic emptying.

7. Teach how to attach outlet on pouch to a bedside urinary drainage container with plastic tubing (at least 5 feet to allow turning) and how to secure tubing to leg to prevent twisting or kinking.

a. Position the drainage bottle lower than the level of the bed to enhance flow by gravity.

b. Clean nighttime drainage equipment with vinegar and water. Rinse well.

8. Advise to drink liberal amounts of fluids to flush the conduit free of mucus and reduce possibility of urinary infection.

9. Teach that the stoma may bleed if it is bumped or rubbed; report bleeding that continues for several hours.

10. Advise carrying spare pouches in handbag or pocket and bringing an extra pouch to every visit with health care provider.

11. Advise wearing cotton (rather than nylon) underwear or the use of specially made underwear for ostomy patients that prevents contact between plastic pouch and skin. Heavy girdles are not allowed because they may cause chafing of the stoma and prevent free flow of urine.

12. Advise reporting problems with peristomal skin or with leakage from the pouch, or the development of fever, chills, pain, change in color of urine (cloudy, bloody), diminishing urine output.

13. For additional information and support, refer to United Ostomy Association, Inc., 19772 MacArthur Blvd., Suite 200, Irvine, CA 92612-2405, 1-800-826-0826; *www.uoa.org.*

For Continent Ileal Urinary Reservoir Patients

1. Teach irrigation of catheter; this must be done every 4 to 6 hours at home.

2. Teach how to change stoma dressing and small urostomy pouch over pelvic drain that will stay in place for 3 weeks after surgery.

3. Instruct in use of leg bag or bedside urinary drainage bag while catheter remains in place.

4. Teach how to catheterize continent urinary diversion when healing is verified:

a. Red rubber or plastic, straight or coudé catheters are used.

b. Apply a small amount of water-soluble lubricant to the tip of the catheter.

c. Use clean technique, wash hands before each catheterization.

d. Maintain schedule of catheterizations during initial "training" period; to gradually allow the pouch to adapt to holding larger amounts of urine (every 2 hours during day and every 3 hours at night; increase by 1 hour each week for 5 weeks).

e. After training period, catheterize four to five times a day, pouch should not hold more than 400 to 500 mL.

f. Irrigate pouch with saline through catheter once a day to clear it of accumulated mucus.

5. Teach patient to report problems such as leakage of urine from stoma between catheterizations.

6. Tell patient to shower or bathe normally, wear normal clothing; only a small dressing or Band-Aid needs to be worn over the stoma.

7. Advise drinking 8 to 10 glasses of water daily.

For Orthotopic Bladder Replacement

1. Teach patient to irrigate Foley catheter that will stay in place for 3 weeks after surgery; irrigate with 30 mL saline every 4 to 6 hours.

2. Instruct in use of leg bag or bedside drainage bag while catheter remains in place.

3. Instruct on how to change dressing or small urostomy pouch over pelvic drain while in place.

4. After healing of pouch is confirmed and catheter is removed, teach patient to "void."

a. Voiding is accomplished by abdominal straining; mucus is expected in voided urine.

b. Voiding schedule must be maintained for first 5 to 6 weeks (every 2 hours during day and every 3 hours at night; increase by 1 hour each week).

c. Incontinence is anticipated after catheter is removed; usually more pronounced when patient is asleep and muscles are relaxed.

5. Teach patient to perform pelvic floor exercises, which must be done faithfully for the rest of life; as pelvic floor sphincter muscles strengthen, incontinence subsides. Most patients continue to have small amounts of nocturnal incontinence.

a. Contract pelvic floor muscles (as if stopping stream of urine or flatus) for 5 seconds, then relax for 5 to 10 seconds.

b. Repeat approximately 15 to 20 times for one set, and do three sets a day.

6. Provide information about absorbent products that may be used temporarily; also preventive skin care.

7. Instruct in clean self-catheterization, which may be needed if urethra becomes obstructed with mucus; pouch should be irrigated with saline if catheterization is necessary.

8. Reassure patient that time, patience, and continued adherence to voiding and exercise schedule will result in continence.

Outcome-Based Evaluation

• Urine draining by way of urinary diversion
• Verbalizes good pain control
• Discusses feelings about change in body image; seeks support through family
• Verbalizes reasonable expectations about sexual function

Prostatic Surgery

Prostatic surgery may be done for BPH or prostate cancer. Surgical approach depends on size of the gland, severity of obstruction, age, underlying health, and prostatic disease.

Surgical Procedures

1. Transurethral resection of the prostate (TUR or TURP)—most common and done without an incision by means of endoscopic instrument
2. Open prostatectomy
   a. Suprapubic—incision into suprapubic area and through bladder wall; frequently done for BPH
   b. Perineal—incision between scrotum and rectal area; may be done for poor surgical risk patients but causes highest incidence of urinary incontinence and impotence
   c. Retropubic—incision at level of symphysis pubis; preserves nerves responsible for sexual function in 50% of patients

Preoperative Management

1. Information about the procedure and the expected postoperative care, including catheter drainage, irrigation, and monitoring of hematuria is discussed.
2. Complications of surgery are discussed.
   a. Incontinence or dribbling of urine may occur for up to 1 year after surgery; pelvic floor (Kegel) exercises help regain urinary control.
   b. Retrograde ejaculation—seminal fluid released into bladder and eliminated in the urine rather than through the urethra during intercourse; impotence is usually not a complication of TUR but often a complication of open prostatectomy.
3. Bowel preparation is given, or the patient is instructed in home administration and fasting after midnight.
4. Optimal cardiac, respiratory, and circulatory status should be achieved to decrease risk of complications.
5. Prophylactic antibiotics are ordered.

Postoperative Management

1. Urinary drainage is maintained and observed for signs of hemorrhage.
2. Wound care is provided to prevent infection.
3. Pain is controlled, and early ambulation is promoted.
4. Surveillance is maintained for complications.
   a. Wound infection and dehiscence
   b. Urinary obstruction or infection
   c. Hemorrhage
   d. Thrombophlebitis, pulmonary embolism
   e. Urinary incontinence, sexual dysfunction

Nursing Diagnoses

• Altered Urinary Elimination related to surgical procedure and urinary catheter
• Risk for Infection related to surgical incision, immobility, and urinary catheter
• Pain related to surgical procedure
• Anxiety related to urinary incontinence, difficulty voiding, and erectile dysfunction

Nursing Interventions
Facilitating Urinary Drainage

1. Maintain patency of urethral catheter placed after surgery.
   a. Monitor flow of three-way closed irrigation and drainage system (Figure 21-3) if used. Continuous irrigation helps prevent clot formation, which can obstruct catheter, cause painful bladder spasms, and lead to infection.

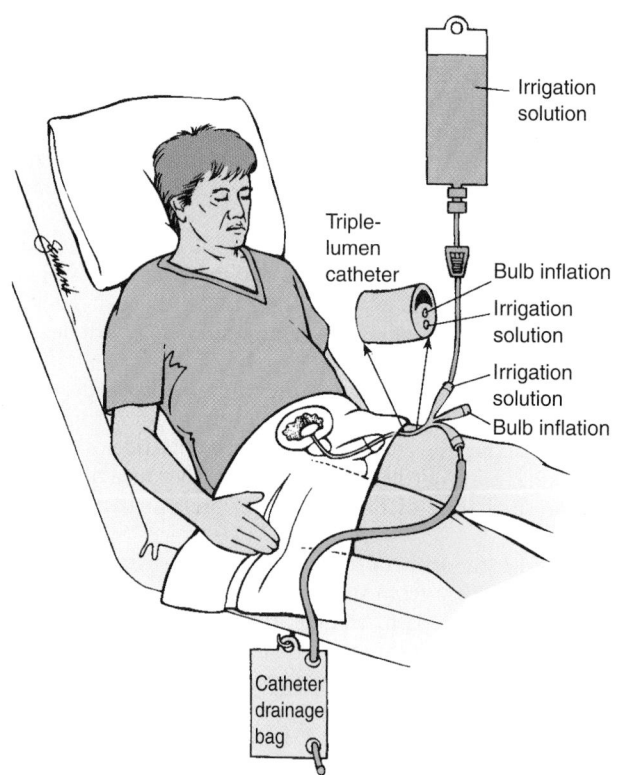

FIGURE 21-3   A three-way system for bladder irrigation.

Irrigation solution

Triple-lumen catheter

Bulb inflation

Irrigation solution

Irrigation solution

Bulb inflation

Catheter drainage bag

b. Perform manual irrigation with 50 mL irrigating fluid using aseptic technique.

c. Avoid overdistention of bladder, which could lead to hemorrhage.

d. Administer anticholinergic medications to reduce bladder spasms, as ordered.

 DRUG ALERT

Anticholinergic medications are contraindicated in patients with narrow-angle glaucoma.

2. Assess degree of hematuria and any clot formation; drainage should become light pink within 24 hours.

a. Report any bright red bleeding with increased viscosity (arterial)—may require surgical intervention.

b. Report any increase in dark red bleeding (venous)—may require traction of the catheter so the inflated balloon applies pressure to prostatic fossa.

c. Prepare for blood transfusion if bleeding persists.

3. Administer IV fluids as ordered, and encourage oral fluids when tolerated to ensure hydration and urine output.

Preventing Infection

1. After open prostatectomy, maintain bed rest for the first 24 hours with frequent monitoring of vital signs, intake and output, and observation of incisional dressing, if present.

2. After 24 hours, encourage ambulation to prevent venous thrombosis, pulmonary embolism, and hypostatic pneumonia.

3. Observe urine for cloudiness or odor, and obtain urine for evaluation of infection as ordered.

4. Administer antibiotics as prescribed.

5. Report any testicular pain, swelling, and tenderness that could indicate epididymitis from spreading infection.

6. Assist with perineal care if perineal incision is present to prevent contamination by feces.

Relieving Pain

1. Administer pain medication, or monitor PCA as directed.

2. Position for comfort, and tell the patient to avoid straining, which will increase pelvic venous congestion and may cause hemorrhage.

3. Administer stool softeners to prevent discomfort from constipation.

4. Make sure catheter is secured to patient's thigh and tubing is not creating traction on catheter, which will cause pain and potential hemorrhage.

NURSING ALERT

 Avoid rectal temperatures, enemas, or rectal tubes postoperatively to prevent hemorrhage or disruption of healing.

Reducing Anxiety

1. Provide realistic expectations about postoperative discomfort and overall progress.

a. Tell patient to avoid sexual intercourse, straining at stool, heavy lifting, and long periods of sitting for 6 to 8 weeks after surgery.

b. Advise follow-up visits after treatment because urethral stricture or bladder neck contracture may occur.

2. Reassure patient that urinary incontinence and frequency, urgency, and dysuria are expected after removal of catheter and should gradually subside.

3. Reassure patient that there may be measures to help.

4. Reinforce the risks for impotence as told by the surgeon. Remind patient that erectile function may not return for as long as 6 months.

5. Encourage patient to express fears and anxieties related to potential loss of sexual function, and to discuss concerns with partner.

6. Advise that options are available to restore sexual function if impotence persists.

Patient Education and Health Maintenance

1. Transurethral prostatectomy is often done on an outpatient basis; the patient may go home the evening of surgery.

2. Open prostatectomy patients may be discharged 2 to 3 days after surgery.

3. Reinforce instructions provided on catheter care, maintaining patency and catheter irrigation.

a. If sent home with catheter, will be removed in about 3 weeks when cystogram confirms healing.

b. Advise that stress incontinence may occur after catheter is removed and is more pronounced when abdominal pressure is increased, such as coughing, laughing, straining.

c. For patients who experienced urgency before surgery, caution that they may have urge incontinence for several weeks postoperatively.

d. Discuss the use of absorbent products to contain urine leakage around catheter, and after catheter is removed.

4. Teach measures to regain urinary control. Teach the patient to correctly perform pelvic floor exercises. Have patient squeeze the pelvic floor muscles (as if stopping stream of urine or flatus) for 5 seconds, and then relax for 5 to 10 seconds. This should be done 15 to 20 times, three times a day. Caution against using abdominal muscles (straining or Valsalva), which increases incontinence.

5. Reinforce availability of options such as medications. Pharmacologic erection programs and penile implants are available to restore sexual function if impotence persists for more than 6 months after surgery.

6. Prostate cancer patients should have a PSA blood test every 3 to 6 months after prostatectomy.

Outcome-Based Evaluation
- Clear yellow drainage by way of catheter
- Incision without drainage; afebrile
- Verbalizes good pain relief
- Verbalizes realistic expectations for urinary and sexual functioning

URINARY DISORDERS

■ Acute Renal Failure

Acute renal failure is a syndrome of varying causation that results in a sudden decline in renal function. It is frequently associated with an increase in BUN and creatinine, oliguria (less than 500 mL urine/24 h), hyperkalemia, and sodium retention.

Pathophysiology and Etiology
Causes
1. Prerenal causes—result from conditions that decrease renal blood flow (hypovolemia, shock, hemorrhage, burns, impaired cardiac output, diuretic therapy)
2. Postrenal causes—arise from obstruction or disruption to urine flow anywhere along the urinary tract
3. Intrarenal causes—result from injury to renal tissue and are usually associated with intrarenal ischemia, toxins, immunologic processes, systemic and vascular disorders

Clinical Course
1. Onset: begins when the kidney is injured and lasts from hours to days.
2. Oliguric–anuric phase (urine volume less than 400 to 500 mL/24 h).
   a. Accompanied by rise in serum concentration of elements usually excreted by kidney (urea, creatinine, organic acids, and the intracellular cations—potassium and magnesium).
   b. There can be a decrease in renal function with increasing nitrogen retention even when the patient is excreting more than 2 to 3 L of urine daily—called nonoliguric or high-output renal failure.
3. Diuretic phase: begins when the 24-hour urine volume exceeds 500 mL and ends when the BUN and serum creatinine levels stop rising.
4. Recovery phase.
   a. Usually lasts several months to 1 year.
   b. Probably some scar tissue remains, but the functional loss is not always clinically significant.

Clinical Manifestations
1. *Prerenal*—decreased tissue turgor, dryness of mucous membranes, weight loss, hypotension, oliguria or anuria, flat neck veins, tachycardia

2. *Postrenal*—obstruction to urine flow, obstructive symptoms of BPH, possible nephrolithiasis
3. *Intrarenal*—presentation based on cause; edema usually present
4. Changes in urine volume and serum concentrations of BUN, creatinine, potassium, and so forth, as described above

Diagnostic Evaluation
1. Urinalysis—reveals proteinuria, hematuria, casts
2. Rising serum creatinine and BUN levels; ratio as high as 41:1
3. Urine chemistry examinations to distinguish various forms of acute renal failure; decreased sodium
4. Renal ultrasonography—for estimate of renal size and to exclude a treatable obstructive uropathy

Management
Preventive Measures
1. Identify patients with preexisting renal disease.
2. Initiate adequate hydration before, during, and after any procedure requiring NPO status.
3. Avoid exposure to nephrotoxins. Be aware that the majority of drugs or their metabolites are excreted by the kidneys.
4. Avoid chronic analgesic abuse—causes interstitial nephritis and papillary necrosis.
5. Prevent and treat shock with blood and fluid replacement. Prevent prolonged periods of hypotension.
6. Monitor urinary output and central venous pressure hourly in critically ill patients to detect onset of renal failure at the earliest moment.
7. Schedule diagnostic studies requiring dehydration so there are "rest days," especially in aged who may not have adequate renal reserve.
8. Pay special attention to draining wounds, burns, and so forth, which can lead to dehydration and sepsis and progressive renal damage.
9. Avoid infection; give meticulous care to patients with indwelling catheters and IV lines.
10. Take every precaution to ensure that the right person receives the right blood—to avoid severe transfusion reactions, which can precipitate renal complications.

Corrective and Supportive Measures
1. Correct any reversible cause of acute renal failure (eg, improve renal perfusion, maximize cardiac output, surgical relief of obstruction).
2. Be alert for and correct underlying fluid excesses or deficits.
3. Correct and control biochemical imbalances—treatment of hyperkalemia.
4. Restore/maintain blood pressure.
5. Maintain nutrition.
6. Initiate hemodialysis, peritoneal dialysis, or continuous renal replacement therapy for patients with progressive renal failure and other life-threatening complications.

Complications

1. Infection
2. Arrhythmias due to hyperkalemia
3. Electrolyte (sodium, potassium, calcium, phosphorus) abnormalities
4. GI bleeding due to stress ulcers
5. Multiple organ systems failure

Nursing Assessment

1. Determine if there is a history of cardiac disease, malignancy, sepsis, or intercurrent illness.
2. Determine if patient has been exposed to potentially nephrotoxic drugs (antibiotics, nonsteroidal anti-inflammatory drugs [NSAIDs], contrast agents, solvents).
3. Conduct an ongoing physical examination for tissue turgor, pallor, alteration in mucous membranes, blood pressure, heart rate changes, pulmonary edema, and peripheral edema.
4. Monitor intake and output.

Nursing Diagnoses

- Fluid Volume Excess related to decreased glomerular filtration rate and sodium retention
- Risk for Infection related to alterations in the immune system and host defenses
- Altered Nutrition: Less Than Body Requirements related to catabolic state, anorexia, and malnutrition associated with acute renal failure
- Risk for Injury related to GI bleeding
- Altered Thought Processes related to the effects of uremic toxins on the central nervous system (CNS)

Nursing Interventions
Achieving Fluid and Electrolyte Balance

1. Monitor for signs and symptoms of hypovolemia or hypervolemia (Table 21-2) because regulating capacity of kidneys is inadequate.
2. Monitor urinary output and urine specific gravity; measure and record intake and output including urine, gastric suction, stools, wound drainage, perspiration (estimate).
3. Monitor serum and urine electrolyte concentrations.
4. Weigh the patient daily to provide an index of fluid balance; expected weight loss is 0.25 to 0.5 kg (½ to 1 lb daily).
5. Adjust fluid intake to avoid volume overload and dehydration.
   a. Fluid restriction is not usually initiated until renal function is quite low.
   b. Give only enough fluids to replace losses during oliguric-anuric phase (usually 400 to 500 mL/24 h plus measured fluid losses).
   c. Fluid allowance should be distributed throughout the day.
   d. Avoid restricting fluids for prolonged periods for laboratory and radiologic examinations because dehydrating procedures are hazardous to patients who cannot produce concentrated urine.
   e. Restrict salt and water intake if there is evidence of extracellular excess (see Table 21-2).
6. Measure blood pressure regularly with patients in supine, sitting, and standing positions.
7. Auscultate lung fields for rales.
8. Inspect neck veins for engorgement and extremities, abdomen, sacrum, and eyelids for edema.
9. Evaluate for signs and symptoms of hyperkalemia (see Table 21-2), and monitor serum potassium levels.
   a. Notify health care provider of value above 5.5 mg/L.
   b. Watch for ECG changes—tall, tented T waves; depressed S–T segment; wide QRS complex.
10. Administer sodium bicarbonate or glucose and insulin to shift potassium into the cells.
11. Administer cation exchange resin (sodium polystyrene sulfonate [Kayexalate]) to provide more prolonged correction of elevated potassium.

TABLE 21-2 Signs and Symptoms of Fluid and Electrolyte Imbalances

	Deficit	Excess
Volume	Acute weight loss (>5%), drop in body temperature, dry skin and mucous membranes, postural hypotension, longitudinal wrinkles or furrows of tongue, oliguria or anuria	Acute weight gain (>5%), edema, hypertension, distended neck veins, dyspnea, rales
Sodium	Abdominal cramps, apprehension, convulsions, fingerprinting on sternum, oliguria or anuria	Dry sticky mucous membranes, flushed skin, oliguria or anuria, thirst, rough and dry tongue
Potassium	Anorexia, abdominal distention, intestinal ileus, muscle weakness, tenderness, and cramps	Diarrhea, intestinal colic, irritability, nausea, parasthesias; flaccid paralysis, cardiac arrhythmias and arrest
Calcium	Abdominal cramps, positive Chovstek's and Trousseau's signs, tingling of extremities, tetany	Anorexia, nausea, vomiting, abdominal pain and distention, mental confusion
Bicarbonate	Deep, rapid breathing (Kussmaul), shortness of breath on exertion, stupor, weakness (metabolic acidosis)	Depressed respirations, muscle hypertonicity, tetany (metabolic alkalosis)
Magnesium	Positive Chovstek's sign, seizures, disorientation, hyperactive deep tendon reflexes, tremor	Hypotension, flushing, lethargy, dysarthria, hypoactive deep tendon reflexes, respiratory depression

12. Watch for cardiac arrhythmia and congestive heart failure from hyperkalemia, electrolyte imbalance, or fluid overload. Have resuscitation equipment on hand in case of cardiac arrest.
13. Instruct patient about the importance of following prescribed diet, avoiding foods high in potassium.
14. Prepare for dialysis when rapid lowering of potassium is needed.
15. Administer blood transfusions *during* dialysis to prevent hyperkalemia from stored blood.
16. Monitor acid–base balance.
    a. Monitor arterial blood gases as necessary.
    b. Prepare for ventilator therapy if severe acidosis is present and/or respiratory problems develop.
    c. Administer sodium bicarbonate for symptomatic acidosis (bicarbonate deficit; see Table 21-2).
    d. Be prepared to implement dialysis for uncontrolled acidosis.

Preventing Infection
1. Monitor for all signs of infection. Be aware that renal failure patients do not always demonstrate fever and leukocytosis.
2. Remove bladder catheter as soon as possible; monitor for urinary tract infection.
3. Use intensive pulmonary hygiene—high incidence of lung edema and infection.
4. Carry out meticulous wound care.
5. If antibiotics are administered, care must be taken to adjust the dosage for renal impairment.

Maintaining Adequate Nutrition
1. Work collaboratively with dietitian to regulate protein intake according to impaired renal function because metabolites that accumulate in blood derive almost entirely from protein catabolism.
    a. Protein should be of high biologic value, rich in essential amino acids (dairy products, eggs, meat), so the patient does not rely on tissue catabolism for essential amino acids.
    b. Low-protein diet may be supplemented with essential amino acids and vitamins.
    c. As renal function declines, protein intake may be restricted proportionately.
    d. Protein will be increased if the patient is on dialysis to allow for the loss of amino acids occurring during dialysis.
2. Offer high-carbohydrate feedings because carbohydrates have a greater protein-sparing power and provide additional calories.
3. Weigh daily.
4. Monitor BUN, creatinine, electrolytes, serum albumin, prealbumin, total protein, and transferrin.
5. Be aware that food and fluids containing large amounts of sodium, potassium, and phosphorus may need to be restricted.
6. Prepare for hyperalimentation when adequate nutrition cannot be maintained through the GI tract.

Preventing Gastrointestinal Bleeding
1. Examine all stools and emesis for gross and occult blood.
2. Administer H_2-receptor antagonist such as cimetidine (Tagamet) or ranitidine (Zantac) or nonaluminum or magnesium antacids as prophylaxis for gastric stress ulcers. If H_2-receptor antagonist is used, care must be taken to adjust the dose for the degree of renal impairment.
3. Prepare for endoscopy when GI bleeding occurs.

Preserving Neurologic Function
1. Speak to the patient in simple orienting statements, using repetition when necessary.
2. Maintain predictable routine, and keep change to a minimum.
3. Watch for and report mental status changes—somnolence, lassitude, lethargy, and fatigue progressing to irritability, disorientation, twitching, seizures.
4. Correct cognitive distortions.
5. Use seizure precautions—padded side rails, airway and suction equipment at bedside.
6. Encourage and assist patient to turn and move because drowsiness and lethargy may prevent activity.
7. Use music tapes to promote relaxation.
8. Prepare for dialysis, which may help prevent neurologic complications.

Patient Education and Health Maintenance
1. Explain that the patient may experience residual defects in kidney function for long period of time after acute illness.
2. Encourage reporting for routine urinalysis and follow-up examinations.
3. Advise avoidance of any medications unless specifically prescribed.
4. Recommend resuming activity gradually because muscle weakness will be present from excessive catabolism.

Outcome-Based Evaluation
- Blood pressure stable, no edema or shortness of breath
- No signs of infection
- Food intake adequate, maintaining weight
- Stools heme negative
- Appears more alert, sleeps less during the day

■ Chronic Renal Failure (CRF, End-Stage Renal Disease, ESRD)

Chronic renal failure is a progressive deterioration of renal function, which ends fatally in uremia (an excess of urea and other nitrogenous wastes in the blood) and its complications unless dialysis or a kidney transplantation is performed.

Pathophysiology and Etiology
Causes
1. Hypertension, prolonged and severe
2. Diabetes mellitus
3. Glomerulopathies

4. Interstitial nephritis
5. Hereditary renal disease, polycystic disease
6. Obstructive uropathy
7. Developmental/congenital disorder

Consequences of Decreasing Renal Function

1. Rate of progression varies based on underlying cause and severity of that condition.
2. Stages: decreased renal reserve → renal insufficiency → renal failure → ESRD.
3. Retention of sodium and water causes edema, congestive heart failure, hypertension, ascites.
4. Decreased glomerular filtration rate (GFR) causes stimulation of renin–angiotensin axis and increased aldosterone secretion, which raises blood pressure.
5. Metabolic acidosis results from kidney's inability to excrete hydrogen ions, produce ammonia, and conserve bicarbonate.
6. Decreased GFR causes increase in serum phosphate, with reciprocal decrease in serum calcium and subsequent bone resorption of calcium.
7. Erythropoietin production by the kidney decreases, causing profound anemia.
8. Uremia affects the CNS, causing altered mental function, personality changes, seizures, and coma.

Clinical Manifestations

1. Gastrointestinal—anorexia, nausea, vomiting, hiccups, ulceration of GI tract, and hemorrhage
2. Cardiovascular—hyperkalemic ECG changes, hypertension, pericarditis, pericardial effusion, pericardial tamponade
3. Respiratory—pulmonary edema, pleural effusions, pleural rub
4. Neuromuscular—fatigue, sleep disorders, headache, lethargy, muscular irritability, peripheral neuropathy, seizures, coma
5. Metabolic and endocrine—glucose intolerance, hyperlipidemia, sex hormone disturbances causing decreased libido, impotence, amenorrhea
6. Fluid, electrolyte, acid–base disturbances—usually salt and water retention but may be sodium loss with dehydration, acidosis, hyperkalemia, hypermagnesemia, hypocalcemia (see Table 21-2)
7. Dermatologic—pallor, hyperpigmentation, pruritus, ecchymoses, uremic frost
8. Skeletal abnormalities—renal osteodystrophy resulting in osteomalacia
9. Hematologic—anemia, defect in quality of platelets, increased bleeding tendencies
10. Psychosocial functions—personality and behavior changes, alteration in cognitive processes

Diagnostic Evaluation

1. Complete blood count (CBC)—anemia (a characteristic sign)
2. Elevated serum creatinine, BUN, phosphorus
3. Decreased serum calcium, bicarbonate, and proteins, especially albumin
4. Arterial blood gases—low blood pH, low CO_2, low bicarbonate (HCO_3)
5. 24-hour urine for creatinine, protein, creatinine clearance

Management

Goal: conservation of renal function as long as possible.

1. Detection and treatment of reversible causes of renal failure (eg, bring diabetes under control; treat hypertension)
2. Dietary regulation—low-protein diet supplemented with essential amino acids or their keto analogues to minimize uremic toxicity and to prevent wasting and malnutrition
3. Treatment of associated conditions to improve renal dynamics
   a. Anemia—recombinant human erythropoietin (Epogen), a synthetic hormone
   b. Acidosis—replacement of bicarbonate stores by infusion or oral administration of sodium bicarbonate
   c. Hyperkalemia—restriction of dietary potassium; administration of cation exchange resin
   d. Phosphate retention—decrease dietary phosphorus (chicken, milk, legumes, carbonated beverages); administer phosphate-binding agents because they bind phosphorus in the intestinal tract
4. Maintenance dialysis or kidney transplantation when symptoms can no longer be controlled with conservative management

Complications

Death

Nursing Assessment

1. Obtain history of chronic disorders and underlying health status.
2. Assess degree of renal impairment and involvement of other body systems by obtaining a review of systems and reviewing laboratory results.
3. Perform thorough physical examination including vital signs, cardiovascular, pulmonary, GI, neurologic, dermatologic, and musculoskeletal systems.
4. Assess psychosocial response to disease process including availability of resources and support network.

Nursing Diagnoses

- Fluid Volume Excess related to disease process
- Altered Nutrition: Less Than Body Requirements related to anorexia, nausea, vomiting, and restricted diet
- Impaired Skin Integrity related to uremic frost and changes in oil and sweat glands
- Constipation related to fluid restriction and ingestion of phosphate-binding agents
- Risk for Injury While Ambulating related to potential fractures and muscle cramps due to calcium deficiency
- Noncompliance With the Therapeutic Regimen related to restrictions imposed by CRF and its treatment

Nursing Interventions
Maintaining Fluid and Electrolyte Balance
See interventions related to acute renal failure, page 711.
Maintaining Adequate Nutritional Status
See interventions related to acute renal failure, page 712.
Maintaining Skin Integrity
1. Keep skin clean while relieving itching and dryness.
   a. "Basis" soap
   b. Sodium bicarbonate added to bath water
   c. Oatmeal baths
   d. Bath oil added to bath water
2. Apply ointments or creams for comfort and to relieve itching.
3. Keep nails short and trimmed to prevent excoriation.
4. Keep hair clean and moisturized.
5. Administer drugs for relief of itching if indicated.
Preventing Constipation
1. Be aware that phosphate binders cause constipation that cannot be managed with usual interventions.
2. Encourage high-fiber diet, bearing in mind the potassium content of some fruits and vegetables.
   a. Commercial fiber supplements (Fiberall, Fiber-Med) may be prescribed.
   b. Use stool softeners as prescribed.
   c. Avoid laxatives and cathartics that cause electrolyte toxicities (compounds containing magnesium or phosphorus).
   d. Increase activity as tolerated.
Ensuring a Safe Level of Activity
1. Monitor serum calcium and phosphate levels; watch for signs of hypocalcemia or hypercalcemia (see Table 21-2).
2. Inspect patient's gait, range of motion, and muscle strength.
3. Administer analgesics as ordered, and provide massage for severe muscle cramps.
4. Monitor x-rays and bone scan results for fractures, bone demineralization, and joint deposits.
5. Increase activity as tolerated—avoid immobilization because it increases bone demineralization.
6. Administer medications as ordered:
   a. Phosphate-binding medications such as sevelamer (Renagel) or calcium carbonate (Oscal) with meals and snacks to lower serum phosphorus
   b. Calcium supplements between meals to increase serum calcium
   c. Vitamin D to increase absorption and utilization of calcium
Increasing Understanding of and Compliance With Treatment Regimen
1. Prepare patient for dialysis or kidney transplantation.
2. Offer hope tempered by reality.
3. Assess patient's understanding of treatment regimen as well as concerns and fears.
4. Explore alternatives that may reduce or eliminate side effects of treatment.
   a. Adjust schedule so rest can be achieved after dialysis.
   b. Offer smaller, more frequent meals to reduce nausea and facilitate taking medication.
5. Encourage strengthening of social support system and coping mechanisms to lessen the impact of the stress of chronic kidney disease.
6. Provide social work referral.
7. Contract with patient for behavioral changes if noncompliant with therapy or control of underlying condition.
8. Discuss option of supportive psychotherapy for depression.
9. Promote decision making by the patient.
10. Refer patients and family members to renal support agencies (see p. 699).

Patient Education and Health Maintenance
To promote adherence to the therapeutic program, teach the following:
1. Weigh self every morning to avoid fluid overload.
2. Drink limited amounts only when thirsty.
3. Measure allotted fluids, and save some for ice cubes; sucking on ice is thirst quenching.
4. Eat food before drinking fluids to alleviate dry mouth.
5. Use hard candy, chewing gum to moisten mouth.

Outcome-Based Evaluation
- Blood pressure stable, no excessive weight gain
- Tolerating small feedings of low-protein, high-carbohydrate diet
- No skin excoriation; reports some relief of itching
- Passing small, firm stool daily
- Ambulating without falls
- Asking questions and reading education materials about dialysis

■ Lower Urinary Tract Infections
A *urinary tract infection* (UTI) is caused by the presence of pathogenic microorganisms in the urinary tract with or without signs and symptoms. Lower urinary tract infections may predominate at the bladder (*cystitis*) or urethra (*urethritis*).

Bacteriuria refers to the presence of bacteria in the urine (10^5 bacteria/mL of urine or greater generally indicates infection).

In *asymptomatic bacteriuria*, organisms are found in urine, but the patient has no symptoms.

Recurrent urinary tract infections may indicate the following:
  Relapse—recurrent infection with an organism that has been isolated during a prior infection
  Reinfection—recurrent infection with an organism distinct from previous infecting organism

Pathophysiology and Etiology
1. Ascending infection after entry by way of the urinary meatus
   a. Women are more susceptible to developing acute cystitis because of shorter length of urethra, anatom-

ical proximity to vagina, periurethral glands, and rectum (fecal contamination), and the mechanical effect of coitus.

b. Women with recurrent urinary tract infections often have gram-negative organisms at the vaginal introitus; there may be some defect of the mucosa of the urethra, vagina, or external genitalia of these patients that allows enteric organisms to invade the bladder.

c. Poor voiding habits may result in incomplete bladder emptying, increasing the risk of recurrent infection.

d. Acute infection in women most often arises from organisms of the patient's own intestinal flora (*Escherichia coli*).

2. In men, obstructive abnormalities (strictures, prostatic hyperplasia) are the most frequent cause.

3. Upper urinary tract disease may occasionally cause recurrent bladder infection.

Clinical Manifestations

1. Dysuria, frequency, urgency, nocturia
2. Suprapubic pain and discomfort
3. Microscopic or gross hematuria

GERONTOLOGIC ALERT

 The only sign of UTI in the elderly may be mental status changes.

Diagnostic Evaluation

1. Urine dipstick may react positively for blood, white blood cells, and nitrates indicating infection.
2. Urine microscopy shows red blood cells and many white blood cells per field without epithelial cells.

NURSING ALERT

Urinalysis showing many epithelial cells is likely contaminated by vaginal secretions in women and is therefore inaccurate in indicating infection. Urine culture may be reported as contaminated, as well. Obtaining a clean-catch, midstream specimen is essential for accurate results, and catheterization may be necessary in some patients.

---

3. Urine culture is used to detect presence of bacteria and for antimicrobial sensitivity testing.

4. Patients with indwelling catheters may have asymptomatic bacterial colonization of the urine without urinary tract infection. In these patients, urinary tract infection is diagnosed and treated in the context of symptoms.

Management

1. Antibiotic therapy according to sensitivity results
   a. A wide variety of antimicrobial drugs are available.
   b. Urinary infections usually respond to drugs that are excreted in urine in high concentrations; a potentially effective drug should rapidly sterilize the urine and thus relieve the patient's symptoms.

2. For uncomplicated infection
   a. Women with uncomplicated cystitis are usually treated with a 2- to 3-day course of antibiotics (trimethoprim–sulfamethoxazole [Bactrim], ciprofloxacin [Cipro], or nitrofurantoin [Macrodantin]). Seven to 10 days of therapy are recommended for women over age 65.
   b. Men are treated with 7 to 10 days of antibiotic therapy.
   c. Follow-up culture to prove treatment effectiveness.
   d. Side effects are nausea, diarrhea, drug-related rash, and vaginal candidiasis.

3. Pregnant women are usually treated for 7 to 10 days.

4. Women with recurrent infections may be treated longer, undergo diagnostic testing to rule out a structural abnormality, or be maintained on a daily dose of antibiotic as prophylaxis.

5. For complicated infection, see treatment of pyelonephritis (p. 718).

6. For severe discomfort with voiding, phenazopyridine (Pyridium) may be ordered three times a day for 2 days.

Complications

1. Pyelonephritis
2. Hematogenous spread resulting in sepsis

Nursing Assessment

1. Determine if patient has a history of urinary tract infections in childhood, during pregnancy, or has had recurrent infections.

2. Question about voiding habits, personal hygiene practices, and methods of contraception (use of diaphragm or spermicides is associated with development of cystitis).

3. Ask if patient has any associated symptoms of vaginal discharge, itching, or irritation—dysuria may be prominent symptom of vaginitis or infection from sexually transmitted pathogens, rather than urinary tract infection.

4. Examine for suprapubic tenderness, as well as abdominal tenderness, guarding, rebound, or masses that may indicate more serious process.

Nursing Diagnoses

- Pain related to inflammation of the bladder mucosa
- Knowledge Deficit related to prevention of recurrent urinary tract infection

Nursing Interventions
Relieving Pain

1. Administer or teach self-administration of antibiotic—eradication of infection is usually accompanied by rapid resolution of symptoms.

2. Encourage patient to take prescribed analgesics and antispasmodics if ordered.

3. Encourage rest during the acute phase if symptoms are severe.

4. Encourage plenty of fluids to promote urinary output and to flush out bacteria from urinary tract.

Increasing Understanding and Practice of Preventive Measures

1. For women with recurrent urinary tract infections, give the following instructions:
   a. Reduce vaginal introital concentration of pathogens by hygienic measures.
   b. Wash genitalia in shower or while standing in bathtub—bacteria in bath water may gain entrance into urethra.
   c. Cleanse around the perineum and urethral meatus after each bowel movement, with front-to-back cleansing to minimize fecal contamination of periurethral area.
2. Drink liberal amounts of water to lower bacterial concentrations in the urine.
3. Avoid bladder irritants—coffee, tea, alcohol, cola drinks, and aspartame.
4. Decrease the entry of microorganisms into the bladder during intercourse.
   a. Void immediately after sexual intercourse.
   b. A single dose of an oral antimicrobial agent may be prescribed after sexual intercourse.
5. Avoid external irritants such as bubble baths, talcum powders, perfumed vaginal cleansers or deodorants.
6. Patients with persistent bacteria may require long-term antimicrobial therapy to prevent colonization of periurethral area and recurrence of urinary tract infection.
   a. Take antibiotic at bedtime after emptying bladder to ensure adequate concentration of drug during overnight period because low rates of urine flow and infrequent bladder emptying predispose to multiplication of bacteria.
   b. Use self-monitoring tests (dipsticks) at home to monitor for urinary tract infection.

Patient Education and Health Maintenance

1. Advise women with simple, uncomplicated cystitis that they do not require follow-up as long as symptoms are completely resolved with antibiotic therapy. Men usually need follow-up cultures and possibly additional testing if more than one episode of infection.
2. Instruct patient to void frequently (every 2 to 3 hours) and to empty bladder completely because this enhances bacterial clearance, reduces urine stasis, and prevents reinfection. Infrequent voiding distends the bladder wall, leading to hypoxia of bladder mucosa, which is then more susceptible to bacterial invasion.
3. Instruct patients who have had urinary tract infections during pregnancy to have follow-up studies.
4. Female patients with uncomplicated but recurrent cystitis may self-administer a 2- or 3-day course of antibiotics when symptoms begin if so prescribed.
5. Recommend self-administration of acidophilus during course of antibiotic therapy to prevent vaginal candidiasis.
6. Cranberry (juice or capsules) may help to prevent cystitis by altering the chemical composition of the urine.

Acidophilus and cranberry capsules are available in health food and vitamin stores.

Outcome-Based Evaluation

- Verbalizes relief of symptoms
- Verbalizes self-care measures to prevent recurrence

◼ Interstitial Cystitis

Interstitial cystitis is a syndrome of chronic, cystitis-like symptoms in the absence of bacterial infection.

Pathophysiology and Etiology

1. The etiology of interstitial cystitis in unknown. Theories include an inflammatory or autoimmune process that alters the normal configuration of cells in the bladder epithelium.
2. The bladder wall is chronically inflamed with no evidence of bacterial infection.
3. Occurs far more frequently in women than in men (9:1).

Clinical Manifestations

1. Extreme urinary urgency.
2. Frequency (as many as 16 times per day) and dysuria.
3. Nocturia (one to two times per night) that increases with duration of symptoms.
4. Continuous bladder pain, may increase during voiding, may be diffuse perineal, vaginal, or suprapubic pain.
5. Symptoms are exacerbated by sexual intercourse and at the time of menstruation.
6. The duration of symptoms is often longer than 9 to 12 months when finally diagnosed.

Diagnostic Evaluation

1. Tender bladder base during pelvic examination, assessed by palpation of the anterior vaginal wall.
2. Cystoscopy under anesthesia with bladder biopsies and bladder distention; presence of bleeding or ulcerations on bladder distention is characteristic of some cases of interstitial cystitis.
3. Urodynamic tests often reveal a small bladder capacity with early sensation of urgency and, in some cases, poor detrusor function with incomplete bladder emptying.
4. Diagnosis is often made by ruling out other potential causes of symptoms, including radiation or chemical cystitis, gynecologic or urologic malignancies, STD, urolithiasis, and so forth.

Management

1. Bladder distention during cystoscopy under general anesthesia relieves symptoms in 30% of patients, although after a 2- to 3-day period of exacerbated symptoms often requiring narcotic analgesia.
2. Oral administration of pentosan polysulfate (Elmiron) relieves symptoms in 40% of patients after 6 to 12 weeks of therapy; many continue this therapy for years.

DRUG ALERT

Pentosan polysulfate (Elmiron) has anticoagulant properties; should not be used by patients taking other anticoagulant drugs or in conditions associated with increased risk of bleeding.

3. Intravesical therapy with various substances including silver nitrate and dimethyl sulfoxide (DMSO) may be mixed with heparin, sodium bicarbonate, or prostaglandins.
4. Oral administration of tricyclic antidepressants (for their analgesic and anticholinergic effects).
5. Surgical intervention in extreme cases; bladder augmentation or cystectomy with urinary diversion.

Complications
1. Psychosocial problems related to pain, urgency, and frequency
2. Secondary bacteriuria

Nursing Assessment
1. Assess voiding patterns including frequency, nocturia, urgency (a voiding diary is helpful). Determine if symptoms increase in relation to menstrual cycle or sexual intercourse.
2. Assess level of pain using a scale of 1 to 10; determine if pain increases during or after voiding and if bladder spasms occur.
3. Perform abdominal and pelvic examination, if indicated, to rule out gynecologic causes and to identify location of pain on palpation.
4. Assess significance of lifestyle alterations.

Nursing Diagnoses
- Chronic Pain related to disease process
- Altered Urinary Elimination related to frequency, urgency, dysuria, and nocturia
- Ineffective Individual Coping related to interruption of lifestyle and chronic, unrelenting symptoms

Nursing Interventions
Controlling Pain
1. Administer pharmacologic agents as ordered to relieve pain; may be given orally or intravesically.
2. Instruct patient in comfort and preventive measures, application of heating pad, avoidance of bladder irritants (caffeine, alcohol, artificial sweeteners), transvaginal pelvic floor stimulation therapy.
3. If prescribed, teach patient self-catheterization and the self-administration of intravesical medications.

Improving Urinary Elimination
1. Encourage patient to use a voiding diary as well as a dietary record to make associations between intake of certain foods or fluids and increase in symptoms.

2. Advise patient to restrict fluids only when necessary due to impending limited access to toilet facilities; normal fluid intake should be encouraged otherwise.
3. Assess patient's response to pharmacologic therapy.

Strengthening Coping
Refer for additional information to agencies such as Interstitial Cystitis Association (ICA), 51 Monroe Street, Suite 1402, Rockville, MD 20850, *www.ichelp.org*.

Patient Education and Health Maintenance
1. Teach patient mechanism of action and side effects of pharmacologic therapies.
2. Teach self-catheterization using clean technique if needed to self-administer medications or accomplish complete bladder emptying.
3. Provide information about food and fluids known to be bladder irritants.
4. Teach patient nonpharmacologic methods to relieve pain.
5. Explore with patient positive coping strategies for self and family in dealing with chronic illness.

Outcome-Based Evaluation
- Verbalizes some relief of pain
- Verbalizes less urgency, frequency, and nocturia
- Seeks additional information and support

Acute Bacterial Pyelonephritis
Bacterial pyelonephritis is an acute infection and inflammatory disease of the kidney and renal pelvis involving one or both kidneys.

Pathophysiology and Etiology
1. Pyelonephritis can result from any of the following sources of bacterial invasion or urinary obstruction:
   a. Enteric bacteria (*E. coli* most common organism)
   b. Secondary to vesicoureteral reflux (incompetence of ureterovesical valve, which allows urine to regurgitate into ureters, usually at time of voiding)
   c. Urinary obstruction/infection
   d. Trauma
   e. Bloodborne infection
   f. Renal disease
   g. Pregnancy
   h. Metabolic disorders
2. Low-grade inflammation with interstitial infiltrations of inflammatory cells may lead to tubular destruction and abscess formation.
3. Chronic pyelonephritis may result in scarred, atrophic, and nonfunctioning kidney(s).

Clinical Manifestations
1. Fever, chills
2. Costovertebral angle tenderness, flank pain (with or without radiation to groin)
3. Nausea, vomiting

Diagnostic Evaluation

1. Urinalysis (dipstick or microscopic) to identify leukocytes, bacteria, or pus in urine; gross or microscopic hematuria
2. Urine culture to identify antibody-coated bacteria in urine; bacteria invading kidney induce an antibody response that coats the bacteria—differentiates renal infection from bladder infection.
3. IVP to evaluate for urinary tract obstruction; other radiologic/urinary tests as necessary.

Management

1. Monitoring and supportive therapy for complications: bacteremia and gram-negative sepsis; papillary necrosis leading to renal failure; renal abscess/perinephric abscess
2. Organism-specific antimicrobial therapy
   a. Usually immediate treatment is started to cover the prevalent gram-negative pathogens; subsequently adjusted according to culture results.
   b. Acute pyelonephritis usually caused by *E. coli* is sensitive to many antimicrobial drugs. A 14-day course of antibiotic therapy is required for acute uncomplicated pyelonephritis. Repeat urine cultures should be performed 5 to 7 days after the start of therapy and 4 to 6 weeks after completion.
3. Parenteral antimicrobial therapy may be necessary if patient cannot tolerate oral intake and is dehydrated; usually admitted to hospital if patient is acutely ill.
4. Complicated pyelonephritis requires at least 21 days of antibiotic therapy. Complicated pyelonephritis occurs when structural or functional abnormalities are present in the upper urinary tract (vesicouretral reflux, ureteral obstruction, and abscesses). There is a 10% to 30% relapse rate after 14 days of therapy; an additional 14-day course is prescribed. In some cases, 6 weeks of antibiotics are necessary with adjustment of antibiotic regimen based on urine culture and sensitivities every 5 to 7 days.

Complications

1. Renal abscess requiring treatment by percutaneous drainage or prolonged antibiotic therapy
2. Perinephric abscess

Nursing Assessment

1. Assess patient for fever, chills, flank pain, nausea, and vomiting.
2. Obtain vital signs; monitor for impending sepsis.
3. Obtain urologic history that could suggest recurrent infections or urinary tract obstruction.

Nursing Diagnoses

- Hyperthermia due to infection
- Pain related to renal swelling and edema

Nursing Interventions

Reducing Body Temperature

1. Administer or teach self-administration of antibiotics as prescribed, and monitor for effectiveness and side effects.
2. Assess vital signs frequently, and monitor intake and output; administer antiemetic medications to control nausea and vomiting.
3. Administer antipyretic medications as prescribed and according to temperature.
4. Use measures to decrease body temperature if indicated; cooling blanket, application of ice to armpits and groins, and so forth.
5. Correct dehydration by replacing fluids, orally if possible, or IV.
6. Monitor urine culture results for resolving infection.

Relieving Pain

1. Administer or teach self-administration of analgesic medications, and monitor their effectiveness.
2. Use comfort measures such as positioning to locally relieve flank pain.
3. Assess patient's response to pain control measures.

Patient Education and Health Maintenance

1. Explain to patient possible causes of pyelonephritis and its signs and symptoms; review also signs and symptoms of lower urinary tract infection.
2. Review antibiotic therapy and importance of completing prescribed course of treatment and having follow-up urine cultures.
3. Explain preventive measures including good fluid intake, personal hygiene measures, and healthy voiding habits.

Outcome-Based Evaluation

- Afebrile
- Verbalizes reduced pain

Acute Glomerulonephritis

Acute glomerulonephritis refers to a group of kidney diseases in which there is an inflammatory reaction in the glomeruli. It is not an infection of the kidney, per se, but rather the result of the immune mechanisms of the body.

Pathophysiology and Etiology

1. Occurs after an infection elsewhere in the body or may develop secondary to systemic disorders.
2. An antigen–antibody reaction produces immune complexes that lodge in the glomeruli, producing thickening of glomerular basement membrane.
3. Eventual scarring and loss of filtering surface may lead to renal failure.

Clinical Manifestations

1. Mild disease is frequently discovered accidentally through a routine urinalysis.
2. History of infection: pharyngitis from group A streptococcus, hepatitis B virus, endocarditis
3. Proteinuria, hematuria, oliguria
4. Puffiness of face, edema of extremities
5. Fatigue and anorexia
6. Hypertension (mild, moderate, or severe), headache
7. Anemia from loss of red blood cells into the urine
8. The clinical course of acute glomerulonephritis proceeds as follows from onset of symptoms to recovery— over 90% of patients regain normal renal function within 60 days:
   a. Diuresis usually starts 1 to 2 weeks after onset of symptoms.
   b. Renal clearances and blood urea concentration return to normal.
   c. Edema decreases, and hypertension lessens.
   d. Microscopic proteinuria or hematuria may persist many months.

Diagnostic Evaluation

1. *Urinalysis*—hematuria (microscopic or gross), proteinuria, red cell casts, white blood cells, renal epithelial cells, and various casts in the sediment.
2. *Blood*—elevated BUN and creatinine levels, low albumin level, high lipid level, increased antistreptolysin titer (from reaction to streptococcal organism).
3. *Needle biopsy* of the kidney reveals obstruction of glomerular capillaries from proliferation of endothelial cells.

Management

1. Management is symptomatic and includes antihypertensives, diuretics, drugs for management of hyperkalemia (due to renal insufficiency), H_2 blockers (to prevent stress ulcers), and phosphate-binding agents (to reduce phosphate and elevate calcium).
2. Antibiotic therapy is initiated to eliminate infection (if still present).
3. Fluid intake is restricted.
4. Dietary protein is restricted moderately if there is oliguria and the BUN is elevated. It is restricted more drastically if acute renal failure develops.
5. Carbohydrates are increased liberally to provide energy and reduce catabolism of protein.
6. Potassium and sodium intake is restricted in presence of hyperkalemia, edema, or signs of congestive heart failure.
7. Therapy for rapidly progressive glomerulonephritis may include:
   a. Plasma exchange
   b. Immunosuppressants (corticosteroids; cyclophosphamide [Cytoxan])
   c. Dialysis—may be considered if fluid retention and uremia cannot be controlled

Complications

1. Hypertension, congestive heart failure, endocarditis
2. Fluid and electrolyte imbalances in the acute phase, hyperkalemia, hyperphosphatemia, hypervolemia
3. Malnutrition
4. Hypertensive encephalopathy, seizures
5. ESRD

Nursing Assessment

1. Obtain medical history; focus on recent infections or symptoms of chronic immunologic disorders (systemic lupus erythematosus, scleroderma).
2. Assess urine specimen for blood, protein, color, and amount.
3. Perform physical examination specifically looking for signs of edema, hypertension, and hypervolemia (engorged neck veins, elevated jugular venous pressure, adventitious lung sounds, cardiac arrhythmia).
4. Evaluate cardiac status and serum laboratory values for electrolyte imbalance.

Nursing Diagnoses

- Altered Renal Tissue Perfusion related to damage to glomerular function
- Fluid Volume Excess related to compromised renal function

Nursing Interventions

Promoting Renal Function

1. Monitor vital signs, intake and output, and maintain dietary restrictions during acute phase.
2. Encourage bed rest during the acute phase until the urine clears and BUN, creatinine, and blood pressure normalize. (Rest also facilitates diuresis.)
3. Administer medications as ordered, and evaluate patient's response to antihypertensives, diuretics, H_2 blockers, phosphate-binding agents, and antibiotics (if indicated).

Improving Fluid Balance

1. Carefully monitor fluid balance; replace fluids according to the patient's fluid losses (urine, respiration, feces) and daily body weight as prescribed.
2. Monitor pulmonary artery pressure and central venous pressure, if indicated.
3. Monitor for signs and symptoms of congestive heart failure: distended neck veins, tachycardia, gallop rhythm, enlarged and tender liver, crackles at bases of lungs.
4. Observe for hypertensive encephalopathy, any evidence of seizure activity.

NURSING ALERT

Hypertensive encephalopathy is a medical emergency, and treatment is aimed at reducing blood pressure without impairing renal function.

Patient Education and Health Maintenance

1. Explain that the patient must have follow-up evaluations of blood pressure, urinary protein, and BUN concentrations to determine if there is exacerbation of disease activity.
2. Encourage patient to treat any infection promptly.
3. Tell patient to report any signs of decreasing renal function and to obtain treatment immediately.

Outcome-Based Evaluation

- Urine output adequate; vital signs stable
- No edema, shortness of breath, or adventitious heart or lung sounds

Nephrotic Syndrome

Nephrotic syndrome is a clinical disorder characterized by marked increase of protein in the urine (proteinuria), decrease in albumin in the blood (hypoalbuminemia), edema, and excess lipids in the blood (hyperlipidemia). These occur as a consequence of excessive leakage of plasma proteins into the urine because of increased permeability of the glomerular capillary membrane.

Pathophysiology and Etiology

1. Seen in any condition that seriously damages the glomerular capillary membrane.
   a. Chronic glomerulonephritis
   b. Diabetes mellitus with intercapillary glomerulosclerosis
   c. Amyloidosis of kidney
   d. Systemic lupus erythematosus
   e. Renal vein thrombosis
   f. Secondary to malignancy (older adults)
2. Hypoalbuminemia results in decreased oncotic pressure, causing generalized edema as fluid moves out of the vascular space.
3. Decreased circulating volume then activates the renin—angiotensin system causing retention of sodium and further edema.
4. Mechanism for increased lipids is unknown.

Clinical Manifestations

1. Insidious onset of pitting edema; weight gain
2. Marked proteinuria—leading to depletion of body proteins
3. Hyperlipidemia—may lead to accelerated atherosclerosis

Diagnostic Evaluation

1. Urinalysis—marked proteinuria, microscopic hematuria, urinary casts, appears "foamy"
2. 24-hour urine for protein (increased) and creatinine clearance (decreased)
3. Needle biopsy of kidney—for histologic examination of renal tissue to confirm diagnosis
4. Serum chemistry—decreased total protein and albumin, normal or increased creatinine, increased triglycerides, and altered lipid profile

Management

1. Treatment of causative glomerular disease
2. Corticosteroids or immunosuppressant agents to decrease proteinuria
3. General management of edema
   a. Sodium and fluid restriction
   b. Diuretics if renal insufficiency is not severe
   c. Infusion of salt-poor albumin
   d. Dietary protein supplements

Complications

1. Hypovolemia
2. Thromboembolic complications—renal vein thrombosis, venous and arterial thrombosis in extremities, pulmonary embolism, coronary artery thrombosis, cerebral artery thrombosis
3. Altered drug metabolism due to decrease in plasma proteins
4. Progression to end-stage renal failure

Nursing Assessment

1. Obtain history of onset of symptoms including changes in characteristics of urine and onset of edema.
2. Perform physical examination looking for evidence of edema and hypovolemia.
3. Assess vital signs, daily weights, intake and output, and laboratory values.

Nursing Diagnoses

- Risk for Fluid Volume Deficit related to disease process
- Risk for Infection related to treatment with immunosuppressants

Nursing Interventions

Increasing Circulating Volume and Decreasing Edema

1. Monitor daily weight, intake and output, and urine specific gravity.
2. Monitor central venous pressure (if indicated), vital signs, orthostatic blood pressure, and heart rate to detect hypovolemia.
3. Monitor serum BUN and creatinine to assess renal function.
4. Administer diuretics or immunosuppressants as prescribed, and evaluate patient's response.
5. Infuse IV albumin as ordered.
6. Encourage bed rest for a few days to help mobilize edema; however, some ambulation is necessary to reduce risk of thromboembolic complications.
7. Enforce mild to moderate sodium and fluid restriction if edema is severe; provide a high-protein diet.

Preventing Infection

1. Monitor for signs and symptoms of infection.
2. Monitor temperature and laboratory values for neutropenia.
3. Use aseptic technique for all invasive procedures and strict handwashing by patient and all contacts; prevent

contact by patient with persons who may transmit infection.

Patient Education and Health Maintenance

1. Teach patient signs and symptoms of nephrotic syndrome; also review causes, purpose of prescribed treatments, and importance of long-term therapy to prevent ESRD.
2. Instruct patient in side effects of prescribed medications and methods of preventing infection if taking immunosuppressants.
3. Carefully review with patient and family dietary and fluid restrictions; consult dietitian for assistance in meal planning.
4. Discuss the importance of maintaining exercise, decreasing cholesterol and fat intake, and changing other risk factors such as smoking, obesity, and stress to reduce risk of severe thromboembolic complications.
5. In patients with severe disease, prepare for dialysis and possible transplantation.

Outcome-Based Evaluation

- Vital signs remain stable; edema decreased
- No signs of infection

Nephrolithiasis and Urolithiasis

Nephrolithiasis refers to renal stone disease; *urolithiasis* refers to the presence of stones in the urinary system. Stones, or calculi, are formed in the urinary tract from the kidney to bladder by the crystallization of substances excreted in the urine. The majority of stones (60%) are composed mainly of calcium oxalate crystals; the rest are composed of calcium phosphate salts, uric acid, struvite (magnesium, ammonium, and phosphate), or the amino acid cystine.

Pathophysiology and Etiology

1. Causes and predisposing factors:
   a. Hypercalcemia and hypercalciuria caused by hyperparathyroidism, renal tubular acidosis, multiple myeloma, and excessive intake of vitamin D, milk, and alkali
   b. Chronic dehydration, poor fluid intake, and immobility
   c. Diet high in purines and abnormal purine metabolism (hyperuricemia and gout)
   d. Genetic predisposition for urolithiasis or genetic disorders (cystinuria)
   e. Chronic infection with urea-splitting bacteria (*Proteus vulgaris*)
   f. Chronic obstruction with stasis of urine, foreign bodies within the urinary tract
   g. Excessive oxalate absorption in inflammatory bowel disease and bowel resection or ileostomy
   h. Living in mountainous, desert, or tropical areas
2. Stones may be found anywhere in the urinary system and vary in size from mere granular deposits (called sand or gravel) to bladder stones the size of an orange.

3. Three of four patients with stones are men; in both sexes, the peak age of onset is between 20 and 40 years.
4. Most stones migrate downward (causing severe colicky pain) and are discovered in the lower ureter. Spontaneous stone passage can be anticipated in 80% of patients with urolithiasis.
5. Some stones may lodge in the renal pelvis, ureters, or bladder neck causing obstruction, edema, secondary infection, and, in some cases, nephron damage.
6. People who have had two stones tend to have recurrences.

Clinical Manifestations

1. Pain pattern depends on site of obstruction (Figure 21-4).
   a. Renal stones produce an increase in hydrostatic pressure and distention of the renal pelvis and proximal ureter causing renal colic. Pain relief is immediate after stone passage.
   b. Large ureteral stones produce symptoms or obstruction as they pass down the ureter (ureteral colic).
   c. Bladder stones produce symptoms similar to cystitis.
2. Obstruction—stones blocking the flow of urine will produce symptoms of urinary tract infection; chills and fever.
3. GI symptoms include nausea, vomiting, diarrhea, abdominal discomfort—due to renointestinal reflexes and shared nerve supply (celiac ganglion) between both the ureters and intestine.

Diagnostic Evaluation

1. IVP—to determine site and evaluate degree of obstruction. Other uroradiologic studies are necessary when stones are radiolucent; retrograde or antegrade pyelography.
2. Spiral CT—special CT technique to assess for stone in ureter.
   a. Requires no preparation and is noninvasive.
   b. Only takes 10 minutes. Can replace IVP.
3. Analysis of available stone material—crystals can be identified by polarization microscopy, x-ray diffraction, and infrared spectroscopy.
4. Urinalysis—hematuria and pyuria; urine culture and drug sensitivity studies.

Management

Extracorporeal Shock Wave Lithotripsy (ESWL)

Noninvasive technique and treatment of choice for stones less than 2 cm (¾ inch) in diameter (80% of stones fall into this category).

1. High-energy shock waves are directed at the kidney stone, disintegrating it into minute particles that pass in the urine. (A *shock wave* is a large, condensed wave of energy produced by high-speed motion.)
2. Patient is placed on specially designed table and immersed in a water bath or placed on an adjustable stretcher positioned over a cushion of water.
   a. In water bath model, shock waves travel through water surrounding the patient.

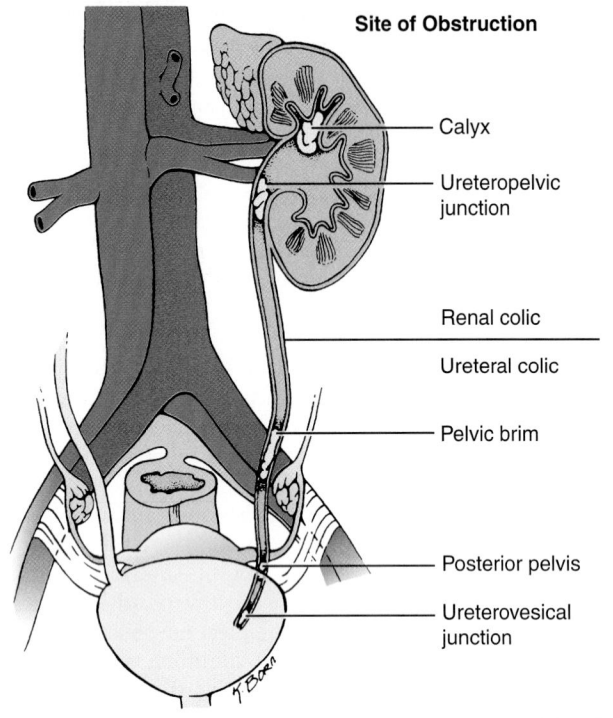

Site of Obstruction

- Calyx
- Ureteropelvic junction
- Renal colic
- Ureteral colic
- Pelvic brim
- Posterior pelvis
- Ureterovesical junction

Clinical manifestations

Flank or CVA pain, hematuria, abdominal distention

Pain at flank or costovertebral angle, migrating to groin and testicle/labia minora

Pain in lateral flank and suprapubic area

Urgency, frequency, genital pain

FIGURE 21-4 Areas where calculi may obstruct the urinary system. The ensuing clinical manifestations depend on the site of obstruction. Stones that have broken loose may obstruct the flow of urine, cause severe pain, and injure the kidney.

b. In cushion model, a layer of gel lies between the stretcher and water; shock waves move through the cushion and gel.

3. Position of the kidney stone is located by fluoroscopy, and the shock waves are targeted directly at the stone. The shock waves do not affect soft tissue.

4. Eliminates need for surgery in majority of patients and can be repeated for recurrent stones with no apparent risk to kidney structure or function.

5. Complications include pain, urinary infection, and temporary bleeding around kidney.

Percutaneous Nephrostolithotomy (PCNL)

For stones larger than 2.5 cm in diameter (Figure 21-5).

1. Under fluoroscopic/ultrasound guidance, a needle is advanced into collecting system; guidewire is advanced into renal pelvis or ureter.

2. Tract is dilated with mechanical dilators or high-pressure balloon dilator until nephroscope can be inserted up against stone.

3. Stones can be broken apart with hydraulic shock waves or a laser beam administered by way of nephroscope; fragments are removed using forceps, graspers, or basket.

4. May be combined with ESWL.

5. Complications include hemorrhage, infection, and extravasation of urine.

Percutaneous Stone Dissolution (Chemolysis)

A multiholed nephrostomy tube (catheter) is placed in kidney; offers a pathway for introduction of solvent (depending on chemical composition of stone) to be infused into stone. A second catheter may be used for drainage.

1. Used for struvite, uric acid, and cystine stones.

2. May be used to shrink large stones before other retrieval methods or to irrigate debris after lithotripsy procedures.

3. Irrigating solution introduced at a continuous rate that patient can tolerate without flank pain or elevation of intrarenal pressure above 25 cm H_2O (most IV infusion pumps can be adapted for use and set to alarm should pressure exceed this level).

4. The patient receives antimicrobial agents before, during, and after procedure to maintain sterile urine.

5. Complications include infection (renal and perirenal abscesses, pyelonephritis, septic shock) and thrombophlebitis and pulmonary embolism (associated with immobilization).

Ureteroscopy

1. Used for distal ureteral calculi; may be used for mid-ureteral calculi.

2. Flexible or rigid ureteroscopes are used in conjunction with baskets or graspers.

3. Electrohydraulic, ultrasonic, or laser equipment may also be used to fragment stone.

4. A stent may be inserted and left in place after surgery to maintain patency of ureter.

Open Surgical Procedures

Indicated for only 1% to 2% of all stones.

1. *Pyelolithotomy*—removal of stones from kidney pelvis

2. *Coagulum pyelolithotomy*—intraoperative injection of certain coagulation factors into the renal pelvis, producing a coagulum that entraps the stones and expedites their removal

3. *Nephrolithotomy*—incision into kidney for removal of stone

A

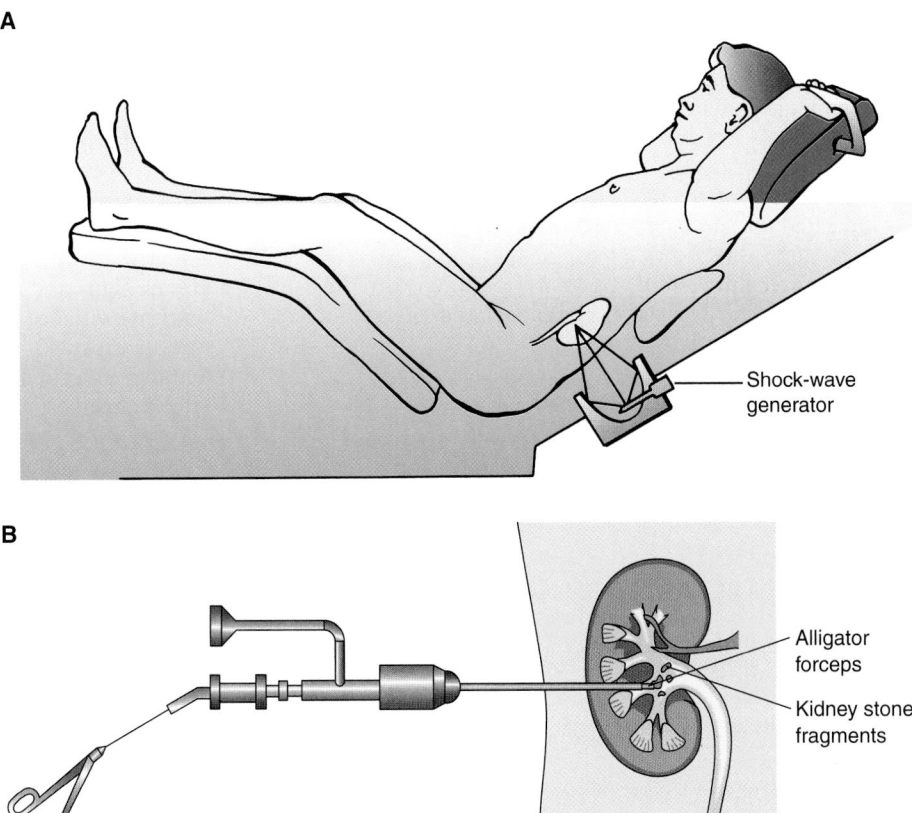

Shock-wave generator

B

FIGURE 21-5 **(A)** Extracorporeal shock wave lithotripsy (ESWL) for kidney stone dissolution. **(B)** A percutaneous nephrostomy tract permits access to the collecting system of the kidney for removal of kidney stones under direct vision via a nephroscope.

Alligator forceps

Kidney stone fragments

4. *Nephrectomy*—removal of kidney; indicated when kidney is extensively and irreparably damaged and is no longer a functioning organ; partial nephrectomy sometimes done
5. *Ureterolithotomy*—removal of stone in ureter
6. *Cystolithotomy*—removal of stone from bladder

Complications
1. Obstruction—from remaining stone fragments
2. Infection—from dissemination of infected stone particles or bacteria resulting from obstruction
3. Impaired renal function—from prolonged obstruction before treatment and removal
4. Perirenal hematoma—from bleeding around the kidney caused by trauma of shock waves or laser treatments

Nursing Assessment
1. Obtain history focusing on family history of stones, episodes of dehydration, prolonged immobility, urinary tract infection, dietary and medication history.
2. Assess pain location and radiation; assess level of pain using a scale of 1 to 10. Observe for presence of associ-

ated symptoms: nausea, vomiting, diarrhea, abdominal distention.
3. Monitor for signs and symptoms of urinary tract infection: chills, fever, dysuria, frequency. Examine urine for hematuria.
4. Observe for signs and symptoms of obstruction: frequent urination of small amounts, oliguria, anuria.

Nursing Diagnoses
- Pain related to inflammation, obstruction, and abrasion of urinary tract by migration of stones
- Altered Urinary Elimination related to blockage of urine flow by stones
- Risk for Infection related to obstruction of urine flow and instrumentation during treatment

Nursing Interventions
Controlling Pain
1. Give prescribed narcotic analgesic (usually IV or IM) until cause of pain can be removed.
   a. Monitor patient closely for increasing pain; may indicate inadequate analgesia.

b. Very large doses of narcotics are often required to relieve pain, so monitor for respiratory depression and drop in blood pressure.
2. Encourage patient to assume position that brings some relief.
3. Reassess pain frequently using pain scale.
4. Administer antiemetics (IM or rectal suppository) as indicated for nausea.

Maintaining Urine Flow

1. Administer fluids orally or IV (if vomiting) to reduce concentration of urinary crystalloids and ensure adequate urine output.

NURSING ALERT

 Avoid overhydration, which may result in increased distention at stone location, causing an increase in pain and associated symptoms.

---

2. Monitor total urine output and patterns of voiding. Report oliguria or anuria.
3. Strain all urine through strainer or gauze to harvest the stone; uric acid stones may crumble. Crush clots, and inspect sides of urinal/bedpan for clinging stones or fragments.
4. For outpatient treatment, the patient may use a coffee filter to strain urine.
5. Assist patient to walk, if possible, because ambulation may help move the stone through the urinary tract.

Controlling Infection

1. Administer parenteral or oral antibiotics as prescribed during treatment, and monitor for side effects.
2. Assess urine for color, cloudiness, and odor.
3. Obtain vital signs, and monitor for fever and symptoms of impending sepsis (tachycardia, hypotension).

Patient Education and Heath Maintenance
Recovery From Surgical Interventions for Stone Disease

1. Encourage fluids to accelerate passing of stone particles.
2. Teach about analgesics that still may be necessary for colicky pain, which may accompany passage of stone debris.
3. Warn that some blood may appear in urine for several weeks.
4. Encourage frequent walking to assist in passage of stone fragments.
5. Teach patient to strain urine through a coffee filter.

Prevention of Recurrent Stone Formation

1. *For patients with calcium oxalate stones*
   a. Instruct on diet—avoid excesses of calcium and phosphorus; maintain a low-sodium diet (sodium restriction decreases amount of calcium absorbed in intestine).
   b. Teach purpose of drug therapy—thiazide diuretics to reduce urine calcium excretion, allopurinol therapy to reduce uric acid concentration.

2. *For patients with uric acid stones*
   a. Teach methods to alkalinize urine to enhance urate solubility.
   b. Instruct on testing urine pH.
   c. Teach purpose of taking allopurinol—to lower uric acid concentration.
   d. Provide information about reduction of dietary purine intake (low protein—red meat, fish, fowl).

3. *For patients with infection (struvite) stone*
   a. Teach signs and symptoms of urinary infection (in patients with neurologic or spinal cord disease, teach use of dipsticks to evaluate urine for nitrites and leukocytes), encourage to report infection immediately; must be treated vigorously.
   b. Try to avoid prolonged periods of recumbency—slows renal drainage and alters calcium metabolism.

4. *For patients with cystine stones*—occur in *cystinuria*, a hereditary disorder of amino acid transport.
   a. Teach patient to alkalinize urine by taking sodium bicarbonate tablets (Soda Mint) to increase cystine solubility; instruct patient how to test urine pH with a pH indicator.
   b. Teach patient about drug therapy with D-penicillamine (Depen)—to lower cystine concentration, or dissolution by direct irrigation with thiol derivatives.
   c. Explain importance of maintaining drug therapy consistently.

5. For *all patients with stone disease*
   a. Explain need for consistently increased fluid intake (24-hour urinary output greater than 2 L)—lowers the concentration of substances involved in stone formation.
      (i) Drink enough fluids to achieve a urinary volume of 2,000 to 3,000 mL or more every 24 hours.
      (ii) Drink larger amounts during periods of strenuous exercise, if patient perspires freely.
      (iii) Take fluids in evening to guarantee a high urine flow during the night.
   b. Encourage a diet low in sugar and animal proteins—refined carbohydrates appear to lead to hypercalciuria and urolithiasis; animal proteins increase urine excretion of calcium, uric acid, and oxalate.
   c. Increase consumption of fiber—inhibits calcium and oxalate absorption.
   d. Save any stone passed for analysis. (Only patients with more than one episode of urolithiasis are advised to have a metabolic evaluation.)

Outcome-Based Evaluation
• Verbalizes reduced pain level
• Urine output adequate with low specific gravity
• Afebrile; urine clear

Renal Cell Carcinoma

Renal cell carcinoma is the most common malignant renal tumor, occurring twice more frequently in men than in women. Most renal cell tumors are found in the renal parenchyma and develop with few (if any) symptoms.

Pathophysiology and Etiology

1. Unknown etiology; weak association with cigarette smoking
2. Most frequently occurs in persons between 40 and 60 years of age
3. Aggressive cancer in which metastasis occurs rapidly, often before diagnosis

Clinical Manifestations

1. Many renal tumors produce no symptoms and are discovered on routine physical examination as a palpable abdominal mass.
2. Weight loss, fever, and night sweats—from systemic effects of renal cancer.
3. Classic triad (late symptoms):
   a. Hematuria—intermittent or continuous, microscopic or gross
   b. Flank pain—from distention of renal capsule, invasion of surrounding structures
   c. Palpable mass in flank

Diagnostic Evaluation

1. Ultrasonography—helpful in differentiating renal cyst from renal tumor.
2. CT or MRI—for patients with urographic findings suggesting tumor; useful for detecting, categorizing, and staging a renal mass.
3. IVP—used as a screening procedure, IVP alone may fail to detect some renal tumors.

Management

Goal: to eradicate the tumor and prevent metastasis.

Radical Nephrectomy

Removal of kidney and associated tumor, adrenal gland, surrounding perirenal fat, Gerota's fascia, and possibly regional lymph nodes—provides maximum opportunity for disease control

1. Performed through a vertical midline, subcostal, thoracoabdominal, or flank incision.
2. See page 702 for care of patient after renal surgery.

Renal Artery Embolization

Preoperative occlusion of renal artery followed by nephrectomy—for patient with large vascular tumor.

1. Catheter is advanced into renal artery.
2. Embolizing material (Gelfoam, steel coils, blood clot) is injected into artery and carried with arterial blood flow to occlude the tumor vessels.
3. Procedure decreases tumor vascularity and minimizes blood loss, relieves pain, and devitalizes the tumor preoperatively, thereby decreasing the chance for tumor cell dissemination at time of surgery.
4. Monitor for postinfarction syndrome (lasts 2 to 3 days)—severe abdominal pain, nausea, vomiting, diarrhea, fever.

5. Complications—arterial obstruction, bleeding, diminution of renal function.

Chemotherapy and Immunotherapy

Renal cell carcinomas are generally refractory to chemotherapeutic agents, radiation, and hormonal manipulation.

1. Interleukin-2 (a lymphokine that stimulates growth of T lymphocytes) may offer some benefit to patients with metastatic renal cancer although toxicity is severe.
2. Interferon is also being investigated for possible beneficial effects in metastatic renal cell cancer.

Complications

Metastasis to the lung, bone, liver, brain, and other areas.

Nursing Assessment

1. Assess for clinical manifestations of systemic disease—fatigue, anorexia, weight loss, pallor, fever—as well as evidence of metastasis.
2. Monitor for side effects and complications of diagnostic tests and treatment.
3. Assess pain control and coping ability.

Nursing Diagnoses

- Anxiety related to diagnosis of cancer and possibility of metastatic disease
- Pain and Hyperthermia related to postinfarction syndrome

Also see page 703 for nursing diagnoses and interventions related to renal surgery.

Nursing Interventions

Reducing Anxiety

1. Explain each diagnostic test, its purpose, and possible adverse reactions. Ensure that informed consent has been obtained as indicated.
2. Assess patient's understanding about diagnosis and treatment options. Answer questions, and encourage more thorough discussion with health care provider as needed.
3. Encourage patient to discuss fears and feelings; involve family and significant others in teaching.

Controlling Symptoms of Postinfarction Syndrome

1. Administer analgesics as prescribed to control flank and abdominal pain.
2. Encourage rest, and assist with positioning for 2 to 3 days until syndrome subsides.
3. Obtain temperature every 4 hours, and administer antipyretics as indicated.
4. Restrict oral intake and provide IV fluids while patient is nauseated.
5. Administer antiemetics as ordered.

Patient Education and Health Maintenance

1. Ensure that patient understands where and when to go for follow-up (surgeon, primary care provider, oncologist, and radiologist for metastatic work-up and treatment).

2. Explain the importance of follow-up for hypertension and renal function, even if patient feels well.
3. Advise patient with one kidney to wear a Medic-Alert bracelet and notify all health care providers because potentially nephrotoxic medications and procedures must be avoided.

Outcome-Based Evaluation
- Asks questions and verbalizes fears
- Afebrile; states reduced pain

◼ Injuries to the Kidney
Trauma to abdomen, flank, or back may produce renal injury. Suspicion is high in a patient with multiple injuries.

Pathophysiology and Etiology
1. *Blunt trauma* (falls, sporting accidents, motor vehicle accidents) can suddenly move the kidney out of position and in contact with a rib or lumbar vertebral transverse process, resulting in injury.
2. *Penetrating trauma* (gunshot and stab wounds) can injure the kidney if it lies in the path of the wound.
3. Renal trauma is classified according to severity of injury (Figure 21-6):
   a. Minor injuries—contusion, minor lacerations, hematomas
   b. Major injuries—major lacerations and rupture of kidney capsule (by expanding hematoma)

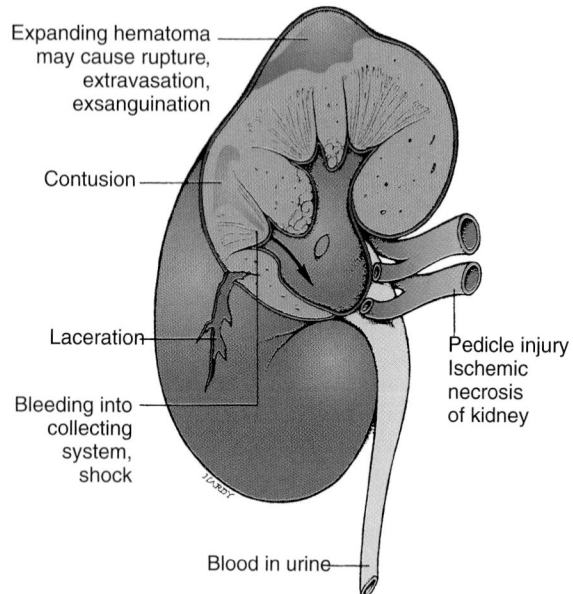

FIGURE 21-6 Types and physiologic effects of renal injuries: contusion, laceration, rupture, and pedicle injury.

Expanding hematoma may cause rupture, extravasation, exsanguination

Contusion

Laceration

Bleeding into collecting system, shock

Pedicle injury
Ischemic necrosis of kidney

Blood in urine

   c. Critical injuries—multiple and severe lacerations and renal pedicle injury (renal artery and vein are torn away from the kidney)
4. 80% of patients with renal trauma will have injuries to other organ systems also necessitating treatment.

Clinical Manifestations
1. Hematuria is common but not indicative of severity of injury.
2. Flank pain; perirenal hematoma.
3. Nausea, vomiting, abdominal rigidity—from ileus (seen when there is retroperitoneal bleeding).
4. Shock—from severe/multiple injuries.

Diagnostic Evaluation
1. History of injury—determine if injury was caused by blunt or penetrating trauma.
2. IVP with nephrotomograms—to define extent of injury to involved kidney and the function of contralateral kidney.
3. CT scan—differentiates between major and minor injuries.
4. Arteriography—if necessary to evaluate the renal artery.

Management
1. Contusions and minor lacerations are managed conservatively with bed rest, IV fluids, and monitoring of serial urines for clearing of hematuria.
2. Major lacerations are surgically repaired.
3. Ruptures are surgically repaired, usually by partial nephrectomy.
4. Renal pedicle injury—this hemorrhagic emergency requires immediate surgical repair and possible nephrectomy.

NURSING ALERT

If there is a history consistent with renal injury and the patient presents in shock, suspect a renal pedicle injury. This is a hemorrhagic emergency requiring immediate treatment of shock and preparation for surgery.

Complications
1. Shock with cardiovascular collapse
2. Hematoma or urinoma formation, abscess formation
3. Hypertension
4. Pyelonephritis
5. Nephrolithiasis

Nursing Assessment
1. Obtain history of traumatic event and any history of renal disease.
2. Inspect for any abrasions, lacerations, or entrance and exit wounds to upper abdomen or lower thorax.

3. Monitor blood pressure and pulse—to assess for bleeding and impending shock; perirenal hemorrhage may cause rapid exsanguination.

4. Assess for presence and degree of hematuria.

NURSING ALERT

Watch for any *sudden* change in the patient's condition—drop in blood pressure, increasing flank or abdominal pain and tenderness, or palpable mass in flank. May indicate hemorrhage, which requires surgical intervention.

Nursing Diagnoses
- Altered Renal Tissue Perfusion related to injury
- Altered Urinary Elimination related to injury
- Pain related to injury

Nursing Interventions

Restoring and Maintaining Renal Perfusion

1. Assess vital signs frequently, including blood pressure, heart rate, and central venous pressure to monitor for hemorrhage and impending shock.

2. Assess abdomen and back for local tenderness and palpable mass, swelling, and ecchymosis, indicating hemorrhage or urine extravasation.

3. Outline original mass with marking pen for future comparison of size.

4. Establish IV access for support of blood pressure with fluids or vasopressors, replacement of blood, and perfusion of kidneys.

5. Monitor serial hematocrit determinations to be certain that continued bleeding is not occurring.

Preserving Urinary Elimination

1. Save, inspect, and compare each urine specimen—to follow the course and degree of hematuria.
   a. Label each specimen with date and time.
   b. If specimen is not grossly bloody, dipstick for blood or send to laboratory for microscopic examination.

2. Monitor intake and output carefully.

3. Give antibiotics as directed to discourage infection from perirenal hematoma or urinoma, or severely contaminated wounds.

4. Monitor for paralytic ileus (lack of bowel sounds) caused by retroperitoneal bleeding.
   a. Keep patient NPO until bowel sounds return.
   b. Administer IV fluids to maintain urine output.

Controlling Pain

1. Administer analgesic medication as prescribed; exercise caution with drugs that may aggravate hypotension or mask complications of hemorrhage.

2. Encourage bed rest and positioning of comfort until hematuria clears to facilitate healing of minor injuries.

3. Expect a low-grade fever with retroperitoneal hematomas as absorption of the clot occurs; administer antipyretics as ordered for comfort.

Patient Education and Health Maintenance

1. Instruct patient not to engage in strenuous activity for at least 1 month after blunt trauma to minimize incidence of delayed or secondary bleeding.

2. Teach patient signs and symptoms of late complications—infection and nephrolithiasis.

3. Advise patient to have blood pressure measured frequently and consistently to monitor self for hypertension.

Outcome-Based Evaluation
- Vital signs stable
- Serial urines clearing
- Reports decreased pain

◼ Injuries to the Bladder and Urethra

Injuries to the bladder and urethra commonly occur along with pelvic trauma or may be due to surgical interventions.

Pathophysiology and Etiology

1. Bladder injuries are classified as follows:
   a. Contusion of bladder
   b. Intraperitoneal rupture
   c. Extraperitoneal rupture
   d. Combination intraperitoneal and extraperitoneal bladder rupture

2. Urethral injuries (occurring almost exclusively in men) are classified as follows:
   a. Partial or complete rupture
   b. Anterior or posterior urethral rupture

3. Injuries to the bladder and urethra are commonly associated with pelvic fractures and multiple trauma.

4. Certain surgical procedures (endoscopic urologic procedures, gynecologic surgery, surgery of the lower colon and rectum) also carry a risk of trauma to the bladder and urethra.

5. Intraperitoneal bladder rupture occurs when the bladder is full of urine and the lower abdomen sustains blunt trauma. The bladder ruptures at its weakest point, the dome. Urine and blood extravasate into the peritoneal cavity.

6. Extraperitoneal bladder rupture occurs when the lower bladder is perforated by a bony fragment during pelvic fracture or with a sharp instrument during surgery. Urine and blood extravasate into the pelvic cavity.

7. Urethral rupture occurs during pelvic fracture (posterior) or when the urethra or penis is manipulated accidentally during surgery or injury (anterior).

Clinical Manifestations

1. Inability to void

2. Hematuria; presence of blood at urinary meatus

3. Shock and hemorrhage—pallor, rapid and increasing pulse rate

4. Suprapubic pain and tenderness
5. Rigid abdomen—indicates intraperitoneal rupture
6. Absence of prostate on rectal examination in posterior urethral rupture
7. Swelling/discoloration of penis, scrotum, and anterior perineum in anterior urethral rupture

Diagnostic Evaluation

1. Retrograde urethrogram—to detect any rupture of urethra

> **NURSING ALERT**
>
> If ruptured urethra is suspected, do not catheterize because catheterization may complete a partial urethral rupture. Urethrogram must be done first to determine patency of urethra.

2. Cystogram—to detect and localize perforation/rupture of bladder
3. Plain film of abdomen—may show associated pelvic fracture
4. Excretory urogram—to survey the kidneys for injury

Management
Bladder Injury

1. Treatment instituted for shock and hemorrhage.
2. Surgical intervention carried out for intraperitoneal bladder rupture. Extravasated blood and urine will first be drained and urine diverted with suprapubic cystostomy or indwelling catheter.
3. Small extraperitoneal bladder ruptures will heal spontaneously with indwelling suprapubic or Foley catheter drainage.
4. Large extraperitoneal bladder ruptures are repaired surgically.

Urethral Injury Management Is Controversial

1. *Immediate repair*—urethra is manipulated into its correct anatomical position with reanastomosis after evacuation of hematoma.
2. *Delayed repair*—suprapubic cystostomy drainage for 6 to 12 weeks allows the urethra to realign itself while hematoma and edema resolve; then surgical reanastomosis.
3. *Two-stage urethroplasty*—reconstruction of the urethra occurs in two separate surgeries with urinary elimination diverted until final procedure.

Complications

1. Shock, hemorrhage, peritonitis
2. Urinary tract infection
3. Urethral stricture disease

Nursing Assessment

1. Obtain vital signs; assess for evidence of shock.
2. Obtain detailed history of injury, if possible.
3. Inspect urinary meatus for evidence of bleeding.
4. Perform physical examination for symptoms of bladder rupture; dullness to palpation; rebound tenderness or rigidity.

Nursing Diagnoses

- Risk for Fluid Volume Deficit related to trauma and resulting hemorrhage
- Altered Urinary Elimination related to disruption of intact lower urinary tract
- Pain related to traumatic injury
- Fear related to traumatic injury and uncertain prognosis

Nursing Interventions
Stabilizing Circulatory Volume

1. Monitor vital signs and central venous pressure frequently as indicated by condition.
2. Establish IV access, and replace blood and fluids as ordered.

Facilitating Urinary Elimination

1. Inspect urethral meatus for blood, and, if present, do not catheterize, but prepare for diagnostic evaluation and suprapubic cystostomy.
2. Obtain urine specimen, if possible, and assess for degree of hematuria and presence of infection.
3. Prepare patient for surgical repair by assisting with preoperative work-up and describing postoperative experiences.
4. Postoperatively, maintain patency and flow of indwelling urinary catheter(s).
5. Inspect suprapubic incision and Penrose drains from perivesical areas for bleeding, extravasation of urine, or signs of infection.

Controlling Pain

1. Administer analgesics as ordered (once the patient's vital signs are stable).
2. Assess patient's response to pain control medications.
3. Position for comfort (usually semi-Fowler's position) if not contraindicated by other injuries, and prevent pulling of catheter tubing.

Relieving Fears

1. Provide information to the conscious patient throughout the stabilization and evaluation phase; prepare for surgery if impending.
2. Keep patient's family or significant others informed of condition and progress.
3. Provide information on long-term outcome of treatment.

Patient Education and Health Maintenance

1. Teach patient to care for indwelling catheters that will remain in place during healing or after surgery.
   a. Empty frequently.
   b. Cleanse catheter and insertion area with soap and water.
   c. Inspect urine for blood, cloudiness, or concentration.
   d. Drink plenty of fluids to keep urine flowing.

2. Teach patient to report signs and symptoms of urinary tract infection.
3. Instruct patient (after surgical repair of bladder rupture) that bladder capacity may be temporarily decreased causing frequency and nocturia; this resolves over time.
4. Explain possibility of recurrent urethral stricture disease to patients with urethral injury; instruct in daily self-catheterization to dilate urethra if prescribed.
5. Inform patient (after severe urethral injury) of chance of impotence or incontinence.

Outcome-Based Evaluation

- Vital signs stable
- Adequate urine output by way of catheter
- Verbalizes relief of pain
- Verbalizes reduction in fear

Cancer of the Bladder

Cancer of the bladder is the second most common urologic malignancy. Approximately 90% of all bladder cancers are transitional cell carcinomas, which arise from the epithelial lining of the urinary tract; transitional cell tumors can also occur in the ureters, renal pelvis, and urethra. The remaining 10% of bladder cancers are adenocarcinoma, squamous cell carcinoma, or sarcoma.

Pathophysiology and Etiology

1. Many bladder tumors are diagnosed when the lesions are superficial, papillary tumors that are easily resected.
2. One fourth of patients with bladder cancer present with nonpapillary, muscle-invasive disease.
3. Bladder tumors tend to be either low-grade superficial tumors or high-grade invasive cancers.
4. Metastases occur in the bladder wall and pelvis; para-aortic or supraclavicular nodes; in liver, lungs, and bone.
5. Although the specific etiology is unknown, it appears that multiple agents are linked to the development of cancer of the bladder, including:
   a. Cigarette smoking—the risk of developing bladder cancer is up to four times higher in smokers.
   b. Prolonged exposure to aromatic amines or their metabolites—generally dyes manufactured by the chemical industry and used by other industries.
   c. Exposure to cyclophosphamide (Cytoxan), radiation therapy to the pelvis, chronic irritation of the bladder (as in long-term indwelling catheterization), and excessive use of the analgesic drug phenacetin, which has been taken off the market.
6. Bladder cancer is the fourth most common cancer in men; it occurs four times more frequently in men; peak incidence occurs in the 6th to 8th decades.

Clinical Manifestations

1. Painless hematuria, either gross or microscopic—most characteristic sign

2. Dysuria, frequency, urgency—symptoms of bladder irritability
3. Pelvic or flank pain—from ureteral obstruction or distant metastases
4. Leg edema—from invasion of pelvic lymph nodes

Diagnostic Evaluation

1. Cystoscopy for visualization of number, location, and appearance of tumors; for biopsy
2. Urine and bladder washing for cytologic study
3. Urine for flow cytometry—uses a computer-controlled fluorescence microscope to scan and image the nucleus of each cell on a slide; based on the fact that cancer cells contain abnormally large amounts of DNA
4. IVP—may reveal filling defect indicative of bladder tumor, also to determine status of upper tracts
5. To evaluate for metastatic disease:
   a. CT or MRI—to evaluate extent of disease and tumor responsiveness
   b. Chest x-ray—to evaluate for pulmonary metastases
   c. Pelvic lymphadenectomy (during cystectomy)—most accurate for staging

Management

Surgery

1. Transurethral resection and fulguration—endoscopic resection for superficial tumors.
   a. May be followed by intravesical chemotherapy to prevent tumor recurrence.
   b. Complications include hemorrhage, infection, bladder perforation, and temporary irritative voiding.
   c. Laser irradiation of bladder tumors is also used to destroy tumors; however, it does not allow for tumor specimen collection for pathologic analysis.
2. Partial cystectomy when lesions are located only in the dome of the bladder, away from the ureteral orifices.
3. Radical cystectomy (removal of bladder) for invasive or poorly differentiated tumors.
   a. Requires diversion of the urinary stream (see p. 704).
   b. In men, includes removal of bladder, prostate and seminal vesicles, proximal vas deferens, and part of proximal urethra.
   c. In women, consists of anterior exenteration with removal of bladder, urethra, uterus, fallopian tubes, ovaries, and segment of anterior wall of the vagina.
   d. May be combined with chemotherapy and radiation.

Intravesical (Within the Bladder) Chemotherapy

1. Instillation of antineoplastic agent such as thiotepa, mitomycin C (Mutamycin), doxorubicin (Adriamycin); allows a high concentration of drug to come in contact with the tumor and urothelium with minimal systemic toxicity.
2. Instillation of immunotherapeutic agent bacillus Calmette-Guérin (BCG) stimulates immune response to prevent recurrence of transitional cell bladder tumors.

3. Patient is instructed as follows:
   a. Minimize fluid intake, and avoid taking diuretic medications for several hours before the instillation period to maximize concentration of drug during treatment period.
   b. Change position as directed during instillation in an effort to have drug contact as much of urothelial surface as possible.
   c. Wash hands and perineal area after voiding the medication to prevent contact dermatitis.
   d. Do not void for 1 to 2 hours after instillation; then increase fluid intake and void frequently.
   e. Course of treatment is weekly instillations for 6 to 8 weeks.
4. Complications from intravesical chemotherapy include urinary tract infection, irritative voiding symptoms, allergic reaction, bone marrow suppression, or systemic BCG reaction. A systemic BCG reaction occurs when fever higher than 100°F (37.7°C) persists for more than 24 hours; treated with antituberculosis agents.

Systemic Chemotherapy

Metastatic bladder cancer is a chemotherapeutically responsive disease; MVAC combination is widely used (methotrexate [Mexate], vinblastine [Velban], doxorubicin [Adriamycin], and cisplatin [Platinol]).

Radiation Therapy

External beam radiation therapy is often used in combination with chemotherapy.

Complications

Regional metastasis through the pelvis as well as metastasis to the lung, liver, and bone

Nursing Assessment

1. Assess for hematuria, irritative voiding symptoms, risk factors (especially smoking history), weight loss, fatigue, and signs of metastasis.
2. Assess coping ability and knowledge of the disease.

Nursing Diagnoses

- Altered Urinary Elimination related to hematuria and transurethral surgery
- Pain related to irritative voiding symptoms and catheter-related discomfort
- Anxiety related to diagnosis of cancer

Nursing Interventions

Maintaining Urinary Elimination After Transurethral Surgery

1. Maintain patency of indwelling urinary drainage catheter; manual irrigation is not recommended due to dangers of bladder perforation; continuous bladder irrigation may be used if necessary.
2. Ensure adequate hydration either orally or IV.

3. Monitor intake and output, including irrigation solution.
4. Monitor urine output for clearing of hematuria.

Controlling Pain

1. Administer analgesic medication for pelvic discomfort.
2. Administer anticholinergic medications or belladonna and opium suppositories to relieve bladder spasms.
3. Ensure patency of catheter drainage; do not irrigate unless specifically ordered.
4. Remove indwelling catheter as soon as possible after procedure.

Relieving Anxiety

1. Allow patient to verbalize fears and concerns.
2. Provide realistic information about diagnostic studies, surgery, and treatments.

Patient Education and Health Maintenance

1. Advise patient that irritative voiding symptoms and intermittent hematuria are possible for several weeks after transurethral resection of bladder tumor(s).
2. Teach patient importance of vigilant adherence to follow-up schedule: cystoscopy every 3 months for 1 year, then every 6 months to 1 year thereafter for the rest of patient's life (70% of superficial tumors will recur).
3. Review purpose and side effects of intravesical chemotherapy treatments (often not given until after recurrence).

Outcome-Based Evaluation

- Urine output adequate and clear
- Verbalizes relief of pain and bladder spasms
- Verbalizes lessened anxiety

CONDITIONS OF THE MALE REPRODUCTIVE TRACT

▪ Urethritis

Urethritis is inflammation of the urethra. It is usually an ascending infection in men. In women, it is usually associated with cystitis (see p. 716) or vaginitis (see p. 765).

Pathophysiology and Etiology

1. Nongonococcal urethritis—urethritis not caused by gonococcus; however, a large number of cases are sexually transmitted by:
   a. *Chlamydia trachomatis*—most clinically significant of the pathogens, accounts for 23% to 55% of cases.
   b. *Ureaplasma urealyticum* and *Mycoplasma genitalium*—responsible for up to one third of cases.
   c. *Trichomonas vaginalis* and herpes simplex virus are other sexually transmitted organisms causing urethritis in both men and women.

d. Incubation period of 1 to 5 weeks depending on the organism; in some cases, infection may be subclinical for a period of time, particularly in men.
2. Gonococcal urethritis—caused by *Neisseria gonorrhoeae*, sexually transmitted; usually most virulent and destructive.
    a. Incubation period usually 3 to 10 days.
    b. Urethritis in homosexual men is more often gonococcal than nongonococcal.
3. Gonococcal and nongonococcal urethritis can both be present.
4. Nonsexually transmitted.
    a. Bacterial urethritis—may be associated with urinary tract infection.
    b. From trauma—secondary to passage of urethral sounds, repeated cystoscopy, indwelling catheter.
5. Postgonococcal urethritis—occurs after treatment for gonococcal urethritis; another pathogen, which was not treated, proliferates.

Clinical Manifestations
1. Often asymptomatic
2. Itching and burning around area of urethra
3. Urethral discharge: may be scant or profuse; thin, clear, or mucoid; or thick and purulent (gonococcal)
4. Dysuria and frequency
5. Penile discomfort

Diagnostic Evaluation
1. Gram's stain—*N. gonorrhoeae* is detected as gram-positive diplococci on microscopic examination of urethral discharge or urine.
2. Culture of urethral discharge on selective medium.
3. Fluorescent antibody stain of urethral discharge—to detect *C. trachomatis* and *N. gonorrhoeae*.
4. Wet mount microscopic examination of fresh urethral discharge—trichomonads may be visible and motile.
5. First voided urine for screening—either positive leukocyte esterase test by dipstick or >10 WBC per high-power field by microscopy indicates urethritis.
6. In rare cases, urethroscopy may be necessary to isolate a lesion such as warts caused by human papillomavirus (HPV).

Management
1. Antimicrobial therapy with tetracycline class, some quinolones, or erythromycin class antibiotics—effective for most cases of nongonococcal urethritis; metronidazole (Flagyl) is used for *Trichomonas*.
2. Penicillinase-resistant penicillins, some cephalosporins, and quinolones may be used to treat gonococcal urethritis; one large-dose treatment is effective.

Complications
Depends on cause, but may include:
1. Prostatitis, epididymitis, urethral stricture, sterility due to vasoepididymal duct obstruction.

2. Rectal infection, pharyngitis, conjunctivitis, skin lesions, arthritis with gonococcal infection.
3. Long-term complications of these infections in women include pelvic inflammatory disease and infertility.

Nursing Assessment
1. Obtain history of unprotected sexual contact.
2. Assess for signs and symptoms involving urinary and reproductive tracts.
3. Perform genital and abdominal examination to assess for extent of infection.

Nursing Diagnoses
• Risk for Infection related to ascending or systemic spread of pathogens
• Risk for Infection Transmission to sexual contacts

Nursing Interventions
Resolving Infection and Preventing Complications
1. Collect urethral swab of discharge, urine, and blood as ordered for laboratory examination.
2. Use universal precautions when handling specimens.
3. Administer antibiotics as prescribed.
    a. Usually ordered based on presumptive diagnosis before test results are back.
    b. Monitor for and advise patient of side effects or allergic reactions.

Preventing Spread of Infection
1. Encourage compliance with antimicrobial regimen for the prescribed time period.
2. Advise abstinence from sexual activity until treatment is complete and cure is established (usually 7 to 10 days).
3. Instruct the patient to avoid sexual activity with previous sexual partner until that person(s) has been tested and treated for infection as well.
4. The use of condoms may prevent transmission, but depends on technique.

Patient Education and Health Maintenance
1. Advise safer sex techniques such as abstinence, mutual monogamy, and use of male or female condom to prevent transmission of sexually transmitted organisms as well as unintended pregnancy.
2. Emphasize the need to return if symptoms persist or return.
3. Advise patient that reporting of gonorrhea to the public health department is required by law in all of the United States and Canada, and reporting of *Chlamydia* is currently required in all states in the United States except New York.
4. Tell patient that he will be called on to name all sexual partners within the past 60 days and that the process will be confidential.

Outcome-Based Evaluation
• Signs of infection resolved
• Reports sexual contacts have been treated

Benign Prostatic Hyperplasia (BPH)

BPH is enlargement of the prostate that constricts the urethra, causing urinary symptoms. One of four men who reach the age of 80 will require treatment for BPH.

Pathophysiology and Etiology

1. The process of aging and the presence of circulating androgens are required for the development of BPH.
2. The prostatic tissue forms nodules as enlargement occurs.
3. The normally thin and fibrous outer capsule of the prostate becomes spongy and thick as enlargement progresses.
4. The prostatic urethra becomes compressed and narrowed, requiring the bladder musculature to work harder to empty urine.
5. Effects of prolonged obstruction cause trabeculation (formation of cords) of the bladder wall, decreasing its elasticity.

Clinical Manifestations

1. In early or gradual prostatic enlargement, there may be no symptoms, because the bladder musculature can initially compensate for increased urethral resistance.
2. Obstructive symptoms—hesitancy, diminution in size and force of urinary stream, terminal dribbling, sensation of incomplete emptying of the bladder, urinary retention.
3. Irritative voiding symptoms—urgency, frequency, nocturia.

Diagnostic Evaluation

1. Rectal examination—smooth, firm, symmetric enlargement of the prostate
2. Urinalysis to rule out hematuria and infection
3. Serum creatinine and BUN—to evaluate renal function
4. Serum PSA—to rule out cancer, but may also be elevated in BPH
5. Optional diagnostic studies for further evaluation:
   a. Urodynamics—measures peak urine flow rate, voiding time and volume, and status of the bladder's ability to effectively contract
   b. Measurement of postvoid residual urine; by ultrasound or catheterization
   c. Cystourethroscopy—to inspect urethra and bladder and evaluate prostatic size

Management

1. Patients with mild symptoms (in the absence of significant bladder or renal impairment) are followed annually; BPH does not necessarily worsen in all men.
2. Pharmacologic management.
   a. α-Adrenergic blockers such as doxazosin (Cardura), tamsulosin (Flomax), terazosin (Hytrin)—relax smooth muscle of bladder base and prostate to facilitate voiding.

> **◆ DRUG ALERT**
>
> Although prescribed for their effect on prostatic smooth muscle, α-adrenergic blockers also have an antihypertensive effect. Dosage is usually titrated up from an initial small dose. It is often recommended that the first dose, or all once-a-day doses, be taken at bedtime.

   b. Finasteride (Proscar)—antiandrogen effect on prostatic cells, reverses or prevents hyperplasia
3. Surgery—TURP, transurethral incision of the prostate (TUIP), or open prostatectomy for very large prostates, usually by suprapubic approach
4. Newer approaches—laser surgery, transurethral electrovaporization, transurethral needle ablation, insertion of intraurethral stents, hyperthermia, and thermotherapy

Complications

1. Acute urinary retention, involuntary bladder contractions, bladder diverticula, and cystolithiasis
2. Vesicoureteral reflux, hydroureter, hydronephrosis
3. Gross hematuria, urinary tract infection

Nursing Assessment

1. Obtain history of voiding symptoms, including onset, frequency of day and nighttime urination, presence of urgency, dysuria, sensation of incomplete bladder emptying, and decreased force of stream. Determine impact on quality of life.
2. Perform rectal (palpate size, shape, and consistency) and abdominal examination to detect distended bladder, degree of prostatic enlargement.
3. Perform simple urodynamic measures—uroflowmetry and measurement of postvoid residual, if indicated.

Nursing Diagnosis

- Altered Urinary Elimination related to obstruction of urethra

Also see page 708 for care of the patient undergoing prostatic surgery.

Nursing Interventions

Facilitating Urinary Elimination

1. Provide privacy and time for patient to void.
2. Assist with catheter introduction with guidewire or by way of suprapubic cystotomy as indicated.
   a. Monitor intake and output.
   b. Maintain patency of catheter.
3. Administer medications as ordered, and monitor for and teach patient about side effects.
   a. α-Adrenergic blockers—hypotension, orthostatic hypotension, syncope (especially after first dose), im-

potence, blurred vision, rebound hypertension if discontinued abruptly

  b. Finasteride (Proscar)—hepatic dysfunction, impotence, interference with PSA testing

4. Assess for and teach patient to report hematuria, signs of infection.

Patient Education and Health Maintenance

1. Explain to patient not undergoing treatment the symptoms of complications of BPH—urinary retention, cystitis, increase in irritative voiding symptoms. Encourage reporting these problems.

2. Advise patients with BPH to avoid certain drugs that may impair voiding (Table 21-3).

3. Advise patient that irritative voiding symptoms do not immediately resolve after relief of obstruction; symptoms diminish over time.

4. Tell patient to avoid sexual intercourse, straining at stool, heavy lifting, and long periods of sitting for 6 to 8 weeks after surgery, until prostatic fossa is healed.

5. Advise follow-up visits after treatment because urethral stricture may occur and regrowth of prostate is possible after TURP.

6. Saw palmetto is an herbal preparation thought to promote "prostate health."

  a. Advise patients that it has shown some efficacy in reducing symptoms of BPH in a number of clinical trials.

  b. The active ingredient in commercial preparations is lipidosterolic extract of *Serenoa repens* (LSESR), and the dosage is 160 mg twice a day.

  c. It should be taken with breakfast and an evening meal to minimize GI side effects.

  d. Although it appears safe and there are no known drug interactions, tell patients they must discuss use of saw palmetto with their health care providers.

Outcome-Based Evaluation

• Voiding adequate without residual urine

Prostatitis

Prostatitis is an inflammation of the prostate gland. It is classified as *bacterial prostatitis* (acute or chronic), *nonbacterial prostatitis*, or *prostatodynia*.

Pathophysiology and Etiology

Acute Bacterial Invasion of Prostate

1. From reflux of infected urine into ejaculatory and prostatic ducts

2. From hematogenous (bloodstream) origin or lymphogenous spread

3. Secondary to urethritis—from ascent of bacteria from urethra

4. May be stimulated by urethral instrumentation or rectal examination of the prostate when bacteria are present

5. Often caused by gram-negative enteric bacteria such as *Pseudomonas* and gram-positive cocci such as *Streptococcus* and *Staphylococcus*

TABLE 21-3 Bladder Function and Drug Actions

Function	Drug Groups	Examples
Detrusor Muscle		
Increased tone and contraction	Cholinergic drugs (stimulate parasympathetic receptors that cause detrusor muscle contraction)	Bethanechol (Urecholine and others)
		Neostigmine (Prostigmin)
Inhibition of detrusor muscle relaxation during filling	β-Adrenergic blocking drugs (block β_2 receptors that cause detrusor muscle relaxation)	Propranolol (Inderal)
Decreased tone	Anticholinergic drugs (block parasympathetic receptors that cause detrusor muscle contraction)	Methantheline (Banthine)
		Propantheline (Pro-Banthine)
		Oxybutynin (Ditropan, Ditropan XL)
		Nifedipine (Adalat, Procardia)
	Calcium-channel blocking drugs (may interfere with influx of calcium to support detrusor muscle tone)	Verapamil (Calan, Isoptin)
		Diltiazem (Cardizem)
		Tolterodine tartrate (Detrol)
Internal Sphincter		
Increased tone	α_1-Adrenergic agonists (activate α receptors that cause contraction of muscles of the internal sphincter)	Phenylephrine (generic)
		Ephedrine (generic)
		Phenylpropanolamine (generic)
Decreased tone	α_1-Adrenergic blocking drugs	Prazosin (Minipress)
		Doxazosin (Cardura)
		Terazosin (Hytrin)
		Tamsulosin (Flomax)
External Sphincter		
Decreased tone	Skeletal muscle relaxants	Baclofen (Lioresal)
		Dantrolene (Dantrium)
		Diazepam (Valium)

Chronic Bacterial Prostatitis

1. From bacteria ascending from urethra in cases of urethritis
2. From hematogenous spread
3. Often caused by gram-negative bacteria such as *E. coli*, *Proteus mirabilis*, *Klebsiella pneumoniae*, and *Pseudomonas aeruginosa*

Nonbacterial Prostatitis

May be complication of urethritis, no bacterial cause may be identified, or may be caused by *C. trachomatis*.

Prostatodynia

Symptoms of prostatitis in the absence of positive cultures or known etiologic cause; difficult to diagnose and manage.

Clinical Manifestations

1. Sudden chills and fever (moderate to high fever) and body aches with acute prostatitis.
2. Symptoms are more subtle with chronic prostatitis.
3. Bladder irritability—frequency, dysuria, nocturia, urgency, hematuria to varying degrees.
4. Pain in perineum, rectum, lower back, lower abdomen, and penile head.
5. Pain after ejaculation, symptoms of urethral obstruction.

Diagnostic Evaluation

1. Culture and sensitivity tests of divided urine specimens.
   a. First 10 to 15 mL voided after cleansing are sent as urethral specimen.
   b. Next 50 to 75 mL of urine are collected as bladder specimen.
   c. Prostate is massaged, and either prostatic fluid drips out by gravity and is collected, or patient voids urine mixed with prostatic fluid.
2. Rectal examination frequently reveals exquisitely tender, painful, swollen prostate, warm to the touch with acute prostatitis.
3. Serum white blood cell count is elevated in bacterial prostatitis.

Management

Acute Bacterial Prostatitis

1. Antimicrobial therapy (10 to 14 days) based on drug sensitivity; IV therapy may be required.
2. Urinary retention is managed with suprapubic cystostomy; urethral catheterization should be avoided.
3. Antipyretic medications to manage fever.

Chronic Bacterial Prostatitis

1. Four weeks of oral antibiotic therapy with ability to diffuse into prostate.
   a. Quinolones such as ciprofloxacin (Cipro), ofloxacin (Floxin), or norfloxacin (Noroxin).
   b. Sulfonamide such as trimethoprim–sulfamethoxazole (Bactrim).
2. Prolonged therapy may be necessary to control symptoms and prevent bacteriuria (12 weeks or more).
3. Oral antispasmodic agents may provide relief from urinary frequency and urgency.

Nonbacterial Prostatitis

1. One to 2 weeks of oral antibiotics including tetracycline (Sumacyn), doxycycline (Vibramycin), or erythromycin (PCE)
2. Symptomatic relief
   a. Prostatic massage (not for acute prostatitis)
   b. Anticholinergics to relieve spasm or anti-inflammatory drugs to relieve inflammation
   c. Hot sitz baths for comfort and to promote penetration of the antibiotic

Prostatodynia

Alpha-adrenergic blockers and skeletal muscle relaxants may provide some relief of symptoms. Aggressive diagnostic intervention should take place to rule out other conditions such as cancer of the prostate or interstitial cystitis.

Complications

1. Bacteriuria, urethritis, epididymitis, prostatic abscess, bacteremia, septicemia
2. Acute urinary retention
3. Constipation

Nursing Assessment

1. Obtain history of previous lower urinary tract infections or STD, recent voiding patterns.
2. Perform examination of genitalia for urethral discharge; rectal examination (except in acute bacterial prostatitis due to tenderness and possibility of disseminating infection) to assess tenderness of prostate.
3. Collect specimens: urine for culture and expressed prostatic secretions.

Nursing Diagnoses

- Hyperthermia related to infectious process
- Pain related to prostatic inflammation
- Chronic Pain related to chronic prostatitis, prostatodynia

Nursing Interventions

Reducing Fever

1. Start antibiotic therapy as soon as specimens obtained for culture.
2. Administer antipyretic medications; use cooling measures if necessary.
3. Keep the patient well hydrated, IV or orally, due to fluid loss through fever; however, avoid overhydration, which increases urine volume and reduces antibiotic concentration in urine.

Relieving Pain

1. Administer analgesic or anti-inflammatory medication as ordered.
2. Maintain bed rest in acute prostatitis to relieve perineal and suprapubic pain.
3. Maintain high-fiber diet and give stool softeners as needed to prevent constipation, which increases pain.

Controlling Chronic Pain

1. Administer or teach self-administration of analgesics, anti-inflammatory agents, α-adrenergic blockers, or skeletal muscle relaxants as ordered.
2. Advise warm sitz baths to relieve pain and promote muscular relaxation of pelvic floor and reduce potential for urinary retention.
3. Perform gentle prostatic massage if indicated (nonbacterial prostatitis only).
4. Assess patient's response to supportive measures and coping with chronic pain.

Patient Education and Health Maintenance

1. Instruct patient to take antibiotic as prescribed; emphasize importance of completing long course of therapy to prevent recurrence and resistance of organisms.
2. Teach patient symptoms of recurrence and of disseminated spread of infection.
3. Instruct patient in comfort measures: sitz baths (10 to 20 minutes) several times daily, continued use of stool softeners, avoid sitting for long periods of time.
4. Advise patient to avoid sexual arousal/intercourse during period of acute inflammation; sexual intercourse may be beneficial in the treatment of chronic prostatitis; chronic prostatic infection is not sexually transmissible.
5. Encourage prescribed follow-up because recurrence is possible.

Outcome-Based Evaluation

- Afebrile
- Verbalizes relief of pain after analgesic
- Verbalizes reduction of chronic pain

◼ Cancer of the Prostate

Cancer of the prostate is the second leading cause of cancer death among American men and is the most common carcinoma in men over 65 years of age.

Pathophysiology and Etiology

1. The incidence of prostate cancer is 30% higher in African-American men.
2. The majority of prostate cancers arise from the peripheral zone of the gland; therefore, most prostatic cancers are palpable on rectal examination.

NURSING ALERT

Annual rectal examination and PSA blood testing are recommended for all men over age 50 by the American Cancer Society. Men who are at high risk for prostate cancer (African Americans or men with a strong family history of prostate cancer) should begin these annual tests at age 40.

3. Prostate cancer can spread by local extension, by lymphatics, or by way of the bloodstream.
4. The etiology of prostate cancer is unknown; there is an increased risk for persons with a family history of the disease.
5. The influences of dietary fat intake, serum testosterone levels, vasectomy, and industrial exposure to carcinogens are under investigation.

Clinical Manifestations

1. Most early-stage prostate cancers are asymptomatic.
2. Symptoms due to obstruction of urinary flow:
   a. Hesitancy and straining on voiding, frequency, nocturia
   b. Diminution in size and force of urinary stream
3. Symptoms due to metastases:
   a. Pain in lumbosacral area radiating to hips and down legs (from bone metastases)
   b. Perineal and rectal discomfort
   c. Anemia, weight loss, weakness, nausea, oliguria (from uremia)
   d. Hematuria (from urethral or bladder invasion, or both)
   e. Lower extremity edema—occurs when pelvic node metastases compromise venous return

Diagnostic Evaluation

1. Digital rectal examination—prostate can be felt through the wall of the rectum; hard nodule may be felt (Figure 21-7).
2. Needle biopsy (through anterior rectal wall or through perineum) for histologic study of biopsied tissue, includes Gleason tumor grade if carcinoma present.
3. Transrectal ultrasonography—a sonar probe placed in rectum.
4. PSA—serologic marker of prostate cancer.
   a. Suspicion of prostate cancer if measures between 4.0 and 10 ng/mL.
   b. Most PSA measurements over 10 ng/mL indicate prostate cancer.
5. Staging evaluation—skeletal x-rays, CT, or MRI and bone scan; analysis of pelvic lymph nodes provides most accurate staging information.

Management
Conservative Measures

1. No treatment may be indicated in men over age 70 because prostate cancer may be slow growing and it is expected that many men will die from other causes. It is

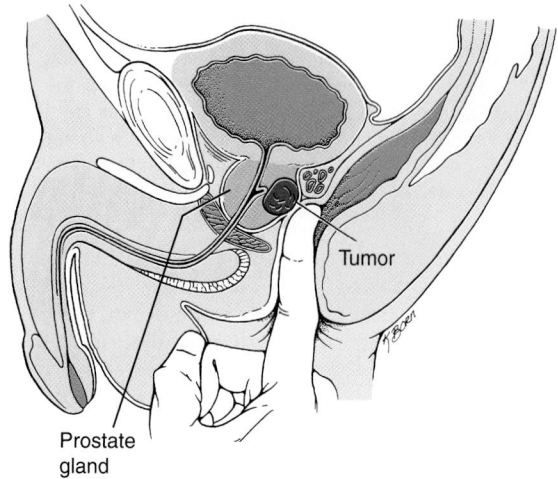

FIGURE 21-7 The prostate gland can be felt through the wall of the rectum. The size of the gland, overall consistency, and the presence of any firm areas and nodules are noted.

often recommended that these patients be followed closely with periodic PSA determinations and examination for evidence of metastases.

2. Symptom control for advanced prostatic cancer in which treatment is not effective:
   a. Analgesics and narcotics to relieve pain.
   b. Short course of radiotherapy for specific sites of bone pain.
   c. IV administration of β-emitter agent (strontium chloride 89) delivers radiotherapy directly to sites of metastasis.
   d. TURP to remove obstructing tissue if bladder outlet obstruction occurs.
   e. Suprapubic catheter placement.

Surgical Interventions (Curative)
1. Radical prostatectomy—removal of entire prostate gland, prostatic capsule, and seminal vesicles; may include pelvic lymphadenectomy.
   a. Complications include urinary incontinence, impotence, and rectal injury.
   b. Newer surgical dissection techniques may preserve sexual potency.
2. Cryosurgery of the prostate freezes prostate tissue, killing tumor cells without removing the gland.

Radiation (Curative)
1. External beam radiation (using linear accelerator) focused on the prostate—to deliver maximum radiation dose to tumor and minimal dose to surrounding tissues.
2. Interstitial radiation—interstitial implantation of radioactive substances (brachytherapy) into prostate, which delivers doses of radiation directly to tumor while sparing uninvolved tissue.

3. Both forms of radiation are used in some patients; external beam followed by brachytherapy.
4. Complications include radiation cystitis (urinary frequency, urgency, nocturia), urethral injury (stricture), radiation enteritis (diarrhea, anorexia, nausea), radiation proctitis (diarrhea, rectal bleeding), impotence.

Hormone Manipulation (Palliative)
1. Prostate cancer is a hormone-sensitive cancer. The aim of hormonal treatment is to deprive tumor cells of androgens or their by-products and thereby alleviate symptoms and retard progress of disease.
2. Bilateral orchiectomy (removal of testes) results in reduction of the major circulating androgen, testosterone. A small amount of androgen is still produced by adrenal glands.
3. Pharmacologic methods of achieving androgen deprivation—also used to reduce tumor volume before surgery or radiation therapy.
   a. Luteinizing hormone-releasing hormone (LHRH) analogues (leuprolide [Lupron], goserelin acetate [Zoladex]) reduce testosterone levels as effectively as orchiectomy.
   b. Antiandrogen drugs (flutamide [Eulexin], bicalutamide [Casodex], nilutamide [Nilandron]) block androgen action directly at the target tissues (testes and adrenals) and block androgen synthesis within the prostate gland.
   c. Combination therapy with LHRH analogues and an anti-androgen blocks the action of all circulating androgen.
4. Complications of hormonal manipulation include hot flashes, nausea and vomiting, gynecomastia, sexual dysfunction.

Complications
1. Bone metastasis—vertebral collapse and spinal cord compression, pathologic fractures
2. Complications of treatment

Nursing Assessment
1. Obtain history of current symptoms; assess for family history of prostate cancer.
2. Palpate lymph nodes, especially in supraclavicular and inguinal regions (may be first sign of metastatic spread); assess for flank pain and distended bladder.

Nursing Diagnoses
• Anxiety related to fear of disease progression and treatment options
• Sexual Dysfunction related to effects of therapy
• Pain related to bone metastases
Also see page 708 for care of the patient after prostatectomy.

Nursing Interventions
Reducing Anxiety
1. Help patient assess the impact of the disease and treatment options on quality of life.

2. Give repeated explanations of diagnostic tests and treatment options; help patient gain some feeling of control over disease and decisions.

3. Help patient/family set reachable goals.

4. Convey a sense of caring and reassurance in your physical care.

Achieving Optimal Sexual Function

1. Although the patient may be ill while experiencing the effects of therapy, he may wonder about sexual function. Give him the opportunity to communicate his concerns and sexual needs.

2. Let patient know that decreased libido is expected after hormonal manipulation therapy and impotence may result from some surgical procedures and radiation.

3. Expect patient's behavior to reflect depression, anxiety, anger, and regression. Encourage ventilation of feelings and communication with partner.

4. Suggest options such as sexual counseling, learning other methods of sexual expression, and consideration of pharmacologic (and other) options for treatment of erectile dysfunction.

 DRUG ALERT

Yohimbine is an herbal preparation sold over the counter as an aphrodisiac and treatment for male erectile dysfunction. Caution patients that it is considered an unsafe herb by the US Department of Agriculture due to its many drug and food interactions and side effects such as hypertension, tachycardia, and tremor.

Controlling Pain

1. Administer and teach self-administration of narcotic analgesics as ordered; oral sustained-release narcotics, sustained-release transdermal patches, and subcutaneous or epidural patient-controlled infusion pumps are among the many options.

2. Encourage patient to take prescribed aspirin (Ecotrin), acetaminophen (Tylenol), or NSAIDs for reduction of mild pain or to supplement narcotic pain control regimen.

3. Be sure that patient is not undermedicated; help family and patient understand that addiction is not a concern.

4. Teach relaxation techniques such as imagery, music therapy, progressive muscle relaxation.

5. Use safety measures to prevent pathologic fractures from falls.

6. Encourage follow-up and palliative treatment such as radiation therapy to bony lesions for pain improvement.

Patient Education and Health Maintenance

1. Teach patient importance of follow-up for check of PSA levels and evaluation for disease progression.

2. Teach IM or subcutaneous administration of hormonal agents as indicated.

3. If bone metastasis has occurred, encourage safety measures around the home to prevent pathologic fractures

such as removal of throw rugs, using hand rail on stairs, using nightlights.

4. Advise reporting of symptoms of worsening urethral obstruction such as increased frequency, urgency, hesitancy, and urinary retention.

5. For additional information and support, refer to agencies such as US TOO International Inc. (network of prostate cancer survivor support groups), 930 N. York Road, Suite 50, Hinsdale, IL 60521, 1-800-808-7866, *www.ustoo.com*; American Foundation for Urologic Disease, 1128 N. Charles Street, Baltimore, MD 21201-5559, 1-800-242-2383.

Outcome-Based Evaluation

- Discusses treatment options, asks questions
- Verbalizes understanding of sexual dysfunction and interest in seeking sexual counseling
- Reports pain relief after narcotic administration

▪ Testicular Cancer

Testicular cancer is a disease that occurs in younger men, between 15 and 35 years of age. It is relatively uncommon—7,400 cases are reported annually. It is the most treatable form of urologic cancer.

Pathophysiology and Etiology

1. The majority of testicular cancers are of germ cell origin; the most common germinal tumors in adults are seminoma, embryonal carcinoma, teratoma, and choriocarcinoma (the latter three are also called nonseminomas).

2. The etiology of testicular tumors is unknown, but there is a relationship between cryptorchidism (failure of the testes to descend into the scrotum) and tumor occurrence.

3. Testicular tumors metastasize to the retroperitoneal lymph nodes with subsequent involvement of the mediastinal lymph nodes, lungs, and liver.

4. Testicular germ cell tumors are considered potentially curable; seminomas are extremely responsive to radiation therapy, nonseminomas are sensitive to platinum-based chemotherapy.

Clinical Manifestations

1. Painless swelling or enlargement of the testis; accompanied by sensation of heaviness in scrotum

2. Pain in the testis (if patient has epididymitis or bleeding into tumor)

3. Symptoms of metastatic disease: cough, lymphadenopathy, back pain, GI symptoms, lower extremity edema, or bone pain

Diagnostic Evaluation

1. Elevated serum markers of human chorionic gonadotropin (HCG) and α-fetoprotein (AFP); assay of tumor markers also used for diagnosis, detection of early recurrence, staging, and monitoring response to therapy.

2. Scrotal ultrasonography—identifies location of lesion and differentiates between solid and cystic lesion

3. Chest film—to seek pulmonary or mediastinal metastases
4. CT scanning of chest, abdomen, and pelvis—to evaluate retroperitoneal lymph nodes and to follow progress of therapy

Management
Choice of treatment depends on tumor histology and stage of disease.

Surgery
1. Inguinal orchiectomy—removal of testis and its tunica and spermatic cord.
2. Retroperitoneal lymph node dissection (RPLND) is usually performed after orchiectomy in nonseminomas for staging and therapeutic purposes.
3. Complications of surgery:
   a. RPLND causes infertility due to ejaculatory dysfunction.
   b. Modified nerve-sparing unilateral lymphadenectomy can be done on selected patients, thus preserving ejaculation.
   c. Unilateral orchiectomy eliminates half of germinal cells, thus reducing sperm count.
   d. Libido and ability to attain an erection are preserved.

Radiation Therapy
1. Radiation therapy to lymphatic drainage pathways (after orchiectomy in seminomas); cure rate is close to 99%.
2. Other testicle is shielded, usually preserving fertility.

Chemotherapy
1. Cisplatin combination therapy is used in treatment of nonseminomatous primary tumor and regional lymphatic metastases and in managing distant metastatic disease.
2. Discomforts of chemotherapy include significant nausea and vomiting, alopecia, myalgia, GI cramping, and mucositis.

Complications
1. Infertility; loss of testicle
2. Retrograde ejaculation after retroperitoneal lymphadenectomy
3. Death from metastatic disease

Nursing Assessment
1. Examine testicular mass; ascertain when it was discovered and if it has changed or enlarged since initial discovery.
2. Examine supraclavicular and inguinal lymph nodes for enlargement.
3. Assess for symptoms of metastatic disease.

Nursing Diagnoses
- Anxiety related to diagnosis of cancer and impending treatments
- Body Image Disturbance related to loss of testicle and fertility
- Risk for Injury related to complications of treatment

Nursing Interventions
Reducing Anxiety
1. Explore with patient the desire to deposit sperm in sperm bank before surgery.
2. Provide realistic information about impending surgery or treatment; dispel myths associated with testicular disease, emphasize positive cure rates.

Preserving Body Image
1. Reassure patient that orchiectomy will not diminish virility, and retroperitoneal lymph node dissection will alter fertility and ejaculation but not libido, erection, and sensation.
2. Advise patient that testicular prosthesis can preserve look and feel of scrotum.
3. Refer the patient for counseling as needed for problems and concerns with relationships, peers, or work life.

Preventing Complications of Treatment
1. Provide routine postoperative care, including early ambulation, respiratory care, and administration of pain medication.
2. After RPLND, monitor for paralytic ileus, which is common after extensive resection.
   a. Auscultate bowel sounds frequently, and observe for abdominal distention.
   b. Withhold oral fluids until bowel sounds have returned.
   c. Report complaints of nausea and any vomiting.
   d. Begin nasogastric decompression, if indicated.
3. For nursing care involving radiation and chemotherapy, see pages 141–154.

Patient Education and Health Maintenance
1. Teach all young men to perform monthly testicular self-examination; after orchiectomy, patient should examine remaining testicle monthly (see Patient Education Guidelines).
2. Review schedule for radiation treatments or chemotherapy; teach patient and family possible side effects; discuss expectations for treatment period.
3. Provide information about retrograde ejaculation after retroperitoneal lymph node dissection and alternatives for fertility.

Outcome-Based Evaluation
- Verbalizes understanding of treatment and complications
- No abdominal distention noted
- Discusses concerns about sexual function with staff and partner

Epididymitis
Epididymitis is an infection of the epididymis that usually spreads from the urethra or bladder to the epididymis by way of the ejaculatory duct and vas deferens.

1. Examine for testicular tumor once a month, at a convenient time such as the first of the month or your birthdate every month, preferably while showering or bathing.
2. Use both hands to feel the testes through the scrotal tissue.
3. Locate the epididymis; this is the irregular cordlike structure on the top and at the back of the testicle that stores and transports sperm. The spermatic cord (and vas) extends upward from the epididymis.
4. Feel each testis between the thumb and first two fingers of each hand. The testes lie freely in the scrotum, are oval shaped, and measure 4–5 cm in length, 3 cm in width, and about 2 cm in thickness.
5. Note size, shape, abnormal tenderness. An abnormality may be felt as a firm area on the front or side of the testicle.
6. Stand in front of mirror and look for changes in size/ shape of scrotum. It is normal to find one testis larger than the other.
7. Report any evidence of a small, pea-size lump or other abnormality.

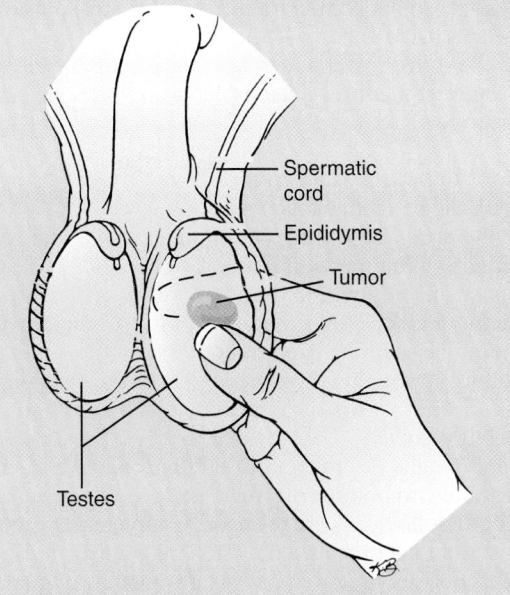

Using the fingertips and thumb, the epididymis, testes, and spermatic cord are located bilaterally.

Pathophysiology and Etiology
1. Occurs as a complication of urinary tract infection, urethral stricture disease, bacterial prostatitis, gonococcal or nongonococcal bacterial urethritis.
2. In men under 35, sexually transmitted organisms are the main etiologic agents, usually *C. trachomatis* and *N. gonorrhoeae*.
3. In homosexual men, *E. coli* is a common cause.
4. In older men, the main causes are bladder outlet obstruction and urinary bacteria (*E. coli*, *P. aeruginosa*).

Clinical Manifestations
1. Unilateral scrotal pain and tenderness
2. Edema, redness, and tenderness of scrotum
3. Dysuria, frequency
4. Fever, nausea, vomiting
5. Pyuria, bacteriuria, leukocytosis

Diagnostic Evaluation
1. Examination (Gram's stain, culture) of initial and midstream urine sample to detect bacteria
2. Examination (Gram's stain, culture, gonorrhea and *Chlamydia* testing) of urethral discharge and expressed prostatic secretions to establish causative organism

Management
1. Antimicrobial therapy after collection of specimens.
   a. Treatment of choice for presumed sexually transmitted infections is combination ceftriaxone (Rocephin) 250 mg IM in a single dose with doxycycline 100 mg orally twice a day for 10 days.
   b. For presumed *E. coli* and other infections, a quinolone such as ofloxacin (Floxin) 300 mg orally twice a day for 10 days is recommended.
2. Analgesics for pain relief.
3. Bed rest with the scrotum elevated on a towel to allow for lymphatic drainage.
4. In some cases, the spermatic cord is injected with a local anesthetic to relieve pain.

Complications
1. Spread of infection to testicle—epididymo-orchitis
2. Infertility; risk is greater when bilateral infection

Nursing Assessment
1. Obtain history of STD (or symptoms); urinary tract infection or prostatitis; recent urologic instrumentation or surgery.
2. Assess for elevated temperature; level of pain; swollen, tender scrotum.

Nursing Diagnosis
• Pain related to scrotal inflammation

Nursing Interventions
Relieving Pain
1. Administer or teach self-administration of analgesics as ordered—often NSAIDs or acetaminophen (Tylenol). Assess patient's response.

2. Encourage bed rest during the acute phase.
3. Apply scrotal support to relieve edema and discomfort, to improve lymphatic drainage, and to take tension off the spermatic cord.
   a. Use rolled towel under scrotum or scrotal bridge.
   b. Suggest a cotton-lined athletic supporter for ambulation.

Patient Education and Health Maintenance
Instruct the patient as follows:
1. Avoid straining (lifting, straining at stool, and sexual activity) until infection is under control.
2. Sexual partners within the past 60 days of patients with chlamydial or gonorrheal urethritis or epididymitis should be examined and treated.
3. Follow up with health care provider as directed—it may take 2 to 4 weeks or longer for epididymitis to completely resolve.
4. Report signs of infection in the reproductive tract immediately to obtain treatment and prevent spread.
5. Obtain follow-up care to ensure complete resolution of infection; uncontrolled infection may impair fertility.
6. Use safer sex practices such as abstinence, mutual monogamy, and condoms to prevent further infection associated with sexual activity.

Outcome-Based Evaluation
• Verbalizes relief of pain

Genital Lesions Caused by Sexually Transmitted Diseases
Genital lesions are ulcerations or other skin or mucous membrane lesions that indicate infection with an STD and may actively shed the infecting organism.

Pathophysiology and Etiology
Causes include:
1. Syphilis—*Treponema pallidum*
2. Chancroid—*Haemophilus ducreyi*
3. Lymphogranuloma venereum (LGV)—specific subtypes of *C. trachomatis*
4. Genital herpes—herpes simplex virus (HSV-2)
5. Condylomata acuminata (genital warts)—specific subtypes of HPV

Clinical Manifestations
See Table 21-4 for clinical manifestations, diagnosis, and treatment of genital lesions.

Patient Education and Health Maintenance
1. Explain transmission of STDs and preventive measures such as male or female condoms, abstinence, and mutual monogamy.
2. Encourage compliance with treatment regimen and follow-up to ensure cure before resuming sexual activity.
3. Explain that some shedding of herpes virus may occur even while asymptomatic, so patient must discuss this

with partner; consider use of condoms at all times; and reduce risk of transmission by abstaining at the first sign of an outbreak (tingling sensation) until 1 to 2 weeks after resolution of symptoms.
4. For additional information and support, refer to STD National Hotline, 1-800-227-8922.

Carcinoma of the Penis
Carcinoma of the penis occurs primarily on the glans of the penis; it is frequently associated with poor personal hygiene and the accumulation of smegma under the skin of an uncircumcised penis. It primarily occurs in men over 60 and represents 0.5% of malignancies in men in the United States.

Pathophysiology and Etiology
1. Several types of penile lesions are potentially premalignant.
   a. Condylomata acuminata
   b. Giant condylomata acuminata (Buschke-Löwenstein tumor)
   c. Kaposi's sarcoma
   d. Leukoplakia
2. Erythroplasia of the glans (erythroplasia of Queyrat) is a carcinoma in situ of the penis and may involve the glans, prepuce, penile shaft, or may spread to the remainder of the genitalia and perineal region.
3. Malignant lesions that ulcerate metastasize quickly to the regional femoral and iliac lymph nodes.
4. Distant metastases occur in the inguinal lymph nodes; in rare cases to lungs, liver, bone, or brain.

Clinical Manifestations
1. Disease process begins with a painless, wartlike growth or ulcer on the glans, prepuce, or coronal sulcus.
2. Phimosis (constriction of foreskin with inability to retract over glans) may obscure a lesion, preventing detection until advanced stages.
3. Lymphadenopathy; secondary infection of lesions.

Diagnostic Evaluation
1. Biopsy of penile lesion
2. Ultrasonography and/or MRI of inguinal lymph nodes
3. Chest x-ray, CT scan (or MRI), bone scan to assess for distant nodal metastases

Management
1. Localized lesions are surgically removed by partial penectomy, laser or cryotherapy or Mohs' micrographic surgery; total penectomy with perineal urethrostomy is necessary for more involved tumors.
2. After other causes of lymphadenopathy are ruled out, bilateral inguinal lymphadenectomy may be performed.
3. Radiation therapy to small superficial tumors and lymph nodes may control the disease.

TABLE 21-4 Characteristics and Management of Genital Lesions Caused by STDs

Disorder and Incubation	Clinical Manifestations	Diagnosis and Treatment
Herpes genitalis—2–7 d	Clustered vesicles on erythematous, edematous base that rupture leaving shallow, painful ulcer that eventually crusts; mild regional lymphadenopathy; recurrent and may be brought on by stress, infection, pregnancy, sunburn.	Diagnostic tests include Tzank smear, viral culture, or antigen test of tissue or exudate from lesion. No cure, but symptomatic period is diminished by acyclovir (Zovirax or other antiherpetic) started with each recurrence; or recurrences greatly reduced or prevented by continuous treatment. Analgesics and sitz baths promote comfort.
Syphilis—10–90 d for primary; up to 6 mo following lesion (chancre) for secondary	*Primary:* Nontender, shallow, indurated, clean ulcer; mild regional lymphadenopathy. *Secondary:* Maculopapular rash including palms and soles, mucous patches, and condylomatous lesions; fever, generalized lymphadenopathy.	VDRL or rapid plasma reagin (RPR) blood test with confirmation by specific treponemal antibody tests. Preferred treatment is benzathine penicillin G (Bicillin LA) 2.4 million units IM in a single dose; doxycycline (Vibramycin), tetracycline (Tetracyn), and possibly erythromycin (Eryc) may be used.
Chancroid—2–10 d	Vesiculopustule that erodes, leaving a tender, shallow or deep, well-circumscribed ulcer with ragged, undermined borders and a friable base covered by purulent exudate; unilateral or bilateral large, tender inguinal lymph nodes (buboes) in 50% of patients.	May be identified on Gram, Giemsa, or Wright stain; must be cultured on special media. Treated with azithromycin (Zithromax), erythromycin (Eryc), or ceftriaxone (Rocephin) IM. Single-dose regimens are available. Apply warm soaks to buboes.
LGV—3–21 d	Small, transient, nontender papule or superficial ulcer precedes firm, adherent unilateral inguinal and femoral lymph nodes (buboes) with characteristic groove in between (groove sign); may suppurate.	Microimmunofluorescence testing of bubo aspirate. Treatment of choice is doxycycline (Vibramycin), but erythromycin (Eryc) may be effective. Incision and excision of buboes should be avoided: aspiration may be helpful.
Condyloma acuminatum—3 wk to 3 mo, possibly years grossly visible	Single or multiple, soft, fleshy, flat or vegetating growth(s) may occur on penis, anal area, urethra; no lymphadenopathy.	Diagnosed by Pap smear or biopsy. Topical therapy with podofilox 0.5% (Condylox) for external warts, podophyllin 10%–25% solution or trichloroacetic acid 80%–90% (TCA). May require multiple applications. Cryotherapy, electrodissection, electrocautery, carbon dioxide laser, and surgical excision may also be done. Recurrence is common.

Complications

1. Disfigurement due to ulceration or treatment
2. Complications of lymphadenectomy—necrosis and infection of skin flap, chronic edema of lower extremities

Nursing Assessment

1. Obtain history of current lesion, history of STDs, and hygiene.
2. Perform genital examination for characteristics of lesion, phimosis, inguinal lymph node enlargement.
3. Assess support system and personal coping mechanisms.

Nursing Diagnoses

- Fear related to diagnosis of cancer
- Body Image Disturbance related to partial or total penectomy

Nursing Interventions

Resolving Fears

1. Provide patient with opportunity to acquire information about causes and prognosis of disease.

2. Interpret diagnostic and staging results to patient.
3. Encourage realistic expectations regarding outcome of treatment.

Enhancing Coping With Body Image Changes

1. Maintain a nonjudgmental approach; allow patient to ventilate feelings about loss of part or all of penis.
2. Provide routine postoperative care confidently, watching for bleeding, monitoring urination, and anticipating pain.
3. Provide opportunity for patient to discuss alternative methods of sexual expression with knowledgeable professional.
   a. About 40% of patients are able to participate in sexual activity and stand to void after partial penectomy.
4. Monitor patient for symptoms of depression requiring intervention.

Patient Education and Health Maintenance

1. Instruct the uncircumcised patient about proper hygiene—importance of daily removal of all retained smegma.

2. Explain expected postoperative function of the penis in patient undergoing partial penectomy.

3. Describe how voiding will occur to the patient undergoing perineal urethroplasty.

4. Provide information about follow-up and monitoring for recurrences, or radiation and chemotherapy as appropriate.

Outcome-Based Evaluation

• Verbalizes understanding and acceptance of diagnosis and treatment plan

• Discusses feelings and interest in seeking counseling

SELECTED REFERENCES

American Cancer Society. (1999). *Cancer facts and figures 1999*. Atlanta, GA: Author.

Blaivas, J. G. (1996). Obstructive uropathy in the male. *Urologic Clinics of North America, 23*(3), 373–384.

Bodner, D. R., Selzman, A. A. & Spirnak, J. P. (1995). Evaluation and treatment of bladder rupture. *Seminars in Urology, 13*(1), 62–65.

Brassil, D. F. (1995) Sexually transmitted diseases. In K. A. Karlowicz (Ed.), *Urologic nursing: Principles and practice* (pp. 199–218). Philadelphia: W. B. Saunders.

Brown, S. L., Persky, L., & Resnick, M. I. (1998). Bladder injury: Intraperitoneal and extraperitoneal. *Atlas of the Urologic Clinics of North America, 6*(2), 59–70.

Carlin, B. I., & Resnick, M. I. (1995). Indications and techniques for urologic evaluation of the trauma patient with suspected urologic injury. *Seminars in Urology, 13*(1), 9–24.

Carraro, J. C., et al. (1996). Comparison of phytotherapy (permixon) with finasteride in the treatment of benign prostate hyperplasia: A randomized international study of 1098 patients. *Prostate, 29*, 231–240.

Centers for Disease Control and Prevention. (1998). Guidelines for treatment of sexually transmitted diseases. *MMWR, 47*(No. RR-1), 1–116.

Crowe, H., & Costello, A. (1994). Laser ablation of the prostate: Nursing management. *Urologic Nursing, 14*(2), 7–40.

Fantyl, J. A., Newman, D. K., Colling, J., et al. (1996, March). *Urinary incontinence in adults: Acute and chronic management*. Clinical Practice Guideline, No. 2, 1996 Update. AHCPR Publication No. 96-0682. Rockville, MD: US Department of Health and Human Services. Public Health Service, Agency for Health Care Policy and Research.

Fetrow, C. W., & Avila, J. R. (1999). *Professional's handbook of complementary and alternative medicines*. Springhouse, PA: Springhouse.

Gallo, M. L., Fallon P. J., & Staskin, D. R. (1997). Urinary incontinence: steps to evaluation, diagnosis and treatment. *The Nurse Practitioner, 22*, 21–44.

Grumet, S. C. & Brunner, D. W. (2000) The identification and screening of men at high risk for prostate cancer. *Urologic Nursing, 20*(1), 15–24, 46.

Haas, M., et al. (2000). Etiologies and outcomes of acute renal insufficiency in older adults: A renal biopsy study of 259 cases. *American Journal of Kidney Disease, 35*(3), 433–447.

Hollander, J. B., & Diokno, A. C. Prostatism: Benign prostatic hyperplasia. *Urologic Clinics of North America, 23*(1), 75–86.

Improte, L. M., & Reilly, N. J. (1995). Management of benign prostatic hyperplasia. *Innovations in Urology Nursing, 5*(4), 54–61.

Jacobs, S. T., Bartlett, J. W., Lim, E., Che, J., Schultz, C., & Kuo, L. B. (1997). Donor and recipient outcomes following laparoscopic donor nephrectomy. Presented at the ASTS 23rd Annual Scientific Meeting, Chicago, IL.

Lancaster, L. (Ed.) (1995). *ANNA core curriculum for nephrology nursing*. Pittman, NJ: A. J. Jannetti.

McConnell, J. D., Barry, M. J., Bruskewitz, R. C., et al. (1994). *Benign prostatic hyperplasia: Diagnosis and treatment*. Clinical Practice Guideline, No. 8. AHCPR Publication No. 94-0582. Rockville, MD: US Department of Health and Human Services, Public Health Service, Agency for Health Care Policy and Research.

Mellinger, B. C. (1994). Human papillomavirus in the male: An overview. *AUA Update Series, 13*(13), 102–107.

Moul, J. W., & Lipo, D. R. (1999). Prostate cancer in the late 1990s: Hormone refractory disease options. *Urologic Nursing, 19*(2), 125–131.

Newman, D. K. (1997). *The urinary incontinence sourcebook*. Los Angeles: Lowell House.

Newton, M., & Kosler, J. H. (1998). Nonsteroidal anti-androgens: Role in treating advanced prostate cancer. *Urologic Nursing, 18*(1), 56–57, 83.

Parker, J. (Ed.). (1998). *Contemporary nephrology nursing*. Pittman, NJ: A. J. Jannetti.

Peters, K. P. (2000) The diagnosis and treatment of interstitial cystitis. *Urologic Nursing, 20*(2), 101–107.

Reilly, N. J. (1995). Cancer of the bladder. In K. A. Karlowicz (Ed.), *Urologic nursing: Principles and practice* (pp. 243–269). Philadelphia: W. B. Saunders.

———. (1995). Genitourinary trauma. In K. A. Karlowicz (Ed.), *Urologic nursing: Principles and practice* (pp. 411–435). Philadelphia: W. B. Saunders.

———. (2000). Assessment and management of acute or transient urinary incontinence. In D. B. Dougherty (Ed.), *Urinary and fecal incontinence: Nursing management* (2nd ed.). St. Louis: Mosby.

Resnick, N. M. (1996). Geriatric incontinence. *Urologic Clinics of North America, 23*(1), 55–74.

Swibold, L. K. (1999). Mainte.nance therapy with bacillus Calmette-Guérin in patients with superficial bladder cancer. *Urologic Nursing, 19*(1), 38–41.

Teloken, C., et al. (1998). Therapeutic effects of high dose yohimbine hydrochloride on organic erectile dysfunction. *Journal of Urology, 159*, 124.

University of Michigan Medical Center, Section of Nephrology. (1999). *Endourological and urological laparoscopy* [On-line], **www.urology.med.umich.edu/clinic/urolap.htm**.

Volk, R. J., Cass, A. R., & Spann, S. J. (1999). A randomized controlled trial of shared decision making for prostate cancer screening. *Archives of Family Medicine, 8*(4), 333–340.

Wald, A., et al. (2000). Reactivation of genital herpes simplex virus type 2 infection in asymptomatic seropositive persons. *New England Journal of Medicine, 342*(5), 844–850.

Walsh, P. C., Retik, A. B., Vaughan, E. D., & Wein, A. J. (Eds.) (1998). *Campbell's urology* (7th ed., vols. 1–3). Philadelphia: W. B. Saunders.

Zaccagnini, M. (1999). Clinical snapshot: Prostate cancer. *American Journal of Nursing, 99*(4), 34–35.

Zellner, K. M. (1999). Acute tubular necrosis. *RN, 62*(10), 42–45.

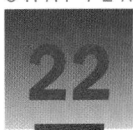
Gynecologic Disorders

GENERAL OVERVIEW

The Menstrual Cycle

The menstrual cycle is the cyclical pattern of ovarian hormone secretion (estrogen and progesterone) under the control of pituitary hormones (luteinizing hormone [LH] and follicle-stimulating hormone [FSH]) that results in thickening of the uterine endometrium, ovulation, and menstruation. Cycle length varies among women.

Phases of the Menstrual Cycle

1. Menstrual or bleeding phase: day 1 of cycle—endometrial sloughing and discharge.
2. Postmenstrual phase: 4 to 5 days after period ends—thin endometrium.
3. Proliferative phase: approximately 14 days before onset of next menstrual period, estrogen increases thickness

of endometrium; includes ovulation, the expulsion of ovum from ovary.
4. Secretory phase: approximately days 16 to 23; corpus luteum forms and then regresses unless pregnancy occurs; thick endometrium because of increased progesterone.
5. Premenstrual phase: days 24 to 28; levels of LH and FSH fall because of increased levels of estrogen and progesterone.

Characteristics of Menstruation
See Table 22-1.

ASSESSMENT

Subjective Data
Explore the patient's symptoms and perform a complete history to elicit important data, such as the following:

TABLE 22-1 Characteristics of Menstruation

Characteristic	Range	Average
Menarche (age at onset)	9–17 y	12.5 y
Cycle length	24–32 d	29 d
Flow—duration	1–8 d	3–5 d
Flow—amount	10–75 mL	35 mL
Menopause—(age at onset)	45–55 y	47–50 y

Irregular Bleeding

1. Characteristics: what is the frequency, duration, and amount of flow? What is the color and consistency of blood? What is the size of clots? Bleeding or spotting between periods, postmenopausal bleeding, or pain with bleeding? What was age at menarche? What was age at menopause?
2. Associated factors: what is the pregnancy and childbirth history? Is the patient sexually active? What method of contraception is used? Is the patient taking hormone replacement or oral contraceptives? Is the patient obese? Is the patient extremely athletic?
3. History: history of tumors or malignancy? Family history of breast or ovarian cancer?
4. Significance: may indicate infection of the vagina or cervix; malignancy of the vulva, vagina, cervix, or uterus; benign tumor of the uterus or ovarian cyst; pregnancy; endometriosis.

Vaginal Discharge

1. Characteristics: what is the color, amount, duration of the discharge? Any odor, itching, urinary symptoms, pain, fever, dyspareunia?
2. Associated factors: what is the sexual history, such as number of partners, type of sexual activity, symptoms in partner? Is barrier method of contraception used?

Is patient menopausal or postmenopausal? Does patient take estrogen replacement? Recent use of antibiotics?
3. History: history of sexually transmitted diseases (STDs)? Diabetes?
4. Significance: may indicate vaginitis, human papillomavirus (HPV), herpes simplex virus (HSV), pelvic inflammatory disease (PID), or genital malignancy.

Pelvic Pain

1. Characteristics: what is frequency, duration, severity, location of pain? Was the onset sudden or gradual? What aggravates and what relieves it? Does it feel like heaviness in the pelvis?
2. Associated factors: fever, nausea, vomiting, dizziness, abnormal bleeding with it? Has there been weight loss? Use of estrogen preparations? Is patient infertile? When was the last menstrual period (LMP)? Did the patient perform a home pregnancy test?
3. History: history of STDs, obstetric trauma, or abdominal surgery? Pregnancy history and history of ectopic pregnancy?
4. Significance: may indicate condition arising from relaxed pelvic muscles, PID, endometriosis, ectopic pregnancy, miscarriage, cervical or uterine cancer.

▪ Physical Examination

Physical examination for a patient with a gynecologic disorder should focus on the abdomen and genitalia. Palpate the lower abdomen for masses or tenderness. Inspect the external genitalia for lesions, discharge, or tissue bulging from the vagina.

The nurse in a gynecologic or obstetric setting may perform a vaginal examination to obtain specimens for diagnostic studies and assess the patient's condition (Procedure Guidelines 22-1).

PROCEDURE GUIDELINES 22-1	VAGINAL EXAMINATION BY THE NURSE

EQUIPMENT

Perineal drape	Sterile gloves	Pap smear equipment
Vaginal specula	Long swab sticks	Adequate lighting
Water-soluble lubricant		

PROCEDURE

PREPARATORY PHASE

1. Have the patient void before assistant positions her on examining table.
2. Position the patient on examining table (slip may be kept on, but other clothing from waist to knees is removed).
   a. Have buttocks at edge of table.
   b. Position feet in stirrups to assume dorsal lithotomy position.
   c. Make the patient as comfortable as possible with a small pillow under her head.
   d. Drape the patient to permit minimal exposure (but adequate for examiner).
3. Encourage the patient to relax; tell her what you are doing and what she may feel.
4. Adjust light for maximum focus.
5. Offer the patient a mirror to watch the examination to teach vulvar self-examination and to teach about contraceptives as appropriate.

PROCEDURE GUIDELINES 22-1   *CONTINUED*

Nursing Action	Rationale

PERFORMANCE PHASE

1. Be gentle and take your time; wash hands; don clean gloves; lubricate fingers.
2. Observe external genitalia for apparent abnormalities, gently separate labia and continue visual inspection.

3. To encourage relaxation in the patient, gently place the tip of one or two fingers into introitus.
4. Identify cervix manually and depress the perineum downward with your fingers.
5. Lubricate speculum with warm water.

6. Gently insert warm speculum horizontally, passing it over your fingers and aiming it toward the cervix.

7. Slowly open the speculum and lock into position. With slow manipulation, the speculum can be turned to permit visualization of the vaginal walls.
8. Inspect the cervix, which should be pink. Normally, the os is a dent, unless the woman has had children, in which case a slit is noted.

9. If Pap test is to be done, follow procedure in accompanying figure. Newer, automated systems can increase the accuracy of Pap results.

1. This promotes relaxation of the patient, making the procedure easier for both.
2. Note any evidence of irritation, infection, or abnormalities such as swelling, bleeding, erythema, discharge (other than clear and odorless).
3. Say to the patient, "Tighten your muscles and squeeze my fingers—try hard—then relax."
4. Downward pressure is away from the more sensitive anterior structures.
5. Any lubricant other than water may interfere with cytology results.
6. If it is preferred not to initially insert gloved fingers, the speculum is introduced vertically using a downward pressure; after entering the vestibule, the speculum is slowly rotated to the horizontal position.
7. Walls normally are pink and moist. A pale white secretion may be noted.

8. If woman is taking an oral contraceptive, the cervix may be deep pink to red. A thread coming out of the cervix would suggest presence of an intrauterine device (IUD). Abnormal cervical signs include erosion, lacerations, and polyps.

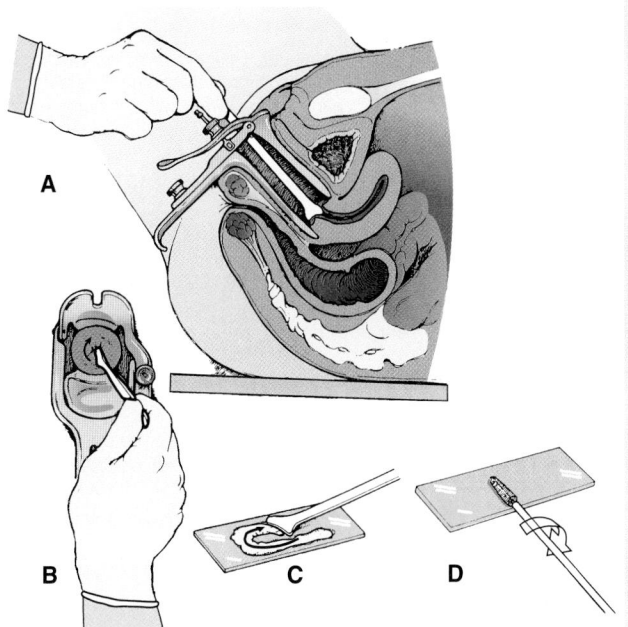

A cervical scrape of secretions for cytology is obtained by using a wooden Ayre spatula. (A) Shows the speculum in place: the Ayre spatula is inserted so that the longer end is placed snugly in the os. (B) A representative sample of secretions is obtained by rotating the spatula. (C) Cervical secretions are gently smeared on a glass slide in a single circular motion. (D) A cytobrush is rotated within the cervical os and smeared onto a glass slide. The slide is placed in the appropriate fixative immediately. Some newer processing systems call for dipping the sample in preservative rather than smearing on a slide.

continued

PROCEDURE GUIDELINES 22-1 — **VAGINAL EXAMINATION BY THE NURSE** *CONTINUED*

Nursing Action	Rationale
10. If indicated, swab cervix with Schiller's iodine solution to detect epithelial change. Or, swab vagina and cervix with acetic acid solution to detect lesions caused by human papillomavirus.	10. Cancer epithelium contains no glycogen and will not absorb iodine as normal epithelium will. Human papillomavirus lesions will be differentiated from normal epithelium by aceto-whitening.
11. When removing speculum, hold it open until cervix is cleared, then withdraw speculum downward, applying pressure to posterior vaginal wall and allowing speculum to close as it is withdrawn.	11. By the time speculum is completely withdrawn, it will be closed.
12. For palpation (bimanual examination), see accompanying figure.	

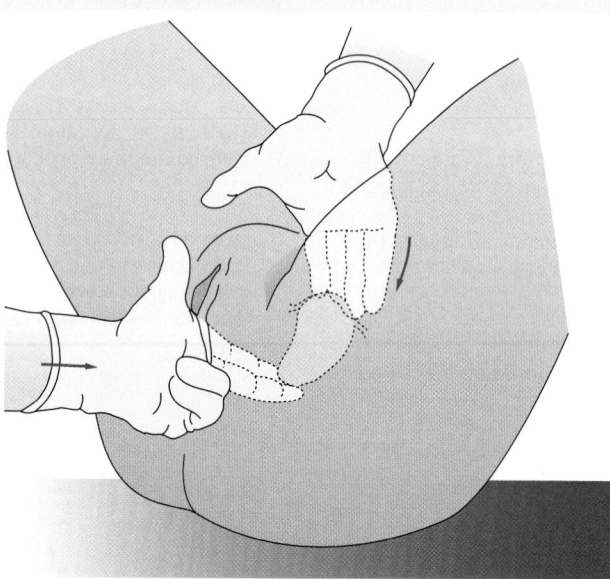

Bimanual examination of the pelvic organs. (1) Insert two fingers of dominant hand into vagina (one finger for virginal introitus). (2) Place second hand over midline lower abdomen. Gently capture the uterus between your two hands to feel contour and size and to elicit tenderness. (3) Move hands to either side of midline to palpate the adnexa, feeling for swelling, masses, or tenderness of the ovaries and fallopian tubes.

FOLLOW-UP PHASE

1. Gently wipe the perineal area with soft tissue or gauze, using firm strokes from the pubic area back to beyond the rectum.	1. This will remove secretions and liquid lubricant.
2. Instruct assistant in carefully helping the patient to remove feet from stirrups.	2. Both feet must be removed at the same time to reduce strain.
3. Elevate the lower third of the examining table to receive legs. Keep the patient covered with a sheet.	3. This permits the patient to assume dorsal recumbent position.
4. Assist the patient in sliding toward head end of table; provide a wide-based stool for her to step on as she gets off table.	4. Do not rush the patient as she is getting off the table, because sudden shifting from recumbent to sitting position may cause a feeling of dizziness.
5. Assist the patient in dressing if necessary. Answer any questions she may have.	

DIAGNOSTIC TESTS

Diagnostic tests for gynecologic disorders include various laboratory tests, radiology or imaging studies, and office or ambulatory surgery procedures. Women with gynecologic disorders, such as endometriosis, may undergo multiple invasive and surgical procedures to fully evaluate the problem.

Laboratory Tests

CA 125
Description
Tumor antigen used as a marker for ovarian cancer.
Nursing and Patient Care Considerations
1. Tell patient a blood test will be taken and the results will be ready in 1 to 3 days.
2. Not a screening test for ovarian cancer, it is better used as a measure of response to treatment.
3. Level may be elevated in benign gynecologic disease, hepatic cirrhosis, and in healthy women.

Cervical Cytology
Description
A Papanicolaou smear of the cervix is obtained during pelvic examination to screen for cervical dysplasia or cancer. May also help to detect endometrial cancer, infections, and endocrine status.
Nursing and Patient Care Considerations
1. Should not be performed during menses.
2. Instruct the patient to avoid douching and sexual intercourse for 24 to 48 hours before the examination.
3. Recommend regular screening based on established guidelines.
   a. American College of Obstetrics and Gynecology (ACOG) and Planned Parenthood—annually; after hysterectomy, every 3 to 5 years if hysterectomy was not for cancer.
   b. American Cancer Society—yearly; less frequent screening following three negative smears in low-risk women
   c. Recommend PAP smears at onset of sexual activity or by 18 years of age.
4. Classification by Bethesda system (preferred) or Papanicolaou number system.
   a. Bethesda system (descriptive diagnosis).
      (i) Infection.
      (ii) Reactive and reparative changes (ie, inflammation).
      (iii) Epithelial cell abnormalities (including atypia, squamous intraepithelial lesion, and squamous cell carcinoma).
      (iv) Nonepithelial malignant neoplasm.
      (v) Hormonal evaluation.
   b. Papanicolaou (original classification system).
      (i) Class 1—without atypical or abnormal cells.
      (ii) Class 2—atypical cytology but no evidence of malignancy.
      (iii) Class 3—cytology suggestive of, but not conclusive for, malignancy.
      (iv) Class 4-cytology strongly suggestive of malignancy
      (v) Class 5—carcinoma in situ.
5. If the patient has an abnormal smear, explain that this is not always conclusive but requires further testing, such as colposcopy, biopsy, or conization. Encourage the patient to return for further testing.

Tests for Gonorrhea and Chlamydia
Description
1. Commonly known as DNA probe or antigen detection tests, a single specimen can detect both STD-causing organisms. Will detect even subclinical infection; can be used as screening test.
2. Can also be done by culture method, but takes longer and requires separate specimens and special processing for each.
3. Screening has also been done in some clinics by urine dipstick test on voided urine specimen for leukocytes, particularly in males. Urine testing for chlamydia by DNA detection is more expensive but may also be used for screening.
Nursing and Patient Care Considerations
1. Explain the procedure to the patient before taking the specimen.
2. Specimens should be taken from the woman without douching for 24 hours, from the man before urinating.
3. Obtain specimen with Dacron-tipped swab from cervical discharge in woman, urethral meatus in man. Small-tipped swabs are available for the urethra.
4. Send swab to laboratory in provided container with preservative.

Radiology and Imaging

Hysterosalpingogram
Description
1. This fluoroscopic x-ray study of the uterus and fallopian tubes is used to determine tubal patency, detect pathology in the uterine cavity, and identify peritoneal adhesions.
2. A bivalve speculum is introduced while the patient is in the lithotomy position, and contrast medium is injected into the uterine cavity; the medium will enter the peritoneum in 10 to 15 minutes if tubes are patent.
Nursing and Patient Care Considerations
1. Determine date of last menstrual period; the test is done a few days after menses ends, before ovulation.
2. Administer enema before procedure to decrease intestinal gas.
3. Administer prescribed medication to reduce anxiety.
4. After procedure, apply perineal pad for drainage of excess contrast medium or blood and instruct patient to

notify health care provider if bloody drainage continues after 3 days or if any signs of infection are present.

5. Inform the patient that pain medication may be necessary for shoulder discomfort because of dye irritation of the phrenic nerve.

Pelvic Ultrasonography
Description
A noninvasive test that uses high-frequency sound waves to form images of the interior pelvic cavity; used to detect uterine, tubal, ovarian, and pelvic cavity pathology, to measure organ size, and to evaluate pregnancy.
Nursing and Patient Care Considerations
1. Inform patient that a full bladder is necessary to discriminate the bladder from the uterus.
2. Drinking 64 oz. of water before the procedure without voiding is recommended. If transvaginal ultrasound will be performed, inform the patient that a vaginal probe will be inserted to obtain more accurate measurements from internal organs.
3. After the procedure, help the patient wipe off ultrasound gel from abdomen and allow her to empty her bladder.
4. Abnormalities are represented as different densities that differentiate solid from cystic masses and can help make a diagnosis; however, explain to the patient that further testing may be necessary.

■ Other Diagnostic Tests
Colposcopy
Description
Examination of the cervix with a bright light and magnification of 10 to 40 times; done to determine distribution of abnormal squamous epithelium and to pinpoint areas from which biopsy tissue can be taken. May be done with cervicography (photographing the cervix).
Nursing and Patient Care Considerations
1. Procedure is preferably done when cervix is least vascular (usually a week after the end of the menstrual flow).
2. Explain that a vaginal speculum will be inserted and that a biopsy may be taken, causing only slight discomfort.
3. Help patient into lithotomy position, drape her appropriately, and provide emotional support throughout the procedure. Provide distraction techniques, such as music and posters (hung on the ceiling), as appropriate.
4. After the cervix and vagina are swabbed with acetic acid solution and inspected through the colposcope, biopsies may be taken. Biopsy tissue is preserved in 10% formalin, labeled, and sent to the laboratory. Saline may be used to rinse the area, and bleeding may be stopped with silver nitrate.
5. After procedure, assist patient to rise slowly and give the following discharge instructions:
   a. Avoid heavy lifting for 24 hours.
   b. There may be some bleeding and cramping; however, more than that of a normal period must be reported to health care provider.
   c. Obtain health care provider's instructions regarding douching and sexual relations.

Conization
Description
Excision of a cone-shaped piece of tissue from the cervix for diagnostic and therapeutic purposes, including the area where the squamous and columnar epithelial tissue meet (transformation zone). The transformation zone is the area of most cervical cancers.
Nursing and Patient Care Considerations
1. Explain to the patient that this test is a minor surgical procedure that requires local anesthesia.
2. After excision, bleeding is controlled by cauterization or suturing and packing.
3. The patient may be observed for several hours after the procedure for excessive bleeding.
4. Advise the patient to avoid tampons, douching, and intercourse for 2 weeks to allow healing.

Culdoscopy
Description
Operative procedure in which an incision is made through the perineum into the posterior vaginal cul-de-sac so that a culdoscope can be inserted to visualize the uterus, tubes, broad ligaments, uterosacral ligaments, rectal wall, sigmoid, and even the small intestine.
Nursing and Patient Care Considerations
1. Prepare patient for any vaginal surgery (see Standards of Care Guidelines).
2. Explain to patient that she will receive local, general, or regional anesthesia and that she will be helped into the knee-chest position.
3. After the procedure, the scope is withdrawn and sutures are placed.
4. The patient will be observed for several hours; make sure follow-up instructions have been given by the health care provider.

Hysteroscopy
Description
Endoscopic visualization of the uterine cavity used to stage endometrial cancer, check tubal patency, determine the cause of uterine bleeding, remove polyps or fibroids, and observe the placement/appearance of intrauterine devices (IUDs).
Nursing and Patient Care Considerations
1. Administer prescribed sedative before the procedure and explain that a local anesthetic will also be injected into the cervix in the operating room.
2. The patient will be assisted into lithotomy position and the perineum and vagina will be cleansed immediately before sterile draping.
3. Explain that sounds are inserted into the cervical canal for dilation before insertion of the hysteroscope. With the scope in place, a concentrated solution of dextran is slowly infused into the endometrial cavity to distend it and allow for viewing.
4. Observe patient for several hours and give discharge instructions.

a. Over-the-counter analgesics may be needed for minor discomfort if analgesic has not been prescribed.
b. Notify the health care provider of severe cramping or bleeding, fever, or unusual discharge.

Endometrial Biopsy
Description
1. Procedure is done with or without local anesthetic to obtain cells from the uterine lining to assist in the diagnosis of endometrial cancer, menstrual disorders, and infertility.

2. During speculum examination, a uterine sound is placed, followed by a curette or suction device to withdraw specimen.

Nursing and Patient Care Considerations
1. Assist patient into dorsal lithotomy position and explain procedure.
2. Administer prostaglandin inhibitor to decrease uterine cramping postoperatively.
3. Label specimen, place in formalin, and send to laboratory.
4. Inform patient that she may experience light bleeding and occasional cramping for a few days.
5. Instruct patient to report fever, chills, and increased bleeding.

Dilation and Curettage
Description
1. This common gynecologic surgery for diagnostic and therapeutic purposes consists of widening the cervical canal with a dilator and scraping the uterine cavity with a curette.
2. Performed to control uterine bleeding, secure endometrial and endocervical tissue for cytologic examination, and treat incomplete abortion.

Nursing and Patient Care Considerations
1. Prepare the patient for the procedure—answer questions, request that she void, administer an enema if ordered, and administer a sedative as directed.
2. Immediately postoperatively, monitor vital signs at frequent intervals—potential for hemorrhage exists.
3. Monitor perineal pads/bed for amount of bleeding; report excessive bleeding.
4. Offer prescribed analgesics for low back and pelvic pain; cramping may occur for 2 to 3 days because of dilation of the cervix.
5. Instruct patient to maintain bed rest for remainder of day to decrease cramping and bleeding.
6. Instruct patient to use perineal pads at home and to report fever, heavy bleeding, and severe cramping.
7. Instruct patient to avoid strenuous activity until bleeding stops.
8. Inform patient that the procedure does not affect sexual functioning, but that she should refrain from sexual intercourse, douching, and tampons for at least 2 weeks, according to preference of health care provider.

Laparoscopy
Description
Endoscopic visualization of the pelvic and abdominal cavities through a small incision below the umbilicus; used to evaluate pelvic pain and infertility, treat endometriosis adhesions, and perform tubal sterilizations (the most common use).

Nursing and Patient Care Considerations
1. Prepare patient by ensuring that she has taken nothing by mouth (NPO), answering questions about the procedure, and administering a sedative and enema if ordered.
2. Inform patient that she may experience shoulder or abdominal discomfort after the procedure from the injection of carbon dioxide given to separate the intestines from

pelvic organs. Elevation of feet higher than shoulders after the procedure helps relieve this.

3. Patient will receive local, general, or regional anesthesia, and will be placed in Trendelenburg position to displace the intestines for better visualization.

4. After procedure, monitor bleeding and vital signs; administer analgesics.

5. Inform patient that passing gas and bowel movements may be difficult initially because of the manipulation of the intestines; ambulation and fluids will be helpful.

6. Advise patient not to have intercourse or to perform strenuous activity for 2 to 3 days and to report bleeding, cramping, or fever.

GENERAL PROCEDURES AND TREATMENT MODALITIES

◼ Fertility Control

Nurses who work with women in the gynecologic setting or in any setting may be involved in contraceptive counseling.

Basic Principles

1. *Contraception* is the prevention of fertility on a temporary basis.

2. *Sterilization* is the permanent prevention of fertility. Both female and male sterilization procedures can be performed. Some procedures can be reversed but with possible complications and variable success rates.

3. Contraception effectiveness depends on motivation, which is a result of education, culture, religion, and personal situation. It is best to include both partners in any contraception decision.

4. Nurses should be familiar with contraceptive methods and educate patients without moral judgment.

5. Failure rate (pregnancy) is determined by experience of 100 women for 1 year and is expressed as pregnancies per 100 woman-years.

Contraceptive Methods
See Table 22-2.

Sterilization Procedures
General Considerations

1. Tubal sterilization is frequently performed for birth control. Hysterectomy and oophorectomy, performed for other reasons, also result in sterility.

2. Male sterilization by vasectomy also has become more common.

3. Informed consent is needed. The couple should be thoroughly counseled about the permanence of the procedure.

Tubal Sterilization

1. Approaches
   a. Abdominal is most frequently used: may be postpartum laparotomy, minilaparotomy, or laparoscopy. Laparoscopy with electrocoagulation is frequently performed. It is a safe and effective procedure.
   b. Vaginal incision in posterior vagina (colpotomy) with the uterine tube pulled through it; higher rate of complications—infection.

2. Techniques vary by surgeon preference.
   a. Electrocoagulation is most common; burn section of tube with or without excision; low reversal rate.
   b. Pomeroy: the tube is tied in midsection and section removed; may be reversed.
   c. Fimbriectomy: the fimbriated end removed and end tied; irreversible.
   d. Cornual resection: removal of the section of tube nearest uterus and suture cornual opening closed.
   e. Silastic bands: plastic or metal clips to occlude tube; may be reversed.

3. Complications
   a. Failure to successfully block the tubes—pregnancy or tubal pregnancy.
   b. Hemorrhage, infection, uterine perforation, damage to bowel or bladder.

4. Nursing interventions
   a. Assess motivation for sterilization and level of knowledge about the procedure. Counsel as necessary.
   b. Teach patient there is no effect on hormones and menstruation will continue.
   c. Teach patient there should not be any adverse effect on sexual response.
   d. Other birth control methods are discontinued immediately before the procedure.
   e. Prepare the patient to expect some abdominal soreness for several days; instruct her to report any bleeding, increasing pain, or fever.
   f. Sexual intercourse and strenuous activity should be avoided for 2 weeks.

Contraceptive Research

1. Vaginal rings that release progestin are becoming available. Placed around the cervix, vaginal rings may be effective for 3 months, are removed during coitus, and require careful vaginal hygiene. Other implantable hormones in various delivery systems to provide contraception for several months to several years are being developed to rival Norplant.

2. RU-486 (Mifepristone) is a progesterone antagonist that prevents implantation and leads to menses. Administered by mouth within 10 days of an expected period, it produces a medical abortion in most patients. If combined with a prostaglandin suppository, it causes an abortion in up to 95% of patients up to 5 weeks after conception. It is widely used in France and other some other countries, but has had difficulty getting FDA approval in the United States.

3. Birth control vaccines are being developed to interfere with hormones and sperm antigens to prevent pregnancy. A male vaccine to interfere with spermatogenesis is a possibility.

◼ Vulvar and Vaginal Irrigation

Vulvar irrigation cleanses the perineal area after urination or a bowel movement to minimize infection after surgery. Vaginal irrigation cleanses or disinfects the vagina and adjacent tissues before surgery and soothes inflamed tissue after surgery (see Procedure Guidelines 22-2 and 22-3).

(*text continues on page 756*)

TABLE 22-2 Contraceptive Methods

Methods	Definition	Procedure	Advantages	Disadvantages
Natural Methods				
1. Periodic abstinence	Abstain from inter-course during fertile period of each cycle.	Determine fertile period by: 1. Calendar method—ovulation occurs 14 d before next menstrual period. 2. Cervical mucus method—increase in mucus at time of ovulation; clear and stringy. 3. Basal body temperature—drops immediately before ovulation and rises 24–72 h after ovulation. 4. Symptothermal method—combines 2 and 3.	1. No health hazards. 2. Inexpensive. 3. May be religiously acceptable. 4. Increased knowledge of cycles.	1. 20% failure rate. 2. Requires consistent record-keeping. 3. Decrease in spontaneity.
2. Coitus interruptus	Withdrawal of penis from vagina when ejac-ulation is imminent.	Must withdraw before ejaculation so that ejaculation occurs away from female genitalia.	1. No cost. 2. No health hazards. 3. Always available.	1. Failure rate of 19%; preejaculatory fluid may contain sperm. 2. Interruption of sexual act.
3. Lactation	Breast-feeding has a contraceptive effect due to prolactin's inhi-bition of luteinizing hormone, which main-tains menstruation.	Breast-feed on demand, around the clock, without formula supplementation.	1. No health hazards. 2. No cost.	1. Unreliable. 2. Need to use other method such as spermicide or barrier, which has no effect on breast milk.
Barrier Methods				
1. Condom	Latex or polyurethane or processed collage-nous tissue sheaths, placed over erect penis to prevent semen from entering vagina. Female condom is placed in the vagina.	1. Place condom over erect penis. 2. Leave dead space at tip of condom (from which air has been expelled) to allow room for ejaculate. 3. Use spermicide on exterior for added protection. 4. Grasp ring around condom at with-drawal to avoid leaving condom in vagina.	1. Failure rate is low with *proper* use (3%). 2. Prevention of STD. 3. Inexpensive. 4. No health hazard. 5. May help premature ejaculation by de-creasing sensitivity. 6. Increases male involvement in contraception.	1. Decreased sensi-tivity. 2. Interruption of sexual act. 3. Sensitivity to latex may be a problem. 4. Failure rate with *typi-cal* use is 12%. 5. Female condoms are more expensive, made of poly-urethane.
2. Diaphragm	Rubber cap shaped like a dome with a flexible rim	1. Check for holes. 2. Place spermicide inside dome. 3. Place diaphragm against and covering cervical opening, behind lower edge of pubic bone.	1. Failure rate with per-fect use is 6%; 18% with typical use. 2. Protection against STDs and possibly cervical neoplasia.	1. Occasional toxic shock or allergic reactions 2. May experience pelvic discomfort. 3. Possible increase in urinary tract infections.

(*continued*)

TABLE 22-2 Contraceptive Methods (Continued)

Methods	Definition	Procedure	Advantages	Disadvantages
		4. Leave in place for at least 6 h after intercourse.		4. Must be properly cleaned with soap and water, dried and stored to preserve integrity of rubber.

NURSING ALERT

Warn patients who use condoms, diaphragms, and the cervical cap that latex sensitivity may be a problem—watch for itching, swelling, generalized reactions.

Methods	Definition	Procedure	Advantages	Disadvantages
3. Cervical cap	Rubber cap, shaped like a cup with a tall dome and flexible rim.	Place spermicide inside cap and place cap over cervical opening prior to intercourse.	1. Failure rate similar to diaphragm. 2. May decrease risk of STDs.	1. Risk of toxic shock, cervicitis, and PID 2. Requires frequent follow-up. 3. Must be properly cleaned with soap and water, dried, and stored.
Spermicides	Nonoxynol-9 or octoxynol-9 available in a variety of forms: foam, jelly, cream, suppository, tablet.	Place next to cervix before intercourse; better if used with a barrier method.	May kill STD agents.	1. Less effective if not, used with barrier method; generally 21% failure rate. 2. Some patients are allergic. 3. May cause birth defects if pregnancy results.
Intrauterine Devices	Small device made of plastic with exposed copper or progesterone-release system; acts to inhibit uterine wall implantation.	1. Healthcare provider inserts device; slowly and usually at time of menses. 2. Check IUD string regularly—at least once a month—or after each intercourse when it is first inserted.	1. Failure rate low, 2% or less. 2. Convenient; permits spontaneous intercourse. 3. Replaced every 10 y.	1. Risk of PID and resultant tubal damage and infertility. 2. May cause spotting, bleeding, or pain. 3. Risk of spontaneous abortion. 4. Risk of uterine rupture.
Hormones 1. Combination oral contraceptives.	Tablets containing estrogen to inhibit ovulation and progestin to make cervical mucus impenetrable to sperm—lowest effective doses are used.	Take for 21 d with 7 d off or 28 d (if 7 d of placebos are included).	1. As low as 0.1% failure rate. 2. Decreased risk of endometriosis, ovarian and endometrial cancer, benign breast disease. 3. Possible decreased risk of PID 4. Aid in menstrual disorders 5. Improves acne	1. Increased risk of cardiovascular disease (higher in women who smoke). 2. Questionable risk of breast, cervical cancer. 3. May experience nausea, vomiting, headache, weight gain. 4. Must remember to take at same time daily.
2. Progestin-only oral contraceptive (Mini-pill).	Smaller doses of progestins than in combined oral contraceptives.	Take daily.	1. As low as 0.5% failure rate. 2. Avoids estrogen-related side effects and possibly cardiovascular risks. 3. May offer protection against PID. 4. Safe in breast-feeding.	1. May cause irregular menses, spotting, amenorrhea.

(continued)

TABLE 22-2 Contraceptive Methods (Continued)

Methods	Definition	Procedure	Advantages	Disadvantages
3. Postcoital contraception (Morning-after pill).	May be combined estrogen and progestin, high-dose estrogen, or progestin.	Must be started within 24–72 h after intercourse.	1. Very effective.	1. May be religiously opposed. 2. Can cause nausea. 3. May cause birth defects.
4. Progesterone implant (Norplant).	Progesterone release system made up of five silastic rods.	Implanted in subcutaneous fat of upper arm.	1. Long-term (up to 5 y). 2. Convenient. 3. Only 0.9% failure rate.	1. May cause irregular bleeding, spotting, amenorrhea, acne, headaches. 2. May be difficult to remove. 3. High initial expense.
5. Progesterone injection (Depo-Provera).	Intramuscular injection of long acting progesterone.	Initial injection within first 5 d of menses, then every 3 mo.	1. Convenient. 2. Only 0.3% failure rate.	1. Requires every 3-mo follow-up. 2. May cause irregular bleeding, spotting, amenorrhea. 3. Long-term effects still unknown. 4. High discontinuation rate in adolescents due to side effects and missed appointments.

PROCEDURE GUIDELINES 22-2   VAGINAL IRRIGATION

EQUIPMENT

Reservoir for irrigating fluid—can or bag.
Irrigating fluid as prescribed (1,000–4,000 mL) at 40.5°–43.3°C (105°–110°F)
Tubing, connecting tubes, and clamp (sterile)

Irrigating vaginal nozzle (sterile)
Bedpan or douche pan
Waterproof pad

Sterile cotton balls, cleansing solution
Gloves

PROCEDURE

Nursing Action	Rationale

PREPARATORY PHASE

1. Check physician's directives for amount and temperature of irrigating fluid. Prepare equipment.
2. Identify patient and explain the procedure. Place patient in dorsal recumbent position with waterproof pad under her.   2. To permit gravity to assist in allowing fluid to reach distal areas of vagina.
3. Wash hands.
4. Have the patient void before beginning irrigation.   4. A full bladder would prevent adequate distention of vagina by solution.
5. Drape the patient   5. To prevent chilling and undue exposure.
6. Arrange irrigating receptacle at a level just above the patient's hips (not more than ½ m, ie, 18 in above hips) so that fluid flows easily but gently.   6. The higher the fluid source, the greater the pressure.

PERFORMANCE PHASE

1. Put on gloves.   1. Clean gloves may be used.
2. Cleanse vulva by separating labia and allowing solution to flow over area; if insufficient, use cotton balls saturated in soap solution, cleanse from front toward anal area.   2. Materials found around vaginal meatus may be introduced into vagina and cervix. This is to be avoided.

continued

PROCEDURE GUIDELINES 22-2   **VAGINAL IRRIGATION** *CONTINUED*

Nursing Action	Rationale
3. Allow some solution to flow through tubing and out over nozzle to lubricate it.	3. Moisture provides lubrication and less resistance when one surface is moved against another.
4. Insert nozzle gently into vagina in a downward and backward direction, approximately 2 in.	4. When the patient is in a dorsal recumbent position, the natural anatomic position of the vagina is in the downward-backward direction.
5. Clamp tubing when solution is almost all used, remove nozzle and permit the patient to sit on bedpan for return flow.	5. Gravity will assist return flow to drain from vaginal tract.

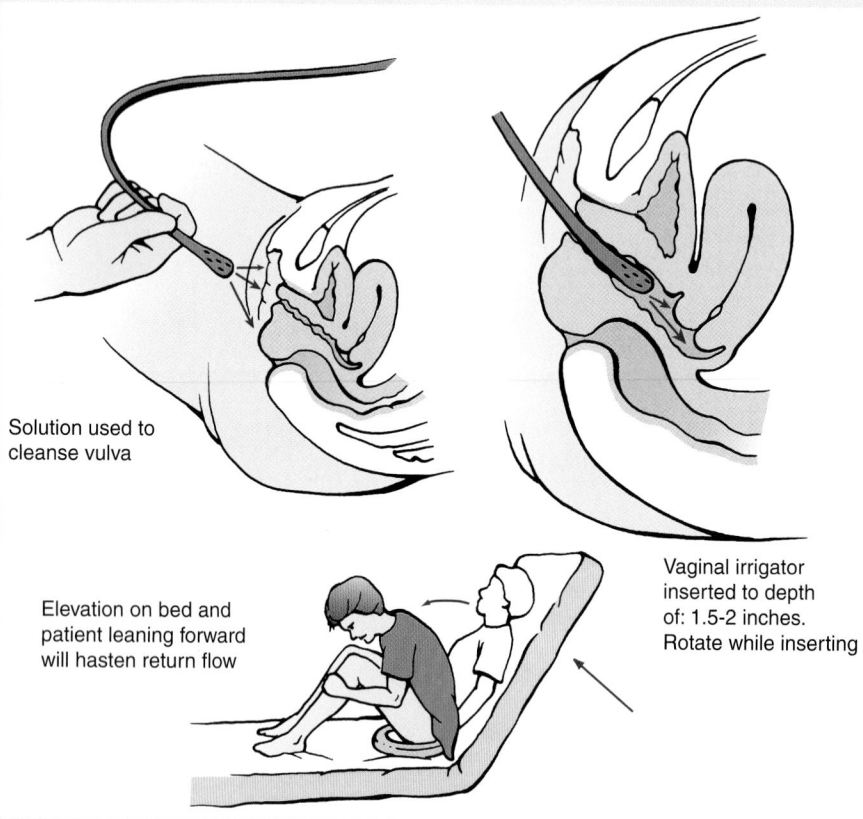

Solution used to cleanse vulva

Elevation on bed and patient leaning forward will hasten return flow

Vaginal irrigator inserted to depth of: 1.5-2 inches. Rotate while inserting

Vaginal irrigation. The nurse wears gloves while doing this procedure.

FOLLOW-UP PHASE

1. Wipe the patient dry, using cotton balls in a front-to-back direction.	1. Drying the area prevents skin excoriation and promotes comfort.
2. Remove bedpan from the patient and apply sterile perineal pad.	2. Perineal pad will absorb any additional drainage or discharge.
3. Remove gloves and wash hands.	
4. Document amount of returned fluid.	

PROCEDURE GUIDELINES 22-3   VULVAR IRRIGATION (PERINEAL CARE)

EQUIPMENT

Container with irrigating fluid (300–500 mL) 40.5°–43.3°C
(105°–110°F) alternately, a squeeze bottle may be used.
Sterile sponge forceps and cotton pledgets
Bedpan

Waterproof pad
Paper bag for cotton pledget disposal
Gloves (optional)

PROCEDURE

NURSING ACTION	RATIONALE

PREPARATORY PHASE

1. Wash hands. Prepare equipment.
2. Place waterproof pad under patient.
3. Place patient on bedpan in dorsal recumbent position with knees flexed and separated.

   3. To expose area to be cleaned.

4. Drape patient with perineal area exposed.
5. Apply gloves (optional).

   5. If forceps is used, hands will not come into contact with body fluids.

PERFORMANCE PHASE

1. Separate labia with nondominant hand. Pour warmed irrigating solution gently over vulva from a sterile pitcher.

   1. Materials will be flushed from perineal area into bedpan.

2. Cleanse perineal area with cotton pledget held in a sponge holder, use a front-to-back direction and discard each sponge in a plastic or paper bag after one use. Use sterile materials if there is an open wound.

   2. Friction facilitates cleansing process and the removal of exudate. Follow aseptic technique, cleanse urethral and vaginal areas first, then external labia, then anus.

3. Dry perineal area using dry cotton pledgets in same fashion as for cleansing.

   3. Cleansing from front to back assists in preventing intestinal organisms from entering vaginal area.

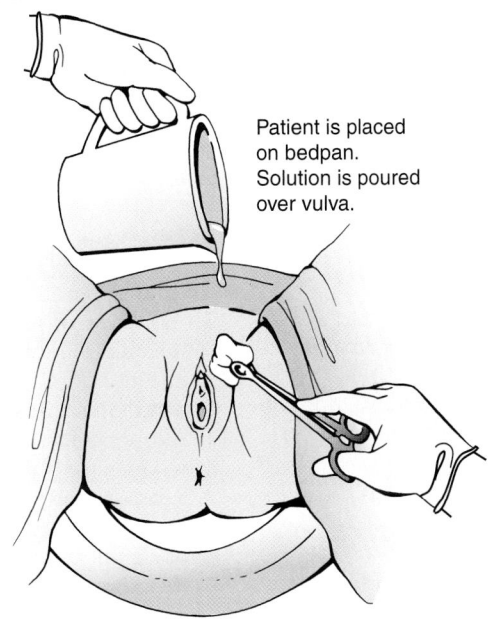

Patient is placed on bedpan. Solution is poured over vulva.

FOLLOW-UP PHASE

1. Apply sterile perineal pad.
2. Wash hands.

   1. To maintain cleanliness and provide comfort for patient.

Hysterectomy

Hysterectomy is the surgical removal of the uterus. Sixty-five percent of these procedures occur during reproductive years.

Types of Hysterectomy

Abdominal

1. Subtotal hysterectomy—corpus of uterus is removed, but cervical stump remains.
2. Total hysterectomy—entire uterus is removed, including cervix; tubes and ovaries remain.
3. Total hysterectomy with bilateral salpingo-oophorectomy—entire uterus, tubes, and ovaries are removed.

Vaginal

Removal of uterus through the cervix and vagina; cervical stump may remain.

Preoperative Management

1. Procedure and reason for hysterectomy, what the procedure involves, and what to expect postoperatively are explained.
2. Patient must remain NPO from midnight the night before surgery and must void before surgery.
3. An enema is administered before surgery to evacuate the bowel and prevent contamination and trauma during surgery.
4. Vaginal irrigation is performed before surgery and ensure that a skin preparation is done if ordered.
5. Preoperative medication is given to help the patient relax.

Postoperative Management

1. Postoperatively, the following assessment is made:
   a. Wound appearance and drainage.
   b. Vital signs, level of consciousness.
   c. Level of pain.
   d. Vaginal drainage (serous, bloody).
   e. Intake and output.
   f. Urge to void, bladder distention, residual urine (if appropriate).
   g. Clarity, color, and sediment of urine.
   h. Homans' sign or impaired circulation.
   i. Return of bowel sounds, passage of flatus, first bowel movement.
2. Exercise and ambulation are encouraged to prevent thromboembolus, facilitate voiding, and stimulate peristalsis.

Complications

1. Incisional/pelvic infection.
2. Hemorrhage.
3. Urinary tract injury.
4. Bowel obstruction.
5. Thrombophlebitis.

Nursing Diagnoses

- Pain related to surgical procedure
- Altered Pattern of Urinary Elimination related to decreased bladder sensation
- Risk for Infection related to surgical procedure
- Self-Esteem Disturbance related to alteration in female organs
- Sexual Dysfunction related to alteration in reproductive organs and function

Nursing Interventions

Relieving Pain

1. Assess pain location, level, and characteristics.
2. Administer prescribed pain medications. Ensure that patient knows how to use patient controlled analgesia pump and is using it properly.
3. Encourage patient to splint incision when moving.
4. Encourage patient to ambulate as soon as possible to decrease flatus and abdominal distention.
5. Institute sitz baths or ice packs as prescribed to alleviate perineal discomfort.
6. Monitor level of sedation related to narcotic administration—may interfere with ambulation and elimination.

Promoting Urinary Elimination

1. Monitor intake and output, bladder distention, signs and symptoms of bladder infection.
2. Maintain patency of indwelling catheter if one is in place.
3. Catheterize patient intermittently if uncomfortable or if she has not voided in 8 hours.
4. Check for residual urine after patient voids; should be less than 100 mL. Continue to check if more than 100 mL or bladder infection may develop.
5. Encourage patient to empty bladder around the clock, not only when feeling the urge, because of loss of sensation of bladder fullness.
6. Encourage fluid intake to decrease risk of urinary infection.

Preventing Infection

1. Assess vaginal drainage amount, color, and odor, incision site, and temperature.
2. Administer antibiotics as prescribed.
3. Assist use of incentive spirometer, coughing and deep breathing, and ambulation to decrease risk of pulmonary infection.

Strengthening Self-Esteem

1. Allow patient to discuss her feelings about herself as a woman.
2. Reassure patient she is still feminine.
3. Encourage patient to discuss her feelings with her spouse or significant other.
4. Reassure patient that she will not go through premature menopause if her ovaries were not removed.

Regaining Sexual Function

1. Discuss changes regarding sexual functioning, such as shortened vagina and possible dyspareunia because of dryness.
2. Offer suggestions to improve sexual functioning.
   a. Use of water-soluble lubricants.

b. Change position—female dominant position offers more control of depth of penetration.

Patient Education and Health Maintenance

1. Advise patient that a total hysterectomy with bilateral salpingo-oophorectomy produces a surgical menopause. Patient may experience hot flashes, vaginal dryness, and mood swings unless hormonal replacement therapy is instituted.
2. Advise her against sitting too long at one time, as in driving long distances, because of the possibility of blood pooling in the lower extremities, causing thromboembolism.
3. Suggest the patient delay driving a car until the third postoperative week because even pressing the brake pedal puts stress on the lower abdomen.
4. Tell the patient to expect a tired feeling for the first few days at home and not to plan too many activities for the first week. She can perform most of her usual daily activities within 4 to 6 weeks, and feel like herself again within 2 to 3 months.
5. Tell the patient not to feel discouraged if at times during convalescence she experiences depression, feels like crying, and seems unusually nervous. This is common, but will not last.
6. Remind the patient to ask her surgeon about any strenuous or lifting activities, which are usually delayed for 4 to 6 weeks.
7. Reinforce instructions given by the surgeon on intercourse, douching, and use of tampons, which are usually discouraged for 4 to 6 weeks. Sexual intercourse should be resumed cautiously to prevent injury and discomfort. Showers are permitted, but tub baths are deferred until healing is sufficient.
8. Instruct the patient to report fever higher than 37.8°C (100°F), heavy vaginal bleeding, drainage, increased pain or cramping, and foul odor of discharge.
9. Emphasize the importance of follow-up visits and routine physical and gynecologic examinations.

Outcome-Based Evaluation

- Verbalizes decreased pain
- Voids every 8 hours of sufficient quantity
- No fever or signs of infection
- Verbalizes positive statements about self and positive outlook on recovery
- Verbalizes understanding of possible changes in sexual functioning and what to do about it

MENSTRUAL CONDITIONS

Dysmenorrhea

Dysmenorrhea is painful menstruation; most common of gynecologic dysfunctions.

Pathophysiology and Etiology

Primary

1. No pelvic lesion; usually intrinsic to uterus.
2. Current research supports increased prostaglandin production by the endometrium as the chief cause.
3. May also be because of hormonal, obstructive, and psychological factors.

Secondary

1. Caused by lesion, such as endometriosis, pelvic infection, congenital abnormality, uterine fibroids, ovarian cyst.

Clinical Manifestations

1. Pain may be caused by increased uterine contractility and uterine hypoxia.
2. Characteristics of pain—colicky or dull, usually in lower midabdominal region, spasmodic or constant.
3. Nausea, vomiting, diarrhea, headache, chills, tiredness, nervousness, and low backache may be experienced.

Diagnostic Evaluation

Tests to rule out underlying lesion:

1. Chlamydia and gonorrhea tests—may show infection.
2. Pelvic ultrasound—may detect tumor, endometriosis, cysts.
3. Serum or urine pregnancy test to rule out ectopic pregnancy.
4. Possibly, hysteroscopy and laparoscopy—primarily to detect endometriosis.

Management

The following measures are for primary dysmenorrhea; treatment of secondary dysmenorrhea is aimed at underlying pathology.

1. Local heat, such as heating pad to increase blood flow and decrease spasms.
2. Exercise to increase endorphin release, which decreases pain perception, and to suppress prostaglandin release.
3. Nonsteroidal anti-inflammatory agents (ibuprofen, naproxen) for their antiprostaglandin action.
4. Oral contraceptives to decrease contractility and menstrual flow.
5. In some cases, dilation and curettage may be helpful.
6. Usually self-limiting without complications.

Nursing Assessment

1. Obtain menstrual and gynecologic history that could suggest underlying pathology.
2. Assess level of pain using scale of 1 to 10; assess patient's emotional response to pain and ability to carry out activities.
3. Obtain vital signs, including temperature, to rule out infection.
4. Perform abdominal and pelvic examination (if indicated) to obtain specimens.

Nursing Diagnosis
- Pain related to menstrual flow

Nursing Interventions
Controlling Pain
1. Administer pharmacologic agents as ordered to control pain and menstrual flow.
2. Apply heating pad to lower back or abdomen as desired by patient.
3. Assess patient's response to pain control measures.

Patient Education and Health Maintenance
1. Explain to patient possible causes of dysmenorrhea.
2. Teach patient nonpharmacologic methods to reduce pain.
   a. Apply heating pad to lower midabdomen or back or take warm tub baths.
   b. Exercise regularly (30 minutes, three times a week).
3. Teach patient to use prescribed medications effectively by taking medication at beginning of discomfort and repeating as necessary, especially on first day of menses.
4. Teach patient side effects of medications.
5. Encourage patient to reduce stress through adequate sleep, good nutrition, exercise, and coping with stressors.
6. Discuss patient's feelings toward menstruation (hygienic issues, inconvenience, female identity).

Outcome-Based Evaluation
- Describes methods to reduce pain and verbalizes reduced pain level

Premenstrual Syndrome

Premenstrual syndrome (PMS) is a group of symptoms that includes headache, irritability, depression, breast tenderness, and bloating that are clearly related to onset of menstruation.

Pathophysiology and Etiology
1. Linked to hormonal imbalances, prostaglandins, endorphins, and psychological factors, such as attitudes and beliefs related to menstruation, and environmental factors, such as nutrition and pollution.
2. Most common in women in their 30s.
3. May occur in 25% to 50% of menstruating women.

Clinical Manifestations
1. Symptoms may begin 7 to 14 days before onset of menstrual flow; may diminish 1 to 2 days after menses begins.
2. Physical—edema of extremities, abdominal fullness, breast swelling and tenderness, headache, vertigo, palpitations, acne, backache, constipation, thirst, weight gain.
3. Behavioral—irritability, fatigue, lethargy, depression, anxiety, crying spells.
4. Diagnosis based on clinical manifestations; usually no diagnostic evaluation is necessary.

Management
1. Restrict sodium, caffeine, tobacco, alcohol, and refined sweets.
2. Aerobic exercise.
3. Vitamin B_6 supplements.
4. Progesterone replacement therapy or oral contraceptives to suppress natural hormones.
5. Prostaglandin inhibitors, such as ibuprofen.
6. Diuretics to decrease fluid retention and weight gain.
7. Anxiolytic agents or selective serotonin reuptake inhibitors (SSRIs), such as paroxetine (Paxil), to control emotional symptoms.
8. Counseling.
9. Calcium supplementation of 1,200 mg elemental calcium per day has been shown to decrease mood swings, irritability, depression, and anxiety.
10. Usually self-limiting without complications.

Nursing Assessment
1. Ask patient to describe symptoms and their onset and means of relief.
2. Assess patient's diet, activity, and rest habits.
3. Assess patient's emotional response to symptoms and methods of coping.

Nursing Diagnosis
- Anxiety related to symptoms and lack of control over condition

Nursing Interventions
Reducing Anxiety
1. Administer medications as ordered; warn patient that diuretics will cause increased urination and anxiolytics may cause drowsiness or cognitive impairment.
2. Provide emotional support for patient and significant others.

Patient Education and Health Maintenance
1. Encourage patient to keep a diary for several consecutive months, which includes dates, cycle days, stressors, symptoms, and their severity to determine if therapy is effective.
2. Instruct patient in the use and side effects of prescribed medications.
3. Teach patient possible causes of syndrome and nonpharmacologic methods to alleviate distress, such as dietary modifications, exercise, and rest.
4. Teach stress reduction techniques, such as imagery and deep breathing.
5. Discuss alternative therapies with patient. Therapies include vitamin preparations, herbal supplements, natural progesterone-based creams, and even a mask with flickering lights that can be worn for 15 minutes per day. None of these has been proved to help a wide range of women with PMS; however, most products are safe in moderation and can be used as adjuncts to conventional therapy.

6. Refer for further resources and support to groups such as PMS Access, P. O. Box 9326, Madison, WI 53715, 1-800-222-4767.

Outcome-Based Evaluation
• Verbalizes reduced anxiety, increased control over condition

Amenorrhea
Amenorrhea is absence of menstrual flow.

Pathophysiology and Etiology
Primary
1. Menarche does not occur by age 16.
2. Caused by chromosomal, hormonal, nutritional, psychogenic disorders, or pregnancy.

Secondary
1. Menstruation stops for 6 months in a woman in whom normal menstruation has been established.
2. May be caused by normal pregnancy or lactation, menopause, psychogenic, hormonal, nutritional, or exercise-related disorders.
   a. Excessive exercise or inadequate nutrition with decreased body fat stores is a significant cause of amenorrhea in young women.
   b. Anovulation secondary to polycystic ovary disease (PCO)—often occurs in obese women. Pituitary tumor and thyroid disease (hyperthyroidism) are hormonal causes.
3. Some medications, such as phenothiazines and oral contraceptives, may also induce amenorrhea.

Diagnostic Evaluation
1. Pregnancy test.
2. Progesterone challenge test.
   a. Positive result—bleeding occurs; chronic anovulation is most likely.
   b. Negative result—no bleeding occurs; may indicate organ failure; other tests are needed.
3. Hormonal levels—LH and FSH—to detect ovarian failure.
4. Prolactin level (elevated) with pituitary tumor.
5. Thyroid stimulating hormone—decreased in hyperthyroidism.
6. Genetic karyotyping to detect chromosome abnormalities.

Management
1. Discontinue causative medications.
2. Nutritional, exercise, or psychological counseling as indicated.
   a. Recommend decreased exercise in athletes to increase body fat stores and decrease stress.
   b. Recommend weight reduction if obese.
3. Hormonal replacement therapy to regulate cycle.

4. Newer medications targeted at insulin resistance are being used for polycystic ovary disease.

Complications
It has been theorized that prolonged amenorrhea may lead to atypia and cancer of the endometrium because of unopposed estrogen stimulation on the endometrium.

Nursing Assessment
1. Assess for signs of chromosomal disorders, such as abnormal genitalia, masculinization, short stature, and characteristic facies.
2. Assess for signs of pituitary tumor, such as headache, visual disturbances, dizziness.
3. Assess weight and body build, change in weight, and nutritional and exercise habits that may indicate anorexia or loss of body fat because of exercise.
4. Assess emotional status, areas of stress, and coping ability.

Nursing Diagnoses
• Altered Nutrition: Less Than Body Requirements related to poor dietary habits and/or rigorous exercise
• Ineffective Individual Coping related to school, job, relationships

Nursing Interventions
Meeting Nutritional Requirements
1. Explore patient's body image, knowledge of the five food groups, behavior regarding meals, and exercise routine; point out misconceptions, dangerous behavior, and ideas for improvement.
2. Monitor weight gain, increase in body fat, and return of menstrual cycles.

Strengthening Coping
1. Provide emotional support for patient and family.
2. Point out ineffective coping mechanisms and teach relaxation techniques and more positive coping mechanisms, such as confrontation.

Patient Education and Health Maintenance
1. Teach patient the physiology of the normal menstrual cycle and possible causes for amenorrhea.
2. Teach proper use and side effects of medications prescribed.
3. Teach the patient to chart menstrual periods on a calendar and maintain regular gynecologic and medical follow-up visits.

Outcome-Based Evaluation
• Verbalizes adequate dietary intake, decreased exercise
• Weight increased and menses resumed

Dysfunctional Uterine Bleeding
Dysfunctional uterine bleeding (DUB) is abnormal uterine bleeding that has no organic cause, such as tumor, infection, or pregnancy.

Pathophysiology and Etiology

1. DUB is frequently caused by immature hypothalamic stimulation in adolescents.
2. DUB is caused by anovulation in any age group, especially in teens and perimenopausal women, because of impaired follicular formation or rupture, or corpus luteum dysfunction.
3. Ovarian failure in perimenopausal women frequently causes DUB.
4. Temporary estrogen withdrawal at ovulation may cause midcycle ovulatory bleeding.
5. Emotional lability, malnutrition, and changes in exercise may cause changes in gonadotropin release at the hypothalamic level, causing altered menstrual pattern.

Clinical Manifestations

1. Abnormal bleeding may occur in any of the following patterns:
   a. *Oligomenorrhea*—significantly diminished menstrual flow; also may be irregular, but consistent periods with long intervals.
   b. *Menorrhagia*—excessive bleeding during regular menstruation; can be increased in duration or amount.
   c. *Metrorrhagia*—bleeding from uterus between regular menstrual periods; significant because it is usually a symptom of disease.
   d. *Polymenorrhea*—frequent menstruation occurring at intervals of less than 3 weeks.

Diagnostic Evaluation

Tests are done to rule out pathologic causes of abnormal bleeding.

1. Pregnancy test.
2. Complete blood count (CBC) to detect anemia and platelet count and coagulation screen to rule out blood dyscrasia.
3. Pap smear to rule out malignancy.
4. Thorough examination to rule out trauma or foreign body.
5. Chlamydia and gonorrhea tests to rule out PID.
6. Pelvic ultrasound to rule out ovarian cysts and tumors and uterine fibroids and tumors.
7. Hysteroscopy to detect uterine fibroids, polyps, and other lesions.
8. Endometrial biopsy to determine hormonal effect on uterus and rule out malignancy.
9. Laparoscopy to evaluate for endometriosis.

Management

1. Treat underlying anemia with iron, possible transfusions (only significant complication).
2. Progesterone therapy to stop acute bleeding.
3. Oral contraceptives to control chronic bleeding.
4. Androgen therapy with a gonadotropin releasing hormone, such as danazol (Danocrine) to reduce menstrual blood loss.

5. Dilation and curettage.
6. Endometrial ablation or hysterectomy may be needed for refractory cases.

Nursing Assessment

1. Ask the patient for menstrual and gynecologic history, sexual activity, and possibility of pregnancy.
2. Assess frequency, duration, and amount of menstrual flow.
3. Assess for other symptoms of underlying pathology, such as pelvic pain, fever, and abdominal masses or tenderness.
4. Assess for signs and symptoms of anemia—fatigue, shortness of breath, pallor, tachycardia.

Nursing Diagnoses

- Fatigue related to excessive blood loss
- Fear of bleeding through clothing related to excessive or unpredictable bleeding

Nursing Interventions

Increasing Energy Level

1. Encourage good dietary intake with increased sources of iron-fortified cereals and breads, meat (especially red meat), and green leafy vegetables.
2. Administer oral iron preparations with meals to prevent nausea. Treat constipation as necessary.
3. Monitor hemoglobin and infuse packed red blood cells as ordered.
4. Help limit patient's exertion and administer oxygen by nasal cannula if ordered.

Relieving Fear

1. Review pattern of menstrual flow with patient and help her plan for excessive bleeding.
2. Suggest wearing double tampons (if able) and double sanitary pads.
3. Tell patient to expect heavy gush of blood on arising from lying or reclining position.
4. Prepare patient to carry an adequate supply of sanitary products and a change of clothing until bleeding is under control.

Patient Education and Health Maintenance

1. Teach the patient the cause of dysfunctional uterine bleeding and about the diagnostic process to rule out pathologic causes of abnormal bleeding.
2. Teach the patient to prevent anemia by eating a diet high in iron, and by consuming vitamin C or citrus fruit to enhance absorption of iron.
3. Teach about hormonal therapy and what side effects to expect, and what to expect of bleeding. Bleeding should stop within 2 to 7 days after short-term progesterone therapy, and should stop within first week of oral contraceptives but should start again in fourth week as regular menstrual period.
4. Advise patient to keep a calendar or log of menses.

Outcome-Based Evaluation
- Verbalizes adequate energy to perform activities
- Verbalizes more confidence in ability to conceal bleeding

Menopause

Menopause is described as the physiologic cessation of menses. Menopause has occurred if menses has not occurred for 12 months.

Pathophysiology and Etiology
1. Menopause is caused by the cessation of ovarian function and decreased estrogen production by the ovary.
2. Climacteric is the transition period (perimenopause) during which the woman's reproductive function gradually diminishes and ceases. It usually occurs at age 50.
3. Artificial or surgical menopause may occur secondary to surgery or radiation involving the ovaries. Some chemotherapeutic agents also cause a chemical menopause.

Clinical Manifestations
1. Genitalia—atrophy of vulva, vagina, urethra results in dryness, bleeding, itching, burning, dysuria, thinning of pubic hair, loss of labia minora, decreased secretions during intercourse.
2. Sexual function—dyspareunia, decreased intensity and duration of sexual response, but can still have active function.
3. Vasomotor—60% to 70% of women experience "hot flashes," which may be preceded by an anxious feeling and accompanied by sweating. These may occur at night, causing a "night sweat."
4. Psychological—insomnia, irritability, anxiety, memory loss, fear, and depression may be experienced.
5. Some women experience palpitations.

Diagnostic Evaluation
Levels of LH and FSH may be increased, and estradiol may be decreased; however, levels may fluctuate during perimenopause, so diagnosis is based on symptoms.

Management
1. Estrogen replacement therapy.
   a. Indicated to reduce symptoms and to prevent osteoporosis and coronary artery disease.
   b. Topical preparations may be used for atrophic vaginitis.
   c. Progesterone preparation also given if uterus is intact to prevent endometrial hyperplasia and possible cancer.
   d. Available as synthetic, animal based, and natural (plant source products).
2. Vaginal lubricants, such as Replens, to decrease vaginal dryness and dyspareunia.
3. Vitamin E and B supplements—to decrease hot flashes.
4. Calcium supplements to prevent bone loss.
5. Dietary supplements (considered natural products by consumers) to take the place of estrogen in relieving menopausal symptoms. Limited data available on efficacy. Patient should discuss with health care provider.

   a. Soy products (isoflavones)—may cause headache, oily skin.
   b. Evening primrose oil—causes slight nausea, headache.
   c. Ginseng—diarrhea, nervousness, palpitations may occur.
   d. Black cohosh—nausea, hypotension, spontaneous abortion.
   e. Dong quai—may cause photosensitivity, bleeding.
   f. Red clover—breast tenderness, stimulates estrogen receptor–positive malignancies.

Complications
1. Osteoporosis has been clearly linked to estrogen depletion in menopause.
2. Coronary artery disease rarely develops in women before menopause and has been associated with the effects of estrogen depletion on blood vessels.
3. Vulvovaginitis or trauma related to a dry, estrogen-depleted epithelium.

Nursing Assessment
1. Obtain history of patient's symptoms and menstrual cycle.
2. Obtain history for other risk factors for coronary artery disease and osteoporosis.
3. Assess genitalia for atrophy, dryness, and elasticity.
4. Assess patient's emotional response to menopause.

Nursing Diagnosis
- Altered Sexual Patterns related to symptoms and psychological impact of menopause

Nursing Interventions
Maintaining Sexuality Patterns
1. Provide patient with information related to estrogen replacement therapy, including dosage schedule, route, side effects, and what to expect of menstrual bleeding. Women who still have a uterus can expect a period at the end of every month if they take hormones cyclically. Another method of hormone replacement, giving estrogen and lower dose progesterone daily, may cause some irregular spotting for 3 months to up to 1 year, after which most women experience no bleeding.
2. Explore with patient her feelings about menopause, clear up misconceptions about sexual functioning, and encourage her to discuss her feelings with her partner.
3. Instruct patient how to use water-based lubricant for intercourse to decrease dryness.

Patient Education and Health Maintenance
1. Teach patient that sexual functioning does not decrease during menopause but may even increase because of loss of fear of pregnancy and increased time if children are grown.
2. Teach patient about foods that are high in calcium—dairy products, broccoli, and some fortified cereals—and encourage her to maintain weight-bearing activities to prevent osteoporosis.

3. Counsel patient on reducing risk factors for coronary artery disease.

4. Encourage patient to keep regular medical and gynecologic follow-up visits.

5. Advise patient that vulvovaginal infection and trauma are possible because of the dryness of the tissue, and to seek prompt evaluation if pain and discharge occur.

6. Encourage patients to talk to their health care providers about concerns, such as breast cancer with HRT. Currently approximately 40% of women who could benefit from HRT use these hormones.

7. Encourage patients to report use of supplements to their health care providers so they can use these preparations appropriately and safely. Caution patients that dehydroepiandrosterone (DHEA) has no proven efficacy in menopause or other condition and may cause significant side effects.

GERONTOLOGIC ALERT

In the postmenopausal woman, if vaginal bleeding not associated with hormone replacement occurs, encourage the patient to see her health care provider immediately because cancer may be suspected.

Outcome-Based Evaluation

• Verbalizes confidence in sexual function and identity, decreased symptoms

---

INFECTIONS AND INFLAMMATION OF THE VULVA, VAGINA, AND CERVIX

Vulvitis

Vulvitis is inflammation of the vulva.

Pathophysiology and Etiology
Causative Factors

1. Infections—*Trichomonas,* molluscum contagiosum, bacteria, fungi.
2. Irritants.
   a. Urine, feces, vaginal discharge.
   b. Close-fitting, synthetic fabrics.
   c. Chemicals, such as laundry detergents, vaginal sprays, deodorants, perfumes.
3. Carcinoma.
4. Chronic dermatologic conditions.

Predisposing Factors

1. Illnesses, such as diabetes mellitus and dermatologic disorders.
2. Atrophy because of menopause.

Clinical Manifestations
1. Pruritus—more acute at night, aggravated by warmth.
2. Reddened, edematous tissue, possible ulceration.
3. Pain, burning, dyspareunia.
4. Exudate—possibly profuse and purulent.
5. Lesions of molluscum contagiosum are multiple, from 1 mm to 1 cm in size, and filled with white caseous material.

Diagnostic Evaluation
1. Vulvar smears and cultures—may show infectious organism.
2. Biopsy of vulvar tissue—may be necessary to rule out malignancy and chronic dermatologic conditions.

Management
1. Oral or topical anti-infectives (antibiotics, antitricomonads, antifungals) to treat infectious agents.
2. Topical steroids to treat inflammation.
3. Topical or systemic estrogen to treat atrophy.
4. Treatment of underlying disorder.
5. Molluscum contagiosum may be treated by scalpel excision or silver nitrate or electrical cautery.

Complications
Scarring and chronic discomfort.

Nursing Assessment
1. Question the patient regarding medical history, symptoms, sexual activity.
2. Determine use of any chemical-containing products on undergarments or directly on vulva.
3. Examine the genitalia and lymph nodes.

Nursing Diagnosis
• Pain related to vulvar inflammation

Nursing Interventions
Relieving Pain

1. Administer prescribed medications and instruct patient on their use, method of application, and side effects.
2. Provide sitz baths or cool compresses to soothe and cleanse vulva.

Patient Education and Health Maintenance
1. Teach patient hygienic principles.
   a. Wipe from front to back after voiding.
   b. Use cotton with warm water and bland soap for cleansing, and pat dry.
   c. Apply nonirritating powder, such as cornstarch.
2. Teach patient to avoid chemical irritants, such as sprays, perfumed soaps, new laundry detergents, static-control dryer sheets.
3. Teach patient to avoid mechanical irritants, such as tight clothing, synthetic fabrics and undergarments; replace these with loose-fitting cotton undergarments. Avoid chronic moisture; change bathing suit after swimming.
4. Teach patient how to use sitz bath and cool compresses at home and to avoid scratching.

5. Teach patient that some infections, such as *Trichomonas* and molluscum contagiosum, are sexually transmitted, so partner needs to seek treatment before intercourse is resumed.

Outcome-Based Evaluation
- Verbalizes increased comfort level

Bartholin Cyst/Abscess

Bartholin cyst or abscess, also called *bartholinitis*, is an infection of the greater vestibular gland, causing cyst or abscess formation.

Pathophysiology and Etiology
1. These glands lie on both sides of the vagina at the base of the labia minora; they lubricate the vagina.
2. If they become obstructed secondary to infection, abscess or cyst formation may occur (Figure 22-1).
3. Abscess or cyst may spontaneously rupture or enlarge and become painful.
4. Most commonly caused by sexual transmission of infection.

Clinical Manifestations
1. Asymptomatic cyst.
2. Pain, erythema, tenderness, swelling.
3. Edema, cellulitis, possible abscess formation.

Diagnostic Evaluation
Take a culture, if draining, to identify infectious organisms.

Management
1. May be treated conservatively with warm soaks or sitz baths; antibiotics used if cellulitis is present.
2. May need incision and drainage; provides immediate relief, but may recur.
3. Marsupialization, for recurrent abscesses.

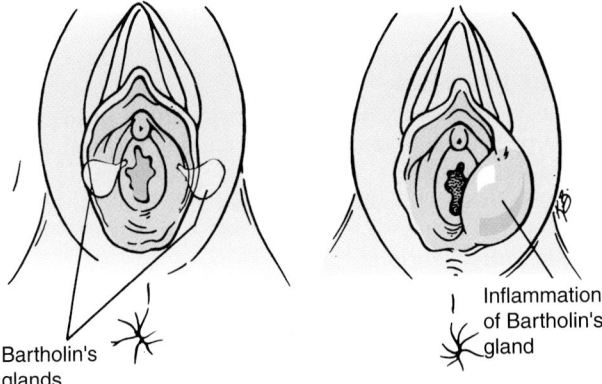

FIGURE 22-1 Site and infection of vestibular gland.

Bartholin's glands

Inflammation of Bartholin's gland

a. Contents are opened and drained, then edges of abscess are sutured to edges of external incision to keep cavity open.
b. Healing occurs from within the area of the abscess.

Complications
Scarring from recurrent infection and rupture

Nursing Assessment
1. Obtain history of sexual activity including new partners, history of STDs.
2. Inspect labia minora for warmth, erythema, swelling.
3. Assess for signs of other STDs—rash, genital ulcers, vaginal discharge.

Nursing Diagnoses
- Pain related to infection, enlargement of gland
- Risk for Infection Transmission related to STD

Nursing Interventions
Relieving Pain
1. Administer pain medications and antibiotics as ordered; explain side effects to patient.
2. Instruct patient to apply warm soaks or to use sitz bath 3 to 4 times a day for 15 to 20 minutes to promote comfort and drainage.
3. Encourage patient to remain in bed as much as possible because pain is exacerbated by activity.
4. Prepare patient for incision and drainage if indicated.
5. For marsupialization: apply ice packs intermittently for 24 hours to reduce edema and provide comfort; thereafter, warm sitz baths or a perineal heat pack or lamp provide comfort.

Preventing Infection Transmission
1. Explain to patient that infection may have been caused by sexually transmitted infection.
2. Tell patient to instruct her partner to be tested for STDs.
3. Advise the patient to abstain from intercourse until cyst or abscess has resolved, partner has been examined and treated, and she has completed all her antibiotics.

Patient Education and Health Maintenance
1. Review principles of perineal hygiene with patient.
2. Discuss STDs and methods of prevention—abstinence, use of female or male condoms.
3. Encourage patient to follow up for recurrent abscess because surgical treatment is often necessary.

Outcome-Based Evaluation
- Verbalizes relief of pain
- At follow-up visit, verbalizes abstinence from intercourse and shows good signs of healing with no recurrence of infection

Vaginal Fistula

A vaginal fistula is an abnormal, tortuous opening between the vagina and another hollow organ (Figure 22-2).

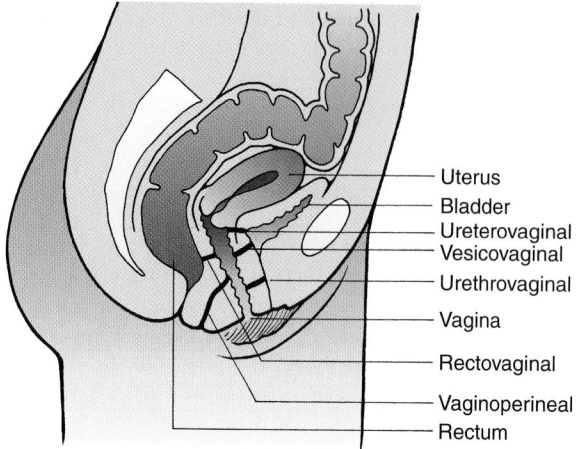

Uterus
Bladder
Ureterovaginal
Vesicovaginal
Urethrovaginal
Vagina
Rectovaginal
Vaginoperineal
Rectum

FIGURE 22-2 Sites of vaginal fistulas.

Pathophysiology and Etiology

Causes
1. Obstetric injury, especially in long labors and in countries with inadequate obstetric care.
2. Pelvic surgery—hysterectomy or vaginal reconstructive procedures.
3. Carcinoma—extensive disease or complication of treatment, such as radiation therapy.

Types
1. *Vesicovaginal* fistula is an opening between the bladder and vagina.
2. *Rectovaginal* fistula is an opening between the rectum and vagina.
3. *Ureterovaginal* fistula is an opening between the ureter and vagina.
4. *Urethrovaginal* fistula is an opening between the urethra and vagina.
5. *Vaginoperineal* fistula is an opening between the vagina and perineum.

Clinical Manifestations
1. Vesicovaginal—most common type of fistula.
   a. Constant trickling of urine into vagina.
   b. Loss of urge to void because bladder is continuously emptying.
   c. May cause excoriation and inflammation of vulva.
2. Rectovaginal.
   a. Fecal incontinence and flatus through the vagina; malodorous.
   b. May present as vulvar cancer.
3. Ureterovaginal fistula—rare.
   a. Urine in vagina but patient still voids regularly.
   b. May cause severe urinary tract infections.
4. Urethrovaginal fistula.
   a. Dysuria
   b. Urine in vagina on voiding
5. Vaginoperineal fistula—pain and inflammation of perineum.

Diagnostic Evaluation
1. Methylene blue test—after instillation of this dye in bladder.
   a. Methylene blue appears in vagina in vesicovaginal fistula.
   b. Methylene blue does not appear in vagina in ureterovaginal fistula.
2. Indigo carmine test—after a methylene blue test shows negative results, indigo carmine is injected intravenously. If dye appears in vagina, this indicates ureterovaginal fistula.
3. Intravenous urography helps detect presence and location of fistula, hydroureter, and hydronephrosis.
4. Cystoscopy—performed to determine number and location of fistulas.

Management
1. Fistulas recognized at time of delivery should be corrected immediately.
2. Treatment of postoperative fistulas may be delayed for 2 to 3 months to allow treatment of infection.
3. Surgical closure of opening via vaginal or abdominal route (when patient's tissues are healthy).
4. Fecal or urinary diversion procedure may be required for large fistulas.
5. Rarely, a fistula may heal without surgical intervention.
6. Medical approach.
   a. Prosthesis to prevent incontinence and allow tissue to heal; done for patients who are not surgical candidates.
   b. Prosthesis is inserted into vagina; it is connected to drainage tubing leading to a leg bag.

Complications
Hydronephrosis, pyelonephritis, and possible renal failure with ureterovaginal fistula.

Nursing Assessment
1. Obtain obstetric, gynecologic, and surgical history.
2. Monitor intake and output and voiding pattern.
3. Assess drainage on perineal pads.
4. Watch for signs of infection, such as fever, chills, flank pain.

Nursing Diagnoses
- Risk for Infection related to contamination of urinary tract by vaginal flora or contamination of the vagina by rectal organisms
- Altered Urinary Elimination related to fistula

Nursing Interventions
Preventing Infection
1. Encourage frequent sitz baths.
2. Perform vaginal irrigation as ordered, and teach patient the procedure.
3. Before repair surgery, administer prescribed antibiotics to reduce pathogenic flora in the intestinal tract.

4. After rectovaginal repair
   a. Maintain patient on clear liquids as prescribed to limit bowel activity for several days.
   b. Encourage rest because of debilitation.
   c. Administer warm perineal irrigations to decrease healing time and increase comfort.

Maintaining Urinary Drainage
1. Suggest the use of perineal pads or incontinence products preoperatively.
2. After versicovaginal repair:
   a. Maintain proper drainage from indwelling catheter to prevent pressure on newly sutured tissue.
   b. Administer vaginal or bladder irrigations gently because of tenderness at operative site.
   c. Maintain strict intake and output records.
3. If medical management is indicated, teach patient the use of prosthetic device.
4. Encourage patient to express feelings about her altered route of elimination, and share them with significant other.

Patient Education and Health Maintenance
1. Teach patient to report signs of infection early.
2. Teach patient to cleanse perineum gently and to follow surgeon's instructions on when to resume intercourse and strenuous activity.
3. Advise patient to keep regular follow-up appointments.

Outcome-Based Evaluation
- No signs of infection—afebrile, no complaints of flank pain or difficulty voiding
- Clear urine flows from catheter postoperatively; patient voids without difficulty after catheter removal

Vaginitis
Vaginitis is inflammation of the vagina caused by infectious pathogens.

Pathophysiology and Etiology
1. May be caused by sexually transmitted organisms or overgrowth of other common organisms.
2. Normal vaginal secretions because of estrogen secretion and acidity inhibit the growth of pathogens.
3. Conditions such as diabetes, pregnancy, stress, coitus, and menopause alter normal vaginal environment.
4. Types of vaginitis (Table 22-3)
   a. Simple (contact)
   b. *Gardnerella*
   c. *Trichomonas*
   d. *Candida albicans*
   e. Atrophic

Clinical Manifestations
1. Vaginal itching, irritation, burning.
2. Odor, increased or unusual vaginal discharge.
3. Dyspareunia, pelvic pain, dysuria.
4. May be asymptomatic.

Diagnostic Evaluation
1. Wet smear for microscopic examination.
   a. Saline slide—discharge mixed with saline; useful in detecting *Gardnerella* and *Trichomonas* organisms.
   b. Potassium hydroxide (KOH); useful in detecting *C. albicans*. If fishy odor is noted when KOH is applied, suspect *Gardnerella* organisms.
2. Vaginal pH (not diagnostic, but may indicate infection)— use Nitrazie paper.
   a. Normal pH—4.0 to 4.5.
   b. *Gardnerella*—5.0 to 5.5.
   c. *Trichomonas*—5.5+.
3. Pap smear—may detect any type of vaginitis.
4. Chlamydia and gonorrhea cultures or DNA probe—to rule out chlamydia or gonorrhea cervicitis.

Management
1. Anti-infectives (oral or vaginal preparations).
2. Estrogen replacement (oral or vaginal preparation) for atrophic vaginitis.

Nursing Assessment
1. Obtain a health history including questions specific to the condition.
   a. Nature of discharge. Cheese-like, frothy, puslike, thick or thin, scant? When was it first noticed? Character, color, odor? Other symptoms: dysuria, itching, dyspareunia?
   b. Menstrual history. Age at menache, menopause; length of cycles, duration and amount of flow, dysmenorrhea, amenorrhea, dysfunctional bleeding?
   c. Disease history. Diabetes mellitus in patient or family? Other debilitating diseases? Control of these? Previous vaginal infections? STDs?
   d. Pregnancy history.
   e. Sexual history. Age of onset of sexual activity, partner(s), how active sexually? Its nature? Urogenital infections in partner? Nature of contraceptives?
   f. Medications being taken. Purpose?
   g. Vaginal hygiene. Use of douches, deodorants, sprays, ointments; types of tampons, bubble bath, shower/bath, nature of clothing (tight fitting)?
2. Perform a physical examination that includes vaginal examination and obtain vaginal discharge specimens as indicated.

Nursing Diagnoses
- Pain related to vaginal irritation
- Impaired Tissue Integrity related to vaginal infection
- Sexual Dysfunction related to abstinence secondary to treatment

Nursing Interventions
Relieving Pain
1. Instruct patient to discontinue use of irritating agents, such as bubble baths, vaginal douches.

TABLE 22-3   Types of Vaginitis

Description	Manifestations	Management
Simple Vaginitis (Contact Vaginitis)		
An inflammation of the vagina, with discharge; this may be due to invading organisms, irritation, poor hygiene. *Urethritis* often accompanies vaginitis because of the proximity of the urethra to the vagina. Predisposing factors: Contact allergens, excessive perspiration, synthetic underclothing, poor hygiene, foreign bodies (tampons, condoms, diaphragms that have been left in too long).	1. Increased vaginal discharge with itching, redness, burning, and edema. 2. Voiding and defecation aggravate the above symptoms.	1. Stimulate the growth of lactobacilli (Döderlein's bacilli) by administering beta-lactose vaginal suppository; this dissolves with body heat, and the sugar then acts. 2. Enhance the natural vaginal flora by administering a weak acid douche, 15 mL of vinegar to 1,000 mL water, (1 T white vinegar to 1 qt water). 3. Foster cleanliness by meticulous care after voiding and defecation. 4. Discontinue use of causative agent.
Gardnerella Vaginitis (Nonspecific or Bacterial)		
An inflammation of the vagina heretofore referred to as "nonspecific vaginitis," because it is not caused by *Trichomonas*, *Candida*, or gonorrhea. It is not considered an STD.	1. Vaginal discharge with odor. 2. Itching and burning may suggest concomitant organisms present. 3. It is benign in that when the discharge is wiped away, underlying tissue is healthy and pink. 4. Vaginal pH is between 5.0 and 5.5. 5. May be asymptomatic.	1. Metronidazole (Flagyl) taken orally for 7 d or topical clindamycin (Cleocin) or metronidazole (Metrogel V). 2. Alcohol intake should be avoided during Flagyl treatment to avoid nausea and vertigo. Flagyl has been associated with teratogenic effects and should not be used in pregnant women during first trimester. 3. Treating partners is controversial unless the condition is recurrent.
Trichomonas Vaginalis		
A condition produced by a protozoan (pear-shaped and motile), that thrives in an alkaline environment. Remissions may occur, but organism remains resistant to treatment in the urinary tract. Is an STD.	1. Copious malodorous discharge; may be frothy and yellow-green in color. 2. May have pruritus, dyspareunia, and spotting. 3. Red, speckled (strawberry) punctate hemorrhages on the cervix. 4. May also have vulvar edema, dysuria, and hyperemia secondary to irritation of discharge.	1. Destroy infective protozoa by taking metronidazole (Flagyl) (orally), usually single dose of 2 g. NOTE: Flagyl is contraindicated in the first trimester of pregnancy. 2. Prevent reinfection by treating male concurrently with Flagyl, even though male is asymptomatic. 3. Avoid alcohol during treatment.
Candida albicans		
A fungal infection caused by *Candida albicans*. Associated factors include: 1. Steroid therapy 2. Obesity 3. Pregnancy 4. Antibiotic therapy 5. Diabetes mellitus 6. Oral contraceptives 7. Frequent douching 8. Chronic debilitative diseases	1. Vaginal discharge is thick and irritating; white or yellow patchy, cheese-like particles adhere to vaginal walls. 2. Itching is the most common complaint. 3. May also experience burning, soreness, dyspareunia, frequency, and dysuria.	1. Eradicate the fungus by applying antifungal vaginal cream, or vaginal suppository for 3 or 4 nights as ordered. 2. Treat the symptomatic or uncircumcised partner by applying antifungal cream under the foreskin nightly for 7 nights. 3. For severe or recurrent cases can use systemic antifungal.
Characteristics 1. *C. albicans* is a normal inhabitant of the intestinal tract and therefore a frequent contaminant of the vagina. 2. Because this fungus thrives in an environment rich in carbohydrates, it is seen commonly in patients with poorly controlled diabetes. 3. This infection is observed in patients who have been on antibiotic or steroid therapy for a while (reduces natural protective organisms in vagina).		

(continued)

TABLE 22-3 Types of Vaginitis (Continued)		
Description	**Manifestations**	**Management**
Atrophic Vaginitis		
This is a common postmenopausal occurrence due to atrophy of the vaginal mucosa secondary to decreased estrogen levels; more susceptible to infection.	1. Vaginal itching, dryness, burning, dyspareunia, and vulvar irritation. 2. May also have vaginal bleeding. **NURSING ALERT** In the postmenopausal woman, if vaginal bleeding occurs, encourage the patient to see her health care provider immediately because bleeding is a warning sign of cancer.	Because this is a manifestation of general body estrogenic depletion, the patient should be treated with oral, water-soluble, natural, conjugated estrogen (Premarin) or estrogen patch. The condition reverses itself under treatment, which must be maintained. If infection is also present, this is treated. Estrogenic vaginal cream may be prescribed. If uterus is intact, progesterone must be added to prevent endometrial hyperplasia due to unopposed estrogen.

2. Suggest patient take cool baths or sitz baths and pat dry or dry with hair dryer on low setting.
3. Encourage patient to wear loose cotton undergarments.
4. Encourage patient to take prescribed steroids and analgesics.
5. Provide emotional support.

Restoring Tissue Integrity
1. Teach patient to cleanse perineum before applying medication.
2. Demonstrate application of prescribed medication.
3. Emphasize importance of taking prescribed medication for full length of therapy and as directed; teach patient side effects.
4. Instruct patient on the proper technique for douching, although douching not usually necessary.
5. Stress importance of follow-up visits.

Restoring Sexual Function
1. Emphasize importance of sexual abstinence and vaginal rest (nothing in vagina) until therapy is complete and sexual partner has been treated, if indicated.
2. Tell patient use of condoms may be protective but may produce irritation during treatment.
3. Instruct patient in the use of water-soluble lubricant if vagina is dry and atrophic.

Patient Education and Health Maintenance
1. Teach causes of vaginitis and its symptoms so patient can seek treatment promptly.
2. Teach patient about all STDs and means of prevention.
3. Teach measures to prevent vaginitis.
   a. Wipe from front to back after toilet use.
   b. Keep area clean and dry.
   c. Wear loose cotton clothing to absorb moisture and provide good circulation.
   d. Change sanitary pads, tampons frequently so they do not become saturated.
   e. Avoid bubble baths, vaginal deodorants, sprays, and douches.
   f. If patient insists on using douches, use a mild vinegar solution (2 tsp. white vinegar to 1 qt. water).

4. For recurrent *Candida* infections, encourage good control if patient has diabetes, or encourage patient to be tested for diabetes. Teach all patients to eliminate concentrated carbohydrates from diet to prevent recurrence.

Outcome-Based Evaluation
- Verbalizes relief of pain
- Vaginal mucosa pink, with normal amount and color of secretions
- Reports safe, satisfying sexual activity

■ Human Papillomavirus Infection
Human papillomavirus infection (HPV) may be asymptomatic but frequently causes Condyloma acuminatum or *genital warts*.

Pathophysiology and Etiology
1. Sexually transmitted; highly contagious.
2. More than 20 types of HPV can infect the genital tract, many are asymptomatic, and multiple types may coexist.
3. Visible genital warts are caused by HPV types 6 and 11.
4. Other types (16, 18, 31, 33, 35) have been strongly associated with cervical dysplasia.
5. Incubation period of up to 8 months.

Clinical Manifestations
1. Single or multiple soft, fleshy painless growths of the vulva, vagina, cervix, urethra, or anal area (Figure 22-3).
2. May be subclinical infection and still contagious.
3. Occasional vaginal bleeding, discharge, odor and dyspareunia.

Diagnostic Evaluation
1. Pap smear—shows characteristic cellular changes (koilocytosis).
2. Acetic acid swabbing on vaginal examination will whiten lesions and make them more identifiable.
3. Anoscopy or urethroscopy may be necessary to identify anal and urethral lesions.

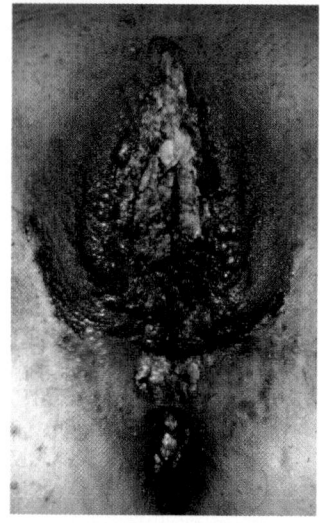

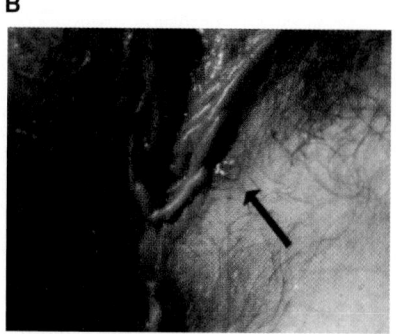

A

B

FIGURE 22-3 Genital lesions. (**A**) Condyloma acuminatum. (**B**) Genital herpes.

4. Viral DNA or RNA tests to detect subclinical cases; however, the significance of positive and negative results has not been determined.

Management
1. External lesions may be treated by patient with multiple applications of a topical preparation.
   a. Podofilox (Condylox)—applied with cotton swab or finger to visible warts twice a day for 3 days, then no treatment for 4 days; may be repeated for up to 4 cycles of therapy.
   b. Imiquimod (Aldara)—applied by finger three times a week for up to 16 weeks; may be washed off 6 to 10 hours after application.
   c. Neither agent should be used during pregnancy.
2. Noncervical lesions may be treated by health care provider with topical preparations, such as podophyllin, trichloroacetic acid, or 5-fluorouracil.
   a. Requires multiple visits for repeat treatments.
   b. May require washing off several hours later.
3. Cryotherapy, electrocautery, laser treatment, or local excision of large or cervical lesions.
4. Highly recurrent, particularly in first 3 months—may require retreatment.

Complications
1. Implicated in cervical intraepithelial neoplasia.
2. May cause neonatal laryngeal papillomatosis if infant born through infected birth canal.
3. Obstruction of anal canal, vagina by enlarging lesions.
4. Scarring and pigment changes if treatment not employed properly.

Nursing Assessment
1. Obtain history of STDs, Pap smear results, sexual partners.

2. Inspect external genitalia for lesions, perform vaginal examination.

Nursing Diagnosis
- Body Image Disturbance related to genital warts

Nursing Interventions
Improving Body Image
1. Explain to patient that the goal of therapy is to remove visible lesions; however, HPV will not be cured or eliminated.
2. Encourage patient to comply with treatment schedule and inspect areas for resolution of lesions or redevelopment of new lesions.
3. Advise patient of high recurrence rate; 3-month follow-up visit is advisable; if lesions redevelop, patient should follow up for retreatment.
4. Advise patient to use condoms to reduce the chance of transmission, although their use does not guarantee protection from HPV. Condom use will protect against other STDs.
5. Encourage female patients to follow up regularly for PAP smears because HPV has been associated with cervical neoplasia.
6. Advise patient of risk to neonate during delivery; patient should receive close prenatal care if pregnant.

Patient Education and Health Maintenance
1. Advise patient to discuss HPV with her partner. He should receive treatment for visible lesions. However, no testing or treatment has been recommended if asymptomatic.
2. Make sure patient realizes that even though lesions may be gone, she may still transmit HPV to new sexual partners. Abstinence and condoms are advisable.

Outcome-Based Evaluation

- Patient presents with no visible lesions at follow-up visit

Herpes Genitalis

Herpes genitalis is a viral infection that causes lesions of the cervix, vagina, and external genitalia.

Pathophysiology and Etiology

1. Caused by HSV, usually type 2.
2. Sexually transmitted.
3. An estimated 40 million people are infected in the United States.
4. Recurrent infection; virus lies dormant in dorsal root ganglia of spinal nerves between outbreaks.

Clinical Manifestations

1. Lesions occur 2 to 10 days after initial exposure, sometimes with fever, malaise, lymphadenopathy and headache for primary infection (see Figure 22-3).
2. Lesions are preceded by sensation of tingling; proceed from vesicles on erythematous, edematous base to painful ulcers that crust and heal without scars.
3. Internal lesions may cause watery discharge, dyspareunia.
4. Recurrent lesions may be stimulated by fever, stress, illness, local trauma, menses, sunburn.
5. Occasionally infection may be asymptomatic.

Diagnostic Evaluation

1. Viral culture—identifies HSV.
2. Pap smear—may show characteristic cellular changes.
3. Tzanck smear—fluid from vesicle or scraping from base of ulcer is stained to show characteristic changes.
4. Antibody tests on genital lesions for screening and diagnosis.

Management

1. Antivirals, such as acyclovir (Zovirax), famciclovir (Famvir), and Valacyclovir (Valtrex) suppress virus and decrease length, severity, and shedding of infection.
   a. Topical treatment (acyclovir) is the least effective.
   b. Oral therapy may be episodic, whenever the first signs of a recurrence are recognized, or continuous to suppress recurrent infection.
   c. Intravenous administration (acyclovir) may be necessary for severe infections or for immunocompromised patients.
   d. Oral therapy given intermittently as soon as occurrence is identified, or continuously in the oral form to suppress recurrences in severe and frequent infections.
2. Pain medication—ranges from acetaminophen and non-steroidal anti-inflammatory drugs to oral narcotics.
3. Local comfort measures, such as lidocaine gel, sitz baths, and compresses.
4. Immunization is under investigation for high-risk people (those who have multiple partners or have a partner with herpes genitalis). Recent phase III clinical trials of an investigational three-stage vaccine proved ineffective.

Complications

1. Meningitis.
2. Neonatal infection if infant born through infected canal.

Nursing Assessment

1. Question patient about frequency and type of sexual activity and discomfort noted.
2. Question patient about pruritus, burning, tenderness, urinary symptoms, unusual discharge.
3. Assess patient's view of herpes, stigmas, misconceptions, fears.
4. Inspect genitalia for lesions, erythema, edema. Use speculum to examine vagina and cervix as indicated.

Nursing Diagnoses

- Pain related to HSV outbreak
- Impaired Skin Integrity related to herpetic lesions
- Self-Esteem Disturbance related to stigma attached to herpes
- Sexual Dysfunction related to potential transmission of herpes

Nursing Interventions

Relieving Pain

1. Demonstrate and encourage the use of warm sitz baths to increase blood supply to the areas and facilitate healing.
2. Instruct patient to keep the area clean and dry. Pat dry with a clean towel or use blow dryer. Wear loose cotton undergarments and loose clothing.
3. Encourage bed rest if case is severe.
4. Administer pain medications as prescribed.
5. Encourage patient to void in a warm sitz bath if urination is painful.
6. Insert indwelling catheter if urination is extremely painful or if retention occurs.
7. Encourage fluid intake.

Restoring Skin Integrity

1. Administer antiviral agent and teach patient its proper use and side effects.
2. Keep lesions clean and dry.
3. Teach patient not to rub or to scratch lesions.
4. Apply moist tea bags to lesions while supine. Tannic acid facilitates healing.

Improving Self-Esteem

1. Explore with patient her feelings about herpes and its effects on relationships.
2. Reiterate that when patient is feeling better physically, her feelings about herself will improve.
3. Discuss effects of stress on future outbreaks. Assist patient to identify stressors in her life and to cope with stress. Review stress reduction methods, such as relaxation, breathing and imagery.
4. Encourage patient to discuss her feelings with family and significant others.

Restoring Satisfying Sexual Function

1. Teach patient to avoid intercourse from first sign of active outbreak to resolution of lesions (at least 2 weeks with primary infection, approximately 1 week with recurrent infections).
2. Teach patient that shedding of virus through genital secretions is possible even during asymptomatic period, so partner must be notified.
3. Inform patient that she and/or partner should use condoms for intercourse, but condoms may not be fully protective.
4. Explore possibility of noncoital aspects of sexual relationship.

Patient Education and Health Maintenance

1. Inform patient that initial outbreak is usually more painful than recurrent outbreaks, and that outbreaks vary from monthly to only a few times per year.
2. Teach patient to recognize precipitating factors.
3. Encourage regular follow-up visit for Pap smears to detect cervical changes early.
4. Remind patient of the effects on a neonate and the importance of notifying her health care provider if she becomes pregnant.
5. Tell patient that oral lesions can occur with HSV-2 because of transmission by oral intercourse, but that most oral cold sores are caused by HSV-1 infection.
6. Refer patient to herpes support groups such as Help (local listings in telephone directory or call 301-369-1323) or the National Herpes Hotline, 919-361-8488.

Outcome-Based Evaluation

- Verbalizes decreased pain
- Skin intact, without signs of secondary infection, scarring
- Verbalizes improved self-esteem
- Reports satisfying sexual activity

Chlamydial Infection

1. Chlamydia infection is a common STD that occurs in both women and men, particularly in adolescents and young adults.
2. Women are asymptomatic or present with cervicitis; men are frequently asymptomatic but may present with urethritis.

Pathophysiology and Etiology

1. Chlamydia infection in women is the result of sexual intercourse, with infection entering the vagina, infecting the cervix, and possibly spreading up through the endometrium and fallopian tubes.
2. *C. trachomatis* is the most common sexually transmitted pathogen in both men and women in the United States, with an incidence of more than 200 cases per 100,000 people.

Clinical Manifestations

1. May be asymptomatic or have vaginal discharge—may be clear mucoid to creamy discharge.
2. May have dysuria and mild pelvic discomfort.
3. Cervix may be covered by thick mucopurulent discharge and be tender, erythematous, edematous, and friable.

Diagnostic Evaluation

1. Antigen detection test on cervical smear.
2. Chlamydia culture from cervical exudate.
3. Screening urinalysis in males for leukocytes; if positive result, confirmed by antigen detection test.
4. Screening test in females by urinalysis is a chlamydia antigen detection test that has proven effective.

Management

1. Antibiotic regimens include:
   a. Azithromycin (Zithromax) 1 g orally in a single dose.
   b. Doxycycline 100 mg orally twice a day for 7 days.
   c. Erythromycin and ofloxacin (Floxin) may also be used.
2. Current or most recent sexual partner(s) should be tested and treated despite test results.

NURSING ALERT

Because chlamydia infection and gonorrhea frequently coexist, especially in teens and young adults, treatment of both STDs is recommended.

Complications

1. Pelvic inflammatory disease (PID).
2. Ectopic pregnancy or infertility secondary to untreated or recurrent PID.
3. Transmission to neonate born through infected birth canal.

Nursing Assessment

1. Obtain history of sexual activity and symptoms or infections in partner.
2. Perform abdominal and pelvic examination for tenderness caused by possible spread to pelvic organs.

Nursing Diagnosis

- Risk for Infection related to sexual activity

Nursing Interventions
Preventing Infection Transmission

1. Advise abstinence from sexual intercourse until treatment has been completed and follow-up culture result is negative.
2. Ensure that partner is treated at the same time; recent partner(s) should receive treatment despite lack of symptoms and negative chlamydia test result.

3. Report case to local public health department (chlamydia is a reportable infectious disease in most of the United States).
4. Ensure that patient begins treatment and will have access to prescription and transportation for follow-up.
5. Explain mode of transmission, complications, and the risk for other STDs.

Patient Education and Health Maintenance
1. Teach about all STDs and their symptoms.
2. Explain the treatment regimen to patient and advise her of side effects.
3. Encourage abstinence, monogamy, or safer sex methods, such as male and female condom use.
4. Stress the importance of follow-up examination and testing to ensure eradication of infection. Recurrence rates are highest in younger patients.
5. For further information on STDs, refer patients to agencies such as: American Social Health Resource Center, 800-230-6039; or CDC National STD Hotline, 800-227-8922.

Outcome-Based Evaluation
- Returns for follow-up, states compliance with abstinence and treatment of partner

Gonnorhea
Gonnorhea is a common STD that affects men and women, causing cervicitis in women and urethritis in men. In women it can easily ascend to the uterus and fallopian tubes if untreated.

Pathophysiology and Etiology
1. Gonorrhea is caused by the gram-positive diplococci *Neisseria gonorrhoeae*.
2. Infection occurs through sexual transmission, causing cervicitis in women, and possible conjunctivitis, pharyngitis, and proctitis.
3. Untreated infection may lead to pelvic inflammatory disease, generalized dissemination, or gonococcal arthritis.
4. Approximately 600,000 new gonococcal infections arise in the United States each year; teens and young adults are the most affected.

Clinical Manifestations
1. Frequently asymptomatic in women.
2. May cause mucopurulent vaginal discharge.
3. Vaginal speculum examination may reveal cervical discharge and inflammation.
4. Cervical motion tenderness and tender pelvic organs on bimanual examination if infection has begun to ascend.

Diagnostic Evaluation
1. Gram's stain of cervical secretions and culture on Thayer Martin agar.

2. DNA testing of cervical secretions (quicker and accurate, can be done simultaneously for chlamydia).
3. Pharyngeal or conjunctival secretions can be tested if pharyngitis or conjunctivitis are suspected.
4. Joint aspiration and blood cultures may be necessary if disseminated infection is suspected.

Management
1. Uncomplicated gonococcal infection of the cervix, urethra (in men), or rectum (in men or women) can be treated with a single-dose antibiotic such as:
   a. Cefixime (Suprax) 400 mg orally.
   b. Ceftriaxone (Rocephin) 125 mg intramuscularly (IM).
   c. Ciprofloxin (Cipro) 500 mg orally.
   d. Ofloxacin (Floxin) 400 mg orally.
2. All of these except cefixime are recommended for pharyngeal infections, and only ceftriaxone is recommended for conjunctival infection.
3. Disseminated infections require IV or IM therapy such as:
   a. Ceftriaxone 1 g IM or IV every 24 hours.
   b. Cefotaxime (Claforan) 1 g IV every 8 hours.
   c. Ciprofloxacin 500 mg IV every 12 hours.
   d. Spectinomycin 2 g IM every 12 hours.
4. For IV or IM therapy, the patient is switched to oral therapy 24 to 48 hours after improvement.
5. In all cases of suspected gonorrhea, concomitant treatment of chlamydia is recommended with appropriate second antibiotic agent. Only if a reliable chlamydia test with negative result is obtained would therapy just be given for gonorrhea.

Complications
1. PID, ectopic pregnancy, and infertility.
2. Disseminated infection.
3. Ophthalmia neonatorum and sepsis (rare) caused by infant born through infected birth canal.

Nursing Assessment
1. Question patient on history of STDs, STD protection, sexual activity, usual women's health care practices.
2. Obtain history of symptoms in patient and partner— incubation period is usually 3 to 7 days in men, but symptoms are often overlooked in women.
3. Assess for ability to change lifestyle practices that may have lead to STD.

Nursing Diagnosis
- Risk for Infection related to STD transmission from partner

Nursing Interventions
Stopping Transmission of STD
1. Administer antibiotics as prescribed, explaining side effects to patient.
2. Ensure that patient can obtain prescription medication at discharge.

3. Monitor for relief of pain, discharge, and other symptoms.
4. Explain importance of sexual abstinence until symptoms are totally resolved and until therapy is complete in patient and partner.

Patient Education and Health Maintenance

1. Teach the patient about all possible STDs, their prevalence, and their mode of transmission.
2. Advise the patient of complications of gonorrhea and chlamydia.
3. Teach protection of STDs by abstinence, monogamous relationships, use of female and male condoms.
4. Encourage follow-up for routine women's health care and periodic STD screening.

Outcome-Based Evaluation

• At follow-up visit, patient reports resolution of symptoms, using condoms

PROBLEMS RESULTING FROM RELAXED PELVIC MUSCLES

▣ Cystocele and Urethrocele

Cystocele is a downward displacement (protrusion) of the bladder into the vagina. *Urethrocele* is a downward displacement of the urethra into the vagina (Figure 22-4).

Pathophysiology and Etiology

1. Associated with obstetric trauma to fascia, muscle, and ligaments during childbirth (results in poor support).
2. Often becomes apparent years later, when genital atrophy associated with aging occurs.
3. May also be caused by congenital defect or may appear after hysterectomy.

Clinical Manifestations

1. May be asymptomatic in early stages.
2. Pelvic pressure or heaviness, backache, nervousness, fatigue.
3. Urinary symptoms—urgency, frequency, incontinence, incomplete emptying.
4. Aggravated by coughing, sneezing, standing for long periods, and obesity, which increase intra-abdominal pressure.
5. Relieved by resting or by lying down.

Diagnostic Evaluation

1. Pelvic examination identifies condition.
2. Urinalysis and culture are done to rule out infection.

Management

1. Vaginal pessary—plastic device inserted into vagina as temporary treatment to support pelvic organs.
   a. Prolonged use may lead to necrosis and ulceration.
   b. Should be removed and cleaned every 1 to 2 months.
2. Estrogen therapy after menopause to decrease genital atrophy.
3. Surgery—if cystocele is large and interferes with bladder functioning.
   a. May do anterior vaginal colporrhaphy (repair of anterior vaginal wall).
   b. Complications of surgery include urinary retention, bleeding (requires vaginal packing).

Complications

Urinary incontinence and infection.

Nursing Assessment

1. Obtain history of obstetric trauma, abdominal surgery, menopause, use of estrogen.
2. Ask about urinary symptoms, pain.
3. Observe perineum while patient bears down or is in upright position for bulge from vagina.

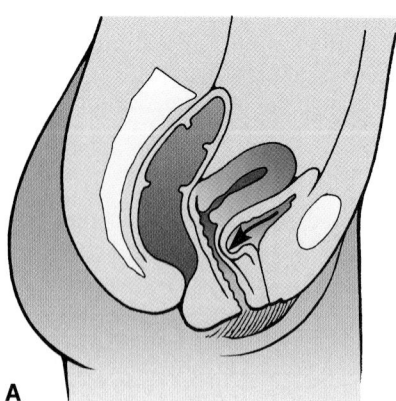 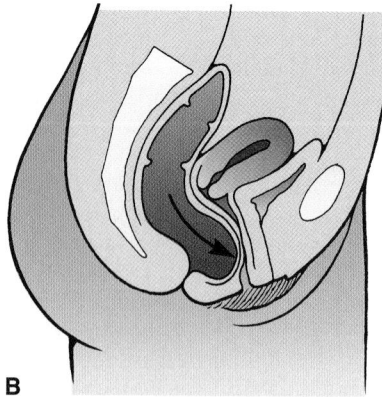 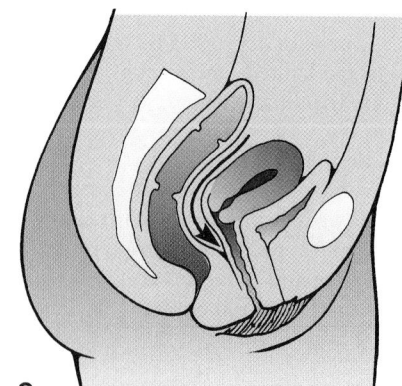

FIGURE 22-4 Pelvic support disorders: (**A**) cystocele, (**B**) rectocele, (**C**) enterocele.

Nursing Diagnoses
- Pain related to pelvic pressure
- Stress Incontinence related to relaxed pelvic muscles, displaced organs
- Urinary Retention related to displaced organs

Nursing Interventions
Relieving Pain
1. Encourage periods of rest with legs elevated to relieve strain on pelvis.
2. Advise use of mild analgesics as necessary.
3. Provide postoperative care.
   a. Encourage voiding every 4 to 8 hours to reduce pressure so that no more than 150 mL will accumulate in bladder—intermittent catheterization or use of an indwelling catheter may be required.
   b. Administer perineal care to the patient after each voiding and defecation.
   c. Use a heat lamp to help dry the incision line and enhance the healing process.
   d. Use available sprays for anesthetic and antiseptic effects.
   e. Apply an ice pack locally to relieve congestion and discomfort.
   f. Administer analgesics as prescribed for relief of pain.

Controlling Incontinence
1. Teach patient Kegel pelvic floor exercises to regain muscle tone.
   a. Practice while voiding by stopping the flow of urine for 3 to 5 seconds, then releasing for 5 seconds.
   b. Patient can tighten pelvic floor muscle at any time, repeat 10 times, three times a day, increase as able.
2. Encourage patient to void frequently, respond to the urge to void promptly.
3. Warn patient to avoid straining to prevent incontinence.

Preventing Urinary Retention
1. Encourage fluids to decrease bacterial flora in the bladder.
2. Catheterize patient if retention is suspected.
3. Obtain urine specimen for culture and sensitivity if infection is suspected.

Patient Education and Health Maintenance
1. Teach women to avoid straining, remain active, avoid obesity, and perform Kegel exercises to minimize pelvic relaxation in their older years.
2. Encourage prompt attention to symptoms of urinary tract infection—dysuria, frequency, foul-smelling urine.

Outcome-Based Evaluation
- Patient verbalizes reduced pain
- Patient reports decreased frequency of incontinence
- Patient voids regularly without symptoms of infection

▧ Rectocele and Enterocele

Rectocele is displacement (protrusion) of the rectum into the vagina. *Enterocele* is displacement of intestine into the vagina (see Figure 22-4).

Pathophysiology and Etiology
1. Posterior vaginal wall becomes weakened, allowing displacement.
2. Weakening caused by obstetric trauma, childbirth, pelvic surgery, aging.

Clinical Manifestations
1. Pelvic pressure or heaviness, backache, perineal burning.
2. Constipation—may have difficulty in fecal evacuation; patient may use fingers into vagina to push feces up so defecation may occur.
3. Incontinence of feces and flatus—if tear between rectum and vagina.
4. Visible protrusion into vagina.
5. Symptoms are aggravated by standing for long periods.

Diagnostic Evaluation
1. Vaginal examination reveals condition.
2. May use Sims speculum to uplift cervix and fully evaluate condition.

Management
1. Pessary—plastic device inserted into vagina to aid pelvic support.
2. Estrogen replacement to prevent atrophy.
3. Surgery, if rectocele is large enough to interfere with bowel functioning: posterior colpoplasty (perineorrhaphy)—repair of posterior vaginal wall.

Complications
1. Total fecal incontinence.

Nursing Assessment
1. Obtain history of childbirth, pelvic surgery, symptoms of bowel function.
2. Observe for bulge into vagina while patient bears down or is in upright position.
3. Monitor bowel movements.

Nursing Diagnoses
- Pain related to pelvic pressure
- Constipation related to displaced rectum/bowel

Nursing Interventions
Relieving Pain
1. Encourage periods of rest with legs elevated to relieve pelvic strain.
2. Encourage use of mild analgesics as needed; avoid narcotics, which may worsen constipation.
3. Postoperative care:
   a. Suggest low Fowler's position to decrease edema and discomfort.
   b. Administer perineal care to the patient after each voiding and defecation.
   c. Use a heat lamp to help dry the incision line and enhance the healing process.
   d. Use ice packs locally to relieve congestion and discomfort.
   e. Administer analgesics and stool softeners as ordered.

Relieving Constipation

1. Teach patient to increase fluid and fiber in diet.
2. Encourage use of stool softeners or bulk laxatives to make passage of stool easier.
3. Use of enema may be necessary to prevent straining.

Patient Education and Health Maintenance

1. Advise patient to avoid straining and obesity, which may cause return of rectocele or enterocele.

Outcome-Based Evaluation

- Verbalizes reduced pain
- Soft stool passed daily

Uterine Prolapse

Uterine prolapse is an abnormal position of the uterus in which the uterus protrudes downward.

Pathophysiology and Etiology

1. Uterus herniates through pelvic floor and protrudes into vagina (prolapse) and possibly beyond the introitus (procidentia).
2. Usually caused by obstetric trauma and overstretching of musculofascial supports.
3. Degrees (Figure 22-5):
   a. First degree—cervix is at the introitus.
   b. Second degree—cervix extends over the perineum.
   c. Third degree—the entire uterus (or most of it) protrudes.

Clinical Manifestations

1. Backache or abdominal pain.
2. Pressure and heaviness in vaginal region.
3. Bloody discharge because of cervix rubbing against clothing or inner thighs.

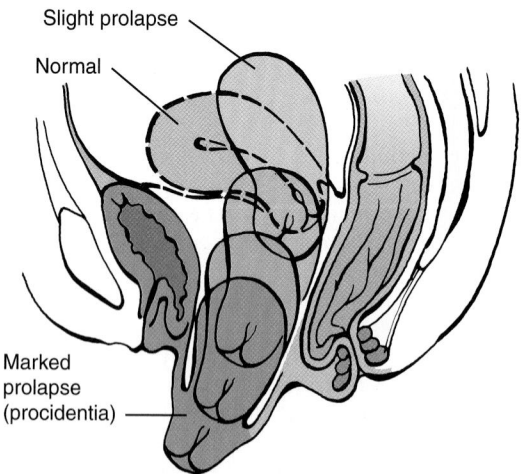

FIGURE 22-5 Degrees of uterine prolapse.

4. Ulceration of cervix.
5. Symptoms are aggravated by obesity, standing, straining, coughing, or lifting a heavy object, because of increased intra-abdominal pressure.

Diagnostic Evaluation

1. Pelvic examination identifies condition.

Management

1. Hysterectomy or surgical correction.
2. Vaginal pessary—plastic device inserted into vagina as temporary or palliative measure if surgery cannot be done.
3. Estrogen cream—to decrease genital atrophy.

Complications

1. Necrosis of cervix, uterus.
2. Infection.

Nursing Assessment

1. Obtain history of childbirth and surgery.
2. Ask about symptoms and aggravating factors.
3. Examine patient in lying or standing position; if cervix not readily visible, spread labia gently, do not attempt to insert speculum.

Nursing Diagnoses

- Pain related to downward pressure and exposed tissue
- Impaired Tissue Integrity related to exposed cervix and uterus
- Sexual Dysfunction related to loss of vaginal cavity

Nursing Interventions

Relieving Pain

1. Administer sitz baths and explain procedure to patient.
2. Provide heating pad for low back or lower abdomen.
3. Administer pain medications as ordered.
4. Check for proper placement of pessary.
5. Increase fluid intake and encourage patient to void frequently to prevent bladder infection.

Maintaining Cervical and Uterine Mucosal Integrity

1. For second- and third-degree prolapse, apply saline compresses frequently.
2. Provide postoperative care.
   a. Administer perineal care to patient after each voiding and defecation.
   b. Use a heat lamp to help dry the incision line and enhance healing process.
   c. If urinary retention occurs, catheterize or use indwelling catheter until bladder tone is regained.
   d. Apply an ice pack locally to relieve congestion.
   e. Promote ambulation but prevent straining to reduce pelvic pressure.

Restoring Sexual Function

1. Discuss with patient noncoital sexual activity before treatment is instituted.
2. Explain to patient that sexual intercourse is possible with pessary; however, vaginal canal may be shortened.

3. Reinforce surgeon's instructions postoperatively about waiting to have vaginal penetration.
4. Encourage patient to explore with partner ways to engage in sexual activity without strain and with greatest comfort.

Patient Education and Health Maintenance

1. Encourage patient with pessary to follow up every 3 months or as directed for removal and cleaning of pessary, and evaluation or any vaginal irritation or trauma.
2. Encourage all patients to report vaginal discharge, pain, or bleeding before or after treatment.

Outcome-Based Evaluation

- Verbalizes reduced pain
- Cervix and uterus without ulceration
- Verbalizes satisfying sexual activity

GYNECOLOGIC TUMORS

■ Cancer of the Vulva

Cancer of the vulva is most commonly carcinoma of the labia majora, labia minora, or clitoris; it may also originate as a urethral tumor.

Pathophysiology and Etiology

1. Most common in women older than 60 years of age; many new cases have increased because of increase in older population.
2. Represents 3% to 5% of gynecologic cancers.
3. The cause is unknown, but associated with history of infections, such as HPV or HSV.
4. Spread primarily through direct extension and lymphatic system; rare distant metastasis.

Clinical Manifestations

1. Lump or mass present for several months—first is leukoplakic (white plaque or mild ulceration); becomes reddened, pigmented, ulcerated.
2. Vulvar pruritus, pain.
3. Discharge or bleeding; may be foul smelling because of secondary infection.
4. Dysuria because of invasion of urethra with bacteria.
5. Edema of tissues.
6. Lymphadenopathy.

Diagnostic Evaluation

Biopsy of lesion and lymph nodes. If small, lesion may be excised at time of biopsy. Most lesions are squamous cell carcinoma.

Management

Choice of surgical methods depends on the site and extent of the primary lesion and the risk of lymph node involvement. The most conservative operation that is consistent with cure of disease is chosen.

1. Precancerous lesions—vulvar intraepithelial neoplasia (VIN).
   a. Simple vulvectomy
   b. Skinning vulvectomy
   c. Local excision
   d. Laser therapy
2. Carcinoma in situ (CIS)-noninvasive
   a. Radical local excision
   b. Radical vulvectomy or modified radical vulvectomy
3. Invasive carcinoma—radical or modified radical vulvectomy with bilateral groin lymph node resection.
   a. Pelvic nodes also may be removed if involvement is suspected.
   b. If cancer is confined to the vulva, there is an 80% to 90% 5-year survival rate after surgery.
4. Advanced carcinoma—pelvic exenteration or surgery and radiation as a palliative measure.
   a. Radiation therapy has an increased role in the preoperative and postoperative management.
   b. Preoperative radiation therapy can decrease the volume of disease and decrease need for radical surgery.
   c. Postoperative radiation therapy is used for patients with positive lymph nodes and close surgical margins.
   d. Long-term outcomes of treatment compared to morbidity associated with treatment are being studied.
5. Chemotherapy alone or in combination with radiation is still under investigation. It may shrink lesion so surgery can be less extensive.

Complications

1. Lymphatic spread.
2. Complications after vulvectomy are common—wound infection, wound breakdown, lymphedema, leg cellulitis, and introital stenosis.

Nursing Assessment

1. Obtain history of lesion, including when the patient first noticed it and any change in appearance.
2. Obtain gynecologic history, especially about past infections.
3. Assess overall health for tolerance of treatment.
4. Assess support systems and personal coping skills.

Nursing Diagnoses

- Fear related to cancer and radical surgery
- Impaired Tissue Integrity related to surgery
- Sexual Dysfunction related to vulvectomy

Nursing Interventions
Preoperative
Relieving Fear

1. Have the patient describe what her understanding is regarding the problem; answer questions and clear up misconceptions.
2. Emphasize the positive outcomes of the prescribed treatment plan; reinforce what the surgeon has already described to her.

3. Prepare patient for surgery and describe to her the post-operative appearance of the wound, use of drains, urinary catheter, etc. (Figure 22-6).
   a. Provide a skin preparation as ordered and cleanse the vulva the night before with hexachlorophene or povidone-iodine shower or scrub if ordered.
   b. Administer bowel preparation as ordered to evacuate intestinal tract before surgery; there will be no bowel movement for 2 to 3 days postoperatively.

Postoperative
Promoting Tissue Healing
1. Maintain drainage and compression of tissues to remove fluid that could cause edema and prevent wound healing. Empty drains as needed (at least every 8 hours).
2. Keep wound clean and dry.
   a. Perform sterile dressing changes as prescribed.
   b. Apply heat lamp if prescribed to increase circulation and healing.
   c. Perform perineal care or sitz baths after each bowel movement or voiding (after catheter removed).
   d. Maintain patency of urinary catheter (approximately 10 days) to prevent wound contamination with urine.
   e. Encourage low Fowler's position to promote comfort and reduce tension on sutures.
   f. Prevent straining with defecation by providing a low-residue diet initially, and stool softeners later, as ordered.
   g. While patient is on bed rest, provide DVT prophylaxis (anticoagulant or sequential compression device) as prescribed and encourage leg exercises to prevent thrombus/embolus formation. Encourage careful ambulation when allowed while preventing perineal tension.

Restoring Sexual Function
1. Encourage patient to ventilate feelings about sexual mutilation, altered functioning.

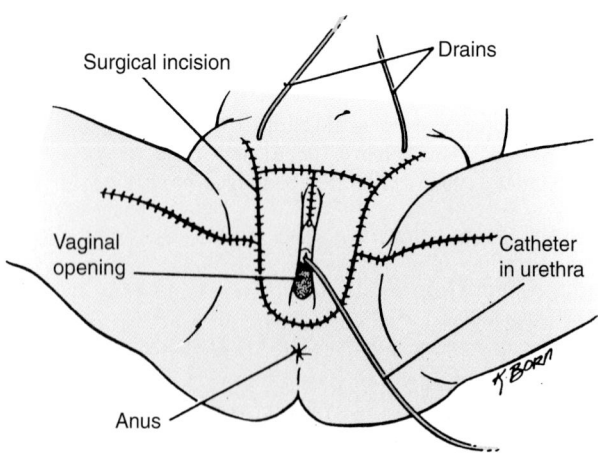

FIGURE 22-6 Postoperative appearance after radical vulvectomy.

2. Tell patient that if vagina is still intact, vaginal intercourse is still possible.
3. Inform patient of changes that may occur because of surgery—loss of sexual arousal if clitoris is removed, shortening of vagina, decreased lubrication.
4. Help patient explore alternate methods of sexual intimacy and encourage her to discuss feelings with her partner.

Patient Education and Health Maintenance
1. Encourage follow-up visits for additional therapy if required.
2. Encourage regular health checkups and screening for cancer and other age-related illness.
3. Encourage early evaluation of any suspicious lesions, bleeding, or discharge.

Outcome-Based Evaluation
- Verbalizes reduced fear
- Perineum healed without complications
- Verbalizes understanding of anatomic changes and sexual function

◼ Cancer of the Cervix
Cancer of the cervix is a common gynecologic malignancy.

Pathophysiology and Etiology
1. Most common between 35 and 55 years of age.
2. Early sexual activity, multiple sexual partners, and history of STDs, especially HPV and HSV, are major risk factors.
3. Incidence is higher in lower socioeconomic status and in blacks.
4. Decreased mortality rate in United States, but most frequent malignancy among women in developing countries.
5. Types:
   a. Dysplasia (precancer)—atypical cells with some degree of surface maturation.
   b. Carcinoma in situ—cytology similar to invasive carcinoma, but confined to epithelium.
   c. Invasive carcinoma—stroma is involved; 90% are of the squamous cell type. Spreads by local invasion and lymphatics to vagina and beyond.

Clinical Manifestations
1. Early disease is usually asymptomatic.
2. Initial symptoms include postcoital bleeding, irregular vaginal bleeding or spotting between periods or after menopause, and malodorous discharge.
3. As disease progresses, bleeding becomes more constant and is accompanied by pain that radiates to buttocks and legs.
4. Weight loss, anemia, and fever signal advanced disease.

Diagnostic Evaluation
1. Pap smear—routine screening measure; abnormal results warrant further diagnostic tests, such as colposcopy and biopsy or conization.

2. Staging is done clinically rather than surgically as with other cancers. Based on physical findings on abdominal and pelvic examination.
3. Supplemental imaging can include chest x-ray, intravenous urogram, colposcopy, cystoscopy, proctosigmoidoscopy, and barium studies of the lower colon and rectum.

Management
Dysplasia to Carcinoma in Situ
1. Techniques to destroy abnormal cells in the cervical transformation zone and penetrate 4–5 mm into cervix.
2. Cryosurgery, laser therapy, electrocautery (loop electrosurgical excision procedure, LEEP), or conization may be performed on outpatient basis.
3. Vaginal discharge, bleeding, pain and cramping result from these procedures in various degrees, but postoperative convalescence is minimal.
Microinvasive Stage
1. Surgical conization—large excision of cervical tissue, may be done under local or general anesthesia.
2. Invasive cervical cancer—extent is staged and treated with hysterectomy, radiotherapy, or chemotherapy.
Other Management
1. Radiotherapy.
   a. Intracavitary (localized for earlier stage) or external (more generalized dosage to pelvis for stages IIB through IVB).
   b. Cisplatin (Platinol), a radiation sensitizer, is used to improve survival.
2. Chemotherapy—cisplatin may be used in combination with radiation for locally advanced disease; or for metastatic disease in which recurrence is common.
3. Surgery.
   a. Simple hysterectomy for stage IA.
   b. Radical hysterectomy and bilateral lymph node resections for stage IB and IIA.
   c. Pelvic exenteration for advanced cases if the patient is a candidate.
      (i) Removal of the vagina, uterus, uterine tubes, ovaries, bladder, rectum, and supporting structures and the creation of an ileal conduit and fecal stoma.
      (ii) Performed for pelvic recurrence after radiation or chemotherapy.

Complications
1. Spread to bladder and rectum; metastasis to lungs, mediastinum, bones, and liver.
2. Complications of intracavitary radiotherapy are cystitis, proctitis, vaginal stenosis, uterine perforation.
3. Complications of external radiation are bone marrow depression, bowel obstruction, fistula.

Nursing Assessment
1. Obtain history of Pap smears, sexual activity, past STDs.
2. Obtain history of symptoms.
3. Assess understanding of disease and responses, such as guilt, fear, denial, anxiety.

Nursing Diagnoses
- Anxiety related to cancer and treatment
- Body Image Disturbance related to surgical treatment

Nursing Interventions
Relieving Anxiety
1. Assist patient to seek information on stage of cancer, treatment options.
2. Prepare patient for hysterectomy or other surgery (see p. 756 for nursing interventions for hysterectomy).
3. Prepare patient for radiation therapy to the uterus (see p. 778 for nursing interventions for radiation therapy).
Enhancing Body Image
1. Provide emotional support during treatment.
2. Encourage patient to take pride in appearance by dressing, putting on makeup, etc. as able.
3. Encourage activity and socialization when patient feels able.

Patient Education and Health Maintenance
1. Explain the importance of life-long follow-up regardless of treatments, to determine the response to treatment and detect spread of cancer.
2. Refer to cancer support group in community.

Outcome-Based Evaluation
- Reports decreased anxiety, increased ability to make decisions
- Reports continued interest in appearance and femininity

Endometrial Cancer
Cancer of the uterus is usually adenocarcinoma of the endometrium of the fundus or body of the uterus.

Pathophysiology and Etiology
1. Most common gynecologic cancer and third leading cancer in women.
2. Most patients are older than 55 years of age.
3. Cause is unknown but associated with increased estrogen stimulation, as in obesity, late menopause, nulliparity, and unopposed estrogen replacement.
4. Hypertension and diabetes mellitus are also risk factors.

Clinical Manifestations
1. Irregular bleeding before menopause or postmenopausal bleeding.
2. Watery, usually malodorous vaginal discharge.
3. Pain, fever, and bowel and bladder dysfunctions are late signs.
4. Anemia secondary to bleeding.

Diagnostic Evaluation
1. Pelvic examination—enlarged uterus may be palpated.
2. Endocervical aspirate—shows abnormal cells.
3. Endometrial biopsy results—may be false negative.
4. Dilation and curettage—most accurate diagnostic tool.

5. Metastatic workup—includes x-ray studies and cystoscopy.

Management

1. Staging for endometrial cancer is based on surgical aspects versus clinical staging.
   a. Emphasis is placed on histologic grade, depth of myometrial invasion, and cervical involvement.
   b. These parameters assist in prediction of lymph node involvement and help determine need for lymph node dissection.
2. Early Stage I requires total abdominal hysterectomy with bilateral salpingo-oophorectomy (BSO) (see p. 756).
3. Advanced Stage I and Stage II require TAH/BSO and selective lymph node dissection.
4. Radiation therapy (intracavitary or external) may be added after surgery or chosen instead of surgery for more advanced stages or for patients who are high-risk surgical candidates.
   a. Acute complications include hemorrhagic cystitis, vaginitis, enteritis, proctitis.
   b. Chronic complications include vaginal dryness, vaginal stenosis, cystitis, bladder dysfunction, proctitis, small bowel obstruction, fistulas, strictures, leg edema.
5. Hormonal therapy—progestational agents may alter receptor sites in endometrium for estrogen and thus decrease growth (for metastatic disease).
6. Chemotherapy—for metastatic and recurrent disease; low response rate of short duration.

Complications

Spread throughout the pelvis; metastasis to lungs, liver, bone, and brain.

Nursing Assessment

1. Obtain history of menses, pregnancy, estrogen replacement.
2. Ask about irregular or postmenopausal bleeding and other symptoms.
3. Assess patient's response to possible diagnosis of cancer—fear, guilt, denial.

Nursing Diagnoses

- Fear related to cancer, treatment options
- Pain related to disease process and surgical treatment

Nursing Interventions

Relieving Fear

1. Support patient through the diagnostic process and reinforce information given by health care provider about treatment options.
2. Prepare patient for radiation therapy, if indicated (see below).
3. Prepare patient for hysterectomy, if indicated (see p. 756).
4. Provide complete and concise explanations for all care you provide; emphasize the positive aspects of patient's recovery.

Relieving Pain

1. Administer pain medications as prescribed and monitor patient's response.
2. Encourage use of relaxation techniques, such as deep breathing, imagery, and distraction to help promote comfort.

Patient Education and Health Maintenance

1. Explain the importance of reporting postmenopausal bleeding.
2. Encourage keeping follow-up visits.
3. Explain that surgery or radiation treatment does not prevent satisfying sexual activity.
4. Refer to local cancer support group.

Outcome-Based Evaluation

- Verbalizes understanding of diagnosis and treatment chosen
- Verbalizes decreased pain

■ Nursing Care of the Patient Receiving Intracavitary Radiation Therapy

Procedural Considerations

1. An applicator (tandems and ovoids) is positioned in the endocervical canal and vagina in the operating room with the patient under anesthesia.
2. On recovery from anesthesia, x-rays are taken to check correct placement.
3. Radiologist inserts radioactive material (radium or cesium) into applicator, which remains in place 24 to 72 hours. Therapy is individualized according to the stage of disease and the patient's response to and tolerance of radiation.
4. External radiation over pelvis may be supplemented to eliminate cancer spread via lymphatic system.

Nursing Interventions

Patient Preparation

1. Patients require a thorough medical evaluation before treatment to evaluate risks/precautions related to pre-existing medical problems or special needs.
2. An enema is given to evacuate the rectal vault before the patient is transferred to the operating room for application.
3. An indwelling catheter is placed in the operating room.
4. Encourage patient to bring diversional activities because she will remain on bed rest during radiation treatment.
5. Instruct patient on radiation safety measures:
   a. Neither patient nor her secretions are radioactive, but the applicator is.
   b. Do not touch source of radiation.
   c. Notify someone immediately if source is dislodged.
   d. When applicators are removed, no radioactivity remains.
   e. Radioactivity is monitored by specially trained personnel.

f. No pregnant women or children younger than 18 years old are allowed to visit.

g. Lead shields may be used to decrease radiation that emanates from the patient.

6. Reinforce that help is readily available.

During Radiation Treatment

1. Maintain patient on strict bed rest on her back with head of bed elevated 15 to 30 degrees. Patient may be log rolled three or four times per day. Use egg crate mattress.
2. Have patient bathe upper body. Perineal care and linen changes are done by the nursing staff.
3. Maintain patient on a low-residue diet to prevent bowel movements, which could dislodge the apparatus. Encourage the patient to eat several small portions rather than few large servings. Medication to induce constipation is given.
4. Inspect indwelling catheter frequently to ensure proper drainage. A distended bladder may cause severe radiation burns.
5. Encourage fluids to prevent bladder infection.
6. Observe for signs and symptoms of radiation sickness—nausea, vomiting, fever, diarrhea, abdominal cramping.
7. Check applicator position every 8 hours, and monitor amount of bleeding and drainage (a small amount is normal).
8. Check patient frequently to minimize anxiety, but minimize time spent at bedside to reduce radiation exposure.
9. Mild sedatives or pain medication may be given for patient comfort.

NURSING ALERT

Long-handled forceps and a lead-lined container are left in the room after loading, in the event the radioactive sources are dislodged.

During Radiation Removal

1. Before removal of the applicator, the patient is medicated with appropriate analgesic.
2. The radioactive sources are removed by radiation personnel and safely stored for transport.
3. The indwelling catheter is removed and then the applicator is removed.
4. The patient is given an enema or suppository to reverse the induced constipation.
5. The patient should be evaluated for safe ambulation because of prolonged bed rest before discharge.

NURSING ALERT

Rules and regulations regarding radiation safety are strictly enforced to protect patients and health care workers.

Myomas of the Uterus

Myomas (fibroids, leiomyomas, fibromyomas) are benign tumors of the uterine myometrium (smooth muscle).

Pathophysiology and Etiology

1. Develop in women 25 to 50 years old.
2. May spontaneously regress after menopause.
3. Unknown cause but occur frequently in all women, most commonly in black women.

Clinical Manifestations

1. Small myomas do not cause symptoms.
2. First indication may be palpable mass.
3. Irregular bleeding—usually menorrhagia.
4. Pain comes form pressure on adjacent organs—possible heavy feeling in pelvis.
5. Secondary symptoms include fatigue because of anemia, urinary disturbances, and constipation.

Diagnostic Evaluation

1. Ultrasound—to identify size and location of myomas.
2. Cytology, dilation and curettage, etc., to rule out cancer.

Management

1. Myomectomy may be done for small tumor, may be done through hysteroscope.
2. Hysterectomy for large or numerous tumors.
3. Gonadotropin-releasing hormone antagonist (Lupron) therapy to create hypoestrogenic environment and to try to shrink tumors.
4. Frequently resolve on own postmenopausally.
5. Uterine artery embolization—transvenous procedure in which the blood supply to the myoma is obstructed and the myoma degenerates.

Complications

Infertility, habitual abortion.

Nursing Assessment

1. Ask about pain, menstrual irregularity, possible urinary symptoms, and constipation.
2. Assess patient's understanding of condition as benign.

Nursing Diagnosis

• Pain related to tumor growth

Nursing Interventions

Relieving Pain

1. Teach patient proper use and side effects of analgesics and use of heating pad as desired.
2. Encourage patient to avoid long periods of standing; rest with pelvis in dependent position periodically to achieve comfort.
3. Encourage patient to void frequently to avoid increased pressure from distended bladder.
4. Advise use of high-fiber diet to prevent constipation.
5. Prepare patient for surgery, if indicated.

Patient Education and Health Maintenance

1. Tell patient to report increased symptoms, and worsening bleeding because myomas may be enlarging and treatment may be indicated.

2. Reassure patient that myomas do not become malignant, but she should keep regular follow-up visits for cancer screening.

Outcome-Based Evaluation
• Verbalizes control of pain

■ Ovarian Cysts

Ovarian cysts are growths arising from ovarian components, usually benign.

Pathophysiology and Etiology
1. Often arise from functional changes in the ovary—from graafian follicle or from persistent corpus luteum.
2. Dermoid cysts may develop from abnormal embryonic epithelium.
3. Frequently found during childbearing years; masses found in women older than age 50 have greater chance of being malignant.

Clinical Manifestations
1. May be asymptomatic or cause minor pelvic pain.
2. Possible menstrual irregularity.
3. Tender, palpable mass.
4. Rupture causes acute pain and tenderness; may mimic appendicitis or ectopic pregnancy.

Diagnostic Evaluation
1. Pelvic sonogram to determine size and characteristics.
2. Pregnancy test to rule out ectopic pregnancy.
3. Biopsy (at time of surgery) is done for suspicious cysts.

Management
1. Functional cysts less than 5 cm wide may be treated with oral contraceptives for 1 to 3 months in attempt to suppress them.
2. Surgery for large, complex, or leaking cyst by laparoscopy or laparotomy.

Complications
Rupture may cause peritoneal inflammation.

Nursing Assessment
1. Obtain history of sexual activity, use of contraception, past episodes of PID to rule out ectopic pregnancy.
2. Obtain history of recent menses—irregular bleeding and spotting often signal follicular cyst; delayed menses and prolonged bleeding signal corpus luteal cyst.
3. Perform abdominal examination for tenderness, guarding, and rebound, which may indicate rupture.

Nursing Diagnoses
• Pain related to abnormal growth
• Risk for Fluid Volume Deficit related to rupture of cyst or postoperative change in intra-abdominal pressure

Nursing Interventions
Relieving Pain
1. Encourage the use of analgesics as prescribed and of heating pad if desired.
2. Teach the patient the proper use of oral contraceptives if prescribed, with side effects; encourage monthly follow-up visits to determine if cyst is resolving.
3. Tell the patient that heavy lifting, strenuous exercise, and sexual intercourse may increase pain.

Maintaining Fluid Volume
1. Monitor for nausea, vomiting, rigid abdomen, and change in vital signs related to rupture of cyst. Administer IV fluids as directed and maintain NPO status until abdominal rigidity resolves.
2. Reassure patient that symptoms will resolve.
3. Prepare the patient with large or nonresponsive cyst for surgery as indicated.
4. Postoperatively monitor vital signs frequently and maintain intravenous (IV) infusion while NPO.
5. Assess frequently for abdominal distention because of fluid and gas pooling in abdominal cavity.
6. Apply abdominal binder to help prevent distention.
7. Place the patient in semi-Fowler's position for greatest comfort and encourage early ambulation to reduce distention (help patient arise slowly to prevent orthostatic hypotension).
8. Administer antiemetics and insert a nasogastric tube as ordered to prevent vomiting.
9. As distention resolves, assess bowel sounds and advance oral intake slowly.

Patient Education and Health Maintenance
1. Reassure patient that in most cases, ovarian function remains, and she remains fertile.
2. Reassure patient about low malignancy rate of cysts.
3. Encourage patient to report recurrent symptoms or worsening of pain if cyst is being treated medically.

Outcome-Based Evaluation
• Verbalizes reduced pain
• Vital signs stable, no orthostasis

■ Ovarian Cancer

Ovarian cancer is a gynecologic malignancy, with high mortality because of advanced disease by time of diagnosis. It is the leading cause of morbidity of gynecologic cancers.

Pathophysiology and Etiology
1. Peak incidence is in fifth decade. One of 70 women will develop ovarian cancer.
2. Cause is unknown but associated with family history of breast or ovarian cancer; high-fat diet; smoking; alcohol use; environmental pollutants; and personal history of breast, colon, or endometrial cancer. Also higher incidence in nulliparous women or women with low parity.

3. Epithelial cell tumors constitute 90%; germ and stromal cell tumors 10%.

Clinical Manifestations
1. No early manifestations.
2. First manifestations—(vague) abdominal discomfort, indigestion, flatulence, anorexia, pelvic pressure, weight gain or loss, ovarian enlargement.
3. Late manifestations—abdominal pain, ascites, pleural effusion, intestinal obstruction.

Diagnostic Evaluation
1. Pelvic examination to detect enlargement, nodularity, immobility of the ovaries.
2. Pelvic sonography and computed tomography (CT) scan not helpful for early detection.
3. Paracentesis or thoracentesis if ascites or pleural effusion is present.
4. Laparotomy to stage the disease and determine effectiveness of treatment.
5. Increase of CA 125 signifies progression, but not useful as diagnostic or screening tool.

Management
1. Total abdominal hysterectomy with BSO and omentectomy is usual treatment because of delayed diagnosis.
2. Chemotherapy is more effective if tumor is optimally debulked; usually follows surgery because of frequency of advanced disease; may be given IV or intraperitoneal.
3. Radiation therapy is not often valuable.
4. Hormonal therapy with tamoxifen (Tamofen), an antiestrogen agent, may be used.
5. Second-look laparotomy may be done after adjunct therapies to take multiple biopsies and determine effectiveness of therapy. Practice is controversial because it does not affect survival.
6. Immunotherapy is being investigated in clinical trials.

Complications
1. Direct intra-abdominal or lymphatic spread

Nursing Assessment
1. Obtain history of irregular menses, pain, postmenopausal bleeding.
2. Ask about vague gastrointestinal-related complaints.
3. Ask about history of other malignancy and family history of breast or ovarian cancer.
4. Assess patient's general health status in terms of tolerating surgical and adjuvant therapy.

NURSING ALERT
A combination of a long history of ovarian dysfunction and persistent undiagnosed gastrointestinal complaints raises the suspicion for ovarian cancer. A palpable ovary in a postmenopausal woman is abnormal and should be evaluated as soon as possible.

Nursing Diagnoses
- Ineffective Coping related to advanced stage of cancer
- Altered Nutrition: Less Than Body Requirements related to nausea and vomiting from chemotherapy
- Body Image Disturbance related to hair loss from chemotherapy
- Pain related to surgery

Nursing Interventions
Strengthening Coping
1. Provide emotional support through diagnostic process; allow patient to ventilate feelings, and encourage positive coping mechanisms.
2. Administer anxiolytic and analgesic medications as prescribed and teach patient and caregivers the potential side effects.
3. Refer patient to cancer support group.

Maintaining Adequate Nutrition
1. Administer or teach patient or caregiver to administer antiemetics as needed for nausea and vomiting.
2. Encourage small, frequent, bland meals or liquid nutritional supplements as able.
3. Assess the need for IV fluids if patient is vomiting.
4. Monitor for passage of gas and bowel movements after surgery. Bowel dysfunction related to surgery may cause nausea and anorexia.

Maintaining Body Image
1. Prepare patient for body image changes with chemotherapy (ie, hair loss).
2. Encourage patient to prepare ahead of time with turbans, wigs, hats, etc.
3. Encourage patient to enhance appearance with makeup, clothing, jewelry, etc., as she is used to doing.
4. Stress the positive effects of patient's treatment plan.

Relieving Pain
1. Prepare patient for surgery as indicated; explain the extent of incision, IVs, catheter, packing, and drain tubes expected (see p. 756 for a discussion of hysterectomy).
2. Postoperatively, administer analgesics as needed and explain to patient she may be drowsy.
3. Reposition frequently and encourage early ambulation to promote comfort and prevent side effects.

Patient Education and Health Maintenance
1. Explain to patient the onset of menopausal symptoms with ovary removal.
2. Tell patient that disease progression will be monitored closely by laboratory tests, and second look laparoscopy may be necessary.
3. Female relatives of patient should notify their doctors; biannual pelvic examinations may be necessary.
4. For women who have not had breast or ovarian cancer, oral contraceptives may decrease the risk of ovarian and endometrial cancer. Multiparity is also protective.

Outcome-Based Evaluation
- Openly discusses prognosis, asks appropriate questions, makes plans for short-term future
- Weight maintained
- Verbalizes satisfaction in appearance with wig
- Verbalizes good control over pain

OTHER GYNECOLOGIC CONDITIONS

Pelvic Inflammatory Disease
Pelvic inflammatory disease is an infection that may involve the fallopian tubes, ovaries, uterus, or peritoneum.

Pathophysiology and Etiology
1. Incidence has been increasing; high recurrence rate because of reinfections.
2. Often polymicrobial; causative agents include *N. gonorrhoeae*, *C. trachomatis*, anaerobes, gram-negative bacteria, and *streptococci*. Cervical infection ascend through the endometrium, into the fallopian tubes, and possibly into the peritoneal cavity.
3. Predisposing factors include multiple sexual partners, early onset of sexual activity, use of IUDs (wick promotes ascension of bacteria), and procedures, such as therapeutic abortion, cesarean sections, and hysterosalpingograms.

Clinical Manifestations
1. Pelvic pain—most common presenting symptom; usually dull and bilateral.

> **NURSING ALERT**
>
> Localized right- or left-lower-quadrant tenderness with guarding, rebound, or palpable mass signifies tubo-ovarian abscess with peritoneal inflammation. Immediate evaluation and surgical intervention are necessary to prevent rupture and widespread peritonitis.

2. Fever—especially with gonococcal infections.
3. Cervical discharge—mucopurulent.
4. Cervical motion tenderness—especially with gonococcal infections.
5. Irregular bleeding.
6. Gastrointestinal symptoms—nausea, vomiting, acute abdomen usually signify abscess.
7. Urinary symptoms—dysuria, frequency.
8. Presentation with chlamydia may be mild.

Diagnostic Evaluation
1. Endocervical DNA testing or culture to identify organisms.
2. CBC shows elevated leukocytes; elevated C-reactive protein; elevated sedimentation rate.
3. Laparoscopy provides direct visualization of the fallopian tubes.

Management
1. Antibiotics—combinations of tetracyclines, penicillins, quinolones, and cephalosporins, orally or parenterally depending on the patient's condition, such as:
   a. Cefotetan (Cefotan) 2 g IV every 12 hours plus doxycycline 100 mg IV or orally every 12 hours.
   b. Clindamycin (Cleocin) 900 mg IV every 8 hours plus gentamycin (Garamycin) 2 mg/kg of body weight IV or IM as loading dose; followed by 1.5 mg/kg every 8 hours as maintenance dosage. (A single daily dose of gentamycin may be substituted.)
   c. Ofloxacin (Floxin) 400 mg orally twice a day plus metronidazole 500 mg orally twice a day for 14 days.
   d. Ceftriaxone 250 mg IM once plus doxycycline 100 mg orally twice a day for 14 days.
2. Parenteral therapy can be switched to oral therapy 24 hours after improvement is shown (reduced fever, decreased pain, resolution of nausea and vomiting).

> **NURSING ALERT**
>
> If patient with PID is to be treated at home, stress the importance of follow-up, usually in 48 hours to determine if oral antibiotic treatment is effective. Advise the patient to report any worsening of symptoms immediately.

3. Inpatient treatment required if uncertain diagnosis; abscess; pregnancy; severe infection with nausea, vomiting, and high fever; cannot take oral fluids; prepubertal or immunodeficient patient; or more aggressive antibiotics required to preserve fertility.
4. Surgical treatment may be necessary to drain abscess or later to treat adhesions or tubal damage.

Complications
1. Abscess rupture and sepsis.
2. Infertility because of adhesions of fallopian tubes and ovaries.
3. Ectopic pregnancy caused by inability of fertilized egg to pass stricture.

Nursing Assessment
1. Obtain history of menstruation, contraception, sexual activity (including number of partners), STD history, symptoms in sexual partner.
2. Assess level of pain, fever, and vital signs for hypotension and increased pulse, indicating hypovolemia.
3. Perform abdominal and pelvic examinations, if indicated; be alert for abdominal tenderness, rebound, guarding, or a mass.
4. Assess patient's feelings about having an STD.

Nursing Diagnoses
- Pain related to pelvic inflammation and infection
- Fluid Volume Deficit related to fever and decreased oral intake

Nursing Interventions
See Nursing Care Plan 22-1.

NURSING CARE PLAN 22-1   Care of the Patient with Pelvic Inflammatory Disease

You are assigned Janice Smith, a 17-year-old with acute PID. From your assessment and your knowledge of PID, you develop your plan of care.

Subjective data: Janice tells you she has severe lower abdominal pain, vaginal discharge, fever, and nausea and vomiting that have made her unable to eat or drink for 2 days. She feels weak and dizzy. She admits to being sexually active with a new partner without condoms. She is on oral contraceptives and her last menstrual period was 1 week ago.

Objective data: Vital signs are—temperature 39°C (102.2°F), pulse 98, BP 94/60, respirations 24. On examination you note lower abdominal tenderness and mild guarding without rebound. On speculum examination, Janice has purulent cervical discharge. On bimanual examination, she has cervical motion tenderness and bilateral adnexal tenderness without masses. The presumptive diagnosis of pelvic inflammatory disorder is made and antibiotic therapy is prescribed.

NURSING DIAGNOSIS   Pain, related to pelvic infection

GOAL/OUTCOME   Pain will be reduced.

Nursing Intervention	Rationale	Outcome-Based Evaluation
1. Administer analgesics as prescribed. Alert patient to side effect of drowsiness.	1. Analgesics provide pain relief. Knowledge of side effects enhances patient compliance.	1. Verbalizes reduced severity of pain after medication.
2. Assist patient to position of pelvic dependence, with head and feet elevated slightly.	2. Promotes drainage of infection without strain on pelvic structures.	2. Resting in pelvic dependent position.
3. Encourage patient to apply heating pad to lower abdomen or low back.	3. Promotes circulation and relief of inflammation, promotes comfort.	3. Uses heating pad properly.

NURSING DIAGNOSIS   Fluid Volume Deficit related to fever and decreased oral intake

GOAL/OUTCOME   Fluid balance will be restored.

Nursing Interventions	Rationale	Outcome-Based Evaluation
1. Maintain IV fluids as ordered.	1. IV fluids replace circulating fluid vol.	1. Denies dizziness. BP 106/64, pulse 88.
2. Administer antiemetics as prescribed.	2. Antiemetics prevent vomiting.	2. No vomiting.
3. Monitor intake and output.	3. Provides feedback on fluid replacement.	3. Intake equals output.
4. Restart oral intake with ice chips and sips of water when vomiting has ceased for 2 h.	4. Will not distend stomach and produce vomiting.	4. Ice chips and sips of water tolerated without vomiting.

NURSING DIAGNOSIS   Risk for Infection Transmission related to sexual activity

GOAL/OUTCOME   Infection will not be transmitted or recur.

Nursing Interventions	Rationale	Outcome-Based Evaluation
1. Advise abstinence until repeat cultures prove cure at follow-up, about 2 w after treatment.	1. Abstinence is the only sure method of preventing transmission of organisms.	1. Reports understanding of abstinence, need for follow-up.
2. Tell patient to advise partner(s) to seek treatment.	2. All partners must receive treatment to break the chain of transmission.	2. Partner has been advised by patient.
3. Teach patient methods of preventing infection with STDs—abstinence, monogamy, proper use of male and female condoms.	3. Safe sexual behavior reduces risk of STDs.	3. Describes proper use of condoms.

Relieving Pain

1. Administer or teach self-administration of analgesics as prescribed.
2. Advise patient to rest in bed for first 1 to 3 days and apply heating pad to pelvis for comfort.
3. Administer or teach self-administration of antibiotics as prescribed. Keep strict dosage schedule and notify health care provider if dose lost through vomiting.

Restoring Fluid Balance

1. Monitor vital signs and intake and output closely.
2. Administer antiemetics as indicated.
3. Maintain IV infusion of fluids until oral intake adequate.
4. Provide clear fluids, and soft, bland diet as tolerated.

Patient Education and Health Maintenance

1. Encourage compliance with antibiotic therapy for full length of prescription.
2. Stress the need for sexual abstinence and pelvic rest (nothing in vagina, including no douching or use of tampons) until follow-up visit and testing ensure cure.
3. Advise testing and possible treatment for all sexual partners. Tell patient that diagnosis of chlamydia or gonorrhea necessitate reporting to public health department and partners will be traced.
4. Educate about safer sexual practice.

Outcome-Based Evaluation

- Verbalizes relief of pain
- Vital signs stable; urine output adequate

◼ Endometriosis

Endometriosis is the abnormal proliferation of uterine endometrial tissue outside the uterus.

Pathophysiology and Etiology

1. May also be found outside the pelvic cavity; an intact uterus is not needed to have endometriosis.
2. Peaks in women aged 25 to 45; may occur at any age. Increased risk in siblings, women with shorter menstrual cycles, and longer duration of flow. More common in whites than blacks, and in women who do not exercise and who are obese.
3. Responds to ovarian hormonal stimulation—estrogen increases it; progestins decrease it.
   a. Bleeds during uterine menstruation, resulting in accumulated blood and inflammation and subsequent adhesions and pain.
   b. Regresses during amenorrhea (ie, pregnancy and menopause) and oral contraceptive and androgen use.
4. Theories of origin:
   a. May be embryonic tissue remnants that differentiate as a result of hormonal stimulation and spread via lymphatic or venous channels.
   b. May be transferred via surgical instruments.
   c. May be caused by retrograde menstruation through fallopian tubes into peritoneal cavity.

Clinical Manifestations

1. Depends on sites of implantation; may be asymptomatic.
2. Pelvic pain—especially during or before menstruation.
3. Dyspareunia.
4. Painful defecation—if implants are on sigmoid colon or rectum.
5. Abnormal uterine bleeding.
6. Persistent infertility.
7. Hematuria, dysuria, flank pain—if bladder involved.

Diagnostic Evaluation

1. Pelvic and rectal examinations—tender, fixed nodules or ovarian mass or uterine retrodisplacement; nodules may not be palpable.
2. Laparoscopy—for definitive diagnosis to view implants and determine extent of disease.
3. Other studies include ultrasound, CT, and barium enema to determine extent of organ involvement.

Management
Medical

1. Danazol (Danocrine)—synthetic androgen suppresses endometrial growth. Contraindicated in pregnancy.
2. Progestins—create a hypoestrogenic environment.
3. Gonadotropin-releasing hormone antagonist (Lupron) injections during a 6-month period—create hypoestrogenic environment.
4. Oral contraceptives—use small amount of estrogen, maximum amount of progestin and androgen effect to decrease implant size.

Surgical

1. Laparoscopic surgery—preferred procedure to remove implants and lyse adhesions; not curative; high recurrence rate.
2. CO_2 laser laparoscopy—for minimal to moderate disease; vaporizes tissue; may be done at same time as diagnosis; good pregnancy rate.
3. Laparotomy—for severe endometriosis or persistent symptoms.
4. Presacral neurectomy—to decrease central pelvic pain; preserves fertility.
5. Hysterectomy—if fertility is not desired and symptoms are severe; ovaries are preserved if not affected.

Complications

1. Infertility.
2. Rupture of cyst—mimics ruptured appendix.

Nursing Assessment

1. Obtain history of symptoms to determine spread and severity of disease.
2. Assess pain—level, location, characteristics.
3. Perform abdominal examination to assess for areas of tenderness, nodules.
4. Assess for impact of endometriosis, infertility on patient, relationship with significant other.

Nursing Diagnoses
- Pain related to hormonal stimulation, adhesions
- Self-Esteem Disturbance related to difficult management of disease, infertility

Nursing Interventions
Reducing Pain
1. Teach use of analgesics, as prescribed, with side effects.
2. Encourage use of heating pad to painful areas, as needed.
3. Teach patient relaxation techniques to control pain, such as deep breathing, imagery, and progressive muscle relaxation.
4. Encourage patient to try position changes for sexual intercourse if experiencing dyspareunia.

Increasing Self-Esteem
1. Include patient in treatment planning; answer questions about drug and surgical treatment so she can make informed choices.
2. Encourage adequate rest and nutrition.
3. Provide emotional support and encourage patient to discuss treatment of infertility with her physician.
4. Prepare patient for surgery as indicated.

Patient Education and Health Maintenance
1. Instruct patient in the side effects of prescribed medication; for example, danazol (Danocrine) may cause voice changes, increased facial hair, acne, weight gain, decreased breast size, and vasomotor reactions.
2. Refer patient to support groups such as Endometriosis Association, 8585 North 76th Place, Milwaukee, WI 53223, 1-800-992-3636.

Outcome-Based Evaluation
- Verbalizes reduced pain
- Verbalizes increased self-esteem

◼ Toxic Shock Syndrome

Toxic shock syndrome (TSS) is a condition caused by a bacterial toxin (*Staphylococcus aureus*) in the bloodstream; it can be life-threatening.

Pathophysiology and Etiology
1. Cause is uncertain, but 70% of cases are associated with menstruation and tampon use.
2. Research studies suggest that magnesium-absorbing fibers in tampons may account for lower levels of magnesium in the body; this contributes to providing an ideal condition for toxin production by the bacteria.
3. TSS does occur in nonmenstruating females and males with conditions such as cellulitis, surgical wound infection, vaginal infections, subcutaneous abscesses, and with the use of contraceptive sponge or diaphragm, and tubal ligation.
4. Oral contraceptives may be protective against TSS by increasing lactobacilli in vaginal flora.

Clinical Manifestations
1. Sudden onset of fever greater than 39°C (102°F).
2. Vomiting and profuse watery diarrhea.
3. Rapid progression to hypotension and shock within 72 hours of onset.
4. Mucous membrane hyperemia.
5. Sometimes, sore throat, headache, and myalgia.
6. Rash (similar to sunburn) that develops 1 to 2 weeks after onset of illness and is followed by desquamation, particularly of the palms and soles.

Diagnostic Evaluation
1. Blood, urine, throat, and vaginal/cervical cultures; possibly cerebrospinal fluid culture to detect/rule out infectious organism.
2. Tests to rule out other febrile illnesses—Rocky Mountain Spotted Fever, Lyme disease, meningitis, Epstein-Barr, or coxsackie virus.
3. CBC, electrolytes, blood urea nitrogen, creatinine, and other tests to monitor condition.

Management
1. Fluid and electrolyte replacement to increase blood pressure and prevent renal failure.
2. Vasopressor medications (ie, dopamine) as needed.
3. Antibiotics (ie, penicillins or cephalosporins) may decrease the rate of relapse.
4. The use of steroids and immunoglobulins is controversial.

Complications
Cardiovascular collapse and renal failure because of shock.

Nursing Assessment
1. Determine menstrual history, use of tampons, or whether there has been recent skin infection, childbirth, or surgery.
2. Determine vital signs and assess temperature and blood pressure as indicated; hemodynamic monitoring may be needed.

Nursing Diagnoses
- Hyperthermia related to infectious process
- Fluid Volume Deficit related to toxin effects
- Impaired Skin Integrity related to latent desquamation

Nursing Interventions
Reducing Fever
1. Administer antipyretics as ordered.
2. Use cooling measures, such as sponge baths and hypothermia blanket, if indicated.
3. Monitor core body temperature frequently.

Restoring Fluid Volume
1. Perform hemodynamic monitoring as indicated (ie, arterial line, central venous pressure, or pulmonary artery pressure).

2. Maintain strict intake and output measurement.
3. Insert indwelling catheter to monitor urine output.
4. Administer IV fluids and vasopressors as ordered to control hypotension.
5. Monitor respiratory status for pulmonary edema and respiratory distress syndrome because of fluid overload from increased fluid replacement.
6. Administer diuretics as ordered if edema results.

Restoring Skin Integrity

1. Tell patient to expect desquamation of skin, as in peeling sunburn.
2. Protect skin and avoid use of harsh soaps and alcohol that cause drying.
3. Tell patient to apply mild moisturizer and avoid direct sunlight until healed.
4. Advise patient that reversible hair loss may occur 1 to 2 months after TSS.

Patient Education and Health Maintenance

1. Tell patient to expect fatigue for weeks to months after TSS.
2. Tell patient not to use tampons in future to reduce risk of recurrence.
3. Encourage follow-up examination and cultures.
4. Teach prevention of TSS.
   a. Alternate use of pads with tampons; avoid super-absorbency tampons.
   b. Change tampons frequently and do not wear one longer than 8 hours—4 hours maximum in heavy discharge time.
   c. Be careful of vaginal abrasions that can be caused by some applicators.
   d. Be alert to symptoms of TSS.

Outcome-Based Evaluation

- Afebrile
- Normotensive, good urine output
- Skin heals without scarring

SELECTED REFERENCES

Allen, K.M. & Phillips, J.M. (1997). *Women's health across the lifespan*. Philadelphia: Lippincott Williams & Wilkins.

Baker, D.A. et al. (1999). Once-daily valacyclovir hydrochloride for suppression of recurrent genital herpes. *Obstetrics and Gynecology, 94,* 103–6.

Centers for Disease Control and Prevention. 1998 Guidelines for Treatment of Sexually Transmitted Diseases. *Morbidity and Mortality Weekly Report, 47*(RR-1), 1–116.

Corey, L. et al. (1999). Recombinant glycoprotein vaccine for the prevention of genital HSV-2 infection. *Journal of the American Medical Association, 282,* 331–340.

Crawford, S.L., et al. (2000). A longitudinal study of weight and the menopause transition: Results from the Massachusetts Women's Health Study. *Menopause, 7*(2), 96–104.

Cullins, V., Dominguez, L., Guberski, T. et al. (1999). Treating vaginitis. *Nurse Practitioner, 24*(10), 46–63.

Davies, J.E. (1998). All that itches is not yeast. *Advance for Nurse Practitioners, 6*(11), 35–38,47,93.

Frezieres, R.G. et al. (1999). Evaluation of the efficacy of a polyurethane condom. *Family Planning Perspectives, 31,* 81–7.

Gaydos, C.A. et al. (1998). Chlamydia trachomatis infections in female military recruits. *New England Journal of Medicine, 339,* 739–42.

Gill, M.A. (1998). Ovarian cancer: It whispers so listen! *Advance for Nurse Practitioners, 6*(11), 48–54.

Jacobs et al. (1999). Screening for ovarian cancer: A pilot randomised controlled trial. *Lancet, 353,* 1207–10.

Keating, N.L., et al. (1999). Use of hormone replacement therapy by postmenopausal women in the US. *Annals of Internal Medicine, 130,* 545–553.

McAllister, M. (1998). Menopause: Providing comprehensive care for women in transition. *Primary Care Practice, 2*(3), 256–270.

Nestler, J.E. et al. (1999). Ovulatory and metabolic effects of D-chiro-inositol in the polycystic ovary syndrome. *New England Journal of Medicine, 340,* 1314–20.

Pilliteri, A. (1999). *Maternal and child health nursing* (3rd ed.). Philadelphia: Lippincott Williams & Wilkins.

Polaneczky, M. & Liblanc, M. (1998). Long-term depot medroxyprogesterone acetate (Depo-Provera) use in inner city adolescents. *Journal of Adolescent Health, 23,* 81–88.

Reeder, S.J., Martin, L.L. & Koniak-Griffin, D. (1997). *Maternity nursing: Family, newborn, and women's health care*. Philadelphia: Lippincott-Raven.

Rhodes, J.C., Kjerulff, K.H., Langenberg, P.W., & Guzinski, G.M. (1999). Hysterectomy and sexual functioning. *Journal of the American Medical Association, 282*(20), 1934–1941.

Ross, R.K., et al. (2000). Effects of hormone replacement therapy on breast cancer risk: Estrogen versus estrogen plus progestin. *Journal of the National Cancer Institute, 92*(3), 328–332.

Schairer, C., et al. (2000). Menopausal estrogen and estrogen-progestin replacement therapy and breast cancer risk. *Journal of the American Medical Association, 282*(2), 485–491.

Scoggin, J. & Morgan, G. (1997). *Practice guidelines for obstetrics and gynecology*. Philadelphia: Lippincott-Raven.

Taffe, A.M. & Cauffield, J. (1998). "Natural" hormone replacement therapy and dietary supplements used in the treatment of menopausal symptoms. *Primary Care Practice, 2*(3), 292–302.

Thys-Jacobs, S. et al. (1998). Calcium carbonate and the premenstrual syndrome: Effects on premenstrual symptoms. *American Journal of Obstetrics and Gynecology, 179,* 444–52.

Wald, A., et al. (2000). Reactivation of genital herpes simplex virus type 2 infection in asymptomatic seropositive persons. *New England Journal of Medicine, 342*(5), 844–850.

Williams, P.A. (1999). Nonscientifically validated herbal treatments for vaginitis. *Nurse Practitioner, 24* (8), 101–104.

Wyatt, K.M. et al. (1999). Efficacy of vitamin B-6 in the treatment of premenstrual syndrome: Systematic review. *British Medical Journal, 318,* 1375–81.

Xu, Y. et al. (1998). Llysophosphatidic acid as a potential biomarker for ovarian and other gynecologic cancers. *Journal of the American Medical Association, 280,* 719–23.

Breast Conditions

ASSESSMENT OF THE BREAST

■ Subjective Data

Obtain a nursing history about specific breast complaints and general health information from the patient to plan care and appropriate patient teaching.

Breast Manifestations

1. Palpable lumps—date noted; affected by menstruation; changes noted since detection.
2. Nipple discharge—date of onset, color, unilateral or bilateral, spontaneous or provoked.
3. Pain or tenderness—localized or diffuse, cyclic or constant, unilateral or bilateral.
4. Date of last mammogram and result.
5. Patient's practice of breast self-examination (BSE).

History
General Information
1. Age.
2. Past medical/surgical history; injuries; bleeding tendencies.
3. Medications, including current or prior use of oral contraceptives/hormones, over-the-counter products, vitamins, and herbal supplements.
Gynecologic and Obstetric History
1. Menarche.
2. Date of last menstrual period.
3. Pregnancies, miscarriages, abortions, deliveries.
4. Lactation history.
5. Prior breast history, including previous history of irradiation involving breast region.
6. Family history of breast cancer.

■ Physical Examination

Perform a breast examination, as outlined in Procedure Guidelines 23-1. Remind all women of the importance of routine checkups with breast examination. BSE is an essential first step in prevention of breast cancer.

Guidelines for Early Detection

The American Cancer Society recommends the following for early detection of breast cancer:
1. BSE—once a month; age 20 and older.
2. Clinical examination—see a health care provider for a physical breast examination.
   a. Age 20 to 40, every 3 years.
   b. Every year after age 40.
3. Mammography—annual screening for women beginning at age 40.

GERONTOLOGIC ALERT

The American Cancer Society has not specified an age at which mammographic screening should be terminated. As long as a woman is in good health, regular screening is recommended.

DIAGNOSTIC TESTS

■ Laboratory Tests
Nipple Discharge Cytology
Description

Secretions are smeared on a slide, fixed, and submitted for cytologic examination. There is a high rate of false-negative test results with this method.

PROCEDURE GUIDELINES 23-1   EXAMINATION OF THE BREAST BY THE NURSE

PURPOSE

1. To detect abnormalities in the breasts
2. To teach a woman how to perform breast self-examination

EQUIPMENT

Good lighting and a private, warm setting

PROCEDURE

Nursing Action	Rationale
	GERONTOLOGIC ALERT Normal breast changes in older patients include drooping, flaccid breasts caused by decreased subcutaneous tissue from decreased estrogen levels. Nipple size and erection are also reduced.

SITTING POSITION

Nursing Action	Rationale
1. Wash your hands under warm water and dry them. Apply powder if they feel "sticky."	1. The breast is sensitive to cold. Powder reduces friction.
2. Have the woman strip to her waist and sit comfortably facing the examiner. Observe breast for abnormalities.	2. This provides an opportunity to observe breasts for lack of symmetry and for gross signs such as redness, irritated nipple, dimpling, orange peel skin.
3. Have patient raise arms overhead.	3. Changes in lower half of breast are more visible.
4. Palpate cervical and supraclavicular area.	4. Note whether lymph nodes are enlarged, fixed, movable, or difficult to locate.
5. Palpate axillary nodes; hold the woman's forearm in your left palm while you check nodes with your right fingertips. Repeat on other side.	5. Same as 4 above.
6. Have patient place hands on hips and press.	6. Flexes pectoral muscles, accentuates skin dimpling or masses.

LYING POSITION

Nursing Action	Rationale
1. Instruct the patient to lie down with her right arm under her head. Place a small pillow under the right shoulder.	1. This will spread breast tissue evenly over chest wall.

2. With the finger pads of two or three fingers, gently palpate breast tissue beginning at the upper outer quadrant.
  a. Proceed in an orderly pattern around the breast and repeat the first quarter examined.
  b. Repeat procedure for other breast.
	2. The sensitive fingers, proceeding in a kneading fashion, can detect thickened, lumpy, or "buckshot" tissue between the patient's skin and chest wall. Because the majority of breast lesions are in the upper outer quadrant, this segment is double checked.

3. Recognize that there is a prolongation of the axillary extension of normal breast tissue that may extend high into axilla.	3. This is normal if symmetrical and may be abnormal if asymmetrical.
4. Check areolar area for crustiness, nipple discharge, signs of infection. If nipple discharge is observed, note if from single or multiple ducts. May hemoccult to check for hidden blood.	4. A nipple discharge may be benign or may be related to cancer.
5. Record findings and report abnormalities to the health care provider.	5. Diagram may be useful for future reference.
6. Instruct the patient in performing self-examination. Encourage her to ask questions; provide her with appropriate literature.	6. Ninety percent of women discover their own abnormalities.

Nursing and Patient Care Considerations

1. Wash nipple area with water and pat dry before obtaining specimen if crusting of drainage is present.
2. Gently milk breast or ask woman to express fluid to obtain a large drop on nipple.
3. Carefully touch slide to drop and draw slide across nipple to obtain smear.
4. Spray with fixative or drop into container with fixative.
5. Inform patient of results promptly to reduce anxiety and explain that other tests may be needed.

Estrogen and Progesterone Receptors
Description

1. Evaluates cancer cells from tissue biopsy to determine receptor sites.
2. If such sites are present, the patient is more likely to respond to endocrine manipulation as adjuvant therapy.
3. Approximately 60% are estrogen-receptor positive. (Positive results—more than 10 fmol/mg protein.)

Nursing and Patient Care Consideration

1. Tell patient that the test may help select appropriate chemotherapy, especially estrogen-blocking agents
2. A negative result is associated with a less favorable prognosis.

Additional Laboratory Tests
Tumor Aggressiveness Tests

Blood tests to evaluate the aggressiveness of a tumor and its potential to regrow.

1. Proliferation/S phase—cell kinetic study that shows percent of cells in S phase in a tumor and gives an indication of proliferative capacity.
2. DNA ploidy—measurement of DNA content of a tumor; interpreted as favorable or unfavorable.
3. Her-2/neu—oncogene that has been demonstrated in 15% to 30% of breast cancers. Found by many investigators to be associated with poorer survival, especially node negative tumors. Scant data on use of this test are available.

Tests to Detect Metastasis

1. Increased values on liver function tests may indicate possible liver metastasis.
2. Increased calcium and alkaline phosphatase levels may indicate possible bony metastasis.
3. The role of biological markers in determining risk of metastasis continues under investigation.

Radiology and Imaging
Mammography
Description

1. Low-dose x-ray of breast used to screen for breast abnormalities or may be used when a lump is found on physical examination. Most sensitive method of early detection of breast cancer; can detect patients with clustered microcalcifications, early in breast cancer.

2. Compression of the breast is used to reduce the amount of radiation absorbed by the breast tissue and separate overlapping tissue.
3. Two views are taken routinely: craniocaudal and mediolateral; other views are done as necessary.
4. Best performed at a facility that is accredited by the American College of Radiology. The machines and staff at these facilities have met specific quality criteria.
5. Mammography is not routinely done if a woman is pregnant.
6. The breasts of young women tend to be extremely dense and are poorly suited to mammography.
7. False-negative results occur even in the best facilities; figure may reach 10%.

Nursing and Patient Care Considerations

1. Recommend regular screening based on established guidelines (see p. 787). Tell women that routine screening mammography has been shown to reduce mortality from breast cancer. Procedure takes approximately 15 minutes.
2. Remind woman not to apply deodorant, cream, or powder to breast, nipple, or underarm areas on examination day.
3. Advise that some discomfort may be felt from compressing the breast.
4. Alert patient that extra views do not imply that the patient has breast cancer.

NURSING ALERT

Fewer than 50% of women obtain regular screening mammograms based on the established guidelines. Because health teaching is an important nursing role, nurses should be educating women about the importance of routine screening.

Ultrasonography
Description

1. Uses high-frequency sound waves to get an image of the breast.
2. Most useful test after mammography; helps determine if a lump is a cyst or a solid mass.
3. May be used if patient is pregnant or is younger than 35 years old.

Nursing and Patient Care Considerations

1. Advise that this test is painless and noninvasive.
2. No preparation is necessary.

Additional Imaging Studies
Galactography

1. A contrast mammogram is obtained by injection of water-soluble contrast medium into a duct for patient with persistent bloody nipple discharge. It is a time-consuming procedure that is not routinely used.
2. It may outline an intraductal papilloma.

3. Its ability to differentiate benign from malignant lesions is limited.

Magnetic Resonance Imaging (MRI)

1. Useful in women with dense breasts and in those with silicone implants. May help in determining extent of disease and multifocality for treatment planning.
2. It is expensive and not useful for generalized screening.
3. MRI and technetium—99m sestamibi imaging are under evaluation and may increase capability for early diagnosis.
4. See p. 438 for description of MRI.

Metastatic workup may include x-rays (ie, chest x-ray), bone scan, or computed tomography (CT) scan to detect metastasis.

▣ Other Tests

In addition to laboratory tests and imaging studies, biopsy methods are commonly used to evaluate breast conditions. A biopsy is the only certain way to learn whether a breast lump or suspicious area seen on a mammogram is cancerous.

Fine Needle Aspiration
Description

1. Uses a thin needle and syringe to collect tissue or to drain lump after using a local anesthetic. If it is a cyst, removing the fluid will collapse it; no other treatment may be needed. Ultrasound may be used to locate a nonpalpable cyst.
2. Normal cyst fluid appears straw-colored or greenish. Fluid should be sent for cytology if it appears suspicious (clear or bloody); otherwise it is discarded.
3. This office procedure uses local anesthetic with results usually within 24 hours.
4. It has limited sensitivity, possibly because of insufficient acquisition of cytologic material.

Nursing and Patient Care Considerations

1. Inform the patient of small risk of hematoma and infection.
2. Band-Aid applied after procedure; usually no discomfort.
3. Solid lesions may warrant an excisional biopsy.

Needle Biopsy
Description

1. Office procedure uses local anesthetic and removes a small piece of breast tissue using a needle with a special cutting edge.
2. For palpable lesions with a high suspicion of malignancy. May provide a tissue diagnosis quickly—usually approximately 24 hours, without doing an excisional biopsy to plan definitive surgery.

Nursing and Patient Care Considerations

1. Inform the patient of small risk of hematoma and infection.
2. Tell patient that several passes may be necessary to obtain specimen, with minor discomfort.
3. Pressure dressing applied after procedure.

4. Recommend use of acetaminophen (Tylenol) or ibuprofen (Advil) for any postprocedure discomfort—usually minimal, if any.

Stereotactic Core Needle Biopsy
Description

1. An x-ray-guided method for localizing and sampling nonpalpable lesions detected on mammography with 90% to 95% sensitivity in detecting breast cancer.
2. Performed as an outpatient procedure with the patient lying prone on a special table using an automated biopsy gun with a vacuum system to draw tissue into a sampling chamber and rotate cutter to excise tissue (Mammotome).
3. After local anesthetic is administered, a needle is placed in the lesion with confirmation of its position on stereotactic x-ray views. Multiple samples are taken from different portions of the lesion. Allows harvesting of larger quantities of tissue with a single needle insertion.
4. The procedure is quicker and less expensive than mammographically guided needle localization followed by surgical excisional biopsy and is an alternative to surgical excisional biopsy.

Nursing and Patient Care Considerations

1. Inform patient that it is a 1-hour outpatient procedure that requires no special preparation.
2. The patient should dress comfortably and will need to remain still during the procedure.
3. Complications may include minor bleeding, hematoma, and infection.
4. Explain that nonspecific, suspicious, or atypical findings may result in proceeding to excisional biopsy.
5. Remind patient that area in question will not be removed, only sampled.

Note: Many nonpalpable abnormalities that require breast biopsy are being identified because of increased use of screening mammography. Large core needle biopsy has become an alternative to surgical excision.

Excisional Biopsy
Description

1. Surgical removal of a palpable or nonpalpable lesion. A frozen section may be done for immediate tissue diagnosis.
2. Excisional biopsy or lumpectomy entails entire removal of a mass; incisional biopsy entails partial removal of a mass.
3. This outpatient procedure may be performed under local or general anesthesia.
4. Curvilinear incision is usually made directly over the mass, which is excised en bloc including a 1-cm grossly free margin of tissue.

Nursing and Patient Care Considerations

1. Pressure dressing is placed, which can be removed in 24 to 48 hours.
2. Inform patient to watch for bleeding, hematoma, and signs of infection.
3. Recommend analgesics for discomfort and a support bra for comfort.

Needle Localization With Biopsy
Description
1. Performed when there is a nonpalpable mammographic finding.
2. Mammogram is used as a guide for placing a needle at the site of the breast change after injecting some local anesthetic.
3. A wire may be left in place for the surgeon and dye may be injected to mark the site.
4. Excisional biopsy is then done (see above).

Nursing and Patient Care Considerations
Inform patient that this may be a tedious procedure because she must remain immobile while the breast is compressed in the mammogram machine and different views are obtained.

Sentinel Lymph Node Biopsy
Description
1. A diagnostic surgical procedure utilizing selective lymph node sampling.
2. Pathologic study of the first (sentinel) axillary lymph node to receive drainage from a tumor; predicts the status of the remainder of the lymph nodes in the axilla.
3. Localization accomplished by injection of a blue dye and/or radioactive particles around a tumor to identify lymph nodes with afferent drainage.
4. The sentinel lymph nodes are subjected to routine pathological examination and immunohistochemical staining.
5. The status of the sentinel lymph node is used to determine whether to proceed with full axillary dissection and/or determine treatment modalities.
6. If the sentinel lymph node tests negative, no further axillary surgery is indicated.
7. If test result is positive, further axillary dissection may be needed.

Nursing and Patient Care Considerations
1. Remind patient that at this time, sentinel lymph node biopsy is not yet standard of care for breast cancer patients. It remains experimental, but its use is increasing. It is an outpatient procedure.
2. There is less morbidity and cost than with axillary dissection.

GENERAL PROCEDURES AND TREATMENT MODALITIES

Breast Self-Examination
BSE is an inexpensive, risk-free method to detect cancer. When lumps are discovered at an early stage, they have a better chance for long-term survival. See Patient Education: Breast Self-Examination.

Patient Education
General Points to Emphasize
1. Examine breasts once a month, just after the menstrual period, because breasts are less engorged and a tumor is easier to detect, and at regular monthly intervals after the cessation of menses.
2. Compare findings with the opposite breast.
3. Remind patient that 90% of breast lumps are not cancer.
4. Do not neglect men when teaching BSE—1% of breast cancers occur in men.

NURSING ALERT

Nurses play an important role in promoting BSE. Women report increased frequency of BSE when taught by a nurse.

Suggestions for Patients Who Find BSE Difficult
1. Tenderness—gentle self-examination may be more effective and less painful than examination by someone else.
2. Cystic breasts—recommend professional examination annually, and instruct patient to compare changes in breasts from one month to the next.
3. Large, pendulous breasts—encourage woman to support her breast with her hand to palpate thoroughly; lying down may help to flatten breasts.

Community Health Education
Implement patient teaching of BSE on a community level by:
1. Teaching BSE to women in the community—schools, churches, women's groups.
2. Reinforcing that early detection is associated with decreased mortality.
3. Helping patients and families establish and maintain support networks.
4. Tailoring patient education messages to patients of different cultures.
5. Knowing the resources available and making people aware of them.
   a. National Cancer Institute—staff can answer questions and send booklets about cancer. Toll-free number is 1-800-4-CANCER.
   b. American Cancer Society—offers many services to patients and their families. Call toll-free number for local information: 1-800-ACS-2345.

Surgery for Breast Cancer
Surgery for breast cancer may involve *mastectomy* or a *breast-preserving procedure*. The objective of breast-preserving procedures is a cosmetically acceptable breast after complete excision of the tumor. Research studies that compare breast conservation with mastectomy have demonstrated equivalent patient survival. See Table 23-1 for surgical approach options available. The following discussion covers mastectomy and axillary node dissection.

Preoperative Management
See p. 112 for routine preoperative care. In addition:
1. The nature of the procedure is explained, along with expected postoperative care that includes drain care, location of the incision, and mobility of the arm.

PATIENT EDUCATION Breast Self-Examination

1. Look for changes.

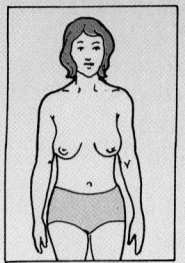 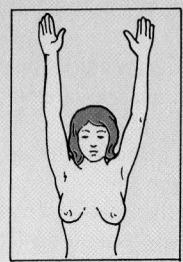 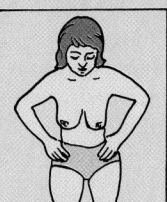

Hands at side.
Compare for symmetry.
Look for changes in:
• shape
• color
Check for:
• puckering
• dimpling
• skin changes
• nipple changes

Hands over head.
Check front and
side view for:
• symmetry
• puckering
• dimpling

Hands on hips,
press down,
bend forward.
Check for:
• symmetry
• nipple direction
• general
  appearance

2. Feel for changes.
3. Check your left breast with your right hand in the same way.

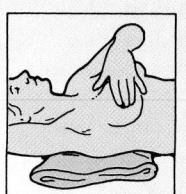 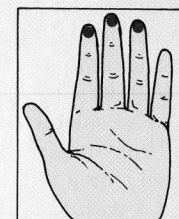 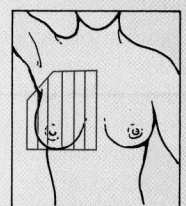

Lie down with a towel
under right shoulder;
raise right arm above
the head.

Use the pads of the
three middle fingers
of the left hand.
Hold hand in
bowed position.
Move fingers in
dime-size circles.

Examine area from:
• underarm to lower
  bra line
• across to breast
  bone
• up to collar bone
• back to armpit

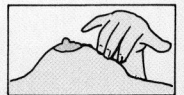 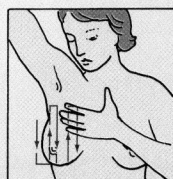

Use three levels
of pressure:
• light
• medium
• firm

Examine entire area
using vertical strip
pattern.

4. If you detect any changes, lumps, or knots, notify your
health care provider immediately.

TABLE 23-1 Types of Surgery for Breast Cancer

Procedure	Description	Indications
Lumpectomy (excisional biopsy)	Removal of tumor and surrounding tissue	For diagnosis of an abnormal mammographic finding or palpable breast lump if needle biopsy not performed. Further surgery may be needed
Quadrantectomy (partial mastectomy)	Removal of a breast quadrant that includes the tumor area and overlying skin	Normal- to large-sized breasts
Axillary dissection	Surgical removal of the axillary lymph nodes	Performed as part of breast-preserving procedure, mainly for prognosis, staging, and local/regional disease control
Simple mastectomy*	Surgical removal of the breast and a few of the axillary lymph nodes close to the breast	Prophylactic: Performed in carefully selected patients who are high risk for developing breast cancer, ie, patients with widespread and/or multifocal ductal carcinoma in situ
Modified radical mastectomy*	Surgical removal of the entire breast and the axillary lymph nodes	Advanced disease, large or multifocal tumors; women with very small breasts in whom local excision of tumor will be cosmetically unacceptable; ineligibility for radiation therapy
Radical mastectomy*	Removal of entire breast, pectoral muscles, axillary nodes	Rarely done today—may be performed for advanced disease

* Mastectomy may be followed by immediate or delayed reconstruction.

2. Information is clarified about diagnosis and possibility of further therapy.
3. Measures are taken to recognize the extreme anxiety and fear that the patient, family, and significant others experience.
   a. Discuss patient's concerns and usual coping mechanisms.
   b. Explore support systems with patient.
   c. Discuss concerns regarding body image changes.
4. The patient's overall medical condition is evaluated to guide preoperative care, help determine how well the patient will tolerate surgery, and help prepare for complications that may occur postoperatively.

GERONTOLOGIC ALERT

 Assessment of preoperative mental status of the older patient will help determine if a cognitive change occurs postoperatively.

Potential Complications

1. Infection.
2. Hematoma, seroma.
3. Lymphedema.
4. Paresthesia, pain of axilla and arm.
5. Impaired mobility of arm.

Postoperative Management and Nursing Care

See p. 116 for routine postoperative care. In addition:
1. Dressing is removed and the wound is assessed for erythema, edema, tenderness, odor, and drainage.
   a. Initial dressing may consist of gauze held in place by elastic, tape, or clear occlusive dressing wrap.
   b. Usually removed within 24 hours.
   c. Incision may remain open to air or Ace wrap may be replaced if patient prefers.
2. Suction drain from wound is maintained.
   a. May have 100 to 200 mL serous to serosanguineous drainage in the first 24 hours.
   b. Report if grossly bloody or excessive in amount.
3. Arm on affected side is observed for edema, erythema, and pain.
4. Patient teaching about drain care, exercises, surgical outcome and BSE occurs.
5. Female relatives, especially sisters, daughters, and mother who may need closer breast cancer surveillance are discussed.

NURSING ALERT

Mastectomy patients may have an elastic wrap bandage that should fit snugly but not so tightly that it hinders respiration. It should fit comfortably and support unaffected breast.

Nursing Diagnoses

- Impaired Physical Mobility related to impaired movement of arm on operative side
- Knowledge Deficit of care of incision, arm, and performance of BSE
- Altered Tissue Perfusion of affected arm related to lymphedema
- Body Image Disturbance related to loss of breast (for mastectomy patient)
- Anxiety related to diagnosis of cancer

PATIENT EDUCATION GUIDELINES   Hand and Arm Care to Help Prevent Lymphedema and Infection

After a mastectomy or axillary dissection, the arm may swell because of the excision of lymph nodes and their connecting vessels. Circulation of lymph fluid is slowed, making it more difficult for the body to combat infection. Special precautions should be taken to prevent lymphedema and infection.

1. Avoid burns while cooking or smoking.
2. Avoid sunburns.
3. Have all injections, vaccinations, blood samples, and blood pressure tests done on the other arm whenever possible.
4. Use an electric razor with a narrow head for underarm shaving to reduce the risk of nicks and scratches.
5. Carry heavy packages or handbags on the other arm.
6. Never cut cuticles; use hand cream or lotion instead.
7. Wear watches or jewelry loosely, if at all, on the operated arm.
8. Wear protective gloves when gardening and when using strong detergents, etc.
9. Use a thimble when sewing.
10. Avoid harsh chemicals and abrasive compounds.
11. Use insect repellent to avoid bites and stings.
12. Avoid elastic cuffs on blouses and nightgowns.

From *Mastectomy: A treatment for breast cancer.* NIH Publication No. 91-658.

- Altered Sexuality Patterns related to loss of breast and diagnosis of breast cancer
- Compromised Family Coping related to diagnosis of cancer

Nursing Interventions

In addition to routine postoperative interventions, provide the following care:

Mobilizing Affected Arm

1. Assess patient's ability to perform self-care and factors impeding performance.
2. Initially encourage wrist and elbow flexion and extension. Encourage use of arm for washing face, combing hair, applying lipstick, and brushing teeth. Encourage patient to gradually increase use of arm.
3. Encourage patient to avoid abduction initially to help prevent seroma formation.
4. Support arm in sling if prescribed to prevent abduction of the arm.
5. Instruct and provide patient with exercises to do when permitted (Table 23-2).

Increasing Knowledge

1. Explain how wound will gradually change and that the newly healed wound may have less sensation because of severed nerves.
2. Instruct patient on signs of infection, hematoma, or seroma formation to be reported.
3. Teach patient to bathe incision gently and to blot carefully to dry, and later, with approval, massage the healed incision gently with cocoa butter to encourage circulation and increase skin elasticity.
4. Teach care of drains, if appropriate; empty contents, measure, and record.
5. Teach care of affected arm (see Patient Education Guidelines).
6. Teach importance of BSE, mammograms, and regular follow-up visits.

7. Encourage discussion with health care provider about pregnancy after breast cancer, if indicated.

GERONTOLOGIC ALERT

Signs and symptoms of infection may not be obvious in older patients. Assess patients for mental status changes or urinary incontinence.

Promoting Lymphatic Drainage

1. Instruct patient in potential problem of lymphedema— at particular risk are patients who undergo axillary node dissection in combination with radiation therapy to axilla.
2. Do not take blood pressure, draw blood, inject medications, or start intravenous lines in affected arm. Post sign over bed.
3. Elevate affected arm on pillows, above level of heart, and hand above elbow to promote gravity drainage of fluid.
4. Teach patient to massage affected arm if prescribed to increase circulation and decrease edema. Treatment for severe lymphedema may also include the application of elastic bandages and/or intermittent pneumatic compression.

Enhancing Body Image

1. Assess mastectomy patient's knowledge of prosthesis and reconstruction options, and provide information as needed.
2. Discuss patient's views on how her body image has been altered.
3. Suggest clothing adjustments to camouflage loss of breast.
4. Assist patient to obtain a temporary prosthesis (may be provided by Reach to Recovery [see below]). First prosthesis should be light and soft to allow incision to heal. She may wear heavier type usually 4 to 8 weeks after surgeon's approval has been secured. Provide informa-

TABLE 23-2 Exercises for the Rehabilitation of the Patient Following Mastectomy

Exercise	Equivalent Daily Activities
1. Stand erect. Lean forward from waist. Allow arms to hang. Swing arms from side to side together; then in opposite direction. Next: swing arms from front to back together; then in opposite direction.	Broom sweeping Vacuum cleaning Mopping floor Pulling out and pushing in drawers Weaving Playing golf
2. Stand erect facing wall with palms of hand flat against wall; arms extended. Relax arms and shoulders and allow upper part of body to lean forward against hands. Push away to original position; repeat.	Pushing self out of bath tub Kneading bread Breast stroke—swimming Sawing or cutting types of crafts
3. Stand erect facing wall with palms of hands flat against wall. Climb the wall with the fingers; descend, repeat.	Raising windows Washing windows Hanging clothes on line Reaching to an upper shelf
4. Stand erect and clasp hands at small of back; raise hands; lower; repeat. Clasp hands back of neck; reach downward; upward; repeat.	Fastening brassiere Buttoning blouse or dress Pulling up a dress zipper Fastening beads Washing the back Drying the back with a bath towel
5. Toss a rope over the shower curtain rod. Hold the ends of the rope (knotted) in each hand and alternately pull on each end. Using a see-saw motion and with arms outstretched, slide the rope up and down over the rod.	Raising and lowering a window blind Closing and opening window drapes
6. Flex and extend each finger in turn.	Sewing, knitting, crocheting Typing, painting, playing piano or other musical instrument

tion regarding where to obtain permanent prosthesis and bras.

5. Encourage patient to discuss feelings with partner.
6. Encourage patient to allow herself to experience the grief process over the loss of her breast and to learn to cope with these feelings.

Reducing Anxiety

1. Familiarize patient with Reach to Recovery (an American Cancer Society program that consists of volunteers who have had mastectomies or breast-preserving procedures, and who visit postoperatively in the hospital to provide support and information) after clearing with patient's health care provider.
2. Discuss patient's usual coping mechanisms.
3. Encourage and assist family to support patient.
4. Assist patient to maintain control by planning care with her and incorporating her usual routines.
5. Refer for postmastectomy support group as needed and desired.
6. Offer list of community resources.
7. Remind patient that stress related to breast cancer and mastectomy may persist for a year or more and to seek help.
8. Include family in supportive interventions and measures to increase coping skills.

Maintaining Sexual Activity

1. Discuss effect of diagnosis and surgery on view of self as a woman.
2. Explore alternative means of sexual activity such as changing position during intercourse to decrease pressure on incision.
3. Encourage patient to discuss concerns with partner.
4. Assist patient and partner to look at incision when ready.

Facilitating Family Coping

1. Allow family members to acknowledge their feelings.
2. Approach family with warmth, respect, and support.
3. Acknowledge family strengths.
4. Involve family in care of patient.
5. Discuss stresses.
6. Direct family to community agencies as indicated.

Community and Home Care Considerations

Because of short stays (1 to 2 days) after mastectomy, many patients can achieve the following benefits from home health care:

1. Assess incision and drain tubes for proper healing and no signs of infection.
2. Teach patient drain tube and dressing care.
3. Support patient with adjustment back into home and community.
4. Monitor for lymphedema and reinforce teaching about arm care and exercises.
5. Other patients may require longer hospitalizations and possibly a short stay in a subacute unit for rehabilitation before going home because of age and comorbid conditions.
6. Goals of home care for these patients are to provide assessment of cardiovascular status and to ensure return of energy and proper healing.

Patient Education and Health Maintenance

1. Advise patient to call surgeon for signs of infection, increased pain, or edema of arm.
2. Ensure that patient knows schedule for follow-up with surgeon.
3. Provide resources for patient for ongoing information and support: American Cancer Society 1-800-ACS-2345.
4. Stress the importance of continued yearly mammogram, clinical breast exam, and monthly BSE.

Outcome-Based Evaluation
- Moves affected arm within prescribed limits
- States care of incision, drains, follow-up guidelines
- No infection or swelling in affected arm
- Expresses positive body image
- Exhibits minimal anxiety
- Reports satisfactory sexual activity and sexuality
- Maintains a functional support system

■ Breast Reconstruction After Mastectomy

Breast reconstruction (mammoplasty) may be performed immediately or as long after surgery as desired. Benefits include improved psychological coping because of improved body image and self-esteem. Demand for postmastectomy reconstruction has been increasing. Cost is usually covered by insurance.

Implants
Indicated for patients with inadequate breast tissue and skin of good quality.

Description
1. Uses prosthetic implants placed in pocket under skin or pectoralis muscle.
2. If opposite breast is ptotic (protruding downward), mastopexy may be necessary for symmetry.
3. Silicone implants are available only to mastectomy patients for reconstruction.
4. Complications include capsular contracture resulting in firmness; may be painful, cause infection.
5. Tissue expanders may be necessary before implants are inserted.
   a. Inflatable envelope is placed under muscle or skin and is filled with saline once incision is healed (about 4 weeks).
   b. Saline is instilled every 1 to 3 weeks until the expander is beyond desired size.
   c. Later, expander is removed and a permanent implant is placed.
   d. Some types of expanders may be left in permanently.
6. Advantages of implant reconstruction over other methods: only one incision; less fibrosis.
7. Disadvantage—may take months.

Nursing and Patient Care Considerations
1. Teach signs and symptoms of infection, hematoma, migration, and deflation.
2. Teach patient to massage breast to decrease capsule formation around implant.
3. Teach patient she may feel discomfort with expanders, if used.

Flap Grafts
Description
1. Transfer of skin, muscle, and subcutaneous tissue from another part of the body to the mastectomy site.

2. Two types:
   a. Latissimus dorsi—skin, fat, and muscles of back between shoulder blades are tunneled under skin to front chest.
   b. Transverse rectus abdominis myocutaneous (TRAM) flap—muscle, fat, skin, and blood supply are tunneled to breast area.
3. Disadvantages include cost, several hospitalizations required, slow process (done in stages), increased morbidity.
4. Complications include flap loss, hematoma, infection, seroma, and abdominal hernia.

Nursing and Patient Care Considerations
1. Assess flap and donor site for color, temperature, and wound drainage.
2. Control pain.
3. Provide support with bra or abdominal binder to maintain position of prosthesis.
4. Teach patient to perform BSE monthly and that she may have some asymmetry.

Nipple-Areolar Reconstruction
1. Usually done at a separate time from breast reconstruction.
2. Uses skin and fat from reconstructed breast for nipple, and upper thigh for areola; tanning or tattoo done to obtain appropriate color.

■ Other Surgeries of the Breast

Reduction mammoplasty may be done for cosmetic purposes or to relieve uncomfortable symptoms. Augmentation mammoplasty is considered a cosmetic procedure.

Reduction Mammoplasty
Description
1. Removal of excess breast tissue, which also involves a reduction in skin and possible transposition of nipple-areolar complex.
2. Used for alleviation of symptoms that may include back and neck pain, muscle spasm, and grooving at the shoulders secondary to bra straps.
3. Complications include hematoma, infection, necrosis of skin flap, and nipple inversion.

Nursing and Patient Care Considerations
1. Explore reasons patient may desire surgery.
2. Discuss postoperative expectations with patient.
3. Nursing interventions are similar to those in the patient undergoing reconstruction.

Augmentation Mammoplasty
Description
1. Enlarging of the breasts with the use of implants.
2. Implants may be made of silicone or saline; currently the FDA has limited use to saline implants only.

3. Complications include hematoma, wound infection, diminished sensation of the nipple, and capsular contracture, resulting in firmness of the breast.

Nursing and Patient Care Considerations

1. Discuss patient's expectations preoperatively.
2. Nursing interventions are similar to those in the patient undergoing reconstruction with implants.

DISORDERS OF THE BREAST

Fissure of the Nipple

A fissure is a type of ulcer that develops in the nipple(s) of a nursing mother.

Etiology and Clinical Manifestations

1. May be caused by lack of preparation of nipples in the prenatal period.

STANDARDS OF CARE GUIDELINES
Problems of the Breast

When caring for any patient undergoing evaluation, diagnostic testing, treatment, or counseling for a breast-related problem, ensure optimal outcome by adhering to the following guidelines:

- Explain the mammogram procedure or other diagnostic test and be sure patient knows when and how she will obtain results.
- Perform breast examination according to American Cancer Society guidelines, and teach procedure to woman.
- Inform health care provider and woman of any suspicious findings on breast examination—asymmetry of breasts, dimpling, skin changes, nipple discharge, fixed or hard mass.
- Inform health care provider and woman of abnormal mammogram or other test result, and ensure that follow-up is arranged.

After surgery for breast cancer:

- Assess for evidence of bleeding from the incision or flaps, including increase in pain, and notify surgeon promptly for increased pain or bleeding.
- Assess drainage from suction drain for amount, color, and odor. Report if grossly bloody, purulent, or excessive in amount (may have 100 to 200 mL in the first 24 hours).
- Assess new reconstructed breast flaps for viability by color, warmth, and wound drainage. Notify surgeon promptly for increased warmth, change in color, purulent or excessive drainage.
- Maintain proper protective positioning (avoid abduction to prevent edema) of arm and follow precautions for lymphedema.
- Assess patient's emotional response and provide support throughout the diagnostic and treatment process.

This information should serve as a general guideline only. Each patient situation presents a unique set of clinical factors and requires nursing judgment to guide care, which may include additional or alternative measures and approaches.

2. Condition aggravated by sucking infant.
3. Nipple appears sore and irritated.
4. Nipple bleeds.
5. Infection may result.

Management and Nursing Interventions

1. Wash nipples with sterile saline solution.
2. Use artificial nipple for nursing.
3. If above does not initiate healing process, stop nursing and use breast pump.
4. Teach proper breast-feeding techniques to prevent fissures.
   a. Wash, dry, and lubricate nipples in prenatal period in preparation for nursing.
   b. Make sure infant's mouth covers areola.
   c. Keep nipple clean by washing and drying after each nursing period.
   d. Use lanolin cream to prevent cracking; must remove before breast-feeding.

Nipple Discharge

Nipple discharge may be serous, serosanguineous, bloody, purulent, or multicolored. It is commonly associated with benign conditions; occasionally malignancy is responsible.

Etiology and Clinical Manifestations

1. Galactorrhea—bilateral, nonspontaneous, multiple duct, milky gray or green discharge usually seen in patients in childbearing years.
   a. Commonly seen after pregnancy and can last for 1 to 2 years.
   b. Also may be secondary to excessive breast manipulation, increased production of prolactin, medication, an endocrine anovulatory syndrome, or pituitary adenoma.
2. Mastitis—usually unilateral, purulent (see below).
3. Discharge containing blood—usually caused by intraductal papilloma (wart) or other benign lesion, but may be malignant.

Diagnostic Evaluation

1. Evaluate with clinical examination, test for occult blood, mammogram if older than age 35.
   a. Use of a hemoccult card gently pressed against the nipple when expressing discharge will help determine if the discharge is bloody, which warrants further workup.
   b. May get prolactin level; if elevated, may indicate pituitary adenoma.
2. Nonspontaneous milky gray or green discharge generally is not of pathologic significance and may not require workup.

Management and Nursing Interventions

1. Nursing interventions are aimed at alleviating anxiety and providing support to patient undergoing diagnostic testing.

a. Reassure woman that nipple discharge rarely indicates cancer.
2. Bromocriptine mesylate (Parlodel) may be given to suppress galactorrhea.
3. Treat for mastitis if purulent (see below).
4. Surgery may be indicated to treat cause of bloody and some other discharge caused by breast lesions.
   a. Most commonly because of wartlike intraductal papilloma in one of larger collecting ducts at edge of areola. May be secondary to fibrocystic changes or duct ectasia.
   b. Excisional biopsy and histologic examination must be done to rule out cancer.
5. Pituitary surgery for excision of adenoma (see p. 818).

◼ Acute Mastitis

Acute mastitis is inflammation of the breast because of infection.

Pathophysiology and Etiology

1. Usually occurs at beginning of lactation in first-time, breast-feeding mothers. May also occur later in chronic lactation mastitis and central duct abscesses.
2. Milk stasis may lead to obstruction, followed by non-infectious inflammation, then infectious mastitis.
3. Source of infection may be from hands of patient, personnel caring for patient, baby's nose or throat, or blood borne.
4. Most common pathogens: *Staphylococcus aureus*, *Escherichia coli*, *Streptococcus*.

Clinical Manifestations

1. Redness, warmth, edema; breast may feel doughy and tough.
2. Patient may complain of dull pain in affected area and may have nipple discharge.
3. Complication is mammary abscess (see below).

Management and Nursing Interventions

1. Diagnosis is usually made by characteristic manifestations.
2. Antibiotics are given—10-day course of penicillinase resistant antibiotic.
   a. Dicloxacillin (Diclox)—250 to 500 mg every 6 hours.
   b. Clindamycin (Cleocin)—150 to 300 mg every 6 hours.
   c. Cephalexin (Keflex)—250 to 500 mg every 6 hours.
3. May or may not have patient stop breast-feeding (controversial).
4. Apply heat to resolve tissue reaction; may cause increased milk production and worsen symptoms.
5. May apply cold to decrease tissue metabolism and milk production.
6. Have the patient wear firm breast support.
7. Encourage the breast-feeding patient to practice meticulous personal hygiene to prevent mastitis.

◼ Mammary Abscess

Mammary abscess is a localized collection of pus in a cavity of breast tissue.

Etiology and Clinical Manifestations

1. May follow acute mastitis if untreated.
2. Patient may have fever, chills, and malaise.
3. Affected area is sensitive and erythematous; may have palpable mass.
4. Pus may be expressed from nipple.

Management and Nursing Interventions

1. May perform needle aspiration if superficial mass.
2. Incision and drainage may be done, if deep.
3. A biopsy of the cavity wall may be done at time of incision and drainage to rule out breast carcinoma associated with abscess.
4. Administer antibiotics and analgesics, if ordered.
5. Apply hot, wet dressings to increase drainage and hasten resolution.

◼ Fibrocystic Changes

Fibrocystic change is a general term that includes various changes in the breast, namely, fibrosis and cystic dilatation of the ducts. May be present in 50% of women.

Pathophysiology and Etiology

1. Pathogenesis is not known, but is related to the cyclic stimulation of the breast by estrogen and represents a change from the normal stimulation and regression pattern of this process.
2. Occurs usually in women between the ages of 35 and 50 and is a source of considerable discomfort in a sizable percentage of women.
3. Hormone replacement therapy may be associated with fibrocystic changes in a woman who had never experienced this previously.

Clinical Manifestations

1. Increased generalized breast lumpiness or excessive nodularity with tenderness, pain, and breast swelling. Symptoms may decrease after a menstrual period.
2. Lumps or cysts—soft or firm, single or multiple, smooth, round, and movable. Cysts may enlarge and become tender and painful. There may be many cysts of different sizes; some may be palpable.
3. Possible nipple discharge—may be milky, yellow or greenish.

Diagnostic Evaluation

1. Physical examination detects changes.
2. Mammography used to rule out calcification associated with malignancy.
3. Aspiration—if a palpable mass exists.
4. Cytology of cyst fluid is not cost effective and rarely of clinical value in fibrocystic breast changes.

Management

Usually geared toward relief of symptoms.

Surgical Management

1. Needle aspiration and conservative medical follow-up if:
   a. The aspirate appears like normal cyst fluid and is not blood-stained.
   b. Cyst completely resolves after aspiration.
   c. No indication of an underlying neoplasm.
2. Surgical excision—indicated if a cyst keeps recurring after several aspirations, or if a single solid discrete lump is present.

Medical Management

1. Sporadic discomfort may be relieved by over-the-counter analgesics.
2. Evening primrose oil, composed of essential fatty acids.
   a. Used in England as initial attempt to control cyclic breast pain. May be obtained over-the-counter in health food stores.
   b. Side effects include bloating and nausea.
3. Bromocriptine (Parlodel), a dopamine agonist.
   a. May help with mastalgia by decreasing serum prolactin levels.
   b. Side effects include nausea, vomiting, headache, dizziness, and fatigue.
4. Contraceptives or supplemental progestins during the secretory phase of the menstrual cycle may help with pain control.
   a. Mastalgia that begins after initiating birth control pills may resolve after a few cycles.
   b. Switching to a lower estrogen/higher progesterone ratio may help.
5. Danazol (Danocrine), a synthetic androgen used for severe fibrocystic changes to decrease hormonal stimulation of the breast by suppressing gonadotropins.
   a. Side effects include menstrual irregularity, weight gain, depression, bloating, and acne.
6. Tamoxifen (Nolvadex) blocks estrogen stimulation; side effects are minimal and may include hot flashes.

Other Measures

1. Diet modifications.
   a. Eliminating caffeine (coffee, tea, cola drinks, and chocolate) from the diet may help reduce symptoms in some women.
   b. Adding vitamin E may help with pain.
   c. Decreasing fat intake may improve swelling, tenderness, and nodularity.
2. Stopping tobacco use has been suggested to relieve symptoms.
3. Prophylactic simple mastectomy—rarely indicated for intractable pain not relieved with medical therapy in women with multiple previous biopsies or biopsy evidence of a precancerous lesion.

Nursing Interventions and Patient Teaching

1. Emphasize the importance of monthly BSE—cysts may mask underlying cancer.
2. Reinforce patient's confidence in BSE by rechecking her findings.
3. Offer suggestions for alternative methods if BSE is difficult to do (ie, tender breasts).
4. Encourage patient to see health care provider regularly for examinations.
5. Recommend that the patient wear a good support bra.
6. Offer emotional support for her anxiety and fear of cancer.
7. Reassure that pain is common to many women and that it is rarely the only presenting sign of cancer.

Benign Tumors of the Breast

Benign tumors of the breast are characterized clinically as benign lesions that are distinct and persistent over time. Approximately 90% are found by women themselves; 90% of breast lumps are benign.

Pathophysiology and Etiology

1. Fibrocystic changes—solid lumps may be fatty or fibrous tissue or fluid-filled cysts (see above).
2. Galactocele—a milk-filled cyst.
3. Fibroadenoma—a benign breast tumor composed of epithelial and stromal components.
   a. Common in young women.
   b. A slight increase in the risk of breast cancer among women with fibroadenomas.
4. Other benign tumors include adenosis, intraductal papillomas, lipomas, and neurofibromatosis that may produce a palpable mass.

Clinical Manifestations

1. Gross cysts—may be tender or nontender. Consistency depends on pressure of fluid within cyst and breast tissue around them; may be soft and fluctuant or may feel like a solid tumor if dense.
2. Galactocele—firm, nontender mass.
3. Fibroadenoma—may be a firm, smooth, movable lump that is usually painless. Size does not usually fluctuate with menstrual cycle changes but tends to enlarge over time.

Diagnostic Evaluation

1. Physical examination, mammography, and ultrasound identify and characterize lesion.
2. Cyst aspiration—diagnostic aspiration is often curative in a galactocele or breast cyst.
3. If a lump does not respond to cyst aspiration, excisional biopsy remains the "gold standard" to rule out cancer.

Management and Nursing Interventions

1. Nonsuspicious or indeterminate masses in young women may be observed through one or two menstrual cycles for resolution of the mass.
2. In general, any distinct and persistent solid lump should have biopsy and possibly excision.
3. Nursing care is directed toward support as woman goes through diagnostic process.

Disorders of the Male Breast

Disorders of the male breast include gynecomastia (benign) and malignant breast cancer.

Clinical Features

Gynecomastia

1. Overdevelopment of breast tissue.
2. Incidence greatest in adolescents and men older than 50 years old.
3. Usually results from hormonal alterations—idiopathic systemic disorders, such as endocrine disorders, disease of the liver, pituitary adenoma; drugs such as cimetidine, phenytoin, reserpine, nifedipine, theophylline; neoplasms such as testicular tumors and in association with lung cancer.
4. Pubertal gynecomastia usually disappears within 4 to 6 months.

Breast Cancer

1. Resembles cancer of the breast in women.
2. One percent of all breast cancers—incidence greatest in men in their 60s.
3. Poor prognosis because men may delay seeking treatment until disease is advanced.
4. Nursing care and treatment is essentially the same as for female breast cancer, including tamoxifen, chemotherapy, and/or radiation therapy.

Cancer of the Breast

Breast cancer or carcinoma is the leading cause of cancer in American women. One of eight women will develop breast cancer.

Pathophysiology and Etiology

1. Most breast cancer begins in the lining of the milk ducts, sometimes in the lobule. Eventually it grows through the wall of the duct and into the fatty tissue. (See Table 23-3 for types of breast cancer.)
2. Family history accounts for approximately 7% of all breast cancers.
   a. Current genetic models attribute 5% to 10% of all breast cancer to dominantly inherited breast cancer susceptibility genes.
   b. BRCA1 and BRCA2—susceptibility gene under study. Prophylactic mastectomy may reduce incidence but is not being recommended at this time. Screening is not warranted for general population.

TABLE 23-3   Types of Breast Cancer

Cell Type	Description	Incidence*	Comments
In situ			
Ductal (DCIS)	Well circumscribed in duct	28% Frequently found in combination with invasive cancer	Considered to be a precancerous condition—majority found by mammogram
Lobular (LCIS)	Solid proliferation of small cells within breast lobules	3–5% More frequent in pre-menopausal women	Nonpalpable mammographic finding. Precancerous. Tends to be bilateral, multicentric
Invasive			
Ductal	Classified on basis of microscopic appearance as ductal or lobular	75%	Characterized by stony hardness on palpation
Lobular	As above	5–10%	Relatively uncommon
Others			
Tubular Medullary Mucinous Papillary Sarcoma	Types frequently associated with above. Cell type must dominate to be assigned	<10% of all breast cancers	Axillary metastasis uncommon in tubular; medullary associated with fast growth rate and favorable prognosis
Inflammatory	Applies to distinctive inflamed appearance of skin. No consistent histologic type	1–4%	Presents with erythema, warmth, tenderness, and edema. May be treated with chemotherapy or radiation therapy first
Paget Disease of Nipple	Usually associated with underlying intraductal or invasive carcinoma	2%	Presents as scaly, erythematous, periareolar eruption

*Percent greater than 100—infiltrating carcinoma frequently includes small areas containing other special types or a combination of in situ and infiltrating carcinoma is seen.

3. Present knowledge does not indicate that carcinogens play an important role in the development of breast cancer.
4. Hormones such as estrogen are not thought to produce cancer; however, they may influence the growth of breast cancer.

Epidemiology of Breast Cancer

Incidence

1. Approximately 182,800 new cases yearly (1,400 male) in the United States, with approximately 41,200 deaths. Breast cancer incidence rates appear to be decreasing primarily in white women and in younger women.
2. There are expected to be 42,600 cases of ductal carcinoma in situ (DCIS) in 2000.

Survival Rates

1. Ten-year overall survival rates:
   Stage 0: 95%
   Stage I: 88%
   Stage II: 66%
   Stage III: 36%
   Stage IV: 7%
2. Lymph node status is the most important prognostic indicator of disease-free survival.
3. Age, staging (tumor size, lymph node status, and distant metastasis), nuclear grade, histologic differentiation, and treatment are important prognostic factors for survival (Tables 23-4 through 23-7).

TABLE 23-4 Staging of Primary Tumor (T) in Breast Cancer, American Joint Committee on Cancer and International Union Against Cancer

TX	Primary tumor cannot be assessed
T0	No evidence of primary tumor
Tis*	Carcinoma in situ: intraductal carcinoma, lobular carcinoma in situ, or Paget's disease of the nipple with no tumor
T1	Tumor 2 cm or less in greatest dimension
	T1a 0.5 cm or less in greatest dimension
	T1b More than 0.5 but not more than 1 cm in greatest dimension
	T1c More than 1 cm but not more than 2 cm in greatest dimension
T2	Tumor more than 2 cm but not more than 5 cm in greatest dimension
T3	Tumor more than 5 cm in greatest dimension
T4†	Tumor of any size with direct extension to chest wall or skin
	T4a Extension to chest wall
	T4b Edema (including peau d'orange) or ulceration of the skin of the breast or satellite skin nodules confined to the same breast
	T4c Both (T4a and T4b)
	T4d Inflammatory carcinoma

* Paget's disease associated with a tumor is classified according to the size of the tumor.
† Chest wall includes ribs, intercostal muscles, and serratus anterior muscle but not pectoral muscle.

TABLE 23-5 Staging of Regional Lymph Nodes (N) in Breast Cancer, American Joint Committee on Cancer and International Union Against Cancer

NX	Regional lymph nodes cannot be assessed (eg, previously removed)
N0	No regional lymph node metastasis
N1	Metastasis to movable ipsilateral axillary lymph node(s)
N2	Metastasis to ipsilateral axillary lymph node(s) fixed to one another or to other structures
N3	Metastasis to ipsilateral internal mammary lymph node(s)

---

4. Mortality rates are declining 1% to 2% annually in countries, such as the United States, that have a higher incidence of breast cancer; this may be related to:
   a. Change in lifestyle, such as diet.
   b. Early diagnosis—increased use of screening mammography.
   c. Improved treatment.

Risk Factors

1. Major—sex, increased age, prior history of breast cancer, and family history (especially mother, sisters). Approximate twofold risk in women with affected sister or mother; this increases if more relatives were affected or if affected close relatives developed breast cancer before menopause.
2. Probable—nulliparity, first child after age 30, late menopause, early menarche, benign breast disease, diagnosis of atypical ductal hyperplasia on biopsy.
3. Controversial—oral contraceptive use (estrogen and progestin may stimulate tumor growth with long-term use), long-term estrogen replacement therapy, alcohol use, obesity, and increased dietary fat intake.
4. Results of breast cancer prevention trials have shown a significant reduction in incidence of breast cancer in high-risk women treated with tamoxifen (Nolvadex) 20 mg per day for 5 years.
5. Studies are underway comparing tamoxifen and relaxofene (Evista).

GERONTOLOGIC ALERT

 Age is the greatest single risk factor for the development of cancer. Cancer warning signals may be unheeded in older women, so thorough history taking and physical examination is essential.

TABLE 23-6 Staging of Distant Metastases (M) in Breast Cancer, American Joint Committee on Cancer and International Union Against Cancer

MX	Presence of distant metastasis cannot be assessed
M0	No distant metastasis
M1	Distant metastasis (includes metastasis to ipsilateral supraclavicular lymph node[s])

TABLE 23-7 Stage Grouping for Breast Cancer, American Joint Committee on Cancer and International Union Against Cancer

Stage 0	Tis	N0	M0
Stage I	T1	N0	M0
Stage IIA	T0	N1	M0
	T1	N1	M0
	T2	N0	M0
Stage IIB	T2	N1	M0
	T3	N0	M0
Stage IIIA	T0	N2	M0
	T1	N2	M0
	T2	N2	M0
	T3	N1, N2	M0
Stage IIIB	T4	Any N	M0
	Any T	N3	M0
Stage IV	Any T	Any N	M1

Clinical Manifestations (Fig. 23-1)

1. A firm lump or thickening in breast, usually painless; 50% located in upper outer quadrant of breast. Enlargement of axillary or supraclavicular lymph nodes may indicate metastasis.
2. Nipple discharge—spontaneous, may be bloody, clear, or serous.
3. Breast asymmetry—a change in the size or shape of the breast or abnormal contours. As woman changes positions, compare one breast to other.
4. Nipple retraction or scaliness, especially in Paget's disease.

5. Late signs—pain, ulceration, edema, orange peel skin (peau d'orange) from interference of lymphatic drainage.

> **NURSING ALERT**
>
> Pain is not usually an early warning sign of breast cancer.

Diagnostic Evaluation

1. Mammography—most accurate method to detect nonpalpable lesion; cancer changes include microcalcifications to visible lesion.
2. Biopsy or aspiration—conclusive for cancer diagnosis and to determine type of breast cancer.
3. Estrogen/progesterone—receptor status, proliferation/S phase study, and other tests of tumor cells used to determine appropriate treatment and prognosis.
4. Laboratory tests to detect metastasis.
   a. Increased values on liver function tests indicate possible liver metastasis.
   b. Increased calcium and alkaline phosphatase levels indicate possible bony metastasis.
5. Additional metastatic workup includes chest x-ray, bone scan, possible brain CT, and possible chest CT.

Management

Based on type and stage of breast cancer, receptors, and menopausal status. For women with localized breast cancer, information from clinical trials indicates that treatment with a breast-preserving procedure has similar survival rates as does modified radical mastectomy.

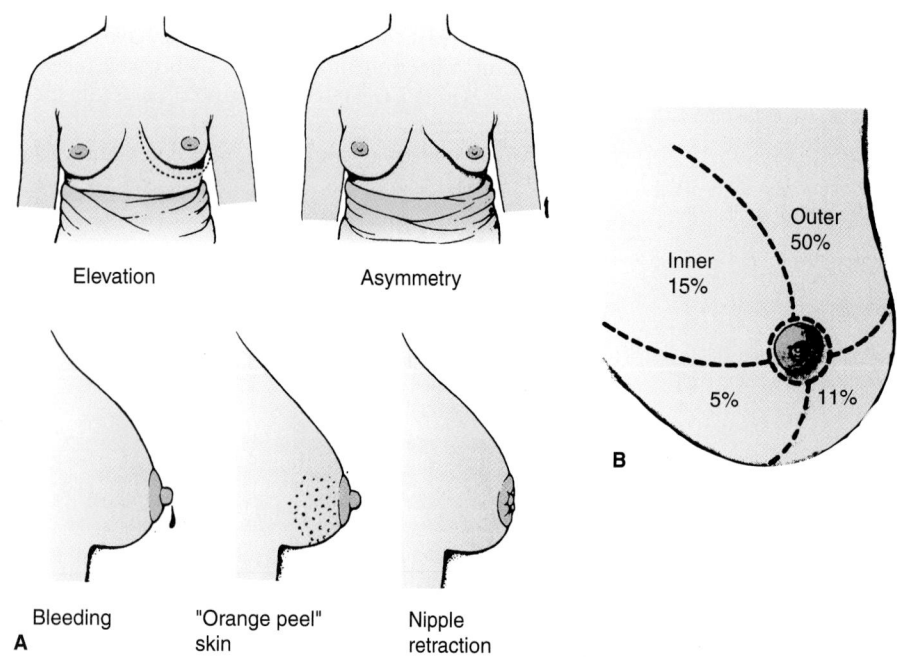

Elevation Asymmetry

Bleeding "Orange peel" skin Nipple retraction

A

B

Inner 15% Outer 50% 5% 11%

FIGURE 23-1 (**A**) Signs of cancer of the breast. (**B**) Distribution of carcinomas in different areas of breast.

Surgery

See p. 791 for a discussion of surgery for breast cancer.

Radiation Therapy

1. In conjunction with breast-preserving procedure as adjuvant (additional) therapy to decrease incidence of local recurrence for both invasive and ductal carcinoma in situ.
2. May be used after a mastectomy in patients with large tumors that involve the chest wall and/or many positive axillary lymph nodes.
3. Contraindications to a breast-preserving procedure include two primary tumors in separate quadrant of the breast, history of previous radiation therapy to the breast, pregnancy, and positive margins.
   a. Also used as primary therapy to shrink a large tumor to operable size.
   b. Also used to alleviate pain in metastatic breast cancer.
4. Radiation directed to breast, chest wall, and remaining lymph nodes.
   a. Usually five treatments a week for 6 or 7 weeks.
   b. A booster or second phase of treatment may be given.
   c. May include implants of radioactive material after external treatment completed.
5. Side effects include mild fatigue, sore throat, dry cough, nausea, anorexia; later, skin will look and feel sunburned. Eventually, the breast becomes more firm. Complications include increased arm edema, decreased arm mobility, pneumonitis, and brachial nerve damage. See p. 151 for care of patient undergoing radiation therapy.

Chemotherapy

1. Major use is in adjuvant treatment postoperatively; usually begins 4 weeks after surgery (stressful for patient who just finished major surgery).
2. Treatments are given every 3 to 4 weeks for 6 to 9 months. Because the drugs differ in their mechanisms of action, combinations of agents are used to treat cancer.
3. Main drugs used for breast cancer include cyclophosphamide (Cytoxan), methotrexate (Mexate), 5-fluorouracil (5-FU), doxorubicin (Adriamycin), and paclitaxel (Taxol). For advanced cancer, docetaxel, vinorelbine, mitoxantrone, fluorouracil by continuous infusion and oral forms of fluorouracil are used.
4. Indications for chemotherapy include:
   a. Large tumors, positive lymph nodes, premenopausal women, and poor prognostic factors. Currently, adjuvant chemotherapy and/or hormonal therapy recommended for all patients with invasive breast cancers 1.0 cm wide or larger.
   b. Recent studies have demonstrated that systemic chemotherapy increased survival in all women regardless of age. This raises questions of whom to treat. No markers are currently available to identify women who will or will not benefit from therapy.
5. Other agents that may be used include:
   a. Herceptin—a monoclonal antibody directed against Her-2/neu oncogene. Patients who express this gene may respond.

   b. Biphosphonates, such as pamidronate and clodronate acid, help to reduce pain and complications from bone metastasis.
6. Side effects include bone marrow suppression, nausea and vomiting, alopecia, weight gain/loss, fatigue, stomatitis, anxiety, depression, and premature menopause (see p. 141 for nursing care of patient undergoing chemotherapy).
7. Chemotherapy may also be used as primary treatment in inflammatory breast cancer and occasionally in large tumors; otherwise, preoperative chemotherapy remains investigational.

Endocrine Therapy

1. Antiestrogens such as tamoxifen (Nolvadex) bind estrogen receptors, thereby blocking effects of estrogen.
   a. Adjuvant systemic therapy after surgery.
   b. Benefits all estrogen receptor-positive patients, regardless of menopausal status.
   c. Given for at least 5 years; oral administration once or twice a day.
   d. Side effects include hot flashes, irregular periods, vaginal irritation, nausea and vomiting, headaches, increased risk for endometrial cancer and thromboembolic events.
2. Raloxifene (Evista) is an estrogen-like drug (an estrogen receptor modulator), with some bone and heart protective benefits. May be used in place of estrogen in breast cancer patients. New findings on this drug are promising.
3. Hormones may be used in advanced disease. Remissions may last months to several years. Agents commonly used include:
   a. Estrogens, such as diethylstilbestrol (DES) or ethinyl estradiol (Estinyl), in high doses to suppress follicle-stimulating hormone (FSH) and luteinizing hormone (LH) and may decrease endogenous estrogen production.
   b. Progestins may decrease estrogen receptors.
   c. Androgens may suppress FSH and estrogen production.
   d. Aminoglutethimide suppresses estrogen production by blocking adrenal steroids; "medical adrenalectomy," especially useful for women with bone and soft tissue metastases.
4. Corticosteroids suppress estrogen/progesterone secretion from the adrenals.
5. Aromatase inhibitors (endocrine sequence blockers), such as anastrozole (Arimidex) block conversion of androstenedione, which is secreted by the adrenal glands and converted into estrogen.

◆ DRUG ALERT

Traditionally, breast cancer survivors have not been considered candidates for estrogen. However, debates and studies continue to be conducted regarding the safety of estrogen in this population.

Bone Marrow Transplant

1. Autologous method after high-dose chemotherapy; may be curative because it allows high doses of drugs.
2. Especially indicated for stage III disease.

Oophorectomy

Removal of ovaries.

1. Treatment for recurrent or metastatic disease in estrogen receptor-positive premenopausal women.
2. Deprives tumor of primary estrogen source—remissions of 3 months to several years.
3. Medical ablation with tamoxifen has been compared to surgical oophorectomy in estrogen receptor-positive postmenopausal women and response rates are similar.
4. Surgical ablation is now considered second choice because of its increased risks.
5. The benefits of tamoxifen in combination with oophorectomy is the subject of ongoing research.

Adrenalectomy

Removal of adrenal glands to eliminate androgen production (which converts to estrogen).

1. Rarely done because of need for long-term steroid replacement therapy.
2. Remissions may last 6 months to several years.
3. Medical ablation with drugs being studied.

Complications

1. Metastasis—most common sites: lymph nodes, lung, bone, liver, and brain.
2. Signs and symptoms of metastasis may include bone pain, neurologic changes, weight loss, anemia, cough, shortness of breath, pleuritic pain, and vague chest discomfort.

Nursing Assessment

1. Assess general health status and underlying chronic illnesses that may have an impact on patient's response to treatment.
2. Identify what the patient and family need to know regarding breast cancer and its treatment, and take measures to decrease their impact. Base education on patient and family needs.
3. Determine level of anxiety, fears, and concerns.
4. Identify coping ability and availability of support systems.

Nursing Diagnoses

See p. 793 for breast surgery care and Chapter 8, Cancer Nursing.

- Anxiety related to diagnosis of cancer
- Knowledge Deficit related to disease process and treatment options
- Ineffective Coping by patient and/or family related to diagnosis, prognosis, financial stress, and/or inadequate support

Nursing Interventions

Reducing Anxiety

1. Realize that diagnosis of breast cancer is a devastating emotional shock to the woman. Support patient through the diagnostic process.
2. Interpret the results of each test in language the patient can understand.
3. Stress the advances made in earlier diagnosis and treatment options.

Providing Information About Treatment

1. Involve patient in treatment planning.
2. Describe surgical procedures.
3. Prepare patient for the effects of chemotherapy; encourage patient to plan ahead for the common side effects of chemotherapy.
4. Educate patient about the effects of radiation therapy.
5. Teach patient about hormonal therapy. Patient may develop hot flashes with the start of hormonal therapy or with the discontinuation of hormonal replacement therapy at the time of diagnosis of breast cancer. Measures that may help with symptoms of hot flashes include:
   a. Clonidine (Catapress) patch, Bellergal-S, antidepressants, soy products, various herbs, and vitamin preparations
   b. Black cohosh and Dong Quai have been used, but have not been rigorously tested.
   c. Progesterone may be helpful, but the possible effect on breast cancer needs further study.

Strengthening Coping

1. Repeat information and speak in calm, clear manner.
2. Display empathy and acceptance of patient's emotions.
3. Explore coping mechanisms.
4. Evaluate where patient is in stages of acceptance.
5. Help patient identify and use support persons.
6. Obtain visit from support group member.
7. Refer for counseling, financial aid, etc.
8. Resources include American Cancer Society (800-ACS-2345) and National Institutes of Health (*www.nci.nih.gov*).

Patient Education and Health Maintenance

1. Encourage patient to continue close follow-up and to report any new symptoms. Most women will be scheduled to be seen every 3 months for the first 2 years, every 6 months for the next 3 years, and once a year after 5 years.
2. Stress importance of continued yearly mammogram.
3. Inform patient that yearly laboratory work, bone scan, and chest x-ray may be performed when clinically indicated.
4. Suggest to patient that psychological intervention may be necessary for anxiety, depression, or sexual problems.

Outcome-Based Evaluation

- Verbalizes less anxiety
- Verbalizes understanding of all treatment options and their side effects
- Identifies appropriate coping mechanisms and support systems

SELECTED REFERENCES

Abramowicz, M. (Ed.) (1996). Drugs of choice for cancer chemotherapy. *Medical Letter*, 39(996), 21–28.

Appling, S.E. (1998). Prevention, early detection, and treatment of breast cancer: a collaborative approach. *Primary Care Practice*, 2(2), 111–118.

Brennan, M.J. & Miller, L.T. (1998). Overview of treatment options and review of the current role and use of compression garments, intermittent pumps, and exercise in the management of lymphedema. *Cancer Supplement, 83*(12), 2821–2827.

Cox, C.E., Haddad, F., & Bass, S. (1998). Lymphatic mapping in the treatment of breast cancer. *Oncology, 12*(9), 1283–1298.

Cummings, S.R. et al. (1999). The effect of raloxifene on risk of breast cancer in postmenopausal women. *Journal of the American Medical Association, 281*, 2189–2197.

Fisher, B. (1999). Highlights from recent national surgical adjuvant breast and bowel project studies in the treatment and prevention of breast cancer. *CA-A Journal for Clinicians, 49*(3), 159–176.

Fisher, B., Brown, A., Wiennd, S., et al. (1997). Effect of preoperative chemotherapy on local-regional disease in women with operable breast cancer: Findings from national surgical adjuvant breast and bowel project B-18. *Journal of Clinical Oncology, 15*(7), 2483–2493.

Fisher, B., Wickerham, D.L., Kavahan, M., et al. (1998). Tamoxifen for prevention of breast cancer: Report of the national surgical adjuvant breast and bowel project P-1 study. *Journal of the National Cancer Institute, 90*(18), 1371–1388.

Fremgen, A.M., Bland, K.I., & McGinnis, L.S. (1999). Clinical highlights from the national cancer data base, 1999. *CA-A Cancer Journal for Clinicians, 49*(3), 158.

Greenlee, R.T., Murray, T., Bolden, S., & Wingo, P.A. (2000), Cancer statistics, 2000. *CA-A Cancer Journal for Clinicians, 50*(1), 7–33.

Hortobagyi, G.N. (1998). Treatment of breast cancer. *New England Journal of Medicine, 339*(14), 974–983.

Karlson, E.W., Hankinon, S.E., Liang, M.H., Sanchez-Guerrero, J., Colditz, G.A., Rosenau, B.J., Speizer, F.E., & Schur, P.H. (1999). Association of silicone breast implants with immunologic abnormalities: A prospective study. *American Journal of Medicine, 106*(1), 11–19.

Leitch, A.M., Dodd, G.D., Costanza, M., et al. (1997). American Cancer Society guidelines for the early detection of breast cancer: Update 1997. *CA-A Cancer Journal for Clinicians, 47*(3), 150–153.

Lippman, M.E. (2000). High dose chemotherapy plus autologous bone marrow transplantation for metastatic breast cancer. *New England Journal of Medicine, 342*(7), 1119–1120.

Mast, M.E. (1998). Survivors of breast cancer: Illness uncertainty, positive reappraisal, and emotional distress. *Oncology Nursing Forum, 25*(3), 555–562.

Mettlin, C. (1999). Global breast cancer mortality statistics. *CA-A Journal for Clinicians, 49*(3), 138–144.

Meyer, J.E., Smith, D.N., Lester, S.C., et al. (1999). Large-core needle biopsy of nonpalpable breast lesions. *Journal of the American Medical Association, 281*(17), 1638–1645.

Morrison, C. (1998). The significance of nipple discharge: Diagnosis and treatment regimens. *Primary Care Practice, 2*(2), 129–140.

Odling, G., Danielson, E., Christensen, S.B., et al. (1998). Living with breast cancer: Care givers' perceptions in a surgical ward. *Cancer Nursing, 21*(3), 187–195.

Oktay, J.S. (1998). Psychosocial aspects of breast cancer. *Primary Care Practice, 2*(2), 149–159.

Price, J., & Purtell, J.R. (1997). Prevention and treatment of lymphedema. *American Journal of Nursing, 97*(9), 34–36.

Ross, R.K., Paganini-Hill, A., Wan, P.C., et al. (2000). Effect of hormone replacement therapy on breast cancer risk: Estrogen versus estrogen plus progestin. *Journal of the National Cancer Institute, 92*, 328–332.

Rosselli Del Turco, M. (1999). Breast cancer update: Encouraging trends...Many new questions. *CA-A Journal for Clinicians, 49*(3), 135–137.

Schairer, C., Lubin, J., Troisi, R., et al. (2000). Menopausal estrogen and estrogen-progestin replacement therapy and breast cancer risk. *Journal of the American Medical Association, 283*, 485–491.

Silverstein, M.J. et al. (1999). The influence of margin width on local control of ductal carcinoma in situ of the breast. *New England Journal of Medicine, 340*, 1455–1461.

Thomas, S., & Greifzu, S.P. (2000a). Breast cancer. *RN, 63*(4), 41–45.

———. (2000b). Breast reconstruction. *RN, 63*(4), 45–47.

Winchester, D.P., & Cox, J.D. (1998). Standards for diagnosis and management of invasive breast carcinoma. *CA-A Journal for Clinicians, 48*(2), 83–107.

Winchester D.P., & Storm, E.A. (1998). Standards for diagnosis and management of ductal carcinoma in situ (DCIS) of the breast. *CA-A Journal for Clinicians, 48*(2), 109–128.

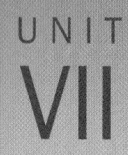

CHAPTER

24

*Endocrine
Disorders*

GENERAL OVERVIEW

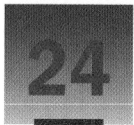 The Function of Hormones

The endocrine system and the nervous system maintain homeostasis. The endocrine glands produce hormones, chemical substances that are secreted into the bloodstream and that exert a stimulatory or inhibitory effect on target tissues or on glands. Hormones achieve their effect by binding with specific receptors located on the membrane on the target cell (eg, catecholamines) or by penetrating the cell membrane and forming a complex that influences cellular metabolism (eg, steroids). The target cell response may be reflected through the production and secretion of a second hormone or through a change in cell metabolism that alters the concentration of electrolytes or other substances in the bloodstream.

General Effects of Hormone Action

1. Regulate the overall metabolic rate and the storage, conversion, and release of energy.
2. Regulate fluid and electrolyte balance.
3. Initiate coping responses to stressors.
4. Regulate growth and development.
5. Regulate reproduction processes.

Regulation of Hormones

1. Hormone secretion is typically controlled through a negative feedback system.

a. Fall in blood concentration of hormone leads to activation of the regulator endocrine gland and to release of its stimulator hormones.

b. Elevations in blood concentration of target cell hormones or of changes in blood composition resulting from target cell activity can cause inhibition of hormone secretion.

2. Endocrine disorders are manifested as states of hormone deficiency or hormone excess. The underlying pathophysiology may be expressed as:

a. *Primary*—the secreting gland releases inappropriate hormone because of disease of the gland itself.

b. *Secondary*—the secreting gland releases abnormal amounts of hormone because of disease in a regulator gland (eg, pituitary).

c. *Tertiary*—the secreting gland releases inappropriate hormone because of hypothalamic dysfunction, resulting in abnormal stimulation by the pituitary.

3. Abnormal hormone concentrations may also be caused by hormone-producing tumors (adenomas) located at a remote site.

ASSESSMENT

History

Patients with diseases of the endocrine system commonly report nonspecific complaints. Often symptoms may reflect changes in general well-being, such as fatigue, weakness, weight change, appetite, sleep patterns, or psychiatric status. A thorough review of systems is necessary to detect changes in various body systems caused by an endocrine disorder (Table 24-1).

Physical Examination

Objective findings may be obvious and related to the patient's complaints or may be "silent signs" of which the patient is completely unaware. Thorough physical examination of all body systems, particularly the skin and cardiovascular and neurologic systems may reveal key findings for endocrine dysfunction.

DIAGNOSTIC TESTS

Various blood tests are available to evaluate endocrine function. These tests may measure the amount of hormone secreted by a specific endocrine gland, determine functioning of the hypothalamic-pituitary-thyroid axis, measure rate of functioning of an endocrine gland, or determine pathologic substances (eg, autoantibodies). Radiologic and imaging studies also evaluate endocrine disorders by measuring function and structure of the glands.

Tests of Thyroid Function
Total Thyroxine (T₄)
Description
1. This is a direct measurement of the concentration of total T_4 in the blood, using a radioimmunoassay technique.

TABLE 24-1 Physical Assessment of Clinical Manifestations of Endocrine Dysfunction

Signs of Symptoms	Possible Causes
Cardiovascular	
Tachycardia or tachyarrhythmia	Hyperthyroidism, Pheochromocytoma
	Adrenal insufficiency
Bradycardia	Hypothyroidism
Orthostatic hypotension	Adrenal insufficiency
	Hyperaldosteronism
	Pheochromocytoma
Hypertension	Pheochromocytoma
	Hyperaldosteronism
	Cushing's syndrome
	Hyperparathyroidism
	Hypothyroidism
Congestive heart failure	Hyperthyroidism
	Hypothyroidism
	Cushing's syndrome
Neurologic	
Fatigue	Adrenal insufficiency
	Hypothyroidism
	Hyperparathyroidism
Nervousness, tremor	Pheochromocytoma
	Hyperthyroidism
Confusion, lethargy, or coma	Diabetic ketoacidosis
	Hypothyroidism
	Syndrome of inappropriate antidiuretic hormone
Paresthesia	Hypothyroidism
	Hypoparathyroidism
	Diabetes mellitus
Headache	Acromegaly
	Pituitary tumor
	Pheochromocytoma
Psychosis	Hyperaldosteronism
	Hypothyroidism
	Hyperthyroidism
	Cushing's syndrome
	Adrenal insufficiency
	Hyperparathyroidism
Chvostek's sign, Trousseau's sign	Syndrome of inappropriate antidiuretic hormone
	Hypoparathyroidism
Increased reflexes	Hyperthyroidism
Decreased reflexes	Hypothyroidism
Gastrointestinal	
Anorexia	Addison's disease
	Hypothyroidism
	Hyperparathyroidism
Peptic ulcer	Cushing's syndrome
Diarrhea	Adrenal insufficiency
Constipation	Hypothyroidism
	Hyperparathyroidism
	Pheochromocytoma
Weight loss	Hyperthyroidism
	Hyperparathyroidism
	Pheochromocytoma
	Diabetes insipidus
Hyperdefecation	Hyperthyroidism
Abdominal pain	Addison's crisis
	Hyperparathyroidism
	Thyroid storm
	Myxedema

(continued)

TABLE 24-1   Physical Assessment of Clinical Manifestations of Endocrine Dysfunction (Continued)

Signs of Symptoms	Possible Causes
Musculoskeletal	
Weakness	Hyperthyroidism
	Hypothyroidism
	Cushing's syndrome
	Adrenal insufficiency
	Hyperparathyroidism
	Hypoparathyroidism
	Hyperaldosteronism
Pathologic fractures	Hyperparathyroidism
Joint pain	Hypothyroidism
	Acromegaly
Bone pain	Hyperparathyroidism
Bone thickening	Acromegaly
Urologic	
Polyuria	Hyperparathyroidism
	Diabetes insipidus
	Diabetes mellitus
	Hyperaldosteronism
Kidney stones	Hyperparathyroidism
	Acromegaly
	Cushing's syndrome
Integumentary	
Hirsutism	Adrenal hyperfunction
	Acromegaly
Hair loss	Hypoparathyroidism
	Hypothyroidism
	Cushing's syndrome
Sparse body hair	Pituitary insufficiency
	Adrenal insufficiency
	Hypogonadism
Hyperpigmentation	Addison's disease
	Hyperthyroidism
	Ectopic corticotropin production
Profuse diaphoresis	Hyperthyroidism
	Pheochromocytoma
Fine skin	Cushing's syndrome
Coarse hair	Hypothyroidism
Fine hair	Hyperthyroidism
Edema	Cushing's syndrome
Reproductive	
Amenorrhea	Hyperthyroidism
	Hypogonadism
	Cushing's syndrome
	Acromegaly
	Pituitary tumor
Gynecomastia	Hypogonadism
	Pituitary tumor
Loss of libido, impotence	Hypogonadism
	Hypothyroidism
	Adrenal insufficiency
	Diabetes mellitus
Ophthalmic/Visual	
Exophthalmos	Graves' disease
Diplopia	Graves' disease
	Pituitary tumor
Visual field deficit	Pituitary tumor
Periorbital swelling	Hypothyroidism
	Graves' disease
Body habitus	
Round face, "buffalo hump"	Cushing's syndrome
Abnormally tall stature	Prepubertal growth
	Hormone excess

2. It is an accurate index of thyroid function when T_4-binding globulin (TBG) is normal.
3. Low plasma-binding protein states (malnutrition, liver disease) may give low values.
4. High plasma-binding protein values (pregnancy, estrogen therapy) may give high values.
5. It is used to diagnose hypo- and hyperfunction of the thyroid and to guide and evaluate thyroid hormone replacement therapy.

Nursing and Patient Care Considerations

1. The test to monitor thyroid hormone therapy should be performed at least 4 weeks after dosage adjustment because of long half-life of T_4.
2. Interpretation of test results:
   a. Hypothyroidism—below normal.
   b. Hyperthyroidism—above normal.
3. Iodides can elevate the results of thyroid tests; therefore, it is important to determine if the patient has had any recent tests that used iodine as a contrast medium.

Free Thyroxine (Free T_4)

Description

1. Direct measurement of free T_4 concentration in the blood using a two-step radioimmunoassay method.
2. Accurate measure of thyroid function independent of the variable influence of thyroid-binding globulin levels.
3. Used to aid in the diagnosis of hyperthyroidism and hypothyroidism.
4. Used to monitor and guide thyroid hormone replacement therapy, particularly with pituitary disease.

Nursing and Patient Care Considerations

1. Interpretation of test results:
   a. Hyperthyroidism—above normal.
   b. Hypothyroidism—below normal.
2. Results best interpreted in conjunction with TSH levels for diagnostic purposes.
3. When used to monitor thyroid hormone replacement therapy, levels only meaningful after 6 to 8 weeks of therapy to evaluate adequacy of dosage, because of long half-life of thyroxine.

Thyroid-Binding Globulin (TBG)

Description

1. This measures the concentration of the carrier protein for T_4 in the blood.
2. Because most T_4 is protein bound, changes in TBG will influence values of T_4.
3. Helpful in distinguishing between true thyroid disease and T_4 test abnormalities caused by TBG excess or deficit.

Nursing and Patient Care Considerations

Determine if the patient is taking estrogen or is pregnant, both of which can elevate TBG; results may be depressed by malnutrition or by liver disease.

Triiodothyronine (T_3)

Description

1. Directly measures concentration of T_3 in the blood using a radioimmunoassay technique.

2. T_3 is less influenced by alterations in thyroid-binding proteins.

3. T_3 has a shorter half-life than T_4 and occurs in minute quantities in the active form.

4. Useful to rule out T_3 thyrotoxicosis, hyperthyroidism when T_4 is normal, and to evaluate effects of thyroid replacement therapy.

Nursing and Patient Care Considerations

1. T_3 can be transiently depressed in the acutely ill patient.

2. Interpretation of test results:
   a. Hypothyroidism—below normal.
   b. Hyperthyroidism—above normal.

T_3 Resin Uptake

Description

1. This is an indirect measure of thyroid function, based on the available protein-binding sites in a serum sample that can bind to radioactive T_3.

2. The radioactive T_3 is added to the serum sample in the test tube.

3. Estrogen and pregnancy produce an increase in binding sites, thus causing a lowered percentage of binding by the available thyroid hormones.

Nursing and Patient Care Considerations

1. Results may be altered if patient has been taking estrogens, androgens, salicylates, or phenytoin.

2. Interpretation of test results:
   a. Hypothyroidism—below normal.
   b. Hyperthyroidism—above normal.

Free Thyroid Index (FTI)

Description

Laboratory estimate of free T_4 concentration with calculated adjustment for variations in patient's TBG concentration.

Nursing and Patient Care Considerations

Interpretation of test results:

1. Below normal in hypothyroidism.

2. Above normal in hyperthyroidism.

Thyrotropin, Thyroid-Stimulating Hormone (TSH)

Description

1. Direct measure of TSH, the hormone secreted by the pituitary gland that regulates the production and secretion of T_4 by the thyroid gland.

2. Blood sample is analyzed by radioimmunoassay.

3. Preferred test differentiates between thyroid disorders caused by disease of the thyroid gland itself and disorders caused by disease of the pituitary or hypothalamus. Also useful to detect early stages of hypothyroidism (subclinical hypothyroidism) and to monitor hormone replacement therapy. Patient must be on stable dose of thyroxine for 6 to 8 weeks for TSH levels to reflect adequacy of treatment accurately.

Nursing and Patient Care Considerations

Interpretation:

1. In primary hypothyroidism, TSH levels are elevated.

2. In secondary hypothyroidism (failure of the pituitary gland), TSH levels are low.

3. In hyperthyroidism, TSH levels are low.

Thyrotropin-Releasing Hormone (TRH) Stimulation Test

Description

1. This test evaluates the patency of the pituitary-hypothalamic axis. Once used primarily to distinguish between primary and central hypothyroidism, this test is rarely used for that purpose with the advent of more sensitive TSH assays. Now, its primary use is to distinguish between secondary and tertiary hypothyroidism and evaluate acromegaly.

2. A baseline sample is drawn, then TRH is injected IV and blood samples are drawn to determine TSH levels at 30, 90, and 120 minutes.

Nursing and Patient Care Considerations

1. Interpretation:
   a. Increased TSH should be seen within 30 minutes.
   b. No rise in secondary hypothyroidism.
   c. Blunted rise in hyperthyroidism.
   d. Delayed rise (90-minute sample) associated with tertiary hypothyroidism.
   e. Elevated growth hormone levels associated with acromegaly.

2. A subnormal response can occur in patients taking L-dopa or cortisol.

Thyroid Autoantibodies

Description

Used to detect selected autoantibodies associated with some thyroid diseases and the titers of those autoantibodies.

1. Thyroid-stimulating antibody (TSAb)—autoantibodies that stimulate the TSH receptor on the thyroid gland, causing hyperfunction of the thyroid. Helpful in the diagnosis of Graves' disease.

2. Thyroid microsomal antibodies (TMAb)—associated with Hashimoto's thyroiditis and Graves' disease.

3. Thyroglobulin antibodies (TgAb)—elevated with Hashimoto's thyroiditis and Graves' disease.

◼ Tests of Parathyroid Function

Parathyroid Hormone (PTH)

Description

1. Test is a direct measurement of PTH concentration in the blood, using radioimmunoassay technique.

2. Results are usually compared with results of total serum calcium to determine likely cause of parathyroid dysfunction.

3. Range of normal values may vary by laboratory and method.

Nursing and Patient Care Considerations

Elevated PTH in hyperparathyroidism; decreased PTH in hypoparathyroidism.

Serum Calcium, Total
Description
1. This is a direct measurement of protein-bound and "free" ionized calcium.
2. Ionized calcium fraction is best indicator of changes in calcium metabolism.
3. Results can be affected by changes in serum albumin, the primary protein carrier.
4. Used to detect alterations in calcium metabolism caused by parathyroid disease or malignancy.

Nursing and Patient Care Considerations
1. Sample should be obtained from fasting patient and should be collected in tube with heparin as anticoagulant.
2. Test should be repeated on three different occasions to confirm parathyroid disease.
3. Elevations in serum calcium can be caused by dehydration, vitamin D intoxication, thiazide diuretics, immobilization, hyperthyroidism, or lithium therapy.
4. Low values may be seen in renal failure, chronic disease states, malabsorption syndrome, and vitamin D deficiency.
5. Interpretation of test results:
   a. Hyperparathyroidism, malignancy—elevated.
   b. Hypoparathyroidism—below normal.

Serum Calcium, Ionized
Description
1. Approximately 45% to 50% of total serum calcium is in biologically active ionized form.
2. This is preferred method of testing changes in calcium metabolism caused by parathyroid disease, malignancy, or neck surgery.

Nursing and Patient Care Considerations
1. Sample should be obtained from fasting patient and should be collected in tube with heparin as anticoagulant.
2. Test should be repeated on three different occasions to confirm parathyroid disease.
   a. Hyperparathyroidism, malignancy—elevated.
   b. Hypoparathyroidism—below normal.

NURSING ALERT

Tourniquet use during blood sample collection for calcium studies should be kept to a minimum. Prolonged constriction will cause migration of plasma proteins into the bloodstream locally; this results in spuriously high serum calcium values, and pseudohypercalcemia.

Serum Phosphate
Description
1. Test measures the level of inorganic phosphorus in the blood.
2. Alteration in parathyroid function tends to have opposite effects on calcium and phosphorus metabolism.
3. Used to confirm metabolic abnormalities that affect calcium metabolism.

Nursing and Patient Care Considerations
Elevated in hypoparathyroidism; low values in hyperparathyroidism.

■ Tests of Adrenal Function
Plasma Cortisol
Description
1. This is direct measure of the primary secretory product of the adrenal cortex by radioimmunoassay technique.
2. Serum concentration varies with circadian cycle so normal values vary with time of day and stress level of patient (8:00 AM levels typically double that of 8:00 PM levels).
3. Useful as an initial step to assess adrenal dysfunction, but further workup is usually necessary.

Nursing and Patient Care Considerations
1. A fasting sample is preferred.
2. Blood specimens should coincide with circadian rhythm with draw time indicated on laboratory slip.
3. Interpretation of test results:
   a. Cushing's syndrome—elevated.
   b. Addison's disease—low values.

24-Hour Urinary Free Cortisol Test
Description
1. Test measures cortisol production during a 24-hour period.
2. Useful to establish diagnosis of hypercortisolism.
3. Less influenced by diurnal variations in cortisol.

Nursing and Patient Care Considerations
1. Instruct patient in appropriate collection technique.
2. Collection jug should be kept on ice and sent to laboratory promptly when collection completed.
3. Interfering factors:
   a. Elevated values—pregnancy, oral contraceptives, spironolactone, stress.
   b. Recent radioisotope scans can interfere with test results.

Dexamethasone Suppression Test (DST)
Description
1. This valuable test is used to evaluate adrenal hyperfunction.
2. Adrenal production and secretion of cortisol is stimulated by corticotropin (ACTH) from the pituitary gland.
3. Dexamethasone is a synthetic steroid effective in suppressing ACTH secretion.
4. In a healthy patient, the administration of dexamethasone will inhibit ACTH secretion and will cause cortisol levels to fall below normal.

Nursing and Patient Care Considerations
1. Explain the procedure to the patient.
   a. Overnight 1 mg DST (used primarily to identify those *without* Cushing's syndrome).
      (i) Administer dexamethasone 1 mg orally at 11:00 PM.

(ii) Draw cortisol level at 8:00 AM before patient rises.

(iii) Expect suppressed cortisol levels (less than 5 μg/dL).

b. High-dose overnight DST (helpful to distinguish Cushing's disease from other forms of Cushing's syndrome).

(i) Give patient dexamethasone 8 mg orally at 11:00 PM.

(ii) Draw cortisol level at 8:00 AM before patient rises.

(iii) Suppressed cortisol levels (less than 50% of baseline value) indicative of patient with ACTH-secreting pituitary adenoma (Cushing's disease).

(iv) Unsuppressed cortisol levels are associated with ectopic ACTH secretion (malignancy) or adrenal tumors.

2. Encourage patient to take dexamethasone with milk because it may cause gastric irritation.

Adrenocorticotropic (ACTH) Stimulation Test
Description
1. ACTH stimulates the production and secretion of cortisol by the adrenal cortex.
2. Demonstrates the ability of the adrenal cortex to respond appropriately to ACTH.
3. This is an important test to evaluate adrenal insufficiency, but may not distinguish primary insufficiency from secondary insufficiency.
4. Useful to determine if hypercortisolism is ACTH-dependent (bilateral hyperplasia) or ACTH-independent (adrenal tumor).

Nursing and Patient Care Considerations
1. Obtain baseline cortisol level.
2. Administer 0.25 mg ACTH (corsyntropin) intravenously (IV) or intramuscularly (IM).
3. Collect cortisol levels at times ordered (usually at 30 and 60 minutes).
4. Interpretation of test results:
   a. Range of normal responses may vary; however, typically a rise in cortisol of double baseline value is considered normal.
   b. Diminished response—adrenal insufficiency with low cortisol values, adrenal tumor with high cortisol values, prolonged glucocorticoid therapy.
   c. Exaggerated response—adrenal hyperplasia with high cortisol values.

Corticotropin Stimulation Test
Description
1. Test measures responsiveness of pituitary gland to corticotropin-releasing factor, a hypothalamic hormone that regulates pituitary secretion of ACTH.
2. Useful to differentiate the cause of excess cortisol secretion when ectopic source of ACTH is suspected.
3. In general, corticotropin will stimulate ACTH secretion in the pituitary, but not in nonpituitary ACTH-secreting tissues.

Nursing and Patient Care Considerations
1. Describe procedure to patient.
   a. Patient is given corticotropin (1 μg/kg or 100 μg) IV.
   b. Blood samples for ACTH test are collected at −15, 0, 15, 30, 60, 90, and 120 minutes.
2. Normal response is a rise in ACTH to at least double the baseline value.
3. Interpretation of test results:
   a. Brisk rise in ACTH double baseline value—Cushing's disease.
   b. No response in ACTH—ACTH-independent Cushing's syndrome (adrenal tumor) or ectopic source of ACTH secretion (ectopic tumor).
   c. Test can produce false-negative response.

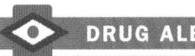

DRUG ALERT

Infusion of corticotropin can cause flushing or slight reduction in blood pressure. Warn patients about these effects, monitor blood pressure, and ensure safety.

Urine Vanillylmandelic Acid (VMA) and Metanephrine
Description
1. Direct measure of metabolites of catecholamines secreted by the adrenal medulla.
2. Metanephrine is a more reliable measure of catecholamine secretion.
3. Preferred method to diagnose pheochromocytoma.

Nursing and Patient Care Considerations
1. Obtain proper urine collection jug with HCl preservative and explain 24-hour urine collection to patient.
2. A wide range of medications and foods may alter test performed by some laboratories. Verify with the laboratory and health care provider the need to hold some medications, such as sympathomimetics and methyldopa, and foods such as coffee, tea, vanilla extract, and bananas before and during urine collection.
3. Interpretation—pheochromocytoma: VMA greater than 10 μg/mg creatinine or greater than 10 mg/24 hours; metanephrine greater than 0.7 μg/mg creatinine or greater than 0.7 mg/24 hours.

Plasma Catecholamines
Description
Direct measure of circulating catecholamines using radioimmunoassay technique; more sensitive test than urine test, but more prone to false-positive results.

Nursing and Patient Care Considerations
1. Collect sample from IV catheter 20 to 30 minutes after venipuncture, if possible, to reduce the rise in catecholamine levels from pain and anxiety.
2. Collect the sample in a heparinized tube.
3. Interpretation—levels greater than 2,000 ng/L diagnostic for pheochromocytoma.

Clonidine Suppression Test

Description

1. Based on the principle that catecholamine production by pheochromocytomas is autonomous, as opposed to other causes of excess catecholamines, which are regulated by the sympathetic nervous system.
2. Clonidine (Catapres), as a central α-adrenergic agonist, suppresses production of catecholamines.
3. Useful to differentiate pheochromocytoma from essential hypertension when test results are inconclusive.

Nursing and Patient Care Considerations

1. Collect baseline catecholamine sample from IV catheter 20 to 30 minutes after venipuncture, if possible, to reduce the rise in catecholamine levels from pain and anxiety.
2. Give clonidine 0.3 mg orally.
3. After 3 hours, collect second catecholamine sample.
4. Interpretation—in patients without pheochromocytoma, a significant drop in catecholamines should be seen at 3 hours (less than 500 pg/mL or reduction of total catecholamines by 50%), whereas in patients with pheochromocytoma, no drop in catecholamines will be evident.

◆ DRUG ALERT

Warn patients not to rise quickly and monitor for orthostatic hypotension after clonidine administration.

Aldosterone (Urine or Blood)

Description

1. Direct measure, using radioimmunoassay technique, of aldosterone, a hormone secreted by the adrenal cortex, which regulates renal control of sodium and potassium.
2. May be measured in the blood or in 24-hour urine collection sample.
3. Urine test is more reliable because it is less influenced by short-term fluctuations in the bloodstream.
4. Useful to diagnose primary aldosteronism.

Nursing and Patient Care Considerations

1. Test results can be elevated by stress, strenuous exercise, upright posture, and medications, such as diazoxide (Hyperstat), hydralazine (Apresoline), and nitroprusside (Nipride).
2. Test results may be decreased by excessive licorice ingestion and the medications fludrocortisone (Florinef) and propranolol (Inderal).

Tests of Pituitary Function

Serum Growth Hormone (GH)

Description

1. Direct radioimmunoassay measurement of human GH, secreted by the anterior pituitary gland; useful to diagnose acromegaly, gigantism, pituitary tumors, or pituitary-related growth failure in children.
2. Because growth hormone secretion is episodic, single fasting samples may not be reliable to detect growth hormone excess or deficiency states.

3. These conditions are best evaluated by using a stimulation test (for deficiency states) or a suppression test (for hormone excess conditions).

Nursing and Patient Care Considerations

1. Blood sample is taken after an overnight fast (caloric intake will lower GH blood levels).
2. Patient should be restful and calm before blood sample collection.
3. Normal range: males—less than 5 ng/mL, females—less than 8 ng/mL.
4. May be elevated by the following medications: alcohol, L-dopa, oral contraceptives, α-antagonists, and β-adrenergic blocking agents.

Serum Prolactin

Description

Direct radioimmunoassay measurement of prolactin, secreted by the anterior pituitary gland; useful to diagnose pituitary tumors.

Nursing and Patient Care Considerations

1. Blood sample is taken after an overnight fast.
2. Normal values: men—1 to 20 ng/mL, women—1 to 25 ng/mL.
3. Values above 300 ng/mL highly suggestive of pituitary tumor.
4. Elevated values may be caused by exercise or by breast stimulation.
5. Medications that will elevate test results include phenothiazines, reserpine (Serpasil), estrogens, and tricyclic antidepressants.

Adrenocorticotropic Hormone (ACTH)

Description

1. Direct measurement of ACTH concentration in the bloodstream by radioimmunoassay technique.
2. One measure of pituitary gland function useful to provide important information regarding adrenal gland dysfunction.
3. Useful to identify cause of adrenal abnormalities when compared with serum cortisol levels.

Nursing and Patient Care Considerations

1. Blood sample should be collected in heparinized tube and put on ice immediately.
2. High stress levels in patient can invalidate results.
3. Interpretation of test results:
   a. Elevated levels with elevated cortisol—Cushing's disease or ectopic production of ACTH.
   b. Elevated levels with low cortisol—Addison's disease.
   c. Low levels with elevated cortisol—adrenal tumor.
   d. Low levels with low cortisol—hypopituitarism.

Insulin Tolerance Test

Description

1. Dynamic test measures pituitary response to induced hypoglycemia, particularly GH secretion and ACTH-stimulated cortisol production by the adrenal gland.

2. Useful to diagnose functional hypopituitarism that is caused by pituitary disease or that appears after pituitary surgery.

3. Considered the "gold standard" for diagnosis of growth hormone deficiency.

Nursing and Patient Care Considerations

1. After overnight fast, insulin 0.1 unit/kg body weight is given IV.

2. Blood samples are collected, usually at baseline, 30, 60, and 90 minutes after insulin dose.

3. The test is considered valid if blood glucose falls to half of baseline or less than 40 mg/dL.

4. Peak response is seen at 60 to 100 minutes.

5. For adrenal response, a rise in cortisol by a factor of at least 1.5 is necessary to show normal response.

6. Growth hormone deficiency is present if growth hormone levels fail to rise above 3 µg/L.

7. This test is contraindicated in people with epilepsy or heart disease. In people with suspected adrenal insufficiency, ACTH stimulation test should be done first.

8. For people in whom the insulin tolerance test is contraindicated, other agents may be used, such as clonidine, arginine, glucagon, L-dopa or GHRH, to stimulate growth hormone secretion.

> **NURSING ALERT**
>
> Test should be performed with health care provider present. Dextrose 50% solution should be available at bedside to treat hypoglycemia, if needed.

Glucose Suppression Test
Description
Postprandial elevations of glucose inhibit the secretion of growth hormone by the pituitary gland. Failure to suppress growth hormone levels after ingestion of glucose suggests a growth-hormone-secreting tumor.

Nursing and Patient Care Considerations

1. Patient should fast for this test.

2. 75 to 100 g of glucola is administered PO.

3. Blood samples are collected at baseline, 30, and 60 minutes.

4. Interpretation of test results:
   a. Growth hormone levels less than 2 µg/L are considered normal in this test.
   b. Growth hormone levels that are not suppressed are suggestive of acromegaly.

5. Failure of growth hormone suppression may also be caused by starvation or protein calorie restriction.

6. Patients may complain of nausea after ingesting Glucola.

Water Deprivation Test
Description
1. Functional test of the adequacy of posterior pituitary secretion of antidiuretic hormone (ADH) and its ability to concentrate urine and to maintain serum osmolality in the face of water deprivation.

2. Useful to determine the diagnosis and etiology of diabetes insipidus (DI).

Nursing and Patient Care Considerations

1. Test is begun by obtaining the patient's weight, serum, and urine osmolality at time 0.

2. Patient weight, urine output volume, and osmolality are determined hourly.

3. Deprivation is continued until urine osmolality "plateaus" as evidenced by a change of less than 30 mOsm/kg during a 3-hour period, if the patient's weight decreases by 3%, or if cardiovascular instability occurs. At this point, serum osmolality is obtained.

4. If urine osmolality remains below that of serum (usually 300 mOsm/kg), the diagnosis of DI is confirmed and the second stage of the test, which distinguishes central and nephrogenic DI, is begun.

5. Artificial ADH (vasopressin 5 IU or DDAVP 1 µg) is given subcutaneously to determine changes in urine osmolality at 30, 60, and 120 minutes in response to the injected hormone.

6. If the highest urine osmolality value obtained after injection is more than 50% higher than the preinjection value, DI is caused by pituitary failure. If the osmolality value is less than 50% of preinjection value, then DI is caused by renal disease.

> **NURSING ALERT**
>
> Patients with suspected DI, who undergo water deprivation test, must be monitored closely because dehydration may occur rapidly in people with severe disease.

◼ Radiology and Imaging
Radioactive ^{131}I Uptake
Description
Measures thyroid uptake patterns of iodine as a whole, or within specified areas of the gland.

Nursing and Patient Care Considerations

1. A solution of sodium iodide 131 is administered orally to the fasting patient.

2. After a prescribed interval, usually 24 hours, measurements of radioactive counts per minute are taken with a scintillator.

3. Normal thyroid will remove 15% to 50% of the iodine from the bloodstream.

4. Hyperthyroidism may result in the removal of as much as 90% of the iodine from the bloodstream (eg, Graves' disease); it may also cause a low uptake with some forms of thyroiditis.

5. Hypothyroidism—reflected in low uptake.

Thyroid Scan
Description
1. Rapid imaging of thyroid tissue, particularly suspicious nodules, as contrast imaging agent is rapidly taken up by functioning tissue.

2. Useful to diagnose thyroid carcinoma.

3. Contrast media is usually administered IV.
   a. Technetium (^{99m}Tc) pertechnetate or ^{123}I is used for best images.
4. Images can be obtained from gamma counter within 20 to 60 minutes.

Nursing and Patient Care Considerations

1. May interfere with serum radioimmunoassay tests; contact laboratory to determine when blood test can be done.
2. Benign adenomas may be visualized as "hot" nodules, indicating increased uptake of iodine, or as "cold" nodules, indicating decreased uptake.
3. Malignant nodules usually take the form of "cold" nodules.

GENERAL PROCEDURES AND TREATMENT MODALITIES

Steroid Therapy

Steroid therapy is a treatment used in some endocrine disorders and in various other conditions. Steroids are hormones that affect metabolism and many body processes.

Classification of Steroids

(By major metabolic effects on body)

Mineralocorticoids

1. Concerned with sodium and water retention and potassium excretion.
2. Example—aldosterone and 11-desoxycorticosterone.

Glucocorticoids (Corticosteroids, Steroids)

1. Concerned with metabolic effects, including carbohydrate metabolism.
2. Example—cortisol.

Sex Hormones

1. Important when secreted in large amounts or when the growth of hormone-sensitive cancers are stimulated.
2. Examples
   a. Androgens—testosterone.
   b. Estrogens—estradiol.
   c. Progestins—progesterone.

Effects of Glucocorticoids

1. Antagonize action of insulin; promote gluconeogenesis, which provides glucose.
2. Increase breakdown of protein (inhibit protein synthesis).
3. Increase breakdown of fatty acids.
4. Suppress inflammation, inhibit scar formation, block allergic responses.
5. Decrease number of circulating eosinophils and leukocytes; decrease size of lymphatic tissue.
6. Exert a permissive action (allow the full effects) on catecholamines.
7. Exert a permissive action on functioning of central nervous system (CNS).
8. Inhibit release of adrenocorticotropin.

9. In summary, glucocorticoids are necessary to resist noxious stimuli and environmental change.

Uses of Steroids

1. Physiologically—to correct deficiencies or malfunction of a particular endocrine organ or system (eg, Addison's disease).
2. Diagnostically—to determine proper functioning of the endocrine system.
3. Pharmacologically—to treat the following:
   a. Asthma and obstructive lung disease.
   b. Acute rheumatic fever.
   c. Blood conditions such as idiopathic thrombocytopenic purpura, leukemia, hemolytic anemia.
   d. Allergic conditions—allergic rhinitis, anaphylaxis (after epinephrine).
   e. Dermatologic problems—drug rashes, contact dermatitis, atopic dermatitis.
   f. Ocular diseases—conjunctivitis, uveitis.
   g. Connective tissue disorders—systemic lupus erythematosus, rheumatoid arthritis.
   h. Gastrointestinal problems—ulcerative colitis.
   i. Organ transplant recipients—as an immunosuppressive agent.
   j. Neurologic conditions—cerebral edema, multiple sclerosis.

Preparing the Patient to Receive Steroid Therapy

1. Determine contraindications/precautions for such therapy.
   a. Peptic ulcer.
   b. Diabetes mellitus.
   c. Viral infections.
2. Administer a tuberculin test, if indicated, before therapy, because steroids may suppress response to the test.
3. Assess the patient's own level of steroid secretion, if possible.
4. Explain the nature of the therapy, what is required of the patient, how long therapy will last, what side effects to watch for, and answer any questions.

Choice of Steroid and Method of Administration

1. May be given by various methods—orally, parenterally, sublingually, rectally, by inhalation, or by direct application to skin or mucous membrane.
2. Combinations of steroids with other drugs should be avoided.
3. To help avoid steroid side effects, alternate-day therapy may be used.
4. May be given in initial high doses, then reduced; if the patient has been taking steroids for several weeks, doses must be tapered gradually to prevent Addisonian crisis.

Nursing Interventions

Preventing Infection

1. Steroids may affect the circulating blood, resulting in decreased eosinophils and lymphocytes, increased red

cells, and increased incidence of thrombophlebitis and infection.

2. Encourage the patient to avoid crowds and the possibility of exposure to infection.
3. Encourage exercise to prevent venous stasis.
4. Be aware that signs of infection/inflammation may be masked—fever, redness, swelling.
5. Practice and encourage good handwashing technique and asepsis.

Preventing Nutritional and Metabolism Complications

1. Determine whether the patient needs assistance in dietary control. Steroids may cause weight gain and an increase in appetite.
2. Encourage a high-protein, high-carbohydrate diet. Since steroids affect protein metabolism, there may be negative nitrogen balance.
3. Encourage the patient to take steroids with milk or with food. Since steroids increase secretion of gastric HCl and have an inhibiting effect on secretion of mucus in the stomach, they may cause peptic ulcer.
4. Be on guard for early evidence of gastric hemorrhage, such as melena, blood in vomitus.
5. Check urine for evidence of glucose.
   a. Steroids precipitate gluconeogenesis and insulin antagonism, which results in hyperglycemia, glucosuria, decreased carbohydrate tolerance.
   b. Temporary insulin injections may be necessary.

Observing for Bone Complications

1. Be on the alert for the possibility of pathologic fractures. Stress safety measures to prevent injury.
   a. Steroids affect the musculoskeletal system, causing potassium depletion and muscular weakness.
   b. Steroids cause increased output of calcium and phosphorus, which may lead to osteoporosis.
2. Administer a diet high in calcium and protein.
3. Recommend a program of activities of daily living and weight-bearing; normal range of motion and safe repositioning for the bedridden.

Avoiding Electrolyte Disturbance

1. Restrict sodium intake and increase potassium intake.
   a. Mineralocorticoids differ from other steroids, resulting in sodium retention and potassium depletion: edema, weight gain.
   b. Lemon juice is high in potassium and low in sodium.
   c. Avoid saline as a diluent in preparing injectable medications.
2. Check blood pressure frequently and weigh the patient daily.
3. Observe for edema.

Monitoring Behavioral Reactions

1. Watch for convulsive seizures (especially in children). Steroids may alter behavior patterns, increase excitability, and may affect the CNS.
2. Avoid overstimulating situations.

3. Recognize and report any mood that deviates from the usual behavior patterns.
4. Report unusual behavior, haunting dreams, withdrawal, or suicidal tendencies.

Preventing Stress Reactions

1. Recommend that the patient carry an identification card that indicates steroid therapy and name of health care provider.
2. Be aware that steroids affect the hypothalamic-pituitary-adrenal system; this affects the patient's ability to respond to stress.
3. Advise the patient to avoid extremes of temperature, infections, and upsetting situations.

Preventing Injury and Promoting Healing

1. Instruct the patient to avoid injury; stress safety precautions. Since steroids interfere with fibroblasts and granulation tissue, altered response to injury results in impaired growth and delayed healing.
2. Observe daily the healing process of wounds, particularly surgical wounds, to recognize the potential for wound dehiscence.

Patient Education and Health Maintenance

1. Teach patient that steroids are valuable and useful medications, but that if taken for longer than 2 weeks, they may produce certain side effects.
   a. Acceptable side effects may include weight gain (due to increased appetite and water retention), acne, headaches, fatigue, and increased urinary frequency.
   b. Unacceptable side effects that are to be reported to the health care provider include dizziness when rising from chair or bed (postural hypotension indicative of adrenal insufficiency), nausea, vomiting, thirst, abdominal pain, or pain of any type.
   c. Additional reportable side effects include convulsive seizures, feelings of depression or nervousness, or development of an infection.
2. Advise patient that a fall or an automobile accident may precipitate adrenal failure. This requires an immediate injection of hydrocortisone phosphate (Solu-Cortef).
3. Tell patients on long-term therapy that they should wear a Medic Alert tag and carry a kit with hydrocortisone as prescribed.
4. Instruct patient to inform any physician, dentist, or nurse about steroid therapy.
5. Tell patient that regular follow-up visits to health care provider are required.

▪ Care of the Patient Undergoing Fine Needle Aspiration Biopsy

Fine needle aspiration biopsy (FNA) is a procedure by which tissue from within a thyroid nodule is removed to detect malignancy. This procedure can easily be performed on an outpatient basis, requires no special patient preparation, and is virtually without complications.

Preparation and Procedure

1. No special patient preparation activities are necessary for this procedure.
2. The procedure is explained to the patient and consent is obtained.
3. The patient is positioned comfortably on the examining table in the supine position with the neck fully exposed.
4. A rolled towel or sheet is placed beneath the patient's shoulder to hyperextend the neck, allowing ease of access to the biopsy site.
5. The biopsy site area is cleansed with alcohol and/or an antibacterial cleansing agent.
6. 1% Lidocaine may be injected intracutaneously for local anesthetic to promote patient comfort.
7. A 25-gauge needle is inserted into the thyroid nodule and manipulated by the physician until a small amount of bloody material is seen on the hub of the needle.
8. The needle is removed and attached to a syringe. The contents of the needle are expressed onto a clean glass slide. A second slide is placed on top of the first slide and then pulled apart quickly to create a thin smear.
9. The slides are placed in a fixative and transported to a cytologist for interpretation.

Postprocedure Management

1. The biopsy site may be dressed with a Band-Aid or other small dressing.
2. Follow-up visit for patient should be arranged to discuss results.

Nursing Interventions

Preventing Infection

1. Ensure that biopsy area is prepped appropriately before procedure.
2. Ensure that instruments are maintained in sterile condition before use.

Reducing Patient Anxiety

1. Encourage patient to verbalize concerns regarding procedure or biopsy results.
2. Employ comfort measures during procedure as necessary.
3. Assure patient that most thyroid nodules are determined to be benign and that most thyroid malignancies have a high cure rate.
4. Encourage support by significant others, nursing staff, social worker, as available.

Patient Education and Health Maintenance

1. Teach patient that some soreness at the biopsy site should be expected for a brief time.
2. Ensure that patient follows up for results and definitive treatment.

◼ Care of the Patient Undergoing Thyroidectomy

Thyroidectomy involves the partial or complete removal of the thyroid gland to treat thyroid tumors, hyperthyroidism, or hyperparathyroidism.

Types of Procedures

1. Thyroidectomy can be total (removal of the entire thyroid gland); subtotal (95% of gland removed)—to prevent damage to the parathyroid glands; and partial (one lobe or isthmus removed)—to treat nodular disease.
2. The parathyroid glands are usually spared to prevent hypocalcemia.
3. Indications for thyroidectomy include Grave's disease, large goiters, adenoma (thyroid cancer), and some nodules.

Preoperative Management

1. The patient must be euthyroid at time of surgery, so thionamides are administered to control hyperthyroidism.
2. Iodide is given to increase firmness of thyroid gland and to reduce its vascularity after blood loss.
3. An attempt is made to counteract the effects of hypermetabolism by maintaining a restful and therapeutic environment and by providing a nutritious diet.
4. The patient is prepared for surgery physically and emotionally in the following ways:
   a. Make a special effort to ensure that patient has a good night's rest preceding surgery.
   b. Explain to the patient that speaking is to be minimized immediately postoperatively and that oxygen may be administered to facilitate breathing.
   c. Explain that postoperatively, fluids may be given IV to maintain fluid, electrolyte, and nutritional needs; IV glucose may also be given in the hours before the administration of anesthetic agents.

Postoperative Management

1. The patient is monitored for bleeding and respiratory distress that indicates laryngeal edema, secondary to swelling in the area of surgery.
2. Signs of hypocalcemia are watched for—irritability, twitching, spasms of hands and feet.
   a. Calcium levels are monitored. If in 48 hours, level falls below 7 mg/100 mL (3 mEq), IV calcium (gluconate, lactate) replacement is given.
   b. IV calcium is used cautiously in patients who have renal disease or who are taking digoxin.
3. Thyroid function is not a concern until several weeks after surgery.

Complications

1. Hemorrhage, edema of the glottis, damage to laryngeal nerve.
2. Hypothyroidism occurs in 5% of patients in first postoperative year; increases at rate of 2% to 3% per year.
3. Hypoparathyroidism occurs in about 4% of patients and is usually mild and transient; requires calcium supplements IV and orally when more severe.

Nursing Diagnoses

• Risk for Injury related to surgery
• Risk for Injury related to possible removal of parathyroid glands

Nursing Interventions

Observing for Hemorrhage and Airway Edema

1. Administer humidified oxygen as prescribed to reduce irritation of airway and to prevent edema.
2. Move the patient carefully; provide adequate support to the head so that no tension is placed on the sutures.
3. Place the patient in semi-Fowler's position, with the head elevated and supported by pillows; avoid flexion of neck.
4. Monitor vital signs frequently, watching for tachycardia and hypotension that indicates hemorrhage (most likely between 12 and 24 hours postoperatively).
5. Observe for bleeding at sides and back of the neck, and anteriorly, when the patient is in dorsal position.
6. Watch for repeated clearing of the throat or for complaint of smothering or difficulty swallowing, which may be early signs of hemorrhage.
7. Watch for irregular breathing, swelling of the neck, and choking—other signs pointing to the possibility of hemorrhage and tracheal compression.
8. Reinforce dressing if indicated.
9. Be alert for voice changes, which may indicate damage to laryngeal nerve.
10. Keep a tracheostomy set in the patient's room for 48 hours for emergency use.

Preventing Tetany

1. Watch for the development of tetany caused by removal or disturbance of parathyroid glands through a progression of signs:
   a. Tingling of toes and fingers and around the mouth; apprehension.
   b. Positive Chvostek's sign—tapping on the cheek over the facial nerve causes a twitch of the lip or facial muscles (Figure 24-1A).
   c. Positive Trousseau's sign—carpopedal spasm induced by occluding circulation in the arm with a blood pressure cuff (see Figure 24-1B).
2. Be prepared to treat hypocalcemic tetany.
   a. Position the patient for optimal ventilation; pillow removed to prevent head from bending forward and compressing trachea.
   b. Keep side rails padded and elevated and position the patient to prevent injury if a seizure occurs; do not use restraints because they only aggravate the patient and may result in muscle strain or fractures.
   c. Have equipment available to treat respiratory difficulties that includes airway suction equipment, tracheostomy, and cardiac arrest equipment.
3. Administer IV calcium as directed.

Patient Education and Health Maintenance

1. Teach patient about complications to look for if discharge occurs within a day or two of surgery.
2. Advise patient to rest at home and to prevent any strain on suture line as directed by surgeon.
3. Advise nutritious diet; report problems swallowing.
4. Encourage follow-up for monitoring and thyroid hormone replacement after surgery.

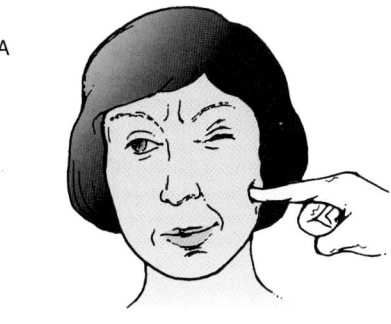

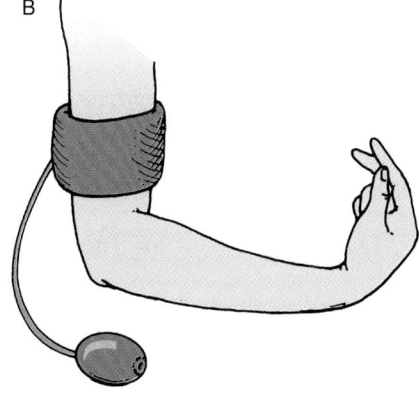

FIGURE 24-1 (**A**) Chvostek's sign. (**B**) Trousseau's sign.

Outcome-Based Evaluation

- No signs of hemorrhage or edema
- No signs of hypocalcemia

Care of the Patient Undergoing Adrenalectomy

Adrenalectomy may be unilateral or bilateral to treat adrenal tumors, Cushing's syndrome, or hyperaldosteronism. It is accomplished through abdominal or flank incision. Careful manipulation of the gland is necessary if surgery is for pheochromocytoma to prevent excessive release of epinephrine causing hypertensive crisis.

Preoperative Management

1. Blood pressure and fluid volume are optimized.
2. Surgery and nursing care are explained to patient. Patient is shown where adrenal glands lie on top of kidneys and where incision may be on abdomen or loin area.
3. Blood pressure will be checked frequently before and after surgery and glucocorticoids will be given to cover period of stress (surgery) because at least one adrenal gland will be removed.
4. Patient is prepared as for major abdominal surgery (see p. 586).

Complications

Hemorrhage, adrenal crisis

Postoperative Management

1. Usual postoperative care for abdominal surgery includes frequent check of vital signs; assessment for hemorrhage; turning, coughing, and deep breathing; early ambulation; slow progression of diet when bowel sounds return; and control of pain with scheduled narcotic administration or patient-controlled analgesia (see p. 586).
2. IV hydrocortisone (Solu-Cortef) is given as directed to prevent adrenal crisis.
3. Nonstressful environment is maintained, rest is promoted, and meticulous care is given to protect the patient from infection and from other complications that could cause adrenal crisis.
4. Serum sodium, potassium, and glucose are monitored for abnormality.
   a. Sodium and potassium may normalize, or potassium may become elevated (because of transient adrenal insufficiency after surgery).
   b. Electrolyte imbalances may persist for 4 to 18 months after surgery.
   c. Hypertension may persist for 3 to 6 months after surgery.
5. Hydrocortisone treatment causes glucose to rise and worsens control in patients with diabetes; may require additional treatment.

Nursing Interventions and Patient Education

1. Assess dressing for leakage initially, and after it has been changed, assess wound for signs of infection.
2. Perform dressing changes, wound care, and teach family how to do wound care at home.
3. Teach patient with bilateral adrenalectomy that glucocorticoid and mineralocorticoid replacement is necessary for rest of life.

4. Administer additional doses IM in times of stress.
5. Administer oral glucocorticoids after unilateral adrenalectomy and teach patient that this treatment will be needed for 6 months to 2 years after surgery until remaining adrenal gland can compensate.
6. Encourage wearing or carrying this information at all times, so that proper treatment can be instituted if patient becomes unconscious.
7. Encourage follow-up to monitor for signs of adrenal insufficiency.

■ Care of the Patient Undergoing Transsphenoidal Hypophysectomy

Procedure

1. Transsphenoidal approach to pituitary removal is carried out through the nasal cavity, sphenoid sinus, and into the sella turcica (Figure 24-2).
2. Advantages over intracranial approach to hypophysectomy include:
   a. No need to shave head.
   b. No visible scar.
   c. Low blood loss, less need for transfusions.
   d. Lower infection rate.
   e. Well tolerated by frail and older patients.
   f. Good visualization of tumor field.
3. Disadvantages include:
   a. Restricted field of surgery.
   b. Potential cerebrospinal fluid (CSF) leak.

Preoperative Management

1. Sinus infection is assessed and treated, if necessary.
2. Hydrocortisone (Cortef) may be given preoperatively because the source of ACTH is being removed.

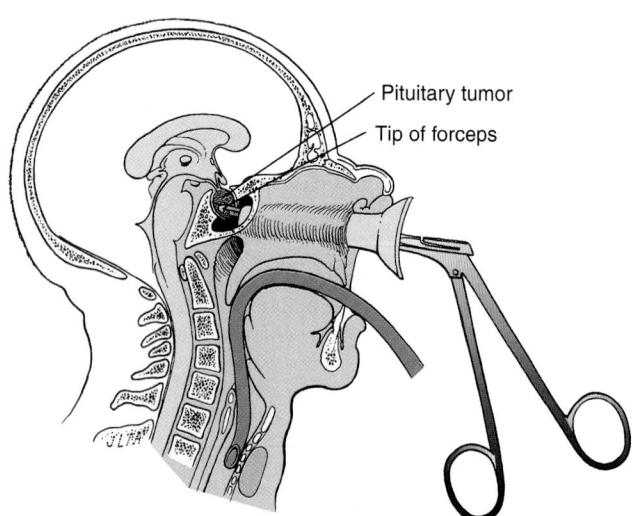

Pituitary tumor

Tip of forceps

FIGURE 24-2 Transsphenoidal approach to the pituitary. A special nasal speculum is used to view the sinus cavity. After the dura is opened, the tumor is removed using microcurettes or other specially designed instruments.

3. The patient is prepared physically and emotionally for surgery.
   a. Deep-breathing exercises.
   b. Avoid coughing and sneezing postoperatively to prevent CSF leak.

Complications
1. CSF leak, meningitis
2. Transient DI.
3. Syndrome of inappropriate ADH secretion (SIADH)

Postoperative Management
1. Vital signs, visual acuity, and neurologic status are monitored.
2. Urine output and specific gravity and serum electrolytes and osmolality are monitored for development of DI or SIADH.
3. Drainage from nose is monitored for signs of infection or cerebrospinal fluid leak (clear fluid).

Patient Education and Health Promotion
1. Monitor vital signs, visual acuity, and neurologic status frequently for signs of increasing intracranial pressure.
2. Monitor fluid intake and output, and report any increase in output and decrease in specific gravity which may indicate DI.
3. Observe for signs of infection. Check incision within inner aspect of upper lip for drainage or bleeding.
4. Assess level of pain and administer analgesic or supervise patient-controlled analgesia.
5. Note frequency of nasal dressing changes and character of drainage. Prepare patient for packing removal one to several days postoperatively.
6. Encourage the use of a humidifier to prevent drying from mouth breathing.
7. Report persistent clear fluid from nose and increasing headache; could signal CSF leak.
8. Teach patient signs of complications and to report them immediately and to follow up as scheduled.

DISORDERS OF THE THYROID GLAND

The thyroid gland affects the metabolic rate of all tissues, including the speed of chemical reactions, the volume of oxygen consumed, and the amount of heat produced. The stimulating effect is through the production and distribution of two hormones:
1. Levothyroxine (T_4)—contains four iodine atoms; maintains body's metabolism in a steady state; T_4 serves as a precursor of T_3.
2. Triiodothyronine (T_3)—contains three iodine atoms; is approximately five times as potent as T_4 is; has a more rapid metabolic action and utilization than T_4 does.

3. Most conversion of T_4 to T_3 occurs at the cellular level in the periphery. Some T_3 is produced in the thyroid gland.

Hypothyroidism
This is a condition that arises from inadequate amounts of thyroid hormone in the bloodstream.

Pathophysiology and Etiology
1. Primary hypothyroidism is the most common form of this condition and is generally caused by (in order of frequency):
   a. Autoimmune disease (Hashimoto's thyroiditis).
   b. Use of radioactive iodine.
   c. Destruction, suppression, or removal of all or some of the thyroid tissue by thyroidectomy.
   d. Dietary iodide deficiency.
   e. Subacute thyroiditis.
   f. Lithium therapy.
   g. Overtreatment with antithyroid drugs.
2. Secondary hypothyroidism is caused by inadequate secretion of TSH caused by disease of the pituitary gland (ie, tumor, necrosis).
3. Inadequate secretion of thyroid hormone leads to a general slowing of all physical and mental processes.
4. General depression of most cellular enzyme systems and oxidative processes occurs.
5. The metabolic activity of all cells of the body decreases, reducing oxygen consumption, decreasing oxidation of nutrients for energy, and producing less body heat.
6. The signs and symptoms of the disorder range from vague, nonspecific complaints that make diagnosis difficult, to severe symptoms that may be life-threatening if unrecognized and untreated.

Clinical Manifestations
1. Fatigue and lethargy.
2. Weight gain.
3. Complaints of cold hands and feet.
4. Temperature and pulse become subnormal; patient cannot tolerate cold and desires increased room temperature.
5. Reduced attention span; impaired short-term memory.
6. Severe constipation; decreased peristalsis.
7. Generalized appearance of thick, puffy skin; subcutaneous swelling in hands, feet, and eyelids.
8. Hair thins; loss of the lateral one-third of eyebrow.
9. Menorrhagia or amenorrhea; may have difficulty conceiving or may experiences spontaneous abortion; decreased libido.
10. Neurologic signs include polyneuropathy, cerebellar ataxia, muscle aches or weakness, clumsiness, prolonged deep tendon reflexes (especially ankle jerk).
11. Hyperlipoproteinemia and hypercholesterolemia.
12. Enlarged heart on chest x-ray.
13. Increased susceptibility to all hypnotic and sedative drugs and anesthetic agents.

Diagnostic Evaluation
1. Low T_3 and T_4 levels.
2. Elevated TSH levels in primary hypothyroidism.
3. Elevation of serum cholesterol.
4. Electrocardiogram (ECG)—sinus bradycardia, low voltage of QRS complexes, and flat or inverted T waves.

Management
Approach
1. Depends on severity of symptoms; may necessitate replacement therapy in mild cases or lifesaving support and treatment in severe hypothyroidism and myxedema coma.
2. As thyroid hormone levels gradually return to normal, the patient is monitored closely to prevent complications resulting from sudden increases in metabolic rate and oxygen requirements.

Restoration of Normal Metabolic State (Euthyroid)
1. Thyroid hormone: T_4-levothyroxine (Synthroid, Levothroid); T_3-liothyronine (Cytomel); T_3 and T_4-thyroglobulin (Proloid) and liotrix (Euthroid, Thyrolar).
   a. Because T_3 acts more quickly than T_4 does, it is given via nasogastric tube if patient is unconscious.
   b. Sodium levothyroxine (Synthroid) is administered parenterally (until consciousness is restored) to restore T_4 level.
   c. Later, the patient is continued on oral thyroid hormone therapy.
   d. With rapid administration of thyroid hormone, plasma T_4 levels may initiate adrenal insufficiency; hence, steroid therapy may be started.
   e. Mild symptoms in the alert patient or asymptomatic cases (with abnormal laboratory results only) require only initiation of low-dose thyroid hormone given orally.
2. Monitoring to anticipate treatment effects:
   a. Diuresis, decreased puffiness.
   b. Improved reflexes and muscle tone.
   c. Accelerated pulse rate.
   d. A slightly higher level of total serum T_4.
   e. All signs of hypothyroidism should disappear in 3 to 12 weeks.
   f. Decreasing TSH level.

GERONTOLOGIC ALERT
When starting thyroid hormone replacement, care must be taken with older patients and with those who have coronary artery disease to avoid coronary ischemia because of increased oxygen demands of the heart. It is preferable to start with much lower doses and increase gradually, taking 1 to 2 months to reach full replacement doses.

Complications
1. Myxedema coma—hypotension, unresponsiveness, bradycardia, hypoventilation, hyponatremia, (possibly) convulsions, hypothermia, cerebral hypoxia.
2. High mortality rate in myxedema coma.

Nursing Assessment
1. Obtain history of symptoms, medication program, and past history of thyroid disease, surgery, or treatment.
2. Perform multisystem assessment, including cardiac, respiratory, neurologic, and gastrointestinal systems.

Nursing Diagnosis
(See Nursing Care Plan 24-1.)
- Decreased Cardiac Output related to decreased metabolic rate and decreased cardiac conduction

Nursing Interventions
Increasing Cardiac Output
1. Monitor vital signs frequently to detect changes in cardiovascular status and ability to respond to stress.
2. Monitor ECG tracings to detect arrhythmias and deterioration of cardiovascular status.
3. Prevent chilling to avoid increasing metabolic rate, which, in turn, places strain on the heart. Provide bed socks, bed jacket, warm environment.
4. Avoid rapid rewarming techniques (warmed IV fluids, hypothermia blanket) because the resulting increased oxygen requirements and peripheral vasodilation may worsen cardiac failure.
5. Administer fluids cautiously, even though hyponatremia is present.
6. Administer all prescribed drugs with caution before and after thyroid replacement begins.
   a. Monitor the effects of sedatives, narcotics, and anesthetics closely because patient is more sensitive to these agents.
   b. After thyroid replacement is initiated, the thyroid hormones may increase the effects of digitalis (monitor pulse) and anticoagulants (watch for signs of bleeding).
7. Report occurrence of angina, and be alert for signs and symptoms of myocardial infarction and cardiac failure.
8. Monitor arterial blood gases to assess cardiopulmonary function.

Patient Education and Health Maintenance
Instruct the patient about the following:
1. The need to receive thyroid hormone replacement therapy for the duration of one's life.
2. How and when to take medications.
3. Signs and symptoms of insufficient and excessive medication; reinforce teaching by providing written instructions.
4. The necessity of having blood evaluations periodically to determine thyroid levels.
5. Energy conservation techniques and the need to increase activity gradually.
6. Fluid intake and use of fiber to prevent constipation.
7. Control of dietary intake to limit calories and reduce weight.
8. Assist patient in identifying sources of information and support available in the community (Table 24-2).

Outcome-Based Evaluation
- Blood pressure and pulse rate stable

TABLE 24-2 Endocrine Internet Resource Web Sites for Patients and Nurses

General
- The Endocrine Society (www.endo-society.org)
- Endocrine Nurses Society (www.endo-nurses.org)
- National Institutes of Health
  (www.NIDDK.nih.gov/health/endo/endo.htm)

Thyroid
- American Thyroid Association (www.thyroid.org/)
- Alt.support thyroid page
  (www.geocities.com/Athens/3626/faqs.html)

Addison's Disease
- National Adrenal Diseases Foundation
  (www.medhelp.org/www/nadf.htm)

Cushing's Syndrome
- Cushing's Support and Research Foundation, Inc.
  (www.world.std.com/~csrf/)

Pituitary Disorders
- Pituitary Tumor Network Association (www.pituitary.com)

■ Hyperthyroidism

This hypermetabolic condition is characterized by excessive amounts of thyroid hormone in the bloodstream.

Pathophysiology and Etiology

1. More common in women than in men; occurs in about 2% of the female population.
2. Graves' disease (most prevalent)—diffuse hyperfunction of the thyroid gland with autoimmune etiology and associated with ophthalmopathy; most common in younger women; may subside spontaneously.
   a. Thyroid-stimulating antibody (TSA_b), an immunoglobulin found in the blood of patients with Graves' disease, is capable of reacting with the receptor for TSH on the thyroid plasma membrane and of stimulating thyroid hormone production and secretion.
   b. May appear after an emotional shock, an infection, or emotional stress.
3. Toxic nodular goiter (single or multiple)—more common in older women with preexisting goiter; will continue to be overactive unless eradicated or kept under suppressive therapy.

NURSING CARE PLAN 24-1   CARE OF THE PATIENT WITH HYPOTHYROIDISM

You see Mrs. White in the clinic. She is a 45-year-old woman with a history of hypothyroidism, who has been treated with L-thyroxine 0.15 mg qd.

From your assessment and knowledge of hypothyroidism, develop your teaching plan.

Subjective data: Mrs. White tells you that she has been feeling tired lately and finds it hard to manage even the simplest of chores around the house. She complains of constipation that gives her a feeling of fullness and affects her appetite. When asked about her medication, she states, "Oh I ran out of those a few months ago and I never refilled the prescription. I was feeling fine, so I didn't see any need to keep taking medicine."

Objective data: Vitals signs are—temperature 36.7°C (98.2°F), pulse 58, BP 100/60, respirations 12. On examination, you notice her skin is cool and dry to touch. She is wearing a sweater although it is a warm day outside. Bowel sounds are hypoactive. Knee jerk reflexes are sluggish.

Laboratory results: T_4—3.4 µg/dL (normal range 5–12 µg/dL)
TSH (thyroid-stimulating hormone) 25 µU/mL (normal range <7 µU/mL)

NURSING DIAGNOSIS   Constipation related to decreased bowel motility caused by hypofunction of the thyroid gland

GOAL/OUTCOME   The patient will resume normal bowel function.

Nursing Intervention	Rationale	Outcome-Based Evaluation
1. Encourage increased intake of fluids.	1. Promotes passage of soft stools.	1. Drinks recommended amount of fluid each day.
2. Recommend foods high in fiber.	2. Increases bulk of stools and promotes more frequent bowel movements.	2. Identifies and consumes foods high in fiber.
3. Recommend patient monitor bowel function by recording frequency and consistency of stool.	3. Documents patient response to nursing interventions.	3. Patient reports bowel pattern has returned to normal.
4. Encourage increased mobility within patient's exercise tolerance.	4. Promotes evacuation of the bowel.	4. Gradually increases exercises.

(continued)

NURSING CARE PLAN 24-1   CARE OF THE PATIENT WITH HYPOTHYROIDISM (Continued)

NURSING DIAGNOSIS   Activity Intolerance related to reduced metabolic rate

GOAL/OUTCOME   Exercise tolerance and participation in activities will increase.

Nursing Intervention	Rationale	Outcome-Based Evaluation
1. Teach patient to space activities to promote rest and exercise as tolerated. 2. Teach patient to keep a record of physical activity, noting duration, intensity, and level of fatigue. 3. Gradually increase level of activity as tolerated.	1. Promotes activity without overly stressing the patient. 2. Promotes patient participation in care and promotes independence. 3. Demonstrates changes in patient activity tolerance.	1. Patient reports increased participation in activities of daily living. 2. Patient provides reports of exercise tolerance and performance in daily activities. 3. Patient reports successful increases in activity tolerance.

NURSING DIAGNOSIS   Knowledge deficit related to self-care needs for thyroid hormone replacement therapy

GOAL/OUTCOME   Patient will demonstrate knowledge appropriate for self-care in thyroid replacement therapy.

Nursing Intervention	Rationale	Outcome-Based Evaluation

1. Teach patient about the nature of chronic hypothyroidism and the purpose of thyroid hormone replacement therapy.
2. Describe effects of thyroid hormone medication to patient.
 	
3. Describe signs and symptoms of underdose and overdose of medication.
  a. Underdosage—fatigue, slow pulse, constipation
  b. Overdosage—increased pulse or palpitations, sweating, difficulty sleeping, feeling jittery
	1. Provides rationale for adherence to prescribed hormone replacement.
	
	2. Allows patient to appreciate benefits of therapy from the standpoint of her current physical complaints.
	3. Allows patient to be an active participant in monitoring her therapy.
		1. Patient describes reason for thyroid hormone replacement therapy and describes regimen correctly.
		
		2. Patient states positive outcomes of thyroid hormone replacement therapy.
		3. Patient identifies signs and symptoms indicative of overdose and underdose that should be reported to her health care provider promptly.

4. Hyperthyroidism is characterized by hypertrophy and hyperplasia of the thyroid gland, which is accompanied by increased vascularity and blood flow and enlargement of the gland.

5. Most of the clinical manifestations result from increased metabolic rate, excessive heat production, increased neuromuscular and cardiovascular activity, and hyperactivity of the sympathetic nervous system.

6. Hyperthyroidism ranges from a mild increase in metabolic rate to the severe hyperactivity known as thyrotoxicosis, thyroid storm, or thyroid crisis.

7. Hyperthyroidism can also be the result of ingestion of excessive amounts of thyroid hormone medication (factitious hyperthyroidism).

Clinical Manifestations

1. Nervousness, emotional lability, irritability, apprehension.
2. Difficulty in sitting quietly.
3. Rapid pulse at rest and on exertion (ranges between 90 and 160); palpitations.

4. Heat intolerance; profuse perspiration; flushed skin (eg, hands may be warm, soft, moist).
5. Fine tremor of hands; change in bowel habits—constipation or diarrhea.
6. Increased appetite and progressive weight loss; frequent stools.
7. Muscle fatigability and weakness; amenorrhea.
8. Atrial fibrillation possible (cardiac decompensation common in older patients).
9. Bulging eyes (exophthalmos)—produces a startled expression.
10. Thyroid gland may be palpable and a bruit may be auscultated over gland.
11. Course may be mild, characterized by remissions and exacerbations.
12. It may progress to emaciation, extreme nervousness, delirium, disorientation, thyroid storm or crisis, and death.
13. Thyroid storm or crisis, an extreme form of hyperthyroidism, is characterized by hyperpyrexia, diarrhea, dehydration, tachycardia, arrhythmias, extreme

irritation, delirium, coma, shock, and death if not adequately treated.

14. Thyroid storm may be precipitated by stress (surgery, infection) or inadequate preparation for surgery in a patient with known hyperthyroidism.

Diagnostic Evaluation

1. Elevated T_3 and T_4.
2. Elevated serum T_3 resin uptake.
3. Radioactive iodine uptake scan may be elevated or below normal depending on the underlying cause of the hyperthyroidism.

Management

Approach to Management

1. Treatment depends on causes, age of patient, severity of disease, and complications.
2. Remission of hyperthyroidism (Graves' disease) occurs spontaneously within 1 to 2 years; however, relapse can be expected in half the patients. Antithyroid drugs, radiation, or surgery may be used for treatment.
3. Nodular toxic goiter—surgery or use of radioiodine is preferred.
4. Thyroid carcinoma—surgery or radiation is used.
5. Goal of therapy is to bring the metabolic rate to normal as soon as possible and to maintain it at this level.

Pharmacotherapy

1. Drugs that inhibit hormone formation:
   a. Thionamides—propylthiouracil (PTU), methimazole (Tapazole).
   b. Act by depressing the synthesis of thyroid hormone by inhibiting peroxidase.
   c. Given in divided daily doses (every 8 hours).
   d. Duration of treatment is determined by clinical criteria.
      (i) Thyroid gland becomes smaller.
      (ii) Uptakes of T_4 and T_3 are measured to determine adequacy of dose.
      (iii) Treatment continued until patient becomes clinically euthyroid; this varies from 3 months to 1 to 2 years; if euthyroidism cannot be maintained without therapy, then radiation or surgery is recommended.
      (iv) Therapy is withdrawn gradually to prevent exacerbation.
2. Drugs to control peripheral manifestations of hyperthyroidism:
   a. Propranolol (Inderal).
      (i) Acts as a β-adrenergic blocking agent.
      (ii) Abolishes tachycardia, tremor, excess sweating, nervousness.
      (iii) Controls hyperthyroid symptoms until antithyroid drugs or radioiodine can take effect.
   b. Glucocorticoids—decrease the peripheral conversion of T_4 to T_3, a more potent thyroid hormone.

Radioactive Iodine

1. Action—limits secretion of thyroid hormone by destroying thyroid tissue.
2. Dosage is controlled so that hypothyroidism does not occur.
3. Chief advantage over thionamides is that a lasting remission can be achieved.
4. Chief disadvantage is that permanent hypothyroidism can be produced.

Surgery

1. Used for those with large goiters, or for those for whom the use of radioiodine or thionamides is contraindicated.
2. Subtotal thyroidectomy involves removal of most of the thyroid gland (see p. 816).

> ◆ **DRUG ALERT**
>
> Observe the patient for evidence of iodine toxicity: swelling of buccal mucosa, excessive salivation, coryza, skin eruptions. If these occur, iodides are discontinued.

Emergency Management of Thyroid Storm

1. Inhibition of new hormone synthesis with thionamides (PTU).
2. Inhibition of thyroid hormone release using iodine (Lugol's solution).
3. Inhibition of peripheral effects of thyroid hormones with propranolol (Inderal), corticosteroids, and thionamides (PTU).
4. Treatment aimed at systemic effects of thyroid hormones and prevention of decompensation.
   a. Hyperthermia—cooling blanket, acetaminophen (Tylenol).
   b. Dehydration—administration of IV fluids and electrolytes.
5. Treatment of precipitating event.

Complications

1. Thionamide toxicity—agranulocytosis may occur suddenly.
2. Hypothyroidism if overtreated with antithyroid medication or if radiation treatment is used.
3. Radiation thyroiditis (a transient exacerbation of hyperthyroidism) may occur as a result of leakage of thyroid hormone into the circulation from damaged follicles.
4. Infiltrative ophthalmopathy
   a. Occurs in 50% of patients with Graves' disease.
   b. Features include exophthalmos, weakness of extraocular muscles, lid edema, lid lag.

Nursing Assessment

1. Obtain history of symptoms, family history of thyroid disease, medications, any recent physical stress, particularly infection.
2. Perform multisystem assessment, that includes cardiac, respiratory, neurologic, and gastrointestinal systems.

3. Closely monitor the patient's temperature for thyroid storm.

Nursing Diagnoses
- Altered Nutrition: Less Than Body Requirements related to hypermetabolic state and fluid loss through diaphoresis
- Risk for Impaired Skin Integrity related to diaphoresis, hyperpyrexia, restlessness, and rapid weight loss
- Altered Thought Processes related to insomnia, decreased attention span, and irritability
- Anxiety related to condition and concern about upcoming surgery/radioiodine treatment

Nursing Interventions
Providing Adequate Nutrition
1. Determine the patient's food and fluid preferences.
2. Provide high-calorie foods and fluids consistent with the patient's requirements.
3. Provide a quiet, calm environment at meals.
4. Restrict stimulants (tea, coffee, alcohol); explain rationale of requirements and restrictions to patient.
5. Encourage/permit the patient to eat alone if embarrassed or if otherwise disturbed by voracious appetite.
6. Monitor IV infusion when prescribed to maintain fluid and electrolyte balance.
7. Monitor fluid and nutritional status by weighing the patient daily and by keeping accurate intake and output records.
8. Monitor vital signs to detect changes in fluid volume status.
9. Assess skin turgor, mucous membranes, and neck veins for signs of increased or decreased fluid volume.

Maintaining Skin Integrity
1. Assess skin frequently to detect diaphoresis.
2. Bathe frequently with cool water; change linens when damp.
3. Avoid soap to prevent drying and use lubricant skin lotions to pressure points.
4. Protect and relieve pressure from bony prominences while immobilized or while hypothermia blanket is used.

Promoting Normal Thought Processes
1. Explain procedures to patient in an unhurried, calm manner.
2. Limit visitors; avoid stimulating conversations or television programs.
3. Reduce stressors in the environment; reduce noise and lights.
4. Promote sleep and relaxation through use of prescribed medications, massage, and relaxation exercises.
5. Minimize disruption of the patient's sleep or rest by clustering nursing activities.
6. Use safety measures to reduce risk of trauma or falls (padded side rails, bed in low position).

Relieving Anxiety
1. Encourage the patient to verbalize concerns and fears about illness and treatment.

2. Support the patient who is undergoing various diagnostic tests.
   a. Explain the purpose and requirements of each prescribed test.
   b. Explain results of tests if unclear to the patient or if questions arise.
3. Clear up misconceptions about treatment options.

Patient Education and Health Maintenance
1. Instruct the patient as follows:
   a. When to take medications.
   b. Signs and symptoms of insufficient and excessive medication.
   c. Necessity of having blood evaluations periodically to determine thyroid levels.
   d. Signs of agranulocytosis (fever, sore throat, upper respiratory infection) or rash, fever, urticaria, or enlarged salivary glands caused by thionamide toxicity.
   e. Signs and symptoms of thyroid storm (ie, tachycardia, hyperpyrexia, extreme irritation) and predisposing factors to thyroid storm (ie, infection, surgery, stress, abrupt withdrawal of antithyroid medications and adrenergic blocking agents).
2. Reinforce teaching by providing written instructions as well.
3. Assist patient in identifying sources of information and support available in the community (see Table 24-2).

Outcome-Based Evaluation
- Food and fluid intake adequate, gaining weight
- Skin cool, dry, and intact
- Maintains concentration, follows conversation, and responds appropriately
- Verbalizes concerns and questions about illness, treatment, and surgery

▩ Subacute Thyroiditis
A self-limiting, painful inflammation of the thyroid gland, usually associated with viral infections.

Pathophysiology and Etiology
1. Affects younger women predominantly.
2. Acute inflammation results in sudden release of preformed T_3 and T_4, often causing symptoms of hyperthyroidism initially.
3. A clinical variant of this disorder, "silent thyroiditis" has been described that is similar to subacute thyroiditis; however, the symptoms may be milder and the thyroid gland is not painful.
4. This disorder has been associated with onset within 6 months of the postpartum period in women.

Clinical Manifestations
1. Pain, swelling, thyroid tenderness lasts several weeks or months, then disappears.
2. Fever, sore throat.

3. Pain referred to the ear, making swallowing difficult and uncomfortable.
4. Fever, malaise, chills.
5. May develop clinical manifestations of hyperthyroidism (irritability, nervousness, insomnia, and weight loss) or hypothyroidism, depending on the point of time in the natural course of the disease when the patient presents.

Diagnostic Evaluation
1. TSH level is low.
2. Radioactive iodine uptake is low.
3. Serum T_3 and T_4 levels are elevated.
4. Erythrocyte sedimentation rate is increased.

Management
1. Analgesics and mild sedatives.
2. The patient may be placed on β-adrenergic blocking medications to reduce the symptoms of thyrotoxicosis.
3. Steroids may be administered for pain, fever, and malaise.
4. Aspirin or nonsteroidal anti-inflammatory agents may be used in mild cases to treat the symptoms of inflammation.

DRUG ALERT

Aspirin should be avoided if the patient exhibits signs of hyperthyroidism, because it displaces thyroid hormone from its binding site and may increase the amount of free circulating hormone, resulting in exacerbation of the symptoms of hyperthyroidism.

Complications
In about 10% of patients, permanent hypothyroidism occurs and long-term T_4 therapy is needed.

Nursing Assessment
1. Assess for signs and symptoms of hyperthyroidism (see p. 822).
2. Assess for level of discomfort.
3. Evaluate patient's coping skills regarding pain.

Nursing Diagnosis
• Pain related to inflammation of thyroid gland

Nursing Interventions
Reducing Pain
1. Explain all tests and procedures to patient/family.
2. Administer or teach self-administration of pain relief medication as prescribed.
3. Provide a restful environment.
4. Assess for degree of pain relief.
5. Notify health care provider if pain relief medications are inadequate for acceptable pain control.

Patient Education and Health Maintenance
1. Explain all medications the patient is to continue at home.
2. Reassure patient that subacute thyroiditis usually resolves spontaneously during weeks to months.

3. Teach patient signs and symptoms of hypothyroidism (ie, fatigue and lethargy, weight gain, cold intolerance) that may be experienced. These should be reported as inflammation of the gland subsides.
4. Assist patient in identifying sources of information and support available in the community (see Table 24-2).

Outcome-Based Evaluation
• Verbalizes acceptable pain relief

Hashimoto's Thyroiditis (Lymphocytic Thyroiditis)
Hashimoto's thyroiditis is a chronic progressive disease of the thyroid gland caused by infiltration of lymphocytes; it results in progressive destruction of the parenchyma and hypothyroidism if untreated.

Pathophysiology and Etiology
1. Cause is unknown; believed to be an autoimmune disease, genetically transmitted and perhaps related to Graves' disease.
2. Ninety-five percent of cases occur in women in their 40s or 50s.
3. Possibly the most common cause of adult hypothyroidism.
4. Appears to be increasing in incidence.

Clinical Manifestations
1. Marked by a slowly developing, firm enlargement of the thyroid gland.
2. Usually no gross nodules.
3. Basal metabolic rate is usually low.
4. Periods of hyperthyroidism caused by large amounts of T_3 and T_4 being released into bloodstream.

Diagnostic Evaluation
1. T_3 and T_4 may be normal but usually become subnormal as the disease progresses.
2. TSH level is usually elevated.
3. Antithyroglobulin antibodies and antimicrosomal antibodies are virtually always present.
4. Normal or high concentration of thyroglobulin-binding protein.

Management
1. Thyroid medications to maintain a normal level of circulating thyroid hormone; this is done to suppress production of TSH, to prevent enlargement of the thyroid, and to maintain a euthyroid state.
2. Surgical resection of goiter if tracheal compression, cough, or hoarseness occur.
3. Careful follow-up to detect and treat hypothyroidism.

Complications
1. Progressive hypothyroidism.
2. Without treatment, Hashimoto's thyroiditis may progress from goiter and hypothyroidism to myxedema.

Nursing Assessment

1. Assess for signs and symptoms of hyperthyroidism and hypothyroidism.
2. Assess size of thyroid gland and symptoms of compression—neck tightness, cough, hoarseness.

Nursing Diagnosis

- Anxiety related to enlargement of neck/thyroid gland

Nursing Interventions
Reducing Anxiety

1. Explain physiology of the disorder and the reason for enlarging gland. Show anatomic pictures of thyroid gland, if possible.
2. Administer or teach self-administration of thyroid hormone to suppress stimulation on gland and possibly reduce size.
3. Reassure regarding slow progression of gland enlargement (during months) and the option of surgical resection if necessary.
4. Suggest wearing loose-necked clothing, avoiding jewelry or scarves around neck, and avoiding excessive neck flexion or hyperextension, which may aggravate feeling of compression.

Patient Education and Health Maintenance

1. Teach signs of tracheal compression that should be reported to health care provider as soon as possible—difficulty breathing, cough, hoarseness.
2. Explain outcome of hypothyroidism and necessity of taking thyroid hormones every day for life.
3. Explain the need for regular medical follow-up visits to monitor thyroid hormone and TSH levels.
4. Assist patient in identifying sources of information and support available in the community (see Table 24-2).

> **GERONTOLOGIC ALERT**
>
> Careful and regular follow-up of older patients with Hashimoto's thyroiditis is especially important because the progression to hypothyroidism is usually subtle in older people and is unlikely to be recognized promptly.

Outcome-Based Evaluation

- Verbalizes reduced anxiety, more relaxed, sleeping better

■ Cancer of the Thyroid

Carcinoma (cancer) of the thyroid is a malignant neoplasm of the gland.

Pathophysiology and Etiology

1. Incidence increases with age. The average age at time of diagnosis is 45 years.
2. There appears to be an association between external radiation to the head and neck in infancy and childhood, and subsequent development of thyroid carcinoma. (Between 1949 and 1960, radiation therapy was often given to shrink enlarged tonsil and adenoid tissue, to treat acne, or to reduce an enlarged thymus.)
3. Papillary and well-differentiated adenocarcinoma (most common).
    a. Growth is slow, and spread is confined to lymph nodes that surround thyroid area.
    b. Cure rate is excellent after removal of involved areas.
4. Follicular (rapidly growing, widely metastasizing type).
    a. Occurs predominantly in middle-aged and older persons.
    b. Brief encouraging response may occur with irradiation.
    c. Progression of disease is rapid; high mortality rate.
5. Parafollicular-medullary thyroid carcinoma (MTC).
    a. Rare, inheritable type of thyroid malignancy, which can be detected early by a radioimmunoassay for calcitonin.
6. Undifferentiated anaplastic carcinoma.
    a. The most aggressive and lethal solid tumor found in humans.
    b. Least common of all thyroid cancers.
    c. Often fatal within months of diagnosis.

Clinical Manifestations

1. On palpation of the thyroid, there may be a firm, irregular, fixed, painless mass or nodule.
2. The occurrence of signs and symptoms of hyperthyroidism is rare.

Diagnostic Evaluation

1. A thyroid scan with ^{99m}Tc will detect a "cold" nodule with little uptake.
2. Fine needle aspiration biopsy.
3. Surgical exploration.

Management

1. Surgical removal is extensive, as required.
    a. Postsurgical radiation therapy is often done to reduce chances of recurrence.
    b. Follow-up includes periodic ^{131}I uptake scan to detect evidence of recurrence.
2. Thyroid replacement.
    a. Thyroid hormone is administered to suppress secretion of TSH.
    b. Such treatment is continued indefinitely and requires annual checkups.
3. For unresectable cancer, patient is referred for treatment with ^{131}I, chemotherapy, or radiation therapy.

Complications

Untreated thyroid carcinoma can be fatal.

Nursing Assessment

Explore patient's feelings and concerns regarding the diagnosis, treatment, and prognosis.

Nursing Diagnosis

- Anxiety related to concern about cancer, upcoming surgery

Nursing Interventions

Also see Care of the Patient Undergoing Thyroidectomy, p. 816.

Allaying Anxiety

1. Provide all explanations in a simple, concise manner and repeat important information as necessary because anxiety may interfere with patient's processing of information.
2. Stress the positive aspects of treatment, high cure rate as outlined by health care provider.
3. Encourage support by significant other, clergy, social worker, nursing staff, as available.

Patient Education and Health Maintenance

1. Instruct the patient on thyroid hormone replacement and follow-up blood tests.
2. Stress the need for periodic evaluation for recurrence of malignancy.
3. Supply additional information or suggest community resources dealing with cancer prevention and treatment.
4. Assist patient in identifying sources of information and support available in the community (see Table 24-2).

Outcome-Based Evaluation

- Discusses concerns with family, hospital clergy

DISORDERS OF THE PARATHYROID GLANDS

The parathyroid glands are small, bean-sized structures embedded in the posterior section of the thyroid gland. Functions include the production, storage, and release of PTH (parathormone) in response to the serum level of ionized calcium. PTH increases serum calcium by decreasing elimination of calcium ions in the urine by the kidney, increasing absorption of calcium ions from the gut, and increasing bone contribution of calcium ions to the plasma.

◼ Hyperparathyroidism

Hyperparathyroidism is hypersecretion of PTH.

Pathophysiology and Etiology

1. Disorder is most common among women older than age 50.
2. Primary hyperparathyroidism.
   a. Single parathyroid adenoma is the most common cause (approximately 80% of cases).
   b. Parathyroid hyperplasia accounts for approximately 20% of cases.
   c. Parathyroid carcinoma accounts for less than 1% of cases.
3. Secondary hyperparathyroidism.
   a. Primarily the result of renal failure.

Clinical Manifestations

1. Decalcification of bones.
   a. Skeletal pain, backache, pain on weight-bearing, pathologic fractures, deformities, formation of bony cysts.
   b. Formation of bone tumors—overgrowth of osteoclasts.
   c. Formation of calcium-containing kidney stones.
2. Depression of neuromuscular function.
   a. The patient may trip, drop objects, show general fatigue, lose memory for recent events, experience emotional instability, have changes in level of consciousness, with stupor and coma.
   b. Cardiac arrhythmias, hypertension, cardiac standstill.

Diagnostic Evaluation

1. Persistently elevated serum calcium (11 mg/100 mL); test is performed on at least two occasions to determine consistency of results.
2. Exclusion of other causes of hypercalcemia—malignancy (usually bone or breast), vitamin D excess, multiple myeloma, sarcoidosis, milk-alkali syndrome, drugs such as thiazides, Cushing's disease, hyperthyroidism.
3. PTH levels are increased.
4. Serum calcium and alkaline phosphatase levels are elevated and serum phosphorus levels are decreased.
5. Skeletal changes are revealed by x-ray.
6. Early diagnosis often is difficult. (Complications may occur before this condition is diagnosed.)
7. Cine computed tomography (CT) will disclose parathyroid tumors more readily than x-ray.

Management

Treatment of Hypercalcemia

1. Hydration (IV saline) and diuretics-furosemide (Lasix) and ethacrynic acid (Edecrin)—to increase urinary excretion of calcium in patients not in renal failure
2. Oral phosphate may be used as an antihypercalcemic agent.
3. Plicamycin (Mithramycin), calcitonin (Cibacalcin), or etidronate disodium (Didronel) are effective in treating hypercalcemia by inhibiting bone resorption.
4. Dietary calcium is restricted, and all drugs that might cause hypercalcemia (thiazides, vitamin D) are discontinued.
5. Dialysis may be necessary in patients with resistant hypercalcemia or those with renal failure.
6. Digitalis is reduced because patient with hypercalcemia is more sensitive to toxic effects of this drug.
7. Monitoring of daily serum calcium, blood urea nitrogen (BUN), potassium, and magnesium levels.
8. Removal of underlying cause.

Treatment of Primary Hyperparathyroidism

Surgery for removal of abnormal parathyroid tissue.

Complications

1. Formation of renal stones, calcification of kidney parenchyma, renal shutdown.
2. Ulceration of upper gastrointestinal tract leading to hemorrhage and perforation.
3. Demineralization of bones, cysts, and fibrosis of marrow leads to fractures, especially of vertebral bodies and ribs.
4. Hypoparathyroidism after surgery.

Nursing Assessment

1. Obtain review of systems and perform multisystem examination to detect signs and symptoms of hyperparathyroidism.
2. Closely monitor patient's input and output and serum electrolytes, especially calcium level. See Standards of Care Guidelines.

Nursing Diagnoses

- Fluid Volume Deficit related to effects of elevated serum calcium levels
- Altered Urinary Elimination related to renal calculi and calcium deposits in the kidneys
- Impaired Physical Mobility related to weakness, bone pain, and pathologic fractures
- Anxiety related to surgery
- Risk for Injury related to hypocalcemia

Nursing Interventions

Achieving Fluid and Electrolyte Balance

1. Monitor fluid intake and output.
2. Provide adequate hydration—administer water, glucose, and electrolytes orally or IV as prescribed.
3. Prevent or promptly treat dehydration by reporting vomiting or other sources of fluid loss promptly.
4. Help patient understand why and how to avoid dietary sources of calcium—dairy products, broccoli, calcium-containing antacids.

Promoting Urinary Elimination

1. Strain all urine to observe for stones.
2. Increase fluid intake to 3,000 mL/day to maintain hydration and prevent precipitation of calcium and formation of stones.
3. Instruct the patient about dietary recommendations for restriction of calcium.
4. Observe for signs of urinary tract infection, hematuria, and renal colic.
5. Assess renal function through serum creatinine and BUN levels.

Increasing Physical Mobility

1. Assist the patient in hygiene and activities if bone pain is severe or if the patient experiences musculoskeletal weakness.
2. Protect the patient from falls or injury.
3. Turn the patient cautiously and handle extremities gently to avoid fractures.
4. Administer analgesia as prescribed.

STANDARDS OF CARE GUIDELINES
Endocrine Disorders

When caring for a patient with an endocrine disorder, remember that important metabolic functions may be disrupted, such as fluid and electrolyte balance, glucose and protein metabolism, energy production, calcium ionization, blood pressure control, thermoregulation, cardiac contractility, intestinal peristalsis, and ability of the body to react to stress.

- Monitor closely for electrolyte imbalance—sodium, potassium, chloride, bicarbonate—by checking laboratory test results, changes in ECG pattern, and signs of particular excess or deficit (see Chapter 21, p. 672).
- Check fingerstick or serum glucose periodically for patients on corticosteroids or for patients with adrenal disease; watch for signs of hyperglycemia (polydipsia, polyphagia, polyuria, blurred vision) or hypoglycemia (nervousness, tremor, difficulty concentrating, lethargy).
- Monitor for hypocalcemia after thyroidectomy, parathyroidectomy, or with hypoparathyroidism by checking serum calcium and phosphorous levels; watch for muscular twitching, anxiety, apprehension, spasms, and tetany. Check Chvostek's sign and Trousseau's sign.
- Monitor vital signs for heart rate, blood pressure, and presence of arrhythmias.
- Monitor temperature and respiratory rate changes in thyroid and adrenal disease.
- Monitor intake and output, weight changes, and edema.
- Maintain a calm, quiet environment and provide meticulous care to prevent infection or dehydration in patients with adrenal hypofunction or patients on corticosteroid replacement.
- After surgery, check for bleeding, signs of infection, changes in vital signs. Monitor respiratory status carefully after thyroidectomy.
- Report worsening condition or development of suspicious signs and symptoms promptly to prevent serious complications, such as myxedema coma, thyroid storm, hypocalcemic tetany, adrenal crisis.
- Provide support and explain care slowly and repeatedly because patient may have mental slowness, confusion, or lethargy because of his or her condition. Ask patient to restate important information to verify understanding.

This information should serve as a general guideline only. Each patient situation presents a unique set of clinical factors and requires nursing judgment to guide care, which may include additional or alternative measures and approaches.

---

5. Assess level of pain and the patient's response to analgesia.
6. Encourage the patient to participate in mild exercise gradually as symptoms subside.
7. Instruct and demonstrate correct body mechanics to reduce strain, backache, and injury.

Relieving Anxiety

1. Encourage patient to verbalize fears and feelings about upcoming surgery.
2. Explain tests and procedures to the patient.

3. Reassure the patient about skeletal recovery.
   a. Bone pain diminishes fairly quickly.
   b. Fractures are treated by orthopedic procedures.
4. Prepare patient for surgery as for thyroidectomy (see p. 816).

Monitoring for Hypocalcemia Postoperatively

1. Monitor ECG to detect changes secondary to hypercalcemia. (During moderate elevations of serum calcium, QT interval is shortened; with extreme hypercalcemia, widening of the T wave is seen.)
2. Monitor serum calcium level and evaluate for signs and symptoms of hypocalcemia and onset of tetany (see p. 817).
   a. Observe calcium levels—if well below normal, and if decline continues into the second week, the skeletal system is absorbing calcium and calcium administration may not be necessary.
   b. If some significant bone involvement was noted before surgery, as evidenced by elevated alkaline phosphatase level, elemental calcium may be ordered.

Patient Education and Health Promotion

1. Instruct the patient about calcium-reducing medications.
   a. Calcitonin (Cibacalcin) is given subcutaneously—teach proper technique.
   b. Etidronate disodium (Didronel)—calcium-rich foods should be avoided within 2 hours of dose; therapeutic response may take 1 to 3 months.
   c. Plicamycin (Mithramycin)—antineoplastic drug that may cause nausea, vomiting, and stomatitis; inspect oral mucosa regularly.
2. Teach signs and symptoms of tetany that the patient may experience postoperatively and should report to health care provider (numbness and tingling in extremities or around mouth).
3. Assist patient in identifying sources of information and support available in the community (see Table 24-2).

Outcome-Based Evaluation

- Output equals intake, normal skin turgor, moist mucous membranes
- No signs and symptoms of kidney stones or urinary tract infection; serum creatinine and BUN levels normal
- Reports less bone and joint pain; using correct body mechanics
- Verbalizes concerns and fears about surgery; appears less anxious
- ECG without QT, T wave changes; no numbness or tingling reported

Hypoparathyroidism

Hypoparathyroidism results from a deficiency of PTH and is characterized by hypocalcemia and neuromuscular hyperexcitability.

Pathophysiology and Etiology

1. The most common cause is accidental removal or destruction of parathyroid tissue or its blood supply during thyroidectomy or radical neck dissection for malignancy.
2. Decrease in gland function (idiopathic hypoparathyroidism); may be autoimmune or familial in origin.
3. Malignancy or metastasis from a cancer to the parathyroid glands.
4. Resistance to PTH action.
5. With inadequate PTH secretion, there is decreased resorption of calcium from the renal tubules, decreased absorption of calcium in the gastrointestinal tract, and decreased resorption of calcium from bone.
6. Blood calcium falls to a low level, causing symptoms of muscular hyperirritability, uncontrolled spasms, and hypocalcemic tetany.
7. In response to decreased serum calcium levels and lack of PTH, the serum phosphate level rises and phosphate excretion by the kidneys decreases.

Clinical Manifestations

1. Tetany—general muscular hypertonia; attempts at voluntary movement result in tremors and spasmodic or uncoordinated movements; fingers assume classic tetanic position.
   a. Chvostek's sign—a spasm of facial muscles that occurs when muscles or branches of facial nerve are tapped.
   b. Trousseau's sign—carpopedal spasm within 3 minutes after a blood pressure cuff is inflated 20 mm Hg above the patient's systolic pressure.
   c. Laryngeal spasm.
2. Severe anxiety and apprehension.
3. Renal colic is often present if the patient has history of stones; preexisting stones loosen and migrate into the ureter.

Diagnostic Evaluation

1. Phosphorus level in blood is elevated.
2. Decrease in serum calcium level to a low level (7.5 mg/100 mL or less).
3. PTH levels are low in most cases; may be normal or elevated in pseudohypoparathyroidism.

Management

IV Calcium Administration

1. A syringe and an ampule of a calcium solution (calcium chloride, calcium gluceptate, calcium gluconate) are to be kept at the bedside at all times.
2. Most rapidly effective calcium solution is ionized calcium chloride (10%).
3. For rapid use to relieve severe tetany, infusion carried out every 10 minutes.
   a. All IV calcium preparations are administered slowly. It is highly irritating, stings, and causes thrombosis; patient experiences unpleasant burning flush of skin and tongue.

 DRUG ALERT

Too-rapid calcium administration may cause cardiac arrest.

b. Typical doses are as follows:
  (i) Calcium chloride—500 mg to 1 g (5 to 10 mL) as indicated by serum calcium; administer at rate of less than 1 mL/min of 10% solution.
  (ii) Calcium gluconate—500 mg to 2 g (10 to 20 mL) at a rate of less than 0.5 mL/min of a 10% solution.
  (iii) Calcium gluceptate—1 to 2 g (5 to 10 mL) at a rate of less than 1 mL/min.
4. A slow drip of IV saline containing calcium gluconate is given until control of tetany is ensured; then intramuscular or oral administration of calcium is prescribed.
5. Later, vitamin D is added to calcium intake—increases absorption of calcium and also induces a high level of calcium in the bloodstream. Thiazide diuretics may also be added because of their calcium-retaining effect on the kidney; doses of calcium and vitamin D may be lowered.
6. Administration of IV calcium seems to cause rapid relief of anxiety.

Other Measures
1. Treat kidney stones.
2. Monitor patient for hypercalciuria. Periodic 24-hour urinary calcium determinations are recommended.
3. Monitor blood calcium level periodically; variations in vitamin D may affect calcium levels.

Complications
1. Acute complications related to hypocalcemia include seizures, tetany, and mental disorders, all of which can be reversed with calcium therapy.
2. If onset of hypocalcemia is acute, the major concerns are laryngeal spasm, acute airway obstruction, and cardiovascular failure.
3. Long-term complications include subcapsular cataracts, calcification of the basal ganglia, and papilledema, (caused by precipitation of calcium out of serum and deposition in tissue); shortening of the fingers and toes, and bowing of the long bones (caused by inadequate PTH and additional genetic abnormalities). Of these complications, only papilledema is reversible.

Nursing Assessment
1. Perform multisystem assessment, focusing on neuromuscular system.
2. Closely monitor patient's input and output and serum electrolytes, especially calcium level.
3. Assess anxiety.

Nursing Diagnosis
• Altered Nutrition: Less Than Body Requirements for calcium

Nursing Interventions
Maintaining Normal Serum Calcium Levels
1. Assess neuromuscular status frequently in patients with hypoparathyroidism and in those at risk for hypocalcemia (patients in the immediate postoperative period after thyroidectomy, parathyroidectomy, radical neck dissection).
2. Check for Trousseau's and Chvostek's signs and notify health care provider if tests results are positive.
3. Assess respiratory status frequently in acute hypocalcemia and postoperatively.
4. Monitor serum calcium and phosphorus levels.
5. Promote high-calcium diet if prescribed—dairy products, green, leafy vegetables.
6. Instruct the patient about signs and symptoms of hypo- and hypercalcemia that should be reported.
7. Use caution in administering other drugs to the patient with hypocalcemia.
  a. The hypocalcemic patient is sensitive to digoxin (Lanoxin); as hypocalcemia is reversed, the patient may rapidly develop digitalis toxicity.
  b. Cimetidine (Tagamet) interferes with normal parathyroid function, especially with renal failure, which increases the risk of hypocalcemia.

Patient Education and Health Maintenance
1. Explain to the patient and family the function of PTH and the roles of vitamin D and of calcium in maintaining good health.
2. Discuss the importance of each medication prescribed for the control of hypocalcemia including vitamin D, calcium, and thiazide diuretic.
  a. Take medications as prescribed.
  b. Do not substitute with over-the-counter preparations without the advice and supervision of the health care provider.
3. Provide the patient with a written list about hypercalcemia and hypocalcemia and advise the patient to contact the health care provider immediately should signs of either condition develop.
4. Advise the patient to wear a Medic Alert tag.
5. Explain the need for periodic medical follow-up for life.

Outcome-Based Evaluation
• Verbalizes understanding of diet and medications; calcium level within normal limits

DISORDERS OF THE ADRENAL GLANDS

The adrenal medulla, or inner portion of the gland, is not necessary to maintain life, but enables a person to cope with stress. It secretes two hormones:
• *Epinephrine* (adrenalin) acts on α and β receptors to increase contractility and excitability of heart muscle, leading to increased cardiac output; facilitates blood flow to muscles, brain, and viscera; enhances blood sugar by stimulating conversion of glycogen to glucose in liver; and inhibits smooth muscle contraction.

- *Norepinephrine* (noradrenaline) acts primarily on α receptors to increase peripheral vascular resistance, leading to increases in diastolic and systolic blood pressure.

    The adrenal cortex, or outer portion of the gland, is essential to life. It secretes adrenocortical hormones—synthesized from cholesterol.
- *Glucocorticoids* (cortisone and hydrocortisone) enhance protein catabolism and inhibit protein synthesis; antagonize action of insulin and increase blood sugar; increase synthesis of glucose by liver; influence defense mechanism of body and its reaction to stress; and influence emotional reaction.
- *Mineralocorticoids* (aldosterone and desoxycorticosterone) regulate reabsorption of sodium; regulate excretion of potassium by renal tubules.
- *Adrenosterones* (adrenal androgens) exert minimal effect on sex characteristics and function.

Primary Aldosteronism

Primary aldosteronism refers to excessive secretion of aldosterone by the adrenal cortex.

Pathophysiology and Etiology

1. Excessive secretion of aldosterone results in the conservation of sodium and excretion of potassium primarily in the renal tubules, but also in the sweat glands, salivary glands, and in the gastrointestinal tract.
2. Usually caused by a cortical adenoma; also caused by bilateral adrenal hyperplasia.
3. Secondary aldosteronism occurs in conjunction with heart failure, renal dysfunction, or cirrhosis of the liver.
4. Women comprise 70% of patients with aldosterone-secreting adenomas and the incidence of primary aldosteronism is four times higher among African Americans than among the general population.

Clinical Manifestations

1. Hypertension (1% to 2% of cases of hypertension are a result of primary aldosteronism, which usually can be treated successfully by surgical removal of the adenoma.)
2. A profound decline in blood levels of potassium (hypokalemia) and hydrogen ions (alkalosis) results in muscle weakness and inability of kidneys to acidify or concentrate urine, leading to excess volume of urine (polyuria).
3. A decline in hydrogen ions (alkalosis) results in tetany, paresthesia.
4. An elevation in blood sodium (hypernatremia) results in excessive thirst (polydipsia) and arterial hypertension.

Diagnostic Evaluation

1. Suspected in all hypertensive patients with spontaneous hypokalemia; also if hypokalemia develops concurrently with start of diuretics and remains after diuretics are discontinued.
2. Salt loading used as screening test—ingestion of at least 200 mEq/d (approximately 12 g salt) for 4 days does

not influence the serum potassium level without aldosteronism, but will cause a decrease of serum potassium to less than 3.5 mEq/L in a patient with aldosteronism.
3. CT scanning to determine and localize cortical adenoma.

Management

1. Removal of adrenal tumor—unilateral adrenalectomy.
2. Management of underlying cause of secondary aldosteronism.
3. Spironolactone (Aldactone) to treat both hypertension and potassium-depleted stages; therapy is needed 4 to 6 weeks before the full effect on blood pressure is seen.
    a. Side effects include reduced testosterone in men (decreased libido, impotence, gynecomastia) and gastrointestinal discomfort.
    b. Amiloride (Midamor) may be used instead in sexually active men or in cases of gastrointestinal intolerance.
    c. Sodium restriction is necessary—no saline infusions, low-sodium diet.
    d. Potassium supplementation is usually necessary, based on severity of deficit.
4. Addition of antihypertensive agent—thiazide diuretic such as triamterene (Dyrenium).

Complications

Long-term effects of untreated hypertension—stroke, renal failure, congestive heart failure.

Nursing Assessment

1. Obtain history of symptoms such as muscle weakness, paresthesia, thirst, and polyuria.
2. Perform multisystem physical examination.
3. Evaluate blood pressure.

Nursing Diagnosis

- Fluid Volume Excess related to sodium retention

Nursing Interventions

See Care of the Patient Undergoing Adrenalectomy, p. 817.

Maintaining Normal Fluid and Sodium Balance

1. Monitor fluid intake and output, daily weights, ECG changes for hypokalemia.
2. Teach low-sodium diet, administration of potassium supplements, as ordered; evaluate serum sodium and potassium results.
3. Monitor blood pressure; administer or teach self-administration of antihypertensives as ordered.
4. Assess for dependent edema; encourage activity, frequent repositioning, and elevation of feet periodically.

Patient Education and Health Maintenance

1. Instruct patient regarding the nature of illness, the necessary treatment, and the need for continued medical care after discharge.

2. Instruct patient on the importance of following prescribed medical treatments.
   a. For medical management, patient must remain on spironolactone (Aldactone) for life.
   b. Patient should report significant side effects that interfere with sexual performance and quality of life.
   c. Glucocorticoid administration may be temporary after subtotal or unilateral adrenalectomy, chronic for bilateral adrenalectomy; dose may need to be increased during times of illness or stress.
3. Teach patient and family members how to take blood pressure readings, if indicated.

Outcome-Based Evaluation

• Intake equals urine output, daily weight stable

■ Cushing's Syndrome

Cushing's syndrome is a condition in which the plasma cortisol levels are elevated, causing signs and symptoms of hypercortisolism.

Pathophysiology and Etiology

1. Occurs 10 times more frequently in women than in men.
2. The normal feedback mechanisms that control adrenocortical function are ineffective, resulting in secretion of adrenal cortical hormones despite adequate amounts of these hormones in the circulation.
3. The manifestations of Cushing's syndrome are the result of excess hormones (glucocorticoids, mineralocorticoids, and adrenal androgens).
4. Excess of one hormone or all the hormones can occur; the predominant hormone secreted in excess (usually glucocorticoids) determines the predominant symptoms.
5. Pituitary Cushing's syndrome (Cushing's disease)—hyperplasia of both adrenal glands caused by overstimulation of the adrenal cortex by ACTH, usually from a pituitary adenoma or hyperplasia.
   a. Most common cause of Cushing's syndrome.
   b. Affects mostly women between 20 and 40 years of age.
6. Adrenal Cushing's syndrome.
   a. Associated with tumors of the adrenal cortex—adenoma or carcinoma.
7. Ectopic.
   a. Results from autonomous ACTH secretion by extrapituitary neoplasms.
   b. Tumors elsewhere in body (such as lung) producing excess ACTH.
8. Iatrogenic Cushing's syndrome caused by exogenous glucocorticoid administration.

Clinical Manifestations

Manifestations Caused by Excess Glucocorticoids
1. Weight gain/obesity (Figure 24-3)
2. Heavy trunk; thin extremities.
3. "Buffalo hump" (fat pad) in neck and supraclavicular area.

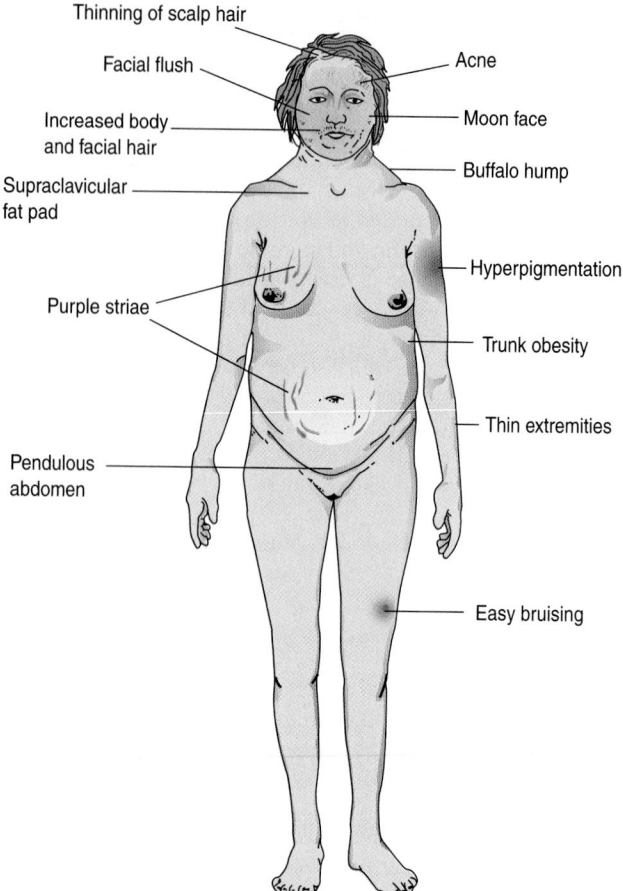

FIGURE 24-3 Clinical manifestations of Cushing's syndrome.

4. Rounded face (moon face); plethoric, oily.
5. Fragile and thin skin, striae and ecchymosis, acne.
6. Muscles wasted because of excessive catabolism.
7. Osteoporosis—characteristic kyphosis, backache.
8. Mental disturbances—mood changes, psychosis.
9. Increased susceptibility to infections.

Manifestations Caused by Excess Mineralocorticoids
1. Hypertension.
2. Hypernatremia, hypokalemia.
3. Weight gain.
4. Expanded blood volume.
5. Edema.

Manifestations Caused by Excess Androgens
1. Women experience virilism (masculinization).
   a. Hirsutism—excessive growth of hair on the face and midline of trunk.
   b. Breasts—atrophy.
   c. Clitoris—enlargement.
   d. Voice—masculine.
   e. Loss of libido.

2. If exposed in utero—possible hermaphrodite.
3. Males—loss of libido.

Diagnostic Evaluation

1. Excessive plasma cortisol levels.
2. An increase in blood glucose levels and glucose intolerance.
3. Decreased serum potassium level.
4. Reduced eosinophils.
5. Elevated urinary 17-hydroxycorticoids and 17-ketogenic steroids.
6. Elevation of plasma ACTH in patients with pituitary tumors.
7. Low plasma ACTH levels with adrenal tumor.
8. Loss of diurnal variation of cortisol secretion.
9. X-rays of the skull detect erosion of the sella turcica by a pituitary tumor.
10. Overnight DST, possibly with cortisol urinary excretion measurement.
    a. Unsuppressed cortisol level in Cushing's syndrome caused by adrenal tumors.
    b. Suppressed cortisol level in Cushing's disease caused by pituitary tumor.
11. CT scan and ultrasonography detect location of tumor.

Management

Surgical and Radiation

Tumor (adrenal or pituitary) is removed or treated with irradiation.

1. The most recent development in the management of pituitary Cushing's syndrome in adults is transsphenoidal adenomectomy or hypophysectomy (pituitary removal) (see p. 818).
2. Transfrontal craniotomy may be necessary when pituitary tumor has enlarged beyond sella turcica (see p. 817).
3. Hyperplasia of adrenals—bilateral adrenalectomy.

Replacement Therapy Postoperatively

1. Adrenalectomy patients require a lifelong replacement therapy with the following:
   a. A glucocorticoid—cortisone (Cortef).
   b. A mineralocorticoid—fludrocortisone (Florinef).
2. After pituitary irradiation or hypophysectomy, patient may require adrenal replacement plus thyroid, posterior pituitary, and gonadal replacement therapy.
3. After transsphenoidal adenomectomy, patient requires hydrocortisone replacement therapy for periods of 12 to 18 months and additional hormones if excessive loss of pituitary function has occurred.
4. Protein anabolic steroids may be given to facilitate protein replacement; potassium replacement is usually required.

Medical Treatment

If patients cannot undergo surgery, cortisol synthesis-inhibiting medications may be used.

1. Mitotane, an agent toxic to the adrenal cortex (DDT derivative)—known as medical adrenalectomy. Nausea, vomiting, diarrhea, somnolence, and depression may occur with use of this drug.
2. Metyrapone (Metopirone) to control steroid hypersecretion in patients who do not respond to mitotane therapy.
3. Aminoglutethimide (Cytadren) blocks cholesterol conversion to pregnenolone, effectively blocking cortisol production. Side effects include gastrointestinal disturbances, somnolence, and skin rashes.

Complications

Possibility of recurrence in patients with adrenal carcinoma.

Nursing Assessment

1. Observe patient for signs and symptoms of Cushing's disease.
2. Perform multisystem physical examination.
3. Monitor input and output, daily weights, and serum electrolytes.

Nursing Diagnoses

- Impaired Skin Integrity related to altered healing, thin and fragile skin, and edema
- Self-Care Deficit related to muscle wasting, osteoporosis, weakness, and fatigue
- Self-Esteem Disturbance related to altered physical appearance and emotional instability
- Anxiety related to surgery
- Risk for Injury related to surgical procedure

Nursing Interventions

Maintaining Skin Integrity

1. Assess skin frequently to detect reddened areas, breakdown or tearing of skin, excoriation, infection, or edema.
2. Handle skin and extremities gently to prevent trauma; protect from falls by use of side rails.
3. Avoid use of adhesive tape to reduce risk of trauma to skin on its removal.
4. Encourage the patient to turn in bed frequently or to ambulate to reduce pressure on bony prominences and areas of edema.
5. Use meticulous skin care to reduce injury and breakdown.
6. Provide foods low in sodium to minimize edema formation.
7. Assess intake and output and daily weights to evaluate fluid retention.

Encouraging Active Participation in Self-Care

1. Assist the patient with ambulation and hygiene when weak and fatigued.
2. Assist the patient in planning schedule to permit exercise and rest.
3. Encourage the patient to rest when fatigued.
4. Encourage gradual resumption of activities as the patient gains strength.
5. Identify for the patient the signs and symptoms indicating excessive exertion.

6. Instruct the patient in correct body mechanics to avoid pain or injury during activities.
7. Use assistive devices during ambulation to prevent falls and fractures.
8. Encourage foods high in potassium (bananas, orange juice, tomatoes), and administer potassium supplement as prescribed to counteract weakness related to hypokalemia.

Increasing Self-Esteem

1. Encourage the patient to verbalize concerns about illness, changes in appearance, and altered role functions.
2. Identify situations that are disturbing to the patient and explore with patient ways to avoid or modify those situations.
3. Be alert for evidence of depression; in some instances this has progressed to suicide; alert health care provider of mood changes, sleep disturbance, change in activity level, change in appetite, or loss of interest in visitors or other experiences.
4. Refer for counseling, if indicated.
5. Explain to the patient who has benign adenoma or hyperplasia that, with proper treatment, evidence of masculinization can be reversed.

Reducing Anxiety

1. Answer questions about surgery and encourage more thorough discussion with health care provider if patient is not well informed.
2. Describe nursing care to expect in postoperative period.
3. Prepare the patient for abdominal surgery (see p. 586) or hypophysectomy (see p. 453) as indicated.

Providing Postoperative Care

1. Provide routine postoperative care for patient with abdominal surgery (see p. 586) or hypophysectomy (see p. 453).
2. Monitor closely for infection because glucocorticoid administration interferes with immune function; maintain aseptic technique, clean environment, and good handwashing.
3. Monitor thyroid function tests and provide hormone replacement therapy as ordered after hypophysectomy.
4. Monitor fluid intake and output and urine specific gravity to detect DI caused by ADH deficiency after hypophysectomy.

Patient Education and Health Maintenance

1. Instruct patient on lifetime hormone replacement therapy and the need to follow up at regular intervals to determine if dosage is appropriate or to detect side effects.
2. Instruct patient in proper skin care and in the prompt reporting of trauma or infection for medical treatment.
3. Teach patient to monitor urine or blood glucose or to report for blood glucose tests as directed to detect hyperglycemia.
4. Help the patient prevent hyperglycemia and obesity by teaching a low-calorie, low-concentrated carbohydrate and fat diet and to increase activity as tolerated.

5. Encourage diet high in calcium (dairy products, broccoli) and weight-bearing activity to prevent osteoporosis caused by glucocorticoid replacement.
6. Assist patient in identifying sources of information and support available in the community (see Table 24-2).

Outcome-Based Evaluation

- Skin intact without evidence of breakdown, excoriation, infection, or trauma
- Participates safely in activities of daily living
- Verbalizes concerns about appearance, interacts well with visitors
- Verbalizes understanding of surgery
- Vital signs stable, pain controlled, no signs of infection

■ Adrenocortical Insufficiency

Adrenocortical insufficiency occurs with inadequate secretion of the hormones of the adrenal cortex, primarily the glucocorticoids and mineralocorticoids.

Pathophysiology and Etiology

1. Primary adrenocortical insufficiency (Addison's disease)—destruction and subsequent hypofunction of the adrenal cortex, usually caused by autoimmune process.
2. Secondary adrenocortical insufficiency—ACTH deficiency from pituitary disease or suppression of hypothalamic-pituitary axis by corticosteroid treatment for nonendocrine disorders causes atrophy of adrenal cortex.
3. Inadequate aldosterone produces disturbances of sodium, potassium, and water metabolism.
4. Cortisol deficiency produces abnormal fat, protein, and carbohydrate metabolism; no cortisol during a period of stress can precipitate Addisonian crisis, an exaggerated state of adrenal cortical insufficiency, and can lead to death.

Clinical Manifestations

1. Hyponatremia and hyperkalemia.
2. Water loss, dehydration, and hypovolemia.
3. Muscular weakness, fatigue, weight loss.
4. Gastrointestinal problems—anorexia, nausea, vomiting, diarrhea, constipation, abdominal pain.
5. Hypotension, hypoglycemia, low basal metabolic rate (BMR), increased insulin sensitivity.
6. Mental changes—depression, irritability, anxiety, apprehension caused by hypoglycemia and hypovolemia.
7. Normal responses to stress lacking.
8. Hyperpigmentation.

Diagnostic Evaluation

1. Blood chemistry—decreased glucose, decreased sodium, increased potassium.
2. Increased lymphocytes on complete blood count.
3. Low fasting plasma cortisol levels; low aldosterone levels.

4. 24-hour urine studies—decreased 17-ketosteroids, 17-hydroxycorticoids, and 17-ketogenic steroids; may be decreased.
5. ACTH stimulation test—no rise in plasma cortisol and urinary 17-ketosteroids.

Management

1. Restoration of normal fluid and electrolyte balance: high-sodium, low-potassium diet and fluids.
2. Treatment of glucocorticoid deficiency with agent such as hydrocortisone (Cortef) or prednisone (Orasone). Patients with chronic obstructive pulmonary disease and congestive heart failure may require preparations with low mineralocorticoid activity, such as methylprednisolone (Solu-Medrol), to prevent fluid retention.
3. Mineralocorticoid deficiency is treated with fludrocortisone (Florinef).

NURSING ALERT

Overtreatment may be manifested by hypertension, edema from sodium and water retention, and weakness caused by potassium loss.

4. Cardiovascular support if indicated.
5. Immediate treatment if Addisonian (adrenal) crisis or circulatory collapse is imminent:
   a. IV sodium chloride solution to replace sodium ions.
   b. Hydrocortisone (Cortef).
   c. Injection of circulatory stimulants, such as atropine sulfate (Atropine), calcium chloride (Calcium), epinephrine (Adrenalin).
6. Diagnosis and treatment of underlying cause of adrenocortical insufficiency or addisonian crisis (eg, antibiotic therapy to treat infection if this is a factor in crisis).

Complications

1. Adrenal crisis—hypotension, nausea, vomiting, weakness, lethargy, and possibly coma.
2. May be precipitated by physiologic stress, such as surgery, infection, trauma, dehydration.

Nursing Assessment

1. Obtain recent or past history of corticosteroid therapy, including length of treatment, dosage, and compliance.
2. Review history for sources of stress, such as surgical procedures, infection, or development of other illness.
3. Perform thorough physical examination for manifestations of adrenocortical insufficiency or contributing factors.

Nursing Diagnoses

• Fluid Volume Deficit related to renal losses of sodium and water
• Risk for Injury related to ineffective stress response
• Activity Intolerance related to decreased cortisol production and fatigue

Nursing Interventions

Achieving Normal Fluid and Electrolyte Balance

1. Assess fluid intake and output and serial daily weights.
2. Monitor vital signs frequently; a drop in blood pressure may suggest an impending crisis.
3. Monitor results of serum sodium and potassium.
4. Assess skin turgor and mucous membranes for dehydration.
5. Encourage diet high in sodium and fluid content; administer or teach self-administration of potassium supplements, if prescribed.
6. Administer or teach self-administration of prescribed glucocorticoids and mineralocorticoids; document response.
7. Administer IV infusions of sodium, water, and glucose as indicated.

Protecting Well-Being

1. Minimize stressful situations.
2. Protect the patient from infection.
   a. Control the patient's contacts so that infectious organisms are not transmitted.
   b. Protect the patient from drafts, dampness, exposure to cold.
   c. Prevent overexertion.
   d. Use meticulous handwashing and asepsis.
3. Assess comfort and emotional status of the patient.
   a. Control the temperature of the room to avoid sharp deviations in the patient's temperature.
   b. Maintain a quiet, peaceful environment; avoid loud talking and noisy radios.
4. Observe and report early signs of Addisonian crisis (sudden drop in blood pressure, nausea and vomiting, fever).

Increasing Activity Tolerance

1. Assist the patient with activities of daily living.
2. Provide for periods of rest and activity to avoid overexertion.
3. Provide for high-calorie, high-protein diet.

Patient Education and Health Maintenance

1. Instruct the patient about the necessity for long-term therapy for adrenocortical insufficiency and medical follow-up visits.
   a. Inform the patient that therapy must be continued throughout the lifespan.
   b. Emphasize the importance of taking more hormones when under stress.
   c. Suggest that the patient carry an identification card that indicates the type of medication being taken and health care provider's telephone number.
2. Instruct the patient about manifestations of excessive use of medications and reportable symptoms.
3. Identify actions to take to avoid factors that may precipitate addisonian crisis (infection, extremes of temperature, trauma).
4. Assist patient in identifying sources of information and support available in the community (see Table 24-2).

Outcome-Based Evaluation
- Normal skin turgor, moist mucous membranes, stable vital signs
- No signs of infection or stress
- Completes daily activities with minimal assistance

Pheochromocytoma

Pheochromocytoma is a catecholamine-secreting neoplasm associated with hyperfunction of the adrenal medulla. It may appear wherever chromaffin cells are located; however, most are found in the adrenal medulla.

Pathophysiology and Etiology

1. Pheochromocytoma can occur at any age, but is most common between the ages of 30 and 60; it is uncommon in people older than age 65.
2. Most pheochromocytoma tumors are benign; 10% are malignant with metastasis.
3. Tumors located in the adrenal medulla produce both increased epinephrine and norepinephrine; those located outside the adrenal gland tend to produce epinephrine only.
4. May occur as component of multiple endocrine neoplasia (MEN) II, an autosomal-dominant syndrome characterized by pheochromocytoma, thyroid carcinoma, hyperparathyroidism, and Cushing's syndrome with excess ACTH.

Clinical Manifestations

1. Variation in signs and symptoms depends on the predominance of norepinephrine or epinephrine secretion and on whether secretion is continuous or intermittent.
2. Excess secretion of norepinephrine and epinephrine produces hypertension, hypermetabolism, and hyperglycemia.
3. Hypertension may be paroxysmal (intermittent) or persistent (chronic).
   a. Chronic form mimics essential hypertension; however, antihypertensives are not effective.
   b. Headaches and visual disturbances are common.
4. The hypermetabolic and hyperglycemic effects produce excessive perspiration, tremor, pallor or face flushing, nervousness, elevated blood glucose levels, polyuria, nausea, vomiting, diarrhea, abdominal pain, and paresthesia.
5. Emotional changes, including psychotic behavior, may occur.
6. Symptoms may be triggered by allergic reactions, physical exertion, emotional upset, or may occur without identifiable stimulus.

Diagnostic Evaluation

1. VMA and metanephrine (metabolites of epinephrine and norepinephrine) are elevated in 24-hour urine sample.
2. Epinephrine and norepinephrine in urine and blood are elevated while patient is symptomatic.
3. CT scan and magnetic resonance imaging (MRI) of the adrenal glands or of the entire abdomen are done to identify tumor.
4. Clonidine suppression test is used to distinguish essential hypertension from pheochromocytoma.

Management
Medical Control of Blood Pressure and Preparation for Surgery

1. α-Adrenergic blocking agents, such as phentolamine (Regitine) or phenoxybenzamine HCl (Dibenzyline), inhibit the effects of catecholamines on blood pressure.
   a. Effective control of blood pressure and blood volume may take 1 or 2 weeks.
   b. Surgery is delayed until blood pressure is controlled and blood volume has been expanded.
2. Catecholamine synthesis inhibitors, such as metyrosine (Demser), may be used preoperatively or for long-term management of inoperable tumors.
   a. Side effects include sedation and crystalluria.

Surgery
Unilateral or bilateral adrenalectomy or other tumor removal.

Complications
Metastasis of tumor.

Nursing Assessment

1. Obtain history of signs and symptoms patient has been experiencing.
2. Assess for predisposing factors that may be triggering signs and symptoms (ie, physical exertion, emotional upset, allergies).
3. Perform thorough physical examination to determine effects of hypertension.

Nursing Diagnoses

- Anxiety related to the systemic effects of epinephrine and norepinephrine
- Altered Tissue Perfusion related to hypotension during the postoperative period

Nursing Interventions
Reducing Anxiety

1. Remain with the patient during acute episodes of hypertension.
2. Ensure bed rest and elevate the head of bed 45 degrees during severe hypertension.
3. Carry out tasks and procedures in calm, unhurried manner when with the patient.
4. Instruct the patient about use of relaxation exercises.
5. Reduce environmental stressors by providing calm, quiet environment. Restrict visitors.
6. Eliminate stimulants (coffee, tea, cola) from the diet.
7. Reduce events that precipitate episodes of severe hypertension—palpation of the tumor, physical exertion, emotional upset.

8. Administer sedatives as prescribed to promote relaxation and rest.
9. Monitor for orthostatic hypotension after administration of phentolamine (Regitine).
10. Encourage oral fluids and maintain IV infusion preoperatively to ensure adequate volume expansion going into surgery.

Maintaining Tissue Perfusion Postoperatively

1. Monitor vital signs, ECG, arterial blood pressure, neurologic status, and urine output closely postoperatively.
2. Assess for and report complications of hypertension, hypotension, and hyperglycemia.
3. Maintain adequate hydration with IV infusion to prevent hypotension. (Because reduction of catecholamines immediately postoperatively causes vasodilation and enlargement of vascular space, hypotension may occur.)
4. Monitor intake and output and laboratory results for BUN, creatinine, and glucose.

Patient Education and Health Maintenance

1. Instruct the patient how and when to take medications. Warn patients who take metyrosine (Demser) of sedation and need to avoid taking other CNS depressants and participating in activities that require alertness; need to increase fluid intake to at least 2,000 mL/day to prevent kidney stones.
2. Inform patient regarding the need for continued follow-up for:
   a. Recurrence of pheochromocytoma.
   b. Assessment of any residual renal or cardiovascular injury related to preoperative hypertension.
   c. Documentation that catecholamines levels are normal 1 to 3 months postoperatively (by 24-hour urine test).
3. Help patient identify sources of information and support available in the community (see Table 24-2).

Outcome-Based Evaluation

- Reports less anxiety during hypertensive episodes
- Blood pressure stable, adequate urine output

DISORDERS OF THE PITUITARY GLAND

The pituitary gland (hypophysis) exerts prime control over the body's hormonal functions. It is located in the sella turcica at the base of the brain. Its function is regulated by the hypothalamus. The pituitary consists of two parts that are structurally and functionally separate, the anterior pituitary and the posterior pituitary. Hypothalamic control of the anterior pituitary is mediated by releasing factors secreted by the hypothalamus; the posterior pituitary is regulated through direct neural stimulation. Hormones of the pituitary gland include:

Hormones	Target Tissue
Anterior Pituitary	
Growth hormone (GH)	Multiple sites
Thyroid stimulating hormone (TSH)	Thyroid gland
Adrenocorticotropic hormone (ACTH)	Adrenal glands
Prolactin	Breasts
Luteinizing hormone (LH)	Ovaries, testes
Follicle stimulating hormone (FSH)	Ovaries, testes
Melanocyte stimulating hormone (MSH)	Melanocytes (skin)
Posterior Pituitary	
Oxytocin	Uterus, breasts
Antidiuretic hormone (ADH)	Kidneys

■ Diabetes Insipidus

Diabetes insipidus (DI) is a disorder of water metabolism caused by deficiency of ADH, also called vasopressin, secreted by the posterior pituitary or by inability of the kidneys to respond to ADH (nephrogenic DI).

Pathophysiology and Etiology

1. Primary: idiopathic.
2. Secondary: head trauma, neurosurgery, tumors (intracranial or metastatic), vascular disease (aneurysms, infarct), infection (meningitis, encephalitis).
3. Nephrogenic DI: longstanding renal disease, hypokalemia, some medications.
4. Deficiency of ADH may be partial or complete.
5. DI may be transient or permanent.

Clinical Manifestations

1. Marked polyuria—daily output of 5 to 20 liters of dilute urine; appearance of urine like that of water, with a specific gravity of 1.000 to 1.005, corresponding to a urine osmolality of 50 to 200 mOsm/kg.
2. Polydipsia (intense thirst)—drinks 4 to 40 liters of fluid daily; has craving for cold water.
3. High serum osmolality (above 295 mOsm) and high serum sodium level (greater than 145 mEq/L).

Diagnostic Evaluation

1. Serum osmolality—high; urine osmolality—low
2. Water deprivation test determines central and nephrogenic DI.
3. Measurements of serum and urine ADH—decreased to absent.

Management

1. Administration of ADH or its derivative.
   a. Vasopressin (Pitressin)—administered IM.
      (i) Effective for 24 to 72 hours.
      (ii) Vial should be warmed and shaken vigorously before administering, to ensure uniform dispersion, because active component settles at bottom of vial.

b. Lypressin (Diapid nasal spray)—absorbed through nasal mucosa.
  (i) Duration of action 4 to 6 hours.
  (ii) May cause chronic nasal irritation.
c. Desmopressin acetate (DDAVP)—vasopressin derivative administered into the nose through a soft, flexible nasal tube.
  (i) Duration of action 12 to 24 hours.
  (ii) For patients who have some residual hypothalamic ADH (determined by low levels of circulating ADH).
d. Chlorpropamide (Diabinese)—potentiates action of vasopressin on renal-concentrating mechanism.
e. Clofibrate (Atromid-S)—probably acts by augmenting ADH secretion from posterior pituitary.
f. Carbamazepine (Tegretol)—potentiates action of endogenous vasopressin.
2. For patients with nephrogenic DI—chlorpropamide (Diabinese) or thiazide diuretics may be of value. Reversible by discontinuing causative medication if cause is drug related.

Complications

1. If untreated, may result in death.
2. Overtreatment of desmopressin (DDAVP) may cause hyponatremia and water intoxication.

> **GERONTOLOGIC ALERT**
>
> Older patients are more sensitive to the effects of desmopressin (DDAVP), so ensure that overdosage does not occur and watch for early signs of hyponatremia and water intoxication—drowsiness, confusion, headache, anuria, weight gain—to prevent seizures, coma, and death.

Nursing Assessment

1. Obtain complete health history to determine possible cause of DI.
2. Assess hydration status.

Nursing Diagnosis

• Risk for Fluid Volume Deficit related to disease process

Nursing Interventions

Maintaining Adequate Fluid Volume
1. Measure fluid intake and output accurately.
2. Obtain daily weights.
3. Monitor hemodynamic status, as indicated, via frequent blood pressure, heart rate, central venous pressure, and other measurements.
4. Provide patient with ample water to drink and administer IV fluids as indicated.
5. Monitor results of serum and urine osmolality and serum sodium tests.

6. Administer or teach self-administration of medication as prescribed and document patient response.

Patient Education and Health Maintenance

1. Inform the patient that metabolic status must be monitored on a long-term basis because the severity of DI changes from time to time.
2. Advise patient to avoid limiting fluids to decrease urinary output; thirst is a protective function.
3. Advise patient to wear a Medic Alert tag stating that the wearer has DI.
4. Teach patient to be alert for signs of dehydration—decreased weight, decreased urine output, increased thirst, dry skin and mucous membranes; and overhydration—increased weight and edema and report these to the health care provider.
5. Tell the patient to consider eliminating coffee and tea from diet—may have an exaggerated diuretic effect.
6. Give written instruction on vasopressin administration. Have the patient demonstrate intranasal and injection technique.

Outcome-Based Evaluation

• Fluid intake equals output, weight stable

■ Pituitary Tumors

Pituitary tumors represent various cell types. Symptoms reflect tumor effects on target tissues or on local structures surrounding the pituitary gland.

Pathophysiology and Etiology

1. The cause of pituitary tumors is unknown.
2. Typically, pituitary tumors are characterized by size and by what hormones, if any, are secreted.
  a. Size.
    (i) Microadenoma—less than 10 mm wide.
    (ii) Macroadenoma—greater that 10 mm wide.
  b. Functional status.
    (i) Hormone secreting—exaggerated hormone activity; may secrete multiple hormones.
    (ii) Nonsecreting—usually diminished hormone activity.
3. Malignancy in pituitary tumors is rare.

Clinical Manifestations

1. "Mass effects"—effects of tumor on surrounding structures.
  a. Headache.
  b. Nausea and vomiting (in some cases).
  c. Impairment of cranial nerves II, III, IV, and VI on testing because of bilateral hemianopsia that results from pressure on the optic chiasm.
  d. Visual disturbances, such as visual field defects and diplopia.
2. Endocrine effects—effects of hormone imbalances caused by tumor (Table 24-3).

TABLE 24-3 Clinical Manifestations Associated With Hormone Effects of Pituitary Tumors

Hormone	Hyperpituitarism (increased secretion)	Hypopituitarism (diminished secretion)
Growth hormone (GH)	Gigantism (child) Acromegaly (adult)	Shortness of stature (child) Silent (adult)
Prolactin	Infertility and galactorrhea (female)	Postpartum lactation failure
Adrenocorticotropic hormone (ACTH)	Cushing's disease	Adrenocortical insufficiency
Thyroid-stimulating hormone (TSH)	Hyperthyroidism	Hypothyroidism
Luteinizing hormone (LH) and follicle-stimulating hormone (FSH)	Gonadal dysfunction	Hypogonadism

Diagnostic Evaluation

1. Skull films (usually normal).
2. CT scan usually enhanced with contrast media, MRI shows mass.
3. Serum hormone levels to identify suspected abnormalities based on clinical evaluation.
4. Provocative testing to detect hormone secretion abnormalities of the pituitary, such as glucose tolerance test and DST.

Management

Hypophysectomy Removal of Pituitary

1. Frontal craniotomy—uncommon approach except where tumor occupies broad area (see p. 453).
2. Transsphenoidal hypophysectomy—direct approach through the sinus and nasal cavity to sella turcica (see p. 818).

Other Methods of Pituitary Ablation

1. Cryogenic destruction or stereotaxic radiofrequency coagulation.
2. Radiation therapy.
3. Drug therapy.
   a. Bromocriptine (Parlodel) for prolactinomas and, in some instances, GH-secreting tumors.
   b. Hormone replacement therapy for hypopituitarism.

Complications

1. Hypothyroidism and adrenocortical insufficiency after ablation, requiring hormone replacement.
2. Menstruation ceases and infertility occurs almost always after total or nearly total ablation.
3. Transient or permanent DI after surgery.
4. Without treatment—death or severe disability caused by stroke, blindness, or imbalances of ACTH, TSH, or ADH.

Nursing Assessment

1. Obtain history of signs and symptoms.
2. Perform thorough neurologic examination and general physical examination to identify signs of hormone deficiency or excess.

Nursing Diagnoses

- Anxiety related to ablation treatment
- Ineffective Management of Therapeutic Regimen postoperatively

Nursing Interventions

See Care of the Patient Undergoing Transsphenoidal Hypophysectomy, p. 818.

Reducing Anxiety

1. Provide emotional support through the diagnostic process and answer questions about treatment options.
2. Prepare patient for surgery or other treatment by describing nursing care thoroughly.
3. Stress likelihood of positive outcome with ablation therapy.

Promoting Management of the Therapeutic Regimen

1. Teach patient the nature of hormonal deficiencies after treatment and the purpose of replacement therapy.
2. Instruct the patient in the early signs and symptoms of cortisol or thyroid hormone deficiency or excess and the need to report them.
3. Describe and demonstrate the correct method of administering prescribed medications.
4. Encourage patient in assuming active role in self-care through seeking information and problem-solving.

Patient Education and Health Maintenance

1. Advise patient on temporary limitations in activities.
2. Teach patient the need for frequent initial follow-up visits and lifelong medical management when on hormonal therapy.
3. If applicable, advise patient on the need for postsurgery radiation therapy and periodic follow-up MRI and visual field testing.
4. Teach patient to notify health care provider if signs of thyroid or cortisol imbalance become evident.
5. Advise patient to wear Medic Alert tag.
6. Help patient identify sources of information and support available in the community (see Table 24-2).

Outcome-Based Evaluation

- States rationale for treatment, asks appropriate questions
- Demonstrates correct medication administration

SELECTED REFERENCES

Allahabadia, A., et al. (2000). Age and gender predict the outcome of treatment for Graves' hyperthyroidism. *Journal of Clinical Endocrinology and Metabolism, 85*(3), 1038–1042.

Baker, J.T. (1997). Adrenal disorders: A primary care approach. *Lippincott's Primary Care Practice 1*(5), 527–536.

Black, E.R., Bordley, D.R., Tape, T.G., & Panzer, R.J. (Eds.) (1999). *Diagnostic strategies for common medical problems* (2nd ed.). Philadelphia: American College of Physicians.

Chabon, S.L. (1997). Identification and evaluation of thyroid nodules. *Lippincott's Primary Care Practice 1*(5), 499–506.

Chipps, E. (1992). Transphenoidal surgery for pituitary tumors, *Critical Care Nurse, 12*, 30.

Consensus Development Panel. (1991). Diagnosis and management of assymptomatic primary hyperparathyroidism consensus conference statement. *Annals of Internal Medicine, 114*, 593.

Edwards, C.R.W. (1995). Primary mineralocorticoid excess syndromes. In DeGroot L.J. et al. (Eds.), *Endocrinology* (3rd ed.). Philadelphia: Saunders.

Elasy, T.A. & Skelly, A.H. (1997). Case study: Patient with hyperparathyroidism. *Lippincott's Primary Care Practice, 1*(5), 563–566.

Elkin, M.K., Perry, A.G., Potter, P.A. (Eds.) (2000). *Nursing interventions and clinical skills* (2nd ed.). St. Louis: Mosby.

Elliott, B. (2000). Diagnosing and treating hypothyroidism. *The Nurse Practitioner, 25*(3), 92–105.

Fishbach, F. (1996). *A manual of laboratory and diagnostic tests.* (5th ed.). Philadelphia: Lippincott-Raven.

Fitzpatrick, L.A. & Arnold, A. (1995). Hypoparathyroidism. In DeGroot L.J. et al. (Eds.), *Endocrinology* (3rd ed.). Philadelphia: Saunders.

Gilkison, C.R. (1997). Thyrotoxicosis: Recognition and management. *Lippincott's Primary Care Practice, 1*(5), 485–498.

Golub, M.D. & Tuck, M.L. (1992). Diagnostic and therapeutic strategies in pheochromocytoma. *Endocrinologist, 2*, 101.

Greenspan F.S., & Strewler, G.J. (Eds.). (1997). *Basic and clinical endocrinology* (5th ed.). Stamford, CT: Appleton & Lange.

Growth Hormone Research Society Workshop Committee. (1998). Consensus guidelines for the diagnosis and treatment of adults with growth hormone deficiency. *Journal of Clinical Endocrinology and Metabolism 83*(2), 379–381.

Hak, A.E., Pols, H.A.P., Visser, T.J., et al. (2000). Subclinical hypothyroidism is an independent risk factor for atherosclerosis and myocardial infarction in elderly women; the Rotterdam Study. *Annals of Internal Medicine, 132*(3)270–278.

Loriaux, D.L. (1995). Tests of adrenocortical function. In Becker, K.L. et al. (Eds.), *Principles and practice of endocrinology and metabolism* (2nd ed.). Philadelphia: Lippincott.

Loriaux, D.L. (1995). Adrenocortical insufficiency. In Becker, K.L. et al. (Eds.), *Principles and practice of endocrinology and metabolism* (2nd ed.). Philadelphia: Lippincott.

Mazzaferri, E.L. (1995). Thyroid cancer. In Becker K.L. et al. (Eds.), *Principles and practice of endocrinology and metabolism* (2nd ed.). Philadelphia: Lippincott.

Orth, D.N. (1995). Cushing's syndrome. *New England Journal of Medicine, 332*(12), 791–803.

Singer, P.A., Cooper, D.S., Levy, E.G., et al. (1995). Treatment guidelines for patients with hyperthyroidism and hypothyroidism. *Journal of the American Medical Association, 273*(10), 808.

Wass, J.A.H. & Besser, M. (1995). Tests of pituitary function. In DeGroot L.J. et al. (Eds.), *Endocrinology* (3rd ed.). Philadelphia: Saunders.

Diabetes Mellitus

GENERAL CONSIDERATIONS

■ Insulin Secretion and Function

1. Insulin is a hormone secreted by the beta cells of the islet of Langerhans in the pancreas.
2. Small amounts of insulin are released into the bloodstream in response to changes in blood glucose levels throughout the day.
3. Increased secretion or a bolus of insulin, released after a meal, helps maintain euglycemia.
4. Through an internal feedback mechanism that involves the pancreas and the liver, circulating blood glucose levels are maintained at a normal range of 60 to 110 mg/dL.
5. Insulin is essential for the utilization of glucose for cellular metabolism as well as for the proper metabolism of protein and fat.
   a. Carbohydrate metabolism—insulin affects the conversion of glucose into glycogen for storage in the liver and skeletal muscles, and allows for the immediate release and utilization of glucose by the cells.
   b. Protein metabolism—amino acid conversion occurs in the presence of insulin to replace muscle tissue or to provide needed glucose (gluconeogenesis).
   c. Fat metabolism—storage of fat in adipose tissue and conversion of fatty acids from excess glucose occurs only in the presence of insulin.
6. Glucose can be used in the endothelial and nerve cells without the aid of insulin.
7. Without insulin, plasma glucose concentration rises and glycosuria results.
   a. Absolute deficits in insulin result from decreased production of endogenous insulin by the beta cell of the pancreas.
   b. Relative deficits in insulin are caused by inadequate utilization of insulin by the cell.

■ Classification of Diabetes

Type 1 Diabetes Mellitus (formerly known as insulin dependent diabetes mellitus, IDDM)

1. Little or no endogenous insulin, requiring injections of insulin to control diabetes and prevent ketoacidosis.
2. Five to 10% of all diabetic patients have type 1.
3. Etiology: autoimmunity, viral, and certain histocompatibility (HLA) antigens, as well as a genetic component.
4. Usual presentation is rapid with classic symptoms of polydipsia, polyphagia, polyuria, and weight loss.
5. Most commonly seen in patients under age 30 but can be seen in older adults.

Type 2 Diabetes Mellitus (formerly known as non-insulin dependent diabetes mellitus, NIDDM)

1. Caused by a combination of insulin resistance and relative insulin deficiency—some individuals have predominantly insulin resistance, whereas others have predominantly deficient insulin secretion, with little insulin resistance.
2. Approximately 90% of diabetic patients have type 2.
3. Etiology: strong hereditary component, often associated with obesity.
4. Usual presentation is slow and often insidious with symptoms of fatigue, weight gain, poor wound healing, and recurrent infection.
5. Found primarily in adults over 30 years of age.
6. Patients with this type of diabetes, but who eventually may be treated with insulin, are still referred to as having type 2 diabetes.

Impaired Fasting Glucose (IFG)

1. A new category defined at the American Diabetes Association's 57th Annual Scientific Sessions in June 1997.
2. Occurs when fasting blood glucose is greater than or equal to 110 but less than 126 mg/dL.

Impaired Glucose Tolerance (IGT)

1. Abnormality in glucose levels intermediate between normal and overt diabetes (formerly called latent or prediabetes).
2. Defined as blood glucose measurement on a glucose tolerance test greater than or equal to 140 mg/dl but less than 200 in the 2-hour sample.
3. Asymptomatic; it can progress to type 2 diabetes or remain unchanged.
4. May be a risk factor for the development of hypertension, coronary heart disease, and hyperlipidemias.

Gestational Diabetes Mellitus (GDM)

1. Defined as carbohydrate intolerance occurring during pregnancy.
2. Occurs in approximately 4% of pregnancies and usually disappears after delivery.
3. Women with GDM are at higher risk for diabetes at a later date.
4. GDM is associated with increased risk of fetal morbidity.
5. Screening for GDM for all pregnant women other than those at lowest risk (less than 25 years old, of normal body weight, have no family history of diabetes, are not a member of an ethnic group with high prevalence of diabetes) should occur between the 24th and 28th weeks of gestation.

Diabetes Associated With Other Conditions

1. Certain drugs can decrease insulin activity resulting in hyperglycemia—corticosteroids, thiazide diuretics, estrogen, phenytoin.
2. Disease states affecting the pancreas or insulin receptors—pancreatitis, cancer of the pancreas, Cushing's disease or syndrome, acromegaly, pheochromocytoma, muscular dystrophy, Huntington's chorea.

DIAGNOSTIC EVALUATION

Laboratory Tests

Laboratory tests include those tests used to make the diagnosis as well as measures to monitor short- and long-term glucose control.

Blood Glucose

Description

Fasting blood sugar (FBS), drawn after at least an 8-hour fast, to evaluate circulating amounts of glucose; postprandial test, drawn usually 2 hours after a well-balanced meal, to evaluate glucose metabolism; and random glucose, drawn at any time, nonfasting.

Nursing and Patient Care Considerations

1. For fasting glucose, ensure that patient has maintained 8-hour fast overnight; sips of water are allowed.
2. Advise patient to refrain from smoking before the glucose sampling because this affects the test results.
3. For postprandial test, advise patient that no food should be eaten during the 2-hour interval.
4. For random blood glucose, note the time and content of the last meal.

5. Interpret blood values as diagnostic for diabetes mellitus as follows:
   a. FBS greater than or equal to 126 mg/dL on two occasions
   b. Random blood sugar greater than or equal to 200 mg/dL and presence of classic symptoms of diabetes (polyuria, polydipsia, polyphagia, and weight loss)
6. Fasting blood glucose result of greater than or equal to 110 mg/dL demands close follow-up and repeat monitoring.

NURSING ALERT

Capillary blood glucose values obtained by finger stick samples tend to be higher than values in venous samples.

Oral Glucose Tolerance Test (OGTT)

Description

Evaluates insulin response to glucose loading. FBS is obtained before the ingestion of a 50- to 200-g glucose load (usual amount, 75 g), and blood samples are drawn at ½, 1, 2, and 3 hours (may be 4- or 5-hour sampling).

Nursing and Patient Care Considerations

1. Advise patient that for accuracy in results, certain instructions must be followed:
   a. Usual diet and exercise pattern must be followed for 3 days before OGTT.
   b. During OGTT, the patient must refrain from smoking and remain seated.
   c. Oral contraceptives, salicylates, diuretics, phenytoin, and nicotinic acid can impair results and may be withheld before testing based on the advice of the health care provider.
2. Diagnostic for diabetes mellitus if 2-hour value is 200 mg/dL or greater.

Glycated Hemoglobin (Glycohemoglobin, HbA1c)

Description

Measures glycemic control over a 60- to 120-day period by measuring the irreversible reaction of glucose to hemoglobin through freely permeable erythrocytes during their 120-day life cycle.

Nursing and Patient Care Considerations

1. No prior preparation, such as fasting or withholding insulin, is necessary.
2. Test results can be affected by red blood cell disorders (eg, thalassemia, sickle cell anemia), room temperature, ionic charges, and ambient blood glucose values.
3. Many methods exist for performing the test, making it necessary to consult the laboratory for normal values.

C-Peptide Assay (Connecting Peptide Assay)

Description

Cleaved from the proinsulin molecule during its conversion to insulin, C-peptide acts as a marker for endogenous insulin production.

Nursing and Patient Care Considerations

1. Test can be performed after an overnight fast or after stimulation with Sustacal, intravenous (IV) glucose, or 1 mg of glucagon subcutaneously.
2. Absence of C-peptide indicates no beta cell function, reflecting possible type 1 diabetes.

Fructosamine Assay

Description

Glycated protein with a much shorter half-life than glycated hemoglobin, reflecting control over a shorter period of time, approximately 14 to 21 days. May be advantageous in patients with hemoglobin variants that interfere with the accuracy of glycated hemoglobin tests.

Nursing and Patient Care Considerations

1. Note if patient has hypoalbuminemia or elevated globulins because test may not be reliable.
2. Should not be used as a diagnostic test for diabetes mellitus.
3. No special preparation or fasting is necessary.

GENERAL PROCEDURES AND TREATMENT MODALITIES

Blood Glucose Monitoring

Accurate determination of capillary blood glucose assists patients in the control and daily management of diabetes mellitus. Blood glucose monitoring helps evaluate effectiveness of medication; reflects glucose excursion after meals; assesses glucose response to exercise regimen; and assists in the evaluation of episodes of hypoglycemia and hyperglycemia to determine appropriate treatment.

Procedure

1. Guidelines for glucose monitoring are included in Procedure Guidelines 25-1.
2. The most appropriate schedule for glucose monitoring is determined by the patient and health care provider.
   a. Medication regimens and meal timing are considered to set the most effective monitoring schedule.
   b. Scheduling of glucose tests should reflect cost effectiveness for the patient. Glucose meter test strips may cost up to $1.00 each.
   c. Glucose monitoring is intensified during times of stress or illness or when changes in therapy are prescribed.
   d. Patients with type 2 DM controlled with oral hypoglycemic agents or a single injection of intermediate-acting insulin may test glucose levels before breakfast and before supper or at bedtime (twice-a-day monitoring).
   e. Patients with type 1 DM using a multiple-dose insulin regimen may test before meals and at bedtime, occasionally adding a 2 to 3 AM test (four to six times daily monitoring).

PROCEDURE GUIDELINES 25-1	BLOOD GLUCOSE MONITORING TECHNIQUE

EQUIPMENT

Blood glucose meter	Lancet/lancing device	2 × 2 gauze or clean tissue
Test strip	Alcohol wipe	*Cotton ball
Disposable gloves		

PROCEDURE

Nursing Action	Rationale
1. Prepare the finger to be lanced by having the patient wash hands in warm water and soap. Dry thoroughly. For convenience, an alcohol wipe may be used to cleanse the finger. Alcohol must dry thoroughly before finger is lanced.	1. Washing in warm water will increase the blood flow to the finger.
2. Don disposable gloves.	2. Complies with CDC standards for blood-borne pathogens.
3. Turn on the glucose meter. Prepare the meter by validating the proper calibration with the strips to be used. (This usually involves matching a code number on the strip bottle to the code registered on the meter.)	3. Errors in glucose readings can result from miscalibrated or improperly coded meters.
4. The meter will indicate its readiness for testing blood glucose by message or symbol. Some meters require that the glucose test strip be inserted at this time.	
5. Prick the patient's finger lateral to the fingertip using lancet/lancing device, obtaining a large, hanging drop of blood. Most inaccurate readings of blood glucose result from insufficient blood samples.	5. This avoids the most sensitive area of the fingertip.

continued

Nursing Action	Rationale
6. Apply the blood carefully to the strip test area (varies by glucose meter model).	6. Some glucose meters require that the test area be covered completely for accurate results. Others use only a small drop of blood inserted at the side of the test strip.

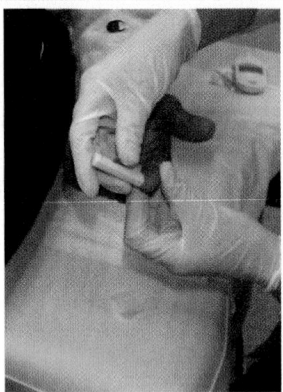

Obtaining blood from a finger using a lancet device

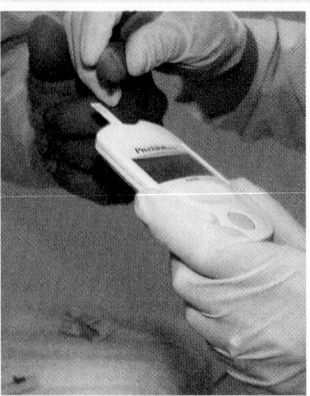

Applying drop of blood to test strip

7. Completing the test
  a. No-wipe system—the blood remains on the strip as the meter times and processes the result.
  b. Meters with a "wipe" system require that the blood be wiped off from the test strip with a firm stroke using a cotton ball at the appropriate end time (usually 60 seconds). The strip is inserted into the meter for the final result/reading.
8. The lanced finger is covered with a gauze or tissue until bleeding subsides. If necessary, an adhesive bandage is then applied.
	
	b. Blood contact time with the test strip can vary with each glucose meter. Precise timing is crucial for accurate results. Consult the glucose meter instruction guide for the timing sequence necessary for your specific product.

*Note: Universal precautions should be used throughout the procedure. All blood-contaminated items should be disposed of properly.

Insulin Therapy

Insulin therapy involves the subcutaneous injection of short-, intermediate-, or long-acting insulin at various times to achieve the desired effect. Short-acting regular insulin can also be given IV. There are about 20 insulins available in the United States, mostly human insulin manufactured synthetically. Only about 6% of diabetics are still using beef or pork insulin due to problems with immunogenicity.

Self-Injection of Insulin

1. Teaching of self-injection of insulin should begin as soon as the need for insulin has been established.
2. Teach both the patient and another family member or significant other.
3. Use written and verbal instructions and demonstration techniques.
4. Teach injection first because this is the patient's primary concern; then teach loading the syringe.
5. See Procedure Guidelines 25-2 for technique.
6. For patients who have difficulty with the injection procedure, newer insulin pens are available that use a pre-filled cartridge that automatically delivers the set dose of insulin by jet stream without a needle.

Community and Home Care Considerations

1. Advise patient to reuse insulin syringe at home until needle is dull (2–10 times). Needle should be recapped by patient and stored in a clean place.
2. Alcohol use to wipe off the top of the vial or prepare the skin is not necessary. It has not proved to result in lower rate of infection and adds cost and time to the procedure. The patient should maintain good hygiene.
3. Storage of the insulin should be in a clean, secure place away from sunlight and heat. Most vials can be kept un-

refrigerated for 1 month. Some insulin pens may need to be discarded weekly; check with manufacturer.

Insulin Regimens

See Figure 25-1.

NPH Only

1. Used alone only in type 2 DM when patients are capable of producing some exogenous insulin as a supplement for better glucose control.
2. Traditionally given as a morning dosage to assist with normalization of glucose during the afternoon and evening.
3. Evening or bedtime dosage can be helpful in controlling early-morning hyperglycemia.
4. NPH can also be given twice daily (morning and bedtime) to eliminate afternoon hypoglycemia yet provide nighttime coverage. Typically $\frac{2}{3}$ to $\frac{3}{4}$ of the daily dosage is given before breakfast and $\frac{1}{3}$ to $\frac{1}{4}$ is given at bedtime.

NPH/Regular or NPH/Lispro

1. Short-acting regular insulin or lispro insulin is added to NPH to promote postprandial glucose control.
2. Short-acting insulin added to morning NPH controls glucose elevations after breakfast.

3. Increased blood glucose levels after supper can be controlled by the addition of short-acting insulin before supper.
4. NPH and regular or lispro insulin given before breakfast and before supper is termed a "split-mix" regimen, providing 24-hour insulin coverage for type 1 DM.

Intensive Insulin Therapy (ITT)

1. Designed to mimic the body's normal insulin responses to glucose.
2. Uses multiple daily injections of insulin.
3. NPH or ultralente insulin is used for basal insulin control.
4. Regular insulin acts as a premeal bolus given 30 minutes before each meal. Lispro insulin may be used instead of regular and is taken with meals.
5. 24-hour insulin coverage designed in this way can be flexible to accommodate mealtimes and physical activity.

Sliding Scale Versus Algorithm Therapy

1. Sliding scale therapy uses regular insulin to retrospectively correct hyperglycemia.
2. Algorithm therapy prospectively determines regular insulin dosages, taking into account meal content and physical activity.
3. Individualization of regular insulin dosages is the most important aspect of sliding scale and algorithm therapy.

NPH Only

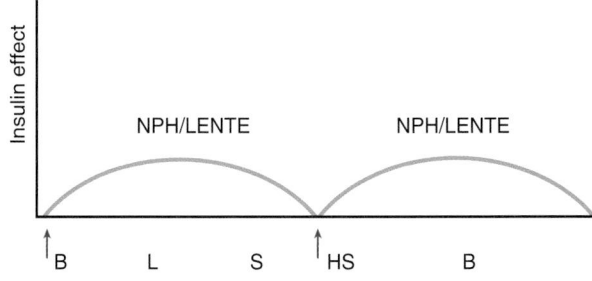

Intensive insulin therapy

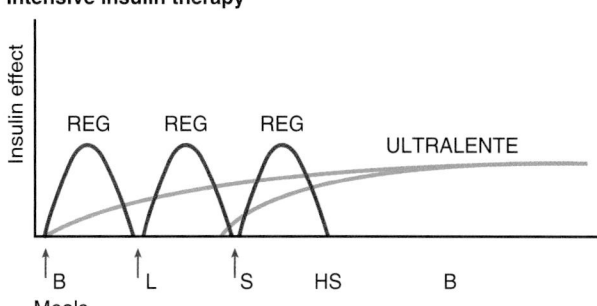

NPH/Regular

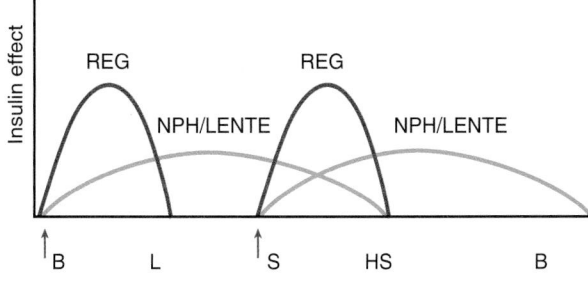

NPH/Lispro

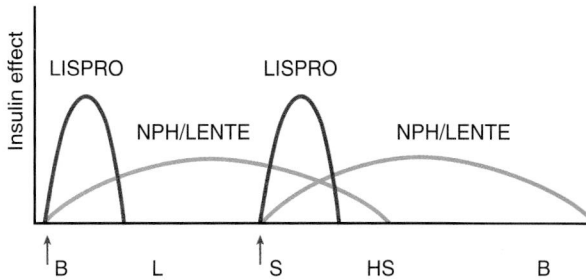

Key

B - Breakfast   S - Supper   B - Bed
L - Lunch   HS - Bedtime snack   ↑ - Time of pre-meal insulin injection

FIGURE 25-1 Insulin regimens.

a. The patient is encouraged to test blood glucoses to analyze insulin dose response.

b. A pattern of increased blood glucose associated with certain foods (eg, pasta, pizza) can help determine the appropriate regimen of insulin dosage.

c. Physical activity, which enhances insulin activity and decreases serum glucose, may indicate the need to reduce the dosage of premeal regular insulin.

Continuous Subcutaneous Insulin Infusion (CSII) and Insulin Pump Therapy

1. Provides continuous infusion of regular insulin via subcutaneous needle inserted in the abdomen.
2. The needle should be replaced every 48 hours or sooner if the site becomes painful or inflamed.
   a. Frequently, the insulin pump is removed for bathing, and tubing and needle are changed at that time.
   b. To reduce tubing and needle blockage, *buffered* regular insulin is used.
3. Intensive insulin management by pump therapy requires patient motivation.
   a. Blood glucose monitoring must be done at least four to six times each day.
   b. Frequent contact with health care team is necessary to adjust insulin dosage.
   c. Careful recordings of diet, insulin, and activity are required to evaluate adjustments.
   d. Increased cost of insulin pump and infusion set compared to usual syringe method.
   e. Heightened risk of hypoglycemia with tighter glucose control.

f. Danger of hyperglycemia exists should insulin pump fail to deliver correct insulin dosage.

g. Increased visibility of diabetes by use of an external device.

4. Advantages of CSII in improving blood glucose control:
   a. Insulin pump can deliver basal insulin at individualized programmed rates throughout a 24-hour period.
   b. Boluses of regular insulin given 30 minutes before eating allow for flexibility in meal content and timing.
   c. Supplements of regular insulin to rapidly correct blood glucoses can be easily given.

Combination Oral Agent and Insulin Therapy

1. Appropriate only in type 2 DM.
2. Intermediate-acting insulin (NPH) is given in the evening and an oral sulfonylurea agent in the morning—called BIDS therapy (bedtime insulin, daytime sulfonylurea).
   a. No oral antidiabetic agent is given at bedtime.
   b. Controlling hepatic glucose production overnight with evening insulin helps to start the day with a lower FBS.
   c. Daytime antidiabetic agent (usually sulfonylurea), along with diet and exercise, controls daytime blood glucose levels.
   d. Some patients may require regular/NPH insulin injected before supper to assist with elevated postprandial evening glucoses.
3. Combination therapy may also include the use of a thiazolidinedione (pioglitazone [Actos], rosiglitazone [Avandia]), metformin (Glucophage), or other agents.

PROCEDURE GUIDELINES 25-2	TEACHING SELF-INJECTION OF INSULIN

EQUIPMENT

Prescribed bottle of insulin
Disposable insulin syringe and needle
Cotton ball and alcohol or alcohol wipe

PROCEDURE

Nursing Action	Rationale
1. Give the patient the syringe containing the prescribed dose of insulin.	
2. Have patient select a clean area of subcutaneous tissue.	
3. Instruct the patient to hold the syringe as he would a pencil.	
4. Show the patient how to select an area of skin from the anterior thighs and form a skin fold by picking up subcutaneous tissue between the thumb and forefinger if the patient is thin.	4. Pinching a skin fold and injecting at 45 degrees is recommended for thin people; injecting at 90 degrees into taut skin is recommended for heavier people. Avoid pinching the skin tightly to avoid trauma.
5. Select areas of upper arms, abdomen, and upper buttocks for injection after patient becomes proficient with needle insertion (see figure).	5. The skin is loose and there is more subcutaneous fat in these areas. Systematic rotation of sites will keep the skin supple and favor uniform absorption of insulin. Use of the same body part for each time of day dosage will make absorption more consistent.

Nursing Action	Rationale

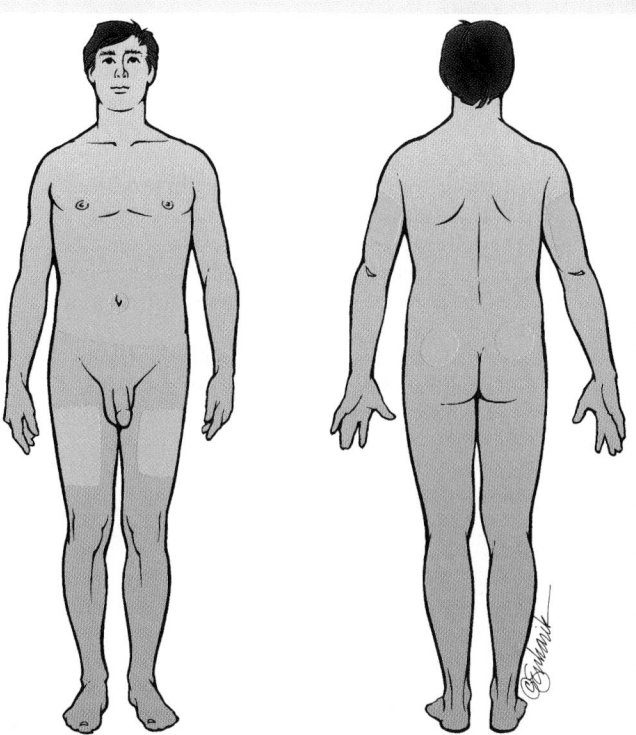

Rotate sites within each body part and use the same body part for the same injection time each day. Absorption is quicker from the abdomen and arms, than the thighs and buttocks. Exercising a body part will hasten insulin absorption, so exercise should be consistent.

Nursing Action	Rationale
6. Assist the patient to insert the needle with a quick thrust to the hub at a 45–90-degree angle to the skin surface.	6. The insulin is injected into deep subcutaneous tissue.
7. Inject the insulin with slow, consistent pressure without aspiration.	7. Aspiration is not necessary.
8. Instruct the patient to release the skin tension and withdraw needle.	8. Prevents painful pulling of the skin as the needle is withdrawn.

TO LOAD THE SYRINGE

1. Shake the bottle of insulin to mix well.	1. May result in air bubbles, but needs to be mixed well.
2. Do not instruct the patient to wipe off the top of the vial with alcohol; instead, ensure that the vial is stored in its original carton and is kept clean.	2. Wiping with alcohol is not necessary as chance of infection is very small.
3. Inject approximately the same volume of air into the insulin vial as the volume of insulin to be withdrawn.	3. Air is injected into the vial to keep its contents under slight positive pressure and to make it easier to withdraw the insulin.

TO FILL A SYRINGE WITH LONG- AND SHORT-ACTING INSULIN MIXTURE

1. Inject air equal to the number of units to be injected into each vial. Use the same sequence each time, for example, always NPH insulin first.	1. Creates positive pressure in vial, so that insulin will be withdrawn from each vial without mixing.
2. After injecting air into the second vial, keep needle in vial and withdraw prescribed amount of that type of insulin, then withdraw needle.	2. There is no real benefit to withdrawing either type of insulin first, as the risk of mixing insulins in the second vial is minimal. It is more important not to switch vials and draw up the wrong dose, so the sequence should always be the same.
3. Withdraw prescribed amount of insulin from the second vial.	3. Positive pressure already created in that vial will make withdrawal of insulin easy.

DIABETES AND RELATED DISORDERS

▦ Diabetes Mellitus

Diabetes mellitus is a metabolic disorder characterized by hyperglycemia and results from defective insulin production, secretion, or utilization.

Pathophysiology and Etiology

1. There is an absolute or relative lack of insulin produced by the beta cell, resulting in hyperglycemia.
2. Defects at the cell level, impaired secretory response of insulin to rises in glucose, and increased nocturnal hepatic glucose production (gluconeogenesis) are seen in type 2 DM.
3. Etiology of type 1 DM is not well understood; viral, autoimmune, and environmental theories are under review.
4. Etiology of type 2 DM involves heredity/genetics and obesity.

Clinical Manifestations

Onset is abrupt with type 1 and insidious with type 2.

Hyperglycemia

1. Weight loss, fatigue
2. Polyuria, polydipsia, polyphagia
3. Blurred vision

Altered Tissue Response

1. Poor wound healing
2. Recurrent infections, particularly of the skin

Diagnostic Evaluation

1. Diabetes can be diagnosed in any of the following ways (and should be confirmed on a different day by any of these tests):
   a. FBS of greater than or equal to 126 mg/dL
   b. Random blood glucose of greater than or equal to 200 mg/dL with classic symptoms (polyuria, polydipsia, polyphagia, weight loss)
   c. OGTT greater than or equal to 200 mg/dL on the 2-hour sample
2. Tests for glucose control over time are glycated hemoglobin and fructosamine assay (see pp. 842–843). These tests are not used for diagnosis.

Management

Diet

1. Dietary control with caloric restriction of carbohydrates and saturated fats to maintain ideal body weight.
2. The goal of meal planning is to control blood glucose and lipid levels (Table 25-1).
3. Weight reduction is a primary treatment for type 2 DM.

TABLE 25-1 Meal Planning Guidelines

Principle	Action
1. Each meal should consist of a balance of carbohydrates, proteins, and fats.	1. a. Carbohydrates should be varied to include fruits, starches, and vegetables. b. Protein selections that are lean will help reduce fat and cholesterol intake. c. Fats should be used sparingly with <10% of total calories derived from saturated fats. High in calories, fats contribute to weight gain in type 2 DM.
2. Consistency in timing of meals and amounts of food eaten on a day-to-day basis help regulate blood glucose levels.	2. a. Avoid skipping or delaying meals. b. Measure portion sizes using a scale or measuring cups. c. Know the equivalent amounts of commonly used foods within a food group, eg, 1 slice of bread = ½ cup cooked pasta.
3. Increase the intake of soluble and insoluble fiber.	3. a. Substitute foods high in fiber for processed foods when possible, eg, whole grain bread in place of white bread. b. Eat fresh fruit and vegetables in place of juices.
4. Avoid salt whenever possible.	4. a. Do not season foods with salt or salt-containing spices. b. Limit use of foods with "hidden" sodium content (eg, crackers, pickled foods, cheese, processed meats). c. Use salt-containing condiments sparingly (ketchup, soy sauce, gravies, bouillon).
5. Prepare foods to retain vitamins and minerals and reduce fats.	5. a. Do not fry foods. b. Bake, broil, or boil foods and discard fat. c. Eat raw fruits and vegetables or steam vegetables to retain fiber. d. Avoid adding calories with butter or cream sauces, fat back, and bacon. e. Trim all visible fat from meat; skim off fat from stews or other prepared dishes.
6. Distribute snacks in the meal plan depending on insulin/medication regimens, physical activity, and lifestyle.	6. a. Smaller, more frequent meals may enhance glucose control in type 2 DM. b. Unplanned activity may call for an additional snack to avoid hypoglycemia.
7. Use alcohol only in moderation.	7. a. Always consume alcohol with food to avoid hypoglycemia. b. Do not omit food from meal plan in exchange for alcohol. c. Limit intake to 1–2 drinks per week (4 oz dry wine, 12 oz beer, or 1.5 oz distilled liquor = 1 alcohol serving).
8. Use alternative nonnutritive, noncaloric sweeteners in moderation.	8. a. Limit "diet" soda intake to 2 L/d. b. Avoid frequent use of foods/beverages with concentrated sucrose.

TABLE 25-2 Oral Antidiabetic Agents

Agent	How Given
Second-Generation Sulfonylureas	
Glyburide (Micronase, Diabeta, Glynase)	0.75–12 mg in single or divided dose with meal
Glipizide (Glibenese, Glucatrol, Glucatrol XL)	2.5–15 mg in single dose or up to 40 mg in two divided doses 30 min. before meal
	5–20 mg in single dose before breakfast
Glimepiride (Amaryl)	1–8 mg in single dose with first main meal
Biguanides	
Metformin (Glucophage)	1700–2500 mg in two–three divided doses with meals
Alpha-glucosidase Inhibitors	
Acarbose (Precose)	150–300 mg in three doses with meals; if <60 kg, max. dose 50 mg three times/d
Miglitol (Glyset)	150–300 mg in three divided doses with meals
Meglitinide Analogue	
Repaglinide (Prandin)	1–16 mg in two–four divided doses within 30 min. of starting meal
Thiazolidinediones	
Rosiglitazone (Avandia)	4–8 mg in one or two divided doses
Pioglitazone (Actos)	15–45 mg once daily in single dose

Exercise

Regularly scheduled exercise to promote the utilization of carbohydrates, assist with weight control, enhance the action of insulin, and improve cardiovascular fitness.

Medication

1. Oral antidiabetic agents for patients with type 2 DM who do not achieve glucose control with diet and exercise only (Table 25-2).
   a. Act by a variety of mechanisms, including stimulation of insulin secretion from functioning beta cells, reduction of hepatic glucose production, enhancement of peripheral sensitivity to insulin, and reduced absorption of carbohydrates from the intestine.
   b. Sulfonylureas and meglitinide analogues may cause hypoglycemic reactions.
   c. Biguanides, alpha-glucosidase inhibitors, and meglitinide analogues may cause significant flatus and gastrointestinal adverse effects.
2. Insulin therapy for patients with type 1 DM who require replacement (Table 25-3).
   a. May also be used for type 2 DM when unresponsive to diet, exercise, and oral antidiabetic therapy.
   b. Hypoglycemia may result, as well as rebound hyperglycemia (Somogyi effect).
   c. Often result in increased appetite and weight gain.

Complications

Acute

1. Hypoglycemia occurs as a result of an imbalance in food, activity, and insulin/oral antidiabetic agent.
2. Diabetic ketoacidosis (DKA) occurs primarily in type 1 DM during times of severe insulin deficiency or illness, producing severe hyperglycemia, ketonuria, dehydration, and acidosis.

3. Hyperglycemic hyperosmolar nonketotic syndrome (HHNKS) affects patients with type 2 DM, causing severe dehydration, hyperglycemia, hyperosmolarity, and stupor.

Chronic (Table 25-4)

1. In type 1 DM, chronic complications usually appear about 10 years after the initial diagnosis.
2. The prevalence of microvascular complications (retinopathy, nephropathy) and neuropathy is higher in type 1 DM.
3. Because of its insidious onset, chronic complications can appear at any point in type 2 DM.

(*text continues on page 852*)

TABLE 25-3 Insulin Onset, Peak, and Duration

Insulin	Onset	Peak	Duration
Immediate-acting (lispro)	0.25 h	0.5–1 h	5 h
Short-acting (regular, semilente)	0.5–1 h	2–4 h	5–7 h
Intermediate-acting (NPH, lente)	1–3 h	6–12 h	18–24 h
Long-acting (ultralente)	4–6 h	10–30 h	24–36 h
Mixed (Regular 30%, NPH 70%)	0.5 h	4–8 h	24 h

> **NURSING ALERT**
>
> Regular insulin is the *only* insulin that may be administered IV; all other insulin formulations are suspensions. Lispro insulin is for subcutaneous injection only.

TABLE 25-4　Chronic Complications of Diabetes Mellitus

Condition	Assessment	Intervention	Prevention/Teaching
MACROANGIOPATHY			
Cerebrovascular Disease Incidence: Twice as frequent in diabetes Hypertension, increased lipids, smoking, and uncontrolled blood glucose increase risk of stroke and transient ischemic attack.	Increased blood pressure Change in mental status Hemiparesis Aphasia Clinical presentation mimics that of nondiabetic patient.	Check blood glucose level to differentiate s/s of stroke vs. hypoglycemia. If stroke is suspected, do *not* give fast-acting carbohydrate as increased levels contribute to recurrence and ↑ mortality rates of strokes in patients with diabetes. Monitor for bleeding if aspirin or other platelet-active medicine is used.	Maintain target goals of blood glucose avoiding severe hypoglycemia and hyperglycemia, which predispose the patient to cerebrovascular accident. In hypoglycemia, increased levels of adrenalin and catecholamines can produce cardiac arrhythmias. Hyperglycemia can lead to dehydration, which affects platelet aggregation.
Coronary Artery Disease Incidence: Increased vessel disease with more vessels affected in diabetes. Higher incidence of "silent" myocardial infarctions. Hyperglycemia contributes to atherosclerosis and vessel deterioration.	Severe coronary artery disease is often asymptomatic, seen only in ECG changes. ECG changes may indicate silent myocardial infarction. Symptoms can also present as pain in the jaw, neck, or epigastric area.	Usual medical treatment for angina prevails—sublingual nitroglycerin, oral nitrates. β-Adrenergic blockers and calcium channel blockers can also be used.	Emphasis must be placed on reducing cardiac risk factors, eg, cigarette smoking, hypertension, hyperlipidemias. Avoid wide fluctuations in blood glucose. Patients with autonomic neuropathy, which can cause orthostatic hypotension, should be carefully monitored when cardiac drug therapies are introduced. β-Adrenergic blockers can blunt or eliminate the clinical signs and symptoms of hypoglycemia.
Peripheral Vascular Disease Incidence: 50% of non-traumatic amputations are related to diabetes. Intermittent claudication, absent pedal pulses, and ischemic gangrene are increased in diabetes.	Physical examination of the lower extremities may reveal changes in skin integrity associated with diminished circulation. Decreased lower leg hair, absent or decreased anterior tibial or dorsal pedis pulses, poor capillary refill of toenails may occur. The extremity may appear pale/cool. Further examination for neurologic changes is indicated.	Any lesion, decrease in peripheral pulses, or change in skin color, temperature or sensation should be evaluated within 24–48 h. To ensure proper healing and prevent infection, treatment should begin as soon as possible and be carefully monitored. Mild antiseptics/antibiotic preparations are used to avoid further damage to the surrounding skin. Avoid the use of surgical tape to skin. Rest affected leg to promote circulation and wound healing.	Foot care guidelines and smoking cessation must be stressed. Safe exercise guidelines and weight reduction as appropriate will further reduce risk of foot injury.
MICROANGIOPATHY			
Retinopathy Incidence: Type 1—10 y post-diagnosis 60% have some degree of retinopathy. Type 2—approximately 20% present with retinopathy at diagnosis, which increases to 60–85% after 15 y. Appearance of hard exudates, blot hemorrhages, and microaneurysms on the retina in background retinopathy.	Usually asymptomatic in the early stages. Symptoms occurring with acute visual problems—"floaters," flashing lights, blurred vision may indicate hemorrhage or retinal detachment. Fundoscopic examination should be done by an ophthalmologist for full retinal visualization.	Laser therapy (photocoagulation) can be helpful in macular edema (focal laser) and proliferative retinopathy (panretinal laser). Reduction of active neovascularization by laser therapy reduces the risk of vitreous hemorrhage. Vitrectomy may be needed to treat retinal detachment or remove vitreous hemorrhage.	Stress importance of annual eye examination with an ophthalmologist (preferably retina specialist). Optimal glucose control can prevent or slow the progression of retinopathy. Maintaining normal blood pressure also reduces the risk of retinopathy.

TABLE 25-4 Chronic Complications of Diabetes Mellitus (Continued)

Condition	Assessment	Intervention	Prevention/Teaching
Progresses to neurovascularization in proliferative diabetic retinopathy.		During the acute phase, before laser therapy, patients must avoid activities that increase the chances of vitreous hemorrhage (eg, weight lifting, high-impact aerobics).	
Nephropathy Incidence: Type 1—with >20 y history of diabetes, approximately 40% will have renal disease. Type 2—5–10 y after diagnosis 5–10% of patients develop nephropathy, with higher incidence in Native Americans, Hispanics, and African Americans. Thickening of the glomerular basement membrane, mesangial expansion, and renal vessel sclerosis are caused by diabetes. Subsequently, diffuse and nodular intercapillary glomerulosclerosis diminishes renal function.	Evidence of ↑ glomerular filtration rate. Microalbuminuria is the first clinical sign of renal disease. Elevation in BUN and creatinine indicate advanced renal disease. Gross proteinuria is further indication of renal deterioration.	Hypertension control, blood glucose control, and reduction of protein and sodium are essential. Angiotensin-converting enzyme inhibitors are the drugs of choice to control blood pressure. Calcium channel blockers may also be used. In end-stage renal disease dialysis or transplantation may be necessary.	Frequent hypertension screening, noting any deviation from patient's normal reading. Early initiation of blood pressure control to prevent kidney damage. Excellent glucose control with insulin/oral agent adjustment to compensate for reduced kidney function, which predisposes the patient to hypoglycemia. Avoidance of nephrotoxic drugs, dyes, or renal procedures that may cause infection. Immediate treatment for any urinary tract infections.
PERIPHERAL NEUROPATHY In general, neuropathy affects 60% of persons with diabetes, with nearly 100% showing signs and symptoms of slowing nerve conduction velocity. It can affect almost every organ system with varying specific symptoms. Distal symmetrical polyneuropathy involving the lower extremities is most commonly seen. In conjunction with peripheral vascular disease, neuropathy to the feet increases susceptibility to trauma and infection. Three clinical syndromes of distal symmetrical polyneuropathy can be seen: acute painful neuropathy, small fiber neuropathy, large fiber neuropathy.	Decreased light touch, vibratory, temperature sensation. Loss of foot proprioception, followed by ataxia, gait disturbances. Diminished ankle jerk response. Formation of "hammer toes," Charcot joint disease, which predispose patient to new pressure point areas. Hypersensitivity or other dysesthetic symptoms are experienced, followed by hypoanesthesia or anesthesia, which is not reversible.	All foot wounds or injuries are immediately evaluated. Culture and sensitivities ordered for any drainage present. Affected foot is elevated—avoid weight-bearing. Wet to dry dressings applied as ordered. Avoid use of caustic chemicals, dressing tapes. Use of systemic antibiotics as needed. Medication for painful neuropathy may include use of the tricyclic antidepressant drugs (eg, amitriptylline—Elavil) or topical application of capsaicin (Zostrix) ointment.	In general, blood glucose control is recommended, avoiding wide fluctuations. In patients who are poorly controlled, care must be taken to correct glucoses slowly to avoid increasing symptoms of neuropathy. Foot care guidelines. Smoking cessation. Frequent evaluation by podiatrist for modified foot wear, eg, orthotics, extra depth shoes. Safe exercise guidelines. Weight reduction as necessary.
AUTONOMIC NEUROPATHY *Gastroparesis* Incidence: Occurs in 25% of people with diabetes Characteristics: Delayed gastric emptying, prolonged pylorospasms and loss of the powerful contractions of the distal stomach to grind and mix foods.	Typical symptoms may include nausea/vomiting, early satiety, abdominal bloating, epigastric pain, change in appetite. Wide fluctuations in blood glucoses and postmeal hypoglycemia caused by poor glucose absorption. Visualiza-	Excellent glucose control to avoid hyperglycemia, which interferes with gut contractility. Avoidance of severe postmeal hypoglycemia by small frequent meals, low fat and low fiber. This diet is also helpful in bloating/early sati-	Maintenance of excellent glucose control. Regular exercise improves/maintains gut motility. Avoid use of laxatives. Small, frequent meals may help.

(continued)

TABLE 25-4 Chronic Complications of Diabetes Mellitus (Continued)

Condition	Assessment	Intervention	Prevention/Teaching
	tion of the gut by upper gastrointestinal barium series may show retained food after an 8–12-h fast.	ety. Medications to improve gut motility include metoclopramide (Reglan) and cisapride (Pepcid).	
Diarrhea Incidence: Approximately 5% of diabetic patients Characteristics: Frequent, watery movements Mild steatorrhea Can be intermittent, persistent, or alternate with constipation.	Diarrhea occurs without warning, frequently at night or after meals. Fecal incontinence may be caused by loss of internal sphincter control and anorectal sensation. Other causes such as celiac sprue, pancreatic insufficiency, lactose intolerance must be investigated. Bacterial overgrowth in the bowel is also suspected.	Dietary changes may include increased fiber, elimination of milk products. Sphincter-strengthening exercises may help. Medications: For diarrhea hydrophilic fiber supplement (Metamucil), cholestyramine (Questran), or synthetic opiates are used. Tetracycline, ampicillin are used for bacterial overgrowth.	Routine bowel elimination habits Maintenance of adequate hydration Excellent blood glucose control reduces dehydration. Inclusion of dietary fiber in the daily diet Daily exercise program that includes walking or swimming has been effective in encouraging bowel regularity.
Impotence/Sexual Dysfunction Incidence is not well documented due to inhibitions about reporting this problem to health care providers. Sexual dysfunction can involve changes in erectile ability, ejaculation, or libido.	Men: History of poor erectile function despite stimulation. Absence of early morning erection in response to increased hormonal levels. Women: May experience decreased vaginal lubrication and dyspareunia. Screening for use of ethanol or other medications associated with impotence (eg, antidepressants, antihypertensives).	Men: Referral to urologist for full examination is indicated. Treatment options may include injection of alprostadel (a prostaglandin), inflatable penile prosthesis, or oral sildenafil (Viagra). Women: Increase lubrication with use of water-based lubricant (K-Y jelly) or estrogen creams, which also may help thicken the vaginal mucosa, affecting dyspareunia.	Reduce consumption of alcohol, which may hasten or contribute to neuropathy. Maintain target ranges of blood glucose control to reduce likelihood of vaginal infections. Discuss alternative ways of maintaining intimacy.
Orthostatic Hypotension One of three syndromes associated with cardiovascular autonomic neuropathy, orthostatic hypotension occurs when the "postural reflex," which increases heart rate and peripheral vascular resistance is dysfunctional.	Patients may report episodes of syncope, weakness, or visual impairment particularly with positional changes. Evaluate blood pressure and pulse in both lying and standing position at each visit. Blood pressure changes that indicate neuropathic involvement: fall in systolic pressure of >30 mm Hg or fall in diastolic pressure of >10 mm Hg with change from lying to standing position.	Improvement in blood glucose control to prevent fluid loss from glycosuria. Moderate amounts of sodium may be used in the diet to encourage fluid retention during hot weather or strenuous exercise. Mechanical devices such as support stockings (full hose to waist) may decrease venous pooling. Drugs to enhance volume expansion may be used. (eg, fludrocortisone—Florine)	Encourage increased fluid intake to maintain hydration. Caution should be used in changing position from lying to standing. "Dangling" is recommended until blood pressure stabilizes. Avoid standing in one position, which may increase venous pooling.

4. Macrovascular complications—in particular cardiovascular disease, occurring both in type 1 and type 2 DM—are the leading cause of morbidity and mortality among persons with diabetes.

Nursing Assessment

1. Obtain a history of current problems, family history, and general health history.
   a. Has the patient experienced polyuria, polydipsia, polyphagia, and any other symptoms?
   b. Number of years since diagnosis of diabetes

   c. Family members diagnosed with diabetes, their subsequent treatment, and complications
2. Perform a review of systems and physical examination to assess for signs and symptoms of diabetes, general health of patient, and presence of complications.
   a. General: recent weight loss or gain, increased fatigue, tiredness, anxiety
   b. Skin: skin lesions, infections, dehydration, evidence of poor wound healing
   c. Eyes: changes in vision—floaters, halos, blurred vision, dry or burning eyes, cataracts, glaucoma
   d. Mouth: gingivitis, periodontal disease

e. Cardiovascular: orthostatic hypotension, cold extremities, weak pedal pulses, leg claudication
f. Gastrointestinal: diarrhea, constipation, early satiety, bloating, increased flatulence, hunger/thirst
g. Genitourinary: increased urination, nocturia, impotence, vaginal discharge
h. Neurologic: numbness and tingling of the extremities, decreased pain and temperature perception, changes in gait/balance

Nursing Diagnoses
- Altered Nutrition (More than Body Requirements) related to intake in excess of activity expenditures
- Fear related to insulin injection
- Risk for Injury (Hypoglycemia) related to effects of insulin, inability to eat
- Activity Intolerance related to poor glucose control
- Knowledge Deficit related to use of oral hypoglycemic agents
- Risk for Impaired Skin Integrity related to decreased sensation and circulation to lower extremities
- Ineffective Coping related to chronic disease and complex self-care regimen

Nursing Interventions
See Standards of Care Guidelines.

Improving Nutrition
1. Assess current timing and content of meals.
2. Advise patient on the importance of an individualized meal plan in meeting weight-loss goals.
3. Discuss the goals of dietary therapy for the patient.
4. Assist the patient to identify problems that may have an impact on dietary adherence and possible solutions to these problems.
5. Explain the importance of exercise in maintaining/reducing body weight.
   a. Caloric expenditure for energy in exercise
   b. Carry-over of enhanced metabolic rate and efficient food utilization
6. Assist patient to establish goals for weekly weight loss and incentives to assist in achieving them.
7. Strategize with the patient to address the potential social pitfalls of weight reduction.

Teaching About Insulin
1. Assist patient to reduce fear of injection by encouraging verbalization of fears regarding insulin injection, conveying a sense of empathy, and identifying supportive coping techniques.
2. Demonstrate and explain thoroughly the procedure for insulin self-injection (see p. 846).
3. Help patient to master technique by taking a step-by-step approach.
   a. Allow patient time to handle insulin and syringe to become familiar with the equipment.
   b. Teach self-injection first to alleviate fear of pain from injection.
   c. Instruct patient in filling syringe when he or she expresses confidence in self-injection procedure.

STANDARDS OF CARE GUIDELINES
Caring for Patients With Diabetes Mellitus

When caring for patients with diabetes mellitus:

- Assess level of knowledge of disease and ability to care for self.
- Assess adherence to diet therapy, monitoring procedures, medication treatment, and exercise regimen.
- Assess for signs of hyperglycemia: polyuria, polydipsia, polyphagia, weight loss, fatigue, blurred vision.
- Assess for signs of hypoglycemia: sweating, tremor, nervousness, tachycardia, light-headedness, confusion.
- Perform thorough skin and extremity assessment for peripheral neuropathy or peripheral vascular disease and any injury to the feet or lower extremities.
- Assess for trends in blood glucose and other laboratory results.
- Ensure that appropriate insulin dosage is given at the right time and in relation to meals and exercise.
- Ensure adequate knowledge of diet, exercise, and medication treatment.
- Immediately report to health care provider any signs of skin or soft tissue infection (redness, swelling, warmth, tenderness, drainage).
- Get help immediately for signs of hypoglycemia that do not respond to usual glucose replacement.
- Get help immediately for patient presenting with signs of either ketoacidosis (nausea and vomiting, Kussmaul respirations, fruity breath odor, hypotension, and altered level of consciousness) or HHNKS (nausea and vomiting, hypothermia, muscle weakness, seizures, stupor, coma).

This information should serve as a general guideline only. Each patient situation presents a unique set of clinical factors and requires nursing judgment to guide care, which may include additional or alternative measures and approaches.

GERONTOLOGIC ALERT

Assess elderly patients for sensory deficits such as impaired vision, hearing, fine touch, and tremors that may have an impact on learning and ability to self-administer insulin. Suggest use of an insulin pen or magnifying glass to assist with drawing up insulin. Pen must be inverted 10 times to ensure mixing.

4. Review dosage and time of injections in relation to meals, activity, and bedtime based on patient's individualized insulin regimen.

Preventing Injury Secondary to Hypoglycemia
1. Closely monitor blood glucose levels to detect hypoglycemia.
2. Instruct patient in the importance of accuracy in insulin preparation and meal timing to avoid hypoglycemia.
3. Assess patient for the signs and symptoms of hypoglycemia.
   a. Adrenergic—sweating, tremor, pallor, tachycardia, palpitations, nervousness from the release of adrenalin when blood glucose falls rapidly

b. Neurologic—headache, light-headedness, confusion, irritability, slurred speech, lack of coordination, staggering gait from depression of central nervous system as glucose level progressively falls

4. Treat hypoglycemia promptly with 10 to 15 g of fast-acting carbohydrates.
   a. Half cup (4 oz) juice, three glucose tablets, four sugar cubes, five to six pieces of hard candy may be taken orally.
   b. Nutrition bar specially designed for diabetics—supplies glucose from sucrose, starch, and protein sources with some fat to delay gastric emptying and prolong effect; may prevent relapse.
   c. Glucagon 1 mg (subcutaneously or intramuscularly) is given if the patient cannot ingest a sugar treatment. Family member or staff must administer injection.
   d. IV bolus of 50 mL of 50% dextrose solution can be given if the patient fails to respond to glucagon within 15 minutes.

5. Encourage patient to carry a portable treatment for hypoglycemia at all times.

NURSING ALERT

If the patient is taking an alpha-glucosidase inhibitor or meglitinide analogue, he or she must use a monosaccharide (glucose tablets) to treat hypoglycemia, since sucrose will not be broken down to an absorbable sugar.

---

6. Assess patient for cognitive or physical impairments that may interfere with ability to accurately administer insulin.

7. Between-meal snacks as well as extra food taken before exercise should be encouraged to prevent hypoglycemia.

8. Encourage patients to wear an identification bracelet or card that may assist in prompt treatment in a hypoglycemic emergency.
   a. Identification bracelet may be obtained from Medic Alert Foundation International, 2323 Colorado, Tarlock, CA 95381.
   b. Identification card may be requested from the American Diabetes Association, 1660 Duke St., Alexandria, VA 22314, 800-676-4065, *www.diabetes.org*.

Improving Activity Tolerance

1. Advise patient to assess blood glucose level before and after strenuous exercise.
2. Instruct patient to plan exercises on a regular basis each day.
3. Encourage patient to eat a carbohydrate snack before exercising to avoid hypoglycemia.
4. Advise patient that prolonged strenuous exercise may require increased food at bedtime to avoid nocturnal hypoglycemia.
5. Instruct patient to avoid exercise whenever blood glucose levels exceed 250 mg/d and urine ketones are present.
6. Counsel patient to inject insulin into the abdominal site on days when arms or legs are exercised.

Providing Information About Oral Antidiabetic Agents

1. Identify any barriers to learning, such as visual or hearing impairments, low literacy, distractive environment.
2. Encourage active participation of the patient and family in the educational process.
3. Teach the action, use, and side effects of oral antidiabetic agents.
   a. Sulfonylurea compounds promote the increased secretion of insulin by the pancreas and partially normalize both receptor and postreceptor defects. Many drug interactions exist, so patient should alert all health care providers of use. Potential adverse reactions include hypoglycemia, photosensitivity, GI upset, allergic reaction, reaction to alcohol, cholestatic jaundice, and blood dyscrasias.
   b. Metformin (Glucophage), a biguanide compound, appears to diminish insulin resistance. It decreases hepatic glucose production and intestinal reabsorption of glucose and increases insulin reception and glucose transport in cells. Many drug interactions exist, so patient should alert all health care providers of its use. Metformin must be used cautiously in renal insufficiency, conditions that may cause dehydration, and hepatic impairment. Potential adverse reactions include GI disturbances, metallic taste, and lactic acidosis (rare).

DRUG ALERT

Lactic acidosis is a rare but potentially fatal complication of metformin. The drug should be discontinued for conditions that predispose to lactic acidosis, including dehydration, alteration in renal function, vomiting and diarrheal illnesses, fasting for surgery and other procedures, imaging studies requiring IV iodinated contrast media, septicemia, heavy alcohol use, and hemodynamic instability.

---

   c. Alpha-glucosidase inhibitors (acarbose [Precose], miglitol [Glyset]) and meglitinide analogues (repaglinide [Prandin]) delay the digestion and absorption of complex carbohydrates (including sucrose or table sugar) into simple sugars such as glucose and fructose, thereby lowering postprandial and fasting glucose levels.
      (i) Alpha-glucosidase inhibitors are contraindicated in inflammatory bowel disease and other conditions of the intestinal tract. They are used cautiously in renal insufficiency and with several other drugs. Flatulence, abdominal pain, and diarrhea are common.
      (ii) Meglitinide analogues interact with many other drugs, must be used cautiously in renal and hepatic dysfunction, and may cause hypoglycemia.
   d. Thiazolidinedione derivatives (rosiglitazone [Avandia] and pioglitazone [Actos]) primarily decrease re-

sistance to insulin in skeletal muscle and adipose tissue without increasing insulin secretion. Secondarily they reduce hepatic glucose production. They should be used cautiously in liver disease and heart failure. Liver function tests should be monitored periodically. Ovulation may occur in anovulatory premenopausal women. Adverse reactions include edema, weight gain, anemia, and elevation in serum transaminases.

 DRUG ALERT

Thiazolidinediones themselves do not cause hypoglycemia; when administered with insulin, however, they increase the risk of hypoglycemia. Be aware that insulin requirements will drop with therapy, so glucose monitoring and insulin adjustments should be done regularly.

Maintaining Skin Integrity

1. Assess feet and legs for skin temperature, sensation, soft tissue injuries, corns, calluses, dryness, hammer toe or bunion deformation, hair distribution, pulses, deep tendon reflexes.
2. Maintain skin integrity by protecting feet from breakdown.
   a. Use heel protectors, special mattresses, foot cradles for patients on bed rest.
   b. Avoid applying drying agents to skin (eg, alcohol).
   c. Apply skin moisturizers to maintain suppleness and prevent cracking and fissures.
3. Instruct patient in foot care guidelines (Procedure Guidelines 25-3).
4. Advise the patient who smokes to stop smoking or reduce if possible, to reduce vasoconstriction and enhance peripheral blood flow. Help patient to establish behavior modification techniques to eliminate smoking in the hospital and to continue them at home for smoking cessation program.

Improving Coping Strategies

1. Discuss with the patient the perceived effect of diabetes on lifestyle, finances, family life, occupation.
2. Explore previous coping strategies and skills that have had positive effects.
3. Encourage patient and family participation in diabetes self-care regimen to foster confidence.
4. Identify available support groups to assist in lifestyle adaptation.
5. Assist family in providing emotional support.

Community and Home Care Considerations

1. A home care/visiting nurse referral can be initiated to follow up on patient education initiated in the hospital or clinic and ensure that the patient has the resources to care for self at home.

2. Patient should be checking fingerstick glucose at home, and glucometer should be checked by home care or clinic nurse periodically to make sure it is properly calibrated and correlates with meter used at clinic or hospital.
3. As long as the home is clean and the patient uses reasonable hygiene, procedures for self glucose monitoring and insulin injection do not need to be sterile. No alcohol preparation of the skin or insulin vial is needed.
4. Insulin syringes may be reused several times, so long as the needle is kept clean and is not dull.
5. Although urine glucose testing is no longer recommended to monitor diabetic condition, the patient may benefit from urine ketone testing, especially when ill. Teach the patient how to test urine with ketone test strip and to notify health care provider if ketosis persists.
6. Ensure that all patients have a handy source of glucose for hypoglycemic episodes. A small tube of glossy decorating gel for cakes, easily carried in a pocket or purse, contains about 15 g glucose and can be squirted in the mouth for fast absorption during a hypoglycemic attack.
7. Draw blood work on a fasting basis (no food or fluids other than water for 8 hours) or ensure that patients attend laboratory appointments for drug monitoring.
   a. For patients taking thiazolidinediones, serum transaminases (AST, ALT) should be monitored every 2 months for a year and then periodically. If levels rise, more frequent monitoring and possibly drug discontinuation will be necessary.
   b. Renal function tests (BUN and serum creatinine) and urine for microalbumin will be monitored periodically.
   c. Fasting plasma glucose and glycated hemoglobin are followed regularly.

Patient Education and Health Maintenance

1. Ongoing education of patient to include advanced skills and rationales for treatment, management.
2. Educational focus—lifestyle management issues, to include sick day management (see Patient Education), exercise adjustments, travel preparations, foot care guidelines, intensive insulin management, and dietary considerations for dining out.
3. For additional information and support, refer to agencies such as American Diabetes Association, Inc., 1660 Duke St., Alexandria, VA 22314, 800-676-4065, *www.diabetes.org*; and American Dietetic Association, 216 West Jackson Blvd., Chicago, IL 60606-6995, 1-800-366-1655.

Outcome-Based Evaluation

- Maintains ideal body weight
- Demonstrates self-injection of insulin with minimal fear
- Hypoglycemia identified and treated appropriately
- Exercises daily
- Verbalizes appropriate use and action of oral hypoglycemic agents
- No skin breakdown
- Verbalizes initial strategies for coping with diabetes

PATIENT EDUCATION GUIDELINES Diabetes Sick Day Guidelines

1. Never omit insulin dosage. Check with health care provider about oral medication. For instance, Glucophage should be withheld if vomiting or in danger of becoming dehydrated.
   - Take, at least, the usual dosage of insulin.
   - Keep regular insulin on hand for supplemental doses as prescribed by health care provider.
2. Monitor blood glucose and urine ketones q 2–4h.
   - Whenever blood glucose is >240 mg/dL, test urine ketones.
   - Record all test results.
3. Drink plenty of fluids.
   - 6–8 oz of fluid every hour is recommended.
   - If unable to eat, drink fluids that contain carbohydrates (eg, fruit juices, regular soda).
4. Contact health care provider if illness becomes severe or unmanageable.
   - Fever, nausea, vomiting, diarrhea increase dehydration
   - Signs and symptoms of infection—redness, swelling, drainage—need immediate attention.
   - Large amount of urine ketones or other signs and symptoms of diabetic ketoacidosis: call health care provider immediately.

PROCEDURE GUIDELINES 25-3   FOOT CARE GUIDELINES

Perform foot care and teach the patient the following guidelines

EQUIPMENT

Mirror (optional)   Moisturizing lotion   Scissors and nail file
Magnifying glass (optional)   Lamb's wool

Teaching Action	Rationale/Comments
1. Inspect the feet carefully and daily for calluses, corns, blisters, abrasions, redness, and nail abnormalities.	1. a. Use a small mirror to check bottom of each foot. b. Use a magnifying glass under good light if eyesight is poor, or have someone else check feet.
2. Bathe the feet daily in warm (never hot) water.	2. a. Do not soak the feet for prolonged periods (soaking is drying). b. Dry feet carefully, especially between the toes.
3. Massage the feet with an absorbable agent.	3. a. Use lanolin, nivea cream, or other cream moisturizers but avoid between the toes to prevent maceration.
4. Prevent moisture between the toes to prevent maceration of the skin.	4. a. Insert lamb's wool between overlapping toes. b. Use foot powder, especially if feet perspire.
5. Wear well-fitting, noncompressive shoes and socks—long enough, wide enough, soft, supple, and low-heeled.	5. a. Buy shoes with a wide toe box for room to wiggle toes without friction. b. Buy shoes in the afternoon—feet are larger in the afternoon than in the morning. c. Have each foot measured before buying shoes—feet enlarge with age. d. Have the measurement taken while standing because foot is larger in the standing position. e. Do not "break in" shoes all at one time. f. Avoid rubber- or plastic-soled shoes, or vinyl shoes, which cause the feet to perspire and aggravate fungal infections. g. Avoid working in soft-soled bedroom slippers or other non-supportive footwear.
6. Go to a podiatrist on a regular basis if corns, calluses, and ingrown toenails are present.	6. a. Cut toenails straight across to prevent ingrown toenails. b. File any rough corners with an emery board.
7. Avoid heat, chemicals, and injuries to the feet.	7. a. Do not go barefoot or expose feet to hot-water bottles, heating pads, caustic solutions, etc. b. Check bath temperature with thermometer or elbow before bathing if neuropathy is present. c. Switch off electric blanket before going to bed; wear socks at night to keep feet warm if necessary. d. Avoid sitting too close to a fire.

PROCEDURE GUIDELINES 25-3   *CONTINUED*

Teaching Action	Rationale
8. Inspect inside of shoes for foreign objects or areas of roughness.	8. a. Inspect seams and lining of shoes for possible areas of pressure or abrasion. b. Avoid the use of constricting sandals, high heels, or boots, which are more likely to cause injury.

9. If an injury occurs to the foot:	9. a. Wash the area with mild soap and water.
	  b. Cover with a dry sterile dressing without adhesive.
	  c. Wear white cotton socks; dye in colored socks and wool may serve as irritants when skin is already irritated.
	  d. Call health care provider.

■ Diabetic Ketoacidosis

Diabetic ketoacidosis (DKA) is an acute complication of diabetes mellitus (usually type 1 DM) characterized by hyperglycemia, ketonuria, acidosis, and dehydration.

Pathophysiology and Etiology

1. Insulin deficiency prevents glucose from being used for energy, forcing the body to metabolize fat for fuel.
2. Free fatty acids, released from the metabolism of fat, are converted to ketone bodies in the liver.
3. Ketone bodies are organic acids that cause metabolic acidosis.
4. Increase in the secretion of glucagon, catecholamines, growth hormone, and cortisol, in response to the hyperglycemia caused by insulin deficiency, accelerates the development of DKA.
5. Osmotic diuresis caused by hyperglycemia creates a shift in electrolytes, with losses in potassium, sodium, phosphate, and water.
6. Caused by inadequate amounts of endogenous or exogenous insulin.
   a. Frequently occurs due to failure to increase the dose of insulin during periods of stress (eg, infection, surgery, pregnancy).
   b. May occur in previously undiagnosed or untreated diabetics.

Clinical Manifestations

Early
1. Polydipsia, polyuria
2. Fatigue, malaise, drowsiness
3. Anorexia, nausea, vomiting
4. Abdominal pains, muscle cramps

Later
1. Kussmaul respiration (deep respirations)
2. Fruity, sweet breath
3. Hypotension, weak pulse
4. Stupor and coma

Diagnostic Evaluation

1. Serum glucose level is usually elevated over 300 mg/dL; may be as high as 1,000 mg/dL.

2. Serum and urine ketone bodies are present.
3. Serum bicarbonate and pH are decreased due to metabolic acidosis, and PCO_2 is decreased as a respiratory compensation mechanism.
4. Serum sodium and potassium levels may be low, normal, or high due to fluid shifts and dehydration, despite total body depletion.
5. Blood urea nitrogen (BUN), creatinine, hemoglobin, and hematocrit are elevated due to dehydration.

NURSING ALERT

 Severity of DKA cannot be determined by serum glucose levels; acidosis may be prominent with glucose level of 200 mg/dL or less.

---

6. Urine glucose is present in high concentration and specific gravity is increased, reflecting osmotic diuresis and dehydration.

Management

1. IV fluids to replace losses from osmotic diuresis, vomiting.
2. IV insulin drip—regular insulin only infused to increase glucose utilization and decrease lipolysis.
3. Electrolyte replacement—sodium chloride and phosphate as required, potassium chloride and bicarbonate based on laboratory results.

Complications

1. Premature discontinuation of IV insulin can result in prolongation of DKA.
2. Too-rapid infusion of IV fluids in cases of severe dehydration can cause cerebral edema and death.
3. Failure to institute subcutaneous insulin injections before discontinuation of IV insulin can result in extended hyperglycemia.

Nursing Assessment

1. Assess skin for dehydration—poor turgor, flushing, dry mucous membranes.
2. Observe for cardiac changes reflecting dehydration, metabolic acidosis, and electrolyte imbalance—hypotension; tachycardia; weak pulse; electrocardiographic

changes, including elevated P wave, flattened T wave or inverted, prolonged QT interval.

3. Assess respiratory status—Kussmaul breathing, acetone breath characteristic of metabolic acidosis.
4. Perform gastrointestinal assessment—nausea, vomiting, extreme thirst, abdominal bloating and cramping, diarrhea.
5. Determine genitourinary symptoms—nocturia, polyuria.
6. Observe for neurologic signs—crying, restlessness, twitching, tremors, drowsiness, lethargy, headache, decreased reflexes.
7. Interview family or significant other regarding precipitating events to episode of DKA.
   a. Patient self-care management before hospitalization
   b. Unusual events that may have precipitated episode (eg, chest pain, trauma, illness)

Nursing Diagnoses
- Fluid Volume Deficit related to hyperglycemia
- Ineffective Management of Therapeutic Regimen related to failure to increase insulin during illness

Nursing Interventions
Restoring Fluid and Electrolyte Balance
1. Assess blood pressure and heart rate frequently, depending on patient's condition; assess skin turgor and temperature.
2. Monitor intake and output every hour.
3. Replace fluids as ordered through peripheral IV line.
4. Monitor urine specific gravity to assess fluid changes.
5. Monitor capillary blood glucoses frequently.
6. Assess for symptoms of hypokalemia—fatigue, anorexia, nausea, vomiting, muscle weakness, decreased bowel sounds, paresthesia, arrhythmias, flat T waves, S-T segment depression.

NURSING ALERT

Electrolyte levels may not reflect the total body deficit of potassium (primarily) and sodium (to a lesser extent) due to compartment shifts and fluid volume loss. Replacement is necessary despite normal to high values.

---

7. Administer replacement electrolytes and insulin as ordered. Flush the entire IV infusion set with solution containing insulin and discard the first 50 mL, because plastic bags and tubing may absorb some insulin and the initial solution may contain decreased concentration of insulin.

DRUG ALERT

Any interruption in insulin administration may result in re-accumulation of ketone bodies and worsening acidosis. Glucose will normalize before acidosis resolves so IV insulin is continued until bicarbonate levels normalize and subcutaneous insulin takes effect and the patient starts eating.

---

8. Monitor serum glucose, bicarbonate, and pH levels periodically.
9. Provide reassurance about improvement of condition and that correction of fluid imbalance will help reduce discomfort.

Preventing Further Episodes of DKA
1. Review with patients precipitating events and causes of DKA.
2. Assist patient in identifying warning signs and symptoms of DKA.
3. Instruct patient in sick day guidelines (see p. 856).

Patient Education and Health Maintenance
1. Ensure that patient and caretakers can demonstrate drawing up and administering insulin in the proper dose, blood glucose monitoring, and urine ketone testing.
2. Ensure that patient and caretakers know whom to notify in the event of hyperglycemia, stressful situation, or symptoms of DKA.

Outcome-Based Evaluation
- Blood pressure and heart rate stable; glucose and bicarbonate levels improving
- Verbalizes sick day guidelines correctly

◼ Hyperglycemic Hyperosmolar Nonketotic Syndrome (HHNKS)

This is an acute complication of diabetes mellitus (particularly type 2 DM) characterized by hyperglycemia, dehydration, and hyperosmolarity, but little or no ketosis.

Pathophysiology and Etiology
1. Prolonged hyperglycemia with glucosuria produces osmatic diuresis.
2. Loss of water, sodium, and potassium results in severe dehydration, causing hypovolemia and hemoconcentration.
3. Hyperosmolarity is a result of excessive blood sugar and increasing sodium concentration in dehydration.
4. Insulin continues to be produced at a level that prevents ketosis.
5. Increased blood viscosity decreases blood flow to the organs, creating tissue hypoxia.
6. Intracellular fluid and electrolyte shifts produce neurologic signs and symptoms.
7. Caused by inadequate amounts of endogenous/exogenous insulin to control hyperglycemia.
   a. Precipitating event may occur, such as cardiac failure, burn, or chronic illness that increases need for insulin.
   b. Use of therapeutic agents that increase blood glucose levels (eg, glucocorticoids, immunosuppressive agents).
   c. Use of therapeutic procedures that cause stress or increase blood glucose levels (eg, hyperosmolar hyperalimenation, peritoneal dialysis).

Clinical Manifestations
Early
1. Polyuria, dehydration
2. Fatigue, malaise
3. Nausea, vomiting
Later
1. Hypothermia
2. Seizures, stupor, coma
3. Muscle weakness

Diagnostic Evaluation
1. Serum glucose and osmolality are greatly elevated.
2. Serum and urine ketone bodies are minimal to absent.
3. Serum sodium and potassium levels may be elevated, depending on degree of dehydration, despite total body losses.
4. BUN and creatinine may be elevated due to dehydration.
5. Urine specific gravity is elevated due to dehydration.

Management
1. Correct fluid and electrolyte imbalances with IV fluids.
2. Provide insulin via IV drip to lower plasma glucose.
3. Evaluate complications, such as stupor, seizures, or shock, and treat appropriately.
4. Identify and treat underlying illnesses or events that precipitated HHNKS.

Complications
1. Too rapid infusion of IV fluids can cause cerebral edema and death.
2. HHNKS is a medical emergency that, if not treated properly, can cause death.
3. Patients who become comatose will need nasogastric tubes to prevent aspiration.

Nursing Assessment
1. Assess level of consciousness.
2. Assess for dehydration—poor turgor, flushing, dry mucous membranes.
3. Assess cardiovascular status for shock—rapid, thready pulse, cool extremities, hypotension, ECG changes.
4. Interview family or significant other regarding precipitating events to episode of HHNKS.
   a. Evaluate patient's self-care regimen before hospitalization.
   b. Determine any events, treatments, or drugs that may have caused the event.

Nursing Diagnoses
- Fluid Volume Deficit related to severe dehydration
- Risk for Aspiration related to reduced level of consciousness and vomiting

Nursing Interventions
Restoring Fluid Balance
1. Assess patient for increasing signs and symptoms of dehydration, hyperglycemia, or electrolyte imbalance.
2. Institute fluid replacement therapy as ordered (usually normal or half strength saline initially), maintaining patent IV line.
3. Assess patient for signs and symptoms of fluid overload and cerebral edema as IV therapy progresses.
4. Administer regular insulin IV as ordered, and add dextrose to IV infusion as blood glucose falls below 300 mg/dL, to prevent hypoglycemia.
5. Monitor hydration status by monitoring hourly intake and output and urine specific gravity.

PREVENTING ASPIRATION
1. Assess patient's level of consciousness and ability to handle oral secretions.
   a. Cough and gag reflex
   b. Ability to swallow
2. Properly position patient to reduce possibility of aspiration.
   a. Elevate head of bed unless contraindicated.
   b. If nausea is present, use side-lying position.
3. Suction as often as needed to maintain patent airway.
4. Withhold oral intake until patient is no longer in danger of aspiration.
5. Insert nasogastric tube as indicated for gastric decompression.
6. Monitor respiratory rate and breath sounds for signs of aspiration pneumonia.
7. Provide mouth care to maintain adequate mucosal hydration.

Patient Education and Health Maintenance
1. Advise the patient and family that it may take 3 to 5 days for symptoms to resolve.
2. Instruct patient and family in signs and symptoms of hyperglycemia and use of sick day guidelines (see p. 856).
3. Explain possible causes of HHNKS.
4. Review any changes in medication, activity, meal plan, or glucose monitoring for home care. It may not be necessary to continue insulin therapy following HHNKS; many patients can be treated with diet and oral agents.

Outcome-Based Evaluation
- Blood pressure stable, dehydration resolved
- No evidence of aspiration

SELECTED REFERENCES
Alberti, K.G., Limmet, P., & DeFronzo, R.A. (Eds.). (1997). *International textbook of diabetes mellitus* (2nd ed.). New York: John Wiley.
American Diabetes Association. (1998). Clinical practice recommendations. *Diabetes Care, 21*(suppl.), s1–99.
Aviles-Santa, L. et al. (1999). Effects of metformin in patients with poorly controlled, insulin-treated type 2 diabetes mellitus: A randomized, double-blinded, placebo-controlled trial. *Annals of Internal Medicine, 131*(15), 182–188.
Bell, S.J. & Forse, R.A. (1999). Nutritional management of hypoglycemia. *The Diabetic Educator, 25*(1), 41–47.

Boland, E. & Savoye, M. (1997). Nutritional strategies for adolescents with insulin-dependent diabetes mellitus. *Lippincott's Primary Care Practice, 1*(3), 270–284.

The Diabetes Control and Complications Trial/Epidemiology of Diabetes Interventions and Complications Research Group. (2000). Retinopathy and nephropathy in patients with type 1 diabetes four years after a trial of intensive therapy. *New England Journal of Medicine, 342*(3), 381–389.

Expert Committee on the Diagnosis and Classification of Diabetes Mellitus. (1997). Report of the expert committee on the diagnosis and classification of diabetes mellitus. *Diabetes Care, 20,* 1183–1197.

Fleming, D.R. (1999). Challenging traditional insulin injection practices. *American Journal of Nursing, 99*(2), 72–74.

Folsom, A.R., Kushi, L.H., & Hong, C.P. (2000). Physical activity and incident diabetes mellitus in postmenopausal women. *American Journal of Public Health, 90*(2), 134–138.

Fonesca, V., et al. (2000). Effects of metformin and rosiglitazone combination therapy in patients with type 2 diabetes mellitus: A randomized controlled trial. *Journal of the American Medical Association,* (7), 1695–1702.

Gu, K., Cowie, C.C., & Harris, M.I. (1999). Diabetes and decline in heart disease mortality in US adults. *Journal of the American Medical Association, 281*(14), 1291–1297.

Gutowski, C. (1999). Understanding new pharmacolgic therapy for type 2 diabetes. *Nurse Practitioner, 24*(6), 15–21.

Halpin-Landry, J.E. & Goldsmith, S. (1999). Feet first: Diabetes care. *American Journal of Nursing, 99*(2), 26–33.

Hannele, Y.J., et al. (1999). Comparison of bedtime insulin regimens in patients with type 2 diabetes mellitus: A randomized, controlled trial. *Annals of Internal Medicine, 130*(5), 389–396.

Ko, G.T., Chan, J.C., Yeung, V.T., Chow, C., Tsang, L.W., Li, J.K., So,W., Wai, H.P. & Cockram, C.S. (1998). Combined use of a fasting plasma glucose concentration and HbA1c or fructosamine predicts the likelihood of having diabetes in high risk subjects. *Diabetes Care, 21*(8), 1221–1225.

Ling, J., Hu, M., Hagerup, T. & Campbell, RK. (1999). Lispro insulin: Absorption and stability in selected intravenous devices. *Diabetes Educator, 25*(2), 237–245.

Lipkin, E. (1999). New strategies for the treatment of type 2 diabetes. *Journal of the American Dietetic Association, 99*(3), 329–334.

Peragallo-Dottko, V. (1995). Aspiration of the subcutaneous insulin injecton: Clinical evaluation of needle size and amount of subcutaneous fat. *Diabetes Educator, 21,* 291–296.

Roper, N.A. & Bilous, R.W. (1998). Resolution of lipohypertrophy following change of short-acting insulin to insulin lispro (Humalog). *Diabetes Medicine, 12,* 1063–1064.

Rosskamp, R. & Park, G. (1999). Long-acting insulin analogs. *Diabetes Care, 22*(suppl. 2), 109–113.

Schoenberg, N.E., Amey, C.H., & Coward, R.T. (1998). Diabetes knowledge and sources of information among African American women. *Diabetes Educator, 24*(3), 319–324.

Sengewaold, J.M. (1999). Update on diabetes medications. *Journal of Emergency Nursing, 25*(1), 28–30.

Spollett, G. (1997). Diet strategies in the treatment of non-insulin dependent diabetes mellitus. *Lippincott's Primary Care Practice, 1*(3), 295–304.

Tamada, J.A., Garg, S., Javonovic, L., Pitzer, K.R., Fermi, M.S., & Potts, R.O. (1999). Noninvasive glucose monitoring: Comprehensive clinical results. *Journal of the American Medical Association, 282*(19), 1839–1844.

Testa, M.A. & Simonson, D.C. (1998). Health economic benefits and quality of life during improved glycemic control in patients with type 2 diabetes mellitus: a randomized controlled, double-blind trial. *Journal of the American Medical Association, 280,* 1490–1496.

Turner, R.C. et al. (1999). Glycemic control with diet, sulfonylurea, metformin, or insulin in patients with type 2 diabetes mellitus: Progressive requirement for multiple therapies (UKPDS 49). *Journal of the American Medical Association, 281,* 2005–2012.

Umeh, L., Wallhagen, M., & Nicoloff, N. (1999). Identifying diabetic patients at high risk for amputation. *Nurse Practitioner, 24*(8), 56–68.

Warren-Boulton, E., Greenberg, R., Lising, M., & Gallivan, J. (1999). An update on primary care management of type 2 diabetes. *The Nurse Practitioner, 24*(12), 14–31.

Winslow, E.H. & Jacobson, A.F. (1999). Saving limbs with the Semmes-Weinstein monofilament. *American Journal of Nursing, 99*(2), 76.

UNIT VIII
Hematologic Health

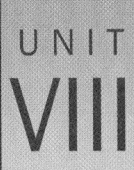

Hematologic Disorders

GENERAL OVERVIEW

Blood, the body fluid circulating through the heart, arteries, capillaries and veins, consists of plasma and cellular components. Plasma, the fluid portion, accounts for 55% of the blood volume and is composed of 92% water, 7% protein, and 1% inorganic salts; nonprotein organic substances such as urea; dissolved gases; hormones; and enzymes. Plasma proteins include albumin, fibrinogen, and globulins. Cellular components include erythrocytes (red blood cells), leukocytes and lymphocytes (white blood cells), and platelets. These cells are derived from pluripotent stem cells in the bone marrow, a process known as hematopoiesis (Figure 26-1). The cellular components of blood account for 45% of the blood volume.

◼ Characteristics of Cellular Components

Blood has multiple functions that are carried out by plasma or the cellular components (Table 26-1).

Erythrocytes (Red Blood Cells)

1. Enucleated, biconcave disc.
2. Approximately 5 million erythrocytes per cubic millimeter of blood.

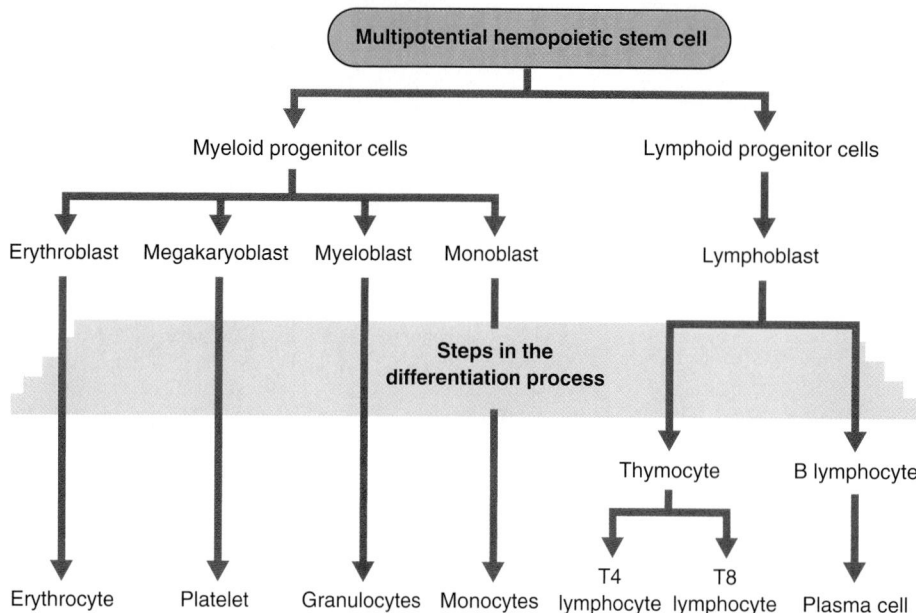

FIGURE 26-1 Steps in differentiation of blood cells.

TABLE 26-1 Functions of Blood		
Function	**Method**	**Cells and Substances Involved**
Oxygen and carbon dioxide transport	Binding to hemoglobin; dissolved in plasma	Erythrocyte Hemoglobin Plasma
Nutrient and metabolite transport	Bound to plasma proteins; dissolved in plasma	Plasma proteins Plasma
Hormone transport	In plasma	Plasma
Transport of waste products to kidneys and liver	In plasma	Plasma
Transport of cells and substances involved in immune reactions	In plasma to site of infection or foreign body	Granulocytes Monocytes Lymphocytes Immunoglobulins Other substances
Clotting at breaks in blood vessels	Hemostasis	Platelets Clotting factors
Maintenance of fluid balance	Blood volume regulation	Water Electrolytes
Body temperature regulation	Peripheral vasoconstriction or dilation	
Maintenance of acid—base balance	Acid-base regulation	Electrolytes

3. Cell contents consist primarily of hemoglobin, essential for oxygen transport. Whole blood contains 14 to 15 g of hemoglobin per 100 mL of blood.
4. Circulate about 115 to 130 days before elimination by reticuloendothelial system, primarily in spleen and liver.

Leukocytes (White Blood Cells) (Table 26-2)
1. Approximately 5,000 to 10,000 leukocytes per cubic millimeter of blood.
2. Classified as granulocytes or mononuclear leukocytes.
   a. Granulocytes account for about 70% of all white blood cells; have abundant granules in cytoplasm; include neutrophils, basophils, and eosinophils.
   b. Mononuclear leukocytes have single-lobed nucleus and granule-free cytoplasm; include monocytes and lymphocytes.

Platelets (Thrombocytes)
1. Approximately 150,000 to 450,000 platelets per cubic millimeter of blood.
2. Small particles without nuclei arise as a result of budding from giant cells (megakaryocytes) in bone marrow.
3. Primary function is to control bleeding through hemostasis.

ASSESSMENT

◼ Subjective Data
The patient who presents with a hematologic disorder may have a disruption of the hematologic, immune, and/or coagulation system, producing a diverse array of symptoms.

TABLE 26-2 Characteristics of White Blood Cells

Cell	Major Function	Physical Characteristics
Neutrophil	Ingest and destroy microorganisms (phagocytosis)	Small cell, multi-lobed nucleus, most plentiful leukocyte
Eosinophil	Host resistance to helminthic infections; also allergic response	Bilobed nucleus; red-staining granules
Basophil	Allergic response	Bilobed nucleus; granules containing heparin and histamine
Monocyte	Phagocytosis	Large cell, kidney-shaped nucleus
B lymphocyte	Produce antibodies (immuno-globulins); humoral immunity	Small, agranular
T lymphocyte	Regulation of immune response; cellular immunity	Small, agranular; include cytotoxic, helper (T4), and suppressor (T8) T cells; identified by surface markers

Patients often present with vague complaints of fatigue, frequent infections, swollen glands, and bleeding tendencies. Characterize these complaints and obtain a review of systems, concentrating on the neurologic, respiratory, cardiovascular, gastrointestinal, genitourinary, and integumentary systems to look for more clues of hematologic dysfunction.

◼ Review of Systems

1. Skin and mucous membranes: Any bruises, infections, drainage, or bleeding from wound sites?
2. Neurologic: Any dizziness, tingling or numbness (paresthesias), headache, forgetfulness or confusion, difficulty walking (disturbance in gait), tiredness (fatigue), weakness?
3. Respiratory: Experiencing shortness of breath, especially on exertion?
4. Cardiovascular: Chest pain or feelings of funny heart beats in your chest (palpitations)?
5. Gastrointestinal: Any bleeding from your gums, abdominal pain, black stools, or blood-streaked vomit (emesis)? How about any mouth sores, rectal pain, or diarrhea?
6. Genitourinary: Describe your menstrual flow. How often do you change pads? For how many days? Any blood in your urine or discomfort on urination?

Key History Questions

1. What are your present medications? Do you take any over-the-counter medications, vitamins, herbals, or nutritional supplements? What else have you taken in the past several months?
2. What medical problems have you had in the past? Any surgery? Ask specifically about partial or total gastrectomy, splenic injury or splenectomy, tendency to bleed (eg, with dental procedures), infectious diseases, human immunodeficiency virus (HIV) infection, cancer.
3. What is your occupation? Ask about exposure to substances such as benzene, pesticides, and ionizing radiation.
4. Do you have a family history of hematologic or malignant disorder?
5. Determine the social history and lifestyle. Do you use recreational drugs or alcohol? What is your pattern of sexual activity?

◼ Physical Examination

Physical examination may produce abnormal assessment findings in various body systems, caused by anemia, uncontrolled bleeding or clotting, or altered immune function that leads to infection in patients with hematologic disorders. Perform a systematic physical examination, paying careful attention to the cardiovascular, respiratory, and integumentary systems.

Key Examination Findings

1. Tachycardia; dyspnea; shiny smooth tongue; ataxia; pallor of conjunctivae, nail beds, lips, and oral mucosa—suggest anemia.
2. Decreased blood pressure, altered level of consciousness, hematuria, tarry stools, petechiae, bleeding sites—suggest altered clotting.
3. Fever; tachycardia; abnormal breath sounds; delirium; oral lesions; erythema, swelling, tenderness, and drainage of the skin—suggest infection.

DIAGNOSTIC TESTS

◼ Laboratory Studies

Laboratory studies routinely done for patients with hematologic disorders include complete blood count (CBC), blood smear, and iron profile. Blood samples for these tests may be obtained by skin puncture or venipuncture (Procedure Guidelines 26-1 and 26-2).

Complete Blood Count
Description

1. Generally includes absolute numbers or percentages of erythrocytes, leukocytes, platelets, hemoglobin, and hematocrit in blood sample.
   a. Erythrocyte (RBC) indices can be done to provide information on the size, hemoglobin concentration, and hemoglobin weight of an average RBC; aids in diagnosis and classification of anemias.

b. Leukocyte (WBC) differential—can be done to determine the percentage of each type of granulocyte (neutrophils, eosinophils, and basophils) and non-granulocytes (lymphocytes and monocytes).
2. Absolute value of each is determined by multiplying the percentage by the total number of WBC.
3. Used to evaluate infection or potential for infection and identify various types of leukemia.

Nursing and Patient Care Considerations

Blood sample can be drawn at any time without fasting or patient preparation; can be obtained by either venipuncture or skin puncture (if only small amount of blood is needed, but values may be lower in capillary blood).

Blood Smear
Description

Blood specimen prepared for microscopic viewing using appropriate stains, allowing visual analysis of numbers and characteristics of cells; can identify abnormal cells of certain anemias, leukemias, and other disorders that affect the blood stream.

Nursing and Patient Care Considerations

Can be done from blood sample drawn for CBC; no additional sample or patient preparation is necessary.

Iron Profile
Description

Test completed on blood sample that generally includes levels of serum ferritin, iron, total iron-binding capacity, folate, vitamin B_{12}, and is used to determine type and severity of anemia.

Nursing and Patient Care Considerations

Recent administration of chloramphenicol, oral contraceptives, iron supplements, and corticotropin (ACTH) may affect results of serum iron and iron-binding capacity. No patient preparation needed.

PROCEDURE GUIDELINES 26-1   **OBTAINING BLOOD BY SKIN PUNCTURE**

EQUIPMENT

Disposable lancet   Alcohol sponges and dry sterile gauze pads
Pipette and tubing   or
Slides   Prepared alcohol prep pads
Disposable gloves

PROCEDURE

Nursing Action	Rationale
PERFORMANCE PHASE	
1. Wash hands and put on gloves.	1. Protects health care worker from possible exposure to blood.
2. Cleanse site (preferably ball of finger) with alcohol and dry with sterile gauze square.	2. If any alcohol remains, it will alter red cell morphology; also, blood will not collect into a compact drop but will run down the patient's finger.
3. Create stasis by pressing on the distal joint of the finger to produce redness at the end of the finger.	
4. Use a sterile disposable lancet or an automated lancet.	4. This avoids the possibility of the transference of blood-borne viral diseases.
5. Prick the skin sharply and quickly with the lancet.	5. Pricking the skin sharply and quickly minimizes pain and produces a free-flowing sample.
6. Release pressure on the finger. Wipe off the first drop of blood.	6. Epithelial or endothelial cells may be found in the first drop of blood and may render the count inaccurate. Also, platelets will begin to clump immediately in the blood at the puncture site.
7. Allow the blood to flow freely with an adequate puncture.	7. Pressing out the blood dilutes it with tissue fluid.
8. Obtain the blood sample:	
a. Fill the pipette or microhematocrit tube.	
b. Make blood slides according to the study required.	b. Gently touch the drop of blood to glass slides or cover slip.
9. Apply pressure over the wound with a dry gauze sponge until bleeding stops.	
10. Remove gloves, wash hands. Dispose of equipment and supplies in approved containers.	10. Protects health care workers from possible exposure to blood.

PROCEDURE GUIDELINES 26-2   OBTAINING BLOOD BY VENIPUNCTURE

EQUIPMENT

70% alcohol
Dry sterile sponges
5- and 10-mL syringe
Disposable gloves

No. 20-gauge needle(s)
or
Vacutainer assembly

PROCEDURE

Nursing Action	Rationale
PERFORMANCE PHASE	
1. Reassure the patient. Explain that relatively little blood will be taken.	1. The patient is reassured when the nurse displays self-assurance and competence in relating to people and when performing technical skills.
2. Wash hands and put on gloves.	2. Protects health care worker from possible exposure to blood.
3. Instruct the patient to extend his arm; the arm should be held straight at the elbow.	
4. Apply the tourniquet directly above the elbow with just sufficient pressure to prevent venous return.	4. A tourniquet increases venous pressure and makes the vein more prominent and easier to enter.
5. Inspect the area to visualize the vein, including the antecubital area, wrist, dorsum (back) of hand, and top of foot (if necessary). Palpate the vein.	5. Select a vein that is visible, palpable, and well fixed to surrounding tissue so that it does not roll away. (Not all veins are visible; some may be deep and can only be palpated.)
6. Cleanse the skin with iodine and alcohol. Dry.	6. Cleansing the skin reduces pathogens.
7. Fix chosen vein with the thumb and draw the skin taut immediately below the site before inserting needle to stabilize the vein.	7. The vein may roll beneath the skin when the needle approaches its outer surface (especially in elderly and extremely thin patients).
8. Hold the syringe between the thumb and last three fingers with the bevel up and directly in line with the course of the vein. Insert the needle quickly and smoothly under the skin and into the vein.	
9. Obtain blood sample by gently pulling back on the plunger.	9. Use minimal suction to prevent hemolysis of blood and collapse of the vein.
10. Release the tourniquet as soon as specimen is obtained.	
11. Withdraw the needle slowly.	11. Slow withdrawal of the needle is less painful.
12. Apply a sterile dry gauze to puncture site and request patient to apply gentle but firm pressure to site for 2–4 min.	12. Firm pressure over the puncture site prevents leakage of blood into surrounding tissues with subsequent hematoma development. Merely flexing the arm may not prevent a hematoma, as the vein can slip to the side of the area where pressure is applied.
13. Make the blood smear from the needle as desired.	
14. Remove the needle from the syringe. As soon as possible after drawing the blood, gently eject the blood sample into a test tube containing an anticoagulant.	14. Slowly transfer the blood into the test tube without forming bubbles.
15. Invert the tube gently several times to mix blood with anticoagulant.	15. For some tests, the blood is allowed to coagulate in the test tube.
16. Label specimens correctly and send to laboratory immediately.	16. Specimens should go to the laboratory with a minimum of delay for optimum reliability.
17. Dispose needle and syringe in appropriate containers to avoid possible spread of blood-borne viral diseases. Clean all spills with 10% bleach solution. Remove gloves and wash hands.	

Other Diagnostic Procedures

Bone Marrow Aspiration

Description

1. Aspiration of bone marrow from the iliac crest or sternum to obtain specimen to examine microscopically and to perform a biopsy (Procedure Guidelines 26-3).
2. Purposes include diagnosis of hematologic disorders; monitoring of course of illness and response to treatment; diagnosis of other disorders, such as primary and metastatic tumors, infectious diseases, and certain granulomas; and isolation of bacteria and other pathogens by culture.

Nursing and Patient Care Considerations

1. Give medication for pain and anxiety before or after the procedure as ordered.
2. Watch for bleeding and hematoma formation after procedure.

Lymph Node Biopsy

Description

1. Surgical excision or needle aspiration usually of a superficial lymph node in the cervical, supraclavicular, axillary, or inguinal region.
2. Performed to determine the cause of lymph node enlargement, to distinguish between benign and malignant lymph node tumors, and to stage metastatic carcinoma.

Nursing and Patient Care Considerations

1. Local anesthetic is usually given.
2. Specimen is placed in normal saline or 10% formaldehyde solution for transportation to the laboratory for cytologic and histologic evaluation.

PROCEDURE GUIDELINES 26-3	BONE MARROW ASPIRATION AND BIOPSY

EQUIPMENT

Bone marrow aspiration tray	Skin antiseptic
Marrow aspiration needles with stylets	Masks and protective eyewear for physician and nurse
Towels	(check institution's policy)
No. 25- and 22-gauge needles	Laboratory equipment
Two 25-mL syringes	Coverslips
Three 5-mL syringes	Microscopic slides
Local anesthetic (1% procaine or xylocaine)	Test tubes (plain and heparinized)
Sterile gauze squares	Scalpel blade and handle
Sterile gloves, drape	

PROCEDURE

Nursing Action	Rationale
PREPARATORY PHASE	
1. Explain the procedure to the patient. Tell patient when the skin will be marked, antiseptic applied, and the needle puncture performed.	1. An explanation helps the patient to cope with anticipated stress. Tactile sensations (pressure, cold) can be misinterpreted as pain unless the patient is forewarned.
2. Give analgesic and/or tranquilizer as requested, 30 min before procedure. May not be necessary for aspiration.	2. Analgesic and/or sedative may minimize pain, discomfort, and anxiety during procedure.
3. Place the patient in prone or supine position.	
4. The following sites are most frequently used:	
a. Posterior superior iliac crest	
b. Anterior iliac crest (if patient is very obese)	
ILIAC CREST ASPIRATION/BIOPSY	
Performance Phase (Nurse Assists Physician)	
1. Position the patient on the abdomen (prone) or on side with top knee flexed.	
a. The posterior iliac crest is located and marked.	a. The iliac crest provides a large marrow cavity at the posterior superior iliac spine away from nearby abdominal organs.
b. The skin area is prepared and draped. The marked area is infiltrated with local anesthetic through the skin and subcutaneous tissue to the periosteum of the bone.	b. Tell the patient he will experience a needle prick followed by a burning sensation. The periosteum is the region of greatest sensitivity.
c. A small incision may be made.	c. The biopsy needle is large, and a small incision facilitates insertion.

PROCEDURE GUIDELINES 26-3   *CONTINUED*

Nursing Action	Rationale
d. The bone marrow needle, with stylet in place, is introduced through the incision.	d. The needle is pointed toward the anterior superior iliac spine and brought into contact with the posterior iliac spine.
e. The needle is advanced and rotated by using firm and steady pressure. When the needle is felt to enter the outer cortex of the bone marrow cavity, the stylet is removed and the syringe attached. Negative pressure is applied, and a small volume of blood and marrow is aspirated.	e. There is usually decreased resistance when the bone marrow cavity is entered. The actual aspiration may cause brief pain, and the patient should be forewarned. Bone marrow appears rusty-red and normally has a thick, fluid-like consistency.
f. A biopsy is taken by using a special needle equipped with a sharp cutting edge and a hollow core.	
g. After removal of needle, apply pressure to site and dressing.	g. Prevents bleeding from puncture site. Dressing keeps site clean and dry until healed.

GENERAL PROCEDURES AND TREATMENT MODALITIES

■ Splenectomy

The spleen is a fist-sized organ located in the upper left quadrant of the abdomen. It includes a central "white pulp" where storage and some proliferation of lymphocytes and other leukocytes occurs, and a peripheral "red pulp" involved in fetal erythropoiesis, and later in erythrocyte destruction and the conversion of hemoglobin to bilirubin. It may be surgically removed because of trauma or to treat certain hemolytic or malignant disorders with accompanying splenomegaly.

Preoperative Management

1. For general aspects of preoperative nursing management, see page 112.
2. Stabilization of preexisting condition:
   a. For trauma: volume replacement with intravenous (IV) fluids, evacuation of stomach via nasogastric tube to prevent aspiration, urinary catheterization to monitor urinary output, assessment for pneumothorax or hemothorax and possible chest tube placement.
   b. For hemolytic or malignant disorder with accompanying thrombocytopenia: coagulation studies, administration of coagulation factors (e.g., vitamin K, fresh frozen plasma, cryoprecipitate), platelet and red cell transfusions.
3. Preoperative pulmonary evaluation and teaching.
4. For patient undergoing elective splenectomy, polyvalent pneumococcal vaccine 10 to 14 days before procedure.

Postoperative Management

1. For general aspects of postoperative nursing management, see page 116.
2. Prevention of respiratory complications: hypoventilation and limited diaphragmatic movement, atelectasis of left lower lobe, pneumonia, left pleural effusion.
3. Monitoring for hemorrhage.
4. Administration of narcotics for pain and observance for side effects.
5. Monitoring for fever.
   a. Postsplenectomy fever—mild, transient fever is expected.
   b. Persistent fever may indicate subphrenic abscess or hematoma; instruct patient to report.
6. Monitoring daily platelet count: thrombocytosis (elevation of platelet count) may appear a few days after splenectomy and may persist during first 2 weeks.

Potential Complications

1. Pancreatitis and fistula formation: tail of pancreas is anatomically close to splenic hilum.
2. Hemorrhage.
3. Atelectasis and pneumonia.
4. Overwhelming postsplenectomy infection (OPSI)—increased risk of developing a life-threatening bacterial infection with encapsulated organisms, such as *Streptococcus pneumoniae*, *Neisseria meningitides*, or *Haemophilus influenzae*.

NURSING ALERT

The risk of OPSI is highest soon after splenectomy and in patients whose splenectomy occurred during childhood or for a malignant disease. Early symptoms include fever and malaise; the infection may progress within hours to sepsis and death, with a mortality rate as high as 50% to 70%. Patient education after splenectomy should include the risks of OPSI, recognition of early symptoms and prompt seeking of medical attention, and the use of vaccinations against these bacteria (such as the polyvalent pneumococcal vaccine), and in some cases, prophylactic antibiotics.

Nursing Diagnoses

• Ineffective Breathing Pattern related to pain and guarding of surgical incision

- Risk for Fluid Volume Deficit related to hemorrhage caused by surgery of highly vascular organ
- Risk for Injury (thromboembolism) related to thrombocytosis
- Risk for Infection related to surgical incision and removal of the spleen
- Pain related to surgical incision

Nursing Interventions
Maintaining Effective Breathing
1. Assess breath sounds and report absent, diminished, or adventitious sounds.
2. Assist with aggressive chest physiotherapy and incentive spirometry.
3. Encourage early and progressive mobilization.

Monitoring for Hemorrhage
1. Monitor vital signs frequently and as condition warrants.
2. Measure abdominal girth and report abdominal distention.
3. Assess for pain and report increasing pain.
4. Prepare patient for surgical reexploration if bleeding is suspected.

Avoiding Thromboembolic Complications
1. Monitor platelet count daily.
2. If elevated, assess for possible thromboembolism.
   a. Assess skin color, temperature, and pulses.
   b. Advise patient to report chest pain, shortness of breath, pain, or weakness.

Preventing Infection
1. Assess surgical incision daily or if increased pain, fever, or foul smell.
2. Maintain meticulous handwashing and change dressings using sterile technique.
3. Teach patient to report signs of infection (fever, malaise) immediately.

Relieving Pain
1. Administer narcotics or teach self-administration, as prescribed and as necessary to maintain level of comfort.
2. Warn patient of side effects, such as nausea and drowsiness; watch for hypotension and decreased respirations.
3. Teach the use of nonpharmacologic methods, such as the use of music, relaxation breathing, progressive muscle relaxation, distraction, and imagery to help to manage pain.
4. Document dosage of medications and response to medication.
5. Ensure patient has analgesics for use postdischarge.

Patient Education and Health Maintenance
1. Teach care of incision.
2. Encourage to gradually increase activity according to guidelines given by surgeon.
3. Advise proper rest, nutrition, and stress avoidance while recovering from surgery.

4. Encourage follow up as directed by surgeon and primary care provider to maintain current pneumococcal vaccination.
5. Encourage patient to seek prompt medical attention for any infections and to contact health care provider immediately for high fever.

Outcome-Based Evaluation
- Respirations unlabored, breath sounds clear
- Vital signs stable, abdominal girth unchanged
- Pulses strong, extremities warm and without pallor or cyanosis
- Afebrile, no purulent drainage from incision
- Verbalizes decreased pain

THE ANEMIAS

Anemia is the lack of sufficient circulating hemoglobin to deliver oxygen to tissues. Anemia has multiple causes, and is often associated with other diseases and disorders (eg, renal disease, cancer, Crohn's disease, alcoholism). Anemia may be caused by inadequate production of red blood cells, abnormal hemolysis and sequestration, or blood loss. Iron deficiency anemia, pernicious anemia, folic acid deficiency, and aplastic anemia are the anemias most often seen in adults.

Iron Deficiency Anemia (Microcytic, Hypochromic)
Iron deficiency anemia is a condition in which the total body iron content is decreased below a normal level, affecting hemoglobin synthesis. Red blood cells appear pale and are small.

Pathophysiology and Etiology
1. The most common cause is insufficient intake (weight loss, inadequate diet), but anemia may also be caused by chronic blood loss (gastrointestinal bleeding, excessive menstrual bleeding, hookworm infestation), iron malabsorption (small bowel disease, gastroenterostomy), or increased requirements (pregnancy, periods of rapid growth).
2. Decreased hemoglobin may result in insufficient oxygen delivery to body tissues.
3. Iron deficiency anemia, the most common type of anemia, is found in 10% to 30% of all adults in the United States. It is a major health problem in developing countries.

Clinical Manifestations
1. Physical—headache, dizziness, tinnitus, palpitations, dyspnea on exertion, pallor of skin and mucous membranes, smooth, sore tongue, cheilosis (lesions at corners of mouth), koilonychia (spoon-shaped fingernails).
2. Behavioral—fatigue, pica (craving to eat unusual substances).

Diagnostic Evaluation

1. CBC and iron profile—decreased hemoglobin, hematocrit, serum iron, and ferritin; elevated red cell distribution width (RDW) and normal or elevated total iron-binding capacity (TIBC).
2. Determination of source of chronic blood loss may include sigmoidoscopy, colonoscopy, upper and lower gastrointestinal studies, stool and urine for occult blood examination.

Management

1. Correction of chronic blood loss.
2. Oral or parenteral iron therapy.
   a. Oral ferrous sulfate preferred and least expensive; treatment continues until hemoglobin level is normalized and iron stores replaced (up to 6 months).
   b. Parenteral therapy may rarely be used when patient cannot tolerate or is noncompliant with oral therapy. May use iron dextran (Imferon) or iron sorbitex (Jectofer).

Complications

1. Severe compromise of the oxygen-carrying capacity of the blood may predispose to ischemic organ damage, such as myocardial infarction or cerebrovascular accident.
2. Anaphylaxis to parenteral iron therapy.

Nursing Assessment

1. Obtain history of symptoms, dietary intake, past history of anemia, possible sources of blood loss.
2. Examine for tachycardia, pallor, dyspnea, and signs of gastrointestinal or other bleeding.

Nursing Diagnoses

- Altered Nutrition: Less Than Body Requirements related to inadequate intake of iron
- Activity Intolerance related to decreased oxygen-carrying capacity of the blood
- Altered Tissue Perfusion related to decreased oxygen-carrying capacity of the blood

Nursing Interventions

Promoting Iron Intake

1. Assess diet for inclusion of foods rich in iron. Arrange nutritionist referral as appropriate.
2. Administer iron replacement as ordered. Technique of parenteral iron administration:
   a. Allow small amount of air in syringe and use new 5-cm (2-inch) needle for injection to avoid tracking medication through subcutaneous tissue and resulting painful induration.
   b. Retract skin over muscle of upper outer quadrant of buttock laterally before inserting needle (Z-track technique) to prevent leakage along track and staining of skin.
   c. Inject deeply and slowly into upper outer quadrant of buttock. Wait a few seconds before withdrawing needle.

DRUG ALERT

Anaphylactic reactions may occur after parenteral iron administration. Monitor patient closely for hypotension, angioedema, and stridor after injection. Do not administer with oral iron. Oral supplements may stain teeth—give with straw.

Increasing Activity Tolerance

1. Assess level of fatigue and normal sleep pattern; determine activities that cause fatigue.
2. Assist in developing a schedule of activity, rest periods, and sleep.
3. Encourage conditioning exercises to increase strength and endurance.

Maximizing Tissue Perfusion

1. Assess patient for palpitations, chest pain, dizziness, and shortness of breath; minimize any activities that cause these symptoms.
2. Elevate head of bed and provide supplemental oxygen as ordered.
3. Monitor vital signs and fluid balance.

Patient Education and Health Maintenance

1. Educate patient on proper nutrition and good sources of iron: select well-balanced diet that includes animal proteins, iron-fortified cereals and bread, green leafy vegetables, dried fruits, legumes, nuts.
2. Teach patient about iron supplementation. Take iron on empty stomach, with full glass of water or fruit juice. Liquid forms may stain teeth; mix well with water/fruit juice and use straw. Anticipate some epigastric discomfort, change in color of stool to green or black, and in some cases nausea, constipation, or diarrhea. Keep iron medications away from children: overdose may be fatal.
3. Encourage follow-up laboratory studies and visits to health care provider.

Outcome-Based Evaluation

- Incorporates several foods high in iron into diet; takes prescribed iron supplementation as ordered
- Tolerates increased activity; obtains sufficient rest
- Vital signs stable without complaints of chest pain, palpitations, or shortness of breath

Megaloblastic Anemia: Pernicious

A megaloblast is a large, nucleated erythrocyte with delayed and abnormal nuclear maturation. Pernicious anemia is a type of megaloblastic anemia associated with *vitamin B$_{12}$ deficiency*.

Pathophysiology and Etiology

1. Vitamin B$_{12}$ is necessary for normal DNA synthesis in maturing RBCs.
2. Pernicious anemia demonstrates familial incidence related to autoimmune gastric mucosal atrophy.

3. Normal gastric mucosa secretes a substance called intrinsic factor, necessary for absorption of vitamin B_{12} in ileum. If a defect exists in gastric mucosa, or after gastrectomy or small bowel disease, intrinsic factor may not be secreted and orally ingested B_{12} not absorbed.

4. Some drugs interfere with B_{12} absorption, notably ascorbic acid, cholestyramine, colchicine, neomycin, cimetidine, and oral contraceptives.

5. Primarily a disorder of older people.

Clinical Manifestations

1. Of anemia—pallor, fatigue, dyspnea on exertion, palpitations, angina pectoris, congestive heart failure.

2. Of underlying gastrointestinal dysfunction—sore mouth, glossitis, anorexia, nausea, vomiting, loss of weight, indigestion, epigastric discomfort, recurring diarrhea or constipation.

3. Of neuropathy (occurs in high percentage of untreated patients)—paresthesia that involves hands and feet, gait disturbance, bladder and bowel dysfunction, psychiatric symptoms caused by cerebral dysfunction.

Diagnostic Evaluation

1. CBC and blood smear—decreased hemoglobin and hematocrit; marked variation in size and shape of RBCs with a variable number of unusually large cells

2. Folic acid (normal) and B_{12} levels (decreased).

3. Gastric analysis—volume and acidity of gastric juice diminished.

4. Schilling test for absorption of vitamin B_{12} uses small amount of radioactive B_{12} orally and 24-hour urine collection to measure uptake—decreased.

Management

Parenteral replacement with hydroxocobalamin or cyanocobalamin (B_{12}) is necessary.

Complications

Neurologic: paresthesia, gait disturbances, bowel and bladder dysfunction, and cerebral dysfunction may be persistent.

Nursing Assessment

1. Assess for pallor, tachycardia, dyspnea on exertion, exercise intolerance to determine patient's response to anemia.

2. Assess for paresthesia, gait disturbances, changes in bladder or bowel function, altered thought processes indicating neurologic involvement.

3. Obtain history of gastric surgery or gastrointestinal disease.

Nursing Diagnoses

- Altered Thought Processes related to neurologic dysfunction in absence of vitamin B_{12}
- Sensory/Perceptual Alterations (Kinesthetic) related to neurologic dysfunction in absence of vitamin B_{12}

Nursing Interventions

Improving Thought Processes

1. Administer parenteral vitamin B_{12} as prescribed.

2. Provide patient with quiet, supportive environment; reorient to time, place, and person if needed; give instructions and information in short, simple sentences and reinforce frequently.

Minimizing the Effects of Paresthesia

1. Assess extent and severity of any sensory or perceptual alterations.

2. Refer for physical therapy/occupational therapy as appropriate.

3. Provide safe, uncluttered environment; ensure personal belongings are within reach; provide assistance with activities as needed.

Patient Education and Health Maintenance

1. Advise patient that monthly vitamin B_{12} administration should be continued for life.

2. Instruct patient to see health care provider approximately every 6 months for hematologic studies and gastrointestinal evaluation; may develop hematologic or neurologic relapse if therapy inadequate. Patients with pernicious anemia have higher incidence of gastric cancer and thyroid dysfunction; periodic stool examinations for occult blood, gastric cytology, and thyroid function tests are done.

Outcome-Based Evaluation

- Oriented, cooperative, and follows instructions
- Carries out activities without injury

▪ Megaloblastic Anemia: Folic Acid Deficiency

Chronic megaloblastic anemia caused by folic acid (folate) deficiency.

Pathophysiology and Etiology

1. Dietary deficiency, malnutrition, marginal diets, excessive cooking of foods; commonly associated with alcoholism.

2. Impaired absorption in jejunum (eg, with small bowel disease).

3. Increased requirements (eg, with chronic hemolytic anemia, exfoliate dermatitis, pregnancy).

4. Impaired utilization from folic acid antagonists (methotrexate) and other drugs (phenytoin, broad spectrum antibiotics, sulfamethoxazole, alcohol, oral contraceptives).

Clinical Manifestations

1. Of anemia: fatigue, weakness, pallor, dizziness, headache, tachycardia.

2. Of folic acid deficiency: sore tongue, cracked lips.

Diagnostic Evaluation

1. Vitamin B_{12} and folic acid level—folic acid will be decreased.
2. CBC will show decreased RBC, hemoglobin, and hematocrit with increased MCV and MCHC.

Management

Oral folic acid replacement.

Complications

Folic acid deficiency has been implicated in the etiology of congenitally acquired neural tube defects.

Nursing Assessment

1. Obtain nutritional history.
2. Monitor level of dyspnea, tachycardia, and development of chest pain or shortness of breath for worsening of condition.

Nursing Diagnosis

- Altered Nutrition: Less Than Body Requirements related to inadequate intake of folic acid

Nursing Interventions

Improving Folic Acid Intake

1. Assess diet for inclusion of foods rich in folic acid: beef liver, peanut butter, red beans, oatmeal, broccoli, asparagus.
2. Arrange nutritionist referral as appropriate.
3. Assist alcoholic patient to obtain counseling and additional medical care as needed.

Community and Home Care Considerations

1. Encourage pregnant patient to maintain prenatal care and to take folic acid supplement.
2. Provide alcoholic patient with information about treatment programs and Alcoholics Anonymous meetings in the community.

Patient Education and Health Maintenance

1. Teach patient to select balanced diet that includes green vegetables (asparagus, broccoli, spinach), yeast, liver and other organ meats, some fresh fruits; avoid overcooking vegetables.
2. Encourage patient to follow up periodically to monitor CBC.

Outcome-Based Evaluation

- Eats appropriate and nutritious diet; takes folic acid supplements as prescribed

Aplastic Anemia

Aplastic anemia is a disorder characterized by bone marrow hypoplasia or aplasia resulting in pancytopenia (insufficient numbers of RBCs, WBCs, and platelets).

Pathophysiology and Etiology

Destruction of hematopoietic stem cells is thought to be through an immune-mediated mechanism.

1. May be idiopathic or caused by exposure to chemical toxins; ionizing radiation; viral infections, particularly hepatitis; certain drugs (e.g., chloramphenicol).
2. May be congenital (Fanconi's anemia).
3. Clinical course is variable and dependent on degree of bone marrow failure; severe aplastic anemia is almost always fatal if untreated.

Clinical Manifestations

1. From anemia: pallor, weakness, fatigue, exertional dyspnea, palpitations.
2. From infections associated with neutropenia: fever, headache, malaise; adventitious breath sounds; abdominal pain, diarrhea; erythema, pain, exudate at wounds or sites of invasive procedures.
3. From thrombocytopenia: bleeding from gums, nose, gastrointestinal or genitourinary tracts; purpura, petechiae, ecchymoses.

Diagnostic Evaluation

1. CBC and peripheral blood smear show decreased RBC, WBC, platelets (pancytopenia).
2. Bone marrow aspiration and biopsy: bone marrow is hypocellular or empty with greatly reduced or absent hematopoiesis.

Management

1. Removal of causative agent or toxin.
2. Allogeneic bone marrow transplantation (BMT)—treatment of choice for patient with severe aplastic anemia (see p. 899). This treatment option provides long-term survival for 75% to 90% of patients, depending on the age of the patient, history of prior blood transfusions, and source of marrow.
3. Immunosuppressive treatment with corticosteroids, cyclosporine (Sandimmune), cyclophosphamide (Cytoxan), antithymocyte globulin (ATG) or antilymphocyte globulin (ALG) as single treatments or in combinations. This treatment option provides long-term survival for 70% to 80% of patients.
4. Androgens (oxymetholone or testosterone enanthate) may stimulate bone marrow regeneration; significant toxicity encountered. They may be used when other treatments have failed.
5. Supportive treatment includes platelet and RBC transfusions, antibiotics, and antifungals.

Complications

1. Untreated severe aplastic anemia is almost always fatal, generally because of overwhelming infection. Even with treatment, morbidity and mortality caused by infections and bleeding are high.

2. Late complications, even after successful treatment, include clonal hematologic diseases such as paroxysmal nocturnal hemoglobinuria (PNH), myelodysplasia, and acute myelogenous leukemia.

Nursing Assessment

1. Obtain thorough history that includes medications, past medical history, occupation, hobbies.
2. Monitor for signs of bleeding and infection.

Nursing Diagnoses

- Risk for Infection related to granulocytopenia secondary to bone marrow aplasia
- Risk for Injury related to bleeding

Nursing Interventions

Minimizing Risk of Infection

1. Care for patient in protective environment while hospitalized—private room with strict handwashing and avoidance of any contaminants (see Patient Education Guidelines).
2. Encourage good personal hygiene including daily shower or bath with mild soap, mouth care, and perirectal care after using the toilet.
3. Monitor vital signs, including temperature, frequently; notify health care provider of oral temperature of 38.3°C (101°F) or higher.

4. Minimize invasive procedures or possible trauma to skin or mucous membranes.
5. Obtain cultures of suspected infected sites or body fluids.

Minimizing Risk of Bleeding

1. Use only soft toothbrush or toothette for mouth care and electric razor for shaving; keep nails short by filing.
2. Avoid intramuscular injections and other invasive procedures.
3. Prevent constipation by use of stool softeners as prescribed.
4. Restrict activity based on platelet count and active bleeding.
5. Monitor pad count for menstruating patient; avoid use of vaginal tampons.
6. Control bleeding by applying pressure to site, using ice packs and prescribed topical hemostatic agents.
7. Administer blood product replacement as ordered; monitor for allergic reaction, anaphylaxis, and volume overload.

Patient Education and Health Maintenance

1. Teach patient how to minimize risk of bleeding: avoid falls or other injury; use electric razor rather than plain razor; use nail clippers or file rather than scissors; avoid blowing nose; use soft toothbrush or toothette for mouth care; use water-soluble lubricants as needed during sexual activity.

PATIENT EDUCATION GUIDELINES   **Preventing, Recognizing, and Treating Infection**

- *What kinds of infections am I at risk for?*

Because some of your white blood cells (called neutrophils) are not present in their normal numbers, you are at risk for infections. Neutrophils attack bacteria and other organisms that cause infections. You are at risk for infections from bacteria (for example, wound infections, urinary tract infections, pneumonia) and some viral infections (for example, cold sores) and fungal infections (for example, thrush, fungal pneumonia).

- *How do I know when I have an infection?*

With low numbers of neutrophils, some of the normal signs of infection, such as pus, may not be present. If you have a fever >100°F you should contact your health care provider immediately. Other signs of infection include chills and sweating, redness near a wound or a catheter, white patches in your mouth, or shortness of breath.

- *How can I protect myself from infection?*

The most important thing you can do is to wash your hands thoroughly after using the bathroom, or after any other "dirty" activity (like taking out the trash). You should keep your mouth clean by brushing your teeth with a soft toothbrush after every meal or snack, and by rinsing with a mild mouthrinse. You should shower daily, using a mild soap.

- *Can I have visitors? Can I go out?*

It is important to ask friends and family not to visit if they are not feeling well. You can certainly go out (unless your doctor or nurse gives you different instructions), but you

should avoid crowded, poorly ventilated places. You may be taught how to wear a special mask when you are outside.

- *Do I need to get rid of my pet?*

If you have pets and gardens, you can still enjoy them. If possible, find someone else who will clean your cat's litter box or scoop your dog's waste. Wear gloves when gardening and be careful not to get cuts and abrasions.

- *Should I stop having sex?*

With your low neutrophil count, you are also at higher risk from sexually transmitted diseases. But this doesn't mean you have to stop having sex! It is important to use a condom and make sure your sexual practice is safe. Depending on your general health, your doctor or nurse may recommend that you avoid sexual intercourse.

- *If I get an infection, how will it be treated?*

A new infection often requires hospital admission to diagnose it and to begin treatment. You may be given many tests to find out exactly what infection you have. Blood will be drawn and examined for infection, x-rays and CT scans may be done, and you may need a lumbar puncture to look for an infection in your spinal fluid. Before the results of all the tests are available, your doctor will begin treatment with IV antibiotics. If your infection does not get better (for example, if you still have a fever in a couple of days), your antibiotics may be changed or other medications may be added. Once your infection begins to improve, it is often possible to go home and continue taking IV or oral antibiotics at home.

2. Teach patient how to minimize risk of infection: wash hands after contact with possible source of infection; immediately cleanse any abrasion or wound of mucous membranes or skin; monitor temperature and report any fever or other sign of infection immediately; avoid crowds and people with illnesses; avoid raw or undercooked foods; use condoms and other safe sex practices.

3. Advise patient to avoid exposure to potential bone marrow toxins: solvents, sprays, paints, pesticides.

4. Teach patient to take only prescribed medications; avoid aspirin and nonsteroidal anti-inflammatory drugs (NSAIDs), which may interfere with platelet function.

5. Resources for patient and family include the Aplastic Anemia Foundation of America, P.O. Box 613, Annapolis, MD 21404, 1-800-747-2820; *www.aamds.org*.

Outcome-Based Evaluation
- Remains afebrile with no signs/symptoms of infection
- Episodes of bleeding are rapidly controlled

MYELOPROLIFERATIVE DISORDERS

Myeloproliferative disorders are disorders of the bone marrow that result from abnormal proliferation of cells from the myeloid line of the hematopoietic system. They include polycythemia vera, acute lymphocytic and acute myelogenous leukemia, and chronic myelogenous leukemia.

Polycythemia Vera

This chronic myeloproliferative disorder involves all bone marrow elements, resulting in an increase in RBC mass and hemoglobin.

Pathophysiology and Etiology
1. Hyperplasia of all bone marrow elements results in:
   a. Increased RBC mass.
   b. Increased blood volume and viscosity.
   c. Decreased marrow iron reserve.
   d. Splenomegaly.
2. Underlying cause is unknown.
3. Usually occurs in middle and later years.

Clinical Manifestations
Result from increased blood volume and viscosity.
1. Reddish purple hue of skin and mucosa, pruritus (especially after bathing).
2. Splenomegaly, hepatomegaly.
3. Epigastric discomfort, abdominal discomfort.
4. Painful fingers and toes from arterial and venous insufficiency, parasthesias.
5. Headache, fullness in head, dizziness, visual abnormalities, altered mentation from disturbed cerebral circulation.

6. Weakness, fatigue, night sweats, bleeding tendency.
7. Hyperuricemia from increased formation and destruction of erythrocytes and leukocytes and increased metabolism of nucleic acids.

Diagnostic Evaluation
1. CBC—elevated RBC and hemoglobin and hematocrit.
2. Bone marrow aspirate and biopsy—hyperplasia.

Management
1. Of hyperviscosity: phlebotomy (withdrawal of blood) at intervals determined by CBC results to reduce RBC mass; generally 250 to 500 mL removed at a time.
2. Of marrow hyperplasia: myelosuppressive therapy, generally using hydroxyurea or IV radioactive phosphorus (^{32}P); biologic response modifier, ie, alpha-interferon.
3. Of hyperuricemia: allopurinol.
4. Of pruritus: antihistamines (cimetidine or cyproheptadine); low-dose acetylsalicylic acid; certain antidepressants (doxepin, paroxetine); phototherapy; cholestyramine.

Complications
1. Thromboembolic events caused by hyperviscosity, including deep vein thrombophlebitis, myocardial and cerebral infarction, transient ischemic attacks (TIA), pulmonary embolism, retinal vein thrombosis, and thrombotic occlusion of the splenic, hepatic, portal and mesenteric veins.
2. Spontaneous hemorrhage caused by venous and capillary distention and abnormal platelet function.
3. Gout caused by hyperuricemia.
4. Congestive heart failure caused by increased blood volume and hypertension.
5. Myelofibrosis or acute leukemia may be terminal complications.

Nursing Assessment
1. Obtain history of symptoms, including changes in skin, epigastric discomfort, bleeding tendencies, circulatory problems, or painful, swollen joints.
2. Monitor for signs of bleeding or thromboembolism.
3. Monitor for hypertension and signs and symptoms of congestive heart failure including shortness of breath, distended neck veins.

Nursing Diagnosis
- Altered Tissue Perfusion (multiple organs) related to hyperviscosity of blood

Nursing Interventions
Preventing Thromboembolic Complications
1. Encourage or assist with ambulation.
2. Assess for early signs of thromboembolic complications—swelling of limb, increased warmth, pain.
3. Monitor CBC and assist with phlebotomy as ordered.

Patient Education and Health Maintenance

1. Educate patient about risk of thrombosis; encourage patient to maintain normal activity patterns and avoid long periods of bed rest.
2. Advise patient to avoid taking hot showers or baths because rapid skin cooling worsens pruritus; use skin emollients; take antihistamines as prescribed; may find starch baths helpful.
3. Instruct patient to take only prescribed medications.
4. Encourage patient to report at prescribed intervals for follow-up blood (hematocrit) studies and phlebotomies.
5. Instruct patient in technique of subcutaneous injection for alpha-interferon.

Outcome-Based Evaluation

- Hematocrit <45% in men and <42% in women; no signs or symptoms of thromboembolism, congestive heart failure, or bleeding

■ Acute Lymphocytic and Acute Myelogenous Leukemia

(See Nursing Care Plan 26-1.)

Leukemias are malignant disorders of the blood and bone marrow that result in an accumulation of dysfunctional, immature cells that are caused by loss of regulation of cell division. They are classified as acute or chronic

(*text continues on page 877*)

NURSING CARE PLAN 26-1   Care of the Patient With Acute Leukemia

You are assigned Charles Wintry, a 48-year-old with acute myelogenous leukemia (AML) who has been admitted with neutropenia and thrombocytopenia following chemotherapy. From your assessment and your knowledge of AML, you develop your plan of care.

Subjective data: Charles tells you he has felt very tired during the past week and has stopped working at his part-time store manager job. Since yesterday evening he has had a low-grade fever and pain in his chest with inspiration. He has also noticed new bruises on his lower legs and abdomen. This morning he had a nosebleed.

Objective data: Vital signs are temperature 38.3°C (101°F), pulse 104, BP 145/90, respirations 32. On examination you notice extensive petechiae; dried blood around the nares and gingival bleeding; warm, dry skin; and crackles heard in the bases of both lungs. CBC reveals 30,000 platelets, 1,200 WBCs with 450 neutrophils, and hematocrit of 32%.

NURSING DIAGNOSIS	Risk for infection related to granulocytopenia secondary to leukemia or its treatment with chemotherapy and/or radiation
GOAL/OUTCOME	Risk of infection will be minimized.

Nursing Intervention	Rationale	Outcome-Based Evaluation
1. Place patient in protected environment (private room) with handwashing precautions strictly enforced.	1. Meticulous handwashing is the single most important method of preventing transmission of endogenous and exogenous nosocomial infections.	1. Staff and visitors comply with handwashing precautions.
2. Avoid exposure to all sources of stagnant water (eg, flower vases, denture cups, water pitchers, humidifiers) and plants.	2. Stagnant water and soil are good media for anaerobic bacterial growth.	2. Sources of possible bacterial growth are eliminated.
3. Encourage or assist with personal hygiene—mouth care, perirectal care, daily shower or bath with mild soap. Inspect skin and mucous membranes daily for possible signs of infection.	3. Skin care and good oral hygiene may help prevent skin, oral, respiratory, and gastrointestinal infections. Signs of infection may be minimal in neutropenic patient.	3. Skin remains clean and lubricated. Oropharynx has no lesions, plaques, or erythema.
4. Monitor vital signs q4h. Obtain baseline pulse oximeter reading (SaO₂)	4. Infections may progress rapidly in immunocompromised patient.	4. Vital signs monitored and changes reported to health care provider.
5. Assess respiratory function q4h while symptoms present, otherwise q8h. Encourage ambulation, deep breathing, and coughing.	5. Neutropenic patient may have significant bacterial or fungal pneumonia with minimal changes on chest x-ray or physical examination.	5. Ambulates and uses incentive spirometer.

(continued)

NURSING CARE PLAN 26-1   Care of the Patient With Acute Leukemia (continued)

Nursing Intervention	Rationale	Evaluation
6. Assess for changes in mental status at least q8h including restlessness, irritability, confusion, headache, or changes in level of consciousness.	6. Mental status changes are often first subtle signs of sepsis.	6. Mental status remains normal.
7. Avoid invasive procedures if possible, eg, urinary catheterization. Use strict aseptic technique if procedure unavoidable.	7. Risk of infection from invasive procedure is high.	7. Invasive procedures minimized. Injections given IV.
8. Prevent rectal trauma by avoiding rectal temperatures, enemas, or suppositories. Use sitz bath and barrier cream for patient with diarrhea and hemorrhoids. Use stool softeners as needed to prevent constipation.	8. Perianal area is high-risk site for infection, including rectal abscesses.	8. Perianal area remains clean and intact.
9. Obtain cultures of suspected infected sites or body fluids.	9. Pus may not be present with neutropenia. Cultures may reveal bacterial, fungal or viral pathogens.	9. Sputum sent for culture.
10. Report: 1) fever ≥ 101°F or 38.3°C; 2) significant change in vital signs, particularly hypotension, tachycardia, and/or tachypnea; 3) chills or rigors; 4) mental status changes.	10. Fever may be only response to infection in neutropenic patient. Patient is at risk for sepsis due to lack of normal immunologic response.	10. Fever reported.
11. Teach patient measures to prevent infection: avoid crowds; avoid raw or undercooked food; use condoms.	11. Potential for infection remains after discharge.	11. Patient states preventative measures.

NURSING DIAGNOSIS   Risk for injury related to bleeding secondary to thrombocytopenia, disseminated intravascular coagulation or leukostasis associated with leukemia

GOAL/OUTCOME   Risk of bleeding will be minimized.

Nursing Intervention	Rationale	Outcome-Based Evaluation
1. Assess for signs of bleeding at least q8h.	1. Overt and covert spontaneous bleeding is possible at platelet counts < 50,000/mm³.	1. No further bleeding noted.
2. Provide soft toothbrush or toothettes and mild mouthwash for mouth care.	2. Minimize damage to mucous membranes.	2. Uses soft toothbrush after meals for gentle cleansing.
3. Use only an electric razor for shaving. Keep fingernails and toenails short and smooth. Lubricate skin with mild lotion.	3. Minimize skin excoriation.	3. Wife brings electric razor from home.
4. Avoid IM injections, invasive procedures, rectal procedures. Use stool softeners to prevent constipation.	4. Minimize risk of bleeding.	4. Invasive procedures minimized. Injections given IV.
5. Restrict activity based on assessment of platelet count and presence of active bleeding.	5. Injury to muscles or spontaneous bleeding may be minimized by restricting activity at lower platelet counts.	5. Ambulates within room with assistance until bleeding controlled and platelet count stabilized.
6. Menstrual suppression may be necessary for females. Monitor pad count/amount. Avoid use of vaginal tampons.	6. Menorrhagia may be severe in thrombocytopenic patient.	6. Menstrual bleeding not exceeding four to five pads per day.

(continued)

NURSING CARE PLAN 26-1   Care of the Patient With Acute Leukemia (continued)

Nursing Intervention	Rationale	Evaluation
7. Control bleeding by applying pressure to site, ice packs, and prescribed topical hemostatic agents such as microfibrillar collagen hemostat (Avitene) or thrombin (Fibrindex, Thrombinar).	7. Topical interventions generally adequate to control most bleeding episodes.	7. No further bleeding episodes.
8. Administer blood product replacement as ordered. Monitor for signs and symptoms of allergic reactions, anaphylaxis, and volume overload.	8. Platelet transfusions may be necessary when platelet count <20,000/mm^3 or with active bleeding. Other blood products (RBCs, fresh frozen plasma, cryoprecipitate) may also be required.	8. Platelet products given q2-3d until thrombocytopenia resolved.
9. Teach patient to avoid activities likely to cause injury (eg, contact sports) and other methods to prevent bleeding.	9. Risk for bleeding remains after discharge.	9. Patient states preventative measures.

NURSING DIAGNOSIS   Pain related to tumor growth, infection, or side effects of chemotherapy

GOAL/OUTCOME   Pain will be controlled.

Nursing Intervention	Rationale	Outcome-Based Evaluation
1. Assess at least q4h for presence, location, intensity, and characteristics of pain.	1. Pain is potentially distressing symptom. Pain may be symptom of infection.	1. Patient rates pain between 1 and 3 on scale 0–10 after first day.
2. Administer analgesics as ordered to control pain. Administer on regular schedule rather than PRN. Avoid aspirin and nonsteroidal anti-inflammatory medications in thrombocytopenic patients. If oral analgesics in optimal doses are not effective or not tolerated, consider IV route.	2. Analgesics on regular schedule at appropriate doses should be used to control pain. Aspirin and non-steroidal anti-inflammatory medications interfere with platelet function. IM and SC injections should be avoided in thrombocytopenia.	2. Oral analgesia (codeine 30 mg q4h) well tolerated.
3. Teach and use nonpharmacologic measures such as the use of music, relaxation breathing, progressive muscle relaxation, distraction and imagery to help manage pain.	3. Nonpharmacologic measures may be useful adjunctive treatments for patients with pain.	3. Heat packs to right chest area provide additional relief.

NURSING DIAGNOSIS   Powerlessness related to diagnosis and perceived lack of support/resources

GOAL/OUTCOME   Patient and family will be empowered to seek appropriate help.

Nursing Intervention	Rationale	Outcome-Based Evaluation
1. Encourage verbalization of feelings regarding diagnosis, treatment plan, and anticipated course of illness.	1. Nurse-patient relationship allows appropriate discussion of concerns.	1. Verbalizes feelings appropriately.
2. Refer as needed to social worker, psychiatric liaison nurse, psychologist.	2. Further assistance and support may be needed.	2. Referred to social worker for assistance with financial concerns.
3. Share information regarding national and local resources.	3. National and local organizations may be significant sources of support for patients and families.	3. Attends American Cancer Society support group after discharge.

based on the development rate of symptoms, and further classified by the predominant cell type. Acute leukemias affect immature cells and are characterized by rapid progression of symptoms. When lymphocytes are the predominant malignant cell, the disorder is *acute lymphocytic leukemia (ALL)*; when monocytes or granulocytes are predominant, it is *acute myelogenous leukemia (AML)*, sometimes called *acute nonlymphocytic leukemia (ANLL)*.

Pathophysiology and Etiology

1. The development of leukemia has been associated with:
   a. Exposure to ionizing radiation.
   b. Exposure to certain chemicals and toxins (eg, benzene, alkylating agents).
   c. Human T-cell leukemia—lymphoma virus (HTLV-1) in certain areas of the world, including the Caribbean and southern Japan.
   d. Familial susceptibility.
   e. Genetic disorders (eg, Down syndrome, Fanconi's anemia).
2. Approximately half of new leukemias are acute. Approximately 85% of acute leukemias in adults are AML. ALL is most common in children, with peak incidence between ages 2 and 9.
3. Childhood ALL is often cured with chemotherapy alone (>75%) whereas only 30% to 40% of adults with ALL are cured.
4. AML is a disease of older people, with a median age at diagnosis of 67 years. Even in the young-old (patients who are younger than 60 years), AML is difficult to treat, with a median survival of 5 to 6 months, despite intensive therapy.

Clinical Manifestations

1. Common symptoms include pallor, fatigue, weakness, fever, weight loss, abnormal bleeding and bruising, lymphadenopathy (in ALL) and recurrent infections (in ALL).
2. Other presenting symptoms may include bone and joint pain, headache, splenomegaly, hepatomegaly, neurologic dysfunction.

Diagnostic Evaluation

1. CBC and blood smear—peripheral WBC count varies widely from 1,000 to 100,000/mm^3 and may include significant numbers of abnormal immature (blast) cells; anemia may be profound; platelet count may be abnormal and coagulopathies may exist.
2. Bone marrow aspiration and biopsy—cells also studied for chromosomal abnormalities (cytogenetics) and immunologic markers to classify type of leukemia further.
3. Lymph node biopsy—to detect spread.
4. Lumbar puncture and examination of cerebrospinal fluid (CSF) for leukemic cells (especially in ALL).

Management

1. To eradicate leukemic cells and allow restoration of normal hematopoiesis.
   a. High-dose chemotherapy given as an induction course to obtain a remission (disappearance of abnormal cells in bone marrow and blood) and then in cycles as consolidation or maintenance therapy to prevent recurrence of disease (Table 26-3).
   b. Leukapheresis (or exchange transfusion in infants) may be used when abnormally high numbers of white cells are present to reduce the risk of leukostasis and tumor burden before chemotherapy.
   c. Radiation, particularly of central nervous system (CNS) in ALL.
   d. Autologous or allogeneic bone marrow transplant.
2. Supportive care and symptom management.

Complications

1. Leukostasis: in setting of high numbers (greater than 50,000/mm^3) of circulating leukemic cells (blasts), blood vessel walls are infiltrated and weakened, with high risk for rupture and bleeding, including intracranial hemorrhage.
2. Disseminated intravascular coagulation (DIC).
3. Tumor lysis syndrome: rapid destruction of large numbers of malignant cells leads to alterations in electrolytes (hyperuricemia, hyperkalemia, hyperphosphatemia, and hypocalcemia).
4. May lead to renal failure and other complications.
5. Infection, bleeding, organ damage.

> **◆ DRUG ALERT**
>
> Allopurinol is commonly used as part of a regimen to prevent tumor lysis syndrome. In rare cases it causes severe, even lethal skin reactions (toxic epidermolysis syndrome). Allopurinol should be discontinued for any patient who develops a new skin rash.

Nursing Assessment

1. Take nursing history, focusing on weight loss, fever, frequency of infections, progressively increasing fatigability, shortness of breath, palpitations, visual changes (retinal bleeding).
2. Ask about difficulty in swallowing, coughing, rectal pain.
3. Examine patient for enlarged lymph nodes, hepatosplenomegaly, evidence of bleeding, abnormal breath sounds, skin lesions.
4. Look for evidence of infection: mouth, tongue, and throat for reddened areas/white patches. Examine skin for breakdown, which is a potential source of infection.

Nursing Diagnoses

- Risk for Infection related to granulocytopenia of disease and treatment
- Risk for Injury related to bleeding secondary to bone marrow failure and thrombocytopenia

TABLE 26-3 Common Chemotherapeutic Drugs Used in Acute Leukemias

Drug	Major Side Effects	Classification	Primary Use
Cytarabine (ARA-C, Cytosar-U)	Bone marrow suppression, nausea and vomiting, pulmonary toxicity, mucositis, lethargy, cerebellar toxicity, dermatitis, kerato-conjunctivitis	Antimetabolite	Induction and consolidation therapy for AML
Daunorubicin (Cerubidine)	Bone marrow suppression, nausea and vomiting, alopecia, cardio-toxicity, vesicant	Antibiotic	Induction and consolidation therapy for AML
Doxorubicin (Adriamycin PFS)	Leukopenia, nausea and vomiting, alopecia, cardiotoxicity, photo-sensitivity, vesicant	Antibiotic	Induction and consolidation therapy for AML
L-asparaginase (Elspar)	Liver dysfunction, nausea and vomiting, hypersensitivity reaction, depression, lethargy	Miscellaneous: enzyme	Induction therapy for ALL
6-Mercaptopurine (6-MP, Purinethol)	Mild bone marrow suppression, gastrointestinal disturbances, hepatotoxicity	Antimetabolite	Maintenance therapy for ALL
Methotrexate (Mexate, Folex)	Bone marrow suppression, stomatitis, nausea, diarrhea, hepatotoxicity, neurotoxicity with intrathecal doses	Antimetabolite	Intrathecal central nervous system treatment and prophylaxis for ALL; maintenance therapy for ALL
Prednisone (Orasone)	Appetite stimulation, mood alteration, Cushing's syndrome, hypertension, diabetes, peptic ulcer	Corticosteroid	Induction therapy for ALL
Vincristine (Oncovin, Vincasar)	Neurotoxicity, alopecia, vesicant	Plant alkaloid	Induction therapy for ALL

ALL, acute lymphocytic leukemia; AML, acute myelogenous leukemia.

Nursing Interventions
Preventing Infection
1. Especially monitor for pneumonia, pharyngitis, esophagitis, perianal cellulitis, urinary tract infection, and cellulitis, which are common in leukemia and which carry significant morbidity and mortality.
2. Monitor for fever, flushed appearance, chills, tachycardia; appearance of white patches in mouth; redness, swelling, heat or pain of eyes, ears, throat, skin, joints, abdomen, rectal and perineal areas; cough, changes in sputum; skin rash.
3. Check results of granulocyte counts. Concentrations less than 500 mm^3 put the patient at serious risk for infection.
4. Avoid invasive procedures and trauma to skin or mucous membrane to prevent entry of microrganisms.
5. Use the following rectal precautions to prevent infection.
   a. Avoid diarrhea and constipation, which can irritate the rectal mucosa.
   b. Avoid rectal thermometers.
   c. Avoid foods that increase bacterial colonization of the gastrointestinal tract, such as fresh fruits, vegetables, raw meat, buttermilk.
   d. Keep perianal area clean.
6. Care for patient in protected environment with strict handwashing practice.
7. Encourage and assist patient with personal hygiene, bathing, and oral care.
8. Obtain cultures and administer antimicrobials promptly as directed.

Preventing and Managing Bleeding
1. Watch for signs of minor bleeding, such as petechiae, ecchymosis, conjunctival hemorrhage, epistaxis, bleeding gums, bleeding at puncture sites, vaginal spotting, heavy menses.
2. Be alert for signs of serious bleeding, such as headache with change in responsiveness, blurred vision, hemoptysis, hematemesis, melena, hypotension, tachycardia, dizziness.
3. Test all urine, stool, emesis for gross and occult blood.
4. Monitor platelet counts daily.
5. Administer blood components as directed.
6. Keep patient on bed rest during bleeding episodes.

Patient Education and Health Maintenance
1. Teach patient and family infection precautions (see p. 872).
2. Teach signs and symptoms of infection and advise whom to notify.
3. Encourage adequate nutrition to prevent emaciation from chemotherapy.

4. Teach avoidance of constipation with increased fluid and fiber, and good perianal care.
5. Teach bleeding precautions, such as use of electric razor, avoidance of aspirin or NSAIDs, avoidance of sharp objects, avoidance of straining at stool or forceful nose-blowing.
6. Encourage regular dental visits to detect and treat dental infections and disease.

7. Provide patient and family with information about resources in the community, such as the Leukemia Society of America and the American Cancer Society (Box 26-1).

Outcome-Based Evaluation
- Afebrile, without signs of infection
- No signs of bleeding

BOX 26-1   Resources for Patients With Hematologic Malignancies

National and Local Organizations

American Cancer Society 1599 Clifton Rd., NE Atlanta, GA 30329 404-320-3333 or 1-800-ACS-2345 www.cancer.org	Patient education materials, CanSurmount and I Can Cope educational and support programs, durable medical equipment loans
Corporate Angel Network, Inc. Westchester County Airport, 1 Loop Road White Plains, NY 10604 914-328-1313 www.corpangelnetwork.org	Use of corporate aircraft to provide free travel to cancer patients going to check-ups, treatments or consultations
Leukemia and Lymphoma Society 600 Third Ave. New York, NY 10016 212-573-8484 or 1-800-955-4572 www.Leukemia-lymphoma.org	Patient education materials, support groups, financial assistance (patient aid) program for patients with leukemia, Hodgkin's and non-Hodgkin's lymphoma and multiple myeloma
National Coalition for Cancer Survivorship 1010 Wayne Ave., Suite 707 Silver Spring, MD 20910 1-888-937-6227 www.cansearch.org e-mail: info@cansearch.org	Network related to survivorship issues, sponsors National Cancer Survivors' Day, publishes Cancer Survivors Almanac of Resources
National Marrow Donor Program www.marrow.org e-mail: webmaster@nmdp.org	Information for patients and volunteer donors regarding unrelated bone marrow transplant
Cancer Information Service National Cancer Institute, Bldg. 31, Rm. 10A24 Bethesda, MD 20892 1-800-4-CANCER www.nci.nih.gov	National telephone hotline for information, patient education materials, research reports
Wellness Centers/Groups (name and address of nearest available from NCI Cancer Information Service at 1-800-4-CANCER)	Psychosocial support including groups, hotlines, patient education materials, social activities

Newsletters and Magazines

Blood and Marrow Transplant Newsletter
2900 Skokie Valley Road
Highland Park, IL 60035
1-888-597-7674
www.bmtnews.org
email:help@bmtnews.org

■ Chronic Myelogenous Leukemia (CML)

This chronic leukemia (ie, involving more mature cells than acute leukemia) is characterized by proliferation of myeloid cell lines, including granulocytes, monocytes, platelets, and occasionally RBCs.

Pathophysiology and Etiology

1. Specific etiology unknown, associated with exposure to ionizing radiation and family history of leukemia. Results from malignant transformation of pluripotent hematopoietic stem cell.
2. First cancer associated with chromosomal abnormality (the Philadelphia [Ph] chromosome), present in more than 90% of patients.
3. Accounts for 25% of adult leukemias and less than 5% of childhood leukemias. Generally presents between the ages of 25 to 60 with peak incidence in mid-40s.
4. With progression of illness, enters terminal phase, resembling an acute leukemia that consists of accelerated phase or blast crisis.

Clinical Manifestations

1. Insidious onset, may be discovered during routine physical examination.
2. Common symptoms include fatigue, pallor, activity intolerance, fever, weight loss, night sweats, abdominal fullness (splenomegaly).

Diagnostic Evaluation

1. CBC and blood smear: large numbers of granulocytes (often more than 100,000/mm^3), platelets may be decreased.
2. Bone marrow aspiration and biopsy: hypercellular, usually demonstrates Ph chromosome.

Management
Chronic Phase

1. Alpha interferon, continued indefinitely, frequently eliminates the Ph chromosome and blasts. It has now become standard firstline therapy, unless condition at diagnosis or other factors intervene. Side effects (most often fatigue and fevers) may be severe.
2. Potentially curative treatment is offered by allogeneic (related or unrelated donor) BMT.
3. Palliative treatment, controlling symptoms, includes chemotherapy with agents such as busulfan (Myleran) or hydroxyurea (Hydrea); irradiation; splenectomy.

Accelerated Phase or Blast Crisis

1. High-dose chemotherapy (usually AML regimens) and leukaphoresis may be used to attempt to regain chronic phase.
2. Supportive care and palliative care, because this phase is usually terminal.

Complications

1. Leukostasis.
2. Infection, bleeding, organ damage.
3. With exception of possible cures using alpha interferon or BMT, CML is a terminal disease with unpredictable survival, on average 3 years.

Nursing Assessment

1. Obtain health history, focusing on fatigue, weight loss, night sweats, activity intolerance.
2. Assess for signs of bleeding and infection.
3. Evaluate splenomegaly, hepatomegaly.

Nursing Diagnosis

- Fear related to disease progression and death
- For patient with CML in blast crisis, see Nursing Care Plan 26-1.

Nursing Interventions
Allaying Fear

1. Encourage appropriate verbalization of feelings and concerns.
2. Provide comprehensive patient teaching about disease, using methods and content appropriate to patient's needs.
3. Assist patient in identifying resources and support (eg, family and friends, spiritual support, community or national organizations, support groups).
4. Facilitate use of effective coping mechanisms.

Patient Education and Health Maintenance

1. Teach patient to take medications as prescribed and monitor for side effects.
2. Teach patient method of subcutaneous injection for self-administration of alpha interferon, and teach strategies for managing side effects such as fatigue and fevers.
3. Provide patient and family with information about resources in the community such as the Leukemia and Lymphoma Society and the American Cancer Society (see Box 26-1).

Outcome-Based Evaluation

- Demonstrates effective coping skills

LYMPHOPROLIFERATIVE DISORDERS

Lymphoproliferative disorders result from proliferation of cells from the lymphoid line of the hematopoietic system. They include chronic lymphocytic leukemia, Hodgkin's disease, non-Hodgkin's lymphomas, and multiple myeloma.

■ Chronic Lymphocytic Leukemia (CLL)

This chronic leukemia (ie, involving more mature cells than acute leukemia) is characterized by proliferation of morphologically normal but functionally inert lymphocytes.

Classified according to cell origin, it includes B cell (accounts for 95% of cases), *T cell*, *lymphosarcoma*, *prolymphocytic leukemia*, and *hairy cell leukemia*.

Pathophysiology and Etiology
1. Specific etiology unknown. Tends to cluster in families, much more common in Western hemisphere. Male hormones may play role.
2. Most common leukemia in United States and Europe. Disease of later years (90% older than 50 years of age). Twice as common in men.
3. May be indolent for years, with gradual transformation to more malignant disease.

Clinical Manifestations
1. Insidious onset, may be discovered during routine physical examination.
2. Early symptoms may include history of frequent skin or respiratory infections, symmetrical lymphadenopathy, mild splenomegaly.
3. Symptoms of more advanced disease include pallor, fatigue, activity intolerance, easy bruising, skin lesions, bone tenderness, abdominal discomfort.

Diagnostic Evaluation
1. CBC and blood smear: large numbers of lymphocytes (10,000 to 150,000/mm^3); may also be anemia, thrombocytopenia, hypogammaglobulinemia.
2. Bone marrow aspirate and biopsy: lymphocytic infiltration of bone marrow.
3. Lymph node biopsy to detect spread.

Management
Symptom Control and Treatments
1. Patient with newly diagnosed CLL is generally observed and followed closely until symptoms develop.
2. Lymphocyte proliferation can be suppressed with chlorambucil (Leukeran), cyclophosphamide (Cytoxan), and prednisone (Orasone).
3. B cell CLL (a particular type) may be treated with fludarabine phosphate (Fludara).
4. Hairy cell leukemia, a distinctive type of CLL with hairlike projections of cytoplasm from lymphocytes, may be successfully treated with alpha interferon.
5. Splenic irradiation or splenectomy for painful splenomegaly or platelet sequestration, hemolytic anemia.
6. Irradiation of painful enlarged lymph nodes.
7. Bone marrow transplant and combinations of alpha interferon and interleukin 2 are also used to treat CLL.

Supportive Care
1. Transfusion therapy to replace platelets and RBCs.
2. Antibiotics, antivirals and antifungals as needed to control infections.
3. IV immunoglobulins or gamma globulin to treat hypogammaglobulinemia.

Complications
1. Thrombophlebitis from venous or lymphatic obstruction caused by enlarged lymph nodes.
2. Infection, bleeding.
3. Median survival depends on severity of disease; varies from 2 to 7 years.

Nursing Assessment
1. Obtain health history, focusing on history of infections, fatigue, bruising and bleeding, swollen lymph nodes.
2. Assess for signs of anemia, bleeding, or infection.
3. Evaluate splenomegaly, hepatomegaly, lymphadenopathy.

Nursing Diagnoses
- Pain related to tumor growth, infection, or side effects of chemotherapy
- Activity Intolerance related to anemia and side effects of chemotherapy

Nursing Interventions
Reducing Pain
1. Assess frequently for pain and administer or teach patient to administer analgesics on regular schedule, as prescribed; monitor for side effects.
2. Teach the use of nonpharmacologic methods, such as the use of music, relaxation breathing, progressive muscle relaxation, distraction, and imagery to help to manage pain.

Improving Activity Tolerance
1. Encourage frequent rest periods alternating with ambulation and light activity as tolerated.
2. Assist with hygiene and physical care as necessary.
3. Encourage balanced diet or nutritional supplements as tolerated.
4. Teach patient to use energy conservation techniques while performing activities of daily living, such as sitting while bathing, minimizing trips up and down stairs, using shoulder bag or push cart to carry articles.

Patient Education and Health Maintenance
1. Teach patient to minimize risk of infection (see p. 872).
2. Teach use of medications as ordered, and possible side effects and their management; also teach patient to avoid aspirin and NSAIDs, which may interfere with platelet function.
3. Provide patient and family with information about resources in the community, such as the Leukemia and Lymphoma Society and the American Cancer Society (see Box 26-1).

Outcome-Based Evaluation
- States free of pain
- Performs activities without complaints of fatigue

Hodgkin's Disease

Hodgkin's disease is a lymphoma. Lymphomas are malignant disorders of the reticuloendothelial system that results in an accumulation of dysfunctional, immature lymphoid-derived cells. They are classified according to the predominant cell type and by the degree of malignant cell maturity (eg, well differentiated, poorly differentiated, or undifferentiated). Hodgkin's disease originates in the lymphoid system and involves predominantly lymph nodes.

Pathophysiology and Etiology

1. Etiology is unknown.
2. Characterized by appearance of "Reed-Sternberg" multinucleated giant cell in tumor. Generally spreads via lymphatic channels, involving lymph nodes, spleen, and ultimately extralymphatic sites.
3. May also spread via bloodstream to sites such as gastrointestinal tract, bone marrow, skin, upper air passages, and other organs.
4. Incidence demonstrates two peaks, at ages 20 to 40 and after age 60.

Clinical Manifestations

1. Common symptoms include painless enlargement of lymph nodes (generally unilateral), fever, chills, night sweats, weight loss, pruritus.
2. Various symptoms may occur with pulmonary involvement, superior vena cava obstruction, hepatic or bone involvement, etc.

Diagnostic Evaluation

Tests are used to determine extent of disease involvement before treatment and followed at regular intervals to assess response to treatment.
1. CBC—determines abnormal cells.
2. Lymph node biopsy determines type of lymphoma.
3. Bilateral bone marrow aspirate and biopsy determine whether bone marrow is involved.
4. Radiographic tests (eg, x-rays, computed tomography [CT], magnetic resonance imaging [MRI]) to detect deep nodal involvement.
5. Gallium-67 scan—detects areas of active disease and may be used to determine aggressiveness of disease.
6. Liver function tests, scan to determine hepatic involvement; liver biopsy may be indicated if results abnormal.
7. Lymphangiogram to detect size and location of deep nodes involved, including abdominal nodes, which may not be readily seen via computed tomography (CT).
8. Surgical staging (laparotomy with splenectomy, liver biopsy, multiple lymph node biopsies)—in selected patients.
9. Lumbar puncture to obtain spinal fluid for cytopathology if meningeal lymphoma is suspected.

Management

Choice of treatment depends on extent of disease, histopathologic findings, and prognostic indicators. Hodgkin's disease is more readily cured than other lymphomas, with a five-year survival of 80%. More than one treatment strategy is available, and combinations of radiation and chemotherapy are commonly used.

Radiation Therapy

1. Treatment of choice for localized disease.
2. Areas of body where lymph node chains are located can generally tolerate high radiation doses.
3. Vital organs are protected with lead shielding during radiation treatments.

Chemotherapy

1. Initial treatment often with MOPP regimen of nitrogen mustard (Mustargen), vincristine (Oncovin), procarbazine (Matulane), and prednisone or ABVD regimen of doxorubicin (Adriamycin), bleomycin (Blenoxane), vinblastine (Valban), and dacarbazine (DTIC).
2. Three or four drugs may be given in intermittent or cyclical courses with periods off treatment to allow recovery from toxicities.

Autologous or Allogeneic Bone Marrow Transplantation (see p. 902)

Complications

1. Side effects of radiation or chemotherapy (see pp. 141–154).
2. Dependent on location and extent of malignancy, but may include splenomegaly, hepatomegaly, thromboembolic complications, spinal cord compression.

Nursing Assessment

1. Obtain health history, focusing on fatigue, fever, chills, night sweats, swollen lymph nodes.
2. Evaluate splenomegaly, hepatomegaly, lymphadenopathy.

Nursing Diagnoses

- Impaired Tissue Integrity related to high-dose radiation therapy
- Altered Oral Mucous Membranes related to high-dose radiation therapy

Nursing Interventions

Maintaining Tissue Integrity

1. Avoid rubbing, powders, deodorants, lotions, or ointments (unless prescribed) or application of heat/cold to treated area.
2. Encourage patient to keep treated area clean and dry, bathing area gently with tepid water and mild soap.
3. Encourage wearing loose-fitting clothes.
4. Advise patient to protect skin from exposure to sun, chlorine, temperature extremes.

Preserving Oral and Gastrointestinal Tract Mucous Membranes

1. Encourage frequent small meals, using bland and soft diet at mild temperatures.
2. Teach patient to avoid irritants such as alcohol, tobacco, spices, extreme food temperatures.
3. Administer or teach self-administration of pain medication or antiemetic before eating or drinking, if needed.

4. Encourage mouth care at least twice a day and after meals using soft toothbrush or toothette and mild mouth rinse.
5. Assess for ulcers, plaques, or discharge that may be indicative of superimposed infection.
6. For diarrhea, switch to low-residue diet and administer antidiarrheals as ordered.

Patient Education and Health Maintenance

1. Teach patient about risk of infection (see p. 872).
2. Teach patient how to take medications as ordered, and instruct about possible side effects, and management.
3. Explain to patients that radiation therapy may cause sterility; men should be given opportunity for sperm banking before treatment; women may develop ovarian failure and require hormone replacement therapy.
4. Reassure patient that fatigue will decrease after treatment is completed; encourage frequent naps and rest periods.
5. Provide patient and family with information about resources in the community, such as the Leukemia and Lymphoma Society and the American Cancer Society (see Box 26-1).

Outcome-Based Evaluation

- Skin intact without erythema or swelling
- Oral mucosa intact, patient eating

◼ Non-Hodgkin's Lymphomas

Non-Hodgkin's lymphomas are a group of malignancies of lymphoid tissue arising from T or B lymphocytes or their precursors.

Pathophysiology and Etiology

1. Association with defective or altered immune system; higher incidence in patients receiving immunosuppression for organ transplant, in HIV-positive people, and with some viruses.
2. Arise from malignant transformation of lymphocyte at some stage during development; level of differentiation and type of lymphocyte influences course of illness and prognosis.
3. Incidence rises steadily from age 40.

Clinical Manifestations

1. Common symptoms include painless enlargement of lymph nodes (generally unilateral), fever, chills, night sweats, weight loss. Unlike Hodgkin's disease, is more likely to be advanced disease at presentation.
2. Various symptoms may occur with pulmonary involvement, superior vena cava obstruction, hepatic or bone involvement, etc.

Diagnostic Evaluation

1. Lymph node biopsy to detect type.
2. CBC, bone marrow aspirate and biopsy to detect bone marrow involvement.

3. X-rays, CT, and MRI to detect deep nodal involvement.
4. Liver function tests, liver scan to detect liver involvement.
5. Lymphangiogram to evaluate lymph system involvement.
6. Surgical staging (laparotomy with splenectomy, liver biopsy, multiple lymph node biopsies).

Management

1. Radiation therapy generally palliative, not curative.
2. Chemotherapy: various regimens available, including CHOP regimen of cyclophosphamide (Cytoxan), doxorubicin (Adriamycin), vincristine (Oncovin), and prednisone (Orasone) or BACOP regimen of bleomycin (Blenoxane), doxorubicin (Adriamycin), cyclophosphamide (Cytoxan), vincristine (Oncovin), and prednisone.
3. Autologous or allogeneic BMT (see p. 902).

Complications

1. Complications of radiation therapy and chemotherapy (see pp. 141–154).
2. Of disease: depends on location and extent of malignancy, but may include splenomegaly, hepatomegaly, thromboembolic complications, spinal cord compression.

Nursing Assessment

1. Obtain health history, focusing on fatigue, fever, chills, night sweats, swollen lymph nodes, and history of illness or therapy causing immunosuppression.
2. Evaluate splenomegaly, hepatomegaly, lymphadenopathy.

Nursing Diagnosis

- Risk for Infection related to altered immune response because of lymphoma and leukopenia caused by chemotherapy or radiation therapy

Nursing Interventions

Minimizing Risk of Infection

1. Care for patient in protected environment with strict handwashing observed.
2. Avoid invasive procedures, such as urinary catheterization, if possible.
3. Assess temperature and vital signs, breath sounds, level of consciousness, and skin and mucous membranes frequently for signs of infection.
4. Notify health care provider of fever greater than 38.3°C (101°F) or change in condition.
5. Obtain cultures of suspected infected sites or body fluids.

Patient Education and Health Maintenance

1. Teach patient infection precautions (see p. 872).
2. Encourage frequent follow-up visits for monitoring of CBC and condition.

3. Provide patient and family with information about resources in the community, such as the Leukemia and Lymphoma Society and the American Cancer Society (see Box 26-1).

Outcome-Based Evaluation
• Remains afebrile with no signs or symptoms of infection

Multiple Myeloma
Multiple myeloma is a malignant disorder of plasma cells.

Pathophysiology and Etiology
1. Etiology unknown; genetic and environmental factors, such as chronic exposure to low levels of ionizing radiation, may play a part.
2. Characterized by proliferation of neoplastic plasma cells derived from one B lymphocyte (clone) and producing a homogeneous immunoglobulin (M protein or Bence Jones protein) without any apparent antigenic stimulation.
3. Plasma cells produce osteoclast-activating factor (OAF) leading to extensive bone loss, severe pain, and pathologic fractures.
4. Abnormal immunoglobulin affects renal function, platelet function, resistance to infection, and may cause hyperviscosity of blood.
5. Generally affects older people (median age at diagnosis is 68 years) and is more common among black men and women.

Clinical Manifestations
1. Constant, often severe bone pain caused by bone lesions and pathologic fractures; sites commonly affected include thoracic and lumbar vertebrae, ribs, skull, pelvis, and proximal long bones.
2. Fatigue and weakness related to anemia caused by crowding of marrow by plasma cells.
3. Proteinuria and renal insufficiency.
4. Electrolyte disturbances, including hypercalcemia (bone destruction), hyperuricemia (cell death, renal insufficiency).

Diagnostic Evaluation
1. Bone marrow aspiration and biopsy—demonstrate increased number and abnormal form of plasma cells.
2. CBC and blood smear—changes reflect anemia.
3. Urine and serum analysis for presence and quantity of abnormal immunoglobulin
4. Skeletal x-rays—osteolytic bone lesions.

Management
1. Chemotherapy, including oral melphalan (Alkeran) or cyclophosphamide (Cytoxan), corticosteroids alone or in combination with chemotherapy.
2. Alpha interferon as maintenance therapy.
3. Plasmapheresis to treat hyperviscosity or bleeding.

4. Radiation therapy for bone lesions.
5. Biophosphanates (eg, pamidronate), potent inhibitors of bone resorption, to treat hypercalcemia and alleviate bone pain.
6. Other supportive care options:
   a. Allopurinol (Zyloprim) and fluids to treat hyperuricemia.
   b. Hemodialysis to manage renal failure.
   c. Surgical stabilization and fixation of fractures.
7. Bone marrow or peripheral blood stem cell transplant in selected cases (usually less than 50 years of age with no renal failure, few bone lesions, and good organ function).

 DRUG ALERT

Pamidronate and other biophosphanates may cause transient temperature elevations, hypophosphatemia, hypomagnesemia, hypocalcemia, and local reactions at the site of intravenous administration, such as thrombophlebitis, pain, and erythema. Biophosphanates are administered as IV infusions, generally during 4 or more hours, rapid IV administration may cause renal failure.

Complications
1. Pathologic fractures, spinal cord compression.
2. Recurrent infections, particularly bacterial.
3. Electrolyte abnormalities (hypercalcemia, hypophosphatemia).
4. Renal failure, pyelonephritis.
5. Bleeding.
6. Thromboembolic complications caused by hyperviscosity.
7. Patients with multiple myeloma have a median survival of 3 to 4 years.

Nursing Assessment
1. Obtain health history, focusing on pain, fatigue.
2. Evaluate for evidence of bone deformities and bone tenderness or pain.
3. Assess patient's support system and personal coping skills.

Nursing Diagnoses
• Pain (bone) related to destruction of bone and possible pathologic fractures
• Impaired Physical Mobility related to pain and possible fracture
• Fear related to poor prognosis
• Risk for Injury related to complications of disease process

Nursing Interventions
Controlling Pain
1. Assess for presence, location, intensity, and characteristics of pain.
2. Administer pharmacologic agents as ordered to control pain. Use adequate doses of regularly scheduled, around-the-clock analgesics.

3. Teach the use of nonpharmacologic methods, such as the use of music, relaxation breathing, progressive muscle relaxation, distraction and imagery to help to manage pain.
4. Assess effectiveness of analgesics and adjust dosage or drug used as necessary to control pain.

Promoting Mobility

1. Encourage patient to wear back brace for lumbar lesion.
2. Recommend physical/occupational therapy consultation.
3. Discourage bed rest to prevent hypercalcemia but ensure safety of environment to prevent fractures.
4. Assist patient with measures to prevent injury and decrease risk of fractures. Advise avoidance of lifting and straining; use walker and other assistive devices as appropriate.

Relieving Fear

1. Develop trusting, supportive relationship with patient and significant others.
2. Encourage patient to discuss medical condition and prognosis with health care provider when patient is ready.
3. Ensure patient that you are available for support, to provide comfort measures, and to answer questions.
4. Encourage use of patient's own support network, religious and community services, and national agencies (see Box 26-1).

Monitoring for Complications

1. Report any sudden, severe pain, especially of back, which could indicate pathologic fracture.
2. Watch for nausea, drowsiness, confusion, polyuria, which could indicate hypercalcemia caused by bony destruction or immobilization. Monitor serum calcium levels.
3. Check results of blood urea nitrogen and creatinine and urine protein tests to detect renal insufficiency, caused by nephrotoxicity of abnormal proteins in multiple myeloma.
4. Increase fluid intake, monitor intake and output, and weigh patient daily.

Community and Home Care Considerations

1. Ensure patient has appropriate housing and equipment to support decreased mobility and risk for pathologic fractures (eg, stair handrails, cane or walker, commode chair, etc.).
2. Inspect home environment for throw rugs, cluttered furnishings, dark hallways, or difficult stairs that may cause a fall and possible fracture.

Patient Education and Health Maintenance

1. Teach patient about risk of infection caused by impaired antibody production (see p. 872).
2. Teach patient to take medications as prescribed and monitor for possible side effects; avoid aspirin and NSAIDs unless prescribed by health care provider, because these drugs may interfere with platelet function.

3. Teach patient to minimize risk of fractures. Use proper body mechanics and assistive devices as appropriate; avoid bed rest, remain ambulatory.
4. Advise patient to report new onset of pain, new location, or sudden increase in pain intensity immediately. Report new onset or worsening of neurologic symptoms (eg, changes in sensation) immediately.
5. Encourage the patient to maintain high fluid intake (2–3 L/d) to avoid dehydration and prevent renal insufficiency; also not to fast before diagnostic tests.
6. Provide patient and family with information about resources in the community, such as the Leukemia and Lymphoma Society and the American Cancer Society (see Box 26-1).

Outcome-Based Evaluation

- States decreased pain
- Ambulates without injury
- Asks questions about disease; contacts support group
- No development of complications

BLEEDING DISORDERS

Bleeding disorders may be congenital or acquired and may be caused by dysfunction in any phase of hemostasis (clot formation and dissolution). Bleeding disorders commonly seen in adults include thrombocytopenia, idiopathic thrombocytopenic purpura (ITP), disseminated intravascular coagulation (DIC), and von Willebrand's disease.

◼ Thrombocytopenia

Thrombocytopenia is a decrease in circulating platelet count (less than $100,000/mm^3$), and is the most common cause of bleeding disorders.

Pathophysiology and Etiology
Classification by Etiology

1. Decreased platelet production—infiltrative diseases of bone marrow, leukemia, aplastic anemia, myelofibrosis, myelosuppressive therapy, radiation therapy; may include inherited disorders such as Fanconi's anemia and Wiskott-Aldrich syndrome.
2. Increased platelet destruction—infection, drug-induced, ITP, DIC.
3. Abnormal distribution or sequestration in spleen.
4. Dilutional thrombocytopenia—after hemorrhage, RBC transfusions.

Clinical Manifestations

1. Usually asymptomatic.
2. When platelet count drops below $20,000/mm^3$:
   a. Petechiae occur spontaneously.
   b. Ecchymoses occur at sites of minor trauma (venipuncture, pressure).

c. Bleeding may occur from mucosal surfaces, nose, gastrointestinal and genitourinary tracts, respiratory system, and within CNS.

d. Menorrhagia is common.

e. Excessive bleeding may occur after procedures (dental extractions, minor surgery, biopsies).

Diagnostic Evaluation

1. CBC with platelet count—decreased hemoglobin, hematocrit, platelets.
2. Bleeding time, prothrombin time (PT), partial thromboplastin time (PTT)—prolonged.

Management

1. Treat underlying cause.
2. Platelet transfusions.
3. Steroids or IV immunoglobulins may be helpful in selected patients.

Complications

Severe blood loss or bleeding into vital organs may be life-threatening.

Nursing Assessment

1. Obtain health history, focusing on prior illnesses and episodes of bleeding, past surgical experiences, exposure to toxins or ionizing radiation, family history of bleeding.
2. Obtain complete list of current and recent medications (including over-the-counter preparations).
3. Perform complete physical examination for signs of bleeding.

Nursing Diagnosis

• Risk for Injury related to bleeding due to thrombocytopenia

Nursing Interventions

Minimizing Bleeding

1. Institute bleeding precautions.
   a. Avoid use of plain razor, hard toothbrush or floss, intramuscular injections, tourniquets, rectal procedures or suppositories.
   b. Administer stool softeners as necessary to prevent constipation.
   c. Restrict activity and exercise when platelet count is less than 20,000/mm³ or when active bleeding occurs.
2. Monitor pad count/amount of saturation during menses; administer or teach self-administration of hormones to suppress menstruation as prescribed.
3. Administer blood products as ordered. Monitor for signs and symptoms of allergic reactions, anaphylaxis, and volume overload.
4. Evaluate urine, stool and emesis for gross and occult blood.

Patient Education and Health Maintenance

1. Teach patient bleeding precautions as described above; also:
   a. Avoid blowing nose.
   b. Take only prescribed medications and avoid use of aspirin and NSAIDs, which may interfere with platelet function.
2. Demonstrate the use of direct, steady pressure at bleeding site if bleeding does develop.
3. Encourage routine follow up for platelet counts.

Outcome-Based Evaluation

• Episodes of bleeding rapidly controlled
• Platelet count maintained at goal (usually 20,000/mm³) by transfusions and therapy

Autoimmune (Idiopathic) Thrombocytopenic Purpura

Autoimmune thrombocytopenic purpura, or idiopathic immune thrombocytopenic purpura, is an acute or chronic bleeding disorder that results from immune destruction of platelets by antiplatelet antibodies.

Pathophysiology and Etiology

1. Autoantibodies of both IgG and IgM subclasses, directed against a platelet-associated antigen, lead to destruction of platelets in spleen, liver.
2. Acute disorder more common in childhood, typically following viral illness; has good prognosis with 80% to 90% recovering uneventfully. Typically lasts 1 to 2 months.
3. Chronic disorder (more than 6-month course) most common at ages 20 to 40, three times more common in women, may last for years or even indefinitely. May be associated with development of systemic lupus erythematosus (SLE) or thyroid disease.

Clinical Manifestations

Bruising, petechiae, bleeding from nares and gums, menorrhagia.

Diagnostic Evaluation

1. CBC demonstrates platelet count less than 20,000/mm³ (acute ITP); 30,000 to 70,000/mm³ (chronic ITP); may also be lymphocytosis and eosinophilia.
2. Bone marrow aspirate shows increased numbers of young megakaryocytes, sometimes increased numbers of eosinophils.
3. Assay for platelet autoantibodies sometimes helpful.

Management

1. Supportive care: judicious use of platelet transfusions, control of bleeding.
2. High dose corticosteroids, IV immunoglobulins (IVIG), danazol (Danocrine), azathioprine (Imuran), vincristine (Oncovin), vinblastine (Velban).

3. Splenectomy (see p. 861) removes potential site for sequestration and destruction of platelets.

Complications

Severe blood loss or bleeding into vital organs may be life-threatening.

Nursing Assessment

1. Obtain history of bleeding episodes, including bruising and petechiae, bleeding of gums, and heavy menses.
2. Perform physical examination for signs of bleeding.

Nursing Diagnosis

• Risk for Injury related to bleeding due to thrombocytopenia

Nursing Interventions

Minimizing Bleeding

1. Institute bleeding precautions (see p. 886).
2. Monitor pad count/amount of saturation during menses; administer or teach self-administration of hormones to suppress menstruation as prescribed.
3. Administer blood products as ordered. Monitor for signs and symptoms of allergic reactions, anaphylaxis, and volume overload.
4. Evaluate all urine and stools for gross and occult blood.

Patient Education and Health Maintenance

1. Teach patient bleeding precautions as outlined above; also avoid blowing nose, take only prescribed medications, avoid use of aspirin and NSAIDs, which may interfere with platelet function.
2. Demonstrate the use of direct, steady pressure at bleeding site if bleeding does develop.
3. Encourage routine follow-up for platelet counts.

Outcome-Based Evaluation

• Episodes of bleeding rapidly controlled

■ Disseminated Intravascular Coagulation

Disseminated intravascular coagulation is an acquired thrombotic and hemorrhagic syndrome characterized by abnormal activation of the clotting cascade and accelerated fibrinolysis. This results in widespread clotting in small vessels of the body with consumption of clotting factors and platelets, so that bleeding and thrombosis occur simultaneously.

Pathophysiology and Etiology

1. A syndrome arising with an underlying disorder or event:
   a. Overwhelming infections, particularly bacterial sepsis.
   b. Obstetric complications: abruptio placentae, eclampsia, amniotic fluid embolism, retention of dead fetus.

   c. Massive tissue injury: burns, trauma, fractures, major surgery, fat embolism.
   d. Vascular and circulatory collapse, shock.
   e. Hemolytic transfusion reaction.
   f. Malignancy: particularly of lung, colon, stomach, pancreas.

Clinical Manifestations

1. Signs of abnormal clotting:
   a. Coolness and mottling of extremities.
   b. Acrocyanosis (cold, mottled extremities with clear demarcation from normal tissue).
   c. Dyspnea, adventitious breath sounds.
   d. Altered mental status.
   e. Acute renal failure.
   f. Pain (eg, related to bowel infarction).
2. Signs of abnormal bleeding:
   a. Oozing, bleeding from sites of procedures, IV catheter insertion sites, suture lines, mucous membranes, orifices.
   b. Internal bleeding leading to changes in vital organ function, altered vital signs.

Diagnostic Evaluation

1. Platelet count—diminished.
2. PT, PTT and TT—prolonged.
3. Fibrinogen—decreased level.
4. Fibrin split (degradation) products—increased level.
5. D-Dimer fibrin degradation product—increased level.
6. Antithrombin III—decreased level.

Management

1. Treat underlying disorder.
2. Replacement therapy for serious hemorrhagic manifestations:
   a. Fresh frozen plasma replaces clotting factors.
   b. Platelet transfusions.
   c. Cryoprecipitate replaces clotting factors and fibrinogen.
3. Supportive measures including fluid replacement, oxygenation, maintenance of blood pressure and renal perfusion.
4. Heparin therapy (controversial) inhibits clotting component of DIC.

Complications

1. Thromboembolic: pulmonary embolism, cerebral, myocardial, splenic or bowel infarction, acute renal failure, tissue necrosis or gangrene.
2. Hemorrhagic: cerebral hemorrhage is most common cause of death in DIC.

Nursing Assessment

1. Be aware that all seriously ill patients are at risk; monitor condition closely.
2. Assess for signs of bleeding and thrombosis, including chest pain, shortness of breath, hematuria, ab-

dominal pain, headache, numbness and coolness of an extremity.

Nursing Diagnoses
- Risk for Injury related to bleeding due to thrombocytopenia
- Altered Tissue Perfusion (all tissues) related to ischemia due to microthrombi formation

Nursing Interventions
Minimizing Bleeding
1. Institute bleeding precautions (see p. 886).
2. Monitor pad count/amount of saturation during menses; administer or teach self-administration of hormones to suppress menstruation as prescribed.
3. Administer blood products as ordered. Monitor for signs and symptoms of allergic reactions, anaphylaxis, and volume overload.
4. Avoid dislodging clots. Apply pressure to sites of bleeding for at least 20 minutes, use topical hemostatic agents. Use tape cautiously.
5. Maintain bed rest during bleeding episode.
6. If internal bleeding is suspected, assess bowel sounds and abdominal girth.
7. Evaluate fluid status and bleeding by frequent measurement of vital signs, central venous pressure, intake and output.

Promoting Tissue Perfusion
1. Keep patient warm.
2. Avoid vasoconstrictive agents (systemic or topical).
3. Change patient's position frequently and perform range of motion exercises.
4. Monitor electrocardiogram and laboratory tests for dysfunction of vital organs caused by ischemia—arrhythmias, abnormal arterial blood gases, increased blood urea nitrogen and creatinine, etc.
5. Monitor for signs of vascular occlusion and report immediately.
   a. Brain—decreased level of consciousness, sensory and motor deficits, seizures, coma).
   b. Eyes—visual deficits.
   c. Bone—bone pain.
   d. Pulmonary vasculature—chest pain, shortness of breath, tachycardia.
   e. Extremities—cold, mottling, numbness.
   f. Coronary arteries—chest pain, arrhythmias.
   g. Bowel—pain, tenderness, decreased bowel sounds.

Patient Education and Health Maintenance
Explain the syndrome and its management to patient and family members as part of reassurance and support during this critical illness.

Outcome-Based Evaluation
- Episodes of bleeding rapidly controlled
- Alert, vital signs stable, urine output adequate, no complaints of chest pain or shortness of breath

von Willebrand's Disease
Inherited (autosomal dominant) or acquired bleeding disorder characterized by decreased level of von Willebrand factor and prolonged bleeding time.

Pathophysiology and Etiology
1. von Willebrand factor synthesized in vascular endothelium, megakaryocytes and platelets; enhances platelet adhesion as first step in clot formation, also acts as carrier of factor VIII in blood.
2. von Willebrand's is most common inherited bleeding disorder; includes multiple subtypes with varying severity.
3. Acquired form is rare, generally appears late in life, often in association with lymphoma, leukemia, multiple myeloma, or autoimmune disorder.

Clinical Manifestations
1. Mucosal and cutaneous bleeding (eg, bruising, gingival bleeding, epistaxis, menorrhagia).
2. Prolonged bleeding from cuts or after dental and surgical procedures.

Diagnostic Evaluation
1. Bleeding time—prolonged.
2. von Willebrand's factor—decreased.
3. Factor VIII—generally decreased.

Management
1. Replacement of factor VIII via infusions of cryoprecipitate.
2. Antifibrinolytic medication (Amicar) to stabilize clot formation before dental procedures and before minor surgery.
3. Desmopressin (DDAVP), a synthetic analogue of vasopressin, may be used to manage mild to moderate bleeding.

Complications
Severe blood loss or bleeding into vital organs may be life-threatening.

Nursing Assessment
1. Obtain history of bleeding episodes, such as menstrual flow.
2. Perform physical examination for signs of bleeding.

Nursing Diagnosis
- Risk for Injury related to bleeding due to decreased level of factor VIII

Nursing Interventions
Minimizing Bleeding
1. Institute bleeding precautions—avoid use of plain razor, hard toothbrush or floss, intramuscular injections, tourniquets, rectal procedures or suppositories; administer stool softeners as necessary to prevent constipation;

restrict activity and exercise when platelet count less than 20,000/mm³ or when active bleeding occurs.

2. Monitor pad count/amount of saturation during menses; administer or teach self-administration of hormones to suppress menstruation as prescribed.

3. Administer blood products as ordered. Monitor for signs and symptoms of allergic reactions, anaphylaxis, and volume overload.

Patient Education and Health Maintenance

1. Teach patient bleeding precautions; also advise to avoid blowing nose, and to take only prescribed medications, avoid use of aspirin and NSAIDs, which may interfere with platelet function.

2. Demonstrate the use of direct, steady pressure at bleeding site if bleeding develops.

Outcome-Based Evaluation

• Episodes of bleeding rapidly controlled

SELECTED REFERENCES

Acevedo, M. (1992). Blood dyscrasias: Polycythemia, idiopathic thrombocytopenic purpura, and thrombotic thrombocytopenic purpura. *Journal of Intravenous Nursing, 15*(1), 52–57.

Ayalew, T. (1998). The Philadelphia chromosome negative chronic myeloproliferative disorders: A practical overview. *Mayo Clinic Proceedings, 73*(12), 1177–1184.

Battaile, R., & Harousseau, J.L. (1997). Medical progress: Multiple myeloma. *New England Journal of Medicine, 336*(23), 1659–1664.

Bean, C.A. (1997). Acute lymphocytic leukemia: Nursing care, psychosocial issues, and discharge education. *Oncology Nursing Forum, 24*(6), 961–962.

Bilodeau, B.A., & Fessele, K.L. (1998). Non-Hodgkin's lymphoma. *Seminars in Oncology Nursing, 14*(4), 273–283.

Callaghan, M. (1998). Hodgkin's disease. *Seminars in Oncology Nursing, 14*(4), 262–272.

Colvin, B.T. (1998). Management of disseminated intravascular coagulation. *British Journal of Haematology, 101*(1S), Supplement, 15–17.

Erickson, J.M. (1996). Anemia. *Seminars in Oncology Nursing, 12*(1), 2–14.

Groenwald, S.L., Frogge, M.H., Goodman, M., & Yarbro, C.H. (Eds.). (1997). *Cancer nursing: Principles and practice* (4th ed.). Boston: Jones and Bartlett.

Griffeth, C.J. (1996). Evaluation and management of anemia: A cost-effective approach. *Advance for Nurse Practitioners, 5,* 29–35.

Huston, C.J. (1994). Disseminated intravascular coagulation. *American Journal of Nursing, 94*(8), 51.

Karpatkin, S. (1997). Autoimmune (idiopathic) thrombocytopenic purpura. *The Lancet, 349*(9064), 1531–1536.

Marsh, J.C.W., & Gordon-Smith, E.C. (1998). Treatment options in severe aplastic anemia. *The Lancet, 9119,* 1830–1832.

Pui, C.H., & Evans, W.E. (1998). Drug therapy: Acute lymphoblastic leukemia. *New England Journal of Medicine, 339*(9), 605–615.

Shelton, B.K., Baker, L., & Stecker, S. (1996). Critical care of the patient with hematologic malignancy. *AACN Clinical Issues, 7*(1), 65–78.

Sheridan, C.A. (1998). Multiple myeloma. *Seminars in Oncology Nursing, 12*(1), 59–69.

Sitton, E. (1992). Early and late radiation-induced skin alterations. Part I: Mechanisms of skin changes. *Oncology Nursing Forum, 19*(5), 801–807.

Sitton, E. (1992). Early and late radiation-induced skin alterations. Part II: Nursing care of irradiated skin. *Oncology Nursing Forum, 19*(6), 907–912.

Skarin, A.T., & Dorfman, D.M. (1997). Non-Hodgkin's lymphomas: Current classification and management. *CA-A Cancer Journal for Clinicians, 47,* 351–372.

Volker, D. (1998). Fever of unknown origin. *Nurse Practitioner Forum, 9*(3), 170–176.

Whedon, M.B., & Wujcik, D. (Eds.). (1997). *Blood and marrow stem cell transplantation: Principles, practice, and nursing insights* (2nd ed.). Boston: Jones and Bartlett.

Yeager, K.A., & Miaskowski, C. (1994). Advances in understanding the mechanisms and management of acute myelogenous leukemia. *Oncology Nursing Forum, 21*(3), 541–548.

Young, N.S., & Maciejewski, J. (1997). Mechanisms of disease: Pathophysiology of acquired aplastic anemia. *New England Journal of Medicine, 336*(19), 1365–1372.

Ziegfeld, C.R., Lubejko, B.G., & Shelton, B.K. (1998). *Manual of cancer care.* Philadelphia: Lippincott-Raven.

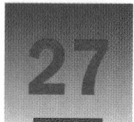
Transfusion Therapy and Blood and Marrow Stem Cell Transplantation

TRANSFUSION THERAPY

🔲 Principles of Transfusion Therapy

Because of the potentially life-threatening consequences of blood type ABO incompatibility and the recent safety concerns about disease transmission through blood products, transfusion therapy has been limited to occasions when it is absolutely necessary. In addition, various transfusion options and stringent screening techniques before transfusion have been instituted. Blood product procurement, storage, preparation, and testing are regulated by the Food and Drug Administration, the American Association of Blood Banks, and the Joint Commission on Accreditation of Healthcare Organizations.

Blood Compatibility
Antigens
1. The surface membrane of the red blood cell (RBC) is characterized by glycoproteins known as antigens.
2. More than 400 different antigens have been identified on the RBC membrane.
3. There are less than a dozen of clinically significant antigens, and of these, only two antigenic systems (ABO and Rh) require routine prospective matching before the transfusion.
4. The ABO blood group system is clinically the most significant because A and B antigens elicit the strongest immune response.
5. The presence or absence of A and B antigens on the RBC membrane determines the person's ABO group

(Table 27-1). The ability to make A or B antigens is inherited.
6. Antibody formation without specific exposure to antigen is unique to the ABO system. Antibody directed against the missing antigen(s) is produced by the age of 3 months in neonates.

Antibodies
1. Antibodies (or immunoglobulins) are proteins produced by B lymphocytes; they consist of two light and two heavy chains that form a Y shape.
2. Antibodies generally have a high degree of specificity, and interact only with the antigen that stimulated their production.
3. The five classes of immunoglobulins are determined by differences in their heavy chains: IgG, IgA, IgM, IgD, IgE.
4. The interaction of antibodies and antigens triggers an immune response, the humoral immune response.
5. Antibodies against the A and B antigens are large IgM molecules. When they interact with and coat the A and B antigens on the RBC surface, the antibody/RBC complexes clump together (agglutinate).
6. Antibody/RBC complexes also activate the complement cascade, resulting in the release of numerous active substances and RBC lysis. The large antibody/RBC complexes also become trapped in capillaries, where they may cause thrombotic complications to vital organs, and in the reticuloendothelial system, where they are removed from circulation by the spleen.
7. The extent of the humoral response elicited by anti-A and anti-B interaction with A and B antigens depends on the quantity of antibody and antigen.

TABLE 27-1 Blood Group Antigens and Antibodies of ABO System

Blood Group	Antigen on RBC	Antibody in Plasma	Approximate Frequency of Occurrence in Population
A	A	anti-B	45%
B	B	anti-A	8%
AB	A and B	none	3%
O	none	anti-A and anti-B	44%

Other Red Blood Cell Antigens

1. Non-ABO RBC antigen–antibody reactions usually do not produce powerful immediate hemolytic reactions, but several have clinical significance.
2. After A and B, D is the most immunogenic antigen. It is part of the Rhesus system, which includes C, D, and E antigens.
   a. D (Rh)-negative people do not develop anti-D without specific exposure, but have a high incidence of antibody development (alloimmunization) after exposure to D.
   b. Two common methods of sensitization to these RBC antigens are by transfusion or fetomaternal hemorrhage during pregnancy and delivery.
   c. Anti-D can complicate future transfusions and pregnancies. For the D (Rh)-negative person, exposure to D should be avoided by the use of Rh-negative blood products. In the case of Rh-negative mother and Rh-positive fetus, prophylaxis for exposure to D uses Rh immunoglobulin, which will prevent anti-D formation.
   d. Exposure to RBC antigens from other antigenic systems (such as Lewis, Kidd, or Duffy) may also cause alloimmunization, which becomes clinically significant in people who receive multiple blood products during long periods of time.

Blood Transfusion Options
Autologous Transfusion

1. Before elective procedures, the patient may donate blood to be set aside for later transfusion.
2. Autologous RBCs can also be salvaged during some surgical procedures or after trauma-induced hemorrhage by use of automated cell-saver devices or by manual suction equipment.
3. Autologous blood products must be clearly labeled and identified.
4. Autologous transfusion eliminates the risks of alloimmunization, immune-mediated transfusion reactions, and transmission of disease, making it the safest transfusion choice.

Homologous Transfusion

1. With the most common option, volunteer donors' blood products are assigned randomly to patients.
2. Before donation, volunteer donors receive information about the process, potential side effects, tests that will be performed on donated blood, postdonation instructions, and education regarding risk for human immunodeficiency virus (HIV) infection and signs and symptoms.
3. Donors are screened against eligibility criteria designed to protect both donor and recipient (Table 27-2).

Directed Transfusion

1. In directed transfusion, blood products are donated by a person for transfusion to a specified recipient.
2. This option may be used in certain circumstances (eg, a parent who provides sole transfusion support for a child), but in general, no evidence exists that directed donation reduces transfusion risks.

Blood Product Screening
Serologic Testing

1. Routine laboratory testing is performed to assess the compatibility of a particular blood product with the recipient before release of the blood product from the blood bank.
   a. ABO group and Rh type: determines the presence of A, B, and D antigens on the surface of the patient's RBCs.

TABLE 27-2 General Blood Donor Eligibility Criteria

Age	Generally 17–66 y.
Weight	Minimum 110 lb.
Vital Signs	Afebrile, normotensive, pulse 50–100.
Hemoglobin	Lower limit for females 12.5 g/dL; for males 13.5 g/dL.
History	Exposure to AIDS evaluated; high-risk groups deferred. International travel to malarial areas is cause for deferral. Pregnancy, recent (<6 wk) delivery, or blood transfusion during prior 6 mo is cause for temporary deferral. History of any hepatitis is cause for deferral.
Immunizations	Attenuated viral vaccines: 2-wk deferral. Rubella vaccine: 1 mo deferral. Rabies vaccine: 1-y deferral. Killed vaccines or toxoids: acceptable if symptom free.
Illnesses	Positive HIV test, diseases of heart, lungs, or liver, abnormal bleeding, or history of cancer are causes for deferral.

b. Direct Coombs' test: determines the antibody attached to the patient's RBCs.

c. Crossmatch (compatibility test): detects agglutination of donor RBCs caused by antibodies in the patient's serum.

d. Indirect Coombs' test: identifies lower molecular weight antibodies (IgG) directed against blood group antigens.

Screening for Infectious Diseases

1. Routine laboratory testing is performed to identify antigens or antibodies in donor blood that may indicate prior exposure to specific blood-borne diseases.

2. Such testing supplements other principles of donation designed to decrease the risk of disease transmission via blood products, including the use of volunteer donors, the exclusion of high-risk populations, and the screening of donors via health and social history.

3. Through the use of donor screening and blood testing the risk of infections transmitted with donated blood is <1%.

4. Specific conditions screened for include:

   a. Hepatitis: tests for the presence of hepatitis B surface antigen and most recently, hepatitis C, the most common non-A, non-B hepatitis.

   b. HIV: tests for the antibody against HIV, which indicates prior exposure to the virus.

      (i) All blood products in the United States have been screened since the test first became available in 1985.

      (ii) Because antibody to the virus is not produced until at least 6 weeks after exposure, donor screening and exclusion of high-risk groups (eg, gay men, intravenous [IV] drug abusers, prostitutes, and sexual partners of high-risk people) remain important parts of preventing transmission of HIV via blood products.

      (iii) A low risk of HIV transmission (estimated to be 1/100,000 units of blood) remains.

   c. Cytomegalovirus (CMV): tests for the antibody against CMV.

      (i) Approximately 50% to 75% of blood donors have been exposed to CMV and 10% to 20% carry CMV virus in white blood cells (WBCs).

      (ii) Patients with impaired immune function (eg, bone marrow and organ transplant recipients, premature babies) are at risk for CMV infection from transfused blood.

   d. Syphilis: tests for the presence of antibody against the spirochete.

   e. Bacteria: contamination of blood products with bacteria may occur during and after collection of blood. This risk is managed by maintenance of sterile technique during phlebotomy and blood processing procedures, correct storage techniques, visual inspection of blood products, and limitation on shelf life.

   f. Other infections that may be transmitted via blood transfusions include malaria, babesios, Chagas' disease, and yersinia.

■ Administration of Whole Blood and Blood Components

Whole blood and blood components are administered to increase the amount of oxygen being delivered to the tissues and organs, to prevent or stop bleeding because of platelet defects or because of deficiencies or coagulation abnormalities, and to combat infection caused by decreased or defective WBCs or antibodies. (See Procedure Guidelines 27-1; also see Standards of Care Guidelines.)

General Considerations

1. A unit of whole blood is usually separated into its various component parts shortly after collection.

2. Less than 3% of the blood collected nationwide is transfused as whole blood.

3. The use of blood components conserves the limited supply of blood, provides optimal therapeutic benefit, and reduces the risk of circulatory overload.

Whole Blood

Description

1. Consists of RBCs, plasma, plasma proteins, and approximately 60 mL anticoagulant/preservative solution in a total volume of approximately 500 mL.

2. Indications include acute, massive blood loss of greater than 1,000 mL, requiring the oxygen-carrying properties of RBCs and the volume expansion provided by plasma. In general, even acute loss of as much as one-third of a patient's total blood volume (1,000–1,200 mL) can be safely and rapidly replaced with crystalline or colloidal solutions.

Nursing and Patient Care Considerations

1. For rapid infusions of large volumes of whole blood, additional steps may be taken to deliver product rapidly and safely.

   a. A small-pore (20-40 μm) filter may be used to remove microaggregates (platelets, WBCs) that have been identified in the lungs of massively transfused patients.

   b. An approved blood warmer may be indicated to prevent hypothermia and cardiac arrhythmias associated with the rapid infusion of refrigerated solutions.

   c. Electromechanical infusion devices to deliver blood at high flow rates can hemolyze RBCs and should be used with caution.

2. Observe closely for the most common acute complication associated with whole blood transfusion—circulatory overload (rise in venous pressure, distended neck veins, dyspnea, cough, crackles at bases of lungs).

3. Reduce the risk of hemolytic reactions by meticulously confirming ABO and Rh compatibility and patient identification before infusion (Table 27-3).

PROCEDURE GUIDELINES 27-1 — ADMINISTERING BLOOD AND BLOOD COMPONENTS

EQUIPMENT

Tourniquet
Iodine-containing skin antiseptic
Needle or venous catheter
Y-type blood infusion set

170-μ filter
Normal saline
Blood product as described

PROCEDURE

Nursing Action	Rationale

PREPARATORY PHASE

1. Inform the patient of the procedure, blood product to be given, approximate length of time, and desired outcome of transfusion.
2. Obtain and record baseline vital signs.

3. Prepare infusion site. Select a large vein that allows patient some degree of mobility. Start the prescribed intravenous infusion.

1. Instruct the patient to report unusual symptoms immediately.

2. If the patient's clinical status permits, delay transfusion if baseline temperature is greater than 38.5°C (101.7°).

3. Antecubital veins are not recommended for lengthy infusions. Prolonged restriction of arm movement is uncomfortable and inconvenient for the patient. In the event of an acute reaction, the intravenous catheter should be maintained with normal saline.

 DRUG ALERT

Crystalloid solutions other than 0.9% saline and all medications are incompatible with blood products. They may cause agglutination and/or hemolysis.

4. Obtain blood product from blood bank. Inspect for abnormal color, cloudiness, clots, and excess air. Read instructions on the product label regarding storage and infusion. Check expiration date.

5. Verify patient identification.
   a. Ask the patient to state his or her full name and compare with name on the wrist band. If the patient is unable to state his or her name, verify identity with an individual familiar with the patient.
   b. Compare the name and ID number on the wristband with the bag tag, transfusion form, and medical order.
   c. Confirm ABO and Rh compatibility by comparing the bag label, bag tag, medical record, and/or transfusion form.
   d. Check bag labels for expiration date and satisfactory serologic testing.

4. Platelets are normally cloudy. If the transfusion cannot begin immediately, return product to blood bank. Blood out of proper storage for more than 30 min (above 10°C [150°F]) cannot be reissued. Never store blood in unauthorized refrigerators, such as those on the nursing unit.

5. The majority of acute fatal transfusion reactions are caused by clerical errors. Patient and product verification is the single most important function of the nurse. It is strongly recommended that two qualified individuals perform this task. Do not proceed with the transfusion if there is any discrepancy. Contact the blood bank immediately.

PERFORMANCE PHASE

1. Start infusion slowly (ie, 2 mL/min). Remain at bedside 15–30 min. If there are no signs of side effect, increase flow to the prescribed rate.

2. Observe the patient closely and check vital signs at least hourly until 1 h after transfusion. Report signs of side effect to health care provider immediately.
3. Record the following information on the patient's chart:
   a. Time and names of persons starting and ending the transfusion.
   b. Names of individuals verifying patient ID.
   c. Unique product identification number.
   d. Product and volume infused.
   e. Immediate response—for example, "no apparent reaction."

1. Institutional policy may vary regarding flow rates and patient monitoring. Signs of a severe transfusion reaction (ie, acute hemolytic, anaphylactic) are usually manifested during infusion of the initial 50–100 mL.

2. Acute reactions may occur at any time during the transfusion.

3. Facts relating to the transfusion should be charted exactly.

   c. It must be possible to trace each transfusion product to the original blood donor.

STANDARDS OF CARE GUIDELINES
Blood Transfusion

When administering whole blood or blood components, ensure the following:

- Follow up on results of CBC and report to health care provider so appropriate blood product can be ordered based on patient's condition.
- Contact the blood bank with health care provider's order and ensure timely delivery of blood product.
- Establish a patent IV line with compatible IV fluid.
- Use appropriate administration set up, filter, warmer, etc.
- Obtain baseline vital signs.
- Ensure proper blood product is given to the right patient.
- Transfuse at prescribed rate during prescribed time, as tolerated by patient.
- Observe for acute reactions—allergic, febrile, septic, hemolytic, air embolism, and circulatory overload—by assessing vital signs, breath sounds, edema, flushing, urticaria, vomiting, headache, back pain.
- Notify patient's health care provider or available house officer if any signs of reaction or other abnormality arise.
- Be aware of delayed reactions and educate patient on risk and what to look for: hemolytic, iron overload, graft versus host disease, hepatitis, and other infectious diseases.

This information should serve as a general guideline only. Each patient situation presents a unique set of clinical factors and requires nursing judgment to guide care, which may include additional or alternative measures and approaches.

Packed Red Blood Cells
Description

1. Consist primarily of RBCs, a small amount of plasma, and approximately 100 mL anticoagulant/preservative solution in a total volume of approximately 250 to 300 mL/unit.
2. Packed RBCs are typically contaminated with WBCs that may increase the risk of minor transfusion reactions and alloimmunization. For patients who receive multiple blood products during a period of time (eg, patients with leukemia or aplastic anemia), packed RBCs may be further manipulated to remove WBCs by washing or freezing the product in the blood bank or by the use of small-pore (20–40 μm) filters during administration.
3. Indications include restoration or maintenance of adequate organ oxygenation with minimal expansion of blood volume.
4. Dosage: average adult dose administered is 2 units; pediatric doses are generally calculated as 5 to 15 mL/kg.

Nursing and Patient Care Considerations

1. Infuse at the prescribed rate. Generally, a unit can be given to an adult in 90 to 120 minutes. Pediatric patients are usually transfused at a rate of 2 to 5 mL/kg per hour.
2. To reduce the risk of bacterial contamination and sepsis, RBCs must be transfused within 4 hours of leaving the blood bank.
3. Observe closely (particularly during first 15 to 30 minutes) for the most common acute complications associated with packed RBCs, allergic and febrile transfusion reactions. Signs and symptoms of the more serious, but rare, hemolytic transfusion reaction are usually manifested during infusion of the first 50 mL.

Platelet Concentrates
Description

1. Consist of platelets suspended in plasma. Products vary according to the number of units (each unit is a minimum of 5.5×10^{10} platelets) and the volume of plasma (50 to 400 mL).
2. Platelets may be obtained by centrifuging multiple units of whole blood and expressing off the platelet-rich plasma (multiple-donor platelets) or from a single volunteer platelet donor using automated cell separation techniques (apheresis). The use of single donor products

---

TABLE 27-3 ABO & Rh Compatibility Chart

WHOLE BLOOD

Recipient	A	B	O	AB	Rh Positive	Rh Negative
					Donor	
A	•					
B		•				
O			•			
AB				•		
Rh Positive					•	•
Rh Negative						•

RED BLOOD CELLS

Recipient	A	B	O	AB	Rh Positive	Rh Negative
					Donor	
A	•		•			
B		•	•			
O			•			
AB	•	•	•	•		
Rh Positive					•	•
Rh Negative						•

PLASMA

Recipient	A	B	O	AB	Rh Positive	Rh Negative
					Donor	
A	•			•		
B		•		•		
O	•	•	•	•		
AB				•		
Rh Positive					•	•
Rh Negative					•	•

The chart above identifies ABO and Rh compatibility when transfusing whole blood, red blood cells, and plasma. Components suspended in plasma, such as platelets and cryoprecipitate, usually follow plasma compatibility rules if the total volume exceeds 120 mL for an adult patient.

decreases the number of donor exposures, thus decreasing the risk of alloimmunization and transfusion-transmitted disease.

3. Patients may become alloimmunized to human leukocyte antigens (HLA) through exposure to multiple platelet products. Apheresis products from HLA-matched platelet donors may be necessary. However, HLA-matched transfusions are often difficult to obtain because of the many possible HLA combinations in the population.

4. Indications include prevention or resolution of hemorrhage in patients with thrombocytopenia or platelet dysfunction.

5. Platelet transfusions are generally contraindicated in heparin-induced thrombocytopenia, where they may precipitate arterial thrombosis, and in thrombotic thrombocytopenic purpura (TTP) where they may worsen this autoimmune destruction of platelets.

6. Dosage: average dose is generally 1 unit of platelets for each 10 kg of body weight; however, patients who are actively bleeding or undergoing surgical procedures may require more.

Nursing and Patient Care Considerations

1. Infuse at the rate prescribed. Generally, the infusion can be completed within 20 to 60 minutes, depending on total volume.

2. Observe closely for the most common acute complications associated with platelet transfusions, allergic and febrile transfusion reactions.

3. Bacterial contamination of platelets, usually skin commensals from the donor's arm, occurs in 4 to 10 per 10,000 units and limits the shelf life of platelet products.

Plasma (Fresh or Fresh Frozen)
Description

1. Consists of water (91%), plasma proteins including essential clotting factors (7%), and carbohydrates (2%). Each unit is the volume removed from a unit of whole blood (200 to 250 mL).

2. May be stored in a liquid state or frozen within 6 hours of collection.

3. Indications include treatment of blood loss or blood clotting disorders related to liver disease and failure, disseminated intravascular coagulation (DIC), over-anticoagulation with warfarin (Coumadin), all congenital or acquired clotting factor deficiencies, and dilutional coagulopathy resulting from massive blood replacement. Storage in liquid state results in the loss of labile clotting factors V and VIII, so that only plasma that has been fresh frozen can be used to treat factor V and VIII deficiencies.

4. Dosage: depends on the clinical situation and assessment of prothrombin time (PT), partial thromboplastin time (PTT), or specific factor assays.

Nursing and Patient Care Considerations

1. Infuse at the rate prescribed. Generally, the infusion can be completed within 15 to 30 minutes, depending on total volume.

2. Observe closely for the most common acute complication associated with plasma infusion, volume overload.

Cryoprecipitate
Description

1. Consists of certain clotting factors suspended in 10 to 20 mL plasma. Each unit contains approximately 80 to 120 units of factor VIII (antihemophilic and von Willebrand factors), 250 mg fibrinogen, and 20% to 30% of the factor XIII present in a unit of whole blood.

2. Indications include correction of deficiencies of factor VIII (ie, hemophilia A and von Willebrand's disease), factor XIII, and fibrinogen (ie, DIC).

3. Dosage: Adult dosage is generally 10 units, which may be repeated every 8 to 12 hours until the deficiency is corrected or until hemostasis is achieved.

Nursing and Patient Care Considerations

Infuse at the rate prescribed. Generally, the infusion can be completed within 3 to 15 minutes.

Fractionated Plasma Products
Description

1. Various highly concentrated plasma protein products are commercially prepared by pooling thousands of single plasma units and by extracting the desired protein. Most techniques involve heat or chemical treatments, which eliminate the risk of transmitting blood-borne viruses, such as hepatitis B and HIV.

2. Colloid solutions provide volume expansion in situations where crystalloid solutions are not adequate, such as therapeutic plasma exchange, shock, and massive hemorrhage. They also may be used in the treatment of acute liver failure, burns, and hemolytic disease of the newborn.
   a. Albumin is available as a 5% solution, which is oncotically equivalent to plasma, and as a concentrated 25% solution.
   b. Plasma protein fraction (PPF) is available as a 5% solution. Rapid infusion of PPF has been associated with hypotension.
   c. Albumin and PPF are pasteurized and carry no risk of viral disease. They do not contain preservatives and should be used immediately after opening.

3. Immune serum globulins (ISGs) are concentrated aqueous solutions of gamma globulin that contain high titers of antibody.
   a. Must be administered by deep intramuscular injection.
   b. Nonspecific ISG is prepared from random donor plasma and is used to increase gamma globulin levels and to enhance general immune response in mild inherited or acquired immune disorders such as hypogammaglobulinemia.
   c. Specific ISG is prepared from donors who have high antibody titers to known antigens and is used to treat specific disorders or conditions. Hepatitis B immuno-

globulin, varicella zoster immunoglobulin, and Rh immunoglobulin are examples of specific ISGs.

   d. ISGs carry no risk of hepatitis B, HIV, or other blood-borne infections.
   e. Problems associated with use include pain at the injection site, limitations on volume administered, loss of IgG into extravascular tissue, or by degradation at the injection site.
4. Intravenous immunoglobulins (IVIGs) are aqueous solutions of immunoglobulins at a higher concentration and are given in larger volumes than ISGs.
   a. Like ISGs, they may be nonspecific or specific.
   b. Indications include chronic replacement therapy in patients with congenital or acquired immunodeficiency syndromes, acute autoimmune disorders such as immune thrombocytopenic purpura (ITP), and the treatment of chronic lymphocytic leukemia (CLL). Also, there are numerous investigational uses, such as Guillain-Barré syndrome, myasthenia gravis, rheumatoid arthritis, and viral infections such as CMV, adenovirus, and influenza. IVIGs also may be used to treat platelet alloimmunization.
   c. IVIGs do not appear to transmit HIV, but have been reported to transmit non-A, non-B hepatitis.
   d. Administration of IVIG should be closely monitored because of the possibility of anaphylactic reactions. Dosage and rate of infusion depend on the manufacturer's formulation.
5. Factor VIII concentrate is a lyophilized concentrate used to treat moderate to severe hemophilia A and severe von Willebrand's disease.
6. Factor IX concentrate is a lyophilized concentrate used to treat factor IX deficiency (Christmas disease).

Nursing and Patient Care Considerations
1. These products may be distributed by the pharmacy rather than by the blood bank.
2. Check order and product insert to ensure proper dosage and administration route.

Granulocyte Concentrates
Description
1. Consist of a minimum of 1×10^{10} granulocytes, variable amounts of lymphocytes (usually less than 10% of the total number of WBCs), 6 to 10 units of platelets, 30 to 50 mL RBCs, and 200 to 400 mL plasma.
2. Obtained via apheresis, generally of multiple donors.
3. Indications include treatment of life-threatening bacterial or fungal infection unresponsive to other therapy in patient with severe neutropenia.
4. Dosage: generally 1 unit daily for approximately 5 to 10 days, discontinuing if no therapeutic response.

Nursing and Patient Care Considerations
1. Product must be ABO compatible and, if possible, Rh compatible, because of the high erythrocyte content.
2. Transfuse granulocytes as soon as they are available. WBCs have a short survival time, and therapeutic benefit is directly related to dose and viability.

3. Premedicate per order to prevent side effects, generally with antihistamine and acetaminophen. Steroids or meperidine may also be required.
4. Begin the transfusion slowly and increase to the rate prescribed and as tolerated. The recommended length of infusion is 1 to 2 hours.
5. Observe the patient closely throughout the transfusion for signs and symptoms of febrile, allergic, and anaphylactic reactions, which may be severe. Have emergency medications and equipment readily available.
6. Agitate the bag approximately every 15 minutes to prevent granulocytes from clumping at the bottom of the bag.
7. Do not administer amphotericin B (Fungizone) immediately before or after granulocyte transfusion because pulmonary insufficiency has been reported with concurrent administration of amphotericin B and granulocytes. Many institutions recommend a 4-hour gap to avoid this risk.

Modified Blood Products
Purpose
1. To reduce the risk of specific transfusion-related complications, blood products may receive further processing or treatment.
   a. Leukocytes are removed from blood products through filtration, washing, and freezing to reduce the risk of febrile, nonhemolytic transfusion reactions, and alloimmunization to HLA antigens.
   b. Function and proliferation of donor lymphocytes are inhibited by irradiation, to decrease the risk of post-transfusion graft-versus-host disease (GVHD) in immunocompromised patients.

Methods
1. Filtration
   a. Standard filters (170 μm) effectively remove gross fibrin clots.
   b. Microaggregate filters (approximately 40 μm) remove microscopic aggregates of fibrin, platelets, and leukocytes that accumulate in RBC products during storage. Their use is recommended during rapid, massive transfusion of whole blood or packed RBCs to prevent pulmonary complications. They may also decrease the incidence of febrile transfusion reactions by removing many of the leukocytes present.
   c. Special leukocyte-depletion filters have been developed for use with platelet products that remove 80% to 95% of leukocytes and that retain 80% of the platelets. These filters may also reduce the risk of CMV transmission.
   d. A product may be filtered before release from the blood bank, but more commonly is released with the appropriate filter that must be attached to the standard infusion set at the bedside per manufacturer's or blood bank's instructions.

2. Washing
   a. Washing RBCs or platelets with a normal saline solution removes 80% to 95% of the WBCs and virtually all of the plasma to reduce the incidence of febrile, nonhemolytic transfusion reactions.
   b. Washing requires an additional hour of processing time, and the shelf life of the product is reduced to 24 hours after this additional manipulation.
3. Freezing
   a. RBCs can be frozen within 7 days of blood collection, and then remain viable for 7 to 10 years.
   b. Removal of the hypertonic freezing preservative (glycerol) before transfusion eliminates all of the plasma and 99% of WBCs.
   c. Thawing and deglycerolization of RBCs requires an additional 90 minutes of preparation time and reduces shelf life to 24 hours after this additional manipulation.
   d. Freezing is also an effective method of storing rare blood types and autologous RBCs.
4. Irradiation
   a. Exposure of blood products to a measured amount of gamma irradiation inhibits lymphocyte function and proliferation without damaging RBCs, platelets, or granulocytes. This eliminates the ability of transfused lymphocytes to engraft in the immunocompromised transfusion recipient and the accompanying risk of posttransfusion GVHD.
   b. Patients at risk for posttransfusion GVHD include bone marrow and peripheral stem cell transplant recipients, premature neonates, and patients with congenital immunodeficiency disorders, Hodgkin's disease, non-Hodgkin's lymphoma, and HIV.

◼ Transfusion Reactions

Every transfusion of blood components can result in a side effect. Reactions can be placed into two general categories: acute and delayed.

Acute Reactions

1. Acute reactions may occur during the infusion or within minutes to hours after the blood product has been infused.
2. Acute reactions include allergic, febrile, septic, and hemolytic reactions, air embolism, and circulatory overload. Patients who also receive multiple blood products within a short time frame may also be at risk for hyperkalemia, hypocalcemia, and hypothermia.
3. Because reactions may exhibit similar clinical manifestations, every symptom should be considered potentially serious and the transfusion should be discontinued until the cause is determined.
4. When a reaction is suspected, the health care provider should be notified immediately and blood bags with tubing from all products recently transfused should be returned to the blood bank for evaluation.

5. The following samples should also be obtained if an acute reaction is suspected.
   a. A clotted blood sample to examine serum for hemoglobin and confirm RBC group and type.
   b. An anticoagulated blood sample for a direct Coombs' test to determine the presence of antibody on the RBCs.
   c. The first voided urine sample to test for hemoglobinuria.
6. Precautions must be taken to avoid the hemolysis of RBCs during venipuncture and sample collection because this could lead to invalid test results. Whenever possible, blood samples should be drawn from a fresh venipuncture and not from existing needles or catheters.
7. If the only symptoms are those resulting from a mild allergic reaction (eg, urticaria), extensive evaluation may not be necessary. In the event of a severe reaction (eg, hypotension, tachypnea), more tests may be required to determine the cause of the reaction.
8. Causes, clinical manifestations, management, and prevention of acute reactions are summarized in Table 27-4.

Delayed Reactions

1. Delayed reactions occur days to years after the transfusion.
2. Delayed reactions include delayed hemolytic reactions, iron overload (hemosiderosis), GVHD, infectious diseases (e.g., hepatitis B, hepatitis C, CMV, Epstein-Barr virus, malaria, HIV).
   Patients who receive multiple blood products also may be at risk for iron overload (hemosiderosis).
3. Symptoms of a delayed reaction can vary from mild to severe. Diagnosis may be complicated by the long incubation period between transfusion and reaction and the complexity of diagnostic tests.
4. Causes, clinical manifestations, management, and prevention of delayed reactions are summarized in Table 27-5.

BLOOD AND MARROW STEM CELL TRANSPLANTATION

Blood and marrow stem cell transplantation are lifesaving treatments with application in many malignant and nonmalignant disorders. Several decades of research have advanced this technology from an experimental treatment of last resort to the preferred method of intervention for selected diseases. Although the basic procedures are now well established, this field continues to grow rapidly through ongoing research in areas such as the use of alternative sources of stem cells (e.g. peripheral blood, umbilical cord blood) and the application of biologic response modifiers to modulate the immune response.

TABLE 27-4   Acute Reactions to Blood Transfusion

Acute Reaction	Cause	Clinical Manifestations	Management	Prevention
Allergic	Sensitivity to plasma protein or donor antibody, which reacts with recipient antigen.	1. Flushing 2. Itching, rash 3. Urticaria, hives 4. Asthmatic wheezing 5. Laryngeal edema 6. Anaphylaxis	1. Stop transfusion immediately. Keep vein open (KVO) with normal saline. Notify health care provider and blood bank. 2. Give antihistamine as directed (diphenhydramine). 3. Observe for anaphylaxis—prepare epinephrine if respiratory distress is severe. 4. If hives are the only clinical manifestation, the transfusion can sometimes continue at a slower rate. 5. Send blood samples and blood bags to blood bank. Collect urine samples for testing.	Before transfusion, ask patient about past reactions. If patient has history of anaphylaxis, alert health care provider, have emergency drugs available, and remain at bedside for the first 30 min.
Febrile, non-hemolytic	Hypersensitivity to donor WBCs, platelets, or plasma proteins.	1. Sudden chills and fever 2. Headache 3. Flushing 4. Anxiety	1. Stop transfusion immediately and KVO with normal saline. Notify health care provider and blood bank. 2. Send blood samples and blood bags to blood bank. Collect urine samples for testing. 3. Check temperature ½ h after chill and as indicated thereafter. 4. Give antipyretics as prescribed—treat symptomatically.	Given antipyretic (acetaminophen or aspirin) before transfusion as directed. Leukocyte-poor blood products may be recommended for future transfusions.
Septic reactions	Transfusion of blood or components contaminated with bacteria.	1. Rapid onset of chills 2. High fever 3. Vomiting, diarrhea 4. Marked hypotension	1. Stop transfusion immediately and KVO with normal saline. Notify health care provider and blood bank. 2. Obtain cultures of patient's blood and return blood bags with administration set to blood bank for culture. 3. Treat septicemia as directed—antibiotics, IV fluids, vasopressors, steroids.	Do not permit blood to stand at room temperature longer than necessary. Warm temperatures promote bacterial growth. Inspect blood for gas bubbles, clotting, or abnormal color before transfusion Complete infusions within 4 h. Change administration set after 4 h of use.
Circulatory overload	Fluid administered at a rate or volume greater than the circulatory system can accommodate. Increased blood in pulmonary vessels and decreased lung compliance.	1. Rise in venous pressure 2. Distended neck veins 3. Dyspnea 4. Cough 5. Crackles at base of lungs	1. Stop transfusion and KVO with normal saline. Notify health care provider. 2. Place patient upright with feet in dependent position. 3. Administer prescribed diuretics, oxygen, morphine, and aminophylline.	Concentrated blood products should be given whenever positive. Transfuse at a rate within the circulatory reserve of the patient. Monitor central venous pressure of patient with heart disease.

(continued)

TABLE 27-4 Acute Reactions to Blood Transfusion (Continued)

Acute Reaction	Cause	Clinical Manifestations	Management	Prevention
Hemolytic reaction	Infusion of incompatible blood products: 1. Antibodies in recipient's plasma attach to transfused RBCs, hemolyzing the cells either in circulation or in the reticuloendothelial system. 2. Antibodies in donor plasma attach to recipient RBCs, causing hemolysis (may result from infusion of incompatible plasma—less severe than incompatible RBCs).	1. Chills; fever 2. Low back pain 3. Feeling of head fullness; flushing 4. Oppressive feeling 5. Tachycardia, tachypnea 6. Hypotension, vascular collapse 7. Hemoglobinuria, hemoglobinemia 8. Bleeding 9. Acute renal failure	1. Stop transfusion immediately—KVO with 0.9% saline. 2. Notify health care provider and blood bank. 3. Treat shock, if present 4. Draw testing samples, collect urine sample. 5. Maintain blood pressure with IV colloid solutions. Give diuretics as prescribed to maintain urine flow, glomerular filtration, and renal blood flow. 6. Insert indwelling catheter to monitor hourly urine output. Patient may require dialysis if renal failure occurs.	Meticulously verify patient identification—from sample collection to product infusion. Begin infusion slowly and observe closely for 30 min—consequences are in proportion to the amount of incompatible blood transfused.

◼ Principles of Blood and Marrow Stem Cell Transplantation

Types of Stem Cell Transplant

The type of transplant selected is contingent on factors, such as the underlying disorder, the availability of a histocompatible (HLA-matched) donor, and the clinical condition of the patient. Stem cells may come from the patient (autologous), and identical twin (syngeneic) or another donor (allogeneic). Stem cells are found in bone marrow, in peripheral blood (especially if the patient is treated to increase the numbers of circulating stem cells), and in umbilical cord blood.

Autologous Bone Marrow Transplantation

1. Bone marrow is removed from the patient during an operative harvesting procedure, frozen, and reinfused after the patient has undergone high-dose chemotherapy and possibly radiotherapy.
2. Advantages: readily available, in most cases lower morbidity and mortality than allogeneic bone marrow transplantation.
3. Disadvantages: operative procedure, marrow must be disease free, sufficient quantity of cellular marrow must be aspirable, in most cases has higher rate of relapse than allogeneic bone marrow transplantation.

Syngeneic Bone Marrow Transplantation

1. Bone marrow is removed from an identical twin during an operative harvesting procedure and infused into the patient, who has undergone high-dose chemotherapy and possibly radiotherapy.
2. Advantages: patient's marrow does not need to be harvestable (as in early relapse, aplastic anemia, CML), generally lower morbidity and mortality than allogeneic bone marrow transplantation.

3. Disadvantages: higher relapse rate than in allogeneic bone marrow transplantation.

Allogeneic Bone Marrow Transplantation

1. Bone marrow is removed from a donor who is most often a sibling or other close relative (related) but may be a volunteer donor (unrelated).
   a. Identical HLA phenotypes are preferred, although one or two mismatches may be used, especially if patient and donor are related.
   b. As with other types of BMT, this is done during an operative harvesting procedure and infused into the patient, who has undergone high-dose chemotherapy and possibly radiotherapy.
   c. Allogeneic bone marrow may be treated in various ways before infusion, including removing RBCs if ABO incompatible and removing T lymphocytes to reduce the risk of GVHD.
2. Advantages: patient's marrow does not need to be harvestable (as in early relapse, aplastic anemia, CML, genetic disorders), lowest rate of relapse (presumed because of a graft-versus-leukemia effect).
3. Disadvantages: risk for GVHD, generally higher morbidity and early mortality than other types of BMT. Unrelated and HLA mismatched transplants have higher risk of GVHD and infectious complications, and risk of graft rejection or failure.

Autologous or Allogeneic Peripheral Blood Stem Cell Transplantation

Although hematopoietic stem cells are primarily found in the bone marrow, they can also be found in the peripheral circulation in smaller numbers. This finding has led to the development of methods to harvest peripheral blood stem cells.

TABLE 27-5   Delayed Reactions to Transfusion Therapy

Delayed Reaction	Cause	Clinical Manifestations	Management	Prevention
Delayed hemolytic reaction	The destruction of transfused RBCs by antibody not detectable during crossmatch, but formed rapidly after transfusion. Rapid production may occur because of antigen exposure during previous transfusions or pregnancy.	1. Fever 2. Mild jaundice 3. Decreased hematocrit	Generally, no acute treatment is required, but hemolysis may be severe enough to cause shock and renal failure. If this occurs, manage as outlined under acute hemolytic reactions.	The crossmatch blood sample should be drawn within 3 d of blood transfusion. Antibody formation may occur within 90 d of transfusion and/or pregnancy.
Iron overload (hemosiderosis)	Deposition of iron in the heart, endocrine organs, liver, spleen, skin, and other major organs as a result of multiple, long-term transfusions (aplastic anemia, thalassemia).	1. Diabetes 2. Decreased thyroid function 3. Arrhythmias 4. CHF and other symptoms related to major organ failure	1. Treat symptomatically. 2. Deferoxamine (Desferal), which chelates and removes accumulated iron through the kidneys; administered IV, IM, or SC.	
Graft-versus-host disease	Engraftment of lymphocytes in the bone marrow of immunosuppressed patients, setting up an immune response of the graft against the host.	1. Erythematous skin rash 2. Liver function test abnormalities 3. Profuse, watery diarrhea	1. Immunosuppression with corticosteroids, cyclosporine A. 2. Symptomatic management of pruritus, pain 3. Fluid and electrolyte replacement for diarrhea	Transfuse with irradiated blood products.
Infectious disease 1. Hepatitis B	Hepatitis B virus transmitted from blood donor to recipient via infected blood products.	1. Elevated liver enzymes (SGPT and SGOT) 2. Anorexia, malaise 3. Nausea and vomiting 4. Fever 5. Dark urine 6. Jaundice	Usually resolves spontaneously within 4–6 wk. Can result in permanent liver damage. Treat symptomatically.	Screen blood donors, temporarily rejecting those who may have had contact with the virus. Those with a history of hepatitis after age 11 are permanently deferred; pretest all blood products (EIA).
2. Hepatitis C (formerly non-A, non-B hepatitis)	Hepatitis C virus transmitted from blood donor to recipient via infected blood products.	Similar to serum B hepatitis, but symptoms are usually less severe. Chronic liver disease and cirrhosis may develop.	Symptoms usually mild and require no treatment.	Pretest all blood donors (ALT, anti-HBc antibody, anti-hepatitis C antibody).
3. Epstein-Barr virus, cytomegalovirus, malaria	Transmitted through infected blood products.	1. Fever 2. Fatigue 3. Hepatomegaly 4. Splenomegaly	Rest and supportive management.	Question prospective blood donors, regarding colds, flu, foreign travel.

(continued)

TABLE 27-5 Delayed Reactions to Transfusion Therapy (Continued)

Delayed Reaction	Cause	Clinical Manifestations	Management	Prevention
4. Acquired immuno-deficiency syndrome	HIV virus transmitted from blood donor to recipient via infected blood products.	1. Night sweats 2. Unexplained weight loss 3. Lymphadenopathy 4. Pneumocystis pneumonia 5. Kaposi's sarcoma 6. Diarrhea	AZT may delay onset of AIDS symptoms. Active disease is treated symptomatically.	Test each donor for HIV anti-body. Reject prospective high-risk donors: males who have had sex with another male since 1977; users of self-injected IV drugs; male or female partners of prostitutes; hemophili-acs or their sexual partners; sexual partners of those with AIDS or high risk for AIDS; immigrants from Haiti or sub-Saharan Africa.
5. HTLV-1 associ-ated myelopathy and tropical spastic parapare-sis (HAM/TSP) Adult T-cell leukemia	Human T-lymphotropic virus type 1 (HTLV-1) transmitted from blood donor to recipient via blood products.	Signs of neuro-muscular disease Signs of T-cell leukemia	HTLV-l-infected individu-als have a low risk of developing disease (3–5%). Incubation pe-riod 10–20 y. Should disease occur, treat symptomatically.	Screen all prospective blood donors for anti-HTLV-I anti-body.
6. Syphilis	Spirochetemia caused by *Treponema pallidum*. Incubation 4–18 wk.	1. Presence of chancre 2. Regional lym-phadenopathy 3. Generalized rash	Penicillin therapy	Test blood before transfusion (rapid plasma reagin—RPF). Organism will not remain viable in blood stored 24–48 h at 4°C.

1. Most peripheral blood stem cell transplantations are autologous, although interest in and research into the use of allogeneic donors continues.
2. Peripheral blood stem cells are collected using one or more apheresis procedures, usually after the patient or donor has been treated to increase the number of circu-lating stem cells by methods such as timed administration of chemotherapy or growth factors. The cells are frozen and stored, and later reinfused into the patient after high-dose chemotherapy and possibly radiotherapy.
3. Advantages: patient's marrow does not need to be har-vestable (as in hypocellular or tumor-contaminated bone marrow); there is no operative risk to the patient or donor. Particularly with adjuvant use of growth factors, peripheral blood stem cell transplantation has a low risk of morbidity and mortality and eliminates lengthy hos-pital stays. The product may be used alone or in con-junction with autologous or allogeneic bone marrow.
4. Disadvantages: this is still a relatively new method and the long-term risks of relapse are not yet known. For al-logeneic donors, the long-term risks of boosting healthy bone marrow production with growth factors, and in some cases chemotherapy, are not yet known.

Umbilical Cord Blood Stem Cell Transplantation

1. Umbilical cord blood is rich in stem cells, and may be stored at birth for later autologous use, related allo-geneic use, or unrelated allogeneic use.

2. Advantages: may provide lifesaving allogeneic stem cells from new sibling to older child, no risk to the donor.
3. Disadvantages: may have higher risk of graft failure than other types of transplants; number of stem cells may be insufficient for older patients.

The Human Leukocyte Antigen System and Transplantation

1. The immune-mediated recognition of the differences in HLA antigens is the first step in the rejection of a trans-planted organ or graft or in GVHD.
2. The HLA antigens are complex proteins expressed on the surface of all nucleated cells (A, B, C antigens) or cells of the immune system (D antigens).
   a. More than a hundred different antigens have been identified.
   b. Antigens are classified according to the locations on chromosome 6, which encodes them.
   c. A person's genetically inherited mixture of antigens expressed on cell surfaces is the phenotype or tissue type of that person.
3. Although considerably more complex, determination of HLA type is similar to that of ABO testing.
   a. Lymphocytes are mixed with antibody directed against known HLA antigens. Lymphocytes will survive if the antigen is absent and will be inactivated if it is present. This method identifies HLA-A, -B, and -C antigens.

b. Donor and recipient lymphocytes are mixed and cultured together. This test, the mixed lymphocyte culture (MLC), identifies HLA-D antigens. Survival of both sources of cells indicates compatibility.

c. New techniques for determining a person's genetic HLA code use DNA probes. These tests are highly accurate, but their use remains limited because of the specialized techniques and high cost.

4. Siblings have a 1 in 4 chance of having identical sets of HLA antigens. With a decreasing national birthrate, however, only 35% of people in the United States can anticipate having an HLA-identical sibling.

5. Because of the complexity of the HLA system, unrelated people have less than a 1 in 5,000 chance of having identical HLA types. The National Bone Marrow Donor Registry, which was established in 1987, maintains a computerized list of potential HLA-typed bone marrow donors and provides assistance to patients who seek an unrelated donor. Information on becoming a volunteer bone marrow donor or on initiating a computerized search for a donor can be obtained by calling the National Marrow Donor Program (see Box 26-1, p. 879, for additional resources for patients undergoing blood and marrow stem cell transplantation).

Indications

1. If an HLA-matched related donor is available, allogeneic bone marrow transplantation is generally considered the treatment of choice in certain disorders, including:
   a. Severe aplastic anemia.
   b. Inherited immunodeficiency disorders, such as severe combined immunodeficiency disease and Wiskott-Aldrich syndrome.
   c. Chronic myelogenous leukemia (CML).
   d. Allogeneic bone marrow transplantation has also been used with varying success in the treatment of other genetic disorders (eg, thalassemia).

2. Allogeneic, syngeneic, and autologous bone marrow transplantation are also widely applied in other malignancies, where success rates depend largely on factors such as the age of the patient, current disease status, the extent of prior treatment, and coexisting morbidity.

3. Autologous peripheral blood stem cell transplantation is widely used in the treatment of solid tumors such as breast cancer and Ewing's sarcoma and in the treatment of leukemias and lymphomas. Allogeneic peripheral blood transplantation is generally used in the treatment of leukemias.

4. Diseases and disorders treated with this technology are summarized in Table 27-6.

Harvesting of Bone Marrow and Peripheral Blood Stem Cells

Evaluation of Recipient

1. Eligibility criteria include age (generally younger than age 55 for allogeneic, younger than age 65 for autologous bone marrow transplantation, and younger than age 70 for peripheral blood stem cell transplantation)

TABLE 27-6 Indications for Bone Marrow Transplantation

Allogeneic	Autologous
Nonmalignant	Acute myeloid leukemia
Aplastic anemia	Acute lymphocytic
Myelofibrosis	leukemia
Wiskott-Aldrich syndrome	Hodgkin's disease
Thalassemia	Non-Hodgkin's lymphoma
Severe combined immuno-	Multiple myeloma
deficiency diseases	Selected solid tumors
Mucopolysaccharidoses	Breast
Osteopetrosis	Lung
Lipid storage diseases	Neuroblastoma
	Testicular/germ cell
	Ovarian
	Colon
Malignant	Melanoma
Acute myeloid leukemia	Sarcomas
Acute lymphocytic leukemia	Gliomas
Chronic myelogenous leukemia	Renal cell
Hodgkin's disease	Pancreatic
Non-Hodgkin's lymphoma	Gastric
Preleukemia	
Burkitt's lymphoma	
Multiple myeloma	
Selected solid tumors	

and availability of suitable bone marrow or peripheral blood stem cell source.

2. Before undergoing transplantation, an extensive workup ensures that the patient's disease is treatable with stem cells and that the patient has no limitations that will increase the risk of mortality.

3. Specific criteria may vary among transplant centers and treatment protocols, but generally include:
   a. Disease-specific evaluation of severity and extent of current disease manifestations.
   b. Adequate cardiac function: generally left ventricular ejection fraction greater than 45%.
   c. Adequate pulmonary function: generally forced expiratory capacity and forced vital capacity greater than 50%.
   d. Adequate renal function: generally creatinine less than 2 mg/dL.
   e. Adequate hepatic function: generally bilirubin less 2 mg/dL.
   f. No active infections (including HIV).
   g. No coexisting severe or uncontrolled medical conditions.

Evaluation of Blood and Marrow Donors

1. Because bone marrow donation for allogeneic or syngeneic BMT is an elective procedure with no benefit to the donor, great care is taken to ensure that the potential donor is fit for surgery and understands the potential risks. Autologous bone marrow donors must generally meet the same criteria. Evaluation includes:
   a. Thorough medical history and physical examination.
   b. Chest x-ray.

c. Electrocardiogram.

d. Laboratory evaluation (complete blood count, chemistry profile, testing for CMV, hepatitis B and C, HIV and syphilis, ABO and Rh determination, coagulation studies).

2. Informed consent including potential donor complications must be obtained.

3. Relatively common complications include:

a. Bruising.

b. Pain at aspiration sites.

c. Mild bleeding.

4. Rare complications include:

a. Side effects of anesthesia (general, spinal, or epidural).

b. Infection of aspiration sites.

c. Persistent pain.

d. Transient neuropathies.

5. Because of the significant loss of blood volume and RBCs during the harvest procedure, donors are advised to give one or two units of autologous blood 1 to 3 weeks before surgery, which may be reinfused during marrow collection if needed.

6. Evaluation of donors for peripheral blood stem cell transplantation is similar, but less stringent. The apheresis procedure is similar to donating platelets.

Stem Cell Collection Procedure

Bone Marrow Harvest (Autologous, Syngeneic, or Allogeneic)

1. Performed under epidural, spinal, or general anesthesia under sterile conditions in operating room.

2. An aspiration needle is used to puncture the skin and puncture the iliac crest multiple times without exiting the skin, removing marrow in 2- to 5-mL aliquots (samples).

3. Marrow is drawn up into heparinized syringes and filtered to remove fibrin clots and other debris.

4. Marrow may be infused immediately, treated and infused, or frozen in a preservative solution containing dimethylsulfoxide (DMSO) until needed.

5. Bone marrow donation is a relatively safe operative procedure with few serious complications. A review of 3,000 cases reported to the International Bone Marrow Transplant Registry found only two donor deaths, neither of which was a result of the harvest procedure itself.

Postharvest Care of the Bone Marrow Donor

1. Procedure is generally done as same-day care, with discharge after recovery from anesthesia.

2. Observe for potential complications (bleeding, hypotension caused by fluid loss).

3. Instruct patient to resume normal activities gradually during the week after donation.

4. Instruct patient to keep aspiration sites clean and dry and observe for signs of infection (redness, swelling, warmth or discharge at sites, fever, malaise).

5. Provide adequate analgesia (frequently acetaminophen with codeine) and instruct patient about pain management.

6. Arrange follow-up appointment with primary care provider in 2 to 3 weeks for complete blood count.

Harvesting of Peripheral Blood Stem Cells

1. Involves donor preparation by "priming" hematopoietic system with timed chemotherapy and sequential growth factors to increase number of circulating stem cells.

2. Large-bore central catheter suitable for apheresis procedures is inserted.

3. One to ten apheresis procedures may be needed to collect sufficient numbers of suitable cells.

4. Cells are frozen in a preservative solution that contains DMSO until needed.

5. Acute complications of apheresis include citrate toxicity, which may be managed by increasing dietary calcium intake 2 to 3 days before procedure and by using calcium-based antacids during procedure. Blood calcium levels should be carefully monitored throughout the procedure and IV calcium given as needed.

Preparation and Performance of the Transplant

Preparation of Recipient

1. A long-term central catheter is inserted for multiple IV treatments, including blood products, total parenteral nutrition, and blood-drawing.

2. High-dose chemotherapy or radiotherapy is administered to:

a. Destroy residual tumor cells.

b. Suppress immune response against new stem cells.

c. Create space within donor marrow for new stem cells.

3. Symptoms immediately associated with high-dose chemotherapy or radiotherapy regimens used in blood and marrow stem cell transplantation may include:

a. Severe nausea and vomiting (with most regimens).

b. Cardiomyopathy, hemorrhagic cystitis (with cyclophosphamide [Cytoxan]).

c. Seizures (with busulfan [Myleran]).

d. Fever, generalized erythema, parotitis (with total body irradiation).

Reinfusion of Bone Marrow or Peripheral Blood Stem Cells

> **NURSING ALERT**
>
> Unlike all other blood products administered to transplant recipients, bone marrow and peripheral blood stem cells should never be irradiated. In addition, infusion pumps and filters should be avoided because they may remove or damage stem cells.

ABO Compatible Untreated Allogeneic Bone Marrow

1. Administered over 2 to 4 hours from large blood infusion bag, generally via large lumen of central catheter.

2. Volume depends on size of recipient and cellularity of bone marrow—generally 500 to 2,000 mL.

3. Potential immediate side effects are generally related to volume overload, allergic reactions (urticaria, chills, fever), or pulmonary compromise (related to fat emboli or clumped aggregates of cells).
4. Emergency medications should be available and the recipient should be closely monitored throughout the infusion.

ABO Incompatible Allogeneic Bone Marrow

1. ABO incompatible bone marrow is processed after harvesting to remove incompatible RBCs and plasma.
   a. Although this processing is highly effective, the recipient should still be considered at risk for intravascular RBC hemolysis.
   b. The recipient should be well hydrated with fluids that contain sodium bicarbonate before and after the infusion to ensure adequate renal perfusion and urine alkalinization.
2. Administered over 2 to 4 hours from blood infusion bag, generally via large lumen of central catheter.
3. Volume after removal of RBCs is usually 200 to 600 mL.
4. Potential immediate side effects are generally related to allergic reactions (urticaria, chills, fever) or intravascular hemolysis (hemoglobinuria, potential anaphylactic reaction).
5. Emergency medications should be available and the recipient closely monitored throughout the infusion.

Treated Allogeneic Bone Marrow (eg, T-cell Depleted)

1. Allogeneic bone marrow may be treated before infusion with various methods to remove T cells as a method of preventing GVHD. Methods include:
   a. Monoclonal antibodies.
   b. Counterflow centrifugation (elutriation).
   c. Positive selection of CD34+ cells.
2. These manipulations may alter total volume and result in RBC and plasma removal.
3. Management of reinfusion incorporates the principles described under allogeneic ABO compatible and incompatible bone marrow reinfusion.

Autologous Bone Marrow

1. Autologous bone marrow is thawed by immersion in a warm water bath immediately before infusion.
2. Administered via slow IV push (if in syringes) or from small infusion bags, generally through large lumen of central catheter.
3. Volume depends on size of recipient and amount of bone marrow harvested; usually 100 to 500 mL.
4. Potential immediate side effects are generally related to use of DMSO as preservative solution and include:
   a. Histamine-release reaction (flushing, feeling of chest tightness, abdominal cramping, nausea).
   b. Cardiac arrhythmias, especially bradycardia.
   c. Anaphylaxis.
5. Emergency medications should be available and the recipient closely monitored throughout the infusion; cardiac monitoring is recommended.

Peripheral Blood Stem Cells

1. Peripheral blood stem cells are thawed by immersion in a warm water bath immediately before infusion.
2. Administered via slow IV push (if in syringes) or from small infusion bags, generally through large lumen of central catheter.
   a. Volume depends on size of recipient and amount of peripheral blood stem cells harvested; often a large volume.
   b. May be administered during the course of several hours because of large volume and high DMSO content.
   c. Recipient may require premedication with antihistamine and antiemetic.
3. Potential immediate side effects are generally related to use of DMSO as preservative solution and include:
   a. Histamine-release reaction (flushing, feeling of chest tightness, abdominal cramping, nausea).
   b. Cardiac arrhythmias, especially bradycardia.
   c. Anaphylaxis.
4. Emergency medications should be available and the recipient should be closely monitored throughout the infusion; cardiac monitoring is recommended.

Post-transplant Care
General Considerations

1. Significant complications that require specialized medical and nursing care may occur during the first few weeks and months after blood and marrow stem cell transplantation.
   a. Risk is highest in mismatched unrelated allogeneic bone marrow transplantation.
   b. Followed by matched unrelated and mismatched related allogeneic bone marrow transplantation.
   c. Followed by matched related allogeneic bone marrow transplantation.
   d. Followed by syngeneic bone marrow transplantation.
   e. Followed by autologous bone marrow transplantation.
   f. Followed by autologous peripheral blood stem cell transplantation.
2. Nursing care is aimed at early identification and treatment of problems, and includes:
   a. Comprehensive physical and psychosocial assessment.
   b. Immediate notification of health care provider of any abnormal assessment parameters found.
   c. Expert symptom management of problems that may occur after blood and marrow stem cell transplantation, such as nausea, vomiting, pain, fatigue, anxiety, delirium.
   d. Prevention of infection.
   e. Prevention of bleeding.

f. Early recognition and intervention for life-threatening complications, such as sepsis, respiratory failure, GI bleeding, renal and hepatic failure, veno-occlusive disease.

Hematopoietic Complications

1. Blood and marrow stem cell transplant patients, particularly allogeneic recipients, are at risk for life-threatening bacterial, viral, and fungal infections because of their profound immunosuppression.
   a. Transplant patients are often cared for in a protective environment, that ranges from single hepafiltered rooms to strict laminar airflow and isolation in sterile environment.
   b. In an ambulatory or home setting, the patient and family must pay strict attention to methods of preventing infection, including wearing high-filtration masks, handwashing, safe food handling, and avoidance of crowded areas and exposure to illnesses.
   c. Additional preventive interventions vary widely and include elaborate disinfection procedures; modified or sterile diets; prophylactic antibiotics, antivirals, and antifungals; surveillance cultures.
2. The megakaryocyte is generally the last cell produced by new stem cells, and platelet counts may take months to return to normal.
   a. Blood and marrow stem cell transplant patients require frequent assessment for signs and symptoms of overt or covert bleeding, protection from injury, and support with platelet products.
3. Anemia is a frequent complication caused by loss of RBCs through aging, destruction, bleeding, and routine phlebotomy. Blood and marrow stem cell transplant patients require frequent RBC transfusions.

Gastrointestinal Complications

1. Mucositis may develop because of high-dose chemotherapy and radiation therapy that destroy rapidly dividing cells, including cells lining the mouth, esophagus, and GI tract. Management includes meticulous oral hygiene, local and systemic analgesia, and antimicrobial therapy.
2. Nausea and vomiting may arise from multiple causes, including high-dose chemotherapy, infection, gastrointestinal bleeding, acute GVHD, and medications. Management includes pharmacologic and nonpharmacologic interventions, replacement of fluids and electrolytes, and support of nutritional requirements.
3. Diarrhea may have multiple causes, including high-dose chemotherapy, infection, gastrointestinal bleeding, GVHD, and medications. Management includes cautious use of antidiarrheals, replacement of fluids and electrolytes, support of nutritional requirements, protection of perirectal skin from excoriation.

Renal and Genitourinary Complications

1. Renal failure may arise from multiple causes, including drug toxicity, infection, and ischemia. Management includes maintenance of fluid and electrolyte balance, monitoring of drug levels, and hemodialysis or continuous veno-venous hemodialysis.

2. Hemorrhagic cystitis may occur as a result of high-dose cyclophosphamide (Cytoxan) or with certain viral infections, such as adenovirus and BK virus. Management includes hydration, blood product support, continuous bladder irrigation, and rare invasive procedures, such as instillation of alum or formalin, or surgery.

Hepatic Complications

Veno-occlusive disease may occur as a result of damage to the liver from high-dose chemotherapy and radiation therapy; incidence is approximately 20%.

1. Signs and symptoms include hepatomegaly (generally painful), bilirubinemia, weight gain.
2. May progress to hepatic encephalopathy, coagulopathies, coma and death in up to 50% of patients with veno-occlusive disease.
3. Management is generally aimed at preventing further damage and at treating symptoms.

Pulmonary Complications

1. Life-threatening pulmonary infections in blood and marrow stem cell transplant patients include bacterial pneumonias, fungal infections, including aspergillosis, CMV pneumonitis (especially in allogeneic recipients), and less commonly, *Pneumocystis carinii* pneumonia (PCP), Legionnaires' disease, toxoplasmosis, and tuberculosis.
   a. Preventive measures include encouragement of exercise, deep breathing, and coughing; administration of CMV-screened blood products, high-dose acyclovir (Zovirax) or ganciclovir (Cytovene), and IVIG for allogeneic BMT patients at high risk for CMV; prophylactic sulfamethoxazole-trimethoprim (Bactrim) for patients at risk for PCP.
   b. Supportive care for symptomatic disease includes oxygen therapy, mechanical ventilation, and pulmonary hygiene.
2. Noninfectious pulmonary disease includes idiopathic pneumonitis, diffuse alveolar hemorrhage, pulmonary fibrosis, and bronchiolitis obliterans.

Graft-Versus-Host Disease

1. Acute GVHD occurs in 40% to 60% of allogeneic recipients even with HLA matching, generally within first 3 months after transplant as a manifestation of the immune response of activated donor T lymphocytes against the recipients cells and organs.
   a. Primarily affects the skin, liver, and gastrointestinal tract; may also affect conjunctivae and lungs.
   b. Severity ranges from mild and self-limited erythematous rash to widespread blistering of skin, profuse watery diarrhea, and liver failure.
   c. Prophylaxis generally includes immunosuppression with medications such as cyclosporin A (Sandimmune), tacrolimus (FK506), and methotrexate (Mexate); may also include T-cell depletion of bone marrow.
   d. Treatment generally includes increased doses of routine immunosuppressive medications and additional drugs, such as corticosteroids, antithymocyte globulin, and monoclonal antibodies.

2. Chronic GVHD occurs in approximately 20% of long-term survivors; usually appears within first year after allogeneic blood and marrow stem cell transplant.
   a. It has many similarities to autoimmune disorders, such as scleroderma.
   b. It affects the skin, mouth, salivary glands, eyes, musculoskeletal system, liver, esophagus, gastrointestinal tract, and vagina.
   c. Treatment generally consists of corticosteroids; may include other immunosuppressive medications, such as thalidomide.
   d. Immune system frequently suppressed beyond the effects of medications; patient is at risk for infections, particularly from encapsulated bacteria, and should receive prophylaxis with suitable antibiotic such as penicillin.

Long-Term Sequelae and Survivorship Issues

1. Long-term, disease-free survival varies from 5% to 10% for patients with resistant, aggressive leukemias or lymphomas to 75% to 80% for aplastic anemia.
2. Long-term complications of blood and marrow stem cell transplantation include:
   a. Relapse of original disease.
   b. Secondary malignancy.
   c. Sterility.
   d. Endocrine dysfunction, including reduced levels of human growth hormone, estrogens and testosterone.
   e. Cataracts (risk increased with radiation therapy, corticosteroids).
   f. Chronic GVHD (allogeneic).
   g. Aseptic necrosis (risk increased with corticosteroids).
   h. Encephalopathy (risk increased with cranial irradiation and intrathecal chemotherapy).
3. Survivorship issues after this intensive and potentially life-threatening treatment include:
   a. Feelings of isolation, guilt, and loss.
   b. Altered family dynamics.
   c. Delayed puberty, decreased libido, early menopause, and other physical problems that have an impact on sexual relationships.
   d. Readjustment to school or work setting.
   e. Financial burden of blood and marrow stem cell transplantation (cost of transplant in the United States in 1999 ranged from approximately $30,000 for an uncomplicated outpatient peripheral blood stem cell transplantation to a minimum of $150,000 for an unrelated allogeneic BMT).
   f. Chronic health problems and fatigue.
   g. Difficulty obtaining adequate health insurance.
4. Despite the complex issues blood and marrow stem cell transplant survivors face as they return to the task of living, several quality-of-life studies have demonstrated that the majority rate their quality of life highly, would choose to undergo transplant again, and frequently state that their experiences have added new dimensions of meaning and purpose to their lives.

SELECTED REFERENCES

Alcoser, P.W. & Burchett, S. (1999). Bone marrow transplantation: Immune system suppression and reconstitution. *American Journal of Nursing, 99*(6), 26–31.

Bensinger, W.I., Buckner, D., & Gahrton, G. (1997). Allogeneic stem cell transplantation for multiple myeloma. *Hematology/Oncology Clinics of North America, 11*(1), 147–157.

Buchsel, P.C., & Whedon, M.B. (Eds.). (1995). *Bone marrow transplantation: Administrative and clinical strategies.* Boston: Jones and Bartlett.

DeWitte, T. (1997). Allogeneic and autologous stem cell transplantation in myelodysplastic syndromes. *Pathologie Biologie, 45*(8), 643–649.

Ernst, D.J. (1999). Reduce your risk when you draw blood. *RN, 62*(12), 65–68.

Forte, K.J. (1997). Alternative donor sources in pediatric bone marrow transplantation. *Journal of Pediatric Oncology Nursing, 14*(4), 213–224.

Gerber, L. (1994). Autologous blood transfusion: Why and how. *Journal of Intravenous Nursing, 17*(2), 65–69.

Greenberg, A.G. (1997). New transfusion strategies. *American Journal of Surgery, 173*(1), 49–52.

Groenwald, S.L., Frogge, M.H., Goodman, M., & Yarbro, C.H. (Eds.). (1997), *Cancer nursing: Principles and practice* (4th ed.). Boston: Jones and Bartlett.

Jarsak, P.F. & Riley, M.B. (1994). Autologous stem cell transplant: An overview. *Cancer Practice, 2*(2), 141–145.

Marsh, J.C.W., & Gordon-Smith, E.C. (1998). Treatment options in severe aplastic anemia. *The Lancet, 9119,* 1830–1832.

Poe, S.S., et al. (1994). A national survey of infection prevention practices on bone marrow transplant units. *Oncology Nursing Forum, 21*(10), 1687–1694.

McDonald, J.C., Stetz, K.M., & Compton, K. (1996). Educational interventions for family caregivers during marrow transplantation. *Oncology Nursing Forum, 23*(9), 1432–1439.

Ringden, O. (1997). Bone marrow transplantation using unrelated donors for hematologic malignancies. *Medical Oncology, 14*(1), 11–22.

Shivnan, J.C. (1998). Bone marrow and peripheral blood stem cell transplantation. In Ziegfeld, C.R., Lubejko, B.G., & Shelton, B.K. (Eds.), *Manual of cancer nursing.* Philadelphia: Lippincott-Raven.

Shivnan, J.C., Ohly, K.V., & Hanson, J. (1995). Bone marrow transplantation. In Nolan, M. & Augustine, S. (Eds.), *Transplantation nursing.* Norwalk, CT: Appleton-Lange.

Shivnan, J.C., Shelton, B.K., & Onners, B.K. (1996). Bone marrow transplantation: Issues for critical care nurses. *AACN Clinical Issues, 7*(1), 95–108.

Wagner, N.D., & Quinones, V.W. (1998). Allogeneic peripheral blood stem cell transplantation: Overview and nursing implications. *Oncology Nursing Forum, 25*(6), 1049–1055.

Walter-Coleman, S. (1996). Transfusion therapy for patients critically ill with cancer. *AACN Clinical Issues, 7*(1), 37–45.

Whedon, M.B., & Wujcik, D. (Eds.). (1997). *Blood and marrow stem cell transplantation: Principles, practice, and nursing insights* (2nd ed.). Boston: Jones and Bartlett.

Wolf, S. (1999a). Another source of stem cells. *RN, 62*(9), 30–33.

Wolf, S. (1999b). Cord blood stem cell banking. *American Journal of Nursing, 99*(8), 60–69.

Wolf, S. (2000). Are you ready for bloodless medicine? *RN, 63*(5), 42–46.

UNDERLYING PRINCIPLES

■ The Allergic Reaction

An allergic reaction results from antigen-antibody re-action on a sensitized mast cell, thus causing the release and synthesis of chemical mediators. The reaction may be characterized by inflammation, increased secretions, and bronchoconstriction.

Definitions

1. Antigen—a protein that stimulates an immune reaction, causing the production of antibodies.
2. Antibody—a globulin (protein) produced by B cells as a defense mechanism against foreign materials.
3. Atopy—a term that refers to the ability to produce IgE antibodies to common allergens.
4. Immunity:
   a. Humoral—the process by which B lymphocytes pro-duce circulating antibodies to act against antigens.
   b. Cell-mediated—that portion of the immune system in which the participation of T lymphocytes and macrophages is predominant.
5. Mast cell—a tissue cell that resembles a peripheral blood basophil and that contains granules with chemi-cal mediators.

6. Hypersensitivity—reaction to an antigen after re-exposure; there are four types; type I (immediate) and type IV (delayed) are considered allergic reactions.

Immunoglobulins

Antibodies that are formed by lymphocytes and plasma cells in response to an immunogenic stimulus comprise a group of serum proteins called immunoglobulins.
1. The abbreviation for immunoglobulin is Ig.
2. Antibodies combine with antigens in special ways (lock-and-key style).
3. There are five major classes of immunoglobulins.
   a. IgM—constitutes 10% of immunoglobulin pool; found mostly in intravascular fluid and primarily engaged in initial defense.
   b. IgG—major immunoglobulin that accounts for 70% to 75% of secondary immune responses and that combats tissue infection.
   c. IgA—15% to 20% of immunoglobulins; predomi-nantly found in seromucous secretions (such as sa-liva, tears) in which it provides a primary defense mechanism.
   d. IgD—less than 1% of immunoglobulin pool; found on many circulating B lymphocytes, but function is unknown.

e. IgE—only a trace found in serum; attaches to surface membrane of basophils and mast cells; responsible for immediate types of allergic reactions.

Immunologic Reactions

See Figure 28-1.

Immediate Hypersensitivity (Type 1)

1. Characterized by:
   a. Allergic reaction.
   b. Occurs immediately after contact with the antigen.
   c. Causes release of chemical mediators.
2. Examples—anaphylaxis, allergic rhinitis, urticaria.

Some Products of Immediate Hypersensitivity (Chemical Mediators)

1. Histamine—a bioactive amine stored in granules of mast cells and basophils.
2. Leukotrienes—newly synthesized potent bronchoconstrictors, cause increased venous permeability.
3. Prostaglandins—potent vasodilators and potent bronchoconstrictors.
4. Platelet-activating factor (PAF)—has many properties; causes the aggregation of platelets.
5. Cytokines—control and/or regulate immunologic functions (eg, interleukins, tumor necrosis factor).
6. Proteases—enzymes, such as tryptase and chymase, increase vascular permeability.
7. ECF-A—causes an influx of eosinophils into the area of allergic inflammation.

Effects of Chemical Mediators and Their Manifestations

1. Generalized vasodilation, hypotension, flushing.
2. Increased permeability.
   a. Capillaries of the skin—edema
   b. Mucous membranes—edema.
3. Smooth muscle contraction.
   a. Bronchioles—bronchospasm.
   b. Intestines—abdominal cramps, diarrhea.

4. Increased secretions.
   a. Nasal mucous glands—rhinorrhea.
   b. Bronchioles—increased mucus in airways.
   c. Gastrointestinal—increased gastric secretions.
   d. Lacrimal—tearing.
   e. Salivary—salivation.
5. Pruritus (itching).
   a. Skin.
   b. Mucous membrane.

Delayed Hypersensitivity (Type IV)

1. Characterized by a cell-mediated reaction between antigens and antigen-responsive T lymphocytes.
2. Maximal intensity occurs between 24 to 48 hours.
3. Usually consists of erythema and induration.
4. Examples—tuberculin skin test; contact dermatitis, such as poison ivy.

ASSESSMENT AND DIAGNOSTIC TESTS

Evaluation of the Patient for Allergy

Evaluation includes:
1. The allergy history (Figure 28-2).
2. Physical examination based on patient presentation and specific allergy condition, usually skin, HEENT, chest.
3. Skin testing (Procedure Guidelines 28-1 and 28-2).
4. Other tests as indicated for specific allergic conditions.

Skin Testing

The purpose of skin testing is to identify antigens responsible for immediate hypersensitivity. The types of skin tests used in clinical allergy are epicutaneous (prick, puncture, or scratch) and intradermal methods. The skin test remains unequaled as a sensitive, specific, and effective test for the diagnosis of allergies.

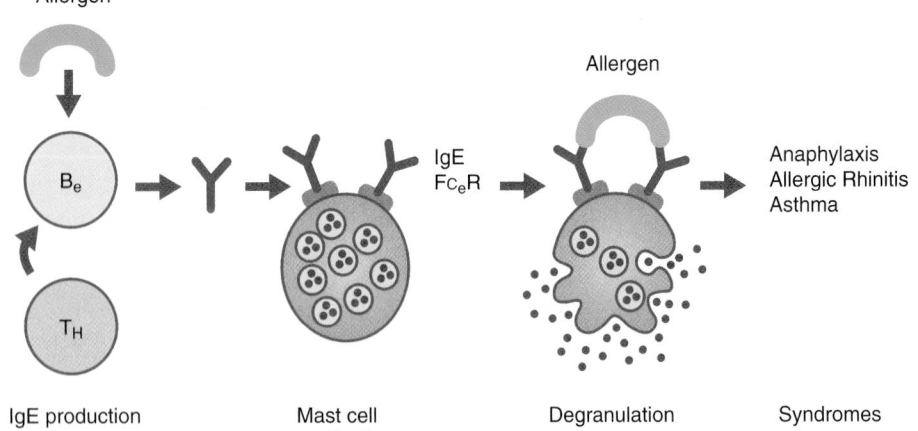

FIGURE 28-1 Type I immediate hypersensitivity. Specific IgE is produced by B cells with T cell help as a result of allergen stimulation. The next step in sensitization is the attachment of the IgE antibody to the mast cell by the E_c receptor. When specific allergen reaches the sensitized mast cell and combines with the two adjacent antibody molecules on the surface of the cell, degranulation occurs, releasing chemical mediators that cause the symptoms associated with type I hypersensitivity.

ALLERGY SURVEY

Name _____ Age _____ Sex _____ Date _____

1. Reason for visit:
2. Do you have any of the following problems?

   _____ Hay Fever   _____ Sinus problems   _____ Eczema
   _____ Asthma   _____ Drug allergy   Other: (please specify)
   _____ Hives   _____ Insect allergy   _____
   _____ Food allergy   _____ Skin rash   _____

3. Does anyone in your family have allergies? _____
4. Have you ever been tested for allergies? _____
   When? _____ Results _____
5. Do you smoke? _____ How much? _____ No. of years _____
6. Exercise habits: _____
7. Other significant past medical history _____
   _____

8. Current symptoms: (Circle one(s) that applies)

   Nasal stuffiness/congestion   Mouth breathing   Shortness of breath
   Sneezing   Snoring   Diminished sense of
   Runny nose   Itching/irritation/redness/   smell
   Itching   tearing of eyes
   Postnasal drip   Cough
   Sinus headaches   Chest tightness
   Sinus infections   Wheezing

9. Do symptoms occur year 'round? _____
10. If not, during what seasons do your symptoms occur?

    Summer   Fall   Winter   Spring

11. Where do symptoms occur? _____

    Home   Office   School   Outdoors   Basement   Bedroom

12. Are symptoms made worse by:

    Smoke   Heat   Humidity   Cold   Pollen   Pollution
    Dust   Exposure to strong odors—ammonia, paint, perfume
    Pets   Exercise   Eating   Drinking   Emotional stress

13. Have you had symptoms after eating? If so, list the foods _____
14. Do you have pets? _____ Dog _____ Cat   Other: _____
15. List any medications that you are currently taking, including over-the-counter drugs:

    Do you know what they are for?

    Are you aware of possible side effects?

16. Can you take aspirin without any adverse reactions?

17. In what way(s) has your health problem affected your lifestyle?

FIGURE 28-2   Allergy survey.

Epicutaneous (Prick) Method

1. Advantages:
   a. Safe—less chance for anaphylaxis because of minimal systemic absorption.
   b. Efficient—results within 15 minutes.
   c. Little discomfort to the patient.
2. Disadvantages:
   a. Less sensitive than the intradermal method.
   b. Old or thick, leathery skin decreases reactivity.
   c. Drops have a tendency to run together, which would affect the accuracy of the test.

Intradermal Method

1. Advantages:
   a. More sensitive than prick testing.
2. Disadvantages:
   a. Less specific than prick testing.
   b. Increased possibility for anaphylactic reactions.

   c. Requires more time and skill to perform.
   d. Increased discomfort to the patient.

Radioallergosorbent Test (RAST)
Description
Measurement of allergen-specific IgE antibodies in serum samples after panel of allergens have been added to samples.
Nursing and Patient Care Considerations

1. Allergy testing without the risk of causing severe allergic reaction.
2. Obtain adequate venous blood for each allergen to be tested.
3. A positive RAST test result depends on the standards for that particular lab.
4. Arrange for a follow-up visit for the patient with the health care provider to discuss test results.

PROCEDURE GUIDELINES 28-1	EPICUTANEOUS SKIN TESTING

EQUIPMENT

Antigens for testing

Controls	Alcohol swabs	Tourniquet
Positive—histamine 1 mg/mL	Paper tissues	Epinephrine 1:1000 aqueous solution
Negative—glycerol saline	Skin marking pencil	for injection for emergency use
Pricking device (sterile needle or lancet)	Millimeter ruler	

PROCEDURE

Nursing Action	Rationale
PREPARATORY PHASE	
1. Explain the procedure to the patient. Ask patient if he or she has taken antihistamines in the past 48–72 h.	1. Oral antihistamines taken 48–72 h before skin testing are likely to prevent a reaction from occurring.
2. Prepare the site (volar surface of forearm or back) by cleansing with alcohol.	2. The forearm is usually preferable because in the event of a significant local or systemic reaction, a tourniquet may be placed proximal to the skin test to slow the diffusion of the antigen into the circulation.
3. Mark the test sites with a skin marking pencil approximately 3–4 cm apart.	3. Sites need to be spaced appropriately so that reactions will remain distinct from one another, thus allowing an accurate reading.
IMPLEMENTATION PHASE	
1. Apply positive (histamine) and negative (glycerol saline) controls next to the appropriate markings. Introduce the tip of the pricking device at a 15–20° angle through each drop, lifting up and tenting the skin until the point pops loose without causing any bleeding. The pricking device must be wiped thoroughly with a paper tissue after each puncture.	1. Because of interpatient variability in cutaneous reactivity, it is necessary to include positive and negative controls whenever skin testing is performed. A response to the positive control confirms an immunologic ability to react. A response to the negative control indicates reactivity to the diluting solution and/or mechanical trauma. Care must be taken to prevent cross-contamination between antigens.
2. Apply small drops of antigens next to the skin markings and prick the drops as described above. Blot (do not rub) skin surface with paper tissue.	2. Rubbing may cause redness and cross-contamination of antigens.
3. Instruct the patient not to scratch the test area during the 15-min waiting interval before the reactions are graded.	3. It is normal for sensitive individuals to have a pruritic sensation at the testing site because of the histamine released by the mast cells.
4. Observe the patient closely for signs of impending anaphylaxis (such as itching, flushing, lump in throat).	4. General systemic or anaphylactic reactions are rare, but do occur. If suspected, apply tourniquet above test site and administer 0.3 mL epinephrine 1:1000 subcutaneously.

PROCEDURE GUIDELINES 28-1 *CONTINUED*

Nursing Action	Rationale
FOLLOW-UP PHASE	
1. Fifteen min after pricking the antigens, measure the extent of induration (wheal) and erythema (flare) in two perpendicular axes through the center of the reaction; record in millimeters (see accompanying figure).	1. Amount of induration indicates the extent of reaction, but erythema is noted as well.

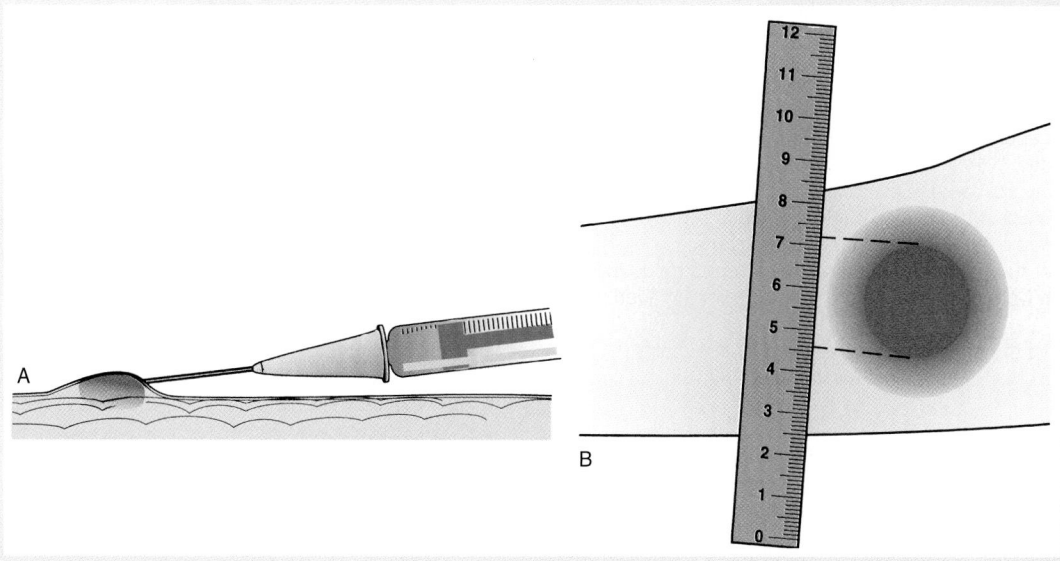

(A) Intradermal injection producing a wheal. (B) Measuring area of induration.

2. Document the procedure, test results, patient tolerance, and any other pertinent observations.

PROCEDURE GUIDELINES 28-2 INTRADERMAL SKIN TESTING

EQUIPMENT

Antigens for testing	Paper tissues
Controls	Skin marking pencil
Positive—histamine 0.1 mg/mL	Millimeter ruler
Negative—human serum albumin	Tourniquet
1-mm tuberculin syringes with 26- or 27-gauge intradermal needle	Gloves
Alcohol swabs	Epinephrine for emergency use

PROCEDURE

Nursing Action	Rationale
PREPARATORY PHASE	
1. Explain the procedure to the patient. Ask the patient if he or she has taken antihistamines in past 48–72 h.	1. Oral antihistamines taken 48–72 h before skin testing are likely to prevent a reaction from occurring.
2. Prepare the site (volar surface of forearm or upper arm) by cleansing with alcohol. Allow to dry.	

continued

PROCEDURE GUIDELINES 28-2   INTRADERMAL SKIN TESTING *CONTINUED*

Nursing Action	Rationale
3. Mark the test sites with a skin marking pencil approximately 3–4 cm apart.	3. Sites need to be spaced appropriately so that reactions will remain distinct from one another, thus allowing an accurate reading.

IMPLEMENTATION PHASE

Nursing Action	Rationale
1. Using sterile technique, draw up 0.05 mL of each testing material. All bubbles must be carefully expelled to avoid "splash reactions," which reduce precision. While wearing gloves, place syringe at a 10°–15° angle to the skin with the bevel up. Stretch the skin taut and insert 0.02 mL of the positive and negative controls. The bevel should penetrate the skin entirely and end between the layers of skin. A bleb approximately 2 mm in diameter should be produced.	1. Gloves should be worn when there is any possibility of exposure to blood or body fluids. Only small amount needs to be deposited into skin—enough to raise a bleb.
2. Inject approximately 0.02 mL of test antigens intradermally next to the skin markings. A different syringe and needle must be used for each antigen.	2. To avoid antigen and microbial contamination.
3. Instruct the patient not to scratch the test area during the 15-min waiting interval before the reaction is graded.	3. It is normal for sensitive individuals to have a pruritic sensation at the testing site because of the histamine released by the mast cells.
4. Observe the patient closely for signs of impending anaphylaxis (itching, flushing, lump in throat).	4. There is an increased possibility of anaphylactic reactions with intradermal skin testing. If suspected, apply tourniquet above test site, and administer 0.3 mL epinephrine 1:1000 subcutaneously.

5. Fifteen minutes after applying antigens, measure the extent of induration (wheal) and erythema (flare) in two perpendicular axes through the center of the reaction and record in millimeters.
  Reactions are graded according to the following:
  0   2 mm or less
  1+   3–5 mm wheal with erythema
  2+   6–10 mm wheal with erythema
  3+   over 11–15 mm wheal without pseudopods*
  4+   wheal over 15 mm with pseudopods

FOLLOW-UP PHASE

Nursing Action	Rationale
1. Document the procedure, test results, patient tolerance, and any other pertinent observations.	
2. Monitor for the following complications during and following testing:	2. Any significant reaction may be anxiety provoking for the patient, but anaphylaxis occurs suddenly and may be life-threatening.

Local Reactions—unusually large 4+ reactions
a. Apply prescribed steroid cream to affected area.
b. If no relief, administer prescribed oral antihistamine.
Vasovagal Reactions—fainting episode
a. Monitor vital signs.
b. Reassure the patient.
c. Finish skin testing if possible.
Systemic Anaphylaxis
a. Stop testing and apply tourniquet above skin testing site.
b. Administer epinephrine subcutaneously.

* Pseudopods—asymmetric extensions of wheal that indicate increased sensitivity.

GENERAL PROCEDURES AND TREATMENT MODALITIES

Immunotherapy

Immunotherapy is the desensitization of the immune system to a known allergen(s) that causes IgE, type I (immediate) hypersensitivity. It is indicated for significant symptoms of allergic rhinitis and asthma that cannot be controlled by avoidance of the allergen.

Although immunotherapy is not a cure, it gives relief to most people. Considerable compliance and time commitment are essential for successful therapy. See Procedure Guidelines 28-3.

Features of Immunotherapy

1. Specific allergen(s) are identified by skin testing or RAST.
2. Serial injections are begun that contain extracts from identified allergens (allergy vaccine).
3. Initially, small amount of dilute allergy vaccine is given, usually at weekly intervals.
4. Amount and concentration are slowly increased to maximum tolerable dose.
5. The maintenance dose is injected every 2 to 4 weeks for a period of one to several years to achieve maximal benefit.
6. Several allergens are now standardized (dust mite, cat, grass pollens).

Precautions and Considerations

1. The danger of anaphylactic reaction exists after injection.
   a. Should only be given in health care facility with epinephrine (Adrenalin), trained personnel, and emergency equipment available. See Standards of Care Guidelines.

   b. Patient should remain in office for 30 minutes after injection, after which the risk of anaphylaxis is greatly reduced.
   c. If large, local reaction (erythema, induration) occurs after an injection, the next dose should not be increased without checking with prescribing health care provider because a systemic reaction may occur.
2. If several weeks are missed, dosage may need to be decreased to prevent a reaction.
3. Medication, such as antihistamines and decongestants, should be continued until significant symptom relief occurs (may take 12 to 24 months).
4. Environmental controls should be maintained to enhance effectiveness of therapy.

PROCEDURE GUIDELINES 28-3	GIVING AN ALLERGY INJECTION

EQUIPMENT

Patient's individualized allergy vaccine   25- to 27-gauge ½ to ⅝-inch needle
1 mL syringe   Alcohol sponges

NURSING ALERT

Because of the risk of anaphylaxis have epinephrine (Adrenalin) 1:1000 readily available for injection.

PROCEDURE

Nursing Action	Rationale
PREPARATORY PHASE	
1. Check record and ask patient about reaction to last injection. Note how many weeks since last shot.	1. Local erythema and induration may have occurred during observation period or later.
2. Check order for prescribed dosage and any special instructions based on reaction history.	2. Significant reaction (greater than 2–3 cm and lasting 24 h) may require injection at same or lower dose. Missed weeks may require dosage adjustment.

continued

PROCEDURE GUIDELINES 28-3   GIVING AN ALLERGY INJECTION *CONTINUED*

Nursing Action	Rationale
3. Draw up dose, checking both strength of allergy vaccine and amount (usually 0.1–0.5 mL).	3. Vaccine will periodically be replaced with a stronger preparation.

PERFORMANCE PHASE

Nursing Action	Rationale
1. Select the appropriate site for subcutaneous injection, usually the lateral upper arms. If two injections are necessary, give in opposite arms.	1. Because injections usually only given once a week, no need to use abdomen or thighs. Using different arms for two injections allows for determining which serum may have caused reaction if one occurs.
2. Cleanse site with alcohol and allow to dry.	2. Disinfects skin.
3. Grasp upper arm with nondominant hand so that tissue is elevated slightly.	3. Secures arm and subcutaneous tissue beneath outer skin.
4. Insert needle at 45°–90°, depending on thickness of subcutaneous tissue at the site.	4. Thickness of subcutaneous tissue varies among individuals.
5. Aspirate for blood return, and if none occurs, inject serum.	5. If blood enters syringe, dispose of it and begin again rather than injecting into a blood vessel.
6. Withdraw syringe, cover site with alcohol sponge, and dispose of needle and syringe. Check site for bleeding or bruising.	6. Follow institution policy; do not resheath needle.

FOLLOW-UP PHASE

Nursing Action	Rationale
1. Have patient wait 30 min before leaving. Check for local reaction periodically and tell patient to report any sudden swelling, itching, or respiratory difficulty.	1. Significant local or systemic reaction may occur; most likely with increased dose.
2. Record amount and concentration of serum; site given; and appearance of site after 30 min.	2. Flow sheet serves as official documentation of medication given and may be reviewed by allergist when evaluating therapy.
3. Dismiss patient with instructions on who to call if reaction occurs and when to return for next injection.	3. May call allergist or primary care provider, or go to emergency room if systemic reaction occurs.

ALLERGIC DISORDERS

◼ Anaphylaxis

Anaphylaxis is an immediate, life-threatening systemic re-action that can occur on exposure to a particular sub-stance. It is a result of a type I hypersensitivity reaction in which chemical mediators released from mast cells affect many types of tissue and organ systems.

> **NURSING ALERT**
>
> With immunotherapy (allergy shots), the risk of systemic reaction is always present. Skin testing can also result in systemic reactions. Have epinephrine 1:1,000 available during these procedures (with syringe and tourniquet) and have patient remain in office or clinic for at least 30 minutes after administration.

Pathophysiology and Etiology

1. May be caused by:
   a. Immunotherapy.
   b. Stinging insects.
   c. Skin testing.
   d. Medications.
   e. Contrast media infusion.
   f. Foods.
   g. Exercise.
   h. Latex.
2. Release of chemical mediators results in massive vaso-dilation; increased capillary permeability, bronchocon-striction, and decreased peristalsis.

Clinical Manifestations

1. Respiratory—laryngeal edema, bronchospasm, cough, wheezing, lump in throat.
2. Cardiovascular—hypotension, tachycardia, palpitations, syncope.
3. Cutaneous—urticaria (hives), angioedema, pruritus, erythema (flushing).
4. Gastrointestinal—nausea, vomiting, diarrhea, abdomi-nal pain, bloating.

> **DRUG ALERT**
>
> Before you administer any drug, ask the patient if he or she has ever had a reaction to it. Do not rely on the chart alone.

Management

Prompt identification of signs and symptoms and immedi-ate intervention are essential; a reaction that occurs quickly tends to be more severe.

Immediate Treatment

1. A tourniquet is applied above site of antigen injection (allergy injection, insect sting, etc.) or skin test site to slow the absorption of antigen into the system.
2. Epinephrine (Adrenalin) 1:1,000, adolescents and adults: 0.3 to 0.5 mL, children 0.01 ml/kg is injected subcutaneously or intramuscularly (IM) into opposite arm; may be repeated every 15 to 20 minutes if necessary—causes vasoconstriction, decreases capillary permeability, relaxes airway smooth muscle, and inhibits mast cell mediator release.
3. Have patient lie in Trendelenburg position.

Subsequent Treatment

1. An adequate airway is established and albuterol is administered by inhalation as needed.
2. Hypotension and shock are treated with fluids and vasopressors.
3. Additional bronchodilators are given to relax bronchial smooth muscle.
4. H_1 antihistamines, such as diphenhydramine (Benadryl) and possibly H_2 antihistamines, such as ranitidine (Zantac), are given to block the effects of histamine.
5. Corticosteroids are given to decrease vascular permeability and diminish the migration of inflammatory cells; may be helpful in preventing late phase responses.

Complications

1. Cardiovascular collapse.
2. Respiratory failure.

Nursing Assessment

1. Quickly assess airway, breathing, and circulation (ABCs) if severe presentation and intervene with cardiopulmonary resuscitation as appropriate.
2. When ABCs are stable, assess vital signs, degree of respiratory distress, and angioedema.
3. Obtain a history of onset of symptoms and of exposure to allergen.

Nursing Diagnoses

- Impaired Breathing Pattern related to bronchospasm and laryngeal edema
- Decreased Cardiac Output related to vasodilation
- Anxiety related to respiratory distress and life-threatening situation

Nursing Interventions

Restoring Effective Breathing

1. Establish and maintain an adequate airway.
   a. If epinephrine has not stabilized bronchospasm, assist with endotracheal intubation, emergency tracheostomy, or cricothyroidotomy as indicated.
   b. Continually monitor respiratory rate, depth, and breath sounds for decreased work of breathing and effective ventilation.
2. Administer nebulized albuterol or other bronchodilators, as ordered. Monitor heart rate (increased with bronchodilators).
3. Provide oxygen via nasal cannula at 2 to 5 L/min or by alternative means, as ordered.
4. Administer aminophylline and corticosteroids intravenously (IV), as ordered.

Increasing Cardiac Output

1. Monitor blood pressure by continuous automatic cuff, if available.
2. Administer rapid infusion of IV fluids to fill vasodilated circulatory system and raise blood pressure.
3. Monitor central venous pressure (CVP) to ensure adequate fluid volume and to prevent fluid overload.
4. Insert indwelling catheter and monitor urine output hourly to ensure kidney perfusion.
5. Initiate and titrate vasopressor, as ordered, based on blood pressure response.

Reducing Anxiety

1. Provide care in a quick, confident manner.
2. Remain responsive to the patient, who may remain alert, but not completely coherent because of hypotension, hypoxemia, and effects of medication.
3. Keep family/significant other(s) informed of patient's condition and the treatment being given.
4. When patient is stable and alert, give simple, honest explanation of anaphylaxis and the treatment that was given.

Community and Home Care Considerations

1. Ensure that patients who have experienced anaphylaxis or severe local reactions obtain a prescription for self-injectable epinephrine (Epi-Pen, Ana-Kit) to have with them at all times.
   a. Instruct the patient and significant other(s) in the injection technique upon exposure to known antigen or at the first signs of a systemic reaction.
   b. Provide the patient with information on epinephrine, including the action of the drug, possible side effects, the importance of prompt administration at the first sign of a systemic reaction, and replacement of outdated syringe.
2. Even if treatment is given successfully at home, the patient should follow up with the health care provider immediately.
3. Ensure that the patient with history of anaphylaxis has access to emergency medical system and does not spend time alone if risk of reaction is present.

Patient Education and Health Maintenance

1. Teach the patient at risk for anaphylaxis about the potential seriousness of these reactions.
2. Educate patients to recognize the early signs and symptoms of anaphylaxis.
3. Persons allergic to bee stings should avoid wearing brightly colored or black clothes, perfumes, and hair spray. Shoes should be worn at all times.
4. For exercise-induced anaphylaxis, patients should exercise in moderation, preferably with another person,

and in a controlled setting, where assistance is readily available.

5. Instruct patients to wear a Medic-Alert bracelet or tag at all times.

6. For potential drug allergies, teach the patient:
   a. Read labels and be familiar with the generic name of the drug thought to cause a reaction.
   b. Discard all unused drugs. Make sure any drug kept in the medicine cabinet is clearly labeled.
   c. Familiarize yourself with drugs that may cross-react with a drug to which you are allergic.
   d. Always know the name of every drug that you take.

7. Advise patient to be extremely careful about everything they eat if there is a known sensitivity to a food product—allergic compounds are often hidden in a preparation (such as monosodium glutamate).

8. Advise that if food is associated with exercise-induced anaphylaxis, wait at least 2 h after eating to exercise.

Outcome-Based Evaluation

- Respirations unlabored with clear lung fields, minimal wheezing
- Blood pressure and CVP within normal range; urine output adequate
- Patient responsive and cooperative

■ Allergic Rhinitis

Allergic rhinitis is an inflammation of the nasal mucosa caused by an allergen that affects 8% to 10% of the population.

Pathophysiology and Etiology

1. Type I hypersensitivity causes local vasodilation and increased capillary permeability.
2. Caused by airborne allergens.
   a. Seasonal—offending allergen is a pollen or mold; symptoms are episodic.
   b. Perennial—offending allergens are dust mites, animal dander, cockroaches, mold; symptoms occur year round.

Clinical Manifestations

1. Nasal—mucous membrane congestion, edema, itching, rhinorrhea with clear secretions, sneezing.
2. Eyes—edema, itching, burning, tearing, redness, dark circles under eyes (allergic) shiners.
3. Ears—itching, fullness.
4. Other—palatal itching, throat itching, nonproductive cough.

Diagnostic Evaluation

1. Skin testing—confirms a hypersensitivity to certain allergens.

2. Nasal smear—an increased number of eosinophils suggests allergic disease.
3. RAST—positive test result for offending allergen(s).
4. Rhinoscopy—allows better visualization of the nasopharynx; useful to rule out physical obstruction (septal deviation, nasal polyps).

Management

Avoidance

1. Patients should minimize contact with offending allergens, regardless of other treatment.
2. Dust mite exposure can be reduced by encasing bed pillows and mattress in allergen-proof encasing and by washing bed linens and stuffed animals in hot water weekly.

Medications: Acute Phase

1. H_1 antihistamines—block the effects of histamine on smooth muscle and blood vessels by blocking histamine receptor sites, thereby relieving the symptoms of allergic rhinitis (oral and topical preparations).
   a. Older, possibly sedating antihistamines (diphenhydramine [Benadryl]; chlorpheniramine [Chlor-Trimeton]) are inexpensive, available over-the-counter, short acting, and effective.
   b. Newer, nonsedating, or less sedating antihistamines (loratadine [Claritin]; fexofenadine [Allegra]; cetirizine [Zyrtec]) are generally more expensive, obtained by prescription, long-acting, and effective.
   c. New topical antihistamine nasal spray available by prescription (azelastine [Astelin]).
2. Decongestants—shrink nasal mucous membrane by vasoconstriction; many available over-the-counter and in combination with antihistamines, pain relievers, and anticholinergics.
3. Anticholinergic agents—inhibit mucous secretions, act as drying agents.

Medications: Preventive Therapy

1. Corticosteroids (oral and intranasal).
   a. Reduce inflammation of nasal mucosa.
   b. Prevent mediator release.
   c. Only given systemically for a short course during a disabling attack.
2. Intranasal cromolyn sodium (Nasalcrom)—mast cell stabilizer; hinders the release of chemical mediators. Mast cell stabilizers now also are available as oral preparation cromolyn (Gastrocrom) and ophthalmic solution cromolyn (Crolom) and lodoxamide (Alomide). These medications are used before and during allergen season.

Immunotherapy

1. Regimen consists of administering subcutaneous injections of increasing amounts of an allergen to which the patient is sensitive to decrease sensitivity and reduce the severity of symptoms.
2. Immunotherapy produces the following immunologic changes:

a. Production of IgG-blocking antibody that combines with antigen before it reacts with IgE antibodies.

b. May decrease IgE antibodies against specific antigens.

c. Modulation from Th2 to Th1 T lymphocytes. (Th2 associated with allergy).

3. Possible side effects of immunotherapy.

a. Systemic reactions—anaphylaxis is rare, but potentially fatal.

b. Local reactions—consist of erythema and induration at the site of injection.

NURSING ALERT

Immunotherapy should not be given to patients who are actively wheezing or receiving β-adrenergic blocking agents. It would be difficult to reverse a systemic reaction, should one occur.

Complications

1. Allergic asthma.
2. Chronic otitis media, hearing loss.
3. Chronic nasal obstruction, sinusitis.

Nursing Assessment

1. Obtain history of severity and seasonality of symptoms.
2. Inspect for characteristic tearing, conjunctival erythema, pale nasal mucous membranes with clear discharge, allergic shiners, and mouth breathing.
3. Auscultate lungs for wheezing or prolonged expiration characteristic of asthma.

Nursing Diagnosis

• Breathing Pattern, Ineffective related to nasal obstruction

Nursing Interventions

Facilitating Normal Breathing Pattern

1. Reassure patient that suffocation will not occur because of nasal obstruction; mouth breathing will occur.
2. Use intranasal saline and increase oral fluid intake to prevent drying of mucous membranes and increased insensible loss through mouth breathing.
3. Administer and teach self-administration of antihistamines, decongestants, and other medications, as directed.

a. Instruct patients on proper use of nasal inhalers— clear mucus from nose first, exhale, flex neck to point nose downward, activate inhaler, and gently sniff while releasing medication.

b. Warn patient to avoid driving or other situations that require alertness if sedating antihistamines, such as diphenhydramine (Benadryl) or chlorpheniramine (Chlor-Trimeton) have been prescribed.

c. Do not use over-the-counter nasal decongestants for more than 2 to 3 days because their effect is short lived and a rebound effect, which causes nasal mucosal edema, often occurs.

DRUG ALERT

Long-term use of nasal corticosteroids may cause nasal septum rupture. Teach patients to direct spray or aerosol away from septum.

Patient Education and Health Maintenance

Immunotherapy

1. Provide information on the purpose, method of administration, time frame of expected results, and possible risks involved (local reactions, anaphylaxis).
2. Inform the patient that close observation for 30 minutes is essential after each injection.
3. Alert patient to the possibility of a delayed reaction that needs to be reported to the nurse or health care provider.

Environmental Control

See Patient Education Guidelines: Environmental Control for Allergic Rhinitis.

Additional Resources

American Academy of Allergy Asthma, and Immunology
611 E. Wells St.
Milwaukee, WI 53202
414-272-6071
www.aaaai.org

American College of Allergy, Asthma and Immunology
800-842-7777
www.allergy.mcg.edu

National Institute of Allergy and Infectious Diseases
NIAID Office of Communications
Bldg. 31, Room 7A-50
31 Center Drive, MSC 2520
Bethesda, MD 20892-2520
301-496-5717
www.niaid.nih.gov

Outcome-Based Evaluation

• Decreased eye and nasal symptoms, mouth breathing; no complaints of dry mouth

▉ Urticaria and Angioedema

Urticaria (hives) may affect 10% of the population at some time. Angioedema is a similar lesion, but involves deep dermis and subcutaneous tissues. Urticaria and angioedema can occur individually or in combination.

Pathophysiology and Etiology

1. Acute urticaria:
   a. Hives that last less than 6 weeks.
   b. A detectable cause is usually determined.
2. Chronic urticaria:
   a. Hives that last 6 weeks or longer.
   b. The cause is undetermined in 75% to 90% of patients.
3. Causes include:
   a. Ingested substances—food, food additives, drugs.
   b. Infections—viral, bacterial, parasitic.

PATIENT EDUCATION GUIDELINES   Environmental Control for Allergic Rhinitis

The following environmental modifications may help reduce symptoms of allergic rhinitis (hay fever):

1. Encase pillows and mattress in allergen-proof covers.
2. Wash all bed linens (mattress pad, sheets, blanket, comforter, bedspread) in hot water weekly.
3. Keep clothing in a closet with door shut.
4. Use wipeable shades and blinds, washable curtains.
5. Avoid stuffed animals and other dust collectors.
6. Vacuum and damp-dust weekly and wear a mask while doing it.
7. If you have severe symptoms of dust allergy, leave the house during cleaning. Allergic reaction is possible for about 30 min after vacuuming because of dust mite feces becoming airborne. Use of fine-filtering face masks may provide some protection.
8. Eliminate upholstered furniture, carpets, and draperies.
9. Use air conditioning and keep windows closed during high pollen and mold season to reduce antigen load indoors.
10. Change furnace/air conditioner filters frequently.
11. Using a high-efficiency air filtering system may help.
12. Avoid smoking and smoke-filled areas.
13. Avoid rapid changes in temperature.
14. If you are allergic to animal danders, you should not have household pets—or you should at least keep them out of the bedroom and run a high efficiency particulate air filter (place on table).
15. Avoid mold growth by dehumidification (<45% R.H.) and use of a fungicide in bathrooms, damp basements, food storage areas, and garbage containers.
16. Avoid outdoor activities when high pollen/pollutants are in the air.

---

c. Physical factors—heat, sun, cold, pressure, emotional stress.
d. Insect stings.

Clinical Manifestations
1. Raised, red, edematous wheals.
2. Intense pruritus.
3. May affect any body region.
4. Diffuse swelling with angioedema, especially of the lips, eyelids, cheeks, hands, and feet.
5. Symptoms may develop within seconds or over 1 to 2 hours and may last up to 24 to 36 hours.

Diagnostic Evaluation
1. Laboratory—serum tryptase is elevated in the acute phase, complement study results can be abnormal, total serum IgE elevated.
2. Challenge testing to determine physical cause.
   a. Exercise challenge.
   b. Ice cube challenge.
   c. Heat challenge.
   d. Pressure challenge.
   e. Dermographism present.

Management
Acute Urticaria
1. Identification and elimination of causative factors.
2. Medications.
   a. H_1 antihistamines, such as diphenhydramine (Benadryl) and cetirizine (Zyrtec).
   b. Epinephrine (Adrenalin) 1:1,000 (0.3-0.5 mL subcutaneously) for extensive urticaria, angioedema.
   c. Corticosteroids—limited to severe cases; unresponsive to antihistamines.

Prolonged Urticaria
1. Elimination diet.
2. Medications.
   a. H_1 antihistamines.
   b. H_2 antihistamines, such as ranitidine (Zantac), may be of some value.
   c. Tricyclic antidepressants, such as doxepin (Adapin), given for antihistaminic effect.
   d. Topical agents to relieve itching (moisturizer or oatmeal baths).

Complications
1. Neurovascular impairment because of swelling.
2. Occasionally edema of the larynx or bronchi may occur.

Nursing Assessment
1. Assess for time frame during which lesions appear and disappear.
2. Assess for triggering factors.
3. Assess for family history of angioedema; may indicate hereditary angioedema rather than allergic reaction.

Nursing Diagnosis
• Sensory and Perceptual Alteration related to pruritus

Nursing Interventions
Relieving Pruritus
1. Administer or teach self-administration of antihistamines, corticosteroids, and additional medications as prescribed.
2. Encourage the proper use of topical and over-the-counter agents, as directed.

3. Advise patient to avoid exposure to heat, exercise, sunburn, and alcohol and to promptly control fever and anxiety—factors that may aggravate reactions caused by vasodilation.
4. Warn patient to avoid identified triggers.
5. Teach relaxation techniques and methods of distraction to enhance coping.
6. Assess effectiveness of therapy.

Patient Education and Health Maintenance
1. Warn the patient to monitor for symptoms of laryngeal edema and to seek medical intervention immediately if respiratory distress occurs.
2. Instruct patients with laryngeal edema how to self-administer epinephrine.

Outcome-Based Evaluation
• Reports relief of pruritus with antihistamines and distraction methods

■ Food Allergies
Food allergies result when the body's immune system overreacts to certain otherwise harmless substances. Food allergies occur in 4% to 6% of children and in 1% to 2% of adults, although the perceived prevalence is much higher because other existing adverse food reactions cause similar symptoms.

Pathophysiology and Etiology
1. Food hypersensitivity—a true food allergy is an IgE-mediated response to a food allergen (protein).
2. Food intolerance—an abnormal physical response to a food or additive; is not immunologic.
   a. Toxicity (poisoning)—caused by toxins contained in foods, microorganisms, or parasites.
   b. Pharmacologic (chemical)—such as caffeine.
   c. Idiosyncratic—etiology unknown.
3. Common food allergens include cow's milk, eggs, shellfish, peanuts, tree nuts, soybean, and wheat.

Clinical Manifestations
1. Respiratory—rhinoconjunctivitis, sneezing, laryngeal edema, wheezing.
2. Cutaneous—urticaria, angioedema, atopic dermatitis.
3. Gastroenteritis—lip swelling, palatal itching, nausea, abdominal cramping, diarrhea.
4. Neurologic—migraine headaches in some patients.

Diagnostic Tests
1. Skin testing.
   a. Limit to those foods suspected of provoking symptoms based on history.
   b. Only epicutaneous testing is done.
   c. Intradermal testing has not been demonstrated to have a high degree of clinical correlation.
2. RAST-positive test result.
3. Oral challenge.

   a. The suspected food is given to the patient to identify the allergen by reproducing the symptoms caused by the initial reaction.
   b. Open—may be used if the suspected food skin test result is negative; suspected food is openly administered and the patient is monitored for a reaction.
   c. Single-blind—the suspected food is disguised in capsules, liquids, or other foods, and administered to the patient in increasing doses at intervals determined by history and may be interspersed with placebo. Some bias exists.
   d. Double-blind placebo-controlled—the most definitive technique to confirm or refute histories of food allergies. The suspected food is administered in capsules or via some other vehicle that masks its identity, and is interspersed with placebo so neither the health care provider/nurse nor patient knows whether the suspected food or placebo is being ingested.
4. Elimination diet.
   a. To determine if the patient's symptoms will stop when certain foods are avoided.
   b. Restrict one or two foods at a time if certain foods are suspected.
   c. If no particular food is suspected, a highly restricted diet for 14 days is preferable.

Management
1. Avoidance of specific foods is the only way of effectively preventing food allergy reactions.
2. Medications:
   a. Antihistamines—may modify IgE-mediated symptoms but will not eliminate them.
   b. Corticosteroids—only used in the treatment of food allergy if associated with eosinophilic gastroenteritis or gastroenteropathy.
   c. Epinephrine (Adrenalin)—if history of anaphylaxis, patient should carry it at all times (Epi-Pen, Ana-Kit).

Complications
1. Anaphylaxis.

Nursing Assessment
1. Assist with assessment for offending foods; encourage the patient to keep a food/symptom diary.
2. Auscultate lungs and document any wheezing.
3. Assess compliance with prescribed diet and relief of symptoms.

Nursing Diagnosis
• Altered Nutrition: Less Than Body Requirements related to restrictive diet

Nursing Interventions
Promoting Adequate Nutrition
1. Consult with dietitian to ensure a balanced diet that excludes identified allergens and incorporates patient's food preferences.

2. Administer dietary supplements as needed.
3. Explain hidden sources of foods to decrease the risk of unexpected exposure to an offending allergen. Encourage label reading.
4. Discuss alternative food preparation techniques and methods of substitution (such as using extra baking powder in place of eggs).
5. Administer and teach self-administration of medications, if necessary, to reduce abdominal cramping and diarrhea, which may deter food intake.
6. Monitor weight.

Patient Teaching and Health Education

1. Instruct the patient with history of anaphylactic reaction about self-injection technique for the administration of epinephrine.
2. Caution highly allergic patients about restaurant food; when eating out, patients should request ingredient information; such brochures are now available in many restaurants, including fast food establishments.
3. Advise patient that most young children and about one-third of older children and adults lose their food sensitivity after 1 to 2 years of avoidance. Compliance with elimination is the key. Sensitivity to shellfish and nuts is rarely lost, however.
4. Provide resource for patient to obtain more information: Food Allergy Network 800-929-4040; Internet website: *www.foodallergy.org*.

Outcome-Based Evaluation

- Decreased frequency and severity of food allergy reactions by log
- Verbalizes acceptance of diet; weight stable

Latex Sensitivity

Latex sensitivity is becoming a major health concern for health care workers, patients, and others at risk by occupation. Allergic reaction may be immediate or delayed. Latex is present in approximately 40,000 medical and other products, including household products and toys. The prevalence of latex sensitivity is estimated to be 1% in the general population, 20% in nurses, and more than 60% in children with spina bifida.

Pathophysiology and Etiology

1. Natural rubber latex, manufactured from the sap of rubber trees, is highly irritating and allergenic in some people.
2. Increased use of latex, in the form of sterile and unsterile gloves, has made latex sensitivity a problem for many health care workers since the inception of Universal Precautions in the 1980s.
3. Three types of reactions to latex may occur:
   a. Irritant dermatitis—not an allergic reaction.
   b. Type IV (cell-mediated, delayed) hypersensitivity—a localized contact allergic reaction.
   c. Type I (IgE mediated, immediate)—a systemic allergic reaction.
4. No predictable pattern exists for the progression of reactions; anaphylaxis may occur at any time.
5. Those at risk include children with spina bifida, health care workers, people with atopic allergies, people with a history of multiple surgeries, and workers in factories that produce latex products.

Clinical Manifestations

1. Irritant dermatitis—may be caused by powder or chemical residue on gloves—erythema and pruritus localized to area of contact; occurs immediately.
2. Type IV (delayed) hypersensitivity—contact allergic reaction—erythema, pruritus, urticaria; possibly flushing, localized edema, rhinitis, coughing, and conjunctivitis. Symptoms occur 1 to 48 hours after contact with product.
3. Type I (immediate) hypersensitivity—urticaria, angioedema, conjunctivitis, dyspnea, pharyngeal edema, arrhythmias, and anaphylaxis. Symptoms are immediate and may be moderate to life-threatening in intensity.

Diagnostic Evaluation

1. History of symptoms gives presumptive diagnosis, but confirmation is difficult because standardized tests are not yet widely available.
2. A crude skin prick test uses a fragment of latex glove soaked in saline for 15 minutes as the solution. This is not standardized, but a positive test result is considered proof of latex sensitivity.
3. A challenge test can be done by having the patient wear a latex glove or fingertip of a glove for 15 minutes; look for a reaction. Latex-free gloves can be used as a control. Severe reactions may occur with this test.
4. Standardized skin testing will become more available pending FDA approval of standardized latex solution, but the threat of anaphylaxis will still exist.
5. RAST testing is safe but expensive, and not as sensitive as skin testing.

Management

1. Avoidance is the key. See Table 28-1 for safety and prevention techniques in the health care workplace.
2. For irritant reactions, changing brands of gloves may be sufficient, or changing to a powder-free glove.
3. Decreasing length of exposure time or wearing cotton liners in gloves may help, but may not solve the problem.
4. Use of latex-free gloves and products is often necessary. Although more hospitals and medical offices are making latex-free products available, a job change may be necessary for some people.
5. A latex-free environment is necessary for treatment.
6. Topical corticosteroid creams for local reactions.
7. Oral antihistamines may be used for mild to moderate reactions.

TABLE 28-1 Safety Measures to Prevent Latex Reactions

Wear gloves only when you need to; follow Universal Precautions.

- Gloves are not a substitute for handwashing.
- Use only water-based hand lotion, if you must use lotion.
- Use powder-free latex gloves to prevent aerosolized latex.
- Dispose of gloves properly; do not leave on counters.
- Wash and dry your hands well after glove removal.
- Avoid touching your eyes and face while wearing gloves.
- If symptoms develop, report them and document according to facility policy.
- Seek medical follow-up as indicated by symptoms.
- Maintain a safe environment for all patients and for all members of the health care team.

(Adapted from Gritter, M. [1997]. Latex allergy. *Primary Care Practice*, 1[2], 150.)

TABLE 28-2 Sources of Latex

Product Containing Latex	Latex-Free Alternatives
Balloons	Mylar balloons
Chewing gum	None
Condoms, diaphragms	Polyurethane condoms (male and female)
Rubber bands	String or clips
Pacifiers	Silicone products
Toys—Koosh, teething rings, dolls	Most Fisher Price, Little Tykes, Discover, and Playschool toys
Feminine hygiene products	Kimberly-Clark products
Adhesive bandages	Cotton pads and plastic tape

(Adapted from Gritter, M. [1997]. Latex allergy. *Primary Care Practice*, 1[2], 149.)

8. Oral or parenteral corticosteroids, IM antihistamines, and IM or subcutaneous epinephrine are given for severe reactions.
9. IV fluids, oxygen, and intubation may be needed for cardiovascular and pulmonary support with severe reactions.

Complications
Unpredictable anaphylaxis and death.

Nursing Assessment
1. Assess patient for history of risk factors and pattern of suspected reactions.
2. Assess skin for erythema, swelling, vesicles, and other lesions.
3. Assess mucous membranes for conjunctivitis, rhinitis, and other lesions.
4. For suspected systemic reactions, assess vital signs for hypotension, tachycardia, arrhythmnia, respiratory distress.
5. Assess respiratory status for stridor caused by laryngeal edema and breath sounds for wheezing.
6. Assess for signs of internal edema with systemic reaction, such as nausea, vomiting, diarrhea.

Nursing Diagnosis
- Knowledge Deficit (sources of latex and how to avoid latex)

Nursing Interventions and Patient Education
Increasing Knowledge on Latex Avoidance
1. Educate patients about the widespread use of latex and some possible alternatives (Table 28-2).
2. Ensure that patients with history of Type I reaction have self-injectable epinephrine and antihistamines on hand at all times to use at first sign of a reaction.
3. Encourage patients who have had moderate to severe reactions to wear a Medic-Alert bracelet.

4. Encourage patients to notify all their health care providers, labs, and clinics before they make a visit, to facilitate the use of latex-free products. These patients should be given the first appointment of the day and all supplies that contain latex should be removed from the room or covered with a cotton cloth. Only latex-free products should be used, and staff members should be careful to avoid wearing or removing latex gloves in the hall while the patient is in the office.
5. Support the patient who has had a severe reaction in the workplace. Remind the patient that the Americans With Disabilities Act (ADA) guarantees workers reasonable modifications to the workplace to accommodate a disability. However, the area of latex sensitivity as a disability is controversial.
6. For further information, contact American Latex Allergy Association, 888-972-5378; or Education for Latex Allergy Support Team and Information Coalition (ELASTIC), *www.latexallergyhelp.com*.
7. Also see care of patient with anaphylaxis, urticaria, and asthma.

▪ Bronchial Asthma
Bronchial asthma is a chronic inflammatory disorder of the airways in which many cells and cellular elements play a role. This inflammation causes episodes of wheezing, breathlessness, chest tightness, and coughing, particularly at night or early in the morning, and airway hyperreactivity to various stimuli. The episodes are usually associated with variable airflow obstruction that is often reversible either spontaneously or with treatment. Few people with persistent asthma will develop irreversible fibrosis of the lining of the airways.

Pathophysiology and Etiology
The basic defect appears to be an abnormality in the host, which intermittently leads to an increased constriction of smooth muscle, hypersecretion of mucus in the bronchial tree, and mucosal edema.

Neuromechanisms (Autonomic Nervous System)

1. Stimulation of the vagus nerve (which is responsible for bronchomotor tone) by viral respiratory infections, air pollutants, and other stimuli causes bronchoconstriction, increased secretion of mucus, and dilation of the pulmonary vessels.
2. β-Adrenergic receptor cells that line the airways are also responsible for bronchomotor tone. Abnormal functioning of these cells predisposes patients to bronchoconstriction.

Antigen-Antibody Reaction

1. Susceptible individuals form abnormally large amounts of IgE when exposed to certain allergens. Most children and half of adults with asthma are sensitized to at least one common inhaled allergen.
2. This immunoglobulin (IgE) fixes itself to the mast cells of the bronchial mucosa.
3. When the person is exposed to certain allergens, the resulting antigen combines with the cell-bound IgE molecules, causing the mast cell to degranulate and release chemical mediators.
4. These chemical mediators act on bronchial smooth muscle to cause bronchoconstriction, on dilated epithelium to reduce mucociliary clearance, on bronchial glands to cause mucus secretion, on blood vessels to cause vasodilation and increased permeability, and on leukocytes to cause a cellular infiltration and inflammation.
5. Late-phase reactions (these occur 4 to 8 hours after the initial response) include the influx of eosinophils, neutrophils, lymphocytes, and monocytes.

Bronchial Inflammation

1. Occurs in both the immediate- and late-phase reactions caused by antigen-antibody response.
2. Factors other than allergens (such as noxious environmental stimuli) cause bronchial inflammation and hyperreactivity by mast cell activation.

Classification

Asthma is classified by severity as mild intermittent, mild persistent, moderate, and severe, as outlined in Table 28-3.

Extrinsic Asthma

1. Hypersensitivity reaction to inhalant allergens (dust mites, animal dander, cockroaches, pollen, mold are the major ones).
2. Mediated by immunoglobulin E (IgE mediated).

Intrinsic Asthma

1. No inciting allergen.
2. Infection, often viral.
3. Environmental stimuli (such as air pollution).

Mixed Asthma

Immediate type I reactivity appears to be combined with intrinsic factors.

Aspirin-Induced Asthma

1. Induced by ingestion of aspirin and related compounds.
2. "Triad" has been described as a combination of aspirin-induced asthma, nasal polyps, and sinusitis.

Exercise-Induced Asthma

Symptoms vary from slight chest tightness and cough to severe wheezing/cough and shortness of breath that usually occur after 5 to 20 minutes of sustained exercise.

TABLE 28-3 Classification of Asthma Severity

Clinical Features Before Treatment*

	Symptoms**	Nighttime Symptoms	Lung Function
STEP 4 Severe Persistent	Continual symptoms Limited physical activity Frequent exacerbations	Frequent	FEV_1 or PEF ≤60% predicted PEF variability >30%
STEP 3 Moderate Persistent	Daily symptoms Daily use of inhaled short-acting beta$_2$-agonist Exacerbations affect activity Exacerbations ≥2 times a week: may last days	>1 time a week	FEV_1 or PEF >60% - <80% predicted PEF variability >30%
STEP 2 Mild Persistent	Symptoms >2 times a week but <1 time a day Exacerbations may affect activity	>2 times a month	FEV_1 or PEF ≥80% predicted PEF variability 20-30%
STEP 1 Mild Intermittent	Symptoms ≤2 times a week Asymptomatic and normal PEF between exacerbations Exacerbations brief (from a few hours to a few days); intensity may vary	≤2 times a month	FEV_1 or PEF ≥80% predicted PEF variability <20%

FEV, forced expiratory volume; PEF, peak expiratory flow.

* The presence of one of the features of severity is sufficient to place a patient in that category. An individual should be assigned to the most severe grade in which any feature occurs. The characteristics noted in this figure are general and may overlap because asthma is highly variable. Furthermore, an individual's classification may change over time.

** Patients at any level of severity can have mild, moderate, or severe exacerbations. Some patients with intermittent asthma experience severe and life-threatening exacerbations separated by long periods of normal lung function and no symptoms.

(From National Asthma Education and Prevention Program [1997]. *Expert Panel Report 2. Guidelines for diagnosis and management of asthma.* NIH Publication No. 97-4051. Bethesda, MD: U.S. Department of Health and Human Services.)

Occupational Asthma

Caused by inhalation of industrial fumes, dust, allergens, and gases.

Clinical Manifestations

1. Episodes of coughing.
2. Wheezing.
3. Dyspnea.
4. Feeling of chest tightness.

 NURSING ALERT

Do not be fooled by lack of wheezing on auscultation when the patient complains of severe shortness of breath. Airflow may be so restricted that wheezing ceases.

Diagnostic Evaluation

1. Pulmonary function testing—>12% decrease in forced expiratory volume in first second of exhalation (FEV_1). Peak flow >20% variability between AM and PM measurements.
2. Laboratory—increased levels of IgE may be seen in atopic asthma.
3. Bronchial methacholine challenge—demonstrates airway hyperreactivity by the inhalation of a cholinergic agent in serial concentrations delivered by nebulization; a positive response is indicated by a 20% decrease in the initial FEV_1 than later challenges.
4. Skin testing to identify causative allergens.
5. Chest x-ray to exclude other lung diseases in new onset asthma in adult.

Management

The goal is to allow the person with asthma to live a normal life. It is important that the patient and his/her family be included in planning management of asthma. The treatment plan should be as simple as possible and individualized to the patient's lifestyle.

Quick-Relief Medications

1. Short-acting bronchodilators by inhalation.
2. β-Adrenergic agonists, such as albuterol (Proventil, Ventolin), metaproterenol (Alupent), and pirbuterol (Maxair).
3. Anticholinergic agent ipratropium bromide (Atrovent).
4. Systemic corticosteroids (short course).

 DRUG ALERT

A short-acting bronchodilator, such as albuterol, is the drug of choice for acute asthma.

Long-Term Controllers

1. Inhaled corticosteroids, such as triamcinolone (Azmacort), beclomethasone (Vaceril, Beclovent), fluticasone (Flovent), budesonide (Pulmicort), flunisolide (AeroBid).
2. Long-acting inhaled β agonists (salmeterol, Serevent).

3. Leukotriene modifiers, such as montelukast (Singulair), zafirlukast (Accolate).
4. Inhaled mast cell stabilizers (cromolyn sodium [Intal], nedocromil [Tilade]).
5. Long-acting oral β-agonists (albuterol extended-release tablets [Volmax]).
6. Oral corticosteroids (maintenance dose).
7. Methylxanthines, such as theophylline (Theo-24, Uniphyl, Theo-Dur).

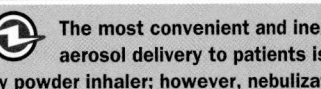 **NURSING ALERT**

The most convenient and inexpensive method of aerosol delivery to patients is the metered-dose or dry powder inhaler; however, nebulization offers better drug delivery.

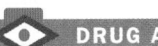 **DRUG ALERT**

Note: β-Blocking agents, such as propranolol (Inderal), have the potential to cause bronchoconstriction and should not be given to patients with asthma.

Other Measures

1. Environmental control (see allergic rhinitis, p. 918).
2. Immunotherapy (see allergic rhinitis, p. 913).
3. Avoidance of foods that contain tartrazine (yellow dye no. 5) in aspirin-sensitive patients.
4. Exercise: Regular aerobic exercise should be encouraged.
5. Use of an inhaled β-agonist or cromolyn taken 15 to 20 minutes before exercise will decrease exercise-induced bronchospasm.
6. Alternative and complementary therapies that include acupuncture, herbal preparations, yoga, and chiropractic treatment have been suggested for acute and chronic asthma control; however, none is a substitute for usual medical treatment.
   a. Chiropractic treatment is based on spinal manipulation to resolve neurologic disturbance that may affect chest wall function and airway tone.
   b. A recent controlled study revealed that 91 children with mild to moderate asthma showed mild improvement in peak expiratory flow and less β-agonist inhaler use in both the control and experimental groups. The experimental group received usual medical care plus chiropractic manipulation; the control group received usual medical care plus *simulated* chiropractic manipulation. The study concluded that chiropractic intervention led to no further benefit than that of usual medical care. Because both control and experimental groups showed improvement, however, there seems to be some benefit from frequent professional attention.

Nursing Assessment

1. Review patient's record: ask about coughing, dyspnea, chest tightness, wheezing, exertional changes, and increased mucous production.

2. Observe the patient and assess the rate, depth, and character of respirations, especially on expiration; observe for hyperinflation.
3. Auscultate the chest for breath sounds/wheezing.
4. Assess for triggers of asthma that include the following:
   a. Allergens.
   b. Respiratory infections.
   c. Inhalation of irritating substances (dust, fumes, gases).
   d. Environmental factors (weather, air pollution, and humidity).
   e. Exercise, particularly in cold weather.
   f. Aspirin and its derivatives.
   g. Sulfite-containing agents used as food preservatives.
   h. Emotional factors.
5. After acute episode subsides, attempt to determine patient's degree of adherence with medications/management regimen.
6. Observe inhalation technique.

Nursing Diagnoses

- Ineffective Breathing Pattern related to bronchospasm
- Anxiety related to fear of suffocating, difficulty in breathing, death

Nursing Interventions

Attaining Relief of Dyspneic Breathing

1. Monitor vital signs, skin color, retraction, and degree of restlessness, which may indicate hypoxia.
2. Provide nebulization and oxygen therapy as prescribed.
3. Monitor airway functioning through peak flow meter or pulmonary function testing to assess effectiveness of treatment.
4. Encourage intake of fluids to liquefy secretions.
5. Instruct patient on positioning to facilitate breathing—sitting upright (leaning forward on a table).
6. Encourage patient to use adaptive breathing techniques (eg, pursued-lip breathing) to decrease the work of breathing.
7. Use chest physiotherapy/postural drainage to mobilize secretions, if ordered.

Relieving Anxiety

1. Explain rationale for interventions to gain patient's cooperation. Provide care in prompt, confident manner.
2. Help patient clarify source(s) of anxiety; suggest measures to reduce anxiety and to control breathing.
3. Encourage active participation and support efforts to adhere to management plan.

Community and Home Care Considerations

1. Initiate peak flow monitoring as ordered by health care provider. This may be done twice daily by the patient with persistent asthma. Provide written and verbal instruction and have the patient demonstrate the procedure.
2. The patient can buy a peak flow meter from a pharmacy or from a medical supply company.

3. Once optimal asthma control is obtained, daily peak flow measurements in the early morning and early afternoon should be used during a 2- to 3-week period to determine the patient's personal best. The personal best peak flow measurement will be used to monitor control and to guide self therapy in an individualized action plan.
4. Teach the patient to obtain peak flow measurement (See Patient Education Guidelines: Obtaining a Peak Flow Measurement).
5. Provide written and verbal instruction on an action plan for self-management of asthma exacerbation as outlined by the health care provider. National Asthma Education and Prevention Program Guidelines suggest the following:
   a. For symptomatic worsening of asthma or asymptomatic decrease in peak flow measurement, use initial inhalation of a short-acting beta agonist by MDI, 2 to 4 puffs for up to 3 treatments at 20 minute intervals, or a single nebulization treatment.
   b. After initial treatment, recheck peak flow; if >80% of personal best and no wheezing or shortness of breath, continue beta agonist every 3 to 4 hours for 24 to 48 hours. If on inhaled corticosteroids, double dose for 7 to 10 days. The patient should contact the health care provider for further instructions.
   c. If peak flow is 50% to 80% of personal best, or if the patient has persistent wheezing and shortness of breath, an oral corticosteroid should be initiated and beta agonist should be continued. The patient should contact the health care provider the same day for further instructions.
   d. If peak flow is <50% of personal best or if the patient has significant wheezing and shortness of breath, an oral corticosteroid should be started, beta agonist should be repeated immediately, and the patient should proceed to the emergency department.

Patient Education and Health Maintenance

1. Provide information on the nature of asthma and methods of treatment.
2. Provide information regarding medications, including the difference between long term controllers and quick relief medications and the proper use of inhalers and spacer devices; stress avoiding overuse of inhalers and nebulizers.
3. Demonstrate the use of MDIs (see Patient Education Guidelines: How to Use an Inhaler and Spacer) and nebulization equipment.
4. Help patient to identify what triggers asthma, warning signs of an impending attack, and strategies for preventing and treating an attack.
5. Teach adaptive breathing techniques and breathing exercises, such as pursed-lip breathing.
6. Discuss environmental control.
   a. Avoid persons with respiratory infections.
   b. Avoid substances and situations known to precipitate bronchospasm, such as allergens, irritants, strong odors, gases, fumes and smoke.

Peak flow measurement can be obtained by:
1. Place the indicator at the base of the numbered scale.
2. Preferably stand, or sit upright.
3. Take a deep breath.
4. Place the meter in mouth and close lips around mouthpiece, with tongue under mouthpiece.
5. Blow out as hard and as fast as possible. Coughing or spitting will result in a falsely elevated level.
6. Note the measurement that the indicator is pointing to on the number scale.
7. Repeat 1–6 twice more and record the highest number.

---

c. Wear a mask if cold weather precipitates bronchospasm.

d. Stay inside when air pollution is high.

e. See Patient Education, Allergic Rhinitis, page 918.

7. Promote optimal health practices, including nutrition, rest, and exercise.

a. Encourage regular exercise to improve cardiorespiratory and musculoskeletal conditioning.

b. Drink liberal amounts of fluids to keep secretions thin.

c. Try to avoid upsetting situations.

d. Use relaxation techniques, biofeedback management.

e. Use community resources for smoking cessation classes, stress management, exercises for relaxation, asthma support groups, etc.

8. Ensure that patient knows whom to follow up with and the frequency of follow-up. Discuss with patient how to overcome any barriers to follow-up, such as transportation, limited office or clinic hours, child care, and work requirements.

9. For additional information and support, refer to American Academy of Allergy, Asthma, and Immunology, 414-272-6071; *www.aaaai.org*.

Outcome-Based Evaluation

- Symptoms (wheezing, coughing, chest tightness) reduced; peak flow improved
- Verbalizes relief of anxiety

Status Asthmaticus

Status asthmaticus is a severe form of asthma in which the airway obstruction is unresponsive to usual drug therapy.

Contributing Factors

1. Infection.
2. Inhalation of air pollutants and allergens to which sensitized.
3. Noncompliance in taking medications, including overuse of bronchodilators.
4. Ingestion of aspirin or related drugs in aspirin-sensitive patient.
5. Aspiration of gastric acid.

Clinical Manifestations

1. Tachypnea, labored respirations, with increased effort on exhalation.

2. Suprasternal retractions, use of accessory muscles of respiration.

3. Diminished breath sounds, decreased ability to speak in phrases/sentences.

4. Anxiety, irritability, fatigue, headache, impaired mental functioning.

5. Muscle twitching, somnolence, diaphoresis—from continued carbon dioxide retention.

6. Tachycardia, elevated blood pressure.

7. Heart failure and death from suffocation.

Management and Nursing Interventions

1. Monitor respiratory rate and oxygen saturation continuously; frequently monitor arterial blood gases, blood pressure, electrocardiogram.

NURSING ALERT

In status asthmaticus, the return to a normal or increasing PCO_2 does not necessarily mean that the patient with asthma is improving—it may indicate a fatigue state that develops just before the patient slips into respiratory failure.

2. Administer repeated aerosol treatments with β_2 agonist bronchodilators, such as albuterol (Ventolin); add anticholinergic ipratropium bromide (Atrovent) as prescribed—administer with caution until the metabolic and respiratory acidosis and hypoxemia have been corrected.

3. Monitor IV therapy.

a. When IV fluids are administered, aminophylline (Aminophyllin) may be prescribed and administered slowly by constant infusion; the clinician must be constantly alert for signs of theophylline toxicity (tachycardia, nausea, vomiting, restlessness, dizziness).

b. Corticosteroids are given to treat inflammation of airways; because these act slowly, their beneficial effects may not be apparent for several hours.

c. Fluids are given to treat dehydration and loosen secretions.

4. Provide continuous humidified oxygen via nasal cannula as prescribed. (Patients with associated chronic obstructive pulmonary disease or emphysema are at risk for depressed hypoxemic ventilatory drive, thus compounding respiratory insufficiency, so use oxygen cautiously.)

PATIENT EDUCATION GUIDELINES   How to Use an Inhaler and Spacer

HOW TO USE AN INHALER

1. Shake the inhaler well before each inhalation.
2. Remove the cap from the mouthpiece.
3. Breathe out through your mouth while standing or sitting upright. Hold the inhaler up to 2 inches away from your open mouth. Alternately, attach a spacer and follow directions at right. Least preferably, used the closed-mouth method by placing the mouthpiece of the inhaler in your mouth and close lips around it tightly.
4. While breathing in deeply and slowly through your mouth, press down firmly on the top of the canister with your index finger. See diagram.
5. Continue to inhale, then try to hold your breath for 5 to 10 seconds. Remove the inhaler from your mouth and release your finger from the canister before breathing out.
6. Wait 1 min and shake the inhaler before you take your next inhalation. Follow the same instructions for your second inhalation as you did for the first.
7. Replace the mouthpiece cap after each use.
8. Clean the inhaler thoroughly and frequently. Remove the metal canister and clean the inhaler and cap at least once a day by rinsing with warm, running water. Dry the inhaler and cap thoroughly with a gentle twisting motion.
9. Discard the canister after you have used the labeled number of inhalations. You should not use it beyond this indicated number because the correct dose amount can no longer be guaranteed.
10. For dry powdered inhalers (DPI), use a forceful, rapid inhalation with closed mouth technique. See specific manufacturer instructions.

HOW TO USE A SPACER

Unless you use your inhaler the right way, much of the medicine can end up on your tongue, on the back of your throat, or in the air. Use of a spacer or holding chamber can help this problem.

1. A spacer or holding chamber is a device that attaches to a metered dose inhaler. It holds the medicine in its chamber long enough for you to inhale it in one or two slow deep breaths. The spacer helps you get your full dose of medicine, prevents you from coughing, and may prevent a yeast infection in your mouth from using a steroid inhaler.
2. There are several different models of spacers or holding chambers that you can purchase through your pharmacist. Ask your health care provider if a spacer would be right for you.
3. Attach the inhaler to the spacer or holding chamber as shown in the product instructions.
4. Shake well.
5. Press the canister on the inhaler. This puts one puff of medicine into the holding chamber.
6. Place the mouthpiece of the spacer into your mouth and inhale slowly.
7. Hold your breath a few seconds and then exhale.
8. If your health care provider has prescribed two or more puffs, wait a minute and then repeat steps 4–7.

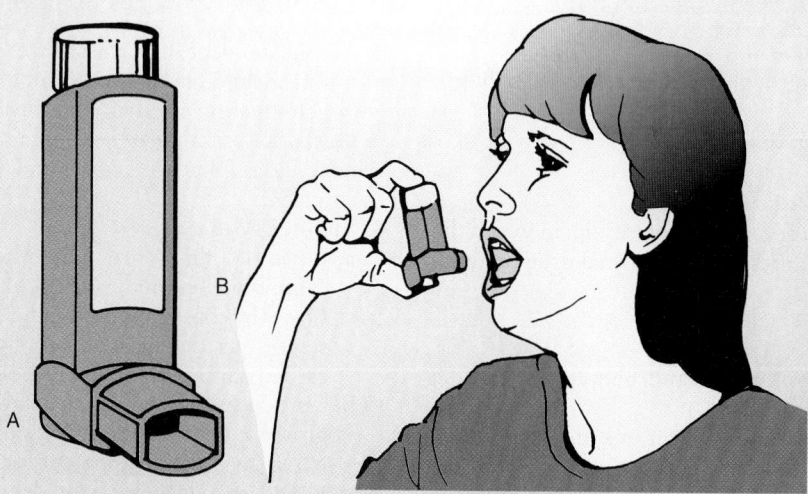

(Adapted from Nettina, S.M. [ed.]. [1997]. Patient education. Using an inhaler and a spacer. *Lippincott's Primary Care Practice, 1*[2], 231–232.)

5. Initiate mechanical ventilation, if necessary.

6. Assist with mobilization of obstructing bronchial mucus.

   a. Perform chest physiotherapy (chest wall percussion and vibration).

   b. Administer expectorant and mucolytic drugs as prescribed.

   c. Remove secretions by suctioning, or prepare for bronchoscopy if needed.

6. Provide adequate hydration.

7. Obtain portable chest x-ray and administer antibiotics as prescribed to treat any underlying respiratory infection.

8. Alleviate the patient's anxiety and fear by acting calmly and by reassuring the patient during an attack. Stay with the patient until the attack subsides.

SELECTED REFERENCES

Autio, L. & Rosenow, D. (1999). Effectively managing asthma in young and middle adulthood. *Nurse Practitioner, 24*(1), 100–111.

Balon, J., Aker, P.K., Crowther, E.R., et al. (1998). A comparison of active and simulated chiropractic manipulation as adjunctive treatment for childhood asthma. *New England Journal of Medicine, 339,* 1013–1020.

Barbarito, C. (1999). Anaphylaxis. *American Journal of Nursing, 99*(1), 33.

Brown, C.S., Parker, N.G., & Stegbauer, C.C. (1999). Managing allergic rhinitis. *Nurse Practitioner, 24*(5), 107–120.

Carrol, P. (1999). Latex allergy. What you need to know. *RN, 62*(9), 41–45.

Crain, E.F., Dercsmar, C., Weiss, K.B., Mitchell, H., & Lynn, H. (1998). Reported difficulties in access to quality care for children with asthma in the inner city. *Archives of Pediatrics & Adolescent Medicine, 152,* 333–339.

Day, J.H., et al. (2000). Onset of action of intranasal budesonide (Rhinocort Aqua) in seasonal allergic rhinitis studied in a controlled exposure model. *Journal of Allergy and Clinical Immunology, 105*(3), 489–494.

Donohoe, M.R. (1997). Approach to therapy: Allergic diseases. *Primary Care Practice, 1*(2), 117–128.

Forbes, H.J. (1997). Practical management of asthma. *Primary Care Practice, 1*(2), 207–216.

Galen, B.A. (1997). Differential diagnosis. Rhinitis. *Primary Care Practice, 1*(2), 129–141.

Gritter, M. (1997). Latex allergy. *Primary Care Practice, 1*(2), 142–151.

Gritter, M. (1998). The latex threat. *American Journal of Nursing, 98*(9), 26–32.

Hessel, P.A., Mitchell, I., Tough, S., Green, F.H., Cockcroft, D., Kepron, W., & Butts, J.C. (1999). Risk factors for death from asthma. *Annals of Allergy, Asthma and Immunology, 83*(5), 362–368.

Jablonski, R.S. (2000). Discovering asthma in the older adult. *The Nurse Practitioner, 25*(3), 1424–1425, 1429–1439.

Matricardi, P.M., et al. (2000). Exposure to foodborne and orofecal microbes versus airborne viruses in relation to atopy and allergic asthma. *British Medical Journal, 320*(3), 412–417.

McGann, E. (1999). Medication compliance in adults with asthma. *American Journal of Nursing, 99*(3), 45–46.

Miller, K.K. & Weed, P. (1998). The latex allergy triage or admission tool: An algorithm to identify which patients would benefit from "latex safe" precautions. *Journal of Emergency Nursing, 24*(4), 145–152.

National Institute for Occupational Safety and Health. (1997). *Preventing allergic reactions to natural rubber latex in the workplace.* (DHHS Pub. No. 97-135). Cincinnati, OH: NIOSH, Department of Health and Human Services.

National Institutes of Health. (1997). *Guidelines for the diagnosis and management of asthma.* NIH publication No. 97-4051, April, 1997.

Owen, C. (1999). New directions in asthma management. *American Journal of Nursing, 99*(3), 26–33.

Tough, S.C., Hessel, P.A., Ruff, M., Green, F.H., Mitchell, I. & Butt, J.C. (1998). Features that distinguish those who die from asthma from community controls with asthma. *Journal of Asthma, 35*(8), 657–665.

HIV Disease and AIDS

TRANSMISSION AND DEVELOPMENT OF HIV INFECTION

Acquired immunodeficiency syndrome (AIDS) is defined as the most severe form of a continuum of illnesses associated with human immunodeficiency virus (HIV) infection. It causes a slow degeneration of the immune system with the development of opportunistic infections and malignancies. HIV disease implies the entire course of HIV infection, from asymptomatic infection and early symptoms to AIDS.

Pathophysiology and Etiology

1. The causative agent is a retrovirus that infects and depletes the "protector" cells of the immune system, called lymphocytes. B lymphocytes secrete antibodies into the body fluids, or humors; this is known as *humoral immunity*. T lymphocytes can penetrate living cells, a process called *cell-mediated immunity*.
2. Monocytes and macrophages, whose role is to present antigen to T cells, thereby initiating the body's immune response, are also infected by HIV.
3. Once HIV has entered the body, it attaches most efficiently to CD4 molecules, which are predominantly located on the cell membrane of T4 helper lymphocytes. HIV destroys the CD4 molecule as it enters to infect the T4 lymphocyte.
4. With progressive invasion of HIV, cellular and humoral immunity declines and opportunistic infections that characterize this disease begin to emerge.
5. Body fluids known to transmit HIV are blood, vaginal secretions, semen, and breast milk.
6. HIV is transmitted by injection of blood or blood components, by sexual contact (vaginal/anal intercourse, oral sex), and perinatally from an infected mother to the child.

High-Risk Groups for HIV Transmission

1. Homosexual or bisexual men
2. Intravenous (IV) drug users
3. Transfusion and blood product recipients (before 1985)
4. Heterosexual contacts of HIV-positive individuals
5. Newborn babies of mothers who are HIV positive

Natural History of HIV Disease
After Exposure to HIV Infection

1. Approximately 80% to 90% of persons will experience a brief flulike illness about 2 to 4 weeks following exposure to HIV—referred to as primary HIV infection (also called acute HIV infection). Typical symptoms include fever, adenopathy, pharyngitis, and rash. Although most patients seek clinical care, few are diagnosed because the symptoms mimic a common flu. It is known that the immune system is compromised by a sudden decrease in T4 helper cells and an increase in viral load for a brief period before returning to baseline.
2. Seroconversion occurs when the person has developed enough antibody to HIV that the serologic test is positive. It takes 3 to 6 months for seroconversion to occur.
3. The Centers for Disease Control (CDC) provides a mechanism to stage HIV disease and to define AIDS using both clinical findings and the CD4 count (Table 29-1). A normal CD4 count is 800 to 1,000/mm^3. Because HIV destroys a CD4 molecule as it enters the T4 lymphocyte, the number of CD4 cells diminishes over time.

Development of AIDS-Related Diseases
Appears years after exposure to HIV (Figure 29-1). Due to declining immunity, frequent infections, severe opportunistic infections, and malignancies develop.

TABLE 29-1 AIDS Surveillance Case Definition for Adolescents and Adults, 1993

	Clinical Categories		
CD4 Cell Categories	A Asymptomatic, or PGL or Acute HIV Infection	B Symptomatic+ (not A or C)	C* AIDS Indicator Condition (1987)
1. >500/mm³ (<29%)	A1	B1	C1
2. 200–499/mm³ (14–28%)	A2	B2	C2
3. <200/mm³ (<14%)	A3	B3	C3

PGL, persistent generalized lymphadenopathy.

*All patients in categories A3, B3 and C1–3 are reported as AIDS, based on the AIDS-indicator conditions and/or a CD4 cell count <200/mm³. AIDS indicator conditions include three new entries: recurrent bacterial pneumonia, invasive cervical cancer, and pulmonary tuberculosis.

+Symptomatic conditions not included in Category C that are (a) attributed to HIV infection or indicative of a defect in cell-mediated immunity, or (b) considered to have a clinical course or management that is complicated by HIV infection. Examples of B conditions include but are not limited to bacillary angiomatosis; thrush; vulvovaginal candidiasis that is persistent, frequent, or poorly responsive to therapy; cervical dysplasia (moderate or severe); cervical carcinoma in situ; constitutional symptoms such as fever (38.5°C) or diarrhea >1 month; oral hairy leukoplakia; Herpes zoster involving two episodes or >1 dermatome; idiopathic thrombocytopenic purpura; listeriosis; pelvic inflammatory disease (especially if complicated by a tubo-ovarian abscess); and peripheral neuropathy.

(From Centers for Disease Control. [1992]. AIDS surveillance case definition for adolescents and adults. *Morbidity and Mortality Weekly Report, 41* [RR-17], 2.)

CLINICAL MANIFESTATIONS

1. Pulmonary manifestations
   a. Persistent cough with and without sputum production, shortness of breath, chest pain, fever
   b. From *Pneumocystis carinii* pneumonia (most common), bacterial pneumonia, *Mycobacterium* tuberculosis, disseminated *Mycobacterium avium complex*, cytomegalovirus (CMV), *Histoplasma*, Kaposi's sarcoma, *Cryptococcus*, Legionella, and other pathogens
2. Gastrointestinal manifestations
   a. Diarrhea, weight loss, anorexia, abdominal cramping, rectal urgency (tenesmus)
   b. From enteric pathogens including *Salmonella, Shigella, Campylobacter, Entamoeba histolytica*, CMV, *M. avium complex*, herpes simplex, *Strongyloides, Giardia, Cryptosporidium, Isospora belli, Chlamydia*, and others
3. Oral manifestations
   a. Appearance of oral lesions, white plaques on oral mucosa, and angular cheilitis from *Candida albicans* of mouth and esophagus

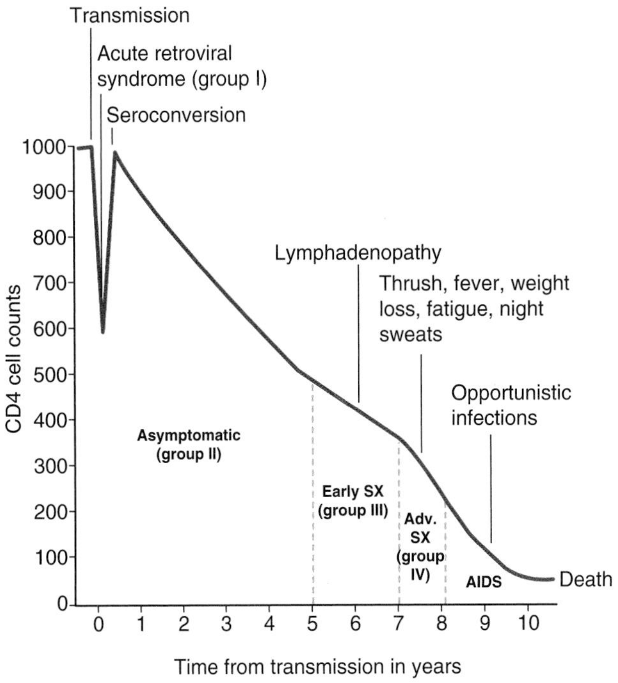

FIGURE 29-1 Natural history of HIV disease.

b. Vesicles with ulceration from herpes simplex virus

c. White, thickened lesions on lateral margins of tongue from hairy leukoplakia

d. Oral warts due to human papillomavirus (HPV) and associated gingivitis

e. Periodontitis progressing to gingival necrosis

4. Central nervous system (CNS) manifestations

  a. Cognitive, motor, and behavioral symptoms (AIDS dementia complex/HIV encephalopathy)

  b. Demonstrated by mental slowing, impaired memory and concentration, loss of balance, lower extremity weakness, ataxia, apathy, and social withdrawal

  c. From CNS toxoplasmosis, cryptococcal meningitis, herpes virus infections, CMV (causing retinopathy and blindness), and CNS lymphoma

6. Malignancies

  a. Kaposi's sarcoma (aggressive tumor involving skin, lymph nodes, gastrointestinal tract, and lungs)

  b. Non-Hodgkin's lymphoma (p. 877) and lymphomas (p. 876)

  c. Cervical carcinoma (p. 774)

Diagnostic Evaluation

1. History of risk factors/high-risk behaviors

2. Positive blood test for HIV

  a. Enzyme-linked immunosorbent assay (ELISA)— serologic test for detecting antibody to HIV

  b. Western blot test—used to confirm a positive result on ELISA test

  c. Once infected with HIV, it can take the body 3 to 6 months to develop enough antibody to HIV for the test result to be positive, resulting in a false-negative test if evaluated early.

  d. Occasionally, a sample that tests reactivity by ELISA may give an indeterminate result by Western blot. The cause of an indeterminate result may be early HIV seroconversion or error during interpretation of the test. The test should be repeated every 2 to 3 months until Western blot becomes positive or there is no longer suspicion of HIV disease.

  e. There are three FDA-approved rapid HIV tests available.They are blood tests that can show a result in about 10 minutes. A negative result is definitely negative, but a positive result must be confirmed positive by the ELISA.

  f. Orasure is an FDA-approved HIV test that uses saliva rather than blood. The results are available in about 3 days.

  g. Calypte HIV-1 Urine EIA is a FDA-approved HIV test that uses urine. A positive result must be confirmed positive by the ELISA.

3. Lymphocyte panel shows decreased CD4 count.

4. A complete blood count (CBC) may show anemia and a low white blood cell count.

5. Presence of indicator disease (e.g., *P. carinii* pneumonia, candidiasis of esophagus, Kaposi's sarcoma, etc.).

6. Diagnostic procedures (biopsies, imaging procedures, etc.) of the organ system involved to confirm opportunistic infection, malignancy, or other causes.

7. Neuropsychological testing—to identify cognitive deficits associated with AIDS dementia complex.

8. Viral load (quantitative HIV RNA) is a measure of the amount of HIV in the blood. A higher number (greater than 750,000) indicates HIV is more active; therefore, it is replicating at a faster rate. This can be predictive of a faster rate of disease progression, which decreases the time between HIV transmission and death. A viral load test result can be undetectable, meaning the amount of virus is less than 150; therefore, the virus could not be found.

Complications

1. Repeated overwhelming opportunistic infections (Table 29-2)

2. Respiratory failure

3. Wasting

MANAGEMENT

Underlying Considerations

1. Treatments are available for the underlying immunodeficiency.

2. HIV vaccine studies are showing initial promise as a treatment to prolong life in those already infected with HIV.

3. Treatment is available for some opportunistic infections and other diseases associated with AIDS. Although individual response to treatment can be variable, treatment of opportunistic infections may suppress the disease for months or for the life of the patient.

4. Management requires the expertise of many specialties: infectious disease, pulmonary medicine, gastroenterology, neurology, obstetrics and gynecology, dentistry, surgery, psychiatry, nursing, nutrition, and social work.

Specific Treatment

1. Antiretroviral therapy (ART) consists of medications that belong to three different classifications because they act to prevent HIV replication at three different points along the replication process. The standard for ART is to take a minimum of three different drugs that come from at least two different drug classifications.

2. Highly active antiretroviral therapy (HAART) refers to any medication regimen that can be expected to decrease the viral load to non-detectable.

3. Classes of antiretroviral drugs:

  a. Nucleoside reverse transcriptase inhibitors (NRTIs) such as zidovudine (AZT), didanosine (ddI), stavudine (d4T) (Table 29-3)

  b. Non-nucleoside reverse transcriptase inhibitors (NNRTIs) such as nevirapine (Viramune), efavirenz (Sustiva)

TABLE 29-2 Opportunistic Infections and Drug Therapies

Name	Clinical Manifestations	Diagnostic Tests	Medications
Pneumocystis carinii pneumonia (PCP)	Cough: dry or scant white sputum production Shortness of breath Low grade fever	Chest x-ray Sputum culture for silver stain Bronchoscopy	Trimethoprim/ sulfamethoxazole (Bactrim) Dapsone (Dapsone) Atovaquon (Mepron) Pentamidine (Pentam) (IV only)
Candida esophagitis	White coating in mouth White coating down throat Sensation of food getting caught in throat while swallowing	Gross observation Microscopy for hyphae Endoscopy	Nystatin (Mycostatin) Clotrimazole (Mycelex) Itaconazole (Sporanox) Fluconazole (Diflucan) Amphotericin B (Fungizone)
Mycobacterium avium complex (MAC)	Weakness Weight loss Diarrhea Fever, chills	Blood culture for acid-fast bacilli	Micobutin (Rifabutin) Ethambutol (Myambutol) Isoniazid (INH) Clarithromycin (Biaxin)

Kaposi's sarcoma	Pink, purple, or brown spots
	Pain, edema of affected area
		Gross observation
		Biopsy
			Local treatment:
			  Liquid nitrogen
			  Vinblastine (Velban)
			  Radiation
			  Laser
			Systematic treatment:
			  Liposomal Daunorubicin (Dauno X)
			  Taxol (Paclitaxel)
			  Bleomycin (Blenoxar)
			  Vincristine (Oncovir)

Toxoplasmosis	Fever Headache Change in mental status Confusion Lethargy Frank psychosis	Computed tomography Magnetic resonance imaging Serum *Toxoplasma* antibodies	Pyrimethamine (Daraprim) Sulfadiazine (Microsulfon) Folic acid
Tuberculosis	Cough: dry or scant frothy white/pink sputum Shortness of breath Fever Lymphadenopathy	Positive purified protein derivative ($\geq$5 mm induration) Chest x-ray Sputum culture for acid-fast bacilli	Isoniazid (INH) Rifampin (Rifadin) Pyrazinamide (Daraprim) Ethambutol (Myambutol)
Cryptosporidium	Severe diarrhea Severe abdominal cramping	Stool culture for *Cryptosporidium*	Octreotide (Somatostatin) Paramomycin (Humatin)
Cryptococcal meningitis	Headache Confusion, memory loss Nausea Seizures Change in mental status Fever Photophobia	Cerebral spinal fluid culture for cryptococcosis	Amphotericin B (Fungizone) Flucytosine (Ancobon) Fluconazole (Diflucan)
Cytomegalovirus (CMV)	Visual changes; floaters/blindness Difficulty swallowing Nausea, vomiting Abdominal cramping	Ophthalmologic examination Blood, urine, tissue culture for CMV	Gancyclovir (Cytorene) Foscarnet (Foscavir) Cidofovir (Vistide) Intraocular gancyclovir release device

HIV encephalopathy/AIDS dementia complex	Early: Inattention
	  Reduced concentration
	  Forgetfulness
	  Slowed movements
	  Clumsiness
	  Ataxia
	  Apathy
	  Agitation
	Late: Paraplegia
	  Mutism
	  Vegetative state
		Computed tomography
		Magnetic resonance imaging
		Cerebral spinal fluid evaluation
			ARTs that penetrate the central nervous system (zidovudine, stavudine hydroxyurea, Abacovir, Nevirapine)

TABLE 29-3   Antiretroviral Therapy

Drug	Dosage	Adverse Reactions	Monitoring
Nucleoside Reverse Transcriptase Inhibitors (NRTIs)			
Zidovudine (AZT, Retrovir)	300 mg twice a day (or with lamivu-dine [Epivir, 3TC] as Combivir, 1 tablet twice a day	Nausea, fatigue (initial month on drug), anemia, myalgias, leukopenia, granulocytopenia	CBC every 4 wk for 3 months, if stable, then every 2 to 3 months
Didanosine (ddi, Videx)	400 mg once a day (weight dependent)	Pancreatitis Peripheral neuropathy	CBC, liver function tests, amylase monthly for 3 months; then every other month if stable
Non-nucleoside Reverse Transcriptase Inhibitors (NNRTIs)			
Nevirapine (Viramune)	200 mg once a day for 14 days, then 200 mg twice a day	Rash Hepatitis	
Efavirenz (Sustiva)	600 mg at bedtime	Dizziness Disconnectedness Somnolence Insomnia Bad dreams Rash	
Protease Inhibitors (PIs)			
Indinavir (Crixivan)	800 mg every 8 hours	Gastrointestinal intolerance Nephrolithiasis Headache	
Saquinavir (Fortovase)	1200 mg three times a day	Gastrointestinal intolerance Headache Increase in liver enzymes	

   c. Protease inhibitors (PIs) such as indinavir (Crixivan), ritonavir (Norvir), and saquinavir (Fortovase)

4. Goals of antiviral therapy:
   a. Prolong life and improve quality of life
   b. Reduce viral load to as low as possible for as long as possible
   c. Increase the CD4 count

5. Indications for antiviral therapy:
   a. Acute retroviral syndrome or less than 6 months since seroconversion
   b. HIV symptoms such as oral thrush
   c. No HIV symptoms but has a CD4 count of 500/mm³ or less and/or a viral load greater than 20,000.

Prevention Therapies

1. Opportunistic infections
   a. *P. carinii* pneumonia (PCP) prophylaxis is started when the CD4 count is less than 200 and the most effective medication is sulfamethoxazole/trimethoprim (Bactrim); others are dapsone, atovaquone (Mepron), and aerosolized pentamidine.
   b. *M. avium complex* prophylaxis is started when the CD4 count is less than 50; medications used are azithromycin (Zithromax) and clarithromycin (Biaxin).

2. Vaccinations
   a. Tuberculosis—all patients should be screened every year with a PPD
   b. Pneumococcal pneumonia—all patients should receive pneumovax every 5 to 6 years
   c. Influenza—patients with a CD4 greater than 200 should receive a flu vaccine each fall.

◆ **DRUG ALERT**

If a patient decides to stop taking antiviral therapy, he or she must stop all antiviral medications at the same time. Taking only some of the antiviral therapies will create resistance to HIV; therefore, the current medications will never be effective treatments for this patient in the future. Resistance can develop within a few days to a few weeks of incorrect dosing.

Supportive Care

1. Treatment of reversible illnesses
2. Nutritional support
3. Palliation of pain
4. Dental management
5. Evaluation and management of psychological and social aspects of AIDS
6. Treatment to relieve symptoms (cough, diarrhea)
7. Antidepressant drugs; psychiatric interventions

▣ Nursing Management of HIV Disease and AIDS

See Standards of Care Guidelines.

Nursing Assessment

1. Obtain history of risk factors, constitutional signs and symptoms, recent infections, positive blood test for HIV antibodies.
2. Review patient's present complaint(s) such as cough, shortness of breath, diarrhea.
3. Evaluate nutritional status by assessing for weight loss, body mass depletion, decreased skin-fold thickness and mid-arm muscle circumference, hypoalbuminemia, decreased iron-binding capacity, selenium deficiency, anemia.
4. Assess respiratory rate and depth and auscultate lungs for breath sounds; assess for skin color and temperature, palpable lymph nodes, and evidence of fever, night sweats.
5. Inspect mouth for lesions; examine skin for rash, sores, Kaposi's sarcoma lesions. Record number, size, and locations.
6. Ask about bowel patterns, changes in habits, constipation, abdominal cramping, number and volume of stools, presence of perianal pain and ulceration.
7. Is patient oriented to time, place, and person? Affect? Any problem with memory and concentration? Headaches? Seizures?
8. How much does the patient know about AIDS? Etiology? Signs and symptoms? Mode of transmission? Methods for limiting exposure?
9. Find out as much as possible about patient's premorbid personality, experience and skills, social support system.
10. Assess the patient's adherence to medications by reviewing all prescribed drugs, the dose, and how often the patient is taking the medication. Ask the patient how many times over the last day/week he or she may have missed a dose.

STANDARDS OF CARE GUIDELINES
HIV/AIDS

When caring for patients with HIV disease and AIDS, ensure that you do the following:

- Utilize universal precautions.
- Protect confidentiality.
- Educate about methods for the prevention of HIV transmission.
- Perform a psychosocial assessment.
- Develop adherence strategies for patients taking antiviral therapy.
- Provide education and interventions for HIV symptom management.

This information should serve as a general guideline only. Each patient situation presents a unique set of clinical factors and requires nursing judgment to guide care, which may include additional or alternative measures and approaches.

 DRUG ALERT

A patient taking antiviral therapy who develops abdominal pain or vomiting should immediately call the provider who ordered the medication. A serious side effect such as pancreatitis must be ruled out. A decision will be made to continue the medication while treating the side effects or to discontinue the therapy.

Nursing Diagnoses

- Fear of disease progression, treatment effects, isolation, and death related to having AIDS
- Risk for Infection related to immunodeficiency and neutropenia secondary to medications/treatment
- Altered Nutrition (Less Than Body Requirements) related to disease/treatment effects
- Altered Oral Mucous Membranes related to opportunistic infection
- Diarrhea related to disease/treatment effects
- Altered Thought Processes (Impaired Cognition and Dementia) related to disease effects
- Hyperthermia related to HIV infection, opportunistic infection, or visceral involvement by Kaposi's sarcoma
- Altered Breathing Pattern related to opportunistic infections and noninfectious disorders (Kaposi's sarcoma of the lung)
- Ineffective Management of Therapeutic Regimen: Individual, based on complicated regimen of medications, treatment plans, clinical appointments, lack of social support, impaired cognitive functioning, substance use, and psychiatric illness

Other nursing diagnoses could include:

- Fatigue related to underlying HIV infection and reactive depression
- Disturbances in Body Image related to rapid body changes from debilitating disease
- Helplessness related to inexperience with illness, sense of loss of control, depression, and vulnerability associated with AIDS
- Pain related to infection, peripheral neuropathies, nodules of Kaposi's sarcoma, diarrhea
- Anticipatory Grieving related to awareness of implications of AIDS, dying and death, unfinished business, multiple bereavements, and changes in lifestyle
- Ineffective Family Coping related to crisis created by AIDS, guilt, fear, overwhelming caretaking responsibilities

---

NURSING ALERT

Never assume the family or loved ones know that the patient is HIV positive. Always ask the patient who knows of the HIV status. Confidentiality regarding HIV infection must be maintained. However, encourage the patient to share the diagnosis to decrease isolation. Offer to be with the patient when the diagnosis is shared with the family; role playing before you meet with family or loved ones can be helpful.

Nursing Interventions

Reducing Fear

1. Maintain nonjudgmental attitude and nonprejudicial approach.
2. Anticipate that the patient may pass through a series of stages: initial crisis, transitional stage, acceptance state, and preparation for death.
3. Allow patient to use denial as a protective mechanism—gives some control over when and how patient will control mortality.
   a. Expect some displaced anger; avoid being personally affronted by patient's anger.
   b. Allow patient to acknowledge reality of the situation without false reassurance.
4. Explain that symptoms of anxiety and depression are common initially but generally improve with time and support.
5. Anticipate that patients with substance use issues may exhibit antisocial behaviors and feelings of alienation and isolation.
6. Provide careful discussion and clarification of treatment options.
7. Help patient set realistic goals and expectations.
8. Offer counseling services, especially when AIDS is initially diagnosed and as patient enters terminal phase of illness.
9. Obtain social service referral for available resources and services such as housekeeping, food shopping, community support services, counseling agencies, Social Security Administration.
10. Help patient identify and strengthen personal resources such as positive coping skills, relaxation techniques, strong support network, and optimistic outlook.
11. Encourage patient to join a support group—helpful in defusing stressful issues and in developing strategies to cope with the disease.
12. Observe for emerging psychiatric problems, especially in persons who are socially isolated, those with guilt about sexuality and lifestyle, and those with poor accommodation.
13. Provide information on advance directives and encourage patient to arrange personal business because cognitive deterioration may make it impossible for patient to act on own behalf at a later date.
14. Allow discussion of nature and management of death—minimizes negative impact of ever-present threat of death.
   a. Assure patient of palliative care, pain control, and help with anxiety and depression.
   b. Respect the right of the patient to participate in treatment decisions (eg, to limit therapy and life-prolonging interventions).

Preventing Infection

1. Have a high index of suspicion for infection even when clinical manifestations are subtle or absent—opportunistic infections may be reactivated at any time during the course of the disease.
2. Follow universal precautions for all patients.
3. Administer prescribed pharmacologic agents; some infections are not treatable with currently available regimens.
4. Administer and teach patient/family good skin care—a break in the skin is a source of secondary infection; use position changes, emollient lotions, special pads and beds, and attend to hydration and nutrition.
5. Maintain cleanliness of environment.
6. Use aseptic techniques when performing invasive procedures.
7. Teach patient to make the most of what remains of the immune system by minimizing the risk of disease.
   a. Avoid exposure to persons with infections—may activate HIV.
   b. Turn, cough, and do breathing exercises, especially when confined to bed.
   c. Avoid continuing injection drug use and unprotected sex with an HIV-positive partner to prevent repeated exposure to HIV.
   d. Instruct visitors about handwashing before entering and leaving the room.
   e. Advise patient/family to wash hands before preparing food and prepare foods on clean surfaces.
   f. Advise patient not to eat raw or undercooked foods.
   g. Tell the patient to have someone else clean a cat box or bird cage; if that is not possible, use rubber gloves.
8. Ensure that the patient is up to date with immunizations.

Improving Nutritional Status

1. Monitor nutritional status by weighing, recording dietary intake and calorie count, taking anthropometric measurements, and evaluating serum albumin, blood urea nitrogen, protein, and transferrin levels.
2. Monitor for sore throat that progresses to dysphagia or odynophagia (pain on swallowing) or persistent heartburn—suggestive of esophageal candidiasis.
3. Consult with dietitian to develop strategies for nutrition care, including additional calories and nutritional supplements to maintain strength, comfort, and level of functioning.
4. Include patient in decision making regarding nutrition care.
5. Alter times of drug administration to improve intake with meals.
   a. Administer or teach patient to administer prescribed antiemetic 30 minutes before meals.
   b. Try to give drug infusions after meals.
6. For patient with oral/esophageal pain from *Candida* esophagitis, herpetic esophagitis, endotracheal Kaposi's sarcoma:
   a. Administer prescribed antifungal therapy.
   b. Avoid highly seasoned or acidic foods.
   c. Offer fluids and blenderized foods to minimize chewing and ease swallowing.
   d. Suggest nutrition-dense supplements such as instant breakfast drinks or protein-fortified juices for home care.

7. Encourage patient to maximize intake during periods when he or she is feeling better.
8. Discourage excessive alcohol intake—has immunosuppressive effect.
9. Make appropriate community referral if patient is unable to shop or prepare meals.
10. Encourage small, frequent meals because these may make best use of limited absorptive capacity.
11. Keep in mind that elemental diets/nutritional supplements may become intolerable to patient as anorexia progresses; prepare patient for enteral or parenteral feedings when necessary.

 DRUG ALERT

Protease inhibitor levels can be affected by grapefruit juice, as can other common medications. Therefore, patients taking any of the antiviral therapies within the protease inhibitor class should be discouraged from consuming grapefruit juice.

Relieving Oral Discomfort
1. Ask about persistent sore throat, dysphagia, and heartburn—these symptoms are suggestive of oral/esophageal candidiasis.
2. Examine mouth for oral candidiasis and other lesions.
3. Administer or teach patient to administer prescribed antifungal mouth rinses or lozenges for oral candidiasis or acyclovir (Zovirax) for herpes simplex.
4. Perform or encourage oral care two to three times a day.

Minimizing the Effects of Diarrhea
1. Keep in mind that gastrointestinal infections and diarrhea decrease absorptive efficiency.
2. Tell patient to monitor stools for blood and try to determine if bleeding is before, with, or after bowel movement to help determine source of bleeding.
3. Monitor intake and output; assess skin and mucous membranes for poor turgor and dryness, indicating dehydration.
4. Administer fluids and electrolytes as prescribed.
5. Advise patient to rest to achieve bowel rest.
6. Use enteric precautions.
7. Plan regimen of skin care, including cleansing/blotting/drying of the anal area, application of ointment or skin barrier cream.
8. Advise patient to eliminate caffeine, alcohol, dairy products, foods high in fats, fresh juices, and acidic juices if diarrhea persists. Drink liquids at room temperature.
9. Advise patient to avoid foods that increase intestinal motility and distention, such as gas-forming fruits and vegetables.
10. Advise patient to report symptoms and signs of increased weakness, dizziness, and continuing weight loss.

Managing Altered Thought Processes
1. Remember that the brain is a critical target organ for HIV infection.
2. Provide daily assessment of mental status; monitor for changes in behavior, memory, concentration ability, and motor system dysfunction—patient may become vegetative and unable to ambulate.
   a. Onset of dementia is usually insidious but may be abrupt, precipitated by acute infection.
3. Reorient patient frequently; use calendar, clock, family/friends' pictures, lists, and structured plan of care.
4. Provide for patient safety: bed rails up, call signal available, articles within patient's reach.
5. Give repeated reassurance.
6. Assess for depressive or suicidal symptoms—AIDS represents a risk for suicide.
7. Anticipate necessity of guardianship, durable power of attorney for health care, and informed consent if patient has AIDS dementia complex, because patient may have poor insight and become indifferent to illness.

Reducing Fever
1. Frequently assess for chills, fever, tachycardia, and tachypnea.
2. Teach patient/caregiver to keep a temperature chart.
3. Encourage high fluid intake to replace insensible water losses incurred by fever/diaphoresis.
4. Administer or teach patient to administer antipyretics as prescribed.
5. Teach patient or caregiver to report a change in fever pattern or significant change in condition.

Improving Breathing Pattern
1. Provide supplemental oxygen as ordered.
2. Watch for sudden change in respiratory function—patient may be developing a secondary infection.
3. Administer or teach patient to administer prescribed narcotic for postinfectious cough, a complication of *P. carinii* pneumonia and viral pneumonia.
4. Encourage smoking cessation to enhance pulmonary ciliary defense.
5. Administer saline nebulization to induce sputum collection for culture and sensitivity.
   a. Wear mask and gloves during sputum collection.
   b. Instruct patient to brush tongue, buccal surfaces, teeth, and palate with water before sputum induction—to remove superficial squamous epithelial cells and their adherent bacteria and foreign material.
   c. Instruct patient to gargle and rinse mouth with tap water.
6. Answer questions and support patient's decision for or against resuscitation and mechanical ventilation.

Improving Patient's Management of Therapeutic Regimen
1. Assess patient's adherence to medications and clinical appointments in the past; if there has been poor adherence in the past, have patient explore what contributed to it.
2. Provide education about prescribed medications before the therapy is started and periodically thereafter; provide education materials that can remain in the home as a resource.

3. Develop a medication schedule for the patient that incorporates his or her usual day's activities; place pills in a medication box according to the schedule.
4. Encourage the involvement of a household member in the education and administration of the patient's medications.

Community and Home Care Considerations

1. If patient is homebound, many agencies offer help specifically for HIV patients and provide home visits for services such as legal counseling, hospice care, respite care, housekeeping, food preparation, care for pets, and "buddies" to decrease time patient is alone.
2. Assist patient/family/significant other to locate these agencies in the community.
3. Assess the home for patient safety and provide durable medical goods that can enhance safety and comfort.
4. Provide latex gloves for the home for handling body fluids of the HIV-positive household member.
5. Explain that routine household cleaning of the bathroom, dishes, and laundry is sufficient to prevent HIV transmission.
6. Explain that the HIV-positive household member should never share toothbrushes or razors because they can provoke bleeding and, therefore, are a potential source of HIV transmission.
7. Establish whether there are persons in the home who will participate in the HIV-positive household member's care; engage these caregivers while attending to the patient. Assess the needs of the caregiver; acknowledge that it is important to have a break from the caregiver role. Provide information about respite services in which the patient can be cared for during the day or for days or weeks at a long-term care facility.

Patient Education and Health Maintenance

1. Indicate that patient is a source of infection to others and should take actions to prevent transmission (no exchange of blood or body fluids).
2. Encourage patient to disclose HIV status to sex and needle-sharing partners.
3. Emphasize to HIV-positive woman that children should be tested for HIV.
4. Discuss family planning with HIV-positive woman; the rate of transmission from mother to newborn is approximately 30% but can be decreased to approximately 5% when antiviral therapy is provided during pregnancy. If she does not want more children, discuss birth control options.
5. Establish a primary care provider for the patient and encourage the need for regular follow-up care, which should include yearly Pap smears for women and routine dental and eye examinations.
6. Teach patient to recognize and report important symptoms:
   a. Change in pattern/magnitude of temperature elevation

   b. Development of a new focal complaint: skin spots, sore mouth, and diarrhea
7. Emphasize to injection drug users that continued use may expose them to additional infection and such infections may activate viral replication.
8. Encourage patient to modify sexual behaviors for safer sex.
   a. Use latex male condoms supplemented by creams and jelly containing a viricidal agent.
   b. If a man will not use a condom, the woman should use a female condom.
   c. Refrain from oral and anal sex.
   d. Encourage patient to read literature from various AIDS action groups on safe sex techniques.
9. If the patient abuses substances (injection drugs, alcohol, pills, etc.):
   a. Enroll in a treatment program.
   b. Do not share needles ("works").
   c. If no access to unused needles, clean needles before using with a bleach/water solution.
10. Teach patient to optimize immune system function by sound dietary practices, exercise, and regular periods of sleep; promote changes in the direction of more healthful living.
11. Some patients may use complementary/alternative therapies such as vitamins, herbs, and teas. Caution the patient to share these additional therapies with the primary provider.

 DRUG ALERT

St. John's Wort is used by many people for depression; however, it interacts with many drugs, including indinavir.

12. Refer patient to resources such as:
    a. National AIDS Hotline, 1-800-342-AIDS (2437); Spanish–1-800-344-7432, TDD service for the deaf–1-800-243-7889: operates 24 hours a day, 7 days a week; offers information on transmission, prevention, testing, and local referrals.
    b. AIDS Action Council, 1875 Connecticut Avenue SW, Suite 700, Washington DC 20009, 1-202-986-1300, 1-202-986-1345 (fax): community outreach, government affairs.
13. The following are resources for both patients and nurses:
    a. CDC National AIDS Clearinghouse, 1-800-458-5231, 1-301-738-6616 (fax), *http://www.cdcnac.org; Gopher: gopher://gopher.cdcnac.org:72*; AIDSNEWS Listserv: listserv@cdcnac.org; File Transfer Protocol: *ftp://ftp.cdcnac.org/pub/cdcnac;* Email: aidsinfo@cdcnac.org: organizational reference and reference service, publication distribution (MMWR, HIV/AIDS Surveillance Report), 24-hour access to CDC NAC online, NAC FAX, Internet services, training and technical assistance.

b. CDC, Division of HIV/AIDS Prevention, *http://www. cdc.gov/nchstp/hivaids/dhap.htm:* general AIDS information, publications, resources, statistics.

c. Johns Hopkins University AIDS Service, *http://www. hopkins-aids.edu:* general AIDS information, content review of recent AIDS conferences, e-mail HIV consult service for providers and patients. The Hopkins HIV Report: mail subscription request to JHU Division of Infectious Diseases, Ross Building, Room 1159, 720 Rutland Avenue, Baltimore, MD 21205, Attn: Newsletter Subscription. This bimonthly publication compiles current HIV information for the clinician. It is free to Maryland residents and costs $20 for non-Maryland residents.

Outcome-Based Evaluation

- Patient speaks openly about HIV disease with health care providers, significant others
- No signs of opportunistic infections
- Patient eats three to four meals a day
- Oral mucosa without lesions
- Patient reports formed stools one to three times a day
- Patient responds appropriately to questions of self, time, and place; verbalizes accurate account of activities
- Afebrile with a normal heart rate
- Respirations unlabored, rate 20/min; no cough or sputum production
- Viral load remains non-detectable

SELECTED REFERENCES

Bartlett, J.G. (1999). *Medical management of HIV infection.* Baltimore: Johns Hopkins Press.

Bartlett, J.G., & Finkbeiner, A.K. (1998). *The guide to living with HIV infection.* Baltimore: Johns Hopkins University Press.

The CASCADE Collaboration. (2000). Survival after introduction of HAART in people with known duration of HIV-1 Infection. *Lancet, 355*(7), 1158–1159.

Casey, K.M., Cohen, F., & Hughes, A. (1996). *ANAC's core curriculum for HIV/AIDS nursing.* Philadelphia: Nursecom, Inc.

Centers for Disease Control. (1987). Public Health Service guidelines for counseling and antibody testing to prevent HIV infection and AIDS. *Morbidity and Mortality Weekly Report, 36*(31), 509–515.

Centers for Disease Control. (1988). Update: Universal precautions for prevention of transmission of human immunodeficiency virus, hepatitis B virus, and other bloodborne pathogens in healthcare settings. *Morbidity and Mortality Weekly Report, 37*(24), 377–382, 387–388.

Centers for Disease Control. (1992). AIDS surveillance case definition for adolescents and adults. *Morbidity and Mortality Weekly Report, 41*(RR-17), 2.

Centers for Disease Control. (1995). HIV counseling and testing. *Morbidity and Mortality Weekly Report, 44*(9), 169–175.

Centers for Disease Control. (1997). U.S. Public Health Service/ Infectious Disease Society of America Guidelines for the prevention of opportunistic infections in persons infected with human immunodeficiency virus. *Morbidity and Mortality Report, 46,* 28–29.

Centers for Disease Control. (1998). Guidelines for the use of antiretroviral agents in pregnant HIV-infected adults and adolescents. *Morbidity and Mortality Weekly Report, 47*(RR-2), 1–30.

Centers for Disease Control. (1999). Update: HIV counseling and testing using rapid tests—United States, 1995. *Morbidity and Mortality Weekly Report, 47*(11), 211–215.

Cohen, F., & Durham, J. (Eds.). (1993). *Women, children, and HIV/ AIDS.* New York: Springer.

Coombs, R.W., Welles, S.L., Hooper, C., Reichelderfer, P.S., D'Aquila, R.T., Japour, A.J., Johnson, V.A., Kuritzkes, D.R., Richman, D.D., Kwok, S., Todd, J., Jackson, J.B., DeGruttola, V., Crumpacker, C.S., & Kahn, J. (1996). Association of plasma human immunodeficiency virus type 1 RNA level with risk of clinical progression in patients with advanced infection. *Journal of Infectious Diseases, 174*(4), 704–712.

Ed-Sadr, W.M., et al. (2000). Discontinuation of prophylaxis for *Mycobacterium avium* complex disease in HIV-1 infected patients who have a response to antiretroviral therapy. *New England Journal of Medicine, 342*(7), 1085–1092.

Elion, R.A., & Cohen, C. (1997). Complementary medicine and HIV infection. In J.L. Randall & J.S. Lazar (Eds.), *Primary care* (pp. 905–919). Philadelphia: W.B. Saunders.

Evans, B.M. (1999). Complimentary therapies and HIV infection. *American Journal of Nursing, 99*(2), 42–45.

Flaskerud, J.H. (1999). *HIV/AIDS: A guide to primary care management.* Philadelphia: W. B. Saunders.

Kosko, D.A., Alexander, C., Benker, K., & Hughes, V.H. (1999). HIV/AIDS. In J.K. Singleton, S.A., Sandowski, C., Green-Hernandez, T.V., Horvath, R.V., DiGregorio, & S.P. Holzemer (Eds.), *Primary care* (pp. 453–479). Philadelphia: Lippincott Williams & Wilkins.

Quinn, T.C., et al. (2000). Viral load and heterosexual transmission of human immunodeficiency virus type 1. *New England Journal of Medicine, 342*(6), 921–929.

Saag, M.S., Holodniy, M., Kuritzkes, D.R., O'Brien, W.A., Coombs, R., Poscher, M.E., Jacobsen, D.M., Shaw, G.M., Richman, D.D., & Volberding, P.A. (1996). HIV viral load markers in clinical practice. *Nature and Medicine, 2*(6), 625–629.

Sande, M.A., & Volberding, P.A. (Eds.). (1997). *The medical management of AIDS* (5th ed.). Philadelphia: W. B. Saunders.

Schmidt, J. (1992). Case management problems and homecare. *Journal of the Association of Nurses in AIDS Care, 3*(3), 37–44.

Theis, S.L., Cohen, F.L., Forrest, J., & Zelewsky, M. (1997). Needs assessment of caregivers of people with HIV/AIDS. *Journal of the Association of Nurses in AIDS Care, 8*(3), 76–84.

Twiname, B. (1993). The relationship between HIV classification and depression and suicidal intent. *Journal of the Association of Nurses in AIDS Care, 4*(4), 28–35.

U.S. Department of Health and Human Services and the Henry J. Kaiser Foundation Panel on Clinical Practices and Treatment of HIV infection. (January 28, 2000). Guidelines for the use of antiretroviral agents in HIV-infected adults and adolescents. *http://www.hivatis.org.*

Williams, A. (1997). Antiretroviral therapy: Factors associated with adherence. *Journal of the Association of Nurses in AIDS Care, 8,* 18–23.

Connective Tissue Disorders

GENERAL OVERVIEW

Connective tissue comprises a large portion of the interstitial tissue of the skin and musculoskeletal system. Structures include bone, cartilage, tendons, ligaments, and the less compact connective tissue of the structures that support and surround organs and cells. These tissues are metabolically active, constantly turning over and replacing their large and molecular components. The interaction between the molecular components and the inflammatory cells (mostly white blood cells [WBCs]) produces chemicals that are important to initiate disease and to determine which connective tissue is affected.

◼ Musculoskeletal and Related Assessment

Assessment for connective tissue disorders focuses on the musculoskeletal system, but also involves remote body systems. Clues to connective tissue disorders may be found in the skin, eyes, lungs, and neurologic system.

Presenting Symptoms

Obtain history of presenting symptoms, including duration and intensity.
1. Musculoskeletal pain—characteristics:
    a. Joint swelling.
    b. Morning stiffness.
2. Constitutional symptoms:
    a. Fever.
    b. Weight loss.
    c. Anorexia.
    d. Fatigue.
3. Involvement of other body symptoms:
    a. Skin.
    b. Ocular.
    c. Pulmonary
    d. Neurologic.
    e. Mucous membranes.
4. Family history of rheumatic or autoimmune disorders.

Physical Examination Findings

1. Musculoskeletal examination:
    a. Pain on palpation or range of motion.
    b. Joint swelling, warmth, or erythema.
    c. Joint motion restriction.
    d. Pain, swelling, or warmth of soft tissues surrounding joints.
2. Skin:
    a. Skin rash or other abnormalities, such as thickening.
    b. Alopecia.
3. Oral mucosa:
    a. Ulcerations.
    b. Dryness.
4. Ocular:
    a. Conjunctival inflammation.
    b. Dryness.
5. Pulmonary:
    a. Adventitious sounds.
    b. Friction rub.
6. Neurologic:
    a. Depression.
    b. Psychosis.
    c. Foot drop.
    d. Muscle weakness.
    e. Strokelike findings.

DIAGNOSTIC TESTS

◼ Laboratory Studies
Antinuclear Antibody (ANA)
Description

A test for antibodies to nucleoprotein (autoantibodies or a heterogeneous group of gamma globulins); highly sensitive for detecting systemic lupus erythematosus (SLE), but is nonspecific (high false-positive rate).

Nursing and Patient Care Considerations
1. Note drug therapy because many drugs may cause false-positive results.

2. Results will be reported in a staining pattern (speckled, homogeneous, peripheral, nucleolar) if positive, which correlates to various types of connective tissue disorders and various subsets of SLE (Table 30-1).

3. Titer will also be reported with positive ANA but does not reflect disease activity or prognosis.

Rheumatoid Factor (RF)

Description

Test for macroglobulin found in the blood of patients with rheumatoid arthritis (RA) and other disorders. RF has properties of an antibody and may be directed against immunoglobulin.

Nursing and Patient Care Considerations

1. It is not a highly sensitive or specific test.

2. May be positive in 30% to 60% of patients with RA, SLE, and Sjögren's syndrome. May be false positive in endocarditis, tuberculosis, syphilis, sarcoidosis, cancer, viral infections, patients with skin or renal allographs, and in some liver, lung, or kidney disease.

3. Negative RF does not exclude the diagnosis of RA.

4. Certain disease manifestations, such as severe joint involvement and extra-articular manifestations may be more frequent in those with high titer RF.

Erythrocyte Sedimentation Rate (ESR)

Description

1. Test determines the rate at which red blood cells (RBCs) fall out of unclotted blood in 1 hour.

2. Based on premise that inflammatory and other disease processes create changes in blood proteins, thus causing aggregation of RBCs that makes them heavier.

Nursing and Patient Care Considerations

1. ESR is generally, but not always, elevated in most rheumatic illnesses.

2. Result may be elevated by pregnancy, menstruation, medications such as heparin and oral contraceptives, and advanced age. Result may be reduced by elevated blood glucose or albumin, high phospholipids, or drugs, such as corticosteroids or high-dose aspirin.

3. Most beneficial in monitoring progress of an inflammatory disease.

Complement

Description

1. Complement is a complex cascade system that activates proteins as part of the body's defense against infection.

2. Specific components include C1q, C2, C3, and C4; measurement helps determine immune complex formation or a gammaglobulinemia.

3. Complement levels are decreased in certain autoimmune diseases because of complement consumption and because of activation of proteolytic enzymes and tissue damage.

Nursing and Patient Care Considerations

1. Obtain venous blood sample and send to laboratory promptly because complement deteriorates at room temperature.

2. Serial measurements may be helpful in monitoring the activity of some rheumatic diseases; decreased levels indicate increased disease activity.

Other Tests

Synovial Fluid Analysis

Description

1. A sample of synovial (joint) fluid is analyzed for several components.
   a. Color.
   b. Clarity/turbidity.
   c. Viscosity.
   d. WBC count with differential.
   e. Crystals and their identification.

2. Arthrocentesis, a sterile procedure, requires antiseptic cleaning agent, local anesthetic, 18-gauge needle, and a 10- to 20-mL syringe.

Nursing and Patient Care Considerations

1. Patients are generally apprehensive about having a needle inserted into a joint. They generally require reassurance and explanation of the importance of information derived from test results.

2. Results help to differentiate infection and inflammation caused by connective tissue disorder or inflammatory arthritis (Table 30-2).

GENERAL PROCEDURES AND TREATMENT MODALITIES

Pharmacologic Agents

Connective tissue disorders may be treated with various drugs to relieve pain and to halt or minimize the disease process. Types of agents include nonsteroidal anti-inflammatory agents (NSAIDs), corticosteroids, immunosuppressive agents, and a group of unrelated drugs known as disease-modifying antirheumatic drugs (DMARDs). Drug therapy may be long-term and may require frequent evaluation for side effects (Table 30-3).

TABLE 30-1 ANA Staining Patterns and Connective Tissue Disorders

ANA Pattern	Connective Tissue Disorder
Peripheral (rim, ring, membranous)	Active SLE, usually with renal disease
Homogenous (diffuse)	SLE, RA
Speckled	SLE, RA, scleroderma, Sjögren's syndrome, mixed connective tissue disorder
Nucleolar	Scleroderma

ANA, antinuclear antibody; RA, rheumatoid arthritis; SLE, systemic lupus erythematosus

TABLE 30-2 Synovial Fluid Analysis

	Color	WBC Count	Viscosity	Crystals
Normal	Clear, yellow	200	Normal	None
Osteoarthritis	Clear, slightly turbid	200–600	Low	None
Gout	Turbid	2,000–75,000	Low	Monosodium urate

Inflammatory arthritis
  RA
  SLE
  Sjögren's
  Psoratic
	Turbid, yellow	2,000–75,000	Low	None

Septic arthritis	Pus, very turbid	Generally 80,000	Low	None

RA, rheumatoid arthritis; SLE, systemic lupus erythematosus; WBC, white blood cell

Physical and Occupational Therapy

Physical and occupational therapy provide a multimodal program to help reduce pain and to improve joint function. Many other measures can be taught to patients for home practice. Components of the program may include:
• Joint conservation.
• Splinting.
• Range-of-motion exercises.
• Application of heat and cold.
• Endurance/aerobic conditioning.
• Energy conservation.
• Modification of home/work environment.

Joint Conservation

Teach or reinforce the following practices:
1. Perform activities using good body mechanics.
2. Maintain ideal body weight—extra weight places undue stress on weight-bearing joints.
3. Use large joints to perform activities—spread the load over as many joints as possible.

TABLE 30-3 Drug Therapy for Connective Tissue Disorders

Drug	Action	Adverse Effects
Anti-inflammatory Agents		
Salicylates Aspirin (may be buffered or enteric coated)	Anti-inflammatory, antipyretic, and analgesic effects	Tinnitus, gastric intolerance or gastrointestinal bleeding and purpuric tendencies

Nonsteroidal anti-inflammatory drugs (NSAIDs)
  Ibuprofen (Motrin)
  Fenoprofen (Nalfon)
  Naproxen (Naprosyn)
  Tolmetin (Tolectin)
  Sulindac (Clinoril)
  Meclofenamate (Meclomen)
  Ketroprofen (Orudis)
  Salsalate (Disalcid)
  Diclofenac (Voltaren)
  Nabumetone (Relafen)
  Ketorolac (Toradol)
  Oxaprozin (Day Pro)
  Flurbiprofen (Ansaid)
  Diflunisal (Dolobid)
  Piroxicam (Feldene)
  Etodolac (Lodine)
  Indomethacin (Indocin)
  Choline magnesium
  Trisalicylate (Trilisate)
	Anti-inflammatory and analgesic effects
	Mechanism of action may be related to inhibition of prostaglandin synthesis (prostaglandins have a role in inflammatory process, pain, and fever)
	Nonsteroidal antirheumatic agents for adjunctive treatment of rheumatoid arthritis
	Sometimes remarkably effective in control of articular symptoms
		Gastrointestinal irritation: nausea, vomiting, epigastric distress, precipitation and reactivation of peptic ulcer, hepatitis
		Hematologic: bone marrow depression, anemia, leukopenia, thrombocytopenia purpura
		Decrease in renal function can precipitate renal failure
		CNS: headache, dizziness, drowsiness, aseptic meningitis
		Cardiovascular: edema, dyspnea palpitations

COX II Inhibitors
  Celecoxib (Celebrex) COX II
  Rofecoxib (Vioxx)
  Meloxicam (Mobic)
	Inhibition causes selective prostaglandin inhibition so that the inflammatory process is reduced without reducing protective prostaglandin effects on gastric mucosa.	Same adverse effects as other NSAIDs, with less risk of gastrointestinal bleeding

(continued)

TABLE 30-3 Drug Therapy for Connective Tissue Disorders (Continued)

Drug	Action	Adverse Effects
Disease-Modifying Agents		

Gold compounds (Chrysotherapy)
  Oral:
    Auranofin (Ridaura)
  Injectable:
    Gold sodium thiomalate (Myocrisine)
    Aurothioglucose (Solganal)
	Mechanism of action unclear
	Anti-inflammatory, anti-arthritic, and immunomodulating effects
		Cutaneous reactions ranging from dermatitis to life-threatening exfoliative dermatitis
		Renal toxicity
		Thrombocytopenia and marrow aplasia
		Nitritoid reaction with IM gold

Antimalarial agents
  Hydroxychloroquine sulfate (Placquenil)
  Chloroquine phosphate (Aralen)
	Remission-induction agents for rheumatoid arthritis
	Used also in certain forms of lupus
		Ocular toxicity (retinopathy that can result in permanent loss of vision; blurred vision, night blindness, scotoma

Chelating agents Penicillamine (Cuprimine; Depen)	Mechanism of action poorly understood Used in active progressive rheumatoid arthritis	Can cause severe toxic reactions: mucocutaneous, renal, gastrointestinal, hepatic, and hematologic toxicities
Leflunomide (Avara)	Pyrimidine synthesis inhibitor	Diarrhea, liver function test abnormalities, alopecia, rash, upper respiratory infection, hypertension
Sulfasalazine (Azulfidine)	Salicylate, sulfonamide	Anorexia, rash, hemolytic anemia
Etanercept (Enbrel)	Tumor necrosis factor blocker	Infection, injection site reaction, dyspepsia
Immunosuppressives		
Methotrexate (Mexate) Azathioprine (Imuran)	Exert anti-inflammatory effect by inhibition of cellular replication Used in patients with inflammatory synovitis refractory to other therapy	Bone marrow suppression, hepatic and pulmonary toxicity, reduced resistance to infection
Cyclophosphamide (Cytoxan)	Alkylating agent that interferes with the growth of rapidly dividing cells	Possibility of a malignancy occurring many years later after initiating therapy can cause sterility, urinary bladder, fibrosis, cystitis
Cyclosporine (Sandimmune)	Inhibition of immunocompetent lymphocytes also inhibits lymphokine production and release	Renal dysfunction, tremor, hypertension, gum hyperplasia

Corticosteroids
  Prednisone (Orasone)
  Prednisolone (Delta-Cortef)
  Triamcinalone (Kenalog)
  Betamethasome (Celestone)
  Hydrocortisone (Cortef)
  Dexamethasone (Decadron)
  Methylprednisolone (Medrol)
	Potent anti-inflammatory drugs may also reduce immune response
	Usually used for short-term management of patients with severe limitations
		Osteoporosis, fractures, avascular necrosis
		Gastric ulcers, infection susceptibility
		Hirsutism, acne, moon facies, abnormal fat deposition, edema, emotional disorders, menstrual disorders
		Hyperglycemia, hypokalemia
		Hypertension, cataracts

4. Perform activities in smooth movements to avoid trauma induced by abrupt movements.

Energy Conservation

Teach or reinforce the following practices:
1. Organize materials, utensils, and tools.
2. Perform lengthy activities in a seated position.
3. Work at an even pace—avoid rushing.
4. Delegate work to others when possible.

Splinting

1. Frequently used for wrists and hands.
2. Ensure proper application.
3. Periodically inspect for skin irritation, neurovascular compromise, or improper fit.
4. Usually worn during acute stage of inflammation to protect joint.

Exercise

Instruct and reinforce correct method of exercise:
1. Avoid exercising inflamed joints—putting these joints through range of motion one to two times per day when inflamed is sufficient.
2. Perform exercises daily as prescribed.
3. Aerobic conditioning exercises may be indicated when disease activity permits.
4. Walking, biking, swimming, and water walking for 30 minutes, three times a week.

Other Measures

1. Reinforce correct use and application of heat and cold.
2. Obtain and teach correct use of assistive devices.
3. Reinforce use of behavior modification and relaxation techniques as adjuncts to therapy.
4. Advise discussion with health care provider about alternative therapies (Box 30-1).

BOX 30-1 Alternative and Complementary Modalities for Patients with Connective Tissue Disorders

A wide variety of alternative therapies may be tried by patients with connective tissue disorders, including the following:

- Antibiotics
- Spa therapy
- Other types of water, mud, and immersion therapies
- Acupuncture
- Homeopathy
- Topical salicylates and nonsteroidal anti-inflammatory drugs
- Capsaicin
- Dimethyl sulfoxide (DMSO)
- Elemental or hypoallergenic diets
- Dietary fatty acids, fish oil
- Vegetarian and vegan diets
- Zen macrobiotic diet
- Ginger

- Collagen Type II
- Shark cartilage
- Dehydroepiandrosterone (DHEA)
- Vitamin E
- Vitamin C
- L-Histidine
- Snake venom
- Bee venom
- Ant venom
- Copper, zinc
- Borage
- Feverfew
- Flax seed
- Selenium

---

5. Advise patient to modify home and work environments as needed, to install safety devices, and to maintain a safe environment.
6. Advise patient to seek counseling regarding sexuality, if joint pain and inflammation are barriers to performance.
7. Reinforce the chronic waxing and waning nature of the illness to lessen susceptibility to quackery.

THE DISORDERS

Rheumatoid Arthritis

Rheumatoid arthritis is a general term used to describe what may be a heterogeneous group of inflammatory diseases that affect joints and other organ systems.

Pathophysiology and Etiology

1. Immunologic processes result in inflammation of synovium, producing antigens and inflammatory by-products that lead to destruction of articular cartilage, edema, and production of a granular tissue called pannus (Figure 30-1).
2. Granulation tissue forms adhesions that lead to decreased joint mobility.
3. Similar adhesions can occur in supporting structures, such as ligaments and tendons, and cause contractures and ruptures that further affect joint structure and mobility.
4. The etiology is unknown but is probably a combined effect of environmental, demographic, infectious, and genetic factors.
5. An infectious agent has not been identified, but many infectious processes can produce a polyarthritis similar to RA.
6. Women are affected more frequently than men.

Clinical Manifestations

1. Arthritis:
   a. Bilateral, symmetric arthritis affects any diarthrodial joint, but most often involves the hands, wrists, knees, and feet (Figure 30-2).

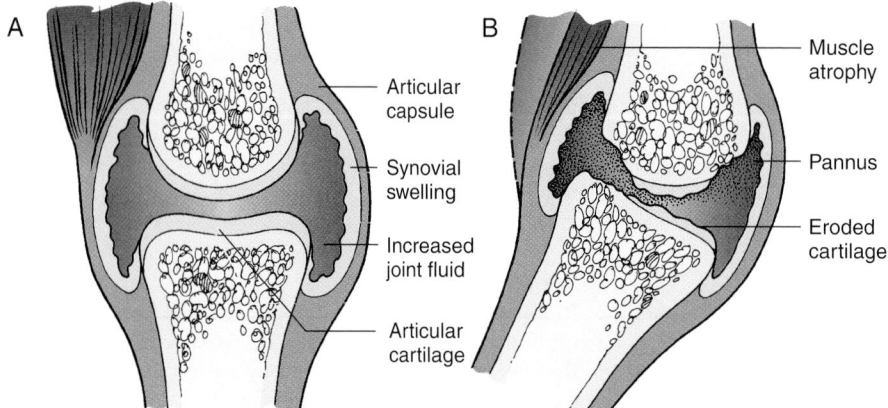

FIGURE 30-1 Pathophysiology of rheumatoid arthritis. (**A**) Joint structure with synovial swelling and fluid accumulation in joint. (**B**) Pannus, eroded articular cartilage with joint space narrowing, muscle atrophy, and ankylosis.

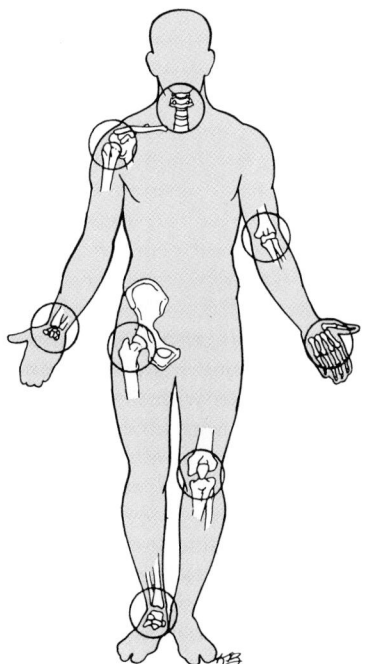

FIGURE 30-2 Rheumatoid arthritis characteristically involves the joints of the hands, wrist, feet, ankles, knees, elbows, and the glenohumeral and acromioclavicular joints and the hips. The articulations of the cervical spine are also affected.

2. Skin manifestations:
   a. Rheumatoid nodules—elbows, occiput, sacrum.
   b. Vasculitic changes—brown, splinterlike lesions in fingers or nail folds.
3. Cardiac manifestations:
   a. Acute pericarditis.
   b. Conduction defects.
   c. Valvular insufficiency.
   d. Coronary arteritis.
   e. Cardiac tamponade—rare.
4. Pulmonary manifestations:
   a. Asymptomatic pulmonary disease.
   b. Pleural effusion.
   c. Interstitial fibrosis.
   d. Laryngeal obstruction caused by involvement of the cricoarytenoid joint—rare.
5. Neurologic manifestations:
   a. Mononeuritis multiplex.
      (i) Wrist drop.
      (ii) Foot drop.
   b. Carpal tunnel syndrome.
   c. Compression of spinal nerve roots.
6. Systemic manifestations:
   a. Fever.
   b. Fatigue.
   c. Weight loss.

Diagnostic Evaluation

1. Complete blood count (CBC)—normochromic anemia.
2. RF—positive in a large percentage of patients.
3. ESR—elevated.
4. Synovial fluid analysis—see Table 30-2.
5. X-rays.
   a. Hands/wrists—marginal erosions of the proximal interphalangeal (PIP), metacarpophalangeal (MCP), and carpal joints; generalized osteopenia.
   b. Cervical spine—erosions that produce atlantoaxial subluxation.
6. Magnetic resonance imaging (MRI)—spinal cord compression that results from C1–C2 subluxation and compression of surrounding vascular structures.
7. Bone scan—increased uptake in the joints involved in RA.
8. Synovial biopsy.
   a. Inflammatory cells associated with RA.
   b. Excludes other causes of polyarthritis by noting the lack of other pathologic findings.

Management

1. Pharmacologic:
   a. NSAIDs to relieve pain and inflammation.
   b. DMARDs to reduce disease activity.
   c. Corticosteroids to reduce inflammatory process.
2. Local comfort measures:
   a. Application of heat and cold.
   b. Use of splints.
   c. Use of transcutaneous electrical nerve stimulation (TENS) unit.
   d. Iontophoresis—delivery of medication through the skin using direct electrical current.
3. Nonpharmacologic modalities:
   a. Behavior modification.
   b. Relaxation techniques.
4. Surgery:
   a. Synovectomy.
   b. Arthrodesis—joint fusion.
   c. Total joint replacement.

Complications

1. Loss of joint function because of bony adhesions and damage of supporting structures.
2. Anemia of chronic disease.

Nursing Assessment

1. Perform joint examination if indicated.
   a. Determine range of motion.
   b. Joint effusions or lack thereof
2. Deformities:
   a. Swan neck—PIP joints hyperextend.
   b. Boutonniere—PIP joints flex.
   c. Ulnar deviation—fingers point toward ulna.
3. Assess pain.
4. Assess functional status.
   a. Class I—no restriction of ability to perform normal activities.

b. Class II—moderate restriction, but adequate for normal activities.

c. Class III—marked restriction, inability to perform most duties of usual occupation or self-care.

d. Class IV—incapacitation or confinement to bed or wheelchair.

5. Assess for signs and symptoms that indicate side effects to medications.

Nursing Diagnoses

- Chronic Pain related to disease process
- Impaired Physical Mobility related to pain and limited joint motion
- Self-Care Deficit related to limitations secondary to disease process
- Ineffective Coping related to pain, physical limitations, and chronicity of RA

Nursing Interventions

Controlling Pain

1. Apply local heat or cold to affected joints for 15 to 20 minutes, three to four times a day. Avoid temperatures likely to cause skin or tissue damage by checking temperature of warm soaks or by covering cold packs with a towel.

2. Administer or teach self-administration of pharmacologic agents.

   a. Advise patient when to expect pain relief, based on mechanism of action of the drug.

3. Encourage use of adjunctive pain control measures.

   a. Progressive muscle relaxation.

   b. TENS.

   c. Biofeedback.

Optimizing Mobility

1. Encourage warm bath or shower in the morning to decrease morning stiffness.

2. Encourage measures to protect affected joints.

   a. Perform gentle range-of-motion exercises.

   b. Use splints.

   c. Assist with activities of daily living if necessary.

3. Encourage exercise consistent with degree of disease activity.

4. Refer to physical therapy and occupational therapy.

Promoting Self-Care

1. Provide pain relief before self-care activities.

2. Provide privacy and an environment conducive to performance of daily activities.

3. Schedule adequate rest periods.

4. Discuss importance of promoting the patient's self-care at an appropriate level with patient and family.

5. Help patient attain appropriate assistive devices, such as raised toilet seats, special eating utensils, and zipper pulls. Contact occupational therapist, social worker, or Arthritis Foundation for information.

Strengthening Coping Skills

1. Be aware of potential job, child care, home maintenance, and social and family functioning problems that may result from RA.

2. Encourage patient to ventilate problems and feelings.

3. Assist with problem-solving approach to explore options and to gain control of problem areas.

4. Reinforce effective coping mechanisms.

5. Refer to social worker or mental health counselor as needed.

Patient Education and Health Maintenance

1. Instruct patient and family in the nature of disease.

   a. Chronic nature of RA with characteristic exacerbations and remissions with time.

   b. Disease can have systemic affects that result in constitutional symptoms and involvement of other organ systems.

   c. Severity of RA is variable, but most patients are *not* confined to bed or wheelchair.

   d. RA has no cure; avoid miracle cures and quackery.

2. Educate about pharmacologic agents.

   a. Medication must be taken consistently to achieve maximum benefit.

   b. Most medications used in the treatment of RA require periodic laboratory testing to monitor for potential side effects.

   c. Advise patient of possible side effects of medications and need to report side effects to health care provider.

   d. Advise patients to discuss the use of any complementary or alternative therapies with their health care provider.

   e. Reinforce to patient the need for lifelong treatment.

3. During periods of remission, encourage patient to exercise regularly, choosing an activity that is inexpensive, convenient, enjoyable, and not dependent on the weather. Suggest dancing, mall walking, use of stationary bicycle in the home, or contacting the local YMCA about special programs for arthritis.

4. To find a local chapter of the Arthritis Foundation, contact the national office at 1330 West Peachtree Street, Atlanta, GA 30309, 404-872-7100; *www.arthritis.org*.

Outcome-Based Evaluation

- Reports reduction in pain
- Wears wrist splints correctly and performs range-of-motion exercises twice a day
- Maintains independent toiletry, bathing, and feeding
- Verbalizes concerns about cleaning and cooking; meets with occupational therapist

■ Systemic Lupus Erythematosus

Systemic lupus erythematosus (SLE) is a chronic, multisystem disease that is most likely a failure of immune regulation.

Pathophysiology and Etiology

1. The T lymphocyte system is affected for unknown reasons, and the failure of its regulatory system may result in an inability to slow or to halt the production of inappropriate autoantibodies.
2. B lymphocyte–stimulating factors are produced and this too may lead to production of autoantibodies.
3. Autoantibodies may combine with other elements of the immune system to activate immune complexes. These immune complexes and other immune system constituents combine to form complement, which is deposited in organs, causing inflammation and tissue necrosis.
4. More women are affected than men.

Clinical Manifestations

1. Skin:
   a. Butterfly-shaped rash, characterized by erythema and edema.
   b. Discoid lesions are ring-shaped, involving the shoulders, arms, and upper back.
   c. Discoid lesions may also result in erythematous, scaly plaques on the face, scalp, external ear, and neck, and alopecia may occur.
2. Arthritis:
   a. Generally bilateral and symmetric, involving the hands, wrists, and other joints.
   b. Can resemble RA and may be mistaken for it especially early in the course of the disease.
   c. Unlike RA, the arthritis is nonerosive; that is, no joint destruction is seen on x-ray.
   d. Tendon involvement is common and may lead to deformities or tendon rupture.
3. Cardiac:
   a. Pericarditis.
   b. Pleural effusion.
   c. Myocarditis.
   d. Endocarditis.
   e. Coronary arteritis—less common.
4. Pulmonary:
   a. Pleuritis.
   b. Pleural effusion.
   c. Lupus pneumonitis.
   d. Pulmonary hemorrhage.
   e. Pulmonary embolism.
5. Gastrointestinal.
   a. Oral ulcers.
   b. Acute or subacute abdominal pain.
   c. Pancreatitis.
   d. Spontaneous bacterial peritonitis.
   e. Bowel infarction.
6. Renal: occurs in 50% of patients with as many as 15% of patients developing renal failure.
   a. Nephritis.
   (i) Mesangial nephritis—mild form, can be reversible, best prognosis.
   (ii) Focal segmental glomerulonephritis—active necrotic or sclerosing lesions.
   (iii) Proliferative—may be focal or diffuse. Diffuse carries good prognosis.
   (iv) Membranous nephritis—may persist for years without serious renal function decline. May present as nephrotic syndrome.
   (v) Sclerosing nephritis—increase in the amount of matrix material in the glomeruli.
   b. Renal thrombosis—rare.
7. Central nervous system:
   a. Neuropsychiatric disorders.
   (i) Depression.
   (ii) Psychosis.
   b. Transient ischemic attacks/stroke.
   c. Epilepsy.
   d. Migraine headache.
   e. Myelopathy.
   f. Guillain-Barré syndrome.
   g. Chorea and other movement disorders.
8. Hematologic:
   a. Hemolytic anemia.
   b. Leukopenia.
   c. Thrombocytopenia.
9. Constitutional:
   a. Fever.
   b. Weight loss.
   c. Fatigue.

Diagnostic Evaluation

1. CBC—leukopenia, anemia (may be hemolytic), thrombocytopenia.
2. ANA—positive in more than 90% of patients with SLE; predominant pattern is homogeneous.
3. ESR—generally elevated.
4. Complement levels—generally decreased when disease is active.
5. Urinalysis—hematuria, proteinuria, and active sediment (RBC casts).
6. 24-hour urine for protein and creatinine clearance.
7. Chest x-ray may show changes.
8. X-ray of hands and wrists—nondestructive arthritis.
9. Computed tomography (CT) scan or MRI.
   a. Brain—to define any neurologic manifestations.
   b. Abdomen—to rule out other abdominal processes in a patient with abdominal pain.
   c. Cerebral arteriogram—to look for evidence of cerebral vasculitis.
   d. Magnetic resonance angiography (MRA).

Management
Pharmacologic

1. NSAIDs—to reduce pain and inflammation.
2. Antimalarials—to decrease disease activity.
3. Corticosteroids—to reduce inflammatory process.
4. Immunosuppressives—to suppress immune process.

Nonpharmacologic

1. Avoid direct exposure to sunlight to reduce the chance of exacerbation.
2. Behavior modification to prevent exacerbations and to reduce symptoms.
3. Joint protection and energy conservation.

Other Management

1. Close follow-up for evaluation of cardiac, neurologic, renal, and other body systems.
2. Referral to specialists for systemic manifestations.

Complications

1. Renal failure.
2. Permanent neurologic impairment.
3. Infection.
4. Death caused by disease process.

Nursing Assessment

1. Obtain clinical history, review systems, and perform physical examination for characteristic findings.
2. Assess for signs and symptoms of infection and other side effects to medications.
3. Assess patient's and family's ability to cope with impact of prolonged disease.

Nursing Diagnoses

- Prolonged Pain related to inflammation of joints and juxta-articular structures
- Powerlessness related to unpredictable course of disease
- Risk for Impaired Skin and Oral Mucous Membrane Integrity related to skin/oral lesions
- Fatigue related to chronic inflammatory process
- Altered Urinary Elimination related to renal involvement

Nursing Interventions

Reducing Pain

1. Administer and teach self-administration of medications to reduce disease activity and of additional analgesics as ordered.
2. Suggest the use of hot or cold applications, relaxation techniques, and nonstrenuous exercise to enhance pain relief.

Increasing Control Over Disease Process

1. Instruct patient to avoid factors that may exacerbate disease.
   a. Avoid exposure to sunlight and ultraviolet light.
      (i) Use sunscreen with sun protection factor (SPF) of 15 or greater. Avoid prolonged sun exposure.
      (ii) Wear protective, lightweight clothing, long sleeves, hats.
      (iii) Avoid use of tanning beds.
   b. Avoid exposure to drugs and chemicals.
      (i) Avoid exposure to hair spray.
      (ii) Avoid exposure to hair-coloring agents.
      (iii) Medications—obtain provider advice before taking any medications or supplements.

2. Teach self-administration of pharmacologic agents to reduce disease activity.
3. Encourage good nutrition, sleep habits, exercise, rest, and relaxation to improve general health and to help prevent infection.
4. Encourage ventilation of feelings, counseling, or referrals to social work, occupational therapy, as needed.

Maintaining Skin and Mucous Membrane Integrity

1. Apply topical corticosteroids to skin lesions as ordered.
2. Suggest alternative hairstyles, scarves, and wigs to cover significant areas of alopecia.
3. Encourage good oral hygiene and inspect mouth for oral ulcers.
   a. Avoid hot or spicy foods that may irritate oral ulcers.
   b. Apply topical agents or analgesics to reduce pain and to promote eating.

Reducing Fatigue

1. Advise patient that fatigue level will fluctuate with disease activity.
2. Encourage patient to modify schedule to include several rest periods during the day; pace activity and exercise according to body's tolerance; use energy conservation techniques in daily activities.
3. Teach relaxation techniques, such as deep breathing, progressive muscle relaxation, and imagery to reduce emotional stress that causes fatigue.

Preserving Urinary Elimination

1. Assist with monitoring of urinary status as indicated by degree of renal involvement.
   a. Monitor intake and output and urine specific gravity.
   b. Measure urine protein, microalbumin, or obtain 24-hour creatinine clearance, as ordered.
   c. Check test results of serum blood urea nitrogen (BUN) and creatinine.
2. See page 651 for the care of patients on dialysis.

Patient Education and Health Maintenance

1. Stress that close follow-up is mandatory, even in times of remission, to detect early progression of organ involvement and to alter drug therapy.
2. Advise on the use of special cosmetics to cover skin lesions.
3. Advise about reproduction.
   a. Avoid pregnancy during time of severe disease activity.
   b. Immunomodulators may have teratogenic effects.
   c. Use of some drugs for treatment of SLE can result in sterility.
4. Stress that any complementary or alternative therapies should be discussed with the health care provider.
5. For additional information and support, refer to agencies such as Lupus Foundation, 1300 Piccard Drive, Suite 200, Rockville, MD 20850-4303, 800-558-0121, *www.lupus.org.*

Outcome-Based Evaluation
- Reports pain reduction
- Verbalizes appropriate use of medications, avoidance of sun and chemicals, and need for nutrition and sleep to minimize disease process
- Reports oral ulcers healing without interference with appetite
- Urine output adequate; specific gravity stable
- Reports resting three times a day, with adequate energy to carry out activities

Systemic Sclerosis

Systemic sclerosis is a generalized disorder of connective tissue, characterized by hardening and thickening of the skin (scleroderma), blood vessels, synovium, skeletal muscles, and internal organs. Fibrotic, degenerative, and inflammatory changes, including vascular insufficiency, result in changes in joints and several organ systems.

Pathophysiology and Etiology
1. The changes seen in the skin and internal organs in systemic sclerosis are most likely caused by overproduction of collagen by fibroblasts.
2. The etiology of systemic sclerosis is unknown.
3. Systemic sclerosis affects three to four times as many women as men.

Clinical Manifestations
Skin
1. Bilateral symmetric swelling of the hands and sometimes the feet.
2. After the edematous phase, the skin becomes hard and thick.
3. Digits, dorsum of hand, neck, face, and trunk are involved.
4. Normal landmarks in skin are absent—no skin folds.
5. Increased or decreased skin pigmentation.
6. Skin changes may regress after several years.
7. Telangiectasia—on tongue, face, fingers, and lips.
8. Areas of calcinosis—late in the course of disease.
9. Raynaud's phenomenon.

Gastrointestinal
1. Esophageal dysmotility—resulting in reflux and dysphagia.
2. Distal esophageal dilation and esophagitis.
3. Barrett's metaplasia—may predispose to adenocarcinoma of the esophagus.
4. Duodenal atrophy dilatation—may cause postprandial abdominal pain, malabsorption, diarrhea, and abdominal distention.
5. Colonic hypomotility—results in constipation.

Musculoskeletal
1. Joint pain.
2. Polyarthritis—large and small joints affected.
3. Carpal tunnel syndrome.
4. Flexion contractures.
5. Inflammatory muscle atrophy.

Cardiac
1. Left ventricular dysfunction.
2. Myocardial involvement—congestive heart failure and atrial and ventricular arrhythmias.
3. Right ventricular involvement—secondary to pulmonary disease.

Pulmonary
1. Interstitial fibrosis.
2. Restrictive lung disease.
3. Pulmonary hypertension.

Renal
Scleroderma renal crisis—rapid malignant hypertension with encephalopathy.

Localized Scleroderma
1. CREST—calcinosis, Raynaud's phenomenon, esophageal dysmotility, sclerodactyly, telangiectasia.
2. Morphea and linear scleroderma—scleroderma lesions appear as streaks or bands in linear scleroderma. Morphea lesions may be several centimeters and may have a purple border.
3. Generally, no visceral involvement exists in localized scleroderma.

Diagnostic Evaluation
1. CBC and ESR—generally normal.
2. RF—positive in approximately 30% of patients.
3. ANA—generally positive with speckled or nucleolar patterns.
   a. Antisclerodermal antibody (Scl-70)—positive in diffuse cutaneous disease.
   b. Anticentromere antibody—highly specific for limited cutaneous disease.
4. X-ray of hands and wrists—muscle atrophy, osteopenia, osteolysis.
5. Barium swallow—esophageal dysmotility.
6. Pulmonary function test—decreased diffusion capacity and vital capacity.
7. Multiple gated image analysis—to determine left ventricular function.
8. Endoscopy—to biopsy for Barrett's metaplasia.
9. Esophageal manometry—to determine contractile capacity of esophageal muscles.

Management
Pharmacologic
1. Penicillamine (Depen) to decrease disease activity.
2. Calcium channel blockers—for Raynaud's phenomenon.
3. NSAIDs—for arthralgias and polyarthritis.
4. H2 blockers and omeprazole (Prilosec)—for reflux.
5. Antibiotics—for malabsorption because of bacterial overgrowth.
6. Antihypertensive agents and drugs for heart failure.
7. Metaclopromide (Reglan)—for intestinal dysmotility.

Nonpharmacologic
1. Skin lubricants.
2. Avoidance of factors associated with exacerbation of Raynaud's phenomenon.
3. Biofeedback.

Complications
1. Skin ulcers.
2. Malabsorption.
3. Esophageal adenocarcinoma.
4. Pulmonary hypertension.
5. Renal failure.
6. Congestive heart failure.
7. Death caused by disease process.

Nursing Assessment
1. Focus physical assessment on:
   a. Skin ulcers, thickening.
   b. Joint examination—flexion contractures.
   c. Heart and lung examination—for signs and symptoms of congestive heart failure, hypertension.
   d. Gastrointestinal function.
2. Determine nutritional status.

Nursing Diagnoses
- Altered Peripheral Tissue Perfusion related to Raynaud's phenomenon
- Risk for Impaired Skin Integrity related to effects of disease process
- Altered Nutrition: Less Than Body Requirements related to impaired swallowing and gastrointestinal involvement
- Body Image Disturbance related to effects of disease

Nursing Interventions
Maintaining Tissue Perfusion
1. Teach patient to identify Raynaud's phenomenon.
   a. Characteristic color change of the fingers—white, blue, red.
   b. Coldness, pallor, numbness, pain.
2. Teach patient to reduce factors associated with precipitation or exacerbation of Raynaud's phenomenon.
   a. Dress warmly—cover head and extremities, keep trunk warm.
   b. Discontinue tobacco usage.
   c. Avoid prolonged exposure to cold.
      (i) Weather.
      (ii) Artificially controlled environments (eg, air conditioning).
      (iii) Limit contact with cold food items, such as frozen foods, ice cube trays—use gloves or tongs.
3. Protect ulcerated digits and observe for signs of infection.

Preserving Skin Integrity
1. Use moisturizers on skin daily.
2. Advise patient to avoid use of drying soaps and detergents.
3. Use protective padding (eg, elbow pads) to protect the skin from friction or trauma.
4. Inspect skin daily for cracking, ulceration, and signs of infection.

Achieving Optimal Nutritional Status
1. Ensure patient is in proper position for meals to avoid aspiration (ie, in chair if possible).
2. Provide smaller, more frequent feedings of well-balanced diet.
3. Encourage patient to remain upright after meals for 45 to 60 minutes and raise head of bed during sleep to avoid reflux.
4. Administer or teach self-administration of medications to prevent nausea and reflux as ordered.
5. Encourage good oral hygiene and frequent dental visits.
6. Advise to use lubricating agents, if necessary, to treat dry mouth and to teach stretching exercises of mouth to maintain aperture.
7. Weigh weekly and ask patient to keep food diary.

Strengthening Body Image
1. Encourage patient to take an active role in treatment plan to feel in control of body changes.
2. Explain that changes may be gradual and slow; although not noticeable, internal organ involvement is even more important than external changes.
3. Suggest continuance of activities that patient enjoys and foster strong support network.
4. Refer for counseling as needed.

Patient Education and Health Maintenance
1. Explain all diagnostic tests and their purpose in detecting gastrointestinal, pulmonary, renal, or cardiac involvement.
2. Teach about drug treatment and side effects.
3. Advise on fluid and sodium restriction if congestive heart failure has been identified.
4. Advise on modifying activity and using oxygen to prevent dyspnea caused by restrictive lung disease.
5. Encourage regular follow-up visits and prompt attention to worsening symptoms.
6. Refer to agencies such as United Scleroderma Foundation, 89 Newbury Street, Suite 201, Danvers, MA 01923, 1-800-722-HOPE; *www.scleroderma.org*.

Outcome-Based Evaluation
- Relates factors that precipitate Raynaud's phenomenon
- Reports no skin cracking or ulceration
- Reports no weight loss
- Reports participating in community and church activities and groups

■ Gout

Gout is a disorder of purine metabolism, characterized by elevated uric acid levels and deposition of urate (usually in the form of crystals) in joints and other tissues.

Pathophysiology and Etiology

Gout results from an overabundant accumulation and subsequent deposition of uric acid in the body. This can occur in one of two ways.

Overproduction of Uric Acid (10% of Cases)

1. Inherited enzyme defects.
2. Certain disease conditions:
   a. Myeloproliferative disorders.
   b. Lymphoproliferative disorders.
   c. Cancer chemotherapy.
   d. Hemolytic anemias.
   e. Psoriasis.

Underexcretion of Uric Acid (90% of Cases)

1. Renal disease.
2. Endocrine disorders.
3. Medications and chemicals:
   a. Diuretics.
   b. Ethanol (alcohol).
   c. Low-dose aspirin.
   d. Pyrazinamide—antituberculosis agent.
   e. Lead.
4. Volume depletion states—nephrogenic diabetes insipidus.

Clinical Manifestations

Acute Gouty Arthritis

1. Generally affects one joint—often the first metatarsophalangeal joint (called podagra).
2. Other joints can be affected, such as ankle, tarsals, knee; upper extremities are less commonly involved.
3. Pain, warmth, erythema, and swelling of tissue surrounding the affected joint.
4. Fever may occur.
5. Onset of symptoms is sudden; intensity is severe.
6. Duration of symptoms is self-limiting; lasts approximately 3 to 10 days without treatment.

Chronic Tophaceous Gout

1. Occurs if acute gout is inadequately treated or if it goes untreated.
2. Characterized by development of tophi or deposits of uric acid in and around joints, cartilage, and soft tissues.
3. Arthritis is more prolonged in nature with discrete attacks less common.
4. Arthritis can produce bone erosions and subsequent bony deformities that can resemble RA.

Renal Disease

1. Caused by hyperuricemia (persistent elevation of uric acid in the blood).
2. Kidney stones are composed of uric acid.
3. Deposition of uric acid in kidney tissue.

Diagnostic Evaluation

1. Synovial fluid analysis.
   a. Identification of monosodium urate crystals under polarized microscopy.
   b. Synovial WBC count can range from 2,000 to 100,000/mm^3.
   c. Culture of synovial fluid to rule out infection.
2. 24-hour urine for uric acid to determine overproduction of uric acid versus underexcretion.
3. ESR—elevated.
4. X-rays of affected joints show changes consistent with diagnosis of gout.

Management

Pharmacologic

1. NSAIDs—for acute attacks to relieve pain and swelling.
2. Colchicine—for prevention of acute attacks and their treatment.
   a. Intravenous (IV) for acute attacks.
   b. Oral at onset of an attack, taken hourly until pain relief or first signs of toxicity (nausea, vomiting, cramping, diarrhea).
3. Corticosteroids.
   a. Intra-articular if attack confined to one joint.
   b. Oral—in short tapering course if other treatments are contraindicated or if attack involves many joints.

Urate-Lowering Agents

1. Uricosuric drugs, such as probenecid (Benamid), interfere with tubular reabsorption of uric acid.
2. Allopurinol (Zyloprim)—interferes with conversion of hypoxanthine and xanthine to uric acid.
   Side effects include skin rash (including exfoliative rashes), hypersensitivity syndrome (fever, eosinophilia, leukocytosis, worsening renal failure, hepatocellular injury, rash); bone marrow depression is rare.

Nonpharmacologic

1. Avoidance of obesity.
2. Avoidance of alcohol.
3. Low-purine diet gives only a minor decrease in serum uric acid levels.

Complications

1. Uric acid kidney stone.
2. Urate nephropathy.
3. Erosive, deforming arthritis.

Nursing Assessment

1. Obtain history for factors predisposing to gout.
2. Perform physical examination.
   a. Inspect involved joint.
   b. Observe for tophi:
      (i) Pinna of ear.
      (ii) Olecranon bursa
      (iii) Achilles tendon.
3. Assess pain and pain relief pattern if attack is acute.

Nursing Diagnoses

• Pain related to acute arthritis
• Impaired Physical Mobility related to arthritis

Nursing Interventions
Relieving Pain
1. Administer and teach self-administration of pain relieving medications as prescribed.
2. Encourage adequate fluid intake to assist with excretion of uric acid and to decrease likelihood of stone formation.
3. Instruct patient to take prescribed medications consistently because interruptions in therapy can precipitate acute attacks.

Facilitating Mobility
1. Elevate and protect affected joint during acute attack.
2. Assist with activities of daily living.
3. Encourage exercise and maintenance of routine activity in chronic gout, except during acute attacks.
4. Protect draining tophi by covering and applying antibiotic ointment as needed.

Patient Education and Health Maintenance
1. Instruct patient and family in nature of disease.
   a. Generally, acute attacks are followed by periods of remission.
   b. Once need for chronic treatment has been determined, it will generally be lifelong.
2. Encourage to avoid alcohol.
3. Avoid rapid weight loss by fasting or crash diets because rapid weight loss results in production of chemicals that compete with uric acid for excretion from the body, resulting in increased uric acid levels.
4. Avoid medications known to increase uric acid levels.
5. Advise prompt treatment of acute attack to reduce joint damage associated with repeated attacks.
6. Instruct in signs and symptoms of allopurinol hypersensitivity syndrome and need to report promptly.
7. Review foods containing purines (sardines, anchovies, shellfish, organ meats) if low-purine diet has been advised.

Outcome-Based Evaluation
- Reports relief of pain
- Performs activities of daily living with minimal assistance

◼ Sjögren's Syndrome
Sjögren's syndrome is a chronic inflammatory autoimmune process that affects the lacrimal and salivary glands. The disease can be primary or secondary. Secondary Sjögren's syndrome is seen most commonly in RA but can be seen in SLE and some other connective tissue diseases.

Pathophysiology and Etiology
1. The etiology of the syndrome is unknown, but is thought to include several factors: genetic predisposition, immunologic, infectious, and hormonal.
2. It is thought that antibodies directed at exocrine glands are produced, leading to disturbed function of the involved tissue.
3. Lymphocytes are found infiltrating affected tissues.
4. Sjögren's syndrome occurs primarily in middle-aged women.

Clinical Manifestations
1. Ocular—decreased tear formation that leads to keratoconjunctivitis, photophobia.
2. Oral—xerostomia (dry mouth) caused by diminished production of saliva, mucosal ulcers, stomatitis.
3. Salivary gland enlargement—unilateral or bilateral.
4. Nasal dryness, epitaxsis, nasal ulcers.
5. Dryness of bronchial tree, hoarseness, recurrent otitis media, pneumonia, and bronchitis.
6. Gastrointestinal—dysphagia, pancreatitis, hypo- or achlorhydria, autoimmune liver disease.
7. Renal—renal tubular acidosis, nephrogenic diabetes insipidus.
8. Skin—xerodermia (dry skin), urticaria, purpura.
9. Neuromuscular—cranial nerve dysfunction, polymyopathy, sensory and motor neuropathy, seizures, multiple sclerosis–like syndrome.
10. Thyroid—autoimmune thyroiditis (Hashimoto's thyroiditis).
11. Cardiovascular—Raynaud's phenomenon, vasculitis, babies born to mothers with Sjögren's syndrome may be born with congenital heart block.
12. Sex organs—vaginal dryness, dyspareunia.
13. Musculoskeletal—nonerosive polyarthritis.

Diagnostic Evaluation
1. CBC—mild anemia, leukopenia present in 30% of patients.
2. ESR—elevated in 90% of patients.
3. RF—positive in 75% to 90% of patients.
4. ANA—positive in 70% of patients; speckled and nucleolar patterns are most common; titer >1:320.
5. Antibodies to SSA/SSB—test to detect antibodies to specific nuclear proteins.
   a. SSA (Ro antibody)—positive in patients with Sjögren's syndrome and SLE.
   b. SSB (La antibody)—positive in patients with Sjögren's syndrome; also in patients with SLE.
6. Organ-specific antibodies—antibodies directed against specific organ tissues have been found.
   a. Gastric.
   b. Thyroid.
   c. Smooth muscle.
   d. Salivary gland.
   e. Lacrimal gland.
7. Salivary scintigraphy—salivary gland function is measured by determining excretion of radioisotope dye.
8. X-rays of affected joints to rule out erosive arthritis.
9. Salivary gland biopsy—to determine lymphocytic infiltration of tissue.

Management
Pharmacologic
1. Corticosteroids—used in severe cases.
2. Cyclophosphamide (Cytoxan)—used in severe cases.
3. Antifungal agents—used for oral candidiasis.
4. Pilocarpine—used orally to improve salivation.

Nonpharmacologic

1. Symptomatic relief of dryness.
   a. Artificial tears, lubricant inserts.
   b. Saliva substitutes—commercially prepared.
   c. Frequent use of nonsugared liquids, gums, and candies.
   d. Vaginal lubricants.
   e. Use of occlusive goggles at bedtime to prevent drying.
2. Dental care.
   a. Frequent brushing and flossing.
   b. Topical fluoride treatments.
   c. Avoidance of high-sucrose foods.

Complications

1. Ocular complications, such as corneal ulceration, corneal opacification, vascularization of the cornea, infection, glaucoma, cataract formation.
2. Tooth loss.
3. Pulmonary fibrosis.
4. Pulmonary hypertension.
5. Obstructive airway disease.
6. Chronic atrophic gastritis.
7. Chronic pancreatitis.
8. Abnormal liver function tests.
9. Primary biliary cirrhosis.
10. Renal tubular function abnormalities and membranous and membranoproliferative glomerulonephritis.
11. Subcortical dementia.

Nursing Assessment

1. Obtain history of signs and symptoms, emphasizing dryness.
2. Perform physical examination that includes oral cavity, eyes, skin, lungs, gastrointestinal, and neurologic systems.
3. Assess nutritional status, because decreased saliva makes eating difficult.

Nursing Diagnoses

- Altered Oral Mucous Membrane related to disease process
- Risk for Impaired Skin Integrity related to dryness
- Altered Nutrition: Less Than Body Requirements related to disturbances in saliva production, taste, and difficulty swallowing
- Sexual Dysfunction related to discomfort of decreased vaginal secretions

Nursing Interventions

Maintaining Mucous Membranes

1. Inspect oral mucosa for oral *Candida*, ulcers, saliva pools, and dental hygiene.
2. Instruct and assist patient in proper oral hygiene.
   a. At least twice daily brushing.
   b. Frequent rinsing with antiseptic mouthwash.
3. Encourage frequent intake of noncaffeinated, nonsugar liquids. Keep pitcher filled with cool water.
4. Promptly report any ulcers or signs of infections.

Protecting Skin Integrity

1. Instruct and assist patient with daily inspection of skin for areas of trauma or for potential breakdown.
2. Apply lubricants to skin daily.
3. Avoid shearing forces and encourage or perform frequent position changes.

Promoting Adequate Nutritional Intake

1. Increase liquid intake with meals.
2. Assist and instruct patient to avoid choosing spicy or dry foods from menu choices.
3. Suggest small, more frequent meals.
4. Weigh weekly and review diet history for deficiency in basic nutrients.

Promoting Optimal Sexual Functioning

1. Encourage patient to discuss sexual difficulty and to explain its relation to disease process.
2. Advise on proper use of water-soluble vaginal lubrication.
3. Suggest alternative positioning and practices to prevent discomfort.
4. Teach patient to report symptoms of vaginitis—discharge, irritation, itching—because infection may result from altered mucosal barrier.

Health Maintenance and Patient Education

1. Advise patient of commercially available artificial saliva preparations, artificial tears, moisturizing nasal sprays, artificial vaginal moisturizers.
2. Encourage frequent dental visits. Dental cavities are more frequent in Sjögren's syndrome.
3. Advise patient to check with health care provider before using any medications because many, such as diuretics, tricyclic antidepressants, and antihistamines, have the side effect of mouth dryness.
4. Advise patient to wear protective eyewear while outdoors.
5. Encourage support through Sjögren's Syndrome Foundation, 366 N. Broadway, Suite PH-W2, Jericho, NY 11753, 516-933-6365; *www.sjogrens.org*.

Outcome-Based Evaluation

- Demonstrates proper oral hygiene
- Reports skin without cracking, scaling, or other lesions
- Maintains weight
- Describes correct use of water-soluble lubricant

▨ Polyarteritis Nodosa

Polyarteritis nodosa (PAN) is a vasculitis that is characterized by an inflammation of small to medium-sized blood vessels. Any organ can be affected; however, the kidney, gastrointestinal system, peripheral nerves, skin, and joints are most commonly involved.

Pathophysiology and Etiology

1. Inflammation caused by deranged immunologic processes results in disruption of the blood vessel walls.
2. The affected vessels may narrow as a result of injury or may develop aneurysms, especially at vessel branching points.

3. Sometimes associated with hepatitis B or hepatitis C infection.
4. Men affected more than women.

Clinical Manifestations

1. Constitutional symptoms—fever, weight loss, fatigue, arthralgias, myalgias.
2. Skin—palpable purpura, ulcers, changes in fingers and toes caused by ischemia.
3. Cardiac—coronary artery aneurysm, congestive heart failure.
4. Gastrointestinal—abdominal pain, hematemesis, melena, thrombosis of mesenteric vessels.
5. Kidneys—proteinuria, hematuria, presence of RBC casts, hypertension.
6. Neurologic—peripheral neuropathy (sensory and motor), seizures (rare).
7. Sex organs—testicular pain.

Diagnostic Evaluation

1. CBC—decreased hemoglobin and hematocrit (normochromic anemia).
2. ESR—generally elevated.
3. Serum albumin—decreased.
4. Complement levels—decreased.
5. Hepatitis B and hepatitis C antigen—found in some patients.
6. RF—sometimes positive.
7. Arteriography—aneurysms.
8. Perform biopsy—to elevate condition of blood vessels. Biopsy site may depend on patient's symptoms.

Management

1. Corticosteroids.
2. Immunosuppressants, such as cyclophosphamide (Cytoxan) and azathioprine (Imuran).

Complications

1. Hypertension.
2. Coronary artery disease.
3. Congestive heart failure.
4. Cerebrovascular disease.
5. Renal failure.
6. Death.

Nursing Assessment

1. Obtain history for constitutional symptoms, vascular changes, and manifestations of internal organ involvement.
2. Perform physical examination that includes the skin, neurologic system, heart and lungs, and measurement of blood pressure.

Nursing Diagnoses

- Risk for Infection related to immunosuppressant therapy
- Altered Peripheral Tissue Perfusion related to vasculitis
- Risk for Injury related to systemic manifestations

Nursing Interventions
Preventing Infection

1. Advise patient to avoid known sources of infection.
2. Advise patient to avoid anyone with a contagious disease.
3. Advise patient to avoid crowds during cold and flu season.
4. Advise patient to avoid stagnant water.
5. Practice and teach frequent handwashing.
6. Report any signs of infection, such as cough, dysuria, sore throat, wound drainage; fever may be absent because of altered inflammatory response caused by medications.
7. Monitor CBC results for leukocyte and absolute neutrophil counts.

Promoting Tissue Perfusion

1. Inspect skin for rash, ulcers, ischemic digits (cold, numb or painful, pale).
2. Protect extremities from trauma and keep warm to enhance blood flow.
3. Administer anti-inflammatory and immunosuppressive agents as ordered, based on patient's response. Stress compliance to maintain response.

Monitoring for Systemic Involvement

1. Be alert for signs of mesenteric ischemia—abdominal pain after meals, vomiting, diarrhea.
2. Provide small, high-caloric meals.
3. Medicate for pain as needed.

NURSING ALERT

Increasing abdominal pain, vomiting, bloody diarrhea, and a developing tender, silent abdomen signal mesenteric infarction. Prompt identification and surgery are necessary to prevent widespread peritonitis and bowel necrosis.

4. Periodically assess the lower extremities for foot drop and decreased sensation.
5. Teach protective measures to prevent injury from hot water, stepping on sharp objects, etc.
6. Monitor renal function through intake and output measurements, urine dipstick, urine specific gravity, and laboratory studies as ordered. Report abnormalities promptly.
7. Administer and teach self-administration of antihypertensive agents as ordered.

Patient Education and Health Maintenance

1. Instruct patient and family in nature of disease.
   a. Course of disease is acute.
   b. Untreated disease has poor survival rate.
   c. Organ destruction and death are not uncommon.
2. Encourage close follow-up.

Outcome-Based Evaluation

- Verbalizes no signs of infection
- Reports fingers without ulceration or signs of ischemia
- Reports no abdominal pain, sensory deficits, signs of renal failure

Fibromyalgia

Fibromyalgia is a syndrome characterized by fatigue, diffuse muscle pain and stiffness, sleep disturbance, and tender points on physical examination.

Pathophysiology and Etiology

The etiology is unknown. Theories have suggested various possible pathophysiologic mechanisms, such as neural-hormonal disturbance, antecedent physical trauma, viral infection, immune dysregulation, psychiatric disturbances, and heightened sensitivity to pain.

Clinical Manifestations

1. Fatigue.
2. Generalized muscle pain and stiffness.
3. Poor or nonrestorative sleep.
4. Irritable bowel syndrome.
5. Tension headaches.
6. Paresthesias.
7. Sensation of swollen hands.
8. Presence of pain in 11 of 18 defined tender point sites (Figure 30-3).

Diagnostic Evaluation

1. To rule out other disorders—tests generally normal in fibromyalgia.
2. Complete history and physical examination.
   a. CBC.
   b. Blood chemistries.
   c. ESR.
   d. TSH.

Management

Pharmacologic

1. NSAIDs, acetaminophen, or tramadol (Ultram) to relieve pain.
2. Selected tricyclic antidepressants to help control chronic pain and depression.

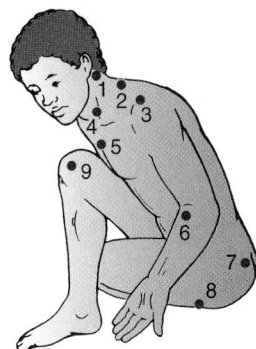

FIGURE 30-3 Fibromyalgia trigger points.

3. Cyclobenzaprine (Flexeril) to relieve muscle tension and spasm.
4. Alprazolam or other antianxiety agent to reduce stress factor.

Nonpharmacologic

1. Cardiovascular fitness training.
2. Electromyogram (EMG) biofeedback.
3. Cognitive behavioral therapy.
4. Hypnotherapy.
5. Electrical stimulation or acupuncture.

Complications

1. Deconditioning.
2. Work disability.
3. Inability to fulfill social role.
4. Unnecessary diagnostic and therapeutic maneuvers.

Nursing Assessment

1. Assess pain level, because it varies during the day/week.
2. Assess functional ability.
3. Assess mood, support system, and coping mechanisms.
4. Assess lifestyle factors that may be impairing well-being—smoking, lack of exercise, poor posture.

Nursing Diagnoses

- Chronic Pain related to disease process
- Sleep Pattern Disturbance related to disease process
- Altered Role Performance related to disabling disease process

Nursing Interventions

Controlling Pain

1. Encourage regular use of analgesics and antidepressants as directed.
2. Encourage regular exercise routine, including stretching, aerobic activity, and muscle strengthening exercises.
3. Suggest referrals to physical therapist or pain specialists for additional pain control modalities as needed.

Improving Sleep

1. Suggest regular nighttime ritual to promote sleep.
2. Discourage staying up late and other erratic sleep habits.
3. Encourage relaxation periods or short nap during day as needed for fatigue.
4. Advise limiting caffeine intake during day and especially after 4 PM.
5. Although sleeping pills are discouraged, advise patient to discuss short-term sleep aid with health care provider.

Strengthening Roles

1. Encourage patient to look at fibromyalgia as a chronic condition that can be controlled.
2. Suggest a fibromyalgia support group.
3. Tell the patient that fibromyalgia is not a progressive debilitating disease and that most people gain control of their symptoms.
4. Help patient plan schedule and pace activities to accomplish routine activities.

Patient Education and Health Maintenance

1. Educate patient and family that fibromyalgia is a real disorder that causes pain and fatigue despite the normal test results and lack of ill appearance.
2. Explain proper use of analgesics and potential side effects.
3. Encourage regular activity as much as possible and avoid physical and emotional stress.
4. Advise patient to discuss all types of alternative and complementary therapy with health care provider.
5. Encourage regular follow-up visits with primary care provider, rheumatologist, and physical therapist as indicated.
6. Suggest further help and information from Fibromyalgia Network, 661-631-1950, or the Arthritis Foundation, *www.arthritis.org.*

Outcome-Based Evaluation

- Patient states pain at 0-2 level
- Sleeping 8 hours per night with 0-1 short awakenings
- Patient going to work, taking care of children

Other Rheumatologic Disorders

Several other conditions affect the joints and periarticular tissue.

Seronegative spondyloarthropathies are inflammatory conditions with negative rheumatoid factor or other autoantibodies, but are associated with HLA-B27 antigen. Seronegative spondyloarthropathies include the following:

1. *Ankylosing spondylitis,* characterized by low back stiffness and possible ocular, cardiac, and pulmonary manifestations.
2. *Reiter's disease,* characterized by the triad of urethritis, arthritis, and conjunctivitis.
3. *Arthritis associated with inflammatory bowel disease.*

Polymyositis (dermatomyositis if rash around eyes is present) is an inflammatory disease of striated muscles that most commonly affects the proximal limb girdle, neck, pharynx, proximal third of the esophagus, and occasionally the heart.

Polymyalgia rheumatica is an inflammatory disease with elevated ESR that affects mostly women older than age 50 and presents with profound stiffness, usually in the shoulder girdle and hips. It responds well to corticosteroids.

Sarcoidosis is a chronic, granulomatous multisystem disorder that most notably affects the lungs but can mimic rheumatic disease by causing fever, arthritis, uveitis, myositis, and rash.

Nursing care for patients with these disorders is similar to that for rheumatoid arthritis.

SELECTED REFERENCES

Abramawicz, M. (Ed.). (2000). Meloxicam (Mobic) for osteoarthritis. *The Medical Letter, 42*(1079), 47–48.

AltMedDex System. Complementary and alternative monographs. *Micromedix, 102.*

Barnett, M., Kramer, J., St. Claire, E.W., et al. (1998). Treatment of rheumatoid arthritis with oral type II collage. *Arthritis and Rheumatism, 41*(2), 290-297.

Bell, M. et al. (1999). Sjögren's syndrome: A critical review of clinical management. *Journal of Rheumatology, 12*(9), 2051–2061.

Bennett, R. (1996). A cost effective approach to the diagnosis and treatment of fibromyalgia. *Rheumatic Disease Clinics of North America, 22*(2), 351–367.

Buchwald, D. (1996). Fibromyalgia and chronic fatigue syndrome: Similarities and differences. *Rheumatic Disease Clinics of North America, 22*(2), 219–243.

Cwynar, D.A., & McNerney, T. (1999). A primer on physical therapy. *Lippincott's Primary Care Practice, 3*(4), 451–459.

Gates, S.J. & Mooar, P.A. (1999). *Musculoskeletal primary care.* Philadelphia: Lippincott Williams & Wilkins.

Gladman, D. (1998). Psoriatic arthritis. *Rheumatic Disease Clinics of North America, 24*(4), 829–844.

Klippel, J.H. (Ed.) (1997). *Primer on rheumatologic disease* (11th ed.). Atlanta: Arthritis Foundation.

McCain, G. (1996). A cost effective approach to the diagnosis and Treatment of fibromyalgia. *Rheumatic Disease Clinics of North America, 22*(2), 323–349.

Moreland, L. (1998). Soluble tumor necrosis factor receptor (P75) fusion protein (Embrel) as a therapy for rheumatoid arthritis. *Rheumatic Disease Clinics of North America, 24*(3), 579–587.

Odell, J. (1999). Treatment of early seropositive rheumatoid arthritis with minocycline. *Arthritis and Rheumatism, 42*(8), 1691–1695.

Panush, R. (Ed.). Complementary and Alternative Therapies for Rheumatic Disease I. *Rheumatic Disease Clinics of North America, 25,*(4).

Petri, M. (1998). Treatment of systemic lupus erythematosus: An update. *American Family Physician, 57*(11), 2753–2760.

Rodgers, E. (1999). Treating pain with COX-2 inhibitors. *Nurse Practitioner, 24*(11), 95–102.

Ryan, L., & Brooks, P. (1999). Disease modifying antirheumatic drugs. *Current Opinion in Rheumatology, 11,* 161–166.

Strand, V. et al. (1996). Biologic agents for the treatment of rheumatoid arthritis. *Rheumatic Disease Clinics of North America, 22*(1), 117–127.

Verhoeven, A.C. et al. (1998). Combination therapy in the treatment of rheumatoid arthritis: Updated systematic review. *British Journal of Rheumatology, 37,* 612–619.

Wallis, W., Furst, D., Strand, B., & Keystone, E. (1998). Biologic agents and immunotherapy in rheumatoid arthritis. *Rheumatic Disease Clinics of North America, 24*(3), 537–560.

Infectious Diseases

GENERAL CONSIDERATIONS

◼ The Infectious Disease Process

The transmission of an infectious agent is accomplished by an infectious source, a vector of spread, and a susceptible host. The six components of the infectious disease process (causative agent, reservoir, portal of exit from reservoir, mode of transmission, portal of entry into host, susceptible host) are known as the chain of infection.

Causative Agent
Types
Bacterium, virus, fungus, parasite, rickettsia, helminth, prion
Characteristics
1. Pathogenicity—ability to cause disease.
2. Virulence—disease severity—and invasiveness—ability to enter and move through tissue.
3. Infectious dose—number of organisms needed to initiate infection.
4. Organism specificity—host preference.
5. Antigenic variations—viral genetic recombinations.
6. Toxogenicity—capacity to produce toxins (poisonous substances).
7. Ability to develop resistance to antimicrobial agents (Table 31-1).

Reservoir
The environment in which the infectious agent can survive.
1. Human—patients, health care workers with disease or colonization.
2. Animal—Rocky Mountain spotted fever from ticks, malaria from mosquitoes, rabies from bats, etc.
3. Environment/fomites—dust, garden soil, contaminated water.

Portal of Exit From Reservoir
Paths by which infectious agent leaves the reservoir.
1. Respiratory tract (most common in humans).
2. Gastrointestinal tract.
3. Genitourinary tract.
4. Open lesions.
5. From bloodstream or tissues by insect bites, hypodermic needles, or surgical instruments.

Mode of Transmission
There are four main routes of transmission.
Contact Transmission
1. Direct contact—person to person.
2. Indirect contact—usually an inanimate object.
3. Droplet contact—large particles from coughing, sneezing, or talking by an infected person.
Common Vehicle Route
(Through Contaminated Items)
1. Food—salmonellosis.
2. Water—shigellosis, legionellosis.
3. Drugs—bacteremia resulting from infusion of a contaminated infusion product.
4. Blood—hepatitis B.
Airborne Transmission
1. Droplet nuclei—residue of evaporated droplets that remain suspended in air.
2. Dust particles in the air containing the infectious agent.
Vector-Borne Transmission
Mechanical or biological spread from vectors such as flies, mosquitoes, ticks, and rats.

Portal of Entry Into Host
Paths by which infectious agent enters the human body.
1. Respiratory tract
2. Gastrointestinal tract
3. Genitourinary tract
4. Direct infection of mucous membranes/break in skin
   a. Parenteral (via blood)
   b. Transplacental—from mother to fetus

Susceptible Host
1. One who lacks effective resistance to infectious agent.
2. Factors influencing susceptibility:

TABLE 31-1 Antibiotic-Resistant Organisms

Organism	Overview and Transmission	Prevention (All)
Methicillin and oxacillin-resistant *Staphylococcus aureus* (MRSA, ORSA)	Found in nasal secretions, on skin. Can produce toxins and invade body tissues. Transmitted primarily via hands of healthcare workers. Only effective antibiotic—vancomycin.	1. Handwashing with antimicrobial soap. 2. Use of gloves and gowns for patient contact.
Vancomycin-resistant *Enterococci* (VRE)	Found in GI tract and female genital tract. Relatively weak pathogen but if infection occurs, treatment options are limited. Transmitted via hands of health care workers and direct contact with contaminated equipment and surfaces.	3. Isolate patient in private room—Contact Isolation. 4. Cohort staff. 5. Use disposable equipment or disinfect reusable items after removal from room.
Vancomycin intermediate-resistant *Staphylococcus aureus* (VISA), also known as glycopeptide-resistant *S. aureus* (GISA)	Transmitted via hands of health care workers and direct contact with contaminated equipment and surfaces. First documented in 1996. Once identified, measures *must* be taken to prevent spread. CDC and state health department must be notified. Strictly follow Contact Precautions and dedicate staff for one-on-one care.	6. Utilize a system for prompt identification and isolation of patients upon readmission.

a. Number of organisms to which host is exposed; duration of exposure.

b. Age, genetic constitution of host, and general physical, mental, and emotional health and nutritional status of host.

c. Status of hematopoietic system; efficacy of reticuloendothelial system.

d. Absent or abnormal immunoglobulins.

e. The number of T lymphocytes and their ability to function.

DIAGNOSTIC TESTS

Collection of Specimens

Proper collection of specimens is important to maximize the outcome of laboratory tests for the diagnosis of infectious diseases. A variety of laboratory tests can be performed to make a presumptive or definitive diagnosis so that therapy can begin. See Standards of Care Guidelines.

Principles

1. It is imperative that specimens be collected and handled very carefully if the causative agent for infection is to be identified correctly.

2. Specimens should be collected during the acute phase of infection and before the initiation of antibiotic therapy, if possible.

3. Obtain an adequate amount of the specimen necessary for tests.

4. Avoid potential contamination of the specimen by using proper collection instruments and containers. Check laboratory guidelines for the correct type of swab and container to use.

5. Label the container properly with the name of the patient, source of the specimen, date, time collected, and test to be performed.

6. Transport the specimen to the laboratory expeditiously or store properly until transported.

Types of Specimen Collection
Blood

1. Normally a sterile body fluid.

2. Specimens obtained by venipuncture are preferred over sampling from vascular catheters.

3. Timing is determined by the patient's clinical condition and should be indicated by the ordering clinician. Usually collection is spaced over 24 hours.

4. Aseptic technique is essential to avoid contaminating the specimen with organisms colonizing the skin.

5. Cleanse the site of venipuncture with povidone-iodine and allow to dry. If the patient is allergic to iodine preparations, use 70% alcohol.

6. The diaphragm tops of the culture bottles are not sterile and must be wiped with povidone-iodine or alcohol before injection of blood.

NURSING ALERT

Do not change needles on the syringe between injections of blood into the culture bottles. The risk of needlestick with a blood-contaminated sharp is too great.

Urine

1. Normally a sterile body fluid.

2. A clean-catch *midstream* urine collection provides the best method for obtaining a specimen to detect a urinary tract infection. The urinary meatus must be cleansed, preferably with povidone-iodine. Patients *must* be thoroughly instructed about how to clean themselves before voiding into sterile specimen containers.

3. Patients who are catheterized should have the specimen withdrawn using a sterile needle and syringe from the catheter sampling port. Clamp the collection tube for about 30 minutes before taking the sample.

4. Urine specimens *must* be transported to the laboratory promptly. If not cultured within 30 minutes of collection, urine must be refrigerated and cultured within 24 hours.

5. Urine specimens that have more than 100,000 colonies of bacteria per milliliter of urine may be indicative of infection.

Stool

1. Obtained to culture organisms that are not part of the normal bowel flora (eg, salmonella, shigella, rotavirus).
2. Patient should defecate into a container. Stool specimens should not contain urine or water from the toilet bowl.
3. Stool specimens can also be obtained directly from the rectum using a sterile swab.

Sputum

1. Specimen needs to be from the lower respiratory tract, not oropharyngeal secretions. The laboratory will perform a Gram stain on all sputum specimens to determine if they are representative of pulmonary secretions. A specimen containing a majority of cells from squamous epithelium will be rejected.
2. The most common method of collection is expectoration from a cooperative patient with a productive cough. Early morning is the optimal time to collect sputum specimens.
3. A sputum specimen can be collected in a sputum trap from patients who have artificial airways and require suctioning.
4. If a patient cannot produce sputum, sputum induction using an aerosol nebulizer may assist with loosening thickened secretions.

5. Bronchoscopy may be required to obtain sputum if induction fails.

Wounds

1. Specimens are cultured for aerobic and anaerobic organisms.
2. Using a sterile cotton-tipped swab, collect as much exudate as possible from the advancing margin of the lesion. Avoid swabbing surrounding skin.
3. Place the swab immediately in appropriate transport culture tube and take to the laboratory.
4. Label with the specific anatomic site.

Throat

1. Use a tongue depressor to hold the tongue down.
2. Carefully yet firmly rub swab over areas of exudate or over the tonsils and posterior pharynx, avoiding the cheeks, teeth and gums.
3. Insert swab into packet and follow directions for handling the transport medium.

■ Laboratory Tests
Microbiologic Evaluation
Microscopy

1. Microscopic examination distinguishes tissue cells from microorganisms.
2. Stains are added to highlight the structural characteristics of microorganisms (eg, Gram stain, acid-fast stains to isolate mycobacteria).
3. Classification is done according to their shape and size: gram-positive versus gram-negative, rods versus cocci, bacteria versus viruses.
4. Results of microscopy are usually available within minutes, which permits the initiation of treatment based on a presumptive diagnosis.

Culture

1. Allows for positive identification of the organism.
2. Different culture media are used for suspected pathogens. A liquid medium is used for blood specimens because fewer microorganisms can be detected. A solid medium will grow polymicrobial cultures.
3. Recovery of the pathogen from cultures will vary based on the type of microorganism, the type of specimen, and the stage of illness. Many common pathogens, such as *Staphylococci*, *Streptococci*, and *Enterococcus* will be identified in 48 hours.
   a. Fungal organisms may take up to 10 days to culture.
   b. Viruses may take weeks to grow in culture.

Antibiotic Susceptibility Testing

1. Used to determine minimal concentration of antibiotics that will inhibit growth of an organism.
   a. Minimum inhibitory concentration (MIC)—amount of drug that will inhibit visible growth—is measured by the size of the zone around the disk in which growth is inhibited.
   b. Results of agar diffusion tests are reported as "resistant" if growth is not altered, "sensitive" if growth is

inhibited, and "intermediate" if results are uncertain or indeterminate.

White Blood Cell Count

1. Nonspecific tests that provide important information about the inflammatory response of a patient as well as the response to therapy.
2. The total number of circulating leukocytes and the differential (given as a percent of the total white blood cell count) may change during a bacterial or viral infection.
3. During an acute bacterial infection, the white blood cell count increases (>11,000/mm^3), accompanied by increased neutrophils and increased bands (immature neutrophils) in the differential. The shift (to the left) in differential reflects phagocytic activity.

Immunologic Tests

1. Pathogens that are antigenic stimulate antibodies that can be detected in the serum of patients.
2. Detection of antibodies is not diagnostic of current infection.
3. Antigen–antibody reactions must be evaluated over a period of time.
4. Immunoglobulin M (IgM) antibody production peaks during active infection and decreases during convalescence.
5. Immunoglobulin G (IgG) antibodies peak during convalescence and persist.
6. A fourfold rise in antibody titer during convalescence indicates concurrent infection.

GENERAL PROCEDURES AND TREATMENT MODALITIES

Immunization

Immunity is the resistance that an individual has against disease. Specific immunity to a particular organism implies that an individual has either generated the appropriate antibody in his or her own body or received ready-made antibodies from another source. Immunity may be natural or acquired, passive or active. (See Table 31-2.)

Natural active immunity occurs when antibodies are acquired naturally following an infection. Antibodies are also acquired through *natural passive immunity,* such as from mother to fetus through the placenta or in breast milk.

Passive artificial immunity is achieved through administration of immune globulin or antitoxin. *Active artificial immunity* occurs when antibodies are produced in response to a vaccine or toxoid.

Prevention of Transmission of Infection in the Health Care Facility

In 1996 the Centers for Disease Control and Prevention issued an isolation guideline for hospitals. It synthesizes the major features of Universal Precautions and Body Substance Isolation into a single set of precautions, called Standard Precautions. *Standard Precautions* apply to (1) blood; (2) all body fluids, secretions, and excretions except sweat, regardless of whether or not they contain visible blood; (3) nonintact skin; and (4) mucous membranes. Standard Precautions are used for the care of *all* patients.

Additional precautions are based on transmission of highly transmissable or epidemiologically important pathogens. These *Transmission-Based Precautions,* designed to reduce the risk of airborne, droplet, and contact transmission in hospitals, are used along with Standard Precautions. There are three types of Transmission-Based Precautions: Airborne Precautions, Droplet Precautions, and Contact Precautions.

Fundamentals of Standard Precautions
Handwashing

1. Handwashing is the single most important measure to reduce the risks of transmitting microorganisms.
2. Washing hands as promptly and thoroughly as possible between patient contacts; after contact with blood, body fluids, secretions, excretions, and contaminated equipment or articles; and after gloves are removed is vital for infection control.
3. It may be necessary to wash hands between tasks on the same patient to prevent cross-contamination of different body sites.

Gloves

1. Gloves are worn to provide a protective barrier and prevent gross contamination of the hands of health care workers and to reduce the transmission of microorganisms to patients.
2. Wearing gloves does *not* replace the need for handwashing because gloves may have small, inapparent defects or may be torn during use, and hands can become contaminated during removal of gloves.
3. Gloves also *must be* changed between patients to prevent infections.

Patient Placement

1. Patient placement is a significant component of isolation precautions. A private room is recommended for a patient with poor hygienic habits or highly transmissible or epidemiologically significant microorganisms.
2. When a private room is not available, two patients infected with the same organism can share a room; this is known as cohorting.
3. A private room with appropriate air handling is important for microorganisms spread by airborne transmission.

Limiting the Movement of Patients

1. Limiting the movement of patients with virulent or epidemiologically important microorganisms reduces transmission.
2. When transport is necessary, appropriate barriers such as masks and impervious dressings are worn by the patient, and personnel in the area to which the patient is to

TABLE 31-2 Guide for Adult Immunization

Population	Vaccination	Dosage
Universally Recommended		
All adults	Tetanus-diphtheria toxoid	One dose administered every 10 years, IM.
All adults aged >50 years	Influenza	One dose administered annually, IM.
All adults aged >65 years	Pneumococcal	One dose, boosters recommended for some high-risk populations, IM or SC.
Recommended for Certain Populations		
Persons aged 15–70 who reside, work, or recreate in areas of high or moderate risk of Lyme disease	Lyme disease vaccine	Three IM doses—initial, second dose 1 month later, third dose 6–12 months after first.
Persons at increased risk for hepatitis A virus (HAV) infection or its consequences, eg, travelers, persons with chronic liver disease	Hepatitis A vaccine	Two IM doses, 6–12 months apart.
Strongly Recommended for Health Care Workers (HCWs)		
HCWs at risk for exposure to blood or body fluids	Hepatitis B recombinant vaccine	Two doses IM 4 weeks apart, third dose 5 months after second. Booster doses not necessary.
HCWs who have contact with patients at high risk for influenza or its complications; HCWs who work in chronic care facilities; HCWs with high-risk medical conditions or aged >50 years	Influenza vaccine	Annual vaccination IM with current vaccine.
HCWs born during or after 1957 who do not have documentation of having received 2 doses of live vaccine on or after the first birthday or a history of physician-diagnosed measles or serologic evidence of immunity, including those born after 1957	Measles, mumps, rubella vaccine (MMR)	One dose SC.
HCWs who do not have either a reliable history of varicella or serologic evidence of immunity	Varicella zoster live-virus vaccine	Two 0.5-mL doses SC 4–8 weeks apart.
Other Vaccines That May Be Indicated for HCWs		
Persons who work with HAV-infected primates or with HAV in a research laboratory setting	Hepatitis A vaccine	Two IM doses 6–12 months apart.
Workers in microbiology laboratories who frequently work with *Salmonella typhi*	Typhoid vaccine, IM, SC, and oral	IM—one dose followed by boosters every 2 years. SC—two doses at least 4 weeks apart followed by boosters every 3 years. Oral—four doses on alternate days; repeat 4-dose series every 5 years.

Abbreviations: IM—intramuscular; SC—subcutaneous.
Note: Some states are considering vaccination of college students for *N. meningitidis*.

be taken are notified. When appropriate, patients are informed how they can assist in preventing transmission.

Masks and Goggles or Face Shields

1. In order to protect the mucous membranes of the eyes, nose, and mouth, masks and goggles or face shields are worn by health care workers during patient care when there is a likelihood of splashes or sprays of blood, body fluids, and secretions.
2. A surgical mask is worn by hospital personnel to provide protection against spread of infectious large-particle droplets during close patient contact.

Air Filters

When caring for patients with known or suspected tuberculosis, health care workers are to wear a N95 respirator, a high-efficiency particulate air (HEPA) filter respirator, or a powered air-purifying respirator (PAPR).

Gowns

1. Gowns are worn to prevent contamination of clothing and to protect the skin of personnel from blood and body fluid exposures.
2. Impermeable gowns, leg coverings, boots, or shoe covers provide greater protection to the skin when splashes or large quantities of infective material are anticipated.
3. Gowns are also worn during the care of patients infected with epidemiologically important pathogens to reduce transmission from patients or items in the environment to other patients. These gowns are removed upon leaving the patient's environment and hands are washed.

Care of Equipment

1. Soiled linen should be handled, transported, and laundered in a manner that avoids transfer of microorganisms to patients, personnel, and environments.

2. No special precautions are needed for dishes, glasses, cups, or eating utensils since the combination of hot water and detergents used in hospital dishwashers is sufficient for decontamination.

3. Patient-care equipment that is soiled with blood, body fluids, secretions, and excretions must be handled in a manner that prevents skin and mucous membrane exposures, contamination of clothing, and transfer of microorganisms to other patients and environments. Reusable equipment must be cleaned and reprocessed appropriately before use for another patient. Single-use items must be discarded properly.

4. Care must be taken to prevent injuries from needles, scalpels, and other sharp objects. Used needles must never be recapped using both hands, removed from syringes, bent, broken, or otherwise manipulated. Used needles and sharps must be disposed of into puncture-resistant containers, which are located as close as is practical to the area of use.

5. Mouthpieces, resuscitation bags, or other ventilation devices are used instead of mouth-to-mouth resuscitation methods.

Transmission-Based Precautions Techniques
Airborne Precautions

1. Designed to reduce the risk of airborne transmission of infectious agents through dissemination of droplet nuclei (small-particle residue of evaporated droplets that may remain suspended in the air for long periods of time) or dust particles containing the infectious agent.

2. Microorganisms carried in this manner can be dispersed widely by air currents and may become inhaled by or deposited on a susceptible host within the same room or over a longer distance from the source patient. Therefore, special air handling and ventilation are required.

3. Examples of illnesses requiring Airborne Precautions: measles, varicella (including disseminated zoster), tuberculosis.

4. Place the patient in a private room that has:
   a. Monitored negative air pressure in relation to the surrounding areas.
   b. Six to 12 air changes per hour.
   c. Appropriate discharge of air outdoors or monitored high-efficiency filtration of room air before recirculation. Keep the room door closed and the patient in the room.

5. Wear respiratory protection when entering the room of a patient with known or suspected pulmonary tuberculosis.

6. Health care workers who are susceptible should not enter the rooms of patients known or suspected to have measles (rubeola) or chickenpox (varicella). If susceptible individuals must enter the room, they should wear a surgical mask. Persons immune to rubeola or varicella need not wear a mask.

7. Limit the transport of the patient from the room to essential purposes only. If transport is necessary, minimize patient dispersal of droplet nuclei by placing a surgical mask on the patient.

Droplet Precautions

1. Designed for care of patients known or suspected to be infected with microorganisms transmitted by droplets (large particles) that can be generated by the patient during coughing, sneezing, talking, or the performance of procedures.

2. Examples of illnesses requiring Droplet Precautions:
   a. Invasive *Haemophilus influenzae* type b disease, including meningitis, pneumonia, epiglotitis, and sepsis.
   b. Invasive *Neiserria meningitidis* disease, including meningitis, pneumonia, and sepsis.
   c. Diphtheria, *Mycoplasma* pneumonia, pertussis, pneumonic plague, streptococcal pharyngitis, pneumonia, or scarlet fever in infants and young children.
   d. Adenovirus, influenza, mumps, Parvovirus B19, rubella.

3. Place the patient in a private room.
   a. When a private room is not available, place patients with the same microorganism together (cohorting).
   b. If neither of these is possible, maintain spatial separation of at least 3 feet between the infected patient and other patients and visitors.

4. Special air handling and ventilation are not necessary, and the door may remain open.

5. Wear a mask when working within 3 feet of the patient.

6. Limit the transport of the patient from the room to essential purposes only. If transport is necessary, minimize dispersal of droplets by masking the patient.

Contact Precautions

1. Used for patients known or suspected to be infected or colonized with epidemiologically important microorganisms that can be transmitted by direct contact with the patient (hand or skin-to-skin contact that occurs when performing patient care activities that require touching the patient's dry skin) or indirect contact (touching) with environmental surfaces of patient care items in the patient's environment.

2. Examples of microorganisms requiring Contact Precautions:
   a. Methicillin (oxacillin)-resistant *Staphylococcus aureus* (MRSA [ORSA]).
   b. Vancomycin-resistant *Enterococcus* (VRE).
   c. Vancomycin-intermediate-resistant *S. aureus* (VISA), also known as glycopeptide-resistant *S. aureus* (GISA).
   d. *Clostridium difficile*.
   e. For diapered or incontinent patients, *Escherichia coli* 0157:H7, Shigella, hepatitis A, rotavirus.
   f. Respiratory syncytial virus, parainfluenza virus, or enteroviral infections in young children; diphtheria; herpes simplex virus.

(*text continues on page 972*)

TABLE 31-3 Selected Infectious Diseases

Disease, Infectious Agent, and Transmission	Clinical Manifestations	Incubation Period	Diagnostic Tests	Management	Complications	Nursing Considerations
Vector-Transmitted Fevers						
Rocky Mountain Spotted Fever *Rickettsia rickettsii* Carried by American dog tick in east and Rocky Mountain wood tick in west	Fever, malaise, myalgia, severe headache, nausea, and vomiting. Rash usually begins on day 4 on wrists and ankles, progresses to palms and soles, then to proximal extremities and trunk as small red or pink macules; blanch with pressure, evolve into petechia and purpura.	Related to the size of the inoculum. Usually 1 week with a range of 1–14 days.	Immunofluorescence of body tissue may identify rickettsiae during the 3rd or 4th day of illness. Serology—increase in antibody titer can usually be detected after 7–10 days of illness, but may be delayed for 4 or more weeks if antibiotic therapy is begun early. Titers wane rapidly in late convalescence.	Doxycycline 100 mg bid or cheoramphenicol 1000 mg qid po or IV for 7 days or for 2 days after afebrile. Supportive therapy including fluid replacement, control of fever, transfusion may be necessary.	Shock Disseminated intravascular coagulation (DIC) Thrombosis and gangrene Cardiac arrhythmias Neurologic sequelae Renal failure Coma and death	1. Not communicable person to person. 2. Instruct patient to report reoccurrence of symptoms immediately; may be relapse. 3. Stress prevention through avoidance of tick-infested areas, wearing protective clothing and tick repellent, inspecting body and clothes for ticks every 3–4 hours. 4. Remove ticks with tweezers or forceps to avoid leaving mouth parts in skin.
Lyme Disease *Borrelia burgdorferi* Tickborne	Erythema migrans (EM), the first manifestation in 60% of patients, is the best clinical marker—an annular skin lesion that appears at the site of the tick bite and expands over a period of days to weeks and develops central clearing. Flulike symptoms—malaise, fever, headache, stiff neck, myalgia. Inflamed painful arthritis and/or lymphadenopathy. Limb weakness. Bell's palsy, cerebellar ataxia.	3–32 days after tick exposure.	IFA, ELISA, and immunoblotting techniques of blood are helpful but not always reliable. Biopsies of skin lesions yield the organism in about 50% of cases.	Doxycycline 100 mg bid or amoxicillin 500 mg tid po for 14–21 days. Ceftriaxone, cefotaxime, penicillin G IV regimens x 3–4 weeks for disseminated infection.	Meningeal irritation leading to meningitis, encephalitis Chorea Atrioventricular block Chronic neurologic manifestations such as encephalopathy, polyneuropathy Chronic arthritis	1. Not communicable person to person. 2. Preventive measures include: (a) vaccine (see Table 32-1); (b) in tick-infested areas, wearing protective clothing; (c) using insect repellent; (d) avoiding tick-infested areas; (e) while working or playing in infested areas, inspection of the body and clothing should be performed every 3–4 hours.

(continued)

TABLE 31-3 Selected Infectious Diseases (Continued)

Disease, Infectious Agent, and Transmission	Clinical Manifestations	Incubation Period	Diagnostic Tests	Management	Complications	Nursing Considerations
						3. Ticks should be removed from the skin with tweezers or forceps, using gentle, steady traction to avoid leaving mouth parts in the skin. Protect hands with gloves, cloth, or tissue when removing ticks.
Viral Infections						
Influenza types A, B and C with many subtypes Airborne	Acute, usually self-limited febrile illness associated with upper and lower respiratory infection. Characterized by a severe and protracted cough, fever, headache, myalgia, coryza, and sore throat.	1–3 days.	Isolation of virus from pharyngeal or nasal secretions or identification of viral antigens in nasopharyngeal cells by fluorescent antibody test or ELISA.	Aspirin or acetaminophen for control of fever. Amantadine or rimantadine as prophylaxis for high-risk persons for influenza type B. Amantadine or rimantadine is given as therapy within 24–48 hours of symptoms of influenza A illness and given for 3–5 days; reduces symptoms. Zanamivir inhalation or oral oseltamivir, started within 36 hours of symptoms and continued for 5 days, can shorten the duration and possibly reduce the incidence of complications. Agent-specific antibiotics for bacterial complications.	Secondary bacterial pneumonia Primary viral pneumonia During major epidemics, severe illness and death occur, primarily among the elderly and chronically ill	1. Highly infectious via aerosolization or droplets from the respiratory tract of infected persons. 2. Best means of prevention—annual influenza vaccination, particularly for high-risk groups and HCWs (see Table 31-2). 3. Maintain bed rest for at least 48 hours after fever subsides. Force fluids. Report symptoms of secondary infection (purulent nasal drainage or sputum, ear pain, increase in fever) to health care provider. 4. Continue antibiotics prescribed for bacterial complications for defined time period (usually 7–10 days).
Mononucleosis *Epstein-Barr virus (EBV)* Direct contact (oropharyngeal)	Fever, exudative pharyngitis, fatigue, splenomegaly, and lymphadenopathy.	4–6 weeks	Lymphocytosis >50%, with more than 10% being atypical lymphocytes, abnormalities in liver function	Supportive therapy to include aspirin or acetaminophen for sore throat and fever, bed rest.	Splenic rupture Thrombocytopenia purpura Hemolytic anemia Pericarditis	1. Person-to-person spread via saliva is prolonged—a year or more after infection.

Disease/Agent/Transmission	Clinical manifestations	Incubation period	Diagnostic tests	Treatment	Complications	Nursing considerations
			tests (AST), or an elevated heterophile antibody titer. Not useful diagnostic tool in children under 5 years of age. If negative, EBV IgM and IgA may be performed.	Surgical removal of the spleen for splenic rupture. Corticosteroids for severe neurologic complications, thrombocytopenia purpura, or hemolytic anemia.	Hepatitis Encephalitis	2. Convalescence may be as long as several months. 3. Patients with splenomegaly should avoid activity that may increase the risk of injury to the spleen, such as contact sports and heavy lifting. 4. Report any excess bruising or bleeding, jaundice, or abnormal CNS functioning.
Cytomegalovirus (CMV) Direct contact with mucous membranes, secretions, and excretions; fetus may be infected in utero or at delivery	Ordinarily asymptomatic, especially in children. Clinical disease in the adult resembles mononucleosis. More extensive organ involvement in the immunosuppressed host—hepatitis, pneumonitis, retinitis may occur. GI tract disorders. Congenital infections are serious and lead to irreversible CNS and liver damage.	3–8 weeks following transplant or transfusion; in neonates 3–12 weeks following delivery-produced infection.	Virus culture. CMV antigen detection. CMV DNA detection by PCR. Serologic studies for CMV-specific IgM antibody or a fourfold rise in titer.	Supportive therapy for control of fever and sore throat. Hyperimmune gamma globulin as a prophylactic agent for patients undergoing marrow transplantation.	Congenital infection leads to neurologic defects (severe mental retardation, microcephaly, psychomotor retardation, hearing loss, and evidence of chronic liver disease). Immunocompromised host—progressive pneumonitis, hemolytic anemia, hepatitis, pericarditis, and GI ulceration	1. Patients with splenomegaly should avoid activity that may increase the risk of injury to the spleen, such as contact sports and heavy lifting. 2. Report any excess bruising or bleeding, jaundice, or abnormal CNS functioning. 3. Pregnant personnel should be counseled about potential risks and urged to practice good hygiene, especially handwashing.
Rabies Rabies virus Direct contact of virus-laden saliva of a rabid animal into a bite or scratch	Initial symptoms nonspecific and consist of malaise, fatigue, headache, and fever. May have pain or paresthesia at the site of exposure. Usually lasts 2–10 days. Progresses to paresis or paralysis, hydrophobia, eventually to delirium and convulsions.	Usually 3–8 weeks. Shorter when the site of the bite is on the head than when it is on an extremity, due to proximity to brain.	Specific FA staining of brain tissue or by virus isolation, or FA staining of frozen skin sections taken from back of neck.	Rabies is a disease best controlled through prevention rather than treatment. Supportive therapy to manage neurologic, respiratory, and cardiac symptoms. Use of high-dose passive rabies immunoglobulin or vaccine after the onset of illness has not been successful.	Almost invariably progresses to death.	1. Contact isolation for respiratory secretions, especially saliva, for duration of illness. 2. Pre-exposure prophylaxis should be offered to persons at high risk for exposure to rabies, such as veterinarians, veterinary students, wildlife (continued)

TABLE 31-3 Selected Infectious Diseases (Continued)

Disease, Infectious Agent, and Transmission	Clinical Manifestations	Incubation Period	Diagnostic Tests	Management	Complications	Nursing Considerations
	Respiratory arrest usually occurs, followed by death.					personnel, park rangers, staff of kennels, and laboratory workers working with rabies.
						3. Bites from animals, particularly dogs and cats, should be thoroughly flushed and cleaned with soap and water immediately. Wounds should not be sutured unless unavoidable.
						4. Domestic dogs and cats should be quarantined for 10 days.
						5. Wild animal carriers include skunk, bat, fox, coyote, raccoon, bobcat, wolf, jackal and other carnivores.
						6. Postexposure prophylaxis must include the use of human rabies immunoglobulin (HRIG) followed by Human Diploid Cell Vaccine (HDCV) unless pre-exposure prophylaxis with HDCV had been administered. HDCV requires 5 doses IM.
Protozoan Infections						
Malaria *Plasmodium vivax, P. falciparum, P. malariae,* and *P. ovale* Vector borne—bite of female Anopheles	Malarial paroxysm characterized by variations of high fever, chills, sweats, headache, rigor, cough, diarrhea, respiratory distress.	Variable depending on the strain.	Diagnosis of malaria rests on the demonstration of parasites in stained peripheral blood smears. Repeated smears may be necessary.	General management should include: IV fluids and electrolytes— restrict fluids in cerebral edema. Assisted ventilation	Shock Acute encephalopathy Renal failure Hepatic failure Cerebral and pulmonary edema	1. Patients with *P. vivax* or *P. ovale* may have recurrence of symptoms and should report them immediately.

Disease / Organism / Transmission	Signs and Symptoms	Incubation	Diagnostic Tests	Complications	Treatment	Nursing Considerations
mosquito; congenital; vehicle—through transfusions or dirty needles	As infection becomes synchronized, fever and paroxysms generally are cyclic. Moderate splenomegaly and tender hepatomegaly.		Leukopenia, hemolytic anemia (normocytic, normochromic), platelets decreased (less than 50,000/mm³). Liver function tests reveal elevated transaminase level and increase in indirect serum bilirubin.	Disseminated intravascular coagulation (DIC) Coma Death	with pulmonary edema. Dialysis in renal failure. Transfusions in anemia. Chemotherapy is based on infecting species, possible drug resistance and severity of disease. Drugs used include chloroquine phosphate, quinidine gluconate, quinine dihydrochloride/sulfate.	2. Travelers to malaria-endemic countries should follow preventive measures: Proper use of mosquito netting at night. Clothing that minimizes contact with mosquitoes. Use of insect repellents. Chemoprophylaxis with suppressive drugs, based on local endemicity and resistance.
Amebiasis *Entamoeba histolytica* Ingestion of fecally contaminated food or water; sexually by oral–anal contact	*Intestinal disease:* May be asymptomatic or mild symptoms such as abdominal distention, flatulence, constipation, and occasionally loose stools. *Nondysenteric colitis:* Recurring episodes of loose stools. Vague abdominal pain. Hemorrhoids with occasional rectal bleeding. *Dysenteric colitis:* Abdominal cramps and diarrhea containing blood and mucus.	Variable—3 days to months or years; usually 2–4 weeks.	Microscopic examination of stool, rectal secretions; positive for trophozoites or cysts of protozoan.	Amebic granulomata of intestinal wall Penile lesions in active homosexuals Abscess of lung or brain Hepatic abscess	Treatment regimens depend on the severity of the illness. Metronidazole followed by iodoquinol, paromomycin, or diloxanide furoate.	1. Instruct patient to wash hands thoroughly after defecating to prevent transmission to others. 2. Household and sexual contacts should seek medical examination and treatment. 3. Instruct patient on safe sexual practices. 4. Travelers to areas where the water supply is not chemically treated or protected from sewage should boil all water used for drinking and cooking. 5. Relapses after treatment are common. Follow-up should be scheduled at 6 weeks and 6 months after treatment.
Giardiasis *Giardia lamblia* Fecal–oral transmission or ingestion of	*Acute:* Explosive, watery diarrheal stool.	1–4 weeks.	Examination of stool; positive for cysts or trophozoites of the *G. lamblia* protozoan.	Chronic diarrhea Malabsorption leading to significant weight	Metronidazole is the drug of choice; 250 mg PO tid for 5 days or 2 g PO qd for 3 days.	1. Instruct patient to wash hands thoroughly after defe-

(continued)

TABLE 31-3 Selected Infectious Diseases (Continued)

Disease, Infectious Agent, and Transmission	Clinical Manifestations	Incubation Period	Diagnostic Tests	Management	Complications	Nursing Considerations
contaminated water or food	Abdominal cramping and flatulence. Nausea. *Chronic:* Intermittent foul-smelling diarrheal stools. Increased flatulence and distention. Anorexia.		Detection of *G. lamblia* antigens by EIA.		loss, failure to thrive, and anemia	cating to prevent transmission to others. 2. Household and sexual contacts should seek medical examination and treatment. 3. Instruct patient on safe sexual practices. 4. Travelers to areas where the water supply is not chemically treated or protected from sewage should boil all water used for drinking and cooking. 5. Relapses after treatment may occur so follow-up should be scheduled.
Hookworm *Ancylostoma duodenale, Necator americanus* Through entry into the skin of soil contaminated with feces from humans, cats, and dogs	Chronic debilitating disease leading to iron-deficiency and hypochromic, microcytic anemia that result from intestinal blood loss to the hookworm.	Symptoms may develop after a few weeks to many months, depending on intensity of infection.	Microscopic examination of cultured stool specimen positive for hookworm eggs.	Mebendazole or pyrantel pamoate. Iron therapy to correct anemia.	Immunosuppressed individuals—septicemia and death In children with heavy, long-term infection—hypoproteinemia, mental and physical retardation	1. Follow-up examination of the stool 2 weeks after therapy is necessary. Repeat therapy if heavy worm burden persists. 2. Nutrition counseling and taking iron supplements is recommended until deficiencies are corrected. 3. Family members and close contacts should be examined and treated for parasites. 4. Educate public about dangers of soil contamination and importance of wearing shoes.

	Clinical Manifestations	Incubation Period	Diagnosis	Treatment	Complications	Nursing Considerations/Prevention
Trichinellosis, trichinosis, *Trichinella spiralis* Ingestion of raw or insufficiently cooked meat, chiefly pork and pork products	Clinical disease highly variable; can range from inapparent infection to a fulminating fatal disease. During first week—abdominal discomfort, nausea and vomiting, diarrhea may occur. Sudden appearance of muscle soreness and pain accompanied by edema of upper eyelids. Ocular signs may progress to subconjunctival, subungual, and retinal hemorrhages; pain; and photophobia. Remittent fever is usual, sometimes as high as 104°F.	5–45 days depending on the number of worms involved; usually 8–15 days after ingestion of infected meat.	Skeletal muscle biopsy not earlier than 10 days after exposure to infection demonstrates the *Trichinella* larvae. Serology; complement fixation, fluorescent antibody—fourfold increase in antibody titer 3 weeks after infection. Differential WBC count—increase in eosinophils to 70%.	Thiabendazole within 24 hours of eating infected meat—25 mg/kg/day for 1 week. Supportive therapy for respiratory, neurologic, and cardiac sequelae.	Cardiac and neurologic—3rd to 6th week Myocardial failure—1st to 2nd or 4th to 8th weeks	1. Instruct patient to thoroughly wash hands after defecation. 2. Proper cooking of pork to 150°F is necessary. 3. Family members and close contacts of patients should be examined and treated for parasites.
Fungal Infections Histoplasmosis *Histoplasma capsulatum* Inhalation of airborne particles from soil or dust that harbor bat, chicken, and/or bird droppings	May be asymptomatic with only hypersensitivity to histoplasmin. Four other forms of disease: 1. *Acute benign respiratory*—mild respiratory illness to temporary flu-like illness. 2. *Acute disseminated*—debilitating fever, GI symptoms, bone marrow suppression, lymphadenopathy; in infants and immunocompromised usually fatal without treatment. 3. *Chronic disseminated*—intermittent fever, weight loss, weakness, hepatosplenomegaly, hematologic abnormalities, focal	Variable, usually 1–3 weeks after exposure.	Complement fixation shows increase in antibodies within 3–4 weeks; fourfold increase suggests disease progression. Fungal culture positive for *H. capsulatum*. Chest x-ray findings: *acute*—transient parenchymal pulmonary infiltrates resembling lobar pneumonia; *chronic*: progressively enlarging areas of necrosis with or without cavitation.	Amphotericin B, ketoconazole, fluconazole. Corticosteroids and diphenhydramine (Benadryl) to minimize the side effects of amphotericin. Bone marrow suppression.	Chronic pulmonary disease Hepatosplenomegaly Death	Investigation for the common source of infection should be done in outbreaks. Educate public to minimize exposure to dust in chicken coops, attics, caves—use protective masks.

(continued)

TABLE 31-3 Selected Infectious Diseases (Continued)

Disease, Infectious Agent, and Transmission	Clinical Manifestations	Incubation Period	Diagnostic Tests	Management	Complications	Nursing Considerations
	disease such as endocarditis, meningitis, mucosal ulcers; usually fatal unless treated. 4. Chronic pulmonary disease—resembles pulmonary tuberculosis with cavitation; occurs most often with underlying emphysema.					
Bacterial Infections Typhoid fever *Salmonella typhi* Ingestion of contaminated food and water	Systemic—insidious onset of fever, severe headache, malaise, anorexia, bradycardia, splenomegaly. Ulceration of the distal ileum; can progress to hemorrhage or perforation.	3 days–3 months, usually 1–3 weeks.	Culture of urine and/or stool positive for *S. typhi* during 2nd week. Culture of blood positive for *S. typhi* during 1st week. Bone marrow culture.	IV fluids and electrolytes. Bed rest. Avoid antispasmodics, laxatives, and salicylates. Chloramphenicol, amoxicillin or TMP-SMX either IV or PO. Immunization is advised for travelers to areas of high endemicity.	Endocarditis Meningitis Pneumonia Pyelonephritis Osteomyelitis Intestinal perforation and hemorrhage Septicemia	1. Transmitted by contaminated food or water and via direct fecal–oral route. 2. Relapses occur in 5–10% of untreated cases and may be more common following antibiotic therapy. Report symptoms immediately. 3. Instruct patient to wash hands thoroughly after defecation and before preparing food. 4. Educate public—control flies, avoid raw shellfish, thoroughly rinse raw fruits and vegetables. 5. Family and close contacts should be examined and treated. 6. Typhoid is communicable for as long as the infective organism is in the feces or urine, which may persist for up to 1 year.

Disease/Organism/Transmission	Signs and Symptoms	Incubation Period	Diagnostic Tests	Treatment	Complications	Nursing Interventions
Botulism *Clostridium botulinum* Foodborne or through contaminated wound	Severe intoxication characterized by visual difficulty, dysphagia, and dry mouth. Followed by descending symmetrical flaccid paralysis. Vomiting and constipation or diarrhea may be present initially.	12–36 hours, sometimes several days after eating contaminated food. Wound—4–14 days after injury.	Culture of *C. botulinum* from stool or stomach contents. Serum positive for botulinal toxins.	IV and IM administration as soon as possible of trivalent botulinum antitoxin, obtained from CDC through state health departments. IV fluids and electrolytes. Intensive care to anticipate and manage respiratory failure: mechanical ventilation. Report to health department immediately.	Death from respiratory failure	1. All patient contacts known to have eaten the same food should have gastric lavage, high enemas, and cathartics and kept under close medical supervision. 2. Instruct patient/patient contacts to wash hands thoroughly after defecation and before handling food. 3. No questionable canned food should ever be tasted.
Tetanus (lockjaw) *Clostridium tetani* Contamination of a wound with organism found in soil; acute disease induced by an exotoxin of the tetanus bacillus	Painful muscular contractions, primarily of the masseter and neck muscles. Abdominal rigidity. Generalized spasms frequently induced by sensory stimuli—opisthotonos (arching of the trunk) and risus sardonicus (distorted grin).	Usually 3–21 days; may range from 1 day to several months; average—10 days.	Organism rarely recovered from the site of infection. No detectable antibody response. Diagnosis is made clinically by excluding other possibilities.	Tetanus immune globulin or tetanus antitoxin. IV metronidazole. Wound care to include cleaning, irrigation, wide debridement. Sedatives and muscle relaxants, sometimes together with tracheostomy or intubation and mechanical ventilation. Cardiac monitoring.	High case fatality rate, up to 90% in infants and elderly. Cardiac arrest. Bacterial shock. Autonomic disturbances.	1. Refer persons with skin injuries for tetanus prophylaxis. 2. Remind adults to receive a tetanus booster every 10 years.
Staphylococci *Staphylococcus aureus* Coagulase-negative staphylococci; *S. epidermidis*, *S. haemolyticus* Direct contact with draining lesions, auto-infection from colonized nares	Skin and soft tissue infections—furuncles (boils), impetigo, carbuncles, cellulitis, abscesses, and infected lacerations. Seeding of the bloodstream may lead to pneumonia, osteomyelitis, septicemia, endocarditis, meningitis, hepatic abscess, splenic abscess, perinephritic abscess.	Variable; usually 4–10 days.	Confirmed by isolation of the organism from culture.	Penicillinase-resistant penicillins (nafcillin) and the cephalosporins (cephalothin). Vancomycin is treatment of choice for methicillin-resistant *S. aureus*. Incision of abscesses to permit drainage of pus. In severe systemic infection, the selection of antibiotics should be governed by results of susceptibility tests on the isolates.	Septicemia Embolic skin lesions Death	1. Monitor patient's response to prescribed therapy. 2. Emphasize meticulous hand washing among patients and visitors. 3. Contain purulent drainage with a dressing. 4. Place soiled dressings in a paper bag before disposal.

(continued)

TABLE 31-3 Selected Infectious Diseases (Continued)

Disease, Infectious Agent, and Transmission	Clinical Manifestations	Incubation Period	Diagnostic Tests	Management	Complications	Nursing Considerations
Streptococci *Streptococcus pyogenes*, group A with approximately 80 serologically distinct types. Large respiratory droplets or direct contact with secretions, ingestion of contaminated food	Streptococcal pharyngitis. Wound and skin infections—impetigo, cellulitis, erysipelas. Scarlet fever (streptococcal sore throat with a rash that occurs if infectious agent produces erythrogenic toxin to which patient is not immune).	Short; usually 1–3 days, rarely longer.	Identification of group A streptococcal antigen in pharyngeal secretions (rapid strep test). Isolation of the organism by culture.	Penicillin is the drug of choice. Therapy should be continued for at least 10 days. Erythromycin for penicillin-allergic patients.	Septicemia Acute glomerulonephritis Rheumatic fever	1. Repeated attacks of sore throat or other streptococcal disease due to different types of streptococci are relatively frequent. 2. Make sure the patient understands the importance of completing the course of antimicrobial therapy. 3. Emphasize the relationship of streptococcal infections to heart disease and glomerulonephritis.
Syphilis *Treponema pallidum*, a spirochete Sexually transmitted; direct contact with infectious exudates	Congenital: can result in stillbirth, hydrops fetalis, prematurity, multisystem abnormalities. Primary: indurated, painless, clean ulcer (chancre). Secondary: generalized macular-papular rash including palms and soles; fever; generalized lymphadenopathy,	Usually 3 weeks, but may be up to 3 months; signs of secondary syphilis develop 6 weeks to 6 months after primary syphilis.	Nonspecific serologic tests such as RPR and VDRL; confirmed by specific antitreponemal antibody tests such as FTA-ABS and MHA-TP; dark-field examination of lesion exudate for organism.	Primary and secondary: parenteral penicillin G; in penicillin allergy, if not pregnant, doxycycline; erythromycin is an inferior substitute in pregnant, penicillin-allergic patients but no proven alternative has been determined. Latent syphilis of longer than 1 year or of unknown duration requires three weekly injections of penicillin G. Tertiary syphilis requires IV penicillin for longer duration.	Tertiary syphilis with cardiac, dermatologic, neurologic, and other systemic manifestations	1. Ensure that sexual activity is not resumed until treatment is complete for both patient and partner. 2. Consider testing for HIV and other sexually transmitted diseases. 3. Encourage follow-up at 3 months for repeat serologic testing.

condylomata, malaise, headache, splenomegaly. Tertiary: aortitis, neurosyphilis, gummatous changes of skin, bone, viscera.

4. All women should be screened serologically for syphilis early in pregnancy.
5. All individuals, including HCWs, who have had close, unprotected contact with patient with early congenital syphilis before or during the first 24 hours of therapy should be examined for lesions in 3 weeks and 3 months.

Prion Disease

Creutzfeldt-Jacob Disease
Prion proteinaceous infectious particles
Unknown in most cases

Potential infectious body fluids include CSF, brain, spinal cord, and eye. Insidious onset with confusion, progressive dementia, ataxia, rigidity.

15 months to more than 30 years.

Brain tissue biopsy. Clinical signs and characteristically periodic EEG.

No treatment, only supportive care.

Fatal degenerative disease

Only infectious agent that requires unique decontamination recommendations. Prion is extremely hardy and resistant to many disinfectants and to normal sterilization practices.
Use disposables as much as possible. Health care facilities should have protocols in place for identification of cases and for instrument reprocessing.

IFA: indirect immunofluorescent antibody; ELISA: enzyme-linked immunosorbent assay; IV: intravenous; bid: twice daily; tid: three times daily; qid: four times daily; WBC: white blood cell; CNS: central nervous system; GI, gastrointestinal; CSF: cerebrospinal fluid; PCR: polymerase chain reaction; RBC: red blood cell; IgM: immunoglobulin class M; FA: direct fluorescent or immunofluorescent antibody test; HIV: human immunodeficiency virus; HCWs: health care workers.

g. Impetigo, major (noncontained) abscesses, cellulitis, or decubiti.

h. Pediculosis, scabies, staphylococcal furunculosis in infants and young children.

i. Zoster

j. Viral hemorrhagic infections (Ebola, Lassa, or Marburg).

3. Place the patient in a private room or in a room with a patient who has the same microorganism.

4. In addition to wearing gloves as outlined under Standard Precautions, wear gloves when entering the room.

a. Change gloves after contact with infective material such as feces and wound drainage.

b. Remove gloves before leaving the patient's environment and wash hands immediately with an antimicrobial soap or waterless antiseptic agent.

c. After glove removal and handwashing, ensure that hands do not touch potentially contaminated environmental surfaces or items in the patient's room.

5. In addition to wearing gloves for Standard Precautions, wear a gown when entering the room if there is likely to be contact with the patient or environmental surfaces, or if the patient has diarrhea, an ileostomy, colostomy, or wound drainage not contained by a dressing.

a. Remove the gown before leaving the patient's environment.

b. After gown removal, ensure that clothing does not contact potentially contaminated surfaces.

6. When possible, dedicate the use of non-critical patient care equipment to a single patient.

7. Thoroughly clean and disinfect reusable equipment before use for another patient.

INFECTIOUS DISORDERS

Infectious disorders are covered throughout the book in a variety of body system chapters. See Table 31-3 for selected infectious disorders. Be aware that new data on infectious diseases are emerging daily. For the latest information on infectious diseases, contact your state public health department or the CDC at *www.cdc.gov.*

■ Emerging Infections

Hantaviral Diseases
Description

1. Hantaviruses infect rodents worldwide.

2. In humans they primarily cause either hemorrhagic fever with renal syndrome or pulmonary syndrome, including acute respiratory distress syndrome (ARDS).

3. Morbidity—50% of reported cases due to pulmonary syndrome.

Transmission

1. Believed to occur through aerosolization of rodent excreta.

2. No person-to-person transmission.

Implications for Nursing

1. Teach prevention through rodent control, proper storage of food, careful wet mop cleaning, and disinfection of rodent-contaminated areas.

Ebola-Marburg Viral Diseases
Description

1. Filoviruses cause severe hemorrhagic fevers, often accompanied by hepatic and renal damage.

2. CNS involvement and shock with multi-organ failure can occur.

3. Mortality—Marburg virus, 25%; Ebola virus, 50% to 90%.

Transmission

Person to person by direct contact with infected blood, secretions, organs, or semen.

Implications for Nursing

1. Strict adherence to Universal/Standard Precautions and Respiratory Precautions and as directed by public health authorities.

West Nile Virus
Description

1. Emerging pathogen in humans.

2. Primarily found in Africa; unknown how it entered U.S.

3. First cases in U.S. in 1999 in New York.

3. Flavivirus may cause encephalitis.

Transmission

1. Bite of infected mosquito that has fed on infected bird.

2. Not transmitted person to person.

Implications for Nursing

1. Teach prevention of mosquito bites by wearing proper clothing and using insect repellent.

SELECTED REFERENCES

Benenson, A.S. (2000). *Control of communicable diseases manual* (17th ed.). Washington, D.C.: American Public Health Association.

Drage, L.A. (1999). Life-threatening rashes: Dermatologic signs of four infectious diseases. *Mayo Clinic Proceedings, 74*(1), 68–72.

Federal Register. (1991). *Occupational exposure to bloodborne pathogens: Final rule.* Washington, D.C.: Occupational Safety and Health Administration, Department of Labor.

Garner, J.S. (1996). Guideline for Isolation Precautions in hospitals. *Infection Control and Hospital Epidemiology, 17,* 53–80.

General recommendations on immunization. (1994). *Morbidity and Mortality Weekly Report, 43,* RR-1.

Immunization of health-care workers. (1997). *Morbidity and Mortality Weekly Report, 46,* RR-18.

Miller, J.M. (1999). *A guide to specimen management in clinical microbiology.* Washington, D.C.: ASM Press.

Peter, G. (Ed.) (2000). *1997 Red Book: Report of the Committee on Infectious Diseases* (25th ed.). Elk Grove Village, IL: American Academy of Pediatrics.

Pugliese, G. (1991). *Universal precautions.* Chicago, IL: American Hospital Publishing.

Vaccine-preventable diseases: Improving vaccination coverage in children, adolescents, and adults. (1999). *Morbidity and Mortality Weekly Report, 48,* RR-8.

CHAPTER

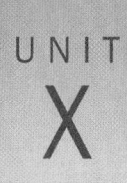

32

Musculoskeletal Disorders

ASSESSMENT

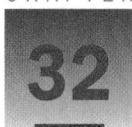 **Subjective Data**

A great deal can be learned about musculoskeletal disorders from subjective data. History of injury, description of symptoms, and associated personal health and family history can give clues to the underlying problem and appropriate care for that problem.

Common Manifestations of Musculoskeletal Problems

Pain

1. Where is the pain located?
   a. Joint(s), as in osteoarthritis (OA)
   b. Muscles or soft tissue, as in contusions, sprains, or strains
   c. Bone, as in fractures or tumors

2. Is it sharp, as in a fracture or sprain, or dull, as in a bone tumor?
3. Does pain radiate?
   a. To buttocks or legs, as in low back pain
   b. To thigh or knee, as in hip fracture
4. What makes the pain increase? What makes it better?

Limited Range of Motion

1. Is stiffness present? How long does it last?
   a. Present in morning for less than 30 minutes with OA
   b. May persist and is associated with acute pain when due to spasm of low back strain
2. Is swelling present and limiting mobility?
   a. May be due to fracture
   b. May be soft tissue injury, such as sprain, strain, or contusion
3. How does limited mobility affect activities of daily living (ADLs)?

Associated Symptoms

1. Any sensory or motor deficits, such as numbness, paresthesias, or weakness, indicating neurovascular compromise?
2. Any weight loss, fever, or malaise, as in bone tumors?
3. Any bony nodules or deformity, as in OA?

History
Mechanism of Injury

1. How did the injury occur? Essential for all trauma, including fractures, contusions, sprains, and strains to help identify the extent of injury.
2. What was the progression of symptoms?
3. If not an acute injury, was there any repetitive movement or strain that may have contributed to problem, as in tendinitis?

Medical History

1. Any history of corticosteroid use that predisposes to osteoporosis?
2. Is the woman postmenopausal? On estrogen replacement? If estrogen deficient, may predispose to osteoporosis.
3. Any history of prostate, breast, or lung cancer, which may metastasize to the bone?
4. What are other chronic conditions that may affect immobility imposed by casting, traction, or surgery?

Social History

1. What is the patient's occupation, which may contribute to low back strain or OA?
2. What activities or sports does the patient participate in, such as running or tennis, that may cause tendinitis?
3. Are there risk factors for osteoporosis, such as smoking, inactivity, or lack of exposure to the sun?
4. Is there a family history of osteoporosis or arthritis?
5. What cultural issues/religious beliefs contribute to this history?

◼ Objective Data

Data on current system condition and functional abilities are secured through inspection, palpation, and measurement. Always compare with contralateral side (one side of the body to the other).

Musculoskeletal System
Skeletal Component

1. Note deviation from normal structure—bony deformities, length discrepancies, alignment, amputations.
2. Identify abnormal motion and crepitus (grating sensation), as found with fractures.

Joint Component

1. Identify swelling that may be due to inflammation or effusion.
2. Note deformity associated with contractures or dislocations.
3. Evaluate stability, which may be altered.
4. Estimate range of motion (ROM), both actively and passively.

Muscle Component

1. Inspect for size and contour of muscles.
2. Assess coordination of movement.
3. Palpate for muscle tone.
4. Estimate strength through cursory evaluation (ie, handshake) or scaled criteria (ie, 0 = no palpable contraction; 5 = normal ROM against gravity with full resistance).
5. Measure girth to note increases due to swelling or bleeding into muscle or decreases due to atrophy (difference of more than 1 cm is significant).
6. Identify abnormal clonus (rhythmic contraction and relaxation) or fasciculation (contraction of isolated muscle fibers).

Additional Assessment
Neurovascular Component

1. Assess circulatory status of involved extremities by noting skin color and temperature, peripheral pulses, capillary refill response, pain.
2. Assess neurologic status of involved extremities by the patient's ability to move distal muscles and description of sensation (eg, paresthesia).
3. Test reflexes of extremities.
4. Compare all to uninjured/unaffected extremity.

Skin Component

1. Inspect traumatic injuries (eg, cuts, bruises).
2. Assess chronic conditions (eg, dermatitis, stasis ulcers).
3. Note hair distribution and nail condition.
4. Inspect for Heberden's or Bouchard's nodes.
5. Assess for warmth or coolness of skin.

DIAGNOSTIC TESTS

◼ Radiologic and Imaging Studies

Many radiologic and imaging studies are helpful in evaluating musculoskeletal problems to rule out fracture or skeletal changes and to differentiate soft tissue injury.

X-rays
Description

1. Of bone—to determine bone density, texture, integrity, erosion, changes in bone relationships
2. Of cortex—to detect any widening, narrowing, irregularity
3. Of medullary cavity—to detect any alteration in density
4. Of involved joint—to show fluid, irregularity, spur formation, narrowing, changes in joint contour
5. Tomogram—special x-ray technique for detailed view of special plane of bone

Nursing and Patient Care Considerations

1. Tell the patient that proper positioning is important to obtain a good x-ray, so cooperation is essential.
2. Advise patient to remove all jewelry, clothing with zippers or snaps, change from pockets, or other items that may interfere with x-ray.

Bone Scan

Description

Parenteral injection of bone-seeking radiopharmaceutical (such as gallium); concentration of isotope uptake revealed in primary skeletal disease (osteosarcoma), metastatic bone disease, inflammatory skeletal disease (osteomyelitis); fracture

Nursing and Patient Care Considerations

1. Advise patient that laxative may be needed before the procedure.
2. Injectable radionuclide may be given 24 to 72 hours before the scan.
3. Reassure patient that there is no pain and that scan will take 1 to 2 hours. Analgesics/sedatives may be ordered for patients for whom lying immobile for any length of time is difficult.
4. Breast-feeding should be discontinued for at least 4 weeks after test to prevent radionuclide exposure to infant.
5. Patients should be told that the exposure to radioactive substances is small, and substances are excreted quickly by the body.
6. Patients should be taught to flush the toilet three times after voiding so the small amount of radioactive material does not stay in the toilet bowl.

Bone Densitometry

Description

A noninvasive study that yields an actual measurement of bone density and is diagnostic for osteoporosis. Simple portable screening tests that analyze the wrist or heel are also available.

Nursing and Patient Care Considerations

1. No special preparation or restrictions.
2. Have patient remove clothing and all jewelry or other metal objects.
3. Advise patient to lie still with hips flexed during test; technician will remain in room.
4. Reassure that radiation exposure is minimal.

Magnetic Resonance Imaging (MRI)

Description

Uses magnetic fields to demonstrate differences in hydrogen density of various tissues. Demonstrates tumors and soft tissue (muscle, ligament, tendon) abnormalities. Although it is more costly than computed tomography (CT) scans, the cost is often validated through the diagnostic accuracy. MRI not only clearly defines internal organs, but also is able to detect nerve damage and changes, such as edema or bruises, of bone. Bone bruises (osseous contusions) with traumatic injuries have some predictive value for future development of post-traumatic arthritis.

Nursing and Patient Care Considerations

1. Prepare patient for need to lie still for about 1 hour; repetitive clanging noise of machine will be heard; patients may feel closed in.
2. Practice relaxation techniques, such as relaxation breathing and imagery, ahead of time.
3. Some patients may need sedation; claustrophobic patients may be unable to undergo procedure or may need open MRI.
4. Contraindicated for patients with metal implants, prosthetic valves, surgical clips, pacemakers, and orthopedic hardware.

NURSING ALERT

 Patients with metal implants, metal braces, or pacemakers are unable to undergo MRI.

Other Tests

1. Arthrogram—injection of radiopaque substance or air into joint cavity to outline soft tissue structures (eg, meniscus) and contour of joint.
2. Myelogram—injection of contrast medium into subarachnoid space at lumbar spine to determine level of disk herniation or site of tumor.
3. Diskogram—injection of small amount of contrast medium into lumbar disk abnormalities.
4. Arthrocentesis—insertion of needle into joint and aspiration of synovial fluid for purposes of examination.
5. Arthroscopy—endoscopic procedure that allows direct visualization of joint structures (synovium, articular surfaces, menisci, ligaments) through a large-bore needle. May be combined with arthrography.
6. Nerve studies—to differentiate nerve root compression, muscle disease (eg, dystrophy, myositis), peripheral neuropathies, central nervous system–anterior horn cell neuropathies, neuromuscular junction problems.
   a. Electromyography (EMG)—measures electrical potential generated by the muscle during relaxation and contraction.
   b. Nerve conduction velocities—measure the rate of potential generation along specific nerves (speed of impulse conduction).

GENERAL PROCEDURES AND TREATMENT MODALITIES

Crutch Walking

Crutches are artificial supports that assist patients who need aid in walking because of disease, injury, or a birth defect.

Preparation for Crutch Walking

Goals: Develop power in the shoulder girdle and upper extremities that bear the patient's weight in crutch walking. Strengthen and condition the patient.

Strengthening the Muscles Needed for Ambulation

Instruct the patient as follows:

1. For quadriceps setting:
   a. Contract the quadriceps muscle while attempting to push the popliteal area against the mattress and raise the heel.

b. Maintain the muscle contracture for the count of 5.

c. Relax for the count of 5.

d. Repeat this exercise 10 to 15 times hourly.

2. For gluteal setting:

   a. Contract or pinch the buttocks together for a count of 5.

   b. Relax for the count of 5.

   c. Repeat 10 to 15 times hourly.

Strengthening the Muscles of the Upper Extremities and Shoulder Girdle

Instruct the patient as follows:

1. Flex and extend arms slowly while holding traction weights; gradually increase poundage of weight and number of repetitions to increase strength and endurance.

2. Do push-ups while lying in a prone position.

3. Squeeze rubber ball—increases grasping strength.

4. Raise head and shoulders from bed; stretch hands forward as far as possible.

5. Sit up on bed or chair.

   a. Raise body from chair by pushing hands against chair seat (or mattress).

   b. Raise body out of seat. Hold. Relax.

Measuring for Crutches

1. When the patient is lying down (an approximate measurement):

   a. Instruct the patient to wear shoes he or she will be using for walking.

   b. Measure from the anterior fold of the axilla to the sole of the foot. Then add 5 cm (2 inches).

   c. Alternatively, subtract 40 cm (16 inches) from the patient's height.

2. When the patient is standing erect:

   a. Stand the patient against the wall with feet slightly apart and away from the wall.

   b. The crutches should be fitted with large rubber suction tips.

   c. The elbow is flexed 30 degrees with the hand resting on the grip.

   d. There should be a two-finger-width insertion between the axillary fold and the underarm piece grip. A foam-rubber pad on the underarm piece will relieve pressure on the upper arm and thoracic cage.

   e. The tip of the crutch is placed 15 to 20 cm (6 to 8 inches) lateral to the forefoot.

Teaching the Crutch Stance

1. Have the patient wear well-fitting shoes with firm soles.

2. Before using the crutches, have the patient stand by a chair on the unaffected leg to achieve balance.

3. Position the patient against a wall with head in a neutral position.

4. Tripod position—basic crutch stance for balance and support.

   a. Crutches rest approximately 20 to 25 cm (8 to 10 inches) in front of and to the side of the patient's toes (Figure 32-1).

   b. Taller patient requires a wider base, whereas shorter patient needs a narrower base.

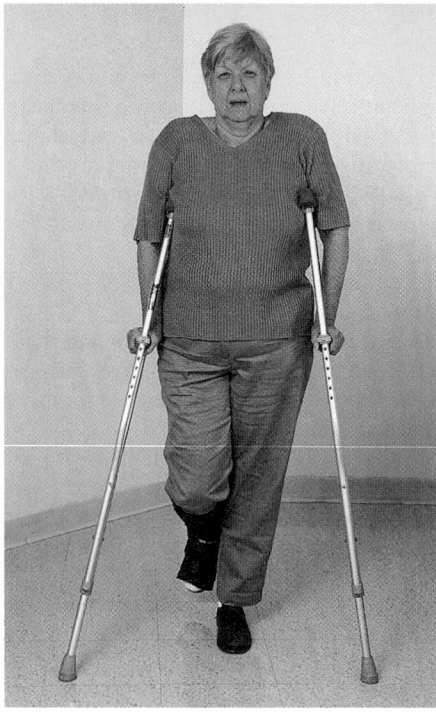

FIGURE 32-1   The tripod position is the basic crutch stance for balance and support.

5. Teach the patient to support weight on hands; weight borne on the axillae can damage the brachial plexus nerves and produce "crutch paralysis."

Teaching the Crutch Gait

1. Crutch walking requires balance, coordination, and a high energy cost; these can be acquired with diligent and regular practice.

2. Practice balancing with crutches while leaning against the wall.

3. Practice shifting body weight in different positions while standing with crutches.

4. The selection of the crutch gait depends on the type and severity of the disability and the patient's physical condition, arm and trunk strength, and/or body balance.

5. Teach the patient at least two gaits—a faster gait to be used for swiftness and a slower one to be used in crowded places.

6. Instruct the patient to change from one gait to another—Relieves fatigue because a different combination of muscles is used.

Crutch Gaits

See Figure 32-2.

Four-Point Gait (Four-Point Alternate Crutch Gait)

1. This is a slow but stable gait; the patient's weight is constantly being shifted.

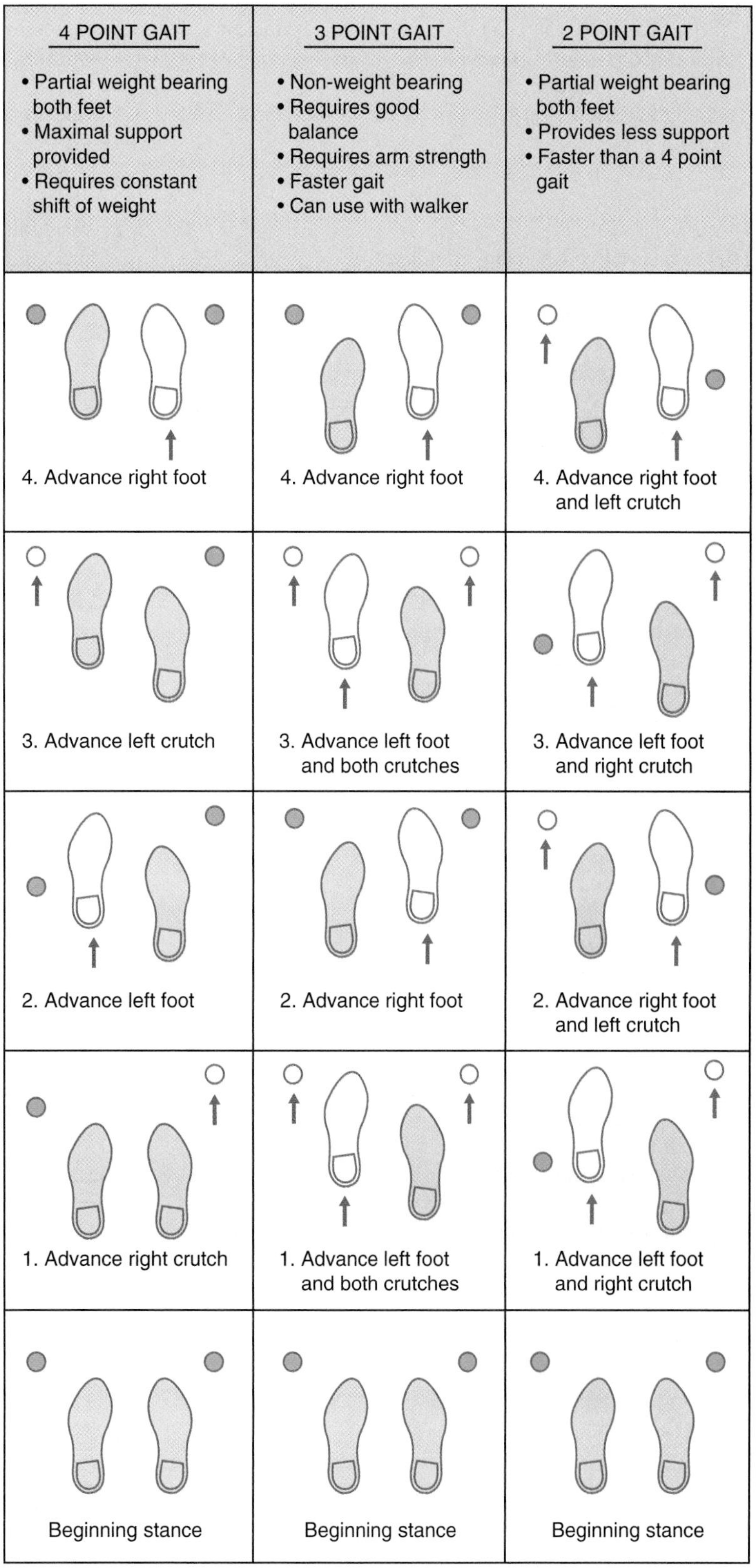

4 POINT GAIT	3 POINT GAIT	2 POINT GAIT
• Partial weight bearing both feet • Maximal support provided • Requires constant shift of weight	• Non-weight bearing • Requires good balance • Requires arm strength • Faster gait • Can use with walker	• Partial weight bearing both feet • Provides less support • Faster than a 4 point gait
4. Advance right foot	4. Advance right foot	4. Advance right foot and left crutch
3. Advance left crutch	3. Advance left foot and both crutches	3. Advance left foot and right crutch
2. Advance left foot	2. Advance right foot	2. Advance right foot and left crutch
1. Advance right crutch	1. Advance left foot and both crutches	1. Advance left foot and right crutch
Beginning stance	Beginning stance	Beginning stance

FIGURE 32-2 Crutch gaits. *Shaded areas* are weight-bearing. *Arrow* indicates advance of foot or crutch.

2. Four-point gait can be used only by patients who can move each leg separately and bear a considerable amount of weight on each of them.
3. *Crutch-foot sequence:*
   a. Right crutch
   b. Left foot
   c. Left crutch
   d. Right foot

Three-Point Gait

This is used when one leg is involved.
   Crutch-foot sequence:
1. Both crutches and the involved lower leg are moved forward simultaneously.
2. Then the stronger lower extremity is moved forward while most of the body weight is put on the crutches.

Two-Point Gait

This is a progression from the four-point gait that allows faster ambulation.
   Crutch-foot sequence:
1. Weight is borne on both lower extremities and both crutches.
2. Advance right foot and left crutch together.
3. Then advance left foot and right crutch together.

Crutch Maneuvering Techniques
See Patient Education Guidelines.

◼ Ambulation With a Walker

A walker provides more support than crutches or a cane for the patient who has poor balance and cannot use crutches.

Technique for Using a Walker
1. Be aware that a walker gives stability but does not permit a natural reciprocal walking pattern.
2. Rolling walkers may assist the patient who has painful joints in the lower extremities, decreased balance, or decreased cardiopulmonary function.
3. Teach the following sequence for a patient using a stationary (nonrolling) walker:
   a. Lift the walker, placing it in front of you while leaning your body slightly forward.
   b. Take a step or two into the walker.
   c. Lift the walker, and place it in front of you again.

◼ Ambulation With a Cane

A cane is used for balance and support. Canes come in a variety of shapes, but the majority have a curved handle and a rubber tip. Tripod canes may offer greater support.

Purposes
1. To assist the patient to walk with greater balance and support and less fatigue
2. To compensate for deficiencies of function normally performed by the neuromuscular skeletal system
3. To relieve pressure on weight-bearing joints

4. To provide forces to push or pull the body forward or to restrain the forward motion of the patient while walking

Principles of Cane Use
1. An adjustable aluminum cane fitted with a 3.75-cm (1½-inch) rubber suction tip to provide traction while walking gives optimal stability to the patient.
2. With bilateral disease, using two canes gives better balance and weight relief.
3. To fit for a cane:
   a. Have patient flex elbow at a 30-degree angle and hold the cane 15 cm (6 inches) lateral to the base of fifth toe.
   b. Adjust the cane so the handle is approximately level with the greater trochanter.
4. Alternatively, while the patient is standing with arms at side, the handle of the cane should line up with the crease in wrist.

Technique for Walking With a Cane
1. Hold the cane in the hand opposite to the affected extremity (ie, the cane should be used on the good side)—allows partial weight-bearing relief because the cane is in contact with the floor at the same time as the affected extremity.
2. Advance the cane at the same time the affected leg is moved forward.
3. Keep the cane fairly close to the body to prevent leaning.
4. If the patient is unable to use the cane in the opposite hand, the cane may be carried on the same side and advanced when the affected leg is advanced.
5. To go up and down stairs:
   a. Step up on unaffected extremity.
   b. Then place cane and affected extremity on the step.
   c. Reverse this procedure for the descending steps.
   d. The strong leg goes up first and comes down last.

◼ Casts

A cast is an immobilizing device made up of layers of plaster or fiberglass (water-activated polyurethane resin) bandages molded to the body part that it encases. See Procedure Guidelines 32-1 and 32-2 for application and removal of a cast.

Purposes
1. To immobilize and hold bone fragments in reduction
2. To apply uniform compression of soft tissues
3. To permit early mobilization
4. To correct and prevent deformities
5. To support and stabilize weak joints

Types of Casts
Short-Arm Cast

Extends from below the elbow to the proximal palmar crease.

Standing Up

1. Move forward to the edge of the chair with the strong leg slightly under the seat.
2. Place both crutches in the hand on the side of the affected extremity.
3. Push down on the hand pieces while raising the body to a standing position.

Sitting in a Chair

Grasp the crutches at the hand pieces for control, and bend forward slightly while assuming a sitting position.

Going Up Stairs

1. Advance the stronger leg first up to the next step.
2. Then advance the crutches and the weaker extremity.

Going Down Stairs

1. Place feet forward as far as possible on the step.
2. Advance crutches to the lower step. The weaker leg is advanced first and then the stronger one—the stronger extremity shares the work of raising and lowering the body weight with the patient's arms.

Note: Strong leg goes up stairs first and down stairs last.

Gauntlet Cast

Extends from below the elbow to the proximal palmar crease, including the thumb (thumb spica).

Long-Arm Cast

Extends from upper level of axillary fold to proximal palmar crease; elbow usually immobilized at right angle.

Short-Leg Cast

Extends from below knee to base of toes.

Long-Leg Cast

Extends from upper thigh to the base of toes; foot is at right angle in a neutral position.

Body Cast

Encircles the trunk stabilizing the spine.

Spica Cast

Incorporates the trunk and extremity.

1. Shoulder spica cast—a body jacket that encloses trunk, shoulder, and elbow.
2. Hip spica cast—encloses trunk and a lower extremity.
   a. Single hip spica—extends from nipple line to include pelvis and extends to include pelvis and one thigh
   b. Double hip spica—extends from nipple line or upper abdomen to include pelvis and extends to include both thighs and lower legs
   c. One-and-a-half hip spica—extends from upper abdomen, includes one entire leg, and extends to the knee of the other

Cast-Brace

External support about a fracture that is constructed with hinges to permit early motion of joints, early mobilization, and independence.

1. Cast bracing is based on the concept that some weight-bearing is physiologic and will promote the formation of bone and contain fluid within a tight compartment that compresses soft tissues, providing a distribution of forces across the fracture site.
2. Cast-brace is applied after initial edema and pain have subsided and there is evidence of fracture stability.

Cylinder Cast

Can be used for upper or lower extremity. Used for fracture or dislocation of knee (lower extremity) or elbow dislocation (upper extremity).

Complications of Casts

1. Pressure of cast on neurovascular and bony structures causes necrosis, pressure sores, and nerve palsies.
2. Compartment syndrome—trauma or surgery affecting an extremity will produce swelling (result of hemorrhage from bone and surrounding tissue and of tissue edema). Vascular insufficiency and nerve and muscle compression due to unrelieved swelling can cause irreversible damage to an extremity.
3. Immobility and confinement in a cast, particularly a body cast, can result in multisystem problems.
   a. Nausea, vomiting, and abdominal distention associated with cast syndrome (superior mesenteric artery syndrome, resulting in diminished blood flow to the bowel), adynamic ileus, and possible intestinal obstruction
   b. Acute anxiety reaction symptoms (ie, behavioral changes and autonomic responses—increased respiratory and heart rate, elevated blood pressure, diaphoresis) associated with confinement in a space
   c. Thrombophlebitis and possible pulmonary emboli associated with immobility and ineffective circulation (eg, venous stasis)
   d. Respiratory atelectasis and pneumonia associated with ineffective respiratory effort
   e. Urinary tract infection—renal and bladder calculi associated with urinary stasis, low fluid intake, and calcium excretion associated with immobility
   f. Anorexia and constipation associated with decreased activity
   g. Psychological reaction (eg, depression) associated with immobility, dependence, and loss of control

Nursing Assessment

1. Assess neurovascular status of the extremity with a cast for signs of compromise.
   a. Pain
   b. Swelling
   c. Discoloration—pale or blue
   d. Cool skin distal to injury

e. Tingling or numbness (paresthesia)
f. Pain on passive extension (muscle stretch)
g. Slow capillary refill; diminished or absent pulse
h. Paralysis
2. Assess skin integrity of casted extremity. Be alert for:
   a. Severe initial pain over bony prominences; this is a warning symptom of an impending pressure sore. Pain increases when ulceration occurs.
   b. Odor
   c. Drainage on cast

> **NURSING ALERT**
>
> Do not ignore the complaint of pain of the patient in a cast. Suspect circulatory complications or a pressure sore. Notify health care provider if symptoms persist. Cast may have to be split or removed.

3. Carefully assess for positioning and potential pressure sites of the casted extremity.
   a. Lower extremity—heel, malleoli, dorsum of foot, head of fibula, anterior surface of patella
   b. Upper extremity—medial epicondyle of humerus, ulnar styloid
   c. Plaster jackets or body spica casts—sacrum, anterior and superior iliac spines, vertebral borders of scapulae
4. Assess cardiovascular, respiratory, and gastrointestinal (GI) systems for possible complications of immobility.
5. Assess psychological reaction to illness, cast, and immobility.

Nursing Diagnoses
- Altered Peripheral Tissue Perfusion related to swelling and constrictive bandage/cast
- Impaired Physical Mobility related to condition and casting
- Risk for Injury related to potential complications

Nursing Interventions
Maintaining Adequate Tissue Perfusion
1. Elevate the extremity on cloth-covered pillow above the level of the heart. Keep the heel off the mattress.
2. Avoid resting cast on hard surfaces or sharp edges that can cause denting or flattening of the cast and consequent pressure sores.
3. Handle moist cast with palms of hands.
4. Turn patient every 2 hours while cast dries.
5. Assess neurovascular status hourly during the first 24 hours, then less frequently as condition warrants and swelling resolves.
6. If symptoms of neurovascular compromise occur:
   a. Notify health care provider immediately.
   b. Bivalve the cast—split cast on each side over its full length into two halves.
   c. Cut the underlying padding—blood-soaked padding may shrink and cause constriction of circulation.
   d. Spread cast sufficiently to relieve constriction.

7. If symptoms of pressure area occur, cast may be "windowed" (hole cut in it) so the skin at the pain point can be examined and treated. The window must be replaced so the tissue does not swell and cause additional pressure problems at window edge (Figure 32-3).

Minimizing the Effects of Immobility
1. Encourage the patient to move about as normally as possible.
2. Encourage compliance with prescribed exercises to avoid muscle atrophy and loss of strength.
   a. Active ROM for every joint that is not immobilized at regular and frequent intervals.
   b. Isometric exercises for the muscles of the casted extremity. Instruct patient to alternately contract and relax muscles without moving affected part.
3. Reposition and turn patient frequently.
4. Avoid pressure behind knees, which reduces venous return and predisposes to thromboembolism.
5. Use antiembolism stockings as prescribed.
6. Administer prophylactic anticoagulants as prescribed.

> **NURSING ALERT**
>
> Persons at high risk for pulmonary emboli include older adults and persons with previous thromboembolism, obesity, congestive heart failure, or multiple trauma. They may require prophylaxis against thromboembolism.

7. Encourage deep-breathing exercises and coughing at regular intervals to prevent atelectasis and pneumonia.
8. Observe for symptoms of cast syndrome—nausea, vomiting, abdominal distention, abdominal pain, and decreased bowel sounds.

> **NURSING ALERT**
>
> Cast syndrome (superior mesenteric artery syndrome) is a rare sequela of body cast application, yet it is a potentially fatal complication. It is important to teach patients about this syndrome, because this can develop as late as several weeks after cast application.

9. Encourage patient to drink liberal quantities of fluid—to avoid urinary infection and calculi secondary to immobility.

Providing Additional Care
1. Encourage balanced nutritional intake.
   a. Assess the patient's food preferences. Serve small meals.
   b. Provide natural bowel stimulants (eg, fiber).
   c. Monitor bowels, and use a bowel program if necessary.
2. If symptoms of cast syndrome develop, report immediately.
   a. Place patient in a prone position, if tolerated, to relieve pressure symptoms.

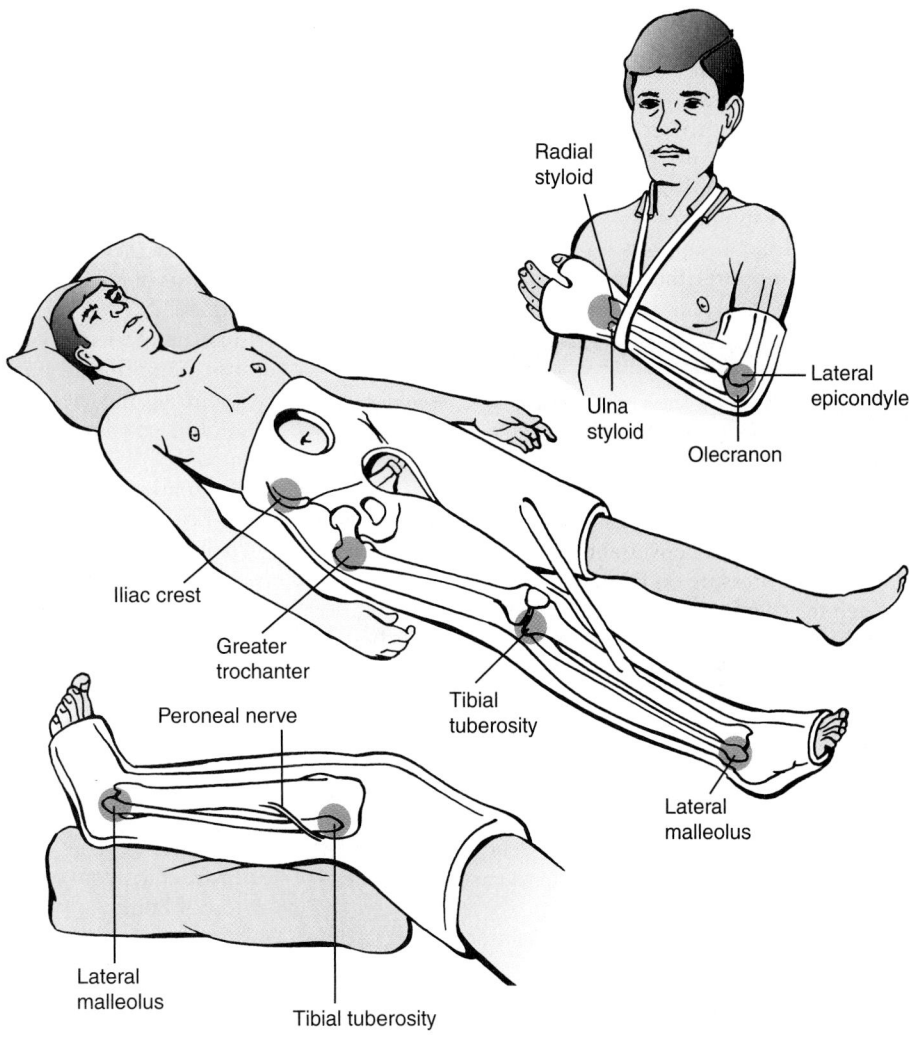

FIGURE 32-3 Pressure areas in different types of casts.

b. Use nasogastric suction as prescribed.

c. Maintain electrolyte balance by intravenous (IV) replacement of fluids as prescribed.

d. Prepare the patient for removal of the cast or surgical relief of duodenal obstruction if necessary.

3. Facilitate patient participation in care planning and activities. Encourage verbalization of feelings and concerns regarding casting.

4. Provide and encourage diversional activities.

Specific Care for Patient in Spica or Body Cast

Positioning

1. Place a bedboard under the mattress for uniform support of the body.

2. Support the curves of the cast with cloth-covered flexible pillows—prevents cracking and flat spots while cast is drying.

a. Place three pillows crosswise on bed for body cast.

b. Place one pillow crosswise at the waist and two pillows lengthwise for affected leg for spica cast. If both legs are involved, use two additional pillows.

3. Encourage the patient to maintain physiologic position by:

a. Using the overhead trapeze.

b. Placing good foot flat on bed and pushing down while lifting himself or herself up on the trapeze.

c. Avoiding twisting motions.

d. Avoiding positions that produce pressure on groin, back, chest, and abdomen.

Turning

1. Move the patient to the side of the bed using a steady, even pulling motion.

2. Place pillows along the other side of the bed—one for the chest and two (lengthwise) for the legs.

3. Instruct the patient to place arms at side or above head.
4. Turn the patient as a unit. Avoid twisting the patient in the cast.
5. Turn the patient toward the leg not encased in plaster or toward the unoperated side if both legs are in plaster.
   a. One nurse stands at other side of bed to receive the patient's shoulders.
   b. Second nurse supports leg in plaster while the third nurse supports the patient's back as he or she is turned.

NURSING ALERT

Do not grasp cross bar of spica cast to move the patient. The purpose of the bar is to maintain the integrity of the cast.

---

   c. Turn the patient in body cast to a prone position twice daily—provides postural drainage of bronchial tree; relieves pressure on back.
6. Keep the cast level by elevating the lumbar sacral area with a small pillow when the head of the bed is elevated.

Hygienic Care
1. Provide hygienic care of the patient.
2. Protect cast from soiling.
   a. Cover perineum with a towel and apply spray (lacquer-type) to perineal area of cast. Tuck 10-cm (4-inch) strips of thin polyethylene sheeting under perineal area of cast and tape to cast exterior. Replace when soiling occurs.
   b. Clean outside of cast with dry cleanser on almost-dry cloth.
3. Roll the patient onto fracture bedpan; use small pillow in lumbosacral area for support.

Skin Care
1. Inspect skin for signs of irritation:
   a. Around cast edge.
   b. Under cast—pull skin taut and inspect under cast, using a flashlight for illumination.
2. Reach up under cast, and massage accessible skin.
3. Protect the toes from the pressure of the bedding.

Patient Education and Health Maintenance
Neurovascular Status
1. Instruct patient to check neurovascular status and to control swelling.
   a. Watch for signs and symptoms of circulatory disturbance, including blueness or paleness of fingernails or toenails accompanied by pain and tightness, numbness, cold or tingling sensation.
   b. Elevate affected extremity, and wiggle fingers/toes.
   c. Apply ice bags as prescribed (one third to one half full) to each side of the cast, making sure they do not make indentations in plaster.

   d. Call health care provider promptly if excessive swelling, paresthesia, persistent pain, pain on passive stretch, or paralysis occurs.
2. Instruct patient to alternate ambulation with periods of elevation to the cast when seated. Encourage the patient to lie down several times daily with cast elevated.

Skin Irritation
Advise patient to prevent skin irritation at cast edge by padding edges of cast with moleskin or "petaling" cast edges with strips of adhesive tape.

Exercise
1. Instruct patient to actively exercise every joint that is not immobilized and to perform isometric exercises (contract muscles without moving joint) of those immobilized to maintain muscle strength and to prevent atrophy.
2. Tell patient to perform hourly when awake.
   a. Leg cast—"Push down on the popliteal (knee) space, hold it, relax, repeat." Move toes back and forth; bend toes down, then pull them back.
   b. Arm cast—"Make a fist, hold it, relax, repeat." Move shoulders.

Cast Care
1. Advise to avoid getting cast wet, especially padding under cast—causes skin breakdown as plaster cast becomes soft.
2. Warn against covering a leg cast with plastic or rubber boots, because this causes condensation and wetting of the cast.
3. Instruct to avoid weight bearing or stress on plaster cast for 24 hours.
4. Instruct to report to health care provider if the cast cracks or breaks; instruct the patient not to try to fix it.
5. Teach how to clean the cast:
   a. Remove surface soil with slightly damp cloth.
   b. Rub soiled areas with household scouring powder.
   c. Wipe off residual moisture.

Teaching Safety Measures
Avoid walking on wet floors or sidewalks, to prevent falls; do not place objects under the cast, to prevent pressure and injury to the skin.

After Cast Is Removed
1. Instruct to cleanse skin with mild soap and water, blot dry, and apply emollient lotion to dry skin.
2. Warn against scratching the skin.
3. Advise to continue prescribed exercises. Gradually resume activities, and elevate extremity to control swelling.

Outcome-Based Evaluation
- No pain, discoloration, or sensory or motor impairment of affected extremity; warm, with good capillary refill
- Ambulating with assistance; performing active ROM and isometric exercises every 1 to 2 hours
- No signs of complications

PROCEDURE GUIDELINES 32-1 | APPLICATION OF A CAST

EQUIPMENT

Plaster or synthetic bandages in desired widths
*Stockinette (tubular knitted material)
*Cast padding (roll padding)
Splints (for reinforcement)
*Cotton, polyester, or polyurethane foam
 padding for bony prominences

Cast knives, scissors
Polyethylene sheeting or newspaper—to protect floor
Disposable gloves—to protect hands of operator
Large, plastic-lined pail of water at room temperature—21°–24°C
 (70°–75°F)—or as recommended by cast material manufacturer
Cast finishing hand cream for synthetic cast as needed

UNDERLYING CONSIDERATIONS

1. The application of a cast requires two to three persons: one to apply the plaster (operator), one to dip and hand the plaster bandages to the operator, and a third person to hold the extremity in correct position. (Body spicas may require additional personnel.)
2. The time required for the cast to become rigid varies with the material used—generally 2–6 minutes.
3. There should be no movement of the extremity while the cast is being applied and set.
4. In general, the joints above and below the involved bone are immobilized.

PROCEDURE

Nursing Action	Rationale
PREPARATORY PHASE	
1. Spread polyethylene sheeting or newspaper on floor.	1. To contain mess.
2. Explain to the patient that there will be a feeling of warmth as the plaster is applied.	2. Heat is produced by crystallization as plaster sets. The reaction of water with plaster of paris liberates heat.
3. Apply stockinette and roll cast padding on the extremity or part to be immobilized.	3. Padding is used to pad the sharp cast margins for patient, comfort and to prevent pressure areas, minimize circulatory problems, and facilitate cast removal. It is applied from the distal to the proximal end of the extremity. When too much padding is used, it may shift and produce pressure areas under the cast.
a. Apply roll padding as smoothly and snugly as possible so each turn overlaps the preceding turn by ½ the width of the roll.	
b. Extra pieces of padding may be placed over bony prominences: olecranon process, malleoli, patella.	
4. While keeping the thumb under the forward edge of the bandage, submerge the plaster bandage vertically in water (room temperature) for a minute or so, or until bubbles cease to rise. Check directions on synthetic cast materials.	4. Water that is too warm will accelerate setting time, may cause a burn, and may result in excessive plaster loss by loosening the adhesive agents that bond the plaster to the fabric.
5. Expel excess water by squeezing (not wringing) toward the center of the bandage; hand bandage to operator with free end hanging loose.	5. The cast will dry more quickly (and thus will acquire maximum strength sooner) if a well-squeezed plaster bandage is used. Maximum strength is achieved by synthetic casts through chemical reaction in about ½ hour.
PERFORMANCE PHASE (BY OPERATOR)	
1. Starting at the distal end, roll the bandage gently and evenly on the extremity overlapping the preceding turn by ½ the width of the roll.	1. Roll inward toward the patient's body for ease of control.
2. Keep the bandage moving and in constant contact with the surface of the extremity. Smooth and rub down successive layers or turns of each bandage into the layers below with the thumbs and thenar eminences (mound on the palm) in circumferential and longitudinal directions.	2. This keeps the cast uniformly thick. Rubbing the plaster as it is applied will form a smooth, solid, and well-fused cast. Avoid indenting the cast with the fingertips because this may produce pressure sores on underlying skin. Handle fresh casts with palms.
3. Take tucks in the lower border of the bandage by lifting the bandage off the surface (without tension) and overlapping it in a V-shaped fashion.	3. Tucking the bandage helps to contour the cast to the changing circumference of the extremity. Do not twist or reverse the bandage to change its direction because this produces sharp cutting edges.

Material needs to be nonabsorbent if non-plaster cast is used.

continued

PROCEDURE GUIDELINES 32-1	APPLICATION OF A CAST *CONTINUED*

Nursing Action	Rationale
4. Trim the cast to size with a sharp knife. Fold stockinette over edges of cast and anchor with cast material.	4. Stockinette produces smooth, comfortable edges on cast. Do not pull too vigorously on the stockinette because this may cause pressure on bony prominences.
5. Finish synthetic cast with cast hand cream as indicated.	5. Smooths rough exterior surface.
6. Ask the patient if there is any discomfort or pain.	6. If a patient complains of pain, it may be due to manipulation of fracture during setting; pain should subside rapidly. If it persists, the cast and encircling dressings are split to avoid constriction, circulatory problems, and pressure sores.

FOLLOW-UP PHASE

Nursing Action	Rationale
1. Support the cast with the palm of the hand while moving the patient. Avoid indentations from tips of fingers.	1. Finger indentation on a fresh cast can produce pressure sores.
2. Expose the cast to warm, circulating, dry air. Or blow air over cast with a circulating fan to increase the evaporation of water.	2. Avoid covering the cast when it is drying because this delays drying time. Usually the plaster cast will reach its maximum temperature 5–15 minutes after it is applied and will then cool rapidly. The ultimate plaster cast strength is obtained after the cast is dry (up to 48 hours, depending on outside temperature and humidity). The synthetic cast strength is maximum within 30 minutes of application and not dependent on being dry.
3. Clean equipment and store ready for use.	

PROCEDURE GUIDELINES 32-2	REMOVAL OF A CAST

EQUIPMENT

Cast cutter—an electric saw with circular blade that oscillates and is connected to a vacuum collector
Cast spreader

Plaster knife
Scissors
Felt-tip pen

PROCEDURE

Nursing Action	Rationale

PREPARATORY PHASE

Nursing Action	Rationale
1. Describe to the patient how and where the cast cutter will be used and the expected sensations.	1. Reassures the patient that the cutter produces vibrations but not pain.
2. Determine whether the cast is padded.	2. An electric plaster cast cutter should not be used on unpadded casts.
3. Determine where the cut will be made. Mark, with a felt pen, the area to be cut.	3. The line should be in front of the lateral malleolus and behind the medial malleolus on a lower extremity cast. An upper extremity cast is usually split along the ulnar or flexor surface.

PERFORMANCE PHASE

Nursing Action	Rationale
1. Inform the patient to shield eyes.	1. Plaster dust may be irritating to the eyes.
2. Grasp the electric cutter as illustrated.	
3. Rest the thumb on the cast.	3. The thumb serves as a depth gauge and acts as a guard in front of the blade.
4. Turn on the electric cutter. Push the blade firmly and gently through the cast while holding the thumb against the cast to steady the blade while cutting through the cast.	
5. As the blade cuts through the plaster, a sudden lack of resistance is felt; plaster will "give" (or "dip") when the cut is completed.	

PROCEDURE GUIDELINES 32-2   *CONTINUED*

Nursing Action	Rationale

6. Lift the cutting blade up a degree (but not out of the cutting groove) and advance the blade at a slightly higher or lower level. The cast is cut by a series of alternating pressure and linear movements along the line of the cut (see accompanying figure).

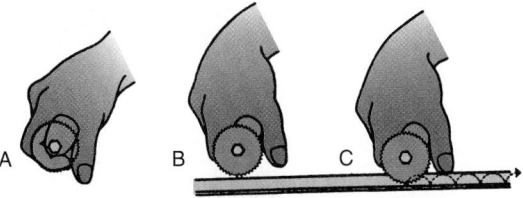

Operating a cast cutter.

7. Avoid drawing the cutting blade along the extremity in a single motion.

7. This will cut the skin. If saw blade is in contact with padding too long, the patient will feel burning sensation on skin from rapidly oscillating blade.

8. Cut the cast on both sides. Then rock the anterior portion of the cast over the posterior portion.

8. This maneuver allows the operator to determine if the cast is completely cut.

9. Insert the blades of the cast spreader in the cut trough. Separate the two halves with the spreader at several sites along the cast split. Separate the cast with the hands.

10. Cut through the padding and stockinette with scissors, keeping the scissor blade that is closest to the skin parallel to the skin.

10. Use bandage scissors; place the flat blade closest to the skin.

11. Lift the extremity carefully out of the posterior portion of the cast. Support the extremity so it is maintained in the same position as when in the cast.

11. When the support of the cast has been removed, stresses and strain are placed on parts that have been at rest.

AFTER REMOVAL OF CAST

1. Cleanse the skin gently with mild soap and water. Blot dry. Apply a skin cream.

1. Explain to the patient that the skin will be scaly and the extremity will appear "thin" from disuse. Reassure him or her that it will take a few weeks to regain normal appearance and function.

2. Emphasize the importance of continuing the prescribed exercises, reporting for physical therapy, and so forth.

2. Exercises are necessary to redevelop and increase strength and function. Pain and stiffness may be expected after cast removal.

◼ Traction

Traction is force applied in a specific direction. To apply the force needed to overcome the natural force or pull of muscle groups, a system of ropes, pulleys, and weights is used. See Procedure Guidelines 32-3.

Purposes of Traction
1. To reduce and immobilize fracture
2. To regain normal length and alignment of an injured extremity
3. To lessen or eliminate muscle spasm
4. To prevent deformity
5. To give the patient freedom for "in-bed" activities
6. To reduce pain

Types of Traction
Running Traction
1. A form of traction in which the pull is exerted in one plane.
2. May use either skin or skeletal traction.
3. Buck's extension traction (Figure 32-4) is an example of running skin traction.

Balanced Suspension Traction
1. Uses additional weights to counterbalance the traction force and floats the extremity in the traction apparatus.
2. The line of pull on the extremity remains fairly constant despite changes in the patient's position.

Application of Traction
Traction may be applied to the skin or to the skeletal system.

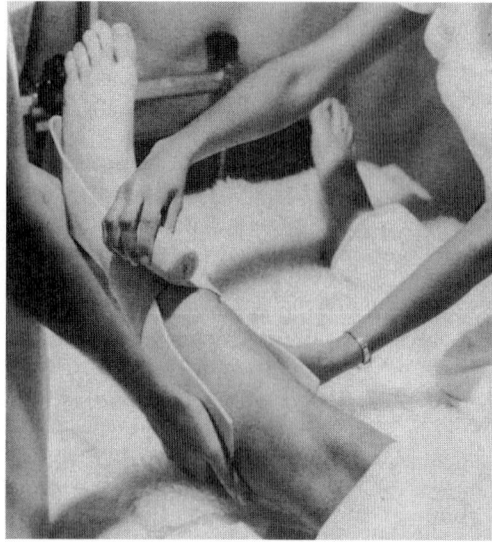
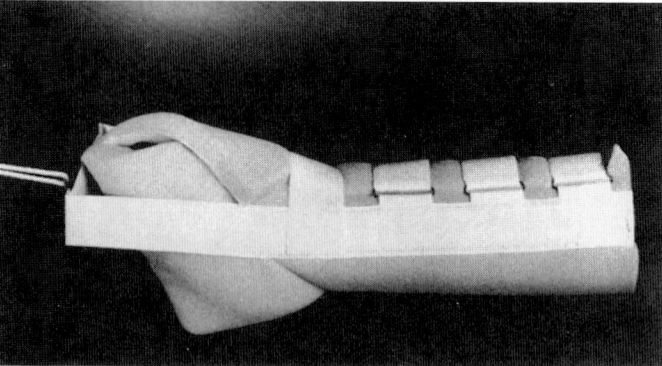

FIGURE 32-4 (*Left*) Applying elastic bandage for Buck's extension traction. (*Right*) Prepadded boot that may be used in Buck's extension. (Photo of boot courtesy of All Orthopedic Appliances.)

Skin Traction

1. Accomplished by applying a light force that pulls on tape, sponge rubber, or special device (boot, cervical halter, pelvic belt) that is in contact with the skin.
2. The pulling force is transmitted to the musculoskeletal structures.
3. Skin traction is used as a temporary measure in adults to control muscle spasm and pain.
4. It is used before surgery in the treatment of hip fracture (Buck's extension) and femoral shaft fractures (Russell's traction).
5. Pelvic and cervical traction are used for treatment of back disorders or injuries. Skin traction may be used definitively to treat fractures in children.

Skeletal Traction

See Figure 32-5.

1. Traction applied by the orthopedic surgeon under aseptic conditions using wires, pins, or tongs placed through bones.
2. Skeletal traction is used most frequently in treating fractures of the femur, humerus (supracondylar fractures), tibia, and cervical spine.

Complications

1. Infection of pin tracts in skeletal traction
2. Skin breakdown and dermatitis under skin traction
3. Complications of immobility
   a. Stasis pneumonia
   b. Thrombophlebitis
   c. Pressure ulcers
   d. Urinary infection and calculi
   e. Constipation

Nursing Assessment

1. Assess for pain, deformity, swelling, motor and sensory function, and circulatory status of the affected extremity.
2. Assess skin condition of the affected extremity, both under skin traction and around skeletal traction, as well as over body prominences throughout the body.
3. Assess for signs and symptoms of complications.
4. Assess traction equipment for safety and effectiveness.
   a. The patient is placed on a firm mattress.
   b. The ropes and the pulleys should be in alignment.
   c. The pull should be in line with the long axis of the bone.
   d. Any factor that might reduce the pull or alter its direction must be eliminated.
      (i) Weights should hang freely.
      (ii) Ropes should be unobstructed and not in contact with the bed or equipment.
      (iii) Help the patient to pull himself or herself up in bed at frequent intervals.

> **NURSING ALERT**
>
> Traction is *not* accomplished if the knot in the rope or the footplate is touching the pulley or the foot of the bed or if the weights are resting on the floor. Never remove the weights when repositioning the patient who is in skeletal traction, because this will interrupt the line of pull and cause the patient considerable pain.

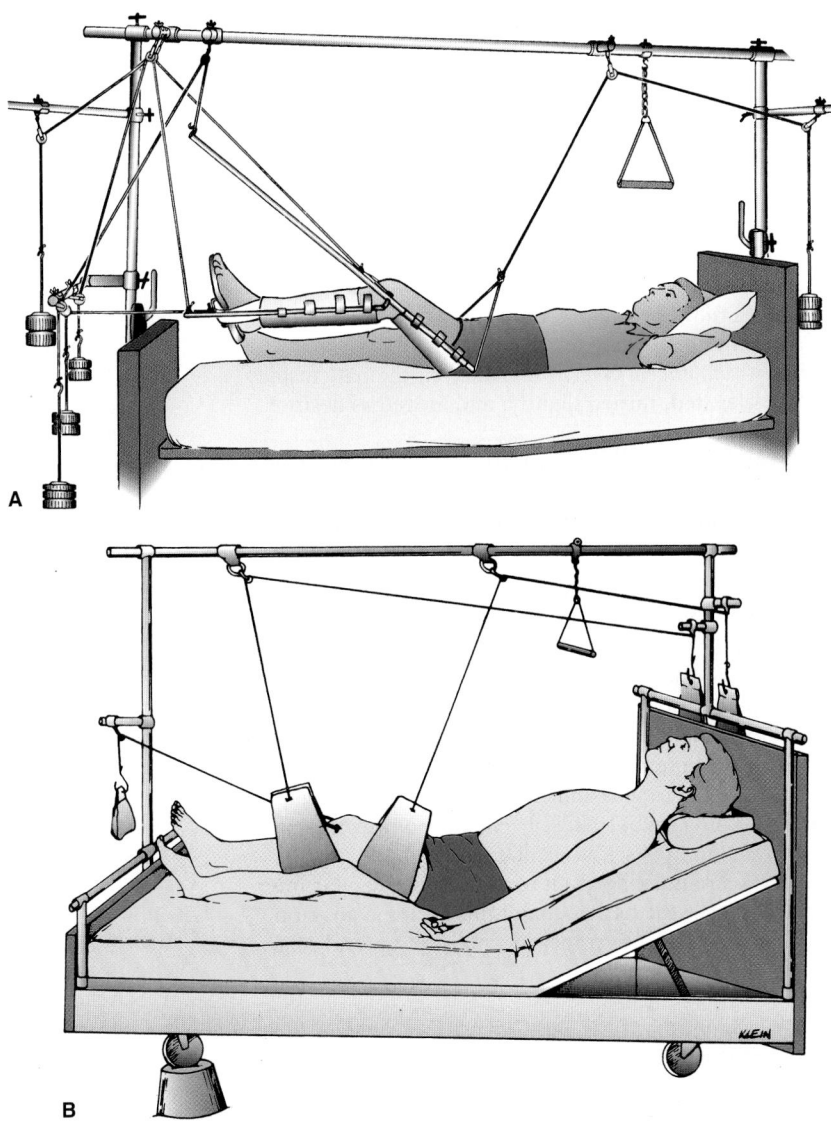

FIGURE 32-5 Balanced skeletal traction using (**A**) Thomas leg splint and Pearson attachment, and (**B**) slings for support and suspension.

e. The amount of weight applied in skin traction must not exceed the tolerance of the skin. The condition of the skin must be inspected frequently.

f. Cover exposed sharp ends of skeletal pins with cork or other pin covering to protect patient and caregivers from injury.

5. Assess emotional reaction to condition and traction as well as understanding of the treatment plan.

Nursing Diagnoses

- Impaired Physical Mobility related to traction therapy and underlying pathology
- Risk for Impaired Skin Integrity related to pressure on soft tissues
- Risk for Infection related to bacterial invasion at skeletal traction site
- Altered Peripheral Tissue Perfusion related to injury or traction therapy

Nursing Interventions

Minimizing the Effects of Immobility

1. Encourage active exercise of uninvolved muscles and joints to maintain strength and function. Dorsiflex feet hourly to avoid development of footdrop and aid in venous return.

2. Encourage deep breathing hourly to facilitate expansion of lungs and movement of respiratory secretions.

3. Auscultate lung fields twice a day.

4. Encourage fluid intake of 2,000 to 2,500 mL daily.
5. Provide balanced high-fiber diet rich in protein; avoid excessive calcium intake.
6. Establish bowel routine through use of diet and/or stool softeners, laxatives, and enemas, as prescribed.
7. Prevent pressure on the calf, and evaluate periodically for the development of thrombophlebitis.
8. Check traction apparatus at repeated intervals—the traction must be continuous to be effective, unless prescribed as intermittent, as with pelvic traction.
   a. With *running traction*, the patient may not be turned without disrupting the line of pull.
   b. With *balanced suspension traction*, the patient may be elevated, turned slightly, and moved as desired.

NURSING ALERT

Every complaint of the patient in traction should be investigated immediately to prevent injury.

Maintaining Skin Integrity

1. Examine bony prominences frequently for evidence of pressure or friction irritation.
2. Observe for skin irritation around the traction bandage.
3. Observe for pressure at traction–skin contact points.
4. Report complaint of burning sensation under traction.
5. Relieve pressure without disrupting traction effectiveness.
   a. Ensure that linens and clothing are wrinkle free.
   b. Use lambs' wool pads, heel/elbow protectors, and special mattresses as needed.
6. Special care must be given to the back at regular intervals, because the patient maintains a supine position.
   a. Have patient use trapeze to pull self up and relieve back pressure.
   b. Provide backrubs.

Avoiding Infection at Pin Site

1. Monitor vital signs for fever or tachycardia.
2. Watch for signs of infection, especially around the pin tract.
   a. The pin should be immobile in the bone, and the skin wound should be dry. Small amount of serous oozing from pin site may occur.
   b. If infection is suspected, percuss gently over the tibia; this may elicit pain if infection is developing.
   c. Assess for other signs of infection: heat, redness, fever.

3. If directed, clean the pin tract with sterile applicators and prescribed solution/ointment—to clear drainage at the entrance of tract and around the pin, because plugging at this site can predispose to bacterial invasion of the tract and bone.

Promoting Tissue Perfusion

1. Assess motor and sensory function of specific nerves that might be compromised.
   a. Peroneal nerve—have patient point great toe toward nose; check sensation on dorsum of foot; presence of footdrop.
   b. Radial nerve—have patient extend thumb; check sensation in web between thumb and index finger.
   c. Median nerve—thumb–middle finger apposition; check sensation of index finger.
2. Determine adequacy of circulation (eg, color, temperature, motion, capillary refill of peripheral fingers or toes).
   a. With Buck's traction, inspect the foot for circulatory difficulties within a few minutes and then periodically after the elastic bandage has been applied.
3. Report promptly if change in neurovascular status is identified.

Patient Education and Health Maintenance

1. Teach the patient the purpose of traction therapy.
2. Delineate limitations of activity necessary to maintain effective traction.
3. Teach use of patient aids (eg, trapeze).
4. Instruct the patient not to adjust or modify traction apparatus.
5. Instruct the patient in activities designed to minimize effects of immobility on body systems.
6. Teach the patient necessity for reporting changes in sensations, pain, movement, and so forth.

Outcome-Based Evaluation

- Exercising as instructed; deep breathing hourly; fluid intake 1,800 mL/24 h; Homans' sign negative
- No signs of skin breakdown under traction bandage or over bony prominences
- No drainage, redness, or odor at pin site
- No motor or sensory impairment; good capillary refill, color, and warmth of extremity

---

PROCEDURE GUIDELINES 32-3	APPLICATION OF BUCK'S EXTENSION TRACTION

Buck's extension skin traction is used as a temporary measure to provide immobility, support, and comfort until definitive treatment is accomplished.

EQUIPMENT

Foam Buck's traction boot or traction tape and 10-cm (4-inch) elastic bandage
Spreader block or metal spreader
Pulley, nylon rope, and weights (2.3–3.1 kg [5–7 lb] is usual [amount of weight is prescribed, generally not more than 10 lb])
Sheepskin pad
Shock blocks or adjustable bed for Trendelenburg's position

PROCEDURE GUIDELINES 32-3 *CONTINUED*

PROCEDURE

Nursing Action	Rationale
PREPARATORY PHASE	
1. Bed position is flat or in Trendelenburg's position. This depends on the size of the patient and the weight applied.	1. Elevating the foot of the bed (counteraction) helps prevent the patient from sliding down toward the foot of the bed.
2. Question the patient to determine previous skin conditions (contact dermatitis). Inspect skin for evidences of atrophy, abrasions, and circulatory disturbances.	2. The skin must be in healthy condition to tolerate skin traction.
3. Make sure the skin of the extremity is clean and dry.	3. Clean, dry skin helps traction tape adherence.
4. Document the neurovascular status of the extremity, any evidence of skin problems or varicosities.	
PERFORMANCE PHASE	
1. Position the patient in center of bed in good alignment.	1. For effective line of pull.
If Traction Tape is Used:	
2. Apply continuous traction tape to medial and lateral aspects of lower leg (below knee and loosely around foot to allow for attachment of spreader).	2. Avoid pressure over malleoli and head of fibula. Pressure sores develop rapidly over bony prominences. Pressure over the region of the fibular head and common peroneal nerve may produce peroneal palsy and footdrop.
3. Have a second person elevate and support the extremity under the ankle and knee while the elastic bandage is applied. Beginning at the ankle, wrap the elastic bandage snugly over the tape up to the tibial tubercle.	3. The elastic bandage holds tape to the skin and helps prevent slipping.
4. Attach a spreader block (or metal spreader) to the distal end of the tape. Attach a rope to the spreader block and pass it over a pulley fastened to the end of the bed and gently apply weights.	4. The spreader block prevents pressure along the side of the foot. The spreader should not be too narrow (causes pressure sores on ankle) or too wide (pulls traction tape away from the heel).
5. Place a sheepskin pad under the leg (or use a commercial heel protector).	5. Sheepskin is used to reduce friction of the heel against the bed.
If Foam Boot is Used:	
1. Apply antiembolitic stockings if prescribed.	1. Prophylactic measure in high-risk population.
2. Place leg in foam boot, adjusting it so the heel is in the heel of the boot.	2. Preventing sore heels is a primary concern.
3. Secure Velcro bootstraps, avoiding excessive pressure on malleoli and fibular head.	3. Pressure over bony prominences causes skin breakdown, and pressure on peroneal nerve may result in footdrop.
4. Attach rope to built-in spreader plate, pass it over pulley, and apply weights gently.	4. The rope should move unobstructed, and the weights should hang free of the bed and not touch the floor.

■ External Fixation

External fixation is a technique of fracture immobilization in which a series of transfixing pins is inserted through bone and attached to a rigid external metal frame (Figure 32-6). The method is used mainly in the management of open fractures with severe soft tissue damage.

Advantages

1. Permits rigid support of severely comminuted open fractures, infected nonunions, and infected unstable joints
2. Facilitates wound care (frequent débridements, irrigations, dressing changes) and soft tissue reconstruction (delayed wound closure, muscle flaps, skin grafts)
3. Allows early function of muscles and joints
4. Allows early patient comfort

Circular Fixators
Purpose
May be used for limb lengthening, correction of angulation and rotation defects, and in treatment of nonunion
Components
1. This fixator apparatus consists of through-the-bone tension wires placed above and below the treatment site.
2. The wires are attached to fixator rings surrounding the limb.
3. The rings are connected to one another by telescoping rods.
Management
1. Adjustments are made daily at about 1 mm/day, stimulating callus and bone formation.
2. Patient compliance is essential.
3. Weight bearing is encouraged.

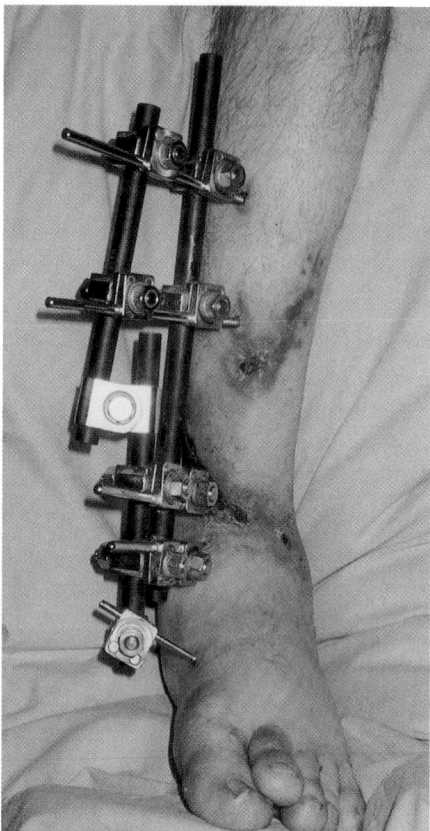

FIGURE 32-6 External fixation device used for reduction and im-mobilization of open fracture, allowing treatment of soft tissue wounds. (Smeltzer, S. & Bare, B. [1999]. *Textbook of medical-surgical nursing* [8th ed.]. Philadelphia: Lippincott Williams & Wilkins.)

4. When the desired length or correction is achieved, the fixator is left in place without further adjustment until bone healing occurs.

Application of External Fixator
1. Under general anesthesia, the skin is cleansed and trans-fixing pins are inserted into the bone through small in-cisions above and below the fracture.
2. After reduction of the fracture, the appliance is stabi-lized by adjusting and tightening the bars connecting the sets of pins.
3. The sharp pin heads are covered with plastic, cork, or rubber covers to protect the other extremity and caregivers.

Nursing Assessment
1. Determine the patient's understanding of procedure and fixation device.
2. Evaluate neurovascular status of involved body part.

3. Inspect each pin site for redness, drainage, tenderness, pain, and loosening of the pin.
4. Inspect open wounds for healing, infection, or devital-ized tissue.
5. Assess functioning of other body systems affected by injury or immobilization.

Nursing Diagnoses
- Anxiety related to appearance of external fixation device and wound
- Risk for Peripheral Neurovascular Dysfunction related to swelling, fixator, and underlying condition
- Risk for Infection related to open injury and skeletal pin insertion
- Impaired Physical Mobility related to presence of fixator and condition

Nursing Interventions
Relieving Anxiety
1. If possible, before placement of the device, reassure the patient that, although the fixator appears clumsy and cumbersome, it should not hurt once it is in place.
2. Emphasize the positive aspects of this device in treating complex musculoskeletal problems.
3. Encourage the patient to verbalize reaction to the device.
4. Inform the patient that greater mobility can be achieved with an external fixation device, thereby minimizing the development of other system problems.
5. Involve the patient in care and in the management of external fixator.

Maintaining Intact Neurovascular Status
1. Assess neurovascular status frequently—every 15 to 60 minutes while swelling is significant and later every 2 to 8 hours.
2. Establish baseline of functioning for comparative mon-itoring. Complex musculoskeletal injuries frequently result in disruption of soft tissue functioning.

NURSING ALERT

 Assess neurovascular status frequently, and record findings.

---

3. Elevate extremity to reduce swelling.
   a. Extremity can be suspended by hanging the fixator directly on the traction frame.
   b. Suspension is for control of edema and not for ap-plication of traction force.
4. Report any change in neurovascular status.

Avoiding Infection
1. Provide site and fixator care.
   a. Cleanse pin sites, and remove crusts with sterile cot-ton applicator, using solution as prescribed, or es-tablished standard of care.
      (i) Crusts formed by serous drainage can prevent fluid from draining and can cause infection.

(ii) A small amount of serous drainage from the pin sites is normal.

b. Note and report inflammation, swelling, tenderness, and purulent drainage at pin site.

c. Note skin tension at pin site—tension can cause discomfort.

d. Report loosened pins.

e. Cleanse fixator with clean cloth and water as needed.

2. Wound care

a. The open wounds at the fracture site are usually treated by daily dressing changes.

b. Use sterile technique.

c. Note wound appearance. Monitor healing. Report signs of infection.

3. Monitor for local and systemic indicators of infection.

Encourage Mobility

1. Encourage the patient to participate in care activities.

2. Assure the patient that pain associated with injury will diminish as tissue reactions to injury and manipulation resolve and healing progresses.

3. Inform the patient that the external fixator maintains the fracture in a very stable position and that the extremity can be moved. Adjustment of the fixator is done by the health care provider. (Patient is taught how to adjust the circular fixator.)

4. To move the extremity, grasp the frame and assist the patient to move. Reassure the patient that the fixator can withstand normal movement.

5. Teach quadriceps exercises and ROM exercises for joints; usually started on first postoperative day.

6. Teach crutch walking when soft tissue swelling has diminished; encourage weight bearing as prescribed.

Patient Education and Health Maintenance

1. Instruct to inspect around each pin site daily for signs of infection and loosening of pins. Watch for pain, soft tissue swelling, and drainage.

2. Teach how to cleanse around each pin daily, using aseptic technique. Do not touch wound with hands.

3. Advise to clean fixator regularly—to keep it free of dust and contamination.

4. *Warn against tampering with clamps or nuts*—can alter compression and misalign fracture.

5. Review weight-bearing and other restrictions associated with injury and treatment regimen.

6. Encourage the patient to follow rehabilitation regimen.

Outcome-Based Evaluation

- Verbalizes understanding of and comfort with fixator device
- Swelling relieved; neurovascular status intact
- No drainage or signs of infection at pin sites; pin tracts remain intact, no loosening of pins
- Ambulating with crutches as directed

Orthopedic Surgery

Types of Surgery

1. Open reduction—reduction and alignment of the fracture through surgical incision

2. Internal fixation—stabilization of the reduced fracture with use of metal screw, plates, nails, or pins

3. Bone graft—placement of autologous or homologous bone tissue to replace, promote healing of, or stabilize diseased bone

4. Arthroplasty—repair of a joint; may be done through arthroscope (arthroscopy) or open joint repair

5. Joint replacement—type of arthroplasty that involves replacement of joint surface(s) with metal or plastic materials

6. Total joint replacement—replacement of both articular surfaces within a joint

7. Meniscectomy—excision of damaged meniscus (fibrocartilage) of the knee

8. Tendon transfer—movement of tendon insertion point to improve function

9. Fasciotomy—cutting muscle fascia to relieve constriction or contracture

10. Amputation—removal of a body part

Note: Joint replacement and amputation will be covered separately.

Preoperative Management and Nursing Care

1. Hydration, protein, and caloric intake is assessed. The goal is to maximize healing and reduce risk of complications by providing IV fluids, vitamins, and nutritional supplements as indicated.

GERONTOLOGIC ALERT

 Many elderly are at risk for poor healing due to undernutrition.

2. If person has had previous corticosteroid therapy, it could contribute to current orthopedic condition (aseptic necrosis of the femoral head, osteoporosis) as well as affect the patient's response to anesthesia and the stress of surgery. May need corticotropin postoperatively.

3. Evaluate for infection (cold, dental, skin, urinary tract infection), which could contribute to development of osteomyelitis after surgery. It is important to determine whether preoperative antibiotics will be necessary.

4. Coughing and deep breathing, frequent vital sign and wound checks, repositioning are described to prepare patient.

5. The patient should practice voiding in bedpan or urinal in recumbent position before surgery. This helps reduce the need for postoperative catheterization.

6. The patient is acquainted with traction apparatus and the need for splint or cast, as indicated by type of surgery.

Postoperative Management and Nursing Care

1. Neurovascular status is monitored, and swelling caused by edema and bleeding into tissues needs to be controlled.
2. The affected area is immobilized and activity limited to protect the operative site and stabilize musculoskeletal structures.
3. Hemorrhage and shock, which may result from significant bleeding and poor hemostasis of muscles that occur with orthopedic surgery, are monitored for.
4. Complications of immobility are prevented through aggressive and vigilant postoperative care.

Complications

1. Compartment syndrome
2. Shock
3. Atelectasis and pneumonia
4. Osteomyelitis, wound infections
5. Thromboembolism
6. Fat embolus

Nursing Diagnoses

- Risk for Fluid Volume Deficit related to hemorrhage
- Ineffective Breathing Pattern related to effects of anesthesia, analgesics, and immobility
- Risk for Peripheral Neurovascular Dysfunction related to swelling
- Pain related to surgical intervention
- Risk for Infection related to surgical intervention
- Impaired Physical Mobility related to immobilization therapy and pain
- Altered Nutrition: Less Than Body Requirements, related to blood loss and the demands of healing

Nursing Interventions

Monitoring for Shock and Hemorrhage

1. Evaluate the blood pressure and pulse rates frequently—rising pulse rate or slowly falling blood pressure indicates persistent bleeding or development of a state of shock.
2. Monitor for hemorrhage—orthopedic wounds have a tendency to ooze more than other surgical wounds.
   a. Measure suction drainage if used.
   b. Anticipate up to 500 mL of drainage in the first 24 hours, decreasing to less than 30 mL per 8 hours within 48 hours, depending on surgical procedure.
   c. Report increased wound drainage or steady increase in pain of operative area.
3. Administer IV fluids and/or blood products as ordered.

Promoting Effective Breathing Pattern

1. Avoid or give respiratory depressant drugs in minimal doses. Monitor respiration depth and rate frequently. Narcotic analgesic effects may be cumulative.
2. Change position every 2 hours—mobilizes secretions and helps prevent bronchial obstruction.
3. Encourage use of incentive spirometer and coughing and deep-breathing exercises every 2 hours.
4. Auscultate lungs for atelectasis and retention of secretions.

Monitoring Peripheral Neurovascular Status

1. Watch circulation distal to the part where cast, bandage, or splint has been applied.
2. Prevent constriction leading to interference with blood or nerve supply.
3. Elevate affected extremity, and apply ice packs as directed to reduce swelling and bleeding into tissues.
4. Observe toes and fingers for healthy color and good capillary refill.
5. Check pulses of affected extremity; compare with unaffected extremity.
6. Note skin temperature.
7. Document observations.

> **NURSING ALERT**
>
> If neurovascular problems are identified, notify surgeon and loosen cast or dressing at once.

Relieving Pain

1. Institute pain relief measures as prescribed.
2. Be aware that muscle spasms may contribute to pain experience.
3. Use patient-controlled analgesia according to standards of care.
4. Principle is to graduate patient from IV medications to PO when tolerated.

Preventing Infection

1. Monitor vital signs for fever, tachycardia, or increased respiratory rate, which may indicate infection.
2. Examine incision for redness, increased temperature, swelling, and induration.
3. Note character of drainage.
4. Evaluate complaints of recurrent or increasing pain.
5. Administer antibiotic therapy as prescribed.
6. Maintain aseptic technique for dressing changes and wound care.

Minimizing the Effects of Immobility

1. Encourage patient to exercise by self with a planned program of exercise as soon as possible after surgery.
2. Have patient flex knee, extend the knee with hip still flexed, and then lower the extremity to the bed.
3. Encourage patient to move fingers and toes periodically.
4. Advise patient to move joints that are not fixed by traction or appliance through their ROM as fully as possible.
5. Suggest muscle-setting exercises (quadriceps setting) if active motion is contraindicated.
6. Apply antiembolism stockings, foot pumps, or sequential compression devices as prescribed by surgeon.
7. Give prophylactic anticoagulants as directed (eg, heparin, warfarin, aspirin).
8. Encourage early resumption of activity.

Providing Appropriate Nutrition

1. Watch for signs and symptoms of anemia, especially after fracture of long bones:
   a. Fatigue
   b. Shortness of breath
   c. Pallor

2. Monitor hemoglobin and hematocrit levels. Report below-normal results to health care provider.
3. Encourage high-iron diet, and administer blood products and iron supplements as directed.
4. Provide a balanced diet, and increase fluids and fiber to reduce incidence of constipation associated with immobility.
5. Avoid giving large amounts of milk to orthopedic patients on bed rest—adds to calcium pool in the body and demands more calcium excretion by the kidneys, predisposing to the formation of urinary calculi.
6. Maintain urinary output and prevent infection and calculi by increased fluid intake.
7. Watch for urinary retention—elderly men with some degree of prostatism may have difficulty in voiding.

Patient Education and Health Maintenance

1. Teach patient activities that will minimize the development of complications (eg, turning, coughing, and deep breathing).
2. Instruct patient in dietary considerations to facilitate healing and minimize development of constipation and renal calculi.
3. Inform patient of techniques that facilitate moving while minimizing associated discomforts (eg, supporting injured area and practicing smooth, gentle position changes).
4. Encourage long-term follow-up and physical therapy (PT) exercises as prescribed to regain maximum functional potential.

Outcome-Based Evaluation

- Blood pressure stable; drainage from wound less than 30 mL
- Respirations, deep; performing effective deep breathing and coughing every 2 hours
- Extremity beyond operative site neurovascularly intact
- Verbalizes decreased pain
- Afebrile; incision without drainage
- Ambulating as directed
- Eating balanced diet high in iron; hemoglobin within normal range

Arthroplasty and Total Joint Replacement

Arthroplasty is reconstructive surgery to restore joint motion and function and to relieve pain. It generally involves replacement of bony joint structure by a prosthesis.

Total joint arthroplasty is the replacement of both articular surfaces with metal or plastic components. The most common types of joint replacement (Figure 32-7) include:

Total hip replacement (total joint arthroplasty)—the replacement of a severely damaged hip with an artificial joint. Although a large number of implants are available, most consist of a metal femoral component topped by a spherical ball fitted into a plastic acetabular socket.

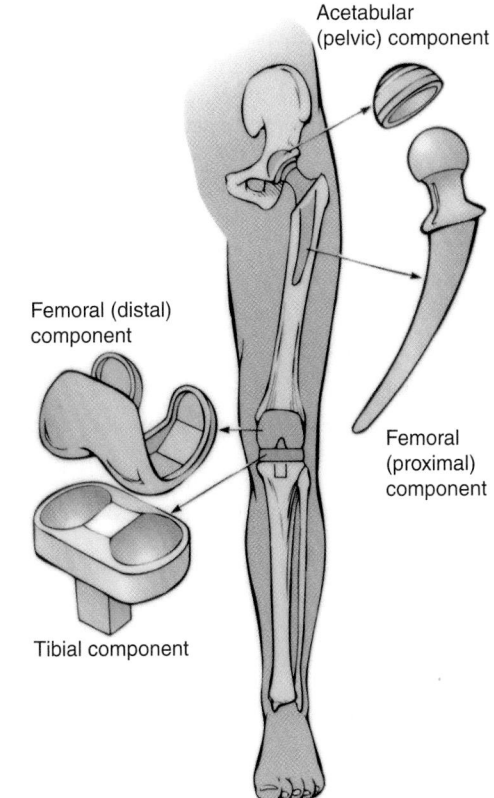

FIGURE 32-7 Hip and knee replacement.

Total knee arthroplasty—an implant procedure in which tibial, femoral, and patellar joint surfaces are replaced because of destroyed knee joint.

Clinical Indications

1. For patients with unremitting pain and irreversibly damaged joints:
   a. Primary degenerative arthritis (OA)
   b. Rheumatoid arthritis (RA)
2. Selected fractures (eg, femoral neck fracture)
3. Failure of previous reconstructive surgery (osteotomy, cup arthroplasty, femoral neck fracture complications—nonunion, avascular necrosis)
4. Congenital hip disease
5. Pathologic fractures from metastatic cancer
6. Joint instability

Considerations

1. The prostheses are of various designs and may be fixed to the remaining bone by cement, press fit, or bone ingrowth.
2. Selection of the prosthesis and fixation technique depends on patient's bone structure, joint stability, and other individual characteristics, including age, weight, and activity level.

3. Arthroplasty is an exacting and meticulous procedure. To reduce the risk of an infected prosthesis, special precautions are carried out in the operating room (impermeable operating room attire, clean air system) to reduce particulate matter and bacterial count of the air.

Preoperative Management and Nursing Care

1. Infections (bladder, dental, skin) are ruled out—potential foci of infection for seeding prosthesis infection.
2. Preoperative patient teaching is provided.
   a. Postoperative regimen (eg, extended exercise program) that will be carried out after surgery is explained; atrophied muscles must be reeducated and strengthened).
   b. Isometric exercises (muscle setting) of quadriceps and gluteal muscles are taught.
   c. Bed-to-wheelchair transfer without going beyond the hip flexion limits (usually 45 degrees) is taught.
   d. Nonweight- and partial weight-bearing ambulation with ambulatory aid (walker, crutches) is taught to facilitate postoperative ambulation.
   e. Abduction splint, knee immobilizer, or continuous passive motion is demonstrated if equipment will be used postoperatively.
3. Antiembolism stockings are applied to minimize development of thrombophlebitis.
4. Skin preparation includes antimicrobial solution to reduce skin microorganisms, a potential source of infection.
5. Antibiotics are administered as prescribed to ensure therapeutic blood level during and immediately after surgery. Antimicrobials usually are given immediately preoperatively, intraoperatively, and postoperatively to reduce incidence of infection.
6. Cardiovascular, respiratory, renal, and hepatic function are assessed, and measures are taken to maximize general health condition.

Postoperative Management
Use of Appropriate Positioning

To prevent dislocation of prosthesis and facilitate healing. Numerous modifications are required in positioning these patients postoperatively.

1. After hip arthroplasty:
   a. The patient is usually positioned supine in bed.
   b. The affected extremity is held in slight abduction by either an abduction splint or pillow or Buck's extension traction to prevent dislocation of the prosthesis.
   c. Avoid acute flexion of the hip.

> **NURSING ALERT**
>
> The patient must not adduct or flex operated hip—may lead to subluxation or dislocation of the hip. Signs of joint dislocation include shortened extremity, increasing discomfort, inability to move joints.

   d. Two nurses turn patient on unoperated side while supporting operated hip securely in an abducted position; the entire length of leg is supported by pillows.
      (i) Use pillows to keep the leg abducted; place pillow at back for comfort.
      (ii) Use overhead trapeze to assist with position changes.
   e. The bed is usually not elevated more than 45 degrees; placing patient in an upright sitting position puts a strain on the hip joint and may cause dislocation.
   f. A fracture bedpan is used. Instruct patient to flex the unoperated hip and knee and pull up on the trapeze to lift buttocks onto pan. Instruct patient NOT to bear down on the operated hip in flexion when getting off the pan.
2. After knee arthroplasty:
   a. The knee may be immobilized in extension with a firm compression dressing and an adjustable soft extension splint or long-leg plaster cast.
   b. Leg is elevated on pillows to control swelling.
   c. Alternatively, continuous passive motion may be started to facilitate joint healing and restoration of joint ROM.

Deterring Complications

1. Provide aggressive care and continuous assessment.
2. Prevent thromboembolism by continuous use of sequential compression devices while patient is in bed. Discontinue when patient is ambulatory.

Promoting Early Ambulation

1. Within 2 days after surgery, short periods of standing may be ordered.
   a. Monitor for orthostatic hypotension.
   b. Weight bearing may be limited with ingrowth prosthesis to prevent disruption of bone growth.
2. Transfers to the chair or ambulation with aids, such as walkers, are encouraged as tolerated and based on patient's condition and type of prosthesis.

Nursing Diagnoses

Also see section titled Orthopedic Surgery, page 991.
• Impaired Physical Mobility related to prosthetic joint

Nursing Interventions

See also page 992.
Promoting Mobility
After hip arthroplasty:

1. Use an abduction splint or pillows while assisting patient to get out of bed.
   a. Keep the hip at maximum extension.
   b. Instruct patient to pivot on unoperated extremity.
   c. Assess patient for orthostatic hypotension.
2. When patient is ready to ambulate, teach him or her to advance the walker and then advance the operated extremity to the walker, permitting weight bearing as prescribed.

3. With increased stability, assist patient to use crutches or cane as prescribed.
4. Encourage practice of PT exercises to strengthen muscles and prevent contractures.

After knee arthroplasty:
1. Assist patient with transfer out of bed into wheelchair with extension splint in place.
2. Ensure that no weight bearing is permitted until prescribed by the orthopedic surgeon.
3. Apply continuous passive motion equipment or carry out passive ROM exercises as prescribed.

Community and Home Care Considerations
1. Encourage patient to continue to wear elastic stockings after going home until full activities are resumed.
2. Ensure that patient avoids excessive hip adduction, flexion, and rotation for 6 weeks after hip arthroplasty (hip precautions).
   a. Avoid sitting in low chair/toilet seat to avoid flexing hip more than 90 degrees.
   b. Keep knees apart; do not cross legs.
   c. Limit sitting to 30 minutes at a time—to minimize hip flexion and the risk of prosthetic dislocation and to prevent hip stiffness and flexion contracture.
   d. Avoid internal rotation of the hip.
   e. Follow weight-bearing restrictions from surgeon.
3. Encourage quadriceps setting and ROM exercises as directed.
   a. Have a daily program of stretching, exercise, and rest throughout lifetime.
   b. Do not participate in any activity placing undue or sudden stress on joint (jogging, jumping, lifting heavy loads, becoming obese, excessive bending and twisting).
   c. Use a cane when taking fairly long walks.
4. Suggest self-help and energy-saving devices:
   a. Handrails by toilet.
   b. Raised toilet seat if there is some residual hip flexion problem.
   c. Bar-type stool for kitchen work.
   d. Occupational therapy (OT) devices for dressing, reaching, and so forth.
5. Advise patient to sleep with two pillows between legs to prevent turning over in sleep. Patient should get out of bed with nonoperative leg.
6. Tell patient to lie prone when able twice daily for 30 minutes to promote full extension of hip.
7. Monitor for late complications—deep infection, increased pain and/or decreased function associated with loosening of prosthetic components, implant wear, dislocation, fracture of components, avascular necrosis or dead bone caused by loss of blood supply; heterotrophic ossification (formation of bone in periprosthetic space).
8. Assess home for safety to prevent falls—long phone cords, scatter rugs, pets that run underfoot, slippery floors.

Patient Education and Health Maintenance
1. Teach patient use of supportive equipment (crutches, canes, raised toilet seat) as prescribed.
2. Advise patient to notify all health care providers about prosthetic joint because prophylactic antibiotic will be needed if undergoing any procedure known to cause bacteremia (tooth extraction, manipulation of genitourinary tract).
3. Avoid MRI studies because of implanted metal component.
4. Advise patient that metal component in hip or knee may set off metal detectors (airports, some buildings). The patient should carry an ID card to explain.
5. New hip or knee is designed for low-impact exercise, such as walking, golf, dancing. High-impact exercises such as jogging may cause the prosthesis to loosen.

Outcome-Based Evaluation
- Maintaining proper positioning without evidence of complications

■ Amputation

Amputation is the total or partial surgical removal of an extremity. Amputation is considered a surgical reconstructive procedure.

Indications
1. Inadequate tissue perfusion, such as results with diabetes mellitus or other peripheral vascular diseases
2. Severe trauma
3. Malignant tumor
4. Congenital deformity

Types of Amputation
Open (Guillotine)
1. Used with infection and patients who are poor surgical risks.
2. Wound heals by granulation or secondary closure in about a week.

Closed (Myoplastic or Flap)
1. Residual limb is covered by a flap of skin.
2. Flap of skin is sutured posteriorly.
3. Most common technique used for vascular disease.

Surgical Considerations
1. The surgeon considers possible limb salvage techniques.
   a. Revascularization
   b. Hyperbaric oxygenation
   c. Tumor resection with bone grafting
2. Determines level for amputation based on level of maximal viable tissue for wound healing.
3. Develops a functional, nontender, pressure-tolerant residual limb.

Types of Dressings
Soft Dressing
1. Secured with elastic bandage.
2. Permits wound inspection.

3. Used with patients who should avoid early weight bearing (eg, those with peripheral vascular disease).

Closed, Rigid Plaster Dressing

1. Applied immediately after surgery
2. Controls edema
3. Supports circulation, promoting healing
4. Minimizes pain on movement
5. Shapes residual limb
6. Permits attachment of prosthetic extension (pylon) and early ambulation

Preoperative Management

1. Hemodynamic evaluation is performed through testing, such as angiography, arterial blood flow, xenon 133—to determine optimal amputation level.
2. Culture and sensitivity tests of draining wounds are done to assist in control of infection preoperatively.
3. Evaluation of sound (contralateral) extremity is performed to determine functional potential postoperatively.
4. Evaluation of cardiovascular, respiratory, renal, and other body systems is necessary to determine preoperative condition of patient and reduce the risks of surgery by optimizing function.

GERONTOLOGIC ALERT

Amputation of the lower extremity can be a life-threatening procedure, especially in patients older than age 60 with peripheral vascular disease. Significant morbidity accompanies above-knee amputations because of associated poor health and disease as well as the complications of sepsis and malnutrition and the physiologic insult of amputation.

---

5. Nutritional status is evaluated and optimized with adequate protein to enhance wound healing.
6. Exercises are taught to strengthen muscles for use of ambulatory aids (lower limb amputee).
   a. Flex and extend arms while holding traction weights.
   b. Do push-ups from a prone position if feasible.
   c. Do sit-ups from a seated position if feasible.
7. Use of ambulatory aids is taught.
   a. Instills confidence in ability.
   b. Maintains mobility.
   c. Prepares for postoperative mobility.
8. Phantom sensation is explained—the patient will continue to "feel" the amputated body part for some time.
9. Emotional support is given.
   a. Support concept of amputation as a surgical reconstructive procedure.
   b. Explore patient's perception of procedure and effect on lifestyle.
   c. Avoid unrealistic and misleading reassurance—management of prosthesis can be slow and painful.

Postoperative Management

1. Complications are monitored for—hemorrhage, infection, unrelieved phantom pain, nonhealing wound.
2. Rehabilitation is initiated through PT and prosthetic fitting (if indicated).
3. Therapy is provided for diabetes mellitus, heart disease, infection, stroke, chronic obstructive pulmonary disease, peripheral vascular disease, and age-related deterioration, which are factors limiting rehabilitation.
4. If wound breakdown, infection, delay in healing of residual limb occur, therapy is provided to prevent delay in rehabilitation.
5. Acceptance of body image change is promoted.

Nursing Diagnoses

- Risk for Fluid Volume Deficit related to hemorrhage from disrupted surgical homeostasis
- Altered Tissue Perfusion related to edema and tissue responses to surgery and prosthesis
- Ineffective Coping related to change in body image and self-care
- Pain related to surgical procedure and phantom sensations
- Impaired Physical Mobility related to amputation, muscle weakness, change in body weight distribution

Nursing Interventions

NURSING ALERT

Prevention of complications associated with a major operation and facilitation of early rehabilitation are essential to prevent prolonged disability. Frequent monitoring of patient's physiologic responses to anesthesia, surgery, and immobility is required.

Monitoring Fluid Balance

1. Monitor patient for systemic symptoms of excessive blood loss—hypotension, tachycardia, diaphoresis, decreased alertness.
2. Watch for excessive wound drainage.
   a. Keep tourniquet (in view) attached to end of bed to apply to residual limb (stump) if excessive bleeding occurs.
   b. Reinforce dressing as required, using aseptic technique.
   c. Measure suction drainage.
   d. Maintain accurate record of bloody drainage on dressing and in drainage system.
3. Monitor intake and output for fluid balance.

Maintaining Adequate Tissue Perfusion

1. Control edema.
   a. Elevate residual limb to promote venous return.
   b. Use air splint if prescribed.
2. Maintain pressure dressing.
   a. Reapply if necessary, using sterile dressing secured with elastic bandage.
   b. Notify surgeon if rigid cast dressing comes off.

Supporting Effective Coping

1. Accept patient responses to loss of body part (ie, depression, withdrawal, denial, frustration).
2. Encourage expression of fears and concerns.
3. Recognize that modification of body image takes time.
4. Encourage participation in rehabilitation planning and self-care.
5. Assist patient to adapt to changes in self-care activities.
   a. Upper extremity amputation—encourage independence in one-handed self-care activities using one-handed aids (eg, one-handed knife) as needed.
   b. Lower extremity amputation—encourage mobility using transfer assistance and ambulatory aids as needed.

Controlling Pain

1. Surgical pain
   a. Assess patient's pain experience.
   b. Administer prescribed medications as needed to control postoperative pain.
   c. Use nonpharmaceutical pain management techniques, such as progressive muscle relaxation and imagery.
   d. Recognize that increasing discomfort may indicate presence of hematoma, infection, or necrosis.
2. Phantom sensations (pain)
   a. Anticipate complaint of pain and sensation located in the missing limb ("phantom pain").
   b. Use physical modalities (eg, wrapping, temperature changes) and transcutaneous electrical nerve stimulation (TENS), if prescribed, in relieving discomfort.
   c. Encourage patient activity to decrease awareness of phantom limb pain.
   d. Reassure patient that phantom limb pain will diminish over time.

Promoting Physical Activity

1. Encourage frequent repositioning in bed.
2. Teach patient to avoid long periods in one position.
   a. Avoids dependent edema.
   b. Avoids flexion deformity.
   c. Avoids skin pressure areas.
3. Prevent deformities.
   a. Lower extremity amputations—hip flexion contracture (avoid placing residual limb on pillow; encourage prone position twice a day) and abduction deformity (use trochanter roll; avoid pillow between legs).
   b. Upper extremity amputations—postural abnormalities (encourage good posture).
4. Encourage active ROM and muscle-strengthening exercises, when prescribed, to:
   a. Minimize muscle atrophy.
   b. Increase muscle strength.
   c. Prepare residual limb for prosthesis.
5. Promote reestablishment of balance (amputation alters distribution of body weight).
   a. Transfer to chair within 48 hours after surgery.
   b. Instruct and guard lower limb amputee during balance exercises (ie, arise from chair; stand on toes holding onto chair; bend knee holding onto chair; balance on one leg without support; hop on one foot while holding onto chair).
6. Supervise ambulation, use of wheelchair, and self-care activities.

Patient Education and Health Maintenance

1. Teach patient and family how to wrap residual limb with elastic bandage to control edema and to form a firm conical shape for prosthesis fitting (Figures 32-8 and 32-9).

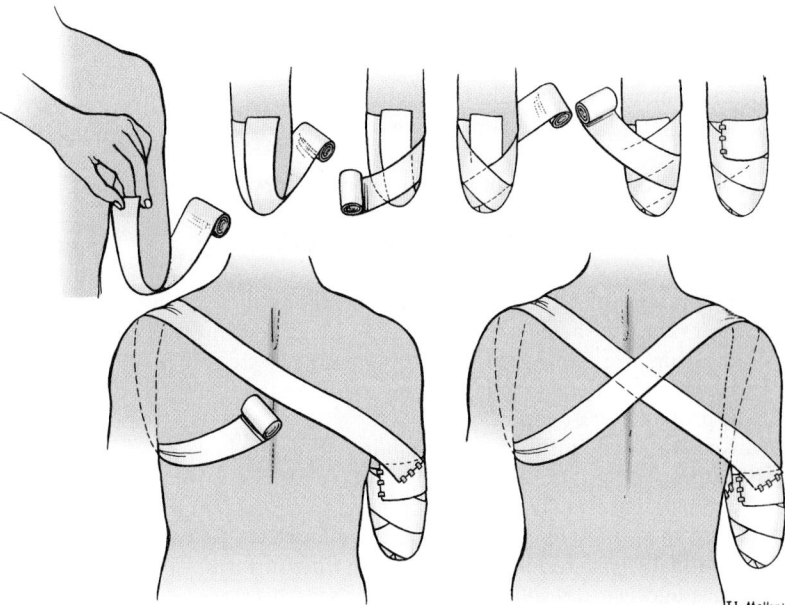

FIGURE 32-8 Wrapping above-elbow residual limb. Elastic bandaging reduces edema and shapes the residual limb for the prosthesis. Bandage may need to be secured by wrapping across back and shoulders.

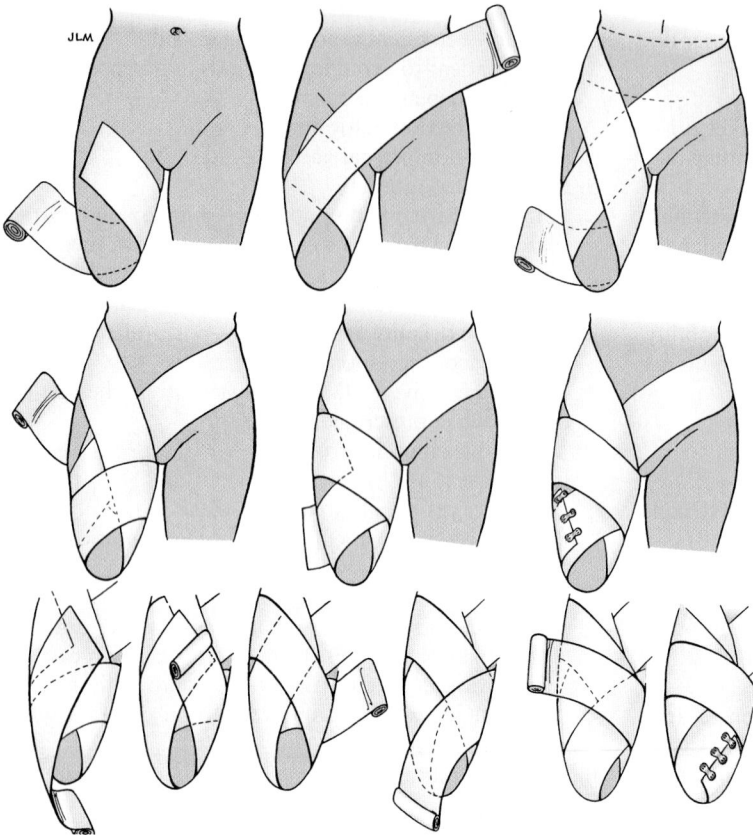

FIGURE 32-9 Wrapping above-knee residual limb. Elastic bandaging reduces edema and shapes the residual limb in a firm conical form for the prosthesis.

a. Wrapping generally begins 1 to 3 days after surgery or after hard plaster dressing is removed.
b. Use diagonal figure-eight bandaging technique.
c. Wrap distal to proximal to maintain pressure gradient and to control edema.
d. Begin wrapping with minimal tension, and increase as wound heals and sutures are removed.
e. Flatten skin at ends of incision to ensure conical stump shape.
f. Rewrap residual limb a couple of times a day and as necessary to achieve a smooth, graded tension dressing.
g. Rewrap if patient complains of more pain—dressing is probably too tight.
h. Keep residual limb wrapped at all times except when bathing.
2. Teach patient residual limb conditioning.
a. Push the residual limb against a soft pillow.
b. Gradually push residual limb against harder surfaces.
c. Massage healed residual limb to soften scar, decrease tenderness, and improve vascularity.

3. Fitting of prosthesis
a. Note residual limb contour.
b. Assess for residual limb contraction.
c. When maximum shrinkage occurs, the prosthetist measures and fits the prosthesis.
d. Adjustments are made by the prosthetist to minimize skin problems.
4. Continuing care of residual limb and prosthesis.
a. Instruct patient to wash and dry limb thoroughly at least twice a day, removing all soap residue, to prevent skin irritation and infection.
b. Avoid soaking residual limb because it results in edema.
c. Inspect residual limb and skin under prosthesis harness daily for pressure, irritation, and actual skin breakdown.
d. Wear residual limb sock/cotton underwear—to absorb perspiration and to avoid direct contact between prosthetic socket/harness and skin.
e. Avoid wrinkles in residual limb sock—potential pressure areas.

f. Wipe socket of prosthesis with a damp cloth when prosthesis is removed for evening.

g. Have prosthesis checked periodically.

5. Teach patient to protect the remaining extremity from injury and to secure prompt treatment of problems.

Outcome-Based Evaluation

- Vital signs stable; dressing reinforced once in 4 hours
- Pressure dressing intact; stump elevated without edema
- Patient participating in plan of care; expressing concerns about independence
- Verbalizes relief of incisional pain; dull phantom sensation tolerable
- Performing ROM actively; transferring to wheelchair with assistance, participating in PT/OT activities

MUSCULOSKELETAL TRAUMA

See Standards of Care Guidelines.

Contusions, Strains, and Sprains

A *contusion* is an injury to the soft tissue produced by a blunt force (blow, kick, or fall). A *sprain* is an injury to ligamentous structures surrounding a joint; it is usually caused by a wrench or twist resulting in a decrease in joint stability. A *strain* is a microscopic tearing of the muscle caused by excessive force, stretching, or overuse.

STANDARDS OF CARE GUIDELINES
Caring for a Patient With Musculoskeletal Trauma, Surgery, Casting, or Immobilization

When caring for a patient with musculoskeletal trauma, surgery, casting, or immobilization, provide the following care as indicated:

- Check neurovascular status of involved extremity(ies).
- Palpate for intact and equal pulses bilaterally.
- Palpate for proper warmth of the skin.
- Check for brisk capillary refill.
- Test sensation to light touch and pain.
- Observe for unusual or increased swelling.
- Ensure that patient can move affected part(s).
- Ensure proper positioning for comfort and alignment.
- Determine pressure points and take precautions to prevent pressure sores.
- Medicate to control pain, particularly before movement, procedures, and physical therapy.
- Provide diversional activities and emotional support during long immobilizations.
- Always document assessments and interventions meticulously, realizing that patient may be involved in Workman's Compensation claim or litigation due to accident and records will be essential to patient's future well-being.

This information should serve as a general guideline only. Each patient situation presents a unique set of clinical factors and requires nursing judgment to guide care, which may include additional or alterative measures and approaches.

Clinical Manifestations

Contusion

1. Hemorrhage into injured part (ecchymosis)—from rupture of small blood vessels; also associated with fractures.
2. Pain, swelling, and discoloration.
3. Hyperkalemia may be present with extensive contusions, resulting in destruction of body tissue and loss of blood.

Strain

1. Hemorrhage into the muscle
2. Swelling
3. Tenderness
4. Pain with isometric contraction
5. May be associated spasm

Sprain

1. Rapid swelling—due to extravasation of blood within tissues
2. Pain on passive movement of joint
3. Increasing pain during first few hours due to continued swelling

Management

1. X-ray may be done to rule out fracture.
2. Immobilize in splint, elastic wrap, or compression dressing to support weakened structures and control swelling.
3. Apply ice for first 24 hours.
4. Analgesics usually include nonsteroidal anti-inflammatory drugs (NSAIDs).
5. Severe sprains may require surgical repair and/or cast immobilization.

Nursing Interventions and Patient Education

1. Elevate the affected part. Maintain splint or immobilization as prescribed.
2. Apply cold compresses for the first 24 hours (20 to 30 minutes at a time)—to produce vasoconstriction, decrease edema, and reduce discomfort.
3. Apply heat to affected area after 24 hours (20 to 30 minutes at a time) four times a day—to promote circulation and absorption.
4. Assess neurovascular status of contused extremity every hour to every 4 hours as patient's condition indicates.
5. Instruct patient on use of pain medication as prescribed.
6. Ensure correct use of crutches or other mobility aid with or without weight bearing, as prescribed.
7. Educate on need to rest injured part for about a month to allow for healing.
8. Teach patient to resume activities gradually.
9. Teach patient to avoid excessive exercise of injured part.
10. Teach patient to avoid reinjury by "warming up" before exercise.
11. Complementary methods such as acupuncture, biofeedback, and imagery may contribute to healing by reducing anxiety and pain.

Tendinitis

Tendinitis is an inflammation of a tendon caused by a lack of sufficient lubrication of the tendon sheath. May be caused by acute stress on tendon structure or by chronic overuse.

Clinical Manifestations

1. Onset of pain may occur immediately after activity or delayed up to a day later. Range-of-motion and resistance testing is painful.
2. Sudden onset of sharp pain in calf and hearing/feeling a "snap" are associated with tendon rupture, as in Achilles tendinitis due to running injuries.
3. Mild swelling occurs, and the tendon sheath is tender to the touch.

Management

1. X-rays not usually diagnostic.
2. Thompson's test helps with diagnosis of Achilles rupture. Patient kneels on chair or lies prone. Examiner squeezes calf of affected leg. Normal response: foot moves downward, denoting intact tendon. If foot does not move, tendon is assumed to be ruptured.
3. Initial treatment includes rest, ice, compression, elevation (RICE).
4. Splinting or casting for up to 6 weeks in functional position usually necessary.
5. Surgical intervention may be necessary if rupture is complete.
6. PT to regain strength and function.

Nursing Interventions and Patient Education

1. Ensure understanding of need for proper immobilization for full time period even though fracture is not present.
2. Encourage the use of warm compresses after 24 hours to relieve pain and inflammation.
3. Advise patient not to return to full activity until strength is equal to unaffected extremity.
4. Teach proper warm-up before exercise/sports activities (stretching of all major tendons).

Bursitis

Bursitis is a painful inflammation of the bursae. Bursae are fluid-filled sacs that are lined with synovium similar to the lining of the joint spaces. Bursae reduce friction between tendons and bones or tendons and ligaments. They are found over joints with bony prominences such as the trochanter, patella, and olecranon. Friction between skin and musculoskeletal tissues may result in bursitis.

Clinical Manifestations

1. Pain around a joint—commonly the knee, elbow, shoulder, and hip.
2. Varying degrees of redness, warmth, and swelling may be visible.
3. There is point tenderness and limited ROM on examination.

Management and Nursing Interventions

1. Rest and immobilization of affected joint
2. Ice for the first 48 hours; moist heat every 4 hours thereafter
3. Non-narcotic analgesics such as NSAIDs
4. Range-of-motion exercises
5. Intra-articular corticosteroid injection
6. Surgery indicated when calcified deposits or adhesions have diminished function

Plantar Fasciitis

Plantar fasciitis is inflammation of the fascia that runs along the bottom of the foot from heel to toes. As the fascia is stretched, microscopic tears develop at the point where fascia attaches to the calcaneus.

Clinical Manifestations

1. Pain along sole of foot, usually unilateral, but may be bilateral
2. Worse upon arising, diminishes with walking
3. Tenderness of heel area

Management and Nursing Interventions

1. Rest—decrease walking, running, exercise, standing.
2. NSAIDs for pain and inflammation.
3. Good supportive footwear.
4. Orthotic devices may be beneficial.
5. Heel cup to cushion the heel (over the counter).
6. Arch support orthotics for pes planus (flat foot).
7. Cushioning of arches for pes cavus (high arch).
8. Steroid injection into painful area.
9. Surgery for release of fascia as last resort.

Traumatic Joint Dislocation

A *dislocation of a joint* occurs when the surfaces of the bones forming the joint are no longer in anatomic contact. This is a medical emergency because of associated disruption of surrounding blood and nerve supplies.

1. Shoulder, fingers, elbow are most common joints to dislocate.
2. Mechanism of injury can be anterior, posterior, lateral, or medial force. Posterior dislocation is the most common.

Clinical Manifestations

1. Pain
2. Deformity
3. Change in the length of the extremity
4. Loss of normal movement
5. X-ray confirmation of dislocation without associated fracture

Management

1. Immobilize part while patient is transported to emergency department, x-ray department, or clinical unit.
2. Secure reduction of dislocation (bring displaced parts into normal position) as soon as possible to prevent

circulatory or nerve impairments; usually performed under anesthesia.

3. Stabilize reduction until joint structures are healed to prevent permanently unstable joint or aseptic necrosis of bone.

Nursing Interventions and Patient Education

1. Assess neurovascular status of extremity before and after reduction of dislocation.
2. Administer or teach self-administration of pain medications, such as NSAIDs.
3. Ensure proper use of immobilization device after reduction.
4. Review instructions for activity restrictions and need for PT and follow-up.

Knee Injuries

The knee ligaments provide stability to the knee joint. These ligaments promote rotational stability (*anterior cruciate ligament [ACL]* and *posterior cruciate ligament*) and prevent varus and valgus instability (*medial and lateral collateral ligaments*). Pieces of cartilage that stabilize the knee internally are known as the medial and lateral menisci. *Anterior cruciate ligament injuries* and *medial meniscus tears* are common due to sports injuries.

Clinical Manifestations

1. Severe stresses are applied to the knee during many sports activities (eg, soccer, skiing, running).
2. Injury to knee structures occurs during rapid position changes involving flexing and twisting of the joint.
3. Torn cartilage (meniscus) causes pain, tenderness, joint effusion, clicking sensations, and decreased ROM.
4. Knee ligaments may be torn, resulting in pain on ambulation, swelling, and joint instability. The patellar tendon may rupture.

Management

1. Special assessment techniques are done to detect anterior cruciate ligament injury (Table 32-1).

2. MRI shows injury to soft tissue involved.
3. Some injuries may be immobilized (splint, brace, or cast) and treated with PT.
4. ACL reconstruction frequently indicated.
   a. Arthroscopic surgery preferred; synthetic ligaments selected where ligaments failed. Graft rejection is a complication.
   b. Postoperative continuous passive motion used.
   c. Postoperative ACL rehabilitation program includes progressive ROM, bracing (not done with synthetic ligaments).
   d. Long-term bracing during sports controversial.
5. Meniscal injury—damaged cartilage removed.
   a. Arthroscopic or open meniscectomy.
   b. Rehabilitation includes progressive ROM and quadriceps strengthening.

Nursing Interventions and Patient Education

1. After arthroscopic surgery, ensure proper use of crutches as indicated and encourage pain control through medications as prescribed and rest, ice, compression, and elevation.
2. For open joint surgery, see care of patient undergoing orthopedic surgery, page 991.
3. Teach patient strengthening exercises for affected extremity.
4. Teach patient to prevent fatigue through rest periods, conservation of energy.
5. Advise on prevention of injuries using proper equipment and footwear for sports.

Fractures

A *fracture* is a break in the continuity of bone. A fracture occurs when the stress placed on a bone is greater than the bone can absorb. Muscles, blood vessels, nerves, tendons, joints, and other organs may be injured when fracture occurs.

Types of Fractures

1. *Complete*—involves the entire cross section of the bone, usually displaced (not normal position)

TABLE 32-1 Assessment Techniques for Anterior Cruciate Ligament Injury

Test	Description	Positive Finding
Anterior drawer test	Place patient supine with knee in 90 degrees of flexion with foot flat on table. Proximal tibia is pulled forward by examiner using two hands.	Tibia subluxes (dislocates) forward on femur.
Lachman test	Place patient supine with knee in 15–20 degrees of flexion. Distal femur is grasped by examiner with one hand while the other hand grasps the proximal tibia and applies forward pressure.	Tibia subluxes forward on femur.
Pivot shift test (evaluates anterolateral rotational stability)	Place patient supine with knee slightly flexed. Examiner grasps patient's ankle in one hand and places palm of other hand over the lateral aspect of the knee distal to the joint. Lower leg is extended and internally rotated, applying a valgus (lateral) stress to knee.	Tibia subluxes and reduces itself ("pivots and shifts")

2. *Incomplete*—involves a portion of the cross section of the bone or may be longitudinal
3. *Closed (simple)*—skin (mucous membranes) not broken
4. *Open (compound)*—skin broken, leading directly to fracture
   a. Grade I—minimal soft tissue injury
   b. Grade II—laceration greater than 1 cm without extensive soft tissue flaps
   c. Grade III—extensive soft tissue injury, including skin, muscle, neurovascular structure, with crushing
5. *Pathologic*—through an area of diseased bone (osteoporosis, bone cyst, bone tumor, bony metastasis)

Patterns of Fracture
See Figure 32-10.
1. *Greenstick*—one side of the bone is broken and the other side is bent.
2. *Transverse*—straight across the bone.
3. *Oblique*—at an angle across the bone.
4. *Spiral*—twists around the shaft of the bone.
5. *Comminuted*—bone splintered into more than three fragments.
6. *Depressed*—fragment(s) are driven inward (seen in fractures of the skull and facial bones).
7. *Compression*—bone collapses in on itself (seen in vertebral fractures).
8. *Avulsion*—fragment of bone pulled off by ligament or tendon attachment.
9. *Impacted*—fragment of bone wedged into other bone fragment.

GERONTOLOGIC ALERT

Osteoporosis is a major risk for fractures, particularly hip and vertebral compression fractures.

10. *Fracture-dislocation*—fracture complicated by the bone being out of the joint.
11. *Other*—described according to anatomic location: epiphyseal, supracondylar, midshaft, intra-articular, and so forth.

Clinical Manifestations
Physical Findings
1. Pain at site of injury
2. Swelling
3. Tenderness
4. False motion and crepitus (grating sensation)
5. Deformity
6. Loss of function
7. Ecchymosis
8. Paresthesia

Altered Neurovascular Status
1. Injured muscle, blood vessels, nerves
2. Compression of structures resulting in ischemia
3. Findings:

a. Progressive uncontrollable pain
b. Pain on passive movement
c. Altered sensations (paresthesia)
d. Loss of active motion
e. Diminished capillary refill response
f. Pallor

Shock
1. Bone is very vascular.
2. Overt hemorrhage through open wound.
3. Covert hemorrhage into soft tissues (especially with femoral fracture) or body cavity, as with pelvic fracture.
4. May be fatal if not detected.

Diagnostic Evaluation
1. X-ray and other imaging studies to determine integrity of bone
2. Blood studies (complete blood count, electrolytes) with blood loss and extensive muscle damage—may show decreased hemoglobin and hematocrit
3. Arthroscopy to detect joint involvement
4. Angiography if associated with blood vessel injury
5. Nerve conduction and electromyogram studies to detect nerve injury

Management
(Emergency management—see p. 1075.)
Principles of Management
1. Factors influencing choice of management include:
   a. Type, location, and severity of fracture.
   b. Soft tissue damage.
   c. Age and health status of patient, including type and extent of other injuries.
2. Goals include:
   a. To regain and maintain correct position and alignment.
   b. To regain the function of the involved part.
   c. To return patient to usual activities in the shortest time and at the least expense.
3. The management process is a three-step process:
   a. *Reduction*—setting the bone; refers to restoration of the fracture fragments into anatomic position and alignment
   b. *Immobilization*—maintains reduction until bone healing occurs (Figures 32-11 and 32-12)
   c. *Rehabilitation*—regaining normal function of the affected part

Approaches to Management
Vary by specific site of fracture (Table 32-2).
1. Closed reduction
   a. Bony fragments are brought into apposition (ends in contact) by manipulation and manual traction—restores alignment.
   b. May be done under anesthesia for pain relief and muscle relaxation.
   c. Cast or splint applied to immobilize extremity and maintain reduction (see section titled Casts, p. 978).

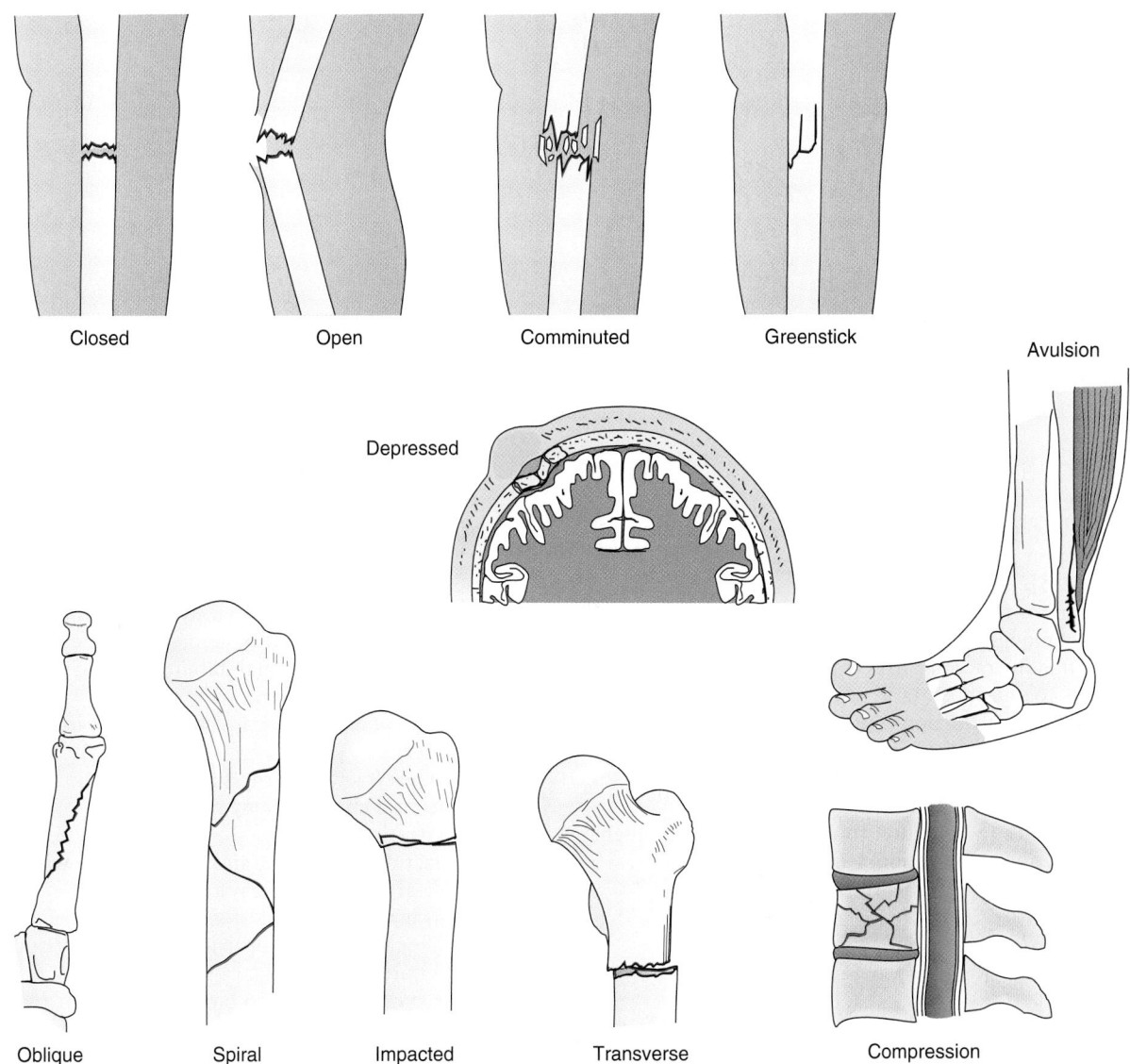

Avulsion—a pulling away of a fragment of bone by a ligament or tendon and its attachment

Closed—a fracture that remains contained; does not break the skin

Comminuted—a fracture in which bone has splintered into several fragments

Compression—a fracture in which bone has been compressed (seen in vertebral fractures)

Depressed—a fracture in which fragments are driven inward (seen frequently in fractures of the skull and facial bones)

Epiphyseal—a fracture through the epiphysis

Greenstick—a fracture in which one side of a bone is broken and the other side is bent

Impacted—a fracture in which a bone fragment is driven into another bone fragment

Oblique—a fracture occurring at an angle across the bone (less stable than transverse)

Open—a fracture in which damage also involves the skin or mucous membranes

Pathologic—a fracture that occurs through an area of diseased bone (bone cyst, Paget's disease, bony metastasis, tumor); can occur without trauma or a fall

Spiral—a fracture twisting around the shaft of the bone

Transverse—a fracture that is straight across the bone

FIGURE 32-10 Patterns of fractures.

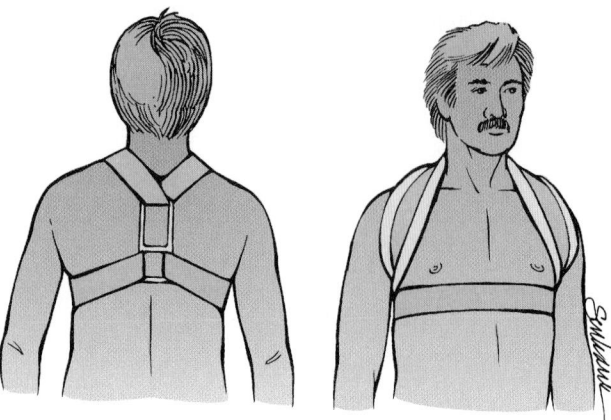

FIGURE 32-11 Method for immobilizing a clavicular fracture with a clavicular strap.

2. Traction
   a. Pulling force applied to accomplish and maintain reduction and alignment (see section titled Traction, p. 985).
   b. Used for fractures of long bones.
   c. Techniques
      (i) Skin traction—force applied to the skin using foam rubber, tape, and so forth
      (ii) Skeletal traction—force applied to the bony skeleton directly, using wires, pins, or tongs placed into or through the bone
3. Open reduction with internal fixation
   a. Operative intervention to achieve reduction, alignment, and stabilization.

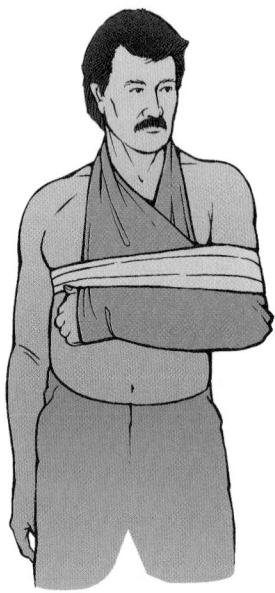

FIGURE 32-12 Immobilization of fracture of upper humerus can be achieved with conventional sling and swathe.

      (i) Bone fragments are directly visualized.
      (ii) Internal fixation devices (metal pins, wires, screws, plates, nails, rods) used to hold bone fragments in position until solid bone healing occurs (may be removed when bone is healed).
      (iii) After closure of the wound, splints or casts may be used for additional stabilization and support.
4. Endoprosthetic replacement
   a. Replacement of a fracture fragment with an implanted metal device.
   b. Used when fracture disrupts nutrition of the bone or treatment of choice is bony replacement.
5. External fixation device
   a. Stabilization of complex and open fracture with use of a metal frame and pin system.
   b. Permits active treatment of injured soft tissue.
      (i) Wound may be left open (delayed primary wound closure).
      (ii) Repair of damage to blood vessels, soft tissue, muscles, nerves, and tendons as indicated.
      (iii) Reconstructive surgery may be necessary (see section titled External Fixation, p. 989).

Complications
Complications Associated With Immobility
1. Muscle atrophy, loss of muscle strength and endurance
2. Loss of ROM—joint contracture
3. Pressure sores at bony prominences or from immobilizing device pressing on skin
4. Diminished respiratory, cardiovascular, GI function, resulting in possible pooling of respiratory secretions, orthostatic hypotension, anorexia, constipation, and so forth

Other Acute Complications
1. Venous stasis and thromboembolism—particularly with fractures of the hip and lower extremities
2. Neurovascular compromise
3. Infection—especially with open fractures
4. Shock—due to significant hemorrhage
5. Pulmonary emboli

TABLE 32-2 Fractures of Specific Sites

Site and Mechanism	Management	Nursing/Patient Care Considerations
Clavicle—fall on shoulder	1. Closed reduction and immobilization with clavicular strap (Figure 32-11), figure-eight bandage, or sling 2. Open reduction with internal fixation for marked displacement, severely comminuted fracture, and extensive soft tissue injury	1. Pad axilla to prevent nerve damage from pressure of immobilizer 2. Assess neurovascular status of arm 3. Teach exercises of elbow, wrist, and fingers 4. Teach shoulder exercises through full range of motion as prescribed
Proximal humerus—fall on outstretched arm; osteoporosis is predisposing factor	1. Many remain in alignment and are supported by a sling and swathe or Belpeau bandage for comfort (Figure 32-12) 2. If displaced, treated with reduction under x-ray control, open reduction, or replacement of humeral head with prosthesis	1. Place a soft pad under the axilla to prevent skin maceration 2. Encourage shoulder range-of-motion exercises after specified period of immobilization to prevent frozen shoulder 3. Instruct patient to lean forward and allow affected arm to abduct and rotate

Shaft of humerus—direct fall, blow to arm, or auto injury; damage to radial nerve may occur	1. Immobilize with sling and swathe, splint, or hanging cast
	2. A hanging cast is applied for its weight to correct displaced fractures with shortening of the humeral shaft
	3. ORIF for associated vascular injury or pathologic fracture, followed by support in sling
		1. Hanging cast must remain unsupported to maintain traction
		   a. Teach patient to avoid supporting elbow in lap or arm on pillow
		   b. Patient should sleep in upright position to maintain 24-h traction.
		2. Encourage exercise of fingers immediately after application of cast
		3. Teach pendulum exercises of arm as prescribed to prevent frozen shoulder

Elbow and forearm—fall on elbow, outstretched hand, or direct blow (sideswipe injury)	1. Treatment depends on specific characteristics of fracture—ORIF, arthroplasty, external fixation, casting 2. Closed drainage system may be used to decrease hematoma formation and swelling	1. Assess neurovascular status of forearm and hand 2. If radial pulse weakens or disappears, report immediately to prevent irreversible ischemia 3. Elevate arm to control edema 4. Encourage finger and shoulder exercises

Wrist—Colles' fracture is common (1.2–2.5 cm above the wrist with dorsal displacement of lower fragment); caused by fall on outstretched palm; often associated with osteoporosis	1. Closed reduction with splint or cast support
	2. Percutaneous pins and external fixator or plaster cast
		1. Elevate arm above level of heart for 48 h after reduction to promote venous and lymphatic return and reduce swelling
		2. Watch for swelling of fingers and check for constricting bandages or cast
		3. Teach finger exercises to reduce swelling and stiffness
		   a. Hold hand above level of heart
		   b. Move fingers from full extension to flexion
		   c. Hold and release
		   d. Repeat at least 10 times every half hour when awake for as long as swelling occurs
		4. Encourage daily prescribed exercises to restore full extension and supination

Hand—caused by numerous injuries	1. Splinting for undisplaced fractures of fingers 2. Débridement, irrigation and Kirchner wire fixation for open fractures 3. Reconstructive surgery may be necessary for complex injuries	1. Provide aggressive care and encouragement with rehabilitation plan to regain maximal function of hand.

Hip (proximal femur)—occur frequently in older adults, women with osteoporosis, and with falls
Types:
1. Intracapsular—femoral neck within joint capsule
2. Extracapsular—femoral neck between greater and lesser trochanter (intertrochanteric) or of femoral shaft
3. Subtrochanteric—of femur just below level of lesser trochanter
	1. Hip fracture identified by shortening and external rotation of affected leg; pain in hip or knee; inability to move leg
	2. Immobilization with Buck's extension traction until surgery
	3. Surgery as soon as medically stable; choice depends on location, character, and patient factors
	   a. Internal fixation with nail, nail–plate combination, multiple pins, screw, or sliding nails
	   b. Femoral prosthetic replacement
	   c. Total hip replacement
		1. Provide constant monitoring and nursing care to reduce the risk of complications, such as pneumonia, thrombophlebitis, fat emboli, dislocation of prosthesis, infection, and pressure sores
		2. Administer aspirin, warfarin (Coumadin), or low-dose subcutaneous heparin as ordered
		3. Use sequential compression devices as ordered
		4. Provide meticulous skin care to prevent breakdown

(continued)

TABLE 32-2 Fractures of Specific Sites (Continued)

Site and Mechanism	Management	Nursing/Patient Care Considerations
		a. Use trapeze for patient to assist with position changes b. Use special bed or mattress as indicated c. Inspect heels daily and use heel protection measures 5. Prevent urinary tract infection by increasing fluids and encouraging frequent voiding 6. Keep affected leg in abduction and neutral rotation 7. Teach quadriceps setting exercise to prevent muscle atrophy of affected leg
Femoral shaft	1. Closed reduction and stabilization with skeletal traction—Thomas leg splint with Pearson attachment; followed by use of orthosis (cast-brace) to allow weight bearing 2. Open reduction with hardware or with bone grafting may be necessary 3. External fixator may be used	1. Marked concealed blood loss may occur; watch for signs of shock initially and anemia later 2. Examine skin under the ring of the Thomas splint for signs of pressure
Knee—direct blow to knee area; involve distal shaft of femur (supracondylar), articular surfaces, or patella	1. Closed reduction and/or immobilization through casting, traction, braces, splints 2. ORIF 3. Goal is to preserve knee mobility	1. Elevate extremity by raising foot gatch of bed 2. Evaluate for effusion—report and loosen pressure dressing if pain is severe; prepare for joint aspiration 3. Teach quadriceps setting exercises and limited weight bearing as prescribed
Tibia and fibula/ankle—distal tibia or fibula, malleoli, or talus fractures generally result from forceful twisting of ankle and often associated with ligament disruption: also high incidence of open fractures of tibial shaft, because tibia lies superficially beneath the skin	1. Closed reduction and toe-to-groin cast for closed fractures, later replaced by short leg cast or orthosis 2. ORIF may be necessary for some closed fractures 3. External fixator for open fracture	1. Elevate lower leg to control edema 2. Avoid dependent position of extremity for prolonged periods 2. Prepare patient for long immobilization period, as union is slow (12–16 weeks, longer for open and comminuted fractures) 3. Prepare patient for stiff ankle joint following immobilization
Foot—metatarsal fracture due to crush injuries of foot	1. Immobilization with cast, splint, or strapping	1. Encourage partial weight bearing as allowed 2. Elevate foot to control edema
Thoracic and lumbar spine—trauma from falls, contact sports, or auto accidents, or excessive loading may cause fracture of vertebral body, lamina, spinous and transverse processes; usually stable compression fractures	1. Suspected with pain that is worsened by movement and coughing and radiates to extremities, abdomen, or intercostal muscles; and presence of sensory and motor deficits 2. Bed rest on firm mattress and pain relief followed by progressive ambulation and back strengthening to treat stable fractures; takes about 6 weeks to heal 3. ORIF with Harrington rod, body cast, or laminectomy with spinal fusion may be necessary for unstable or displaced fractures	1. Use log roll technique to change positions 2. Monitor bowel and bladder dysfunction, as paralytic ileus and bladder distention may occur with nerve root injury 3. Assist patient to ambulate when pain subsides, no neurologic deficit exists, and x-rays reveal no displacement 4. Teach proper body mechanics and back preservation techniques 5. Encourage weight reduction 6. Teach patient with osteoporosis the importance of safety measures to avoid falls

Pelvis—sacrum, ilium, pubic, ischium, and coccyx fractures may occur from auto accidents, crush injuries, and falls; most are stable fractures that do not involve the pelvic ring and have minimal displacement	1. Emergency management to treat multiple trauma, shock from intraperitoneal hemorrhage, and injury to internal organs is necessary (see p. 1076–1082)
	2. Bed rest for several days followed by progressive weight bearing for stable fracture
	3. Prolonged bed rest, external fixation, ORIF, skeletal traction, or pelvic sling are options for unstable fracture
		1. Monitor and support vital functions as indicated
		2. Observe urine output for blood indicating genitourinary injury
		3. Do not attempt to insert urethral catheter until patency of urethra is known; incidence of urethral injury in males is high with anterior fractures
		4. Assist the patient being treated in pelvic sling
		  a. Fold sling back over buttocks to enable the patient to use bedpan
		  b. Reach under sling to give skin care; line sling with sheepskin
		  c. Loosen sling only as directed

Fat Emboli Syndrome

1. Associated with embolization of marrow or tissue fat or platelets and free fatty acids to the pulmonary capillaries, producing rapid onset of symptoms
2. Clinical manifestations
   a. Respiratory distress—tachypnea, hypoxemia, crackles, wheezes, acute pulmonary edema, interstitial pneumonitis
   b. Mental disturbances—irritability, restlessness, confusion, disorientation, stupor, coma due to systemic embolization, and severe hypoxia
   c. Fever
   d. Petechiae in buccal membranes, hard palate, conjunctival sacs, chest, anterior axillary folds, due to occlusion of capillaries

> **NURSING ALERT**
>
> Restlessness, confusion, irritability, and disorientation may be the first signs of fat embolism syndrome. Confirm hypoxia with arterial blood gas analysis. Young adults (20 to 30 years old) and older adults (60 to 70 years old) with multiple fractures or fractures of long bones or pelvis are particularly susceptible to development of fat emboli.

Bone Union Problems

1. *Delayed union* (takes longer to heal than average for type of fracture)
2. *Nonunion* (fractured bone fails to unite)
3. *Malunion* (union occurs but is faulty—misaligned)

Nursing Assessment

1. Ask patient how the fracture occurred—mechanism of injury important in determining possible associated injuries.
2. Ask patient to describe location, character, and intensity of pain to help determine possible source of discomfort.
3. Ask patient to describe sensations in injured extremity—to aid in evaluation of neurovascular status.
4. Observe patient's ability to change position—to assess functional mobility.
5. Note patient's emotional status and behavior—indicators of ability to cope with stress of injury.

> **NURSING ALERT**
>
> Change in behavior and/or cerebral functioning may be an early indicator of cerebral anoxia from shock or pulmonary or fat emboli.

6. Assess patient's support system; identify current and potential sources of assistance/caregiving.
7. Review findings on past and present health status—to aid in formulating plan of care.
8. Conduct physical examination.
   a. Examine skin for lacerations, abrasions, ecchymosis; note areas of swelling and edema.
   b. Auscultate lungs to establish baseline assessment of respiratory function.
   c. Assess pulses and blood pressure; assess peripheral tissue perfusion, especially in injured extremity, to establish circulatory status baseline.
   d. Determine neurologic status (sensations and movement) of extremity distal to injury.
   e. Note length, alignment, and immobilization of injured extremity.
   f. Evaluate behavior and cognitive functioning of patient to determine ability to participate in care planning and patient education activities.

> **GERONTOLOGIC ALERT**
>
> Assessment of patient's health and functional abilities before fracture and available support system facilitates development of realistic rehabilitation and discharge goals.

Nursing Diagnoses

- Risk for Fluid Volume Deficit related to hemorrhage and shock
- Impaired Gas Exchange related to immobility and potential pulmonary emboli or fat emboli
- Risk for Peripheral Neurovascular Dysfunction
- Risk for Injury related to thromboembolism
- Pain related to injury
- Risk for Infection related to open fracture or surgical intervention
- Bathing and Hygiene Self-Care Deficit related to immobility
- Impaired Physical Mobility related to injury/treatment modality
- Risk for Disuse Syndrome related to injury and immobilization
- Post-Trauma Response

Nursing Interventions

Evaluating for Hemorrhage and Shock

1. Monitor vital signs as frequently as clinical condition indicates, observing for hypotension, elevated pulse, cold clammy skin, restlessness, pallor.
2. Watch for evidence of hemorrhage on dressings or in drainage containers.
3. Review laboratory data; report abnormal values.
4. Administer prescribed fluids/blood to maintain circulating volume.
5. Monitor intake and output.

Monitoring for Impaired Gas Exchange

1. Evaluate changes in mental status and restlessness that may indicate hypoxia.
2. Review diagnostic evaluation data—especially arterial blood gas values and chest x-ray.
3. Position to enhance respiratory effort.
4. Encourage coughing and deep breathing to promote lung expansion and diminish pooling of pulmonary secretions.
5. Administer oxygen as prescribed.
6. Report any sudden or progressive changes in respiratory status.

Preventing Neurovascular Compromise

1. Monitor neurovascular status for compression of nerve, diminished circulation, development of compartment syndrome.
   a. Pain—progressive, localized, deep throbbing, persistent, unrelieved by immobilization and medications
   b. Pain—on passive stretch
   c. Weakness progressing to paralysis
   d. Altered sensation, hypothesia, paresthesia
   e. Poor capillary refill response
   f. Skin color—pale, cyanotic
   g. Elevated compartment pressure—palpable tightness of muscle compartment, elevated measured tissue pressure
   h. Pulselessness

> **NURSING ALERT**
>
> Monitoring the neurovascular integrity of the injured extremity is essential. Development of compartment syndrome (increased tissue pressure causing hypoxemia) leads to permanent loss of function in 6 to 8 hours. This situation must be identified and managed promptly.

2. Reduce swelling.
   a. Elevate injured extremity (unless compartment syndrome is suspected—may contribute to vascular compromise).
   b. Apply cold to injury if prescribed.
3. Relieve pressure caused by immobilizing device as prescribed (such as bivalving cast, rewrapping elastic bandage, or splinting device).
4. Relieve pressure on skin to prevent development of pressure sore.
   a. Frequent repositioning
   b. Skin care
   c. Special mattresses

Preventing Development of Thromboembolism

> **GERONTOLOGIC ALERT**
>
> Older adults with fractures, trauma, immobility, obesity, or history of thrombophlebitis are at high risk for developing thromboembolism.

1. Encourage active and passive ankle exercises.
2. Use elastic stockings, foot pumps, or sequential compression devices, as prescribed.
3. Elevate legs to prevent stasis, avoiding pressure on blood vessels.
4. Encourage mobility; change position frequently; encourage ambulation.
5. Administer anticoagulants as prescribed.
6. Monitor for development of thrombophlebitis.
   a. Note complaint of pain and tenderness in calf.
   b. Report calf pain.
   c. Report increased size and temperature of calf.

Relieving Pain

1. Secure data concerning pain.
   a. Have patient describe the pain, location, characteristics (dull, sharp, continuous, throbbing, boning, radiating, aching, and so forth).
   b. Ask patient what causes the pain, makes the pain worse, relieves the pain, and so forth.
   c. Evaluate patient for proper body alignment, pressure from equipment (casts, traction, splints, appliances).
2. Initiate activities to prevent or modify pain.
   a. Assist patient with pain-reduction techniques—cutaneous stimulation, distraction, guided imagery, TENS, biofeedback, and so forth.
   b. Immobilize injured part.
   c. Position patient in correct alignment.
   d. Support splinted fracture above and below fracture when repositioning or moving patient.
   e. Reposition patient with slow and steady motion; use additional personnel as needed.
   f. Elevate painful extremity to diminish venous congestion.
   g. Apply heat or cold modalities as prescribed.
   h. Modify environment to facilitate rest and relaxation.
3. Administer prescribed pharmaceuticals as indicated. Encourage use of less potent drugs as severity of discomfort decreases.
4. Establish a supportive relationship to assist patient to deal with discomfort.
5. Encourage patient to become an active participant in rehabilitative plans.

Monitoring for Development of Infection

1. Cleanse, débride, and irrigate open fracture wound as prescribed as soon as possible to minimize chance of infection.
   a. Open fractures are contaminated.
   b. Begin prescribed antibiotic therapy promptly after wound culture obtained.
2. Use sterile technique during dressing changes to minimize infection of wound, soft tissues, and bone.
3. Evaluate patient for elevation of temperature at regular intervals.
4. Note elevated white blood cell (WBC) counts.
5. Report areas of inflammation and swelling around incision or open wound.
6. Report purulent drainage.
7. Obtain specimens for culture and sensitivity to determine causative organism.
8. Administer antibiotic therapy as prescribed.

Promoting Self-Care Activities

1. Encourage participation in care.
2. Arrange patient area and personal items for patient convenience to promote independence.
3. Modify activities to facilitate maximum independence within prescribed limits.
4. Allow time for patient to accomplish task.
5. Teach safe use of mobility and other aids.

6. Assist with ADLs as needed.

7. Teach family how to assist patient while promoting independence in self-care.

Promoting Physical Mobility

1. Perform active and passive exercises to all nonimmobilized joints.

2. Encourage patient participation in frequent position changes, maintaining supports to fracture during position changes.

3. Minimize prolonged periods of physical inactivity, encouraging ambulation when prescribed.

4. Administer prescribed analgesics judiciously to decrease pain associated with movement.

Preventing Development of Disuse Syndrome

1. Teach and encourage isometric exercises to diminish muscle atrophy.

2. Encourage use of immobilized extremity within prescribed limits.

Promoting Positive Psychological Response to Trauma

1. Monitor patient for symptoms of post-trauma stress disorder.
   a. Memory of event; anger, helplessness, vulnerability, mood swings, depression, cognitive impairment, sleep disturbance, increased dependency, social withdrawal.

2. Assist patient to move through phases of post-traumatic stress (outcry, denial, intrusiveness, working through, completion).

3. Establish trusting therapeutic relationship with patient.

4. Encourage patient to express thoughts and feelings about traumatic event.

5. Encourage patient to participate in decision making to reestablish control and overcome feelings of helplessness.

6. Teach relaxation techniques to decrease anxiety.

7. Encourage development of adaptive responses and participation in support groups.

8. Refer patient to psychiatric liaison nurse or refer for psychotherapy, as needed.

Community and Home Care Considerations

1. Assist patient to actively exercise joints above and below the immobilized fracture at frequent intervals.
   a. Isometric exercises of muscles covered by cast—start exercise as soon as possible after cast application.
   b. Increase isometric exercises as fracture stabilizes.

2. After removal of immobilizing device (eg, cast, splint), have patient start isotonic exercises and continue with isometric exercises.

3. Assess the home for any safety hazards for falls when patient ambulates.

4. Obtain PT/OT consultation for assistance with ADLs, transferring technique, gait strengthening, and conditioning after lengthy immobilization, as needed.

5. Assess orthostatic blood pressure when patient begins to ambulate to prevent falls.

Patient Education and Health Maintenance

1. Explain basis for fracture treatment and need for patient participation in therapeutic regimen.

2. Promote adjustment of usual lifestyle and responsibilities to accommodate limitations imposed by fracture.

3. Instruct patient on exercises to strengthen upper extremity muscles if crutch walking is planned.

4. Instruct patient in methods of safe ambulation—walker, crutches, cane.

5. Emphasize instructions concerning amount of weight bearing that will be permitted on fractured extremity.

6. Discuss prevention of recurrent fractures—safety considerations, avoidance of fatigue, proper footwear.

7. Encourage follow-up medical supervision to monitor for union problems.

8. Teach symptoms needing attention, such as numbness, decreased function, increased pain, elevated temperature.

9. Encourage adequate balanced diet to promote bone and soft tissue healing.

Outcome-Based Evaluation

- Vital signs stable; urine output adequate
- Respirations unlabored; alert and oriented
- No signs of neurovascular compromise
- No calf pain reported: Homans' sign negative
- Reports decreased pain with elevation, ice, and analgesic
- Afebrile; no wound drainage
- Performing hygiene and dressing practices with minimal assistance
- Performing active ROM correctly
- Using affected extremity for light activity as allowed
- Denies acute symptoms of stress; reports working through feelings about trauma

OTHER MUSCULOSKELETAL DISORDERS

Low Back Pain

Low back pain is characterized by an uncomfortable or acute pain in the lumbosacral area associated with severe spasm of the paraspinal muscles, often with radiating pain.

Pathophysiology and Etiology

Multiple causes:

1. Mechanical (joint, muscular, or ligamentous sprain)
2. Degenerative disk disease; acute herniation of disk(s)
3. Lack of physical activity and exercise; weakness of musculature of back
4. Arthritic conditions
5. Diseases of bone (osteoporosis, vertebral fracture, Paget's disease, metastatic carcinoma)
6. Congenital disorders
7. Systemic diseases
8. Infections of disk spaces or vertebrae
9. Spinal cord tumors
10. Referred pain from other areas

Clinical Manifestations

1. Pain localized or radiating to buttocks or to one or both legs
2. Paresthesias, numbness, and/or weakness of lower extremities
3. Spasm in acute phase
4. Bowel/bladder dysfunction in cauda equina syndrome

Diagnostic Evaluation

1. X-rays of lumbar spine are usually negative.
2. CT of spine—to detect arthritic changes, degenerative disk disease, tumor, and other abnormalities.
3. Myelography—to confirm and localize disk herniation.
4. MRI—to detect any pathology: disk herniation, soft tissue injury, and so forth.
5. Electromyography of lower extremities—to detect nerve changes related to back pathology.
6. Diskogram—to detect herniated disk.

Management

For management of herniated disk, see page 502. For management of spinal cord tumors, see page 494.

1. Rest in bed in a supine to semi-Fowler's position with hips and knees flexed—to relieve painful muscle and ligament sprain, heal soft tissue injury, remove stress from lumbar sacral area, relieve tension on sciatic nerves, and open the posterior part of the intervertebral spaces.
   a. Acute spasm and pain should subside in 3 to 7 days if there is no nerve involvement or other serious underlying disease.
   b. Isometric exercises should be done hourly while on bed rest, if possible.
2. Heat or ice used to relax muscle spasm and relieve discomfort. Follow heat with massage.
3. Medications
   a. Oral analgesic and anti-inflammatory agent—usually NSAID is first-line agent, unless contraindicated due to history or high risk of GI bleeding, renal insufficiency, or allergy.
   b. Painful trigger points may be injected with hydrocortisone/xylocaine for pain relief.
   c. Pain may be treated with narcotic when severe; may be sedating.
   d. Muscle relaxant to relieve spasm/tense muscles; may be sedating.
4. Lumbosacral support may be used—provides abdominal compression and decreases load on lumbar intervertebral disks.
5. TENS may be helpful in relieving chronic pain.
6. Psychiatric intervention may be needed for patient with chronic depression, anxiety, and low back syndrome.
   a. Psychotropic medication may be used for treatment of depression and anxiety, which potentiate pain.
   b. Focus on getting back to functional state after long disability.

Complications

1. Spinal instability, infection, sensory and motor deficits
2. Chronic pain
3. Malingering and other psychosocial reactions

Nursing Assessment

1. Obtain history to determine when, where, and how the pain occurs, aggravating or relieving factors, relationship of pain to specific activities, presence of numbness or paresthesia.
2. Perform physical examination of neurologic system—spots localized weakness of extremities and reflex and sensory loss.
3. Perform musculoskeletal examination for changes in strength, tone, and ROM.
4. If condition chronic, assess coping ability of patient and family/significant others.
5. Assess effect of illness on daily living—work, school, and so forth.

Nursing Diagnoses

- Pain related to injury
- Impaired Physical Mobility related to pain

Nursing Interventions

Relieving Pain

1. Advise patient to rest in bed on firm mattress to provide immobilization and relieve strain on back muscles, ligaments, and other structures.
2. Keep pillow between flexed knees while in side-lying position—minimizes strain on back muscles.
3. Apply heat (moist towels; hydrocollator packs) or ice, as prescribed.
4. Administer or teach self-administration of pain medications and muscle relaxants, as prescribed.
   a. Give NSAIDs with meals to prevent GI upset and bleeding.
   b. Muscle relaxants may cause drowsiness.

Promoting Mobility

1. Encourage ROM of all uninvolved muscle groups.
2. Suggest gradual increase of activities and alternating activities with rest in semi-Fowler's position.
3. Avoid prolonged periods of sitting.
4. Encourage patient to discuss problems that may be contributing to backache.
5. Encourage patient to do prescribed back exercises. Exercise keeps postural muscles strong, helps recondition the back and abdominal musculature, and serves as an outlet for emotional tension.

Patient Education and Health Maintenance

Instruct patient to avoid recurrences as follows:

1. Standing, sitting, lying, and lifting properly are necessary for a healthy back.
2. Alternate periods of activity with periods of rest.
   a. Avoid prolonged sitting (intradiskal pressure in lumbar spine is higher during sitting), standing, and driving.

b. Change positions and rest at frequent intervals.

c. Avoid assuming tense, cramped positions.

d. Sit in a straight-back chair with the knees slightly higher than the hips. Use a footstool if necessary.

e. Flatten the hollow of the back by sitting with the buttocks "tucked under." Pelvic tilt (small of back is pressed against a flat surface)—decreases lordosis.

f. Avoid knee and hip extension. When driving a car, have the seat pushed forward as necessary for comfort. Place a cushion in the small of the back for support.

3. When standing for any length of time, rest one foot on a small stool or platform to relieve lumbar lordosis.

4. Avoid fatigue, which contributes to spasm of back muscles.

5. Use good body mechanics when lifting or moving about.

6. Daily exercise is important in the prevention of back problems (see Patient Education Guidelines).

a. Do prescribed back exercises twice daily—strengthens back, leg, and abdominal muscles.

b. Walking outdoors (progressively increasing distance and pace) is recommended.

c. Reduce weight if necessary—decreases strain on back muscles.

Outcome-Based Evaluation

• Verbalizes relief of pain with rest and medication
• Performs back exercises correctly

Osteoarthritis

Osteoarthritis, or *degenerative joint disease*, is a chronic, noninflammatory, slowly progressing disorder that causes deterioration of articular cartilage. It affects weight-bearing joints (hips and knees) as well as joints of the distal interphalangeal and proximal interphalangeal joints of the fingers.

Pathophysiology and Etiology

1. Changes in articular cartilage occur first; later, secondary soft tissue changes may occur.

2. Progressive wear and tear on cartilage leads to thinning of joint surface and ulceration into bone.

3. Leads to inflammation of the joint and increased blood flow and hypertrophy of subchondral bone.

4. New cartilage and bone formation at joint margins results in osteophytosis (bone spurs), altering the size and shape of bone.

5. Generally affects adults age 50 to 90; equal in males and females.

6. Cause is unknown, but aging and obesity are contributing factors. Previous trauma may cause secondary OA.

Diagnostic Evaluation

1. No specific laboratory examination.

2. X-rays of affected joints show joint space narrowing, osteophytes, and sclerosis.

3. Radionuclide imaging (bone scan)—shows increased uptake in affected bones.

4. Analysis of synovial fluid differentiates OA and RA.

Management
Conservative Management

Includes PT and OT to maintain function while preserving the joints.

Pain management using non-narcotic analgesics such as acetaminophen; NSAIDs mostly for analgesic affects; and potentially narcotics such as oxycodone, codeine, or hydrocodone, possibly in combination with non-narcotic analgesics.

1. Two agents called viscosupplements have been approved by the FDA. These are hyaluronate (Hyalgan) and hylan G-F 20 (Synvisc). These are intra-articular injections into the knee administered over time.

a. They relieve pain and are most effective for people with mild to moderate knee OA.

b. After the injection, patient is instructed to avoid prolonged weight-bearing activities for 48 hours.

c. Contraindicated for patients with allergies to hyaluronate preparations, joint infections, and allergies to avian proteins, bird feathers and/or eggs.

2. A new type of NSAID known as cyclooxygenase-2 (COX-2) inhibitors has been approved by the FDA. It includes celecoxib (Celebrex), refecoxib (Vioxx), and meloxicam (Mabic). COX-2 inhibitors mainly block the prostaglandins involved in inflammation.

a. They are generally safer for the stomach and provide a new treatment option for people with RA and OA who cannot take NSAIDs due to GI upset or risk for GI bleeding.

b. They can be used in patients taking warfarin, because bleeding time and platelet aggregation are not affected.

c. Celecoxib is contraindicated in people with known allergies to sulfonamides and a history of asthma, urticaria, or allergic reaction to other NSAIDs.

d. They can cause renal impairment, so renal function should be monitored with long-term use.

3. Weight loss, if necessary, to relieve stress on joints.

4. Proper nutrition, sleep, and stress reduction to improve well-being.

5. Over-the-counter supplements glucosamine and chondroitin sulfate are common alternative remedies that have potential cartilage-rebuilding effects, but clinical trials in humans have been scant up to this point.

Surgical Intervention

Surgical intervention is considered when the pain becomes intolerable to patient and mobility is severely compromised. Options include osteotomy, débridement, joint fusion, arthroscopy, and arthroplasty.

Complications

1. Limited mobility

2. Neurologic deficits associated with spinal involvement

PATIENT EDUCATION GUIDELINES   Taking Care of Your Lower Back

Almost everyone has low back pain at some time. Chronic pain will develop in some, and a few will become disabled because of it. Risk factors for chronic low back pain include being overweight, being deconditioned (out of shape), having poor posture, and having poor abdominal muscle tone. You can relieve pain and avoid disability by adhering to the following instructions:

Do Back Exercises Every Day

1. Lie on your back on the floor or a firm mattress. Bend one knee, and bring that leg up toward your chest. Hold it against your chest a few seconds. Then repeat with the other leg. Alternate legs several times.
2. Lie on your back with your knees bent and feet flat on the floor. Tighten your abdomen and buttocks and push your lower back to the floor. Hold for a few seconds, then relax. Repeat several times.
3. Lie on your back with knees bent and feet flat on the floor. Do a partial sit-up by crossing your arms on your chest and lifting your shoulders off the floor 6 to 12 inches. Repeat several times.

Protect Your Back While Sitting and Standing

1. Avoid sitting in soft, cushioned chairs too long.
2. If you sit for long periods at work, make sure your knees are level with your hips. Use a step stool if necessary.
3. If you stand for long periods, try to put one foot up on a stool, then the other. Walk around and change position periodically.
4. Adjust your car seat so there is a bend in your knees. Do not stretch.
5. Put a firm pillow behind your low back if it does not feel supported while you are sitting.

Stay Active and in Good Health

1. Take a walk every day wearing comfortable, low-heeled shoes.
2. Eat a balanced, low-fat diet with plenty of fruits and vegetables to avoid constipation.
3. Get plenty of sleep on a firm mattress.
4. See your health care provider promptly for worsening pain or new injury.

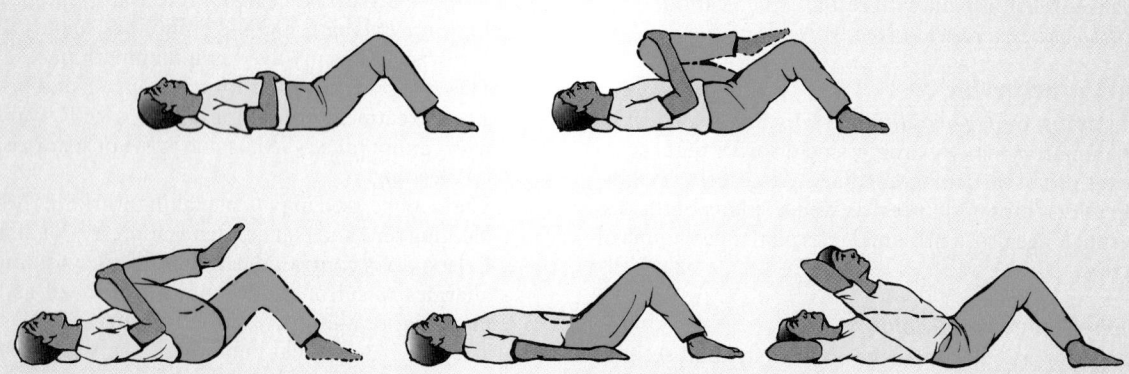

Back exercises to strengthen abdominal and postural muscles, to stretch contracted back muscles, and to maintain flexibility.

Be Careful How You Lift

1. Move your body close to an object before picking it up.
2. Bend at the knees, not the back, to pick up an object that is low.
3. Hold the object close to your abdomen and chest.
4. Bend at the knees again to put down an object.
5. Avoid reaching, twisting, or turning your back as you lift or carry an object.

Nursing Assessment

1. Obtain history of pain and its characteristics—which joint(s) involved.
2. Evaluate ROM and strength.
3. Assess effect on ADLs and emotional status.

Nursing Diagnoses

- Pain related to joint degeneration and muscle spasm
- Impaired Physical Mobility related to pain and limited joint motion
- Self-Care Deficits (feeding, bathing/hygiene, dressing/ grooming, toileting) related to pain and limited joint movement

Nursing Interventions

Relieving Pain

1. Advise patient to take prescribed NSAIDs or over-the-counter analgesics as directed to relieve inflammation and/or pain. May alternate with narcotic analgesic, if prescribed.

> **GERONTOLOGIC ALERT**
>
> Elderly patients are at greater risk for GI bleeding associated with NSAID use. Encourage administration with meals, and monitor stool for occult blood.

2. Provide rest for involved joints—excessive use aggravates the symptoms and accelerates degeneration.
   a. Use splints, braces, cervical collars, traction, lumbosacral corsets as necessary.
   b. Have prescribed rest periods in recumbent position.
3. Advise patient to avoid activities that precipitate pain.
4. Apply heat as prescribed—relieves muscle spasm and stiffness; avoid prolonged application of heat—may cause increased swelling and flare symptoms.
5. Teach correct posture and body mechanics—postural alterations lead to chronic muscle tension and pain.
6. Advise sleeping with a rolled terrycloth towel under the neck—for relief of cervical OA.
7. Provide crutches, braces, or cane when indicated—to reduce weight-bearing stress on hips and knees.
8. Teach use of cane in hand on side opposite involved hip/knee.
9. Advise wearing corrective shoes and metatarsal supports for foot disorders—also help in the treatment of arthritis of the knee.
10. Encourage weight loss to decrease stress on weight-bearing joints.
11. Support patient undergoing orthopedic surgery for unremitting pain and disabling arthritis of joints (see p. 991).

Increasing Physical Mobility

1. Encourage activity as much as possible without causing pain.
2. Teach ROM exercises to maintain joint mobility and muscle tone for joint support, to prevent capsular and tendon tightening, and to prevent deformities. Avoid flexion and adduction deformities.
3. Teach isometric exercises and graded exercises to improve muscle strength around the involved joint.
4. Advise putting joints through ROM after periods of inactivity (eg, automobile ride).

Promoting Independence in Activities of Daily Living

1. Suggest performing important activities in morning, after stiffness has been abated and before fatigue and pain become a problem.
2. Advise on modifications, such as wearing looser clothing without buttons, placing bench in tub or shower for bathing, sitting at table or counter in kitchen to prepare meals.
3. Help with obtaining assistive devices, such as padded handles for utensils and grooming aids, to promote independence.
4. Refer to OT for additional assistance.

Patient Education and Health Maintenance

1. Suggest swimming or water aerobics (offered by the YMCA) as a form of nonstressful exercise to preserve mobility.
2. Encourage adequate diet and sleep to enhance general health.
3. Advise patients that the Arthritis Foundation does not recommend the use of alternative therapies such as glucosamine and chondroitin sulfate at this time due to lack of evidence; encourage patients to discuss their use with their health care provider.
4. Refer for additional information and support to local chapter of The Arthritis Foundation, 1-800-933-0032, *www.arthritis.org.*

Outcome-Based Evaluation

- Reports reduction in pain while ambulatory
- Performs ROM exercises
- Dresses, bathes self, and grooms with assistive devices

Neoplasms of the Musculoskeletal System

Musculoskeletal neoplasms include primary *sarcomas, metastatic bone disease,* and benign tumors (*osteoma, chondroma, osteoclastoma*) of the bone. Over 60% of bone neoplasms are metastatic from other sites of cancer.

Pathophysiology and Etiology

Benign Bone Tumors

Osteoid osteoma, chondroma, and osteoclastoma (benign giant cell tumor) are examples of benign bone tumors. Malignant transformation occurs with some.

Malignant Bone Tumors

1. Chondrosarcoma and osteosarcoma are examples of primary malignant bone tumors.
   a. Tumors develop in areas of rapid growth.

b. Risk factors include Paget's disease, previous radiation therapy to the bone, and other bone diseases.

c. Hematogenous spread to the lung occurs.

2. Multiple myeloma is a malignant neoplasm arising from the bone marrow.

Metastatic Bone Tumors

1. Metastatic bone tumors are most frequently associated with cancers of the breast, prostate, and lung (primary malignancy site).

2. Bone metastasis most frequently occurs in the vertebrae and results in pathologic fracture.

Clinical Manifestations

1. Pain in the involved bone—from effects of tumor (destruction, erosion, and expansion of tumor).

   a. Generally mild to constant pain, which may be worse at night or with activity.

   b. Pain will be acute with fracture.

   c. Neurologic symptoms may present with nerve root compression.

2. Swelling and limitation of motion and joint effusion.

3. Physical findings.

   a. Palpable, tender, fixed bony mass.

   b. Increase in skin temperature over mass.

   c. Superficial veins dilated and prominent.

Diagnostic Evaluation

1. X-ray will usually reveal bone tumor; may show increased or decreased bone density. Tomograms may be helpful for some benign osseous lesions.

2. CT and/or MRI demonstrate soft tissue involvement and location of tumor(s).

3. Bone scan—helpful in detecting initial extent of malignancy, planning therapy, defining level of amputation, and following course of radiation/chemotherapy.

4. Serum alkaline phosphatase—usually increased.

5. Bence Jones protein in urine with multiple myeloma.

6. Biopsy of bone—to confirm suspected diagnosis.

7. Chest x-ray and lung scan—to determine if metastases are present.

8. Arteriography—to assess soft tissue involvement.

Management

A multidisciplinary approach in a cancer center is often preferred. The basic objective is to halt the progression of the tumor by destroying or removing the lesion. Treatment depends on the type of tumor. Combinations of chemotherapy, surgery, and/or radiation may be indicated as most appropriate for specific type of tumor.

Surgery

1. Tumor curettage or resection with bone grafting may be used.

2. Limb-salvaging procedures involve resection of affected bone and surrounding normal muscle tissue and reconstruction using metallic prostheses or allografts for bone/joint replacement and skin grafting, as needed.

3. Amputation is necessary in some cases.

Chemotherapy

May be used as preoperative, adjunctive, and palliative treatment.

1. Chemotherapy may be administered before (to shrink the tumor) and after (to destroy metastases) surgery.

2. Chemotherapy used in combination to achieve a greater patient response at a lower toxicity rate and to minimize potential problems of drug resistance and may be given in varying courses separated by rest periods.

Radiotherapy

1. Tumor irradiation may be used.

2. Prophylactic lung irradiation may be performed—to suppress metastases.

Other Therapies

1. Immunotherapy—interferon.

2. Hormone therapy may be used with metastatic tumors of the breast and prostate.

3. If pathologic fracture occurs, the fracture is managed with open reduction and internal fixation or other fracture treatment method.

Complications

1. Lack of tumor control and metastases

2. Pathologic fracture

3. Hypercalcemia from bone destruction

Nursing Assessment

1. Obtain history of progression of disease; presence of pain, fever, weight loss, malaise.

2. Examine for painless mass.

3. Review records for evidence of pathologic fracture.

4. Assess knowledge of cancer, experiences with family or others, and present coping.

Nursing Diagnoses

• Pain related to effects of tumor

• Risk for trauma related to altered bone structure

• Ineffective Individual Coping related to diagnosis and treatment options

Nursing Interventions

See also sections titled Orthopedic Surgery, page 991, and Amputation, page 995.

Relieving Pain

1. Use multiple approaches to reduce discomfort.

2. Administer pain medications ½ hour before ambulation or other uncomfortable movement.

3. Support painful extremities on pillows.

Preventing Pathologic Fractures

1. Assist patient in movement with gentleness and patience.

2. Avoid jarring patient or bed.

3. Support joints when repositioning patient.

4. Guard patient to avoid falls.

5. Create a hazard-free environment.

Strengthening Coping Abilities

1. Create a supportive environment.

2. Use psychological support services as needed.

3. Answer questions and clear up misconceptions about treatment options.

Patient Education and Health Maintenance

1. Teach about particular treatment selected. See page 141 for information on chemotherapy, and page 151 for radiation therapy information.
2. Encourage appropriate follow-up and diagnostic testing for recurrence.
3. Refer for additional information and support to American Cancer Society, 19 West 56th Street, New York, NY 10019, 212-586-8700; *www.cancer.org.*

Outcome-Based Evaluation

- Reports decreased pain with ambulation
- No signs or symptoms of fractures
- Verbalizes understanding of treatment options and strength to make decisions

Osteomyelitis

Osteomyelitis is a severe pyogenic infection of the bone and surrounding tissues that requires immediate treatment. Generally three routes:

Bloodstream (hematogenous spread)

Adjacent soft tissue infection (contiguous focus)

Direct introduction of microorganisms into the bone

Pathophysiology and Etiology

1. Bacteria lodge and multiply in bone.
2. Pressure increases as pus collects in confined rigid bone, contributing to ischemia, vascular occlusion, and leading to bone necrosis.
3. *Staphylococcus aureus* is the most common infecting microorganism, although others are prevalent: *Escherichia coli, Pseudomonas, Klebsiella, Salmonella,* and *Proteus.*
4. Hematogenous osteomyelitis is the most common method of spread in prepubescent children.

Clinical Manifestations

1. Infection of long bones with acute pain and signs of sepsis.
2. Localized pain and drainage.
3. Symptoms vary in adult and children according to the site of involvement.

Diagnostic Evaluation

1. Acute osteomyelitis diagnosis made on initial clinical signs (history, physical examination, CBC, ESR).
2. Aerobic and anaerobic cultures of bone and tissue to identify the organism.
3. ESR elevated, WBC and hemoglobin decreased.
4. Radiographic evidence of osteomyelitis lags behind symptoms by 7 to 10 days.
5. Plain film evidence of infection 3 to 4 weeks later.
6. Bone necrosis seen 10 to 14 days on x-rays.

7. Radionuclide bone scans used to diagnose early acute osteomyelitis.
8. MRI used increasingly—distinguishes between soft tissue and bone marrow.

Management

1. Acute: full recovery possible with minimal loss of function
2. Chronic: develops with inadequate or ineffective course of antibiotics or delayed treatment

Surgical Intervention

1. Needle aspiration or needle biopsy done initially.
2. Surgical intervention may be needed to obtain culture and sensitivity of specimen.
3. Surgical decompression considered when patient does not improve after 36 to 48 hours of antimicrobial therapy.
4. Débridement may be done, or antibiotic-impregnated beads used in wound (removed after 2 to 4 weeks and replaced with bone graft).

Pharmacologic Intervention

1. Employed quickly after presentation of symptoms to avoid chronicity
2. Parental antimicrobial therapy based on blood/wound cultures
3. Medications depend on organism, but include:
   a. Penicillins (Pen G, Pen V)
   b. Semisynthetic penicillins (nafcillin, oxacillin, methicillin)
   c. Extended-spectrum penicillins (ampicillin, carbenicillin, amoxicillin)
   d. Beta-lactam agents (Imipenem)
   e. Tetracyclines
   f. Cephalosporins
   g. Aminoglycosides

Complications

1. Nonhealing wound
2. Sepsis
3. Immobility
4. Amputation

Nursing Assessment

1. Obtain detailed history of injury.
2. Assess pain and functional deficits.
3. Be aware that systemic symptoms are acute in children, but vary in intensity with adults.
4. Perform general systemic assessment because adults with long bone involvement generally have more systemic septic symptoms.

Nursing Diagnoses

- Pain/Chronic Pain related to inflammatory process
- Knowledge Deficit: Disease and medications
- Impaired Physical Mobility related to rest of affected part

Nursing Interventions
Relieving Pain
1. Administer opioids for acute pain; non-narcotics for chronic pain.
2. Administer medications around the clock (ATC) vs prn to establish a consistent blood level.
3. Report any increase in pain that may indicate worsening infection.

Increasing Knowledge
1. Describe the infectious process and rationale for prolonged treatment with osteomyelitis.
2. Explain IV antibiotic therapy, potential side effects, and reactions.
3. Explain strict adherence to infection control practices (sterile technique, handwashing, selection of roommate, and so forth) to prevent spread of infection in some cases.

Promoting Rest Without Complications
1. Support the affected extremity (splint, traction) to minimize pain.
2. If patient is on bed rest, prevent hazards of immobility (passive ROM, position changes, cough and deep breathing, and so forth).
3. Encourage distraction activities.

Patient Education and Health Maintenance
1. Advise patient to adhere to infection control principles—proper handwashing, disposal of wound drainage, dressings to prevent reinfection or transmission of infection at home.
2. Stress adherence to medication regimen, which may be prolonged, with frequent follow-up visits.
3. Teach care of indwelling device for medication delivery (such as Hickman catheter).

Outcome-Based Evaluation
- Pain managed with non-narcotic analgesics
- Infectious process minimized
- Functional status of affected joint intact

Paget's Disease (Osteitis Deformans)

Paget's disease of the bone is a skeletal disorder resulting from excessive osteoclastic activity, affecting the long bones, pelvis, lumbar vertebrae, and the skull predominantly.

Pathophysiology and Etiology
1. The cause of this disease is unknown, although there is evidence of familial tendency (25% to 40% have at least one relative with it).
2. More common in men than women.
3. Rare before age 40, and increases as age does—12% after age 80.
4. May be caused by infection from bloodborne viruses. After acute viremia, osteoclasts become chronically infected, stimulating osteoclastic proliferation.

Clinical Manifestations
1. Generally, asymptomatic.
2. Most common symptoms are pain and predisposition to fracture.
3. Pagetic lesions can lead to OA, joint destruction, spinal deformity.
4. Decrease in hearing as a result of skull enlargement.
5. Tinnitus or vertigo may also occur.
6. Rarely, CHF, hypertension, atherosclerosis, and aortic valve calcification.
7. Malignant bone tumor.

Diagnostic Evaluation
1. Elevated serum alkaline phosphatase.
2. Serum calcium, phosphorus and albumin levels usually normal.
3. Generally confirmed with radiologic examinations.
4. Bone scans can evaluate pagetic activity.
5. Bone biopsy.

Management
1. No treatment for asymptomatic Paget's.
2. Pain management—NSAIDs, aspirin.
3. Medications—calcitonin is the main medication used for this disease.
4. Other medications used to block bone resorption—etidronate disodium (Didronel), alendronate sodium (Fosamax), plicamycin, pamidronate disodium.
5. Tibial osteotomy done to realign knees and relieve pain.

Nursing Assessment
1. Assess pain and functional ability.
2. Observe for bowing (legs) or complaint that hats feel tight.
3. Assess for cardiovascular complications.
4. Assess for auditory symptoms—tinnitus, vertigo, and hearing loss.

Nursing Diagnoses
- Pain related to pathophysiologic process
- Risk for Injury due to falls

Nursing Interventions
Reducing Pain
1. Administer and teach self-administration of analgesics.
2. Avoid sedation through use of narcotics, which may increase risk of falls.

Preventing Injury
1. Establish exercise protocols through a PT consult to maintain physical abilities and prevent falls.
2. Teach safe transferring, and make sure patient can alert nurses if needs help.
3. Assist patient with activities as necessary.
4. Provide function and mobility aids such as heel lifts, walking aids as needed, through an OT consult.

Patient Education and Health Maintenance

1. Teach safety measures in the home—removal of loose rugs and obstacles to prevent falls, good lighting, and so forth.
2. Provide education about the disease process and medication treatment.
3. Ensure that patient knows how to use mobility aids.
4. Initiate home care referral as indicated.
5. Provide information about The Paget Foundation, 1-800-23-PAGET, *www.paget.org*. Email: pagetfdn @aol.com.
6. Encourage follow-up for periodic hearing tests and blood work.

▣ Hallux Valgus

Also called *bunion, hallux valgus* is a deformity of the foot involving the first metatarsal and great toe. Occurs in females more frequently than males, and incidence increases with age; may have a genetic predisposition. Often occurs with other deformities of the feet such as hammer toe, mallet toe, and claw toe.

Clinical Manifestations

1. Pain
2. Possible callus of skin overlying bunion and accompanying toe deformities
3. Diminished ROM
4. Generally associated with irritating footwear

Management and Nursing Interventions
Conservative Management

1. Wearing footwear made of soft leather with a wider toe-box, rounded rather than pointed, and with low heel.
2. Special orthoses can be ordered.
3. Steroid injections to relieve pain.

Surgical Management

Surgical alignment of the great toe by osteotomy of metatarsal or proximal phalanx of the great toe or fusion of the metatarsal–metatarsophalangeal joint

Postoperative Care

1. Elevation of the foot to reduce pain
2. Initial nonweight bearing, with very gradual progress in activity
3. Crutch walking initially, followed by wooden shoe immobilizer for several weeks
4. NSAIDs and narcotic analgesics for pain
5. Bandages changed by surgeon initially

SELECTED REFERENCES

Adalberth, T., Roos, H., Laur'en, M., et al. (1997). Magnetic resonance imaging, scintography, and arthroscopic evaluation of traumatic hemarthrosis of the knee. *American Journal of Sports Medicine, 25,* 231–232.

Childs, S. (1999). Acute ankle injuries. *Primary Care Practice, 3*(4), 428–437.

Corbett, J. V. (1998). Laboratory test and diagnostic procedures in orthopaedic nursing practice. *Nursing Clinics of North America, 33*(4), 685–700.

Crowther, C. L. (1999). Cox-2 inhibitors. *Lippincott's Primary Care Practice, 3*(4), 394–396.

Doyle, G. D., et al. (2000). Effectiveness of manual physical therapy and exercise in osteoarthritis of the knee. *Annals of Internal Medicine, 132*(3), 173–181.

Dunkin, M. A. (1999). Drug guide. *Arthritis Today, 13*(4), 27–48.

Haynes, K. (1998). Neoplasms of the musculoskeletal system. In Maher, A., Salmond, S., & Pellino, T. (Eds.), *Orthopaedic nursing* (2nd ed., pp. 769–803). Philadelphia: W. B. Saunders.

Herzberg, M. A. (1997). *Osteoporosis independent study.* Pitman, NJ: National Association of Orthopaedic Nurses.

Kupecz, D. (1999). Treating pain with COX-2 inhibitors. *The Nurse Practitioner, 24*(11), 95–102.

Kunkler, C. E. (1999). Neurovascular assessment. *Orthopaedic Nursing Journal, 18*(3), 63–71.

La Prade, R. F., & Swiontkowski, M. F. (1999). New horizons in the treatment of osteoarthritis of the knee. *Journal of the American Medical Association, 281*(10), 876–878.

Leeb, B. F., et al. (2000). A meta-analysis of chondroitin sulfate in the treatment of osteoarthritis. *Journal of Rheumatology, 27*(1), 205–211.

Leslie, M. (1999). Hyaluronic acid treatment for osteoarthritis of the knee. *The Nurse Practitioner, 24*(7), 38–48.

Lewis, T., Tesh, A. S., & Lyles, K. W. (1999). Caring for the patient with Paget's disease of the bone. *The Nurse Practitioner, 24*(7), 50–65.

Maher, A., Salmond, S., & Pellino, T. (Eds.). (1998). *Orthopaedic nursing* (2nd ed.). Philadelphia: W. B. Saunders.

Mangini, M. (1998). Physical assessment of the musculoskeletal system. *Nursing Clinics of North America, 33*(4), 643–652.

McAlindon, T. E., et al. (2000). Glucosamine and chondroitin for treatment of osteoarthritis: A systematic quality assessment and meta-analysis. *Journal of The American Medical Association, 283*(5), 1469–1475.

Moon, L. B. & Backer, J. (2000). Relationships among self-efficacy, outcome expectancy, and postoperative behaviors in total joint replacement patients. *Orthopaedic Nursing, 19*(2), 77–86.

Palmer, L. M. (1999). Management of the patient with a total joint replacement: The primary care practitioner's role. *Primary Care Practice, 3*(4), 419–427.

Peloso, M. (2000). NSAIDs: A Faustian bargain. *American Journal of Nursing, 100*(6), 34–40.

Ridge, R. & Goodson, A. (2000). The relationship between multidisciplinary discharge outcomes and functional status after total hip replacement. *Orthopaedic Nursing, 19*(1), 71–82.

Rodts, M. F. (Ed.). (1991). Orthopaedic nursing, sports nursing. *Nursing Clinics of North America, 26*(1).

Salmond, S., Mooney, N. E., & Verdisco, L. (Eds.). (1996). *Core curriculum for orthopaedic nursing* (3rd ed.). Pitman, NJ: National Association of Orthopaedic Nurses.

Towhead, T. E. & Anastassiades, T. P. (2000). Glucosamaine and chondroitin for treating symptoms of osteoarthritis: Evidence is widely touted but incomplete. *Journal of the American Medical Association, 283*(5), 1483–1484.

Williamson, V. (1998). Amputation. In Maher, A., Salmond, S., & Pellino, T. (Eds.), *Orthopaedic nursing* (2nd ed., pp. 718–745). Philadelphia: W. B. Saunders.

Wolfe, F., et al. (2000). Preference for nonsteroidal antiinflammatory drugs over acetaminophen by rheumatic disease patients. *Arthritis and Rheumatism, 43*(2), 378–385.

Yarnold, B. D. (1999). Hip fracture. Caring for a fragile population. *American Journal of Nursing, 99*(2), 36–40.

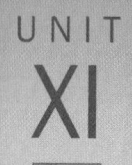

CHAPTER

33

Dermatologic Disorders

GENERAL OVERVIEW

Description of Skin Lesions

Dermatologic conditions are usually described by the types of lesions that appear on the skin, their shape, and configuration. See Figure 33-1 for types of skin lesions.

Primary Lesions

1. Macula—flat, circumscribed discoloration of skin; may have any size or shape.
2. Papule—solid, elevated lesion less than 1 cm wide (0.4 in.).
3. Nodule—raised, solid lesion larger than 1 cm wide (0.4 in.).
4. Vesicle—circumscribed elevated lesion less than 1 cm (0.4 in.) that contains fluid.
5. Bulla—a vesicle or blister larger than 1 cm wide (0.4 in.).
6. Pustule—circumscribed raised lesion that contains pus; may form as a result of purulent changes in a vesicle.
7. Wheal—elevation of the skin that lasts less than 24 hours, caused by edema of the dermis; may be surrounded by erythema or blanching.
8. Plaque—solid, elevated lesion on the skin or mucous membrane, larger than 1 cm (0.4 in.) in its largest diam-

eter; psoriasis is commonly manifested as plaques on the skin; leukoplakia is an example of plaques on mucous membranes.
9. Cyst—soft or firm mass in the skin, filled with semisolid or with liquid material contained in a sac.

Secondary Lesions

Secondary lesions involve changes that take place in primary lesions that modify them.

1. Scale—heaped-up, horny layer of dead epidermis; may develop as a result of inflammatory changes.
2. Crust—covering formed by the drying of serum, blood, or pus on the skin.
3. Excoriation—linear scratch marks or traumatized areas of skin.
4. Fissure—cracks in the skin, usually from marked drying and longstanding inflammation.
5. Ulcer—lesion formed by local destruction of the epidermis and by part or all of the underlying dermis.
6. Lichenification—thickening of skin accompanied by accentuation of skin markings.
7. Scar—new formation of connective tissue that replaces the loss of substance in the dermis as a result of injury or disease.

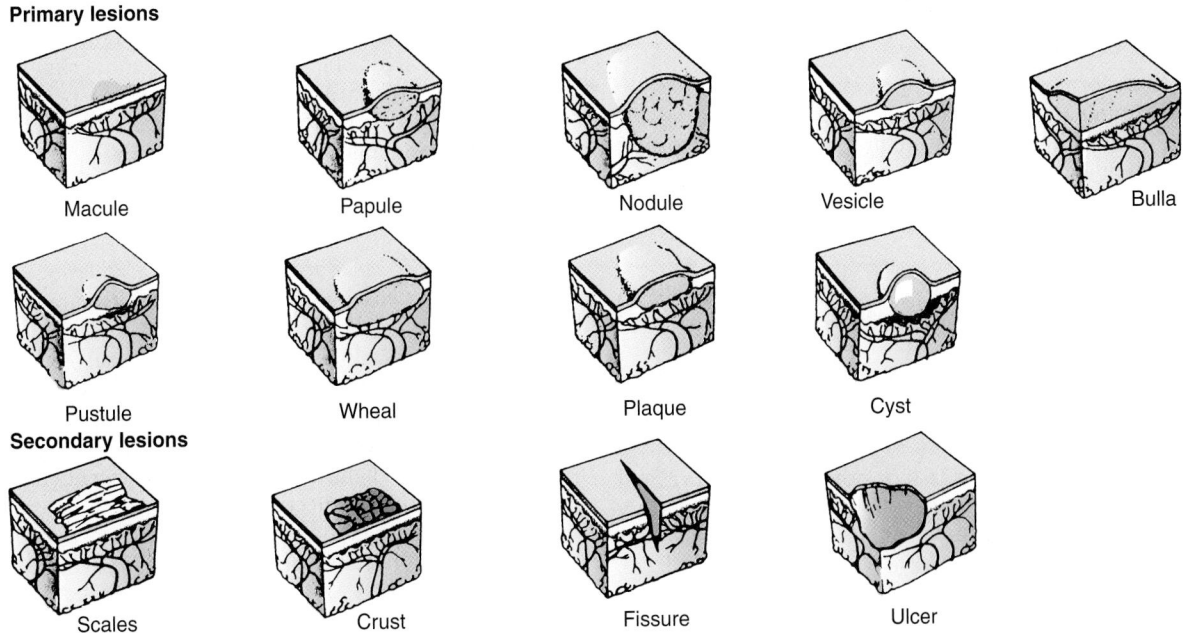

Primary lesions

Macule Papule Nodule Vesicle Bulla

Pustule Wheal Plaque Cyst

Secondary lesions

Scales Crust Fissure Ulcer

FIGURE 33-1 Types of skin lesions.

8. Atrophy—diminution in size or in loss of skin cells that causes thinning of the skin.

Shape and Configuration

After the type of lesion is identified, the shape, configuration or arrangement (in relation to each other), and pattern of distribution is noted (Figure 33-2). The following are descriptions frequently used:

1. Annular—ring-shaped
2. Circinate—circular
3. Confluent—lesions run together or join
4. Discoid—disk-shaped
5. Discrete—lesions remain separate
6. Generalized—widespread eruption
7. Grouped—clustering of lesions
8. Guttate—droplike

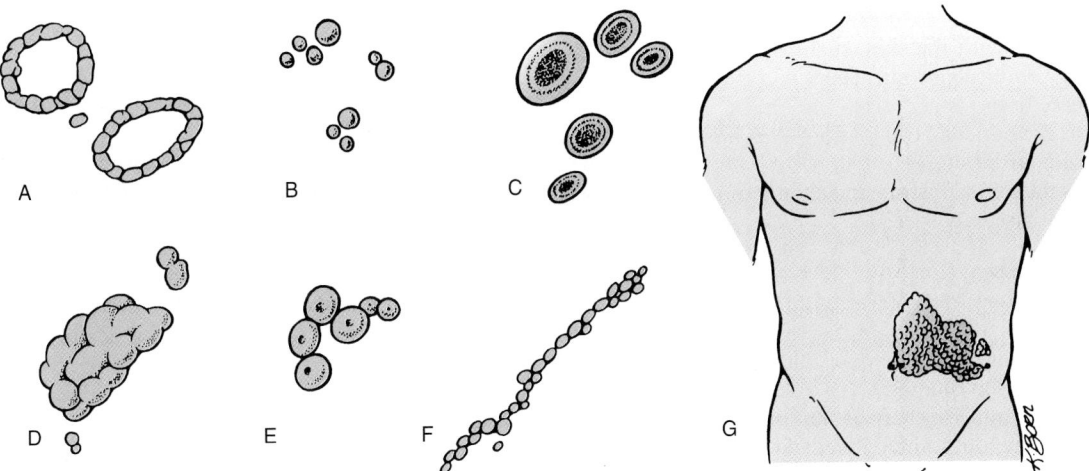

FIGURE 33-2 Shape and arrangement of skin lesions: (**A**) annular, (**B**) grouped, (**C**) iris, (**D**) confluent, (**E**) herpetiform, (**F**) linear, (**G**) zosteriform.

9. Herpetiform—grouped vesicles
10. Iris—ring or a series of concentric circles
11. Linear—in lines
12. Multiform—more than one kind of skin lesion
13. Nummular—coin-shaped
14. Polymorphous—occurring in several or many forms
15. Reticulated—lacelike network
16. Serpiginous—snakelike or creeping eruption
17. Telangiectasia—tiny, superficial, dilated cutaneous vessel; can be seen as a red thread or line
18. Zosteriform or dermatomal—bandlike distribution, limited to one or more dermatomes of skin

ASSESSMENT

History

By obtaining a history of rash or other complaints related to dermatologic conditions, you will understand characteristics of the problem and their effects on the patient that will help in planning care.

Characteristics of Rash

1. When did the rash first occur? Was the onset sudden or gradual?
2. What site was first affected? Describe the spread and its severity.
3. What was the initial color and configuration of the rash? Has it changed?
4. Is there associated itching, burning, tingling, pain, or numbness?
5. Has it been constant or intermittent?

Associated Factors

1. What makes the rash worse or better? Is it seasonal? Is it affected by stress?
2. What medications are being taken? What topical products have been used? What effect did they have?
3. What skin products are used? What chemicals have come into contact with the skin, such as laundry detergent, cleaning products, insecticides?
4. Has there been pet contact?
5. What is the patient's occupation? Any hobbies, such as gardening or hiking?
6. What is the sexual history and chance of sexually transmitted disease exposure?

Medical History

1. Is there a history of hay fever, asthma, hives, eczema, or allergies?
2. Has the patient had this particular rash or had other skin disorders in the past?
3. What is the family history of skin disorders?
4. Are there any longstanding medical problems?

Physical Examination

1. Focus your examination on the skin, hair, and nails. Some dermatologic conditions affect other body systems; so, perform a general physical exam as indicated.

2. Ask the patient to show you the area of concern and examine the skin surface under good lighting conditions. You may have to examine the entire skin if the condition is generalized.
3. Note the distribution and configuration of skin lesions. Compare right and left sides of the body.
4. Note the shape, border, texture, and surface of the lesions.
5. Palpate the lesions for texture, warmth, and tenderness.
6. Use a metric ruler to determine size of lesions and to serve as a baseline for comparison with subsequent measurements.
7. Examine the scalp, nails, and oral mucosa.
8. Perform diascopy—gently press a glass slide or Lucite rule over a skin lesion to detect blanching (caused by dilated blood vessels).
9. Use a Wood's light to inspect for fluorescent changes with some fungal infections.
10. For dark-skinned individuals, look for black, purple, or gray lesions, and palpate carefully to determine if rash is present.

DIAGNOSTIC TESTS

Laboratory Tests

Some dermatologic conditions can be evaluated by laboratory tests of microscopy and culture.

Microscopy
Description

1. A sample is taken by scraping, swabbing, or aspirating a skin lesion and transferred to a glass slide for direct observation or staining.
   a. Direct visualization of scrapings mixed with mineral oil for visualization of scabies, mites, or the nits of lice that cling to hair.
   b. A Tzanck smear is obtained from vesicular fluid or a moist ulcer and stained to detect characteristics of herpes simplex virus, herpes zoster, and varicella (chicken pox).
   c. Potassium hydroxide may be added to skin scrapings on a glass slide and heated to dissolve skin cells to detect hyphae and spores in fungal infections.
   d. Gram stain may be performed to tentatively identify bacteria in certain skin infections.

Nursing and Patient Care Considerations

1. Use the side of a glass slide or a scalpel held at a 45-degree angle to gently scrape the skin of a dry lesion or of an inflamed area; only mild discomfort and pinpoint bleeding should occur.
2. For moist or semimoist ulcerations or crusted lesions, roll a saline-soaked cotton or Dacron-tipped swab over the lesion; for weeping lesions, use a dry swab.
3. For intact vesicles, aspirate fluid from the edge with a 25-gauge sterile needle; if vesicle is partially broken, gently unroof with forceps and obtain fluid on a swab.

PATIENT EDUCATION GUIDELINES   Patch Testing

Patch testing is a process used to determine what substances may be causing allergic reactions in your skin. Your dermatologist will decide which substances he or she wants tested. The goal of patch testing is to reproduce the skin rash on a small controlled area of the skin. The patch test will identify materials such as preservatives, fragrances, dyes, and chemicals that come in contact with your skin and that result in an allergic reaction. Since patch testing does not break the skin barriers, the following are not identified: allergies to food, inhalants, and oral medication.

What to Expect

1. The nurse will tape aluminum disks that contain a small amount of each chemical or allergen to your upper back. The upper back is used because the strongest responses are seen in this area.
2. Each patch test strip contains ten small discs. Your dermatologist or health care provider will choose one or more specially prepared patch test kits for the nurse to apply.
3. A positive reaction will occur when small areas of skin (only the skin that comes in contact with disc) reacts visibly. This redness or rash may itch and persist for several days or even for several weeks. Your dermatologist/health care provider will advise you which allergens are to be avoided.
4. Initial visit: This visit takes approximately 30 min. The nurse applies the patches to your back.
5. 48 hours later: The nurse will remove the patches, mark your skin, and do the first reading. You will have to wait 30 min before the reading is done by the nurse.
6. 96 hours later: The final reading is done. A copy of your test results will be given at this visit.

Do's and Don'ts

1. DO wear loose or high neck clothing throughout the day. HINT: Wear a tee shirt to bed to avoid catching the edges of the tape on the bedsheets.
2. DO apply tape to patch edges if they become loose.
3. DO contact your health care provider immediately if a patch test area burns severely or if you are unable to carry out normal daily activities. NOTE: some itching will occur if you are having a positive reaction; you do not need to call your dermatologist.
4. DO NOT wet the patches for the entire testing period. No showers. Sponge baths are allowed.
5. DO NOT engage in strenuous activities. Exercise may result in excess sweating, thus causing the tape to loosen.
6. DO NOT expose your back to the sun for 2 weeks prior to patch testing.
7. DO NOT discontinue antihistamine therapy (these agents do not affect test results).
8. DO NOT use nonmedicated creams and lotions on your back for at least 24 hours before testing (lotions and creams keep patches from sticking).

Culture
Procedure

1. Drainage from lesions may be cultured on specific media to detect causative organism and sensitivity to antimicrobial therapy; also, portions of skin, hair, and nails may be submitted for fungal culture.
2. Usually takes 24 to 48 hours for results; fungal cultures may take 4 to 5 weeks.

Nursing and Patient Care Considerations

1. Obtain specimen with cotton or Dacron-tipped swab and send to laboratory in culturette or viral culture container; refrigerate viral culture if laboratory pickup is delayed.

2. To obtain specimen for fungal culture, scrape or clip the affected skin, hair, or nails.

Other Tests
Patch Testing

Patch testing is an office procedure done in dermatology to determine if patients are allergic to contact materials. Materials are applied in patches to the skin and checked for reaction 48 hours after application and possibly again later. Erythema, swelling, papules, and vesicles indicate an allergic contact dermatitis rather than an irritant contact dermatitis or no reaction.

See Procedure Guidelines 33-1 and Patient Education Guidelines.

PROCEDURE GUIDELINES 33-1   PATCH TESTING

Patch testing is an essential diagnostic tool used to differentiate irritant versus allergic contact dermatitis. Patients who present with dermatitis or eczema are potential candidates for patch testing.

EQUIPMENT

Finn chambers (strips of 10 shallow aluminum cups or chambers 8 mm wide)
Allergens (5-mm ribbons of petrolatum-base allergen or discs with filter paper dampened with aqueous solution).
Standard tray includes:

1. Benzocaine 5%
2. Meraptobensothiasole 1%
3. Colophony 20%
4. p-Phenylenediamine 1%
5. Imidazolidinyl urea 2%
6. Cinnamic aldehyde 1%

continued

PROCEDURE GUIDELINES 33-1   PATCH TESTING *CONTINUED*

7. Lanolin alcohol 30%
8. Carba mix 3%
9. Neomycin sulfate 20%
10. Thiuram mix 1%
11. Formaldehyde 1%
12. Ethylenediamine dihydrochloride 1%
13. Epoxy resin 1%

14. Quaternium-15 2%
15. P-tert-Bulyllphenol formaldehyde resin 1%
16. Mercapto mix 1%
17. Black rubber mix 0.6%
18. Potassium dichromate 0.25%
19. Balsam of Peru
20. Nickel sulfate

 DRUG ALERT

Patients should not currently be on oral corticosteroids; topical corticosteroids should have been discontinued 1–2 weeks before testing to prevent a weak reaction or false-negative results.

Nursing Action	Rationale
1. Prepare Finn chambers with allergen. Aqueous allergens come in prefilled syringes that should be kept refrigerated.	
2. Apply strip to patient's back.	
a. Avoid hairy areas and areas affected by dermatitis and sunburn.	a. Should be a large area of skin unaffected by friction and free from interfering skin lesions so that results will be clear. Hair may interfere with tape adhesion.
b. Preferred area is upper back.	b. Skin on upper back is most sensitive to reaction.
3. Number the discs 1–10 to match the allergen placed on the disk. If the patient is having several strips applied, draw a diagram on the patient's file to record which tray is placed in which location.	3. To ensure that results are interpreted correctly.
4. Apply additional tape as required to keep patches secure.	4. Sweating and activity may reduce adherence in some people.
5. Instruct the patient to keep area dry, not to scratch or remove the patches unless they become unbearable (severe burning, stinging, or pruritus).	5. Area may become uncomfortable with positive reaction, but removal or disruption of patch will invalidate results.
6. When patient returns in 48 hours for the first reading, mark the outline of the patch strip on the patient's back, then remove the strip. A skin marker or an ultraviolet skin pen marker may be used.	6. Outline serves as a reference point to interpret results.
7. Wait 30 min, then do the first reading. Document as follows:	7. The skin may be red from the application of the tape and a false reading may occur if read too soon.
1+ Weak reaction. Nonvesicular, but with erythema, induration, possible papules	
2+ Strong reaction. Edematous and vesicular, with erythema, edema, papules, and vesicles.	
3+ Extreme reaction. Spreading, bullous, ulcerative.	
IR Irritant reaction.	
- Negative reaction	
Not tested	
Patches fell off	
8. Instruct patient to keep the area dry after removal of the patches and return again in 24–72 hours (usually 48 hours) for additional reading.	8. Though the initial 48-hour reading may be negative, positive results may be seen at the 96-hour reading because of delayed reaction.
9. A final reading is done on the last visit, results are recorded, and counseling is given on negative or positive results.	
10. If the results are positive, the nurse discusses avoidance of allergens and gives the patient written information regarding the allergens to be avoided.	

GENERAL PROCEDURES AND TREATMENT MODALITIES

■ Baths and Wet Dressings

A therapeutic bath is used to apply medication to the entire skin surface and is useful in treating widespread eruptions and general pruritus. Baths soothe, soften, and reduce inflammation, and relieve itching and dryness. See Table 33-1 for types and desired effects. Wet dressings and soaks are damp compresses that contain water, normal saline solution, aluminum acetate solution, or magnesium sulfate solution. They may be sterile or clean, or warm or cool, depending on the skin condition and the area to which they are applied.

Therapeutic Baths
Indications
1. Vesicular, bullous, and ulcerative disorders.
2. Acute inflammatory conditions.
3. Erosions and exudative, crusted surfaces.

Nursing and Patient Care Considerations
1. Prepare the bath or teach the patient to prepare a warm bath at 32°C to 38°C (90°F to 100°F); with the tub half full, add the prescribed quantity of medication, and mix thoroughly to prevent sensitivity reaction.
2. Do not rub the skin. Soaking for at least 15 minutes will promote removal of loosened scales.
3. Keep the room and water at comfortable temperatures and limit bathing to 20 to 30 minutes; the bath area should be well ventilated if tars are used, because they are volatile.
4. Tell the patient to use a bath mat inside the tub and to use a rug outside the tub when bathing at home, because medication may make the tub and wet surfaces slippery.

TABLE 33-1 Therapeutic Baths

Bath Solution and Medication	Desired Effect
Water	To remove crusts and relieve inflammation
Saline	Used for widely disseminated lesions
Colloidal—oatmeal or Aveeno	Antipruritic and demulcent
Sodium bicarbonate	Cooling
Starch	Soothing
Tar baths (follow package directions) Alma-Tar, Balnetar, Lavatar, Polytar	Tar baths are used for psoriasis and chronic eczematous conditions
Bath oils Alpha-keri, Lubath Nutraderm Bath Oil	Bath oils are used for antipruritic and emollient soothing properties Used for acute and subacute eczematous eruptions

5. Blot skin dry with a towel and apply emollient or topical medication to moist skin, if prescribed.

Open Wet Dressings
Indications
1. Bacterial infections that require drainage.
2. Inflammatory and pruritic conditions.
3. Oozing and crusting conditions.

Nursing and Patient Care Considerations
1. Apply dressing to affected area or teach patient to apply and moisten to the point of slight dripping; remoisten as necessary.
2. Apply ice cubes to solution if cooling is desired; use warm tap water if warming is desired.
3. Rewarm or recool every 5 minutes, because compresses reach body temperature quickly.
4. Apply for 15 minutes three to four times a day, unless otherwise indicated.
5. Keep the patient warm and do not treat more than one-third of body at a time, because open wet dressings can cause chilling and hypothermia.
6. Teach patients to prevent burns by measuring temperature of solution with a bath thermometer or by testing tap water on wrist before applying compress. Advise them not use microwave ovens to warm dressings, because uneven heating can occur.

■ Dressings for Skin Conditions

Occlusive Dressing
An occlusive dressing is formed by an airtight plastic or vinyl film applied over medicated areas of skin (usually with corticosteroids) to enhance absorption of medication and to promote moisture retention.

Indications
Skin conditions with thick scaling, such as psoriasis.

Nursing and Patient Care Considerations
1. Wash area and pat dry.
2. Apply medication while skin is still moist.
3. Cover with plastic wrap, vinyl gloves, plastic bag.
4. Seal with paper tape at edges or cover with other dressing to hold in place.

> **◆ DRUG ALERT**
>
> **Excessive use of occlusive dressings that contain corticosteroids may cause skin atrophy, striae, telangiectasia, folliculitis, nonhealing ulceration, erythema, and systemic absorption of corticosteroids.**

5. Do not apply to ulcerated or abraded skin, remove within 12 to 24 hours, or apply with high-potency corticosteroids.

Other Dressings
Other dressing materials may be used as dry dressings to protect the skin, keep affected areas clean, absorb drainage, or to cover medication or to hold occlusive dressings in place.

Nursing and Patient Care Considerations

1. Apply dry gauze dressing using clean technique (unless sterile technique is indicated by open wounds).
2. Wrap extremities with elastic or cotton-rolled bandages, or apply tape.
3. Alternative dressing materials can be used for home care, such as disposable gloves for the hands, cotton socks for the feet, sheets or towels for large areas, disposable diapers or towels folded in diaper fashion for the groin, washcloths for the axilla, cotton T-shirt or cotton pajamas for the trunk, turban or plastic shower cap for the scalp, or mask made from gauze for the face, with holes cut for the eyes, mouth, and nose.

Skin Biopsy

Description

1. Removal of a piece of skin by shave, punch, or excision technique to detect malignancy or other characteristics of skin disorders.
2. Types of biopsy.
   a. Shave biopsy—scalpel used to remove raised lesions, leaving lower layers of dermis intact.
   b. Punch biopsy—special instrument used to remove round core of lesion, containing all layers of skin. Core is usually closed with sutures.
   c. Excisional biopsy—scalpel and scissors used to remove entire lesion; suturing required.

Nursing and Patient Care Considerations

1. Position the patient comfortably with the site exposed; explain that a local anesthetic will be given. Check if the patient has any known allergies to local anesthetics. Ask the patient what current medication he or she is taking. Aspirin or blood thinners may cause increased postoperative bleeding.
2. Explain the procedure.
3. Obtain written consent.
4. After the biopsy, apply pressure to the site to stop bleeding if required and apply an appropriate dressing. Pressure dressing may be required for larger wounds or wounds that are bleeding.
5. Place the biopsy specimen in a clearly labelled container with 10% formaldehyde and transport it to the lab.

Patient Education

1. Keep the bandage on surgery site for 24 to 48 hours. During this time, keep site clean and dry.
2. After this time, remove the bandage and do the following daily:
   a. Wash the incision with soap and water.
   b. Dry the incision well.
   c. Apply antibiotic ointment as prescribed 1 to 4 times a day, keeping the incision moist at all times.
3. After a few days the dressing is no longer needed, but still apply antibiotic ointment 1 to 4 times a day.

4. Do not apply makeup directly to the stitches.
5. Repeat wound care for 2 or 3 days after stitches have been removed, unless otherwise instructed.

Wound Coverage: Grafts and Flaps

Wound coverage, using grafts and flaps, is a type of reconstructive (plastic) surgery performed to improve the skin's appearance and function.

Description
Skin Graft

1. A section of skin tissue is separated from its blood supply and transferred as free tissue to a distant (recipient) site; it must obtain nourishment from capillaries at the recipient site.
2. In dermatology, skin grafting is used to repair defects that result from excision of skin tumors and to cover areas of denuded skin.
3. Definitions.
   a. Autografts—grafts done with tissue transplanted from the patient's own skin.
   b. Allografts—involve the transplant of tissue from one individual of the same species; these grafts are also called allogenic or homografts.
   c. Xenograft or heterograft—involve the transfer of tissue from another species.
4. Classification by thickness.
   a. Split thickness (thin, intermediate, or thick)—graft that is cut at varying thicknesses and is used to cover large wounds, because its total potential donor area is virtually unlimited..
   b. Full thickness—graft consists of epidermis and all of the dermis without the underlying fat; used to cover wounds that are too large to close primarily. They are used frequently to cover facial defects, because they provide a better contour match and less postoperative contracture.

Skin Flaps

1. A flap is a segment of tissue that has been left attached at one end (called a base or pedicle); the other end has been moved to a recipient area. It is dependent for its survival on functioning arterial and venous blood supplies and on lymphatic drainage in its pedicle or base.
   a. Free flap or free-tissue transfer—one that is completely severed from the body and is transferred to another site; receives early vascular supply from microvascular anastomosis with vessels at recipient site.
2. Flaps may consist of skin, mucosa, muscle, adipose tissue, omentum, and bone.
3. Used for wound coverage and to provide bulk, especially when bone, tendon, blood vessels, or nerve tissue are exposed.
4. Flaps offer the best aesthetic solution, because a flap retains the color, texture, and thickness match of the donor area.

5. Flaps are classified according to the method of movement, composition, location, or function.

Procedure for Skin Grafts

1. Split-thickness skin graft is obtained by razor blade, skin-grafting knife, electric, or air-powered dermatome/drum dermatome. Most commonly obtained from the inner aspect of the upper arm or outer thigh.
2. A full-thickness skin graft is primarily excised, defatted, and tailored to fit accurately over the defect area.
3. Skin is taken from the donor or host site and applied to the wound/defect site, called the recipient site or graft bed.
4. Process of revascularization and reattachment of the skin graft to the recipient bed is referred to as a take. A bolster (pressure) dressing is applied to the graft to enhance the survival of the skin graft by providing stable approximation of the graft to the recipient bed.
5. The bolster dressing is left in place for 1 week.
6. The donor site is maintained clean and dry.
   a. If Scarlet Red (a single layer dressing impregnated with epithelial growth promoter) is used on the donor site for split-thickness grafts, it is left in place for 2 to 3 weeks to allow the wound to heal.
   b. Occlusive dressings, such as Omniderm or Allevyn, may also be used to decrease pain, alleviate frequent wound care, and speed healing.
   c. Daily wound care and dressing change with an antimicrobial ointment and nonstick dressing may also be used.

NURSING ALERT

Patients usually find the donor site more painful than the graft site.

Preoperative Management and Nursing Care

1. Aspirin and nonsteroidal anti-inflammatory drugs (NSAIDs) and vitamin E are discontinued 14 days before the procedure. Coumadin should be held for several days before the procedure and prothrombin time (PT) and International normalized ratio (INR) should be measured before the procedure as ordered.
2. Efforts should be made to enhance wound healing several months to several weeks before the procedure, such as smoking cessation, alcohol avoidance, and proper nutrition.
3. Medical history and examination should be evaluated, particularly for latex sensitivity, cardiovascular problems requiring endocarditis antibiotic prophylaxis, bleeding problems, and high blood pressure.
4. The procedure is usually done under local anesthetic, so no meals are withheld.
5. The operative site should be free of makeup.

6. The patient should have someone available to drive home after surgery unless otherwise notified.

Postoperative Management and Nursing Care

Educate the patient with a skin graft on the following care:

1. Initial pressure dressing will be left in place for 24 to 48 hours.
2. If your wound begins to ooze apply firm pressure for 10 to 15 minutes (without peeking). If bleeding persists, contact your surgeon.
3. Do not take aspirin or aspirin-containing medication for pain. You may take 1 to 2 acetaminophen tablets every 4 to 6 hours as needed.
4. Most skin grafts are held in place by a bolster dressing (cotton ball or foam). Do not remove the bolster dressing during the next week.
5. You may clean site and apply ointment to the surrounding area of the bolster dressing.
6. *Do not* get the bolster dressing wet.
7. Once the bolster dressing is removed you may shower, but DO NOT let the water directly hit the graft.
8. Keep the graft edges moist with antibiotic ointment.
9. Protect the graft from the sun. The sun will cause pigmentation changes in the graft. A sunscreen may be used in 2 to 3 weeks.
10. Skin grafts to the lower leg must be kept elevated, because the new capillary connections are fragile, and excess venous pressure may cause rupture. Keep your leg elevated as much as possible during the next week.
11. Inspect the dressing daily. Report unusual drainage or signs of an inflammatory reaction.
12. After 2 to 3 weeks, any water-based moisturizer may be applied to the skin donor site for split thickness skin grafts.
13. Expect some loss of sensation in the grafted area for a time.
14. Avoid strenuous exercise (jogging, lifting heavy objects). Anything that causes your face to flush will raise your blood pressure, cause bleeding, and impair healing.

Aesthetic Procedures (Cosmetic Surgery)

Aesthetic procedures are a type of reconstructive (plastic) surgery performed to reconstruct or to alter congenital or acquired defects or to restore or improve the body's appearance.

Types of Procedures

1. Rhytidectomy—(face lift) done through various techniques and incisions to alleviate skin folds and wrinkles to improve the appearance of the aging face.
2. Blepharoplasty—done by scalpel or carbon dioxide laser excision to remove excess skin or fat from the upper and lower eyelids.

3. Dermabrasion—(skin planing) uses a special instrument to abrade the skin and remove the epidermis and superficial dermis to improve the appearance.

4. Body contouring—(liposuction) reduces localized deposits of fat not amenable to weight loss, with a cannula aided by suction or fitted to a syringe; may be done on the face, neck, breasts, abdomen, flanks, hips, buttocks, and extremities.

General Preoperative Management and Nursing Care

1. Local or general anesthetic will be administered. For local anesthetic, patient may eat and drink before surgery. For general anesthetic:
   a. Preoperative assessment may be necessary, depending on health status and patient's age.
   b. Patient should not eat or drink for several hours before surgery.
   c. Patient should have someone to escort him or her home and must be reminded not to drive home alone after surgery.
2. Review patient's allergies and medication before surgery.
3. Instruct patient to cleanse skin with antiseptic agent the night before surgery, if prescribed.
4. Make sure patient thoroughly understands procedure and has discussed the risks and benefits with the health care provider before surgery.
5. Ensure that consent form is signed before any procedure.
6. Ensure that aspirin, warfarin (Coumadin), and NSAIDs have been discontinued for 2 weeks before surgery, unless otherwise indicated.

Postoperative Management and Nursing Care
Rhytidectomy
1. Rest for 24 to 48 hours after the procedure, and avoid exercise that causes the face to flush, because blood pressure rises and increases the chance of bleeding.
2. Elevate the head at night for 2 weeks after the procedure. Avoid bending and lifting, which may increase edema and provoke bleeding.
3. Expect the face or affected part to be swollen, bruised, and numb for several days to weeks.
4. Be aware that complications include bleeding and hematoma, sloughing of skin, and possible facial nerve damage. Notify surgeon if the areas become increasingly red or swollen or if they become more tender or painful.

Blepharoplasty
1. Apply iced gauze compresses to eyes for 10 minutes 4 to 6 times daily, to reduce edema after surgery.
2. Avoid strenuous exercise for 1 week.
3. Watch for complications that include eyelid hematomas, ocluar mobility dysfunction, postsurgical ectropian (eversion of eyelid).

Dermabrasion
1. Do not pluck at crusts, because new epithelium will be injured; soak face several times a day, and apply emollient as directed.
2. Keep areas treated clean and moist.
3. Avoid sun on treated areas. Apply sunscreen with sun protection factor (SPF) of 15 to 30 when outdoors.
4. Complications include pigment alteration, scarring, infection.

Liposuction
1. After liposuction, increased fluids are required.
2. Aspirin and NSAIDs should be avoided for at least 1 week to prevent bleeding.
3. Wear compression garment as instructed.
4. Notify the surgeon if increased swelling develops; could indicate development of a seroma.
5. Expect blood-tinged fluid from cannula injection sites for 2 to 3 days.
6. Keep sutured areas moist with ointment as instructed.
7. Avoid jarring exercise as instructed.
8. Complications include development of seromas, lumpiness in treated areas, excessive bruising.

NURSING ALERT

Advise all postoperative patients to notify the health care provider if sudden pain, swelling, or bruising develop; these suggest hematoma or abscess. Do not take aspirin for postoperative discomfort; follow surgeon's orders.

DERMATOLOGIC DISORDERS

Cellulitis

Cellulitis is an inflammation of the subcutaneous tissue of the skin that results from an infectious process.

Pathophysiology and Etiology
1. Caused by infection with group A beta-hemolytic streptococci, *Staphylococcus aureus, Haemophilus influenzae,* or other organisms.
2. Usually results from break in skin.
3. Infection can spread rapidly through lymphatic system.

Clinical Manifestations
1. Tender, warm, erythematous, and swollen area that is well demarcated.
2. Tender, warm, erythematous streak that extends proximally from the area, indicating lymph vessel involvement.
3. Possible fluctuant abscess or purulent drainage.
4. Possible fever, chills, headache, malaise.

Diagnostic Evaluation
1. Gram stain and culture of drainage.
2. Blood cultures.

Management

1. Oral antibiotics (penicillinase-resistant penicillins, cephalosporins, or quinolones) may be adequate to treat small localized areas of cellulitis of legs or trunk.
2. Parenteral antibiotics may be needed for cellulitis of the hands, face, or lymphatic spread.
3. Surgical drainage and debridement for suppurative areas.

Complications

1. Tissue necrosis.
2. Septicemia.

Nursing Assessment

1. Obtain history of trauma to skin, needle stick, insect bite, or wound.
2. Observe for expanding borders and lymphatic streaking; palpate for fluctuance of abscess formation.
3. Watch for signs of antibiotic sensitivity—shortness of breath, urticaria, angioedema, maculopapular rash, or severe skin reaction, such as erythema multiforme, or toxic epidermal necrolysis.
4. Assess for patient and caretaker ability to provide care at home, keep affected area clean, and adhere to medication prescribed.

Nursing Diagnoses

- Risk for Impaired Skin Integrity related to infectious process
- Pain related to inflammation of subcutaneous tissue

Nursing Interventions

Protecting Skin Integrity

1. Administer, or teach patient to administer, antibiotics as prescribed; teach dosage schedule and side effects.
2. Maintain intravenous infusion or venous access to administer intravenous antibiotics, if indicated.
3. Elevate affected extremity to promote drainage from area.
4. Administer warm soaks to relieve inflammation and to promote drainage.
5. Prepare patient for surgical drainage and debridement, if necessary.

Relieving Pain

1. Encourage comfortable position and immobilization of affected area.
2. Administer, or teach patient to administer, analgesics as prescribed; monitor for side effects.
3. Use bed cradle to relieve pressure from bed covers.

Patient Education and Health Maintenance

1. Ensure that patient understands dosage schedule of antibiotics and the importance of complying with therapy to prevent complications.

2. Advise patient to notify health care provider immediately if condition worsens; hospitalization may be necessary.
3. Outpatient-treated cellulitis should be observed within 48 hours of starting antibiotics to determine adequacy of treatment.
4. Teach patients with impaired circulation or with impaired sensation proper skin care and how to inspect skin for trauma.

Outcome-Based Evaluation

- Skin is normal color and temperature, nontender, nonswollen, and intact
- Patient actively moving extremity; verbalizes no pain

■ Necrotizing Fasciitis

Necrotizing fasciitis is a type of necrotizing infection of the soft tissue that spreads rapidly along fascia. It rapidly progresses toward death if not treated quickly.

Pathophysiology and Etiology

1. Usually caused by group A *Streptococcus,* known as flesh-eating bacteria, but may also be clostridia or polymicrobial infection.
2. May result postoperatively or from local injury with superficial or deep infection.
3. More common in patients with diabetes, drug abusers, and other immunocompromised populations.
4. Spreads along fascia, causing extensive necrosis of skin and subcutaneous tissue.

Clinical Manifestations

1. Increasing pain or pain out of proportion to local infection or injury.
2. Fever, rapid pulse.
3. Tissue appears darkened under skin.
4. Possible bullae or petechiae, or appears hemorrhagic.
5. May be foul odor and drainage (late).

Diagnostic Evaluation

1. Surgical excision and debridement is diagnostic to determine the extent as well as therapeutic.
2. Gram stain and culture from deep tissue to determine exact etiology.
3. Blood cultures to rule out septicemia.

Management

1. Immediate hospitalization with intensive care support.
2. Prompt and repeated surgical debridement.
3. Intravenous antibiotic regimen using multiple agents including clindamycin, penicillin G, erythromycin, ceftriaxone, and others.

Complications

1. Muscle gangrene—requires amputation.
2. Loss of tissue and function.
3. Death.

Nursing Assessment

1. After trauma, surgery, or with cellulitis, frequently assess for increasing pain, fever, and changes in skin appearance, which may indicate necrotizing fasciitis.

> **NURSING ALERT**
>
> Call health care provider immediately if pain is out of proportion to injury or if progressive skin changes occur.

2. The patient should be assessed for necrotizing fasciitis.
3. Be aware of underlying immunocompromise, such as diabetes, alcoholism, malnutrition, IV drug use, cancer, and cancer treatment, which increases the risk and worsens the course of necrotizing fasciitis.
4. Monitor vital signs frequently for any change (rise or fall in blood pressure, temperature, pulse, and respirations) that may indicate worsening condition.
5. Monitor would dressings after debridement for amount, color, and odor of drainage. Wounds will usually be left open to heal by second intention.

Nursing Diagnoses

- Hyperthermia related to infectious process
- Pain related to necrosis

Nursing Interventions

Normalizing Body Temperature

1. Administer antipyretics as directed.
2. Encourage oral fluids as able and administer IV fluids as directed.
3. Monitor intake and output to ensure adequate hydration in light of fluid loss through fever and insensible loss.
4. Provide cool compresses, sponge baths, and clothing and linen changes as comfort measures.

Relieving Pain

1. Administer analgesics as directed and based on pain assessment; however, be alert for sedation that may mask signs of worsening condition.
2. Assist patient to position of comfort that will not place pressure on affected area.
3. Administer analgesic 30 to 60 minutes before wound care and dressing changes.

Patient Education and Health Maintenance

1. Ensure that patient can complete wound care at home and will follow up as directed.
2. May require home care.
3. Teach patient signs of infection to notify health care provider immediately—increasing pain, fever, redness, swelling, warmth, increased and odorous drainage.
4. Advise patient to eat a balanced diet rich in vitamin C, iron, and zinc for wound healing.

Outcome-Based Evaluation

- Core temperature 97.6° to 98.8°F
- Patient turning in bed, verbalizing minimal pain

Toxic Epidermal Necrolysis

Toxic epidermal necrolysis is a severe, potentially fatal skin disease associated with erythema and epidermal sloughing.

Pathophysiology and Etiology

1. Exact mechanism is unknown, but can be induced by various drugs, including sulfonamides, anticonvulsants, NSAIDs, and vaccines.
2. Resembles second-degree burns, with sloughing of skin at epidermal/dermal junction.

Clinical Manifestations

1. Malaise, fatigue, vomiting, and diarrhea may be prodromal symptoms.
2. Sudden onset of urticaria and erythema, then large bullae appear.
3. Within hours coma may develop; fever may develop.
4. Bullae become confluent and slough in large sheets, leaving moist, erythematous surface.
5. Positive Nikolsky's sign (desquamation of skin on light pressure).
6. Ulceration of lips and buccal mucosa; conjunctivitis.

Diagnostic Evaluation

1. Skin biopsy to determine level of separation.
2. Possible cultures of blood and body fluids to differentiate infection.

Management

1. Treatment in intensive care unit or regional burn center, because toxic epidermal necrolysis has similar pathophysiologic characteristics to those of extensive burns.
2. Treatment of affected skin:
   a. Wounds are cleansed in operating room under anesthesia; loose skin and blisters are removed, necrotic areas are debrided to prevent infection.
   b. Temporary biologic dressings (porcine cutaneous xenographs, amnion, collagen-based skin substitute, or plastic semipermeable dressings) applied to prevent secondary skin infection while awaiting re-epithelialization.
3. All nonessential drugs are stopped immediately.
4. Fluid replacement therapy, as necessary, and possible enteral nutrition if extensive oral involvement.
5. Topical antimicrobial dressings to enhance reepithelialization.
6. Ophthalmologic examination and removal of corneal adhesions as necessary.

Complications

1. Sepsis.
2. Pneumonia.
3. Blindness.

Nursing Assessment

1. Obtain medication and immunization history.
2. Monitor vital signs and level of consciousness closely, because condition is rapidly progressive.
3. Monitor fluid and nutritional status through daily weight, vital signs, and laboratory test results (electrolytes, blood urea nitrogen, creatinine, albumin, and total protein).

Nursing Diagnoses

- Impaired Skin Integrity related to sloughing
- Risk for Fluid Volume Deficit related to transudation of fluid into bullae
- Pain related to exposed dermal nerve endings
- Altered Oral Mucous Membranes related to oral lesions

Nursing Interventions

Restoring Skin Integrity

1. Place patient on warmed air-fluidized bed to distribute weight with minimal shearing forces.
2. Use extreme care in handling patient, because skin is very fragile; obtain assistance to move patient.
3. Gently apply warm, wet compresses of prescribed antiseptic solution to reduce bacterial population of wound surface.
4. Inspect xenograft several times daily for dislodgement or purulence; these will require new xenograft.
5. Watch for new areas of toxic epidermal necrolysis; note and record progression of skin slough and chart progress.
6. Patient should be in private room on reverse isolation to prevent infection.
7. Provide nutritional supplements through enteral feeding to ensure healing.

Maintaining Fluid Balance

1. Monitor vital signs for falling blood pressure or for rising pulse that indicates hypovolemia; use an indwelling arterial catheter to provide continuous measurement while avoiding cuff pressure on the skin.
2. Measure hourly urine output.
3. Weigh patient daily.
4. Give intravenous fluids as prescribed.
5. Assess bowel sounds and give oral or enteral fluids as tolerated.

Reducing Pain

1. If patient cannot verbalize, watch for facial expressions, guarding, or for increased pulse and respirations to indicate pain.
2. Administer analgesics as prescribed and as required, possibly around the clock; monitor for side effects and document effectiveness.
3. Provide distraction through music or other measures to promote relaxation.
4. Provide emotional support and encouragement.

Protecting Mucous Membranes

1. Use meticulous oral hygiene:
   a. Inspect oral cavity daily; note any changes.
   b. Rinse mouth with normal saline, diluted hydrogen peroxide, or other solution to remove debris and to cleanse ulcerations.
   c. Apply petroleum jelly or other lubricant/protectant to cracked, swollen lips.
2. Assess urethral, vaginal, and anal regions for ulcerations or bleeding.
3. Inspect eyes and remove crusts from eyelid margins, using damp compresses or saline-soaked swabs; apply eyedrops as prescribed.

Patient Education and Health Maintenance

1. Encourage follow-up appointments with plastic surgeon and other health care providers as indicated.
2. Encourage compliance with physical therapy as indicated, to restore function.
3. Advise patient to use sunscreen of at least 15 SPF, avoid direct sunlight during the healing phase, and continue to use sunscreen.
4. Advise patient to avoid suspected medication in the future.

Outcome-Based Evaluation

- New epithelium noted without scarring
- Output equals input; weight and vital signs remain stable
- Patient verbalizes reduced pain
- Oral mucosa intact

Herpes Zoster

Herpes zoster (shingles) is an inflammatory condition in which a virus produces a painful vesicular eruption along the distribution of the nerves from one or more dorsal root ganglia. The prevalence increases with age.

Pathophysiology and Etiology

1. Caused by a varicella-zoster virus, which is a member of a group of DNA viruses.
2. Virus is identical to the causative agent of varicella (chicken pox). After the primary infection, the varicella-zoster virus may persist in a dormant state in the dorsal nerve root ganglia. The virus may emerge from this site in later years, either spontaneously or in association with immunosuppression, to cause herpes zoster.

Clinical Manifestations

1. Eruption may be accompanied or preceded by fever, malaise, headache, and pain; pain may be burning, lancinating, stabbing, or aching.

2. Inflammation is usually unilateral, involving the cranial, cervical, thoracic, lumbar, or sacral nerves in a bandlike configuration.
3. Vesicles appear in 3 to 4 days.
   a. Characteristic patches of grouped vesicles appear on erythematous, edematous skin.
   b. Early vesicles contain serum; they later rupture and form crusts; scarring usually does not occur unless the vesicles are deep and they involve the dermis.
   c. If ophthalmic branch of the facial nerve is involved, patient may have a painful eye.
   d. In healthy host, lesions resolve in 2 to 3 weeks.
4. A susceptible person can acquire chicken pox if he or she comes in contact with the infective vesicular fluid of a zoster patient. A person with a history of chicken pox is immune and thus is not at risk from infection after exposure to zoster patients.

> **NURSING ALERT**
>
> Varicella-zoster virus may be a life-threatening condition to the patient who is immunosuppressed, who is receiving cytotoxic chemotherapy, or who is a bone marrow transplant recipient.

Diagnostic Evaluation
1. Usually diagnosed by clinical presentation.
2. Culture of varicella-zoster virus from lesions or detection by fluorescent antibody techniques, including viral detection that uses monoclonal antibodies (Micro-Trak), may be done to confirm diagnosis.

Management
1. Antiviral drugs, such as acyclovir (Zovirax), famcylovir (Famvir), and valacyclovir (Valtrex), interfere with viral replication; may be used in all cases, but especially for treatment of immunosuppressed and/or debilitated patients.
2. Corticosteroids early in illness—given for severe herpes zoster if symptomatic measures fail; given for anti-inflammatory effect and for relief of pain. Controversial.
3. Pain management; aspirin, acetaminophen, NSAIDs, narcotics—useful during the acute stage, but not generally effective for postherpetic neuralgia.

Complications
1. Chronic pain syndrome (postherpetic neuralgia), characterized by constant aching and burning pain or by intermittent lancinating pain or hyperesthesia of affected skin after it has healed.
2. Ophthalmic complications with involvement of ophthalmic branch of trigeminal nerve with keratitis, uveitis, corneal ulceration, and possibly blindness.
3. Facial and auditory nerve involvement, resulting in hearing deficits, vertigo, and facial weakness.
4. Visceral dissemination—pneumonitis, esophagitis, enterocolitis, myocarditis, pancreatitis.

Nursing Diagnoses
- Pain related to inflammation of cutaneous nerve endings
- Impaired Skin Integrity related to rupture of vesicles

Nursing Interventions
Controlling Pain
1. Assess patient's level of discomfort and medicate as prescribed; monitor for side effects of pain medications.
2. Teach patient to apply wet dressings for soothing effect.
3. Encourage distraction techniques, such as music therapy.
4. Teach relaxation techniques, such as deep breathing, progressive muscle relaxation, and imagery, to help control pain.

Improving Skin Integrity
1. Apply wet dressings to cool and dry inflamed areas by means of evaporation.
2. Administer antiviral medication in dosage prescribed (usually high dose); warn the patient of side effects, such as nausea.
3. Apply antibacterial ointments (after acute stage) as prescribed, to soften and separate adherent crusts and prevent secondary infection.

Patient Education and Health Maintenance
1. Teach patient to use proper handwashing technique, to avoid spreading herpes zoster virus.
2. Advise patient not to open the blisters, to avoid secondary infection and scarring.
3. Reassure that shingles is a viral infection of the nerves; nervousness does not cause shingles.
4. A caregiver may be required to assist with dressings and meals. In older persons, the pain is more pronounced and incapacitating. Dysesthesia and skin hypersensitivity are distressing.

Outcome-Based Evaluation
- Patient verbalizes decreased pain
- Reepithelialization of skin without scarring

◼ Pemphigus
Pemphigus is a serious autoimmune disease of the skin and of the mucous membranes, characterized by the appearance of blisters (bullae) of various sizes on apparently normal skin and mucous membranes (mouth, esophagus, conjunctiva, vagina) (Figure 33-3). Familial benign chronic pemphigus (Hailey-Hailey disease) is a familial type of pemphigus that appears in adults, affecting particularly the axillae and groin.

Pathophysiology and Etiology
1. The cause is unknown.
2. Certain drugs, other autoimmune diseases, and genetics may play a role in its development.
3. Many variants of pemphigus exist.

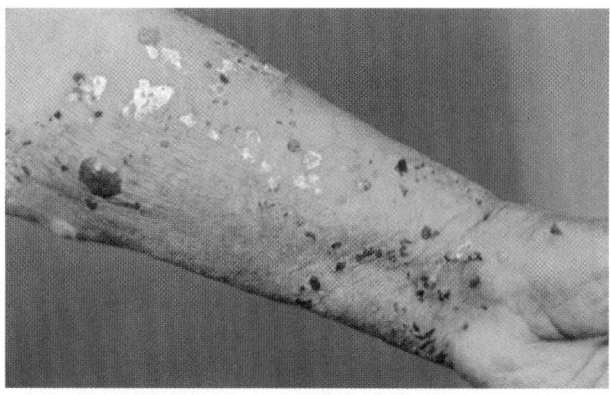

FIGURE 33-3 Pemphigus vulgaris blisters on the forearm.

Clinical Manifestations

1. Initial lesions may appear in oral cavity; flaccid blisters (bullae) may arise on normal or erythematous skin.
   a. The bullae enlarge and rupture, forming painful, raw, and denuded areas that eventually become crusted.
   b. The eroded skin heals slowly; eventually, widespread areas of the body may become involved.
   c. In the mouth, the blisters are usually multiple, of varying size and irregular shape, painful, and persistent. Oral lesions may appear initially, with lesions of the mucous membranes of the pharynx and esophagus; the conjunctivae, larynx, urethra, cervix, and rectum may become affected as well.
2. An offensive odor may emanate from the bullae.
3. Positive Nikolsky's sign—separation of epidermis when minimal pressure is applied to the skin. Downward pressure on a bulla will cause it to expand laterally.

Diagnostic Evaluation

1. Skin biopsies of blisters and surrounding skin—demonstrate acantholysis (separation of epidermal cells from each other).
2. Immunofluorescent studies of serum—reveal circulating antibodies (pemphigus antibodies).

Management

1. Corticosteroids in large doses to control the disease and keep skin free of blisters.
2. Immunosuppressive agents, such as cyclophosphamide (Cytoxin) and azathioprine (Imuran), are used alone or in combination with steroids, for immunosuppressive and steroid-sparing effect.
3. Plasmapheresis—reinfusion of specially treated plasma cells; temporarily decreases serum level of antibodies.
4. Treatment of denuded skin.

Complications

1. Infections (skin, pneumonia, septicemia).
2. Psychosis.

3. Side effects from acute and chronic corticosteroids; gastrointestinal bleeding, secondary infection, psychosis, hyperglycemia, and others.

Nursing Assessment

1. Assess for odor or drainage from lesions, which may indicate infection.
2. Assess for fever and signs of systemic infection.
3. Assess for side effects of corticosteroids, such as abdominal pain, white patches in mouth that indicate *Candida* infection, and emotional changes.

Nursing Diagnoses

- Altered Oral Mucous Membrane related to ruptured bullae
- Impaired Skin Integrity related to ruptured bullae
- Risk for Fluid Volume Deficit related to transudation of fluid into bullae
- Body Image Disturbance related to widespread or chronic skin lesions

Nursing Interventions

Restoring Oral Mucous Membrane Integrity

1. Inspect oral cavity daily; note and report any changes—oral lesions heal slowly.
2. Keep oral mucosa clean and allow regeneration of epithelium.
3. Give topical oral therapy as directed.
4. Offer prescribed mouthwashes through a straw, to rinse mouth of debris and to soothe ulcerative areas.
5. Teach patient to apply petrolatum to lips frequently.
6. Use cool-mist therapy to humidify environmental air.

Restoring Skin Integrity

1. Keep skin clean and eliminate debris and dead skin—the bullae will clear if epithelium at the base is clean and not infected.
2. Obtain swab of bullous fluid for cultures—most common organism is *S. aureus*.
3. Administer cool, wet dressings and/or baths or teach patient to administer, to soothe and cleanse skin. Large areas of blistering have a characteristic odor that is lessened when secondary infection is under control.
   a. After the bath, dry and cover with talcum powder as directed; this enables the patient to move more freely in bed. Large amounts are necessary to keep clothes and sheets from sticking.
4. The nursing management of patients with blistering or with bullous skin conditions is similar to that of the patient with a burn (see p. 1056).

Achieving Fluid Balance

1. Evaluate for fluid and electrolyte imbalance—extensive denudation of the skin leads to fluid and electrolyte imbalance.
   a. Monitor serum albumin and protein levels.
   b. Monitor vital signs for hypotension or tachycardia.
   c. Weigh patient daily.
   d. Monitor intake and output.

2. Administer intravenous saline solutions as directed.
3. Encourage the patient to maintain hydration; suggest cool nonirritating fluids.
    a. Suggest soft, high-protein, high-calorie diet, or liquid supplements (Ensure, Sustacal, eggnogs, milkshakes) that will not be irritating to oral mucosa but will replace lost protein.

Promoting Positive Body Image
1. Develop a trusting relationship with the patient.
2. Educate patient and family about the disease and its treatment; this reduces uncertainty and clears up misconceptions.
3. Encourage expression of anxieties, embarrassment, discouragement.
4. Encourage patient to maintain social contacts and activities among support network.

Patient Education and Health Maintenance
Instruct the patient as follows:
1. The disease may be characterized by relapses that require continuing therapy to maintain control.
2. Long-term administration of immunosuppressive drugs is associated with numerous side effects and risks—hyperglycemia, osteoporosis, psychosis, adrenal suppression, and increased risk of cancer. Report for health care follow-up visits regularly.
3. Monitor skin/mouth for recurrence of pemphigus activity.

Outcome-Based Evaluation
- Oral mucous membranes pink with healing lesions and no signs of infection
- Skin with intact bullae, healing lesions, and no signs of infection
- Vital signs stable; urine output adequate
- Patient expresses concerns and plans activities

Psoriasis
Psoriasis (Figure 33-4) is a chronic inflammatory disorder in which epidermal turnover occurs 6 to 9 times faster than normal.

Pathophysiology and Etiology
1. Affects 1% to 3% of people.
2. Classified as mild if <2% of body affected; moderate if 2% to 10% affected; severe if >10%.
3. Types of psoriasis include:
    a. Plaque—most common type, occurs on knees, elbows, scalp, and other areas.
    b. Guttate—occurs on trunk, arms, legs; triggered by streptococcal infection.
    c. Inverse—affects flexural areas, such as axilla and groin.
    d. Erythrodermic—severe form that affects most of body.
    e. Pustular—blisters contain pus-like material on hand and feet or on widespread area.

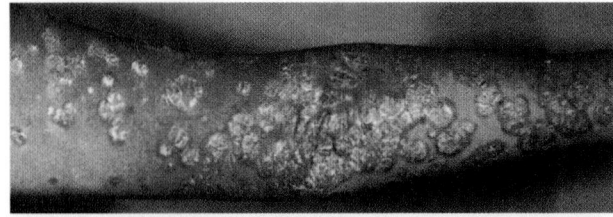
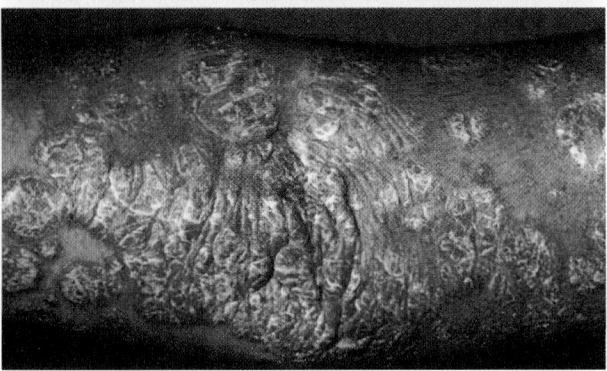

FIGURE 33-4 The lesions of psoriasis appear as red, raised patches of skin covered with silvery scales that in time coalesce, forming irregularly shaped patches.

f. Psoriatic arthritis—arthritis and other abnormalities accompany skin involvement.
4. Formerly considered idiopathic, now thought to be genetically linked and immune system modulated.
    a. May be caused by some antigenic stimuli that activate cytokines and T cells, thus causing an extreme dermal response.
    b. Genes are being identified that may predispose a person to developing psoriasis.
5. Condition tends to be lifelong, with flareups and remissions. May be exacerbated by infection; drugs, such as lithium, beta blockers, angiotensin converting enzyme inhibitors, antimalarial drugs, and indomethacin; stress; and injury.

Clinical Manifestations
1. Erythematous, raised patches with silvery scales.
2. Symmetric involvement.
3. May be pruritic and painful.
4. Characteristic pitting of nails.
5. Arthritis in approximately 10% of patients.

Management
1. Diagnosed by clinical features; rarely, a biopsy may be needed.
2. Coal tar and anthralin preparations inhibit excessive skin turnover.
    a. Applied topically, with no system side effects.
    b. Application may be messy, odorous, and may stain clothing.

3. Topical corticosteroids are used for short periods, because of their side effects (striae, thinning of the skin, adrenal suppression). They may cause tachyphylaxis and pustular psoriasis.

4. Topical calcipotriene, a vitamin D derivative, used for mild to moderate psoriasis; is generally without side effects.

5. Other topical preparations include a receptor selective retinoid (tazarotene), which is teratogenic, and a topical formation of methotrexate is being studied.

6. Phototherapy—20 to 30 short treatments. Narrow band UVB light is now safer than full-spectrum UVB light, which carries the risk of sunburn and skin cancer.
   a. Photochemotherapy—ingestion of a photosensitizer (psoralen compound) before light therapy.
   b. Cataracts, nausea, and malaise are possible side effects.

7. Oral methotrexate, acitretin (a retinoid), and cyclosporine also are used for severe cases.
   a. Hepatotoxicity may occur with methotrexate.
   b. Acitretin is not teratogenic like other retinoids, unless alcohol is consumed with its use or for 2 months after. Women are still cautioned not to become pregnant with use or for 3 years after ceasing therapies.
   c. Hypertension and renal failure may occur with cyclosporine.

 DRUG ALERT

Cyclosporine is contraindicated in patients with renal disease, uncontrolled hypertension, active infection, internal malignancy, immune deficiency, gout, hepatic disease, and concomitant use of nephrotoxic drugs. Serum creatinine must be followed closely throughout treatment.

Nursing Interventions and Patient Education

1. Assist patient with daily tub bath to soften scales and plaques; may gently rub with bath brush.

2. Apply topical preparations after bath and scale removal.

3. Warn patient that coal tar and anthralin preparations may stain clothing; let dry before dressing.

4. Advise patient to wear goggles for phototherapy, to prevent cataracts and to follow up with periodic eye exams.

5. Encourage patient to follow up closely with primary care provider or with dermatologist and to report for blood work, to check renal function and liver function tests as indicated.

6. Reinforce to women of childbearing age that retinoids and methotrexate are teratogenic; woman must be using birth control.

7. Encourage patients to try to identify triggers that may cause flareups and to practice avoidance techniques, such as relaxation therapy, to avoid stress.

8. Teach patients to avoid direct sun exposure by wearing protective clothing and sunscreen, especially after photochemotherapy.

9. Advise patients to use good lubricants to prevent drying and cracking of skin, which can lead to hyperkeratinization.

10. For more information, contact the National Psoriasis Foundation at *www.psoriasis.org,* 6600 SW 92nd Avenue, Suite 300, Portland, OR, 97223—7195, 800-723-9166; fax: 503-245-0626.

Benign Tumors

Benign tumors are common skin growths. Most do not require any treatment but are important to recognize to differentiate malignant lesions.

Characteristics of Benign Tumors
Seborrheic Keratoses
Tumors are benign, wartlike lesions of varying size and color, ranging from light tan to black; they are the most common skin tumors in middle-aged and older people.
Actinic (Solar) Keratoses
Premalignant skin lesions appearing as rough, scaly patches with underlying erythema, which develop as a consequence of prolonged exposure to ultraviolet rays.

1. Develop in areas of body that experience prolonged sun exposure; may gradually transform into squamous cell carcinoma.

2. Many available treatments, including topical fluorouracil (Effudex), liquid nitrogen cryosurgery, and curettage.
Verrucae (Warts)
Common, benign skin tumors caused by human papilloma virus.

1. Warts often do not need treatment, because they tend to disappear spontaneously.

2. Treatment options:
   a. Freezing with liquid nitrogen—destroys wart and spares rest of skin.
   b. Area may be treated surgically with curettage or electrodesiccation.
   c. Application of salicylic acid, topical fluorouracil, topical vitamin A acid, or other irritants may be helpful, especially for flat warts.
Angiomas (Birthmarks)
Benign vascular tumors involving the skin and subcutaneous tissue.

1. May occur as flat, violet-red patches (port-wine angiomas) or as raised, bright-red nodular lesions (strawberry angiomas). Strawberry angiomas may involute spontaneously, whereas port-wine angiomas usually persist indefinitely.

2. Most patients use masking cosmetics (Covermark) to camouflage the defect.

3. Laser is being used with good success.
Pigmented Nevi (Moles)
Common skin tumors of various sizes and shapes, ranging from yellowish to brown to black.

1. May be flat, macular lesions, elevated papules, or nodules that occasionally contain hair.
2. Most pigmented nevi are harmless; however, in rare cases, malignant changes supervene and a melanoma develops at the site of the nevus.
3. Treatment:
   a. Nevi at sites subject to repeated irritation from clothing or jewelry can be removed for comfort.
   b. Nevi that show change in size or color, become symptomatic (itch or bleed), or develop notched borders should be removed to determine if malignant changes have occurred. This is especially true for nevi with irregular borders or variations of red, blue, and/or blue-black colors.

Keloids
Benign overgrowths of connective tissue at site of scar or trauma in predisposed individuals.
1. More prevalent among blacks.
2. Usually asymptomatic—may cause disfigurement and cosmetic concern.
3. Management—intralesional corticosteroid therapy, surgical removal, radiation.

Cancer of the Skin
Skin cancer is the most common malignancy. Basal and squamous cell carcinomas are easily curable because of early diagnosis and slow progression. These cancers are locally invasive and tend not to metastasize. Conversely, malignant melanomas are less common and metastasize eventually.

Pathophysiology and Etiology
1. Most basal and squamous cell carcinomas are located on sun-exposed areas and are directly related to ultraviolet radiation. *Sun damage is cumulative.*
2. Risk factors for skin cancer include:
   a. Fair complexion, blue eyes, blond or red hair.
   b. Working outdoors.
   c. Older people with sun-damaged skin.
   d. History of x-ray treatment of skin conditions.
   e. Exposure to certain chemical agents (arsenicals, nitrates, tar and pitch, oils, and paraffins).
   f. Burn scars, damaged skin in areas of chronic osteomyelitis, fistulae openings.
   g. Long-term immunosuppressive therapy.
   h. Genetic susceptibility.
   i. Multiple dysplastic nevi—moles that are larger, irregular, more numerous, or variable colors—or family history of dysplastic nevi.
   j. Congenital nevi.
3. Types of skin cancer:
   a. Basal cell carcinoma—arises from basal layers of the epidermis or hair follicle; most common type, rarely metastasizes.
   b. Squamous cell carcinoma—arises from the epidermis; metastasis occurs more often than with basal cell carcinoma.
   c. Malignant melanoma—arises from nevocytic cells in the upper dermis; can metastasize.

Clinical Manifestations
Basal Cell Carcinoma
1. Lesions often begin as small nodules with a rolled, pearly, translucent border with telangiectasia, crusting, and occasionally ulceration (Figure 33-5A).
2. Appear most frequently on sun-exposed skin, frequently on face between hairline and upper lip.
3. If neglected, may cause local destruction, hemorrhage, and infection of adjacent tissues, producing severe functional and cosmetic disabilities.

Squamous Cell Carcinoma
1. Appears as reddish rough, thickened, scaly lesion with bleeding and soreness—may be asymptomatic; border may be wider, more indurated, and more inflammatory than basal cell carcinoma (Figure 33-5B).
2. May be preceded by leukoplakia (premalignant lesion of mucous membrane) of the mouth or tongue, actinic keratoses, scarred or ulcerated lesions.
3. Seen most commonly on lower lip, rims of ears, head, neck, and backs of the hands.

Malignant Melanoma
See Figure 33-6.
1. Melanoma in situ. Earliest phase, difficult to recognize because clinical changes are minimal.
2. Superficial spreading melanoma (most common).
   a. Circular, with irregular outer portions; the margins may be flat, or elevated and palpable.
   b. Has combination of colors—hues of tan, brown, and black mixed with gray, bluish black, or white.
   c. May be dull pink-rose color in a small area within the lesion.
   d. Occurs anywhere on body; usually affects middle-aged persons.

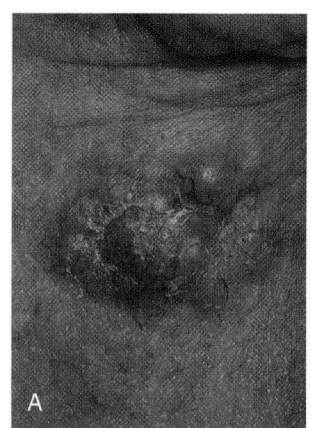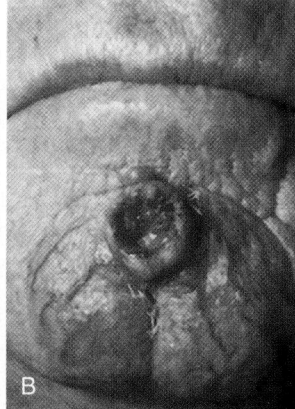

FIGURE 33-5 Basal cell carcinoma, squamous cell carcinoma.

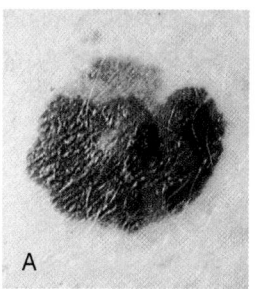 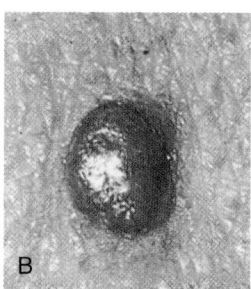 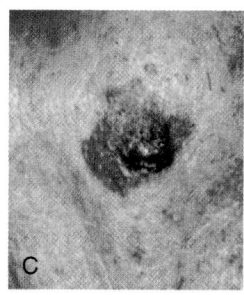

FIGURE 33-6 (**A**) Superficial spreading melanoma; note irregular border. (**B**) Nodular melanoma. (**C**) Lentigo-maligna melanoma; note irregular pigment pattern.

3. Nodular melanoma.
   a. Spherical blueberry-like nodule with relatively smooth surface and relatively uniform blue-black, blue-gray, or reddish blue color.
   b. May be polypoidal and elevated, with smooth surface of rose-gray or black color.
   c. Occurs commonly on torso and extremities.
   d. Invades directly into the subjacent dermis (vertical growth) and hence has a poorer prognosis.
4. Lentigo malignant melanoma.
   a. First appears as tan, flat macule—malignant degeneration is manifested by changes in color, size, and topography.
   b. Evolves slowly; occurs on exposed skin surfaces of persons in the 5th or 6th decade of life.
5. Acrolentiginous melanoma (uncommon).
   a. Irregular pigmented macules, which develop nodules; may become invasive early.
   b. Occurs commonly on palms, soles, nail beds, and rarely on mucous membranes.
   c. Most common type of melanoma in blacks.

Diagnostic Evaluation
Excisional biopsy (for histopathologic diagnosis) and microstaging determination of thickness and level of invasion; helps determine treatment and prognosis.

Management
Method of treatment depends on tumor location, cell type (location and depth), history of previous treatment, and whether it is invasive, or if metastasis has occurred.
1. Curettage followed by electrodesiccation—usually done on small tumors of basal or squamous cell type (less than 1 cm).
2. Surgical excision for larger lesions or for those in areas more likely to recur (around nose, eyes, ears, lips); may be followed by simple closure, flap, or graft.
3. Moh's surgery, a microscopically controlled excision, with immediate examination of frozen or chemically fixed sections for evidence of cancer cells. Layers are removed until a reasonable cancer-free margin is achieved.
4. Radiation therapy—can be done for cancer of eyelid, tip of nose, in or near vital structures, such as facial nerve or where tissue sparing is difficult with other

forms of treatment; also used for extensive malignancies where goal is palliation, or when other medical conditions contraindicate other forms of therapy.
5. Regional perfusion—chemotherapeutic agent may be perfused directly into area that contains melanoma by mechanically controlling arterial and venous blood flow; allows higher concentration of cytotoxic drug to be delivered to site, with less systemic toxicity.
6. Systemic chemotherapy—generally used for recurrence of metastasis or palliation; may be combined with autologous bone marrow transplantation or several agents used in combination.
7. Other therapeutic regimens—topical fluorouracil, interferon, retinoids, photoradiation.

Complications
Local invasion, regional or systemic metastasis (frequently central nervous system).

Nursing Assessment
1. Have a high index of suspicion for persons at risk.
2. Ask about sunbathing habits. Question patient about pruritus, tenderness, pain, or bleeding, which are not features of a benign nevus (mole).
3. Ask about changes in preexisting moles or about development of a new pigmented lesion.
4. Use a magnifying lens in a brightly lit room to look for variegated color and irregular border and surface in the mole. Use side lighting to assess subtle elevation.
5. Examine entire skin surface, including scalp, genital area, gluteal folds, and soles of feet.
6. Examine diameter of mole; melanomas are often larger than 6 mm; look for lesions situated near the mole.

NURSING ALERT

 Any skin lesion that changes in size or color, that bleeds, that ulcerates, or that becomes infected may be skin cancer.

Nursing Diagnoses
- Knowledge Deficit related to risk factors for skin cancer
- Anxiety related to diagnosis of cancer

Nursing Interventions

Increasing Knowledge and Awareness

1. Encourage follow-up skin examinations and instruct the patient to examine skin monthly as follows:
   a. Use a full-length mirror and a small hand mirror to aid in examination.
   b. Learn where moles/birthmarks are located.
   c. Inspect all moles and other pigmented lesions; report any change in color, size, elevation, thickness, or development of itching or bleeding.
2. Teach the patient to use a sunscreen with SPF of at least 15 routinely for the rest of life and *to never become sunburned.*
   a. Sunlight permanently damages the skin and can be cumulative.
   b. Do not try to tan if skin burns easily, never tans, or tans poorly.
   c. Avoid unnecessary exposure to the sun, especially during times when ultraviolet radiation is most intense (10:00 AM to 3:00 PM).
   d. Wear protective clothing (long sleeves, broad-brimmed hat, high collar, long pants, etc.). However, clothing does not provide complete protection; up to 50% of sun's damaging rays can penetrate clothes.
   e. Do not use sunlamps for indoor tanning; avoid commercial tanning salons.

Reducing Anxiety

1. Provide dressing changes and wound care while teaching patient to take control, as directed after surgical intervention.
2. Administer chemotherapy with attention to possible side effects, as directed.
3. Allow patient to express feelings about the seriousness of diagnosis.
4. Answer questions, clarify information, and correct misconceptions.
5. Emphasize use of positive coping skills and support system.

Patient Education and Health Maintenance

1. Encourage lifelong follow-up appointments with dermatologist and/or primary care provider with examinations every 6 months.
2. Encourage all individuals to have moles removed that are accessible to repeated friction and irritation, congenital, or suspicious in any way.
3. Teach all individuals the importance of sun-avoidance measures; teach proper use of sunscreen:
   a. Sunscreens with a sun protection factor of 15 or greater offer good protection.
   b. Sunscreens should be used from infancy through old age.
   c. Sunscreens should be applied, before going outdoors, to all areas that may be exposed, preferably before dressing. They should be applied liberally to achieve the stated SPF.
   d. Newly developed sunscreens are more resistant to removal by water, clothing, sweating, etc.; however, periodic reapplication is necessary when spending prolonged periods outdoors, especially when swimming.
   e. Protect lips with a lip balm that contains a sunscreen with the highest SPF.
4. For more information, refer patients to agencies such as The Skin Cancer Foundation, 245 Fifth Avenue, Suite 1403, New York, NY 10016, 212-725-5176, *www.skincancer.org.*

Outcome-Based Evaluation

- Patient using high SPF sunscreen, wearing protective clothing, and performing monthly skin examinations
- Patient verbalizes decreased anxiety

■ Other Dermatologic Disorders

See Table 33-2.

(*text continues on page 1043*)

TABLE 33-2 Other Dermatologic Disorders

Name/Description	Clinical Manifestations	Management	Nursing/Patient Care Considerations
Bacterial Infections			
Folliculitis—inflammation of the hair follicle	1. Single or multiple papules or pustules. 2. Commonly seen in the beard area of men and on women's legs from shaving.	1. Twice daily cleansing with antibacterial soap. 2. Topical antibiotic ointment. 3. Systemic antibiotics for recurrent or recalcitrant cases.	1. Advise warm compresses to relieve inflammation.
Furunculosis—perifollicular abscess (boil) caused by *Staphylococcus aureus;* Carbuncles are two or more confluent furuncles	1. Tender, circumscribed, erythematous area whose center may become fluctuant and suppurate. 2. Commonly occur on the back of neck, axillae, buttocks.	1. Warm compresses to reduce inflammation and to promote drainage. 2. When area becomes fluctuant, incision and drainage can be performed, followed by packing.	1. Encourage the use of warm compresses. 2. Warn patient not to squeeze or incise the lesion.

(continued)

TABLE 33-2 Other Dermatologic Disorders (Continued)

Name/Description	Clinical Manifestations	Management	Nursing/Patient Care Considerations
		3. Furuncles of the ear canal, nares, upper lip, and nose may require systemic antibiotic treatment, because these areas drain directly into cranial venous sinuses.	3. If severe or recurrent, look for underlying immunosuppression by disorders such as diabetes, AIDS, alcoholism, or malnutrition.
Paronychia—inflammation of skin folds surrounding the fingernail	1. Tender, purulent, erythematous swelling of nail border. 2. Chronic and recurrent paronychia cause horizontal ridges at base of nail.	1. Incision and drainage for acutely inflamed paronychia. 2. Fungicidal or bactericidal ointment for chronic paronychia. 3. Systemic antibiotic treatment usually is necessary. 4. Prevention of trauma and maceration.	1. Encourage soaking in warm water for 10–15 minutes 3–4 times a day while acutely inflamed to relieve pain and promote drainage. 2. Identify persons with work-related chronic paronychia (bartenders, dishwashers, housekeepers) and recommend use of rubber gloves over thin cotton gloves when working around moisture.
Erysipelas—streptococcal infection involving the superficial dermal lymphatics of head or extremities, may be *S. aureus* of the face.	1. Prodromal—malaise, fever, chills, headache, vomiting, joint pain. 2. Local—redness, warmth, swelling, and characteristic raised indurated border. 3. Leukocytosis. 4. Advancing edge of the patch with extension. 5. May vessiculate.	1. Oral, IM, or IV antibiotics, usually penicillianase-resistant penicillin derivatives; cephalosporin or macrolide antibiotic may be used.	1. Ice or cold compresses may be soothing. 2. Prompt treatment required in diabetic to prevent extensive spread and necrotizing fasciitis.
Intertrigo—superficial inflammation and secondary infection where two skin surfaces are in apposition	1. Erythematous and mascerated rash. 2. There may be erosions, fissures, and drainage. 3. Burning and itching.	1. Topical antibacterial and antifungal agents.	1. Teach patient to prevent skin maceration by separating opposing skin surfaces with gauze or cotton material. 2. Skin surfaces should be dried thoroughly after bathing with a hair dryer on low setting. 3. Talcum powder can be applied lightly to the area after drying. 4. Loose, airy clothing should be worn.

Mycotic (fungal) Infections

Name/Description	Clinical Manifestations	Management	Nursing/Patient Care Considerations
Tinea pedis—ringworm of the foot; Tinea corporis—ringworm of the body; Tinea cruris—ringworm of the groin; Tinea capitis—ringworm of the scalp	1. Caused by the dermatophyte *Trichophyton, Epidermophyton,* or *Microsporum.* 2. Erythematous, inflamed, and vesicular lesions of feet. 3. Scaling erythematous patches of body or head with central clearing. 4. Dull red or brownish rash of upper inner thighs and groin with scaling borders. 5. Itching and irritation.	1. Examination of rash under Wood's light differentiates erythrasma, which will fluoresce; most tinea patches will not. 2. Skin scraping from leading edge shows characteristic spores and hyphae with KOH preparation under microscope. 3. Treat with topical antifungals or systemic antifungals for severe cases.	1. Advise washing 1–2 times daily with water and mild soap, then applying talc powder or cornstarch to well-dried area. 2. Use hair dryer set on low temperature to dry tender areas. 3. Encourage wearing cotton socks and underwear and light, airy clothing to promote evaporation.

(continued)

TABLE 33-2 Other Dermatologic Disorders (Continued)

Name/Description	Clinical Manifestations	Management	Nursing/Patient Care Considerations
		4. Reduction of moisture in groin, between toes.	4. Warn about contamination from feet to groin or other areas of the body by hands or clothing. 5. Encourage use of open shoes or canvas sneakers and avoidance of plastic or rubber soled shoes or boots and tight shoes with tinea pedis. 6. Wash contaminated clothing in hot water.
Tinea vesicolor—superficial fungal infection by *Malassezia furfur*	1. Patchy macular or mildly scaly rash of upper trunk and upper arms; yellowish or brownish in light skinned people, hypopigmented in dark skin. 2. Mild itching and scaling.	1. On Wood's light examination, may fluoresce and will show hypopigmented patches. 2. Microscopic examination with KOH preparation of skin scraping shows characteristic "spaghetti and meatballs" appearance of hyphae and spores. 3. Treat with selenium sulfide shampoo (leave on for 40 minutes before showering) daily for 1 week. 4. Topical or systemic antifungal may be used.	1. Common in high temperature, high humidity environments. 2. Advise patient that discoloration may persist after fungus have been eradicated; lost pigmentation will resolve with sun exposure. 3. Tell patient that recurrence is common after 2–12 weeks if prophylactic treatment is not given periodically.
Onychomycosis (tinea unguium)—infection of the nail by fungus	1. Discoloration (white, yellow, or darkened) of the nail. 2. Nail becomes brittle, cracked, irregular, loosened. 3. May be some inflammation and pain.	1. Identification of offending fungus by microscopic examination of shavings with KOH or by culture. 2. Treatment with appropriate antifungal, either topical or systemic, for prolonged period—usually at least 6 weeks for fingernails and at least 12 weeks for toenails. 3. Surgical removal of nail may be necessary	1. Encourage patient to comply with lengthy treatment, as fungal infections of the nail are difficult to treat. 2. Examine patient for other areas of tinea infection (feet, groin), encourage treatment, and teach patient that infection may be spread from fingernails by scratching. 3. After nail removal, advise patient to keep hand or foot elevated for several hours, and change dressing daily by applying gauze and antibiotic ointment or other prescribed medication until nail bed is dry.

 DRUG ALERT

Oral antifungal agents are associated with significant drug interactions with such agents as warfarin, simvastatin, lovastatin, triazolam, cisapride, digoxin, cyclosporine, phenytoin, cimetidine, and rifampin. Ketoconazole requires frequent liver function test monitoring.

(continued)

TABLE 33-2 Other Dermatologic Disorders (Continued)

Name/Description	Clinical Manifestations	Management	Nursing/Patient Care Considerations
Parasitic Infections			
Pediculosis capitis—head lice; Pediculosis corporis—body lice; Pediculosis pubis—crab louse infestation of the genital region	1. Itching is primary complaint. 2. Lice and nits may be seen in seams of clothing (body lice) or clinging to hairs (pubic lice). 3. Skin excoriation in affected area. 4. Erythematous macules or wheals may appear at puncture sites. 5. Gray-blue macules may appear on trunk or inner thighs with pediculosis pubis.	1. Treatment for pediculosis corporis involves washing with soap and water and washing all infested clothing and linens with hot water. Alternatively, clothes may be dry-cleaned or ironed, paying close attention to the seams. 2. Pediculosis capitis and pubis are treated with a topical antiparasitic preparation such as lindane (Kwell) or permethrin (Nix). 3. Manual removal of nits (eggs) may be performed, and retreatment in 3–7 days is recommended. 4. Petroleum may be applied to eyelashes, then lice and nits removed with swab or tweezers or pilocarpine drops can be used to paralyze the lice. 5. Items that cannot be washed or dry cleaned can be stored for 30 days without use.	1. Advise patient that pediculosis pubis is considered a sexually transmitted disease; partners must be examined and treated. 2. Teach patient the proper use of medication: a. Apply lotion or cream after bathing to affected hairy and adjacent areas, wash off after 8–12 hours. b. Alternatively, apply shampoo to affected hairy areas and lather for 4–5 min, rinse and let hair dry. c. Use fine-tooth comb to remove nits. 3. Urge patient to wash all clothing, towels, linens, combs, and hair items by soaking in hot water for 10 min. 4. Advise patient not to use antiparasitic preparations more frequently than recommended and not to use at all if pregnant.
Scabies—superficial infestation by itch mite; transmitted by close personal contact	1. Itching, more intense at night. 2. Small erythematous papules and short, wavy burrows are seen on skin surface. 3. Frequently seen between fingers or in groin area. 4. Spares head and scalp except in children under 1 year of age.	1. Parasite identified by microscopic examination of skin scraping. 2. Treated with antiparasitic such as lindane (Kwell) or crotamiton (Eurax). 3. Machine wash and dry clothing and linens on hot cycle. 4. Topical or systemic steroids may be needed to treat symptoms of allergic reaction to mites.	1. Teach proper use of medication: a. Apply thin layer from neck downward, with particular attention to hands, feet, and intertriginous areas; every inch of skin must be treated because mites are migratory. Apply to dry skin. (Wet skin allows more penetration and the possibility of toxicity.)

 GERONTOLOGIC ALERT

Infestation with scabies may be a problem in nursing homes, particularly among debilitated patients who require extensive hands-on care.

	5. Atypical scabies may be found in immune compromised people and may be resistant to standard treatment.		b. Leave medication on for 8–12 hours but no longer, as this will irritate the skin. Then wash thoroughly.

(continued)

TABLE 33-2 Other Dermatologic Disorders (Continued)

Name/Description	Clinical Manifestations	Management	Nursing/Patient Care Considerations
			2. Advise patient to avoid close contact for 24 hours after treatment to prevent transmission. 3. Encourage treatment of sexual and close contacts simultaneously. 4. Tell patient that itching may persist for days to weeks following treatment due to an allergic reaction to mites; retreatment is not necessary.
Viral Infections Herpes simplex—acute vesicular eruption caused by herpes simplex virus type 1 or 2	1. Prodromal pain, burning, or tingling, possible fever and malaise. 2. Tiny vesicles appear on erythematous, swollen base; they rupture, forming painful ulcers, crusting, and eventual healing. 3. Can occur anywhere, especially near mucocutaneous junctions. 4. Viral shedding may occur between symptomatic periods, leading to transmission of the infection.	1. Tzanck smear from scraping of ulcer or fluid from vesicle shows characteristic giant cells with intranuclear inclusions; also diagnosed by fluorescent antibody detection or viral culture. 2. Antiviral treatment with acyclovir (Zovirax), famciclovir (Famvir), or valcyclovir (Valtrex) for acute infection or continuous suppressive therapy to prevent or lessen recurrence. 3. Analgesics may be needed for widespread and genital eruptions.	1. Teach patient that herpes simplex can be transmitted by close and sexual contact; good personal hygiene and hand washing are required for facial cases; sexual abstinence or condom use is required for genital cases. 2. Recurrence may be brought on by fever, illness, emotional stress, menses, pregnancy, sunlight, and other factors. 3. Advise patients with active herpes simplex infection to avoid contact with immunosuppressed individuals (diabetes, HIV disease, cancer or cancer treatment, alcoholism, malnutrition, etc.), because herpes simplex infection can be severe in these individuals. 4. Tell patients that lesions usually resolve in 1–2 weeks without scarring.
Other Conditions Contact dermatitis—inflammatory condition caused by exposure to irritating or allergenic substances, such as plants, cosmetics, cleaning products, soaps and detergents, hair dyes, metals and rubber	1. Itching, burning, erythema, and vesiculation at point of contact. 2. Progresses to weeping, crusting, drying, fissuring, and peeling. 3. Lichenification (thickening of skin) and pigmentation changes may occur with chronicity.	1. Topical or oral steroids, depending on severity. a. Oral steroids usually given in tapered dose—start with high dose and gradually decrease to provide greatest antiinflammatory effect without adrenal suppression. 2. Removal or avoidance of causative agent. 3. Antipruritics—systemic or topical antihistamines or topical calamine preparations.	1. Take thorough history to determine causative agent or contributing factors; have patient keep log of activities and symptoms if unsure of irritant. 2. Teach patient to use allergen-free products, wear gloves and protective clothing, wash and rinse skin thoroughly, and wash clothing after contact. 3. Advise patient that rash is not contagious, not even oozing lesions of poison ivy; however, contami-

(continued)

TABLE 33-2 Other Dermatologic Disorders (Continued)

Name/Description	Clinical Manifestations	Management	Nursing/Patient Care Considerations
		4. Desensitization to poison ivy and other substances may be accomplished for those who have severe reactions and cannot avoid contact.	nated clothing may cause spread of poison ivy in those who are sensitive. 4. Advise patient to perform patch test by applying substance behind ear or on inside of wrist before trying new cosmetics, soaps, or hair products.
Exfoliative dermatitis—chronic extensive scaling and inflammation of the skin; may be idiopathic or related to preexisting skin conditions, drug reactions, or underlying malignancy	1. Starts as patchy erythema, with possible fever, chills, and malaise. 2. Rapid spread until whole integument is involved. 3. Skin color changes to scarlet, desquamates, and may ooze serous fluid. 4. Pruritus, hair loss, secondary infection.	1. Discontinuation of offending drug or treatment of underlying condition. 2. Systemic corticosteroids should control most cases. 3. Supportive treatment—bed rest, warm environment, fluid and electrolyte replacement. 4. Soothing baths and topical emollients for symptomatic relief. 5. Possible use of immunosuppressants—azathioprine (Imuran), methotrexate (Mexate), and cyclophosphamide (Cytoxan).	1. Monitor fluid balance and electrolyte values 2. Watch for signs of secondary infection and reports to antimicrobial therapy can be started. 3. Watch for signs of heart failure caused by chronically increased cutaneous blood flow. 4. Teach patient how to relieve itching with oatmeal baths and emollient creams. 5. Tell patient to avoid environments with temperature fluctuations to avoid chilling. 6. Advise patient to avoid all irritants.
Alopecia—hair loss, may be idiopathic (alopecia areata), male-pattern, physiologic, or due to hair pulling (trichotillomania); also due to scarring from other skin or systemic disorders	1. Patterned, patchy, or diffuse hair loss. 2. Inflammation and scarring with some types. 3. Physiologic alopecia may be associated with hormonal changes (childbirth), nutritional factors, or toxin exposure.	1. Treatment of underlying cause. 2. Minoxidil (Rogaine) may cause fine hair regrowth in male-pattern baldness and alopecia areata. Finasteride (Propecia), an oral agent, can be used by men only, with good results. 3. Other methods of hair replacement—surgical grafting of hair follicles, hair weaving, hair pieces.	1. Explain that alopecia areata and physiologic loss are usually temporary and self-limiting. 2. Encourage women to change hairstyle or wear hairpieces or turbans until hair grows back after childbirth. 3. Counsel men on the slow, limited effects of minoxidil treatment and stress that effects reverse when treatment is stopped.
Seborrheic dermatitis—chronic, superficial inflammatory skin disorder	1. Crusted pinkish or yellow patches. 2. Loose scales that may be dry, moist, or greasy. 3. Mild itching. 4. Affects the scalp, eyebrows, eyelids, nasolabial creases, lips, ears, chest, axillae, umbilicus, groin.	1. Selenium sulfide (Selsun), tar (Pentrax), zinc, or resorcinol shampoo to scalp several times a week. 2. Corticosteroid lotions or creams. 3. For eyelid margin involvement (blepharitis), daily debridement with cotton-tipped applicator and baby shampoo, and ophthalmic steroid ointment or lotion. 4. Zinc soap or selenium lotion for washing once controlled.	1. Advise patient of chronic nature of seborrhea and that condition may be exacerbated by perspiration, neuroleptic drugs, and emotional stress; also seen more frequently in persons with Parkinson's disease, HIV disease, diabetes mellitus, malabsorption syndromes, and epilepsy. 2. Teach patient to apply topical preparations as prescribed.

(continued)

TABLE 33-2 Other Dermatologic Disorders (Continued)

Name/Description	Clinical Manifestations	Management	Nursing/Patient Care Considerations
		5. For external ear canal involvement, corticosteroid cream.	3. Advise baby shampoo use only and gently rubbing with swab near eyes to prevent irritation of conjunctiva in seborrheic blepharitis.
Hidradenitis suppurativa—chronic plugging and secondary infection of the apocrine glands of the groin and axilla	1. Development of tender red nodules that enlarge, rupture, and suppurate. 2. Sinus tracts develop with recurrent lesions, leading to continuous inflammation and drainage.	1. Initial treatment involves prolonged antibiotics (2 months or greater) such as tetracycline, clindamycin, or erythromycin and systemic or intralesional corticosteroids; however, progression of the condition is likely. 2. Surgical treatment necessary when chronic suppuration and fistulas develop: a. Incision and drainage or laser stripping b. Cauterization of sinus tracts c. Exteriorization with curretage and electrodissection d. Excision with possible skin grafting. 3. Isotretinon (Accutane), antiandrogens, and intralesional or systematic steroid therapy may be helpful but not curative.	1. Advise patient to use antibacterial soap and keep axilla and groin dry to reduce bacterial colonization of the skin. 2. Advise patient to avoid shaving of hair in affected area to prevent trauma and possible infection. 3. Advise patient to avoid use of deodorant or other chemicals on affected area. 4. Teach patient the signs of bacterial infection—purulent drainage, odor, pain—that call for notification of health care provider and treatment with antibiotics. 5. Encourage use of warm compresses to relieve inflammation.
Bullous pemphigoid—chronic bullous disease of the elderly of unknown etiology, probably autoimmune	1. Tense vesicles and bullae arise on normal or erythematous skin, rupture, and heal without scarring. 2. Occurs on flexor aspects of the body, axilla, inguinal areas, abdomen, and occasionally on mucous membranes.	1. Systemic corticosteroid treatment if widespread involvement. Intralesional corticosteroid therapy if limited lesions. Immunosuppressant for resistant cases. 2. Condition may remit within 2–4 years even without treatment.	1. Keep skin clean and dry to reduce chances of secondary infection. 2. If patient is immobilized, encourage positioning to prevent undue pressure on lesions; may cause premature rupture and secondary infection. 3. Be sure to differentiate from early pressure sore development and treat pressure sores appropriately. 4. Advise patient that lesions usually heal without scarring.
Acne vulgaris—obstruction and inflammation of sebaceous glands and follicles	1. Closed comedones (whiteheads). 2. Open comedones (blackheads). 3. Papules, pustules, nodules, cysts, or abcesses may develop. 4. Primary sites are face, chest, upper back, and shoulder.	1. Topical benzoyl peroxide—antibacterial and comedolytic. 2. Topcal retinoic acid (retin-A)—comedolytic, or adapalene (Differin)—a synthetic retinoid that is more potent.	1. Advise patient to wash face gently with mild soap and water 1–2 times daily. 2. Teach proper application of topical preparation—use sparingly and decrease frequency if irritation and redness develop.

(continued)

TABLE 33-2 Other Dermatologic Disorder (Continued)

Name/Description	Clinical Manifestations	Management	Nursing/Patient Care Considerations
		3. Topical antibiotics—suppress growth of *Propionibacterium acnes* and produce decrease in comedones, papules, and pustules without systemic side effects. 4. Azelaic acid (Azelex), a topical agent with multiple anti-acne effects. 5. Systemic antibiotics—long-term, low-dose therapy for more inflammatory and extensive causes. 6. Retinoid therapy—(Accutane) inhibits sebum production and secretion; for severe, disfiguring cystic acne. 7. Estrogen therapy—anti-androgenic effect decreases sebum production. 8. Intralesional steroid injection—for inflamed lesions. 9. Dermabrasion—surgical planing or chemical peels to smooth surface configuration of old scars.	3. Teach side effects of systemic antibiotics. 4. Ensure that women of childbearing potential are using contraceptives and that a negative pregnancy test has been obtained before starting Accutane therapy. 5. Encourage follow-up and monitoring of laboratory tests while on Accutane for elevated liver enzymes, cholesterol and triglycerides, and decreased HDL. 6. Advise patient on Accutane to notify health care provider of persistent headache—could signal pseudotumor cerebri. 7. Tell patient that initiation of therapy may worsen symptoms for several weeks, but to continue treatment. 8. Advise not to squeeze pimples and avoid friction around face. 9. Advise use of water-based and hypoallergenic cosmetics. 10. Encourage balanced diet and avoidance of foods believed to aggravate acne.
Rosacea—an erythematous, pustular eruption of the butterfly area of the face, most common in adults 40–60 years of age; unknown cause	1. Diffuse redness, papules, and pustules develop over butterfly region of face. 2. Later, dilated blood vessels and flushing are seen. 3. Rhinophyma (hypertrophic, bulbous nose) may develop.	1. Topical metronidazole gel applied bid. 2. Oral tetracycline. 3. Treatment necessary for 4–6 weeks and repeated if recurrence. 4. Avoid exercise, stress, hot beverages, spicy foods.	1. Teach patient to avoid flushing by reducing stress, replacing strenuous exercise with low-intensity workouts, staying cool, and avoiding the sun. 2. Advise contacting the National Rosacea Society at *www.rosacea.org*.

HDL: high-density lipoprotein; AIDS: acquired immunodeficiency syndrome; IM: intramuscular; IV: intravenous; HIV: human immunodeficiency virus; KOH: potassium hydroxide.

SELECTED REFERENCES

Arndt, K., Robinson, J., Leboit, P., & Wintroub, B. (1996). *Cutaneous medicine and surgery: An integrated program in dermatology, Vol. 2.* Philadelphia: W.B. Saunders.

Ashcroft, D.M., et al. (2000). Systematic review of comparative efficacy and tolerability of calcipotriol in treating chronic plaque psoriasis. *British Medical Journal, 320*(7), 963–967.

Autier, P., Dore, J.F., Cattaruzza, M.S., et al. (1998). Sunscreen use, wearing clothes, and number of nevi in 6-7 year old European children. *Journal of National Cancer Institute, 90*, 1873–1880.

Barone, E.J, Jones, J.C., & Schaefer, J.E. (2000). *Skin disorders.* Philadelphia: Lippincott Williams & Wilkins.

Brown, T.J., & Nelson, B.R. (1999). Melanoma: A clinical review. *American Journal of Medicine, 63*(5), 275–284.

DeVilley, R.L., Jacobs, J.P., Szpumar, C.A., et al. (1994). Androgenital alopecia in the female: Treatment with 2% topical minoxidil solution. *Archives of Dermatology, 130*(3), 303–307.

Drugge, R. (Ed.). (2000). *The electronic textbook of dermatology.* Internet Dermatology Society, Inc., *www.telemedicine.org/stamford.htm*

Duke, D., & Grevelink, J.M. (1998). Care before and after laser skin resurfacing: A survey and review of the literature. *Dermatologic Surgery, 24,* 201–206.

Feldman, S.R, & Clark, A.R. (1998). Psoriasis. *Medical Clinics of North America, 82,* 1135–1144.

Fisher, A.A. (1996). *Contact dermatitis.* Philadelphia: Lea & Febiger.

Gianoulis-Alissandratos, G. (1999). Common dermatologic conditions. In Singleton, J.K. et al. *Primary care.* Philadelphia: Lippincott Williams & Wilkins.

Hall, J.C. (2000). *Sauer's manual of skin diseases* (8th ed.). Philadelphia: Lippincott Williams & Wilkins.

Hoang, M.R. & Eichenfield, L.F. (2000). The rising incidence of melanoma in children and adolescents. *Dermatology Nursing, 12*(3).

Landis, B.J. (1994). Facial cosmetic surgery: A primary care perspective. *Nurse Practitioner, 19*(11), 71–76.

Lesher, J.L. (1999). Oral therapy of common superficial fungal infections of the skin. *Journal of the American Academy of Dermatology, 40*(6, part 2), S31–S34.

Marks, J.G., & DeLeo, V.A. (1997). *Contact and occupational dermatology.* St. Louis: Mosby-Year Book.

Nicol, N.H. & Baumeister, L.L. (1997). Topical corticosteroid therapy: Considerations for prescribing and use. *Lippincott's Primary Care Practice, 1*(1), 62–69.

Resnick, B. (1997). Dermatologic problems in the elderly. *Lippincott's Primary Care Practice, 1*(1), 14–30.

Ringel, E.W. (1998). The morality of cosmetic surgery for aging. *Archives of Dermatology, 134,* 427–431.

Robinson, N.D, Hashimoto, T., Amagai, M., & Chan, L. (1999). The new pemphigus variants. *Journal of the American Academy of Dermatology, 40*(5), 649–671.

Scher, R.K. (1999). Onychomycosis: Therapeutic update. *Journal of the American Academy of Dermatology, 40*(6, part2), s21–s26.

Sinnni-McKeehen, B. (1997). Scaling skin disorders. *Lippincott's Primary Care Practice, 1*(1), 3–13.

Swartz, S.M., et al. (1993). The technique of patch testing: Role of the office staff. *Dermatology Nursing, 5*(2), 133–137.

Thiers, B.H. (1998). Psoriasis therapy update. *Western Journal of Medicine, 1169,* 221–222.

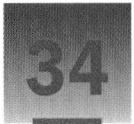
Burns

ETIOLOGY AND PHYSIOLOGY OF BURNS

Burns are a form of traumatic injury caused by thermal, electrical, chemical, or radioactive agents.

Inhalation injury and associated pulmonary complications are a significant factor in mortality and morbidity from burn injury (50% to 60% of fire deaths are secondary to inhalation injury).

▓ Etiology and Incidence

1. More than 2 million injuries and 7,000 to 9,000 deaths occur as a result of fire and burns each year in the United States.
2. Most accidents occur at home. The second most frequent place of injury is at work.
3. Flame injury is the leading cause of accidents for adults, and scalding is the leading cause of accidents for children.
4. Teenage boys have a high incidence of electrical injuries.
5. The very young and the elderly are at greatest risk for burn injuries.
6. Smoking, often combined with alcohol intake, is associated with at least half of major fire injuries and deaths.
7. Males are more commonly injured by burns than are females.

Pathophysiology
Burn Injury
1. A burn injury usually results from energy transfer from a heat source to the body. The type of burn injury may be flame/flash, contact, scald (water, grease, etc.), chemical, electrical, inhalation, or any thermal source. Many factors alter the response of body tissues to these sources of heat.
   a. Local tissue conductivity—bone is most resistant to the heat source accumulation. Lesser resistance is seen in nerves, blood vessels, and muscle tissue.
   b. Adequacy of peripheral circulation.
   c. Skin thickness, insulating material of clothing, or dampness of the skin.
2. Physiologic reaction to a burn is similar to the inflammatory process.
   a. Adjacent intact vessels dilate, causing redness and blanching with pressure.
   b. Platelets and leukocytes begin to adhere to the vascular endothelium as an early event in the inflammatory process.
   c. Increased capillary permeability produces wound edema.
   d. An influx of polymorphonuclear leukocytes and monocytes occurs at the injury site.
   e. Eventually, new capillaries, immature fibroblasts, and newly formed collagen fibrils appear within the wound. This supports the regenerating epithelium or forms a granulating tissue bed to accept a skin graft.
3. Burns may be partial or full thickness (Figure 34-1).
   a. Partial-thickness burn injuries involve the epidermis and upper portions of the dermis. Some of the dermal appendages remain, from which the wound can spontaneously re-epithelialize.
   b. In full-thickness injuries, all layers of the skin and sometimes underlying tissues are destroyed. Grafting usually is required to close the wound.
4. Burn depth is directly related to the temperature of the burning agent and the duration of contact with body tissue.
   a. Below 44°C (112°F), no local damage occurs unless exposure is for a protracted period.
   b. At 49°C (120°F), it takes 5 minutes' exposure to create a full-thickness burn.
   c. At 52° degrees C (125°F) the time requirement is 2 minutes, and at 60°C (140°F) only 6 seconds are required.
   d. At 70°C (159°F) it takes 1 second to create a full-thickness burn in a healthy adult—less time or temperature in children or the elderly.

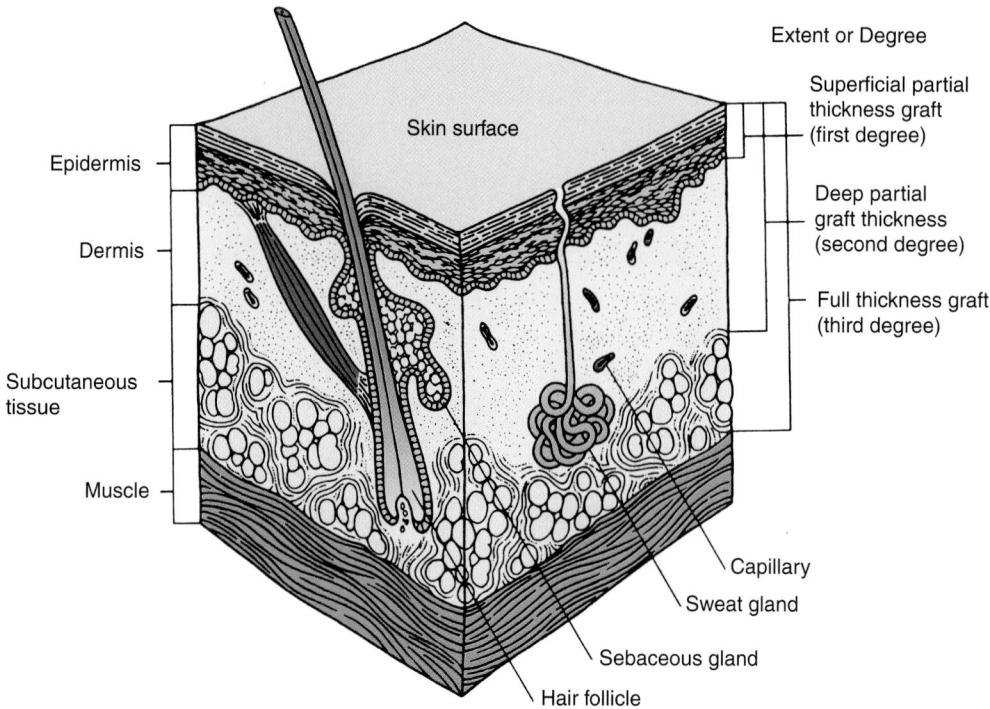

Skin surface

Epidermis

Dermis

Subcutaneous
tissue

Muscle

Extent or Degree

Superficial partial
thickness graft
(first degree)

Deep partial
graft thickness
(second degree)

Full thickness graft
(third degree)

Capillary

Sweat gland

Sebaceous gland

Hair follicle

FIGURE 34-1   Cross-section of skin depicting blood supply, depth of burn, and relative thickness of skin grafts. (From The Burn Patient, Ethicon.)

Inhalation Injury

1. May be upper airway (supraglottic) and incur injury in minutes to hours or may involve the lower airway and cause adult respiratory distress syndrome (ARDS). This can occur in as little as 4 hours. Thermal injury can be seen in the lower airway with steam or drug activity, such as free basing. Adult respiratory distress syndrome is most simply described as pulmonary edema of noncardiac origin. It may also be seen in children.
2. Carbon monoxide (CO) is a colorless, odorless, tasteless, nonirritating gas produced from incomplete combustion of carbon-containing materials.
3. Affinity of hemoglobin for CO is 200 times greater than for oxygen.
4. Toxicity depends on concentration of CO in inspired air and the length of time of exposure.
   a. A carboxyhemoglobin level of less than 10 ppm is not a cause for alarm.
   b. From 10 to 20 ppm bears watching and should be correlated with the spirometry results. (Smokers have been known to have carboxyhemoglobin levels of 15 to 18 ppm.)
   c. Levels of 20 to 50 ppm can produce fatigue, irritability, cardiac dysrhythmias, ataxia, vomiting, syncope, possible coma, increased blood pressure, tinnitus, dystopia, ventricular dysrhythmias, severe alterations

of consciousness, neurologic compromise, loss of consciousness, deep coma, hypertension, convulsions, paralysis, and areflexia. This is considered a severe to lethal exposure.
5. Sulfur dioxide and nitrous oxide are toxic agents inhaled in soot. In the presence of water, they form corrosive acids and alkalis that are extremely toxic.
6. Toxic fumes from burning plastic are more dangerous than smoke.
   a. Noxious gases include hydrogen cyanide, hydrochloric acid, sulfuric acid, halogens, and perhaps phosgene.
7. Restrictive pulmonary complications can occur because of the tourniquet effect of edema seen with circumferential chest burns. Lung compliance and alveolar gas exchange can also be decreased because of noncardiogenic pulmonary edema (ARDS).

Systemic Changes in Major Burns

Major burns involve more than 25% of total body surface area (TBSA).

Fluid Shifts

1. In addition to changes in the local burned area, there are alterations and disruptions in the vascular and other systems of the body.
2. The water-vapor barrier for the body is the outermost layer of epidermis. When it is rendered nonfunctioning, severe systemic reactions from fluid losses can occur.

3. Fluid volume deficit is directly proportional to the extent and depth of burn injury.
4. Capillary permeability increases, permitting fluid and protein to move from vascular to interstitial spaces (edema results) for the first 24 to 36 hours, peaking at 12 hours postburn. Protein-rich fluid is lost in blebs of the burned tissues as well as by weeping of second-degree wounds and surface of full-thickness wounds. With reduced vascular volume, the patient will go into shock if untreated.
5. Capillary permeability starts to change in about 48 hours, but protein lost in interstitial spaces may remain there for 5 days to 2 weeks before returning to the vascular system.
   a. When fluid mobilizes (moves from interstitial spaces back to vascular compartment), patients with good cardiac and renal function will diurese.
   b. Patients with impaired cardiac or renal function are in danger of fluid overload and pulmonary edema at this time.
6. Red blood cell mass is also diminished because of thrombosis, sludging, and red blood cell death from thermal injury; as fluid escapes from capillary walls, however, blood concentrates and the hematocrit rises, causing sluggish flow (Figure 34-2).
7. Capillary stasis may cause ischemia and even necrosis.
8. The body attempts to compensate for losses of plasma volume.
   a. Constriction of vessels.
   b. Withdrawal of fluid from undamaged extracellular space.
   c. The patient is thirsty. (Oral fluids are not given until bowel sounds are heard or until patient is no longer intubated.)

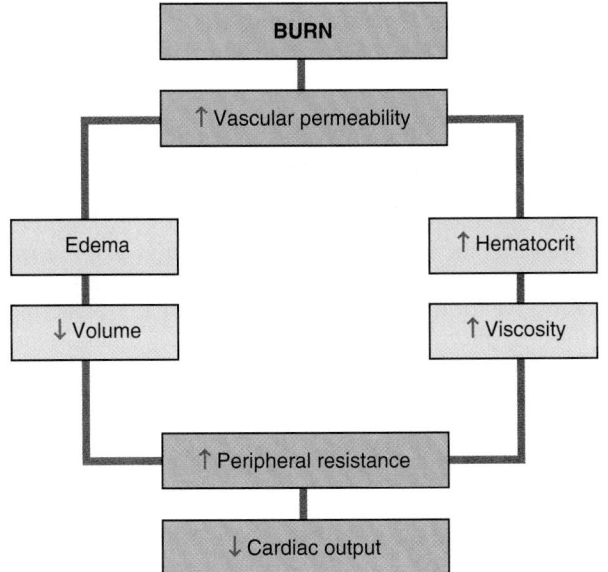

FIGURE 34-2 Hemodynamic changes in burn injury.

Hemodynamics
1. Lessened circulating blood volume results in decreased cardiac output initially and increased pulse rate.
2. There is a decreased stroke volume as well as a marked rise in peripheral resistance (due to constriction of arterioles and increased hemoviscosity).
3. This results in inadequate tissue perfusion, which may in turn cause acidosis, renal failure, and irreversible burn shock.
4. Electrolyte imbalance may also occur.
   a. Hyponatremia usually occurs during the 3rd to 10th day due to fluid shift.
   b. The burn injury also causes hyperkalemia initially due to cell destruction, followed by hypokalemia as fluid shifts occur and potassium is not replaced.

Metabolic Demands
1. Catecholamine release appears to be the major mediator of the hypermetabolic response to burn injury.
2. "Burn fever" is common and is dependent on depth of burn and percentage of TBSA involved. Temperatures of 102°F to 103°F (38.8°C to 39.4°C) are common as "fever spikes."
3. Healing a large surface area requires much energy; glucose is the primary metabolic fuel.
4. Because total body glucose stores are limited and stored liver and muscle glycogen is exhausted within the first few days postburn, hepatic glucose synthesis (gluconeogenesis) increases.
5. Insulin levels decrease early postburn, and patients develop hyperglycemia. They continue to be hyperglycemic when insulin levels increase, probably due to increased gluconeogenesis.
6. Skeletal and visceral protein is mobilized to meet increased nutritional demands.
7. With adequate fluid resuscitations, the patient's weight will increase during the first few days. Fluid mobilization will result in weight loss, as will the catabolic response. Nutritional support in the form of enteral and/or total parenteral nutrition may be necessary. Weight loss from fluid mobilization usually starts within 3 to 4 days postresuscitation.
8. Despite all nutritional support, it is almost impossible to counteract a negative nitrogen balance; the sooner a burn wound is closed, the more rapidly a positive nitrogen balance is reached.
9. The resting metabolic expenditure increases linearly with amount of TBSA; a burn of 40% to 50% TBSA has a metabolic rate almost twice normal.
10. The adult burn patient may require 3,000 to 5,000 calories or more per day.
    a. A burn of less than 10% usually requires minimal supplementation.
    b. A high-protein, high-calorie diet is necessary for a 10% to 20% burn.
    c. Between 20% and 30%, enteral feedings are generally necessary.

d. TBSA burns of 30% to 40% may require total parenteral nutrition. However, the current trend is to meet nutritional needs enterally, if possible.

Renal Needs

1. Glomerular filtration may be decreased in extensive injury.
2. Without resuscitation or with delay, decreased renal blood flow may lead to high output or oliguric renal failure and decreased creatinine clearance.
3. Hemoglobin and myoglobin, present in the urine of patients with deep muscle damage often associated with electrical injury, may cause acute tubular necrosis and call for a greater amount of initial fluid therapy and osmotic diuresis.

Pulmonary Changes

1. Hyperventilation and increased oxygen consumption are associated with major burns.
2. The majority of deaths from fire are due to smoke inhalation.
3. Overzealous fluid resuscitation and the effects of burn shock on cell membrane potential may cause pulmonary edema, contributing to decreased alveolar exchange. Therefore, with an inhalation injury, it may be necessary to keep the patient slightly less hydrated.
4. Initial respiratory alkalosis resulting from hyperventilation may change to respiratory acidosis associated with pulmonary insufficiency as a result of major burn trauma.

Hematologic Changes

1. Thrombocytopenia, abnormal platelet function, depressed fibrinogen levels, inhibition of fibrinolysis, and a deficit in several plasma clotting factors occur postburn.
2. Anemia results from the direct effect of destruction of red blood cells due to burn injury, reduced life span of surviving red blood cells, overt or (more commonly) occult blood loss from duodenal or gastric ulcers, and blood loss during diagnostic and therapeutic procedures.

Immunologic Activity

1. The loss of the skin barrier and presence of eschar favor bacterial growth.
2. Granulation tissue, richly vascular, resists bacteria.
3. Abnormal inflammatory response after burn injury causes a decreased delivery of antibiotics, white blood cells, and oxygen to the injured area.
4. Hypoxia, acidosis, and thrombosis of vessels in the wound area impair host resistance to pathogenic bacteria.
5. Several major immunoglobulins, complement, and serum albumin are decreased soon after the burn occurs.
6. Depressed cellular immunity is reflected by lymphocytopenia, impaired delayed skin sensitivity, decreased allograft rejection potential, depletion of thymus-dependent lymphoid tissue, and increased susceptibility to fungi, viruses, and gram-negative organisms.
7. Burn wound sepsis
   a. After colonization of the burn wound surface by bacteria, subeschar and intrafollicular colonization develop. Intraeschar and subeschar colonization may progress to invasion of subadjacent, nonburned, previously viable tissue.
   b. A bacterial count of 10^5 per gram of tissue as determined by burn wound biopsy indicates burn wound sepsis.
   c. The wound is fully colonized in 3 to 5 days.
8. Seeding of bacteria from the wound may give rise to systemic septicemia.

Gastrointestinal

1. As a result of sympathetic nervous system response to trauma, peristalsis decreases and gastric distention, nausea, vomiting, and paralytic ileus may occur.
2. Ischemia of the gastric mucosa and other etiologic factors put the burn patient at risk for duodenal and gastric ulcers, manifested by occult bleeding and, in some cases, life-threatening hemorrhage.

■ Assessment and Diagnostic Evaluation

As with all trauma victims, a primary and secondary trauma survey, including assessment of airway, breathing, and circulation as well as vital signs, is done. Other assessment parameters specific to the burn injury focus on the extent and severity of burn injury and inhalation injury.

Severity of Burns

Severity of burns is determined by:
1. Depth—first, second (partial thickness), third degree (full thickness).
2. Extent—percentage of TBSA.
3. Age—the very young and very old have a poor prognosis; the prognosis alters for adults after age 45.
4. Area of the body burned—face, hands, feet, perineum, and circumferential burns require special care.
5. Medical history and concomitant injuries and illness.
6. Inhalation injury.

Assessment for Inhalation Injury

1. If victim was burned in a closed area, there should be a high index of suspicion that smoke inhalation has occurred.
2. Evaluate all patients in closed-space fires for symptoms of carbon monoxide poisoning: headache, visual changes, confusion, irritability, decreased judgment, nausea, ataxia, and collapse.
3. Question the patient about types of things that burned in this room—type of carpet, vinyl articles, synthetics.
4. Observe for upper body burns, erythema or blistering of lips, buccal mucosa or pharynx, singed nasal hair, soot in oropharynx, dark gray or black sputum (Figure 34-3).
5. Listen for hoarseness and crackles. Increasing hoarseness, stridor, and/or drooling are indicators of increasing need for intubation.
6. Obtain arterial blood gases (ABGs), carboxyhemoglobin levels, and spirometry.
7. Direct visualization of the vocal cords may be necessary. Further visualization may be accomplished through bronchoscopy if necessary.
8. A chest x-ray should be obtained as a baseline.

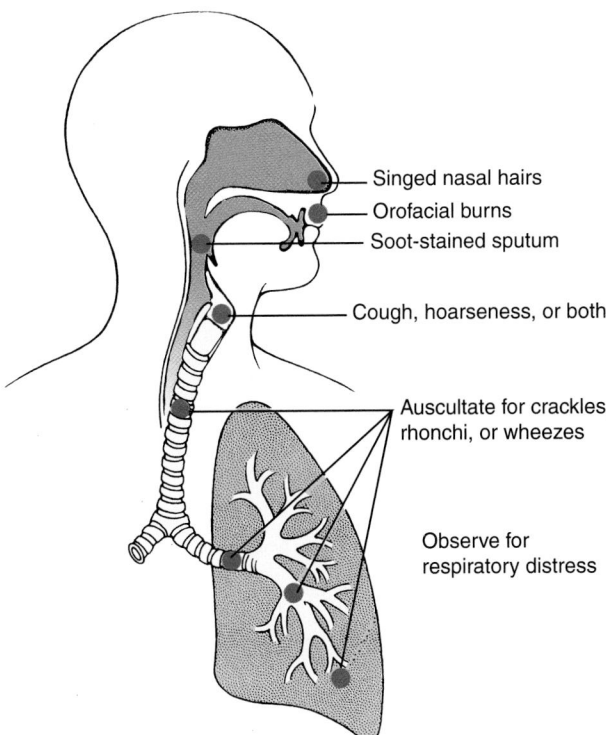

FIGURE 34-3 In the nursing history, determine whether the victim was in a closed area during the fire and whether he or she lost consciousness. If any of the above physical findings are noted in addition to the nursing history data, the victim should be taken to the hospital or burn center for further evaluation. Baseline arterial blood gas measurements (to detect hypoxemia) should be taken immediately on admission.

Signs and Symptoms of Toxicity From Carbon Monoxide

CO Blood Level	Manifestations
0–10%	None Smokers may normally have 10% CO level
10%–20%	Headache, visual disturbance, angina in patients with cardiovascular disease, slowed mental function
20%–40%	Tight feeling in head, rapid fatigue from muscular effort, decreased muscular co-ordination, confusion, irritability, ataxia, nausea, vomiting, increased pulse rate, decreased blood pressure, dysrhythmias
40%–60%	Pulmonary and cardiac dysfunction, collapse, coma, convulsions
Over 60%	Often fatal

With the increasing use of synthetics, toxicity from aldehydes, cyanide, and other substances are increasing and must be considered.

Extent of Body Surface Burned

1. Anatomic location—burns affecting hands, feet, face, and perineum require specialized care. Circumferential burns also require special attention and may require escharotomy.
2. Determination is based on the use of tables for this purpose, such as the "rule of nines" (Figure 34-4), the Lund and Browder chart, or the rule of the palm. The patient's palm (including the fingers) is approximately 1% of the TBSA burned. Calculation of the percentage of TBSA burned serves as a guide for fluid therapy.
3. Repeat assessment may be performed on the 2nd or 3rd day to verify demarcation of burned areas.

Depth of Burn and Triage Criteria

1. It may be difficult to differentiate between second- and third-degree wounds initially. If the areas appear wet and are particularly sensate, then a second-degree (partial-thickness) injury is likely. If the area is less painful or insensate, the hairs are easily pulled out, and the area appears dry and is firm to touch, then it is most likely a third-degree (full-thickness) burn (Table 34-1).
2. Reassess daily for the first few days because second-degree burn can convert to a third-degree injury.

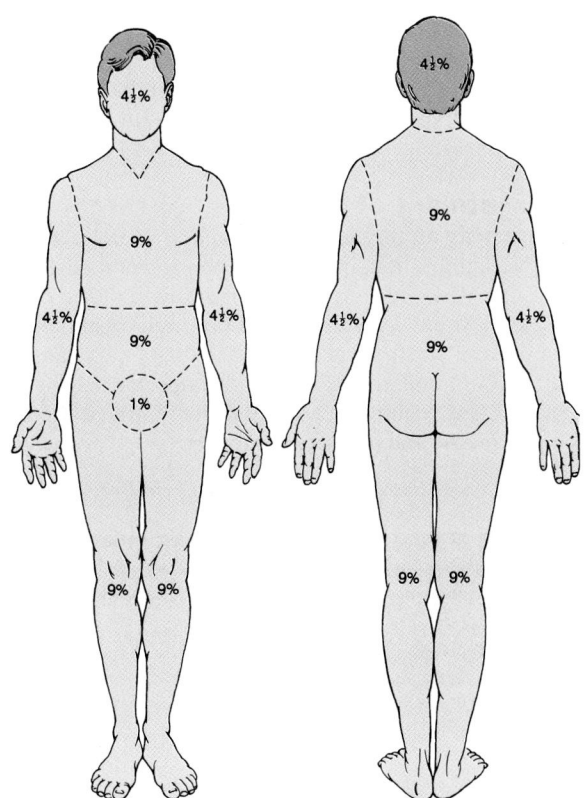

FIGURE 34-4 Rule of nines for calculating total burn surface area (TBSA).

TABLE 34-1   Assessment of Burn Injury

Extent or Degree	Assessment of Extent	Reparative Process
First degree	Pink to red: slight edema, which subsides quickly. Pain may last up to 48 hours; relieved by cooling. (Sunburn is a typical example.)	In about 5 days, epidermis peels, heals spontaneously. Itching and pink skin persist for about a week. No scarring. Heals spontaneously if it does not become infected within 10 days–2 weeks.
Second degree	*Superficial:* Pink or red; blisters form (vesicles); weeping, edematous, elastic. Superficial layers of skin are destroyed; wound moist and painful.	Takes several weeks to heal. Scarring may occur.
	Deep dermal: Mottled white and red: edematous reddened areas blanch on pressure. May be yellowish but soft and elastic—may or may not be sensitive to touch; sensitive to cold air. Hair does not pull out easily.	Takes several weeks to heal. Scarring may occur.
Third degree	Destruction of epithelial cells—epidermis and dermis destroyed. Reddened areas do not blanch with pressure. Not painful; inelastic; coloration varies from waxy white to brown; leathery devitalized tissue is called *eschar.* Destruction of epithelium, fat, muscles, and bone.	Eschar must be removed. Granulation tissue forms to nearest epithelium from wound margins or support graft. For areas larger than 3–5 cm, grafting is required. Expect scarring and loss of skin function. Area requires debridement, formation of granulation tissue, and grafting.

3. Second- and third-degree burns of certain extent, chemical burns, electrical burns, burns of certain areas of the body, and any airway or inhalation injury should be triaged to a regional burn center (Table 34-2).

Treatment of Burns

Management of the acute burn injury includes hemodynamic stabilization, metabolic support, wound debridement, use of topical antibacterial therapy, biologic dressings, and wound closure. Prevention and treatment of complications, including infection and pulmonary damage, and rehabilitation are also of major importance. The patient will also require physical and occupational therapy and psychiatric and nutritional support.

TABLE 34-2   Triage Criteria for Determining When It Is Advisable to Transfer a Patient to a Burn Center

Burned area second degree and third degree
  (age <10 or >50): 10%
Burned area second degree and third degree
  (age >10 or <50): 20%
Burned area third degree: >5% at any age
Chemical burn
Electrical injury
Burn of face, hands, feet, or perineum or circumferential burns
Burn accompanied by airway or inhalation injury

Hemodynamic Stabilization
Intravenous Fluid Therapy

1. Immediate intravenous (IV) fluid resuscitation is indicated for:
   a. Adults with burns involving more than 15% to 20% of TBSA.
   b. Children with burns involving more than 10% to 15% of TBSA.
   c. Patients with electrical injury, the elderly, or those with cardiac or pulmonary disease and compromised response to burn injury. These patients require meticulous monitoring and may require a modification of fluid requirements.
2. The goal is to give sufficient fluid to allow perfusion of vital organs without overhydrating the patient and risking later complications and circulatory overload.
3. Generally a crystalloid (Ringer's lactate) solution is used initially. Colloid is used during the 2nd day (5% albumin, plasmate, or hetastarch).
4. One of several formulas may be used to determine the amount of fluid to be given in the first 48 hours.
   a. The Parkland formula is most commonly used.
   b. The Brooks and Evans formulas may also be used.
5. Parkland formula:
   a. First 24 hours—4 mL of Ringer's lactate × weight in kg × % TBSA burned.
   b. One-half amount of fluid is given in the first 8 hours, calculated from the time of injury. If the starting of

fluids is delayed, then the same amount of fluid is given over the remaining time. Remember to deduct any fluids given in the prehospital setting.

c. The remaining half of the fluid is given over the next 16 hours. Example:
Patient's weight: 70 kg; % TBSA burn: 80%
$4\text{ mL} \times 70\text{ kg} \times 80\%\text{ TBSA} = 22,400\text{ mL}$ of Ringer's lactate
1st 8 hours = 11,200 mL or 1,400 mL/hour
2nd 16 hours = 11,200 mL or 700 mL/hour

d. Second 24 hours:
0.5 mL colloid × weight in kg × TBSA + 2,000 mL 5% dextrose in water run concurrently over the 24-hour period. Example:
$0.5\text{ mL} \times 70\text{ kg} \times 80\% = 2,800\text{ mL}$ colloid + 2,000 mL 5% D/W yields
117 mL colloid/hour
84 mL 5% D/W per hour

e. Boluses of crystalloid or colloid may be necessary to keep a urinary output of 0.5 to 1 mL/kg/hour.

Additional Interventions

1. Enzymatic agents applied to the burn wound may be used for more rapid debridement of eschar.
2. In surgical excision, primary or tangential, all nonviable tissue is removed down to a viable base, which is covered with biologic dressings: heterograft, homograft (both temporary), or autograft.
3. Fluids may be titrated to achieve a urinary output of 30 to 50 mL/hour (0.5 mL to 1.0 mL/kg/hour in an adult and approximately 1 mL/kg/hour in a child).
4. An indwelling urinary catheter is needed to monitor response to fluid therapy.
5. Weigh the patient on admission and then daily.
6. Elevate extremities.
7. Monitor peripheral pulses.
8. Administer humidified oxygen through a nasal cannula, mask, or ventilator support.

Metabolic Support

1. Initially, keep the patient on nothing-by-mouth (NPO) status until bowel sounds return (1 to 2 days). However, small amounts (5 to 10 mL/hour) of isotonic enteral tube feedings are often started within 24 hours to help maintain a functioning gastrointestinal tract. Small amounts of erythromycin may be used to encourage gastrointestinal motility.
2. Reduce metabolic stress by allaying pain, fear, and anxiety and maintaining a warm environment.
3. Nutritional management must be aggressive to combat acute nutritional deficiency and weight loss; a positive nitrogen balance should be the goal throughout the postburn care.
4. When bowel sounds return, administer oral fluids and advance diet as tolerated.
5. Offer more solid food after 2 to 3 days postburn as tolerance to food improves.

a. Build up daily caloric intake to match daily caloric expenditure.
b. Provide 3 g protein/kg body weight: 20% of needed calories in form of fats; remainder in carbohydrates.
6. When caloric requirements cannot be met by enteral feedings, it may be necessary to initiate total parenteral nutrition (amino acids, carbohydrates, and fat emulsions).
7. Provide potassium and vitamin and mineral supplements (zinc, iron, vitamin C).

Wound Cleansing and Debridement

Treatment of the burn wound includes daily or twice-daily wound cleansing with debridement, or hydrotherapy (tubbing) and dressing changes. Early excision of deep second- and third-degree burns is the goal.

1. Burn wounds must be cleansed initially and usually daily with a mild antibacterial cleansing agent and saline solution or water.
   a. This may be done in the hydrotherapy tub, in the bathtub or shower, or at the bedside.
   b. See Hydrotherapy, below.
2. Nonviable tissue (eschar) may be removed through natural, enzymatic, mechanical, and/or surgical debridement.
3. Burn eschar will begin to separate from the underlying viable tissue by a natural process of bacterial growth, which causes a lysis of protein at the viable–nonviable tissue interface.
4. Eschar can be removed through daily or twice-daily dressing changes and use of forceps and scissors at time of wound cleansing.
5. Enzymatic agents applied to the burn wound may be used for more rapid debridement of eschar.
6. In surgical excision, facial or tangential, all nonviable tissue is removed to a viable base or fascia and is then covered with a biologic dressing, that is, xenograft, allograft, or autograft. This may be a temporary or permanent covering procedure.

Hydrotherapy

Hydrotherapy ("tubbing," "tanking," or "showering") is the bathing of the burn patient in a tub of water or with a water shower to facilitate cleansing and debridement of the burned area.

Advantages

1. Topical medications, adherent dressings, and eschar are more easily removed.
2. Provides an opportunity for the patient to practice range-of-motion exercises.
3. Total assessment of the burn area is facilitated; total body cleansing can be achieved.

Disadvantages

1. Loss of body heat; loss of sodium.
2. Uncomfortable and at times painful for the patient.
3. Maintenance of IV lines and ventilator care may be difficult during tubbing.

4. The patient's anxiety level often increases, and there is often a fear of drowning as well as the discomfort of the experience.

Interventions

1. Describe the procedure to the patient who is experiencing hydrotherapy for the first time.
2. Select the time for future tubbings in collaboration with the patient; administer a pain-control medication, if prescribed, before the treatment so that maximum benefit is realized. Use nursing activities to assist patient with the pain experience.
3. If the patient has an indwelling catheter, drain and plug it or maintain a closed system to avoid contamination.
4. Aseptic technique is adhered to as closely as possible in preparing the patient for hydrotherapy, during hydrotherapy, and in redressing the patient's wounds after therapy.
5. During hydrotherapy, after cleansing of the wounds, debride wound, shave adjacent areas at health care provider's direction, shampoo hair, and gently wash normal skin.
6. Limit hydrotherapy to as brief a time as possible to decrease the loss of body temperature and subsequent chilling.
7. Never leave the patient unattended in the tub.
8. Respect the patient's feelings and expressions of stress, pain, cold, and fatigue.
9. After treatment, the patient may be weighed before being carefully dressed and returned to the unit.
10. Document significant data, including status of the wound.

Topical Antimicrobials

Topical medications are used to cover burn areas and to reduce the number of organisms.

Principles

1. They are applied directly to the burn area as ointments, creams, or solutions, or they may be incorporated in single-layer dressings that do not stick to the wound but permit drainage.
2. Dressings may take the form of commercial multilayered pads, standard 4 × 4 gauze pads, or several layers of stretch bandage (Kerlex type).
3. If gauze or pads are used, they may be held in place by stretch gauze or net tube dressings.
4. When wet dressings are used, that is, after a surgical procedure, then the same dressings are maintained. They are remoistened every 4 to 6 hours, as ordered. Heat loss may be prevented by limiting evaporative loss with a dry blanket and by warming the bed or using a heat cradle.
5. When wet dressings are used, 20-ply gauze will help retain solution at the proper concentration if rewet every 4 hours. A dry top layer of stockinette or a cotton bath blanket prevents evaporative heat loss.
6. Desired characteristics in a topical antimicrobial:

a. Demonstrates action against a broad spectrum of bacteria.
b. Has the ability to diffuse through the wound and penetrate the eschar.
c. Nontoxic and noninjurious to body tissue.
d. Inexpensive, pleasant to use, odorless or has pleasant odor, will not stain skin or clothing.
e. Will not cause resistant strains of pathogenic organisms to develop.

7. Generally, all of the previously applied topical cream should be removed and the wound gently cleansed before applying new cream with each dressing change. Extremity dressings should be wrapped distally to proximally, taking care to avoid circulatory compromise when edema occurs or dressing is too tight.
8. There is no "ideal" topical antimicrobial.

Types of Topical Antimicrobial Agents

See Table 34-3.

Surgical Management

Early excision and grafting is the basic goal.

Tangential Excision

1. A special blade is used to slice off thin layers of damaged skin until live tissue is evidenced by capillary bleeding.
2. Commonly used with deep partial-thickness burns and followed with immediate coverage with a biosynthetic or biologic dressing or an autograft.

Fascial (Primary) Excision

1. The skin, lymphatics, and subcutaneous tissue are removed down to fascia, with either immediate autografting or temporary coverage with biologic or biosynthetic dressings.
2. This is repeated until all the deep burn areas are removed.

General Consideration

1. Early surgical intervention reduces the potential for wound infection and speeds the course of hospital care.
2. Operative excision is very stressful metabolically and incurs heavy blood loss; therefore, more conservative measures may be indicated for some patients.
3. As a general consideration, up to 190 mL of blood may be lost per 1% of burn excised in the adult patient.

Burn Wound Coverings

For types of burn wound coverings, see Table 34-4.

Biologic Dressings

1. Biologic dressings are used to cover large surfaces of the body. Usually they are split-thickness grafts harvested either from human cadavers or from other mammalian donors, such as pigs. Human amnion may also be used.
2. An allograft is a graft of skin taken from a person other than the burn victim and applied to a burn wound temporarily (a cadaver is the most common source).
3. A xenograft or heterograft is a segment of skin taken from an animal, such as a pig. It is useful in preparing debrided area for grafting and is really a biologic dressing.

TABLE 34-3 Topical Antimicrobial Agents for Burns

Topical Agent	Description and Indications	Disadvantages	Nursing Implications
Silver sulfadizane 1% (Silvadene SSD)	A white, crystalline, highly insoluble compound in an opaque, odorless, water-miscible cream Exerts antimicrobial effect at level of cell membrane and cell wall against gram-negative and gram-positive bacteria and yeasts Penetration of silver sulfadiazine into wound is intermediate between silver nitrate and mefenide Systemic toxicity is rare Most widely used agent and least common incidence of side effects	May cause transient leukopenia that disappears afer 2–3 days of treatment May increase possibility of kernicterus and should not be used in pregnant women in last trimester, premature infants, or neonates <2 months Impairment of hepatic and renal function that results in decreased excretion of drug constituents may preclude therapeutic benefits of continued silver sulfadiazine administration Exposure to sunlight produces gray discoloration Crystalluria and methemoglobinemia are rare toxic effects Protracted use may be associated with emergence of sulfadiazine resistance	Use with either open treatment, light or occlusive dressings Apply with sterile gloved hand directly to wound or applied to gauze dressing 0.16 cm (1/16 in.) thick, once or twice daily after thorough wound cleansing Silver sulfadiazene will be discontinued if WBC are less than 1,500 in an adult or less than 2,000 in a child. WBC count usually recovers in 2–4 days and application may be resumed.
Mafenide acetate 10% cream or 5% solution (Sulfamylon)	Usually supplied in water-miscible, hydroscopic cream base Active against most gram-positive organisms and particularly Clostridia sp. Active against common gram-negative burn wound pathogens but has little antifungal activity Not significantly bound by protein and wound exudate Good penetrating power and useful for control of established invasive burn wound infection	Painful during and for a while after application A potent carbonic anhydrase inhibitor resulting in metabolic acidosis therefore not used if > 20% TBSA Brisk alkaline diuresis and inappropriate polyuria may result when used on patients with a large burn surface area Compensatory hyperventilation and pulmonary failure may ensue if mafenide is not discontinued Hemolytic anemia is a rare complication	Cream is applied with or without dressing if possible. Must be reapplied every 12 hours to maintain therapeutic effectiveness Therapeutic solution concentration is maintained with bulky wet dressings, rewet every 2–4 hours Application is associated with significant pain Hypersensitivity evidenced by maculopapular rash; is treated with antihistamines and/or discontinuing use Requires careful monitoring of pulmonary status and acid-base and fluid balance
Silver nitrate (0.5% solution)	Clear solution with low toxicity and significant antimicrobial effect against common burn wound pathogens Minimal absorption occurs because of the insolubility of its chloride and other salts Nonallergenic and not usually painful on application Best use is prophylaxis against infection	Can cause electrolyte abnormalities by depleting serum sodium, chloride, potassium, and magnesium Methemoglobinemia is a rare complication Stains everything (including normal skin) brown or black	Monitor electrolyte balance carefully; supplementation with sodium and potassium salts is routinely needed for patients with extensive burns Use bulky dressings, rewet every 2–4 hours, to maintain therapeutic concentration Maintain patient warmth and minimize transcutaneous evaporative water loss with dry top layer, such as stockinette or bath blanket

Other topical agents
Cerium nitrate (1.74% solution)
Cerium nitrate combined with silver sulfadiazine cream
Povidone-iodine (1% cream; also in foam and solution forms) (Betadine)
Gentamicin (0.1% ointment) (Garamycin)
Nitrofurazone (0.2% ointment) (Furacin)
Polymixin B-bacitracin ointment (Polysporin)
Bibiotic solution (Bacitracin powder 5,000 units and polymixin powder 200,000 units to 1 liter of 0.9% saline solution

TABLE 34-4 Burn Wound Coverings

Description	Indications	Source or Form	Nursing Considerations
Amnion (rarely used)			
Amnionic and chorionic membranes collected from human placentas under sterile conditions	To protect partial-thickness burns To temporarily cover granulation tissue awaiting autograft	Obstetric department frees membranes from placenta and processes for short-term storage	Apply to clean wounds Change every 48 hours; wound may be left open to air or redressed immediately
Allograft/Homograft			
Human cadaver skin, about 0.015-in. thick Preferred biologic dressing	To debride untidy wounds To protect granulation tissue after escharotomy To cover excised wound immediately To serve as test graft before autograft	Fresh, cryopreserved homografts available from tissue banks throughout U.S.	Remember that length of time dressing is left in place varies greatly Observe for exudate; also, watch for local and systemic signs of infection and rejection
Xenograft Heterograft			
Pigskin similar to human skin, harvested after slaughter, then cryopreserved or lyophilized for long-term storage	Same as for homograft To cover meshed autografts To protect exposed tendons To cover partial-thickness burns that are eschar-free and clean or only slightly contaminated	Available in fresh, frozen, or lyophilized form, in rolls or sheets; also available meshed and impregnated with silver sulfadiazine	Change every 2–5 days; wound may be dressed or left open Observe for signs of infection
Biobrane			
Nylon fabric bonded to silicon rubber membrane, containing collagenous porcine peptides Elastic and durable; adheres to wound surface until removed or sloughed by spontaneous reepithelialization	To cover donor graft sites To protect clean, superficial, partial-thickness burns and excised wounds awaiting autografts To cover meshed autografts	Individually packaged sterile sheets of various sizes; also in glove-shaped form for hand burns	Remember that Biobrane is useful for wounds awaiting autograft because it can be left in place 3–14 days or longer and it is permeable to antimicrobials, which can be applied over it
Duo-Derm			
Hydroactive dressing that interacts with moisture on skin, creating bond that makes it adhere Interacts with wound exudate to produce soft, moist gel, facilitating removal	To cover small partial-thickness burns To prevent bacterial contamination	Individual, peelable, "blister" packages containing sheets of various sizes (from 3 × 3 to 8 × 12 in.)	Use size that allows dressing to extend beyond wound onto healthy skin Be careful to distinguish pus from liquefied material that normally remains in wound Used until it falls off, usually 7–10 days
Op-Site			
Thin, transparent elastic film that adheres to dry surfaces, conforms to body contours, and stretches with movement Occlusive and waterproof; permeable to moisture, vapor, and air	To cover clean partial-thickness burns and clean donor sites and to reduce pain from these wounds To provide moist environment for reepithelialization	Individual, sterile, peelable packages of sheets in various sizes	Maintain closed dressing; if exudate forms, drain aseptically with needle and syringe; seal hole with Op-Site patch Check for pooling of exudate in dependent areas Used until it falls off, usually 7–10 days
N-terface			
Surface material used between burn and outer dressing Translucent, nonabsorbent, and nonreactive; permeable to air and fluid	To cover partial-thickness burns and newly applied autografts To eliminate shearing of epithelium and protect healing tissue	Sterile, individually packaged strips, sheets, or rolls of various sizes	Remember that N-terface will shorten time it normally takes to change dressing, eliminating soaking and other steps required with conventional gauze dressing Changed with each dressing

(continued)

TABLE 34-4 Burn Wound Coverings (Continued)

Description	Indications	Source or Form	Nursing Considerations
Vigilon Colloidal suspension on a polyethylene mesh support Permeable to gases and water vapor; provides moist environment Compatible with topical preparations	To clean small partial-thickness burns	Individual sterile or nonsterile sheets in various sizes	For occlusive use, remove one polyethylene film backing and place uncovered side on wound; for non-occlusive use, remove both backings and secure over wound with gauze or tape Change daily
Integra Artificial Skin*	Permanent bilayer membrane composed of a dermal portion that consists of a porous lattice of fibers of cross-linked bovine collagen and glycos-aminoglycan composite and an epidermal layer of synthetic polysiloxane polymer. To create a template for dermal regeneration by formation of a "neodermis." Provides an immediate post-excisional physiologic wound closure. Allows for use of a thinner autograft.	Sterile, individual sheets	Remember that the dermal regeneration layer is very soft and fragile. No hydrotherapy immersion should occur while the silicone layer is still in place. Outer dressing is changed every 4–5 days. Removal of the silicon layer is usually in 14–21 days.
Acticoat†	Temporary covering of a nano-crystalline film of pure ionic silver. To provide a temporary layer with optimal antimicrobial protection. May be used for immediate wound coverage as well as for post graft site coverage. May also be used as donor site coverage.	Sterile individual sheets	It is important to remember that Acticoat must be moistened immediately before application. It must also be moistened with sterile water every 4–6 hours. Do not apply any topical antimicrobial over or onto the silver sheeting.

*Integra LifeSciences Corporation. P.O. Box 688, 105 Morgan Ln., Plainsboro, NJ 08536.
† Westaim Corporation Biomedical Products. 10102 14th St., Fort Saskatchewan, Alberta, Canada T8L, 3W4.
(Adapted with permission from Bayley, E. & Smith, G. [1987]. The three degrees of burn care. *Nursing 87, 17*[3], 34–41.

Donor Criteria
1. Skin color is unimportant because it is only a temporary graft.
2. Donor should be an adult, free of infection.

Purpose and Benefits
1. Decreases heat, fluid, and protein losses.
2. Reduces bacterial proliferation.
3. Closes wound temporarily; enhances production and protection of granulation tissue.
4. Protects exposed neurovascular and muscle tissue as well as tendons.
5. Reduces pain and facilitates patient comfort.
6. Acts as a test graft to determine when granulating wounds will accept autograft successfully.
7. Provides an effective donor-site dressing.

Clinical Procedures
1. Allograft (cadaver) skin is the most popular temporary biologic dressing.
2. Devitalized tissue is first removed surgically or enzymatically.
3. Allograft is applied directly (shiny side down) to the denuded area. Before applying, it may be dipped in saline solution. It may be trimmed to fit the wound.
4. The grafts are usually secured with Steri-Strips. Staples or sutures may be used as well. The graft is covered with wet Adaptic (bibiotic solution or saline) and covered with stretch gauze; this is again wet down with the appropriate solution.
5. The wound remains unchanged initially for 3 to 5 days, during which time it is wet down every 4 to 6 hours.

6. After the initial takedown, dressings are changed daily.
7. If allograft or xenograft is used, the wound bed may be prepared for permanent autografting.

Biosynthetic Dressings

1. Temporary biosynthetic dressings help prevent bacterial contamination.
2. Used when permanent autograft is unavailable or unnecessary (as when partial-thickness wounds will heal spontaneously over time).
3. Biobrane (Woodruff Laboratories) consists of a custom-knit nylon fabric mechanically bonded to an ultrathin silicone rubber membrane, to which collagenous peptides of porcine skin are covalently bonded.
   a. Has a longer shelf life and lower cost than biologic dressings, such as pigskin.
   b. Is widely used for coverage of shallow wounds awaiting epithelialization, excised wounds awaiting autografts, widely meshed autografts until closure of interstices, and donor sites awaiting healing.

Artificial Dermis

1. Method being studied in selected burn centers to improve survival of patients with massive burns and little donor skin available.
2. Composed of a porous collagen-chondroitin 6-sulfate fibrillar mat covered with a thin Silastic sheet.
3. Used with an epidermal graft to provide a permanent cover that is at least as satisfactory as other available grafting techniques.
4. Used with donor sites that are thinner and that heal faster; seems to result in less hypertrophic scarring than the usual grafting methods.

Wound Closure

1. Skin grafting is usually required or preferred with full-thickness burns greater than 3 to 5 cm in diameter or in deep partial-thickness wounds or in areas of function.
2. After gradual eschar removal and development of a base of granulating tissue or in the presence of viable tissue after excision, grafts of the patient's own skin (autografts) are applied.
3. Sheet grafts or meshed grafts, providing wider expansion from donor sites, may be used.
4. Blood flow is established by the 3rd or 4th day, and by the 7th to 10th day postgrafting, vascular continuity, and wound closure have been established.
5. Cultured epithelial autografts may be used for patients with large burns and little available donor skin.
   a. Biopsies of unburned skin are cultured in a specialized laboratory to yield confluent sheets of epithelial cells suitable for grafting in about 3 weeks.
   b. Available donor sites can be used for coverage of the most functional or posterior surfaces, and the more delicate cultured epithelial autografts can be used to cover other large areas.
   c. Additional experience is needed to determine the long-term durability of cultured epithelial autografts, which may be life-saving treatment for the severely burned.

6. Many partial-thickness burn wounds will heal spontaneously within a few weeks, provided they are protected from infection.
7. The donor site requires meticulous care and may be covered with a synthetic dressing (Biobrane, etc.), scarlet red, or an antimicrobial cream. If a cream is used, the wound must be dressed.

Prevention and Treatment of Complications

Primary causes of morbidity and mortality in burn victims are those related to infection and pulmonary problems.

1. Intravenous antibiotics may be given prophylactically to prevent gram-positive infection.
2. Topical antibacterial agents help to retard the proliferation of pathogenic organisms until wound closure occurs spontaneously or through surgical intervention.
3. Broad-spectrum antibiotics may be necessary to treat systemic gram-positive and gram-negative infections and sometimes fungal infection.
4. Critical diagnostic parameters include observing for signs of burn-wound sepsis, obtaining quantitative and qualitative wound biopsy, checking for signs of systemic septicemia, and taking blood for cultures.
5. Meticulous pulmonary care is essential, because pneumonia (especially if patient remains intubated) is common.
6. Severe inhalation injury, including ARDS, can contribute significantly to mortality, even though the burn wound size may be small.

◼ Nursing Management of the Burn Patient

Nursing Assessment

1. Obtain a thorough history, including:
   a. Causative agent—hot water, chemical, gasoline, flame, etc.
   b. Duration of exposure.
   c. Circumstances of injury, including whether in closed or open space, accidental or intentional, or self-inflicted.
   d. Age.
   e. Initial treatment, including first aid, prehospital emergency care (including fluids, intubation, etc.), or care rendered in another facility (emergency department, etc.).
   f. Preexisting medical problems—heart disease, diabetes, ulcers, alcoholism, chronic obstructive pulmonary disease, epilepsy, psychosis.
   g. Current medications.
   h. Concomitant injuries (eg, from fall, explosions, assaults).
   i. Evidence of inhalation injury.
   j. Allergies.
   k. Tetanus immunization status.
   l. Height and weight.
2. Take photograph of burned area (with patient permission) for medical record of extent of burn.

3. Perform ongoing assessment of hemodynamic and respiratory status, condition of wounds, and signs of infection.

Nursing Diagnoses
- Impaired Gas Exchange related to inhalation injury
- Ineffective Breathing Pattern related to circumferential chest burn, upper airway obstruction, or ARDS
- Decreased Cardiac Output related to fluid shifts and hypovolemic shock
- Altered Peripheral Tissue Perfusion related to edema and circumferential burns
- Risk for Fluid Volume Excess related to fluid resuscitation and subsequent mobilization 3 to 5 days postburn
- Impaired Skin Integrity related to burn injury and surgical interventions (donor sites)
- Altered Urinary Elimination related to indwelling catheter
- Ineffective Thermoregulation related to loss of skin microcirculatory regulation and hypothalamic response
- Risk for Infection related to loss of skin barrier and altered immune response
- Impaired Physical Mobility related to edema, pain, skin and joint contractures
- Altered Nutrition: Less Than Body Requirements related to hypermetabolic response to burn injury
- Risk for Injury related to decreased gastric motility and stress response
- Pain related to injured nerves in burn wound and skin tightness
- Ineffective Individual Coping related to fear and anxiety
- Body Image Disturbance related to cosmetic and functional sequelae of burn wound

Nursing Interventions
Achieving Adequate Oxygenation and Respiratory Function
1. Provide humidified 100% oxygen until carbon monoxide level is known. (*Caution:* Adjust oxygen flow rate for patient with chronic obstructive pulmonary disease as prescribed.) If the patient is stable, try to get the initial ABG on room air.
2. Assess for signs of hypoxemia (anxiousness, tachypnea, tachycardia), and differentiate this from pain.
3. Suspect respiratory injury if burn occurred in an enclosed space.
4. Observe for and report erythema or blistering of buccal mucosa; singed nasal hairs; burns of lips, face, or neck; increasing hoarseness.
5. Monitor respiratory rate, depth, rhythm, cough.
6. Auscultate chest and note breath sounds.
7. Note character and amount of respiratory secretions. Report carbonaceous sputum, tracheal tissue.
8. Observe for signs of inadequate ventilation and begin serial monitoring of ABGs and oxygen saturation.
9. Provide mechanical ventilation, continuous positive airway pressure, or positive end-expiratory pressure if requested.

10. Keep intubation equipment nearby, and be alert for signs of respiratory obstruction.
11. In mild inhalation injury:
    a. Provide humidification of inspired air.
    b. Encourage coughing and deep breathing.
    c. Maintain pulmonary toilet.
12. In moderate to severe inhalation injury:
    a. Initiate more frequent bronchial suctioning.
    b. Closely monitor vital signs, urinary output, and ABGs.
    c. Administer bronchodilator treatments as ordered.
    d. For additional respiratory problems, it may be necessary to have patient intubated and placed on mechanical ventilation.

Maintaining Adequate Tidal Volume and Unrestricted Chest Movement
1. Observe rate and quality of breathing; report if progressively more rapid and shallow.
2. Assess tidal volume; report decreasing volume to health care provider.
3. Encourage deep breathing and incentive spirometry (may use sigh control on ventilator as needed).
4. Place patient in semi-Fowler's position to permit maximal chest excursions if there are no contraindications, such as hypotension or trauma.
5. Ensure that chest dressings are not constricting.
6. Prepare the patient for escharotomy and assist as indicated.

Supporting Cardiac Output
1. Position the patient to increase venous return.
2. Give fluids as prescribed.
3. Monitor vital signs, including apical pulse, respirations, central venous pressure, pulmonary artery pressures, and urine output at least hourly.
4. Determine cardiac output as requested.
5. Monitor sensorium.
6. Document all observations, and particularly note trends in vital sign changes.

Promoting Peripheral Circulation
1. Remove all jewelry and clothing.
2. Elevate extremities.
3. Monitor peripheral pulses hourly. Use Doppler as necessary.
4. Prepare the patient for escharotomy if circulation is impaired.
5. Monitor tissue pressure.

Facilitating Fluid Balance
1. Titrate fluid intake as tolerated. The initial resuscitation formula is only a base.

GERONTOLOGIC ALERT

 The elderly and those with impaired renal function, cardiovascular disease, and pulmonary disease are more likely to develop fluid overload. Proceed with caution.

---

2. Maintain accurate intake and output records.
3. Weigh the patient daily.

4. Monitor results of serum potassium and other electrolytes.
5. Be alert to signs of fluid overload and congestive heart failure, especially during initial fluid resuscitation and immediately afterward, when fluid mobilization is occurring.
6. Administer diuretics as ordered.

Protecting and Reestablishing Skin Integrity

1. Cleanse wounds and change dressings twice daily. Use an antimicrobial solution or mild soap and water. Dry gently. This may be done in the hydrotherapy tank, bathtub, shower, or at the bedside.
2. Perform debridement of dead tissue at this time. May use gauze, scissors, or pickups or forceps as appropriate. Try to limit time to 20 to 30 minutes depending on the patient's tolerance. Additional analgesia may be necessary.
3. Apply topical bacteriostatic agents as directed. Cream or ointment is applied ⅛ inch thick.
4. Dress wounds as appropriate, using conventional burn pads, gauze rolls, or any combination. Dressings may be held in place as necessary with gauze rolls or netting.
5. For grafted areas, use extreme caution in removing dressings; observe for and report serous or sanguineous blebs or purulent drainage. Redress grafted areas according to protocol.
6. Observe all wounds daily and document wound status on the patient's record.
7. Promote healing of donor sites by:
   a. Preventing contamination of donor sites that are clean wounds.
   b. Opening to air for drying postoperatively if gauze or impregnated gauze dressing is used. If exudate occurs after the first 24 hours, swab the area for culture and apply an antimicrobial topical cream. If the culture is positive, treatment will be in accord with sensitivities.
   c. Following health care provider's or manufacturer's instructions for care of sites dressed with synthetic materials.
   d. Allowing dressing to peel off spontaneously.
   e. Cleansing healing donor site with mild soap and water once dressings are removed; lubricating site twice daily and as needed.

Preventing Urinary Infection

1. Maintain closed urinary drainage system and ensure patency.
2. Observe color, clarity, amount of urine frequently.
3. Empty drainage bag frequently.
4. Provide catheter care, such as washing with soap and water.
5. Encourage removal of catheter and use of urinal, bedpan, or commode as soon as frequent urine output determinations are not required.

Promoting Stable Body Temperature

1. Be efficient in care; do not expose wounds unnecessarily.
2. Maintain warm ambient temperatures.
3. Use radiant warmers, warming blankets, or adjustment of the bed temperature to keep the patient warm.
4. Obtain urine, sputum, and blood cultures for temperatures greater than 38.9°C (102°F) rectal or core temperature or if chills are present.
5. Provide a dry top layer for wet dressings to reduce evaporative heat loss.
6. Warm wound cleansing and dressing solutions to body temperature.
7. Use blankets in transporting patient to other areas of the hospital.
8. Administer antipyretics as prescribed.

Avoiding Wound and Systemic Infection

1. Wash hands with antibacterial cleansing agent before and after all patient contact.
2. Use barrier garments—isolation gown or plastic apron—for all care requiring contact with the patient or the patient's bed.
3. Cover hair and wear mask when wounds are exposed or when performing a sterile procedure.
4. Use sterile examination gloves for all dressing changes and all care involving patient contact.
5. Maintain proper concentration of topical antibacterial agents used in wound care.
6. Be alert for reservoirs of infection and sources of cross-contamination in equipment, assignment of personnel, etc.
7. Check history of tetanus immunization and provide passive and/or active tetanus prophylaxis as prescribed.
8. Change IV tubing and lines according to Centers for Disease Control and Prevention recommendations.
9. Administer antibiotics as prescribed and be alert for toxic effects and incompatibilities.
10. Assess wounds daily for local signs of infection—swelling and redness around wound edges, purulent drainage, discoloration, loss of grafts, etc.
11. Be alert for early signs of septicemia, including changes in mentation, tachypnea, and decreased peristalsis as well as later signs, such as increased pulse, decreased blood pressure, increased or decreased urine output, facial flushing, increased and later decreased temperatures, increasing hyperglycemia, and malaise. Report to health care provider promptly.
12. Promote optimal personal hygiene for the patient, including daily cleansing of unburned areas, meticulous care of teeth and mouth, shampooing of hair every other day, shaving of hair in or near burned areas, and meticulous care of IV and urinary catheter sites.
13. Inspect skin carefully for signs of pressure and breakdown.
14. Observe for and report signs of thrombophlebitis or catheter-induced infections.
15. Prevent atelectasis and pneumonia through chest physical therapy, postural drainage, meticulous pulmonary technique, and, if indicated, tracheostomy care.

Promoting Range of Motion and Ability to Perform Activities of Daily Living

1. Ensure consultation with physical and occupational therapists, who will exercise the patient at least once or twice daily as necessary.
2. Encourage the patient to be as active as possible and to perform active range-of-motion exercises throughout the day.
3. Maintain splints in proper position as prescribed by occupational therapist; remove splints on regular schedule and observe for signs of skin irritation before reapplying.
4. Position the patient to decrease edema and avoid flexion of burned joints.
5. Coordinate pain management and other care to allow optimal effort during periods of physical exercise.
6. Initiate passive and active range-of-motion and breathing exercises during early postburn period.
7. Plan with therapists for a conditioning regimen that gradually increases energy expenditure and tolerance for activity.
8. Act as advocate for the patient's need for rest by coordinating the patient's therapeutic and social activities and prioritizing interventions and visits.
9. Help the patient achieve adequate relaxation and sleep through medication and environmental measures.

Ensuring That Nutritional Intake Meets Metabolic Demands

1. Weigh the patient daily with dressings removed.
2. Obtain consultation from dietitian for calculation of nutritional needs based on age, weight, height, and burn size. Two of the more popular formulas used to estimate nutritional needs are the Harrison-Benedict and Curreri formulas.
3. Administer vitamins and mineral supplements as prescribed.
4. Minimize metabolic stress by allaying fears, pain, and anxiety and by maintaining a warm environmental temperature.
5. Generally, for burns less than 10% TBSA, a well-balanced diet with emphasis on protein intake is necessary. For 10% to 20% TBSA, a high-protein, high-calorie diet is ordered. From 20% to 30% TBSA, supplementary enteral nutrition is necessary. Between 30% and 40% TBSA, total parenteral nutrition may be implemented.
6. When the patient is ready for oral fluids, observe tolerance. If there are no problems, advance the diet as tolerated.
7. Provide nasogastric tube feedings as prescribed, using caution to prevent aspiration by checking tube placement before each feeding and checking amount of gastric aspirate.
8. Administer IV hyperalimentation and fat emulsions prescribed with usual nursing precautions.
9. Keep record of caloric intake.
10. Encourage the patient to feed self.
11. Supplement meals with between-meal high-protein, high-calorie snacks, such as milkshakes or foods brought from home according to patient's preference.

Preventing Paralytic Ileus and Stress Ulcer

1. Keep on nothing-by-mouth (NPO) status until bowel sounds resume.
2. Assess bowel sounds every 2 to 4 hours while acutely ill. (Decreased peristalsis may be an early sign of septicemia.)
3. Decompress stomach with nasogastric tube on low intermittent suction until bowel sounds resume.
4. Recent practice now encourages small amounts of tube feedings, 5 to 10 mL/hour, immediately following the initial injury to help preserve the function of the gut and prevent paralytic ileus or stress ulcer.
5. Check amount and pH of gastric drainage or aspirate and report change.
6. Administer histamine-2 blockers and antacids as prescribed. This will help prevent or diminish the occurrence of stress (Curling's) ulcers.
7. Heed complaints of nausea while intubated by checking for abdominal distention, tube placement, residual aspirate.
8. Provide mouth care every 4 hours while intubated.
9. Test stools for occult bleeding.

Reducing Pain

1. Assess for pain periodically; do not wait for complaints of pain to intervene.
2. Determine previous experience with pain, the patient's response, and coping mechanisms.
3. Offer analgesics before wound care or before particularly painful treatments.
4. Change the patient's position when possible, supporting extremities with pillows.
5. Reduce anxiety by approaches such as sensory-oriented explanations of procedures.
6. Teach relaxation techniques, such as imagery, breathing exercises, and progressive muscle relaxation, to help the patient cope with pain.
7. Allow the patient to make choices regarding care whenever possible, thus allowing some measure of input and control in care.

Enhancing Effective Coping Strategies

1. Assess the patient's coping mechanisms from past history and current behavior.
2. Provide opportunities for the patient to express thoughts, feelings, fears, and anxieties regarding injury.
3. Explore with the patient alternative mechanisms for coping with the burn injury and its consequences.
4. Assure the patient of the normality of responses and the effect that time and healing will likely have on current concerns.
5. Interpret patient behavior to concerned family members and significant others.
6. Respect current coping mechanisms and discourage them only when an appropriate alternative can be provided.

7. Support family and friends' communications and visits if this is noted to help the patient.
8. Assess need for mental health consultation.
9. Offer antianxiety medications as prescribed.

Preserving Positive Body Image
1. Gather data on the patient's preburn self-image and life-style.
2. When ready, encourage the patient to express concerns regarding changes in self-image or life-style that may result from burn injury.
3. Be honest, but positive, in responding to the patient and family.
4. Positively reinforce appropriate, effective coping mechanisms.
5. Arrange for the patient to see face (if burned) with appropriate supportive personnel before being placed/transferred to a room with access to a mirror.
6. Arrange for the patient to talk with other patients who have had a similar injury and are progressing satisfactorily.
7. Encourage participation in a burn survivor's group, such as the Phoenix Society or other local support group.
8. Use and emphasize the concept of being a burn survivor. Survivors continue onward. Avoid the use of the term "burn victim" because it enhances the sick role.

Community and Home Care Considerations
1. Demonstrate and explain wound care procedures to be continued after discharge:
   a. Wash hands.
   b. Cleanse small open wounds with mild soap in tub or shower.
   c. Rinse well with tap water.
   d. Pat dry with clean towel.
   e. Apply prescribed topical agent and/or dressing.
2. Assess for and teach patient to observe for local signs of wound infection:
   a. Increased redness of normal skin around burn area.
   b. Increased or purulent drainage.
   c. Increased pain, foul odor in burn area.
   d. Elevated body temperature.
3. Coordinate physical therapy consultation and encourage patient to develop a schedule to incorporate exercise regimen as prescribed by physical therapist.
   a. Suggest scheduling exercises immediately after wound cleansing and application of topical agent, because skin may be more pliable and less sensitive to stretching then.
4. Instruct the patient in use and care of splints and pressure garments.
   a. Cleanse with mild soap and rinse well daily.
   b. Keep away from heat; dry garment by laying it flat on towels.
   c. Wear garment as prescribed. This is usually 23 out of 24 hours/day. The garment is usually worn for 1 to 1-½ years.

d. Small open wounds should be covered with a light dressing under splints or pressure garments.
   e. Small superficial wounds smaller than 1.5 cm are usually treated with an antiseptic drying agent, such as merbromin 4% or 10%, twice a day.
   f. Observe for signs of skin breakdown. Reassure the patient that small blister formation is normal and generally lessens after the first year.
   g. Wear/bring splints and pressure garments to follow-up visits to be checked for proper fit.

Patient Education and Health Maintenance
Health education is closely related to rehabilitation as the burn patient prepares to return to a productive place in society. Functional and cosmetic reconstruction is accomplished, and the patient attempts to integrate a new self-concept into social realities. Broadly viewed, health education focuses on biologic, psychological, and social parameters.
1. Assist the patient in transition from dependence on the health team to independence by assisting the patient to communicate needs and functional abilities to others.
2. Guide the patient in thinking positively about self. Promote ability to redirect others' attention from the scarred body to the self within.
3. Instruct the patient in measures to lubricate and enhance comfort of healing skin:
   a. After cleansing, use moisturizers such as cocoa butter, Nivea, Absorbase, Eucerin, or other nonperfumed hand lotion at least twice a day or more frequently as needed.
   b. Wear clean white underwear and clothing free of irritating dyes until wounds are well healed.
   c. Take antipruritics as prescribed.
   d. Stay in a cool environment if itching occurs.
   e. Protect skin from further trauma; use a sunscreen numbered 24 or higher.
   f. Discuss summer precautions, which should include a hat with a full, wide brim if there were facial or neck burns. Also limit exposure to sun, because the affected areas will sunburn more easily and tan more deeply.
   g. Advise the patient that if wearing a pressure vest with or without sleeves or tights, the Occupational Safety and Health Administration standards for work in a hot environment should be used. The patient should also be aware of the need for oral fluid replacement.
4. Review with the patient and family common emotional responses during convalescence (depression, withdrawal, grieving, dreaming, anxiety, guilt, excessive sensitivity, emotional lability, insomnia, fear of future), and discuss usual temporary nature of these as well as effective coping mechanisms.
   a. There may be some psychological sequelae that will require long-term intervention, such as image adjustment disorders or post-traumatic stress issues.

b. Make sure that the patient has a phone number or referral to the counselor should he or she want to make follow-up appointments.

5. Ensure that information has been given about follow-up evaluations and home health care services, as needed, in the interim.

6. For additional information and support, contact agencies such as the American Burn Association, 625 N. Michigan Ave., Suite 1530, Chicago, IL 60613, 312-642-9260, *www.ameriburn.org* or the Phoenix Society for Burn Survivors, 22153 Wealthy St. SE #215, East Grand Rapids, MI 49506, (616) 458-2773. The Phoenix Society is a national foundation with local chapters whose primary function is support of other burn survivors. It has a toll-free number that burn survivors may use: (800) 888-BURN (2876).

Outcome-Based Evaluation

- Carboxyhemoglobin below 10, ABGs within normal limits, respiratory rate 12 to 28
- Tidal volume within normal limits
- Pulse 110 or below, blood pressure stable
- Peripheral pulses strong
- Weight stable, no edema, lungs clear
- Wounds clean and granulating
- Catheter patent, urine clear and quantity sufficient
- Temperature normal to low-grade fever, no chills
- No signs of infection
- Normal range of motion achieved and performing activities of daily living independently
- Less than 5% weight loss from baseline
- No gastric distention, aspirate and stool hemoccult negative
- Reports minimal pain after analgesic administration
- Using appropriate coping mechanisms
- Verbalizing fears and concerns after viewing self in mirror

SELECTED REFERENCES

Carrougher, G. L. (Ed.) (1998). *Burn care and therapy*. St. Louis: Mosby.

Davey, R. B. (1997). The use of contact media for burn scar hypertrophy. *Journal of Wound Care, 6*(2), 80–82.

Eadie, P. E. (1995). Thirty-five years of paediatric scalds: Are lessons being learned? *British Journal of Plastic Surgery, 48;* 103–105.

McGill, V., et al. (1995). The impact of substance use on mortality and morbidity from thermal injury. *Journal of Trauma, 38,* 931–934.

Pessina, M. A., & Ellis, S. M. (1997). Burn management. *Nursing Clinics of North America, 32*(2), 365–374.

Shiozak, T. et al. (1995). Difference in body temperature change during dressing change in surviving and non-surviving burned patients. *British Journal of Surgery, 82,* 784–786.

Staley, M. J., & Richard, R. L. (1997). Management of the acute burn wound: An overview. *Advances in Wound Care, 10*(2), 39–44.

Ward, R. S., & Saffle, J. R. (1995). Topical agents in burn and wound care. *Physical Therapy, 75*(6), 526–538.

UNIT XII

Emergency Nursing

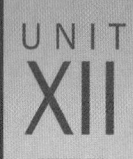

CHAPTER

35

Emergent Conditions

BASIC APPROACH TO EMERGENCY CARE

Emergency care can be defined as the episodic and crisis-oriented care provided to patients with serious or potentially life-threatening injuries or illnesses. The philosophy of emergency care includes the concept that an emergency is whatever the patient or family considers it to be. See Standards of Care Guidelines.

Emergency Assessment

A systematic approach to the assessment of an emergency patient is essential. Often, the most dramatic injury is not the most serious. The primary and secondary survey provide the emergency nurse with a methodical approach to help identify and prioritize patient needs.

Primary Assessment

1. The initial rapid assessment of the patient is meant to identify life-threatening problems (airway, breathing,

and circulation). If conditions are identified that present an immediate threat to life, appropriate interventions are required before proceeding to the secondary assessment.

2. The first step in the primary assessment is to determine if the patient is conscious. If the patient is conscious, the primary assessment can be performed at a glance.
   a. A patient who is alert and talking indicates that there is breathing and circulation.
   b. A conscious patient also indicates that circulation is adequate and enough blood is being circulated to the brain.
   c. If, however, the patient is not fully conscious, the primary assessment should proceed step by step.
3. In seriously injured or ill patients, it is recommended to add two more letters to the primary survey: D—disability, and E—expose.
4. **Airway:** Does the patient have an open airway?
5. **Breathing:** Is the patient breathing?
6. **Circulation:** Is circulation in immediate jeopardy?
   a. Is there a pulse?
   b. Is there profuse bleeding?
7. **Disability**—Assess level of consciousness and pupils (a more complete neurologic survey will be completed in the secondary survey).
   a. Assess level of consciousness using the AVPU scale:
      (i) A—Is the patient alert?
      (ii) V—Does the patient respond to voice?
      (iii) P—Does the patient respond to painful stimulus?
      (iv) U—The patient is unresponsive even to painful stimulus.

8. **Expose**—Undress the patient to look for clues to injury or illness, such as wounds or skin lesions.

Secondary Assessment

The secondary survey is a systematic, brief (2 to 3 minutes) examination of the patient from head to toe. The purpose is to detect and prioritize additional injuries or to detect signs of underlying medical conditions.

History

1. If possible, a brief history of the chief complaint, accident, or illness is taken from the patient or an accompanying person—relative, prehospital provider.
   a. What is the mechanism of injury—the circumstances, forces, location, and time of injury?
   b. When did the symptoms appear?
   c. Was the patient unconscious after the accident?
   d. How did the patient reach the hospital?
   e. What was the health status of the patient before the accident or illness?
   f. Is there a history of illness?
   g. Is the patient currently taking any medications?
   h. Does the patient have any allergies?
   i. Is the patient under a health care provider's care (name of provider)?
   j. Was treatment attempted before arrival at the hospital—home remedies, over-the-counter medication, or prehospital emergency medical services care?

NURSING ALERT

To obtain a good descriptive history, do not ask questions that can be answered with a yes or no.

Vital Signs

1. Routinely includes temperature, pulse rate, respiratory rate, blood pressure, and pain scale.
2. When obtained early in the assessment, they help to establish complete baseline information.

Head-to-Toe Assessment

1. General appearance
   a. Position/posture/gait
   b. Level of consciousness—restlessness is a danger signal
   c. Behavior and degree of distress
   d. Cooperation
   e. Skin condition and color
2. Head/scalp
   a. Bleeding
   b. Deformity and depressions
   c. Facial symmetry
3. Ears
   a. Blood
   b. Clear fluid (cerebrospinal fluid [CSF])
   c. Battle's sign (bluish discoloration of the mastoid area)
4. Eyes
   a. Pupil size and reaction to light
   b. Extraocular motions
   c. Orbital ecchymosis
   d. Gross vision
   e. Conjunctivae—examine for pallor or cyanosis

5. Nose
   a. Blood
   b. Clear fluid (CSF)
6. Mouth
   a. Missing teeth
   b. Cyanosis of the lips
   c. Foreign material/vomitus
7. Neck
   a. Tracheal deviation
   b. Jugular distention
   c. Tenderness
8. Chest
   a. Symmetry
   b. Tenderness/pain
   c. Ecchymosis
   d. Subcutaneous emphysema
   e. Soft tissue injuries
   f. Breath sounds
   g. Heart sounds
9. Abdomen
   a. Distention/rigidity
   b. Tenderness/pain
   c. Guarding
   d. Bowel sounds
   e. Soft tissue injuries
10. Pelvis
    a. Stability
    b. Tenderness
11. Genitalia
    a. Bleeding
    b. Wounds/trauma
    c. Priapism
    d. Rectal tone
    e. Pain
12. Extremities
    a. Pain
    b. Deformity and bruises
    c. Pulses
    d. Sensation and strength
    e. Soft tissue injury
    f. Capillary refill
    g. Edema
13. Posterior (observe cervical spine precautions in trauma patients)
    a. Soft tissue injury
    b. Spinal tenderness
    c. Pain or tenderness

Focused Assessment

1. A more detailed assessment of deviations from normal or problems identified in the secondary survey.
2. If more then one focused assessment is necessary, any problem identified with the pulmonary system, cardiovascular system, or neurologic system should be assessed first.

■ Triage

Triage is a French verb meaning "to sort." Most patients entering an emergency department are greeted by a triage nurse. The role of the triage nurse is to do a brief evaluation of the patient to determine a level of acuity or priority of care. Thus, the triage nurse acts as a gatekeeper, sorting patients into categories, ensuring that the more seriously ill are treated first.

Priorities of Care and Triage Categories

Standardized triage categories are usually developed within each emergency department. Most common triage systems consist of three levels of acuity.

Emergent I

1. Conditions requiring immediate medical interventions. Any delay in treatment is potentially life or limb threatening.
2. Includes conditions such as:
   a. Airway compromise
   b. Cardiac arrest
   c. Severe shock
   d. Cervical spine injury
   e. Multisystem trauma
   f. Altered level of consciousness
   g. Eclampsia

Urgent II

1. Patients who present as stable but whose condition requires medical intervention within a few hours. There is no immediate threat to life or limb for these patients.
2. Conditions include:
   a. Fever
   b. Minor burns
   c. Minor musculoskeletal injuries
   d. Dizziness
   e. Lacerations

Nonemergent III

1. Patients who present with chronic or minor injuries. There is no danger to life or limb by having these patients wait to be seen. These patients are in no obvious distress.
2. Conditions include:
   a. Chronic low back pain
   b. Routine medication refills
   c. Dental problems
   d. Missed menses

■ Psychological Considerations

Body trauma is an insult to physiologic and psychological homeostasis; it requires both physiologic and psychological healing.

Approach to the Patient

1. Understand and accept the basic anxieties of the acutely traumatized patient. Be aware of the patient's fear of death, mutilation, and isolation.
   a. Personalize the situation as much as possible. Speak, react, and respond in a warm manner.
   b. Give explanations on a level that the patient can grasp. An informed patient can cope with psychological/physiologic stress in a more positive manner.
   c. Accept the rights of the patient and family to have and display their own feelings.

d. Maintain a calm and reassuring manner—helps the emotionally distressed patient or family to mobilize their psychological resources.

2. Understand and support the patient's feelings concerning loss of control (emotional, physical, and intellectual).

3. Treat the unconscious patient as if conscious. Touch, call by name, and explain every procedure that is done. Avoid making negative comments about the patient's condition.
   a. Orient the patient to person, time, and place as soon as he or she is conscious; reinforce by repeating this information.
   b. Bring the patient back to reality in a calm and reassuring way.
   c. Encourage the family, when possible, to orient the patient to reality.

4. Be prepared to handle all aspects of acute trauma; know what to expect and what to do—alleviates the nurse's anxieties and increases the patient's confidence.

Approach to the Family

1. Inform the family where the patient is, and give as much information as possible about the treatment he or she is receiving.

2. Recognize the anxiety of the family and allow them to talk about their feelings. Allow expressions of remorse, anger, guilt, and criticism.

3. Allow the family to relive the events, actions, and feelings preceding admission to the emergency department.

4. Deal with reality as gently and quickly as possible; avoid encouraging and supporting denial.

5. Assist the family to cope with sudden and unexpected death. Some helpful measures include the following:
   a. Take the family to a private place.
   b. Talk to all of the family together so they can mourn together.
   c. Assure the family that everything possible was done; inform them of the treatment rendered.
   d. Avoid using euphemisms, such as "passed on." Show the family that you care by touching, offering coffee, and so forth.
   e. Allow family to talk about the deceased—permits ventilation of feelings of loss. Encourage family to talk about events preceding admission to the emergency department.
   f. Encourage family to support each other and to express emotions freely—grief, loss, anger, helplessness, tears, disbelief.
   g. Avoid volunteering unnecessary information (patient was drinking, and so forth).
   h. Avoid giving sedation to family members—may mask or delay the grieving process, which is necessary to achieve emotional equilibrium and prevent prolonged depression.
   i. Be cognizant of cultural and religious beliefs and needs.
   j. Encourage family members to view the body if they wish—to do so helps to integrate the loss (cover mutilated areas).
      (i) Go with family to see the body.
      (ii) Show acceptance of the body by touching to give family permission to touch and talk to the body.
      (iii) Spend a few minutes with the family, listening to them.

6. Encourage the emergency department staff to discuss among themselves their reaction to the event to share intense feelings for review and for group support.

CARDIOPULMONARY RESUSCITATION AND AIRWAY MANAGEMENT

Cardiopulmonary resuscitation (CPR) is a technique of basic life support for the purpose of oxygenating the brain and heart until appropriate, definitive medical treatment can restore normal heart and ventilatory action. Management of foreign-body airway obstruction or cricothyroidotomy may be necessary to open the airway before CPR can be performed.

▨ Cardiopulmonary Resuscitation

See Procedure Guidelines 35-1: Cardiopulmonary Resuscitation.

Indications

1. Cardiac arrest
   a. Ventricular fibrillation
   b. Ventricular tachycardia
   c. Asystole
   d. Pulseless electrical activity
2. Respiratory arrest
   a. Drowning
   b. Stroke
   c. Foreign-body airway obstruction
   d. Smoke inhalation
   e. Drug overdose
   f. Electrocution/injury by lightning
   g. Suffocation
   h. Accident/injury
   i. Coma
   j. Epiglottitis

Assessment

1. Immediate loss of consciousness
2. Absence of breath sounds or air movement through nose or mouth
3. Absence of palpable carotid or femoral pulse; pulselessness in large arteries

Complications

1. Postresuscitation distress syndrome (secondary derangements in multiple organs)
2. Neurologic impairment, brain damage

NURSING ALERT

The patient who has been resuscitated is at risk for another episode of cardiac arrest.

PROCEDURE GUIDELINES 35-1   CARDIOPULMONARY RESUSCITATION

EQUIPMENT

Trained personnel   Intravenous (IV) setup
Arrest board   Defibrillator
Oral airway   Emergency cardiac drugs
Bag and mask device   Electrocardiograph machine

PROCEDURE

Nursing Action	Rationale
RESPONSIVENESS/AIRWAY	
1. Determine unresponsiveness: tap or gently shake patient while shouting, "Are you OK?"	1. This will prevent injury from attempted resuscitation on a person who is not unconscious.
2. Activate emergency medical service (EMS; call local emergency telephone number or 911) if outside hospital.	
3. Place patient supine on a firm, flat surface. Kneel at the level of the patient's shoulders. If the patient has suspected head or neck trauma, the rescuer should move the patient only if absolutely necessary.	3. This enables the rescuer to perform rescue breathing and chest compression without moving the knees.
4. Open the airway.	
a. *Head-tilt/Chin-lift Maneuver:* Place one hand on the patient's forehead and apply firm backward pressure with the palm to tilt the head back. Then, place the fingers of the other hand under the bony part of the lower jaw near the chin and lift up to bring the jaw forward and the teeth almost to occlusion.	a. In the absence of sufficient muscle tone, the tongue and/or epiglottis will obstruct the pharynx and larynx. This supports the jaw and helps tilt the head back.
b. *Jaw-thrust Maneuver:* Grasp the angles of the patient's lower jaw and, lifting with both hands, one on each side, displace the mandible forward, while tilting the head backward.	b. The jaw-thrust technique without head tilt is the safest method for opening the airway in the presence of suspected neck injury.
BREATHING	
Determine presence or absence of spontaneous breathing.	
1. Place ear over patient's mouth and nose while observing the chest, *look* for the chest to rise and fall, *listen* for air escaping during exhalation, and *feel* for the flow of air.	1. Keep maintaining an open airway.
2. Perform rescue breathing—mouth-to-mouth: While keeping the airway open, pinch the nostrils closed using the thumb and index finger of the hand that is on the forehead. Take a deep breath, open mouth wide, and place it outside of the patient's mouth, creating an airtight seal.	2. This prevents air from escaping from the patient's nose.
Ventilate the patient with two full breaths (1–1½ seconds each breath), taking a breath after each ventilation. If the initial ventilation attempt is unsuccessful, reposition the patient's head and repeat rescue breathing.	Adequate ventilation is indicated by seeing the chest rise and fall, feeling the air escape during ventilation and hearing the air escape during exhalation.
CIRCULATION	
Determine pulselessness.	
1. While maintaining head-tilt with one hand on the forehead, palpate the carotid or femoral pulse. If pulse is not palpable, start external chest compressions.	1. Cardiac arrest is recognized by pulselessness in the large arteries of the unconscious, breathless patient. If there is a palpable pulse, but no breathing present, initiate rescue breathing at rate of 12 times per minute (once every 5 seconds) after initial two breaths.

Nursing Action	Rationale
External Chest Compressions Consist of serial, rhythmic applications of pressure over the lower half of the sternum.	
1. Kneel as close to side of patient's chest as possible. Place the heel of one hand on the lower half of the sternum, 3.8 cm (1½ inches) from the tip of the xiphoid. The fingers may either be extended or interlaced but must be kept off the chest.	1. The long axis of the heel of the rescuer's hand should be placed on the long axis of the sternum; thus the main force of the compression will be on the sternum and decrease the chance of rib fracture.
2. While keeping your arms straight, elbows locked, and shoulders positioned directly over your hands, quickly and forcefully depress the lower half of the patient's sternum straight down, 3.8–25 cm (1½–2 inches).	
3. Release the external chest compression completely and allow the chest to return to its normal position after each compression. The time allowed for release should equal the time required for compression. Do not lift the hands off the chest or change position.	3. Release of the external chest compression allows blood flow into the heart.
4. Use 80 compressions per minute (100 if possible). For one rescuer, do 15 compressions at a rate of 80–100 per minute and then perform two ventilations; re-evaluate the patient.	4. Rescue breathing and external chest compressions must be combined. Check for return of carotid pulse. If absent, resume CPR with two ventilations followed by compressions. For CPR performed by health professionals, mouth-to-mask ventilation is an acceptable alternative for rescue breathing.
5. For CPR performed by two rescuers, the compression rate is 80–100 per minute. The compression–ventilation ratio is 5:1 with a pause for ventilation (1–1½ seconds)	
6. While resuscitation proceeds, simultaneous efforts are made to obtain and use special resuscitation equipment to manage breathing and circulation and provide definitive care.	6. Definitive care includes defibrillation, pharmacotherapy for dysrhythmias and acid–base disturbances, and ongoing monitoring and skilled care in an intensive care unit.

Adapted from Guidelines for cardiopulmonary resuscitation and emergency cardiac care. (1992). *Journal of the American Medical Association,* 268(16),2172–2198. Guideline 2000 for Cardiopulmonary Resuscitation and Emergency Cardiovascular Care was published by the American Heart Association in August 2000. Changes in CPR and life support are not included in this chapter because they were not yet implemented in clinical practice at the time of publication. Contact *www.americanheart.org* for more information.

■ Foreign-Body Airway Obstruction

Foreign-body obstruction of the airway may be either partial or complete.

The Heimlich maneuver (subdiaphragmatic abdominal thrusts) is recommended for relieving foreign-body airway obstruction in the adult. See Procedure Guidelines 35-2.

Assessment

1. Weak, ineffective cough
2. High-pitched noises on inspiration
3. Respiratory distress
4. Inability to speak or breathe
5. Cyanosis

PROCEDURE

Emergency Action	Rationale
HEIMLICH MANEUVER WITH CONSCIOUS PATIENT SITTING OR STANDING	
1. Stand behind the patient; wrap your arms around waist and proceed as follows: a. Make a fist with one hand, placing the thumb side of the fist against the patient's abdomen in the midline, slightly above the navel and well below the xiphoid process. Grasp the fist with the other hand.	

continued

PROCEDURE GUIDELINES 35-2	MANAGEMENT OF FOREIGN-BODY AIRWAY OBSTRUCTION *CONTINUED*

Nursing Action	Rationale
b. Press your fist into the patient's abdomen with a quick upward thrust. Each new thrust should be a separate and distinct maneuver.	b. A subdiaphragmatic abdominal thrust, by elevating the diaphragm, can force air from the lungs to create an artificial cough intended to move and expel an obstructing foreign body in the airway.

HEIMLICH MANEUVER WITH UNCONSCIOUS PATIENT LYING DOWN

1. Position patient supine with face up.
2. Kneel astride the patient's thighs, facing head.
3. Place the heel of one hand against the patient's abdomen in the midline slightly above the navel and well below the tip of the xiphoid; place the second hand directly on top of the first.
4. Press into the abdomen with a quick upward thrust.

Finger Sweep

1. Open patient's mouth by grasping both the tongue and lower jaw between the thumb and fingers and lift the mandible (tongue–jaw lift).
2. Insert the index finger of the other hand down along the inside of the cheek and deeply into the throat to the base of the tongue.
3. Use a hooking action to dislodge the foreign body and maneuver it into the mouth for removal.

1. This maneuver is to be used only in the unconscious patient. This action draws the tongue away from the foreign body that may be lodged there.

3. Take care not to force the object deeper into the throat.

CHEST THRUST WITH CONSCIOUS PATIENT STANDING OR SITTING

1. Stand behind the patient with arms under axillae to encircle the patient's chest.
2. Place thumb side of your fist on middle of patient's sternum, taking care to avoid xiphoid process and rib cage margins.
3. Grasp your fist with the other hand and perform backward thrusts until the foreign body is expelled or patient becomes unconscious.

1. This technique is to be used only in advanced stages of pregnancy or in markedly obese person.

3. Each thrust is administered with the intent of relieving the obstruction.

CHEST THRUST WITH UNCONSCIOUS PATIENT LYING DOWN

1. Place the patient on back and kneel close to the side of body.
2. Place the heel of your hand on the lower half of the sternum.
3. Deliver each chest thrust slowly and distinctly with the intent of relieving the obstruction.

This maneuver is used only in the advanced stages of pregnancy or when the rescuer cannot apply the Heimlich maneuver effectively to the unconscious, markedly obese person.

Adapted from Guidelines for cardiopulmonary resuscitation and emergency care. (1992). *Journal of the American Medical Association, 268*(16),2172–2198.

◼ Cricothyroidotomy

Cricothyroidotomy is the puncture or incision of the cricothyroid membrane to establish an emergency airway in certain emergency situations when endotracheal intubation or tracheostomy is not possible or is contraindicated. See Procedure Guidelines 35-3.

Indications

1. Compromised airway and inability to intubate or perform tracheostomy:
   a. Foreign-body obstruction
   b. Trauma to head and neck
2. Allergic reaction causing laryngeal edema

PROCEDURE GUIDELINES 35-3   CRICOTHYROIDOTOMY

EQUIPMENT

No. 11 gauge needle or scalpel with No. 11 scalpel blade

PROCEDURE

Nursing Action	Rationale
1. Extend the neck. Place a towel roll beneath the shoulders.	1. So the cricothyroid membrane can be palpated readily.
2. Identify the prominent thyroid cartilage (Adam's apple) and allow your finger to descend in the midline to the depression between the lower border of the thyroid cartilage and the upper border of the cricoid cartilage (see accompanying figure).	2. This depression represents the cricothyroid membrane.

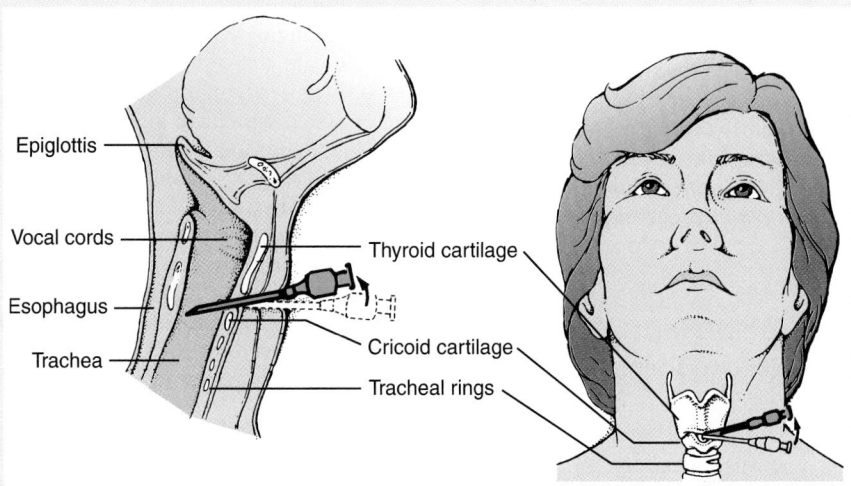

Cricothyroidotomy, or cricothyroid membrane puncture.

3. Insert a needle or any sharp instrument at a 10- to 30-degree caudal direction in the midline just above the upper part of the cricoid cartilage.	
4. Listen for air passing back and forth through the needle synchronously with the patient's respirations.	
5. Direct the needle downward and posteriorly.	5. To avoid injury to the vocal cords (located cephalad to the cricothyroid membrane).
6. Tape the needle with adhesive for stability.	6. To prevent laceration or perforation of the posterior tracheal wall.
7. An alternate method is to make a transverse incision overlying the cricothyroid membrane and a similar incision through the membrane itself. The membrane incision is spread, and a tracheostomy tube is inserted and directed into the trachea.	
8. Prepare for endotracheal intubation/tracheostomy.	8. After the patient is stabilized, a more permanent means of ventilatory support is implemented.
9. Potential complications: bleeding, aspiration.	

INJURIES TO THE HEAD, SPINE, AND FACE

Head Injuries

Head injuries can include fractures to the skull and face, direct injuries to the brain (as from a bullet), and indirect injuries to the brain (such as a concussion, contusion, or intracranial hemorrhage). Any time the skull is fractured, the patient is said to have an *open head injury*. If the skull is intact, the term *closed head injury* is used. Head injuries commonly occur from motor vehicle accidents, assaults, or falls.

Concussion: A temporary loss of consciousness that results from a transient interruption of the brain's normal functioning.

Contusion: A bruising of the brain tissue. Actual small amounts of bleeding into the brain tissue.

Intracranial hemorrhage: Significant bleeding into a space or a potential space between the skull and the brain. This is a serious complication of a head injury with a high mortality rate due a rising intracranial pressure and the potential for brain herniation. Intracranial hemorrhages can be classified as *epidural hematomas*, *subdural hematomas*, or *subarachnoid hemorrhages*, depending on the site of bleeding.

> **NURSING ALERT**
>
> Assume a cervical spine fracture for any patient with a significant head injury, until proven otherwise.

Primary Assessment

1. Airway: assess for vomitus, bleeding, and foreign objects.
2. Breathing: assess for abnormally slow or shallow respirations. An elevated PCO_2 can worsen cerebral edema.
3. Circulation: assess pulse and bleeding.

Primary Interventions

1. Open the airway using the jaw-thrust technique without head tilt. Oral suction equipment (to handle heavy vomitus) should be at hand.
2. Administer high-flow O_2: the most common cause of death from head injury is cerebral anoxia.
3. Assist inadequate respirations with a bag-valve mask. In general, head-injured patients should be hyperventilated with a respiratory rate of 20 to 25 breaths per minute. Hyperventilation lowers the $PaCO_2$, causing cerebral vasoconstriction and minimizing cerebral edema. Close monitoring of PaO_2 and $PaCO_2$ are necessary to prevent further ischemia to the injured brain tissue.
4. Control bleeding—do not apply pressure to the injury site. Apply a bulky, loose dressing. Do not attempt to stop the flow of blood or CSF from the nose or ears; apply a loose dressing if needed.
5. Initiate an intravenous (IV) line to run at a keep-vein-open rate.

Subsequent Assessment

1. History
   a. Mechanism of injury
   b. Duration of loss of consciousness
   c. Memory of the event
   d. Position found
2. Level of consciousness
   a. Change in the level of consciousness is the most sensitive indicator of a change in the patient's condition.
   b. Glasgow Coma Score (see p. 446).
3. Vital signs
   a. Hypertension and bradycardia indicate an increasing intracranial pressure.
   b. Head-injured patients may have associated cardiac dysrhythmias, noted by an irregular pulse or a fast pulse.
   c. Changing patterns of respiration or apnea may indicate a head injury.
   d. Elevated temperature—high temperatures are associated with head injury.
4. Unequal or unresponsive pupils
5. Confusion or personality changes
6. Impaired vision
7. One or both eyes appear sunken
8. Seizure activity
9. Battle's sign—a bluish discoloration behind the ears (indicates a possible basal skull fracture)
10. Rhinorrhea or otorrhea (indicative of leakage of CSF)
11. Periorbital ecchymosis (indicates anterior basilar fracture)

> **NURSING ALERT**
>
> If basilar skull fracture or severe midface fractures are suspected, a nasogastric tube is contraindicated. An orogastric tube may be considered for insertion.

General Intervention

1. Keep the neck in a neutral position with the cervical spine immobilized.
2. Hyperventilation to reduce intracranial pressure as indicated.
3. Establish an IV line of normal saline or Ringer's lactate—fluid volume should be restricted.
4. Be prepared to manage seizures—if seizures occur, they should be controlled immediately.
5. Maintain normothermia.
6. Pharmacologic interventions.
   a. Diazepam (Valium)—to control seizures.
   b. Steroids—to reduce swelling and brain cell oxygen requirements.
   c. Mannitol (Osmitrol)—to reduce cerebral edema and decrease intracranial pressure.
   d. Barbiturate coma.
   e. Antibiotics.
7. Prepare for immediate surgical intervention if patient shows evidence of neurologic deterioration.

▣ Cervical Spine Injuries

Injuries to the cervical spine are serious, because the crushing, stretching, and rotational shear forces exerted on the cord at the time of trauma can produce severe neurologic deficits. Edema and cord swelling contribute further to the loss of spinal cord function.

Any person with a head, neck, or back injury or fractures to the upper leg bones or to the pelvis should be suspected of having a potential spinal cord injury until proven otherwise.

Primary Assessment

1. Provide immediate immobilization of the spine while performing assessment.
2. Airway.
3. Breathing.
   a. Intercostal paralysis with diaphragmatic breathing indicates cervical spinal cord injury.
   b. In conscious patient, observe for increased respiratory rate and difficulty in speaking due to shortness of breath.
4. Circulation.

Primary Interventions

1. Immobilize the cervical spine.
2. Open the airway using the jaw-thrust technique without head tilt.
3. If the patient needs to be intubated, it may be done nasally.
4. If respirations are shallow, assist with a bag-valve mask.

Subsequent Assessment

1. Assess the position of the patient when found.
   a. Forearms flexed across the chest—C-6 injury.
   b. Arms stretched out above head—cervical injury.
2. Hypotension and bradycardia accompanied by warm, dry skin—suggests spinal shock.
3. Neck and/or back pain/extremity pain or burning sensation to the skin.
4. History of unconsciousness.
5. Total sensory loss and motor paralysis below level of injury.
6. Loss of bowel and bladder control; usually urinary retention and bladder distention.
7. Loss of sweating and vasomotor tone below level of cord lesion.
8. Priapism—persistent erection of penis.
9. Hypothermia—due to the inability to constrict peripheral blood vessels and conserve body heat.
10. Loss of rectal tone.

General Interventions

> **NURSING ALERT**
>
> A spinal cord injury can be made worse during the acute phase of injury, resulting in permanent neurologic damage. Proper handling is an immediate priority.

1. Monitor blood gas values serially.
2. Prepare for nasotracheal intubation—to prevent regurgitation and aspiration from gastric dilation and ileus.
3. Initiate IV access.
4. Insert an indwelling urinary catheter to avoid bladder distention.
5. Monitor for hypotension, hypothermia, and bradycardia.
6. Continue with repeated neurologic examinations to determine if there is deterioration of the spinal cord injury.
7. Be prepared to manage seizures.
8. Pharmacologic interventions:
   a. High-dose steroids.
   b. Diazepam (Valium)—for seizure control.

▣ Maxillofacial Trauma

Injuries to the head frequently result in facial lacerations and fractures to the facial bones (ie, nasal fractures, orbital fractures, maxillary fractures, and mandibular fractures).

Primary Assessment

1. Initiate immobilization of the spine while performing assessment.
2. Airway obstruction can occur due to tongue swelling (fractured jaw), bleeding, or broken or missing teeth.
3. Breathing—may be impaired due to an obstructed airway.
4. Circulation—control bleeding.

Primary Interventions

1. Establish and maintain an airway. This includes having high-flow suction available, inserting an oral airway, or assisting with intubation. A nasopharyngeal airway should only be used if there is no evidence of nasal fractures or CSF leakage from the nose.
2. Control bleeding—do not apply pressure to the injury site. Apply a bulky, loose dressing. Do not attempt to stop the flow of blood or CSF from the nose or ears; apply a loose dressing if needed.

Subsequent Assessment

1. Examine the mouth for broken or missing teeth.
2. Assess for a potential eye injury, vision loss, double vision, or pain in the eye.
3. Examine the eye for dysconjugate gaze—discoordination of eye movements.
4. Paralysis of the upward gaze is indicative of an inferior orbit fracture (blowout fracture).
5. Crepitus or a crackling feeling on palpation around the nose usually indicates a nasal fracture.
6. Malocclusion of the teeth is indicative of a maxilla or mandible fracture.
7. A palpable flattening of the cheek and a loss of sensation below the orbit may indicate a zygoma (cheekbone) fracture.
8. Spasms of the jaw (trismus) and mobility of the jaw indicate a maxilla fracture.
9. Rhinorrhea or otorrhea (indicative of leakage of CSF).

General Interventions

1. Gently apply ice to areas of swelling or ecchymosis. This may reduce further swelling and pain. However, if you suspect an injury to the eye itself, do not apply ice.
2. If other injuries permit, elevate the head of the bed.
3. Possible pharmacologic interventions:
   a. Morphine (Duramorph)—pain management
   b. Diazepam (Valium)—sedation
4. With the potential for a CSF leak, the patient should be instructed not to blow the nose, cough, or sneeze because of the potential for transmitting infection to the brain or eyes.

INJURIES TO SOFT TISSUE, BONES, AND JOINTS

Soft Tissue Injuries

Soft tissue injuries involve the skin and underlying subcutaneous tissue and muscles. They can be classified as open or closed injuries. A *closed wound* is an injury to the soft tissue but without a break in the skin. Closed wounds include:

1. *Contusion*—bleeding beneath the skin into the soft tissue. The bleeding can be minor or extensive. Extensive bleeding can cause severe pain and swelling, leading to a compromise of vital structures.
2. *Hematoma*—well-defined pocket of blood and fluid beneath the skin.

An *open wound* is an injury to soft tissue with a break in the skin. Generally, they are more serious than closed injuries due to the potential for blood loss and infection. Open wounds include:

1. *Abrasion*—superficial loss of skin resulting from rubbing or scraping the skin over a rough or uneven surface.
2. *Laceration*—tear in the skin. Can be a partial or full thickness cut. Can be defined as incisional or jagged.
3. *Puncture*—occurs when the skin is penetrated by a pointed object. Can be penetrating (entrance wound only) or perforating (entrance and exit wound). Generally, puncture wounds do not cause serious external bleeding, but there may be significant internal bleeding and damage to vital organs.
4. *Avulsion*—involves a tearing off or loss of a flap of skin.
5. *Amputation*—traumatic cutting or tearing off of a finger, toe, arm, or leg.

Primary Assessment

1. Always ensure the adequacy of airway, breathing, and circulation before initiating treatment.
2. If the bleeding from the injury has been significant, be aware of the clinical symptoms and signs of shock.
   a. Skin pale, mottled, cold, and/or diaphoretic.
   b. Tachycardia (rapid, weak pulse).
   c. Tachypnea (rapid, shallow breathing).
   d. Hypotension (falling blood pressure is a late sign of shock).
   e. Restlessness, confusion, and anxiety.
3. Assess for arterial or venous bleeding. Arterial bleeding is bright red and usually spurts from the wound. Venous bleeding is darker red and will flow steadily from a wound.

Primary Interventions

The primary goal and nursing intervention are to control severe bleeding.

> **NURSING ALERT**
>
> Wounds that result in severe arterial bleeding should be considered life threatening, and treatment is second only to CPR.

Direct Pressure

1. Most external bleeding can be controlled by direct pressure.
2. Cover the injury with sterile dressings.
3. Apply firm direct pressure to the site of injury.
4. Pressure should be maintained until the bleeding stops, a pressure dressing is applied, or definitive treatment is undertaken.
5. If the dressing becomes saturated, reinforce the dressing; do not remove the dressing.
6. After bleeding has stopped, apply a pressure dressing.
   a. A pressure bandage is made by securing several gauze pads over the injury with a rolled gauze bandage.
   b. A pressure dressing allows the nurse freedom to continue assessing the patient or attend to other injuries.
   c. After applying a pressure dressing, always ensure that the patient has a pulse distal to the dressing. If no pulse is present, the dressing may be too tight.

Elevation

1. Elevating the injured area while applying direct pressure helps to control bleeding. This measure uses gravity to slow the blood flow and to promote clotting.
2. If possible, the injured area should be elevated above the level of the heart.
3. Do not raise a limb if a fracture is suspected or if elevation causes the patient pain or discomfort.

Pressure Points

1. Pressure points are used when direct pressure and elevation cannot control bleeding alone or when direct pressure cannot be applied to a bleeding site due to a protruding bone or an embedded object.
2. Pressure points are located between the site of injury and the heart where a main artery passes over a bone or underlying muscle mass (Figure 35-1).
3. Locate the pressure point and apply firm, steady pressure with the fingers or the heel of the hand.
4. If heavy bleeding still is not controlled and the patient may exsanguinate, a tourniquet may be used or a vas-

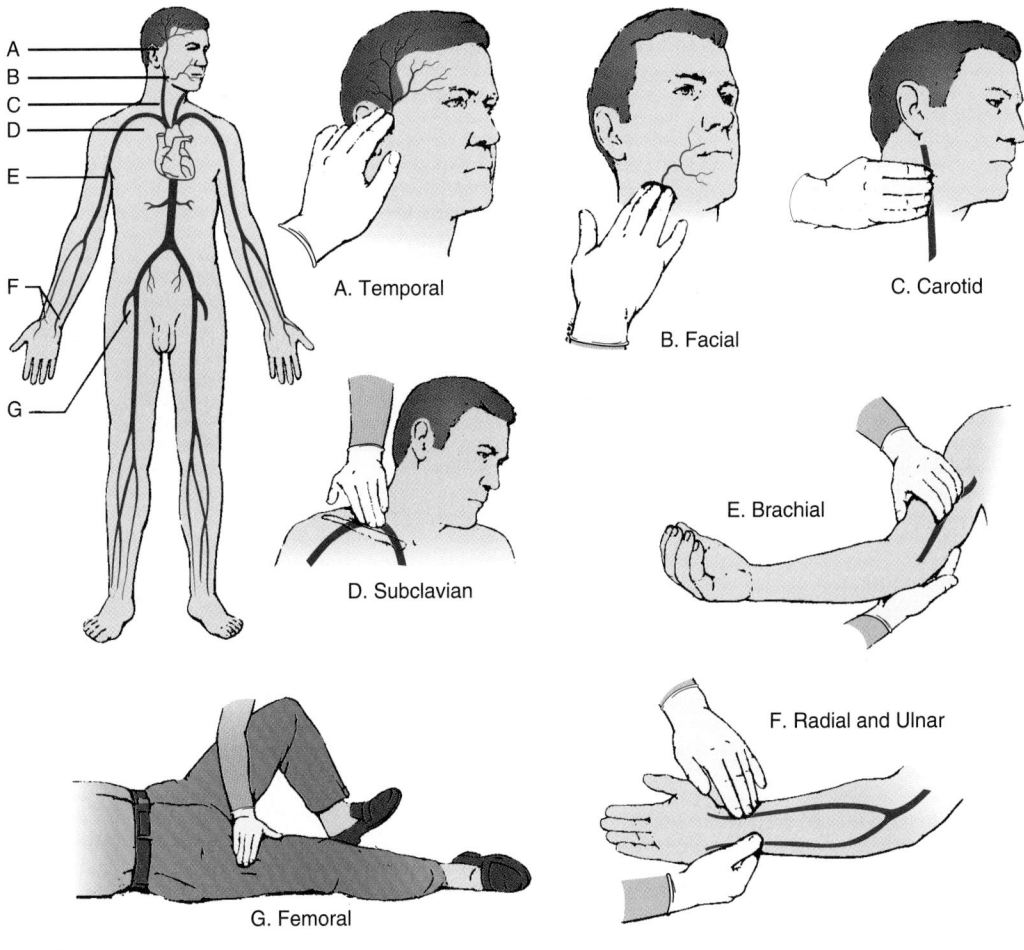

A

B

C

D

E

F

G

A. Temporal

B. Facial

C. Carotid

D. Subclavian

E. Brachial

F. Radial and Ulnar

G. Femoral

FIGURE 35-1 Pressure points for control of hemorrhage.

cular clamp can be applied to the artery. Apply a tourniquet only as a last resort.

Subsequent Assessment

1. Expose the wound; cut away clothing if necessary. Do not remove any impaled objects.
2. Assess for the presence of concomitant injuries.
3. Assess vascular status distal to the injury, and compare it to the uninjured extremity.
   a. Color of the injured extremity—pallor suggests poor arterial perfusion, and cyanosis suggests venous congestion.
   b. Test capillary refill time by depressing the fingernail until it blanches and seeing how long until the nail bed returns to pink. A capillary refill time greater than 2 seconds suggests decreased arterial capillary perfusion.
   c. Test pulses distal to the injury—generally, they should be full and strong.

4. Perform a neurologic assessment of the injured extremity to determine peripheral nerve insult, possibly caused by direct injury, compression, or edema.
   a. Sensory function—while the patient's eyes are closed, lightly touch the area distal to the injury.
   b. Motor function—have patient move extremity distal to the injury.
5. Determine tetanus immunization status.
6. History of the injury, including when and how the wound occurred. Any wound that is more than 6 hours old is considered at high risk for infection, and primary closure by suturing may not be an option.
7. Allergies to local anesthesia, epinephrine, and antibiotics.

General Interventions
Wound Preparation

1. Shave the area surrounding area of the wound, but only shave what is necessary. Eyebrows are never shaved.

2. Irrigate gently and copiously with isotonic sterile saline solution or sterile water to remove dirt and debris.
   a. A catheter-tip syringe may be used to create a hydraulic action.
   b. General rule—irrigate with 50 mL per inch of wound per hour of age of wound. Use more irrigant for grossly contaminated wounds.
   c. If the wound is grossly contaminated, the wound may need to be cleaned with a surgical scrub sponge and then irrigated.
   d. The wound may be anesthetized first if the patient cannot tolerate the wound irrigation and cleaning.
3. The wound is infiltrated with local anesthetic intradermally through the wound margins or by regional nerve block.
4. Devitalized tissue and foreign matter are removed—Devitalized tissue inhibits wound healing and enhances chance of bacterial infection.

Wound Closure

1. Closure by primary intent
   a. Wound is repaired without delay after the injury; yields the fastest healing.
   b. Primary closure may be with sutures, skin tapes, staples, or tissue adhesives.
2. Closure by secondary intent
   a. Wound is allowed to granulate on its own without surgical closure.
   b. Wound is cleansed and covered with a sterile dressing.
3. Closure by secondary intent with delayed closure
   a. Wound is cleansed and dressed.
   b. Patient returns in 3 to 4 days for definitive closure.

Wound Dressing

1. Dressing should be applied in three layers.
   a. The first layer is the contact layer. This should consist of a nonabsorbent hydrophilic dressing that will allow exudate to pass through to the second layer without wetting the contact layer. Examples of contact layer dressings are Adaptic, petroleum gauze, and Xeroform gauze.
   b. The second layer is the absorbent layer and is usually constructed of surgical dressing pad or 4 × 4 gauze dressings.
   c. The third layer is the outer wrap that holds the dressing in place. The outer wrap may consist of rolled gauze and tape.

Pharmacologic Interventions

1. Give antimicrobial treatment as directed, depending on how the injury occurred, age of wound, presence of soil—infection potential.
2. Give tetanus prophylaxis as indicated, based on patient's immunization status and wound. For inadequate primary immunization, both tetanus toxoid and tetanus immune globulin are given.

Tetanus Prophylaxis in Routine Wound Management—United States

History of Adsorbed Tetanus Toxoid (Doses)	Clean, Minor Wounds		All Other Wounds*	
	Td†	TIG	Td†	TIG
Unknown or < three	Yes	No	Yes	Yes
≥ Three†	No§	No	No‖	No

* Such as, but not limited to, wounds contaminated with dirt, feces, soil, saliva, etc.; puncture wounds; avulsions; and wounds resulting from missiles, crushing, burns, and frostbite.

† For children under 7 years old, DTP (DT, if pertussis vaccine is contraindicated) is preferred to tetanus toxoid alone. For persons 7 years old and older, Td is preferred to tetanus toxoid alone.

‡ If only three doses of *fluid* toxoid have been received, a fourth dose of toxoid, preferably an adsorbed toxoid, should be given.

§ Yes, if more than 10 years since last dose.

‖ Yes, if more than 5 years since last dose. (More frequent boosters are not needed and can accentuate side effects.)

(From *MMWR, Morbidity and Mortality Weekly Report*. [1986]. 34,405.)

Patient Education

1. Inform the patient that pain should subside in 24 hours.
2. Acetaminophen (Tylenol) or prescribed analgesic to be taken for the first 24 hours after a simple laceration.
3. If pain reappears, a wound infection may be suspected.
4. Recommend that the wound be elevated to limit accumulation of fluid in the wound's interstitial spaces.
   a. Elevate extremity for first 48 hours.
   b. Sleep with the head elevated if facial lacerations are present.
   c. Advise that health care provider be contacted if there is sudden or persistent onset of pain, fever/chills, bleeding, rapid swelling, foul odor, purulent fluid, or redness surrounding the wound.

Injuries to Bones and Joints

Injuries to bones and joints are common injuries. They are usually obvious injuries and may be dramatic in nature. However, rarely are these injuries life threatening. *Fractures* may be caused by direct trauma (eg, projectiles, crush injuries) or by indirect trauma (ie, bones being pulled apart or rotational forces). In addition, bones may be fractured due to pathologic reasons. A pathologic fracture is due to a weakness in the bone secondary to a disease process, such as metastatic cancer. For the classification of fractures, see p. 1001.

Other injuries include:

1. *Dislocation*—complete displacement or separation of a bone from its normal place of articulation. It may be associated with a tearing of the ligaments. The shoulder, elbow, fingers, hips, and ankles are the joints most frequently affected.
2. *Subluxation*—partial disruption of the articulating surfaces.

3. *Sprains*—injuries in which ligaments are partially torn or stretched. These types of injuries are usually caused by a twisting of a joint beyond its normal range of motion. The severity can range from mild to severe. The more seriously injured ligaments may resemble a fracture.
4. *Strains*—stretching or tearing of muscle and tendon fibers. Usually caused by overexertion or overextension.

Primary Assessment

1. Always ensure the adequacy of airway, breathing, and circulation before initiating treatment.
2. Occult blood loss into a closed space from the fracture may be significant enough to produce hypovolemic shock. Death by exsanguination can occur from pelvic and femoral fractures. Estimated blood loss from closed fractures in liters:
   a. Tibia—1.5 L
   b. Femur—2 L
   c. Pelvis—6 L
   d. Humerus—2 L
3. A fractured cervical spine, pelvic fracture, or fractured femur may produce life-threatening injuries. Posterior dislocations of the hip are life- and limb-threatening emergencies due to the potential for blood loss and the disruption in blood supply to the head of the femur. Unless this dislocation is promptly reduced, the patient may develop avascular necrosis of the femoral head and subsequently may require a hip replacement.

Primary Interventions

1. Support airway, breathing, and circulation if compromised.
2. Initiate IV line, and treat for shock if evident.
3. Protect injured part from movement or further trauma.

Subsequent Assessment

1. Seek information on the mechanism of injury.
   a. How did the injury occur?
   b. In what position was the limb after the injury?
   c. Did the person fall? How many feet did the person fall?
   d. What was the direction and amount of force? Certain musculoskeletal injuries commonly occur together.
2. Assess for the presence of concomitant injuries.
   a. A fractured calcaneus as the result of a fall from a great height may also include a compression fracture of the spine.
   b. A person with a fractured patella from a motor vehicle accident may also have a fractured or dislocated femur.
   c. A fractured pelvis may occur with lumbosacral spine fractures and bladder injuries.
3. Perform a neurovascular assessment to include the area above and below the injury.
   a. Assess for ischemia to the extremity.

(i) Pallor suggests poor arterial perfusion.
(ii) Cyanosis suggests venous congestion.
(iii) A capillary refill time greater than 2 seconds suggests decreased arterial capillary perfusion.
(iv) Palpate the pulse distal to the extremity—it should be full and strong.
(v) Loss of a pulse or coldness of the extremity distal to the injury indicates pressure on an artery and may require immediate medical intervention.
   b. Assess neurologic supply of the injured extremity to determine peripheral nerve insult. Damage to a peripheral nerve can be the result of a direct injury, compression, or edema.
   (i) Test sensory function—with the patient's eyes closed, lightly touch the area distal to the injury.
   (ii) Test motor function—have patient move extremity distal to the injury.
   (iii) Numbness or paralysis indicates pressure on the nerves and may require immediate medical interventions.
4. Examine the bones and joints adjacent to the injury. If there was enough force to produce one injury, there may be other injuries.
5. Signs and symptoms of fractures:
   a. Pain and tenderness over the fracture site.
   b. A grating or crepitus over the fracture site.
   c. Swelling, due to internal bleeding and edema.
   d. Deformity, unnatural position, or movement where there is no joint.
   e. Loss of use or guarding.
   f. Discoloration due to bleeding into the surrounding tissue.
   g. Shortening of an extremity or rotation of the extremity.
6. Signs and symptoms of dislocations:
   a. Loss of joint motion—the joint may appear "frozen."
   b. Obvious deformity—lump, ridge, or excavation.
   c. Severe pain.
7. Signs and symptoms of sprains:
   a. Pain in the joint area.
   b. Swelling.
   c. Limited use or movement.
   d. Discoloration.
8. Signs and symptoms of strains:
   a. Pain located in a muscle or its tendon, not a bone or a joint.
   b. Swelling is usually minimal.
9. Closely monitor vital signs.

General Interventions
Interventions for the Severely Injured Patient

1. Initiate an IV line, and start volume replacement with Ringer's lactate.
2. Immobilize the injury—this will prevent further damage and will help to relieve the pain.

3. Prepare the patient for the operating room for open reduction, closed reduction, internal fixation, and/or wound care.
4. Antibiotics may be started.

Other Interventions

1. Elevate to prevent or limit swelling.
2. Apply ice packs or cold compresses; ice should not be placed directly on the skin.
3. Cover open fractures with a sterile dressing.
4. Splint the extremity in as good alignment as possible until definitive care is complete. Immobilize the joint above and below the fracture.
5. Handle the part gently and as little as possible.
6. Provide pain management.

NURSING ALERT

If compartment syndrome is suspected, do not elevate limb above the level of the heart. This may decrease perfusion to the compromised extremity.

Assess for Compartment Syndrome

1. Increased pressure within an extremity resulting from bleeding and swelling into a closed space, causing pressure on vital structures.
2. The six P's (signs and symptoms) of compartment syndrome are:
   a. *Pain*—development of a different type of pain or the return of pain after treatment/splinting had caused pain relief
   b. *Pallor*—deterioration in skin color and an increase in the capillary refill time
   c. *Pulselessness*
   d. *Paresthesias*
   e. *Paralysis*—late sign
   f. *Puffiness*—late sign

SHOCK AND INTERNAL INJURIES

■ Shock

Shock is the common denominator in a wide variety of disease processes that presents as an immediate threat to life. Simply defined, *shock* is inadequate tissue perfusion. This inadequate tissue perfusion is the result of failure of one or more of the following: (1) the heart—pump failure, (2) blood volume, (3) arterial resistance vessels, and (4) the capacity of the venous beds. Any condition that significantly affects any of the above may precipitate a shock state.

Shock is classified as:
1. *Hypovolemic shock*—occurs when a significant amount of fluid is lost from the intravascular space. This fluid may be blood, plasma, or electrolyte solution. May result from hemorrhage, burns, or fluid shifts.
2. *Cardiogenic shock*—occurs when the heart fails as a pump. Primary causes of this failure are myocardial infarction, serious cardiac dysrhythmias, and myocardial

depression. Secondary causes include mechanical restriction of cardiac function or venous obstruction, such as occurs with cardiac tamponade, vena cava obstruction, or tension pneumothorax.
3. *Septic shock*—occurs as the result of bacteria and their products circulating in the blood. The primary cause is the vasoactive mediators released by gram-negative bacteria affecting almost every physiologic system. Any septic focus has the potential to produce septic shock.
4. Other types—include *spinal shock, neurogenic shock, anaphylactic shock,* and *hypoglycemic shock.*

Primary Assessment and Interventions

1. Rapid recognition and prompt intervention are essential to increase the chance of survival, because a downward spiral of physiologic responses will occur if shock is not treated.
2. The initial priorities in the assessment are the same for all types of shock.
   a. Is the airway open?
   b. Is the patient breathing?
   c. Is there a circulation problem?
3. Initiate immediate interventions as indicated.
   a. Resuscitate as necessary.
   b. Administer oxygen to augment oxygen-carrying capacity of arterial blood.
   c. Start cardiac monitoring.
   d. Control hemorrhage.

Subsequent Assessment

1. Assess level of consciousness.
   a. Important indicator of shock because it reflects cerebral perfusion.
   b. Changes may include:
      (i) Confusion
      (ii) Irritability
      (iii) Anxiety
      (iv) Agitation
      (v) Inability to concentrate
   c. Watch for increasing lethargy progressing to obtundation and coma, indicating progression of shock.
2. Monitor arterial blood pressure.
   a. If the patient can compensate for the shock state, the blood pressure may initially rise approximately 20%. A significant change in blood pressure may not occur until late.
   b. Narrowing pulse pressure—early in shock, the diastolic pressure may rise due to an initial vasoconstriction produced by release of catecholamines from the sympathetic nervous system.
   c. Fall in the systolic pressure—there is no absolute value in blood pressure that indicates a shock state. It is the deviation from normal that is important. However, it is generally accepted that a systolic pressure below 80 mm Hg or a mean arterial pressure below 60 mm Hg is indicative of shock.

3. Pulse quality and rate change.
   a. The rate usually is increased.
   b. Weak, thready pulse due to decreased cardiac output and increased peripheral vascular resistance.
4. Assess urinary output.
   a. A decrease in renal blood flow or pressure will result in decreased urinary output.
   b. Ideally in an adult, the urine output should be 50 mL/h. An output of less than 25 mL/h may indicate shock.
5. Assess capillary perfusion.
   a. Pale, ashen, mottled, cold, and sweaty skin indicates potent vasoconstriction.
   b. A capillary refill time greater than 2 seconds indicates vasoconstriction.
6. Also assess for:
   a. Subjective feeling of impending doom.
   b. Metabolic acidosis due to anaerobic metabolism within the cells.
   c. Excessive thirst.
   d. Hyperthermia if septic shock.

General Interventions

1. Administer O_2 to maintain the PaO_2 at 80 to 100 torr. This will augment oxygen-carrying capacity of arterial blood.
   a. One hundred percent oxygen by nonrebreather face mask.
   b. Intubation if the patient is unable to manage secretions or is ventilating poorly.
   c. If intubated, the patient may be hyperventilated to help control the acidosis.
2. Fluid resuscitation.
   a. Two large-bore IV lines should be established.
   b. Ringer's lactate is the initial fluid choice. Normal saline is the second choice, because hyperchloremic acidosis may develop if massive amount of normal saline is infused.
   c. Rate of infusion depends on severity of blood loss and clinical evidence of hypovolemia.
   d. Fresh whole blood is infused when there is massive blood loss.
   e. Additional platelets and coagulation factors are given when large amounts of blood are needed, because replacement blood is deficient in clotting factors.
   f. Warm the blood (commercial warmer or basin of warm water)—massive blood replacement has a cooling effect that can cause cardiac dysrhythmias, paradoxical hypotension, decreased oxyhemoglobin dissociation, or cardiac arrest.
3. Insert an indwelling urinary catheter.
   a. Record urinary output every 15 to 30 minutes.
   b. Urinary volume reveals adequacy of kidney and visceral perfusion.
4. Apply pneumatic antishock garment, also known as military antishock trousers (MAST), per local protocol—to control internal bleeding and to facilitate blood flow to vital areas (Figure 35-2). (Its primary use is for hypovolemic shock secondary to bleeding in the lower part of the body.)
5. Maintain patient in supine position with the legs elevated. (This position is contraindicated in patients with head injuries.)

6. Electrocardiogram (ECG) monitoring—dysrhythmias may contribute to shock.
7. Maintain ongoing nursing surveillance of total patient—blood pressure, heart rate, respiratory rate, skin temperature, color, central venous pressure, arterial blood gases, urinary output, ECG, hematocrit, hemoglobin, coagulation profiles, and electrolytes—to assess patient response to treatment.
8. Immobilize fractures to minimize blood loss.
9. Maintain normothermia.
   a. Too much heat produces vasodilatation, which counteracts the body's compensatory mechanism of vasoconstriction and also increases fluid loss through perspiration.
   b. A patient who is in septic shock should be kept cool, because high fever will increase the cellular metabolic effects of shock.
10. Pharmacologic interventions:
    a. Inotropes are used in cardiogenic shock.
       (i) Isoproterenol (Isuprel)
       (ii) Digoxin (Lanoxin)
       (iii) Dobutamine (Dobutrex)

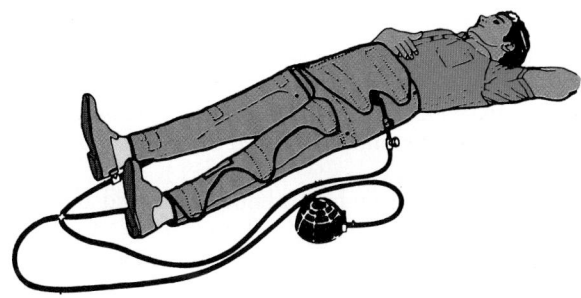

FIGURE 35-2 The military anti-shock trouser (MAST) is a garment designed to correct internal bleeding and hypovolemia by the application of counter pressure around the legs and abdomen. This creates an artificial peripheral resistance and helps sustain coronary perfusion. It should be applied as soon as possible after injury, preferably before the patient is transferred to the emergency department. (Courtesy of David Clark Co., Inc., Worcester, MA.)

b. Vasopressors.
   (i) Dopamine (Intropin)
   (ii) Norepinephrine (Levophed)
   (iii) Metaraminol (Aramine)
c. Antibiotics—broad spectrum for septic shock.

Abdominal Injuries

Abdominal injuries account for a large percentage of trauma-related injuries and deaths. The visceral organs contained within the abdomen can be classified as either hollow or solid. Damage to a hollow organ can result in acute peritonitis leading to shock within a few hours, and damage to a solid organ can result in lethal hemorrhage. Abdominal injuries may be classified as either penetrating or blunt.

Penetrating abdominal injury—usually the result of gunshot wounds or stab wounds. The mechanism that caused the penetrating abdominal trauma may cross the diaphragm and enter the chest. The opposite can also occur.

Blunt abdominal injury—usually caused by motor vehicle accidents or falls. Trauma to the abdomen is frequently associated with extra-abdominal injuries (ie, chest, head, and extremity injuries) and severe concomitant trauma to multiple intraperitoneal organs. Causes more delayed complications, especially if there is injury to liver, spleen, or blood vessels, which can lead to substantial blood loss into the peritoneal cavity.

Primary Assessment and Interventions

1. Assess airway, breathing, and circulation.
2. Initiate resuscitation as indicated.
3. Control bleeding, and prepare to treat shock.
4. If there is an impaled object in the abdomen, leave it there. Stabilize the object in place with bulky dressings along the sides of the object.

Subsequent Assessment

1. Obtain a history of the mechanism of the injury, type of weapon, and estimated amount of blood loss.
   a. If the patient was stabbed, how long was the blade?
   b. Was the person who stabbed the patient a man or a woman?
      (i) Men usually hold a knife underhand and stab/thrust upward.
      (ii) Women usually will stab/thrust downward with an overhand motion.
   c. Time of onset of symptoms.
   d. Passenger location (driver frequently sustains spleen/liver rupture).
2. Inspect the abdomen for obvious signs of injury (penetrating injury, bruises).
3. Evaluate for signs and symptoms of hemorrhage—frequently accompanies abdominal injury, especially if the liver and spleen have been traumatized.

4. Note tenderness, rebound tenderness, guarding, rigidity, and spasm.
   a. Press the area of maximal tenderness (let the patient point to the area).
   b. Remove the fingers quickly to check for rebound tenderness; pain at suspected point indicates peritoneal irritation.
5. Ask about referred pain: Kehr's sign—pain radiating to the left shoulder is a sign of blood beneath the left diaphragm; pain in right shoulder can result from laceration of liver.
6. Look for increasing abdominal distention. Measure abdominal girth at umbilical level early in assessment—serves as a baseline from which changes can be determined.
7. Auscultate for bowel sounds—a silent abdomen accompanies peritoneal irritation.
8. Auscultate for loss of dullness over solid organs (liver, spleen)—indicates presence of free air; dullness over regions normally containing gas may indicate presence of blood.
9. Look for chest injuries, which frequently accompany intra-abdominal injuries.
10. Cullen's sign, a slight bluish discoloration around the navel, is a sign of hemoperitoneum.
11. Pain is a poor indicator of the extent of the abdominal injury. Rebound tenderness and boardlike rigidity are indicative of a significant intra-abdominal injury.
12. A rectal examination should be done on all patients and a pelvic examination on all female patients. The presence of blood on a gloved hand is indicative of trauma.
13. Continually assess vital signs, urinary output, central venous pressure readings, hematocrit values, and neurologic status. Tachypnea, tachycardia, and hypotension may be clues to intra-abdominal bleeding.

General Interventions

1. Goals are to control bleeding, maintain blood volume, and prevent infection.
2. Keep the patient quiet and on the stretcher, because movement may fragment or dislodge a clot in a large vessel and produce massive hemorrhage.
3. Cut the clothing away from the wound.
4. Count the number of wounds.
5. Look for entrance and exit wounds.
6. If the patient is comatose, immobilize the cervical spine until after cervical films are taken and cleared.
7. Apply compression to external bleeding wounds and occlusion of chest wounds.
8. Insert two large-bore IV lines and infuse Ringer's lactate. If possible, one of the lines should be in a central venous location.

9. Insert a nasogastric tube to decompress the abdomen. This will serve to empty the stomach, relieve gastric distention, and facilitate abdominal assessment. In addition, if blood is found, it may indicate stomach injury or esophageal injury.

10. Cover protruding abdominal viscera; do not attempt to replace the protruding organs into the abdomen. Use sterile saline dressings to protect viscera from drying.

11. Cover open wounds with dry dressings.

12. Withhold oral fluids to prevent increased peristalsis and vomiting.

13. Insert an indwelling urethral catheter to ascertain the presence of hematuria and to monitor urinary output. If a fracture of the pelvis is suspected, a catheter should not be placed until the integrity of the urethra is ensured.

14. Pharmacologic interventions
    a. Tetanus prophylaxis.
    b. Broad-spectrum antibiotics, because bacterial contamination is a frequent complication (depending on history and nature of wound).

15. Prepare for peritoneal lavage when there is uncertainty about intraperitoneal bleeding. See Procedure Guidelines 35-4.

16. Prepare for surgery if the patient shows evidence of unexplained shock, unstable vital signs, peritoneal irritation, bowel protrusion or evisceration, significant penetrating injury, significant gastrointestinal bleeding, or peritoneal air.

17. Prepare the patient for diagnostic procedures.
    a. Catheterization and urinalysis—as a guide to possible urinary tract injury and to monitor urine output.
    b. Serial hemoglobin and hematocrit levels—their trend reflects presence or absence of bleeding.
    c. Complete blood count—white blood cell count is generally elevated with trauma.
    d. Serum amylase elevation usually indicates pancreatic injury or perforations of gastrointestinal tract.
    e. Computed tomography scans permit detailed evaluation of abdominal and retroperitoneal injuries.
    f. Abdominal and chest x-rays may reveal free air beneath diaphragm, indicating ruptured hollow viscus.

PROCEDURE GUIDELINES 35-4   PERITONEAL LAVAGE

Peritoneal lavage is a technique of irrigation of the peritoneal cavity and examination of the irrigating fluid to evaluate the effects of trauma to the abdomen.

EQUIPMENT

Peritoneal dialysis tray
Sterile solution (lactated Ringer's solution)
IV tubing; IV pole

Peritoneal dialysis catheter (multiple perforations)
Local skin anesthetic; sterile gloves

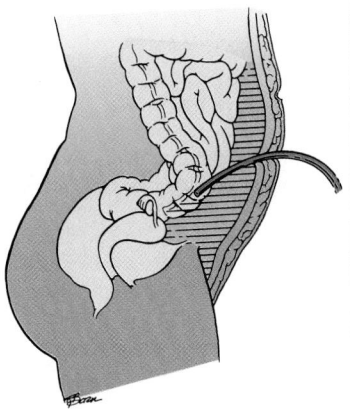

Peritoneal lavage.

continued

PROCEDURE GUIDELINES 35-4   PERITONEAL LAVAGE *CONTINUED*

PROCEDURE

Nursing Action	Rationale
PREPARATORY PHASE	
1. Explain the procedure to the patient; see that the consent form has been signed.	
2. Insert indwelling catheter into the bladder.	2. To prevent puncture of urinary bladder.
3. Prepare the abdomen as for surgery.	3. To minimize or eliminate surface bacteria and decrease the possibility of wound contamination and infection.
4. Place the patient in a supine position.	
5. Fill the IV tubing with solution using aseptic technique.	
PERFORMANCE PHASE (BY THE PHYSICIAN)	
1. The skin is infiltrated 2–3 cm (0.7–1.2 inches) below the umbilicus in the midline with local anesthetic.	1. The midline area is relatively avascular. Epinephrine may be injected with local anesthetic to produce capillary constriction and prevent a false-positive tap.
2. A small vertical incision is made at the chosen site.	
3. Bleeding vessels are carefully ligated.	3. Ligation of vessels helps avoid a false-positive lavage.
4. The peritoneum is opened under direct vision and the peritoneal catheter is inserted into the peritoneal cavity, *OR*	4. There are various methods (open or percutaneous) of introducing the catheter into the peritoneal space.
5. A needle is passed intra-abdominally, a flexible wire is passed through the needle, and a catheter is guided over the wire.	
6. A syringe is attached to the catheter, and the peritoneal cavity is aspirated.	6. If more than 10 mL of blood is obtained or the fluid contains bile, feces, or particulate matter, the test is considered positive and the patient is prepared for immediate laparotomy (incision into abdominal cavity).
7. If no blood (or less than 10 mL) is present, the catheter is attached to the IV tubing; 500–1000 mL of solution is infused into the peritoneal cavity through the IV tubing attached to the dialysis catheter.	7. If not contraindicated by the patient's condition, he or she may be turned from side to side to ensure that the solution reaches all parts of the abdominal cavity.
8. After the solution is infused, the empty IV bag is removed from the pole and lowered below the abdominal level (near the floor).	8. Lowering the bag creates a siphon effect to drain the excess fluid. As much of the fluid as possible is siphoned out of the peritoneal cavity by gravity.
9. The peritoneal dialysis catheter is removed, and the wound is closed (unless laparotomy is necessary).	
10. The fluid recovered from the peritoneal cavity is examined visually and is usually sent to the laboratory for cell counts and microscopic inspection of spun-down sediment.	
INTERPRETATION OF LAVAGE FLUID	
1. Clear fluid indicates a lack of significant intraperitoneal bleeding.	1. This indicates a negative test.
2. Criteria for positive results: Aspiration of free blood from peritoneal cavity Red blood cells > 100,000 per mm³ White blood cells > 500 per mm³ Amylase > 110 IU/dL Presence of bile, bacteria, or fecal or food particles in lavage fluid	2. If the test is positive, a laparotomy is usually done. Indeterminate or equivocal results merit monitoring and investigation.
FOLLOW-UP PHASE	
1. Assess the patient for complications.	1. Complications include visceral perforation, wound hematoma, perforated bowel, puncture of bladder, laceration of major vessels, infection.
2. Watch the patient closely for any type of deterioration.	2. Repeated physical examinations of the abdomen should be performed when intra-abdominal injury is suspected.

Multiple Injuries

The patient with multiple injuries requires rapid and definitive interventions during the first hour after the trauma to increase chance of survival; this first hour has been called the "golden hour." During this time, multiple assessments and interventions may be performed simultaneously by the health care team.

Primary Assessment and Interventions

Airway

1. Assume a cervical spine injury, and open the airway using the jaw-thrust technique without head tilt.
2. Apply suction to clear the trachea and bronchial tree. Remove debris from mouth (ie, broken teeth, mucus).
3. Insert an oropharyngeal airway—to prevent occlusion by the tongue, avoid flexing the head.
4. Prepare for endotracheal intubation if adequate airway cannot be maintained.
5. If upper airway trauma or edema exists, a cricothyroidotomy may be indicated.

Breathing

1. Note the character and symmetry of chest wall motion and pattern of breathing. Assess for open wounds, deformity, and flail segments.
2. Auscultate the lungs, and assess for tracheal deviation. If a tension pneumothorax is present, the trachea will shift from the midline.
3. Ask the conscious patient if experiencing difficulty in breathing or chest pain with breathing.
4. Administer oxygen by 100% nonrebreather mask, or assist the patient's ventilations by bag-valve mask to alleviate hypoxia.
5. Suspect serious intrathoracic injuries if respiratory distress continues after adequate airway has been established.
6. Assess the overall effectiveness of ventilations.

Circulation

1. Assess cardiac function, and treat cardiac arrest (hypoxia, metabolic acidosis, and chest trauma may precipitate cardiac arrest).
   a. For cardiac arrest, start closed chest compression and ventilation.
   b. If the chest wall is unstable (flail chest), emergency thoracotomy and manual compression may be necessary.
2. Control hemorrhage.
   a. Apply pressure over bleeding points if hemorrhage is overt.
   b. Expect significant blood loss in patients with fractures to the shaft of the femur, multiple fractures, or pelvic trauma.
   c. Use tourniquet(s) for massive arterial bleeding from extremities that cannot be halted with pressure.
   d. Prepare for immediate surgical intervention if patient is bleeding internally.

3. Palpate the carotid pulse, and note its rate and quality. In addition, assess the femoral and radial pulses to determine an approximate systolic pressure.
   a. If the carotid pulse is present, the systolic pressure is at least 60 mm Hg.
   b. If the femoral pulse is present, the systolic pressure is at least 70 mm Hg.
   c. If the radial pulse is present, the systolic pressure is at least 80 mm Hg.
4. Prevent and treat hypovolemic shock.
   a. Insert at least two (sometimes four) IV lines, one above diaphragm and one below. Use venous cutdown if necessary.
   b. Initiate a central venous catheter to monitor the patient's response to fluid infusion—to prevent fluid overload and as a route for fluid infusion.
   c. Fluid resuscitation—Ringer's lactate or normal saline is given for volume replacement until blood is available.
   d. Administer blood—massive transfusions have a cooling effect that can cause cardiac irritability and arrest; blood should be warmed.
5. Note presence or absence of pulses in fractured extremities.

Neurologic

1. Assess level of responsiveness, pupil size and reactivity, motor power, and reflexes.
2. Determine a Glasgow Coma Score as a baseline (see p. 446).
3. If signs of increased intracranial pressure exist, intracranial pressure monitoring may be instituted.

Subsequent Assessment and Interventions

1. The goals are rapid determination of the extent of the injuries and treatment prioritization.
2. Monitor ECG—to detect life-threatening dysrhythmias.
3. Insert indwelling urethral catheter, and monitor urinary output to aid in diagnosis of shock and monitor effectiveness of therapy. Do not force the catheter—the patient may have a ruptured urethra.
4. Perform an ongoing clinical evaluation to observe for improvement or deterioration, such as changes in vital signs, improvement in level of responsiveness, skin warmth, and speed of capillary filling.
5. Prepare for immediate surgical intervention if the patient does not respond to fluids or blood. Inability to restore blood pressure and circulatory volume in the patient usually indicates major internal bleeding.
6. Splint fractures to prevent further trauma to soft tissues and blood vessels and to relieve pain.
7. Examine the patient for abdominal pain, muscular rigidity, tenderness, rebound tenderness, diminished bowel sounds, hypotension, and shock.
8. Prepare for peritoneal lavage to assess for intraperitoneal bleeding.

9. Draw blood for laboratory studies (type and crossmatching, hemoglobin, hematocrit, baseline complete blood count, electrolytes, blood urea nitrogen (BUN), glucose, prothrombin time).
10. Insert a nasogastric tube to prevent vomiting and aspiration.
11. Prepare for laparotomy if the patient shows continuing signs of hemorrhage and deterioration.
12. Continue to monitor urinary output every 30 minutes—reflects cardiac output and state of perfusion of vital organs.
13. Assess for hematuria and oliguria.
14. Evaluate the patient for other injuries, and institute appropriate treatment, including tetanus immunization.
15. Perform a more thorough physical examination after resuscitation and management of the aforementioned priorities.

ENVIRONMENTAL EMERGENCIES

■ Heat Exhaustion

Heat exhaustion is the inadequacy or the collapse of peripheral circulation due to volume and electrolyte depletion. Heat exhaustion is one condition in the spectrum of heat-related illnesses, including heat rash, heat edema, heat cramps, and heat syncope. Untreated heat exhaustion may progress to heatstroke.

Primary Assessment and Interventions

1. Expect the patient to be alert without significant cardiorespiratory or neurologic compromise.
2. If vital functions are significantly impaired, suspect secondary condition, such as myocardial infarction or stroke.

Subsequent Assessment

1. Obtain history of headache, fatigue, dizziness, muscle cramping, and nausea.
2. Inspect skin—usually pale, ashen, and moist.
3. The temperature may be normal, slightly elevated, or as high as 104°F (40°C).
4. Measure vital signs for hypotension, orthostatic changes, tachycardia, and tachypnea.
5. The patient will be awake but may give a history of syncope or confusion.
6. Laboratory analysis will show hemoconcentration and hyponatremia (if sodium depletion is the primary problem) or hypernatremia (if water depletion is the primary problem).
7. The ECG may show dysrhythmias without evidence of infarction.

General Interventions

1. Move the patient to a cool environment, and remove all the clothing.
2. Position the patient supine with the feet slightly elevated.

3. If the patient complains of nausea or vomiting, do not give fluids by mouth.
4. Start an IV line with Ringer's lactate or normal saline until electrolyte results are confirmed.
5. Monitor the patient for changes in the cardiac rhythm and vital signs. Vital signs should be taken at least every 15 minutes until the patient is stable.
6. Provide fans and cool sponge baths as cooling methods.
7. Provide patient education.
   a. Advise the patient to avoid immediate reexposure to high temperatures; the patient may remain hypersensitive to high temperatures for a considerable length of time.
   b. Emphasize the importance of maintaining an adequate fluid intake, wearing loose clothing, and reducing activity in hot weather.
   c. Athletes should monitor fluid losses, replace fluids, and use a gradual approach to physical conditioning, allowing sufficient time for acclimatization.

> **NURSING ALERT**
>
> **Identify those at increased risk for heat exhaustion and heatstroke so preventive measures can be taken.** Risk factors include such underlying conditions as cardiovascular disease, alcohol abuse, malnutrition, diabetes, skin diseases, and major burn scarring; very young or very old age; such drugs as anticholinergics, phenothiazines, diuretics, antihistamines, antidepressants, and beta blockers; and such behaviors as working outdoors, wearing inappropriate clothing, inadequate fluid intake, and living in poor environmental conditions.

■ Heatstroke

Heatstroke is a medical emergency that can result in significant morbidity and mortality. It is defined as the combination of hyperpyrexia (105°F [40.6°C]) and neurologic symptoms. It is caused by a shutdown or failure of the heat-regulating mechanisms of the body.

Primary Assessment and Interventions

1. Assess airway, breathing, and circulation.
2. Level of consciousness may be altered.
3. Expect to intervene immediately if cardiovascular collapse occurs.

Subsequent Assessment

1. Obtain a history from accompanying person about environmental conditions, activity, underlying health, and medications that may have contributed to heatstroke.
2. Perform a neurologic assessment.
   a. Initially, the patient may exhibit bizarre behavior or irritability. This may progress to confusion, combativeness, deliriousness, and coma.
   b. Other central nervous system (CNS) disturbances include tremors, seizures, fixed and dilated pupils, and decerebrate or decorticate posturing.

3. Assess vital signs.
   a. Temperature greater than 105°F (40.6°C).
   b. Hypotension.
   c. Rapid pulse; may be bounding or weak.
   d. Rapid respirations.
4. The skin may appear flushed and hot; in early heatstroke, the skin may be moist, but, as the heatstroke progresses, the skin will become dry as the body loses its ability to sweat.
5. Arterial blood gases show metabolic acidosis.

General Interventions

> **NURSING ALERT**
>
> Once the diagnosis of heatstroke is made or suspected, it is imperative to reduce patient's temperature.

1. Provide cooling measures.
   a. Reduce the core (internal) temperature to 102°F (39°C) as rapidly as possible.
   b. Evaporative cooling is the most efficient. Spray tepid water on the skin while electric fans are used to blow continuously over the patient to augment heat dissipation.
   c. Apply ice packs to neck, groin, axillae, and scalp (areas of maximal heat transfer).
   d. Soak sheets/towels in ice water and place on patient, using fans to accelerate evaporation/cooling rate.
   e. Immerse patient in cold water (controversial because it may result in peripheral vasoconstriction and may decrease the body's heat loss).
   f. If the temperature fails to decrease, initiate core cooling: iced saline lavage of stomach, cool fluid peritoneal dialysis, cool fluid bladder irrigation, or cool fluid chest irrigations.
   g. Place the patient on a hypothermia blanket.
   h. Discontinue active cooling when the temperature reaches 102°F (39°C). In most cases, this will reduce the chance of overcooling, because the body temperature will continue to fall after cessation of cooling.
2. Oxygenate patient to supply tissue needs that are exaggerated by the hypermetabolic condition: 100% nonrebreather mask or intubate the patient if necessary to support a failing cardiorespiratory system.
3. Monitor condition.
   a. Monitor and record the core temperature continually during cooling process to avoid hypothermia; also, hyperthermia may recur spontaneously within 3 to 4 hours.
   b. Monitor the vital signs continuously, including ECG, central venous pressure, blood pressure, pulse, and respiratory rate.
   c. Perform frequent (every 30 minutes) neurologic assessments.
4. Replace fluids.

   a. Start IV infusion using Ringer's lactate to replace fluid losses, maintain adequate circulation, and facilitate cooling.
   b. At least one IV line should be a central line.
   c. Fluid replacement is based on the patient's response and laboratory results.

> **GERONTOLOGIC ALERT**
>
> Vigorous fluid replacement in the elderly or those with underlying cardiovascular disease may cause pulmonary edema.

5. Other measures:
   a. Dialysis for renal failure.
   b. Diuretics such as mannitol (Osmitrol) to promote diuresis.
   c. Anticonvulsant agents to control seizures.
   d. Potassium for hypokalemia and sodium bicarbonate to correct metabolic acidosis, depending on laboratory results.
   e. Antipyretics are not useful in treating heatstroke. They may contribute to the complications of coagulopathy and hepatic damage.
   f. Intense shivering may be controlled by diazepam (Valium). Shivering will generate heat and increase the metabolic rate.
   g. Patients with depleted clotting factors may be treated with platelets or fresh frozen plasma.
6. Insert a Foley catheter with a urimeter, and measure urinary output at least hourly—acute tubular necrosis is a complication of heatstroke.
7. Perform continuous ECG monitoring and frequent cardiovascular assessments for possible ischemia, infarction, and dysrhythmias.
8. Perform serial laboratory testing (clotting parameters, electrolytes, glucose, and serum enzymes).
9. The patient should be admitted to an intensive care unit; complications can occur including heart failure, cardiovascular collapse, hepatic failure, renal failure, disseminated intravascular coagulation, and rhabdomyolysis.
10. Monitor the patient for the development of seizures, and provide for a safe environment in case of seizures.

Frostbite

Frostbite is trauma due to exposure to freezing temperatures that cause actual freezing of the tissue fluids in the cell and intracellular spaces, resulting in vascular damage. The areas of the body most likely to develop frostbite are the earlobes, cheeks, nose, hands, and feet. Frostbite may be classified as frostnip (initial response to cold, reversible), superficial frostbite, and deep frostbite.

Primary Assessment and Interventions

1. If not alert, assess airway, breathing, and circulation.
2. Deficits may indicate coexisting hypothermia or underlying condition.

3. Protect frostbitten tissue while performing other interventions.

Subsequent Assessment
Frostnip
1. History of gradual onset.
2. Skin appears white.
3. Numb, painfree.

Superficial Frostbite
1. Damage is limited to the skin and subcutaneous tissue.
2. The skin will appear white and waxy.
3. On palpation, the skin will feel stiff but the underlying tissue will be pliable, soft, and have its normal "bounce."
4. Sensation is absent.

Deep Frostbite
1. Skin will appear white, yellow-white, or mottled blue-white.
2. On palpation, the surface will feel frozen and the underlying tissue will feel frozen and hard.
3. The affected part is completely insensitive to touch.

General Interventions
1. Frostnip may be treated by placing a warm hand over the chilled area.
2. Leave the frostbitten area alone until definitive rewarming is undertaken. Pad the extremity to prevent damage from trauma.

> **NURSING ALERT**
>
> Once definitive rewarming of a frostbitten extremity has started, it must not be stopped. Refreezing of a partially thawed extremity reverses ice crystal formation in tissues and increases tissue damage and loss.

3. Handle the part gently to avoid further mechanical injury.
4. Remove all constricting clothing that can impair circulation, including watchbands and rings.
5. Rewarming:
   a. Rewarm the extremity by controlled and rapid rewarming. Rewarm with a temperature of 98.6°F to 104°F (37°C to 40°C) in a fairly large tepid water bath where the part can be fully immersed without touching the side or bottom. If clothing, socks, or gloves are frozen to the extremity, they should be left on and removed after rewarming.
   b. More warm water may be added to the container by removing some cooled water and adding warm water.
   c. Slow rewarming is less effective and may increase tissue damage.
   d. Dry heat is not recommended for rewarming.
   e. The rewarming procedure may take 20 to 30 minutes.
   f. Rewarming is complete when the area is warm to the touch and pink or flushed.
   g. Do not rub or massage a frostbitten extremity. The ice crystals in the tissue will lacerate delicate tissue.
6. Pharmacologic interventions:
   a. Narcotics for pain control.
   b. Antibiotics if there is an open wound.
   c. Tetanus prophylaxis.
7. Protect the thawed part from infection. Large blisters may develop in 1 hour to a few days after rewarming; these blisters should not be broken.
8. Place sterile gauze or cotton between affected fingers/toes to absorb moisture.
9. Use strict aseptic technique during dressing changes. Frostbite injuries make the patient susceptible to infection. Make sure any dressings are loosely applied.
10. Elevate the part to help control swelling.
11. Use a foot cradle to prevent contact with bedding if the feet are involved—prevents further tissue injury.
12. Perform a physical assessment to look for concomitant injury (soft tissue injury, dehydration, alcohol coma, fat embolism due to fracture, immobility).
13. Restore electrolyte balance; dehydration and hypovolemia occur frequently in frostbite victims.
14. Whirlpool bath for the affected extremity—to aid circulation, débride dead tissue, and help prevent infection.
15. Escharotomy (incision through the eschar)—to prevent further tissue damage, allow for normal circulation, and permit joint motion.
16. Fasciotomy (incision in fascia to release pressure on the muscles, nerves, blood vessels)—to treat compartment syndrome.
17. Encourage hourly active motion of the affected digits to promote maximum restoration of function and to prevent contractures.
18. Advise patient not to use tobacco because of the vasoconstrictive effects of nicotine, which further reduce the already deficient blood supply to injured tissues.
19. Perform serial laboratory testing (urinalysis and serum enzymes) to monitor for the complications of rhabdomyolysis and subsequent renal failure.

Hypothermia

Hypothermia is a condition in which the core (internal) temperature of the body is less than 95°F (35°C) as a result of exposure to cold. In response to a decreased core temperature, the body will attempt to produce or conserve more heat by (1) shivering, which produces heat through muscular activity; (2) peripheral vasoconstriction, to decrease heat loss; and (3) raising the basal metabolic rate. Hypothermia may be classified as mild, moderate, or severe.

> **GERONTOLOGIC ALERT**
>
> The elderly are at greater risk for hypothermia due to altered compensatory mechanisms.

Primary Assessment and Interventions

NURSING ALERT

Extreme caution should be used in moving or transporting hypothermia patients, because the heart is near fibrillation threshold.

1. Assess airway and breathing
   a. Spontaneous respirations may be extremely slow and imperceptible.
   b. Assist breathing and oxygenation with supplemental O_2 at 100% or a bag-valve mask device.
   c. If intubation is necessary, extreme caution should be used, because ventricular fibrillation may be precipitated.
2. Assess circulation.
   a. If the body temperature falls below 86°F (30°C), the heart sounds may not be audible even if the heart is still beating. Tissues conduct sound poorly at low temperatures.
   b. Blood pressure readings may be extremely difficult to hear, because cold tissue conducts sound waves poorly.
   c. Pupil reflexes may be blocked by a decrease in cerebral blood flow, so the pupils may appear fixed and dilated.
   d. A patient with a heartbeat may present like a patient in cardiac arrest with fixed dilated pupils, no pulse, and no blood pressure. Provide CPR until further evaluation through ECG and hemodynamic monitoring.

Subsequent Assessment

1. There is progressive deterioration marked by apathy, poor judgment, ataxia, dysarthria, drowsiness, and, eventually, coma.
2. Speech is slow and may be slurred.
3. Shivering may be suppressed below a temperature of 90°F (32.2°C).
4. Cardiac dysrhythmias—cold disrupts the conduction system of the heart, and a variety of dysrhythmias may be seen. A hypothermic heart is extremely susceptible to ventricular fibrillation. Very cold hearts do not respond to drugs or defibrillation.
5. The heartbeat and the blood pressure may be so weak that the peripheral pulsations become undetectable.
6. Urine output may increase in response to peripheral vasoconstriction—cold diuresis.
7. Initial tachypnea followed by slow and shallow respirations, possibly two or three a minute in severe hypothermia.
8. Fruity or acetone odor to the breath, because the body may be metabolizing fat as a result of decreased insulin levels.

General Interventions

Goal: rewarm without precipitating cardiac dysrhythmias.

Supportive Measures

1. Handle the patient carefully and gently—to avoid triggering ventricular fibrillation.
2. Continuously monitor core temperatures with a low reading rectal thermometer.
3. Continuously monitor ECG. Because you may be unable to obtain a pulse due to the hypothermia, rely on the cardiac monitor to determine the need for CPR.
4. Monitor the patient's condition through vital signs, central venous pressure, urinary output, arterial blood gas values, and blood chemistry determinations.
5. Maintain an arterial line for recording blood pressure and to facilitate blood sampling—allows rapid detection of acid–base disturbances and assessment of adequacy of ventilation and oxygenation.
6. Start IV therapy with normal saline. Ringer's lactate is not recommended, because the cold liver may not be able to metabolize the lactate.

Rewarming Techniques

The type of rewarming depends on the degree of hypothermia. Rewarming should continue until the core temperature is 93.2°F (34°C). If the patient is in cardiac arrest, rewarming should continue until a temperature of 89.6°F (32°C) has been reached. Death in hypothermia is defined as a failure to revive after rewarming.

1. Passive external rewarming (temperature above 82.4°F [28°C]).
   a. Remove all the wet or cold clothing, and replace with warm clothing.
   b. Provide insulation by wrapping the patient in several blankets.
   c. Provide warmed fluids to drink.
   d. Disadvantage: slow process.
2. Active external rewarming (temperature above 82.4°F [28°C]).
   a. Provide external heat for the patient—warm hot water bottles to the armpits, neck, or groin. (Do not apply hot water bottles directly to the skin.)
   b. Warm water immersion.
   c. Disadvantages:
      (i) Causes peripheral vasodilation, returning cool blood to the core, causing an initial lowering of the core temperature.
      (ii) Acidosis due to the "washing out" of lactic acid from the peripheral tissues.
      (iii) An increase in the metabolic demands before the heart is warmed to meet these needs.
3. Active core rewarming (temperature below 82.4°F [28°C]).
   a. Inhalation of warmed, humidified oxygen by mask or ventilator.
   b. Warmed IV fluids.
   c. Warmed gastric lavage.
   d. Peritoneal dialysis with warmed standard dialysis solution.
   e. Mediastinal irrigation through open thoracotomy has been used successfully but has serious complications.

f. Cardiopulmonary bypass.

g. Disadvantage of active core rewarming is the invasiveness of the procedures.

TOXICOLOGIC EMERGENCIES

Toxicology is the study of the harmful effect of various substances on the body. Poisons are substances that are harmful to the body no matter how much or in what manner they enter the body. Drugs become toxic when they are taken in excess quantities or manners that are not therapeutic. Alcohol is considered a drug. The treatment goals of toxicologic emergencies are first, supportive; second, to prevent or minimize absorption; third, to provide an antidote.

▮ Ingested Poisons

Ingested poisons can produce immediate or delayed effects. Immediate injury is caused when the poison is caustic to the body tissues (ie, a strong acid or a strong alkali). Other ingested poisons must be absorbed into the bloodstream before they become harmful. Ingested poisoning may be accidental or intentional.

Primary Assessment and Interventions

1. Maintain an open airway—some ingested substances may cause soft tissue swelling of the airway.
2. Attain control of the airway, ventilation, and oxygenation; in the absence of cerebral or renal damage, the patient's prognosis depends largely on successful management and support of vital functions.

Subsequent Assessment

1. Identify the poison.
   a. Try to determine the product taken: where, when, why, how much, who witnessed the event, time since ingestion.
   b. Call the poison control center in the area if an unknown toxic agent has been taken or if it is necessary to identify an antidote for a known toxic agent.
2. Continue the focused assessment, observing any significant deviations from normal. Different poisons will affect the body in different ways.
3. Obtain blood and urine tests for toxicology screening. Gastric contents may also be sent for toxicology screening in serious ingestions.
4. Monitor neurologic status, including mentation; monitor the course of vital signs and neurologic status over time.
5. Monitor for fluid and electrolyte imbalance.

General Interventions
Supportive Care

1. Initiate large-bore IV access.
2. Administer oxygen for respiratory depression.
3. Monitor and treat shock.

4. Prevent aspiration of gastric contents by positioning (on side with head down), use of oropharyngeal airway, and suctioning.
5. Give supportive care to maintain vital organ systems.
6. Insert an indwelling urinary catheter to monitor renal function.
7. Support the patient having seizures; many poisons excite the CNS, or the patient may convulse from oxygen deprivation.
8. Monitor and treat for complications: hypotension, coma, cardiac dysrhythmias, and seizures.
9. Psychiatric evaluations may be done after the patient is stabilized.

Minimizing Absorption

1. The primary method for preventing or minimizing absorption is to administer activated charcoal with a cathartic to hasten excretion. Newer superactivated charcoals can reduce absorption of a toxic substance by as much as 50%. Administering activated charcoal plus a cathartic is just as effective or more effective than gastric lavage.
   a. Administration of oral-activated charcoal—absorbs the poison on the surface of its particles and allows it to pass with the stool. Multiple doses may be administered.
   b. Activated charcoal is usually mixed in tap water to make a slurry.
2. The secondary method for preventing or minimizing absorption is induction of emesis with syrup of ipecac. This procedure should be done only if the patient is conscious and has a good gag reflex. It is most effective within 30 minutes of ingestion of poison.
   a. Syrup of ipecac, 30 mL by mouth followed by two glasses of water is the usual adult dose.
   b. For children between age 1 and 12, give 15 mL followed by 8 to 16 oz of water.

NURSING ALERT

⊘ **Do not induce emesis after ingestion of caustic substances, hydrocarbons, iodides, silver nitrates, strychnine, or petroleum distillates; to a patient having seizures; or to pregnant patients.**

3. Gastric lavage for the obtunded patient (see Procedure Guidelines 35-5). Save gastric aspirate for toxicology screens.
4. Procedures to enhance the removal of the ingested substance if the patient is deteriorating.
   a. Forced diuresis with urine pH alteration—to enhance renal clearance.
   b. Hemoperfusion (process of passing blood through an extracorporeal circuit and a cartridge containing an adsorbent, such as charcoal, after which the detoxified blood is returned to patient).
   c. Hemodialysis—used in selected patients to purify blood and accelerate the elimination of circulating toxins.

d. Repeated doses of charcoal—for binding nonabsorbed drugs/toxins.

e. Gastric lavage may be used in conjunction with activated charcoal and a cathartic to maximize elimination of the substance.

Providing an Antidote

1. An antidote is a chemical or physiologic antagonist that will neutralize the poison.
2. Administer the specific antidote as early as possible to reverse or diminish effects of the toxin.

PROCEDURE GUIDELINES 35-5   ASSISTING WITH GASTRIC LAVAGE

Gastric lavage is the aspiration of the stomach contents and the washing out of the stomach by means of a gastric tube.

PURPOSES

1. To remove unabsorbed poison after poison ingestion.
2. To diagnose and treat gastric hemorrhage and for the arrest of hemorrhage.
3. To cleanse the stomach before endoscopic procedures.
4. To remove liquid or small particles of material from the stomach.

EQUIPMENT

Large-bore orogastric tubes or large-bore Ewald tube
Large irrigating syringe with adapter
Large plastic funnel with adapter to fit gastric tube
Water-soluble lubricant

Lavage fluid (warm saline or other prescribed solution)
Bucket for aspirate
Nasotracheal or endotracheal tubes with inflatable cuffs if patient is unconscious
Containers for specimens

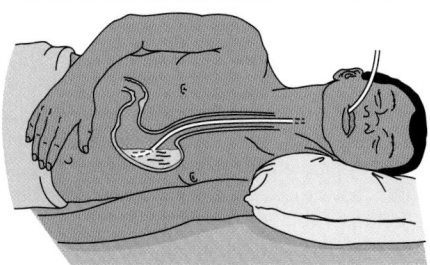

Gastric lavage.

PROCEDURE

Emergency Department/Team Action	Rationale
1. Remove dental appliances and inspect oral cavity for loose teeth.	1. To prevent accidental aspiration.
2. Measure the distance on the lavage tube between the bridge of the nose and the xiphoid process. Mark with indelible pencil or tape.	2. This is a rule-of-thumb measurement of the distance the tube is passed to reach the stomach; avoids curling/kinking of excess tubing.
3. Lubricate the tube with water-soluble lubricant.	
4. If the patient is comatose, he or she is intubated with a cuffed nasotracheal or endotracheal tube.	4. A cuffed endotracheal tube prevents aspiration of gastric contents.
5. Place the unconscious patient in a left lateral position with the head (lowered approximately 15 degrees downward), neck, and trunk forming a straight line.	5. This position decreases passage of gastric contents into the duodenum during lavage and minimizes the possibility of aspiration into lungs.
6. Pass the tube by way of the oral (or nasal) route while keeping the head in a neutral position. Pass the tube to the adhesive marking or about 50 cm (20 inches). After the lavage tube is passed, the head of the table is lowered. Have standby suction available.	6. The depth of insertion of the tube will vary with the height of the patient. If the tube enters the larynx instead of the esophagus, the patient will experience coughing and dyspnea.
7. Submerge free end of tube below water level at the moment of the patient's exhalation or auscultate the stomach during injection of air with a syringe to confirm gastric location.	7. If tube is inadvertently in the lungs, the water will bubble with each exhalation.

continued

PROCEDURE GUIDELINES 35-5   ASSISTING WITH GASTRIC LAVAGE *CONTINUED*

Emergency Department/Team Action	Rationale
8. Aspirate the stomach contents with syringe attached to the tube before instilling water or antidote. Save the specimen for analysis.	8. Aspiration is performed to remove the stomach contents. Initial gastric aspirates are saved for toxicologic analysis.
9. Remove syringe. Attach funnel to the stomach tube or use 50-mL syringe to put lavage solution in gastric tube. Volume of fluid placed in the stomach should be small.	9. Overfilling of the stomach may cause regurgitation and aspiration or force the stomach contents through the pylorus.
10. Elevate funnel above the patient's head and pour approximately 150–200 mL of solution into funnel.	10. The lavage fluid is left in place about 1 minute and then allowed to drain.
11. Lower the funnel and siphon the gastric contents into the bucket.	11. The fluid should flow in freely and drain by gravity.
12. Save samples of first two washings.	12. Keep track of fluid input/output to be sure that most of fluid is being removed.
13. Repeat lavage procedure until the returns are relatively clear and no particulate matter is seen.	13. This usually requires a total volume of at least 2 L; some clinicians advocate 5–20 L.
14. At the completion of lavage: a. Stomach may be left empty. b. An adsorbent (powder form of activated charcoal mixed with water to form a slurry, the consistency of thick soup) may be instilled in the tube and allowed to remain in the stomach. c. A saline cathartic may be instilled in the tube.	b. Activated charcoal adsorbs a variety of drugs and toxic agents onto its surface and is used to prevent gastrointestinal absorption of various substances. It renders the poison inaccessible to the circulation, thereby reducing its toxicity. c. A cathartic facilitates the transit of the charcoal and remains of the ingested substance through the intestinal tract.
15. Pinch off tube during removal or maintain suction while tube is being withdrawn.	15. Pinching off the tube prevents aspiration and the initiation of the gag reflex. Keeping the patient's head lower than the body also gives this protection.
16. Give the patient a cathartic if prescribed. Warn the patient that stools will turn black from the charcoal.	16. A cathartic may be given if the poison has no corrosive action on the bowel. The cathartic will help remove unabsorbed material from the intestine.

■ Carbon Monoxide Poisoning

Carbon monoxide poisoning is an example of an inhaled poison and is the result of the inhalation of the products of incomplete hydrocarbon combustion. It may occur as an industrial or household accident or as an attempted suicide. Carbon monoxide exerts its toxic effect by binding to circulating hemoglobin to reduce the oxygen-carrying capacity of the blood. The affinity between carbon monoxide and hemoglobin is 200 to 300 times that between oxygen and hemoglobin. (Carbon monoxide combines with hemoglobin to form carboxyhemoglobin.) As a result, tissue anoxia occurs.

Primary Assessment
1. Assess airway and breathing.
   a. Respiratory depression may be present.
   b. If the carbon monoxide poisoning is due to smoke inhalation, stridor (indicative of laryngeal edema due to thermal injury) may be present.

Primary Interventions
1. Provide 100% oxygen by tight-fitting mask. (The elimination half-life of carboxyhemoglobin, in serum, for a person breathing room air is 5 hours 20 minutes. If the patient breathes 100% oxygen, the half-life is reduced to 80 minutes; 100% oxygen in a hyperbaric chamber will reduce the half-life to 23 minutes.)
2. Intubate if necessary to protect the airway.

Subsequent Assessment
1. A thorough history is important: determine the type and length of exposure as well as possible other fumes inhaled. An underlying anemia, cardiac disease, or pulmonary disease may place a person at higher risk.
2. Determine level of consciousness—the patient may appear intoxicated from cerebral hypoxia; confusion may progress rapidly to coma.
3. Assess complaints of headache, muscular weakness, palpitation, dizziness.
4. Inspect skin: may be pink, cherry red, or cyanotic and pale—skin color is not a reliable sign.
5. Monitor vital signs: increased respiratory and pulse rates are generally present. Be alert for altered breathing patterns and respiratory failure.
6. Listen for rales or wheezes in the lungs (with smoke inhalation, indicates adult respiratory distress syndrome).

7. Obtain arterial blood samples for carboxyhemoglobin levels.
   a. Normal is less than 12%.
   b. Severe carbon monoxide poisoning is present when levels are greater than 30% to 40%.

General Interventions

1. History of exposure to carbon monoxide justifies immediate treatment.
2. Goals are to reverse cerebral and myocardial hypoxia and hasten carbon monoxide elimination.
3. Give 100% oxygen at atmospheric or hyperbaric pressures to reverse hypoxia and accelerate elimination of carbon monoxide. Patients should receive hyperbaric oxygen for CNS or cardiovascular system dysfunction.
4. Use continuous ECG monitoring, treat dysrhythmias, and correct acid–base and electrolyte abnormalities.
5. Observe the patient constantly—psychoses, spastic paralysis, visual disturbances, and deterioration of personality may persist after resuscitation and may be symptoms of permanent CNS damage.

Insect Stings

Insect stings or bites are injected poisons that can produce either local or systemic reactions. Local reactions are characterized by pain, erythema, and edema at the site of injury. Systemic reactions usually begin within minutes and produce mild to severe and life-threatening reactions.

Primary Assessment and Interventions

1. Assess airway, breathing, and circulation.
2. Anaphylactic reactions may produce unconsciousness, laryngeal edema, and cardiovascular collapse.
3. Epinephrine is the drug of choice—the amount and route depend on the severity of the reaction.
4. Administer a bronchodilator to help relieve the bronchospasm.
5. Initiate an IV with Ringer's lactate.
6. Prepare for CPR.

Subsequent Assessment

1. Obtain history of insect sting, previous exposure, and allergies.
2. Inspect skin for local reaction—erythema, edema, pain at site of injury—as well as generalized pruritus, urticaria, and angioedema.
3. Continue to monitor blood pressure and respiratory status for dyspnea, wheezing, and stridor.

General Interventions

1. Apply ice packs to site to relieve pain.
2. Elevate extremity with large edematous local reaction.
3. Administer oral antihistamine for local reactions.
4. Clean the wound thoroughly with soap and water or an antiseptic solution.
5. Administer tetanus prophylaxis if not up to date.
6. Provide patient education.

   a. Always have epinephrine on hand (EpiPen).
   b. Wear medical emergency bracelets indicating hypersensitivity.
   c. Instructions when sting occurs:
      (i) Take epinephrine immediately if stung.
      (ii) Remove stinger with one quick scrape of fingernail.
      (iii) Do not squeeze venom sac, because this may cause additional venom to be injected.
      (iv) Report to nearest health care facility for observation.
   d. Avoid exposure.
      (i) Avoid locales with stinging insects (camp and picnic sites).
      (ii) Stay away from insect feeding areas—flower beds, ripe fruit orchards, garbage, fields of clover.
      (iii) Avoid going barefoot outdoors—yellow jackets may nest on ground.
      (iv) Avoid perfumes, scented soaps, bright colors—attract bees.
      (v) Keep car windows closed.
      (vi) Spray garbage cans with rapid-acting insecticide, and keep areas meticulously clean.

Snakebites

The majority of snakes in the United States are not poisonous. The poisonous varieties are pit vipers (rattlesnakes and copperheads) and coral snakes. Bites by these snakes may result in envenomation, an injected poisoning.

Primary Assessment and Interventions

1. Assess airway, breathing, and circulation if patient is not alert.
2. Severe envenomation may lead to neurotoxicity with respiratory paralysis, shock, coma, and death.
3. Be prepared to resuscitate and provide advanced life support.

Subsequent Assessment

1. Get a description of the snake, the time of the snakebite, and the location of the bite. Bites to the head and trunk may progress more rapidly and be more severe.
   a. Pit vipers have triangular heads, vertical pupils, indentations between the eyes and nostrils, and long fangs.
   b. Coral snakes are small, brightly colored, with short fangs and teeth behind them, and with a series of bands of yellow, red, yellow, and black (in that order).
2. Assess for local reactions—burning, pain, swelling, and numbness at the site. Local reactions to coral snakebites may be delayed several hours and may be very mild.
3. A few hours after the bite, hemorrhagic blisters may occur at the site, and the entire extremity may become edematous.
4. Watch for signs of systemic reactions, including nausea, sweating, weakness, lightheadedness, initial euphoria followed by drowsiness, difficulty in swallowing, paralysis

of various muscle groups, signs of shock, seizures, and coma.

5. Monitor vital signs closely, because tachycardia or bradycardia may develop.

General Interventions

1. Keep the patient calm and at rest in a recumbent position with the affected extremity immobilized.
2. Administer oxygen.
3. Start an IV line with normal saline or Ringer's lactate.
4. Administer antivenin and be alert to allergic reaction (antivenin is horse serum based).
5. Administer vasopressors in the treatment of shock.
6. Monitor for bleeding, and administer blood products for coagulopathy.

■ Drug Intoxication

Substance abuse includes the use of specific substances that are intended to alter mood or behavior.

Drug abuse is the use of drugs for other than legitimate medical purposes. There is a growing tendency among drug users to take a variety of drugs simultaneously (polydrug abuse), including alcohol, sedatives, hypnotics, and marijuana, which may have additive effects. The clinical manifestations may vary with the drug used (Table 35-1), but the underlying principles of management are essentially the same.

Overdose refers to the toxic effects that occur when a drug is taken in a larger than normal dose.

Primary Assessment and Interventions

1. Assess the presence and adequacy of respirations.
2. Attain control of the airway, ventilation, and oxygenation.
3. Intubate and/or provide assisted ventilation in severe respiratory-depressed patients or in patients lacking gag or cough reflexes. If possible, intubation should be held off until a trial dose of naloxone (Narcan) is given.
4. Begin external cardiac compression and ventilation in the absence of heartbeat.

Subsequent Assessment

1. Do a thorough physical examination to rule out insulin shock, meningitis, head injury, stroke, or trauma.
2. If the patient is unconscious, consider all possible causes of loss of consciousness.
3. Monitor level of consciousness continuously.
4. Monitor vital signs frequently—some drugs will cause depressed vital signs; others will elevate the vital signs.
5. Monitor the pupils: Extreme miosis (pinpoint pupils) may indicate narcotic overdose.
6. Look for needle marks and external evidence of trauma.
7. Perform a rapid neurologic survey: Level of responsiveness, pupil size and reactivity, reflexes, and focal neurologic findings.

8. Keep in mind that many drug abusers take multiple drugs simultaneously.
9. Be aware that there is a high incidence of human immunodeficiency virus (HIV) and infectious hepatitis among drug users.
10. Examine the patient's breath for characteristic odor of alcohol, acetone, and so forth.
11. Try to obtain a history of the drug experiences (from the person accompanying the patient or from the patient).

General Interventions

1. Goals:
   a. Support the respiratory and cardiovascular functions.
   b. Give definitive treatment for drug overdose.
   c. Prevent further absorption, enhance drug elimination, and reduce its toxicity.
2. Measure arterial blood gases for hypoxia due to hypoventilation or for acid–base derangements.
3. Continuously monitor ECG.
4. Draw blood samples for testing glucose, electrolytes, blood urea nitrogen, creatinine, and appropriate toxicologic screen.
5. Initiate IV fluids.
6. Administer oxygen.
7. Pharmacologic interventions:
   a. Give specific drug antagonist if drug is known.
   b. Naloxone hydrochloride (Narcan) for CNS depression due to narcotics.
   c. Dextrose 50% IV to rule out hypoglycemic coma.
8. If the drug was taken by mouth, the primary method for preventing or minimizing absorption is to administer activated charcoal with a cathartic to hasten excretion. Mix activated charcoal with water to make a slurry. Follow with a cathartic. Multiple doses may be administered.
9. Vomiting may be induced if the patient is seen early after ingestion; save vomitus for toxicologic study.
10. Use gastric lavage if the patient is unconscious or if there is no way to determine when the drug was ingested; save gastric aspirate. In patients lacking gag or cough reflexes, perform this procedure only after intubation with cuffed endotracheal tube to prevent aspiration of stomach contents.
11. Take rectal temperature—extremes of thermoregulation (hyperthermia/hypothermia) must be recognized and treated.
12. Treat seizures with diazepam (Valium).
13. Assist with hemodialysis/peritoneal dialysis for potentially lethal poisoning.
14. Catheterize the patient, because the drug or metabolites are excreted by the urine.
15. Do not leave the patient alone, because there is a potential for the patient to harm self or emergency department staff.

TABLE 35-1 Specific Drug Overdose Presentations and Interventions

Type of Drug	Presentation	Interventions
CNS stimulants Amphetamines Designer drugs (MDA, Ecstasy, Ice, Eve) Cocaine (can be smoked in freebase or crack form, snorted, or injected)	Palpitations, feeling of impending doom, tachycardia, hypertension, dysrhythmia, myocardial ischemia/infarction; euphoria, agitation, combativeness, confusion, hallucinations, paranoia, aggressive or violent behavior, suicide attempts, hyperpyrexia, seizures. When the drug wears off—depression, exhaustion, irritability, sleeplessness.	Secure airway, breathing, and circulation. Monitor ECG and provide oxygen for ischemia. Sedate as necessary. Administer antiarrhythmics for ventricular dysrhythmia. Administer diazepam (Valium) for seizures. Closely monitor hemodynamic status and provide IV fluids as indicated.
Hallucinogens Lysergic acid diethylamide (LSD) Phencyclidine HCl (PCP) Mescaline Psilocybin mushrooms Jimson weed seeds	Marked anxiety bordering on panic, confusion, incoherence, hyperactivity, hallucinations, hazardous behavior, convulsions, coma, circulatory collapse, death. Flashbacks may occur months to years after initial drug use.	Try to talk the patient down by understanding what patient is going through, reducing fears, and establishing contact with reality. Reduce sensory stimuli, encourage patient to keep eyes open, and stay with patient. Monitor for hypertensive crisis and evidence of trauma. Sedate if hyperactivity cannot be controlled, and place patient in a protected environment.
Narcotics Heroin (may be cut with other ingredients in 20:1 to 200:1 ratio) Morphine and its derivatives Codeine and its derivatives	Hypotension, respiratory depression leading to apnea, miosis, drowsiness progressing to stupor and coma.	Administer naloxone (Narcan) 0.4 to 2 mg IV or by endotracheal tube (effective in 1–2 minutes). Maintain an open airway but defer intubation until naloxone given, if possible. Monitor for reappearance of symptoms and readminister naloxone or provide continuous infusion, as necessary. Protect the patient from harm (may be combative on awakening).
Sedatives Barbiturates such as amobarbital (Amytal) and secobarbital (Seconal) Benzodiazepines such as diazepam (Valium) and flurazepam (Dalmane) Other sedative/hypnotics such as chloral hydrate (Noctec) and glutethimide (Doriden)	Incoordinations, ataxia, impaired thinking and speech, lethargy to coma, early miosis; later, fixed and dilated pupils, hypoventilation, hypotension, hypothermia, decreased reflexes.	Administer flumazenil (Romazicon) to reverse or diminish effects of benzodiazepines. Administer activated charcoal. Protect the airway. For hypotension, infuse with Ringer's lactate and give vasopressors.
Alcohol Intoxication generally occurs with blood levels greater than 100 mg/dL. Levels over 400 mg/dL are due to rapid consumption of alcohol and represent a medical emergency.	Slurred speech, incoordination, ataxia, belligerent behavior ranging to stupor and coma; odor of alcohol on breath and clothing; respiratory depression.	Protect the airway. Closely monitor for CNS and respiratory depression. Draw blood for ethanol concentration, electrolytes, glucose, and drug screen using nonalcohol skin cleanser. Assess for head injury and other trauma and organic disease. Administer IV fluids, magnesium sulfate (to reduce risk of seizures), thiamine (to prevent Wernicke-Korsakoff syndrome), and glucose (to treat hypoglycemia).

CNS: central nervous system; ECG: electrocardiogram.

16. Anticipate complications—sudden death from cerebral hypoxia, dysrhythmias, seizures, respiratory arrest, myocardial infarction.
17. Always suspect mixtures of medications and alcohol.

Alcohol Withdrawal Delirium

Alcohol withdrawal delirium (delirium tremens, or alcoholic hallucinosis) is an acute toxic state that follows a prolonged bout of steady drinking or sudden withdrawal from prolonged intake of alcohol. It may be precipitated by acute injury or infection. Symptoms can begin as early as 4 hours after a reduction of alcohol intake and usually peak at 24 to 48 hours, but may last up to 2 weeks.

NURSING ALERT

Alcohol withdrawal delirium is a serious complication and is life threatening.

Primary Assessment and Interventions
1. Patient will present alert, unless experiencing a seizure.
2. If the patient is having a seizure, ensure the airway.

Subsequent Assessment
1. Assess for major symptoms—may occur independently or in combination.
   a. Shakes
   b. Seizures
   c. Hallucinations
2. Obtain drinking history, including the severity of past withdrawal episodes and any recent drug intake. Be aware that alcoholics tend to underestimate drinking habits.
3. Assess complaints of nausea and vomiting, malaise, weakness, anxiety, or fear.
4. Perform thorough examination for signs of autonomic hyperreactivity—tachycardia, diaphoresis, elevated temperature, dilated but reactive pupils—as well as any coexisting illnesses or injuries (head injury, pneumonia, metabolic disturbances).
5. Observe behavior for talkativeness, restlessness, agitation, or preoccupation.

General Interventions
1. Protect the patient from injury. The hallucinations may be visual, tactile, or auditory and are frequently of a frightening nature.
2. Take a breath analyzer reading—indicates where patient is in the withdrawal process.
3. Using a nonalcohol skin preparation, draw blood for measurement of ethanol concentration, toxicologic screen for other drugs of abuse, and other tests as directed.
4. Pharmacologic interventions:
   a. Diazepam (Valium) or chlordiazepoxide (Librium) for sedation. Sedate the patient with sufficient dosage of medication to produce adequate relaxation and to reduce agitation, prevent exhaustion, and promote sleep.
   b. Diazepam (Valium) or phenytoin (Dilantin) for seizure control.
5. Monitor vital signs every 30 minutes.
6. Place the patient in a private room where close observation can take place.
7. Maintain electrolyte balance and hydration through oral or IV route—fluid losses may be extreme because of profuse perspiration, vomiting, and agitation.
8. Assess respiratory, hepatic, and cardiovascular status of patient—pneumonia, liver disease, and cardiac failure are complications.
9. Observe for hypoglycemia, and treat appropriately. Hypoglycemia may accompany alcoholic withdrawal because alcohol depletes liver glycogen stores and impairs gluconeogenesis; many patients also suffer from malnutrition.
   a. Administer thiamine followed by parenteral dextrose if liver glycogen is depleted.
   b. Give orange juice, Gatorade, or other carbohydrates to stabilize blood sugar and to counteract tremulousness.

BEHAVIORAL EMERGENCIES

A *behavioral emergency* is an urgent, serious disturbance of behavior, affect, or thought that makes the patient unable to cope with his or her life situation and interpersonal relationships.

A patient presenting with a psychiatric emergency may be overactive or violent, depressed, or suicidal.

■ Violent Patients
Violent and aggressive behavior is usually episodic and is a means of expressing feelings of anger, fear, or hopelessness about a situation.

Assessment
1. Assess for overactivity, aggression, or anger out of proportion to the circumstances.
2. Determine risk factors for violence, including:
   a. Intoxicated with drugs/alcohol.
   b. Going through drug or alcohol withdrawal.
   c. Acute paranoid schizophrenic states, acute organic brain syndrome, acute psychosis, paranoia, or borderline personality.

General Interventions
1. Goals are to bring violence under control and protect patient and staff from harm.
2. Establish control.
   a. Keep the door of the room open, and be in clear view of the staff.
   b. Help the patient bring violence under control.

(i) Give the patient space. Do not make any sudden movement.

(ii) Avoid touching an agitated patient or standing too close.

(iii) Ask if he or she has a weapon. Request that it be placed in a neutral area.

(iv) If the patient will not surrender weapon, leave the room and allow security personnel/police to handle the situation.

  c. Try not to leave the patient alone; this may be interpreted as rejection or the patient may try to harm self.

  d. Adopt a calm, nonconfrontational approach, and remain in control of the situation. External calm and structure may help the patient gain control.

3. Provide emotional support.

  a. Talk and listen to the patient.

  b. Crisis intervention is best done with an attitude of interest in the patient's well-being and with an attempt to "tune in" to the patient while remaining firm.

  c. Acknowledge the patient's state of agitation (eg, "I want to work with you to relieve your distress").

  d. Give the patient the opportunity to ventilate anger verbally; avoid challenging the delusional state.

  e. Try to hear what the patient is saying.

  f. Convey the expectation of appropriate behavior, and make the patient aware that help is available for him or her to gain control.

  g. Administer prescribed tranquilizer to reduce anxiety and hyperactivity, if verbal management techniques fail to attenuate the patient's tension.

4. Secure assistance.

  a. Allow security personnel/police to intervene if patient does not become calm.

  b. Use restraints when absolutely necessary but with minimal force.

  c. Have a specific plan and enough well-trained personnel available when applying restraints; if patient is intoxicated, restrain in a left lateral position and monitor closely for aspiration.

  d. Talk reassuringly while applying restraints; use empathic and supportive verbal interactions.

  e. Monitor patient continuously after restraints are applied; check circulation of restrained extremities.

Depression

Depression may be seen as the presenting condition at the health care facility or may be masked by the presentation of anxiety and somatic complaints.

Assessment

1. Observe for sadness, apathy, feelings of worthlessness, self-blame, suicidal thoughts, desire to escape, worsening of mood in morning, anorexia, weight loss, sleeplessness, lessening interest in sex, reduction of activity, or ceaseless activity.

2. The agitated, depressed person may exhibit motor restlessness and severe anxiety.

General Interventions

1. Listen to the patient in a calm, unhurried manner.

2. The patient will benefit from ventilation of feelings.

3. Give the patient an opportunity to talk about problems.

4. Anticipate that the patient may be suicidal.

5. Attempt to find out if the patient has thought about or attempted suicide.

  a. "Have you ever thought about taking your own life?"

  b. The patient is generally relieved because of the opportunity to discuss feelings.

6. Find out if there is an illness, perceived or real.

7. Assess whether there has been sudden worsening of depression.

8. Notify relatives about a seriously depressed patient. Do not leave the patient alone, because suicide is usually an act committed in solitude.

9. Give antidepressant and antianxiety agents as prescribed.

10. Point out to the patient that depression is treatable.

11. Be aware of crisis and supportive services in the community: telephone counseling and referral, suicide prevention centers, group therapy, marital and family counseling, drug/alcohol counseling, adolescent counseling, or befriending programs.

12. Refer for psychiatric consultation or to psychiatric unit.

Suicide Ideation

Suicide is the eighth leading cause of death in the United States and the second most lethal killer of young people.

Assessment

1. Assess for risk factors:

  a. Associated psychiatric illness (affective disorders and substance abuse in adults; conduct disorders and depression in young people).

  b. Personality traits such as aggression, impulsivity, depression, hopelessness, borderline personality disorder, or antisocial personality.

  c. Persons who have experienced early loss, decreased social support, chronic illness, or recent divorce.

  d. Genetic and familial factors: family history of suicide, certain psychiatric disorders or alcoholism; alcohol and substance abuse.

2. Determine whether patient has communicated suicidal intent, such as preoccupation with death or talking of someone else's suicide.

3. Determine whether patient has ever attempted suicide— the risk is much greater in these people.

4. Determine whether there is a specific plan for suicide and a means to carry out the plan.

General Interventions

1. Use crisis intervention (a form of brief psychotherapy) to determine suicide potential, discover areas of depression and conflict, find out about the patient's support

system, and determine whether hospitalization, psychiatric referral, and so forth is warranted.
2. Treat the consequences of the suicide attempt (eg, gunshot wound, drug overdose).
3. Prevent further self-injury—a patient who has made a suicide gesture may do so again.
4. Admit to intensive care unit (if condition warrants), arrange follow-up care, or admit to psychiatric unit, depending on assessment of suicide potential.

SEXUAL ASSAULT

Rape

Rape is defined as unlawful carnal knowledge of a female forcibly and against her will. *Carnal knowledge* is defined as penetration of genitalia, no matter how slight, by the penis. Rape is also committed if intercourse occurs while the female is sleeping, unconscious, or under the influence of alcohol or drugs. A male who is sexually assaulted is sodomized. Sodomy is oral or anal penetration.

> **NURSING ALERT**
>
> The management of the sexual assault is important, but immediate physical health should be ensured first. A complete primary and focused assessment should take place, being alert for signs of internal hemorrhage, shock, or respiratory distress. If the victim has suffered trauma in the form of physical assault (eg, head or abdominal trauma), the trauma should be managed in the order of established priorities.

Assessment
Initiating a Supportive Relationship
1. The manner in which the patient is received and treated in the emergency department is important to the future psychological well-being of the patient.
   a. Call the rape crisis intervention counselor (if available), who will meet the patient/family in the emergency department.
   b. Do not leave patient alone. Accept the emotional reactions of the patient (hysteria, stoicism, overwhelmed feeling, and so forth).
2. Emotional trauma may be present for weeks, months, or years. Patient's reaction to rape has been called the "rape trauma syndrome." Patients may go through phases of psychological reactions:
   a. Acute phase (disorganization)—shock, disbelief, fear, anxiety, guilt, humiliation, suppression of feelings—may last for months to years.
   b. Phase of denial and unwillingness to talk about incident, followed by phase of heightened anxiety, fear, flashbacks, sleep disturbances, hyperalertness, and psychosomatic reactions.
   c. Phase of reorganization—putting incident into perspective.

Interviewing the Patient
1. Consent should be obtained for the examination, the collecting of cultures/evidence, and for release of information to law enforcement agencies.

> **NURSING ALERT**
>
> Most emergency departments have commercially prepared rape evidence collection kits as well as written protocols for treatment of injuries, legal documentation, and sexually transmitted disease and pregnancy prevention.

2. Record history of event in the patient's own words.
3. Ask if the patient has bathed, douched, gargled or brushed teeth, changed clothes, or urinated or defecated since attack—may alter interpretation of subsequent findings.
4. Record time of admission, time of examination, date and time of sexual assault, and the general appearance of the patient.
   a. Document any evidence of trauma—discoloration, bruises, lacerations, secretions, torn and bloody clothing.
   b. Record emotional state.

Interventions
Preparing for Physical Examination
1. Assist the patient to undress over a sheet/large piece of paper to obtain debris.
2. Place each item of clothing in a separate paper bag (plastic bags promote moisture retention, which may lead to formation of mold and mildew, which can destroy evidence).
3. Label bags appropriately; give to appropriate law enforcement authority.
4. Advise the patient of the nature and necessity of each procedure; give the rationale for each question asked.

Physical Examination
1. Examine the patient (from head to toe) for injuries, especially to the head, neck, breasts, thighs, back, and buttocks.
2. Assess for external evidence of trauma (bruises, contusions, lacerations, stab wounds).
3. Assess for dried semen stains (appearing as crusted, flaking areas) on the patient's body.
4. Inspect fingers for broken nails and tissue and foreign materials under nails.
5. Assist in conducting oral examination to determine secretion status of patient compared with that of assailant.
   a. Obtain a saliva specimen.
   b. Take prescribed cultures of gum and tooth areas.
6. Document evidence of trauma with body diagrams or photographs.

Pelvic and Rectal Examinations
1. Examine perineum and thighs with an ultraviolet light (Wood's lamp); areas that are found to fluoresce may indicate semen stains. Urine and other stains may also fluoresce.
2. Note color and consistency of any discharge present.

3. Use water-moistened vaginal speculum for examination; do not use lubricant (contains chemicals that may interfere with later forensic testing of specimens and acid phosphatase determinations).

Obtaining Laboratory Specimens

1. Collect vaginal aspirate, which is examined for presence or absence of motile/nonmotile sperm.
2. Use sterile swab to draw from vaginal pool for acid phosphatase, blood group antigen of semen, and precipitin test against human sperm and blood.
3. Obtain separate smears from the oral, vaginal, and anal areas.
4. Obtain swabs of body orifices for gonorrhea and chlamydia testing (to determine preexisting infection or new infection if patient is not presenting immediately).
5. Trim areas of pubic hair suspected of containing semen; obtain several pubic hairs with follicles; place in separate containers and identify these as patient's pubic hairs.
6. Obtain blood serum for syphilis; a sample of serum may be frozen and saved for future testing.
7. Collect foreign material (leaves, grass, dirt), and place in appropriate container.
8. Examine rectum for signs of trauma, blood, and semen stains.
9. Conduct a pregnancy test if there is possibility that patient is pregnant.
10. Label all specimens with name of patient, date, time of collection, body area from which specimen was obtained, and names of personnel collecting specimens to preserve chain of evidence; give to designated person (crime laboratory, etc.), and obtain an itemized receipt.
11. Photographs are taken by designated person.

Other Interventions

1. Treat physical trauma as with any patient.
2. Protect patient against sexually transmitted diseases.
   a. Specimens obtained for sexually transmitted diseases, including gonorrhea, cannot be immediately obtained (positive cultures taken in the immediate post-rape period will only reflect existing disease).
   b. In addition, follow-up visits cannot be ensured, so some health care providers may treat the patient as if they have been exposed to a known case of gonorrhea or chlamydia.
   c. Antibiotic choices include single-dose oral or injectable and oral treatment for 7 days of the following:
      (i) Cephalosporins, such as ceftriaxone (Rocephin) or cefoxitin (Mefoxin)
      (ii) Tetracyclines, such as doxycycline (Vibramycin)
      (iii) Quinolones, such as ciprofloxacin (Cipro) or ofloxacin (Floxin)
      (iv) Erythromycins or macrolides, such as azithromycin (Zithromax)
3. Protect patient against pregnancy.
   a. It is important to determine whether pregnancy existed before the attack.
   b. Negative pregnancy test should be obtained before administering postcoital therapy.
   c. Hormonal treatment to prevent pregnancy—morning after pill as indicated.
4. Allay fear of human immunodeficiency virus (HIV) or acquired immunodeficiency syndrome (AIDS). Consider prophylactic treatment for HIV.
5. Possible prophylactic scabies treatment.
6. Provide the patient with cleansing facilities, including a cleansing douche, shower, and mouthwash.

Providing for Follow-Up Services

1. Make an appointment for follow-up surveillance for pregnancy, sexually transmitted disease, and HIV counseling.
2. Inform the patient of counseling services to prevent long-term psychological effects; counseling services should be made available to the family.
3. Encourage the patient to return to previous level of functioning as soon as possible.
4. The patient should be accompanied by a family member or friend when leaving the health care facility.

SELECTED REFERENCES

American Health Consultants (1999). Are sexual assault victims getting the proper treatment in your ED? *ED Nursing, 2*(8), 101–107.

American Heart Association (1997–1999). *Basic life support for health care providers.* Dallas, TX: Author.

Anderson, R. J., & Taliaferro, E. H. (1998). Violence: Recognition, prevention & management. *Journal of Emergency Medicine, 16*(3). 487–498.

Barry, P. (1994). *Mental health and mental illness.* Philadelphia: J. B. Lippincott.

Chochesy, J. M., Breau, C., Cardin, S., Whittaker, A., & Rudy, E. B. (1996). *Critical care nursing.* Philadelphia: W. B. Saunders.

Emergency Nurses Association. (1998). *Emergency nurse pediatric core course provider manual* (2nd ed.). Des Plaines, IL: Author.

———. (1998). *Sheehy's emergency nursing principles and practice* (4th ed.). St. Louis: Mosby.

———. (1995). *Trauma nursing core course provider manual* (4th ed.). Des Plaines, IL: Author.

Ledray, L., & Arndt, S. (1994). Examining the sexual assault victim: A new model for nursing care. *Journal of Psychosocial Nursing, 32*(2), 712.

Lisanti, P. (1998). Barbiturate overdose. *American Journal of Nursing, 98*(10), 38.

Luckman, J. (1997). *Saunders manual of nursing care.* Philadelphia: W. B. Saunders.

Mankin, S. L. (1998). Stab wound. *American Journal of Nursing, 98*(9), 49.

Mattera, C. J. (1998). Spinal trauma: New guidelines for assessment and management in the out of hospital environment. *Journal of Emergency Nursing, 24*(6), 523–534.

Moore, A. (1999). Emergency contraceptive options. *RN, 62*(12), 43–45.

Neff, J., & Stinson Kidd, P. (1993). *Trauma nursing: The art and science.* St. Louis: Mosby.

Springhouse (1993). *Responding to patients in crisis.* Springhouse, PA: Springhouse.

Worf, N. (2000). Tetanus—still a problem. *RN, 63*(6), 44–48.

Maternity and
Neonatal Nursing

Maternal and Fetal Health

INTRODUCTION TO MATERNITY NURSING

Providing care to childbearing families is aimed at the ideal of having every pregnancy result in a healthy mother, baby, and family unit. The nurse today faces many evolving and challenging issues in achieving this goal. Such advances as in vitro fertilization and embryo freezing have afforded people opportunities once never thought possible. An increasing number of high-risk pregnancies results from such factors as drug abuse, acquired immunodeficiency syndrome (AIDS), late or no prenatal care, teenage pregnancies, and pregnancies in women older than 35 years. Technologic advances in high-risk obstetric units, fetal monitoring, sonography, and neonatal intensive care units are now providing the means to improve maternal health and save fetuses and infants who would not have survived years ago.

Regionalization of obstetric services is being implemented so that childbearing families have access to the technologic advances and skilled personnel capable of managing pregnancy or neonatal complications. Childbearing families are also being offered alternative types of care in birthing centers; labor, delivery, recovery rooms (LDRs); labor, delivery, recovery, postpartum rooms (LDRPs); home deliveries; alternative methods used during delivery, including hydrotherapy; and changes in hospital policies, such as having children and others present during labor and delivery.

Economic changes in the health care climate are also affecting the practice of nursing as cost-containment considerations have shortened the hospital length of stay. Some hospitals have adopted a practice of 12- to 24-hour discharge after delivery coordinated with home health care follow-up.

This combination of advancing technology, pregnancy risk factors, and changing economics challenges the nurse to be a highly skilled clinician and outstanding communicator.

Terminology Used in Maternity Nursing

1. Gestation—pregnancy or maternal condition of having a developing fetus in the body.
2. Embryo—conceptus up to the 10th week of gestation (8th week postconception).
3. Fetus—human conceptus from 10th week of gestation (8th week postconception) until delivery.
4. Viability—capability of living, usually accepted as 24 weeks, although survival is rare.
5. Gravida (G)—woman who is or has been pregnant, regardless of pregnancy outcome.
6. Nulligravida—woman who is not now and never has been pregnant.
7. Primigravida—woman pregnant for the first time.
8. Multigravida—woman who has been pregnant more than once.
9. Para (P)—refers to past pregnancies that have reached viability.
10. Nullipara—woman who has never completed a pregnancy to the period of viability. The woman may or may not have experienced an abortion.
11. Primipara—woman who has completed one pregnancy to the period of viability regardless of the number of infants delivered and regardless of the infant being live or stillborn.
12. Multipara—woman who has completed two or more pregnancies to the stage of viability.
13. Living children—refers to the number of living children a woman has delivered regardless of whether they were live births or stillborn births.

A woman pregnant for the first time is a primigravida and is described as Gravida 1 Para 0 (or G1P0). A woman who delivered one fetus carried to the period of viability and who is pregnant again is described as Gravida 2, Para 1. A woman with two pregnancies ending in abortions and no viable children is Gravida 2, Para 0.

Obstetric History

TPAL

In some obstetric services, a woman's obstetric history is summarized by a series of four digits, such as 5-0-2-5. These digits correspond with the abbreviation TPAL.

1. **T** represents full-term deliveries, 37 completed weeks or more.
2. **P** represents preterm deliveries, 20 to less than 37 completed weeks.
3. **A** represents abortions, elective or spontaneous loss (miscarriage) of a pregnancy before the period of viability.
4. **L** represents the number of children living. If a child has died, further explanation is needed for clarification.

If, for example, a particular woman's history is summarized as G 7, P 5-0-2-5, then she has been pregnant seven times, had five term deliveries, zero preterm deliveries, two abortions, and five living children.

GTPALM

In some institutions, a woman's obstetric history can also be summarized as GTPALM.

1. **G** represents gravida.
2. **T** represents full-term deliveries, 37 completed weeks or more.
3. **P** represents preterm deliveries, 20 to less than 37 completed weeks.
4. **A** represents abortions, elective or spontaneous loss of a pregnancy before the period of viability.
5. **L** represents the number of children living. If a child has died, further explanation is needed for clarification.
6. **M** represents the number of multiple gestations and births (not the number of neonates delivered).

If, for example, a particular woman's history is summarized as G 5, P 5-0-0-6-1, then she has been pregnant five times, had five term deliveries, zero preterm deliveries, zero abortions, six living children, and one multiple gestation/birth.

THE EXPECTANT MOTHER

Manifestations of Pregnancy

Pregnancy may be determined by cessation of menses, enlarged uterus, and a positive result on a pregnancy test. These and the many other manifestations of pregnancy are classified into three groups: presumptive, probable, and positive.

Presumptive Signs and Symptoms

Physical signs and symptoms that suggest, but do not prove, pregnancy.

1. Abrupt cessation of menses—pregnancy is suspected if more than 10 days have elapsed since the time of the expected onset in a healthy woman who previously had predictable menstrual periods.

2. Breast changes:
   a. Breasts enlarge and become tender. Veins in breasts become increasingly visible.
   b. Nipples become larger and more pigmented. Nipple tingling may also be present.
   c. Colostrum, a thin, milky fluid, may be expressed in the second half of pregnancy.
   d. Montgomery's glands, small elevations on the areolae, may appear.
3. Skin pigmentation changes:
   a. Chloasma/melasma gravidarum (the mask of pregnancy)—brownish pigmentation appearing on the face in a butterfly pattern in 50% to 70% of women. It is usually symmetric and is distributed on the forehead, cheeks, and nose. The mask of pregnancy is more common in dark-haired, brown-eyed women and is progressive throughout the pregnancy.
   b. Linea nigra—dark vertical line on the abdomen between the sternum and the symphysis pubis.
   c. Abdominal striae (striae gravidarum)—reddish or purplish linear marks sometimes appearing on the breasts, abdomen, buttocks, and thighs because of the stretching, rupture, and atrophy of the deep connective tissue of the skin.
4. Nausea and vomiting (morning sickness)—occurs mainly in the morning but may occur at any time of the day, lasting a few hours. Begins between 2 and 6 weeks after conception and usually disappears spontaneously near the end of the first trimester (12 weeks).
5. Frequency of urination:
   a. Caused by pressure of the expanding uterus on the bladder
   b. Decreases when the uterus rises out of the pelvis (around 12 weeks)
   c. Reappears when the fetal head engages in the pelvis at the end of pregnancy
6. Fatigue—characteristic of early pregnancy in response to increased hormonal levels.

Probable Signs and Symptoms

Objective findings detected by 12 to 16 weeks of gestation.

1. Enlargement of abdomen—at about 12 weeks' gestation, the uterus can be felt through the abdominal wall, just above the symphysis pubis.
2. Changes in shape, size, and consistency of the uterus:
   a. Uterus enlarges, elongates, and decreases in thickness as pregnancy progresses. The uterus changes from a pear shape to a globe shape.
   b. Hegar's sign—lower uterine segment softens 6 to 8 weeks after the onset of the last menstrual period.
3. Changes in cervix:
   a. Chadwick's sign—bluish or purplish discoloration of cervix and vaginal wall.
   b. Goodell's sign—softening of the cervix; may occur as early as 4 weeks.

c. With inflammation and carcinoma during pregnancy, the cervix may remain firm.
4. Intermittent contractions of the uterus (Braxton Hicks contractions)—painless, palpable contractions occurring at irregular intervals, more frequently felt after 28 weeks. They usually disappear with walking or exercise.
5. Ballottement—sinking and rebounding of the fetus in its surrounding amniotic fluid in response to a sudden tap on the uterus (occurs near midpregnancy).
6. Changes in levels of human chorionic gonadotropin (HCG) in maternal plasma and urine.
7. Leukorrhea—increase in vaginal discharge.
8. Quickening (sensations of fetal movement in the abdomen)—occurs between the 16th and 20th week after the onset of the last menses.
9. Positive HCG—laboratory (urine or serum) test for pregnancy.

Positive Signs and Symptoms
Diagnostic of pregnancy.
1. Fetal heart tones (FHTs)—usually heard between 16th and 20th week of gestation with a fetoscope or the 10th and 12th week of gestation with a Doppler stethoscope.
2. Fetal movements felt by the examiner (after about 20 weeks' gestation).
3. Outlining of the fetal body through the maternal abdomen in the second half of pregnancy.
4. Sonographic evidence (after 4 weeks' gestation) using vaginal ultrasound. Fetal cardiac motion can be detected by 6 weeks' gestation.

Maternal Physiology During Pregnancy
Duration of Pregnancy
1. Averages 280 days or 40 weeks (10 lunar months; 9 calendar months) from the 1st day of the last normal menstrual period.
2. Duration may also be divided into three equal parts, or trimesters, of slightly more than 13 weeks or 3 calendar months each.
3. Estimated date of confinement is calculated by adding 7 days to the date of the 1st day of the last menstrual period and counting back 3 months (Nägele's rule).
   a. For example, if a woman's last menstrual period (LMP) began on September 10, 1999, her estimated date of confinement (EDC) would be September 10, 1999, plus 7 days = September 17, 1999, minus 3 months = June 17, 1999. If the date of the woman's LMP begins after March 31, an additional year must be added to give a correct EDC. Thus, an additional year would be added to the above date making the correct EDC = June 17, 2000.
   b. Another method of calculating the EDC is McDonald's rule: after 24 weeks' gestation, the fundal height measurement will correspond to the week of gestation plus 2 to 4 weeks.

Changes in the Reproductive Tract
Uterus
1. Enlargement during pregnancy involves stretching and marked hypertrophy of existing muscle cells secondary to increased estrogen and progesterone levels.
2. In addition to an increase in the size of the uterine muscle cells, there is an increase in fibrous tissue and elastic tissue. The size and number of blood vessels and lymphatics increase.
3. Enlargement and thickening of the uterine wall is most marked in the fundus.
4. By the end of the 3rd month (12 weeks), the uterus is too large to be contained wholly within the pelvic cavity—it can now be palpated suprapubically.
5. As the uterus rises out of the pelvis, it rotates somewhat to the right because of the presence of the rectosigmoid on the left side of the pelvis.
6. By 20 weeks' gestation, the fundus has reached the level of the umbilicus.
7. By 36 weeks, the fundus has reached the xiphoid.
8. By the end of the 5th month, the myometrium hypertrophy ends and the walls of uterus become thinner, allowing palpation of the fetus.
9. During the last 3 weeks, the uterus descends slightly because of fetal descent into the pelvis.
10. Changes in contractility occur—from the first trimester, irregular painless contractions occur (Braxton Hicks contractions). In latter weeks of pregnancy, these contractions become stronger and more regular.
11. There is a progressive increase in uteroplacental blood flow during pregnancy.

Cervix
1. Pronounced softening and cyanosis—due to increased vascularity, edema, hypertrophy, and hyperplasia of the cervical glands.
2. Endocervical glands secrete a thick mucus that forms a cervical plug and obstructs the cervical canal. This plug prevents bacteria and other substances from entering and ascending into the uterus.
3. Erosions of cervix, common during pregnancy, represent an extension of proliferating endocervical glands and columnar endocervical epithelium.
4. Evidence of Chadwick's sign, the bluish, purplish coloring of the cervix. This sign is due to the increased vascularity and hyperemia caused by increased estrogen levels.

Ovaries
1. Ovulation ceases during pregnancy; maturation of new follicles is suspended.
2. One corpus luteum functions during early pregnancy (first 10 to 12 weeks), producing mainly progesterone. However, small levels of estrogen and relaxin are also produced by the corpus luteum.
3. After 8 weeks' gestation, the corpus luteum remains the source for the hormone relaxin. However, relaxin is not required for a successful outcome and normal delivery.

Vagina and Outlet

1. Increased vascularity, hyperemia, and softening of connective tissue in skin and muscles of perineum and vulva.
2. Vaginal walls prepare for labor: mucosa increases in thickness, connective tissue loosens, and small-muscle cells hypertrophy. Secretions are thick, white, and acidic in nature and play a major role in the prevention of infections.
3. Vaginal secretions increase; pH is 3.5 to 6—because of increased production of lactic acid from glycogen in the vaginal epithelium by *Lactobacillus acidophilus*. (Acid pH probably aids in keeping vagina relatively free of pathogenic bacteria.)
4. Hypertrophy of the structures, along with fat deposits, causes the labia majora to close and cover the vaginal introitus (vaginal opening).

Changes in the Abdominal Wall

1. Striae gravidarum (stretch marks) may develop—reddish, slightly depressed streaks in the skin of abdomen, breast, and thighs (become glistening silvery lines after pregnancy).
2. Linea nigra may form—line of dark pigment extending from the umbilicus down the midline to the symphysis. Often during the first pregnancy, the linea nigra occurs at the height of the uterus. During subsequent pregnancies, the entire line may be present early in gestation.
3. Diastasis recti may occur as muscles (rectus) separate. If severe, a part of the anterior uterine wall may be covered only by a layer of skin, fascia, and peritoneum.

Breast Changes

1. Tenderness and tingling occur in early weeks of pregnancy.
2. Increase in size by 2nd month—hypertrophy of mammary alveoli. Veins become more prominent, and striae may develop as the breasts enlarge.
3. Nipples become larger, more deeply pigmented, and more erectile early in pregnancy.
4. Colostrum, a yellow secretion rich in antibodies, may be expressed by second trimester.
5. Areolae become broader and more deeply pigmented. The depth of pigmentation varies with the person's complexion.
6. Scattered through the areola are a number of small elevations (glands of Montgomery), which are hypertrophic sebaceous glands.

Metabolic Changes

Numerous and intensive changes occur in response to rapidly growing fetus and placenta.

Weight Gain Average

11.5 to 16 kg (25 to 35 lb)

Area	Kg	Lb
Fetus	3.2–3.4	7.0–7.5
Placenta	0.5–0.7	1.0–1.5
Amniotic fluid	0.9	2.0
Uterus	1.1	2.5
Breast tissue	0.7–1.4	1.5–3.0
Blood volume	1.6–2.3	3.5–5.0
Maternal stores	1.8–4.3	4.0–9.5

Water Metabolism

1. The average woman retains 6 to 8 L of extra water during the pregnancy secondary to hormonal influence.
2. Approximately 4 to 6 L of fluid cross into the extracellular spaces. This creates a physiologic increase in blood volume (hypervolemia).
3. Many pregnant women experience the normal accumulation of fluid in their legs and ankles at the end of the day. This is most common in the third trimester and is referred to as *physiologic edema.*
4. Sodium excretion in the normal pregnant woman is similar to the nonpregnant woman.
5. Sodium retention is usually directly proportional to the amount of water accumulated during the pregnancy. However, pregnancy lends itself toward sodium depletion, making sodium regulation more difficult.
6. Additional sodium is required during pregnancy to meet the need for increased intravascular and extracellular fluid volumes and to maintain a normal isotonic state.

NURSING ALERT

The limitation of sodium is discouraged in pregnancy because it can result in decreased kidney function, resulting in decreased urine output. As a result, the pregnancy outcome could also be adversely affected.

Protein Metabolism

1. Fetus, uterus, and maternal blood are rich in protein rather than in fat or carbohydrates.
2. At term, fetus and placenta contain 500 g of protein or approximately half of the total protein increase of pregnancy.
3. Approximately 500 g more of protein is added to the uterus, breasts, and maternal blood in the form of hemoglobin and plasma proteins.

Carbohydrate Metabolism

1. Carbohydrate metabolism during pregnancy is controlled by glucose levels in the plasma and the metabolism of glucose in the cells.
2. The liver controls the plasma glucose level. Not only does it store glucose as glycogen, but it also converts it into glucose when the woman's blood glucose levels are low.
3. Early in pregnancy, the effects of estrogen and progesterone can induce a state of hyperinsulinemia. As pregnancy advances, there is increased tissue resistance coupled with increased hyperinsulinemia.

4. Approximately 2% to 3% of all women will develop gestational diabetes mellitus (GDM—type 3) during pregnancy regardless if they have a prior history of carbohydrate intolerance.
5. Pregnant women with preexisting diabetes mellitus (type 1 or 2) may experience a worsening of the disease attributed to hormonal changes occurring with pregnancy.
6. During pregnancy, there is a "sparing" of glucose used by maternal tissues and a shunting of glucose to the placenta for use by the fetus.
7. Human placental lactogen (placental hormone) promotes lipolysis, increases plasma free fatty acids, and thereby provides alternative fuel sources for the mother.
8. Human placental lactogen, estrogen, progesterone, and cortisol oppose the action of insulin during pregnancy and promote maternal lipolysis as well.

Fat Metabolism
1. Lipid metabolism during pregnancy causes an accumulation of fat stores, mostly cholesterol, phospholipids, and triglycerides.
2. This accumulation of fat stores has no negligible effect on the fetus.
3. Fat storage occurs before the 30th week of gestation. After 30 weeks' gestation, there is no further fat storage, only fat mobilization that correlates with the increased utilization of glucose and amino acids by the fetus.
4. The ratio of low-density proteins (LDL) to high-density proteins (HDL) is increased during pregnancy.

Nutrient Requirements
Caloric Requirements
1. Additional calories are usually not required during the first trimester due to the limited metabolic demands.
2. An additional 300 kcal/dL are required during the second and third trimester over the nonpregnant woman. However, due to variety of women and their individualized needs, the exact caloric requirements need to be established on an individual basis.
3. Caloric expenditure varies throughout pregnancy. There is a slight increase in early pregnancy and a sharp increase near the end of the first trimester, which continues throughout pregnancy.

Protein Requirements
1. Protein is required for adequate amino acids to accommodate the normal development of the fetus, blood volume expansion, and growth of maternal breast and uterine tissue.
2. An additional requirement of 10 g of protein per day is recommended over the nonpregnant intake.

Carbohydrate and Fat Requirements
1. As in the nonpregnant woman, carbohydrates should supply 55% to 60% of calories in the diet. This intake should be in the form of complex carbohydrates, such as whole-grain cereal products, starchy vegetables, and legumes.

2. Fat intake should not exceed 30% of the diet. Saturated fats should not exceed 10% of the total calories.

Iron Requirements
1. Total circulating red blood cells (RBCs) increase about 40% to 50% during pregnancy; therefore, iron requirements are increased to 20 to 40 mg daily. This often exceeds dietary intake.
2. Supplemental iron is valuable and necessary during pregnancy and for several weeks after pregnancy or lactation.
3. During the last half of pregnancy, iron is transferred to the fetus and stored in the fetal liver. This store lasts 3 to 6 months.

Changes in Cardiovascular System
Heart
1. Diaphragm is progressively elevated during pregnancy; heart is displaced to the left and upward, with the apex moved laterally.
2. Heart sounds—exaggerated splitting of the first heart sound; a loud, easily heard third sound.
3. Heart murmurs—systolic murmurs are common and usually disappear after delivery.

Blood Volume Changes
1. Cardiac volume increases by 40% to 50% (1450 to 1750 mL) by 32 weeks' gestation, causing slight hypertrophy of the heart and increased cardiac output.
2. Cardiac output increases by 30% to 50% above normal within the first 13 weeks of pregnancy and reaches a volume of 6 to 7 L/min by term.
3. In the supine position, the large uterus compresses the venous return from the lower half of the body to the heart. This may cause arterial hypotension, referred to as the *supine hypotensive syndrome*. Cardiac output increases by 25% to 30% with an increase in uterine and renal blood flow when the woman turns from her back to lateral position (either left or right side).
4. Femoral venous pressure increases—because of retardation of blood flow from lower extremities as a result of pressure of enlarged uterus on pelvic veins and inferior vena cava.
5. Increased cutaneous blood flow dissipates excess heat caused by increased metabolism of pregnancy.
6. Plasma volume increases 20% to 30% (250 to 450 mL), resulting in hemodilution, more commonly referred to as *physiologic anemia of pregnancy* or *physiologic dilutional anemia*. This "anemic" state is not a true pathologic state and does decrease the risk of thrombosis.

Blood Pressure Changes
1. Blood pressure—during the first half of pregnancy, there is a slight (5 to 10 mm Hg) decrease in systolic and diastolic blood pressure, with the lowest point occurring in the second trimester. By the third trimester, the blood pressure gradually returns to prepregnancy levels.
2. Maternal position influences blood pressure: the highest reading is obtained in the sitting position, the lowest

reading is obtained in the left lateral position, and an intermediate reading is obtained in the supine position.

3. Maternal blood pressure will also rise with uterine contractions and returns to the baseline level after the uterine contraction is over.

Hematologic Changes

1. Total volume of circulating RBCs increases 18% to 30%; hemoglobin concentration at term averages 12 to 16 g/dL; hematocrit concentration at term averages 37% to 47%.
2. Average leukocyte (WBC) count in the third trimester is 5 to 12,000/mm³. WBC count can be elevated as high as 25,000 or more during labor—cause unknown; probably represents the reappearance in the circulation of leukocytes previously shunted out of active circulation.
3. Pregnancy is a hypercoagulable state due to the increased levels of a number of essential coagulation factors. These factors include factor I (fibrinogen by 50%), factor V (proaccelerin or labile factor), factor VII (proconvertin or serum prothrombin conversion accelerator), factor VIII (antihemophilic factor or antihemophilic globulin), factor IX (plasma thromboplastin component or Christmas factor), factor X (Stuart or Prower factor), and factor XII (Hageman or glass or contact factor). Factor II (prothrombin) increases slightly, whereas factors XI (plasma thromboplastin antecedent) and XIII (fibrin-stabilizing factor) decrease during pregnancy.
4. There is no significant change in the number, appearance, or function of platelets. Average platelet count is 140,000 to 400,000, which increases the risk to the pregnant woman for venous thrombosis.

Changes in the Respiratory Tract

1. Diaphragm is elevated during pregnancy—chiefly by the enlarging uterus that decreases the length of the lungs.
2. Thoracic cage expands its anteroposterior diameter causing flaring of the ribs—result of increased mobility of rib attachments.
3. Breathing is more diaphragmatic than costal.
4. Hyperventilation occurs—increase in respiratory rate, tidal volume (amount of air inspired and expired with normal breath) increases 30% to 40%, and minute ventilation (amount of air inspired in 1 minute) increases 40%.
5. Increased total volume lowers blood PCO_2, causing mild respiratory alkalosis that is compensated for by lowering of the bicarbonate concentration.

6. Increased respiratory rate and reduced PCO_2 are probably induced by progesterone and estrogen to a lesser degree on the respiratory center.
7. Oxygen consumption increases 15% to 20% and as much as 300% in labor. This increase leads to increased maternal alveolar and arterial PO_2 levels.
8. Approximately 60% to 70% of pregnant women experience shortness of breath; the cause is unknown.
9. Nasal stuffiness and epistaxis (nosebleeds) are also common during pregnancy, secondary to vascular congestion caused from the increased estrogen levels.

Changes in Renal System

1. Ureters become dilated and elongated during pregnancy because of mechanical pressure and perhaps the effects of progesterone. When the uterus rises out of the uterine cavity, it rests on the ureters, compressing them at the pelvic brim. Dilation is greater on the right side—left side is cushioned by the sigmoid colon.
2. Glomerular filtration rate (GFR) increases 50% by the second trimester, and the increase persists almost to term. Renal plasma flow increases early in pregnancy and decreases to nonpregnant levels in the third trimester. These changes may be due to placental lactogen.
3. Glucosuria may be evident—because of the increase in glomerular filtration without increase in tubular resorptive capacity for filtered glucose.
4. Excreted protein may be increased due to the increased GFR, but is not considered abnormal until the level exceeds 250 mg/dL. Slight amounts of protein may be excreted during or just after vigorous labor.
5. Toward the end of pregnancy, pressure of the presenting part impedes drainage of blood and lymph from the bladder base, often leaving the area edematous, easily traumatized, and more susceptible to infection.

Changes in Gastrointestinal Tract

1. Gums may become hyperemic and softened and may bleed easily.
2. A localized vascular swelling of the gums may appear—called *epulis of pregnancy.*
3. Stomach and intestines are displaced upward and laterally by the enlarging uterus. Heartburn (pyrosis) is common, caused by reflux of acid secretions in the lower esophagus.
4. Tone and motility of gastrointestinal tract decrease, leading to prolongation of gastric emptying due to large amount of progesterone produced by the placenta. Decreased motility, mechanical obstruction by the fetus, and decreased water absorption from the colon leads to constipation.
5. Hemorrhoids are common because of elevated pressure in veins below the level of the large uterus and constipation.
6. Distention and hypotonia of the gallbladder are common, which can cause stasis of bile. Additionally,

there is a decrease in emptying time and thickening of bile, resulting in hypercholesterolemia and gallstone formation.

7. Liver function tests are altered. With pregnancy, bilirubin, AST (SGOT), and ALT (SGPT) values are unchanged; prothrombin time may show a slight increase or be unchanged. Liver size and morphology are unchanged.

8. Peptic ulcer formation or exacerbation is uncommon during pregnancy due to decreased hydrochloric acid (caused by increased estrogen levels).

9. The appendix is pushed superiorly.

Changes in Endocrine System

1. Anterior pituitary gland enlarges slightly; posterior pituitary gland remains unchanged.

2. Thyroid is moderately enlarged because of hyperplasia of glandular tissue and increased vascularity.
   a. Basal metabolic rate increases progressively during normal pregnancy (as much as 25%)—because of metabolic activity of fetus.
   b. Level of protein-bound iodine and thyroxine rises sharply and is maintained until after delivery—because of increased circulatory estrogen and HCG.
   c. Hyperthyroidism during pregnancy is rare.

3. Parathyroid gland size and concentration of parathyroid hormone increase and peak between 15 and 35 weeks' gestation.

4. Adrenal secretions considerably increased—amounts of aldosterone increase as early as 15th week to accommodate for the increased sodium excretion.

5. Pancreas—because of the fetal glucose needs for growth, there are alterations in maternal insulin production and usage.
   a. Estrogen, progesterone, cortisol, and human placental lactogen (HPL) decrease maternal utilization of glucose.
   b. Cortisol also increases maternal insulin production.
   c. Insulinase, an enzyme produced by the placenta, deactivates maternal insulin.
   d. These changes result in an increased need for insulin, and the islets of Langerhans increase their production of insulin.

Changes in Integumentary System

1. Pigmentary changes occur because of melanocyte-stimulating hormone, the level of which is elevated from the 2nd month of pregnancy until term.

2. Striae gravidarum appear in later months of pregnancy as reddish, slightly depressed streaks in the skin of the abdomen and occasionally over the breasts and thighs.

3. A brownish black line of pigment is often formed in the midline of the abdominal skin—known as *linea nigra.*

4. Brownish patches of pigment may form on the face—known as *chloasma/melasma* or *"mask of pregnancy."*

5. Angiomas (vascular spider nevis), minute red elevations commonly on the skin of the face, neck, upper chest, legs, and arms, may develop.

6. Reddening of the palms (palmar erythema) may also occur.

7. There is also an increased warmth to the skin and increased nail growth.

Changes in Musculoskeletal System

1. The increasing mobility of sacroiliac, sacrococcygeal, and pelvic joints during pregnancy is a result of hormonal changes, specifically relaxin.

2. The center of gravity shifts secondary to increased weight gain, fluid retention, lordosis, and mobile ligaments. This mobility and the change in the center of gravity contribute to alteration of maternal posture and to back pain.

3. Late in pregnancy, aching, numbness, and weakness in the upper extremities may occur because of lordosis and paresthesia, which ultimately produces traction on the ulnar and median nerves.

4. Separation of the rectus muscles due to pressure of the growing uterus creates a diastasis recti. If this is severe, a portion of the anterior uterine wall is covered by only a layer of skin, fascia, and peritoneum.

Changes in Neurologic System

1. Usually no system changes.

2. Mild frontal headaches are common in the first and second trimester related to tension or hormonal changes.

3. Dizziness is common and is related to vasomotor instability, postural hypotension, or hypoglycemia after long periods of standing or sitting.

4. Tingling sensations in the hands are common and are due to excessive hyperventilation decreasing maternal P_{CO_2} levels.

> **NURSING ALERT**
>
> Severe headaches after 20 weeks' gestation may be associated with hypertensive disorders of pregnancy. If these occur accompanied with visual changes, elevated blood pressure, and facial edema, the woman should be seen immediately by her health care provider for further evaluation.

Changes in Hormonal Responses
Steroid Hormones

1. Estrogen:
   a. Is secreted by the ovaries in early pregnancy, but by 7 weeks' gestation over half of the estrogen is secreted by the placenta.
   b. The three classic estrogens during pregnancy are estrone, estradiol, and estriol. More than 90% of the estrogens secreted during pregnancy is estriol.
   c. Estrogens also ensure uterine growth and development, maintenance of uterine elasticity and contractility, maintenance of breast growth and its ductal structures, and enlargement of the external genitalia.

2. Progesterone:
   a. Is initially secreted by the corpus luteum and then by the placenta.
   b. Plays critical role in the maintenance of the pregnancy by suppressing the maternal immunologic response to the fetus and the rejection of the trophoblasts.
   c. Progesterone also helps to maintain the endometrium, inhibits uterine contractility, helps in the development of breast lobules for lactation, stimulates the maternal respiratory center, and relaxes smooth muscle.

Placental Protein Hormones

1. Human chorionic gonadotropin (HCG):
   a. Secreted by the syncytiotrophoblasts and stimulates the production by the corpus luteum of progesterone and estrogen until the fully developed placenta takes over.
   b. In multiple gestations, HCG can be twice as high as a singleton pregnancy.
   c. HCG levels peak around 10 weeks' gestation (50,000 to 100,000 mIU/mL) then decrease to 10,000 to 20,000 mIU/mL by 20 weeks' gestation.
2. Human placental lactogen (HPL):
   a. Also referred to as *human chorionic somatomammotropin*. Produced by the syncytiotrophoblasts of the placenta; detected in maternal serum as early as 6 weeks' gestation.
   b. Serum HPL levels rise concomitantly with placental growth.
   c. HPL is an antagonist of insulin, increases the amount of free fatty acids available to the fetus for metabolic needs, and decreases the maternal metabolism of glucose allowing for protein synthesis. This allows the fetus to have the needed nutrients when the woman has not or is not eating.

Other Hormones

1. Prostaglandins:
   a. Exact function is still unknown.
   b. Affect smooth muscle contractility and some potent vasodilators.

c. Essential for the cardiovascular adaptation to pregnancy, cervical ripening, and initiation of labor.
   d. Increased levels of prostaglandins may lead to vasodilatation.
2. Relaxin:
   a. Secreted primarily by the corpus luteum. Can be secreted in small amounts by the decidua and the placenta.
   b. Inhibits uterine activity, decreases the strength of uterine contractions, softens the cervix, and remodels collagen.
3. Prolactin:
   a. Released from the anterior pituitary gland.
   b. Responsible for sustaining milk protein, casein, fatty acids, lactose, and the volume of milk secretion during lactation.

Structure of the Pelvis

Bones of the Pelvis

The pelvis is composed of four bones:
1. Two innominate bones (hip bones) form the sides and front.
2. Sacrum and coccyx form the back. Pelvic bones are held together by fibrocartilage of the symphysis pubis and several ligaments.

Divisions of the Pelvis

1. False pelvis—lies above an imaginary line called the *linea terminalis* or *pelvic brim* (Figure 36-1). Function of the false pelvis is to support the enlarged uterus.
2. True pelvis lies below the pelvic brim or linea terminalis; it is the bony canal through which the infant must pass. It is divided into three planes: the inlet, the midpelvis, and the outlet.
   a. Inlet:
      (i) Upper boundary of true pelvis—bounded by upper margin of symphysis pubis in front, linea terminalis on sides, and sacral promontory (first sacral vertebra) in back.
      (ii) Largest diameter of inlet is transverse (Figure 36-2).

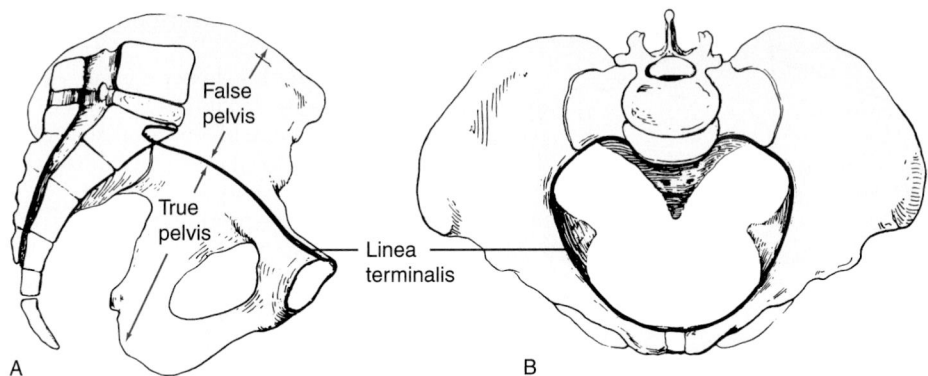

FIGURE 36-1 (**A**) Side view of the true and false pelvis. (**B**) Front view showing linea terminalis (pelvic brim).

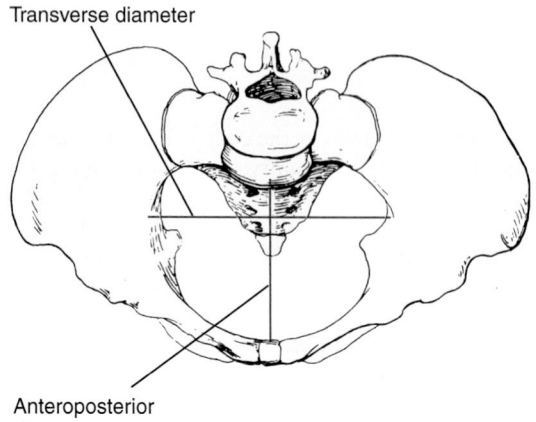

FIGURE 36-2   Inlet of normal female pelvis showing transverse and anteroposterior diameters.

(iii) Smallest diameter of inlet is anteroposterior.
(iv) Anteroposterior diameter is most important diameter of inlet: measured clinically by diagonal conjugate—distance from lower margin of symphysis to the sacral promontory (usually 13.5 cm) (Figure 36-3).
(v) Obstetric (true) conjugate—distance between inner surface of symphysis and sacral promontory measured by subtracting 1.5 to 2 cm (thickness of symphysis) from the diagonal conjugate. Adequate diameter is usually 11.5 cm. This is the

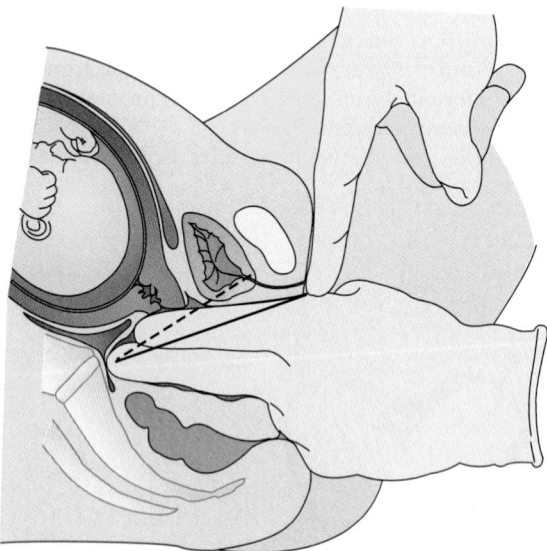

FIGURE 36-3   Measurement of diagonal conjugate diameter. *Straight line* shows diagonal conjugate; *dotted* line shows true conjugate.

shortest anteroposterior diameter through which the fetus must pass.
b. Midpelvis:
  (i) Bounded by inlet above and outlet below—true bony cavity. Contains the narrowest portion of the pelvis.
  (ii) Diameters cannot be measured clinically.
  (iii) Clinical evaluation of adequacy is made by noting the ischial spines. Prominent spines that protrude into the cavity indicate a contracted midpelvic space. The interspinous diameter is approximately 10 cm.
c. Outlet:
  (i) Lowest boundary of the true pelvis.
  (ii) Bounded by lower margin of symphysis in front, ischial tuberosities on sides, tip of sacrum posteriorly.
  (iii) Most important diameter clinically is distance between the tuberosities (>10 cm).

Shapes of the Pelvis
There are four main types of pelvic shapes (Figure 36-4).
1. Gynecoid (normal female pelvis); optimal diameters in all three planes; 50% of all women.
2. Android (normal male pelvis); posterior segments are decreased in all three planes; deep transverse arrest of descent of the fetus and failure of rotation of the fetus are common; 20% of all women.
3. Anthropoid (apelike pelvis with long anterioposterior diameter); may allow for easy delivery of an occiput-posterior presentation of the fetus; 25% of all women.
4. Platypelloid (flat female pelvis with wide transverse diameter); arrest of fetal descent at the pelvic inlet is common; labor progress can be poor; 5% of all women.

Structure of the Uterus
1. Located behind the symphysis pubis between the bladder and the rectum.
2. Uterine size increases after childbirth.
3. Consists of four parts:
  a. Fundus—upper rounded segment that extends above the insertion of the fallopian tubes; fetal growth is measured by fundal height.
  b. Body (corpus)—main portion between cervix and fundus.
  c. Isthmus (neck)—lower uterine segment.
  d. Cervix—divided into two sections:
    (i) Supravaginal—portion that extends inside the uterus; contains internal os that opens into the uterine cavity.
    (ii) Vaginal—portion that extends outside the uterus into the vagina; contains the external os that is the visible opening of the cervix; portion that is felt during vaginal examination in assessing cervical dilatation.
4. Consists of three layers:
  a. Parietal peritoneum—serous coat; covers most of uterus except cervix and anterior portion of body.

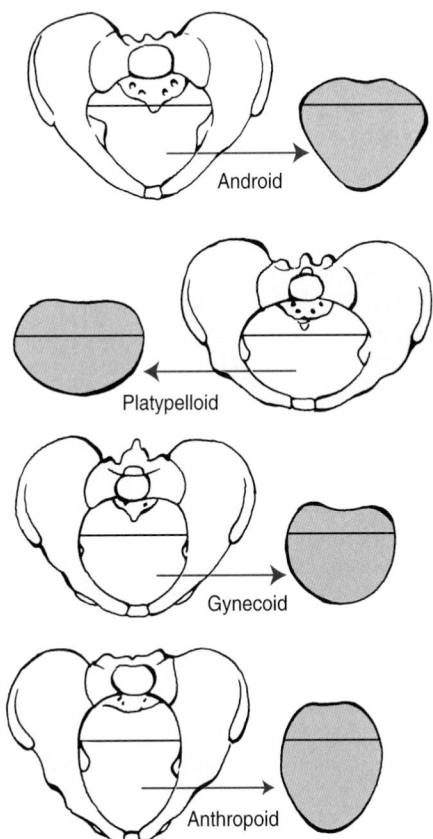

FIGURE 36-4 The four types of female pelvis. Android—male-type pelvis. Platypelloid—broad pelvis with shortened anteroposterior diameter and flattened, oval, transverse shape. Gynecoid—typical female pelvis in which inlet is round instead of oval. Anthropoid—pelvis in which anteroposterior diameter is equal to or greater than the transverse diameter.

b. Myometrium—three layers:
    (i) Outer layer—provides power to expel the fetus.
    (ii) Middle layer—provides contractions after childbirth to control blood loss.
    (iii) Inner layer—provides sphincter action to help keep cervix closed during pregnancy.
c. Endometrium—highly vascular mucous membrane; responds to hormonal stimulation with hypertrophy and secretion; sloughs if pregnancy does not occur.

◼ Prenatal Assessment
Health History
Age
1. Adolescents (younger than 19 years of age) have an increased incidence of anemia, pregnancy-induced hypertension (PIH), preterm labor (PTL), small-for-gestational-age (SGA) infants, intrauterine-growth-restricted (IUGR) infants, cephalopelvic disproportion (CPD), and dystocia.

2. Women of advanced maternal age (over 35 years of age) have an increased incidence of hypertension, pregnancies complicated by underlying medical problems such as diabetes, multiple gestation, and infants with genetic abnormalities,

Family History
1. Includes maternal and paternal history
2. Congenital disorders, hereditary diseases, multiple pregnancies, diabetes, heart disease, hypertension, mental retardation, renal disease, use of diethylstilbestrol (DES)

> **NURSING ALERT**
>
> Daughters born to mothers who sustained their pregnancies with DES may have uterine anomalies that increase their risk of preterm labor (PTL) or uterine hyperstimulation.

Woman's Medical History
1. Childhood diseases, especially rubella. Others to consider are measles and chicken pox.
2. Major illnesses, surgery (especially of the reproductive tract), blood transfusions.
3. Drug, food, and environmental sensitivities.
4. Urinary infections, heart disease, diabetes, hypertension, endocrine disorders, anemias.
5. Use of oral or other contraceptives.
6. History of sexually transmitted diseases.
7. Menstrual history (start of menarche, length, amount, regularity, and pain [dysmenorrhea] of menstrual cycle). Also, assess bleeding between periods.
8. Use of medications (prescription and over-the-counter), other drugs, alcohol, tobacco, and caffeine.
9. History of tuberculosis, hepatitis, group B beta streptococcus, or human immunodeficiency virus (HIV).

Woman's Past Obstetric History
1. Problems of infertility, date of previous pregnancies, and deliveries—dates; infant weights; length of labors; types of deliveries; multiple births; abortions; and maternal, fetal, and neonatal complications.
2. Woman's perception of past pregnancy, labor, and delivery for herself and effect on her family.

Woman's Present Obstetric History
1. Gravidity, parity.
2. Date of last menstrual period.
3. Estimated date of birth—expected date of confinement.
4. Signs and symptoms of pregnancy—amenorrhea, breast changes, nausea and vomiting, fetal movement, fatigue, urinary frequency, skin pigmentary changes. Expectations for her present pregnancy, labor, and delivery.
5. Rest and sleep patterns—length, quality, and regularity of rest and sleep.
6. Activity and employment—exercise patterns, type and hours of employment, exposure to hazardous material (occupational hazards), plans for continued employment.
7. Sexual activity—sexual satisfaction, frequency and positions during intercourse, alternative practices used to achieve sexual satisfaction.

8. Diet history—weight gain, eating patterns (times and frequency of eating daily), social or cultural dietary habits, number of servings of food from five food groups (Table 36-1), calories, protein, vitamins, and minerals consumed daily, history of eating disorders (obesity, bulimia, anorexia nervosa).
9. Psychosocial status—emotional changes she is experiencing, woman's and family's reactions to present pregnancy, support system—family's and friends' willingness to provide support, woman's present coping with lifestyle changes caused by the pregnancy.

Laboratory Data
Urinalysis
1. Urine is tested for glucose, ketones, and protein. Urine is usually collected by way of clean catch midstream (CCMS).
2. Glucose may be present in small amounts because the glomerular filtration rate is increased without the same increase in kidney tubular reabsorption. It should be investigated to rule out diabetes.
3. Protein in the urine that exceeds 250 mg/dL should be reported because it may be a sign of a hypertensive disorder of pregnancy, renal problems, or urinary tract infection.
4. Ketones in the urine should be reported because it may be a sign of excessive weight loss, dehydration, or electrolyte imbalance, often secondary to nausea and vomiting of pregnancy.
5. If the urine is cloudy and bacteria or leukocytes are present (>4 leukocytes per high-powered field), a urine culture is done.

6. The presence of bilirubin is indicative of liver or gallbladder disease or breakdown of RBCs.
7. The presence of blood in the urine (hematuria) is suggestive of urinary tract infection, kidney disease, or vaginal contamination.

Blood
1. Determination of hematocrit and hemoglobin levels and description of the morphology of the RBCs are done to find evidence of anemias, such as sickle cell or Mediterranean anemia.
2. Hemoglobin levels average 12 to 16 g/dL.
3. Blood type, Rh factor, and antibody screen—if the woman is found to be Rh negative or to have a positive antibody screen, her partner is screened and a maternal antibody titer is drawn as indicated.
   a. Coombs' test—retested at 28 weeks in the Rh-negative woman for detection of antibodies.
   b. Rh0(D) immune globulin (RhoGAM) given at 28 weeks as indicated.
   c. Given within 72 hours of birth of Rh0(D) mom or Du– and without antibodies and neonate is $Rh_1(D)$ or Du+ with negative Coombs' test.
4. Glucose—diabetic screening done at 24 to 28 weeks. One hour 50-g glucose load test.
5. Alpha-fetoprotein—done at 15 to 18 weeks. High maternal levels after 18 weeks may indicate a neural tube defect in the fetus; however, this test has high false-positive results.

Infection
1. Venereal Disease Research Lab (VDRL) test or Fluorescent Treponemal Antibody Absorption Test (FTA-ABS)

TABLE 36-1 Recommended Dietary Allowances of Selected Nutrients for Pregnancy and Lactation

Nutrient	11–14 Years (101 lb—62 in.)	15–18 Years (120 lb—64 in.)	19–22 Years (120 lb—64 in.)	23–50 Years (120 lb—64 in.)	Added for Pregnancy	Added for Lactation
Protein (g)	46	46	44	44	+30	+20
Fat-soluble vitamins						
Vitamin A (µg RE)	800	800	800	800	+200	+400
Vitamin D (µg)	10	10	7.5	5	+5	+5
Vitamin E (mg αTE)	8	8	8	8	+2	+3
Water-soluble vitamins						
Vitamin C (mg)	50	60	60	60	+20	+40
Thiamine (mg)	1.1	1.1	1.1	1.0	+0.4	+0.5
Riboflavin (mg)	1.3	1.3	1.3	1.2	+0.3	+0.5
Niacin mg NE	15	14	14	13	+2	+5
Vitamin B_6 (mg)	1.8	2.0	2.0	2.0	+0.6	+0.5
Folacin (µg)	400	400	400	400	+400	+100
Vitamin B_{12} (µg)	3.0	3.0	3.0	3.0	+1.0	+1.0
Minerals						
Calcium (mg)	1200	1200	800	800	+400	+400
Phosphorus (mg)	1200	1200	800	800	+400	+400
Magnesium (mg)	300	300	300	300	+150	+150
Iron (mg)	18	18	18	18	30 to 60 mg of supplemental iron is recommended	
Zinc (mg)	15	15	15	15	+5	+10
Iodine (µg)	150	150	150	150	+25	+50

From Food and Nutrition Board, National Academy of Sciences—National Research Council.

for syphilis is done on the initial visit; repeat VDRL at 32 weeks as indicated.

2. Gonorrhea—cervical cultures are usually done at the initial visit and when symptoms are present.
3. Herpes—all possible lesions are cultured, and the cervix is cultured weekly beginning 4 to 8 weeks before delivery.
4. Chlamydia—done at the initial visit and when symptoms are present.
5. Rubella titer—if nonimmune, less than 1:8, immunize postpartum.
6. Hepatitis B surface antigen.
7. HIV—screen is done on high-risk women.

Other Tests

1. Toxoplasmosis—done as indicated for women at risk.
2. Tuberculin skin tests—done as indicated.
3. Papanicolaou smear—done unless recent results available.
4. Maternal serum alpha-fetoprotein (MsAFP)—done to detect open neural tube defects or open abdominal wall defects; offered to all women and usually drawn between 16 and 18 weeks' gestation.
5. Sickle cell screen—done to detect presence of sickle hemoglobin in at-risk women.
6. Group B beta streptococcus (cervical and pharyngeal swabs)—done to detect carriers or active group B beta streptococcus.

Physical Assessment

General Examination

1. The woman is asked to empty her bladder before the examination so during vaginal examination her uterus and pelvic organs may be readily palpated.
2. Evaluation of the woman's weight and blood pressure.
3. Examination of eyes, ears, and nose—nasal congestion during pregnancy may occur as a result of peripheral vasodilatation.
4. Examination of the mouth, teeth, throat, and thyroid—gums may be hyperemic and softened because of increased progesterone.
5. Inspection of breasts and nipples—breasts may be enlarged and tender; nipple and areolar pigment may be darkened.
6. Auscultation of heart.
7. Auscultation and percussion of the lungs.

Abdominal Examination

1. Examination for scars or striations, diastasis (separation of the rectus muscle), or umbilical hernia.
2. Palpation of the abdomen for height of the fundus (palpable after 13 weeks of pregnancy); measurement recorded and used as guideline for subsequent calculations.
3. Palpation of the abdomen for fetal outline and position (Leopold maneuvers)—third trimester.
4. Check of FHT—FHTs are audible with a Doppler after 10 to 12 weeks and at 18 to 20 weeks with a fetoscope.
5. Record fetal position, presentation, and FHTs.

Pelvic Examination

1. The woman is placed in lithotomy position.
2. Inspection of external genitalia.
3. Vaginal examination—done to rule out abnormalities of the birth canal and to obtain cytologic smear (Papanicolaou and, if indicated, smears for gonorrhea, vaginal trichomoniasis, candidiasis, herpes, group B beta streptococcus, and chlamydia) (Figure 36-5).
4. Examination of the cervix for position, size, mobility, and consistency. Cervix is softened and bluish (increased vascularity) during pregnancy.
5. Identification of the ovaries (size, shape, and position).
6. Rectovaginal exploration to identify hemorrhoids, fissures, herniation, or masses.
7. Evaluation of pelvic inlet—anteroposterior diameter by measuring the diagonal conjugate.
8. Evaluation of midpelvis—prominence of the ischial spines.
9. Evaluation of pelvic outlet—distance between ischial tuberosities and mobility of coccyx.

Subsequent Prenatal Assessments

1. Uterine growth and estimated fetal growth (Figure 36-6).
   a. Fundus at symphysis pubis indicates 12 weeks' gestation.
   b. Fundus at umbilicus indicates 20 weeks' gestation.
   c. Fundal height corresponds with gestational age between 22 and 34 weeks.
   d. Fundus at lower border of rib cage indicates 36 weeks' gestation.
   e. Uterus becomes globular, and drop indicates 40 weeks' gestation.
2. A greater fundal height suggests:
   a. Multiple pregnancy
   b. Miscalculated due date
   c. Polyhydramnios (excessive amniotic fluid)
   d. Hydatidiform mole (degeneration of villi into grapelike clusters; fetus does not usually develop)
   e. Uterine fibroids
3. A lesser fundal height suggests:
   a. Intrauterine fetal growth restriction
   b. Error in estimating gestation
   c. Fetal or amniotic fluid abnormalities
   d. Intrauterine fetal death
   e. Small for gestational age (SGA)
4. FHTs—palpate abdomen for fetal position.
   a. Normal—110 to 160 bpm.
5. Weight—major increase in weight occurs during second half of pregnancy; usually between 0.22 kg (0.5 lb)/week and 0.44 kg (1 lb)/week. Greater weight gain may indicate fluid retention and hypertensive disorder.
6. Blood pressure—should remain near woman's prepregnant baseline.

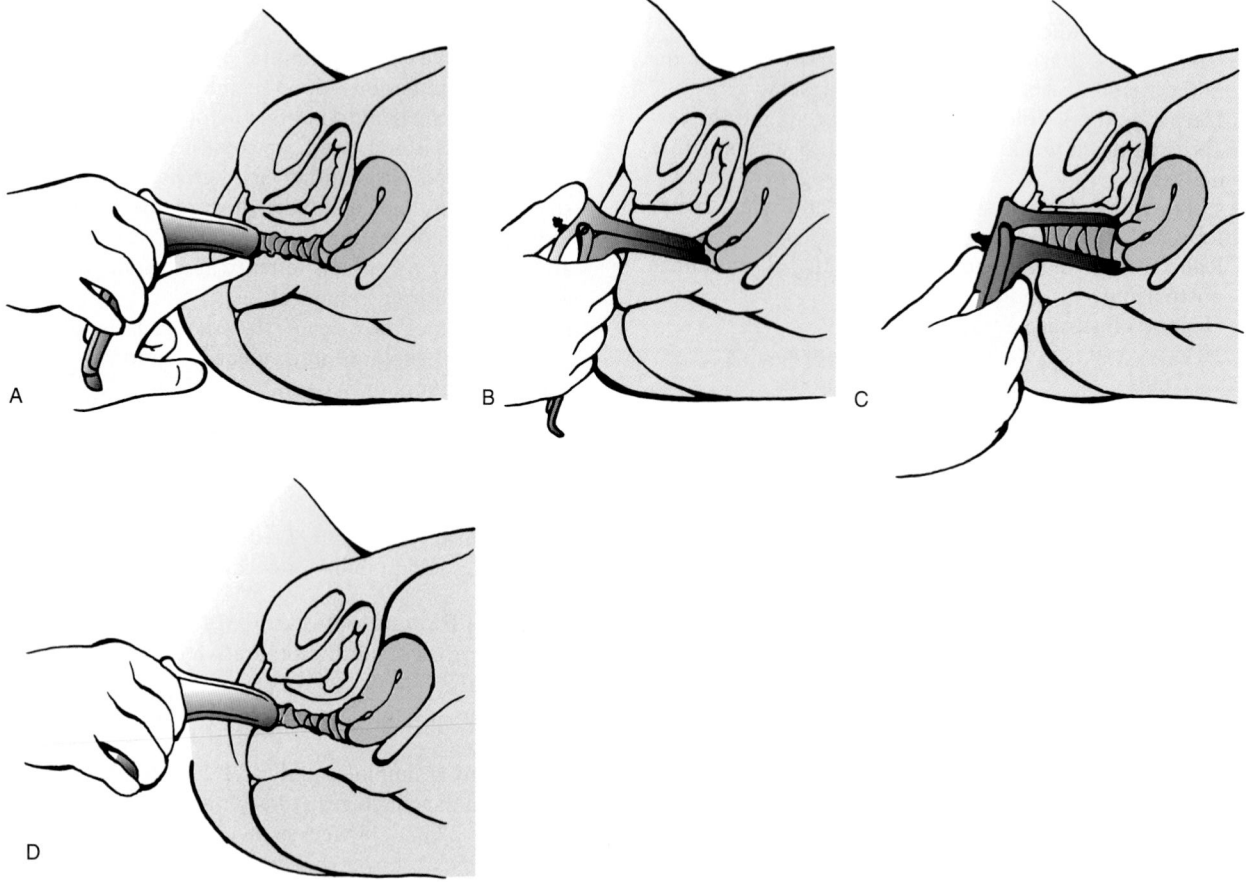

FIGURE 36-5 Vaginal speculum examination. (**A**) Blades held obliquely on entering the introitus. (**B**) Blades rotated to horizontal position and pushed toward cervix. (**C**) Blades separated to encircle cervix. (**D**) Blades removed with gentle pulling.

7. Complete blood count (CBC) at 28 and 32 weeks' gestation; VDRL—rechecked at 36 to 40 weeks' gestation.
8. Antibody serology screen if Rh negative at 36 weeks' gestation.
9. Culture smears for gonorrhea, chlamydia, group B beta streptococcus, and herpes, as indicated; usually at 36 and 40 weeks' gestation.
10. Urinalysis—for protein, glucose, blood, and nitrates.
11. Alpha-fetoprotein—done at 15 to 20 weeks.
12. Diabetic screening—done at 24 to 28 weeks.
13. Administer RhoGAM as indicated at 28 weeks.
14. Edema—check the lower legs, face, and hands.
15. Evaluate discomforts of pregnancy—fatigue, heartburn, hemorrhoids, constipation, and backache.
16. Evaluate eating and sleeping patterns, general adjustment and coping with the pregnancy.
17. Evaluate concerns of the woman and her family.
18. Evaluate preparation for labor, delivery, and parenting. See Patient Education Guidelines.

▪ Health Education and Intervention
Nursing Diagnoses
- Pain (backache, leg cramps, breast tenderness) related to physiologic changes of pregnancy
- Altered Nutrition: Less Than Body Requirements related to morning sickness and heartburn and lack of knowledge of requirements in pregnancy
- Altered Urinary Elimination (frequency) related to increased pressure from the uterus

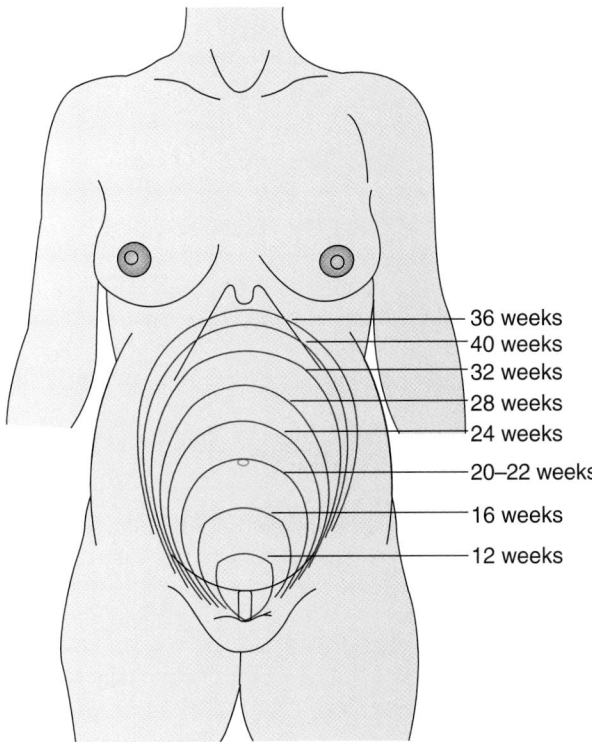

FIGURE 36-6 Height of fundus.

— 36 weeks
— 40 weeks
— 32 weeks
— 28 weeks
— 24 weeks
— 20–22 weeks
— 16 weeks
— 12 weeks

- Constipation related to physiologic changes of pregnancy and pressure from the uterus
- Impaired Tissue Integrity related to pressure from the uterus and increased blood volume
- Anxiety/Fear related to the birth process and infant care

- Altered Role Performance related to the demands of pregnancy
- Activity Intolerance related to physiologic changes of pregnancy and enlarging uterus

Nursing Interventions
Minimizing Pain

1. Teach the woman to use good body mechanics—wear comfortable, low-heeled shoes with good arch support; try the use of a maternity girdle.
2. Instruct the woman in the technique for pelvic rocking exercises.
3. Encourage the woman to take rest periods with her legs elevated.
4. Inform the woman that adequate calcium intake may decrease leg cramps.
5. Instruct the woman to dorsiflex the foot while applying pressure to the knee to straighten the leg for immediate relief of leg cramps.
6. Instruct the woman to wear a fitted, supportive brassiere.
7. Instruct the woman to wash her breasts and nipples with water only.
8. Instruct the woman to apply vitamin E or lanolin cream to the breast and nipple area. Lanolin is contraindicated for women with allergies to lamb's wool.

Minimizing Morning Sickness and Heartburn and Maintaining Adequate Nutrition

1. Encourage the woman to eat low-fat protein foods and dry carbohydrates, such as toast and crackers.
2. Encourage the woman to eat small, frequent meals.
3. Instruct the woman to avoid brushing her teeth soon after eating.
4. Instruct the woman to get out of bed slowly.

PATIENT EDUCATION GUIDELINES   Prenatal Care

1. It is important to keep scheduled prenatal care appointments:
   - Weeks 1–28: Every month
   - Weeks 28–36: Every 2 weeks
   - Weeks 36–delivery: Every week
2. Expect the following discomforts of pregnancy, and speak with your nurse or health care provider about strategies for relief:
   - Back pain, leg cramps, breast tenderness
   - Morning sickness, heartburn
   - Frequent urination
   - Constipation
   - Swelling of legs, varicose veins
   - Fatigue
3. Follow healthy, balanced diet with three meals a day, and take prenatal vitamin as directed by your health care provider.

4. Get regular exercise, and use proper body mechanics to avoid injury.
5. Be aware of danger symptoms of pregnancy—require prompt reporting to health care provider:
   - Visual disturbances—blurring, spots, or double vision
   - Vaginal bleeding, new or old blood
   - Edema of the face, fingers, and sacrum
   - Headaches—frequent, severe, or continuous
   - Fluid discharge from vagina; unusual or severe abdominal pain
   - Chills, fever, or burning on urination
   - Epigastric pain (severe stomachache)
   - Muscular irritability or convulsions
   - Inability to tolerate food or liquids, leading to severe nausea and/or hyperemesis

5. Encourage the woman to drink soups and liquids between meals to avoid stomach distention.

6. Instruct the woman in the use of antacids; caution against the use of sodium bicarbonate because it results in the absorption of excess sodium and fluid retention.

7. Teach the woman the importance of good nutrition for herself and her fetus. Review the basic food groups with appropriate daily servings.
   a. Seven servings of protein-rich foods, including one serving of a vegetable protein
   b. Three servings of dairy products or other calcium-rich foods
   c. Seven servings of grain products
   d. Two or more servings of vitamin C-rich vegetable or fruit
   e. Three servings of other fruits and vegetables
   f. Three servings of unsaturated fats
   g. Two or more servings of other fruits and vegetables

8. If the woman is a vegetarian, inform her of appropriate intake. Assess type of vegetarian and food intake.
   a. Two broad groups of vegetarians:
      (i) Traditional—cultural or religious affiliation prescribes their diet.
      (ii) New—adopted vegetarian dietary patterns as a personal or philosophical choice.
   b. Subgroups exist within the above two groups.
      (i) Vegan—eat no animal foods.
      (ii) Lacto—eat milk/dairy products, but eat no meat, poultry, fish, seafood, or eggs.
      (iii) Lacto-ovo—eat milk/dairy products and eggs, but eat no meat, poultry, fish, or seafood.
   c. Partial vegetarians may exclude a specific type of animal food, usually meat, but may consume fish and poultry.
   d. Recommend iron and folic acid supplements.

9. Inform the woman that average weight gain in pregnancy is 25 to 35 lb. About 2 to 5 lb are gained in the first trimester and about 1 lb per week for the remainder of the gestation.
   a. Average weight gain for obese women is 15 lb (6.8 kg).
   b. Adolescent weight gain should be about 5 lb more than for adult women if within 2 years of starting menses.
   c. Women with a multiple pregnancy should gain between 35 and 45 lb.
   d. Average weight gain for underweight women is 28 to 40 lb.

10. Advise the woman to limit the use of caffeine.

11. Inform the woman that alcohol should be limited or eliminated during pregnancy; no safe level of intake has been established.

12. Inform the woman that smoking should be eliminated or severely reduced during pregnancy; risk of spontaneous abortion, fetal death, low birth weight, and neo-natal death increases with increased levels of maternal smoking.

13. Inform the woman that ingesting any drug during pregnancy may affect fetal growth and should be discussed with her health care provider.

Minimizing Urinary Frequency/Urinary Tract Infection (UTI)

1. Instruct the woman to limit fluid intake in the evening.
2. Instruct the woman to void before going to bed.
3. Encourage the woman to void after meals.
4. Encourage the woman to void when she feels the urge and after sexual intercourse.
5. Encourage the woman to wear loose-fitting cotton underwear.
6. Cranberry or blueberry juice (Vaccimium family) is recommended to help prevent UTIs.

Avoiding Constipation

1. Instruct the woman to increase fluid intake to at least eight glasses of water a day. One to two quarts of fluid a day is desirable.
2. Teach the woman that foods high in fiber should be eaten daily.
3. Encourage the woman to establish regular patterns of elimination.
4. Encourage daily exercise, such as walking.
5. Inform the woman that over-the-counter laxatives should be avoided and that bulk-forming agents may be prescribed if indicated.

Maintaining Tissue Integrity

1. Encourage the woman to take frequent rest periods with her legs elevated.
2. Instruct the woman to wear support stockings and wear loose-fitting clothing for leg varicosities.
3. Instruct the woman to rest periodically with a small pillow under the buttocks to elevate the pelvis for vulvar varicosities.
4. Instruct the woman to avoid constipation, apply cold compresses, take sitz baths, and use topical anesthetics, such as Tucks, for the relief of anal varicosities (hemorrhoids).
5. Provide reassurance that varicosities will totally or greatly resolve after delivery.

Reducing Anxiety and Fear and Promoting Preparation for Labor, Delivery, and Parenthood

1. Encourage the woman/couple to discuss their knowledge, perceptions, and expectations of the labor and delivery process.
2. Provide information on childbirth education classes, and encourage them to attend.
3. Encourage a tour of the birth facility.
4. Discuss coping and pain control techniques for labor and birth.
5. Inform the woman/couple of common procedures during labor and birth.
6. Provide guidelines for coming to the birth facility.

7. Encourage the woman/couple to discuss their perceptions and expectations of parenthood and their "idealized child."
8. Discuss the infant's sleeping, eating, activity, and response patterns for the first month of life.
9. Discuss physical preparations for the infant, such as a sleeping space, clothing, feeding, changing, and bathing equipment.
10. Discuss plans for returning to work and child care arrangements.
11. Discuss the importance of planning time for themselves and each other apart from the newborn.
12. Provide information and encourage attendance at baby care, breast-feeding, and parenting classes.
13. Answer any questions the woman/couple may have.

Enhancing Role Changes
1. Encourage discussion of feelings and concerns regarding the new role of mother and father.
2. Provide emotional support to the woman/couple regarding the altered family role.
3. Discuss physiologic causes for changes in sexual relationships, such as fatigue, loss of interest, and discomfort from advancing pregnancy. Some women experience heightened sexual activity during the second trimester.
4. Teach the woman/couple that there are no contraindications to intercourse or masturbation to orgasm provided the woman's membranes are intact, there is no vaginal bleeding, and she has no current problems or history of premature labor.
5. Teach the woman/couple that female superior or side-lying positions are often more comfortable in the latter half of pregnancy.

Minimizing Fatigue
1. Teach the woman reasons for fatigue, and have her plan a schedule for adequate rest.
   a. Fatigue in the first trimester is due to increased progesterone and its effects on the sleep center.
   b. Fatigue in the last trimester is due mainly to carrying increased weight of the pregnancy.
   c. About 8 hours of rest are needed at night.
   d. Inability to sleep may be due to excessive fatigue during the day.
   e. In the latter months of pregnancy, sleeping on the side with a small pillow under the abdomen may enhance comfort.
   f. Frequent 15- to 30-minute rest periods during the day are important to avoid overfatigue.
   g. Whenever possible, the woman should work while sitting with her legs elevated.
   h. The woman should avoid standing for prolonged periods of time, especially during the third trimester.
      (i) To promote placental perfusion, the woman should not lie flat on her back—left lateral position provides the best placental perfusion; however, either side is acceptable.
2. Help the woman plan for adequate exercise.
   a. In general, exercise during pregnancy should be in keeping with the woman's prepregnancy pattern and type of exercise.
   b. Activities or sports that have a risk of bodily harm (skiing, snowmobiling, skating, roller blading, horseback riding) should be avoided.
   c. During pregnancy, endurance during exercise may be decreased.
   d. Exercise classes for pregnant women that concentrate on toning and stretching have resulted in enhanced physical condition, increased self-esteem, and greater social support as a result of being in the exercise group.

Community and Home Care Instructions
1. Community and home care is prevention-oriented care.
2. Case management coordinates health care management collaboratively.
3. Search out and register for prepared childbirth classes. Preferable to attend those associated with the family's intended delivery hospital.
4. Social support available from Women, Infants, and Children's (WIC) Special Supplemental Feeding Program, breast-feeding groups (La Leche), and father support groups.
5. Prenatal education should focus on nutrition, sexuality, stress reduction, lifestyle behaviors, and hazards at home or work.
6. Consider cultural practices because they have important implications for the provision of nursing care.

Alternative Therapies
General Measures
1. Alternative therapies range from nutrition and lifestyle changes to mind and body programs.
2. Encourage woman to discuss options with her health care provider.
3. Physical activities—maintaining an active lifestyle and healthy diet. Some use macrobiotic diets and isometric exercise.
4. Attitudinal activities—maintaining a positive attitude, positive self-image, and have fun and laugh.
5. Relational activities—maintaining social relationships—friends, pets, and family.
6. Spiritual activities—having faith, hope, prayer, music, and meditating as an active part of daily life.
7. Self-caring activities—taking care of self; balancing life, personal integrity, knowing and trusting self, and own time management.
8. Help-seeking activities—seeking assistance in health care ranging from prescribed treatments to biomedicine (self-healing touch). Help-seeking activities include ethnomedicine (Chinese herbal medicine and acupuncture), structure/energy therapies (therapeutic touch and osteopathy), pharmacologic/biologic treatments (antioxidants), biofeedback, guided imagery, music therapy, meditation, and prayer.

Alternative Therapies Specific to the Prenatal Period

1. Therapeutic touch.
2. Yoga.
3. Cranberry or blueberry juice for UTI prevention.
4. Nausea is sometimes attributed to vitamin B deficiencies, but does not always improve with simple vitamin supplements. The woman can take red raspberry or peppermint tea, ginger root, and ginger ale to alleviate the nausea. To increase the effectiveness of red raspberry tea, add alfalfa to the tea.
5. Catnip, fennel, lobelia, papaya, spearmint, and wild yams decrease colic stomach cramps, gas, and heartburn, and improve the appetite.
6. Many herbs are available to be used during pregnancy including the labor and delivery process. It is essential that the woman and her family discuss the use of herbs with her primary care provider before use. Herbs come in different forms—capsules, tablets, extracts, tinctures, powders, dried and prepared as teas or juices, in combinations, and as external preparations. Become familiar with the local distributor and ask questions. Although herbs are natural, they can be harmful if misused. Herbs should be used with the same respect as medications. It is also important to realize that there are few herbal therapies that are FDA approved. They include:
   a. Aloe as a laxative
   b. Capsicum or cayenne pepper (chili pepper; red pepper) as topical analgesic; marketed as a cream and used topically
   c. Cascara (sacred bark; bitter bark) as a laxative
   d. Psyllium (plantago seed) as a laxative
   e. Senna as a laxative
   f. Slippery elm (red elm) as oral demulcent; marketed as throat lozenges
7. Despite the fact that few herbs are FDA approved, many other herbs are sold on the market and used by millions of women, both pregnant and nonpregnant. Many herb formulas contain substances that are refined or synthesized by pharmaceutical companies and marketed as acceptable treatments by the medical and nursing communities.
8. Herbs can be used alone or in conjunction with traditional medicine. Women should be offered traditional and alternative therapies. If herbal therapy is desired, refer woman to a knowledgeable herbalist.

Outcome-Based Evaluation

- Verbalizes understanding of proper body mechanics and wears low-heeled shoes
- Identifies the basic food groups and describes meals to include needed servings for pregnancy
- Reports limited fluid intake in the evening
- Describes foods high in fiber
- Wears support stockings and loose-fitting clothing
- Discusses expectations for labor, delivery, and parenthood and attends educational classes
- Verbalizes an understanding of the physiologic causes that may change the sexual relationship
- Reports engaging in regular exercise

Psychosocial Adaptation of Pregnancy

Rubin's Framework for Maternal Role Assumption

1. Attainment of motherhood role occurs with each pregnancy.
2. Involves a series of cognitive operations.
   a. Mimicry—woman begins observing and modeling her behavior after other pregnant women.
   b. Role-play—woman begins acting out behaviors of a mother. For example, the woman will rock a baby to sleep.
   c. Searching for a role "fit"—woman has perceptions of how the motherhood role will be. She observes others' behaviors to determine how well they fit with her expectations of the motherhood role.
   d. Grief work—woman experiences a sense of loss of her "old" self as she prepares to begin her new role as a mother.
3. Maternal task—often divided by trimesters.
   a. First trimester (first 3 months):
      (i) Acceptance of pregnancy—progressive movement from a state of conflict and ambivalence to one of acceptance of the pregnancy, the child, and the motherhood role.
      (ii) Realignment of roles—expectant parents begin to realign their roles and responsibilities as they relate to the child.
      (iii) Safe passage—although the mother seeks to ensure a safe passage for her fetus and self throughout her pregnancy, the main focus during this trimester is on self-safety.
   b. Midtrimester (second 3 months):
      (i) Safe passage—in this trimester, the mother's main focus is on appropriate nutrition and exercise.
      (ii) Acceptance by others—acceptance of this child by each family member.
      (iii) Binding-in to the child—maternal perception of the child as a real person.
   c. Last trimester (last 3 months):
      (i) Safe passage—during this trimester, the main focus is on the safety of the fetus and is inseparable from self-safety.
      (ii) Giving of oneself—the most complex task, in which the mother is learning to give to the unborn child and placing the unborn child's need in relation to her own needs.
      (iii) Critical to this trimester is the preparation of the nursery because it solidifies the acceptance of the unborn child.

Rubin's Framework for Paternal Role Assumption
1. The fatherhood role can also be attained with the pregnancy.
2. Paternal tasks can also be divided by trimesters.
   a. First trimester (first 3 months):
      (i) Announcement and realization of the pregnancy—father will exhibit excitement over the announcement of the pregnancy and is more interested in maternal changes. Often, he will insist on accompanying the mother to each prenatal appointment.
      (ii) Some fathers will even begin to experience the same signs and symptoms of pregnancy experienced by the mother. This is more commonly referred to as *couvadé*.
   b. Midtrimester (second 3 months):
      (i) Anticipation—father anticipates and adapts to the role of fatherhood.
      (ii) Fantasy and exploration—along with the mother, the father begins to imagine what his child will look like and may also begin to explore the talents and attributes of the unborn child.
      (iii) Adjustment of sexual expression to accommodate the pregnancy.
   c. Last trimester (last 3 months):
      (i) Preparation—now, serious preparation for the forthcoming child includes preparation of the nursery and childbirth education courses to prepare for labor and delivery.
      (ii) Reassurance—provided by the father to ease the anxious mother's fears regarding labor and delivery.

THE FETUS

◼ Fetal Growth and Development

Previously, methods used to determine how well the fetus was growing and maturing consisted of evaluating uterine growth and listening to fetal heart sounds. Advances in knowledge and technology have provided newer methods for assessing fetal well-being and maturity. Improved methods for assessment and diagnosis enable early intervention for improved outcome.

Stages of Growth and Development

The growth and development of the fetus is often divided into three stages.

Preembryonic Stage: Fertilization to 2 to 3 Weeks
1. Rapid cell division and differentiation
2. Develop embryonic membranes and germ layers

Embryonic Stage: 4 to 8 Weeks' Gestation
1. Most critical stage of physical development
2. Organogenesis

Fetal Stage: 9 Weeks to Birth
1. Every organ system and external structure present.
2. Refinement of fetus and organ function occurs. See Figure 36-7.

Development by Month

First Lunar Month
1. Fertilization to 2 weeks of embryonic growth.
2. Implantation is complete.
3. Primary chorionic villi forming.
4. Embryo develops into two cell layers (trophoblast and blastocyst).
5. Amniotic cavity appears.

Second Lunar Month
1. 3 to 6 weeks of embryonic growth.
2. At the end of 6 weeks of growth, the embryo is approximately 1.2 cm long.
3. Arm and leg buds are visible; arm buds are more developed with finger ridges beginning to appear.
4. Rudiments of the eyes, ears, and nose appear.
5. Lung buds are developing.
6. Primitive intestinal tract is developing.
7. Primitive cardiovascular system is functioning.
8. Neural tube, which forms the brain and spinal cord, closes by the 4th week.

Third Lunar Month
1. 7 to 10 weeks of growth.
2. The middle of this period (9 weeks) marks the end of the embryonic period and the beginning of the fetal period.
3. At the end of 10 weeks of growth, the fetus is approximately 6.1 cm from crown to rump and weighs 14 g.
4. Appearance of external genitalia.
5. By the middle of this month, all major organ systems have formed.
6. The membrane over the anus has broken down.
7. The heart has formed four chambers (by 7th week).
8. The fetus assumes a human appearance.
9. Bone ossification begins.
10. Rudimentary kidney begins to secrete urine.

Fourth Lunar Month
1. 11- to 14-week-old fetus.
2. At the end of 14 weeks of growth, the fetus is approximately 12 cm crown–rump length and 110 g.
3. Head erect; lower extremities well developed.
4. Hard palate and nasal septum have fused.
5. External genitalia of male and female can now be differentiated.
6. Eyelids are sealed.

Fifth Lunar Month
1. 15- to 18-week-old fetus.
2. At the end of 18 weeks of growth, the fetus is approximately 16 cm crown–rump length and 320 g.
3. Ossification of fetal skeleton can be seen on x-ray.
4. Ears stand out from head.
5. Meconium is present in the intestinal tract.

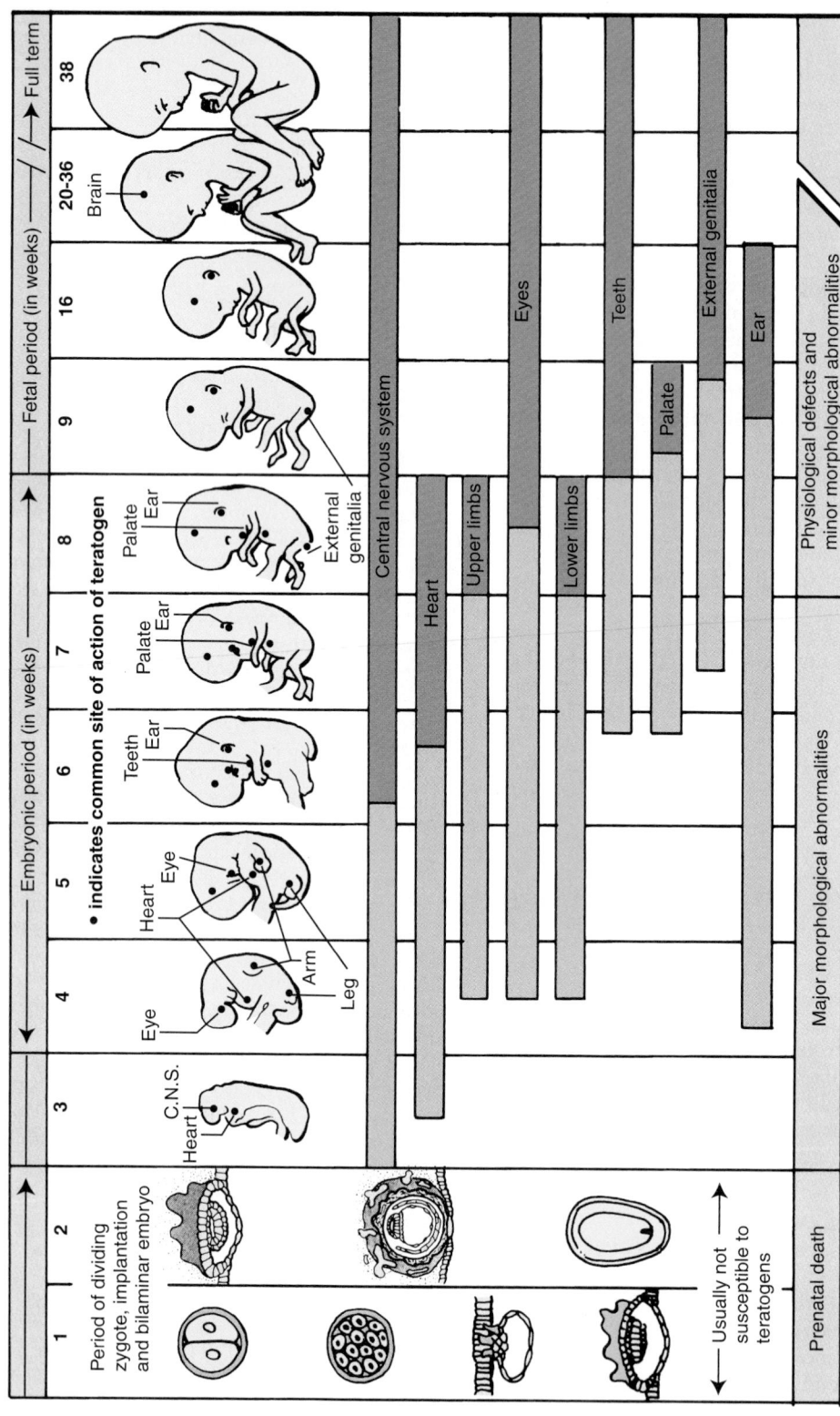

FIGURE 36-7 Schematic illustration of the sensitive or critical periods in human development. During the first 2 weeks of development, the embryo is usually not susceptible to teratogens. During these predifferentiation stages, a substance either damages all or most of the cells of the embryo, resulting in its death, or damages only a few cells, allowing the embryo to recover without developing defects. The left (*shaded*) sides of the bars denote highly sensitive periods; the right sides indicate stages that are less sensitive to teratogens. (Moore, K.L. *The developing human: Clinically oriented embryology* [4th ed.]. Philadelphia: W.B. Saunders.)

6. Fetus makes sucking motions and swallows amniotic fluid.
7. Fetal movements may be felt by the mother (end of month).

Sixth Lunar Month
1. 19- to 22-week-old fetus.
2. At the end of 22 weeks of growth, the fetus is approximately 21 cm crown–rump length and 630 g.
3. Vernix caseosa covers the skin.
4. Head and body (lanugo) hair visible.
5. Skin is wrinkled and red.
6. Brown fat, an important site of heat production, is present in neck and sternal area.
7. Nipples are apparent on the breasts.

Seventh Lunar Month
1. 23- to 26-week-old fetus.
2. At the end of 26 weeks of growth, the fetus is approximately 25 cm crown–rump length and 1,000 g.
3. Fingernails present.
4. Lean body.
5. Eyes partially open; eyelashes present.
6. Bronchioles are present; primitive alveoli are forming.
7. Skin begins to thicken on hands and feet.
8. Startle reflex present; grasp reflex is strong.

Eighth Lunar Month
1. 27- to 30-week-old fetus.
2. At the end of 30 weeks of growth, the fetus is approximately 28 cm crown–rump length and 1,700 g.
3. Eyes open.
4. Ample hair on head; lanugo begins to fade.
5. Skin slightly wrinkled.
6. Toenails present.
7. Testes in inguinal canal, begin descent to scrotal sac.
8. Surfactant coats much of the alveolar epithelium.

Ninth Lunar Month
1. 31- to 34-week-old fetus.
2. At the end of 34 weeks of growth, the fetus is approximately 32 cm crown–rump length and 2,500 g.
3. Fingernails reach fingertips.
4. Skin pink and smooth.
5. Testes in scrotal sac.

Tenth Lunar Month
1. 35- to 38-week-old fetus; end of this month is also 40 weeks from onset of last menstrual period.
2. End of 38 weeks of growth, fetus is approximately 36 cm crown–rump length and 3,400 g.
3. Ample subcutaneous fat.
4. Lanugo almost absent.
5. Toenails reach toe tips.
6. Testes in scrotum.
7. Vernix caseosa mainly on the back.
8. Breasts are firm.

Fetal Circulation
See Figure 36-8.

Assessment of Fetal Maturity and Well-Being
Maternal History and Examination
History
1. The woman's family medical history, the woman's medical history, and reproductive health history
2. Comprehensive physical examination, history of current pregnancy, and identified risk factors
3. Health during previous pregnancies
4. Outcome of previous pregnancies
5. Routine prenatal labs
6. Fetal assessment after first trimester and individualized fetal surveillance as indicated

Fetal Heart Tones
Description
FHTs are representative of the fetal heart rate (FHR) and are an indicator of oxygen perfusion to the fetal brain, heart, and adrenals. The evaluation of FHTs is indicated in routine assessment of fetal well-being, in determining gestational age, and in cases of threatened abortion or other abnormalities. FHTs can be heard using techniques that amplify sound.
1. Doppler at approximately 10 to 12 weeks' fetal gestation.
2. Fetoscope (fetal stethoscope) at approximately 18 to 20 weeks' fetal gestation.
3. Electronic fetal monitoring testing is usually done when the fetus is considered viable; around 24 weeks' gestation.
4. Rate—between 110 and 160 bpm.
5. In latter months of pregnancy, fetal heart sounds found.
   a. Near the woman's midline in fetal occipitoanterior positions
   b. Lateral to midline in fetal occipitotransverse positions
   c. In the woman's flank in fetal occipitoposterior positions
   d. Below the woman's umbilicus in cephalic presentations
   e. At or above the woman's umbilicus in breech presentations
6. Failure to hear FHTs at the expected time may be due to maternal obesity, polyhydramnios, error in date calculation, or fetal death.

Nursing and Patient Care Considerations
1. Explain equipment, purpose, and procedure to the woman.
2. Assist the woman to a side-lying or semi-Fowler's position. Position may affect the ability to clearly hear the heart tones. Perform Leopold's maneuvers.
3. Document findings on the woman's chart and/or monitor strip along with date, time, activity level, medications, and other information per health care facility's guidelines.
4. Discontinue electronic fetal monitoring as indicated according to guidelines.
5. Communicate appropriate information to the woman and other personnel.

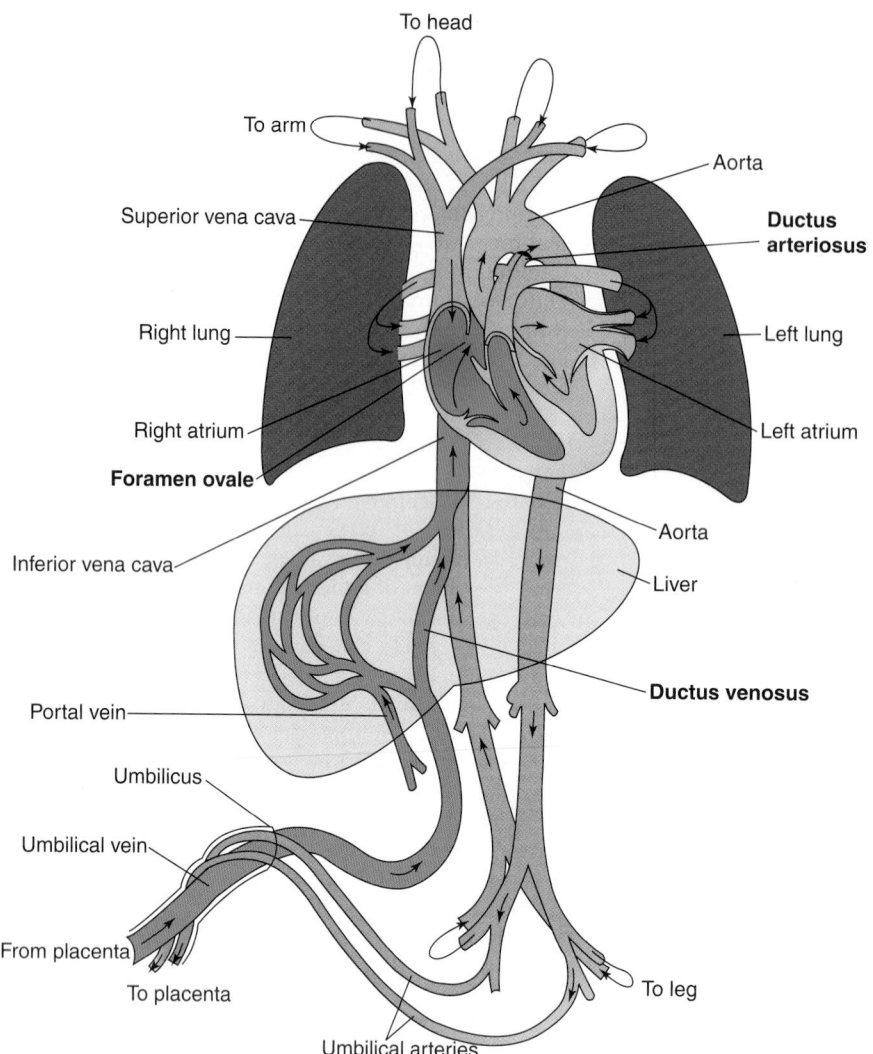

To head

To arm

Aorta

Superior vena cava

Ductus arteriosus

Right lung

Left lung

Right atrium

Left atrium

Foramen ovale

Aorta

Inferior vena cava

Liver

Ductus venosus

Portal vein

Umbilicus

Umbilical vein

From placenta

To leg

To placenta

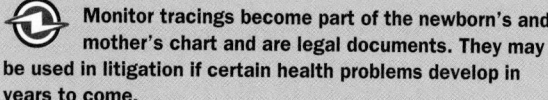

Umbilical arteries

FIGURE 36-8 Diagram of the fetal circulation shortly before birth. *Arrows* indicate course of blood.

NURSING ALERT

Monitor tracings become part of the newborn's and mother's chart and are legal documents. They may be used in litigation if certain health problems develop in years to come.

Fetal Movement
Description
Fetal movements or "kick counts" may be evaluated daily by the pregnant woman to provide reassurance of fetal well-being. Several methods proposed; however, neither the ideal number of kicks nor the ideal interval for movement counting has been defined. There are two methods defined in the literature.
1. Cardiff Count-to-Ten:
   a. Assess fetal movement once a day at the same time each day.
   b. Less than 10 fetal movements in 10 hours for 2 consecutive days or no fetal movement in a 10-hour period must be reported to the primary care provider.
2. Sadovsky:
   a. Assess fetal movement three times each day at the same time.
   b. Less than 4 fetal movements in 2 hours must be reported to the primary care provider.

Nursing and Patient Care Considerations
1. Instruct the woman to lie on her side in a quiet place with no distractions. Have her place her hands on the largest part of her abdomen and concentrate on fetal movement.
2. Instruct the woman to use a clock and record the movements felt.
3. Instruct the woman that fetal movements are best assessed after meals, after or with light abdominal massage, and after short walks.

4. Instruct the woman that the fetus can sleep for up to 40 minutes.
5. Request the woman to explain the procedure so her understanding is ensured.

Maternal Serum Alpha-Fetoprotein
Description
Maternal serum alpha-fetoprotein (MsAFP) levels are analyzed at 15 to 20 weeks' gestation to identify certain birth defects and chromosomal abnormalities during pregnancy. Alpha-fetoprotein is a major protein produced in the fetal yolk sac during the first trimester and in the fetal liver during late term.

1. Elevated AFP levels are associated with birth defects and chromosomal abnormalities such as open neural tube defects, open abdominal defects, and congenital nephrosis. Also associated with Rh isoimmunization, multiple gestation, maternal diabetes mellitus, and fetoplacental dysfunction.
2. Decreased levels are associated with Down syndrome and other chromosome anomalies (eg, gestational trophoblastic disease).
3. Follow-up for abnormal high or low levels includes ultrasound examination and amniocentesis.

Nursing and Patient Care Considerations
1. Obtain health and pregnancy history, including the date of the woman's last menstrual period and risk factors. Accurate dating of the pregnancy is crucial to interpret the results of the serum levels.
2. Explain the purpose and procedure for the test.
3. Discuss the woman's concerns.

Ultrasound
Description
Ultrasound is a noninvasive, safe technique that uses reflected sound waves as they travel in tissue to produce a picture. A clear gel is applied to the woman's abdomen or transducer, and the transducer is moved along the abdomen by the examiner producing images on a screen.

1. Uses in the first trimester of pregnancy include:
   a. Early confirmation of pregnancy and determination of the estimated date of confinement
   b. Diagnosis of an ectopic pregnancy
   c. Detection of an intrauterine device
   d. Evaluation of placental location
   e. Diagnosis of a multiple gestation
   f. Guidance for chorionic villus sampling (CVS)
2. Uses in the second and third trimester include:
   a. Evaluation of fetal growth, weight, and gestational age
   b. Evaluation of the placenta for placenta previa or separation associated with vaginal bleeding
   c. Evaluation of fetal presentation and position
   d. Evaluation of fetal abnormalities
   e. Evaluation of fetal viability
   f. Determination of the Biophysical Profile (BPP) Score

g. Evaluation of amniotic fluid volume
h. Guidance for amniocentesis or fetal blood sampling

Nursing and Patient Care Considerations
1. Explain the purpose and procedure to the woman, emphasizing the need to remain still.
2. Inform the woman of the need for a full bladder before the procedure.
3. Instruct the woman to drink three to four glasses of water if the bladder is not full.
4. Instruct the woman not to void until the procedure is over.
5. Remove the lubricant from the woman's abdomen after the procedure.

Note: Nurse can perform ultrasound if credentialed in limited ultrasound.

Amniocentesis
Description
Amniocentesis is a procedure needing informed consent, in which amniotic fluid is removed from the uterine cavity by insertion of a needle through the abdominal and uterine walls and into the amniotic sac. The procedure, usually performed between 16 and 18 weeks' gestation, is used in prenatal diagnosis of genetic or metabolic diseases, fetal lung maturity, and in the treatment of polyhydramnios. Risks associated with the procedure are very low.

1. In determination of genetic or metabolic diseases, the procedure is performed between 16 and 18 weeks' gestation. It is useful for women 35 years of age or older, family history of metabolic disease, previous child with a chromosomal abnormality, family history of chromosomal abnormality, patient or husband with a chromosomal abnormality, or a possible female carrier of an X-linked disease.
2. In determination of lung maturity, the lecithin/sphingomyelin (L/S) ratio of the amniotic fluid is analyzed.
   a. When the L/S ratio is 2:1 or greater, the fetal lung is considered mature and the incidence of respiratory distress syndrome in the newborn is low.
   b. Results may be less reliable with maternal diabetes or if the fluid is contaminated with blood or meconium.
3. The presence of phosphatidylglycerol (PG), one of the last lung surfactants to develop, is the most reliable indicator of fetal lung maturity. PG is not present until 36 weeks' gestation and is measured as being present or absent. PG is not affected by hypoglycemia, hypoxia, or hypothermia like L/S is.
4. A Triple Marker Screening (TMS) can also be used for the evaluation of trisomy 18 and 21 and neural tube defects. This test is costly when compared to MsAFP, thus is limited in its use. The TMS evaluates unconjugated estriol and HCG: Down syndrome shows increased HCG and decreased estriol levels; trisomy *18* shows decreased HCG and decreased estriol levels.
5. In the treatment of polyhydramnios (2,000 mL amniotic fluid or >25 cm amniotic fluid index [AFI]),

amniocentesis may be performed to drain excess fluid and relieve pressure. Polyhydramnios is associated with specific fetal abnormalities, such as trisomy 18, anencephaly, spina bifida, and esophageal atresia or tracheoesophageal fistula (TEF).

Nursing and Patient Care Considerations

1. Reduce anxiety related to the procedure.
   a. Reduce the parents' anxiety by determining their understanding of the procedure and the meaning it holds for them.
   b. Reexplain the procedure before it begins, and answer any questions they have. Ensure informed consent is signed.
   c. Provide explanations during the procedure, correct misinformation they may have, and make sure they know when the results will be available and how they may obtain the results as soon as possible.
2. Reduce pain and discomfort related to the procedure.
   a. Reduce discomfort by having the mother lie comfortably on her back with her hands and a pillow under her head. Relaxation breathing may help.
   b. Ensure adequate time between infiltration of local anesthetic and introduction of needle into the amniotic sac.
   c. Start IV fluids in accordance with institutional policy. Administer terbutaline SQ or IV or ritodrine IV per institutional policy.
3. Reduce potential for traumatic injury to fetus, placenta, or maternal structures.
   a. Have the woman empty her bladder if the fetus is more than 20 weeks' gestation to avoid injury to the woman's bladder. If the fetus is less than 20 weeks' gestation, the woman's full bladder will hold the uterus steady and out of the pelvis. The placenta is localized with the use of ultrasound.
   b. Obtain maternal vital signs and a 20-minute fetal heart rate tracing to serve as a baseline to evaluate possible complications.
   c. Monitor the woman during and after the procedure for signs of premature labor or bleeding.
   d. Tell the woman to report signs of bleeding, unusual fetal activity or abdominal pain, cramping, or fever while at home after the procedure.

Chorionic Villus Sampling (CVS)
Description
CVS involves obtaining samples of chorionic villus (placental tissue [fetal origin]) to test for genetic disorders of the fetus. CVS is performed between 9 and 12 weeks' gestation.
1. Using an ultrasound picture, a catheter is passed vaginally into the woman's uterus, where a sample of chorionic villus tissue is snipped off or obtained by suction.
2. Results from CVS are available in 1 to 2 weeks.
3. Complications include rupture of membranes, intrauterine infection, spontaneous abortion, hematoma, fetal trauma, or maternal tissue contamination.
4. Incidence of fetal loss is about 2% to 5%.

Nursing and Patient Care Considerations
1. Obtain maternal vital signs.
2. Instruct the woman to void.
3. Reduce woman's anxiety as related to the procedure.
4. Inform the woman that a small amount of spotting is normal, but heavy bleeding or passing clots or tissue should be reported.
5. Instruct the woman to rest at home for a few hours after the procedure.

Percutaneous Umbilical Blood Sampling (PUBS)
Description
PUBS, or cordocentesis, involves a puncture of the umbilical cord for aspiration of fetal blood under ultrasound guidance.
1. It is used in the diagnosis of fetal blood disorders, infections, Rh isoimmunization, metabolic disorders, and karyotyping.
2. Transfusion to the fetus may be done with this procedure.
3. Using ultrasound picture, the provider inserts a needle (guided by ultrasound) for insertion into one of the umbilical vessels. A small amount of blood is withdrawn.
4. Can also be used for fetal therapies such as RBC and platelet transfusion.

Nursing and Patient Care Considerations
1. Explain the procedure to the woman.
2. Provide support to the woman during the procedure.
3. Monitor the woman after the procedure for uterine contractions and the fetal heart rate for distress.

Nonstress Test (NST)
Description
The NST is used to evaluate FHR accelerations that normally occur in response to fetal activity in a fetus in good condition. Accelerations are indicative of an intact central and autonomic nervous system and a sign of fetal well-being.
1. Maternal indications include postdates, Rh sensitization, maternal age 35 or older, chronic renal disease, hypertension, collagen disease, sickle cell disease, diabetes, premature rupture of membranes, history of stillbirth, trauma, vaginal bleeding in the second and third trimesters.
2. There are no contraindications for the NST.
3. Fetal indications include decreased fetal movement, intrauterine growth restriction, fetal evaluation after an amniocentesis, oligohydramnios or polyhydramnios.
   a. Criteria for a reactive NST in a fetus >37 weeks include two accelerations within 20 minutes, each lasting at least 15 seconds with a FHR increased by 15 bpm above baseline in response to fetal activity. The test period should be a minimum of 20 minutes to allow for fetal rest cycle patterns. A reactive NST is associated with a normal baseline fetal heart rate (FHR) and average long-term variability (LTV).

b. Criteria for a reactive preterm NST include two accelerations within 60 to 90 minutes, each lasting at least 10 seconds with a FHR increased by 10 bpm above baseline in response to fetal activity.

c. In a nonreactive NST, the above criteria are not met.

d. In an equivocal NST there are:
   (i) Less than two accelerations in 20 minutes
   (ii) Accelerations not meeting the 15×15 criteria (15 bpm above the FHR baseline lasting for 15 seconds from time heart rate leaves the baseline until the time it returns to the baseline) for term, or 10×10 criteria for preterm
   (iii) Minimal or decreased LTV
   (iv) Quality of the tracing is not adequate for interpretation

Significance/Management

1. Reactive NST—suggests <1% chance of fetal death within 1 week of the NST.
2. Nonreactive NST—suggests fetus may be compromised and there needs to be further follow-up with Biophysical Profile (BPP), Contraction Stress Test (CST), or Oxytocin Challenge Test (OCT).
3. Equivocal NST—needs to be repeated in 2 to 3 hours or follow-up with CST, OCT, or BPP.

Nursing and Patient Care Considerations

1. Explain the procedure and equipment to the woman. Ensure the woman has had adequate nutrition and fluid intake and, if a smoker, has not been smoking within the last 2 hours.
2. Assist the woman to a semi-Fowler's position in bed. Perform Leopold's maneuvers, and apply the external fetal and uterine monitors.
3. Event markers do not need to be used unless the fetal movement is not observed on the fetal monitor. If fetal movement not observed, instruct the woman to make a mark on the monitor strip each time fetal movement is felt. The nurse will do this if the woman cannot.
4. Evaluate the response of the fetal heart rate immediately after fetal activity.
5. Monitor the woman's blood pressure and uterine activity for deviations during the procedure.

Vibroacoustic Stimulation Test (VST)

Description

Vibroacoustic stimulation (VAS), using an artificial larynx, is an additional method of fetal assessment. It is used to stimulate the fetus and assess its reaction to the sound

1. This test may be as good a screening tool as the NST, because the loud noise stimulates the fetus and notes ability to respond to the noise by increasing heart rate.
2. Professional interpretation of its use during labor and its role in the intrapartum period are controversial; however, it is being examined as an alternative to fetal scalp sampling.
3. Interpretation depends on individualized institutional guidelines. Usually:

a. Reactive—two accelerations meeting 15×15 criteria
b. Nonreactive—no accelerations
c. Equivocal—one acceleration or accelerations not meeting the 15×15 criteria or uninterpretable/unreadable fetal tracing

4. Tachycardic rate may result from stimulus and may last >1 hour. If this occurs, observe FHR for normal baseline characteristics, other than the tachycardia, until the FHR returns to the prestimulus rate.

Nursing and Patient Care Considerations

1. Explain procedure, equipment, and purpose to the woman.
2. Assist woman to a semi-Fowler's position in bed.
3. Apply external fetal monitors to the woman.
4. Demonstrate how the stimulus may feel on the woman's forearm or leg.
5. Observe for reactivity.

Oxytocin Challenge Test (OCT) or Contraction Stress Test (CST)

Description

This test is used to evaluate the ability of the fetus to withstand the stress of uterine contractions as would occur during labor.

1. The test is usually used when a woman has a nonreactive NST or equivocal VST.
2. The test is contraindicated in women with third trimester bleeding, multiple gestation, incompetent cervix, placenta previa, previous classic uterine incision, hydramnios, history of preterm labor (PTL), or premature rupture of membranes (PROM).
3. CST is endogenously produced oxytocin by way of nipple or breast stimulation.
4. OCT is exogenous oxytocin administered by way of IV administration.

Nursing and Patient Care Considerations

1. Obtain maternal vital signs, especially blood pressure.
2. Instruct the woman to void.
3. Assist the woman to a semi-Fowler's or side-lying position in bed.
4. Obtain a 20-minute strip of the fetal heart rate and uterine activity for baseline data.
5. For CST:
   a. Apply warm packs to the breasts for 10 minutes before the CST.
   b. Instruct the mother on nipple stimulation (four cycles of 2 minutes on [stimulating] and 2 minutes off [not stimulating].
      (i) If no uterine contractions after four cycles, wait 10 minutes, then restimulate.
      (ii) If no uterine contractions after the second four cycles, stop the stimulation, notify physician, and prepare for OCT or BPP.
   c. Stop the stimulation if:
      (i) Three or more contractions within 10 minutes of >40 seconds.
      (ii) Tetanic uterine contractions or hyperstimulation.

6. For OCT: follow 1 through 4 above. In addition:
   a. Administer diluted oxytocin through an IV line infusion pump as indicated until three contractions occur within 10 minutes and last >40 seconds. Maintain mainline IV fluids in accordance with institutional policy.
   b. Discontinue the infusion when:
      (i) Criteria are met.
      (ii) Hyperstimulation occurs.
      (iii) Prolonged deceleration or bradycardia occurs.
      (iv) Persistent late decelerations are present.

Interpretation for CST/OCT

1. Negative (normal)—three uterine contractions in 10 minutes without late decelerations.
2. Positive (abnormal)—persistent late decelerations or late decelerations with >50% of uterine contractions even if frequency is <3 contractions in 10 minutes; usually associated with minimal or decreased LTV.
3. Suspicious (equivocal)—late decelerations with <50% of uterine contractions or significant variables.
4. Unsatisfactory—quality of tracing inadequate to assess or <3 contractions in 10 minutes.
5. Hyperstimulation:
   a. Contractions more frequent than every 2 minutes or lasting >90 seconds or hypertonus.
   b. If no late decelerations with hyperstimulation, it is interpreted as "negative."
   c. If late decelerations with hyperstimulation, it is interpreted as "unsatisfactory" and classified as "hyperstimulation."

Significance/Management of CST/OCT

1. Negative—reassuring.
2. Positive—nonreassuring.
3. Suspicious—repeat in 24 hours.
4. Unsatisfactory—repeat in 24 hours.
5. Hyperstimulation—repeat in 2 hours.

Biophysical Profile (BPP)

Description

The BPP uses ultrasonography and NST to assess five biophysical variables in determining fetal well-being. A BPP is performed over a 30-minute time frame.

1. Nonstress test—looking for acceleration in relation to fetal movements.
2. Amniotic fluid index volume—assessing for one or more pockets of amniotic fluid measuring 2 cm or more in two perpendicular planes.
3. Fetal breathing movements—one or more episodes lasting at least 30 seconds.
4. Gross fetal body movements—three or more body or limb movements, to include rolling, in 30 minutes.
5. Fetal muscle tone—one or more episodes of active extension with return to flexion of spine, hand, or limbs.
   For each variable, if the criteria are met, a score of 2 is given. For an abnormal observation, a score of 0 or 1 is given. A score of 8 to 10 is considered normal, 6 is equivocal, and 4 or less is abnormal.

Nursing and Patient Care Considerations

1. Explain the purpose and procedure to the woman.
2. Inform the woman that a full bladder may be necessary.
3. Instruct the woman to drink three to four glasses of water if the bladder is not full.
4. Remove the lubricant from the woman's abdomen after the procedure.
5. Instruct the woman to void after the procedure.

Modified BPP

Description

The modified BPP consists of an NST and an AFI check. Research has found that modified BPP provides the same viable information as a full BPP.

Nursing and Patient Care Considerations

1. Explain NST and AFI check in accordance with previously stated guidelines as noted in this chapter.
2. Document findings in woman's prenatal record.

SELECTED REFERENCES

Anderson, C. A. (1997). What is nursing anyhow? *Nursing Outlook, 45,* 249–250.

Astin, J. A., Marie, A., Pelletier, K. R., Hansen, E., & Haskell, W. L. (1998). A review of the incorporation of complementary and alternative medicine by mainstream physicians. *Archives of Internal Medicine, 158,* 2203–2310.

Association of Women's Health, Obstetric, and Neonatal Nurses (AWHONN) (1997). *Fetal heart monitoring principles and practices.* Dubuque, IA: Kendall-Hunt.

Borrie, M. M., et al. (1994). *Foundations of maternal newborn nursing.* Philadelphia: W. B. Saunders.

Carpenito, L. J. (1993). *Handbook of nursing diagnosis* (5th ed.). Philadelphia: J. B. Lippincott.

Carrington, B. W., et al. (1993). The need for family planning services for women delivering with little or no prenatal care [editorial]. *Woman and Health, 20*(1), 1–9.

Cogswell, M. E., et al. (1995). Gestational weight gain among average weight and overweight women—What is excessive? *American Journal of Obstetrics and Gynecology, 172*(2), 705.

Creasy, R. K., & Resnik, R. (1999). *Maternal–fetal medicine principles and practice* (4th ed.). Philadelphia: W. B. Saunders.

Cunningham, F. G., et al. (1998). *Williams' obstetrics* (20th ed.). Norwalk, CT: Appleton and Lange.

Dickason, E. J., et al. (1994). *Maternal–infant nursing care* (2nd ed.). St. Louis: Mosby–Year Book.

Di Iorio, C., et al. (1992). Patterns of nausea during first trimester of pregnancy. *Clinical Nursing Research, 1*(2), 127–140, discussion 141–143.

Eisenberg, D. (1997). Advising patients who seek alternative medical therapies. *Annals of Internal Medicine, 127*(1), 61–69.

Fried, P. (1993). Prenatal exposure to tobacco and marijuana: Effects during pregnancy, infancy, and early childhood. *Clinical Obstetrics and Gynecology, 36*(2), 319–337.

Kane, K. (1997). Herbal medicine and childbirth—Do they mix? *International Journal of Childbirth Education, 12*(2), 22–24.

Luke, B. (1994). Maternal–fetal nutrition. *Clinical Obstetrics and Gynecology, 37*(1), 93–109.

Maloni, J. A. (1998). *Antepartum bedrest: Case studies, research, and nursing care.* Washington, DC: AWHONN.

May, K. A., & Mahlmeister, L. R. (1994). *Maternal and neonatal nursing—Family centered care* (3rd ed.). Philadelphia: J. B. Lippincott.

Mayberry, L. (1999). *Management of the second stage of labor.* Washington, DC: AWHONN.

McFarland, G. K., & McFarlane, E. A. (1993). *Nursing diagnosis and intervention* (2nd ed.). St. Louis: Mosby–Year Book.

National Academy of the Sciences. (1990). *Nutrition during pregnancy.* Washington, D.C.: National Academy Press.

Newman, V., et al. (1993). Clinical advances in the management of severe nausea and vomiting during pregnancy. *Journal of Obstetric, Gynecologic, and Neonatal Nursing, 22,* 483–490.

Randall, B. P. (1993). Growth versus stability: Older primiparous woman as a paradigmatic case for persistence. *Journal of Advanced Nursing, 18*(4), 518–525.

Simpson, K. R., & Creehan, P. A. (1996). *Perinatal nursing.* Philadelphia: Lippincott-Raven.

Stephens, S. (1997). Body work and childbirth, proven wonders. *International Journal of Childbirth Education, 12*(4), 20–21.

Worthington, R., et al. (1993). *Nutrition in pregnancy and lactation* (5th ed.). St. Louis: Mosby–Year Book.

Youngkin, E. Q., & Israel, D. S. (1996). A review and critique of common herbal alternative therapies. *Nurse Practitioner, 21*(10), 39–60.

Nursing Management During Labor and Delivery

THE LABOR PROCESS

From the initial prenatal visits, the nurse needs to emphasize that labor and delivery are normal physiologic processes. The pregnant woman often approaches the time of delivery with major concerns of her personal well-being, that of her unborn child, and fear of a difficult and painful labor. Addressing these concerns and minimizing her discomfort should be of paramount importance to all participants involved in the care of the mother and her fetus.

■ General Considerations

Prepared Childbirth

Previously, the term *natural childbirth* was used to describe one approach to giving birth. To some, natural childbirth meant delivery without analgesic or anesthesia, whereas to those who had developed the approach it simply meant being prepared for childbirth through prenatal education and training. This preparation gave the woman a method of coping with the discomforts of labor and delivery. To avoid the suggestion that analgesia or anesthesia is unavailable to the woman during labor and delivery should she need it, the term *prepared childbirth* is now used instead of natural childbirth.

Method of Grantly Dick-Read

1. This method is based on the idea that fear and anticipation of pain arouse natural protective tensions in the body, both psychic and muscular.
2. Fear stimulates the sympathetic nervous system and causes the circular muscle of the cervix to contract.
3. The longitudinal muscles of the uterus then have to act against increased cervical resistance, causing tension and pain.

4. Tension and pain aggravate fear, which produces a vicious cycle of tension, pain, and fear.
5. A minor degree of pain, magnified by fear, becomes unbearable.
6. According to Dick-Read, prenatal courses and training reduce fear, overcome ignorance, and build a woman's self-confidence. Included in this method are:
   a. Explanations of fetal development and childbirth.
   b. Descriptions of methods available to relieve pain.
   c. Exercises that strengthen certain muscles and relax others.
   d. Breathing techniques that will enable the woman to relax in the first stage of labor and work effectively with muscles used during delivery.
   e. Explanations of the value of improved physical health and emotional stability for childbirth.
   f. The woman is not told that labor and delivery will be painless; analgesia and anesthesia are available if needed or desired.
   g. The woman is given empathic understanding and support during labor by her partner, the nurse, and the health care provider.

Psychoprophylactic or Lamaze Method

1. Psychoprophylactic childbirth has a rationale based on Pavlov's concept of pain perception and his theory of conditioned reflexes (the substitution of favorable conditioned reflexes for unfavorable ones). The Lamaze method is an example of this technique.
2. The woman is taught to replace responses of restlessness, fear, and the loss of control with more useful activity. A high level of activity can excite the cerebral cortex efficiently to inhibit other stimuli, such as pain in labor.

3. The mother-to-be is taught exercises that strengthen the abdominal muscles and relax the perineum.
4. Breathing techniques to help the process of labor are practiced.
5. The woman is conditioned to respond with respiratory activity and disassociation or relaxation of the uninvolved muscles, while controlling her perception of the stimuli associated with labor.
6. One method of control consists of breathing normally while silently mouthing the words to a song and simultaneously tapping the rhythm with the fingers.
7. Similarity between the Dick-Read and Lamaze methods:
   a. Fear, which enhances the perception of pain, may diminish or disappear when the woman understands the physiology of labor.
   b. Because psychic tension enhances perception of pain, relaxation is achieved more easily in a calm, agreeable atmosphere with supportive people nearby.
   c. Muscular relaxation and a specific type of breathing diminish or abolish the pains of labor.

The Bradley Method of Delivery
1. Commonly referred to as "husband-coached childbirth," although the coach is not necessarily the husband of the woman.
2. Involves the concepts of leading, guiding, supporting, caring, and fostering specific skills and confidence.
3. Coaches attend classes and learn to help the woman long before pregnancy begins.
4. The coach serves as a conditioned stimulus using the sound of his or her voice, use of particular words, and repetition of practice.
5. Medications are not encouraged for pain relief. Relaxation is the core component. Increased tolerance to pain is accomplished by decreased mental anxiety and fear, which ultimately decreases the awareness of the pain stimulus. Occurs with cognitive and physical rehearsal.

The Leboyer Method of Delivery
1. The Leboyer method is based on the premise that the infant suffers psychological shock at the time of delivery. An effort is made to reduce the contrast between the intrauterine environment and the outside world.
2. Gentle, controlled delivery—prenatal education, support from family and personnel to decrease anxiety, fear, and tension.
3. Emphasis on providing protection to the craniosacral axis by gently supporting the newborn infant's head, neck, and sacrum. The craniosacral axis is completely relaxed, and lost body heat is restored in a warm water bath.
4. Avoiding overstimulation of the newborn sensorium—the infant is allowed to breathe spontaneously; cutting the cord is delayed to permit placental blood transfusion for improved respiration.
5. Importance of maternal–infant bond—skin-to-skin contact with mother is provided, and infant is fondled and stroked.

Home Delivery
1. Home delivery, although controversial, has won increasing support in recent years.
2. Motivations for home delivery:
   a. Belief that home birth has significant advantages for the family and the newborn infant.
   b. Objection to the impersonal and authoritarian atmosphere of the hospital environment with enforced separation of woman and family.
   c. Desire to avoid such practices as routine cesarean delivery for breech presentation, episiotomy, forceps delivery, oxytocin stimulation, routine monitoring of the fetal heart tones, and other practices associated with hospitals.
   d. Risk of in-hospital infections; belief that infant is immune to own-home bacteria.
   e. Rising costs of hospitalization.
3. Contraindications:
   a. High-risk indications for infant and mother.
   b. Patient with history of premature or postdate delivery in previous pregnancy.
   c. Woman with medical or emotional complications.
   d. Patient who cannot be quickly transported to a hospital.
4. Alternatives
   a. Alterations of hospital setting to a family-centered approach.
   b. Birthing centers with adequate facilities for emergency care for low-risk women.
   c. Properly educated and motivated support personnel.

Initiation of Labor
The exact mechanism that initiates labor is unknown. Theories include:
1. Uterine stretch theory—uterus becomes stretched and pressure increases, causing physiologic changes that initiate labor.
2. As pregnancy progresses, there is a gradual rise in the amount of circulating oxytocin.
3. As pregnancy advances, progesterone is less effective in controlling rhythmic uterine contractions that normally occur. In addition, there also may be an actual decrease in the amount of circulating progesterone.
4. There is increased production of prostaglandins by fetal membranes and uterine decidua as pregnancy advances.
5. In later pregnancy, the fetus produces increased levels of cortisol that inhibit progesterone production from the placenta.

Factors Affecting Labor
Successful labor and delivery depend on adequate pelvic dimensions, adequate fetal dimensions and presentation, and adequate uterine contractions.

Pelvic Dimensions
1. Adequate pelvic inlet (anteroposterior diameter; normal shape).

2. Adequate midpelvis (ischial spines do not protrude into bony canal).
3. Adequate outlet (adequate distance between tuberosities; mobile coccyx).
4. Adequacy of pelvic dimensions determined by pelvic examination during pregnancy and again with the onset of labor.

Fetal Dimensions

Important fetal dimensions influenced by fetal size, posture, lie, and presentation. Fetal position is also an important factor in successful labor.

1. Fetal size—with excessive size, fetal skull bones may not be able to override enough to be accommodated in the bony pelvic cavity.
2. Fetal posture—fetus assumes a characteristic posture in later pregnancy to accommodate to the uterine cavity. The fetal head is flexed, back is rounded, and extremities are flexed. Flexed head allows smallest diameter of fetal head (occiput) to present and pass through the birth canal (Figure 37-1).
3. Fetal lie—fetus assumes a lie (comparison of the fetal long axis to the long axis of the woman) that is either transverse, longitudinal, or oblique. In a longitudinal lie (99% of all births), the fetal head will present (cephalic presentation) or the buttocks or feet will present (breech presentation). In a transverse lie, the shoulder presents. In an oblique lie, the fetus is in an angle off the transverse lie.
4. Fetal presentation—whichever portion of the fetus is deepest in the birth canal and is felt on vaginal examination is referred to as the presenting part; this determines fetal presentation. Presentation can be cephalic (occiput, sinciput, brow, face, or chin [mentum]), breech (frank, complete, or footling [single or double]), shoulder, or compound (hand/arm presenting same time as vertex [head] or hand presenting same time as breech).
5. Fetal position—designation of landmark of fetal presenting part (occiput, mentum, sacrum, scapula) to right or left, and anterior, posterior, or transverse portion of the woman's pelvis. For example, a fetus presenting by the vertex with occiput on the left anterior part of the woman's pelvis would have presentation and position described as LOA, or left occiput anterior (Figure 37-2). The first and third letters relate to the pelvis, and the second letter relates to the fetus.

Fetal Head

In approximately 95% of all births, the fetal head presents first. The sutures and fontanelles provide important landmarks for determining fetal position during a vaginal examination (Figure 37-3).

1. Bones of the fetal skull:
   a. Occipital bone posteriorly.
   b. Two parietal bones on the sides.
   c. Two temporal bones anteriorly.
   d. Two frontal bones anteriorly.
2. Sutures of the fetal skull—membranous spaces between the bones of the fetal skull:
   a. Frontal suture—between the two frontal bones.
   b. Sagittal—between the two parietal bones.

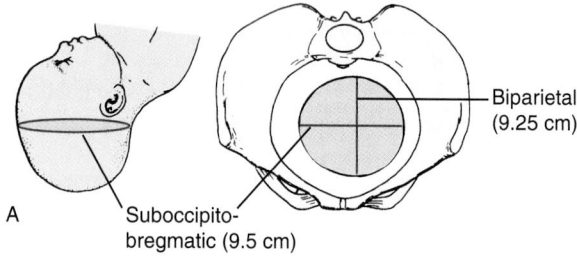

A — Suboccipito-bregmatic (9.5 cm) / Biparietal (9.25 cm)

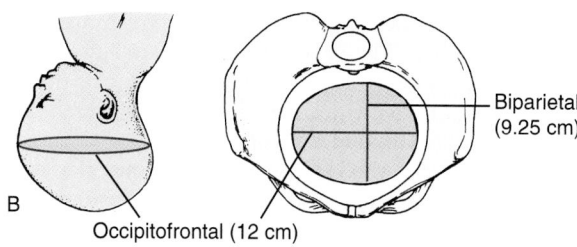

B — Occipitofrontal (12 cm) / Biparietal (9.25 cm)

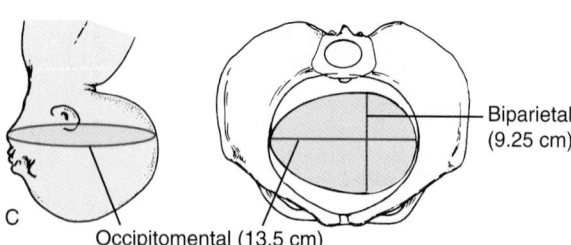

C — Occipitomental (13.5 cm) / Biparietal (9.25 cm)

FIGURE 37-1 (**A**) Complete flexion allows smallest diameter of head to enter pelvis. (**B**) Moderate extension causes larger diameter to enter pelvis. (**C**) Marked extension forces largest diameter against pelvic brim, but head is too large to enter pelvis.

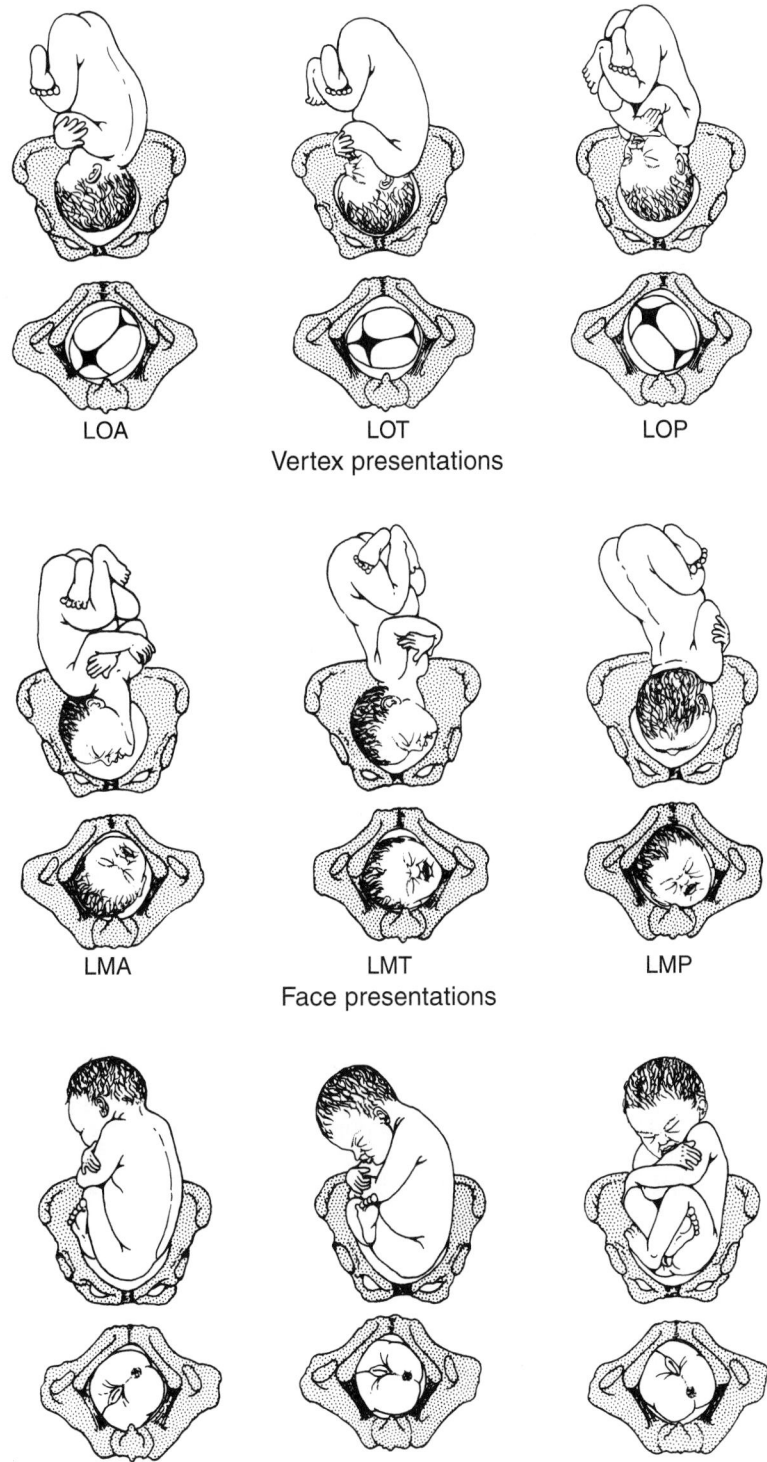

FIGURE 37-2 Standard landmarks for the fetal presenting part. A three-letter abbreviation is used to describe the relationship of the presenting part to the maternal pelvis:

1. Identify which side the presenting part is facing in the pelvis: R (right) or L (left).

2. Identify the landmark that is presenting: O (occiput, or head), S (sacrum), Sc (scapula, or shoulders), M (mentum, or chin).

3. Identify the direction the presenting part is facing in the pelvis: A (anterior, or front), P (posterior, or back), or T (transverse).

(From Benson, R.C. *Handbook of obstetrics and gynecology*. Los Altos, CA: Lange Medical Publication.)

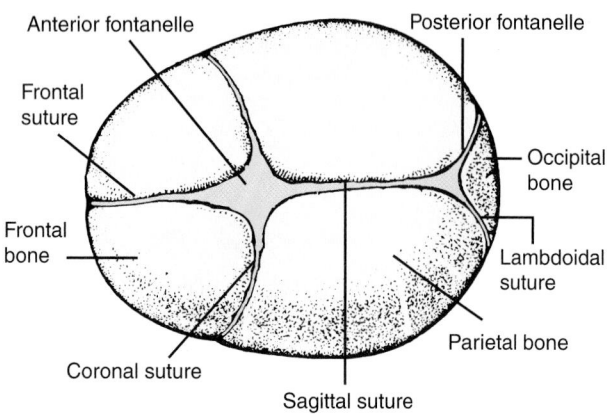

FIGURE 37-3 Fetal head.

c. Coronal—between the frontal and parietal bones.

d. Lambdoidal—between the back of the parietal bones and the margin of the occipital bone.

3. Fontanelles—irregular spaces formed where two or more sutures meet. Sutures and fontanelles allow fetal skull bones to overlap in order to pass through the maternal pelvis.

    a. Anterior fontanelle—largest fontanelle; junction of the sagittal, frontal, and coronal sutures—Closes by 18 months of age; "diamond" shaped.

    b. Posterior fontanelle—located where the sagittal suture meets the lambdoidal (smaller than anterior)—Closes at 6 to 8 weeks of age; "triangle" shaped.

Uterine Contractions

Successful labor also depends on uterine contractions occurring at regular intervals and having adequate intensity.

1. Uterine contractions are involuntary, rhythmic, and intermittent.

2. Uterine contractions cause vasoconstriction of the umbilical cord vessels; considered normal.

3. Uterine contractions increase in intensity, frequency, and duration as labor progresses due to stretching of the cervix.

4. During uterine contractions, the active upper portion of the uterus becomes thicker, whereas the lower uterine segment stretches and becomes thinner (referred to as fundal dominance).

5. At the completion of a contraction, the upper uterine segment retains its shortened, thickened cell size and, with each succeeding contraction, becomes thicker and shorter. As a result, the upper uterine segment never totally relaxes during labor. Cells of the lower uterine segment become thinner and longer with each contraction. This mechanism is greatly responsible for the progress of the fetus through the birth canal.

6. The differentiation point between the upper and lower uterine segment is known as the "physiologic retraction ring."

Events Preliminary to Labor

1. Lightening (the settling of the fetus in the lower uterine segment) occurs 2 to 3 weeks before term in the primigravida and later, during labor, in the multigravida.

    a. Breathing becomes easier as the fetus falls away from the diaphragm.

    b. Lordosis of the spine is increased as the fetus enters the pelvis and falls forward. Walking may become more difficult; leg cramping may increase.

    c. Urinary frequency occurs because of pressure on the bladder.

2. Vaginal secretions may increase.

3. Mucous plug is discharged from the cervix along with a small amount of blood from surrounding capillaries—Referred to as "show" ("bloody show").

4. Cervix becomes soft and effaced (thinned).

5. Membranes may rupture.

6. False labor contractions may occur (Table 37-1).

7. Backache may increase.

8. Diarrhea may occur.

9. Weight loss of 1 to 3 lb.

10. Sudden burst of energy is experienced by some women.

Stages of Labor

First Stage of Labor (Stage of Cervical Dilation)

1. Begins with the first true labor contractions and ends with complete effacement and dilation of the cervix (10 cm dilation).

2. The first stage of labor averages about 13.3 hours for a nullipara and about 7.5 hours for a multipara.

3. Latent phase (early):

    a. Dilates from 0 to 3 cm.

    b. Contractions are usually every 5 to 20 minutes, lasting 20 to 40 seconds, and of mild intensity.

    c. The contractions progress to about every 5 minutes and establish a regular pattern.

TABLE 37-1 True and False Labor Contractions

True Labor Contractions	False Labor Contractions
Result in progressive cervical dilation and effacement	Do not result in progressive cervical dilation and effacement
Occur at regular intervals	Occur at irregular intervals
Interval between contractions decreases	Interval between contractions remains the same or increases
Intensity increases	Intensity decreases or remains the same
Located mainly in back and abdomen	Located mainly in lower abdomen and groin
Generally intensified by walking	Generally unaffected by walking
Not affected by mild sedation	Generally relieved by mild sedation

4. Active phase:
   a. Dilates from 4 to 7 cm.
   b. Contractions are usually every 2 to 5 minutes; lasting 30 to 50 seconds and of mild to moderate intensity.
   c. After reaching the active phase, dilation averages 1.2 cm/h in the nullipara and 1.5 cm/h in the multipara.
5. Transitional phase:
   a. Dilates from 8 to 10 cm.
   b. Contractions are every 2 to 3 minutes, lasting 50 to 60 seconds and of moderate to strong intensity. Some contractions may last up to 90 seconds.

Second Stage of Labor (Stage of Expulsion)

1. Begins with complete dilation and ends with birth of the baby.
2. The second stage may last from 1 to 4 hours in the nullipara and from 20 to 45 minutes in the multipara.

Third Stage of Labor (Placental Stage)

1. Begins with delivery of the baby and ends with delivery of the placenta.
2. The third stage may last from a few minutes to 30 minutes.

Fourth Stage

Lasts from delivery of the placenta until the postpartum condition of the woman has become stabilized (usually 1 hour after delivery).

Mechanisms of Labor

1. If the woman's pelvis is adequate, size and position of the fetus are adequate, and uterine contractions are regular and of adequate intensity, the fetus will move through the birth canal.
2. The position and rotational changes of the fetus as it moves down the birth canal will be affected by resistance offered by the woman's bony pelvis, cervix, and surrounding tissues.
3. The events of engagement, descent, flexion, internal rotation, extension, external rotation, and expulsion overlap in time (Figure 37-4).

Engagement

When biparietal diameter (BPD) of fetal head has passed through pelvic inlet:
1. Primigravidas—occurs up to 2 weeks before onset of labor.
2. Multigravidas—usually occurs with onset of labor.
3. Because BPD is the narrowest diameter of fetal head and anteroposterior diameter is the narrowest of pelvic inlet, the fetal head usually enters pelvis in a transverse position.
4. Cardinal movements—the remaining movements are known as "cardinal movements," which are the passive adjustments of position the fetus makes as it descends through the pelvis during labor.

Descent

Occurs throughout labor and is the downward movement of the fetus; occurs simultaneously with engagement.
1. Accomplished by force of uterine contractions on fetal portion in fundus and pressure of the amniotic fluid; during second stage of labor, bearing down increases intra-abdominal pressure, thus augmenting effects of uterine contractions. In addition, the extension and straightening of the fetal body assists with its descent.
2. Station is the relationship of the level of the presenting part to the ischial spines. The degree of descent is described as:
   a. Floating—fetal presenting part is not engaged in pelvic inlet (Figure 37-5).
   b. Fixed—fetal presenting part has entered pelvis.
   c. Engagement—fetal presenting part (usually BPD of fetal head) has passed through pelvic inlet.
   d. Stations that are −1, −2, −3, or −4 occur when the presenting part is 1, 2, 3, or 4 cm above the level of the ischial spine (Figure 37-6).
   e. Station 0 occurs when the presenting part is at the level of the ischial spine.
   f. Station +1, +2, +3, or +4 is when the presenting part is 1, 2, 3, or 4 cm below the ischial spines. A station of +4 indicates that the presenting part is on the pelvic floor (on the perineum).

Flexion

Resistance to descent causes head to flex so the chin is close to the chest; this causes the smallest fetal head diameter, the suboccipitobregmatic, to present through the canal. This puts the posterior fontanelle at almost the center of the cervix, making it easily palpable on vaginal examination. Flexion begins at the pelvic inlet and continues until the fetal head (or presenting part) reaches the pelvic floor.

Internal Rotation

In accommodating the birth canal, the fetal occiput rotates 45 or 90 degrees from its original position toward the symphysis. The rotation is usually anteriorly but if the pelvis cannot accommodate the occiput anteriorly due to a narrow forepelvis, it will rotate posteriorly, resulting in an OP (occiputoposterior) position of the fetus. This movement results from the shape of the fetal head, space available in the midpelvis, and contour of the perineal muscles. The ischial spines project into the midpelvis, causing the fetal head to rotate anteriorly to accommodate to the available space.

Extension

As the fetal head descends further, it meets resistance from the perineal muscles and is forced to extend. The fetal head becomes visible at the vulvovaginal ring; its largest diameter is encircled (crowning), and the head then emerges from the vagina.

External Rotation

Initial phase is called *restitution*. It is simply the fetal head returning to its normal relations with the shoulders. After restitution, the second phase of external rotation occurs as the body rotates so that the shoulders are in the anteroposterior diameter of the pelvis.

Expulsion

After delivery of the infant's head and internal rotation of the shoulders, the anterior shoulder rests beneath the symphysis pubis. The posterior shoulder is born, followed by the anterior shoulder and the rest of the body.

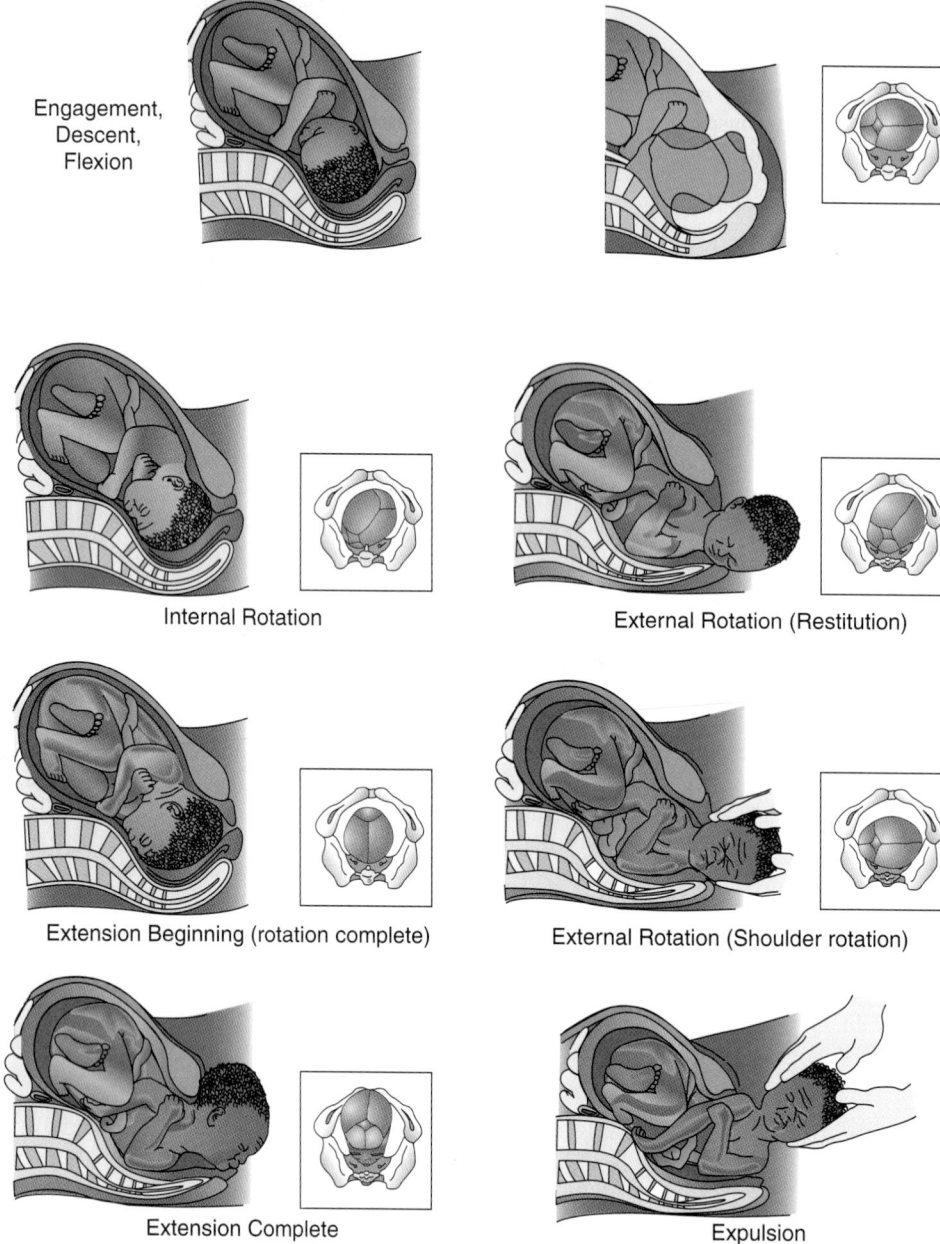

Engagement, Descent, Flexion

Internal Rotation

External Rotation (Restitution)

Extension Beginning (rotation complete)

External Rotation (Shoulder rotation)

Extension Complete

Expulsion

FIGURE 37-4 Mechanism of delivery for a vertex presentation.

NURSING ASSESSMENT AND INTERVENTIONS

When Labor Begins

Nursing responsibilities when labor begins include history taking, performing a vaginal examination as indicated, and initiating fetal monitoring evaluation. Additionally, the nurse needs to assess the membrane status. (See Standards of Care Guidelines.)

History and Baseline Data

1. Introduce yourself; maintain eye contact; ask for name of woman's health care provider, if he or she has been notified that the woman was coming to the hospital or birth center, and presenting complaints/concerns.
2. Establish baseline information.
   a. Assess gravidity, parity, expected date of delivery or confinement.
   b. When did contractions begin? How far apart are they? How long do they last? Intensity level?

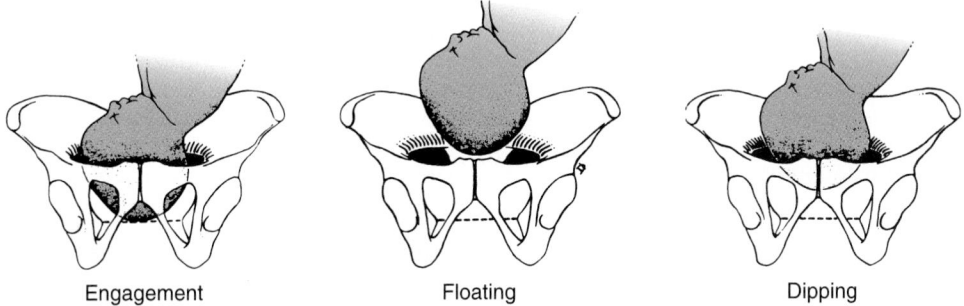

FIGURE 37-5 Engagement, floating, and dipping. (Oxom, H. & Foote, W.R. *Human labor and birth.* New York: Appleton-Century-Crofts.)

c. Have the membranes ruptured? Time of rupture? Color? Consistency? Amount of fluid? Odor?

d. Is there any bloody show?

e. How much discomfort is the woman experiencing?

f. What, if any, problems has the woman had in this pregnancy? Problems in past pregnancies?

g. Blood type and Rh? RhoGAM?

h. Last meal/drink? What type of food/drink?

i. Medications—nonprescription/prescription/illicit?

j. Support system?

3. Establish baseline maternal and fetal vital signs.

a. Temperature—elevation above 99.6°F (37.6°C) suggests a possible infection or dehydration.

b. Pulse—evaluate between contractions; may be slightly elevated over the resting rate.

c. Respirations—evaluated between contractions.

d. Blood pressure—evaluated between contractions.

(i) A slight elevation over baseline may be attributed to anxiety.

(ii) A blood pressure with a systolic elevation of 30 mm Hg or greater than 140 mm Hg and a diastolic elevation of 15 mm Hg or greater than 90 mm Hg suggests hypertension and requires further evaluation.

e. Assess the fetal heart rate (FHR); if a fetal monitor is to be used, run a 20- to 30-minute strip for baseline data.

f. Assess reflexes and clonus.

STANDARDS OF CARE GUIDELINES
Labor and Delivery

1. Establish a baseline history for the woman in labor, including maternity history, labor events thus far, last meal, medications, allergies, and support systems available.

2. Determine fetal presentation and notify health care provider if fetus is not in vertex presentation.

3. Assess fetal heart tones periodically and after rupture of membranes.

4. Assess uterine contractions at intervals.

5. Assess cervical dilation and effacement. If ROM, do not perform vaginal examination.

6. Initiate and continue fetal monitoring according to health care provider orders and institution protocol.

7. Ensure that licensed health care provider is available if oxytocin is being used.

8. Administer oxygen and change mother's position for the following:
   a. Nonreassuring and/or repetitive variable decelerations
   b. Repetitive late decelerations
   c. Prolonged decelerations or bradycardia

9. Notify health care provider for the following:
   a. Abnormal maternal vital signs
   b. Nonreassuring fetal tracing

10. Assist the woman with breathing and pain control techniques during contractions.

11. Assess woman and partner/significant others for coping, and work with them to carry out the birth plan.

This information should serve as a general guideline only. Each patient situation presents a unique set of clinical factors and requires nursing judgment to guide care, which may include additional or alternative measures and approaches.

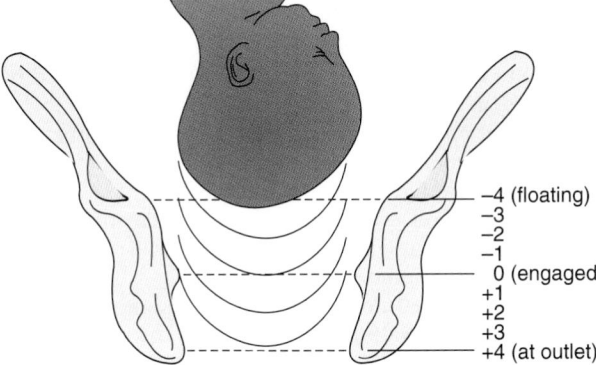

-4 (floating)
-3
-2
-1
0 (engaged)
+1
+2
+3
+4 (at outlet)

FIGURE 37-6 Stations of presenting part. The location of the presenting part in relation to the level of the ischial spines is designated station and indicates the degree of advancement of the presenting part through the pelvis. Stations are expressed in centimeters above (minus) or below (plus) the level of the ischial spines (zero).

4. Obtain a urine specimen—test the urine for glucose and protein. Protein results may be positive if the membranes have ruptured.

Methods for Determining Fetal Presentation
Vaginal Examination and Determination
of Fetal Landmarks Presenting (see p. 1133)

Leopold's Maneuvers

Determined by abdominal palpation (Figure 37-7).

1. First maneuver (see Figure 37-7A)—to determine fetal presentation or the part of the fetus (fetal head or breech) that is in the upper uterine fundus. While facing the woman, place the hands on top of the uterus (fundus) and palpate. Head feels smooth, hard/firm, and round, freely movable and ballotable. A breech feels irregular, rounded, softer, and is less mobile.
2. Second maneuver (see Figure 37-7B)—to determine the fetal position or identify the relationship of the fetal back and the small parts to the front, back, or sides of the maternal pelvis. Still facing the woman, place hands on either side of the abdomen. While one hand stabilizes the one side of the uterus, the other hand palpates the opposite side to identify the location of the back and small parts. Palpation begins in the midline and continues down the side of the uterus. Then the other side of the uterus is stabilized and palpated. Palpate, applying gentle but deep pressure. The back is long, smooth, and a hard continuous structure; fetal body parts (extremities) will feel knobby, irregular, and may be moving.
3. Third maneuver (see Figure 37-7C)—to determine the portion of the fetus that is presenting. While facing the woman, grasp the lower uterine segment between the thumb and fingers of one hand just above the symphysis pubis. Pay close attention to the size, contour, and consistency of the presenting part. The head will feel firm and globular. If not engaged into the pelvis, the presenting part is movable. If immobile, engagement has occurred. The head is at the inlet or in the pelvis in 90% of women.
4. Fourth maneuver (see Figure 37-7D)—to determine fetal attitude or the greatest prominence of the fetal head over the pelvic brim. In this maneuver, the examiner faces the woman's feet. Using the tips of the first three fingers of each hand, the examiner presses deep in the direction of the pelvic inlet (toward the symphysis pubis). The fingers should come in contact with a bony cephalic prominence. If the prominence is located on the opposite side from the back, it is usually the fetus' brow, and the head is in flexion. If the prominence is located on the same side as the back, it is the occiput, and the head is in extension.

Ultrasonography
See page 1119.

Assessing Fetal Heart Tones

Fetal heart tones (FHT; also referred to as fetal heart rate [FHR]) are auscultated with a DeLee-Hillis fetoscope or Pinard stethoscope. However, in practice, the term *auscultation* is often used to refer to the assessment of the fetal heart sounds by means of a hand-held Doppler device or ultrasound monitor.

1. Determine the position and presentation of the fetus by palpation using Leopold's maneuvers. As internal rotation and descent occur, the location of the FHR changes, swinging gradually from the lateral to the medial area and dropping until immediately before birth, when it is above the pubic bone (Figure 37-8).
2. Place the fetoscope or Doppler on the abdomen over the back or chest of fetus. Avoid friction noises caused by fingers on the abdominal surface area.
3. Differentiate between fetal heart tone and other abdominal sounds.
   a. FHR—a rapid crisp or ticking sound.
   b. Uterine bruit—a soft murmur, caused by the passage of blood through dilated uterine vessels; is synchronous with maternal pulse.
   c. Funic souffle (uterine souffle)—a hissing sound produced by passage of blood through the umbilical arteries; it is synchronous with the FHR.
4. Palpate the maternal radial pulse to differentiate the maternal heart rate from the FHR.
5. Count the FHR during auscultation to clarify the relationship between the FHR and uterine contractions.
6. Listen and count the FHR for 6 seconds and multiply by 10; note the location and character when counting.

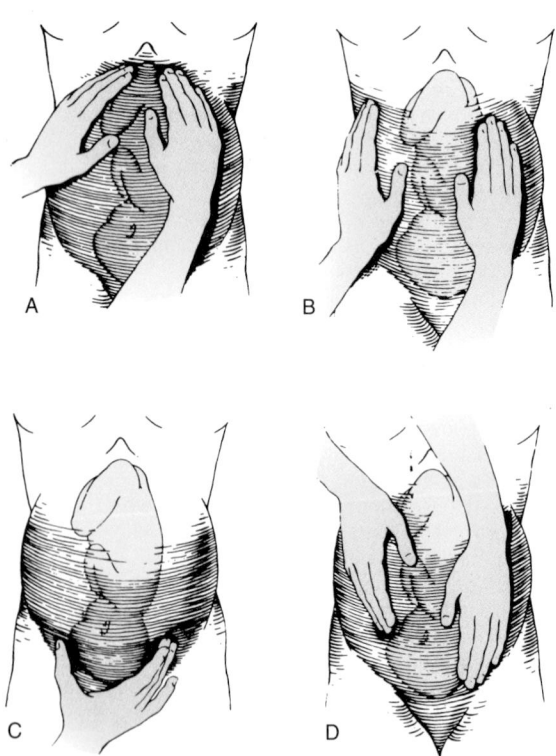

FIGURE 37-7 Leopold's maneuvers.

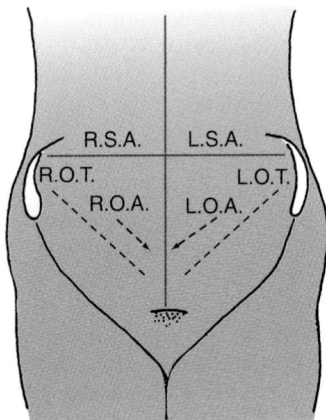

FIGURE 37-8 Fetal heart tone locations on the abdominal wall indicating possible corresponding fetal positions and the effects of the internal rotation of the fetus.

7. Count the FHR between uterine contractions for at least 30 to 60 seconds to identify baseline rate.
8. While auscultating the FHR, identify the baseline FHR, rhythm of the FHR (whether regular or irregular), and any increases or decreases in the FHR.
9. Check the FHR immediately after the rupture of membranes; a sudden release of fluid may cause a prolapse of the umbilical cord.

> **NURSING ALERT**
>
> If decreases are heard in the FHR during auscultation, the patient should be turned to her side and placed on external electronic fetal monitoring (EFM) to verify the fetal tracing. Once placed on EFM, if the decreases are interpreted as variable or late deceleration patterns, notify the health care provider and continue with applicable interventions (see page 1138).

Assessing Uterine Contractions

Intensity, frequency, duration:
1. Place fingertips gently on the fundus.
2. As contraction begins, tension will be felt under the fingertips. Uterus will become harder, then slowly soften.
3. The intensity may be described as follows:
    a. Mild—the uterine muscle is somewhat tense. Feels like the tip of the nose.
    b. Moderate—the uterine muscle is moderately firm. Feels like the chin.
    c. Strong (hard)—the uterine muscle is so firm that it seems almost boardlike. Feels like the forehead.
4. The frequency is measured in minutes—represents the time from the beginning of one contraction until the beginning of the next.
5. Duration of a contraction is timed in seconds or minutes from the moment the uterus first begins to tighten until it relaxes again.

6. As labor progresses, the character of the contractions changes and they last longer until the second stage of labor.
7. When the cervix becomes completely dilated (end of first stage, beginning of second stage), the contractions may initially stop, then become very strong, last for 60 seconds, and occur at 2- to 3-minute intervals.

> **NURSING ALERT**
>
> If any contraction lasts longer than 90 seconds and is not followed by a period of uterine muscle relaxation, notify the health care provider immediately. Uterine rupture and fetal hypoxia may occur if the pattern persists without intervention.

Vaginal Examination

See Figure 37-9.
1. Explain the procedure to the woman. Place her in a lithotomy position.
2. Conduct examination gently, under aseptic conditions.
3. Evaluate the following:
    a. Condition of cervix
        (i) Hard or soft (in labor, cervix is soft).
        (ii) Effaced and thin or thick and long (in labor, cervix is thin and effaced). Measured in percentages from 0% to 100%.
        (iii) Easily dilatable or resistant.
        (iv) Closed or open (dilated); degree of dilation. Measured in centimeters from 1 cm to 10 cm. Before reaching 1 cm, the cervix is closed or fingertip; 10-cm dilation is also referred to as *complete dilation.*
    b. Presentation
        (i) Breech, cephalic (head), or shoulder.
        (ii) Caput succedaneum (edema occurring in and under fetal scalp) present (small or large).
        (iii) Station identified: engaged, floating.
    c. Position
        (i) Cephalic presentation (identification of the sagittal suture and of its direction).
        (ii) Location of posterior fontanelle.
    d. Membranes—intact or ruptured
        (i) Amount of fluid.
        (ii) Passage of meconium; color.
        (iii) Odor.
        (iv) Bulging.
        (v) Rupture usually increases frequency and intensity of uterine contractions.
        (vi) Contraindicated in presence of vaginal bleeding, premature labor, or abnormal fetal presentation or position.
    e. Perineum—assess for ulcerations or vesicles that might indicate sexually transmitted disease, such as syphilis or genital herpes. *Note:* If these are present, stop the examination and notify the primary care provider.

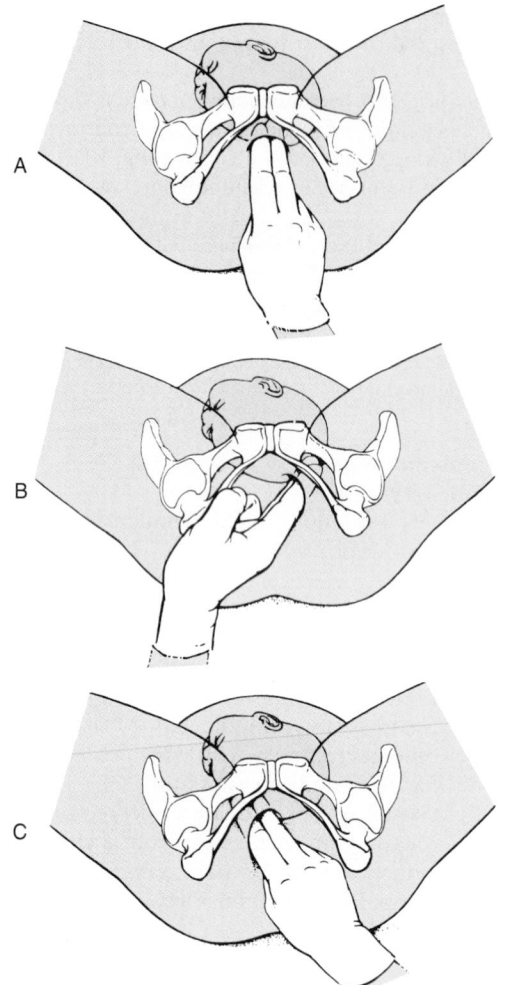

FIGURE 37-9 Vaginal examination. (**A**) Determining the station and palpating the sagittal suture. (**B**) Identifying the posterior fontanelle. (**C**) Identifying the anterior fontanelle.

Sterile Speculum Examination

In some situations (eg, premature rupture of membranes [PROM] or rupture of membranes [ROM] without labor), a vaginal examination is deferred and a sterile speculum examination (SSE) is done instead.

1. Explain the procedure to the woman.
2. Ask her to empty her bladder.
3. Have her remove all clothing from the waist down, and give her a sheet to cover herself.
4. Place her in a lithotomy position. Place a pillow under her head and place her feet in the stirrups. To ensure the woman is not on her back, place a hip roll under her left hip.
5. Drape her legs and the abdomen (optional).
6. Position a lighted gooseneck lamp to light the perineum. Ensure it is not touching the woman. Position a stool at the end of the examination table.

7. Select a sterile speculum. Using aseptic technique, open the package.
8. Put on sterile gloves.
9. Sitting on the stool, ask the woman to gently spread her legs as far as possible.
10. Explain to the woman that anytime she becomes upset or experiences pain during the SSE to let you know. If that occurs, stop the examination, but do not remove your fingers, just hold your hand still. Also explain to the woman that she will occasionally feel vaginal pressure during the SSE.
11. With the nondominant hand, place two fingers just inside the introitus and gently press down on the base of the vagina. Then insert the closed speculum past the fingers at a 45-degree downward angle.
12. Using no lubricant, grasp the speculum with the dominant hand.
13. After the speculum is in the vagina, remove your fingers. Turn the blades of the speculum into a horizontal position, maintaining a moderate downward pressure.

> **NURSING ALERT**
>
> If you cannot visualize the cervix, sweep the blades slowly upward by gently pressing on the handle. If still cannot visualize, close the blades, withdraw the speculum a little, and move the blades toward the back of the vagina and try again.

14. When the cervix is in view, tighten the thumbscrew to keep the blades open.
15. When the examination is completed, release the thumbscrew. Hold the blades apart by pressing on the thumb piece and begin withdrawing the speculum until the cervix is released from between the blades.
16. Release the thumb piece, allowing the blades to close. Rotate the speculum sideways, exerting a downward pressure, and remove the blade.
17. Wipe any moisture or discharge from the perineal area.

Assessing the Woman's or Couple's Expectations and Concerns

1. What are their concerns?
2. How anxious are they?
3. What has been their preparation for labor (type, by whom, and when)?
4. What is their understanding of the labor process?
5. What are their expectations of the labor and delivery process (prepared childbirth, anesthesia, analgesics, use of birthing room, and so forth)?
6. How well are they coping and how well are they communicating with each other?
7. Review written birth plan with the couple.

■ Fetal Heart Monitoring

The goal of fetal heart monitoring (FHM) was originally to identify the fetal heart rate (FHR) changes that may indicate a fetus at risk for asphyxia.

Now, after more than 2 decades of research and experience using electronic FHM, considerable information exists about the nature and implications of the alterations seen in the FHR. The purpose of FHM is now believed to be both the identification of a fetus experiencing well-being and the identification of a fetus experiencing compromise. FHM during labor can be accomplished either externally, internally, or a combination of the two. FHM uses nonelectronic or electronic methods of monitoring of the FHR and uterine activity (UA).

Risk Identification Factors

1. Historical and current pregnancy risk factors:
   a. Anemia and other hemoglobinopathies
   b. Gravidity and parity
   c. Cardiopulmonary disease
   d. Intrauterine growth restriction (IUGR)
   e. Rh sensitization
   f. Preeclampsia/eclampsia
   g. Diabetes
   h. Postterm gestation (>42 weeks' gestation)
2. Intrapartum risk factors:
   a. Term PROM
   b. Preterm premature rupture of membranes (PPROM)
   c. Prolonged ROM
   d. Postterm gestation
   e. Preterm gestation (<37 full weeks' gestation)
   f. Low-birth-weight infant
   g. Pitocin induction/augmentation (especially if macrosomic or dysfunctional labor pattern)
   h. Fetal macrosomia
   i. Fetal malpresentation
   j. Amniotic fluid abnormalities (oligohydramnios, polyhydramnios, intra-amniotic infection)
   k. Meconium-stained amniotic fluid
   l. Bleeding (maternal or fetal)
   m. Dysfunctional labor

Nonelectronic Techniques of FHM

Nonelectronic techniques of FHM include auscultation and palpation.

Auscultation

1. Methods:
   a. Fetoscope—detects the auditory signal of the opening and closing of the heart valves.
   b. Doptone (hand-held Doppler ultrasound)—detects cardiac motion.
   c. In practice, a hand-held Doppler or external ultrasound monitor is more frequently used, although the use of the fetoscope is increasing.
2. Detects:
   a. FHR baseline.
   b. FHR rhythm.
   c. Increases and/or decreases in FHR.
   d. Differentiation of fetal and maternal heart rates—eliminates error due to monitor misplacement or fetal demise.

   e. Verification of FHR dysrhythmias visualized on EFM tracing (fetoscope only).
   f. Clarification of halving or doubling on the EFM tracing (fetoscope only).
3. Limitations:
   a. Does not detect long-term variability (LTV) or short-term variability (STV).
   b. Does not offer a continuous recording.
   c. Does not offer a permanent record.
   d. Requires education, practice, skill, and a one-to-one nurse/patient ratio.
   e. Disrupted by uterine contractions.
   f. Assessment may be limited by position and/or movement of the mother and the fetus and maternal size.
4. Benefits:
   a. Noninvasive.
   b. Widespread application.
   c. Comparable to EFM.
5. Application:
   a. Check maternal pulse.
   b. Perform Leopold's maneuvers finding fetal back. Apply fetoscope or Doppler device over fetal back. If fetus is OP, apply auscultation device over fetal chest. Count for 6 seconds and multiply by 10.
   c. Auscultate during uterine contractions and, if possible, for 30- to 60-second intervals after the contraction.
   d. Recommended (by American College of Obstetricians and Gynecologists [ACOG] and Association of Women's Health, Obstetric, and Neonatal Nurses [AWHONN]) frequency of intermediate auscultation during labor for low-risk patients: active phase of labor—every 30 minutes; second stage of labor—every 15 minutes. For high-risk patients: active phase of labor—every 15 minutes; second stage of labor—every 5 minutes.
   e. Recommendations by Society of Obstetricians and Gynecologists for Canada (SOGC) differ slightly. The SOGC recommends: latent phase of labor—every 30 minutes; active phase of labor—every 15 to 30 minutes; second stage of labor—every 5 minutes.

NURSING ALERT

 The external monitoring of uterine contractions is not accurate for intensity or resting tone. External monitoring of FHR is not accurate for short-term variability.

Abdominal Palpation

1. Methods:
   a. Palpation using fingertips placed over fundal area to feel uterus contract.
   b. Often used in conjunction with Leopold's maneuvers.
2. Assesses:
   a. Length of uterine contraction.
   b. Duration of uterine contraction.

c. Intensity of uterine contraction—subjective. Description based on indentation of uterine muscle.
  (i) Mild—feels like tip of nose.
  (ii) Moderate—feels like chin.
  (iii) Strong—feels like forehead.
3. Benefits:
  a. Noninvasive.
  b. Ruptured membranes not required.
  c. Allows freedom of movement for patient.
  d. Patient feels touch from care provider.
4. Limitations:
  a. Cannot adequately assess intensity and resting tone of uterine contraction.
  b. Subjective in assessment.
  c. No graphic record for review/collaboration.
  d. Maternal movement and intolerance may interfere with assessment.

Electronic Techniques of FHM
Uterine Assessment by Tocodynamometer
1. Benefits:
  a. Noninvasive.
  b. Provides information on uterine contraction frequency, duration, and configuration.
  c. Can be used antepartally or intrapartally with intact or ruptured membranes.
  d. More sensitive to onset and duration of uterine contractions than palpation, especially in obese or restless mothers.
  e. Less personnel intensive than palpation.
2. Limitations:
  a. Unable to detect uterine contraction intensity and resting tone.
  b. Unable to accurately detect exact frequency and duration in some cases such as obesity and preterm labor.
  c. Location sensitive.
  d. Sensitive to maternal and fetal movement—may be superimposed over contraction waveform.
  e. Needs to be reapplied over the fundus as the fetus and uterus descend during labor.

Uterine Assessment by Intrauterine Pressure Catheter (IUPC)
Fluid-Filled Catheter
1. Benefits:
  a. Accurate method of assessing uterine pressure during contractions and at rest; measured in mm Hg.
  b. More accurate timing of FHR changes with uterine activity.
  c. Can perform aspiration of amniotic fluid to assess for chorioamnionitis or fetal lung maturity.
  d. Can perform amnioinfusion.
2. Limitations:
  a. Requires rupture of membranes and adequate cervical dilatation.
  b. Invasive procedure—risk of infection and uterine perforation increased.
  c. Requires careful attention to technique for insertion and calibration.

d. Risk of catheter wedging preventing pressure data or producing a distorted, damped, or truncated pressure wave.
e. Catheter tip placement may affect pressure readings (in relation to external uterine monitoring).
f. Catheter may become obstructed with meconium, vernix, or blood.
g. Contraindicated in women with human immunodeficiency virus (HIV) or herpes simplex II (genital).
h. Pressure readings may be lower than with sensor-tipped catheter.

Sensor-Tipped Catheter
1. Benefits:
  a. Can be zeroed to atmospheric pressure easily; capable of rezeroing during monitoring.
  b. Pressure artifacts avoided due to design (no kinking/air collection).
  c. Provides accurate assessment of uterine activity.
  d. Allows for amnioinfusion.
  e. Allows for aspiration of amniotic fluid as needed.
2. Limitations:
  a. Rigidity of catheter requires greater degree of caution/expertise in placement.
  b. Maternal position change may change hydrostatic pressure in uterus, altering readings. (Need to assess baseline resting tone in left, right, tilt positions.)
  c. Pressure readings higher than fluid-filled catheters.
  d. Same limitations as noted above with fluid-filled catheters.

Fetal Heart Assessment by Ultrasound
1. Benefits:
  a. Noninvasive.
  b. No need for ruptured membranes.
  c. Determines LTV.
  d. Relatively consistent recordings if placed correctly.
  e. Graphic display for review and collaboration.
  f. Less personnel intensive than auscultation.
2. Limitations:
  a. Restricts patient's freedom of movement.
  b. Measures cardiac motion, thus cannot be used to differentiate dysrhythmias.
  c. Ultrasound reflections may be weak/absent, producing false FHR patterns.
  d. Episodic maternal and fetal movement may interfere with recording.
  e. Half counting of FHR may occur, especially with tachycardic FHR >240 bpm.
  f. Double counting of FHR may occur, especially with first or second generation monitors and cases of complete heart block (FHR <30 to 60 bpm).
  g. Artifact may affect the appearance of variability; autocorrelation producing false STV readings.
  h. Maternal size may limit ability to assess FHR.
  i. Small risk of uterine perforation, separation of undiagnosed placenta previa, or bleeding due to excessive cervical manipulation.

3. Placement
   a. The ultrasonic transducer device should be applied over the area of the abdomen where the sharpest fetal heart sound is heard.
   b. Lubricate the face of the transducer with a thin layer of ultrasonic gel to aid in the transmission of sounds.
   c. The transducer will need to be readjusted when the fetus changes positions.

Fetal Heart Assessment by Fetal Spiral Electrode (FSE)

1. Benefits:
   a. Depicts STV changes in FHR along with LTV.
   b. Allows for increased patient movement.
   c. May detect dysrhythmias.
   d. Continuous detection of FHR.
2. Limitations:
   a. Rupture of membranes/cervical dilation necessary.
   b. Small risk of fetal hemorrhage or infection.
   c. Small risk of maternal endometritis.
   d. Electronic interference and artifact may occur.
   e. Produces a maternal heart rate in presence of fetal demise.
   f. Fetal arrhythmias may be missed if logic or ECG activation switch is on.
   g. A moist environment is necessary for FHR detection.

Indications for Internal Techniques of FHM

IUPC
1. Labor dystocia.
2. Previous uterine scar.
3. Patient undergoing oxytocin (Pitocin) induction and augmentation when external methods of assessing uterine activity are inadequate.
4. Amnioinfusion.
5. Need for accurate correlation between FHR and contractions.
6. Need for amniotic fluid sampling.
7. Labor abnormalities including prolonged labor; arrested labor.
8. Suspected cephalopelvic disproportion (CPD).
9. Previous cesarean sections attempting vaginal birth after a cesarean (VBAC).
10. Uterine anomalies (bicornuate uterus, fibroleiomyoma).

FSE
1. Unable to accurately detect FHR with external monitoring.
2. Maternal or fetal movement interfering with tracing.
3. Need to accurately assess FHR periodic/nonperiodic (episodic) changes.
4. Patient undergoing oxytocin (Pitocin) induction and augmentation when external methods of assessing uterine activity are inadequate.

Contraindications for Internal Techniques of FHM

IUPC
1. Presence of placenta previa.
2. Uterine bleeding of unknown origin.
3. Presence of infections such as active herpes simplex II (genital) or HIV.
4. Certain presentations/stations such as shoulder or footling breech presentations and floating or ≥+3 stations.

FSE
1. Should not be applied to fetal face, fontanelles, or genitalia.
2. Presence of placenta previa.
3. Presence of active herpes simplex, HIV, group B strep (institution/provider-dependent), or gonorrhea.
4. Mother is confirmed carrier of hemophilia, and status of fetus is unknown.

Interpretation

Baseline Rate
1. Fetal heart rate is initially evaluated for the baseline rate and is established over a 10-minute period and rounded by 5 bpm.
2. A minimum of 2 minutes of interpretable baseline is needed, excluding periodic or episodic changes, marked variability, or differences in baseline >25 bpm.
3. Baseline rate is the FHR when the mother is not in labor, when the fetus is not moving, between contractions, and when the fetus is not being stimulated.
4. Commonly accepted baseline FHR is 110 to 160 bpm.
5. FHR between 110 and 120 bpm is considered normal after 40 weeks' gestation.
6. Variations from the normal baseline rate are tachycardia, bradycardia, and undulating patterns.

Tachycardia
1. FHR of 160 or more for at least 10 minutes.
2. Etiology—maternal causes:
   a. Fever
   b. Infection
   c. Dehydration
   d. Hyperthyroidism
   e. Anxiety
   f. Anemia
   g. Medicine or drug response
      (i) Betasympathomimetics (terbutaline, ritodrine)
      (ii) Parasympathomimetics (epinephrine)
      (iii) Inotropic agents
      (iv) Illicit drugs
3. Etiology—fetal causes:
   a. Infection
   b. Prolonged fetal activity or stimulation
   c. Compensatory response to hypoxemia
   d. Chronic hypoxemia
   e. Supraventricular tachycardia
   f. Prematurity
   g. Congenital anomalies

Bradycardia
1. A baseline FHR below 110 for at least 10 minutes.
2. Fetal bradycardia above 90 bpm in the second stage of labor is not considered abnormal unless there is a loss of variability.

3. Etiology—maternal causes:
   a. Position
   b. Drug response
   c. Connective tissue disease (systemic lupus erythema)
   d. Prolonged maternal hypoglycemia
   e. Hypotension
4. Etiology—fetal causes:
   a. Mature parasympathetic nervous system (PSNS)
   b. Decompensated fetus
   c. Cardiac conduction or structural defect
   d. Excessive PSNS tone caused by chronic head compression in the vertex, OP, or transverse presentation
   e. Vagal stimulation
   f. Prolonged umbilical cord occlusion
   g. Hypothermia

Undulating

1. Undulating patterns have a characteristic repetitive shape in the form of a sine wave.
2. The baseline rate is usually within the normal range.
3. Referred to as *sinusoidal* or *pseudosinusoidal*.
   Sinusoidal:
   a. Uniform wavelike pattern.
   b. Undulations smooth, uniform, and persistent.
   c. Characteristics: no STV, no accelerations, no response to uterine contractions.
   d. Serious pattern; associated with:
      (i) Rh isoimmunization.
      (ii) Severe fetal anemia.
      (iii) Placental abruptio placentae.
      (iv) Severe fetal acidosis.
      (v) Fetal–maternal hemorrhage.
   Pseudosinusoidal:
   a. Less uniform wavelike pattern.
   b. "Saw-toothed" appearance and intermittent.
   c. Characteristics: periods of normal variability (STV/LTV), accelerations, shows periodic changes in response to uterine contractions.
   d. Associated with:
      (i) Narcotic administration or ingestion.
      (ii) Analgesic administration or ingestion.
      (iii) Thumb sucking of the fetus in utero.
      (iv) Unknown cause.

Variability

1. Beat-to-beat changes in FHR that result from the interplay between the sympathetic and parasympathetic nervous systems.
2. Variability indicates normal neurologic function in relation to heart rate and also fetal reserve.
3. Fluctuations are irregular in amplitude and frequency.
4. Fluctuations in baseline FHR ≥2 cycles/minute.
5. STV—beat-to-beat fluctuation in FHR due to slightly different periods between R waves of the ECG in normal fetus.
6. LTV—either amplitude excursions or frequency of the longer-term unidirectional changes of FHR that occupy a cycle of <1 minute.

7. STV may exist independently of LTV, but LTV cannot exist independently of STV.
8. Overview of variability
   a. Absent variability—amplitude range undetectable
   b. Minimal variability—amplitude range > undetectable to ≤5 bpm
   c. Moderate variability—amplitude range 6–25 bpm
   d. Marked variability—amplitude range >26 bpm

Periodic Fetal Heart Rate Changes/Patterns

1. Acceleration or deceleration of FHR in direct relation to uterine activity.
2. Acceleration—increases in the FHR.
   a. Physiology—most often fetal movements or fetal stimulation in direct response to uterine contractions; also seen with breech presentations, OP presentations, and uterine contractions.
   b. Characteristics—may or may not resemble the shape of the uterine contraction; can be either biphasic or triphasic. Visually abrupt increase above baseline FHR.
      (i) For term: acme ≥15 bpm and lasts ≥15 seconds from onset to return to baseline
      (ii) For preterm (<32 weeks): acme ≥ 10 bpm and lasts ≥10 seconds from onset to return to baseline
   c. Prolonged accelerations last at least 2 minutes but <10 minutes.
   d. Treatment—none required; reassuring pattern.
   e. Double-peaked accelerations have been associated with minor cord compressions; might require position change.
3. Early decelerations
   a. Physiology—gradual decelerations in response to head compression from uterine contractions, vaginal examination, scalp stimulation; also seen as a reflex vagal response during the second stage of labor with pushing; higher association seen with CPD, unengaged presenting part in early labor, or with persistent OP presentation. Not associated with the level of fetal oxygenation.
   b. Characteristics—mirror image of the contraction, and all look the same. Uniform shape. Gradual decrease in FHR.
      (i) Onset begins early in the contraction, with the onset to peak in ≤30 seconds. Nadir (lowest point) usually reached at the same time as the peak of the uterine contraction.
      (ii) Returns to baseline by the end of the contraction.
   c. Treatment not required; benign pattern.
   d. Maternal position changes do not usually alter the pattern.
4. Late decelerations
   a. Physiology—gradual decelerations in response to uteroplacental insufficiency (decreased uterine blood flow) with uterine contractions.
   b. Characteristics—uniform in shape often with a reverse mirror image of the contraction phase; often re-

flects the intensity of the uterine contractions. Smooth and symmetrical.

  (i) Onset is late in the contraction, usually after the acme of the contraction with the nadir of the deceleration occurring well after the acme. Onset to peak in ≤30 seconds.

  (ii) Returns to baseline after the end of the contraction. Baseline FHR may be increased with repetitive late decelerations.

c. Nadir commonly decreases 5 to 30 bpm and rarely decreases 30 to 40 bpm below the baseline FHR.

d. Variability may be moderate, minimal, or absent.

e. Treatment—aimed at increasing uteroplacental perfusion by correcting cause.

  (i) Change maternal position to a lateral position (right or left)

  (ii) Correct any hypotension through increasing the maintenance intravenous (IV) fluids.

  (iii) Discontinue uterine stimulation (discontinue oxytocin [Pitocin]).

  (iv) Administer oxygen by snug face mask at 8 to 10 L/min.

  (v) Consider tocolytic administration.

  (vi) Provide support and decrease anxiety.

f. Reflex lates—late decelerations with average LTV or present STV often caused by acute physiologic insult (ie, supine hypotension, epidural anesthesia) without resulting severe fetal hypoxia.

5. Variable decelerations

a. Physiology—visually abrupt decelerations in response to cord compression that can result from maternal position, prolapsed cord, cord around a fetal part, second stage labor, decreased amniotic fluid volume (AFV), a short cord, and a true knot in the cord.

b. Characteristics—shape is variable in depth and duration; frequently are shaped like a "U," "V," or "W." "W"-shaped variable decelerations are more common when the cord is long or wrapped around the fetal body.

  (i) Onset is variable. Onset to peak in ≤30 seconds. May include an acceleration phase that precedes or follows the deceleration pattern and is a component of the variable deceleration pattern. Shoulders generally increase in rate <20 bpm and lasting <20 seconds. These are referred to as "shoulders" and are not associated with poor outcome.

  (ii) Decrease in FHR below baseline is ≥15 bpm, lasting ≥15 seconds and <2 minutes from onset to return to baseline.

  (iii) Usually abrupt and decelerate abruptly; may be in combination with other pattern types.

  (iv) Recovery occurs rapidly, often followed by a shoulder. Overshoots may also be present after the deceleration pattern. Overshoots are compensatory accelerations that only follow the deceleration with an increase in rate generally >20 bpm and lasting >20 seconds. When repetitive and accompanied with absent STV is considered "nonreassuring."

c. Treatment involves observing that the return occurs quickly and that there is no loss of variability.

  (i) Change maternal position.

  (ii) Vaginal examination for prolapsed umbilical cord or imminent delivery.

  (iii) Amnioinfusion.

  (iv) Provide oxygen at 8 to 10 L/min by snug face mask.

  (v) Provide information and decrease anxiety.

d. Atypical features of variables (Figure 37-10)

  (i) Described by Krebs, Petres, and Dunn.

  (ii) Identified as characteristics more commonly associated with hypoxemia.

  (iii) Include:

    (a) Loss of variability

    (b) Loss of secondary acceleration (shoulder)

    (c) Biphasic

    (d) Prolonged secondary acceleration (overshoot)

    (e) Slow return to baseline FHR

    (f) Continuation of baseline FHR at lower level

    (g) Loss of initial acceleration (shoulder)

e. Reassuring variables:

  (i) Lasting no more than 30 to 45 seconds

  (ii) Rapid return to baseline FHR

  (iii) Accompanied by normal baseline FHR and variability

f. Nonreassuring variables:

  (i) Prolonged return to baseline FHR

  (ii) Presence of overshoots

  (iii) Rising baseline FHR

  (iv) Absence or loss of STV and/or LTV

  (v) Persistent to <70 bpm and >60 seconds

6. Combined deceleration patterns may result when more than one physiologic mechanism causes a combination of "single" decelerations. These patterns contain characteristics of both "single" patterns in regard to shape and timing. Most patterns are not combined. They are described as:

a. Late variable decelerations

b. Early variable decelerations

c. Variable decelerations with late components

NURSING ALERT

Regardless of the pattern, it is important to recognize the existing physiology and intervene to correct the pattern based on the physiology.

Episodic FHR Changes/Patterns

1. Accelerations or decelerations of the FHR not in direct relation to uterine activity.

2. Acceleration—increase in the FHR.

a. Physiology—response to environmental stimuli or fetal activity that is not associated with uterine ac-

SIGNIFICANCE

1st   Loss of variability
2nd   Loss of secondary acceleration ONLY if accompanied by #1
3rd   Biphasic deceleration
4th   Prolonged secondary acceleration
5th   Slow return to baseline
6th   Continuation of baseline at lower level
7th   Loss of initial acceleration

FREQUENCY

6th
3rd
5th
4th
2nd
7th
1st

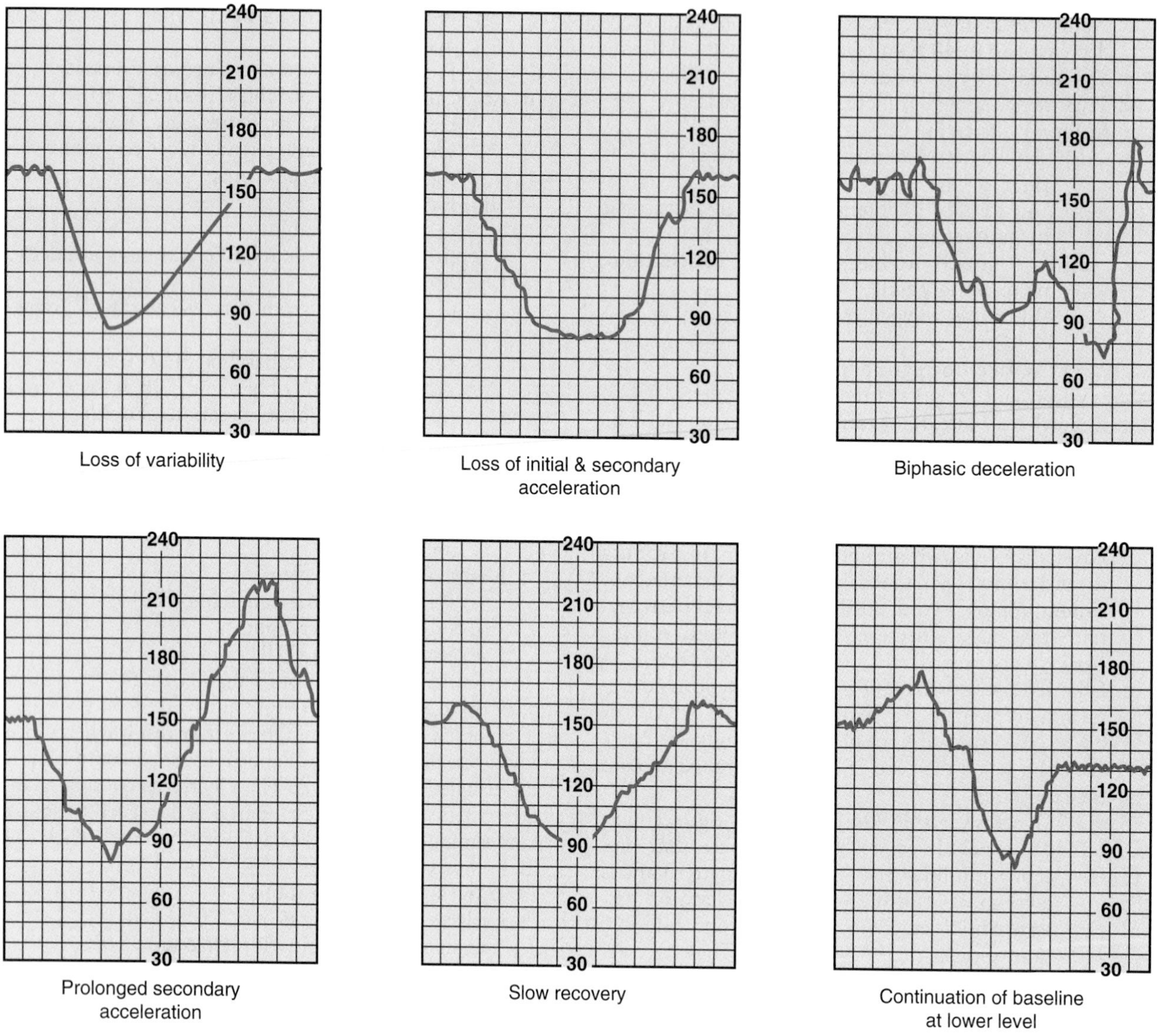

FIGURE 37-10   Atypical features of variable decelerations.

tivity (contractions); associated with nonacidotic, oxygenated, active fetus.
   b. Characteristics—same as periodic accelerations.
   c. Treatment—none required; reassuring pattern.
3. Variable deceleration.
   a. Physiology—same as periodic variable deceleration; associated with decreased amniotic fluid volume or umbilical cord entanglement; more often associated

with fetal movement or cord entanglement. May be found with chronic condition or changes associated with decreased amniotic fluid index (AFI), especially in a postmature fetus.
   b. Characteristics—resembles periodic variable deceleration; may be of shorter duration or less depth than periodic variable deceleration.
   c. Treatment—same as periodic variable deceleration.

4. Prolonged deceleration.
  a. Physiology—depends on precipitating cause; may be in response to profound changes in fetal environment such as placentae abruptio, uterine hypertonus or hyperstimulation, drug reactions, terminal fetal conditions, maternal death, and umbilical cord accidents. Can also be in response to hypotension of vagal stimulation from rapid fetal descent, vaginal examination, fetal blood sampling, or application of internal fetal monitoring methods. Less frequent cause associated with umbilical cord impingement, umbilical cord prolapse, uterine rupture, maternal seizures, status asthmaticus, or maternal cardiorespiratory collapse.
  b. Characteristics—visually abrupt decrease with onset to peak in ≤30 seconds. Decrease in FHR baseline is ≥15 bpm, lasting ≥2 minutes but ≤10 minutes from onset to return to baseline. Transient fetal tachycardia and loss of FHR variability may be associated with profound episodes.
  c. Treatment
    (i) Maternal position change
    (ii) Vaginal examination to check for prolapsed cord or imminent delivery
    (iii) Assess blood pressure for hypotension
    (iv) Discontinue uterine stimulation
    (v) Provide fluid bolus
    (vi) Provide oxygen 8 to 10 L/min by snug face mask
    (vii) Provide tocolytics
    (viii) Perform amnioinfusion
    (ix) Provide support and decrease anxiety

▣ First Stage of Labor—Latent Phase (0 to 3 cm)

Nursing Diagnoses
- Altered Nutrition: Less Than Body Requirements related to food restriction during labor
- Fluid Volume Deficit related to decreased oral intake
- Anxiety related to concern for self and the fetus
- Pain related to uterine contractions and/or position of the fetus

Nursing Interventions
Maintaining Nutrition and Hydration
1. Provide clear liquids and ice chips as allowed.
2. Evaluate urine for ketones and glucose.
3. Administer IV fluids as indicated.

Relieving Anxiety
1. Establish a relationship with the woman/couple.
2. Provide information on the health care facility's policies and procedures.
3. Inform the woman/couple of maternal status and fetal status and labor progress.
4. Explain all procedures and equipment used during labor.
5. Answer any questions the woman/couple have.
6. Review the birth plan and make appropriate revisions.

7. Monitor maternal vital signs. Remember the individual patient condition is used to determine frequency of vital signs and FHR assessment. Adjust as needed.
  a. Temperature every 2 to 4 hours, unless elevated or membranes ruptured, then every 1 to 2 hours.
  b. Pulse and respirations as indicated by institutional policy, medical condition, or medications being administered (eg, oxytocin or $MgSO_4$).
  c. Blood pressure every hour unless hypertension or hypotension exists or woman has received pain medication or anesthesia. Then evaluate more frequently based on findings or as indicated.
8. Monitor FHR
  a. Frequency of monitoring is established by institutional policy. The frequency may vary from every 1 to 2 hours depending on policy, provider's orders, or patient condition.
  b. Evaluate immediately after rupture of the membranes.

Controlling Pain
1. Encourage ambulation as tolerated regardless of membrane status as long as presenting part is engaged. (This may vary according to health care provider.)
2. Encourage diversional activities, such as reading, talking, watching TV, playing cards, listening to music.
3. Review, evaluate, and teach proper breathing techniques.
  a. Slow chest breathing (slow paced/Lamaze)—relax, take one deep cleansing breath, and exhale slowly and completely. Breathe deeply, slowly, rhythmically throughout contraction. Follow with another deep, complete cleansing breath. Take about six to nine breaths a minute. Breathe slowly and deeply in through the nose and out through nose or slightly pursed lips.
  b. Modified-paced breathing—used when slow chest breathing no longer effective. Take one deep breath, and exhale slowly and completely. Breathe regularly at more shallow level. When stronger contraction occurs, breathe more quickly with very light breaths. Then take deep breath, and exhale slowly. Rate not to exceed twice woman's average respiratory rate.
  c. Patterned-paced breathing (pant-blow breathing/ Lamaze)—concentrate on breathing in controlled manner. Take a deep breath, and exhale slowly and completely. At beginning of contraction, take a fairly deep cleansing breath. Then take four shallow breaths through the mouth making a "hee" or "heh" sound. Blow out through the mouth at the end of the shallow breaths—short puffs, not prolonged exhalation. Keep even, steady rhythm; rate not to exceed one breath per minute. Rhythm can vary from two pants, one blow to three pants, one blow, or even six pants, one blow—whatever rhythm feels comfortable for the woman. Take cleansing breath at end of uterine contraction. This breathing pattern is most often used during transition.
4. Effleurage—light massage over abdomen with fingertips; can be used with slow chest and modified-paced

breathing; start at pubic bone and move hands slowly up sides of abdomen in wide circular sweep; during exhaling, move fingertips down center of abdomen. Usually done by the laboring mother, but can be done with one hand if side-lying or the coach can do (Figure 37-11).

5. Encourage a warm shower. Laboring woman can sit on a chair in the shower with the water running continuously over her lower back.
6. Encourage relaxation techniques.
7. Provide comfort measures.
   a. Give back rubs.
   b. Assist the woman to change position. Walking, squatting, semi-sitting, hands and knees, kneeling, standing, side-lying, or sitting on the toilet are positions that help to accommodate the descending fetus and relieve pain of uterine contractions. Side-lying position with the woman lying on the opposite side of the fetal occiput or on hands and knees will help rotate a persistent OP position to an anterior position.
   c. Reposition external monitors as needed.

Alternative Therapies
Birthing Balls
Sturdy inflatable vinyl balls approximately 2½ feet in diameter used by the laboring woman. The laboring woman can sit on the ball and sway from side to side, or she may

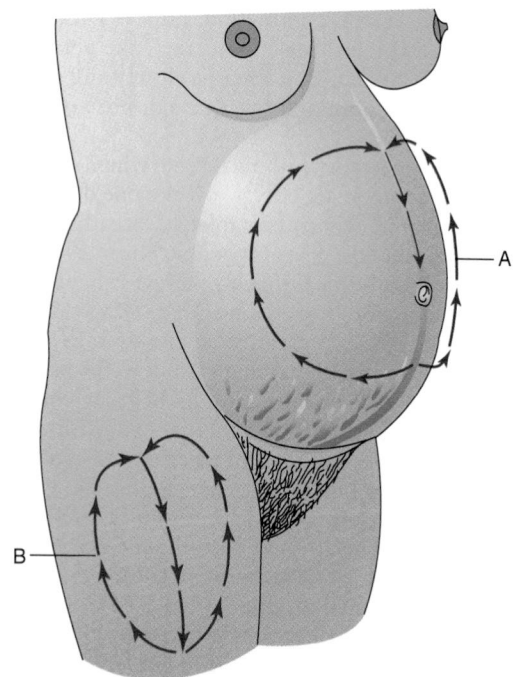

FIGURE 37-11 Effleurage. **(A)** During uterine contractions, a woman creates the pattern on her bare abdomen with her fingers. **(B)** If electronic fetal monitoring is being used, effleurage may be performed on the thigh.

kneel and lean forward resting on the birthing ball to assist in fetal descent.

Self-Hypnosis
Women are trained to rehearse the birth mentally and to control physical reactions like blood pressure, pulse, or pain. The American Psychotherapy and Medical Hypnosis Association (*http://APMHA.com*) can provide referrals.

Acupuncture
Although there are no current U.S. studies on acupuncture, the practice is active in this country and is said to relieve as much as 90% of the pain in early labor and 60% of the pain during transition. Referrals can be made to the American Academy of Medical Acupuncture; 5820 Wilshire Boulevard, Los Angeles, CA 90036; 323-937-5514; *www.medicalacupuncture.org*.

Herbal Therapies
Although many of the herbs used are not FDA approved, they have been researched and found to be effective in laboring women and are documented in a myriad of medical and nursing references.

1. Evening primrose oil—rubbed on abdomen in prelabor to stimulate uterine activity.
2. Corn silk—stimulates sluggish labor.
3. Nutmeg—enhances uterine contractions; if added, cayenne and bayberry help with bleeding after delivery.
4. Nutmeg with yarrow, mistletoe, and corn silk—utilized as a treatment for hemorrhage postpartum.

> **NURSING ALERT**
>
> Although red raspberry is effective when used to expel retained placenta, it should not be used during labor—only for immediate postpartum period. Avoid licorice, mistletoe, thyme, and slippery elm during labor because they can significantly increase uterine tone.

Community and Home Care Considerations
1. Consider mother's birthing plan.
2. Many alternative therapies or pain relief strategies can be done at home with skilled provider in attendance.
3. If hospital birth is desired, woman can stay at home until pain is uncontrollable despite all pain relief interventions or if rupture of membranes occurs. Before coming to the hospital, woman or significant other should notify the hospital and/or the primary care provider.
4. If home birth is desired, woman needs to notify her primary care provider and prepare for delivery at home. Woman should always have an emergency birth plan to prepare for unexpected emergencies and needed operative intervention.

Outcome-Based Evaluation
- Tolerates fluids well and urine negative for ketones and glucose
- Verbalizes positive statements about self and fetus
- Reports pain decreased from comfort strategies

■ First Stage of Labor—Active and Transition Phase

Nursing Diagnoses

- Anxiety related to concern for self and fetus
- Pain related to uterine contractions and/or nausea and vomiting
- Altered Urinary Elimination related to epidural anesthesia or from pressure of the fetus
- Ineffective Individual Coping related to discomfort
- Risk for Infection related to rupture of the membranes
- Impaired Physical Mobility related to medical interventions and/ or discomfort
- Ineffective Breathing Pattern related to pain and fatigue

Nursing Interventions

Relieving Anxiety

1. Monitor maternal vital signs and FHR, and keep the woman/couple informed of the maternal and fetus status.
   a. Maternal temperature every 2 to 4 hours unless elevated or membranes ruptured, then every 1 hour.
   b. Blood pressure, pulse, respirations usually every 30 to 60 minutes or as indicated by institutional policy.
   c. Evaluate FHR every 30 minutes if low-risk patient or every 15 minutes if high-risk patient regardless if monitoring is continuous or intermittent.
2. Provide encouragement and support.
3. Involve the support person in the woman's care.

Minimizing Pain

1. Encourage position changes for comfort.
2. Assist the woman with breathing and relaxation techniques as needed.
3. Provide back, leg, and shoulder massage as needed.

> ### NURSING ALERT
>
> Leg massage should only be light stroking of the legs, not deep leg massage, to avoid possible dislodgement of embolism, if present.

4. Administer prescribed analgesia as needed (Table 37-2).
   a. Confirm that the woman has no known allergies to the drug.
   b. Describe effects of the drug, such as making the woman feel sleepy, relaxed, and more comfortable.
   c. Evaluate cervical status by way of vaginal examination before drug administration.
   d. Evaluate vital signs after drug administration.
   e. Observe for signs and symptoms of a drug reaction.
   f. Evaluate FHR pattern. Decreased variability and a pseudosinusoidal or sinusoidal pattern are sometimes seen after narcotic administration to the mother.
   g. Maintain IV fluids as indicated.
5. Assist with regional anesthesia (epidural) if needed.
   a. Administer IV fluid bolus of Ringer's lactate as indicated.

   b. Assist with positioning the woman to either side-lying or sitting position.
   c. Monitor the FHR during the procedure, and assess for a nonreassuring pattern.
   d. Monitor the woman's blood pressure, pulse, and respirations every 2 to 3 minutes after the procedure, then every 15 minutes thereafter or as indicated.
   e. Observe for hypotension, nausea and vomiting, and lightheadedness after the procedure. If these occur, notify primary care provider and anesthesia provider and:
      (i) Increase the rate of the IV fluid.
      (ii) Flatten the head of the bed and put patient in Trendelenburg's position if necessary.
      (iii) Turn the woman to her side.
      (iv) Administer oxygen by face mask at 8 to 10 L/min.
      (v) Have ephedrine available.
   f. Provide safe environment.
   g. Document on the woman's record and monitor strip according to institutional policy.

Encouraging Bladder Emptying

1. Encourage the woman to void every 2 hours at least 100 mL.
2. Palpate the lower abdomen, and evaluate for a distended bladder.
3. Assist with enabling the woman to void by providing time and privacy, running the sink water gently, providing a perineal bottle of warm water for the woman to squirt against her perineum.
4. Catheterize (in and out) when necessary or as directed by primary care provider.
5. Monitor intake and output, especially if on Pitocin or $MgSO_4$ drips.

Strengthening Coping With Active Labor and Transition

1. Assist the woman with breathing and relaxation techniques.
2. Encourage a positive attitude.
3. Encourage the labor coach to assist with coping strategies.
4. Provide comfort measures, which may include:
   a. Back rubs and leg stroking.
   b. A cool cloth to face, neck, abdomen, or back.
   c. Ice chips to moisten mouth.
   d. An emesis basin.
   e. Clean pads and linens as needed.
   f. A quiet environment.
   g. Repositioning, either side is preferable, with pillow and blanket. Supports as needed.
5. Encourage the woman to deal with one contraction at a time.
6. Provide reassurance and encouragement during each contraction.
7. Provide information on the contraction's ascent, peak, and descent.
8. Encourage resting between contractions.
9. Encourage the woman not to push with feelings of rectal pressure until complete cervical dilation has occurred. Assisting her with panting may be helpful.

TABLE 37-2 Obstetric Analgesia and Anesthesia

Drug	Comment
Narcotic Analgesics/Parenteral Opioids Meperidine (Demerol) Butorphanol (Stadol) Nalbuphine (Nubain) Fentanyl (Sublimaze) Pentazocine (Talwin)	Decreases fear and anxiety, promotes physical relaxation and rest between contractions; may cause nausea and vomiting; respiratory depression is the main side effect and is seen primarily in the newborn. Most commonly given IV or IM every 3 to 4 hours.
Tranquilizers Promethazine (Phenergan) [ataractic] Hydroxyzine (Vistaril) [ataractic] Propiomazine (Largon) [ataractic]	May be used in combination with narcotics; potentiates narcotics; may be used as an antiemetic. Used in latent and first stage of labor to relieve anxiety, increase sedation/rest, and decrease nausea and vomiting.
Sedatives Sodium secobarbital (Seconal) [barbiturate] Sodium pentobarbital (Nembutal) [barbiturate] Sodium phenobarbital (Luminal)	Produces sedation and hypnosis. Used for latent stage of labor to decrease anxiety, inhibit uterine contractions, and allow for rest. Does not relieve pain. Given orally or IM.
Epidural Anesthesia/Analgesia Epidural narcotics (walking epidural)	Used with a local anesthetic to provide pain relief with a decreased motor block in labor. Used postoperatively to promote long-acting analgesia.
Epidural block	Used for labor to provide a sensory block up to the T10–T12 level. Medication is given through the epidural catheter. Used for cesarean section and postpartum tubal ligation by increasing the level of anesthesia up to T4–T6.
Subarachnoid block (spinal/intrathecal)	Used for such surgical procedures as a cesarean section and postpartum tubal ligation. The procedure is quicker and easier to perform. There is no catheter for the procedure. Medication lasts for a finite period of time.
Local anesthesia	Used for pain control of the perineal area for an episiotomy or repair during a vaginal delivery.
Pudendal block	Used during the second stage of labor just before delivery to numb the lower vaginal canal, vulva, and the perineum for delivery. May also be used to provide pain relief for a forceps delivery if the woman doesn't have an epidural and for perineal repair.
General anesthesia	Used for emergency delivery involving cesarean section; if the woman refuses regional anesthesia; if regional anesthesia cannot be performed.

◆ **DRUG ALERT**

Seconal, Nembutal, Sparine, and Phenergan can cause the following fetal and/or neonatal complications: fetal tachycardia, decreased long-term variability, absent short-term variability, hypotonia, hypothermia, generalized drowsiness, and a reluctance to feed in the first days of life.

Demerol, Fentanyl, Morphine, Nubain, Stadol, and Talwin can cause subtle effects on neonatal behavior in the first 24 hours secondary to these drugs crossing the placenta. General anesthesia is contraindicated in situations where the fetus is already compromised and delivery cannot be anticipated within minutes of anesthetic administration.

Preventing Intrauterine Infection

1. Take the woman's temperature, and record every 2 hours if not ruptured. If ruptured, take and record temperature every 1 hour.
2. Change the pads and linens when wet or soiled.
3. Provide perineal care after voiding and as needed.
4. Discourage the use of perineal pads, because they create a warm, moist environment for bacteria.
5. Minimize vaginal examinations.
6. Observe for fetal tachycardia.
7. Assess complete blood count (CBC) as indicated.

Maintaining Mobility

1. Provide information regarding limitations and opportunities for movement with electronic fetal monitoring.
2. Encourage the woman to be out of bed ambulating and/or sitting in a chair while being monitored, if indicated.
3. Encourage position change in bed every hour or as indicated.

4. Assist with back rubs, leg stroking (lightly), and leg exercises while in bed.

Encouraging Effective Breathing Techniques

1. Assist the woman with altering her breathing and relaxation techniques as needed to maintain control.
2. Inform the woman that the urge to push is common during transition and is usually due to rapid fetal descent, the dilating cervix, and uterine contractions. Pushing with feelings of rectal pressure before complete cervical dilation should be avoided due to risks of increasing cervical edema and lacerations.
3. Assist the woman to avoid pushing prematurely by:
   a. Maintaining close eye contact during breathing.
   b. Breathing with the woman, having her blow out strong, short breaths.
4. Awaken the woman before the beginning of each contraction so she can gain control of her breathing if she has partial amnesia between contractions.

Outcome-Based Evaluation

- Verbalizes positive statements about self and fetus
- Reports pain decreased from comfort strategies and medical interventions
- Bladder remains undistended, and the woman voids or bladder is emptied for 100 mL or more
- Directs strategies for decreasing discomfort
- Absence of fever and signs of infection
- Changes position during labor
- Uses breathing techniques during contractions

◼ Second Stage of Labor

Nursing Diagnoses

- Fear/Anxiety related to impending delivery
- Pain related to descent of the fetus
- Risk for Infection related to episiotomy and/or tissue trauma

Nursing Interventions

Minimizing Fear and Anxiety

1. Monitor maternal vital signs as follows:
   a. Blood pressure—every 5 to 15 minutes depending on the woman's status.
   b. Pulse and respirations—every 15 to 30 minutes.
   c. Temperature—every 1 hour once membranes have ruptured.
2. Monitor FHR and uterine contractions every 15 minutes in low-risk women and every 5 minutes in high-risk women.
   a. Early decelerations and some fetal bradycardia may occur due to head compression.
   b. There is normally no loss of variability during pushing.
   c. Contractions may become less frequent, but intensity does not decrease.
3. Explain procedures and equipment during pushing and delivery.
4. Keep the woman/couple informed of their status.

5. Provide frequent, positive encouragement.
   a. Use of a mirror often allows the woman to see her progress.
6. Assist and instruct the woman in the pushing technique.
   a. Take a full, cleansing breath, in through the nose and out through the mouth, at the beginning and end of each contraction.
   b. Push only during contractions when mother feels the urge to push. If anesthetized with epidural anesthesia, have mother push at the peak of the contraction as evidenced by the uterine monitor.
   c. Push down toward the perineum with the abdominal muscles, and try to keep the rest of the body relaxed.
   d. Pushing techniques include:
      (i) Closed glottis—cleansing breath; hold breath up to the count of 8; end with cleansing breath; a minimum of three pushes in this pattern for each contraction. This style of pushing increases the maternal blood pressure initially; then it falls as the breath holding continues. Ultimately, there is an increased catecholamine release that decreases uterine activity. This method also causes the fetal blood pressure to fall (due to mother's falling blood pressure), decreases oxygen to the fetus (due to mother not inhaling enough oxygen), and increases fetal carbon dioxide (due to breath holding). It is not uncommon to see FHR changes such as variable or late decelerations with this pushing style.
      (ii) Open glottis—pushing while exhaling. Pushing is done in short 6- to 7-second periods with the mother pushing only with the urge to push. There is minimal change in maternal blood pressure, thus minimal, if any, change in the FHR pattern. This method also relaxes the perineum, allowing the gentle delivery of the fetal head.
      (iii) Tug-of-war—uses the natural bearing down effort of the abdominal muscles. Take a gown or short sheet, and tie a knot in both ends. (Alternative way is to tie knot in one end and tie other end to squat bar of labor bed.) When mother has the urge to push, she grabs one end of the gown or sheet and pulls as much as she can. (If not tied to the squat bar, the other end is given to the coach to pull in the opposite direction from the mother). This method also causes minimal change in the maternal blood pressure, relaxes the perineum, and has been found to decrease the second stage of labor as much as 20 minutes.

Promoting Comfort

1. Assist the woman to a comfortable position.
   a. Left or right lateral, squatting, hand and knees, or semisitting positions may be used.
   b. Assist the woman with pulling her legs back so her knees are flexed.

c. Teach the woman to put her chin to her chest so her body forms a "C" shape while pushing.

2. Evaluate bladder fullness, and encourage voiding or catheterize as needed.

3. Evaluate effectiveness of anesthesia as indicated.

Preventing Infection and Promoting Safety

1. Prepare the birthing room or delivery room using aseptic technique, allowing ample time for setup before delivery.

2. Prepare the infant resuscitation area for delivery.

3. Prepare necessary items for newborn care.

4. Notify necessary personnel to prepare for delivery.

5. If delivery room is to be used, transfer the primigravida to the delivery room when the fetal head is crowning. The multigravida is taken earlier depending on fetal size and speed of fetal descent.

6. Place all side rails up before moving. Instruct the woman to keep her hands off the rails, and move from the bed to the delivery table between contractions.

7. If delivering in LDR (Labor, Delivery, Recovery) or LDRP (Labor, Delivery, Recovery, Postpartum) room, prepare labor bed for delivery in accordance with manufacturer's instructions. Prepare infant warmer and remainder of room for delivery.

8. Position the woman for delivery using a large cushion for her head, back, and shoulders. Elevate the head of the bed. Stirrups or footrests may be used for leg or foot support. Pad the stirrups. Place both legs in the stirrups at the same time to avoid ligament strain, backache, or injury.

9. Cleanse the vulva and perineal areas once the woman is positioned for delivery.

   a. Cleanse from the lower abdomen to the mons.
   b. Then cleanse the groin to the inner thigh on each side.
   c. Then cleanse each labia.
   d. Finally, cleanse the introitus.

10. Guide the woman step by step during the delivery process.

    a. When the fetal head is encircled by the vulvovaginal ring, an episiotomy may be performed to prevent tearing.
    b. When the head is delivered, mother is instructed to stop pushing. Mucus is wiped from the infant's face, and the mouth and nose are aspirated with a bulb syringe. If thick or particulate meconium amniotic fluid is present, the mouth and nose are suctioned on the perineum with deep suction before the delivery of the body.
    c. If loops of umbilical cord are found around the infant's neck, they are loosened and slipped from around the neck. If the cord cannot be slipped over the head, it is clamped with two clamps and cut between the two clamps.
    d. After this step, the woman is asked to give a gentle push so the infant's body may be quickly delivered.

e. After delivery of the infant's body and cutting of the cord, the infant is shown to the parents and then placed on the maternal abdomen or taken to the radiant warmer for inspection and identification procedures.

11. Practice universal precautions during labor and delivery.

Outcome-Based Evaluation

- Verbalizes positive statements about delivery outcome
- Reports decreased pain from proper positioning
- No infection results

■ Third Stage of Labor

Nursing Diagnosis

- Impaired Tissue Integrity related to placental separation
- Risk for Injury related to potential hemorrhage

Nursing Interventions

Promoting Tissue Integrity

1. Ask the woman to bear down gently. Fundal pressure is never applied to facilitate delivery of the fetus or the placenta (Figure 37-12). Observe for the signs of placental separation:

   a. The uterus rises upward in the abdomen.
   b. The umbilical cord lengthens.
   c. Trickle or spurt of blood appears.
   d. The uterus becomes globular in shape.

2. Evaluate the placenta for size, shape, and cord site implantation. Evaluate placenta for Duncan or Schultze presentation.

   a. Schultze—central region of the placenta separates first with the shiny surface of the placenta (fetal side) appearing first. Commonly referred to as shiny Schultze.
   b. Duncan—periphery of the placenta separates first with the dull, irregular surface of the placenta (maternal side) appearing first. Commonly referred to as dirty Duncan.

NURSING ALERT

Duncan placental separation carries a slightly increased risk of retained placental fragments due to incomplete separation. As a result, the woman carries an increased risk of postpartum hemorrhage. Delivery of the placenta should take no more than 30 minutes. Watch the time closely, and notify the provider as necessary.

Preventing Hemorrhage

1. Ensure accurate measurement of intake and output maintained throughout labor and delivery.

2. Immediately after delivery of the placenta, administer oxytocin (Pitocin) either IV piggyback (IVPB) or intramuscularly (IM) as directed by institutional policy and provider. Infuse as bolus initially, then titrate to uterus (ie, if uterus is firm, decrease the infusion; if boggy, leave as bolus). Pitocin should never be administered IV push.

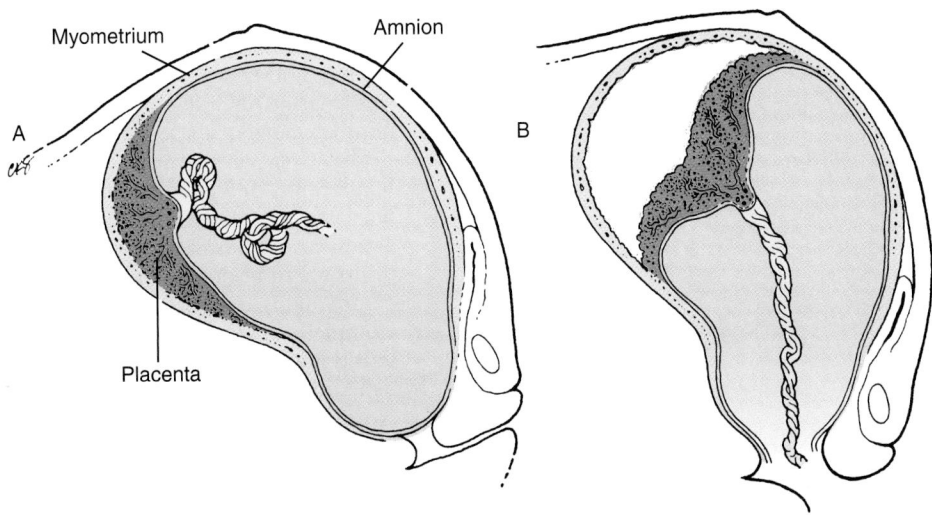

FIGURE 37-12   Placental separation. (**A**) Placenta attached to uterine wall. (**B**) Placenta separated from uterine wall.

3. Immediately after initiating Pitocin, massage uterine fundus until firm. Uterine massage is done with two hands, one anchored at the lower uterine segment above the symphysis pubis and the other hand gently massages the fundus.
4. Check to see that the placenta and membranes are complete.
5. Evaluate and massage the uterine fundus until firm.
6. Evaluate vaginal bleeding. If bleeding continuously and uterus is boggy, prepare Methergine IM or Hemabate (Prostin, Prostaglandin F$_2$ Alpha) IM for injection. Administer as directed. Increase IV fluids. Monitor vital signs, especially blood pressure and pulse.

DRUG ALERT

Methergine is contraindicated in women with hypertension. Hemabate is contraindicated in women with asthma.

7. If bleeding continues and uterus is firm, notify health care provider for evaluation of lacerations or retained placental fragments. Inspection and repair of lacerations of the vagina and cervix are made by the health care provider.
8. If still no relief, notify health care provider and prepare patient for possible surgery (dilation and curettage [D&C]).

Outcome-Based Evaluation
• An intact placenta is delivered
• Blood loss will be controlled and hemorrhage prevented

Immediate Care of the Newborn
Nursing Diagnoses
• Ineffective Airway Clearance related to nasal and oral secretions from delivery
• Ineffective Thermoregulation related to environment and immature ability for adaptation
• Risk for Injury related to immature defenses of the newborn

Nursing Interventions
Promoting Airway Clearance and Transitioning of the Newborn
1. Wipe mucus from the face and mouth and nose. Aspirate with a bulb syringe.
   a. If meconium is present before the delivery, mechanical suctioning of the nasopharynx with an 8 or 10 French catheter is done.
   b. Suctioning is done by the birth attendant when the head is delivered.
2. Clamp the umbilical cord approximately 2.5 cm (1 inch) from the abdominal wall with a cord clamp.
   a. Cord clamping is done by the birth attendant.
   b. Count the number of vessels in the cord—fewer than three vessels has been associated with renal and cardiac anomalies.
3. Evaluate the newborn's condition by the Apgar scoring system (Table 37-3) at 1 and 5 minutes after birth.
   a. Newborns scoring 7 to 10 are free of immediate stress.
   b. Newborns scoring 4 to 6 are moderately depressed.
   c. Newborns scoring 0 to 3 are severely depressed.

TABLE 37-3   Apgar Scoring Chart

Sign	0	1	2
Heart rate	Absent	Slow (less than 100)	Over 100
Respiratory effort	Absent	Slow, irregular	Good, crying
Muscle tone	Flaccid	Some flexion of extremities	Active motion
Reflex irritability	No response	Cry	Vigorous cry
Color	Blue, pale	Body pink, extremities blue	Completely pink

d. Apgar scores <7 at 5 minutes are to be repeated every 5 minutes until 20 minutes have passed, the infant is intubated, or two successive scores of >7 occur.

Promoting Thermoregulation

1. Dry the newborn immediately after delivery, remove wet towels, and place infant on warm dry towels. A wet, small newborn loses up to 200 cal/kg/min in the delivery room through evaporation, convection, conduction, and radiation. Drying the infant cuts this heat loss in half.
2. Cover the newborn's head with a cotton stocking cap to prevent heat loss.
3. Wrap the newborn in warm blankets.
4. Place the newborn under a radiant heat warmer, or place the newborn on the mother's abdomen with skin-to-skin contact.
5. Provide a warm, draft-free environment for the newborn.
6. Take the newborn's axillary temperature—a normal temperature is between 36.4°C and 37.2°C (97.5°F–99.0°F).

Preventing Injury and Infection

1. Administer prophylactic treatment against ophthalmia neonatorum (gonorrheal or chlamydial).
   a. Treatment may be with erythromycin or tetracycline antibiotic ophthalmic ointment or drops. Given within 1 hour after birth.

DRUG ALERT

Excessive ophthalmic ointment should be wiped away with a sterile pad or cotton ball at least 1 minute after installation.

   b. If the mother has a positive gonococcal or chlamydial culture, the newborn will require further treatment.
   c. Treatment is mandatory in all states.
2. Administer a prophylactic injection of vitamin K. This is done to prevent a neonatal hemorrhage during the first few days of life before the infant begins to produce its own vitamin K.
3. Place matching identification bracelets on the mother and the newborn.
   a. Bracelets are placed on the newborn's ankle and wrist.
   b. A similar bracelet is placed on the mother. The father or significant other may also wear a bracelet matching the mother's.
   c. Information includes the mother's name, hospital number, newborn's sex, race, and date and time of birth.
   d. Fingerprints of the mother and footprints of the newborn may also be done for the family. But it is not used as a means of hospital identification protocol. If footprints are to be done, remove all vernix from the foot before inking to improve the quality of the footprint.
   e. Complete all identification procedures before the infant is taken from the delivery room.
4. Weigh and measure the infant.
   a. Normal newborn weight is 2,700 to 4,000 g (6 to 9 lb).
   b. Normal newborn length is 48 to 53 cm (19 to 21 inches).
5. Administer hepatitis B vaccine.
   a. Vaccination of all infants born in the United States is recommended regardless of mother's hepatitis status. It is given within 12 hours after birth for the prevention of acute and chronic hepatitis B infection.
   b. If mother is hepatitis B positive, infant will also receive hepatitis B immunoglobulin (HBIG). Additionally, infants of hepatitis-positive mothers will receive HBIG at 1 month and 6 months of age.

Community and Home Care Considerations

1. Issues regarding promoting airway clearance, transitioning the newborn, and promoting thermoregulation are essentially unchanged for home births, although Apgar scores are sometimes not given at home deliveries.
2. Eye prophylaxis is unchanged; parents may choose to not use prophylaxis.
3. Vitamin K administration is not a requirement for home deliveries. Vitamin K levels naturally increase at 7 days of life. If infant is a boy, and parents desire circumcision, the procedure is withheld until after day 7.
4. Ensure attendants are familiar with neonatal resuscitation and emergency numbers/procedures are readily available.
5. Identification procedures are not required for home births, although required state paperwork must be completed by the health care provider.

Outcome-Based Evaluation

- Newborn transitions appropriately as evidenced by Apgar score between 7 and 10
- Temperature remains between 36.4°C and 37.2°C (97.5°F–99.0°F)
- Identification bracelets on newborn and initial newborn care complete

Fourth Stage of Labor

Nursing Diagnoses

- Risk for Injury related to uterine atony and hemorrhage
- Fluid Volume Deficit related to decreased oral intake, bleeding, and diaphoresis

- Pain/Fatigue related to tissue trauma and birth process
- Altered Urinary Elimination related to epidural or spinal anesthesia and tissue trauma
- Sensory/Perceptual Alterations (tactile) related to effects of regional anesthesia
- Altered Parenting related to the newborn and/or inexperience

Nursing Interventions
Promoting Uterine Contraction and Controlling Bleeding

1. Monitor blood pressure, pulse, and respirations every 15 minutes for 1 hour, then every ½ hour to 1 hour until stable or transferred to the postpartum unit.
2. Take temperature every 4 hours unless elevated, then every 2 hours.
3. Evaluate the following at the time vital signs are taken initially then every 4 hours or more frequently as indicated for 12 to 24 hours or per institutional policy:
   a. Uterine fundal tone, height, and position. The uterus should be firm around the level of the umbilicus, at the midline. If deviated to the side (usually the right side), it is indicative of a full bladder; have the mother empty her bladder and the uterus should return to midline.
   b. Amount of vaginal bleeding.
      (i) Scant—blood only on tissue when wiped or less than 1-inch stain on perineal pad within 1 hour.
      (ii) Small/light—less than 4-inch stain on perineal pad within 1 hour.
      (iii) Moderate—less than 6-inch stain on perineal pad within 1 hour.
      (iv) Heavy—saturated perineal pad within 1 hour.
   c. Perineum for edema, discoloration, bleeding, or hematoma formation.
   d. Episiotomy for intactness and bleeding.

Maintaining Fluid Volume

1. Maintain IV fluids as indicated.
2. Provide oral fluids and a snack or meal as tolerated.
3. Encourage drink and food before assisting the woman out of bed.

Relieving Discomfort and Fatigue

1. Apply a covered ice pack to the perineum for an episiotomy, perineal laceration, or edema.
2. Administer analgesics as indicated.
3. Assist the woman in finding comfortable positions.
4. Assist the woman with a partial bath and perineal care, and change linens and pads as necessary.
5. Allow for privacy and rest periods between postpartum checks.
6. Provide warm blankets, and reassure the woman that tremors are common during this period.

Encouraging Bladder Emptying

1. Evaluate the bladder for distention.
2. Encourage the woman to void.
   a. Provide adequate time and privacy.
   b. The sound from a running faucet may stimulate voiding.
   c. Gently squirting tepid water against the perineum in a perineal bottle may help.
3. Catheterize the woman (in and out) if the bladder is full and she is unable to void.
   a. Birth trauma, anesthesia, and pain from lacerations and episiotomy may reduce or alter the voiding reflex.
   b. Bladder distention may displace the uterus upward and to the side.

Assessing Return of Sensation

1. Evaluate mobility and sensation of the lower extremities.
2. Evaluate vital signs.
3. Remain with the woman, and assist her out of bed for the first time. Evaluate her ability to support her weight and ambulate.
4. Do not provide hot fluids if sensation is decreased.

Promoting Parenting

1. Show the newborn to the mother and father or support person immediately after birth when possible.
2. Encourage the mother and/or father to hold the baby as soon as possible.
3. Teach the mother/parents to hold the newborn close to their faces, about 8 to 12 inches, when talking to the baby.
4. Have the mother/parents look at and inspect the baby's body to familiarize themselves with their child.
5. Assist the mother with breast-feeding during the first 30 minutes, then 2 hours, after birth. This is often a period of quiet alert time for the newborn, and he or she will often readily take to the breast.
6. Provide quiet alone time in a low-lighted room for the family to become acquainted.
7. Observe and record the reaction of the mother/parents to the newborn.

Outcome-Based Evaluation

- Vital signs remain stable, vaginal bleeding remains light to moderate, and uterus remains firm at the midline
- Tolerates fluids well after delivery
- Verbalizes decreased perineal pain and feeling more rested
- Voids greater than 100 mL within 6 hours of delivery
- Ambulates without problems
- Interacts with the newborn

SPECIAL CONSIDERATIONS

Newborn Resuscitation

This procedure is most effective when there is a simple, organized, and efficient system established in the birth area.

Causes

Asphyxia is the main reason for newborn resuscitation. When the infant is deprived of oxygen, an initial period of rapid respirations occur followed by the cessation of respirations, decreased heart rate, decreased neuromuscular tone, and the infant enters into primary apnea.

Primary Apnea

1. Intrauterine asphyxia may result in passage of meconium, fetal tachycardia, loss of variability, late decelerations, or prolonged bradycardia.
2. Infants born with primary apnea will need sensory stimuli (tactile or positive-pressure ventilation) to initiate respirations.
3. May occur in utero or after birth.

Secondary Apnea

1. Secondary apnea occurs when primary apnea is unresolved. The heart rate drops, the blood pressure drops, the infant becomes flaccid, and spontaneous gasps occur.
2. May occur in utero or after birth.
3. At birth, these infants are pale, flaccid, and bradycardiac. Spontaneous respirations will not occur with sensory stimuli because of the biochemical, neurologic, and circulatory changes that have occurred.

> **NURSING ALERT**
>
> When the infant is apneic at birth, it is difficult to distinguish between primary and secondary apnea; therefore, you must assume it is secondary apnea and resuscitation must begin immediately.

Steps in Newborn Resuscitation

1. Call for assistance if needed.
2. Place the infant in a warm radiant warmer.
3. Suction the mouth, then the nose with a bulb syringe or wall suction.
4. Stimulate the infant, dry off the trunk with warmed towels, dispose of wet towels, and attempt to keep the infant warm.
5. Assess respiratory and cardiac status.
6. If no respirations, begin bag and mask ventilation using 100% oxygen.
   a. Use an inspiratory pressure of 30 to 40 cm water for initial breath. Then use 15 to 20 cm water for normal lungs or 20 to 30 cm water for diseased lungs at a rate of 40 to 60 breaths/min.
   b. Observe chest movement, and auscultate for air movement in all lung fields.
7. Begin chest compressions at a rate of 90 to 120 compressions/min if, after 15 to 30 seconds of positive pressure ventilation with 100% oxygen, heart rate <60 bpm or if heart rate is between 60 and 80 bpm and is not increasing.
8. Assist with endotracheal intubation if needed.
9. Assist with insertion of an umbilical venous line for administration of medications and fluids if needed.
10. Transport when stable.

■ Emergency Delivery and Delivery in Absence of Health Care Provider

In delivery under emergency conditions, consider the woman and infant as a unit; work to prevent infection, injury, and hemorrhage in woman and infant and to establish respirations in the newborn.

Interventions

1. Provide reassurance and instruct the woman in a calm, controlled manner. Have the mother feather blow or pant-blow unless told to push. Do not break down the birthing bed.
2. Instruct the woman to assume a lithotomy position.
3. Wash hands, don gloves, and cleanse perineum. This should be done by the birth attendant if time permits.
4. Exert gentle pressure against the head of the fetus, using pads of thumb, index finger, and middle fingers or cupped palm of hand, to control its progress and prevent too rapid a delivery.
   a. Use a clean or sterile towel. Maintain flexion of fetal head.
   b. This prevents undue stretching of the perineum.
   c. This prevents sudden expulsion through the vulva with subsequent infant and maternal complications.
5. Encourage the woman to pant at this time to prevent bearing down.
6. Rupture the membranes by tearing them at the nape of the infant's neck. This is done if membranes have not ruptured by the time the head is delivered.
7. Wipe the infant's face and mouth with a clean towel. Suction the mouth and nose with a bulb syringe if available.
8. Check to see whether the cord is wrapped around the infant's neck or other body part. If the cord is too tight to permit slipping it over the infant's head, it must be clamped in two places and cut between the clamps before the rest of the body is delivered.
9. Allow head to restitute. Hold the infant's head with flats of both hands and gently exert downward pressure toward the floor, thus slipping the anterior shoulder under the symphysis pubis.
10. As soon as the anterior shoulder is delivered, provide upward, outward traction to the head to deliver the posterior shoulder.
11. Support the infant's body and head in the lower hand. As the body is delivered, slide the upper hand down the back to grasp the infant's feet.
12. Hold the infant with the head down to help drain mucus; wipe away excess mucus from the mouth and nose; gentle rubbing of the back may stimulate breathing.
13. Double clamp the cord. Cut the cord between the clamps. If clamps are unavailable, tie off the cord with suitable material.
14. Place the infant on the mother's abdomen where she can see him or her after the infant cries.
15. Avoid touching the perineal area to prevent infection.
16. Avoid pulling on the cord, which might break and cause hemorrhage.
17. Watch for signs of placental separation.

18. Check fundal contractions; massage if indicated. Putting the baby to breast may help the uterus to contract.
19. Place identification of some kind on the mother and infant.
20. Give the woman fluids.
21. Assist the woman to a suitable environment, if she is not in a bed or in a place where she can lie down.
22. Do not leave the woman alone.
23. Teach the woman to massage her fundus; explain why the cord has not been cut.
24. Record the time and date of birth.
25. Assist and transport as necessary.

SELECTED REFERENCES

Aldrich, C. J., et al. (1995). Late fetal heart decelerations and changes in cerebral oxygenation during the first stage of labour. *British Journal of Obstetrics and Gynecology, 102*(1), 9–13.

American Academy of Pediatrics (AAP)/ACOG. (1995). *Neonatal resuscitation.* Elk Grove Village, IL: Author.

American College of Obstetricians and Gynecologists (ACOG). (1995). *FHR patterns: Monitoring, interpreting, and management.* ACOG Technical Bulletin #207. Washington, D.C.: Author.

Association of Women's Health, Obstetric, and Neonatal Nurses (AWHONN) (1997) *Fetal heart monitoring principles and practices* (2nd ed.). Dubuque, IA: Kendall-Hunt.

Avery, G., et al. (1994). *Neonatology pathophysiology and management of the newborn* (4th ed.). Philadelphia: J. B. Lippincott.

Beischer, N. A., Mackay, E. V., & Colditz, P. B. (1997). *Obstetrics and the newborn* (3rd ed.). Philadelphia: W. B. Saunders.

Blackburn, S. T., & Loper, D. L. (1992). *Maternal, fetal and neonatal physiology: A clinical perspective.* Philadelphia: W. B. Saunders.

Cabaniss, M. (1993). *Fetal monitor interpretation.* Philadelphia: J. B. Lippincott.

Cassidy, J. (1993). A picture-perfect birth. *RN, 56*(6), 45–46.

Collins, C. (1998). Yoga; Intuition, preventive medicine, & treatment. *Journal of Obstetric, Gynecologic, and Neonatal Nursing, 98*, 563–568.

Creasy, R. K., & Resnik, R. (1999). *Maternal–fetal medicine principles and practice* (4th ed.). Philadelphia: W. B. Saunders.

Davis, C. A. (1992). The effects of music and basic relaxation instruction on pain and anxiety of women undergoing in-office gyn procedures. *Journal of Music Therapy, 29*(4), 202–216.

Dickason, E. J., et al. (1994). *Maternal–infant nursing care* (2nd ed.). St. Louis: Mosby–Year Book.

Engebretson, J. (1996). Comparison of nurses & alternative healers. *Image—The Journal of Nursing Scholarship, 28*(2), 95–99.

Freeman, R. K., Garite, T. J., & Nageotte, M. P. (1991). *FHR monitoring* (2nd ed.). Baltimore: Williams & Wilkins.

Gorrie, T. M., et al. (1994). *Foundations of maternal newborn nursing.* Philadelphia: W. B. Saunders.

Kane, A. (1998). Childbirth and aromatherapy. *International Journal of Childbirth Education, 12*(1), 14–15.

Koontz, K. (1998). Why having baby just got better. *Redbook, 74,* 78.

Kreiger, D. (1990). Therapeutic touch: Two decades of research, teaching, and clinical practice. *NSNA Imprint, 37*(3), 83, 86–88.

Lucas, V. A. (1993). Birth: Nursing's role in today's choices. *RN, 56*(6), 38–44.

Malinowski, J., Pedigo, C., & Phillips, C. (1993). *Nursing care during the labor process* (3rd ed.). Philadelphia: F. A. Davis.

Martin, J. E. (1996). *Intrapartum management modules* (2nd ed.). Philadelphia: Williams & Wilkins.

Mattson, S., & Smith, J. E. (1993). *Core curriculum for maternal–newborn nursing.* Washington, D.C.: AWHONN.

May, K. A., & Mahlmeister, L. R. (1994). *Maternal and neonatal nursing: Family centered care* (3rd ed.). Philadelphia: J. B. Lippincott.

Merenstein, G. B., & Gardner, S. L. (1993). *Handbook of neonatal intensive care* (3rd ed.). St. Louis: Mosby–Year Book.

Morrison, J. C., et al. (1993). Monitoring by auscultation or electronic means. *American Journal of Obstetrics and Gynecology, 168*(Pt 1), 63–66.

Murray, M. (1996). *Antepartum and intrapartum fetal monitoring.* Albuquerque, NM: Learning Resources International.

NAACOG. (1990). *Fetal heart rate auscultation; OGN Nursing Practice Resource.* Washington, D.C.: Author.

Naef, R., Morrison, J., Washburn, J., McLaughlin, B., Perry, K., & Roberts, W. (1994). Assessment of fetal well-being using nonstress test in home setting. *Obstetrics and Gynecology, 84*(3), 424–426.

Olson, S. (1998). Bedside musical care: Applications in pregnancy, childbirth, & neonatal care. *Journal of Obstetric, Gynecologic, and Neonatal Nursing, 98,* 569–575.

Parer, J. (1997). *Handbook of fetal heart monitoring* (2nd ed.). Philadelphia: W. B. Saunders.

Rickford, F. (1993). Choice in childbirth. *Nursing Times, 89*(13), 19.

Sadler, C. (1993). Baby brainwave [news]. *Nursing Times, 89*(3), 18–19.

Schifrin, B. S., & Clement, D. (1990). Why fetal monitoring remains a good idea. *Contemporary OB/GYN, 35,* 70–86.

Simpson, K. R., & Creehan, P. (1996). *Perinatal nursing: Care of the childbearing woman and the neonate.* Philadelphia: Lippincott-Raven.

Simpson, K. R., & Poole, J. H. (1998). *Cervical ripening and induction and augmentation of labor.* Washington, D.C.: AWHONN.

Spencer, J. A. (1992). Current methods of continuous fetal heart rate monitoring. *Professional Nurse, 8*(3), 173–175.

Starn, J. R. (1998). Energy healing with women & children. *Journal of Obstetric, Gynecologic, and Neonatal Nursing, 98,* 576–583.

Stein, D. (1995). *Essential Reiki: A complete guide to an ancient healing art.* Freedom: The Crossing Press.

Thomson, A. M. (1993). Pushing techniques in the second stage of labor. *Journal of Advanced Nursing, 18*(2), 171–177.

Tiedje, L. B. (1998). Alternative health care: An overview. *Journal of Obstetric, Gynecologic, and Neonatal Nursing, 98,* 557–562.

Wolfson, I. S. (1984). Therapeutic touch and midwifery. In K. Brown & R. Skillman (Eds.), *The many facets of touch* (pp. 166–172). Brunswick, NJ: Johnson & Johnson.

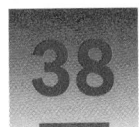

Care of Mother and Newborn During the Postpartum Period

NURSING CARE OF THE MOTHER

The Puerperium

The puerperium is the period beginning after delivery and ending when the woman's body has returned as closely as possible to its prepregnant state. The period lasts approximately 6 weeks. (See Standards of Care Guidelines.)

Physiologic Changes of the Puerperium

1. Uterine changes.
   a. The fundus is usually midline and approximately at the level of the woman's umbilicus after delivery. Within 12 hours of delivery, the fundus may be 1 cm above the umbilicus. After this, the level of the fundus descends approximately 1 finger breadth (or 1 cm) each day, until by the 10th to the 14th day, it has descended into the pelvic cavity and can no longer be palpated (Figure 38-1).
   b. After delivery, lochia, a vaginal discharge that consists of fatty epithelial cells, shreds of membrane, decidua, and blood, is red (lochia rubra) for approximately 2–4 days. It then progresses to a paler or more brownish color (lochia serosa), followed by a whitish or yellowish color (lochia alba) in the 7th to 10th day. Lochia usually ceases by 3 weeks, and the placental site is completely healed by the 6th week.
   c. Immediately after delivery of the placenta, the cervix has little tone or resemblance to the prepregnant state. In approximately 2–3 days, it appears more like the prepregnant state and is dilated to 2–3 cm. The cervical opening is more slit-like than the prepregnant dimple and remains that way. The cervical opening does not return to the prepregnant dimple following delivery unless the cervix has never been dilated.

2. The vaginal walls, uterine ligaments, and muscles of the pelvic floor and abdominal wall regain most of their tone during the puerperium. Immediately after delivery, the vaginal walls are smooth and swollen because the vaginal rugae are absent. Rugae reappears approximately 3 weeks postpartum. At approximately 6 weeks postpartum, involution of the vagina is complete.

3. Postpartum diuresis occurs between the 2nd and 5th postpartum days, as extracellular water accumulated during pregnancy is excreted. Diuresis may also occur shortly after delivery if urinary output was obstructed, because of the pressure of the presenting part, or if intravenous fluids were given to the woman during labor.

4. Breasts
   a. With loss of the placenta, circulating levels of estrogen and progesterone decrease and levels of prolactin increase, thus initiating lactation in the postpartum woman.
   b. Colostrum, a yellowish fluid that contains more minerals and protein but less sugar and fat than mature breast milk, and has a laxative effect on the infant, is secreted for the first 2 days postpartum.
   c. Mature milk secretion is usually present by the third postpartum day, but may be present earlier if a woman breast-feeds immediately after delivery.
   d. Breast engorgement with milk, venous and lymphatic stasis, and swollen, tense, and tender breast tissue may occur between day 3 and day 5 postpartum.

STANDARDS OF CARE GUIDELINES
Postpartum Care

- Perform assessment regularly for BUBBLERS—breasts, uterus size and consistency, bladder distention, bowel elimination, lochia, episiotomy, emotional response, and Homans' sign.
- Notify health care provider immediately for any abnormalities.
  - a. Increased respiration and pulse, decreased blood pressure, and orthostatic changes with may indicate hemorrhage.
  - b. Excessive vaginal bleeding (saturation of peri-pad within 1 hour for 2 or more hours), expulsion of large clots, or steady increase in vaginal bleeding, which indicates hemorrhage.
  - c. Boggy uterine fundus that does not become firm and remain firm with massage, indicating uterine atony.
  - d. Inability to void and bladder distention, which may displace uterus, leading to uterine atony.
  - e. Decreased urine output, which may indicate hemorrhage.
  - f. Elevated temperature, increased pain, swelling, and redness from incisions, indicating infection.
  - g. Calf tenderness, swelling, redness, or warmth, which may indicate a blood clot.
  - h. Excessive irritability, crying, moodiness, withdrawal, insomnia, and loss of interest in activities, which may indicate postpartum depression.
- Encourage rest, nutrition, and bonding with the infant.
- Provide education on feeding, bathing, changing, safety measures, signs of illness, and when to call infant's pediatric care provider with questions.

This information should serve as a general guideline only. Each patient situation presents a unique set of clinical factors and requires nursing judgment to guide care, which may include additional or alternative measures and approaches.

5. Endocrine/metabolic function
   a. Thyroid levels are normal by 4–6 weeks postpartum.
   b. Glucose levels are low secondary to decreased human placental lactogen and decreased growth hormone.
6. Ovarian function
   a. Estrogen and progesterone levels decrease rapidly after the placenta delivers.
   b. Estrogen reaches the follicular phase by 3 weeks after birth, as long as the woman is not lactating.
   c. Ovulation may occur as early as 27 days after delivery. The average time is 70–75 days postdelivery and 190 days postdelivery if breast-feeding.
   d. The start of menses after delivery is individualized. Usually, the first menses occurs approximately 3 months after delivery, although breast-feeding women may not start their first menses until 8 months.
7. Kidneys and bladder function
   a. Mild proteinuria is common for 1–2 days after delivery in 50% of postpartum women.
   b. Bladder tone returns between 5 and 7 days postpartum.
   c. Stress incontinence is common during the first 6 weeks postpartum.

NURSING ALERT

Hematuria immediately after normal spontaneous vaginal birth is usually indicative of bladder trauma. If hematuria occurs after the first 24 hours, it is indicative of urinary tract infection (UTI).

8. Neurologic function
   a. Discomfort and fatigue are common.
   b. Afterpains and discomfort from the delivery, lacerations, episiotomy, and muscle aches are common.

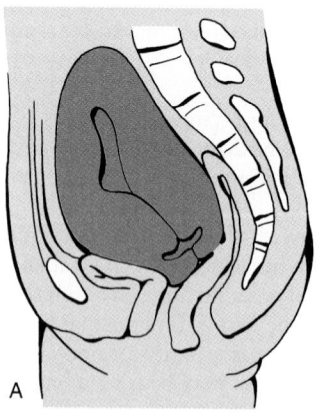
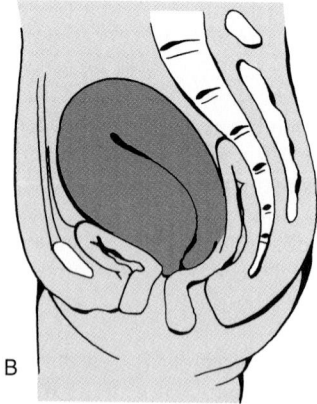
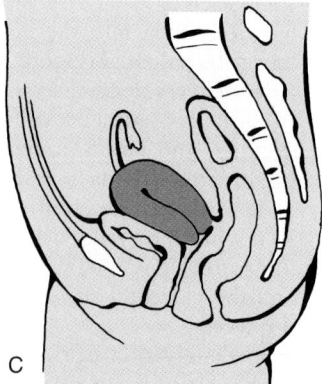

FIGURE 38-1   Changes in uterine size and shape following delivery. (**A**) Uterus after delivery. (**B**) Uterus at sixth day. (**C**) Nongravid uterus.

c. Frontal and bilateral headaches are common and are caused by fluid shifts in the first week postpartum.

d. Non-REM sleep is absent after birth and increases during the next 2 weeks. REM sleep decreases as non-REM sleep increases.

9. Cardiovascular function
   a. Most dramatic changes occur in this system.
   b. Cardiac output decreases rapidly and returns to normal by 2–3 weeks postpartum.
   c. Hematocrit increases and increased RBC production stops.
   d. Leukocytosis with increased WBCs common during the first postpartum week.

10. Respiratory function
   a. Returns to normal by approximately 6–8 weeks postpartum.
   b. Basal metabolic rate increases for 7–14 days postpartum, secondary to mild anemia, lactation, and psychological changes.

11. Gastrointestinal/hepatic function
   a. Gastrointestinal tone and motility decreases in early postpartum period, causing constipation.
   b. Normal bowel function returns approximately 2–3 days postpartum.
   c. Liver function returns to normal approximately 10–14 days postpartum.
   d. Gall bladder contractility increases to normal, allowing for expulsion of small gallstones.

12. Musculoskeletal function
   a. Generalized fatigue and weakness is common.
   b. Decreased abdominal tone is common.
   c. Diastasis recti heals and resolves by the 4th to 6th week postpartum. Until healing is complete, abdominal exercises are contraindicated.

NURSING ALERT

A positive Homans' sign is indicative of thrombophlebitis and should be reported to the primary care provider. The woman should be instructed not to massage her legs.

---

13. Integumentary function
   a. Stria lightens and melasma is usually gone by 6 weeks postpartum.
   b. Hair loss can increase for the first 4–20 weeks postpartum and then regrowth will occur, although the hair may not be as thick as it was before pregnancy.

14. A good method to remember how to check the postpartum changes is the use of the acronym BUBBLERS:
   a. B = breast.
   b. U = uterus.
   c. B = bladder.
   d. B = bowel.
   e. L = lochia.
   f. E = episiotomy.
   g. R = emotional response.
   h. S = Homans' sign.

Emotional and Behavioral Status

1. After delivery, the woman may progress through Rubin's stages of taking in, taking hold, and letting go.
   a. Taking in:
      (i) May begin with a refreshing sleep after delivery.
      (ii) Woman exhibits passive, dependent behavior.
      (iii) Woman is concerned with sleep and the intake of food, mainly for herself.
   b. Taking hold:
      (i) Woman begins to initiate action and to function more independently; occurs usually on days 2 to 7.
      (ii) Woman may require more explanation and reassurance that she is functioning well, especially in caring for her infant.
      (iii) Openness to teaching on care of self and newborn.
   c. Letting go:
      (i) Begins near end of the first week.
      (ii) Re-establishment of couple relationship.
      (iii) As the woman meets success in caring for the newborn, her concern extends to other family members and to their activities.

2. Some women may experience euphoria in the first few days after delivery and set unrealistic goals for activities after discharge from the birthing place.

3. Many women may experience temporary mood swings during this period because of the discomfort, fatigue, and exhaustion after labor and delivery, and because of hormonal changes after delivery.

4. Some mothers may experience postpartum blues at approximately the third postpartum day and may exhibit irritability, poor appetite, insomnia, tearfulness, or crying. This is a temporary situation. Severe or prolonged depression is usually a sign of a more serious condition.

5. Nursing research findings indicate that new mothers identified the postpartum needs listed below. Coping with:
   a. The physical changes and discomforts of the puerperium, including a need to regain their prepregnancy figure.
   b. Changing family relationships and meeting the needs of family members, including the infant.
   c. Fatigue, emotional stress, feelings of isolation, and being tied down.
   d. A lack of time for personal needs and interests.

■ Nursing Assessment

Immediate Postpartum Assessment

The first hour after delivery of the placenta (fourth stage of labor) is a critical period; postpartum hemorrhage is most likely to occur at this time (see p. 1215).

Subsequent Postpartum Assessment

1. Check firmness of the fundus at regular intervals. Perform fundal massage if the uterus is boggy (not firm) (Figure 38-2).

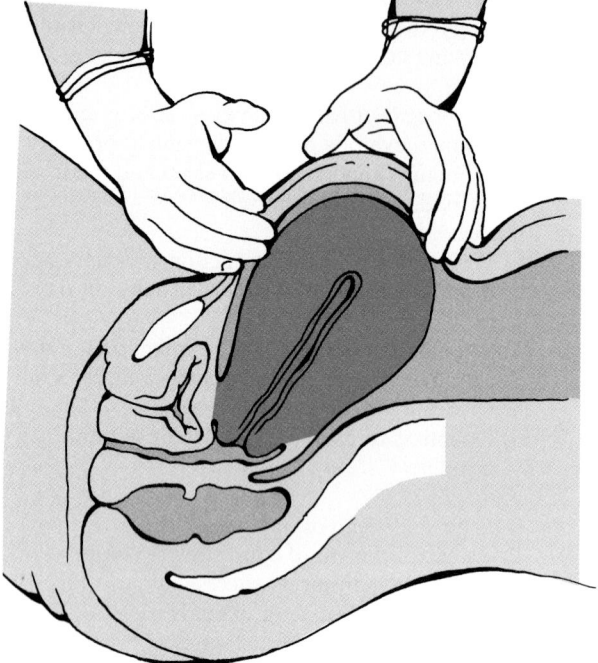

FIGURE 38-2 Fundal massage. With hands correctly positioned, gentle fundal massage stimulates the uterine muscles to contract, helping to restore normal tone and control bleeding.

2. Inspect the perineum regularly for frank bleeding.
   a. Note color, amount, and odor of the lochia (Figure 38-3).
   b. Count the number of perineal pads that are saturated in each 8-hour period.
3. Assess vital signs at least twice daily and more frequently if indicated.
4. Assess bowel and bladder elimination.
5. Evaluate interaction and care skills of mother and family with infant.
6. Assess for breast engorgement and condition of nipples if breast-feeding.
7. Inspect legs for signs of thromboembolism, and assess Homans' sign.
8. Assess incisions for signs of infection and healing.
9. If a patient is Rh negative, evaluate the need for $Rh_o(D)$ immune globulin (RhoGAM). If indicated, administer the RhoGAM within 72 hours of delivery.
10. If the woman is not rubella immune, a rubella vaccination may be given, and pregnancy must be avoided for at least 3 months.

Nursing Management

Nursing Diagnoses

- Risk for Fluid Volume Deficit related to blood loss and effects from anesthesia
- Altered Urinary Elimination related to birth trauma

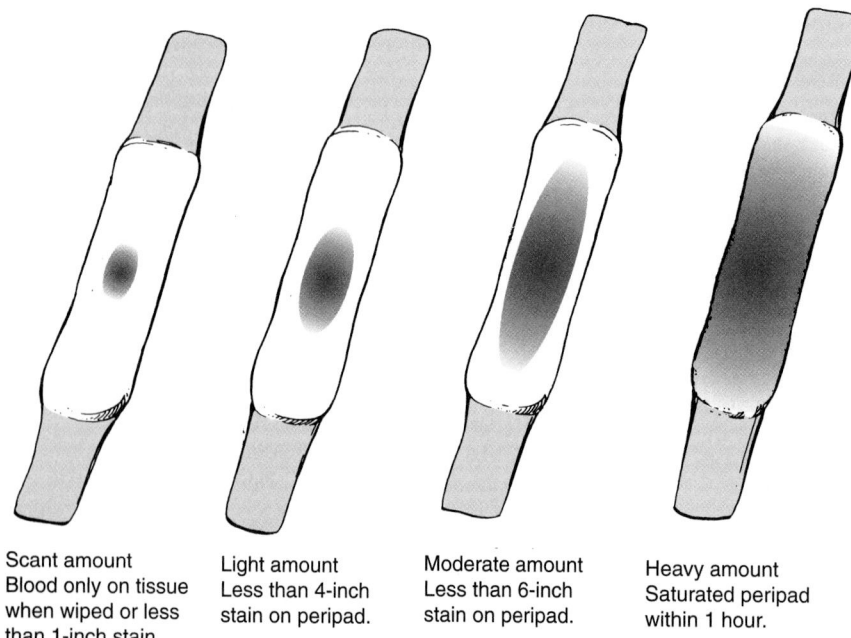

Scant amount
Blood only on tissue
when wiped or less
than 1-inch stain
on peripad.

Light amount
Less than 4-inch
stain on peripad.

Moderate amount
Less than 6-inch
stain on peripad.

Heavy amount
Saturated peripad
within 1 hour.

FIGURE 38-3 Assessing the volume of lochia by peri-pad saturation.

- Colonic Constipation related to physiologic changes from birth
- Risk for Infection related to birth process
- Fatigue related to labor
- Pain related to perineal discomfort from birth trauma, hemorrhoids, and physiologic changes from birth
- Altered Health Maintenance related to lack of knowledge of postpartum care
- Altered Health Maintenance related to lack of knowledge of newborn care
- Ineffective Breast-feeding related to lack of knowledge and inexperience

Nursing Interventions
Monitoring for Hypotension and Bleeding
1. Monitor vital signs every 4 hours during the first 24 hours, then every 8–12 hours or as delineated by institutional policy. Observe for the following:
   a. Decreased respiratory rate below 14–16 breaths per minute may occur after receiving epidural narcotics or narcotic analgesics.
   b. Increased respiratory rate greater than 24 breaths per minute may be caused by increased blood loss, pulmonary edema, or a pulmonary embolus.
   c. Increased pulse rate greater than 100 beats per minute (bpm) may be present with increased blood loss, fever, or pain.
   d. Decrease in blood pressure 15–20 mm Hg below baseline pressures may indicate decreased fluid volume or increased blood loss.
2. Assess the woman for light-headedness and dizziness when sitting upright or before ambulating.
   a. Evaluate orthostatic blood pressures.
   b. Have the woman lie in bed if symptoms exist.
3. Assess vaginal discharge for clots and amount.
4. Evaluate lower extremity sensory function and motor function before ambulation if the woman had regional anesthesia.
5. Encourage food and drink as tolerated.
6. Maintain intravenous line as indicated.
7. Monitor postpartum hemoglobin and hematocrit.

Encouraging Bladder Emptying
1. Observe for the woman's first void within 6–8 hours after delivery.
2. Palpate the abdomen for bladder distention if the woman cannot void or if she complains of fullness after voiding.
   a. Uterine displacement from the midline suggests bladder distention.
   b. Frequent voidings of small amounts of urine suggest urinary retention with overflow.
3. Catheterize the woman (in and out) if indicated.
4. Instruct the woman to void every several hours and after meals to keep her bladder empty. An undistended bladder may help decrease uterine cramping.

Promoting Proper Bowel Function
1. Teach the woman that bowel activity is sluggish because of decreased abdominal muscle tone, anesthetic effects, effects of progesterone, decreased solid food intake during labor, and prelabor diarrhea.
2. Inform the woman that pain from hemorrhoids, lacerations, and episiotomies may cause her to delay her first bowel movement.
3. Review the woman's dietary intake with her.
4. Encourage daily, adequate amounts of fresh fruit, vegetables, fiber, and at least eight glasses of water.
5. Encourage frequent ambulation.
6. Administer stool softeners as indicated.

Preventing Infection
1. Observe for elevated temperature above 38°C (100.4°F).
2. Evaluate episiotomy/perineum for redness, ecchymosis, edema, discharge (color, amount, odor) and approximation of the skin.
3. Assess for pain, burning, and frequency on urination.
4. Administer antibiotics as ordered.

Reducing Fatigue
1. Provide a quiet and minimally disturbed environment.
2. Organize nursing care to keep interruptions to a minimum.
3. Encourage the woman to minimize visitors and phone calls.
4. Encourage the woman to sleep while the baby is sleeping, specifically to nap or lie down and get off her feet at least 30 minutes per day.

Minimizing Pain
1. Instruct the woman to apply ice packs to the perineal area for the first 24 hours for perineal trauma or edema.
   a. Take breaks between applications to prevent tissue damage.
   b. Commercial or handmade packs of ice chips in a glove may be used.
   c. Place a thin barrier between ice pack and skin.
2. Initiate the use of sitz baths for perineal discomfort after the first 24 hours.
   a. Use three times a day for 15–20 minutes.
3. Instruct the woman to contract her buttocks before sitting to reduce perineal discomfort.
4. Assist the woman in the use of positioning cushions and pillows while sitting or lying.
5. Teach the woman to use a perineal bottle and squirt warm water against her perineum while voiding.
6. Provide pads, such as Tucks, or topical creams or ointments as indicated.
7. Administer pain medication as indicated.
8. Check breasts for signs of engorgement (swollen, tender, tense, shiny breast tissue).
   a. If breasts are engorged and the woman is breast-feeding:
      (i) Allow warm-to-hot shower water to flow over the breasts to improve comfort.
      (ii) Hot compresses on the breasts may improve comfort.
      (iii) Express some milk manually or by breast pump to improve comfort and make nipple more available for infant feeding.

(iv) Nurse the infant.

(v) A mild analgesic may be used to enhance comfort.

b. If breasts are engorged and the mother is bottle-feeding:

(i) Teach the woman to wear a snug, supportive bra night and day.

(ii) Teach the woman to avoid handling her breasts, because this stimulates more milk production.

(iii) Suggest ice bags to the breasts to provide comfort.

(iv) Moderately strong analgesics may be needed to provide comfort.

Promoting Postpartum Health Maintenance

1. Teach the woman to perform perineal care—warm water over the perineum after each voiding and after each bowel movement several times a day to promote comfort, cleanliness, and healing.

2. Promote sitz baths for the same purpose.

3. Teach the woman to apply perineal pads by touching the outside only, thus keeping clean the portion that will touch her perineum.

4. Assess the condition of the woman's breasts and nipples. Inspect nipples for reddening, erosions, or fissures. Reddened areas may be improved with A & D ointment, a lanolin cream, and air drying for 15 minutes, several times a day.

5. Teach the woman to wash her breasts with warm water WITHOUT soap, which prevents the removal of the protective skin oils.

6. Teach the woman to wear a bra that provides good support night and day.

7. Instruct the breast-feeding woman to add between 500 and 750 additional calories daily for milk production. Inform her that she also needs 2–3 quarts of liquid per day; 20 g more protein than before pregnancy; and additional calcium, phosphorus, vitamins D, A, C, E, B, and B_2; and additional niacin, zinc, and iodine.

8. Instruct the woman in postpartum exercises for the immediate and later postpartum period.

a. Immediate postpartum exercises can be performed in bed.

(i) Toe stretch (tightens calf muscles)—while lying on your back, keep your legs straight and point your toes away from you, then pull your legs toward you and point your toes toward your chest. Repeat 10 times.

(ii) Pelvic floor exercise (tightens perineal muscles)—contract your buttocks for a count of 5 and relax. Contract your buttocks and press thighs together for a count of 7 and relax. Contract buttocks, press thighs together, and draw in anus for a count of 10 and relax.

(iii) Kegel exercises (tightens vaginal muscles)—contract vaginal muscles as if stopping stream of urine. Do 15 per day, increasing 5 more each week to a maximum of 40 per day. Once conditioned, patient can do 4 or 5 Kegel's per day for maintenance.

(iv) Abdominal breathing—lie on back, knees bent, hands on belly, feet flat. Suck in your belly, trying to pull your navel toward your spine. Hold 5 seconds; release. When you can do 10 (this can take a week), add a head lift. Suck in your belly, then hold it as you lift head toward chest, counting slowly to 4. Lower head for 4 slow counts; release belly. Muscles are working if fingers move down when you suck in belly, not up. Work up to 10 repetitions.

(v) Arm circles—stand with feet approximately 12 inches apart, arms at sides. Keeping arms at sides, draw large circles with your shoulders by moving them forward, up, and back, and finish with a press down. Do 10–20 repetitions. Next, extend both arms as you reach forward, up, back, and down. Move slowly, breathe deeply for 5–10 repetitions.

(vi) Short walks—start with 5 minutes at first, then increase 5 minutes per day as desired.

(vii) Shoulder-side roll—lying on back, fold left arm across chest. Lift right arm and cross it over to left side. Feel as if your right arm is pulling you over so your right shoulder lifts and you roll to left. Continue to spiral movement as rib cage turns, then hips. Use left arm to take pressure off breasts, which may feel full. Lying on your left side, roll hips back toward right, followed by ribs, then shoulders until you are on your back. Repeat, other side. Five slow repetitions each side.

b. Exercises for the later postpartum period can be done after the first postpartum visit (1–2 weeks postpartum.)

(i) Bicycle (tightens thighs, stomach, and waist)—lie on your back on the floor, arms at sides, palms down. Begin rotating your legs as if you were riding a bicycle, bringing the knees all the way in toward the chest and stretching the legs out as long and as straight as possible. Breathe deeply and evenly. Do the exercises at a moderate speed and do not tire yourself.

(ii) Buttocks exercise (tightens buttocks)—lie on your stomach and keep your legs straight. Raise your left leg in the air, then repeat with your right leg (feel the contraction in your buttocks). Keep your hips on the floor. Repeat 10 times.

(iii) Twist (tightens waist)—stand with legs wide apart. Hold your arms at your sides, shoulder level, palms down. Twist your body from side to front and back again. Feel the twist in your waist.

(iv) Back bridge—begin by doing a pelvic tilt while lying on the back and flattening the lower back against the floor. Then continue to push your hips forward, lifting them off the floor. Hold the pelvic tilt for 4 seconds so that your back is flat, supporting your weight with your upper back. Lower your body slowly for 4 seconds so that upper back touches floor first, then waist touches, then pelvis.

(v) All fours—begin on your hands and knees. First do a pelvic tilt, tucking in your buttocks and sucking in your belly. Do not allow your back to arch. Next, keeping your pelvic tilt, lift your left leg out behind you and extend your right arm in front of you. Slowly lower arm and leg. At first you will have to work hard to keep your balance.

(vi) Lift and laugh—this is a fun exercise to do with your body. Sit with legs crossed, back straight, belly sucked in. Cradle your baby in your folded arms and lift until your elbows are at shoulder height. Laugh and cuddle as you hold for 2 seconds. Slowly lower your baby, keeping shoulders even, if possible. Do 5–10 repetitions.

NURSING ALERT

Inform mother to listen to her body. Avoid pain and fatigue. If pain and/or fatigue occur, instruct mother to stop exercises. She may consult her primary care provider if desired.

Promoting Health Maintenance of the Newborn

1. Encourage the parents to participate in daily care of the infant.
2. Advise the parents to attend parenting and baby care classes offered during their stay at the birth facility.
3. Teach the parents to bathe and diaper the infant, perform circumcision care, and initiate either breast or bottle feeding (Table 38-1).
4. Foster bonding by encouraging skin-to-skin contact with the infant, eye contact, and talking to and touching the infant.
5. Instruct the parents to contact the infant's health care provider for the following:
   a. Fever above 37.2°C (100°F).
   b. Loss of appetite for two consecutive feedings.
   c. Inability to awaken baby to his or her usual activity state.
   d. Vomiting all or part of two feedings.
   e. Diarrhea—three watery stools.
   f. Extreme irritability or inconsolable crying.
6. Inform the parents that by law, infants and young children in cars are required to be in a car safety seat that is located in the back seat and that faces the back of the seat. Demonstrate and review the proper technique for use of the car seat.
7. Provide positive reinforcement and reassurance to the parents.
8. Provide written instructions and educational material on discharge.

Promoting Breast-Feeding

1. Assist the woman and infant in the breast-feeding process.
   a. Have the mother wash her hands before feeding to help prevent infection.
   b. Encourage the mother to assume a comfortable position, such as sitting upright, tailor sitting, lying on her side.
   c. Have the woman hold the baby so that he or she is facing the mother. Common positions for holding the baby are the cradle hold, with the baby's head and body supported against the mother's arm, with buttocks resting in her hand; the football hold, in which the baby's legs are supported under the mother's arm, and the head is at the breast, resting in the mother's hand; lying on the side with the baby lying on his/her side facing the mother.
   d. Teach the woman to bring the baby close to her, to prevent back, shoulder, and arm strain.
   e. Have the woman cup the breast in her hand in a C position, with bottom of the breast in the palm of her hand and the thumb on top.
   f. Have the woman place her nipple against the baby's mouth, and when the mouth opens, guide the nipple and the areola into the mouth. If the baby has latched on to the nipple only, take the baby off the breast by putting the tip of the mother's finger in the corner of the baby's mouth to break the suction, and then reposition on the breast to prevent nipple pain and trauma.
   g. Encourage the woman to alternate the breast she begins feeding with at each feeding to ensure emptying of both breasts and stimulation for maintaining milk supply.
   h. Advise the mother to use each breast at each feeding. Begin with approximately 10 minutes at each breast, then increase the time at each breast, allowing the infant to suck until he or she stops sucking actively. Pinning a safety pin to the bra as a reminder of which breast to start with at the next feeding is helpful.

TABLE 38-1	Typical Pattern of Infant Feedings		
Age of Infant	**Number of Feedings**	**Volume per Feeding**	**Total**
Birth–2 wk	6–10	2–3 oz (60–90 mL)	12–30 oz (360–900 mL)
2 wk to 1 mo	6–8	3–4 oz (90–120 mL)	18–32 oz (540–960 mL)
1–3 mo	5–6	5–6 oz (150–180 mL)	25–36 oz (750–1080 mL)
3–7 mo	4–5	6–7 oz (180–210 mL)	25–36 oz (750–1080 mL)
7–12 mo	3–4	7–8 oz (210–240 mL)	25–36 oz (750–1080 mL)

(Taken from May, K. A., & Mahlmeister, L. R. [1994]. *Maternal and neonatal nursing—Family centered care* (3rd ed.). Philadelphia: J. B. Lippincott.).

i. Have the mother breast-feed frequently and on demand (every 2–4 hours) to help maintain the milk supply.

j. Have the mother air dry her nipples for approximately 15–20 minutes after feeding to help prevent nipple trauma.

k. Have the mother burp the infant at the end of the feeding to help release the air in the stomach and to make the infant less fretful.

2. Alert the mother that uterine cramping may occur, especially in multiparous women, because of the release of oxytocin, which can be worse in women with lessened uterine tone. Commonly referred to as after pains.

3. Teach the mother to provide for adequate rest and to avoid tension, fatigue, and a stressful environment, which can inhibit the letdown reflex and make breast milk less available at feeding.

4. Advise the woman to avoid taking medications and drugs without provider approval, because many substances pass into the breast milk and may affect milk production or the infant.

Outcome-Based Evaluation

- Vital signs within normal limits; decreasing color and amount of lochia
- Voids freely and without discomfort
- Lack of constipation; eats high-fiber foods and uses stool softeners
- Afebrile, no abnormal redness of perineum, no purulent discharge or foul odor of lochia
- Verbalizes feeling rested
- Verbalizes decreased pain
- Incorporates postpartum care into activities of daily living
- Demonstrates confidence in performing infant care; shows signs of maternal-child bonding
- Demonstrates successful breast-feeding; breasts and nipples intact and without redness or cracks

Postpartum Patient Education

1. Advise the woman that healing occurs within 2–4 weeks; however, evaluation by the health care provider during the follow-up visit is necessary.

2. Inform the woman that intercourse may be resumed when perineal and uterine wounds have healed and when vaginal bleeding has stopped. Review methods of contraception. Sexual arousal may cause milk to leak from breasts. Breastfeeding is not a reliable method of contraception.

3. Inform the woman that menstruation usually returns within 4 weeks to 8 weeks if bottle-feeding; if breast-feeding, menstruation usually returns within 4 months, but may return between 2–18 months postpartum. Nursing mothers may ovulate even if experiencing amenorrhea, so a form of contraception should be used if pregnancy is to be avoided.

4. Counsel the woman to rest for at least 30 minutes after she arrives home from the hospital and to rest several times during the day for the first few weeks.

5. Advise the woman to confine her activities to one floor if possible and to avoid stair climbing as much as possible for the first several days at home.

6. Counsel the woman to provide quiet times for herself at home, and to help her establish realistic goals for resuming her own interests and activities.

7. Encourage the couple to provide times to reestablish their own relationship and to renew their social interests and relationships.

NURSING CARE OF THE NEWBORN

◼ Physiology of the Newborn

The first 24 hours of life constitute a highly vulnerable time, during which the infant must make major physiologic adjustments to extrauterine life.

Transitional Stages

During the period of postnatal transition, six overlapping stages have been identified:

- Stage 1. Receives stimulation (during labor) from the pressure of the uterine contractions and from changes in pressure when the membranes rupture.
- Stage 2. Encounters various foreign stimuli—light, cold, gravity, and sound.
- Stage 3. Initiates breathing.
- Stage 4. Changes from fetal circulation to neonatal circulation.
- Stage 5. Undergoes alteration in metabolic processes, with activation of liver and gastrointestinal tract for passage of meconium.
- Stage 6. Achieves a steady level of equilibrium in metabolic processes (production of enzymes, increased blood oxygen saturation, decrease in acidosis associated with birth, and recovery of the neurologic tissues from the trauma of labor and delivery).

Respiratory Changes
Factors Initiating Respiration

1. Mechanical—pressure changes from intrauterine life to extrauterine life produce stimulation to initiate respirations.

2. Chemical—changes in the blood, as a result of transitory asphyxia, include:
   a. Lowered oxygen level.
   b. Increased carbon dioxide level.
   c. Lowered pH—if asphyxia is prolonged, depression of the respiratory center (rather than stimulation) occurs, and resuscitation is necessary.

3. Sensory—light (visual), sound (auditory), olfactory, and tactile stimulation, beginning in utero with uterine contraction and when the infant is touched and dried, contribute to the initiation of respiration.

4. Thermal—a drop in environmental temperature from 37°C (98.6°F) to 21°–24°C (70°–75°F).
5. First breath—maximum effort is required to expand the lungs and to fill the collapsed alveoli.
   a. Surface tension in the respiratory tract and resistance in lung tissue, thorax, diaphragm, and respiratory muscles must be overcome.
   b. First active inspiration comes from a strong contraction of the diaphragm, which creates a high negative intrathoracic pressure, causing a marked retraction of the ribs and distention of the alveolar space. (Any remaining fluid is reabsorbed rapidly if the pulmonary capillary blood flow is adequate, because the fluid is hypotonic and passes easily into the capillaries.)

Character of Normal Respirations
1. First period of reactivity occurs immediately after birth. Vigorous, diffuse, purposeless movements alternate with periods of relative immobility/inactivity.
2. Respirations are rapid, as frequent as 80 breaths/minute, accompanied by tachycardia, 140–180 breaths/minute.
3. Relaxation occurs and the infant usually sleeps; he or she then awakes to a second period of activity. Oral mucus may be a major problem during this period.
4. Respirations are reduced to 35–50 breaths/minute and become quiet and shallow; respiration is carried out by the diaphragm and abdominal muscles.
5. Period of dyspnea and cyanosis may occur suddenly in an infant who is breathing normally; this may indicate an anomaly or a pathologic condition.
6. Apnea is normal in the neonatal period and lasts 10–15 seconds.

Circulatory Changes
Anatomic Changes (see p. 1118)
Blood Volume
Blood volume is 85–100 mL/kg at birth. Factors that influence blood volume:
1. Maternal blood volume (affected by maternal diseases and iron intake).
2. Placental function.
3. Uterine contractions during labor.
4. Amount of blood loss associated with delivery.
5. Placental transfusion at birth—increase in blood volume of 60% if cord is clamped and cut after pulsation ceases.

Peripheral Circulation
Residual cyanosis in hands and feet for 1–2 hours after birth because of sluggish circulation. This is commonly referred to as acrocyanosis.

Pulse Rate
1. Generally follows pattern similar to that of respiration.
2. Apical pulse rate is more accurate.
3. Normal rate 80–160 bpm.
4. May rise to 180 bpm when the infant is crying or drop to 70 bpm during deep sleep.

Blood Pressure
1. Blood pressure is 70/45 at birth; 100/50 by 10th day.
2. Blood pressure rises with crying.
3. Blood pressure in the leg will be slightly higher.
4. Pulse pressure is 25–30 mm Hg at term.

NURSING ALERT

A systolic blood pressure in the upper extremities that is 20 mm Hg greater than in the lower extremities strongly suggests coarctation of the aorta.

Blood Coagulation
Coagulability is temporarily diminished because of lack of bacteria in the intestinal tract that contributes to the synthesis of vitamin K.
1. Coagulation time is 3–4 minutes.
2. Bleeding time is 2–4 minutes.
3. Prothrombin 50%, decreasing to 20%–30%.

Blood Elements
Values for blood components in the neonate:
1. Hemoglobin, 16–22 g.
2. Reticulocytes, 2.5–6.5%.
3. Leukocytes, 15,000–20,000 mm³.

Temperature Regulation
1. Mechanism not fully developed; heat production low.
2. Infant responds readily to environmental heat and cold stimuli.
3. Heat loss of 2°C–3°C may occur at birth by evaporation, convection, conduction, and radiation.
   a. Radiation—transfer of heat from neonate to cooler object not in direct contact with the infant.
   b. Convection—transfer of heat when flow of cool air passes over infant's skin.
   c. Evaporation—loss of heat when water on infant's skin is converted to vapor.
   d. Conduction—transfer of heat when neonate comes into direct contact with cooler surface/object.
4. Decreased adipose tissue, thinner skin, blood vessels closer to the skin results in increased heat loss.
5. Infant develops mechanisms to counterbalance heat loss.
   a. Vasoconstriction—blood directed away from skin surfaces.
   b. Insulation—from subcutaneous adipose tissue.
   c. Heat production—by nonshivering thermogenesis (brown fat metabolism) elicited by the sympathetic nervous system's response to decreased temperatures; activated by adrenaline.
   d. Fetal position—by assuming a flexed position.

Basal Metabolism
1. Surface area of infant is large in comparison to weight.
2. Basal metabolism per kilogram of body weight is higher than that of an adult.
3. Calorie requirements are high—117 calories per kilogram of body weight per day.

Renal Function
Low arterial blood pressure and increased renal vascular resistance lead to the following effects:

1. Decreased ability to concentrate urine because of low tubular resorption rate and low levels of antidiuretic hormone.
2. Limited ability to maintain water balance by excretion of excess water or retention of needed water.
3. Decreased ability to maintain acid-base mechanism; slower excretion of electrolytes, especially sodium and the hydrogen ions, results in accumulation of these substances, which predisposes the infant to dehydration, acidosis, and hyperkalemia.
4. Excretion of large amount of uric acid during newborn period—appears as brick dust stain on diaper.

Hepatic Function
Function limited because of lack of gastrointestinal tract activity and limited blood supply; consequences include the following:
1. Decreased ability to conjugate bilirubin (rationale for physiologic jaundice).
2. Decreased ability to regulate blood glucose concentration (rationale for neonatal hypoglycemia).
3. Deficient production of prothrombin and other coagulation factors that depend on vitamin K for synthesis (rationale for neonate's predisposition to hemorrhage).

Endocrine Function
Endocrine glands are better organized than other systems; disturbances are most often related to maternally provided hormones. This can cause the following:
1. Vaginal discharge (and/or bleeding [pseudomenstruation]) in female infants.
2. Enlargement of mammary glands (breast engorgement) in both sexes—related to increased estrogen, luteal, and prolactin activity. Milky secretions may be present (witch's milk).
3. Disturbances related to maternal endocrine pathology (eg, mother with diabetes or mother with inadequate iodine intake).

Gastrointestinal Changes
The newborn's intestinal tract is proportionately longer than the adult's; however, elastic tissue and musculature are not fully developed, and neurologic control is variable and inadequate.
1. Most digestive enzymes are present, with the exception of pancreatic amylase and lipase. Protein and carbohydrates are easily absorbed, but fat absorption is poor.
2. Limitations relate primarily to anatomic structures and neutrality of the gastric contents.
3. Imperfect control of the cardiac and pyloric sphincters and immaturity of neurologic control cause mild regurgitation or slight vomiting.
4. Irregularities in peristaltic motility slow stomach emptying.
5. Peristalsis increases in the lower ileum, resulting in stool frequency—one to six stools per day. No stool within 48 hours after birth is indicative of intestinal obstruction.

Neurologic Changes
Neurologic mechanisms are immature; they are not fully developed anatomically or physiologically. As a result, uncoordinated movements, labile temperature regulation, and poor control over musculature are characteristic of the infant. Reflexes are important indicators of infant neural development (see p. 1167).

Nursing Assessment
Pertinent Maternal History
1. Mother's age, socioeconomic status, ethnic or cultural group, educational level, marital status.
2. Mother's/family's past medical history.
3. Mother's past obstetric history.
4. Mother's prenatal history with this pregnancy.
5. Labor and delivery.

Physical Assessment Findings and Physiologic Functioning
Posture
1. Full-term newborn assumes symmetric posture; face turned to side; flexed extremities; hands tightly fisted with thumb covered by fingers.
2. Asymmetric posture may be caused by fractures of clavicle or humerus or by nerve injuries commonly of the brachial plexus.
3. Infants born in breech position may keep knees and legs straightened or in frog position, depending on the type of breech birth.

Length
Average length of full-term newborn is 51 cm (20 in.); range, 46–56 cm (18–22 in.).

Weight
Average weight of male infants is 3,400 g (7 1/2 lb.); female infants, 3,200 g (7 lb.). Range of 80% of full-term newborns is 2,900–4,100 g (6 lb 5 oz–9 lb 2 oz).

Skin
Examine under natural light for:
1. Hair distribution—term infant will have some lanugo over back; most of the lanugo will have disappeared on extremities and other areas of the body.
2. Turgor—term infant should have good skin turgor, ie, after gently pinching small portion of skin and releasing it, the skin should return to its original position.
3. Color
   a. Cyanosis—acrocyanosis, bluish color in palms of hands and soles of feet, is common, because of immature peripheral circulation. This is exacerbated by cold temperatures.
   b. Pallor—may indicate cold, stress, anemia, or cardiac failure.
   c. Plethora—reddish (ruddy) coloration may be caused by high level of red blood cells to blood volume from intrauterine intravascular transfusion (twins), cardiac disease, or diabetes in the mother.
   d. Jaundice—physiologic jaundice caused by immaturity of liver is common beginning on day 2, peaking

at 1 week and disappearing by the 2nd week. First appears in skin over face or upper body, then progresses over larger area; can also be seen in conjunctivae of eyes.

   e. Meconium staining—staining of skin, fingernails, and umbilical cord indicates passage of meconium in utero (possibly caused by fetal hypoxia in utero).

4. Dryness/peeling—marked scaliness and desquamation are signs of postmaturity.
5. Vernix—in full-term infants, most vernix is found in skin folds under the arms and in the groin under the scrotum (in males) and in the labia (in females).
6. Nails—should reach end of fingertips and be well developed in the full-term infant. There should be no evidence of pits, ridges, aplasia, or hypertrophy.
7. Edema—some edema may occur over buttocks, back, and occiput if the infant has been supine; pitting edema may be caused by erythroblastosis, heart failure, electrolyte imbalance.
8. Ecchymosis—may appear over the presenting part in a difficult delivery; may also indicate infection or bleeding problem.
9. Petechiae—pinpoint hemorrhages on skin caused by increased intravascular pressure, infection, or thrombocytopenia; regresses within 48 hours.
10. Erythema toxicum (newborn rash)—small white, yellow, or pink to red papular rash that appears on trunk, face, and extremities; regresses within 48 hours.
11. Hemangiomas—vascular lesions present at birth; some may fade, but others may be permanent.
   a. Strawberry—bright red, raised, lobulated tumor that occurs on the head, neck, trunk, or extremities; soft, pressible, with sharp demarcated margins; increases in size for approximately 6 months, then regresses after several years.
   b. Cavernous—larger, more mature vascular elements; involves dermis and subcutaneous tissues; soft, pressible, with poorly defined margins; increases in size the first 6–12 months, then involutes spontaneously.
12. Telangiectatic nevi (stork bites)—flat red or purple lesions most often found on back of neck, lower occiput, upper eyelid, and bridge of nose; regress by 2 years of age, although the ones on the neck may persist through adulthood.
13. Milia—enlarged sebaceous glands found on nose, chin, cheeks, brow, and forehead; regress in several days to a few weeks. They appear as multiple yellow or pearly white papules, approximately 1 mm wide. When found in the mouth, they are referred to as Epstein pearls.
14. Mongolian spots—blue-green or gray pigmentation on lower back, sacrum, and buttocks; common in blacks (90%), Asians, and infants of southern European heritage; regress by 4 years of age.
15. Café-au-lait spots—tan or light brown macules or patches. When less than 3 cm in length and less than 6 in number, there is no pathologic significance; if

greater than 3 cm or more than 6 in number, may indicate cutaneous neurofibromatosis.
16. Harlequin color change—when on side, dependent half turns red, upper half pale; caused by gravity and vasomotor instability.
17. Abrasions or lacerations can result from internal monitoring and instruments used at birth.
18. Cutis marmorata—bluish mottling or marbling of skin in response to chilling, stress, or overstimulation.
19. Port wine nevus (nevus flammeus)—flat pink or reddish purple lesion consisting of dilated, congested capillaries directly beneath the epidermis; does not blanch.

Head

1. Examine head and face for symmetry, paralysis, shape, swelling, movement.
   a. Caput succedaneum—swelling of soft tissues of the scalp because of pressure; swelling crosses suture lines.
   b. Cephalohematoma—subperiosteal hemorrhage with collection of blood between periosteum and bone; swelling does not cross suture lines.
   c. Molding—overlapping of skull bones, caused by compression during labor and delivery (disappears in a few days).
   d. Examine symmetry of facial movements.
   e. Forceps marks—U-shaped bruising usually on cheeks after forcep delivery.
2. Measure head circumference—33–35 cm (13–14 in.), approximately 2 cm (1 in.) larger than chest. Measure just above the eyebrows and over the occiput.
3. Fontanelles—area where more than two skull bones meet; covered with strong band of connective tissue; also called soft spot.
   a. Enlarged or bulging—may indicate increased intracranial pressure.
   b. Sunken—often indicates dehydration.
   c. Size—posterior may be obliterated because of molding; generally closes in 2–3 months. Anterior is palpable; generally closes in 12–18 months.
4. Sutures—junctions of adjoining skull bones.
   a. Overriding—caused by molding during labor and delivery.
   b. Separation—extensive separation may be found in malnourished infants and with increased intracranial pressure.

Face

1. Eyes—examine the following:
   a. Color—sclera in most full-term infants are white; blue sclera is indicative of osteogenesis imperfecta. Eye color usually slate-gray, brown, or dark blue; final eye color is evident by 6–12 months.
   b. Hemorrhagic areas—subconjunctival hemorrhages may appear as a red band from pressure during delivery; regress within 2 weeks.
   c. Edema—edema of the eyelids may be caused by pressure on the head and face during labor and delivery.
   d. Conjunctivitis or discharge—may be caused by instillation of silver nitrate (if still used) or infections

from organisms, such as staphylococcus or gono-coccus. Tear formation does not usually begin until 2–3 months of age.

e. Jaundice—may be seen in sclera because of physiologic jaundice or, if severe, blood group incompatibility.

f. Pupils—equal in size and should constrict equally in bright light.

g. Infant can see and discriminate patterns; limited by imperfect oculomotor coordination and inability to accommodate for varying distances.

h. Red reflex—red-orange color seen when light from an ophthalmoscope is reflected from the retina. No red reflex indicates cataracts.

i. Brushfield's spots—white or yellow pinpoint areas on iris that may indicate trisomy 21 or even a normal variant.

j. Abnormal placement of eyes or small eye openings can signify a syndrome or chromosomal anomaly.

k. Strabismus—cross-eyed appearance that is common; nystagmus (constant, rapid, involuntary movement of the eye) is also common and disappears by 4 months of age.

2. Nose—examine the following:

a. Patency—necessary because infants breathe through the nose, not the mouth.

b. Nasal flaring—abnormal and may indicate respiratory distress. Check for appropriate size and shape of the nose; should be placed vertically midline in face.

c. Discharge—stuffiness is normal unless chronic nasal discharge is present; may be caused by possible infection.

d. Sense of smell—infants will turn toward familiar odors and away from noxious odors.

e. Septum should be midline; low nasal bridge with broad base may be associated with Down's syndrome.

f. Periodic sneezing is common.

3. Ears—examine the following:

a. Formation—large, flabby ears that slant forward may indicate abnormalities of kidney or other parts of urinary tract.

b. Position in relation to eye—helix (top of ear) on same plane as eye; low-set ears may indicate chromosomal or renal abnormalities.

c. Cartilage—full-term infant has sufficient cartilage to make ear feel firm.

d. Hearing—auditory canals may be congested for a day or two after birth; the infant should hear well in a few days.

e. Observe for skin tags; preauricular sinus located in front of ear may be normal or associated with genetic disorders.

4. Mouth—examine the following:

a. Size—small mouth found in trisomy 18 and 21; corners of mouth turn down (fish mouth) in fetal alcohol syndrome. Mucous membranes should be pink.

b. Palate—examine hard and soft palate for closure.

c. Size of tongue in relation to mouth—normally does not extend much past the margin of gums. Excessively large tongue seen in congenital anomalies, such as cretinism and trisomy 21.

d. Teeth—predeciduous teeth are found on rare occasions; if they interfere with feeding, they may be removed.

e. Epstein's pearls—small white nodules found on sides of hard palate (often mistaken for teeth); regress in a few weeks.

f. Frenulum linguae—thin ridge of tissue running from base of tongue along undersurface to tip of tongue, formerly believed to cause tongue-tie; no treatment necessary. True congenital ankyloglossia (tongue-tie) is rare.

g. Sucking blisters (labial taberales)—thickened areas on midline of upper lip that may be filled with fluid or callous; no treatment necessary.

h. Infections—thrush, caused by *Candida albicans*, may appear as white patches on tongue and/or insides of cheeks that do not wash away with fluids; treated with nystatin suspension.

Neck

Examine the following:

1. Mobility—infant can move head from side to side; palpate for lymph nodes; palpate clavicle for fractures, especially after a difficult delivery.

2. Torticollis—appears as a spasmodic, one-sided contraction of neck muscles; generally from hematoma of sternocleidomastoid muscle; usually no treatment required.

3. Excessive skin folds may be associated with congenital abnormalities, such as trisomy 21.

4. Stiffness and hyperextension may be caused by trauma or infection.

5. Clavicle—for intactness.

6. Observe for masses, such as cystic hygroma—soft and usually seen laterally or over clavicle.

Chest

1. Circumference and symmetry—average circumference is 30 cm to 33 cm (12–13 in.), approximately 2 cm smaller than head circumference.

2. Breast.

a. Engorgement—may occur at day 3 because of withdrawal of maternal hormones, especially estrogen; no treatment required. Regresses in 2 weeks.

b. Nipples and areolae—less formed and pronounced in preterm infants.

Respiratory System

1. Rate—normally between 40–60 breaths/minute; influenced by sleep-wake status, when last fed, drugs taken by mother, and room temperature.

2. Rhythm—respirations may be shallow with irregular rhythm.

a. Respiratory movements are symmetric and mainly diaphragmatic because of weak thoracic muscles. For example, the lower thorax pulls in and the abdomen bulges with each respiration.

b. Periodic breathing—resumption of respiration after 5- to 15-second period without respiration; decreases with time; more common in preterm infants. Substernal retractions if accompanied by gasps or stridor is indicative of upper airway obstruction.

c. Observe for abnormal respiratory signs.

3. Breath sounds—determined by auscultation.

   a. Bronchial sounds are heard over most of the chest.

   b. Rales may be heard immediately after birth.

   c. Expiratory grunting is indicative of respiratory distress syndrome (RDS).

Cardiovascular System

1. Rate—normal between 110–160 bpm (80–110 normal with deep sleep); influenced by behavioral state, environmental temperature, medication; take apical count for 1 min.

2. Rhythm—common to find periods of deceleration followed by periods of acceleration.

3. Heart sounds—second sound higher in pitch and sharper than first; third and fourth sounds rarely heard; murmurs common, majority are transitory.

4. Pulses—examine equality and strength of brachial, radial, pedal, and femoral pulses; lack of femoral pulses indicative of inadequate aortic blood flow.

5. Cyanosis—examine for cyanosis. Acrocyanosis of distal extremities is common; record location of any cyanosis, color changes with time, and when crying.

6. Blood pressure—newborns who weigh more than 3 kg have systolic blood pressure between 60–80 mm Hg; diastolic, between 35–55 mm Hg. Blood pressure is usually higher in the lower extremities than in the upper extremities. Routine blood pressure screening is no longer recommended by the American Academy of Pediatrics for all newborns. It is reserved for infants who show signs of distress.

Abdomen

1. Shape—cylindrical, protrudes slightly, moves synchronously with chest in respiration.

2. Distention may be caused by bowel obstruction, organ enlargement, or infection.

3. Palpate abdomen for masses; gap between rectus muscles is common; palpate liver and spleen.

   a. Liver has decreased ability to conjugate bilirubin (rationale for physiologic jaundice).

   b. Liver has decreased production of prothrombin and factors that depend on vitamin K for synthesis (rationale for neonate's predisposition to hemorrhage).

4. Auscultate abdomen in all four quadrants for bowel sounds; usually bowel sounds occur an hour after delivery.

5. Kidneys—palpate kidneys for size and shape.

   a. Infant has decreased ability of kidney to concentrate urine, excrete a solute load, maintain water and electrolyte balance.

   b. Urine may contain uric acid crystals, which appear on diaper as reddish blotches; uric acid crystals may yield false-positive result when the infant's urine is tested for protein.

6. Umbilical cord

   a. Normally contains two arteries, one vein; single artery sometimes associated with renal and other congenital abnormalities.

   b. Signs of infection around insertion into abdominal wall-redness, discharge.

   c. Meconium staining—associated with intrauterine compromise or postmaturity.

   d. By 24 hours, becomes yellowish brown; dries and falls off in approximately 10–14 days.

   e. Umbilical hernia—defect in abdominal wall.

7. Genitalia

   a. Female

      (i) Labia majora cover labia minora and clitoris in full-term female infants.

      (ii) Hymenal tag (tissue) may protrude from vagina—regresses within several weeks.

      (iii) Vaginal discharge—white mucous discharge common; pink-tinged mucous discharge (pseudomenstruation) may be present because of the drop in maternal hormones; no treatment necessary.

   b. Male

      (i) Full-term—testes in scrotal sac; scrotal sac appears markedly wrinkled due to rugae.

      (ii) Edema may be present in scrotal sac if the infant was born in breech presentation; a frank collection of fluid in the scrotal sac is a hydrocele—regresses in approximately a month.

      (iii) Examine glans penis for urethral opening—normally central; opening ventral (hypospadias); opening dorsally (epispadias); abnormally adherent foreskin (phimosis).

   c. Check for patent anus—infant should stool within 24 hours after delivery. If passed meconium in utero, patent anus has been established.

Back

1. Examine spinal column for normal curvature, closure, and pilonidal dimple or sinus; also for tufts of hair or skin disruptions that would indicate possible spina bifida.

2. Examine anal area for anal opening, response of anal sphincter, fissures.

Musculoskeletal System

1. Examine extremities for fractures, paralysis, range of motion, irregular position.

2. Examine fingers and toes for number and separation: extra digits, polydactyly; fused digits, syndactyly.

3. Examine hips for dislocation—with the infant in supine position, flex knees and abduct hips to side and down to table surface; clicking sound indicates dislocation (Ortolani's sign).

4. Asymmetrical gluteal folds also indicate congenital hip dislocation.

5. Examine feet for structural and positional deformities, ie, club foot (talipes equinovarus) or metatarsus adductus (inward turning of the foot).

Neurologic System

1. Neurologic mechanisms are immature anatomically and physiologically; as a result, uncoordinated movements, labile temperature regulation, and lack of control over musculature are characteristic of the infant.
2. Examine muscle tone, head control, and reflexes.
3. Two types of reflexes are present in the newborn:
   a. Protective in nature (blink, cough, sneeze, gag)—remain throughout life.
   b. Primitive in nature (rooting/sucking, moro, startle, tonic neck, stepping, and palmar/plantar grasp)—either disappear within months or become highly developed and voluntary (sucking and grasping) (Figure 38-4).

Behavioral Assessment

Response to Stimulation

1. Newborns exhibit predictable, directed responses in social interactions with nurturing adults or in response to attractive auditory or visual stimuli.
2. Newborn responses are influenced by states of consciousness, such as:
   a. Quiet, deep sleep (sleep state)—no spontaneous activity, eyes closed, respirations regular, with delayed response to external stimuli.
   b. Light, active sleep (sleep state)—random startles, eyes closed, rapid eye movements, frequent change of state with response to stimulation.
   c. Drowsy awake (transitional state)—eyes open or closed, appearing dull and heavy lidded, eyelids flutter, variable activity level, mild startles periodically, delayed response to stimulation.
   d. Quiet alert (awake state)—eyes open, little motor activity, focuses on source of stimulation. Interacts most with environment; respirations regular.
   e. Alert active (awake state)—eyes open, less bright and attentive, much motor activity, increase in startles in response to stimulation.
   f. Crying (awake state)—intense crying that is difficult to interrupt with stimulation; increased motor activity and color changes.

Sleeping Pattern

1. Length of sleep cycles (rapid eye movement, active and quiet sleep) changes with maturation of the central nervous system.
2. Quiet sleep should increase with time in relation to rapid eye movement sleep.
3. Newborns usually sleep 20 hours per day.

Feeding Pattern

1. Most newborns eat 6–8 times per day with 2–4 hours between feedings; establish fairly regular feeding patterns in approximately 2 weeks.
2. Caloric requirements are high—110–130 calories/kg of body weight daily.

3. Most digestive enzymes are present at birth.
4. Imperfect control of cardiac and pyloric sphincters; immaturity results in regurgitation.

Pattern of Elimination

1. Stool
   a. Meconium is usually passed in 24 hours.
   b. Passage of meconium (tarry green-black stools) continues for 48 hours, followed by transitional stools (combination of meconium and yellow or milk stools). Milk stools (yellow) are passed by day 5.
   c. Newborn has up to six stools per day in the first weeks after birth.
2. Voiding
   a. Newborn voids within first 24 hours.
   b. After first few days, infant voids from 10–15 times a day.

Temperature Regulation

1. Infant's body responds readily to changes in environmental temperature.
2. Heat loss at birth may occur through evaporation, convection, conduction, and radiation.
3. Physiologic mechanisms to avoid heat loss include:
   a. Vasoconstriction.
   b. Nonshivering thermogenesis elicited by sympathetic nervous system in response to decreased temperature.
   c. Adipose tissue and brown fat—the latter contains many small blood vessels, fat vacuoles, and mitochondria and is a site of heat production. Brown fat is found between scapulae, around neck and thorax, behind sternum, and around kidneys and adrenals.
   d. Flexed position of full-term newborn.

Metabolic Screening Tests

1. Phenylketonuria (PKU)—inability of the infant to metabolize phenylalanine; scheduled after 48 hours of protein feedings.
2. Galactosemia—inborn error of carbohydrate metabolism, in which galactose and lactose cannot be converted to glucose.
3. Hypothyroidism—thyroid hormone deficiency.
4. Maple sugar urine disease (MSUD)—inability to metabolize leucine, isoleucine, and valine.
5. Homocystinuria—inborn error of sulfur amino acid metabolism.
6. Sickle cell anemia—abnormally shaped red blood cells with lower oxygen solubility.

Community and Home Care Considerations

1. The American Academy of Pediatrics (AAP) and the American College of Obstetricians and Gynecologists (ACOG) have established guidelines and have suggested criteria for discharging childbearing women within 24 hours after birth.
   a. Mother with uncomplicated vaginal birth after normal term antepartum course and immediate postpartum course.

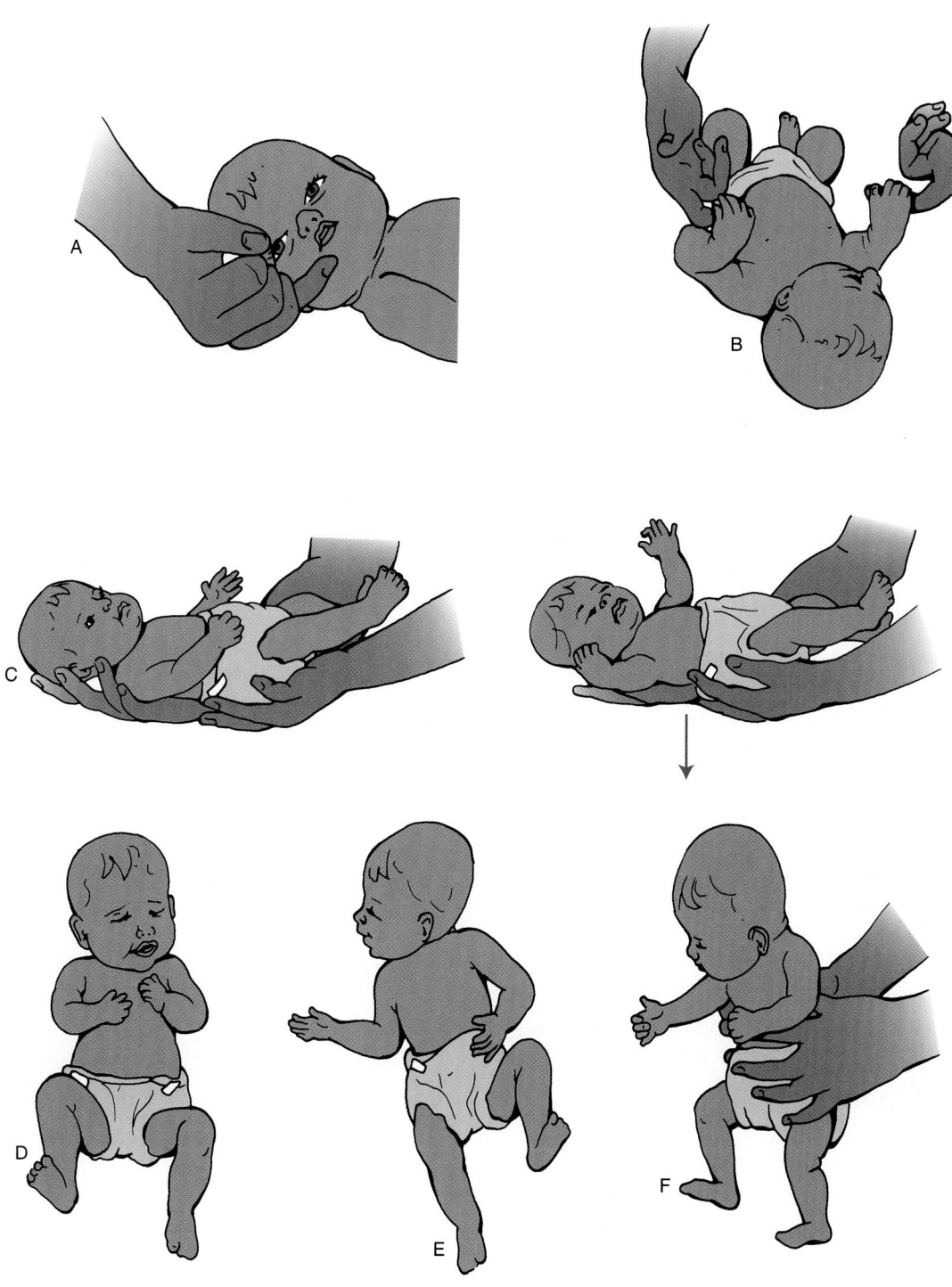

FIGURE 38-4   Newborn reflexes. (**A**) Rooting. (**B**) Grasp. (**C**) Moro. (**D**) Startle. (**E**) Tonic neck.
(**F**) Stepping.

b. Pertinent lab data within normal limits (WNL) for mother and newborn.

c. Newborn stable, maintaining thermal homeostasis, and feeding well.

d. Family members and support persons available at home for next several days.

e. Mother aware of complications for self and newborn.

f. Institution has in place mechanisms to address patient questions after discharge.

2. The first visit at home by the perinatal home care personnel is the longest because a complete physical of mother and the newborn is completed. Subsequent visits are shorter.

3. Listening is important. The approach for care is a collaborative one.

4. Nurse needs to have a thorough knowledge base in:
   a. Normal postpartum and newborn care.
   b. Potential complications in the postpartum and newborn periods.
   c. Nursing interventions for postpartum and newborn complications.

5. Personal safety is also a concern. There should be a mechanism in place to locate the home care personnel if needed. Staff should also be trained in actions to take when encountering potentially unsafe situations. It is recommended that home care personnel leave their purse and other pertinent information in their vehicle or at home. Do not carry it on your person should quick escape be necessary.

◼ Nursing Management

See Procedure Guidelines 38-1.

In caring for the newborn, the nurse establishes an ongoing plan of care for the infant and the family until discharge. The nurse's assessment of the newborn includes observing and recording vital signs, daily weight gain or loss, bowel and bladder function, activity and sleep patterns, and thermoregulation. Observation for potential problems in the newborn, ensuring safety, and the prevention of infection are main goals of nursing care.

Another main component of caring for the newborn is to assist with establishing a healthy family unit. Because so much of the baby's time is spent with parents, the nurse has the opportunity to assist them with promoting health maintenance by teaching feeding methods and by demonstrating baby care techniques, such as diapering, bathing, and circumcision care. The nurse provides health counseling and education and answers questions to enable the parents to gain confidence, control, and satisfaction in caring for their child at home.

PROCEDURE GUIDELINES 38-1	NEWBORN CARE

EQUIPMENT

Cotton balls or disposable washcloths	Petrolatum gauze
Neutral soap	Protective ointment
70% alcohol	

PROCEDURE

Nursing Action	Rationale
WEIGHT, TEMPERATURE, AND BLOOD PRESSURE	
1. Weigh infant and record weight.	1. Infant may lose 5%–10% of birth weight because of minimal intake of nutrients and fluid and loss of excess fluid.
2. Take axillary temperature by placing thermometer in axilla and pressing infant's arm gently but firmly against it for 10 min. Prevent undue exposure; provide warm environment (24°–27°C [75°–80°F]).	2. Use of rectal thermometer predisposes to irritation of rectal mucosa.
3. Take blood pressure, if indicated.	3. Hypotension may be present and require remedial action.
BATHING TECHNIQUE (BATH WATER (37°–38°C [98°–100°F])	
1. Use cotton balls or soft, disposable washcloths to wipe eyes, face, and outer ears. Eyes are wiped from inside corner outward.	1. Start from cleanest areas to most soiled.
2. Use a neutral soap—check pH. Clear water may be used if infant's skin is dry.	2. Prevents irritation of skin. The use of hexachlorophene to prevent staphylococcal infection is controversial. Hexachlorophene may cause brain damage if a sufficient quantity is absorbed through the skin.
3. Wash infant's head, using gentle circular motions.	3. Prevents cradle cap from forming, especially over the frontal areas.
4. Tilt head back to cleanse neck.	4. Exposes neck folds for more thorough cleansing.
5. Bathe torso and extremities quickly.	5. Prevents unnecessary exposure and chilling.

NURSING ACTION	**RATIONALE**
6. Inspect umbilical cord. Check area for bleeding or foul odor. A drying agent, such as 70% alcohol or merthiolate, may be applied several times daily (according to institutional policy). Do not cover with diaper. Dressings are not used.	6. Minimizes colonization by bacteria.

7. Cleanse genital area of male infants.
  a. Cleanse penis without retracting foreskin.
 	
  b. Circumcision care—keep area clean. Place sterile petrolatum gauze over area for first 24 hrs; change after voiding. Observe hourly for bleeding. Position infant and diaper to avoid friction.
	7.
	  a. Edema and constriction of the penis may result if foreskin is retracted.
	  b. Prevents infection and promotes healing. Bleeding can be controlled by pressure or by application of adrenaline solution. Prevents discomfort.

8. Cleanse genital area of female infants.
  a. Wash vulva from front to back.
  b. Wipe vulva with cotton ball, using 1 stroke in a front-to-back direction.
	8.
	  a. Removes vernix and other discharge.
	  b. Front-to-back cleansing prevents contamination of vagina.

9. Bathe buttocks, using a gentle, patting motion. Keep area clean and dry to prevent diaper rash. If rash does occur, protective ointment (zinc oxide or A & D) may be used. Exposure of buttocks to air or heat lamp is helpful.	9. Area is susceptible to skin breakdown because of acid reaction of urine and feces.

STOOL OBSERVATION

1. Observe stool pattern—meconium during first 2–3 d.	1. Material composed of epithelial and epidermal cells, lanugo, and bile pigments.
2. Transitional stools—change from tarry black to greenish black, to greenish brown to brownish yellow to greenish yellow.	2. Changes reflect intake of milk—stools are composed of both meconium and milk stools.

3. Number, color, and consistency are recorded daily.	3. For early identification of abnormalities.
	  a. No stool within 48 hrs indicates an intestinal obstruction.
	  b. Passage of meconium only (without other stool) suggests obstruction in the ileum.
	  c. Thick, putty-like meconium may indicate cystic fibrosis.
	  d. Diarrhea may be caused by overfeeding or by gastroenteritis.
	  e. Blood in the stool is an indication of intestinal bleeding.

NUTRITIONAL CONSIDERATIONS

1. Provide for nutritional intake.	1. Infants vary in their readiness to feed.
2. Promote feeding method of choice.	2. Although recommendations may be made, family decisions should be respected and continuity of care provided.
3. Test blood glucose using enzymatic strip test (according to institutional policy).	3. Infant may be hypoglycemic and require feeding sooner than usual 4–6-h wait.

4. Instruct the parent in technique of bottle-feeding.
  a. Hold baby in semiupright position.
  b. Position bottle so that neck of bottle is filled.
  c. Insert nipple into baby's mouth so that baby's tongue is under nipple.
  d. Burp during feeding by holding infant upright.
	4.
	  a. Gravity assists flow of milk into stomach.
	  b. Prevents the baby from swallowing air.
	  c. Sucking and swallowing reflexes are used in feeding.
	
	  d. Allows air to escape from stomach, preventing distention or milk regurgitation.

COMMUNITY AND HOME CARE CONSIDERATIONS

1. Preparation for home care: instruction is given concerning infant bathing and care, preparation of formula, and infant feeding. Written formula with instructions for preparation is provided to parents.	1. Instruction for infant care is a combined responsibility of the medical and nursing staffs.
2. Provide ample opportunity for parent contact and care of infant while nursing support is available. Take every opportunity to teach.	2. Early attachment results in improved parent-child relationships.
3. Arrange home visits as necessary.	

PROBLEMS OF INFANTS

■ Premature Infant

The premature infant is an infant born before the completion of 37 weeks' gestation.

A low birth weight (LBW) infant is one whose birth weight is less than 2,500 g (5 lb. 8 oz.), regardless of gestational age.

A very low birth weight (VLBW) infant is one whose birth weight is below 1,500 g, regardless of gestational age.

Pathophysiology and Etiology

1. There is a wide range of maternal factors associated with prematurity, including poor nutrition, diabetes, drug abuse, chronic disease, being a multigravida mother younger than 18 years of age, or a primigravida mother older than 40 years of age.
2. Complications of pregnancy associated with prematurity include, but are not limited to:
   a. Pregnancy-induced hypertension (PIH).
   b. Bleeding.
   c. Placenta previa or abruptio placentae.
   d. Incompetent cervix.
   e. Premature rupture of membranes (PROM).
   f. Polyhydramnios/oligohydramnios.
   g. Chorioamnionitis.
3. Fetal factors associated with prematurity include:
   a. Chromosomal abnormalities.
   b. Anatomic abnormalities, such as tracheoesophageal atresia or fistula (TEF) and intestinal obstruction.
   c. Fetoplacental unit dysfunction.
4. Premature labor may occur idiopathically.
5. The premature infant has altered physiology because of immature and often poorly developed systems. The severity of any problem that occurs depends somewhat on the gestational age of the infant. Systems and situations that are most likely to cause problems in the premature infant include:
   a. Respiratory system.
   b. Digestive system.
   c. Thermoregulation.
   d. Immune system.
   e. Neurologic system.

Nursing Assessment and Interventions

1. Notice physical characteristics of the premature infant:
   a. Hair—lanugo, fluffy.
   b. Poor ear cartilage.
   c. Skin—thin; capillaries are visible (may be red and wrinkled).
   d. Lack of subcutaneous fat.
   e. Sole of foot is smooth.
      (i) 36 weeks' gestation—anterior ⅓ of foot is creased.
      (ii) 38 weeks' gestation—⅔ of foot is creased.
   f. Breast buds 5 mm.
      (i) 36 weeks' gestation—none.
      (ii) 38 weeks' gestation—3 mm.
   g. Testes—undescended.
   h. Labia majora—undeveloped.
   i. Rugae of scrotum—fine.
   j. Fingernails—soft.
   k. Abdomen—relatively large.
   l. Thorax—relatively small.
   m. Head—appears disproportionately large.
   n. Muscle tone poor, possibly weak reflexes.
2. Obtain accurate body measurements.
   a. Head circumference—frontal-occipital circumference (FOC) one finger above eyebrows, using parallel lines of tape around head.
   b. Abdominal girth—one finger above umbilicus, mark location.
   c. Heel–crown.
   d. Shoulder to umbilicus—used to calculate proper length of catheter for umbilical arterial catheter placement.
   e. Weight in grams.
3. Assess gestational age (Figure 38-5) using a tool such as the Ballard scoring system (recommended by Committee of Fetus and Newborn of American Academy of Pediatrics):
   a. Observation of physical and neurologic characteristics that change predictably with growth and maturation. Ideally done in the first 12 to 24 hours of life.
   b. Later, adjusted, or corrected age will be determined once the infant reaches term (40 weeks after conception). Chronologic age is adjusted for prematurity by taking gestational age – 40 plus chronologic age = developmental or corrected age. This is the age the infant would have been if he had been born at 40 weeks' gestation.
4. Assist with laboratory testing as indicated for blood gases, blood glucose, CBC or Hbg and Hct, electrolytes, calcium, bilirubin.
5. Monitor closely for respiratory or cardiac complications.
   a. Respirations above 60 min. during a time frame may be indicative of respiratory difficulty.
   b. Expiratory grunting, retractions, chest lag, or nasal flaring should be reported immediately (Figure 38-6).
   c. Watch for cyanosis (other than acrocyanosis—coldness and cyanosis of hands and feet) and other signs of respiratory distress.
   d. Increased (more than 180/bpm) or irregular heart rate may indicate cardiac or circulatory difficulties.
   e. Muscle tone and activity should be evaluated.
   f. Hypotension, indicated by blood pressure measurement, may be caused by hypovolemia.
   g. Hypoglycemia may result from inadequate glycogen stores, respiratory distress, and cold stress.

SKIN	0	1	2	3	4	5
SKIN	gelatinous red, transparent	smooth pink, visible veins	superficial peeling &/or rash, few veins	cracking pale area, rare veins	parchment, deep cracking, no vessels	leathery, cracked, wrinkled
LANUGO	none	abundant	thinning	bald areas	mostly bald	
PLANTAR CREASES	no crease	faint red marks	anterior transverse crease only	creases ant. 2/3	creases cover entire sole	
BREAST	barely percept.	flat areola, no bud	stippled areola, 1–2 mm bud	raised areola, 3–4 mm bud	full areola, 5–10 mm bud	
EAR	pinna flat, stays folded	sl. curved pinna, soft with slow recoil	well-curv. pinna, soft but ready recoil	formed & firm with instant recoil	thick cartilage, ear stiff	
GENITALS Male	scrotum empty, no rugae		testes descending, few rugae	testes down, good rugae	testes pendulous, deep rugae	
GENITALS Female	prominent clitoris & labia minora		majora & minora equally prominent	majora large, minora small	clitoris & minora completely covered	

	0	1	2	3	4	5
Posture						
Square Window (Wrist)	90°	60°	45°	30°	0°	
Arm Recoil	180°		100°–180°	90°–100°	<90°	
Popliteal Angle	180°	160°	130°	110°	90°	<90°
Scarf Sign						
Heel to Ear						

Score	Wks
5	26
10	28
15	30
20	32
25	34
30	36
35	38
40	40
45	42
50	44

FIGURE 38-5 Ballard assessment of gestational age criteria.

6. Institute cardiac monitoring and care for infant in isolette or radiant heater. Omit bath until infant's temperature has stabilized.

7. Observe for early signs of jaundice and check maternal history for any any blood incompatibilities. Also be aware of maternal factors that can lead to additional complications, such as drug use, diabetes, and infection.

8. Once the infant is admitted to the nursery, be aware that the first 24–48 hours after birth is a critical time, often requiring constant observation and intensive care management. Make the following observations:

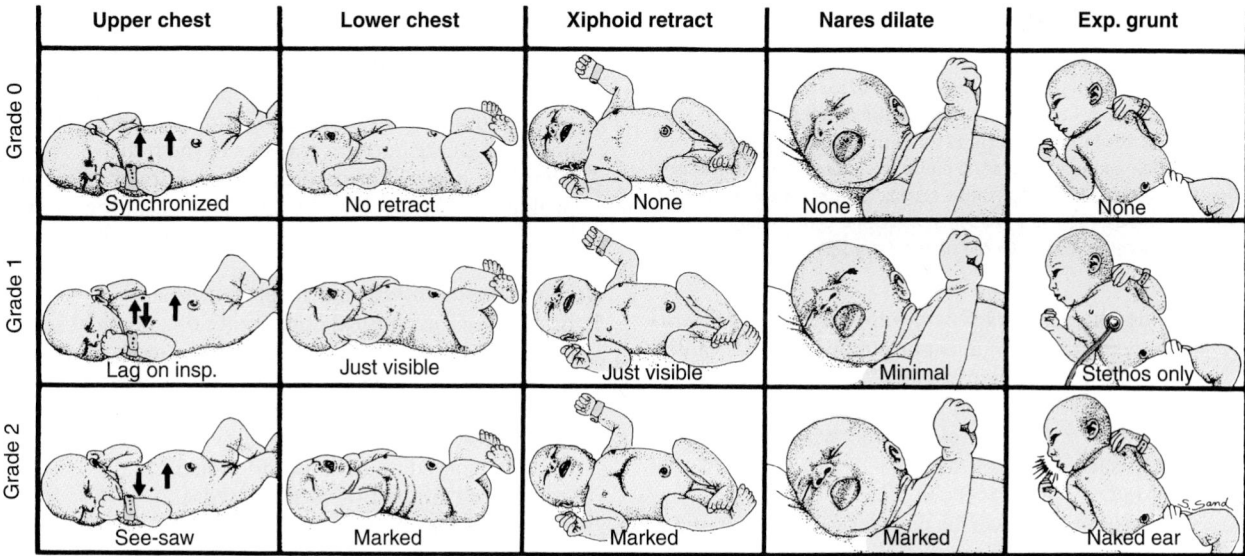

FIGURE 38-6 Observation of retractions.

a. Note bleeding from the umbilical cord—apply pressure, and notify health care provider.

b. Note first voiding—may occur up to 36 hours after birth; after first voiding, report any 4–6 hour period when voiding does not occur.

c. Note stools—abdominal distention and lack of stool may indicate intestinal obstruction or other intestinal tract anomalies. Measure abdominal girth at regular intervals.

d. Note activity and behavior—look for sucking movement, and hand-to-mouth maneuver, which can help to determine oral feeding initiation.

e. Observe for a tense and bulging fontanelle; feel suture lines, noting separation or overriding—may indicate intracranial hemorrhage. Be alert to twitching and seizures.

f. Note color skin for cyanosis and jaundice, rashes, paleness, ruddiness.

g. Carefully monitor, record, and report vital signs.

9. Have available resuscitative equipment, oxygen, and suction apparatus.

a. A rubber ear bulb syringe is often all that is necessary for clearing the mouth.

b. Frequent suctioning of the pharynx may not be necessary.

10. Position infant to allow for easy ventilation, paying careful attention to maintaining body alignment and facilitating hand-to-mouth positioning.

a. Elevate head and trunk to decrease pressure on diaphragm from abdominal organs.

b. Change position from side to side.

NURSING ALERT

Prone positioning has been shown to increase the risk of sudden infant death syndrome (SIDS). The American Academy of Pediatrics recommends that all healthy infants be positioned supine for sleep. Prone positioning offers some advantage for oxygenation in preterm infants with respiratory compromise. During the initial phase of illness, these infants are cared for with cardiorespiratory monitoring and may be placed prone according to institutional policy. Before discharge, these infants should become accustomed to sleeping supine and supine positioning should be reinforced with the infant's care providers.

---

11. Provide oxygen therapy with moisture in the percentage necessary to maintain appropriate blood gas values.

a. Monitor oxygen with analyzer continuously to ensure consistency in percentage used.

b. Pulse oximeter correlates well with oxygenation (O_2 saturation of arterial hemoglobin) of the blood.

12. Monitor for apnea versus periodic breathing (regular repetition of breathing pauses of less than 15 seconds, alternating with breaths of regularly increasing then decreasing amplitude for 10–15 seconds). Theophylline may be given to reduce apneic episodes.

13. Protect the infant from infection by following scrupulous handwashing policy, minimizing infant's contact with unsterile equipment, and minimizing the number of people who come in contact with the infant.

14. Provide good skin care using water for bathing, an approved emollient for the skin, avoiding adhesives, and providing adequate hydration.

15. Avoid cranial deformity by using gel head pillow, frequent turning, and upright position.

16. Protect the infant's eyes from bright lights.

17. Continue to provide IV and oral feedings according to infant's needs. Assist the mother with breast pumping as needed, and encourage both parents to hold and feed infant.

18. Continue to monitor for complications, such as hypoglycemia, hyperglycemia, respiratory distress syndrome (see p. 1360), apnea, infection, hypocalcemia, cardiac abnormalities, necrotizing enterocolitis, intracranial hemorrhage, and hyperbilirubinemia. Long-term complications may include retinopathy of prematurity, chronic lung disease, hearing loss, learning disabilities.

19. Do not neglect the needs of the parents. Instead, make every effort to include them in the infant's care and update them frequently on the infant's condition.

Postmature Infant

The postmature infant is one whose gestation is 42 weeks or longer and who may show signs of weight loss with placental insufficiency.

Pathophysiology and Etiology

1. Cause is not known in many cases. Maternal factors associated with postmaturity include primigravida and high-parity mother at any given age, and prolonged gestation in preceding pregnancies.

2. The postmature infant appears to have suffered from intrauterine malnutrition and hypoxia. Before the termination of the pregnancy, but at the point when the birth should have occurred, the placental function begins to diminish, resulting in impaired oxygen exchange and inadequate nutrient transfer to the fetus.

3. There are stages of postmaturity—severity of associated problems is determined by length of gestation (ie, the longer the gestation, the more severe the problems).

Nursing Assessment and Interventions

1. Be alert for the physical appearance of a postmature infant. The following characteristics are most often seen in an infant of 44 weeks' gestation or more:

a. Reduced subcutaneous tissue—loose skin, especially of buttocks and thighs.

b. Long, curved fingernails and toenails.

c. Reduced amount of vernix caseosa.

d. Abundant scalp hair.

e. Wrinkled, macerated skin; possibly pale, cracked, parchment-like skin.

f. Having the alert appearance of a 2 week- to 3-week-old infant after delivery.

g. Greenish-yellow staining of skin, fingernails or cord, indicating fetal distress.

2. Determine gestational age by physical examination. Measure weight, length, and head circumference, and plot on Colorado intrauterine growth chart. Compare percentiles.

3. Determine blood sugar; below 40 mg/100 mL indicates hypoglycemia.

4. Assess for asphyxia neonatorum by Apgar score and blood gas analysis.

5. Be alert for meconium aspiration; signs include:
   a. Thick meconium in amniotic fluid at delivery.
   b. Tachypnea, increasing signs of cyanosis; difficulty breathing, with need for ventilation.
   c. Tachycardia.
   d. Inspiratory nasal flaring and retraction of chest.
   e. Expiratory grunting.
   f. Increased anteroposterior diameter of the chest.
   g. Palpable liver.
   h. Crackles and rhonchi on chest auscultation.
   i. Concomitant cerebral irritation—jitteriness, hypotonia, seizures.
   j. X-ray—classic coarse, patchy, irregular pulmonary infiltrates ranging in severity.
   k. Additional signs: metabolic acidosis, hypotension, hypoglycemia, hypocalcemia.

6. Provide supportive treatment for meconium aspiration.
   a. Warmth—maintain thermally neutral environment so the infant uses fewer calories and less oxygen.
   b. Adequate oxygenation and humidification to maintain PaO_2 at 50–70 mm Hg.
   c. Respiratory support with ventilator; extracorporeal membrane oxygenation (ECMO) may be needed if persistent pulmonary hypertension of the newborn develops.
   d. Adequate administration of calories and fluid.
   e. Accurate monitoring of intake and output—assess possible alteration in kidney function caused by hypoxia.
   f. Administration of antibiotics prophylactically.

NURSING ALERT

Some cases of meconium aspiration can be prevented if meconium is removed from the mouth and trachea by proper suctioning, before the infant takes his or her first breath (just after head delivery).

7. Provide oral feeding or IV glucose soon after birth to treat or prevent hypoglycemia. If oral feedings are not contraindicated, they can begin 1–2 hours after birth. Monitor blood sugar every hour until condition stabilizes.

8. Be alert for persistent pulmonary hypertension of the newborn (PPHN)—physiologic disorder characterized by severe, labile cyanosis arising from persistent or return to suprasystemic pulmonary vascular resistance and pressure normally found in the fetus.

a. Cyanosis, pronounced respiratory distress, murmur, and/or congestive heart failure.
b. Treatment is aggressive respiratory support in a tertiary care nursery.

9. Provide psychological support to the parents. Long-term sequelae common in the postmature infant are central nervous system problems.

Infant of Mother Who Has Diabetes

A mother may have overt diabetes or gestational diabetes. The severity of infant problems depends on the severity of the maternal diabetes. Also known as infant of diabetic mother (IDM).

Pathophysiology and Etiology

Hyperinsulinemia in utero, secondary to elevated maternal glucose levels, results in the following in the infant:

1. Macrosomia—increased amount of body fat, not edema.
   a. Total body water is somewhat reduced at birth
   b. High urinary output during first 2 days of life, probably from freeing of intracellular water.

2. Hypoglycemia
   a. Occurs within first ½–12 hours of life; may occur within minutes after birth.
   b. The infant's response to glucose is excessive (ie, insulin blood level has a slight elevation, will drop and then peak within 1 hour). This is probably caused by maternal hyperglycemia.
   c. The infant's cord insulin levels may not be higher than in a normal infant unless a large amount of glucose is given.
   d. Infant may be symptomatic or asymptomatic, with blood sugars less than 20 mg/100 mL.

3. Hypocalcemia
   a. Associated with prematurity, difficult labor and delivery, asphyxia at birth, and/or decreased functioning of parathyroid glands.
   b. Generally occurs during the first 24–72 hours of life.

4. Hyperbilirubinemia
   a. Most likely to occur within 48–72 hours after birth.
   b. Immature liver results in inability to conjugate bilirubin.
   c. Hct is higher on the 3rd day after birth and extracellular volume is decreased.
   d. Because of large size, birth trauma may increase risk of enclosed hemorrhage.
   e. Prematurity.
   f. May be premature or small for gestational age when associated with placental insufficiency in some cases.
   g. Respiratory function is similar to that of other premature infants. Thus, infant is prone to respiratory distress syndrome.

5. Polycythemia
   a. Venous hematocrit greater than 65% or venous hemoglobin 22 g/100 ml.

b. Polycythemia increases the risks of occurrence of renal vein thrombosis, respiratory distress, hypoglycemia, and hypocalcemia.

6. Congenital anomalies
   a. Increased incidence of congenital anomalies may be caused by:
      (i) Divergent gene pattern.
      (ii) Glucose homeostasis in utero.
      (iii) Episodes of ketoacidosis in early pregnancy.
   b. Common anomalies are renal and CNS anomalies, caudal regression syndrome, facial clefts, patent ductus arteriosus (PDA), transposition of the great vessels, ventricular septal defect (VSD), and small colon syndrome.

7. Infection
   a. Prematurity and lowered passive immunity.
   b. Possible maternal urinary tract infection and bacteria crossing the placenta.

Nursing Assessment and Interventions

1. Be alert for typical appearance of IDM—macrosomia, cardiomegaly, hepatomegaly, large umbilical cord and placenta, plethora, full-face, tendency to be large for gestational age (some may be normal weight or small for gestational age [SGA]), abundant fat, abundant hair, extensive vernix caseosa, and hypertrichosis pinnae.

2. Assist with diagnostic evaluation of the infant.
   a. Maternal history of diabetes.
   b. Physical assessment of infant and determination of gestational age.
   c. Laboratory tests—serum glucose, calcium, phosphorus, magnesium, electrolytes, bilirubin, arterial blood gas analysis, blood hemoglobin, and hematocrit.

3. Monitor for hypoglycemia.
   a. Monitor serum glucose levels every 30–60 minutes beginning immediately after birth for 24 hours every 4–8 hours until stabilized.
   b. May be asymptomatic or may show signs of jitteriness, tremors, convulsions, sweating, cyanosis, weak or high-pitched cry, refusal to eat, hypotonia, apnea, temperature instability.
   c. Hypoglycemia may be prevented or treated by early feedings of 10% glucose or formula by nipple or gavage, if blood sugar 20–40. If less than 20, will require a IV solution with appropriate glucose concentration.

4. Monitor infant closely for changes in acid-base status, respiratory distress, temperature instability, hypocalcemia, and sepsis.

5. Observe for hyperbilirubinemia.
   a. Infants of mothers with diabetes have a higher incidence of hyperbilirubinemia. Levels will be elevated 48–72 hours after birth.
   b. The infant may need an exchange transfusion at relatively lower bilirubin levels (as in the premature infant) to prevent kernicterus. Phototherapy may need to be initiated early.

6. Monitor intake and output, ensure adequate fluid intake, and assess for dehydration.

7. Observe for possible cardiac anomalies and secondary congestive heart failure.

8. Observe for other complications, including respiratory distress syndrome, renal vein thrombosis, infection, hypermagnesemia or hypomagnesemia, birth injuries (encephalohematomas, facial nerve paralysis, fractured clavicles, brachial nerve plexus injuries), prematurity, asphyxia neonatorum, and organomegaly.

9. Support the family, especially the mother, who may feel guilty about being responsible for the infant's problems.

■ Jaundice in the Newborn (Hyperbilirubinemia)

Hyperbilirubinemia (jaundice) in the newborn is an accumulation of serum bilirubin above normal levels. Onset of clinical jaundice seen when serum bilirubin levels are 5–7 mg/100 dL. Kernicterus is a yellow discoloration of specific areas of brain tissue by unconjugated bilirubin; can be confirmed only by death and autopsy. Bilirubin encephalopathy best describes the occurrence of the syndrome and the accompanying neurologic sequela in neonates.

Pathophysiology and Etiology
Causes

1. Increased bilirubin load.
   a. Hemolytic disease—Rh and ABO incompatibility.
   b. Morphologic abnormalities of red blood cells.
   c. Red blood cell enzyme defects.
   d. Physiologic jaundice (see p. 1175).
   e. Sepsis.

2. Extravascular blood.
   a. Cephalohematoma.
   b. Pulmonary or cerebral hemorrhage.
   c. Any enclosed occult blood.

3. Decrease or inhibition of bilirubin conjugation.
   a. Inherited bilirubin conjugation defect: Crigler-Najjar syndrome (deficiency of glucuronyl transferase).
   b. Acquired bilirubin conjugation defect: breast-milk jaundice, Lucey-Driscoll syndrome, infant of mother with diabetes, asphyxiated infant with respiratory distress.

4. Increased extrahepatic circulation.
   a. Intestinal obstruction.

5. Polycythemia.
   a. Twin–twin transfusion.
   b. Maternal–fetal transfusion.
   c. Infant of mother with diabetes.
   d. Small for gestational age infant.

6. Hypothyroidism.

7. Familial, transient—associated with inhibiting factor in plasma.

8. Unknown.

9. Obstructive disorders.

10. Intrauterine infection.

Physiologic Jaundice

1. Increased load of bilirubin on liver cells.
   a. Increased bilirubin production—more rapid hemolysis because of higher level of circulating RBCs per kg of body weight and a shorter RBC life span.
   b. Enterohepatic circulation—reabsorption of unconjugated bilirubin.
2. Decreased clearance of bilirubin from plasma.
   a. Predominant bilirubin-binding protein in liver cells may be deficient in the first days of life.
   b. Glucuronyl transferase enzyme activity may be decreased, resulting in impaired conjugation of bilirubin.
   c. Liver may show decreased ability to excrete large amounts of conjugated bilirubin.
   d. Poor portal blood supply may decrease the liver's capacity to act effectively.
3. Physiologic jaundice occurs 3–5 days after birth.
   a. Increase in unconjugated bilirubin levels; levels must not exceed 5 mg/100 dL per day.
   b. Full-term peak levels are reached 48–72 hours after birth; clinical jaundice declines in 1 week.
   c. Premature peak levels are reached by 4–6 days of age; clinical jaundice declines in 2 weeks.

Erythrocyte Destruction

1. Erythroblastosis fetalis (isoimmunization caused by Rh factor or ABO incompatibility).
   a. Immune hemolysis or Rh/ABO blood group incompatibility; the mother's and fetus's blood are different. Rh factor; different ABO blood groups (see Coombs' test, page 1108).
   b. Mother produces antibodies against the antigen of the fetus's blood. Fetal cells frequently cross the placenta.
   c. Antibodies of the mother's blood are in the infant's blood at birth, causing hemolysis of the infant's red blood cells, leading to a rising level of indirect bilirubin.
2. Glucose-6-phosphate dehydrogenase (G-6-PD) deficiency—nonimmune hemolytic disease (erythrocyte biochemical factor).
   a. Deficiency results in reduced stability to oxidative destruction from substances that act as oxidizing agents (ie, vitamin K, naphthalene, salicylates).
   b. X-linked recessive disease that affects primarily black and Mediterranean-Asian groups.
   c. Screen maternal blood for carrier state and screen neonate blood in high-risk groups.
3. Other conditions associated with increased erythrocyte destruction:
   a. Infection—bacterial, viral, and/or protozoan.
   b. Structural abnormal erythrocyte.
   c. Sequestered blood (ie, cephalohematoma, ecchymoses).

Nursing Assessment and Interventions

1. Be alert for signs and symptoms of jaundice:
   a. Sclerae appears yellow before skin appears yellow.
   b. Skin appears light to bright yellow.
   c. Lethargy.
   d. Dark amber, concentrated urine.
   e. Poor feeding.
   f. Dark stools.
2. Make observations in daylight, sunlight, or white fluorescent light.
   a. Blanch the skin during the observation to clear away capillary coloration: forehead, cheeks, and clavicle sites allow for clear view.
   b. Be alert to the infant's age in connection with the appearance of jaundice.
3. Assist with treatment.
   a. Fluids—ensure adequate hydration.
   b. Exchange transfusion—mechanically remove bilirubin.
   c. Phototherapy—allow for utilization of alternative pathways for bilirubin excretion.
   d. Enzyme induction agent—reduce bilirubin levels by inducing hepatic enzyme system involved in bilirubin clearance (ie, phenobarbital).
4. Provide nursing care related to phototherapy.
   a. Photoisomerization of tissue bilirubin occurs when the baby is exposed to 420–460 nm of light.
   b. Check light intensity for therapeutic range daily. Use commercial Bililight.
   c. Have the infant completely undressed so entire skin surface is exposed to light.
   d. Keep the infant's eyes covered, unless using a bili-blanket, to protect from constant exposure to high-intensity light, which may cause retinal injury.
   e. Shield gonads.
   f. Develop a systematic schedule of turning infant so all surfaces are exposed (ie, every 2 hours).
   g. Maintain thermo-neutrality—light affects the ambient temperature.
   h. Shield the infant (by Plexiglas) from direct exposure of lights.
   i. Obtain bilirubin levels as directed. The diminishing icterus (ie, the lowering of unconjugated bilirubin from cutaneous tissue) does not reflect the serum bilirubin concentration. Lights should be turned off when blood is being collected to eliminate false-low bilirubin levels.
   j. If possible, remove the infant from under the lights, remove eye covers, and encourage parents to hold the infant for feedings.

NURSING ALERT

If priapism occurs during phototherapy, turn the infant on his abdomen for short periods of time, and this will cease.

Septicemia Neonatorum

Septicemia neonatorum (sepsis of the newborn) is a generalized infection that may occur in the neonate and is characterized by the proliferation of bacteria in the bloodstream and frequently involves the meninges (as distinguished from simple bacteremia, congenital infection, septicemia after major diseases or surgery, or major congenital anomalies). High mortality rate.

Pathophysiology and Etiology

1. The distribution of etiologic agents varies from year to year and from institution to institution.
   a. Gram-negative organisms include *E. coli, Klebsiella* (enterobacteriaceae), *Pseudomonas, Proteus, Salmonella, H. influenzae.*
   b. Gram-positive organisms include Group B beta-hemolytic *Streptococcus, Listeria monocytogenes, S. aureus* (coagulase-negative and coagulase-positive), *S. epidermides, Streptococcus pneumoniae, Streptococcus faecalis.*
2. Fungal infections from the organism *Candida albicans* are increasing in incidence, especially in the low-birth-weight infant.
3. Predisposing factors include a wide range of maternal perinatal complications; iatrogenic factors, such as use of catheters, oxygen, and resuscitative equipment; and infant complications, such as prematurity, congenital anomalies, respiratory distress syndrome, skin infections, and asphyxia.
4. Infection occurs because of a temporary breakdown or depression of the infant's defense mechanism for unknown reason.

Nursing Assessment and Interventions

1. Be alert for early signs of sepsis, which are usually vague and subtle.
   a. Poor feeding; gastric retention; weak sucking.
   b. Lethargy, limpness; weak crying.
   c. Temperature alteration—generally hypothermia, but infant may have hyperthermia.
   d. Hypo- or hyperglycemia.
2. Assist with diagnostic tests.
   a. Cultures from the blood, urine, spinal fluid, skin lesions, nose, throat, rectum, gastric fluid.
   b. WBC and differential, hemoglobin, hematocrit.
   c. Blood chemistries—glucose, calcium, pH, electrolytes.
   d. C-reactive protein and erythrocyte sedimentation rate.
   e. Acid-base studies (acidosis).
   f. Bilirubin.
   g. TORCH (toxoplasmosis-rubella-cytomegalic inclusion virus-herpes-other) detect antibodies against common intrauterine-infective agents.
   h. Arterial blood gases.
   i. Chest x-ray—may demonstrate pulmonary infection.
   j. Urinalysis.

3. Assist with treatment.
   a. Before the specific organism is identified, and after cultures have been obtained, the antibacterial therapy is based on the more common causative agents and their anticipated susceptibilities.
   b. Supportive therapy includes: observation, isolation, hydration, nutrition, oxygen, regulation of thermal environment, blood transfusion to correct anemia and shock, and protection from further infection.
4. Observe for complications, such as meningitis (very common), shock, adrenal hemorrhage, disseminated intravascular coagulation, PPHN, metabolic derangements, seizures, pneumonia, urinary tract infection, and congestive heart failure.

Infant of Substance-Abusing Mother

Maternal abuse of substances such as drugs, alcohol and tobacco may have an impact on the growth, development, and well-being of her fetus or newborn.

Pathophysiology and Etiology

1. Drugs and alcohol cross the placental barrier and enter the fetal circulation. The supply to the infant is abruptly terminated at delivery, causing withdrawal symptoms.
2. Fetal alcohol syndrome is direct ethanol toxicity to developing fetus. Additional effects on the fetus come from maternal malnutrition, maternal hypoglycemia, smoking, and alcohol-induced illness (ie, gastric hemorrhage, cirrhosis of liver).
3. Cocaine is a CNS stimulant that results in increased norepinephrine levels, which leads to vasoconstriction, tachycardia, hypertension, and uterine contractions; may lead to cerebral hemorrhage.
4. The long-term biologic effects on the infant of a drug-dependent mother are not fully known. These children may have:
   a. Abnormal psychomotor development associated with intrauterine growth retardation.
   b. Behavioral disturbances, such as hyperactivity, brief attention spans, temper tantrums.
   c. These infants often suffer from intrauterine growth retardation (IUGR), fetal anoxia and meconium aspiration, prematurity, and a wide variety of complications.
5. Infants and children with fetal alcohol syndrome may develop intellectual impairment, poor fine motor control, difficulty feeding, hyperactivity, delay of gross motor skills, and brain dysfunction.
6. Complications of cocaine abuse include spontaneous abortion, premature labor, abruptio placenta, uterine rupture, meconium staining, and congenital anomalies.

Nursing Assessment and Interventions

1. Obtain maternal history of drug, dosage, time of last dose. Be alert for onset of symptoms of narcotic withdrawal.

a. Heroin—several hours after birth to 3–4 days of life.

b. Methadone—7–10 days after birth to several weeks of life.

c. Cardinal signs of neonatal narcotic withdrawal include coarse, flapping tremors; irritability; hyperactivity; hypertonicity; persistent high-pitched cry; restlessness; sleepiness.

2. Be alert for fetal alcohol syndrome.
   a. Difficulty establishing respirations.
   b. Metabolic problems.
   c. Irritability.
   d. Increased muscle tone, tremulousness.
   e. Lethargy.
   f. Opisthotonos.
   g. Poor sucking reflex.
   h. Abdominal distention.
   i. Seizure activity.
   j. Facial abnormalities.

3. Be alert for infant born to mother of cocaine abuse—does not appear to experience classic neonatal abstinence syndrome. Instead, may exhibit:
   a. Mild tremulousness.
   b. Increased irritability and startle response.
   c. Muscular rigidity.
   d. Difficulty in being consoled.
   e. Pronounced state of lability.
   f. Tachycardia and tachypnea.
   g. Poor tolerance for oral feedings, diarrhea.
   h. Disturbed sleep pattern.

4. Collect urine for toxicology screen within 24 hours after birth. Obtain blood gases, blood glucose, and other laboratory tests as indicated, including meconium stool sent for toxicology screen.

5. Administer medications as directed.
   a. Narcotic antagonist, such as naloxone (Narcan) for narcotic-induced respiratory depression at birth. There has been a report of seizures secondary to acute opioid withdrawal after administration to a baby born to an opioid user, so use with caution.
   b. Drug therapy for alleviation of signs of narcotic withdrawal. Duration of therapy using decreasing dosages may be from 4–40 days.
      (i) Paregoric (camphorated tincture of opium) orally.
      (ii) Phenobarbital, orally.
      (iii) Chlorpromazine (Thorazine) orally.
      (iv) Diazepam (Valium) intramuscularly.
      (v) Methadone.

6. Provide nursing care to support infant and to relieve symptoms.
   a. Irritability and restlessness, high-pitched crying.
      (i) Loosely swaddle (may increase infant's temperature).
      (ii) Minimize handling.
      (iii) Decrease environmental stimuli (ie, light, noise).
      (iv) Organize care to allow for periods of uninterrupted sleep.
      (v) Prone positioning may help the infant organize motor movements.
      (vi) Give medications with meals unless patient vomits; then 30 minutes before.
   b. Floppy tremors—protect skin from irritation and abrasions.
      (i) Change position frequently.
      (ii) Give good, frequent skin care—keep the infant clean and dry.
   c. Frantic sucking—give pacifier between feedings; protect the infant's hands from excoriation.
   d. Poor feeding—give small, frequent feedings; maintain caloric and fluid intake requirement for the infant's desired weight.
   e. Vomiting/diarrhea—position the infant to prevent aspiration; provide good skin care to areas exposed to vomitus or stool.
   f. Muscle rigidity, hypertonicity.
      (i) Change position frequently to minimize development of pressure areas.
      (ii) Use sheepskin and provide good skin care.
   g. Increased salivation and/or nasal stuffiness.
      (i) Aspirate nasopharynx; suction tracheal mucus.
      (ii) Provide frequent nose and mouth care.
      (iii) Note respiration rate and characteristics and infant's color.
   h. Tachypnea.
      (i) Note onset and severity of accompanying signs of respiratory distress; place the infant on respiratory monitor.
      (ii) Position the infant for easier ventilation—semi-Fowler's position; tilt head back slightly.
      (iii) Minimize handling.
      (iv) Have resuscitative equipment available.
      (v) Tachycardia and hypertension—monitor vital signs closely; cardiopulmonary monitor may be indicated.

7. Assist mother in learning to care for infant, in efforts to promote bonding, and in her own alcohol or drug rehabilitation efforts.

8. Obtain further information and resources from March of Dimes Birth Defects Foundation, Community Services Department, 1275 Mamaroneck Avenue, White Plains, NY 10605, (914) 428-7100, *www.modimes.org*.

SELECTED REFERENCES

Als, H. et al. (1994). Individualized developmental care for the very-low-birth-weight preterm infant: medical and neurofunctional effects. *Journal of the American Medical Association, 272*(11), 854–858.

American Heart Association Regulatory Advisory. (1999). *Newborns and Mothers Health Protection Act: The interim final rule.* Washington DC: Author.

American Academy of Pediatrics/American College of Obstetricians and Gynecologists. (1998). *Guidelines for perinatal care.* Washington DC: Author.

American Academy of Pediatrics. (1994). Provisional committee for quality improvement and subcommittee on hyperbilirubinemia.

Practice parameter: Management of hyperbilirubinemia in the healthy term newborn. *Pediatrics, 94,* 558–565.

Avery, G., et al. (1994). *Neonatology pathophysiology and management of the newborn* (4th ed.). Philadelphia: J.B. Lippincott.

Ballard, J.L. et al. (1991). New Ballard score expanded to include extremely premature infants. *Journal of Pediatrics, 119,* 417–423.

Bear, K., et al. (1993). Management strategies for promoting successful breastfeeding. *Nursing Practice, 18*(6), 50, 53–54, 56–58.

Bell, G., & Lau, K. (1995). Perinatal and neonatal issues of substance abuse. *Pediatric Clinics of North America, 42*(2), 261–281.

Buchi, K. (1998). The drug exposed infant in the well baby nursery. *Clinical Perinatology, 25*(2), 335–348.

Canadian Pediatric Society. (1999). Approach to management of hyperbilirubinemia in term newborn infants. *Pediatric Child Health, 4,* 161–164.

Church, M.W., & Abel, E.L. (1998). Fetal alcohol syndrome. Hearing, speech, and vestibular disorders. *Obstetrics and Gynecology Clinics of North America, 36*(2), 255–266.

D'Apolito, K. (1998). Substance abuse: Infant and childhood outcomes. *Journal of Pediatric Nursing, 13*(5), 307–316.

Faller, H.S., et al. (1993). Sibling visitation: How far should the pendulum swing? *Journal of Pediatric Nursing, 8*(2), 92–99.

Furmon, L. (1993). Breastfeeding and full-time maternal employment: Does the baby lose out? *Journal of Human Lactation, 9*(1), 1–2.

Gowie, T.M., et al. (1994). *Foundations of maternal newborn nursing.* Philadelphia: W.B. Saunders.

Hadson, P. (1992). Health visitors, preventing postnatal illness. *Nursing Times, 88*(43), 68, 70.

Hagedorn, M.I., & Gardner, S.L. (1999). Hypoglycemia in the newborn. Part 1: Pathophysiology and nursing management. *Mother Baby Journal,* 15–24.

Hall, W.A., et al. (1993). Managing the early discharge experience: Taking control. *Journal of Advanced Nursing, 18*(4), 574–582.

Johnson and Johnson Consumer Products, Inc. (1996). *Compendium of postpartum care.* Skilman, NJ: Author.

Kaltenbach, K., Berghella, V., & Finnegan, L. (1998). Opioid dependence during pregnancy. Effects and management. *Obstetric and Gynecology Clinics of North America, 25*(1), 139–151.

Konrad, C. & Norton, J. (1998). Newborn temperature regulation: Challenges for mother–baby nurses. *Mother Baby Journal, 3*(4), 12–16.

Lockridge, T. (1999). Persistent pulmonary hypertension of the newborn. *Mother Baby Journal, 4*(2), 19–32.

Maisels, M.J., & Newman, T.B. (1995). Kernicterus in otherwise healthy breast-fed term newborns. *Pediatrics, 96*(4), 730–733.

May, K.A., & Mahlmeister, L.R. (1994). *Maternal and neonatal nursing: Family centered care* (3rd ed.). Philadelphia: J.B. Lippincott.

Parkin, P.C., et al. (1993). Randomized controlled trial of three interventions in the management of persistent crying of infancy. *Pediatrics, 92*(2), 197–201.

Peterec, S. (1995). Management of neonatal Rh disease. *Clinical Perinatology, 22*(3), 561–592.

Plessinger, M.A., & Woods, J.R. (1998). Cocaine in pregnancy. *Obstetric and Gynecology Clinics of North America, 25*(1), 99–118.

Reece, E.A., Sivan, E., Francis, G., & Homko, C. (1998). Pregnancy outcomes among women with and without diabetic microvascular disease (White's classes B to FR) versus non-diabetic controls. *American Journal of Perinatology, 15*(9), 549–555.

Schlosser, S.P. (1996). Yes, you can still exercise. *Childbirth planner.* Washington DC: Association of Women's Health, Obstetrics, and Neonatal Nurses (AWHONN).

Schlosser, S.P. (1996). Getting back into shape. *Childbirth planner.* Washington DC: AWHONN.

Simpson, K.R. & Creehan, P.A. (1996). *Perinatal nursing.* Philadelphia: J.B. Lippincott.

Tapero, E. & Honeyfield, M.E. (1996). *Physical assessment of the newborn* (2nd ed.). Petaluma, CA: NICU Ink.

Taeusch, H.W., & Ballard, R.A. (1998). *Avery's diseases of the newborn.* Philadelphia: W.B. Saunders.

Tyrala, E.E. (1996). The infant of the diabetic mother. *Obstetrics and Gynecology Clinics of North America, 23*(1), 221–240.

Wagner, C.L., Katikaneni, L.D., Cox, T.H., & Ryan, R.M. (1998). The impact of prenatal drug exposure on the neonate. *Obstetrics and Gynecology Clinics of North America, 21*(1), 169–194.

Watters, N.E., et al. (1995). The evaluation of combined mother/infant versus separate postnatal nursing care. *Research in Nursing, 18* (1), 17–26.

Complications of the Childbearing Experience

OBSTETRIC COMPLICATIONS

> **NURSING ALERT**
>
> Many obstetric complications involve the possibility of hemorrhage requiring blood replacement. Determine the patient's feelings and beliefs regarding the possibility of transfusions, and notify health care providers if transfusion is refused.

■ Ectopic Pregnancy

Ectopic pregnancy is any gestation located outside the uterine cavity. Often referred to as "tubal" pregnancy.

Pathophysiology and Etiology

1. The fertilized ovum implants outside the uterus.
   a. The most common site of implantation is the fallopian or uterine tube (Figure 39-1).
   b. Other sites include the abdomen and the ovaries.
2. Structural factors that prevent or delay the passage of the fertilized ovum include adhesions of the tube, salpingitis, congenital and developmental anomalies of the fallopian or uterine tube, previous ectopic pregnancy, use of an intrauterine device (IUD) for >2 years, and multiple induced elective abortions.
3. Functional factors include menstrual reflux and decreased tubal motility.
4. Contributing factors may include:
   a. History of pelvic inflammatory disease (PID)
   b. Endometriosis
   c. Previous tubal surgery
   d. Uterine curettage
   e. Maternal age and race
   f. Renal disease and/or transplant

Clinical Manifestations

1. Intermittent abdominal or pelvic pain.
2. Amenorrhea—in 75% of the cases.
3. Irregular vaginal bleeding—usually scanty and dark.
4. Uterine size is usually similar to what it would be in a normally implanted pregnancy.
5. Abdominal tenderness on palpation.
6. Shoulder pain.
7. Increased pulse and anxiety.
8. Nausea, vomiting, faintness, or vertigo and syncope with abdominal pain may develop. Pelvic examination reveals a pelvic mass, posterior or lateral to the uterus, adnexal tenderness, and cervical pain on movement of the cervix.

> **NURSING ALERT**
>
> Pain may become severe if a tubal rupture occurs, and clinical presentation will be that of shock.

Diagnostic Evaluation

1. Serum β-human chorionic gonadotropin (β-HCG)—when done serially, will not show characteristic rise as in intrauterine pregnancy
2. Ultrasound—may identify tubal mass, absence of gestational sac within the uterus

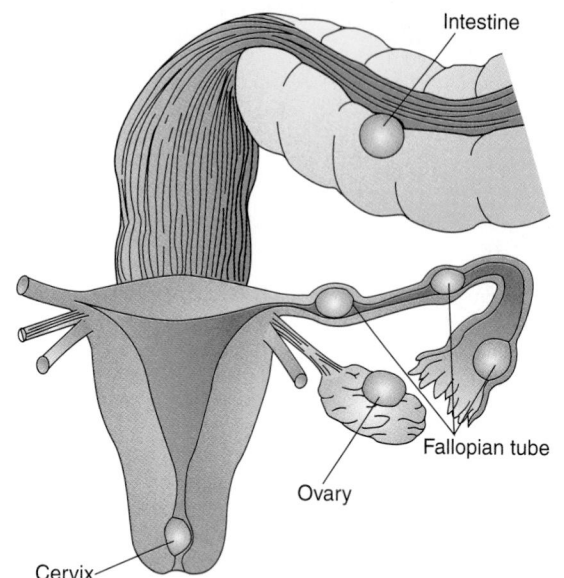

FIGURE 39-1 Sites of ectopic pregnancy.

3. Culdocentesis—bloody aspirate from the cul-de-sac of Douglas indicates intraperitoneal bleeding from tubal rupture
4. Laparoscopy—visualization of tubal pregnancy
5. Laparotomy—indication for surgery if there is any question about the diagnosis

Management
1. Conservative therapy is chosen should the patient desire future childbearing. Treatment with methotrexate is fast becoming the standard of care for ectopic therapy. Goal of treatment is to remove ectopic pregnancy and preserve productive function.
   a. Single-dose methotrexate intramuscular (IM) administration. Often given on outpatient basis. Must meet criteria as set forth by ACOG:
      (i) Ectopic size 3 cm or less.
      (ii) Desire for future fertility.
      (iii) Stable or rising hCG levels with peak values below 15,000 mIU/mL (IRP).
      (iv) Tubal serosa intact.
      (v) No active bleeding.
      (vi) Ectopic pregnancy fully visualized at laparoscopy.
      (vii) Selected cases of cervical and cornual pregnancy.
   b. Eliminates side effects caused by multiple dosing: gastritis, stomatitis, increased hepatic transaminase levels, leukopenia, and thrombocytopenia.
   c. Increased safety and patient acceptance.
   d. Requires less medication, thus decreases patient follow-up and cost of treatment.
   e. Contraindications:

(i) Poor patient compliance.
(ii) History of active herpes or renal disease.
(iii) Presence of fetal cardiac activity.
(iv) Abnormal serum creatinine or serum glutamic oxalacetic transaminase (SGOT).
(v) Active peptic ulcer disease.
(vi) Blood leukocyte count of <3000 or a platelet count of <100,000.

2. If woman does not consent to or meet criteria for methotrexate and she desires future fertility, surgical intervention is instituted. The surgical procedure depends on the extent of tubal involvement and if rupture has occurred. The surgery of choice used to preserve future fertility is a salpingostomy. Should a woman not desire future fertility, the surgery of choice is salpingectomy. Other surgeries range from removal of ectopic pregnancy with tubal resection, salpingostomy (removes conceptus leaving tube intact, yet scarred), and possibly salpingo-oophorectomy.
3. Treat shock and hemorrhage if necessary.
4. Administer RhIG (immune globulin) per institutional policy if woman is Rh negative.

Nursing Assessment
Evaluate the following to determine pregnancy and to monitor for changes in patient's status, such as rupture or hemorrhage:
1. Maternal vital signs
2. Presence and amount of vaginal bleeding
3. Amount and type of pain
4. Presence of abdominal tenderness on palpation/shoulder pain
5. Date of last menstrual period
6. Presence of positive pregnancy test
7. Rh type

Nursing Diagnoses
- Risk for Fluid Volume Deficit related to blood loss from ruptured tube
- Pain related to ectopic pregnancy or rupture and bleeding into the peritoneal cavity
- Anticipatory Grieving related to loss of pregnancy and potential loss of childbearing capacity

Nursing Interventions
Maintaining Fluid Volume
1. Establish an intravenous (IV) line with a large-bore catheter, and infuse fluids and blood products as prescribed.
2. Obtain blood samples for complete blood count (CBC) and type and screen for whole blood, as directed.
3. Monitor vital signs and urine output frequently, depending on condition.

Promoting Comfort
1. Administer analgesics as needed and prescribed.
2. Encourage the use of relaxation techniques.

Providing Support During Grief

1. Be available to patient and provide emotional support.
2. Listen to concerns of patient and significant others.
3. Be aware that family may be experiencing denial or other stage of grieving.
4. Suggest referrals such as social worker, psychiatrist, and clergy, as appropriate. Suggest grief counseling.

   Note: The term *family* may refer to a nontraditional group of persons, such as the patient and significant other, friend, sibling, parent, or grandparent.

Patient Education and Health Maintenance

1. Teach signs and symptoms related to ectopic pregnancy to women at risk including increased vaginal bleeding, severe abdominal pain, shoulder pain, nausea, and/or vomiting.
2. Instruct woman to report to her primary care provider should any signs and symptoms be present or to emergency room if condition is severe.
3. Instruct woman to bring support person(s) with her when she comes to the hospital/clinic.
4. Encourage grief counseling and supportive care at home.
5. Teach signs of postoperative infection including fever, abdominal pain, and increased or malodorous vaginal discharge.
6. Reinforce that chances of another ectopic pregnancy are increased and that subsequent conception potential may be decreased, based on health care provider's explanation.
7. Discuss contraception.
8. Teach signs of recurrent ectopic pregnancy—abnormal vaginal bleeding, abdominal pain, menstrual irregularity.

Outcome-Based Evaluation

- Vital signs stable
- Verbalizes pain relief
- Patient and support person express sorrow over their loss

Hydatidiform Mole

Hydatidiform mole (gestational trophoblastic disease) is an abnormal pregnancy resulting from a developmental anomaly of the placenta. It is characterized by the conversion of the chorionic villi into a mass of clear vesicles. There may be no fetus, or a degenerating fetus may be present.

Pathophysiology and Etiology

1. It is believed to be derived from genetic abnormalities as the paternal haploid, X-carrying set of chromosomes that reaches 46 XX by its own duplication. Not all moles have the 46 XX chromosomal makeup.
2. It arises in fetal rather than maternal tissue.
3. Large amounts of hCG are present secondary to the proliferation of chorionic tissue. Assay values of β-hCG are elevated in the condition.
4. Contributing factors may include chromosomal abnormalities, malnutrition, hormonal imbalance, age under 20 or over 40, and low economic status.

Clinical Manifestations

1. First trimester vaginal bleeding
2. Absence of fetal heart tones and fetal structures
3. Rapid enlargement of the uterus; size greater than dates
4. β-hCG titers greater than expected for gestational age
5. Expulsion of the vesicles
6. Hyperemesis (severe nausea and vomiting)
7. Signs of pregnancy-induced hypertension (PIH) before 24 weeks' gestation

Diagnostic Evaluation

1. β-hCG levels—elevated
2. Ultrasound—shows a characteristic picture of the mole in most cases

Management

1. Suction curettage is the method of choice for immediate evacuation of the mole with possibility of laparotomy.
2. Follow-up for detection of malignant changes because a complication is the development of choriocarcinoma of the endometrium.
3. Administer RhIG (RhoGAM) per institutional policy if woman is Rh negative.

Nursing Assessment

1. Monitor maternal vital signs; note presence of hypertension.
2. Assess the amount and type of vaginal bleeding; note the presence of any other vaginal discharge.
3. Assess the urine for the presence of protein.
4. Palpate uterine height; if above the umbilicus, measure the fundal height.
5. Determine date of last menstrual period and date of positive pregnancy test.
6. Rh type.

Nursing Diagnoses

- Potential for Fluid Volume Deficit related to maternal hemorrhage
- Anxiety related to loss of pregnancy and medical interventions

Nursing Interventions

Maintaining Fluid Volume

1. Obtain blood samples for type and screen, and have 2 to 4 units of whole blood available for possible replacement.
2. Establish and maintain IV line; start with a large needle to accommodate possible transfusion and large quantities of fluid.
3. Assess maternal vital signs, and evaluate bleeding.
4. Monitor laboratory results to evaluate patient's status.

Decreasing Anxiety

1. Prepare the patient for surgery. Explain preoperative and postoperative care along with intraoperative procedures.

2. Educate patient and family on the disease process.
3. Allow the family to grieve over the loss of the pregnancy.

Patient Education and Health Maintenance
1. Advise the woman on the need for continuous follow-up care.
2. Provide reinforcement of follow-up procedures:
   a. Measure hCG levels every 1 to 2 weeks until normal—then begin monthly testing for 6 months, then every 2 months for a total of 1 year.
   b. Consider chemotherapy or hysterectomy if β-hCG levels rise or begin to plateau or there is evidence of metastasis.
3. Encourage ongoing discussion of care with health care provider.

Outcome-Based Evaluation
- Vital signs stable; laboratory work within normal limits
- Verbalizes concerns about self and related procedures; describes follow-up care and its importance

▣ Spontaneous Abortion

Spontaneous abortion is the unintended termination of pregnancy at any time before the fetus has attained viability (20 weeks' gestation or fetal weight of <500 g [1.1 lb]). See Table 39-1. For a discussion of therapeutic or voluntary abortion, see Box 39-1.

Pathophysiology and Etiology
1. Cause frequently unknown, but 50% are due to chromosomal anomalies
2. Exposure or contact with teratogenic agents.
3. Poor maternal nutritional status.
4. Maternal illness with virus such as rubella, cytomegalovirus (CMV), active herpes, and toxoplasmosis, or specific bacterial microorganisms that put the pregnancy at risk.
5. History of diabetes, thyroid disease, anticardiolipin antibodies, or lupus erythematosus.
6. Smoking or drug abuse or both.
7. Immunologic factor by which the mother and father are genetically similar, with similar major antigens that cause the maternal immune system to reject the embryo.
8. Luteal phase defect.
9. Postmature sperm or ova.
10. Abnormal uterine development or structural defect in the maternal reproductive system (including an incompetent cervix).
11. Imperfect sperm or ova.
12. Environmental factors such as drugs, radiation, or trauma.

Clinical Manifestations
1. Uterine cramping, low back pain.
2. Vaginal bleeding usually begins as dark spotting, then progresses to frank bleeding as the embryo separates from the uterus.

TABLE 39-1 Types of Spontaneous Abortions

Classification	Clinical Manifestations	Management
1. Threatened	Vaginal bleeding or spotting Mild cramps Tenderness over uterus, simulates mild labor or persistent low backache with feeling of pelvic pressure Cervix closed or slightly dilated Symptoms subside or develop into inevitable abortion	Vaginal examination Bed rest (some clinicians will not limit activity in belief that the embryo will be aborted anyway) Pad count
2. Inevitable	Bleeding more profuse Cervix dilated Membranes rupture Painful uterine contractions	Embryo delivered, followed by dilatation and curettage (D&C)
3. Habitual	Spontaneous abortion occurs in successive pregnancies (three or more)	D&C Treatment of possible causes: hormonal imbalance, tumors, thyroid dysfunction, abnormal uterus, incompetent cervix; with treatment, 70% to 80% carry a pregnancy successfully Hysterogram to rule out uterine abnormalities, infections Surgical suturing of the cervix if incompetent cervix is a causative factor
4. Incomplete	Fetus usually expelled Placenta and membranes retained	D&C
5. Missed	Fetus dies in utero and is retained Maceration No symptoms of abortion, but symptoms of pregnancy regress (uterine size, breast changes)	Real time ultrasound, and if second trimester, fetal monitoring to determine if fetus is dead If fetus is not passed after diagnosis, oxytocin induction may be used. Retained dead fetus may lead to development of disseminated intravascular coagulation or infection Fibrinogen concentrations should be measured weekly

BOX 39-1   Therapeutic or Voluntary Abortion

Therapeutic abortion is the termination of pregnancy before fetal viability for the purpose of safeguarding the woman's health. Elective abortion is the termination of a pregnancy before fetal viability as a choice of the woman.

Procedures

- First-trimester abortions can be managed by dilation and curettage (D&C) or dilation and suction.
- Second-trimester abortions can be managed using prostaglandin E_2 vaginal suppositories or by IM injection of F_2 analogs. Laminaria or magnesium sulfate tents may be used before prostaglandin induction to "soften" the cervix and assist with dilatation.
- Late second-trimester abortions can be done using intra-amniotic saline injection, hysterotomy, or hysterectomy.

Complications

- Retained products of conception
- Hemorrhage
- Prostaglandin complications including fever, diarrhea, nausea and vomiting, tachycardia, and bronchoconstriction
- Surgical complications including uterine perforation, bowel trauma, cervical laceration

Nursing Considerations

- Review the woman's knowledge of her choice and the options available in regard to childbearing to allow for informed decision making.
- Ensure that patient understands the possible benefits and risks of a therapeutic or voluntary abortion.
- Encourage patient to have support person accompany her and drive her home after the procedure.
- Teach that cramping and bleeding, similar to a regular menstrual period, can be expected. Length of bleeding varies, but it usually subsides in 3 to 4 days.
- Discuss the need for contraception, and advise when to begin again.
- Inform that a normal menstrual cycle should resume in 4 to 6 weeks.
- Discuss the need for pelvic rest, as ordered (usually 2 to 3 weeks), to prevent infection, consisting of avoidance of sexual intercourse, douching, inserting tampons, and so forth.
- Teach signs of infection (fever, pelvic pain, increased bleeding), and advise to report them to health care provider immediately.
- Arrange for follow-up appointment and counseling, if necessary.

---

3. β-hCG levels may be elevated for as long as 2 weeks after loss of the embryo.

Diagnostic Evaluation

1. Ultrasonic evaluation of the gestational sac or embryo
2. Visualization of the cervix; presence of dilation or tissue evaluated

Complications

1. Hemorrhage
2. Uterine infection
3. Septicemia
4. Disseminated intravascular coagulation (DIC) in a missed abortion

Nursing Assessment

1. Evaluate the amount and color of blood that is present; determine the time the bleeding began and any precipitating factors.
2. Determine whether a positive pregnancy test has previously been obtained, also the date of the last menstrual period.
3. Monitor maternal vital signs for indications of complications such as hemorrhage, infection.
4. Evaluate any blood or clot tissue for the presence of fetal membranes, placenta, or fetus.

Nursing Diagnoses

- Risk for Fluid Volume Deficit related to maternal bleeding
- Anticipatory Grieving related to loss of pregnancy, cause of the abortion, future childbearing

- Risk for Infection related to dilated cervix and open uterine vessels
- Pain related to uterine cramping and possible procedures

Nursing Interventions

Maintaining Fluid Volume

1. Report any tachycardia, hypotension, diaphoresis, or pallor, indicating hemorrhage and shock.
2. Draw blood for type and screen for possible blood administration.
3. Establish and maintain an IV with large-bore catheter for possible transfusion and large quantities of fluid replacement.
4. Inspect all tissue passed for completeness.

Providing Support Through the Grieving Process

1. Assess the reaction of patient and support person, and provide information regarding current status, as needed.
2. Encourage the patient to discuss feelings about the loss of the baby; include effects on relationship with the father.
3. Do not minimize the loss by focusing on future childbearing; rather acknowledge the loss and allow grieving.
4. Provide time alone for the couple to discuss their feelings.
5. Discuss the prognosis of future pregnancies with the couple.
6. If the fetus is aborted intact, provide an opportunity for viewing, if parents desire.
7. Refer to chaplain or social worker if indicated or requested.

Preventing Infection

1. Evaluate temperature every 4 hours if normal, and every 2 hours if elevated.

2. Check vaginal drainage for increased amount and odor, which may indicate infection.
3. Instruct on and encourage perineal care after each urination and defecation to prevent contamination.

Promoting Comfort
1. Instruct patient on the cause of pain to decrease anxiety.
2. Instruct and encourage the use of relaxation techniques to augment analgesics.
3. Administer pain medications as needed and as prescribed.

Community and Home Care Considerations
1. Teach patient with threatened abortion signs and symptoms of hemorrhage.
2. Discuss emergency access to care with patient and support personnel.
3. If the woman should pass anything through her vagina, instruct her not to discard it, but to bring it to the hospital/clinic with her for evaluation.
4. Explain to woman to bring her support person(s) with her to the hospital/clinic.

Patient Education and Health Maintenance
1. Provide the names of local support groups for couples who have experienced an early pregnancy loss. Resolve groups may be available through a local hospital.
2. Discuss with the couple the methods of contraception to be used.
3. Explain the need to wait at least 3 to 6 months before attempting another pregnancy.
4. Teach the woman to observe for signs of infection (fever, pelvic pain, change in character and amount of vaginal discharge), and advise to report them to provider immediately.
5. Provide information regarding genetic testing of the products of conception if indicated; send the specimen according to policy.

Outcome-Based Evaluation
- Vital signs remain normal; minimal blood loss
- Expresses feelings regarding the loss of the pregnancy by demonstrating normal signs of grief
- No signs of infection, temperature normal, performs perineal care
- Verbalizes relief of pain

◼ Hyperemesis Gravidarum
Hyperemesis gravidarum is exaggerated nausea and vomiting during pregnancy. Hyperemesis gravidarum can be experienced with or without food intake at any time of the day.

Pathophysiology and Etiology
1. Occurs during the first 16 weeks' gestation. Cause unknown but may possibly result from high levels of hCG or estrogen.
2. Accompanied by appetite disturbances that are intractable in nature.

3. Psychological factors including neurosis or altered self-concept may be contributory.
4. Seen in molar pregnancies, multiple gestation, and history of hyperemesis in previous pregnancies.
5. Slowed gastric motility occurs.
6. The persistent vomiting may result in fluid and electrolyte imbalances, dehydration, jaundice, and elevation of serum transaminase.

Clinical Manifestations
1. Persistent vomiting; inability to tolerate anything by mouth.
2. Dehydration—fever, dry skin, decreased urine output.
3. Weight loss (up to 5% to 10% of body weight).
4. Severity of symptoms increases as the disease progresses.

Diagnostic Evaluation
1. Tests may be done to rule out other conditions causing vomiting (cholecystitis, appendicitis), pancreatitis, or hepatitis.
2. Liver function studies—elevated alanine aminotransferase (ALT) and aspartate aminotransferase (AST) up to four times normal in severe cases.
3. Prothrombin time, partial thromboplastin time usually normal.
4. Blood urea nitrogen (BUN) and creatinine—may be slightly elevated.
5. Serum electrolytes—may be hypokalemia, hypo- or hypernatremia; loss of hydrogen and chloride.
6. Urine for ketones—positive.

Management
1. Try withholding food and fluid for 24 hours, or until vomiting stops and appetite returns; then restart small feedings.
2. Control of vomiting may require antiemetics such as:
   a. Prochlorperazine (Compazine) in injectable or rectal suppository form.
   b. Metoclopramide (Reglan).
   c. Meclizine (Antivert).
   d. Ondansetron (Zofran)—expensive and used less frequently.
3. Control of dehydration through IV fluids—often 1 to 3 L of dextrose solution with electrolytes and vitamins, as needed. Bicarbonate may be given for acidosis.
4. Most women respond quickly to restricting oral intake and giving IV fluids, but repeated episodes may occur.
5. Rarely, total parenteral nutrition is needed.
6. Rarely, complications of hepatic or renal failure or coma could result from disease progression.

Nursing Assessment
1. Evaluate weight gain or loss pattern. Compare the prepregnant weight with the current weight.
2. Evaluate 24- or 48-hour dietary recall.
3. Evaluate environment for factors that may affect the woman's appetite. Determine if woman is ingesting nonfood substances (known as pica) such as starch, clay, or toothpaste.

4. Monitor vital signs for tachycardia, hypotension, and fever due to dehydration.

5. Assess skin turgor and mucous membranes for signs of dehydration.

Nursing Diagnoses

• Risk for Fluid Volume Deficit, Electrolyte Imbalance related to prolonged vomiting
• Altered Nutrition: Less Than Body Requirements related to prolonged vomiting
• Ineffective Individual Coping related to stress of pregnancy and illness
• Fear related to concerns for fetal well-being

Nursing Interventions

Maintaining Fluid Volume

1. Establish an IV line, and administer IV fluids as prescribed.
2. Monitor serum electrolytes, and report abnormalities.
3. Medicate with antiemetics as prescribed. Administer intramuscularly (IM) or by rectal suppository to avoid loss of dose through vomiting.
4. Maintain NPO status except for ice chips until vomiting has stopped.
5. Assess intake and output, urine specific gravity and ketones, vital signs, skin turgor, and fetal heart tones as indicated by condition.

Encouraging Adequate Nutrition

1. Advise the woman that oral intake can be restarted when emesis has stopped and appetite returns.
2. Begin small feedings. Suggest or provide bland solid foods; serve hot foods hot and cold foods cold; do not serve lukewarm.
   a. Avoid greasy, gassy, and spicy foods.
   b. Provide liquids at times other than meal times.
3. Suggest or provide an environment conducive to eating.
   a. Keep room cool and quiet before and after meals.
   b. Keep emesis pan handy, yet out of sight.

Strengthening Coping Mechanisms

1. Allow patient to verbalize feelings regarding this pregnancy.
2. Encourage patient to discuss any personal stress that may have a negative effect on this pregnancy.
3. Refer to social service and counseling services as needed.

Allaying Fears

1. Explain the effects of all medications and procedures on maternal as well as fetal health.
2. Accentuate the positive signs of fetal well-being.
3. Praise mother for attempts at following nutritious diet and healthy lifestyle.

Patient Education and Health Maintenance

1. Educate the woman about proper diet and nutrition in pregnancy.
2. Educate the woman about healthy weight gain in pregnancy.
3. Educate the woman on the need for child care during the periods of severe nausea and vomiting.

4. Encourage the woman to move slowly, avoiding quick changes of position. Quick changes of position can cause vertigo and then nausea and vomiting.
5. Educate the woman on the need to take antiemetics during the nausea phase, before vomiting occurs.
6. Educate the woman on tips to assist with hyperemesis gravidarum.
   a. Eat dry toast or crackers before rising from bed or anytime nausea begins.
   b. Get fresh, outside air daily; lie down in a semiprone position.
   c. Drink spearmint or peppermint tea.
   d. Take vitamin B_6 50 to 100 mg daily.
   e. Avoid food odors.
   f. Eat smaller, frequent meals.
7. Educate the woman that if all interventions fail, contact her primary care provider.

Outcome-Based Evaluation

• Demonstrates signs of normal hydration with no ketosis 6 hours after treatment initiated. Urine output adequate; urine specific gravity within normal limits; blood pressure stable
• Tolerates small, bland feedings without vomiting
• Verbalizes concerns and stresses related to pregnancy
• Mother expresses confidence in baby's well-being

▨ Placenta Previa

Placenta previa is the abnormal implantation of the placenta in the lower uterine segment, partially or completely covering the internal cervical os (Figure 39-2). Classified as total (implantation totally obstructs the cervical os), partial (implantation partially obstructs the cervical os), marginal (placental edge approaches the cervical os), or low-lying (implantation is in the lower part of uterus rather than upper); however, during labor, classification may change as the cervix dilates. Placenta previa occurs in 3 to 6 per 1,000 pregnancies.

Pathophysiology and Etiology

1. The cause is unknown.
2. One possible theory states that the embryo will implant in the lower uterine segment if the decidua in the uterine fundus is not favorable or delayed implantation.
3. About 80% of placenta previa episodes occur in multiparas.
4. Seen more often with history of abortion, cesarean section, uterine scarring, or prior placenta previa.
5. Age greater than 35 years of age.
6. Conditions that yield abnormally large placentas such as multifetal gestation or Rh isoimmunization.

Clinical Manifestations

1. Cardinal sign is painless vaginal bleeding, which usually appears near the end of the second trimester or later. Bleeding appears without warning.

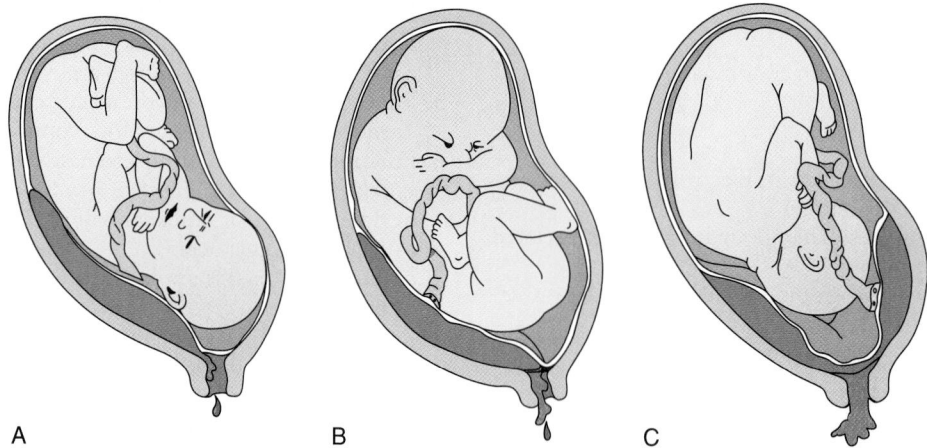

FIGURE 39-2 Degrees of placenta previa. (**A**) Low implantation. (**B**) Partial placenta previa. (**C**)Total placenta previa.

2. Initial episode is rarely fatal and usually stops spontaneously, with subsequent bleeding episodes occurring spontaneously; each episode is more profuse than the previous one.
3. Bleeding from placenta previa may not occur until cervical dilation occurs and the placenta is loosened from the uterus.
4. With a complete placenta previa, the bleeding will occur earlier in the pregnancy and be more profuse.

Diagnostic Evaluation
1. Transabdominal ultrasound is the method of choice to show location of the placenta.
2. If findings are questionable, transvaginal ultrasound can improve the accuracy of diagnosis. Due to bleeding tendencies, however, this must be done by a highly skilled technician.
3. Sterile speculum examination can also confirm placenta previa.

Management
1. Conservative management with bed rest and hospitalization until fetus is mature and delivery can be accomplished as usual.
2. If woman is discharged, she needs availability of immediate transport to the hospital for recurrent bleeding.
3. IV access and at least 2 units of blood should be available at all times.
4. Continuous maternal and fetal monitoring.
5. Amniocentesis may be done to determine fetal lung maturity for possible delivery.
6. Cesarean section is often indicated if the degree of previa is >30% or if there is excessive bleeding. The cesarean section may be performed immediately.
7. Vaginal delivery may sometimes be attempted in a marginal previa without active bleeding.

8. A pediatric specialty team may be needed at delivery due to prematurity and other neonatal complications.

Complications
1. Fetal mortality resulting from hypoxia in utero and prematurity
2. Immediate hemorrhage, with possible shock and maternal death
3. Postpartum hemorrhage resulting from decreased contractility of uterine muscle

Nursing Assessment
1. Determine the amount and type of bleeding; also, review any history of bleeding throughout this pregnancy.
2. Inquire as to the presence or absence of pain in association with the bleeding.
3. Record maternal and fetal vital signs.
4. Palpate for the presence of uterine contractions.
5. Evaluate laboratory data on hemoglobin and hematocrit status.
6. Assess the fetal status with fetal monitoring.

NURSING ALERT

 Never perform a vaginal examination on anyone who is bleeding until a previa has been ruled out. This may puncture the placenta.

Nursing Diagnoses
- Altered Tissue Perfusion, Placental, related to excessive bleeding causing fetal compromise
- Fluid Volume Deficit related to excessive bleeding
- Risk for Infection related to excessive blood loss and open vessels near cervix
- Anxiety related to excessive bleeding, procedures, and possible maternal–fetal complications

Nursing Interventions
Promoting Tissue Perfusion
1. Frequently monitor mother and fetus.
2. Administer IV fluids, as prescribed.
3. Position on side to promote placental perfusion.
4. Administer oxygen by face mask, as indicated.
5. Prepare for emergency delivery, as needed.

Maintaining Fluid Volume
1. Establish and maintain a large-bore IV line, as prescribed, and draw blood for type and screen for blood replacement.
2. Position in a sitting position to allow the weight of fetus to compress the placenta and decrease bleeding.
3. Maintain strict bed rest during any bleeding episode.
4. If bleeding is profuse and delivery cannot be delayed, prepare the woman physically and emotionally for a cesarean delivery.
5. Administer blood or blood products protocol per institutional policy.

NURSING ALERT

Women who have had a placenta previa are at risk for postpartum hemorrhage because of the decreased contractility of the lower uterine segment and the large space the placenta occupied.

Preventing Infection
1. Use aseptic technique when providing care.
2. Evaluate temperature every 4 hours unless elevated; then, evaluate every 2 hours.
3. Evaluate white blood cell (WBC) and differential count.
4. Teach perineal care and handwashing techniques.
5. Assess odor of all vaginal bleeding or lochia.

Decreasing Anxiety
1. Explain all treatments and procedures, and answer all related questions.
2. Encourage verbalization of feelings by patient and family.
3. Provide information on a cesarean delivery, and prepare patient emotionally.
4. Discuss the effects of long-term hospitalization or prolonged bed rest.

Community and Home Care Considerations
1. Can care for placenta previa and other antenatal bleeding disorders at home with the following criteria:
   a. No active bleeding.
   b. No signs and symptoms of preterm labor (PTL).
   c. Home close to medical facility—maximum of 15 to 20 minutes away.
   d. Emergency support readily available.
2. Teach the woman signs and symptoms of hemorrhage. Woman is to report to Labor and Delivery immediately if bleeding occurs.
3. Monitor vaginal discharge and bleeding after each urination and bowel movement.
4. Instruct the woman on doing home uterine activity monitoring (HUAM) daily by way of palpation or electronic telemetry units.
5. Instruct the woman on fetal movement counts (kick counts) to be performed on daily basis.
6. Perform daily or twice weekly nonstress test (NST) or home visits and daily provider contact.
7. Instruct the woman to have support person(s) readily available.
8. Instruct the woman that there is to be nothing in the vagina. Discuss alternative methods of sexual gratification.

Patient Education and Health Maintenance
1. Educate the woman and her family about the etiology and treatment of placenta previa.
2. Educate the woman to inform medical personnel about her diagnosis and not to have vaginal examinations.
3. Educate the woman who is discharged from the hospital with a placenta previa to avoid intercourse or anything per vagina, to limit physical activity, to have an accessible person in the event of an emergency, and to go to the hospital immediately for repeat bleeding or uterine contractions >6 per hour.

Outcome-Based Evaluation
- Fetal condition stable
- Absence of shock, stable vital signs, absence of bleeding
- Does not develop any symptoms of an infection
- Verbalizes concerns and understanding of procedures and treatments

▦ Abruptio Placentae

Abruptio placentae is premature separation of the normally implanted placenta. It may be classified as partial, complete, or marginal. Hemorrhage can be either occult or apparent. With an occult hemorrhage, the placenta separates centrally, and a large amount of blood is accumulated under the placenta. When an apparent hemorrhage is present, the separation is along the placental margin, and blood flows under the membranes and through the cervix (Figure 39-3).

Pathophysiology and Etiology
1. Frequently, the etiology is unknown.
2. Women at risk for developing abruptio placentae include those with history of hypertension or previous abruptio placentae; those who have rapid decompression of the uterine cavity, short umbilical cord or presence of a uterine anomaly or tumor; preterm premature rupture of membranes (PPROM) at <34 weeks' gestation, uterine fibroids, increased parity (>6), or multiple gestation.
3. Additional risk occurs in existing pregnancies complicated by blunt abdominal trauma, supine hypotension, pregnancy-induced hypertension (PIH), alcohol, cigarette smoking, and cocaine or amphetamine abuse.
4. Hemorrhage occurs into the decidua basalis.

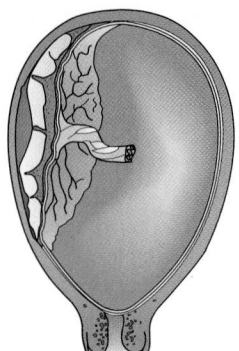 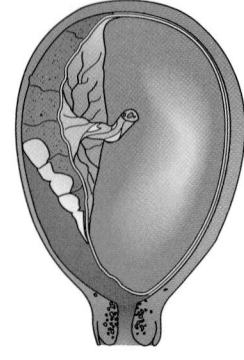 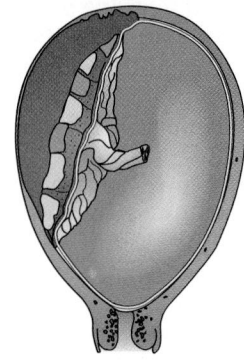

FIGURE 39-3 Abruptio placentae—premature separation of the placenta.

Partial Separation (Concealed Hemorrhage)

Partial Separation (Apparent Hemorrhage)

Complete Separation (Concealed Hemorrhage)

5. The decidua basalis then forms a hematoma.
6. This hematoma can expand as the bleeding increases, causing the hematoma to increase in size and further detach the placenta from the uterine wall.

Clinical Manifestations

1. Sudden onset, intense, localized, uterine pain/tenderness with (external) or without (occult) vaginal bleeding.
2. Uterine contractions may be low amplitude and high frequency.
3. Fetal heart rate (FHR) may change, depending on the degree of hemorrhage; increased FHR (tachycardia), late decelerations, and/or decreased variability.
4. Abdominal pain is often present due to increased uterine activity.
5. Abruptio placentae grades:
   a. Grade 0 (mild)—small retroplacental clot or small rupture of marginal sinus; <100 mL blood
   b. Grade 1 (moderate)—small retroplacental clot; detachment <50%; >100 mL but <500 mL blood
   c. Grade 2 (moderate to severe)—significant retroplacental clot; detachment approaches 50%; blood loss approaches 500 mL
   d. Grade 3 (moderate to severe)—significant retroplacental clot; detachment >50%; >500 mL blood loss

Diagnostic Evaluation

1. Based on woman's history, physical examination, laboratory studies, and signs and symptoms, including vaginal bleeding, abdominal pain, uterine contractions, uterine tenderness, fetal distress. Not all may be seen in every case.
2. Ultrasound is done but is not always sensitive enough to rule out the diagnosis.
3. Laboratory screen for APT on mother's blood to check for fetal hemoglobin.

Management

Management depends on the maternal and fetal status and degree of bleeding.

1. Mild—conservative management with bed rest, tocolytics, and evaluation of fetus with fetal assessment methods until fetal lung maturity can be established and delivery accomplished.
2. Moderate—augment labor if stable and decreased blood loss. Vaginal delivery is accomplished if cervix dilates. If fetal or maternal status deteriorates and/or blood loss is excessive, cesarean delivery is performed.
3. Moderate to severe—restore and maintain maternal physiologic status; IV/blood replacement.
4. Management of hemorrhagic shock with fluid resuscitation.
5. A pediatric specialty team may be necessary at delivery due to prematurity and neonatal complications.

Complications

1. Maternal shock
2. DIC
3. Amniotic fluid embolism (AFE)
4. Postpartum hemorrhage
5. Prematurity
6. Maternal/fetal death
7. Adult respiratory distress syndrome (ARDS)
8. Sheehan's syndrome (postpartum pituitary necrosis)
9. Renal tubular necroses
10. Rapid labor and delivery

Nursing Assessment

See Table 39-2.

1. Determine the amount and type of bleeding and the presence or absence of pain.
2. Monitor maternal and fetal vital signs, especially maternal blood pressure, pulse, FHR, and FHR variability.
3. Palpate the abdomen.
   a. Note the presence of contractions and relaxation between contractions (if contractions are present).
   b. If contractions are not present, assess the abdomen for firmness.
4. Measure and record fundal height to evaluate the presence of concealed bleeding.
5. Prepare for possible delivery.

TABLE 39-2 Characteristics of Abruptio Placentae and Placenta Previa

Characteristic	Abruptio Placentae	Placenta Previa
Onset	Third trimester	Third trimester (commonly in 8th month)
Bleeding	May be concealed, external dark hemorrhage, or bloody amniotic fluid	Mostly external, small to profuse in amount, bright red
Pain and uterine tenderness	Usually present; irritable uterus, progresses to board-like consistency	Usually absent; uterus soft
Fetal heart tone	May be irregular or absent	Usually normal
Presenting part	May or may not be engaged	Usually not engaged
Shock	Moderate to severe depending on extent of concealed and external hemorrhage	Usually not present unless bleeding is excessive
Delivery	Immediate delivery, usually by cesarean section	Delivery may be delayed, depending on size of fetus and amount of bleeding

Nursing Diagnoses
- Altered Placental Tissue Perfusion related to excessive bleeding, hypotension, and decreased cardiac output
- Fluid Volume Deficit related to excessive bleeding
- Fear related to excessive bleeding, procedures, and unknown outcome

Nursing Interventions
Maintaining Tissue Perfusion
1. Evaluate amount of bleeding by weighing all pads. Monitor CBC results and vital signs.
2. Position in the left lateral position, with the head elevated to enhance placental perfusion.
3. Administer oxygen through a face mask at 8 to 12 L. Maintain oxygen saturation level above 90% if using pulse oximetry monitoring.
4. Evaluate fetal status with continuous external fetal monitoring.
5. Encourage relaxation techniques.
6. Prepare for possible cesarean delivery should maternal or fetal compromise be evident.

Maintaining Fluid Volume
1. Establish and maintain large-bore IV line for fluids and blood products as prescribed.
2. Evaluate coagulation studies.
3. Monitor maternal vital signs and contractions.
4. Monitor vaginal bleeding, and evaluate fundal height to detect an increase in bleeding.

Decreasing Fear
1. Inform the woman and her family about the status of both herself and the fetus.
2. Explain all procedures in advance when possible or as they are performed.
3. Answer questions in a calm manner, using simple terms.
4. Encourage the presence of a support person.

Patient Education and Health Maintenance
1. Provide information to the woman and her family regarding etiology and treatment for abruptio placentae.
2. Encourage involvement from the neonatal team regarding education related to fetal/neonatal outcome.
3. Teach high-risk women the signs and symptoms of placental abruption and increased uterine activity.
4. Instruct woman to report to Labor and Delivery immediately should excessive bleeding and/or pain occur at home.
5. Instruct woman to have emergency plan in place for transport to medical facility expediently. Important to have support person(s) aware of procedures as well.

Outcome-Based Evaluation
- FHR within normal range, without a loss of variability
- Absence of shock, demonstrated by stable maternal vital signs after initiation of treatment
- Demonstrates concern; asks questions

Hypertensive States of Pregnancy
Hypertensive states of pregnancy encompass distinct clinical groups. These states are classified as such:
1. *Pregnancy-induced hypertension* (PIH) is a disorder occurring during pregnancy after the 20th week of gestation. It occurs in 5% to 10 % of all pregnancies. PIH is further divided into three distinctive clinical groups.
   a. Hypertension without proteinuria and/or edema.
   b. *Preeclampsia*—hypertension with proteinuria, edema, or both. Further classified as mild or severe.
   c. *Eclampsia*—hypertension with convulsions and/or coma occurs in the absence of an underlying neurologic condition. *Note:* Eclampsia was previously referred to as *toxemia* because it was thought to be caused by toxins. Currently, the term *eclampsia* is more commonly used.
2. Chronic hypertension/coincidental hypertension

3. Preeclampsia/eclampsia superimposed on chronic hypertension
4. Transient hypertension

Pathophysiology and Etiology

1. Actual cause is unknown.
2. Theories of the etiology include the exposure to chorionic villi for the first time, or in large amounts, along with immunologic, genetic, and endocrine factors.
3. The disease is primarily seen in primagravidas.
4. Chronic hypertension, hydatidiform mole, multiple gestation, polyhydramnios, preexisting vascular disease, and diabetes mellitus may predispose to PIH.
5. Adolescents (<17 years of age) and women over 35 years of age are at higher risk.
6. Multisystem disease with widespread vasospasms occur and result in increased resistance in vascular flow, increasing the arterial blood pressure and causing endothelial damage. Stimulates platelet and fibrinogen use, causing hypoxic damage to vulnerable organ systems.
7. Increased sensitivity to angiotensin II occurs before the onset of hypertension.
8. Hemoconcentration occurs due to the vasoconstriction or as a result of increased vascular permeability or a combination of both. Will see increased hematocrit (not consistent with normal pathophysiology of pregnancy where hematocrit decreases).
9. Decreased placental production of prostacyclin and increased thromboxane A_2.

> **NURSING ALERT**
>
> The risk of PIH is increased, and similar to being a primagravida, for multigravida women if they have a new partner (father of the baby different than the previous children) due to new genetic makeup of the fetus.

Clinical Manifestations

1. Hypertension sustained at ≥140/90 mm Hg on at least two occasions 6 hours apart.
2. Proteinuria—300 to 500 mg/24 h or 1+ to 2+ on qualitative assessment (urine dipstick).
3. Edema—clinically evident swelling or sudden rapid weight gain of 1 lb/week in the second trimester or 2 lb/week in the third trimester. The sudden weight gain often occurs before the edema is present.
4. Mild preeclampsia—blood pressure ≥140/90 mm Hg on at least two occasions ≥6 hours apart.
5. Severe preeclampsia—the presence of one or more of the following is classified as severe preeclampsia:
    a. Systolic blood pressure ≥160/110 mm Hg or diastolic blood pressure ≥110 mm Hg on two occasions at least 6 hours apart with the patient on bed rest.
    b. Proteinuria—≥5 g/24 h or 3+ to 4+ on qualitative assessment (urine dipstick).

c. Oliguria—≤400 to 500 mL/24 h.
    d. Cerebral or visual disturbances (altered level of consciousness, headache, scotomata, or blurred vision).
    e. Epigastric pain or right upper quadrant (RUQ) pain.
    f. Pulmonary edema or cyanosis.
    g. Impaired liver function of unclear etiology.
    h. Thrombocytopenia (platelet count <150,000).
    i. Development of eclampsia.
6. Eclampsia
    a. Seizures and/or coma without underlying neurologic or febrile origin in patient with preeclampsia.
    b. Third trimester and 48 hours postpartum are the most common times for eclampsia to occur.
7. Chronic hypertension—any of the three occur:
    a. Hypertension predates pregnancy.
    b. Diagnosed before 20 weeks' gestation.
    c. Continues beyond 42nd week postpartum.
8. Preeclampsia/eclampsia superimposed on chronic hypertension—women with preexisting hypertension who develop preeclampsia or eclampsia.
9. Transient hypertension
    a. Development of mildly elevated blood pressure during pregnancy or in first 24 hours postpartum without any other signs of chronic disease or preeclampsia.
    b. Usually resolves after delivery but may reoccur with subsequent pregnancies.
    c. Diagnosis can be made only after the postpartum period is complete.

Diagnostic Evaluation

1. A 24-hour urine for protein of 300 mg or greater
2. Serum BUN and creatinine to evaluate renal function
3. Sonogram, NST to evaluate placenta and fetus
4. Deep tendon reflexes (DTRs) and clonus evaluation to assess level of disease process
5. Blood pressure changes meeting criteria for diagnosis

Management

Directed toward decreasing the maternal blood pressure through the use of inpatient hospitalization or conservative management and antihypertensive medications along with increase in dietary protein and an increase in calories, if indicated.

Seizure Prevention and Treatment

1. Magnesium sulfate ($MgSO_4$) may be given either IV or IM.
    a. A 4- to 6-g loading dose of 50% $MgSO_4$ is usually given IV over 15 to 30 minutes followed by a maintenance dose (secondary infusion) of 1 to 4 g/h.
    b. IM injection of 10 g (5 g in each buttock) as a loading dose is usually given, followed by 5 g every 4 hours.
    c. If seizures develop and the patient is not on $MgSO_4$, 4 g is given over 5 minutes; if seizures continue, an additional 2 g is given over 3 to 5 minutes; if seizures

still continue, paralytic agents need to be given and the patient mechanically ventilated.

   d. If seizures develop and patient is already on MgSO₄, an additional 2 g of MgSO₄ may be given or amobarbital sodium may be used.

   e. Actions: decreases neuromuscular irritability and blocks the release of acetylcholine at the neuromuscular junction; depresses vasomotor center; depresses central nervous system (CNS) irritability.

2. Calcium gluconate is kept at bedside as a reversal agent for magnesium toxicity.

   a. Dosage is 1 g (10 mL of 10% solution) by slow IV push.

   b. Signs of MgSO₄ toxicity include loss of knee-jerk reflex, respiratory depression, oliguria, respiratory arrest, and cardiac arrest.

Antihypertensive Drug Therapy

May be used when the diastolic pressure reaches or exceeds 110 mm Hg or when cerebrovascular accident is impending.

1. Hydralazine (Apresoline) is the drug of choice.

   a. Hydralazine relaxes the arterioles and stimulates cardiac output.

   b. Dosage: 5 mg IV push followed by 5 to 10 mg IV no more often than every 20 minutes to a total acute dose of 30 to 40 mg.

   c. If desired response not obtained after 30 to 40 mg, change agents and consider hemodynamic monitoring.

   d. Side effects of hydralazine include flushing, headache, maternal and fetal tachycardia, palpitations, uteroplacental insufficiency with subsequent fetal tachycardia, late decelerations, and worsening hypertension (if hypertension due to elevated cardiac output). Rebound hypotension is possible if drug given too frequently.

2. Labetalol—used in place of hydralazine.

   a. Contraindicated in women with asthma and second- or third-degree heart block.

   b. Alpha/beta adrenergic blocker that decreases systemic vascular resistance (SVR) without reflex tachycardia.

   c. Administered either IV bolus or titrated drip.

     (i) If IV bolus: initial dose 10 mg; subsequent doses progressively increase (20, 30, 40 mg) every 10 minutes. Maximum dose is 300 mg.

     (ii) If titrated/continuous infusion, start at 1 to 2 mg/min until therapeutic goals achieved, then decrease to 0.5 mg/min or stop.

   d. Onset of action is 1 to 2 minutes.

   e. Side effects of labetalol include transient fetal and neonatal hypotension, bradycardia, and hypoglycemia. Small doses excreted in breast milk.

3. Nifedipine (Procardia)—third-line agent; protocols for administration vary.

   a. Calcium channel blocker that decreases blood pressure by blocking the intracellular pathways of calcium movement causing smooth muscle relaxation and vasodilatation.

   b. Adverse effects include hypotension, palpitations, nausea, headache, fetal acidosis related to uteroplacental insufficiency.

   c. Cautious administration with MgSO₄ due to potential for exaggerated hypotensive response. Avoid concurrent use of beta blockers.

4. Sodium nitroprusside (Nipride)—used only when all other agents have failed and the patient has life-threatening hypertension.

   a. Given in titrated drip only with onset of action occurring in 15 to 30 seconds.

     (i) Initial dose started at 0.25 µg/kg/min and titrate to desired effect.

     (ii) Maintenance dose is increased by 0.25 µg/kg/min every 5 minutes.

     (iii) Average dose is 3 µg/kg/min with the range being 0.5 to 10 µg/kg/min.

   b. Actions: potent vasodilator with direct effect on arterial and venous smooth muscle.

   c. Contraindicated for antepartum use because it crosses the placenta and causes fetal cyanide toxicity.

   d. Side effects include nausea, diaphoresis, anxiety, headache, bradycardia, ECG changes, tachycardia, raised intracranial pressure, decreased reflexes, blurred vision, crosses placenta, and cyanide toxicity.

   e. Dilute in D5W only, and do not mix with any other drug.

   f. Continuous blood pressure monitoring with arterial line and ECG monitoring, along with central hemodynamic monitoring should be considered.

   g. Arterial blood gases (ABGs) need to be monitored for metabolic acidosis, which may be an early sign of cyanide toxicity.

NURSING ALERT

 Sodium nitroprusside solution is light sensitive and should be covered in foil and changed every 24 hours.

---

5. Nitroglycerin—indicated for hypertension refractory to conservative pharmacologic therapy.

   a. Dosage: initial dose is 5 to 10 µg/min; subsequent doses titrated to the desired response by increasing the dose 5 µg/min every 3 to 5 minutes.

   b. Actions: relaxes predominantly venous, but also arterial, vascular smooth muscle; decreases preload at low doses and afterload at high doses.

   c. Must be diluted before administration in D5W or normal saline (NS).

   d. Requires central hemodynamic monitoring (central venous pressure [CVP], pulmonary artery pressure, and pulmonary artery wedge pressure).

   e. FHR variability may be decreased with this drug, and fetal stress may occur when mean arterial pressure (MAP) is <106 mm Hg.

f. Hypovolemia must be corrected before use.

g. Side effects include hypotension, tachycardia, nausea, vomiting, pallor, sweating, headache, flushing of skin, methemoglobinemia (with IV doses >7 μg/kg/min).

Correction of Hypovolemia

1. Important to correct hypovolemia before initiation of antihypertensive therapy.
2. To avoid abrupt and often profound drops in blood pressure.
3. Maintain diastolic blood pressure between 95 and 100 diastolic to maintain uteroplacental perfusion.

Complications

Complications of PIH affect many body systems, including cardiovascular, renal, hematologic, neurologic, hepatic, and uteroplacental systems.

1. Abruptio placentae
2. DIC
3. HELLP syndrome (Box 39-2)
4. Prematurity
5. Intrauterine growth restriction (IUGR) from decreased placental perfusion
6. Maternal/fetal death
7. Hypertensive crisis
8. Pulmonary edema; cerebral edema
9. Oliguria; acute renal failure
10. Thrombocytopenia
11. Hemorrhage; cerebrovascular accident (CVA)
12. Blindness
13. Fetal intolerance of labor
14. Hypoglycemia
15. Hepatocellular dysfunction; hepatic rupture

BOX 39-2 HELLP Syndrome

HELLP syndrome is a severe complication of pregnancy-induced hypertension. It comprises hemolysis of RBCs, elevated liver enzymes, and low platelets (<100,000).

- These findings are frequently associated with DIC and, in fact, may be diagnosed as DIC.
- The hemolysis of erythrocytes is seen in the abnormal morphology of the cells.
- The elevated liver enzyme measurement is associated with the decreased blood flow to the liver as a result of fibrin thrombi.
- The low platelet count is related to vasospasm and platelet adhesions.
- Treatment is similar to treatment for PIH with close monitoring of liver function and bleeding.
- These women are at increased risk for postpartum hemorrhage.
- Complaints range from malaise, epigastric pain, and nausea and vomiting to nonspecific viral syndrome–like symptoms.

Nursing Assessment

1. Evaluate blood pressure with patient in a sitting position and in the left lateral position.
2. Check the protein level of a spot urine specimen.
3. Evaluate edema, carefully noting the presence after 12 hours or more of bed rest. Measure weight.
4. Evaluate deep tendon reflexes and clonus.
5. Evaluate fetal status with NST, fetal movement (kick) counts, biophysical profile (BPP), and contraction stress test (CST).
6. Evaluate uterine activity for high-frequency, low-intensity uterine contractions.
7. Observe for signs and symptoms of disease escalation.
8. Monitor for signs of $MgSO_4$ toxicity—absent knee-jerk reflex, respiratory depression, oliguria. Discontinue $MgSO_4$, and notify health care provider (see Box 39-2).

Nursing Diagnoses

- Fluid Volume Excess related to pathophysiologic changes of PIH and increased risk of fluid overload
- Altered Tissue Perfusion, Fetal Cardiac and Cerebral, related to altered placental blood flow caused by vasospasm and thrombosis
- Risk for Injury related to convulsions
- Anxiety/Knowledge Deficit related to diagnosis and concern for self and fetus
- Diversional Activity Deficit related to prolonged bed rest
- Decreased Cardiac Output related to decreased preload or antihypertensive therapy

Nursing Interventions
Maintaining Fluid Balance

1. Control IV fluid intake using a continuous infusion pump.
2. Monitor intake and output strictly; notify health care provider if urine output is <30 mL/h.
3. Monitor hematocrit levels to evaluate intravascular fluid status.
4. Monitor vital signs every hour.
5. Auscultate breath sounds every 2 hours, and report signs of pulmonary edema (wheezing, crackles, shortness of breath, increased pulse rate, increased respiratory rate).

Promoting Adequate Tissue Perfusion

1. Position on side, preferably the left side to promote placental perfusion.
2. Monitor fetal activity.
3. Evaluate NST to determine fetal status.
4. Increase protein intake to replace protein lost through kidneys.

Preventing Injury

1. Instruct on the importance of reporting headaches, visual changes, dizziness, and epigastric pain.
2. Instruct to lie down on left side if symptoms are present.
3. Keep the environment quiet and as calm as possible.
4. If patient is hospitalized, side rails should be padded and remain up to prevent injury if seizure occurs.

5. If patient is hospitalized, have oxygen and suction setup, along with a tongue blade and emergency medications, immediately available for treatment of seizures.

 DRUG ALERT

Keep calcium gluconate at bedside as the reversal agent for magnesium toxicity. Dosage is 1 g (10 mL of a 10% solution) slow IV push. Be cautious with concurrent administration of narcotics, CNS depressants, calcium channel blockers, and beta blockers.

Decreasing Anxiety/Increasing Knowledge

1. Explain the disease process and treatment plan including signs and symptoms of the disease process.
2. Explain that PIH does not lead to chronic hypertension.
3. Explain that PIH usually does not occur with subsequent pregnancies.
4. Discuss the effects of all medications on the mother and fetus.
5. Allow time to ask questions and discuss feelings regarding the diagnosis and treatment plan.

Promoting Diversional Activities

1. Explain the need for bed rest to the woman and her support person(s).
2. Explore woman's hobbies/diversional activities.
3. Instruct family to arrange for easy access to TV, phone, and stereo to limit woman getting out of bed.
4. Instruct family to arrange for community support (eg, church, woman's groups, and so forth).

Maintaining Cardiac Output

1. Control IV fluid intake using a continuous infusion pump.
2. Monitor intake and output strictly; notify primary care provider if urine output is <30 mL/h.
3. Monitor maternal vital signs, especially mean blood pressure and respirations.
4. Assess edema status, and report pitting edema of ≥+2 to primary care provider.
5. Monitor oxygenation saturation levels with pulse oximetry. Report oxygenation saturation rate of <90% to primary care provider.

Community and Home Care Considerations

Mild PIH may be treated at home.

1. Ensure that patient meets criteria set forth by ACOG for home management:
   a. Gestational age >20 weeks.
   b. Blood pressure <150/100 mm Hg sitting position or <140/90 mm Hg lateral position.
   c. No headache or visual disturbances present.
   d. No epigastric pain, marked edema, clonus, or DTRs >+2.
   e. Must have available blood pressure equipment.
2. Ensure that patient has daily phone contact with primary care provider.
3. Make periodic home visits, either daily or twice weekly.
4. Teach woman signs and symptoms of disease progression.

5. Teach woman at-home blood pressure monitoring for two to four times daily in the same arm and the same physical position (eg, on left side, on right side, and so forth).
6. Obtain daily weights at the same time each day.
7. Assess urine protein status daily on the first voided urine and/or obtain 24-hour urine each week.
8. Teach woman to assess daily fetal movement (kick) counts; arrange for weekly NST.

Patient Education and Health Maintenance

1. Teach the woman the importance of bed rest in helping to control symptoms.
2. Encourage the support of family and friends while on bed rest.
3. Provide and suggest diversional activities while on bed rest.
4. Provide information on tests and procedures to evaluate maternal–fetal status, such as laboratory tests, sonogram, NST.
5. Include support of the neonatal team for discussion of fetal prognosis with the woman and her family.

Outcome-Based Evaluation

- No evidence of pulmonary edema; urine output adequate
- FHR within normal range; reactivity present
- No seizure activity
- Expresses concern for self and the fetus
- Maintaining bed rest and pursuing diversional activities
- Blood pressure and other vital parameters stable

Polyhydramnios

Polyhydramnios or *hydramnios* is an excessive amount of amniotic fluid in the amniotic sac. At 36 weeks of pregnancy, there is usually about a liter of fluid present. The amount of amniotic fluid normally decreases after this time. The amount of amniotic fluid present is controlled in part by fetal urination and swallowing.

Pathophysiology and Etiology

1. The etiology is often unclear.
2. Normal amniotic fluid volume at term is 500 to 1,000 mL. The volume in polyhydramnios exceeds 2,000 mL.
3. Anomalies causing impaired fetal swallowing or excessive micturition may contribute to the condition.
4. It is associated with maternal diabetes, multiple gestation, Rh isoimmunization, anomalies of the CNS including spina bifida and anencephaly, or anomalies of the gastrointestinal tract including tracheoesophageal fistula.

Clinical Manifestations

1. Excessive weight gain, dyspnea.
2. Abdomen may be tense and shiny.
3. Edema of the vulva, legs, and lower extremities.
4. Increased uterine size for gestational age usually accompanied by difficulty in palpating fetal parts and in auscultation of fetal heart.

Diagnostic Evaluation

1. A diagnosis is made based on the present symptoms and ultrasound evaluation revealing amniotic fluid index (AFI) >25 cm.
2. Ultrasound evaluation will show large pockets of fluid between the fetus and uterine wall or placenta.
3. Difficult to palpate fetus and/or hear FHR.
4. Fundal height (FH) > age of gestation (AOG).

Management

1. Depends on the severity of the condition and the cause; hospitalization is indicated for maternal distress or for intervention regarding fetal prognosis.
2. If impairment of maternal respiratory status occurs, amniocentesis for removal of fluid may be performed.
   a. The amniocentesis is performed under ultrasound for location of the placenta and fetal parts.
   b. The fluid is then slowly removed.
   c. Rapid removal of the fluid can result in a premature separation of the placenta.
   d. Usually 500 to 1,000 mL of fluid is removed.

Complications

1. PTL
2. Dysfunctional labor with increased risk for cesarean section
3. Postpartum hemorrhage due to uterine atony from gross distention of the uterus
4. AFE
5. Acute fetal hypoxia secondary to prolapsed cord or trauma if associated with diabetes (macrosomia)

Nursing Assessment

1. Evaluate maternal respiratory status; frequently present with dyspnea.
2. Inspect abdomen and evaluate uterine height and compare with previous findings.
3. Evaluate for abdominal pain, edema, varicosities of lower extremities and vulva.

Nursing Diagnoses

- Ineffective Breathing Pattern related to pressure on the diaphragm
- Altered Tissue Perfusion, Placental, related to pressure from excess fluid
- Impaired Physical Mobility related to edema and discomfort from the enlarged uterus
- Anxiety related to fetal outcome
- Risk for Injury related to overdistention of the uterus and possible hemorrhage

Nursing Interventions
Promoting Effective Breathing

1. Position to promote chest expansion with head elevated.
2. Provide oxygen by face mask, if indicated.
3. Limit activities and plan for frequent rest periods.
4. Maintain adequate intake and output.

Promoting Placental Tissue Perfusion and Oxygen to Fetus

1. Position on side if possible, with head elevated. If unable to position on side, use a wedge to displace the uterus to either side.
2. Encourage passive or active assisted range of motion to the lower extremities.
3. Monitor FHR as directed and assess for abnormal FHR pattern: decreased or absent variability, tachycardia, prolonged, variable, or late decelerations
4. Provide good fluid intake and a diet adequate in protein, iron, and fluids.
5. Administer oxygen at 8 to 12 L/min per snug face mask as needed.

Promoting Mobility

1. Assist the woman with position changes and ambulation as needed.
2. Advise on alternating activity with rest periods for legs.
3. Instruct the woman to wear loose-fitting clothing and low-heeled shoes with good support.

Decreasing Anxiety

1. Explain the cause of hydramnios, if known.
2. Encourage the patient and family to ask questions regarding any treatment or procedures.
3. Encourage expression of feelings.
4. Prepare patient for the type of delivery that is anticipated and for the expected finding at the time of delivery.
5. Encourage presence of support person.

Improving Labor Curve and Reducing Risk of Hemorrhage

1. Use Friedman's curve to assess labor status.
2. Follow augmentation and induction protocol per orders/institutional policy.
3. Notify primary care provider of inadequate or abnormal labor curve.
4. Keep woman well hydrated and nourished.
5. Administer oxytocin (Pitocin) immediately after delivery of placenta.
6. Observe for changing vital signs indicating excessive blood loss: decreasing blood pressure and increasing pulse.
7. Have other ergotrate drugs available should oxytocin not be effective (eg, Methergine, Hemabate).

Patient Education and Health Maintenance

1. Instruct the woman to notify her health care provider if she experiences respiratory distress.
2. Teach the woman signs of PTL and the need to report them to health care provider.

Outcome-Based Evaluation

- Respirations at normal rate of 18 to 20 and unlabored
- FHR within normal limits without fetal compromise
- Verbalizes improved comfort; moves freely
- Discusses realistically the pregnancy outcome; questions regarding treatment for self and fetus
- Labor progresses, and involution occurs without hemorrhage

Oligohydramnios

Oligohydramnios is the marked decrease of amniotic fluid in the amniotic sac. Usually, the fluid is extremely concentrated. Cord compression and fetal compromise may occur and lead to a poor outcome. Often, the infant will suffer from pulmonary hypoplasia and skeletal abnormalities due to a lack of fluid in the terminal air sacs if oligohydramnios occurs in the first or second trimester.

Pathophysiology and Etiology
1. Frequently related to fetal problems such as obstruction in the urinary tract, renal agenesis, and IUGR
2. Associated with premature rupture of membranes (PROM) and severe preeclampsia where there is a significant decrease in fetal vascular volume causing decreased urine output
3. Frequently seen in postdate pregnancies
4. Placental insufficiency
5. Premature separation of placenta from the uterus
6. Twin-to-twin transfusion

Clinical Manifestations
1. Prominent fetal parts on palpation of the abdomen
2. Small-for-date uterine size

Diagnostic Evaluation
1. Ultrasound evaluation of the AFI—amniotic fluid of <5 cm total in all four vertical plane quadrants of the uterus is associated with lower perinatal mortality. AFI between 5 and 8 cm is considered borderline with treatment being provider driven.
2. Fundal height (FH) < age of gestation (AOG).

Management
1. Frequent evaluation of fetal status through NST, CST, or OCT as indicated.
2. Ultrasound is also done to further evaluate fetal renal and urinary systems along with fetal growth.
3. Amnioinfusion (the installation of fluid into the amniotic cavity to replace normal volumes of amniotic fluid) during labor.
   a. Protocols vary; usually begin with 800-mL bolus followed by a maintenance continuous infusion.
   b. Fluid used is either NS or Ringer's lactate (RL).
   c. Assess for fluid returning during infusion.
   d. Monitor uterine activity and FHR during the infusion.
   e. No requirement for warming the fluid; however, recommendation is made to warm the fluid if
      (i) Fetus is preterm.
      (ii) There is fetal compromise.
      (iii) Infusion rate is >600 mL/h.

NURSING ALERT

Contraindications to amnioinfusion include suspected or diagnosed abruptio placentae, acute fetal compromise, fetal head is engaged and tightly applied to the cervix, or the inability to measure intrauterine pressures.

---

4. Delivery may be indicated for conditions such as IUGR or fetal compromise.

Complications
1. Umbilical cord compression
2. Passage of meconium
3. Fetal/neonatal death
4. PTL

Nursing Interventions and Patient Education
1. Evaluate fetal status by way of fetal monitoring.
2. Evaluate maternal vital signs for signs of infection, especially if oligohydramnios is secondary to PROM.
3. Assist with an amnioinfusion as indicated.
4. Inform health care provider of fetal compromise, assist the woman to a side-lying position, and treat as indicated.

Multiple Gestation

Multiple gestation or *multifetal pregnancy* results when two or more fetuses are present in the uterus at the same time.

Etiology
1. Types of twinning (Figure 39-4)
   a. Dizygotic—occurs when two separate ova are fertilized. Dizygotic twins do not have the same genetic makeup and are as similar as other brothers and sisters.
   b. Monozygotic—occurs when one ovum divides early in gestation and two embryos develop. Monozygotic twins are identical in genetic makeup. Etiology unclear for spontaneous monozygotic twins.
2. Artificially induced ovulation as well as in vitro fertilization where multiple embryos are transferred into the uterus increase the chances of multiple gestation.
3. Increasing maternal age and parity increase the chance of twinning.

Clinical Manifestations
1. Usually, the uterus is large for gestational age (FH > AOG) during the second trimester.
2. Auscultation of two distinct and separate fetal hearts may occur with a Doppler late in the first trimester or with a fetoscope after 20 weeks' gestation.
3. Ultrasound is the best screening test at present. It may identify separate gestation sacs.

Complications
1. Spontaneous abortion
2. IUGR
3. PTL and/or birth
4. Polyhydramnios; oligohydramnios with twins common
5. PIH
6. Umbilical cord problems such as entwinement, cord prolapse, or vasa previa
7. Placenta accidents such as abruptio placentae or placenta previa

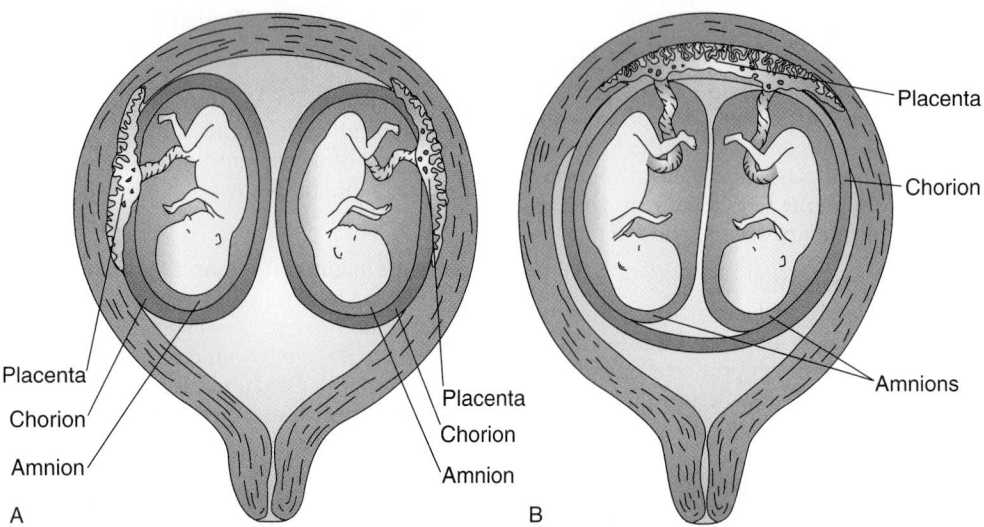

FIGURE 39-4   Multiple gestations. (**A**) Dizygotic twins showing two placentas, two chorions, and two amnions. (**B**) Monozygotic twins with one placenta, one chorion, and two amnions.

Management and Nursing Interventions

1. Nutrition counseling—stress increased caloric and protein intake as well as vitamin supplements to meet the demands of multiple gestation.
2. Fetal evaluation—encourage follow-up for serial sonograms during the pregnancy to evaluate growth and development and to detect IUGR. Explain NST, biophysical profile, and amniocentesis for detection of fetal lung maturity. Percutaneous umbilical cord sampling may be used to establish fetal well-being if twin-to-twin transfusion is suspected.
3. Evaluate the woman for signs and symptoms of PIH, which is more common in multiple gestation.
4. PTL prevention—explain that hospitalization may be necessary for signs and symptoms of PTL.
   a. Encourage bed rest and hydration.
   b. Institute fetal monitoring and assist with tocolytic therapy, if ordered (see section titled Tocolytic Therapy, in next section).
5. Explain to the woman that mode for delivery depends on the presentation of the twins, maternal and fetal status, and gestational age. Delivery of multiples other than twins is done by cesarean section.
6. Intrapartum management
   a. Establish IV access to be prepared for emergency birth or other complications.
   b. Provide for electronic fetal monitoring for each fetus.
   c. Double set-up is recommended for delivery.
   d. Pitocin induction/augmentation may be required secondary to hypotonic labor.
   e. Postpartum hemorrhage may occur due to uterine atony.
7. Emotional support—encourage family to discuss feelings about multiple births and identify ways in which they will need help. Refer to resources such as National Organization of Mothers of Twins Clubs, Inc., 12404 Princess Jeanne NE, Albuquerque, NM 87112-4640, 877-540-2200.

Community and Home Care Considerations

1. Discuss with woman and support person(s) the warning signs of PTL.
2. Teach the woman uterine self-palpation. Woman is to evaluate uterine activity twice daily.
3. Engage in home visits recommended for NST and/or FHR assessment as needed.
4. Ensure weekly provider phone contact by patient.

COMPLICATIONS OF LABOR

▣ Preterm Labor

Preterm labor is defined as uterine contractions occurring after 20 weeks' gestation and before 37 completed weeks of gestation. It occurs in up to 10% of all pregnancies. Contractions are less than 10 minutes apart, resulting in progressive cervical changes or cervical dilation of 2 cm or effacement of 75%.

Pathophysiology and Etiology

The exact etiology for PTL remains unknown. However, certain changes in the body occur with the onset of spontaneous labor. Cervical "ripening" occurs, which includes softening and shortening of the cervix. Oxytocin receptors are present in the myometrium. Prostaglandin levels in the amniotic fluid are increased.

A number of risk factors are associated with PTL. Risk factors are divided into three categories:

1. Medical/obstetric predating the pregnancy
   a. Prior preterm birth
   b. Previous second-trimester abortion/miscarriage

c. Cervical incompetence

d. Uterine/cervical abnormalities

e. Hypertension

f. Diethylstilbestrol (DES) exposure

2. Current pregnancy related

a. Anemia

b. Multiple gestation

c. Placenta previa

d. Abruptio placentae

e. Fetal anomaly

f. Hydramnios (polyhydramnios, oligohydramnios)

g. Abdominal surgery

h. Maternal infection

i. Maternal bleeding

j. Cervical effacement >50% or dilatation >1 cm by 32 weeks' gestation

k. Previous PTL

l. Uterine distention

m. Cervical incompetence

3. Demographic and behavioral

a. Maternal age <20 or >35 years of age

b. Nonwhite

c. Low socioeconomic status

d. Single parent

e. Smoker

f. Chemical (drug) use or dependence

g. Prepregnancy weight ≤100 lb

h. Poor weight gain

i. Inadequate prenatal care

j. Psychological stress

Clinical Manifestations

1. Uterine cramps

2. Uterine contractions ≥ every 10 to 15 minutes

3. Low abdominal pressure

4. Low backache

5. Any vaginal bleeding

6. Increased vaginal discharge of clear or tan fluid

7. Feeling that "something" is in the vagina

8. Abdominal cramping with or without nausea, vomiting, or diarrhea

9. Intermittent or persistent thigh pain

Management

The focus of treatment is prevention of delivery of a preterm infant. The method depends on the cervical dilatation and contraction pattern. If contractions are detected early and treatment is begun early, there is a higher rate of stopping labor.

Conservative Treatment

1. Treatment is begun early with the use of bed rest in a left lateral position.

2. Hydration with IV fluids and continuous monitoring of fetal status and uterine contraction pattern are instituted.

3. If this stops the contractions, tocolytic therapy is not needed.

Tocolytic Therapy

If conservative therapy is not successful, tocolytic therapy is instituted. These drugs should be used only when the potential benefit to the fetus outweighs the potential risk.

1. Betamimetic agents such as ritodrine (Yutopar) and terbutaline (Brethine)

a. These drugs stimulate the β_2 receptors, which causes uterine relaxation.

b. Ritodrine is administered IV or orally; terbutaline may be administered IV, subcutaneously, or orally.

> **NURSING ALERT**
>
> Ritodrine is the only drug FDA approved for the treatment of PTL. However, due to the increased maternal and fetal side effects, its use has dramatically decreased.

c. Frequent monitoring is necessary to observe for side effects of increased pulse, shortness of breath, chest pain, decreased blood pressure, hypervolemia, decreased potassium concentration, hyperglycemia, and hyperinsulinemia.

d. Before administration of these medications is begun, the following laboratory tests should be done and a baseline ECG should be obtained for ritodrine use: CBC with differential, electrolytes, glucose, BUN, creatinine, prothrombin time, and partial thromboplastin time.

2. $MgSO_4$

a. $MgSO_4$ interferes with smooth muscle contractility. The exact action is not clear.

b. Administration is IV on an infusion pump.

c. During administration, the woman is monitored for pulmonary edema, loss of deep tendon reflexes, decreased respirations, hypotension.

d. Serum magnesium levels are monitored.

e. Calcium gluconate is the antidote for $MgSO_4$ and should be at the bedside.

f. If used, protocol is the same as for PIH (see p. 1190).

3. Indomethacin (Indocin)

a. Indomethacin is a prostaglandin inhibitor that inhibits contractions.

b. Administration is oral or rectal.

c. It is usually well tolerated by the woman.

4. Nifedipine (Procardia)

a. Nifedipine is a calcium channel blocker that relaxes smooth muscle by inhibiting the transport of calcium.

b. Administration is sublingual or oral.

c. Side effects include headache, nausea, and flushing from vasodilatation.

5. Oxytocin antagonists (Atosiban)

a. Competes with oxytocin at the receptor sites and inhibits uterine contractions.

b. Still under investigation and used rarely.

c. Side effects minimal at this point.

Acceleration of Fetal Lung Maturity for <32 Weeks' Gestation

1. Corticosteroid administration
   a. Decreases intraventricular hemorrhage (IVH), necrotizing enterocolitis (NEC), and respiratory distress syndrome (RDS).
   b. Given before delivery to mother; try to postpone delivery for 48 hours.
   c. Usually, IM administration of betamethasone with initial dose followed by second dose 24 hours later.
2. Artificial surfactant therapy
   a. Decreases ventilatory days for infants with RDS.
   b. Given after delivery to infant directly into lungs by way of endotracheal tube

Complications

1. Prematurity and associated neonatal complications, such as lung immaturity
   a. IVH
   b. RDS
   c. Patent ductus arteriosus (PDA)
   d. NEC
   e. Financially costly
2. Long-term tocolytic use
   a. Terbutaline—neonatal cardiovascular toxicity and myocardial necrosis
   b. Indomethacin—pulmonary hypertension and premature closure of PDA
   c. MgSO$_4$—hypotonia, neonatal bone abnormalities, and decreased calcium levels

Nursing Assessment

During tocolytic therapy, assess the following:
1. Fetal status by way of electronic fetal monitoring
2. Uterine activity pattern
3. Respiratory status (pulmonary edema is a common side effect)
4. Muscular tremors
5. Palpitations
6. Dizziness/lightheadedness
7. Urinary output
8. Patient education to signs and symptoms of PTL
9. Patient education to signs and symptoms of infection

Nursing Diagnoses

• Anxiety related to medication and fear of outcome of pregnancy
• Diversional Activity Deficit related to prolonged bed rest
• Risk for Injury to fetus secondary to prematurity
• Risk for Injury secondary to betasympathomimetic tocolytics
• Ineffective Family Coping: Compromised, secondary to hospitalization

Nursing Interventions

Decreasing Anxiety
1. Provide accurate information on the status of the fetus and labor (contraction pattern).
2. Allow the woman and her support person to verbalize their feelings regarding the episode of PTL and the treatment.
3. If a private room is not used, do not place the woman in a room with a woman who is in labor or who has lost an infant.
4. Encourage relationship with other patients who are also experiencing PTL.

Promoting Diversional Activities
1. Determine quiet craft activities that can be done in bed.
2. Provide radio, books, and television.
3. Encourage visits from family, especially other children and friends. If possible, encourage them to bring in favorite foods for the woman and to dine as a family.

Minimizing Injury to Fetus
1. Monitor fetal status and labor progress.
2. Assist with delivery of infant as needed.
3. Notify provider of dysfunctional (protracted) labor curve.

Minimizing Risk of Drug-Related Injury
1. Maintain accurate intake and output.
2. Discontinue infusion if side effects occur; notify primary care provider.
3. Educate the woman on side effects of tocolytic therapy.

Promoting Maternal–Family Coping
1. Encourage private time for woman and partner.
2. Allow visitation with other children as tolerated by woman.
3. Comment on strengths of the family unit.
4. Encourage other family activities, such as helping with homework. This will assist on maintaining the family unit.

Community and Home Care Considerations

1. Use home uterine activity monitoring (HUAM) for home management of PTL.
   a. Some evidence exists to support its use.
   b. Patient education is paramount.
2. Ensure that woman meets following criteria for home management of PTL:
   a. No evidence of active PTL.
   b. No evidence of intra-amniotic infection.
   c. Cervical dilatation <3 cm.
3. Ensure that protocols or orders are in place for each of the following:
   a. Warning signs for PTL.
   b. Demonstration of uterine self-palpation by woman.
   c. Twice-daily uterine activity assessment.
   d. Monitoring vaginal discharge; signs of spontaneous rupture of membranes.
   e. Assessment of urine frequency, signs and symptoms for urinary tract infection (UTI); diarrhea, pelvic heaviness/pressure, maternal temperature, uterine cramping/tenderness.
   f. Frequent home visits; NST, FHR assessment, and vaginal examination evaluation necessary.
   g. Daily provider-initiated phone consult.

Patient Education and Health Maintenance

1. Educate the woman about the importance of continuing the pregnancy until term or until there is evidence of fetal lung maturity.
2. Encourage the need for compliance with a decreased activity level or bed rest, as indicated.
3. Teach the woman the importance of proper nutrition and the need for adequate hydration—at least 8 glasses of fluids a day.
4. Instruct the woman not to engage in sexual activity if diagnosed with PTL.
5. Teach the woman the signs and symptoms of infection and to report them immediately.

Outcome-Based Evaluation

- Demonstrates concern about treatment and pregnancy outcome
- Participates in diversional activities
- No fetal compromise noted
- Adequate fluid intake and output
- Family focused on woman's well-being

Premature Rupture of Membranes

Premature rupture of membranes (PROM) is defined as rupture of the membranes after 37 completed weeks' gestation before the onset of spontaneous labor. PROM occurs in 2 of 18 pregnancies.

Pathophysiology and Etiology

1. The exact etiology of PROM is not clearly understood. PROM at term may result from stretching of the membranes and fetal movements that cause the membranes to weaken.
2. PROM is manifested by a large gush of amniotic fluid or leaking of fluid per vagina, which usually persists.

Diagnostic Evaluation

1. Sterile speculum examination for identification of "pooling" of fluid in the vagina.
2. Nitrazine test—positive test will change pH paper strip from yellow-green to blue in the presence of amniotic fluid taken from the vaginal canal.
3. Fern test—positive test will reveal "ferning" on a slide viewed under a microscope. A swab of the posterior vaginal fornix is taken to obtain amniotic fluid.

Management

1. Once PROM is confirmed, the woman is admitted to the hospital and usually remains there until delivery.
2. The woman is evaluated to rule out labor, fetal compromise, and infection and to establish gestational age. If all factors are ruled out, the woman is managed expectantly.
3. Management of PROM at 36 weeks' gestation or greater focuses on delivery.
4. Vaginal examinations are kept to a minimum to prevent infection.

Complications

1. PTL
2. Prematurity and associated complications
3. Maternal infection—chorioamnionitis
4. Fetal or neonatal infection

Nursing Assessment

1. Evaluate maternal blood pressure, respirations, pulse, and temperature every 2 to 4 hours. If temperature or pulse is elevated, continue monitoring every 1 to 2 hours as indicated.
2. Monitor the amount and type of amniotic fluid that is leaking, and observe for purulent, foul-smelling discharge.
3. Evaluate daily CBC with differentials, noting any shift to the left (ie, increase of immature forms of neutrophils).
4. Evaluate fetal status every 4 hours or as indicated, noting fetal activity and heart rate and uterine activity.
5. Determine if uterine tenderness occurs on abdominal palpation.

Nursing Diagnosis

- Risk for Infection related to ascending bacteria

Nursing Interventions
Preventing Infection

1. Evaluate amount and odor of amniotic fluid leakage.
2. Do not perform vaginal examinations without consulting the health care provider.
3. Place patient on disposable pads to collect leaking fluid, and change pads every 2 hours or more frequently as needed.
4. Review the need for good handwashing technique and hygiene after urination and defecation.
5. Monitor FHR and fetal activity every 4 hours or as indicated.
6. Monitor maternal temperature, pulse respirations, blood pressure, and uterine tenderness every 4 hours or as indicated.

Outcome-Based Evaluation
- No signs of infection

Preterm Premature Rupture of Membranes

Preterm premature rupture of membranes (PPROM) is defined as rupture of membranes before 37 completed weeks' gestation with or without the onset of spontaneous labor.

Pathophysiology and Etiology

1. Exact cause is unknown.
2. In PPROM, risk factors include:
   a. Infection (amnionitis; group B beta *Streptococcus*)
   b. Previous history of PROM or preterm birth
   c. Hydramnios (polyhydramnios/oligohydramnios)
   d. Incompetent cervix

e. Increased intrauterine volume (multiple gestation, fibroids, polyhydramnios)

f. Abruptio placentae

g. Cigarette smoking

h. Fetal anomalies

i. Coitus (intercourse)

j. Vaginal colonization with group B beta *Streptococcus*

k. Prenatal vaginal bleeding in more than one trimester

Diagnostic Evaluation

1. Same as PROM.
2. Ultrasound to assess amniotic fluid volume.
3. Amniocentesis to inject indigo carmine or Evans blue dye. Watch for vaginal leakage of blue fluid to assess for ruptured membranes.

Management

1. For PPROM, tocolytics, corticosteroids (to decrease the severity of RDS in the premature neonate), and prophylactic antibiotics are used.
2. Management is influenced by gestational age.
3. Initial management:
   a. Confirm rupture of membranes (ROM).
   b. Determine if bacterial infection is present at time of rupture by way of vaginal/cervical cultures.
   c. Document age of gestation.
   d. Determine fetal lung maturity by way of amniocentesis or vaginal culture.
4. Active management:
   a. Tocolytic therapy.
   b. Antibiotic therapy.
   c. Corticosteroid administration.
   d. Amnioinfusion.
5. Conservative management:
   a. Bed rest.
   b. Vital signs per institutional policy and patient condition.
   c. Monitor fetal well-being daily or more often as dictated by institutional policy and patient condition.

Complications

1. Maternal
   a. Increased risk of intrauterine infection
   b. Postpartum endometritis
   c. Placental abruption
2. Fetal—infection
3. Neonatal—RDS, infection, death

Nursing Assessment

1. Evaluate maternal vital signs every 2 to 4 hours to include fetal assessment. If temperature or pulse is elevated, continue monitoring every 1 to 2 hours as indicated.
2. Monitor for fetal tachycardia.
3. Monitor for maternal chorioamnionitis (purulent, foul-smelling vaginal discharge, increased temperature, increased uterine activity).

4. Minimize infection with decreased or no vaginal examinations, aseptic techniques, and appropriate pericare.
5. Strict bed rest with or without bathroom privileges.
6. Evaluate daily CBC with differentials, noting any shift to the left.
7. Supportive care for woman and her family.

Nursing Diagnosis

• Risk for Infection related to ascending bacteria
   Also see section titled Preterm Labor, page 1196.

Nursing Interventions
Preventing Infection

1. Evaluate amount and odor of amniotic fluid leakage.
2. Do not perform vaginal examinations without consulting the primary health care provider.
3. Place patient on disposable pads to collect leaking fluid, and change pads every 2 hours or more frequently as needed.
4. Review the need for good handwashing technique and hygiene after urination and defecation.
5. Monitor FHR and fetal activity every 4 hours or as indicated.
6. Monitor maternal temperature, pulse respirations, blood pressure, and uterine tenderness every 4 hours or as indicated.
7. Administer antibiotics as prescribed.

Outcome-Based Evaluation

• Free from signs of infection

▧ Induction of Labor

Induction of labor refers to measures used for the deliberate initiation of uterine contractions before their spontaneous onset. Augmentation of labor refers to assisting labor that has started spontaneously to be more effective.

Indications

When the woman's life or well-being is in danger, or if the fetus may be compromised by remaining in the uterus any longer.

1. Maternal:
   a. Hypertension
   b. Diabetes mellitus
   c. Renal disease
   d. PROM
   e. Placental insufficiency
   f. Chorioamnionitis
   g. Abruptio placentae
   h. History of rapid labors and living a long distance from birth center
2. Fetal:
   a. Postmaturity
   b. Erythroblastosis
   c. Macrosomia
   d. Fetal anomaly

e. Nonreassuring FHR

f. Fetal hydrops

g. IUGR

h. Intrauterine fetal demise (IUFD)

Contraindications

1. Active genital herpes
2. Vaginal bleeding, known placenta previa or vasa previa
3. Abnormal fetal lie
4. Classic uterine incision
5. Known cephalopelvic disproportion (CPD)
6. Severe fetal compromise
7. Invasive cervical carcinoma
8. Pelvic abnormalities
9. Fundal uterine scar

Relative Contraindications

1. Grand multipara (greater than 6)
2. Overdistended uterus
   a. Polyhydramnios
   b. Multifetal gestation
   c. Uterine fibroids

Management

Amniotomy (Artificial Rupture of Membranes [AROM])

1. Vulva is cleansed, vaginal examination done, amniohook is inserted through the cervix, and membranes are ruptured after the fetal presentation is evaluated. Fluid should be clear or cloudy without odor.
2. Should make contractions stronger.
3. Fetal heart tones are assessed continually for at least the next 20 minutes.
4. Complications include umbilical cord prolapse or compression, maternal or fetal infection, and/or distorted fetal head.

Oxytocin

1. Fetal monitoring is instituted. If membranes have ruptured, an intrauterine catheter and internal scalp electrode may be used but this is not required. A reactive NST is required by ACOG guidelines before the start of oxytocin.
2. An IV is mixed with 10 units of oxytocin and piggybacked into the primary IV at the port of entry nearest the skin insertion.
3. The oxytocin is given only with an infusion pump and when constant monitoring of maternal and fetal status is available (with either nonelectronic or electronic methods of fetal assessment).
4. The dose is increased as indicated by institution policy as designated by provider-driven ACOG guidelines.
5. The goal is to establish a regular labor pattern—contractions occurring every 2 to 3 minutes lasting 45 to 60 seconds and an intensity of 50 mm Hg (moderate) or Montevideo Units (MVUs) >180.
6. Complications include uterine hyperstimulation (more than five contractions in 10 minutes), uterine hypertonus

(uterine resting tone ≥20 to 25 mm Hg), contractions >90 seconds in duration, coupling of contractions, fetal distress, increased incidence of cesarean section, and neonatal hyperbilirubinemia possibly from red blood cell trauma from intense contractions or decreased maturity of the neonate.

> **◆ DRUG ALERT**
>
> Administration of oxytocin requires strict intake and output, especially IV fluid monitoring. A major side effect of oxytocin is water toxicity, which can lead to congestive heart failure. Symptoms of water toxicity include headache, nausea and vomiting, mental confusion, decreased urine output, hypotension, tachycardia, and cardiac arrhythmia.

Prostaglandin E$_2$ (PGE$_2$)

1. PGE$_2$ is primarily used before induction of labor for cervical ripening.
2. If labor results from administration of PGE$_2$, it is similar to spontaneous labor.
3. Prostaglandins are administered intracervically or vaginally.
   a. May be inserted in solid (Cervidil), tablet (Cytotec), or gel (Prepidil) form.
   b. PGE$_2$ gel is given by way of a catheter or diaphragm in doses ranging from 0.5 to 5 mg.
   c. Cervidil is a solid, time-released suppository placed into the vagina. The suppository is 10 mg that releases 0.3 mg/h. Requires continuous fetal monitoring as evidenced by manufacturer and research guidelines.
   d. Misoprostol (Cytotec) is a tablet containing prostaglandins. Misoprostol is used usually for IUFD removal, although recent research studies have shown success with one quarter tablet (25 mcg) intracervically to induce labor.

> **◆ DRUG ALERT**
>
> Side effects of misoprostol include shivering, backache, vomiting, diarrhea, shortness of breath, uterine hypertonus, or uterine rupture.

4. Uterine hyperstimulation is a complication.

Stripping the Membranes

1. Separating the membranes from the lower uterine segment without rupturing the membranes
2. Usually done during vaginal examination
3. Membranes and amniotic fluid now act as a wedge to dilate cervix.
4. Complications include maternal/fetal infection, PPROM, umbilical cord prolapse, and personal discomfort.

Active Management of Labor

1. Augmentation protocol directed toward reducing cesarean deliveries due to dystocia in nulliparous woman.
2. Goal is to have birth within 12 hours after admission to Labor and Delivery.
3. Criteria for active management of labor:

a. Nulliparity.

b. Greater than 37 weeks' gestation.

c. Singleton pregnancy.

d. Spontaneous labor (uterine contractions every 5 minutes/100% effacement).

e. AROM within 2 hours after admission.

f. Oxytocin if no cervical change.

g. Dosage is 6 μu/min, increase by 6 μu/min every 15 minutes to a maximum of 36 to 40 μu/min.

Nursing Assessment

> **NURSING ALERT**
>
> Make sure that patient is aware of the procedures to be used and all questions have been answered. Ensure that the provider has given the woman informed consent and the consent form is signed and witnessed before the start of the procedure.

Before Induction

1. Obtain a 20-minute NST to assess fetal well-being.

2. Evaluate maternal vital signs.

3. Evaluate the patency of the IV site, if IV ordered.

After the Administration of Oxytocin

1. Continuously monitor FHR and uterine activity, especially uterine resting tone.

2. Assess maternal vital signs in accordance with institutional policy. Temperature is taken every 2 to 4 hours unless an amniotomy has been performed and then every 1 to 2 hours.

3. Limit vaginal examinations, especially after the membranes have ruptured.

4. Maintain intake and output records, and watch for signs of water intoxication—dizziness, headache, confusion, nausea, vomiting, hypotension, tachycardia, decreased urine output.

5. Evaluate IV site for patency and rate control for correct rate at least hourly.

Nursing Diagnoses

- Anxiety related to planned childbirth and outcome
- Altered Tissue Perfusion, uteroplacental, with altered oxygen to fetus related to strength of uterine contractions
- Pain related to uterine activity

Nursing Interventions
Decreasing Anxiety

1. Teach or review the use of relaxation and distraction techniques.

2. Before beginning any new procedure, explain the procedure to the woman and her support person.

3. Answer questions that the family and woman may have.

Promoting Tissue Perfusion and Oxygen Supply to Fetus

1. Assess fetal status and uterine contractions through the use of a monitor or auscultation/palpation. Assess for signs of uteroplacental insufficiency (decreased variability, abnormal baseline FHR, late decelerations).

2. Position on the left side to enhance placental perfusion.

3. Have oxygen set up with a mask ready, and administer as prescribed (8 to 12 L/min by way of snug face mask) if decelerations occur.

4. If hyperstimulation of the uterus or fetal compromise (late decelerations, nonreassuring variable decelerations, or absent STV) occurs, discontinue the infusion, maintain the primary IV, and notify the health care provider immediately.

5. Administer adequate fluid volume.

Controlling Pain

1. Encourage use of breathing techniques, distraction, and nonpharmacologic comfort measures.

2. Administer analgesia/anesthesia as prescribed.

3. Maintain positive outlook and support as labor progresses.

Outcome-Based Evaluation

- Verbalizes understanding of the induction process
- No evidence of hyperstimulation or fetal compromise
- Labor progressing with pain controlled

◼ Dystocia

Dystocia, or difficult labor, refers to abnormal progress in labor. Maternal psychological factors such as fear, anxiety, and exhaustion may play a role in dystocia. Often, more than one cause exists at a time.

Pathophysiology and Etiology
Contraction Abnormalities

1. Contractions that are not strong enough or frequent enough to produce a normal labor pattern will not result in dilatation and effacement or fetal descent within a normal time frame. Cause is unknown, although common causes are increased uterine tone, abnormal contraction pressure, hypotonic labor (prolonged latent phase, protracted or arrested active phase, or prolonged second stage of labor), and abnormal contraction pressure.

2. Problems with the force of labor will result in ineffective contractions or ineffective bearing down (pushing) during the second stage of labor.

3. Etiology of abnormalities in the force of labor include:

   a. Early or excessive use of analgesia

   b. Overdistention of the uterus

   c. Excessive cervical rigidity

   d. Grand multiparity (>6)

   e. Mild pelvic contraction

   f. Postmature and large infants

Passageway Abnormalities

1. Abnormalities in the passageway may be the result of problems in the pelvis or soft tissues of the reproductive tract.

2. Most often problems with the passageway are a result of pelvic abnormalities that interfere with the engagement, descent, and expulsion of the fetus.
   a. The size and shape of the pelvis are important.
   b. Obstruction may result from problems of the soft tissue such as a uterine or ovarian fibromyoma.
3. Contractions of the inlet are noted when the anteroposterior diameter is less than 10 cm or the greatest transverse diameter is less than 12 cm. Contracted inlets may be of genetic origin or a result of rickets.
4. Midpelvic contractions occur when the distance between the ischial spines is less than 9 cm. Often, this is not detected early in labor because the fetal head has engaged, and molding along with caput formation gives the suggestion that the head has descended further than it has.
5. A contracted pelvic outlet is diagnosed when the distance between the ischial spines is less than 8 cm. When the pelvis is contracted and the fetus cannot fit through the pelvis, CPD exists.

Fetal Passage Abnormalities

1. Normal fetal passage.
   a. Normally, the fetus enters the pelvic inlet transversely and then rotates to an occiput anterior position, allowing for the smallest diameter of the fetal head to pass through the pelvis.
   b. When the fetal head enters the pelvis posteriorly, it must rotate to the anterior position. This is done usually without problems if the fetus is of average size and well flexed and the contractions are a good quality.
   c. Synclitism—the position of the fetal head in relation to the anteroposterior diameter of the maternal pelvis. Refers specifically to the position of the fetal head when the sagittal suture is halfway between the sacral promontory and symphysis pubis. If synclitism exists, the planes of the pelvis and the fetal skull are parallel with the same space all around the fetal head.
2. Asynclitism.
   a. Either posterior or anterior.
   b. Posterior—position of the fetal head when the sagittal suture is closer to the sacral promontory.
   c. Anterior—position of the fetal head when the sagittal suture is closer to the symphysis pubis.
3. If the fetus does not turn, then it remains in the posterior position and may slow down the progress of descent.
   a. If the pelvis is large enough, the baby can be born in the posterior position (occiput posterior).
   b. If the pelvis is borderline and the contractions ineffective, a cesarean section may be necessary.
4. Breech presentations occur in approximately 3% of all deliveries.
   a. This presentation is more common in multiple gestations, increased parity, hydramnios, congenital dislocated hip, placenta previa, and preterm infants.
   b. Usually, the method of choice for delivery is a cesarean section.

5. Shoulder presentation (transverse lie) occurs when the infant lies crosswise in the uterus. The infant is delivered by cesarean section, if external cephalic version (ECV) is unsuccessful.
6. A large fetus has an increased risk of trauma in its attempt to fit through a normal size pelvis. A large infant may not fit through the pelvis, and CPD may result.

Diagnostic Evaluation

1. Inadequate progress of cervical effacement, dilatation, or descent of the presenting part as determined by vaginal examination
2. Evaluation of labor progress by recording and assessing serial vaginal examinations using Friedman's curve
   a. Using Friedman's curve, a prolonged latent phase in the primigravida is >20 hours and in the multigravida it is >14 hours.
   b. During the active phase, the cervix of a primagravida will normally dilate at least 1.2 cm/h, and the multigravida 1.5 cm. In addition, the fetus should be descending through the birth canal. In the primagravida, the rate of descent is 1 cm/h, and 2 cm/h for the multigravida.

Management

1. Treatment for contraction abnormalities involves stimulation of labor through the use of oxytocin. An intrauterine pressure catheter may be used.
2. Management for maternal passageway or fetal passage problems involves delivery in the safest manner for the mother and fetus.
   a. If the problem is related to the inlet or midpelvis, a cesarean delivery is indicated.
   b. If the size of the outlet is the problem, a forceps delivery is usually performed.

Complications

1. Maternal exhaustion
2. Infection
3. Fetal distress
4. Postpartum hemorrhage
5. Fetal or maternal trauma from instrumented delivery

Nursing Assessment

1. Perform Leopold's maneuvers, and evaluate fetal presentation, position, and size.
2. Using Friedman's labor curve, evaluate progress of labor, noting dilations and effacement in relation to time of labor along with descent of the fetal head.
3. Monitor FHR and contraction status in accordance with standards of care and institutional policy according to the stage of labor and risk status of woman.
4. Monitor maternal vital signs in accordance with institutional policy.
5. Assess bladder fullness.

Nursing Diagnoses
- Pain related to physical and psychological factors of difficult labor
- Anxiety related to threat of change in the health status of self and fetus

Nursing Interventions
Promoting Comfort
1. Review relaxation techniques.
2. Encourage use of breathing techniques learned in prenatal classes.
3. Encourage frequent change of position.
4. Encourage voiding every 1 to 2 hours.
5. Provide back rubs and sacral pressure as needed.
6. Offer ice chips as needed to combat a dry mouth, if permitted.
7. Provide a quiet room.
8. Provide frequent encouragement to the woman and her support person.
9. Administer pain medication for analgesia, as ordered.
10. Assist with the administration of anesthesia, as indicated.

Decreasing Anxiety
1. Provide anticipatory guidance regarding the use of medication, equipment, and procedures.
2. Educate the woman about the administration of oxytocin (Pitocin).
3. Discuss with the woman the nature of the contractions associated with an induced labor (ie, short acceleration, intense plateau, short deceleration, increased strength/intensity).
4. Prepare the family for cesarean delivery, if necessary.

Outcome-Based Evaluation
- Verbalizes increased comfort
- Verbalizes understanding of procedures

■ Shoulder Dystocia

Shoulder dystocia is the arrest of spontaneous delivery of shoulders secondary to impaction of the anterior shoulder against the symphysis pubis.

Pathophysiology and Etiology
1. Prepregnancy risk factors:
   a. Maternal birth weight
   b. Prior shoulder dystocia
   c. Prior macrosomic infant
   d. Preexisting maternal diabetes
   e. Obesity
   f. Multiparity
   g. Advanced maternal age (≥35 years of age)
2. Prepartum factors:
   a. Glucose intolerance of pregnancy
   b. Excessive weight gain
   c. Diagnosed or suspected fetal macrosomia
   d. Abnormal pelvic size or shape
   e. Postdatism
3. Intrapartum factors:
   a. Prolonged second stage of labor
   b. Protracted or arrest of descent
   c. Pronounced fetal head molding
   d. Need for midpelvic forceps delivery

Management
1. Identification by evidence of the Turtle sign—fetal head descends down with pushing and then rescinds back to original position when pushing is done.
2. Prevention is the key because shoulder dystocia is difficult to predict.
   a. Early identification and treatment of gestational diabetes mellitus (GDM).
   b. Good diabetic control for patients with insulin-dependent diabetes mellitus (IDDM).
   c. Recorded estimated fetal weight measurements.
   d. Prevent postdated deliveries.
   e. Prevent abnormal progression of labor.
   f. Prevent excessive maternal weight gain.
3. No fundal pressure or traction on the fetal head.
4. Anticipation with plan of action.
   a. Utilize available personnel.
   b. Step stool at the bedside to allow for appropriate suprapubic pressure.
   c. Have resuscitation equipment/personnel readily available.
5. Nursing procedures:
   a. McRobert's maneuver—exaggerated flexion of the mother's legs on her abdomen
   b. Suprapubic pressure
6. Health care provider procedures:
   a. Rotation of the anterior shoulder to oblique position
   b. Delivery of posterior arm
   c. Rubin's maneuver—displacement of the posterior shoulder anteriorly, with respect to fetus, from behind; use with suprapubic pressure
   d. Wood's screw maneuver—rotation of the anterior shoulder 180 degrees to posterior
   e. Zavanelli maneuver—replacement of the head into the vagina and delivery by cesarean delivery

Complications
1. Fetal:
   a. Asphyxia—most immediate danger
   b. Brachial plexus injury
   c. Fractured clavicle/humerus
   d. Intracranial hemorrhage
   e. Torticollis
2. Maternal:
   a. Postpartum hemorrhage—major maternal risk
   b. Vaginal lacerations

c. Lower uterine segment laceration
d. Uterine rupture
e. Vulvar and vaginal hematomas
f. Puerperal infection, especially with intrauterine manipulation

Nursing Assessment

1. Continuously evaluate labor curve evaluating cervical dilation, effacement, and fetal descent.
2. Observe for Turtle sign during second stage of labor. Notify primary care provider if shoulder dystocia is suspected.
3. Continue fetal monitoring after the fetal head is delivered to ascertain time between delivery of head and delivery of body. Keep provider aware of time frame.

Nursing Diagnoses

- Fear and Anxiety related to inability to deliver fetus
- Pain associated with operative/instrumented procedures or uterine manipulation
- Risk for Injury to fetus and/or mother secondary to instrumented delivery

Nursing Interventions

Reducing Fear and Anxiety

1. Give brief explanation to the woman and her support person about procedures being performed.
2. Keep voice calm and situation in delivery/labor room controlled.
3. Limit numbers of personnel in the room during delivery should shoulder dystocia occur.

Decreasing Pain

1. Ensure appropriate anesthesia/analgesia available for woman.
2. Provide woman with appropriate anesthesia/analgesia after delivery.

Reducing and Identifying Trauma

1. Do not perform fundal pressure.
2. Perform critical assessment of neonate after delivery—Moro reflex, cord gases, range of motion.
3. Monitor labor curve, and notify primary care provider if the normal labor curve is not met.

NURSING ALERT

Fundal pressure is never applied for the treatment of shoulder dystocia. It can lead to further impaction of the anterior shoulder, irreversible brachial plexus injury, fetal neurologic injury secondary to hypoxia, and even fetal death.

Outcome-Based Evaluation

- Patient verbalizes understanding of situation and is cooperative with plan
- Patient verbalizes control of pain
- No neonatal distress or injury

▨ Uterine Rupture

Uterine rupture is a spontaneous or traumatic rupture of the uterus. Rupture occurs in about 1 in 15,000 births with about 50% infant mortality.

Pathophysiology and Etiology

1. Rupture of the scar from a previous cesarean delivery or hysterotomy
2. Uterine trauma related to manipulation with instrumentation (ie, curet) or abdominal trauma resulting from sharp objects (eg, knives, bullets), or accidents
3. Uterine congenital anomaly
4. Injudicious use of oxytocin; hyperstimulation
5. Breech extraction
6. Midforceps delivery
7. Multiple gestation or polyhydramnios causing uterine overdistention
8. Perforation from placement of intrauterine pressure catheter
9. Grand multipara (> six pregnancies)
10. Obstructed labor maneuvers within the uterus

Clinical Manifestations

Complete Rupture

Extends through entire uterine wall, and contents extrude into abdominal cavity. Clinical manifestations usually represent traumatic or violent rupture.

1. Sudden sharp abdominal pain during contractions
2. Abdominal tenderness
3. May have cessation of contractions, but not always
4. Bleeding into the abdominal cavity and sometimes into the vagina
5. Fetus easily palpated in the abdominal cavity; fetal heart tones cease
6. Signs of shock—rapid, weak pulse; cold, clammy skin; pale color; flaring of nostrils due to air hunger
7. Chest pain from diaphragmatic irritation due to bleeding into the abdomen

Incomplete Rupture

Extends through endometrium and myometrium only; often associated with dehiscence (separation of old scar with fetus remaining in the uterus).

1. Asymptomatic; usually will not have pain unless extends beyond scar tissue.
2. Contractions continue, but cervix fails to dilate.
3. Vaginal bleeding may be present.
4. Rising pulse rate and skin pallor.
5. Loss of fetal heart tones or fetal distress.
6. Little or no change noted in intrauterine pressure catheter.

Management

1. Immediate preparation for surgery, including blood and fluid replacement.
2. Oxytocin is given to contract the uterus and control bleeding.

3. The fetus is extracted as soon as possible, and the uterus is repaired, if possible.
4. A hysterectomy is done if bleeding cannot be controlled.
5. After surgery, additional blood and fluid replacement is continued along with antibiotic therapy.

Complications
1. Maternal—hypovolemic shock, peritonitis
2. Fetal—anoxia, death

Nursing Assessment
1. Continuously evaluate maternal vital signs; especially note an increase in the rate and depth of respirations, an increase in pulse, or a drop in blood pressure indicating status change.
2. Observe for signs and symptoms of impending rupture (ie, lack of cervical dilatation, tetanic uterine contractions, restlessness, anxiety, severe abdominal pain, fetal bradycardia, and/or late or variable decelerations of the FHR).
3. Assess fetal status by way of monitoring.
4. Speak with family, and evaluate their understanding of the situation.

Nursing Diagnoses
- Fluid Volume Deficit related to active fluid loss from hemorrhage
- Altered Tissue Perfusion, Maternal Vital Organ and Fetal, related to hypovolemia
- Fear related to surgical outcome for fetus and mother

Nursing Interventions
Maintaining Fluid Volume
1. Start or maintain an IV as prescribed. Use a large-gauge catheter when starting the IV for blood and large quantities of fluid replacement.
2. Maintain CVP and arterial lines, as indicated for hemodynamic monitoring.
3. Maintain bed rest to decrease metabolic demands.
4. Insert Foley catheter, and monitor urine output hourly or as indicated.
5. Obtain and administer blood products as indicated.

Maintaining Maternal and Fetal Tissue Perfusion
1. Administer oxygen using a face mask at 10 L/min or as ordered to provide high oxygen concentration.
2. Apply pulse oximeter, and monitor oxygen saturation as indicated.
3. Monitor ABGs and serum electrolytes as indicated to assess respiratory status, observing for hypoventilation and electrolyte imbalance.
4. Continually monitor maternal and fetal vital signs to assess pattern because progressive changes may indicate profound shock.

Reducing Fear
1. Give a brief explanation to the woman and her support person before beginning a procedure.
2. Answer questions that the family and woman may have.
3. Maintain a quiet and calm atmosphere to enhance relaxation.

4. Remain with the woman until anesthesia has been administered; offer support as needed.
5. Keep the family members aware of the situation while the woman is in surgery and allow time for them to express feelings.

Patient Education and Health Maintenance
1. Provide information and support regarding the possibility for future pregnancies.
2. Encourage the support of family and friends.
3. Inform the woman that, postoperatively, diet will be advanced with the return of bowel sounds.
4. Educate the woman about the importance of ambulation to prevent intestinal gas and other postoperative complications.

Outcome-Based Evaluation
- Vital signs stable; no evidence of shock
- ABGs within normal limits; FHR within normal limits
- Verbalizes concerns about self and her fetus

◼ Anaphylactic Syndrome of Pregnancy

Anaphylactic syndrome of pregnancy, previously known as *amniotic fluid embolism (AFE)*, is the escape of amniotic fluid containing debris such as meconium, lanugo, and vernix caseosa into the maternal circulation, usually resulting in deposition of fluid or debris in the pulmonary arterioles, resulting rapidly in respiratory distress, shock, and the possible development of DIC. Anaphylactic syndrome of pregnancy is rare (1 in 8,000 births), nonpreventable, and often fatal.

Pathophysiology and Etiology
1. The exact mechanism causing AFE is unclear.
2. It can occur in the intrapartum or postpartum period.
3. Myometrial vessels are exposed, usually at the placental site, and contractions are especially forceful. A thromboplastinlike substance is found in amniotic fluid, which causes defibrination leading to DIC.
4. Predisposing conditions include abruptio placentae; uterine rupture; intrauterine fetal demise; advanced maternal age (>35 years of age); polyhydramnios; short, tumultuous labor; Pitocin induction; and high parity.

Clinical Manifestations
1. Sudden dyspnea and chest pain
2. Cyanosis, tachycardia
3. Pulmonary edema
4. Vomiting
5. Seizures
6. Shaking chills; diaphoresis
7. Increasing restlessness and anxiety
8. Coughing with frothy, pink sputum
9. Profound shock due to:
   a. Anaphylaxis, which causes vascular collapse
   b. Uterine bleeding with development of hypofibrinogenemia

Diagnostic Evaluation

1. Clinical picture of rapidly developing dyspnea, tachypnea, and cyanosis
2. DIC confirmed by coagulation studies (prolonged thrombin time, prothrombin time, and partial prothrombin time, decreased factor V, VIII, X; decreased platelets; increased fibrin split products)

Management

1. Transfer to tertiary care center if woman is not in one
2. Endotracheal intubation
3. Administration of IV crystalloid fluids
4. Administration of blood products and heparin to combat DIC
5. Establishment of CVP line
6. Immediate delivery of the fetus
7. Initiation of cardiopulmonary resuscitation, if needed

Complications

The maternal–fetal mortality rate is estimated to be greater than 85% due to DIC and cardiopulmonary collapse, especially if the syndrome occurs within 10 to 32 minutes after delivery and/or ROM.

Nursing Assessment and Interventions

1. Be alert to signs and symptoms of potential AFE.
2. Monitor maternal vital signs to assess for signs of shock.
3. Monitor FHR for signs of distress.
4. Administer oxygen by way of face mask to assist respiratory status.
5. Alert medical staff immediately, and assist with emergency procedures such as delivery and with the cardiopulmonary resuscitation as needed.
6. Provide information and comfort to the family or support persons. If unable to do this personally due to the emergent needs of the woman, delegate another member of the staff to stay with the family or support persons.

■ Prolapsed Umbilical Cord

A prolapsed umbilical cord slips in front of or alongside the fetal presenting part. Types of cord prolapse include:

Complete—the cord can be felt on vaginal examination and be seen in the vaginal canal; membranes are ruptured. Changes in the FHR are evident.

Occult—the cord cannot be felt on vaginal examination or be seen. The cord lies between the presenting part and the maternal pelvis; membranes can be intact or ruptured. Changes in the FHR are evident.

Forelying—the cord can be felt on vaginal examination, but cannot be seen; usually contained within intact membranes. The cord lies in front of the presenting part.

Pathophysiology and Etiology

A fetal cord prolapse may occur when there is adequate room between the fetal parts and the maternal pelvis. Predisposing factors include:

1. ROM, before the presenting part is not engaged in the pelvis
2. More common in abnormal fetal positions like shoulder and foot presentations
3. Prematurity—small fetus allows more space around presenting part
4. Polyhydramnios—causes greater amount of fluid to be released with greater force when membranes rupture
5. Multifetal gestation
6. Fetopelvic disproportion (ie, CPD)
7. Abnormally long umbilical cord
8. Result of interventions or maneuvers (ie, external cephalic version [ECV] or amniotomy)

Clinical Manifestations

1. Cord may be seen protruding from vagina or palpated in the vagina or cervix.
2. With compression, FHR pattern may show variable decelerations with contractions or between contractions; often fetal bradycardia is present.

 NURSING ALERT

Prolapsed cord should be suspected with FHR deceleration after ROM.

Management

1. Delivery of the fetus as soon as possible.
2. Relief of pressure from the umbilical cord immediately.
3. Change maternal position—usually in knee–chest position to relieve pressure of presenting part.
4. Prepare for emergent delivery.

Complications

Maternal

1. Infection
2. Risk for hemorrhage from emergency delivery
3. Risk for increased perineal trauma from emergency vaginal forceps delivery
4. Uterine atony related to anesthesia effect

Fetal

1. Prematurity
2. Hypoxia
3. Meconium aspiration
4. Fetal death if delayed or undiagnosed

Nursing Assessment and Interventions

1. Observe for prolonged FHR deceleration.
2. Identify complete or forelying cord prolapse with a vaginal examination by a qualified nurse or health care provider. If the cord is exposed to cold room air, there may be a reflex constriction of the umbilical blood vessels that further restricts the oxygen flow to the fetus.
3. Do not pinch or squeeze the umbilical cord because it may cause the cord to spasm, which decreases umbilical blood flow and fetal oxygen leading to fetal hypoxia.

4. Explain procedures as much as possible to the woman during this emergent situation.
5. Administer oxygen by face mask at 8 to 10 L/min.
6. Relieve pressure from the presenting part of the fetus off the umbilical cord by manually pushing the presenting part upward with a gloved hand. Pressure must be relieved until the fetus is delivered by way of cesarean or vaginally. Do not remove hand until delivery is imminent (Figure 39-5).
7. Provide constant support to the woman and her support persons.
8. Encourage the woman to talk about her feelings regarding herself and the baby after delivery.

Community and Home Care Considerations

1. If prolapsed cord occurs at home with ROM, have the mother or significant other look or feel in the vagina for the protruding cord. If the cord is visible or felt, lift the fetal presenting part off the cord. Call 911.
2. Feel the uterus for increased (above normal) fetal activity.
3. Have mother lie on floor or bed with hips elevated above level of her head (Trendelenburg's position).

Inversion of the Uterus

Inversion of the uterus is a potentially life-threatening complication in which the uterus turns inside out during the third stage of delivery. Inversion may be:

    Spontaneous—occurs with increased abdominal pressure, as seen with forceful coughing or bearing down
    Forced—occurs with pulling on the umbilical cord
    Complete—uterus totally inverts into the vagina

    Partial—fundus of uterus partially inverts but not beyond the cervical os

Pathophysiology and Etiology

Inversion is more commonly seen with fundal placental implantation and with a thin uterine wall at the site of implantation. Predisposing factors include:

1. Excessive traction on the cord while the placenta is still attached to the uterine wall
2. Lax or thin uterine wall
3. Fundal pressure
4. Spontaneous inversion
5. Delivery of an infant with a short umbilical cord
6. Uterine atony
7. Leiomyomas
8. Placenta accreta or increta

Clinical Manifestations

1. Primary sign is hemorrhage and sudden agonizing pelvic pain.
2. Maternal bleeding and shock, with symptoms often seeming out of proportion for the blood loss.
3. A complete inversion may appear protruding from vagina.
4. Inability to palpate fundus in association with clinical manifestations.
5. Confirmed with bimanual examination.

Management

1. Prevention is the most effective therapy.
2. Goal is to restore the uterus to its normal position, manually.

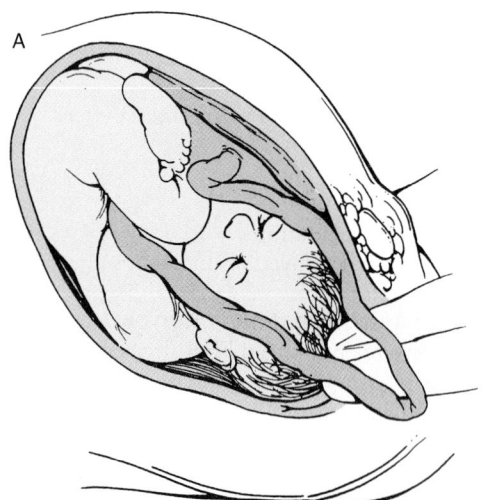 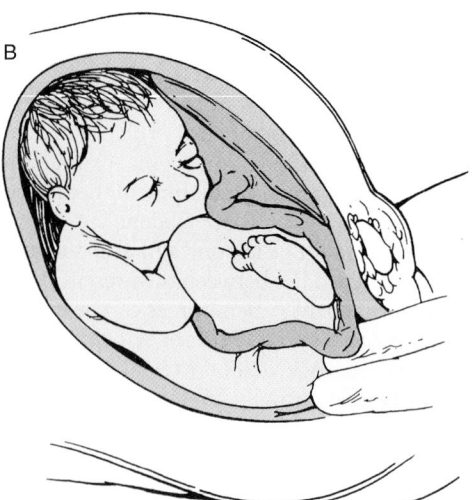

FIGURE 39-5 Prolapsed cord. Reduction of cord compression using gloved examiner's hand in vagina to elevate presenting part. (**A**) Vertex. (**B**) Breech.

3. Often involves the use of general anesthesia and tocolytic therapy (terbutaline or $MgSO_4$).

4. In addition, blood replacement therapy may be instituted to correct the shock.

5. After the uterus has been restored to its normal position, oxytocin is given to contract the uterus.

6. Abdominal or vaginal surgery may be necessary. Additionally, the woman is treated with broad-spectrum antibiotics.

Complications

1. Infection, anemia
2. Potential for a hysterectomy if uterus cannot be returned to its normal position
3. Potential for paralytic ileus

Nursing Assessment and Interventions
Before Correction of the Inversion

1. Check maternal vital signs and evaluate for blood loss.
2. Place the woman flat in bed in Trendelenburg's position so that pelvis is higher than head.
3. Administer oxygen by face mask at 8 to 12 L/min.
4. Establish an IV line with a 16- or 18-gauge catheter for administration of fluids, blood products, and medications. Two IV lines will be needed.
5. Apply a pulse oximeter to determine oxygen saturation.
6. If replacement of the uterus is unsuccessful, prepare the woman and her support persons for emergency surgery.

After Correction of the Inversion

1. Check maternal vital signs, and monitor CBC for signs of bleeding, infection.
2. Administer oxytocin and other uterine tonics, as ordered
3. Measure and record accurate intake and output.
4. Evaluate uterine fundus for position and firmness.
5. Evaluate lochia for amount of blood loss.
6. Evaluate for transfusion reactions (ie, itching, wheezing, anaphylaxis).
7. Administer antibiotics, as ordered, to minimize risk of infection.
8. Provide support to the woman, and encourage her to express her feelings.

OPERATIVE OBSTETRICS

■ Episiotomy

An episiotomy is an incision of the perineum during delivery to:

  Substitute a straight surgical incision for the laceration that may otherwise occur

  Facilitate repair of laceration and promote healing

  Spare the infant's head from prolonged pressure and pushing against the rigid perineum, which may result in brain damage, especially in the premature infant

  Shorten the second stage of labor

Types of Episiotomies
See Figure 39-6.
Median (Midline)

1. Incision is made in the middle of the perineum and directed toward the rectum.
2. This method is believed to heal with few complications, is more comfortable for the woman during healing, is easy to repair, and is associated with minimal blood loss.
3. If a larger incision is needed during delivery, however, it may necessitate incision into anal sphincter.

Mediolateral

1. Incision is made laterally in the perineum.
2. This method avoids the anal sphincter if enlargement is needed.
3. Women find it extremely uncomfortable during healing.
4. Associated with increased blood loss.
5. Necessitates longer wound healing time.

Management

1. Pain relief
   a. The stretching of the perineum and pressure from the fetal head may provide a natural numbing effect.
   b. Local perineal infiltration with lidocaine provides anesthesia for performing and repairing the episiotomy.
   c. A pudendal block provides anesthesia to the lower two thirds of the perineum and vagina using lidocaine injection into the vaginal walls.
   d. Epidural anesthesia provides anesthesia from the level of the umbilicus to the midthigh area.
2. The episiotomy is performed when the fetal head is about 3 to 4 cm visible with a contraction.

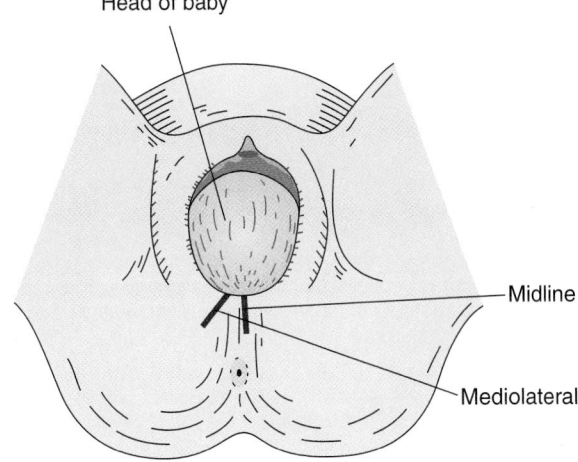

FIGURE 39-6 Position of episiotomy incision in a woman during second stage of labor. Baby's head is presenting to vaginal outlet (crowning).

3. The repair of the episiotomy usually begins after the delivery of the placenta.

Complications
1. Infection
2. Increased risk of blood loss
3. Third- and fourth-degree lacerations
4. Episiotomy pain
5. Risk for hematoma
6. Dyspareunia (pain during intercourse), which may last up to 6 months

Nursing Assessment
During the recovery period, the episiotomy should be evaluated every 15 minutes and three times a day after this.
1. Describe and document the degree of healing.
2. Assess for infection, which may be indicated by edema, redness, purulent drainage at the site; increased temperature.
3. Notify health care provider of bleeding at site, other than slight oozing.
4. Monitor for hematoma formation.

Nursing Diagnoses
- Risk for Infection related to traumatized tissue
- Pain related to surgical procedure

Nursing Interventions
Preventing Infection
1. Instruct the woman to cleanse from the front to the back.

2. Provide instructions on techniques used for perineal care.
   a. Provide a peri-bottle, and teach the woman to squirt the water gently on her perineum after using the toilet.
3. Explain the importance of changing the perineal pad each time after urination and defecation and of not touching the inner surface of the pad.
4. Explain the importance of proper handwashing before and after perineal care.
5. Explain that perineal care should be carried out after urination and defecation and at least every 4 hours during the day.
6. Encourage a diet that is high in protein and vitamin C and encourage at least 2,000 mL of fluid each day.

Promoting Comfort
1. Apply ice packs to the perineal area for the first 24 hours after delivery. The ice packs should not remain in place longer than 30 minutes at a time to get the maximum benefit for the treatment.
2. Encourage sitz baths with either warm or cool water. The warm water is soothing, whereas the cool water helps to decrease pain sensation and edema. See Procedure Guidelines 39-1.
3. Administer pain medication and topical anesthetics as ordered.
4. Instruct the woman to tighten her buttocks and perineal muscles before sitting in a chair and to release the muscles once seated.

Outcome-Based Evaluation
- No evidence of infection; afebrile
- Demonstrates increase in comfort

PROCEDURE GUIDELINES 39-1 | SITZ BATH

A sitz bath aids the healing of the perineum through application of moist heat.

EQUIPMENT
Sitz bath basin, bag, and tubing
Towel
Perineal pad

PROCEDURE

Nursing Action	Rationale
1. Assess patient's condition, pain level, and ability to ambulate to bathroom.	1. Effects of childbirth, pain medication, and lost sleep may make patient lightheaded, fatigued, or drowsy, impairing her ability to ambulate and tolerate sitting on toilet without support.
2. Wash hands.	2. To prevent spread of germs onto clean equipment.
3. Fill sitz bath basin with warm water and place on toilet bowl (with toilet seat up). Fill bag with warm water at a temperature of 105 to 110°F (40 to 43°C) and attach tubing to basin.	3. Warm water is soothing and results in vasodilation to enhance healing, but should not create thermal injury.

Nursing Action	Rationale

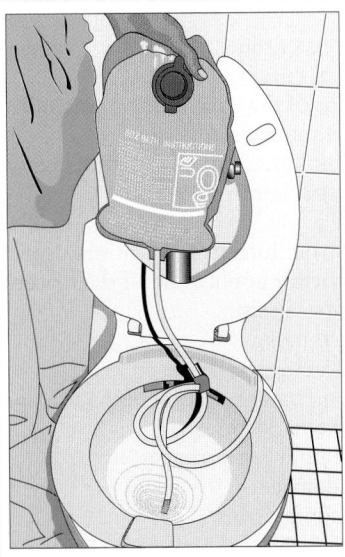

4. Hang bag overhead so a steady stream of water will flow from the bag, through the tubing, into the basin.

5. Assist patient with removal of peri-pad from front to back and positioning on sitz basin.

6. Instruct patient to use clamp on tubing to control water flow. Ensure that she has robe or blanket to prevent chilling and that she can call for assistance if necessary.

7. Allow patient to sit for 20 minutes, then assist her with drying and applying a clean peri-pad (avoid touching front of pad).

8. Assist patient back to bed, noting tolerance of the procedure.

9. Document tolerance of procedure, pain, and appearance of the perineal area.

4. Flow of water in the basin continuously replenishes warm water and enhances cleansing and circulation of the perineum, reducing inflammation and enhancing healing.

5. Removal of peri-pad from front to back prevents rectal contamination of incision.

6. Adequate circulation of water enhances comfort and healing, but too brisk a flow will drain water too quickly to achieve benefit. Privacy should be protected.

7. Beneficial effects of heat are lost after 20 minutes due to vasoconstriction. Contamination of front of peri-pad might result in infection of healing tissue.

8. Use of warm water and prolonged sitting in one position may result in lightheadedness on arising.

9. Decreased swelling, redness, and drainage and complete healing are the goals.

■ Forceps Delivery

Obstetric forceps (Table 39-3) are designed for rotating or extracting the fetal head. Forceps consist of two pieces: a right blade, which is slipped into the right side of the mother's pelvis, and a left blade, which is slipped into the left side. Each piece consists of four parts:

Handle—used to hold the forceps.

Shank—the piece between the handle and the blade. It contributes to the length of the forceps.

Lock—keeps the two pieces of forceps together.

Blade—fits around the fetal head.

Types of Forceps Deliveries
Outlet Forceps
1. Scalp visible at the introitus; labia not separated
2. Fetal skull at pelvic floor

3. Sagittal suture in anteroposterior diameter or right-to-left occiput anterior or posterior position
4. Fetal head at or on perineum
5. Rotation not more than 45 degrees

Low Forceps
1. Leading point of fetal skull is at station greater than or equal to +2 cm, and not on the pelvic floor.
2. Rotation less than or equal to 45 degrees (left or right occiput anterior to occiput anterior, or left or right occiput posterior to occiput posterior)
3. Rotation greater than 45 degrees
4. Mid-forceps station above +2 cm; head engaged

Indications for Forceps Delivery
General Criteria
1. Pelvis should be adequate, with no disproportion.
2. Fetal head must be engaged—preferably deeply engaged.

TABLE 39-3   Representative Types of Forceps*

Major Classifications	Use
1. Simpson— separated shanks (DeLee forcep is one example)	Extract fetus with elongated, molded head; commonly used with nulliparas who have long labors
2. Elliot—overlapping shanks (Tucker–McLean is one example)	Extract fetus with unmolded, rounder heads; commonly used with multiparas who have briefer labors
3. Specialized types	
a. Piper	Deliver aftercoming head in a breech presentation
b. Kielland	Rotate head from transverse or posterior position to an anterior position; used to deliver women with anthropoid pelves
c. Barton	Rotate head from transverse to an anterior position; designed for use in women with flat pelves

*There are more than 600 types of forceps.

3. Cervix must be completely dilated.
4. Accurate diagnosis of position and station must be made.
5. Membranes must be ruptured.
6. Some form of anesthesia should be used.
7. Rectum and bladder should be empty.

Fetal Indication
1. Fetal compromise
2. Cord prolapse
3. Malposition of the head
4. Abruptio placentae

Maternal Indications
1. Maternal indications for shortening the second stage of labor
   a. Heart disease
   b. Acute pulmonary edema
   c. Maternal exhaustion
2. Intrapartum infections
3. Maternal hemorrhage
4. Eclampsia
5. Epidural or spinal anesthesia
6. Arrest of labor during second stage of labor
7. Elective low pelvic delivery

Contraindications
1. Confirmed CPD
2. Face or brow presentation
3. Incompletely dilated cervix
4. Unengaged fetal head
5. Preterm infant

Management
1. The woman is placed in the lithotomy position.
2. The bladder is usually emptied by catheterization.
3. Regional anesthesia is most frequently used; pudendal block can also be used.

4. The pediatric/neonatal staff is in attendance at delivery.
5. An episiotomy is usually performed.

Complications
Maternal
1. Lacerations of the vulva, cervix, vagina, and rectum
2. Fracture of coccyx
3. Extensions of the episiotomy to include the rectum
4. Bladder trauma, uterine rupture
5. Postpartum infection, postpartum hemorrhage secondary to uterine atony

Fetal
1. Bruising from forceps application, cephalohematoma
2. From incorrect application of the forceps:
   a. Facial paralysis
   b. Brachial palsy
   c. Skull fracture
3. From incorrect application of the forceps or from compromised fetal status:
   a. Intracranial hemorrhage
   b. Brain damage
   c. Cord compression

Nursing Assessment
1. After application of the forceps, the FHR should be evaluated continuously or at least every 5 minutes.
2. Evaluate maternal sensation.
3. Evaluate bladder fullness—bladder should be empty before the application of the forceps.
4. Ensure aseptic technique is maintained.

Nursing Diagnoses
• Anxiety related to fetal outcome
• Pain related to procedures

Nursing Interventions
Decreasing Anxiety
1. Explain how the forceps are applied.
2. Explain that a sensation of pressure rather than pain will be felt.
3. Answer any questions that the woman and her support persons might have.
4. Stay with the woman, and provide guidance during the delivery process.

Promoting Comfort
1. Encourage use of breathing and relaxation techniques.
2. Make sure bladder is completely empty.
3. Encourage relaxation between contractions and use of abdominal muscles and pushing with the contractions.
4. Use blankets and pillow supports when positioning the woman for delivery.

Outcome-Based Evaluation
• Verbalizes concerns regarding forceps; responds to instructions
• Demonstrates increased level of comfort

Vacuum Extraction

A vacuum extractor applies suction to the fetal head with a suction cup, thus allowing adequate traction for delivery of the infant's head.

Indications

1. Indications for a vacuum delivery are the same as for a forceps delivery.
2. Contraindications for vacuum delivery are the same as for a forceps delivery and also include breech presentations, profound fetal compromise/maternal distress.
3. Advantages include ease of application and ability to perform procedure without requiring extra space in birth canal, as with forceps.

Management

1. Fetus is in vertex presentation.
2. Membranes must be ruptured.
3. The woman is in the lithotomy position.
4. The bladder is usually catheterized.
5. Evaluate progress with suction.
6. Anesthesia may be indicated.
7. Unsuccessful extraction is followed by a cesarean section.
8. Pediatric/neonatal staff is in attendance at delivery.

Complications

Complications are usually less frequent and less severe with vacuum extraction than with forceps.
Maternal
Lacerations of the cervix or vagina
Fetal
1. Cephalohematoma
2. Caput succedaneum (swelling of the scalp) from the vacuum
3. From improper technique or from compromised fetal status:
   a. Intracranial hemorrhage
   b. Retinal hemorrhage
4. Abrasions

Nursing Assessment

1. After application of the vacuum extractor, the FHR should be evaluated at least every 5 minutes or continuously.
2. Evaluate maternal sensation.
3. Evaluate bladder fullness—bladder should be empty before the application of the vacuum extractor.
4. Ensure aseptic technique is maintained.
5. Monitor the vacuum pressure of the equipment according to institution protocol.

Nursing Interventions

Same as for a forceps delivery.

Cesarean Birth

Cesarean birth or delivery is the surgical removal of the infant from the uterus through an incision made in the abdominal wall and an incision made in the uterus. About 25% of all births are cesarean.

Types of Cesarean Delivery
Uterine Incisions
1. Low segment transverse—incision made transversely in lower segment of uterus.
   a. Incision is made in thinnest portion so blood loss is minimal and uterus is easier to open.
   b. Lower segment is area of least uterine activity.
   c. Postoperative convalescence is more comfortable.
   d. Possibility of later rupture is lessened.
   e. Incidence of postoperative adhesions and danger of intestinal obstruction are reduced.
   f. It is the incision of choice.
2. Classic—vertical incision is made directly into the wall of the body of the uterus; usually done in emergency situations only .
   a. Useful when bladder and lower segment are involved in extensive adhesions.
   b. Selected when anterior placenta previa or emergency situation exists.
   c. Useful when fetus is in a transverse lie.
   d. Increased blood loss with classic cesarean.
   e. Increased risk of uterine rupture in subsequent deliveries.
3. Low vertical (used rarely).
   a. May be extended upward into a classic incision if extra room is needed for delivery.
   b. May extend downward and cause trauma to the cervix, vagina, and bladder.

Abdominal Incisions
1. Pfannenstiel—a horizontal incision right above the pubic hair line
   a. Cosmetic advantage of not being seen because pubic hair covers incision
   b. Decreased chance of dehiscence or hernia formation
2. Vertical—a vertical incision made in the midline of the abdomen below the umbilicus to the pubis
   a. Quicker procedure to perform
   b. Provides better uterine visualization
   c. Cosmetically less appealing
   d. Greater chance of wound dehiscence and hernia formation

Indications for Cesarean Delivery
1. CPD
2. Uterine dysfunction, inertia, inability of cervix to dilate
3. Neoplasm obstructing birth canal or pelvis
4. PIH
5. Severe diabetes mellitus
6. Uteroplacental insufficiency and oligohydramnios
7. Malposition and malpresentation

8. Previous uterine surgery (cesarean delivery, myomectomy, hysterotomy) or cervical surgery—evaluated on an individual basis
9. Complete or partial placenta previa
10. Abruptio placentae
11. Prolapse of the umbilical cord
12. Fetal compromise
13. Active genital herpes simplex
14. Breech or shoulder presentation
15. Multiple gestation more than three fetuses
16. Conjoined twins
17. Indications for cesarean hysterectomy:
    a. Ruptured uterus
    b. Intrauterine infection
    c. Hemorrhage due to uterine atony that does not respond to oxytocin, prostaglandin, or massage
    d. Laceration of major uterine vessel
    e. Severe dysplasia or carcinoma in situ of the cervix
    f. Placenta accreta
    g. Gross multiple fibromyomas

Management
1. NPO (except possible ice chips) during labor.
2. A blood sample should be typed and screened and available to be crossmatched if needed; a CBC is obtained.
3. Anesthesia, regional or general, depends on the indication for surgery.
4. Permit signed/witnessed; informed consent confirmed.
5. A large-bore IV is established, and Foley catheter is inserted.
6. An antacid is administered to reduce gastric acidity and the risk of aspiration pneumonia.
7. Antibiotics may be given prophylactically.
8. An abdominal prep is done, and a grounding pad for electrocautery is applied.

Complications
1. Increase in morbidity and mortality compared with a vaginal birth
2. Hemorrhage, endometritis
3. Paralytic ileus, intestinal obstruction
4. Pulmonary embolism, thrombophlebitis
5. Anesthesia accidents
6. Bowel or bladder injury
7. Respiratory depression of the infant from anesthetic drugs
8. Possible delay in maternal–infant bonding
9. Amniotic fluid or air embolism (rare occurrence)

Nursing Assessment
Before Delivery
1. Assess knowledge of procedure.
2. Ensure informed consent obtained, permits signed/witnessed.
3. Monitor maternal and fetal vital signs.

4. Determine maternal blood type and Rh.
5. Determine last time the woman ate or drank.
6. Identify drug allergies.
7. Identify other allergies (eg, latex, betadine, tape).

After Delivery
1. Assess maternal vital signs every 15 minutes the first hour, every 30 minutes the second hour, and then hourly until she is transferred to the postpartum/LDR(P) unit or per institutional protocol.
2. Evaluate fundal position and firmness along with vital signs.
3. Evaluate amount and type of lochia along with vital signs.
4. Assess condition of the incision line or dressing.
5. Monitor urine output, presence of bowel sounds.
6. Assess level and presence of anesthesia or pain.
7. Auscultate lung sounds, maternal oxygen saturation.
8. Assess maternal–infant bonding.

Nursing Diagnoses
- Anxiety related to cesarean delivery
- Pain related to surgical procedure
- Risk for Infection related to traumatized tissue
- Risk for Ineffective Parent/Infant Attachment related to interruption in bonding process

Nursing Interventions
Relieving Anxiety
1. Explain the reason for the cesarean delivery.
2. Answer any questions the woman and her support person may have regarding a cesarean delivery.
3. Explain all procedures before doing them.
4. Allow the support person to attend the birth.
5. Explain that a sensation of pressure will be felt during the delivery, but that little pain will occur. Instruct that any pain should be reported to the nurse.

Promoting Comfort
1. Encourage use of relaxation techniques after medication has been given for pain.

NURSING ALERT

Do not administer parenteral narcotics if patient is receiving epidural narcotics unless ordered by anesthesiologist/nurse anesthetist.

2. Monitor for respiratory depression up to 24 hours after epidural narcotic administration.
3. Monitor/instruct patient on use of PCA pump.
4. Use a back rub and a quiet environment to promote the effectiveness of the medication.
5. Support/splint the abdominal incision when moving or coughing and deep breathing.
6. Encourage frequent rest periods, and plan for them after activities; also, place a "Do Not Disturb" sign on the door during rest and sleep periods.

7. To reduce pain caused by gas, encourage ambulation, use of rocking chair, and lying as much on stomach as possible/tolerated.

Preventing Infection

1. Although shaving the skin before delivery is no longer a standard of practice, it is still carried out in some institutions. If skin preparation includes shaving, shave skin carefully, avoiding any nicks in the skin. Then, carry out surgical skin preparation correctly.
2. Postoperatively, use aseptic technique when changing dressings.
3. Provide perineal care along with vital signs every 4 hours or as needed.
4. Provide routine postoperative care measures to prevent urinary or pulmonary infection.

Promoting Effective Bonding

1. Encourage the woman and her support person to discuss their feelings regarding the cesarean birth both before and after the delivery.
2. When talking of the birth, refer to it as a cesarean birth or delivery, to imply it is just another method of birth, not a surgical experience.
3. Encourage mother–child bonding as soon as possible.
4. Emphasize that adjustments to parenting under any circumstances are necessary and normal.

Patient Education and Health Maintenance

1. Teach the woman the "football hold" for breast-feeding so the infant is not lying on her abdomen.
2. Teach the woman to observe for signs of infection (foul-smelling lochia, elevated temperature, increased pain, redness and edema at the incision rate) and to report them immediately.
3. Assist the woman in planning for the assistance of friends, family, or hired help at home during the period immediately after discharge.

Outcome-Based Evaluation

- Verbalizes an understanding of the cesarean birth procedure and postdelivery care
- Reports relief of pain
- Has no signs of infection
- Participates in care of self and infant

POSTPARTUM COMPLICATIONS

Postpartum Infection

Postpartum (puerperal) infection is a postpartum infection of the genital tract, usually of the endometrium (endometritis), that may remain localized or may extend to various parts of the body such as the connective tissue by way of lymphatic spread (parametritis). The main pathway for spread of the infection is the broad ligament.

Pathophysiology and Etiology

The most common cause is polymicrobial ascent to the uterus from the lower genital tract. Hematogenous bacterial spread may also occur.

1. Prolonged labor or ROM, PPROM
2. Number of vaginal examinations
3. Infection elsewhere in the body; wound infection, UTI, pneumonia, mastitis
4. Anemia, malnutrition
5. Size and number of perineal lacerations
6. Intrauterine manipulation
7. Retained placental fragments of membranes
8. Lapse in aseptic technique
9. Poor perineal hygiene
10. Cesarean delivery
11. Instrumented delivery; forceps or vacuum extraction
12. Pelvic thrombophlebitis
13. NEC

Clinical Manifestations

Diagnosis is made by sustained fever of 38°C (100.4°F) or higher occurring on any two of the first 10 days postpartum, excluding the first 24 hours. Symptoms depend on site and extension of infection.

Endometritis Postpartum

Infection involving the endometrium

1. Uterus usually larger than expected for postdelivery day; uterus tender.
2. Lochia may be profuse, bloody, and foul smelling.
3. Chills, malaise, and fever occur if lochial discharge is obstructed by clots.
4. WBC >20,000/mm^3 with increased neutrophils.
5. Infection may spread to myometrium (endomyometritis), parametrium, uterine (fallopian) tubes, peritoneum, and blood.

Parametritis (Pelvic Cellulitis)

Infection of the pelvic connective tissue spread by the lymphatic system within the uterine wall. Often a result of an infected wound in the cervix, vagina, perineum, or lower uterine segment.

1. Chills, fever (38.8° to 40.0°C [102° to 104°F]), tachycardia
2. Severe unilateral or bilateral pain in lower abdomen
3. Enlarged and tender uterus
4. Uterine position may become fixed as it is displaced by the exudate along the broad ligament

Management

1. Antibiotic therapy is instituted after cultures are obtained and causative agent identified. Broad-spectrum antibiotics are the treatment of choice including penicillins, cephalosporins (cefoxitin, cefazolin), clindamycin (Cleocin) and aminoglycosides (gentamicin, tobramycin). Antibiotics are given until the woman is afebrile for 48 hours.

2. Supportive therapy is used to control pain and to maintain hydration and nutritional status.
3. Drainage is indicated for abscess development.
4. Administration of single-dose ampicillin or cephalosporins after umbilical cord clamping is considered effective prophylaxis for nonelective cesarean delivery.

> **◈ DRUG ALERT**
>
> Clindamycin/gentamicin treatment is successful in only 75% to 92% of cases and is associated with renal toxicity. It is not effective against enterococci—ampicillin is the drug of choice in this instance.

Complications

1. Thrombophlebitis may result from postpartum infection spread along the veins.
   a. Femoral thrombophlebitis—appears 10 to 20 days after delivery as pain in calf, positive Homans' sign (pain with foot flexion), fever, edema; affected leg circumference 2 cm greater than unaffected leg.
   b. Pelvic thrombophlebitis—infection of the veins of uterine wall and broad ligament usually caused by anaerobic streptococci; presents about 2 weeks after delivery with severe repeated chills and wide range of temperature changes.
   c. Treatment includes strict bed rest, anticoagulants, and antibiotics.
2. Pulmonary embolus may occur—dyspnea and chest pain.
3. Peritonitis—spread of infection through lymphatic channels.

Nursing Intervention and Patient Education

1. Perform postpartum assessment, noting uterine tenderness on palpation and the color, amount, and odor of lochia.
2. Monitor vital signs every 4 hours for signs of infection.
3. Assess knowledge and skill of perineal hygiene; teach proper technique and assist, if necessary.
4. Provide for adequate rest periods.
5. Increase fluid intake.
6. Position in high Fowler's position to promote drainage.
7. Administer antibiotics and analgesics, as ordered.
8. Explain the benefit of perineal washing or sitz baths and demonstrate setup.
9. Explain the need for good handwashing technique and how contamination of vagina from the rectum occurs.
10. Show how to place perineal pads and medications; encourage to change pads with each voiding, bowel movement, or every 4 hours while awake.
11. Encourage minimal separation from the infant and continuation of breast-feeding, as able.
12. Promote good handwashing technique for the mother before contact with the infant.
13. Observe for signs of septic shock: tachycardia >120 bpm, hypotension, tachypnea, changes in sensorium, and decreased urine output.

14. If pulmonary embolism in question, elevate the head of the bed and provide oxygen.

▩ Postpartum Hemorrhage

Postpartum hemorrhage involves a loss of 500 mL or more of blood; it occurs early (first 24 hours) or late (after 24 hours and <6 weeks after birth). The greatest risk is during the first hour after birth. Hemorrhage is defined as a decrease in the hematocrit of at least 10%.

Note: For each 450 to 500 mL of blood loss, there will be a decrease in the hematocrit of 2% to 4% and a decrease in the hemoglobin of 1 to 1.5 g/dL.

Pathophysiology and Etiology

See Figure 39-7.

Early Postpartum Hemorrhage

1. Main cause is uterine atony—relaxation of the uterus secondary to:
   a. Overdistention of uterus secondary to multiple pregnancy or polyhydramnios
   b. High parity (more than six pregnancies)
   c. Prolonged labor with maternal exhaustion
   d. Large doses of drugs—oxytocin, $MgSO_4$, tocolytics, anesthetics
   e. Fibromyomata—prevents uterus from contracting
   f. Retained placental fragments—result from manual removal of placenta, succenturiate (additional) lobe, abnormal adherent placenta (placenta accreta), or spontaneous Shultze placenta (periphery detaches first instead of central [Duncan] detachment)

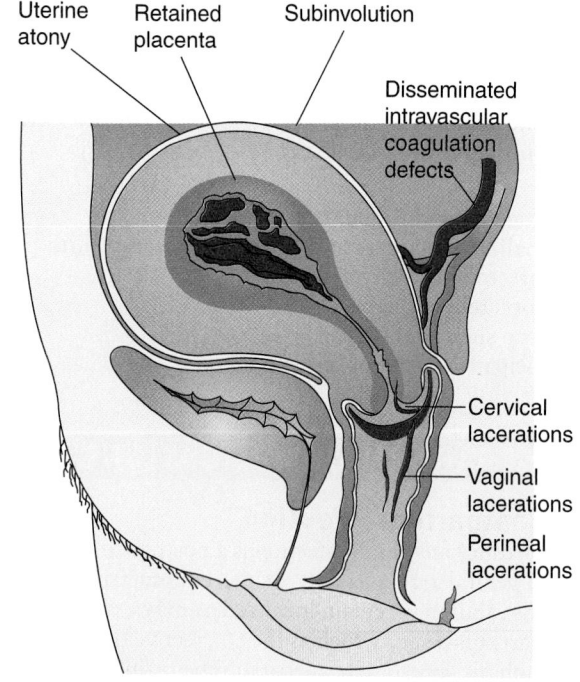

FIGURE 39-7   Common causes of postpartum hemorrhage.

2. Uterine inversion
3. Bleeding disorders, such as DIC
4. Laceration of the vagina, cervix, or perineum secondary to:
   a. Forceps delivery, especially rotation forceps
   b. Large infant
   c. Multiple pregnancy

Late Postpartum Hemorrhage
1. Main cause is retained placental fragments
2. Infection
3. Subinvolution (delayed healing) of placental site

Clinical Manifestations
Early Postpartum Hemorrhage
1. With uterine atony, uterus is soft or boggy, often difficult to palpate, and will not remain contracted; excessive vaginal bleeding occurs.
2. Lacerations of the vagina, cervix, or perineum care cause bright red, continuous bleeding even when the fundus is firm.

Late Postpartum Hemorrhage
1. Uterus is soft or boggy.
2. Slow, reddish oozing or heavy bleeding (first 6 weeks postdelivery)
3. Low persistent backache
4. Abdominal pain or tenderness
5. Fatigue
6. Loss of appetite

Management
1. For uterine atony, IV administration of oxytocin (Pitocin), IM administration of methylergonovine (Methergine), or prostaglandins administered IM or directly into myometrium.
2. Bimanual massage of the uterus.
3. Pain medication may be needed to counter uterine contractions.
4. If placental fragments have been retained, curettage of the uterus is indicated.
5. Lacerations may need to be repaired.
6. Emergency hysterectomy may be necessary.

Nursing Assessment
1. Assess maternal history for etiology of previous postpartum hemorrhage (eg, rapid or prolonged labor, uterine distention [macrosomia, polyhydramnios, or multiple gestation], use of tocolytics or halogenated anesthesia, operative birth, high parity, chorioamnionitis/intra-amniotic infection, placental abnormalities, or previous uterine surgery).
2. Assess blood loss; evaluate presence of clots; note number of pads saturated in 1 hour or shorter time frame if applicable. Note that a saturated pad contains about 25 to 50 mL of blood.
3. Assess vital signs every 15 minutes, especially mean arterial pressure (MAP).
4. Assess intake and output.

5. Assess for hypotension, tachycardia, change in respiratory rate, decrease in urine output, and change in mental status—may indicate hypovolemic shock.
6. Assess location and firmness of uterine fundus.
7. Percuss and palpate for bladder distention, which may interfere with contracting of the uterus.
8. Inspect for intactness of any perineal repair.

> **NURSING ALERT**
>
> In cases of postpartum hemorrhage, remember the acronym ORDERS:
> - **O**xygen
> - **R**estore circulation
> - **D**rugs to stop hemorrhage
> - **E**valuate interventions
> - **R**emedy problems
> - **S**upport emotionally

Nursing Diagnoses
- Anxiety related to unexpected blood loss and uncertainty of outcome
- Fluid Volume Deficit related to blood loss
- Risk for Infection related to blood loss and vaginal examinations

Nursing Interventions
Decreasing Anxiety
1. Maintain a quiet and calm atmosphere; provide emotional support.
2. Provide information about the situation and explain everything as it is done; answer questions that the woman and her family ask.
3. Encourage the presence of a support person.

Maintaining Fluid Volume
1. Maintain or start a large-bore IV line if vaginal bleeding becomes heavy.
2. Monitor and maintain accurate intake and output; use of Foley catheter provides accurate output measurements.
3. Ensure that crossmatched blood is available.
4. Provide additional oxygen by way of face mask; monitor oxygen saturation with pulse oximetry.
5. Infuse oxytocin (Pitocin), methergine, carboprost tromethamine (Hemabate) or Prostin $F_2\alpha$, IV fluids, and blood products at prescribed rate.
6. Apply correct uterine massage.
7. Monitor CBC for anemia.
8. D&C (may be needed for late postpartum hemorrhage)

> **NURSING ALERT**
>
> Avoid Trendelenburg's position for shock because it interferes with the cardiac and respiratory function by increasing pressure on the chemoreceptor and baroreceptors, which ultimately decreases lung expansion. The best thing to do is elevate the legs 20 to 30 degrees.

Preventing Infection
1. Maintain aseptic technique.
2. Evaluate for symptoms of infection, chilling, and elevated temperature, changes in WBC, uterine tenderness, and odor of lochia.
3. Administer antibiotics as prescribed.
4. Maintain adequate rest and proper nutrition.

Patient Education and Health Maintenance
1. Educate the woman about the cause of the hemorrhage.
2. Teach the woman the importance of eating a balanced diet and taking vitamin supplements.
3. Advise the woman that she may feel tired and fatigued and to schedule daily rest periods.
4. Teach woman and family signs and symptoms of hemorrhage to watch for during the puerperium.
5. Ensure woman has emergency procedures/numbers readily available.
6. Advise the woman to notify her health care provider of increased bleeding or other changes in her status.

Outcome-Based Evaluation
- Verbalizes concerns about her well-being
- Vital signs stable, urine output adequate, hematocrit stable
- Remains afebrile, WBC count within normal limits

Postpartum Hematomas

Postpartum hematomas are localized collections of blood in loose connective tissue beneath the skin that covers the external genitalia, beneath the vaginal mucosa, or in the broad ligaments. Occurs usually without laceration of the overlying tissue. Most commonly found in perineal and vaginal area, but can be elsewhere.

Pathophysiology and Etiology
1. Trauma during spontaneous labor
2. Trauma during forceps application or delivery
3. Inadequate suturing of an episiotomy
4. Delayed homeostasis/difficult or prolonged second stage of labor or both

Clinical Manifestations
1. Complaints of pressure and pain, often noting that the pain is excruciating.
2. Discolored skin that is tight, full feeling, and painful to touch. This may be the first sign seen.
3. Possible decrease in blood pressure, tachycardia.
4. Absence of lochia flow if the vaginal tract is impeded.

Management
1. Small hematomas (<3 cm) are left to resolve on their own—ice packs may be applied.
2. Large hematomas (>3 cm) may require evacuation of the blood and ligation of the bleeding vessel.
3. Analgesics and broad-spectrum antibiotics may be ordered (due to increased chance of infection).

Complications
1. Hypovolemia and shock from extreme blood loss
2. Anemia, infection
3. Increased length of postpartum recovery period
4. Sepsis/death
5. Calcification/scar tissue
6. Dyspareunia (painful intercourse)

Nursing Interventions and Patient Education
1. Inspect perineal and vulva area for signs of a hematoma when woman complains of pain or pressure after delivery.
2. Inspect the vaginal area for signs of a hematoma if woman is unable to void after anesthesia has worn off.
3. Monitor vital signs at least every 10 to 15 minutes, and evaluate for signs of shock.
4. Relieve pain of a hematoma by applying an ice bag to perineal area, medicating with mild analgesics, and positioning for comfort to decrease pressure on the affected area.
5. Help relieve voiding problems by assisting to bathroom to void if able to ambulate. If patient is unable to ambulate, then assist her to sit on bedpan with legs hanging over side of bed. Provide privacy, and run water while the woman is attempting to void.
6. If she is unable to void, catheterize.
7. Teach the woman the importance of eating a balanced diet and to include food high in iron.
8. Encourage the woman to take vitamin supplements and to take medications as ordered.
9. Instruct the woman in the use of the sitz bath to provide perineal comfort after the first 24 hours and at home.

Postpartum Depression

There still is no consensus regarding the classification of postpartum depression. The most common conditions are often identified as:
1. Maternity blues; postpartum blues; baby blues; mother's blues; or 3rd-, 4th-, or 10th-day blues
2. Postpartum or postnatal depression
3. Postpartum or puerperal psychosis
4. Postpartum panic disorder
5. Postpartum obsessive compulsive disorder
   Social, cultural, physiologic, and psychological factors experienced may contribute to postpartum depression.

Clinical Manifestations
1. Confusion
2. Exaggerated and prolonged periods of irritability, moodiness, hostility, fatigue
3. Ineffective coping
4. Withdrawal and inappropriate response to the infant or family
5. Loss of interest in activities
6. Insomnia/sleep disturbances
7. Headache

8. Constipation or other gastrointestinal difficulty
9. Hair loss
10. Dysmenorrhea
11. Difficulties with lactation
12. Decreased sexual responsiveness

Evaluation and Management

Signs and symptoms may be overlooked, making the diagnosis of depression difficult. There are several assessment tools designed to screen for women who may need further evaluation for postpartum depression. The Postpartum Depression Checklist (PDC) (Table 39-4) can be used by the nurse or health care provider as a means of communication to bring out the woman's thoughts and feelings after having a baby. Questions should be worded empathically and nonjudgmentally to bring out honest answers.

Counseling with a mental health professional, medication, and continuous support from family and friends may be helpful in managing the depressed patient. If untreated, the woman may not fully recover and may possibly harm the infant or others.

DRUG ALERT

The use of psychotropic medications during breast-feeding remains a controversial issue. All of the major classes of psychotropic drugs are expressed in breast milk.

NURSING ALERT

Any indication of suicide or harm to baby requires immediate referral to mental health professional.

Nursing Interventions and Patient Education

1. Listen to the woman regarding her adjustment to role of mother, and observe for any clinical manifestations suggesting depression.

2. Ask the woman about the infant's behavior. Negative statements about the infant may suggest that the woman is having difficulty coping.

3. Consult/refer woman to health care provider and other resources skilled in postpartum depression as necessary.

4. Provide support, and encourage family and friends to support and assist with the infant and mother. Physical support as well as emotional support may be indicated.

5. Educate the woman that treatment may help alleviate her symptoms and allow her to better care for herself and infant.

6. Encourage the woman to engage in activities that enhance attachment: rooming-in, breast-feeding, becoming involved in the medical examination of the newborn.

7. Realize that effective attachment behaviors differ from culture to culture and do not necessarily indicate maladaptive parenting behaviors.

SELECTED REFERENCES

American College of Obstetricians and Gynecologists (1990). *Ectopic pregnancy.* ACOG Technical Bulletin #150. Washington, D.C.: Author.

Beck, C. T. (1999). *Postpartum depression: Case studies, research, & nursing care.* Washington, DC: Association of Women's Health, Obstetric, and Neonatal Nurses.

Buckley, K., & Kulb, N. (1993). *High risk maternity nursing manual* (2nd ed.). Baltimore: Williams & Wilkins.

Burrow, G. N., & Ferris, T. F. (1995). *Medical complications during pregnancy* (4th ed.). Philadelphia: W. B. Saunders.

Creasy, R. K., & Resnick, R. (1999). *Maternal–fetal medicine principles and practice* (4th ed.). Philadelphia: W. B. Saunders.

Danforth, D. N., & Scott, J. R. (1994). *Danforth's obstetrics and gynecology* (7th ed.). Philadelphia: J. B. Lippincott.

DeCherney, A. H., & Agel, A. O. (1997). *Ectopic pregnancy. Clinical gynecology* (Vol. 1, pp. 1–20). Washington, D.C.: ACOG.

Dickason, E. J., et al. (1994). *Maternal–infant nursing care* (2nd ed.). St Louis: Mosby–Year Book.

Gilbert, E. S., & Harmon, J. S. (1993). *Manual of high risk pregnancy and delivery.* St Louis: Mosby–Year Book.

Gorrie, T. M., et al. (1994). *Foundations of maternal newborn nursing.* Philadelphia: W. B. Saunders.

James, D. K., et al. (1994). *High risk pregnancy management options.* Philadelphia: W. B. Saunders.

Johnson & Johnson Consumer Products, Inc. (1996). *Compendium of postpartum care.* Skillman, NJ: Author.

Mandeville, L. K., & Troiano, N. H. (1999). *High-risk and critical care intrapartum nursing* (2nd ed.). Philadelphia: Lippincott Williams & Wilkins.

May, K. A., & Mahlmeister, L. R. (1994). *Maternal and neonatal nursing—Family centered care* (3rd ed.). Philadelphia: J. B. Lippincott.

Pillitteri, A. (1999). *Maternal and child health nursing* (3rd ed.). Philadelphia: Lippincott Williams & Wilkins.

Queenan, J. T. (1994). *Management of high-risk pregnancy* (3rd ed.). Cambridge, MA: Blackwell Science.

Reeder, S. J., Martin, L. L., & Koniak-Griffin, D. (1997). *Maternity nursing* (18th ed.). Philadelphia: Lippincott-Raven.

Simpson, K. R., & Creehan, P. A. (1996). *Perinatal nursing.* Philadelphia: Lippincott-Raven.

Stoval, T. G., & Ling, F. W. (1993). Single-dose methotrexate: An expanded clinical trial. *American Journal of Obstetrics and Gynecology, 168*(6), 1759–1765.

TABLE 39-4 Postpartum Depression Checklist (PDC)

The PDC can be administered by the caregiver using questions about the following list of symptoms:

Symptoms	Yes	No
Lack of concentration		
Loss of interest		
Loneliness		
Insecurity		
Obsessive thinking		
Lack of positive emotions		
Loss of self		
Anxiety attacks		
Loss of control		
Guilt		
Contemplating death		

Pediatric Nursing

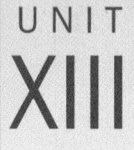
Pediatric Growth and Development

GROWTH AND DEVELOPMENT

◼ Basic Concepts

Growth and development begins with birth. As infants and children grow and mature, they pass through predictable stages of development. Knowledge and assessment of growth and development help the nurse provide screening for physical and emotional problems; offer anticipatory guidance to parents and caregivers; develop a rapport with the child to enhance the provision of health care; and provide education to the family to build a healthy lifestyle for the future. For assessment of the newborn see Chapter 38, p. 1162. This chapter will cover the beginning of infancy (1 month) to adolescence (12 to 14 years old).

◼ Infant to Adolescent Growth and Development

See Table 40-1.

◼ Developmental Screening Tools

Developmental screening tools have been created to determine the overall developmental age of the child or to detect specific areas of development that are lacking.

Goodenough-Harris Draw-a-Person Test

This test provides one of the methods of measuring the level of mental development of children generally between 3 and 10 years. Results of this test correlate well with intelligence quotient (IQ) test.

Procedure

The child is supplied with a pencil (preferably a No. 2 with eraser) and a sheet of blank paper and instructed to "Draw a person" or "Draw the best person you can."

No additional directions are necessary. Encouragement may be supplied if necessary. Under no condition should the examiner suggest that the child's picture needs to be supplemented or changed in any way—the only exception being a drawing of the stick figure. In this case the examiner is permitted to encourage the child to "draw a whole person."

Scoring

The child receives one point for each detail present according to the following scoring guides:

Goodenough-Harris Scoring			
General:	☐ Head present	**Proportion:**	☐ Head: 10% to 50% of trunk area
	☐ Legs present		☐ Arms: Approx. same length as trunk
	☐ Arms present		
Trunk:	☐ Present		☐ Legs: 1–2 times trunk length; width less than trunk width
	☐ Length greater than breadth		
	☐ Shoulders		☐ Feet: to leg length
Arms/ legs:			☐ Arms and legs in two dimensions)
	☐ Attached to trunk		
	☐ At correct point		☐ Heel

(*text continues on page 1233*)

TABLE 40-1   Infant to Adolescent Growth and Development

Age and Physical Characteristics	Behavior Patterns	Nursing Implications/ Parental Guidance
Birth–4 weeks (1 month) Much neurologic disorganization Strong Moro reflex Sleep cycle disorganized Gastrointestinal system too immature for solid foods	**Motor Development** Momentary visual fixation on objects and adult face. Eyes follow bright moving objects. Lies awake on back with head averted. Immediately drops objects placed in hands. Responds to sounds of bell and other similar noises. Keeps hands fisted. **Socialization and Vocalization** Mews and makes throaty noises. Shows interest in human face. **Cognitive and Emotional Development** Reflexive. External stimuli are meaningless. Responses are generally limited to tension states or discomfort. Gains satisfaction from feeding and being held, rocked, fondled, and cuddled. Has an intense need for sucking pleasure. Quiets when picked up.	**Play Stimulation** Use human face—smile and talk. Dangle bright and moving object in field of vision (mobile). Hold, touch, caress, fondle, kiss. Rock, pat, change position. Play soft music or have infant listen to ticking clock, sing. Talk to infant, call by name. **Parental Guidance** Begin to expose infant to different household sounds. Change crib location in room. Use bright-colored clothing and linen. Keep infant nearby. Allow infant to sleep. Play with infant when awake. Hold during feeding.
4–8 weeks (2 months) Crossed extensor reflex disappears. Tonic neck reflex begins to fade.	**Motor Development** Reflexive behavior is slowly being replaced by voluntary movements. Turns from side to back. Begins to lift head momentarily from prone position. Shows eye coordination to light and objects. If bell is sounded nearby, infant will stop activity and listen. Eyes follow better, both vertically and horizontally. Focuses well. **Socialization and Vocalization** Begins vocalization—coos, especially to a voice. Crying becomes differentiated. Visually looks for sounds. May squeal with delight when stimulated by touching, talking, or singing. Begins social smile. Eyes follow person or object more intently. **Cognitive and Emotional Development** Recognizes familiar face. Becomes more aware and interested in environment. Anticipates being fed when in feeding position. Enjoys sucking—puts hand in mouth.	**Play Stimulation** Arrange mobile over crib so infant's movement will set it in motion. Hang wind chimes near infant. Hang bright-colored pictures on wall (yellow and red-colored stripes, for example). Use cradle gym and infant seat. Use rattles. Hold infant and walk around room. Allow freedom of kicking with clothes off. **Parental Guidance** Talk to infant and smile; get excited when baby coos. Place infant seat near mother's activities but where it cannot fall off or tip over. Put in prone position in bed or on floor. Expose infant to different textures. Exercise infant's arms and legs. Sing to infant. Provide tactile experience during bathing, diapering, feeding.
8–12 weeks (2–3 months) Landau reflex appears at 3–4 months. Positive support reflex disappears. Posterior fontanelle closes. Increase in body fluids—real tears appear, drooling, and gastrointestinal juices increase.	**Motor Development** When prone, will rest on forearms and keep head in midline—makes crawling movements with legs, arches back, and holds head high; may get chest off surface. Indicates preference for prone or supine position. Discovers hands—strikes at objects while watching hands. Holds objects in hands and brings to mouth. Has fairly good head control.	**Play Stimulation** Encourage socialization, smiling, laughing. Place on mat on floor. Continue to introduce new sounds. **Parental Guidance** Take on daily outing as weather permits. Bounce on bed. Play with infant during feeding. Rattles can be used effectively for visual following and for hand play.

(continued)

TABLE 40-1   Infant to Adolescent Growth and Development (Continued)

Age and Physical Characteristics	Behavior Patterns	Nursing Implications/ Parental Guidance
	Socialization and Vocalization Smiles more readily. Babbles and coos. Stops crying when mother enters room or when caressed. Enjoys playing during feeding. Stays awake longer without crying. Turns head to follow familiar person. **Cognitive and Emotional Development** Shows active interest in environment. Recognizes familiar faces and objects. Focuses and follows objects. Shows repetitiveness in play activity. Is aware of strange situations. Derives pleasure from sucking—purposefully gets hand to mouth. Begins to establish routine preceding sleep.	Encourage older siblings to "make faces" and sing and talk to baby.
12–16 weeks (3–4 months) Moro reflex fades. Stepping reflex disappears. Rooting reflex disappears. By 4–5 months infant's weight approximately doubles birth weight. Average weekly weight gain, 140–200 g (4–7 oz). Average monthly height gain, 2.5 cm (1 inch). Pulse rate slows to 100–140 Respirations, 20–40/min Grasp becomes voluntary. Sucking becomes voluntary.	**Motor Development** Eyes focus on small objects, may pick a dangling ring. Holds head up (when being pulled to sitting position). Becomes more interested in environment. Hand comes to meet rattle. Listens—turns head to familiar sound. Sits with minimal support. Intentional rolling over, back to side. Reaches for offered objects. Grasps objects with both hands, and everything goes into mouth. **Socialization and Vocalization** Laughs and chuckles socially. Demands social attention by fussing. Recognizes mother. Begins to respond to "No, no." Enjoys being propped in sitting position. **Cognitive and Emotional Development** Actively interested in environment. Enjoys attention; becomes bored when alone for long periods of time. Recognizes bottle. More interested in mother. Indicates increasing trust and security. Sleeps through night; has defined nap time.	**Play Stimulation** Encourage mirror play. Provide soft squeeze toys in vivid colors of varying texture. Allow infant to splash in bath. Infant still enjoys holding and playing with rattles. Enjoys old-fashioned clothespins and playing pat-a-cake, peek-a-boo. **Parental Guidance** Be certain button eyes on toys and other small objects cannot be pulled off. Hold rattle and let infant reach and grasp it. When baby is in high chair, strap in. Move mobile out of reach—baby may grab it and cause injury. Repeat child's sounds. Talk in varying degrees of loudness. Begin looking at and naming pictures in book. Begin roughhousing play by both parents. Give space in playpen or on sheet on floor to practice rolling over.
16–26 weeks (4–7 months) By 5–6 months, tonic neck reflex disappears. By 6–7 months, palmar grasp disappears. By 7–9 months, develops eye-to-eye contact while talking; engages in social games. Two central lower incisors erupt. Spine "C shaped"—lacks lordotic and lumbar curves. Eustachian tube short and horizontal making baby prone to ear infections.	**Motor Development** Shows momentary sitting with hand support. Bounces and bears some weight when held in standing position. Transfers and mouths objects in one hand. Discovers feet. Bangs objects together. Rolls over well. May begin some form of mobility. **Socialization and Vocalization** Discriminates between strangers and familiar figures.	**Play Stimulation** Enjoys social games, hide-and-seek with adult, toys, large blocks. Likes to bang objects. Plays in bounce chair, walker. Enjoys large nesting toys (round rather than square). Likes to drop and retrieve things. Likes metal cups, wooden spoons, and things to bang with. Loves crumpled paper. Enjoys squeeze toys in bath. Likes peek-a-boo, bye-bye, and pat-a-cake. *(continued)*

TABLE 40-1   Infant to Adolescent Growth and Development (Continued)

Age and Physical Characteristics	Behavior Patterns	Nursing Implications/ Parental Guidance
Gastrointestinal system maturing enough for solid foods.	**Crows and squeals.** Starts to say "Ma," "Da." Self-play is self-contained. Laughs out loud. Makes "talking" sounds in response to others' talking. Begins fear of strangers, 8½–10 months **Cognitive and Emotional Development** Secures objects by pulling on string. Searches for lost objects that are out of sight. Inspects objects; localizes sounds. Likes to sit in high chair. Drops and picks up objects. Displays exploratory behavior with food. Exhibits beginning fear of strangers. Becomes fretful when mother leaves. Shows much mouthing and biting.	**Parental Guidance** Will play as long as you can. Tie toys to chair with short string. Let play with extra spoon at feeding. Give soft finger foods. Because infant puts everything in mouth, *use safety precautions.* Keep small items away from infant; could choke on them. Show excitement at achievements. Supply kitchen items for toys.
26–40 weeks (7–10 months) 4 upper incisors erupt around 7–9 months. By 9–12 months, plantar reflex disappears. By 9–12 months, neck-righting reflex disappears. 6–12 months Average weekly weight gain, 85–140 g (3–5 oz). Average monthly height gain, 1.25 cm (½ inch).	**Motor Development** Sits without support. Recovers balance. Manipulates objects with hands. Unwraps objects. Creeps. Pulls self upright at crib rails. Uses index finger and thumb to hold objects. Rings a bell. Can feed self a cracker and can hold bottle. Chewing reflex develops. Can control lips around cup. Does not like supine position. Can hold index finger and thumb in opposition. **Socialization and Verbalization** Claps hands on request. Responds to own name. Is very aware of social environment. Imitates gestures, facial expressions, and sounds. Smiles at image in mirror. Offers toy to adult, but does not release it. Begins to test parental reaction during feeding and at bedtime. Will entertain self for long periods of time. **Cognitive and Emotional Development** Begins to imitate. Shows more interest in picture books. Enjoys achievements. Has strong urge toward independence— locomotion, feeding, dressing.	**Play Stimulation** Encourage use of motion toys—rocking horse, stroller. Water play. Imitate animal sounds. Allow exploration outdoors. Provide for learning by imitation. Offer new objects (blocks). Child likes freedom of creeping and walking, but closeness of family is important. Good toys: plastic milk carton; bean bag for tossing; fabric books; things to move around, fill up, empty out; pile-up and knock-down toys. **Parental Guidance** Do things with infant. Protect from dangerous objects—cover electrical outlets, block stairs, remove breakable objects from tables. Have child with family at mealtime. Offer cup.
10–12 months (1 year) Developing lordotic and lumbar curves to make walking possible. By 12–24 months, Landau reflex disappears. Weight should approximately triple birth weight. 2 lower lateral incisors appear. 4 first molars appear by 14 months.	**Motor Development** Cruises around furniture. Beginning to stand alone and toddle. Turns pages in book. Tries tossing object. Shows hand dominance. Navigates stairs; climbs on chairs. Builds a tower of 2 blocks. Puts balls in box. May use spoon. Can release objects at will. Has regular bowel movements.	**Play Stimulation** Ball play Cloth doll Motion objects and toys Transporting objects Name and point to body parts. "Put-in" and "take-out" toys Sand box with spoons and other simple objects. Blocks Music *(continued)*

TABLE 40-1 Infant to Adolescent Growth and Development (Continued)

Age and Physical Characteristics	Behavior Patterns	Nursing Implications/ Parental Guidance

Child Development Theories
Freudian: Behavior
  Birth–1 year—Oral Stage
Eriksonian: Emotion/Personality
  Birth–1 year—Sense of Trust vs. Mistrust
Piagetian: Intellectual Activity (Thought Process)
  Birth–2 years—Sensorimotor Period
	Socialization and Verbalization
	Uses jargon.
	Points to indicate wants.
	Loves give-and-take game.
	Responds to music.
	Enjoys being center of attention and will repeat laughed-at activities.
	
	Cognitive and Emotional Development
	Shows fear, anger, affection, jealousy, anxiety, and sympathy.
	Experiments to reach new goals.
	Displays intense determination to remove barriers to action.
	Begins to develop concepts of space, time, and causality.
	Has increased attention span.
		Parental Guidance
		Allow self-directed play rather than adult-directed play.
		Continue to expose to foods of different textures, taste, smell, substance.
		Offer cup.
		Show affection and encourage child to return affection.
		Safety teaching: Child gets into everything within reach. Place medications in safe, locked place. Create a safe environment for child. Have ipecac syrup at home; stair guards; faucet protectors, drawer locks.

12–18 months *NOTE:* Between 1 and 3 years the child is called a "toddler." Anterior fontanelle closes. Abdomen protrudes, arms and legs lengthen. Big muscles become well developed. 4 cuspids appear by 18 months. Fine muscle coordination begins to develop. Average yearly weight gain, 2–3 kg (4½–6½ lb). Average height gain during second year, 12 cm (4¾ inches).	**Motor Development** Walks up stairs with help, creeps downstairs. Walks without support and with balance. Falls less frequently. Throws ball. Stoops to pick up toys, look at bug. Turns pages of book. Holds and lifts cup. Builds 3-block tower. Picks up and places small beads in container. Begins to use spoon. **Cognitive and Emotional Development** Has vocabulary of 10 words that have meanings. Uses phrases, imitates words. Points to objects named by adult. Follows directions and requests. Imitates adult behavior. Retrieves toy from several hiding places. **Psychosocial Development** Develops new awareness of strangers. Wants to explore everything in reach. Plays alone, but near others. Is dependent on parents, but begins to reach out for autonomy. Finds security in a blanket, toy, or thumb-sucking.	**Play Stimulation** Allow unrestricted motor activity (within safety limits). Offer push-pull toys. Child selects favorite toy. Child likes blocks, pyramid toys, teddy bears, dolls, pots and pans, cloth picture books with colorful large pictures, telephone, musical top, nested blocks. **Parental Guidance** Begin to teach tooth brushing to establish good dental habits. Limits need to be set that give toddlers sense of security, yet encourage exploration. Identify behavior changes common in toddler. Reinforce safety teaching.
1½–2 years Protruding abdomen less noticeable. Landau reflex disappears. During first 2 years 35 cm (14–15 inches) are added to height. Slight bowing of legs with a wide-based walk. Handedness may become apparent.	**Motor Development** Walks up and down stairs. Opens doors; turns knobs. Has steady gait. Holds drinking cup well with 1 hand. Uses spoon without spilling food (may prefer fingers). Kicks a ball in front of him without support. Builds a tower of 4–6 blocks. Scribbles. Rides tricycle or kiddie car (without pedals). **Cognitive Development** Has 200–300 words in vocabulary. Begins to use short sentences.	**Play Stimulation** Shows parallel play, although he enjoys having other children around. Has very short attention span. Enjoys same toys as child of 18 months. Likes doll play, ball. Imitates parents in domestic activities. Likes swing, hammering, paper, large crayons. **Parental Guidance** Has need for peer companionship, although displays immaturity by inability to share and take turns.

(continued)

TABLE 40-1 Infant to Adolescent Growth and Development (Continued)

Age and Physical Characteristics	Behavior Patterns	Nursing Implications/ Parental Guidance
	Refers to self by pronoun. Obeys simple commands. Does not know right from wrong. Begins to learn about time sequences. **Psychosocial Development** Uses word "mine" constantly. Is possessive with toys. Displays negativism—uses "no" as assertion of self. Routine and rituals are important. May begin cooperation in toilet training. Resists restrictions on freedom. Has fear of parents' leaving. Shows parallel play. Dawdles. Resists bedtime—uses transitional objects (blanket, toy). Vacillates between dependence and independence.	A decrease in appetite normally occurs at this stage. Toilet training should be started (each child follows own pattern). Begin to have child eat meals with family if not already doing so. Begin to read to child; child likes storybooks with large pictures.
2–3 years Height approximates half adult height. Legs are about 34% of body length. Begins 2 + kg (5 lb) weight gain per year until 5 years old. At 2½ years has full set (20) of baby teeth. 4 second molars appear by 2½ years. Height gain, 6–8 cm (2⅜–3¼ inches). Lordosis and protuberant abdomen of toddler disappear	**Motor Development** Throws objects overhead. Pedals tricycle. Walks backward. Washes and dries hands. Begins to use scissors. Can string large beads. Can undress himself. Feeds himself well. Tries to dance. Jumps in place. Builds tower of 8 blocks. Balances on one foot. Swings and climbs. Can eat an ice cream cone. Drinks from a straw. Chews gum without swallowing it. **Cognitive Development** Shows increased attention span. Gives first and last name. Begins to ask "why." Is egocentric in thought and behavior. Beginning ability to reflect on own behavior. Talks in short sentences. Uses plurals. May attempt to sing simple songs. Has vocabulary of 900 words. Begins fantasy. Begins to understand what it means to take turns. Can repeat 3 numbers. Shows interest in colors.	**Play Stimulation** Plays simple games with other children. Enjoys story-telling and dress-up play. Plays "house." Colors. Uses scissors and paper. Rides tricycle. Read simple books to child. Will assist in developing memory skills, visual discrimination skills, and language. **Parental Guidance** From 2–3 years, the child develops a seeming maturity; do not expect more than child is able to do. Arrange first visit to the dentist to have teeth checked. Be aware that negativistic and ritualistic behavior is normal. Be consistent in discipline. Control temper tantrums. Begin to teach traffic safety. Supervise outdoor play.

Child Development Theories
Freudian:
  1–3 years—Anal Stage
Eriksonian:
  1–3 years—Sense of Autonomy vs. Shame and Doubt
	Psychosocial Development
	Negativism grows out of child's sense of developing independence—says "no" to every command.
	Ritualism is important to toddler for security (follows certain pattern, especially at bedtime).	

(continued)

TABLE 40-1 Infant to Adolescent Growth and Development (Continued)

Age and Physical Characteristics	Behavior Patterns	Nursing Implications/ Parental Guidance
Piagetian: 2–7 years—Preoperational Period; shows egocentrism and centering	Temper tantrums may result from toddler's frustration in wanting to do everything for self. Shows parallel play as well as beginning interaction with others. Engages in associative play. Fears become pronounced. Continues to react to separation from parents but shows increasing ability to handle short periods of separation. Has daytime bladder control and is beginning to develop nighttime bladder control. Becomes more independent. Begins to identify sex (gender) roles. Explores environment outside the home. Can create different ways of getting desired outcome.	
3–4 years *NOTE:* Between 3 and 5 years, the child is called a "preschooler." May appear "knock kneed."	**Motor Development** Drawings have form and meaning, not detail. Copies a circle and a cross. Buttons front and side of clothes. Laces shoes. Bathes self, but needs direction. Brushes teeth. Shows continuous movement going up and down stairs. Climbs and jumps well. Attempts to print letters. **Cognitive Development** Awareness of body is more stable; child becomes more aware of own vulnerability. Is less negativistic. Learns some number concepts. Begins naming colors. Can identify longer of 2 lines. Has vocabulary of 1500 words. Uses mild profanities and name-calling. Uses language aggressively. Asks many questions. May not be abstract enough to understand body parts that cannot be seen or felt. Can be given simple explanation as to cause and effect. Thinks very concretely; demonstrates irreversibility of thought. Immature concept of death—believes it is reversible. Has beginning understanding of past and future. Is egocentric in thought. **Psychosocial Development** Is more active with peers and engages in cooperative play. Performs simple tasks. Frequently has imaginary companion. Dramatizes experiences. Is proud of accomplishments. Exaggerates, boasts, and tattles on others. Can tolerate separation from mother longer without feeling anxiety. Is keen observer.	**Play Stimulation** Plays and interacts with other children. Shows creativity. Likes ring-around-the rosy. "Helps" adults. Likes costumes and enjoys dramatic play. Toys and games: record player, nursery rhymes, housekeeping toys, transportation toys (tricycle, trucks, cars, wagon), blocks, hammer and peg bench, floor trains, blackboard and chalk, easel and brushes, clay, crayon and finger paints, outside toys (sandbox, swing, small slide), books (short stories, action stories), drum, scrapbook. **Parental Guidance** Base your expectations within child's limitations. Provide limited frustrations from environment to assist in coping. Give small errands to do around the house (putting silverware on table, drying a dish). Expand child's world with trips to the zoo, to the supermarket, to restaurant, etc. Prevent accidents. Provide for brief nonthreatening separation from parents and home. Reinforce correct use of language. Use opportunities for simple sexual education as child's needs arise. Accept masturbation as a normal phenomenon to be discouraged in public. Provide consistent discipline, motivated by love not anger. Consider nursery school.

(continued)

TABLE 40-1 Infant to Adolescent Growth and Development (Continued)

Age and Physical Characteristics	Behavior Patterns	Nursing Implications/ Parental Guidance
	Has good sense of "mine" and "yours." Behavior still frequently ritualistic. Becomes curious about life and sex. Often indulges in masturbation	
4–5 years By 2–5 years adds 25 cm (9–10 inches) to height. At age 4, legs comprise about 44% of body length. **Child Development Theories** Freudian: 3–6 years—Phallic Stage Eriksonian: 3–6 years—Sense of Initiative vs. Guilt Piagetian: 2–7 years—Preoperational Period; shows egocentrism and centering	**Motor Development** Hops 2 or more times. Dresses without supervision. Has good motor control—climbs and jumps well. Walks up stairs without grasping handrail. Walks backward. Washes self without wetting clothes. Prints first name and other words. Adds 3 or more details in drawings. Draws a square. **Cognitive Development** Has 2100-word vocabulary. Talks constantly. Uses adult speech forms. Participates in conversations. Asks for definitions. Knows age and residence. Identifies heavier of two objects. Knows weeks as time units. Names days of week. Begins to understand kinship. Knows primary colors. Can count to 10. Can copy a triangle. Has high degree of imagination. Questioning is at a peak. Begins to develop power of reasoning. **Psychosocial Development** May have an imaginary companion. Has a sense of order (likes to finish what was started). Is obedient and reliable. Is protective toward younger children. Begins to develop an elementary conscience with some influence in governing behavior. Has increased self-confidence. Accepts responsibility for acts. Is less rebellious. Has dreams and nightmares. Is cooperative and sympathetic. Shows generosity with toys. Begins to question parents' thinking. Identifies strongly with parent of same sex.	**Play Stimulation** Demonstrates gross motor activity—likes to jump rope, skip, climb on jungle gyms, etc. Prefers group play and cooperates in projects. Plays simple letter, number, form, and picture games. Plays with cars and trucks. Still likes being read to. Continues to enjoy fantasy play. **Parental Guidance** Child no longer takes an afternoon nap. Prepare child for kindergarten. Tell him stories. Provide opportunities and reassurance for group play; have his friends visit for lunch and an afternoon of playing. Prevent accidents. Encourage child's participation in household activities.
Middle Childhood (5–9 years) Growth rate is slow and steady. Child gains an average of 3.18 kg (7 lb) per year. Height increases approximately 6.25 cm (2½ inches) per year. Among children there is considerable variation in height and weight. Child appears taller and slimmer. Early lordosis disappears.	**Motor Development** 6 years Is active and impulsive. Balance improves. Uses hands as manipulative tools in cutting, pasting, hammering. Can draw large letters or figures. 7 years Has lower activity level. Capable of fine hand movements; can print sentences.	**Parental Guidance** Family atmosphere continues to have impact on child's emotional development and future response within the family. The child needs ongoing guidance in an open, inviting atmosphere. Limits should be set with conviction. Deal with only one incident at a time. When punishment is necessary, the child should not be humiliated. Child should know that it was

(continued)

TABLE 40-1 Infant to Adolescent Growth and Development (Continued)

Age and Physical Characteristics	Behavior Patterns	Nursing Implications/ Parental Guidance
Child begins to lose baby teeth; permanent teeth appear at a rate of about 4 teeth per year from 7–14 years. Neuromuscular and skeletal development allows improved coordination. Eyes become fully developed; vision approaches 20/20. Handedness should be well developed. **Child Development Theories** Freudian: 5–9 years—Beginning of Latency Period Eriksonian: 5–9 years—Industry vs. Inferiority Piagetian: 5–9 years—Enters Stage of Concrete Operations	Nervous habits such as nail biting are common. Muscular skills such as ball throwing have improved. 8 years Moves with less restlessness. Has developed grace and balance, even in active sports. Has developed coordination of fine muscles, allowing child to write in script. 9 years Uses both hands independently Has become skillful in manual activities because of improved eye–hand coordination. **Cognitive Development** 6 years Begins to learn to read. Defines objects in terms of use. Time sense is as much in past as present. Is interested in relationship between home and neighborhood; knows some streets. Uses sentences well; uses language to share others' experiences; may swear or use slang. Distinguishes morning from afternoon. 7 years More reflective and has deeper understanding of meanings. Interested in conclusions and logical endings. Begins to have scientific interests in cause and effect. More responsible in relation to time, is more punctual. Sense of space is more realistic; child wants some space of own. Knows value of coins. Concept of death becoming mature—includes idea of irreversibility. 8 years Thinking is less animistic. Is aware of impersonal forces of nature. Begins to understand logical reasoning, conclusions, implications. Less self-centered in thinking. Personal space is expanding; goes places on own. Aware of time; plans events of day. Understands right from left. 9 years Intellectually energetic and curious. Realistic; reasonable in thinking. Able to plan in advance. Breaks complex activities into steps. Focuses on detail. Sense of space includes the entire earth. Participates in family discussions. Likes to have secrets. **Psychosocial Development** (The following characteristics apply to the child in the 5–9-year group.)	the *act* that the adult found undesirable, not the child. Needs assistance in adjusting to new experiences and demands of school. Should be able to share experiences with family. Parents need to have communication with the teacher to work together for the health of the child. Convey love and caring in communication. The child understands language directed at feelings better than at intellect. Get down to eye level with the child. Focus attention on child's abilities and accomplishments rather than shortcomings and limitations. Child is sex-conscious. Child should be able to discuss questions at home rather than with friends. Requires simple, honest answers to questions. Common problems include teasing, quarreling, nail biting, enuresis, whining, poor manners, swearing, lying, cheating, stealing. These are usually fleeting phases and should not be handled negatively. The causes for such behavior should be investigated and dealt with constructively. The child needs order and consistency to help in coping with doubts, fears, unacceptable impulses, and unfamiliar experiences. Encourage peer activities as well as home responsibilities and give recognition to child's accomplishments and unique talents. Television may stimulate learning in several spheres, but should be monitored. Accidents are a major cause of disability and death. Safety practices should be continued. (Refer to section on safety, p. 1277). Exercise is essential to promote motor and psychosocial development. The child should have a safe place to play and simple pieces of equipment. A school health program should be available and concerned with the child's physical, emotional, mental, and social health. This should be augmented by information and example at home. Medical supervision should continue with yearly examination to detect developmental delay, disease. Appropriate immunizations should be administered. Child frequently has "quiet days"—periods of shyness, which should be tolerated as part of growing up and deciding who he or she is. Child may be subject to nightmares, a situation that requires reassurance and understanding.

(continued)

TABLE 40-1 Infant to Adolescent Growth and Development (Continued)		
Age and Physical Characteristics	**Behavior Patterns**	**Nursing Implications/ Parental Guidance**
	Still requires parental support, but pulls away from overt signs of affection.	Parents, teachers, and health professionals should be available and able to provide information and answer questions about the physical changes that occur.
	Peer groups provide companionship in widening circle of persons outside the home. Child learns more about self as he learns about others.	
	"Chum" stage occurs at about 9–10 years of age. Child chooses a special friend of same sex and age in whom to confide. This is usually child's first love relationship outside of home, when someone becomes as important to him as himself.	
	Play teaches the child new ideas and independence. Child progressively uses tools of competition, compromise, cooperation, and beginning collaboration.	
	Body image and self-concept are fluid because of rapid physical, emotional, social changes.	
	Latency-stage sexual drive is controlled and repressed. Emphasis is on the development of skills and talent.	
	Patterns of Play	
	6–7 years	
	Child acts out ideas of family and occupational groups with which he has contact.	
	Painting, pasting, reading, simple games, watching television, digging, running games, skating, riding bicycle, and swimming are all enjoyed activities.	
	8 years	
	Child enjoys collections; loosely formed, short-lived clubs; table games; card games; books; television; records.	
Late Childhood (9–12 years) Vital signs approach adult values. Loses childish appearance of face and takes on features that will characterize individual as an adult. Growth spurt occurs, and some secondary sex characteristics appear: in girls, at age 10–12 years; in boys, at age 12–14 years. Physical changes of puberty: Increased height and weight, increased perspiration and activity of sebaceous glands; vasomotor instability; increased fat deposition. Physical changes in girls: Pelvis increases in transverse diameter; hips broaden; tenderness in developing breast tissue; enlargement of areola diameter; appearance of pubic hair. Physical changes in boys: Size of testes increases; scrotum color changes; breasts enlarge, temporarily; height and shoulder breadth increase	**Motor Development** Energetic, restless, active movements such as finger-drumming or foot-tapping appear. Has skillful manipulative movements nearly equal to those of adults. Works hard to perfect physical skills. **Cognitive Development** 10 years Likes to reason, enjoys learning. Thinking is concrete, matter of fact. Wants to measure up to challenge. Likes to memorize, identify facts. Attention span may be short. Space is rather specific (ie, where things are). Can write for relatively long time with speed. 11 years Likes action in learning. Concentrates well when working competitively. Can understand relational terms such as weight and size. Perceives space as nothingness that goes on forever. Able to discuss problems.	**Parental Guidance** Continue appropriate interventions related to early childhood. Continue sex education and preparation for adolescent body changes. Understanding is important. Encourage participation in organized clubs, youth groups. Democratic guidance is essential as child works through a conflict between dependence (on parents) and independence. Child needs realistic limits set. Needs help channeling energy in proper direction—work and sports. Requires adequate explanation of body changes. Special understanding required for the child who lags in physical development. Continue consistent disciplinary style.

(continued)

TABLE 40-1   Infant to Adolescent Growth and Development (Continued)

Age and Physical Characteristics	Behavior Patterns	Nursing Implications/ Parental Guidance

Appearance of lightly pigmented hair at base of penis.
Increase in length and width of penis.
 	
Child Development Theories
Freudian:
  9–12 years—Latency Period continues
Eriksonian:
  9–12 years—Industry vs. Inferiority continues
Piagetian:
  9–12 years—Stage of Concrete Operations continues
	Can conceptualize symbolically enough to understand body parts.
	Can describe some abstract terms.
	12 years
	  Enjoys learning.
	  Considers all aspects of a situation.
	  Motivated more by inner drive than by competition.
	  Able to classify, arrange, generalize.
	  Likes to discuss and debate.
	  Begins conceptual thinking.
	  Verbal, formal reasoning now possible.
	  Can recognize moral of a story.
	  Defines time as duration; likes to plan ahead.
	  Understands that space is abstract.
	  Can be critical of own work.
	
	Psychosocial Development
	Gang becomes important, and gang code takes precedence over nearly everything. Often gang codes are characterized by collective action against the mores of the adult world. Here, children begin to work out own social patterns without adult interference. Early gangs may include both sexes; later gangs are separated by sex.
	May strive for unreasonable independence from adult control.
	Often interested in religion, morality.
	Has increased interest in sexuality.
	May reach puberty; resurgence of sexual drives causes recapitulation of Oedipal struggle.
	
	Patterns of Play
	Continues to enjoy reading, TV, table games.
	More interested in active sports as a means to improve skills.
	Creative talents may appear; may enjoy drawing, modeling clay. By age 10, sex differences in play become profound.
	Occasional privacy is important.
	Begins to have vocational aspirations.	

Early Adolescence (12–14) Phase of development begins when reproductive organs become functionally operative; phase ends when physical growth is completed. Skeletal system grows faster than supporting muscles. Hands and feet grow proportionately faster than rest of body. Large muscles develop more quickly than small muscles. Girls: Physical changes include appearance of menarche; growth of axillary and perineal hair; deepened voice; ovulation; further development of breasts.	**Motor Development** Often uncoordinated; has poor posture. Tires easily. **Cognitive Development** Mind has great ability to acquire and use knowledge. Abstract thinking is sufficient to learn multi-variable ideas such as the influence of hormones on emotions. Categorizes thoughts into usable forms. May project thinking into the future. Is capable of highly imaginative thinking. **Psychosocial Development** Interest in opposite sex increases. Often revolts from adult authority to conform to peer-group standards.	**Parental Guidance** Stresses frequently result from conflicting value systems between generations. Parents may need help to see that the adolescent is a product of the times and that actions reflect what is happening around the youngster. Parents' limits and rules should be realistic and consistent. They should convey the love and concern of parents and should be a source of comfort and reassurance, protecting the child from activities for which he is not ready. The home should be an accepting, emotionally stable environment. Continue sex education, including discussion of ovulation, fertilization, menstrua-

(continued)

TABLE 40-1 Infant to Adolescent Growth and Development (Continued)

Age and Physical Characteristics	Behavior Patterns	Nursing Implications/ Parental Guidance

Nutritional need for iron and calcium increase dramatically.
Boys:
  Physical changes include growth of axillary, perineal, facial, chest hair; deepening of voice; production of spermatozoa; nocturnal emissions.
 	
Child Development Theories
Freudian:
  12–14 years—Begins Stage of Sexuality
Eriksonian:
  12–14 years—Identity vs. Role Diffusion
Piagetian:
  12–14 years—Begins Stage of Formal Operations
	Continues to rework feelings for parent of opposite sex and unravel the ambivalence toward parent of same sex.
	Affection may turn temporarily to an adult outside of the family (for example, crush on family friend, neighbor, or teacher).
	Uses peer-group dialect—highly informal language or specially coined terminology.
	Peer groups are especially important and help adolescent to define own identity, to adapt to changing body image, to establish more mature relationships with others, and to deal with heightened sexual feelings. Cliques may develop.
	Dating generally progresses from groups of couples to double dates and finally single couples.
	Teenage "hangouts" become important centers of activity.
	Begins questioning existing moral values.
		tion, pregnancy, contraception, masturbation, nocturnal emissions, and hygiene.
		Adolescents have an increased need for rest and sleep because they are expending large amounts of energy and are functioning with an inadequate oxygen supply.
		Recreational interests should be fostered. Favorite activities include sports, dating, dancing, reading, hobbies, and television. Talking on the telephone, listening to records are favorite pastimes.
		Adolescent health problems that require preventive education are accidents, obesity, acne, pregnancy, sexually transmitted disease, drug abuse.
		Allow adolescent to handle own affairs as much as possible, but be aware of physical and psychosocial problems that may require help. Encourage independence but allow child to lean on parents for support when frightened or unable to attain goals.
		Adolescents with special problems should have access to specialists such as adolescent clinics and psychologists.
		Requires reassurance and help in accepting changing body image. Parents should make the most of child's positive qualities.
		Give gentle encouragement and guidance regarding dating. Avoid strong pressures in either direction.
		Understand conflicts as child attempts to deal with social, moral, and intellectual issues.

Goodenough-Harris Scoring (Continued)

Neck: □ Present
□ Outline of neck continuous with head, trunk, or both

Face: □ Eyes
□ Nose
□ Mouth
□ Nose and mouth in two dimensions
□ Nostrils

Hair: □ Present
□ On more than circumference; nontransparent

Motor coordination: □ Lines firm and well connected
□ Firmly drawn with correct joining
□ Head outline
□ Trunk outline
□ Outline of arms and legs
□ Features

Ears: □ Present
□ Correct position and proportion

Clothing: □ Present
□ Two articles; nontransparent
□ Entire drawing nontransparent (sleeves and trousers)
□ Four articles
□ Costume complete

Fingers: □ Present
□ Correct number
□ Two dimension; length, breadth
□ Thumb opposition
□ Hand distinct from fingers and arm

Eye detail: □ Brow or lashes
□ Pupil
□ Proportion
□ Glance directed front in profile drawing

Chin: □ Present; forehead
□ Projection

Profile: □ Not more than one error
□ Correct

Joints: □ Elbow, shoulder or both
□ Knee, hip, or both

(Siberry, G. K. & Iannone, R. [Eds.] [2000]. *The Harriet Lane handbook* [15th ed.]. St. Louis: Mosby.)

GOODENOUGH AGE NORMS

Age (yr)	3	4	5	6	7	8	9	10	11	12	13
Points	2	6	10	14	18	22	26	30	34	38	42

Developmental Milestones

A method of evaluation has been developed by using an interview technique asking parents a list of questions regarding milestones in achievements that most will remember. Developmental quotient (DQ) can be determined. A DQ less than 70% signifies a delay requiring further evaluation.

Denver II Developmental Screening Test
Directions for Administration

1. Try to get child to smile by smiling, talking or waving. Do not touch him/her.
2. Child must stare at hand several seconds.
3. Parent may help guide toothbrush and put toothpaste on brush.
4. Child does not have to be able to tie shoes or button/zip in the back.
5. Move yarn slowly in an arc from one side to the other, about 8" above child's face.
6. Pass if child grasps rattle when it is touched to the backs or tips of fingers.
7. Pass if child tries to see where yarn went. Yarn should be dropped quickly from sight from tester's hand without arm movement.
8. Child must transfer cube from hand to hand without help of body, mouth, or table.
9. Pass if child picks up raisin with any part of thumb and finger.
10. Line can vary only 30 degrees or less from tester's line.
11. Make a fist with thumb pointing upward and wiggle only the thumb. Pass if child imitates and does not move any fingers other than the thumb.

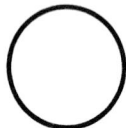 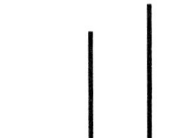 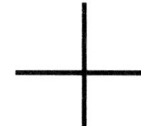 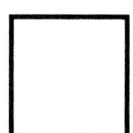

12. Pass any enclosed form. Fail continuous round motions.
13. Which line is longer? (Not bigger.) Turn paper upside down and repeat. (pass 3 of 3 or 5 of 6)
14. Pass any lines crossing near midpoint.
15. Have child copy first. If failed, demonstrate.

When giving items 12, 14, and 15, do not name the forms. Do not demonstrate 12 and 14.

16. When scoring, each pair (2 arms, 2 legs, etc.) counts as one part.
17. Place one cube in cup and shake gently near child's ear, but out of sight. Repeat for other ear.
18. Point to picture and have child name it. (No credit is given for sounds only.)
    If less than 4 pictures are named correctly, have child point to picture as each is named by tester.

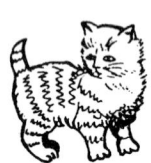 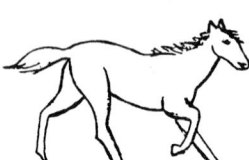 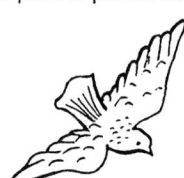 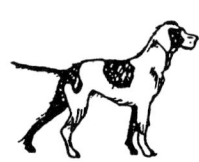 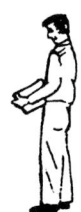

19. Using doll, tell child: Show me the nose, eyes, ears, mouth, hands, feet, tummy, hair. Pass 6 of 8.
20. Using pictures, ask child: Which one flies?... says meow?... talks?... barks?... gallops? Pass 2 of 5, 4 of 5.
21. Ask child: What do you do when you are cold?... tired?... hungry? Pass 2 of 3, 3 of 3.
22. Ask child: What do you do with a cup? What is a chair used for? What is a pencil used for?
    Action words must be included in answers.
23. Pass if child correctly places <u>and</u> says how many blocks are on paper. (1, 5).
24. Tell child: Put block **on** table; **under** table; **in front of** me, **behind** me. Pass 4 of 4.
    (Do not help child by pointing, moving head or eyes.)
25. Ask child: What is a ball?... lake?... desk?... house?... banana?... curtain?... fence?... ceiling? Pass if defined in terms of use, shape, what it is made of, or general category (such as banana is fruit, not just yellow). Pass 5 of 8, 7 of 8.
26. Ask child: If a horse is big, a mouse is __? If fire is hot, ice is __? If the sun shines during the day, the moon shines during the __? Pass 2 of 3.
27. Child may use wall or rail only, not person. May not crawl.
28. Child must throw ball overhand 3 feet to within arm's reach of tester.
29. Child must perform standing broad jump over width of test sheet (8 1/2 inches).
30. Tell child to walk forward, ⚬⚬⚬⚬➔ heel within 1 inch of toe. Tester may demonstrate.
    Child must walk 4 consecutive steps.
31. In the second year, half of normal children are non-compliant.

OBSERVATIONS:

Scoring

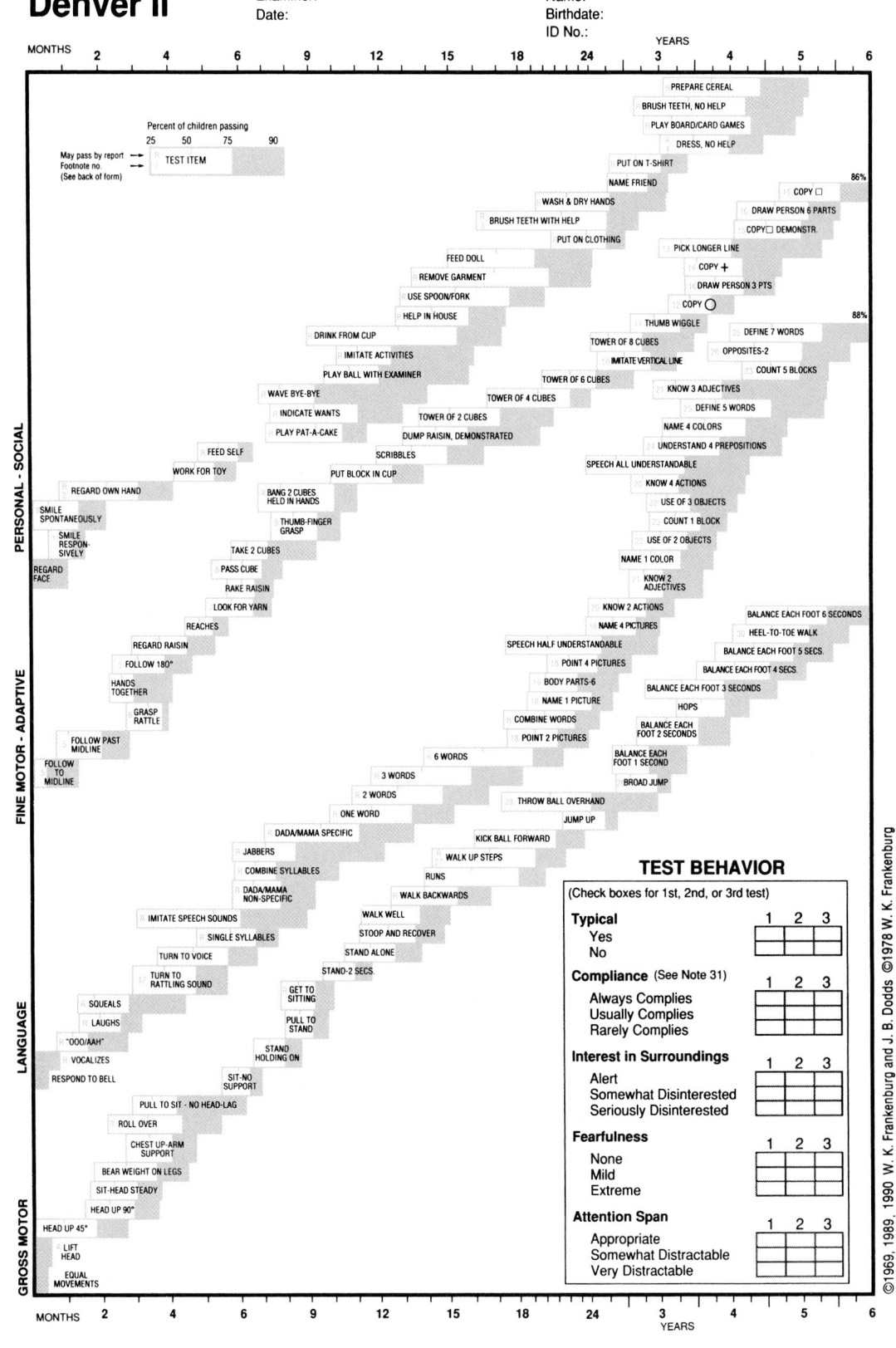

DEVELOPMENTAL MILESTONES

Age	Gross Motor	Visual-Motor/ Problem-Solving	Language	Social/Adaptive	Age
1 mo	Raises head slightly from prone, makes crawling movements	Birth: visually fixes 1 mo: has tight grasp, follows to midline	Alerts to sound	Regards face	1 mo
2 mo	Holds head in midline, lifts chest off table	No longer clenches fist tightly, follows object past midline	Smiles socially (after being stroked or talked to)	Recognizes parent	2 mo
3 mo	Supports on forearms in prone, holds head up steadily	Holds hands open at rest, follows in circular fashion, responds to visual threat	Coos (produces long vowel sounds in musical fashion)	Reaches for familiar people or objects, anticipates feeding	3 mo
4 mo	Rolls front to back, supports on wrists and shifts weight	Reaches with arms in unison, brings hands to midline	Laughs, orients to voice	Enjoys looking around environment	4 mo
5 mo	Rolls back to front, sits supported	Transfers objects	Says 'ah-goo,' razzes, orients to bell (localizes laterally)		5 mo
6 mo	Sits unsupported, puts feet in mouth in supine position	Unilateral reach, uses raking grasp	Babbles	Recognizes strangers	6 mo
7 mo	Creeps		Orients to bell (localized indirectly)		7 mo
8 mo	Comes to sit, crawls	Inspects objects	'Dada' indiscriminately	Fingerfeeds	8 mo
9 mo	Pivots when sitting, pulls to stand, cruises	Uses pincer grasp, probes with forefinger, holds bottle, throws objects	'Mama' indiscriminately, gestures, waves bye-bye, understands 'no'	Starts to explore environment; plays gesture games (e.g., pat-a-cake)	9 mo
10 mo	Walks when led with both hands held	—	'Dada/mama' discriminately; orients to bell (directly)	—	10 mo
11 mo	Walks when led with one hand held	—	One word other than 'dada/mama,' follows 1-step command with gesture	—	11 mo
12 mo	Walks alone	Uses mature pincer grasp, releases voluntarily, marks paper with pencil	Uses two words other than 'dada/mama,' immature jargoning (runs several unintelligible words together)	Imitates actions, comes when called, cooperates with dressing	12 mo
13 mo	—	—	Uses three words	—	13 mo
14 mo	—	—	Follows 1-step command without gesture	—	14 mo
15 mo	Creeps up stairs, walks backwards	Scribbles in imitation, builds tower of 2 blocks in imitation	Uses 4–6 words	15–18 mo: uses spoon, uses cup independently	15 mo
17 mo	—	—	Uses 7–20 words, points to 5 body parts, uses mature jargoning (includes intelligible words in jargoning)	—	17 mo
18 mo	Runs, throws objects from standing without falling	Scribbles spontaneously, builds tower of 3 blocks, turns 2–3 pages at a time	Uses 2-word combinations	Copies parent in tasks (sweeping, dusting), plays in company of other children	18 mo
19 mo	—	—	Knows 8 body parts	—	19 mo
21 mo	Squats in play, goes up steps	Builds tower of 5 blocks	Uses 50 words, 2-word sentences	Asks to have food and to go to toilet	21 mo
24 mo	Walks up and down steps without help	Imitates stroke with pencil, builds tower of 7 blocks, turns pages one at a time, removes shoes, pants, etc.	Uses pronouns (I, you, me) inappropriately, follows 2-step commands	Parallel play	24 mo
30 mo	Jumps with both feet off floor, throws ball overhand	Holds pencil in adult fashion, performs horizontal and vertical strokes, unbuttons	Uses pronouns appropriately, understands concept of '1,' repeats 2 digits forward	Tells first and last names when asked; gets self drink without help	30 mo

(continued)

DEVELOPMENTAL MILESTONES (Continued)

Age	Gross Motor	Visual-Motor/Problem-Solving	Language	Social/Adaptive	Age
3 yr	Can alternate feet when going up steps, pedals tricycle	Copies a circle, undresses completely, dresses partially, dries hands if reminded	Uses minimum 250 words, 3-word sentences; uses plurals, past tense; knows all pronouns; understands concept of '2'	Group play, shares toys, takes turns, plays well with others, knows full name, age, sex	3 yr
4 yr	Hops, skips, alternates feet going down steps	Copies a square, buttons clothing, dresses self completely, catches ball	Knows colors, says song or poem from memory, asks questions	Tells 'tall tales,' plays cooperatively with a group of children	4 yr
5 yr	Skips alternating feet, jumps over low obstacles	Copies triangle, ties shoes, spreads with knife	Prints first name, asks what a word means	Plays competitive games, abides by rules, likes to help in household tasks	5 yr

(From Siberry, G. K. & Iannone, R. [Eds.] [2000]. *The Hamet Lane handbook* [15th ed.]. St. Louis: Mosby.)

SELECTED REFERENCES

Barnes, P. (1995). *Personal, social and emotional development of children*. Boston: Blackwell Publishers.

Burns, C.E. (2000). *Pediatric primary care: A handbook for nurse practitioners*. Philadelphia: W.B. Saunders.

Capute, A.J., & Biehl, R.F. (1973). Functional development evaluation: Prerequisite to habilitation. *Pediatric Clinics of North America, 20, 3.*

Capute, A.J., & Accardo, P.J. (1978). Linguistic and auditory milestones during the first two years of life. *Clinical Pediatrics, 17, 847.*

Capute, A.J., Shapiro, B.K., Wachtel, R.C., Gunther, V.A., & Palmer, F.B. (1986). The clinical linguistic and auditory milestone scale (CLAMS). *American Journal of Disabilities of Children, 140, 694.*

Capute, A.J., Palmer, F.B., Shapiro, B.K., Wachtel, R.C., Schmidt, S., & Ross, A. (1986). Clinical linguistic and auditory milestone scale: Prediction of cognition in infancy. *Developmental Medicine and Children's Neurology, 28,762.*

Collins, W.A. & Laursen, B.P. (1999). *Relationships as developmental contexts*. Princeton, NJ: Lawrence Erlbaum Associates.

Davies, D. (1999). *Child development: A practitioner's guide*. New York: Guilford Press.

Dixon, S.D. (1992). *Encounters with children: Pediatric behavior and development*. St. Louis: Mosby—Year Book.

Fox, J.A. (2000). *Primary health care of children*. St. Louis: Mosby.

Fuller, J., & Schaller-Ayers, J. (2000). *Health assessment: A nursing approach*. Philadelphia: Lippincott Williams & Wilkins.

Green, M. (1994). *Bright futures: Guidelines for health supervision of infants, children, and adolescents*. Arlington, VA: National Center for Education in Maternal and Child Health.

Goldstein, J.H. (1994). *Toys, play and child development*. New York: Cambridge University Press.

Lamb, M.E. (1997). *The role of the father in child development*. New York: Wiley.

Marsten, A.S. (1999). *Cultural processes in child development*. Princeton, NJ: Lawrence Erlbaum Associates.

McMillan, J.A. (Ed.). (1999). *Oski's principles and practice of pediatrics*. Philadelphia: Lippincott Williams & Wilkins.

Pillitteri, A. (1999). *Maternal and child health nursing* (3rd ed.). Philadelphia: Lippincott Williams & Wilkins.

Schuster, C.S., & Ashburn, S.S. (1992). *The process of human development*. Philadelphia: J.B. Lippincott.

Siberry, G.K., & Iannone, R. (Eds.) (2000). *The Harriet Lane handbook* (15th ed.). St. Louis: Mosby.

Taylor, E. (1961). *Psychological appraisal of children with cerebral defects*. Boston: Harvard University Press.

Pediatric Physical Assessment

HISTORY

▣ Obtaining a History

A history of the child is obtained to establish a relationship with the child and family; to assess what a family understands about its child's health; to formulate an individual plan of care; and to correct any misinformation the family may have.

Focus on specific topics in the history, depending on the child's age, including:

- Infant—prenatal and postnatal history, nutrition, development.
- Toddler—home environment, safety issues, development, parent's response.
- School age—school, friends, reaction to previous hospitalizations.
- Adolescent—alcohol, drugs, friends, sexual history, relationships with parents, identity.

Identifying Information

Type of Information Needed

1. Date and time.
2. Health care provider's name and telephone number, if known. Insurance data.
3. Patient's name, address, telephone number, birth date.
4. Referring health care source (eg, school, other health care provider, clinic).

Note: Permission from the legal guardian must be obtained to treat the child.

Method of Collecting Data

1. Identify the care person in charge of the patient by name and relationship to the patient; obtain relative's or care person's address, and home and work telephone numbers, if different from those of the patient.
2. To make the informant feel more at ease, the questions should begin in a friendly, nonthreatening manner. Questions addressed to the parent should be phrased appropriately.

3. Casual, friendly responses or remarks on the part of the interviewer may also help break the ice:
   a. "Whoever takes care of this baby certainly does a good job."
   b. "That's a lovely outfit the baby is wearing." (Remember that families will often put a new dress or suit on a baby for a visit to a health care agency.)
4. Sometimes repeat the information to verify data. This will give you a better judgment of the care person's cooperation and reliability.
5. If age appropriate, get some data directly from child.

Chief Complaint

Method of Recording

1. Write an exact description of the complaint.
2. Use quotation marks to clearly indicate that the informant's words are being used. It is helpful to explain:
   a. "I'll write it down so there will be no mistake."
   b. "Let me read this back to you to be sure it is correct."
3. Quotation of the care person's exact words may give an indication of how he or she feels about the symptoms; it may reflect fear, guilt, defensiveness, etc.

Method of Collecting Information

1. Begin with a helpful open-ended question. That is the first overture made to this patient:
   a. "How have things been going?"
   b. "Please tell me the reason for your coming here today."
   c. "What do you think is wrong with the baby?"
2. Then proceed to more specific questions.

Duration of Complaint

1. The information obtained may indicate the natural history of the disease, if one is present, and its gradual evolution. Pursue the information with a series of probing questions.
   a. "How long has the baby (child) had this problem?"
   b. If the informant cannot remember, try another route: "When did he (or she) last act well?"; "Do you

remember last Christmas? Did the baby have the trouble then?"

2. Write down the responses; try to assess, as more questions are asked, how accurate the informant's answers may be.

History of Present Illness
Type of Information Needed
When the patient is an infant or a preverbal child, information will consist mainly of what the informant has been able to observe. Having established what the chief complaint is, identify further problems, if any. Obtain the following information for each problem:
1. Body location—of pain, itching, weakness, etc.
2. Quality and quantity of complaint—both type (a burning pain) and severity (knifelike, comes and goes).
3. Degree of symptom—(eg, pain, how severe; cough, day and night; eye drainage, amount).
4. Chronology—indicate time sequence and whether problem is episodic (lasts for a while and then clears up completely).
5. Environment or setting—where and when the symptoms occur.
6. Aggravating and alleviating factors—what makes the pain worse or better?
7. Associated manifestations or symptoms—accompanied by vomiting, blurred vision, etc.

Importance of Detail
1. Frequently, a carefully written description of a symptom will be the source of a future diagnosis and will serve all who are involved in helping the patient.
2. Do not worry about how many notes you have to take at first.
3. You will be able to recheck this information when you do the review of systems.

Family History
1. Family members—mother's age and state of health, father's age and health, siblings (who is at home with you?).
2. Family health history—any of the following conditions:
   a. Eyes, ears, nose, throat—nose bleeds, sinus problems, glaucoma, cataracts, myopia, strabismus, other problems of eyes, ears, nose, throat.
   b. Cardiorespiratory—tuberculosis, asthma, hay fever, hypertension, heart murmurs, heart attacks, strokes, rheumatic fever, pneumonia, emphysema, other problems.
   c. Gastrointestinal—ulcers, colitis, vomiting, diarrhea, other problems.
   d. Genitourinary—kidney infections, bladder problems, congenital abnormalities.
   e. Musculoskeletal—congenital hip or foot problems, muscular dystrophy, arthritis, other problems.
   f. Neurologic—seizures, epilepsy, nervous disorder, mental retardation, emotional problems, comas, headaches, others.
   g. Chronic disease—diabetes, liver disease, cancer, tumors, anemia, thyroid problems, congenital disorder.
   h. Special senses—anyone deaf or blind?
   i. Miscellaneous—any other medical problem not mentioned.
3. Family social history:
   a. Residence—apartment or house, how large? Yard, stairs, proximity to transportation, shopping, playground, school, safe neighborhood? City water?
   b. Financial situation—who works, where employed, occupation, welfare, food stamps.
   c. Outside help—baby sitters, day-care center.
   d. Family interrelationships—happy, cooperative, antagonistic, chaotic, multiproblem, violent, etc.

Past History
Prenatal
1. Pregnancy—planned or not; source of care; approximate date of seeking care; birth order of this pregnancy, including miscarriages. This area of the history may be one of great sensitivity. Try to make the questions gentle and supportive:
   a. "Did you plan a baby around this time?"
   b. "When did you manage to get your first checkup for the pregnancy?"
   c. "Were there any unusual problems related to your pregnancy or delivery?"
2. Maternal health—includes illnesses and dates, abnormal symptoms (eg, fever, rash, vaginal bleeding, edema, hypertension, urine abnormalities, sexually transmitted disease). Avoid technical words, if possible.
   a. "Were the doctors or nurses worried about your health?"
   b. "Were your rings tight?"
   c. "Do you know if your blood pressure went up?"
   d. "Did you have trouble with your urine?"
3. Weight gain—validate by trying to get a figure for nonpregnant weight and weight at delivery.
4. Medicines taken—eg, vitamins, iron, calcium, aspirin, cold preparations, tranquilizers ("nerve medicine"), antibiotics; use of ointments, hormones, injections during pregnancy, special or unusual diet; radiation exposure; sonography; and amniocentesis.
5. Quality of the fetal movements: when felt?

Natal
1. Expected date of delivery and approximate duration of pregnancy.
2. Place of delivery and name of person who conducted the delivery.
3. Labor—spontaneous or induced, duration, and intensity.
4. Analgesia or anesthesia.
5. Presentation—vaginal, breech, or vertex; cesarean delivery, forceps.
6. Complications (eg, need for blood transfusion, delay in delivery, etc.)

Neonatal

1. Condition of infant.
2. Color (if seen) at delivery.
3. Activity of infant.
4. Type of crying heard.
5. Breathing abnormality.
6. Birth weight and length.
7. Problems that occurred immediately at birth.

Postnatal

1. Duration of hospitalization of the mother and infant.
2. Problems with baby's breathing or feeding.
3. Need of supportive care (eg, oxygen, incubator, special care nursery, isolation, medications).
4. Weight changes, weight at discharge if known.
5. Color—cyanosis or jaundice.
6. Bowel movements—when.
7. Problems—seizures, deformities identified, consultation required.
8. Mother's contact with the baby and her first impression:
   a. "What was it like when you first saw your baby?"
   b. "What did the baby do when you were first together?"

Nutrition

1. Breast- or bottle-fed? What formula? How prepared?
2. Amounts offered and consumed.
3. Frequency of feeding—weight gain.
4. Addition of juice or solid foods.
5. Food preferences or allergies.
6. Feeding problems—variations in appetite.
7. Age of weaning.
8. Vitamins—type, amount, regularity.
9. Pattern of weight gain.
10. Current diet—frequency and content of meals.

Growth and Development

1. Past weights and lengths if available.
2. Milestones—sat alone unsupported; walked alone; used words, then sentences.
3. Teeth—eruption, difficulty, cavities, brushing, flossing.
4. Toilet training.
5. Current motor, social, and language skills.
6. Sexual development.
   a. Infant—swollen breast tissue, vaginal discharge, hypertrophy of the labia.
   b. Toddler or school-aged child—early development of breasts or pubic hair.
   c. Prepubertal or pubertal child—in girls, time of development of breasts and pubic hair and onset of menstruation. In boys, time of enlargement of testes and penis, development of pubic and facial hair, and voice changes.

Health Maintenance

1. Immunizations—rubella, rubeola, mumps, polio, diphtheria, pertussis, tetanus toxoid, varicella, pneumococcal, bacille Calmette-Guérin (BCG), influenza, *Haemophilus influenzae* b (HIB), hepatitis B. Indicate number and dates.
2. Screening procedures—hematocrit or hemoglobin, urinalysis tuberculin testing, visual and auditory acuity color vision; rubella antibodies, syphilis testing, gonorrhea screen, Papanicolaou smear.
3. Dental care—source and frequency of care, dental hygienist visits, fillings, or extractions.

Acute Infectious Diseases

Rubella, rubeola, mumps, chickenpox, scarlet fever, rheumatic fever, hepatitis, infectious mononucleosis, sexually transmitted disease, tuberculosis. Recent exposure to communicable disease.

Hospitalizations and Operations

1. Dates, hospital, physician.
2. Indications, diagnosis, procedures.
3. Complications.
4. Reactions to previous hospitalizations.

Injuries

1. Emergency department visits—frequency and diagnosis.
2. Fractures—location and treatment.
3. Trauma, burns, bruises.
4. Ingestions.

Medications

1. For general use, such as vitamins, antihistamines, laxatives.
2. Special or fad diets.
3. Recent antibiotics.
4. Routine use of aspirin.
5. Oral contraceptives—types, dose, duration.
6. Drugs, narcotics, marijuana, hallucinogens, mood elevators, tranquilizers, alcohol.
7. Determine when last dose of medication was taken; is medication with patient? How does the child take the medication?
8. Allergy to medication?

Method of Collecting Data

1. Straightforward questions to a child (eg, "What grade are you in?"; "Who are your friends?").
2. Three wishes offered to the child:
   a. "If Christmas were here, what would you ask for?"
   b. "If you had your way, whom would you like to be?"
   c. "What would be the best thing that could happen to you?"
3. "Who's your best friend?"
4. Questions to parents: "How does that seem to you?"
5. Adolescents—may want to interview without parents present, but parents must be included in some way.

School History

Type of Information Needed

1. Present and past schooling, grade, and performance.
2. Favored and least favored subjects.
3. School-related behavior—anxious to go, anxious to stay home.
4. General attitude toward school and career plans; attitude toward peer groups.
5. Gang dress or behavior.

Method of Collecting Data

Emphasize the positive (eg, "What's your best subject?"; "Have you repeated a grade?"; "Do you see your friends after school?")

Social History

Type of Information Needed

1. Environment—rural, urban.
2. Housing—type, location, heating, sewage, water supply, family pets, other animal exposure.
3. Parents' occupations (employment) and marital status.
4. Number of individuals living in home, sleeping arrangements.
5. Religious affiliations.
6. Previous utilization of social agencies.
7. Health insurance and usual source of care.

Method of Collecting Data

Parents are proud, so be careful with some of the questions. Ask permission.

1. "Can you tell me a little bit about your home?"
2. "I need to know more about how you live to help you with your child's problem."

Personal History

Type of Information Needed

1. Hygiene, exercise.
2. Sleep habits.
3. Elimination habits.
4. Activities, hobbies, special talents.
5. Friends, teacher relationships.
6. Sibling and parent relationships.
7. Expression of emotions.
   a. Blows up easily.
   b. Quiet.
8. Idiosyncratic behavior and habits (eg, thumb sucking, nail biting, temper tantrums, head banging, pica, breath holding, rituals, tics, etc.).

Review of Systems

Type of Information Needed

1. General—activity, appetite, affect, sleep patterns, weight changes, edema, fever, behavior.

2. Allergy—eczema, hay fever, asthma, hives, food or drug allergy, sinus disorders.
3. Skin—rash or eruption, nodules, pigmentation or texture change, sweating or dryness, infection, hair growth, itching.
4. Head—headache, head trauma, dizziness.
5. Eyes—visual acuity, corrective lenses, strabismus, lacrimation, discharge, itching, redness, photophobia.
6. Ears—auditory acuity, earaches (frequency, ages, response to specific medications), infection, drainage.
7. Nose—colds and runny nose (frequency), infection, drainage.
8. Teeth—hygiene practices, general condition, cavities, malocclusions.
9. Throat—sore throat, tonsillitis, difficulty swallowing.
10. Speech—peculiarity of or change in voice, hoarseness, clarity, enunciation, stammering, development of articulation, vocabulary, use of sentences.
11. Respiratory—difficulty breathing, shortness of breath, chest pain, cough, wheezing, croup, pneumonia, tuberculosis or exposure, wheezing.
12. Cardiovascular—cyanosis, fainting, exercise intolerance, murmurs.
13. Hematologic—pallor, anemia, tendency to bruise or bleed.
14. Gastrointestinal—appetite (amount, frequency, cravings), nausea, vomiting, abdominal pain, abnormal size, bowel habits and nature of stools, parasites, encopresis (incontinence of feces), colic.
15. Genitourinary—age of toilet training, frequency of urination, straining, dysuria, hematuria (or unusual color or odor of infant's soiled diaper), previous urinary tract infection, enuresis (age of onset; day or nighttime); urethral or vaginal discharge. Girls and young women: last menses, cramps, changes in interval, and duration.
16. Musculoskeletal—deformities, fractures, sprains, joint pains or swelling, limitation of motion, abnormality of nails.
17. Neurologic—weakness or clumsiness, coordination, balance, gait, dominance, fatigability, tone, tremor. Seizures or paroxysmal behavior. Personality changes.

PHYSICAL EXAMINATION

■ General Principles

1. Establish the order of all data collection according to the needs of the patients. For example:
   a. An exhausted parent with a screaming baby will not give a careful, comprehensive history.
   b. Alternative care may not be available for preschoolers when the newborn comes in for the first checkup.
2. If the parent has come in with more than one child, try to organize some supervision of the other children so that you can have a little time with the parent alone.
3. Remember that the safest place for a young child is on the parent's knee. Privacy may not be possible when other children are present.
4. Attempt to develop rapport with the young patient from the moment you first see or meet him or her.
5. Explain to the school-aged child or teenager what you are looking for as you proceed with the examination.

Approach to the Patient

1. Offer the young child a choice of being examined on parent's lap or on your "special table."
2. To evaluate the chest properly, you need to listen through 10 heartbeats when the child is not screaming; therefore, the chest is a good place to begin the examination.
3. The part to be examined should be completely exposed, but if an apprehensive child objects to having clothes removed, slip your stethoscope under the shirt.
4. After listening to the heart, begin with parts of the body that are already exposed.
5. Start with either the head or the toes and work thoroughly and systematically toward the other end.
6. Gradually remove the child's clothes; look for asymmetry very carefully in the bodies of all children.
7. Develop a pattern appropriate to the patient's age.
   a. With infants it may be wise to leave the diaper area until last.
   b. Adolescents and school-aged children are often embarrassed at the genital examination—you may want to leave this until last.
8. Using a cold stethoscope may result in a frightened and screaming child, so warm the stethoscope before bringing it into contact with the child.
9. Some children are less frightened if allowed to hold the examining equipment first.
10. Show the child the procedure by demonstrating on the parent first.
11. Many young children enjoy listening to their own hearts.
12. Toddlers and preschoolers enjoy blowing your otoscope light out.

Technique	Findings

Vital Signs

1. Obtain temperature, pulse rate, respiratory rate, and blood pressure as often as thought necessary, based on child's condition.

Temperature
Oral 36.4°–37.4°C. (97.6°–99.3°F.)
Rectal 36.2°–37.8°C. (97°–100°F.)
Axillary 35.9°–36.7°C. (96.6°–98°F.)

Pulse and Respiratory Rates

Age	Pulse	Respirations
Newborn	70–170	30–50
11 mos	80–160	26–40
2 yrs	80–130	20–30
4 yrs	80–120	20–30
6 yrs	75–115	20–26
8 yrs	70–110	18–24
10 yrs	70–110	18–24
Adolescence	60–110	12–20

Blood Pressure
Varies with age, height, and weight of child

2. Measure core temperature, whenever possible, via rectal or ear route. Leave mercury thermometer in place 3–5 min. for rectal reading, longer for oral or axillary.
3. Obtain apical pulse rate on an infant or small child; radial, temporal, or carotid pulse may be measured with an older child. Pulse may be counted for 30 seconds and multiplied by 2.
4. Count respirations on an infant for 1 full minute; observe the chest as well as the abdomen. Respirations may be counted for 30 seconds and multiplied by 2 in an older child.
5. Obtain blood pressure by auscultatory method, rather than palpation method, whenever possible. Make sure the cuff covers no less than ½ and no more than ⅔ the length of the upper arm or leg.

Technique   Findings

Standing Height, Head Circumference, and Chest Circumference

1. Use tape measure to obtain accurate head circumference. Measure widest part of head.

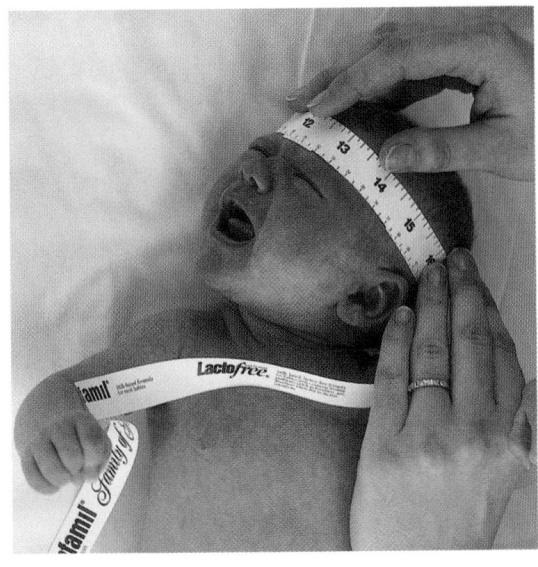

Head and Chest Circumference				
Age	Head Circumference		Chest Circumference	
Yr Mo	Inch	Cm	In	Cm
Birth	13.8	35.0	13.0	33.0
3	15.9	40.4	15.8	40.2
6	17.1	43.4	17.1	43.4
9	17.8	45.3	18.0	45.7
1–0	18.3	46.6	18.6	47.3
1–6	18.9	47.9	19.4	49.2
2–0	19.3	48.9	19.8	50.4
3–0	19.6	49.8	20.6	52.5
3–6	—	—	20.8	52.8
4–0	19.8	50.4	21.0	53.4
5–0	20.0	50.8	21.5	54.6

(From Studies at Harvard School of Public Health.)

2. Measure chest at level of the nipples.
3. Record height and weight at each visit. Plot on growth chart.

3. Trends in growth are as important as the basic measurements.

General Appearance

1. Begin observations with the first contact with the patient, taking into account that there are at least two people to observe (child and parent).
2. The patient's interaction with the caretaker, whether it be the mother, father, a babysitter, an older sibling, or a friend of the family, is vital in the assessment of the child. As you observe for race, sex, general physical development, nutritional state, mental alertness, evidence of pain, restlessness, body position, clothes, apparent age, hygiene, and grooming, remember that many of these things are part of the parent's caretaking.

1. If the child is easily distracted or sleepy, it may be naptime.

2. Careful observation of the general state of the child will provide many clues about the child's relationship to the family and its response to the child.

Skin and Lymphatics

Examine as you move through each body region (include hair and skin).

Inspection

Inspection of the skin is the same as for the adult.

1. Observe for skin color, pigmentation, lesions, jaundice, cyanosis, scars, superficial vascularity, moisture, edema, color of mucous membranes, hair distribution.

1. In young babies, the skin is soft, smooth, and velvety in texture.

Technique	Findings
2. Describe any variation in color, particularly in children with increased pigmentation. No pigment, or vitiligo, in darker children can be noted.	2. Pigmentations vary in children, depending on race, and will change as the child gets older.
3. Birthmarks of any type are recorded. (May change as child grows older.)	3. A suntan, freckles, small, light-brown patches or café-au-lait spots may occur.
4. Bruises or unusual marks of any kind, wounds or insect bites, scratch marks, scars, etc., may have particular significance.	4. Bruises are particularly important because of the possibility of child abuse.
5. Draw a picture of anything unusual such as a scar, and measure the dimensions of the lesion when recording the findings.	5. If you have difficulty describing something, use ordinary words, rather than inaccurate technical terms.
6. To ascertain suspected jaundice, take the child to the window to get a true picture of the color of the skin. (A room with yellow walls and artificial lighting may create a wrong impression when jaundice is suspected.)	6. Carotenemia, which causes the nose and palms of the hands to have a yellowish tinge, may lead the parents to suspect jaundice; however, carotenemia is caused by eating many yellow vegetables (carrots, sweet potatoes, squash, etc.). In carotenemia, the sclerae are clear; this is not so in jaundice.
7. The skin of newborn infants will still be covered with vernix caseosa, the oily material that covers the fetus's body while in utero.	7. Swollen sebaceous glands over the nose and chin are frequently seen right after birth and are called *milia*.
8. Postmature infants may have scaliness that persists for several weeks after birth, particularly around the feet. The color of the skin may change as the child gets a little older.	8. The blotchy, pink patches over the eyelid, bridge of the nose, and the back of the neck may persist until the child is almost 2 years of age.
9. Note striae.	9. May indicate rapid weight gain.
10. Dark skinned children may have Mongolian spots on base of spine or elsewhere.	10. Important to distinguish from child abuse.

Palpation

1. Use the tips of the fingers to palpate—fingertips are more sensitive.
2. Feel the tension of the skin by pinching up a fold of skin—normal skin quickly falls back, but dehydrated skin remains in pinched position.

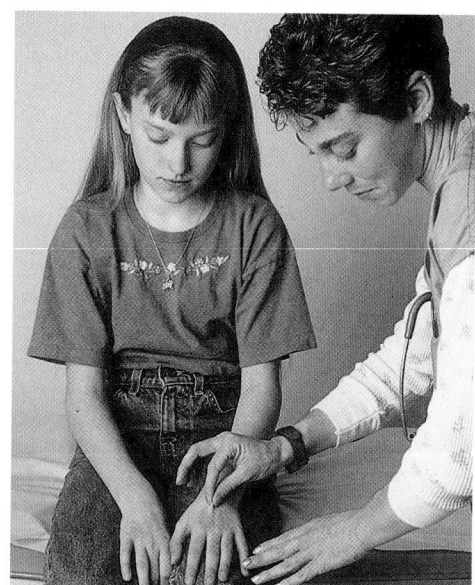

3. Feel the skin for texture, moisture, temperature, turgor, elasticity, masses, tenderness.

3. Skin that is rough and dry in texture may actually have a discrete rash that can be felt but not seen.

Technique	Findings

Lymph

1. Observe and palpate for lymph node enlargement in lymph chain areas.
   a. Neck.
   b. Axilla.
   c. Inguinal.
   d. Epitrochlear.
2. Note tenderness, size, and consistency.

1. May be large or readily palpable, but should be non-tender and spongy.

Nails

1. Observe for color, shape, irregularities in surface, and general nail care; cleanliness, evidence of biting, etc.
2. Palpate the skin around the fingernails for firmness. Palpate any part that appears inflamed.

1. Nail beds should be pink, nails convex.

2. General care of the child is frequently reflected in good care of nails.

Hair

1. Observe for color and distribution.
   a. Note according to the age of the child and race.
   b. Be aware that tufts of hair over the spine or sacral area may mark an underlying abnormality.
2. Note any change in pigmentation.

3. Palpate the hair for texture and thickness.

4. Examine to see if there are patches where hair is missing on the head.

5. Separate thick hair on the head to get a good view of the scalp. Check for dandruff or scaliness in older children.
6. Check scalp for any signs of lice infestation.

7. Inspect in the axillae and over the pubis and the extremities for hair and its quantity, to gauge the development and level of puberty.

1. *Newborn:* Normally varies from no hair to a thick bush. *Infant:* Consists of lanugo, a soft, downy covering frequently seen over the shoulders, back, arms, face, and sacral area, especially in dark-skinned children.
2. Remember, children frequently experiment with mother's hair dye or rinse.
3. Texture may be thick or thin, coarse or fine, straight or curly.
4. May denote underlying skin infection; however, some children pull their hair out; sometimes the hair is braided so tightly that it falls out.
5. Look carefully for broken hairs, for scaliness on the scalp or cradle cap in infants.
6. Nits (louse eggs) appear on the hair as little white dots. Lice may be seen on the scalp; they move quickly and may jump.
7. The child need not be totally undressed; a prepubertal child will usually be embarrassed if all clothes are removed.

◼ Head and Neck

1. Unless specifically requested otherwise, examine the eyes and ears at the very last, especially in the younger child.
2. Also, examine the throat toward the last, unless the child exhibits concern about the "throat stick." It is then best to examine the throat right away to "get it over with." If a child cries you may be able to avoid using a tongue blade.
3. To avoid frightening the child when palpating the head, make a game out of it—ask, "Where's your nose?" "Where are your eyes?"

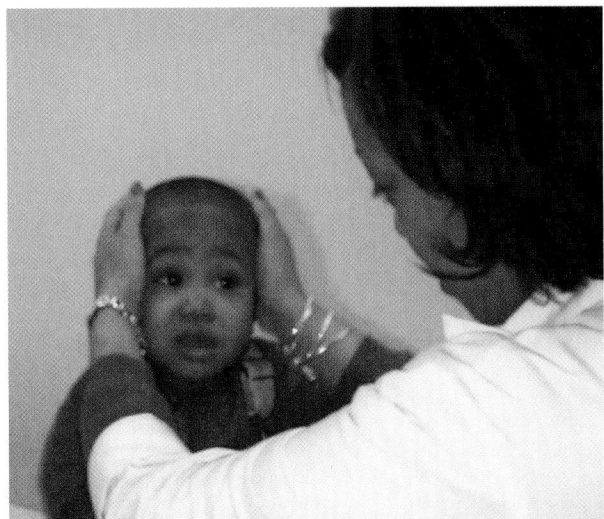

Technique	Findings

Inspection

1. Observe the face and skull for asymmetry, deformity, and abnormal or limited movements.

2. Closely observe facial expressions, blinking, etc., if the child is not crying. This may be one of your few moments to see the child when he or she is not crying. If you are examining a crying baby, watch particularly for asymmetry of the face.

3. Observe the movement of the head on the neck as the baby looks around. When turning an infant over, observe the head for control, position, and movement.

4. Because an infant's neck is often short and there are often several folds of skin under the chin, it is necessary to lift the chin a little to observe the skin completely—to see that it is clear and free of perspiration rash or irritation.

1. A baby's head may be asymmetrical because of pressure during pregnancy and delivery. The rounded head of the baby born by breech delivery contrasts with the long, pointed head of a baby who is a firstborn and whose head was moulded during a prolonged labor.

2. In a baby born by forceps delivery, there may be signs of weakness of the facial nerve caused by pressure of the forceps over the front of the ear where the facial nerve emerges. When the baby cries, the involved side will show weakness and downturning of the mouth.

3. There should be very little head lag beyond the age of 3 months.

4. In the back, the neck should be free of webbing or of extra folds of skin extending from just beneath the ear toward the shoulder.

Palpation

1. Palpate the skull for the suture lines. Feel the face for masses, noting size, consistency, surface, temperature, and tenderness.

2. Palpate the anterior and posterior fontanelles.

1. The suture lines of the skull may be felt to override as a result of the pressure applied when contractions occurred during labor. This is usually most marked between the frontal and the parietal bone, where the coronal suture is located.

2. The fontanelles are soft and flat. Tense or bulging fontanelles may indicate hydrocephalus. Depressed fontanelles are often a sign of dehydration. The fontanelles usually close by 18 months.

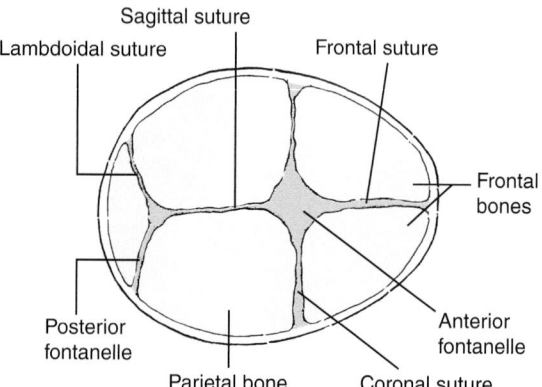

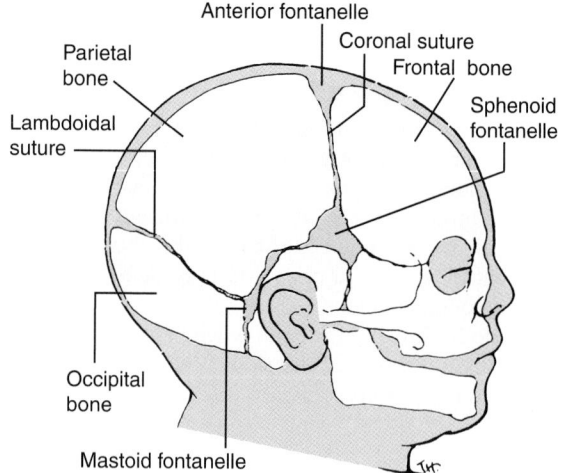

3. Palpate along the lambdoidal suture at the back of the head between the parietal bones and the occipital bone.

4. Palpate the neck for swollen lymph nodes, noting tenderness, mobility, location, and consistency.

4. Palpation of the lymph nodes may reveal slightly enlarge nodes in the anterior cervical chain secondary to sore throat.

Technique	**Findings**

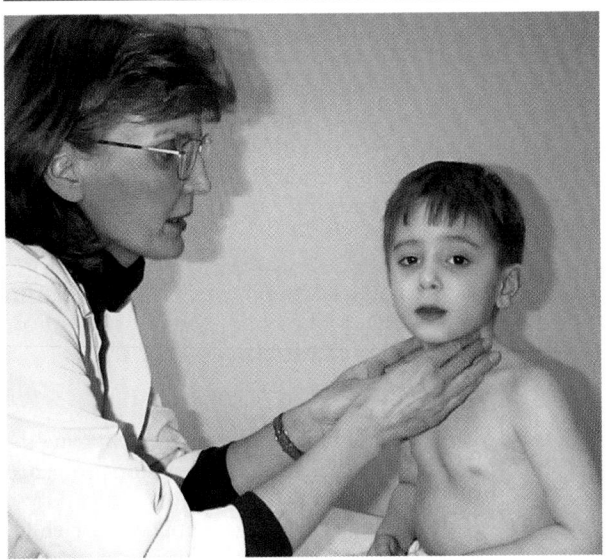

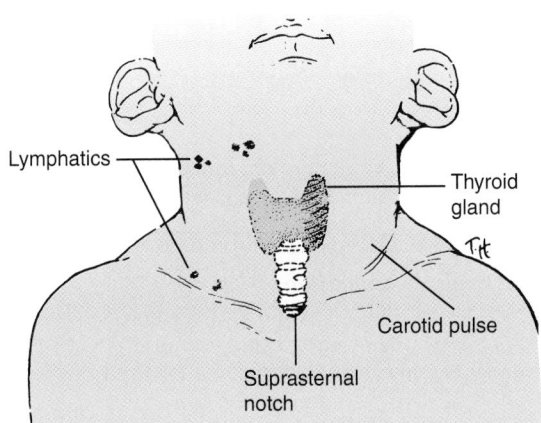

Lymphatics — Thyroid gland — Carotid pulse — Suprasternal notch

5. Note that there are other nodes, which are normally not palpable.

5. These include the pre- and postauricular, the posterior cervical (behind the sternomastoid), the submental and submandibular (under the jaw), and the occipital nodes (along the prominence of the occiput).

6. Feel the pulses in the neck for location, strength, and equality.
7. Check the thyroid for enlargement, position, texture, and tenderness.
8. Locate the trachea in the suprasternal notch for position in the center of the neck.
9. Palpate sternocleidomastoids, making sure they are equal in size.

Percussion
1. Percussion of the face may elicit tenderness over the sinuses.
2. Percuss over the head and neck directly with the fingertips, usually the middle finger of the right hand.

3. Percuss over the forehead for tenderness in the sinuses and across the zygoma, or cheekbone.

1. Tenderness may be caused by a tooth cavity or by a sinus infection.
2. Gentle tapping over the skull elicits a typical noise when the sutures are open, and elicits a different sound when the sutures are closed.
3. This determines underlying tenderness in the frontal or maxillary sinus.

Auscultation
Auscultate the skull and carotid arteries in the neck.

To determine bruits.

Eyes and Vision
Equipment
Ophthalmoscope and penlight. Be sure batteries are new and lights are bright.

Inspection
(Similar to adult examination; see pp. 54–56)
1. Pay particular attention to the lacrimal duct and excessive tearing.

1. Discharge from the eyes along the lower lid or from the lacrimal duct can occur as a result of infection or reaction to silver nitrate administered to the neonate.

Technique	Findings
2. Note the distance between the eyes and the distribution of the eyebrows.	2. Hypertelorism denotes a wider area between the eyes than normal. Excessively long and full eyebrows that meet in the midline and extra-long eyelashes may signify a developmental abnormality.
3. Test the eyes for light perception.	3. It is difficult to prevent children from blinking their eyes or closing them when testing light response.
4. Do cover/uncover test.	4. To discover strabismus.

Palpation

If the child is old enough, have him squeeze eyes tightly (not possible in younger children) while you try to open them.

Weakness of the muscles around the eyes is difficult to demonstrate in the young child. Muscle strength or weakness can be evaluated when the child cries.

Fundoscopic Examination

1. Check to see that the child's eyes move in conjugate fashion. Ask the mother if she has noticed any signs of squinting, especially when the child is tired.
2. This is a difficult examination to conduct because children tend to watch the light and stare directly at you, which constricts their pupils. If the child cannot cooperate, it may be necessary to dilate the pupil to see the fundus. It is often not necessary to do a fundoscopic examination on children.
3. Start your examination at about $\frac{1}{3}$ m (1 ft) from the patient. Look for the red reflex, which should be readily observable.
4. Look for any opacities and then slowly approach the patient, turning the ophthalmoscopic dial to the smaller plus (+) numbers. Start originally at +8 to +10.

5. To help guide your gaze, put your hand on top of the child's head or at the side, with your thumb at the corner of the eye at the outer edge. If you lose the fundus, you can return to your thumb and get your bearings by directing your gaze medial to the tip of your thumbnail.

1. Loss of vision can occur if the eyes are not working together properly. Squinting can indicate vision problems.

2. A picture can be pinned to the wall opposite the child, who is then instructed to look at the picture during the examination. If the child is examined while lying down, a picture can be placed on the ceiling.

4. The red reflex is diminished if there is something obstructing your view. A cataract or an opacity in the retina can cause this, as would a tumor filling the posterior chamber. If there is any paleness in the red reflex or difficulty in identifying it, a consultation should be sought immediately.

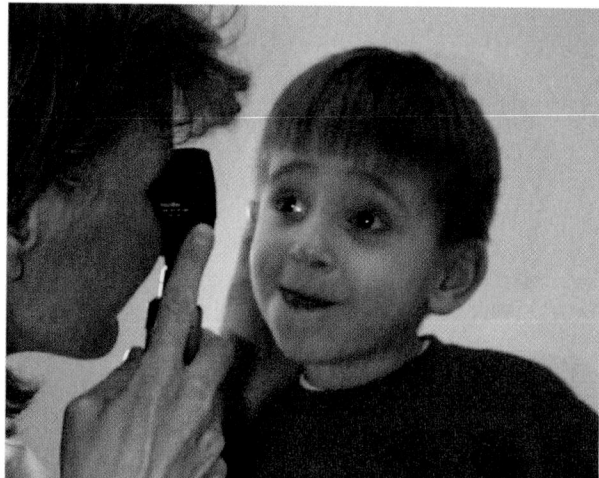

Ears and Hearing

Equipment

Otoscope with pneumatic bulb
Small speculum for child's ear
Fresh batteries to ensure a bright light

Technique	Findings

Inspection

1. When examining the external ear, the auricle, or the pinna, be sure to note the position of the ear.

   The top of the ear should cross an imaginary line drawn between the edge of the eye and the back of the occiput. If the ear is positioned more obliquely or is low-set, some underlying abnormality, particularly of the genitourinary system, may be present.

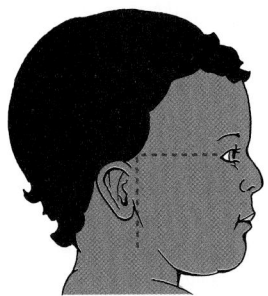

2. If you cannot get the child to cooperate by offering an explanation or by playing a game, the child will have to be restrained. Many children will enjoy watching the light on their leg or seeing the red glow of their finger with the light shining through or blowing the light out. If restraint is needed:

   a. The child can be seated on the parent's knee with the child's legs wedged between the parent's knees and the head held firmly with one hand while the child's hands are controlled with the other hand.

   b. An older child may be held in a supine position, with the parent holding the child's arms above the head and controlling the head.

   c. If the child is very restless and apprehensive, examine the child from the top while the parent leans over the child's body, holds the arms down with her elbows, and at the same time grasps the child's head with her hands.

2. If the child is in a supine position, be sure to remove the shoes, because some children will kick when frightened.

Inspection with Otoscope

1. Hold the otoscope gently with the handle between the thumb and forefinger. This will enable you to control the head of the otoscope while keeping your hand steady on the child's head.

1. Small children will jerk about, so be careful not to push the speculum into the eardrum.

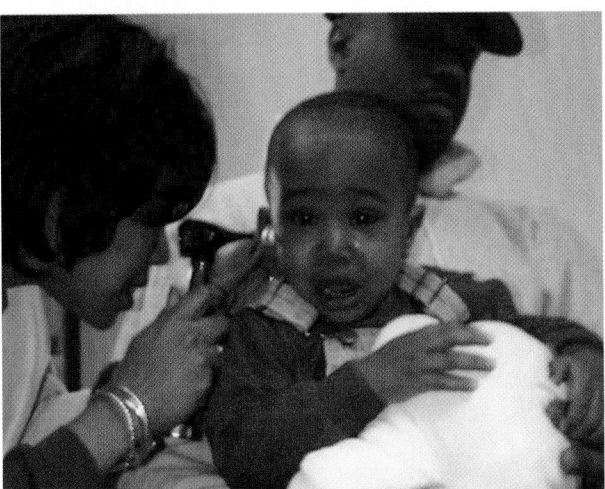

2. With your free hand, pull the pinna back and slightly upward to straighten the canal. Examine the canal.

2. Cerumen or wax may interfere with your view of the eardrum. You may need to remove the wax with an ear curette or hydrogen peroxide instillation.

Technique	Findings

3. Inspect the eardrum and test for mobility by means of the pneumatoscope (the tube attachment of the otoscope).

3. The normal eardrum moves slightly when air is introduced into the ear canal.

Palpation
Palpate behind the ear over the mastoid process.

Tenderness behind the ear denotes infection. Sometimes a lymph node can be felt in this area.

Special Testing
1. Most children will be able to respond to a test of gross hearing.

1. A small bell, such as the kind found in the Denver kit, can be used to determine hearing ability by noting if the child stops moving when the bell is rung and turns head toward the sound.

2. More specific tests using an electric screening device are used before school age.

Nose and Sinuses
Equipment
Nasoscope, small speculum

Inspection
1. Observe for general deformity.
2. With nasoscope, examine nasal septum, mucous membranes and turbinates, and for discharge and nasal obstruction (see Adult Physical Examination, p. 58).
3. Check for presence of any foreign body. Always remember that any child who has a "strange" odor may have a foreign body in the nose or ear. (In a female child, do not forget the vagina.)
4. Observe for nasal flaring.

2. Dry mucous membranes may bleed and cause clots of blood to form in the nares. Scratches may also occur if child picks at nose or scratches when itching occurs.
3. A foreign body in the nose will cause a foul odor, purulent discharge, and may possibly cause bleeding.

Palpation
Palpate the sinuses, remembering the order of development.

Sinuses develop in a set order; the ethmoid and maxillary sinuses are present at birth. It was believed that the frontal sinus develops at around 7 years of age, and the sphenoid after puberty. These times of development are probably earlier than originally believed.

Mouth and Throat
Equipment
Penlight, tongue depressor
1. Shining the light into the mouth or around the lips and teeth is not a threatening gesture.
2. However, the tongue blade, which is used to press against the inside of the cheek to allow for examination of the mucous membranes, and which is also used to push the tongue out of the way, is a threatening instrument.
3. When the tongue depressor is placed on the tongue, it can have the unpleasant effect of making the child gag.
4. To avoid this unpleasant occurrence, encourage the child to stick out his tongue, breath deeply, and say "ah." This may allow for easy visualization of the palate and uvula without need for the "stick."

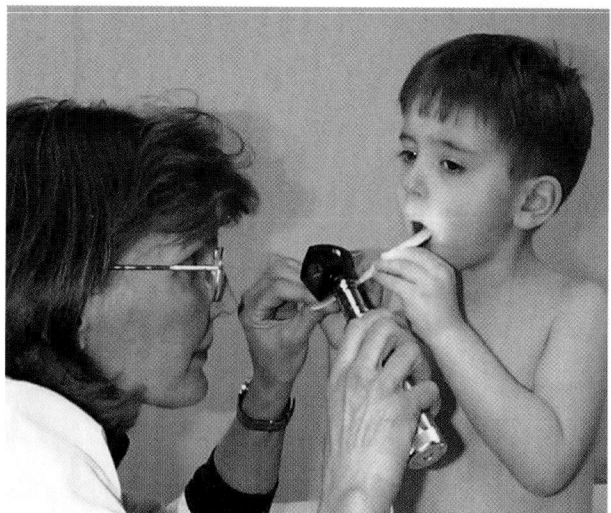

Technique	Findings

5. If these steps are not feasible, then the child may need to be restrained. If such is the case, examining the throat should be left to last, so as not to frighten the child.

A child may also be allowed to place the tongue blade directly on own tongue while you guide with your hand.

Inspection

1. Observe the lips, noting the color. (Remember that cyanosis is difficult to detect in a black child.)

1. *Infants:* There may be a protuberance on the upper lip, the so-called "sucking blister."
   Children: May have dry lips and redness around the lips caused by allergy.

2. Count the teeth (see p. 1252) and note any extra or missing teeth, and any evidence of caries, staining, tartar, and malocclusion.
3. Check the gums for swelling and signs of easy bleeding. Also note mouth odor.
4. Check the tongue for movement, color, and taste buds on the surface. Check to see that the frenulum under the tongue is of the proper length.

4. If the frenulum is too short, the child may be tongue-tied (meaning that the baby cannot advance the tip of the tongue beyond the lips), although this is not thought to interfere with sucking or speech.

5. As the gag reflex is elicited, note how the palate moves upward and the uvula springs into view.
6. Examine the roof of the mouth.

5. It should be midline and single, although occasionally it will be divided or bifurcated.
6. The roof of the mouth at the junction of the hard and soft palate will frequently reveal whitish lesions, or Epstein's pearls, which persist through infancy.

7. Inspect the height of the arch of the palate.

7. With experience, an unusually high arch is easily recognizable.

8. Note the tonsils on each side of the uvula and immediately posterior to it for position, surface, size, equality, and color.

8. Any coating with pus or ulcers or a pocket or cryptic appearance should be recorded.

9. As the baby cries, note the odor of the breath and any hoarseness of the voice; note difficulty on inspiration, as in croup, or wheezing on expiration.

9. These signs may indicate throat and chest disturbances.

Palpation

1. Palpate the lips and cheeks manually using a finger cot or glove.
2. Note any evidence of swelling.
3. Palpate for submucous cleft.

1. By comparing one side with the other, differences caused by abnormality can be detected.

3. Submucous cleft may indicate a genetic disposition toward cleft palate.

Technique   Findings

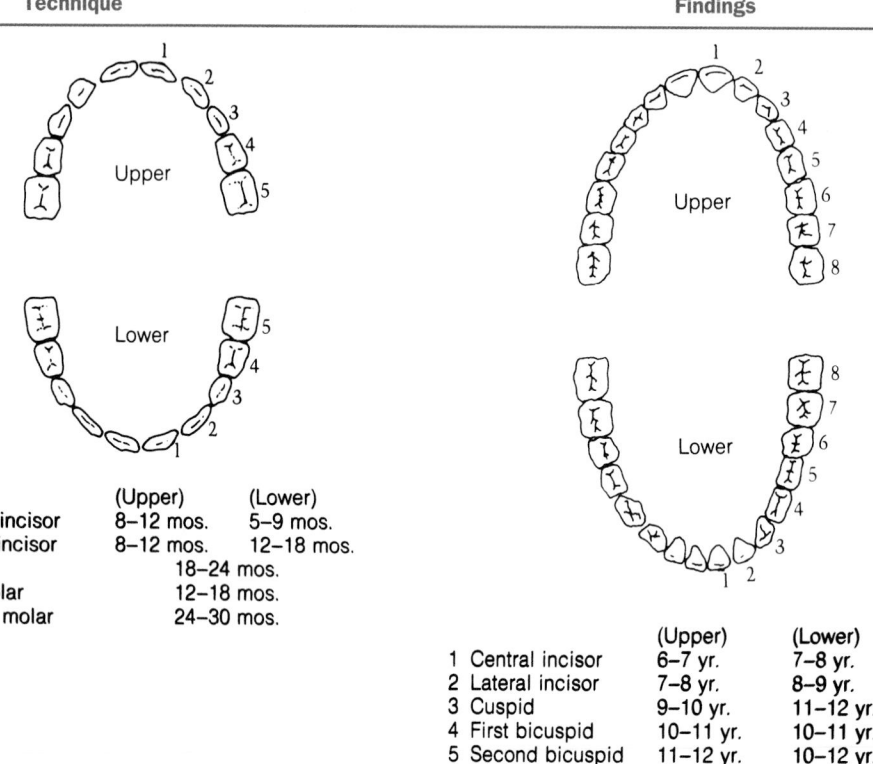

	(Upper)	(Lower)
1 Central incisor	8–12 mos.	5–9 mos.
2 Lateral incisor	8–12 mos.	12–18 mos.
3 Cuspid		18–24 mos.
4 First molar		12–18 mos.
5 Second molar		24–30 mos.

	(Upper)	(Lower)
1 Central incisor	6–7 yr.	7–8 yr.
2 Lateral incisor	7–8 yr.	8–9 yr.
3 Cuspid	9–10 yr.	11–12 yr.
4 First bicuspid	10–11 yr.	10–11 yr.
5 Second bicuspid	11–12 yr.	10–12 yr.
6 First molar	6–7 yr.	6–7 yr.
7 Second molar	11–13 yr.	12–13 yr.
8 Third molar	17 yr.	17–18 yr.

Breast

1. Sometimes young children object to having their clothes removed.
2. The following approaches may overcome this problem:
   a. Distract the child by having him or her listen to a few heartbeats.
   b. Have the parent (while the child is on his or her knee) remove the underclothing while you stand by.
   c. For an older child entering puberty, provide an examining sheet or gown.

Inspection

1. Check to see if there are any small extra nipples present.

2. In the newborn infant, the nipples appear a little darker than normal, and breast tissue underneath may form a small knot with occasional leakage of milk.
3. In the child, a lump found under the nipple in either male or female may cause some concern for cancer.

4. Occasionally, the breasts begin to develop earlier than normal, at approximately 5 or 6 years of age.

1. These would appear along a line extending from the anterior axillary line through the normal nipple down toward the symphysis pubis.
2. This leakage is a secondary effect of the hormone level in the mother; instruct the mother not to try to express the milk, because of the danger of infection.
3. Such lumps are usually secondary to hormone stimulation and occur toward puberty or during the newborn period.
4. This should be a reason for referral to a physician.

Technique	Findings

◼ Thorax

Inspection

1. Observe the entire thorax as the child breathes; note symmetry and equal expansion of both sides as the lungs inflate.

2. Confirm the respiratory rate as you observe the child with his or her shirt off.
3. Observe for substernal, suprasternal, and intercostal retractions.

1. In babies (especially an infant lying on the parent's knee) and young children diaphragm excursion is more marked than intercostal expansion. Thus, the abdomen goes up and down more than the chest expands.

Percussion

Percussion of the child's chest is difficult. Because the underlying structures are crowded, not too much is elicited. The heart edge is difficult to outline.

Light percussion is necessary; a hyperresonant note may be elicited over air, particularly of a stomach bubble that projects up into the left side of the chest.

Palpation

1. Use warmed hands as you palpate the shape and angle of the sternum. Note if there is depression of the sternum.

2. Palpate the costochondral junctions for tenderness and enlargement.
3. As you palpate, vibration may be felt through your hands as the child cries.

4. Vocal fremitus is difficult to elicit in the smaller child since it is difficult to have him or her make repetitive sounds on command.

1. The shape of the sternum may vary, although there may be a depression of the sternum (funnel sternum) that may cause subsequent trouble because of pressure on underlying structures. This should be referred to the pediatrician.
2. May suggest an underlying inflammatory response.

3. Normal inspiration and expiration do not give a sensation under the fingers, except for the expansion of the chest.
4. In the older child, it is worth trying to obtain transmission of sound through the lung tissue (see p. 66).

Auscultation

1. Try to examine a baby before he or she begins crying.
2. Warm the stethoscope before using by rubbing it between your hands.
3. Be aware that breathing is louder in younger children with slightly increased length of inspiration, almost to the point of bronchovesicular breathing in the adult.
4. Crackles (discontinuous; interrupted, explosive sounds) may be heard more easily in children.

5. Wheezes.

1. Note, however, that crying increases lung expansion.
2. A cold stethoscope will startle the child.

3. Bronchial breathing with equal inspiration and expiration is very loud and easy to hear if the patient has pneumonia.
4. Added coarse-quality sounds in the chest are commonly associated with mucus in the trachea or even in the back of the nose.
5. Recurrent airway disease is an important finding in children.

◼ Heart

Inspection

In thin children, the apical beat or the point of maximal impulse (PMI) can easily be seen, particularly if you look obliquely across the chest wall.

As in all areas of the pediatric examination, measurement and documentation of the distance from the midline and the exact rib space are worth noting.

Palpation

The apical beat may be felt in the 6th intercostal space about 5 cm (2 inches) from the midline in the school-aged child. It is more difficult to feel in the baby, particularly a

The apical beat will be deviated to the left with cardiac enlargement or a collapsed lung on that side. The apical pulse could be pushed toward the right by a tumor or a collapsed

Technique	Findings

plump child, and would not be so far out toward the anterior axillary line.

Auscultation

1. Identify the first heart sound (S_1) (occurs during systole).
   a. Locate the apical beat (closing of the mitral valve) by placing the stethoscope over the maximum impulse area, concentrating on the first heart sound. (As the ventricle on the left contracts, pushing the blood up into the aorta, the sound of the mitral valve closing is heard.)
   b. That sound can be identified by placing the thumb on the carotid pulse of the neck, which will coincide very closely with the heart sounds.

2. Identify the second heart sound (S_2).
   a. Move the stethoscope up toward the sternum and to the left.
   b. At the base of the heart, both over the aortic and pulmonic areas, S_2 is louder than S_1.

3. Move the stethoscope in small jumps from the apical area medially toward the sternum. Go up to the left side of the sternum, listening at each interspace next to the sternum.
4. Move next to the patient's right second intercostal space—again next to the sternum.
5. Listen to only one sound; concentrate on that to the exclusion of all others. Can you identify this sound? Is it clear? Compare it with your own heart sound or that of the parent.
6. If there is question of a heart murmur or added sounds, refer to the physician.
7. As you listen to the heart sounds, you are also listening to the rhythm to confirm your findings on pulse.
   a. If child breathes in and out deeply, the sinus arrhythmia will be obvious.
   b. If a child holds his breath, the sinus arrhythmia will disappear.
8. Be sure to count a rapid heart that is heard even when the child is quiet.
9. In the infant, heart sounds are just a series of taps; they occur so fast that it is impossible to make out which sound is S_1.

lung on the right. Pneumothorax under tension will push the heart away from the side of the increased pressure.

1. Consists of the "lub" portion of the "lub-dub" heart sound.

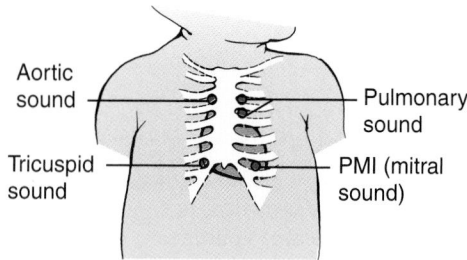

2. Represents the "dub" portion of the "lub-dub" heart sound.

   b. In a child, S_2 can be heard as two heart sounds because the two valves in the aorta and pulmonary vessels do not close at quite the same time. This split will increase with inspiration and decrease with expiration.
3. This represents the area of maximum intensity of sound of the pulmonary vessels.

4. It is at this area that you will hear the aortic sound best.

5. The child will enjoy this comparison if allowed to listen.

7. The typical rhythm of a child is called *sinus arrhythmia*. As the heart speeds up, the child is breathing in; the heart slows down on expiration.

8. This may be indicative of a tachycardia that requires further investigation.
9. In the infant, the S_1 and S_2 are equal in intensity.

■ Abdomen

1. For examination of the abdomen, the child should be lying down, relaxed, and not crying. Placing a small child, particularly around the age of 1–3 years, on a high table on cold paper can be very frightening; as a result, the abdomen will not be relaxed.

Technique	Findings

2. Babies up to 1 year of age do not seem to be perturbed and will often lie down and play very nicely as long as they can see the parent, who should be stationed at the head of the child while you examine the abdomen.
3. Having the child lie across the parent's knees with the legs dangling on one side and the head cradled in his or her arms, will enable you to feel the abdomen quite well.
   a. You may find that with the baby's head in the parent's left arm, you can use your left hand to examine the baby's abdomen on the right, feeling up under the right costal margin and into the right hypochondrium.
   b. You may need to turn the baby around and use your right hand to examine the left side of the child's abdomen.

Inspection

1. Observe the abdomen for contour and any markings both while the child is standing and when lying down. As you inspect, you may see some abdominal movement with respiration. (Remember that the diaphragm, as it goes up and down, will move the contents of the abdomen.)
2. Check for early signs of puberty as evidenced by pubic hair over the symphysis pubis.

3. Carefully inspect the umbilicus for cleanliness and the presence of any scar tissue.

1. Sometimes superficial veins are seen on the abdomen, particularly in a very blond infant. Striae are often noticed on the flank following rapid loss or gain of weight.

2. Early pubic hair in younger children (8–10 years) may appear long and silky. This will ultimately become curly toward the onset of puberty.
3. A deep umbilicus may be difficult to keep clean. Immediately after the cord has dropped off, a granuloma may occur.

Auscultation

1. Because percussion and palpation will stimulate the small bowel and increase bowel sounds, auscultation should precede these two techniques.
2. To obtain the child's cooperation, you can conduct a running commentary as you listen, saying such things as, "I can hear the Cheerios in there."

1. Bowel sounds are heard as tinkling, irregular sounds that indicate that fluid is moving from one section of the bowel to the next.
2. In a quiet baby who has just eaten, not many bowel sounds will be heard. In a hungry child, noisy bowel sounds can be heard, even without a stethoscope.

Percussion

1. On the right side, percuss for the liver. Confirm on palpation.
2. Percuss over the left upper quadrant.

3. Percuss the lower abdomen, particularly above the symphysis pubis.

1. Liver dullness can frequently be outlined to determine size of the liver.
2. Percussion over a gas-filled bowel or stomach gives a high-pitched, hollow sound.
3. Above the symphysis pubis, a filled bladder can produce a duller sound, as does a pregnant uterus. (A mass in the abdomen of a girl over 10 years of age may be a fetus.)

Palpation

1. Divide the abdomen into imaginary quadrants, palpating each with the fingertips.
2. In the right upper quadrant, palpate for the liver edge.
   a. Although the liver is easily palpable in most children, you may have to press quite firmly.

a. The liver is frequently felt about 1 cm (3/8 inch) below the right costal margin and in some instances as low as 2 cm (3/4 inch). This is a common finding in the newborn and through the early school-age years.

Technique	Findings
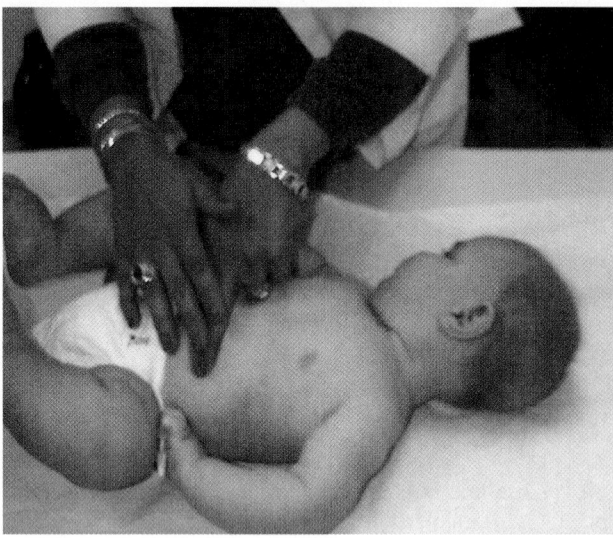	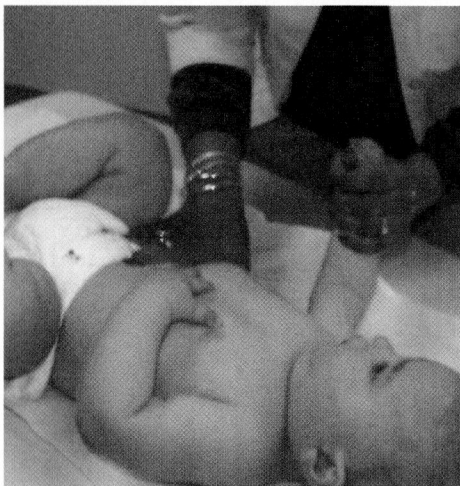

3. In the left upper quadrant, palpate for the spleen. Less resistance is encountered as you feel up under the left costal margin.

4. In the upper quadrants also try to palpate for the kidneys. Deep palpation for both kidneys should routinely be a part of the examination to make sure there is no enlargement of the kidney. Normally, the kidney is not palpable.

5. In the iliac fossa or the left lower quadrant, palpate for the descending bowel.

6. Palpate on the right lower quadrant (RLQ) where the appendix is located.

7. If the child has pain in any area or has pointed to the umbilicus when asked to show where the pain is, avoid the area demonstrated and leave it until last. Note whether the pain is with pressure or rebound.

8. Palpate around the umbilicus for any masses that may indicate a hernia, especially in black children. As you press over the protruding hernia you can feel the sensation of gurgling under your fingers as the bowel returns to the abdomen.

3. Only the tip of the spleen can be felt in the upper outer left quadrant, in the early months of life and in very thin children of preschool age.

4. Kidney palpation is difficult, but during the newborn period, the lower pole of the right kidney can frequently be felt and sometimes the left as well. (This applies to the period immediately after delivery, when the infant's abdomen is relaxed and the bowel is not distended.)

5. The descending colon can be felt, particularly if filled with firm stool. It may be slightly tender, but it should not cause severe pain on gentle palpation.

6. In the RLQ, usually the only sensation is that of gas-filled bowel. Tenderness in this area could be related to an inflamed appendix.

7. If the painful area is palpated first, the child may tense up when the other areas of the abdomen are examined.

8. Most of these hernias heal naturally by the age of 6 years. A hernia above the umbilicus can be revealed by asking the child to lift his head from the table. (Widening of the muscles above the umbilicus is called *diastasis recti*.)

Rectum and Anus

1. Rectal examinations are rarely necessary in infants and young children.

2. If the child will be examined by a health care provider, it is not necessary to duplicate this part of the examination.

3. Rectal examinations are embarrassing and uncomfortable for most children. Explain the procedure before performing the examination.

Technique	Findings

4. Positioning for a rectal examination:
   a. Infants can be placed on their abdomens, sides, or backs with the legs raised to the chest.
   b. Young children and teenagers can be positioned on their sides.

Inspection

1. When examining a baby or toddler, place the child on a flat surface so that the weight is evenly distributed on the front of the pelvis. As the baby moves about on the abdomen, observe the entire back, the lower back, the upper thigh, and the tightening of the buttocks.
2. Notice particularly the lower part of the back for hairiness or a mass.
3. As the child moves away, part the buttocks and look at the cleft between them.

4. Pay careful attention to the outer appearance of the anus and the perineum, the underside of the scrotum in the male, and the labia majora in the female.

Palpation

1. Consider the child's age and feelings; ask the mother to assist if need be. This part of the examination is not always necessary.
2. Start by parting the buttocks with the left hand and introducing a well-lubricated finger (with finger cot) into the anus.
3. Gently apply pressure on the anal sphincter to allow the muscles to relax and the fingertip to slide into the rectum.
4. Gently palpate the inner ring, feeling for areas of thickening and tenderness and simultaneously judging the sphincter tone.
5. If the rectum is full of feces, it will be impossible to feel any other mass.

6. Palpate the walls of the rectum.

7. In the male, gently turn your finger through 180° and feel the posterior surface of the prostate. Note size, consistency, tenderness, and contour.
8. In the female, perform a bimanual examination and palpate the cervix.

■ Examining Male Genitalia

1. This part of the examination requires a direct, matter-of-fact approach. Acknowledge that it is normal to feel embarrassed during an examination of the genitals. Explain what you are looking for as you proceed through the examination with a teenager.
2. Reassure the child after the examination that his genitals are normal. This decreases anxiety.

(Findings column)

1. If one buttock is larger than the other, you will see that side projected above the other. Weakness of one side will be obvious as the baby moves around, although a child in the early stages of crawling will tend to use one knee as a predominant leader, dragging the other behind.
2. This may indicate an underlying abnormality of the vertebrae in spina bifida.
3. A pilonidal dimple or sinus may be seen over the lower back. This is a common finding, but parents should be told about it for cleaning purposes. Be sure there is no drainage.
4. The anus is inspected for blood, fissures, or splitting in the external tissue, redness, swelling, or pads of extra flesh. On occasion, small white pinworms may be seen adhering to the anal skin.

2. When an infant is being examined, the small finger should be used.

3. Apply pressure with pulp of the finger rather than jab at the anus with the fingertip.
4. As the perianal area is pressed on from the inside, tenderness will be elicited if a deep fissure exists or if an infection has occurred around a fissure.
5. In the young child, particularly the infant, dilatation provided by the finger may result in a bowel movement. In the older child, a suppository or even an enema may be required.
6. Within the rectum, the mucosal walls should be smooth, and deep palpation should elicit mild tenderness and no acute pain.

Technique	Findings

3. When examining the testes in a young child, you may need to block the canals to prevent them from retracting into the abdomen.

Scrotum and Testes
Inspection

1. Before touching the child, determine by observation of the testes whether they are in the scrotum.

2. Observe the skin over the scrotum for color and surface appearance, noting the presence of wrinkles, or rugae.

1. Retraction of the testes into the abdomen occurs very frequently in young children; the development of the scrotum depends on the presence of the testes.
2. The skin over the scrotum varies in color, being a darker brown to black in the more pigmented races and reddish in the fair-skinned. The wrinkles, or rugae, are more developed as the child grows older.

Palpation

1. Check the scrotum wall for swelling or sensitivity. Gently feel the testes, palpating across the upper pole and feeling for the epididymis. (Remember the scrotum is extremely sensitive to pressure.)
2. Estimate the size of the testes and identify the spermatic cord, tracing it from the testis up toward the groin.

3. Make a special effort to locate the testis in a young child whose testes may be retracted into the abdomen via a hyperactive cremasteric reflex. You may have to have the child in a sitting or standing position. Occasionally you may have to ask a parent to check at home with the child sitting in a warm bathtub.
   a. If the testes cannot be felt in the scrotum, gently run the skin of the upper scrotum between your fingers, moving superiorly and approaching the external inguinal ring.
   b. Try to milk the testis down toward the scrotum from above with your hand.
   c. If this fails, have the child sit cross-legged to abolish the reflex of the cremaster muscle.
4. When examining a boy in the early stages of puberty, it is important to note the size of the testis as well as the greater number of rugae on the scrotum and the appearance of pubic hair around the penis.

1. The epididymis is a ridge of soft, bumpy tissue extending from the superior pole and running down and behind the testis.
2. The spermatic cord, with the vas deferens, feels firm and is accompanied by softer nerves, arteries, veins, and a few muscle fibers.
3. The presence of the testes in the scrotum is vital in the preschool or early school-age child. Nondescent of the testes requires that the child be referred to a health care provider.

During this period the testis is about 1.5–2 cm ($\frac{1}{2}$–$\frac{3}{4}$ inch) in length.
In the quiescent period before puberty, the male genitalia remain fairly infantile.

4. In early puberty, the testes start to grow. Onset of puberty varies, occurring in some boys by age 10 and in others as late as age 14. In most teenagers, the findings are similar to those in adults.

Penis

1. Evaluate the penis on all sides by lifting up the shaft.

2. If the child is not circumcised, partially retract the foreskin to observe the glans and meatus.

3. Observe the position of the meatus and evert the lips of the meatus to reveal an adequate orifice.

4. In the older child, inspect the penis for ulcers, sores, or discharge from the meatus.

1. The shaft of the penis contains the urethra on the under, or ventral surface and is easily palpable.
2. The foreskin may adhere to the glans for the first few years of life. It is not necessary for the parent to "stretch" the foreskin by retraction.
   Whitish discharge around the glans under the foreskin is normal and not a sign of infection. The foreskin should completely encircle the glans.
3. The meatus may be positioned off center. Refer the child to a health care provider if the meatus is located on the dorsal or ventral surface of the shaft.
4. Consider sexually transmitted diseases in the older child and teenager.

Technique	**Findings**

Inguinal Area

1. Palpate for hernia over the external inguinal ring. Have the child cough to enhance your observation.

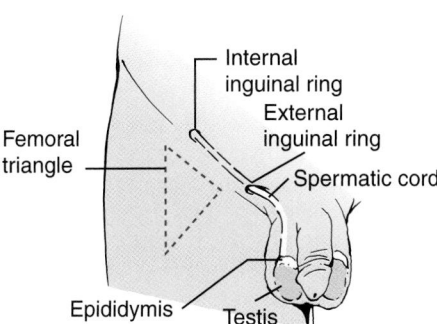

2. An increased cough reflex or swelling in the area should be checked by carefully placing the finger on the scrotal skin and invaginating the skin over your fingers toward the external ring. You are trying to follow the course of a hernia that would descend into the scrotum while you feel the external ring from below. A hernia in the inguinal region presents as a bulge that can be either seen or felt from below by placing the finger in the scrotum pointing up toward the external inguinal ring.
3. Also palpate for the inguinal lymph nodes.

1. Having the child stand either with the parent holding him or placing him against his or her knee will help you in locating a hernia in the inguinal area.

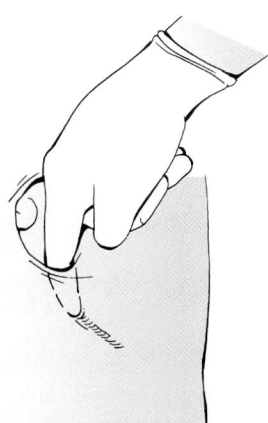

3. The inguinal lymph nodes in an infant are palpable as small and "shotty." Anything more than this should alert you to possible infection, since the perianal area drains into the superficial inguinal lymph nodes. Thus, any signs of diaper rash will explain enlargement of the lymph nodes, which should be noted and reported.

Femoral Area

Palpate the femoral triangle carefully for a hernia and for lymph nodes.

In the femoral area, a swelling that can be reduced with a gurgling sound is an unusual finding.

Auscultation

If you are trying to reduce a mass, listen over the scrotum to see if there is a gurgling sound.

This will locate the bowel for you and confirm a hernia.

Transillumination

1. To locate the testis, darken the room and shine a bright light from behind the scrotum. In a normal child, the testis will stand out as the darker area.
2. Transilluminate any suspicious mass to help locate a hernia.

1. Testes that are swollen by fluid (hydrocele) will transilluminate. Fluid around the testes or cord must be differentiated from a hernia.
2. Any mass in this area must be reported to a health care provider immediately.

■ Examining Female Genitalia

1. If the child will be examined by a health care provider, it is not necessary to duplicate this part of the examination.
2. Place the infant or toddler on the table or on the parent's knee while she holds the knees in an abducted and flexed position.

Technique	Findings

3. A preschool child can be allowed to lean over her parent's knee. However, remember that the structures are being visualized upside down.
4. The older child or teenager should be draped as an adult would and should be placed in a lithotomy position with the aid of stirrups.

Equipment

Disposable gloves, speculum, light source

1. Carefully inspect the perineal area for cleanliness, inflammation, and abnormality.
2. Fold back the labia majora and note the labia minora.

3. Part the labia and note the clitoris and the meatus at the anterior end. (The clitoris is a hook-like structure that extends over the opening of the urethral meatus.) The meatus appears as a slit that is slightly darker in color against the pink of the mucosa about 2 cm (¾ inch) posterior to the clitoris.
4. Having parted the labia, check for any signs of inflammation, discharge, tenderness, or infection. Include the urethral meatus, periurethral glands, the vagina, and the greater vestibular glands (Bartholin's). (Tenderness of these glands is unusual in young children, but may occur in adolescents.)

1. This includes the mons pubis, clitoris, labia, urethra, and perineum.
2. The labia minora are seen as two slender folds of tissue inside the labia majora.
3. In some instances, adhesions of the labia minora occur because of the lack of natural hormones. The opening of the vagina is obscured by the two lateral flaps, which stick together, sometimes to the degree that urination is difficult because the urethral meatus is covered. This should be referred to a health care provider.
4. Inflammation and puslike discharge from the urethra may be noted on palpation. The periurethral glands may be tender because of infection—possibly due to gonococci. If discharge is collected from the vagina, it should be cultured.

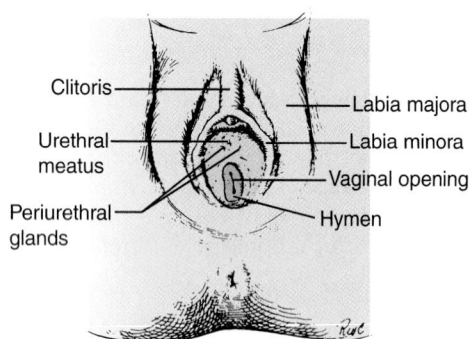

5. If the mother of a newborn infant has noted a bloody discharge from the infant's vagina during the first few days of life, reassure her that this is not an uncommon occurrence; the discharge will disappear, as will any swelling of the labia majora and clitoris and any enlargement of the infant's breasts.
6. Note the vaginal opening, which may vary in size because of the presence of a thin membrane, the hymen. The hymen varies in appearance according to the age of the child.

7. In the young child, it is usually unnecessary to examine inside the vagina. Should you suspect a foreign

5. Hormone stimulation from the mother's body accounts for this occurrence. The discharge usually stops once the hormones are excreted. The bloody appearance on the diaper may be confused with the presence of urates, which are also orange-red and which appear quite normally in the urine.
6. The lack of an opening into the vagina may result in the retention of menstrual fluid when the child reaches puberty. In the sexually active adolescent, vestigial remains on the hymen may appear as small particles (caruncles) at the fringe of the vagina.
   If there is possibility of sexual abuse, this examination should be referred to specialist in sexual abuse.
7. A foreign body may be suspected if there is vaginal discharge (of any quantity) that is blood-tinged or has an

Technique	Findings

body, insert a finger into the rectum and milk anteriorly to allow you to feel the lower part of the cervix and any firm foreign body within the vagina.

8. In an older child, the little finger can be inserted gently into the vagina and anterior pressure applied.

9. Turn the finger gradually, sweeping down the right side of the vagina, back over the rectum, and up on the left side of the vagina. Turn your finger, arm, and wrist so that undue pressure is not made on the child's tissues.

10. Once the genitalia are examined, lower the child's legs somewhat so that the femoral and inguinal areas can be palpated the same way as in the male.

odor. In the older child, vaginal discharge of this type may be due to gonorrhea.

8. Anterior pressure and milking downward palpates the urethra toward the meatus. The periurethral glands are located on each side of the urethra.

10. Enlargement of the lymph nodes in a hernia in the femoral triangle may be found. Similarly, enlargement of the inguinal nodes may occur.

▣ Musculoskeletal System

1. Evaluation of the musculoskeletal system can be done both in an informal manner while watching the child at rest, and at play, and in a formal manner as specific findings are methodically checked.

2. In the newborn, observe the position of the extremities during sleep and the quality of movement when the infant is awake.

3. Various aspects of size, shape, and movement are evaluated as the baby is observed pushing up on arms and turning head toward mother.

4. The infant in the early stages of walking offers many opportunities for evaluation of muscle strength and movement.

5. At the same time, rapport with the mother can be reinforced by your admiring the baby's ability and by inquiring if she is concerned about the manner in which the baby is walking.

6. A more mobile child can be evaluated as you watch him play and explore the room.

7. Having the older child reach for crayons, run after a ball, or walk around the room enables you to evaluate the musculoskeletal system and the child's sense of balance.

Upper Extremities

1. In the infant, evaluate the status of the clavicles when examining the skull and neck.

2. Carefully examine the hands to note shape of the hand, shape and length of the fingers, changes in the nails, and creases on the palms.

1. During a difficult delivery, the clavicle that has been exposed to traction may snap. A lump can be felt on the bone at about 3 weeks of age.

2. Variation in the hands or unusual length of the fingers should be noted. An incurved little finger or low-set thumb with the single simian crease may reflect Down's syndrome.

Lower Extremities

1. Examine the appearance of the infant's foot, noting arch formation.

2. Inspect the angle of the foot and lower leg and then manipulate the ankle to evaluate the range of motion.

1. The foot of an infant is usually flat and appears broad because the arch on the inside of the foot is covered by a fat pad. Parents may need reassurance in this regard.

2. Full flexibility of the foot (plantar flexion) rules out underlying abnormality. The foot should return to the neutral position after manipulation. Frequently, the foot will turn in, or adduct. Such a finding should be recorded.

Technique	Findings

3. Place the legs together and see how far the ankles and knees are separated.

3. The toddler has normally bowed legs, but with ankles touching, knees should be no more than 2 finger breaths apart.
The preschooler has a normally knock-kneed walk, but with knees touching, ankles should be no more than 2 finger breaths apart.

4. Evaluate the baby's ability to walk, noting the appearance of the legs and foot placement. Remember to look at the child's shoes and see which side of the sole is worn down.

4. When babies first start to walk, their legs appear bow-legged. The feet are kept wide apart and turn slightly in so that the ankles seem curved when viewed from behind.

Hip

1. When examining children under 1 year of age, check to see if there are signs of hip dislocation.

1. Any difficulties with hip examination call for immediate medical consultation because of possible congenital dislocation of the hip.
In the normal infant, the lateral aspect of each knee will touch the examining table without difficulty.

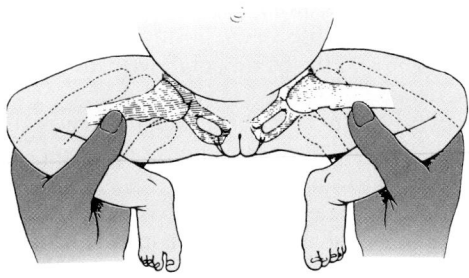

Spine

1. Check the spine for any signs of abnormal curvature.

1. The normal child has a curve inward at the lumbar region (lordosis), but this should not be exaggerated. It is normally more exaggerated in black children.
Kyphosis: Forward curvature of the shoulders.
Scoliosis: Side-to-side curvature of the spine.

2. Observe the child from the side and back in the standing position to see forward curving of the shoulders.
3. Have the child bend forward with the arms hanging down. A unilateral rib prominence will be seen in children with scoliosis.

2. These appear most often during school years and adolescence.

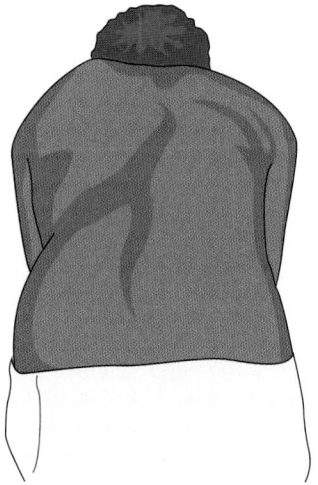

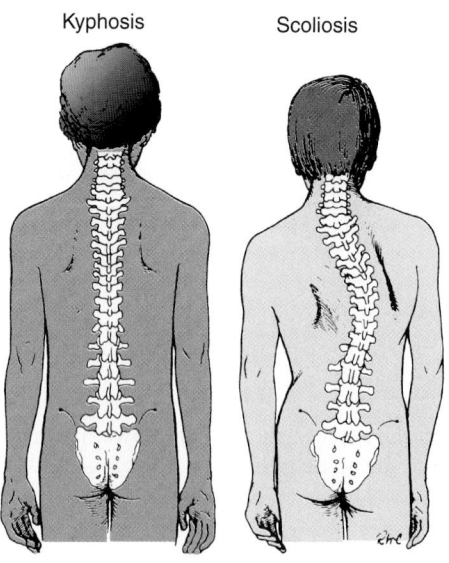

Kyphosis   Scoliosis

Technique	Findings

◼ Neurologic Examination

1. The neurologic system at birth is different from that of the baby of a few months. There is an even greater contrast between the baby and children and adults.
2. The central nervous system at birth is underdeveloped and the functions tested are below the level of the cortex.

Equipment

Flashlight, noisemaker, ophthalmoscope, tongue depressor, tuning fork

Procedure for the Newborn and Young Infant

(See pp. 1166–1167.)

1. Observe the newborn for general appearance, positioning, activity, crying, and alertness. Take note of the posture—including head, neck, and extremities.
2. Note the pitch, volume, and character of the cry.

3. Observe the infant's facial expression and the symmetry of the face when crying or sucking.

4. Most of the cranial nerves are difficult to check at this early age.

Automatic Reflexes

1. *Blinking reflex due to loud noise.*
   Clap your hands or produce a loud clicking noise, being careful not to clap near the baby so that a wave of air causes blinking of eyes anyway.
2. *Blinking reflex due to bright light*
   Shine a bright light into the infant's eyes to elicit blinking reflex.
3. *Cranial nerve 10* can be checked by using a tongue depressor to gag the infant.
4. *Palmar grasp reflex*
   Place your fingers across the baby's palm from the ulnar side. The baby needs to be in a relaxed position with his head in a central position. Reinforcement may be offered by having the baby suck on the bottle at the same time.
5. *Rooting reflex*
   Touch the edge of the baby's mouth.

6. *Incurving of the trunk*
   Hold the baby horizontally and prone in one arm while using the other hand to stimulate one side of the infant's back from the shoulders to the buttocks.
   The trunk curves toward the stimulated side as the shoulders and pelvis move toward the stroking hand (persists until infant is about 2 months old).

Findings

1. Stiffness of the neck or marked attraction of the head will cause a position of opisthotonos and necessitates referral.
2. The high-pitched cry of the infant who has intracranial irritation is very distinctive.
3. Poor sucking, with dribbling, is abnormal. Transient weakness of the mouth caused by 7th cranial nerve paralysis is frequently seen as a result of a forceps delivery in which the forceps is pressed on the facial nerve where it emerges from the ear.

1. Lack of a blink in response to a loud noise may indicate deafness.

2. Failure to blink may indicate blindness.

3. Palate moves.

4. Both hands will flex and can be compared for strength. Weakness on one side may be indicated by a failure to grasp when the palm is stimulated.

5. The baby's mouth will open, and the head will turn toward the side stimulated. This reflex is marked during the early weeks of life.

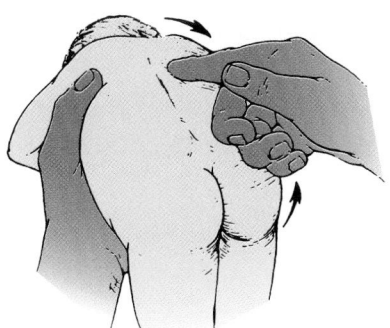

Technique	Findings

7. *Vertical suspension position*
Place your hands under the baby's axillae with thumbs supporting the back of the head and hold the baby upright.

7. The legs flex at the hips and knees (persists for about 4 months).

8. *Stepping response*
Hold the baby under its axillae with thumbs supporting the back of the head. Allow baby's foot to touch firm surface.

8. Normally the baby responds by lifting one knee and hip into a flexed position and moving the opposite leg forward—making a series of stepping movements (*A*).
   a. Difficulty with the stepping reflex and stiffness or spasticity connected with crossing of the feet and scissoring (*B*) is indicative of spastic paraplegia or diplegia.
   b. It should be noted that the stepping response may be affected by breech delivery. (It may also be affected by weakness.)
   c. The stepping response is evident toward the end of the first week and persists for a variable time.

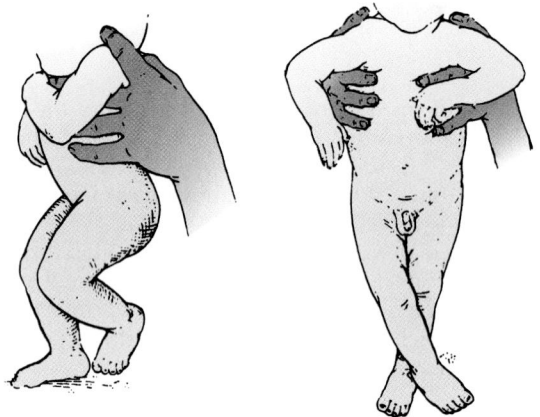

9. *Tonic neck reflex*
Hold the baby in a supine position with the head turned to one side and the jaw held in place over the shoulder.

9. a. The arm and leg on the side to which the head is turned will extend, whereas those on the other side will flex (the so-called "bow and arrow position").
   b. This reflex persists for about 6 months; it may be present at birth or delayed until the baby is 6 or 8 weeks old.
   c. Persistence beyond 6 months suggests major cerebral damage.

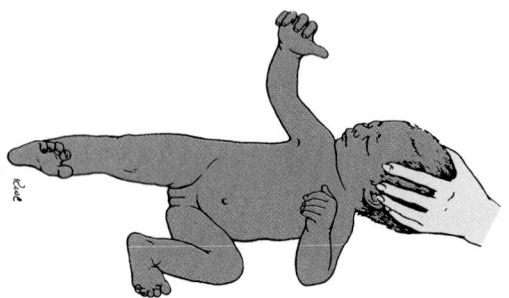

10. *Mass reflexes* (Moro or startle reflex)
Hold the baby along your arm with the other hand below the lower legs. Lower the feet and body in a sudden motion.

10. The arms will spring up and out, abducting and extending; the fingers are also extended. The arms then return forward over the body with a clasping motion. At the same time, the legs flex slightly and the hips abduct.
   a. The Moro reflex is present at birth and disappears at approximately the end of the third month. Persistence beyond 6 months is significant.
   b. Asymmetric response may be caused by paralysis of the arm after difficult delivery, tension and injury to the brachial plexus, or a fracture of the clavicle or humerus. A dislocated hip would produce an asymmetrical response in the lower extremities.

Technique	Findings

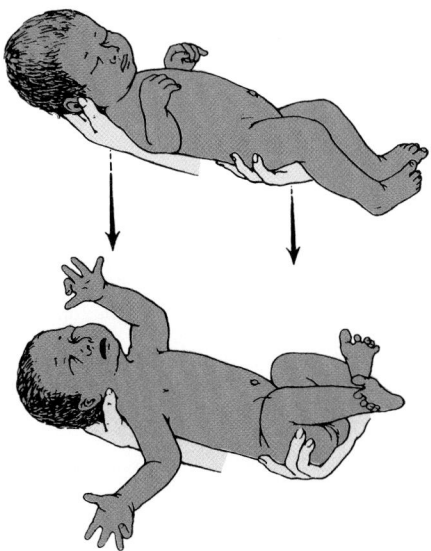

11. *Perez reflex*

Hold the baby in a prone position along your arm; place the thumb of the other hand on the sacrum and move it firmly toward the head, along the entire length of the spine.

11. The head and spine will extend and the knees will flex upward.

Summary

1. Some of the jerking and shaking movements seen in infants are normal, but they should be rechecked frequently during the first few weeks of life.
2. Variants in the findings caused by the baby's sleepiness or hunger should be taken into account and reevaluations should be carried out under different conditions.
3. Severe neurologic damage may be completely asymptomatic and impossible to detect during the first few weeks of life.

Neurologic Examination of the Toddler and Early School-Aged Child

1. The neurologic examination for the toddler and the early school-aged child is similar to that for the adult.
2. The Draw-A-Person Test and the Denver Developmental Assessment are both excellent methods for testing areas in the development of the child (see pp. 1222, 1234).
3. Beyond the newborn period, specific gross and fine motor coordination testing, accompanied by appropriate evaluation of the Denver test, will assist in assessing the child's level of development.
4. These tests also assess social and language development and are important screening devices.
5. Interview techniques can also be useful in assessing development in the preschool child (see p. 1236).

SELECTED REFERENCES

Barness, L. A. (1998). *Handbook of pediatric physical diagnosis.* Philadelphia: Lippincott-Raven.

Bickley, L. S., & Hoekelman, R. A. (1999). *Bates's guide to physical examination and history taking* (7th ed.). Philadelphia: Lippincott Williams & Wilkins.

Bickley, L. S., & Hoekelman, R. A. (2000). *Bates's pocket guide to physical examination and history taking* (3rd ed.). Philadelphia: Lippincott Williams & Wilkins.

Behrman, R. E., & Kliegman, R. (Eds.) (1998). *Nelson's essentials of pediatrics.* Philadelphia: W.B. Saunders.

Engel, J. (1997). *Pocket guide to pediatric assessment* (3rd ed.). St. Louis: Mosby.

Fletcher, M. A. (1998). *Physical diagnosis in neonatology.* Philadelphia: Lippincott-Raven.

Fuller, J., & Schaller-Ayers, J. (2000). *Health assessment: A nursing approach.* Philadelphia: Lippincott Williams & Wilkins.

Gartner, J. C., & Zitelli, B. J. (1997). *Common and chronic symptoms in pediatrics: A companion to the atlas of pediatric physical diagnosis.* St. Louis: Mosby.

Giardino, A. P., Christian, C. W., & Giardino, E. R. (1997). *A practical guide to the evaluation of child physical abuse and neglect.* Thousand Oaks: SAGE Publications.

Green, M. (1998). *Pediatric diagnosis* (5th ed.). Philadelphia: W. B. Saunders.

Heger, A. (1999). *Evaluation of the sexually abused child: A medical textbook and photographic atlas.* New York: Oxford University Press.

McMillan, J. A. (Ed.) (1999). *Oski's pediatrics: Principles and practice of pediatrics.* Philadelphia: Lippincott Williams & Wilkins.

Najarian, S. P. (1999). Infant cranial molding deformation and sleep position: Implications for primary care. *Journal of Pediatric Health Care, 13,* 178.

Pillitteri, A. (1999). *Maternal and child health nursing* (3rd ed.). Philadelphia: Lippincott Williams & Wilkins.

Siberry, G. K. & Iannone, R. (Eds.) (2000). *The Harriet Lane handbook* (15th ed.). St. Louis: Mosby.

Tappero, E. P. (1996). *Physical assessment of the newborn: A comprehensive approach to the art of physical examination.* Petaluma, CA: NICU Ink Book Publishers.

Zitelli, B. J., & Davis, H. W. (1997). *Atlas of pediatric physical diagnosis.* St. Louis: Mosby-Wolfe.

Pediatric Primary Care

HEALTH MAINTENANCE

Pediatric primary care includes health promotion and disease prevention interventions that will positively affect the well-being of children and their families. The goal of pediatric primary care is to achieve physical, emotional, and developmental health for all children. Primary prevention through immunizations, proper nutrition, and safety counseling are essential components of pediatric health care.

Immunizations

Disease prevention through immunizations has significantly reduced childhood morbidity and mortality from infectious diseases. However, despite effective immunizations, vaccine-preventable diseases are still present in the United States and continue to pose significant public health problems. Nurses are in a vital position to promote child health by assessing, recommending, and administering immunizations. A review of immunizations and administration of vaccines needed should be done at every health care visit.

General Considerations
Requirements of National Childhood Vaccine
Injury Act (Effective 1988)

1. Childhood-mandated vaccines include diphtheria, tetanus toxoid, pertussis (DTP); oral polio virus vaccine (OPV) or inactivated polio virus vaccine (IPV); measles, mumps, rubella (MMR); and *Haemophilus influenzae* type b (Hib) vaccines and any combination.
   a. Hepatitis B vaccine (HBV) and *Varicella* (Var) are recommended.
   b. Pneumococcal and influenza vaccines are available but not part of the regular schedule for all children at this time.
2. Patient, parent, or legal guardian should be informed about the benefits and risks of immunizations. They must be provided with the Vaccine Information Statement (VIS), developed by the Centers for Disease Control and Prevention (CDC), before the administration of the vaccine. Health care providers must record the name of the vaccine VIS publication (eg, polio), date of VIS publication, and the date the VIS was given to the patient/family on the child's medical record.
3. Federal law mandates that all health care providers must record the following information in the patient's permanent medical record: month, day, and year of administration; vaccine or other biologic administered; manufacturer; lot number and its expiration date; site and route of administration; name, address, and title of the health care provider administering the vaccine.
4. Health care providers are required to report selected events occurring after vaccination to the Vaccine Adverse Events Reporting System (VAERS).

Immunization Schedules
1. Immunizations may be started at any age. If an immunization program is not begun in infancy, a slightly different schedule may be followed, depending on the child's age and the prevalence of specific diseases at the time.
2. An interrupted primary series of immunization need not be restarted; it need only be continued, regardless of the length of time that has elapsed.
3. The recommended schedule for immunization is detailed in Tables 42-1 and 42-2.
4. The immunoresponse is limited in a significant proportion of young infants, and the recommended booster doses are designed to ensure and maintain immunity.

Contraindications
It is important to read the manufacturer's insert for each vaccine before administration.
1. All vaccines
   a. Anaphylactic reaction to a vaccine or a vaccine constituent
   b. Moderate or severe illnesses with or without a fever
2. All live virus vaccines (OPV, MMR, *Varicella*)
   a. Pregnancy

TABLE 42-1 Recommended Routine Schedule for Healthy Infants and Children

Birth to 2 months	HBV #1	Give 12 hours after birth to infants with HbsAg (+) mothers, second dose at least 1 month after the first dose.
1 to 4 months	HBV #2	In HbsAg (−) mothers, infant can receive first HBV vaccine at 2 months, second at 4 months.
2 months	DTaP #1, Hib #1, IPV #1	DTaP is preferred, although whole cell DTP is acceptable.
4 months	DTaP #2, Hib #2, IPV #2	Combination vaccines are available and may be used to decrease the number of injections.
6 months	DTaP #3, Hib #3	Hib #3 is not needed if first two doses were PRP-OMP.
6 to 18 months	HBV #3, IPV or OPV #3	Infants born to HbsAg (+) mothers should get HBV #3 at 6 months of age.
12 to 15 months	MMR #1, Hib #3 or #4, Var #1	MMR must be given after first birthday.
15 to 18 months	DTaP #4	If Var and MMR are not given on the same day, space them ≥ 28 days apart.
4 to 6 years	DTaP #5, MMR #2, OPV or IPV #4	Repeat Td every 10 years.
11 to 12 years	Td #1	Give MMR, Var, and HBV if not immunized earlier in life.

Notes:
Nurses should carefully read all packet insert instructions before administering vaccinations.
Vaccine abbreviations: HBV, hepatitis B virus vaccine; DTap, diphtheria, tetanus toxoid and acellular pertussis vaccine; DTP, diphtheria, tetanus toxoid and whole cell pertussis vaccine; Hib, *Haemophilus influenzae* type B vaccine; IPV, inactive polio vaccine; OPV, live oral polio vaccine; MMR, live measles, mumps and rubella vaccine; Var, live varicella virus vaccine; Td, tetanus toxoid and diphtheria vaccine.
HbsAg is hepatitis B surface antigen. All pregnant women are screened for the presence of HBsAg before birth.

b. Immunosuppression or immunodeficiency
c. Some vaccines are contraindicated in children with household or close contact with people who are immunosuppressed or immunodeficient
3. DTP/DTaP—encephalopathy within 7 days of administration of previous dose of DTP/DTaP

4. IPV—anaphylactic reaction to neomycin, streptomycin, or polymyxin B
5. MMR and *Varicella*—anaphylactic reactions to neomycin or gelatin
6. Influenza—anaphylactic reaction to eggs or egg protein
7. Hepatitis B—anaphylactic reaction to baker's yeast

TABLE 42-2 Recommended Schedule for Healthy Infants and Children Not Vaccinated on Routine Schedule

Visit Number	Minimal Timing From Initial Visit	Vaccines	Comments
Child >4 months and <7 years old			
1	Initial visit	DTaP, IPV, Hib, HBV, MMR, Var	DTP may be substituted for DTaP.
2	28 days or greater	DTaP, IPV, Hib, HBV	Var and MMR must be given at
3	2 months	DTaP, OPV or IPV, Hib,	>12 months of age.
4	8 months	DTaP, HBV, HIB	Hib vaccine recommendations vary.
5	4 to 6 years of age	DTaP, OPV or IPV, MMR	Check packet insert for correct
6	11 to 12 years of age	Td if > 5 years since last dose	schedule/administration.
Child >7 years old			Hib not needed for child ≥ 5 years; if
1	Initial visit	HBV, OPV or IPV, MMR, Td	child > 15 months give only 1 dose
2	2 months	HBV, OPV or IPV, Td	of Hib.
3	8 to 14 months	HBV, OPV or IPV, Td	Give HBV, Var, and MMR at 11 to
4	11 to 12 years of age	MMR, Td if > 5 years since last dose	12 years if not already received. Repeat Td every 10 years.

Notes:
Nurses should carefully read all packet insert instructions before administering vaccinations.
Pneumococcal vaccine: A new recommendation for the PCV7 vaccination was released by the American Academy of Pediatrics (AAP) for the prevention of pneumococcal infections in infants and children. Each dose should contain 0.5 mL of PVC7 and should be administered intramuscularly to all children 23 months and younger at 2, 4, 6 and 12–15 months. For infants and children not immunized according to the routine schedule, catch-up schedule can be found at the AAP website (*www.aap.org*).
Vaccine abbreviations: HBV, hepatitis B virus vaccine; DTaP, diphtheria, tetanus toxoid and acellular pertussis vaccine; DTP, diphtheria, tetanus toxoid and whole cell pertussis vaccine; Hib, *Haemophilus influenzae* type B vaccine; IPV, inactive polio vaccine; OPV, live oral polio vaccine; MMR, live measles, mumps and rubella vaccine; Var, live varicella virus vaccine; Td, tetanus toxoid and diphtheria vaccine.

Misconceptions Concerning Vaccine Contraindications

1. Some health care providers inappropriately consider certain conditions or circumstances to be contraindications to vaccination. Conditions most often inappropriately regarded as such include:
   a. Mild acute illness with low-grade fever or mild diarrheal illness in an otherwise well child
   b. Current antimicrobial therapy or the convalescent phase of illness
   c. Reaction to a previous DTaP dose that involved only soreness, redness, swelling in the immediate vicinity of the vaccination site, or temperature of less than 105°F (40.5°C).
   d. Prematurity
   e. Person using aerosolized steroids, short course of oral steroids (<14 days), or topical steroid preparations
   f. Pregnancy of mother or other household contact
   g. Recent exposure to an infectious disease
   h. Breast-feeding
   i. History of nonspecific allergies or relatives with allergies
   j. Allergies to penicillin or any other antibiotic, except anaphylactic reactions to neomycin or streptomycin
   k. Allergies to duck meat or duck feathers
   l. Family history of convulsions in people considered for pertussis or measles vaccination
   m. Family history of sudden infant death syndrome in children considered for DTaP vaccination
   n. Family history of an adverse event, unrelated to immunosuppression, after vaccination
   o. Malnutrition
2. In most cases, children with the above conditions can still be immunized.

Vaccine Administration Considerations

1. Strict adherence to the manufacturer's storage and handling recommendation is vital. Failure to observe these precautions and recommendations may reduce the potency and effectiveness of vaccines.
2. Health care personnel administering vaccines should be immunized against measles, mumps, rubella, hepatitis B, influenza, tetanus, and diphtheria. Gloves should be worn when administering vaccines. Good handwashing technique is mandatory before and after vaccine administration.
3. Sterile, disposable needles and syringes should be discarded promptly in appropriate biohazardous containers. Do not recap needles.
4. Parenteral vaccines should be administered in the anterolateral aspect of the upper thigh in infants and in the deltoid area of the upper arm in older children and adolescents. Recommended routes of administration are included in the package inserts of vaccines.
5. Before administering a subsequent dose of any vaccine, question patients and parents about side effects and possible reactions from previous doses.

6. Routine vaccines can be safely and effectively administered simultaneously.

Specific Immunization
DTP and DTaP

1. DTaP (diphtheria, tetanus toxoid, and acellular pertussis) is the preferred vaccine for all doses; however, whole cell DTP is an acceptable alternative. Fewer side effects and local reactions will occur with the DTaP vaccine compared with the DTP.
2. A time lapse of 8 weeks is recommended between the first three DTP/DTaP injections for desirable maximum effects.
3. The combination of depot antigens is preferred because it is more immunogenic.
4. Administration of acetaminophen at the time of immunization and at 4 and 8 hours after immunization decreases the incidence of febrile and local reactions.
5. Because of the increased risk of possible reactions to either diphtheria or pertussis antigen, Td (adult-type tetanus and diphtheria toxins) is recommended for children over 7 years of age.
6. For contaminated wounds, a booster dose of tetanus should be given if more than 5 years have elapsed since the last dose.
7. Protection of infants against pertussis should begin early.
8. In newborn infants, the best protection against pertussis is avoidance of household contacts by adequate immunization of older siblings.
9. Children who have recovered from culture-proven pertussis do not need pertussis immunization.
10. If the fourth dose of pertussis vaccine is given after the fourth birthday, no further doses are needed.

Tuberculin Test

1. It is recommended that the tuberculin test be given before or at the time of measles, mumps, and rubella (MMR). Measles vaccine can temporarily suppress tuberculin reactivity if given 4 to 6 weeks before a tuberculin test.
2. The frequency of repeated tuberculin testing depends on the following:
   a. Risk of tuberculosis exposure to the child
   b. Prevalence of tuberculosis in the population group
   c. Presence of underlying host factors in the child (immunosuppressive conditions or HIV infection)

Measles Vaccine

1. Usually given at 12 to 15 months of age but should be given at 12 months in high-risk areas.
2. Second dose is recommended at 4 to 6 years of age.
3. During an outbreak, infants as young as 6 months of age can be immunized. A second dose should be given at 12 to 15 months and again at age 11 or 12 years or at school entry.
4. Mild postimmunization symptoms include transient skin rashes and fever, which can occur up to 2 weeks after vaccination.
5. Immunoglobulin preparations will interfere with the serologic response to measles vaccine; therefore,

wait the specified time after administration for vaccination.

Mumps Vaccine

1. Usually administered in combination with measles and rubella vaccine (MMR) at 12 to 15 months of age.
2. Second dose administered as MMR is important because a substantial number of cases have occurred in people with previous immunizations.
3. Important to immunize susceptible children approaching puberty, adolescents, and adults.

Rubella Vaccine

1. Two doses of rubella vaccine are recommended to avoid consequences such as congenital rubella syndrome.
2. Important to immunize postpubertal individuals, especially college students and military recruits.
3. Women should avoid pregnancy within 3 months of vaccine due to the theoretical risk to the fetus.

Polio Vaccine

1. Two types of trivalent vaccine are available—live oral polio virus vaccine (OPV) and inactivated polio virus vaccine (IPV), given parenterally. Both are effective in preventing poliomyelitis.
2. To reduce the risk of vaccine-induced polio with OPV, IPV is the vaccine of choice for most children.
3. OPV should not be given to infants and children living in households with an immunodeficient person. Live OPV is excreted in the stool for up to a month after vaccination. Vaccine-induced polio is a risk to both the vaccinated child and any immunosuppressed contact.

H. influenzae Type B (Hib) Vaccine

1. Incidence of invasive disease caused by Hib has declined dramatically since the introduction of conjugate vaccine.
2. Several different types of Hib vaccines are available. Different vaccines have different schedules.
3. Minimal adverse reactions (pain, redness, or swelling at immunization site for less than 24 hours).

Hepatitis B Vaccine (HBV)

1. There are two schedules for this vaccine. Infants born to hepatitis B surface antigen (HBsAg)–negative mothers should receive the routine schedule. Infants born to HBsAg-positive mothers should be on an accelerated vaccination schedule.
2. Recommended for all infants born to HBsAg-negative mothers. Three-dose schedule is initiated in newborn period or by 2 months of age; second doses given 1 to 2 months later; third dose 6 to 18 months later.
3. All infants born to HBsAg-positive mothers, including premature infants, should receive hepatitis B immunoglobulin and vaccine within 12 hours after birth. The second dose is at 1 to 2 months of age; third dose at 6 months of age.
4. Preterm infants weighing less than 2 kg may have lower seroconversion rates. Initiation of HBV should be delayed until just before hospital discharge if the infant weighs 2 kg or more or until approximately 2 months of age when other routine immunizations are given.
5. All children and adolescents who have not had HBV should be immunized.

Rotavirus Vaccine

1. In 1998, rotavirus vaccine, which prevents the most common cause of diarrhea in childhood, was licensed for use in the United States.
2. About 7 months after licensure, rotavirus vaccine recommendations were suspended and later rescinded, and the vaccine was taken off the market because of an increased incidence of intussusception in vaccinated infants.

◼ Nutrition in Children

The nutritional status of the child is an important aspect of health maintenance. A balanced diet influences child growth and psychosocial development. Feeding provides emotional and psychological benefits in addition to nutritional needs. In the United States, obesity in childhood has become a major problem. Good eating habits and proper foods introduced early in life could prevent morbidity from childhood obesity. Table 42-3 presents nutritional guidelines based on age and developmental maturation.

Breast-Feeding

1. Breast-feeding is the natural and ideal nourishment that will supply an infant with adequate nutrition as well as immunologic and anti-infection properties. With breast milk being at the proper temperature, it may prevent other gastrointestinal (GI) disturbances as well. The development of allergies is decreased in breast-fed babies.
2. Breast-feeding provides psychological and emotional satisfaction for the infant and mother and can promote bonding. The physical closeness may also provide comfort after a frightening or painful procedure.
3. Breast-feeding can be continued through most illnesses and hospitalizations of the infant. In times of stress, the infant may cope with breast-feeding better than bottle-feeding. Because breast milk is more easily and quickly digested, shorter periods of NPO both preoperatively and postoperatively may be necessary. Attempts should be made to maintain the breast-feeding bond and routines of the child and mother.
   a. Supplemental artificial formula can be given to the infant if the mother is not available.
   b. The mother can pump her breasts so that milk can be given to the infant by way of bottle when she is not available.
   c. Breast milk can be frozen for up to 6 months (check the facility's specific policy).
   d. Thaw frozen breast milk for use in tepid water. Do not use microwave, which may destroy vitamins and nutritional properties.
4. Stress of new motherhood or illness in the infant or mother may decrease the mother's milk supply and inhibit her "let-down" reflex, as well as increase or decrease the infant's desire to suckle. Care may be initiated to help stimulate the mother's milk supply through pumping. An electronic pump may be necessary if prolonged pumping is expected or if manual pumping is not successful.
5. Education and encouragement should be offered to all new mothers and those having difficulty or concerns about breast-feeding (see Patient Education Guidelines).

TABLE 42-3 Nutrition in Children

Age and Developmental Influence on Nutritional Requirements and Feeding Patterns	Feeding Pattern/Diet	Nursing Implications/Parental Guidance

Neonate:
 	
Birth–4 wk
Newborn's rapid growth makes infant especially vulnerable to dietary inadequacies, dehydration, and iron deficiency anemia.
Feeding process is basis for infant's first human relationship, formation of trust. Feeding reinforces mother's sense of "motherliness."
Because of limited nutritional stores, neonates require vitamin and mineral supplements.
Neonates require more fluid relative to their size than do adults.
Sucking ability is influenced by individual neuromuscular maturity.
	Breast milk or formula is generally given in 6 to 8 feedings per day, spaced 2 to 4 h apart.
	Feeding schedules should be individualized according to infant's needs.
		Provide information to help parents make decision concerning breast- or bottle-feeding.
		Support parents in their decision.
		Breast-fed infant:
		
		1. Help mother assume comfortable and satisfying position for self and baby.
		2. Help mother to determine schedule, timing, and when infant is satisfied.
		3. Provide specific information about the following:
		  a. Feeding technique: position, "bubbling"
		  b. Care of breasts
		  c. Manual expression of milk from breast
		  d. Maternal diet
		
		Bottle-fed infant:
		
		1. Provide specific information concerning
		  a. Type of formula
		  b. Preparation of formula: measuring and sterilization
		  c. Equipment—types of bottles, nipples, and so forth.
		  d. Sterilization of equipment
		  e. Technique of feeding: position, "bubbling"
		2. Help mother to determine when infant is satisfied; develop schedule for feeding.
		
		Provide information concerning normal characteristics of stools, signs of dehydration, constipation, colic, milk allergy.
		Discuss need for vitamin supplements and how to administer.
		Discuss need for additional fluids during periods of hot weather, and with fever, diarrhea, and vomiting.
		Observe for evidence of common problems and intervene accordingly:
		
		1. Overfeeding
		2. Underfeeding
		3. Difficulty digesting formula because of its particular composition.
		4. Improper feeding technique; holes in nipples too large or too small; formula too hot or too cold; uncomfortable feeding position; failure to "bubble"; improper sterilization; bottle propping.
		5. Bottles should never be given to infants to take to bed.

Infant 3 mo–1 y Increased neuromuscular development allows infant to make transition from a totally liquid diet to a diet of milk and solid foods as well as to more active participation in the feeding process. 3–6 mo Sucking reflex becomes voluntary and chewing action begins; infant can approximate lips to rim and cup and may begin drinking from cup at 6 mo.	Number of feedings per day decreases through the first year. By 4–6 mo of age, generally ready to begin strained foods. The usual sequence of foods is cereal followed by fruits, and vegetables. Meats may be started at 8–9 mo. Sequence may vary according to preferences of family and health care provider.	The person feeding should be calm, gentle, relaxed, and patient in approach. When the child is first offered puréed foods with a spoon, he expects and wants to suck. The protrusion of the tongue, which is needed in sucking, makes it appear that he is pushing the food out of mouth. This response should not be interpreted as dislike for the food; it is a result of immature muscle coordination and surprise at the taste and feel of the new food. The baby foods selected should be high in nutrients without providing excessive calories. Personal and cultural preferences should be considered. Iron-fortified formulas and cereals are needed to prevent physiologic anemia.

(continued)

TABLE 42-3 Nutrition in Children (Continued)

Age and Developmental Influence on Nutritional Requirements and Feeding Patterns	Feeding Pattern/Diet	Nursing Implications/Parental Guidance
6–12 mo Loses maternal iron stores at 6 mo; first tooth erupts at 6–9 mo; eyes and hands can work together; infant is able to sit without support and has developed grasp; able to feed self a biscuit; bangs objects on table; able to hold own bottle at 9–12 mo; can "pincer" grasp food; able to be weaned from bottle as child becomes developmentally able to take sufficient fluids from the cup. Food provides the infant with a variety of learning experiences; motor control and coordination in self-feeding; recognition of shape, texture, color; stimulation of speech movement through use of mouth muscles. Mealtime allows the infant to continue development of trust in a consistent, loving atmosphere. The infant is forming lifetime eating habits; it is therefore important to make mealtime a positive experience.	Mashed table foods or junior foods generally are started at 6–8 mo, when infant begins chewing action. Infant begins to enjoy finger foods at 10–12 mo. The transition from iron-fortified formula or breast milk to cow's milk is usually advised at about 12 mo of age. By 1 y of age, most infants are satisfied with three meals and additional fluids throughout the day.	New foods should be offered one at a time and early in the feeding while the infant is still hungry. Allow 3–5 days between new foods. Infants should be observed for allergic reactions when new foods are added. Common allergies are to citrus juices, egg white, cow's milk, and peanut butter. These foods should be avoided until 12 mo of age. Also avoid honey until 12 mo due to the risk of infantile botulism. Finger foods should be selected for their nutritional value. Good choices include teething biscuits, cooked vegetables, bananas, cheese sticks, and enriched cereals. Avoid nuts, raisins and raw vegetables, which can cause choking. Parents can be taught to prepare their own strained or junior foods using a commercial baby food grinder or blender. Weaning is a gradual process. 1. Assist parents to recognize indications of readiness. 2. Do not expect the infant to completely drop old pattern of behavior while learning a new one; allow overlap of old and new techniques. 3. Evening feedings usually the most difficult to eliminate, because the infant is tired and in need of sucking comfort. 4. During illness or household disorganization, the infant may regress and return to sucking to relieve his discomfort and frustration. **NURSING ALERT** Obtain a thorough nursing history for the hospitalized infant that includes the following: feeding pattern and schedule; types of foods that have been introduced; likes and dislikes; breast or bottle fed, type of bottle; temperature at which infant prefers foods and fluids.
Toddler **1–3 y** Growth slows at the end of the first year. The slower growth rate is reflected in a decreased appetite. The toddler has a total of 14 to 16 teeth, making him more able to chew foods. Increased self-awareness causes the toddler to want to do more for self. Refusals of food or of assistance in feedings are common ways in which the toddler asserts himself. Because body tissues, especially muscles, continue to grow quite rapidly, protein needs are high.	Appetite is sporadic; specific foods may be favored exclusively or refused from time to time. Child may be ritualistic concerning food preferences, schedule, manner of eating, and so forth. Diet should include a full range of foods: milk, meat, fruits, vegetables, breads, and cereals. Iron-fortified dry cereals (rice, barley) are an excellent source of iron during the second year of life. Older toddler can be expected to consume about one half the amount of food that an adult consumes. Whole milk is recommended up to 2 years of age.	Provide foods with a variety of color, texture, and flavor. Toddlers need to experience the feel of foods. Offer small portions. It is fun for the child to ask for more. It is more effective to give small helpings than to insist that he eat a specific amount. Maintain a regular mealtime schedule. Provide appropriate mealtime equipment: 1. Silverware scaled to size. 2. Dishes—colorful, unbreakable; shallow, round bowls are preferable to flat plates. 3. Plastic bibs, placemats, and floor coverings permit a relaxed attitude toward child's self-feeding attempts. 4. Comfortable seating at good height and distance from table. Adults who help toddlers at mealtime should be calm and relaxed. Avoid bribes or force feeding because this reinforces negative behavior and may lead to a dislike for mealtime. Encourage independence, but provide assistance when necessary. Do not be concerned about table manners.

(continued)

TABLE 42-3 Nutrition in Children (Continued)

Age and Developmental Influence on Nutritional Requirements and Feeding Patterns	Feeding Pattern/Diet	Nursing Implications/Parental Guidance
		Avoid the use of soda or "sweets" as rewards or between-meal snacks. Instead, substitute fruit, juice, or cereal. Toddlers who show little interest in eggs, meat, or vegetables should not be permitted to appease their appetite with carbohydrates or milk because this may lead to iron-deficiency anemia. Milk should be limited to approximately 16 oz/d. **NURSING ALERT** Nursing history for the hospitalized toddler should include the following: feeding pattern and schedule; food likes and dislikes; food allergies; special eating equipment and utensils; whether child is weaned; what child is fed when ill.
Preschooler 3–5 y of age Increased manual dexterity enables child to have complete independence at mealtime. Psychosocially, this is a period of increased imitation and sex identification. The preschooler identifies with parents at the table and will enjoy what parents enjoy. Additional nutritional habits are developed that become part of the child's lifetime practices. Slower growth rate and increased interest in exploring his environment may decrease the preschooler's interest in eating. Eating assumes increasing social significance. Mealtime promotes socialization and provides the preschooler with opportunities to learn appropriate mealtime behavior, language skills, and understanding of family rituals.	Appetite tends to be sporadic. Child requires the same basic four food groups as the adult, but in smaller quantities. Generally likes to eat one food from plate at a time. Likes vegetables that are crisp, raw, and cut into finger-sized pieces. Often dislikes strong-tasting foods.	Emphasis should be placed on the quality rather than the amount of food ingested. Foods should be attractively served, mildly flavored, plain, as well as being separated and distinctly identifiable in flavor and appearance. Nutritional foods (eg, crackers and cheese, yogurt, fruit) should be offered as snacks. Desserts should be nutritious and a natural part of the meal, not used as a reward for finishing the meal or omitted as punishment. Unless they persist, periods of overeating or not wanting to eat certain foods should not cause concern. The overall eating pattern from month to month is more pertinent to assess. Frequent causes of insufficient eating: 1. Unhappy atmosphere at mealtime 2. Overeating between meals 3. Parental example 4. Attention-seeking 5. Excessive parental expectations 6. Inadequate variety or quantity of foods 7. Tooth decay 8. Physical illness 9. Fatigue 10. Emotional disturbance Measures to increase food intake: 1. Allow child to help with preparations, planning menu, setting table, and other simple chores. 2. Maintain calm environment with no distractions. 3. Avoid between-meal snacks. 4. Provide rest period before meal. 5. Avoid coaxing, bribing, threatening. **NURSING ALERT** Consider cultural differences. Allow parents to bring in favorite foods or eating utensils from home for the hospitalized preschooler. Encourage family members to be present at mealtime.

(continued)

TABLE 42-3 Nutrition in Children (Continued)

Age and Developmental Influence on Nutritional Requirements and Feeding Patterns	Feeding Pattern/Diet	Nursing Implications/Parental Guidance
		Place children in small groups, preferably at tables during mealtime. Use nursing history to determine likes and provide simple foods in small portions. Peanut butter and jelly sandwiches are often favorites. Allow and encourage children to feed themselves. Do not punish children who refuse to eat. Offer alternative foods.
School-Age Child Slowed rate of growth during middle childhood results in gradual decline in food requirements per unit of body weight. The preadolescent growth spurt occurs about age 10 in girls and about age 12 in boys. At this time, energy needs increase and approach those of the adult. Intake is particularly important, because reserves are laid down for the demands of adolescence. The child becomes dependent on peers for approval and makes food choices accordingly. The child experiences increased socialization and independence through opportunities to eat away from home (eg, at school and homes of peers).	By this time, food practices are generally well established, a product of the eating experiences of the toddler and preschool period. Many children are too busy with other affairs to take time out to eat. Play readily takes priority unless a firm understanding is reached and mealtime is relaxed and enjoyable.	Nutrition education should help the child to select foods wisely and to begin to plan and prepare meals. Parental attitudes continue to be important as the child copies parental behavior (eg, skipping breakfast, not eating certain foods). Most children require a nutritious breakfast to avoid lassitude in late morning. Mealtime should continue to be relaxed and enjoyable. Diversions such as television should be avoided. Calcium and vitamin D intake warrant special consideration. They must be adequate to support the rapid enlargement of bones. Parents and health professionals should be alert to signs of developing obesity. Intake should be altered accordingly. Table manners should not be overemphasized. The young child often stuffs his mouth, spills foods, and chatters incessantly while eating. Time and experience will improve his habits. Provide some companionship and conversation at the child's level during meals. Peers should be invited occasionally for meals.

> **NURSING ALERT**
>
> Nursing history of the hospitalized child should include the following: food preferences; mealtime patterns and snacks; food allergies; food preferences when ill. Provide opportunities for children to eat in small groups at tables. Consider cultural differences. Allow parents to bring in favorite foods from home. Allow child to order own meal.

Adolescent 11–17 y of age Dietary requirements vary according to stage of sexual maturation, rate of physical growth, and extent of athletic and social activity. When rapid growth of puberty appears, there is a corresponding increase in energy requirements and appetite. Menstruating teen is particularly susceptible to iron-deficiency anemia.	Previously learned dietary patterns are difficult to change. Food choices and eating habits may be quite unusual and are related to the adolescent's psychological and social milieu. Generally, a significant percentage of the daily caloric intake of the adolescent comes from snacking.	Continue nutrition education, with special emphasis on the following: 1. Selecting nutritious foods high in iron. 2. Nutritional needs related to growth. 3. Preparing favorite "adolescent foods." 4. Foods and physical fitness. Informal sessions are generally more effective than lectures on nutrition. Special problems requiring intervention: Obesity Excessive dieting Extreme fads—eccentric and grossly restricted diets Anorexia nervosa/bulimia Adolescent pregnancy Iron deficiency anemia

TABLE 42-3 Nutrition in Children (Continued)

Age and Developmental Influence on Nutritional Requirements and Feeding Patterns	Feeding Pattern/Diet	Nursing Implications/Parental Guidance
		Provide nutritious foods relevant to the adolescent's lifestyle. Discourage cigarette smoking, which may contribute to poor nutritional status by decreasing appetite and increasing the body's metabolic rate. **NURSING ALERT** **Allow hospitalized adolescent to choose own foods, especially if on a special diet. Provide a refrigerator in the recreation room for snacks, or utilize a snack cart. Serve foods that appeal to adolescents. Use a nursing history similar to that for the school-age child.**

PATIENT EDUCATION GUIDELINES Breast Feeding

Breastfeeding is the best possible source of nutrition for your infant. It provides an immunologic boost for the infant, protects against breast cancer, hastens postpartum healing, and serves as a wonderful bond between the infant and mother.

1. You should begin breastfeeding in a quiet, comfortable place that is free of interruption. You may need a pillow to help support the baby and a footstool to use to elevate your leg.
2. Make sure the infant is awake and dry before the feeding is started. If awake and comfortable, the infant will settle down and feed better. The infant should also be hungry.
3. Dress the infant appropriately so that he or she is not too warm or too cool during the feeding. If too warm, the infant may fall asleep after the first few sucks of milk. A sleepy baby will not nurse well. If too cool, infant may be fussy and restless.
4. Position the baby at breast by placing him or her in a semi-sitting position with face close to the breast and supported by one of your arms and hand. A pillow may be used under the baby for support. You may need to support your breast with your other hand. Proper positioning will provide the infant with comfort and security and make it easier to suck and swallow. This makes the nipple more easily accessible to the infant's mouth and prevents obstruction of nasal breathing.
5. When the feeding is to start, let the breast touch the infant's cheek. Do not hold cheek, but try to help the infant find the nipple. The rooting reflex will take over and the infant will turn head toward the breast with mouth open. If cheek is touched with a hand, infant will become confused, perhaps turning toward the hand.
6. The infant's lips should be out over the areola and not just around the nipple before beginning to suck. Because the nipple is so small, suction cannot be achieved merely by grasping it. The areola must be in the infant's mouth to establish suction and make the suck effective.
7. You may notice the "let-down" reflex during the nursing period. Milk flowing from the other breast during nursing is quite normal.
8. The length of feeding time may vary from 5 to 30 minutes. Let the infant nurse until satisfied. When the infant is satisfied and has nursed well, he or she is relaxed and usually falls asleep. Infant will stop sucking.
9. Burp the baby during and at the end of the feeding to prevent abdominal distention or regurgitation from air swallowed during the feeding.
10. One or both breasts may be used at each feeding. It makes no difference as long as the baby is satisfied at the end of the feeding and one breast is completely emptied at the feeding. If both breasts were used, the second breast is not usually emptied and should be used first at the next feeding. Regular and complete emptying of the breast is the only stimulation for the production of milk.
11. Once the infant has stopped sucking, he or she likes to cling to the breast. To break this suction, insert a finger to the corner of the baby's mouth and gently pull.
12. When the infant has finished feeding, change diaper if it is wet or soiled. Position infant on right side in bed. Note whether baby appears satisfied or still seems to be hungry.
13. To continue successful breastfeeding, get adequate rest and nutrition.
14. For more information and support, contact LaLeche League International, 1400 N. Meacham Road, Schaumburg, IL 60173, 847-519-7730; or read their publication *The Womanly Art of Breastfeeding* (6th ed.).

Bottle-Feeding

1. Bottle-feeding is a method of supplying nutrition to the infant by oral feedings, using a bottle and nipple set-up.
2. Bottle-feeding can supplement breast-feeding with formula or water, or can be the sole means of nutritional intake for the infant.
3. Bottle-feeding can also provide intermittent feedings of expressed breast milk when the mother is unable to be present at the time of the feeding.
4. Bottle-feeding can be a time of bonding between the mother and infant. The father or other capable members of the family should be taught bottle-feeding technique as well (see Procedure Guidelines 42–1).

PROCEDURE GUIDELINES 42-1 | **BOTTLE FEEDING**

EQUIPMENT

Sterile nipple and bottle
Sterile formula or breast milk

PROCEDURE

Nursing Action	Rationale
PREPARATORY PHASE	
1. Baby should be awake and hungry. Change wet or soiled diaper.	1. A sleepy baby will not feed well. A dry diaper will provide comfort so that the baby will settle down and eat more easily.
2. Prepare formula according to manufacturer's instructions. Check formula for correct type and amount.	2. To prevent error.
3. Some babies prefer warmed formula, *not* hot.	3. Check temperature of formula on inner wrist before feeding.
4. Sit in a comfortable chair. Cradle baby with one hand and arm, while supporting baby against your body or lap.	4. Proper position will provide the baby with comfort and security and will make it easier to suck and swallow. Holding infant will enhance trust-building and provide sensory stimulation.
PERFORMANCE PHASE	
1. Let the baby root for the nipple by touching the corner of mouth with the nipple. When infant opens mouth, insert the nipple.	1. Place the nipple on top of the tongue and far enough in mouth so suction can be created when the infant sucks.
2. Hold the bottle at an angle to completely fill the nipple with fluid.	2. This prevents the baby from sucking and swallowing excessive amounts of air.
3. NEVER prop the bottle or leave the baby unattended during feeding.	3. This is unsafe. Should vomiting occur, aspiration is more likely.
4. Handle the bottle carefully so as not to contaminate the nipple or fluid.	4. Contamination will increase the chances of gastrointestinal disturbances.
5. Baby's feeding time will vary from 10 to 25 minutes. Position baby so eye contact can be established (en face) during feeding. Soothing talk and fondling can provide additional comfort to the baby.	5. The length of time will depend on the age of the baby and how vigorously he or she sucks.
6. Burp the baby at least once during the feeding and at the end of the feeding.	6. Most babies swallow some air during feeding. These positions aid in expelling air and thus prevent abdominal distention, discomfort, and regurgitation. Vigorous handling or patting may result in the infant spitting up or regurgitating feeding.
a. Place the baby in sitting position in lap, tilt slightly forward, and gently rub or pat back or abdomen.	
b. Place the baby in prone position on shoulder and gently pat or rub back.	
c. Place the baby in prone position on lap and gently rub or pat back.	
FOLLOW-UP PHASE	
1. After final burping, change wet or soiled diaper and place baby in crib on right side.	1. This position aids in emptying the stomach and prevents regurgitation.
2. Check baby in a few minutes. If restless, pick baby up and burp. Note if any spitting-up has occurred.	2. Some babies relieve themselves of air when in the crib and also bring up small amounts of formula at the same time.

PROCEDURE GUIDELINES 42-1 ⟨ *CONTINUED* ⟩

NURSING ALERT

When feeding a premature infant, infant will tire more easily and fall asleep. Allow frequent rest periods and use a soft nipple so that less energy is needed to suck. To stimulate this infant to suck, the nurse can brush the infant's cheek with finger, place thumb or finger under the infant's chin, or move the nipple slowly back and forth in mouth. Feeding time should not exceed 30 minutes. Keep the infant warm during feeding.

■ Safety

Safety is an important aspect of child health and well-being. Injuries are the leading cause of death for children in the United States. Additionally, injury is a significant cause of childhood morbidity. Although childhood deaths from other causes have decreased, deaths from injuries remain constant.

Role of the Nurse

1. Identify environmental hazards, and act to reduce or eliminate them.
2. Identify behavioral characteristics of individual children that may be related to accidental liability, and caution parents accordingly. Pay particular attention to children who show the following:
   a. Characteristics that increase exposure to hazards, such as excessive curiosity, inability to delay gratification, hyperactivity, and daringness
   b. Characteristics that reduce the child's ability to cope with hazards, such as aggressiveness, stubbornness, poor concentration, low frustration threshold, lack of self-control
3. Provide anticipatory guidance about child development as it relates to accidents. Direct preventive teaching toward individuals or groups, toward children or adults.
4. Participate in policy setting for accident prevention with great emphasis on effective public health measures.

Principles of Safety

1. The type of accident likely to occur is influenced by the child's age and developmental level. Parents who have knowledge of their own child's typical behavior patterns may foresee potential accident situations.
2. Children are naturally curious, impulsive, and impatient. The young child needs to touch, feel, and investigate. Consistent adult supervision will enable children to learn in a safe environment.
3. Children copy the behavior of their parents and absorb parental attitudes. Parents and other adults should be a role model for using proper and safe methods.
4. Children become less careful and less willing to listen to warnings and to observe routine safety precautions when they are tired or hungry.
5. An estimated 90% of all accidents are preventable.

General Areas of Adult Responsibility for Child Safety

Motor Vehicle

1. Automobiles should be in good mechanical condition.
2. Use properly fitted and installed car seats and seat belts. Be aware of the guidelines for restraints based on the child's age and weight.
3. Infants riding in a rear-facing car seat should never be placed in the front seat equipped with an air bag.
4. The center rear seat is the safest seat for a child.
5. Driver should look carefully in front and back of the car before getting into the car.
6. Lock all car doors.
7. Never leave young children in a car alone.
8. Do not place heavy or sharp objects on the same seat with a child.

Sports and Recreation

1. Keep equipment in good condition and proper working order.
2. Encourage the routine use of bike helmets (Figure 42-1).
3. Wear appropriate clothing and safety equipment for the activity (Figure 42-2).
4. Do not attempt activities beyond one's physical endurance.
5. Keep firearms and ammunition locked up.

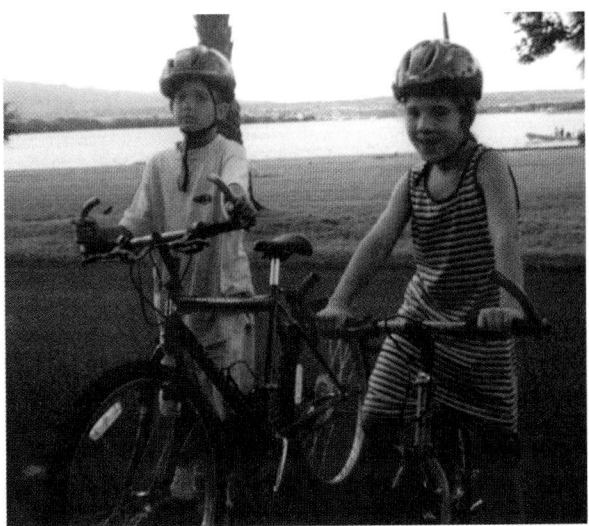

FIGURE 42-1　Use of bike helmets by all children for safety.

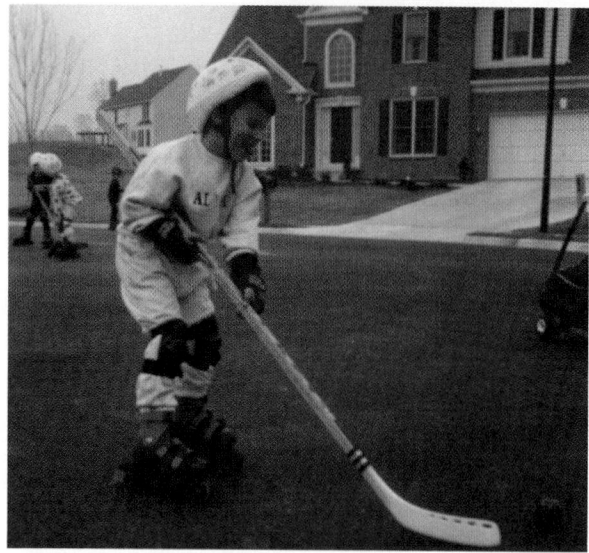

FIGURE 42-2 Use of appropriate pads and helmets for safety.

Electrical and Mechanical Equipment

1. Only underwriter-approved devices should be installed; they should be inspected periodically.
2. Dry hands before touching appliances. Keep radios, transportable heaters, and hair dryers out of the bathroom.
3. Disconnect appliances after each use and before attempting minor repairs.
4. Keep garden equipment and machinery in a restricted area. Teach proper use of the equipment as soon as the child is old enough.
5. Avoid overloading electrical circuits.
6. Discourage children from playing with or being in area where appliances or power tools (eg, washing machine, clothes dryer, saw, lawn mower) are in operation.

Prevention of Falls

1. Keep stairs well lighted and free from clutter.
2. Provide sturdy railings.
3. Anchor small rugs securely.
4. Use rubber mats in the bathtub and shower.
5. Use only sturdy ladders for climbing.

Poisonings and Ingestions

1. Do not mix bleaches with ammonia, vinegar, and other household cleaners.
2. See section on ingested poisons and pediatric poisoning (p. 1282).
3. Become familiar with telephone number for poison control centers where available.
4. Label poisonous household materials, and keep them out of child's reach.

Fire

1. Maintain an adequate fire escape plan, and routinely conduct home fire drills. Teach children escape routes as soon as they are old enough.
2. Keep a pressure-type, hand-held fire extinguisher on each floor. Instruct all family members who are old enough in its use.
3. Fit fireplaces with snug fireplace screens.
4. Store gasoline and other flammable fluids in tightly covered containers that are clearly labeled and away from heat and sparks.
5. Dispose of paint- and oil-soaked cloth quickly.
6. Use flame-retardant sleepwear.
7. Mark children's rooms so they are obvious to fire-fighters.
8. Teach children about the danger of smoke inhalation.
9. Teach children to stop, drop, and roll if their clothing catches fire.
10. Maintain smoke detectors in working order.
11. Keep lighters and matches out of reach of children.
12. Keep children away from heated oven, stovetop, and outdoor grill.

Swimming Pools

1. Completely enclose pool with a fence that complies with local regulations. The gate should be self-closing and have a lock.
2. Indicate water depth with numbers on the edge of the pool. Place a safety float line where the bottom of the slope begins to deepen.
3. Install at least one ladder at each end of the pool. Ladders should have handrails on both sides, and the diameter of the rails should be small enough for a child to grasp.
4. Use nonslip materials on ladders, deck, and diving boards.
5. If the pool is used at night, install underwater lighting as well as outdoor lights.
6. Install a ground fault circuit interrupter on the pool circuit to cut off electrical power and thus prevent electrocutions should electrical fault occur.
7. Instruct children about safety rules such as not swimming alone, no running around the pool, and no pushing others. Avoid using radios or other electrical appliances around the pool.
8. Keep essential rescue devices and first-aid equipment close to the pool.

Emergency Precautions

1. Record emergency telephone numbers in an obvious and easily accessible place.
2. Keep a well-stocked first-aid kit immediately available for emergencies.
3. Give instruction in principles of first aid to all family members who are old enough.
   a. Responsible adults should enroll in first-aid courses offered by the American Red Cross, adult education programs, and so forth.
   b. Be aware of first-aid procedure for:
      • Burns
      • Electrical shock
      • Poisoning
      • Bites and stings
      • Cuts, scrapes, and punctures

- Near drowning
- Fractures
- Cardiopulmonary arrest

  c. Teach children safety precautions concerning bicycles, answering telephone or door, strangers outside the home, street safety.
4. Know the location of gas, water, and electrical switches and how to turn them off in an emergency.
5. Teach children their address and telephone number and how to dial 911 in case of emergency.

Miscellaneous

1. Take advantage of preventive health care.
   a. Obtain recommended immunizations.
   b. Have regular physical and dental examinations.
2. Seek immediate treatment of all diseases and health problems.
3. Balance periods of work, rest, and exercise in daily living.

PEDIATRIC CARE TECHNIQUES

▣ Nursing Management of the Child With Fever

Fever is any abnormal elevation of body temperature. Prolonged elevation of temperature above 40°C (104°F) may produce dehydration and harmful effects on the central nervous system (CNS).

General Considerations

1. Consider basic principles related to temperature regulation in pediatric patients.
   a. Usually an infant's temperature does not stabilize before 1 week of age. A newborn's temperature varies with the temperature of the environment.
   b. The degree of fever does not always reflect the severity of the disease. A child may have a serious illness with a normal or subnormal temperature.
   c. Febrile seizures may occur in some children when the temperature rises rapidly.
   d. The range for normal temperature varies widely in children. A common explanation for "fever" is misinterpretation of a normal temperature reading.
   e. A child's temperature is influenced by activity and by the time of day; temperatures are highest in late afternoon.
2. Temperature interpretation depends on accurate temperature measurement in a child. The mode should be appropriate for the child's age and condition, and the thermometer should be left in place for the required time period. Parents or caregivers should be taught the appropriate assessment of temperature as the child grows.

Causes of Fevers in Children

1. Infection
2. Inflammatory disease
3. Dehydration
4. Tumors
5. Disturbance of temperature-regulating center
6. Extravasation of blood in the tissues
7. Drugs or toxins

Nursing Assessment

1. Assess history of present illness for source of fever origin.
   a. Age of the child
   b. Pattern of the fever
   c. Length of the illness
   d. Change in normal patterns of eating, elimination, recreation, and so forth
   e. Other symptoms—poor feeding, cough, earache, diarrhea, vomiting, rash, and so forth
   f. Exposure to any illness
   g. Recent immunizations or drugs
   h. Treatment of fever and effectiveness of treatment
   i. Previous experiences with fever and its control
2. Assess the general appearance of the child.
3. Perform a systematic physical assessment.
   a. Inspection of the skin for rashes, sores, flushed appearance
   b. Inspection of eyes, ears, nose, and throat for redness and drainage
   c. Auscultation of lungs for abnormal sounds
   d. Neurologic observation for changes in state of consciousness, pupillary reaction, strength of grip, abnormal muscle movement, or lack of movement
   e. Inspection of the external genitals for redness and drainage
   f. Presence of abdominal or flank tenderness
4. Assist with laboratory tests as indicated. Initial tests frequently include complete blood count; urinalysis; cultures of the throat, nasopharynx, urine, blood, spinal fluid; and chest x-ray.
5. Attempt to identify the pattern of the fever. Take the child's temperature by the same method every hour until stable, then every 2 hours until normal, then every 4 hours for 24 hours.

Nursing Measures to Reduce Fever

Fever does not necessarily require treatment. The presence of fever should not be obscured by the indiscriminate use of antipyretic measures. However, if the child is uncomfortable or appears toxic because of fever, an attempt should be made to reduce it by any of the following nursing measures or by a combination of these measures:

1. Increase the child's fluid intake to prevent dehydration.
2. Expose the skin to the air by leaving the child lightly dressed in absorbent material. Avoid warm, binding clothing and blankets.
3. Administer antipyretic drugs as prescribed.
4. Use tub bath or a hypothermia blanket.

▣ Administering Medications to Children

Administration of medication is often traumatic for children. Proper approach to administration can facilitate the process and enhance the child's understanding of the importance of taking medications.

Important Considerations

1. The manner of approach should indicate that the nurse firmly expects the child to take the medication. This manner often convinces the child of the necessity of the procedure.
2. Establishing a positive relationship with the child will allow expression of feelings, concerns, and fantasies regarding medications.
3. Explanation about medication should appeal to the child's level of understanding (ie, through play or comparison to something familiar).
4. The nurse must mask his or her own feelings regarding the medication.
5. Always be truthful when the child asks, "Does it taste bad?" or "Will it hurt?" Respond by saying, "The medication does not taste good, but I will give you some juice as soon as you swallow it," or "It will hurt for just a minute, like a mosquito bite."
6. It is often necessary to mix distasteful medications or crushed pills with a small amount of carbonated drink, cherry syrup, ice cream, or applesauce.
7. Never threaten a child with an injection when refusing oral medication.
8. Do not mix medications with large quantities of food or with any food that is taken regularly (eg, milk).
9. Avoid giving medications to a child at mealtime unless specifically prescribed.
10. For each medication administered, the nurse should know the common use, safe dose based on the child's weight, contraindications, side effects, and toxic effects.
11. The child must be accurately identified before medication is given.
12. When preparing intramuscular (IM) injections, draw 0.2 mL of air in addition to the correct amount of medication. This clears the medication from the needle on injection and prevents backflow and the depositing of medication in subcutaneous fat when the needle is withdrawn.

Calculating the Pediatric Dosage

General Principles

1. The nurse is responsible for knowing the safe dosage range for the medication he or she administers.
2. Factors determining the amount of drug prescribed include:
   a. Action of the drug, absorption, detoxification, excretion are related to the maturity and metabolic rate of the child.
   b. Neonates and premature infants require a reduced dosage because of:
      (i) Deficient or absent detoxifying enzymes
      (ii) Decreased effective renal function
      (iii) Altered blood–brain barrier and protein-binding capacity
   c. Dosage recommendations based on age groups are not satisfactory because a child may be much smaller or larger than the average child in the age group.
   d. Dosages based on child's weight are more accurate; however, these calculations have limitations.
3. Be alert to a prescription that would be inappropriate for a child.
4. Consult drug literature for recommended dosage and other information.

Calculating by Body Surface Area

The following formulas are used to estimate the pediatric dosage based on the child's body surface area (BSA). BSA calculations are generally preferred because many physiologic processes in the child (eg, blood volume, glomerular filtration) are related to BSA.

1. Surface area in square meters × Dose per square meter = Approximate child dose
2. Surface area of child/surface area of adult × Dose of adult = Approximate child dose
3. Surface area of child in square meters/1.75 × Adult dose = Child dose

Calculating by Clark's Rule

The following rule may be used as an estimate of the pediatric dosage based on the child's weight in respect to the adult dose of the drug:

Child's weight in pounds/150 × Adult dose = Approximate dose for child

---

NURSING ALERT

 Always check a child's identification bracelet with medication card before administering a medication. Ask the older child his or her name.

Oral Medications

Infants

1. Draw up medication in a plastic dropper or disposable syringe.
2. Elevate infant's head and shoulders; depress chin with thumb to open mouth.
3. Place dropper or syringe on the middle of the tongue and slowly drop the medication on the tongue.
4. Release thumb, and allow child to swallow.
5. Once the correct amount of medication has been measured, it can be placed in a nipple and the infant can suck the medication through the nipple.
6. If the nurse feels comfortable managing the infant in his or her lap, it is acceptable to hold the infant for medication administration.

Toddlers

1. Draw up liquid medications in syringe or measure into medicine cup. Medications may be placed in medicine cup or spoon after being measured accurately in a syringe.

2. Elevate the child's head and shoulders.
3. Squeeze cup and put it to the child's lips, or place the syringe (without needle) in the child's mouth, positioning the syringe tip in space between cheek mucosa and gum, and slowly expel the medicine. Child may prefer using a familiar teaspoon.
4. Allow the child time to swallow.
5. Allow the child to hold the medicine cup if able and to drink it at his or her own pace. (This may be a more agreeable method.) Offer a favorite drink as a "chaser," if not contraindicated.
6. The small, safe medicine cups can be given to the child for play.

School-Aged Children

1. When a child is old enough to take medicine in pill or capsule form, teach the child to place the pill near the back of the tongue and immediately swallow fluid such as water or fruit juice. If swallowing of the fluid is emphasized, the child will no longer think about the pill.
2. Always praise a child after taking medication.
3. If the child finds it particularly difficult to take oral medications, express understanding and offer help.

Intramuscular Medications
General Considerations for Intramuscular Injections

1. After the medication is drawn from vial, draw up additional 0.2 to 0.3 mL of air into a syringe, thus clearing needle of medication and preventing medication seepage from the injection site.
2. When injecting less than 1 mL of medication, use a tuberculin syringe for accuracy.
3. Cleanse site thoroughly, using friction with an antiseptic solution; let site dry.
4. Establish anatomic landmarks (Figure 42-3). Alternate injection site, and keep record at bedside or on medication card.

5. After penetrating site, aspirate to check for blood vessel puncture. If this occurs, withdraw needle and discard medicine and start again.
6. After injection, massage site (unless contraindicated). The complication of fibrosis and contracture of the muscle can be diminished by massage, warm soaks, and range-of-motion exercises to disrupt and stretch immature scar tissue when multiple injections are being administered.

Infants

1. Acceptable site selection includes rectus femoris (mid anterior thigh), vastus lateralis (middle third), or ventrogluteal. These are relatively free of major nerves and blood vessels. The gluteus maximus and deltoid muscles are underdeveloped in the infant, and use of these sites can result in nerve damage.
2. Rectus femoris injection
   a. Place the child in a secure position to prevent movement of the extremity.
   b. Do not use a needle more than 2.5 cm (1 inch).
   c. Use upper quadrant of the thigh.
   d. Insert needle at 45-degree angle in a downward direction, toward the knee.
3. Vastus lateralis injection
   a. Place the child in a prone or supine position.
   b. Area is a narrow strip of muscle extending along a line from the greater trochanter to lateral femoral condyle below.
   c. Insert needle perpendicular to skin, 2 to 4 cm deep—needle parallel to floor.
4. Ventrogluteal injection.
   a. This site provides a dense muscle mass that is relatively free of the danger of injuring the nervous and vascular systems.
   b. The disadvantage is that the injection site is visible to the child.

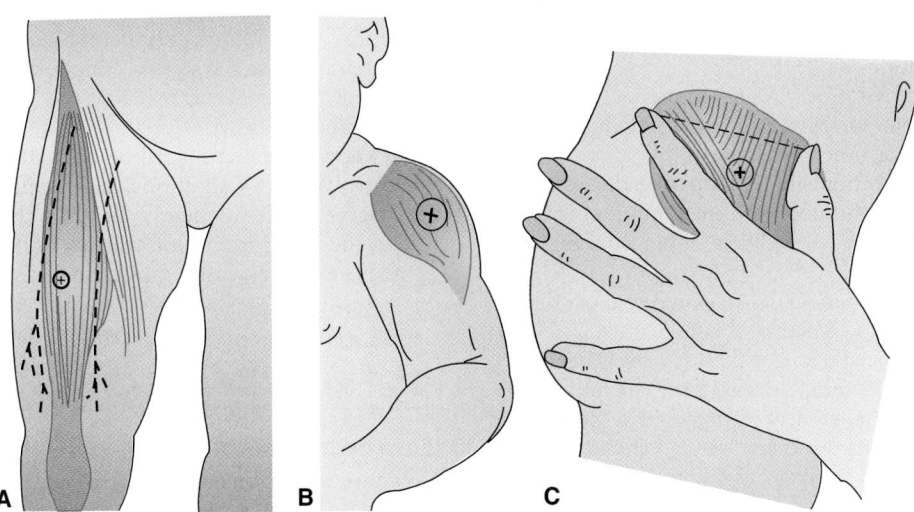

FIGURE 42-3 Sites for IM injections in children: (**A**) rectus femoris, (**B**) deltoid, (**C**) ventrogluteal.

c. Administration
 (i) Place the child on back.
 (ii) Place the index finger on the anterosuperior spine.
 (iii) With the middle finger moving dorsally, locate the iliac crest; drop finger below the crest. The triangle formed by the iliac crest, index finger, and middle finger is the injection site.
 (iv) Inject needle perpendicular to the surface on which the child is lying.
5. After administration of medication, hold and cuddle infant.

Toddlers and School-Aged Children

1. Posterogluteal injection—upper outer quadrant
 a. Gluteal muscles do not develop until a child begins to walk; they should be used only when the child has been walking for 1 year or more. Complications include sciatic nerve injury or subcutaneous injury due to medication being injected, and poor absorption.
 b. Upper outer quadrant of the young child's buttock is smaller in diameter than that of an adult; thus accuracy in determining the area comprising the upper outer quadrant is essential.
 c. Administration
 (i) Do not use a needle longer than 2.5 cm (1 inch).
 (ii) Position the child in a prone position.
 (iii) Place thumb on the trochanter.
 (iv) Place middle finger on the iliac crest.
 (v) Let index finger drop at a point midway between the thumb and middle finger to the upper outer quadrant of the buttock. This is the injection site.
 (vi) Insert needle perpendicular to the surface on which the child is lying, not to the skin.
2. Ventrogluteal injection
 a. May be used for the older child who is difficult to restrain.
 b. See description and administration (p. 1281).
3. Deltoid injection
 a. May be used for older, larger children.
 b. Inaccurate site injection can result in damage to the radial nerve or brachial artery.
 c. Determine injection site by palpating the acromion process of the shoulder and imagining an inverted triangle 2.5 to 5 fingerbreadths down from the acromion process.
 d. Inject needle perpendicular to skin 2 to 3 cm deep.
4. Lateral and anterior aspect of the thigh
 a. Do not use a needle longer than 2.5 cm (1 inch).
 b. Use the upper outer quadrant of the thigh.
 c. Insert needle at 45-degree angle in a downward direction, toward the knee.
5. Nursing support of toddlers and older children
 a. Explain to the child where you are going to give the injection (site) and why you are giving it.
 b. Allow the child to express fears.
 c. Carry out procedure quickly and gently. Have needle and syringe completely prepared and ready before contact with child.
 d. Numb site of injection by rubbing skin firmly with cleansing swab or with ice (older children may assist with this). Minimize pain of IM injection by injecting needle into muscle with a quick, darting motion.
 e. Always secure the assistance of a second nurse to help immobilize the child and divert attention as well as to offer support and comfort.
 f. Praise the child for behavior after the injection. Often, allowing the child to assist with applying a Band-Aid will give some feeling of comfort.
 g. Also encourage activity that will use the muscle site of the injection—promotes dispersal of medication and decreases soreness. This can also be done by firmly massaging muscle after injection, unless contraindicated.
 h. Record accurately the injection site to ensure proper site rotation.

Intravenous Medications

1. Administration of intravenous (IV) medications may be done through a variety of techniques, including piggyback, through a heparin lock, through a volume control set, or through an implantable port. See pages 89 to 91 for information on these techniques.
2. Prepare mixtures aseptically (laminar-flow hood), and use sterile technique when violating the line. (Sepsis is a constant threat when a child is receiving IV medications.)
3. Be aware that an exaggerated pharmacologic effect may exist with IV medications. As with any medication, know the use, side effects, and toxic effects of the drug, as well as the pharmacologic effect on the body.
4. Dilute IV medications and inject slowly—never less than 1 minute (this allows peripheral blood flow through the entire circulating system to dilute the medication and prevent high concentrations of the drug from reaching the brain and heart).
5. Be knowledgeable regarding compatibilities of drugs, electrolytes in IV solutions, and the fluid itself.
6. Observe IV site frequently. Restrain child, as needed, to prevent infiltration. Infiltration of fluids containing medications can cause rapid and severe tissue necrosis.

SPECIAL CONSIDERATIONS IN PEDIATRIC PRIMARY CARE

■ Acute Poisoning

Exposure to poisons can occur by ingestion, inhalation, or skin or mucous membrane contact. This section focuses on the most common poisoning, toxic ingestions.

Poisoning by ingestion refers to the oral intake of a harmful substance that, even in small amount, can damage tissues, disturb bodily functions, and possibly cause death. The substances may include medications such as *acetaminophen* and *iron*; household products; and plants. More than 80% of poisonings occur in the home. Poisoning accounts for approximately 10% to 20% of emergency department visits, of which a high majority are pediatric patients.

Pathophysiology and Etiology
1. Improper or dangerous storage of potentially toxic substances.
2. Poor lighting—causes errors in reading.
3. Human factors:
   a. Failure to read label properly
   b. Failure to return poisons to their proper place
   c. Failure to recognize the material as poisonous
   d. Lack of supervision of the child
   e. Purposeful use of poison
4. Toxin is ingested and may have limited local effects or continue to a stage of absorption and interference with metabolic processes and organ function.
5. Most often occurs in children under 5 years of age, with a peak incidence at 2 years of age.
6. Acute poisoning may result in arrhythmias or permanent multiorgan damage due to initial loss of airway, breathing, circulation, and specific organ toxicity.

Poisoning With Acetaminophen
Acetaminophen is a common drug-poisoning agent in children due to its replacement of salicylates. Ingestion by adolescents is frequently intentional.
Clinical Manifestations
1. Acetaminophen is toxic to the liver, resulting in cell necrosis and possibly cell death.
2. First 24 hours after ingestion:
   a. May be asymptomatic
   b. Anorexia
   c. Nausea and vomiting
   d. Diaphoresis
   e. Malaise
   f. Pallor
3. 24 to 48 hours:
   a. Above symptoms diminish or disappear
   b. Right upper quadrant pain due to liver damage
   c. Elevated liver function tests
   d. Oliguria
4. Days 3 to 8:
   a. Peak liver function abnormalities
   b. Anorexia, nausea, vomiting, and malaise may reappear
5. Days 4 to 14:
   a. Blood chemistry returns to normal

Diagnostic Evaluation
1. Serum acetaminophen level 4 hours after ingestion
Note: Children under 6 years of age are unlikely to develop significant toxicity even with large doses of acetaminophen. Adolescents have higher incidences of toxic acetaminophen levels with markedly elevated liver enzymes.
2. Serial liver function tests
Management
1. Syrup of ipecac
2. Gastric lavage
3. Charcoal
4. n-Acetylcysteine (Mucomyst) as antidote—if charcoal is given, lavage it out before giving Mucomyst.
5. As with all poisons, airway, breathing, circulation, and treatment of shock are always the priority in management.

Iron Poisoning
This occurs frequently in childhood due to the prevalence of iron-containing preparations. The severity of iron poisoning is related to the amount of elemental iron absorbed. The range of potential toxicity is approximately 50 to 60 mg/kg.
Clinical Manifestations
1. 30 minutes to 2 hours after ingestion:
   a. Local necrosis and hemorrhage of GI tract
   b. Nausea and vomiting, including hematemesi.
   c. Abdominal pain
   d. Diarrhea, often bloody
   e. Severe hypotension
   f. Symptoms subside after 6 to 12 hours
2. 6 to 24 hours—period of apparent recovery
3. 24 to 40 hours:
   a. Systemic toxicity with cardiovascular collapse, shock, hepatic and renal failure, seizures, coma, and possible death
   b. Metabolic acidosis
4. 2 to 4 weeks after ingestion:
   a. Pyloric and duodenal stenosis
   b. Hepatic cirrhosis
Diagnostic Evaluation
1. Measurement of serum free iron
   a. Total serum iron
   b. Total serum iron-binding capacity
2. Abdominal x-ray to visualize iron tablets
Management
1. Administration of ipecac to induce vomiting
2. Gastric lavage
3. Administration of deferoxamine (Desferal) for severe cases—binds with iron

Primary Assessment in Acute Poisoning
1. Initial assessment should include level of consciousness, vital signs, and neurologic assessment.

2. Assess for symptomatic effects of poisoning by systems.
   a. GI—common in metallic acid, alkali, and bacterial poisoning. These may include nausea and vomiting, diarrhea, abdominal pain or cramping, and anorexia.
   b. CNS—may include convulsions (especially with CNS depressants such as alcohol, chloral hydrate, barbiturates) and behavioral changes. Dilated or pinpoint pupils may be noted.
   c. Skin—rashes, burns to the mouth, esophagus and stomach, eye inflammation, skin irritations, stains around the mouth, lesions of the mucous membranes. Cyanosis may be visible, especially with cyanide and strychnine.
   d. Cardiopulmonary—dyspnea (especially with aspiration of hydrocarbons) and cardiopulmonary depression or arrest.
   e. Other—odor around the mouth.
3. Identify the poison when possible.
   a. Determine the nature of the ingested substances from the child's history or by reading the label on the container. Nursing intervention may need to be implemented immediately after this assessment.
      (i) Call the nearest poison control center or toxicology section of the medical examiner's office to identify the toxic ingredient and obtain recommendations for emergency treatment.
      (ii) Save vomitus, stool, and urine for analysis once the child reaches the hospital.

Primary Interventions
Assisting the Family by Telephone Management
1. Calmly obtain and record the following information:
   a. Name, address, and telephone number of caller
   b. Evaluation of the severity of the ingestion
   c. Age, weight, and signs/symptoms of the child, including neurologic status
   d. Route of exposure
   e. Name of the ingested product, approximate amount ingested, and time of ingestion
   f. Brief past medical history
   g. Caller's relationship to victim
2. Instruct the caller regarding appropriate emergency actions.
3. Direct the patient to the nearest emergency department. Dispatch an ambulance if necessary.
4. Instruct the caller to clear the child's mouth of any unswallowed poison.
5. Identify what treatments have already been initiated.

6. Instruct the parents to save vomitus, unswallowed liquid or pills, and the container and to bring them to the hospital as aids in identifying the poison.
7. Identify whether other children were involved in the poisoning to initiate treatment for them also.
8. If treatment is at home, follow-up phone calls should be made at ½, 1, and 4 hours after exposure.

Intervening Related to the Patient's Condition
Support airway, breathing, and circulation as needed.
Removing the Poison From the Body
1. Dilute with 6 to 8 oz of water if advised, by having patient drink water.
2. For skin or eye contact, remove contaminated clothing and flush with water for 15 to 20 minutes.
3. For inhalation poisons, remove from the exposed site.
4. Induce vomiting unless contraindicated.

   a. For children over 6 months of age, administer syrup of ipecac according to the directions on the label.
   b. If no vomiting occurs after 20 to 30 minutes, repeat this process one time only.
   c. Position the child with head down or on side to prevent aspiration of vomitus.

5. Administer gastric lavage. (This is indicated when vomiting is impossible because of the child's condition or age, when induction of vomiting has been unsuccessful, or when the poison is one that is rapidly absorbed [eg, cyanide].)
6. Follow lavage with a cathartic and activated charcoal to hasten removal of the poison from the GI tract. Use cautiously with young children.
7. Be aware of the dangers associated with lavage.
   a. Esophageal perforation—may occur in corrosive poisoning

b. Gastric hemorrhage

c. Impaired pulmonary function resulting from aspiration

d. Cardiac arrest

e. Convulsions—may result from stimulation in strychnine ingestion

Reducing the Effect of the Poison by Administering an Antidote

1. An antidote may either react with the poison to prevent its absorption or counteract the effects of the poison after its absorption.

2. Not all poisons have specific antidotes.

3. Information regarding appropriate antidotes for specific poisons is available through all poison control centers. Antidotes for the most common poisons should be listed in the emergency department of the hospital.

4. Effectiveness of the antidote usually depends on the amount of time that elapses between ingestion of the poisons and administration of the antidote.

5. Activated charcoal absorbs all poisons except cyanide, if given within 1 hour of poisoning and after vomiting has occurred, in a dose of 30 to 50 g in a child and 50 to 100 g in an adolescent in 175 to 250 mL (6 to 8 oz) of water with sweetener.

6. Charcoal inactivates ipecac; therefore, administer charcoal only after ipecac has induced vomiting.

Eliminating the Absorbed Poison

1. Force diuresis.

   a. Administer large quantities of fluid either orally or IV.

   b. Carefully monitor intake and output.

2. Assist with kidney dialysis, which may be necessary if the child's own kidneys are not functioning effectively.

3. Assist with exchange transfusion if this method is indicated for removing the poison.

Providing Emotional Support

1. Remain calm and efficient while working rapidly.

2. Reassure child and family that therapeutic measures are being taken immediately.

3. Discourage anxious parents from holding, caressing, and overstimulating child.

Subsequent Nursing Assessment and Interventions

Observing the Child for Progression of Symptoms

1. CNS involvement

   a. Observe for restlessness, confusion, delirium, seizures, lethargy, stupor, or coma.

   b. Administer sedation with caution—to avoid CNS depression and masking of symptoms.

   c. Avoid excessive manipulation of the child.

   d. See nursing care of the child with seizures, page 1417.

   e. See nursing care of the unconscious patient, Chapter 15.

2. Respiratory involvement

   a. Observe for respiratory depression, obstruction, pulmonary edema, pneumonia, or tachypnea.

   b. Have artificial airway and tracheostomy set available.

   c. Be prepared to administer oxygen and provide artificial respiration.

   d. Other nursing concerns:

      (i) Nursing care for mechanical ventilation, page 1371.

      (ii) Procedures for administration of oxygen, page 1373.

      (iii) Procedure for cardiopulmonary resuscitation, page 1336.

3. Cardiovascular involvement

   a. Observe for peripheral circulatory collapse, disturbances of heart rate and rhythm, or cardiac failure.

   b. Maintain IV therapy as directed to prevent shock. Assess for complications of overhydration.

   c. Be prepared for cardiac arrest.

4. GI involvement

   a. Observe for nausea, pain, abdominal distention, and difficulty swallowing.

   b. Maintain IV therapy to replace water and electrolyte losses.

   c. Offer a diet that is easily swallowed and digested.

      (i) Begin with clear liquids.

      (ii) Progress to full liquids, soft foods, and then a regular diet as the child's condition improves.

5. Kidney involvement

   a. Observe the child for decreased urine output. Record oral and IV intake and urine output exactly.

   b. Observe for hypertension.

   c. Insert indwelling catheter if necessary for urinary retention.

   d. Administer appropriate amounts of fluids and electrolytes.

   e. See nursing care of child with renal failure, page 1011.

   f. Correct and monitor acid–base balance.

Providing Supportive Care

1. Maintain adequate caloric, fluid, and vitamin intake. Oral fluids are preferable if they can be retained.

2. Avoid hypothermia or hyperthermia. (Control of body temperature is impaired in many types of poisoning.) Monitor the child's temperature frequently.

3. Observe closely for inflammation and tissue irritation.

   a. This is especially important in ingestion of kerosene or other hydrocarbons, which cause chemical pneumonitis.

   b. Isolate the patient from other children, especially those with respiratory infections.

   c. Administer antibiotics as prescribed by the physician.

4. Counsel parents who often feel guilty about the accident.

   a. Encourage parents to talk about the poisoning.

   b. Emphasize how their quick action in getting treatment for the child has helped.

   c. Discuss ways that they can be supportive to their child during the hospitalization.

d. Do not allow prolonged periods of self-incrimination to continue. Refer parents to a psychologist for assistance in resolving these feelings if necessary.
5. Involve the young child in therapeutic play to determine how he or she views the situation.
   a. The child often sees nursing measures as punishments for misdeed involving the poisoning.
   b. Explain treatment and correct misinterpretations in a manner appropriate for child's age.
6. Initiate a community health nursing referral for any childhood poisoning incident. A home assessment should be made to identify problems and provide proper poisoning prevention interventions and education.

Family Education and Health Maintenance
Stressing Prevention

1. Information concerning poison prevention should be available on every hospital pediatric unit and during every child health care visit.
   a. Many free booklets and home safety checklists are available from sources such as insurance companies and drug companies.
   b. Teaching may be done with any parent regardless of the reason for the child's hospitalization or office visit.
2. Teach the following precautions:
   a. Keep medicines and poisons out of reach of children.
   b. Provide locked storage for highly toxic substances; select cabinet that is higher than child can reach or climb.
   c. Do not store poisons in the same areas as foods.
   d. Be certain all containers are properly marked and labeled. Keep medicines, drugs, and household chemicals in their original containers.
   e. Do not discard poisonous substances in receptacles where children can reach them, but do discard used containers of poisonous substances.
   f. Teach children not to taste or eat unfamiliar substances.
   g. Clean out medicine cabinets periodically.
   h. Keep medications in childproof containers that are securely closed.
   i. Read all labels carefully before each use.
   j. Do not give medicines prescribed for one child to another.
   k. Never refer to drugs as candy or bribe children with such inducements.
   l. Never give or take medications in the dark.
   m. Encourage parents not to take medication in front of young children because children role-play adult behavior.
   n. Suggest that mothers avoid keeping medications in their purses or on the kitchen table.
   o. Keep baby creams and ointments away from young children.
   p. Never puncture or burn aerosol containers.
   q. Store lawn and garden pesticides in a separate place under lock and key outside of the house; do not store large quantities of cleaning products, pesticides, and so forth.
3. Advise parents to keep a 30-mL (1-oz) bottle of ipecac syrup in the home and become familiar with how to use it. Their day care providers and babysitters should do the same.
4. Tell family to keep a list of emergency telephone numbers including the poison control center, health care provider's number, nearest hospital, and ambulance service.
5. Reinforce the need for vigilance and consistent supervision of infants and young children due to their increased mobility, increased curiosity, and increased dexterity.

Teaching Emergency Actions

1. Suspect poisoning with the occurrence of sudden, bizarre symptoms or peculiar behavior in toddlers and preschoolers.
2. Read label on the ingested product, or call the health care provider, hospital, or poison control center for instructions regarding treatment for the poisoning. Give all relevant information about the child, condition, and substance taken.
3. Maintain an adequate airway in a child who is convulsing or who is not fully conscious.
4. Dilute the poison with 6 to 8 oz of water if advised.
5. Make the child vomit if so directed. Do not induce vomiting if any of the following occurs:
   a. The child is unconscious or convulsing.
   b. Ingested poison was a strong corrosive such as lye or drain cleaner.
   c. Ingested poison contains gasoline, kerosene, or other petroleum distillates.
6. Directions for making the child vomit:
   a. Administer 1 tablespoon of ipecac syrup with 250 mL (1 cup) of warm water.
   b. If vomiting does not occur in 20 minutes, this dose may be repeated once only.
7. Transport the child promptly to the nearest medical facility.
   a. Wrap the child in a blanket to prevent chilling.
   b. Bring the container and any vomitus or urine to the hospital with the child.
8. Avoid excessive manipulation of the child.
9. Act promptly but calmly.
10. Do not assume the child is safe simply because the emesis shows no trace of the poison or because the child appears well. The poison may have produced a delayed reaction or may have reached the small intestine where it is still being absorbed.

■ Lead Poisoning

There are approximately 1 million children with elevated blood lead levels (>10 μg/dL) in the United States. Lead poisoning, referred to as *plumbism,* results from some form of lead consumption. Blood lead levels that exceed 10 µg/dL can affect intellectual functioning in children.

Millions of children live in housing built before 1950, which contains the highest surface soil level and internal household dust contaminated with lead. Normal hand-to-mouth activities of children may introduce leaded household dust, soil, and nonfood items into their GI tract. Pica (eating nonfood substances, particularly leaded paint chips) is generally associated with more severe degrees of poisoning.

Pathophysiology and Etiology
Etiologic Factors
1. Multiple episodes of chewing on, sucking, or ingestion of nonfood substances (pica).
   a. Toys, furniture, windowsills, household fixtures, and plaster painted with lead-containing paint

> **NURSING ALERT**
>
> Legislation stipulates that toys, children's furniture, and the interior of homes be painted with lead-free paint; however, the problem arises when deeper layers of paint and plaster on older products are contaminated with lead. One paint chip contains much more lead than is considered safe.

   b. Cigarette butts and ashes
   c. Acidic juices or foods served in lead-based earthenware pottery made with lead glazes
   d. Colored paints used in newspapers, magazines, children's books, matches, playing cards, and food wrappers
   e. Water from lead pipes
   f. Fruit covered with insecticides
   g. Dirt containing lead fallout from automobile exhaust
   h. Antique pewter, especially when used to serve acidic juices or foods
   i. Lead weights (curtain weights, fishing sinkers)
   j. Continuous proximity to lead-processing center
   k. Occupations or hobbies that use lead
2. Inhalation of fumes containing lead (less common cause in children).
   a. Leaded gasoline
   b. Burning storage batteries
   c. Dust containing lead salts
   d. Dust in the air at shooting galleries and in enclosed firing ranges with poor ventilation
   e. Cigarette smoke
3. Highest incidence in children between 1 and 6 years of age, especially those between 1 and 3 years.
   a. High incidence in individuals living in old homes or deteriorated housing conditions
   b. No significant difference in incidence by sex
   c. High incidence among siblings

4. Symptomatic lead poisoning occurs most frequently in summer months.

Systemic Effects
1. Lead absorption from GI tract is affected by age, diet, and nutritional deficiency. Young children absorb 40% to 50% and retain 20% to 25% of dietary lead.
2. It takes the body twice as long to excrete lead as it does to absorb lead.
3. Lead is stored in two places in the body:
   a. Bone
   b. Soft tissue
4. Principal toxic effects occur in nervous system, bone marrow, and kidneys.
5. Nervous system.
   a. Brain—increased capillary permeability results in edema, increased intracranial pressure, and vascular damage; destruction of brain cells causes seizures, mental retardation, paralysis, blindness, and learning disabilities.
   b. Neurologic damage cannot be reversed.
   c. CNS of young children and fetuses is most sensitive to lead.
6. Bone marrow.
   a. Lead attaches to red blood cells.
   b. Inhibition of a number of steps in the biosynthesis of heme, thus reducing the number of red blood cells, increasing fragility, and reducing half-life.
   c. The decreased production of hemoglobin results in anemia and respiratory distress.
7. Kidneys—injury to the cells of the proximal tubules, causing increased excretion of amino acids, protein, glucose, and phosphate.
8. Recurrence rate is high, especially if lead is not removed from the home environment.

Clinical Manifestations
Symptoms in young children may develop insidiously and may abate spontaneously.
1. GI—anorexia, sporadic vomiting, intermittent abdominal pain (colic), constipation
2. CNS—hyperirritability; decreased activity; personality changes; loss of recently acquired developmental skills; falling, clumsiness, loss of coordination (ataxia); local paralysis; peripheral nerve palsies
3. Hematologic—anemia, pallor
4. Cardiovascular—hypertension, bradycardia

Diagnostic Evaluation
1. Detailed history with emphasis on the presence or absence of clinical symptoms, evidence of pica, family history of lead poisoning, possible source of exposure to lead, recent change in behavior, developmental delay, or behavior problems, recent change of address, or recent renovations in the home.
2. Assess serum lead level and repeat confirmatory levels (Table 42-4).

TABLE 42-4 Interpretation of Blood Lead Test Results and Follow-up Activities

Class	Blood Lead Concentrations ($\mu g/dL$)	Comment
I	≤9	A child in class I is not considered to be lead poisoned.
IIA	10–14	Many children (or a large proportion of children) with blood lead levels in this range should trigger community-wide childhood lead poisoning prevention activities. Children in this range may need to be rescreened more frequently.
IIB	15–19	A child in class IIB should receive nutritional and educational interventions and more frequent screening. If the blood level persists in this range, environmental investigation and intervention should be done.
III	20–44	A child in class III should receive environmental evaluation and remediation and a medical evaluation. Such a child may need pharmacologic treatment of lead poisoning.
IV	45–69	A child in class IV will need both medical and environmental interventions, including chelation therapy.
V	≥70	A child with class V lead poisoning is a medical emergency. Medical and environmental management must begin immediately.

(From Centers for Disease Control. [1991]. *Preventing lead poisoning in young children.* Atlanta, GA: US Department of Health and Human Services, Public Health Service.)

3. Hematologic evaluation for iron deficiency anemia.
4. Flat plate of abdomen—may reveal radiopaque material if lead has been ingested during the preceding 24 to 36 hours.
5. Erythrocyte protoporphyrin level—not sensitive enough for identifying lead levels below approximately 25 mg/dL. Can be used to follow levels after medical and environmental interventions for poisoned children have occurred. A progressive decline in erythrocyte protoporphyrin levels indicates management is successful.
6. 24-hour urine—more accurate than a single voided specimen in determining elevated urinary components that correspond with elevated blood lead levels.
7. Radiologic examination of long bones—unreliable for diagnosis of acute lead poisoning; may provide some indication of past lead poisoning or length of time poisoning has occurred.
8. Edetate calcium disodium provocation chelation test—used only in selected medical centers treating large numbers of lead-poisoned children; demonstrates increased lead levels in urine over an 8-hour period after injection of edetate disodium.

Management
Removal of Lead From the Environment
1. Remove leaded paint/paint chips or objects containing lead from the child's environment.
2. Remove child from environment during lead abatement process.
Low-Fat, High-Iron Diet
1. Iron supplements may be needed to correct associated anemia.
2. Reduced fat diet and small frequent meals will reduce the GI absorption of lead.

Chelation Therapy
1. Chelation therapy is indicated in children with blood lead levels (BPb) between 45 and 70 µg/dL. Children with 70 BPb or higher levels should be hospitalized immediately and started on the most aggressive chelation therapy available.
2. Ethylenediaminetetraacetic acid (EDTA), British anti-Lewisite (BAL), and succimer (Chemet) bind with lead in the blood to form nontoxic compounds that are excreted by bowel and kidney.
3. Effectiveness of therapy depends on degree and duration of lead poisoning.
4. BAL is given first to decrease the chance of seizures.
   a. Used alone in patients with encephalopathy.
   b. Do not give with iron supplements, and avoid in patients with plant allergies.
   c. Avoid in patients with glucose-6-phosphate dehydrogenase (G6PD) deficiency due to potential for hemolysis.
   d. Administered deep IM—results in pain and tissue necrosis at the injection site.
5. EDTA may be toxic to the kidneys.
   a. Monitor urinary output as well as renal and liver function studies.
   b. Administer IV.
6. Chemet—approved for use in 1991.
   a. Not given to patients with encephalopathy.
   b. Administer orally.
   c. Monitor hematologic parameters.
7. Dosage—depends on individual drug, the child's weight, severity of poisoning, prior history, and whether other chelating agents are being used simultaneously.

8. Chelating drugs are usually given every 4 hours for 5 days. A second course of therapy may be needed if there is a rebound in the blood lead level.

9. Increased oral and IV fluids are given to enhance excretion, except if increased intracranial pressure is present.

10. d-Penicillamine (Depen), another drug that chelates heavy metals, may be given for long-term chelation only if current exposure to lead is definitely excluded. If this drug is used, it should be given on an empty stomach, 2 hours before breakfast.

Additional Treatment

1. Supplemental calcium, phosphorus, and vitamin D to help lead move from the blood (where it is toxic) to the bones (where it is nontoxic).

2. For the child with encephalopathy, corticosteroids are given and intensive care management is maintained until acute stage is resolved.

Complications

1. Severe and often permanent mental, emotional, and physical impairment

2. Neurologic deficits
   a. Learning disabilities
   b. Mental retardation
   c. Seizures
   d. Encephalopathy

Nursing Assessment

1. Partake in primary prevention through screening for lead poisoning—should target high-risk groups. This includes children:
   a. Who live in homes built before 1950
   b. With iron deficiency anemia
   c. Who are exposed to contaminated dust or soil
   d. Who have developmental delays
   e. Who are victims of abuse or neglect
   f. Whose parents are exposed to lead
   g. Who live in low-income families

2. Also universal screening of children who live in communities with >27% houses built before 1950 or in populations where ≥12% of the children have elevated lead levels.

3. Assess all children for signs of lead toxicity, including hyperactivity, developmental delay, constipation, anorexia, colicky abdominal pain, clumsiness, and pallor.

4. Inquire about presence of pica behavior in all children under 6 years of age.

5. Assess the child's level of development. The Denver Developmental Screening Test (DDST) may be useful for this purpose (see p. 1234) and will help detect delays possibly caused by lead poisoning.

Nursing Diagnoses

• Risk for Injury related to seizures and encephalopathy
• Pain related to chelation therapy injections

• Altered Growth and Development related to the effects of chronic lead exposure
• Compromised Family Coping related to guilt and concern for child

Nursing Interventions

Protecting the Child With Seizures and Encephalopathy

1. Maintain seizure precautions.
   a. Crib or bed rails elevated and padded
   b. Tongue blade and suction equipment at bedside

2. Be aware that encephalopathy may occur 4 to 6 weeks after first symptoms:
   a. Sudden onset of persistent vomiting
   b. Severe ataxia
   c. Altered state of consciousness
   d. Coma
   e. Seizures
   f. Massive cerebral edema in younger children

3. Observe for signs of increased intracranial pressure in the child with encephalopathy:
   a. Rising blood pressure
   b. Papilledema
   c. Slow pulse
   d. Seizures
   e. Unconsciousness

4. Provide supportive care to maintain vital functions.

Reducing Pain Associated With Chelation Therapy

1. Plan appropriate play activities to prepare the child for the injections and as an outlet for pain and anger child feels.

2. Implement measures to decrease pain at injection site.
   a. Rotate sites of injection.
   b. Apply warm packs to site to decrease pain.
   c. Move painful areas slowly.

3. Provide diversion activities, fluids, and meals between injections.

4. Monitor intake and output and blood studies such as electrolytes and liver and kidney function tests as directed.

Promoting Growth and Development

1. Provide and encourage activities that will help the child to learn and progress from present developmental state to meet next appropriate milestone.

2. Initiate appropriate referrals in cases of obvious developmental delays or learning difficulties. Such referrals may be to such professionals as psychologists, psychiatrists, and specialists in early child education.

3. Share the results of developmental testing with the parent(s), and discuss ways to provide stimulation for the child at home.

Strengthening Family Coping

1. Use sensitivity in interviewing and teaching to avoid causing or increasing guilt feelings about the poisoning and to establish a positive, trusting relationship between the family and the health care facility.

2. Explain the treatment and its purpose because parents are frequently faced with putting an asymptomatic child through painful treatments.
3. Encourage frequent visits by parents and siblings, and facilitate family involvement.

Community and Home Care Considerations

1. Coordinate community care efforts to return the child to a safe home. Communicate with community outreach workers so that environmental case management is conducted. Lead abatement must be conducted by experts, not untrained parents, property owners, or contractors.
2. Suggest periodic, focused household cleaning to remove the lead dust; use a wet mop.
3. Encourage handwashing before meals and at bedtime to eliminate lead consumption from normal hand-to-mouth activity.
4. Observe the child and other children in the home for pica.
   a. Observe and record the child's eating habits and food preferences.
   b. Report any attempted eating of nonfood substances.
   c. Encourage the caregivers to provide regular meals and make mealtime a pleasurable time for the child.
   d. Teach the caregivers to discourage oral activity and substitute activity that contributes to play, social skills, and ego development.
   e. Refer the family for additional social or psychiatric casework if indicated to reduce the economic and other factors that result in pica in the child.
5. Screen siblings and playmates of known cases immediately.
6. Make certain that the family is able to provide close supervision of the child or assist them to make arrangements to ensure that the child is adequately supervised at home.

Family Education and Health Maintenance
Ensuring Long-Term Follow-Up

1. Teach the parents why long-term follow-up is important. Tell them that residual lead is liberated gradually after treatment and:
   a. May result in the renewal of symptoms
   b. May increase serum lead to a dangerous level
   c. May cause additional damage to the CNS, which may not become apparent for several months
2. Stress that acute infections must be recognized and treated promptly because these may reactivate the disease.
3. Teach that iron supplementation may be continued to treat anemia. Advise on administration and side effects and periodic complete blood count monitoring.

Preventing Reexposure of the Child to Lead

1. Advise parents that the single most important factor in managing childhood lead poisoning is reducing the child's reexposure to lead.

NURSING ALERT

Children should not return home until their home environment is lead free.

2. Instruct parents regarding the seriousness of repeated lead exposure.
3. Initiate referrals to home health nursing and community agencies as indicated.

Providing Community Education

1. Initiate and support educational campaigns through schools, day care centers, and news media to alert parents and children to hazards and symptoms of lead poisoning.
2. Provide in clinics, waiting rooms, and other appropriate settings literature stressing the hazards of lead, sources of lead, and signs of lead intoxication.
3. Support legislation to study the nature and extent of the lead poisoning problem and to eliminate the causes of lead poisoning.
4. Include the topic of pica and lead poisoning in nutritional teaching.
5. For additional information, contact the state or local health department or Centers for Disease Control and Prevention (*www.cdc.gov*).

Outcome-Based Evaluation

- Seizure precautions maintained; no signs of increased intracranial pressure
- Tolerating chelation therapy injections; expressing anger through doll play
- Parents providing appropriate play and stimulation for development
- Family involved in care; providing support to the child

Communicable Diseases

With the dramatic success of immunizations, many childhood diseases have decreased in frequency. However, a number of communicable diseases still cause significant morbidity in children (Table 42-5).

Child Abuse and Neglect

Child abuse is any type of maltreatment of children or adolescents by their parents, guardians, or caretakers. Child abuse includes physical or emotional abuse, injury, trauma, neglect, or sexual abuse of a child that is intentional and nonaccidental. Abuse includes:

- Battering—physical injury
- Drug abuse—intentional administration of harmful drugs, especially during pregnancy
- Sexual abuse
- Sexual assault or molestation (non-family member)
- Incest (family offender)
- Emotional abuse—scapegoating, belittling, humiliating, lack of mothering

Neglect is omission of certain appropriate behaviors, with such omission having detrimental physical or psychological effects on development. Neglect includes:
- Child abandonment
- Lack of provision of the basic needs of survival: shelter, clothing, stimulation, medical care, food, love, supervision, education, attention, emotional nurturing, and safety

Etiology and Incidence

The cause of child abuse and maltreatment is multidimensional. The abuse may be related to the combined presence of three factors: special kind of child, special kind of parent or caretaker, special circumstances of crisis. Abuse occurs in all ethnic, geographic, religious, educational, occupational, and socioeconomic groups.
1. In 1996, 3 million cases were reported, and 1 million child abuse cases were confirmed.
2. The most common type of abuse is neglect (60% of cases), followed by physical abuse (23%), sexual abuse (9%), emotional maltreatment (4%), and other forms of abuse (4%).
3. Each year, 4,000 children die from abuse.

Contributing Factors

1. Incidents of child abuse may develop as a result of disciplinary action taken by the abuser who responds in uncontrolled anger to real or perceived misconduct of the child. The parents may confuse punishment with discipline. "Good parenting" may be equated with physical contact to eradicate child behavior. The abuser may be a stern, authoritarian disciplinarian.
2. Incidents of child abuse may develop out of a quarrel between caretakers. The child may come to the aid of one parent, may find himself or herself in the midst of the quarrel; marital discord is common.
3. The abuser may be under a great deal of stress because of life circumstances (debt, poverty, illness) and may thus resort to child abuse. Crisis and stress may be ongoing. The abuser may have a low frustration tolerance level and may not have well-developed means of coping with stress in general.
4. The abuser may be intoxicated with alcohol or drugs at the time of the abuse; only 10% of abusers have a history of mental illness.
5. Child abuse frequently occurs while the mother is away from the home and the child is left in the care of a babysitter or boyfriend.
6. Lack of effective parenting, inappropriate parent–child bonding, and punitive treatment as a child may contribute to the parent becoming an abuser.
7. Specific characteristics evident in many abusing parents include:
   a. Low self-esteem—a sense of incompetence in role, unworthiness, unimportance, have difficulty controlling aggressive impulses, and often live in social isolation.
   b. Unrealistic attitudes and expectations of child, little regard for the child's own needs and age-appropriate abilities, lack of knowledge related to parenting skills.
   c. Fear of rejection—a deep need to feel wanted and loved, but a feeling of rejection when love is not obvious; a crying infant may elicit a feeling of rejection.
   d. Inability to accept help—isolation from the community, loneliness.
   e. Unhappiness due to unsatisfactory relationships; may look to child for satisfaction of own emotional needs.
   f. Child abusers are often the children of abuse or victims of spousal abuse.
8. Incidents of child abuse may develop from a general attitude or resentment or rejection on the part of the abuser toward the child.
9. Atypical child behavior (eg, hyperactivity or a technology-dependent child who needs additional care) may unintentionally provoke the abuser.
10. The degree of the family crisis is not usually in proportion to the degree of abuse.

Clinical Manifestations
Characteristics of the Child
That Should Raise Suspicion

1. Child usually under 3 years of age. School-aged children and adolescents are also subject to abuse. The average age of a sexually abused child is 9 years.
2. General health of child indicates neglect (diaper rash, poor hygiene, malnutrition, unattended physical problem).
3. Characteristic distribution of fractures (scattered over many parts of body).
4. Disproportionate amount of soft tissue injury.
5. Evidence that injuries occurred at different times (healed and new fractures, resolving and fresh bruises).
6. Cause of recent trauma in question.
7. History of similar episodes in the past.
8. No new lesions occurring during the child's stay in hospital.
9. May show a wide range of reactions—may be either very withdrawn or overactive. The child may be anxious, tense, or nervous.
10. Child may show unusual affection for strangers or may be overly fearful of adults and avoid any physical contact with them.
11. For sexual abuse: child may fear no one will believe him or her; may experience self-blame; most know their abuser.
12. Children may not "tell" about abuse from parents, fearing loss of security; "a bad parent is better than no parent at all."

TABLE 42-5 Childhood Diseases

Disease	Incubation (I) and Communicability (C) Periods	Symptoms
Chickenpox a. Varicella-zoster b. Highly communicable; acquired in direct contact, droplet spread and airborne transmission c. 2–9 y; January to May Diagnostic tests: Tzanck smear shows multinucleated giant cells.	I: 11–21 d after exposure C: Onset of fever (1–2 d before first lesion) until last vesicle is dried (5–7 d)	a. General malaise, low-grade fever and anorexia for 24 h b. Rash—macules to papules and vesicles to crusts within several hours c. Pruritis of lesions may be severe, and scratching may cause scarring. Rash characteristics: Rash appears first on head and mucous membranes, then becomes concentrated on body and sparse on extremities, papulovesicular eruption.
Streptococcal pharyngitis a. β-Hemolytic streptococcus group A strain b. Direct or indirect contact with nasopharyngeal secretion of infected person or recently established carrier c. Rare under 3 y of age; 5–16 y; incidence higher in winter and spring Diagnostic tests: Nasopharyngeal (throat) culture; rapid diagnostic test.	I: 2–5 d C: Greatest during initial phase of illness	a. Onset is generally acute; high fever, headache, vomiting, chill b. After 12–24 h—some sore throat of varying degrees of severity, dry throat, anterior cervical lymphadenopathy, white tongue coating that becomes strawberry-red tongue, exudate on tonsils, scarlatina rash initially in axilla, groin, and neck area that becomes generalized.
Rubella (German 13-d measles) a. Rubella virus; RNA toga virus b. Oral droppler or transplacentally c. School age, young adults, spring, winter Diagnostic tests: Tissue culture of throat, blood or urine; latex agglutination, enzyme immunoassay, passive hemagglutination, fluorescent immunoassay tests Passive immunity: Birth to 6 months of age from maternal antibodies	I: 14–21 d after exposure C: Virus can be passed from 7 d before to 5 d after rash appears.	Enlarged lymph nodes in postauricular, auricular suboccipital, and cervical areas 24 h before rash develops Eranthem: discrete rose spots on soft palate Exanthem: variable, begins on face, spreads quickly over entire body; usually maculopapular; clears by third day.
Roseola Infantum (exanthem subitum) a. Human herpes virus-6 b. Transmission not known c. 6–18 months; late fall to early spring	I: 5–15 d C: Not known—believed not to be highly contagious	Fever of 39.4°–41.2°C (103°–106°F), either intermittent or sustained 3–4 d with no clinical findings Fever suddenly drops and macular or maculopapular rash develops on trunk, spreading to arms and neck; mild involvement of face and legs; rash fades quickly.
Rubeola (hard, red, 7-d measles) a. Measles virus, RNA-containing paramyxovirus b. Direct contact with droplets from infected persons, respiratory route Diagnostic tests: Serologic procedures not routinely done Passive immunity: Birth to 4–6 mo of age if mother is immune before pregnancy c. 5–10 y, adolescents; spring	I: 10–12 d C: 5th day of incubation to 4th day of rash	Fever, lethargy, cough, coryza, and conjunctivitis 2–3 d later; Koplik's spots on buccal pharyngeal mucosa (grayish white spots with reddish areolae), which disappear within 12–18 h 2 d later: maculopapular rash appears at hairline and spreads to feet in 1 d; rash begins to clear after 3–4 d.
Mumps a. Mumps virus, paramyxovirus b. Direct contact, airborne droplets, saliva, and possibly urine c. School age; all seasons but slightly more frequent in late winter and early spring	I: 14–21 d C: 7 d before to 9 d after swelling appears; virus in saliva greatest just before and after parotitis onset.	a. Headache, anorexia, generalized malaise; fever 1 d before glandular swelling; fever lasts 1–6 d. b. Glandular swelling usually of parotid—one side or bilaterally.

Treatment	Complications	Special Considerations
Symptomatic: Shorten fingernails to prevent scratching Daily antiseptic baths Oral antihistamines to decrease pruritus Treatment of itching: Baking soda (sodium bicarbonate) or oatmeal baths, Calamine lotion to lesions Isolation until all lesions have crusted Acyclovir (Zovirax) PO within first 24 h Avoid salicylates.	Complications are rare in normal children. Secondary bacterial infection of lesions Hemorrhagic varicella, pneumonia, encephalitis, and thrombocytopenia are not common, but they can occur. Reye's syndrome	Severe in neonate and pregnant women VZIG is available from American Red Cross for high-risk susceptible children who have been exposed to varicella zoster. High-risk children include those receiving corticosteroids or antimetabolites. Varicella vaccine is recommended for all children 12 months and older.

Isolation for 1 d while starting prescription
Antibiotic therapy:
  Penicillin G—IM
  Penicillin V—PO
Erythromycin (Pediazole)—if allergic to penicillin
Cephalosporins PO
	Acute glomerulonephritis, 1–2 wk after acute stage
	Rheumatic fever, 2–3 wk after acute stage
	Peritonsillar abscess, cervical adenitis
	Pneumonia, otitis media, meningitis, sinusitis, mastoiditis
	Erythrogenic toxin responsible for rash (scarlet fever). After 5–7 d, rash may subside but desquamation of skin on face, trunks, hands, and feet may persist for 4–6 wk.
		Throat cultures are considered for entire household when others are symptomatic concurrently or within past 3 wk; frequent or relapsing infections. Repeat throat cultures are recommended after treatment if child has history of rheumatic fever. Nonsymptomatic carriers have low risk for rheumatic fever and do not require treatment.

Symptomatic—isolation	In adolescent females: arthritis; arthralgias Encephalitis Thrombocytopenia	Exposure of nonimmune pregnant women in first trimester results in high percentage of affected fetuses and infants born with various birth defects: cataracts, deafness, growth retardation, congenital heart disease, mental retardation.
Symptomatic—antipyretic	Convulsions due to high fever Encephalitis (rare)	

Symptomatic:
  Sedatives
  Antipyretic
  Bed rest in humid, comfortably warm room
  Dark room for photophobia
  Adequate fluid
	Otitis media
	Pneumonia, laryngitis
	Mastoiditis, encephalitis
	Appendicitis	

Isolation until swelling has subsided
Symptomatic
  Analgesics
  Hydration
  Alimentation
  Antipyretics
  Rest
	Meningoencephalitis
	Orchitis, epididymitis
	Auditory nerve involvement, resulting in unilateral deafness	

(continued)

TABLE 42-5 Childhood Diseases (Continued)

Disease	Incubation (I) and Communicability (C) Periods	Symptoms
Diagnostic tests: Cell culture from saliva, urine, spinal fluid or blood Passive immunity: Birth to 6 mo of age if mother is immune before pregnancy		c. Enlargement and reddening of Wharton's duct and Stensen's duct d. Subclinical infection may occur.
Diphtheria a. *Corynebacterium diphtheriae* b. Acquired through secretions of carrier or infected individual by direct contact with contaminated articles and environment c. Incidence increased in autumn and winter Diagnostic tests: Cultures of nose and throat	I: 2–4 d C: 2–4 wk untreated; 1–2 d with antibiotic treatment	Nasal diphtheria (1) Coryza with increasing viscosity, possibly epistaxis, low-grade fever (2) Whitish gray membrane may appear over nasal septum. Pharyngeal and/or tonsillar diphtheria (1) General malaise, low-grade fever, anorexia (2) 1–2 d later, whitish gray membranous patch on tonsils, soft palate, and uvula (3) Lymph node swelling, fever, rapid pulse "bull neck" Laryngeal diphtheria (1) Usually spread from pharynx to larynx (2) Fever, harsh voice, stridor barking cough; respiratory difficulty with inspiratory retraction Nonrespiratory diphtheria: affects eye, ear, genitals, or, rarely, skin
Pertussis (Whooping Cough) a. *Bordetella pertussis* b. Direct contact or respiratory droplet spread c. Infants and young children; females > males Diagnostic tests: Culture of nasopharyngeal mucus	I: 3–12 d; mean of 7 d C: 7 d after exposure (greatest just before catarrhal stage) to 3 wk after onset of paroxysms or until cough has ceased	Stage I (catarrhal stage) (1) Lasts 1–2 wk (2) Rhinorrhea, conjunctival injection, lacrimation, mild cough and low-grade fever Stage II (paroxysmal stage) (1) Lasts 2–4 wk or longer (2) Frequent severe, violent coughing attacks occurring in clusters leading to vomiting, cyanosis, and exhaustion Stage III (convalescent stage) (1) Lasts 2 wk to several months (2) Coughing attacks decrease, but may return with each respiratory infection Duration: 9 mo to 2 y
Staphylococcal Scaled Skin Syndrome (Ritter Disease) Group II phage type *Staphylococcus aureus* Disseminated from a primary infection site (usually nose or around eyes) Infants and children under 10 y Diagnostic tests: Cultures of skin, conjunctiva, nasopharynx, stools and blood. Biopsy of exfoliated epidermis.	I: Few days C: Onset of rash until after antibiotics initiated	Malaise, fever, irritability or asymptomatic Rash develops in three phases: (1) Erythematous—macular involving face, neck, axilla, and groin (2) Exfoliative—upper layer of epidermis becomes wrinkled and can be removed by light stroking (Nikolsky sign); crusting around eyes, mouth, and nose produce characteristic "sunburst," radial pattern; irritable due to extreme tenderness of skin. (3) Desquamative—epidermis peels away leaving moist areas that dry quickly and heal in 10–14 d.
Poliomyelitis (polio) Virus serotypes 1, 2, and 3; incidence is higher in summer and fall Virus is harbored in gastrointestinal tract and is transmitted through saliva, vomitus, and feces.	I: 7–14 d, paralytic or nonparalytic; 3–5 d for prodromal or minor illness C: Increases around onset when virus is in throat and is excreted in feces; virus	Nonparalytic polio (1) Headache, lethargy, anorexia, vomiting, fever (2) Muscle pain and stiffness of posterior muscles, neck, and limbs

Treatment	Complications	Special Considerations

Diphtheria antitoxin IV
Antibiotic therapy (penicillin, erythromycin)
Supportive treatment:
  Respiratory support
  Isolation until three cultures are
    negative after antibiotic therapy is
    completed
  Bed rest for 2–3 wk
  Hydration
  Immunization with diphtheria toxoid
    after recovery
	Myocarditis
	Neuritis
	Paralysis
	Toxic neurosis and hyaline degeneration of
	  heart, liver, adrenal glands, and kidneys
	Gastritis, hepatitis
	Nephritis
		Identify close contacts and monitor for ill-
		  ness; culture nose, throat, and cutaneous
		  lesions, and administer prophylactic anti-
		  microbial therapy.

Specific:
  Erythromycin estolate
Supportive:
  Antipyretics
  Bed rest
  Quiet environment to reduce coughing
  Gentle suctioning
  Increase fluid intake
  Oxygen
	Respiratory: pneumonia, atelectasis,
	  emphysema, aspiration pneumonia,
	  pneumothorax
	CNS: convulsions, encephalopathy, coma
		Pertussis disease eliminates the need for
		  pertussis immunization.
		Erythromycin should be given to all close
		  and household contacts for 14 days.

Specific
  Therapy with penicillinase-resistant
    penicillin PO, IM, or IV
Symptomatic:
  Gentle cleansing of skin
    with compresses
	Excessive fluid loss, electrolyte imbal-
	  ance, pneumonia, septicemia, cellulitis	

Nonparalytic: Supportive (ie, relief of pain)
  Analgesics, heat
  Enteric isolation
  Bed rest
	Respiratory paralysis
	Hypertension
		Most cases of polio in the United State are
		  vaccine-induced; therefore, experts recom-
		  mend the inactive polio vaccine be used to
		  vaccinate all children.

(continued)

TABLE 42-5 Childhood Diseases (Continued)

Disease	Incubation (I) and Communicability (C) Periods	Symptoms
Young children; peaks in August, September, and October, in temperate zones Diagnostic tests: Isolation of polio virus from feces and throat	Is present in throat 1 wk after onset, in stool 3–4 wk after.	Paralytic polio (1) Same as nonparalytic type, lasting about 1 wk (2) Then 1–2 d of CNS symptoms: loss of deep tendon reflexes, positive Kernig's and Brudzinski's signs, lethargy (3) 1–2 d later, weakening of muscles and paralysis
Erythema Infectiosum (Fifth Disease/ Slapped Check) a. Parovirus B 19 b. Respiratory route c. School-aged children Diagnostic tests: Not widely available; IgM antibody test, polymerase chain reaction detection test	I: 6–14 d C: Until rash develops	Mild fever, chills, fatigue or asymptomatic rash develops in three stages: (1) Sudden appearance of bright erythema on cheeks (2) Erythematous, maculopapular rash on trunk and extremities (3) Rash on body fades with central clearing giving a lacy or reticulated appearance Rash lasts 2–39 d; frequently pruritic without desquamation Occasional joint arthropathy
Rotavirus a. Reoviridae group A—Most common agent responsible for infantile diarrhea b. Fecal–oral route c. 6 mo to 2 y of age; most common in winter in temperate climates Diagnostic tests: Enzyme-linked immunosorbent assay	I: 1–3 d C: Until 2–5 d after diarrhea	Fever Vomiting Profuse, watery, non–foul-smelling diarrhea

a. Agent
b. Mode of transmission
c. Age when most common

13. Behavior problems, depression, and acting-out behaviors may result.
14. For abuse that occurs in school or day care, the child may exhibit fear of the teacher, have nightmares, decrease school attendance, or develop psychosomatic illnesses.

Injuries or Types of Abuse That May Occur
1. Bruises, welts (linear or looplike)
2. Abrasions, contusions, lacerations (most common)
3. Wounds, cuts, punctures
4. Burns (cigarette, radiator, and so forth), scalding—stocking or glove distribution
5. Bone fractures
6. Sprains, dislocations
7. Subdural hemorrhage or hematoma; "shaken baby syndrome"
8. Brain damage
9. Internal injuries
10. Drug intoxication
11. Malnutrition (deliberately inflicted)
12. Freezing, exposure
13. Whiplash-type injury

14. Eye injuries, periorbital injuries, ear bruises
15. Dirty, infected wounds or rashes
16. Unexplained coma in infant
17. Failure to thrive—developmental delay; malnutrition with decreased muscle mass; decreased interaction with environment and with others; dental caries; listless; behavior problems
18. Sexually transmitted diseases—genital trauma, recurrent urinary tract infection, pregnancy

Management
1. The goal of treatment is to ensure the physical and emotional safety of the child. Therefore, treatment is inclusive of other family members and caretakers and is often focused on the parents. A team approach is employed to determine the most effective use of community resources to protect the child and help the parents.
2. It is estimated that 80% to 90% of abusing parents can be rehabilitated. The ideal approach is to return the child to biologic parents.
3. Counseling is offered to help parents do the following:
   a. Understand and redirect their anger

Treatment	Complications	Special Considerations

Paralytic: Hospitalize
  Fluid and electrolytes
  Rest
  Relief of muscle pain and spasms
  Respiratory support
  Minimize skeletal deformity		

No treatment is needed for healthy children. Immunoglobulin for immunocompromised patients	Complications are rare among healthy children. Children with abnormal red blood cells (sickle cell disease, hereditary sphero-cytosis, thalassemia, etc.) can develop transient aplastic anemia and may require multiple transfusions. Immunocompromised patients may develop severe, chronic anemia.	
Oral fluid and electrohydrate solution	Isotonic dehydration with acidosis. Malnourished infants may develop malabsorption dehydration and die.	Excellent hygiene (handwashing) is necessary to avoid spreading disease.

    b. Develop an adequate parent–child relationship
    c. See their child as an individual with own needs and differences
    d. Understand child development and normal behaviors of developing children
    e. Learn about effective discipline techniques
    f. Enjoy the child
    g. Develop realistic expectations of their child
    h. Decrease their use of criticism
    i. Increase their own sense of self-esteem and confidence
    j. Establish supportive relationships with others
    k. Improve their economic situation (if appropriate)
    l. Show progress toward physical, emotional, and intellectual development of their child

Nursing Assessment

1. Identify family or child at risk.
    a. Alcohol/drug abuser
    b. Adolescent parent
    c. Low-income, single-parent family
    d. Multiple births
    e. Unwanted child
    f. Sickly and more demanding child
    g. Premature child with long separation from mother at birth
2. Inspect for evidence of possible abuse.
    a. Describe completely on the medical record all bruises, lacerations, and similar lesions as to location and state of healing. Look carefully at areas generally covered with clothing (ie, buttocks, underarms, behind knees, bottom of feet).
    b. Ask how injuries occurred and record descriptions of the injury, including the date, time, and place of the event.
3. Collect any necessary specimens for identification of organisms, sperm, or semen.
4. Take color photographs as indicated.
5. Assess developmental level of the child.
6. Observe for behaviors common in abusing or neglecting parent(s). Be aware that not all abusing parents exhibit these behaviors but be alert for parent(s) who:
    a. Anxiously volunteers information or withholds information related to an injury.

b. Gives explanation of the injury that does not fit the condition or gets story confused concerning the injury.

c. Shows inappropriate reaction or concern to severity of injury.

d. Becomes irritable about questions being asked.

e. Seldom touches or speaks to the child; does not respond to child. May be critical or indicate unreal expectations of child (or may be oversolicitous to child).

f. Delays seeking medical help; refuses to sign permit for diagnostic studies; frequently changes hospitals or health care providers.

g. Shows no involvement in care of the hospitalized child; does not inquire about the child.

h. Obtains little or no prenatal care and shows inappropriate response to newborn; acts disinterested or unhappy with child.

7. Assess the parent–child relationship in the areas of appropriate involvement in care, show of affection, reaction to arrival and leaving, expectations, role portrayal.

8. Assess for signs of sexual abuse. Sexual abuse should be suspected when the young, prepubertal child presents with:

a. Genital trauma not readily explained

b. Gonorrhea, syphilis, or other sexually transmitted organisms

c. Blood in urine or stool

d. Painful urination or defecation

e. Penile or vaginal infection or itch

f. Penile or vaginal discharge

g. Report of increased, excessive masturbation

h. Report of increased, unusual fears

i. Trauma to genitalia, inner thigh, breast

9. Establish a relationship with the child based on mutual respect, empathy, and sensitivity to facilitate further investigation.

a. Consideration of the child's emotions in conjunction with a good relationship may encourage the child to express feelings either verbally or through drawings or play.

b. Prepare the child both physically and psychologically for the necessary physical and pelvic examination.

c. Talk with the child without the presence of the parents, especially when incest is possible.

NURSING ALERT

If the alleged sexual abuse occurred within 72 hours of health care visit, or if trauma or bleeding is present, an immediate physical examination should be done. If more than 72 hours have passed since the alleged sexual abuse, the physical examination might be delayed. Once child abuse has been reported, additional children in the family may be examined as well.

10. Report suspicion of child abuse based on your assessment. All states (as well as the District of Columbia) have mandatory reporting laws based on Public Law 94-247 (Child Abuse and Neglect Act, 1973). All states provide statutory immunity for those who report real or suspected child abuse. There is no immunity from civil or criminal liability for failure to report such. Notify the appropriate officials.

NURSING ALERT

Every nurse is morally and legally responsible to report and provide protective services for the abused child. Become familiar with laws, procedures, and protective services in your community and state.

Nursing Diagnoses
- Fear of adults related to experiences with abuse
- Altered Parenting related to abusive treatment of child

Nursing Interventions
Relieving Fear and Fostering Trust

1. Be aware that some of these children have never learned how to trust an adult; they are fearful of giving affection for fear of rejection.

2. Assign one nurse to care for the child over a period of time.

3. Make no threatening moves toward the child. The child will indicate readiness and awareness of the environment by verbal or facial expressions.

4. Touch the child gently.

5. Provide nonthreatening physical contact (hold and frequently cuddle child). Pick up and carry child around; encourage any exploration of your face, hair, and so forth.

6. Provide appropriate opportunities for play.

7. Set limits for child.

8. Provide therapeutic play to allow the child to express fears and anger in a nonverbal manner; be nonjudgmental and supportive with expression of feelings; correct misconceptions.

9. Provide additional help in the following areas:

a. Having ambivalent feelings toward parent(s) or any adult caretaker

b. Overcoming low self-image and the fear that something is wrong with him or her

c. Fearing future abuse on return home or for misbehavior in the hospital

Providing Support in Parenting

1. Assume a nonjudgmental attitude that is neither punitive nor threatening. Convey a desire to help parents through the healing process.

2. Refrain from questioning them about the incident of abuse. The health care provider, the social worker, and the investigative authority will interview the suspected abuser.

3. Include the parents in the hospital experience (ie, orient them to the unit and to any procedure to be done to the child). Serve as a role model in the management of the child's behavior as well as their own. Try to give the parents as much information as possible about the care of their child. Listen to what they are saying.

4. Refrain from challenging all the information they may give.

5. Express appropriate concern and kindness. Remain objective yet empathic. This will help foster the parents' self-respect and improve their self-image and dignity.

6. Discuss the reporting to the authorities with them because of the widespread nature of the problem and the need for education and assistance.

7. Support the parents who may have feelings of guilt, anger, and helplessness. Explain to them the extent of trauma, and educate them. Allow them to ventilate their feelings. Support their parental role in handling the child (eg, allow the child to talk about or play out the incident, but do not force it).

8. Build a relationship by working with the parents' strengths rather than their weaknesses. Use compliments as positive reinforcement.

9. Assist parents to learn safe and appropriate parenting skills.
   a. Remember that many of these parents were abused as children and have no role models or personal experience with nurturing behaviors.
   b. Foster attachment between child and parents, not between child and nurse, when the parents are present; the latter would increase their feelings of incompetence in the parenting role.
   c. Correct erroneous expectations as to what is appropriate behavior for a particular age group.
   d. Encourage parents to take time out from caring for their children to meet their own needs; assist them in identifying safe and appropriate resources for their child's care.

10. Provide the parent with psychological support and reinforcement for appropriate parenting behaviors.

11. Work with parent in planning for the child's future care.

12. Determine in what areas the parent needs help. Does the baby cry often? How does this make the parent feel? How does parent comfort child? Is there someone the parents can call for help?

2. Understand the dynamics of child abuse and neglect. This crisis is due to the stress with which the parents are unable to cope and to the deprivations they have themselves suffered in the past.

Community and Home Care Considerations

Nurses often provide home care visits as part of a multidisciplinary team engaging in extensive community follow-up. Education and continued assessment are the focus.

1. Teach the parents about normal growth and development (see Chapter 40).
   a. Give specific information about and examples of the types of behavior to expect at the various stages of development. Point out in a nonthreatening way normal behavior exhibited by their child.
   b. Give specific strategies on dealing with this behavior.
   c. Serve as a role model and teacher; minimize intensity when the parents become threatened.

2. Teach the parents how to use discipline without resorting to physical force.
   a. Discipline must be consistent. Offer suggestions for alternative ways of handling undesirable behavior (time-out).
   b. Suggest using a reward system for acceptable behavior (eg, a trip to the zoo, staying up later than usual for a special television show, a special treat).
   c. Instruct parents to withhold rewards for unacceptable behavior.

3. Teach children how to avoid being the victims of abuse.
   a. Teach them about "good touch" and "bad touch."
   b. Emphasize that they can say no to anyone who wants to touch their body.
   c. Provide names or places where they can go if they feel they are being abused.
   d. Assist them in dealing with their fears that their parents will be sent to jail or that they will be removed from the home.

4. Be alert for signs of abuse in the school. If a teacher is suspected of being the abuser, the child may:
   a. Display increased fear of the teacher
   b. Decrease school attendance
   c. Develop psychosomatic symptoms during school days
   d. Develop nightmares
   e. Worry excessively over school performance

Family Education and Health Maintenance

1. Teach both parents and child (if age is appropriate) any specific instructions relative to injury and follow-up care.

2. Ensure that family knows where and when to follow up.

3. Review schedule for well-child visits and immunizations so family can keep up with routine care.

4. Make known to parents your continued concern and your availability as a source of help. Help them to use resources in the community including home health nurse, social worker, and therapists.

5. Refer those interested in learning more about abuse to the following agencies: Prevent Child Abuse America, 332 South Michigan Ave., Suite 1600, Chicago, IL 60604, 1-800-55NCPCA; National Clearinghouse on Child Abuse and Neglect Information, P.O. Box 1182, Washington, DC 20013-1182, 1-800-FYI-3366, *www.calib.com/nccanch.*

Outcome-Based Evaluation

- Child exhibiting appropriate developmental behavior
- Both parents participating in feeding and playing with child

SELECTED REFERENCES

American Academy of Pediatrics. (1999). Policy statement. Guidelines for the evaluation of sexual abuse in children: Subject review (RE9819). *Pediatrics, 103*(1), 186–191.

———. (1999). Poliomyelitis prevention: Revised recommendations for use of inactive and live oral poliovirus vaccines (RE9853). *Pediatrics, 103*(1), 171–172.

———. (1998a). Prevention of rotavirus disease: Guidelines for use of rotavirus vaccine (RE9840). *Pediatrics, 102*(6), 1483–1491.

———. (1998b). Screening for elevated blood levels (RE9815). *Pediatrics, 101*(6), 1072–1078.

———. (1995). Treatment guidelines for lead exposure in children (RE9529). *Pediatrics, 96*(1), 155–160.

Atkinson, W., Humiston, S., Wolfe, C., & Nelson, R. (1999). *Epidemiology and prevention of vaccine preventable diseases* (5th ed.). Washington, DC: US Department of Health and Human Services, Public Health Service.

Behrman, R. (1996). *Nelson textbook of pediatrics* (15th ed.). Philadelphia: W. B. Saunders.

Bell, K. K., & Rawlings, N. L. (1998). Promoting breast-feeding by managing common lactation problems. *Nurse Practitioner, 23*(6), 102–104, 106, 109–110.

Browne, K. (1995). Preventing child maltreatment through community nursing. *Journal of Advanced Nursing, 21*(1), 57–63.

Cheung, K. (1999). Identifying and documenting findings of physical child abuse and neglect. *Journal of Pediatric Health Care, 13*(3), 142–143.

Cohen, B. A. (1993). *Atlas of pediatric dermatology.* Baltimore: Wolfe.

Greenfield, L., Marcuse, E., & Bibus, D. (1998). Calling the shots: A guide to immunization resources. *Contemporary Pediatrics, 15*(4), 125–138.

Hay, W. W., Jr., Groothius, J. R., Hayward, A. R., & Levin, M. J. (Eds.). (1995). *Current pediatric diagnosis and treatment* (12th ed.). Norwalk, CT: Appleton & Lange.

Immunization Action Coalition. (1999). *Needle tips and the hepatitis B coalition news.* St. Paul, MN: Author.

Levenberg, P. B. (1998). GAPS: An opportunity for nurse practitioners to promote the health of adolescents through clinical preventive services. *Journal of Pediatric Health Care, 12*(1), 2–9.

Lovelady, C. A., Garner, K. E., Moreno, K. L., & Williams, J. P. (2000). The effect of weight loss in overweight, lactating women on the growth of their infants. *New England Journal of Medicine, 342*(7), 449–453.

Maffeis, C., Provera, S., Filippi, L., Sidoti, G., Schena, S., Pinelli, L., & Tato, L. (2000). Distribution of food intake as a risk factor for childhood obesity. *International Journal of Obesity and Related Metabolic Disorders, 24*(1), 75–80.

Markowitz, M., Rosen, J., & Clemente, I. (1999). Screened for lead poisoning. *American Journal of Public Health, 89*(7), 1088–1090.

Matte, T. (1999). Reducing blood lead levels. Benefits and strategies. *Journal of the American Medical Association, 281*(4), 2340–2341.

Moody, C. (1999). Male child sexual abuse. *Journal of Pediatric Health Care, 13*(3), 112–119.

Murphy, J. M. (1998). Child passenger safety. *Journal of Pediatric Health Care, 12*(3), 130–138.

Niederhauser, V. P. (1999). Varicella: The vaccine and the public health debate. *Nurse Practitioner, 24*(3), 74–76, 79, 83–84.

———. (1997). Prescribing for children: Issues in pediatric pharmacology. *Nurse Practitioner, 22*(3), 16–18, 23, 26–28.

Olds, D. L., Eckenrode, J., Henderson, C. R., Jr., Kitzman, H., Powers, J., Cole, R., Sidora, K., Morris, P., Pettitt, L. M., & Luckey, D. (1997). Long-term effects of home visitation on maternal life course and child abuse and neglect. Fifteen-year follow-up of a randomized trial [comment]. *Journal of the American Medical Association, 278*(8), 637–643.

Ott, M., & Aruda, M. (1999). Hepatitis B vaccine. *Journal of Pediatric Health Care, 13*(5), 211–216.

Peter, G. (Ed.). (1994). *1997 Red Book: Report of the Committee on Infectious Diseases* (24th ed.). Elk Grove Village, IL: American Academy of Pediatrics.

Sibbery, G. K. & Iannone, R. (Eds.) (2000). *The Harriet Lane handbook* (15th ed.). St. Louis: Mosby.

Thomas, D. D. (1995). Fever in children: Friend or foe? *RN, 58*(4), 42–47.

US Department of Health and Human Services. (1994). *Clinician's handbook of preventative services.* Washington, DC: US Department of Health and Human Services, Public Health Services.

Winston, F. K., et al. (2000). The danger of premature graduation to seat belts for young children. *Pediatrics, 105*(6), 1179–1183.

CHAPTER

43

Care of the Sick or Hospitalized Child

GENERAL PRINCIPLES OF CARE

■ Family-Centered Care

Family-centered care provides a framework for health care providers to ensure all aspects of care and the care environment are designed and focused toward family needs and concerns. The patient and family members are active members of the care team. The family is recognized and cares for the hospitalized child with full information, support, and respect.

The goal of family-centered care is to maintain or strengthen the roles and ties of the family with the hospitalized child to promote normality of the family unit.

Benefits for Parents and Child
1. Care and teaching are in keeping with specific family needs and strengths.
2. Family roles and close family interactions during time of stress are enhanced.
3. Minimizes separation anxiety.
4. Decreases reactions of protest, denial, and despair.
5. Increases sense of security for the child.
6. Family needs to care for their child physically and emotionally are fulfilled.
7. Parents feel useful and important, rather than dependent and peripheral.
8. Decreases parental guilt feelings.
9. Increases parents' competence and confidence in caring for the sick child.
10. Families of children with special needs share comfort and support from one another.
11. Greater absorption of staff teaching by the family.
12. Diminishes posthospitalization reactions.

Implementation Strategies
Implementation of family-centered care will depend on regulations of the particular health care setting as well as the capabilities of the individual family unit. Review the policies and regulations regularly with the input of children/adolescents and family members. Examples of activities that can facilitate and strengthen family ties include:
1. Taking a family history and listening for specific family/cultural needs and preferences
2. Allowing rooming-in for parents of young children
3. Having parents participate in the child's physical care
4. Acknowledging that parents are not "visitors"; having flexible visiting regulations for family members, including siblings
5. Having pictures of family members available at the hospital
6. Encouraging telephone contact
7. Using family tape recordings

Role of the Nurse

1. To create an environment conducive to maintaining family strength, integrity, and unity. The nurse should:
   a. Help to maintain a positive nurse–parent–child relationship. Avoid actions that may cause parents to feel threatened by the nurse.
   b. Facilitate a supportive marital relationship, allowing for differences in style and needs.
   c. Include siblings in planning and intervention as appropriate to their age and the situation.
   d. Supplement the family abilities and role in achieving the common goal of the child's welfare.
2. To assist parents with decision making about when to stay with their child and when to be away.
   a. Parents' presence is especially important if the child is 5 years or younger, especially anxious, upset, or in medical crisis.
   b. The parents' decision is influenced by needs of other family members, as well as by job, home responsibilities, and personal needs.
   c. The nurse should try to alleviate guilty feelings of parents who are unable to stay with their child.
3. To develop trusting, goal-directed relationships with families.
   a. Obtain a thorough nursing history that provides information to assess broad consideration of strengths, relationships, and concerns; include family and individual stage of development, cultural, spiritual, social, material, and financial areas.
   b. Plan with the family toward mutual, realistic goals.
   c. Recognize and acknowledge the care and consideration the child receives from parents.
4. To observe the parent–child relationship and be able to:
   a. Evaluate the degree of participation and effectiveness of the parents in physical and emotional care.
   b. Observe parents' attitudes, skills, and techniques and the child's behavior and response to them.
   c. Assess what teaching needs to be done.
   d. Detect and respond to actual and potential problems in parent–child relationship.
5. To teach parents knowledge, understanding, and skills necessary to function effectively with the hospitalized child. The nurse should:
   a. Carefully assess and address the learning needs, learning styles, and potential barriers to understanding and skill development.
   b. Perform nursing techniques safely and efficiently.
   c. Mutually with parents, assess and interpret the behavior of the hospitalized child, so appropriate understanding and intervention are reached.
   d. Assess the child's and parents' understanding of essential medical care and wellness-focused information.
   e. Interpret and reinforce what health care providers have told parents. Answer questions thoroughly and honestly as knowledge and nurse role permits. Refer core questions about diagnosis and prognosis to the provider most involved with the specific question being asked.
   f. Explain medical procedures and diagnostic tests and the preprocedure preparations required.
   g. Provide health teaching and anticipatory guidance concerning medically related information and wellness behaviors, parenting and child-rearing matters, and crisis intervention and community resources.
6. To help parents adapt to the situation and to develop their own feeling of value by coping with the child's illness and deriving meaning through the difficult experiences they are facing.
   a. Be aware of common parental reactions to the stress experienced by families of children who have severe or chronic illness; respond or refer to other discipline as indicated.
   b. Be aware that defense mechanisms, if used in moderation, are constructive and may facilitate optimal coping.
   c. Help parents recognize and value their own feelings and the feelings of significant others.
   d. Identify parental support systems as well as adaptive and maladaptive coping.
   e. Be perceptive of parents' physical and emotional needs and limitations.
      (i) As possible, help prevent parents becoming fatigued.
      (ii) Encourage parents to leave and take a break.
7. To assist families, as appropriate, in dealing with normative family developmental tasks.
   a. Be aware that the child's hospitalization is often only one of many stresses a family experiences at a given time. Others may include:
      (i) Interpersonal problems
      (ii) Debt, unemployment, job change
      (iii) Recent changes in dwelling place and consequent disruption
      (iv) Problems associated with child care and discipline
      (v) Concurrent illness of other family members
   b. Keep in mind that the family unit and family members individually have strengths and resources to be discovered and contributed.
   c. Consciously identify and separate your feelings and judgments about the situation from those of the child and family; the goal is to draw on individual and family strengths to meet needs and solve problems as a family unit.

■ Settings of Pediatric Illness Care Delivery

The ill child benefits from being at home or in a homelike environment, and this setting is preferred when possible. Many additional factors influence the increasing use of nonhospital care for sick children, even seriously ill children and children dependent on medical technology: Family preference, community health services, availability of programmable intravenous (IV) pumps and other devices, shortened length of hospital stays, insurance benefits.

Home Care

1. Anticipatory guidance, planning, and teaching are strategies used to prepare the child and family for care at home during acute or chronic illness.
2. The quality of care and family life is enhanced by a general knowledge of the child's:
   a. Condition
   b. Treatment regimens
   c. Medical equipment
   d. Signs of complications
   e. Resources: who and when to call for assistance
3. Specific issues and skill development depend on the age and condition of the child, the home situation, family resources and abilities, as well as the community environment and resources.

Office and Clinic Services

1. Conditions that were previously diagnosed and treated in the hospital are now managed on an outpatient basis.
2. Increased early discharge of hospitalized children with outpatient follow-up require more care by family.
3. This leads to an increased role of the office nurse to:
   a. Assess a child's and family's coping with home care
   b. Provide education and support
   c. Administer treatments in an outpatient setting

School or Day Care

1. Children and youth with chronic and/or ongoing health concerns are able to remain in school and participate in activities with their peers.
2. Adaptive education and medical technology are bringing new opportunities that foster development and socialization for children with special needs.
3. Assessment of changing health, wellness counseling, health teaching, referral, and skilled care are among the roles of a school nurse.
4. Interventions may include medication administration, urinary catheterization, tube feedings, and initial crisis intervention.

Camp

1. Summer camp is an exciting experience for children.
2. They learn about nature and themselves; they experience independence and group living; they get a change of pace from their usual routines.
3. Many camps are set up for children with chronic or handicapping conditions where the special needs are met and they have an opportunity to learn, play, and socialize with other people who are much like themselves.

4. In these settings, the nurse serves the role of camp counselor, confidant, and provider of care.

Hospital or Extended-Care Facility

1. Inpatient facilities have special programs to facilitate the age-related needs of infants, children, and youth.
2. Nursing care is directed toward the child patient and family members.
3. Where the facility is not wholly dedicated to children, attention is given to ensure pediatric standards of care are met throughout the continuum of care: laboratory, diagnostic imaging, surgery, physical therapy, emergency department.

▪ Impact of Prolonged Illness or Hospitalization on the Child's Stage of Development

The child has the same basic emotional and social needs during a prolonged illness or hospitalization as a child not challenged by these circumstances. Both prolonged illness and hospitalization can retard growth and development and cause adverse reactions in the child based on stage of development.

Neonate (Birth to 1 Month)
Primary Concerns

1. Bonding—prolonged illness and hospitalization interrupt the early stages of the development of a healthy mother–child relationship and family integration, thus early stages of the development of trust are missing.
2. Sensory and motor deprivation—tactile, visual, auditory, kinesthetic.
3. Sensory overload.

Reactions

1. Impairment of parent–infant attachment/bonding
2. Impairment of infant's ability to respond to parents/family members
3. Impairment of parent's ability to love and care for the baby
4. Risk of infant emotional and physical well-being
5. Risk of stress within the family constellation

Nursing Interventions

1. Provide care within a family-centered context.
2. Provide for continual contact between baby and the parents (eye contact, touch, talk).
3. Minimize isolation and strangeness by explaining and re-explaining equipment, procedures to parents.
4. Actively involve parents in caring for their baby—provide for rooming-in.
5. Foster neonate–sibling relationships as appropriate.
6. Identify areas of infant deprivation or overstimulation. Plan a schedule of appropriate stimulation (ie, hold and rock every 3 to 4 hours, eye contact).
7. Provide sensory-motor stimulation as appropriate.
8. Allow individuality to begin to emerge.
9. Provide consistent caretaker.

Young Infant (1 to 4 Months)
Primary Concerns
1. Separation—mother and father are learning to identify and meet the needs of their infant. Infant is learning to make his or her needs known and to trust the mother to meet them.
2. Sensory-motor deprivation.
3. Needs—security, motor activity, comforting measures.
Reactions
1. Separation anxiety is different from that of older child, because for the infant, the mother seems to be a part of him or her.
2. Development of trust is disturbed when infant is separated from mother and when illness or hospitalization interferes with meeting the infant's needs.
3. Interference with development of a basic sense of trust has lifelong implications.
Nursing Interventions
1. Encourage mother to balance her responsibilities and minimize separation, staying with infant and providing care for her baby.
2. When mother is absent, meet the baby's basic needs promptly and give infant attention and appropriate handling from a limited number of personnel.
3. Provide opportunity for sensory stimulation, motor development, and social responsiveness appropriate to infant's age and condition.
4. Help parents to see the infant as a unique individual with needs and personal style, to acquire infant care skills and to work through their anxieties about parenting and the infant's condition. Remember, parental touch communicates comfort and calm or discomfort and stress to the infant.

Mid-Aged Infant (4 to 8 Months)
Primary Concerns
1. Separation from mother and family members, as the infant now recognizes mother as a separate person from self. Infant rejects strangers.
2. Development of self-quieting behaviors.
Reactions
1. Separation anxiety—crying, terror, somatic upset, blank facial expression, extreme preoccupation
2. Emotional withdrawal and depression
3. Interference with development of basic trust
4. Interference with growth and achievement of developmental milestones
Nursing Interventions
1. Encourage mother's presence and nurturing of her baby.
2. Foster mother's confidence and competence in this new role.
3. Encourage mother/family to adjust schedule and home routines.
4. Become friends with the infant through the mother; avoid overshadowing the parents.
5. The infant is beginning to develop purposeful activities and to strive toward independence. Provide opportuni-

ties and encouragement for this development to continue, and provide ways for infant to use newly acquired skills.

Older Infant (8 to 12 Months)
Primary Concerns
1. Beginning definition of self—infant is aware of a growing ability to influence his or her environment.
2. Separation—infant becomes more possessive of mother and clings to her at the time of separation.
Reactions
1. Passivity toward environment
2. Separation anxiety—tolerance is limited; fear of strangers, excessive crying, clinging, and overdependence on mother
Nursing Interventions
1. Have the mother stay and care for her child.
2. Relieve some of tensions and loneliness with "transference" object (ie, blanket, toy).
3. Prepare the child for procedures. The procedures should be performed in another room or a treatment room; let the mother soothe the child afterward.
4. Provide for sensory stimulation and motor development appropriate for age. Provide opportunities for child to continue using acquired skills, such as feeding self and drinking from a cup.
5. Child needs opportunity to foster increased independence, curiosity and exploration, locomotion, and language skills. Use infant seats, swing; give room to move around in crib, playpen, or floor; use color, texture, and sound; physical stroking, rocking, and talking.

Toddler (1 to 3 Years)
Primary Concerns
1. Separation anxiety—relationship with mother is intense. Separation represents the loss of family and familiar surroundings, resulting in feeling of insecurity, grief, anxiety, and abandonment. The toddler's emotional needs are intensified by the mother's absence.
2. Changes in rituals and routines, all of which are important to sense of security, become a source of concern.
3. Inability to communicate—beginning use and understanding of language affords child limited communication between self and the world. Child has limited capacity to understand reality, passage of time.
4. Loss of autonomy and independence—egocentric view of life helps child develop a sense of autonomy. Child sees self as a separate being with some potential control of own body and environment.
5. Body integrity—incomplete and inaccurate understanding of the body results in fear, anxiety, frustration, and anger.
6. Decrease in mobility—restricting mobility causes frustration. Child wants to keep moving for the pleasure it gives as well as for the feeling of independence, the opportunity to learn about the world, and the route it pro-

vides for coping with frustrations that cannot be verbally expressed. Physical interference with this freedom results in a sense of helplessness.

Reactions

1. Protest
   a. Has urgent desire to find mother.
   b. Expects that she will answer cries, "I want mommy."
   c. Frequently cries and shakes crib.
   d. Rejects attention of nurses.
   e. When with mother, child shows signs of distrust with anger or tears.
2. Despair
   a. Feels increasingly hopeless about seeing mother.
   b. Becomes apathetic, anorectic, listless; looks sad.
   c. May cry continuously or intermittently.
   d. Uses comfort measures—thumbsucking, fingering lip, tightly clutching a toy.
3. Denial
   a. Represses all feelings and images of mother.
   b. Does not cry when she leaves.
   c. May seem more attached to nurses—will go to anyone.
   d. Finds little satisfaction in relationships with people.
   e. Accepts care without protest.
4. Regression—temporarily ceases use of newly acquired skills in an attempt to retain or regain control of a stressful situation.

Nursing Interventions

1. Provide rooming-in, unlimited visiting. Parental visits provide:
   a. Opportunity for child to express some of feelings about the situation
   b. Assurance that parents are not abandoning or punishing child
   c. Periods of comfort and reassurance that allow for the reestablishment of family bonds
2. Attempt to continue routines used at home, especially with regard to sleeping, eating, and bathing. Reestablish trust through body contact and comfort.
3. Set limits.
4. Obtain from parents key words in communicating with child. Find out about nonverbal behavior as well. Familiar toys, blankets, pillow cases, and family pictures can reinforce the child's sense of security.
5. Allow child to make choices when possible. Arrange physical setting to encourage independence. Allow child to explore environment. Ensure an age-appropriate safe environment. No latex balloons.
6. A Band-Aid may give the child a security of wholeness after an injection.
7. Replace lost mobility with another form of motion, such as moving about in a wheelchair, cart, or bed. Exercise restrained extremity. Provide opportunity for the child to release energy suppressed by decreased mobility (ie, by pounding, throwing). Provide opportunity to continue learning about world through sensory modalities such as water play and diversional play.

8. Discharge—if rooming-in has not occurred during hospitalization, parents must be prepared for the possible posthospital behavior of their toddler. They will need support in understanding and handling these behaviors. The child may do any of the following:
   a. Show lack of affection or resist close physical contact. Parents may interpret this as rejection.
   b. Regress to an earlier stage of development.
   c. Cling to mother, unable to tolerate any separation from her; show excessive need for love and affection.
9. Appropriate parental response to the child's behavior is vital if relationships are to be reestablished.
   a. Extra love and understanding will help restore the child's trust.
   b. Hostility and withdrawal of love will cause the child's further loss of trust, self-esteem, and independence.

Preschool Child (3 to 5 Years)
Primary Concerns

1. Separation—although cognitive and coping capabilities have increased and the child responds less violently to separation from parents, separation and hospitalization represent stress beyond the coping mechanisms and adaptive capabilities of the preschool child. Loneliness and insecurities are experienced. Language is important; although children may not verbally express what they are feeling, there is an attempt at this in 4- to 5-year-old children.
2. Unfamiliar environment—this requires coping with a change in daily routine and represents a loss of control and security.
3. Abandonment and punishment—fantasies and thoughts may contain vengeful wishes for other persons, for which the child expects retribution. Illness may be interpreted as punishment for thoughts. Enforced parental separation may be interpreted as loss of parental love and represents abandonment by them.
4. Body image and integrity—hospitalization and intrusive procedures provide a multitude of threats of both bodily mutilation and loss of identity, which are just beginning to develop along with the acquisition of autonomy.
5. Immobility—mobility is the child's dominant form of self-expression and adaptation to the environment. The child has great urge for locomotion and exercise of large muscles. It represents the main expression of emotion and release of tension.
6. Loss of control—this influences the preschooler's perception of and reaction to separation, pain, and illness.

Reactions

1. Regression—child temporarily stops using newly acquired skills in an attempt to retain or regain control of a stressful situation. Preschooler may return to behavior of infant or toddler.
2. Repression—child may attempt to exclude the undesirable and unpleasant stresses from consciousness.

3. Projection—preschooler may transfer own emotional state, motives, and desires to others in environment.

4. Displacement/sublimation—emotions are permitted to be directed and expressed in other situations such as art or play.

5. Identification—the child assumes characteristics of the aggressor in an attempt to reduce fear and anxiety and to feel in control of the situation.

6. Aggression—hostility is direct and intentional; physical expression takes precedence over verbal expression.

7. Denial and withdrawal—the child is able to ignore interruptions and disavow any thought or feeling that would result in a painful experience.

8. Fantasy—a mental activity to help the child bridge the gap between reality and fantasy because of lack of experience.

9. The preschooler may simply show similar behaviors (protest, despair, denial) to those of the toddler although the stage of protest is usually less aggressive and direct.

Nursing Interventions

1. Minimize stress of separation by providing for parental presence and participation in care. Strive to shorten the hospital stay. Help parents understand what hospitalization means to the child.

2. Identify defense mechanisms apparent in the child and help child through the stressful situation by accepting, showing love and concern, and being alert to readiness to relinquish them.

3. Set limits for the child. Let child know that someone is there. Help the child become master of something in the situation.

4. Provide opportunity and encouragement for child to verbalize.

5. Careful preparation for all procedures should be done on the child's level of development and comprehension. Provide privacy during these procedures.

6. Be sure the child has opportunities for play. Play is one important medium through which the child can overcome fear and anxiety. A body outline, doll, and simple visual aids are appropriate teaching tools. Provide self-expression, role reversal through puppets, dolls, drawings.

7. Encourage activities with other children.

8. Provide consistency in nursing personnel and approach to care.

9. Encourage the child to participate in own care and hygiene as appropriate.

10. Deal specifically with castration and mutilation fears. If the child is having surgery, describe exactly which body part will be repaired.

11. Whenever appropriate, reassure the child that no one is to blame for the illness or hospitalization.

12. Discourage parents from reinforcing negative feelings to the child—"If you're not good, I'll leave you here" or "I'll have the nurse give you a shot."

School-Aged Children (5 to 12 Years)
Primary Concerns

1. Many fear loss of recently mastered skills.

2. Many worry about separation from school and peers. They may fear loss of former roles.

3. Mutilation fantasies are common.

4. Some may believe that they or their parents magically caused the illness merely by thinking that the event would occur.

5. Often, they have increased concerns related to modesty and privacy.

6. The imposed passivity may be interpreted as punishment for being bad.

7. Children may feel their body no longer is their own but rather is controlled by doctors and nurses.

Reactions

1. Regression

2. Separation anxiety—especially early school-aged period

3. Negativism

4. Depression

5. Tendency to be phobic (normal)
   a. Fears include that of the dark, doctors, hospitals, surgery, medication, and death.
   b. Unrealistic fears are commonly attached to needles, x-ray procedures, and blood.

6. Conscious attempts at mature behavior

7. Suppression or denial of symptoms

Nursing Interventions

1. Help parents to prepare the child for elective hospitalizations.

2. Obtain a thorough nursing history, including information regarding health and physical developments, hospitalizations, social and cultural background, and normal daily activities. Use this information to plan care.

3. Provide order and consistency in the environment whenever possible.

4. Establish and enforce reasonable policies to protect the child and to increase sense of security in the environment.

5. Arrange the environment to allow for as much mobility as possible (ie, make sure articles are appropriately placed; move the bed if the child is immobilized).

6. Respect the child's need for privacy, and respect modesty during examinations, bathing, and other activities.

7. Use treatment rooms whenever possible when performing painful or intrusive procedures. Keep the room as "safe" territory.

8. Help young children identify problems and questions (often through play). Then help them find the answers.

9. Provide information about the illness and hospitalization based on assessment of what facts the child needs and wants and how this information can be made readily understandable.

10. View all nursing care activities as teaching situations. Explain the function of equipment, and allow the child

to handle it. Teach scientific terminology for body parts, procedures, and equipment.

11. When explaining a procedure, make sure that the child knows its purpose, what will be done, and what will be expected. Reassure the child during the procedure by continuing the explanations and support.

12. Reassure the child having surgery; explain where the organ to be removed or repaired is located and that no other body part will be removed.

13. Carefully assess pain, and provide appropriate relief.

14. Use play whenever appropriate to provide information about the hospital experience and to identify and decrease the child's fantasies and fears.

15. Reassure the child that he or she or parents are not to blame for illness.

16. Facilitate discharge of energy and aggression through appropriate play activities or through sharing aspects of ward management.

17. Encourage the child's participation in care and self-hygiene.

18. Support intellectual potential through the use of games, puzzles, school work, and drawings.

19. Assist the family to understand the child's reactions to illness and hospitalization so family members can facilitate positive coping patterns.

20. Let the child know that his or her normal status as a family member remains intact during hospitalization. Encourage a consistent visiting pattern and allow sibling visits.

21. Help parents to deal with their own anxieties about hospitalization, and assist them to help their child cope with the situation.

22. Encourage parental participation in the child's care when appropriate.

23. Encourage written communication with peers, and allow peer visiting when appropriate.

24. Begin discharge planning early, including plans for physical and emotional needs. Alert families to possible behavioral changes, including phobias, nightmares, regression, negativism, and disturbances in eating and learning.

Adolescent
Primary Concerns

1. Physical illness, exposure, and lack of privacy may cause increased concern about body image and sexuality.

2. Separation from security of peers, family, and school may cause anxiety.

3. Interference with struggle for independence and emancipation from parents is a concern.

4. The adolescent may be threatened by helplessness and may see illness as a punishment for feelings not mastered or for breaking rules imposed by parents or physicians.

5. Illness and hospitalizations may interfere with peer associations, self-concept, sexuality, and independence.

Reactions

1. Anxiety or embarrassment related to loss of control.

2. Insecurity in strange environment.

3. Intellectualization about disease details to avoid addressing actual concerns. They may know others with the same chronic type of illness who have died; may fear the future or feel guilty they have survived.

4. Rejection of treatment measures, even if previously accepted.

5. Anger (may be directed toward parents or staff) because goals are being thwarted.

6. Depression.

7. Increased dependency on parents, staff.

8. Denial or withdrawal.

9. Demanding or uncooperative behavior (usually an attempt to assert control).

10. Capitalization on gains from illness or pain.

Nursing Interventions

1. Help parents to prepare the adolescent for elective hospitalization.

2. Assess the impact of illness on the adolescent by considering factors such as timing, nature of illness, new experiences imposed, changes in body image, and expectations for the future. Be aware of misconceptions.

3. Introduce the adolescent to the hospital staff and to regular routines soon after admission.

4. Obtain a thorough nursing history that includes information about hobbies, school, family, illness, hospitalization, food habits, sexuality, and recreation.

5. Encourage adolescents to wear their own clothes, and allow them to decorate their beds or rooms to express themselves.

6. Have drawers and closets available to store personal items.

7. Allow the adolescent access to a telephone.

8. Allow adolescents control over appropriate matters (ie, timing of bath, selection of food, and so forth).

9. Respect their need for periodic isolation and privacy.

10. Have a supervised recreational and activities program available that is planned by a professional child care worker.

11. Accept adolescent's level of performance. Allow regression with expectation of growth.

12. Involve adolescent patients in planning care so they will be more accepting of restrictions and receptive to health teaching. Focus on capabilities rather than limitations. Adolescent should be accepted as a vital member of the health care team. The adolescent's consent should be obtained for procedures and surgery.

13. Explain clearly all procedures, routines, expectations, and restrictions imposed by illness. If necessary, clarify the adolescent's interpretation of illness and hospitalization. Plan separate teaching sessions for parents.

14. Facilitate verbal rejection of treatment measures to protect the adolescent from harming himself physically by stopping treatment.

15. Assess the adolescent's intellectual skills, and provide necessary information to allow for problem solving to deal with illness and hospitalization.

16. Recognize positive and negative coping behaviors as attempts to adjust to a threatening situation. Attempt to deal with feeling that caused the behavior as well as with the behavior itself.

17. Be a good listener. Maintain a sense of humor. Be honest and respectful with the adolescent and family.

18. Provide opportunities such as writing, art work, and recreational activities to allow nonverbal adolescents to express themselves.

19. Foster interaction with other hospitalized adolescents and continuation of peer relationships with outside friends.

20. Establish regular group meetings to allow patients to meet with staff members and with each other to comment and ask questions about their hospital experiences.

21. Set necessary limits to encourage self-control and ensure the rights of others.

22. Help adolescents work through sexual feelings. Avoid behavior that could be interpreted as provocative or flirtatious. Masturbation, unless excessive, may be considered a psychologically healthy way to discharge sexual tension.

23. Describe and interpret the needs and reactions of hospitalized adolescents to parents. Emphasize the adolescent's need to be respected as a unique individual, separate from parents.

24. Assist parents to cope with the illness and hospitalization as well as to deal effectively with the adolescent's response to related stress.

25. Encourage continuation of education.

26. Stress the confidential nature of conversations between nurse and patient, physician and patient.

Pediatric Acute Care Nursing

Refer to the previous section on the impact of hospitalization on the developmental stage of the child. In addition to the stress of hospitalization and the illness itself, the child must deal with multiple providers and the noxious environment: high noise level, loss of sleep, bright lights, random and unpredictable procedures, and the drastic change from normal routine.

The parental role changes once their child is admitted to the ICU, from that of parents of a well child to one of parents of a critically ill child. To ease this transition, parents need to be informed about their child's current condition, plan of care, and the future. They also need to feel needed and vital in their child's recovery.

Emotional Support to Child

1. If possible, familiarize the child with the setting/unit before admission.

2. Provide immediate physical care that communicates competence, caring, and strength and facilitates trust.

3. Be alert to behavioral changes that may indicate physical distress.

4. Facilitate parent–child interaction; facilitate frequent family visits.

5. Ask parents about the child's own way of responding to emotional stress. Use particular comforts that are most soothing to the child.

6. Support parents so they will be best able to support their child.

7. Foster rest and prolonged periods of sleep. Time activities to reduce interruptions; dim lights to allow for adequate sleep; whenever possible, cluster caregiving activities.

8. Do everything possible to reduce the amount of pain the child must endure; anticipate and prevent anxiety and pain; provide comfort measures and therapeutic distractions as appropriate. Administer anxiety-reducing or pain-reducing medications as ordered, and determine effectiveness. Consider conscious-sedation, and assist according to standards and procedures.

9. Provide age-appropriate stimulation when indicated by the child's condition (TV, games, books, toys, and so forth).

10. Provide opportunities for the child to express fears and concerns.

11. If possible, avoid exposing an alert child to the death or resuscitation of another child. If the child is exposed, provide adequate explanation. The child must also be helped to express own feelings and work through the experience.

12. Prepare the child and family for transfer from the intensive care unit (ICU) by implementing a nursing care plan similar to one that the child will experience on a regular unit (eg, decrease frequency of monitoring of vital signs, encourage independence). Give a thorough report to the receiving nurse during transfer.

Emotional Support to Family

1. Orient parents to the unit and its waiting areas. Clarify visiting policies and hospital expectations.
   a. If the admission to the ICU is expected, familiarize the parents with the ICU before the admission.
   b. If the admission is unexpected and sudden, the experience can be traumatic for the family. Care to reduce fears, stress, and anxiety is of prime importance for the family.

2. Encourage liberal visiting hours and unlimited phone calls from parents to the ICU.

3. Assure parents that everything possible is being done for their child. Whenever possible, allow them to see child receiving treatment.

4. Make certain that parents are informed of important changes in the child's clinical status. If parents are leaving the unit, exchange telephone numbers to ensure contact if needed. Reinforce medical interpretations.

5. Explain special equipment and changes in nursing management.

6. Provide opportunities for parents to ask questions and have them answered.

7. Encourage parents to keep a journal of their hospital experience. It is a very real way for parents to confront their feelings, especially if they are not expressing them to the hospital team.

8. Encourage parents to interact verbally and physically with their child. Support them in this endeavor.

9. Facilitate expression of parental grief.

10. Provide opportunities for parents to talk to a person with whom they can share their concerns and fears. Be sure this person can see them as often as they require.

11. Provide opportunities for parents to meet together to share experiences and offer mutual support. Encourage parents not to compare progress of other patients to their child. It can set them up to be quickly disappointed. Focus on each child and situation as unique.

12. Be sensitive to parents' additional commitments to family as well as to their need to remain with their child. Whenever possible, allow visiting at mutually convenient time.

13. Help parents provide anticipatory guidance for siblings and extended family members.

14. Refer parents to appropriate community resources for help for financial, environmental, or psychological problems.

15. Offer follow-up contact to parents if appropriate.

16. Guide families in the use of the Internet, and help connect them with support groups for information and peer support. Candlelighters Childhood Cancer Foundation can be reached at 800-366-2223 or *www. candlelighters.org.*

◼ Therapeutic Play and Child Life Programs

Play is a central mechanism in which children cope. Through play, children communicate, learn, and master a traumatic experience such as hospitalization.

Many hospitals have established programs with a specially trained staff whose job it is to concern themselves solely with the social and emotional welfare of every pediatric patient. Such programs are called by a variety of names, including "Child Life," "Children's Activities," "Recreational Therapy," "Play Therapy," and others.

Collaboration between nurses and child life specialists extends the benefits of these approaches across time and settings of care.

Goals of Child Life Programs

1. To prevent some of the emotional pain and fear associated with illness and hospitalization
   a. Child life workers may assume primary responsibility or a supportive role in the preparation of patients for hospitalization, surgery, or particular procedures.

   b. In many hospitals, child life workers arrange preadmission tours, puppet shows, and similar activities to which all children who are planned pediatric admissions are invited.

2. To provide a comfortable, accepting, and nonthreatening environment where the child may play and interact with other children and with an adult who is not involved with health care
   a. Ideally, there is a separate child life playroom in every unit. However, there may be only an open area at the end of the corridor or in the middle of the unit.

   b. Generally, there is a specific regulation that no medical procedures (even a relatively benign one such as taking child's temperature) are to be carried out in the play area.

   c. In many settings, children are encouraged to have their meals in the playroom. Generally, they not only enjoy the opportunity to eat with others, but also seem to eat better.

3. To provide the child with an opportunity for choice
   a. The child may choose whether he or she wishes to come to the playroom. Once there, child may choose what to do.

   b. A variety of craft and play materials, including real and miniature medical equipment, are available.

   c. Should the child choose to sit and watch or be held and rocked, these activities are seen as acceptable choices.

4. To provide a continuing educational program
   a. In some settings, teachers are paid by the hospital and are an integral part of the child life program. In others, teachers are provided by the local public schools, and they work in close cooperation with the child life department.

   b. In most hospitals, the educational program includes special activities for preschoolers and toddlers as well as a program of infant stimulation that may be in collaboration with physical and/or occupational therapists.

◼ Pain Management

General Considerations

1. Pain experienced by infants and children is not effectively identified or managed in many cases.

2. There are still misunderstandings about the ways pain is experienced and expressed by infants and children.

3. Behavioral and physiologic cues are used to assess pain in infants. Special rating tools are available to involve children in assessing the intensity of their pain, including the Pain Experience Inventory, CRIES Neonatal Postoperative Pain Measurement Scale, Oucher Pain Rating Scale, Numerical or Visual Analog Scale, and the FACES Pain Rating Scale (Figure 43-1).

4. Pain caused by a condition is not always proportional to the seriousness of the illness or injury. For example, a relatively minor illness, such as an earache, is a very

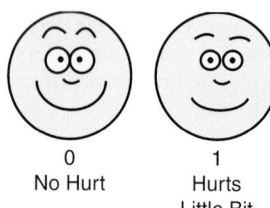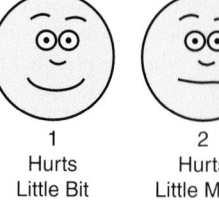

0	1	2	3	4	5
No Hurt	Hurts Little Bit	Hurts Little More	Hurts Even More	Hurts Whole Lot	Hurts Worst

FIGURE 43-1 FACES pain rating scale. (Whaley, L. & Wong, D. [1997]. *Essentials of pediatric nursing* [5th ed.]. Copyright by Mosby-Year Book. Used with permission.)

painful experience, whereas an enlarging tumor may not cause pain in early stages.

5. It is important to consider pain when a child is paralyzed, noncommunicative, or intubated.

6. It is equally important to consider pain when a child requires an injection, blood test, noninvasive or invasive diagnostic test.

7. Consider parents when assessing and managing the pain of their child. It is well documented that parents are important influences on their children.
   a. Consider the way in which parents view the situation experienced by the child, and work with them to intervene effectively.
   b. Presence of parents during a procedure can be very positive, especially when the family has been prepared.
   c. At other times, it is recommended that parents mutually agree to wait in a nearby area.
   d. Arbitrary rules against parental presence are often designed to meet the needs of staff, not the needs of the child and parents.

Nursing Interventions

1. Anticipate pain and intervene early.
2. Use a rating scale that the child can understand, and use it consistently with that child for initial pain assessment and to determine the effectiveness of interventions.
3. Use self as therapeutic presence to help ease pain.
4. Teach self-regulation and self-control techniques.
5. Utilize distraction by sounds, music, audio images, and movies.
6. Consider referral for self-hypnosis and conscious relaxation techniques.
7. Utilize medication delivered by way of noninvasive routes where possible.
8. Administer premedication—anesthetizing, antianxiety, and antiemetic medications as indicated.
9. Assist with conscious sedation when indicated, following standards of practice related to assessment, staffing, care, and documentation.

■ The Child Undergoing Surgery

Psychological Preparation and Support

Such preparation and support will minimize stress and will help the child and family cope with fears.

1. Potential threats for the hospitalized child anticipating surgery are:
   a. Physical harm—bodily injury, pain, mutilation, death
   b. Separation from parents, and peers for the older child/adolescent
   c. The strange and unknown—possibility of surprise
   d. Confusion and uncertainty about limits and expected behavior
   e. Relative loss of control of their world, loss of autonomy
   f. Fear of anesthesia
   g. Fear of the surgical procedure itself
   h. Misinterpretation of medical jargon (eg, dye–die)

2. The attitudes of the parents toward hospitalization and surgery largely determine the attitudes of their child.
   a. The experience may be emotionally distressing.
   b. Parents may have feelings of fear or guilt.
   c. The preparation and support should be integrated for parent, child, and family unit.
   d. Give individual attention to parents; explore and clarify their feelings and thoughts; provide accurate information and appropriate reassurance.
   e. Stress parents' importance to the child. Help mother understand how she can care for her child.

Preoperative Teaching

1. All preparation and support must be based on the child's age, developmental stage and level; personality; past history and experience with health professionals and hospitals; background including religion, socioeconomic circumstances, culture, and family attitudes.
2. Inquire as to what information the child has already received.
3. Determine what the child knows or expects; identify family myths and possible misunderstandings.
4. Additional guidelines in preparation include:
   a. Use illustration or model of a child's body, concrete examples, and simple terms (not medical jargon).
   b. Identify changes that may occur as a result of the procedure, both in body and daily routine.
   c. Give explanations slowly and clearly, saving anxiety-producing aspects until the end. Repeat as needed.
   d. Make use of child's creative ability and logical thinking powers to aid in preparation for procedures.
   e. Involve parents, as indicated, depending on the situation.

f. Allow and encourage the child to participate as able.

g. Suggest ways for the child to cope—crying is okay.

h. Offer constant reassurance; speak in a calm manner.

5. Orient patient and family to the unit, room, location of playroom, operating room, and recovery room, and introduce them to other children, parents, and some personnel. Make arrangements for the child to meet anesthesiologist as well as the operating room nurse and recovery room nurse.

6. Allow and encourage questions. Give honest answers.

a. Such questions will give the nurse a better understanding of the child's fears and perceptions of what is happening.

b. Infants and young children need to form a trusting relationship with those who care for them.

c. The older the child the more reassuring information can be.

7. Provide opportunity for child and parent to work out concerns and feelings (play, talk). Such supportive care should result in less upset behavior and more cooperation.

8. Prepare child for what to expect postoperatively (ie, equipment to be used or attached to child, different location, how child will feel, what child will be expected to do, diet, new caregivers).

Physical Preparation

1. Assist with necessary laboratory studies. Explain to child what is going to happen before procedure and how he or she can respond. Give continual support during procedure.

2. See that patient has nothing by mouth (NPO). Explain to child and parents what NPO means and the importance of it.

3. Assist with fever reduction.

a. Fever will result from some surgical problems (eg, intestinal obstruction).

b. Fever increases risk of anesthesia and need for fluids and calories.

4. Administer appropriate medications as prescribed. Sedatives and drugs to dry the secretions are often given on the unit.

5. Establish good hydration. Parental therapy may be necessary to hydrate the child, especially if child is NPO, vomiting, or febrile.

Immediate Postoperative Care

1. Maintain a patent airway and prevent aspiration.

a. Position the child on side or abdomen to allow secretions to drain and to prevent tongue from obstructing pharynx.

b. Suction any secretions present. Avoid causing a gag reflex or spasm during suctioning.

2. Make frequent observations of general condition and vital signs. Postoperative protocols may vary per procedure and facility.

a. Take vital signs every 15 minutes until child is awake and condition is stable.

b. Note respiratory rate and quality, pulse rate and quality, blood pressure, skin color.

c. Watch for signs of shock.

(i) All children in shock have signs of pallor, coldness, increased pulse, and irregular respiration.

(ii) Older children have decreased blood pressure and respiration.

d. Change in vital signs may indicate airway obstruction, hemorrhage, or atelectasis.

e. Restlessness may indicate pain or hypoxia. Medication for pain is not usually given until anesthesia has worn off.

f. Check dressings for drainage or constriction and pressure.

3. See that all drainage tubes are connected and functioning properly. Gastric decompression relieves abdominal distention and decreases the possibility of respiratory embarrassment.

4. Monitor parenteral fluids as prescribed.

5. Be physically near as child awakens to offer soothing words and a gentle touch. Reunite parents and child as soon as possible after the child recovers from anesthesia. If a language barrier exists, the parents should be with the child during recovery from anesthesia.

After Recovery From Anesthesia

After undergoing simple surgery and receiving a small amount of anesthesia, the child may be ready to play and eat in a few hours. More complicated and extensive surgery debilitates the child for a longer period of time.

1. Continue to make frequent and astute observations in regard to behavior, vital signs, dressings or operative site, and special apparatus (IV lines, chest tubes, oxygen).

a. Note signs of dehydration—dry skin and membranes; sunken eyes; poor skin turgor; sunken fontanelle in infant.

b. Record any passage of flatus or stool, bowel sounds. Observe for intestinal ileus because crying children swallow air, which may cause gastric distention.

c. Record vomiting time, amount, characteristics.

2. Assess behavior for signs of pain, and medicate appropriately.

3. Record intake and output accurately.

a. Parenteral fluids and oral intake.

b. Drainage from gastric tubes or chest tubes, colostomy, wound, and urinary output.

c. Parenteral fluid is evaluated and prescribed by considering output and intake. It is usually maintained until the child is taking adequate oral fluids.

4. Advance diet as tolerated, according to the child's age and the health care provider's directions.

a. First feedings are usually clear fluids; if tolerated, advance slowly to full diet for age. Note any vomiting or abdominal distention.

b. Because anorexia may occur, offer what the child likes, in small amounts and in an attractive manner.

5. Prevent infection.
   a. Keep the child away from other children or personnel with respiratory or other infections.
   b. Change the child's position every 2 to 4 hours; prop infants with a blanket roll.
   c. Encourage the child to cough and breathe deeply; let the infant cry for short periods of time, unless contraindicated.
   d. Keep operative site clean—change dressing as needed; keep diaper away from wound.
6. Provide good general hygiene, and opportunities for exercise and diversional activity; encourage sleep and rest.
7. Provide emotional support and psychological security. Reassure child that things are going well. Talk about going home, if appropriate.
8. Begin early to prepare for discharge: teach special procedures, provide written instructions, and arrange for community nurse referral.

◼ The Dying Child

The nursing role is to assist the child and family to cope with the experience in such a way that it will promote growth rather than destroy family integrity and emotional well-being.

Recognize the Stages of Dying
See Table 43-1.
1. Be aware that dying children, their families, and the staff will all progress through these stages, not necessarily at the same time.
2. Children experience the stages with much variation. They tend to pass more quickly through the stages and may merge some of these stages.
3. The nursing goal is to accept the child and family at whatever stage they are experiencing, not to push them through the stages.

4. Understand the meaning of illness and death at various stages of growth and development (Table 43-2).
5. Be aware of other factors that influence a child's personal concept of death. Of particular importance are:
   a. The amount and type of direct exposure a child has had to death
   b. Cultural values, beliefs, and patterns of bereavement
   c. Religious beliefs about death and an afterlife

Communicate With Child About Death
Research indicates that children generally can cope with more than adults will allow and that children appreciate the opportunity to know and understand what is happening to them. It is important that the child's questions be answered simply, but truthfully, and that they be based on the child's particular level of understanding. The following responses have been suggested by Easom in *The Dying Child* and may be useful as a guide:

Preschool-Aged Child
1. When the child at this age is comfortable enough to ask questions about illness, questions should be answered. When death is anticipated at some future time and the child asks, "Am I going to die?" a response might be, "We will all die someday, but you are not going to die today or tomorrow."
2. When death is imminent and the child asks, "Am I going to die?" the response might be, "Yes, you are going to die, but we will take care of you and stay with you."
3. When the child asks, "Will it hurt?" the response should be truthful and factual.
4. Death may be described as a form of sleep—a sleep where he will be secure in the love of those around. However, some children may fear sleep as the result of this type of explanation. Anesthesia is sometimes called a "special sleep" so it is not currently recommended to refer to death as "sleep."

TABLE 43-1 Stages of Dying as Identified by Dr. Elizabeth Kübler-Ross

Stage	Nursing Implications
I. Denial, shock, disbelief.	Accept denial, but function within a reality sphere. Do not tear down the child's (or family's) defenses. Be aware that denial usually breaks down in the early morning when it may be dark and lonely. Be certain that it is the child or family who is using denial, not the staff.
II. Anger, rage, hostility.	Accept anger and help the child express it through positive channels. Be aware that anger may be expressed toward other family members, nursing staff, physicians, and other persons involved. Help families to recognize that it is normal for children to express anger for what they are losing.
III. Bargaining (from "No, not me," to "Yes, me, but . . .")	Recognize this period as a time for the child and family to regain strength. Encourage the family to finish any unfinished business with the child. This is the time to do things such as take the promised trip or buy the promised toy.
IV. Depression. (The child and/or family experiences silent grief and mourns past and future losses.)	Recognize this as a normal reaction and expression of strength. Help families to accept the child who does not want to talk and excludes help. This is a usual pattern of behavior. Reassure the child that you can understand his or her feelings.
V. Acceptance.	Assist families to provide significant loving human contact with their child and one another.

TABLE 43-2 Stages in the Development of a Child's Concept of Death

Age of Child	Stage of Development
Child up to 3 y	At this stage, the child cannot comprehend the relationship of life to death because child has not developed the concept of infinite time. The child fears separation from protecting and comforting adults. The child perceives death as a reversible act.
Preschool child	At this age, the child has no real understanding of the meaning of death; child feels safe and secure with parents. The child may view death as something that happens to others. The child may interpret the separation that occurs with hospitalization as punishment; the painful tests and procedures that child is subjected to support this idea. The child may become depressed because of not being able to correct these wrongdoings and regain the grace of adults. The concept may be connected with magical thoughts of mystery.
School-aged child	The child at this age sees death as the cessation of life; child understands that he or she is alive and can become "not alive"; child fears dying. The child differentiates death from sleep. Unlike sleep, the horror of death is in pain, progressive mutilation, and mystery. The child is vulnerable to guilt feelings related to death because of difficulty in differentiating death wishes and actual event. The child believes death may be caused by angry feelings or bad thoughts. The child learns the meaning of death from own personal experiences, such as pets, and the death of family members, political figures, and so forth. Television and movies have contributed to concept of death and understanding of the meaning of illness. There may be more knowledge in the meaning of the diagnosis and an awareness that death may occur violently.
Adolescent	The adolescent comprehends the permanence of death as the adult does although may not comprehend death as an event occurring to persons close to self. Adolescent wants to live—sees death as thwarting pursuit of goals: independence, success, achievement, physical improvement, and self-image. Adolescent fears death before fulfillment. The adolescent may become depressed and resentful because of bodily changes that may occur, dependency, and the loss of social environment. The adolescent may feel isolated and rejected because own adolescent friends may withdraw when faced with impending death of friend. The adolescent may express rage, bitterness, and resentment; especially resents the fact that fate is to die.

5. Parents can express to the child the fact that they do not want child to go and that they will miss the child very much; they feel sad, too, that they are going to be separated.

School-Aged Child

1. Responses to the school-aged child's questions about death should be answered truthfully. The child looks for support from those he or she trusts.
2. The school-aged child should be given a simple explanation of diagnosis and its meaning; child should also receive an explanation of all treatments and procedures.
3. The child should be given no specific time in terms of days or months because each individual and each illness is different.
4. When the school-aged child asks, "Am I going to die?" and death is inevitable, child should be told the truth. The school-aged child does have the emotional ability to look to parents and those he or she trusts for comfort and support.
5. The school-aged child believes in parents. The child should be allowed to die in the comfort and security of family.

6. The school-aged child knows death means final separation and knows what will be missed. The child must be allowed to mourn this loss. The dying child may be sad and bitter and demonstrate aggressive behavior. The child must be allowed the opportunity to verbalize this if able to do so.

Adolescent

1. The adolescent should be given an explanation of illness and all necessary treatment and procedures.
2. The adolescent feels deprived and reasonably resentful regarding illness because he or she wants to live and reach fulfillment.
3. As death approaches, the adolescent becomes emotionally closer to family.
4. The adolescent should be allowed to maintain emotional defenses—including absolute denial. The adolescent will indicate by questions what kind of answers are desired.
5. If the adolescent states, "I am not going to die," he or she is pleading for support. Be truthful and state, "No, you are not going to die right now."
6. The adolescent may ask, "How long do I have to live?" Adolescents are able to face reality more directly and

can tolerate more direct answers. No absolute time should be given because that blocks all hope. If an adolescent has what is felt to be a prognosis of approximately 3 months, the response might be, "People with an illness like yours may die in 3 to 6 months, but some may live much longer."

Support Parents' Adaptation to Child's Death

1. Develop a plan of care that includes the following approach:
   a. The primary responsibility for communicating with the parents should be designated to one nurse.
   b. Information regarding the parents' concerns should be communicated to all staff members.
2. Accept parental feelings about the child's anticipated death, and help parents deal with these feelings.
   a. It is not unusual for parents to reach the point of wishing the child dead and to experience guilt and self-blame because of this thought.
   b. The parents may withdraw emotional attachments to the child if the process of dying is lengthy. This occurs because the parents complete most of the mourning process before the child reaches biologic death. They may relate to the child as if he or she were already dead.
3. Provide anticipatory guidance regarding the child's actual death and immediate decisions and responsibilities afterward.
   a. Describe what the death will probably be like and how to know when it is imminent. This is necessary to dispel the horrifying fantasies that many parents have. Reassure the parent that the child will be kept comfortable at the time of death.
   b. Clarify the parents' wishes about being present at the child's death, and respect their desires. See if they want to hold the child—before, during, or after the death.
   c. If appropriate, allow the parents to discuss their feelings about issues such as autopsy and organ donation in order that they may make appropriate decisions. Do not make them feel guilty if they do not consent.
   d. If necessary, assist the parents to think about funeral arrangements.
4. Be aware of factors that affect the family's capacity to cope with fatal illness, especially social and cultural features of the family system, previous experiences with death, present stage of family development, and resources available to them.
5. Contact the appropriate clergy if the family desires. Contact other extended family members for support if they wish.
6. During final hours, do not leave the family alone, unless they request it.
7. Encourage parents and siblings to share their thoughts with the dying child.
8. Provide information on bereavement support groups, usually available through hospital or church.

PEDIATRIC PROCEDURES

Restraints

Protective measures to limit movement are mechanisms for restraining children (Figure 43-2). They can be a short-term restraint to facilitate examination and minimize the child's discomfort during special tests, procedures, and specimen collections. Restraints can also be used for a longer period of time to maintain the child's safety and protection from injury.

General Considerations

1. Protective devices should be used only when necessary and after all other considerations are exhausted, never as a substitute for careful observation of the child.
2. Protective devices cannot be used on a continuous basis without an order. Continuous use requires justification and full documentation of the type of restraint used, reason for use, and the effectiveness of the restraint used. Ongoing monitoring, documentation, and renewal of the order are required.
3. The reason for using the protective device should be explained to the child and parents to prevent misinterpretation and to ensure their cooperation with the procedure. Children often interpret restraints as punishment.
4. Any protective device should be checked frequently to make sure it is effective. It should be removed periodically to prevent skin irritation or circulation impairment. Provide range of motion and skin care routinely.
5. Protective devices should always be applied in a manner that maintains proper body alignment and ensures the child's comfort.
6. Any protective device that requires attachment to the child's bed should be secured to the bed springs or frame, never the mattress or side rails. This allows the side rails to be adjusted without removing the restraint or injuring the child's extremity.
7. Any required knots should be tied in a manner that permits their quick release. This is a safety precaution.
8. When a child must be immobilized, an attempt should be made to replace the lost activity with another form of motion. For example, although restrained, a child can be moved in a stroller, wheelchair, or in bed. When arms are restrained, the child may be allowed to play kicking games. Water play, mirrors, body games, and blowing bubbles are helpful replacements.

NURSING ALERT

 A health care provider's order is needed to initiate continuous restraints. Proper documentation is required when restraints are in use. Do not secure restraints to bed rails or mattresses. Hourly assessment of the restrained extremity is needed to ensure there has been no impairment of circulation and constriction or respiratory compromise with chest restraints.

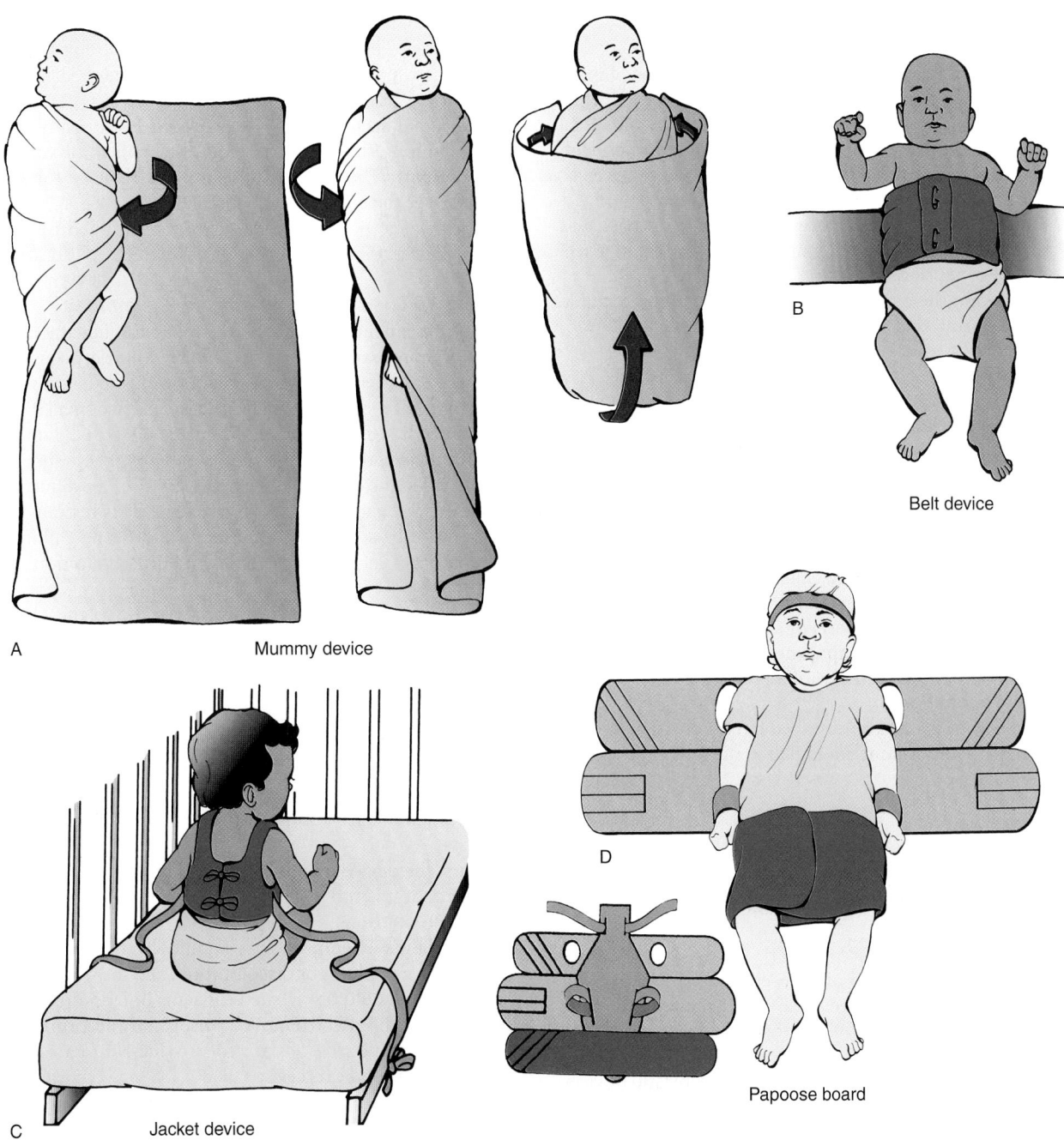

A   Mummy device

B   Belt device

C   Jacket device

D   Papoose board

FIGURE 43-2 Types of restraints.

Mummy Device

The mummy device involves securing a sheet or blanket around the child's body in such a way that the arms are held to the sides and leg movements are restricted (see Figure 43-2). This short-term type of restraint is used on infants and small children during treatments and examinations involving the head and neck.

Equipment
Small sheet or blanket
Nursing Action
1. Place the blanket or sheet flat on the bed.
2. Fold over one corner of the blanket.
3. Place the child on the blanket with neck at the edge of the fold.

4. Pull the right side of the blanket firmly over the child's right shoulder.
5. Tuck the remainder of the right side of the blanket under the left side of the child's body.
6. Repeat the procedure with the left side of the blanket.
7. Separate the corners of the bottom portion of the sheet, and fold it up toward the child's neck.
8. Tuck both sides of the sheet under the infant's body.
9. Secure by crossing one side over the other in the back and tucking in the excess, or by pinning the blanket in place.

Special Precautions

Make certain the child's extremities are in a comfortable position during this procedure.

Jacket Device

The jacket device is a piece of material that fits the child like a jacket or halter. Long tapes are attached to the sides of the jacket (see Figure 43-2). Jacket device restraints are used to keep the child in a wheelchair, high chair, or crib.

Nursing Action

1. Put the jacket on the child so the opening is in the back.
2. Tie the strings securely.
3. Position the child in high chair, wheelchair, or crib.
4. Secure the long tapes appropriately:
   a. Under the arm supports of a chair
   b. Around the back of the wheelchair or high chair
   c. To the springs or frame of a crib

Special Precautions

Children in cribs must be observed frequently to make certain they do not become entangled in the long tapes of the jacket device.

Belt Device

The belt device is exactly like the jacket method of restraining, except that the material fits the child like a wide belt and buckles in the back (see Figure 43-2).

Elbow Device

The elbow device consists of a piece of material into which tongue depressors have been inserted at regular intervals. It is especially useful for infants receiving a scalp vein infusion, those with eczema or cleft lip repair, and children having eye surgery. Some companies have plastic devices that fit around the arm at the elbow bend and are secured with Velcro straps. This type of restraint prevents flexion of the elbow.

Equipment

1. Elbow cuff
2. Tongue depressors
3. Safety pins, tapes, string or commercial plastic elbow restraint

Nursing Action

1. Insert tongue depressors into the appropriate places in the elbow cuff.
2. Place the child's arm in the center of the elbow cuff.
3. Wrap the cuff around the child's arm.
4. Secure the cuff with pins, tapes, or string.

Special Precautions

1. The tongue depressors should be cut to about 10 cm (4 inches) in length if the elbow cuff is to be used for an infant for greatest comfort.
2. Additional security may be provided by dressing the child in long-sleeved shirt before the application of the elbow cuff. The ends of the shirt can then be turned back over the cuff and pinned securely.
3. If the plastic device is used, it may be applied over a shirt sleeve or padded to prevent sweating.

Devices to Limit Movement of the Extremities

Many different kinds of devices are available to limit motion of one or more extremities. One commercial variety consists of a piece of material with tapes on both ends to be secured to the frame of the bed. The material also has two small flaps sewn to it for securing the child's ankles or wrists. Similar devices are available that use sheepskin flaps. These should be used when the device will be necessary over a prolonged period or for children with sensitive skin. This restraining device may be used to restrain infants and young children for procedures such as IV therapies and urine collection.

Equipment

1. Extremity restraint of appropriate size for the child (small, medium, or large)
2. Several safety pins
3. Cotton wadding covered with gauze

Nursing Action

1. Secure the device to the crib frame.
2. Pad the extremities to be restrained with cotton wadding, gauze, or other suitable material.
3. Pin the small flaps securely around the child's ankles or wrists.
4. Adjust the device by pinning a tuck in the center of the material if it is too large.

Special Precautions

1. The infant's fingers or toes should be observed frequently for coldness or discoloration, and the skin under the device should be checked for signs of irritation.
2. The device should be removed periodically according to policy or standards of care to provide skin care and range-of-motion exercises.

Abdominal Device

The abdominal device is used for restraining a small child in a crib. It operates exactly like the method described for limiting the movements of extremities. However, the strip of material is wider and has only one wide flap sewn in the center for fastening around the child's abdomen.

Clove-Hitch Device

The clove-hitch device is a mechanism for restraining an extremity by tying gauze strips or a diaper in a special way.

Equipment

1. Cotton wadding covered with gauze
2. Gauze bandage cut in lengths of 1.37 m (1½ yd)

Nursing Action

1. Pad the extremity to be restrained with cotton wadding that is covered with gauze or other suitable material.
2. Spread out the gauze strip.
3. Make a figure-eight loop in the center of the gauze strip.
4. Place the child's wrist or ankle in the loop of the device.
5. Pull the ends of the device to the desired tightness.
6. Tie the ends to the crib springs or frame.
7. Check the device to make certain it does not tighten when both ends are pulled taut or slip over the child's hand or foot.

Mitts

Mitts are used to prevent a child from injuring self with hands. They are especially useful for children with dermatologic conditions, such as eczema or burns. Mitts can be purchased commercially or made by wrapping the child's hands in Kling gauze.

> **NURSING ALERT**
>
> Mitts should be removed at least every 4 hours to permit skin care and to allow the child to exercise fingers.

Crib Top Device

A crib top device is used to prevent an infant or small child from climbing over the crib sides. Several types of commercial devices are available, including nets, plastic tops, and domes. A crib top device should be applied to the crib of an infant capable of climbing over the crib sides.

> **NURSING ALERT**
>
> In all instances, it is essential to be certain that the crib sides are kept all of the way up and latched securely. There should be no space between the top of the crib sides and the bottom of the crib top device.

Papoose Board

A papoose board is the most cumbersome restraint device that may be used for procedures of the head, chest, and abdomen. Straps restrain the child or infant at the forehead, lower arms, and thighs. (See Figure 43-2.)

■ Specimen Collection

Evaluation of specimens such as blood, urine, and stool is important in determining the status of the child. The nurse should be adept in the techniques for obtaining specimens, as well as meticulous in labeling and recording them.

For blood collection procedure, see Procedure Guidelines 43-1.

For urine specimen collection, see Procedure Guidelines 43-2.

For percutaneous suprapubic bladder aspiration, see Procedure Guidelines 43-3.

For stool collection, see Procedure Guidelines 43-4.

(text continues on page 1322)

PROCEDURE GUIDELINES 43-1	ASSISTING WITH BLOOD COLLECTION

EQUIPMENT

No. 23–19-gauge short needle or scalp vein needle   Smaller tourniquet (rubber band may be used with infant)
Smaller volume or micro blood-collecting tubes   Gloves per standard (universal) precautions

PROCEDURE

Nursing Action	Rationale
PREPARATORY PHASE	
1. Immobilize the child by placing in a mummy restraint if necessary (see p. 1315).	1. Infants and young children squirm. Immobilizing them allows easier access to the venipuncture site. It also helps keep the infant warm.
2. Position the patient.	2. These positions allow for optimal visualization and stabilization of the patient.
a. *Femoral venipuncture*: Place the child on back with legs in froglike position. Nurse places hands on child's knees.	a. Cover perineum to protect site and operator should infant void.
b. *External jugular venipuncture:* Place the child in mummy restraint and lower head over the side of the bed or table. Turn head to side and stabilize. See accompanying figure.	b. Crying will make external jugular vein visible and causes blood to flow more readily.
c. *Antecubital fossa venipuncture:* Place the child in a supine position. The nurse stands on the side opposite the site to be used (across from the person drawing the specimen). The nurse positions right arm across the upper part of the child's chest and grasps the shoulder at the axilla position. Nurse's left arm is placed across the lower part of the child's chest and is used to extend the child's arm at the wrist (see accompanying figure).	c. Nurse's hands are used to straighten and hold child's arm still; arms are used to maintain stability of child's upper body.

continued

PROCEDURE GUIDELINES 43-1   **ASSISTING WITH BLOOD COLLECTION** *CONTINUED*

Nursing Action   **Rationale**

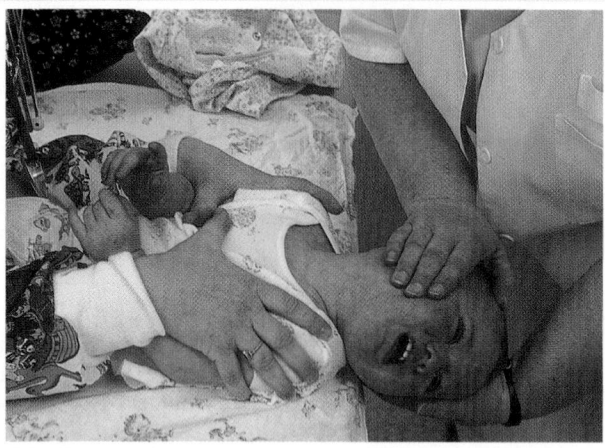

Assisting with jugular venipuncture.

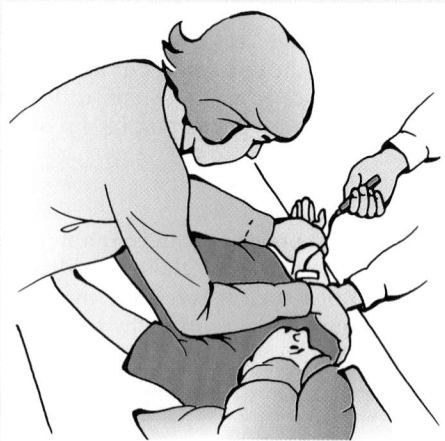

Assisting with antecubital fossa venipuncture.

   d. *Infant—heel, toe, or digital puncture:* warm area with warm compress for 5–10 minutes.

   d. This dilates vessels allowing blood to flow more freely.

PERFORMANCE PHASE

1. a. *Capillary:* Clean area with antiseptic and dry with dry sterile 2 × 2 gauze. Hold heel firmly, and with free hand quickly puncture with microlancet or sterile No. 21-gauge needle on most medial or lateral part of plantar surface. Puncture deeply enough to get free-flowing blood—never deeper than 2.4 mm. Discard first drop of blood; rapidly collect specimen in proper capillary tube.

1. Universal precautions. Both persons holding the infant and drawing the blood should wear gloves.

2. After the specimen is collected and the needle is removed, apply pressure to the site with dry gauze for 3–5 minutes.

   a. *Jugular venipuncture:* While applying pressure to the site, place the patient in an upright sitting position. Do not apply excessive pressure that may compromise circulation or respiration.

2. Both the femoral and jugular veins are large vessels. Because intravascular pressure is great, bleeding, oozing, and hematoma formation may result. External pressure prevents this from happening.

3. When the bleeding has been stopped, soothe and comfort the child before leaving.

3. Crying and thrashing about may initiate bleeding.

FOLLOW-UP PHASE

1. Check the patient frequently for 1 hour after the procedure for oozing, bleeding, or evidence of a hematoma.

1. Reapply pressure and report if oozing continues.

2. Record carefully and accurately:
   a. Site of venipuncture
   b. How the patient tolerated procedure
   c. Bleeding stopped or continued and for how long
   d. For what test the specimen was collected, time and place sent.

PROCEDURE GUIDELINES 43-2 COLLECTING A URINE SPECIMEN FROM THE INFANT OR YOUNG CHILD

EQUIPMENT

Collecting device—plastic, disposable urine bag or collector (Hollister, U-Bag, double chamber)

Cleansing agent
Wiping material—4 × 4s or cotton balls
Clean or sterile water

Containers for solutions
Specimen container
Gloves

PROCEDURE

Nursing Action	Rationale
PREPARATORY PHASE	
1. Offer the young child choice of fluids to drink 30–60 min before procedure, if no contraindications.	1. To increase urine production.
2. Position the patient so genitalia are exposed by placing on back with legs in froglike position. Assistance may be needed to hold the legs of the young child in proper position.	2. Proper positioning will facilitate cleansing and allow for proper placement of collection device.
3. When small samples of urine are needed for pH, Clinitest, and so forth to be done by the nurse, urine can be extracted from the diaper using a syringe or dropper.	
PERFORMANCE PHASE	
1. Wear gloves.	1. Universal precautions.
2. Cleanse genital area.	2. This method of cleansing the female will prevent contamination of the genitalia from the anus, and will prevent contamination of the urine specimen obtained. During the cleansing, be gentle to avoid any injury or possible stimulation of urination.
a. *Female:* Using cotton balls, dip into cleansing agent, wipe labia majora from top to bottom (clitoris to anus) only once with each cotton ball. Repeat this once more. Wipe again with clear water. Then spread labia apart with one hand while wiping the labia minora in the same manner with other hand. Wipe area dry.	
b. *Male:* Wipe tip of penis in circular motion down toward the scrotum. Be certain to retract foreskin if present. Wipe first with cleansing agent two to three times, then clear water. Dry the area.	
3. Apply collecting bag firmly so the opening is exposed to receive urine.	3. If collecting bag is properly and securely placed, the procedure will not have to be repeated.
a. *Female:* Stretch perineum taut during application. Attach bag to perineum first, then proceed up to symphysis.	a. This should ensure leak-proof contact.
b. *Male (small boys):* Place penis inside bag.	

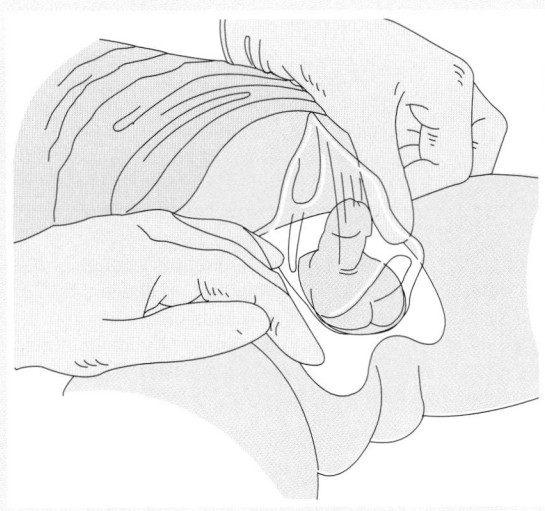

Urine collector for male infants.

continued

PROCEDURE GUIDELINES 43-2	COLLECTING A URINE SPECIMEN FROM THE INFANT OR YOUNG CHILD *CONTINUED*

Nursing Action	Rationale
4. Apply diaper and comfort patient; possibly give additional clear fluids.	
5. Elevate head of bed or place child in an infant seat if appropriate.	5. To aid flow of urine by gravity.
6. Check the patient frequently (30–45 minutes) to see if he or she has voided. When the patient has voided, remove bag gently. Cleanse area and reapply diaper to the child. If child has not voided within 45 minutes, procedure must be repeated.	6. The adhesive on the collecting bag may tend to be sticky. Careful removal of the bag will prevent skin injury on and around genitalia. Also avoid spilling urine out of the bag during removal. Reapplication of bag will decrease the possibility of unreliable test results.

FOLLOW-UP PHASE

Nursing Action	Rationale
1. Pour specimen into proper collecting container. Send specimen to the laboratory within 30 minutes or refrigerate.	1. Prompt delivery of specimen to the laboratory will prevent growth of organisms in an uncontrolled environment and distortion of the test results.

2. Accurately chart and describe the following in the nurse's notes:
   a. Time specimen collection was started and ended
   b. Amount of urine voided
   c. Color of urine (cloudy, clear, any sediment)
   d. Type of test to be done
   e. Condition of skin of perineal area
	2. Guideline for weighing diaper, excluding weight of dry diaper, 1 g = 1 mL urine.

Note: If 24-hour urine collection is needed, use a collection bag that has a long tube attachment to facilitate frequent emptying of urine every 1–2 hours. Place urine in receptacle in refrigerator. Adherence of bag to skin can be improved by applying a thin coating of tincture of benzoin to skin and allowing this to dry before attaching collection bag.

PROCEDURE GUIDELINES 43-3	ASSISTING WITH A PERCUTANEOUS SUPRAPUBIC BLADDER ASPIRATION

EQUIPMENT

Antiseptic skin cleansing solution
Band-Aid
Sterile 4 × 4s
Gloves
Needle, No. 20–22 gauge, 3.7 cm (1½ inches) long
Syringe, 20 mL
Specimen container

PROCEDURE

Nursing Action	Rationale

PREPARATORY PHASE

Nursing Action	Rationale
1. Check diaper for wetness. If the child has just voided, report this or report last voiding time. At least 1 hour should pass without voiding.	1. To perform a successful bladder aspiration, enough urine must be present to distend the bladder up above the pubic symphysis—so bladder is accessible.
2. Position the child on back on the examining table. Head should be toward nurse, feet toward the health care provider. Spread legs apart in a froglike position. Place hands on child's knees and thumbs along sides at the hip level.	2. This position allows the nurse to stabilize the child. It also gives a full view of the child, making it easier to observe, talk to him, and soothe the child.
3. Ensure that the skin over the puncture site is cleansed in an antiseptic manner.	3. To prevent infection from being introduced into the bladder by inserting the needle through unclean skin, which would contaminate the specimen.

PROCEDURE GUIDELINES 43-3 *CONTINUED*

Nursing Action	Rationale
PERFORMANCE PHASE	
1. Both the health care provider and nurse should wear gloves.	1. Universal precautions.
2. While the procedure is being performed, note the condition of the patient and any signs of distress. Comfort child by talking and smiling.	2. Report any changes in color or respiration rate or other signs. Soothing the child will promote relaxation and decreased movement. Crying increases the muscle tone of the lower abdomen, making it more difficult to insert the needle.
3. To prevent urination during procedure, compress the infant's urethra: a. *Male:* Pressure on penis. b. *Female:* Digital pressure upward on urethra from rectum.	
4. When urine has been obtained or the procedure is discontinued and the needle is removed, apply pressure over the puncture site with a 4 × 4 and gloved fingers.	4. This prevents any bleeding from occurring either internally or externally. Pressure should be maintained about 3 minutes or until oozing ceases and coagulation has taken place.
5. Apply a Band-Aid if necessary. Reapply diaper. Hold and comfort child for a few minutes.	5. Holding the child will help to restore and maintain a good nurse–patient relationship and will help the child to relax after a frightening and painful procedure.
FOLLOW-UP PHASE	
1. Check the child periodically for 1 hour after procedure to see that bleeding or oozing has not occurred.	1. This is not likely if pressure was applied properly after procedure and the patient was left quiet.
2. Note time of first voiding after procedure. Note color of urine (it may be pink). Bloody urine should be reported to the health care provider.	2. It is important to note any changes in voiding pattern after the procedure because change might indicate injury. The first voided urine may be bloody because of a small amount of local capillary bleeding at the time of the procedure.
3. Accurately describe and chart the procedure, including: a. Time of procedure b. Whether or not a specimen was obtained c. How the patient tolerated the procedure d. Description and amount of urine obtained e. Patient's condition and activity after the procedure.	

PROCEDURE GUIDELINES 43-4 COLLECTING A STOOL SPECIMEN

EQUIPMENT

Diaper	Tongue blade
Cellophane or plastic liner (used when stool is loose or watery)	Specimen container
	Gloves

Note: Collecting a stool specimen from an older child who is toilet-trained is the same as collecting such a specimen from an adult.

PROCEDURE

Nursing Action	Rationale
PREPARATORY PHASE	
1. If a specimen is needed from a patient whose stools are loose or watery enough to be absorbed in the diaper, line the diaper with a piece of cellophane or plastic. Place this liner between the diaper and the skin. Then apply diaper to the child and position so head is slightly elevated. If stools are soft or formed, apply diaper.	1. The liner and position will allow the loose stool specimen to collect in the liner and not be absorbed by the diaper.

continued

PROCEDURE GUIDELINES 43-4	COLLECTING A STOOL SPECIMEN *CONTINUED*

Nursing Action	Rationale
PERFORMANCE PHASE	
1. Wear gloves.	1. Universal precautions.
2. Check the child frequently to see if stooling has occurred.	2. A fresh specimen should be obtained so test results will not be distorted by time lapse. This will also decrease the chance of contamination of the stool with urine and will prevent skin irritation from the stool.
3. Remove soiled diaper from child. Clean perineal area, apply clean diaper, and leave the child comfortable.	
4. Remove small amount of stool from diaper with the tongue blade and place it in the specimen container.	
5. Send labeled specimen to the laboratory promptly.	5. Prompt delivery to the laboratory will prevent changes from occurring in the specimen that could alter the test results.
FOLLOW-UP PHASE	

1. Accurately describe and record the following:
  a. Time specimen was collected
  b. Color, amount, and consistency of stool (note any foul smell)
  c. Type of specimen collected
  d. Nature of test for which the specimen was collected
  e. Condition of the skin	

Feeding and Nutrition

Nutritional requirements of the infant or child may increase while ill, but the ability to feed naturally may be impaired by illness or the child's response to illness. If existing feeding patterns cannot be maintained, alternate methods may be necessary.

Gavage Feeding

Refer to Procedure Guidelines 43-5.
1. Gavage feeding is a means of providing food by way of a catheter passed through the nares or mouth, past the pharynx, down the esophagus, and into the stomach, slightly beyond the cardiac sphincter. Feedings may be continuous or intermittent.
2. Gavage feedings can provide a method of feeding or administering medications that require minimal patient effort when the infant is unable to suck or swallow adequately (ie, premature infants under 32 weeks' gestation or under 1,560 g).
3. Gavage feedings provide a route that allows adequate calorie or fluid intake, and they can provide supplemental or additional calories.
4. Gavage feedings can prevent fatigue or cyanosis that is apt to occur from bottle-feeding. They can provide supplement for an infant who is a poor bottle-feeder.
5. Gavage feedings can provide a safe method of feeding a limp, listless patient, a patient experiencing respiratory distress (respiratory rate greater than 60/min), or intubated patients, debilitated patients, or those with anomalies of the digestive tract.

Gastrostomy Feeding

Refer to Procedure Guidelines 43-6.
1. Gastrostomy feeding is a means of providing nourishment and fluids by way of a tube that is surgically inserted through an incision made through the abdominal wall into the stomach. It is the method of choice for those requiring tube feedings for an extended period of time.
2. Gastrostomy feedings provide a safe method of feeding a hypotonic patient or one who cannot tolerate alternative methods. Specific indications may include duodenal atresia, tracheoesophageal fistula, and omphalocele. Gastrostomy feedings may provide a route that allows adequate calorie or fluid intake in a child with chronic lung disease or in one who does not have continuity of the gastrointestinal (GI) tract, such as in esophageal atresia, chronic reflux, or aspiration processes.
3. Gastrostomy tubes can also allow better decompression of the stomach (because of the large tube size) after a surgical procedure.

Community and Home Care Considerations

Gastrostomy feedings often are maintained for an extended period of time. If a child is receiving these tube feedings at home, nursing responsibilities include the following:
1. Teach the child (if age appropriate) and family about gastrostomy feedings.
   a. Anatomy of tube placement
   b. Amount and timing of feedings

c. Signs and symptoms of problems—tube obstruction or displacement, distended stomach, infection

d. Appropriate actions to be taken if problems occur—call home care nurse or health care provider

2. Teach the use of equipment: syringes, feeding bag, feeding tubing.

3. Teach the use of control pump (for continuous feedings).

4. Teach care of the gastrostomy tube—how to clamp, observe for leakage.

5. Stoma care—clean with soap and water, observe for breakdown, apply skin barrier.

6. Instruct about formula—proper mixing if not reconstituted; need to refrigerate if opened; discard any unused, nonrefrigerated formula after 4 hours.

7. Teach measures to take in an emergency.

a. Procedure to follow if the tube falls out—cover site with sterile gauze dressing, and call health care provider or proceed to emergency room.

b. Troubleshooting for nonfunctioning equipment—ensure that pump is plugged in and turned on, tubing is unclamped, tubing is not kinked, abdomen is not distended.

c. Proper phone numbers available to have as a resource or to obtain assistance

8. Perform regular home visits to assess nutritional and hydration status of the child, check tube placement and stoma site, and modify plan of care as needed.

Nasojejunal Feeding/Nasoduodenal Feedings

Refer to Procedure Guidelines 43-7.

1. Nasojejunal (N-J) or nasoduodenal (N-D) feedings are means of providing full enteral feedings by way of a catheter passed through the nares, past the pharynx, down the esophagus, bypassing the stomach through the pylorus into the duodenum or jejunum.

2. Duodenal or jejunal feedings decrease the risk of aspiration because the feeding bypasses the pylorus; can minimize regurgitation and gastric distention.

3. N-D and N-J feedings provide a route that allows for adequate calorie or fluid intake (a full enteral feeding) by way of intermittent or continuous drip.

4. N-D or N-J feedings may also provide a route for administration of oral medications.

5. N-D or N-J feedings can provide a method of feeding that requires minimal patient effort when the child or infant is unable to tolerate alternative feeding methods (low birth weight, persistent respiratory effort in the intubated patient).

(*text continues on page 1329*)

PROCEDURE GUIDELINES 43-5 | **GAVAGE FEEDING**

EQUIPMENT

Sterile rubber or plastic catheter, rounded-tip, size 5–12 (French Argyle feeding tube)	Syringe	Tape—hypoallergenic
Clear, calibrated reservoir for feeding fluid	Stethoscope	Feeding fluid, room temperature
	Water for lubrication	Pacifier

PROCEDURE

Nursing Action	Rationale
PREPARATORY PHASE	
1. Position the infant on side or back with a diaper roll placed under shoulders. A mummy restraint may be necessary to help maintain this position.	1. This position allows for easy passage of the catheter, facilitates observation, and helps avoid obstruction of the airway.
2. Measure feeding catheter and mark with tape; measure distance from tip of nose to ear to xiphisternum.	2. Premeasuring the catheter provides a guideline as to how far to insert catheter.
3. Have suction apparatus readily available.	3. Suctioning clears the airway and prevents aspiration if regurgitation occurs.
PERFORMANCE PHASE	
1. Lubricate catheter with sterile water or saline.	1. Do not use oil because of danger of aspiration.
2. Stabilize the patient's head with one hand; use the other hand to insert catheter.	
a. *Insertion through nares:* Slip the catheter into nostril and direct toward the occiput in a horizontal plane along floor of nasal cavity. Do not direct the catheter upward. Observe for respiratory distress.	a. This direction will follow the nares' passageway into the pharynx. Positioning in nares may cause partial airway obstruction. Avoid this route if there is critical airway compromise.
b. *Insertion through the mouth:* Pass the catheter through the mouth toward the back of the throat. Depress anterior portion of tongue with forefinger, insert catheter along forefinger, and tilt head slightly forward.	

continued

PROCEDURE GUIDELINES 43-5   **GAVAGE FEEDING** *CONTINUED*

Nursing Action	Rationale
3. If the patient swallows, passage of the catheter may be synchronized with the swallowing. Do not push against resistance. Gently try rotating the tube if resistance is met.	3. Swallowing motions will cause esophageal peristalsis, which opens the cardiac sphincter and facilitates passage of the catheter. Perforation occurs with very little pressure.
4. If there is no swallowing, insert the catheter smoothly and quickly.	4. Because of cardiac sphincter spasm, resistance may be met at this point. Pause a few seconds, then proceed.
5. In the infant, especially, observe for vagal stimulation (ie, bradycardia [slow heart rate] and apnea).	5. The vagus nerve pathway lies from the medulla through the neck and thorax to the abdomen. Above the stomach, the left and right branches unite to form the esophageal plexus. Stimulation of these nerve branches with the catheter will directly affect the cardiac and pulmonary plexus.
6. Once the catheter has been inserted to the premeasured length, tape the catheter to the patient's face (see accompanying figure).	6. This prevents movement of catheter from the pre-measured, preestablished correct position. Alternative method; loop narrow cloth tape around tube just below nostril, then secure it above lip or nose with tape. Some movement of tube may be seen with swallowing.

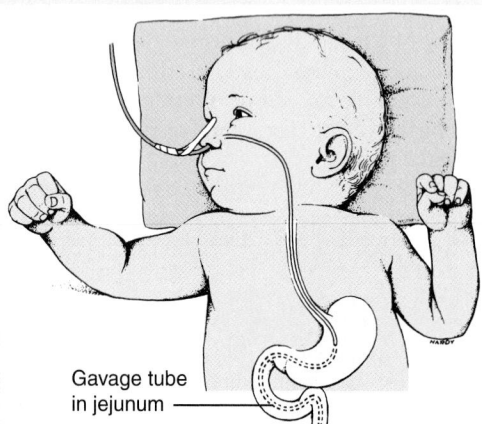

Gavage tube in jejunum

Gavage tube in jejunum

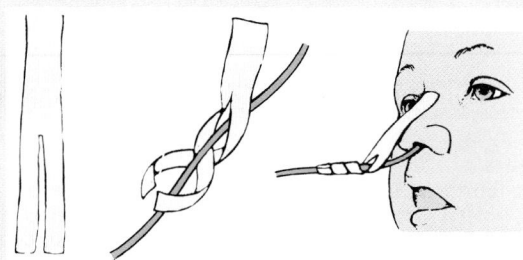

Steps in preparing adhesive tape to retain gavage tube.

7. Test for correct position of the catheter in the stomach: a. Inject 0.5–5 mL air into the catheter and stomach. At the same time, listen to the typical growling stomach sound with a stethoscope placed over the epigastric region.	a. Aids in ensuring proper location of catheter.
b. Aspirate injected air from the stomach.	b. This prevents abdominal distention.
c. Aspirate small amount of stomach content and test acidity by pH tape.	c. Failure to obtain aspirate does not indicate improper placement; there may not be any stomach content or the catheter may not be in contact with the fluid.
d. Observe and gently palpate abdomen for tip of catheter. Avoid inserting catheter into the infant's trachea. (An infant's anatomy makes it relatively difficult to enter the trachea because esophagus is behind the trachea.)	d. If improper placement occurs and the catheter enters the trachea, the patient may cough, fight, and become cyanotic. Remove the catheter immediately and allow the patient to rest before attempting to insert tube again.
8. The feeding position should be right-side-lying, with head and chest slightly elevated. Attach reservoir to catheter and fill with feeding fluid. Encourage infant to suck on pacifier during feeding. Hold infant when possible.	8. This position allows the flow of fluid to be aided by gravity. The use of the pacifier will relax the infant, allowing for easier flow of fluid as well as provide for normal sucking needs. Sucking will help develop muscles and provide a positive association between sucking and relief of hunger.

PROCEDURE GUIDELINES 43-5   *CONTINUED*

Nursing Action	Rationale

9. Aspirate tube before feeding begins.
   a. If over half the previous feeding is obtained, withhold the feeding.
   b. If small residual of formula is obtained, return it to stomach and subtract that amount from the total amount of formula to be given.
	9. This is done to monitor for appropriate fluid intake, digestion time, and overfeeding that can cause distention. Note an increase in gastric residual contents.

10. The flow of the feeding should be slow. Do not apply pressure. Elevate reservoir 15–20 cm (6–8 inches) above the patient's head.	10. The rate of flow is controlled by the size of the feeding catheter; the smaller the size, the slower the flow. If the reservoir is too high, the pressure of the fluid itself increases the rate of flow.
11. Food taken too rapidly will interfere with peristalsis, causing abdominal distention and regurgitation.	11. The presence of food in the stomach stimulates peristalsis and causes the digestive process to begin. Also, when tube is in place, incompetence of the esophageal–cardiac sphincter may result in regurgitation.
12. Feeding time should last approximately as long as when a corresponding amount is given by nipple, 5 mL/5–10 min or 15–20 minutes total time.	
13. When the feeding is completed, the catheter may be irrigated with clear water. Before the fluid reaches the end of the catheter, clamp it off and withdraw it quickly or keep in place for next feeding.	13. Clamp the catheter before air enters the stomach and causes abdominal distention. Clamping also prevents fluid from dripping from the catheter into the pharynx, causing the patient to gag and aspirate.
14. Discard feeding tube and any leftover solution.	

> **NURSING ALERT**
>
> Intermittent gavage feeding is often preferred to indwelling gavage feeding. An indwelling catheter may coil and knot, perforate the stomach, and cause nasal airway obstruction, ulceration, irritation of the mucous membranes, incompetence of esophageal–cardiac sphincter, and epistaxis. However, if intermittent intubation is not well tolerated and the indwelling method is used, the catheter should be clamped to prevent loss of feeding or entry of air and changed every 48–72 hours. (Use alternate sides of the nares.) Constant alertness to the above problems should be stressed. Indwelling method may be preferred with older infant or child.

FOLLOW-UP PHASE

1. Burp the patient.	1. Adequate expulsion of air swallowed or ingested during feeding will decrease abdominal distention and allow for better tolerance of the feeding.
2. Place the patient on right side for at least 1 hour.	2. To facilitate gastric emptying and minimize regurgitation and aspiration.
3. Observe condition after feeding; bradycardia and apnea may still occur.	3. Because of vagal stimulation as mentioned above.
4. Note any vomiting or abdominal distention.	4. Due to overfeeding or too rapid feeding. Regurgitation of 1–2 mL may occur in the premature infant as the musculature of the sphincter of the gastrointestinal tract is relaxed and allows for easy reflex.
5. Note infant's activity.	5. Fatigue or peaceful sleep offers insight as to tolerance of the feeding.
6. Accurately describe and record procedure, including time of feeding, type of gavage feeding, type and amount of feeding fluid given, amount retained or vomited, how the patient tolerated feeding, and activity before, during, and after feeding.	6. Observe for readiness of the infant to feed by nipple—note sucking activity and sleep–wake cycle in relation to feeding.

PROCEDURE GUIDELINES 43-6   GASTROSTOMY FEEDING

EQUIPMENT

Warm feeding fluid	Reservoir syringe or funnel
Pacifier	Syringe for aspirating

PROCEDURE

Nursing Action	Rationale
PREPARATORY PHASE	

1. Gastrostomy tube may be in one of three positions between feedings:
  a. Lowered and open to start drainage.
  b. Open, connected to reservoir (funnel, syringe) that is elevated 10–12 cm (4–43/4 inches).
  c. Clamped.
	a. Constant decompression.
	  b. To serve as safety valve outlet to prevent esophageal reflux and increased stomach pressure.
	  c. Most "normal" physiologic setup, preparation for home care or tube removal.

2. The nurse may be directed to check residual stomach contents before any feeding.
  a. Attach syringe and aspirate stomach contents.
  b. Measure.
  c. Residual fluid may be returned to stomach or discarded, depending on amount.
	2. This is done to monitor for appropriate fluid intake, digestion time, and overfeeding that can cause distention.

3. A Y-tube that is connected at the point where reservoir and gastrostomy tube join may be used during feeding.	3. To provide simultaneous decompression during feeding.
4. When feeding is about to begin, infant/child should be placed in comfortable position in bed—either flat or with head slightly elevated. If condition permits, the nurse should hold the infant. A pacifier can be given.	4. When the infant/child is comfortable and relaxed, feeding fluid will flow more easily into stomach. Pacifier will satisfy normal sucking activity, provide exercise for jaw muscles, and relax musculature as well as provide pleasure normally associated with feeding.

Note: Gastrostomy tube feeding button:

The child may have a gastrostomy tube feeding button, in which case insert the special tube into the button and follow the feeding procedure in the Performance Phase.

Nursing Action	Rationale
PERFORMANCE PHASE	
1. Attach reservoir syringe to tube (if not already open to continuous elevation), and fill reservoir with feeding fluid unclamping tube.	1. Prevents air from entering tube (and then stomach), which may cause distention.
2. Elevate tube and reservoir to 10–12 cm (4–43/4 inches) above abdominal wall. Do not apply any pressure to start flow.	2. This elevation level will allow for slow, gravity-induced flow. Pressure may cause a backflow of fluid into the esophagus.

3. Feed slowly, taking 20–45 minutes. Fill reservoir with remaining fluid before it is empty to avoid instillation of air.	3. Too rapid a feeding will interfere with normal peristalsis and will cause abdominal distention and backflow into reservoir or esophagus.
	  a. This rinses tubing and will prevent clogging.
	  b. Feeding fluid is allowed to return to reservoir if infant cries or changes position, and thus decreases pressure on the stomach.

4. Continue to provide infant with pleasant feelings associated with feeding.	

5. When feeding is completed:
  a. Instill clear water (10–30 mL, or 0.3–1 oz) if tube is to be clamped. Apply clamp before water level reaches end of reservoir.
  b. Leave tube unclamped and open to continuous elevation.	

6. Often when oral feedings are started, they are given simultaneously with gastrostomy feedings.	6. This allows the infant to learn or reestablish the sucking-swallowing process as well as to build up tolerance to eating without compromising nutritional intake.

PROCEDURE GUIDELINES 43-6 *CONTINUED*

Nursing Action	Rationale

FOLLOW-UP PHASE

1. Check dressing and skin around point of tube entry for wetness. Clean skin and apply skin barrier (petrolatum, Maalox, aluminum paste, etc.). See that there is no pull on tube.

2. Leave the infant dry and comfortable. If unable to hold infant during feeding, this may be a good time to hold, fondle, and provide warmth and love. Place on right side or in Fowler's position.

3. Accurately describe and record procedure, including time of feeding, type and amount of feeding fluid given, amount and characteristics of residual (if any) and what was done with it, how the patient tolerated feeding, any abdominal distention, activity after feeding.

1. Skin breakdown is caused by continued exposure to stomach contents that may be leaking out around tube causing excoriation and infection. Constant pulling on tube can cause widening of skin opening and subsequent leakage.

2. To promote relaxation and improved digestion of feeding.

 NURSING ALERT

Should infant pull out gastrostomy tube, cover ostomy site with sterile dressing and tape, notify health care provider and accurately record events.

PROCEDURE GUIDELINES 43-7 **NASOJEJUNAL (N-J) AND NASODUODENAL (N-D) FEEDINGS**

EQUIPMENT

Sterile radiopaque silicone or polyvinyl nasojejunal (N-J) or nasoduodenal (N-D) tube, 1 m (39 inches) (appropriate size for child); may or may not have weighted tip
Tape
pH paper
Reservoir for feeding

Possibly an infusion pump
Three-way stopcock
Syringe—0.5 mL normal saline or sterile water
Equipment for nasogastric (N-G) tube insertion;
   introducer catheter

PROCEDURE

Nursing Action	Rationale

PREPARATORY PHASE

1. Attach cardiac monitor to infant.

2. Tube is generally inserted by a health care provider.
   a. Measure from glabella (prominent point between eyebrows) to the heel for estimated length.
   b. Measure and mark the remaining length of tubing and record.

3. Place the infant on right side with hips slightly elevated. Gentle restraint or soft mittens may have to be applied.

1. To allow for continuous monitoring of heart rate and rhythm. The vagus nerve pathway lies from the medulla through the neck and thorax to the abdomen. Above the stomach, the left and right branches unite to form the esophageal plexus. Stimulation of these nerve branches with the catheter will directly affect the cardiac and pulmonary plexus.

   b. This serves as a double-check to ensure that tube has not advanced farther than intended.

3. Facilitates passage of tube. Restraints prevent infant from pulling out tube before the tip passes the pylorus. Do not place on left side.

continued

PROCEDURE GUIDELINES 43-7   NASOJEJUNAL (N-J) AND NASODUODENAL (N-D) FEEDINGS
CONTINUED

Nursing Action	Rationale
4. Tube is inserted by threading the N-J or N-D vinyl catheter into a No. 10 French feeding catheter and introducing both through the nostril into the stomach. The feeding tube is then withdrawn, and the N-D/N-J feeding tube is allowed to advance through the pylorus.	4. Oral insertion may cause increased salivation, air swallowing, and regurgitation. The N-G acts as an introduction catheter and may not be needed because N-D or N-J catheters come with an internal guidewire to aid in placement.
5. Check intestinal aspirate for pH every 1–2 hours. Infant may be positioned on right side, back, or abdomen. Once the tube is past the pylorus, abdominal posteroanterior and lateral x-rays are taken to confirm that tip of catheter is at the ligament of Treitz. Remove the guidewire.	5. When aspiration fluid reaches a pH of 5–7 or bile-colored fluid is obtained, the tip of the tube has passed the pylorus and duodenum into the jejunum.
6. A small N-G feeding tube may be passed through the other nostril at this time and left indwelling. This is used to check stomach for residual fluid and regurgitation through the pylorus.	6. If gastric residual is significant, it will interfere with prescribed feeding. Notify health care provider. (4 mL/kg reflux in stomach is usually tolerated.) Do not remove N-G tube because it will adhere to N-J tube during withdrawal and pull out N-J tube also.
7. N-D/N-J feedings can generally be started following this progression: a. D$_s$W initially b. Half-strength formula with low osmolality for 6–12 hours. Higher osmolarity formulas for older children. c. Full-strength, low-osmolality formula for infants and high-osmolality formula for older children. d. The volume of feeding is increased at a slow rate until daily calorie and fluid requirements are being administered.	 b. Low-solute formulas include SMA, Similac, Enfamil (20 cal/30 mL). c. Low-osmolality formula is used to prevent loss of fluid into intestine and possible necrotizing enterocolitis. d. 150 mL/kg fluid requirement is generally used (130–150 cal/kg).
8. Medications may be given by way of the N-D/N-J tube if prescribed. A three-way stopcock will have to be placed at the connection of the N-J tube and the line from the feeding fluid. Alternative method for administering oral medications is by passing an oral–gastric or nasogastric feeding tube; in this way, the stomach and process of digestion and absorption are not bypassed.	8. Flush tubing with small amounts of normal saline solution or sterile water after medication is administered to ensure that infant receives entire dosage prescribed and to prevent any sediment from remaining in tubing or prevent tube clogging. Pills should be crushed finely.

PERFORMANCE PHASE

Nursing Action	Rationale
1. N-J feedings can be given as follows: a. Intermittently (ie, q 1–3 h) b. In a continuous slow drip.	 b. Generally, the preferred method to minimize the satiety–hunger cycle and large-volume instillation.
2. If intermittent feeding is the method used, the feeding techniques are the same as for nasogastric (gavage) feeding.	2. Feeding is given at room temperature. Avoid cold fluid, which may cause infant discomfort. If breast milk is used, gently rotate reservoir periodically to mix settled-out fat content.
3. If slow continuous drip method is used, the set-up used is similar to the pediatric IV infusion using an infusion pump and small (100–250 mL) closed chamber for reservoir. a. Reservoir chamber and tubing should be changed q8–24 h. b. Record input every hour. Fill reservoir as needed, with no more than 3 hours worth of feeding fluid.	 a. To prevent growth of bacteria. b. To ensure a constant flow and minimize overinfusion directly into the jejunum/duodenum.

FOLLOW-UP PHASE

Nursing Action	Rationale
1. Be constantly alert for mechanical problems: a. Check for abdominal distention resulting from the infant's inability to handle ingested amount of fluid by: • Palpating abdomen • Observing for ripple of intestines	1. Tube clogging due to inadequate rinsing. Tube advancing too far into jejunum; check protruding tube measurement. Fluid overload, causing aspiration.

PROCEDURE GUIDELINES 43-7   *CONTINUED*

Nursing Action	Rationale

• Measuring abdominal girth q3–8 h
    • Checking residual formula in jejunum q3–8 h
    • Discarding or refeeding residual formula as prescribed.
  b. Check stools for occult blood and pH, and urine for glucose every voiding or 4–8 hours to determine tolerance of feeding fluid.
  c. Check emesis for blood and report to physician immediately—may be a sign of necrotizing enterocolitis.
2. Position child/infant in recumbent position.
3. Observe child/infant closely to avoid potential dangers as tube passes the pylorus.
  a. Close attention to amount, type, concentration, and osmolality of feeding fluid is stressed.
  b. Check heart rate and blood pressure.
4. Hold, fondle, and give positive stimulation to the child/infant if conditions permit.
 	
5. Accurately describe and record condition of infant and procedure, including type and amount of feeding given, amount of residual and characteristics, any signs of impending infant distress or problems.
	
	2. Less likely for "dumping syndrome" to occur.
	3. Diarrhea; as the tube passes through the pylorus, it (the tube) becomes stiff because of the change in pH. A stiff tube has been reported to cause intestinal perforation. If tube becomes clogged or dislodged, it must be removed.
	
	4. This procedure limits the normal pleasures associated with feeding. Infant needs some attention to psychological needs to thrive.

Fluid and Electrolyte Balance

Basic Principles

1. Infants and small children have different proportions of body water (Table 43-3) and body fat than do adults.
   a. The body water of a newborn infant approaches 80% of body weight compared with that of an average adult man, which approaches 60%.
   b. The normal infant demonstrates a rapid physiologic decline in the ratio of body weight to body water during the immediate postpartum period.
   c. Proportion of body water declines more slowly throughout infancy and reaches the characteristic value for adults by approximately 2 years of age.
2. Compared with adults, a greater percentage of the body water of infants and small children is contained in the extracellular compartment.

   a. Infants—approximately one half of the body water is contained in the cell.
   b. Adults—approximately two thirds of the body water is contained in the cell.
3. Compared with adults, the water turnover rate per unit of body weight is three or more times greater in infants and small children.
   a. The child has more body surface in relation to weight.
   b. The immaturity of kidney function in infants may impair their ability to conserve water.
4. Electrolyte balance depends on fluid balance and cardiovascular, renal, adrenal, pituitary, parathyroid, and pulmonary regulatory mechanisms (Table 43-4).
5. Infants and children are more vulnerable to disorders of hydration than are adults.
   a. The basic principles relating to fluid balance in children make the magnitude of fluid losses considerably greater in children than adults.
   b. Children are prone to severe disturbances of the GI tract that result in diarrhea and vomiting.
   c. Young children cannot independently respond to increased losses by increased intake. They depend on others to provide them with adequate fluid.

Common Fluid and Electrolyte Therapy

1. Repair of preexisting deficits that may occur with prolonged or severe diarrhea or vomiting.
   a. Deficits are estimated and corrected as soon and as safely as possible.

TABLE 43-3 Body Fluids Expressed as Percentage of Body Weight

Fluid	Adult		Infant (%)
	Male (%)	Female (%)	
Total body fluids	60	54	75
Intracellular	40	36	40
Extracellular	20	18	35

TABLE 43-4 Common Abnormalities of Fluid and Electrolyte Metabolism

Substance	Major Function	Abnormality	Cause	Clinical Manifestation	Laboratory Data
Water	Medium of body fluids, chemical changes, body temperature, lubricant	Volume deficit	1. Primary—inadequate water intake 2. Secondary—loss following vomiting, diarrhea, gastrointestinal obstruction, and so forth	Oliguria, weight loss, signs of dehydration including dry skin and mucous membranes, lassitude, sunken fontanelles, lack of tear formation, increased pulse rate, decreased blood pressure	Concentrated urine, azotemia, elevated hematocrit, hemoglobin and erythrocyte count
		Volume excess	1. Failure to excrete water in presence of normal intake such as in congestive heart failure, renal disease 2. Water intake in excess of output	Weight gain, peripheral edema, signs of pulmonary congestion	Variable urine volume, low specific gravity of urine, decreased hematocrit
Potassium	Intracellular fluid balance, regular heart rhythm, muscle and nerve irritability	Potassium deficit	1. Excessive loss of potassium due to vomiting, diarrhea, prolonged cortisone, ACTH or diuretic therapy, diabetic acidosis 2. Shift of potassium into the cells such as occurs with the healing phase of burns, recovery from diabetic acidosis	Signs and symptoms variable, including weakness, lethargy, irritability, abdominal distention, and eventually cardiac arrhythmias	Low plasma K^+ level (may be normal in some situations); hypochloremic alkalosis; ECG changes
		Potassium excess	Excessive administration of potassium-containing solutions, excessive release of potassium due to burns, severe kidney disease, adrenal insufficiency	Variable, including listlessness, confusion, heaviness of the legs, nausea, diarrhea, ECG changes, ultimately paralysis and cardiac arrest	Elevated potassium plasma level
Sodium	Osmotic pressure, muscle and nerve irritability	Sodium deficit	Water intake in excess of excretory capacity, replacement of fluid loss without sufficient sodium; excessive sodium losses	Headache, nausea, abdominal cramps, confusion alternating with stupor, diarrhea, lacrimation, salivation, later hypotension; early polyuria, later oliguria	Sodium plasma level may be high, low, or normal
		Sodium excess	Inadequate water intake especially in the presence of fever or sweating; increased intake without increased output; decreased output	Thirst, oliguria, weakness, muscular pain, excitement, dry mucous membranes, hypotension, tachycardia, fever	Elevated Na^+ plasma level, high plasma volume
Bicarbonate	Acid–base balance	Primary bicarbonate deficit	Diarrhea (especially in infants), diabetes mellitus, starvation, infectious disease, shock or congestive heart failure producing tissue anoxia	Progressively increasing rate and depth of respiration—ultimately becoming Kussmaul respiration, flushed, warm skin, weakness, disorientation progressive to coma	Urine pH usually <6 Plasma bicarbonate <20 mEq/L Plasma pH <7.35
		Primary bicarbonate excess	Loss of chloride through vomiting, gastric suction, or the use of excessive diuretics, excessive ingestion of alkali	Depressed respiration, muscle hypertonicity, hyperactive reflexes, tetany and sometimes convulsions	Urine pH usually >7, plasma bicarbonate >25 mEq/L (30 mEq/L in adults), plasma pH >7.45

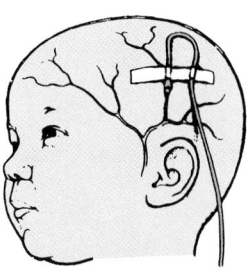

Venipuncture of scalp vein

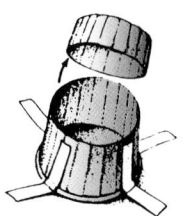

Paper cup taped over venipuncture site for protection. A clear plastic cup may also be used.

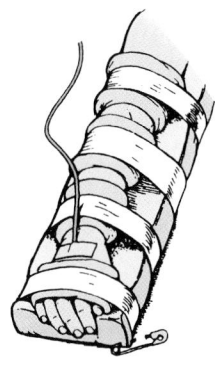

Restraint of arm when hand is site of infusion

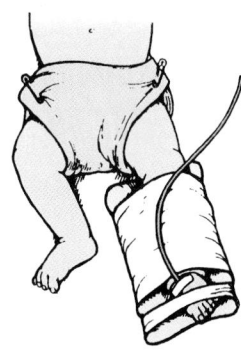

Infant's leg taped to sandbag for immobilization (IV site should be visible)

FIGURE 43-3   IV fluid therapy.

b. Initial therapy is aimed at restoring blood and extra-cellular fluid volume to relieve or prevent shock and restore renal function.

c. Intracellular deficits are replaced slowly over an 8- to 12-hour period after the circulatory status is improved.

2. Provision of maintenance requirements.

   a. Maintenance requirements occur as a result of normal expenditures of water and electrolytes due to metabolism.

   b. Maintenance requirements bear a close relationship to metabolic rate and are ideally formulated in terms of caloric expenditure.

3. Correction of concurrent losses that may occur by way of the GI tract as a result of vomiting, diarrhea, or drainage of secretions.

4. Replacement should be similar in type and amount to the fluid being lost.

5. Replacement is usually formulated as milliliters of fluid and milliequivalents of electrolytes lost.

Intravenous Fluid Therapy

IV therapy refers to the infusion of fluids directly into the venous system. This may be accomplished through the use of a needle or by venous cutdown and insertion of a small catheter directly into the vein (Figure 43-3). IV therapy is used to restore and maintain the child's fluid and electrolyte balance and body homeostasis when oral intake is inadequate to serve this purpose. Refer to Procedure Guidelines 43-8.

1. Infusion pumps are often used in pediatrics to provide a controlled, constant rate of infusion.

2. Because infants and children are vulnerable to fluid shifts, the rates need to be controlled carefully.

3. During an IV infusion, every hour, check:

   a. Delivery rate

   b. Volume delivered

c. For infiltration, because many pumps will continue to infuse solution even if infiltration has occurred See Standards of Care Guidelines.

(text continues on page 1335)

STANDARDS OF CARE GUIDELINES
Pediatric IV Therapy

When caring for a child undergoing IV therapy,

- Check IV apparatus and site hourly, noting skin color, evidence of swelling. Compare to opposite extremity or look for asymmetry. Feel area for sponginess. Observe for leakage.
- Record reading on the container or reservoir, amount of fluid absorbed in the hour, rate flow.
- Check for blood return in tube by stopping IV fluid flow.
- Make certain child is adequately and safely restrained.
- Check function of pump rate set versus amount infused.
- Maintain accurate intake and output record and 24-hour totals
- Describe consistency of all stools and vomitus.
- Weigh child at regular intervals using same scale each time. An increase or decrease of 5% body weight in a relatively brief period of time is usually significant.
- Monitor electrolytes (see Table 43-4, p. 1330).
- Report evidence of electrolyte imbalances: decreased skin turgor, marked increase or decrease in urination, fever, sunken or bulging fontanelles, sudden change in vital signs, diarrhea, weakness, lethargy, apathy, pyrogenic reactions.
- If child is experiencing severe reactions, IV should be discontinued and solution saved for possible analysis.
- Change the IV container and tubing q24h or as per hospital policy.
- If infiltration occurs, remove IV, apply heat to site, restart IV at alternative site, and notify health care provider if irritation develops or toxic medication has infiltrated.

This information should serve as a general guideline only. Each patient situation presents a unique set of clinical factors and requires nursing judgment to guide care, which may include additional or alternative measures and approaches.

PROCEDURE GUIDELINES 43-8	INTRAVENOUS FLUID THERAPY

EQUIPMENT

A. NEEDLE METHOD

IV solution
  The kind of solution is specified by the health care provider.
  For small children, 250-mL bottles should be used for purposes of safety.
IV pole, pump device
IV administration set, pump tubing
Micropore filter
Syringe, 5 or 10 mL—approximately ½–⅔ filled with normal saline
Butterfly needle or catheter of appropriate gauge
  The size of the needle depends on the age and size of the child and the type of fluid to be administered
Alcohol sponges, dry sponges
Betadine or other antibacterial cleansing solution
Normal saline
Small tourniquet or rubber band
Hypoallergenic tape, 1.2 cm (½ inch), 2.5 cm (1 inch), 5 cm (2 inches)
Padded armboard
Gauze bandage for securing the extremity to the armboard
Restraining devices—bath blanket, extremity restraint, covered sandbags
  The type of restraint depends on the child's age, his level of cooperation, and the kind of IV to be started.
Safety razor (if scalp vein is to be used)

B. CUTDOWN METHOD

IV solution, IV pole, IV administration set
Alcohol sponges
Hypoallergenic tape, 1.2 cm (½ inch), 2.5 cm (1 inch), 5 cm (2 inches)
Padded armboard
Dry sponges
Gauze bandage
Sterile cutdown tray
  The tray should include the following equipment: medicine cups, treatment towels, wound towel, syringe, No. 25 gauge 1.5-cm (⅝-inch) needle, No. 1–20 gauge 2.5-cm (1-inch) needle, knife handle and No. 15 blade, forceps, scissors, gauze sponges, 4-0 black silk suture, needle holder
Assorted sizes of sterile polyethylene tubing and Luer adapters
5-0 black silk suture with a straight eye needle
1%–2% procaine
Normal saline
Tourniquet
Sterile gloves
Restraining devices

PROCEDURE

Nursing Action	Rationale
PREPARATORY PHASE	
1. Obtain the IV solution.	1. Although the type of solution and the rate of flow are prescribed, the nurse should be aware of the composition of common parenteral solutions and should know how to calculate maintenance therapy.
2. Check the IV fluid for sediment or contaminant by holding the container up to the light.	2. Contaminant is most easily identified with the container in this position. If sediment is observed, the solution should be discarded.
3. Check the container for cracks.	3. If a flash of light can be seen through the bottle, it has a razor-thin crack and should be discarded.

PROCEDURE GUIDELINES 43-8	*CONTINUED*

Nursing Action	**Rationale**
4. Attach a micropore filter to the end of the infusion tubing that attaches to the needle. Use aseptic technique.	4. A 0.45-μm filter prevents entry into the vein of larger particles, air emboli, and most bacterial and fungal organisms except some *Pseudomonas* organisms. A 0.22-μm filter prevents entry of any organisms but requires the use of an IV pump.
5. Remove the metal seal from the IV container without touching the rubber top.	5. Do not use the solution if the seal has been broken. It is not necessary to cleanse the sterile, rubber top with alcohol unless it has been accidentally contaminated.
6. Following product information, insert the end of the administration set into the container's opening. Fill the tubing with solution.	

7. Promote the cooperation of the child.
  a. *Infant:* Provide with a pacifier.
  b. *Older child:* Explain the procedure and its purpose.
	7. The procedure will be least traumatic if child is able to cooperate and is not frightened or resistant.

8. Position the child for comfort.	
9. Restrain the child as necessary.	9. Protective devices may be necessary to prevent the child from dislodging the IV needle. The type and size of such devices should be appropriate for the child's age and the position of the IV.
a. *Infant or young child:* Restraints may include mummy wrappings, jacket or elbow restraints, or small sandbags.	
b. *Older child:* The extremity to be used should be comfortably restrained on the armboard. Free extremities may also require light restraints to remind the child not to move.	b. Toes and fingers should be visible to avoid compromising blood flow. The restraint board must be padded and the main pressure points (heel, palm) padded with gauze. Before strapping an extremity to the armboard, back the adhesive with tape or gauze wherever it touches the skin.

PERFORMANCE PHASE

1. The persons starting the IV and holding the infant should wear gloves.	1. Universal precautions.
2. Assist as necessary.	2. The nurse may insert the IV, based on institution policy.
3. When applying the tourniquet, a second rubber band is placed crosswise under it. To remove the tourniquet, grasp the unstretched rubber band, pull up, and cut the tourniquet (see accompanying figure).	3. To ensure easy and rapid removal of tourniquet.

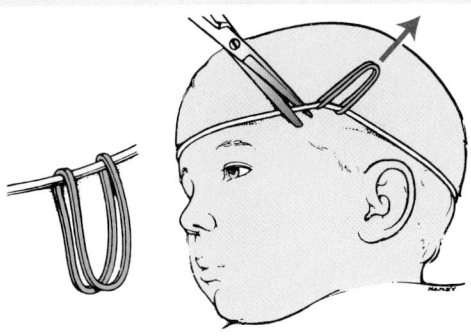

Applying the tourniquet for IV therapy.

continued

PROCEDURE GUIDELINES 43-8   **INTRAVENOUS FLUID THERAPY** *CONTINUED*

Nursing Action	Rationale
4. Check the restraints at intervals, and adjust them as necessary.	4. The restraints may become loose after a period of time and must be secured to ensure the child's safety. They may also become too tight and require loosening to maintain adequate circulation.

FOLLOW-UP PHASE

Nursing Action	Rationale
1. Comfort and reassure the child.	1. The procedure is usually disturbing for the child. This should be acknowledged. If crying and upset, the child should be reassured that his behavior is acceptable.
2. Regulate the IV rate by way of pump	2. Pump infusion devices are more often than not used in IV rate regulation of infants and children.
3. Record: Type of solution being used Reading on the container or reservoir Rate of flow Time that the infusion began Name of the physician or nurse who started the IV Site of administration Reaction of the child to the procedure	
4. Return the child to room.	

IRRIGATING AN IV

PERFORMANCE PHASE

Nursing Action	Rationale
1. Irrigate the IV as necessary.	1. Irrigation may be required to dislodge small clots in the needle or to maintain the infusion rate of a sluggish IV.
2. Gather equipment: Syringe with 1–3 mL normal saline solution Several alcohol wipes	
3. Clamp off the IV solution.	
4. Disconnect the IV tubing at the needle insertion site. Keep it sterile.	
5. Remove the needle from the syringe.	
6. Connect the syringe to the tubing at the needle insertion site or stopcock.	
7. Slowly inject the normal saline solution.	7. Great force of injector should be avoided because this may cause the vein to rupture or the needle to become dislodged from the vein.
8. Disconnect the syringe, and reconnect the IV tubing to the needle insertion site.	
9. Unclamp the IV, and regulate the flow of the solution.	
10. Check frequently to make certain that the IV is functioning properly.	

REMOVAL OF AN IV LINE

PERFORMANCE PHASE

1. Disconnect the IV when prescribed or if it has obviously infiltrated.
2. Gather equipment:
   Scissors
   4 × 4 gauze square
   Band-Aid
3. Explain the procedure to the child, depending on age.
4. Clamp off the flow of the IV fluid.
5. Determine the location of the needle.
6. Loosen the tape around the needle, holding the needle firmly in position so it does not slip out.

Nursing Action	Rationale
7. Hold the 4 × 4 lightly over the insertion site, and remove the needle quickly and carefully.	7. Alcohol sponges should not be used for removing IV needles because the stinging of alcohol on the puncture site causes unnecessary discomfort.
8. Apply pressure to the site immediately and hold until bleeding stops. 9. Apply Band-Aid.	9. The Band-Aid should not be applied until all bleeding has stopped to minimize the possibility of prolonged or unnoticed bleeding.
10. Remove the tape and armboard from the extremity.	10. If the intracath or plastic needle is not intact, notify the health care provider.
11. Comfort the child as required. 12. Note the fluid level on the container or reservoir, and complete recordings. 13. Record that the IV was discontinued.	

For additional information relating to IV therapy, including criteria for selecting a suitable vein for venipuncture, guidelines for administering an infusion using the antecubital fossa, and complications of intravenous therapy, refer to Chapter 6, IV Therapy.

■ Cardiac and Respiratory Monitoring

Cardiac and respiratory monitoring refers to electrical surveillance of heart and respiratory rates and patterns. It is indicated in all patients whose conditions are unstable.

Nursing Management

1. Select a monitor that is appropriate for the child's needs. This will depend on the child's age, ability to cooperate, purpose for monitoring, information desired, and equipment available.
2. Stabilize the device to reduce the amount of mechanical noise and for safety considerations.
3. Reduce the child's anxiety:
   a. Provide age-appropriate explanations of the equipment.
   b. When possible, involve the child in care, including change of electrodes.
4. Select lead placement sites according to equipment specifications:
   a. Cardiac monitors frequently use three leads located at:
      (i) Right upper lateral chest wall below clavicle
      (ii) Left lower chest wall in the anterior axillary line
      (iii) Upper left chest wall
   b. Respiratory monitors frequently use three electrodes located:
      (i) On either side of the chest (anterior axillary line in fourth or fifth intercostal space)
      (ii) A reference electrode placed on the manubrium or other suitable distal point
5. Apply electrodes by:
   a. Cleaning the appropriate areas on the chest with alcohol.
   b. Place pregelled, disposable electrodes.
   c. Apply the electrode firmly to completely dry skin.
6. Plug the leads into the lead cable at appropriate insertion points.
7. Be certain that the monitor alarms are in the "on" position. High and low alarm limits should be set according to the child's age and condition so apnea, tachypnea, bradycardia, and tachycardia can be readily detected.
8. Avoid skin breakdown by changing lead placement sites as needed. Clean and dry old sites, and expose them to air.
9. Check integrity of the entire system at least once each shift.
   a. Carefully inspect lead wires and cable for breaks and proper attachment.
   b. If malfunction is suspected, change equipment and notify the engineering department or manufacturer immediately.
10. Continue to count respiratory and apical rates at frequent intervals.
    a. Compare with monitor rates to verify accuracy of equipment.
    b. It must be remembered that monitors cannot substitute for close observation of the child.
11. Apnea mattresses or pads that use sensing devices may be used for infants, eliminating the need for electrodes.

a. Although less susceptible to cardiovascular artifact, these devices may record physical impact, vibrations, or body movements as breaths.

b. In addition, older infants can easily roll or crawl off the pad.

▣ Cardiopulmonary Resuscitation

Cardiopulmonary resuscitation (CPR) involves measures instituted to provide effective ventilation and circulation when the patient's respiration and heart have ceased to function. In children, more often the initial cause is of a respiratory nature.

Underlying Considerations
Cardiac Arrest
1. Signs—absence of heartbeat and absence of carotid and femoral pulses
2. Causes—asystole, ventricular fibrillation, or cardiovascular collapse related to arterial hypotension

Respiratory Arrest
1. Signs—apnea and cyanosis
2. Causes—obstructed airway, depression of the central nervous system, neuromuscular paralysis

Emergency Preparation
1. Every hospital should have a well-defined and organized plan to be carried out in the event of cardiac or respiratory arrest.
2. Emergency carts should be placed in strategic locations in the hospital and checked daily to ensure that all equipment is available.

Equipment
1. Emergency cart—assembled and ready for use
2. Positive pressure breathing bag with nonrebreathing valve and universal 15-mm adapter
3. Mask (premature infant, child, adult sizes)
4. Oropharyngeal airways, sizes No. 0 to No. 4
5. Laryngoscope with blades of various sizes
6. Extra batteries and light bulbs for laryngoscope
7. Endotracheal tubes with connectors (complete sterile set, 2.5-8.0 mm inner diameter)
8. Portable suction equipment and sterile catheters of various sizes
9. Bulb syringe, DeLee trap
10. Oxygen source—portable supply gauge and tubing, masks of various sizes
11. Cardiac board (30×50 cm)
12. Emergency drugs:
13. Sodium bicarbonate
14. Epinephrine (Adrenalin)
15. Isoproterenol (Isuprel)
16. Saline solution (for dilution)
17. Diphenhydramine hydrochloride (Benadryl)
18. Diazepam (Valium)
19. Hydrocortisone sodium succinate (Solu-Cortef)
20. Digoxin (Lanoxin)
21. Naloxone (Narcan)
22. Calcium gluconate
23. Calcium chloride 10%
24. Dextrose 50%
25. Lidocaine (Xylocaine)
26. Atropine
27. Phenytoin sodium (Dilantin)
28. Insulin
29. Procainamide (Pronestyl)
30. Propranolol (Inderal)
31. Dopamine (Intropin)
32. Bretylium tosylate (Betylol)
33. Volume expanders
34. Ringer's lactate—Hespan
35. Intracardiac needles, No. 20 and 22 gauge, 6 to 8 cm ($2\frac{3}{8}$ to $3\frac{1}{8}$ inches) long
36. IV equipment
37. Fluids
38. Infusion set
39. Tourniquet
40. Armboards
41. Tape
42. Scalp vein needles of various sizes
43. Nasogastric tubes of various sizes
44. Other equipment
45. Syringes of various sizes
46. Needles of various sizes
47. Intraosseous needles
48. Longdwell catheters of various sizes
49. Three-way stopcock
50. Cutdown set
51. Pole
52. Labels
53. Alcohol wipes
54. Tongue blades
55. Sterile 4×4 gauze sponges
56. Sterile hemostat
57. Sterile scissors
58. Blood specimen tubes
59. Electrocardiograph and monitor
60. Lubricating jelly
61. Defibrillator and paddles (pediatric and adult)

Artificial Ventilation
Mouth-to-Mouth Technique
1. Infants and young children
   a. Slightly extend neck by gently pulling chin up and forward and the head back (chin lift or jaw thrust). Place a rolled towel or diaper under the infant's shoulder, or use one hand to support the neck in an extended position. Do not hyperextend the neck because this narrows the airway.
   b. Check the mouth and throat, and clear mucus or vomitus with finger or suction, if necessary.

c. Take a breath.

d. Make a tight seal with your mouth over the infant's mouth and nose.

e. Gently blow air from the cheeks, and observe for chest expansion.

f. Remove your mouth from infant's mouth and nose, and allow the infant to exhale.

g. If spontaneous respiration does not return, continue breathing at a rate and volume appropriate for the size of the infant (usually 20 times/min or 1 breath every 3 seconds).

2. Older children and adolescents

a. Clear mouth of mucus or vomitus with fingers or suction.

b. Hyperextend neck with one hand or a rolled towel (head tilt, chin lift, or jaw thrust).

c. Clamp the nostrils with the fingers of one hand, which also continues to exert pressure on the forehead to maintain the neck extension.

d. Take a deep breath.

e. Make a tight seal with your mouth over the child's mouth.

f. Force air into the lungs until the chest expansion is observed.

g. Release your mouth from the child's mouth, and release nostrils to allow the child to exhale passively.

h. Repeat approximately 12 to 15 times/min or 1 breath every 4 to 5 seconds.

Hand-Operated Ventilation Devices

1. Remove secretions from mouth and throat, and move mandible forward.

2. Appropriately extend the neck with one hand or place a diaper roll behind the neck.

3. Select an appropriate size mask to obtain an adequate seal, and connect mask to bag.

4. Hold the mask snugly over the mouth and nose, holding the chin forward and the neck in extension.

5. Squeeze the bag, noting inflation of the lungs by chest expansion.

6. Release the bag, which will expand spontaneously. The child will exhale, and the chest will fall.

7. Repeat 12 to 20 times/min (depending on size of the child).

8. Because this technique is often difficult to master, it should be practiced in advance, under supervision.

Indications of Effective Technique

1. Victim's chest rises and falls.

2. Rescuer can feel in own airway the resistance and compliance of the victim's lungs as they expand.

3. Rescuer can hear and feel the air escape during exhalation.

4. Victim's color improves.

Management of Complications

1. Gastric distention (occurs frequently if excessive pressures are used for inflation)

a. Turn victim's head and shoulders to one side.

b. Exert moderate pressure over the epigastrium between the umbilicus and the rib cage.

c. A nasogastric tube may be used to decompress the stomach.

2. Vomiting

a. Turn patient on side for drainage.

b. Clear the airway with fingers or suction.

c. Resume ventilations.

Artificial Circulation

General Principles Related to Artificial Circulation

See Table 43-5 and Figure 43-4.

1. A backward tilt of the head lifts the back in infants and small children. A firm support beneath the back is therefore essential if external cardiac compression is to be effective.

2. A supine position on a firm surface is mandatory. Only in this position can chest compression squeeze the heart against the immobile spine enough to force blood into the systemic circulation.

3. External cardiac compression must always be accompanied by artificial ventilation for adequate oxygenation of the blood.

4. Compressions must be regular, smooth, and uninterrupted. Avoid sudden or jerking movements.

5. Relaxation must immediately follow compression; relaxation and compression must be of equal duration.

6. Between compression, the fingers or heel of the hand must completely release their pressure but should remain in constant contact with the chest.

7. Fingers should not rest on the patient's ribs during compression. Pressure with fingers on the ribs or lateral pressure increases the possibility of fractured ribs and costochondral separation.

8. Never compress the xiphoid process at the tip of the sternum. Pressure on it may cause laceration of the liver.

9. Indications of effective technique include:

a. A palpable femoral or carotid pulse

b. Decrease in size of pupils

c. Improvement in the patient's color

Nursing Management in Cardiopulmonary Resuscitation

1. Recognize cardiac and respiratory arrest.

2. Send for assistance and note time.

3. If alone:

a. First ventilate the child's lungs rapidly two times, using appropriate technique, then palpate the carotid or brachial pulse. If a pulse is palpated, continue ventilatory support.

b. If no pulse is felt, institute artificial circulation using appropriate technique.

c. For an infant or child, interpose 1 breath after each series of 5 compressions. For an adolescent,

TABLE 43-5 Technique of Artificial Circulation

Size of Child	Preparatory Phase	Action Phase	Distance of Compression	Rate
Neonate, premature, or small infant	1. Place in supine position. 2. Encircle the chest with the hands, with thumbs over the midsternum *or* Use method for a larger infant, at a rate of 100–120/min.	1. Compress midsternum with both thumbs, gently but firmly.	⅔ distance to the spine or 1.3–1.8 cm (½–¾ inch)	100/min
Larger infant	1. Place on a firm, flat surface. 2. Support the back with one hand or use a small blanket under the shoulders. 3. Place the tips of the index and middle fingers of one hand over the midsternum.	Compress the midsternum with the tips of the index and middle fingers.	1.3–2.5 cm (½–1 inch)	≥100/min
Small child	1. Place on a firm, flat surface. 2. Support the back by slipping one hand beneath it, or use a small blanket. 3. Place the heel of one hand over the midsternum, parallel with the long axis of the body.	1. Apply a rapid downward thrust to the midsternum, keeping the elbow straight. 2. Hold for approximately 0.4 seconds. 3. Instantly and completely release the pressure so the chest wall can recoil. 4. Do not remove the heel of the hand from the chest.	2.5–3.8 cm (1–1½ inches)	80–100/min
Larger child, adolescent	1. Place on a flat, firm surface, or place a board under the thorax. 2. Place the heel of one hand on the lower half of the sternum, about 2.5–3.8 cm. (1–1½ inches) from the tip of the xiphoid process and parallel with the long axis of the body. 3. Place the other hand on top of the first one (may interlock fingers). 4. Place shoulders directly over child's sternum, in order to use own weight in application of pressure.	1. Exert pressure vertically downward to depress lower sternum, keeping elbows straight. 2. Hold for approximately 0.4 seconds. 3. Instantly and completely release the pressure so the chest wall can recoil. 4. Do not remove the hands from the chest.	3.8–5 cm (1½–2 inches)	80–100/min

Note: Changes in CPR and life support have been recommended by the American Heart Association, but are not included in this chapter because they were not yet implemented at the time of publication. Contact *www.americanheart.org* for more information.

interpose 2 breaths after each series of 15 compressions.

d. Continue repeating this cycle until help arrives.

4. When help arrives:
   a. One rescuer performs mouth-to-mouth resuscitation or institutes bag breathing.
   b. Another rescuer performs cardiac compressions.
   c. A ratio of 3 compressions to 1 breath is maintained for both infants and children (small) and 5 compressions to 1 breath for older children.
   d. Cardiac compression should not be stopped for respiration. Breaths should be interposed on the upstroke of each fifth cardiac compression.

5. Anticipate and assist with emergency procedures and medications.
   a. Assist with intubation, monitoring, placement of cutdown, administration of IV fluids, defibrillation, and other definitive measures.
   b. Prepare and administer emergency medications as prescribed. Record dose and time.

6. After resuscitation:
   a. Care for the child as required.
   b. Determine if family members have been notified and are being cared for.
   c. Record all events.
   d. Restock emergency cart.

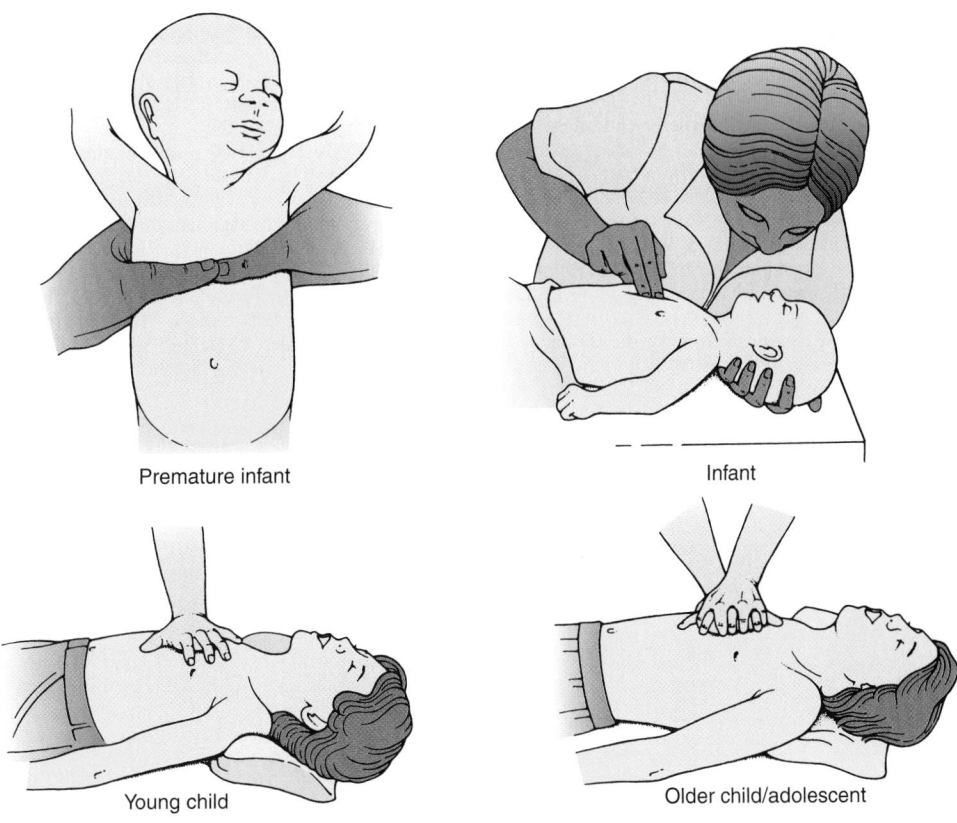

Premature infant

Infant

Young child

Older child/adolescent

FIGURE 43-4 Cardiopulmonary resuscitation in children. In the young child, the heel of the hand is placed over the lower sternum. In older children and adolescents, both hands are used.

SELECTED REFERENCES

Adams, R. A., et al. (1999). Maternal stress in caring for children with feeding disabilities: Implications for health care providers. *Journal of the American Dietetic Association, 99*(8), 962–966.

Aehlert, B. (1996). *Pediatric advanced life support study guide.* St. Louis: Mosby.

Als, H., & Gilkerson, L. (1997). The role of relationship-based developmentally supportive newborn intensive care in strengthening outcome of preterm infants. *Seminars in Perinatology, 21*(3), 178–189.

American Heart Association. (1996). *Pediatric basic life support.* Product #70-1109. Dallas: Author.

Avery, G., et al. (1999). *Neonatology and management of the newborn* (5th ed.). Philadelphia: Lippincott Williams & Wilkins.

Barrett, B., et al. (1998). Hmong/medicine interactions: Improving cross-cultural health care. *Family Medicine, 30*(3), 179–184.

Batshaw, M. L. (1997). *Children with disabilities* (4th ed.). Baltimore: Paul H. Brookes.

Bindler, R. M. (1997). *Pediatric drugs and nursing implications.* Stamford, CT: Appleton & Lange.

Blackburn, S. (1998). Environmental impact of the NICU on developmental outcomes. *Journal of Pediatric Nursing, 13*(5), 279–289.

Boie, E. T. (1999). Do parents want to be present during invasive procedures performed on their children in the emergency department? *Annals of Emergency Medicine, 34*(1), 70–74.

Boynton, R. W., et al. (1998). *Manual of ambulatory pediatrics.* Philadelphia: Lippincott-Raven.

Braver, E. R., et al. (1998). Seating positions and children's risk of dying in motor vehicle crashes. *Injury Prevention, 4*(3), 181–187.

Chestnut, M. A. (1998). *Pediatric home care manual.* Philadelphia: Lippincott-Raven.

Cox, T. H. (1995). An evaluation of post-operative pain management in pediatric patients at a university teaching hospital. *Hospital Pharmacy, 30*(11), 980–992.

Davies, B., et al. (1998). Experiences of mothers in five countries whose child died of cancer. *Cancer Nursing, 21*(5), 301–311.

Grollman, E. (1993). *Straight talk about death for teenagers—how to cope with losing someone you love.* Boston: Beacon Press.

Guilden, D. J. (1997). Ask the expert: Conscious sedation. *Journal of the Society of Pediatric Nursing, 2*(3), 143–147.

Hazinski, M. F. (1999). *Manual of pediatric critical care.* St. Louis: Mosby.

Klaus, M. H. (1999). *Care of the high risk infant* (4th ed.). Philadelphia: W. B. Saunders.

Kopecky, E. A., et al. (1997). Review of a home-based palliative care program for children with malignant and non-malignant diseases. *Journal of Palliative Care, 13*(4), 28–33.

Kubler–Ross, E. (1997). *On death and dying.* New York: Scribner.

Larson, E. (1998). Re-framing the meaning of disability to families: The embrace of paradox. *Social Science and Medicine, 47*(7), 865–875.

Lewin, D. S., & Dahl, R. E. (1999). The importance of sleep in the management of pediatric pain. *Journal of Developmental and Behavioral Pediatrics, 20*(4), 244–252.

Leyden, C. G. (1998). Consumer bill of rights: Family-centered care. *Pediatric Nursing, 24*(1), 72.

Madigan, C. K., et al. (1999). Development of a family liaison model during operative procedures. *MCN: American Journal of Maternal and Child Nursing, 24*(4), 185–189.

Manley, L. (1997). Easing pain in children. *Journal of Trauma Nursing, 3*(4), 130–133.

McIntier, T. M. (1995). Nursing the family when a child dies. *RN, 58*(2), 50–54.

Palm, M. L. (1999). *Clinical simulations in pediatric nursing.* CD-ROM (Windows). Philadelphia: Lippincott Williams & Wilkins.

Pillitteri, A. (1999). *Child health nursing: Care of the child and family.* Philadelphia: Lippincott Williams & Wilkins.

Pressdee, D., et al. (1997). The use of play therapy in the preparation of children undergoing MR imaging. *Clinical Radiology 52*(12), 944–945.

Purcell, C. (1997). Withdrawing treatment from a critically ill child. *Intensive Critical Care Nursing, 3*(2), 103–107.

Rushton, C. H., et al. (1996). Therapeutic boundaries as patient advocates. *Pediatric Nursing, 22*(3), 185–189.

Schmitt, B. D. (2000). *Pediatric telephone protocols* (8th ed.). Littleton, CO: American Academy of Pediatrics.

Siberry, G. K., & Iannone, R. (Eds.) (2000). *The Harriet Lane handbook.* St. Louis: Mosby.

Skadberg, B. T., et al. (1998). Abandoning prone sleeping: Effect on the risk of SIDS. *Journal of Pediatrics, 132*(2), 340–343.

Weir, R., & Peters C. (1997). Affirming the decisions adolescents make about life and death. *Hastings Center Report, 27*(6), 29–40.

Whaley, L., & Wong, D. (1999). *Nursing care of infants and children* (6th ed.). St. Louis: Mosby–Year Book.

Whittam, E. (1993). Terminal care of the dying child: Psychosocial implications of care. *Cancer, 71*(10 suppl), 3450–3462.

Wong, D., & Whaley, L. (2000). *Wong and Whaley's clinical manual of pediatric nursing* (5th ed.). St. Louis: Mosby.

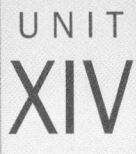

UNIT XIV

Pediatric Health

CHAPTER

44

Pediatric Respiratory Disorders

THE DISORDERS

Common Pediatric Respiratory Infections

Respiratory tract infection is a frequent cause of acute illness in infants and children. Many pediatric infections are seasonal. The child's response to the infection will vary based on the age of the child, causative organism, general health of the child, existence of chronic medical conditions, and degree of contact with other children. Information about specific respiratory infections, including bacterial pneumonia, viral pneumonia, *Pneumocystis* pneumonia, *Mycoplasma* pneumonia, bronchiolitis, croup, and epiglottitis, may be found in Figure 44-1 and Table 44-1.

Nursing Assessment

Determine the severity of the respiratory distress that the child is experiencing. Make an initial nursing assessment.

1. Observe the respiratory rate and pattern. Count the respirations for 1 full minute, document and note level of activity, such as awake or asleep. Determine if the rate is appropriate for age (see p. 1242).
2. Observe respiratory rhythm and depth. Rhythm is described as regular, irregular, or periodic. Depth is normal, hypopnea or too shallow, hyperpnea or too deep.
3. Auscultate breath sounds over all lung fields. Note airflow and presence of adventitious sounds such as crackles, wheeze, or stridor.
4. Observe degree of respiratory effort, normal, difficult, or labored. Normal breathing is effortless and easy.
5. Document character of dyspnea or labored breathing; continuous, intermittent worsening or sudden onset. Note relation to activity such as, rest, exertion, association with pain, positioning, or orthopnea.
6. Note presence of additional signs of respiratory distress: nasal flaring, grunting, retractions. Note location of retractions (Figure 44-2) and character (mild, moderate, or severe).
7. Observe for head bobbing usually noted in a sleeping or exhausted infant. The infant is held by caregiver with head supported on the caregiver's arm at the suboccipital area. The head bobs forward with each inspiration.
8. Observe the child's color. Note presence and location of cyanosis—peripheral, perioral, facial, and trunk. Note degree of color changes, duration, and association with activity such as crying, feeding, sleeping.
9. Observe presence of cough, type, and duration, such as dry, barking, paroxysmal, productive. Note any pattern, such as time of day, night, association with activity, physical exertion, or feeding.

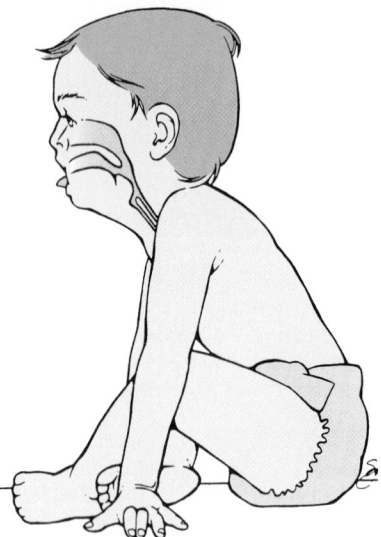

FIGURE 44-1 Characteristic posture of a child with acute epiglottitis: sitting forward on hands, in the "tripod" position; mouth open, tongue out, head forward and tilted up in a sniffing position in an effort to relieve the acute airway obstruction secondary to swollen epiglottis.

10. Note presence of sputum, color, amount, consistency, and frequency.
11. Observe child's fingernails and toenails for cyanosis and presence and degree of clubbing, which indicates underlying chronic respiratory disease (Figure 44-3).
12. Evaluate the child's degree of restlessness, apprehension, and muscle tone.

Nursing Diagnoses
- Ineffective Airway Clearance related to inflammation, obstruction, secretions, or pain
- Ineffective Breathing Pattern related to inflammatory process or pain
- Fluid Volume Deficit related to fever, decreased appetite, vomiting
- Fatigue related to increased work of breathing
- Anxiety related to respiratory distress and hospitalization
- Parental Role Conflict related to hospitalization of the child

Nursing Interventions
Promoting Effective Airway Clearance
1. Provide a humidified environment enriched with oxygen to combat hypoxia and to liquefy secretions (Procedure Guidelines 44-1, p. 1373).
   a. Use a croup tent with cool mist or ultrasonic mist in tent to moisten airway, minimize fluid loss from lungs, liquefy and mobilize respiratory secretions, and allow for oxygen therapy up to 40% concentration.

2. Advise parents to use ultrasonic nebulizer at home and encourage fluids as tolerated.
3. Keep nasal passages free of secretions. Infants are obligate nose breathers.

> **NURSING ALERT**
>
> At no time should the mist be allowed to become so dense that it obscures clear visualization of the patient's respiratory pattern.

Improving Breathing Pattern
1. Place the child in a comfortable position to promote easier ventilation.
   a. Semi-Fowler's—use pillows, infant seat, or elevate head of bed.
   b. Occasional side or abdominal position will aid drainage of liquefied secretions. Do not place infant in prone position.
   c. Do not position the child in severe respiratory distress in a supine position. Allow the child to assume a position of comfort.
2. Provide measures to improve ventilation of affected portion of the lung.
   a. Change position frequently.
   b. Provide postural drainage if prescribed.
   c. Relieve nasal obstruction that contributes to breathing difficulty. Instill saline solution or prescribed nosedrops, and apply nasal suctioning.
   d. Quiet prolonged crying, which can irritate the airway, by soothing the child; however, crying may be an effective way to inflate the lungs.
   e. Realize that coughing is a normal tracheobronchial cleansing procedure, but temporarily relieve coughing by allowing the child to sip water; use extreme caution to prevent aspiration.
   f. Insert a nasogastric tube as ordered to relieve abdominal distention, which can limit diaphragmatic excursion.
3. Ensure that compressed air or oxygen is supplied when using a mist tent to avoid excess CO_2 concentrations and increased respiratory rate.
4. Administer appropriate antibiotic or antiviral therapy.
   a. Observe for drug sensitivity.
   b. Observe the child's response to therapy.
5. Be aware that ribavirin (Virazole) inhalation is considered controversial and is currently recommended in limited cases such as coexisting congenital heart disease, chronic lung disease, immunosuppression, and other cases of very ill, hospitalized infants and young children.
6. If the decision is made to initiate ribavirin therapy, appropriate precautions should be implemented to protect personnel and visitors.
   a. Information should be provided about the potential but unknown risk of exposure to ribavirin.

(text continues on page 1351)

TABLE 44-1 Common Pediatric Respiratory Infections

1. Bacterial Pneumonia:

Bacterial infection of the lung parenchyma.
General Considerations: In the normal child, bacterial pneumonias are not common. A viral respiratory infection often occurs before the bacterial pneumonia. The initial viral infection alters the lungs' defense mechanisms.

Condition and Causative Agent	Age and Incidence	Clinical Manifestations	Diagnostic Evaluation	Treatment	Nursing Considerations	Complications
A. *Pneumococcal pneumonia:* The most common causative agent is *Streptococcus pneumoniae.*	Responsible for the majority of bacterial pneumonias in ages 1 month through 6 years. However, it is seen in all age groups. The incidence has declined due to the use of the vaccine. Winter and spring.	*Infants:* Mild URI of several days' duration, poor feeding, decreased appetite. Abrupt onset of fever 39°C (102.2°F) or higher; restless, respiratory distress, air hunger, pallor, often cyanosis, nasal flaring, retractions, grunting, tachypnea, tachycardia, irritable; may see abdominal distention due to swallowed air or ileus. *Older child:* Mild URI, followed by fever up to 40.5°C, shaking chills, headache, decreased appetite, vomiting, drowsiness, restlessness, dry hacking cough, increased respirations, anxiety, occasionally circumoral cyanosis, pleuritic pain, diminished breath sounds, may develop a pleural effusion or empyema.	Chest x-ray: Often does not correspond to clinical findings. *Infants:* Patchy, diffuse areas follow a bronchial distribution, many limited areas of consolidation around smaller airways. *Young and older child:* Lobar or segmental consolidation; pleural fluid may be present. WBC elevated, arterial blood gases indicate hypoxemia. Cultures: Sputum, nasopharyngeal secretions, pleural fluid, blood.	Oxygen. Penicillin G; penicillin allergy: erthromycin, trimethoprim-sulfamethoxazole, alternately amoxicillin, ampicillin, cefuroxime, cefotaxime, ceftriaxone, clindamycin, chloramphenicol. Due to the increased incidence of penicillinase-resistant pneumococci, all pneumococcal isolates should be tested for resistance. Vancomycin has been recommended for penicillin-resistant strains. Bronchodilators.	Bed rest, monitor fluids, intake and output. Give oral fluids cautiously to avoid aspiration. Do not give oral fluids to a child in respiratory distress. Administer oxygen with humidification. Perform frequent, thorough respiratory assessment. Administer antipyretics as prescribed. Change position frequently. Isolation procedures as ordered or per policy.	Rare, but include bacteremia, empyema, pleural effusion, otitis media, sinusitis, meningitis, hemolytic uremic syndrome.

(continued)

TABLE 44.1 Common Pediatric Respiratory Infections (Continued)

Condition and Causative Agent	Age and Incidence	Clinical Manifestations	Diagnostic Evaluation	Treatment	Nursing Considerations	Complications
B. *Streptococcal pneumonia* Beta-hemolytic *Streptococcus* group A	3–5 year old. Uncommon, serious. An endemic influenza predisposes to streptococcal pneumonia and tracheobronchitis.	Sudden onset, high fever, chills, worsening cough, pleuritic pain, respiratory distress, grunting, retractions, altered mental status, signs of shock, decreased capillary refill, tachycardia. May be insidious, mildly ill, low-grade fever. Severe group A *Streptococcus pneumoniae*, toxic shock syndrome, skin involvement—erythematous rash, desquamation, hypotension, hepatic dysfunction, renal involvement, vomiting/diarrhea, hematologic abnormalities, acute respiratory distress syndrome.	Initial chest x-ray may be normal or slightly abnormal. Within 24 hours, CXR worsens. Unilateral lobar disease, bilateral diffuse infiltrates with severe disease. Blood cultures, nasopharyngeal secretions cultured, throat swab, culture pleural fluid/lung aspirate. Leukocytosis, sedimentation rate increased, elevated serum antistreptolysin (ASO) titer.	Penicillin G	Administer antipyretics. Provide humidified oxygen as needed. Rest. Monitor intake and output.	Empyema, toxic shock syndrome, severe respiratory compromise, pneumatoceles. Can be life threatening.
C. *Staphylococcal pneumonia Staphylococcus aureus*, gram-positive	Most common in children 6 months to 1 year old. Oct.–May	Predisposing factors: cystic fibrosis, maternal infection, immunodeficiency. Usually preceded by a viral URI. Changes abruptly to high fever, cough, respiratory distress, tachypnea, grunting, nasal flaring, cyanosis, retractions. Anxiety, lethargic, occasionally vomiting, diarrhea, anorexia, abdominal distention, toxic appearance.	*Older infant/child:* Leukocytosis, elevated WBC, especially polymorphonuclear cells. *Young infant:* WBC may be normal, mild to moderate anemia. Cultures—pleural fluid, lung aspirate, sputum, gastric aspirate, blood. If pulmonary fluid is purulent and of a large amount, closed chest drainage may be utilized. Chest x-ray: Patchy infiltrate, may involve entire lobe, or	Thoracentesis Naficillin, oxacillin, methicillin, cefzolin, clindamycin, vancomycin. Methicillin-resistant *S aureus* (MRSA) exists, especially in long-term care facilities, or patients with a prolonged hospital stay.	Isolation per policy, check for MRSA, prevent nosocomial infection. Rapid treatment is important. Administer antibiotics as soon as possible. Monitor for signs of tension pneumothorax. Monitor fluid status closely. Strict handwashing.	Empyema, tension pneumothorax, abscess, fibrothorax, bronchiectasis, osteomyelitis, staphylococcal pericarditis. Consider screening infants for CF and immunodeficiency.

Causative agent	Epidemiology	Clinical manifestations	Diagnosis	Medical treatment	Nursing considerations	Complications
D. *Haemophilus influenzae*, type B	Majority of children less than 4 years old. Infants and children who are not immunized. Winter and spring.	Preceded by a URI typically. Associated with otitis media, epiglottitis, and meningitis; appears toxic. Insidious onset; cough, febrile, tachypneic, nasal flaring, retractions.	Chest x-ray: Usually lobar infiltrates; however, segmental, single or multiple lobe infiltrates are also seen. Pleural effusion, pneumatocele. CBC: Elevated WBC, lymphopenia. Cultures: blood, pleural fluid, lung aspirates, and nasal secretions. In the absence of a positive urine culture, a positive urine latex agglutination can confirm diagnosis. If atelectasis is present, bronchoscopy to rule out foreign body.	Patients may present receiving antibiotics for otitis media. Ceftriaxone and other cephalosporins, ampicillin, chloramphenicol.	Administer antibiotics on time. Ensure adequate hydration. Monitor for signs of upper respiratory impairment, drooling, stridor, and dusky color. Respiratory isolation until 24 hours after appropriate antibiotic therapy is initiated. Rifampin prophylaxis should be considered for close household contacts if there are: • Incomplete or unvaccinated members under 48 months of age. • Immunocompromised child. • Daycare setting with two or more cases of invasive disease within 2 months and incompletely vaccinated children in attendance.	hemithorax. Right lung involvement common; bilateral involvement is also seen. Pleural effusion, empyema, pyopneumothorax, pneumatoceles, pneumothorax, lung abscesses. Frequently in young infants, bacteremia, pericarditis, cellulitis, empyema, meningitis, pyarthrosis.
II. Viral Pneumonia Respiratory syncytial virus (RSV); parainfluenza virus types 1, 2, 3; Adenoviruses types 1, 2, 5, 6; and types 3, 7, 11, 21; Influenza A and B.	Peak age for bronchiolitis is within the first year of life. Peak age for viral pneumonia is 2–3 years of age. Typically seen in the winter months.	Usually preceded by URI with symptoms of cough, rhinitis, and mild fever. Progressing to tachypnea, poor feeding in infants, retractions, intercostals, subcostal, suprasternal, and nasal flaring. Along with use of	Chest x-ray shows patchy infiltrates, transient lobal infiltration, and hyperinflation. CBC: Slightly elevated WBC. Cultures: Blood and nasopharyngeal secretions. Viral antigens for rapid diagnosis.	If bacterial pneumonia is suspected, administer antibiotics. Supportive measures: Intravenous fluids, CPT, antipyretics, humidified oxygen, assisted ventilation. Avoid aspirin due to risk of Reye's syndrome.	Monitor closely for signs of respiratory fatigue or distress. Monitor oxygen saturation levels and response to oxygen therapy if hypoxic. Monitor for adequate hydration and nutritional status. Prop infants up to an	Influenza: severe fulminant pneumonia with hemorrhagic exudate. Death may result. Severe disease may be seen in children with cardiopulmonary disease, cystic fibrosis, bronchopulmonary *(continued)*

TABLE 44-1 Common Pediatric Respiratory Infections (Continued)

Condition and Causative Agent	Age and Incidence	Clinical Manifestations	Diagnostic Evaluation	Treatment	Nursing Considerations	Complications
		accessory muscles, wheeze, severe cough, cyanosis, and respiratory fatigue. A viral infection may present with a primary bacterial pneumonia. Adenovirus types 3, 7, 11, and 21 may cause severe necrotizing pneumonia in infants.		Amantadine for influenza A.	angle of 10–30 degrees to ease breathing. Infants and children who require mechanical ventilation require close supervision and frequent monitoring. Institute isolation measures as directed by policy; prevent nosocomial infections. Prevention: influenza vaccine.	dysplasia, and neurovascular disease. Type A and B may cause myocarditis. Type B—myositis
Respiratory syncytial virus—RSV subgroup A (more virulent), RSV subgroup B	In infants, RSV is the most common cause of pneumonia, bronchiolitis, and hospitalizations. Severity of RSV infection decreases with age and subsequent infections. Peak age is 2–7 months, October to April.	Typically begins with URI, rhinorrhea, fever usually less than 39°C (102°F), otitis media, and conjunctivitis. Progressing to coughing, wheeze, tachypnea, greater than 70 bpm, intercostals and subcostal retractions, hypoxia, poor air exchange, decreased breath sounds, cyanosis, listless apenic episodes, lethargy, and irritability. Infants will present with poor feeding, inability to suck and breathe.	Nasopharyngeal secretions for rapid antibody or assay for RSV antigen detection. Chest x-ray: chest hyperexpanded, air trapping, multiple lobe infiltrates, atelectasis, RML/RUL.	Supportive ribavirin in selected patients (controversial due to effectiveness, cost, duration, and toxicity). IV RSV immunoglobin: Used to prevent infection in children without congenital heart disease, children with BPD, and those with a history of prematurity (less than 35 weeks gestational age). IM RSV monoclonal antibody: used to prevent infection in children with BPD, and for premature infants of less than 35 weeks' gestation.	Prevent nosocomial spread. Institute contact isolation. Strict handwashing. RSV-positive patients should not be in contact with other high-risk patients, such as those with chronic cardiac or respiratory illness, immunocompromised patients. Assess frequently for signs of respiratory failure. Use noninvasive oxygen monitoring. In tachypneic patients and those in respiratory distress, oral fluids are contraindicated due to risk of aspiration.	RSV may be life threatening in patients with chronic cardiac and respiratory diseases, premature infants, and those with underlying neuromuscular or immunologic diseases. Respiratory failure, intubation, and mechanical ventilation. In older children with asthma, RSV can cause an acute asthmatic episode.

III. Pneumocystis carinii Pneumonia

Condition and Causative Agent	Age and Incidence	Clinical Manifestations	Diagnostic Evaluation	Treatment	Nursing Considerations	Complications
P carinii is a fungus with similarities to a protozoa. The organism exists in three forms in the tissues: trophozoite, sporozoite, and cyst.	Most healthy humans are infected before age 4 years and are asymptomatic. Life-threatening pneumonia is seen in the immunosuppressed host. P carinii pneu-	Slow onset, tachypnea, retractions, and nasal flaring cyanosis. Sporadic form in imunocompromised patients. Signs may vary, onset	Chest x-ray: Bilateral, diffuse, alveolar disease with a granular pattern, initially perihilar densities, which progress to peripheral and apical areas.	P carinii pneumonia is fatal within 3–4 weeks without treatment. If treated early there is a 70% to 90% survival rate. Trimethoprim-sulfamethoxazole,	Close monitoring of respiratory status, hydration, and nutrition. Monitor for adverse reactions to therapy: Vomiting, nausea, rash.	

monia in severely immunocompromised children with acquired or congenital immunodeficiency disorders, malignancies, organ transplant recipients, and debilitated, malnourished, and premature infants.		may be acute or fulminant. Fever, tachypnea, dyspnea cough, nasal flaring, cyanosis, subacute, diffuse pneumonitis with dyspnea at rest, tachypnea and decreasing oxygen saturation. Extrapulmonary sites rarely occur and are usually asymptomatic.	Organism cannot be cultured from routine specimens. Open lung biopsy is the most reliable method. Bronchoalveolar lavage is also utilized to obtain samples. Needle aspiration of the lung. IgM–ELISA: elevated. CBC: mild leukocytosis, moderate eosinophilia.	rate of adverse reactions high in HIV-infected patients. Pentamidine, parenterally or aerosolized. Corticosteroids recommended for children older than 13 years, may be used in younger children.	Respiratory isolation should be instituted for 48 hours after initiation of therapy. PCP prophylaxis (see p. 1554).

⚡ **NURSING ALERT**

Pentamidine is associated with a high incidence of adverse reactions: pancreatitis, renal dysfunction, hypoglycemia, hyperglycemia, hypotension, fever, and neutropenia. Pentamidine should not be used with didanosine, which also causes pancreatitis.

IV. Mycoplasma Pneumonia

Mycoplasma pneumoniae, microorganisms with properties between bacteria and viruses.	Fall/winter. Crowded living conditions. Seen in 6–18 year olds, peak age 8–10 years.	Slow onset; 2- to 3-week incubation period. Coryza, malaise, headache, anorexia, low-grade fever, sore throat, muscle pain, vomiting, subacute tracheobronchitis, shortness of breath, bronchitic productive cough, mild chest pain, wheezing.	Chest x-ray: bronchopneumonic, diffuse bilateral infiltrates. Complement fixation test: increased. Cold agglutinins: increased. Positive sputum culture.	Erythromycin, azithromycin	Children should be on secretion precautions. Monitor fever. Assess need for use of cough suppressants.

V. Bronchiolitis

Inflammation of the bronchioles. Causative agents: RSV, adenovirus, parainfluenza type 1 or 3, influenza virus and *M pneumoniae*.	Winter and spring. Most common in infants younger than 6 months old, may occur up to 2 years of age. Greater incidence in males than females. Increased in day care centers.	Gradual onset after exposure to an individual with URI. Coryza, tachypnea, respiratory rate greater than 50 bpm, retractions, wheeze, paroxysmal cough, fever, cyanosis, dehydration, poor feeding, vomiting, tachycardia, irritability, dyspnea. Apnea may be first sign in infants with RSV. Decreased breath sounds with prolonged expiratory phase. Hypoxemia may persist for 4 to 6 weeks.	Chest x-ray: Patchy or peribronchial infiltrates, hyperinflation of lungs with flattening of diaphragms. Some will present with a normal chest x-ray. Viral cultures: Nasopharyngeal. Serologic studies for specific organisms. Arterial blood gases for children with respiratory distress.	A broad-spectrum antibiotic until causative organism is identified. Humidified oxygen, ventilatory assistance as needed. Bronchodilators by way of nebulizer.	Avoid high-density humidity; may cause bronchospasm. Monitor fluid and electrolyte balance closely. Place infant on apnea monitor. Keep nasal passages free of secretions, infants are obligate nose breathers. Position patient upright to facilitate breathing. Monitor closely for signs of impending respiratory failure. There is a high risk of cross-contamination to noninfected children. Institute	Increasing respiratory distress resulting in the need for mechanical ventilation. Secondary bacterial infection. Pneumothorax and pneumomediastinum. Apneic episodes, may be life threatening in children with chronic respiratory or cardiac disease. Some infants demonstrate abnormal lung functions months after infection.

(continued)

TABLE 44-1 Common Pediatric Respiratory Infections (Continued)

Condition and Causative Agent	Age and Incidence	Clinical Manifestations	Diagnostic Evaluation	Treatment	Nursing Considerations	Complications
					contact and respiratory isolation. Monitor oxygenation levels with noninvasive monitoring.	

VI. Croup Syndromes

Croup syndromes refer to infections of the supraglottis, glottis, subglottis and trachea.

Condition and Causative Agent	Age and Incidence	Clinical Manifestations	Diagnostic Evaluation	Treatment	Nursing Considerations	Complications
A. *Acute laryngo-tracheobronchitis* (subglottic croup) Parainfluenza types 1, 2, 3, RSV, influenza A and B, adenovirus, measles.	3 months to 5 years of age. Peak age 1–2 years old. Greater incidence in males than females. Late autumn, early winter.	Usually a preceding URI is seen. Initially, a mild brassy or barking cough, hoarse, intermittent stridor, progresses to continuous stridor. Nasal flaring, suprasternal, infrasternal, intercostals, retractions. Breathing labored, prolonged expiratory phase. Temperature slightly elevated. Crying and agitation aggravate signs. Child prefers to be held upright or sit up in bed. Symptoms are worse at night. Severe croup: restlessness, air hunger, decreased breath sounds, hypoxemia, hypercapnia, and tachycardia.	Diagnosis is made by clinical evaluation and careful history. A croup score may be assigned to grade severity. Lateral neck x-ray: subglottic edema, narrowing with normal supraglottic structures. A/P neck film: steeple sign.	Cool, humidified oxygen. If placement of the child in a mist tent causes increased anxiety, it is not necessary. Racemic epinephrine nebulized with oxygen. Monitor pulse and cardiac rhythm. Levorotatory form of epinephrine may be used outside the United States. Dexamethasone. Severe airway edema may require intubation.	Maintain a calm environment, avoid agitating the child, and disturb as little as possible. Monitor oxygenation with noninvasive pulse oximeter. Monitor respiratory status closely and frequently. Closely observe response to racemic epinephrine. Have intubation equipment at bedside and available during transport. Increasing tachypnea may be first sign of hypoxia. If severe distress does not respond to initial treatment, ABG should be obtained. In a hypoxic, pale, cyanotic, or obtunded patient, do not manipulate larynx, do not examine with a tongue depressor, it may lead to sudden cardiopulmonary arrest.	Dehydration, intubation, airway obstruction, death.

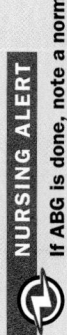 **NURSING ALERT**

If ABG is done, note a normal P_{CO_2} may not indicate decreased severity. By the time hypercapnia is seen, intubation will be required.

Condition	Age/Epidemiology	Clinical Findings	Diagnosis	Treatment	Complications
B. Spasmodic croup/acute spasmodic laryngitis No infectious agents seen. Thought to be related to spasm of laryngeal muscle. Cause may be viral in a few cases, allergic or psychological. Gastroesophageal reflux (GER) may be a triggering event.	1–3 years old	Similar to acute laryngotracheobronchitis. Symptoms are sudden, in the evening or night. Afebrile, barking, brassy cough, hoarse, stridor. Breathing is noisy on inspiration, slow and labored, respiratory distresses. Tachycardia. Skin cool, moist. Dyspnea is worse with excitement. Cyanosis is rare; severity decreases over time. Patient appears well in the morning, may cough or sound hoarse. The symptoms may recur for subsequent nights; however, they will be less severe.	CBC is normal, x-ray: subglottic narrowing. Endoscopic exam: Inflammation of the arytenoids cartilage, epithelium intact, pale mucosa.	Treatment of GER, mist, occasionally racemic epinephrine, occasionally steroids.	Same as acute laryngotracheobronchitis. Allow parent to hold child, remain in upright position.
B. Bacterial tracheitis (pseudomembranous croup) Tracheal inflammation in the subglottic region. S aureus, H. influenzae, streptococci, group A and B, Escherichia coli, Klebsiella, Moraxella catarrhalis, Pseudomonas, Chlamydia trachomatis, Corynebacterium diphtheriae should be considered in the nonvaccinated patient.	No season variation. Age is variable, 1 month to 6 years old, however most are under 3 years old.	Usually follows a viral illness. Slow or sudden deterioration, child appears toxic. High fever, stridor, hoarse, respiratory distress. Thick, purulent, copious airway secretions. Mucosal necrosis, brassy or barking cough. Epiglottitis may coexist. May cause life-threatening airway obstruction.	Neck x-ray: subglottic narrowing, large epiglottis, thick arytenoepiglottic folds, pseudomembrane in trachea. Tracheal culture. Laryngoscopy, CBC, leukocytosis, bandemia.	Humidified oxygen as required, mist, antibiotic therapy, cephalosporin. Admit to ICU, intubation and frequent suctioning. Racemic epinephrine ineffective.	Airway obstruction, death, tracheostomy, pneumothorax, toxic shock syndrome.
C. Acute epiglottitis: Supraglottitis, inflammation of the epiglottis and edema of the arytenoepiglottic folds.	Range 2–7 years old; peak age 3–5 years. Autumn and winter. Incidence significantly decreased due to the routine use of	Sudden fulminating course, high fever, toxic appearance, sore throat, drooling, dysphagia, aphonia, cough pro-	Clinical evaluation and history, determining the onset of symptoms. Monitor oxygen saturation level.	Medical emergency. Establish a stable artificial airway first. Approach child in a calm manner; emotional upset and agi-	Airway obstruction, death, pneumothorax, pulmonary edema.

(continued)

TABLE 44-1 Common Pediatric Respiratory Infections (Continued)

Condition and Causative Agent	Age and Incidence	Clinical Manifestations	Diagnostic Evaluation	Treatment	Nursing Considerations	Complications
H influenzae type B, most common. *S pneumoniae*, *S aureus*, group A. Beta-hemolytic streptococcus, *Streptococcus pyogenes*, *Moraxella catarrhalis*, *Candida albicans* (in the immunocompromised).	the *H influenzae* vaccine.	gresses to stridor, retractions, air hunger, anxious, tachycardia, hoarseness, irritability, restlessness, rapid progression to respiratory distress. Sitting forward, neck hyperextended, mouth open, tongue protruding. Older child will sit in tripod position. Complete fatal airway obstruction and death may occur within hours if not treated. In group A. beta-hemolytic streptococcus and *H influenzae*, patient will present with acute respiratory distress. Stridor and breath sounds decrease as child begins to tire. A brief episode of air hunger with restlessness and agitation may rapidly progress into increasing cyanosis, coma, and death.	Lateral neck films: swollen epiglottis. Direct exam or laryngoscopy: large, swollen cherry-red epiglottis, edema of arytenoepiglottic folds. CBC, cultures, intravenous catheters must be done after intubation.	tation may result in complete airway obstruction. Allow parent to hold child. Proceed to OR or ICU with physician skilled and equipped to intubate or perform a percutaneous tracheostomy. Lateral neck films should be done in OR or ICU after airway is established. Antibiotics: intravenous cefotaxime, ceftriaxone, ampicillin with sulbactam. Supplemental humidified oxygen; mechanical ventilation if necessary. If epiglottitis is strongly suspected, examination of the throat is contraindicated; due to reflex laryngospasm, acute airway obstruction, aspiration and cardiopulmonary arrest during or immediately after examination of the pharynx with a tongue blade.	Allow child to maintain position of comfort (not supine). Equipment for intubation and tracheostomy must remain with patient at all times. A physician skilled in intubation and tracheostomy procedures must accompany child to OR or ICU. After intubation, the child should remain in the ICU with frequent assessment of oxygenation levels and need for mechanical ventilation. Prevent self-extubation; use arm boards/restraints to prevent arm movements, extubation, and death. After intubation, administer sedation as needed. When decision is made to extubate child, emergency tracheostomy and intubation equipment must be at bedside.	

> **NURSING ALERT**
>
> Do not place the child in the supine position. It will increase agitation, and positional change of the epiglottis will cause airway obstruction.

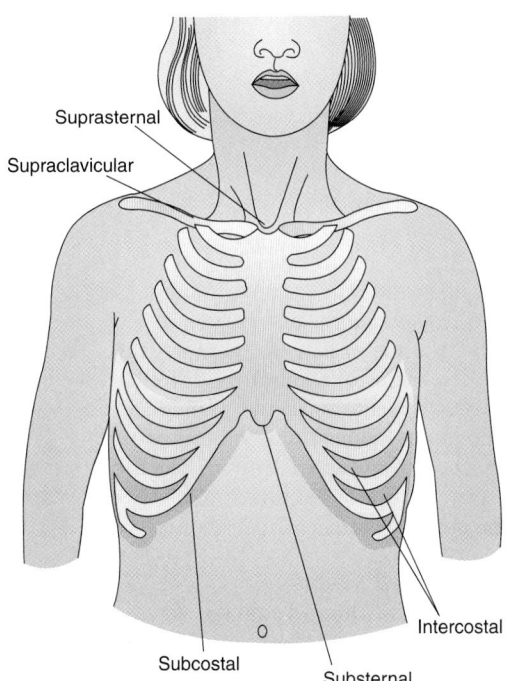

FIGURE 44-2 Sites of respiratory retractions.

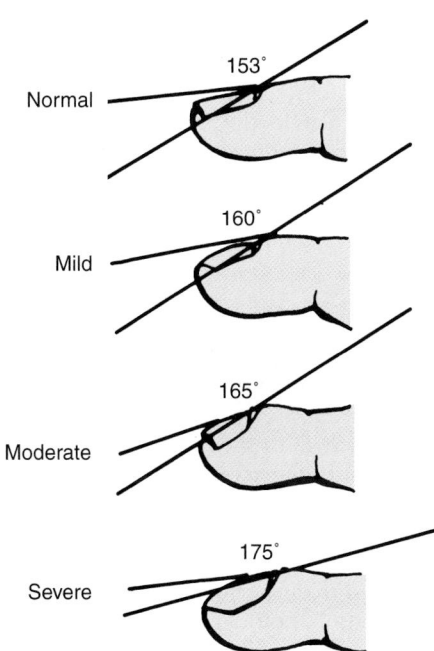

FIGURE 44-3 Clubbing of the fingernails. (Whaley, L., & Wong, D. [1999]. *Nursing care of infants and children* [6th ed.]. St. Louis: Mosby Year Book. Used with permission.)

b. Pregnant women should be advised to refrain from providing direct care to patients who are receiving ribavirin therapy.

c. Methods to reduce environmental exposure to ribavirin should be employed:

  (i) Stop aerosol administration before opening hood or tent.

  (ii) Use room with adequate ventilation of at least six air exchanges per hour.

  (iii) Consider the use of scavenger devices to help decrease the escape of ribavirin into the air.

NURSING ALERT

To minimize spasm and sudden blockage of airway, avoid the following: making the child lie flat, forcing the child to drink, and looking down the child's throat.

---

7. For cases of severe respiratory distress, assist with intubation or tracheostomy and mechanical ventilation.

a. Tracheostomy and endotracheal tubes are generally not cuffed for infants and small children because the tube itself is big enough relative to the size of the trachea to act as its own sealer.

b. Position the infant with a tracheostomy with neck extended by placing a small roll under the shoulders to prevent occlusion of the tube by the chin. Support the head and neck carefully when moving the infant to prevent dislodgement of the tube.

c. When feeding, cover the tracheostomy with a moist piece of gauze, or use a bib for older infants or young children.

d. See p. 1371 in this chapter, as well as Chapter 10, for care of the patient on mechanical ventilation.

NURSING ALERT

Infants with a history of very low birth weight and bronchopulmonary dysplasia (BPD) have chronic compensated carbon dioxide retention. Careful attention must be given to oxygen administration in order to avoid respiratory depression by suppressing their hypoxic drive.

Promoting Adequate Hydration

1. Administer intravenous (IV) fluids at the prescribed rate.

2. To prevent aspiration, withhold all oral food and fluids if the child is in severe respiratory distress.

3. Offer the child small sips of clear fluid when the respiratory status improves.

a. Note any vomiting or abdominal distention after the oral fluid is given.

b. As the child begins to take more fluid by mouth, notify the health care provider and modify the IV fluid rate to prevent fluid overload.

c. Do not force the child to take fluids orally, because this may cause increased distress and possibly vomiting. Anorexia will subside as the condition improves.

4. Assist in the control of fever to reduce respiratory rate and fluid loss.
   a. Give antipyretics as prescribed.
   b. Increase evaporation from skin with tepid sponges.
5. Record the child's intake and output, and monitor urine specific gravity.

Promoting Adequate Rest

1. Disturb the child as little as possible by organizing nursing care, and protect child from unnecessary interruptions.
2. Be aware of the age of the child, and be familiar with the level of growth and development as it applies to hospitalization.
3. Encourage the parents to stay with the child as much as possible to provide comfort and security.
4. Provide opportunities for quiet play as the child's condition improves.

Reducing Anxiety

1. Explain procedures and hospital routine to the child as appropriate for age.
2. Provide a quiet, stress-free environment.
3. Observe the child's response to the oxygen therapy environment, and reassure the child.
   a. The child may experience fear of confinement or suffocation.
   b. Vision is distorted through the plastic.
   c. The environment is noisy and damp.
   d. Physical and diversional activities are restricted.
   e. Parental contact is decreased.
   f. The environment is often uncomfortable.
4. Provide frequent change of clothing and linen for a child in a mist tent to promote comfort; provide socks, booties, cap, if necessary, to keep child warm (temperature in mist tent is usually 6°F to 15°F below room temperature).
5. Avoid the use of sedatives and opiates, which may obscure restlessness. Restlessness is a sign of increasing respiratory distress or obstruction.
6. Allow the child to assume position of comfort.

Strengthening the Parents' Role

1. Help parents understand the purpose of the mist tent and how to work with it.
2. Discuss their fears and concerns about the child's therapy.
3. Include the parents in planning for the child's care. Promote their participation in caring for the child.
4. Recognize that the parents will need rest periods. Encourage them to take breaks and eat on a regular basis.

Family Education and Health Maintenance

1. Teach the importance of good hygiene. Include information on handwashing and appropriate ways to handle respiratory secretions at home.
2. Teach the family when it is appropriate to keep the child home from school (any fever, coughing up secretions, significant runny nose in toddler or younger child).
3. Teach methods to keep the ill child well hydrated.
   a. Provide small amounts of fluids frequently.
   b. Offer clear liquids, such as Pedialyte.
   c. Offer Popsicles and Jello.
   d. Avoid juices with a high sugar content.
4. Teach ways to assess the child's hydration status at home.
   a. Decreased number of wet diapers or number of times the child urinates in a day
   b. Decreased activity level
   c. Dry lips and mucous membranes
   d. No tears when the child cries
5. Teach parents when to contact their health care provider—signs of respiratory distress, recurrent fever, decreased appetite and activity, and signs of dehydration.
6. Teach about medications and follow-up.
7. If tracheostomy was required, teach care of the tracheostomy, use of equipment, safety, and referral for home nursing care before discharge.

Outcome-Based Evaluation

- Breath sounds clear and equal
- Easy, regular, unlabored respirations on room air (or back to baseline if child is on oxygen)
- Mucous membranes moist; urine output adequate
- Bathing and feeding tolerated well
- Child calm and interacting appropriately with family and staff
- Parents participating in the child's care

■ Disorders Requiring Surgery of the Tonsils and Adenoids

Tonsillectomy and *adenoidectomy* are the surgical removal of the adenoidal and tonsillar structures, part of the lymphoid tissue that encircles the pharynx. These are the most frequently performed surgical procedures in the child. The most common disease processes that require tonsillectomy and adenoidectomy are *obstructive sleep apnea,* chronic persistent *otitis media,* and chronic, persistent *tonsillitis* or *adenoiditis.*

Pathophysiology and Etiology

Function of Tonsils and Adenoids

1. They are a first line of defense against respiratory infections.
2. Because the growth of the tonsils and adenoids in the first 10 years of life exceeds general somatic growth, these structures appear especially large in the child.
3. The natural process of involution of tonsillar and adenoidal lymphoid tissue in prepubertal years is associated with decreased frequency of throat and ear infections.

Obstructive Sleep Apnea

1. Adenotonsillar hypertrophy causes airway obstruction during sleep leading to persistent hypoventilation during sleep.
2. Peak incidence in children is 3 to 6 years.
3. Incidence is increased in children with Down syndrome.

Tonsillitis and Adenoiditis

1. In tonsillitis/adenoiditis, structures that are already large become inflamed due to an infectious agent and cause airway obstruction, decreased appetite, and pain.
2. Infection is caused by bacterial or viral organisms, with viral organisms most commonly implicated.
3. Group A beta-hemolytic *Streptococcus* is the most common bacterial cause.
4. Enlarged adenoids may block nasal passages, resulting in persistent mouth breathing.
5. Chronic adenoiditis without tonsillitis is most often seen in children younger than 4 years.

Otitis Media

1. Bacterial infection caused most commonly by *Streptococcus pneumoniae* or *Haemophilus influenzae.*
2. Chronic infection may be associated with enlarged adenoids that block drainage from the eustachian tubes.

Clinical Manifestations

Obstructive Sleep Apnea

1. Loud snoring or noisy breathing in sleep
2. Excessive daytime sleepiness
3. Mouth breathing

Chronic Infection of Tonsils and Adenoids

1. Mouth breathing or difficulty breathing
2. Frequent sore throat
3. Anorexia, decreased growth velocity
4. Fever
5. Obstruction to swallowing/breathing
6. Nasal, muffled voice
7. Night cough
8. Offensive breath

Chronic Otitis Media

1. Ear pain or general irritability in young children
2. Alterations in hearing
3. Fever
4. Enlarged lymph nodes
5. Anorexia

Diagnostic Evaluation

1. Thorough ears, nose, and throat examination and appropriate cultures to determine presence and source of infection
2. Preoperative blood studies to determine risk of bleeding—clotting time, smear for platelets, prothrombin time, partial thromboplastin time

Treatment

Appropriate antibiotics are given, and the decision to perform surgery is made. Tonsillectomy and adenoidectomy may be performed together or separately. Controversy exists over indications for and benefits of surgery.

Indications for Tonsillectomy

1. Conservative
   a. Recurrent or persistent tonsillitis with documented streptococcal infection four times in 1 year
   b. Marked hypertrophy of tonsils, which distorts speech, causes swallowing difficulties, and causes subsequent weight loss
   c. Tonsillar malignancy
   d. Diphtheria carrier
   e. Cor pulmonale due to obstruction
2. Controversial
   a. Peritonsillar abscess or retrotonsillar abscess
   b. Suppurative cervical adenitis with tonsillar focus
   c. Persistent hyperemia of anterior pillars
   d. Enlarged cervical lymph nodes

Indications for Adenoidectomy

1. Conservative
   a. Adenoid hypertrophy resulting in obstruction of airway leading to hypoxia, pulmonary hypertension, and cor pulmonale
   b. Hypertrophy with nasal obstruction accompanied by breathing difficulty and severe speech distortion
   c. Hypertrophy associated with chronic suppurative or serous otitis media and sensorineural or conductive hearing loss, chronic mastoiditis, or cholesteatoma
   d. Mouth breathing due to hypertrophied adenoids
2. Controversial
   a. Enlarged adenoids, chronic otitis media, and no evidence of complications

Contraindications to Surgery

1. Bleeding or coagulation disorders
2. Uncontrolled systemic disorders (eg, diabetes, rheumatic fever, cardiac or renal disease)
3. Child younger than 4 years, unless life-threatening situation
4. Presence of upper respiratory infection in child or immediate family
5. Specific for adenoidectomy—certain palate abnormalities (ie, cleft palate or submucous cleft palate)

Complications

1. If untreated, obstructive sleep apnea in the child may result in pulmonary hypertension, cor pulmonale, failure to thrive, respiratory failure, attention deficit disorders, cardiac arrhythmias.
2. Untreated chronic tonsillitis may result in failure to thrive, peritonsillar or retropharyngeal abscess, difficulty swallowing, poor eating.
3. Untreated chronic otitis media may result in hearing loss, scarring of the eardrum (tympanosclerosis), mastoiditis, meningitis.
4. Complications of surgery include hemorrhage, reactions to anesthesia, otitis media, bacteremia.

Nursing Assessment

Preoperative Assessment

1. Assess child's developmental level.
2. Assess parents' and child's understanding of the surgical procedure.
3. Assess psychological preparation of the child for hospitalization and surgery.

a. Does the child understand what will happen?

b. Do the parents know the importance of telling the child the truth and have a good understanding of the procedure?

c. Does the child have preconceived ideas from peers that may pose a threat?

NURSING ALERT

The preschool child is especially vulnerable to psychological trauma as a result of surgical procedures or hospitalization.

---

4. Obtain thorough nursing history from the parents to gather any pertinent information that would impact child's care.

   a. Has the child had a recent infection? It is desirable for the child to be free of respiratory infection for at least 2 to 3 weeks.

   b. Has the child recently been exposed to any communicable diseases?

   c. Does the child have any loose teeth that may pose the threat of aspiration?

   d. Are there any bleeding tendencies in the child or family?

5. Obtain the child's baseline vital signs along with height and weight.

6. Assess the child's hydration status.

Postoperative Assessment

1. Assess pain on a frequent basis.

2. Assess ability to maintain adequate oral intake.

3. Assess frequently for signs of postoperative bleeding. Monitor vital signs.

4. Assess for indications of negative psychological sequelae related to the surgery and hospitalization.

Nursing Diagnoses

- Fear related to painful procedure, unfamiliar environment
- Parental Anxiety related to concept of surgery
- Risk for Fluid Volume Deficit related to reduced intake postoperatively and blood loss
- Ineffective Airway Clearance related to pain and effects of anesthesia
- Pain related to surgical incision

Nursing Interventions
Reducing Fear

1. Prepare the child and parents by encouraging participation in hospital tours and preadmission programs specifically for children.

2. Prepare the child specifically for what to expect postoperatively, using techniques appropriate to the child's developmental level (books, dolls, drawings). Include the following:

   a. Where child will wake up

   b. Temporary sore throat, emesis of blood, position, foul taste and smell in mouth

c. Ice collar, medications

d. Fluid regimen

3. Talk to the child about the new things to be seen in the operating room, and clear up any misconceptions. Whenever possible, allow the child to see, touch, and examine equipment, such as thermometers, beds, tubings, suction equipment, and so forth.

Relieving Parental Anxiety

1. Help the parents prepare the child by talking at first in general terms about surgery and progressing to more specific information.

2. Reassure parents that complication rates are low and that recovery is usually swift.

3. Encourage parents to stay with child and help provide care.

Maintaining Adequate Fluid Volume

1. Assess frequently for bleeding postoperatively. Check all secretions and emesis for presence of fresh blood. Indications of hemorrhage include the following:

   a. Increased pulse

   b. Frequent swallowing

   c. Pallor

   d. Restlessness

   e. Clearing of throat and vomiting of blood

   f. Continuous slight oozing of blood over a number of hours

   g. Oozing of blood in back of throat

2. Have suction equipment and packing material readily available in case of emergency.

3. Provide adequate fluid intake.

   a. Give ice chips 1 to 2 hours after awakening from anesthesia.

   b. When vomiting has ceased, advance to clear liquids cautiously.

   c. Offer cool fruit juices without pulp at first because they are best tolerated; then offer Popsicles, cool water for first 12 to 24 hours. Avoid red/brown fluids.

   d. There is some controversy regarding intake of milk and ice cream the evening of surgery. It can be soothing and can reduce swelling, but it does coat the mouth and throat, causing the child to clear throat more often, which may initiate bleeding.

Promoting Effective Airway Clearance

1. Assist the child in maintaining a patent airway by draining secretions and preventing aspiration of vomitus.

2. Assess for signs and symptoms of airway obstruction and respiratory distress, which may result due to edema, or accumulation of secretions: stridor, drooling, restlessness, agitation, tachypnea, and cyanosis

   a. Place the child prone or semiprone with head turned to side while still under the effects of anesthesia.

   b. Allow the child to assume a position of comfort when alert. (Parent may hold the child.)

   c. The child may vomit old blood initially. If suctioning is necessary, avoid trauma to oropharynx.

   d. Remind the child not to cough or clear throat unless necessary.

Improving Comfort

1. Provide ice collar to neck, if desired. (Remove ice collar if child becomes restless.)
2. Give analgesics as ordered, parenteral or rectally.
3. Rinse mouth with cool water or alkaline solution.
4. Keep child and environment free from blood-tinged drainage to help decrease anxiety.
5. Encourage the parents to be with the child when the child awakens. This is the most important comfort measure the nurse can provide for the child.
6. When parents must leave, reassure the child that they will return.

Family Education and Health Maintenance

1. Explain and write instructions concerning the care of the child at home after discharge.
   a. Diet should still consist of large amounts of fluids and soft, cool, nonirritating foods. (Supply list of suggestions.)
   b. Eating helps promote healing because it increases the blood supply to tissues.
   c. Bed rest should be maintained for 1 to 2 days and then daily rest periods for about 1 week. Resume normal eating and activities within 2 weeks after surgery.
   d. Avoid contact with people with infections.
   e. Discourage the child from frequent coughing and clearing of throat.
   f. Avoid gargling. Mouth odor may be present for a few days after surgery; only mouth rinsing is acceptable.
2. Advise when to call health care provider. (Ensure that parents have phone number of health care provider and emergency department.)
   a. Earache accompanied by fever
   b. Any bleeding, often indicated only by frequent swallowing; most common about 5th to 10th day when membrane sloughs from surgical site
3. Teach about medications prescribed or suggested for pain relief.
4. Discuss with the parents what results they can expect from the surgery.
   a. Decreased number of sore throats
   b. Lessened evidence of obstructive symptoms
   c. Decreased incidence of cervical lymphadenitis
   d. Improvement in nutritional status
   e. No improvement in nasal allergies
   f. No improvement in secretory otitis media
5. Guide parents in helping the child think of the experience as a positive one once surgery is over to make subsequent health care experiences easier.
   a. Talk about what happened and the positive outcomes.
   b. Let the child play out his or her feelings.

Outcome-Based Evaluation

- Child acting out surgery with dolls, asking questions
- Parents interacting with the child, asking appropriate questions
- Taking fluids well; no signs of bleeding
- No vomiting; breathing without difficulty
- Verbalizes reduced pain

◼ Asthma

Also see Chapter 28 for complete discussion of asthma.

Asthma is the most common chronic disease of childhood. Symptoms typically begin before age 8 with a decrease in symptoms or severity during adolescence in some children. Of those, approximately half will continue to have asthma. A significant number of those who believe they have outgrown their asthma experience asthma symptoms later in life. Etiology and pathophysiology are the same as in adults (see p. 921), and presentation may be gradual or sudden. In addition, cough variant asthma is most often seen in children, where cough (especially at night) is the principal symptom. The child may never wheeze. Although symptoms are chronic and often mild in many children, severe exacerbations (attacks) may arise, even resulting in respiratory failure and death.

Factors Identified for Increased Risk of Asthma Death

1. Adolescence, African-American ethnicity
2. Previous exacerbation requiring hospitalization within the last year, history of intensive care unit (ICU) admission, history of intubation for asthma
3. Hospitalization two or more times within the year, three or more emergency department visits in the last year
4. Use of two canisters per month of short-acting inhaled beta-2 agonist
5. Current use of steroids; recent withdrawal from oral steroids
6. Poor perception of airflow obstruction or its severity
7. Low socioeconomic status, poor access to health care
8. History of depression, psychological problems, or psychiatric disease
9. Sensitivity to *Alternaria* (outdoor mold).
10. Illicit drug use

Management of Acute Exacerbation

1. Be alert for severe asthma exacerbation. In a severe exacerbation, the child is short of breath, audibly wheezing with a prolonged expiratory phase, restless, apprehensive, anxious, diaphoretic; color may be pale or flushed. Lips may be dark red or cyanotic. Cyanosis of lips and nail beds is an ominous sign. There are signs of respiratory distress, such as nasal flaring, use of accessory muscles, retractions, hypoxemia, and respiratory alkalosis progressing to respiratory acidosis. Also seen are tachypnea, tachycardia, one- to two-word dyspnea (speaking in short phrases), decreased level of consciousness. Young child will assume tripod position; older child will sit upright with shoulders hunched.
2. The goals of emergency management are to quickly reverse airflow obstruction, to reduce likelihood of recurrence, and to correct hypoxemia.
3. Assess peak expiratory flow (PEF) rate or FEV_1 upon arrival; assess degree of respiratory distress or fatigue.

4. Obtain an oxygen saturation level; maintain levels of 95% or greater.
5. Obtain arterial/capillary blood gas in infants with a oxygen saturation of <90%, and in a child with moderate to severe respiratory distress.

> ### NURSING ALERT
>
> **Absence of wheezing with decreased breath sounds and inability to blow a PEF indicates minimal air exchange. Situation requires immediate, swift attention to prevent respiratory failure.**

6. Obtain a brief history and physical, focus on prior treatment and possible triggers of the episode such as respiratory infection or lack of medication.
7. Administer short-acting inhaled beta-2 agonist, such as albuterol, every 20 to 30 minutes for three treatments. Repeat assessment after first and third dose of inhaled beta-2 agonist (Table 44-2).

> ### ◆ DRUG ALERT
>
> **Anticholinergics such as ipratropium bromide, 0.25 mg for children, may be added to albuterol in nebulizer. It has been shown to improve bronchodilation in some patients, especially those with severe airflow obstruction.**

8. Administer corticosteroids, oral or IV as prescribed.
   a. Steroids are recommended early in the episode for infants. Monitor oxygen saturation levels, and maintain at >95%.
   b. Assess infant's level of airway obstruction/signs of serious respiratory distress by observing for use of accessory muscles, paradoxical breathing, cyanosis, respiratory rate >60, oxygen saturation level ≤91%. Assess for improvement.
9. Obtain arterial blood gas (ABG) for patients with severe distress, suspected hypoventilation, or FEV_1 or PEF ≤30% of predicted after treatment.
10. Children in severe status asthmaticus unresponsive to above therapy may require:
    a. Intubation and mechanical ventilation with 100% oxygen for impending or actual respiratory distress, decreased mental alertness, increased fatigue, PCO_2 greater than or equal to 42 mm Hg
    b. Nebulized beta-2 agonist, hourly or continuously
    c. Anticholinergic, such as ipratropium
    d. IV steroid
    e. Admission to ICU
    f. Pharmacologic paralysis to ventilate effectively
    g. Cardiopulmonary monitoring of the child's response to treatment
    h. Placement of an arterial line for blood monitoring
11. Therapies not recommended for treating an exacerbation, based on the 1997 National Heart, Lung, and Blood Institute Expert Panel Report:

a. Subcutaneous beta-2 agonist provides no advantage over inhaled medication.
b. Theophylline/aminophylline is not recommended in the emergency department. It does not provide additional benefit to short-acting beta-2 agonists; it may produce adverse effects.
c. Chest physical therapy (CPT) and mucolytics.
d. Antibiotics are not recommended for asthma treatment. However, antibiotics may be needed in patients with fever, purulent sputum, and evidence of bacterial pneumonia.
e. Anxiolytic and hypnotic drugs are contraindicated.
f. Aggressive hydration is not recommended in older children. Assess fluid status; make corrections as needed for infants and young children to decrease risk of dehydration.

Long-Term Management

1. As the child becomes stabilized, begin to develop a home/school management plan. Components of the plan should include:
   a. Use of quick-relief medications (inhaled beta agonists); expected effect, side effects
   b. Use of long-term controllers (usually inhaled anti-inflammatories, leukotriene modifiers, mast cell stabilizers); desired effect, side effects
   c. Inhalation technique with nebulizer or multidose inhaler with spacer (Figure 44-4)
   d. Peak flow and symptom monitoring
   e. Use of PEF zone system if indicated (see below)
   f. Identification of triggers (eg, mold, pollen, exercise, weather change, infection, allergen exposure)
   g. Environmental control by removal of suspected stimuli
   h. Hydration, nutrition, rest, and exercise regimens
   i. Emergency action plans
2. Plan a team conference involving child, parents, school nurse, and teacher if possible. Ideally, the plan should be clear and easy for the child and family to follow, adapted to their lifestyle, using the least amount of medications necessary to control and prevent the child's asthma symptoms. A written action plan should be submitted to the school, including information on self-medication, identified triggers, steps in an emergency plan, and emergency contact information. A copy of this form can be found in *Guidelines for the Diagnosis and Management of Asthma,* NIH Publication No. 97-4051A.
3. Stress that, without exception, no smoking should be permitted in the home or car of a child with asthma. Even if the child is out of the home, the residual odor will cause symptoms. Opening windows, sprays, air cleaners, and so forth are not acceptable alternatives.
4. Encourage parents to pay particular attention to environmental control in the child's bedroom, including elimination of dust, not allowing any pets, and avoidance of any strong smells or sprays.

TABLE 44-2 Drugs Used in the Treatment of Pediatric Asthma

Drug	Available Forms	Action	Nursing Implications
Short-acting Beta-2 Agonists, Inhaled			
Albuterol (Ventolin, Proventil, Ventolin Rotocaps, Airet)	Metered-dose inhaler (MDI), nebulizer solution, dry powder inhaler	Bronchodilator; relaxes smooth muscles. May decrease release of substances that cause inflammatory response from mast cells.	This is drug of choice for initial treatment of acute exacerbation. It may be given as a continuous nebulization in status asthmaticus. Ensure that the drug is being delivered properly, child is sitting upright, and mask is applied correctly. Use of spacer attachment is recommended for all MDI. Check child technique periodically. Onset of action is 5–15 min. Duration: 4–6 hours. Some research suggests that chronic regular use may result in development of tolerance or airway hyperresponsiveness. If administering by way of nebulizer for acute exacerbation, oxygen is generally used.
Metaproterenol (Alupent)	MDI, nebulizer solution.	Bronchodilator; relaxes airway smooth muscles.	This has more cardiovascular effects than albuterol (increased heart is primary effect).
Terbutaline (Brethine, Brethaire)	MDI, nebulizer solution, also available in injectable and intravenous form	Bronchodilator; relaxes airway smooth muscles.	More cardiovascular effects than albuterol. Acute, severe exacerbations that do not respond to conventional treatment may be treated with subcutaneous injection or continuous IV infusion.
Bitolterol (Toralate)	Nebulizer, MDI	Bronchodilator	Nebulizer solution is not recommended for children under age 12 years old. Duration: 5–8 hours. If asthma symptoms become worse, or if patient does not respond to usual dose, contact health care provider. Do not increase dose.
Beta-2 Agonists, Oral			
Albuterol (Alupent), terbutaline	Oral		Onset of action 30 minutes. Not indicated for treatment of acute episodes. Great likelihood of adverse effects when compared to inhaled form.
Long-Acting Beta-2 Agonists			
Salmeterol (Serevent)	MDI	Bronchodilator	Duration: 12 hours. Used to help prevent asthma symptoms. Not for immediate relief of symptoms during an acute episode. During an acute episode, patient must use a short-acting beta-2 agonist, and continue the regular schedule of salmeterol. Salmeterol should not be taken more than, two times a day. It should not be used in place of anti-inflammatory therapy. It is not recommended for children under 12 years old. Patient education on the proper use of this MDI is important to avoid serious effects of overuse or misuse in the presence of an acute asthmatic episode. Patient should be given restrictions on the number of doses of a short-acting beta-2 agonist, which can be taken safely within a 24-hour period.
Anti-inflammatory, Corticosteroids			
Prednisone (Orasone), prednisolone (Pediapred), methylprednisone (Medrol)	Parenteral, oral	Thought to decrease inflammatory response by interfering with prostaglandin and arachadonic acid production; may increase responsiveness of airways to beta agonists.	A short, 4- to 5-day course of oral steroids is frequently used in acute exacerbation. A taper is not needed for a short oral course of the drug. Onset of action is 3 hours. Side effects may include increased appetite, increased activity or mood change, increased serum glucose levels, facial swelling, hypertension, peptic ulcer, and necrosis of the hip. Prolonged use: osteoporosis, Cushing's syndrome, cataracts, muscle wasting, fragile skin, petechiae, impairment of immune system, potassium loss, hypothalamic-pituitary suppression, slower growth. Take with food to avoid stomach irritation. Monitor child's growth. Ophthalmology exams every 1–2 years. Close monitoring, frequent assessment with a goal of changing to inhaled steroids. Long-term side effects may be minimized by a single AM alternate-day dose.

(continued)

◆ **DRUG ALERT**

Prolonged oral corticosteroid treatment is used only in cases of very severe asthma. The child should be followed by a pediatric pulmonologist and pediatric allergist.

TABLE 44-2 Drugs Used in the Treatment of Pediatric Asthma (Continued)

Drug	Available Forms	Action	Nursing Implications
Beclomethasone (Beclovent, Vanceril), triamcinolone (Azmacort), flunisolide (Aerobid), fluticasine (Flovent)	Inhaled steroids, MDI	Same as above.	Used to prevent symptoms and episodes. Dose per inhalation varies between preparations, for example, beclomethasone delivers 43 µg/puff, triamcinolone delivers 100 µg/puff. Inhaled steroids have fewer side effects than oral steroids. The lowest dose possible to maintain control symptoms should be used. There is a potential but small risk of adverse effect on linear growth from the use of inhaled steroids. The effect appears to be dose related. Inhaled steroids may cause oral candidiasis. This can be prevented by the use of a spacer, and rinsing of the mouth after use. Cough due to upper airway irritation may be seen with use of corticosteroid MDI.
Nonsteroidal Anti-inflammatory Drugs			
Cromolyn (Intal)	MDI, nebulizer solution	Thought to stabilize mast cell membranes, preventing the release of inflammatory substances.	Administered prophylactically, especially for patients with exercise-induced asthma (EIA), or triggers due to allergies. It may take 4–6 weeks before maximum benefit is seen. This drug is not used for the treatment of acute asthma.
Nedocromil sodium (Tilade)	MDI	Similar to Intal. Inhibits activation and release of inflammatory mediators, eosinophils, neutrophils, macrophages.	Used to prevent asthma symptoms. Do not use to treat an acute episode. Recommended for children 12 years of age and older. Rinse mouth with water after use/brush teeth to decrease unpleasant taste. Do not place canister in water.
Methylxanthines			
Theophylline (Slo-Bid, Theo-Dur)	Syrup, sustained-released tablets or capsules, intravenous (aminophylline)	Bronchodilator; may increase respiratory muscle contractions.	Often used to treat nocturnal asthma. Aminophylline is a theophylline salt and is about 80% available theophylline. When the patient is converted from IV to oral theophylline, the dose must be adjusted and levels monitored. Metabolism is decreased in infants younger than 6 months and increased in children compared with adults. Metabolism of the drug is increased by administration of many antibiotics and decreased in fever. Many drugs have interactions with theophylline. Be aware of all the drugs patient is receiving. Levels should be monitored regularly. Signs and symptoms of theophylline toxicity include cardiac arrhythmias, restlessness, nausea, vomiting, and seizures. Many children experience GI upset with this drug.
Leukotriene Modifiers			
Zafilukast (Accolate), zileuton (Zyflo)	Tablet	Compete for leukotriene receptor sites, blocking inflammatory action. Additional research needed for long-term efficacy and tolerance.	Not recommended for children under 12 years old. A new class of anti-asthma drugs with properties of both anti-inflammatory and bronchodilators. Have been found to modify bronchospasm with exercise, decrease pulmonary reaction to aspirin sensitivity, improve airflow obstruction, and decrease symptoms. Used as an option in children and adults with mild to moderate asthma who are not controlled with inhaled steroids.

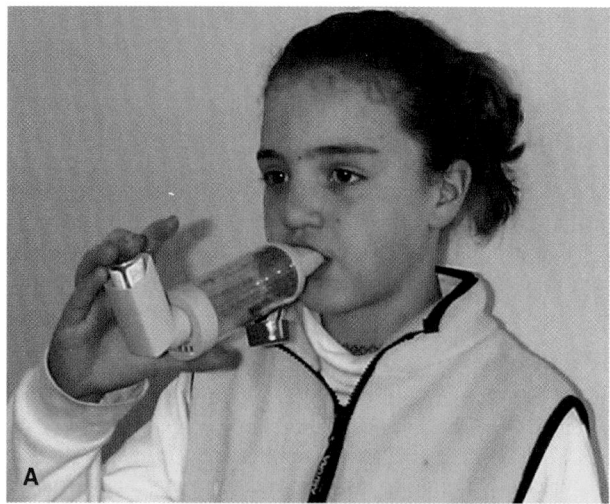

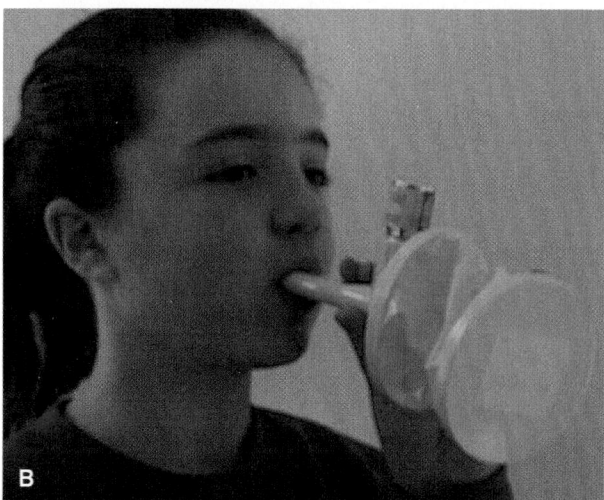

FIGURE 44-4 Multidose inhaler use with spacers. (**A**) Aero Chamber; (**B**) Inspirease.

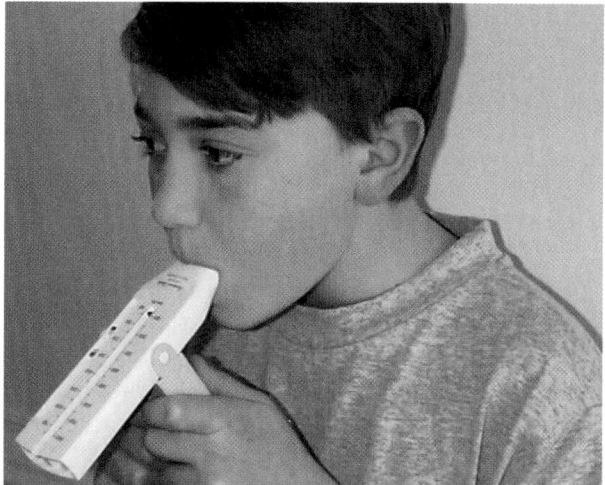

FIGURE 44-5 Peak flow monitoring.

5. Obtain more information from The National Asthma Education Program, PO Box 30105, Bethesda, MD 20824; The American Association of Allergy and Asthma, *www.aaai.org*; or the American Lung Association at *www.lungusa.org*.

Peak Expiratory Flow Monitoring and the Zone System

1. Teach family and child the importance of PEF monitoring at home (Figure 44-5). It is one of the most important tools in asthma education. PEF monitoring, along with an asthma diary, is of paramount importance for newly diagnosed patients and those with labile or persistent symptoms. It assists the family with the following:
   a. Identification of individual triggers
   b. Appreciation of varying degrees of airflow obstruction
   c. Recognition and treatment of early symptoms
   d. Active participation in asthma management plan
   e. Increases self-confidence and assists in decision-making skills
   f. Increases compliance
2. A PEF meter measures the PEF rate that can be produced during a forced expiration. It measures airflow through the large airways; the result is effort dependent. PEF measurements can be initiated in children as young as 5 years of age. Given time and practice, consistent readings will be produced. (See p. 925 for directions on use of PEF meter.)
3. A table of predicted PEF values should be included in the packaging of the home PEF meter. These values are based on age and height. A few patients may find their reading is above or below the published values. Therefore, each child should establish his or her personal best PEF value. Ideally, this should be implemented during a time when the child is symptom free. If PEF readings are consistently below predicted values, the health care provider should be contacted and additional medications may be necessary.
4. Use of the PEF zone system along with a home asthma management plan assists families in the proper use of medications, and assists in decision making regarding the degree of airflow obstruction. Once the personal best PEF value is identified, teach the patient that subsequent PEF measurements can be classified into three zones that will dictate a home management plan.
   a. Green Zone = 80% to 100% of personal best. No asthma symptoms are present. Continue usual medications.
   b. Yellow Zone = 50% to less than 79% of personal best. Signals caution. May be experiencing an asthma

episode, or day-to-day control is suboptimal. Need to use short-acting inhaled beta-2 agonist, follow emergency plan, and contact health care provider for further instructions.

c. Red Zone = less than 50% of personal best value. This zone signals danger. Must take a short-acting inhaled beta-2 agonist immediately, and, if PEF does not return to yellow or green zone, contact health care provider or proceed to emergency department immediately.

■ Respiratory Distress Syndrome (Hyaline Membrane Disease)

Respiratory distress syndrome (RDS), formerly known as hyaline membrane disease, is a syndrome of premature infants that is characterized by a progressive and frequently fatal respiratory failure resulting from atelectasis and immaturity of the lungs. RDS occurs most frequently in premature infants (primarily weighing between 1,000 and 1,500 g [2.2 to 3.3 lb]) and between 28 and 37 weeks' gestation. In infants ≤28 to 30 weeks' gestation, the incidence is 50% to 70%, and increases with degree of prematurity.

Pathophysiology and Etiology

1. Adequate pulmonary function at birth depends on the following:
   a. Adequate amount of surfactant (a lipoprotein mixture) lining the alveolar cells, which allows for alveolar stability and prevents alveolar collapse at the end of expiration
   b. Adequate surface area in air spaces to allow for gas exchange (ie, sufficient pulmonary capillary bed in contact with this alveolar surface area)
2. RDS is ultimately the result of decreased pulmonary surfactant, incomplete structural development of lung, and a highly compliant chest wall.
3. Contributing factors are any factor that decreases surfactant, such as the following:
   a. Prematurity and immature alveolar lining cells
   b. Acidosis
   c. Hypothermia
   d. Hypoxia
   e. Hypovolemia
   f. Diabetes
   g. Elective cesarean section
   h. Fetal or intrapartum stress that compromises blood supply to fetal lungs: vaginal bleeding, maternal hypertension, difficult resuscitation associated with birth asphyxia. (Some situations, such as steroid therapy and heroin-addicted mother, result in the acceleration of surfactant.)
   i. Unknown factors
4. Surfactant production is deficient by type II alveolar cells. (Although some surfactant may be present at birth, it may not be regenerated at adequate rate.) Surfactant production may be reduced due to the following:

a. Extreme immaturity of alveolar lining cells
b. Diminished or impaired production rate resulting from fetal or early neonatal stress
c. Impairment of release mechanism for phospholipid from type II alveolar cells
d. Death of many of these cells responsible for decreased surfactant production

5. Intra-alveolar surface tension is increased, and alveoli are unstable and collapse at the end of expiration. Functional reserve capacity—the amount of air left in the lungs after expiration—is decreased; thus, the next breath requires almost as much effort as the first breath after birth.
6. More oxygen and energy are required to expand the alveoli with each breath, causing fatigue.
7. The number of alveoli that expand progressively decreases, leading to alveolar instability and atelectasis.
8. Pulmonary vascular resistance increases, causing hypoperfusion of lung.
9. Persistence of fetal circulation right-to-left shunt results, leading to hypoxemia and hypercapnia, which lead to respiratory and metabolic acidosis.
10. Hypoxemia and pulmonary vascular pressure cause ischemia in the alveoli, leading to transudate into the alveoli and formation of membranous layer (Figure 44-6).
11. Gas exchange becomes inhibited. Lungs become stiff (decreased compliance), requiring more pressure to expand them.
12. Airway obstruction leads to increased hypoxia and vasoconstriction, and the cycle continues.
13. RDS is usually a self-limited disease, and symptoms peak in about 3 to 4 days, at which time surfactant synthesis begins to accelerate, and pulmonary function and clinical appearance begin to improve.
    a. Moderately ill infants or those who do not require assisted ventilation usually show slow improvement by about 48 hours and rapid recovery over 3 to 4 days with few complications.
    b. Severely ill and very immature infants who require some ventilatory assistance usually demonstrate rapid deterioration. Ventilatory assistance may be required for several days, and chronic lung disease and other complications are common.

Clinical Manifestations

Symptoms are usually observed soon after birth and may include the following:
Primary Signs and Symptoms

1. Expiratory grunting or whining (when infant is not crying)
2. Sternal, suprasternal, substernal, and intercostal retractions progressing to paradoxical seesaw respirations
3. Inspiratory nasal flaring
4. Tachypnea >60 bpm
5. Hypothermia

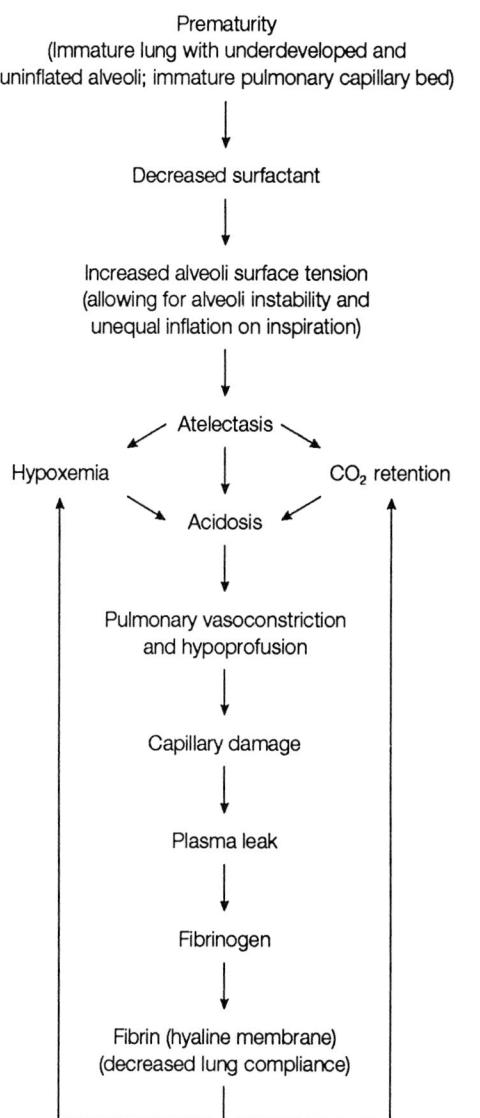

FIGURE 44-6 Schematic outline of hyaline membrane disease.

6. Cyanosis when child is in room air (infants with severe disease may be cyanotic even when given oxygen), increasing need for oxygen
7. Decreased breath sounds and dry "sandpaper" breath sounds
8. As the disease progresses:
   a. Seesaw retractions become marked with marked abdominal protrusion on expiration.
   b. Peripheral edema increases.
   c. Muscle tone decreases.
   d. Cyanosis increases.
   e. Body temperature drops.
   f. Short periods of apnea occur.
   g. Bradycardia may occur.

   h. Changes in distribution of blood throughout body result in pale gray skin color.
   i. Diminished breath sounds.

Secondary Signs and Symptoms
1. Hypotension
2. Edema of hands and feet
3. Absent bowel sounds early in the illness
4. Decreased urine output

Diagnostic Evaluation
1. Laboratory tests
   a. P_{CO_2}—elevated
   b. P_{O_2}—low
   c. Blood pH—low due to metabolic acidosis
   d. Calcium—low
   e. Serum glucose—low
2. Chest x-ray—diffuse, fine granularity; "whiteout," very heavy, uniform granularity reflecting fluid-filled alveoli and atelectasis of some alveoli, surrounded by hyperdistended bronchioles; "ground glass" appearance with prominent air bronchogram extending into periphery of lung fields
3. Pulmonary function studies—stiff lung with a reduced effective pulmonary blood flow

Treatment
Early recognition is imperative so treatment may be instituted immediately. Transportation to a facility providing specialized care is desirable when possible.
Supportive
1. Maintenance of oxygenation—PaO_2 at 60 to 80 mm Hg to prevent hypoxia; frequent arterial pH and blood gas measurements, and use of a pulse oximeter
2. Maintenance of respiration with ventilatory support, if necessary—intermittent mandatory ventilations plus positive end-expiratory pressure (PEEP) or continuous positive airway pressure (CPAP)
3. Maintenance of normal body temperature
4. Maintenance of fluid, electrolyte, and acid–base balance—metabolic acidosis buffered with $NaHCO_3$
5. Maintenance of nutrition—IV dextrose 10% usually required
6. Antibiotics as needed to treat infection
7. Constant observation for complications—pneumothorax, disseminated intravascular coagulation (DIC), patent ductus arteriosus (PDA) with heart failure, chronic lung disease
8. Care appropriate for small, premature infant
9. Prevent hypotension
10. Maintain a hematocrit (hct) of 40% to 45%
Aggressive (Offered in Tertiary Care Centers)
1. Administration of exogenous surfactant into lungs early in the disease.
   a. Especially beneficial in the very low birth weight (VLBW) infant
   b. May be given preventively to VLBW infants at birth

c. Available preparations: bovine (Survanta) and synthetic (Exosurf) surfactant

d. Administered into the endotracheal tube

2. Surfactant replacement therapy.

a. Prophylactic surfactant therapy: infants at increased risk for RDS, infants of less than 30 weeks' gestational age, infants with a birth weight of less than 1,250 g.

b. Treatment initiated after infant is stabilized in the delivery room or within 30 minutes of life.

c. Rescue surfactant therapy: infants with moderate to severe RDS, requiring ventilatory assistance, with an oxygen requirement of greater than 40%.

d. Benefits of surfactant: decreased oxygen requirement and mean airway pressure; decreases pulmonary leaks.

e. Complications observed in surfactant administration: pulmonary hemorrhage, PDA.

f. Nursing assessment with surfactant administration: suctioning delayed for 1 hour or as indicated by protocol. Assist with delivery of surfactant, collection and monitoring of ABG, meticulous monitoring of oxygenation status with pulse oximeter/transcutaneous monitor (TcpCO$_2$).

g. Assess infant's tolerance of the procedure: increase in respiratory compliance, which will require adjustments of the ventilator.

3. High-frequency ventilation—mechanical ventilation that uses rapid rates (can be greater than 900 bpm) and tidal volumes near and often less than anatomical dead spaces.

a. Jet ventilator delivers short burst of gases at high flow.

(i) Exhalation is passive.

(ii) Necrotizing tracheitis is a significant complication, along with hypotension and pneumopericardium.

b. Oscillator ventilator delivers gases by vibrating columns of air.

(i) Exhalation is active.

(ii) The child appears to shake on the bed, which may be frightening for parents.

4. Extracorporeal membrane oxygenation (ECMO)—indicated in infants with reversible cardiac or respiratory failure. ECMO is a modified heart–lung bypass machine used to allow gas exchange outside the body.

a. Blood is removed from the venous system by a catheter placed in the internal jugular vein or right atrium.

b. Oxygen is added and carbon dioxide removed with a membrane oxygenator.

c. Oxygenated blood is returned by way of the right common carotid (in venoarterial ECMO) or the femoral vein (in venovenous ECMO).

d. The infant must be heparinized for the procedure, increasing the risk of intraventricular hemorrhage. For this reason, VLBW infants or infants of decreased gestational age are usually not candidates for the procedure.

e. One nurse and one perfusionist must be present at the bedside at all times to monitor the patient and equipment. The patient will receive paralytic agents as well as analgesia and sedation; therefore, diligent continuous monitoring is required.

f. Cannula dislodgement or tubing separation will result in immediate hemorrhage. Tubing and cannula must be secured and visible.

Complications

1. Complications related to respiratory therapy

a. Air leak: pneumothorax, pneumomediastinum, pneumopericardium, and pneumoperitoneum

b. Pneumonia, especially gram-negative organisms

c. Pulmonary interstitial emphysema

2. PDA

3. Intraventricular hemorrhage—most often seen in infants weighing less than 1,500 g (3.3 lb)

4. DIC

5. Chronic problems associated with long-term use of oxygen

a. BPD—cystic-appearing lungs with hyperinfiltration, obstructive bronchiolitis, dysplastic changes, and pulmonary fibrosis

b. Chronic respiratory infections

6. Necrotizing enterocolitis

7. Tracheal stenosis

8. Retinopathy of prematurity (retrolental fibroplasia)

9. Other complications related to prematurity

Nursing Assessment

1. Review the birth history.

a. Apgar scores 1 and 5 minutes after birth

b. Type of resuscitation required

c. Any treatment or medication administered

d. Any medication or anesthesia administered to the mother during labor

e. Estimated gestational age

f. Maternal history—contributing factors or complications

2. Carefully assess the infant's respiratory status to determine the degree of respiratory distress.

a. Determine the degree and severity of retractions.

b. Count the respiratory rate for 1 full minute, note level of activity, and determine if they are regular or irregular.

c. Identify any periods of apnea, length, and type of stimulation necessary.

d. Listen for expiratory grunting or whining sounds from the infant when quiet. This indicates an attempt to maintain PEEP and prevent alveoli from collapse.

e. Note any nasal flaring.

f. Note any cyanosis—location, improvement with oxygen.

g. Auscultate chest for diminished breath sounds and presence of crackles.

3. Determine the infant's cardiac rate and rhythm.

a. Count the apical pulse for 1 full minute.

b. Note any irregularity in the rate or bounding pulses.

4. Observe the infant's general activity.

a. Lethargic or listless

b. Active and responds to stimuli

c. Infant's cry

5. Assess skin for cyanosis, jaundice, mottling, paleness or grayness, and edema.

Nursing Diagnoses

- Impaired Gas Exchange related to disease process
- Altered Nutrition: Less Than Body Requirements related to prematurity and increased energy expenditure on breathing
- Ineffective Thermoregulation related to immaturity
- Altered Parenting related to separation from the newborn due to hospitalization

Nursing Interventions

Promoting Adequate Gas Exchange

1. Have emergency equipment readily available for use in the event of cardiac or respiratory arrest.

2. Institute cardiorespiratory monitoring to monitor continuously heart and respiratory rates.

3. Administer supplemental oxygen.

a. Incubator with oxygen at prescribed concentration

b. Plastic hood with oxygen at prescribed concentration when using radiant warmer

c. CPAP, if indicated, using nasal prongs or endotracheal tube

4. Assist with endotracheal intubation, and maintain mechanical ventilation as indicated.

5. Measure oxygen concentration every hour and record.

6. Monitor ABG as appropriate. Obtain sample through indwelling umbilical line, arterial puncture, or capillary puncture. (Capillary gas analysis for monitoring P_{CO_2} and pH but not P_{O_2}.)

7. Institute pulse oximetry, if available, for continuous monitoring of oxygen saturation of arterial blood (Sa_{O_2}).

a. Avoid using adhesive to secure the sensor when infant is active. Wrap it snugly enough to reduce sensitivity to movement but not tight enough to constrict blood flow.

b. If transcutaneous P_{O_2} monitor (Tc_{PO_2}) is used, reposition the probe every 3 to 4 hours to avoid burns caused by heating the probe to achieve sufficient arterialization.

8. Observe the infant's response to oxygen.

a. Observe for improvement in color, respiratory rate and pattern, and nasal flaring.

b. Note response by improvement in arterial or capillary blood gas.

c. Observe closely for apnea.

9. Stimulate infant if apnea occurs. If unable to produce spontaneous respiration with stimulation within 15 to 30 seconds, initiate resuscitation.

10. Position the infant to allow for maximal lung expansion.

a. Prone position provides for a larger lung volume because of the position of the diaphragm, decreases energy expenditure, and increases time spent in quiet sleep, but it may be contraindicated due to placement of umbilical catheter. The risk for SIDS is increased, but the infant is continuously monitored.

b. Change position frequently.

11. Suction as needed because the gag reflex is weak, and cough is ineffective.

12. Try to minimize time spent on procedures and interventions, and monitor effects on respiratory status. (Infants undergoing multiple procedures lasting 45 minutes to 1 hour have shown a moderate decrease in P_{O_2}.)

13. The decision to suction should be based on assessment of the infant, such as auscultation of chest, decrease in oxygenation, excessive moisture in the endotracheal tube, and irritability.

a. Nasopharyngeal, tracheal, or endotracheal tube suctioning should be done gently, quickly, 5 seconds or less, with intermittent suction applied as the catheter is withdrawn.

b. To prevent hypoxemia, observe oximeter before, during, and after procedure.

c. Suctioning of the endotracheal tube (ETT) is done to maintain a patent airway. The practice of inducing a catheter into the tube until resistance is met, and then withdrawn has been shown to cause trauma to the tracheal wall. Instead, the suction catheter should be premeasured according to the size of the infant's ETT length and documented. When suctioning, do not insert the catheter beyond this predetermined length. This will prevent damage to the mucosa.

14. Observe for complications of suctioning: bronchospasm, vagal nerve stimulation/bradycardia, hypoxia, increased intercranial pressure, trauma to airway, infection and pneumothoraces.

15. Percussion and vibration techniques are not tolerated in extremely low birth weight babies, and VLBW babies.

NURSING ALERT

Prone position may present several problems: turning head to side can compromise upper airway and increase air flow resistance; observation of chest is obstructed, and retractions are more difficult to detect; and abdominal distention is more difficult to recognize.

Promoting Adequate Nutrition and Hydration

1. Administer IV fluids or enteral feeding as ordered, and observe infusion rate closely to prevent fluid overload.

2. Observe IV sites for infiltration or infection; use meticulous technique to prevent sepsis.

3. If umbilical artery catheter is in place, observe for bleeding.

4. Provide adequate caloric intake (80 to 120 kcal/kg/24 h) through the following:

a. Nasojejunal tube (best tolerated by VLBW infants)

b. Nasogastric tube

c. Parenteral nutrition—D10W or hyperalimentation fluid usually required

5. Monitor for hypoglycemia, which is especially common during stress. Maintain serum glucose >45 mg/dL.

6. Monitor intake and output closely.

a. Include amount of blood drawn (small infants can become anemic due to frequent blood sampling).

b. Apply urine collection bag to obtain sample of urine, and measure specific gravity periodically.

7. Weigh infant daily.

Maintaining Thermoregulation

1. Provide a neutral thermal environment to maintain the infant' s abdominal skin temperature between 97° and 98°F (36° and 36.5°C) to prevent hypothermia, which may result in vasoconstriction and acidosis.

2. Adjust Isolette or radiant warmer to obtain desired skin temperature. For the infant weighing less than 1,250 g, the radiant warmer should be used with caution because of increased water loss and potential for hypoglycemia.

3. Prevent frequent opening of Isolette.

4. Ensure that O_2 is warmed to 87.6° to 93.2°F (32° to 34°C) with 60% to 80% humidity.

Encouraging Parental Attachment

1. Identify any factors prohibiting parents' visitation and communication: geographic distance, lack of transportation, care of siblings, employment restrictions, economic issues, lack of telephone in the home, fear. Refer to social services for assistance and intervention.

2. If the infant has been transported to tertiary care center immediately after birth, send a photograph of the baby to the mother.

3. Call the parents daily to update them on the infant's condition until they are able to visit the child. Emphasize positive aspects of the infant's status.

4. Refer to the child by his or her first name when speaking with the parents.

5. Prepare the parents for the neonatal intensive care unit (NICU) environment and how their child will appear before their first visit.

6. Assist the parents to participate in the child's care as appropriate.

7. Demonstrate for the parents how they can touch and speak to the child while the child is in an Isolette.

8. Allow the parents to hold the infant as soon as possible.

9. If the mother plans to breast-feed, assist her with pumping, and use the breast milk to feed the infant when enteral feedings are initiated.

10. If the infant has siblings, provide the parents with information on how to discuss the infant's illness with them.

11. If unit policies allow and the situation is appropriate, encourage sibling visitation with adequate preparation.

12. Provide the parents with information concerning the disease process, expected outcomes, and usual course of the NICU stay. Encourage the parents to ask questions and participate in the plan of care.

13. Help parents work through their grief at the birth of a premature child.

Family Education and Health Management

1. Prepare the family for long-term follow-up as appropriate. Infants with BPD may eventually go home on oxygen therapy.

2. Stress the importance of regular health care, periodic eye examinations, and developmental follow-up with the parents.

3. Ensure that the family receives information on routine well-baby care.

4. Before discharge, parents should feel comfortable in their abilities to care for infant, referrals for home nursing visits are completed, and a physician is identified for follow-up care.

Outcome-Based Evaluation

- Respiratory rate within norms for age; pattern regular and unlabored
- Tolerating enteral feedings well; weight gain noted
- Temperature maintained within normal limits
- Parents interacting with infant, participating in care, and asking appropriate questions

■ Cystic Fibrosis

Cystic fibrosis (CF) is a generalized multisystem disorder affecting the exocrine glands so the substances they secrete are abnormally viscous, affecting primarily pulmonary and gastrointestinal function. Incidence is estimated to be 1:3200 live births in Caucasians, 1:9500 in Hispanics, 1:15,000 in African Americans, and much lower in Asians. About 4% to 5% of the white population are carriers. Slightly more males than females are affected. The average life expectancy for a child born with CF in the 1990s is projected to be into the forties.

Pathophysiology and Etiology

1. CF is inherited as an autosomal mendelian recessive trait.

2. Chloride channel functioning is affected, resulting in a decreased ability of cell membranes to transport water and electrolytes.

3. The secretions of the exocrine glands are thick and sticky rather than thin and slippery.

4. Pulmonary involvement includes:

a. Decreased ciliary action

b. Metaplasia and hyperplasia of squamous cells of mucus-secreting glands, leading to increased production of thick secretions (increased risk of infection)

c. Plugged bronchi and bronchioles, resulting in bronchiectasis and bronchiolitis

d. Atelectasis and hyperinfiltration of lungs; irreversible fibrotic changes in lungs

5. Gastrointestinal and pancreatic involvement includes:

a. Acini and ducts of pancreas become filled with thick mucus and are obstructed.

b. Trypsin, chymotrypsin, lipase, and amylase do not reach the small intestine.

c. Digestion is impaired. Interruption of the enterohepatic circulation of bile acids probably results in interference with normal pancreatic lipolysis and fat absorption through the intestinal wall.

d. Stools are abnormal and indicate malabsorption syndrome.

e. Meconium ileus often occurs in infant, indicating that bowel is obstructed by thick intestinal secretions.

f. Biliary cirrhosis occurs because the intrahepatic biliary tract is obstructed by thick secretions.

6. Sweat gland involvement includes:

a. Secretions contain excessive amount of sodium and chloride, leading to excessive loss, especially with hot weather, fever, or exertion.

b. Saliva also contains an excess of sodium and chloride.

Clinical Manifestations

1. Presentation usually occurs younger than 6 months of age but may occur at any age.

2. Typically the child will have symptoms of:

a. Pancreatic enzyme deficiency due to duct blockage

b. Progressive chronic obstructive lung disease associated with infection and intestinal obstruction

c. Sweat gland dysfunction

3. Symptoms and severity of the disease vary and change over time as the disease progresses.

a. Mild form of CF—limited digestive and respiratory problems

b. Severe forms of CF—life-threatening pulmonary disease with severe malabsorption

c. Pancreatic insufficiency without pulmonary disease

d. Pulmonary disease without pancreatic insufficiency

4. Gastrointestinal signs and symptoms:

a. Meconium ileus found in newborns

b. Failure to thrive/failure to gain weight in the presence of a good appetite

c. Abdominal distention

d. Vomiting, dehydration, electrolyte imbalance

e. Maldigestion, steatorrhea (fatty stools, loss of fat-soluble vitamins)

5. Respiratory signs and symptoms include:

a. Recurrent pulmonary infections

b. Cough, dry to productive

c. Wheezing

d. Dyspnea

e. Barrel-shaped chest (increased anteroposterior chest diameter)

f. Cyanosis

g. Clubbing of fingers and toes

h. Nasal polyps

6. Thin extremities, sallow skin, wasted buttocks

7. Hyperglycemia, glucosuria, polyuria, weight loss

8. Other signs may include:

a. Salty taste when parents kiss skin

b. Sterility in males

c. Obstructive jaundice

d. Hypoproteinemia/anemia

e. Bleeding diathesis

f. Hyponatremia/heat prostation

Diagnostic Evaluation

1. Sweat chloride test to measure sodium and chloride level in sweat

a. Chloride level of >60 mEq/L is virtually diagnostic.

b. Chloride of 40 to 60 mEq/L is borderline and should be repeated.

c. Sodium level >60 mEq/L is diagnostic.

2. Measurement of trypsin concentration in duodenal secretions; absence of normal concentration virtually diagnostic

3. Analysis of digestive enzymes (trypsin and chymotrypsin) in stool—reduced, used for initial screening for CF

4. Chest x-ray—may be normal initially; later shows increased areas of infection, overinflation, bronchial thickening and plugging, atelectasis, and fibrosis and obstructive emphysema

5. Analysis of stool for steatorrhea

6. BMC (Boehringer-Mannheim Corporation) meconium strip test for stool includes lactose and protein content; used for screening

7. Pulmonary function studies (after 4 years old)

a. Decreased vital capacity and flow rates

b. Increased residual volume or increased total lung capacity

8. Diagnosis made when a positive sweat test is seen in conjunction with one or more of the following:

a. Positive family history for CF

b. Typical chronic obstructive lung disease

d. Documented exocrine pancreatic insufficiency

e. Failure to thrive

f. History of frequent respiratory infections

9. Prenatal diagnostic tests—prenatal genetic screening for families affected with CF

a. Chorionic villus sampling at approximately 12 weeks' gestation

b. DNA probes

c. Microvillar enzymes

Treatment

Goals of treatment are to prevent and minimize pulmonary complications, ensure adequate nutrition for growth, and assist family and child to adapt to chronic disease.

Pulmonary Interventions

1. Antimicrobial therapy as indicated for pulmonary infection

a. Oral antibiotics may be given prophylactically or when symptomatic.

b. IV antibiotics are given when the child fails to respond to oral antibiotics; this may be inpatient or at-home therapy.

c. Inhaled antibiotics, such as gentamicin (Garamycin) or tobramycin (Nebcin), may be used for severe lung disease or colonization of organisms. Recently, some practitioners advocate using nebulized antibiotics earlier in therapy.
d. Patients with CF metabolize antibiotics rapidly; drug dosage is higher than normal, monitor for signs of toxicity.

2. Bronchodilators and vasoconstrictors for relief of bronchospasm
3. Aerosol, expectorants, and mucolytic agents to decrease viscosity of secretions
4. CPT for bronchial drainage, especially during acute exacerbations
   a. Postural drainage (Figure 44-7 and Procedure Guidelines 44-2, p. 1376)
   b. Coughing and deep breathing exercises, huffing helps move secretions from smaller airways.
5. Bronchopulmonary lavage—treatment of atelectasis and mucoid impaction using large volumes of saline (used in some institutions in the United States)
6. Lobectomy—resection of symptomatic lobar bronchiectasis to retard progression of lesion to total lung involvement

Gastrointestinal Interventions

1. Pancreatic enzyme supplementation is provided with each feeding.
   a. Favored preparation is pancrelipase (Pancrease).
   b. Occasionally, antacid is helpful to improve tolerance of enzymes.
   c. Favorable response to enzymes is based on tolerance of fatty foods, decreased stool frequency, absence of steatorrhea, improved appetite, and lack of abdominal pain.
2. Provide a high-energy diet by increasing carbohydrates, protein, and fat (possibly as high as 40%). Increases in dietary intake should consider growth and repair, infection, the work of breathing and energy expenditure for coughing, malabsorption, and physical activity.
3. Provide zinc and iron supplements and water-soluble and fat-soluble vitamins.
4. Ensure adequate fluid and salt intake.

Controversial and Experimental Treatment

1. Administration of aerosolized recombinant human deoxyribonuclease
   a. Enzyme that breaks down DNA in leukocytes is present in thick pulmonary secretions.
   b. The goal of treatment is to reduce viscosity of sputum, making the sputum easier to clear from the airways and decreasing the incidence of infection.
   c. Early trials show improvement in forced vital capacity and forced expiratory volume.
2. Heart–lung, double-lung, or single-lung transplantation for end-stage lung disease
   a. This treatment is limited by availability of donor organs.

b. Survival rate is similar to survival rates in patients without CF.
c. Bilateral lobar transplantation using a new method called bipartitioning of a single donor lung is under study. This method could result in increasing the availability of donor organs.

3. Gene therapy
   a. Phase 1 clinical trials in the United States were started in 1993.
   b. Therapy is based on somatic gene correction; an attempt to correct the defect in the cells of the individual is made by adding the correct gene sequence to the cells.
   c. One trial method will use a virus carrying DNA with the appropriate gene sequence, which will be introduced into the affected lung cells by nebulization.
   d. A second method being investigated is the introduction into the lungs of DNA by nebulization with the appropriate gene sequence suspended in liposomes.
   e. It is thought that the treatment will need to be repeated at regular intervals.
4. Physical exercise—stimulates mucous secretions and may be used as a substitute for CPT; also improves self-esteem.

Complications

1. Pulmonary infections
   a. Most frequently caused by *Pseudomonas aeruginosa, Staphylococcus aureus, H. influenzae, Burkholderia cepacia. Pseudomonas* is the most difficult organism to treat.
   b. Bronchiectasis and bronchiolitis

> **NURSING ALERT**
>
> *Burkholderia cepacia* affects 5% to 10% of CF patients, is associated with a rapid decline in pulmonary function, and is multiple antibiotic–resistant. Twenty percent of colonized patients develop fulminant septicemia and necrotizing pneumonia leading to death.

2. Other pulmonary complications, including emphysema, atelectasis, pneumothorax, and hemoptysis (primarily seen in adolescents) and pulmonary hypertension
3. Biliary cirrhosis, leading to portal hypertension, esophageal varices, and splenomegaly
4. Pancreatic fibrosis with islets of Langerhans involvement, resulting in glucose intolerance, diabetes mellitus
5. Cor pulmonale
6. Chronic sinusitis
7. Rectal polyps (3 months to 3 years)
8. Rectal prolapse
9. Intussusception (younger than 2 years)
10. Pancreatitis
11. Hypertrophic pulmonary osteoarthropathy (HPO). Arthritis, clubbing, periosteitis. The long tubular bones are most commonly involved.

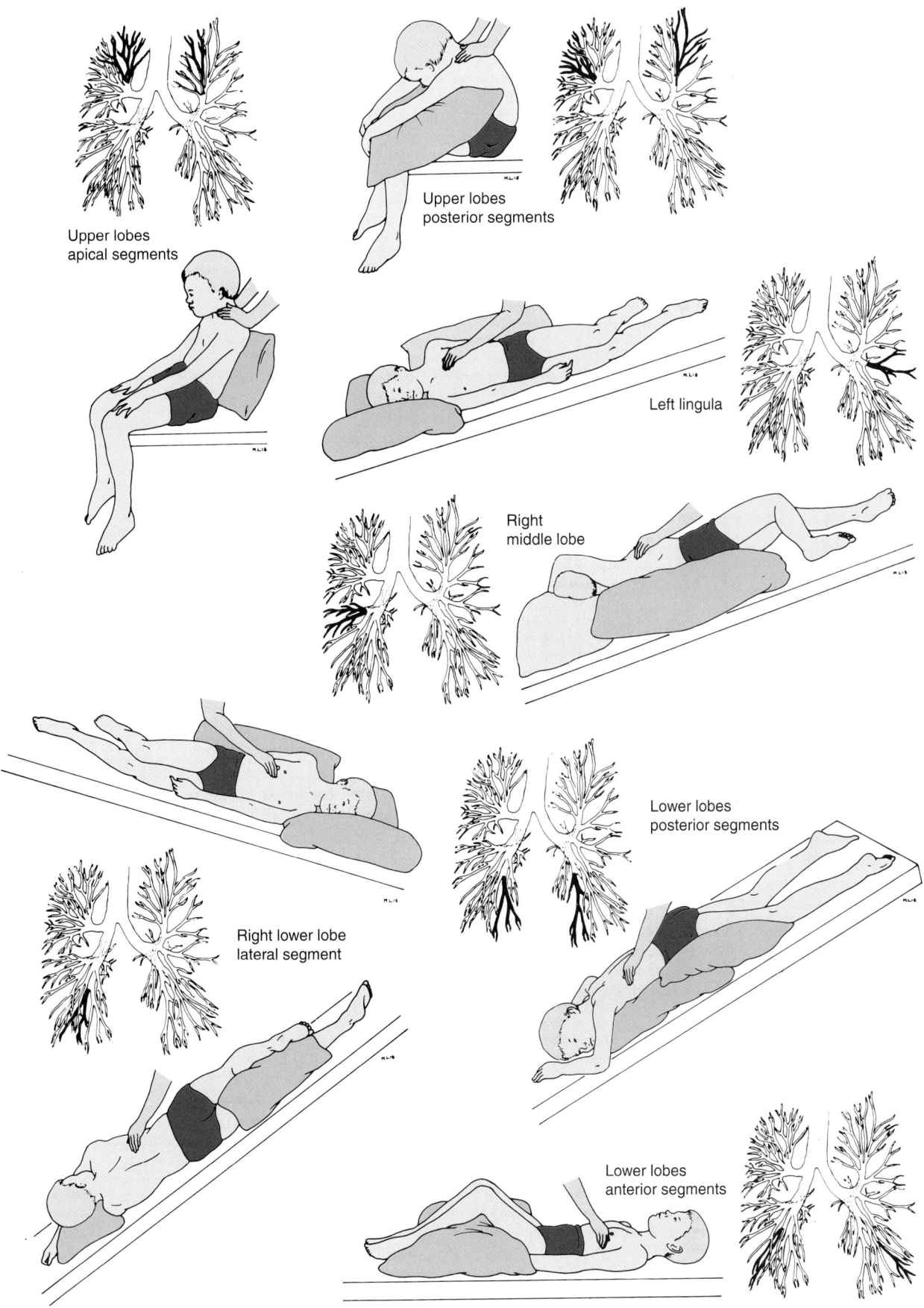

FIGURE 44-7 Positions for postural drainage.

Upper lobes
apical segments

Upper lobes
posterior segments

Left lingula

Right
middle lobe

Lower lobes
posterior segments

Right lower lobe
lateral segment

Lower lobes
anterior segments

12. Heat prostration
13. Fibrosis of epididymis and vas deferens in male; aspermia
14. Growth retardation
15. Gastroesophageal reflux
16. Allergic bronchopulmonary aspergillosis
17. Respiratory failure and death

Nursing Assessment

1. Check for family history of CF, failure to thrive, and unexplained infant death; check the child's history and physical condition. Carefully listen for subtle information that may suggest CF.
2. Assess respiratory status.
   a. Increased work of breathing
   b. Quality of breath sounds by auscultation
   c. Child's perception of respiratory status
   d. Ability to participate in activities of daily living
3. Assess nutritional status and characteristics of stool.

Nursing Diagnoses

- Ineffective Airway Clearance related to thick pulmonary secretions
- Risk for Infection related to thick, tenacious secretions
- Altered Nutrition: Less Than Body Requirements related to decreased appetite or inadequate absorption
- Body Image Disturbance related to chronic disease process
- Altered Family Processes related to the child with a chronic disease

Nursing Interventions

Promoting Airway Clearance

1. Use intermittent aerosol therapy three to four times a day when child is symptomatic.
   a. Use prior postural drainage.
   b. Administer bronchodilators and other medications, diluted in normal saline, in aerosol form to penetrate respiratory tract.

NURSING ALERT

Mist therapy is no longer recommended because water droplets may cause bronchospasm in some patients, and the equipment required to deliver the therapy is frequently contaminated with opportunistic organisms.

---

2. Perform CPT three to four times a day after aerosol therapy; perform more frequently if infection is present.
   a. Perform 1 hour after eating to prevent vomiting or discomfort.
   b. Place child in position that gives greatest access to affected lobes of lung and facilitates gravity drainage of mucus from specific lung areas.
3. Help the child to relax to cough more easily after postural drainage.
4. Suction the infant or young child when necessary if not able to cough.
5. Teach child breathing exercises using pursed lips to increase duration of exhalation.

6. Maintain cautious oxygen therapy due to chronic CO_2 retention.
7. Monitor for signs and symptoms of pneumothorax, such as tachypnea, tachycardia, pallor, dyspnea, and cyanosis.
8. Monitor for hemoptysis, which requires immediate treatment and may be life threatening.
9. Provide treatment of hemoptysis: bed rest, cough suppressants, antibiotics. Bronchoscopy is used to locate site, cauterize or embolize. Administer vitamin K.

Preventing Infection

1. Provide good skin care and position changes to prevent skin breakdown of malnourished child.
2. Change diapers promptly to prevent diaper rash and superimposed infection.
3. Provide frequent mouth care to reduce the chance of infection because mucus is present.
4. Restrict contact with people with respiratory infection.
5. Administer antibiotics as prescribed to treat specific organisms when child is symptomatic.

Promoting Adequate Nutrition

1. Encourage diet composed of foods high in calories and protein and moderate to high in fat because absorption of food is incomplete. Provide 120% to 150% of recommended dietary allowances because only 80% to 85% of intake is absorbed.
2. Administer fat-soluble vitamins in water-miscible solution in two to three times the normal dose, as prescribed, to counteract malabsorption.
   a. Give vitamins A, D, and E on a daily basis.
   b. Give vitamin K when the child has an infection or is being treated with antibiotics.
3. Administer pancreatic enzymes with each meal and snack.
   a. Mix capsule, granules, or powder with small portion of food for infant or small child; do not mix with formula (may not be finished).
   b. Offer the older child capsules or tablets.
   c. Withhold enzymes, as ordered, if child is taking only clear liquid diet or enteral feedings.
   d. Beads should not be chewed or crushed.
4. Increase salt intake during hot weather, fever, or excessive exercise to prevent sodium depletion and cardiovascular compromise.
5. To prevent vomiting, allow ample time for feeding, especially if irritable because of not feeling well and coughing.
6. Check weights at least weekly to assess nutritional interventions. Document and plot height and weight every 3 months.
7. Infants who are breast-fed will need enzyme supplementation. If supplementation with formula is necessary, choose a high-calorie preparation.
8. Administer supplemental parenteral or enteral feedings as required.
9. Constipation, due to malabsorption, decreased gastric motility, viscous intestinal secretions may be treated with laxatives, stool softeners, or rectal administration of Gastrografin or Mucomyst.

Enhancing Self-Esteem and Body Image

1. Explain each procedure, medication, and treatment to the child as appropriate for age.
2. Allow child to show frustrations, fears, and feelings by talking, complaining, or crying.
3. Support and comfort the child by talking to and holding him or her.
4. Provide diversional activities related to child's interests, and praise child for accomplishments.
5. Encourage older child to take responsibility for treatments and be involved in care plan.
6. Help child to identify strengths and limitations and to feel good about self.
7. If child resists CPT due to anger, fear, or frustration, help to redirect those feelings.
8. Encourage regular exercise and activity to foster sense of accomplishment and independence and improve pulmonary function.

Enhancing Family Processes

1. Provide opportunities for parents to learn all aspects of care for the child.
2. Provide education and support during hospitalization to make home care easier.
3. Encourage maintenance of family activities and involvement with other children.
4. Initiate social work referral as needed.
5. Encourage information sharing about CF with friends, teachers, and relatives. Explain that one of the most important things people can do to help a child with CF is to treat him or her just as they would any other child.
6. Help family share and interpret feelings about CF and its impact on all of their lives.

Family Education and Health Maintenance

1. Teach parents to have a thorough understanding of the dietary regimen and special need for calories, fat, and vitamins. Consultation with a registered dietitian is recommended.
2. Discuss need for salt replacement and free access of the child to salt, as well as the increased need for salt during hot weather or in the presence of fever, vomiting, or diarrhea.
3. Help the parents to become skilled at CPT and other pulmonary treatments. Demonstrate and explain procedures, and evaluate their return demonstration.
4. Help the family to schedule care for the child within the framework of family life.
   a. CPT should be done at least 1 hour after meals.
   b. Aerosol treatments should be done before CPT.
   c. Mild exercise and activity are beneficial to the child.
   d. Vacations and major family outings can be planned for remissions of the child's symptoms.
5. Help the parents to provide emotional support to their child. The child needs love, understanding, and security, not overprotection.
6. Stress the importance of regular medical care.
   a. Routine immunizations
   b. Prompt attention to infection
   c. Continued evaluation and supervision in home management
   d. Attention to developments through research that may change therapy
   e. Prevention or early detection of complications
7. Discuss with parents limitations and expectations for the child.
   a. With proper care, the child will most likely live to adulthood but may be smaller and shorter than peers.
   b. Play and school participation depends on severity of illness.
   c. Involve teachers and school nurses in planning of the child's day.
8. Suggest parents and child meet other CF families. Investigate location and participation in summer camps for children with CF.
9. Investigate home care options for families, especially respite services for caregivers.
10. After the diagnosis is confirmed, refer the parents to genetic counseling. It is important for the parents to realize that the affected child inherits the defective gene from both parents. Each pregnancy has a 1:4 chance of resulting in a child with CF.
11. Refer families for additional information and support to agencies such as Cystic Fibrosis Foundation, 6931 Arlington Road, Bethesda, MD 20814-3205, (800)-FIGHT CF, *www.cff.org*. Most areas have local chapters of the organization.
12. As the child with CF approaches adolescence, the pediatric health care team should discuss with the patient and parents the concept of eventual transitioning of care from a pediatric CF center to an adult CF center. Facilitate a planned, efficient, and smooth transition by:
    a. Encouraging the patient to gradually assume responsibility for health care.
    b. Encouraging parents to foster adolescent's independence.
    c. Providing patient and family time to adjust and educate themselves about the transitioning process.
    d. Identifying and introducing the patient and family to members of the adult care team.
    e. Advocating for the patient in regard to any restrictions superimposed by the patient's health insurance plan.
13. Sadly, at some point, it will become apparent to the health care team that the time has arrived to discuss end-of-life issues. Use a family-centered approach to provide care for the child and family facing a life-threatening illness or death. Discuss hospice care and other available services with the family (see p. 1312).

Apnea of Infancy and Apparent Life-Threatening Event (ALTE)

Apnea of infancy is the cessation of breathing for more than 20 seconds, or a shorter episode associated with bradycardia, cyanosis, or pallor. It may be identified during infancy, usually between 2 weeks and 6 months of age, because of an unexplained frightening respiratory or cardiac event, usually occurring while the infant is asleep, termed *apparent life-threatening event (ALTE)*. Apnea is a clinical sign, not a diagnosis, and is a risk factor for *sudden infant death syndrome* (SIDS), but there is not a strong link between the two. SIDS is the sudden death of any infant more than 37 weeks' gestation, or young child, which is unexplained by history, and in which a thorough postmortem examination fails to demonstrate an adequate cause of death (Box 44-1).

Pathophysiology and Etiology

1. Cause is often unknown—may result from many different pathologic processes; may be idiopathic.
2. Apnea may be related to organic disorders, such as seizure disorders, sepsis, severe infection, hypoglycemia, and impaired regulation of breathing.
3. Apnea of prematurity is related to immaturity of respiratory control.

Clinical Manifestations

1. The infant may be found by parents or caretaker to be limp, cyanotic, and pale, with no respiration. Skin is cool to touch.
2. Some form of resuscitation may be required.
3. The infant usually exhibits symptoms when asleep, although the syndrome may occur during waking hours.
4. Types of sleep apnea include:
   a. Central or diaphragmatic—chest movement ceases, absence of airflow.
   b. Obstructive—chest and diaphragm move, but there is no air exchange.
   c. Mixed—cessation of air flow and chest movement, followed by respiratory effort without air flow.

Diagnostic Evaluation

Complete history, physical examination, and diagnostic tests are aimed at ruling out other medical problems that could result in respiratory failure as a secondary cause.

1. Complete blood count with differential, serum glucose, electrolytes, calcium, phosphate, magnesium, ABG, as indicated.
2. Chest x-ray.
3. Electrocardiogram.
4. Electroencephalogram (may not be routine) and neurologic examination.
5. Respiratory studies—a 12- to 24-hour pneumogram recording of small changes in electrical resistance with each breath or respiratory pattern; multichannel sleep test with continuous printout, monitoring heart rate, chest impedance, nasal airflow, and oxygen saturation.
6. Continuous cardiac and apnea monitoring for recurrence of event, prolonged apnea, or bradycardia.
7. Barium swallow for gastroesophageal reflex.
8. Because of hypoxemia that may have occurred, child should be assessed for learning difficulties (hearing, eye-

sight), discrete neurologic impairments, personality disorders, and so forth.
9. Polysomnograph—records brain waves, eye movements, esophageal manometry, and end tidal CO_2.

Management

1. Cardiopulmonary monitoring is critical; hospitalization if ALTE has occurred.
2. Specific treatment of the underlying cause, if identified.
3. Theophylline (Theolair) may be used to decrease apneic episodes (therapeutic levels of 6 to 10).
4. Long-term follow-up for physiologic and neurologic behavioral functions.
5. Prevention of SIDS: the most effective method of prevention is public education to avoid prone sleeping. More education is needed, with an emphasis on poorer, underserved areas.

NURSING ALERT

Infants who have experienced apnea may be at risk for recurrent apnea, hypoxia, and sudden death and should be monitored closely. Research has shown that SIDS is more likely in infants sleeping prone. It is now recommended that all infants be put to sleep on their backs or sides.

Nursing Assessment

1. Obtain a nursing history, including the parents' description of the events that preceded the hospitalization, and their understanding of prolonged apnea.
   a. This information may provide clues for factors to observe during hospitalization and provides data for the development of a teaching plan.
   b. It allows for the correction of misinformation and misconceptions.
2. Have the parents describe sleep patterns, feeding habits, prior health problems, immunizations, and medications; this may provide data regarding possible influencing factors or causes of the condition.
3. Have the parents describe a typical day in the life of the infant and the family unit. This provides important data on how home monitoring may affect family life, and contributes to the effective development of home management and family teaching plans; it also provides a basis for continuity of care for the infant.

Nursing Diagnoses

- Ineffective Breathing Pattern related to periods of apnea
- Parental Anxiety related to life-threatening event
- Knowledge Deficit regarding home monitoring

Nursing Interventions
Maintaining Breathing Pattern

1. Be prepared for the infant's admission, and have all equipment, including apnea monitor, ready for use. Continuous cardiac monitoring is also recommended.

a. Select a room that is clearly visible from the nursing station; the room should be quiet to reduce sensory stimulation, which may reduce the likelihood of a recurring episode.

b. Be aware that the family has just experienced the extreme stress of feeling that their infant has almost died. Reassure them with empathy and efficiency at the time of admission.

2. Continuously monitor respirations. Document any apnea along with state of consciousness; sleep state; color; position of infant; muscle tone; respiratory effort before, during, and after event; relationship to activity (eg, feeding); and intervention necessary (nothing, gentle stimulation, vigorous stimulation, resuscitation).

3. Administer theophylline, if prescribed. Observe for signs of toxicity: Apical rate above 200, vomiting, and agitation. Concentration of theophylline for apnea is lower than the concentration for bronchospasm.

4. Continue the infant's normal activities whenever possible (eg, holding him or her for feedings, playing with him or her, disconnecting from monitor for bathing); allow for continuation of usual eating or sleeping patterns. Simulating the home environment as much as possible will encourage deep-sleep patterns, which may stimulate apnea and provide valuable diagnostic information.

Minimizing Anxiety

1. Encourage parents to continue involvement in infant care during hospitalization.
2. Clarify any misconceptions about apnea and SIDS.
3. Allow ventilation of feelings and concerns.
4. Assess family dynamics for any conflicts or maladapted responses; intervene or refer as appropriate.
5. Use anticipatory guidance in preparing parents for emotional responses to home monitoring.
   a. Increased anxiety or tension
   b. Constant worry about the alarm even when it does not go off
   c. Fatigue
   d. Financial and emotional burdens encountered by the family
   e. Perceived loss of "normal, healthy child"; parents may grieve when given the diagnosis

Increasing Confidence in Home Monitoring

1. Demonstrate operation and maintenance of the monitor. Reinforce teaching by equipment supplier. Provide information on contacting a monitor technician. Teach parents proper electrode/belt placement and skin care.
2. Identify the presence of a telephone in the home and, if not, an alternative plan in the event of an emergency situation.
3. Describe how to record apnea in relation to activity and position and when to report apnea to health care provider.
4. Teach methods of responding to alarms; what to observe and document in diary (eg, color, presence or absence of breathing) and how to respond (gentle versus vigorous stimulation, CPR).

5. Discuss the necessary adjustments in daily living, and anticipated changes.
   a. Emphasize that responsibility must be shared by family members.
   b. Discuss the possible impact on siblings.
   c. Advise the parents to eliminate noises that would interfere with their ability to hear the alarm (eg, showering, vacuum cleaning). Someone must always be available to hear and respond to the alarm.
   d. Avoid traveling long distances alone with infant.
   e. Encourage the parents to enlist the assistance of a third person who is willing to learn CPR and to help care for the infant and provide the parents with an opportunity for respite time.
6. Emphasize the healthy aspects of the infant. Encourage the parents to continue as many usual routines as possible. Provide specific things parents can do to encourage normal development and a healthy parent–child relationship.
7. Encourage the parents to provide total care for their infant 24 hours before discharge so they regain confidence in caring for their child.

Family Education and Health Maintenance

1. Advise family to keep emergency numbers near telephone or set on speed dial.
2. Educate about feeding precautions: frequent burping, no bottle in bed, upright position after feeding, positioning infant on back or side, not abdomen.
3. Have parents contact local emergency service to inform them about their infant, and to be certain that they have infant resuscitation equipment. Arrange for notification of the utility company in order to plan for the event of a power outage.
4. Instruct the parents in the administration of any new medications.
5. Teach CPR to all those involved in providing care for the infant.
6. Refer family to home care agency for home nursing visits, additional teaching and support.

Outcome-Based Evaluation

- Monitoring maintained; respirations regular without apnea
- Parents verbalize concern over infant's well-being
- Parents demonstrate correct operation of respiratory monitor and response to alarms

PEDIATRIC RESPIRATORY PROCEDURES

Mechanical Ventilation

Available ventilators for pediatric use have a wide range of capabilities, versatility, and clinical application. Some are more suitable for use with infants, others with older

BOX 44-1 Sudden Infant Death Syndrome (SIDS)

SIDS is sudden, unexplained death in infancy. Typically, the infant is well when put to bed for the night or a nap and is found dead several hours later. Postmortem exam finds no real cause for death. Peak incidence is 2 weeks to 1 year of life. Fortunately, the incidence of SIDS has decreased dramatically since the American Academy of Pediatrics recommended putting all infants to sleep on their backs or sides rather than prone.

Current theories relating to the cause of SIDS include prolonged sleep apnea, chronic oxygen deficiency, and enzyme abnormalities. Although many believe that some infants with sleep apnea are at risk for SIDS, a definitive causal relationship between the two has not been established scientifically. Characteristics that may identify infants at risk for SIDS include prematurity, male gender, low birth weight/height, not breastfeeding, previous ALTE, and twin sibling of SIDS victim.

Maternal risk factors include prenatal/postnatal smoking, young maternal age (<20 years old), less prenatal care, and poverty. Approximately three fourths of all SIDS victims are not associated with a high-risk group, however.

The psychosocial devastation that occurs to the mother and family after SIDS can be alleviated through grief counseling and support groups. Parents should be reassured that it was not their fault, and siblings should be comforted that SIDS will not affect them. Refer families to organizations such as:

National Sudden Infant Death Syndrome Foundation (NSIDF)
1314 Bedford Avenue, Suite 210
Baltimore, MD 21208
1-800-638-7437
www.sidsalliance.org

New York City Information and Counselling Program for Sudden Infant Death
520 First Avenue, Room 419
New York, NY 10016
212-686-8854

children. Nurses must be well acquainted with the characteristics of the particular machine being used and the meaning of the settings and alarms on the machine.

Nursing Management

Refer to Procedure Guidelines 10-22 (p. 252). In addition, the nurse who is caring for a pediatric patient should remember the following.

Setting Controls

In setting controls, inspiratory flow rate will be less, and the respiratory rate will be greater than in the adult pa-

tient. These depend on the patient's size and condition and are determined by the health care provider or respiratory therapist.

Humidification

1. Because of their small diameters, pediatric endotracheal tubes are easily obstructed by thick secretions. Therefore, adequate humidification must be maintained to keep secretions loose.
2. During ventilation of an infant in an incubator, the amount of ventilator tubing outside the incubator should be kept to a minimum. The warm temperature inside the incubator helps decrease the amount of condensation in the tubing and thus provides higher water content in the inspired gas.

Oxygen Concentration

1. In infants, inspired concentrations of oxygen should always be kept as low as possible (while still providing for physiologic requirements) to prevent the development of retrolental fibroplasia or pulmonary O_2 toxicity.
2. The oxygen concentration should be checked periodically with an analyzer.

Blood Gases

1. The arterialized capillary sample method is inaccurate for infants in respiratory distress because the constricted peripheral circulation may not reflect the ABG accurately.
2. An umbilical artery catheter is most frequently used to obtain arterial blood samples.

Sterile Precautions

The newborn has only those antibodies transferred across the placenta from the mother. Therefore, sterile precautions are essential.

1. Ventilator tubing should be changed every 24 hours.
2. Routine cultures should be taken after intubation; there should be daily Gram's staining of secretions.
3. Suctioning requires aseptic technique.

Tubing Support

1. Special frames are available to support ventilator tubing; this helps prevent accidental decannulation in infants and small children.
2. Infants may require folded diapers or padding on either side and at the top of their heads to decrease mobility and take up space between the head and the frame.

Monitoring the Ventilator

1. Pressure gauges should be checked at frequent intervals because this gives an indication of changing compliance or increased airway resistance.
2. Volume measurements are difficult to obtain in infants because most spirometers incorporated into ventilators and meters do not read accurately at low volumes and flows. However, they are helpful with older children.
3. Measure respiratory rates of the machine and the patient at least every hour.

PROCEDURE GUIDELINES 44-1 | **OXYGEN THERAPY FOR CHILDREN**

PROCEDURE

Nursing Action | **Rationale**

1. Explain the procedure to the child and allow him or her to feel the equipment and the oxygen flowing through the tube, mask, and so forth.
2. Maintain a clear airway by suctioning, if necessary.
3. Provide a source of humidification.

4. Measure oxygen concentrations every 1–2 hours when a child is receiving oxygen through incubator hood, tent, or Croupette.
   a. Measure when the oxygen environment is closed.
   b. Measure the concentration close to the child's airway.
   c. Record oxygen concentrations and simultaneous measurements of the pulse and respirations.

5. Observe the child's response to oxygen.

6. Organize nursing care so interruption of therapy is minimal.
7. Periodically check all equipment during each tour of duty.

8. Clean equipment daily, and change it at least once each week. (Tubing and nebulizer jars should be changed daily.)
9. Keep combustible materials and potential sources of fire away from oxygen equipment.
   a. Avoid using oil or grease around oxygen connections.
   b. Do not use alcohol or oils on a child in an oxygen tent.
   c. Do not permit any electrical devices in or near an oxygen tent.
   d. Avoid the use of wool blankets and those made from some synthetic fibers because of the hazards resulting from static electricity.
   e. Prohibit smoking in areas where oxygen is being used.
   f. Have a fire extinguisher available.
10. Terminate oxygen therapy gradually.
    a. Slowly reduce liter flow.
    b. Open air vents in incubators.
    c. Open zippers or flip a section of the canopy over the top of the tent.
11. Continually monitor the child's response during weaning. Observe for restlessness, increased pulse rate, respiratory distress, cyanosis.

Rationale

1. The child will be reassured if he or she understands the procedure and knows what to expect.

2. The delivery of oxygen requires a clear airway.
3. Oxygen is a dry gas and requires the addition of moisture to prevent drying of the tracheobronchial tree and thickening and consolidating secretions.
4. It is desirable to keep the oxygen concentration as low as possible while still providing for physiologic requirements. This minimizes the danger of the child's developing retrolental fibroplasia or pulmonary oxygen toxicity. (Desired oxygen concentrations are determined by the arterial oxygen tension measurement.) The oxygen analyzer itself should be calibrated daily on both room air and 100% oxygen. The concentration of oxygen within the space is determined by the liter flow, the efficiency of the equipment, and the frequency with which it is opened to the external environment.
5. Desired response includes
   a. Decreased restlessness
   b. Decreased respiratory distress
   c. Improved color
   d. Improved vital sign values
6. Interruption of therapy may result in the return of anoxia and defeat the goals of therapy.
7. For optimal functioning, the equipment should be clean, undamaged, and in good working order.
8. Unclean equipment may be a source of contamination.

9. Oxygen supports combustion.

10. This allows the child to adjust to normal atmospheric oxygen concentrations.

11. These are indications that the child is unable to tolerate reduced oxygen concentration.

OXYGEN BY NASAL CANNULA OR CATHETER

1. Refer to Procedure Guidelines 10–14: Administering Oxygen by Nasal Canula, p. 235.
2. Nasal cannulas are available in a variety of sizes for neonates, infants, and children.
3. Low flow meters are available to titrate oxygen at levels under 1 Lpm.

continued

PROCEDURE GUIDELINES 44-1   OXYGEN THERAPY FOR CHILDREN *CONTINUED*

Nursing Action	Rationale

OXYGEN BY MASK

1. Choose an appropriate size mask that covers the mouth and nose but not the eyes.

2. Use a mask that is capable of delivering the desired oxygen concentration.

3. Place the mask over the child's mouth and nose so it fits securely. Secure the mask with an elastic head grip.

4. Remove the oxygen mask at hourly intervals; wash the face and dry.
5. Do not use masks for comatose infants or children.

6. For additional information, refer to Procedure Guidelines 10–16: Administering Oxygen by Venturi Mask (p. 238) and Procedure Guidelines 10-15: Administering Oxygen by Face Mask (p. 236).

1. Extra space under the mask and around the face is added dead space and decreases the effectiveness of the therapy.
2. Venturi masks, available for use in pediatrics, deliver low to moderate concentrations of oxygen: 24%, 28%, 35%, or 40%.
3. Make sure the mask is adjusted properly over the mouth and nose. Do not allow the oxygen to blow in child's eyes. Small pieces of cotton may be placed above the ears to help relieve pressure and discomfort caused by the head strap.
4. Makes the patient feel more comfortable.

5. Such children are more likely to vomit. The risk of aspiration may be increased with mask therapy because of obstruction of the flow of vomitus.

FACE TENT

1. Face tents are available in the adult size only. They can be used effectively in pediatric patients if inverted to create a smaller reservoir and better fit.
2. A flow of 8–10 L should be used to flush the system and provide a stable oxygen concentration.

1. Face tents combine the positive qualities of aerosol masks and mist tents. The child is accessible and may continue to play without feeling confined.
2. Larger children will require higher flows.

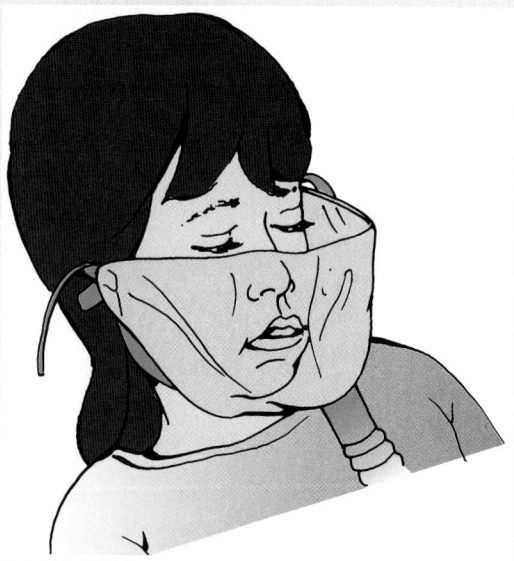

A child receiving humidity and oxygen by way of an aerosol face tent.

T-BARS AND TRACHEOSTOMY MASKS

1. These devices are used to deliver oxygen to intubated patients.
2. The flow rate must be set to meet the minute volume requirements of the child and to provide a 100% source of gas.

2. T-bars require a short, flexible tube on the distal end to act as a reservoir and prevent room-air entrapment.

PROCEDURE GUIDELINES 44-1   *CONTINUED*

Nursing Action	Rationale

OXYGEN TENT

1. Select the smallest tent and canopy that will achieve the desired concentration of oxygen and maintain patient comfort.
2. Pad the metal frame that supports the canopy.
3. Analyze and record the tent, atmosphere every 1–2 hours. Concentrations of 30%–50% can be achieved in well-maintained tents.
4. Maintain a tight-fitting canopy. Whenever possible, provide nursing care through the sleeves or pockets of the tent.

5. Make certain the crib sides are up. Check child frequently.
6. Select toys that retard absorption, are washable, and will not produce static electricity.
7. Check child's temperature routinely.

(Rationale)

1. This increases the efficiency of the unit.

2. This protects the child from injury.
3. The concentration varies with the efficiency of the tent, the rate of flow of oxygen, and the frequency with which the tent is opened to the outside environment.
4. This prevents oxygen leakage and disruption of the tent atmosphere.
   a. If the child is extremely restless or uncooperative, it may be useful to permit a parent to hold the child's hand through a small opening in the zipper of the canopy.
5. The canopy, when tucked into the mattress, often gives the illusion of a safe, confined environment.
6. The child needs toys for stimulation and diversion. They should be safe and practical.
7. Moisture accumulation may result in hypothermia.

CROUPETTE

1. This is an oxygen tent equipped with a high-humidification system (refer to procedure under "Oxygen Tent" above).
2. Change the child's clothing and bed linen when damp. Cover the child with a cotton blanket.
3. Check the child frequently.

4. If possible, remove the child from the mist periodically.

5. Promote postural drainage, and suction the child as necessary.
6. Observe the small infant for signs of overhydration.

(Rationale)

1. If the child's condition requires high humidity but not oxygen, the unit can be operated with compressed air.
2. This prevents chilling in an environment of cooled, super-saturated, aerated mist.
3. Condensation on the canopy may make it difficult to see the child.
4. This prevents maceration of the skin. Mist may be delivered through nebulizer tubing or mask during these periods.
5. Rapid mobilization of secretions may follow initiation of mist tent therapy.
6. This occasionally results from intensive use of an ultrasonic nebulizer, especially if a saline solution is nebulized. Cannot reliably maintain Fio_2 of greater than 40% to 50%.

CLOSED INCUBATOR/ISOLETTES

1. The incubator is used to provide a controlled environment for the neonate.
2. Adjust the oxygen flow to achieve the desired oxygen concentration.
   a. An oxygen limiter prevents the oxygen concentration inside the incubator from exceeding 40%.
   b. Higher concentrations (up to 85%) may be obtained by placing the red reminder flag in the vertical position.

(Rationale)

1. The unit is able to provide precise environmental control of temperature, oxygen, humidity, and isolation.
2. Refer to table below.

   a. This is desirable because it reduces the hazard of the child's developing retrolental fibroplasia.
   b. This operates by reducing the air intake.

Incubator Oxygen Therapy

Red Flag in Horizontal Position		Red Flag in Vertical Position	
Flow of Oxygen (L/min)	Concentration of Oxygen (%)	Flow of Oxygen (L/min)	Concentration of Oxygen (%)
4	28–31	4	Flow not sufficient for high concentration
6	32–36	8	70–75
8	37–40	10	75–80
		12	80–85

(From Lough, M. D., & Doershuk, C.F. [1995]. Oxygen therapy. In M. D. Lough, C. F. Doershuk, & R. C. Stern [Eds.] *Pediatric respiratory therapy.* Chicago, IL: Year Book Medical Pub. Used with permission.)

continued

Nursing Action	Rationale
3. Secure a nebulizer to the inside wall of the incubator if mist therapy is desired.	3. This should be cleaned and autoclaved daily. Sterile solutions are used to keep the bacteria count at a minimum.
4. Keep sleeves of incubator closed to prevent loss of oxygen.	4. When incubator or sleeves are opened, supply supplemental oxygen with oxygen mask to face and nose.
5. Periodically analyze the incubator atmosphere.	5. Be certain the child is receiving the desired concentration of oxygen.
6. Drain and fill reservoirs with sterile water at least every 24 hours.	6. To decrease risk of *Pseudomonas* contamination.

OXYGEN HOOD

Nursing Action	Rationale
1. Warmed, humidified oxygen is supplied through a plastic container that fits over the child's head.	1. This is especially useful when high concentrations of oxygen are desired. The hood may be used in an incubator or with a warming unit. Oxygen should not be allowed to blow directly into the infant's face.

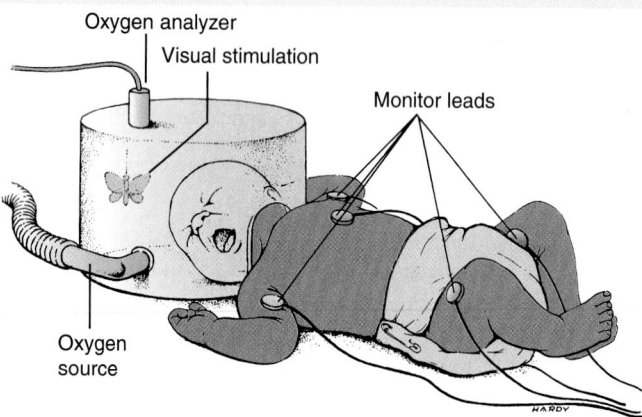

Oxygen hood.

Nursing Action	Rationale
2. Continuously monitor the oxygen concentration, temperature, and humidity inside the hood.	2. Oxygen should be warmed to 31°–34°C. (87.8°–93.2°F) to prevent a neonatal response to cold stress, including oxygen deprivation, metabolic acidosis, rapid depletion of glycogen stores, and reduction of blood glucose levels.
3. Open the hood or remove the baby from it as infrequently as possible.	3. This prevents fluctuations of heat and oxygen, which may further debilitate the young infant.
4. Several different designs are available for use. The manufacturer's directions should be carefully followed.	4. This is a safety consideration.

PROCEDURE GUIDELINES 44-2   PROMOTING POSTURAL DRAINAGE IN THE PEDIATRIC PATIENT

Postural drainage is the positioning of the patient so gravity will assist in the movement of secretions from the smaller bronchial airways to the main bronchus and trachea, from which the secretions can be removed by coughing or suctioning.

PROCEDURE

Nursing Action	Rationale
PREPARATORY PHASE	

1. Assess the child's respiratory status.
    a. Obtain a baseline respiratory rate.
    b. Observe for respiratory distress, retractions, nasal flaring, and so forth.
	1. This is necessary to evaluate the effectiveness of the therapy.

2. Identify the involved portion(s) of the lung by auscultation, percussion, or review of the x-ray report (see Figure 44-5).	2. The positions selected for drainage will depend on what portion of the lung is involved.

Nursing Action	**Rationale**

3. Explain the procedure to the child or the parent.

    3. This allays anxiety and helps to secure the child's cooperation.

4. Make the child comfortable.
   a. Remove constricting clothes.
   b. Flex the child's knees and hips.

       b. To assist in relaxing and decreasing strain on the abdominal muscles during coughing.

   c. Have tissues and an emesis basin available.
   d. Have several pillows available.

       c. To collect mucus.
       d. To facilitate positioning.

5. Provide bronchodilator or nebulization therapy before the procedure if indicated.

    5. It is easier to raise mucus mechanically after the bronchi are dilated and the secretions are thinned.

PERFORMANCE PHASE

1. Place the child in a series of appropriate positions.
   a. The area to be drained should be elevated and its respective bronchus placed in a vertical position.
   b. The spine should be as straight as possible to permit optimal expansion of the rib cage.

    1. The positions are selected and modified according to the lung area involved, the child's age and general condition, and equipment such as IV, tracheostomies, monitors, ventilators.
       b. Infants are positioned on the nurse's lap, in the isolette, or in the crib; older children may be treated on a tilt board or in bed.

2. Unless contraindicated, cup the chest wall for 1–2 minutes.

    2. More secretions can be raised in a shorter period of time when cupping and vibration are added to posturing.

3. Have the child inhale deeply; then, as he exhales, vibrate the chest wall during three to five exhalations.
4. Encourage the child to cough.
5. Allow the child to rest for a minute, then repeat cupping, vibration, and coughing until no more mucus is produced or the child's condition indicates that the procedure should be stopped.

    4. Infants and young children may require suctioning.
    5. Total treatment time should generally not exceed 20–30 minutes.
       a. In acute conditions such as atelectasis, postural drainage may be done for 5 minutes of every hour.
       b. In chronic conditions such as cystic fibrosis, postural drainage may be done two to five times per day for 15–30 minutes.

 NURSING ALERT

Do not place very-low-birth-weight infants in Trendelenburg's position.

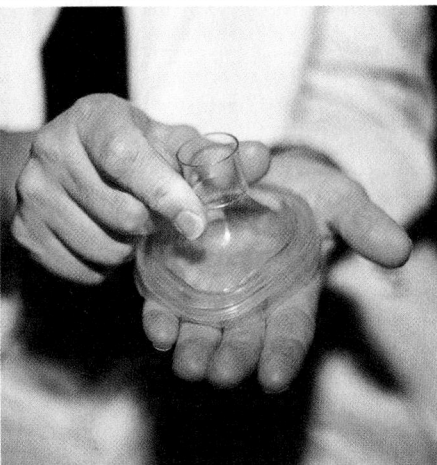

To assist with percussing an infant or small child, an alternative percussion device may be used, such as a mask from a manual resuscitation bag.

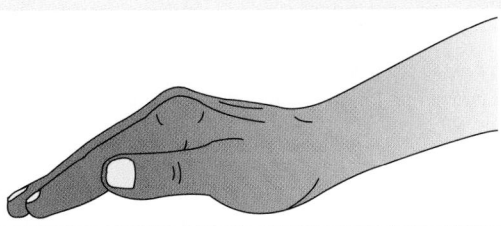

Cupping the chest.

 NURSING ALERT

Postural drainage should not be done immediately after meals because it may induce vomiting.

6. Provide for patient safety.

    6. Stay with the child during the procedure, especially when he or she is in a head-down position.

SELECTED REFERENCES

American Academy of Pediatrics, Committee on Children with Disabilities. (1995). Guidelines for home care of infants, children, and adolescents with chronic disease. *Pediatrics, 99*(1), 161–164.

American Academy of Pediatrics, Committee on Infectious Diseases. (1996). Reassessment of the indications for ribavirin therapy in respiratory syncytial virus infections. *Pediatrics, 97*(1), 137–140.

American Academy of Pediatrics, Committee on Infectious Diseases and Committee on Fetus and Newborn. (1997). Respiratory syncytial virus immune globulin intravenous: Indications for use. *Pediatrics, 99*(4), 645–650.

American Academy of Pediatrics, Committee on Pediatric AIDS. (1997). Evaluation and medical treatment of HIV-exposed infant. *Pediatrics, 99*(6), 909–917.

Armitage, J. M., Kurland, G., Michaels, M., et al. (1995). Critical issues in pediatric lung transplantation. *Journal of Thoracic and Cardiovascular Surgery, 109*(1), 60–64.

Avila, P. C. (1998). Differential diagnosis of wheezing in children. *Lippincott's Primary Care Practice, 2*(6), 559–577.

Behrman, R., Kliegman, R., & Arvin, A. (Eds.). (1996). *Nelson's textbook of pediatrics* (15th ed.). Philadelphia: W. B. Saunders.

Chernick, V., & Boat, T. (Eds.). (1998). *Kendig's disorders of the respiratory tract in children* (6th ed.). Philadelphia: W. B. Saunders.

Coakley, A. (2000). Leukotrienes: New therapies and their influence in asthma. *British Journal of Nursing, 9*(12), 741–781.

Conway, S. P. (1998). Transition from pediatric to adult orientated care for adolescents with cystic fibrosis. *Disabilities and Rehabilitation, 20*(6–7), 209–216.

Couetil, J. P., Tolan, M. J., et al. (1997). Pulmonary bipartitioning and lobar transplantation: A new approach to donor organ shortage. *Journal of Thoracic and Cardiovascular Surgery, 113*(3), 529–537.

Coune, I. T. (1997). Chronic illness: The importance of support for families caring for a child with cystic fibrosis. *Journal of Clinical Nursing, 6*(2), 121–129.

Czarnecki, M., & Kaucic, C. (1999). Infant nasal-pharyngeal suctioning: Is it beneficial? *Pediatric Nursing, 25*(2), 193–196.

Deutsch, E. S. (1996). Tonsillectomy and adenoidectomy. Changing indications. *Pediatric Clinics of North America, 43*(6), 1319–1338.

Driver, L., & Oertel, M. (1999). Synagis: An anti-RSV monoclonal antibody. *Pediatric Nursing, 25*(5), 527–530.

Egan, T. M., & Detterbeck, F. C. (1998). Lung transplantation for cystic fibrosis: Effective and durable therapy in a high risk group. *Annals of Thoracic Surgery, 66*(2), 337–346.

Friedrich. B. (2000). Pediatric asthma: A clinical management update. *Journal of Pediatric Nursing, 15*(3), 189–190.

Gries, D., Moffit, D., Pulos, E., & Carter, E. (2000). A single dose of intramuscularly administered dexamethasone acetate is as effective as oral prednisone to treat asthma exacerbations in young children. *Journal of Pediatrics, 136*(3), 298–302.

Groothuis, J. R., et al. (1995). Respiratory syncytial virus infection in preterm infants and the protective effects of RSV immune globulin (RSVIG): Respiratory Syncytial Virus Immune Globulin Study Group. *Pediatrics, 95*(4), 467–476.

Hazinski, M. F. (Ed.). (1992). *Nursing care of the critically ill child* (2nd ed.). Philadelphia: Mosby–Year Book.

Henskens, J., & Von Nessen, S. (2000). *Burkholderia cepacia* in cystic fibrosis: Implications for nursing practice. *Pediatric Nursing, 26*(3), 325–327.

The Impact RSV Study Group. (1998). Palivizumab, a humanized respiratory syncytial virus monoclonal antibody, reduces hospitalization from respiratory syncytial virus infection in high risk infants. *Pediatrics, 122*(3), 531–537.

Johnson, C. A., Butler, S. M, Konstan, M. W., et al. (1999). Estimating effectiveness in an observational study: A case study of doe-

nase alfa in cystic fibrosis. The investigators and coordinators of the Epidemiologic Study of Cystic Fibrosis. *Journal of Pediatrics, 134*(6), 734–739.

Johnson, D. W., Jacobson, S., et al. (1998). A comparison of nebulized beudesonide, intramuscular dexamethasone, and placebo for moderately severe croup. *New England Journal of Medicine, 339*(8), 498–503.

Leversha, A., Campanella, S., Arckin R., & Asher, M. (2000). Costs and effectiveness of spacer versus nebulizer in young children with moderate and severe acute asthma. *Journal of Pediatrics, 136*(4), 497–502.

McNamara, F., & Sullivan, C. (2000). Obstructive sleep apnea in infants: Relation to family history of sudden infant death syndrome, apparent life threatening events, and obstructive sleep apnea. *Journal of Pediatrics, 136*(3), 318–323.

McNaughton, S., Shepherd, R., et al. (2000). Nutritional status of children with cystic fibrosis measured by total body potassium as a marker of body cell mass: Lack of sensitivity of anthropometric measure. *Journal of Pediatrics, 136*(2), 188–194.

Melnyk, B. (1999). Building a case for evidence-based practice: Inhalers vs. nebulizers. *Pediatric Nursing, 25*(1), 102–103.

National Heart, Lung, and Blood Institute. (1997). *Highlights of the Expert Panel Report 2. Guidelines for the diagnoses and management of asthma.* Publication No. 97-4051A. Washington, DC: US Department of Health and Human Services.

———. (1997). *Practical guide for the diagnosis and management of asthma.* Publication No. 97-4053. Washington, DC: US Department of Health and Human Services.

———. (1995). *Nurses: Partners in asthma care.* Publication No. 95-3308. Washington, DC: US Department of Health and Human Services.

———. (1991). *Executive summary: Guidelines for the diagnoses and management of asthma.* Publication No. 91-304A. Washington, DC: US Department of Health and Human Services.

Nield, T., Langenbacher, D. et al. (2000). Neurodevelopmental outcome 3.5 years of age in children teated with extracorporeal life support: Relationship to primary diagnosis. *Journal of Pediatrics, 136*(3), 338–344.

Peter, G. (Ed.). (1997). *Red Book: Report of the Committee on Infectious Diseases* (24th ed.). Elk Grove Village, IL: American Academy of Pediatrics.

Rizos, J. D., DiGravio, B. E., et al. (1998). The disposition of children with croup treated with racemic epinephrine and dexamethasone in the emergency department. *Journal of Emergency Medicine, 12*(4), 535–539.

Robinson, W. M., Ravilly, S., Berde, C., & Whole, M. E. (1997). End of life care in cystic fibrosis. *Pediatrics, 100*(2), 205–209.

Schneiderman-Walker, J., Pollock, S., et al. (2000). A randomized controlled trial of 3-year home exercise program in cystic fibrosis. *Journal of Pediatrics, 136*(3), 304–310.

Sitzman, S. J., & Fiechtner, H. B. (1998). Treatment of croup with glucocorticoids. *Annals of Pharmacotheraputics, 32*(9), 973–974.

Tan, T., Mason, E., & Barson, W. (1998). Clinical characteristics and outcome of children with pneumonia attributable to penicillin susceptible and penicillin nonsusceptible *Streptococcus pneumoniae*. *Pediatrics, 102*(6), 1369–1375.

Taussig, L., & Landau, L. (Eds.). (1999). *Pediatric respiratory medicine.* St. Louis: Mosby.

Wang, E., Law, B., et al. (1999). Pediatric investigators collaborative network on infections in Canada. Study of the role of age, and respiratory syncytial virus illness in patients with underlying heart disease. *Pediatrics, 99*(e9).

Whaley, L., & Wong, D. (1999). *Nursing care of infants and children* (6th ed.). St. Louis: Mosby–Year Book.

Pediatric Cardiovascular Disorders

CONGENITAL HEART DISEASE

Congenital heart disease (or defects) (CHD) are uncommon. They involve all chambers, valves, and great vessels arising from the heart (Figure 45-1). Box 45-1 presents a list of abbreviations that describe CHD.

In most cases, the cause of CHD is not known. Some infants and children with CHD may appear perfectly healthy, whereas others may be critically ill. Most infants and children with CHD can be successfully managed with medications and surgeries.

Etiology and Incidence

1. Congenital heart disease (CHD) affects 8 of every 1,000 newborns.
2. Exact cause of CHD is unknown in 90% of cases.
3. The heart begins as a single cell and develops into a four-chambered pumping system during the third to eighth weeks of gestation.
4. Associated factors for CHD include:
   a. Fetal or maternal infection during the first trimester (rubella).
   b. Chromosomal abnormalities (Trisomy 21, 18, 13).
   c. Maternal insulin-dependent diabetes.
   d. Teratogenic effects of drugs and alcohol.
5. Syndromes with associated CHD:
   a. Marfan's syndrome: mitral valve prolapse, dilated aortic root.
   b. Turner's syndrome: aortic valve stenosis, coarctation of the aorta.
   c. Noonan's syndrome: dysplastic pulmonary valve.
   d. William's syndrome: supravalve stenosis.
   e. DiGeorge syndrome: interrupted aortic arch (IAA), truncus arteriosis, transposition of great arteries (TGA), tetralogy of Fallot (TOF).

Common Congenital Heart Malformations

Congenital heart defects can be classified into three categories: obstruction to blood flow, increased pulmonary blood flow (acyanotic lesions), and decreased pulmonary blood flow (cyanotic lesions).

1. Obstructive lesions:
   a. Aortic valve stenosis.
   b. Coarctation of the aorta.
   c. Pulmonary valve stenosis.
2. Increased pulmonary blood flow (acyanotic):
   a. Patent ductus arteriosis (PDA).
   b. Atrial septal defect (ASD).
   c. Ventricular septal defect (VSD).
   d. Atrioventricular canal (AVC).
3. Decreased pulmonary blood flow (cyanotic):
   a. Tetralogy of Fallot (TOF).
   b. Tricuspid atresia (TA).
   c. Total anomalous pulmonary venous return (TAPVR).
   d. Transposition of great arteries.
   e. Truncus arteriosis.
   f. Hypoplastic left heart syndrome (HLHS).

◼ Aortic Valve Stenosis

Congenital aortic valve stenosis may be caused by a bicuspid aortic valve with fused commissures that does not open completely, or by a hypoplastic aortic valve annulus. The result is turbulent blood flow across the aortic valve and into the ascending aorta. Patients with abnormal aortic valves must be evaluated for additional left heart obstructive lesions that include subaortic stenosis, coarctation of the aorta, and mitral valve stenosis.

Aortic valve stenosis is the most common form of left ventricular outflow tract obstruction. Aortic valve stenosis may occur at any age, and it occurs more often in boys than in girls. In most children, it is a progressive lesion that creates left ventricular outflow tract obstruction (LVOTO).

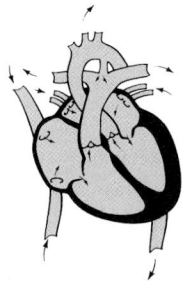

Patent Ductus Arteriosus (PDA)

The PDA is a vascular connection that, during fetal life, short circuits the pulmonary vascular bed and directs blood from the pulmonary artery to the aorta. Functional closure of the ductus normally occurs soon after birth. If the ductus remains patent after birth, the direction of blood flow in the ductus is reversed by the higher pressure in the aorta.

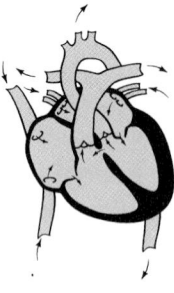

Ventricular Septal Defect (VSD)

A VSD is an abnormal opening between the right and left ventricle. VSDs vary in size and may occur in either the membranous or muscular portion of the ventricular septum. Due to higher pressure in the left ventricle, a shunting of blood from the left to right ventricle occurs during systole. If pulmonary vascular resistance produces pulmonary hypertension, the shunt of blood is then reversed from the right to the left ventricle, with cyanosis resulting.

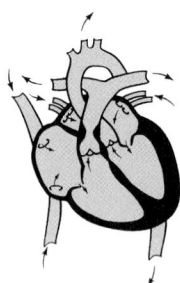

Pulmonary Stenosis

Pulmonary stenosis refers to any lesion that obstructs the blood flow from the right ventricle to the pulmonary artery. The right ventricular pressure increases and can cause right ventricular hypertrophy and eventual right-sided heart failure.

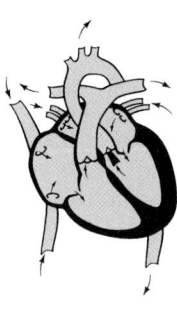

Subaortic Stenosis

In many instances, the stenosis is valvular with thickening and fusion of the cusps. Subaortic stenosis is caused by a fibrous ring below the aortic valve in the outflow tract of the left ventricle. At times, both valvular and subaortic stenosis exist in combination. The obstruction presents an increase workload for the normal output of the left ventricular blood and results in left ventricular enlargement.

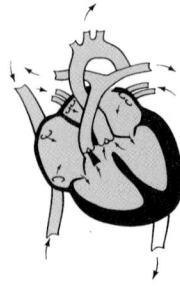

Tetralogy of Fallot

Tetralogy of Fallot is characterized by the combination of four defects: 1) pulmonary stenosis, 2) ventricular septal defects, 3) overriding aorta, 4) hypertrophy of right ventricle. It is the most common defect causing cyanosis in patients surviving beyond 2 years of age. The severity of symptoms depends on the degree of pulmonary stenosis, the size of the ventricular septal defect, and the degree to which the aorta overrides the septal defect.

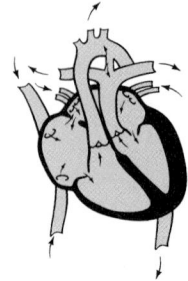

Complete Transposition of Great Vessels

This anomaly is an embryologic defect caused by a straight division of the bulbar trunk without normal spiraling. As a result, the aorta originates from the right ventricle and the pulmonary artery from the left ventricle. An abnormal communication between the two circulations must be present to sustain life.

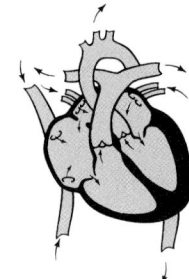

Atrial Septal Defects (ASD)

An ASD is an abnormal opening between the right and left atria. Basically, three types of abnormalities result from incorrect development of the atrial septum. An incompetent foramen ovale is the most common defect. The high ostium secundum defect results from abnormal development of the septum secundum. Improper development of the septum primum produces a basal opening known as an ostium primum defect, frequently involving the atrioventricular valves. In general, left-to-right shunting of blood occurs in all ASDs.

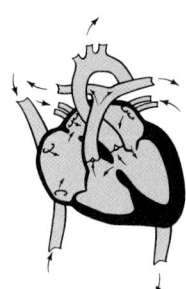

Tricuspid Atresia

Tricuspid valvular atresia is characterized by a small right ventricle, large left ventricle, and usually a diminished pulmonary circulation. Blood from the right atrium passes through an ASD into the left atrium, mixes with oxygenated blood returning from the lungs, flows into the left ventricle, and is propelled into the systemic circulation. The lungs may receive blood through one of three routes: 1) an VSD, 2) PDA, 3) bronchial vessels.

FIGURE 45-1 Congenital heart abnormalities.

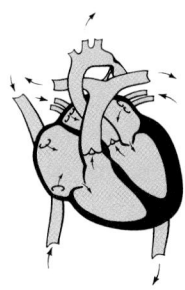

Coarctation of the Aorta
Coarctation of the aorta is characterized by a narrowed aortic lumen. It exists as a preductal or postductal obstruction, depending on the position of the obstruction in relation to the ductus arteriosus. Coarctations exist with great variation in anatomic features. The lesion produces an obstruction to the flow of blood through the aorta causing an increased left ventricular pressure and workload.

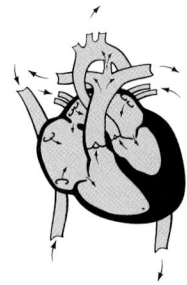

Hypoplastic Left Heart
A collection of complex congenital heart lesions results in the abnormal development of the left side of the heart. The right ventricle pumps blood through the pulmonary and systemic circulations. A patent foramen ovale allows a left-to-right shunt, and blood is shunted from left atrium back to right atrium. A PDA is the sole supply of blood to the system.

FIGURE 45-1 (Continued)

Pathophysiology and Etiology

1. Blood flows at an increased velocity across the obstructive valve and into the aorta.
2. During systole, left ventricular pressure rises dramatically to overcome the increased resistance at the aortic valve.
3. Myocardial ischemia may occur because of an imbalance between the increased oxygen requirements related to the hypertrophied left ventricle (LV) and the amount of oxygen that can be supplied.
4. Left ventricular failure results in an increased LV end diastolic pressure that is reflected back to the left atrium and pulmonary veins.

Clinical Manifestations

Newborn with Critical Aortic Stenosis

1. Severe congestive heart failure (CHF).
2. Metabolic acidosis.
3. Tachypnea.
4. Faint peripheral pulses, poor perfusion, poor capillary refill, cool skin.
5. Poor feeding.

BOX 45-1 Abbreviations Used for Congenital Heart Disease (CHD)

AoS	Aortic stenosis
ASD	Atrial septal defect
AV canal	Atrioventricular canal
CHF	Congestive heart failure (also known as heart failure)
CoA	Coarctation of the aorta
HLHS	Hypoplastic left heart syndrome
IAA	Interrupted aortic arch
PA	Pulmonary artery
PDA	Patent ductus arteriosus
PS	Pulmonary stenosis
PVR	Pulmonary vascular resistance
TA	Tricuspid atresia
TAPVR	Total anomalous pulmonary venous return
TGA	Transposition of great arteries
TOF	Tetralogy of Fallot
VSD	Ventricular septal defect

Child and Adolescent

1. Chest pain on exertion, decreased exercise tolerance.
2. Dyspnea, fatigue, shortness of breath.
3. Syncope, lightheadedness.
4. Palpitations.
5. Sudden death.

Diagnostic Evaluation

1. Auscultation.
   a. Systolic ejection murmur heard best at right upper sternal border, radiates to neck.
   b. Ejection click.
   c. Single S2.
2. ECG: left ventricular hypertrophy (LVH).
3. Chest x-ray (CXR): increased cardiac silhouette, increased pulmonary vascular markings.
4. Echocardiogram: two-dimensional echocardiogram with Doppler study and color flow mapping to visualize the anatomy and to estimate the gradient across the valve.

Management

The Neonate

1. Stabilize with prostaglandin E_1 (PGE$_1$) infusion to maintain cardiac output through the PDA.
2. Inotropic support as needed.
3. Intubation and ventilation as needed.
4. Cardiac catheterization → aortic balloon valvuloplasty.
5. Surgical valvotomy.

The Child and Adolescent

1. Medical management with close follow-up to monitor increasing gradient across the aortic valve.
2. Restrict intense exercise and anaerobic exercise (eg, weight lifting).
3. Aortic balloon valvuloplasty
4. Surgical intervention.
   a. Valvotomy.
   b. Aortic valve replacement.
      (i) Mechanical prosthesis (St. Jude valve).
      (ii) Ross procedure (pulmonary autograft).

Complications
1. Congestive heart failure and pulmonary edema.
2. Dizziness, light-headedness, and/or syncope.
3. Palpitations, arrhythmias.
4. Bacterial endocarditis.
5. Sudden death.

■ Coarctation of the Aorta

Coarctation of the aorta is a discrete narrowing or a long segment hypoplasia of the aortic arch, usually distal to the left subclavian artery.

Pathophysiology and Etiology
1. The discrete narrowing or hypoplastic segment of the aorta increases the workload of the left ventricle (increased LV systolic pressure).
2. In a newborn with critical coarctation of the aorta, the lower body blood flow pattern is: right ventricle (RV) → PA → PDA → Ao.
3. In the older child, collateral vessels grow and bypass the coarctation to perfuse the lower body.

Clinical Manifestation
1. The newborn with critical coarctation of the aorta (ductal dependent lesion):
   a. Asymptomatic until the patent ductus arteriosis begins to close.
   b. After PDA closure: severe CHF, poor perfusion, tachypnea, acidosis, absent femoral pulses.
2. The child or adolescent with CoA:
   a. Usually asymptomatic—normal growth and development.
   b. Hypertension in the upper extremities, with absent or weak femoral pulses.
   c. Nosebleeds, headache, leg cramps.

Diagnostic Evaluation
1. Auscultation—varies; nonspecific systolic murmur.
2. CXR—varies.
3. ECG—varies; normal or left and right ventricle hypertrophy.
4. Two-dimensional echocardiogram with Doppler study and color flow mapping identifies area of aortic arch narrowing and associated lesions (bicuspid aortic valve, VSD, PDA).
5. Magnetic resonance angiography (MRA).
6. Invasive studies (cardiac catheterization) usually not needed to make the initial diagnosis; may need aortic angiography to identify collateral vessels before surgery.

Management
Critical Coarctation in the Neonate
1. Medical management.
   a. Resuscitation and stabilization with PGE$_1$ infusion (0.025–0.05 mcg/kg/min); monitor for complications related to PGE$_1$ therapy (fever, apnea).
   b. Intubation and ventilation as needed.
   c. Assess renal, hepatic, and neurologic function.
   d. Refer for surgical intervention.
2. Surgical intervention: usually performed as soon as the diagnosis is made.
   a. Subclavian flap repair (Waldhausen procedure).
   b. End-to-end anastomosis.

Coarctation in the Child or Adolescent
1. Surgical intervention.
   a. End-to-end anastomosis.
   b. Dacron patch.
2. Medical management for hypertension (beta blockers).

Recurrent Coarctation in the Newborn or Child
1. Balloon angioplasty.
2. Redo surgical intervention.

Complications
1. Hypertension.
2. CHF.
3. Cerebral hemorrhage.
4. Endocarditis.

■ Pulmonary Valve Stenosis

The pulmonary valve opens during systole to let blood flow from the right ventricle into the main pulmonary artery. Obstruction to flow can occur at three levels: subvalvular, valve, and/or supravalvular level. The most common cause of RV outflow tract obstruction is pulmonary valve stenosis.

Pathophysiology and Etiology
1. Critical pulmonary stenosis (PS) in the newborn: blood flows into the right atrium, across a patent foramen ovale into the left heart; pulmonary blood flow comes from a left-to-right shunt through a patent ductus arteriosis.
2. Right ventricular pressure increases to pump blood across the obstructive pulmonary valve.
3. Right ventricular hypertrophy develops in response to the increased pressure gradient across the pulmonary valve.
4. Signs of right-sided heart failure include hepatic congestion, neck vein distention, elevated central venous pressure (CVP).

Clinical Manifestations
Critical PS in the Newborn
1. Hypoxia.
2. RV failure.

Mild to Moderate PS in the Child and Adolescent
1. Asymptomatic.
2. Decreased exercise tolerance, fatigue, dyspnea.
3. Chest pain.

Diagnostic Evaluation
1. Auscultation: systolic ejection murmur heard best at the left upper sternal border; ejection click.
2. ECG: right ventricular hypertrophy.

3. CXR: varies; may show right ventricular enlargement; post-stenotic dilation of pulmonary artery.
4. Two-dimensional echocardiography with Doppler study and color flow mapping to visualize the site(s) of obstruction, observe the degree of RV hypertrophy, and estimate the pressure gradient across the valve.
5. Cardiac catheterization is usually not needed for the initial diagnosis.

Management
Newborn with Critical PS
1. Medical management:
   a. Stabilize and improve oxygen saturations with PGE$_1$ infusion.
   b. Intubation and ventilation as needed.
   c. Inotropic support as needed.
2. Intervention:
   a. Pulmonary balloon valvuloplasty.
   b. Blalock-Taussig shunt.

Child and Adolescent with PS
1. Medical management:
   a. Monitor and record RV to PA gradient; assess RV function.
   b. Assess exercise tolerance.
   c. Bacterial endocarditis precautions.
   d. Refer for intervention when RV pressure is greater than two-thirds of the systemic pressures.
2. Intervention:
   a. Balloon pulmonary valvuloplasty in the cardiac catheterization laboratory.
   b. Surgical valvotomy or partial valvectomy for dysplastic pulmonary valve.

Complications
1. Cyanosis (critical PS in the newborn).
2. Arrhythmia; sudden death.
3. CHF.

■ Patent Ductus Arteriosus

The ductus arteriosus is a normal fetal connection between the pulmonary artery and the aorta. During fetal life, blood flow is shunted away from the lungs through the PDA and directly into the systemic circulation. PDAs are common in premature infants who weigh less than 1,500 grams.

Pathophysiology and Etiology
1. During fetal life, the ductus arteriosus allows blood to bypass the pulmonary circulation (fetus receives oxygen from the placenta) and flow directly into the systemic circulation.
2. After birth, the ductus arteriosus is no longer needed. The PDA usually closes in the first few days of life.
3. When the ductus arteriosus fails to close, blood from the aorta (high pressure) flows into the low-pressure pulmonary artery, resulting in pulmonary overcirculation.
4. Increased pulmonary blood flow leads to a volume-loaded LV.

Clinical Presentation
Small to Moderate-Size PDA
Usually asymptomatic.
Large PDA
1. CHF, tachypnea.
2. Poor weight gain, failure to thrive.
3. Feeding difficulties.
4. Decreased exercise tolerance.

Diagnostic Evaluation
1. Auscultation: continuous murmur heard best at left upper sternal border.
2. Wide pulse pressure; bounding pulses.
3. CXR: varies; normal or cardiomegaly with increased pulmonary vascular markings.
4. ECG: varies or left atrial dilation and left ventricular hypertrophy.
5. Two-dimensional echocardiogram with Doppler study and color flow mapping to visualize the PDA with left-to-right blood flow.
6. Cardiac catheterization is not needed for the initial diagnosis.

Treatment
1. In the symptomatic premature neonate: indomethacin (0.1 to 0.25 mg/kg/dose intravenous [IV] over 30 minutes every 12 to 24 hours up to a total of three doses.)
2. Medical management:
   a. Monitor growth and development.
   b. Reassess for spontaneous PDA closure.
   c. Increase caloric intake as needed for normal weight gain.
   d. Diuretics: furosemide (Lasix), spironolactone (Aldactone).
   e. Cardiac catheterization → for small PDAs: coil occlude; for larger PDAs a closure device may be used.
3. Surgical management:
   PDA ligation via a lateral thoracotomy (closed heart procedure).

Complications
1. CHF, pulmonary edema.
2. Bacterial endocarditis.
3. Pulmonary hypertension/pulmonary vascular occlusive disease.

■ Atrial Septal Defect

An atrial septal defect (ASD) is an abnormal communication between the left and right atrias. ASDs account for 9% of congenital heart defects. There are three types:
1. Ostium secundum ASD: the most common type of ASD; abnormal opening in the middle of the atrial septum.
2. Ostium primum ASD: abnormal opening at the bottom of the atrial septum; increased association with cleft mitral valve and atrioventricular defects.
3. Sinus venosus ASD: abnormal opening at the top of the atrial septum; increased association with partial anomalous pulmonary venous return.

Pathophysiology and Etiology

1. Blood flows from the higher-pressure left atrium across the ASD into the lower-pressure right atrium (left to right shunt).
2. Increased blood return to the right heart leads to right ventricular volume overload and right ventricular dilation.
3. Increased pulmonary blood flow leads to elevated PA pressures.

Complications

1. CHF (rare).
2. Bacterial endocarditis.
3. Embolic CVA.
4. Pulmonary hypertension.

Clinical Manifestations

1. Ostium secundum and sinus venous ASDs—usually asymptomatic
2. Ostium primum ASD—clinical symptoms vary depending on type of associated defects
   a. CHF.
   b. Frequent URIs.
   c. Poor weight gain.
   d. Decreased exercise tolerance.

Diagnostic Evaluation

1. Auscultation: ostium secundum ASD—soft systolic flow murmur heard best at the left upper sternal border; widely split, fixed second heart sound; ostium primum ASD—systolic murmur heard best at the lower left sternal border because of mitral regurgitation.
2. CXR: varies; normal to right atrial and ventricular dilation, increased pulmonary markings.
3. ECG: ostium secundum ASD—right ventricular volume load; incomplete right bundle branch block (RBBB); ostium primum—superior axis.
4. Two-dimensional echocardiogram with Doppler study and color flow mapping to identify the site of the atrial septal defect and associated lesions and document left to right flow across the atrial septum.
5. Cardiac catheterization usually not needed for initial diagnosis.

Treatment

Ostium Secundum ASD

1. Monitor and reassess: small spontaneous closure rate (up to age 2).
2. Medical management: usually none.
3. Refer for surgical closure in early childhood to protect future cardiovascular health.
   a. Primary repair: suture closure of the ASD.
   b. Pericardial patch repair of the ASD.

Ostium Primum ASD

1. Monitor growth and development.
2. Medical management: CHF.
3. Refer for surgical closure: timing of repair dependent on associated lesions and degree of CHF.

Sinus Venosus ASD

1. Medical management: usually none.
2. Refer for surgical closure in early childhood.

▪ Ventricular Septal Defect

A ventricular septal defect is an abnormal communication between the right and left ventricles. It is the most common type of congenital heart defect, accounting for approximately 25% of all CHDs. VSDs vary in the size (small and restrictive to large and nonrestrictive defect), number (single versus multiple), and type (perimembranous or muscular).

Pathophysiology and Etiology

1. Blood flows from the high-pressure left ventricle across the VSD into the low-pressure right ventricle and into the pulmonary artery, resulting in pulmonary over-circulation.
2. A left-to-right shunt because of a VSD results in increased right ventricular pressure and increased pulmonary artery pressure.
3. The increased pulmonary venous return to the left side of the heart results in left atrial dilation.
4. Long-standing pulmonary overcirculation causes a change in the pulmonary arterial bed, leading to increased pulmonary vascular resistance. High pulmonary vascular resistance (PVR) can reverse the blood flow pattern that leads to a right-to-left shunt across the VSD (Eisenmenger's syndrome), resulting in cyanosis. Once this develops, the child is no longer a candidate for surgical repair.

Clinical Manifestations

1. Small VSDs—usually asymptomatic; high spontaneous rate during the first year of life.
2. Large VSDs.
   a. Tachypnea, tachycardia, excessive sweating associated with feeding, hepatomegaly.
   b. Frequent upper respiratory infections.
   c. Poor weight gain, failure to thrive.
   d. Feeding difficulties.

Diagnostic Evaluation

1. Auscultation: grade III-IV/VI harsh systolic murmur heard best at the lower left sternal border; increased PVR associated with loud second heart sound (P2); S3 (gallop).
2. CXR: varies; normal cardiac silhouette to cardiomegaly and increased pulmonary vascular markings.
3. ECG: varies; normal to biventricular hypertrophy.
4. Two-dimensional echocardiogram with Doppler study and color flow mapping to identify the size, number, and site of the defect(s), estimate PA pressure, and identify associated lesions.
5. Cardiac catheterization usually not needed for initial diagnosis; may be needed to calculate the size of the shunt and/or to assess pulmonary vascular resistance.

Treatment

Small VSD

1. Usually no medical management is needed.
2. Surgical repair indicated for cardiac catheterization results showing Qp:Qs >2.0.
3. Bacterial endocarditis precautions.

Large VSD

1. CHF management: digoxin and diuretics (furosemide, spironolactone) and afterload reduction.
2. Avoid oxygen; oxygen is a potent pulmonary vasodilator and will increase blood flow into the pulmonary artery.
3. Increase caloric intake: fortify formula or breast milk to make 24 to 30 cal/oz formula; supplemental nasogastric feeds as needed.
4. Refer for surgical intervention.
   a. Usually repaired before first year of life.
   b. One-stage approach: preferred surgical plan; patch closure of VSD (open heart).
   c. Two-stage approach: first surgery is to band the pulmonary artery (closed heart) to restrict pulmonary blood flow; second surgery is to patch close the VSD and remove the PA band.

Long-Term Follow-Up

1. Monitor ventricular function.
2. Monitor for subaortic membrane and double-chamber RV.

Complications

1. CHF.
2. Frequent upper respiratory infections (URIs).
3. Failure to thrive; poor weight gain.
4. Bacterial endocarditis.
5. Eisenmenger's syndrome.

Tetralogy of Fallot

Tetralogy of Fallot (TOF) is the most common complex congenital heart defect; it accounts for 6% to 10% of all CHDs. The four abnormalities of TOF include the following:

1. A large, nonrestrictive VSD
2. Aortic override
3. Right ventricular outflow tract obstruction
4. Right ventricular hypertrophy

Pathophysiology and Etiology

1. Degree of cyanosis depends on the size of the VSD and the degree of right ventricular outflow tract obstruction (RVOTO).
2. Obstruction of blood flow from the right ventricle to the pulmonary artery results in deoxygenated blood being shunted across the VSD and into the aorta (right-to-left shunt → cyanosis).
3. Right ventricular outflow tract obstruction can occur at any or all of the following three levels: pulmonary valve stenosis, infundibular hypertrophy, or supravalvular stenosis.
4. The right ventricle becomes hypertrophied as a result of the increased gradient across the RVOT.
5. Minimal RVOTO results in a pink TOF variant, with the physiology behaving more like a large, nonrestrictive VSD.

Clinical Manifestations

1. Clinical manifestations are variable and depend on the size of the VSD and the degree of RVOTO.
2. Cyanosis.
   a. Newborns may have normal oxygen saturations; as the infants grow, the RVOTO increases and the oxygen saturations fall.
   b. Newborns with unacceptably low oxygen saturations need PGE_1 infusion to maintain ductal patency and adequate oxygen saturations.
   c. Cyanosis may initially be observed only with crying and with exertion.
3. Polycythemia.
4. A common clinical manifestation years ago was squatting, a posture characteristically assumed by older children to increase systemic vascular resistance and to encourage increased pulmonary blood flow. Squatting is very rarely seen currently, because TOF is now surgically repaired during the first year of life.
5. Tet spell: a life-threatening hypoxic event with a dramatic decrease in oxygen saturations; mechanism is usually infundibular spasm, which further obstructs pulmonary blood flow and increases right-to-left flow across the VSD.
   a. Typical hypoxic spells occur in the morning soon after awakening; during or after a crying episode; during or after a feeding; during painful procedures such as blood draws.
   b. Typical scenario includes tachypnea, irritability, and increasing cyanosis, followed by flaccidity and loss of consciousness.
   c. Home treatment for the caregiver: soothe the baby and place him or her in a knee–chest position; notify the health care provider immediately.
   d. Hospital treatment includes knee–chest position, sedation (morphine), beta blockers (propranolol, esmolol) to relax the infundibulum, and administration of medications to increase systemic vascular resistance (phenylephrine).
   e. Oxygen administration is of limited value; the problem is decreased pulmonary blood flow.
   f. Tet spells usually prompt the cardiologist to refer for surgical intervention.

Diagnostic Evaluation

1. Auscultation: harsh systolic ejection murmur heard best at the upper left sternal border (RVOT murmur); single second heart sound; during a Tet spell the murmur disappears.
2. CXR: varies; normal cardiac silhouette; decreased pulmonary vascular markings.
3. ECG: right ventricular hypertrophy.
4. Two-dimensional echocardiogram with Doppler study and color flow mapping to identify the structural

abnormalities, estimate the degree of RVOTO and assess the coronary artery pattern.

5. Cardiac catheterization is usually not needed for the initial diagnosis.

Management
Medical Management
1. Monitor oxygen saturations.
2. Monitor growth and development.
3. Monitor for hypoxic spells (many spells go unnoticed by parents).

Surgical Intervention: Palliative Versus Definitive Repair
1. Many centers prefer definitive, one-stage repair.
2. Potential obstacles for one-stage repair: abnormal coronary artery distribution (LAD arises from RCA and crosses RVOT); multiple VSDs; hypoplastic branch pulmonary arteries; small infant < 2.5 kg.
3. Palliative surgery: modified Blalock-Taussig shunt (BT shunt); tube graft between the left subclavian artery and the pulmonary artery: increased pulmonary blood flow results in higher oxygen saturations.
4. Definitive surgery: patch closure of VSD, relief of right ventricular outflow tract obstruction; with or without transannular patch across PV.

Long-Term Follow-Up
1. Assess RV outflow tract, monitor degree of PR.
2. Monitor RV function and exercise tolerance.
3. Monitor for arrhythmias.

Complications
1. Hypoxia.
2. Tet spells.
3. Polycythemia.
4. CHF: rare; associated with pink TOF.

■ Transposition of the Great Arteries

Transposition of the great arteries (TGA) occurs when the pulmonary artery arises off the left ventricle and the aorta arises off the right ventricle. It accounts for 5% to 10% of congenital heart defects. Associated lesions include VSD, ASD, PDA, pulmonary stenosis, and coarctation of the aorta.

Pathophysiology and Etiology
1. This defect results in two parallel circulations:
   a. The right atrium receives deoxygenated blood from the IVC and SVC; blood flow continues through the tricuspid valve into the right ventricle and is pumped back to the aorta.
   b. The left atrium receives richly oxygenated blood from the pulmonary veins; blood flow continues through the mitral valve into the left ventricle and is pumped back into the pulmonary artery.
2. To sustain life, there must be an accompanying defect that allows mixing of deoxygenated blood and oxygenated blood between the two circuits.

3. Shunting occurs at one or more of the following levels: PDA, ASD or patent foramen ovale (PFO) and VSD.
4. Infants born with transposition of the great arteries with an intact ventricular system are usually more cyanotic and sicker than infants born with TGA with a VSD.

Clinical Manifestations
Symptoms evident soon after birth; clinical scenario is influenced by the extent of intercirculatory mixing.
1. Cyanosis.
2. Tachypnea.
3. Metabolic acidosis.

Diagnostic Evaluation
1. Auscultation: varies—no murmur, or a murmur related to an associated defect, single S2.
2. CXR: varies—newborn CXR often normal; cardiomegaly with a narrow mediastinum and increased pulmonary markings; or decreased pulmonary markings with pulmonary stenosis.
3. ECG: biventricular hypertrophy.
4. Two-dimensional echocardiogram with Doppler study and color flow mapping identifies the structural abnormalities: transposed vessels, coronary artery pattern, and degree of mixing across the atrial septum plus associated lesions.

Treatment
Medical Management
1. Stabilize with PGE_1 infusion.
2. Severe hypoxia → balloon atrial septostomy (Rashkind) to improve atrial level mixing.
3. Treat pulmonary overcirculation with diuretics as needed.
4. Refer for surgical intervention.

Surgical Management
1. Arterial switch operation (Jatene)—procedure of choice:
   a. Ideally performed during the first week of life.
   b. The aorta and pulmonary artery are switched back to their anatomically correct ventricle
   c. Coronary arteries are transferred to the new aorta.
   d. Associated lesions are also repaired at this time.
2. Rastelli operation—performed for TGA, VSD, and PS.
   a. Repaired during the first year of life.
   b. VSD patch repaired to include LV to Ao outflow continuity with pulmonary blood flow provided via a RV to PA homograft.
3. Atrial switch operation: Mustard or Senning procedure:
   a. Rerouting of atrial blood flow: RA → baffle → mitral valve (MV) → LV → PA and LA → baffle → tricuspid valve (TV) → RV → Ao
   b. Restores oxygenated blood into the systemic system and deoxygenated blood guided to the pulmonary system.
   c. Disadvantages:
      (i) RV is left as the systemic ventricle—will develop RV dysfunction.

(ii) Increased incidence of atrial dysrhythmias and baffle obstruction.

Complications
1. Severe hypoxia.
2. Multiorgan ischemia.

Tricuspid Atresia

When tricuspid atresia (TA) occurs, there is no communication between the right atrium and right ventricle. Associated lesions include:
1. Obligatory PFO/ASD.
2. PDA.
3. VSD.
4. Hypoplastic RV.

Pathophysiology and Etiology
1. With TA, systemic venous return enters the right atrium and cannot continue into the RV; blood flows across an atrial septal opening into the left atrium.
2. Pulmonary blood flow occurs by way of:
   a. Ao → PDA → PA, or
   b. LV → VSD → RV → PA.

Clinical Manifestations
1. Cyanosis.

Diagnostic Evaluation
1. Auscultation: murmurs vary depending on the associated lesions; single second heart sound
2. CXR: pulmonary markings related to the amount of pulmonary blood flow; normal to slightly increase cardiac silhouette
3. ECG: superior axis; right and left atrial hypertrophy; LV hypertrophy.
4. Two-dimensional echocardiogram identifies the atretic tricuspid valve and hypoplastic RV; Doppler study and color flow mapping documents the right-to-left atrial shunt.

Management
Medical Management
1. Stabilize with PGE_1 infusion.
2. Intubate and ventilate as needed.
Surgical Management
1. First surgery—newborn:
   a. Too little pulmonary blood flow → BT shunt.
   b. Too much pulmonary blood flow → pulmonary artery band.
   c. Balanced pulmonary blood flow → do nothing.
2. Second surgery: 6 to 9 months:
   a. Bi-directional Glenn shunt: end-to-side anastomosis of the SVC to the right PA.
3. Third surgery: 2 to 5 years:
   a. Fontan completion: IVC to PA connection (extracardiac conduit or intracardiac baffle).

Complications
Cyanosis

Hypoplastic Left Heart Syndrome

Hypoplastic left heart syndrome (HLHS) is a constellation of left heart abnormalities that include the following:
1. Critical mitral stenosis or atresia.
2. Hypoplastic LV.
3. Critical aortic stenosis or atresia.
4. Hypoplastic ascending aorta with severe coarctation of the aorta.

Pathophysiology and Etiology
1. The left side of the heart is underdeveloped and essentially nonfunctional.
2. The right ventricle supports both the pulmonary and systemic circulations.
3. An atrial septal defect allows blood to flow from the left atrium into the right heart.
4. Blood flows right to left across the patent ductus arteriosus and into the descending aorta to deliver oxygen and nutrients to the body.

Clinical Manifestations
1. Newborn may appear completely well.
2. Once the PDA begins to close:
   a. CHF and tachypnea.
   b. Decreased urine output.
   c. Poor feeding.
   d. Lethargic; change in level of alertness.
   e. Pallor; gray color.
   f. Weak peripheral pulses.

Diagnostic Evaluation
1. Auscultation: single S2; systolic murmur.
2. CXR: cardiac silhouette varies (normal to increased size); increased pulmonary markings.
3. ECG: RV hypertrophy; decrease electrical forces in V5 and V6.
4. Two-dimensional echocardiogram with Doppler study and color flow mapping identifies the structural abnormalities and the altered blood flow patterns.

Management
Medical Management
1. Resuscitation and stabilization with PGE_1 infusion.
2. May need balloon atrial septostomy to allow unrestrictive LA to RA blood flow.
3. Inotropic support as needed (dopamine, dobutamine).
4. Assess hepatic, renal, and neurologic function.
5. Refer for surgical intervention.
Surgical Management
1. Palliative, staged repair:
   a. Stage I Norwood (neonate): reconstruction of the hypoplastic aorta, using the pulmonary artery and homograft; repair of the coarctation and creation of a BT shunt.

b. Stage II: bidirectional Glenn shunt (6 to 9 months): transect the SVC off the right atrium and directly suture end to side to right PA; ligate BT shunt.

c. Stage III: Fontan (18 months to 5 years): IVC to PA connection.

2. Cardiac transplantation.

Complications
1. Metabolic acidosis.
2. Cardiovascular collapse.
3. Multisystem failure.
4. Death.

■ Nursing Care of the Child With Congenital Heart Disease

Nursing Assessment
1. Obtain a thorough nursing history.
2. Discuss the care plan with the health care team (cardiologist, cardiac surgeon, nursing case manager, social worker, nutritionist).
3. Measure and record height and weight. Plot on a growth chart.
4. Record vital signs and oxygen saturations.
    a. Measure vital signs at a time when the infant/child is quiet.
    b. Choose appropriate size blood pressure cuff.
    c. Check four extremity blood pressure × 1.
5. Assess and record:
    a. Skin color: pink, cyanotic, mottled.
    b. Mucous membranes: dry, cyanotic.
    c. Extremities: check peripheral pulses for quality and symmetry; dependent edema; capillary refill; cool.
6. Assess clubbing (cyanotic heart disease).
7. Assess chest wall for deformities; prominent precordial activity.
8. Assess respiratory pattern.
    a. Before disturbing the child, stand back and count the respiratory rate.
    b. Loosen or remove clothing to directly observe chest movement.
    c. Assess for signs of respiratory distress: increased respiratory rate, grunting, retractions, nasal flaring.
    d. Auscultate for crackles, wheezing, congestion, stridor.
9. Assess heart sounds.
    a. Determine rate (bradycardia, tachycardia, or normal for age) and rhythm (regular or irregular).
    b. Identify murmur.
10. Assess fluid status.
    a. Daily weights.
    b. Strict intake and output (number of wet diapers; urine output).
11. Assess and record the child's level of activity.
    a. Observe the child at play. Is play interrupted to rest? Ask the parent if the child keeps up with peers while at play.

b. Observe the infant while feeding. Does the infant need frequent breaks or does he or she fall asleep during feeding? Assess for sweating, color change, or respiratory distress while feeding.

c. Assess and record findings relevant to the child's developmental level: age appropriate behavior, cognitive skills, gross and fine motor skills.

Nursing Diagnoses
- Impaired Gas Exchange related to altered pulmonary blood flow or pulmonary congestion
- Decreased Cardiac Output related to decreased myocardial function
- Activity Intolerance related to hypoxia or decreased myocardial function
- Altered Nutrition: Less Than Body Requirements related to excessive energy demands required by increased cardiac work load
- Risk for Infection related to chronic illness
- Fear and Anxiety related to life-threatening illness

Nursing Interventions
Relieving Respiratory Distress
1. Position the child in a reclining, semi-upright position.
2. Suction oral and nasal secretions as needed.
3. Identify target oxygen saturations and administer oxygen as prescribed.
4. Administer prescribed medications and document response to medications (improved, no change, or worsening respiratory status).
    a. Diuretics.
    b. Bronchodilators.
5. May need to change oral feedings to nasogastric feedings because of increased risk of aspiration with respiratory distress.

Improving Cardiac Output
1. Organize nursing care and medication schedule to provide periods of uninterrupted rest.
2. Provide play or educational activities that can be done in bed with minimal exertion.
3. Maintain normothermia.
4. Administer medications as prescribed.
    a. Diuretics (furosemide, spironolactone):
        (i) Give the medication at the same time each day. For older children, do not give a dose right before bedtime.
        (ii) Monitor the effectiveness of the dose: measure and record urine output.
    b. Digoxin:
        (i) Check heart rate for 1 minute. Hold the dose and notify the physician for bradycardia.
        (ii) Lead II rhythm strip. Measure P-R interval. Hold dose and notify the physician for first degree heart block.
        (iii) Give medication at the same time each day. For infants and children, digoxin is usually divided and given twice a day.

(iv) Monitor electrolytes. Increased incidence of digoxin toxicity associated with hypokalemia.
c. Afterload-reducing medications (captopril, enalapril):
   (i) When initiating a new medication: check blood pressure immediately before dose and 1 hour after dose.
   (ii) Monitor for signs of hypotension: syncope, lightheadedness, faint pulses.
   (iii) Hold medication and notify the physician according to ordered parameters.

Improving Oxygenation and Activity Tolerance

1. Place pulse oximeter probe (continuous monitoring or measure with vital signs) on finger or toe.
2. Administer oxygen as needed.
3. Titrate amount of oxygen to reach target oxygen saturations.
4. Assess response to oxygen therapy: increase in baseline oxygen saturations, improved work of breathing, and change in patient comfort.
5. Explain to the child how oxygen will help. If possible, give the child the choice for face mask oxygen or nasal cannula oxygen.

Providing Adequate Nutrition

1. For the infant:
   a. Small, frequent feedings.
   b. Fortified formula or breast milk (up to 30 cal/oz).
   c. Limit oral feeding time to 15 to 20 minutes (infant).
   d. Supplement oral feeds with nasogastric feeds as needed to provide weight gain (ie, continuous nasogastric feeds at night with ad lib PO feeds during the day).
2. For the child:
   a. Small, frequent meals.
   b. High-calorie, nutritional supplements.
   c. Determine child's likes and dislikes and plan meals accordingly.
3. Report feeding intolerance: nausea, vomiting, diarrhea.
4. Document daily weight (same time of day, same scale, same clothing).
5. Record accurate I & Os; assess for fluid retention.
6. Fluid restriction not usually needed for children; manage excess fluid with diuretics.

Preventing Infection

1. Maintain routine childhood immunization schedule.
2. Administer yearly influenza vaccine.
3. Prevent exposure to communicable diseases.
4. Good handwashing.
5. Report fevers.
6. Report signs of upper respiratory infection: runny nose, cough, increase in nasal secretions.
7. Report signs of gastrointestinal illness: diarrhea, abdominal pain, irritability.

Reducing Fear and Anxiety

1. Educate the patient and family.
2. Provide the family with contact phone numbers: how to schedule a follow-up visit; how to reach a cardiologist during the work week, evenings, weekends, and holidays.

Family Education and Health Maintenance

1. Instruct the family in necessary measures to maintain the child's health:
   a. Complete immunization.
   b. Adequate diet and rest.
   c. Prevention and control of infections.
   d. Regular medical and dental checkup. The child should be protected against infective endocarditis when undergoing certain dental procedures.
   e. Regular cardiac checkups.
2. Teach the family about the defect and its treatment.
   a. Signs and symptoms of CHF (see below).
   b. Signs of hypoxic spells associated with cyanotic defects and need to place child in knee-chest position and administer oxygen.
   c. Need to prevent dehydration, which increases risk of thrombotic complications.
   d. Emergency precautions related to hypoxic attacks, pulmonary edema, cardiac arrest (if appropriate).
   e. Special home care equipment, monitors, oxygen.
3. Encourage the parents and other people (teachers, peers, etc.) to treat the child in as normal a manner as possible.
   a. Avoid overprotection and overindulgence.
   b. Avoid rejection.
   c. Promote growth and development with modifications. Facilitate performance of the usual developmental tasks within the limits of the child's physiologic state.
   d. Prevent adults from projecting their fears and anxieties onto the child.
   e. Help family deal with its anger, guilt, and concerns related to the disabled child.
4. Initiate a community health nursing referral if indicated.
5. Stress the need for follow-up care.

Outcome-Based Evaluation

- Improved oxygenation evidenced by easy, comfortable respirations
- Improved cardiac output demonstrated by stable vital signs and adequate peripheral perfusion
- Increased activity level
- Maximal nutritional status demonstrated by weight gain and increase in growth curve percentile
- No signs of infection
- Parents discuss diagnosis and treatment together and with child

■ Congestive Heart Failure

Congestive heart failure (CHF), also known as heart failure, occurs when the cardiac output cannot meet the metabolic demands of the body.

Pathophysiology and Etiology

1. May result from the following:
   a. Congenital heart defects with a left-to-right shunt or atrioventricular valve regurgitation.
   b. Acquired heart disease: myocarditis, cardiomyopathy, acute rheumatic fever.

c. Chronic pulmonary disease (cor pulmonale).
d. Anemia.
e. Iatrogenic fluid overload.
2. In an attempt to meet the metabolic needs of the body, the heart rate increases to increase cardiac output (CO).
a. Cardiac output (CO) = Heart rate × Stroke volume.
b. Stroke volume is the amount of blood (cc) ejected from the heart with each heart beat; it depends on preload and vascular resistance.
3. Preload (CVP) increases as the failing heart contracts poorly.
4. With decreased cardiac output, the systemic vascular resistance increases to maintain blood pressure. This increase in afterload limits CO.
5. With decreased blood flow to the kidneys, the glomerular filtration rate decreases as tubular reabsorption increases sodium and water retention, resulting in a decreased urine output.
6. Long term, these compensatory mechanisms are detrimental to the failing myocardium. The chronic increase in preload and afterload contributes to chamber dilation and myocardial hypertrophy, leading to progressive heart failure.

Clinical Manifestations

1. Impaired myocardial function.
a. Tachycardia, S3.
b. Poor peripheral perfusion: weak peripheral pulses, cool extremities.
c. Pallor.
d. Exercise or activity intolerance.
2. Pulmonary congestion.
a. Tachypnea.
b. Cyanosis.
c. Retractions, nasal flaring, grunting.
d. Cough.
3. Systemic venous congestion.
a. Hepatomegaly.
b. Peripheral edema: scrotal and orbital.
c. Water weight gain.
d. Decreased urine output.

Diagnostic Evaluation

1. Palpation:
a. Weak peripheral pulses; cool extremities.
b. Poor capillary refill.
c. Liver edge palpable below right costal margin.
d. Increased precordial activity.
2. Auscultation:
a. Heart.
(i) Gallop rhythm (S3).
(ii) Systolic flow murmur.
(iii) Tachycardia.
b. Lungs.
(i) Tachypnea.
(ii) Crackles, wheezing.

3. CXR:
a. Cardiomegaly.
b. Pulmonary congestion.

Management

1. Diuretics to reduce intravascular volume (furosemide, spironolactone).
2. Digoxin to increase myocardial contractility.
3. Afterload reduction to decrease the work load of the ailing myocardium (ACE inhibitors: captopril, enalapril, lisinopril).
4. Beta blockers to counteract the increased sympathetic activity and reduce systemic vascular resistance (metoprolol, carvedilol).

Complications

1. Pulmonary edema.
2. Metabolic acidosis.
3. Failure to thrive.
4. Upper respiratory infections.
5. Arrhythmia.
6. Death.

Nursing Assessment

1. Assess response to medical treatment plan.
2. Document vital signs and oxygen saturations.
3. Observe infant or child during feeding or activity. Assess for diaphoresis, need for frequent rest periods, and inability to keep up with peers.

Nursing Diagnoses

- Decreased Cardiac Output related to myocardial dysfunction
- Fluid Volume Excess related to decreased cardiac contractility and decreased excretion from the kidney
- Impaired Gas Exchange related to pulmonary venous congestion
- Activity Intolerance
- Risk for Infection related to pulmonary congestion
- Altered Nutrition (Failure to Thrive) related to increased metabolic demands with decreased caloric intake
- Anxiety related to child's diagnosis and prognosis

Nursing Interventions
Improving Myocardial Efficiency
1. Administer digoxin as prescribed.
a. Measure heart rate. Hold medication and notify physician for bradycardia.
b. Check most recent potassium level. Hold medication and notify health care provider for hypokalemia.
c. Run Lead II ECG. Measure P-R interval. Hold medication and notify health care provider for first degree AV block.
d. Report signs of possible digoxin toxicity: vomiting, nausea, visual changes, bradycardia.

e. Double-check dose of digoxin with another nurse before administering the dose.

2. Administer afterload reduction medications as prescribed.
   a. Measure blood pressure before and after giving the patient the medication. Hold the medication and notify the health care provider for low BP (greater than a 15-mm Hg drop from baseline).
   b. Observe for other signs of hypotension: dizziness, light-headedness, syncope.

Maintaining Fluid and Electrolyte Balance

1. Administer diuretics as prescribed.
   a. Obtain daily weights.
   b. Keep strict intake and output record.
   c. Monitor serum electrolytes. Provide potassium supplements as needed.
2. Sodium restriction: not usually needed; provide dietary assistance as needed.
3. Fluid restriction: not usually needed.

Relieving Respiratory Distress

1. Administer oxygen therapy as prescribed.
2. Elevate head of bed; infants may be more comfortable in an upright infant seat.

Reducing Energy Requirements

1. Organize nursing care to provide periods of uninterrupted sleep/rest.
2. Avoid unnecessary activities.
3. Respond efficiently to a crying infant. Provide comfort and treat the source of distress: wet/dirty diaper, hunger.
4. Provide diversional activities that require limited expenditure of energy.
5. Provide small, frequent feedings.

Decreasing Risk of Infection

1. Ensure good handwashing by everyone.
2. Avoid exposure to ill children or caretakers.
3. Monitor signs of infection: fever, cough, runny nose, diarrhea, vomiting.

Providing Adequate Nutrition

1. For the older child: provide nutritious foods that the child likes, along with supplemental high-calorie snacks (milkshake, pudding).
2. For the infant:
   a. High-calorie formula (24 to 30 cal/oz).
   b. Supplement oral intake with nasogastric feeds. Allow ad lib oral intake through the day with continuous nasogastric feeds at night.

Reducing Anxiety

1. Communicate the care plan to the child and family.
2. Educate the family.
3. Encourage questions; answer questions as able or refer to another member of the health care team.

Family Education and Health Maintenance

1. Teach the signs and symptoms of CHF.
2. Teach medications: brand name and generic name, expected effects, side effects, dose.
3. Demonstrate medication administration.
4. With the family, design a medication administration time schedule.
5. Provide guidelines for when to seek medical help.
6. Teach infant and child cardiopulmonary resuscitation (CPR) as needed.
7. Reinforce dietary guidelines; provide a recipe to the parent on how to make high-calorie formula.
8. Reinforce ways to prevent infection.
9. Referral for skilled home nursing visits as needed.
10. Contact primary medical caregiver. Continue with well child care issues/needs.
11. Schedule follow-up visit.

Outcome-Based Evaluation

- Heart rate within normal range for age; adequate urine output
- No unexpected weight gain
- Clear lungs; normal respiratory rate and effort
- Participating in quiet diversional activities
- No signs of infection
- Adequate intake of small, frequent feedings
- Parents express understanding of disease process and treatment

ACQUIRED HEART DISEASE

Note: Kawasaki disease is discussed in Chapter 53.

Acute Rheumatic Fever

Acute rheumatic fever (ARF) is an acute autoimmune disease that occurs as a sequelae of group A beta hemolytic streptococcal infection. It is characterized by inflammatory lesions of connective tissue and endothelial tissue, primarily affecting the joints and heart.

Pathophysiology and Etiology

1. Most first attacks of ARF occur 2 to 3 weeks after a streptococcal infection of the throat or of the upper respiratory tract.
2. Peak incidence occurs in children 6 to 15 years of age. Incidence after a mild streptococcal pharyngeal infection is 0.3% and after a severe streptococcal infection is 1% to 3%.
3. Streptococcal infection abates with or without treatment; however, autoantibodies attack the myocardium, pericardium, and cardiac valves.
   a. Aschoff bodies (fibrin deposits) develop on the valves, possibly leading to permanent valve dysfunction, especially of the mitral valve.
   b. Severe myocarditis may cause dilation of the heart and heart failure.
4. Inflammation of the large joints causes a painful arthritis that may last 6 to 8 weeks.
5. Involvement of the nervous system causes chorea (sudden involuntary movements).

Clinical Manifestations

Documented or undocumented group A beta hemolytic streptococcal infection is usually followed in several weeks by fever, malaise, and anorexia. Major symptoms of ARF may appear several weeks to several months after initial infection.

Major Manifestations

1. Carditis—manifested by systolic murmur, prolonged PR and QT intervals on ECG, and possibly by signs of heart failure (see p. 1390).
2. Polyarthritis—pain and limited movement of two or more joints; joints are swollen, red, warm, and tender.
3. Chorea—purposeless, involuntary, rapid movements often associated with muscle weakness, involuntary facial grimaces, speech disturbance, and emotional lability.
4. Erythema marginatum—nonpruritic pink, macular rash mostly of the trunk with pale central areas; migratory.
5. Subcutaneous nodules—firm, painless nodules over the scalp, extensor surface of joints, such as wrists, elbows, knees, and vertebral column.

Minor Manifestations

1. History of previous rheumatic fever or evidence of pre-existing rheumatic heart disease.
2. Arthralgia—pain in one or more joints without evidence of inflammation, tenderness, or limited movement.
3. Fever—temperature greater than 38°C (100.4°F).
4. Laboratory abnormalities—elevated erythrocyte sedimentation rate (ESR), positive C-reactive protein, elevated white blood cell count.
5. ECG changes—prolonged PR interval.

Diagnostic Evaluation

1. Diagnosed clinically through use of the Jones criteria from the American Heart Association—presence of two major manifestations or one major and two minor manifestations (as listed above), with supporting evidence of a recent streptococcal infection.
2. ECG done to evaluate PR interval and other changes.
3. Laboratory tests listed above. In addition, group A streptococcal culture and/or antistreptolysin O (ASO) titer to detect streptococcal antibodies from recent infection.
4. CXR for cardiomegaly, heart failure.

Management

1. Course of antibiotic therapy to completely eradicate streptococcal infection (may be given despite previous treatment).
   a. Usually benzathine penicillin is given intramuscularly (IM) in a single dose.
   b. Oral erythromycin may be used for children who are allergic to penicillin.
2. Oral salicylates (aspirin) or nonsteroidal anti-inflammatory drugs (naproxen sodium) usually used to control pain and inflammation of arthritis.
3. Corticosteroids used in severe cases to try to control cardiac inflammation.
4. Phenobarbital, diazepam, or other neurologic agent to control chorea.
5. Bed rest during the acute phase (until ESR decreases, C-reactive protein becomes negative, and pulse rate returns to normal) to rest the heart.
6. Mitral valve replacement may be necessary in some cases.
7. Secondary prevention of recurrent ARF:
   a. Risk of recurrence greatest within first 5 years, with multiple episodes of ARF, and with rheumatic heart disease. Prophylactic antibiotic treatment may be lifelong.
   b. For those at low risk for recurrence, antibiotic prophylaxis may be continued for 5 years or longer.
   c. Antibiotic regimens may include:
      (i) Benzathine penicillin intramuscularly (IM) every 3 to 4 weeks.
      (ii) Penicillin V or erythromycin 250 mg twice a day.
      (iii) Sulfisoxazole (Pediazole) 0.5 to 1 g once a day (depending on weight).

Complications

1. Heart failure.
2. Pericarditits, pericardial effusion.
3. Aortic or mitral regurgitation.
4. Permanent cardiac damage.

Nursing Assessment

1. Assess for signs of cardiac involvement by auscultation of the heart for murmur and cardiac monitoring for prolonged PR interval.
2. Monitor pulse for 1 full minute to determine heart rate.
3. Assess temperature for elevation.
4. Observe for involuntary movements: stick out tongue or smile; garbled or hesitant speech when asked to recite numbers or the ABCs; hyperextension of the wrists and fingers when trying to extend arms.
5. Assess child's ability to feed self, dress, and do other activities if chorea or arthritis present.
6. Assess pain level using scale appropriate for child's age.
7. Assess parent's ability to cope with illness and care for child.

Nursing Diagnoses

- Decreased Cardiac Output related to carditis
- Pain related to arthritis
- Risk for Injury related to chorea

Nursing Interventions
Improving Cardiac Output

1. Explain to the child and family the need for bed rest during the acute phase (approximately 2 weeks) and as long as heart failure is present. In milder cases, light indoor activity is allowed.
2. In severe cases, organize care so that the child will not have to exert self and will have hours of uninterrupted rest.

3. Maintain cardiac monitoring if indicated.

4. Administer course of antibiotics as directed. Be alert to side effects, such as nausea and vomiting and GI distress.

5. Administer mediations for heart failure as directed. Monitor blood pressure, intake and output, and heart rate.

Relieving Pain

1. Administer anti-inflammatory medication, analgesics, and antipyretics as directed.
   a. Monitor for signs of aspirin toxicity such as tinnitus, nausea and vomiting, and headache.
   b. Monitor for signs of corticosteroid use—gastrointestinal distress, acne, weight gain, emotional disturbances—or long-term effects, such as rounded face, ulcer formation, and decreased resistance to infection.
   c. Administer all anti-inflammatory medications with food to reduce gastrointestinal injury.
   d. Be aware that anti-inflammatories may not alter the course of myocardial injury.

2. Teach family the importance of maintaining dosage schedule, continuing medication until all signs and symptoms of the ARF have gone, and tapering the dose as directed by health care provider.

3. Assist child with positioning for comfort and protecting inflamed joints.

4. Suggest diversional activities that do not require use of painful joints.

Protecting the Child With Chorea

1. Use padded side rails if chorea is severe.

2. Assist with feeding and other fine motor activities as needed.

3. Assist with ambulation if weak.

4. Avoid the use of straws and sharp utensils if chorea involves the face.

5. Ensure that child consumes nutritious diet with recommended vitamins, protein, and calories.

6. Be patient if speech is affected, and offer emotional support.

7. Protect the child from stress.

8. Administer phenobarbital or other medication for chorea as directed. Observe for drowsiness.

Family Education and Health Maintenance

1. Teach the appropriate administration of all medications, including prophylactic antibiotic.

2. Encourage all family and household members to be screened for streptococcus and receive the appropriate treatment.

3. Instruct on additional prophylaxis for endocarditis with dental procedures and surgery as indicated.

4. Encourage following activity restrictions, resuming activity gradually, and resting whenever tired.

5. Encourage keeping appointments for follow-up evaluation by cardiologist and other health care providers.

6. Advise the parents that child cannot return to school until health care provider assesses that all disease activity is gone. Parents may need to discuss with teachers how the child can catch up with school work.

7. Instruct on follow-up with usual health care provider for immunizations, well child evaluations, hearing and vision screening, and other health maintenance needs.

8. Provide general health education about early identification and treatment seeking for any possible streptococcal infection (fever, sore throat). Compliance with 10 to 14 days of antibiotics can greatly reduce the risk of ARF and other poststreptococcal sequelae.

Outcome-Based Evaluation

• Heart rate and PR interval within normal range for age; no signs of heart failure

• Compliant with anti-inflammatory therapy; reports pain as 1 to 2 on scale of 1 to 10

• Can feed self, wash face and hands, and ambulate to bathroom without injury

■ Cardiomyopathy

According to the type of myocardial changes, cardiomyopathy (CAM) can be classified into three categories: dilated, restrictive, and hypertrophic. The most common type in children is dilated cardiomyopathy.

Pathophysiology and Etiology

1. Familial (family history, genetic predisposition) tendency.

2. Idiopathic in most cases.

3. May be related to:
   a. Nutritional deficiency (carnitene or selenium)
   b. Viral infection (myocarditis), human immunodeficiency virus (HIV).
   c. Collagen vascular disease (systemic lupus erythematosus [SLE]).
   d. Cardiotoxic drugs (doxorubicin [Adriamycin]).
   e. Cocaine abuse.
   f. Postpartum.
   g. Sustained tachycardia (ectopic atrial tachycardia).
   h. Catecholamine surge; hyperthyroidism.

4. Dilated CAM involves dilatation of one or both ventricles associated with normal septal and LV free wall thickness.

5. Decreased systolic function (contractility) results in CHF.

6. Increasing end-systolic dimension results in AV valve regurgitation, further worsening CHF.

Clinical Manifestations

1. Tachycardia, tachypnea, dyspnea.

2. Hepatosplenomegaly.

3. Decreased exercise tolerance, fatigue, sweating.

4. Poor weight gain, nausea, abdominal tenderness.

5. Ventricular arrhythmia.

6. Chest pain.

7. Syncope.

Diagnostic Evaluation

1. ECG: tachycardia, abnormal ST segments, arrhythmia, ectopic atrial tachycardia.
2. CXR: cardiomegaly, pulmonary congestion.
3. Two-dimensional echocardiogram: poor ventricular systolic function, dilated heart chambers; AV valve insufficiency.
4. Cardiac catheterization: not needed for initial diagnosis; endomyocardial biopsy; assess PVR.

Management

1. Identify and treat the underlying cause.
2. Maximize caloric intake: fortify formula; supplemental nasogastric feeds.
3. Supplemental oxygen as needed.
4. Pharmacologic treatment for dilated CAM to treat systolic dysfunction:
   a. Diuretics: furosemide, spironolactone.
   b. Inotropics: digoxin.
   c. Afterload reduction: captopril, enalapril, lisinopril.
   d. Anticoagulation: warfarin, low molecular weight heparin (enoxaparin).
   e. Antiarrhythmics.
5. Pharmacologic treatment for hypertrophic CAM to treat diastolic dysfunction:
   a. Beta blockers.
   b. Calcium channel blockers.
   c. AV sequential pacing.
   d. Myomectomy or myotomy.
6. Pharmacologic treatment for restrictive CAM to treat diastolic dysfunction:
   a. Diuretics to decrease volume.
7. Activity restriction (usually self-imposed by the younger child and infant).
8. Cardiac transplantation.

Complications

1. Severe CHF.
2. Increased pulmonary vascular resistance.
3. Intracardiac thrombus.
4. Embolus.
5. Malignant arrhythmias.
6. Sudden death.

Nursing Assessment

Perform a thorough nursing assessment as for congenital heart disease (see p. 1388).

Nursing Diagnoses

- Decreased Cardiac Output related to impaired systolic or diastolic ventricular function
- Altered Nutrition: Less Than Body Requirements related to increased metabolic demands and poor feeding from dyspnea, fatigue, and poor appetite
- Ineffective Family Coping related to chronic illness

Nursing Interventions

Maximizing Cardiac Output

1. Monitor vital signs; notify physician for hypotension, tachycardia, arrhythmia; increasing tachypnea.
2. Administer oxygen therapy as prescribed.
3. Administer medications as prescribed.
   a. Maintain bleeding precautions for anticoagulated patients.
   b. Document response to diuretics; monitor intake and output.
4. Monitor electrolytes.
5. Restrict level of activity.

Providing Maximal Nutritional Support

1. Encourage frequent, small meals. Provide foods the child likes.
2. Provide high-calorie supplements (milkshakes, pudding).
3. Administer supplemental tube feedings if nutritional needs are not being met.
4. Administer parenteral hyperalimentation and intralipids as directed (rarely needed).

Promoting Effective Coping and Control Within the Family

1. Organize a family meeting with various members of the health care team to review the child's medical condition and to explain the treatment plan.
2. Allow the child and family to express their questions, fears, and concerns.
3. Identify support systems and services for the child and family: extended family members, clergy, support groups, community resources.

Family Education and Health Maintenance

1. Teach child and family medication administration: purpose of the drug, drug dosage, drug schedule, and side effects.
2. Help family design a realistic medication schedule.
   a. Identify usual wake-up time and bedtime. Schedule medications accordingly.
   b. Do not give a diuretic right before bedtime or nap time.
   c. If possible, avoid having to give medications at school.
3. Teach bleeding precautions if the child is on anticoagulation agents (Coumadin).
   a. Monitor prothrombin INR regularly.
   b. Observe for signs of bleeding.
4. Give guidelines for notifying the physician.
   a. Worsening shortness of breath.
   b. Irregular pulse; palpitations.
   c. Syncope, dizziness, or lightheadedness.
   d. Increasing fatigue.
5. Teach infant and child CPR.

Outcome-Based Evaluation

- Stable vital signs
- Maximal nutritional status as evidenced by weight gain and growth
- Compliance with the treatment plan and follow-up visits

CARDIAC PROCEDURES

Cardiac Catheterization

Cardiac catheterization is an invasive procedure used to identify cardiac anatomy; measure intracardiac pressures, shunts, and oxygen saturations; and calculate systemic and pulmonary vascular resistance.

Procedure

1. Catheter insertion sites include femoral vein or artery, umbilical vein or artery, brachial vein, or internal jugular vein.
2. Under fluoroscopy, catheters are guided through the heart, collecting pressure measurements and oxygen saturations.
3. Contrast dye is injected through the catheters to visualize blood flow patterns and abnormalities.
4. Cardiac catheterization is usually an outpatient procedure for children who undergo an elective procedure. After interventional procedures, some children are observed in the hospital for 24 hours.

Indications

1. To confirm or establish the diagnosis.
2. To measure cardiac output.
3. To measure pressures and oxygen saturations.
4. To calculate intracardiac shunting, and pulmonary and systemic vascular resistance.
5. To visualize coronary arteries.
6. To intervene:
   a. Balloon atrial septostomy (Rashkind) for restrictive atrial septum.
   b. Balloon valvuloplasty (AoS, PS) and angioplasty (recurrent CoA).
   c. Endomyocardial biopsy.
   d. To occlude vessels (coil embolization) or defects (ASD closure devices; PDA closure devices).
   e. To stent vessels open (branch PA stenosis, recurrent CoA).

Complications

1. Arrhythmias (usually catheter induced).
2. Infection.
3. Bleeding at catheter insertion site; large hematoma.
4. Allergic reaction to contrast material.
5. Loss of pulse in the extremity used for cannulation.
6. Perforation.
7. Cerebrovascular accident.
8. Death.

Nursing Diagnoses

- Fear related to surgical procedure
- Knowledge Deficit regarding surgical procedure and associated nursing care
- Risk for Injury related to complications of cardiac catheterization

Nursing Interventions

Preoperatively:

Reducing Fear in Child and Parents

1. Provide specific instructions in nonthreatening manner:
   a. Day and time of the procedure.
   b. NPO guidelines.
   c. Sedation versus general anesthesia.
   d. Site of the planned arterial and venous puncture.
   e. Routine postprocedure care.
2. Provide appropriate teaching geared toward the child's age and level of cognitive development. Use diagrams and models as appropriate.
3. Provide parents an opportunity, without the child present, to discuss the procedure, risks, benefits, and alternative choices.
4. Give child opportunity to express fears and ask questions.

Explaining and Providing Nursing Care

1. Obtain baseline set of vital signs: heart rate (HR), blood pressure (BP), respiratory rate (RR), and oxygen saturation.
2. Measure and record child's height and weight.
3. Note time of last oral intake: solids and liquids.
4. Identify known allergies.
5. List current medications and note time last taken.
6. Help child change into a hospital gown.
7. Start peripheral IV as needed.
8. Administer sedation as prescribed.

Postoperatively:

Observe for and Prevent Complications

1. Monitor and record routine vital signs (q 15 mins × 4, q 30 mins × 2, then q 1 hr); extremity pulse check with vital signs.
2. Notify health care provider for:
   a. HR, RR, or BP outside normal parameters for age.
   b. Bleeding or increasing hematoma at puncture site.
   c. Change in oxygen saturations.
   d. Fever.
   e. Cool, pulseless extremity.
3. Observe puncture site for redness, pain, swelling, or induration.
4. Maintain the child in a reclining position for 2 to 3 hours after the procedure.
5. Offer fluids as soon as the child is ready.

Family Education and Health Maintenance

1. Provide discharge information:
   a. Care of the incision or puncture site (keep dry for 48 hours).
   b. Activity restrictions (usually for 48 hours).
   c. Observe for and report late complications: redness, swelling, drainage from puncture site.
   d. Follow-up medical care.
2. If cardiac catheterization was a preoperative procedure, use the recovery time to teach the child and family about upcoming hospital stay.

Outcome-Based Evaluation
- Child describes procedure in own words; parents and child discuss procedure and ask appropriate questions
- Child cooperative with preoperative nursing care
- Insertion site intact without drainage, redness, or hematoma; no complications

◼ Cardiac Surgery

The ultimate goal of treatment of cardiovascular disease in children is to restore normal structure and function of the heart. Most types of congenital heart defects can be palliated or definitively repaired.

Procedures
Closed-Heart Surgery
1. Surgical approach: lateral thoracotomy or mediastinal incision.
2. Indications:
   a. PDA ligation.
   b. Pulmonary artery banding.
   c. Coarctation of the aorta.
   d. Vascular rings.

Open-Heart Surgery
1. Mediastinal incision is the more common technique, although a lateral thoracotomy can be done for uncomplicated cardiac surgery (simple ASD repair).
2. With the use of cardiopulmonary bypass, the surgeon can stop the heart and operate inside to repair the defects.
3. Deep hypothermia with circulatory arrest allows the surgeon to safely stop cardiopulmonary bypass and remove arterial or venous cannulas to better visualize and repair the defects.
4. Indications:
   a. ASD, VSD, atrioventricular canal.
   b. Aortic stenosis, pulmonary stenosis.
   c. TOF.
   d. TGA.
   e. Tricuspid atresia.
   f. TAPVR.
   g. Truncus arteriosus.
   h. Hypoplastic left heart syndrome (HLHS).
   i. Complex single ventricle.

Potential Complications of Specific Surgeries
1. PDA ligation: laryngeal nerve damage, phrenic nerve damage, diaphragm paralysis, thoracic duct injury.
2. Coarctation of the aorta: rebound hypertension, mesenteric arteritis (abdominal pain), coarctation restenosis.
3. Aorta-pulmonary shunt (BT shunt): shunt occlusion, PA distortion, pulmonary overcirculation.
4. ASD: atrial arrhythmias, sinoatrial (SA) node dysfunction.
5. VSD: transient or permanent heart block, residual VSD, ventricular dysfunction.
6. TOF: low cardiac output, residual RVOTO or VSD, ectopic junctional tachycardia/arrhythmias, thoracic duct injury.
7. TGA: arterial switch operation—coronary artery injury, ventricular dysfunction, suprapulmonary stenosis.
8. TGA: atrial switch operation—baffle obstruction, RV failure, atrial arrhythmias.
9. Valvotomy (for valve stenosis): valve insufficiency.
10. Bidirectional Glenn shunt: SVC syndrome, low cardiac output, hypoxia, pleural effusions.
11. Fontan completion: low cardiac output, pleural effusions, ventricular dysfunction.

Cardiac Transplant Surgery
Cardiac transplantation is the last treatment option for children with progressive heart failure not amenable to conventional medical-surgical therapy. Children who cannot grow and meet developmental milestones or who have unacceptable quality-of-life issues may benefit from cardiac transplant surgery. Not all children activated for transplant will receive a donor organ. Approximately one in four children die while waiting. Those children who receive a donor heart must take lifelong immunosuppression medications to prevent organ rejection.

Indications for Cardiac Transplantation
1. End-stage cardiomyopathy.
2. Untreatable complex congenital heart disease.
3. Malignant arrhythmia.
4. Retransplant for cardiac graft failure.

Immunosuppressive Medications
1. Cyclosporine (Neoral).
2. Azathioprine (Imuran).
3. Tacrolimus (FK 506, Prograf).
4. Prednisone.
5. OKT3.

Complications
1. Organ rejection: routine surveillance endomyocardial biopsies are performed to assess for rejection.
   a. With mild to moderate rejection, children may initially be asymptomatic.
   b. With severe rejection, children are usually symptomatic with hemodynamic instability.
2. Infection.
3. Accelerated diffuse coronary artery disease.

Routine Follow-Up
1. Routine well-child care visits to primary care provider.
   a. Transplant children should not receive any live virus immunizations (oral polio, measles-mumps-rubella [MMR], varicella). Monitor for side effects of chronic steroids and immunosuppressive medications.
2. Routine cardiology clinic visits.
   a. Laboratory studies: chemistry, hematology, therapeutic drug levels.
   b. Vital signs.
   c. ECG.
   d. Echocardiography.
3. Serial cardiac catheterizations and endomyocardial biopsies.

4. Yearly coronary angiography or dobutamine stress echo-cardiography.

Nursing Assessment
Baseline Assessment on Day of Surgery
1. Measure and record height and weight.
2. Document vital signs: HR, RR, BP, and oxygen saturation.
3. Assess for preoperative infection: fever, signs of URI (cough, runny nose, crackles), vomiting or diarrhea that might delay surgery.
4. Document last oral intake.
5. Void on call to the operating room (OR).

Nursing Diagnoses
- Fear of surgical procedure
- Risk for Injury caused by complications of surgery
- Impaired Adjustment after surgery

Nursing Interventions
Preoperatively:
Preparing the Child and Family and Reducing Fear
1. Be honest and use nonthreatening language the child can understand.
2. The following are frequently asked questions from parents. Address them with the parents:
   a. What to tell the child.
   b. When to tell the child.
   c. What to bring to the hospital.
   d. Anticipated hospital course: how long in the operating room; how many days in the intensive care unit (ICU); how many days on the general care unit; visiting policy, rooming-in accommodations.
3. Review preoperative instructions.
   a. NPO guidelines.
   b. Where to report on the day of the surgery.
   c. Time to arrive at the hospital; time of surgery.
   d. Preoperative medications (injection, liquid, inhalation).
   e. What the OR looks like; what the people wear in the OR (hats, gowns, and masks, etc.).
4. Explain the preoperative period.
   a. Change into a hospital gown.
   b. Parents stay with the child.
   c. Transportation to the operating room (walking, wheelchair, or stretcher).
5. Explain the operative period.
   a. OR waiting room.
   b. Updates during the surgery will come from the surgical scrub nurses.
   c. Surgeon will meet the family after surgery to review the surgical findings and to describe the operation.
6. Explain the postoperative period. Use models and diagrams.
   a. Pediatric ICU routines and procedures.
   b. Monitoring lines and equipment.
   c. Ventilators, oxygen therapy.
   d. Protective restraints.
7. Offer medical equipment to handle and play with (ECG leads, face mask, blood pressure cuff), age-appropriate books about surgery and hospital stays, and tour of ICU and surgical area as available.
8. Prehospital tour of the pediatric ICU and general pediatric care unit.
9. Allow an opportunity for the child and family to ask questions, express their concern, or to ask for more detail.

Postoperatively:
Observing for and Preventing Complications
1. Assess respiratory status and maintain respiratory support.
   a. Maintain ventilatory support as needed.
   b. Maintain patent airway with routine endotracheal suctioning.
   c. Auscultate breath sounds frequently. Decreased breath sounds may indicate pleural effusions, atelectasis, pneumothorax, hemothorax.
   d. Report results of routine CXR.
   e. Perform frequent position changes: side–back–side.
   f. Monitor arterial blood gases (ABGs) and oxygen saturations.
   g. Assess chest tube drainage.
   h. Extubate when hemodynamically stable and when patient meets extubation criteria.
   i. Administer oxygen therapy as needed after extubation.
2. Assess cardiac status.
   a. Monitor vital signs and oxygen saturations.
   b. Maintain continuous ECG monitoring.
      (i) Daily 12-lead ECG to assess rhythm.
      (ii) Temporary epicardial pacemaker wires available for pacing as needed.
   c. Continuous BP monitoring (arterial line).
   d. Monitor intracardiac pressures (CVP, LA, PA).
   e. Monitor peripheral perfusion, capillary refill, toe temperature.
   f. Titrate vasopressors (dopamine, dobutamine, milrinone) as prescribed.
3. Assess fluid status.
   a. Record hourly intake (IV fluids, blood products, fluid boluses).
   b. Record hourly output (urine, chest tube drainage, nasogastric drainage).
   c. Perform daily weights.
   d. Administer diuretics as prescribed.
4. Assess neurologic status.
   a. Monitor level of responsiveness, response to verbal commands, and response to pain.
   b. Check pupil size and reactivity to light.
   c. Document movement of all extremities.
   d. Monitor all invasive lines for air bubbles and potential air embolism.
   e. Observe for signs of neurologic injury related to hypoperfusion or embolism.

5. Monitor for potential specific complications related to particular surgery for CHD.
6. Assess for postoperative pain.
   a. Monitor level of responsiveness, agitation.
   b. Implement pediatric pain scale rating to assist the child in identifying the severity of pain.
   c. Administer pain medication as prescribed: continuous IV infusion and/or IV boluses prn.
   d. Utilize patient-controlled analgesia (PCA) continuous pump as appropriate.
7. Assess serum electrolyte balance. Obtain blood tests and report results. Treat deficits with supplements.
8. Assess packed cell volume, platelet count and coagulation studies.
   a. Low hematocrit (<30): consider directed donor transfusion or blood bank transfusion.
   b. Low platelet count: continue to monitor; if bleeding persists, transfuse platelets.
   c. Prolonged coagulation studies: continue to monitor; if bleeding or oozing persists → protamine, fresh frozen plasma.

Enhancing Adjustment Postoperatively

1. Provide continuity of care (primary nursing and consistent medical team).
2. Explain all procedures and routines to the child and parents to minimize fear.
3. Explain to the parents a child's typical reactions to stressful events.
   a. Regression—temporary loss of developmental milestones.
   b. Fear of any medical personnel (white coat anxiety).
   c. Sibling jealousy that one child is receiving a lot of attention.
   d. Withdrawal—related to stimulation overload and lack of undisturbed sleep.
   e. Nightmares.
   f. Increased dependency; clinging behavior.
4. Suggest parent support groups, community resources, and counseling as needed.

Family Education and Health Maintenance

1. Provide the child and family with oral and written discharge instructions and recommendations.
   a. Medications.
   b. Activity restrictions.
      (i) No strenuous activity or contact sports for 6 to 8 weeks after surgery.
      (ii) Most children are ready to return to school at least part time, about 2 weeks after surgery.
      (iii) If child needs prolonged recovery time at home, may need to consider home tutoring.
      (iv) No gym class until full recovery.
   b. Care of the incision.
   c. Dietary recommendations.
   d. Bathing or showering guidelines.
2. Provide the child and family with a list of potential signs of complications and instructions to notify the health care provider.

   a. Fever greater than or equal to 101.5°F.
   b. Any redness, swelling, or drainage from chest incision.
   c. Partial opening of the chest incision.
   d. Poor appetite, nausea, vomiting.
   e. Breathing difficulties, shortness of breath.
3. Provide the family with the names and phone numbers of people to call for questions and emergencies.
4. Make follow-up appointments for the child to be seen by his or her primary care provider 2 to 3 days after discharge from the hospital and 10 to 14 days to be seen by their pediatric cardiologist.
5. Review American Heart Association's recommendations for endocarditis prophylaxis: standard general prophylaxis for children at risk: amoxicillin 50 mg/kg (maximum dose = 2 g) given orally 1 hour before the procedure.

Community and Home Care Considerations

1. Arrange skilled home nursing visits as needed to:
   a. Review medications.
   b. Assess wound healing.
   c. Monitor vital signs and oxygen saturations.
   d. Assess oral intake; nutritional supplements.
   e. Resource for family.
2. Make referral to community agencies as needed (infant and toddler program).
3. Arrange for home medical equipment (oxygen, feeding pump, and supplies) as needed.
4. Review safety precautions in the home:
   a. Child-proof medication bottles.
   b. Poison control phone number for accidental medication overdose.
   c. Infant and child CPR techniques.
   d. Bleeding precautions for children on anticoagulation therapy. No aspirin products. Be sure to read the labels on over-the-counter cold and cough syrups. Avoid activities with high risk of injury. All head injuries need to be evaluated by a physician. Signs of bleeding:
      (i) Blood in the urine.
      (ii) Black tarry stools.
      (iii) Prolonged nosebleeds.
      (iv) Bleeding gums.
      (v) Bruising for no known trauma.
      (vi) Spitting or coughing up blood.
      (vii) Any unusual swelling or pain.
   e. Medic-Alert bracelet or tags.
5. Discuss developmental issues with the family.
   a. A child on diuretics may have difficulty with toilet training.
   b. Disciplining, establishing behavioral expectations, and setting limits in a child with CHD should be similar to those for a child without CHD.
6. Discuss the need for home schooling or tutoring during recovery time. Return to the classroom as soon as the child is ready.
7. Discuss infants with CHD in daycare situations— address each case individually. Daycare programs usu-

ally have increased risk of upper respiratory infections and other childhood communicable diseases.

8. Encourage routine dental visits to prevent dental caries (dental caries predispose the child to bacteremia and endocarditis).

9. Encourage heart healthy eating and exercise routines.

10. Encourage age appropriate activities. A few children will need exercise restrictions. Children with CHD should be allowed to participate in activities with rest periods as needed. Children with pacemakers and children on anticoagulation therapy should refrain from participating in contact sports.

11. Maintain standard childhood immunization schedule. Delay vaccines around the perioperative time until fully recovered from surgery.

12. Encourage yearly influenza vaccine for children with unrepaired or complex congenital heart disease.

Outcome-Based Evaluation

- Child describes procedure without fear; parents and child discuss procedure and ask appropriate questions
- Vital signs stable, no signs of infection
- Parents offer support to child

SELECTED REFERENCES

Bove, E.L., Mosca, R.S. (1996). Surgical repair of hypoplastic left heart syndrome. *Progress Pediatric Cardiology, 5*, 23–35.

Emmanouilides, G.C., Allen, H.D., Riemenschneider, T.A., & Gutgesell, H.P. (1998). *Clinical synopsis of Moss and Adams' heart disease in infants, children and adolescents.* Baltimore: Williams & Wilkins.

Hawkins, J.A., Minich, L.L., Tani, L.Y., Day, R.W., Judd, V.E., Shaddy, R.E., & McGough, E.C. (1998). Late results and reintervention after aortic valvotomy for critical aortic stenosis in neonates and infants. *Annals of Thoracic Surgery, 65*, 1758–62.

Hoffman, T.M., Wernovsky, G., Wieand, T.S., et al. (1999). Predictors of arrhythmias in a pediatric cardiac intensive care unit. *Journal of the American College of Cardiology, 33*, 539A.

Jackson, P.L., & Vessey, V.A. (1996). *Primary care of the child with a chronic condition.* St. Louis: Mosby.

Kanter, K.R., Tam, V.K., Vincent, R.N., Cuadrado, A.R., Raviele, A.A., & Berg, A.M. (1999). Current results with pediatric heart transplantation. *Annals of Thoracic Surgery, 68*, 527–31.

Moloney-Harmon, P.A., & Smith, J.B. (1996). *Critical care nursing of infants and children.* Philadelphia: W.B. Saunders.

Mullins, C.E., & Mayer, D.C. (1994). *Congenital heart disease: A diagrammatic atlas.* New York: John Wiley.

Nichols, D.G., Cameron, D.E., Greeley, W.J., Lappe, D.G., Ungerleider, R.M., & Wetzel, R.C. (1995). *Critical heart disease in infants and children.* St. Louis: Mosby.

Snider, A.B., Serwer, G.A., & Ritter, S.B. (1997). *Echocardiography in pediatric heart disease.* St Louis: Mosby.

Pediatric Neurologic Disorders

NEUROLOGIC AND NEUROSURGICAL DISORDERS

◼ Cerebral Palsy

Cerebral palsy is a comprehensive diagnostic term used to designate a group of nonprogressive disorders resulting from malfunction of the motor centers and pathways of the brain. Although there are varying degrees and clinical manifestations of cerebral palsy, it is generally characterized by paralysis, weakness, incoordination, or ataxia. Cerebral palsy occurs in approximately 2 per 1,000 live births. It is a major cause of disability among children.

Pathophysiology and Etiology
Prenatal Factors (Most Common)
1. Infection, such as rubella, toxoplasmosis, herpes simplex, and cytomegalovirus
2. Maternal anoxia, anemia, placental infarcts, abruptio placentae
3. Prenatal cerebral hemorrhage, maternal bleeding, maternal toxemia, Rh or ABO incompatibility
4. Prenatal anoxia, twisting or kinking of the cord
5. Genetic factors
6. Miscellaneous—toxins, drugs

Perinatal Factors
1. Anoxia from any cause
   a. Anesthetic and analgesic drugs administered during labor
   b. Prolonged labor
   c. Placenta previa or abruptio placentae
   d. Respiratory obstruction
2. Cerebral trauma during delivery
3. Complications of birth
   a. "Small for date" babies, prematurity, immaturity, postmaturity, low birth weight (especially <1,500 g)
   b. Hyperbilirubinemia
   c. Hemolytic disorders
   d. Respiratory distress
   e. Infections
   f. Electrolyte disturbances (hypoglycemia, hypocalcemia)

Postnatal Factors
1. Head trauma
2. Infections
   a. Meningitis
   b. Encephalitis
   c. Brain abscess
3. Vascular accidents
4. Anoxia
5. Neoplastic and late neurodevelopmental defects

Types of Cerebral Palsy (Table 46-1)
1. Spastic type—defect in the cortical motor area or pyramidal tract causes abnormally strong tonus of certain muscle groups.
   a. Attempt to move a joint causes muscles to contract and block the motion.
   b. Permanent contractures develop without muscle training.
2. Dyskinetic type—lesions of the extrapyramidal tract and basal ganglia cause involuntary, uncoordinated, uncontrollable movements of muscle groups.
3. Ataxia—disturbances of balance result from cerebellar involvement.

Clinical Manifestations
Early Signs
Early signs may include one or more of the following:
1. Asymmetric movements
2. Listlessness or irritability
3. Difficulty in feeding or swallowing or poor sucking with tongue thrust
4. Excessive, high-pitched, or feeble cry

TABLE 46-1 Classification of Cerebral Palsy

Type	Characteristics
Classification by Clinical Type	

Spasticity—40%–50%; usually appears by 6 mo	1. Persistent primitive reflexes; delay of normal posture control, spastic paresis
	2. Arms pressed against body with forearm bent at right angle and hand flexed against forearm; in milder cases, fingers overextended and rotation of wrist on reaching
	3. Legs usually more involved than arms, but may be less involved
	   a. Mild cases—wide-based gait on walking
	   b. Moderate cases—slow and labored movements; walking jerky; balance poor
	   c. Severe cases—unable to sit or walk unsupported
	   d. Bilateral leg involvement—contractures cause scissoring (legs crossing and toes pointing out)

Dysthnesia—20%–25%; accentuated by emotional stress	1. Involuntary extraneous motor activity known as athetosis 2. Jerky, irregular, twisting movements of any or all extremities, especially the fingers and wrists, except when sleeping 3. Walk writhing, lurching, stumbling with incoordination of the arms 4. Improvement when well rested and calm
Ataxia—1%–10%	1. Difficulty achieving and maintaining balance, gross or fine motor incoordination 2. High-stepping, stumbling, or lurching gait 3. Nystagmus
Topographical Classification	
Hemiplegia—35%–40%	1. Findings limited to one side of the body 2. Arm usually involved more than leg
Diplegia—10%–20%	1. Similar parts of both sides of body involved 2. Legs usually involved more than arms
Paraplegia—10%–20%	1. Legs only involved
Quadriplegia—15%–20%	1. All four extremities involved 2. Upper and lower extremities affected equally
Monoplegia—rare	1. Only one extremity involved
Triplegia—rare	1. Three extremities involved
Classification by Degree of Severity	
Mild	1. Impairment of only fine precision movement
Moderate	1. Gross and fine movements and speech impaired 2. Able to perform usual activities of living
Severe	1. Inability to perform adequately the usual activities of living (walking, using hands, communicating verbally)

5. Long, thin infants who are slow to gain weight
6. Poor head control

Late Signs

Late signs may include one or more of the following:

1. Failure to follow normal pattern of motor development. Delayed gross motor development is a universal manifestation of cerebral palsy.
2. Persistence of infantile reflexes
3. Weakness
4. Preference for one hand before the infant is 12 to 15 months old
5. Abnormal postures
6. Delayed or defective speech
7. Evidence of mental retardation

Common Associated Findings

1. Seizures
2. Hearing deficiency
3. Visual defect
4. Perceptual disorders
5. Mental retardation
6. Language disorders
7. Growth disorders
8. Gastroesophageal reflux
9. Behavioral problems

Diagnostic Evaluation

1. Thorough evaluation of prenatal, perinatal, and postnatal factors; Apgar scores
2. Computed tomography (CT) scan or magnetic resonance imaging (MRI) and blood testing to rule out presence of toxins, infectious processes, neoplasms
3. Psychological testing to determine cognitive functioning

Treatment

1. Correction or alleviation of specific neuromotor deficits or associated disabilities

a. Administration of antispasticity medications, such as dantrolene (Dantrium) or diazepam (Valium)

b. Administration of antireflux medications, such as metoclopramide (Reglan) or bethanechol (Duvoid)

c. Orthopedic management of scoliosis, contractures, dislocations

d. Selective dorsal rhizotomy in an attempt to decrease spasticity

2. Developmental enrichment experiences

a. Development of prevocational, vocational, and socialization skills

b. Emotional, behavioral, and social adjustments

3. Family's ability to carry out supportive and participant roles in rehabilitation—key determinant of the success of any comprehensive management program

Complications

Contractures

Nursing Assessment

1. Perform a functional assessment; determine ability to perform activities of daily living.

2. Perform a developmental assessment; use Denver developmental (p. 1234) or other screening tool.

3. Evaluate ability to protect airway—gag reflex, swallowing.

4. Assess nutritional status—growth, signs of deficiency.

5. Assess neuromuscular function and mobility—range of motion, spasticity, coordination.

6. Assess speech, hearing, vision.

7. Evaluate parent–child interactions.

8. Determine parents' understanding of and compliance with treatment plan.

Nursing Diagnoses

- Impaired Physical Mobility related to altered neuromuscular functioning
- Altered Growth and Development related to the nature and extent of the disorder
- Altered Family Processes related to the nature of the defect, the demands of daily management, and resultant changes in family life
- Risk for Injury related to deficit in motor activity and coordination

Nursing Interventions

Increasing Mobility and Minimizing Deformity

1. Carry out and teach the parents to carry out appropriate exercises under the direction of the physical therapist.

2. Use splints and braces to facilitate muscle control and improve body functioning.

a. Apply as directed.

b. Remove for recommended time.

c. Inspect underlying skin for redness and irritation, signs of improper application, or poor fit.

3. Use assistive devices, such as adapted grooming tools, writing implements, and utensils, to enhance independence. Handles of toothbrushes, spoons, and forks can be built up with sponges or specially curved to make holding easier.

4. Encourage self-dressing with easy pull-on pants, large sweatshirts, and other loose clothing.

5. Use play, such as board games, ball games, peg boards, and puzzles, to improve coordination.

6. Maintain good body alignment to prevent contractures.

7. Provide adequate rest periods.

a. Avoid exciting events before rest or bedtime.

b. Administer or teach parents to administer muscle relaxants or anticonvulsants as prescribed.

c. Schedule physical therapy after child has rested, and avoid stress and frustration during physical therapy.

Maximizing Growth and Development

1. Evaluate the child's developmental level and then assist with tasks within that level.

2. Provide for continuity of care at home, day care, therapy centers, and the hospital.

a. Obtain a thorough history from the parents regarding the child's usual home routines, weaknesses and strengths, and likes and dislikes.

b. Communicate with representatives from all disciplines involved in the child's care.

c. Formulate a consistent care plan that incorporates the goals of all related disciplines and meets the needs of the child and family. Include in the care plan guidelines for the following:

(i) Feeding

(ii) Sleeping

(iii) Physical therapy

(iv) Play

(v) Other ways to foster growth and development

(vi) Special interests and emotional needs, such as use of security objects

3. During feeding, maintain a pleasant, distraction-free environment.

a. Provide a comfortable chair.

b. Serve the child alone, initially. After the child begins to master the task of eating, encourage the child to eat with other children.

c. Do not attempt feedings if the child is very fatigued.

d. Find the eating position in which the child can be most self-sufficient.

e. Allow the child to hold the spoon even if self-feeding is minimal.

f. Stand behind and reach over the child's shoulder to guide the spoon from the plate to the child's mouth.

g. Serve foods that stick to the spoon, such as thick applesauce or mashed potatoes.

h. Encourage finger foods that the child can handle alone.

i. Provide appropriate assistive devices for independent feeding, such as spoon and fork with special handles, plate and glass holders, and special feeding chair.

j. Disregard "messy" eating; use a large plastic bib, smock, or towel to protect the child's clothes.

4. If the child must be fed, do so slowly and carefully. Be aware of any difficulty sucking and swallowing due to poor muscle control.
   a. Cut solid foods into small pieces.
   b. Place the food back on the tongue for ease in swallowing.

5. Be alert for associated sensory deficits that delay development and could be corrected.
   a. Hearing, speech, vision
   b. Squinting, failure to follow objects, or bringing objects very close to the face

Strengthening Family Processes

1. Encourage the parents to express their feelings about the child and cerebral palsy, and help them to deal with these feelings.
2. Assist the parents to appraise the child's assets so they may capitalize on these positive features.
   a. Early recognition of the extent of the child's disability and realistic direction for obtainable goals are essential.
   b. Help the parents to recognize immediate needs and identify short-term goals that can be integrated into the long-range plan.
3. Acknowledge the numerous challenges of daily care of a child with cerebral palsy, and allow the parents to express frustration over the many demands and limited resources for such care.
4. Provide positive feedback for effective parenting skills and positive approaches to caring for the child.
5. Assist the parents to deal with siblings' responses to the disabled child.
   a. Encourage parents to find time to spend with each sibling separately.
   b. Encourage family to maintain contacts with friends and community and engage in outside activities as much as possible.
   c. Suggest family counseling.
6. Assist the parents to secure respite care to provide a break from the day-to-day care of the child with cerebral palsy when needed.
7. Assist parents to find local resources to help in the child's care.
   a. Look in phone book for county social service agency.
   b. Contact hospital social worker or discharge planner.
   c. Contact local United Way or Catholic Charities office.
   d. Visit public library to look up specific community service programs.

Protecting the Child From Injury

1. Evaluate the child's need for specific safety measures, such as suction machine, safety helmet, or seizure precautions, and modify the environment as appropriate to ensure the child's safety.
2. Select toys that are safe.

Community and Home Care Considerations

1. Assess the home environment for safety. Stairs should be gated, clear paths available for walking with assistive devices.
2. Query parents about keeping health maintenance visits, immunizations, and so forth. Help with transportation if needed.
3. Assess whether infant/child is getting social and play time. Work with physical therapy (PT)/occupational therapy (OT) to help parents choose appropriate toys.
4. If in school, participate in the development of the child's Individual Education Plan (IEP). Ensure regular updates.
5. Reinforce parental knowledge and performance of exercises, contracture prevention, and infection prevention.
6. Assess the family unit for signs of stress, and help them arrange for respite care as needed.
7. Check all adaptive equipment, braces, walkers, and so forth for correctness of fit. Arrange for replacement as needed.
8. Provide care and teach family about surgical procedures as indicated.

Family Education and Health Maintenance

1. Instruct the parents in all areas of the child's physical care.
2. Encourage regular medical and dental evaluations.
   a. The child should receive all regular immunizations.
   b. Dental visits should occur every 6 months, starting at the age of 2 years.
3. Advise parents that the child needs discipline to feel secure and relaxed.
   a. Set realistic limits within which the child can function successfully.
   b. Be firm but not rejecting.
4. Refer parents to agencies such as The United Cerebral Palsy Association of America, Inc., 1660 L St. NW, Suite 700, Washington, DC 20036, 800-872-5827; *www.ucp.org.*

Outcome-Based Evaluation

- Dressing and feeding independently; no contractures noted
- Consistent growth curve maintained; sequential developmental milestones consistent with condition achieved
- Participation in school and community activities; use of respite care once a week, as needed
- Child wearing bicycle helmet while playing outdoors; no injury reported
- Child attending school, with IEP in place, and progress reported at each assessment

◼ Hydrocephalus

Hydrocephalus is a condition of altered production, flow, or absorption of cerebrospinal fluid (CSF). It is characterized by an abnormal increase in CSF volume within the intracranial cavity and by enlargement of the head in infancy.

Occurs in approximately 3 to 4 cases per 1,000 births, including those associated with spina bifida.

Pathophysiology and Etiology

1. Noncommunicating hydrocephalus—obstruction in the system between the source of CSF production (ventricles) and the area of its reabsorption (the subarachnoid space).
   a. May be partial, intermittent, or complete.
   b. Occurs in the majority of cases.
   c. Caused by congenital defects such as Arnold-Chiari malformation, Dandy-Walker cyst (etiology largely unknown), aqueductal stenosis (neurofibromatosis).
   d. Also caused by acquired conditions such as infections, trauma, spontaneous intracranial bleeding, and neoplasms.
2. Communicating hydrocephalus:
   a. Failure in the absorption system; cause unknown.
   b. Excessive production of CSF—tumor or unknown causes (rare).
3. The ventricular system becomes greatly distended.
   a. The increased ventricular pressure results in thinning of the cerebral cortex and cranial bones, especially in the frontal, parietal, and temporal areas.
   b. The floor of the third ventricle commonly bulges downward, compresses the optic nerves, dilates the sella turcica, and often compresses the hypophysis cerebri.
   c. The basal ganglia, brain stem, and cerebellum remain relatively normal but compressed.
   d. The choroid plexus is usually atrophied to some degree.

Clinical Manifestations

May be rapid, slow and steadily advancing, or remittent. Clinical signs depend on the age of the child, whether the anterior fontanelle has closed, whether the cranial sutures have fused, and the type and duration of hydrocephalus.

Infants

1. Excessive head growth (may be seen up to 3 years of age)
2. Delayed closure of the anterior fontanelle
3. Fontanelle tense and elevated above the surface of the skull
4. Signs of increased intracranial pressure (IICP; Box 46-1)
5. Alteration of muscle tone of the extremities, including clonus or spasticity
6. Later physical signs:
   a. Forehead becomes prominent ("bossing").
   b. Scalp appears shiny with prominent scalp veins.
   c. Eyebrows and eyelids may be drawn upward, exposing the sclera above the iris.
   d. Infant cannot gaze upward, causing "sunset eyes."
   e. Strabismus, nystagmus, and optic atrophy may occur.
   f. Infant has difficulty holding head up.
   g. Child may experience physical or mental developmental lag.

> **BOX 46-1 Signs and Symptoms of IICP in Infants and Children**
>
> Vomiting
> Restlessness and irritability
> High-pitched, shrill cry (infants)
> Rapid increase in head circumference (infants)
> Tense, bulging fontanelle (infants)
> Changes in vital signs:
>   Increased systolic blood pressure
>   Decreased pulse
>   Decreased and irregular respirations
>   Increased temperature
> Pupillary changes
> Papilledema
> Possible seizures
> Lethargy, stupor, coma
> Older children may also experience:
>   Headache, especially on awakening
>   Lethargy, fatigue, apathy
>   Personality changes
>   Separation of cranial sutures (may be seen in children up to age 10)
>   Visual changes such as double vision

Older Children

Older children have closed sutures and present with signs of IICP.

Diagnostic Evaluation

1. Infant's head transilluminates, indicative of abnormal fluid collection.
2. Percussion of the infant's skull may produce a typical "cracked pot" sound (Macewen's sign).
3. Ophthalmoscopy may reveal papilledema.
4. CT scan is the diagnostic tool of choice.
5. With ventriculography (rarely used), abnormalities are visualized in the ventricular system or the subarachnoid space.
6. Skull x-rays show widening of the fontanelle and sutures and erosion of intracranial bone.

Treatment

Hydrocephalus can be treated through a variety of surgical procedures, including direct operation on the lesion causing the obstruction, such as a tumor; intracranial shunts for selected cases of noncommunicating hydrocephalus to divert fluid from the obstructed segment of the ventricular system to the subarachnoid space; and extracranial shunts (most common) to divert fluid from the ventricular system to an extracranial compartment, frequently the peritoneum or right atrium.

Extracranial Shunt Procedures

1. Ventriculoperitoneal shunt (V–P shunt; Figure 46-1):
   a. Diverts CSF from a lateral ventricle or the spinal subarachnoid space to the peritoneal cavity.

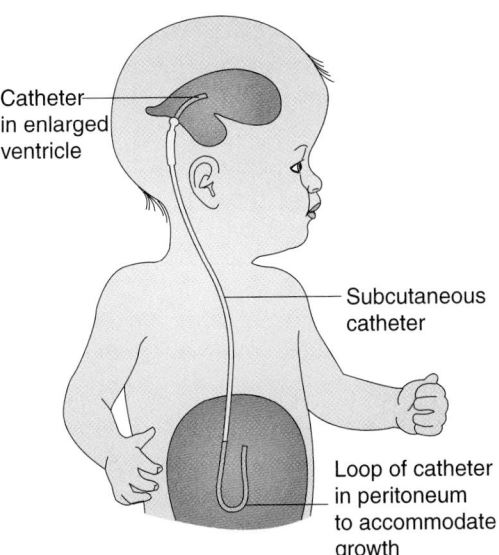

Catheter in enlarged ventricle

Subcutaneous catheter

Loop of catheter in peritoneum to accommodate growth

FIGURE 46-1 A ventriculoperitoneal shunt removes excessive cerebrospinal fluid from the ventricles and shunts it to the peritoneum. A one-way valve is present in the tubing behind the ear.

b. A tube is passed from the lateral ventricle through an occipital burr hole subcutaneously through the posterior aspect of neck and paraspinal region to the peritoneal cavity through a small incision in the right lower quadrant.

2. Ventriculoatrial shunt (V–A shunt):
   a. A tube is passed from the dilated lateral ventricle through a burr hole in the parietal region of the skull.
   b. It then is passed under the skin behind the ear and into a vein down to a point where it discharges into the right atrium or superior vena cava.
   c. A one-way pressure sensitive valve will close to prevent reflux of blood into the ventricle and open as ventricular pressure rises, allowing fluid to pass from the ventricle into the bloodstream.

3. Ventriculopleural shunt:
   a. Diverts CSF to the pleural cavity
   b. Indicated when the V–P or V–A route cannot be used

4. Ventricle–gall bladder shunt:
   a. Diverts CSF to the common bile duct
   b. Used when all other routes are unavailable

5. Most shunts have the following components:
   a. Ventricular tubing
   b. A one-way or unidirectional pressure sensitive flow valve
   c. A pumping chamber
   d. Distal tubing

Shunt Complications

1. Need for shunt revision frequently occurs because of occlusion, infection, or malfunction.

2. Shunt revision may be necessary because of growth of the child. Newer models, however, include coiled tubing to allow the shunt to grow with the child.

3. Shunt dependency frequently occurs. The child rapidly manifests symptoms of IICP if the shunt does not function optimally.

4. Children with V–A shunts may experience endocardial contusions and clotting, leading to bacterial endocarditis, bacteremia, and ventriculitis or thromboembolism and cor pulmonale.

Prognosis

1. Prognosis depends on early diagnosis and prompt therapy.

2. With improved diagnostic and management techniques, the prognosis is becoming considerably better.
   a. Many children experience normal motor and intellectual development.
   b. The severity of neurologic deficits is directly proportional to the interval between onset of hydrocephalus and the time of diagnosis.

3. Hydrocephalus due to meningitis might spontaneously resolve due to gradual disappearance of adhesions.

4. Approximately two thirds of patients will die at an early age if they do not receive surgical treatment.

Complications

1. Seizures
2. Herniation of the brain
3. Spontaneous arrest due to natural compensatory mechanisms, persistent IICP, and brain herniation
4. Developmental delays

Nursing Assessment

Infants

1. Assess head circumference.
   a. Measure at the occipitofrontal circumference—point of largest measurement.
   b. Measure the head at approximately the same time each day.
   c. Use a centimeter measure for greatest accuracy.

2. Palpate fontanelle for tenseness, bulging.
3. Assess pupillary response.
4. Assess level of consciousness.
5. Evaluate breathing patterns and effectiveness.
6. Assess feeding patterns and patterns of emesis.
7. Assess motor activity.
8. Determine attainment of developmental milestones.

Older Child

1. Measure vital signs for signs of IICP.
2. Assess patterns of headache, emesis.
3. Determine pupillary response.
4. Evaluate level of consciousness.
5. Assess motor function.
6. Evaluate attainment of milestones, school performance.
7. Obtain parents' report of recent behavior.

Nursing Diagnoses

- Altered Cerebral Tissue perfusion related to IICP prior to surgery
- Altered Nutrition: Less Than Body Requirements related to reduced oral intake and vomiting
- Risk for Impaired Skin Integrity related to alterations in level of consciousness and enlarged head
- Anxiety (of parents) related to child undergoing surgery
- Risk for Injury related to malfunctioning shunt
- Risk for Fluid Volume Deficit related to CSF drainage, decreased intake postoperatively
- Risk for Infection related to bacterial infiltration of the shunt
- Ineffective Family Coping related to diagnosis and surgery

Nursing Interventions

Maintaining Cerebral Perfusion

1. Observe for evidence of IICP, and report immediately.

> **NURSING ALERT**
>
> Brain stem herniation can occur with IICP and is manifested by opisthotonic positioning (flexion of head and feet backward). This is a grave sign and may be followed by respiratory arrest. Obtain help, and prepare for ventricular tap. Have emergency equipment on hand for resuscitation.

2. Assist with diagnostic procedures to determine cause of hydrocephalus and indication for surgical intervention.
   a. Explain the procedure to the child and parents at their levels of comprehension.
   b. Administer prescribed sedatives 30 minutes before the procedure to ensure their effectiveness.
   c. Organize activities so the child is permitted to rest after administration of the sedative.

> **DRUG ALERT**
>
> Sedatives are contraindicated in many cases because IICP predisposes the child to hypoventilation or respiratory arrest. If they are administered, the child should be observed very closely for evidence of respiratory depression.

   d. Observe closely after ventriculography for the following:
      (i) Leaking of CSF from the sites of subdural or ventricular taps. These tap holes should be covered with a small piece of gauze or cotton saturated with collodion.
      (ii) Reactions to the sedative, especially respiratory depression
      (iii) Changes in vital signs indicative of shock
      (iv) Signs of IICP, which may occur if air has been injected into the ventricles

Providing Adequate Nutrition

1. Be aware that feeding is often a problem because the child may be listless, anorectic, and prone to vomiting.

2. Complete nursing care and treatments before feeding so the child will not be disturbed after feeding.

3. Hold the infant in a semisitting position with head well supported during feeding. Allow ample time for bubbling.

4. Offer small, frequent feedings.

5. Place the child on side with head elevated after feeding to prevent aspiration.

Maintaining Skin Integrity

1. Prevent pressure sores (pressure sores of the head are a frequent problem) by placing the child on a sponge rubber or lamb's wool pad or an alternating-pressure or egg-crate mattress to keep weight evenly distributed.

2. Keep the scalp clean and dry.

3. Turn the child's head frequently; change position at least every 2 hours.
   a. When turning the child, rotate head and body together to prevent strain on the neck.
   b. A firm pillow may be placed under the child's head and shoulders for further support when lifting the child.

4. Provide meticulous skin care to all parts of the body, and observe skin for the effects of pressure.

5. Give passive range-of-motion exercises to the extremities, especially the legs.

6. Keep the eyes moistened with artificial tears if the child is unable to close the eyelids normally. This prevents corneal ulcerations and infections.

Reducing Anxiety

1. Prepare the parents for their child's surgery by answering questions, describing what nursing care will take place postoperatively, and explaining how the shunt will work.

2. Encourage the parents to discuss all the risks and benefits with the surgeon. Help them to understand the prognosis and what to expect of the child's neurologic and cognitive development.

3. Prepare the child for surgery by using dolls or other forms of play to describe what interventions will occur.

Improving Cerebral Tissue Perfusion

Postoperatively

1. Monitor the child's temperature, pulse, respiration, blood pressure, and pupillary size and reaction every 15 minutes until stable; then monitor every 1 to 2 hours.

2. Avoid hypothermia or hyperthermia.
   a. Provide appropriate blankets or covers, an Isolette or infant warmer, or hypothermia blanket.
   b. Administer a tepid sponge bath or antipyretic medication for temperature elevation.

3. Aspirate mucus from the nose and throat as necessary to prevent respiratory difficulty.

4. Turn the child frequently.

5. Promote optimal drainage of CSF through the shunt by pumping the shunt and positioning the child as directed.
   a. If pumping is prescribed, carefully compress the valve the specified number of times at regularly scheduled intervals.

b. Report any difficulties in pumping the shunt.

c. Gradually elevate the head of child's bed to 30 to 45 degrees as ordered. Initially, the child will be positioned flat to prevent excessive CSF drainage.

6. Assess for excessive drainage of CSF.
   a. Sunken fontanelle, agitation, restlessness (infant)
   b. Decreased level of consciousness (older child)

7. Assess closely for IICP, indicating shunt malfunction.
   a. Note especially change in level of consciousness, change in vital signs (increased systolic blood pressure, decreased pulse rate, decreased or irregular respirations), vomiting, pupillary changes.
   b. Report these changes immediately to prevent cerebral hypoxia and possible brain herniation.

8. Prevent excessive pressure of skin overlying shunt by placing cotton behind and over the ears under the head dressing and avoiding positioning the child on the area of the valve or the incision until the wound is well healed.

Maintaining Fluid Balance

1. Accurately measure and record total fluid intake and output.

2. Administer intravenous (IV) fluids as prescribed; carefully monitor infusion rate to prevent fluid overload.

3. Use a nasogastric tube if necessary for abdominal distention.
   a. This is most frequently used when a V–P shunt has been performed.
   b. Measure the drainage, and record the amount and color.
   c. Monitor for return of bowel sounds after nasogastric suction has been disconnected for at least 30 minutes.

4. Give frequent mouth care while the child is to have nothing by mouth (NPO).

5. Begin oral feedings once the child is fully recovered from the anesthetic and displays interest.
   a. Begin with small amounts of 5% dextrose water.
   b. Gradually introduce formula.
   c. Introduce solid foods suitable to the child's age and tolerance.
   d. Encourage a high-protein diet.
   e. Observe for and report any decrease in urine output, increased urine specific gravity, diminished skin turgor, dryness of mucous membranes, or lethargy, indicating dehydration.

Preventing Infection

1. Assess for fever (temperature normally fluctuates during the first 24 hours after surgery), purulent drainage from the incision, or swelling, redness, and tenderness along the shunt tract.

2. Administer prescribed prophylactic antibiotics.

Strengthening Family Coping

1. Begin discharge planning early, including specific techniques for care of the shunt and suggested methods for providing daily care.
   a. Turning, holding, and positioning
   b. Skin care over shunt

c. Exercises to strengthen muscles—incorporated with play
   d. Feeding techniques and schedule
   e. Pumping the shunt

2. Accompany all instructions with reassurance necessary to prevent the parents from becoming anxious or fearful about assuming the care of the child.

3. Encourage the parents to treat the child as normally as possible, providing him or her with appropriate toys and love.

4. Help the parents to assist siblings to understand hydrocephalus and the child's special needs. Encourage parents to spend individual time with siblings and not to neglect their needs as well. Suggest family counseling if needed.

5. Assist parents in locating additional resources.
   a. Social worker, discharge planner, or department of social services
   b. Visiting or home health nurses or aides
   c. Parent groups
   d. Community agencies
   e. Special programs at school

Community and Home Care Considerations

1. Follow the Community and Home Care Considerations listed under Cerebral Palsy on p. 1403. Check shunt functioning regularly, and reinforce parental performance of shunt checks and assessment for shunt malfunction and IICP.

2. Perform total physical assessment regularly, looking for signs of trauma or skin breakdown.

3. Patient should wear a Medic-Alert bracelet, once he or she starts to attend school or day care.

4. Ensure that parents/caregivers are certified in CPR.

Family Education and Health Maintenance

1. Stress the importance of recognizing symptoms of IICP and reporting them immediately.

2. Advise parents to report shunt malfunction or infection immediately to prevent IICP.

3. Teach parents that illnesses that cause vomiting and diarrhea or that prevent an adequate fluid intake are a great threat to the child who has had a shunt procedure. Advise parents to consult with the child's health care provider about immediate treatment of fever, control of vomiting and diarrhea, and replacement of fluids.

4. Tell the parents that few restrictions are required for children with shunts and to consult with the health care provider about specific concerns.

5. Alert parents that additional information and support are available from the Hydrocephalus Association, 870 Market Street, Suite 705, San Francisco, CA 94102, 415-732-7040, *www.hydroassoc.org*.

Outcome-Based Evaluation

- No changes in vital signs, level of consciousness, or head size; no vomiting; pupils equal and responsive

- Feeding every 4 hours without vomiting; no significant weight loss
- No erythema, blanching, or skin breakdown; wound healing evident
- Parents verbalizing purpose and type of operative procedure, risks, and benefits
- Shunt pumping without resistance; stable level of consciousness and vital signs
- Urine output less than intake; skin turgor normal; electrolytes within normal limits
- Afebrile; no drainage from shunt site
- Parents actively seeking resources, showing affection for patient and siblings

Spina Bifida

Spina bifida, also called spinal dysraphia, refers to a malformation of the spine in which the posterior portion of the laminae of the vertebrae fails to close. It occurs in approximately 1 per 1,000 live births in the United States and is the most common developmental defect of the central nervous system (CNS). It is more common in white than in nonwhite people.

Several types of spina bifida are recognized, of which the following three are most common (Figure 46-2):

Spina Bifida Occulta

The defect is only in the vertebrae. The spinal cord and meninges are normal.

Meningocele

The meninges protrude through the opening in the spinal canal. This forms a cyst filled with CSF and covered with skin.

Myelomeningocele (or Meningomyelocele)

Both the spinal cord and cord membranes protrude through the defect in the laminae of the vertebral column. Myelomeningoceles are covered by a thin membrane.

Pathophysiology and Etiology

1. Unknown etiology but generally thought to result from genetic predisposition triggered by something in the environment.
   a. Certain drugs, including valproic acid, have been known to cause neural tube defects if administered during pregnancy.
   b. Women who have spina bifida and parents who have one affected child have an increased risk of producing children with neural tube defects.
2. Involves an arrest in the orderly formation of the vertebral arches and spinal cord that occurs between the 4th and 6th week of embryogenesis.
3. Theories of causation include:
   a. There is incomplete closure of the neural tube during the 4th week of embryonic life.
   b. The neural tube forms adequately, then ruptures.

> ◆ **DRUG ALERT**
>
> Maternal periconceptional use of folic acid supplementation reduced by 50% or more the incidence of neural tube defects in pregnancies at risk.

4. In spina bifida occulta, the bony defect may range from a very thin slit separating one lamina from the spinous process to a complete absence of the spine and laminae.
   a. A thin, fibrous membrane sometimes covers the defect.
   b. The spinal cord and its meninges may be connected with a fistulous tract extending to and opening onto the surface of the skin.
5. In meningocele, the defect may occur anywhere on the cord. Higher defects (from thorax and upward) are usually meningoceles.

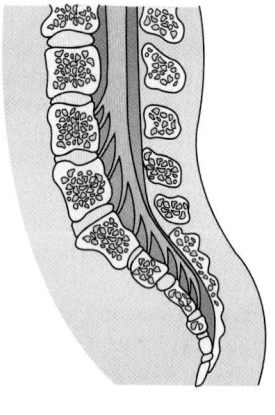 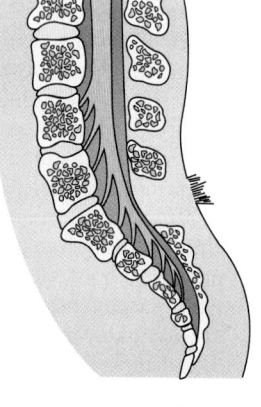 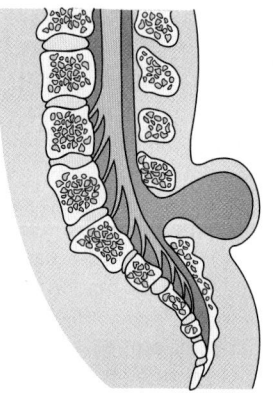 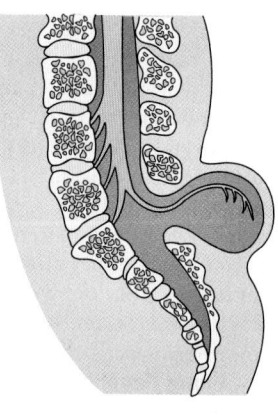

| A | B | C | D |

FIGURE 46-2 Spina bifida. (**A**) Normal spine. (**B**) Spina bifida occulta. (**C**) Spina bifida with meningocele. (**D**) Spina bifida with myelomeningocele.

a. Surgical correction is necessary to prevent rupture of the sac and subsequent infection.

b. Prognosis is good with surgical correction.

6. In myelomeningocele (meningomyelocele), the lesion contains both the spinal cord and cord membranes.

a. A bluish area may be evident on the top because of exposed neural tissue.

b. The sac may leak in utero or may rupture after birth, allowing free drainage of CSF. This renders the child highly susceptible to meningitis.

c. Occurs four to five times more frequently than meningocele.

Clinical Manifestations

Spina Bifida Occulta

1. Most patients have no symptoms.

a. They may have a dimple in the skin or a growth of hair over the malformed vertebra.

b. There is no externally visible sac.

2. With growth, the child may develop foot weakness or bowel and bladder sphincter disturbances.

3. This condition is occasionally associated with more significant developmental abnormalities of the spinal cord, including syringomyelia and tethered cord.

Meningocele

1. An external cystic defect can be seen in the spinal cord, usually in the midline.

a. The sac is composed only of meninges and is filled with CSF.

b. The cord and nerve roots are usually normal.

2. There is seldom evidence of weakness of the legs or lack of sphincter control.

Myelomeningocele

1. A round, raised, and poorly epithelialized area may be noted at any level of the spinal column. However, the highest incidence of the lesion occurs in the lumbosacral area.

2. Clinical problems due to myelomeningocele include the following:

a. Arnold-Chiari malformation

(i) Associated malformation involving the brain stem and cerebellum

(ii) Causes a block in the flow of CSF through the ventricles and leads to failure in the reabsorption mechanism of CSF

(iii) Produces significant hydrocephalus in approximately two thirds of children with myelomeningocele

b. Loss of motor control and sensation below the level of the lesion can occur. These conditions are highly variable and depend on the size of the lesion and its position on the cord.

(i) A low thoracic lesion may cause total flaccid paralysis below the waist.

(ii) A small sacral lesion may cause only patchy spots of decreased sensation in the feet.

c. Contractures may occur in the ankles, knees, or hips. Hips may be pulled out of the sockets.

(i) Nature and degree of involvement depend on size and location of lesion.

(ii) This occurs because some fibers of innervation do get through. One side of a hip, knee, or ankle may be innervated while the opposing side may not be. The unopposed side then becomes pulled out of position.

d. Clubfeet are a common accompanying anomaly. This anomaly is thought to be related to the position of paraplegic feet in the uterus.

e. Bladder dysfunction can occur.

(i) Almost all lesions affect the sacral nerves that innervate the bladder.

(ii) The bladder fails to respond to normal messages that it is time to void and simply fills and overflows, causing incontinence and susceptibility to urinary tract infections because of incomplete emptying.

f. Fecal incontinence and constipation are caused by poor innervation of the anal sphincter and bowel musculature.

3. Developmental disabilities include the following:

a. Most children have average intellectual ability despite hydrocephalus.

b. Most children are able to learn in a "mainstreamed" school environment, provided they are able to overcome other barriers (architectural and attitudinal).

c. The most significant problems are secondarily handicapping conditions that develop when a child has a disability of this degree.

Diagnostic Evaluation

1. Prenatal detection is now possible through amniocentesis and measurement of alpha-fetoprotein (AFP). This testing should be offered to all women at risk (women who are affected or have had other affected children).

2. Diagnosis is primarily based on clinical manifestations.

3. CT scan and MRI may be performed to evaluate further the brain and spinal cord.

Treatment

Surgical Intervention

1. Procedure: laminectomy and closure of the open lesion or removal of the sac usually can be done soon after birth.

2. Purpose:

a. To prevent further deterioration of neural function

b. To minimize the danger of rupture and infection, especially meningitis

c. To improve cosmetic effect

d. To facilitate handling of the infant

Multidisciplinary Follow-Up for Associated Problems

1. A coordinated team approach will help maximize the physical and intellectual potential of each affected child.

2. The team may include a neurologist, neurosurgeon, orthopedic surgeon, urologist, primary care provider, social worker, physical therapist, a variety of community-based and hospital staff nurses, and the child and family.
3. Numerous neurosurgical, orthopedic, and urologic procedures may be necessary to help the child achieve maximum potential.

Prognosis

1. Influenced by the site of the lesion and the presence and degree of associated hydrocephalus. Generally, the higher the defect, the greater the extent of neurologic deficit and the greater the likelihood of hydrocephalus.
2. In the absence of treatment, most infants with meningomyelocele die early in infancy.
3. Surgical intervention is most effective if it is done early in the neonatal period, preferably within the first few days of life.
4. Even with surgical intervention, infants can be expected to manifest associated neurosurgical, orthopedic, or urologic problems.
5. New techniques of treatment, intensive research, and improved services have increased life expectancy and have greatly enhanced the quality of life for most children who receive treatment.

Complications

1. Hydrocephalus associated with meningocele; may be aggravated by surgical repair
2. Scoliosis, contractures, and joint dislocation
3. Skin breakdown in sensory denervated areas and under braces

Nursing Assessment

1. Assess sensory and motor response of lower extremities.
2. Assess ability to void spontaneously, retention of urine, symptoms of urinary tract infection.
3. Assess usual stooling patterns, need for medications to facilitate elimination.
4. Assess mobility and use of braces, casts, and other special equipment.

Nursing Diagnoses
Neonatal Period (Preoperative)

- Risk for Impaired Skin Integrity related to impaired motor and sensory function
- Risk for Infection related to contamination of the myelomeningocele site
- Altered Urinary Elimination related to neurologic deficits
- Altered Cerebral Tissue Perfusion related to potential hydrocephalus
- Fear (parents) related to neonate with neurologic disorder and to surgery

Infancy and Childhood (Postoperative)

- Ineffective Thermoregulation following surgery
- Reflex Incontinence related to sacral denervation

- Bowel Incontinence/Constipation related to impaired innervation of anal sphincter and bowel musculature
- Body Image Disturbance related to the child's appearance, difficulties with locomotion, and lack of control over excretory functions

Nursing Interventions
Neonatal Period
Protecting Skin Integrity

1. Avoid positioning on the infant's back to prevent pressure on the sac. Check position at least once every hour.
2. Do not place a diaper or other covering directly over the sac.
3. Observe the sac frequently for evidence of irritation or leakage of CSF.
4. Use prone positioning with hips only slightly flexed to decrease tension on the sac.
5. Place a foam rubber pad covered with a soft cloth between the infant's legs to maintain the hips in abduction and to prevent or counteract subluxation. A diaper roll or small pillow may be used in place of the foam rubber pad.
6. Allow the infant's feet to hang freely over the pads or mattress edge to prevent aggravation of foot deformities.
7. Provide meticulous skin care to all areas of the body, especially ankles, knees, tip of nose, cheeks, and chin.
8. Provide passive range-of-motion exercises for muscles and joints that the infant does not use spontaneously. Avoid hip exercises because of common hip dislocation, unless otherwise recommended.
9. Use a foam or fleece pad to reduce pressure of the mattress against the infant's skin.
10. Avoid pressure on infant's back during feeding by holding the infant with your elbow rotated to avoid touching the sac, or feeding while infant is lying on side or prone on your lap. Encourage parents to use these positions to provide infant stimulation and bonding.

Preventing Infection

1. Be aware that infection of the sac is most commonly caused by contamination by urine and feces.
2. Keep the buttocks and genitalia scrupulously clean.
   a. Do not diaper the infant if the defect is in the lower portion of the spine.
   b. Use a small plastic drape taped between the defect and the anus to help to prevent contamination.
3. Apply a sterile gauze pad or towel or a sterile, moistened dressing over the sac as directed.
   a. When the sterile covering is used, it should be changed frequently to keep the area free of exudate and to maintain sterility.
   b. Care must be taken to prevent the covering from adhering to and damaging the sac.
4. Monitor and report immediately any signs of infection.
   a. Oozing of fluid or pus from the sac
   b. Fever

c. Irritability or listlessness

d. Seizure

Promoting Urinary Elimination

1. Use the Credé method for emptying the bladder (unless contraindicated by vesicoureteral reflux), and teach parents the technique.
   a. Apply firm, gentle pressure to the abdomen, beginning in the umbilical area and progressing toward the symphysis pubis.
   b. Continue the procedure as long as urine can be manually expressed.
2. Ensure fluid intake to dilute the urine.
3. Administer prescribed prophylactic antibiotics.
4. Monitor and report concentrated or foul-smelling urine.

Maintaining Cerebral Tissue Perfusion

1. Monitor for signs of hydrocephalus, and report immediately.
   a. Irritability
   b. Feeding difficulty, vomiting, decreased appetite
   c. Temperature fluctuation
   d. Decreased alertness
   e. Tense fontanelle
   f. Increased head circumference

Reducing Fear

1. Encourage parents to express feelings of guilt, fear, lack of control, or helplessness.
2. Provide accurate information about spina bifida and what to expect postoperatively.
3. Include the parents in all of infant's care, and encourage private bonding time.

Infancy and Childhood
Maintaining Thermoregulation
and Preventing Complications

1. Frequently monitor temperature, pulse, respirations, color, and level of responsiveness postoperatively, based on the infant's stability.
2. Use an Isolette or infant warmer to prevent temperature fluctuation.
3. Prevent respiratory complications.
   a. Periodically reposition the infant to promote lung expansion.
   b. Watch for abdominal distention, which could interfere with breathing.
   c. Have oxygen available.
4. Maintain hydration and nutritional intake.
   a. Administer IV fluids as ordered; keep accurate intake and output log.
   b. Administer gavage feedings as ordered.
   c. Begin bottle feeding when infant is responsive and tolerating feedings. Give small, frequent feedings slowly so air can be expelled naturally without bubbling.
5. Keep the surgical dressing clean and dry, and observe for drainage. Avoid pressure to the area and diapers that cover the incision until well healed.

6. Monitor for and teach parents to recognize signs of hydrocephalus. Report immediately.
7. Limit or prevent direct contact of the child to products routinely used that contain latex, due to risk of latex allergy and severe reaction. Latex products include blood pressure cuffs, tourniquets, tape, Foley catheters, gloves, and IV tubing injection ports. Develop protocols specifying modification of care for children at risk for latex allergy.

NURSING ALERT

Be aware that children with spina bifida have a far greater risk for latex allergy than the general population, estimated at up to 20% of spina bifida patients. Symptoms include hives, itching, wheezing, and anaphylaxis. Incidence increases with time and may be related to repeated exposure to products containing latex.

Achieving Continence

1. Teach parents that continence can usually be achieved with clean, intermittent self-catheterization.
   a. Children can generally be taught to catheterize themselves by the age of 6 to 7 years.
   b. Parents can catheterize younger children.
2. Teach the following procedure:
   a. Gather equipment: catheter, water-soluble lubricant, soap and water, urine collection container.
   b. Wash hands.
   c. Clean the area around the urethral meatus.
   d. Lubricate the catheter tip.
   e. Insert the catheter until urine starts to flow.
   f. Remove catheter when urine is drained from bladder.
   g. Clean off any lubricant from child.
   h. Dispose of urine.
   i. Wash hands.
3. Teach about the action of medications, such as imipramine hydrochloride (Tofranil) and ephedrine sulfate (Ephed II), if prescribed, which are used to help children retain urine rather than dribbling. When used with self-catheterization, many children can stay dry for 3 to 4 hours at a time.
4. Teach the signs of urinary tract infection (concentrated, foul-smelling urine; irritability; pain or burning; and fever) and the proper administration of antibiotics either prophylactically or when prescribed for infection.
5. For children who cannot achieve urinary continence through intermittent catheterization, provide information about options, such as surgically implanted mechanical urinary sphincters and bladder pacemakers, indwelling catheters, external collecting devices, and urinary diversion (may be necessary in some cases).

Achieving Regular Bowel Elimination

1. Assist with bowel training program to compensate for decreased sacral sensation.
   a. Children are placed on a toileting schedule and are taught to push.

b. Medications, such as stool softeners, suppositories, or enemas, may be used initially to help determine scheduling.

2. To prevent constipation and enhance fecal control, encourage intake of high-fiber, high-fluid diet. Medications such as psyllium (Metamucil) may be used to increase bulk or soften stool.

Fostering Positive Body Image

1. Emphasize rehabilitation that makes use of the child's strengths and minimizes disabilities.
2. Continually reassess functional abilities, and offer suggestions to increase independence. Periodically consult with physical or occupational therapists to help maximize function.
3. Encourage the use of braces and specialized equipment to enhance ambulation while minimizing the appearance of the equipment. For example, wear pants instead of dresses or shorts to cover leg braces; choose a compact wheelchair that can be decorated or personalized for the child.
4. Encourage participation with peer group and in activities that build on strengths, such as cognitive abilities, interest in music, or art.
5. Periodically, reassess bowel and bladder programs. The ability to stay dry for reasonable time intervals is one of the greatest factors in enhancing self-esteem and positive body image.

Community and Home Care

1. Follow the Community and Home Care Considerations listed under Cerebral Palsy on p. 1403.
2. Survey the home environment for latex, and substitute products obtained, if possible. Toys and equipment for children, such as nipples, pacifiers, and elastic on the legs of disposable diapers, also contain latex. Teach the parents how to recognize latex allergy and to notify the child's health care provider.
3. Teach the family how to clean and reuse urinary catheters. The catheter should be washed in warm, soapy water and rinsed well in warm water. The catheter should be air dried and, when completely dried, placed in a clean jar or plastic bag. A catheter should be replaced when it becomes dry, cracked, stiff, or if the child develops a urinary tract infection.
4. Instruct the parents to notify the health care provider for signs of associated problems, such as hydrocephalus, meningitis, urinary tract infection, and latex sensitivity.

Family Education and Health Maintenance

1. Prepare the parents to feed, hold, and stimulate their infant as naturally as possible.
2. Teach the parents the special techniques that may be required for holding and positioning, feeding, caring for the incision, emptying the bladder, and exercising muscles.

3. Alert the parents to safety needs of the child with decreased sensation, such as protection from prolonged pressure, the risk of burns due to bath water that is too warm, and avoidance of trauma from contact with sharp objects.
4. Urge continued follow-up and health maintenance, including immunizations and evaluation of growth and development.
5. Advise parents that children with paralysis are at risk for becoming overweight due to inactivity, so they should provide a low-fat, balanced diet; control snacking; and encourage as much activity as possible.
6. For additional resources, refer families to agencies such as The Spina Bifida Association of America, 4590 MacArthur Blvd. NW, Suite 250, Washington, DC 20007, 800-621-3141; *www.sbaa.org*.

Outcome-Based Evaluation

- No signs of meningeal sac or skin breakdown
- Afebrile, alert, and active
- Clear urine without odor; adequate elimination; no infection
- Fontanelle soft; head circumference stable
- Parents asking questions about surgery, showing affection for infant
- Vital signs stable; incisional dressing dry and intact
- Parents/child demonstrate proper catheterization technique
- Passing stool once a day; adequate elimination; no constipation
- Child verbalizes participation in chorus, Girl or Boy Scouts, or school activities

Muscular Dystrophy

Muscular dystrophy (MD) is a group of genetically determined, progressive, degenerative myopathies affecting a variety of muscle groups. Many MD patients are children. Most with Duchenne MD rarely survive beyond 20 to 25 years of age.

Pathophysiology and Etiology

1. Inherited; may be X-linked, autosomal dominant, or recessive.
2. Genetic coding defect causes abnormal muscle development and function.
3. Loss of skeletal muscle fibers but no associated structural abnormalities in peripheral nerves or spinal cord.
4. Marked reduction of dystrophin, a protein vital to muscle function.

Clinical Manifestations

1. Progressive muscular weakness (Table 46-2).
2. Gower's sign is a hallmark feature of Duchenne MD, characterized by a child's difficulty rising from floor.

TABLE 46-2 Clinical Manifestations of Muscular Dystrophies

Disorder	Genetics	Onset	Clinical Manifestations
Duchenne's muscular dystrophy	Autosomal recessive (X-linked)	3–6 years	Progressive weakness and atrophy of iliopsoas, gluteal, and quadriceps muscles; pseudohypertrophy of the calves; waddling gait, difficulty walking and climbing stairs; later, weakening of pretibial, pectoral girdle, and upper limbs; heart abnormalities; death due to pulmonary infections before 20 years Etiology: genetic defect in which gene coding for "dystrophin" is absent
Becker's muscular dystrophy	X-linked	11 years	Similar to Duchenne's dystrophy except that course is more benign; dystrophin is abnormal
Emery-Dreifuss syndrome	X-linked	Childhood–adulthood	Upper arm and pectoral girdle weakness; distal muscles spared; severe cardiomyopathy
Facioscapulohumeral dystrophy	Autosomal dominant	6–20 years	Inability to raise arms over head, close eyes firmly, and purse the lips; scapular winging; "Popeye" effect of arms (forearms large and upper arm slim)
Limb-girdle (scapulohumeral and pelvifemoral) dystrophy	X-linked; autosomal recessive		Facial muscles spared; absence of pseudohypertrophy of the calves
Progressive external ophthalmoplegia	Familial	Childhood	Ptosis and ophthalmoparesis without strabismus or diplopia
Oculopharyngeal dystrophy	Autosomal dominant	40–50 years	Bilateral ptosis and dysphagia
Myotonic dystrophy	Autosomal dominant; genetically linked to a marker on chromosome 19 with high penetrance	Third decade	Weakness of levator palpebrae, facial, masseter, pharyngeal, laryngeal muscles, sternomastoid (weakness results in "swan neck" deformity), forearm, hand, pretibial, and cardiac muscles, myotonia of muscles; can bring out with forced eyelid closure or clenching the fist Changes in nonmuscular tissues: frontal baldness blue-green cataracts, testicular atrophy, increased insulin response to glucose
Congenital myotonic dystrophy		Birth	Profound hypotonia, facial diplegia, ptosis, tented upper lip and open jaw; difficulty in sucking and swallowing and respiratory distress
Late-onset distal muscular dystrophy (Milhorat and Wolff: Welander)	Autosomal dominant	Middle adult	Weakness and wasting of muscles of hands, forearms, and lower legs

(From Kelley, W.N. [Ed.]. [1994]. *Essentials of internal medicine.* Philadelphia: J. B. Lippincott.)

The child must take the following steps to assume a standing position:
  a. Roll onto hands and knees.
  b. Bear weight with legs by creating a wide base of support, while using hands on floor to support some weight.
  c. Use arms to climb up legs.
  d. Push torso to an upright stance with legs remaining wide apart.
3. Heart muscle weakens, and tachycardia develops.
4. Respiratory muscles weaken, causing ineffective cough and frequent infections.

Diagnostic Evaluation
1. NCT and EMG show abnormalities
2. Serum creatinine kinase (CK)—elevated
3. DNA analysis of blood
4. Muscle biopsy—for definitive diagnosis

Management
1. Goals of treatment are directed toward maintaining mobility, quality of life, and prevention of complications.
2. Medications to control symptoms such as antiarrhythmics and bronchodilators.
3. Promotion of ambulation in calipers after loss of ability to walk; wheelchair when appropriate.
4. Provision of spinal orthotic supports.
5. Surgical tendon releasing to treat contractures.
6. Physical therapy such as passive stretching to preserve function.
7. Vigorous respiratory therapy, such as chest percussion, inspirometry, and assisted cough.

8. Pulmonary function monitoring.
9. Carrier detection and genetic counseling to explain implications of Duchenne MD to parents and detect sibling carriers.

Complications

1. Infections (pulmonary, urinary, systemic)
2. Cardiac dysrhythmias
3. Respiratory insufficiency and failure secondary to weakness of diaphragm and chest muscles
4. Aspiration pneumonia due to oropharyngeal dysfunction
5. Depression
6. Orthopedic deformities—contractures, lordosis, scoliosis
7. Learning and behavioral disorders

Nursing Assessment

1. Assess muscle strength, atrophy, gait, age-related motor development.
2. Evaluate respiratory and cardiac status—breath sounds, heart sounds, pulse rate and rhythm.
3. Evaluate ADL skills.
4. Identify psychosocial issues, such as altered self-concept, decreased socialization, and family discord.

Nursing Diagnoses

• Ineffective Breathing Pattern related to muscle weakness
• Impaired Physical Mobility related to disease process
• Decreased Cardiac Output related to cardiac muscle involvement
• Impaired Swallowing related to muscle weakness
• Diversional Activity Deficit related to weakness

Nursing Interventions

Maintaining Breathing Pattern

1. Encourage upright positioning to provide for maximum chest excursion.
2. Encourage energy-conservation techniques and avoidance of exertion.
3. Teach deep-breathing exercises to strengthen respiratory muscles.
4. Assess rate, depth, and pattern of respirations; listen to breath sounds; and report any change in condition.
5. Note results of arterial blood gases, sputum cultures, and chest x-rays.
6. Encourage coughing and deep breathing or perform chest physiotherapy as indicated.

Preserving Optimal Motor Function

1. Refer to physical therapy for stretching and strengthening exercise to optimize remaining motor function.
2. Perform range-of-motion exercises to preserve mobility and prevent atrophy.
3. Schedule activity with consideration to energy highs throughout the day.
4. Consult with occupational therapist for assistive devices to maintain independence.

5. Apply braces and splints to prevent contractures.

Improving Cardiac Output

1. Monitor vital signs, cardiac rhythm, and signs of congestive heart failure, such as edema, adventitious breath sounds, and weight gain.
2. Monitor intake and output, and maintain IV or oral fluid intake as ordered.

Monitoring Swallowing Function

1. Assess cranial nerve function for swallowing (gag reflex) and chewing.
2. Provide a diet that the patient can handle; blenderizing food may be necessary.
3. Diet should be high protein and controlled calories to provide optimal nutritional value.
4. Encourage eating in upright position without talking and in small, more frequent meals.
5. Administer alternative enteral feeding if gag reflex is diminished.

Encouraging Diversional Activities

1. Encourage diversional activities that prevent overexertion and frustration, but discourage long periods of bed rest and inactivity, such as TV watching.
2. If upper extremities are mostly affected, suggest walking or riding a stationary bike; if lower extremities are mostly affected, encourage use of a wheelchair to promote mobility and performing simple crafts.
3. Discuss patient's interests, and assist with preferred activities.
4. Investigate with the patient various methods of stress management to deal with frustration.
5. Administer analgesics and antidepressants as ordered to facilitate participation in activities.

Community and Home Care Considerations

1. Follow the Community and Home Care Considerations listed under Cerebral Palsy on p. 1403.
2. Obtain services and devices that will promote maximal functioning, such as wheelchair ramp, wheelchair van for transportation, assistive devices.
3. Explore physical and recreational activities with family, such as Special Olympics.
4. Assess child's educational progress and ability to attend school versus home schooling.
5. Collaborate with patient and family to establish daily plan of activities that incorporates patient's interest, ability, and need for rest periods.

Family Education and Health Maintenance

1. Offer genetic counseling, if indicated, to determine options of family planning.
2. Instruct the patient and family in range-of-motion exercises, pulmonary care, and methods of transfer and locomotion.
3. Refer to community respite and counseling services.
4. Stress the importance of fluids to decrease risk of urinary/pulmonary infection.

5. Advise patient or family to report signs of respiratory infection immediately to obtain treatment and prevent congestive heart failure.
6. Refer patient/family to agencies such as The Muscular Dystrophy Association, 3300 East Sunrise Drive, Tucson, AZ 85718, 520-529-2000, *www.mdausa.org*.

Outcome-Based Evaluation

- Deep, unlabored respirations with clear breath sounds
- Ambulating unassisted, no contractures noted
- Vital signs stable, no edema
- Tolerating small blenderized feedings without aspiration
- Out of bed most of day, engages in diversional and social activities

Bacterial Meningitis

Bacterial meningitis is an inflammation of the meninges that follows the invasion of the spinal fluid by a bacterial agent. Most cases are seen in children younger than 5 years.

Pathophysiology and Etiology

1. The proportion of cases due to a specific organism varies from year to year; there also is considerable geographic difference. The organisms most commonly causing bacterial meningitis in different age groups follow:
   a. Birth to 3 months—*Escherichia coli, Streptococcus,* group B, *Listeria monocytogenes*
   b. 3 months to 6 years—*Streptococcus pneumoniae, Neisseria meningitidis, Haemophilus influenzae*
   c. 6 to 16 years—*S. pneumoniae, N. meningitidis, Mycobacterium tuberculosis*
2. Bacterial meningitis is frequently preceded by an upper respiratory infection, which is complicated by bacteremia. Bacteria in the circulating blood then invade the CSF.
   a. Less commonly, bacterial meningitis may occur as an extension of a local bacterial infection, such as otitis media, mastoiditis, or sinusitis.
   b. Bacteria also may gain direct entry through a penetrating wound, spinal tap, surgery, or anatomic abnormality.
3. The infective process results in inflammation, exudation, and varying degrees of tissue damage in the brain.

Clinical Manifestations

1. Signs and symptoms are variable, depending on the patient's age, the etiologic agent, and the duration of the illness when diagnosed. Onset may be insidious or fulminant.
2. Infants younger than 2 months usually display irritability, lethargy, vomiting, lack of appetite, seizures, high-pitched cry, fever, or hypothermia.
3. Infants up to 2 years of age manifest symptoms similar to those of the young infant and may have altered sleep patterns, fever, tenseness of the fontanelle, nuchal rigidity, positive Kernig's or Brudzinski's signs.

4. Children older than 2 years initially have vomiting, headache, mental confusion, lethargy, and photophobia. Later symptoms include nuchal rigidity within 12 to 24 hours after onset, positive Kernig's or Brudzinski's sign, seizures, and progressive decline in responsiveness.
5. Petechiae or purpura may develop.
   a. Characteristic skin lesions are most often observed in cases of meningococcal or *Pseudomonas* infection.
   b. Hemorrhagic rashes may occur in any child with overwhelming bacterial sepsis because of disseminated intravascular coagulation.
6. Septic arthritis suggests either meningococcal or *H. influenzae* infection.

Diagnostic Evaluation

1. Diagnosis is usually established by performance of a lumbar puncture and examination of the CSF.
   a. Cloudy or turbid appearance
   b. Elevated CSF pressure
   c. High cell count with mostly polymorphonuclear cells
   d. Low glucose level
   e. Elevated protein level (also may be normal)
   f. Positive Gram's stain and cultures (identifies the causative organism)
2. Additional laboratory studies include the following:
   a. Complete blood count—total white blood cell count often increased, with a preponderance of young neutrophils in the differential blood count
   b. Blood, urine, and nasopharyngeal cultures to look for source of infection
   c. Platelet count, serum electrolytes, glucose, blood urea nitrogen (BUN) and creatinine, and urinalysis usually done to monitor critically ill patient

Treatment

1. IV administration of the appropriate antimicrobial agents to promote rapid destruction of the bacteria and to suppress the emergence of resistant strains. The first dose of antibiotics should be administered as soon as possible.
2. Recognition and treatment of hyponatremia caused by syndrome of inappropriate antidiuretic hormone secretion (SIADH).
3. Supportive management of the comatose child or the child with seizures.
4. Appropriate prophylactic treatment provided for contacts when indicated.

Complications

1. Acute—seizures, cerebral edema and IICP, shock, SIADH.
2. Long-term—sensorineural hearing loss, hydrocephalus, blindness, learning disabilities/developmental delays

Nursing Assessment

1. Obtain a history from the parents about recent upper respiratory or other infection.

2. Assess level of consciousness and neurologic status.
   a. Evaluate for *Kernig's sign*—with the child in the supine position and knees flexed, flex the leg at the hip so the thigh is brought to a position perpendicular to the trunk. Attempt to extend the knee. If meningeal irritation is present, this cannot be done, and attempts to extend the knee result in pain.
   b. Evaluate for *Brudzinski's sign*—flex the patient's neck. Spontaneous flexion of the lower extremities indicates meningeal irritation.
3. Monitor breathing pattern and circulatory status.

Nursing Diagnoses
- Altered Cerebral Tissue Perfusion related to endotoxin release into the cerebrospinal fluid
- Hyperthermia related to infectious process
- Pain related to neurologic effects from the disease process
- Risk for Infection Transmission related to bacterial agents
- Altered Cerebral Tissue Perfusion related to complications of infectious process
- Anxiety of parents related to severity of illness and hospitalization

Nursing Interventions
See Standards of Care Guidelines.
Maintaining Cerebral Tissue Perfusion
1. Administer antimicrobial agents at specified time intervals to obtain optimal serum levels. Obtain bloodwork for peak and trough levels as ordered.
2. Maintain patent IV line for medication administration; observe for signs of infiltration and phlebitis.
3. Monitor closely for signs of complications affecting cerebral perfusion.
   a. Monitor vital signs, level of consciousness, and neurologic status at frequent intervals.
   b. Monitor intake and output, weight, and head circumference daily to assess for hydrocephalus.
   c. Be especially alert for lethargy or subtle changes in condition, which may indicate cerebral edema.
   d. Accurately chart child's behavior and clinical signs.
Reducing Fever
1. Administer antipyretics, tepid sponge baths, and hypothermia blanket as ordered to reduce fever. Fever increases metabolic rate and energy requirements by the brain; this may lead to hypoxemia and brain damage in the child with cerebral vascular compromise.
2. Monitor for seizures and use seizure precautions in the febrile child.
   a. There is an increased potential for seizures in the febrile child.
   b. Ensure safety by using padded bed or crib rails and having airway and suction equipment on hand.
Relieving Pain and Irritability
1. Reduce the general noise level around the child, and prevent sudden loud noises.
2. Organize nursing care to provide for periods of uninterrupted rest.

> ### STANDARDS OF CARE GUIDELINES
> ### Caring for a Child With Neurologic Dysfunction
>
> - Monitor vital signs, level of consciousness, pupillary reaction, and behavior as indicated and observe for signs of increased intercranial pressure (IICP); report significant changes immediately.
> - Ensure that the patient receives all seizure medications and antibiotics as directed, and that any deviation from dosage schedule or change in therapeutic serum drug levels is reported immediately.
> - Assess for adequate elimination: ability for the child to urinate or caregiver or child to do catheterization. Report deviation from normal pattern and take measures to prevent constipation and stool impaction.
> - Assess for signs of secondary infection: postoperative incision infection; shunt malfunction and infection; pneumonia; skin breakdown. Report abnormality in timely fashion.
> - Monitor for seizures, and maintain safety. Document and report all seizures, including type, time of onset, duration, and behavior afterward. Administer p.r.n. medications per protocol or orders.
> - Ensure that any assistive devices fit adequately to avoid tissue breakdown. Check more frequently if child is restless.
> - Observe/assist with ambulation for safety.
> - Train all caregivers in standards of home safety, including CPR, seizure control, and accident prevention.
> - Ensure that the patient/family is aware of all community resources, including respite and support groups, educational assistance, and social services.
> - Teach caregivers to do range-of-motion exercises to prevent contractures. Utilize physical therapy/occupational therapy as needed.
> - Encourage regular health maintenance visits to monitor growth, development, and general health.
>
> This information should serve as a general guideline only. Each patient situation presents a unique set of clinical factors and requires nursing judgment to guide care, which may include additional or alternative measures and approaches.

3. Keep general handling of the child at a minimum. When necessary, approach the child slowly and gently.
4. Maintain subdued lighting as much as possible.
5. Speak in a low, well-modulated tone of voice.
6. Medicate for pain as ordered, avoiding narcotics that cause CNS and respiratory depression.
Preventing Transmission of Infection
1. Use precautions until at least 24 hours after initiation of appropriate antibiotic therapy.
2. Practice careful handwashing technique.
3. Ensure that personnel with colds or other infections avoid contact with infants with meningitis, and wear a mask when it is necessary to enter the nursery.
4. Teach parents and other visitors proper handwashing and gown technique.
5. Maintain sterile technique for procedures when indicated.
6. Identify close contacts of the child with meningitis caused by *H. influenzae* or *N. meningitidis* who might benefit from prophylactic treatment.

Avoiding Complications

1. Monitor for and report any of the following:
   a. Decreased respirations, decreased pulse rate, increased systolic blood pressure, pupillary changes, or decreased responsiveness, which may indicate IICP.
   b. Decreased urine volume and increased body weight, which may indicate SIADH.
   c. Sudden appearance of a skin rash and bleeding from other sites, which may indicate disseminated intravascular coagulation
   d. Persistent or recurring fever, bulging fontanelle, signs of IICP, focal neurologic signs, seizures, or increased head circumference, which may indicate subdural effusion
   e. Hearing disturbances and apparent deafness, indicating cranial nerve involvement
2. Observe for episodes of apnea, and initiate measures to stimulate respiration.
   a. Institute respiratory monitoring.
   b. Stimulate the infant when apnea does occur.
      (i) Pinch feet and provide more vigorous stimulation if necessary.
      (ii) When spontaneous respiration does not occur within 15 to 20 seconds, provide bag, valve, or mask ventilation.
   c. Report any periods of apnea.
   d. Record length of apnea episode and response to stimulation.

Allaying Parental Anxiety

1. Encourage the parents to engage in quiet activities with their child, such as reading or listening to soft music.
2. Provide the parents with an opportunity to express their concerns and answer questions they may have regarding the child's progress and care.
3. Engage the parents in the supportive care of the child so they may feel some control over the situation.

Family Education and Health Maintenance

1. Provide parents with appropriate information if they and other family members are to receive antibiotic prophylaxis, usually one dose of rifampin (Rifadin).
2. Discuss symptoms for which the parents should watch as signs of possible latent complications, especially hydrocephalus.
3. Give specific instruction regarding medications to be administered at home.
4. Encourage regular health maintenance visits to chart growth and development and assess for any delays.
5. Parents can obtain more information about meningitis at the Centers for Disease Control and Prevention's website at *www.cdc.gov*.

Outcome-Based Evaluation

- Alert without signs of IICP
- Fever below 101°F (38.4°C), no subsequent infection
- Resting comfortably, verbalizing reduced pain
- Precautions maintained
- Vital signs stable; breathing pattern regular without apnea
- Parents participating in child's care, asking questions

Seizure Disorders (Convulsive Disorders, Epilepsy)

Seizure disorder is a term used to encompass a number of varieties of episodic disturbances of brain function. Seizures should not be regarded as one specific disease, but as a symptom of an underlying disorder. They are relatively common in children, being more prevalent during the first 2 years than at any other time in life. Incidence of epilepsy is estimated at 15 cases per 100,000 population. Of individuals with seizure disorders, 90% are diagnosed before the age of 20.

Pathophysiology and Etiology

Etiologic Factors

Seizure disorders are idiopathic or related to a variety of contributing factors.

1. Prenatal factors include genetic predisposition, congenital structural anomalies, fetal infections, maternal diseases.
2. Perinatal factors include trauma, hypoxia, jaundice, infection, prematurity, drug withdrawal.
3. Postnatal factors include:
   a. Primary infection of the CNS
   b. Infectious diseases of childhood with encephalopathy
   c. Head trauma
   d. Circulatory diseases
   e. Toxic encephalopathy
   f. Allergic encephalopathy
   g. Metabolic encephalopathy
   h. Degenerative diseases
   i. Cerebral neoplasms
   j. Renal disease
   k. Anoxia

Altered Physiology

1. The basic mechanism for all seizures appears to be prolonged depolarization, causing brain cells to become overactive and to discharge in a sudden, violent, disorderly manner.
2. This paroxysmal burst of electrical energy spreads to adjacent areas of the brain or may jump to distant areas of the CNS, resulting in a seizure.
3. The biochemical basis of seizures is incompletely understood, but some seizures appear to occur under the influence of a triggering factor.
   a. Hormonal factors, such as those related to the menstrual period, menarche, and menopause
   b. Nonsensory factors, such as hyperthermia, hyperventilation, metabolic disorders, sleep deprivation, emotional disturbances, and physical stress
   c. Sensory factors, such as those related to vision, hearing, touch, the startle reaction, and those that are self-induced

Clinical Manifestations: Types of Seizures
Generalized Seizures (Tonic-Clonic)
1. Onset is abrupt.
   a. May occur at night.
   b. An aura (peculiar sensation, often dizziness) occurs in about one third of epileptic children before a generalized seizure.
2. Tonic spasm:
   a. The child's entire body becomes stiff.
   b. The child loses consciousness.
   c. The face may become pale and distorted.
   d. The eyes are frequently fixed in one position.
   e. The back may be arched with head held backward or to one side.
   f. Arms are usually flexed and hands clenched.
   g. If standing, the child falls to the ground.
   h. The child may utter a peculiar, piercing cry.
   i. The child is often unable to swallow saliva.
   j. Breathing is ineffective, and cyanosis results if spasm includes the muscles of respiration.
   k. The pulse may become weak and irregular.
3. Clonic phase:
   a. Characterized by rhythmic, jerking movements that follow the tonic state.
   b. Usually start in one place and become generalized, including the muscles of the face.
   c. The child may be incontinent and may bite the tongue or cheek. (This occurs because of sudden forceful contraction of the jaw and abdominal muscles.)
4. Duration varies from a few seconds to 30 minutes or longer; usually seizures cease after a few minutes.
5. Postictal (postconvulsive) state:
   a. Usually is sleepy or exhausted.
   b. May complain of headache.
   c. May appear to be in a dazed state.
   d. Often performs relatively automatic tasks without being able to recall the episode.

Status Epilepticus
1. State of continuing or recurring seizures that last longer than 30 minutes or occur in a series without the patient's regaining consciousness between attacks.
2. Transient postictal signs and symptoms include ataxia, aphasia, and mental sluggishness.
3. Damage to cerebral tissue may occur secondary to prolonged cerebral hypoxia or hypoglycemia, not the seizure itself.
4. This condition should be treated as a medical emergency.

Absence Seizures
1. Rarely appears before 5 years of age. Previously referred to as petit mal seizures.
2. Clinical signs:
   a. The child will lose contact with the environment for a few brief seconds.
   b. The child may appear to be staring or daydreaming.
   c. If reading or writing, the child will suddenly discontinue the activity and may resume it when the seizure has ended.

   d. Atypical absence seizure—minor manifestations include rolling of the eyes, nodding of the head, slight hand movements, and smacking of the lips.
3. Duration is usually 5 to 10 seconds.
4. Frequency varies from one or two per month to several hundred each day.
5. Precipitating factors include hyperventilation, fatigue, hypoglycemia, and stress.
6. Postseizure state:
   a. Child appears normal.
   b. Child is not aware of having had a seizure.

Partial Seizures—Psychomotor
1. Occur most frequently in children 3 years through adolescence.
2. Seizure discharge usually originates in the temporal lobe and may be referred to as "temporal lobe seizures."
3. Clinical signs include the following:
   a. The child frequently experiences a sense of fullness rising from the abdomen to the thorax.
   b. Aura, if present, often includes bad odor or taste.
   c. The child may experience complex auditory or visual hallucinations, déja vu feeling, or strong sense of fear and anxiety.
   d. Perceptual alterations may occur.
   e. Dysphagia or aphasia may be present.
   f. Most common motor symptom is drawing or jerking of the mouth and face.
   g. The child may perform coordinated but inappropriate movements repeatedly in a stereotypical manner (eg, clutching, kicking, picking at clothes, walking in circles, chewing, licking, spitting).
   h. Consciousness may be impaired but is rarely completely lost.
4. Duration is brief, usually from 30 seconds to 5 to 10 minutes.
5. Postictal state is usual after an attack. Confusion and amnesia are common.
6. These seizures may be confused with tics.

Partial Seizures—Focal Motor
1. Clinical signs:
   a. Sudden jerking movements occur in a particular area of the body, such as the face, thumb, or toe.
   b. Consciousness may or may not be disturbed.
   c. Clonic movements occasionally begin in one area of the body and spread to adjacent areas on the same side in a fixed progression (Jacksonian seizures).
2. Prognosis—may become more extensive as the child matures, leading to generalized seizures

Partial Seizures—Focal Sensory
1. Sensations occur, such as numbness, tingling, and coldness, in the part of the body controlled by the area of the brain cell overactivity.
2. Rare in children.

Infantile Spasms (Myoclonic Seizures, Massive Myoclonic Spasms)
1. These seizures occur in infants; they are second in incidence only to generalized seizures in this age group.

2. Peak incidence is in children between 4 and 8 months; onset after 2 years is rare.
3. Clinical signs include the following:
   a. Sudden, forceful, myoclonic contractions involving the musculature of the trunk, neck, and extremities.
      (i) Flexor type—the infant adducts and flexes the extremities, drops the head, and doubles on himself or herself.
      (ii) Extensor type—the infant extends neck, spreads arms out, and bends body backward in a position described as "spread eagle."
      (iii) Mixed—a combination of the above two types occurring in clusters or volleys of each.
   b. A cry or grunt may accompany severe attacks.
   c. The infant may grimace, laugh, or appear fearful during or after the attack.
4. Duration is momentary (usually less than 1 minute).
5. Frequency varies from a few attacks per day to hundreds per day.
6. Almost always associated with cerebral abnormalities. Mental retardation usually accompanies this disorder.
7. Usually this type of seizure disappears spontaneously by the time the child reaches 4 years of age. Subsequent generalized or other types of seizures often develop.

Diagnostic Evaluation
Electroencephalogram
1. The electroencephalogram (EEG) shows characteristic abnormalities during seizures and with generalized seizures, between seizures as well.
2. A normal EEG does not preclude the diagnosis of epilepsy.

Laboratory Studies
1. Serum electrolytes, magnesium, calcium, and fasting blood sugar.
2. Toxicology screen—drug overdoses may cause seizures.
3. Blood cultures—fever and CNS infections may cause seizures.
4. Lumbar puncture may be done if fever is present.
5. Serum levels of seizure medications should follow therapy.

Treatment
General Principles Related to the Administration of Medications
1. Selection of the most effective drug(s) depends on correct identification of the clinical seizure type.
2. A desirable drug level is one that will prevent seizures without producing undesirable side effects.
3. Dosages are adjusted according to blood level and clinical signs.
4. Accurate timing is essential to prevent seizures. This is especially true when the child tends to have seizures at a certain time each day.
5. Enteric-coated tablets, which have a delayed effect, should be used for children who are prone to attacks during sleep.

6. Most anticonvulsants are available in liquid form and in capsules or tablets. Some drugs are less well absorbed in liquid form.
7. It may take several months to find the best combination of medications and the best dosages of each to control the child's seizures. Single-drug therapy is attempted initially. If this is not successful, a second drug may be tried or added on.
8. Symptoms may not be controlled 100% in every patient.
9. Dosage adjustment may be required from time to time because of the child's growth.
10. Blood counts, urinalyses, and liver function studies are done at regular intervals in children receiving certain anticonvulsants.
11. Medication is often not discontinued until 2 to 3 years after the last attack.
12. Weaning from medication should always be gradual, with stepwise reduction of dosage and withdrawal of one drug at a time.
13. There is some evidence to suggest that long-term use of some antiepileptic agents may cause intellectual impairment in children with epilepsy.

Drugs Used for the Control of Seizures in Children
See Table 46-3.

Surgical Management
1. Surgical removal is the appropriate treatment for an identified lesion, such as a hematoma or brain tumor.
2. Surgical treatment, such as hemispherectomy, nontemporal lobe resection, or corpus callostomy, may be performed in children with severe, medically intractable seizure disorders.

Diet Therapy
1. The ketogenic diet may be used for seizure control and consists of precisely calculated portions of protein and fat without carbohydrates. This diet causes the child to become ketotic because fats are used for fuel rather than carbohydrates. It is thought that ketones may inhibit seizures.
   a. Children on this diet should not be given IV fluids with dextrose.
   b. All medications should be in sugar-free suspensions.
   c. The child will be on strict fluid restriction.
   d. This diet must be carefully monitored by a licensed dietitian.
2. The mechanism of action of this treatment is unknown.
3. There is some evidence that this diet may put the child at increased risk of developing kidney stones.

General Prognosis
1. General prognosis depends on type and severity of seizure disorder, coexisting mental retardation, organic disorders, and the type of medical management.
2. Medically treated seizures—spontaneous cessation of seizures may occur. Drugs may be gradually discontinued when the child has been free from attacks for an extensive period and the EEG pattern has reverted to normal.

TABLE 46-3 Drugs Used to Treat Seizures in Children

Drugs and Dosage	Advantages	Adverse Reactions	Special Considerations
Phenobarbital (Luminal) Maintenance dosage: 3–5 mg/kg/d given qd or bid Status epilepticus: 10–20 mg/kg, may repeat to maximum 40 mg/kg	Relatively safe and inexpensive	Excitement, hyperactivity, rash, gastrointestinal (GI) distress, dizziness, ataxia, worsening of psychomotor seizures, drowsiness; toxicity causing respiratory depression, circulatory collapse, and renal impairment	This is contraindicated in hepatic or renal dysfunction, hypersensitivity. IM or IV loading dose can be given. IV rate should not exceed 1 mg/kg/min.
Phenytoin (Dilantin) Loading dose: 20 mg/kg Maintenance 3–9 mg/ kg/d given qd or bid	Safest drug for psychomotor seizures; does not cause drowsiness	Hypertrophy of gums, hirsutism, rickets, nystagmus, ataxia, rash; may accentuate absence seizures; toxicity may cause blood dyscrasias and liver damage	May interact with a wide variety of drugs due to extensive protein binding. Daily gum massage may prevent gum disease, Avoid IM administration. If given IV, do not exceed rate of 0.5 mg/kg/min. Drug must be given with normal saline to prevent precipitation.
Ethosuximide (Zarontin) Maintenance: 20–40 mg/ kg/d given qd by oral route only	Used for absence seizures	Drowsiness, GI distress, lethargy, euphoria; may aggravate generalized seizures; toxicity causes blood dyscrasias and psychiatric symptoms	This is contraindicated in hepatic or renal disease. Dosage should not be increased more often than every 4–7 days
Primidone (Mysoline) children younger than 8 years: 10–25 mg/ kg/d given tid or qd Children older than 8 years: 750–1,500 mg/d tid or qid by oral route only	May control generalized seizures not responsive to treatment by other drugs	Ataxia, vertigo, GI symptoms; megaloblastic anemia as a rare idiosyncratic reaction; drowsiness in breastfed infants of treated mothers; Stevens-Johnson syndrome, gum hypertrophy, night terrors	This is contraindicated in those hypersensitive to phenobarbital and those with porphyria. It is often used with other drugs for mixed seizures. Dosage increases are usually done weekly until effect is seen.
Diazepam (Valium) IV dosage: 0.04–0.2 mg/ kg to maximum of 10 mg if ≥ 5 y old; maximum of 5 mg if < 5 y old Rectal dosage: 0.5 mg/kg	Used IV, IM, or rectally for status epilepticus or as adjunct therapy	Ataxia, drowsiness, fatigue, venous thrombosis or phlebitis at injection site, confusion, depression, headache; tonic status epilepticus when given IV for absence seizures; toxicity may cause somnolence, confusion, diminished reflexes, hypotension, coma, apnea, cardiac arrest	If administered IV, give no faster than 1 mg/min. Drug used cautiously in children with limited pulmonary reserve. Monitor respirations closely.
Carbamazepine (Tegretol) 20–30 mg/kg/d tid or qid Maximum dose of 1,000 mg/d if > 12 y old; 100 mg bid if 6–12 y old; 20 mg/kg/d if < 6 y old	Especially useful for major motor and psychomotor seizures	Most likely to occur during initiation of therapy: dizziness, drowsiness, nausea and vomiting; toxicity may cause bone marrow depression (fever, sore throat, oral ulcers, easy bruising)	Administration with phenytoin reduces half-life of phenytoin; higher dose of phenytoin may be needed. This is contraindicated in previous bone marrow depression and is used cautiously in patients with cardiac, hepatic, or renal problems. Erythromycin increases plasma levels. Give with food.
Lorazepam (Ativan) 0.1 mg/kg/dose q 10–15 min Maximum dose: 4 mg and may be repeated once	Used IV or rectally for status epilepticus; longer acting; may cause less respiratory depression	Sedation, dizziness, respiratory depression, hypotension, ataxia, weakness	Use with caution in patients with hepatic or renal dysfunction. Monitor respiratory status closely.
Valproic acid (Depakene) 10 mg/kg/d loading Maximum dose: 30–60 mg/kg/d tid or qid	Adjunct for poor seizure control, some success with behavioral problems	Nausea, vomiting, anorexia, amenorrhea, sedation tremor, weight gain, alopecia, hepatotoxicity	Caution with hepatic dysfunction. Increases serum levels of phenytoin, phenobarbital, and primidone

3. Nontreated epilepsy—seizures tend to become more numerous.

Complications
1. Apnea/hypoventilation
2. Hypoglycemia in status epilepticus
3. Injuries sustained during a seizure

Nursing Assessment
1. During a seizure, assess the following:
   a. Any indications of difficulties with airway or breathing
   b. Significant preseizure events, such as noise, excitement, lethargy
   c. Behavior before the seizure, aura
   d. Types of movements observed
   e. Time seizure began and ended
   f. Site where twitching or contraction began
   g. Areas of the body involved
   h. Movements of the eyes and changes in pupil size
   i. Incontinence
   j. Color change—pallor, cyanosis, flushing
   k. Mouth—teeth clenched, abnormal movements, tongue bitten
   l. Apparent degree of consciousness during the seizure
2. After a seizure, assess the following:
   a. Degree of memory for recent events
   b. Types of speech
   c. Coordination, paralysis or weakness
   d. Length of time the child is postictal
   e. Pupillary reaction
   f. Vital signs

Nursing Diagnoses
- Risk for Injury during a seizure
- Ineffective Breathing Pattern related to spasms of respiratory musculature
- Social Isolation related to the child's feelings about seizures or public fears and misconceptions
- Self-Esteem Disturbance related to lack of control over seizures

Nursing Interventions
Ensuring Safety During a Seizure
1. Use preventive measures.
   a. Remove hard toys from the bed.
   b. Pad the sides of the crib or side rails of the bed.
   c. Have a suction machine available to remove secretions during a seizure.
   d. Have an emergency oxygen source in the room in case of sudden respiratory difficulty.
2. Make sure the child can be readily observed.
3. During a seizure, monitor vital signs and assess neurologic status frequently.
4. After a seizure, check the child frequently and report the following:

a. Behavior changes
b. Irritability
c. Restlessness
d. Listlessness

Preventing Respiratory Arrest and Aspiration
1. During a seizure, take the following emergency actions:
   a. Clear the area around the child.
   b. Do not restrain the child.
   c. Loosen the clothing around the neck.
   d. Turn the child on side so saliva can flow out of the mouth.
   e. Place a small, folded blanket under the head to prevent trauma if the seizure occurs when the child is on the floor.
2. Suction the child, and administer oxygen as necessary.
3. Do not give anything by mouth or attempt to place anything in the mouth.
4. After the seizure, place the child in a side-lying position.

Promoting Socialization
1. Advise the parents that the child should be in an environment that is as normal as possible.
2. Encourage regular attendance at school after the school nurse and teachers have been notified, and emergency treatment of seizures is understood.
3. Encourage the child to participate in organizations and outside activities with limited restrictions.
   a. Each child must be treated individually; the kind of activity depends on the degree of control.
   b. Generally, children with seizure disorders should not be allowed to climb in high places or to swim alone.
   c. Responsible adults should be made aware of the child's disorder.
   d. Children with seizures should wear a Medic-Alert bracelet at all times.

Strengthening Self-Esteem
1. Offer reassurance and praise to the parents and child for coping effectively with seizures.
2. Observe the parent–child interactions for evidence of rejection or overprotection.
   a. Tell the parents that the child should not be made to feel that he or she can never be left alone.
   b. Advise the parents that the child needs to be disciplined as any other child and should not gain attention directly or indirectly by having seizures.
3. Help the child gain more control by providing education about seizure disorders.
   a. Include the child in treatment planning.
   b. Allow the opportunity to ask questions, and answer them honestly.
   c. Make sure the child is aware of restrictions and can deal with them.
   d. Encourage parents gradually to give the child responsibility for taking medications.
4. Help the older child or adolescent to achieve independence.

a. Encourage the parents to give the older child the opportunity for privacy to discuss concerns with the physician.

b. Encourage parents to allow the older child to use his or her own judgment in making decisions.

c. Help the older child to develop realistic educational and career goals.

5. Help parents deal with a noncompliant child. Fantasies that "there is nothing wrong with me" or the refusal to take medications requires prompt intervention. This is most often seen during adolescence. Family counseling may be necessary.

Community and Home Care Considerations

1. Follow Community and Home Care Considerations listed under Cerebral Palsy on p. 1403.

2. Ensure that the home environment is safe, especially where the child sleeps and plays. Remove toys with sharp edges or parts or small pieces the child could choke on if they are put in the mouth, and cover very hard surfaces, such as the floor, against which the child could fall.

3. Reinforce parents' knowledge and ability to dispense seizure medications.

4. Help the family acquire a Medic-Alert tag that the child should wear at all times, especially once attending day care or school.

5. Ensure that parents and caregivers are trained in CPR and seizure management.

6. Ensure that a portable or disposable airway is available for emergencies at all times.

Family Education and Health Maintenance

1. Describe completely any examinations, evaluations, treatments that the child is receiving.

2. Provide information regarding the disease itself.
   a. Epilepsy is not contagious, is seldom dangerous, and does not indicate insanity or mental retardation.
   b. Most children with epilepsy have infrequent seizures and with medications can completely control their convulsions.
   c. The child may have normal intelligence and can live a useful and productive life.
   d. The child's medication is not addicting when used as prescribed. It should in no way cause him or her to become a drug addict.

3. Prepare the parents for the fact that it may take several months of regulating drug dosages before adequate control is obtained.

4. Encourage parents and older children to obtain genetic counseling.
   a. People with epilepsy can marry and have children.
   b. There is no proof that epilepsy is hereditary, although there may be a tendency to transmit a low convulsive threshold.

c. It is impossible to predict accurately the possibility of the seizure disorder appearing in siblings or offspring of the affected child.

5. Teach the parents and child factors that may precipitate a seizure.
   a. The child should be kept in optimal physical condition with routine immunizations, medical care, dental care, and eye care, and should receive prompt evaluation and treatment of infections.
   b. Excessive fatigue, overhydration, and hyperventilation should be avoided.
   c. Irregular, fluctuating schedules are detrimental. A routine of daily living should be encouraged.

6. For additional resources, refer families to agencies such as The Epilepsy Foundation of America, 4351 Garden City Drive, Landover, MD 20785-2267, 800-332-1000; *www.epilepsyfoundation.org.*

Outcome-Based Evaluation

- Padded bed rails in place; suction machine and airway at bedside; only stuffed animals in crib; no injury reported
- Breathing unlabored after seizure, with lungs clear
- Parents and child verbalize understanding of child's ability to participate in activities
- Child participating in treatment plan, taking medications as ordered without reminders; serum drug levels are therapeutic

▨ Febrile Seizures

Febrile seizures refer to seizures that occur in the context of a febrile illness in a previously normal child. The seizures are brief and generalized. They should be distinguished from focal or prolonged seizures, which occur in a child with an underlying seizure disorder that is exacerbated by fever. Febrile seizures occur in approximately 2% to 4% of all children. Most first febrile seizures occur in children between the ages of 6 months and 3 years and are unusual after 5 years.

Boys are more likely to have febrile seizures than girls.

Pathophysiology and Etiology

1. Seizures accompany intercurrent infections, especially viral illness, tonsillitis, pharyngitis, and otitis.

2. They appear to occur in a familial pattern, although exact pattern of inheritance is incompletely understood. Children with a positive family history of febrile seizures have a greater risk of recurrent febrile seizures.

3. It is unclear whether the seizure is triggered by a rapid rise in temperature or the actual temperature attained.

4. Most febrile seizures consist of generalized tonic-clonic seizures (see above).

Clinical Manifestations

1. Seizures generally last less than 15 minutes.

2. Fever is usually more than 101.8°F (38.8°C) rectally.

3. Seizures usually occur near the onset of fever rather than after prolonged fever.

Diagnostic Evaluation

Measures are directed toward delineating the cause of any seizure as precisely as possible so its implications and prognosis may be discussed with the parents. Diagnostic methods may include the following:

1. CSF examination to detect CNS infection
2. Complete blood count and urinalysis to detect signs of infection
3. Cultures of nasopharynx, blood, or urine as appropriate to determine cause of fever
4. Blood glucose, calcium, and electrolyte levels to detect abnormalities that may cause seizures
5. EEG (for atypical seizures or for a child at risk for epilepsy)
   a. Demonstrates mild, postictal slowing soon after the attack.
   b. Pattern is generally normal after a few days.

Treatment

The goals of treatment are to control seizures and decrease temperature.

1. Administration of antipyretics and other cooling measures.
2. Administration of medications to control seizures.
   a. The advisability of long-term anticonvulsant medications in normal children with simple febrile seizures is controversial. Recommendations vary among health care providers from no medication to maintenance therapy with phenobarbital (Luminal).
   b. Intermittent therapy with phenobarbital during febrile episodes is apparently of no value because of the length of time required to achieve therapeutic serum levels of the drug.
3. Airway management as required.
4. Prognosis—febrile seizure recurrence is about 33% for a second febrile seizure.
   The younger the child is at the time of the first seizure, the greater the risk for additional febrile seizures.
5. The risk for development of nonfebrile seizures is relatively low (about 5%). At risk are children who demonstrate the following characteristics:
   a. Prolonged or complex febrile seizures
   b. Abnormal or suspected abnormal development before the first seizure
   c. Family history of nonfebrile seizures
   d. Persistent EEG abnormalities

Complications

Injury may occur during seizure.

Nursing Assessment and Interventions

Nursing assessment and interventions are the same as for seizure disorders, p. 1421.

Family Education and Health Maintenance

1. Reinforce realistic, reassuring information, such as the following:
   a. A seizure does not necessarily imply that the underlying disease is serious.
   b. The prognosis depends on the cause of the seizure.
      (i) A single febrile seizure does not indicate later chronic epilepsy.
      (ii) Children who have a tendency to develop febrile seizures usually lose it as they grow older.
      (iii) Occasional, brief seizures have no adverse effects on the child's ultimate development.
2. Discuss and demonstrate emergency management of seizures.
3. Stress that medical evaluation is indicated as soon as the child develops a fever.
   a. Review technique of temperature measurement.
   b. Prompt administration of antipyretic measures is necessary when the child is febrile but may not prevent a febrile seizure.
4. Review administration schedule, adverse reactions, and appropriate follow-up in regard to anticonvulsant therapy.

◼ Subdural Hematoma

Subdural hematoma refers to an accumulation of fluid, blood, and its degradation products within the potential space between the dura and arachnoid (subdural space). Subdural hematomas are classified as acute or chronic, depending on the time between injury and the onset of symptoms.

Also see Chapter 15 for care of unconscious patient, ICP monitoring, and other neurologic care.

Pathophysiology and Etiology
Causes

1. Direct or indirect trauma to the head:
   a. Birth trauma
   b. Accidental causes
   c. Purposeful violence, as in cases of child abuse
2. Meningitis

Classification

1. Acute syndrome—presents as an acute problem, closely related to the time of presumed injury.
2. Chronic:
   a. Signs and symptoms are nonlocalizing and subacute.
   b. This is the most common type of subdural hematoma in children.
   c. It is often difficult to delineate the exact time and type of injury, because the precipitating episode may appear relatively insignificant.

Altered Physiology

1. Trauma to the head causes tearing of the delicate subdural veins, resulting in small hemorrhages into the subdural space. (Bleeding may be of arterial origin in cases of acute subdural hematoma.)

2. As the blood breaks down, there is an increased capillary permeability and effusion of blood cells and protein into the subdural space.
3. The breakdown products of blood stimulate the growth of connective tissue and capillaries largely from the dura.
4. A membrane is formed that usually extends frontally and laterally over the hemispheres, surrounding the clot.
5. Fluid accumulates within the membrane and increases the width of the subdural space.
6. Further hemorrhages occur.
7. The lesion enlarges, compressing the brain and expanding the skull, and, if unrelieved, ultimately causes cerebral atrophy or death from compression and herniation.
8. The lesion may arrest spontaneously at any point.
9. Further bleeding may occur into an already existing sac and may increase symptoms.
10. In long-standing subdural hematoma, the fluid may disappear, leaving a constricting membrane that prevents normal brain growth.

Clinical Manifestations
Acute
1. Often present with continuous unconsciousness from the time of injury, but child may present with a lucid interval.
2. Ensuing manifestations include deterioration of level of consciousness, progressive hemiplegia, focal seizures, and signs of brain stem involvement and herniation (pupillary enlargement, changes in vital signs, decerebrate posturing, and respiratory failure; Figure 46-3).

Chronic
This has a slow, gradual onset; symptoms are variable and are related to the age of the child.
1. Infants—early signs:
    a. Anorexia, difficulty feeding, vomiting
    b. Irritability
    c. Low-grade fever
    d. Retinal hemorrhages
    e. Failure to gain weight
2. Infants—later signs:
    a. Enlargement of the head
    b. Bulging and pulsation of the anterior fontanelle
    c. Tight, glossy scalp with dilated scalp veins
    d. Strabismus, pupillary inequality, ocular palsies (rare)
    e. Hyperactive reflexes
    f. Seizures
    g. Retarded motor development
3. Older children—early signs:
    a. Lethargy, anorexia
    b. Symptoms of IICP (vomiting, irritability, headache)
4. Older children—later signs (also may occur immediately if bleeding takes place rapidly):
    a. Seizures
    b. Coma

Diagnostic Evaluation
1. CT scan is the procedure of choice for diagnosing subdural hematomas.
2. Bilateral subdural taps may provide the diagnosis and immediate relief of IICP.
3. Skull films may be obtained if abuse is suspected.

Treatment
Acute Subdural Hematoma
This requires evacuation of the clot through a burr hole or craniotomy.
Chronic Subdural Hematoma
1. Repeated subdural taps are done to remove the collecting fluid.
    a. In infants, the needle can be inserted through the fontanelle or suture line.

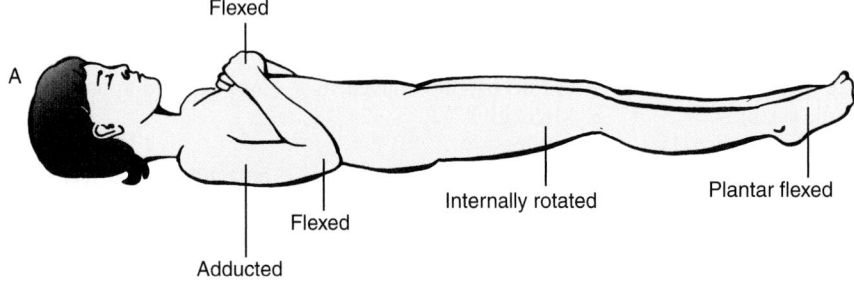
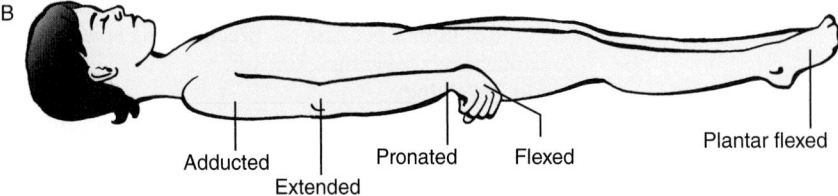

FIGURE 46-3 Primitive posturing in unconscious states due to loss of motor control. (**A**) Decorticate posturing occurs when cortical loss is present. (**B**) Decerebrate posturing occurs when the midbrain is involved.

b. In older children, burr holes into the skull are necessary before the needle can be inserted.

c. Subdural taps may be the only treatment required if the fluid disappears entirely, and symptoms do not recur.

d. Concurrently, treatment is instituted to correct anemia, electrolyte imbalance, and malnutrition.

2. Shunting procedure may be indicated if repeated taps fail to reduce significantly the volume or protein content of the subdural collections. Shunting is usually to the peritoneal cavity.

Prognosis

1. Treatment is usually successful when the diagnosis is made before cerebral atrophy and a fixed neurologic deficit have occurred. In such cases, subsequent development is normal.

2. Prognosis depends on the effect of the initial trauma on the brain and the effect of continued fluid collection.

3. Mortality in massive, acute subdural bleeding is very high, even if promptly diagnosed.

Complications

1. Mental retardation
2. Ocular abnormalities
3. Seizures
4. Spasticity, paralysis
5. Brain stem herniation and death

Nursing Assessment

Assess the child's neurologic status to evaluate the effectiveness of treatment or to identify disease progress.

1. Observe general behavior, especially irritability, lethargy, and evidence of personality changes. It is important to obtain a thorough history from the parents regarding normal behavior and level of functioning so abnormalities can be more easily recognized.

2. Evaluate appetite and feeding difficulties, including vomiting.

3. Assess for signs of IICP.

a. Vital signs, including pulse, respiration, and blood pressure, should be monitored frequently.

b. Be alert for the following:
   (i) Increased systolic blood pressure
   (ii) Widened pulse pressure
   (iii) Decreased pulse or irregularities
   (iv) Changes in respiratory rate or difficulty breathing

4. Assess level of consciousness; describe response explicitly, including what type of stimulus was required to elicit a response.

5. Assess pupillary and visual changes, especially dilated pupil, double vision, lack of response to light, alterations in visual acuity, and nonsymmetric or abnormal eye movements.

6. Monitor for seizures.

7. Evaluate motor function, including ability to move all extremities. The ability to grasp should be checked and compared bilaterally.

8. Inspect for drainage of CSF from the nose or ears indicating fractured skull with CSF leak.

Nursing Diagnoses

- Altered Cerebral Tissue Perfusion related to disease process
- Impaired Physical Mobility related to decreased level of consciousness
- Altered Nutrition: Less Than Body Requirements related to decreased level of consciousness
- Ineffective Family Coping: Compromised related to hospitalization of child

Nursing Interventions
Maintaining Cerebral Tissue Perfusion

1. Avoid additional increase in intracranial pressure.

a. Maintain a quiet environment.

b. Avoid sudden changes in position.

c. Organize nursing activities to allow for long periods of uninterrupted rest.

d. Carefully regulate fluid administration to avoid danger of fluid overload.

e. Measure urine output, and record specific gravity.

f. Administer laxatives or suppositories to prevent straining during a bowel movement.

2. Assist with subdural taps.

a. Protect and restrain the child as needed (see p. 1314).

b. Hold the child securely to avoid injury caused by sudden movement.

c. Apply firm pressure over the puncture site(s) for a few minutes after the tap has been completed to prevent fluid leakage along the needle tract.

d. Observe the child frequently after the procedure for shock or drainage from the site of the tap.

e. Note whether there is serous drainage or frank blood.

f. Reinforce the dressing as needed to prevent contamination of the wound.

g. Monitor temperature frequently, and monitor for signs of developing infection.

h. Report purulent drainage from the site of the subdural tap.

3. Avoid discussing the child's condition near the bed. Even though comatose, the child may be able to hear.

4. Have emergency equipment available for resuscitation.

Preventing Complications of Immobility

1. Change the child's position frequently, and provide meticulous skin care to prevent hypostatic pneumonia and decubitus ulcers.

2. Prevent contractures.

a. Apply passive range-of-motion exercises to all extremities.

b. Place pillows appropriately to support the child's body in good alignment.

c. Use splints designed by physical therapy as instructed.

3. Suction the child as necessary to remove secretions in the mouth and nasopharynx.

4. Observe for signs of respiratory or urinary infection related to stasis.
5. Keep the child's eyes well lubricated to prevent corneal damage.

Maintaining Nutritional Status

1. Provide nutrition and fluids through nasogastric feedings as ordered. Observe for gastric distention.
2. Monitor urine output and specific gravity daily.
3. Monitor electrolyte and protein levels on laboratory work.
4. Do not neglect mouth care, even if child is not eating.

Strengthening Family Coping

1. Encourage the parents to hold and cuddle the infant as much as possible.
2. Encourage the parents to bring diversional activities from home.
   a. Infants—mobiles or musical toys
   b. Older children—quiet games, books, dolls
3. Provide emotional support to the parents.
   a. Encourage as much parental participation in the child's care as possible.
   b. Reassure the parents that the prognosis is favorable with adequate treatment.
4. Act nonjudgmental in cases caused by intentional or accidental trauma.
   a. Attempt to alleviate their guilt feelings if present.
   b. Ensure that cases of suspected child abuse have been reported to the appropriate agency and that parents have been referred for counseling.
5. Encourage visitation by siblings.

Community and Home Care Considerations

1. Follow Community and Home Care Considerations listed under Cerebral Palsy on p. 1403.
2. Perform periodic developmental assessments, and reinforce the need to report any signs of developmental delay to the health care provider.
3. Discuss return-to-play criteria for contact sports with parents, coaches, and teachers, to prevent a second injury after any type of head injury.
   a. Grade I or mild concussion (confusion without amnesia or loss of consciousness)—minimum time to return to play is 20 minutes; symptoms must be resolved.
   b. Grade II or moderate concussion (confusion and transient amnesia without loss of consciousness)—minimum time to return to play is 1 week; symptoms must be resolved for at least 1 week.
   c. Grade III or severe concussion (confusion, amnesia, and loss of consciousness)—minimum time to return to play is 1 month; symptoms must be resolved for at least 1 week.

Family Education and Health Maintenance

1. Reinforce explanations in the following areas:
   a. The condition
   b. Causes of the child's specific symptoms
   c. Need and rationale for treatment
   d. Postoperative and recovery expectations
2. Encourage parents to keep all follow-up appointments for medical evaluation and physical and occupational therapy.
3. Teach parents safety measures to prevent injuries in the future.
4. Assist parents in seeking additional support and resources through social work department, church groups, community agencies, or private counseling.

Outcome-Based Evaluation

- Drowsy but responsive to verbal stimuli; pupils equal and reactive to light; vital signs stable; ventricular tap site without drainage
- Skin without signs of erythema or breakdown; full range of motion of all joints; functional position maintained
- Tolerating nasogastric feedings without distention; urine output sufficient
- Parents participating in child's care, holding and reading to child; parents receiving counseling

■ Reye's Syndrome

Reye's syndrome is a rare illness characterized by acute encephalitis with accompanying fatty infiltration of the liver, heart, lungs, pancreas, and skeletal muscles that occurs in children of all ages. Cause is unknown but has generally occurred after a viral infection such as varicella or upper respiratory infection. There is a strong association with the use of aspirin for symptom relief in viral infection and the development of Reye's syndrome. Therefore, acetaminophen is highly preferred to the use of aspirin for fever and pain of viral infections in children. The incidence of Reye's syndrome has greatly decreased since acetaminophen has become widely used (from 555 cases in 1980 to 6 or less cases per year from 1994 to 1999).

The child with Reye's syndrome is often in a coma. Care is similar to care of the child with subdural hematoma. Cardiac and respiratory support are primary features. Prevention is the key, however, so every parent and caretaker should be taught the appropriate use of antipyretics. Children on aspirin therapy for arthritis and Kawasaki's disease may still be at risk for Reye's syndrome, so they should be vaccinated against varicella and influenza. These parents should be taught the early signs of Reye's syndrome—nausea, vomiting, muscle weakness, lethargy, and neurologic impairment—to seek medical attention immediately.

SELECTED REFERENCES

Allan, W. C., et al. (1997). Antecedents of cerebral palsy in a multicenter trial of indomethacin for intraventricular hemorrhage. *Archives of Pediatric and Adolescent Medicine, 151*(6), 580–585.

American Academy of Pediatrics, Committee on Genetics (1999). *Folic acid for the prevention of neural tube defects* [position statement]. Elk Grove Village, IL: American Academy of Pediatrics.

Baird, C. et al. (2000). Late shunt infections. *Pediatric Neurology, 31*(5), 269–273.

Baker, S., et al (1995). Cerebral palsy. *Paediatric Nursing, 7*(10), 31–35.

Belay, E. D., Bresee, J. S., Holman, R. C., Khan, A. S., Shahriari , A., & Schonberger, L. B. (1999). Reye's syndrome in the United States from 1981 through 1997. *New England Journal of Medicine, 340*(18), 1377–1382.

Boaz, J. C., et al. (1999). Hydrocephalus in children: Neurosurgical and neuroimaging concerns. *Neuroimaging Clinics of North America, 9*(1), 73–91.

Bourgeois, M., et al (1999). Epilepsy in children with shunted hydrocephalus. *Journal of Neurosurgery, 90*(2), 274–281.

Comstock, C. P., et al. (1998). Scoliosis in total-body-involvement cerebral palsy. Analysis of surgical treatment and patient and caregiver satisfaction. *Spine, 23*(12), 1412–1424.

Cornell, S. (1998). Pediatric infectious disease: Updates on the three top offenders. *Advanced Nursing Practice, 6*(4), 70–72.

Cremer, R., et al. (1998). Longitudinal study on latex sensitization in children with spina bifida. *Pediatric Allergy and Immunology, 9*(1), 40–43.

DelGiudice, E., et al. (1999). Gastrointestinal manifestations in children with cerebral palsy. *Brain Development, 21*(5), 307–311.

Dias, M. S., et al. (1998). Pediatric neurosurgical disease. *Pediatric Clinics of North America, 45*(6), 1539–1578.

———. (1998). Split cord malformations. *Neurosurgery Clinics of North America, 6*(2), 339–358.

Egelhoff, J. C. (1999). MR imaging of congenital anomalies of the pediatric spine. *Magnetic Resonance Imaging Clinics of North America, 7*(3), 459–479

Fleisher G. R., & Ludwig, S. (Eds.). (1999). *Textbook of pediatric emergency medicine* (4th ed.). Philadelphia: Williams & Wilkins.

Freeman, G. L. (1997). Cooccurrence of latex and fruit allergies. *Allergy and Asthma Proceedings, 18*(2), 85–88.

Freeman, J., et al (1996). *The epilepsy diet treatment: An introduction to the ketogenic diet* (2nd ed.). New York: Demos Vermande.

Frim, D. M., et al. (1998). Surgical management of neonatal hydrocephalus. *Neurosurgery Clinics of North America, 9*(1), 105–110.

Futagi, Y., et al. (1997). Prognosis of infants with ankle clonus within the first year of life. *Brain Development, 19*(1), 50–54.

Grabb, P. A., et al. (1999). Ventral brain stem compression in pediatric and young adult patients with Chiari I malformations. *Neurosurgery, 44*(3), 520–527.

Hickey, J. V. (1997). *The clinical practice of neurological and neurosurgical nursing* (4th ed.). Philadelphia: Lippincott-Raven.

Hill, A. (2000). Neonatal Seizures. *Pediatrics in Review, 21*(4), 117–121.

Hirtz, D. G. (1997). Febrile seizures. *Pediatrics in Review, 18*(1), 5–8.

Johnson, K. B. (Ed.). (1999). *The Harriet Lane handbook* (15th ed.). Philadelphia: Mosby–Year Book.

Ketelaar, M., et al. (1998). Functional motor abilities of children with cerebral palsy: A systematic literature review of assessment measures. *Clinical Rehabilitation, 12*(5), 369–380.

Lawton, K. H., et al. (1997). Current practices and advances in pediatric neurosurgery. *Nursing Clinics of North America, 32*(1), 73–96.

Madikians, A., et al. (1997). Cerebrospinal fluid shunt problems in pediatric patients. *Pediatric Annals, 26*(10), 613–620.

Mazon, A., et al. (1997). Factors that influence the presence of symptoms caused by latex allergy in children with spina bifida. *Journal of Allergy and Clinical Immunology, 99*(5), 600–604.

McLone, D. G. (1998). Care of the neonate with a myelomeningocele. *Neurosurgery Clinics of North America, 9*(1), 111–120.

McMillan, J. A., DeAngelis, C. D., Feigin, R. D., & Warshaw, J. B. (Eds.). (1999). *Oski's pediatrics: Principles and practice* (3rd ed.). Philadelphia: Lippincott Williams & Wilkins.

Michaud, L. J. (1993). Traumatic brain injury in children. *Pediatric Clinics of North America, 40*(3), 553–565.

Monsen, R. B. (1999). Mother's experiences of living worried when parenting children with spina bifida. *Journal of Pediatric Nursing, 14*(3), 157–163.

Niggeman, B. & Breiteneder, H. (2000). Latex allergy in children. *International Archives of Allergy and Immunology, 121*(2), 98–107.

Pillitteri, A. (1999). *Maternal and child health nursing* (3rd ed.). Philadelphia: Lippincott Williams & Wilkins.

Rekate, H. L. (1997). Recent advances in the understanding and treatment of hydrocephalus. *Seminars in Pediatric Neurology, 4*(3), 167–178.

Roland, E. H. (2000). Muscular dystrophy. *Pediatrics in Review, 21*(7), 223–238.

Ryan, J. A., et al. (1999). Hydrocephalus and shunts in children with brain tumors. *Journal of Pediatric Oncology Nursing, 2*(4), 223–229.

Segelson, J. E., & Haun, S. E. (1996). Status epilepticus in children. *Pediatric Annals, 25*(7), 380–386.

Sheeran, T., et al. (1997). Mothers' resolution of their child's diagnosis and self-reported measures of parenting stress, marital relations, and social support. *Journal of Pediatric Psychology, 22*(2), 197–212.

Shemie, S., et al. (1997). Acute obstructive hydrocephalus and sudden death in children. *Annals of Emergency Medicine, 29*(4), 524–528.

Sood, B. A., Kim, S., Ham, S. D., Canady, A. I., & Greninger, N. (1993). Useful components of the shunt tap test for evaluation of shunt malfunction. *Child's Nervous System, 9*, 157–162.

Staudt, C. A., & Peacock, W. J. (1995). Dorsal rhizotomy for spasticity. *Western Journal of Medicine, 162*(3), 260.

White, M., & Williams, J. (1992). A good start to a full life. Managing continence in children with spina bifida and hydrocephalus. *Professional Nurse, 7*(7), 474–477.

Wildrick, D. (1997). Intraventricular hemorrhage and long-term outcome in the premature infant. *Journal of Neuroscience Nursing, 29*(5), 281–289.

Williams, P. D., et al. (1997). Outcomes of a nursing intervention for siblings of chronically ill children: A pilot study. *Journal of Sociology and Pediatric Nursing, 2*(3), 127–137.

Zaferiou, D. I., et al. (1999). Characteristics and prognosis of epilepsy in children with cerebral palsy. *Journal of Child Neurology, 14*(5), 289–294.

———. (1996). Adrenocorticotropic hormone and vigabatrin treatment of children with infantile spasms underlying cerebral palsy. *Brain Development, 18*(6), 450–452.

CHAPTER

47

Pediatric Eye and Ear Problems

CONDITIONS OF THE EYE

Also see Chapter 16 for additional information on eye problems.

Infectious Processes

Infectious processes of the eye include *conjunctivitis, orbital* or *periorbital cellulitis,* and *hordeolum.* They are characterized by inflammation and tissue damage caused by microbes, such as bacteria, viruses, or *Chlamydia trachomatis.* Conjunctivitis is a common problem, affecting almost all children at some time or another.

Pathophysiology and Etiology

1. Microbes are usually introduced into the eye or surrounding tissues by direct contact with infected objects. Periorbital cellulitis is often associated with infection in nearby tissues, eg, sinusitis or dental abscess.
2. This initiates an inflammatory response that includes dilation of blood vessels, swelling, antibody production, and destruction of the offending agent by white blood cells.
3. Common bacterial agents include *Staphylococcus, Streptococcus pneumoniae, and Haemophilus influenzae.* Adenovirus and, less commonly, herpes virus may occur.
4. Because the infecting agents are easily spread from person to person, conjunctivitis may occur in outbreaks in which several children in the same family, classroom, or community are affected.

Clinical Manifestations

These depend on the part of the eye that is infected.

Redness is characteristic, and must be differentiated from the red eye of noninfectious processes (Table 47-1).

Conjunctivitis

1. Redness of the eye caused by dilation of the blood vessels of the conjunctiva.
2. Excessive tearing and/or exudate.
3. Photophobia.
4. Vision may be cloudy because of exudate, but is not impaired.

Orbital or Periorbital Cellulitis

1. Swelling and inflammation of soft tissues surrounding the eye.
2. Tenderness/pain.
3. Increased temperature of affected areas.
4. Vision is not impaired.

Hordeolum (Stye)

1. Pustule in area of eyelash follicle.
2. Tenderness/pain.
3. Localized swelling and erythema.

Diagnostic Evaluation

1. Culture of exudate for bacteria or virus or antigen testing for *Neisseria gonorrheae* or *C. trachomatis.* Different media are required for cultures of each, but one swab may be sent for antigen testing. The most likely agents are tested, based on the history and physical findings.
2. Screening vision exam may be done; a thorough visual and ocular exam may be done if vision is impaired or if internal involvement is suspected.
3. A dendritic ulcer caused by herpes virus can be visualized by instilling fluorescein dye and examining the cornea with a cobalt-filtered blue light.

NURSING ALERT

A child who has a painful red eye should be referred immediately for medical evaluation, because this may indicate herpetic infection or damage to the cornea.

Treatment

1. Antibiotic eye drops or ointment, such as erythromycin, trimethoprim sulfate and polymyxin B, sulfacetamide, ciprofloxacin, or tobramycin, will shorten the course of bacterial conjunctivitis and will make the child more comfortable.

TABLE 47-1 Common Causes of Eye Redness in Children

Cause	Associated Symptoms	Management
Conjunctivitis		
Viral	Often associated with other symptoms of generalized viral illness	Hygiene, rest
Bacterial	Yellow, green, or white pus, photophobia	Antibiotic eye drops or ointment, hygiene
Chlamydial	Cough, history of maternal infection	Systemic antibiotic
Herpetic	Pain, photophobia, skin lesions	Evaluation by specialist, antiviral agents
Allergic	Itching, seasonal onset of symptoms, other allergic symptoms, watery discharge	Antihistamine, eye drops, avoidance of allergens
Chemical	Watery discharge, onset of symptoms when exposed to cigarettes or other irritants	Avoidance of irritating substances
Trauma	Pain, photophobia, increased tear production	Eye patch, referral to specialist
Congenital Glaucoma	Increased tear production, cloudiness of cornea	Referral to specialist

2. Systemic antibiotic treatment is indicated for orbital cellulitis. These children may be admitted to the hospital for close observation and aggressive management.
3. Hordeolums will usually resolve without antibiotic treatment. Warm compresses are recommended, and incision and drainage may be necessary.

Complications
1. Permanent scarring of the cornea and visual impairment with herpetic infection.
2. Spread of orbital cellulitis to the central nervous system.

Nursing Assessment
1. Assess nature and extent of symptoms and their effect on child's activities.
2. Assess visual acuity.
3. Determine resources available to family for treatment.

Nursing Diagnoses
- Risk for Infection (transmission) related to hand-to-hand or hand-to-object contact
- Pain, Acute related to tissue swelling, inflammation, and light sensitivity

Nursing Interventions
Preventing Infection
1. Perform or teach proper cleansing of drainage.
   a. Use warm water or saline and a disposable applicator, such as cotton balls or gauze.
   b. Use a separate applicator for each eye.
   c. Wipe from inner to outer canthus to avoid contamination.
2. Teach self-care measures to prevent spread of disease to others.
   a. Observe good handwashing practices.
   b. Wipe eyes and nose with tissues and dispose promptly.
3. Administer and teach proper instillation of eye drops or ointment (see p. 1115).

4. Administer oral or IV (intravenous) antibiotics as indicated.

Minimizing Pain
1. Apply warm compresses to affected area.
2. Suggest darkened room and sunglasses for patients with photophobia.
3. Administer analgesics as indicated.

Family Education and Health Maintenance
1. Advise of ways to prevent transmission to others.
   a. Do not share washcloths or towels.
   b. Avoid swimming until infection is resolved.
   c. The child may return to school after having received antibiotic treatment for 24 hours.
   d. Dispose of contaminated items in proper receptacles.
2. Advise parents of indications for reevaluation by health care provider.
   a. Lack of response to antibiotic treatment.
   b. Increase in swelling and tenderness.
   c. Eye pain.
   d. Worsening of visual acuity.
   e. Development of additional symptoms, such as fever.
3. Encourage routine follow-up visits.

Outcome-Based Evaluation
- Parents performing treatment correctly; hygiene procedures followed
- Patient verbalizes less pain; tolerates bright light

Congenital Problems
Congenital problems of the eye include structural defects present at birth or developing soon thereafter. These are often genetically transmitted. They include *cataract, dacryostenosis, glaucoma, ptosis,* and *strabismus.* See Table 47-2 for pathophysiology, clinical manifestations, and management of each.

TABLE 47-2 Congenital Eye Problems

Condition and Description	Clinical Manifestations	Management
Congenital cataract—opacity of the lens. Possible causes include abnormal embryonic development, infection during pregnancy, disturbance of carbohydrate metabolism, metabolic disorders, retinopathy of prematurity. Incidence is 1 in 250 newborns.	Absence of red reflex Visible clouding of lens Varying impairment of vision, depending on size, location, and density of cataract May result in amblyopia	Surgical removal within first 3 months, followed by contact lens in affected eye to correct vision. Postoperative care: sedation for first 24 hours to prevent crying, vomiting and increased intraocular pressure; antibiotic and steroid ointments to prevent infection; eye patch and shield for several days.
Dacryostenosis—relatively common obstruction of the nasolacrimal duct caused by incomplete duct development and persistence of membrane at lower end of duct. Tears cannot exit via the duct into the nasal cavity and continuously spill over onto the cheek. May be unilateral or bilateral.	Excessive tearing and spilling onto cheek Crusted eyelashes and lids Excoriated cheek Normal-appearing eye structures and vision Possible episodes of secondary conjunctivitis and lacrimal duct infection	Resolves spontaneously in 90% of infants in first year of life. Some recommend gentle massage of lacrimal duct, but effectiveness has not been documented. Topical antibiotics for secondary infection. Surgical probing of duct if persists beyond 12 months of age; more complex surgery if probing unsuccessful.
Glaucoma—rare congenital or acquired abnormality in which the balance between aqueous fluid production and outflow is disrupted. Increased pressure of fluid in anterior chamber causes damage to the retina, cornea, and other structures.	Haziness of the cornea Photophobia Excessive tearing Decreased visual acuity (symptoms present in 35% at birth) Permanent loss of vision and amblyopia may result without treatment	Tonometry is done to determine intraocular pressure (IOP). Surgical intervention is often necessary to normalize IOP. Postoperatively, a patch and shield may be worn for several days to protect sutures.
Ptosis—drooping of the eyelid caused by weakness of levator palpebrae or, less frequently, Muller's muscle. May be congenital or acquired; affecting either the muscle or the nerve that innervates it.	Drooping is visible on inspection Vision may be impaired if eyelid covers the pupil May be unilateral or bilateral If unilateral, amblyopia may result without treatment	Surgical correction to raise the eyelid and increase visual field. Patching not necessary postoperatively.
Strabismus—malalignment of the eyes caused by muscle imbalance or by paralysis, which prevents both eyes from focusing correctly on the same image. Occurs in 3% of the population.	Asymmetric pupillary light reflexes Asymmetric extraocular movements Diplopia, impaired depth Tendency to close one eye or tilt head during vision testing Amblyopia may result without treatment	Patching of the stronger eye may correct latent strabismus by exercising the muscles of the weaker eye. Surgical repositioning of the extraocular muscles for severe or fixed cases. Postoperatively: antibiotic ointment, no eye patch.

Nursing Assessment

1. Assess for red light reflex, especially in newborns. Absence or asymmetry of the red light reflex may indicate congenital cataract or an intraocular tumor.
2. Inspect the eyes for redness of conjunctiva, cloudiness of the cornea, excessive tearing, eyelids that partially occlude the pupil, or obvious misalignment, which provide clues to congenital eye problems.
3. Assess visual acuity routinely in infants and children. Changes in acuity may be the first manifestation of a problem or indication of effectiveness of treatment.
4. Perform Hirschberg's test for symmetry of the pupillary light reflexes to help detect strabismus. Normally, the light reflexes are in the same position in each pupil, but will not be with strabismus (positive Hirschberg's test).
5. Perform the cover-uncover test to detect latent strabismus caused by weak eye muscles. When covered, the lazy eye drifts out of position and snaps back quickly when uncovered.

Nursing Diagnoses

- Sensory/Perceptual Alterations (Visual), related to reduction in visual acuity
- Body Image Disturbance related to the need for patch or glasses
- Risk for Injury related to reduced visual acuity and modified depth perception
- Altered Growth and Development related to altered visual stimulation and possible overprotective behavior of parents

Nursing Interventions
Minimizing Effects of Vision Loss

1. Participate in visual acuity problem identification and encourage prompt treatment to minimize functional impairment.
   a. Newborns should be examined in the nursery to detect congenital eye problems.
   b. All children should be screened for visual acuity and strabismus. In young children, this is accomplished by physical examination and assessment of developmental milestones (ie, looks at mother's face, smiles responsively, reaches for objects). By 3 to 5 years of age, most children can cooperate for performance of accurate visual acuity screening tests.
2. Encourage and assist parents in obtaining corrective lenses for child.
3. Encourage and assist parents in providing normal experiences for child to achieve maximum potential:
   a. Assist parents in locating and accessing resources, such as financial assistance, special education in braille, or parent support groups.
   b. Advise parents of their child's right to a public education.

Minimizing Body Image Disturbance

1. Encourage parents to focus on normalization rather than on overprotection. This means having expectations based on the child's abilities rather than disabilities, providing opportunities for interaction with peers, and making the child's life as normal as possible.
2. Encourage acceptance of appearance and emphasize the positive aspects of treatment.

Preventing Injury

1. Encourage the family to be aware of safety in the home, school, and community.
   a. Suggest the use of impact-resistant eyeglasses and devices to keep eyeglasses from falling off.
   b. Advise the family to maintain a consistent and uncluttered furniture arrangement; notify child of planned changes.
   c. Instruct child in the use of a cane or other assistive device.
   d. Teach traffic safety and personal security measures.
2. Orient visually impaired children in the hospital to the placement of furniture and other objects in their room.
   a. Orient child to food placement on meal trays.
   b. Assist child with ambulation and use side rails on bed or crib to prevent falls.

Promoting Normal Growth and Development

1. Encourage parents to provide many sensory opportunities, such as manipulating objects, hearing various sounds, noting the smells in the environment, and tasting an assortment of substances.
2. Allow child to perform activities of daily living as independently as possible.

Family Education and Health Maintenance
Postoperative Teaching

1. Teach about instillation of medications and use of eye shield to prevent injury to eye after surgery.
2. Teach about activity restrictions after glaucoma surgery.
   a. Bed rest may be required immediately postoperatively.
   b. Older children should not engage in strenuous activity or contact sports for 2 weeks.
3. Advise that activity is usually not restricted for surgery for strabismus or ptosis.
4. After cataract surgery, encourage behaviors to reduce the risk of damage to sutures from increased intraocular pressure:
   a. Avoid overfeeding to prevent vomiting.
   b. Minimize crying.
5. Encourage parents to remove eye discharge or crusts on lashes regularly by washing the eyes with warm water. Separate washcloths should be used for each child. Moist cotton balls may be used to clean the affected child's eyes. A separate one should be used for each eye.

Other Concerns

1. Advise of indications for reevaluation by health care provider:
   a. Worsening of visual acuity.
   b. Evidence of infection, such as pain, redness, swelling, drainage, and increased temperature.
2. Refer family for information on eye disease and safety measures to Prevent Blindness America, 500 East Remington Road, Schaumburg, IL 60173, 800-331-2020, *www.preventblindness.org.*

Outcome-Based Evaluation

- Child wearing glasses as prescribed; vision improved
- Parents and child report involvement in activities, satisfactory school performance, and positive peer interactions
- No injuries reported
- Age-appropriate developmental milestones achieved

▧ Eye Trauma

Eye trauma causes structural damage to the eye and is produced by mechanical force or contact with a corrosive chemical. Some common types of eye trauma are *corneal abrasions, blunt trauma, perforating injuries,* and *chemical injuries.* Eye injuries are common among children and are usually related to their involvement in vigorous play activities.

Pathophysiology and Etiology
Corneal Abrasion

1. Produced when an area of the cornea is scratched.
2. This may happen when a foreign object becomes lodged in the eye, a contact lens rubs against the eye because of inadequate tear production, or a fingernail or other sharp object enters the eye and scrapes the cornea.

Blunt Trauma

1. This occurs when the eye and/or surrounding tissues are struck by a blunt object, such as a ball.
2. The resulting injury includes tissue swelling and seepage of blood into the surrounding tissues.
3. The bony structures surrounding the eye may be fractured.
4. The lens may become dislodged or the retina may separate from the back of the eye.

Perforating Injury

1. When an object penetrates the eyeball, there may be loss of vitreous material and/or damage to the internal structures of the eye.
2. Bacteria may also be introduced into the interior of the eye, causing infection.

Chemical Injuries

1. Corrosive chemicals burn the delicate tissues of the cornea and may penetrate into deeper layers of the eye.
2. Healing may occur with scarring.

Clinical Manifestations

1. Pain—because the delicate tissues of the eye contain many nerve endings.

NURSING ALERT

At times, pain may be useful in distinguishing a serious eye problem from a self-limiting condition.

2. Increased tear production—one of the eye's defenses against injury or irritation.
3. Injection of the blood vessels of the cornea—increase of blood flow to the cornea is another protective mechanism; most likely to be seen with foreign bodies, abrasions, or chemical burns that affect the cornea.
4. Impaired visual acuity caused by:
   a. Swelling of the cornea, reducing its clarity.
   b. Swelling of the soft tissues surrounding the eye, causing the eye to partially or completely close.
   c. Excessive tear production, impairing vision.
   d. Damage to internal structures of the eye, altering or obstructing visual pathways.
5. Visible signs of injury—bruising, swelling, or a foreign object visible in the eye.

Diagnostic Evaluation

1. Thorough inspection of the eye, including eversion of the upper lid to inspect for a foreign object.
2. Fundoscopic examination may detect abnormalities, such as a dislodged lens, retinal hemorrhage, retinal detachment, or papilledema with increased intraocular pressure.
3. Staining with fluorescein dye will reveal lesions of the cornea, such as abrasions.
4. Assessment of eye function, including near and far acuity, extraocular movements, and visual field testing.

Management

Most childhood injuries are not severe and will resolve spontaneously with no adverse long-term consequences. It is important, however, to identify and obtain prompt treatment for significant injuries.

Corneal Abrasion

1. If the abrasion was caused by a contact lens or foreign body, removal of the offending body is indicated.
2. Patching of the affected eye, usually for 24 hours, will control pain.
3. Antibiotic eye drops or ointment prevent infection.

Blunt Trauma

1. Application of cold compresses may help control pain and swelling.
2. The head should be elevated 30 degrees to avoid increased intraocular pressure.
3. Surgery may be required because of damage to underlying bones or eye structures.

Perforating Injury

1. Surgery is usually necessary to remove the object and reconstruct damaged tissues.

NURSING ALERT

Never remove a penetrating object from the eye. It should be stabilized and the eye should be shielded with no pressure applied. The other eye should be patched and the patient transported by stretcher. The head should be elevated 30 degrees to avoid increased intraocular pressure, and the child should be kept on NPO (nothing-by-mouth) orders in preparation for surgery.

Chemical Injuries

1. Gentle flushing of the affected eye(s) with water will help remove the offending chemical. This should be done from the inner aspect of eye to the outer to prevent contaminated water from flowing into the other eye.
2. Antibiotics may be prescribed to prevent infection.
3. Further management depends on the nature and extent of the injury.

Complications

1. Infection.
2. Extensive tissue damage may result in permanent visual impairment.
3. Disfigurement may result from severe or extensive tissue damage.

Nursing Assessment

1. Obtain history of injury, including the child's account of how the injury occurred, and a description of symptoms experienced by him or her.
2. Inspect for location and extent of swelling and/or bruising, asymmetry, or abnormality in appearance of any part of the eye.

3. Assess visual acuity and compare with baseline. This should include near and far acuity in each eye. If the patient cannot see well enough to read a Snellen chart, assess ability to count fingers or perceive light.

Nursing Diagnoses
- Pain, Acute related to inflammation, photophobia, or trauma to eye tissue
- Risk for Injury related to impaired vision and side effects of pain medications
- Self-Care Deficits (feeding, bathing/hygiene, toileting, dressing/grooming, and instrumental) related to impaired vision and side effects of pain medications

Nursing Interventions
Minimizing Pain
1. Apply cold compresses to the affected area to help reduce swelling and discomfort.
2. Keep the child's room as dark as possible to help reduce pain for photophobic patients.
3. Administer or teach parents to administer analgesics as prescribed.

Preventing Injury
1. Enforce safety measures:
   a. Use of side rails.
   b. Assistance with ambulation.
   c. Observe closely.

Maintaining Activities of Daily Living
1. Provide assistance with eating, bathing, toileting, and other activities of daily living, as needed.
2. Teach child location of self-care items and positioning of food on tray to promote independence.
3. Encourage child to attempt self-care, and offer praise even if unsuccessful.

Family Education and Health Maintenance
1. Teach indications for reevaluation by health care provider.
   a. Increase in swelling, tenderness, discoloration, or pain.
   b. Worsening of visual acuity.
   c. Development of additional symptoms, such as fever, alteration in sensorium, or other indications of neurologic injury.
2. Provide safety education to all families to prevent common causes of injury. In particular, encourage families to use protective eyewear when participating in sports activities.
3. Provide families with information and support as they cope with having a visually impaired child in the home. The American Academy of Ophthalmology has patient information and a list of helpful resources at its web site: *http://www.eyenet.org/*.

Outcome-Based Evaluation
- Demonstrates decreased pain
- No injuries reported
- Dressing and feeding self with minimal assistance

▪ Functional Problems

Functional problems of the eye involve impairment of the vision because of *refractive errors* or disuse of visual pathways resulting in *amblyopia*. Abnormal vision screening with referral occurs in 1.2% of 5-year-old patients and increases to 9.1% by the time the child is 13 years old. Amblyopia affects 1% to 3% of the population.

Pathophysiology and Etiology
1. Refractive errors are usually caused by a genetic predisposition to shortened or elongated eyeballs or by individual variations in growth.
   a. In an elongated or shortened eyeball, the visual image is focused either in front of or behind the retina, resulting in unclear images.
   b. The nearsighted (myopic) child can see near objects, such as print in schoolbooks, but cannot focus clearly on far objects, such as writing on the blackboard.
   c. The farsighted (hyperopic) child can see far objects clearly, but has difficulty seeing near objects.
   d. The problem may be unilateral or bilateral.
2. Amblyopia may result from any condition that causes the two retinas to receive different images.
   a. Diplopia caused by strabismus.
   b. Significant difference in acuity of the two eyes.
   c. Cataract.
   d. Unilateral ptosis.
3. When a discrepancy exists between images received on the two retinas, the more unclear image is suppressed.
   a. Over time, a young child will become permanently unable to use the visual pathways of the suppressed eye.
   b. Although the visual pathways are structurally normal, the child is visually impaired in that eye.

Clinical Manifestations
Children often do not complain that they cannot see well, but may exhibit other signs of vision problems, including the following.
1. Poor academic performance or behavioral problems in school.
2. Dislike for reading.
3. Head tilting.
4. Squinting.
5. Sitting close to the television or holding reading materials close to the face.
6. Refusal or resistance to covering one eye during vision screening.

Diagnostic Evaluation
1. Standardized vision screening tests, such as the Snellen chart, the Titmus machine, or the H:O:T:V matching symbol test, may be used for distance acuity screening.
   a. Tests can be administered to children as young as 3 years of age.
   b. Each eye should be tested separately.

2. Near vision may be tested by having the child read or by standardized vision screening tests, such as the Titmus machine. Each eye should be tested separately.
3. Muscle balance can be tested using the cover test and the Titmus machine.

Management

1. Most visual acuity problems can be treated by the use of corrective lenses or refractive surgery.
2. Amblyopia is treated with glasses and patching of the weaker eye. New pharmacologic treatments are becoming available but are not in widespread use. Optimal outcome is accomplished when treatment is begun early in life, while visual pathways are still developing. However, some visual function may be recovered even if the problem is treated in adolescence or adulthood. Ideally, the problem can be prevented by early identification and treatment of factors that may cause it.

Complications

1. Injuries caused by visual impairment.

Nursing Assessment

1. Begin visual acuity screening early, in the preschool years, and whenever a child displays behaviors suggestive of acuity problems.
2. Assess Hirschberg's test for symmetry of the pupillary light reflexes routinely, beginning at birth.
3. Perform the cover-uncover test as part of routine eye assessment as soon as the child can cooperate (as young as 3 years of age).
4. Assess the effect of the functional deficit on the child's overall function, including academic progress, self-esteem, and safety.

Nursing Diagnoses

- Sensory/Perceptual Alterations (Visual) related to reduced acuity or inability to use one eye
- Risk for Injury related to impaired visual acuity or lack of depth perception
- Self-Esteem Disturbance related to lowered performance caused by poor vision

Nursing Interventions

Minimizing Effects of Sensory Deficits

1. Encourage the consistent use of corrective lenses as prescribed.
2. Teach the parents ways to help develop the child's skills in interpreting information through the senses of hearing, smell, and touch.
   a. Familiarize the child with common sounds and smells in the environment. Also orient the child to traffic sounds and sounds associated with danger, such as animals and speeding vehicles, and instruct the child how to respond.
   b. Use voice or touch, rather than facial expressions or gestures, to express emotion.
   c. Speak to the child before touching to reduce startling.
   d. Allow the child to touch and handle unfamiliar objects to learn about them.
   e. Have the child practice such things as retelling stories and giving the home telephone number and address.
   f. Explain unfamiliar sounds and smells to the hospitalized child.

Preventing Injury

1. Recommend the use of shatterproof eyeglasses with flexible frames.
2. Recommend the use of eye protection on a routine basis, because eye trauma can occur unexpectedly. This is especially important for children who rely on only one eye.
3. Suggest extra protection, such as shatterproof goggles or shields, when participating in contact or ball sports and activities.
4. Maintain a stable arrangement of furniture in the home, adequate lighting, and an uncluttered environment to minimize falls.
5. Orient hospitalized children to the hospital room and offer assistance when walking.

Promoting a Positive Sense of Self-Esteem

1. Provide opportunities for mastery of developmentally appropriate activities.
2. Encourage interactions with sighted children to decrease feelings of isolation. Also suggest interactions with children with similar alterations in vision.
3. Encourage the child to discuss feelings and strategies for coping with negative peer reactions, such as teasing.
4. Encourage independence in self-care activities to promote autonomy, such as dressing, feeding, and use of bathroom.
5. Assist the patient and family with effective coping mechanisms to promote family stability.

Community and Home Care Considerations

1. Perform a safety inspection of the home environment and make changes as necessary to help prevent falls and other injuries.
2. Assist family access to financial and social resources as needed.
3. Ensure that child is receiving specialized educational resources as needed.

Family Education and Health Maintenance

1. Teach the importance of wearing corrective lenses as prescribed, and their proper care.
2. Refer families of blind children to community resources that can help their child learn special skills, such as reading braille, using a cane, or developing self-care skills. Information can be obtained from agencies such as the American Foundation for the Blind, 11 Penn Plaza, Suite 300, New York, NY (212) 502-7600, *www.afb.org*.

Outcome-Based Evaluation

- Child identifies common sounds
- No injury reported; wears protective eyeglasses
- Reports good school performance and participation in extracurricular activities; can eat and dress independently

CONDITIONS OF THE EAR

Also see Chapter 17 for additional information on ear, nose, and throat problems.

Eustachian Tube Dysfunction

Eustachian tube dysfunction (ETD) comprises disorders that arise from closure of the eustachian tube, which ventilates the middle ear to equalize pressure on both sides of the tympanic membrane. ETD leads to middle ear effusion. ETD may present as otitis media with effusion (OME), also known as serous otitis; acute otitis media (AOM); and recurrent otitis media. Approximately 91% of children experience one or more episodes of middle ear effusion by the time they are 24 months of age.

Pathophysiology and Etiology

1. Swelling of the eustachian tube lining is caused by an acute upper respiratory tract infection or an allergic response.
   a. Infected secretions may pass through the tube from the nasal area into the middle ear.
   b. When swelling causes the eustachian tube to close, the passage of air into and out of the middle ear is prevented.
   c. The air in the middle ear is absorbed into the middle ear lining and a vacuum is created.
   d. The vacuum is filled by serous fluid that seeps out of the middle ear lining.
   e. The warm, moist environment of the middle ear and nutrients in the serous fluid are conducive to the growth of viruses and/or bacteria that may be present in the middle ear cavity.
2. Children between the ages of 6 months and 24 months are predisposed to the development of acute otitis media because their short, relatively straight eustachian tubes more easily allow the passage of infected nasal secretions into the middle ear cavity. Risk factors include:
   a. More frequent episodes of upper respiratory tract infections in younger children.
   b. Nasal allergies.
   c. Genetics—in some families, children's eustachian tubes tend to be floppy and to close easily.
   d. Native American or Eskimo heritage.
   e. Craniofacial abnormalities.
   f. Down's syndrome.
   g. Lower socioeconomic status.
   h. Exposure to cigarette smoke.
3. Most common bacterial agents include:
   a. *S. pneumoniae.*
   b. *Haemophilus influenzae.*
   c. *Moraxella catarrhalis.*
4. Barotrauma, caused by rapid changes in atmospheric pressure, may also lead to closure of the eustachian tube and to development of serous otitis. This is less likely to involve introduction of microorganisms through infected nasal secretions; development of acute otitis media is less common.

Clinical Manifestations

1. Decreased hearing—temporary conductive hearing loss; usually resolves when tympanic membrane mobility is restored.
2. Sensation of fullness in the affected ear(s).
3. Popping sensations in the affected ear(s) may be experienced as the eustachian tube begins to open and admit air into the middle ear cavity.
4. Ear pain.
5. Signs of infection—fever, irritability, or decreased appetite.

Diagnostic Evaluation

1. Otoscopic examination.
   a. OME—yellowish effusion, prominent bony landmarks, a diffuse light reflex, and decreased mobility of tympanic membrane.
   b. Acute otitis media—inflamed tympanic membrane with decreased or absent mobility; bulging of the tympanic membrane may obscure the bony landmarks and light reflex.
2. Tympanometry—quick and simple way to assess tympanic membrane mobility (Figure 47-1).
   a. A probe occludes the ear canal while pressure is varied and a test sound is emitted. The test produces a graphic display that shows the mobility of the tympanic membrane at various air pressures.
   b. A normal reading has a distinct peak in the middle of the graph (see Figure 47–1A).
   c. A flat tympanogram (no peak) indicates lack of mobility of the tympanic membrane, usually caused by serous otitis or acute otitis media (see Figure 47–1B).
   d. A peak to the left of the center indicates negative pressure in the middle ear (see Figure 47–1C).
3. Acoustic reflectometry—useful in infants older than age 3 months of age.
   a. A probe held at the opening of the ear canal measures reflected sound waves from the middle ear.
   b. Reduction in reflected sound is an indication of middle ear effusion.

Management

OME

1. Usually resolves spontaneously.
2. Treatment of underlying predisposing factors, eg, allergies, may provide some relief.

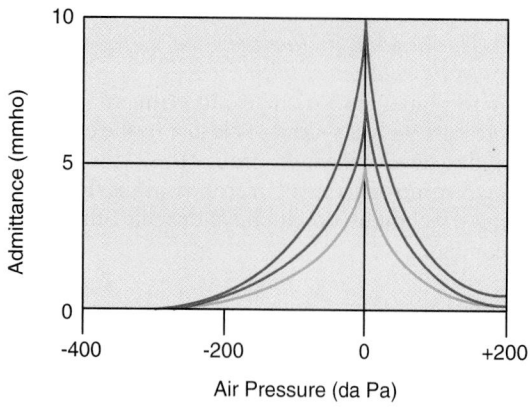

A

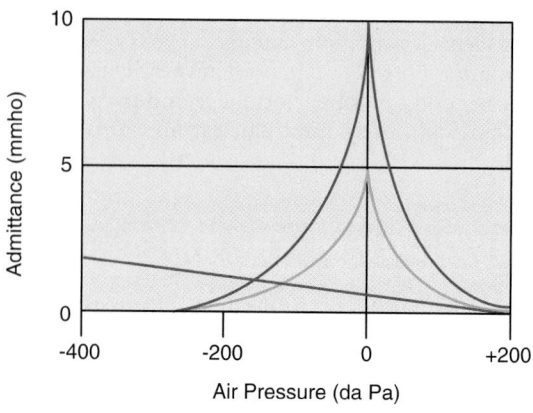

B

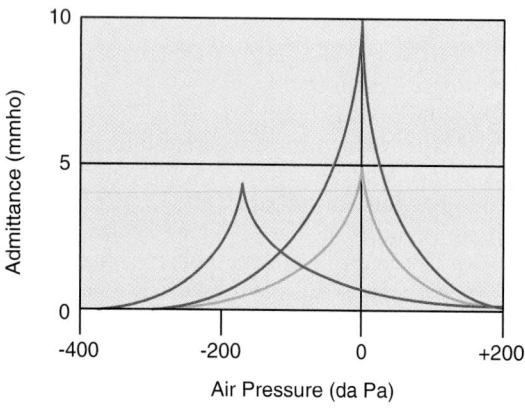

C

FIGURE 47-1 (**A**) Type A tympanogram: This is the normal pattern showing mobility of the tympanic membrane with a peak mobility at the 0 point (the point at which there is neither positive nor negative pressure in the external ear canal). (**B**) Type B tympanogram: This pattern shows a low level of mobility with no peak. It is characteristic of impaired mobility due to the presence of fluid in the middle ear. (**C**) Type C tympanogram: This pattern shows a distinct peak in the mobility level of the tympanic membrane, but the peak occurs when there is negative pressure in the external ear canal. This indicates eustachian tube dysfunction causing negative pressure in the middle ear cavity. Negative pressure in the external ear canal equalizes pressure on both sides of the tympanic membrane and allows for maximum mobility. (Dershewitz, R. A. [1988]. *Ambulatory pediatric care*. Philadelphia: J. B. Lippincott.)

3. Placement of ventilating tubes may be considered for effusions that persist for 3 or more months with bilateral hearing loss of 20 or more decibels.
4. Adenoidectomy may benefit some children.

Acute Otitis Media

1. Systemic antibiotic treatment—usually an oral preparation is taken for 5 to 10 days.
2. Amoxicillin remains the drug of choice, although higher doses are now given (80–90 mg/kg) because of growing prevalence of resistant bacteria (*S. pneumoniae*).
   a. Those at risk for resistance are children younger than age 2, those treated with antibiotics within the past 2 months, and those who attend day care.
   b. Some authorities recommend treating only symptomatic cases.
3. Alternative antibiotics for treatment failures include amoxicillin-clavulanate (Augmentin) or cefuroximine exetil (Ceftin) or ceftriaxone (Rocephin) IM (intramuscularly).
4. Placement of ventilating tubes by myringotomy (incision into the tympanic membrane) may be considered

for children who experience three or more episodes in 6 months or four or more episodes per year (Figure 47-2).

Recurrent Otitis Media
1. Placement of ventilating tubes in the tympanic membrane allows fluid to drain through the ear canal rather than to become trapped in the middle ear.
2. Antibiotic prophylaxis is controversial. Many do not recommend it because it may contribute to the problem of antibiotic-resistant bacteria.

Complications
1. Permanent hearing loss, perforations of the tympanic membrane, scarring because of healed perforations, or damage to the ossicles of the middle ear.
2. Delayed speech and language development.
3. Mastoiditis, meningitis, lateral sinus thrombosis, or intracranial abscess; spread of bacterial infection.

Nursing Assessment
1. Assess for etiologic factors that contribute to eustachian tube dysfunction.
2. Assess for symptoms of serous otitis and acute otitis media to identify and to document the nature and severity of the illness.
3. Assess hearing after the middle ear effusion is resolved. Promptly identify any hearing loss that may have social and educational consequences.
4. Assess speech and language development in children who experience recurrent or prolonged infections to determine deficits.

NURSING ALERT

Prompt identification of speech and language delays is important in young children, because speech and language development is quite rapid at this time. Young children may demonstrate rapid regression or failure of progression.

---

5. Assess for effects of illness on family, such as sleep deprivation of parents caused by staying up with child at night or decreased attendance at work caused by keeping child out of school.

Nursing Diagnoses
- Pain, Acute, related to increased pressure in the middle ear
- Sensory/Perceptual Alterations (Auditory), related to reduced sound wave conduction
- Impaired Verbal Communication caused by conductive hearing loss

Nursing Interventions
Minimizing Discomfort
1. Administer and teach parents to administer antibiotics. Provide instruction in:
   a. Measurement of correct dosage.
   b. Time of doses.
   c. Importance of administering all doses.
   d. Proper storage and disposal of unused medication.
   e. Side effects.
2. Administer acetaminophen as directed for pain or fever.
3. Apply warm compresses to the external ear.
4. Administer analgesic otic drops, if prescribed; usually indicated when no perforation of the tympanic membrane exists.
5. Advise elevation of head to facilitate drainage of fluid from the middle ear into the pharynx.
6. Teach older children to stimulate opening of their eustachian tubes by yawning or performing Valsalva's maneuver.

Minimizing Hearing Loss
1. Teach parents to recognize early signs of otitis and to seek prompt treatment.
2. Provide preoperative and postoperative teaching if ventilation tubes are indicated (see p. 212).
3. Stress the importance of the follow-up visit to ensure that otitis has resolved.

Facilitating Verbal Communication
1. Assess hearing, speech, and language development regularly.
2. Alert parents to immediately report signs of hearing difficulty or delayed speech to ensure early intervention.
3. Refer to a specialist for evaluation and treatment, if necessary.

Family Education and Health Maintenance
1. Teach parents that episodes of otitis may be minimized by:
   a. Breast-feeding.
   b. Placing older, bottle-fed infants in a sitting position during feeding.
   c. Using specially designed bottles to allow upright feeding.
   d. Identifying and eliminating allergens, such as particular foods, molds, and dust.
   e. Not exposing the child to cigarette smoke.

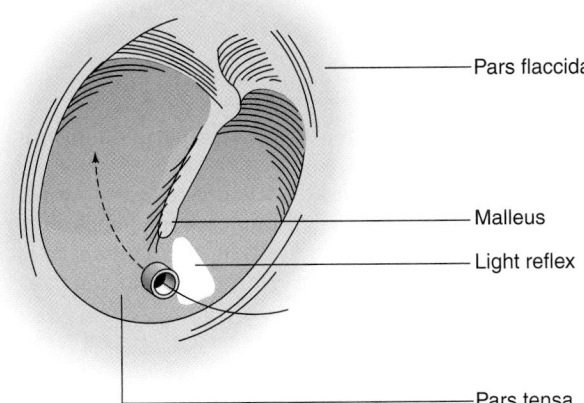

FIGURE 47-2 A ventilating (myringotomy) tube provides air to the middle ear to prevent otitis media.

Pars flaccida
Malleus
Light reflex
Pars tensa

2. Teach the importance of taking antibiotic at prescribed times for the indicated length of therapy to prevent partial treatment and the development of resistance.

3. Teach all parents the difference between viral and bacterial infections and that overuse of antibiotics for viral infections contributes to the development of resistant bacteria. Encourage all parents to consult with health care provider before starting antibiotic therapy for presumed infection.

4. If ventilating tubes are placed, instruct parents to do the following.
   a. Avoid water or other fluids from entering the ear canal. Encourage use of earplugs when the child is bathing or swimming.
   b. Discourage instillation of eardrops or other medications in the external ear.
   c. Tubes will come out of the ear spontaneously, usually in 6–12 months.

5. Encourage families to discuss herbal therapy with health care provider if interested.
   a. Echinacea is used by some to enhance immune function.
   b. Ear drops with mullein, St. John's wort, and garlic are available to alleviate pressure in the middle ear during acute ear infections.
   c. Goldenseal is said to have antimicrobial activity. High amounts may cause gastrointestinal discomfort and possibly nervous system effects.

Outcome-Based Evaluation

- Demonstrates improved comfort; family states proper treatment regimen
- Follow-up visits maintained; effusion resolved
- Speech and language development appropriate for age; reports regular assessment; receives therapy from specialist, if indicated

■ External Otitis

External otitis is inflammation in the external ear canal. It is frequently unilateral but may be bilateral.

Pathophysiology and Etiology

1. Caused by bacteria or fungi. Common pathogens include:
   a. *Pseudomonas aeruginosa.*
   b. *Enterobacter aerogenes.*
   c. *Proteus mirabilis.*
   d. *Staphylococcus epidermidis.*
   e. Fungi (candida, aspergillus).
2. Risk factors include:
   a. Frequent swimming, especially in chlorinated pools. Chlorine destroys the normal ear flora.
   b. Insertion of objects, eg, cotton swabs, into the ear canals.
   c. Acute otitis media with perforation of the tympanic membrane.
   d. Ventilation tubes with drainage.

3. When water remains in the external ear canal, a warm, moist environment is created.
4. Skin lining the canal is irritated, causing breakdown of its protective barrier.
5. Bacteria and/or fungi overgrow in the conducive environment and cause symptoms of inflammation and infection in 1–2 days.
6. Breakdown of protective barrier and introduction and proliferation of infectious organisms can also occur through trauma to the ear canal, such as cleaning the ear with an inappropriate object or using an inappropriate technique.

Clinical Manifestations

1. Ear pain, itching, and white, yellow, or greenish drainage.
2. Inflammation of the external ear canal and structures.
3. Pain when the ear pinna is manipulated.

Diagnostic Evaluation

1. Otoscopic examination; may be difficult because of severe pain and swelling; shows redness, swelling, and drainage in canal; tympanic membrane appears normal.
2. Cultures usually not necessary.

Treatment

1. Acetic acid solution (VoSol) to dry and modify the pH of the ear canal.
2. Topical antibiotic solution, possibly combined with a steroid to reduce significant discomfort and swelling.
3. Ear canal may require irrigation to remove drainage.
4. A medication-soaked wick may be applied to facilitate medication administration.

Nursing Assessment

1. Assess severity of symptoms and need for pain relief.
2. Assess ear hygiene and the need for earplugs.

Nursing Diagnosis

- Pain, Acute, related to inflammation and irritation of drainage

Nursing Interventions
Relieving Pain

1. Administer eardrops, or teach parents administration, as prescribed.
   a. Have child lie on side with affected ear upward.
   b. Instill drops, using caution not to contaminate dropper.
   c. Have child maintain position for 5 minutes to facilitate penetration of medication into ear canal.
   d. Repeat on other side, if ordered.
2. Administer analgesics, such as acetaminophen (Tylenol), as directed.
3. Suggest application of warm or cold compresses to outer ear to relieve discomfort.
4. Frequently cleanse drainage from area surrounding opening of ear canal to relieve irritation.

Family Education and Health Maintenance

1. Teach proper ear hygiene.
   a. Insert nothing into ear canal for cleaning or scratching.
   b. Cleanse the outer area with a washcloth only.
   c. Drain water promptly from ear by leaning the child over and pulling auricle slightly downward and outward.
2. Instruct in the use of well-fitting earplugs, if necessary.
3. Instruct in the use of routine acetic acid solution instillation after water activity, if prescribed.

Outcome-Based Evaluation

- Reports pain relieved; uses compresses and analgesics, if necessary

■ Functional Hearing Disorders

These conditions arise from problems in the function of the ear. In a quiet environment, the healthy child can hear tones between 0 and 25 decibels. Categories of hearing impairment include slight, 15–25 decibels; mild, 25–40 decibels; moderate, 40–65 decibels; severe, 65–95 decibels; and profound, 95 or more decibels. Congenital hearing loss occurs in approximately 1:600 live births.

Pathophysiology and Etiology

1. Hearing loss may be conductive or sensorineural.
2. Conductive loss occurs when there is impaired transmission of sound through the outer and/or middle ear, caused by impaction of cerumen in the external ear canal, fluid in the middle ear cavity, or scarring of the tympanic membrane.
   a. A mechanical obstruction, such as cerumen or a foreign object blocking the external ear canal, may block the passage of sound waves to the tympanic membrane.
   b. With otitis media or OME, fluid in the middle ear cavity does not transmit sound as well as air.
   c. A scarred or perforated tympanic membrane has lost its normal mobility and does not transmit sound as well as a normal one.
   d. Most cases of conductive hearing loss in children are reversible and produce no permanent effect.
3. Sensorineural hearing loss results from damage to the cochlea or auditory nerve and congenital defects of the cochlea. Examples include damage caused by ototoxic drugs, damage resulting from prenatal infections, and damage caused by prolonged exposure to loud noise.
   a. Damage to the auditory nerve prevents transmission of sound impulses to the brain for interpretation.
   b. Damage to the hair cells of the cochlea may be caused by prolonged exposure to loud noise, resulting in hearing loss. This is especially pronounced for high-pitched sounds.
   c. Sensorineural problems are usually irreversible.

Clinical Manifestations

Children often do not complain that they cannot hear well. They may exhibit other signs of hearing problems, including the following.

1. Poor academic performance or behavior problems in school.
2. Lack of response to sounds.
3. Delayed language development.
4. Listening to the television or radio at a loud volume.
5. Speaking loudly.

Diagnostic Evaluation

1. Assess all infants for their response to sound and achievement of developmental speech language milestones.
2. High-risk infants should be screened by an audiologist.
3. Routine audiometric screening should be done beginning as soon as the child can cooperate and follow instructions (between ages 3 and 5 years).

Management

1. Treatment of the underlying problem, such as impacted cerumen or otitis media.
2. Hearing aids may be helpful for both conductive and sensorineural hearing loss.
3. Cochlear implants help some children with sensorineural hearing loss.
   a. Consists of an external microphone and speech processor, which sends radio signals to an internal electrode array implanted in the cochlea.
   b. Most effective in the young child who has had shorter hearing deprivation, but requires a long period of rehabilitation.
4. If the problem cannot be corrected, the focus of treatment is on development of adaptive skills through special education, sign language, or technical devices for the hearing impaired.

Complications

1. Speech and language delays.
2. Inadequate social development.

Nursing Assessment

1. Periodically assess hearing in the child with an identified hearing impairment, to follow up promptly on changes in ability to hear.
2. Assess speech and language development frequently so that children may obtain special assistance, as indicated.
3. Assess social development and academic progress periodically so that counseling and intervention can be instituted.

Nursing Diagnoses

- Sensory/Perceptual Alterations (Auditory), related to limited ability to hear
- Impaired Verbal Communication related to inability to hear and imitate speech sounds

- Risk for Injury related to inability to hear warning sounds of impending danger
- Self-Esteem Disturbance related to social and academic difficulties

Nursing Interventions

Minimizing Effects of Hearing Loss

1. Face the child, use appropriate facial expressions, and make sure the child can see your face clearly when communicating.
2. Approach the child so that you can be seen; touch the deaf child on the shoulder to get attention.
3. Assist the child in utilizing hearing aid as prescribed.

Promoting Effective Communication

1. Determine usual method of communication: ability to write, using verbal cues, or reading lips. Do not depend on gestures to communicate with child or with a third party who does not know sign language.
2. Obtain an interpreter, when necessary, for children who communicate using sign language. Adequate communication is especially important when providing health education or when treating children who may have been abused.
3. Help the parents of a young child to stimulate and communicate with him or her.
   a. Teach them to use gestures, mime, and nonverbal communication.
   b. Teach them to help the infant to develop watching behavior by rewarding him or her with pleasure and praise.
   c. Teach them to talk to the child while looking directly into his or her eyes and using appropriate facial expressions.

Preventing Injury

1. Advise parents that home safety devices, such as smoke detectors, may require visual or tactile alarms (flashing lights or vibration) rather than auditory alarms.
2. Encourage the use of other senses to compensate for inability to hear. For example, the child should be especially careful to look in all directions when crossing the street.
3. Do not leave the child alone in an unfamiliar environment without means of communication.
4. Provide close surveillance and frequent visual contact for the hospitalized child.

Increasing Self-Esteem

1. Inform families of the child's right to a public education.
2. Encourage interaction with both hearing and nonhearing children to promote integration.
3. Encourage mastery of developmental milestones and skills through self-care activities and play.
4. Help parents understand that the child may not be able to express anxiety or frustration and may act out instead.

5. Teach them to be consistent in their use of discipline and to provide alternative ways for the child to gain attention or to relieve stress.
6. Praise the child for accomplishments and attempts at social interaction.

Family Education and Health Maintenance

1. Encourage families to learn sign language and alternative methods of communication with the child.
2. Advise on proper cleaning and maintenance of hearing aids.
3. Encourage attention to health maintenance needs, such as immunizations and well-child visits.
4. For additional support and information, refer to agencies such as the American Speech-Hearing Association, 10801 Rockville Pike, Rockville, MD 20852, 800-638-TALK, *www.asha.org*.

Outcome-Based Evaluation

- Responds appropriately to environmental stimuli
- Communicates effectively through sign language, interpreter, and visual cues
- No injuries reported
- Reports adequate progress in school and participation in extracurricular activities

SELECTED REFERENCES

American Academy of Pediatrics (1997). Environmental tobacco smoke. A hazard to children. *Pediatrics, 99*(4), 639–642.

Campos, E. C. (1997). Future directions in the treatment of amblyopia. *The Lancet, 349*(9060), 1190.

Carpenito, L. J. (1997). *Nursing diagnosis: Application to clinical practice* (7th ed.). Philadelphia: Lippincott-Raven.

Clemens, C. J., et al. (2000). The false positive in universal newborn hearing screening. *Pediatrics, 106*, e7. (*http://www.pediatrics.org/cgi/content/full/106/1/e7*)

Damoiseaux, R. A., van Balen, F. A., Hoes, A. W., Verheij, T. J., & de Melker, R. A. (2000). Primary care based randomized, double blind trial of amoxicillin versus placebo for acute otitis media in children age under 2 years. *British Medical Journal, 320*(7231), 350–354.

Daw, N. W. (1998). Critical periods and amblyopia. *Archives of Ophthalmology, 116*(4), 502–505.

Donahue, S. P., Khoury, J. M., & Kowalski, R. P. (1996). Common ocular infections: A prescriber's guide. *Drugs, 52*(4), 526–540.

Gwiazda, J., Ong, E., Held, R., & Thorn, F. (2000). Myopia and ambient night-time lighting. *Nature, 404*, 144.

Hodges, S. C., Stratford, K. J., & Moore, D. R. (1997). Duration and recurrence of otitis media with effusion from birth to 3 years: Prospective study using monthly otoscopy and tympanometry. *British Medical Journal, 314*(7077), 350–353.

Kanra, G., Scemeer, G., Gonc, E. N., Ceyhan, M., & Ecevit, Z. (1996). Periorbital cellulitis: A comparison of different treatment regimens. *Acta Paediatrica Japonica, 38*(4), 339–42.

Lee, J., Adams, G., Sloper, J., & McIntyre, A. (1998). Future of preschool vision screening. Cost effectiveness of screening for amblyopia is a public health issue. *British Medical Journal, 316*(7135), 937–938.

Nelson, J. D. (1998). *1998 pocket book of pediatric antimicrobial therapy* (13th ed.). Baltimore: Williams & Wilkins.

Orlando, R. G., & Doty, J. H. (1996). Ocular sports trauma. A private practice study. *Journal of the American Optometric Association, 67*(2) 77–80.

Paradise, J. L. (1995). Managing otitis media. A time for change. *Mayo Clinic Proceedings, 96*(4), 712–715.

Pillitteri, A. (1998). *Maternal and child health nursing* (3rd ed.). Philadelphia: Lippincott Williams & Wilkins.

Quinn, G. E. (1999). Myopia and use of night lights in infancy. *Nature, 399,* 113–114.

Recurrent Ear Infections. *www.vitaminbuzz.com/Concern/ Ear_Infections.htm.*

Rittichier, K. K., Roback, M. G., & Bassett, K. E. (2000). Are signs and symptoms associated with persistent corneal abrasions in children? *Archives of Pediatrics and Adolescet Medicine, 154*(4), 370–374.

Siberry, G. K., & Iannone, R. (Eds.) (2000). *The Harriet Lane Handbook* (15th ed.). St. Louis: Mosby.

Swanson, J. A., & Hoecker, J. L. (1996). Otitis media in young children. *Mayo Clinic Proceedings, 71*(2), 179–183.

Tigges, B. B. (2000). Acute otitis media and pneumococcal resistance: Making judicious management decisions. *Nurse Practitioner, 25*(1), 69–80, 85.

Wagner, R. S. (1997). Eye infections and abnormalities: Issues for the pediatrician. *Contemporary Pediatrics, 14*(8), 137–153.

Woodruff, G. (1995). Amblyopia. Could we do better? *British Medical Journal, 310*(6988), 1153–1154.

Yawn, B. P., Lydick, E. G., Epstein, R., & Jacobsen, S. J.(1996). Is school vision screening effective? *Journal of School Health, 66*(5), 171–175.

Young, J. D. H, & MacEwen, C. J. (1997). Fortnightly review: Managing congenital lacrimal obstruction in general practice. *British Medical Journal, 315*(7103), 293–296.

Young, N. (1994). Cochlear implants in children. *Current Problems in Pediatrics, 24,* 131–138.

COMMON PEDIATRIC GASTROINTESTINAL DISORDERS

◼ Cleft Lip and Palate

Cleft lip and palate are congenital anomalies resulting in structural facial malformation. They are usually apparent at birth and may be associated with any of over 150 syndromes (Table 48-1). One in 700 newborns is affected by cleft lip and/or palate in the United States. Cleft lip (with or without cleft palate) occurs more frequently in boys, and isolated cleft palate is more frequent in girls. They are most prevalent among Native Americans (3.6 per 1,000 births) and less common in Asians (1.7 to 2.1 per 1,000 births), Caucasians (1 per 1,000 births), and African Americans (0.3 per 1,000 births).

Combination of cleft lip and palate occurs in approximately 50% of cases; cleft lip along occurs in about 25% of cases; and cleft palate alone occurs in about 25% of cases.

Pathophysiology and Etiology
1. A failure of embryonic development occurs, but cause is not known.
2. Hereditary factor.
3. May be related to mutant genes, chromosomal abnormalities, teratogens, or environment. Most often, it is multifactorial inheritance.

Types of Defect
1. Development of lip and palate independent; thus, can have any combination of defects and degree of involvement
2. Cleft lip—prealveolar cleft:

   a. Varies from a notch in the lip to complete separation of the lip into the nose
   b. May be unilateral or bilateral
   c. Failure of maxillary process to fuse with nasal elevations on frontal prominence; normally occurs during 5th and 6th week of gestation
   d. Merging of upper lip at midline complete between 7th and 8th week of gestation
3. Isolated cleft palate—postalveolar cleft:
   a. Cleft of uvula
   b. Cleft of soft palate
   c. Cleft of both soft and hard palate through roof of mouth
   d. Unilateral or bilateral
   e. Failure of mesodermal masses of lateral palatine process to meet and fuse; normally occurs between 7th and 12th week of gestation
4. Submucous cleft:
   a. Muscles of soft palate not joined
   b. Not recognized until child talks; cannot be seen at birth
5. Pierre Robin syndrome—cleft palate, glossoptosis (tongue back on pharynx), and micrognathia (underdeveloped mandible):
   a. This causes feeding difficulties, potential airway obstruction by tongue, slow weight gain, and ear infections.
   b. By 3 to 4 months of age, the mandible has grown enough to accommodate the tongue, and respiratory difficulty is greatly diminished.

Clinical Manifestations
1. Physical appearance of cleft lip or palate:
   a. Incompletely formed lip—varies from slight notch in vermilion to complete separation of lip.

TABLE 48-1 Most Common Syndromes Associated With Cleft Lip and Palate

Syndrome	Features (in addition to cleft lip or palate)
Ectrodactyly-ectodermal dysplasia-clefting (EEC)	Claw hands and feet
Hay-Wells	Adhesions of eyelids; dystrophic nails; coarse, sparse hair
Meckel-Gruber	Polydactyly, polycystic kidneys, encephalocele
Opitz G	Hypertelorism (increased distance between two organs, such as eyes), hypospadias
Rapp-Hodgkin	Ectodermal dysplasia
Trisomy 13	Polydactyly, microcephaly, congenital heart disease
Van der Woude's	Lower lip pits
Waardenburg's	Telecanthus (increased distance between eyes), heterochromia (diversity of color of iris), deafness
Crouzon's	Shallow eye sockets; curved, parrot-like nose; hearing loss
Velocardiofacial	Long face with maxillary excess, mandibular retrusion; thin upper lip; ventricular septal defect; learning disabilities
Goldenhar syndrome	Facial asymmetry, preauricular skin tags, middle ear deformity
Treacher Collins	Downslanting eyes, malformed ears, hearing loss
Pierre Robin	Micrognathia, glossoptosis (tongue falls into throat), narrow airway

b. Opening in roof of mouth felt with examiner's finger on palate.
2. Eating difficulty:
   a. Suction cannot be created for effective sucking.
   b. Food returns through the nose.
3. Nasal speech.

Diagnostic Evaluation
1. Prenatal ultrasonography enables many cleft lips and some cleft palates to be identified in utero.
2. Magnetic resonance imaging (MRI) to evaluate extent of abnormality before treatment.
3. Photography to document the abnormality.
4. Serial x-rays before and after treatment.
5. Dental impressions for expansion prosthesis.
6. Genetic evaluation to determine recurrence risk.

Treatment
Interdisciplinary approach begins early and continues into late adolescence. Craniofacial team consists of a plastic surgeon, otolaryngologist, pediatric dentist, prosthodontist, orthodontist, feeding specialist, speech pathologist, audiologist, geneticist, psychologist, and community health nurse. Each team member has a role at some point in the child's care.
1. General management is focused on closure of the cleft(s), prevention of complications, habilitation, and facilitation of normal growth and development of the child.
2. The cleft lip is generally repaired before the palate defect.
   a. Immediate repair—several hours to several weeks after birth.
   b. Intraoral or extraoral prosthesis to prevent maxillary collapse, stimulate body growth, and aid in feeding and speech development; may be used before surgical repair.
   c. Later repair when infant is 6 to 12 weeks old, hemoglobin 10 g/dL, steady weight gain seen—10 lb or WBC count normal.

3. Cleft palate repair may be done any time between 6 months and 5 years; it is based on degree of deformity, width of oropharynx, neuromuscular function of palate and pharynx, and surgeon's preference.
   a. Repair at 9 to 18 months may be preferred because speech patterns have not been set, yet growth of involved structures allows for improved surgical repair.
   b. If repair is delayed to age 4 or 5 years, a special denture palate is used to help occlude the cleft and aid in establishing speech patterns.

Nursing Assessment
1. If cleft lip is visualized, assess for cleft palate by direct visualization and palpation with finger.
2. Obtain family history of cleft lip or palate.
3. Evaluate feeding abilities.
   a. Effectiveness of suck and swallow
   b. Amount taken
4. Observe for other syndromic features.

Nursing Diagnoses
- Altered Nutrition: Less Than Body Requirements related to eating difficulties
- Risk for Infection related to open wound created by malformation
- Impaired Adjustment to infant related to malformation and special care needs
- Risk for Aspiration related to tongue and palate deformities in Pierre Robin syndrome
- Knowledge Deficit related to home management of infant with cleft malformation

Nursing Interventions
Maintaining Adequate Nutrition
1. Administer gavage feedings if nipple feeding is to be delayed to prevent spread of a cleft lip.

2. If sucking is permitted, use a soft nipple with crosscut to facilitate feeding. Note that nipples can be softened by boiling them.
3. If sucking is ineffective due to inability to create a vacuum, try alternate oral feeding methods.
   a. Feeding devices include preemie nipple, crosscut nipple, NUK nipple, Ross Cleft Palate Nurser, Haberman Feeder, or palatal obturator.
   b. Avoid enlarging nipple holes due to infant's inability to control flow of milk, which will result in choking. Crosscut nipples allow milk to flow only when infant squeezes the crosscut open.
   c. Using a squeezable bottle (eg, Mead Johnson Cleft Palate Nurser) or plastic liner can be helpful by applying rhythmic pressure along with the infant's normal sucking and swallowing.
   d. Rubber-tipped asepto syringe or dropper; the rubber extension should be long enough to extend back into the mouth to prevent regurgitation through the nose. Direct tip to side of mouth, and feed slowly.
4. Feed baby in an upright, sitting position to decrease possibility of fluid being aspirated or returned through the nose or back to the auditory canal.
   a. Feeding is often easier if the nipple is angled to the side of the mouth away from the cleft so the baby's tongue can press the nipple against the upper gum or dental arch.
   b. Feed slowly over approximately 18 to 30 minutes. Feedings longer than 45 minutes expend too many calories and tire infant.
   c. Smaller but more frequent feedings may be necessary if the infant tires or requires extended time to eat.
   d. Bubble frequently during feeding to decrease amount of air swallowed.
   e. Avoid repeated removal of nipple due to fear of choking. This may only frustrate the infant, causing crying and increasing chances of aspiration.
   f. Feed infant before he or she becomes too hungry. If the infant is too agitated, feeding becomes a problem.
5. Advance diet as appropriate for age and needs of baby. Eating often improves when solids are introduced because they are easier for the baby to manipulate.
6. Encourage the mother to begin feeding the baby as soon as possible to enhance bonding and to strengthen the oral structures needed later for mastication and speech production.
7. Assist and support mother with breast-feeding if this is preferred.
   a. Suggest the use of a breast pump before nursing to stimulate the let-down reflex.
   b. Hold the infant in a semiupright, straddle, or football hold position.
8. Nursing may need to be maintained and facilitated by using a breast pump and then bottle-feeding the pumped milk.

Preventing Infection

1. Protect child from infection so that surgery will not be delayed.
   a. Use and teach good handwashing practice.
   b. Avoid patient contact with anyone who has an infection.
2. Change the baby's position frequently.
3. Clean the cleft after each feeding with water and a cotton-tipped applicator.
4. Observe for fever, irritability, redness, or drainage around cleft, and report promptly.
5. Monitor vital signs; report temperature >101°F.

Promoting Acceptance and Adjustment

1. Show acceptance of the baby; maintain composure, and do not show negative emotion when handling the infant. The manner in which the nurse handles the baby can make a lasting impression on the parents.
2. Support parents when showing a newborn baby for the first time. Demonstrate acceptance of both the baby and the parents' feelings. Parents may be grieving about the infant's cosmetic imperfections and may harbor ambivalent feelings about this baby.
3. Offer information and answer any questions in a simple, matter-of-fact manner. The better informed the family, the easier it will be for them to see the baby as a normal child with a physical difference that will require surgery, dental work, and possibly speech therapy.
4. Be aware that the normal sequence of parental responses may include shock, disbelief, worry, grief, and anger, and then proceed to a state of equilibrium and reorganization.
5. Encourage parental involvement in infant's care: frequent holding, cuddling, and playing.

Preventing Aspiration and Airway Obstruction

1. When feeding the infant with Pierre Robin syndrome, consideration must be given to respiratory effort, flaccid tongue, and cleft palate. Generally, feeding can be done with a nursing bottle (feeding techniques similar to those used for cleft palate).
   a. Use orthopneic position—vertical and slightly forward; this allows infant to push jaw forward to suck and allows the feeder a clear view of the infant.
   b. Use gentle finger pressure at mandibular attachment to bring the jaw forward.
   c. Feed slowly.
2. Prevent respiratory obstruction by the tongue, especially on inspiration and when the infant is quiet.
   a. Place the infant in prone position so tongue and jaw fall forward.
   b. Tilt head back as tolerated by the infant, and slightly elevate upper trunk.
   c. Place stockinette cap on infant's head and suspend from an overhead support to assist the infant to maintain a position for easy ventilation.
   d. Suction nasopharynx as needed.

e. If the tongue is sutured to pull it forward, observe for slipping, cut tongue, and infection.

3. Observe closely for respiratory compromise.

Preparing for Home Management

1. Prepare family for home feedings by providing several days to practice feeding and to become familiar with the baby's feeding pattern.
2. Alert caregiver to difficulties with feeding and how to manage them.
   a. Nasal regurgitation: feed in more upright position and/or stop feeding and allow the infant a few seconds to cough or sneeze and clear the airway.
   b. Respiratory distress: feed slowly, and observe for aspiration.
   c. Longer feeding times: feed more frequently so infant does not tire.
3. Suggest that about 1 week before scheduled admission for surgery, the mother begin using feeding techniques preferred by surgeon for postoperative feeding.
   a. Side of spoon
   b. Rubber-tipped dropper
   c. Toddler cup
4. Encourage the parents to prepare siblings at home for the arrival of this baby. Suggest a picture of the new baby.
5. Offer parents available literature about children with cleft lip and palate.
6. Encourage parental involvement with local self-help groups that provide information and parent-to-parent contact.
7. Initiate referrals, as indicated, for additional support and financial assistance and early intervention programs.
8. Describe and reinforce surgical treatment plans to the parents to promote communication and hope.
9. Stress compliance with follow-up care with the pediatrician, plastic surgeon, dentist, orthodontist, psychologist, and speech therapist to prevent chronic otitis media, hearing loss, speech impairment, and emotional problems.
10. Initiate a community nurse referral to continue emotional support and teaching progress at home.

Nursing Care of the Child Undergoing Surgery
Preoperative Care

1. Prepare the infant or toddler for the postoperative experience to decrease fear and increase cooperation.
   a. Practice the feeding measure that will be used postoperatively—cup, side of spoon, or syringe.
   b. Use elbow restraints for short periods of time; allow the child to play with them and the caregiver to use them.
   c. Explain that jacket restraint may be necessary in older child to prevent rolling over and rubbing suture line against sheets.

d. Place child on back or side to familiarize with these positions.
   e. Demonstrate and practice mouth irrigation as it will be done postoperatively for cleft palate repair; allow the child to assist if age appropriate.
2. Prepare the parents emotionally for the postoperative appearance of the child.
   a. Explain the use of the Logan bow (a curved metal wire that prevents stress on the suture line) and restraints.
   b. Encourage a parent to be with the child, especially when awakening from anesthesia, to offer security and comfort.

Postoperative Care

1. Apply elbow restraints to prevent hands from reaching the mouth while still allowing some freedom of movement.
   a. Pad restraint, and place it from the axilla to inner aspect of the wrist.
   b. Remove restraints occasionally, one at a time, to exercise the arms.
   c. Consider pinning restraints or cuff of shirt to the bed to decrease chances of the infant rubbing lip with his upper arm.
2. Check Logan bow, butterfly-type adhesive, or Band-Aid placed cheek-to-cheek across top of lip to prevent lateral tension on cleft lip incision.
   a. Prevent wetting tape, or it will loosen.
   b. Observe for and report bleeding.
3. Prevent the child from crying, blowing, sucking, talking, and laughing, which increase tension on the suture line.
   a. Encourage the mother to hold and cuddle the child.
   b. Keep the child dry, fed, and comfortable.
4. Position the child on back or propped on side to keep from rubbing lip on the sheets. An infant seat may be useful for variation of position, comfort, entertainment, and to prevent interference with suture line.
   a. Provide for appropriate diversional activity, hanging toys, mobiles, and so forth.
   b. If only cleft palate was repaired, child may lie on abdomen.
5. Do not allow child to put anything in mouth, such as straw, eating utensils, or fingers.
6. Monitor respiratory effort after cleft palate repair.
   a. Be aware that breathing with a closed palate is different from the child's customary way of breathing; the child also must contend with increased mucus production.
   b. Provide for croup tent with mist to decrease occurrence of respiratory problems and provide moisture to mucous membranes that may become dry from mouth breathing.
7. Clean suture line after every feeding.
   a. Gently wipe lip incision with cotton-tipped applicator and solution of choice, such as water, saline,

or hydrogen peroxide. Gently pat dry, and apply antibiotic ointment or petroleum jelly if ordered.

   b. Rinse the mouth with water, or offer a drink of water after each feeding.

   c. Irrigate the mouth with normal saline solution or water after cleft palate repair. Direct a gentle stream over the suture line using an ear bulb syringe with the child in a sitting position with head forward.

   d. Keep the mouth moist to promote healing and provide comfort.

8. Accomplish feeding without tension on the suture line for several days after lip repair.

   a. Use dropper or syringe with a rubber tip, and insert from the side to avoid suture line or to avoid stimulating sucking.

   b. Use side of spoon. Never put spoon into the mouth.

   c. Perform nasogastric gavage; usually this is last treatment of choice.

   d. Advance slowly to nipple feeding as directed. The infant should be able to suck more efficiently with the lip repaired.

9. After palate repair, feed the child in the manner used preoperatively (cup, side of spoon, or rubber-tipped syringe). Never use straw, nipple, or plain syringe.

   a. Diet progresses from clear liquids to full liquids to soft foods.

   b. Soft foods are usually continued for about 1 month after surgery, at which time a regular diet is started, excluding hard food.

10. Check weight periodically to see if adequate nutrition is being maintained.

11. Administer antibiotics as prescribed because the mouth and suture line are constantly contaminated.

Community and Home Care Considerations

1. As the patient's advocate, alert members of the craniofacial team when a family is overwhelmed by too many appointments and interventions. Act as liaison and case manager as indicated.

2. Continue to assess weight gain, feeding behavior, overall development, parent–child bonding and interactions.

3. Advise the parents to discuss the child's problem with the teacher and other responsible adults in close contact with the child.

   a. Aesthetic touch-up and bone graft surgery performed later may interfere with schooling.

   b. Speech differences require early identification and intervention.

   c. Monitor for reading and learning problems related to speech and language delays.

   d. Hypernasality may develop at age 10 to 14 due to normal shrinkage of adenoid tissue occurring at this time.

4. Assess the child's self-perception and coping skills. Assess the family's support systems and coping mechanisms.

5. Help school-aged children deal with teasing (as a result of being "different" from their peers) by allowing them to express their feelings and guiding their response: ignoring the remark, responding with a joke or good-natured tease, or educating the teaser.

6. Encourage the child to perceive self as a person born with a birth defect, not a "cleft person." Those who do not consider the defect a main ingredient of their personalities will experience fewer social problems.

7. The school nurse assists by performing frequent hearing evaluations, organizing an assembly or class discussion dealing with disabilities and individual differences, working with the teacher in regard to a hearing impairment (teaching position, classroom seating).

Family Education and Health Maintenance

1. Instruct on continued protection of the mouth after surgery. Child cannot put anything in mouth, including lollipops.

2. Demonstrate how to rinse mouth after eating.

3. Advise parents on the introduction of solid foods; semiupright position or upright position; avoid spicy or acidic foods, which may irritate the oral and nasal cavities; avoid hard, sharp foods such as raw carrots or potato chips.

4. Advise on increased risk of ear infections and need to seek medical attention for colds, ear pain, fever, or other signs and symptoms. Frequent hearing screens and tympanometry should be done to monitor the effects of middle ear pathology. *Note:* Hearing should be monitored at least every 6 months during the first year of life and then annually to prevent hearing impairment.

5. Encourage modeling "good speech" by providing a stimulating language environment, and encourage spontaneous imitations of sounds at home.

6. Stress the importance of speech therapy and practicing exercises as directed by the speech therapist.

7. Encourage thorough brushing of teeth, regular dental examinations and fluoride treatment as indicated due to risk of tooth decay related to defective enamel and abnormally positioned teeth with clefts.

8. Advise the parents on current therapies available: bone grafting providing permanent teeth support, dental implants to replace missing teeth, speech prosthesis for incomplete velopharyngeal closure.

9. Help the parents realize that, although rehabilitation is extensive, their child can live a normal life.

10. For additional information and support, refer patients and family to The Cleft Palate Foundation, 104 South Estes Drive, Suite 204, Chapel Hill, NC 27514, 800-242-5338, *www.cleftline.com*.

Outcome-Based Evaluation

- Infant feeding with appropriate feeding device in small amounts every 1 to 2 hours
- No signs of infection
- Parents holding and talking to infant

- Prone position maintained; no airway obstruction
- Parents demonstrate proper feeding technique
- Parents understand preoperative care instructions
- Parents express understanding and demonstrate post-operative home care procedures

▣ Esophageal Atresia With Tracheoesophageal Fistula

Esophageal atresia is failure of the esophagus to form a continuous passage from the pharynx to the stomach during embryonic development. Tracheoesophageal fistula (TEF) is the abnormal connection between the trachea and esophagus. These disorders occur in 1 in 3,500 births, frequently associated with prematurity and low birth weight.

Pathophysiology and Etiology

1. Cause unknown in most cases. Possible influences include:
   a. Inheritable genetic factor
   b. Teratogenic stimuli
   c. Environmental factors
2. Failure of proper separation of the embryonic channel into the esophagus and trachea occurring during the 4th and 5th weeks of gestation.
3. Esophageal atresia can be classified as (Figure 48-1):
   a. *Type I* (10% to 15% of cases; second most common): proximal and distal segments of esophagus are blind; there is no connection to trachea.
   b. *Type II* (rare): proximal segment of esophagus opens into trachea by a fistula; distal segment is blind.
   c. *Type III* (80% to 90% of cases; most common; discussion is limited to this type): proximal segment of esophagus has blind end; distal segment of esophagus connects into trachea by a fistula.
   d. *Type IV* (rare): esophageal atresia with fistula between both proximal and distal ends of trachea and esophagus.
   e. *Type V* (not usually diagnosed at birth): both proximal and distal segments of esophagus open into trachea by a fistula; no esophageal atresia (H-type).
4. With TEF, child is unable to swallow effectively.
   a. Saliva or formula accumulates in upper esophageal pouch and is aspirated into airway.
   b. Gastric acid is regurgitated through distal fistula.
   c. Abdominal distention occurs as a result of air entering the lower esophagus through the fistula and passing into the stomach, especially when the child is crying.
   d. Gastric distention may be severe enough to cause respiratory distress by elevation of the diaphragm.

Clinical Manifestations

These appear soon after birth.
1. Excessive secretions
   a. Constant drooling
   b. Large amount of secretions from nose

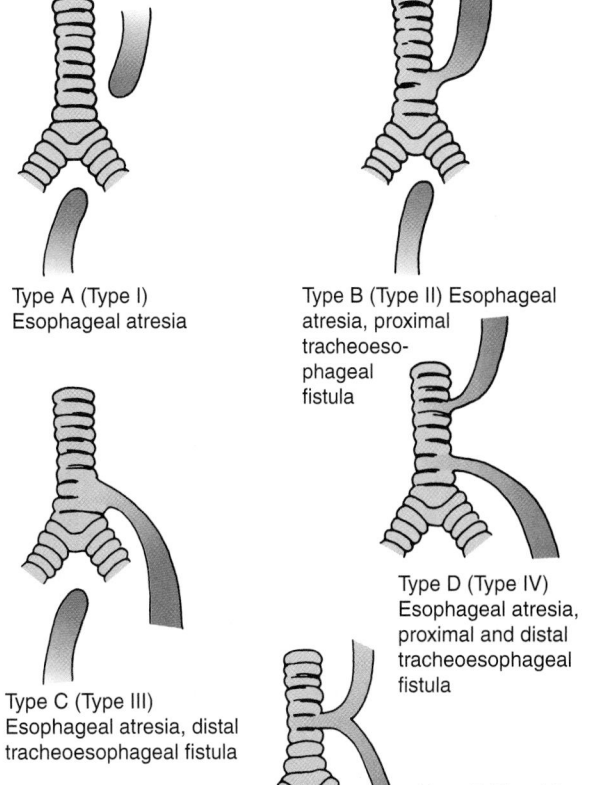

Type A (Type I)
Esophageal atresia

Type B (Type II) Esophageal atresia, proximal tracheoeso-phageal fistula

Type C (Type III)
Esophageal atresia, distal tracheoesophageal fistula

Type D (Type IV)
Esophageal atresia, proximal and distal tracheoesophageal fistula

Type E (Type V)
Tracheoesophageal fistula (H-type)

FIGURE 48-1 Types of esophageal atresia: esophageal atresia and tracheoesophageal fistula (TEF).

2. Intermittent unexplained cyanosis; laryngospasm caused by aspiration of accumulated saliva in blind pouch
3. Abdominal distention
4. Violent response after first or second swallow of feeding
   a. The infant coughs and chokes.
   b. Fluid returns through nose and mouth.
   c. Cyanosis occurs.
   d. The infant struggles.
5. Poor feeding
6. Inability to pass catheter through nose or mouth into stomach; tip of catheter stops at blind pouch, or atresia. *Note:* Be aware of coiling of catheter; coiling may make catheter appear to be descending into stomach.
7. Infant often premature and pregnancy complicated by polyhydramnios

Diagnostic Evaluation

1. Ultrasound scanning techniques enable TEF to be identified in utero for some infants.

2. Failure to pass an 8F catheter into the stomach through nose or mouth. Catheter is left in situ while an x-ray confirms the diagnosis.
3. Litmus paper may be used to test for acid reaction.
4. X-ray flat plate of abdomen and chest may reveal presence of gas in stomach and catheter coiled in the blind pouch. Barium x-ray may be used in some cases.
5. Electrocardiogram and echocardiogram are performed because there is a high association with cardiac anomalies.

Treatment
Immediate Treatment
1. Propping infant at 30-degree angle to prevent reflux of gastric contents.
2. #8 nasogastric tube remains in situ and suctioned very frequently to prevent aspiration until put on low suction.
3. Pouch is washed out with normal saline to prevent thick mucus from blocking the tube.
4. Gastrostomy to decompress stomach and prevent aspiration; later used for feedings.
5. Nothing by mouth (NPO); intravenous (IV) fluids.

Appropriate Treatment of Any Existing Pathologic Processes
These processes are either acquired complications, such as pneumonitis, or complications from concomitant lesions, such as congestive heart failure.

Supportive Therapy
Supportive therapy includes meeting nutritional requirements, IV fluids, antibiotics, respiratory support, maintaining thermally neutral environment.

Surgery
1. Prompt primary repair: fistula found by bronchoscopy is divided, followed by esophageal anastomosis of proximal and distal segments if infant is greater than 2,000 g and is without pneumonia.
2. Short-term delay: subsequent primary repair is used to stabilize infant and prevent deterioration when the patient's condition contraindicates immediate surgery.
3. Staging: initially, fistula division and gastrostomy are performed with later secondary esophageal anastomosis or colonic transplant performed approximately 1 year later to effect total repair. Approach may be used with a very small, premature infant or a very sick neonate or when severe congenital anomalies exist.
4. Circular esophagomyotomy may be performed on proximal pouch to gain length and allow for primary anastomosis at initial surgery.
5. Cervical esophagostomy: when ends of esophagus are too widely separated, esophageal replacement with segment of intestine is done at 18 to 24 months of age.
6. Postoperative complications occur in 5% to 10%:
   a. Leak at anastomosis site
   b. Recurrent fistulas
   c. Esophageal strictures
   d. Abnormal function of distal esophagus sphincter (gastroesophageal reflux [GER]) and esophagitis

   e. Tracheomalacia
   f. Feeding problems with the older child

Complications of Tracheoesophageal Fistula
1. Death from asphyxia
2. Pneumonitis secondary to:
   a. Salivary aspiration
   b. Gastric acid reflux
3. Concomitant lesions (approximately 40% to 50%):
   a. Congenital heart disease
   b. Gastrointestinal (GI) anomalies, particularly imperforate anus
   c. Skeletal and muscular deformities
   d. Renal anomalies
   e. Vertebral defects (possibility of Vater syndrome—vertebral defects, anal atresia, TEF, and radial limb dysfunction)
4. Prematurity
5. Dehydration and electrolyte imbalance

Nursing Assessment
Assessment begins immediately after birth.
1. Be alert for risk factors of polyhydramnios and prematurity.
2. Suspect in infant with the following:
   a. Excessive amount of mucus
   b. Difficulty with secretions
   c. Cyanotic episodes (unexplained)
3. Report suspicion to health care provider immediately.

Nursing Diagnoses
Preoperative Care
- Risk for Aspiration related to structural abnormality
- Risk for Fluid Volume Deficit related to inability to take oral fluids
- Anxiety of parents related to critical situation of newborn

Postoperative Care
- Ineffective Airway Clearance related to surgical intervention
- Altered Nutrition: Less Than Body Requirements related to restricted oral intake and increased nutritional needs for healing
- Pain related to surgical procedure
- Impaired Tissue Integrity related to postoperative drainage
- Risk for Injury related to complex surgery
- Risk for Altered Parent/Infant Attachment related to prolonged hospitalization

Nursing Interventions
Preoperative
Preventing Aspiration
1. Position the infant with head and chest elevated 20 to 30 degrees to prevent or decrease reflux of gastric juices into the tracheobronchial tree.
   a. This position also may ease respiratory effort by dropping the distended intestines away from the diaphragm.

b. Prone position will allow gastric juices to pool anteriorly away from the esophagus.

c. Turn frequently to prevent atelectasis and pneumonia.

2. Perform intermittent nasopharyngeal suctioning or maintain indwelling Repogle tube (double-lumen tube) or sump tube with constant suction to remove secretions from esophageal blind pouch.

a. Tip of tube is placed in the blind pouch.

b. Replogle or sump tube allows air to be drawn in through a second lumen and prevents tube obstruction by mucous membrane of pouch.

c. Maintain indwelling tube patency by irrigating with 1 mL normal saline solution frequently.

d. Ensure that indwelling tube is changed as needed and at least once every 12 to 24 hours (by the health care provider); alternate nostrils. Prevent necrosis of nostrils from pressure by catheter.

3. Place the infant in an Isolette or under a radiant warmer with high humidity to aid in liquefying secretions and thick mucus. Maintain the infant's temperature in thermoneutral zone, and ensure environmental isolation to prevent infection by using Isolette.

4. Administer oxygen as needed.

5. Suction mouth to keep clear of secretions and prevent aspiration. Provide mouth care.

6. Be alert for indications of respiratory distress.

a. Retractions

b. Circumoral cyanosis

c. Restlessness

d. Nasal flaring

e. Increased respiration and heart rate

7. Maintain NPO status.

8. Administer antibiotics as ordered to prevent or treat associated pneumonitis.

9. Observe infant carefully for any change in condition; report changes immediately.

a. Check vital signs, color and amount of secretions, abdominal distention, and respiratory distress.

b. Evaluate for complications that can occur in any neonate or premature infant.

10. Be available, and recognize need for emergency care or resuscitation.

a. Have resuscitation equipment on hand.

b. Accompany the infant to other departments and the operating room in Isolette with portable oxygen and suction equipment.

11. Monitor for signs or symptoms that may indicate additional congenital anomalies or complications.

12. Gastrostomy tube may be placed before definitive surgery to aid in gastric decompression and prevention of reflux. Maintain gastrostomy tube to straight gravity drainage, and do not irrigate before surgery.

Preventing Dehydration

1. Administer parenteral fluids and electrolytes as prescribed.

2. Monitor vital signs frequently for changes in blood pressure and pulse, which may indicate dehydration or fluid volume overload.

3. Record intake and output, including gastric drainage (if gastrostomy tube for decompression is present).

Reducing Parental Anxiety

1. Explain procedures and necessary events to parents as soon as possible.

2. Orient parents to hospital and intensive care nursery environment.

3. Allow family to hold and assist in caring for infant.

4. Offer reassurance and encouragement to family frequently. Provide for additional support by social worker, clergy, and counselor as needed.

Postoperative

Maintaining Patent Airway

1. Keep endotracheal tube patent by frequent lavage and suction. *Note:* Reintubation could damage the anastomosis.

2. Suction frequently; every 5 to 10 minutes may be necessary, but at least every 1 to 2 hours.

3. Observe for signs of obstructed airway. Ventilatory support is continued until clinically stable (usually 24 to 48 hours)

4. Request that the surgeon mark a suction catheter, indicating how far the catheter can be safely inserted without disturbing the anastomosis (usually 2 to 3 cm).

5. Administer chest physiotherapy as prescribed.

a. Change the infant's position by turning; stimulate crying to promote full expansion of lungs.

b. Elevate head and shoulders 20 to 30 degrees.

c. Use mechanical vibrator 2 to 3 days postoperatively (to minimize trauma to anastomosis), followed by more vigorous physical therapy after the 3rd day.

NURSING ALERT

 Care should be taken not to hyperextend the neck, causing stress to the operative site.

---

6. Continue use of Isolette or radiant warmer with humidity.

7. Be prepared for an emergency: have emergency equipment available, including suction machine, catheter, oxygen, laryngoscope, endotracheal tubes in varying sizes.

Providing Adequate Nutrition

Feedings may be given by mouth, by gastrostomy, or (rarely) by a feeding tube into the esophagus, depending on the type of operation performed and the infant's condition. The gastrostomy is generally attached to gravity drainage for 3 days postoperatively, then elevated and left open to allow for air to escape and gastric secretions to pass into the duodenum before feedings are begun.

1. Administer IV solutions until gastrostomy feedings can be started.

2. Begin gastrostomy feedings as soon as ordered because adequate nutrition is an important factor in healing.
   a. Give the infant a pacifier to suck during feedings, unless contraindicated.
   b. Use care to prevent air from entering the stomach, thereby causing gastric distention and possible reflux.
   c. Continue gastrostomy feedings until the infant can tolerate full feedings orally.

Providing Comfort Measures

1. Position comfortably.
2. Avoid restraints when possible.
3. Administer mouth care frequently.
4. Offer pacifier frequently.
5. Administer analgesics as ordered. Wean as soon as possible so ventilator can be discontinued without risk.
6. Caress and speak or sing to infant frequently. Handling should be kept to a gentle minimum.

Maintaining Chest Drainage

1. Assess type of chest drainage present (determined by surgical approach). Report saliva or hemorrhage.
   a. Retropleural—small tube in posterior mediastinum; may be left open for drainage
   b. Transthoracic—chest tube placed in pleural space and connected to suction
2. Keep tubing patent: free from clots, unkinked, and without tension.
3. If a break occurs in the closed drainage system, immediately clamp tubing close to the infant to prevent pneumothorax.

Observing for Complications

1. Inspect for leak at the anastomosis, causing mediastinitis, pneumothorax, and saliva in chest tube: hypothermia or hyperthermia, severe respiratory distress, cyanosis, restlessness, weak pulses.
2. Continue to monitor for complications during the recovery process.
   a. Stricture at the anastomosis: difficulty in swallowing, vomiting, or spitting up of ingested fluid; refusing to eat; fever secondary to aspiration and pneumonia
   b. Recurrent fistula: coughing, choking, and cyanosis associated with feeding; excessive salivation; difficulty in swallowing associated with abnormal distention; repeated episodes of pneumonitis; general poor physical condition (no weight gain)
   c. Atelectasis or pneumonitis: aspiration, respiratory distress
3. Provide meticulous care for cervical esophagostomy— artificial opening in the neck that allows for drainage of the upper esophagus.
   a. Keep the area clean of saliva.
   b. Wash with clear water.
   c. Place an absorbent pad over the area.
4. As soon as possible, allow the infant to suck a few milliliters of milk at the same time gastrostomy feeding is being done. Advance the infant to solid foods as appropriate if esophagostomy is maintained for a few months.
   a. Encourage sucking and swallowing.
   b. Familiarize the infant with food so that when able to eat orally, infant will be used to it.
5. Begin oral feedings 10 to 14 days postoperatively after anastomosis as directed.
   a. Feed slowly to allow the infant time to swallow.
   b. Use upright sitting position to avoid risk of regurgitation.
   c. Bubble frequently.
   d. Use demand feedings rather than strictly scheduled feedings.
   e. Do not allow the infant to become overtired at feeding time. Note cardiac rate.
   f. Try to make each feeding a pleasant experience for the infant. Use a consistent approach and patience. Encourage parental involvement.

Stimulating Parent–Infant Attachment

1. Gently hold and cuddle the infant for feedings and after feedings.
2. Encourage parents to cuddle and talk to the infant.
3. Provide for visual, auditory, and tactile stimulation as appropriate for the infant's physical condition and age.
4. Provide opportunities for the parents to learn all aspects of care of their infant.
5. Encourage the parents to talk about their feelings, fears, and concerns.
6. Help to develop a healthy parent–child relationship through flexible visiting, frequent phone calls, and encouraging physical contact between child and parents.

Community and Home Care Considerations

1. Teach carefully and thoroughly all procedures to be done at home. Show the parents how to do them, and then watch return demonstration of the following procedures:
   a. Gastrostomy feedings and care
   b. Esophagostomy care with feeding technique
   c. Suctioning
   d. Identifying signs of respiratory distress
2. Advise parents that swallowing and gastric reflux will be affected for many years, due to the narrowed abnormal esophagus emptying slowly and tension on the stomach from the anastomosis.
3. Monitor weight gain and developmental progress.
4. Observe parental feeding technique.
5. Encourage parents to discuss child's condition with day care workers, teachers, school nurse, or other responsible adults in close contact with the child so they will be able to recognize possible problems and reinforce good eating habits.
6. To compensate for altered motility, encourage cutting food into small pieces, chewing food well, swallowing food with fluid, and sitting upright while eating.
7. Observe parent–child interaction to assess for overprotection and appropriate coping skills.

Family Education and Health Maintenance

1. Help the parents understand the psychological needs of the infant for sucking, warmth, comfort, stimulation, and affection. Suggest that activity be appropriate for age.
2. Encourage the parents to continue close medical follow-up, and help them learn to recognize possible problems.
   a. Eating problems may occur, especially when solids are introduced.
   b. Repeated respiratory tract infection should be reported.
   c. Occurrence of stricture at site of anastomosis weeks to months later may be recognized by difficulty in swallowing, spitting of ingested fluid, and fever.
   d. Dilatation of esophagus may be necessary to treat stricture at the site of the anastomosis.
   e. Signs of fistula leakage are dusky color or choking with feeding.
3. Monitor for signs and symptoms of gastroesophageal reflux. Feeds may be thickened with rice cereal if symptomatic. Notify health care provider if emesis is persistent.
4. Help the parents understand the need for good nutrition and the need to follow the diet regimen suggested by the health care provider.
5. Reassure parents that an infant's raspy cough is normal and will gradually diminish as the infant's trachea becomes stronger over 6 to 24 months (most infants have some tracheomalacia).
6. Teach parents to guard against the child swallowing foreign objects.
7. Help and support can be given by introducing the parents to other parents of children with TEF.
8. For additional information and support, refer parents to EA/TEF Child and Family Support Connection, Inc., 111 West Jackson Boulevard, Suite 1145, Chicago, IL 60604-3502, 312-987-9085; email: eatef2@aol.com.

Outcome-Based Evaluation

- No cyanosis or respiratory distress
- Hydrated; urine output adequate
- Parents holding infant; expressing concerns
- Postoperatively, tolerating gastrostomy feedings without distention or regurgitation
- Thriving infant with adequate weight gain
- Infant sleeping and resting without irritability
- Chest tube in place with minimal drainage
- Feeding without regurgitation 12 days postoperatively
- Parents holding and talking to baby

Gastroesophageal Reflux

Gastroesophageal reflux (GER) is a malfunction of the distal end of the esophagus, antireflux barrier, permitting return of acid stomach content into the esophagus. GER is a common problem during the first year of life, affecting about 3% of newborns.

Pathophysiology and Etiology

1. Cause undetermined in most patients. Possible causes include:
   a. Delayed neuromuscular development
   b. Cerebral defects
   c. Obstruction at or just below the pylorus
   d. Physiologic immaturity
   e. Complication of esophageal surgery
   f. Increased abdominal pressure; obesity
2. Mechanisms of GER may involve an interplay of:
   a. Esophageal motility
   b. Lower esophageal sphincter activity
   c. Gastric emptying
   d. Physiologic immaturity
   e. Complication of esophageal surgery
3. The lower esophageal sphincter is a physiologic rather than an anatomic segment that forms an antireflux barrier.
   a. The segment is 2 to 5 cm in length.
   b. The segment is characterized by a pressure greater than that found proximally in the esophagus or distally in the stomach.
   c. Constitutes an effective barrier to protect the esophageal mucosa from damage by gastric contents (acid, pepsin, bile salts).
   d. GER is a consequence of incompetence or malfunctioning of this lower esophageal sphincter.
4. Associated conditions that cause reflux include:
   a. Coughing and wheezing from cystic fibrosis, bronchopulmonary dysplasia, asthma
   b. Indwelling oronasogastric feeding tube
   c. Mechanical ventilation
   d. Medications: theophylline and bronchodilators, which affect lower sphincter and increase gastric acidity
   e. Position: supine, chest physical therapy positions

Clinical Manifestations
Infant

1. Vomiting (unexplained).
   a. Immediately after feeding, especially when the infant is placed in a prone position
   b. Usually regurgitation rather than projectile vomiting
2. Onset usually over 2 months of age. Referral to pediatric specialist is warranted for infants less than 2 months of age.
3. Weight loss or failure to gain weight; rumination.
4. Refusal to eat.
5. Dehydration.
6. Recurrent respiratory symptoms; cough, wheeze, stridor, pneumonia.
7. Irritability, excessive crying.
8. Sleep disturbances.
9. Arching, stiffening.

10. Sandifer's syndrome—dystonic posturing caused by reflux; possible therapeutic effect with improved esophageal motility and clearance.
11. Eructation.

Older Child
1. Noncardiac chest discomfort
2. Upper abdominal discomfort; pressure or "squeezing" feeling
3. Chronic cough stridor
4. Nocturnal asthma, especially after a large meal
5. Dysphagia as evidenced by irritability during eating
6. Anemia
7. Hematemesis or melena (blood in stools)

Diagnostic Evaluation
1. History of infant's or child's feeding habits.
2. Barium swallow or upper GI series (not extremely reliable).
3. Esophageal pH monitoring to document frequency and severity of reflux. Considered gold standard for reflux; however, requires day of admission for reliable recording.
4. Technetium scintigraphy to document frequency and duration of postprandial reflux and define gastric emptying. Used most often by primary health care providers.
5. Esophageal manometry to measure the peristalsis of the esophagus.
6. Endoscopy most useful in older children evaluated for reflux esophagitis.
7. Esophageal histology and suction biopsies.

Complications
Complications result from frequent and sustained reflux of gastric contents into lower esophagus.
1. Recurrent pulmonary disease; aspiration pneumonia
2. Chronic esophagitis
3. Failure to thrive
4. Anemia
5. Cyanotic episodes may be associated with choking
6. Apnea
7. Near-miss sudden infant death syndrome (SIDS)
8. Esophageal stricture from scarring; esophagitis
9. Asthma
10. Hiatal hernia frequently associated with a chalasia (reflux; relaxation or incompetence of lower esophageal sphincter)
11. Barrett's esophagus

Treatment
Goal of treatment is to alleviate and relieve symptoms and prevent complications. May be treated medically or surgically.

Medical Management
1. Positioning—based on premise that gravity will help reduce amount of reflux; should be maintained as much as possible

a. Infants younger than 6 months:
  (i) Prone—improved gastric emptying.

NURSING ALERT

Careful monitoring of prone infant is imperative based on SIDS research.

  (ii) Infant on side (especially right lateral, which speeds gastric emptying) is recommended position while asleep.
  (iii) Raise head of crib at least 6 inches.
  (iv) Infant may also be held upright.
  (v) Postprandial use of infant seat is discouraged due to poor truncal control causing increased intra-abdominal pressure.
b. Older infant—placement in a walker with parental instruction about safety and continuous monitoring of infant.
c. Older child:
  (i) Raise head of bed with blocks or foam wedge to maintain 30- to 45-degree angle.
  (ii) Avoid postprandial recumbency for at least 3 hours after a meal.
2. Feeding
a. Infant:
  (i) Thickened feedings, such as dry rice cereal or commercial thickening agent.
  (ii) May cause a decrease in the number of episodes; however, the duration of reflux episodes is increased, thus increasing the risk of complications.
  (iii) Small, frequent feedings followed by positioning.
  (iv) Small frequent feeding must be weighed against the more frequent stimulation of stomach acid with introduction of food.
b. Older child:
  (i) Nothing to eat 2 hours before bedtime.
  (ii) Low-fat diet (fats slow gastric emptying and should be avoided).
  (iii) Avoid spicy and acidic foods (onions, citrus products, apple juice, tomatoes), esophageal irritants (chocolate, caffeinated beverages, peppermint, and second-hand smoke), and carbonated beverages.
  (iv) Should remain upright while awake.
  (v) Chew gum (stimulates parotid secretions, which augments esophageal clearance and provides buffering effect).
  (vi) Prevent obesity.
  (vii) Avoid tight or constrictive clothing.
  (viii) Avoid nonsteroidal anti-inflammatory drugs (NSAIDs), especially at bedtime.
3. Medication—may be used alone or in combination
a. Antacids—buffer existing acids and also increase serum gastrin levels, leading to increase in lower esophageal sphincter pressure (symptomatic relief).

b. H$_2$ receptor antagonists—act by reducing hydrochloric acid and pepsinogen secretion by blocking histamine receptors on the parietal cells, such as cimetidine (Tagamet) and ranitidine (Zantac).

c. Prokinetic agents—promote the transport of material through the GI tract, such as metoclopramide (Reglan).

d. Proton pump inhibitors—block all gastric acid secretion by binding to the +K+ATPase, such as omeprazole (Prilosec). Reserved for older children with very resistant esophagitis.

 DRUG ALERT

Cimetidine may potentiate other drugs such as phenytoin (Dilantin) and theophylline. Cisapride (Propulsid) has been taken off the market in the U.S. due to the association of abnormal heart rhythms due to prolonged Q–T interval.

Omeprazole may alter absorption of pH-dependent drugs such as amoxicillin.

Surgical Management

1. Reserved for severe cases refractory to 3- to 6-month course of medical management or for intractable respiratory disease.
2. Fundoplication is the wrapping of the fundus around the lower esophageal sphincter. The most commonly used method is the Nissen, a 360-degree wrap that completely prevents reflux episodes.
3. Other types of fundoplication (Thal, Toupet, and laparoscopic) prevent reflux less completely.
4. Antroplasty or pyloroplasty (gastric emptying procedure) may also be performed.
5. Simultaneous gastrostomy may be performed in neurologically abnormal children for feeding purposes or temporarily to decompress the stomach, avoiding gastric distention.
6. Complications include inability to burp or vomit, dysphagia, retching with feeding, watery diarrhea, growth retardation, small bowel obstruction, and dumping syndrome. Dumping syndrome usually occurs 30 minutes after meal and includes symptoms such as diaphoresis, palpitations, weakness, syncope, abdominal fullness, nausea, and diarrhea.
7. Nursing care is similar to care of child after surgery for pyloric stenosis (see p. 1458).

Nursing Assessment

1. Obtain history of infant's or child's eating habits.
2. Observe infant's or child's feeding behaviors.
3. Assess general appearance, skin integrity, and growth and development.

Nursing Diagnoses

- Risk for Aspiration related to reflux of gastric contents
- Altered Nutrition: Less Than Body Requirements related to decreased oral intake

- Risk for Fluid Volume Deficit related to frequent vomiting
- Fear of eating due to distress

Nursing Interventions
Preventing Aspiration

1. Administer medications such as metoclopramide 30 minutes before feeding and before sleep for best effect.
2. Maintain infant or child upright 30 to 40 degrees at all times whether awake or asleep. Gravity will help reduce reflux and help clear esophagus more readily.

 NURSING ALERT

Avoid slouching position because this may change angle of esophagus in relation to stomach, increase intra-abdominal pressure, and facilitate reflux of stomach contents.

3. Use infant "antireflux" saddle—covered, padded wedges with a sling designed for infant to straddle face down at elevated angle.
   a. Observe for lower leg edema, flattening of parietal skull, and torticollis (muscle contraction of neck).
   b. Turn infant's head frequently.
   c. Elevate infant's legs before eating or bathing.
4. Use cardiac and apnea monitors for infants and children with severe reflux.
   a. Observe for apneic periods of more than 20 seconds or accompanied by cyanosis, pallor, or bradycardia.
   b. Document apnea episodes, associated symptoms, and recovery efforts.
5. Provide chest physiotherapy before, rather than after, meals.
6. Avoid supine position with mechanical ventilation use.

Maintaining Adequate Nutrition

1. Thicken formula for each feeding.
   a. Add 1 teaspoon to 1 tablespoon of rice cereal to each ounce of formula.
   b. Enlarge nipple hole by cross-cutting it so formula can be more easily extracted.
2. Prop infant upright.
3. Reduce crying before and after meals, which increases intra-abdominal pressure and swallowing of air, increasing the likelihood of reflux.
4. Use a pacifier for non-nutritive sucking after eating only when infant is seated upright, because use of pacifier while prone increases reflux.
5. Handle the infant gently, with minimal movement during and after feeding.
6. Bubble frequently during and after feeding.
7. Record accurately activity of infant.
   a. Amount of feeding taken; whether retained
   b. Emesis: estimated amount, type, occurrence in relation to feeding
   c. Any change in behavior as a result of feeding technique
8. If breast-feeding, feeding modifications must be made (ie, express milk and thicken with cereal).

9. Ensure that older children avoid caffeine-containing food and beverages (such as chocolate) to reduce gastric acid production. Also maintain a low-fat diet because fat delays gastric emptying, and discourage eating 2 to 4 hours before bedtime.
10. Monitor weight frequently to evaluate progress.

Maintaining Fluid and Electrolyte Balance

1. Monitor vital signs, and assess skin turgor for signs of dehydration.
2. Observe and record accurately urinary output.
   a. Amount, frequency, color, and concentration
   b. Specific gravity
3. Monitor IV therapy if ordered.
4. Monitor serum electrolytes, and replace sodium and potassium as ordered.
5. Promote good skin care to prevent lesions of dry and delicate tissues.
   a. Change position frequently.
   b. Change soiled diapers often.
   c. Apply lotion, and gently massage any reddened areas.

Reducing Fear of Eating

1. Thickened feedings: use 1 tablespoon of rice cereal to each ounce of formula. This meal will be more satisfying to the infant than formula alone.
2. Identify and attempt to reduce stress, especially around meal time.
3. Feed the child in a quiet, calm environment.
4. Children like routines; try and feed around the same time and by the person with whom the child is familiar and comfortable.
5. For the older child, encourage participation in family dinner time so the child observes eating as a pleasurable experience.
6. Advise parents that clinical specialists in feeding disorders are available.

Community and Home Care Considerations

1. Recommend careful feeding and behavioral diary to monitor symptoms and improvements.
2. Recognize with older children that school and community activities may affect compliance with management strategies.
3. Advise parents to discuss medication and lunch time behaviors with teacher and school nurse so consistency can be maintained.
4. Assess need for community services such as respite care, especially for single parent.

Family Education and Health Maintenance

1. Plan a program of intensive parental teaching on how to handle and care for the infant. Explain rationale to parents. Ensure that they have proper equipment for propping the infant. Help the parents understand that it is not necessary to keep infant in infant seat or propped up at all times.
   a. Bathe or play with the infant before feeding.
   b. Change position about 1 hour after feeding.
   c. During the night after feeding, the infant can sleep in an upright position.
   d. Expect occasional small amounts of vomiting.

2. Offer clear, concise instructions. Focus on parental fears. Discuss techniques to promote developmental tasks of infants while facilitating bonding and normal parental behavior.
3. Help parents to understand that GER is self-limited; symptoms usually disappear within 12 months.
4. If a temporary gastrostomy is done, ensure that the parents know how to use, clear, and replace the tube. Tube and vent should be elevated to avoid gastric distention.
5. Help the parents understand the importance of follow-up of weight gain and development.
6. Assist with community resource planning (eg, education, advocacy, and financial assistance). Identify support groups.
7. Instruct parents and caregivers in cardiopulmonary resuscitation training before discharge of infant, if indicated.
8. Provide written and verbal instructions as to medications and side effects.
9. Advise parents on when to call their health care provider in regard to their child's symptoms.
10. Encourage family to contact their health care provider immediately with treatment concerns or problems.

Outcome-Based Evaluation

• Mild regurgitation immediately after feeding; no apnea or cyanosis noted
• Taking 3 to 4 oz thickened formula every 2 hours; weight gain
• Urine output adequate
• Child exhibits pleasure in eating

STANDARDS OF CARE GUIDELINES
Care of Child With Gastrointestinal or Nutritional Disorder

When caring for a child with a gastrointestinal or nutritional disorder:

• Monitor weight.
• Monitor urinary and bowel elimination.
• Monitor intake and output.
• Assess developmental milestone attainment.
• Provide and teach appropriate feeding products and techniques.
• Use most efficient position for feeding.
• Facilitate a calm, pleasant environment for feeding.
• Avoid foods that may inhibit absorption of nutrients or cause symptoms such as gas.
• Encourage and support parental involvement in care and feeding of the child.
• Encourage and support normal play and other activities for the child as condition allows.
• Identify and respond to signs and symptoms that may indicate lack of adequate nutrition or sign of complications.

This information should serve as a general guideline only. Each patient situation presents a unique set of clinical factors and requires nursing judgment to guide care, which may include additional or alternative measures and approaches.

Failure to Thrive

Failure to thrive (FTT) is the inadequate physical development of an infant or child manifested as a deceleration in weight gain, a low weight/height ratio, or as a low weight/height/head circumference ratio. The exact prevalence is unknown, although research suggests FTT accounts for 3% to 5% of pediatric hospital admissions.

Pathophysiology and Etiology

1. FTT is a nutritional disorder having both organic and nonorganic components.
   a. Organic FTT implies a major illness or organ system dysfunction as the etiology of the growth failure. It occurs equally in all populations and accounts for approximately 25% of FTT cases.
   b. Nonorganic FTT is the result of multiple psychosocial factors including disturbances in parent–child interaction. This type accounts for 50% of cases of FTT and is most common among the psychosocially and economically deprived.
   c. The remaining 25% of cases represent mixed etiology.
2. Organic FTT has pathophysiologic cause that reduces the availability of nutrients for maintenance and growth and is best divided into three categories:
   a. Genetic, congenital, and chromosomal abnormalities such as fetal alcohol syndrome (FAS), palatal anomaly, Pierre Robin syndrome, trisomy 21, Turner's or Noonan's syndrome, and dwarfing disorders.
   b. Excessive loss of nutrients or malabsorptive disorders such as chronic ileocecal intussusception, GER, lactose intolerance, malrotation of the colon, hypoplastic stomach, necrotizing enterocolitis with short bowel syndrome, pancreatic insufficiency, pyloric stenosis, and acquired immunodeficiency syndrome (AIDS).
   c. Interaction of poor nutrition, excessive catabolism, and endocrine disorders as in congenital heart disease, neurologic lesions, hydronephrosis, adrenal hyperplasia, diabetes insipidus, chronic or recurrent urinary tract infection (UTI), and hypothyroidism.
3. Nonorganic FTT occurs in the absence of GI, endocrine, congenital, or chronic diseases. It is usually associated with psychological deprivation, but can also be related to behavioral or economic problems. Multiple features of the parents, child, and environment interact over time resulting in a parent–child interaction that ultimately leads to undernutrition and undernurturance of the child.

Clinical Manifestations

Organic FTT

1. Retarded growth accompanied by manifestations of the underlying disease.
2. Weight loss in early stages. If poor intake continues, linear growth slows down or ceases. In latent stage, head circumference growth is retarded, indicating compromised brain development.
3. Developmental delays; parental distress.
4. Infant stress—irritability, fussiness, jitteriness.
5. Feeding disorders—ineffective sucking, difficulty chewing, difficulty swallowing.

Nonorganic FTT

1. Retarded growth
2. Infant stress—irritability, fussiness, jitteriness
3. Vomiting
4. Feeding disorders—ineffective sucking, difficulty chewing, difficulty swallowing
5. Reduced energy level
6. Difficult temperament
7. Fitful sleep
8. Reduced responsiveness and interaction with the environment
9. Social isolation, lack of vocalization
10. Spasticity or rigidity when touched
11. Inability to make eye contact or smile
12. Refusal to eat; rejection of foods
13. Spits up, gags, coughs with feeding

Parental Characteristics

1. No social support systems
2. Maladaptive relationships
3. Frequent history of alcoholism or drug abuse
4. History of anxiety or depression
5. Inadequate formal education
6. Lack of parental skills
7. Increased stress within family
8. Family crisis—marital discord, loss of employment, death in family
9. Low socioeconomic level
10. Father is frequently absent or not involved

Diagnostic Evaluation

1. FTT suggested if a child is falling off a previously established growth curve or falls below the 5th percentile. If FTT is of recent onset, weight but not height will fall below accepted standards. Depression of both weight and height indicates chronic malnutrition.
2. Technique for evaluating growth—look at growth percentage of the median for that age. Divide the actual value of height or weight by median value for that age. For example, 12-month-old female weighs 15 lb; the median for age is 21.5 lb. Child is 70% of median for age.

NURSING ALERT

Children whose weights are <60% of the median value for age or <70% for height are in acute danger of severe morbidity and malnutrition.

---

3. Complete health and dietary history—feeding, eating patterns, 24-hour intake recall
4. Physical examination for evidence of organic causes, with particular attention to ears, facial structure, mouth, heart, lungs, abdomen, and neurologic system

5. Developmental assessment
6. Family assessment—family short stature syndrome, family dynamics
7. Other tests to rule out secondary complications or organic problems:
   a. CBC with differential and indices, sedimentation rate to rule out anemia or hematologic or inflammatory cause
   b. Urinalysis and urine culture as baseline for bladder and renal function
   c. Thyroid-stimulating hormone and free T4 to rule out hypothyroidism
   d. Blood chemistry: provide data on electrolyte balance, renal function, and skeletal disorders
   e. Stool tests for pH, blood, and fat to determine carbohydrate intolerance or inflammatory bowel disease
   f. Radiologic studies including upper GI series, barium swallow, scintiscan, and airway films to rule out structural abnormalities

Treatment

1. Immediate treatment is directed at reversing malnutrition.
2. Nutritional treatment is aimed at providing sufficient calories to support "catch-up" growth to restore deficits in weight and height. Protein and energy requirements for normal and FTT children are outlined in Table 48-2.
3. Multivitamin supplementation containing zinc and iron is often recommended.
4. If cause is organic, the underlying disease entity is treated or managed.
5. In nonorganic FTT, hospitalization is avoided (unless the child is in imminent danger) because it further disrupts the parent–child relationship. Therefore, frequent home or clinic visits are necessary.
6. Developmental interventions through occupational and physical therapy are instituted, if necessary, to prevent further delay.
7. Support, education, and financial assistance is offered to the family.

Complications

1. Anemia, fatigue
2. Vulnerability to infection
3. Delayed healing
4. Behavior problems, poor academic performance

TABLE 48-2 Protein and Energy Requirements

| | Normal Children | | FTT Children | |
Age (years)	Protein (g/kg)	Energy (kcal/kg)	Protein (g/kg)	Energy (kcal/kg)
0–0.5	2.2	.08	3.2	150–250
0.5–1	1.6	98	3.2	150–250
1–3	1.2	102	2.5	150–250
4–6	1.1	90	2.5	150–250
7–10	1.0	70	2.5	150–250

5. Developmental, speech, and language delays
6. Perceptual difficulties

Nursing Assessment

1. Obtain accurate anthropometric measurements.
   a. Weights on children <36 months old should be done unclothed in a supine position using a calibrated beam scale. Children older than 36 months should be done standing on a standard scale wearing same clothing each time. Effort should be made to use the same scale each time.
   b. Heights should be recumbent up to 2 years of age. All children should be measured without shoes.
   c. Head circumference is measured each visit until 2 years old with a nonstretchable tape placed firmly from maximal occipital prominence to just above the eyebrow.
   d. All measurements need to be corrected for prematurity up to the second birthday by subtracting the number of weeks premature from the chronologic age.
   e. Measurements should be plotted on growth chart using a straight edge or plot grid.
2. Obtain nutritional history regarding eating patterns; nutritional beliefs for food allocation; 24-hour recall; who normally feeds the child; the type, amount, and frequency of feedings; the amount of time and effort required for meals; the child's reactions (physiologic and psychological) to feedings; food likes and dislikes; and environmental factors.
3. Observe parent–child interactions such as sensitivity to child's needs, eye-to-eye contact, if and how the infant is held, and how the parent speaks to the child.
4. If possible, observe the parent feed the child. Assess child's overall tone, sucking pattern, oral sensitivity (gag reflex), lip and tongue function, and swallowing ability. A videotape of the child eating in the home can be reviewed later to reduce the chance of observer distraction.
5. Assess neurologic and cardiovascular status for alertness, attentiveness, developmental delays, cardiac arrhythmias or murmurs.

Nursing Diagnoses

- Altered Nutrition: Less Than Body Requirements related to FTT process
- Altered Growth and Development related to malnutrition
- Altered Parenting related to inability to meet the needs of the FTT child

Nursing Interventions

Promoting Adequate Nutrition

1. If hospitalized, provide a primary core of staff to feed the child. Ask the parents to do so when present, in a nonthreatening manner.
2. Develop individualized teaching plan to instruct parents of child's dietary needs. Specify type of diet, essential nutrients, serving sizes, and method of preparation.
3. Provide a quiet, nonstimulating environment for eating.

4. Demonstrate proper feeding techniques including details on how to hold and how long to feed the child.
5. Administer multivitamin supplements as prescribed.
6. Encourage nutritious, high-calorie, and fortified fluids to increase nutrient density. For infants, use 24 to 30 cal/oz rather than 20 cal/oz. For older children, suggest fruit smoothies using whole milk and ice cream.
7. Refeed as necessary, with caution.
8. Gradually increase nutrients, and use small, frequent feedings with adequate fluids to ensure hydration.

NURSING ALERT

Be alert for signs of dehydration due to sudden change to a high-calorie, high-protein diet. A dramatic increase in protein can increase renal solute load to the point that a child is at risk of dehydration.

9. Monitor intake and output.
10. Maintain high-nutrient diet until weight is appropriate for height (usually 4 to 9 months).
11. Advise family that some nutritional intervention will be continued until appropriate height for age is reached.

Promoting Adequate Growth and Development

1. Obtain accurate weight at every visit or every day if hospitalized.
2. Assess child's growth by using age- and gender-appropriate growth charts.
3. Assess child's development using developmental screening tests such as the Denver II (p. 1235) or CAT/CLAMS (p. 1608).
4. Observe interactions between parents and child and among family members including eye contact, communications patterns, coping ability.
5. Provide the infant with visual and auditory stimulation by exposing to bright colors, shapes, and music. Provide the older child with age-appropriate stimulation such as books, games, and toys. Place the infant prone on the floor to encourage trunk control.
6. Encourage periods of scheduled rest and sleep.

Promoting Effective Parenting

1. Teach the parents (especially the mother) normal parenting skills by demonstrating proper holding, stroking, feeding, and communication using age-appropriate words and gestures.
2. If hospitalized, encourage and facilitate the parents to spend as much time as possible with the child.
3. Educate the parents to recognize and respond to the child's distress and hunger calls.
4. Help the parents to develop organizational skills—write down daily schedule with meal times, time for shopping, and so forth.
5. Refer for counseling, if necessary, to help parents overcome feelings of mistrust or neglect resulting from adverse personal childhood experiences.
6. Refer to social services to help resolve any social and financial difficulties that might interfere with providing a nurturing environment.

7. Monitor parents' progress and provide positive reinforcement.

Community and Home Care Considerations

1. Make regular home visits to:
   a. Observe for continued parent–child interaction.
   b. Encourage continued developmentally appropriate play.
   c. Monitor feeding status and assess intake amount.
   d. Determine frequency of voiding and stooling.
   e. Assess child's weight, height, and head circumference.
   f. Monitor vital signs, and watch for signs of dehydration.
   g. Auscultate bowel sounds.
   h. Assess muscle tone and vigor of activity.
   i. Assess family dynamics and use of support systems.
2. Inform parents of community resources such as WIC program, food banks, parenting groups.
3. Ensure that day care providers can meet child's special needs in terms of diet, feeding, and developmentally appropriate play. Day care may be beneficial in the presence of family dysfunction by providing structure.
4. Make referrals to social work and occupational or physical therapy as needed.

Family Education and Health Maintenance

1. Reinforce the need for a quiet, nonthreatening, nurturing environment.
2. Encourage the parents to be consistent with feedings. Although forced feeding is avoided, strict adherence to appropriate feeding is essential for growth.
3. Advise the parents to introduce new foods slowly and follow the child's rhythm of feeding.
4. Review the importance of providing a routine rest schedule in an environment that is conducive to sleep.
5. Review development, stressing need for visual, auditory, and tactile stimulation and age-appropriate toys for continued development.
6. Reinforce the need for follow-up care, well-child visits, and immunizations.

Outcome-Based Evaluation

- Weight steadily increasing
- Attaining developmental milestones at appropriate age
- Parents participating in child's care, using appropriate feeding technique

■ Hypertrophic Pyloric Stenosis

Hypertrophic pyloric stenosis is an acquired, progressive hypertrophy of the muscle of the pylorus, causing partial or total obstruction of the stomach outlet (pyloric sphincter). It is the second most common condition (after inguinal hernia) requiring surgery, which rarely occurs before 2 weeks or later than 5 months of age. Incidence is 1 in

250 live births and is predominant in males (5:1) and more common in first-born males. Incidence peaks in spring and fall. It is more likely to affect a full-term infant than a premature infant.

Pathophysiology and Etiology
1. Unknown cause. Maternal stress in last trimester, elevated prostaglandins, deficiency of nitric acid, immature pyloric ganglion cells with abnormal muscle innervation, and breast-feeding have been identified as possible etiologic factors.

 DRUG ALERT

A cluster of infants treated with erythromycin for pertussis exposure developed pyloric stenosis at an unusually high rate. A possible link between oral erythromycin use in the newborn and the development of pyloric stenosis is being investigated. Erythromycin should be used cautiously in infants less than 1 month old.

2. Increase in size of the circular musculature of the pylorus with thickening (size and shape of an olive). The pylorus muscle becomes elongated and thickened and is enlarged to about twice the usual size.
3. Hypertrophy of the pylorus musculature occurs with narrowing of the pyloric lumen.
4. Constriction of the lumen of the pyloric canal (at the distal end of the stomach) causes the stomach to become dilated.
5. Gastric emptying is delayed.

Clinical Manifestations
Onset is usually between 3 and 12 weeks after birth.
1. Cardinal sign is projectile, nonbilious vomiting.
   a. Initially, occasional regurgitation (similar to GER) may be present, but eventually vomiting increases in frequency and intensity.
   b. Vomitus contains milk and gastric juices; however, it may be blood streaked or "coffee ground" in appearance.
   c. Emesis occurs just after or near the end of a feeding.
2. Constipation or decreased quantity of stools.
3. Loss of weight or failure to gain weight.
4. Epigastric distention.
5. Visible gastric peristaltic waves, left to right, seen just after baby vomits.
6. Excessive hunger—willingness to eat immediately after vomiting.
7. Dehydration—electrolyte disturbance with alkalosis.
8. Decreased urinary output.
9. Palpable pyloric mass in upper right quadrant of abdomen, to the right of the umbilicus and best felt during feeding or immediately after vomiting.
10. Jaundice.

Diagnostic Evaluation
1. Palpation of pyloric mass ("olive") in conjunction with persistent, projectile vomiting is pathognomonic.
2. Ultrasound evaluation—broadly used, noninvasive method to evaluate the length and diameter of the pyloric muscle.
3. Barium upper GI series—indicated if ultrasound is inconclusive.
4. Flat film of abdomen—dilated, air-filled stomach; nondilated pyloric canal.
5. Tests for metabolic alkalosis (seen in less than 10% due to more prompt diagnosis over the past 20 years).
6. Urinalysis—urine alkaline and concentrated.
7. Blood hemoglobin and hematocrit—elevated due to hemoconcentration.

Treatment
Considered a medical, not a surgical, emergency.
1. Initial treatment.
   a. Rehydrate to correct electrolytes.
   b. Correct alkalosis.
2. Surgical—Ramstedt pyloromyotomy is procedure of choice, performed through a short transverse incision or laparoscopically.
   a. Other surgical approaches, such as supraumbilical skin-fold incision and umbilical incision, are used with better cosmetic results.
   b. Hypertrophy of the pyloric muscle regresses to normal size by about 12 weeks postoperatively.
   c. Persistent emesis after surgery suggests incomplete pyloromyotomy, gastritis, hiatal hernia, or obstruction.
   d. Postoperative complications includes duodenal perforation, small bowel obstruction, or GER.

Complications
1. Starvation
2. Dehydration
3. Severe electrolyte imbalance
4. Hematemesis

Nursing Assessment
1. Obtain a thorough history of infant's feeding behaviors and history of vomiting.
2. Assess hydration status and for signs and symptoms of electrolyte imbalance (p. 1330).
3. Assess and chart growth and development parameters.

Nursing Diagnoses
Preoperative
- Fluid Volume Deficit related to frequent vomiting
- Altered Nutrition: Less Than Body Requirements (failure to thrive) related to vomiting
- Pain related to gastric distention
- Anxiety of parents related to illness, hospitalization, and impending surgery of child

Postoperative
- Risk for Injury related to postoperative complications
- Risk for Fluid Volume Deficit after surgery
- Impaired Tissue Integrity related to surgical incision

Nursing Interventions
Preoperative
Maintaining Fluid and Electrolyte Balance
1. Administer IV therapy as ordered to treat dehydration, metabolic alkalosis, and electrolyte deficiency.
2. Carefully monitor output, including amount, and characteristics of urine (check specific gravity), vomiting, and stools.
3. Accurately measure daily weight as a guide for calculating need for parenteral fluid.
4. Monitor laboratory data for serum electrolytes.
5. Apply appropriate restraints on infants to prevent interference with fluid therapy.
6. Provide pacifier for infants who are NPO.
7. Monitor vital signs as indicated by condition. Watch for tachycardia, hypotension, change in respirations.

NURSING ALERT

 Irregular respiratory rate with apnea is a sign of severe alkalosis.

Maintaining Nutrition
1. Emphasize rehydration, electrolyte balance, and replacement of body fat and protein stores. This depends on severity of depletion and may require total parenteral nutrition for several days or weeks before surgery to improve surgical risk.
2. Maintain NPO status with indwelling nasogastric tube (inserted to remove any residual barium and retained formula) as ordered. Ensure placement, position, and patency. Record drainage type, color, and amount.
3. If oral feedings are to be continued, do the following:
   a. Provide small, frequent feedings, given slowly.
   b. Bubble frequently before, during, and after feeding.
   c. Thicken formula if ordered.
   d. Allow breast-feeding as tolerated.
4. Prop the patient in upright position (Figure 48-2).
   a. Elevate head of bed, mattress, or infant seat at a 75- to 80-degree angle.
   b. Place slightly on right side to aid in gastric emptying.
   c. Handle gently and minimally after feeding.

Providing Comfort
1. Provide mouth care, and wet lips frequently if NPO.
2. Let the infant suck on a pacifier.
3. Provide for physical contact or nearness without excessive stimulation.
4. Provide for audio and visual stimulation that may be soothing.
5. Do not palpate pyloric "olive" to decrease risk of postoperative wound infection from bruising abdominal wall and excoriating tissue in operative site.
6. Administer analgesics as ordered.

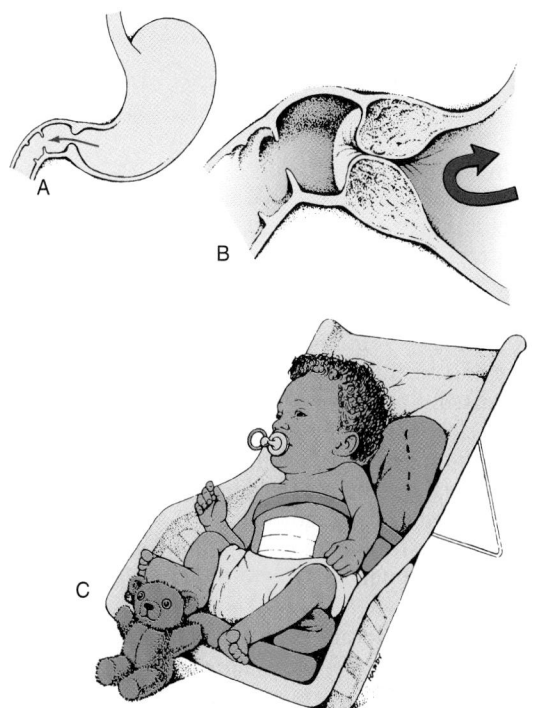

FIGURE 48-2 Pyloric stenosis. (**A**) Normal passage through pyloric sphincter. (**B**) Stoppage of flow due to stenotic sphincter. (**C**) Postoperative treatment: child propped upright, slightly on right side, aids in gastric emptying.

Alleviating Parental Anxiety
1. Assess understanding of diagnosis and plan of care.
2. Help minimize guilt feelings by providing adequate, specific information and clarifying any misconceptions.
3. Prepare the parents for the surgery of their child.
   a. Be honest with them.
   b. Prepare them for the expected postoperative appearance of the infant.
   c. Show them where the operating room and recovery room are located and where to wait during surgery.
4. Allow them to hold the infant to maintain bonding.
5. Encourage them to rest to care better for the infant postoperatively.
6. Accept and explore negative displays of emotion, which may be due to fatigue and frustration because of the extensive care given to the child before hospitalization.
7. Reassure them that surgery is considered curative, and normal feeding should resume shortly afterward.

Postoperative
Preventing Complications
1. Assess vital signs to evaluate for fluid and electrolyte imbalances.
2. Assess skin and mucous membranes for hydration status.
3. Weigh daily to assess gain or loss.
4. Elevate head slightly.

5. Maintain patent nasogastric tube to prevent gastric distention. Record losses.
6. Monitor blood glucose levels to prevent hypoglycemia.

Maintaining Hydration

1. Administer IV fluids until adequate intake has been established.
2. Resume oral feeding 2 to 8 hours after surgery when infant is alert or as ordered.
3. Start with small, frequent feedings of glucose water, and slowly advance to full-strength formula and regular diet as tolerated.
4. Report any vomiting—amount and characteristics. Feeding schedule may be withheld 4 hours and then restarted.
5. Feed slowly, and bubble frequently.
6. Note how feeding is taken and if it is retained.
7. Increase the amount of feeding as the time interval between feedings is lengthened.
8. Allow breast-feeding to resume as tolerated, beginning with limited nursing of 5 to 8 minutes and gradually increase.
9. Continue to elevate the infant's head and shoulders after feeding for 45 to 60 minutes for several feedings after surgery. Place on right side to aid gastric emptying.
10. Expect that regurgitation may continue for a short period after surgery. Nasogastric tube may be maintained for length of time, as determined by provider.

Promoting Healing

1. Provide analgesia and comfort measures, such as a pacifier, rocking, and other soothing stimulation to keep infant quiet and prevent tension on incision.
2. Involve parents in care of infant postoperatively to prepare them for care of wound after discharge.
3. Observe for drainage or signs of inflammation at incision site, and provide care to incision as ordered.
4. Note that poor nutritional status may delay wound healing.

Community and Home Care Considerations

1. Teach proper care of the operative site.
   a. Check for signs and symptoms of inflammation.
   b. Observe for drainage.
   c. Provide specific care of site as ordered by provider.
2. Monitor weight and feeding behavior.
3. Observe for signs of delayed gastric emptying or GER.
4. Assess parent–infant interaction and parental coping.

Family Education and Health Maintenance

1. Teach feeding technique to be continued at home; length of feeding technique varies depending on wound healing, nutritional status, and growth.
2. Provide written and verbal instructions as to infant's care and follow-up schedule.
3. Review with family when medical attention is needed and appropriate resource:

a. Signs of infection
b. Frequent vomiting, vomiting longer than 5 days, or poor feeding with signs of dehydration
c. Abdominal distention

Outcome-Based Evaluation

- Vital signs stable; urine output adequate
- Tolerating 1- to 2-oz feedings in upright position without vomiting
- Quietly resting with pacifier
- Parents verbalizing understanding of surgery and postoperative care
- Vital signs stable; blood glucose within normal limits
- No signs of dehydration
- Incision healing without signs of infection

Celiac Disease

Celiac disease, also called *gluten-sensitive enteropathy* or *celiac sprue,* is a disease of the small intestines characterized by a permanent inability to tolerate dietary gluten. The ingestion of gluten produces an immune response that damages the villi of the small intestine, decreasing the surface area, causing malabsorption, and giving a cobblestone appearance to the surface. Occurs most frequently in Caucasians and among females by 2:1 over males. Incidence is highest in Europe with 1 in 250 children in Italy. It may be underdiagnosed in America with 1 in 4,700 children.

Pathophysiology and Etiology

1. The cause is unknown; although it appears to require interaction between a number of intrinsic factors (genetic susceptibility, activation of the immune system) and extrinsic factors (gluten and possibly other environmental factors). Both cellular immunity and humoral immunity are implicated. There is a familial tendency with association of specific HLA antigens.
2. The disease can be triggered by surgery, pregnancy, viral infection or severe emotional stress. IgA-deficient children are 20 times more likely to develop celiac disease.
3. Characteristics of celiac disease include the following:
   a. Impaired intestinal absorption
   b. Histologic abnormalities of the small intestine
   c. Clinical and histologic improvement with wheat-, rye-, barley-, and possibly oat-free diet
   d. Recurrence of clinical manifestations and histologic changes after reintroduction of dietary gluten
4. Histologic changes in mucosa of small bowel, especially duodenum and jejunum, resulting from dietary gluten include the following:
   a. Irregularity of epithelial cells
   b. Loss of normal villous pattern
   c. Obliteration of intervillous spaces that are infiltrated with plasma cells and eosinophils
   d. Loss of epithelial cell brush border

5. Mucosal damage results in the following:
   a. Disaccharidase deficiency
   b. Depression of peptidase activity
6. Subsequent malabsorption probably results from the following:
   a. Decreased area of absorption in small bowel
   b. Impaired enzyme activity
7. The body is unable to absorb fats, fat-soluble vitamins (A, D, E, and K), minerals, and some protein and carbohydrates.
8. The severity of symptoms depends on the extent of histologic intestinal changes.
   a. The extent of affected intestine is variable.
   b. When most or all of the small intestine mucosa is involved, symptoms are severe and malabsorption is generalized. If involvement is focal and limited to the proximal bowel, GI symptoms may be absent.

Clinical Manifestations

The age and mode of presenting signs and symptoms are extremely variable. Diagnosis is most commonly made by 6 to 24 months of age; however, it can be made in the adult.

3 to 9 Months of Age
1. Irritability
2. Acutely ill; severe diarrhea and vomiting
3. Possibly failure to thrive

9 to 18 Months of Age
"Typical" celiac appearance is seen.
1. Impaired growth
   a. Normal growth during early months of life
   b. Slackening of weight followed by weight loss
2. Abnormal stools
   a. Pale
   b. Soft
   c. Bulky
   d. Offensive odor
   e. Greasy—steatorrhea
   f. May increase in number
3. Abdominal distention
4. Anorexia
5. Muscle wasting—most obvious in buttocks and proximal parts of extremities
6. Hypotonia
7. Mood changes—ill humor, irritability, temper tantrums, shyness
8. Mild clubbing of fingers
9. Vomiting—often occurring in evening
10. Seizures
11. Tooth discoloration or loss of enamel
12. Pale sores on inside of mouth called "aphthus ulcers"
13. Painful skin rash called "dermatitis herpetiformis"

Older Child
Symptoms diminish or disappear in adolescence and reappear in early adulthood.

1. Signs and symptoms often related to nutritional or secondary deficiencies resulting from disease
2. May have abnormal stools and growth impairment
3. May have colicky abdominal pain with constipation and large, pale stools
4. Missed menstrual period due to increased weight loss
5. Fingerprint changes; ridge atrophy

Manifestations Secondary to Malabsorption
1. Anemia, vitamin deficiency
2. Hypoproteinemia with edema
3. Hypocalcemia, hypokalemia, hypomagnesemia
4. Hypoprothrombinemia resulting from impaired vitamin K absorption
5. Disaccharide intolerance—with acid sugar-containing stools (secondary to the altered small bowel mucosa)
6. Low bone density, osteoporosis secondary to decreased calcium absorption

Diagnostic Evaluation
1. Thorough history, including dietary patterns, and general status of the child.
2. Elevated endomysial antibodies and presence of antigliadin antibodies. Serum immunoglobulin IgG and IgA antigliadin antibodies assess the activity of the disease.
3. Endoscopy with small bowel biopsy demonstrating flattened villi.
4. Diagnostic criteria:
   a. Severely damaged or flat, villous lesions
   b. Clinical response to gluten elimination
   c. Histologic recovery after gluten elimination
   d. Histologic recurrence of villous injury within 2 years of gluten reintroduction—not considered essential if findings on intestinal biopsy are characteristic of disease and if clear-cut remission on strict gluten-free diet without symptoms
5. D-xylose absorption—less than 20 to 25 mg/dL at 60 minutes.
6. Biochemical changes include low serum albumin, protein, and magnesium in malnourished patients.
7. Other abnormal blood values include decreased folic acid, decreased hemoglobin, decreased prothrombin time, and hypochromia on red blood count smear.
8. 24-hour stool collection for fecal fat times three—increased.
9. Radiologic studies—skeletal x-rays.
   a. Demineralization
   b. Retarded bone age
10. Sweat test and pancreatic function studies to rule out cystic fibrosis.

Complications
1. Possible predisposition to malignant lymphoma and adenocarcinoma of small intestine at later age if dietary restrictions are terminated
2. Refractory sprue

3. Associated disorders
   a. Dermatitis herpetiformis
   b. Insulin-dependent diabetes mellitus
   c. Cystic fibrosis
   d. Thyroid disease
   e. Systemic lupus erythematosus
   f. Liver disease
   g. Collagen vascular disease
   h. Rheumatoid arthritis
   i. Sjögren's syndrome
4. Impaired growth, inability to fight infection, electrolyte disturbances, and blood clotting
5. Osteoporosis at a later age due to poor calcium absorption
6. Seizures related to inadequate absorption of folic acid and buildup of calcium deposits on the brain

Treatment
1. Lifelong gluten-free diet
   a. Avoid all foods containing wheat (including spelt, triticale, and kamut), rye and barley gluten. The exclusion of oats is controversial; it appears to require a much larger intake of oats to bring about an equivalent effect. Therefore, it is best to err on the safe side and omit oats or consume in very small quantities.
   b. The small intestinal mucosa will always respond abnormally to dietary gluten, although clinical signs may not be immediately evident.
   c. Biopsy reverts to normal with appropriate diet.
   d. Clinical signs of improvement should be seen days to weeks after proper diet is initiated.
2. Adequate caloric intake
3. Supplemental vitamins and minerals
   a. Folic acid for 1 to 2 months
   b. Vitamins A and D because not absorbed
   c. Iron for 1 to 2 months if anemic
   d. Vitamin K if evidence of hypoprothrombinemia and bleeding
   e. Calcium if milk is restricted
4. Reduction of fat intake (rare)
5. Possible elimination of lactose and sucrose from diet for 6 to 8 weeks based on reduced disaccharidase activity

Nursing Assessment
1. Obtain family dietary history as it relates to onset of symptoms.
2. Assess child's nutritional status.
3. Check for signs of infection.
4. Assess growth and development.

Nursing Diagnoses
- Altered Nutrition: Less Than Body Requirements related to malabsorption of nutrients, diarrhea, and vomiting
- Risk for Infection related to malnourishment and anemia
- Altered Parenting related to inability to control behavioral problems

Nursing Interventions
Providing Adequate Nutrition and Dietary Restrictions
1. Ensure that initial diet is high in protein, relatively low in fat, and free of starch.
   a. Provide mild protein or skim milk that is sweetened with banana powder.
   b. Watch for fat intolerance in infants and young children.
2. Advise adding proteins and sugars gradually.
   a. Add individual foods one at a time at several-day intervals, such as lean meat, cottage cheese, egg white, and raw ground apple.
   b. Add starchy foods to diet last.
3. Restrict wheat, rye, and barley from diet.
4. Maintain NPO status during the initial treatment of celiac crisis or during diagnostic testing. Take special precautions to ensure proper restriction if the child is ambulatory.
5. Encourage small, frequent, appetizing meals, but do not force eating if the child has anorexia.
6. Note the child's reaction to food. Close observation of the child's responses to food may reveal other intolerances. Note and record the following:
   a. Foods taken and those refused
   b. Appetite
   c. Change in behavior after eating
   d. Characteristics and frequency of stools
   e. General disposition—behavior improvement often seen within 2 to 3 days after diet control is initiated
7. Be prepared to temporarily eliminate new food introduced if symptoms increase.
8. Assist with gluten-challenge diet if used to evaluate histologic and clinical response during therapy.
   a. Be aware that, after an extended time on dietary regimen, the child may dislike gluten-containing foods.
   b. Assess for mild GI symptoms (eg, loose stools, vague abdominal pain) that may be related to anxiety rather than gluten intolerance.
   c. Support the family and provide reassurance. The gluten-challenge diet may last 3 to 4 months.

Preventing Infection
1. Advise parents to avoid exposing the child to anyone with an infection.
2. Teach parents that the child usually perspires freely and has a subnormal temperature with cold extremities; prevent dampness and chilling, and encourage appropriate clothing.
3. Prevent upper respiratory infection by position changes, good hygiene, and clearance of secretions.
4. Teach and practice good handwashing.
5. Assess for fever, cough, irritability, or other signs of infection.

Promoting Effective Parenting
1. Teach the parents to develop an awareness of the child's behavior; recognize changes, and care for child accordingly.

2. Explain that diet and eating have a direct effect on behavior and that behavior may indicate how the child is feeling.
3. Help the parents recognize and understand mood swings, from having temper tantrums to being very timid, nervous, or unstable.
4. Advise the parents to allow the child to express feelings freely through safe and age-appropriate media.
   a. Encourage parents to define limits of behavior for the child and convey them to all family members.
   b. Avoid conflict or emotional upset in the child's presence when possible. These may precipitate diarrhea, vomiting, and celiac crisis.
5. Encourage patience, routines, and consistency.
6. Advise parents to record changes in behavior, especially in relation to eating and diet to document effectiveness of therapy.
7. Help the parents to maintain a balance between the child with celiac disease, the other family members, and additional rules and responsibilities.
8. If the child is withdrawn, advise providing opportunity for play with other children, especially when the child begins to feel better.
9. Explain that the toddler may cling to infantile habits for security. Allow this behavior; it may disappear as physical condition improves.
10. Suggest offering the child other sensory stimulation to compensate for lack of eating pleasure.
11. Help the parents to understand that, after initial rapid weight gain, further improvement may be slow.
12. Provide emotional support for the child and parents.
13. Refer for counseling if indicated.

Family Education and Health Maintenance

1. Teach parents about celiac disease and how it is controlled by diet.
   a. Provide a specific list of restricted and acceptable foods.
   b. Teach the parents how to read labels on foods to identify those containing wheat, rye, and oat glutens, thus avoiding them.
      (i) Advise any ingredient of unspecified grain origin should be assumed to contain gluten.
      (ii) Advise medications should also be checked; filler and excipients such as alcohol in cough medication may be wheat based.
      (iii) Advise gluten is found in many manufactured products as a filler or thickener, such as gravy powder.
   c. Provide substitutes for wheat, rye, barley, and oats, such as corn, rice, soybean flour, and gluten-free starch.
   d. Help the parents become comfortable in situation problem solving (eg, supplying gluten-free cupcakes for birthday party to which child has been invited).
   e. Initiate referral with dietitian.
   f. Emphasize the importance of the vitamin regimen.
   g. Discuss the importance of continued adherence to diet, even though the child is feeling well, eating well, and has normal stools. Advancing diet too rapidly may result in a setback. Encourage child to become involved in diet.
   h. Adolescent compliance may be variable. Encourage support and understanding.
   i. Alteration in diet may have significant cultural, ethnic, and religious implications. Help parents identify how adjustments can be made.
2. Advise parents on eating out—inform friends before visiting, question waiter or chefs at restaurants about possible hidden sources of gluten, or, if in doubt, avoid it and fill up on vegetables, potatoes, and rice. Advise parents to discuss child's dietary needs with other parents, especially at sleepovers.
3. Work with the school nurse and school dietitian or provide homemade condiments to be kept in school refrigerator to be added to the child's lunch.
4. Advise parents of support groups, recipes, and food companies that offer gluten-free products.
5. Tell parents that common problems with long-term gluten-free diet are constipation due to low dietary fiber intake and weight gain due to now normal absorption; therefore, encourage regular physical activity and avoidance of high-calorie foods.
6. Impress on the parents the importance of regular medical follow-up.
7. Encourage the parents to practice good hygiene to prevent infection because this child is especially prone to infection because of malnutrition and anemia.
8. Help the parents to understand that the emotional climate in the home and around the child is vitally important in maintaining the child's medical and physical stability. Stress the importance of not making the child feel abnormal or a nuisance to the family. Family support is invaluable in facilitating acceptance of the diet.
9. Stress that the disorder is lifelong; however, changes in the mucosal lining of the intestine and the general clinical condition of their child are reversible when dietary gluten is avoided.
10. Due to heredity nature of the disease, encourage other family members to be tested.
11. For additional information and support, refer to Celiac Sprue Association, P.O. Box 31700, Omaha, NE 68131-0700, 402-558-0600, *www.csaceliacs.org*; Canadian Celiac Association, *www.celiac.ca*; or Celiac Disease Foundation, *www.celiac.org*.

Outcome-Based Evaluation

- Tolerating starch-free diet well without pain or vomiting
- No signs of infection
- Parents setting limits with child and documenting behavior in relation to meals

Diarrhea

Diarrhea is an excessive loss of water and electrolytes that occurs with passage of one or more unformed stools. It is a symptom of many conditions and may be caused by many diseases (Table 48-3). Often, the cause is difficult to determine; occasionally, it is unknown.

Pathophysiology and Etiology
Mechanisms of Diarrhea

1. Secretory—decreased absorption, increased secretion
2. Osmotic—maldigestion, transport defects, ingestion of unabsorbable solute
3. Increased motility—decreased transit time or stasis (bacterial overgrowth)
4. Decreased surface area—decreased functional capacity
5. Mucosal invasion (motile or secretory)—inflammation, decreased colonic reabsorption, increased motility

Physiologic Effects of Diarrhea

1. Dehydration (extracellular fluid loss)
   a. Large loss of fluid and electrolytes in watery stools
   b. Losses with repeated vomiting; decreased fluid intake
   c. Increased insensible fluid losses from skin and lungs resulting from fever and rapid respirations
   d. Continued urine excretion
2. Electrolyte imbalance
   a. Potassium—varies
   b. Chloride; sodium; hypotonic, isotonic, or hypertonic dehydration
3. Acid–base imbalance—metabolic acidosis
   a. From large losses of potassium, sodium, and bicarbonate in stools
   b. From impaired renal function
4. Monosaccharide intolerance and protein hypersensitivity

Pathogens

1. Bacteria—*Escherichia coli* 0157:H7, *Salmonella*, *Shigella*, *Yersinia enterocolitica*, *Campylobacter jejuni*, *Clostridium difficile*, dysentery, cholera
2. Viral—rotavirus (most common; peaks during winter months), enteroviruses (echovirus), adenoviruses, human reoviruslike agent, Norwalk virus
3. Normal intestinal tract inhabitants that act as pathogens in certain circumstances (eg, after ingestion of antibiotics)

TABLE 48-3 **Differential Diagnosis of Diarrhea**		
	Infant	Child	Adolescent
Acute			
Common	Gastroenteritis Systemic infection Antibiotic associated Overfeeding	Gastroenteritis Food poisoning Systemic infection Antibiotic associated	Gastroenteritis Food poisoning Antibiotic associated
Rare	Primary disaccharidase deficiency Hirschsprung's toxic colitis Adrenogenital syndrome	Toxic ingestion	Hyperthyroidism
Chronic			
Common	Postinfectious secondary lactase deficiency Cow's milk/soy protein intolerance Chronic nonspecific diarrhea of infancy Celiac disease Cystic fibrosis AIDS enteropathy	Postinfectious secondary lactase deficiency Irritable bowel syndrome Celiac disease Lactose intolerance Giardiasis Inflammatory bowel disease AIDS enteropathy	Irritable bowel syndrome Inflammatory bowel disease Lactose intolerance Giardiasis Laxative abuse (anorexia nervosa)
Rare	Primary immune defects Familial villous atrophy Secretory tumors Acrodermatitis enteropathica Lymphangiectasia Abetalipoproteinemia Eosinophilic gastroenteritis Short bowel syndrome Intractable diarrhea syndrome Autoimmune enteropathy	Acquired immune defects Secretory tumors Pseudo-obstruction	Secretory tumor Primary bowel tumor Gay bowel disease

AIDS = acquired immunodeficiency syndrome.

4. Fungal—*Candida* enteritis
5. Parasitic—*Giardia lamblia, Cryptosporidium parvum*
6. Protozoal

Noninfectious Etiologic Factors

1. Malabsorption—lactase deficiency, cow's milk protein intolerance, wheat protein allergy, celiac disease, cystic fibrosis of the pancreas
2. Inflammatory bowel disease—ulcerative colitis, Crohn's disease
3. Immune deficiency—severe combined immunodeficiency, IgA deficiency
4. Infant exposed to overeating
5. Child exposed to excessive stress, emotional excitement, and fatigue
6. Direct irritation of GI tract by foods
7. Inappropriate use of laxatives and purgatives
8. Mechanical disorders—malrotation, incomplete small bowel obstruction, intermittent volvulus
9. Congenital anomalies (eg, Hirschsprung's disease)

Acute Diarrhea

1. Sudden change in frequency of stools
2. Usually self-limited, but can result in dehydration

Chronic or Persistent Diarrhea

1. Passage of more than three liquid stools in a day for more than 2 weeks' duration.
2. Associated with disorders of malabsorption, anatomic defects, abnormal bowel motility, hypersensitivity reaction, or a long-term inflammatory response.

NURSING ALERT

Infants and young children in day care centers may be at increased risk for diarrhea due to *Shigella*, *Salmonella*, rotavirus, endopathogenic *E. coli*, and giardiasis. This is known as "day care diarrhea," and handwashing is the major preventive measure.

Risk Factors for Diarrhea

1. Age—the younger the child, the greater the susceptibility and severity.
   a. Extracellular fluid volume is proportionately larger in the infant and young child.
   b. Nutritional reserves are relatively smaller in the young child.
2. Impaired health—susceptibility is increased in the malnourished or debilitated child.
3. Climate—susceptibility is increased in warm weather.
4. Environment—frequency is increased where there is overcrowding, poor sanitation, inadequate refrigeration of food, and inadequate health care and education.
5. Virulence of a potential pathogen affects severity.
6. Internationally adopted child.

Clinical Manifestations

Symptoms vary with severity, specific cause, and type of onset (insidious versus acute).

1. Low-grade fever to 41.1°C (100°F)
2. Anorexia
3. Mild and intermittent to severe vomiting
4. Stools
   a. Appearance of diarrhea from a few hours to 3 days
   b. Loose and fluid consistency
   c. Greenish or yellow-green
   d. May contain mucus, pus, or blood
   e. Frequency varies from 2 to 20 per day
   f. Expelled with force; may be preceded by pain
5. Behavioral changes
   a. Irritability and restlessness
   b. Weakness
   c. Extreme prostration
   d. Stupor and convulsions
   e. Flaccidity
6. Physical changes
   a. Little to extreme loss of subcutaneous fat
   b. Up to 50% total body weight loss
   c. Poor skin turgor; capillary refill >2 seconds
   d. Dry mucous membranes and dry cracked lips
   e. Pallor
   f. Sunken fontanelles and eyes
   g. Petechiae seen with bacterial infections
7. Vital sign/output changes
   a. Low blood pressure
   b. High pulse
   c. Respirations rapid and hyperpneic
   d. Decreased or absent urinary output
   e. Collapse imminent

Diagnostic Evaluation
Studies to Evaluate Condition

1. Thorough history and physical examination to determine hydration status

---

NURSING ALERT

A postural change in heart rate is a useful clue in assessing the fluid state of a toddler. An increase greater than 20 beats per minute when moving from lying to standing is an indicator of hypovolemia.

---

2. Electrolyte and kidney function tests—serum sodium, chloride, potassium, and blood urea nitrogen variable
3. Acid–base balance—serum CO_2; arterial pH and CO_2 possibly abnormal
4. Complete blood count to determine plasma volume by hematocrit; infection by WBC and differential
5. Sedimentation rate—elevated in infection and inflammation

Studies to Determine Cause

1. Thorough history to determine recent contact or exposure, travel to at-risk countries, antibiotic therapy, and possible immunosuppression.

2. Rotazyme (rapid test for rotavirus).
3. Stool and rectal swab cultures and stool for ova and parasites can detect specific pathogens. Must specify *Giardia* profile, *Cryptosporidium*, and *E. coli* 0157:H7 serotyping when ordering tests.
4. Stool for white blood cell count to rule out invasive bacterial disease.
5. Stool and rectal swab cultures and stool for ova and parasites can detect specific pathogens.
6. Stool pH, reducing substances—decreased pH may indicate various noninfectious causes; acid stool containing sugar is characteristic of disaccharide intolerance.
7. Blood cultures can rule out septicemia.
8. Serologic studies can detect viral pathogens.
9. Breath hydrogen test can determine carbohydrate malabsorption and bacterial overgrowth.
10. Urinalysis can exclude UTI as cause of nonspecific diarrhea.

Treatment

Treatment is based on the degree of dehydration; mild (<5%), moderate (5% to 10%), and severe (>10% weight loss; Table 48-4)
1. Prevent spread of disease; suspect disease to be communicable until proven otherwise. Use enteric isolation precautions.
2. For mild to moderate dehydration (5%): maintain hydration and electrolyte balance with oral rehydration solution (WHO solution, Pedialyte, Infalyte) and BRATS (bananas, rice cereal, applesauce, dry toast and saltine crackers) diet.
   a. For oral rehydration, administer 100 mL/kg over 4 hours, with additional fluids after each liquid bowel movement.
   b. Candidates for oral rehydration include mild to moderate (<10%) dehydration, >4 months old, no persistent vomiting, and probable gastroenteritis.
3. For moderate to severe dehydration (10%): administer IV fluid and electrolyte replacement as ordered (usually 20 mL/kg over 20 minutes).
4. Provide supportive care; monitor and record oral or IV fluids, weights, fluid loss from diarrhea, urine, and vomiting. Provide good mouth care.
5. Administer specific antimicrobial therapy.
   a. Complications include dehydration, protracted diarrheal state, transient lactose intolerance.

Complications

1. Severe dehydration and acid–base derangements with acidosis
2. Shock

Nursing Assessment

1. Obtain accurate history of signs and symptoms: nature and frequency of stools, type of onset, length of illness, associated symptoms.
2. Assess degree of dehydration (see Table 48-4).

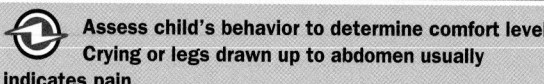

NURSING ALERT

Assess child's behavior to determine comfort level. Crying or legs drawn up to abdomen usually indicates pain.

Nursing Diagnoses

• Fluid Volume Deficit related to diarrhea and extracellular fluid loss
• Risk for Infection transmission to others related to infectious diarrhea

---

TABLE 48-4 Assessment for Dehydration in Children

Clinical Signs	Degree of Dehydration		
	Mild	**Moderate**	**Severe**
General:			
• Infants	• Thirsty, alert, restless	• Restless or lethargic; irritable to touch	• Limp, drowsy; cyanotic extremities
• Older children	• Thirsty, alert, restless	• Thirsty, alert; postural hypotension	• Usually conscious; cyanotic extremities
Respirations	Slightly increased	Increased	Deep and rapid
Pulse	Slightly increased	Increased	Rapid
Blood pressure	Normal	Decreased	May be unrecordable
Capillary refill	< 2 seconds	2–3 seconds	> 3 seconds
Skin turgor	Normal	Slightly reduced	Reduced
Skin color	Pale	Gray	Mottled
Weight loss	Up to 5%	Up to 10%	Up to 15%
Mucous membrane	Tacky	Tacky/dry	Parched
Anterior fontanelle	Flat	Slightly depressed	Sunken
Urine volume	Small	Oliguria	Oliguria/anuria
Specific gravity	<1.020	>1.030	>1.035

(Adapted from Eliason, B., & Lewan, R. [1998]. Gastroenteritis in children: Principles of diagnosis and treatment. *American Family Physician, 58*[8], 1769–1776; Straughn, A., & English, B. [1996]. Oral rehydration therapy: A neglected treatment for pediatric diarrhea. *American Journal of Maternal Child Nursing, 21*[3], 144–147.)

- Risk for Impaired Skin Integrity related to irritation by frequent stools
- Altered Nutrition: Less Than Body Requirements related to malabsorption
- Anxiety and Fear related to hospitalization and illness

Nursing Interventions
Restoring Fluid Balance
1. Monitor amount and rate of IV fluid therapy, which have been calculated by the health care provider. Fluid needs are based on fluid deficit, ongoing losses, and body weight.
2. Prevent overload of circulatory system.
   a. Check flow rate and amount absorbed hourly and totally.
   b. Adhere to prescribed volume carefully when oral feedings are given in conjunction with IV fluid.
   c. Never administer IV fluids to pediatric patient without safeguard of a volume-control infusion device or pump.
   d. Observe for signs of fluid overload: edema, increased blood pressure, bounding pulse, labored respirations, and crackles in lung fields.
3. Check IV site for infiltration or improper flow so site can be changed as necessary.
4. Use appropriate protective devices to prevent the child from injuring involved extremity or causing IV to malfunction.
5. Weigh the patient daily as a guide for fluid needs and patient status.
6. Monitor urine output, and keep accurate intake and output record, including vomitus and liquid stools.
7. If NPO, provide frequent mouth care and non-nutritive sucking with a pacifier. Continue to bubble infant to expel air swallowed while crying or sucking.
8. If oral rehydration solution is used, reassess hydration status every 2 to 4 hours, once rehydrated, continue for 8 to 12 hours, then resume breast-feeding with increased frequency of feedings or formula at full strength or increased frequency if half strength.

   Note: Unless severe vomiting, do not deprive of nutrition for longer than 1 to 2 days.

NURSING ALERT

Diluted fruit juices and soft drinks are not recommended. High-carbohydrate content aggravates diarrhea by osmotic effect.

Preventing Spread of Infection
1. Ensure adherence to good handwashing and gown technique protocols for all people having contact with infant or child.
2. Follow policy as to care of diapers.
3. Handle specimens collected using universal precautions, and transport to laboratories in appropriate containers per policy.
4. Teach good hygiene measures to older children.

Preventing Skin Impairment
1. Protect infant's diaper area from becoming excoriated by making frequent diaper changes.
2. Expose to air and light as much as possible.
3. Avoid commercial baby wipes, which contain alcohol and may sting inflamed or excoriated diaper area. Use mild soap and water, place infant in tub of water or baking soda bath (soothing and neutralizing) for cleaning.
4. Prevent scratching or rubbing of irritated area. Holding infant on parent's protected lap may provide comfort and stimulation for parent and infant.
5. Use protective barrier creams, such as zinc oxide (Desitin) or karaya powder; completely remove after each stool for thorough cleansing.
6. Leave diaper area open to air until thoroughly dried.

Resuming Adequate Nutritional Intake
1. After rehydration, advance slowly from clear liquids, such as Pedialyte, to half-strength formula, to regular diet.
   a. Contrary to widespread belief and practice, lactose-based milk does not have to be eliminated.
   b. In older infants and children, rice cereal, bananas, potatoes, or other nonlactose, carbohydrate-rich foods should be offered shortly after successful rehydration.
2. As diet is advanced, note any vomiting or increase in stools, and report it immediately. Oral feedings should not be resumed too early or advanced too rapidly, because diarrhea may recur.

Reducing Fear and Anxiety
1. Acknowledge that hospitalization is frightening, especially when it is sudden, as with diarrhea.
2. Many treatments and procedures may be painful. Give reassurance to the child before, during, and after treatment.
   a. Talk to the child.
   b. Hold and comfort child after the procedure.
   c. Explain in age-appropriate language.
   d. Include family in care and treatments when possible.
3. Explain to family that intermittent abdominal cramps may be painful, and provide support.
4. Provide some means of pleasant stimulation, entertainment, or diversion, especially while child remains in bed.
   a. Infant—mobile, musical toy
   b. Young child—books, tapes
   c. Older child—television, videos
5. Provide physical closeness to provide comfort, if child displays interest.
   a. Petting, stroking
   b. Holding, rocking

Community and Home Care Considerations
1. Infants and young children in day care centers may be at increased risk for diarrhea due to *Shigella, Salmonella,* rotavirus, *E. Coli, Cryptosporidium, Campylobacter, C. difficile,* and *Giardia.* This is known as "day care diarrhea," and good handwashing is the major preventive measure. This is especially important with rotavirus

because it can be excreted for 21 days or for as long as 57 days in some cases.
2. If infectious agent is identified, other children may be at risk and should be reported.
    a. Encourage parents to contact the child care center and report.
    b. A child with diarrhea containing blood or mucus should be excluded from day care until the diarrhea resolves.
    c. Stool cultures positive for *E. coli* 0157:H7 or *Shigella* are reportable illnesses, and the child should be excluded until the diarrhea resolves and two cultures are negative for these organisms.
3. Assess sanitation and hygiene practices in the home or day care center for overcrowding, number of working toilets in the home for number of people, availability of working sinks with soap and towels in the bathrooms and their proximity to food preparation areas, disposal of diapers, and handwashing practices of caregivers and children.
4. Because most treatment for diarrhea is done on an outpatient basis, nurses in the community need to be available to answer questions.

Family Education and Health Maintenance

1. After the cause of the diarrhea is determined, it may be necessary to teach proper hygiene, formula or food preparation, handling, and storage.
    a. Use handwashing before bottle and food preparation.
    b. Use disposable bottles, or sterilize or use dishwasher for reusable bottles.
    c. Refrigerate reconstituted formula and all other fluids between uses. Milk may become contaminated within 1 hour if left out at room temperature; juice becomes contaminated within several hours.
    d. Discard small amounts of food or fluid from containers already used.
2. Explain the fecal–oral mode of transmission of infectious diarrheal illnesses.
3. Explain the early symptoms of a diarrheal illness and of dehydration, which requires notification of the health care provider.
4. Discourage the use of antiemetics and antidiarrheal medications for infants and children with gastroenteritis; they have little effect on infantile diarrhea, may cause toxicity, and can mask signs and symptoms of more serious illness.

> **◆ DRUG ALERT**
>
> **Bismuth subsalicylate, an over-the-counter drug that is readily available, has shown only modest beneficial effects in children and may increase the risk of Reye's syndrome due to salicylate absorption.**

5. Advise parents when traveling internationally with their children to eat and drink cleanly boiled, bottled, or carbonated water, be aware of drinks with ice cubes, food rinsed with water, and make sure all food is well cooked.
6. Help parents understand the importance of medical care and general good hygiene.
7. For additional information and support, refer to National Institute of Diabetes and Digestive and Kidney Diseases, *www.niddk.nih.gov*.

Outcome-Based Evaluation

- Vital signs stable; urine output adequate
- Family, staff members handwashing properly and frequently
- No redness or excoriation of diaper area
- Tolerating small feedings of clear liquids without diarrhea or vomiting
- Child playing quietly

■ Hirschsprung's Disease

Hirschsprung's disease (congenital aganglionic megacolon) is a congenital absence of the parasympathetic ganglion nerve cells from within the muscle wall of the intestinal tract, usually at the distal end of the colon. Occurs in 1 in 5,000 live births with no racial predilection. It is three times more common in males. Approximately 10% of children with Hirschsprung's disease have Down syndrome.

Pathophysiology and Etiology

1. An arrest in embryologic development affecting the migration of parasympathetic nerves (innervation) of the intestine, occurring before the 12th week of gestation. There is a genetic cause.
2. The parasympathetic ganglion cells in Auerbach's plexus within the intestinal tract muscle wall are absent or reduced in number, usually at the distal end of the colon and the rectum.
    a. Most commonly affected site is the rectosigmoid colon (referred to as short segment disease).
    b. Less common (long segment disease) extends to the upper descending colon and possibly the transverse colon.
3. No peristalsis occurs in the affected portion of intestine (ie, spastic and contracted).
    a. This section is usually narrow; therefore, no fecal material passes through it.
    b. The intestine above the affected section has an accumulation of fecal material.
4. Proximal to the narrow affected section, the colon is dilated.
    a. Filled with fecal material and gas.
    b. Hypertrophy of muscular coating.
    c. Ulceration of mucosa may be seen in newborn.
5. The internal rectal sphincter fails to relax, and evacuation of fecal material and gas is prevented. Abdominal distention and constipation result.

Clinical Manifestations

Clinical manifestations vary depending on degree of involved bowel.

1. Newborn—symptoms appearing at birth or within first weeks of life.
   a. No meconium passed in the first 48 hours of life.
   b. Vomiting—bile-stained or fecal
   c. Abdominal distention
   d. Constipation—occurs in 100% of patients
   e. Overflow-type diarrhea
   f. Dehydration; failure to thrive
   g. Temporary relief of symptoms with enema
2. Older child—symptoms not prominent at birth. Short segment disease commonly presents later.
   a. History of obstipation at birth
   b. Progressive abdominal distention
   c. Peristaltic activity observable
   d. Absence of retentive posturing
   e. Constipation—unresponsive to conventional remedies
   f. Absence of encopresis (common feature of functional constipation)
   g. Ribbonlike, fluidlike, or pellet stools
   h. Failure to grow—loss of subcutaneous fat; appears malnourished, stunted growth
   i. Presentation insidious or catastrophic as with enterocolitis
3. Enterocolitis—consists of severe toxemia and a proliferation of bacteria in the colonic lumen.
   a. Abdominal distention
   b. Explosive diarrhea
   c. Vomiting
   d. Fever
   e. Lethargy
   f. Rectal bleeding
   g. Shock

Diagnostic Evaluation

1. Supportive findings on history and physical examination for Hirschsprung's disease.
2. Digital rectal examination—reveals an anal canal and a rectum that are narrow and empty of stool (in long segment disease). In short segment disease, rectal impaction may be present; removal of finger may be associated with a rush of stool as the obstruction is relieved.
3. Plain films—show severe gaseous distention of the bowel, with absence of air in the rectum.
4. Radiopaque markers, ingested, measure intestinal transit time. Children with short segment disease retain the markers in the rectum for long periods.
5. Barium enema—used to demonstrate a transition zone between the proximal dilated, normal innervated colon, and the distal, narrow, aganglionic colon.
   a. May be nondiagnostic in young infants who have not had sufficient time to develop a transition zone.
   b. Delayed passage of barium is suggestive, but not definitive for Hirschprung's disease.

6. Anorectal manometry—demonstrates failure of the intestinal sphincter to relax in response to transient rectal distention. Requires cooperation of the child.
7. Full thickness or suction rectal biopsy—absence or reduced number of ganglion nerve cells; definitive diagnosis.

Treatment

Definitive treatment is removal of the aganglionic, nonfunctioning, dilated segment of the bowel, followed by anastomosis, and improved functioning of internal rectal sphincter.

1. Initially, a colostomy or ileostomy is performed to decompress intestine, divert fecal stream, and rest the normal bowel.
2. Definitive surgery includes the following reconstructive procedures:
   a. Swenson—abdominoperineal pull-through
   b. Duhamel—retrorectal transanal pull-through
   c. Soave—endorectal pull-through
      (i) Procedure can be done laparoscopically.
      (ii) May be delayed until 9 to 12 months old or until child is 6. 8 to 9 kg (15 to 20 lb).
3. In older child when symptoms are chronic but not severe, treatment may consist of isotonic enemas, stool softeners, and low-residue diet.
4. Treatment of enterocolitis.
   a. Colonic irrigation with saline solution is initial emergency treatment.
   b. Surgical decompression colostomy.
   c. At least 1 month after, abdominal perineal pull-through.

Complications

1. Before primary surgery
   a. Enterocolitis—a major cause of death
   b. Hydroureter or hydronephrosis
   c. Water intoxication from tap water enemas
   d. Cecal perforation
2. Postoperative
   a. Enterocolitis, typically within 2 years of surgery
   b. Leaking of anastomosis and pelvic abscess
   c. Temporary sudden inability to evacuate colon
   d. Long-term: intestinal obstruction from adhesions, volvulus, intussusception
3. Postoperative—colostomy
   a. Abdominal distention
   b. Respiratory distress
   c. Infection
   d. Hemorrhage, shock

Nursing Assessment

1. Observe neonate for constipation.

NURSING ALERT

Diagnosis should be suspected in any infant who fails to pass meconium within the first 24 hours and requires repeated rectal stimulation to induce bowel movements.

2. Obtain parents' history, especially on infant's bowel and feeding habits.
   a. Onset of constipation
   b. Character of stools (ribbonlike or fluid-filled)
   c. Frequency of bowel movements
   d. Enemas needed
   e. Suppositories or laxatives needed
3. Observe for irritability, feeding difficulty, distended abdomen, and signs of malnutrition (pallor, muscle weakness, thin extremities, fatigue).

Nursing Diagnoses
Preoperative
- Ineffective Breathing Pattern related to abdominal distention
- Pain related to intestinal obstruction
- Altered Nutrition: Less Than Body Requirements related to poor intake
- Constipation due to pathophysiologic process

Postoperative
- Risk for Injury related to postoperative course
- Risk for Infection of Surgical Incision
- Risk for Injury related to decreased peristalsis postoperatively
- Ineffective Family Coping related to care of child with colostomy

Nursing Interventions
Preoperative
Improving Breathing Pattern
1. Monitor for respiratory embarrassment that may result from abdominal distention; watch for rapid, shallow respirations; cyanosis; sternal retractions.
2. Elevate head and chest of infant by tilting mattress.
3. Administer oxygen as ordered to support respiratory status.

Relieving Pain
1. Note degree of abdominal tenderness.
   a. Legs of infant drawn up
   b. Chest breathing
2. Note color of abdomen and presence of gastric waves; take sequential measurements of abdominal girth for evidence of changes.
3. Assist in emptying the bowel by giving repeated enemas and colonic irrigations.
   a. Procedure for enema in an infant is similar to that in an adult, except that less fluid and pressure are used.
   b. Physiologic saline solution (warmed) should be used for irrigations. Tap water may result in large quantities of water being absorbed and in water intoxication.
4. Administer medications (antibiotics) to reduce the bacterial flora of the bowel.
5. Note any change in degree of distention before and after irrigation. Record if location of distention changes (ie, upper or lower abdomen).

6. Record all intake and output of irrigant and drainage. Report marked discrepancies in retention or loss of fluid.
7. Insert rectal tube for escape of accumulated fluid and gas as ordered.
8. If abdominal distention is not relieved by enemas and discomfort is significant, insert a nasogastric tube as ordered.
   a. Note drainage from nasogastric tube, and chart characteristics.
   b. Check for patency; saline irrigations may be requested. Carefully record intake and output.
   c. Give frequent mouth care.
   d. Alternate nares when changing nasogastric tube every 24 hours, and use minimal amount of tape to prevent skin irritation.
9. Offer pacifier for non-nutritive sucking if on parenteral fluids.
10. Encourage parents to hold and rock infant.
11. Maintain position of comfort with head elevated. Offer soothing stimulation (eg, music, touch, play therapy).

Providing Adequate Nutrition
1. Obtain a dietary history regarding food and eating habits.
   a. This will contribute to planning dietary alterations.
   b. Explain to parents that eating problems are common with Hirschsprung's disease.
2. Monitor IV fluids appropriately. Measure all output.
3. Offer small, frequent feedings. (Low-residue diet will aid in keeping stools soft.)
   a. Feed child slowly.
   b. Provide as comfortable a position as possible for child during feedings.
4. Inform parents that defect can be corrected, but it may take some time for their child's physical status and feeding habits to improve.
   a. Feeding may cause additional discomfort because of distention and nausea.
   b. Parenteral nutrition may be necessary.

Controlling Constipation in the Older Child
1. Be aware that older children who present with milder forms of the disorder may be treated medically (rare).
2. Note and record frequency and characteristics of stools (constipation is likely to occur).
3. Provide demonstration and written and verbal instructions to family for saline enema administration and use of stool softeners.
4. Obtain dietary consultation for teaching of low-residue diet.

Postoperative
Preventing Complications
1. Monitor vital signs and respiratory status closely.

NURSING ALERT

 Prevent injury to rectal mucosa by taking axillary or external ear temperature.

2. Monitor for proper functioning of colostomy, if present.
   a. Note drainage from colostomy: characteristics, frequency, fecal material, or liquid drainage.
   b. Note abdominal distension.
   c. Measure fluid loss from colostomy because the amount will affect fluid replacement.
3. Report signs of obstruction from peritonitis, paralytic ileus, handling bowel, or swelling.
   a. No output from colostomy
   b. Increased tenderness
   c. Irritability
   d. Vomiting
   e. Increased temperature
4. Place child in a lateral position on a flat or only slightly elevated bed. When head of bed is elevated, the residual CO_2 in the child's abdominal cavity causes referred pain in neck and shoulder.
5. Differentiate type and cause of pain to determine appropriate pain management interventions. Proper positioning, patent catheters and tubes, and timely administration of analgesics are key to ensuring patient comfort.
6. "Nothing per rectum" sign should be placed at head of bed so no rectal temperatures, rectal medications, or digital rectal examinations are done.

Preventing Wound Infection

1. Change wound dressing using sterile technique. If done laparoscopically, wound is minimal.
2. Prevent contamination from diaper.
   a. Apply diaper below dressing.
   b. Change diaper frequently.
3. Prevent perianal and anal excoriation by thorough cleansing sitz baths and application of oxide paste and karaya after soiling.
4. Use careful handwashing technique.
5. Report any wound redness, swelling or drainage, evisceration, or dehiscence immediately.
6. Suction secretions frequently to prevent infection of the tracheobronchial tree and lungs.
7. Encourage frequent coughing and deep breathing to maintain respiratory status.
8. Allow the infant to cry for short periods to prevent atelectasis.
9. Change infant's position frequently to increase circulation and allow for aeration of all lung areas.

Preventing Abdominal Distention

1. Maintain patency of nasogastric tube immediately postoperatively.
   a. Watch for increasing abdominal distention; measure abdominal girth.
   b. Measure fluid loss because amount will affect fluid replacement .
2. Maintain NPO status until bowel sounds return and the bowel is ready for feedings as determined by provider.
3. Administer fluids to maintain hydration and replace lost electrolytes.
4. Provide frequent oral hygiene while NPO.

5. Begin oral feedings as ordered.
   a. Avoid overfeeding.
   b. Bubble frequently during feeding.
   c. Turn head to side or elevate after feeding to prevent aspiration.

Supporting the Parents

1. Acknowledge that even a temporary colostomy can be a difficult procedure to accept and learn to manage.
   a. Initiate ostomy referral.
   b. Support the parents when teaching them to care for the colostomy.
   c. Include them soon after surgery in dressing changes and any other appropriate activities.
   d. Assist and encourage them to treat the baby or child as normally as possible.
   e. Reassure parents that colostomy will not cause delay in the child's normal development.
2. Encourage the parents to talk about their fears and anxieties. Anticipating future surgery for resection may be confusing and frightening.
3. Initiate community-nurse referral to help the parents care for the child at home away from the comforting situation of the hospital, and obtain necessary equipment.
4. Initiate a genetic counseling referral, especially if parents plan to have more children.

Ostomy Care in Children

Care of the colostomy and ileostomy in the infant and young child is based on the same principles and is essentially the same as that for an adult (see Chapter 18), with the following exceptions:

1. Colostomy irrigation is not part of management in small children. Irrigation is primarily for the purpose of regulating the colostomy to empty at regular intervals. Because children have bowel movements at more frequent intervals, this type of control is not feasible. Irrigation should be done only in preparation for tests or surgery and occasionally for the treatment of constipation.
2. Dehydration occurs quickly in the infant or small child; therefore, it is particularly important to observe drainage for amount and characteristics. Drainage should be measured to provide an accurate basis for computation of fluid replacement.
3. Prevention and treatment of skin excoriation around the stoma is of primary concern. With the advent of better skin shields and equipment designed especially for the pediatric patient, keeping an ostomy appliance in place is now less difficult. Through careful application and trying different types of pouches until a proper fit is obtained, most children can be kept clean and dry for at least 24 hours between changes. This is a significant factor in preventing skin breakdown and subsequent infections in the peristomal area. Remember, however, that infant dressings must be checked frequently.
   a. Check ostomy bag for leakage every 2 hours, and change bag as soon as leakage is suspected.

b. Teach the parents the importance of emptying the bag when it is ¼ to ⅓ full.

c. Skin breakdown is more frequent. Reinforce to parents to treat breakdown with method and products recommended by ostomy nurse.

d. Be aware that infant elimination is more frequent than in the older child.

4. For older children with ostomies:

a. "Potty training" can be achieved for ostomy pouch emptying.

b. Pouching optimizes socialization and developmental activities.

c. Encourage a matter-of-fact and accepting attitude to help build child's self-confidence. Encourage the child to participate in ostomy care.

d. Encourage child to join age-appropriate ostomy support group.

5. Refer families for additional help and information to the United Ostomy Association, 800-826-0826, *www.uao.org.*

6. For ostomy supplies, refer families to the following:

Able Medical Aids
1280 N. Missouri Ave.
Largo, FL 33770
800-831-9099
www.ablemedical.com/ostomy.html

C. R. Bard Inc.
713 Central Avenue
Murray Hill, NJ 07974
908-277-8000
www.crbard.com

Hollister, Inc.
2000 Hollister Dr.
Libertyville, IL 60048
800-323-4060
www.hollister.com

Community and Home Care Considerations

1. Begin early teaching about the colostomy (preoperatively, before discharge, and at home) including how it works, and how to care for it and the child. Explanations should be thorough and in accordance with family readiness. Encourage care of the ostomy as part of normal activities of daily living.

2. Arrange frequent home visits to carry out comprehensive teaching plan. Consult with ostomy nurse as needed for any skin breakdown or other ostomy problems.

3. Involve the entire family in teaching colostomy care to enhance acceptance of body change of the child. An older child should become totally responsible for own colostomy care.

4. Assess family's self-care of the ostomy including procedures such as preparation of skin, application of collecting appliance, care of appliance, and control of odor.

5. Observe for and teach family about signs of stomal complications include ribbonlike stool, diarrhea, failure of evacuation of stool or flatus, and bleeding.

6. If ordered, practice and teach dilatation of stoma with finger or soft rubber rectal tube.

7. Assess hydration status, and teach increased fluid intake because colon absorption is decreased.

8. Review gastrostomy feeding techniques if ordered.

9. Assist family to discuss the child's needs with day care workers, teachers, and school nurse as applicable. Review care of ostomy with child's care providers.

10. Assist with preoperative preparation for colostomy closure when the time comes.

Family Education and Health Maintenance

1. Instruct the parents to serve small, frequent meals to the child and be alert for and eliminate foods that cause gas and diarrhea, such as cabbage, spicy foods, beans, Brussels sprouts, fruits, and fruit juices.

2. Advise parents that colds or viruses may cause loose stools, which increases risk of dehydration, especially in long segment disease, so to increase fluids.

3. Alert parents of common postoperative problems including bacterial overgrowth, colitis or enterocolitis, and lactose intolerance. Therefore, parents need to contact their health care provider if persistent diarrhea, abdominal distention, abdominal pain, or constipation occurs.

4. Encourage parents to practice all procedures long before the infant is to be discharged.

5. Emphasize the importance of treating the child as normally as possible to prevent behavior problems later.

6. Teach the basics of good nutrition and diet. Involve the dietitian as necessary.

7. Encourage close medical follow-up and general good health and hygiene.
a. Safety
b. General growth and development
c. Immunizations

8. Advise older children without colostomies that fecal staining may occur, but this will improve with time.

9. For additional information and support, refer to American Pseudo-Obstruction and Hirschsprung's Disease Society, 158 Pleasant Street, North Andover, MA 01845, 978-685-4477; *www.tiac.net/users/aphs.*

Outcome-Based Evaluation

- Respiratory rate normal for age and unlabored; no cyanosis
- Abdominal girth decreased; resting comfortably
- Tolerating 1- to 2-oz feedings every hour
- Having stool every 2 days spontaneously or after enema
- Vital signs within normal limits, afebrile, no abdominal distention
- Wound pink without drainage, redness, warmth, and tenderness
- Bowel sounds present, nasogastric tube discontinued
- Parents listening and asking questions about care of child

Intussusception

Intussusception is the invagination or telescoping of a portion of the intestine into an adjacent, more distal section of the intestine. It is the most common cause of bowel obstruction in the first year of life and most commonly occurs in the 6- to 18-month age range. It is twice as common in male infants as in female infants. Incidence in the United States is 2.4 cases per 1,000 births.

Pathophysiology and Etiology

1. Cause usually unknown.
2. May be due to increased mobility of intestine and hyperperistalsis present in young children especially during viral illness.
3. Possible contributing causes in older child include:
   a. Meckel's diverticulum
   b. Polyps, cysts in the bowel
   c. Malrotation of intestines
   d. Acute enteritis
   e. Abdominal injury
   f. Abdominal surgery; intestinal intubation
   g. Cystic fibrosis
   h. Celiac disease
4. Lymphoid hyperplasia (Peyer's patches) act as lead point of the proximal intussusception segment.
5. Mesentery pulled into intestine when invagination occurs.
6. Progression to obstruction.
   a. Intestine becomes curved, sausagelike; blood supply is cut off.
   b. Bowel begins to swell; hemorrhage may occur.
   c. Complete intestinal obstruction results; necrosis of involved segment occurs.
7. Classification of location:
   a. Ileocecal (most common): ileum invaginates into ascending colon.
   b. Ileocolic: ileum invaginates into colon.
   c. Colocolic: colon invaginates into colon.
   d. Ileo-ileo (enteroenteric): small bowel invaginates into small bowel.

Clinical Manifestations

1. Paroxysmal abdominal pain:
   a. "Attacks of pain" that awake child from sleep; inconsolable.
   b. Cyclic repetition of symptoms at approximately 5- to 30-minute intervals.
   c. Between episodes, child may act normal.
2. Currant jelly–like stools:
   a. Blood and mucus present in stool.
   b. Controversy exists whether use of this term is counterproductive; any gross blood in the stool should raise suspicion of intussusception.
3. Vomiting—eventually becomes bilious.
4. Bowel sounds are diminished, absent, or high pitched.
5. Increasing absence of stool.
6. Increasing abdominal distention and tenderness.
7. Sausage-like mass palpable in abdomen. Pathognomonic is Dance's sign—elongated mass in the right upper quadrant of the abdomen with absence of bowel sounds in the right lower quadrant.

8. Unusual-looking anus; may look like rectal prolapse.
9. Dehydration, fever, lethargy; shocklike state with rapid pulse, pallor, marked sweating.

Diagnostic Evaluation

1. X-ray examination.
   a. Flat plate of abdomen reveals staircase pattern. (Invagination appears like stair steps on x-ray—"coiled spring.")
   b. Barium enema under fluoroscopy shows coil-like appearance of bowel.
   c. Air enema—also exhibits "coiled spring" appearance; exposes patient to less fluoroscopic radiation.

> **NURSING ALERT**
>
> Enemas are contraindicated in cases involving clinical findings of peritonitis, shock, or signs of perforation on abdominal radiograph.

2. Ultrasonogram to locate area of telescoped bowel.
3. Color Doppler sonography used more recently to determine whether reducible or not. Absence of blood flow (color) indicates ischemia, and, therefore, enema reduction should be avoided.

Treatment

1. Pneumatic reduction or telescoped bowel with air enema recommended treatment during first 24 hours after onset and may reduce intussusception in 94% of patients.
2. Hydrostatic reduction of telescoped bowel with barium enema may reduce intussusception in 78% of patients and carries a lower safety profile than air enemas, especially with perforation.
3. Surgical reduction of intussusception may be necessary when radiologic reduction is unsuccessful, a pathologic lead point or peritonitis is suspected, or with multiple recurrence.
4. Surgery involves a laparotomy, manual milking out of the intussuscepted segment, followed by resection of the nonviable bowel.

Complications

1. Perforation
2. Peritonitis

Nursing Assessment

1. Obtain careful history of infant's or child's physical and behavioral symptoms, including any recent or chronic illness.

> **NURSING ALERT**
>
> Report of episodic, severe, colicky abdominal pain combined with vomiting suggests intussusception.

2. Perform physical examination, which may reveal a well-developed, well-nourished, afebrile infant with abdominal tenderness and distention.
3. Observe for dehydration, may be mild or severe.

    Assess capillary refill, mental status, urinary output, because these are reliable indicators of shock in children.

Nursing Diagnoses
Preoperative
- Pain related to paroxysmal abdominal pain, fever, and treatments
- Risk for Fluid Volume Deficit related to vomiting
- Ineffective Breathing Pattern related to abdominal distention
- Anxiety related to hospitalization, knowledge deficit of illness, surgery, and treatments

Postoperative
- Risk for Injury related to postoperative course

Nursing Interventions
Preoperative
Minimizing Pain
1. Observe behavior as indicator of pain; the infant may be irritable and very sensitive to handling or lethargic or unresponsive. Handle very gently.
2. Encourage family to participate in comfort measures. Explain cause of pain, and reassure parents as to purpose of diagnostic tests and treatments.
3. Administer medications as prescribed.

Maintaining Fluid and Electrolyte Balance
1. Monitor fluids, and maintain NPO status.
2. Restrain infant as necessary for IV therapy.
3. Monitor intake and output.

Promoting Effective Breathing
1. Be alert for respiratory distress because of abdominal distention. Watch for grunting or shallow and rapid respirations if in shocklike state.
2. Insert nasogastric tube if ordered to decompress stomach.
    a. Irrigate at frequent intervals.
    b. Note drainage and return from irrigation.
3. Maintain NPO status as ordered.
    a. Wet lips, and give mouth care.
    b. Give infant pacifier to suck.
4. Continually reassess condition because increased pain and bloody stools may indicate perforation.

> ### NURSING ALERT
> **Passage of one normal brown stool may occur, clearing the colon distal to the intussusception. Passage of more than one normal brown stool may indicate that the intussusception has reduced itself. Report any stools immediately to the provider.**

Preparing for Surgery
1. Offer support to the parents during time of crisis and fear.
2. Offer specific teaching to parents

    a. Compare intussusception to a collapsible telescope or antenna or by drawing a picture.
    b. Visual aids, such as a rubber glove with one finger into itself, may be helpful. Reduction can be demonstrated by filling glove with water until inverted finger resumes its normal position.
3. Children need brief, simple explanations in age-appropriate language.

Postoperative
Preventing Postoperative Complications
1. Monitor vital signs and general condition, notify health care provider of any change or unexpected trend.
2. Assess temperature and administer antipyretics and other cooling measures. Fever is usually present from absorption of bacteria through the damaged intestinal wall.
3. Assess for abdominal tenderness, bowel sounds, and distention of abdomen. Maintain nasogastric suction as ordered.
4. Assess pain and level of consciousness.
5. When able to take fluids, assess tolerance carefully and advance intake slowly.

Family Education and Health Maintenance
1. Explain that recurrences are rare and usually occur within 36 hours after reduction. Review signs and symptoms with parents.
2. Review activity restrictions with parents (eg, positioning on back or side, quiet play, and avoidance of water sports until wound heals).
3. Encourage follow-up care.
4. Provide anticipatory guidance for developmental age of child.
5. Encourage awareness of symptoms that require prompt medical attention among day care centers and other child care providers (eg, paroxysmal abdominal pain, blood or mucus in stool).

Outcome-Based Evaluation
- Less irritable, dozing
- Urine output adequate
- Respirations unlabored; abdominal distention relieved
- Parents verbalize understanding of condition and surgery
- Postoperative vital signs stable; audible bowel sounds; passes stool on 4th postoperative day; abdominal distention relieved

Imperforate Anus (Anorectal Malformations)

The term *imperforate anus* is used to describe all congenital abnormalities of the anorectal canal or in the location of the anus within the perineum. Incidence is 1 in 4,000 to 1 in 5,000 live births with a slight male predominance.

Pathophysiology and Etiology

1. An arrest in embryologic development of the anus, lower rectum, and urogenital tract at the 8th week of embryonic life; however, cause is unknown.
2. Approximately 40% of infants with anorectal malformations have associated major anomalies including:
   a. Down syndrome
   b. Congenital heart disease
   c. Renal abnormalities
   d. Cryptorchidism
   e. Esophageal atresia
   f. Malformation of the spine
3. Abnormal development of the terminal hindgut ranges from mild anal stenosis, corrected by simple dilatation, to complex deformities, such as rectal atresia and fistula.
4. Defect is classified as high or low depending on where the normal caliber bowel ends.
   a. Ninety percent of children with low anal anomaly achieve bowel continence.
   b. Thirty percent of high anomalies or anomalies associated with genitourinary fistula achieve continence.

Types (Figure 48-3)

1. Anal stenosis:
   a. Anal opening is very small.
   b. Defecation is difficult.
   c. Stools may be ribbon-like.
   d. This accounts for 10% of anomalies.
2. Imperforate anal membrane:
   a. Infant fails to pass meconium.
   b. Greenish, bulging membrane is seen.
   c. Bowel and sphincter return to normal after excision.
3. Anal agenesis:
   a. Anal dimple is present.
   b. Stimulation of the perianal area leads to puckering (indicative of external sphincter).
   c. Intestinal obstruction occurs if no associated fistula.
   d. Fistulas may be perineal or vulvar in the female and perineal or urethral in male.
4. Rectal agenesis:
   a. Fistulas are usually present.
   b. Fistulas in male may communicate with posterior urethra; in females, fistula ends high in vagina.
   c. Associated major congenital malformations are common.
   d. Accounts for 75% of anomalies.
5. Rectoperineal fistula:
   a. Small orifice located in the perineum.
   b. Anterior to the center of the external sphincter.
   c. Close to scrotum in the male or vulva in the female.
6. Rectovaginal fistula—rectum communicates with the vagina.

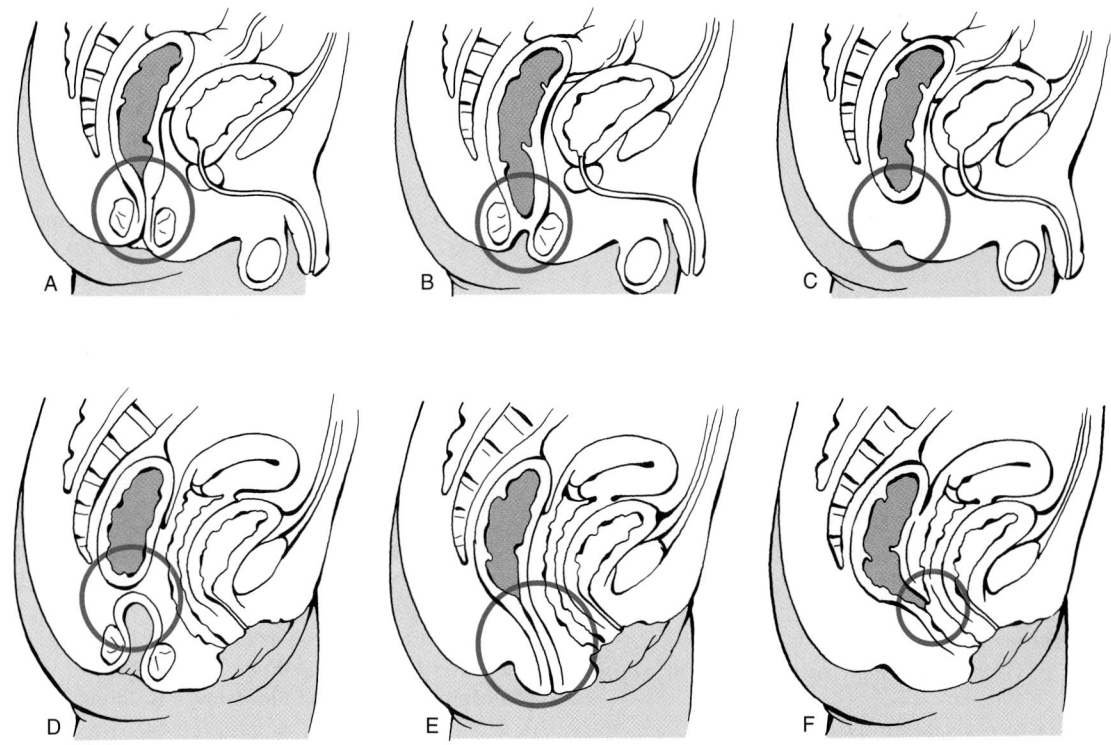

FIGURE 48-3 Anorectal malformations. (**A**) Anal stenosis. (**B**) Imperforate anal membrane. (**C**) Anal agenesis. (**D**) Rectal agenesis. (**E**) Rectoperineal fistula. (**F**) Small orifice located in the perineum. (Adapted with permission from Wong D.L. [1995]. *Whaley and Wong's nursing care of infants and children* [5th ed.]. St. Louis: Mosby.)

Clinical Manifestations

Condition is usually discovered immediately after birth or within several hours.

1. Absence of anal opening.
2. Misplaced anal opening.
3. Anal opening near vaginal opening in female.
4. Thermometer, small finger, or rectal tube cannot be inserted into the rectum.
5. Meconium stool is absent.
6. Stool passed by way of the vagina or urethra may appear as green-tinged urine.
7. Progressive abdominal distention.
8. Fistula is likely to be present.
9. Vomiting if infant is fed.

Diagnostic Evaluation

1. Urine examination for presence of meconium and epithelial debris indicates presence of fistula.
2. Voiding cystourethrogram shows abnormality.
3. Wangensteen-Rice x-ray (upside-down position):
   a. Limited accuracy in locating rectal pouch
   b. Useful only after infant is 24 hours of age
4. Sonography locates rectal pouch.

Treatment

1. Low—female:
   a. Decompression of bowel with catheter irrigations
   b. Dilatation of fistula for 8 to 12 months thereafter
   c. Definitive repair
2. Low—male:
   a. Rectal cutback anoplasty or Y-V plasty
   b. Local dilatation of fistula
3. High—male:
   a. Colostomy for decompression
   b. Definitive pull-through surgery; deferred until about 1 year of age or when child attains 6.75 to 9 kg (15 to 20 lb)
4. High—female:
   a. Colostomy
   b. Definitive repair done when infant is 1 year of age or 6.75 to 9 kg (15 to 20 lb)

Complications

1. Infection
2. Intestinal obstruction
3. Loss of sphincter control

Nursing Assessment

1. Perform physical assessment of newborn for abnormalities.
   a. Presence of perineal fistula
   b. Meconium coming from vagina or presence of meconium-stained urine
   c. No anal opening or inability to pass thermometer into rectum

2. Perform thorough examination for other congenital anomalies.

 NURSING ALERT

A newborn who does not pass a stool in the first 24 hours after birth requires further assessment.

3. Assess parents' level of understanding of condition and ability to cope with infant's surgery.

Nursing Diagnoses

Preoperative
• Risk for Injury of infant with anomalies before surgery

Postoperative
• Risk for Infection related to surgical incision of anoplasty
• Risk for Impaired Skin Integrity related to ostomy
• Risk for Fluid Volume Deficit related to restricted intake
• Family Coping: Potential for Growth related to increased needs of infant
• Risk for Injury after definitive repair surgery

Nursing Interventions

Preoperative
Maintaining Stability Before Surgery
1. Withhold feedings. Note any vomiting: color and amount.
2. Minimize energy expenditure due to altered nutritional status.
3. Maintain nasogastric tube passed to decompress the stomach. Measure abdominal girth.
4. Observe the patient carefully for any signs of distress, and report. Check vital signs frequently.
5. Use an Isolette or radiant warmer to maintain temperature stability.
6. Minimal handling; cluster procedures together to encourage rest and sleep.
7. Keep fistula area clean.
8. Administer good oral care.

Postoperative
Preventing Infection of Suture Line
1. After anoplasty, do not put anything in rectum.
2. Expose perineum to air.
3. Position the infant for easy access to perineum for cleansing and minimal irritation to site (ie, place the infant on abdomen, possibly with hips elevated, to prevent pressure on perineal surfaces; turn side-to-side).
4. Observe for redness, drainage, poor healing.

Preventing Skin Breakdown (see p. 267)
Maintaining Fluid and Electrolyte Balance
1. Start oral feedings as ordered (usually within hours after an anoplasty).
2. Monitor for return of peristalsis. When primary repair is done, nasogastric suction may be maintained until feedings are started.

3. Monitor parenteral fluids, and discontinue when oral intake is sustained.
4. Report any vomiting or stooling.

Strengthening Coping

1. Ensure the parents that colostomy is temporary.
2. Encourage the parents to participate in care of the child and to provide emotional security for the child.
3. Provide thorough teaching program for special care needed at home.
   a. Colostomy care
   b. Anal dilatation to prevent a stricture at site of anastomosis from scar tissue (after instructions by health care provider)
4. Initiate referral to community nurse, especially if the parents are particularly anxious about caring for the child at home.
5. Encourage the parents to talk about their concerns.
6. Enlist help of enterostomal therapy, enterostomal therapy nurse, or provide support for anticipated home care needs.
7. If mother prefers to breast-feed, encourage frequent pumping to establish milk supply.

Providing Appropriate Care for Definitive Pull-Through Surgery

1. Carry out perineal care as stated previously.
2. Provide proper care of gastrostomy or nasogastric tube used to decompress the GI tract until peristalsis returns.
3. Provide proper care of bladder catheter, if used, and measure urinary output accurately.
4. Observe carefully for abdominal distention, bleeding from perineum, and respiratory embarrassment.

Family Education and Health Maintenance

1. Review special care and procedures to be continued at home. Involve parents and other caregivers in teaching. Advise parents to make day care providers, teachers, and school nurse aware of child's needs.
2. Help the parents to understand situations that may be encountered as a result of imperforate anus as the baby gets older.
   a. Fecal impaction due to lack of sensation to defecate
   b. Future surgery if primary repair was not done
   c. Toilet training—may be delayed, especially after a pull-through procedure
   d. Inability to control fecal seepage from rectum
3. Provide some practical guidelines to help parents cope.
   a. Fecal control may not be achieved until age 10 years; however, about 80% of children achieve normal or socially acceptable continence.
   b. Encourage bowel habit training or patterning of defecation (eg, after breakfast).
   c. Promote diet modifications; teach foods that produce laxative effect (plums, prunes, chocolate, nuts, corn) and foods that have binding effect (peanut butter, hot cereal, cheese).

   d. Stool softeners and at other times antidiarrheal medications may be effective, especially Imodium.
   e. Rectal inertia may cause fecal impaction in rectosigmoid colon with soiling from fluid overflow. Bisacodyl suppository or cleansing enema provides assistance in management.
4. Antegrade continence enema procedures may allow for continence in children without anal sphincter function.
5. Encourage mutual support from other families who have a child with an anorectal malformation.
6. For additional information and support, refer the parents to National Organization for Rare Disorders, Inc., P.O. Box 8923, New Fairfield, CT 06812-8923, 203-746-6518.

Outcome-Based Evaluation

- Vital signs stable, abdominal girth stable
- No signs of infection of suture line
- Skin intact surrounding ostomy
- Bowel sounds present; oral feeding tolerated without vomiting
- Family discussing plans for home care with enterostomal therapist
- Bowel sounds present, nasogastric tube discontinued

SELECTED REFERENCES

Ault, D., & Schmidt, D. (1998). Diagnosis and management of gastroesophageal reflux in infants and children. *The Nurse Practitioner, 23*(6), 78–100.

Balasubrahmanyam, G., Scherer, N., Martin, J., & Michael, M. (1998). Cleft lip and palate: Keys to successful management. *Contemporary Pediatrics, 15*(11), 133–151.

Bomback, D. (1998). Intussusceptions current concepts. *Emergency and Office Pediatrics, 11*(4), 133–135.

Borkowski, B. (1994). Common pediatric surgical problems. *Nursing Clinics of North America, 29*(4), 551–562.

Chestnut, M. A. (1998). *Pediatric home care manual*. Philadelphia: Lippincott-Raven.

Cleft Palate Foundation. (1998). *Cleft lip and cleft palate: The first four years* (3rd ed.) [Brochure].

Edmondson, R., & Reinbartsen, D. (1998). The young child with cleft lip and cleft palate: Intervention needs in the first three years. *Infants and Young Children, 11*(2), 12–20.

Eliason, B., & Lewan, R. (1998). Gastroenteritis in children: Principles of diagnosis and treatment. *American Family Physician, 58*(8), 1769–1776.

George, C., Hammes, M., & Schwarz, D. (1995). Laparoscopic Swenson pull-through procedure for congenital megacolon. *AORN Journal, 62*(5), 727–736.

Henderson, D., Thomas, D., & Ladebauche, P. A. (1992). Intussusception in pediatric patients. *Journal of Emergency Nursing, 18*(3), 275–277.

Hill, I., Fasana, A., Schwartz, R., et al. (2000). The prevalence of celiac disease in at-risk groups of children in the United States. *Journal of Pediatrics, 136*, 86–90.

Hyman, P. (1994). *Pediatric gastrointestinal motility disorders*. New York, NY: Academy Professional Information Services.

Johnson, D. (1997). Gastroesophageal disease. Long-term management strategies. *Consultant, 37*(7), 1833–1844.

———. (1997). Gastroesophageal reflux disease: Short-term management strategies. *Consultant, 37*(5), 1329–1348.

Lifschitz, C. (1997). Treatment of acute diarrhea in children. *Current Opinion in Pediatrics, 9*(5), 498–501.

Mahan, K. L. & Escott-Stumps, S. (2000). *Krause's food, nutrition, and diet therapy* (10th ed.). Toronto: W.B. Saunders.

McCance, K., & Huether, S. (1998). *Pathophysiology: The biologic basis for disease in adults and children* (3rd ed.). New York: Mosby.

Nowicki, M., & Bishop, P. (1999). Organic causes of constipation in infants and children. *Pediatric Annals, 28*(5), 293–300.

Papadakis, K., Chen, E., Luks, F., Lessin, M., Wesselhoeft, C., & DeLuca, F. (1999). The changing presentation of pyloric stenosis. *American Journal of Emergency Medicine, 17*(1), 67–69.

Schwartz, R., & Abeggien, J. A. (1996). Failure to thrive: An ambulatory approach. *Nurse Practitioner, 21*(15), 19–35.

Siberry, G. K. & Iannone, R. (eds.). (2000). *The Harriet Lane handbook* (15th ed.). St. Louis: Mosby.

Stark, S. (1999). Living with celiac disease. *American Journal of Nursing, 99*(3), 24B–24D.

Straughn, A., & English, B. (1996). Oral rehydration therapy: A neglected treatment for pediatric diarrhea. *American Journal of Maternal Child Nursing, 21*(3), 144–147.

Trier, J. (1993). Diagnosis and treatment of celiac sprue. *Hospital Practice, 28*(4A), 41–48.

CHAPTER

49

Pediatric Renal and Genitourinary Disorders

ACUTE DISORDERS

■ Acute Glomerulonephritis

Acute glomerulonephritis is a broad term used to describe several disease processes that result in glomerular injury. The glomerular injury is the result of antigen-antibody deposits within the glomeruli. It occurs most frequently in school-aged children, is rare in children younger than 2 years of age, and occurs more frequently in boys than in girls (2:1).

Pathophysiology and Etiology

1. Presumed cause—antigen-antibody reaction secondary to an infection elsewhere in the body.
2. The initial infection is usually either an upper respiratory infection or a skin infection.
3. Most frequent causative agent—nephritogenic strains of group A β-hemolytic streptococcus.
4. It is speculated that the streptococcal infection is followed by the release of a membrane-like material from the organism into the circulation.
5. Antibodies produced to fight the invading organism also react against the glomerular tissue, thus forming immune complexes.
6. The immune complexes become trapped in the glomerular loop and cause an inflammatory reaction in the affected glomeruli.
7. Changes in the glomerular capillaries reduce the amount of the glomerular filtrate, allow passage of blood cells and protein into the filtrate, and reduce the amount of sodium and water that is passed to the tubules for reabsorption.
8. General vascular disturbances, including loss of capillary integrity and spasm of arterioles, are secondary.

Clinical Manifestations

Onset
1. Usually 7–21 days after acute pharyngitis. In streptococcal skin infections, the latency period may be as long as 6 weeks.
2. May be abrupt and severe, or mild and detected only by laboratory measures.

Signs and Symptoms
1. Urinary symptoms:
   a. Decreased urine output
   b. Bloody or brown-colored urine
2. Edema
   a. Present in most patients
   b. Usually mild
   c. Often manifested by periorbital edema in the morning
   d. May appear only as rapid weight gain
   e. May be generalized and influenced by posture
3. Hypertension
   a. Present in more than 50% of patients
   b. Usually mild
   c. Rise in blood pressure may be sudden
   d. Usually appears during the first 4 to 5 days of the illness
4. Malaise
5. Mild headache
6. Gastrointestinal disturbances, especially anorexia and vomiting

Diagnostic Evaluation

1. Urinalysis:
   a. Decreased output—may approach anuria
   b. Microscopic or gross hematuria
   c. Specific gravity—moderately elevated
   d. Proteinuria may be mild to severe
   e. Microscopic—red blood cells, leukocytes, epithelial cells, and casts

2. Serum complement level—usually reduced.
3. Blood urea nitrogen (BUN) and creatinine—often mildly to moderately elevated; normal in 50% of the patients.
4. Antistreptolysin-O (ASO) titer—elevated.
5. DNAase B antigen titer—elevated.
6. Erythrocyte sedimentation rate (ESR)—elevated.
7. Complement C3—depressed.
8. Chest x-ray—may show pulmonary congestion, cardiac enlargement during the edematous phase.

Management

1. Antibiotic therapy if any concern that streptococci are still present.
2. Other management is mostly symptomatic; in most patients, spontaneous recovery is expected. Hospitalization is usually not necessary.
3. Salt and fluid intake should be restricted during the acute phase of the disease.
4. Diuretics should be administered if significant edema or hypertension develops.
5. A renal biopsy may be indicated if the child does not recover from apparent acute poststreptococcal glomerulonephritis.

Complications

(Occur infrequently)
1. Hypertensive encephalopathy
2. Congestive heart failure
3. Uremia
4. Anemia

Nursing Assessment

1. Obtain history regarding recent streptococcal infection.
2. Obtain appropriate culture(s) and assess for current infection.
3. Measure urine output and degree of hematuria and proteinuria.
4. Weigh child and document areas and extent of edema.
5. Obtain baseline blood pressure reading to assess for hypertension.

Nursing Diagnoses

- Altered Urinary Elimination related to glomerular dysfunction
- Fluid Volume Excess related to impaired renal function
- Diversional Activity Deficit related to focus on fluid restriction
- Knowledge Deficit regarding acute glomerulonephritis and its management

Nursing Interventions

Promoting Normal Urinary Pattern

1. Monitor daily intake and output.
2. Test and record urine for hematuria and proteinuria as ordered. Note color of urine.
3. Monitor daily weights.

Reducing Excess Fluid Volume

1. Provide a no-added-salt diet during the acute phase of the illness. Other restrictions may be indicated if renal function is impaired. Protein intake is not usually restricted because of the possible risk of malnutrition.
2. Restrict fluids in children with hypertension, edema, congestive failure, or renal failure.
3. Place a sign that indicates dietary restrictions on the child's bed, so that staff and visitors will be aware of special needs.
4. With fluid restrictions, offer small amounts of fluids spaced at regular intervals throughout the day and evening. Use an appropriate size of cup for the amount of fluid being offered.
5. Check blood pressure as ordered or needed and observe for signs of hypertension. Administer antihypertensive drugs as ordered by health care provider.

Promoting Diversional Activity

1. Explain fluid restriction at an age-appropriate level and direct the child's focus away from restrictions.
2. Provide the child with diversional activity/play therapy.
3. Encourage activity as tolerated.

Providing Information

1. Explain all aspects of the diagnostic tests and treatment in terms the family can understand.
2. Explain the purpose of all medications and the restricted diet, including a review of high-sodium foods to avoid and sample menus.
3. Encourage family participation in the child's care.
4. Help the family plan for adaptation of the child's nursing care to the home environment.
5. Arrange for appointments for continued medical supervision and initiate referrals when appropriate.

Family Education and Health Maintenance

1. Reinforce medical explanation of the disease process.
   a. Emphasize the need for medical evaluation and culture of all sore throats for all family members.
   b. Alert the family to signs and symptoms of disease recurrence.
2. Reinforce activity recommendation; usually not restricted.
3. Advise that tonsillectomy or other oral surgery is not recommended for several months after the acute phase of glomerulonephritis.
   a. If this type of surgery is necessary, penicillin may be recommended before and after the procedure to prevent bacterial infection.
   b. Obtain information regarding drug allergies before administering penicillin.

Outcome-Based Evaluation

- Output remains adequate
- Weight remains stable
- Child can do age-appropriate activities as tolerated and does not complain of thirst
- Parents and child can state rationale for treatment

Nephrotic Syndrome

Nephrotic syndrome is characterized by heavy proteinuria, hypoalbuminemia, and edema with hyperlipidemia. The syndrome can be subdivided into congenital, primary (idiopathic), and secondary types. Approximately 80% to 90% of primary cases in children are minimal change nephrotic syndrome (MCNS) and are associated with minimal histologic change in the glomeruli. Nephrotic syndrome annually afflicts approximately 2 to 7 children per 100,000 younger than the age of 16 years in the United States; it is slightly more frequent in Asian children and in girls than in boys. Mean age at onset is 2.5 years of age.

Pathophysiology and Etiology

Primary (idiopathic, minimal change, childhood) nephrotic syndrome

1. Underlying defect is thought to be caused by the loss of charge selectivity of the glomerular basement membrane (GBM), which permits negatively charged proteins, primarily albumin, to pass easily through the capillary walls into the urine.
2. Excessive urinary loss of protein and catabolization by the kidney of circulating albumin leads to a decrease in serum protein (hypoalbuminemia).
3. The colloidal osmotic pressure that holds water in the vascular compartments is reduced because of the decrease in the amount of serum albumin. This allows fluid to flow from the capillaries into the interstitial spaces, thus producing edema.
4. The shift of fluid from the plasma to the interstitial spaces reduces the vascular fluid volume (hypovolemia), which in turn stimulates the renin-angiotensin system and the secretion of antidiuretic hormone and aldosterone.
5. Tubular reabsorption of sodium and water is increased to increase intravascular volume.
6. The loss of proteins, particularly immunoglobulins, predisposes the child to infection.

Clinical Manifestations

1. Onset is insidious—thought to be caused by immune system disturbances, because it often occurs after a mild upper respiratory infection.
2. Edema is often the presenting symptom.
   a. Edema may be minimal or massive.
   b. Edema is usually first apparent around the eyes.
   c. Dependent edema occurs in areas of the body, such as the hands, ankles, feet, and genitalia.
   d. Fluid that accumulates in the body spaces may give rise to ascites and/or pleural effusions.
   e. Striae may appear on the skin from overstretching.
3. Profound weight gain caused by edema; the child may actually double normal weight.
4. Decreased urine output during the edematous phase—urine appears concentrated and frothy.
5. Pallor, irritability, lethargy, and fatigue.
6. Gastrointestinal disturbances, including vomiting, diarrhea, and/or anorexia caused by edema of intestinal mucosa.

Diagnostic Evaluation

1. Urinalysis:
   a. Protein—2+ or greater
   b. Blood—absent or transient
2. 24-hour urine protein—frequently greater than 2 g/m^2 per day.
3. Blood:
   a. Total protein—reduced
   b. Albumin—less than 2 g/dL
   c. Cholesterol—greater than 200 mg/dL with edema
4. Renal biopsy is indicated if patient is steroid resistant (has failed to achieve remission after 28 days of steroid therapy).

Management
Steroid Therapy

Preferred approach to treatment.

1. Prednisone is usually the drug of choice because it is less likely to induce salt retention and potassium loss and is the least expensive.
2. No standard program of therapy exists, but most children receive 60 mg/m^2 per day for induction of remission.
   a. The steroid dosage may also be calculated on ideal body weight with an equivalent dose being 2 mg/kg per day.
   b. Practice varies; however, the maximum steroid dosage is up to 80 mg/day for 4 weeks.
3. After daily steroid therapy, the prednisone should be discontinued slowly to avoid complications of steroid withdrawal, particularly benign intracranial hypertension.

   Practice varies; however, most centers recommend tapering using alternate-day prednisone over 6–8 weeks.
4. Children with nephrotic syndrome may respond to steroid therapy in several ways:
   a. Steroid sensitive: achieving a remission within 28 days of the start of prednisone therapy for the initial presentation of nephrotic syndrome.
   b. Steroid dependent: two consecutive relapses, occurring during prednisone therapy, or within 14 days after its cessation.
   c. Steroid resistant: failure to achieve response in spite of 4 weeks of prednisone therapy at 60 mg/m^2 per day.
5. Children with steroid-responsive MCNS have a favorable long-term prognosis.

Alternative Drug Therapies

1. Should be considered when children relapse frequently (4–6 per year), become steroid resistant or steroid dependent, or demonstrate unacceptable side effects of steroid therapy (steroid toxicity). The decision to use alternative therapy in conjunction with steroids should be made by an experienced pediatric nephrologist.

a. Levamisole (Ergamisol)
b. Cyclophosphamide (Cytoxan, Neosar)
c. Cyclosporin A (Neoral, Sandimmune)

Intravenous (IV) Albumin 25%

1. To shift fluid from interstitial space into the vascular system.
2. This is only a temporary treatment to relieve edema but may be used in severe cases of edema that causes respiratory distress or severe discomfort due to edema.
3. Diuretic therapy is used in combination with IV albumin to help relieve edema. In cases of hypovolemia, diuretics may not be indicated.

Complications

1. Infections:
   a. Peritonitis, caused by *Streptococcus pneumoniae*
   b. Gram-negative septicemia
   c. Staphylococcal cellulitis
2. Thrombosis
3. Hyperlipidemia
4. Acute renal failure

Nursing Assessment

1. Obtain history of onset of illness and symptoms.
   a. Precipitating events
   b. Recent immunizations
   c. Recent upper respiratory tract infections
   d. Flulike symptoms
   e. Time of onset and location of edema
   f. Urinary pattern changes
2. Perform physical examination focusing on vital signs; auscultation of breath sounds to determine adventitious sounds; areas and extent of edema, especially periorbital region, extremities, genitalia, abdomen; and peripheral perfusion, including pulses, color, warmth of extremities.

Nursing Diagnoses

- Fluid Volume Excess related to fluid accumulation in tissues
- Risk for Infection related to urinary loss of proteins and/or chronic steroid use
- Altered Nutrition: Less Than Body Requirements related to loss of proteins through urine and anorexia
- Altered Family Processes related to childhood illness

Nursing Interventions
Relieving Excess Fluid

1. Administer corticosteroids as recommended by the health care provider.
   a. Observe for side effects and complications of therapy, such as Cushing's syndrome—increased body hair (hirsutism), rounding of the face ("moon face"), abdominal distention, striae, increased appetite with weight gain, and aggravation of adolescent acne.

b. Stress that these physical changes are not harmful or permanent and that they will disappear after the steroid treatment is stopped.
c. Observe for serious side effects and uncommon complications of corticosteroids (see p. 814).

NURSING ALERT

No vaccinations or immunizations should be given during active episodes of nephrosis or while the child receives immunosuppressive therapy.

2. Administer immunosuppressive drugs as prescribed.
   a. Ensure that patient and parents understand the desired and side effects of therapy.
   b. Observe for complications of therapy, such as decreased white blood count, increased susceptibility to infection, hair loss, hemorrhagic cystitis.

DRUG ALERT

Administer cyclophosphamide in the morning, with large volumes of fluid, to prevent concentration of the drug in the urine and increased susceptibility to cystitis.

3. Administer diuretics as prescribed.
   a. Be aware of those diuretics that may cause potassium depletion.
   b. Offer foods high in potassium, such as orange juice, bananas, grapes, and milk.
   c. Administer supplemental potassium chloride as ordered and if the urine output is adequate.
4. Encourage activity as tolerated.
5. Restrict fluids as ordered (usually only during the extreme edematous phases).
   a. Restriction is carefully calculated at frequent intervals, based on the urine output of the previous day plus estimated insensible losses.
   b. Offer small amounts of fluids spaced at regular intervals throughout the day and evening. Use a cup of appropriate size for the amount of fluid being offered.
   c. Measure fluids accurately in graduated containers. Do not estimate fluid intake or output.
   d. Place a sign on the child's bed to ensure that no urine is accidentally discarded and that all intake is recorded.
   e. Determine total intake and output every 8 hours. In children who are not toilet trained, a fairly accurate record of output can be obtained by weighing diapers before and after voiding.
   f. Record other causes of fluid loss, such as the number of stools per day, perspiration, etc.
6. Assist with abdominal paracentesis; this may be required because of marked ascites. During the procedure, fluid is withdrawn from the peritoneal cavity to relieve pressure symptoms and respiratory distress.

Protecting the Child From Infection

1. Monitor complete blood count for decreased white cell count and neutropenia.
2. Closely observe the child who takes corticosteroids for signs of infection. Be aware that fever and other symptoms may be masked.
3. Provide meticulous skin care to the edematous areas of the body.
   a. Bathe the child frequently and apply powder. Areas of concern are moist parts of the body and edematous male genitalia. Support the scrotum with a cotton pad held in place by a T-binder, if necessary, for the child's comfort.
   b. Position the child so that edematous skin surfaces are not in contact. Place a pillow between the child's legs when lying on side, etc.
   c. Elevate the child's head to reduce edema.
4. If possible, avoid invasive procedures, such as femoral venipunctures and intramuscular injections, to decrease the chance of introducing pathogens. Venipuncture of the lower extremities may also predispose the child to thromboembolism because of the hypovolemia, stasis, and increased plasma concentration of clotting factors.
5. Educate parents regarding signs and symptoms of possible infections.

Enhancing Nutritional Status

1. Assess nutritional intake, growth, and development as appropriate for age.
2. Provide a diet low in sodium, fat and sugar. Place a sign on the child's bed that indicates dietary restrictions, so that everyone will be aware of special needs.
3. Provide food choices that appeal to the child and that are easy to eat according to stage of development.
4. Provide nutritional supplements as needed.

Providing Emotional Support

1. Encourage frequent visiting and allow as much parental participation in the child's care as possible. Hospitalization, if necessary, is usually brief.
2. Allow the child as much activity as tolerated.
   a. Balance periods of rest, recreation, and quiet activities during the convalescent phase.
   b. Allow the child to eat meals with family or other children.
3. Encourage the child and family to verbalize fears, frustrations, and questions.
   a. Be aware that young children frequently fear abandonment by their parents.
   b. Allow parents to express frustrations regarding the uncertainties associated with the cause of the disease, the clinical course, and prognosis.
   c. Explain the difference between nephritis and nephrosis if parents have questions.
4. Help the child adjust to changes in body image, such as cushingoid appearance, by explaining changes ahead of time.

5. Discuss the problems of discipline with the parents. Encourage them to set consistent limits and reasonable expectations of their child's behavior.
6. Suggest parents get involved with a support group for families of children with chronic illnesses, as needed.

Family Education and Health Maintenance

1. Prepare the family for home management of the child's care plan.
   a. Have the dietitian discuss special diets with the parents.
   b. Teach the parents about the child's medication.
   c. Demonstrate urine testing.
   d. Initiate a community health nursing referral if necessary for reassessment and reinforcement of teaching.
2. Encourage continued medical follow-up visits.
3. Emphasize the necessity of taking medication according to the prescribed schedule and for an extended time. Discuss complications encountered with steroid therapy.
4. Teach prevention and recognition of signs and symptoms of infection.
5. Advise family on activity restrictions necessary.
6. Teach signs and symptoms of relapse (increased edema, decreased urine output) and whom and when to call with questions.
7. Teach signs and symptoms of fluid imbalances (excess or dehydration).

Outcome-Based Evaluation

- Decrease in fluid volume excess as demonstrated by reduction in edema and ascites and adequate urine output
- Child exhibits no signs of infection
- Family can verbalize and follow dietary restrictions as demonstrated by appropriate weight gain/loss
- Family can verbalize concerns regarding child's illness as demonstrated by open communication with staff and other family members

Urinary Tract Infection

A urinary tract infection (UTI) is defined as bacteria that exists anywhere between the renal cortex and the urethral meatus. Because it is often difficult to determine the exact location of the infection, the term UTI is used to explain microorganisms anywhere within the urinary tract. The female-to-male ratio of UTI incidence during childhood is 10:1.

Pathophysiology and Etiology

1. Causative organisms—*Escherichia coli* (80%)
2. Route of entry:
   a. Ascent from the urethra (most common)
   b. Circulating blood
3. Contributing causes:
   a. Urinary stasis
   b. Obstruction, usually congenital

c. Vesicoureteral reflux
d. Infections elsewhere in the body—upper respiratory, gastrointestinal, diarrhea
e. Poor perineal hygiene
f. Short female urethra
g. Catheterization and instrumentation
h. Entrance of an irritant into the bladder
i. Inherent defect in the ability of the bladder mucosa to protect it from microbial invasion
j. Chronic or intermittent constipation
k. Local inflammation
l. Antimicrobial use for other infections that cause resistance
m. Dysfunctional voiding
n. Congenital renal anomalies (male infant)
4. Inflammatory changes occur in the affected portions of the urinary tract, including kidneys, ureters, and/or bladder/urethra.
5. Clumps of bacteria may be present.
6. Inflammation results in urinary retention and stasis of urine in the bladder.
7. Backflow of urine into the kidneys may occur through the ureters; this is called reflux.
8. Inflammatory changes in the renal pelvis, and throughout the kidney, occur when this organ is involved.
9. Scarring of the kidney parenchyma occurs in chronic infection and interferes with kidney function, particularly with the ability to concentrate urine.
10. If left untreated, the kidney may become small, tissue may be destroyed, and renal function could fail.

Clinical Manifestations

1. Onset may be abrupt or gradual; may be asymptomatic.
2. Fever.
   a. May be moderate or severe.
   b. May fluctuate rapidly.
   c. May be accompanied by chills or convulsions.
3. Anorexia and general malaise.
4. Urinary frequency, urgency, dysuria, dribbling.
5. Daytime or nocturnal enuresis.
6. Foul odor or change in the appearance of urine.
7. Abdominal or suprapubic pain.
8. Tenderness over one or both kidneys.
9. Irritability.
10. Vomiting.
11. Failure to thrive in infancy.

Diagnostic Evaluation

1. Urine culture:
   a. Documentation of pathogenic organisms in the urine is the only means of definitive diagnosis.
   b. A urine culture, demonstrating more than 100,000 bacteria per mL, indicates significant bacteriuria.
   c. A catheterized urine specimen, with growth greater than 100 colonies of bacteria per mL, is considered significant.

2. Urinalysis:
   a. Leukocytes.
   b. Casts, especially white cell casts, may be present and are indicative of intrarenal infection.
   c. Hematuria—occurs occasionally.
3. Renal concentrating ability—decreased.
4. Urologic and radiologic studies to identify anatomic abnormalities or renal changes that stem from recurrent infections—renal ultrasound, voiding cystourethrogram, intravenous pyelogram (IVP), and dimercaptosuccinic acid (DMSA).

Management

See Table 49-1.
1. Oral antibiotic therapy for uncomplicated UTI.
2. Repeat culture may be necessary before treatment is discontinued.

Complications

1. A tendency for recurrent infection exists.
2. Children with obstructive lesions of the urinary tract and those with severe vesicoureteral reflux are at highest risk for kidney damage.

Nursing Assessment

1. Obtain history to determine if UTI is initial or recurrent and to determine if there may be other disease processes contributing to this infection.
2. Focus assessment on identifying clinical manifestations and determining location of infection, such as presence and appearance of urethral discharge, high-grade fever (more common with upper UTI), or low-grade fever (more common with lower UTI).
3. Determine urinary pattern (ie, amount and frequency) and associated discomfort.

Nursing Diagnoses

• Altered Urinary Elimination related to infection
• Pain related to inflammatory changes and fever
• Self-Esteem Disturbance related to exposure and manipulation of the genitourinary tract

Nursing Interventions
Promoting Urinary Elimination

1. Obtain a clean urine specimen for urinalysis or culture.
   a. Obtain freshly voided early morning specimen, if possible (most accurate). This urine is usually acid and concentrated, which tends to preserve the formed elements.
   b. Provide fluids to help the child void.
   c. Perform catheterization, if necessary, to obtain a sterile specimen; however, this procedure may cause emotional trauma and the accidental introduction of additional bacteria.
   d. Send urine to the laboratory immediately or refrigerate to avoid a falsely high bacterial count.

TABLE 49-1 Antimicrobial Agents Commonly Used in the Management of Childhood Urinary Tract Infection

Drug	Side Effects	Nursing Considerations
Amoxicillin (Amoxil)	Occasional nausea, vomiting, diarrhea Hypersensitivity reactions of skin	Readily absorbed. May be taken with food.
Ampicillin (Omnipen)	Diarrhea, urticaria Anaphylactic reaction	Contraindicated in penicillin-sensitive children. Package insert should be consulted regarding reconstitution, administration, and storage of IM and IV preparations. Absorption of oral preparations may be decreased with food. Dose must be repeated q6h to ensure therapeutic blood levels.
Cephalexin (Keflex)	Diarrhea, nausea, vomiting	May be taken with food. Dose should be reduced if renal function is impaired.
Gentamicin (Garamycin)	Renal and auditory toxicity; respiratory paralysis	Toxic effects can be minimized by slow IV infusion (over 1 hour).
Nitrofurantoin (Macrodantin)	Fever, nausea, vomiting, peripheral neuropathy	Recommended for prolonged use. Give with food or milk to decrease gastrointestinal side effects. May cause urine to be amber or brown in color. Contraindicated in renal failure and in infants younger than 3 months of age.
Sulfasoxazole	Nausea, vomiting, drug fever, rashes, photosensitivity	Keep the child well hydrated to avoid crystallization of the drug in the urine. Contraindicated if known drug sensitivity and in infants younger than 2 months of age.
Trimethoprim-sulfamethoxazole (Bactrim, Septra)	Same as with sulfasoxazole	Commonly used if bacterial resistance is anticipated or the child fails to respond to initial therapy.

2. Administer antibiotics as ordered by the health care provider (after specimen has been obtained for culture).
   a. Antibiotic therapy is generally determined by the results of the urine cultures and sensitivities and by the child's response to therapy; however, empirical therapy may be started before culture results are back.
   b. Become familiar with toxic effects of antimicrobial agents and assess the child regularly for any of the signs and symptoms.

Maintaining Comfort and Providing Symptomatic Relief
1. Administer analgesics and antipyretics as ordered.
2. Maintain child on bed rest while febrile.
3. Encourage fluids to reduce the fever and dilute the concentration of the urine. (Water is the best clear fluid.)
4. Administer IV fluids if necessary.

Protecting Self-Esteem
1. Reinforce medical explanations of the disease and its therapy.
2. Explain all diagnostic tests and procedures to the child, allowing time for questions and answers.
3. Encourage verbalizing. Correct any misconceptions and particularly address concerns about the functioning of the urinary tract and sexual function. Reassure the child that he or she did not cause the problem.
4. Maintain privacy for the child as much as possible.
5. Provide an environment that is as close to normal as possible during hospitalization. Include opportunities for the child to play.

6. Prepare the child and family for discharge and begin discussions of rest, fluids, and medications.

Family Education and Health Maintenance
1. Review long-term antibiotic therapy, if prescribed, to prevent recurrence of UTI. Schedules for prolonged therapy vary from several months to continuous prophylaxis.
2. Encourage scheduled follow-up visits because of the possibility of disease recurrence.
   a. Emphasize that even though this disease may have few symptoms, it can lead to serious, permanent disability.
   b. Advise family that subsequent suspected UTIs should be assessed and followed by health care provider.
3. Teach measures of prevention:
   a. Minimize spread of bacteria from the anal and vaginal areas to the urethra in female children by cleansing the perianal area from the urethra back toward the anus.
   b. Avoid bubble baths because of the bladder-irritant effect of these solutions.
   c. Encourage adequate fluid intake, especially water.
   d. Avoid carbonated/caffeinated beverages because of their irritative effect on bladder mucosa.
   e. Encourage the child to void frequently and to empty the bladder completely with each voiding (double voiding).
   f. Encourage a high-fiber diet to avoid constipation.

Outcome-Based Evaluation

- Voiding regularly in adequate amounts
- No complaints of pain during or after voiding; afebrile
- Shows less anxiety about hospitalization; appears more relaxed about appearance, body image, tests

ABNORMALITIES OF THE GENITOURINARY TRACT THAT REQUIRE SURGERY

■ Exstrophy of the Bladder

Exstrophy of the bladder is part of a spectrum of anomalies that involve the urogenital tract, the musculoskeletal system, and sometimes the intestinal tract. It occurs in approximately 1 in 40,000 to 50,000 deliveries, with the male-to-female ratio 3:1.

Pathophysiology and Etiology

1. Results from failure of the abdominal wall and its underlying structures to fuse in utero.
2. The anterior surface of the bladder lies open on the lower part of the abdomen, allowing constant passage of urine to the outside.

Clinical Manifestations

1. Urine dribbles constantly.
2. Infection and ulceration of the bladder mucosa may occur.
3. Genitalia may be ambiguous.
4. Affected children may walk with a waddling or an unsteady gait.

Diagnostic Evaluation

1. Inspection is the most important tool in evaluation. The obvious anomaly may involve multiple systems.
2. Diagnostic procedures, such as radiography, ultrasound, cystoscopic examination, urodynamic testing, and IVP determine extent of the anomaly.

Management

1. Surgical closure of bladder within first 48 hours.
2. Complete correction by school age by means of staged reconstructive and orthopedic surgery.
3. Urinary diversion may be necessary.

Complications

1. Skin excoriation
2. Infection
3. Trauma to bladder mucosa

Nursing Assessment

1. Assess the child for growth and development during the reconstructive process.
2. Assess the family for coping ability.

Nursing Diagnoses

- Risk for Injury related to abnormal urinary elimination
- Risk for Injury related to complications of surgery

Nursing Interventions

Providing Care Before Reconstruction to Prevent Complications

1. Protect the bladder area from trauma and infection.
   a. Keep the infant in an Isolette to avoid irritation from clothing and blankets. Position the infant on back or side.
   b. Humidity to exposed bladder using hood: may cover area with wet gauze, when out of Isolette, for feeding.
   c. Change bed linen frequently to maintain skin integrity.
2. Observe the infant closely for signs of infection.
3. Involve other members of the health care team for parental support because of the psychosocial implications of a child who has special needs.
4. Assist the parents in dealing with their emotional reactions regarding the child's defect.
5. Prepare child and parents for the proposed surgery (see p. 1488).

Providing Postoperative Care to Prevent Complications

1. Provide care for the ureteral and urethral catheters. Observe and record the amount of urinary drainage, catheter positions, and bladder spasms.
2. Care for the child, who is placed in a body cast for several weeks (see p. 981) or in a traction system (see p. 985).
3. Provide care and instruction for an ileal conduit as necessary (see p. 664).
4. Observe for complications.
   a. Urinary or incisional infections
   b. Fistulae in the suprapubic or penile incisions
5. Recommend long-term support for children and families to help them deal with such fears as appearance of genitalia, potential inability to reproduce, rejection by peers, and sexual function. Ongoing discussion groups for parents and children may be helpful.
6. Teach the parents how to care for the child at home and make appropriate referrals.

Family Education and Health Maintenance

1. For more information and support, refer families to the following resources:
   a. Newsletter—Association of Bladder Exstrophy Children (ABC) Update, P.O. Box 1472, Wake Forest, NC 27588; 919-554-3088; *www.bladderexstrophy.com.*
   b. Book—*Living with Bladder Exstrophy: A book for Families*, Murrey and Schremmer, 1996. Available through ABC.

■ Obstructive Lesions of the Lower Urinary Tract

Obstruction of the lower urinary tract may be caused by structural lesions, such as urethral valves, bladder neck obstruction, meatal stricture, and urolithiasis; or by functional lesions, such as neuromuscular dysfunction. The effect of obstruction on ureteral and renal function depends on the degree and duration of obstruction, on the rate of urine formation, and whether infection exists.

Pathophysiology and Etiology
Types of Obstruction
1. Urethral valves:
   a. Filamentous valves that obstruct urine flow
   b. Most commonly found in urethra
2. Congenital narrowing of the urethra.
3. Bladder neck obstruction—most common site of lower urinary tract obstruction.
4. Meatal stricture.
5. Neuromuscular dysfunction.
6. Severe phimosis (rare).
7. Inflammatory processes.
8. Neoplasia.
9. Urolithiasis (calculi) can occur after reconstructive bladder surgery.
10. Trauma.

Effects of Obstruction
1. Urinary tract becomes distended, proximal to the point of obstruction.
2. The bladder dilates and hypertrophies.
3. Stasis of urine occurs.
4. The ureters become elongated, dilated, and tortuous.
5. Hydronephrosis and destruction of kidney tissue inevitably result.

Clinical Manifestations
1. Abnormal urination.
   a. Dysuria, frequency
   b. Enuresis, dribbling
   c. Reduced force of urine stream
   d. Difficulty starting urine stream
   e. Straining during urination
   f. Abrupt cessation during urination
2. Signs of infection—fever, pain, irritability.

Diagnostic Evaluation
1. Physical examination may reveal abdominal mass.
2. Laboratory findings depend on the degree that renal function is compromised.
3. IVP may show hydronephrosis.
4. Renal and bladder ultrasound.
5. Radionuclide scanning.
6. Endoscopic examination.
7. Ureteroscopy.
8. Urodynamic examination.

Management
1. Prevention or eradication of infection with antibiotics
2. Dilation of urethral stenosis or stricture
3. Surgical relief of the obstruction

Complications
1. Urinary stasis could lead to renal failure.
2. Severe and recurrent UTI.
   See Care of the Child Who Undergoes Urologic Surgery, p. 1488.

◼ Obstructive Lesions of the Upper Urinary Tract

Obstructive lesions of the upper urinary tract include ureteropelvic junction obstruction, ureterovesical junction obstruction, ureteral stricture, congenital absence or duplication of a ureter, and urolithiasis. These obstructive lesions are primarily congenital.

Pathophysiology and Etiology
1. Congenital anomalies develop in the upper urinary tract.
   a. Ureteropelvic junction obstruction
   b. Ureterovesical junction obstruction.
   c. Stricture of a ureter
   d. Congenital absence of one ureter
   e. Duplication of the ureter of one kidney
2. Urolithiasis (renal calculi) is rare in children but may be associated with metabolic disease, such as cystinosis or oxalosis.

Clinical Manifestations
1. Hydronephrosis may present as an abdominal mass.
2. Often asymptomatic (seldom any problem with voiding).
3. Vague symptoms, such as failure to thrive, may be present.
4. UTIs may be frequent.
5. Hypertension may occur.

Diagnostic Evaluation
1. Laboratory tests to determine renal function.
2. IVP, renal ultrasound, radionuclide imaging, and ureteroscopy to determine the extent of the lesion.

Management
1. Prevention or eradication of infection
2. Surgical correction of the obstruction

Complications
Renal failure

◼ Hypospadias

Hypospadias is a malposition of the urethral opening that may be associated with other urogenital tract abnormalities. It is a rare congenital defect, more common in boys than in girls.

Pathophysiology and Etiology
1. Possibly caused by decreased testosterone production in early gestation.

2. In males, the urethra opens on the ventral aspect of the penis, anywhere along the shaft of the penis, and may deflect the penis downward (chordee).
3. In females, the urethra opens into the vagina (rare).
4. Undescended testicle or inguinal hernia may be associated.
5. There is an increased chance for incidence with future male siblings.

Clinical Manifestations
1. Inability to void with the penis in the normal elevated position.
2. In females, urine dribbling from vagina.

Diagnostic Evaluation
1. Usually not difficult to diagnose because of visual anomaly. Assess glans penis for possible hypospadias before circumcision.
2. Severe cases require genotypic/phenotypic sex determination, chromosomal, and hormonal studies.
3. Renal ultrasound, IVP, voiding cystourethrography to determine associated defects.

Treatment
Surgical reconstruction before 1 year of age.

Complications
Severe forms interfere with reproductive ability. See Care of the Child Who Undergoes Urologic Surgery.

■ Cryptorchidism (Undescended Testicle)
Cryptorchidism refers to the failure of one or both testes to descend through the inguinal canal to the normal position in the scrotum. It is more common in premature infants and is the most common surgical problem in pediatric urology.

Pathophysiology and Etiology
1. Possibly caused by delayed descent, prevention of descent by mechanical lesion, or endocrine disorder (rare).
2. Testicular and ductal development are abnormal. It is unclear whether this is because of congenital dysplasia or because of underdevelopment.
3. Degeneration of the sperm-forming cells occurs after puberty because of the higher temperatures of the abdomen, compared with normal location in the scrotum.

Clinical Manifestations
Testicle nonpalpable within the scrotum.

Diagnostic Evaluation
1. Ultrasonography may reveal undescended testicle.
2. Serum testosterone measurements may be decreased.

Treatment
1. Orchiopexy surgery to achieve permanent fixation of the testis in the scrotum. Surgery should be performed between the ages of 1 and 3 years to prevent damage to the tissues and to lessen emotional concerns related to body image.
2. Plastic surgery in patients with one testicle.
3. Administration of human chorionic gonadotropin (HCG) has produced descent of the testicles in some children. Testicles may have descended spontaneously in many of these cases.

Complications
1. Testicular torsion
2. Associated hernias
3. Emotional disturbances
4. Significant increase in sterility and malignancy later in life
   See Care of the Child Who Undergoes Urologic Surgery (below).

■ Care of the Child Who Undergoes Urologic Surgery
Also, see Chapter 21 for a discussion of kidney surgery and urinary diversion.

Nursing Assessment
1. Obtain history from prenatal and birth record, family, and child.
2. Assess feeding and crying patterns, indicating potential obstruction or abdominal pain.
3. Assess urinary elimination pattern to determine degree of disorder.
4. Assess for associated congenital defects.
5. Assess for failure to thrive.
6. Determine family's response to body image changes. Expect anxieties regarding sterility and homosexuality and perceptions of the child as defective or inadequate.
7. Measure and record vital signs, height, weight, abdominal girth, and compare with previous measurements, if available. Renal insufficiency may alter growth. Fever may be indicative of infection.
8. Visually and manually inspect genitalia and record abnormalities (eg, if bladder mucosa is visible, describe signs of irritation).
9. Palpate abdomen; note masses.
10. Obtain urine for culture and sensitivity. Note color, amount, odor, degree of cloudiness.
11. Review results of all laboratory and diagnostic procedures.

Nursing Diagnoses
- Knowledge Deficit related to surgery
- Altered Urinary Elimination related to the condition and surgical intervention
- Body Image Disturbance related to appearance of genitalia

- Risk for Infection related to surgical incision and drainage tubes
- Risk for Fluid Volume Deficit related to surgical losses
- Pain related to surgical incision and drainage tubes

Nursing Interventions

Promoting Understanding of Surgical Treatment

1. Determine the child's expectation regarding illness and hospitalization through discussion and play therapy.
2. Explain the anatomy and physiology of the urinary system in terms the child can understand.
   a. Use a body outline appropriate for the age of the child.
   b. Explain how the child differs from the normal. Relate defect to symptoms whenever possible.
3. Explain all diagnostic tests before their occurrence. These may include urinalysis, 24-hour urine collections, IV and retrograde pyelography, angiography, and cystoscopy. Descriptions should include such information as:
   a. Preparation required—fasting, enemas, etc.
   b. Location of the test—operating room, radiology department, etc.
   c. Appearance and attire of personnel
   d. Positioning
   e. Anesthesia
   f. Pain or discomfort
   g. Expectations after the procedure—diet, rest, urine collections, etc.
4. Determine the child's understanding of the procedure.
   a. Ask simple, direct questions.
   b. Allow child to perform the procedure on a doll or to demonstrate it on a diagram.
5. Explain the surgical procedure, including the following:
   a. Preparation required—fasting, enemas, etc.
   b. Description of the operating room, including the appearance of the personnel
   c. Anesthesia
   d. Postoperative appearance—urinary drainage tubing and collection devices, appearance of urine, sutures, bandages, IV infusion
6. Determine the child's understanding of surgery and reinforce teaching when necessary.
7. Emphasize additional points:
   a. The child is in no way to blame for illness.
   b. No other part of the body will be operated on.

Promoting Normal Urinary Pattern

1. Monitor daily intake and output.
2. Encourage adequate fluids and monitor daily weights.
3. Care for all catheters and urinary tubes according to hospital policy. Maintain appropriate position of tubes.
4. Observe and record amount and appearance of urinary drainage, occurrence of bladder spasms, symptoms of urinary or incisional infection.

Providing Emotional Support Regarding Body Image

1. Continue reassurance about appearance of genitalia.
2. Maintain discussions regarding reactions. This may need to be done with patient and family alone, as well as a family unit.

3. Discuss plans for interim period from initial surgery until secondary or reconstructive procedures can be performed.
4. Initiate independence of care.
5. Focus on activities the child can perform and accomplish.

Preventing Infection

1. Administer antibiotics and IV fluids as ordered.
2. Maintain patency of catheter(s). Provide catheter care as directed.
3. Administer wound care using aseptic technique. Inspect incision for drainage or signs of infection.

Maintaining Fluid Volume

1. Administer fluids as ordered.
2. Monitor vital signs for hypotension or tachycardia.
3. Assess patient's skin turgor and mucous membranes for signs of dehydration.
4. Measure and record accurate intake and output.

Promoting Comfort

1. Administer analgesics as ordered and according to assessment of complaints of pain, restlessness, crying, or withdrawal.
2. Administer antispasmodics as ordered for bladder spasm.
3. Provide distraction and comfort measures.

Family Education and Health Maintenance

1. Advise the family about follow-up appointments, additional surgeries, or procedures.
2. Teach care of incision, signs of infection.
3. Advise on avoidance of straddle toys for 6 weeks to promote healing.
4. Encourage good nutrition to promote healing and to prevent infection.

Outcome-Based Evaluation

- Child and family verbalize understanding of surgery
- Clear urine draining via catheter
- Child and family verbalize relief that defects can be surgically repaired and reconstructed
- Incision without drainage or signs of infection
- Vital signs stable; urine output adequate
- Decreased crying and increased restful periods and sleep noted

RENAL FAILURE AND DIALYSIS

Acute Renal Failure

Acute renal failure is a sudden, usually reversible deterioration in normal renal function. This results in fluid and electrolyte imbalance and accumulation of metabolic toxins. Nursing care of children with acute renal failure is generally the same as that of adults (see p. 670), although there are special considerations for pediatric patients.

Pathophysiology and Etiology

1. Causes are divided into *prerenal* (problem occurs in blood supply to the kidneys), *intrarenal* (problem is

within the kidney or kidneys), and *postrenal* (problem occurs in urinary system after the kidneys).

   a. Prerenal causes: conditions causing hypovolemia (dehydration, shock, trauma, or burns) cause decreased blood flow to the kidneys.

   b. Intrarenal causes: conditions causing a reduction in glomerular filtration rate (GFR), renal ischemia, and tubular damage. May be due to vascular diseases (hemolytic uremic syndrome, thrombosis), tubular nephropathies (myoglobinuria, hemoglobinuria, toxins), or interstitial nephritis (penicillins, allergies). These are the largest group to require extended medical management.

   c. Postrenal causes: conditions causing obstruction to urine flow. Uncommon, except for obstructive uropathies in the first year of life. Renal function is restored with relief of the obstruction.

2. The exact pathophysiology of acute renal failure is not always known. Three phases of acute renal failure are recognized in children:

   a. Initiating phase: begins when kidney is injured and lasts from hours to days. Signs and symptoms of renal impairment are present.

   b. Oliguric phase: usually lasts 5 to 15 days but can persist for weeks; shorter in infants and children (3–5 days) and longer in older children and adolescents (10–14 days).

   c. Diuretic phase: highly variable, from mild and lasting only a few days to profound.

3. Trauma, burns, and nephrotoxic agents may cause acute tubular necrosis and temporary cessation of renal function. Myoglobin (a protein released from muscle when injury occurs) and hemoglobin are released, causing renal toxicity, ischemia, or both.

4. Severe transfusion reactions may result in hemoglobin that filters through the kidney glomeruli. This becomes concentrated in the kidney tubules. Resulting precipitation interferes with the excretion of urine.

5. Nonsteroidal anti-inflammatory drugs interfere with prostaglandins that normally protect renal blood flow, decreasing glomerular filtration rate (GFR).

 DRUG ALERT

Nephrotoxic agents include aminoglycosides, penicillins, cephalosporins, and sulfonamides. Chemicals that contain arsenic and mercury are also nephrotoxic.

Clinical Manifestations
1. Nausea and vomiting
2. Diarrhea
3. Decreased tissue turgor
4. Dry mucous membranes
5. Lethargy
6. Difficulty in voiding; changes in urine flow
7. Steady rise in serum creatinine
8. Fever
9. Edema

Diagnostic Evaluation
1. Serum creatinine level—the most reliable measure of the GFR, found to be rising.
2. Radionuclide studies to evaluate GFR and renal blood flow and distribution.
3. Urinalysis—reveals proteinuria, hematuria, casts.
4. Ultrasonography to determine anatomic abnormalities.

Management
1. 75% of children with acute renal failure attain complete recovery.
2. Treatment is directed toward the underlying cause.
3. Correction of any reversible cause of acute renal failure (ie, surgical relief of obstruction).
4. Correction and control of fluid and electrolyte imbalances.
5. Restoration and maintenance of stable vital signs.
6. Maintenance of nutrition with low-sodium, low-potassium, low-phosphate, moderate-protein diet.
7. Initiation of dialysis for patients with life-threatening complications.

Complications
1. Fluid and electrolyte imbalance, especially hyperkalemia—when glomerular filtration rate is reduced, patient cannot excrete potassium.
2. Metabolic acidosis, caused by decreased acid excretion and bicarbonate regeneration.
3. Insufficient nutritional intake because of metabolic abnormalities and symptoms, such as nausea and vomiting.

Nursing Assessment
1. Obtain history of all medications, recent and past illnesses or injuries, allergies, and potential exposure to toxic substances.
2. Measure intake and output. Insert indwelling urinary catheter as indicated.
3. Monitor vital signs. Institute cardiac monitoring as indicated.
4. Monitor urine specific gravity as directed. Fixed specific gravity of 1. 010 indicates the kidneys' inability to concentrate or dilute urine.

Nursing Diagnoses
- Risk for Fluid Volume Imbalance related to inability of the kidneys to maintain fluid balance
- Risk for Injury related to hyperkalemia

Nursing Interventions
Maintaining Fluid Volume
1. Administer IV fluids slowly to prevent heart failure.
2. Maintain fluid restriction as ordered.
3. Keep strict intake and output records.

4. Weigh child daily.

5. Promptly report signs of heart failure—edema, bounding pulse, third heart sound, shortness of breath, and adventitious breath sounds.

Preventing Harm From Severe Electrolyte Disturbance

1. Monitor blood test results (creatinine, BUN, electrolytes, calcium) and notify health care provider promptly of abnormal levels.

2. Watch for signs of hyperkalemia—weak, irregular pulse, abdominal cramps, muscle weakness.

3. Do not administer IV fluids with potassium while renal function is impaired.

4. Maintain low-protein, low-potassium, low-sodium, and high-carbohydrate diet.

5. Administer treatments for hyperkalemia as ordered, such as IV sodium bicarbonate, IV glucose, and insulin, which both drive potassium into cells and temporarily out of the blood stream.

6. Administer cation exchange enemas to reduce potassium as ordered.

7. Watch for signs of hypocalcemia—muscle twitching and tetany.

Family Education and Health Maintenance

1. Explain all steps of the diagnostic and treatment process to the family.

2. Teach about dialysis if this becomes necessary.

3. Explain that as kidney function resumes, diuresis may occur to eliminate excess fluid the body was storing.

4. Educate about prompt medical attention for illnesses that may cause dehydration to prevent renal injury in future.

Outcome-Based Evaluation

• No signs of heart failure
• Potassium remains within upper range of normal

◼ Chronic Renal Failure

Chronic renal failure is irreversible destruction of nephrons, so that they are no longer capable of maintaining normal fluid and electrolyte balance. Nursing care of children with chronic renal failure is similar to that of adults (see p. 672). The following considerations are important for pediatric patients.

Pathophysiology and Etiology

1. Congenital renal and urinary tract abnormalities (most common cause younger than 5 years of age).

2. Most common causes from 5 to 15 years:
   a. Glomerular disease
   b. Hereditary renal disease
   c. Renal vascular disorders

3. Similar progression regardless of cause.
   a. Nephron damage that results in hypertrophy and hyperplasia of remaining nephrons.

b. Overload results in decreased ability for nephrons to excrete effectively.

c. Results in azotemia and clinical uremia.

d. Inability of kidney to excrete phosphate causes hypocalcemia, which results in osteodystrophy.

e. Kidneys cannot synthesize vitamin D, thus impairing calcium absorption. Bones may become so calcium depleted that growth halts and bones become brittle (renal rickets).

f. Kidneys cannot synthesize erythropoietin, thus resulting in anemia.

g. Excretion of nitrogenous waste through sweat causes pruritus.

h. Overload of fluid results in edema and hypertension.

4. Severity of chronic renal failure is indicated by GFR. The lower the GFR, the greater the loss of renal function.

Clinical Manifestations

Variable and not chronological.

1. Decreased appetite and energy level.

2. Initial polyuria caused by kidney's inability to concentrate urine; later oliguria and anuria.

3. Bone or joint pain.

4. Dryness and itching of skin.

Diagnostic Evaluation

1. Serum studies:
   a. Decreased hematocrit, hemoglobin, Na+, Ca++; increased K+ and phosphorus.
   b. As renal function declines, BUN, uric acid, and creatinine values continue to climb.

2. Urine studies:
   a. Specific gravity—increased or decreased.
   b. 24-hour urine for creatinine clearance is decreased (increased creatinine in urine), thus reflecting decreased GFR.
   c. Changes in total output.

3. Many other tests may be ordered to evaluate other systems and extent of disease (eg, chest x-ray, electrocardiogram).

Management

1. Correction of calcium-phosphorus imbalance. Administer activated vitamin D to increase calcium absorption, and calcium phosphate binders with meals, to bind phosphate in the gastrointestinal tract.

2. Correction of acidosis with buffers, such as Bicitra.

3. Diets should meet caloric needs of the child and contain adequate protein for development (1.0–1.5 g/kg per day).

4. Correction of anemia through the use of erythropoietin (Epogen) administered subcutaneously at home.

5. Growth retardation should be evaluated for possible use of growth hormone.

6. Treatment options for end-stage renal disease are hemodialysis, peritoneal dialysis, and transplantation.

7. Dialysis, while renal transplant work-up is in progress.

Complications

1. Growth retardation.
2. Delayed or absent sexual maturation.
3. Severe anemia—kidneys cannot stimulate erythropoietin; uremic toxins deplete erythrocytes; nutritional deficiencies.
4. Hypertension—renal ischemia stimulates renin-angiotensin system.
5. Congestive heart failure.
6. Azotemia/uremia—nitrogen waste products accumulate in blood. Toxic levels manifest themselves in many ways, such as coma, headache, gastrointestinal disturbances, neuromuscular disturbances.
7. Metabolic acidosis.
8. Electrolyte imbalance—hypocalcemia, hyperkalemia.

Nursing Assessment

1. Perform a comprehensive, multisystem assessment to help in planning care.
2. Assess growth and developmental status.
3. Assess coping, support systems, and other resources.

Nursing Diagnoses

Children with chronic renal failure are in multisystem physiologic crises. The nursing diagnoses throughout the chapter are applicable, but focus may be:

• Risk for Injury related to hypocalcemia
• Risk for Fluid Volume Imbalance related to renal failure and dialysis
• Altered Nutrition: Less Than Body Requirements related to gastrointestinal disturbances and diet restrictions
• Activity Intolerance related to fatigue and anemia
• Coping, Ineffective, related to changes in lifestyle and body image on dialysis

Nursing Interventions

Ensuring Safety

1. Protect the child from the effects of decreased level of consciousness and involuntary movements, by maintaining crib or bed side rails up and padded, as necessary.
2. Monitor for seizure activity and have airway or tongue blade and suction equipment on hand.
3. Monitor BUN, creatinine, electrolyte, and calcium levels, and report abnormalities promptly.

Promoting Fluid Balance

See Acute Renal Failure, p. 1489.

Ensuring Adequate Nutrition

1. Ensure adequate protein in diet, but explain importance of restriction.
2. Encourage appropriate fluid intake between meals, so child does not feel denied.
3. Discourage drinking milk if recommended, because of high phosphate, sodium, and potassium content. Instead, administer feedings of low-protein, low-electrolyte formula as directed.

Increasing Activity Tolerance

1. Plan activities when child is rested.
2. Encourage activity as tolerated, but excessive exercise should be avoided to reduce nitrogenous waste from metabolism.
3. Administer blood transfusions as ordered.

Enhancing Coping With Chronic Renal Failure

1. Because numerous issues may interfere with the child's psychological and social development and education, help the child and family to cope with:
   a. Uncertainty regarding the course of the disease and ultimate prognosis
   b. Abnormal lifestyle necessitated by dialysis
   c. Burden of dialysis and continuous administration of medications
   d. Problems of adjustment related to growth failure
   e. Fear of death, present in most children, adolescents, and family members
   f. Possible kidney transplantation, involving major surgery and prolonged hospitalization, followed by altered body image that is caused by high-dose steroids and potential for rejection, which may threaten survival

Family Education and Health Maintenance

1. Teach child to avoid high-sodium foods, such as chips, pretzels, and popcorn; luncheon meats; canned foods; and fast foods, if sodium is restricted.
2. Encourage follow-up as advised by kidney specialist and primary health care provider.
3. Encourage family to keep up with regular dental care, immunizations, and health assessments to help prevent infections, problems with growth, and more severe childhood diseases.
4. Teach about medications and support child who may be taking multiple medications—calcium, phosphate binder, acid neutralizer, and others.
5. Advise the family about support services and media resources available, for example, *It's Just a Part of My Life—a Kid's View of Dialysis*, by the National Kidney Foundation, 30 E. 33rd Street, New York, NY, 10016, 212-889-2210, *www.kidney.org*.

◼ The Child Who Undergoes Dialysis

Dialysis is the passage of a solute through a semipermeable membrane. The purpose of dialysis is to preserve life by replacing some of the normal kidney functions. See p. 697 for a complete description of different types of dialysis.

General Considerations

The following principles should be considered by the nurse who works with pediatric patients:

1. Peritoneal dialysis:
   a. Because of the child's small size, the volume of dialysate is 30 to 50 mL/kg or 1,000 to 1200 mL/m².

b. The child can be expected to participate at a developmentally appropriate level with his or her own care.

2. Hemodialysis:
   a. When possible, subcutaneous or intramuscular injections are avoided because the child is anticoagulated with heparin.
   b. Blood pressure cuff and tourniquets should not be applied to a limb with a fistula.

3. Specific care for the child during dialysis is generally provided by specially trained personnel in a dialysis unit. However, the following considerations should be noted:
   a. Choice for vascular access depends on patient size and availability of peripheral blood vessels of suitable size (Figure 49-1).
   b. Extracorporeal blood volume (blood outside of the body at any given time) should be as small as possible. It should not exceed 8% to 10% of the child's total blood volume.
   c. Efficiency or adequacy of the dialyzer, relative to the child's weight, should be noted and blood pump speed adjusted accordingly.
   d. External catheter should be secured to ensure catheter is not traumatized.

Nursing Care of the Child Who Undergoes Dialysis

1. Prepare the child for the procedure. Dialysis is threatening to most children and may evoke fears of pain, mutilation, immobilization, helplessness, and dependency. Many children have fears of losing all of their blood in this process. A child who is well prepared will be less frightened and better able to cooperate during the procedure.
   a. Explain the procedure in terms that the child can understand.
   b. Allow the child to handle equipment similar to that which will be used during dialysis.
   c. Encourage the child to express fears so that misinterpretations can be corrected.
   d. Provide simple pictures and diagrams, if appropriate.
   e. Allow the child to talk with peers who have undergone dialysis.

2. Explain the procedure to family members and answer questions so that they will be in the best position to support the child.

3. Protect the child from infection.
   a. Keep the dressings and area around the catheter clean and dry.
   b. Use aseptic technique throughout the dialysis procedure.
   c. Provide supplemental vitamins because diet may be low in vitamins.
   d. Provide meticulous daily hygiene.

4. Maintain appropriate nutritional and fluid modifications. Because anorexia is often seen in chronic renal failure, provide small frequent meals.

5. Restrict fluids and sodium to prevent fluid overload in children who are hypertensive or who have minimal urine output. Potassium is limited to prevent complications related to hyperkalemia. The child may see dietary restrictions as a punishment and must be helped to realize the purpose of restrictions.

6. Do not restrict protein, which is vital to allow for normal growth and development. Peritoneal dialysis is a continual treatment and therefore can constantly dialyze metabolic waste and fluids off.

7. Maintain careful records of intake and output, vital signs, blood pressure, and daily weights. These provide valuable information about the effectiveness of the therapy.

8. Support the child during the dialysis procedure.
   a. Provide symptomatic relief of nausea, vomiting, malaise, or headache. Notify the health care provider if these symptoms are severe.
   b. Involve the child in diversional activities, such as play therapy, crafts, television, books, etc.
   c. Encourage the family to bring in articles that will make the child's room appear more homelike (ie, pictures, posters, etc.).
   d. Encourage the child to be as independent as possible in daily care.

9. Help the child to keep up with schoolwork by initiating a referral to a tutor, providing study times, etc.

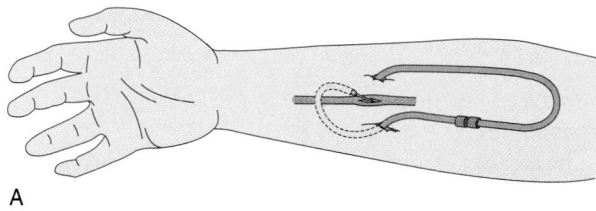

A

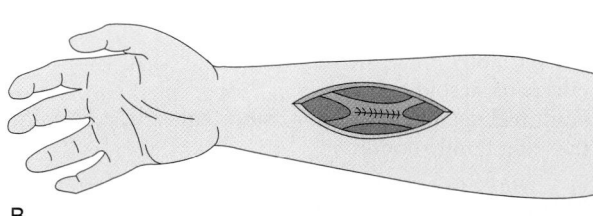

B

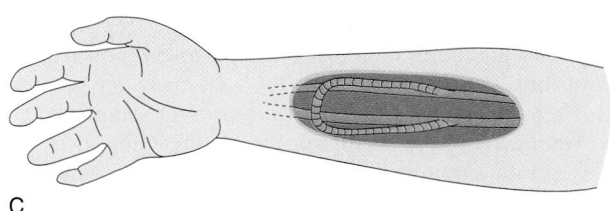

C

FIGURE 49-1 Vascular access devices for hemodialysis. (**A**) An external arteriovenous shunt. (**B**) An internal arteriovenous fistula. (**C**) An internal arteriovenous graft.

Community and Home Care Considerations

1. Be aware that although life is preserved, it is by no means normal during the time on dialysis or between dialyses. These measures may increase the child's feeling of self-esteem and diminish regression and social isolation. By serving as role models, health professionals may encourage parents to recognize and foster the normal, healthy aspects of the child's daily life.
2. Offer appropriate support to the family.
   a. Provide opportunity for family members to discuss their feelings, fears, and frustrations and to ask questions.
   b. Allow family members to become involved in the child's care.
   c. Provide for continuity of personnel.
   d. Initiate appropriate referrals. These may include referrals to a social worker, psychiatrist, dietitian, community health agency, or other families who are coping with dialysis.
3. Be aware that families often need extensive support from many health professionals to cope with the physical, psychological, financial, and logistical aspects of renal failure and dialysis. Attention must be focused on siblings and parents because sibling relationships are often strained and difficult.
4. Teach the child and family about all of the important aspects of renal failure and dialysis, including the following:
   a. Protection from infection
   b. Dietary restrictions and recommendations; ways of incorporating the special diet into the family meal plan
   c. Dialysis schedule
   d. Medications
   e. Emergency procedures
   f. Reintegration into the community and school
5. Empower the family to care for the child at home. Learning about the child's care also helps restore some sense of control in a frightening situation.

▇ Renal Transplant

Renal (kidney) transplantation is the optimal therapeutic modality for end-stage renal disease in the pediatric age group. With successful transplantation, there is a greater likelihood of optimum rehabilitation than with any form of dialytic therapy. The potential for normal growth and pubertal development is significantly increased after transplantation. However, it should be noted that post-transplant growth is affected by many variables: age of onset of chronic renal disease, caloric intake, corticosteroid dosage, bone age at transplantation, transplant function, and rejection episodes. Requirements of preoperative management and nursing care of children or teens for renal transplantation are similar to that of adults (see p. 702). However, they are also more exhaustive because both the recipient and parent(s) must be included. The emotional, psychological, and financial needs of both the recipient

and the family must be evaluated. An appropriate care plan must then be designed to address identified needs; this care plan must be appropriate for the developmental age of the recipient.

Evaluation of Recipient

The major issues that must be evaluated when considering renal transplantation in children are the following:
1. Patient age
2. Primary renal disease
3. Psychological status
4. Live versus cadaveric donor allograft
5. Optimal immunosuppressive regimen
6. Maximization of growth and pubertal development

Donor Selection (by Priority)

A tissue-compatible transplantation from a relative is 90% successful.
1. Identical twin sibling
2. Sibling—siblings cannot be used as donors until they are of legal age to give consent for removal of a kidney
3. Parent
4. Aunt or uncle
5. Unrelated live donor (more commonly used)
6. Cadaver donor

Operative Procedure

Children often receive the kidney of an adult, if the child weighs more than 10 kg. Kidney replacement occurs within the abdomen, with vessel anastomosis to the aorta and superior vena cava.

Potential Emotional Concerns of Children With Transplants

1. The concept of a foreign body, especially a cadaver kidney, inside one's own body may be disturbing.
2. Fear that the kidney may wear out sooner if it is from an older person.
3. Altered body image because of growth failure and the effects of steroid therapy.
4. Guilt feelings if a live donor transplant fails, especially that of a family donor.

Nursing Interventions

Also see kidney transplantation, page 703.
1. Support the child and family through the preoperative phase, including diagnostic testing and blood transfusions.
2. After surgery, maintain strict infection precautions.
3. Administer immunosuppressants as directed.
4. Continue support through hemodialysis as necessary.
5. Monitor urine output, blood work results, and urine specific gravity.
6. Watch for signs of rejection—fever, oliguria, proteinuria, weight gain, hypertension, and tenderness over transplanted kidney. Acute rejection usually occurs in the first

3 months after transplant. Chronic rejection may develop at any time, and the kidney gradually loses function during 6 or more months.

Community and Home Care Considerations

The practice of discharging patients from an in-hospital setting as quickly as possible is also true for the pediatric transplant recipient. Community and/or home care nurses must have:

1. The knowledge to care for a child who receives intravenous medications
2. The ability to access and heparinize central venous lines and peripheral intravenous catheters (PICs)

Family Education and Health Maintenance

1. Teach families about the signs of rejection.
2. Encourage close follow-up for proper dosing of immunosuppressants.
3. Advise family that close medical surveillance will always be necessary, because the incidence of malignant disease is 6 times more likely in transplant recipients than in the general population.
4. Teach parents not to overprotect the child. Once the child has healed from surgery, regular activity can be resumed.

SELECTED REFERENCES

Alexander, S. (1990). Controversies in pediatric renal transplantation. *American Kidney Foundation Nephrology Letter, 7*(2), 5–21.

Couser, W.G. (1999). Glomerulonephritis. *The Lancet, 353,* 1509–1515.

Danovitch, G.M. (1996). *Handbook of kidney transplant.* Boston: Little, Brown.

Downs, S.M. (1999). Technical report: Urinary tract infections in febrile infants and young children. The Urinary Tract Subcommittee of the American Academy of Pediatrics Committee on Quality Improvement. *Pediatrics, 103*(4), e54.

Harmon, W.E. (1999). *Pediatric nephrology* (4th ed.). Philadelphia: Lippincott Williams & Wilkins.

Kaysen, G.A. (1988). Albumin metabolism in the nephrotic syndrome: The effect of dietary protein intake. *American Journal of Kidney Diseases, 12*(6), 461–480.

Kelsch, R.C., & Sedman, A.B. (1993). Nephrotic syndrome. *Pediatrics in Review, 14*(1), 30–38.

Neumann, M. (1997). Evaluation of the pediatric renal transplant recipient. *ANNA Journal, 24*(5), 515–538.

Pan, C.G. (1997). Glomerulonephritis in childhood. *Current Opinions in Pediatrics, 9*(2), 154–159.

Report of a Workshop by the British Association for Paediatric Nephrology and Research Unit, Royal College of Physicians (1994). Consensus statement of management and audit potential for steroid responsive nephrotic syndrome. *Archives of Disease in Childhood, 70,* 151–157.

Rodrigo, R., Bravo, I., & Pino, M. (1996). Proteinuria and albumin homeostasis in the nephrotic syndrome: Effect of dietary protein intake. *Nutrition Reviews, 54*(11), 337–347.

Salvatierra, O., Alfrey, E., Tanney, D.C., Mak, R., Hammer, G.B., Krane, E.J., So, S.K.S., Lemley, K., Orlandi, P.D., & Conley, S.B. (1997). Superior outcomes in pediatric renal transplant. *Archives of Surgery, 132,* 842–849.

Schrier, R.W., & Gottschalk, C.W. (1997). *Diseases of the kidney* (6th ed.). Boston: Little, Brown.

Siberry, G. k. & Iannone, R. (2000). *The Harriet Lane handbook* (15th ed.). St. Louis: Mosby.

Takeda, A., Ohgushi, H., Niimura, F., & Matsutani, H. (1998). Long-term effects of immunosuppressants in steroid-dependent nephrotic syndrome. *Pediatric Nephrology, 12,* 74–750.

Tenbrock, K., Muller-Berghaus, J., Fuchshuber, A., Michalk, D., & Querfeld, U. (1998). Levamisole treatment in steroid-sensitive and steroid-resistant nephrotic syndrome. *Pediatric Nephrology, 12,* 459–462.

Van Gool, J.D., Hjalmas, K., Tamminen-Mobius, T., & Olbing, H. (1992). Historical clues to the complex of dysfunctional voiding, urinary tract infection and vesicoureteral reflux. The International Reflux Study in Children. *Journal of Urology, 148*(5 Pt. 2), 1699–1702.

Washizawa, K., Kasai, S., Mori, T., Komiyama, A., & Shigematsu, H. (1993). Ultrastructural alteration of glomerular anionic sites in nephrotic patients. *Pediatric Nephrology, 7,* 1–5.

Watson, A.R., & Coleman, J.E. (1993). Dietary management in nephrotic syndrome. *Archives of Disease in Childhood, 69*(2), 179–180.

Wong, C.S., et al. (2000). The risk of the hemolytic-uremic syndrome after antibiotic treatment of *Escherichia coli* 0157: H7 infections. *New England Journal of Medicine, 342,* 1930–1936.

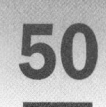

CHAPTER

50

Pediatric Metabolic and Endocrine Disorders

ASSESSMENT

■ Common Nursing Assessment for Growth and Development

Endocrine dysfunction in children frequently leads to altered growth and development. Accurate nursing assessment can help detect variations in growth and developmental patterns, identify factors such as diet and medications that may have an impact on growth and development, and obtain information about compliance and understanding of treatment.

Evaluation of Growth Patterns

1. Perform frequent and accurate measurements of both height and weight.
2. Accurately plot measurements on growth curve for absolute chronologic age.
3. Assess growth pattern for any deviation from the child's percentile or from the parallel of the growth curve for age (includes both an upward as well as a downward deviation).
4. Calculate growth velocity—take the difference of current height from previous height and divide by the time period. Growth rate for a pre-pubertal child should be 2 to 3 inches on an annual basis.
5. Report any child whose pattern deviates from the expected pattern for age to health care provider.

General Health History

1. Dietary history—what is the child's meal frequency, volume, and food preferences? Be especially critical in the history of a child when anorexia may be possible—growth velocity will usually be low, in addition to poor weight gain.

2. History of major illnesses or surgeries that have impacted on growth and development.
3. Clothing—outgrowing clothing and shoes?
4. Social history relative to friendships.
5. Academic/school performance—recent changes?
6. Activity—activities the child participates in? Intensity and type of exercise?

Medication History and Compliance

1. Is child on any steroidal medications (such as prednisone) that would suppress growth?
2. When pubertal signs are present on physical examination, does child have access to any gonadal steroids (ie, birth control pills, anabolic steroids)?
3. Are child and family compliant with treatment medications according to dose, frequency, and route? Is medication stored properly?
4. Do child and family know what the medications are and their indications?
5. If taking oral medication, is it being taken with food if indicated? If pills are being chewed, are teeth being brushed soon after, which could be rinsing out the medications?
6. If injectable, are injection sites being rotated appropriately? Review technique.

Physical Examination Relative to Development

1. Dental development—eruption of teeth and presence of permanent teeth (see p. 1252)
2. Pubertal development—Tanner staging of pubic hair and gonadal development (Table 50-1)
3. Presence of genetic dysmorphology—such as short-limbed dwarfism and various atypical stigmata

TABLE 50-1 Tanner Staging of Puberty

Boys' Genital Development	Girls' Breast Development	Both Sexes: Pubic Hair

Stage 1

Preadolescent. Testes, scrotum, and penis are of about the same size and proportion as in early childhood.

Preadolescent. Elevation of papilla only.

Preadolescent. The vellus over the pubis is not further developed than that over the abdominal wall, ie, no pubic hair.

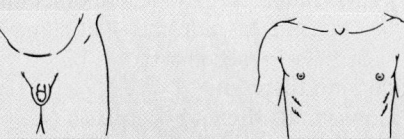 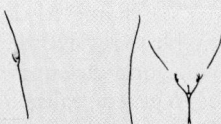 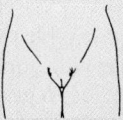 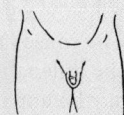

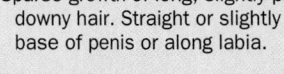

Stage 2

Enlargement of scrotum and testes. Skin of scrotum reddens and changes in texture. Little or no enlargement of penis at this time.

Breast bud stage. Elevation of breast and papilla as small mound. Enlargement of areola diameter.

Sparse growth of long, slightly pigmented downy hair. Straight or slightly curled at base of penis or along labia.

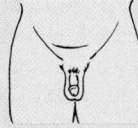 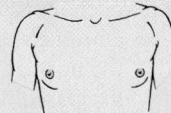 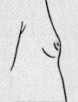 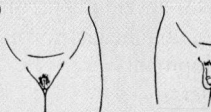

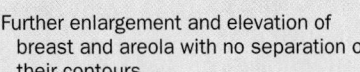 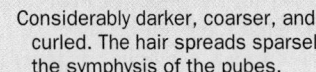

Stage 3

Enlargement of penis that occurs at first mainly in length. Further growth of testes and scrotum.

Further enlargement and elevation of breast and areola with no separation of their contours.

Considerably darker, coarser, and more curled. The hair spreads sparsely over the symphysis of the pubes.

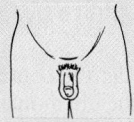 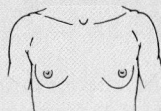 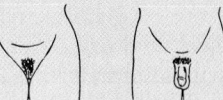

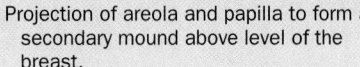 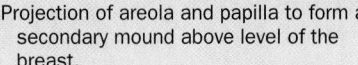 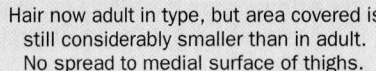

Stage 4

Increased size of penis with growth in breadth and development of glans. Testes and scrotum larger; scrotal skin darkened.

Projection of areola and papilla to form a secondary mound above level of the breast.

Hair now adult in type, but area covered is still considerably smaller than in adult. No spread to medial surface of thighs.

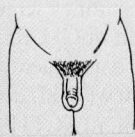 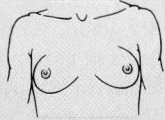 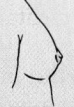 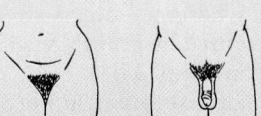

Stage 5

Genitalia adult in size and shape.

Mature stage: projection of papilla only, due to recession of the areola to the general contour of the breast.

Adult in quantity and type; distribution of the horizontal (or classically "feminine") pattern. Spread to medial surface of thighs or above base of the inverse triangle occurs late (stage 6).

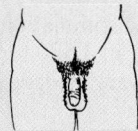 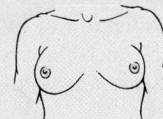 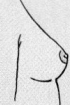 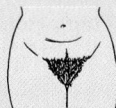 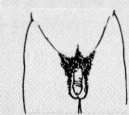

(Adapted from Tanner, J. M. [1975]. Growth and endocrinology of the adolescent. In Gardner, L. [Ed.]. *Endocrine and genetic diseases of childhood and adolescence* [2nd ed.] Philadelphia: W. B. Saunders.)

Causes of Disorders of Growth and Stature

It is important to realize that growth and stature problems are caused by a wide variety of factors. Thorough history, physical examination, and diagnostic testing can help reveal the underlying cause. Many of the disorders are associated with other anomalies such as mental retardation, cardiac problems, and secondary sex characteristic abnormalities. The cause may be treatable to resolve the growth problem, be amenable to growth hormone supplementation, or may be untreatable due to genetic cause.

Short Stature and Growth Failure
Genetic Causes
1. Familial short stature—short stature relative to U.S. standards; however, growth rate is normal.
2. Constitutional delay—normal growth rate with delayed onset of pubertal development. Short stature relative to peers; however, final height normal upon completion of pubertal development.
3. Genetic disorders:
   a. Dwarfisms—multiple types and causes relative to chondrodysplasias (see p. 37)
   b. Turner syndrome—occurs in about 1 in 2,500 female births. Characterized by short stature, ovarian dysgenesis (underdeveloped, degenerate ovaries), and, in some cases, unusual physical appearance (see p. 36)
   c. Russell-Silver syndrome—characterized by unilateral poor growth, short stature, characteristic facies, mental delays. Whenever unilateral change in growth is presented, abdominal tumor needs to be ruled out.
   d. Prader-Willi syndrome—rare syndrome characterized by below-normal intelligence; small stature; small, slow growth of hands; small penis; cryptorchidism (see p. 36)
   e. Down syndrome—occurs in 1 in 700 live births; characterized by growth retardation and mental retardation (see p. 35)
   f. Cystic fibrosis—occurs in 1 in 2000 live births. In addition to respiratory and gastrointestinal symptoms, growth retardation occurs (see p. 1364).

Endocrine Disorders
1. Hypothyroidism
2. Growth hormone insufficiency
3. Glucocorticoid excess—Cushing syndrome

Non-endocrine Disorders
1. Glucocorticoid (prednisone) therapy for asthma, prevention of transplant rejection, etc.
2. Nutritional deficiency
3. Psychosocial issues
4. Other medical problems—chronic disease, renal failure, heart disease, etc.
5. Medical interventions—eg, surgical tumor resections, radiation for brain tumors, etc.

Tall Stature and Excessive Growth
Genetic Causes
1. Familial tall stature—tall stature relative to U.S. standards; however, normal for family. Growth rate is usually normal.
2. Genetic disorders:
   a. Marfan syndrome—tall, long extremities, long fingers and toes; cardiac and other anomalies
   b. Klinefelter's syndrome—tall, slim, underweight, small testicles, gynecomastia

Endocrine Disorders
1. Congenital adrenal hyperplasia (see p. 1506)
2. Precocious puberty (see p. 1510)
3. Hyperthyroidism (see p. 1503)
4. Acromegaly—overproduction of growth hormone usually related to pituitary tumors; very rare in children (see p. 839)

Non-endocrine Disorders
1. Exogenous use of androgens (ie, testosterone injections):
   a. Although stature and growth will initially be above the normal expected for age, ultimate height will be decreased due to undue advance of bone maturation at growth plate.
   b. The child will ultimately end up shorter than genetically determined.

DISORDERS OF THE ANTERIOR PITUITARY

The anterior pituitary is under the control of the hypothalamus and secretes six specific hormones: growth hormone (GH), thyroid-stimulating hormone (TSH), adrenocorticotropic hormone (ACTH), luteinizing hormone (LH), follicle-stimulating hormone (FSH), and prolactin. GH is the only hormone that does not have a target gland to induce further hormonal secretion. Hypopituitarism is a deficiency of one, some, or all of the hormones secreted by the pituitary gland. With the exception of GH, decreased secretion results in hypofunction of the consequential target gland.

Thyroid stimulating hormone (TSH) deficiency, adrenocorticotropic hormone deficiency (ACTH), and leutenizing hormone/follicle stimulating hormone deficiency are discussed under disorders of the thyroid gland, disorders of the adrenal glands, and disorders of gonadal function, respectively.

Growth Hormone Insufficiency

Insufficient secretion of GH is caused by lack of pituitary production or hypothalamic stimulation on the pituitary. Incidence is approximately 1 in 3,500 for classic GH insufficiency and is unknown for varying degrees of insufficiency.

Pathophysiology and Etiology
1. The lack of GH impairs the body's ability to perform the following functions:

a. Protein metabolism—growth through increased protein synthesis; nitrogen, phosphorus, and potassium storage

b. Fat metabolism—increases lipolysis and oxidation of fat

c. Carbohydrate metabolism—decreases conversion of glucose to fat in adipose tissue

2. Organic etiology:
   a. Intracranial cyst
   b. Central nervous system (CNS) tumor (adenoma)
   c. Craniopharyngioma
   d. CNS irradiation
   e. Exogenous (head trauma, infection)
   f. Histiocytosis X
   g. Septo-optic dysplasia (abnormal forebrain development)

3. Idiopathic causes:
   a. Isolated GH deficiency
   b. Traumatic birth or breech delivery
   c. Genetic (GH gene deletion)
   d. Aplasia

4. Genetic cause—Turner syndrome:
   a. The pituitary and hypothalamus are not abnormal in Turner syndrome, and growth hormone secretion measurement is usually normal; however, growth hormone is bioinactive due to binding problems.
   b. Hypothyroidism is common with Turner syndrome.
   c. Growth rate usually declines within the first year of life.
   d. Treatment with growth hormone is a commonly accepted therapy to restore growth.

Clinical Manifestations

1. Hypoglycemia (usually in the newborn)
2. Growth velocity usually less than the 5th percentile for chronologic age
3. Delayed skeletal maturation—bone age at least 1 year delayed from chronologic age
4. "Pudgy" when the weight age (50% for weight) exceeds the height age (50% for height)
5. Frequently delayed eruption of primary and secondary teeth (not as severe as in hypothyroidism)
6. Delayed or lack of sexual development
7. In young adulthood after epiphyseal fusion, the following symptoms may develop, requiring evaluation from an adult endocrinologist:
   a. Altered body composition (increased fat mass, decreased lean body mass)
   b. Reduced aerobic exercise capacity or performance
   c. Decreased muscle strength
   d. Abnormal blood lipid (fat and cholesterol) concentrations
   e. Decreased bone mineral density or content
   f. Impaired cardiac function
   g. Impaired health-related quality of life (low energy level, decreased physical mobility, difficulties with concentration and memory, increased emotional lability, irritability, difficulty relating to others, or increased social isolation)

Diagnostic Evaluation

1. Rule out organic, non-endocrine causes of short stature (ie, chronic illness, nutritional deficiencies, genetic disorders, psychosocial factors).
2. Calculate growth velocity (does growth pattern parallel or deviate from the growth curve?).
3. Bone age assessment—ascertain age of physical development—it is usually delayed.
4. General physical examination—physical development that of a younger-appearing child?
5. If a girl, tests to rule out Turner syndrome.
6. Thyroid function tests to rule out hypothyroidism.
7. GH secretion laboratory indicators: IGF-1, IGF-binding protein 3 are decreased.
8. Subnormal secretion of GH in response to two provocative stimuli:
   a. Insulin-induced hypoglycemia
   b. Stimulatory response to arginine infusion, L-dopa, clonidine, or glucagon—all of which have specific actions resulting in GH secretion from pituitary
   c. Administration of stimulus followed by blood sample for growth hormone
9. In the newborn with hypoglycemia, GH release is reduced at time of documented hypoglycemia (concomitant GH level relative to documented hypoglycemia is abnormally low).

NURSING ALERT

In newborn with hypoglycemic episode, always draw blood for cortisol and growth hormone *before* initiating corrective action for the hypoglycemia. Early detection and diagnosis will protect child from future episodes if related to hypopituitarism.

---

10. Computed tomography (CT) scanning or magnetic resonance imaging (MRI) of head to rule out lesion etiology.

Treatment

1. Goal of treatment is to restore normal growth and development as well as to maximize growth potential and prevent hypoglycemia.
2. Replacement of deficiency uses recombinant DNA-derived GH given as subcutaneous injection.
3. Typical dose is 0.2 to 0.3 mg/kg per week divided in 3, 6 or 7 doses weekly until final height is achieved. In treatment of Turner syndrome, dose is generally 0.375 mg/kg per week divided in doses as above.
4. Therapy is being recommended for adult replacement. Depending upon the degree of insufficiency, continued treatment into adulthood may be useful. Dosing recommendations range from less than 0.006 mg/kg/day to as high as 0.0125 mg/kg/day after epiphyseal fusion has occurred.

Complications

1. Altered carbohydrate, protein, and fat metabolism
2. Hypoglycemia—seizures/death in newborns

Nursing Assessment

1. See common nursing assessment for growth and development, page 1496.
2. Obtain family history related to parental heights and ages of pubertal maturation.

Nursing Diagnoses

• Altered Growth and Development related to lack of GH
• Social Isolation related to short stature and peer acceptance
• Self-Esteem Disturbance related to discordant expectations by peers and adults

Nursing Interventions

Patient Teaching

1. Teach method of injecting GH through written and verbal instructions. Give demonstration and encourage return demonstration.
2. Encourage rotation of sites in the subcutaneous tissue of the upper arms or thighs if irritation occurs.
3. Document growth at regular intervals.
4. If poor growth response, evaluate for appropriate dose, compliance, and injection technique. There may be initial "catch-up" growth that will be exhibited by a growth velocity above normal.

 DRUG ALERT

Assess for allergic response or reaction to diluents used in reconstitution of lypholized GH preparations. Local redness or swelling may occur at injection site. Also assess for headaches (may be related to pseudotumor cerebri) and leg or hip pains (possible slipped capital femoral epiphysis).

Encouraging Social Interaction

1. Encourage the child to verbalize feelings regarding short stature.
2. Have the child describe what he or she likes about certain people to help the child understand that friendships and social value are based on personality traits rather than absolute height.
3. Suggest involvement in activities that do not use height as an advantage, such as music, art, and gymnastics.
4. Ask the child to identify behaviors that may deter socialization (may or may not be related to short stature) and find ways to change behavior.

Strengthening Self-Esteem

1. Help child and parents to identify age-appropriate behaviors and develop a plan for maintaining consistent behaviors both in the home and socially.
2. Make sure parents have realistic expectations of child.
3. Encourage the use of positive feedback rather than punishment.

Community and Home Care Considerations

1. Become familiar with the growth hormone preparation being used and develop a teaching plan for home injection (mixing and injection technique). Provide periodic evaluation and ongoing support.
2. If home injections are difficult relative to family learning or parental availability, attempt to include school nurse in administering daily injections.
3. Review storage and stability of GH product relative to manufacturer's specifications for the home as well as use in travel.

Family Education and Health Maintenance

1. Tell child and family that short stature is not a "disease." It is the symptom of growth failure.
   a. Growth catch-up to peers usually occurs when peers have stopped growing.
   b. After initial start-up of treatment, growth rate should be in the 2- to 3-inch/year rate.
   c. Treatment is not to make child tall; it is to restore normal growth that is reflected in height achievement.
2. Review medication dosage and injection technique periodically.
3. Tell family to think of GH as a replacement rather than a medication; therefore, it should always be given regardless of illness or other medication therapies.
4. Encourage regular follow-up for growth evaluation and maintenance of therapy.
5. Discuss potential life-long therapy, which may be necessary depending on the degree of insufficiency. Many hypopituitary patients require life-long replacement therapy.
6. Counseling about infertility for girl with Turner syndrome. This should be done with a genetic counselor if available.

Outcome-Based Evaluation

• The child or parent demonstrates appropriate injection technique
• Growth rate is restored to normal; 1 inch growth over past 6 month; child reports interest in school activities and playing with friends
• Parents report more positive behavior relative to self-esteem

DISORDERS OF THE POSTERIOR PITUITARY

The posterior pituitary is under the control of the hypothalamus and secretes two hormones, vasopressin (antidiuretic hormone—ADH) and oxytocin. Abnormality of ADH function is the most common disorder seen in children. The function of ADH is to conserve water at the distal tubules and collecting ducts of the kidney and to act on smooth muscle to increase blood pressure.

Diabetes Insipidus

Diabetes insipidus (DI) is failure of the body to conserve water due to a deficiency of ADH, decreased renal sensitivity to ADH, or suppression of ADH secondary to excessive ingestion of fluids (primary polydipsia).

Pathophysiology and Etiology

1. The function of water metabolism in the body is to maintain a constant plasma osmolality near the mean level of 287 mOsm/kg.
2. Intake and output of water are governed by the centers in the hypothalamus to control thirst and synthesis of ADH.
3. Thirst ensures adequate intake of water, and ADH prevents water loss through the kidney.
4. Patients with DI are unable to produce appropriate levels or action of ADH, leading to polyuria, increased plasma osmolality, and increased thirst.
5. Classified as central or nephrogenic DI:
   a. Central DI—low levels of ADH; may be congenital or acquired
      (i) Congenital causes—CNS defects, hereditary
      (ii) Acquired causes—CNS tumors, head trauma, infections, vascular disorders, idiopathic
   b. Nephrogenic DI—renal unresponsiveness to vasopressin; usually caused by chronic renal disease

Clinical Manifestations

1. Sudden onset of excessive thirst and polyuria.
2. In infants:
   a. Excessive crying—quieted with water more than milk feeding
   b. Rapid weight loss—caloric loss due to water preference over feedings
   c. Constipation
   d. Growth failure—failure to thrive
   e. Sunken fontanel with dehydration
3. In children:
   a. Excessive thirst and drinking
   b. Polyuria with nocturia and enuresis
   c. Pale, dry skin with reduced sweating

Diagnostic Evaluation

Tests document inability to produce ADH in the face of hyperosomolality of plasma.

1. Urine specific gravity, sodium, and osmolality are decreased.
2. Serum osmolality and sodium are elevated.
3. Serum measurement of ADH is low in conjunction with high plasma osmolality.
4. Water deprivation test (potentially dangerous):
   a. Fluids are restricted, and the urinary volumes and concentrations are monitored hourly along with the child's weight.
   b. Test is terminated if child loses more than 3% to 5% of body weight. Serum sodium and osmolality are measured at completion of test and are high; urine osmolality remains lower.
   c. Test is completed by giving the child a dose of ADH, which should stop the abnormal diuresis. If it does not, child may have nephrogenic DI (renal unresponsiveness).
5. Assess for underlying cause:
   a. MRI or CT scan of hypothalamic-pituitary region
   b. High incidence of associated anterior pituitary disorders

Treatment

1. Daily replacement of ADH using desmopressin (DDAVP), a synthetic analogue.
2. Available as a metered nasal spray , measured insufflation (nasal) tube, or tablets. In children with cleft lip and palate, sublingual administration has been shown to be effective.
3. Thiazide diuretics in nephrogenic DI.

Complications

1. Dehydration
2. Hypernatremia

Nursing Assessment

1. Assess children with complaints or behaviors of polyuria and polydipsia for dehydration.
2. Obtain a thorough history of symptoms and behaviors—specific attention to changes in sleep patterns (may be caused by enuresis) and choices of fluids, including sources of water (eg, does child drink from toilet bowls or dog dishes?).
3. Evaluate height and weight—assess for weight loss related to possible decrease in calories due to excessive drinking, which cuts appetite.
4. For the child on treatment, assess for hydration status. Obtain history of fluid intake and output from the parents to assess appropriate dosage, frequency, and administration of medication.

Nursing Diagnoses

- Fluid Volume Deficit related to disease process
- Altered Nutrition: Less Than Body Requirements due to fluid preference over food
- Sleep Pattern Disturbance related to nocturia and enuresis

Nursing Interventions

Regaining Fluid Balance

1. Assess for and teach parents assessment of dehydration—dry mucous membranes, weight loss, increased pulse, listlessness or irritability, sunken fontanelle in infants, fever, poor skin turgor.
2. Administer intravenous (IV) fluid as ordered if acutely dehydrated.
3. Monitor intake and output and teach parents to maintain record of fluid intake and output in child. Reduced

output may require restriction of fluids if overdosage of DDAVP is suspected.

4. Keep record of daily weights.

> **NURSING ALERT**
>
> Watch for and report signs of water intoxication due to excess free water and hyponatremia—drowsiness, listlessness, headache, confusion, anuria, weight gain. Hold DDAVP to prevent seizures, coma, and death.

5. Administer and teach proper administration of DDAVP. Proper management should eliminate symptoms.
6. Teach parents to provide free access to fluid (water) sources at all times. However, caution parents that child is unprotected from water excess.
7. Calculate rough estimated total daily fluid requirements based on body size to assess fluid replacement versus excess: 100 mL/kg for first 10 kg of body weight, 50 mL/kg for second 10 kg of body weight, 20 mL/kg for each additional kilogram.

Maintaining Adequate Nutrition
1. Ensure that adequate formula is ingested between plain water bottles.
2. For older child, provide liquid nutritional supplements.
3. Stress to parents or caregivers the importance of providing nutritional requirements with fluids to ensure meeting caloric demands for growth.
4. Consult with dietitian about need for vitamin or other supplements.
5. Monitor length and weight and developmental milestones at regular intervals.

Normalizing Sleep Pattern
1. Ensure adequate evening administration of DDAVP to prevent nighttime water craving and enuresis.
2. Suggest the use of diapers at night and plastic padding on bed to make bedwetting easier until optimum management of condition is attained.
3. Encourage easy access to fluids and toilet or commode for older child during night.

Family Education and Health Maintenance
1. Teach family insufflation method (for infants and young children):
   a. Correct dose is measured and drawn up into catheter.
   b. Catheter is inserted into patient's nostril.
   c. Parent or patient inserts other end of catheter into mouth and gently blows.
   d. Older children may be able to inhale the solution.
2. Advise that nostrils should be as clear as possible before administration of dose.
3. Advise that, if dose is thought to be swallowed, do not readminister due to potential overdosage. Split the dose into both nares if swallowing is occurring.
4. Tell family to store drug away from heat and direct light and moisture (not in bathroom).
5. Advise parents that children should wear Medic Alert bracelet for DI.

6. Tell parents that school personnel should be aware of condition and symptoms needing attention (water intoxication).
7. Advise routine follow-up; treatment may be temporary or life-long, depending on cause.

Outcome-Based Evaluation
- No signs of dehydration, intake equals output
- No weight loss, growth curve maintained
- Child sleeping through night

DISORDERS OF THE THYROID GLAND

Under hypothalamic-pituitary regulation, the thyroid gland secretes thyroxine (T4) and triiodothyronine (T3). The action of these hormones promotes cellular growth and differentiation, protein synthesis, and lipid metabolism (cholesterol turnover). Disorders of the thyroid gland are broadly classified as hypothyroidism and hyperthyroidism.

▪ Hypothyroidism
Hypothyroidism is low circulating level of thyroid hormone (T4). Congenital hypothyroidism occurs in 1 in 4,000 live births.

Pathophysiology and Etiology
1. Circulating levels of T4 are dependent on hypothalamic-pituitary stimulation (TRH/TSH) of the thyroid gland.
2. Low levels of T4 cause a rise in TSH.
3. Absent or decreased levels of T4 result in abnormal development of the CNS of the newborn.
4. In older children, hypothyroidism results in a decrease in metabolism, growth, and physical maturation.
5. Congenital causes:
   a. Thyroid agenesis or dysgenesis
   b. Hormone synthesis defect
   c. Maternal thyroid antibodies crossing placenta
   d. Iodine deficiency
   e. Drug-induced destruction (thionamides for treatment of hyperthyroidism, iodide excess)
   f. Peripheral T4 resistance
6. Acquired (postnatal) causes:
   a. Autoimmune thyroiditis (Hashimoto's disease or chronic lymphocytic thyroiditis)
   b. Radiation
   c. Surgical ablation (thyroidectomy)
   d. Antithyroid drugs
   e. Iodine deficiency
   f. Central hypothyroidism (TRH/TSH deficiency)

Clinical Manifestations
Newborn
1. Very subtle physical signs, if any
2. Markedly open posterior fontanelle

3. Prolonged physiologic jaundice
4. Feeding difficulties
5. Skin cool to touch/mottled
6. Poor muscle tone—hypotonia, umbilical hernia

After 6 Months
1. Growth failure
2. Large, protruding tongue
3. Coarse facial features
4. Poor feeding and constipation

Acquired Cases
1. Growth retardation—slow growth rate, increased weight gain
2. Lethargy—obedient, nonaggressive, somnolent
3. Cold intolerance
4. Possible poor school performance
5. Constipation

Diagnostic Evaluation

1. Neonatal screening of T4 and TSH. Elevation of TSH or a low T4 may indicate congenital hypothyroidism.
2. Thyroid nuclear scan—reduced uptake
3. Abnormal growth rate
4. Bone age x-ray; delayed
5. Blood studies:
   a. Free T4, T4, T3 resin uptake may be decreased; TSH elevated
   b. Thyroid antibodies—elevated in autoimmune thyroiditis

Treatment

1. Replacement of thyroid hormone: levothyroxine (Synthroid, Levothroid).
2. Treatment must not be delayed.
3. Therapy goal is to maintain normalcy of thyroid function tests (free T4, T4 and T3 concentrations).

Complications

1. Mental retardation in newborn who is undiagnosed or untreated
2. Short stature, growth failure, and delayed physical maturation and development in the older child

Nursing Assessment

1. Assess newborn for clinical manifestations listed above.
2. Perform behavioral assessment to include sleeping, eating, bowel patterns, level of alertness, and school performance.
3. Assess growth patterns: growth velocity (rate of growth over time), weight gain, and head circumference.

Nursing Diagnoses

- Altered Growth and Development related to effects of hypothyroidism
- Knowledge Deficit regarding hypothyroidism and its treatment

Nursing Interventions

Promoting Growth and Development
1. Administer or teach parents to administer thyroid hormone replacement daily.
2. Discourage mixing thyroid medication with liquid in bottle that may not be completely finished during a feeding; instead mix with small amount of fluid and give with dropper or syringe, or crush tablet and place in teaspoon of baby food.
3. If thyroid pill is being chewed rather than swallowed, have patient avoid brushing teeth immediately after to protect against rinsing away dose.
4. Monitor growth and developmental milestones at regular intervals.

Increasing Knowledge
1. Encourage the parents to verbalize feelings about child and the condition.
2. Educate the parents as to the importance of the therapy so child will grow and develop normally.
3. Stress that with replacement therapy, the child can participate in all usual activities.

Family Education and Health Maintenance

1. Encourage follow-up for blood studies and evaluation of neurologic development to ensure adequate treatment and prevent mental retardation.
2. Make sure the family understands that therapy is lifelong.
3. Support the parents and refer child for special testing and therapy if mental retardation is suspected.
4. Teach family the importance of avoiding overdosage of levothyroxine and of being alert for signs of overdosage (weight loss, restlessness, heat intolerance, fatigue, muscle weakness, tachycardia).

Outcome-Based Evaluation

- Growth curve and developmental milestones appropriate for age
- Parents verbalize understanding and acceptance of therapy

◼ Hyperthyroidism

Hyperthyroidism is a disorder of the thyroid gland in which a high circulating level of T4 results in abnormally increased body metabolism (thyrotoxicosis). Graves' disease is the most common cause in children, affecting 1% to 2% of school-aged children.

Pathophysiology and Etiology

1. May be caused by autoimmune process—thyrotropin receptor antibodies of a stimulating nature are produced.
   a. Graves' disease—most common cause of hyperthyroidism in children
   b. Chronic thyroiditis—Hashimoto's disease; usually short-term hyperthyroidism before developing hypothyroidism

2. Autoantibodies stimulate thyroid gland to produce and secrete T4.
3. Elevated circulating thyroid hormone increases the body's metabolic rate, causing an increase in excitability of the neuromuscular, cardiovascular, and sympathetic nervous systems.
4. May also be caused by ingestion or overdosage of thyroid medication (iatrogenic) or pituitary adenoma (TSH initiated).

Clinical Manifestations

1. Thyromegaly—enlargement of the thyroid, possibly with a bruit
2. Polyphagia with weight loss
3. Exophthalmos, proptosis, lid retraction
4. Hyperactivity—restlessness, nervousness, hand tremors, sleeping disturbances, emotional lability
5. Heat intolerance, excessive diaphoresis
6. Fatigue, muscle weakness
7. Tachycardia, wide pulse pressure
8. Tall stature, underweight for height

Diagnostic Evaluation

1. Serum thyroid function tests—elevated T4, T3 resin uptake with a suppressed TSH
2. Microsomal antibodies—positive
3. Thyroid radionuclide scan of goiter—rule out cold nodules that could indicate thyroid carcinoma

Treatment

1. Propranolol (Inderal), a β-adrenergic blocking agent, for cardiac effects.
2. Inorganic iodide preparation, such as propylthiouracil (PTU) or methimazole (Tapazole), to block release of thyroid hormone. Side affects include headache, nausea, diarrhea, skin rash, itching, jaundice, arthralgia, and rarely agranulocytosis (severe leukopenia).
3. Radioactive ablation of thyroid gland using radioiodine—preferred over thyroidectomy. This is chosen when medical management is ineffective. Results in permanent hypothyroidism that requires treatment.

Complications

1. Development of a goiter (glandular enlargement due to overstimulation)
2. Cardiac problems of tachycardia and hypertension
3. Exophthalmos—abnormal protrusion of the eyeball

Nursing Assessment

1. Perform physical assessment to include temperature, heart rate, blood pressure, height, and weight.
2. Obtain history of symptoms specific to onset and subsequent development of symptoms.
3. Elicit history of any changes in behavior, school performance, emotions, or sleep patterns.

4. Assess for presence of goiter—pain with swallowing or talking, palpation of thyroid.

Nursing Diagnoses

- Activity Intolerance related to effects of excessive metabolic activity
- Altered Nutrition: Less Than Body Requirements due to increased metabolic demand
- Sleep Pattern Disturbance related to high metabolic rate
- Fear related to radioiodine ablation of gland if therapy choice

Nursing Interventions

Improving Activity Tolerance

1. Administer and teach parents to administer medications and comply with treatment to gradually lower the metabolic rate and improve activity tolerance.
2. Assess activity tolerance periodically. Ascertain if fatigue is present at rest, with activities of daily living, or with exercise. Promote relaxation and rest between activities.
3. Avoid overactivity.

Ensuring Adequate Diet

1. Encourage high-calorie, nutritious diet to try to maintain weight.
2. Advise parents that effective treatment will lower metabolic rate and facilitate appropriate weight gain.
3. Periodically assess growth and development parameters.

Normalizing Sleep Pattern

1. Assess sleep pattern, including naps and sleeping through the night.
2. Adjust schedule to allow maximum amount of rest until sleeping through the night.
3. Allow short naps as needed.

Reducing Fear

1. Encourage parents and child to verbalize fears related to the thyroid ablation.
2. Teach them about the procedure and clear up misconceptions.
   a. Ablation is accomplished through radioactive destruction of thyroid tissue by administration of a radioactive iodine pill.
   b. The thyroid gland is the only tissue in the body that absorbs iodine; therefore, the radiation only destroys thyroid tissue.
   c. Radiation will be eliminated through the child's urine and feces; precautions for disposal must be followed according to nuclear medicine department policies.
3. Tell them that the resultant effect will most likely be hypothyroidism, which can be managed with life-long treatment of T4 replacement.

Family Education and Health Maintenance

1. Review prescribed medications and their function. Stress the importance of compliance.
2. Advise about periodic blood testing and monitoring for side effects of antithyroid medication.

DRUG ALERT

Antihyperthyroid medications may cause agranulocytosis (severe leukopenia), thrombocytopenia, and aplastic anemia. Periodic blood testing is necessary to monitor blood counts. Agranulocytosis may present with sore throat and fever. Drug should be discontinued immediately and health care provider notified.

3. Educate family about possibility of oversuppression, from which hypothyroidism could develop.
4. If mid-day dose of medication is necessary, have family contact school nurse to coordinate dosing.
5. If gland is radioactively ablated, be certain family and other caregivers are appropriately instructed on storage and disposal of human waste after ablative therapy.
6. Encourage follow-up to monitor treatment through blood tests, growth and development evaluation, and size of thyroid gland.

Outcome-Based Evaluation
- The child can play normally without early fatigue
- No weight loss noted
- The child displays normal sleep patterns both through the night as well as naps
- Parents and child verbalize understanding of radiation procedure and its rationale

DISORDERS OF CALCIUM METABOLISM

Calcium and phosphorus homeostasis depends on the function of parathyroid hormone (PTH) and vitamin D.

Parathyroid hormone is secreted by the parathyroid glands primarily for regulation of calcium. The target tissues are bone for mobilization of calcium and phosphorus and kidney for excretion of phosphorus and reabsorption of calcium.

Vitamin D is absorbed from the intestine or produced in the skin through sunlight ultraviolet photochemical conversion, primarily for regulation of phosphorus. Target tissues are the intestine for absorption of calcium from the diet, bone for normal growth and mineralization via incorporation of intestinal calcium into bone matrix, and kidney for absorption of phosphorus and inverse regulation of calcium.

Disorders of calcium metabolism are caused by dysfunction of the parathyroid glands or a target organ. Hypoparathyroidism is impaired synthesis and secretion of PTH or target organ resistance to the effects of PTH (pseudohypoparathyroidism). Management is similar to that of adults (see p. 829). Hyperparathyroidism is overactivity of the parathyroid glands resulting in excess secretion of PTH. Management is similar to that of adults (see p. 827).

Rickets

Rickets is undermineralization of the cartilaginous epiphyseal growth plate and reduction in mineralization of bone (osteomalacia) due to vitamin D deficiency.

Pathophysiology and Etiology
1. Reduced serum phosphate concentration due to either vitamin D deficiency or renal wasting.
2. Results in lower than needed optimal mineralization for bone development.
3. Lack of vitamin D impairs function of PTH at bone.
4. Vitamin D deficiency may be caused by:
   a. Nutritional deprivation/malabsorption
   b. Inadequate sun exposure
   c. Anticonvulsant therapy that causes increased hepatic elimination of vitamin D
   d. Renal disease
5. Hypophosphatemic rickets may be caused by:
   a. Proximal renal tubular phosphate wasting (primary hypophosphatemic rickets)
   b. Fibrous tumors or dysplasias of bone
   c. Fanconi syndrome—complex proximal renal tubular dysfunction
6. Other causes include distal renal tubular acidosis, end-organ resistance to vitamin D, and decreased synthesis of vitamin to metabolites.

Clinical Manifestations
1. Development of osseous manifestations: proliferation of uncalcified cartilage, frontal bossing, thickening of the wrist, palpable swelling of the costochondral junction (rachitic rosary), bowing of the legs (genu varum)
2. Walking problem in toddlers
3. Latent signs of hypocalcemia if severe enough

Diagnostic Evaluation
1. Growth evaluation
2. Reduced serum phosphate concentration
3. Irregular mineralization on x-ray

Treatment
1. Primary hypophosphatemia:
   a. Phosphate supplementation (Neutra-Phos, Neutra-Phos-K, or K-Phos)
   b. Active vitamin D metabolite, calcitriol (Rocaltrol)
2. Vitamin D deficiency:
   a. Vitamin D or one of the metabolites with varying doses, depending on the condition

 DRUG ALERT

Phosphorus replacement frequently causes severe gastric upset. Different preparations may be tried if child is having difficulty tolerating current therapy.

Complications

1. Hypocalcemia
2. Secondary hyperparathyroidism
3. Hypophosphatemia

Nursing Assessment

1. Assess growth and development—important to include measurement of head circumference.

NURSING ALERT

If child has leg bowing, standing heights may exaggerate bowing and thus decrease absolute height. Recumbent measurements may be more accurate, even in the older child.

2. Determine familial history of rickets.
3. Assess dietary habits, sun exposure, medication history, and chronic disease such as renal disease.
4. Assess for rachitic deformities, leg bowing, flaring of wrists, frontal bossing.

Nursing Diagnoses

• Impaired Physical Mobility related to skeletal deformities
• Noncompliance related to difficult dosage schedule for phosphorus
• Diarrhea related to phosphorus replacement

Nursing Interventions
Promoting Mobility

1. Along with growth and developmental evaluation, assess walking ability in young child at regular intervals.
2. Encourage referral for orthopedic evaluation and bracing if bowing is severe or interferes with functional ability.
3. Stress to parents and child the importance of investing in their therapy now to prevent future leg and mobility problems. Encourage and support a child in braces.
4. Share with parents the x-ray findings of the skeletal deformities—specifically the "roughened" epiphyseal plates and the correction, if present, due to their therapeutic management at home.

Improving Compliance

1. Teach the family about the physiology of bone growth and maturation with respect to phosphorus, calcium, and vitamin D, and explain the chronicity of the condition.
2. Stress to caregivers that early growth and bone formation are critical in the young child. Constantly reinforce that treatment is prevention.
3. Suggest use of school nurse to administer mid-day dose if needed.

Controlling Diarrhea

1. Advise family that phosphorus replacement upsets gastrointestinal function. Stress need to give medication with food.
2. Assess frequency and consistency of stools. Assess for dehydration, indicating inadequate fluid replacement.
3. Suggest alternative supplementation if diarrhea persists.

Family Education and Health Maintenance

1. Continue to stress that focused, consistent treatment with respect to the medication replacement will prevent future skeletal problems.
2. Encourage follow-up to evaluate bone growth and proper development.
3. Advise parents that treatment is usually life-long, with close follow-up through the growth years.
4. If vitamin D is given, teach parents to watch for signs of vitamin D toxicity—bone pain, weakness.

Outcome-Based Evaluation

• Child can walk effectively with leg braces
• Parents report compliance with medication
• Loose, formed stools no more than 3 times a day

DISORDERS OF THE ADRENAL GLANDS

The adrenal glands are responsible for the life-sustaining production of mineralocorticoids (aldosterone) for sodium retention, glucocorticoids (cortisol) for blood glucose regulation, and androgens (DHEA, androstenedione) for phallic and secondary sex characteristic development (adrenarchy).

Adrenocortical insufficiency is the inability of the adrenal gland to produce aldosterone and cortisol due to adrenal failure or lack of adrenal stimulation. With the exception of congenital adrenal hyperplasia (discussed below), pediatric adrenocortical insufficiency is similar in adults (see p. 834).

Hyperadrenalism, although rare in children, does occur, causing tissue to be exposed to excessive glucocorticoids (cortisol). This is commonly called Cushing's syndrome. Additionally, hyperfunction of the adrenal medulla, in which epinephrine, norepinephrine, and other catecholamines are secreted, is commonly seen in the disorder of pheochromocytoma. See pages 832 and 836 for a discussion of these conditions.

Congenital Adrenal Hyperplasia

Congenital adrenal hyperplasia (CAH) is the most common type of adrenocortical insufficiency in children. Adrenal dysfunction is a result of an enzyme deficiency in the steroid pathway to aldosterone, cortisol, or androgen production. The most common form of the condition is life threatening and requires diagnosis and treatment soon after birth.

Pathophysiology and Etiology

1. Production of adrenal mineralocorticoids and glucocorticoids is blocked by an enzyme deficiency in the steroid pathway. "Blocks" may be severe or partial.
   a. Deficiency of 21-hydroxylase (90%–95% of CAH cases)—insufficiency in cortisol and usually aldosterone production

b. Deficiency of 11-β-hydroxylase (5%–8%)—insufficiency of cortisol and aldosterone; however, precursor block to aldosterone is a potent mineralocorticoid.

c. Deficiency of 3-β-hydroxysteroid dehydrogenase (5%)—insufficiency in cortisol, aldosterone, and androgen production

2. Due to lack of feedback suppression, ACTH and renin are secreted to stimulate adrenal gland production, causing hyperplasia of the gland.

3. Aldosterone insufficiency results in fluid and electrolyte imbalance.

   a. Loss of sodium at the kidney results in loss of fluid and an increase in serum potassium (cation exchange).

   b. Depletion of extracellular fluid leads to decreased blood pressure.

   c. Low blood pressure stimulates renin in the kidney to activate the adrenal aldosterone pathway.

4. Cortisol insufficiency results in diminished hepatic gluconeogenesis and tissue glucose uptake.

   a. Diminished production/secretion results in low blood sugar levels—more pronounced in times of stress.

   b. Low blood sugar, stress, or low cortisol stimulates feedback to hypothalamic-pituitary axis to release ACTH to stimulate adrenal activity, which also stimulates the release of melanocyte-stimulating hormone (MSH).

   c. Constant ACTH stimulation of gland causes overproduction and "backup" of blocked steroid pathways, resulting in "spillover" production of adrenal androgens.

5. Depending on etiology, overproduction of androgens will virilize female external genitalia or underproduction of androgens will block virilization of male external genitalia.

Clinical Manifestations

1. Ambiguous female genitalia—varying degrees of virilization due to exposure of androgens during development in utero:

   a. Clitoromegaly (may be penile shaped)

   b. Labial fusion (partial or complete)

   c. Rugated labia appearing scrotal

   d. Vagina may be incomplete, ending in a blind pouch

2. Ambiguous male genitalia (3-β-dehydrogenase)—incomplete virilization development of external genitalia:

   a. Small phallic development

   b. Incomplete scrotal fusion

3. Hyperpigmentation (due to MSH secretion)

4. Dehydration

5. Vomiting/poor feeding

6. Shock

7. Latent signs—basal cortisol levels are normal due to compensated chronic ACTH stimulation:

   a. Weakness, fatigue

   b. Anorexia, nausea, diarrhea

   c. Weight loss (failure to thrive)

   d. Hyperpigmentation—no bathing suit lines

   e. Hypotension/postural dizziness

   f. Rapid growth rate—adrenal androgen effect

   g. Premature adrenarche—pubic hair, axillary hair, acne, body odor

Diagnostic Evaluation

Newborns

1. Pelvic ultrasound for identification of uterus, ovaries, or testes to determine true sex (internal development of gender-specific organs depends on presence or absence of Y chromosomal activity; external genital development depends on the presence or absence of androgens)

2. Karyotyping

3. Serum electrolytes—sodium depletion

4. Serum glucose levels—hypoglycemia

5. Serum 17-hydroxyprogesterone (most common precursor to 21-hydroxylase)—elevated

Latent Diagnosis

1. Rapid growth velocity, premature adrenarche

2. Advanced bone age x-ray for chronologic age

3. Elevated serum 17-hydroxyprogesterone

4. Elevated plasma renin activity—compensated prevention of salt loss

Treatment

1. Glucocorticoid replacement—physiologic production of cortisol is 15 to 20 mg/m^2 per day. Doses are individually dependent. Replacement is with hydrocortisone (Cortef) twice or three times a day or prednisone (Orasone) once daily when final growth has been achieved.

2. Mineralocorticoid replacement—aldosterone is replaced with fludrocortisone (Florinef) tablets at 0.05 to 0.20 mg daily.

> ◆ **DRUG ALERT**
>
> Overdosage of chronic corticosteroid use will result in growth failure. If child fails to grow and exhibits excessive hunger, corticosteroid dosing should be reviewed.

3. Added salt to the diet of newborns if salt loss is severe.

4. Surgical correction of ambiguous genitalia—can require multiple corrections over time.

Complications

1. Aldosterone insufficiency:

   a. Hyponatremia, hyperkalemia

   b. Hypotension

   c. Shock

   d. Hypertension in 11-β-hydroxylase insufficiency where aldosterone precursor is potent mineralocorticoid

2. Cortisol insufficiency—hypoglycemia

Nursing Assessment

Newborns

1. Assess genitalia for ambiguity.

NURSING ALERT

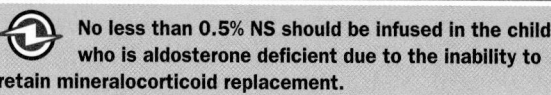 In male-appearing genitals, at least one testis must be palpated; if not, assumption must be that child is female with severe virilization. Notify health care provider so diagnostic evaluation can be initiated.

---

2. Assess for signs of hypoglycemia, hyponatremia, and hyperkalemia (Table 50-2).
3. Assess feeding pattern of newborn.
4. Look for hyperpigmentation—may be subjective.

Latent Diagnosis or Child on Treatment
1. Assess growth and development.
2. Monitor vital signs; include sitting and recumbent blood pressure for orthostatic changes.
3. Assess skin for hyperpigmentation.
4. Obtain history to include level of activity/fatigue, dietary history, salt craving, behavior, and school performance.

Nursing Diagnoses
- Fatigue related to hypoglycemia and electrolytic imbalances
- Risk for Fluid Volume Deficit related to aldosterone deficiency
- Risk for Injury related to stress and deficiency of corticosteroids
- Anxiety of parents related to gender, sexual ambiguity, and chronic illness

Nursing Interventions
Minimizing Fatigue
1. Administer glucocorticoids and emphasize compliance to increase energy level.
2. Encourage frequent rest periods and prevent overactivity.
3. Assess activity tolerance to determine adequacy of replacement therapy.
4. Tell family that child's activity level as well as growth rate should be normalized on therapy. If growth rate is too high, review corticosteroid dose and compliance with family. If growth rate is too low, overdosage of corticosteroid should be suspected. Review dosing with family.

Maintaining Fluid Balance
1. Assess for fluid status and review history of fluid intake and output for appropriate volumes. Assess hydration status of child.
2. If child is vomiting and unable to take oral fluids and mineralocorticoids, administer IV fluids. Start with D5NS and monitor serum sodium level.

NURSING ALERT

No less than 0.5% NS should be infused in the child who is aldosterone deficient due to the inability to retain mineralocorticoid replacement.

---

3. Emphasize compliance with mineralocorticoid replacement.

Preventing Acute Adrenocortical Insufficiency
1. Identify times of stress, such as acute infections, surgical procedures, or extreme emotional stress, that require increased corticosteroid replacement.
2. Teach the parents how to use and give intramuscular injection of hydrocortisone (Solucortef) for stress management when oral supplementation is not possible due to vomiting.
3. Ensure that child is evaluated by the primary care provider and treated for the cause of stress.

Reducing Anxiety
1. Encourage parents to verbalize feelings regarding diagnosis, gender decisions or changes, and treatment plans.
2. Explain to the parents that the ambiguity is a result of the development process not being completed, rather than being a "mistake."

Family Education and Health Maintenance
1. Stress and reinforce the function of and need for constant replacement of adrenal steroid therapy to maintain normal daily activities.
2. Encourage parents to obtain a Medic Alert bracelet, which indicates steroid dependency, for the child.
3. Facilitate instructions to school nurse to notify parents and health care provider of signs of illness and for emergency injection of hydrocortisone should it become necessary.
4. Explain to parents and child why pubic hair may be developing and encourage discussion with teachers, etc., to prevent embarrassment of child in the locker room and other situations.

Outcome-Based Evaluation
- Parents report child is more active
- No signs of dehydration
- Parents verbalize understanding when to call health care provider or when to use emergency hydrocortisone in-

---

TABLE 50-2   Manifestations of Hyponatremia and Hyperkalemia

Hyponatremia	Hyperkalemia
Caused by dilution of Na when water intake exceeds output. Signs and symptoms occur when Na level falls below 120 mEq/L. Gradual fall: anorexia, apathy, mild nausea and vomiting Rapid fall: headache, mental confusion, muscular irritability, delirium, convulsions	Caused by a shift of K out of cells to compensate for decreased Na caused by an oliguric state. Usually asymptomatic except for ECG changes. ECG characteristics: (progressive) shortened QT interval tall, peaked T waves, ventricular arrhythmias, degeneration of QRS complex, ventricular asystole or fibrillation

jection; parents also demonstrate correct technique for hydrocortisone injection
- Parents verbalize understanding of disorder and need for reconstructive surgery

DISORDERS OF GONADAL FUNCTION

Proper gonadal function is necessary for developing sexual maturation (puberty). The process involves the hypothalamic release of gonadotropin-releasing hormone (GnRH), which in turn stimulates the pituitary to release LH and FSH. In turn, these stimulate the gonads to produce and release the gonadal steroid of testosterone from the testes in males or estrogen from the ovaries in females. The actions of these steroids lead to the development of secondary sexual characteristics and maturation.

Delayed Sexual Development

Delayed sexual development is the lack of pubertal development or progression.

Pathophysiology and Etiology

1. Lack of production or secretion of gonadal steroids from the testes (testosterone) or ovaries (estrogen), due either to the lack of pituitary stimulation (secondary delayed sexual development) or to gonad dysfunction (primary delayed sexual development).
2. Primary delayed sexual development—absence or dysfunction of the gonads.
   a. 45 XO Turner syndrome (chromosomal variants)
   b. Sporadic gonadal dysgenesis
   c. Bilateral gonadal failure due to radiation, chemotherapy, infection, defect in gonadal steroid synthesis, trauma
3. Secondary delayed sexual development—lack of hypothalamic-pituitary stimulation to gonads.
   a. Hypothalamic lesions due to infections, trauma, irradiation, or isolated deficiency of GnRH (Kallmann's syndrome)
   b. Pituitary lesions due to infection, trauma, or irradiation; also hypopituitarism or isolated LH and FSH deficiencies
4. Failure of end organs to respond to circulating gonadal steroid—androgen insensitivity.
5. Other causes include chronic illness, anorexia nervosa, and autoimmune atrophy.
6. Resultant effect is failure to achieve sexual maturity.

Clinical Manifestations

1. Females—lack of breast development by age 13 to 13.5 years or failure to progress through puberty
2. Males—lack of testicular enlargement by age 13.5 to 14 years or failure to progress through puberty
3. Emotional lability

Diagnostic Evaluation

1. Bone age x-ray to determine physical age—pubertal delay is not consistent with bone age
2. Laboratory measurement of sex steroids (testosterone and estrogen) and gonadotropins (LH, FSH)
   a. Gonadal failure will show elevated LH and FSH with low estrogen.
   b. No good test is available to distinguish isolated gonadotropin deficiency (LH or FSH).
   c. End organ insensitivity (lack of gonadal steroid receptor)—both sex steroid and gonadotropins will be elevated. Hypothalamic receptors for feedback inhibition are the same as the end organ receptors; therefore, there is no hypothalamic "shut-off."
4. Abdominal ultrasound to view internal organ structure and development

Treatment

1. Replacement of gonadal steroid—should be as close to the physiologic level as possible; however, maximal adult height may be compromised due to potential side effect of acceleration of skeletal maturation.
   a. Boys—testosterone supplement; 50 to 100 mg monthly by injection until final height is achieved, then 200 mg monthly
   b. Girls—conjugated estrogen (Premarin); 0.3 to 0.625 mg daily by oral tablet. When appropriate, a progestational agent is added to the therapy for normal periods to occur. An alternative is the use of birth control pills that have the combination of estrogen and progesterone.
2. There is no pituitary or hypothalamic agent for use in secondary gonadal failure.

Complications

1. Sterility
2. Ambiguity—in androgen insensitivity, male genital development does not respond to circulating level of testosterone from testes; may result in mistaken gender assignment.
3. Potential for dysfunctional dormant gonad to become malignant

Nursing Assessment

1. Assess growth and development, particularly height.
2. Assess sexual development at regular intervals.

Nursing Diagnoses

- Altered Growth and Development related to lack of sexual development
- Body Image Disturbance related to delayed sexual maturation
- Self-Esteem Disturbance related to delayed sexual maturation

Nursing Interventions
Promoting Sexual Development
1. Administer or teach self-administration of medication as prescribed.
2. Teach technique for intramuscular injections of testosterone enanthate (Testone LA). Watch return demonstration.
3. Stress compliance with prescribed dose and not to exceed recommended dose. Excessive use of testosterone will stunt potential statural growth.

Improving Body Image
1. Discuss strategies for improving appearance through hair style, clothing, makeup, and minimizing delay in sex characteristics.
2. Stress the importance of cautious therapy to prevent loss of potential height, therefore making sexual development a slow process.

Improving Self-Esteem
1. Encourage child to discuss self-concept; list positive and negative characteristics.
2. Explore ways to strengthen and add to positive characteristics.
3. Encourage participation in age-appropriate activities and social functions.

Family Education and Health Maintenance
1. Teach the patient about side effects of testosterone replacement—possible behavioral changes (aggressiveness, moodiness) and an increase in acne.
   a. Suggest over-the-counter acne products or referral to dermatologist if indicated.
   b. Alert family to report behavioral changes to the health care provider.
2. Teach the patient taking estrogen replacement the importance of daily compliance. Missed doses could result in breakthrough bleeding/spotting due to drop in circulatory estrogen levels. Alert patient to notify health care provider if spotting does occur with estrogen replacement.
3. In both treatments, stress to child not to exceed prescribed dose to prevent loss of final adult height.

Outcome-Based Evaluation
- At follow-up visit, there is an increase in height and progression of sexual development
- Child verbalizing improved feelings of body image
- Child lists more positive concepts of self

■ Advanced Sexual Development and Precocious Puberty

Advanced sexual development is secondary sexual development earlier than the normal timing for a child's maturation. There is abnormal early production and secretion of the gonadal steroids or adrenal androgens. Normal pubertal development occurs abnormally early. Skeletal maturation is also advanced under presence of sex steroids and adrenal androgens.

Pathophysiology and Etiology
Central Precocious Puberty (CPP)
1. Early activation of the hypothalamic-pituitary gonadotropin axis
2. May be idiopathic or caused by:
   a. Tumors of hypothalamus/pituitary
   b. Cranial irradiation
   c. Trauma
   d. Infection—meningitis
   e. Hydrocephalus
3. Most common form of precocious puberty

Peripheral Precocious Puberty (PPP)
1. Sex hormone production at the glandular level independent of central stimulation
2. Ovarian PPP caused by estrogen-producing tumors or cysts
3. Testicular PPP caused by androgen- and estrogen-producing tumors or autonomous production of testosterone
4. Adrenal PPP caused by enzyme defects (CAH) or androgen- and estrogen-producing tumors

Other Causes
1. Hypothyroidism
2. Exogenous estrogen or androgen exposure

Clinical Manifestations
1. Boys:
   a. Testicular enlargement (4 mL): under age 8.5 years
   b. Tanner stage II pubic hair: under age 9.0 years
   c. Tanner stage III pubic hair: under age 10.0 years
2. Girls:
   a. Breast bud (stage II): under age 8.0 years
   b. Tanner stage III pubic hair: under age 8.5 years
   c. Menarche: under age 9.5 years
3. In both sexes, rapid growth (increased growth velocity) is evident.

Diagnostic Evaluation
1. Physical assessment: Tanner staging:
   a. If adrenarche is present without thelarche (breast development) or testicular enlargement, adrenal cause is likely.
   b. In girls, if thelarche is only present, ovarian or exogenous estrogen involvement is likely.
   c. If both adrenarche and pubarche (gonadal signs) are present, central cause is likely.
2. Skeletal x-ray for bone age—usually advanced. Pubertal stage development is often commensurate with bone age maturation.
3. Laboratory analysis:
   a. Gonadal steroids—may be elevated; however, secretion is diurnal early in development.
   b. Elevated gonadotropins to GnRH (Factrel) stimulation if CPP. Basal levels are frequently unreliable. Lack of elevation of gonadotropins may indicate peripheral source.
   c. Thyroid function to rule out hypothyroidism.

4. MRI and CT of head to rule out central etiology.
5. Ultrasound of abdomen, pelvis, testes for presence of cysts or tumors.

Treatment

For CPP, most common form of advanced sexual development in children.
1. Goal is to inhibit puberty to preserve psychosocial well-being and to delay epiphyseal closure to maximize adult height.
2. GnRH agonist—down-regulates GnRH receptors of the pituitary against endogenous GnRH
   a. Nafarelin (Synarel)—intranasal spray, twice daily
   b. Leuprolide (Lupron)—daily subcutaneous injection
   c. Depot-leuprolide (Lupron Depot, Lupron Depot-Ped)—monthly intramuscular injection
   d. Histrelin (Supprelin)—subcutaneous daily injection

 DRUG ALERT

Intramuscular injections of Lupron have had rare reports of sterile abscesses. The site should not be reused and the health care provider notified immediately if abscess occurs.

3. Progestins
   a. Medroxyprogesterone injections (Depo-Provera)—biweekly intramuscular injections
   b. Medroxyprogesterone tablets (Cycrin)—oral daily dosing

Complications

1. Complications of underlying tumor
2. Behavioral problems
3. Short stature for final height due to early epiphyseal closure

Nursing Assessment

1. Assess sexual development using Tanner scale.
2. Obtain history of when signs and symptoms began with specific attention to chronology of events.
3. Perform psychosocial assessment relative to peer relations.
4. While child is on treatment, perform ongoing assessment of height and sexual characteristics.

Nursing Diagnoses

- Body Image Disturbance related to early presence of secondary sexual characteristics
- Knowledge Deficit regarding maturing body and sexuality
- Personal Identity Disturbance due to societal height expectations versus appropriate age-related expectations

Nursing Interventions

Fostering Positive Body Image

1. Encourage the child to verbalize concerns regarding body development changes.

2. Stress to child that the changes are normal events that peers will go through; however, they are occurring abnormally early.
3. Teach the child that therapy will halt the process and soon peers will catch up.

Reducing Fear

1. Assist and encourage parents to teach the child about sexual development to reduce fear of the unknown.
2. Encourage proper hygiene practices for body odor, hair growth, and menses.
3. Teach administration techniques for medication treatment, including intranasal, intramuscular, or subcutaneous administration as indicated.
4. In GnRH-agonist treatment in girls, instruct child and parents that it takes 10 to 12 days to fully down-regulate the pituitary receptors. The suppression results in a fall of estrogen and may cause breakthrough bleeding or even a period to occur. This will only happen once if child remains suppressed on therapy.

Promoting Sense of Identity

1. Encourage the child and parents to discuss normal age-related behaviors and identify inappropriate behaviors that are associated with society's expectations of advanced height and development.
2. Encourage the child to wear age-appropriate clothing, participate in age-appropriate activities, and socialize with peers.
3. Suggest counseling as needed.

Family Education and Health Maintenance

1. Encourage follow-up at regular intervals while on treatment and, if condition is not treated, to monitor progress and address behavioral issues.
2. Discuss with parents that child may act out relative to advancing pubertal development (this may include masturbation). This behavior needs to be dealt with in an understanding way, not necessarily through punishment.
3. Encourage parents to meet with school personnel regarding potential embarrassment in a locker room situation; alternatives to changing clothes in front of peers may be necessary.
4. Prepare family for the start of menstruation if puberty is advanced. The school nurse may need to assist with feminine hygiene during the cycle. Parents may need to meet with the nurse to plan for assistance during school days.
5. Teach family to inspect injection sites and notify health care provider immediately upon noticing a hard, painful, reddened area, which may be a sterile abscess from Lupron injections and require treatment.
6. Teach family to maintain strict adherence to hormonal therapy. Failure to maintain suppression of gonadotropins can result in relative rise in estrogen. Subsequent suppression may cause breakthrough bleeding.

Outcome-Based Evaluation
- Child accepts body changes through verbalization at follow-up visits
- Parents and/or child gives adequate return demonstration of intramuscular injection; verbalizes understanding of sexual development
- Child participates in school activities and socializes with peers of same age

DISORDERS OF THE PANCREAS

The pancreas manufactures powerful enzymes for digestion as well as the hormones insulin and glucagon. These hormones are manufactured and secreted from cell clusters called the islets of Langerhans. Both glucagon and insulin regulate the amount of sugar that is present in the bloodstream. Glucagon is a potent counter-regulatory hormone that raises the blood sugar by fostering the release of glucose from stores in the liver. Insulin stimulates glucose uptake by peripheral tissues, inhibits lipolysis, and inhibits hepatic glucose production.

Type 1 Diabetes Mellitus
Diabetes mellitus (DM) is a disorder of glucose intolerance caused by a deficiency in insulin production and action, resulting in hyperglycemia and abnormal carbohydrate, protein, and fat metabolism. In pediatrics, particularly younger and school-aged children, most cases are type 1, formerly called juvenile onset or insulin-dependent diabetes mellitus (IDDM). Type 1 DM affects as many as 1 in 500 children.

Type 2 diabetes mellitus (formerly called adult onset or non-insulin dependent diabetes mellitus [NIDDM]) was formerly found in only about 2% of cases of diabetes in children and adolescents. This is rapidly changing, and Type 2 diabetes now accounts for up to 40% of cases of diabetes diagnosed in adolescents. Etiology suggests morbid obesity, sedentary lifestyle, high caloric intake, and family history of diabetes. There is also an increased risk in African-American, Hispanic, and Native American populations. The onset of pubertal development and the insulin resistance that is characteristic of puberty may be a factor in the onset of Type 2 diabetes in susceptible adolescents. Type 2 DM is discussed on page 841.

Pathophysiology and Etiology
1. Etiology suggests genetic and environmental or acquired factors, association with certain HLA types, and abnormal immune responses, including autoimmune reactions.
2. Autoimmune destruction of the islets of Langerhans in the pancreas (which secrete insulin) results.
3. Since insulin facilitates glucose transport into cells, glucose builds up in the bloodstream, causing hyperglycemia.
4. As the kidneys attempt to lower blood glucose levels, glycosuria and polyuria result, along with electrolyte excretion.
5. Since the body cells are unable to use glucose for energy, protein and fat are broken down.
6. Fat metabolism results in a buildup of ketones and acidosis.

Clinical Manifestations
1. Rapid onset (usually over a period of a few weeks)
2. Major symptoms:
   a. Increased thirst
   b. Increased urination, enuresis
   c. Increased food ingestion
   d. Weight loss
   e. Fatigue
3. Minor symptoms:
   a. Skin infections
   b. Dry skin, poor wound healing
   c. Monilial vaginitis in adolescent girls
4. Diabetic ketoacidosis (DKA)
   a. Precomatose state:
      (i) Drowsiness
      (ii) Dryness of skin
      (iii) Cherry-red lips
      (iv) Increased respirations
      (v) Nausea
      (vi) Vomiting
      (vii) Abdominal pain
   b. Comatose state:
      (i) Extreme hyperpnea (Kussmaul breathing)
      (ii) Acetone breath
      (iii) Soft, sunken eyeballs
      (iv) Rigid abdomen
      (v) Rapid, weak pulse
      (vi) Decreased temperature
      (vii) Decreased blood pressure
   c. Circulatory collapse and renal failure may follow, resulting from the combination of lowered pH, electrolyte deficiency, and dehydration.

Diagnostic Evaluation
1. Presence of symptoms
2. Glycosuria on routine examination
3. Random blood glucose higher than 200 mg/dL
4. Ketonuria
5. Metabolic acidosis (pH less than 7.3 and bicarbonate less than 14 mEq/L)

Treatment
1. Fluid therapy in DKA—treat dehydration, increase peripheral perfusion, and replace sodium and potassium loss due to osmotic diuresis.
2. Insulin therapy—to reduce hyperglycemia and inhibit lipolysis and ketogenesis (Table 50-3).
   a. Subcutaneous insulin may be given twice a day at a dose usually of a 2:1 ratio of NPH to regular (or lispro) and a 2:1 ratio for morning to evening dose. Initially short-acting insulin is often given four times a day.

TABLE 50-3 Types of Insulin and Their Effects

Type of Insulin	Onset (hours)	Maximal Activity (hours)	Duration (hours)
Lispro (Humalog)	10–30 min	1–2	2–4
Regular	½–1	2–4	6–8
Semi-Lente	½–1	2–4	10–12
NPH	2	4–12	24
Lente	2	8–10	24
Ultralente	4–8	14–20	36

b. Dosage needs are based on the child's size, diet, and level of activity. Dosages are adjusted through daily monitoring of blood glucose levels.
c. DKA treatment—low-dose continuous IV infusion of regular insulin only (Box 50-1)
d. Insulin pump therapy, consisting of a continuous subcutaneous infusion of insulin that can be programmed to give bolus and basal rates, may be used by some children.

3. Research is ongoing to develop alternative routes for insulin administration. Most promising is intranasal insulin.
4. Balanced diet with controlled carbohydrates and adequate protein and fat to meet energy and growth requirements.

Complications
Acute
1. Usually reversible
2. Diabetic ketoacidosis (DKA) accounts for 70% of diabetes-related deaths in children under 10 years of age
3. Cerebral edema—related to treatment correction. Thought to be due to a rapid decline in blood glucose causing a fluid shift.
4. Hyperglycemia (untreated or undertreated)
5. Hypoglycemia (insulin reaction)
Subacute
1. Develops over short period of time
2. Lipohypertrophy (localized tissue build-up from giving injections in the same site)—repeated injections in the same area; can cause abnormal absorption
3. Skeletal and joint abnormalities—limited joint mobility

BOX 50-1 Treatment of Diabetic Ketoacidosis

Initiate IV Fluids
1. Start with 0.9% NS.
2. Estimate fluid deficit by amount of weight loss (1 kg [2.2 lb] equals 1 L fluid). Infuse fluids to replace one-half of estimated loss plus maintenance needs (10–20 mL/kg) over first 8–12 hours; second half plus maintenance needs over next 16–36 hours.

NURSING ALERT
Avoid infusion of hypertonic solutions because ketoacidosis is accompanied by a profound free water deficit. Replace fluids slowly to prevent rapid decline in serum osmolarity, which may precipitate cerebral edema.

3. When blood glucose falls below 250 mg/dL, change to 5% glucose in 0.45% NS.
4. Closely monitor vital signs, ECG, and intake and output, and obtain laboratory values, including urine and blood glucose, electrolytes, BUN and creatinine, serum osmolarity, arterial or venous pH, serum and urine ketones, calcium and phosphorus every 1–4 hours as condition warrants.

Administer Insulin
1. Give IV bolus of 0.1 unit/kg of regular insulin if no intermediate-acting insulin has been given in the last 6–8 hours. Lispro insulin (another short-acting insulin) may be used.
2. Provide continuous IV drip of regular insulin at rate of 0.1 unit/kg/hour.

NURSING ALERT
Flush IV tubing with insulin solution before infusion and change tubing with each bag because insulin will bind to the plastic tubing, changing concentration.

3. Continue IV insulin until metabolic acidosis is corrected (pH greater than 7.3 and bicarbonate greater than 13–15) and bowel sounds have returned and can take oral fluids.
4. When meals are tolerated, begin subcutaneous regular insulin dose of 0.25–1 unit/kg divided in four doses, before meals and at bedtime.
5. When stabilized, return to previous insulin regimen or determine twice-daily dosing of NPH and regular insulin.

Potassium and Bicarbonate Replacement
1. Initial serum K levels will be normal or high even though intracellular levels are low. Serum levels will fall as insulin therapy drives K into the cells.
2. Begin replacement of K when urine output and renal function have been established.
3. Add KCl 20–40 mEq to each liter of fluid.
4. Monitor T waves on ECG for peaking (hyperkalemia) or flattening (hypokalemia).
5. Bicarbonate administration is controversial in correcting acidosis but may be indicated for respiratory depression, decreased myocardial contractility, or refractory, severe acidosis.

(Adapted from Wheeler, M.D. [1991]. Care of the child in diabetic ketoacidosis. In *Proceedings of the 7th annual conference on pediatric critical care nursing* (pp. 210–216). Danville, CA: Contemporary Forum; and Alario, A.J. [1997]. *Practical guide to the care of the pediatric patient.* St. Louis: Mosby.)

4. Growth failure and delayed sexual maturation due to underinsulinization

Chronic

1. Very rarely seen in children
2. Retinopathy/cataracts—may cause blindness
3. Neuropathy—peripheral and autonomic
4. Nephropathy—proteinuria/renal failure
5. Cardiopathy—congestive cardiac failure

Nursing Assessment

1. Prediagnosis/treatment:
    a. Obtain history of onset of signs and symptoms of clinical manifestations.
    b. Assess for levels of dehydration and weight loss with level of appetite.
    c. Check for sores that are slow to heal.
    d. Identify any fruity smell to breath—acetone breath due to ketosis.
    e. Assess abdominal pain—may mimic appendicitis.
2. Initial diagnosis/treatment (DKA):
    a. Assess for potential cerebral edema (diminished level of consciousness) when fluid replacement is initiated.
    b. Assess cardiac function—tachycardia with dehydration, arrhythmias related to potassium imbalances.
    c. Assess renal function—urinary output with intake and output, ketonuria, glucosuria.
    d. Watch for hypoglycemia—overtreatment of insulin; glucose level correction should be slow. IV replacements frequently contain glucose to prevent large osmotic fluid shifts leading to cerebral edema.
3. During treatment/routine follow-up:
    a. Assess growth parameters—excessive weight gain may indicate overtreatment of insulin (child eats due to constant hunger). Loss or lack of weight gain may indicate underinsulinization (losing calories that are not metabolized).
    b. Review blood glucose diaries for level of control and need for insulin adjustments (check for appropriate adjustments of insulin made by parents).
    c. Obtain history of any hypoglycemic reactions—be specific to time of day, dietary record, and exercise/activity.
    d. Assess injection sites—look for signs of lipohypertrophy.
    e. Assess for signs of hyperglycemia—polyuria, polydipsia. Does child need to get up in the night to go to the bathroom?

Nursing Diagnoses

• Fluid Volume Deficit related to osmotic diuresis and vomiting
• Altered Nutrition: Less Than Body Requirements due to metabolic catabolism due to lack of insulin
• Knowledge Deficit related to insulin management
• Knowledge Deficit related to blood glucose monitoring
• Risk for Injury related to hypoglycemia

• Fear/Anxiety of child and family related to diagnosis, treatment, and management procedures

Nursing Interventions

Restoring Fluid Balance

1. Administer IV fluids as ordered.
2. Monitor intake and output, blood pressure, serum electrolyte results, and daily weights.
3. Report abnormal sodium and potassium result promptly.
4. Assess for signs of dehydration—dry skin and mucous membranes, constipation.
5. Encourage oral fluids when able.

Meeting Nutritional Requirements

1. Provide an adequate diet for the child and teach the family about the diet.
    a. The most common meal plan is one based on carbohydrate counting. This type of meal plan offers flexibility and a wide variety of choice. Total carbohydrate requirements will be calculated, then labels can be read and charts consulted to determine grams of carbohydrate per serving of food eaten.
    b. Occasionally a more rigid, strictly controlled diet is necessary.
    c. The diet should be composed of approximately 55% carbohydrate, 30% fat, and 15% protein.
        (i) Some diets are restricted in carbohydrates, saturated fats, and cholesterol and may be based on the exchange method as recommended by the American Diabetes Association.
        (ii) Approximately 70% of the carbohydrate content should be derived from complex carbohydrates such as starch.
        (iii) Foods with high fiber content should be encouraged.
        (iv) All diets must supply sufficient caloric intake for activity and growth, sufficient protein for growth, and the required vitamins and minerals.
    d. Foods are distributed throughout the day to accommodate varying peak action of insulin. Distribution may be adjusted for increased or decreased amounts of exercise.
    e. Include fluids containing sugar (sodas, juices, milk) in carbohydrate count.
2. Determine the child's usual dietary habits so that adherence to the controlled diet will be easier.
3. Include the child and parents in meal planning as soon as possible.
4. Allow the child normal activity while hospitalized so that the observed result of the dietary control will be valid. Because the child's activity level usually decreases during the hospital stay, the child and family must understand that the insulin and dietary needs will alter on discharge.
5. Allow the child to eat with other children.
6. Make certain that the child adheres to the prescribed diet and understands the rationale for it.

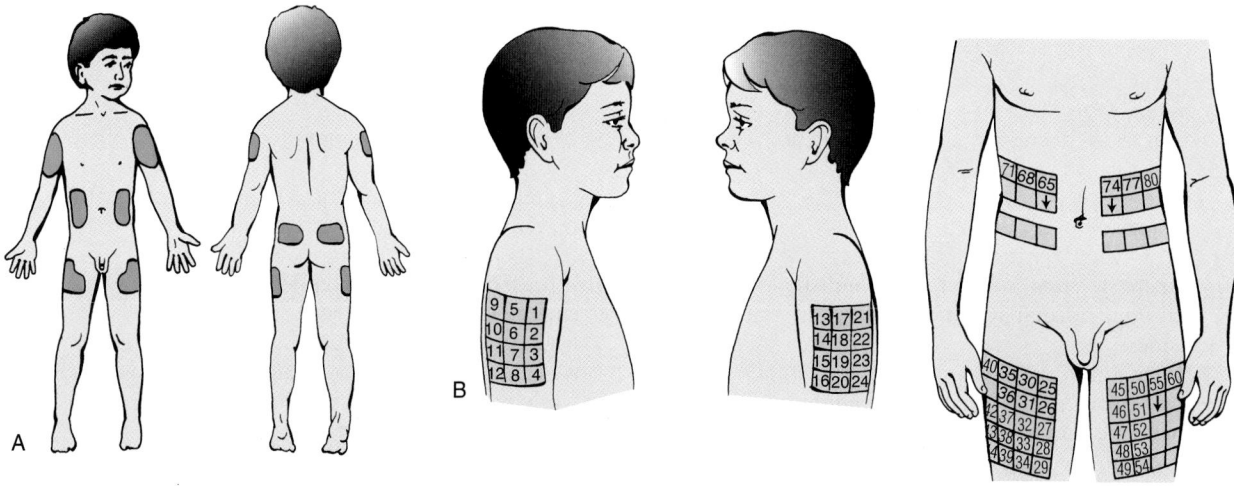

FIGURE 50-1 (**A**) Insulin injection sites are the upper outer portions of the arms, the thighs, and the abdominal area. (**B**) Injection sites are rotated, with subsequent injections given about 2.5 cm (1 inch) apart.

7. Refer family to a dietitian for additional planning and education.

Increasing Knowledge About Insulin Administration

1. Insulin should be given as directed. Lispro (Humalog) insulin begins to work immediately and should be given right before the meal. If taking regular insulin, the child should wait 20 to 30 minutes before eating.
2. Be aware of the major types of insulin and their effects.
3. Develop a systematic plan for injections that emphasizes rotation of sites (Figure 50-1).
   a. The upper arms and thighs are the most acceptable sites for injection in children, but the outer areas of the abdomen or hips may also be used.
   b. Subsequent injections are given about 2.5 cm (1 inch) apart.
   c. Guidelines for site location:
      (i) Arms—begin below the deltoid muscle and end one hand breadth above the elbow. Begin at the midline and progress outward laterally, using the external surface only.
      (ii) Thighs (Figure 50-2)—begin one hand breadth below the hip and end one hand breadth above the knee. Begin at the midline and progress outward laterally, using only the outer, anterior surface.
      (iii) Abdomen—avoid the beltline and 1 inch around the umbilicus.
      (iv) Buttocks—use the upper outer quadrant of the buttocks.
4. Be certain that the measuring scale of the syringe matches the unit strength on the bottle of insulin. U-100 insulin is preferred because it allows the smallest possible amount to be given. Other concentrations of insulin are rarely used.

5. Use insulin that is at room temperature.
   a. The bottle in use may be kept at room temperature for approximately 1 month without losing appreciable strength.
   b. Extra bottles should be stored in the refrigerator.
6. Mix the solution thoroughly by shaking the bottle (rolling may not be effective).
7. Administer insulin subcutaneously.

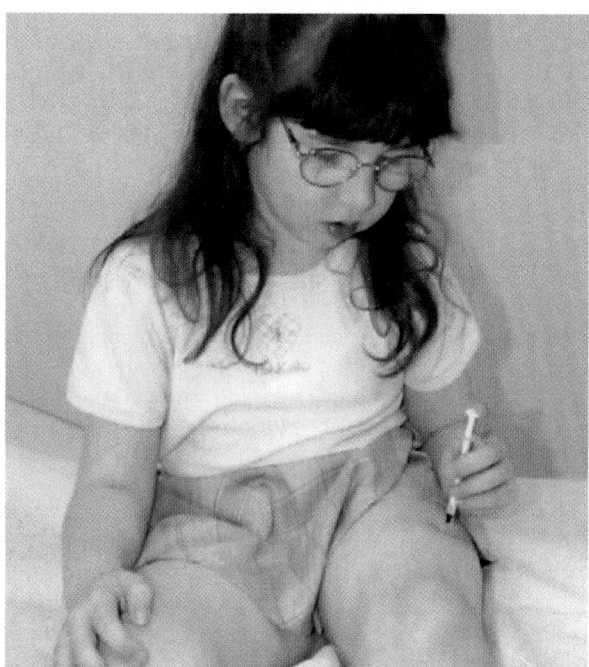

FIGURE 50-2 Insulin injection by a child.

8. Observe the skin closely for signs of irritation. Avoid the injection site for several weeks if signs of local irritation are observed.

9. Observe the skin for a rash indicating an allergic reaction to the insulin (rare with newer preparations). Notify the health care provider immediately if there is an allergic reaction.

10. Be aware of factors that vary the need for and utilization of insulin, particularly exercise and infection.
    a. Exercise tends to lower the blood sugar level. Encourage normal activity, regulated in amount and time.
    b. Infection or illness increases the child's insulin requirement (insulin is still administered during illness). Be alert for signs of infection and dehydration.

11. Encourage the child to express feelings about the injections. The child may be helped to master fear of injections by gaining control of the situation through play and active participation in the procedure.

Providing Information About
Blood Glucose Monitoring

1. Teach child and parents the chosen method for blood glucose monitoring.
2. The procedure requires a drop of blood (obtained by finger stick), a reagent strip, and a glucometer.
3. Specific instructions for performing the procedure vary with the equipment being used and must be followed explicitly.
4. Blood glucose measurements are usually made four times a day—before meals and at bedtime.
5. Additional blood tests are helpful during episodes of hypoglycemic symptoms or other problem situations.
6. Urine tests for ketones should be performed if the child is ill or if blood glucose level is greater than 240 mg/100 mL.
7. Record the results of blood glucose testing accurately.
    a. Use a standard form for recording so that the information will be clear and readily available.
    b. Help the child to understand how the disease is controlled by teaching the child to test his or her own blood, record results, and report information to health care personnel or parents.

Identifying and Controlling Hypoglycemia

1. Have glucagon available for injection if hypoglycemic reaction occurs and the child is unconscious or combative. Administer 0.5 to 1 mg intramuscularly or subcutaneously and assess response.
2. Teach family the causes, signs and symptoms, and treatment for hypoglycemia.
    a. Common causes:
        (i) Overdose of insulin
        (ii) Reduction in diet or increased exercise without sufficient caloric coverage
    b. Symptoms:
        (i) Trembling, shaking, dizziness
        (ii) Sweating, apprehension
        (iii) Tachycardia

        (iv) Hunger, weakness
        (v) Drowsiness, unusual behavior
        (vi) Mental confusion
        (vii) Seizures, coma
    c. Be prepared to give orange juice, sugar cubes, or another food containing readily available simple sugars.
3. Watch for a pattern of activity or time of day that precedes hypoglycemic reactions and work with family to alter behavior to prevent reactions.
4. If prescribed, teach the child and family how to use an emergency glucagon injection kit.
5. If glucagon cannot be given and the child is unresponsive, honey or corn syrup can be rubbed inside a cheek while positioning the child to prevent aspiration.

Reducing Fear and Anxiety

1. Explain the need and purpose of every test to child and parents. Allow child to vent feelings and cry if fearful. When appropriate, demonstrate procedures on yourself first (eg, finger sticks for glucose testing, allowing parent to give saline injection for practice of insulin injection).
2. Teach family the pathophysiology of diabetes. Understanding the disease process aids in understanding the treatment, signs, and symptoms. Assess knowledge level of teaching by having family verbalize knowledge of disease management.
3. Allow parents to verbalize feelings related to the expectations of their performance. Stress that the learning is through the actual "hands-on" management. Assist the parents in performing the needed tasks (finger sticks, insulin injections) to build their confidence. Give the parents clear objectives and directions for home management.
4. Stress that the child's condition is now the family's condition as well. Only foods appropriate for the child should be in the home.
5. Caution the parents that the focus on the child may cause sibling rivalry. Encourage involvement by all family members in making the home a healthy one and urge the parents to give individual attention to the nondiabetic children as well.
6. Explain to child that he or she did not cause the disease to occur—young children often blame themselves for "bad" things that happen to them. Help the child understand that good management is the key to participating in all usual activities. The perspective should be that he or she is a "child with diabetes," not a "diabetic child."

Community and Home Care Considerations

1. Perform home assessment for adequate nutritional resources.
2. Reteach and assess family's adherence to insulin administraton and blood glucose monitoring.
3. Reteach and assess family's ability to respond to hypoglycemia.

4. Ensure that school is able to follow through with management plan for insulin administration, planned exercise and meal times, and responding to hypoglycemia.

5. When child is ill, evaluate for dehydration, hyperglycemia, and ketonuria. Teach family how to monitor condition, maintain insulin coverage, and notify the health care provider. (See Sick Day Guidelines, p. 856.)

Family Education and Health Maintenance

Patient or parental education is one of the most important aspects in the nursing care of the child with diabetes. Thorough instruction is essential in the following areas:

1. Influence of exercise, emotional stress, and other illnesses on both insulin and diet needs

2. Recognition of the symptoms of insulin shock and diabetic acidosis and knowledge of related emergency management

3. Prevention of infection:
   a. Attend to regular body hygiene, with special attention to foot care.
   b. Report any breaks in the skin. Treat them promptly.
   c. Use only properly fitted shoes; do not wear vinyl or plastic, which do not permit ventilation. Avoid calluses and blisters.
   d. Dress the child appropriately for the weather.
   e. See that the child receives regular dental checkups and maintenance every 6 months.
   f. Follow routine immunizations according to the recommended schedule.

4. Precautionary measures:
   a. Have the child carry an identifying card that states that he or she has diabetes and includes name, address, telephone number, and health care provider's name and telephone number.
   b. Suggest a simple, convenient source of sugar that can be easily carried by the child or parents in a pocket, purse, or backpack to have available for hypoglycemic symptoms. A good example is five sugar cubes or cake decorating gel that comes is a tube, such as Cake Mate.
   c. Help the family discuss the child's disease with the school nurse and other responsible adults who are in close contact with the child (eg, teachers, Scout leaders, etc.).
   d. Advise parents that vials of insulin should be kept on one's person when traveling because baggage may be subjected to extreme temperatures and pressures incompatible with the stability of insulin. If necessary, a thermos can be used to keep the insulin at the appropriate temperature.

5. Follow up with primary care provider or pediatrician for immunizations, all regular health check-ups, and growth and development evaluations.

6. For additional information and support, refer to agencies such as American Diabetes Association, 1660 Duke Street, Alexandria, VA 22314, 1-800-676-4065, *www.diabetes.org*; and Juvenile Diabetes Foundation International, 120 Wall Street, New York, NY 10005, 1-800-JDF-CURE, *www.jdf.org*.

Outcome-Based Evaluation

- Intake equals output, blood pressure stable, sodium and potassium within normal limits
- Parents and child describe a meal plan that is followed consistently
- Child and parents demonstrate correct insulin administration technique
- Child and parents demonstrate correct glucose monitoring technique
- Child and parents verbalize causes, signs and symptoms, and treatment for hypoglycemia
- Child and parents speak openly about diabetes, ask appropriate questions, display no crying

SELECTED REFERENCES

Aarskog, D. (1991). Rickets and growth. *Growth: Genetics and Hormones, 7*(4), 1–3.

Ahern, J.A. (1997). Insulin-dependent diabetes mellitus in children. *Lippincott's Primary Care Practice, 1*(5), 555–558.

American Association of Clinical Endocrinologists (1998). Clinical practice guidelines for growth hormone use in adults and children. *Endocrine Practice, 4*, 165–173.

Alario, A. (1997). *Practical guide to the care of the pediatric patient.* St. Louis: Mosby.

August, G. P. (1993). Hypogonadism and cryptorchidism. In *A current review of pediatric endocrinology—April 28–May 2, 1993* (pp. 57–64). Norwell, MA: Serono Symposia, USA.

Boland, E. & Savoye, M. (1997). Nutritional strategies for adolescents with insulin-dependent diabetes mellitus. *Lippincott's Primary Care Practice, 1*(3), 270–284.

Carpenter, T. O. (1993). Vitamin D metabolism and phosphate homeostasis: Physiology and clinical application. In *A current review of pediatric endocrinology—April 28–May 2, 1993* (pp. 213–222). Norwell, MA: Serono Symposia, USA.

Chrousos, G. P. (1993). Adrenal insufficiency. In *A current review of pediatric endocrinology—April 28–May 2, 1993* (pp. 73–84). Norwell, MA: Serono Symposia, USA.

Clemons, R. D., Kappy, M. S., Stuart, T. E., Perelman, A. H., & Hoekstra, F. T. (1992). Long-term effectiveness of depot gonadotropin-releasing hormone analogue in the treatment of children with central precocious puberty. *American Journal of Diseases of Children, 147*, 653–657.

Fleming, D. R. (1999). Challenging traditional insulin injection practices. *American Journal of Nursing, 99*(2), 72–74.

Freeland, B. S. (1998). Diabetic ketoacidosis. *American Journal of Nursing, 98*(8), 52.

Glaser, N. & Jones, K. L. (1995). Non-insulin dependent diabetes diabetes in childhood. *Pediatric Research, 37*, 89A.

Glaser, N. S. (1997). Non-insulin dependent diabetes mellitus in childhood and adolescents. *Pediatric Clinics of North America, 44*, 307–337.

Howie, J. (1991). Congenital adrenal hyperplasia. In *The fourth annual conference of the Pediatric Endocrinology Nursing Society* (pp. 9–14). Norwell, MA: Serono Symposia, USA.

Jackson, D. B., & Saunders, R. B. (Eds.) (1993). *Child health nursing: A comprehensive approach to the care of children and their families.* Philadelphia: J. B. Lippincott.

Kaplan, S. L. (Ed.) (1990). *Clinical pediatric and adolescent endocrinology.* Philadelphia: W. B. Saunders.

Kappy, M. S., Blizzard, R. M., & Migeon, C. J. (Eds.). (1994). *The diagnosis and treatment of endocrine disorders in childhood and adolescence* (4th ed.). Springfield, IL: Charles C. Thomas.

Kaufman, F. R. (1998). Diabetes in children and adolescents. *Medical Clinics of North America, 82,* 721–737.

Lawson Wilkins Pediatric Endocrine Society (1995). *A current review of pediatric endocrinology.* Norwell, MA: Serano Symposia USA.

Lifshitz, F. (Ed.) (1996). *Pediatric endocrinology.* New York: Marcel Dekker.

Moore, W. V. (1993). Disorders of growth hormone secretion and action. In *A current review of pediatric endocrinology—April 28–May 2, 1993* (pp. 9–14). Norwell, MA: Serono Symposia, USA.

Pillitteri, A. (1999). *Maternal and child health nursing* (3rd ed.). Philadelphia: Lippincott Williams & Wilkins.

Pinhas-Hamiel, O., Dolan, L. M., Daniels, S. R., Standiford, D., Khoury, P. R., & Zeitler, P. (1996). Increased incidence of non-insulin dependent diabetes mellitus amoung adolescents. *Journal of Pediatrics, 128,* 608–615.

Pinhas-Hamiel, O., Dolan, L. M., & Zeitler, P. (1997). Diabetic ketoacidosis among obese African-American adolescents with NIDDM. *Diabetes Care, 20,* 484–486.

Porterfield, S. P.(1997). *Endocrine physiology.* St. Louis: Mosby-Year Book.

Rosebloom, A. L., Joe, J. R., Young, R. S., & Winter, W. E. (1999). Emerging epidemic of type 2 diabetes in youth. *Diabetes Care, 22,* 345–354.

Rosenfield, R. L. (1993). Precocious puberty. In *A current review of pediatric endocrinology—April 28–May 2, 1993* (pp. 51–56). Norwell, MA: Serono Symposia, USA.

Shalet, S. M., Toogood, A., Rahim, A.,& Brennan, B. M. D (1998). The diagnosis of growth hormone deficiency in children and adults. *Endocrine Reviews, 19*(2), 203–223.

Siberry, G. K. & Iannone, R. (Eds.) (2000). *The Harriet Lane handbook* (15th ed.). St. Louis: Mosby.

Strowig, S. (1995). Insulin therapy. *RN, 58*(6), 30–36.

Vance, M. L. (1994). Hypopituitarism. *New England Journal of Medicine, 330,* 1651–1662.

Vance, M. L. & Mauras, N. (1999). Growth hormone therapy in adults and children. *New England Journal of Medicine,* October 14, 1206–1216.

Wheeler, M. D. (1991). Care of the child in diabetic ketoacidosis. In *Proceedings of the 7th annual conference on pediatric critical care nursing.* Danville, CA: Contemporary Forums.

Pediatric Oncology

Cancer is the second leading cause of death from disease in children from 1 to 14 years of age. It affects approximately 14/100,000 children annually in the United States. The incidence of specific cancers is related to age, sex, and ethnic background.

Common types of cancer in children (in order of frequency) include leukemia, central nervous system (CNS) cancers, lymphoma, neuroblastoma, rhabdomyosarcoma, Wilms' tumor, bone cancer, and retinoblastoma. Treatment modalities include surgery, radiation, and chemotherapy, transplant, immunotherapy, and gene therapy (see Chapter 8, p. 137). See Chapter 43, p. 1301 for general nursing care of the sick or hospitalized child.

PEDIATRIC ONCOLOGY DISORDERS

Acute Lymphocytic Leukemia

Acute lymphocytic leukemia (ALL) is a primary disorder of the bone marrow in which the normal marrow elements are replaced by immature or undifferentiated blast cells. When the quantity of normal marrow is depleted below the level necessary to maintain peripheral blood elements within normal ranges, anemia, neutropenia, and thrombocytopenia occur. ALL is the most common malignancy in children, occurring in nearly 4/100,000 children younger than 15 years of age. It is more common among white children and more common in boys than in girls.

Pathophysiology and Etiology
1. The exact cause of ALL is unknown.
2. Environmental factors, such as viral agents, genetic factors, and chromosomal abnormalities, are suspected in some cases.
3. ALL results from the growth of an abnormal type of nongranular, fragile leukocyte in the blood-forming tissues, particularly in the bone marrow, spleen, and lymph nodes.
4. The abnormal lymphoblast has little cytoplasm and a round, homogeneous nucleus (Figure 51-1).
5. ALL is classified according to the cell type involved: T cell, B cell, early pre-B, and pre-B.
6. Normal bone marrow elements may be displaced or replaced in this type of leukemia.
7. The changes in the blood and bone marrow result from the accumulation of leukemic cells and from the deficiency of normal cells.
   a. Red blood cell precursors and megakaryocytes from which platelets are formed are decreased, causing anemia, prolonged and unusual bleeding, tendency to bruise easily, and petechiae.
   b. Normal white blood cells are significantly decreased, predisposing the child to infection.
   c. The bone marrow is hyperplastic, with a uniform appearance caused by leukemic cells.
8. Leukemic cells may infiltrate into lymph nodes, spleen, and liver, causing diffuse adenopathy and hepatosplenomegaly.
9. Expansion of marrow or infiltration of leukemic cells into bone causes joint pain.
10. Invasion of the CNS by leukemic cells may cause headache, vomiting, cranial nerve palsies, convulsions, coma, papilledema, and blurred or double vision.
11. Weight loss, muscle wasting, and fatigue may occur when the body cells are deprived of nutrients because of the immense metabolic needs of the proliferating leukemic cells.

Clinical Manifestations
1. Manifestations depend on the degree to which the bone marrow has been compromised and the location and extent of extramedullary infiltration.
2. Presenting symptoms:
   a. Fatigability
   b. General malaise, listlessness
   c. Persistent fever of unknown cause
   d. Recurrent infection

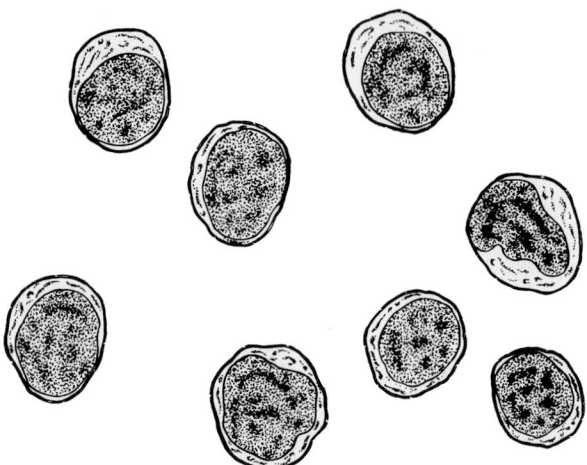

FIGURE 51-1 Abnormal lymphoblast in acute lymphocytic leukemia (ALL).

e. Petechiae, purpura, and ecchymoses after minor trauma
f. Pallor
g. Generalized lymphadenopathy
h. Abdominal pain caused by organomegaly
i. Bone and joint pain
j. Headache and vomiting (with CNS involvement)
3. Presenting symptoms may be isolated or in any combination or sequence.

Diagnostic Evaluation
1. May have altered peripheral blood counts. Blood studies may show the following:
   a. Low hemoglobin, red blood cell count, hematocrit, and platelet count
   b. Decreased, elevated, or normal white blood cell count
2. Bone marrow examination and stained peripheral smear examination show large numbers of lymphoblasts and lymphocytes.
3. Lumbar puncture determines CNS involvement.
4. Renal and liver function studies determine contraindications or precautions for chemotherapy.
5. Chest x-ray determines whether a mediastinal mass or pneumonia is present.
6. Varicella and cytomegalovirus titer determine risk of infection.

Treatment
Supportive Therapy
To control disease complications such as hyperuricemia, infection, anemia, bleeding, and pain.
Specific Therapy
To eradicate malignant cells and to restore normal marrow function.

1. Chemotherapy is used to achieve complete remission, with restoration of normal peripheral blood and physical findings.
2. No universally accepted standard therapy for the treatment of children with ALL exists, but most centers have similar protocols that use a combination of drugs.
3. Components of therapy:
   a. Induction, the initial course of therapy designed to achieve a complete remission, usually includes a combination of vincristine (Oncovin) and prednisone (Orasone). A third drug, such as 6-mercaptopurine (Purinethol), L-asparaginase (Elspar), daunorubicin (Cerubidine), doxorubicin (Adriamycin), or cytosine arabinoside (Cytosar-U), may be added.
   b. CNS prophylaxis generally consists of intrathecal administration of methotrexate (Mexate) alone or in combination with hydrocortisone (Cortef) and cytarabine (Ara-C). Craniospinal irradiation also may be used.
   c. Consolidation treatment, a period of intensified treatment immediately after remission induction, attempts total eradication of leukemic cells. It usually includes a combination of methotrexate (Mexate), 6-mercaptopurine (Purinethol), teniposide (M-26, Vumon), etoposide (VP-16, VePesid), cytosine arabinoside (Cytosar-U), cyclophosphamide (Cytoxan), prednisone (Orasone), vincristine (Oncovin), L-asparaginase (Elspar) and doxorubicin (Adriamycin) or daunorubicin (Cerubidine).
   d. Maintenance or continuation therapy prevents reappearance of the disease (usually continued for approximately 2.5 to 3 years). It usually includes daily oral administration of 6-mercaptopurine (Purinethol) and weekly oral or intramuscular administration of methotrexate (Mexate) with intermittent administration of other drugs, such as vincristine (Oncovin), prednisone (Orasone), cyclophosphamide (Cytoxan), cytosine arabinoside (Cytosar-U), or daunorubicin (Cerubidine).
   e. Reinduction therapy induces remissions if relapse occurs and usually includes the same initial drugs. Sometimes additional agents are added.

◆ DRUG ALERT

Assess patient and monitor vital signs after chemotherapy administration for signs of anaphylaxis. Have emergency drugs and equipment at the bedside (oxygen, epinephrine, antihistamines, and steroids).

   f. If testicular relapse occurs, radiation therapy to the testicles is administered.
4. An indwelling central venous catheter or an implantable port is usually inserted to administer chemotherapy.

5. Ongoing research determines the optimal method of inducing and maintaining remission with the least risk to the patient.
6. Bone marrow transplantation has been used successfully for treating children who fail to respond to conventional treatment.

Prognosis

1. At least 95% of children with ALL can be expected to achieve an initial remission if treated in a specialized center.
2. Overall cure rate is 65% to 75%.
3. The prognosis becomes poorer with each relapse the child experiences.
5. Relapse is rare after 7 years from diagnosis.
6. Factors associated with prognosis: (a) initial WBC (higher WBC has worse prognosis); (b) age (<2 and >10 have poorer prognosis with infants >1 having worse prognosis); (c) extramedullary involvement; (d) type of leukemia; (e) cytogenetic factors; and (f) immunophenotype.

Complications

1. Infection—most frequently occurs in the blood, lungs, gastrointestinal tract, or skin
2. Hemorrhage—usually caused by thrombocytopenia
3. CNS involvement
4. Bony involvement
5. Testicular involvement
6. Urate nephropathy
7. Acute complications of treatment (eg, cardiomyopathy)
8. Late effects of treatment

Nursing Assessment

1. Obtain a history.
   a. When taking the history, focus on symptoms that led to the diagnosis and previous symptoms for the past 2 weeks. For example, inquire about fatigue, headache, nausea, vomiting, pallor, bleeding, pain, or fever.
   b. Ask about past history of varicella zoster infection (chickenpox), which could lead to disseminated infection if acquired during immunosuppression.
2. Perform a physical examination, including:
   a. Examination of skin for petechiae, purpura, and ecchymoses
   b. Palpation of lymph nodes for enlargement, tenderness, and mobility
   c. Palpation of spleen and liver for enlargement
   d. Examination of fundi to detect papilledema with CNS disease
   e. Inspection of skin for areas of infection, including indwelling catheter sites
   f. Auscultation of lungs for rales or rhonchi, indicative of pneumonia
   g. Temperature for fever
3. Assess family coping mechanisms and use of resources, such as support systems.

Nursing Diagnoses

- Anxiety of parents related to learning of diagnosis
- Risk for Infection and hemorrhage related to bone marrow suppression caused by chemotherapy and disease
- Body Image Disturbance related to alopecia associated with chemotherapy
- Altered Nutrition: Less Than Body Requirements related to anemia, anorexia, nausea, vomiting, and mucosal ulceration secondary to chemotherapy or radiation
- Pain related to diagnostic procedures, progression of the disease, and side effects of treatment
- Activity Intolerance related to fatigue that results from the disease and treatment
- Anxiety of child related to hospitalization and diagnostic and treatment procedures

Nursing Interventions

Decreasing Parental Anxiety

1. Be available to the parents when they want to discuss their feelings.
2. Offer kindness, concern, consideration, and sincerity toward the child and parents; be a source of consolation.
3. Contact the family's clergyman or the hospital chaplain.
4. Obtain the services of a social worker, as appropriate, to help the family use appropriate community resources.
5. Offer hope that therapy will be effective and will prolong life.
6. Have parents speak with parents of a child currently on therapy.
7. Encourage parents to participate in activities of daily living to help them feel a part of their child's care.
8. Assess family dynamics and coping mechanisms and plan interventions accordingly.
9. Assist the parents to deal with anticipatory grief.
10. Assist the parents to deal with other family members, especially siblings and grandparents, and friends.
11. Encourage the parents to discuss concerns about limiting their child's activities, protecting child from infection, disciplining child, and having anxieties about the illness.
12. Facilitate communication with the clinic nurse or clinical specialist who may interact with the child during the entire course of illness.

Preventing Infection and Hemorrhage

1. Monitor complete blood count (CBC) as ordered.
2. Provide adequate hydration.
   a. Maintain parenteral fluid administration.
   b. Offer small amounts of oral fluids if tolerated.

3. Observe renal function carefully.
   a. Measure and record urinary output.
   b. Check specific gravity.
   c. Observe the urine for any evidence of gross bleeding.
   d. Use labsticks to determine if occult urinary bleeding is present.
4. Protect the child from sources of infection.
   a. Never use a rectal thermometer when caring for a neutropenic patient.
   b. Family, friends, personnel, and other patients who have infections should not visit or care for the child.
   c. Do not place a child with an infection in the room with a child with leukemia.
   d. Good handwashing is the most important way to control infection.
   e. Observe the child closely and be alert for signs of impending infection.
      (i) Observe broken skin or mucous membrane for signs of infection.
      (ii) Report fever more than 101°F (38.4°C).
      (iii) Assess central line site for redness or tenderness.
   e. Administer growth factors, such as granulocyte colony-stimulating factor (G-CSF), to stimulate the production of neutrophils and to decrease the incidence of severe infections in the child after intense chemotherapy.
   f. Administer intravenous (IV) antibiotics as ordered.
   g. Administer trimethoprim-sulfamethoxazole (Bactrim), if ordered, twice daily three times per week to prevent infection with *Pneumocystis carinii*.
5. Record vital signs and report any changes that may indicate hemorrhage.
   a. Tachycardia
   b. Lowered blood pressure
   c. Pallor
   d. Diaphoresis
   e. Increasing anxiety and restlessness
6. Observe for gastrointestinal bleeding and hematest all emesis and stool.
7. Move and turn the child gently because hemarthrosis may occur and may cause pain.
   a. Handle the child in a gentle manner.
   b. Turn frequently to prevent pressure sores.
   c. Place the child in proper body alignment, in a comfortable position.
   d. Allow the child to be out of bed in a chair if this position is more comfortable.
8. Avoid intramuscular (IM) injections if possible.
9. Handle catheters and drainage and suction tubes carefully to prevent mucosal bleeding.
10. Protect the child from injury by monitoring activities and environmental hazards.
11. Be aware of emergency procedures for control of bleeding:
    a. Apply local pressure carefully so as not to interfere with clot formation.

   b. Administer leukocyte-poor packed red blood cells and platelets as ordered.

Promoting Acceptance of Body Changes

1. Prepare the patient for potential changes in body image (alopecia, weight loss, muscle wasting, etc.) and help child cope with related feelings.
2. Contact the school nurse and teacher to help them prepare for the child's return to school. Discuss the bodily changes that have occurred and that may happen in the future.

Promoting Optimal Nutrition

1. Provide a highly nutritious diet as tolerated by the child.
   a. Determine the child's likes and dislikes.
   b. Offer frequent, small meals.
   c. Offer supplemental feedings high in calories and protein.
   d. Encourage the parents to assist at mealtime.
   e. Allow the child to eat with a group at a table if his or her condition allows this.
   f. Avoid foods high in salt while child is taking steroids.
2. Give careful oral hygiene; the gums and mucous membranes of the mouth may bleed easily.
   a. Use a soft toothbrush.
   b. If the child's mouth is bleeding or painful, clean the teeth and mouth with a moistened cotton swab or toothette.
   c. Use a nonirritating rinse for the mouth (no alcohol-containing mouthwash or hydrogen peroxide).
   d. Apply petroleum to cracked, dry lips.
   e. Assess for mucositis and provide appropriate mouth rinse.
3. Be alert for nausea and vomiting.
   a. Administer antiemetic drugs on a round-the-clock, regular schedule (eg, ondansetron, dexamethasone).
   b. Become knowledgeable about all chemotherapeutic agents and adjust antiemetic therapy for those drugs with delayed nausea and vomiting.
   c. Monitor strict intake and output.
   d. Maintain parental fluid administration and assess for signs of dehydration or overhydration.
   e. Administer antiemetic drugs for patients who receive radiation to the chest, abdomen, pelvis, or craniospinal axis.
   f. Suggest relaxation techniques or guided imagery for patients who experience anticipatory nausea/vomiting.

Relieving Pain

1. Position the child for comfort. Water beds and bean bag chairs are often helpful.
2. Administer medications on a preventive schedule before pain becomes intense. Continuous infusion pumps for narcotic administration are used.
3. Manipulate the environment as necessary to increase the child's comfort and to minimize unnecessary exertion.
4. Prepare the child for treatment and diagnostic procedures.
   a. Use knowledge of growth and development to prepare the child for procedures, such as bone marrow

aspirations, spinal taps, blood transfusions, and chemotherapy.

   b. Provide a means for talking about the experience. Play, storytelling, or role playing may be helpful.

   c. Convey to the child an acceptance of fears and anger.

   d. Use EMLA cream for local anesthesia at spinal tap, injection, and bone marrow sites to decrease pain.

   e. Administer conscious sedation before procedures and monitor pulse, blood pressure, respirations, and pulse oximetry during and after procedures.

Conserving Energy

1. Assess the child's energy level and space needed activities accordingly. Allow the child to rest, if necessary.
2. Encourage the child to lie down and rest after diagnostic procedures, such as bone marrows and spinal taps.

Reducing the Child's Anxiety

1. Provide for continuity of care.
2. Encourage family-centered care (see p. 1301).
3. Facilitate play activities for the child and use opportunities to communicate through play.
4. Maintain some discipline, placing calm limitations on unacceptable behavior.
5. Provide appropriate diversional activities.
6. Encourage independence and provide opportunities that allow the child to control the environment.
7. Explain the diagnosis and treatment in terms the child can understand.

Community and Home Care Considerations

1. Begin to develop a home care plan before the patient leaves the hospital.
2. Communicate with health care provider, hospital nurses, family, and others familiar with the case to gather information about the child's illness, treatment plan, and specific needs in the home.
3. Arrange schedule for blood drawing and how results will be managed.
4. Contact the child's school and arrange a meeting with the school nurse, principal, and appropriate teachers to explain child's diagnosis, treatment, and potential time away from school.
5. Discuss with patient the possibility of making a visit to the classroom; explain about cancer and the side effects of chemotherapy to facilitate school re-entry.
6. Collaborate with primary care provider regarding immunization schedule and the contraindication for children on immunosuppressive therapy who receive live vaccines.
7. Ensure that parents can demonstrate the proper technique for care of venous access, such as dressing changes, daily flushing, and assessing for infection.

Family Education and Health Maintenance

1. Teach parents about normal CBC values and expected variations caused by therapy.
2. Instruct parents about leukemia and side effects of chemotherapy.
3. Inform parents to call if child has a fever more than 101°F (38.4°C), bleeding, signs of infections, and exposure to chickenpox if the child has not had it. Immunosuppressed children are in danger of developing disseminated varicella and may be treated prophylactically with varicella immune globulin.
4. Teach parents the importance of detecting and reporting fever in the child with leukemia. Unlike other children, immunosuppressed children rarely develop fever. A fever over 101°F (38.4°C) may indicate overwhelming infection and impending septic shock.
5. Teach preventive measures, such as handwashing and isolation from children with communicable diseases.
6. Reinforce that parents *never* use a rectal thermometer.
7. Refer parents to agencies such as Candlelighters, 3910 Warner St. Kensington MD 20895, 1-800-366-2223, *www.candlelighters.org;* or Leukemia and Lymphoma Society, 1-800-955-4572, *www.leukemia-lymphoma.org.*

Outcome-Based Evaluation

- Parents discuss their feelings about the child's diagnosis and treatment
- Afebrile, no signs of localized infection or bleeding
- Maintains a positive body image; does not become overly self-conscious or shy about appearance
- Eats at mealtime; takes between-meal feedings
- Experiences relief from pain (no crying or expression of pain)
- Rests at intervals
- Child acts out feelings in play; participates in age-appropriate activities
- Parents call and bring child in at appropriate time (eg, fever, exposure to illness)

■ Brain Tumors in Children

Brain tumors are expanding lesions within the skull. Approximately 20% of the malignant tumors that occur in children are brain tumors. Four main types of brain tumors appear in children. *Cerebellar astrocytoma*, a slow-growing, often cystic type of tumor of the cerebellum, accounts for approximately 10% to 20% of all pediatric brain tumors. *Medulloblastoma* is a highly malignant, rapidly growing tumor, usually found in the cerebellum. Medulloblastoma is the single most common tumor of the CNS in children, with a 2:1 male to female ratio. *Brain stem glioma*, a tumor of the brain stem, accounts for approximately 15% of brain tumors in children. *Ependymoma* is a tumor derived from the ependyma, or lining of the central canal of the spinal cord and cerebral ventricles. It frequently arises on the floor of the fourth ventricle, causing obstruction of the flow of cerebrospinal fluid (CSF). Ependymomas represent approximately 5% to 10% of all primary childhood CNS tumors.

Pathophysiology and Etiology

1. The etiology of brain tumors is unknown.
2. Cerebellar astrocytoma produces slowly increasing intracranial pressure. It is classified according to its malig-

nancy, from grade I (least malignant) to grade IV (most malignant).

3. Medulloblastoma grows rapidly and produces evidence of increased intracranial pressure progressing during several weeks. As the tumor grows, it seeds along CSF pathways.

4. Through its growth, brain stem glioma interferes early with the function of cranial nerve nuclei, pyramidal tracts, and cerebellar pathways.

5. Ependymomas grow with varying speed. Because of location, tumors can invade the cardiorespiratory center, cerebellum, and spinal cord. They are graded according to degree of differentiation, as are the astrocytomas.

Clinical Manifestations
Cerebellar Astrocytoma
Insidious onset and slow course.

1. Evidence of increased intracranial pressure—especially headache, visual disturbances, papilledema, and personality changes
2. Cerebellar signs—ataxia, dysmetria (inability to control the range of muscular movement), nystagmus
3. Behavioral changes
4. Seizures

Medulloblastoma
Fast growing, malignant, and invasive.

1. Similar to manifestations of cerebellar astrocytoma, but condition develops more rapidly.
2. The child may present with unsteady gait, anorexia, vomiting, and early morning headache; may later develop ataxia, nystagmus, papilledema, drowsiness, and increased head circumference.

Brain Stem Glioma
1. Cranial nerve palsies
   a. Strabismus
   b. Weakness, atrophy, and fasciculations of the tongue
   c. Swallowing difficulties
2. Hemiparesis
3. Cerebellar ataxia
4. Signs of increased intracranial pressure (advanced disease)

Ependymoma of the Fourth Ventricle
1. Signs of increased intracranial pressure
   a. Nausea or vomiting
   b. Headache
2. Unsteady gait/ataxia; dysmetria
3. Focal motor weakness, visual disturbances, seizures

Diagnostic Evaluation
Determined by the type of tumor that is suspected; usually includes many or all of the following procedures to localize and determine extent of the tumor:

1. Computed tomography (CT)
2. Magnetic resonance imaging (MRI)
3. Myelogram
4. Positron emission tomography (PET)
5. Lumbar puncture with CSF cytologic evaluation
6. Angiography (occasional)

Treatment
1. Surgery is performed to determine the type of the tumor, to assess the extent of invasiveness, and to excise as much of the lesion as possible.
2. Radiation therapy is usually initiated as soon as the diagnosis is established and the surgical wound is healed.
3. Chemotherapy is used in children younger than age 4 who have medulloblastoma to avoid early radiation and in children with ependymomas.
4. A ventriculoperitoneal shunt is often necessary for children who develop hydrocephalus.
5. The use of immunotherapy or gene transfer therapy has potential for future treatment.
6. Prognosis is improved in cases that involve early diagnosis and adequate therapy. Five-year survivors are increasing, especially in children with low-grade astrocytomas or ependymomas.

Complications
1. Brain stem herniation
2. Hydrocephalus

Nursing Assessment
Assess the child's neurologic status to help locate the site of the tumor and the extent of involvement; identify signs of disease progression.

1. Obtain a thorough nursing history from the child and parents, particularly data related to normal behavioral patterns and presenting symptoms.
2. Perform portions of the neurologic examination as appropriate. Assess muscle strength, coordination, gait, and posture.
3. Observe for the appearance or disappearance of any of the clinical manifestations previously described. Report these to the health care provider and record each of the following in detail:
   a. Headache—duration, location, severity
   b. Vomiting—time of occurrence, whether projectile
   c. Seizures—activity before seizure, type of seizure, areas of body involved, behavior during and after seizure
4. Monitor vital signs frequently, including blood pressure and pupillary reaction.
5. Monitor ocular signs. Check pupils for size, equality, reaction to light, and accommodation.
6. Observe for signs of brain stem herniation—should be considered a neurosurgical emergency.
   a. Attacks of opisthotonos (Figure 51-2)
   b. Tilting of the head; neck stiffness
   c. Poorly reactive pupils
   d. Increased blood pressure; widened pulse pressure
   e. Change in respiratory rate and nature of respirations
   f. Irregularity of pulse or lowered pulse rate
   g. Alterations of body temperature

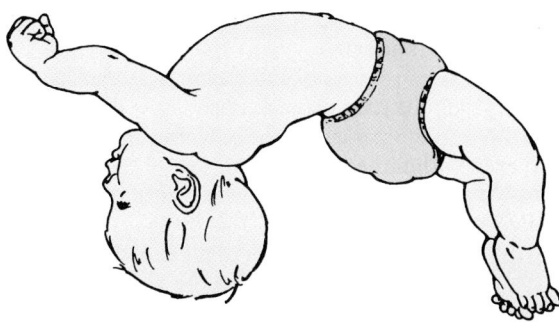

FIGURE 51-2 Opisthotonos, a sign of brainstem herniation.

NURSING ALERT

Signs of brain stem herniation, especially opisthotonos, are ominous. The health care provider should be called immediately and the child should be prepared for ventricular tap to relieve pressure. Have resuscitation equipment on hand.

Nursing Diagnoses

- Anxiety of parents related to the nature of the diagnosis and the need for surgery
- Anxiety of child related to hospitalization and to diagnostic and treatment procedures
- Pain related to increased intracranial pressure and surgery
- Altered Nutrition: Less Than Body Requirements related to nausea and vomiting associated with increased intracranial pressure, chemotherapy, and radiation
- Risk for Infection postoperatively
- Body Image Disturbance related to appearance of the incision, shaved head, or changes caused by radiation, chemotherapy, and steroids

Nursing Interventions
Reducing Parents' Anxiety
See page 1521.

1. Encourage the parents to ask questions and to understand fully the risks and benefits of surgery.
2. Prepare the parents for the postoperative appearance of their child and for the fact that he or she might be comatose immediately after surgery.
3. Continue supporting the parents during the postoperative period. They may be frightened and upset by the appearance of their child and by necessary emergency procedures.
4. Facilitate the return of normal parent–child relationships.
   a. The parents may be overprotective.
   b. Help the parents to see the child's increasing capabilities and encourage them to foster independence.

Reducing Child's Anxiety
See page 1523.

1. Prepare the child for surgery in realistic terms, but at the appropriate developmental level.
2. Determine the plan regarding shaving of the child's head, bandages, and other procedures. Prepare the child accordingly.
3. Prepare the child for postoperative expectations (eg, may feel sleepy or have a headache and will need to remain flat).

Reducing Pain Postoperatively

1. Administer narcotics as ordered in the immediate postoperative period, assessing the child's level of consciousness before administration.
2. Keep the child as comfortable as possible by repositioning.

Maintaining Nutritional Status

1. Feed the child after he or she vomits. (Vomiting is not usually associated with nausea.)
2. Allow the child to participate in the selection of foods and the preparation of tray.
3. Maintain IV hydration or hyperalimentation and intralipids if indicated.
4. As the child recovers, encourage child to eat progressively larger meals.
5. If the child cannot eat, provide tube feedings. A gastrostomy tube may be inserted.

Preventing Infection and Other Complications Postoperatively

1. Position the child according to surgeon's request—usually on unaffected side with head level.
   a. Raising the foot of the bed may increase intracranial pressure and bleeding.
   b. Post a sign above the bed, noting the exact position of the head.
2. Check the dressing for bleeding and for drainage of CSF.
3. Monitor the child's temperature closely.
   a. A significant rise in temperature may be caused by trauma, disturbance of the heat-regulating center, or intracranial edema.
   b. If hyperthermia occurs, administer antipyretics and sponge baths as ordered. Temperature should not be reduced too rapidly.
4. Observe child closely for signs of shock, increased intracranial pressure, and alterations in level of consciousness.
5. Assess the child for edema of the head, face, and neck.
6. Carefully regulate fluid administration to prevent increased cerebral edema.
7. Change the child's position frequently and provide meticulous skin care to prevent hypostatic pneumonia and pressure sores.
   a. Move the child carefully and slowly, being certain to move the head in line with the body.
   b. Support paralyzed or spastic extremities with pillows, rolls, or other means.
8. Have equipment readily available for cardiopulmonary resuscitation, respiratory assistance, oxygen inhalation, blood transfusion, ventricular tap, and other potential emergency situations.

9. Report fever or sign of infection.
10. If the child is receiving chemotherapy or radiation, instruct the parents to call if child has a fever of more than 101°F (38.4°C) or nausea and vomiting unrelated to chemotherapy.

Promoting Acceptance of Body Changes

1. Encourage the child to express feelings regarding the threat to body image.
2. Reassure the child that a wig or a hat can be worn after recovery.
3. If the child's hair has not been totally shaved, comb it so that the area of baldness is not evident.
4. Reassure the child that hair will grow back.

Family Education and Health Maintenance

1. Provide parents with written information regarding the child's needs—medications, activity, care of the incision, and follow-up appointments.
2. Teach the parents about radiation and chemotherapy and their side effects.
3. If a child has a ventriculoperitoneal shunt, teach parents to report fever, nausea, vomiting, irritability, or a bulging anterior fontanelle.
4. Initiate a referral to a community health nurse to reinforce teaching and to maintain therapeutic support for the family.
5. Encourage parents to contact the child's teacher and the school nurse before the child returns to school so that they can prepare classmates for child's return and help them to deal with their feelings.
6. Provide the parents with the phone number of the clinic or nursing unit so that they may call if questions occur to them after discharge.
7. For additional resources, refer family to agencies such as American Brain Tumor Association, 2720 River Road, Des Plaines, IL 60018, 800-886-2282, *www.abta.org*, or Candlelighters (see p. 1523).

Outcome-Based Evaluation

- Parents discuss feelings about the child's diagnosis and surgery
- Child demonstrates lessened anxiety through verbalization, play, or other age-appropriate activities
- Child verbalizes relief from pain
- Eats three meals, no weight loss noted
- Afebrile, lungs clear, vital signs stable
- Child verbalizes acceptance of appearance with hat, desire to visit with friends

Neuroblastoma

Neuroblastoma refers to a malignant tumor that arises from the sympathetic nervous system. It is the most common extracranial solid tumor of childhood, with an annual incidence of less than 1 in 10,000 children. It primarily affects infants and young children and occurs slightly more frequently in boys.

Pathophysiology and Etiology

1. Etiology is unknown.
2. Tumors arise from embryonic neural crest cells anywhere along the craniospinal axis.
3. Histologic picture varies greatly from tumor to tumor and even within the same tumor.
4. Tumors are staged primarily by extent of disease.
   a. Evans staging system:
      (i) Stage I (tumor confined to the organ or structure of origin) to stage IV (remote disease involving the skeleton, parenchymal organs, soft tissue, distant lymph nodes, or bone marrow).
      (ii) Stage IV-S refers to cases that would otherwise be stage I or II but that have remote disease confined to one or more sites, such as the liver, skin, or bone marrow, without evidence of skeletal metastasis.
   b. Pediatric Oncology Group Staging Stages A-D—evaluates regional lymph nodes for disease.
5. Neuroblastoma is one of the few tumors that may demonstrate spontaneous remission.

Clinical Manifestations

1. Symptoms depend on the location of the tumor and the stage of the disease.
2. Most tumors are located within the abdomen and present as firm, nontender, irregular masses that cross the midline.
3. Other common signs:
   a. Bowel or bladder dysfunction that results from compression by a paraspinal or pelvic tumor
   b. Neurologic symptoms because of compression by the tumor on nerve roots or because of tumor extension
   c. Supraorbital ecchymosis, periorbital edema, and exophthalmos that results from metastases to the skull bones and retrobulbar soft tissue
   d. Lymphadenopathy, especially in the cervical area
   e. Bone pain with skeletal involvement
   f. Swelling of the neck or face, wheezing, dyspnea and cough with thoracic masses
   g. Symptoms of bone marrow failure, such as anemia, bleeding, or infection
   h. General symptoms of pallor, anorexia, weight loss, and weakness with widespread metastasis

Diagnostic Evaluation

Workup done to document the extent of the disease throughout the body:

1. Chest and skeletal x-rays
2. Bone scan
3. Bone marrow aspiration and biopsy
4. CBC, platelet count, ferritin
5. 24-hour urine collection—elevated excretion of homovanillic acid (HVA) and vanillylmandelic acid (VMA)
6. Liver and kidney function tests

7. Histologic confirmation
8. Additional studies:
   a. CT scan of primary site and chest
   b. MRI—areas above diaphragm
   c. Ultrasound examination
   d. Liver/spleen scan
9. *N-myc* oncogene—multiple copies associated with a poor prognosis

Treatment

1. Surgery—role is both diagnostic and therapeutic. Either primary (before chemotherapy or radiation) or delayed/secondary (after therapy).
2. When complete surgical resection of a stage I tumor is possible, this may be the only treatment required.
3. Children with other than stage I disease generally receive a combination of surgery, radiation therapy, and chemotherapy. Drugs of choice include vincristine (Oncovin), dacarbazine (DTIC-Dome), cyclophosphamide (Cytoxan), doxorubicin (Adriamycin), cisplatin (Platinol), carboplatin (Paraplatin), ifosfamide (Ifex) and VM26 (teniposide).
4. Overall survival rate is approximately 30% to 35%, with almost all recurrences or deaths occurring within the first 2 years after diagnosis.
5. Influencing factors for prognosis:
   a. Stage of disease—the earlier the stage, the better the prognosis.
   b. Age—infants younger than 1 year of age demonstrate the best survival.
   c. Site of primary tumor—children with tumors above the diaphragm appear to do better than children with abdominal tumors.
   d. Pattern of metastasis—children with metastases to the bone marrow, liver, and skin have better prognosis than those with radiographic bone involvement.
6. Neuroblastoma is one of few childhood tumors that has not responded dramatically to modern antitumor therapy.
7. The use of newer chemotherapy drugs and other techniques, such as immunotherapy and bone marrow transplant, may improve survival rates for these children.

Complications

Metastasis to the liver, soft tissue, bones, lymph nodes, bone marrow and skin.

Nursing Assessment

1. Obtain a history.
   a. Inquire about when symptoms began. Focus on decrease in appetite, weakness, pain, abdominal distention, or change in bowel and bladder function.
   b. Symptoms exhibited depend on the location of the primary tumor.
2. Perform a physical examination, including the following:
   a. Examination of skin for signs of increased bruising or petechiae
   b. Palpation of liver and spleen for enlargement
   c. Palpation of abdominal mass or other primary site of tumor
   d. Auscultation of lungs
   e. Palpation of lymph nodes
   f. Blood pressure for detection of hypertension
   g. Temperature for fever caused by infection or disease
   h. Assessment of bones and joints for pain or swelling
   i. Neurologic examination for signs of compression by tumor. Nerves involved depend on location of tumor.
3. Assess coping mechanisms of family.

Nursing Diagnoses

- Anxiety of parents related to learning of diagnosis
- Fear of child related to diagnostic procedures and surgery or biopsy
- Activity Intolerance related to fatigue from tumor growth and bone marrow suppression
- Potential Constipation or Bowel and Bladder Incontinence related to pressure of tumor
- Risk for Infection related to bone marrow suppression from chemotherapy and radiation
- Pain related to tumor, surgery, or progression of disease
- Body Image Disturbance related to hair loss

Nursing Interventions

Reducing Parents' Anxiety
See page 1521.
Reducing Child's Fear
See page 1523.
Increasing Activity Tolerance
See page 1523.
Regaining Normal Bowel and Bladder Function
1. Assess normal elimination patterns the child had before the illness began.
2. Keep careful intake and output records.
3. Assess for urinary overflow incontinence and loss of bowel function, depending on the age of the child.
4. Notify health care provider if these should occur.
Preventing Infection
See page 1521.
   Observe the surgical incision for erythema, drainage, or separation of the incision. Report any of these changes.
Relieving Pain
See page 1522.
Promoting Acceptance of Body Changes
See page 1526.

Family Education and Health Maintenance

1. Teach parents about the laboratory tests and x-rays needed at diagnosis and periodically throughout therapy.
2. Instruct parents about chemotherapy medications used and their potential side effects.

3. Inform parents about potential treatment methods, such as radiation therapy and bone marrow transplant.
4. Advise parents to use good handwashing and to prevent exposure to children with communicable diseases.
5. Refer families to resources such as Candlelighters (see p. 1523).

Outcome-Based Evaluation

- Parents and child discuss their feelings about diagnosis and treatment
- Child participates in play and expresses feelings through play
- Activity level normal
- Voiding and stooling according to normal pattern
- Afebrile, lungs clear, no signs of localized infections
- Child rests without crying or guarding surgical incision
- Child interacts with others, seems comfortable with self

Rhabdomyosarcoma

Rhabdomyosarcoma is a highly malignant soft tissue tumor that arises from the embryonic mesenchymal cells that form striated muscle. Most common soft tissue tumor in persons younger than age 21. Accounts for 5% to 8% of all malignant disease in children younger than 15 years of age. Peak incidence is during the first decade of life.

Pathophysiology and Etiology

1. Etiology is unknown in most cases.
2. Certain genetic and environmental factors have been associated.
3. Classified in six pathologic categories based on histologic characteristics.
4. Tumor spreads either by local extension or by metastasis via the venous and lymphatic system.
5. The lung is the most common site of metastasis.
6. Tumor staging is based on the extent of the disease:
   a. Stage I: localized tumor, completely resected
   b. Stage II: local tumor resected, microscopic residual disease
   c. Stage III: localized disease, with gross residual disease after resection
   d. Stage IV: metastatic disease at diagnosis

Clinical Manifestations

1. Often presents as an asymptomatic lump noted by the patient or parent.
2. Signs and symptoms are variable and reflect the location of the tumor and metastases.
   a. Orbit—ptosis, ocular paralysis, exophthalmos
   b. Nasopharynx—epistaxis, pain, dysphagia, nasal voice, airway obstruction
   c. Sinuses—swelling, pain, discharge, sinusitis
   d. Middle ear—pain, chronic otitis, facial nerve palsy
   e. Neck—hoarseness, dysphagia
   f. Truncal, extremities, testicular areas—enlarging soft tissue masses
   g. Prostate, bladder—urinary tract symptoms
   h. Retroperitoneal tumors—gastrointestinal and urinary tract obstruction, weakness, paresthesia, pain
   i. Vaginal—abnormal vaginal bleeding or mass

Diagnostic Evaluation

To document the extent of the disease and to provide objective criteria for measuring response to therapy:
1. Open biopsy of the primary tumor—definitive diagnostic procedure
2. CT scan of the chest and primary lesion
3. MRI
4. Bone marrow aspiration and biopsy
5. Bone scan or skeletal survey
6. Ultrasound
7. Chest x-ray
8. CBC, liver and renal function tests, electrolytes, serum calcium and phosphorus, uric acid
9. Monoclonal antibody assays
10. Urinalysis
11. Lumbar puncture—for children with cranial lesions

Treatment

1. Surgery—to biopsy the lesion, determine the stage of the disease, and completely remove or reduce the primary tumor. Increasingly, chemotherapy/radiation therapy is used before surgery to avoid the disability associated with radical surgery for selected anatomic sites (head, neck, and pelvis).
2. Radiation—high-dose radiation is generally recommended for the primary tumor and metastasis.
3. Chemotherapy.
   a. Used for all patients, usually in combination with irradiation.
   b. Commonly used drugs include dactinomycin (Actinomycin D), vincristine (Oncovin), cyclophosphamide (Cytoxan), doxorubicin (Adriamycin), cisplatin (Platinol), etoposide (VP-16, VePesid), ifosfamide (Ifex), methotrexate (Mexate), and melphalan (Alkeran).
   c. Promising new agents include topetecan, paclitaxel (Taxol), and docetaxel (Taxotere).
4. Survival rates have improved considerably in recent years, and overall survival is approximately 70%.
5. Prognosis is related to the stage of the disease at diagnosis, the location of the primary tumor and the age at diagnosis.

Complications

1. Direct tumor extension to CNS with cranial nerve palsy, brain stem compromise with bradypnea and bradycardia.
2. Metastasis to bone, bone marrow, lung.

Nursing Assessment

1. Obtain a history.
   a. Inquire about recent illness history and when the child became symptomatic.

b. Obtain review of systems, to help identify the primary tumor and any metastases present.

2. Perform a physical examination, including the following:
   a. Palpation of lymph nodes for enlargement, tenderness, and mobility
   b. Palpation of the liver and spleen to detect hepatosplenomegaly
   c. Palpation of primary site of tumor and suspected areas of metastasis
   d. Auscultation of lungs to assess breath sounds or abnormality caused by the spread of the tumor
3. Assess family coping, resources, and emotional state of child and parents.

Nursing Diagnoses

- Anxiety of parents related to learning of diagnosis
- Anxiety of child related to diagnostic procedures and surgery or biopsy
- Altered Nutrition: Less Than Body Requirements related to anemia, anorexia, nausea, vomiting, and mucosal ulceration secondary to chemotherapy or radiation
- Pain related to surgery or possible progression of disease
- Body Image Disturbance related to alopecia associated with chemotherapy
- Risk for Infection related to bone marrow suppression from chemotherapy or radiation

Nursing Interventions

Reducing Parents' Anxiety
See page 1521.

Reducing Child's Anxiety
See page 1523.

Improving Nutritional Intake
See page 1522.

Relieving Pain
See page 1522.

Maintaining Positive Body Image
See page 1526.

Preventing Infection
See page 1521.

Family Education and Health Teaching

1. Teach parents about laboratory diagnostic tests that will be done periodically to follow the child's condition.
2. Instruct parents about treatment methods, including chemotherapy and radiation protocols postoperatively, and their side effects.
3. Stress the importance of follow-up, so that any recurrence can be detected early and appropriate treatment can be instituted.
4. Refer families to resources such as Candlelighters (see p. 1523).

Outcome-Based Evaluation

- Parents verbalize understanding of diagnosis
- Child plays, interacts with others and asks questions
- Eats three small meals and snacks
- Child verbalizes reduced pain
- Child verbalizes acceptance of self; looks in mirror
- Afebrile, no signs of localized infection

Wilms' Tumor

Wilms' tumor is a malignant renal tumor and is the most common renal neoplasm in children. It constitutes approximately 30% of all pediatric renal masses and 7% of all childhood tumors. Incidence is 1 in 10,000. Seventy-five percent of cases occur before the child is 5 years of age. Most commonly a unilateral disease, but in 5% to 10%, both kidneys are involved.

Pathophysiology and Etiology

1. The etiology of Wilms' tumor is not known.
2. Genetic inheritance has been documented in a small percentage of cases.
3. Children with Wilms' tumor may have associated anomalies.
4. Wilms' tumor has a capacity for rapid growth and usually grows to a large size before it is diagnosed.
5. The effect of the tumor on the kidney depends on the site of the tumor.
6. In most cases, the tumor expands the renal parenchyma, and the capsule of the kidney becomes stretched over the surface of the tumor.
7. The tumor is often exceedingly vascular, soft, mushy, or gelatinous in character.
8. Wilms' tumors present various histologic patterns.
9. The neoplasms metastasize either by direct extension or by way of the bloodstream. They may invade perirenal tissues, lymph nodes, the liver, the diaphragm, abdominal muscles, and the lungs. Invasions of bone and brain are less common.
10. Staging of Wilms' tumor is done based on clinical and anatomic findings. It ranges from group I (tumor is limited to the kidney and is completely resected) to group IV (metastases are present in the liver, lung, bone, or brain). Group V includes those cases that include bilateral involvement, either initially or subsequently.

Clinical Manifestations

1. A firm, nontender upper quadrant abdominal mass is usually the presenting sign; it may be on either side. (It is frequently observed by the parents.)
2. Abdominal pain, which is related to rapid growth of the tumor, may occur. As the tumor enlarges, pressure may cause constipation, vomiting, abdominal distress, anorexia, weight loss, and dyspnea.
3. Less common are hypertension, fever, hematuria, and anemia.
4. Associated anomalies.
   a. Hemihypertrophy of the vertebrae
   b. Aniridia (without the iris)
   c. Genitourinary anomalies

Diagnostic Evaluation

1. Abdominal ultrasound—to demonstrate the tumor and to assess the status of the opposite kidney.
2. Radiography of chest to identify metastases.
3. CBC and peripheral smear—for baseline data.
4. Urinalysis for hematuria.
5. Blood chemistries, especially serum electrolytes, uric acid, renal function tests (blood urea nitrogen and creatinine), and liver function tests (bilirubin, alanine aminotransferase [ALT], aspartate aminotransferase [AST], lactic dehydrogenase [LDH], total protein, albumin, and alkaline phosphatase) may show abnormalities.
6. Urinary VMA and HVA to distinguish from neuroblastoma.
7. MRI or CT scan of the abdomen to evaluate local spread to lymph nodes or adjacent organs.
8. Real-time ultrasonography.

Treatment

1. Surgical removal of primary tumor remains the cornerstone of therapy. Accurate staging and assessment of tumor spread is also done.
2. Radiation and/or chemotherapy may be administered preoperatively to patients with massive tumors or risky intravascular extension to reduce tumor burden.
3. Radiation therapy is given to the tumor bed postoperatively to render nonviable all cells that have escaped locally from the excised tumor. Children who have stage III and IV Wilms' tumor, or who have an unfavorable histology, usually receive this treatment.
4. Whole lung radiation is used to treat stage IV tumors with lung metastasis.
5. Late effects of radiation therapy to the abdomen include scoliosis and underdevelopment of soft tissues.
6. Chemotherapy is initiated postoperatively to achieve maximal killing of tumor cells.
7. Overall survival rates for Wilms' tumor are the highest among all childhood cancers—greater than 85%.
8. Prognosis is based on histologic tumor features, lymph node involvement, age, tumor size, and possible chromosomal factors.

Complications

1. Metastasis to the lungs, lymph nodes, liver, bone, and brain.
2. Complications from radiation therapy include bowel obstruction, hepatic damage, nephritis, sterility in girls, interstitial pneumonia, scoliosis.
3. Approximately 15% of children who survive will develop a soft tissue sarcoma, bone tumor, or leukemia in 5 to 25 years because of radiation.

Nursing Assessment

1. Obtain a history.
   a. Inquire about how tumor was first discovered.
   b. Ask whether the child has history of any other genitourinary anomalies or whether there is a family history of any type of cancer.
   c. Determine whether the child has had hematuria, dysuria, constipation, abdominal pain, decreased appetite, or fever before hospitalization and ask how these were treated.
2. Perform a physical examination that includes the following.
   a. Assessment for associated anomalies: aniridia, hemihypertrophy of the spine, or cryptorchidism
   b. Palpation of lymph nodes for enlargement, tenderness, and mobility
   c. Palpation of the liver and spleen for enlargement
   d. Palpation of the abdomen to determine the size and location of the tumor
   e. Auscultation of the lungs to assess breath sounds or abnormality because of spread of tumor
3. Assess coping, resources, and emotional state of the family.

NURSING ALERT

Avoid indiscriminate manipulation of the abdomen both preoperatively and postoperatively to decrease the danger of metastasis. Because the tumor is soft and highly vascular, seeding may occur because of excessive palpation or handling of the child's abdomen.

Nursing Diagnoses

- Anxiety of parents related to learning of diagnosis
- Anxiety of child related to surgery and diagnostic tests
- Risk for Fluid Volume Deficit postoperatively
- Pain related to surgery and possible progression of the disease.
- Altered Nutrition: Less Than Body Requirements related to anemia, anorexia, nausea, vomiting, and mucosal ulceration secondary to chemotherapy or radiation
- Body Image Disturbance related to alopecia associated with chemotherapy
- Activity Intolerance related to fatigue that results from the size of the tumor and treatment
- Risk for Infection and hemorrhage related to bone marrow suppression caused by chemotherapy

Nursing Interventions

Reducing Parents' Anxiety

See page 1521.

Reducing Child's Anxiety

See page 1523.

Preventing Fluid Volume Deficit and Other Complications

1. Insert a nasogastric tube as ordered. Many children require gastric suction postoperatively to prevent distention or vomiting.
2. Monitor gastric output accurately and replace it with the appropriate IV fluids as ordered.

3. When bowel sounds have returned, begin with small amounts of clear fluids.

4. Keep accurate intake and output record.

5. Monitor vital signs as the child's condition warrants and check the surgical dressing frequently for drainage.

Controlling Pain
See page 1522.

Promoting Adequate Nutrition
See page 1522.

Promoting Acceptance of Body Changes
See page 1526.

Increasing Activity Tolerance
See page 1523.

Preventing Infection
See page 1521.

Family Education and Health Maintenance

1. Teach parents that children who have only one kidney should not play rough contact sports, to avoid injuring the remaining kidney.

2. Inform parents to call if child has a fever of more than 101°F (38.4°C), bleeding, signs of infections, or exposure to chickenpox if the child has not had it.

3. Teach measures to prevent infection, such as handwashing and isolation from children with communicable disease.

4. Refer families to resources such as Candlelighters (see p. 1523).

Outcome-Based Evaluation

- Parents discuss their feelings about diagnosis and treatment
- Child expresses feelings during play and participates in playroom activities
- No abdominal distention or vomiting, vital signs stable
- Child verbalizes relief from pain
- Eats three meals, nausea relieved by antiemetics
- Child plays with others without notice to alopecia
- Participates in all normal daily activities without fatigue
- Afebrile, no signs of local infection

Osteogenic Sarcoma

Osteogenic sarcoma is a malignant tumor of the bone. Most frequent malignant bone cancer in children, with approximately 11 cases per million adolescents. Occurs as 50% of second malignancy sarcomas in survivors of retinoblastoma. Most common at the peak of the adolescent growth spurt. The male-to-female ratio is 1.5:1; it is rare in African-Americans.

Pathophysiology and Etiology

1. Etiology is unknown.

2. Presumably arises from bone-forming mesenchyme tissue.

3. Produces malignant spindle-cell stroma, which gives rise to malignant osteoid tissue.

4. Common sites of occurrence—distal femur, proximal tibia, and proximal humerus. Less common sites include the pelvis, phalanges, and jaw.

5. Most commonly metastasize to lungs and other bones.

Clinical Manifestations

1. Pain in the affected site, frequently causing limp or limitation of motion.

2. Palpable, tender, fixed bony mass.

3. Additional symptoms related to site of metastasis, if present.

Diagnostic Evaluation

1. Radiographic examination of lesion—to visualize the tumor.

2. Biopsy of lesion—to confirm the diagnosis and to provide histologic date for the selection of a treatment plan.

3. CT and MRI—to determine local tumor extent before surgery.

4. Bone scan—helpful in detecting initial extent of malignancy, planning therapy, and evaluating effects of treatment.

5. Renal and liver function tests.

6. Arteriography—possibility if limb salvage procedure is a consideration.

Treatment

1. Surgery—procedures fall into two categories.
   a. Radical amputation of the affected extremity, and often the joint proximal to the involved area, is required in most cases
   b. Limb salvage procedure

2. The decision on the type of surgery depends on tumor location, size, extramedullary extent, distant metastasis, age, skeletal development, and lifestyle preference.

3. Chemotherapy is advocated for 1 to 3 years after surgery. It is also used preoperatively for patients who undergo resectional surgery and for the treatment of metastatic disease.

4. Survival has greatly improved with the aggressive use of multimodal therapy.

5. Approximately 50% to 60% of patients who undergo surgery followed by chemotherapy can expect to be disease-free after 3 years.

6. Most important prognostic factor is extent of disease at diagnosis. Other factors include age, sex and serum LDH.

7. Limb-saving surgery has improved the quality of life for many survivors.

Complications

1. Metastasis to lung and bones
2. Later metastasis to CNS and lymph nodes

Nursing Assessment

1. Obtain a history.
   a. Inquire about how symptoms first presented and the duration of symptoms.

b. Determine whether the child has pain or limitation of motion in the affected area.

2. Perform a physical examination, including the following:
   a. Palpation of the mass to determine the size and location. Determine whether the mass is tender or is fixed to the bone.
   b. Palpation of other bones to check for metastases.
   c. Auscultation of the lungs to assess breath sounds or other abnormalities caused by spread of tumor.
3. Assess family coping, resources such as support systems, and emotional state of adolescent and parents.

Nursing Diagnoses

- Anxiety of parents related to learning of diagnosis
- Anxiety of child or adolescent related to surgery, diagnostic tests, and treatment
- Body Image Disturbance related to surgery and possible amputation and alopecia associated with chemotherapy
- Pain related to surgery and possible progression of the disease
- Altered Nutrition: Less Than Body Requirements related to anemia, anorexia, nausea, vomiting, and mucosal ulceration caused by chemotherapy
- Risk for Infection related to surgery or bone marrow suppression secondary to chemotherapy

Nursing Interventions
Reducing Parents' Anxiety
See page 1521.
Reducing Adolescent's Anxiety
1. Incorporate the adolescent's developmental level and develop a teaching program to include diagnostic tests and postoperative care.
2. Support and prepare the child for routine surgical care or care of the amputated limb. Involve the parents in teaching plan and make sure they all know what to expect before going to surgery.
3. If an amputation is going to be done, teach the child about the need for physical therapy for exercises and to learn crutch walking and the need for a prosthesis.
4. Nursing care of the adolescent with osteogenic sarcoma is the same as care of the adult (see p. 1014).

Promoting Acceptance of New Self-Image
1. Understand that adolescents need time and support to accept the diagnosis and the surgery and to grieve for their lost body part if an amputation is done.
2. Try to introduce the adolescent to another adolescent with the same diagnosis who has undergone similar treatment.
3. Suggest the selection of clothing that will camouflage the prosthesis and that is fashionable and appealing.
4. Suggest wigs, scarves, or hats for adolescents who experience hair loss because of chemotherapy.
5. Encourage visits by peers and help the child to deal with questions and reactions from peers.

Relieving Pain
See page 1522.
Promoting Adequate Nutrition
See page 1522.
Preventing Infection and Hemorrhage
See page 1521.

Community and Home Care Considerations
1. Assess the home for accessibility of adolescent who has had an amputation.
2. Educate parents about changes that may need to be made in the home.
3. Encourage the parents to contact the school system to arrange for a tutor for student who needs to remain out of school for lengthy time.
4. Assist the parents in contacting the school nurse to facilitate reentry into the classroom.

Family Education and Health Maintenance
1. Teach adolescent and parents about infection control measures, such as good handwashing and preventing exposure to children with communicable diseases, because chemotherapy is usually long term.
2. Parents and adolescents should be instructed about chemotherapy medications used and their potential side effects.
3. Teach parents and adolescents about the radiation procedure and effects.
4. Advise the adolescent to protect a leg that has received radiation treatment by avoiding excessive pressure on the leg through sports.
5. Refer families to resources such as Candlelighters (see p. 1523).

Outcome-Based Evaluation
- Parents discuss feelings about surgery and chemotherapy treatments
- Child verbalizes feelings about surgery and asks questions
- Child looks in mirror, touches amputation site
- Child verbalizes relief from pain
- Eating pattern adequate, nausea relieved by antiemetics
- Afebrile, vital signs stable, no signs of bleeding

■ Retinoblastoma

Retinoblastoma is a malignant, congenital tumor, arising in the retina of one or both eyes. Occurs in approximately 11 per million children younger than age 5, or approximately 200 children in the United States each year. Incidence is increasing because of prolonged survival of affected children, with transmission of the tumor to their offspring, and increased exposure to mutagenic agents. Median age of diagnosis is 2 years of age.

Pathophysiology and Etiology
1. Most cases appear sporadically, though an inherited form of the disease has been discovered.
2. Nonhereditary somatic mutations account for approximately 60% of all retinoblastomas. Always demonstrate unilateral involvement.

3. Hereditary germinal mutations:
   a. Account for approximately 40% of all retino-blastomas.
   b. May be bilateral or unilateral.
   c. Mode of inheritance is autosomal dominant.
4. Can be associated with chromosomal aberrations.
5. Usually arise in multiple foci rather than a single tumor from any of the nucleated retinal layers.
6. Some tumors (endophytic type) arise in the internal nuclear layers of the retina and grow forward into the vitreous cavity.
7. Some tumors (exophytic type) arise in the external nuclear layer and grow into the subretinal space, with detachment of the retina.
8. Most tumors have a combination of endophytic and exophytic growth.
9. Extension of the tumor may occur into the choroid, the sclera, and optic nerve.
10. Hematogenous spread of the tumor may occur to the bone marrow, skeleton, lymph nodes, and liver.
11. Tumor staging reflects the extent of the disease and the probability of preserving useful vision in the affected eye, from group I (favorable) to group V (unfavorable).

Clinical Manifestations

1. Signs and symptoms of an intraocular tumor depend on its size and position.
2. "Cat's eye reflex"—whitish appearance of the pupil, represents visualization of the tumor through the lens as light falls on the tumor mass—most common sign.
3. Strabismus—second most common presenting sign.
4. Other occasional presenting signs.
   a. Orbital inflammation
   b. Hyphema
   c. Fixed pupil
   d. Heterochromia iridis—different colors of each iris or in the same iris
5. Vision loss is not a symptom because young children do not complain of unilaterally decreased vision.
6. Symptoms of distant metastasis—anorexia, weight loss, vomiting, headache.

Diagnostic Evaluation

1. Bilateral indirect ophthalmoscopy under general anesthesia.
2. Ultrasonography and CT scan or MRI of head and eyes to visualize tumor.
3. Bone marrow aspiration and lumbar puncture under anesthesia to determine metastasis.

Complications

1. Spread to brain and other eye
2. Metastasis to bone, bone marrow, liver, and lymph nodes

Treatment

1. Depends on the stage of the disease at the time of diagnosis.

2. Unilateral tumors in stages I, II, or III are usually treated with external beam irradiation.
   a. Goal of treatment is to eradicate the tumor(s) and to preserve useful vision.
   b. Radiation is usually administered during 3 weeks to 4 weeks.
3. Surgery (enucleation) is the treatment of choice for advanced tumor growth, especially with optic nerve involvement when no hope exists for useful vision.
4. Bilateral disease often requires enucleation of the severely diseased eye and irradiation of the least affected eye.
   a. Every attempt is made to salvage whatever vision there may be.
   b. Bilateral enucleation is indicated with extensive bilateral retinoblastoma when no hope of vision exists.
5. Radioactive applicators, light coagulation, and cryotherapy are sometimes used to treat small, localized tumors.
6. Intraocular penetration of systemic drugs is poor, so chemotherapy is used for cases of extraocular disease, regional or distant metastases. Generally, chemotherapy response has been of short duration; however, a phase II trial of etoposide and carboplatin has provided an 85% response rate for children with extraocular disease.
7. Overall survival rate is high (90%).
8. Heritable retinoblastoma and bilateral retinoblastoma are associated with a high incidence of spontaneous and radiation-related new tumors, particularly sarcomas.

Nursing Assessment

1. Obtain a history.
   a. Ask about a family history that is positive for retinoblastoma or other types of cancer.
   b. Inquire about when symptoms began and strabismus, cat's eye reflex (leukocoria), orbital inflammation, vomiting, or headache.
2. Perform a physical examination.
   a. Assess pupils for reactivity of light, size, and leukocoria.
   b. Evaluate the strabismus when checking muscle balance.
   c. Assess eyes for associated signs, such as erythema, inflammation of the orbit, hyphema, and heterochromia iridis.
3. Assess family's ability to cope, to use support systems, and to communicate feelings.

Nursing Diagnoses

- Anxiety of parents related to the diagnosis, treatment, and genetic implications of the diagnosis
- Impaired Tissue Integrity related to skin changes, loss of lashes, fat atrophy, impaired bone growth, and dryness caused by radiation
- Fear of child related to hospitalization and to diagnostic and treatment procedures
- Body Image Disturbance and Ineffective Coping related to enucleation and need for an eye prosthesis

- Sensory/Perceptual Alteration (Vision) related to disease process or enucleation

Nursing Interventions
Decreasing Parental Anxiety and Guilt
1. Listen to the parental feelings of guilt about transmitting the disease to the child or because they did not notice symptoms earlier.
2. Discuss the benefit of consultation about the probability of having another affected child.
   a. Risk ranges from approximately 1% to 10%, depending on family history and whether the affected child had unilateral or bilateral disease.
   b. The reportedly high lifelong cancer burden among retinoblastoma patients may also be important to parents in making informed decisions.
   c. Support parental decisions regarding future pregnancies.
3. Encourage the parents to seek genetic counseling for the affected child when he or she reaches puberty.
   a. The risk to offspring is from 1% to 50%, depending on family history and whether disease was unilateral or bilateral.
   b. Among affected offspring, there is a high probability (greater than 50%) of bilateral disease.

Preserving Tissue Integrity
1. Administer sedatives for radiation, if necessary.
   a. Administer the medication in a timely manner so that sedation is adequate for positioning of the child.
2. Observe for possible side effects of irradiation and prepare the parents for their occurrence.
   a. Skin changes at the temples.
      (i) Use soap sparingly in these areas.
      (ii) Avoid exposure to the sun.
      (iii) Apply a nonirritating lubricant.
   b. Loss of lashes.
   c. Fat atrophy with ptosis.
   d. Delayed wound healing.
   e. Dry eye.
   f. Permanent radiation dermatitis.
   g. Impaired bone growth.

Allaying the Child's Fear
See also page 1523.
1. Encourage the parents to "room-in" and participate in the child's care, to minimize separation anxiety.
2. Prepare the child and parents for all diagnostic procedures.
3. Describe the surgery and anticipated postoperative appearance of the child. Draw pictures or use a doll, if one is available.
   a. A surgically implanted sphere maintains the shape of the eyeball.
   b. The child's face may be edematous and ecchymotic.
4. Offer the family the opportunity to talk with another parent who has gone through the experience or to see pictures of another child with an artificial eye.
5. See nursing management of eye enucleation on page 521.

Promoting Acceptance of Prosthesis
1. Explain to child the changes in terms of losing diseased eye, having a bandaged orbit until it heals after surgery, and receiving a prosthetic eye.
2. Explain that the prosthesis will be made for him or her and will look like the removed eye.
3. Tell parents to expect the child to grieve the loss and to help him or her by talking about it, but to treat the child as the same person.

Minimizing Effects of Vision Loss
1. Maintain a safe, uncluttered environment for the child.
2. Hold the child frequently and stand close, within child's field of vision, while speaking or providing care.
3. Encourage the use of touch and other senses for exploring.
4. Set environmental limits so the child feels safe and can obtain help easily.

Family Education and Health Maintenance
1. Teach care of the orbit.
2. Teach care of the prosthesis—initial instructions are provided by the ocularist and should be reinforced by the nurse.
3. Advise protection of the remaining eye from accidental injury, such as wearing safety glass for sports, not putting sharp objects near eye, treating eye infections promptly.
4. Encourage maintenance of routine checkups for eye and medical care.
5. Stress need to have subsequent children carefully evaluated for retinoblastoma.
   a. An ophthalmologic examination under anesthesia is usually recommended at approximately 2 months of age.
   b. The child should receive frequent examinations thereafter until judged safe from developing retinoblastoma, usually approximately age 3 years.
6. Refer families to resources such as Candlelighters (see p. 1523).

Outcome-Based Evaluation
- Parents discuss their feelings openly, show affection to the child
- Parents describe possible side effects of radiation and how to care for skin around eyes
- Child demonstrates lessened anxiety by participating in age-appropriate activities
- Child shows acceptance of the prosthesis and not inhibited in behavior
- Child moves about environment with ease

SELECTED REFERENCES
Altman, A.J., & Quinn, J.J. (1995). Cancer in infancy. *Contemporary Pediatrics, 12*(2), 39–63.
Broxmeyer, H.E. (1995). Cord blood as an alternative source for stem and progenitor cell transplantation. *Current Opinion in Pediatrics, 7*(1), 47–55.

Ching-Hon Pui (1997). Acute lymphocytic leukemia. *Pediatric Clinics of North America, 44*(4), 831–846.

Goede, I., & Betcher, D. (1994). EMLA. *Journal of Pediatric Oncology Nursing, 11*(1), 38–41.

Hinds, P.S., et al. (1997). Decision making by parents and healthcare professionals when considering continued care for pediatric patients with cancer. *Oncology Nursing Forum, 24*(9), 1523–1528.

Hinds, P.S. et al. (1996). Coming to terms: Parents' response to a first cancer recurrence in their child. *Nursing Research, 45*(3), 148–153.

Jones, P.D., Henry, R.L., Stuart J., & Francis, L. (1998). Suspected infection in children with cancer. *Journal of Quality in Clinical Practice, 18*(4), 275–84.

Keeley, K., & Lange, B. (1997). Oncologic emergencies. *Pediatric Clinics of North America, 44*(4), 809–30.

Kennedy, L., & Diamond, J. (1997). Assessment and management of chemotherapy-induced mucositis in children. *Journal of Pediatric Oncology Nursing, 14*(3), 164–74.

Kun, L. (1997). Brain tumors: Challenges and directions. *Pediatric Clinics of North America, 44*(4), 907–18.

Lyos A.T., et al. (1996). Soft tissue sarcomas of the head and neck in children and adolescents. *Cancer, 77*(1) 193–200.

Macpherson, C.F. & Lundblad, L.A. (1997). Conscious sedation of pediatric oncology patients for painful procedures. Development and implementation of a clinical practice protocol. *Journal of Pediatric Oncology Nursing, 14*(1), 33–42.

Mandel, I.D. (1994). Antimicrobial mouthrinses: Overview and update. *Journal of the American Dental Association, 125*(supp 2), 2S–10S.

Meyers, P., & Gorlick, R. (1997). Osteosarcoma. *Pediatric Clinics of North America, 44*(4), 973–89.

Nichols, M.L. (1995). Social support and coping in young adolescents with cancer. *Pediatric Nursing, 21*(3), 235–240.

Notis C.M., et al. (1996). Parents with unilateral retinoblastoma and their affected children. *British Journal of Opthamology, 80*(3), 197–99.

Papadatou, D. (1997). Training health professionals in caring for dying children and grieving families. *Death Studies, 21*(6), 575–600.

Parker S.L., et al. (1997). Cancer statistics. *CA: A Cancer Journal for Clinicians, 47*(1), 5–27.

Petruzzi, M.J., & Green, D. (1997). Wilms' tumor. *Pediatric Clinics of North America, 44*(4), 949–954.

Pillitteri, A. (1999). *Maternal and child health nursing* (3rd ed.). Philadelphia: Lippincott Williams & Wilkins.

Pizzo, P., & Poplach, D. (1997). *Principles and practice of pediatric oncology* (3rd ed.). Philadelphia: Lippincott-Raven.

Poliquin, C.M. (1997). Overview of bone marrow and peripheral blood stem cell transplantation. *Clinical Jounral of Oncology Nursing, 1*(1), 11–17.

Rhiner, M., Ferrell, B.R., Shapiro, B., & Dierkes, M. (1994). The experience of pediatric cancer pain, Part II: Management of pain. *Journal of Pediatric Nursing, 9*(6), 380–7.

Rhodes, V.A., et al. (1995). Nurses perceptions of antiemetic effectiveness. *Oncology Nursing Forum, 22*(8), 1243–52.

Ridgeway, D., & Wolfff, L.J. (1993). Active immunization of children with leukemia and other malignancies. *Leukemia and Lymphoma, 9*(3), 177–92.

Schonfeld, D. (1993). Talking with children about death. *Journal of Pediatric Health Care, 7*(6), 269–274.

Shiminski-Maher, T. (1993). Brain tumors in childhood: Implications for nursing practice. *Journal of Pediatric Health Care, 4*(3), 122–130.

Tyc, V.L., Bieberich, A.A., Hinds, P., & Sifford, L. (1998). A survey of pain services for pediatric oncology patients: Their composition and function. *Journal of Pediatric Oncology Nursing, 15*(4), 207–15.

Van Dongen-Melman, J.E., et al. (1995). Late psychological consequences for parents of children who survived cancer. *Journal of Pediatric Psychology, 20*(50), 567–86.

Whaley, L.F., & Wong, D.L. (1999). *Nursing care of infants and children* (6th ed.). St. Louis: Mosby.

Pediatric Hematologic Disorders

PEDIATRIC HEMATOLOGIC DISORDERS

■ Anemia

Anemia refers to a deficit of red blood cells (RBC) or hemoglobin in the blood, resulting in decreased oxygen-carrying capacity. It is the most frequent hematologic disorder encountered in children.

Pathophysiology and Etiology

1. RBCs and hemoglobin are normally formed at the same rate at which they are destroyed. Whenever formation of RBCs or hemoglobin is decreased or their destruction is increased, anemia results. The ability of hemoglobin to carry oxygen to the tissues and remove carbon dioxide for excretion by the lungs is decreased.
2. May be caused by blood loss related to:
   a. Trauma and ulceration
   b. Decreased production of platelets
   c. Increased destruction of platelets
   d. Decreased number of clotting factors
3. May be caused by impairment of RBC production caused by nutritional deficiency.
   a. Iron deficiency—most common type of anemia in all age groups; approximately 3% of all children
   b. Folic acid deficiency
   c. Vitamin B_{12} deficiency
   d. Vitamin B_6 deficiency
   e. Lead poisoning
4. May be caused by decreased erythrocyte production.
   a. Pure RBC anemia
   b. Secondary hemolytic anemias associated with chronic infection, renal disease, and drugs. In anemia of

chronic infection and inflammation, the life span of the RBC is moderately decreased and the ability of the bone marrow to produce RBCs is significantly decreased.
   c. Bone marrow depression—leukemia, aplastic anemias, transient erythocytopenia of childhood
5. May be caused by increased erythrocyte destruction.
   a. Extrinsic factors:
      (i) Drugs and chemicals
      (ii) Infections—parovirus (fifth disease)
      (iii) Antibody reactions—passively acquired antibodies against Rh, A, or B isoimmunization, autoimmune hemolytic anemia, burns, poisons (including lead poisoning)
   b. Intrinsic factors:
      (i) Abnormalities of the RBC membrane
      (ii) Enzymatic defects—glucose-6-phosphate dehydrogenase deficiency (G6PD)
      (iii) Abnormal hemoglobin synthesis—sickle cell disease, thalassemia syndromes
   c. In hemolytic anemias, the RBCs are destroyed at abnormally high rates, primarily by the spleen.
      (i) The activity of the bone marrow increases to compensate for the shortened survival time of the RBCs.
      (ii) Bone marrow hypertrophies and occupies a larger than normal share of the inner structure of bones.
      (iii) Products of RBC breakdown increase with hemolysis.
      (iv) Jaundice results when the liver cannot clear the blood of the pigment that results from the breakdown of hemoglobin from destroyed RBCs.
      (v) Iron builds up (hemosiderosis) and may deposit on body tissues.

Clinical Manifestations

1. Condition may be acute or chronic.
2. Early symptoms:
   a. Listlessness
   b. Fatigability
   c. Anorexia related to decreased energy
3. Late symptoms:
   a. Pallor
   b. Weakness
   c. Tachycardia
   d. Palpitations
   e. Tachypnea; shortness of breath on exertion
   f. Jaundice (with hemolytic anemias)

Diagnostic Evaluation

1. Complete blood count (CBC) with indices and reticulocytes—vary with types of anemia (Table 52-1).
2. Serum iron and total iron-binding capacity—ratio of less than 0.2.
3. Serum ferritin—less than 12 g/dL.
4. Lead—greater than 20 g/dL.
5. Free erythrocyte protoporphyrin—greater than 35 g/dL.
6. B_{12}, B_6, folate levels—may be decreased.
7. Hemoglobin electrophoresis—may show hemoglobin S or other abnormality.
8. Parovirus B_{19} titer—may be elevated in transient erythroblastopenia.

Management

Iron Deficiency Anemia

1. Oral iron at a dose of 6 mg elemental iron/kg per day given between meals.
2. Dietary: decrease milk intake to 16 oz/day; include iron-fortified cereals and bread products; increase consumption of red meat; include foods rich in vitamin C.
3. Currently, iron is rarely given intramuscularly because of high incidence of allergic reactions. If administered intramuscularly, it is given by Z-track method.

Anemia of Chronic Lead Poisoning (see p. 1287)

1. Early detection of high lead levels through screening questionnaires and blood tests.
2. Maintenance of a well-balanced diet, high in calcium and vitamin D.
3. Administration of chelating agents ethylenediaminetetraacetic acid (EDTA) or dimercaprol (BAL) according to recommendations of the Centers for Disease Control and Prevention.
4. Use of lead-free paints, gasoline, etc.
5. Testing of house and soil.
6. Removal of individuals from unsafe environment.

Megaloblastic Anemia

1. Folate deficiency—administration of folic acid orally.
2. B_{12} deficiency—administration of B_{12} (cyanocobalamin [Cyanoject]) intramuscularly.

Hemoglobinopathies

1. Sickle cell anemia (see p. 1539)
2. Thalassemia (see p. 1545)

Transient Erythroblastopenia of Childhood

1. For hemoglobins of less than 5 g or cardiac failure, usually a transfusion of packed RBCs.
2. Usually, unless cardiac failure occurs, supportive care, not therapy, is provided.

Complications

1. Mental sluggishness, as a result of decreased oxygen and energy for normal neural activity; usually associated with a decreased attention span, deceased intelligence, and lethargy.
2. Growth retardation related to anorexia and decreased cellular metabolism.
3. Delayed puberty related to growth retardation.
4. Cardiac enlargement related to muscle hypertrophy because of increased strain on the heart, attempting to compensate for increased oxygen demand by the tissues; eventually results in congestive heart failure.
5. Death from cardiac failure related to circulatory collapse and shock.

Nursing Assessment

1. Obtain history of potential causes.
   a. Dietary history, including the amount of milk and meat consumed
   b. Medications
   c. Persistent infection, fever, or chronic disease
   d. Exposure to drugs, poisons, etc.
   e. Pica—craving and consuming nonfood items (eg, paint chips, ice, paper, etc.)
2. Obtain a baseline assessment.
   a. Observe skin and mucous membranes for pallor.
   b. Obtain height and weight and plot on growth curve.

TABLE 52-1	Blood Tests in Anemia by Cause				
	MCV	**MCHC**	**Reticulocyte**	**Ferritin**	**FEP**
Iron deficiency	Low	Low	Low	Low	High
Lead poisoning	Low	Low	Low	Normal	High
β-Thalassemia	Low	Low	Low	Normal	Normal
Folate deficiency	High	Normal	Low	Normal	Normal
B_{12} deficiency	High	Normal	Low	Normal	Normal
Sickle cell disease	Normal	Normal	High	Normal	Normal

FEP, free erythrocyte protoporphyrin; MCHC, mean corpuscular hemoglobin concentration; MCV, mean corpuscular volume.

c. Measure vital signs, including blood pressure.
d. Assess child's functional level—level of exercise tolerance, mental functioning.
e. Assess attainment of developmental milestones.
3. Observe for fatigue, listlessness, irritability, etc.
4. Observe for blood loss: bruising, bleeding, hematuria, or hematochezia (blood in stool).

NURSING ALERT

Be alert for children at risk for iron deficiency anemia—children in rapid growth stages (toddlers and adolescents) and pregnant or lactating adolescents.

Nursing Diagnoses

- Fatigue related to decreased ability of blood to transport oxygen to the tissues
- Altered Nutrition: Less Than Body Requirements of recommended daily dietary allowances
- Risk for Infection related to debilitated state
- Anxiety related to hospitalization and painful diagnostic procedures (venipunctures, finger sticks, etc.)
- Altered Growth and Development related to decreased energy

Nursing Interventions

Minimizing Fatigue

1. Plan nursing care to allow for lengthy periods when the child is not disturbed by hospital routines, procedures, treatments, etc.; set priorities.
2. Observe for early signs of fatigue, such as irritability, hyperactivity, listless, etc.
3. Encourage sedentary rather than active projects.
4. Administer oxygen and position upright if dyspnea present.
5. Do not always encourage self-care.
6. Provide finger foods that are easy to chew to conserve energy.

Providing Adequate Nutritional Intake

1. Be aware of the child's food preferences and plan diet accordingly.
2. Offer small amounts of food at frequent intervals.
3. Reward the child for positive attempts to eat.
4. Allow the child to participate in selection of foods and in preparation of meal tray.
5. Avoid tiring activities and unpleasant procedures at mealtime.
6. Make mealtime as pleasurable as possible.
7. Provide iron-rich food and vitamins when necessary.
8. If iron is ordered, give between meals and with orange juice (iron is absorbed best in acidic environment).
9. Limit milk and milk products to 16 oz to 24 oz/day. Milk products inhibit the absorption of oral iron.
10. Administer liquid iron with a dropper or straw or dilute with water or fruit juice to prevent staining of the teeth.
    a. If administered by dropper, ensure that liquid iron is deposited in the back of the mouth.

b. Dental stains can be removed by brushing the teeth with sodium bicarbonate or hydrogen peroxide and then rinsing with water after each administration.
11. Be alert for side effects of iron supplements—gastric distress, colic pain, diarrhea, or constipation; may call for decreased dose.
12. Advise family that child's stool may turn dark green or black.
13. Stress the importance of continuing iron therapy according to health care provider's directions, even though the child may not appear to be ill.
14. Inform parents that iron overdoses can be harmful or fatal.

Preventing Infection

1. Teach and assist with good hygiene practices, such as handwashing and mouth care.
2. Avoid exposure to others with colds, infections, etc.
3. Ensure that staff, family, and visitors always wash hands thoroughly.
4. Report any temperature elevation or other signs of infection.

Reducing Anxiety

1. Allow the child to handle equipment used for tests and procedures (tourniquets, syringes, etc.).
2. Explain all procedures and the treatment plan to the child in a way that child can understand.
3. Allow the older child to look through a microscope at a blood smear, if interested and if appropriate for child's age.
4. Permit the child to cleanse the area for a venipuncture or a finger stick and to choose the finger.

Promoting Normal Growth and Development

1. Ensure that nutrition is adequate for age and activity level.
2. Encourage participation in age-related activities.
3. Encourage doing homework and tutored activities.
4. Encourage peer socialization.
5. Promote age-appropriate play and therapeutic play.
6. Perform periodic growth chart evaluation and developmental testing.
   a. Share results with parents and explain the association between diet/anemia and growth and development.
   b. Notify health care provider and make referrals as indicated.

Family Education and Health Maintenance

1. Stress to the parents the importance of continuing the iron therapy according to the provider's directions even though the child may not appear ill.

DRUG ALERT

Much variation exists in the elemental iron content of commercially available liquid preparations that contain iron. To avoid confusion, the dosage should be expressed in terms of elemental iron and then converted to the proper amount of the therapeutic agent selected.

2. Initiate and reinforce good dietary habits.
   a. Foods rich in iron include dark green leafy vegetables, fortified cereals, dried fruits, nuts, and red meats.
   b. Do not allow the child to drink excessive quantities of milk to the exclusion of other foods that contain more iron. Limit milk intake to 16 oz to 24 oz/day.
   c. Provide vitamin supplements if necessary. Vitamin C appears to enhance the absorption of iron.
   d. Explain the reasons for diet change to parents in language they can understand. Visual aids and pictures may be helpful.
   e. Assist the parents to select iron-rich foods that are acceptable to the child, within the family's food budget, and culturally acceptable.
3. Discuss with parents any of the social, economic, and environmental problems that may contribute to the child's disease.
4. Emphasize to the parents the benefits of a referral to a community health nurse if it appears that the family will need support in dealing with the child's chronic disease.
5. Discuss general health measures, including adequate rest, diet, sunshine, and fresh air activity.
6. Encourage regular medical and dental evaluations. Emphasize the need for appropriate follow-up visits.
7. Explain that infection may be prevented by dressing the child according to the weather and by keeping away from persons with colds, sore throats, and other infections.
8. Teach the parents how to administer medication.
9. Alert the parents to signs of disease progression—increased fatigue, pallor, weakness, developmental delays, and poor performance in school and activities.

Outcome-Based Evaluation

- Increasing activity noted
- Eats frequent small feedings of cereal, bread, red meat, vegetables; tolerating iron supplement without side effects
- Remains free of infection; normal temperature
- Cooperates with frequent blood sampling
- Maintains growth curve; manages age-appropriate developmental activities

◼ Sickle Cell Disease (Sickle Cell Anemia)

Sickle cell disease is a severe, chronic, hemolytic anemia occurring in persons who are homozygous for the sickle gene. The clinical course is characterized by episodes of pain caused by the occlusion of small blood vessels by sickled RBCs. Persons heterozygous for the sickling gene are said to possess sickle cell trait, which is associated with a benign clinical course. Found almost entirely in blacks and persons of Arabic northern Mediterranean ancestry. Approximately 8% of blacks have sickle cell trait. Approximately 1 of every 600 black infants born in the United States has sickle cell anemia.

Pathophysiology and Etiology

1. Genetically determined, inherited disease—autosomal recessive.
2. Each person inherits one gene from each parent, which governs the synthesis of hemoglobin (Table 52-2).
3. Normally each hemoglobin molecule consists of four molecules of heme folded into one molecule of globin. Each globin molecule consists of two α chains and two β chains.
4. The amino acid sequence on the chain is altered in sickle cell hemoglobin—valine is substituted for glutamic acid in the sixth position of the 574 amino acids that make up the globin fraction of hemoglobin.
5. Sickle cell hemoglobin aggregates into elongated crystals under conditions of low oxygen concentration, acidosis, and dehydration.
6. This distorts the membrane of the RBC, causing it to assume a crescent or sickle shape. The cells easily become entangled and enmeshed, leading to increased blood viscosity, vessel occlusion, and tissue necrosis.
7. Sickled RBCs are fragile and are rapidly destroyed in the circulation; they live 6 to 20 days versus 120 days for normal RBCs.
8. Anemia results when the rate of destruction of RBCs is greater than the rate of production.
9. Increased sequestration of RBCs occurs in the spleen.

Clinical Manifestations

Children are rarely symptomatic until late in the first year of life, related to increased amounts of fetal hemoglobin (HgF). Clinical manifestations are sporadic; the child may be asymptomatic for several months. Periods of crisis occur at variable intervals.

Signs of Anemia

May last 1 to 2 weeks and subside spontaneously.

1. Hemoglobin—6 g/dL to 9 g/dL
2. Loss of appetite
3. Paleness
4. Weakness
5. Fever
6. Irritability
7. Jaundice; increased hemolysis results in hemosiderosis (increased iron storage in the liver)

TABLE 52-2 Transmission of Sickle Cell Disease			
	Probability of Abnormal Hemoglobin in Offspring		
Genotype of Parents	Normal	Trait	Disease
1 parent with trait	50%	50%	0
Both parents with trait	25%	50%	25%
1 parent with trait; 1 parent with disease	0	50%	50%
Both parents with disease	0	0	100%

Precipitating Factors of Crisis
1. Dehydration
2. Infection
3. Trauma
4. Strenuous physical exertion
5. Extreme fatigue
6. Cold exposure
7. Hypoxia
8. Acidosis

Sickle Cell (Vaso-occlusive) Crisis
Most common form of crisis.
1. Small blood vessels are occluded by the sickle-shaped cells, causing distal ischemia and infarction (Figure 52-1).
2. Extremities:
   a. Bony destruction—related to erythroid hyperplasia of marrow, leading to osteoporosis or ischemic necrosis.
   b. Bone pain; painful and swollen large joints.
   c. Dactylitis ("hand-foot" syndrome)—aseptic infarction of metacarpals and metatarsals, causing symmetrical swelling and pain; often first vaso-occlusive event seen in infants and toddlers.
3. Spleen:
   a. Abdominal pain.
   b. Splenomegaly—initially increases in size because of increased activity as site of RBC hemolysis; increased size results in discomfort.

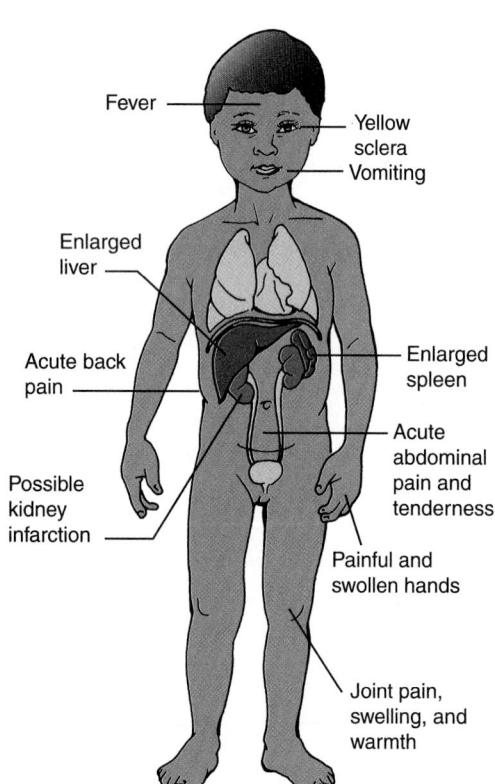

Fever
Yellow sclera
Vomiting
Enlarged liver
Acute back pain
Enlarged spleen
Acute abdominal pain and tenderness
Possible kidney infarction
Painful and swollen hands
Joint pain, swelling, and warmth

FIGURE 52-1 Sickle cell crisis signs and symptoms.

c. After multiple episodes of splenic vaso-occlusion, the spleen becomes fibrotic and atrophied.
   d. Decreased splenic function increases the risk of infection.
4. Cerebral occlusion:
   a. Strokes.
   b. Hemiplegia.
   c. Retinal damage, leading to blindness.
   d. Seizures.
5. Pulmonary infarction.
6. Altered renal function: enuresis, hematuria.
7. Impaired liver function.
8. Priapism—abnormal, recurrent, prolonged, painful penile erection.

Splenic Sequestration Crisis
1. Large amounts of blood become pooled in the spleen.
2. Spleen becomes massively enlarged.
3. Great decrease in RBC mass occurs within hours.
4. Signs of circulatory collapse develop rapidly.
5. Frequent cause of death in infants with sickle cell disease.

Aplastic Crisis
1. Bone marrow ceases production of RBCs only.
2. Results in low reticulocyte counts.

Chronic Symptoms
Chronic organ damage results in organ dysfunction.
1. Jaundice.
2. Gallstones.
3. Progressive impairment of kidney function.
4. Fibrotic spleen, resulting in high susceptibility to *Haemophilus influenzae* and *Streptococcus pneumoniae* infections, osteomyelitis, and pneumococcal septicemia.
5. Growth retardation of the long bones and spine deformities.
6. Delayed puberty.
7. Cardiac decompensation related to chronic anemia.
8. Chronic, painful leg ulcers related to decreased peripheral circulation and unrelated to injury; may take months to heal or may not heal without intense therapy, including blood transfusions and grafting.
9. Decreased life span.
10. Altered bony structures—aseptic necrosis of the bones, especially the femoral and humoral heads.

Diagnostic Evaluation

> **NURSING ALERT**
>
> In 1987, the National Institutes of Health issued guidelines for all infants born in the United States to be mandatorily tested for sickle cell disease. This is done before discharge, using the sickle cell prep from a heel stick.

1. Sickle cell prep (sickling test):
   a. Done by finger or heel stick.
   b. Oxygen is removed from a drop of blood.
   c. The blood is observed under the microscope for sickle-shaped cells.

d. Test does not distinguish between persons with sickle cell trait and disease or other sickle hemoglobinopathies.

2. Sickledex:

a. Done by finger stick.

b. A small amount of blood is placed in a solution containing a chemical reducing agent.

c. Sickle hemoglobin is indicated if the solution turns cloudy.

d. Test also does not distinguish between persons with sickle cell trait and disease or other sickle hemoglobinopathies.

3. Hemoglobin electrophoresis:

a. Requires venipuncture.

b. Hemoglobin is subjected to an electric current that separates the various types and determines the amounts present.

c. Test is used to diagnose both sickle cell trait and sickle cell disease if two types of hemoglobin are demonstrated in approximately equal amounts.

d. A person is diagnosed as having sickle cell anemia if most hemoglobin is sickle hemoglobin (hemoglobin S). This may also diagnose other sickle hemoglobinopathies including sickle C, sickle-β-thalassemia, or other hemoglobin variants.

4. Antenatal diagnosis is available to the high-risk group through amniocentesis and gene mapping.

Management
Prevent Sickling

1. Promote adequate oxygenation and hemodilution.

a. Encourage increased intake of fluids—150 mL/kg per day or 2,250 mL/m2 per day.

b. Avoid high altitudes and other low-oxygen environments.

c. Avoid strenuous physical exertion.

d. Administer oxygen for pulse oximetry of 90% or less.

e. Avoid extreme heat or cold.

Crisis Episodes

Supportive and symptomatic care depend on type.

1. Aplastic episode—usually requires a blood transfusion starting at 10 mL/kg.

2. Splenic sequestration—usually requires a blood transfusion to release trapped RBCs in severe cases. Plasma volume expanders may also be used to correct hypovolemia. One or more episodes may require splenectomy.

3. Hemolytic episode—usually requires only hydration. May occur with splenic sequestration, aplastic, and painful episodes, which are then treated accordingly. Transfusions are required if a significant drop in hemoglobin occurs.

4. Vaso-occlusive or painful episode—must be individualized; must determine if the painful event is a manifestation of an underlying illness (infection) or of an inflammatory condition. Most often caused by increased sickling, resulting from hypoxia and acidosis.

a. Hydration—to reverse dehydration that may have been caused by decreased fluid intake, increased insensible loss, hyposthenuria, and hyperthermia (fever). This is accomplished by increased oral and parenteral fluid intake of up to one and a half or twice fluid maintenance needs.

b. Electrolyte and pH balance must be closely monitored.

c. Analgesics—administered on fixed schedule, not to extend beyond the duration of the pharmacologic effect. Intravenous (IV) narcotics such as morphine are preferred for severe pain, either as a continuous infusion or on a patient-controlled analgesia (PCA) pump to reach desired effects. Other agents, such as nonsteroidal anti-inflammatory drugs (NSAIDs) and acetaminophen (Tylenol) are used for milder pain or to increase the analgesic effects of narcotics.

d. Alternative pain management techniques—behavior modification programs, relaxation therapy, hypnosis, music therapy, massage, and transcutaneous electrical nerve stimulation (TENS).

e. New research on butyrate and hydroxyurea (Hydrea), which increase fetal hemoglobin and prevent sickling, is being conducted, with promising results.

f. Those with chronic or severe vaso-occlusive crises may benefit from monthly blood transfusions, which will improve their anemia and decrease their total amount of sickle hemoglobin.

5. Infection—major cause of morbidity and mortality.

a. Most serious include *S. pneumoniae, H. influenzae, Neisseria meningitidis,* Salmonella species, *Mycoplasma pneumoniae, Staphylococcus aureus, Escherichia coli,* and *Streptococcus pyogenes.*

b. Infection of any type is more difficult to eradicate in patients with sickle cell and often exacerbates crises such as aplastic episodes caused by parvovirus (fifth disease), increases the rate of hemolysis, and precipitates vaso-occlusive episodes.

c. Prevention is most important—give usual primary immunizations as well as pneumococcal, *Haemophilus* b conjugate, hepatitis, meningococcal, and trivalent influenza vaccines.

d. Antibiotic prophylaxis—prevents bacteremia and reduces nasopharyngeal colonization.

e. Fever of 102°F (38.9°C), with minimal clinical signs, should be treated with broad-spectrum antibiotics, such as cefuroxime (Kefurox) 100 mg/kg per day, to prevent septicemia. The choice of subsequent antibiotics can be guided by results of cultures and clinical course.

Complications

1. Chronic hemolytic anemia.

2. Greatest risk of death is in children younger than 5 years of age, mainly from overwhelming sepsis or sequestration.

3. Episodes of splenic sequestration, hemolysis, aplasia, vaso-occlusion.

4. Life expectancy is variable; however, it is improving with new forms of treatment.

Nursing Assessment

1. Obtain history for possible dehydration, hypoxia, infection, or other precipitating event.
2. Obtain history and characterization of pain.
3. Observe for pallor and jaundice, changes in vital signs (elevated temperature, tachycardia, hypotension, tachypnea), change in mental status, swelling of extremities, ulcers or skin lesions, or signs of dehydration (decreased elasticity of skin, dry mucous membranes, decreased urine output, increased urine concentration and specific gravity).
4. Examine for enlarged liver and spleen, tenderness of hands or feet.
5. Evaluate growth and development.

Nursing Diagnoses

• Pain related to tissue anoxia from disease process
• Altered Tissue Perfusion related to increased blood viscosity
• Risk for Infection related to fibrotic changes in the spleen
• Impaired Gas Exchange related to effects of narcotics, anesthesia, and blood loss of surgery
• Activity Intolerance related to anemia
• Altered Family Process related to frequent medical care, hospitalization, and chronic illness

Nursing Interventions

Also see Nursing Care Plan 52-1: Painful Vaso-occlusive Crisis

Relieving Pain

1. Identify and use effective measures to alleviate pain, such as:
    a. Carefully position and support painful areas.
    b. Hold or rock the infant; handle gently.
    c. Distract the child by singing, reading stories, providing play activities.
    d. Provide familiar objects; encourage visits by familiar persons.
    e. Bathe the child in warm water, applying local heat or massage.
    f. Give prescribed medications. Do not give aspirin because it enhances acidosis.
    g. Maintain bed rest during crisis.
2. Share effective methods of reducing pain with other staff members and family.

Increasing Tissue Perfusion

1. Administer blood for severe anemia and vaso-occlusion.
2. Administer oxygen via tent, face mask, or nasal cannula, depending on age.

Reducing Infection

1. Administer antibiotics as prescribed.
2. Give meticulous care to leg ulcers and other open wounds.

3. Use good handwashing and meticulous technique in all procedures.

Preventing Hypoxia

1. Monitor for and prevent respiratory depression caused by narcotics.
    a. Check respiratory rate and depth frequently.
    b. Encourage coughing and deep breathing.
    c. Use incentive spirometry.
    d. Obtain pulse oximetry reading as indicated.
    e. Raise side rails and supervise ambulation if drowsiness occurs.
2. Help reduce the risks of anesthesia and blood loss during surgery.
    a. Administer preoperative blood transfusion(s) as prescribed to suppress the formation of new sickle cells and to reduce the threat of anoxia.
    b. Maintain adequate hydration before and after surgery.
    c. Observe the child closely for signs of infection, especially of the respiratory tract.
    d. Inform anesthesia department of child's disease status.
    e. Monitor vital signs frequently and obtain pulse oximetry readings.

Improving Activity Tolerance

1. Maintain bed rest during crisis, then increase activity gradually to increase endurance.
2. Encourage rest periods, alternating with activity.
3. Encourage good eating habits, sleep, and relaxation.

Normalizing Family Processes

1. Encourage parents to talk about their child, the illness, and how they feel about it.
2. Expect such feelings as guilt, shock, frustration, depression, and resentment.
3. Accept negative feelings, but try to build on positive coping mechanisms.
4. Provide factual information to child and parents about their concerns.
5. Encourage role playing and play activities to identify fears.
6. Assure adolescents that although sexual development is delayed, they will eventually catch up with their peers.
7. Stress the normalcy of the child despite sickle cell.
    a. Sickle cell disease does not affect intelligence; the child should go to school and keep up with class work while stable.
    b. Between periods of crisis the child can usually participate in peer group activities, with the exception of some strenuous sports.
    c. The child needs discipline as do other children in family.

Community and Home Care Considerations

Home care nurses and school nurses can be instrumental in the care of patients with sickle cell anemia, by assuring that their primary health care needs are met.

1. Because of the child's predisposition to infections, be sure that the following are carried out routinely:
   a. Ophthalmology exams every 1 to 2 years after the age of 10.
   b. Hearing tests yearly after the age of 3 years of age.
   c. A TB skin test every 2 to 3 years (every year in endemic areas). Any positive findings should be followed up promptly.
   d. All routine childhood immunizations, as well as the hepatitis B series, pneumococcal, meningococcal, *Haemophilis* type B, and yearly trivalent influenza.
   e. Dental checkups and teeth cleaning every 6 months.
2. Educate parents, teachers, and day care providers involved in the care of children with sickle cell disease about their common problems and special needs:
   a. Frequent absences because of pain and illness.
   b. Fatigue and inattention, caused by anemia or ischemia of CNS tissue.
   c. Inability to concentrate urine, requiring frequent restroom breaks.
   d. Permanent learning disabilities or delays, requiring individualized teaching plans.
   e. Need for a controlled environment to prevent sickling, avoiding temperature extremes, dehydration, and excessive stress.
   f. Need for moderate physical exercise, with avoidance of rough contact sports and activities.
   g. Desire to feel "normal" and have opportunities and environmental stimulation similar to other children their age.
3. Assess the child's home environment for protection from infection and injury, adequate nutritional resources, transportation to medical appointments, and emotional support. Initiate social service and other referrals as needed.

Family Education and Health Maintenance

1. Discuss the genetic implications of sickle cell disease and offer genetic counseling to the family.
2. Instruct the parents in ways that they can help their child to avoid sickling episodes.
   a. Do not allow the child to become chilled or to wear tight clothing that might impede circulation.
   b. Provide adequate fluids and notify health care provider if excessive fluids are lost through vomiting, diarrhea, fever, excessive sweating.
3. Instruct parents how to recognize signs of dehydration (dry skin and mucous membranes, decreased urine output; irritability or listlessness in the infant).
4. Encourage parents to seek prompt treatment of cuts, sores, mosquito bites, etc., and to notify the health care provider if the child is exposed to a communicable disease.
5. Encourage good dental hygiene and frequent dental checkups to avoid dental infections.

6. Instruct on preventive care, including all the recommended childhood immunizations and screening tests.
7. Teach the child to avoid undue emotional stress.
8. Warn against trips to the mountains or against trips in unpressurized airplanes that will decrease oxygen concentration.
9. Provide sexually active adolescents with information on contraception and sexually transmitted disease.
10. Teach signs of a mild crisis:
    a. Fever
    b. Decreased appetite
    c. Irritability
    d. Pain or swelling in abdomen, extremities, back
    e. Teach parents to palpate spleen.
11. Instruct on home management of mild crisis.
    a. Push fluids.
    b. Administer antipyretic medications, as directed by health care provider familiar with condition.
    c. Encourage rest.
    d. Keep the child warm.
    e. Apply warm compresses to the painful area.
    f. Hospitalization may be required for the child if pain becomes severe or if IV hydration is required.
12. Teach the signs of severe crises and whom to notify:
    a. Pallor
    b. Lethargy and listlessness
    c. Difficulty in awakening
    d. Irritability
    e. Severe pain
    f. Fever of 102°F (38.9°C)—report immediately
13. Instruct the parents to have emergency information available to those involved in the child's care (school nurse, teacher, babysitter, family members, etc.).
    a. Name and phone number of health care provider or clinic.
    b. Closest emergency facility and ambulance phone number.
    c. Child's blood type, allergies, medications, and medical records number.
    d. Name of informed neighbor or relative to be notified in an emergency.
14. Stress the benefit of wearing a Medic-Alert tag.
15. For additional information and support, refer to Sickle Cell Foundation, 5110 West Goldleaf Circle, #150, Los Angeles, CA 90056, 323-299-3600, *www.scdfc.org*.

Outcome-Based Evaluation

- Appears more comfortable and does not cry or complain of pain
- Less pallor noted with oxygen use
- Afebrile with no signs of infection
- No change in respirations; uses incentive spirometer hourly
- Ambulates 20 minutes four or five times a day
- Parents verbalize concerns about chronic illness

NURSING CARE PLAN 52-1   Painful Vaso-occlusive Crisis

You are assigned Danielle, a 6-year-old with sickle cell anemia, who has been admitted with a fever of 38.9°C (102°F), chest pain, bilateral leg pain, and an oxygen saturation of 90%.

Subjective Data: Danielle complains of bilateral leg pain, states that it hurts to breathe, and says that she has the chills. She felt tired and had much pain yesterday and was unable to go to school. Mom was giving her some pain medication at home, but when she spiked a fever, she was brought to the emergency room and was admitted to your unit.

Objective Data: Vital signs—temperature of 38.2°C (100.7°F), pulse 120, BP 90/52, and respirations of 34. You notice that her legs are warm and swollen, tender to touch. Respiratory evaluation reveals bilateral crackles at the lung bases, labored respirations with O_2 mask on, and pallor.

Laboratory data:
1. CBC—WBC, 15.4; HgB, 6.5; Hct, 20.1; and platelets, 636,000
2. Pulse oximetry—90%
3. Chest x-ray—bilateral lower lobe pneumonia
4. Electrolytes—Na, 131; Cl, 110; K, 4.8
5. Blood, urine, and throat cultures are pending.

You know that hypoxia, dehydration, and acidosis may have been caused by the underlying respiratory infection and can all precipitate vaso-occlusive crisis. You develop your plan of care to focus on resolution of these factors and to support the patient through crisis.

NURSING DIAGNOSIS   Impaired Gas Exchange related to pneumonia

OUTCOME/GOAL   Oxygenation will be enhanced and respiratory acidosis will be prevented.

Nursing Interventions	Rationale	Outcome-Based Evaluation
1. Administer oxygen via face mask to relieve dyspnea and promote oxygenation.	1. Secretion-filled aveoli impair gas exchange leading to hypoxemia	1. Respirations 34, shallow, and with sternal retractions on face mask. Pulse oximetry 88%. Changed to Venturi mask at 40%.
a. Obtain pulse oximetry reading frequently and correlate with arterial blood gas results.	a. Pulse oximetry serves as guide to improving or worsening oxygenation. Arterial blood gases should be done for correlation and to evaluate acid-base status.	
b. Assess respiratory rate, use of accessory muscles and depth of respirations.	b. Increasing rate, decreasing depth, and increased effort of breathing may lead to respiratory failure.	
2. Administer bronchodilator nebulization treatments q3h, followed by cough and deep breathing exercises. Auscultate lungs hourly.	2. Will promote opening of airways and expectoration of secretions. Frequent auscultation of lungs will help evaluate effectiveness of therapy and determine the need for corticosteroids to reduce inflammation and open the airways further.	2. Lungs clearer following nebulization and coughing.
3. Administer IV antibiotics, as ordered.	3. To resolve pneumonia.	3. Antibiotic infusing via peripheral line.

NURSING DIAGNOSIS   Pain related to tissue anoxia caused by abnormal hemoglobin and clumping of sickled cells within the small vessels

OUTCOME/GOAL   Pain will be relieved.

Nursing Interventions	Rationale	Outcome-Based Evaluation
1. Use nonpharmacologic strategies to help manage pain; distraction, relaxation, guided imagery, positive self-talk, cutaneous stimulation (warm soaks, massage, etc), behavioral contracting.	1. Will limit the amount of analgesia, which may depress respirations.	1. Child uses blowing, looks at magic wand, listens to relaxation tapes and videos; states that they help.

(continued)

NURSING CARE PLAN 52-1 Painful Vaso-occlusive Crisis (Continued)

Nursing Intervention	Rationale	Outcome-Based Evaluation
a. Involve parent and child in selecting strategies.	a. Child will be more receptive to own choices and allows participation in care.	
b. Institute and teach selected strategies before pain becomes severe.	b. If pain is severe, child may not be able to concentrate on these strategies if not practiced.	
2. Administer prescribed analgesia around the clock. Avoid PRN orders when pain is predictable and continuous.	2. To maintain a steady state of analgesic and prevent clock watching.	2. Receives medication q4h without breakthrough pain reported.

> **⊘ NURSING ALERT**
>
> **Avoid IM analgesia if possible because children associate great deal of pain with shots and may deny pain to avoid getting shot.**

Nursing Intervention	Rationale	Outcome-Based Evaluation
3. Assess pain relief and increase or decrease dose or time interval of medication for adequate control.	3. To maximize analgesia with minimal side effects.	3. No breakthrough pain with increased time interval (6 hours) between doses.
a. Avoid placebo.	a. If expected effect is not received by placebo, child may lose trust in caretakers.	
b. Assess for respiratory depression, hypotension, and drowsiness with narcotics.	b. Narcotics may cause CNS depression, shallow respirations, and hypotension in large or frequent dosing.	b. Alert, respirations 24 and deep, BP 96/56

NURSING DIAGNOSIS Fluid Volume Deficit related to fever, insensible loss through mouth breathing and increased respiratory rate, and increased blood viscosity

OUTCOME/GOAL Hydration will be promoted.

Nursing Interventions	Rationale	Outcome-Based Evaluation
1. Administer IV fluids as ordered based on calculation of recommended daily fluid intake requirements plus estimated loss.	1. Child should consume approximately 1,500 mL/m². Loss may be established by decrease in body weight (1 kg equals 1 liter of fluid).	1. D₅NS infusing via peripheral IV volumetric pump.
2. Encourage child to drink by providing fluids preferred.	2. Intake will be enhanced by using preferences.	2. Sipping juices at intervals.
3. Monitor intake and output. Monitor urine specific gravity.	3. To determine fluid balance and hydration status.	3. Intake and output equal; urine specific gravity 1.020.
4. Administer acetaminophen for fever over 38°C (100.4°F) and maintain bed rest.	4. To reduce fluid loss through perspiration due to fever or exertion.	4. Temperature 37.5°C (99.5°F)

■ Thalassemia Major (Cooley's Anemia)

Thalassemia major is the most severe of the beta-thalassemia syndromes and represents the homozygous form of the disease. Beta-thalassemia (β-thalassemia) refers to an inherited hemolytic anemia, characterized by a reduction or absence of the β-globulin chain in hemoglobin synthesis. This RBC has a decreased amount of hemoglobin, resulting in a fragile RBC with a short life span. Most prevalent in the Mediterranean basin, Middle East, Southeast Asia, and Africa. In the United States, it is most common in children of Italian, Greek, and Southeastern Asian ancestry. About 1,400 people in the United States are affected.

Pathophysiology and Etiology

1. Genetically determined, inherited disease—autosomal recessive pattern of inheritance.
2. Insufficient β-globin chain synthesis allows large amounts of unstable chains to accumulate.

3. The precipitates of α chains that form cause RBCs to be rigid and easily destroyed, leading to severe hemolytic anemia and resultant chronic hypoxia.
4. Erythroid activity is significantly increased in an attempt to overcome the increased rate of destruction, resulting in enormous expansion of bone marrow, thinning of bony cortex leading to:
   a. Skeletal deformities: frontal and maxillary bossing
   b. Growth retardation
   c. Pathologic fractures
5. Rapid destruction of defective RBCs, decreased production of hemoglobin, and increased absorption of dietary iron caused by the body's response to anemia result in an excess supply of available iron (hemosiderosis), which deposits iron on organ tissues, resulting in decreased function (especially cardiac).
6. In response to the low level of adult hemoglobin, large concentrations of HgF, which does not contain α chains, are produced; HgF does not hold oxygen well.

Clinical Manifestations
1. Onset is usually insidious, with symptoms noted toward the end of the first year of life.
2. Symptoms are primarily related to the progressive anemia, expansion of the marrow cavities of the bone, and the development of hemosiderosis.
3. Early symptoms often include progressive pallor, poor feeding, and lethargy.
4. Further signs of progressive anemia include headache, bone pain, exercise intolerance, jaundice, and protuberant abdomen caused by hepatosplenomegaly.

Diagnostic Evaluation
1. Hemoglobin level—decreased.
2. RBCs—increased number.
3. Low mean corpuscular volume (MCV) and mean corpuscular hemoglobin concentration (MCHC)—microcytosis and hypochromia.
4. Peripheral blood smear—many anisopoikilocytes, nucleated RBCs.
5. Reticulocyte count—low, usually less than 10%.
6. Hemoglobin electrophoresis—elevated levels of HgF and HgA2; limited amount of HgA.

Management
1. Frequent and regular blood transfusions of packed RBCs to maintain hemoglobin levels above 10 g/dL.
   a. Washed, packed RBCs are usually used to minimize the possibility of transfusion reactions. If unavailable, leukofiltered cells can be substituted.
   b. The frequency and amount of transfusions depend on the size of the child, usually 10 mL to 15 mL packed RBC per kg body weight every 2 to 3 weeks.
2. Iron chelation therapy with deferoxamine (Desferal) reduces the toxic side effects of excess iron; increases iron excretion through urine and feces.

a. IV infusion of 100 to 150 mg/kg per day given in hospital during blood transfusion or for child with high ferritin level and poor compliance with home chelation therapy.
   b. Subcutaneous infusion of 50 mg/kg per day usually infused 12 hours during night for home therapy.
3. Splenectomy.
4. Supportive management of complications.
5. Bone marrow transplants are a possibility; however, the survival rate is poor. Young patients with few complications are good candidates.
6. Prognosis is poor because of no known cure; often fatal in late adolescence or early adulthood.

Complications
1. Splenomegaly—usually requires splenectomy; overwhelming postsplenectomy infection rate seen in 25% of these patients.
2. Growth retardation in second decade.
3. Endocrine abnormalities:
   a. Delayed development of secondary sex characteristics—most boys fail to undergo puberty; most girls experience alteration in menstruation.
   b. Diabetes mellitus is often seen in older patients, related to iron deposits on the pancreas.
   c. Hypermetabolic rate results in increased temperature and lethargy.
4. Skeletal complications—become less common because of early transfusion therapy and maintenance of hemoglobin levels above 10 g/dL:
   a. Frontal and parietal bossing (enlarging)
   b. Maxillary hypertrophy, leading to malocclusion
   c. Broad ribs
   d. Premature fusion of epiphyses of long bones
   e. Generalized skeletal osteoporosis
   f. Pathologic fractures of the long bones and vertebral collapse
5. Cardiac complications:
   a. Fibrosis and hypertrophy
   b. Pericarditis
   c. Congestive heart failure—usual cause of death
6. Liver enlargement—fibrosis, coagulation abnormalities, and eventually cirrhosis.
7. Gallbladder disease—gallstones are common by late adolescence; may require cholecystectomy.
8. Megaloblastic anemia—caused by sporadic folic acid deficiency from increased use by hyperplastic marrow.
9. Skin—bronze pigmentation caused by iron deposits in the dermis; jaundice.
10. Leg ulcers.

Nursing Assessment
1. Obtain family history of thalassemia or unexplained anemia or heart failure.
2. Perform whole body examination to assess for anemia and systemic complications of thalassemia.
3. Measure growth and development parameters.

Nursing Diagnoses

- Altered Tissue Perfusion related to abnormal hemoglobin
- Chronic Pain related to progression of disease in bone
- Activity Intolerance related to bone pain, cardiac dysfunction, and anemia
- Risk for Infection related to progressive anemia and splenectomy
- Knowledge Deficit related to iron chelation therapy
- Body Image Disturbance related to endocrine and skeletal abnormalities
- Ineffective Family Coping related to poor prognosis

Nursing Interventions

Maximizing Tissue Perfusion

1. Administer blood transfusions as ordered.
   a. Observe for signs of transfusion reaction (increased chance caused by frequency) including allergic, febrile, septic, circulatory overload, and hemolytic reactions.
   b. Allergic reactions usually occur within 15 to 20 minutes of start of the transfusion.
   c. Be aware that delayed reactions may occur up to several months later.
2. Monitor cardiovascular status for complications.
   a. Monitor apical pulse, blood pressure, and respirations.
   b. Assess for edema.
   c. Auscultate heart sounds for gallop and lungs for rales.
   d. Assess extremities for ulcer formation.
3. Refer to care of the child with congestive heart failure (see p. 1389).

Relieving Bone Pain

1. Monitor CBC as ordered and report hemoglobin levels of less than 10 g/dL.
2. Elevate lower extremities.
3. Provide warm baths or soaks.
4. Administer or teach proper administration of NSAIDs, such as ibuprofen (Motrin) or naproxen (Naprosyn). Use carefully and monitor liver enzymes in patients with liver complications.

Minimizing Activity Intolerance

1. Encourage participation in activities that do not require significant strenuous activity. Full participation in some activities, especially with peers, will increase self-esteem.
2. Facilitate physical and occupational therapy consultation to develop an acceptable exercise plan.
3. Assist the parents in contacting the child's school and develop a plan of gym activities, classes, and rest periods that allow the greatest level of participation and slowly develop endurance. Advise parents that during the week of the scheduled transfusion, the fatigue will be greatest, so gym and other exertional activities should be modified.
4. Suggest that driving the child to school and providing adequate rest at home will provide him or her with more energy for school activities.
5. Discourage participation in contact or other sports that increase the child's risk for a fracture (skateboarding, football, soccer, etc.).

Preventing Infection

1. Explain to parents that after splenectomy, child has increased susceptibility to infection and should be maintained on oral penicillin prophylaxis.
2. Ensure that child has been vaccinated against *H. influenzae*, pneumococcal, and meningococcal infections before splenectomy, and encourage yearly trivalent influenza vaccination.
3. Encourage prompt medical attention for fever or signs of infection. Fever of 102°F (38.9°C) should be reported immediately and IV broad-spectrum antibiotics, such as ceftriaxone (Rocephin), started.

Promoting Understanding and Compliance

1. Explain to family that deferoxamine (Desferal) is used as a chelating (binding) agent to decrease iron deposits in tissues and to increase iron excretion through urine and feces.
2. Administer IV deferoxamine as ordered.
   a. Infuse slowly, during 8 to 24 hours, through peripheral line or implanted infusion device, via volumetric pump.
   b. Have emergency resuscitation equipment nearby in case severe allergic reaction occurs.
3. Teach administration of subcutaneous deferoxamine and initiate referral for home infusion therapy.
   a. Infuse during 12 hours, usually overnight.
   b. Pick a site in the subcutaneous tissue in the abdomen, thigh, or arm, and insert a small subcutaneous needle attached to a syringe pump.
   c. EMLA, a topical anesthetic, may be used to decrease pain at the insertion site.
   d. Infusion site may become red, hard, and painful; must rotate sites. Warm soaks to area are helpful.
   e. Because allergic reaction may occur, instruct parents to give antihistamine, and if necessary, epinephrine.
4. Be alert for visual and hearing deficits associated with use of deferoxamine and encourage follow-up visits for periodic visual and audiometric testing.

> **NURSING ALERT**
>
> Because of the excess iron deposition in children with thalassemia, dietary iron should be decreased as much as possible.

Improving Body Image

1. Explore the child's feelings of being different from other children.
2. Encourage the child to express feelings through the use of play: art, role playing, etc.
3. Give positive reinforcement regarding appearance.
4. Encourage socialization and peer interaction.
5. Suggest endocrine consultation for delayed growth and puberty and craniofacial specialist for bony abnormalities.
6. Encourage the use of makeup, clothing, hair styles that will make the adolescent appear older.

7. Suggest support group or individual counseling as needed.

Improving Family Coping Strategies

1. Alleviate the child's anxieties about illness by providing explanation in a way he or she can understand.
2. Use role playing and play activities to identify concerns.
3. Assist parents in strengthening coping mechanisms, such as support network, problem solving, and planning ahead.
4. Help identify resources for financial support, medical supplies, respite care, etc.
5. Encourage parents to continue education of child and obtain vocational planning, if realistic.
6. Encourage parents to set limits and to provide discipline for child that is consistent with that for other children in family.
7. Provide supportive care to the dying child (see p. 1312).
8. Encourage bereavement support for parents, siblings, and family.

Family Education and Health Maintenance

1. Discuss the genetic implications of thalassemia and refer for genetic counseling.
2. Provide detailed instruction regarding:
   a. Prevention and prompt treatment of infections
   b. Medications
   c. Home chelation therapy
   d. Dietary modifications to limit iron intake
   e. Activity restrictions, including avoidance of activities that increase the risk of fractures
   f. Signs of complications
3. Encourage parents to provide information about the child's condition to significant adults who are involved with the child (teacher, school nurse, babysitter, Scout leader, etc.).
4. For additional information and support, refer to Cooley's Anemia Foundation, 129-09 26th Ave., Room 203, Flushing, NY 11354, 718-321-2873, *www.thalassemia.org*.

Outcome-Based Evaluation

- Blood pressure stable; no edema; no leg ulcers
- Verbalizes better tolerance of pain
- Reports increased participation in activity, less fatigue
- Afebrile; immunizations current

- Parents verbalize purpose of chelation therapy, treatment of allergic reaction, how to treat site; demonstrating correct technique for infusion
- Verbalizes interest in appearance and positive statements about self
- Parents seek help from support group and social worker; discuss illness with child and siblings

Hemophilia

Hemophilia is usually an inherited, congenital bleeding disorder characterized by a lack of blood clotting factors, especially factors VIII and IX. It appears primarily in males but is transmitted by females. Occurs in 1 in 5,000 males. There is no racial predilection, and hemophilia is found in all ethnic groups.

- Eighty percent to 85% have factor VIII deficiency or hemophilia A (classic hemophilia).
- Fifteen percent to 20% have factor IX deficiency or hemophilia B (Christmas disease).
- Few have factor XI deficiency or hemophilia C.

Pathophysiology and Etiology

1. Hereditary (approximately 80% of patients).
   a. Sex-linked, recessive trait—caused by a gene carried on the X chromosome.
   b. Transmitted by asymptomatic females (Table 52-3).
   c. Appears in males who have the hemophilic gene on their only X chromosome.
   d. Affected males may pass the gene to female offspring, making them carriers.
   e. May appear in females if a female carrier bears offspring with a male hemophiliac.
2. Spontaneous mutations may cause the condition when the family history is negative for the disease (about 20% of patients).
3. The basic defect is in the intrinsic phase of the coagulation cascade. The blood clotting factors are necessary for the formation of prothrombin activator, which acts as a catalyst in the conversion of prothrombin to thrombin.
   a. The rate of formation of thrombin from prothrombin is almost directly proportional to the amount of prothrombin activator available.
   b. The rapidity of the clotting process is proportional to the amount of thrombin formed.

TABLE 52-3 Transmission of Hemophilia

	Probability of Abnormality in Offspring				
	Female			Male	
Genotype of Parents	Normal	Carrier	Hemophiliac	Normal	Hemophiliac
Female carrier/normal male	50%	50%	0	50%	50%
Noncarrier female/hemophiliac male	0	100%	0	100%	0
Female carrier/hemophiliac male	0	50%	50%	50%	50%

4. The result is an unstable fibrin clot.
5. Platelet number and function are normal; therefore, small lacerations and minor hemorrhages are usually not a problem.

Clinical Manifestations

1. Seldom diagnosed in infancy unless excessive bleeding is observed from the umbilical cord or after circumcision.
2. Usually diagnosed after the child becomes active.
3. Varies in severity, depending on the plasma level of the coagulation factor involved.
   a. Level of less than 1% of normal—severe hemophilia; often severe clinical bleeding, with a tendency for spontaneous bleeds.
   b. Level of 1% to 5% of normal—moderately afflicted; may be free of spontaneous bleeding and may not manifest severe bleeding until trauma occurs.
   c. Level of 6% to 30% of normal—mildly afflicted; patients usually lead normal lives and bleed only with severe injury or surgery.
   d. Degree of severity tends to be constant within a given family.
4. Signs and symptoms of abnormal bleeding include:
   a. History of prolonged bleeding episodes, such as after circumcision
   b. Easily bruised
   c. Prolonged bleeding from the mucous membranes of the nose and mouth from lacerations
   d. Spontaneous soft tissue hematomas
   e. Hemorrhages into the joints (hemarthrosis)—especially elbows, knees, and ankles, causing pain, swelling, limitation of movement
   f. Spontaneous hematuria
   g. Gastrointestinal bleeding
   h. Cyclic bleeding episodes may occur with periods of little bleeding, followed by periods of severe bleeding.
   i. Head trauma, resulting in intracranial hemorrhage

Diagnostic Evaluation

1. Prothrombin time and bleeding time are normal.
2. Partial thromboplastin time—prolonged.
3. Prothrombin consumption—decreased.
4. Thromboplastin—increased.
5. Assays for specific clotting factors—abnormal.
6. Gene analysis—to detect carrier state, for prenatal diagnosis.

Management

1. Prompt, early, appropriate treatment is the key to preventing most complications.
2. Must replace missing coagulation factor (VIII or IX) through the administration of type-specific coagulation concentrates during bleeding episodes.
   a. Factor VIII—made from cryoprecipitate that has been viral inactivated, monoclonal or solvent detergent purified. The monoclonal concentrates are the cleanest because most viruses and extraneous proteins have been removed. Since 1993, recombinant factor VIII concentrates are available for use. The factor VIII molecule has been sequenced and placed in a mammalian cell culture to produce recombinant factor VIII, which is free of all viruses.
   b. Factor IX—made from fresh frozen plasma that has been viral inactivated by solvent detergent; monoclonal, heptane vapor; or affinity chromatography. The purest factor IX products are those that have gone through the monoclonal process or the affinity chromatography process, which removes most viruses and any other extraneous proteins and other factors. These are known as factor IX coagulation concentrates.
3. No viral inactivated concentrate exists for hemophilia C; fresh frozen plasma is given to supply factor XI.
4. Mild and moderate factor VIII—deficient hemophiliacs may respond to desmopressin (DDAVP), which causes the release of factor VIII from the endothelial stores. It is given in a dose of 0.3 µg/kg per dose, usually every 24 hours.
5. Antifibrinolytics, such as aminocaproic acid (Amicar) and tranexamic acid (Cyklokapron), are given as adjunctive therapy for mucosal bleeding to prevent clot breakdown by salivary proteins.
6. Activated prothrombin complex concentrates that have activated factors VII, X, and IX are used when inhibitors (autoantibodies) have developed, to bypass factor VIII or IX. In the case of factor VIII inhibitors, porcine factor VIII may also be given.
7. Supportive therapies:
   a. NSAIDs are used to decrease inflammation and arthritic-like pain associated with chronic hemarthroses. Must be used with caution because some types and higher doses interfere with platelet adhesion.
   b. Physical therapy to prevent contractures and muscle atrophy. This includes exercise, whirlpool, and icing.
   c. Orthotics to prevent injury to affected joint and help to resolve hemorrhages.
8. Synovectomy—orthopedic surgical intervention to remove damaged synovium in chronically involved joints.
   a. Open procedure provides direct visualization of joint and removal of damaged tissue.
   b. Arthroscopic—visualization and removal of the joint synovium through the use of an arthroscope.
   c. Radionucleotide—instillation of ^{32}P, which removes damaged synovium; usually done through a needle.
9. Research into gene therapy—genetic copies of sequenced factor VIII and IX molecules are inserted into the body via some type of vector cell to find their way into the human host genetic machinery and begin to produce either factor VIII or factor IX in deficient patients.

Complications

1. Airway obstruction caused by hemorrhage into the neck and pharynx.

2. Repeated hemorrhages may produce degenerative joint changes with osteoporosis and muscle atrophy.

3. Intestinal obstruction caused by bleeding into intestinal walls or peritoneum.

4. Compression of nerves with paralysis caused by hemorrhaging into deep tissues; known as compartment syndrome.

5. Intracranial bleeding, resulting in serious neurologic impairments.

6. Death may result from exsanguination after any serious hemorrhage, such as intracranial, airway, or other highly vascular areas.

7. Contaminated cryoprecipitate, fresh frozen plasma, and concentrates have resulted in chronic active hepatitis and secondary cirrhosis.

8. Acquired immunodeficiency syndrome (AIDS) and human immunodeficiency virus (HIV)–related infections in patients receiving transfusions before 1985 with nontested IV-contaminated blood products.

9. Uncertain life span for many hemophiliacs as a result of complications from hemorrhage or blood-borne viruses (hepatitis/AIDS). However, as a result of advances in therapy, viral inactivation of human plasma-derived factor concentrates and the new recombinant factor VIII concentrate, a normal life span is now possible.

10. It has been estimated that 20% of patients with hemophilia will develop an inhibitor or an autoantibody to the infused factor replacement. This results in more serious hemorrhages as a result of the difficulty in treating these patients to control the hemorrhage.

Nursing Assessment

1. Obtain history of and observe for unusual bleeding—eccyhmosis, prolonged bleeding from mucous membranes and lacerations, hematomas, hemarthroses, hematuria, rectal and gastrointestinal bleeding.

2. Assess joints for swelling, warmth, tenderness, range of motion, contractures, and surrounding muscle atrophy.

3. Assess family resources and coping skills.

Nursing Diagnoses

- Risk for Fluid Volume Deficit related to hemorrhage
- Altered Protection related to inability of blood to clot
- Impaired Physical Mobility related to repeated hemarthroses
- Pain related to bleeding into joints and muscles
- Ineffective Family Coping related to disabling and life-threatening disease

Nursing Interventions
Preventing Hypovolemia Through
Control of Bleeding

1. Provide emergency care for bleeding.
   a. Apply pressure and cold on the area for 10 to 15 minutes to allow clot formation. This should be done especially after venipuncture or injection.

b. Place fibrin foam or absorbable gelatin foam in the wound.
   c. Suturing and cauterization should be avoided.

2. Immobilize the affected part and elevate above the level of the heart.

3. Administer recombinant factor VIII or factor IX coagulation concentrate.
   a. Avoid rapid administration to minimize the possibility of transfusion reaction; usually 2 to 3 mL/min; consult package inserts.
   b. Cryoprecipitate and fresh frozen plasma are not recommended because of their lack of viral inactivation treatment.
   c. Stop the transfusion if hives, headaches, tingling, chills, flushing, or fever occurs.

4. Apply fibrinolytic agents to wound for oral bleeding.

5. Keep child quiet during treatment to decrease pulse and rate of bleeding.

6. Monitor vital signs and treat for shock if child becomes hypotensive (see p. 1076).

Providing Protection Against Bleeding

1. Avoid rectal temperatures; insert thermometer probe gently and use axillary, oral (if age appropriate), or external ear route.

2. Avoid injections if possible.
   a. Administer medications orally whenever possible.
   b. Subcutaneous route is preferred over intramuscular.
   c. Apply pressure to injection site for 10 to 15 minutes. Then apply a pressure dressing with self-adhesive gauze (Coban).

 DRUG ALERT

Children with hemophilia should not receive aspirin or compounds containing aspirin because this medication affects platelet function and prolongs bleeding time.

3. Maintain a safe environment and teach parents safety measures.
   a. Pad crib or bed rails.
   b. Inspect toys for sharp or rough edges.
   c. Offer finger foods and fluids in plastic or paper containers.
   d. Supervise small children when they are ambulatory.
   e. Use protective devices that the child brings from home. (Many children wear helmets and knee and elbow pads.)
   f. Continually assess environment for potential hazards.
   g. No straws or sharp eating utensils.
   h. No hard candy, suckers, or candy canes.

Preserving Mobility

1. Treat hemarthrosis or muscle bleed as soon as possible.

2. Provide supportive care for hemarthrosis.
   a. Immobilize the joint in a position of slight flexion.
   b. Elevate the affected part above the level of the heart.

c. Apply ice packs. Later, after active bleeding has stopped, apply heat to promote absorption of blood.

3. For severe hemarthroses, continue immobilization through casting, if necessary, and prevent weight bearing on the affected limb.

4. For less severe hemarthroses, begin gentle, passive exercise 48 hours after the acute phase to prevent joint stiffness and fibrosis. Progress to active exercises.

5. Administer short course of corticosteroids as ordered to relieve inflammation.

6. Refer for physical therapy if persistent deformity or if crutches, braces, splints, or specialized treatments are needed.

Relieving Pain

1. Be aware that increased pain usually means that bleeding continues and further replacement therapy may be needed.

2. Assess for further swelling of joints and limitation of movement.

3. Administer or teach administration of acetaminophen (Tylenol) during acute phase. NSAIDs may be used for chronic pain, but cautiously to prevent interference with platelet function.

4. Administer narcotics sparingly, as ordered for severe, acute pain.

5. For chronic pain consider alternatives such as hypnosis, biofeedback, relaxation techniques, and TENS.

Enhancing Family Coping

1. Help parents understand that no one is to blame.

2. Allow the child and other family members to handle equipment used in care.

3. Use play to help the young child and siblings adjust to illness by "transfusing" teddy bear, etc.

4. Encourage the parents to allow the child to participate in as many normal activities as possible within the realm of safety.

5. Encourage the child's continuing education. Parents fear sending the child to school, but safety issues can be addressed through discussions with the school nurse, teachers, and principal. Home or hospital tutoring should be continued while child is away from school.

6. Refer to social worker for counseling and identification of resources for financial concerns, etc.

7. Encourage avoidance of overprotection—this can be more disabling than the disease itself.
   a. Promote a sense of independence and self-care within the patient's limitations.
   b. Encourage healthful activity and reasonably aggressive pursuits. Reinforce self-judgment of child or teenager in selection of safe physical activities.
   c. Participate in as many age-appropriate activities as possible.
   d. Help parents understand the importance of vocational guidance for their child—emphasis given to occupations using intellect or skills rather than physical effort.

8. Encourage involvement in support group.

Community and Home Care Considerations

1. Perform a home safety survey to identify potential hazards to the hemophiliac child, such as cluttered furniture the child may bump into, sharp edges on furniture or other objects, loose rugs that promote falls, slippery tub or floor surfaces, rocks or holes in backyard, or concrete play areas.

2. Provide teaching and referrals to initiate an infusion therapy program at home when hemorrhage begins. Assist with teaching the following:
   a. How to assess the child to determine if and what treatment is needed
   b. Storage and preparation of replacement factors
   c. Venipuncture technique
   d. Transfusion management
   e. Record keeping
   f. Awareness of signs of transfusion reaction and its management
   g. Recognition of indications of need for subsequent transfusions

3. Ensure that primary health care needs are being met by facilitating the following:
   a. Regular visits to their primary care provider for preventative health maintenance, to address growth and development, behavior, and psychosocial issues.
   b. Dental exams and teeth cleaning every 6 months.
   c. All the recommended childhood immunizations, plus hepatitis A and B series, to prevent infection from bloodborne pathogens.

4. Provide education to family and all caregivers about recognizing and treating bleeds appropriately.

5. Provide emotional support through the provision of educational materials, information about support groups, and a list of resources within the community.

6. Educate teachers and other school faculty about the child's special needs.
   a. These children can have permanent mental or physical disabilities from old hemorrhages, necessitating individualized plans.
   b. They must avoid all rough or contact sports and activities; they do better with individual or calm group activities.
   c. All injuries must be taken seriously. The school nurse should be notified so that proper first aid and treatment can be initiated.
   d. Although they have a chronic illness, these children have a need to be "normal," with the same opportunities and environmental stimulation as other children.

Family Education and Health Maintenance

1. Review safety measures to prevent or minimize trauma.

2. Encourage education by parents to teachers, babysitters, and others involved of child's care so that they can be responsive in an emergency.

3. Advise wearing a Medic-Alert bracelet.

4. Remind parents not to administer aspirin to the child.

5. Teach emergency treatment for hemorrhage.
    a. Immobilize the part with splints or an elastic compression bandage. (These materials should be immediately available in the home.)
    b. Apply ice packs. Parents should keep two or three plastic bags of ice immediately available in the freezer.
    c. Consult the child's health care provider and initiate additional recommended therapy.
6. Encourage regular medical and dental supervision.
    a. Preventive dental care is important. Soft-bristled or sponge-tipped toothbrushes should be used to prevent bleeding. Factor replacement therapy is necessary for extensive dental work and extractions.
    b. Hepatitis B vaccine is necessary to protect against hepatitis from blood transfusions.
7. Teach healthy diet to avoid overweight, which places additional strain on the child's weight-bearing joints and predisposes to hemarthroses. Also, teach child to avoid sharp utensils, hard candy, suckers, and other foods with sharp edges that may cause mucosal lacerations.
8. Assist the parents in teaching the child to understand the exact nature of the illness as early as possible. Special attention should be given to the signs of hemorrhage, and the child should be told of the need to report even the slightest bleeding to an adult immediately.
9. Advise families that genetic counseling and family planning are available for parents and adolescent patients.
10. Educate regarding hepatitis B and C and HIV disease, risks of treatment.
11. For additional information and support, refer to Hemophilia Association, 104 East 40th St., Suite 506, New York, NY 10016, 212-682-5510.

Outcome-Based Evaluation

- Bleeding controlled; blood pressure stable
- Needle sticks avoided; staff and parents observe safety precautions
- Performs passive range of motion without pain
- Verbalizes relief of pain with acetaminophen
- Parents participate in care, play with child

SELECTED REFERENCES

Aiello, J. (2000). Tools for analyzing trends in anemia management, case study of the anemic patient. *Nephrology Nursing Journal, 27*(1), 57–60.

Beyer, J.E., et al. (1999). Practice guidelines for the assessment of children with sickle cell pain. *Journal of the Society of Pediatric Nursing, 4*(2), 61–73.

Buchanon, G.R. (1999). The tragedy of iron deficiency during infancy and early childhood. *Journal of Pediatrics, 135*(4), 413–415.

Holman, C.F. (1997). Management of the child with sickle cell disease within the school setting. *Journal of School Nursing, 13*(5), 29–34.

Horan, J. & Lerner, N. (2000). Prediction of adverse outcomes in children with sickle cell disease. *New England Journal of Medicine, 342*(21), 1612–1615.

Hoyer, L. (1994). Hemophilia A. *New England Journal of Medicine, 330,* 38–47.

Jacobs, R.F., & Schutze, G.E. (1995). What's causing the hyperbilirubinemia? *Patient Care, 28*(20), 127–128.

Kalif-Ezra, J., Zibis, A., Chaliassos, N., Hatzikonstantinon, I., & Karantanas, A. (2000). Body composition in homozygous beta-thalassemia. *Annals of the New York Academy of Science, 904,* 621–624.

Kline, N.E. (1996). A practical approach to the child with anemia. *Journal of Pediatric Health Care, 10*(3), 99–105.

Lusher, J., Arkin, S., Abildgard, C., & Schwartz, R. (1993). Blood coagulation factor 8. *New England Journal of Medicine, 328*(7), 453–459.

Martin, M., & Butler, R. (1993). Understanding the basics of β-thalassemia major. *Pediatric Nursing, 19*(2), 143–145.

Mitchell, R. (1999). Sickle cell anemia. *American Journal of Nursing, 99*(5), 36–37.

Nathan, D., & Oski, F. (1993). *Hematology of infancy and childhood* (3rd ed.). Philadelphia: W.B. Saunders.

Oni, L., & Bent, S. (1998). Sickle cell disease. *Nursing Times, 94*(37), 50–53.

Pillitteri, A. (1999). *Maternal and child health nursing* (3rd ed.). Philadelphia: Lippincott Williams & Wilkins.

Platt, O.S. (2000). The acute chest syndrome of sickle cell disease. *New England Journal of Medicine, 342*(25), 1904–1907.

Preiss, D.J. (1998). The young child with sickle cell disease. *Advanced Nursing Practice, 6*(6), 32–39.

Protonotarion, A. A., & Tolis, G.J. (2000). Reproductive health in female patients with beta-thalassemia major. *Annals of the New York Academy of Sciences, 900,* 119–124.

Quintero, C. (1993). Blood administration in pediatric Jehovah's Witnesses. *Pediatric Nursing, 19*(1), 46–48.

Richardson, L.C., et al. (2000). Risk of hepatitis A virus infection in persons receiving plasma derived products. *Transfusion Medicine Reviews, 14*(1), 64–73.

Riske, B. (1995). *Hemophilia nursing handbook.* New York: Hemophilia Foundation.

Siberry, G. K. & Iannone, R. (Eds.) (2000). *The Harriet Lane handbook* (15th ed.). St. Louis: Mosby.

Simon, K., Lobo, M.L., & Jackson, S. (1999). Current knowledge in the management of children and adolescents with sickle cell disease: Part 1, Physiological issues. *Journal of Pediatric Nursing, 14*(5), 281–295.

Thomas, V.N., Wilson-Barrett, J., & Goodhart, F. (1998). The role of cognitive-behavioral therapy in the management of pain in patients with sickle cell disease. *Journal of Advanced Nursing, 27*(5), 1002–1009.

Tigner, R. (1998). Handling a sickle cell crisis. *RN, 61*(7), 32–35.

Vichinsky, E. P., et al. (2000). Causes and outcomes of the acute chest syndrome in sickle cell disease. *New England Journal of Medicine, 342,* 1855–1865.

Vidler, V. (1999). Teaching parents advanced clinical skills. *Haemophilia, 5*(5), 349–353.

Pediatric Immunologic Disorders

IMMUNODEFICIENCY

Pediatric HIV Disease

Pediatric human immunodeficiency virus (HIV) disease is represented by a continuum of health conditions ranging from asymptomatic disease to conditions that define the child as having acquired immunodeficiency syndrome (AIDS). A child infected with HIV will, over time, show signs of impaired immune function, although the severity of the impairment can vary widely from mildly abnormal laboratory markers of immune function to full-blown AIDS-defining illnesses.

Epidemiology

1. HIV is transmitted by sexual contact, through exposure to blood and blood components, perinatally from an infected mother to the child, and through breast-feeding from an HIV-infected mother to her infant.
2. Perinatal transmission accounts for at least 90% of all pediatric HIV disease in the United States.
3. In the U. S., the perinatal transmission rate has dramatically decreased from about 25% to as low as 3% to 5%. This reflects concerted efforts to provide voluntary HIV testing for pregnant women and the use of zidovudine administered during pregnancy, labor, and delivery, and for the first 6 weeks of life of the HIV-exposed newborn. Combination antiretroviral regimens and cesarean birth prior to rupture of membranes are also considered effective.
4. Perinatal transmission can be in utero, intrapartum, or postpartum (through breast milk). Most perinatal transmission probably occurs late in pregnancy or during birth.
5. An HIV-infected mother can have a child who is also infected and have future children who are not infected.

Likewise, one twin or triplet can be infected while the other is not.
6. As of December 1999, 8718 children younger than 13 years of age had been reported to the Centers for Disease Control and Prevention (CDC) using laboratory and diagnostic criteria updated in 1994.
7. Two general patterns of illness in HIV-infected children have been observed. About 10% to 20% of children develop serious disease in the first year of life; most of these "rapid progressors" die by age 4 years. The remaining 80% to 90% of HIV-infected children have a slower rate of disease progression; many may not develop serious symptoms until school age or later.

Pathophysiology and Etiology

1. The causative agent is a retrovirus that damages the immune system by infecting and depleting the CD4 lymphocytes (T4-helper cells). These CD4 lymphocytes play a central role in the regulation of the immune system.
2. There are also abnormalities in the function of cellular and humoral immunity (B cells, CD8 cells, natural killer cells, monocytes, macrophages, and specific antibodies).
3. Progressive destruction of the immune system leads to:
   a. Increased incidence of serious bacterial infections such as bacteremias, bacterial pneumonias, osteomyelitis
   b. Opportunistic infections, which commonly include *Pneumocystis* pneumonia (PCP), esophageal candidiasis, and *Mycobacterium avium* infection.
   c. More aggressive forms of viral infections such as severe varicella, disseminated zoster, cytomegalovirus pneumonitis
   d. Cancers, especially lymphomas
   e. Wasting syndromes and encephalopathy
4. Multisystem organ involvement results in cardiomyopathies, nephropathies, neurologic impairment, gastro-

intestinal dysfunction, dermatologic manifestations, musculoskeletal abnormalities, ocular impairments, ear, nose, and throat problems, and hematologic disorders.

Clinical Manifestations

1. Generalized lymphadenopathy, especially in less common sites such as epitrochlear and axillary areas
2. Persistent, recurrent oral candidiasis
3. Failure to thrive
4. Developmental delays or loss of previously acquired milestones
5. Hepatomegaly
6. Splenomegaly
7. Persistent diarrhea
8. Hyper- or hypogammaglobulinemia (elevated IgG, IgM, IgA)
9. Parotitis
10. Unexplained anemias, thrombocytopenia
11. Unexplained cardiac or kidney disease
12. Recurrent serious bacterial infections

Diagnostic Evaluation

1. Neonatal testing with enzyme-linked immunosorbent assay (ELISA) is not indicated because this is only testing for the presence of circulating maternal antibodies to HIV and is not an indication of the child's infection status.
2. Polymerase chain reaction (PCR) and virus culture are the most sensitive and specific assays for detecting HIV infection in a child younger than 15 months of age. A standard P24 antigen assay, while less sensitive than viral culture or PCR, is also available. Two or more negative viral diagnostic tests obtained at more than 1 month of age and more than 4 months of age establishes a low probability of HIV infection for the HIV-exposed infant.
3. After 18 months of age, ELISA can be used for testing. As with adults, a reactive ELISA must be followed by a confirmatory Western blot test.
4. Additional laboratory studies important to follow on the HIV-exposed infant include complete blood count (CBC) with differential to monitor for anemia and neutropenia and lymphocyte subsets (CD4s). For a known

infected child, CBC, platelet counts, serum chemistries, serial CD4s, and HIV PCR should be done every 3 to 6 months (depending on previous results and the stage of disease). In addition, a baseline echocardiogram and chest x-ray should be done and repeated yearly.

5. In known infected children or at-risk infants (those born to an HIV-infected mother but whose own status is still indeterminate), computed tomography scanning or magnetic resonance imaging of the head is indicated if there is evidence of neurologic impairment, falling rate of head growth, or developmental delays or regression.

Management

1. Initiation of PCP prophylaxis when indicated by low CD4 counts, with the exception being that all infants born to HIV-infected women should be started on PCP prophylaxis at 4 to 6 weeks of age, regardless of their CD4 count (Table 53-1).
   a. The first drug of choice is trimethoprim-sulfamethoxazole (Bactrim).
   b. Pentamidine and dapsone are alternative choices.
   c. PCP prophylaxis should be discontinued among infants in whom infection has been reasonably excluded on the basis of two or more negative viral diagnostic tests performed at more than 1 month and more than 4 months.
2. Aggressive antiretroviral therapy should be initiated in all infants infected with HIV younger than 1 year of age regardless of clinical manifestations, immune parameters, or viral load. Antiretroviral therapy is recommended for HIV-infected children with clinical symptoms of HIV or evidence of immune suppression regardless of the age of the child or HIV PCR level (viral load).
   a. Clinical trial data from both adults and children have demonstrated that antiretroviral therapy in symptomatic patients slows clinical and immunologic disease progression and reduces mortality.
   b. Three types of antiretrovirals have been approved for use in children: nucleoside reverse transcriptase inhibitors, non-nucleoside reverse transcriptase inhibitors, and protease inhibitors.

TABLE 53-1 Recommendations for PCP Prophylaxis and CD4+ Monitoring for Human Immunodeficiency Virus (HIV)–Exposed Infants and HIV-Infected Children, by Age and HIV-Infection Status

Age/HIV-Infection Status	PCP Prophylaxis	CD4+ Monitoring
Birth to 4–6 weeks, HIV exposed	No prophylaxis	1 month
4–6 weeks to 4 months, HIV exposed	Prophylaxis	3 months
4–12 months, HIV infected or indeterminate	Prophylaxis	6, 9, and 12 months
Under 4–12 months, HIV infection reasonably excluded	No prophylaxis	None
1–5 years, HIV infected	Prophylaxis if: CD4+ count is <500 cells/(L or CD4+ percentage is <15%	Every 3–4 months
6–12 years, HIV infected	Prophylaxis if: CD4+ count is <200 cells/(L or CD4+ percentage is <15%	Every 3–4 months

(Adapted from Centers for Disease Control and Prevention [1995]. 1995 revised guidelines for prophylaxis against *Pneumocystis carinii* pneumonia for children infected with or perinatally exposed to human immunodeficiency virus. *MMWR, 44* [RR-4], 1–11.)

c. Combination therapy is now recommended with special emphasis on adherence as viral resistance (particularly to protease inhibitors) develops rapidly with even slight fluctuations in drug levels.

 DRUG ALERT

Lack of adherence to prescribed antiretroviral regimens and subtherapeutic drug levels increase the possibility that resistant virus will develop. Strict adherence to combination regimens is critical in ensuring sustained response to treatment.

3. Use of intravenous immune globulin (IVIG) in infected children who have had two or more serious bacterial infections within 1 year or for the treatment of HIV-related thrombocytopenia.
4. Use of antifungal drugs such as nystatin, ketoconazole (Nizoral), fluconazole (Diflucan), and clotrimazole (Mycelex) for persistent or recurrent oral candidiasis.
5. Use of antivirals such as acyclovir (Zovirax), famciclovir (Famvir), valacyclovir (Valtrex), ganciclovir (Cytovene), and cidofovir (Vistide) for suppression or treatment of recurrent viral infections.
6. Aggressive, prompt assessment and treatment of febrile illnesses.
7. Nutritional support.
8. Evaluation and treatment of developmental delays and regression.
9. Adequate pain management in advanced or end-stage disease.
10. Support and interventions for both the child and family (including caretakers for the child in the event of maternal death) with issues of disclosure, parental guilt, and long-term care.

NURSING ALERT

 Families can find out about clinical treatment trials available for their child by calling 1-800-TRIALS-A.

Complications
1. Repeated, overwhelming infections and certain cancers, particularly lymphomas
2. Hearing loss, tooth and gum disease, acute and chronic ENT infections
3. Drug-related toxicities
4. Opportunistic infections
5. Reactive airway disease
6. Cardiomyopathy
7. Failure to thrive, malabsorption, wasting
8. Chronic atopic dermatitis and other skin reactions
9. Nephropathy
10. Developmental delay
11. Neuropathy, myopathy
12. Anemia, thrombocytopenia, neutropenia
13. Psychological challenges for children and caregivers, including multiple loss, issues of disclosure, and isolation
14. Death

Nursing Assessment
1. Review maternal records to identify newborn infants who may be at risk for HIV disease.
2. Review records of at-risk or known infected children to determine nutritional status, growth and development, frequency of serious bacterial infections, presence of or risk for opportunistic infections, laboratory values, and immunization status.
3. Assess growth, development, lymph nodes, hepatomegaly, splenomegaly, and oropharynx for presence of oral candidiasis.
4. Assess the family's understanding of the child's condition, care needs, prognosis, and medical plan of care.
5. Assess the family's coping mechanisms, comfort with disclosure issues, and long-term plans for care (including plans for respite and permanent alternative caretakers).
6. Assess the child's understanding of health condition.
7. In children with advanced or end-stage disease, assess the level of pain and discomfort.
8. Assess the child's coping and response to the frequent painful and invasive procedures experienced as part of the ongoing diagnosis and management of the disease.

Nursing Diagnoses
- Risk for Infection related to immunodeficiency, neutropenia
- Altered Nutrition: Less Than Body Requirements related to malabsorption, anorexia, and pain
- Altered Oral Mucous Membranes related to candidiasis and herpes stomatitis
- Diarrhea related to enteric pathogens, disease process, and medications
- Hyperthermia related to HIV infection and secondary infection
- Altered Growth and Development related to HIV CNS infection
- Ineffective Family Coping related to parental guilt and nature of disease
- Ineffective Individual Coping by child related to unresolved issues around disclosure, hospitalization, and losses
- Pain related to advanced or end-stage HIV disease
- Fear related to frequent invasive procedures

Nursing Interventions
Preventing Infection
1. Have a high index of suspicion for secondary infection even when clinical manifestations are subtle or absent.
2. Administer or teach caretaker to administer prescribed pharmacologic agents that may help prevent serious bacterial infections, prevent opportunistic infections, and treat infections that occur.
3. Monitor total white count and absolute neutrophil counts, which may drop significantly as a side effect of antiretroviral drugs.
4. Maintain cleanliness of the environment and teach family members the essentials of environmental sanitation.
5. Use aseptic techniques when performing invasive procedures.

6. Administer and teach the family good skin care—a break in the skin is a source of secondary infection.

7. Teach the family the importance of safe food preparation, including use of safe water, to avoid introducing pathogens through contaminated or undercooked food.

8. Monitor immunization status and advise families of the need to complete all recommended childhood immunizations. In general, live virus vaccines (oral polio and varicella) should not be administered to children with immunosuppression. The measles, mumps, rubella (MMR) vaccine is the exception and is recommended for HIV-infected children who are not severely immunocompromised. Yearly influenza vaccine and every 3 to 5 year pneumococcal vaccine are also recommended in addition to the standard childhood immunization schedule.

9. Children infected with HIV and those noninfected children living with HIV-infected parents or siblings should not receive the oral polio vaccine, but rather the inactivated polio vaccine, which is an injectable vaccine. This is due to the prolonged shedding of the virus from the live oral vaccine, which may prove to be hazardous for immunocompromised individuals.

10. Provide appropriate chemoprophylaxis following exposure to communicable diseases such as varicella.

Maintaining Adequate Nutrition

1. Carefully monitor growth parameters (height, weight, head circumference).

2. Consult with a dietitian to develop strategies for nutritional care, including additional calories and nutritional supplements.

3. Teach the family to prepare high-calorie, nutritious meals that are pleasing and acceptable to children.

4. As age appropriate, involve the child in meal planning.

5. Encourage small, frequent meals if the child is experiencing absorption problems.

Maintaining Oral Mucosa Integrity

1. Include regular examinations of the oral mucosa in the physical assessment of the child.

2. Administer prescribed antifungal and antiviral therapy.

3. Offer fluids and blenderized foods to minimize chewing and facilitate swallowing.

4. Avoid highly seasoned or acidic foods.

Minimizing Effects of Diarrhea

1. Monitor for the presence or development of diarrhea.

2. Monitor daily weights when diarrhea is present.

3. Monitor intake and output and assess skin and mucous membranes for turgor and dryness.

4. Use enteric precautions.

5. Avoid foods that increase intestinal motility.

6. Administer IV hydration as indicated.

7. Plan a regimen of skin care, including cleansing/blot drying of the anal area and application of ointment or skin barrier cream.

8. Teach the family safe food preparation techniques to minimize contamination of food.

9. Administer medications as directed for relief of severe diarrhea and enteric infections.

Detecting and Controlling Fever

1. Monitor for fever and report any core temperature over 101°F (38.4°C).

2. Institute comfort measures such as sponge baths, dry clothing and linens, and antipyretics as ordered.

3. Teach the family how to accurately monitor the child's rectal temperature.

4. Teach the family to promptly report any febrile episode over 101°F (38.4°C) rectally.

5. Administer antipyretics.

Promoting Developmental Goals

1. Assess the child's developmental status on a regular basis.

2. Report any regression or delay in achieving developmental milestones.

3. Make appropriate referrals for more in-depth developmental evaluation when delays and regression are noted.

4. Teach the family appropriate developmental stimulation activities for their child.

5. Implement any recommendations for developmental stimulation (including school-based programs) and assist the family in doing likewise.

Promoting Effective Family Coping

1. Assess the family's coping mechanisms, strengths, and weaknesses.

2. Provide emotional support to the family.

3. Refer the family to appropriate community resources for grief counseling and legal assistance (such as with wills, custody issues).

4. Help the family set realistic goals and expectations for the child.

5. Maintain a nonjudgmental attitude and nonprejudicial approach.

6. Allow the family to use denial as a protective mechanism—this gives them some sense of control.

7. Explain all care and treatment plans to the family.

8. Involve the family in planning for the care and management of their child.

9. Refer the family to community resources for home care, respite care, day care of other siblings, transportation services, school-based services, and hospice.

Strengthening Coping Skills of the Child

1. Introduce the subject of disclosure of diagnosis to the child with the family. Offer the family guidelines as to age-appropriate approaches.

2. Accept that some families may not be able to disclose the nature of the disease to their child, even after much support and guidance.

   a. Explore with these families how they want you to address questions the child may present to you, the nurse.

   b. The illness and the impact of the illness can be effectively dealt with without actually telling the child that he or she has HIV disease or AIDS, if the family refuses to disclose.

3. Answer the child's questions as honestly as possible within parental constraints that may be present.

4. Actively involve the child in as much of the care as possible, such as by having the child decide where to place

the intravenous (IV) line, cleaning off skin for needle insertion, and so forth.

5. Use therapeutic play techniques (age appropriate) such as drawing, playing with dolls, playing with medical equipment, and storytelling to allow the child to express himself or herself in less verbal ways.

6. Refer the child and family for counseling if the child's coping skills do not progress or there appears to be regression in how he or she is handling the issue of illness and chronic health care needs. Signs indicating possible need for additional in-depth interventions include more acting out by the child, withdrawn behavior, and difficulty in school (either behaviorally or academically).

7. Recommend and facilitate peer support groups.

Minimizing Discomfort

1. Assess for signs of pain in the child. In the infant or nonverbal child such signs include restlessness, crying, withdrawn behavior, and changes in vital signs.

2. Discuss concerns over pain issues with the primary health care provider and team providing care for the child. Initiate or request referral to a pain management team if the child does not experience relief.

3. Stress to the parent or guardian the need for adequate pain management in children; many people do not acknowledge that infants or children suffer from pain and that this needs to be alleviated.

4. Use appropriate techniques to assess the level of pain or discomfort a child is experiencing.

Minimizing Fear

1. Ensure that all painful and invasive procedures are done in a location other than the child's bed in hospital.

2. Monitor central line if used for venous access. A central line access may be less traumatic over time than repeated peripheral access attempts. Some children with HIV will need long-term, probably lifelong, IV therapies and blood monitoring, and a central line greatly eliminates the pain and anxiety associated with these procedures.

3. Ensure that the parent/caregiver realizes that most clinic visits will involve blood tests so that they do not falsely reassure the child that "no needle sticks" will occur.

4. Use diversionary techniques, such as bubble blowing, for distraction during painful procedures. Practice first with the child and tell him or her this is an activity that you will help with during the procedure. Children can also be taught other relaxation techniques.

5. Offer small rewards (such as stickers, small toy items, etc.) after painful procedures to reduce anxiety. Such rewards should be given regardless of how the child reacted. The reward is not for "not crying" but acknowledges difficulty in going through painful and invasive procedures on a regular basis.

6. Involve the child in the procedure as much as possible (age appropriate). Such involvement can include selecting a possible site for accessing or receiving IV medications, cleaning the site, selecting a special bandage for after procedure, etc. Use topical anesthetic.

Community and Home Care Considerations

1. Assess home environment for resources such as nutritious foods and safe food preparation; adequate water, heat, electricity, and space; developmentally appropriate toys; and supplies needed for care and hygiene.

2. Assess caretaker's/child's correct administration of medications.

3. Draw blood samples using universal precautions and careful transport of blood and used equipment.

4. Perform developmental assessment periodically.

5. Act as liaison between family, specialists, school, and other team members.

Family Education and Health Maintenance

1. Teach families and other caretakers of the child universal precautions. In caring for HIV-infected infants and children, gloves are recommended when handling potentially contaminated body fluids (such as blood) but are not considered necessary for routine diaper changing unless bloody diarrhea or hematuria exists.

2. Facilitate supply of adequate numbers of latex gloves to families to use as indicated.

3. Offer guidance as to how to initiate discussion of their child's HIV status with schools and day-care settings. The "need to know" principle serves as a guideline when deciding to whom disclosure should be made (generally the principal, school nurse, and classroom teacher). It is not currently required that schools and day-care centers be advised but is generally encouraged because this alerts the school to notify the parent promptly in the event of an outbreak of infectious disease that could pose a threat to the HIV-infected child (such as varicella).

4. Give families concrete guidelines as to when to notify health care providers about their child's condition. Signs and symptoms of illnesses require prompt notification, all fevers over 101°F (38.4°C) should be reported, and any adverse experiences or suspected adverse experiences with medications need prompt reporting.

5. Assess whether the parents are receiving care for themselves. Often times parents will neglect their own care to provide for their child. As a result, the parents' immune status may become more quickly compromised.

6. Refer families to a social worker or social services agency. Children with HIV may qualify for certain entitlement programs that help with their health care and the family's financial situation. Many states have initiated case management programs for people with HIV.

7. Provide guidance using a childhood chronic illness model that addresses psychosocial issues such as disclosure and parental guilt as well as medical issues such as multi-organ involvement and likelihood of exacerbations of a variety of related conditions (eg, infections and nutritional deficiencies).

8. Assist parents in obtaining the latest information regarding treatment protocols of pediatric HIV. Such information can be obtained by calling 1-800-TRIALS-A.

Outcome-Based Evaluation
- Absolute neutrophil count within normal limits; aseptic technique maintained
- Eating small meals and snacks; growth curve maintained
- Oral mucous membranes without ulceration
- Two to three loose stools per day; perianal skin without irritation
- Afebrile; mother demonstrates accurate monitoring of temperature
- Assessment using Denver developmental tool appropriate for age; child with delay receiving appropriate services
- Mother assisting with care and seeking help through community resources (home care, respite, day care, school, hospice)
- Child asking questions and participating in care
- Child reporting increase in comfort level
- Child practicing distraction techniques during procedures

CONNECTIVE TISSUE DISORDERS

Juvenile Rheumatoid Arthritis

Juvenile rheumatoid arthritis (JRA) is a chronic inflammatory, generalized, systemic disease that involves a wide spectrum of manifestations, including joint, connective tissue, and visceral lesions throughout the body. JRA affects about 250,000 children in the U. S.

Pathophysiology and Etiology
1. The cause of JRA is unknown.
2. Current hypotheses:
   a. Infection from an unidentified organism
   b. Autoimmune process or hypersensitivity to unknown stimuli
   c. Some subtypes have genetic predisposition
3. In the early stages, one or more joints show signs of inflammation.
4. The inflammation is initially localized in a joint capsule, primarily in the synovium. The tissue becomes thickened from congestion and edema.
5. A characteristic inflammatory response develops in the interior of the joint.
6. The articular cartilage may become adherent and deprived of nutrition.
7. By starvation and invasion, this inflammatory tissue slowly destroys the articular cartilage.
8. Inflamed and overgrown synovial tissue eventually fills the joint space, leading to narrowing, fibrous ankylosis (fusion), and bony fusion.
9. Growth centers next to inflamed joints may undergo either premature epiphyseal closure or accelerated epiphyseal growth.
10. Tendons and tendon sheaths may develop inflammatory changes similar to the synovial tissues.
11. Inflammation of muscle may occur.
12. Eventually there is deformity, subluxation, and fibrous or bony ankylosis of joint(s).

Clinical Manifestations
1. Characterized by exacerbations and remissions. Infections, injuries, or surgical procedures often precipitate exacerbations (Table 53-2).
2. Involved joints become inflamed with morning stiffness (gelling), swelling, warmth, pain, and impaired movement. This may occur gradually or suddenly and lead to joint destruction, dislocation, deformity, or fusion.
3. Symptoms of iridocyclitis include eye redness, pain, photophobia, decreased visual acuity, and nonreactive pupil(s). It can be unilateral or bilateral.
4. Rheumatoid nodules are uncommon in children.

Diagnostic Evaluation
Of limited value; however, helps to differentiate subtypes.
1. Elevated erythrocyte sedimentation rate (ESR)
2. Leukocytosis
3. High total serum proteins
4. Positive C-reactive protein
5. Possible positive serum antinuclear antibodies (ANA) and rheumatoid factor
6. Possible alteration in serum proteins (increased α and γ; decreased albumin)
7. Changes in bone, demonstrated by x-rays—initially nonspecific
8. Slit-lamp examinations of eye to rule out iridocyclitis

Management
1. Although this is a painful disease of long duration, the outlook for remission is good (70%).
2. There is no specific cure; treatment is supportive.
3. The goal of drug therapy is to reduce inflammation and relieve pain.
4. Nonsteroidal anti-inflammatory drugs (NSAIDs), such as aspirin, tolmetin sodium (Tolectin), ibuprofen (Motrin), and naproxen (Naprosyn), are used.
   a. Daily dose usually is divided into two to four doses.
   b. Aspirin is the drug of choice, preferably enteric-coated to avoid gastrointestinal complications.
   c. Serum levels of aspirin are monitored (keep at 20–30 mg/dL) for anti-inflammatory effectiveness and to avoid toxicity. Therapeutic response may take weeks or even months.
   d. Signs of toxicity may include rapid or deep breathing or tinnitus.

◆ DRUG ALERT

Because of the increased association of aspirin treatment during a viral illness and the development of Reye's syndrome, advise the family to contact the health care provider when the child has a viral illness. Aspirin may be discontinued and another treatment for JRA substituted until the viral illness is over.

5. Cimetidine, a histamine-2-receptor antagonist that decreases the amount of hydrochloric acid in the stom-

TABLE 53-2 Clinical Manifestations of Juvenile Rheumatoid Arthritis by Subgroups

	Polyarticular (−) RF	Polyarticular (+) RF	Pauciarticular Type I	Pauciarticular Type II	Systemic-Onset
Percentage of JRA Patients	20–25	5–10	35–40	10–15	20
Age at Onset	Throughout child-hood	Late childhood	<10	>10	1–3 and 8–10
Sex	90% girls	80% girls	80% girls	90% boys	60% boys
Joints Involved	>4; any joints—usually affects small joints of fingers and hands symmetrically	>4; any joints—usually affects small joints symmetrically	<5 (usually large joints: knee, ankle, elbow) nonsymmet-rical	<5 (few large joints—hip) nonsymmetrical	Any joints
Lab Tests: *CRP/ESR*	Elevated	Elevated	Elevated	Elevated	Elevated with severe anemia and leuko-cytosis
RF	Negative	Positive	Negative	Negative	Negative
Serum ANA	25% positive	75% positive	90% positive	Negative	Negative
HLA studies	?	+HLA DR4	+HLA DRW5, DRW6, DRW8	+HLA B27	?
Other Symptoms	Minimal systemic signs such as low-grade fever, malaise, lymph-adenopathy	Minimal systemic signs such as low-grade fever, malaise, lymph-adenopathy	Chronic iridocyclitis (eye inflammation) low-grade fever, malaise	Sacroiliitis, iridocycli-tis, few systemic manifestations	High intermittent fever (102°), malaise, macu-lar rash, pleuri-tis, pericarditis, splenomegaly, hepatomegaly, lymphadenop-athy
Prognosis	10–15% severe arthritis; 1:4 remission	>50% severe arthri-tis; 1:4 remission	Blindness (10%) Poly-arthritis (20%) 2:3 remission	Ankylosing spondylitis 2:3 remission	25% severe arthritis; 1–2% mortality

ANA, antinuclear antibody; CRP/ESR, C-reactive protein and erythrocyte sedimentation rate; HLA, human leukocyte antigen (indicating genetic predisposition); RF, rheumatoid factor.

ach, is often used to prevent mucosal irritation during NSAID therapy.

6. Disease-modifying antirheumatic drugs (DMARDs) such as gold sodium thiomalate (Myochrysine) or auro-thioglucose (Solganal), D-penicillamine (Depen), or hydroxychloroquine (Plaquenil) may be added to the regimen when NSAIDs have been ineffective.

   a. Injectable gold salts are used sparingly because of the high risk of toxic side effects, such as skin rash, nephritis with hematuria or proteinuria, thrombo-cytopenia, neurotoxicity, gastric upset, leukopenia, anemia, and mucosal ulcers.

   b. An oral gold, auranofin (Ridaura), is being studied for use in children.

   c. Hydroxychloroquine (Plaquenil) or chloroquine (Aralen), used mainly for polyarticular disease. They may cause gastric upset, retinal toxicity, and corneal and retinal changes leading to blindness.

7. Immunosuppressant cytotoxic drugs, such as cyclo-phosphamide (Cytoxan), azathioprine (Imuran), chlor-ambucil (Leukeran), and methotrexate (Mexate), are reserved for patients with severe debilitating disease and those who have responded poorly to NSAIDs and DMARDs. Methotrexate is an immunopressant drug that is often used in conjunction with an NSAID such as naproxen. It is introduced sooner in the course of the disease. It has been discovered to be effective in many children with relatively few side effects.

8. Corticosteroids are the most potent anti-inflammatory agents available; used for life-threatening disease, in-capacitating systemic disease that has been unrespon-sive to other anti-inflammatory therapy, and irido-cyclitis.

   a. Administered in the lowest effective dose, on alternate days (rather than daily). Their use does not prevent complications of severe arthritis or influence ultimate prognosis.

   b. Tuberculin test should be done before starting steroid therapy because corticosteroids can blunt skin test results.

  c. Monitor for glucosuria and other side effects such as weight gain, edema, acne, and fatigue.
9. Gamma globulin has been used with good effect on some children with the systemic type of juvenile arthritis.
10. Monoclonal antibodies are being investigated.
11. Exercise program is instituted to promote joint movement.
12. Surgery may be necessary.
  a. Synovectomy—to maintain function when extensive synovitis develops, especially around wrists
  b. Joint replacement—with severe destructive arthritis (ankylosing spondylitis)

Complications

1. Bony deformities—crippling from progressive polyarthritis
  a. Growth disturbance
  b. Failure to thrive—short stature
  c. Cervical spine and temporomandibular jaw problems (micrognathia—receding chin)
  d. Leg length discrepancies
2. Psychological and social reactions to this chronic illness
3. Iridocyclitis—leading to cataracts, glaucoma, or blindness
4. Pericarditis

Nursing Assessment

1. Focus history on child's general health, onset of symptoms, activity impairment, level of pain, and treatments used at home.
2. Focus physical examination on the clinical manifestations that differentiate the subtypes of JRA, such as extent of joint involvement, as well as vital signs and growth and development.
3. Gather data for psychosocial assessment about impact of this chronic, painful disease on the child and family.

Nursing Diagnoses

• Pain related to joint inflammation
• Impaired Physical Mobility related to joint destruction and pain
• Self-Care Deficit related to pain and immobility
• Altered Family Processes related to caring for a child with a chronic/painful illness

Nursing Interventions

Minimizing Discomfort

1. Administer and teach parents to administer analgesic and anti-inflammatory drugs as prescribed and based on child's response.
2. Provide daytime heat to joints through the use of tub baths, whirlpools, paraffin baths, warm moist pads, and soaking; provide nighttime warmth through the use of a sleeping bag, thermal underwear, or heated waterbed.
3. Immobilize any acutely inflamed joints with pillows, splints, or slings.

Preserving Joint Mobility

1. Encourage compliance with physical therapy regimen to strengthen muscles and mobilize joints. Assist with range-of-motion exercises as indicated.
2. Splint joints to maintain proper position (joint extension) and decrease pain and deformity.
3. Encourage prone position with thin or no pillow and firm mattress.
4. Encourage therapeutic play (swimming, throwing, riding bike).
5. Encourage child to do own activities of daily living to maintain joint mobility.

Promoting Self-Care

1. Refer to occupational therapy for provision of adaptation devices to facilitate completion of daily activities (Velcro closures, utensils and self-care implements with enlarged handles).
2. Reward child for task completion.
3. Schedule rest periods to maximize energy; discourage bed rest and lengthy inactivity because they increase stiffness.
4. Offer pain medications and treatments before daily activities (tub baths, dressing, feeding).

Normalizing Family Processes

1. Refer to community resources and support groups.
2. Encourage child and family to verbalize feelings.
3. Encourage attendance in school, participation in activities, and socialization with peers as much as possible.
4. Remind parents to devote time to other children, themselves, and each other because the disease affects the whole family.

Community and Home Care Considerations

1. Assess home for safety in ambulating.
2. Assist with obtaining adaptive devices for bathing and transporting the child in the home.
3. Keep school nurse informed of condition so individual educational plan can be updated.
4. Reevaluate need for physical and occupational therapy periodically.

Family Education and Health Maintenance

1. Educate and motivate parents and child in continuing program of treatment at home. This is a chronic disease and has an unpredictable course; however, compliance with prescribed treatment will minimize crippling and allow the child to grow and develop to his or her full potential. Avoid unorthodox and unproven treatments.
2. Teach the family that daily exercise, such as swimming, helps to maintain full range of motion. Avoid exercises that cause overtiring and joint pain.
3. Urge the parents to keep the school nurse informed of the child's condition so that there will be continuity of care even at school. Tell the parents to inform child's teacher of need for hourly movement, side effects of medications, and application of special equipment.

4. Teach the family about a nutritionally balanced diet to prevent obesity, which puts additional stress on joints.
5. Stress the need for routine follow-up care, ophthalmologic evaluation, and prompt attention to infections or other illness that may prompt exacerbations.
6. Encourage routine well-child visits with immunizations, including the influenza vaccine each year, to decrease stress caused by the flu and the chance of Reye's syndrome from salicylate intake.
7. Refer family to agencies such as the Arthritis Foundation, 404-872-7100, *www.arthritis.org;* or JRA World at *http://jraworld.arthritisinsight.com.*

Outcome-Based Evaluation
• Child reports decreased pain
• Range of motion of all joints intact
• Child completes self-care with minimal assistance
• Parents seek additional resources

Systemic Lupus Erythematosus

Systemic lupus erythematosus (SLE) is a chronic inflammatory disease of the connective tissue with vascular and perivascular fibrinoid changes that may involve any organ or system. A number of clinical variants of SLE have been identified, including discoid lupus (usually affects only the skin), subacute cutaneous lupus erythematosus (skin and mild systemic manifestations), neonatal lupus (transient skin lesions, heart block, and hematologic abnormalities), and drug-induced lupus (lupus-like syndrome that resolves when drug is discontinued).

The incidence is higher in females than in males (8:1) and is most common during the childbearing period (15–44 years). However, it can affect children 5 to 15 years of age. It is generally more acute and severe in children than in adults. It is more prevalent in African American, Hispanic, or Asian populations. It is no longer thought that the course of childhood onset SLE is more severe than that seen in adult-onset SLE.

Pathophysiology and Etiology
1. Cause is unknown. General theory of etiology is altered immune regulation. Etiologic factors include:
   a. Genetic predisposition—genetic markers within human leukocyte antigen (HLA) system have been demonstrated.
   b. Viral—nonspecific antibody rise as part of general immunologic hyperactivity.
2. Possible factors that trigger or unmask initial symptoms:
   a. Exposure to sunlight; snow on bright day
   b. Injury, infection
   c. Stress, extreme fatigue
   d. Radiation therapy
   e. Vaccination
   f. Antioxidants
   g. Other drugs such as anticonvulsants, sulfonamides
3. Connective tissue in different organs develops nonspecific aberrations such as fibrinoid change in collagen and cellular infiltration, either in the walls of small blood vessels or elsewhere.

4. Alteration of collagen and subendothelial thickening of small blood vessels obstruct the flow of blood. These changes may be widespread or limited in distribution.
5. Neonate born to a known SLE-afflicted mother:
   a. Positive ANA and lupus erythematosus factor transmitted transplacentally.
   b. Infant may have clinical or nonclinical evidence of lupus erythematosus.
   c. Discoid lesions may be present.
   d. Other infants may have no clinical symptoms.
   e. Symptoms usually resolve in 3 to 4 months; however, the child has a small chance of developing SLE later in life.

Clinical Manifestations
1. Onset may be gradual with vague symptoms or acute with significant manifestations.
2. General characteristic signs and symptoms may include:
   a. Malar erythema (butterfly rash), which usually spreads over bridge of nose; rash may vary from a faint blush to scaly erythematous papules and may be photosensitive. Rash spreads from face and scalp to neck, chest, and extremities.
   b. Acute polyarthritis, arthralgia
   c. Fever
   d. Fatigue, malaise
   e. Anorexia, weight loss
3. Cardiac involvement—pleurisy or pericarditis most diagnostic.
4. Nephritis—at onset or during course of disease. Clinically evident nephritis occurs in at least 75% of patients and is even more frequent and of greater severity in children than adults. It usually develops within 2 years of onset.
   a. Routine monitoring of urine is essential in management of children with SLE.
   b. Hematuria, proteinuria, hypertension may be evident.
5. Central nervous system (CNS) involvement during course of disease:
   a. Behavior disturbances, convulsions, coma
6. Splenomegaly, hepatomegaly, lymphadenopathy
7. Anemia, thrombocytopenia, hypoglobulinemia
8. Raynaud's phenomenon
9. Pulmonary involvement with pleural effusion and lupus pneumonitis.

Diagnostic Evaluation
1. Diagnosis is made largely by clinical manifestations (Box 53-1).
2. Antibody studies:
   a. ANA—nonspecific but positive in 90% of people with SLE
   b. Other antibodies such as anti-dsDNA, anti-ssDNA, anti-RNP, anti-Ro, and anti-La if diagnosis is unclear or to identify clinical variant
3. ESR—elevated.
4. Serum complement studies—decreased.

BOX 2-1 American Rheumatism Association Criteria for Diagnosis of Systemic Lupus Erythematosus

The presence of four or more criteria must be documented to diagnose SLE.

1. Malar rash
2. Discoid rash
3. Photosensitivity
4. Oral ulcers
5. Arthritis of two or more joints
6. Serositis—pleuritis or pericarditis
7. Renal disorder—persistent proteinuria or cellular casts
8. Neurologic disorder—seizures or psychosis
9. Hematologic disorder—hemolytic anemia, leukopenia, lymphopenia, or thrombocytopenia
10. Immunologic disorder—positive lupus erythematosus preparation or anti-DNA antibody or anti-Sm antibody or false-positive serologic test for syphilis
11. Positive antinuclear antibody (ANA)

---

5. CBC—leukopenia and mild to moderate anemia; can be hemolytic anemia, thrombocytopenia.
6. Serologic test for syphilis—false positive.
7. Serum chemistry and urine studies to detect kidney and other body system involvement.
8. Renal biopsy—verifies lupus nephritis.

Management

1. Course is unpredictable, often progressive, and may terminate in death if untreated. Therapy is based on the extent and severity of disease. To simplify therapy, SLE is classified as mild (fever, arthritis, pleurisy, pericarditis, or rash) or severe (hemolytic anemia; thrombocytopenic purpura; massive pleural or pericardial involvement; significant renal, gastrointestinal, or CNS involvement).
2. Goal of medication therapy is to control symptoms and decrease inflammation.
3. Salicylates and NSAIDs are used to relieve joint symptoms, fever, fatigue, pain.
4. Antimalarials such as hydroxychloroquine (Plaquenil) to relieve joint symptoms and skin rash.
5. Steroids such as prednisone (Orasone) are used when there is renal or neurologic involvement or hemolytic anemia.
   a. Intravenous steroids are used to treat severe SLE.
   b. Provides rapid response but little effect on long-term course.
   c. Indications: acute CNS involvement, pulmonary disease, hemolytic anemia, severe nephritis.
   d. Children with deteriorating renal function and severe immunologic abnormalities have been reversed.

NURSING ALERT

Intravenous glucocorticoid "pulse" therapy has been known to cause hypertension or hypotension, tachycardia, blurring of vision, flushing, sweating, and metallic taste in mouth. Close monitoring of temperature, pulse rate, respiratory rate, and blood pressure is indicated.

---

6. Immunosuppressive agents such as azathioprine (Imuran), cyclophosphamide (Cytoxan), and chlorambucil (Leukeran)—used in severe disease, especially with nephritis or steroid-resistant patients.
7. Dialysis and renal transplantation as adjunctive therapy for severe lupus nephritis.
8. Supportive therapy:
   a. Rest
   b. Adequate nutrition; avoid obesity because of joint problems
   c. Treatment of existing complications with antibiotics, antihypertensives, and anticonvulsants
   d. Early identification and treatment of opportunistic infection
   e. Topical steroid preparations—may help suppress cutaneous lesions

Complications

1. Sepsis—primarily resulting from steroid and immunosuppressive therapy
2. Renal failure
3. Cardiac complications
4. Growth retardation related to steroids and immunosuppressive therapy

Nursing Assessment

1. Obtain a review of systems to determine involvement of other body systems.
2. Perform a complete physical examination, focusing on vital signs that might indicate renal or cardiac involvement, auscultation of the chest for heart and lung involvement, abdominal examination, and evaluation of the skin and extremities for vascular or cutaneous lesions.
3. Assess psychosocial status to evaluate child's and family's coping with chronic illness, school performance, and socialization.

Nursing Diagnoses

- Fatigue related to disease process
- Pain related to arthritis
- Hyperthermia related to disease process
- Risk for Injury related to CNS involvement (seizures)
- Risk for Injury related to IV glucocorticoid therapy
- Altered Urinary Elimination related to kidney involvement
- Altered Nutrition: Less Than Body Requirements related to anorexia and oral ulcers
- Body Image Disturbance related to manifestations of disease or drugs

Nursing Interventions
Minimizing Fatigue

1. Intersperse periods of rest between activities.
2. Provide opportunities for nonexertional therapeutic play.
3. Schedule procedures and activities after rest.

Promoting Comfort

1. Administer or teach parents to administer analgesics, NSAIDs, or steroids as prescribed and according to child's response.
2. For child on steroids, monitor for glycosuria and check blood test results for hyperglycemia and hypokalemia.
3. Provide diversional activities such as listening to music and quiet games.

Controlling Fever

1. Monitor temperature every 4 hours and document pattern.
2. Administer or teach parents to administer antipyretics as prescribed; note results.
3. Give tub or sponge bath to help reduce fever if necessary.
4. Encourage increased fluids by mouth when feverish.
5. Monitor for signs of dehydration such as dry skin and mucous membranes, poor skin turgor, decreased urine output, and thirst.
6. Administer IV fluids as ordered if dehydration develops.

Protecting From Injury Due to Seizures

1. Institute seizure precautions if indicated:
   a. Padded crib or bed rails
   b. Safe play area with no sharp toys or surfaces
   c. Airway and suction equipment on hand
2. Encourage protective environment and equipment such as bicycle helmet if prone to seizures.
3. Monitor condition during seizure and behavior after seizure.

Protecting From Adverse Reactions

1. While administering IV glucocorticoid therapy, monitor pulse and blood pressure every 15 minutes for 1 hour, then every 30 minutes for 1 hour.
2. Slow the rate or discontinue infusion if there are significant changes in blood pressure or pulse.
3. Notify the health care provider and continue to monitor vital signs frequently until they return to normal.

Maintaining Urinary Elimination

1. Monitor laboratory work for signs of renal abnormalities (blood urea nitrogen [BUN], creatinine, urine specific gravity, proteinuria, etc.).
2. Monitor intake and output.
3. Monitor blood pressure; watch for development of edema.

Maintaining Weight

1. Allow child to help in selecting and preparing foods. Give finger foods to smaller children.
2. Encourage small meals with snacks in between.
3. Apply topical medication to oral ulcers or give analgesics before meals.
4. Monitor food intake and weight.

Improving Self-Image

1. Encourage contact with peers and family.
2. Allow child to ventilate feeling about bodily changes and chronic illness.
3. Allow child to be involved in planning care and making decisions.
4. Structure play therapy to reduce fears and anxiety, promote interaction with other children, and allow child to gain control and master some tasks.
5. Refer to peer groups.

Community and Home Care Considerations

See Juvenile Rheumatoid Arthritis, p. 1560.

Family Education and Health Maintenance

1. Teach ways to prevent exacerbations and complications of the disease. Important "do's" include:
   a. Get enough rest.
   b. Avoid anxiety and tension.
   c. Follow treatment plan and medication schedule; understand medication side effects (especially with salicylates and steroids).
   d. Avoid contact with persons with infectious diseases; get pneumococcal and flu vaccine and keep routine immunizations up to date.
   e. Follow prescribed diet, especially when receiving steroids.
   f. Seek medical attention at times of illness or stress.
   g. Recognize warning signs of exacerbation such as chills, anorexia, fever, and fatigue.
   h. Become knowledgeable about SLE.
2. Important "don'ts" include:
   a. Do not overexert.
   b. Do not alter prescribed medications.
   c. Do not use over-the-counter drugs.
   d. Do not alter treatment plan.
   e. Do not expose self to sun and reflected sun through clouds, on snow, water, or white concrete or to fluorescent lighting. When exposure cannot be avoided, use sunscreen with 15–30 SPF.
   f. Do not use unproven therapies.
3. Teach parents about normal growth and development, emphasizing normal problems such as adolescent body image and peer relationships and how chronic illness can affect the child and the family.
4. Teach the importance of continual medical follow-up.
   a. Disease progress needs reevaluation, especially renal function, and drug therapy and laboratory results need frequent monitoring to prevent complications.
   b. Prognosis varies widely depending on the organ involvement and the intensity of the inflammatory reaction. Some children have milder SLE with little organ involvement. Prolonged spontaneous remission is unusual in children. The 5-year survival rate is 90%.
5. Advise family that child on hydroxychloroquine (Plaquenil) requires frequent ophthalmologic evaluation for corneal and retinal changes to prevent blindness. Retinitis is usually reversible, but the total period of treatment should not exceed 2 years.
6. Refer to agencies such as the Lupus Foundation, 1300 Piccord Drive, Suite 200, Rockville, MD 20850, 1-800-558-0120, *www.lupus.org*.

Outcome-Based Evaluation

- Plays for 45 minutes without fatigue
- Reporting reduced level of pain
- Afebrile
- Seizure precautions maintained
- No changes in vital signs during glucocorticoid infusion
- Urine output adequate
- Eating three small meals and two snacks; weight stable
- Interacting with siblings and peers

▮ Henoch-Schönlein Purpura

Henoch-Schönlein purpura (*anaphylactoid purpura, Schönlein-Henoch vasculitis*) is a diffuse disease resulting from inflammatory reaction around capillaries and arterioles involving the skin, intestines, joints, kidneys, and nervous system. There is a higher incidence in boys than in girls (2:1). Onset is between ages 2 and 8 years; it is seen most often in winter and can occur in clusters.

Pathophysiology and Etiology

1. Cause is unknown; however, theories include an allergic reaction to a variety of antigenic stimuli such as infection (eg, streptococci), airborne allergens, insect bites, food, and drugs.
2. Acute vasculitis develops.
   a. Swelling and edema of capillaries, small venuoles, and arterioles
   b. Fibrin is deposited in the glomeruli of the kidney
3. Vasculitis results in skin manifestations (nonthrombocytopenic purpura), arthritis, and gastrointestinal symptoms.

Clinical Manifestations

1. Rash—sudden onset may precede or follow other manifestations.
   a. Typical rash begins with itching and urticarial wheals and then proceeds to maculopapular erythematous lesions.
   b. These lesions become less raised and more petechial or purpuric in character and do not fade with pressure. They blanch initially, then progress to ecchymotic areas until they fade.
   c. Several stages of the rash may be present at one time.
   d. Rash appears primarily on buttocks, lower back, extensor aspects of arms, legs, and face, then disappears.
2. Arthritis of knee and ankle joint develops.
   a. The condition is moderately severe, with painful swelling due to periarticular edema and migrating arthritis.
   b. Movement is limited, but there is no permanent damage or deformity.
3. Angioedema—especially of scrotum
4. Colicky abdominal pain—from submucosal hemorrhage
5. Nausea, vomiting, malaise, low-grade fever
6. Proteinuria
7. Microscopic hematuria
8. Symptoms may appear acutely or gradually and vary in intensity and duration.

Diagnostic Evaluation

1. Blood studies (not diagnostic, but support clinical evidence):
   a. IgA may be elevated.
   b. Coagulation studies and platelet count are normal in presence of purpura.
   c. ESR and white blood cell count are elevated.
   d. Anemia is possible.
   e. Elevated BUN and creatinine with severe kidney involvement.
2. Urine studies show proteinuria, microscopic hematuria, and casts.
3. Stools show occult or gross blood.

Management

Treatment is primarily symptomatic and supportive.

1. Encourage bed rest until the child is able to ambulate and can do so without increasing edema of feet.
2. Remove allergen if it is known.
3. Give antibiotic therapy if acute episode was preceded by infection, especially streptococcal.
4. Manage complicating abdominal or renal involvement and arthritis.
   a. Steroids such as prednisone (Orasone) may relieve abdominal symptoms and prevent intussusception from bowel edema.
   b. Immunosuppressive therapy such as azathioprine (Imuran) or cyclophosphamide (Cytoxan) may be given to stabilize persistent renal involvement.
   c. High-dose immune globulin has been recommended for severe cases.
5. Provide comfort measures and analgesics. Salicylates are not particularly effective; NSAIDS are given.

Complications

1. Acute nephritis or nephrosis that may lead to chronic nephritis
2. Intussusception
3. Neurologic vasculitis with headaches, seizures, and neuropathies

NURSING ALERT

Be alert for signs of intussusception—sudden onset of paroxysmal abdominal pain, currant jelly–like stools, vomiting, increasing abdominal distention and tenderness—and report immediately.

Nursing Assessment

1. Obtain a complete history, checking for recent upper respiratory infection, medications, and allergen exposure.

2. Perform physical assessment of renal, integumentary, musculoskeletal, and gastrointestinal systems.
3. Determine impact of illness on the psychosocial well-being of the child and family.

Nursing Diagnoses

- Pain related to arthritis and abdominal pain
- Activity Intolerance related to fatigue and pain
- Risk for Impaired Skin Integrity related to rash and itching
- Altered Urinary Elimination related to renal involvement
- Fear related to discomfort, hospitalization, and lack of knowledge

Nursing Interventions
Reducing Discomfort

1. Monitor pain level and location. Nonverbal behavior may be the most important source of information in the small child.
2. Administer or teach parents to administer pain medications as prescribed and according to the child's response.
3. Apply warm or cool compresses to joints or abdomen for 30-minute periods to help soothe painful areas.
4. Provide diversional activities such as listening to music, coloring, and quiet games.
5. Place in position of comfort; elevate affected limbs.

Increasing Participation in Activities

1. Monitor completion of daily and diversional activities.
2. Alternate activities with rest periods.
3. Allow child to choose activities.
4. Modify play to be nonexertional and done while sitting.

Maintaining Skin Integrity

1. Assess skin condition and turgor.
2. Maintain adequate fluids.
3. Provide loose, comfortable clothing.
4. Administer or teach parents to administer antipruritics such as hydroxyzine (Atarax) by mouth, or topical products as needed.
5. Avoid soap, scratching, or dry skin that may exacerbate rash.

Maintaining Urinary Output

1. Record intake and output, vital signs, weight, specific gravity, and level of edema.
2. Check urine for protein, hematuria, and color.
3. Report or teach parents to report changes promptly.

Alleviating Fear

1. Allow child and family to verbalize feelings about hospitalization and illness.
2. Monitor anxiety level of child and family.
3. Offer realistic encouragement. The long-term outlook is good when renal involvement is minimal.
4. Encourage the family and peers to visit the hospitalized child and bring in familiar articles from home.
5. Allow child to make some age-appropriate decisions and become involved in planning care.

Family Education and Health Maintenance

1. Reassure the parents that symptoms are self-limiting.
2. Ensure that parents and child understand the disease and the need to report changes in urine or signs of intussusception.
3. Encourage the parents to comply with follow-up. Urinalysis will be evaluated 6 and 12 months following the acute episode because of possible delayed renal damage.

Outcome-Based Evaluation

- Child reports relief of pain
- Child participating in activity for longer period each day
- Rash resolved, skin intact
- Urine output adequate, negative protein
- Child playing, interacting with others

■ Kawasaki Disease

Kawasaki disease (*mucocutaneous lymph node syndrome*) is a multisystem vasculitis identified by a febrile illness with several distinguishing features that compromise vital body systems. It is the leading cause of acquired heart disease in children in the U. S. Peak age of occurrence is in the toddler; 80% of patients are under age 5. It seldom occurs in children over 8 years old. It is most frequently seen in Japan and in children of Japanese heritage and is slightly more common in boys than girls. Seasonal epidemics usually occur in late winter and early spring. The long-term prognosis is still unknown.

Pathophysiology and Etiology

1. Cause is unknown, although exposure to rug shampoos and infectious agents such as retrovirus, *Propironibacteriae*, and Group A streptococcus have been implicated. Hypersensitivity reactions from exposure to environmental or infectious agents are being investigated.
2. Although vasculitis is a multisystem disease, the cardiovascular system seems to be primarily involved.
3. Initially: stage I
   a. Perivasculitis of arterioles, venules, and capillaries
   b. Coronary arteries are included—pancarditis
4. As disease progresses: stages II and III
   a. Panvasculitis and perivasculitis of coronary arteries
   b. Aneurysm formation, coronary thrombosis, pericarditis, myocarditis, endocarditis, and phlebitis may result
5. Stage IV
   a. Coronary arterial scarring, stenosis, calcification
   b. Myocardial fibrosis and endocardial fibroelastosis
   c. Healing begins

Clinical Manifestations
Acute Febrile Phase—Stage I

1. The child appears severely ill and irritable (days 1–11).
2. Major criteria according to CDC as diagnostic of Kawasaki disease:

a. High, spiking fever for 5 or more days
b. Bilateral conjunctival infection
c. Oropharyngeal erythema, "strawberry" tongue, red and dry lips
d. Indurative edema of hands and feet, erythema of palms and soles, general edema, or periungual desquamation
e. Erythematous rash
f. Cervical lymphadenopathy—at least one lymph node greater than 1.5 cm

3. Carditis—pericarditis, myocarditis, cardiomegaly, congestive heart failure, pleural effusion
4. Iridocyclitis and aseptic meningitis

Subacute Phase—Stage II

1. Acute symptoms of stage I subside as temperature returns to normal. The child remains irritable and anorectic (days 11–21).
2. Dry, cracked lips with fissures
3. Desquamation of toes and fingers
4. Arthralgia, arthritis (temporary)
5. Coronary thrombosis, aneurysms

Convalescent Phase—Stage III

1. The child appears well (days 21–60)
2. Transverse grooves of fingers and toenails (Beau's lines)
3. Coronary thrombosis; aneurysms (may occur)

Diagnostic Evaluation

1. The CDC requires that fever and four of the six other criteria listed above in stage I be demonstrated.
2. Electrocardiogram, echocardiogram, cardiac catheterization, and angiocardiography may be required to diagnose cardiac abnormalities.
3. Although there are no specific laboratory tests, the following may help support diagnosis or rule out other diseases:
   a. CBC—leukocytosis during acute stage
   b. ESR—elevated during acute stage
   c. Erythrocytes and hemoglobin—slight decrease
   d. C-reactive protein—positive
   e. Platelet count—increased during second to fourth week of illness and beta-1-antitripylin increased
   f. IgM, IgA, IgG, and IgF—transiently elevated
   g. Urine—protein and leukocytes present
   h. Elevated transaminases

Management

1. Although treatment is considered controversial, goals are amelioration of symptoms and prevention of coronary thrombosis, coronary aneurysm, and death.
2. Single dose of immune globulin (gamma globulin) IV therapy—IVGG (2 g/kg per day)—is initiated during stage I over an 8- to 10-hour infusion to reduce the incidence of coronary artery abnormalities.

DRUG ALERT

Infusion of IVGG has been known to cause a precipitous drop in blood pressure, possibly due to rate of infusion, which may mimic anaphylaxis. Monitor blood pressure and heart rate at the start of infusion, after 15 minutes, 30 minutes, and then hourly until infusion is complete. Slow the infusion and have the patient evaluated for any drop in blood pressure. Keep epinephrine on hand to use for an anaphylactic reaction.

NURSING ALERT

The effectiveness of live vaccinations such as measles, mumps, and rubella may be reduced after IVGG infusion. MMR immunizations should be postponed until 5 months after IVGG infusion.

3. Aspirin therapy:
   a. Anti-inflammatory dose (80–100 mg/kg per day) divided into 4 doses during acute stage of illness
   b. Antiplatelet dose (3–5 mg/kg per day) as a single dose after fever is controlled and continued for 2 to 3 months after illness (when the echocardiogram is normal) or until ESR and platelet count are normal, to reduce risk of spontaneous coronary thrombosis. It may be continued indefinitely if there are coronary abnormalities.

DRUG ALERT

Risk of Reye's syndrome exists for children on aspirin therapy if they develop varicella or influenza. For children who have not had chickenpox, parents need to notify health care provider urgently if child has been exposed. Aspirin may be withheld.

4. Thrombolytic therapy may be required during the acute phase or during convalescence. Dipyridamole (Persantine) may be given as a platelet aggregation inhibitor if aneurysms are present.
5. Supportive measures:
   a. Maintain fluid and electrolyte balance; give nutritional support.
   b. Provide comfort.
6. Cardiac follow-up by pediatric cardiologist with serial two-dimensional echocardiograms, angiography, and cardiac isoenzymes is indicated.

Complications

1. Fifteen percent to 20% of patients develop cardiac complications (coronary arteritis, aneurysmal thrombosis or rupture, myocardial infarction, congestive heart failure, coronary insufficiency, and ischemia).
2. Aspirin toxicity.
3. Mortality rate is less than 0.3%.

Nursing Assessment

1. Focus history on gathering data that support the diagnosis of Kawasaki disease, such as fever and skin manifestations.
2. Perform physical examination, concentrating on the cardiovascular system.

Nursing Diagnoses

- Pain related to conjunctival inflammation and arthritis
- Decreased Cardiac Output related to vasculitis and aneurysms
- Altered Oral Mucous Membrane related to disease process
- Risk for Impaired Skin Integrity related to edema, dehydration, desquamation, and bed rest
- Fluid Volume Deficit related to hyperthermia, anorexia, and oral ulcer
- Fear of parents and child related to severity of illness and hospitalization

Nursing Interventions

Reducing Discomfort

1. Allow the child periods of uninterrupted rest. Offer pain medication routinely rather than PRN during acute phase. Monitor effectiveness of analgesic measures.
2. Perform comfort measures related to the eyes.
   a. Conjunctivitis can cause photosensitivity; darken the room, offer sunglasses.
   b. Apply cool compresses.
   c. Discourage rubbing of eyes.
   d. Instill artificial tear drops to soothe conjunctiva.
3. Perform comfort measures related to joint pain and tender lymph nodes.
   a. Use passive range-of-motion exercises every 4 hours while the child is awake because movement may be restricted.
   b. Allow and encourage the child to move about freely under supervision.
   c. Provide soft toys and quiet play and encourage use of hands and fingers.
   d. Monitor pain level and child's response to analgesics.
4. Provide quiet, peaceful environment with diversional activity such as listening to music.

Maintaining Cardiac Output

1. Institute continual cardiac monitoring and assessment for complications.
   a. Take vital signs and blood pressure every 2 hours; report abnormalities.
   b. Ensure proper functioning of cardiac monitor; observe for and report any arrhythmia.
   c. Assess the child for signs of myocarditis (tachycardia, gallop rhythm, chest pain).
   d. Monitor the child for congestive heart failure (dyspnea, nasal flaring, grunting, retractions, cyanosis, orthopnea, crackles, moist respirations, distended neck veins, edema).
2. Closely monitor intake and output and administer oral and IV fluids as ordered.

3. If administering IVGG, monitor blood pressure and heart rate at the start of the infusion, after 15 minutes, after 30 minutes, and then hourly until infusion is complete. Slow the infusion and contact the health care provider to evaluate the child for any drop in blood pressure. Keep epinephrine on hand to use for an anaphylactic reaction.
4. Prepare the child for cardiac surgery or thrombolytic therapy as indicated (see p. 1396).

Preserving Oral Mucous Membranes

1. Offer and encourage frequent cool liquids (ice chips and popsicles).
2. Progress to soft, bland foods.
3. Give mouth care every 1 to 4 hours with special mouth swabs; use soft toothbrush only after healing has occurred.
4. Apply petroleum to dried, cracked lips.
5. Observe the mouth frequently for signs of infection.

Improving Skin Integrity

1. Avoid the use of soap because it tends to dry skin and makes it more likely to break down.
2. Elevate edematous extremities.
3. Use sheepskin, egg-crate mattress, and smooth sheets.
4. If clothes are used, encourage use of soft flannel or terry cloth that fits loosely.
5. Apply emollients to skin, as ordered.
6. Protect peeling skin; observe for signs of infection.

Maintaining Fluid Balance

1. Monitor temperature every 4 to 8 hours—every 2 hours if elevated. Maintain temperature graph chart.
   a. Give tub or sponge baths for temperature over 101°F (38.3°C).
   b. Administer antipyretics as ordered.
   c. Use a cooling blanket for higher temperatures not responsive to antipyretics, as needed.
   d. Monitor for febrile seizures.
2. Offer clear liquids every hour when child is awake.
3. Monitor hydration status by checking skin turgor, weight, urinary output, presence of tears and moist mucous membranes, and specific gravity.
4. Infuse IV fluids as ordered through a volume control device if dehydration is present, and check the site and amount hourly.
5. Monitor and document fluid volumes and intake and output.
6. Encourage the child to eat a balanced diet, including good protein sources to prevent hypoalbuminemia, which will result in intravascular fluid volume deficit.

Reducing Fear

1. Use play therapy (both passive and active) to help the child express feelings.
2. Explain all procedures to the child and family.
3. Provide respite for parents during irritable stage of illness when child may be inconsolable. Provide emotional support as necessary.
4. Encourage the parents and child to verbalize their concerns, fears, and questions.

5. Practice relaxation techniques with child such as relaxation breathing, guided imagery, and distraction.
6. Keep family informed of progress and reinforce information about stages and prognosis.

Family Education and Health Maintenance

1. Teach parents about disease process, possible complications, medications, and side effects.
2. Ensure that the family understands the medications, follow-up tests, and level of physical activity that have been prescribed for the child based on specific categories. For long-term follow-up care, children can be categorized into one of three groups: those with no cardiac involvement, those with small coronary aneurysms, and those with aneurysms greater than 8 mm.
3. Teach parents that long-term care after discharge is critical because complications can occur during the period of convalescence or months after acute illness.
4. Provide written instructions about cardiac complications and stress the need to report the development of symptoms.
5. Encourage family members to learn cardiopulmonary resuscitation, if indicated.
6. Teach parents to report the possible development of salicylate toxicity—tinnitus, nausea and vomiting, gastrointestinal distress, blood in stool, increased respirations.
7. Provide anticipatory guidance about child's behavior.
   a. Do not overprotect the child. Discuss with parents the grief and mourning process of denial, anger, bargaining, depression, and acceptance they may be going through because of the chronic illness.
   b. Allow child to be as active as desired unless the stress test is abnormal or the child is on anticoagulants. Try to protect the child from injury if he or she is taking anticoagulants (no sharp toys, no contact sports).
   c. Discuss regression that might occur as a result of hospitalization or the disease process and how to deal with these changes.
8. Refer for additional information to agencies such as American Heart Association, 7272 Greenville Ave., Dallas, TX 75231-4596, 214-373-6300, *www.americanheart.org*.

Outcome-Based Evaluation

- Child reporting less pain; minimal crying noted
- Vital signs stable, no edema noted
- Taking fluids by mouth well; no signs of oral infection
- Mild peeling of skin, no signs of infection
- Skin and mucous membranes moist, urine output adequate
- Child and parents asking appropriate questions; child using relaxation breathing

SELECTED REFERENCES

American Academy of Pediatrics (1997). *Report of the Committee on Infectious Diseases* (24th ed.). Elk Grove Village, IL: AAP.

American Academy of Pediatrics, Committee on Pediatric AIDS. (1999) Disclosure of illness status to children and adolescents with HIV infection (RE9827). *Pediatrics, 103*(1), 164–166.

Applegate, B. (1995). Kawasaki syndrome: An important consideration in the febrile child. *Postgraduate Medicine, 97*(2), 121–126.

Baumeister, L. & Nicol, N. H. (1994). Pediatric lupus and the role of sun protection. *Pediatric Nursing, 20*(4), 371–375.

Belkengren, R. & Sapala, S. (1997). Pediatric management problems. *Pediatric Nursing, 23*(4), 404–405.

Cassidy, J. & Petty, R. (1995). *Textbook of pediatric rheumatology* (3rd ed.). Philadelphia: W. B. Saunders.

Centers for Disease Control and Prevention. (1999). Recommended childhood immunization schedule—United States. *MMWR, 48*(1), 12–16.

Centers for Disease Control and Prevention (1996). AIDS among children—United States. *MMWR, 45*(46).

Centers for Disease Control and Prevention (1995). 1995 revised guidelines for prophylaxis against *Pneumocystis carinii* pneumonia for children infected with or perinatally exposed to human immunodeficiency virus. *MMWR, 44*(RR-4).

Centers for Disease Control and Prevention (1994a). 1994 revised classification system for human immunodeficiency virus infection in children less than 13 years of age. *MMWR, 43*(RR-12).

Centers for Disease Control and Prevention (1994b). Recommendations for the use of zidovudine to reduce perinatal transmission of human immunodeficiency virus. *MMWR, 43*(RR-11).

Connor, E.M., Sperling, R.S., Gelbert, R., et al. (1994). Reduction of maternal-infant transmission of human immunodeficiency virus type 1 with zidovudine treatment: Pediatric AIDS Clinical Trials Group protocol 076 study group. *New England Journal of Medicine, 331*, 1173–1180.

Driscoll, S.W. et al. (1994). Juvenile rheumatoid arthritis. *Physical Medicine and Rehabilitation Clinics of North America, 5*(4), 763–783.

The International Perinatal HIV Group, Read, J. S. (Ed.) (1999). The mode of delivery and the risk of vertical transmission of human immunodeficiency virus type 1. *New England Journal of Medicine, 340*(13), 977–987.

Landesman, S.H., Kalish, L.A., Burns, D.N., et al. (1997). Obstetrical factors and the transmission of human immunodeficiency virus type 1 from mother to child. *New England Journal of Medicine, 334*, 1617–1623.

Lux, K.M. (1991). New hope for children with Kawaski disease. *Journal of Pediatric Nursing, 6*(3), 159–165.

Melish, M.E. (1996). Kawaski syndrome. *Pediatrics in Review, 17*(5), 153–162.

Newshan, G. (1997). Pain in human immunodeficiency virus disease. *Seminars in Oncology Nursing, 13*, 36–41.

Pahl, E. (1997). Kawaski disease: Cardiac sequelae and management. *Pediatric Annals, 26*(2), 112–115.

Pizzo, P.A. & Wilfert, C.M. (Eds.) (1998). *Pediatric AIDS: The challenge of HIV infection in infants, children, and adolescents* (3rd ed.). Baltimore: Williams & Wilkins.

Shulman, S.T., Di Inocenio, J., & Hirsh, R. (1995). Kawaski disease. *Pediatric Rheumatology, 42*(5), 1205–1222.

Singsen, B. & Goldbach-Mansky, R. (1997). Methotrexate in the treatment of juvenile arthritis and other pediatric rheumatic and nonrheumatic disorders. *Rheumatic Disease Clinics of North America, 23*(4).

Tsubata, S. et al. (1995). Successful thrombolytic therapy using tissue-type plasminogen activator in Kawasaki disease. *Pediatric Cardiology, 16*, 186–189.

U.S. Public Health Service Task Force (2000). Recommendations for the use of antiretroviral drugs in pregnant women infected with HIV-1 for maternal health and for reducing perinatal HIV-1 transmission in the United States. *http://www.hivatis.org*

White, P.H. (1994). Pediatric systemic lupus and neonatal lupus. *Rheumatic Disease Clinics of North America, 20*(1), 19–125.

Working Group on Antiretroviral Therapy: National Pediatric HIV Resource Center (2000). Guidelines for the use of antiretroviral agents in pediatric HIV infection. *http://www.hivatis.org*

Working Group on Antiretroviral Therapy: National Pediatric HIV Resource Center (1998). 1998 guidelines for use of antiretroviral agents in pediatric HIV infection. *MMWR, 47*(RR-4).

Pediatric Orthopedic Problems

COMMON ORTHOPEDIC DISORDERS IN CHILDREN

▣ Fractures

A fracture is a break or disruption in the continuity of bone. Fractures in children differ from those in adults. The anatomy, biomechanics, and physiology of the child's skeleton are different from those of the adult. The incidence of musculoskeletal injuries sustained by children and adolescents has increased significantly in the last 2 decades.

Pathophysiology and Etiology

1. Most fractures in children are a result of low-velocity trauma, such as a fall.
   a. Up to age 2, most fractures are sustained as a result of the child being injured by another person.
   b. Fractures in newborns and infants are often the result of child abuse. Abuse should be suspected when treating fractures in this age group.
2. A bone fractures when the force applied to it exceeds the amount the bone can absorb.
   a. Children's long bones are more resilient than those of adults. They are able to withstand greater deflection without fracturing.
   b. Children's bones also have thick periosteum.
3. Unique to fractures in children is the involvement of growth plates. Cartilaginous growth plates are present at each end of the long bones and at one end of metacarpals and metatarsals. The plate is weaker than surrounding ligaments, tendons, and joint capsules and is disrupted before these tissues are injured.
   a. Damage to the growth plate may result in cessation of or a disturbance in bone growth (depending on the extent of damage sustained at the growth plate).
   b. On the other hand, there is often acceleration in bone growth after a fracture in the long bones of children.
4. Children's fractures heal more rapidly than adult fractures. The younger the child, the more rapidly bone heals.
5. Children's fractures remodel more completely and actively than adult fractures, and usually result in less and disability.

Common Sites of Fractures in Children
Epiphyseal Injuries
1. Fifteen percent to 30% of all childhood fractures involve the physis (growth plate).
2. The most frequent site of physeal injuries (excluding phalangeal fractures) is the distal radius and ulna.
3. The 11- to 15-year-old age group tends to sustain the majority of physeal injuries to the distal radius and ulna.
4. The mechanism of injury is usually a fall on an outstretched arm.
Forearm Fractures
1. Most common site of fracture in children.
2. Account for more than half of all fractures in children.
3. Seventy-five percent of forearm fractures occur in the distal third of the radius and ulna.
4. Most common cause is from a fall on an outstretched arm.
Humerus Fractures
1. The mechanism of injury for the majority of humeral fractures is a fall onto an outstretched arm or hand.
2. Less than 1% of fractures occur at the proximal humerus.
3. Ten percent of all humeral fractures occur at the shaft of the humerus; they account for less than 2% of all pediatric fractures.
   a. Humeral shaft fractures are usually a result of twisting injuries in infants and toddlers (child abuse is a common cause of these fractures in this age group).

b. Direct trauma to the humeral shaft is the most common mechanism of injury in older children.

4. Supracondylar fractures account for 60% of all elbow fractures in children. There is a high incidence of neurovascular injury with supracondylar fractures, 8% of which sustain a neurologic injury.

5. Twenty percent of distal humeral injuries occur in the lateral condyle; this ranks as the second most common elbow fracture in children.

6. Medial epicondyle fractures are the third most common elbow fracture in children, accounting for 5% to 10% of all pediatric elbow fractures.

Spinal Fractures

1. Rare in children.

2. Mechanism of injury is due to significant trauma such as an automobile accident, fall from a significant height, or pedestrian versus motor vehicle accident.

Pelvis and Hip Fracture

1. Pelvic fractures are uncommon in children and adolescents.

2. Pelvic fractures are often the result of high-energy trauma or a crush-type injury.

3. Damage to the abdominal wall and pelvic organs may occur in association with the pelvic fracture.

4. Hip fractures account for less than 1% of all fractures in children.

5. Seventy-five percent of hip fractures in children result from high-energy trauma such as motor vehicle accidents, bicycle accidents, and falls from significant heights.

6. Half of children who sustain a hip fracture have been involved in a motor vehicle accident or pedestrian versus motor vehicle accident; these children usually have other injuries.

7. Child abuse is the most common cause of hip fracture in children under the age of 3 years.

Femur Fractures

1. Common in children.

2. The midshaft of the femur is the most common location for femoral fractures in children.

3. Usually the result of high-energy trauma such as a motor vehicle accident or fall from a significant height.

4. Seventy percent of femur fractures in children under 1 year of age are associated with child abuse.

Tibial Fracture

1. The most common lower extremity fracture in children occurs in the tibial and fibular shaft.

2. A rotational mechanism of injury to the lower leg is the most common cause of tibial fractures in children under the age of 3 years (toddler's fracture).

3. Greater force is required to injure the tibia in older children; motor vehicle accidents and sports injuries are the most common causes of tibial fractures in children and adolescents.

Ankle Fracture

1. Common in children and adolescents.

2. Often involve the growth plate.

3. Greatest incidence is in boys between 10 and 15 years of age.

4. Usually the result of direct trauma.

Foot Fracture

1. Metatarsal fractures are most common.

2. Mechanism of injury is usually a direct or indirect trauma such as falls, jumping from heights, and twisting injuries.

Classification of Fractures

1. Open fractures: underlying fracture in bone communicates with an external wound.

2. Closed fractures: underlying fracture with no open wound.

3. Plastic deformation: a bending of the bone in such a manner as to cause a microscopic fracture line that does not cross the bone. When the force is removed, the bone remains bent. Unique to children and most common in the ulna (Figure 54-1A).

4. Buckle (torus) fractures: fracture on the tension side of the bone near the softer metaphyseal bone; crosses the bone and buckles the harder diaphyseal bone on the opposite side, causing a bulge (see Figure 54-1B).

5. Greenstick fracture: the bone is bent and the fracture begins but does not entirely cross through the bone (see Figure 54-1C).

6. Complete fractures (see Figure 54-1D):
   a. Spiral–from a rotational force
   b. Oblique—diagonally across the diaphysis

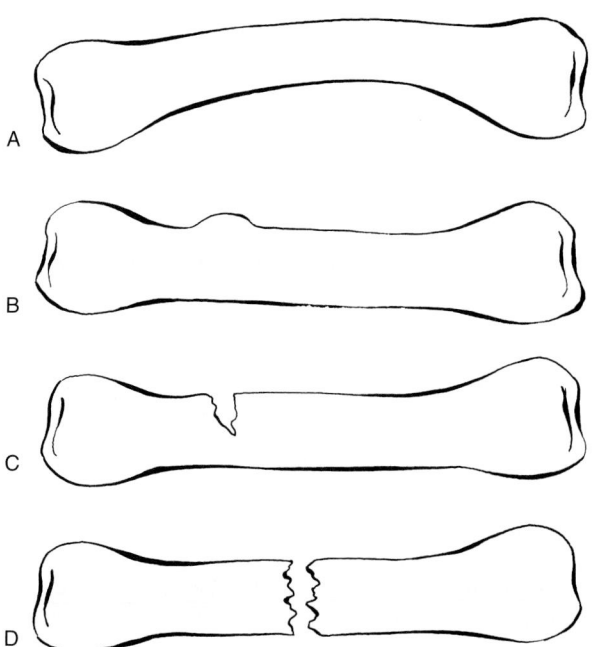

FIGURE 54-1 Common fractures in children. (**A**) Plastic deformation (bend). (**B**) Buckle (torus). (**C**) Greenstick. (**D**) Complete.

c. Transverse—usually diaphyseal
d. Epiphyseal—through the physis

Clinical Manifestations

1. Inability to stand, walk, or use injured part.
2. Limb deformity (visible or palpable).
3. Ecchymosis.
4. Pain.
5. History of injury or trauma (may not be the case with pathologic fractures).
6. Spontaneous onset of pain (usually seen with pathologic fractures).
7. Local swelling and marked tenderness.
8. Movement between bone fragments.
9. Crepitus or grating.
10. Muscle spasm.

Diagnostic Evaluation

1. X-rays of suspected limb fractures should include the joint above and below the injured part.
   a. Should always include a minimum of two views at 90-degree angles to each other (AP and lateral).
   b. Comparison views of the opposite extremity are frequently needed. They help to distinguish the fracture line from the growth plate.
   c. In some situations oblique x-rays are warranted in order to help identify a fracture that is difficult to detect.
2. Further radiologic studies may be indicated in certain instances to evaluate a fracture: tomography, CT scan, MRI, bone scan, fluoroscopy.
3. Vascular assessment may include the use of:
   a. Doppler studies
   b. Compartment pressure monitoring
   c. Angiography

Management

Treatment is dependent upon the type of fracture, its location, and the age of the child.

1. Treatment may consist of:
   a. Immobilization by cast, splint, or brace
   b. Closed reduction followed by a period of immobilization in a cast or splint
   c. Open reduction with or without internal fixation and usually followed by a period of immobilization in a cast or splint
   d. Closed reduction and percutaneous pinning followed by a period of immobilization
   e. Closed or open reduction and application of an external fixator
   f. Traction (skin, skeletal) followed by a period of immobilization
2. Most children's fractures heal in 12 weeks or less. Simple fractures that are closed and nondisplaced can heal enough to be free from immobilization within 3 weeks.

Complications

1. Infection, avascular necrosis
2. Delayed union, nonunion, malunion
3. Shortening—epiphyseal arrest (deformities in angulation or limb length)
4. Vascular injuries
5. Nerve injuries—palsies
6. Visceral injuries
7. Tendon and joint injuries
8. Fat embolism
9. Compartment syndrome
10. Osteoarthritis (later)
11. Reflex sympathetic dystrophy

Nursing Assessment

1. Follow the basic assessment for the trauma victim (see p. 1062).
2. Obtain history from child, parents, and others to include accident or trauma details, noting the position of the extremity at impact.
3. Perform physical exam for location of deformity, swelling, ecchymosis, and pain; vital signs; and neurovascular assessment.
4. Assess child's support mechanisms/social situation with consideration of discharge needs.

Nursing Diagnoses

- Pain related to tissue trauma and reflex muscle spasms secondary to fracture
- Altered Peripheral Tissue Perfusion related to swelling and/or immobilization
- Impaired Skin Integrity related to mechanical trauma (eg, fixation device, traction, casts, other orthopedic devices)
- Ineffective Coping related to separation from family and home
- Impaired Physical Mobility related to fracture and external immobilization device (eg, cast, splint, external fixator)
- Self-Care Deficit related to external devices (eg, cast, splint)
- Risk for Infection related to trauma (fracture) and surgery
- Risk for Peripheral Neurovascular Dysfunction related to restrictive envelope secondary to cast or splint

Nursing Interventions

Also see page 991 for orthopedic surgery.

Promoting Comfort

1. Monitor and assess pain level using an age-appropriate pain scale (eg, Oucher or Faces scale).
2. Properly position, align, and support affected body part.
3. Administer analgesics as indicated and monitor effectiveness of analgesia.
4. Use nontraditional methods of pain relief—music therapy, diversionary activities, relaxation techniques, therapeutic touch, play therapy.

Maintaining Tissue Perfusion

1. Frequently assess perfusion to limb by checking temperature, color, sensation, and pulses.
2. Elevate extremity above heart level to prevent edema.
3. Encourage movement of digits on affected limb.
4. Remove compressive bandages (eg, elastic bandages, splints) that restrict flow of circulation.

Maintaining Skin Integrity

1. Assess for and relieve pressure caused by tight bandages, casts, and/or splints.
2. Provide periodic cleaning, thorough drying, and lubrication to pressure points if in traction.
3. Encourage frequent position changes as allowed.
4. Assess skin condition on a regular basis.
5. Massage healthy skin around affected area to stimulate circulation.
6. Protect skin at risk with special dressings or products (eg, barrier cream, moisture-permeable dressing).
7. Promote a diet high in protein and carbohydrates.

Promoting Effective Coping

1. Assess child's and parent's response to events.
2. Explain condition, treatment, and rehabilitation goals as indicated.
3. Provide reassurance and emotional support when needed.
4. Refer to community-based support agencies (eg, social services, United Way) if indicated.
5. Structure the child's day with routine, activities, and therapy to keep him or her busy.
6. Encourage the child and parents to verbalize feelings.
7. Encourage child to express feelings and emotions through writing (eg, journal), drawing, or play therapy.

Promoting Mobility

1. Encourage exercise of uninvolved limbs regularly throughout day.
2. Teach appropriate ambulation techniques using aids such as crutches, walkers, or wheelchairs as indicated.
3. Teach safety precautions when using an ambulatory aid.

Attaining Independence

1. Assess family situation for ability to care for child at home.
2. Allow child to care for self when able.
3. Encourage parents and siblings to assist only as needed.
4. Encourage child to participate in care as much as possible.
5. Evaluate child's ability to participate in self-care activities.

Preventing Infection

1. Assess wounds frequently for warmth, erythema, swelling, tenderness, or purulent drainage.
2. Report signs of infection.
3. Provide appropriate wound care for open injuries and surgical wounds.
4. Administer antibiotics as ordered.
5. Encourage child to eat and maintain good caloric and protein intake to promote healing.
6. Teach good handwashing technique to child and parents.

Preventing Peripheral Neurovascular Dysfunction

1. Assess the neurovascular status of affected limb every hour for the first 24 hours (or as indicated by hospital protocol)—compare with unaffected limb.
2. Assess for nerve injury (eg, abduct all fingers, touch thumb to small finger, plantar flexion, dorsiflexion).
3. Assess for presence of numbness, tingling, "pins and needles," excessive pain (disproportionate to injury and analgesia administered).
4. Encourage range-of-motion exercises in fingers, toes, and unaffected limbs.
5. Teach child and parents signs and symptoms of neurovascular compromise and what to do.

Community and Home Care Considerations

A home care visit may be necessary in the initial postoperative stage to ensure that the family is coping with the care of their immobilized child. Often reinforcement is needed to help reassure the parents that they are able to care for their child. Make certain that the family has a way of contacting a nurse after home care visits have been discontinued.

1. Assess coping ability of family members.
2. Assess skin of child for signs of breakdown.
3. Assess condition of the hip spica cast, especially around perineal area.
4. Assess neurovascular status of affected limb.
5. Assess child's coping ability—participation in self-care.
6. Assess traction device to ensure it is intact and maintained.
7. Assess child's nutritional status.
8. Assess child's bowel and bladder routine.
9. Answer questions parents may have about care of their immobilized child.
10. Teach patient and family about care of their child's external fixation device (pin site care).
11. Have the family do a return demonstration so as to assess their skill and ability to care for their child's pin sites.
12. Teach the child and family about signs and symptoms of infection and whom to contact should an infection occur.

Family Education and Health Maintenance

1. Teach proper care of casts, splints, and immobilization devices (see Patient Education Guidelines).
2. Teach safety measures and prevention of further injuries.
   a. Advise use of bicycle helmets and knee, elbow, and wrist pads.
   b. Emphasize importance of supervising young children while playing.
   c. Teach safety measures such as placing gates at stairs and installing top-opening windows on second floors.
3. Teach family and child the natural history of fracture healing (eg, presence of fracture bump, gradual recovery of range of motion, predicted time frame for healing).

1. Keep the casted body part elevated on a pillow for the first few days to decrease swelling.
2. Avoid touching the cast until it is fully dry to avoid denting it.
3. Watch the body part below the cast for swelling or blueness.
4. Move the body part below the cast at least every 4 hours for the first 24 hours.
5. Avoid strenuous activity such as roughhousing or sports while the cast is in place, but remain active with usual activities.
6. Do not put anything inside the cast.
7. Keep the cast dry; cover with plastic bag to shower; do not swim or submerge cast in water.
8. If itching occurs under the cast, blow some cool air into it from a hair dryer.
9. Develop a plan for carrying out usual activity, such as dressing, walking up and down steps, carrying books, etc.
10. Call your health care provider if there is pain, blueness, swelling, or inability to move the body part.
11. Be sure to keep follow-up appointments.

Outcome-Based Evaluation

- Child reports acceptable level of comfort
- Extremity warm with good color sensation, pulses, and capillary refill
- No skin breakdown noted
- Parents comforting child; child responding appropriately
- Using aids and ambulating independently
- Bathing and feeding self with minimal assistance
- No signs of infection surrounding wound
- Denies numbness and tingling; good range of motion

Osteomyelitis

Osteomyelitis is a pyogenic infection of the bone and/or surrounding soft tissues. It may occur at any age but is primarily a disease of growing bones. Long bones are frequently involved, and the characteristic site of involvement is the metaphyseal region. Boys are afflicted three times as often as girls.

Pathophysiology and Etiology

1. Usually bacterial in origin; causative agents include:
   a. *Staphylococcus aureus*—responsible for 90% of acute hematogenous osteomyelitis.
   b. Streptococcus.
   c. Group B streptococcus—common in infants and young children.
   d. *Escherichia coli*—frequently found in young children and neonates.
2. Three methods of inoculation:
   a. Hematogenous (through the bloodstream)—occurs often in children after blunt trauma to long bones.
   b. Contiguous infection (direct spread from adjacent tissue)—occurs after surgery or from a primary infection.
   c. Direct inoculation (through puncture or stab wounds)—occurs with open fractures or surgical wounds.
3. Risk factors include:
   a. External fixation device.
   b. Urinary drainage—Foley catheters
   c. Central or peripheral IV lines
4. Once the site is inoculated, there is an inflammatory and immunologic response:
   a. Pus formation
   b. Edema
   c. Vascular congestion
5. Vascular occlusion leads to ischemia and bone necrosis.
6. Infection spreads through bone via Volkmann's and haversian canals, causing further vascular occlusion.
7. Ischemia allows necrotic bone to separate from living bone, forming sequestra.
8. Sequestra enlarge, spreading toward and breaching the cortex and forming a subperiosteal abscess, further interfering with the vascular supply.
9. If the vascular supply remains sufficient to maintain life of the bone tissue, new bone is created and bone healing occurs.
10. If vascular supply is diminished below that necessary to maintain life of bone tissue:
    a. Bone dies and becomes inert. Small pieces of dead bone may be completely destroyed by granulation tissue from contiguous living tissue.
    b. Large pieces of dead bone cannot be completely destroyed.
    c. Central residual remains as a sequestrum composed of cancellous or cortical bone or combination.
    d. New bone is laid down beneath the elevated periosteum and tends to form an encasement (involucrum) around the sequestrum.
    e. Numerous channels through which pus may escape from the inside puncture the involucrum.
    f. Pockets of infection are walled off in which organisms can lie dormant for long periods.
    g. Chronic sinuses may form that eventually reach the surface and drain.
    h. Drainage continues until infection quiets once more.

Channels become plugged with granulations and remain closed until the pressure of the pus builds up and causes the sinuses to reopen or reach the surface through new channels (chronic osteomyelitis).

11. Complete healing takes place only when all the dead bone has been destroyed, discharged, or excised.

Clinical Manifestations

1. Localized pain (becomes progressive with severity)
2. Swelling, erythema, warmth
3. Fever
4. History of local injury/trauma (found in about 50% of children)
5. Pre-existing bacterial infection (skin, upper respiratory tract)
6. Tenderness on palpation
7. Limitation in range of motion
8. Malaise, irritability
9. Generalized signs of sepsis

Diagnostic Evaluation

1. Blood cultures should be obtained before initiation of antibiotic therapy to help make definitive diagnosis.
2. Needle aspiration of bone may be done if necessary to identify the causative agent.
   a. Gram stain, culture and sensitivity of specimen once obtained
   b. Negative aspirate does not always rule out infection
3. Complete blood count—marked leukocytosis, low hemoglobin.
4. Erythrocyte sedimentation rate (ESR)—elevated.
5. X-ray may be negative in early stages.
   a. Rules out fracture
   b. Will eventually demonstrate changes
6. Bone scan to rule out soft tissue involvement is sometimes indicated.
7. MRI to differentiate soft tissue from bone marrow involvement.

Management

1. Intravenous antibiotics.
   a. Broad-spectrum antibiotics until organism sensitivity obtained
   b. Intravenous antibiotics for a minimum of 3 to 4 weeks
   c. Usually requires placement of a central intermittent infusion catheter (eg, midline or PICC line)
   d. Additional 4 to 8 weeks of oral antibiotics at completion of IV therapy is recommended (depending on sedimentation rate)
2. If abscessed, surgical incision and drainage are performed.
3. Bed rest.

Complications

1. Chronic osteomyelitis
2. Pathologic fracture
3. Joint destruction (contracture)
4. Skeletal deformities, limb length discrepancy
5. Abscess formation, septic arthritis
6. Systemic infection—life threatening if unrecognized and untreated

Nursing Assessment

1. Obtain a detailed history, including recent infections (ear, tonsils, chest, urinary tract), trauma, and onset of symptoms.
2. Obtain history of current or recent antibiotic therapy to help determine resistance of organism.
3. Perform physical assessment for signs of primary infection as well as osteomyelitis.
4. Assess coping mechanisms and resources of family.

Nursing Diagnoses

- Pain related to swelling, hyperthermia and infectious process of bone
- Hyperthermia related to inflammatory response secondary to osteomyelitis
- Impaired Physical Mobility related to pain in affected limb secondary to inflammatory response and/or surgical treatment
- Ineffective Management of Therapeutic Regimen related to insufficient knowledge of pharmacologic therapy

Nursing Interventions

Maintaining Comfort

1. Assess pain characteristics and use age-appropriate pain-measurement tools.
2. Maintain rest and immobilization of affected part.
3. Administer analgesics as indicated and monitor effectiveness of analgesics.

Reducing Temperature

1. Assess temperature every 4 hours.
2. Increase fluid intake to prevent dehydration.
3. Administer antipyretics as indicated.

Preventing Complications of Immobility

1. Instruct on allowable activities—generally no weight bearing on affected limb and bed rest during acute phase.
2. Encourage usage and exercise of unaffected limbs and joints through play.
3. Provide ambulation aid if indicated (eg, crutches).

Promoting Compliance With Therapeutic Regimen

1. Instruct patient and family on need for maintaining serum levels of antibiotics after discharge, even after signs and symptoms improve.
2. Initiate appropriate home care referrals for reinforcement and monitoring of IV therapy and wound care.
3. Encourage evaluation of response to treatment through periodic laboratory tests (ESR, serum drug levels) and follow-up.
4. Teach family about proper maintenance and care of vascular access device (eg, midline, PICC line).

Community and Home Care Considerations

Many visits may be necessary to ensure parents are comfortable with medication administration through a venous access device and maintenance of the device. Parents will also need extra coaching about wound care.

1. Teach parents and child (if appropriate) about signs and symptoms of an infection.
2. Teach parents how to prepare the antibiotic for administration.
3. Teach parents how to administer the IV antibiotic.
4. Teach parents about the antibiotic being administered.
5. Teach parents and child about maintenance of the vascular access device.
6. Teach parents and child how to care for the child's wound.
7. Assess parents' coping ability.
8. Reinforce teaching to parents on a frequent basis. Employ the use of return demonstrations to assess parental ability to administer IV antibiotics and/or care for their child's wound.
9. Provide the family with the number of a contact nurse to whom they can turn for concerns and/or advice after hours.

Family Education and Health Maintenance

1. Instruct in signs and symptoms of recurrent or chronic infection.
2. Stress the importance of compliance with treatment.
3. Encourage early medical intervention for subsequent infections.

Outcome-Based Evaluation

- Reports reduced pain or no pain
- Afebrile
- Exercising unaffected limbs
- Surgical wounds without signs of infection
- Child and parents demonstrate proper techniques for IV therapy and/or dressing care

■ Developmental Dysplasia of the Hip

Previously referred to as congenital dislocation of the hip, this term is now the accepted means of describing those conditions involving the abnormal development of the proximal femur and/or acetabulum. The variability in presentation has spawned the need for a more accurate way of referring to this group of disorders. It may be associated with other congenital anomalies.

Incidence is 1.5 in 1000 live births, but is geographically variable. Bilateral involvement occurs in more than 50% of cases, and the left hip is more frequently involved than the right hip. Females are afflicted eight times more often than males.

Pathophysiology and Etiology

1. Caused by genetic and environmental factors.
2. Acetabulum tends to be shallow and extremely oblique.
3. Head of the femur tends to be smaller than normal.
4. Ossification centers are delayed in appearance.
5. Degrees of developmental hip dysplasia include:
   a. Dysplasia—shallow acetabulum, acetabular roof slants upward.
   b. Subluxation—acetabular surface of the femoral head is in contact with shallow dysplastic acetabular surface, but the head slides laterally and superiorly.
   c. Dislocation—articular cartilage of completely displaced femoral head does not contact acetabular articular cartilage.

Clinical Manifestations

Physical findings change as the child ages; the presence of one or more of the following should be noted:

1. Thigh asymmetry or thigh gluteal folds (present in 10% or normal infants)
2. Limitation in abduction of the hip
3. Positive Barlow's test and positive Ortolani's test (Figure 54-2)
4. Shortening of affected femur
5. Abnormal gait patterns
6. Trendelenburg's sign—downward tilt of pelvis on affected side
7. Pain in older children

Diagnostic Evaluation

1. X-rays— cartilaginous femoral head is difficult to visualize in the newborn. As the child ages, the ossification center can be better viewed and the efficiency of this exam increases, usually after 6 months of age. It can be useful in ruling out other pelvic, spinal, and femoral anomalies.
2. Ultrasound examination—yields a high degree of accuracy in diagnosing with a skilled technician.
3. CT—helpful after operative intervention such as reduction and casting, because plain x-rays have difficulty penetrating the casting material and visualizing the femoral head.
4. Arthrograms—can be useful to outline the cartilaginous portions of the acetabulum and femoral head.
5. MRI—is costly, often requires the child to be sedated, and provides little in the way of additional information.

Management

To restore as closely as possible the anatomic alignment of the hip. Methodology depends on the age of the child at presentation.

Birth to Age 6 Months

1. Subluxable hips:
   a. Observe for 3 weeks.
   b. If persistent, treat in Pavlik harness (Figure 54-3).
2. Dislocated or dislocatable hips:
   a. Pavlik harness—frequent follow-up is needed to check position, make strap adjustments, and determine hip stability.

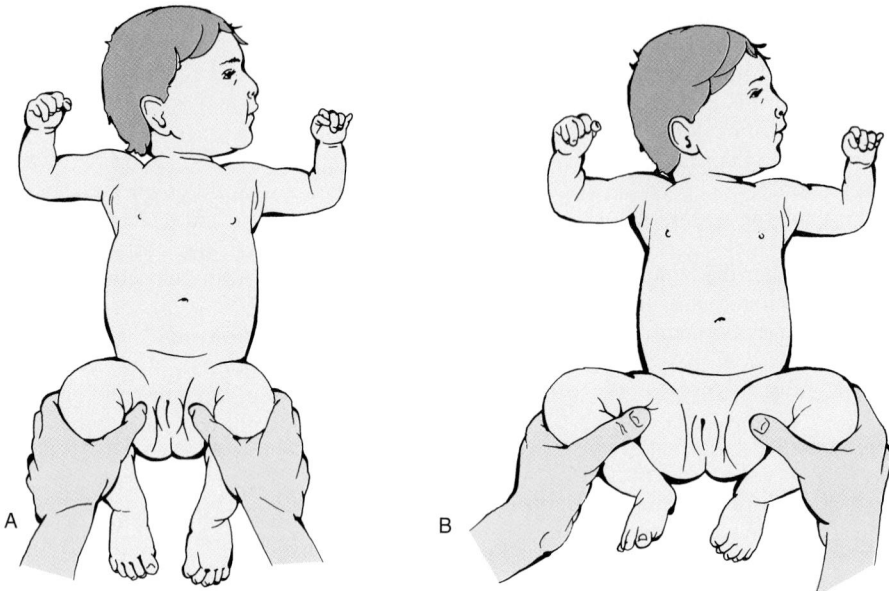

FIGURE 54-2   Assessing for Barlow's and Ortalani's signs. Place the child supine on a firm surface. Be gentle, not forceful. (**A**) Barlow's test—used to detect hip instability. The located hip is subluxed or dislocated during the maneuver. The examiner's fingers are placed over the child's greater trochanters. Holding the hips and knees at 90 degrees of flexion, a backward pressure is applied while adducting the hips. The femoral head is felt slipping out of the acetabulum posterolaterally when the test is positive. (**B**) Ortolani's sign—present when the hip is dislocated. The maneuver relocates the femoral head. With the examiner's fingers on the child's greater trochanters, the hips and knees are flexed to 90 degrees. The hips are then abducted while applying upward pressure over the greater trochanter. A positive sign is detected when a "clunk" is felt as the femoral head reenters the acetabulum.

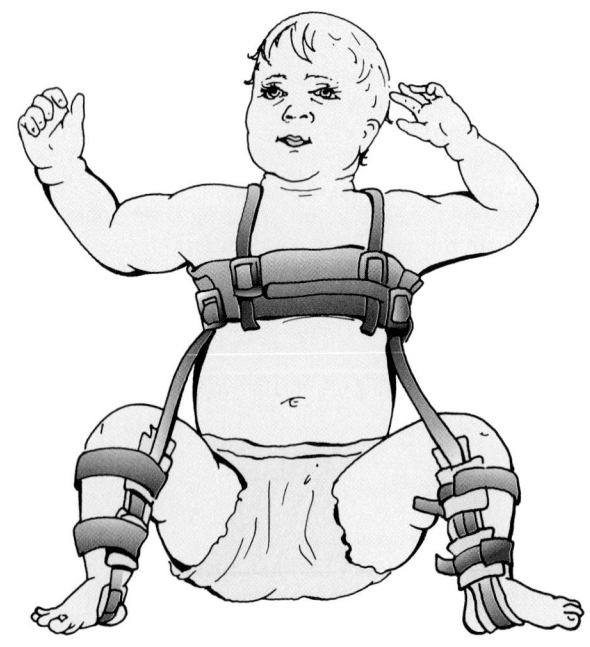

FIGURE 54-3   Pavlik harness.

  b. Ultrasound to determine if hip was reduced.
  c. Infant will wear harness on a full-time basis until clinical and radiographic examinations are normal.

Age 6 Months to 18 Months

1. Hip subluxation and dislocation in children between 6 and 9 months:
   a. Pavlik harness—followed on a frequent basis.
   b. Treatment in the Pavlik harness may continue for 4 months or until the child is able to stand in the harness.
   c. Once standing, the harness is exchanged for an abduction brace until the hip is normal.
   d. Traction and closed reduction if harness treatment is unsuccessful.
2. Hip subluxation and dislocation in children 9 to 18 months.
3. Follow-up continues until age of skeletal maturity.

Age 18 Months to 36 Months

1. Dislocated hip:
   a. Traction and closed reduction (under general anesthesia)
   b. Application of hip spica cast for 3 months to maintain the reduction

2. Failure of closed reduction and casting:
   a. Open reduction and innominate osteotomy
   b. Hip spica cast application
   c. Abduction bracing
3. Follow-up continues until age of skeletal maturity.

3 Years of Age and Older
1. Subluxation or dislocation of hip—treated surgically by open reduction.
2. Follow-up continues until age of skeletal maturity.

Adolescents
1. Acetabular dysplasia:
   a. Use of NSAIDS and ambulation device (eg, crutches, cane) to limit weight bearing on the affected limb.
   b. Usually need for surgical correction.

Complications
1. Avascular necrosis
2. Redislocation or subluxation
3. Loss of range of motion
4. Leg length discrepancy
5. Early osteoarthritis
6. Recurrent dislocation or unstable hip
7. Femoral nerve palsy
8. Iatrogenic hip dislocation

Nursing Assessment
1. Obtain a family history, including hip pathology.
2. Obtain an obstetric history for presence of risk factors such as breech presentation and first-born status.
3. Perform a physical assessment for range of motion, appearance of Trendelenburg's sign, Barlow's test, Ortolani's sign, and asymmetric thigh folds.
4. Assess family's response to the problem.

Nursing Diagnoses
- Risk for Altered Parenting related to ineffective adaptation to stressors associated with a diagnosis of DDH and the prescribed therapeutic regimen
- Risk for Impaired Skin Integrity related to perineal soiling secondary to confinement in an orthopedic device (eg, Pavlik harness, hip spica cast)
- Impaired Physical Mobility related to external device (eg, hip spica cast)

Nursing Interventions
Promoting Effective Parenting
1. Explain the condition and treatment in terms the family can understand.
2. Encourage holding the child with abduction of the hips while handling and avoiding swaddling as an infant.
3. Reassure parents that effective outcome depends on early intervention and compliance.
4. Demonstrate application of Pavlik harness and ensure that parents know and feel comfortable in applying it.
5. Stress importance of keeping follow-up appointments and strict compliance with prescribed treatment.

6. Provide parents with the name and number of a contact person if they have concerns about their child's care.

Maintaining Skin Integrity
See page 1572.

Preventing Complications of Immobility
1. Stimulate the child with games and activities to exercise upper body and feet as able.
2. Turn the child frequently and encourage ambulation as able. Support the head and legs to reposition.
3. Encourage deep-breathing exercises at intervals to prevent atelectasis and hypostatic pneumonia. Children can blow bubbles, party favors, and cotton balls across the table as appropriate.
4. Encourage fluids and a high-fiber diet to prevent constipation.

Community and Home Care Considerations
1. An initial home care visit may be required to assess the child in a Pavlik harness.
2. For children in a hip spica cast, see the "Community and Home Care Considerations" section under Fractures, page 1572.
3. Carefully assess parental role development and educate them on normal care of infant as well as special care needed by their child, such as safety measures and positioning.

Family Education and Health Maintenance
1. If the child is to be treated with an abduction splint, explain its purpose and demonstrate its application and removal to the parents.
   a. Instruct the parents as to if and when the device can be removed.
   b. Instruct the parents to check fit of abduction splint at every diaper change.
   c. Allow the parents to demonstrate their ability to properly place the device on the child.
   d. Follow this with written instructions whenever possible.
2. Instruct on skin care and reporting any skin breakdown or disruption of the cast, brace, or splint.
3. Encourage regular follow-up evaluations and regular health maintenance visits.

Outcome-Based Evaluation
- Parents holding child and participating in care (eg, applying Pavlik harness)
- No perineal skin breakdown
- Lungs clear with good aeration bilaterally

▨ Congenital Clubfoot (Talipes Equinovarus)

Clubfoot is a congenital anomaly characterized by a three-part deformity of the foot, consisting of inversion of the heel (varus), adduction and supination of the forefoot, and ankle equinus. Other congenital disorders of the foot and ankle occur but are less common. Incidence of clubfoot is 1 to 3 in 1000 live births. It is bilateral in 50% of afflicted children and occurs in boys twice as often and girls.

Pathophysiology and Etiology
1. Foot is plantar flexed at the ankle and subtalar joints.
2. Hind foot is inverted.
3. Midfoot and forefoot are adducted and inverted.
4. Contractures of the soft tissues maintain the malalignments.
5. Exact etiology is unknown. Suggested contributing factors include:
   a. Intrauterine positioning
   b. Primary arrest in fetal development
   c. Familial tendency (about 10% of cases)
   d. Neuromuscular defect

Clinical Manifestations
1. Deformity usually is obvious at birth with varying degrees of rigidity and ability to correct position.
2. Deformity becomes fixed if untreated, which can lead to:
   a. Child bearing weight on lateral border of foot.
   b. Awkward gait.
   c. Callosities and bursae may develop over the lateral side of the foot.

Diagnostic Evaluation
1. Clinical presentation and physical examination.
2. X-rays have been used to determine bony anatomy and assess treatment efficiency.

Management
Should begin as soon after birth as possible, with the goal to establish a functional, pain-free foot that can be fit with standard footwear.
Initial—Nonoperative
1. Serial manipulation followed by immobilization in a plaster cast, taping, or strapping started at the time of diagnosis.
2. Done daily (parents taught by physiotherapist—can be done at home).
3. After the initial period (age 2 to 6 months), evaluation will determine the need to continue with manipulation and casting, proceeding to corrective shoes with or without a Dennis-Browne bar or the more recent Wheaton brace or Bebax shoe.
Surgical Treatment
1. Usually performed at 4 to 9 months of age so that the child is free of postoperative immobilization before beginning walking.
2. The child who presents late or has a recurrent or residual deformity may require an aggressive surgical procedure to stabilize the bony structures and balance the muscle and tendons by a combination of fusions, releases, lengthenings, and transfers.

3. Postoperative routines usually include a period of cast immobilization of up to 12 weeks, followed by a brace (ankle-foot orthosis) or corrective shoe for a period of 2 to 4 years.

Complications
1. "Rocker bottom" deformity from excessive dorsiflexion and a "breaking through" the midtarsal bones
2. Disturbances in epiphyseal plates from over-aggressive manipulation
3. Recurrent or residual deformity

Nursing Assessment
1. Obtain a family history of foot deformities.
2. Obtain an obstetric history for risk factors.
3. Perform a physical assessment for presence of other anomalies and classic foot position and range of motion. If late presentation, perform a thorough neurologic exam to rule out causative factors.
4. Assess family coping and resources available for lengthy treatment.

Nursing Diagnoses
• Risk for Altered Parenting related to ineffective adaptation to stressors associated with a diagnosis of clubfoot and the therapeutic regimen
• Risk for Impaired Skin Integrity related to serial casting
• Altered Tissue Perfusion (Peripheral) related to postoperative edema and/or casting
• Pain related to tissue and muscle trauma secondary to surgery

Nursing Interventions
Promoting Effective Parenting
1. Provide an accurate description of deformity and the importance of treatment in terms the parents can understand.
2. Provide opportunity for parents to verbalize questions and concerns.
3. Reinforce causative factors and the fact that it was not anyone's fault.
4. Encourage parents to hold and play with child and participate in care.
5. Provide parents with a contact family that has been through the treatment process for support.
Protecting Skin Integrity
1. Assess fit of cast, splint, orthotic device, or special shoes. Teach parents that due to rapid growth rate of infant, device may need to be replaced to prevent skin breakdown.
2. Assess and teach assessment of excessive pressure on skin—redness, excoriation, foul odor from underneath cast, or pain.
Preserving Tissue Perfusion
1. Perform frequent neurovascular assessments after surgery, including color, warmth, sensation, capillary refill, pulses, and presence of pain.

2. Elevate the extremity to prevent edema.
3. Protect and assess foot for injury.

Relieving Pain

1. Assess for signs of discomfort such as irritability, crying, poor feeding and sleeping, tachycardia, and increased blood pressure.
2. Administer analgesics regularly for 24 to 48 hours after surgery.
3. Provide comfort measures such as soft music, pacifier, teething ring, rocking and cuddling with parent.
4. Encourage parents to administer analgesics after discharge from hospital (when needed). Discuss dosage and administration and dispel misconceptions about addiction.

Family Education and Health Maintenance

1. Teach parents to remove cast at home before weekly manipulation and recasting by soaking in water and vinegar mixture to avoid anxiety and possible abrasions from using cast saw.
2. Teach the parents when orthotic devices may be removed—usually for bathing. Stress that devices must be worn as prescribed.
3. Advise parents that infant's sleep may be disturbed initially due to wearing brace at night and that he or she may be irritable while awake due to fatigue.
4. Instruct parents on providing a safe environment for the ambulatory child.
5. Discuss the importance of long-term and frequent follow-up, and assist parents with special needs such as transportation, flexible appointment times, and financing orthotic equipment.
6. Teach parents to check color, warmth, capillary refill, movement of toes, and position of cast (ensure cast does not slip to hide toes).

Outcome-Based Evaluation

- Parents holding infant, participating in care
- No signs of skin breakdown
- Neurovascular status of affected foot intact
- Resting and feeding well

■ Legg-Calvé-Perthes Disease

Legg-Calvé-Perthes disease is a self-limiting condition of the proximal femur characterized by avascular necrosis of the femoral head. It occurs most frequently in children between the ages of 3 to 11 years. Ratio of occurrence in males to females is 5 : 1, and it is frequently found in Caucasians and Asians. It is bilateral in 15% of cases.

Pathophysiology and Etiology

1. Etiology is unknown.
2. Interruption of the vascular supply to the femoral head leads to the death of bone. Deformity can occur with loss of the spherical nature of the femoral head during the disease process. The disease progresses through identifiable stages.

Stage I (Avascularity)

1. Spontaneous interruption of the blood supply to the upper femoral epiphysis.
2. Bone-forming cells in the epiphysis die and bone ceases to grow.
3. Slight widening of the joint space.
4. Swelling of the soft tissues around the hip.

Stage II (Revascularization)

1. Growth of new vessels supplies the area of necrosis; bone resorption and deposition take place.
2. The new bone lacks strength, and pathologic fractures may occur.
3. Abnormal forces on the weakened epiphysis may produce progressive deformity.

Stage III (Reossification)

1. The head of the femur gradually reforms.
2. Nucleus of the epiphysis breaks up into a number of fragments with cystlike spaces between them.
3. New bone starts to develop at the medial and lateral edges of the epiphysis, which becomes widened.
4. Dead bone is removed and is replaced with new bone, which gradually spreads to heal the lesion.

Stage IV (Postrecovery)

1. Without treatment:
   a. Head of the femur flattens and becomes mushroom shaped.
   b. Incongruity between the head of the femur and the acetabulum persists and worsens.
2. With treatment:
   a. Head of femur remains near spherical.
   b. Acetabulum appears normal.
   c. Width of the neck of the femur is normal.

Clinical Manifestations

1. Synovitis causing limp and pain in the hip (may be intermittent initially)
2. Referred pain to knee, inner thigh, and groin
3. Limited abduction and internal rotation of the hip
4. Mild to moderate muscle spasm

Diagnostic Evaluation

1. Early x-ray findings may be normal.
2. X-ray findings are related to the stage of the disease process.
3. MRI has been useful in demonstrating the pathologic process.
4. Bone scans can detect avascular state early.
5. Arthrograms may be useful in evaluating sphericity of the femoral head.

Management

Goal: to maintain as normal a shape to the femoral head as possible.

1. Restore motion—initial relief of synovitis, muscle spasm, and pain in the joint:
   a. Salicylates/anti-inflamatory medications
   b. Limitation of activities, bed rest with or without skin traction

2. Prevent deformity—primarily of femoral head by containing it within the acetabulum:
   a. Non-weight-bearing abduction cast or brace (Petrie casts)
   b. Weight-bearing abduction brace (Scottish Rite orthosis)
   c. Surgical intervention by means of an osteotomy of the proximal femur or acetabulum (Salter innominate) or a combination of these

Complications
1. Early degenerative joint disease
2. Residual deformity
3. Loss of motion and/or function of involved hip
4. Persistent pain and gait disturbance

Nursing Assessment
1. Obtain a detailed history, including onset of symptoms and characteristics of pain.
2. Perform a physical assessment to include evaluation of gait, range of motion, and presence of any contractures.

Nursing Diagnoses
- Alteration in Comfort related to pain secondary to disease process
- Impaired Physical Mobility related to external immobilization device (eg, cast)
- Self-Care Deficit related to pain and immobilization device
- Ineffective Management of Therapeutic Regimen related to insufficient knowledge of condition and activity restrictions

Nursing Interventions
Promoting Comfort
1. Monitor and assess pain level using age-appropriate pain measurement tool.
2. Instruct child and parents as to which activities can be continued and which to avoid (eg, contact sports, high-impact running).
3. Administer analgesics as indicated and monitor effectiveness.

Promoting Mobility
1. Encourage activities to maintain range of motion (eg, swimming, bicycle riding).
2. Encourage parents to allow activities that involve unaffected body parts within restriction guidelines.
3. Provide equipment to assist with mobility (eg, wheelchair, walker).

Promoting Participation in Self-Care
1. Assess parents' ability to care for child at home. Provide community-based referral to assist if indicated.
2. Teach parents and siblings to assist only as needed.
3. Encourage child to identify aspects of care that he or she can perform.
4. Evaluate ability of child to participate in self-care activities.

5. Provide an opportunity for child to express fears and emotions. Offer support when needed.

Promoting Compliance With Treatment
1. Explain the disease process to parents and child, emphasizing compliance with treatment.
2. Allow child to voice concerns and ask questions about his or her treatment.
3. Encourage attendance at regular follow-up appointments.

Family Education and Health Maintenance
1. Teach proper care of casts/braces and the need to remain compliant with usage.
2. Stress need to remain active within restrictions and to promote positive body image.
3. Reinforce to child that he or she is only temporarily restricted. Stress remaining positive aspects of activity.

Outcome-Based Evaluation
- Child free from pain
- Child participating in self-care
- Parents understand disease process and assist child as needed
- Range of motion and function maintained

◼ Structural Scoliosis

Scoliosis is lateral curvature of the spine. There are many different types of scoliosis that vary by age of onset and structure of the spine.

Pathophysiology and Etiology
1. Idiopathic scoliosis—exact etiology is unknown. Classified into three groups (based on age at time of diagnosis):
   a. Infantile—presentation before 3 years of age
   b. Juvenile—presentation between the ages of 3 and 10 years
   c. Adolescent—presentation after age 10
      (i) Partially familial
      (ii) 25 per 1000 in adolescents with curve less than 10 degrees (Cobb angle)
      (iii) Curves greater than 10 degrees—prevalence decreases
      (iv) Progressive curves are more prevalent in females than males (7:1 females to males for curves greater than 25 degrees)
      (v) Overall incidence less than 1%
2. Congenital scoliosis—exact etiology unknown; represented as malformation of one or more vertebral bodies that results in asymmetric growth.
   a. Type I—failure of vertebral body formation (eg, isolated hemivertebra, wedged vertebra, multiple wedged vertebrae, multiple hemivertebrae).
   b. Type II—failure of segmentation (eg, unilateral unsegmented bar, bilateral block vertebra).
   c. Often associated with other congenital anomalies (eg, Klippel-Feil syndrome, 25%; genitourinary tract abnormalities, 30%; cardiac abnormalities, 12%;

cervical spine anomalies, 15%; and intraspinal anomalies, 15%).

3. Neuromuscular scoliosis—child has a definite neuromuscular condition that directly contributes to the deformity.
   a. Most severe in non-ambulatory patients
   b. Occurs in children with cerebral palsy, Duchenne and Becker muscular dystrophy, spina bifida, syringomyelia, spinocerebellar degeneration, Charcot-Marie-Tooth syndrome)

4. Additional but less common causes of scoliosis are osteopathic conditions such as fractures, bone disease, arthritic conditions, and infections.

5. Miscellaneous factors that can cause scoliosis include spinal irradiation, endocrine disorders, post-thoracotomy, and nerve root irritation.

6. In all types of scoliosis, the vetebral column develops lateral curvature.
   a. The vertebrae rotate to the convex side of the curve, which rotates the spinous processes toward the concavity.
   b. Vertebrae become wedge shaped.
   c. Disk shape is altered, as are the neural canal and posterior arch of the vertebral body.

7. As the deformity progresses, changes in the thoracic cage increase, with eventual respiratory and cardiovascular compromise.
   a. Changes in the thoracic cage, ribs, and sternum lead to further characteristic deformities such as the "rib hump."
   b. Neurologic compromise in idiopathic scoliosis is rare.

Clinical Manifestations

1. Physical characteristics:
   a. Poor posture
   b. Increased or decreased thoracic kyphosis or lumbar lordosis
   c. Leg length discrepancy
   d. Shoulder asymmetry
   e. Scapular prominence
   f. Truncal imbalance (relationship of trunk over pelvis)
   g. Lump (rib hump) on back
   h. Uneven waistline
   i. Uneven breast size

2. Visualization of deformity

3. Back pain may be present but is not a routine finding in idiopathic scoliosis. The adolescent who presents with back pain and scoliosis warrants close consideration to rule out a distinct pathologic condition such as a tumor, disk disease, or intraspinal anomalies.

Diagnostic Evaluation

1. Adams forward bending test
2. Thorough neurologic evaluation
3. X-rays of the spine in the upright position, preferably on one long (36-inch) cassette—show characteristic curvature

4. MRI, myelograms, tomograms, CT with or without three-dimensional reconstruction may be indicated for those children with severe curvatures who have a known or suspected spinal column anomaly before management decisions are made.

5. Pulmonary function tests for compromised respiratory status.

6. Clinical photographs to assist with documenting the appearance of the spine over time. (Note: Consent for photographs must be obtained from the child's legal guardian.)

7. Workup for associated renal abnormalities with a congenital scoliosis due to a high correlation between the two.

Management

Goal: to stop progression of the existing curve with non-operative management. When this fails, the goal of operative management should be to correct the scoliosis as much as possible and stabilize the spine by fusion to prevent further progression.

Medical Management

1. Observation—periodic physical and radiographic examinations to detect curve progression.
   a. Child is not skeletally mature
   b. Curves less than 25 degrees

2. Brace management—goal is to prevent progression of the curve.
   a. Requires faithful compliance on the part of the child for success.
   b. Some curves progress despite brace wear.
   c. Recommended wearing time is 23 hours per day.
   d. Bracing is for skeletally immature children with curves that are about 25 to 40 degrees.

3. Types of braces include:
   a. Boston orthosis for low thoracic and thoracolumbar curves. This is an underarm molded orthosis.
   b. Milwaukee brace for thoracic or double major curves. Standard brace has neck ring with chin rest.
   c. Charleston bending brace has been tried for night-time usage in selected patients. Results have been positive in some centers, but widespread acceptance has not occurred.

4. Exercise therapy has been promoted to help maintain flexibility in the spine and prevent muscle atrophy during prolonged bracing.

Surgical Correction

1. Stabilization of the spinal column is the goal. This is usually accomplished with a spinal fusion and one of several methods of instrumentation.

2. Indications for surgical correction vary, but generally accepted principles are:
   a. Progression of the curve over a short period in a curve greater than 45 degrees despite bracing
   b. Skeletal immaturity
   c. Bracing is not possible
   d. Cosmesis

3. Preoperative traction or casting may be used to help gain correction and increase flexibility.
4. Postoperative protection of the fusion mass by means of a cast may be required.
5. Surgical approach and techniques may be anterior or posterior with various instrumentation methods such as:
   a. Harrington instrumentation and posterior spinal fusion
   b. Multiple-level (segmental fusion) systems such as the Texas Scottish Rite Hospital (TSRH) system or the Cotrel-Dubousset system (Figure 54-4)
   c. Luque technique, which includes dual rods with sublaminar wire segmental fixation (usually reserved for those children with existing neurologic compromise due to increased risk of neurologic damage with the use of sublaminar wires)
   d. Anterior procedures, which include staple and cable or rod systems such as the Dwyer or anterior TSRH

Nursing Assessment

1. Assess respiratory, cardiovascular, and neurologic systems.
2. Perform a physical exam in the upright and forward-bending positions and observe physical characteristics such as leg lengths, gait, and overall development.

Nursing Diagnoses

- Body Image Disturbance related to negative feelings about spinal deformity and appearance in brace
- Risk for Impaired Skin Integrity related to mechanical irritation of brace

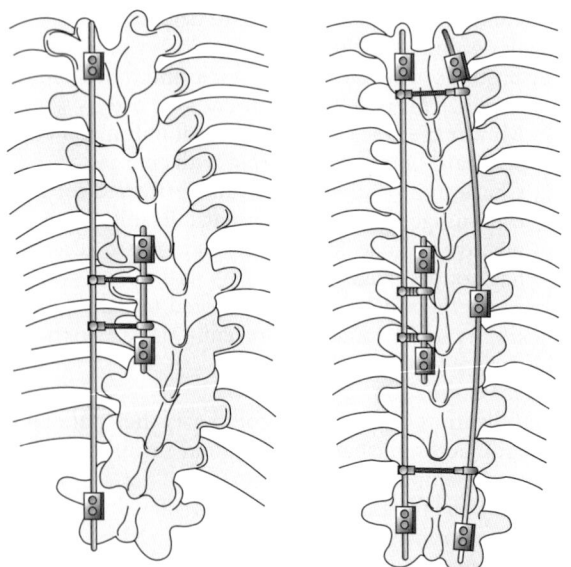

FIGURE 54-4 Cotrel-Dubousset rods to correct scoliosis. A short distraction rod is linked to a longer one to correct the major curve.

- Risk for Injury related to postoperative complications
- Ineffective Management of Therapeutic Regimen (Family) related to chronicity and complexity of treatment regimen

Nursing Interventions

Promoting Positive Body Image

1. Encourage child to express feelings and concerns about body image.
2. Encourage child to express concerns about wearing a brace.
3. Discuss options for brace wearing (eg, wear baggy clothes).
4. Encourage child to discuss scoliosis with his or her peers, including disease process and treatment.
5. Provide a peer support person when possible so the child can associate positive outcomes and expressions from others.

Preserving Skin Integrity

1. Assess skin integrity and fit of brace at every follow-up appointment.
2. Assess for proper fit of brace/cast.
3. Teach proper skin care to patient and/or family.
4. Instruct patient to wear cotton shirt under brace to avoid rubbing.

Preventing Postoperative Complications

1. Prepare the patient for surgery by teaching deep breathing exercises, explaining positioning, and explaining patient-controlled analgesia or another method of pain control.
2. Following surgery, keep patient flat and log roll only to prevent any flexion of back.
3. Perform frequent neurovascular assessments and monitor vital signs frequently.
4. Monitor drainage or bleeding from incision site.
5. Maintain indwelling catheter for first couple of days, until patient is out of bed. Monitor intake and output.
6. Assist patient with ambulation slowly, when allowed, to avoid orthostatic hypotension from position change.

Promoting Compliance With Treatment

1. Explain scoliosis and the treatment options to the child in language she or he can understand.
2. Explain the importance of complying with treatment and possible outcomes with noncompliance.
3. Encourage the child and family to discuss concerns and questions they may have about scoliosis and the prescribed treatment.
4. Assist with social service referral for financial, transportation, and other needs.

Family Education and Health Maintenance

1. Provide adequate information on condition and treatment.

2. Instruct to examine brace daily for signs of loosening or breakage. Instruct to contact orthotist when repairs are needed.
3. Teach family to inspect skin for any irritation under brace.
4. Suggest to family to discuss child's treatment with teachers and school officials, so child can receive tutoring or home schooling in order to keep up with grade requirements if out for surgery.

Outcome-Based Evaluation
- Child making positive comments about self
- Skin without signs of breakdown
- Wearing brace as prescribed
- Neurovascular status intact; no bleeding noted

■ Slipped Capital Femoral Epiphysis

Slipped capital femoral epiphysis (SCFE), also known as coxa vara, is the most common hip disorder in adolescents. It is characterized by a slipping of the epiphysis and metaphysis due to weakening of the perichondral ring of the physis. The epiphysis slips downward and backward. Incidence is 2 to 3 per 100,000, and it is three times more common in boys than girls.

Pathophysiology and Etiology
1. Skeletally immature and obese adolescents are at greatest risk.
2. Left hip is most frequently affected—30% of adolescents will also have a slip in the opposite hip.
3. Exact etiology is unknown; risk factors include:
   a. Mechanical stress
   b. Trauma
   c. Endocrine and immunologic abnormalities
   d. Body build (eg, obesity, hypogenitalism, Froelich syndrome)
4. Perichondral ring of the physis weakens.
5. Epiphysis and metaphysis displace from each other.
6. The epiphysis slips downward and backward.
7. Classified by duration of symptoms:
   a. Acute—sudden onset; symptoms for less than 3 weeks
   b. Chronic—symptoms lasting more than 3 weeks
8. Eighty-five percent of children have stable slips.

Clinical Manifestations
1. Pain in groin, medial thigh, or knee
2. Decreased range of motion in affected hip
3. Sudden onset of pain (acute SCFE)
4. Decreased range of motion in hip—inability to bear weight (acute SCFE)
5. Limp when walking (usually found with chronic cases)
6. Intermittent pain
7. Trendelenburg gait
8. External rotation of the lower limb

Diagnostic Evaluation
1. X-rays confirm diagnosis—AP and frog leg lateral views.
2. Bone scan—rules out presence of avascular necrosis.
3. CT scan—helps to define extent of slip.

Treatment
1. Goal is to prevent progressive slippage and minimize deformity while avoiding necrosis of cartilage (chondrolysis) and avascular necrosis.
2. Treatment is surgical—percutaneous cannulated screw fixation.
   a. One screw usually used for stable hips
   b. Two screws used for unstable hips
3. External fixation may be used.

Complications
1. Chondrolysis over femoral head resulting in permanent loss of range of motion
2. Avascular necrosis of femoral head

Nursing Assessment
1. Obtain a detailed history, including onset of symptoms and characteristics of pain.
2. Perform a physical assessment and include evaluation of gait and range of motion in hips.

Nursing Diagnoses
- Pain related to disease process
- Impaired Physical Mobility related to disease process
- Diversional Activity Deficit related to activity restriction

Nursing Interventions
Promoting Comfort
1. Monitor and assess pain level using age-appropriate pain-measurement tools.
2. Instruct child and parents as to which activities can be continued and which to avoid (eg, contact sports, high-impact running).
3. Administer analgesics as indicated and monitor effectiveness.

Promoting Mobility
1. Facilitate bed rest or other activity restriction as directed.
2. Provide equipment to assist with mobility (eg, wheelchair, crutches).
3. For home care, encourage parents to allow activities that involve unaffected body parts within restriction guidelines.

Promoting Diversional Activities
1. Be alert to the needs of adolescents to socialize with peers. Encourage liberal phone calls, visitation, and communication with friends and family.
2. Encourage family to provide books, magazines, games, and electronics for the adolescent to use.

3. Provide support for the family and reinforce the importance of following activity restrictions to prevent permanent damage to femur.

Family Education and Health Maintenance

1. Assess parents' ability to care for child at home. Provide community-based referral to assist if indicated.
2. Teach proper use of mobility devices (eg, crutches).
3. Stress need to maintain activity within restrictions and to promote positive body image.
4. Encourage follow-up during active treatment and following surgery. About 30% of children later develop the same condition in the opposite hip, so careful attention is paid to both legs at follow-up.

Outcome-Based Evaluation

- Child reports feeling little or no pain
- Child following activity restriction
- Child maintaining socialization with friends and partaking of hobbies in room

ORTHOPEDIC PROCEDURES

▣ Immobilization: Casts, Braces, and Splints

Casting, bracing, and splinting are all means of immobilizing an injured or diseased body part. The length of time can vary from a few days to several months, depending on the nature of the problem. The management of children who are immobilized differs little from that of the adult; however, age-appropriate changes must be considered. See Procedure Guidelines 54-1.

Complications of Immobilization

1. Peripheral neurovascular compromise
2. Alteration in skin integrity due to pressure or friction
3. Loss of efficient use of affected extremity due to noncompliance

---

PROCEDURE GUIDELINES 54-1	CARE OF THE CHILD WITH A CAST, SPLINT, OR BRACE

EQUIPMENT

Casting materials or immobilization device   Cotton padding material, plastic padding

PROCEDURE

Nursing Action	Rationale
1. Prepare child for procedure by showing materials to be used and describing the procedure in age-appropriate terms.	1. Reduces fear and enlists cooperation.
2. Assess the need for pain medication, sedation, distraction techniques, or restraint and administer as ordered.	2. Manipulation of the affected part may be painful, so pharmacologic preparation is often necessary.
3. Obtain baseline neurovascular assessment, including discoloration or cyanosis, impaired movement, loss of sensation, edema, absent pulses, and pain disproportionate to injury or not relieved by analgesics.	3. Will serve as a baseline to compare subsequent assessments after immobilization.
4. Assist with application of the immobilization device as indicated.	
5. If a cast or plaster splint was applied, help facilitate drying. a. Keep the child and/or affected part still until thoroughly dry. b. Support the curves of the cast with pillows. c. Avoid excessive handling of the cast, and use palms of hands when handling it.	5. About 24–48 hours are required for drying. Dries from the outside inward, so may appear dry but is still moldable with movement or pressure.
6. Assess the skin around edges of the device daily for signs of skin irritation. Teach child or parents to look for and report redness, skin breakdown, localized pain, foul odor that may indicate open wounds under device.	6. Pressure or friction may disrupt skin integrity. May be readily visible or occur under the device and not detected until advanced. Braces can be altered if skin irritation becomes apparent.
7. Try to prevent skin breakdown by padding edges of device and telling child to avoid placing anything inside the device.	
8. Assess neurovascular status frequently after application of device, then daily to detect compromise.	8. Initial swelling from the injury may contribute to vascular insufficiency and/or nerve compression.
9. If child is in hip spica cast, prevent skin breakdown from frequent soiling around perineum. a. Line cast edges around the perineum with a plastic covering to prevent soiling of cast. b. Use a fracture bedpan or urinal to facilitate toileting.	9. Soiled edges of the cast may contribute to skin irritation or begin to disintegrate.

PROCEDURE GUIDELINES 54-1 *CONTINUED*

Nursing Action	Rationale
c. If not toilet trained, use a small diaper or perineal pad tucked under the edges of the cast, covered by a larger diaper, and change diapers as soon as soiled. d. Wash the perineum frequently and dry thoroughly. e. If the cast is synthetic and becomes soiled, clean it with a damp cloth and small amount of detergent.	e. Plaster casts cannot be washed because they absorb water and soften.

CAST REMOVAL

Nursing Action	Rationale
1. Prepare the child for cast removal by describing the sensation (warmth, vibration) and demonstrating the cast cutter by touching it lightly to your palm.	1. Children are frightened by the loud noise and believe that the cast cutter will cut through their skin or extremity.
2. Provide and teach care of skin after cast, brace, or splint removal.	2. An accumulation of dead skin and sebaceous secretions causes the skin to appear brown and flaky.
a. Wash with soapy warm water.	
b. Soak the area daily with warm water to facilitate removal of desquamated skin and secretions.	
c. Advise child to avoid scratching; instead apply lotion or oil to relieve itching.	c. Excessive rubbing may cause trauma.
d. Encourage exercise as prescribed to regain strength and function.	d. May initially be weak and stiff due to lack of use.

■ Traction

Traction is the application of a pulling force to an injured or diseased part of the body or an extremity while a counter traction pulls in the opposite direction. Traction may be used to reduce fractures or dislocations, maintain alignment and correct deformities, decrease muscle spasms and relieve pain, promote rest of a diseased or injured body part, and promote exercise. See Procedure Guidelines 54-2.

Types of Traction

1. Manual—direct pulling on the extremity or body part. Usually used to reduce fractures before treatment or immobilization.
2. Skin—force is applied directly to the skin by means of traction strips or tapes secured by Ace bandages or by means of traction boots. Usually of short-term duration and often used in children in whom small amounts of force are required.
3. Skeletal—force is applied to the body part through fixation directly into or through bone by means of a traction pin or screw. Allows for greater force over longer periods of time or used when skin traction is not feasible, as in soft tissue injury or damage.
4. Continuous or intermittent—traction forces should only be disrupted in accordance with the health care provider's orders.

Complications of Traction

1. Neurovascular compromise to extremity
2. Skin and soft tissue injury
3. Pin or screw tract infection, osteomyelitis (with skeletal traction)

PROCEDURE GUIDELINES 54-2 CARE OF A CHILD IN TRACTION

EQUIPMENT

Traction tapes	Elastic bandages	Spreader blocks, ropes, weights, pulleys
Adhesive tape	Tincture of Benzoin/other adhesive agent	Traction bars, slings

PROCEDURE

Nursing Action	Rationale
1. Explain the procedure to the child and parents.	1. If the traction is to be effective, it is essential that the parents understand and cooperate while the child is in traction.

continued

PROCEDURE GUIDELINES 54-2   **CARE OF A CHILD IN TRACTION** *CONTINUED*

Nursing Action	Rationale
2. Maintain even, constant traction.	2. Traction must be kept constant to achieve the desired results.
a. Do not add or remove weights unless ordered.	
b. Allow the weights to hang free at all times.	
c. Be certain that the ropes are in the wheel grooves of the pulleys.	c. To maintain proper alignment.
d. Keep the weights out of the child's reach.	d. To prevent loosening or undoing of traction knots.
e. Wrap knotted areas of the ropes with adhesive tape to prevent slipping.	
f. Do not elevate the head or foot of the bed without consulting health care provider.	f. May disrupt traction forces.
g. Supervise the child's position so that the purpose of the traction is accomplished.	
3. Check for disturbance of circulation by observing the following:	3. Compare the affected extremity with the unaffected one.
a. Skin color—for redness, pallor, cyanosis	a. May indicate neurovascular compromise.
b. Joint motion restriction	
c. Skin temperature—warmth	
d. Tingling, numbness	
e. Swelling, edema	
4. Provide skin care.	4. Immobilized children readily develop areas of pressure unless meticulous skin care is provided.
a. Pad bony prominences (ankles) with cotton padding before wrapping with elastic bandages.	a. Protects skin from injury.
b. Wash and dry all exposed areas thoroughly.	
c. Massage the child's back and sacral area frequently.	c. Stimulates microcirculation.
d. Inspect the heels, ankles, popliteal space, and top of the foot for signs of pressure from elastic bandages.	d. These are the areas most prone to breakdown.
e. Keep the linen free from wrinkles and food crumbs.	e. This prevents undue pressure areas.
f. Do not allow the traction cords to dig into the child's skin.	f. This is a safety measure.
g. Use a fracture bedpan.	g. This is less awkward and more comfortable for the child.
5. Plan for short periods of muscle exercise every day.	5. Disuse of muscles can result in atrophy, contractures, and deformities.
a. Encourage use of unaffected extremity.	
b. Assist the child to exercise unaffected joints.	
c. Provide for diversionary activities that require movement of unaffected joints and muscles.	
6. Encourage deep breathing exercises.	6. Prevents respiratory complications of prolonged immobilization.
7. Record the intake and output.	7. Prolonged immobilization renders the child prone to urinary retention and renal calculi.
8. Encourage a diet high in fiber and fluids.	8. Helps to prevent constipation and urinary calculi.
9. Provide daily diversion and encourage family visitation.	9. This helps prevent boredom and assists the child to cope with immobilization.
a. Suspend or place favorite toys within easy reach of child.	
b. Provide for continuing education for school-age children.	b. Length of immobilization in traction may be considerable.
c. Encourage activities that will allow for diversion: drawing, coloring, videogames.	c. Activities that can be done while remaining in traction.
d. Immobilized patients should be roomed together if possible.	d. Encourages peer support.
10. If not contraindicated, provide the child with an overhead trapeze.	10. This will assist with movement and self-help.

PROCEDURE GUIDELINES 54-2   *CONTINUED*

Nursing Action	Rationale
11. Document the following: a. Color, temperature, and appearance of the affected limb b. Skin condition c. Body alignment d. Functioning of traction system e. Response of child to treatment.	11. Proper documentation facilities communication between health care providers. c. Proper alignment facilitates proper extremity positioning and maintains proper traction force.
12. Ensure countertraction is provided. a. Foot of bed may need to be raised or placed on "shock blocks" to prevent child from being pulled to foot of bed.	12. The child's body is the usual counterweight. a. Frequently the child's weight is insufficient to maintain proper alignment of the extremity.
13. Do not alter the traction system.	13. Notify the health care provider if adjustment is indicated.
14. Avoid sudden movement or jarring of bed.	14. This can cause pain to the child and disturb alignment.
15. Do not allow weights to hang over the child's bed.	15. This is a safety precaution.

SKIN TRACTION

1. Do not apply over an open wound or over damaged skin.	1. The skin must be intact for the pull of the traction to be effective. Prevents contamination of the wound and further skin breakdown.
2. Prepare the skin with an adhesive agent before application of traction tapes.	2. Adhesive agents allow the traction tapes to adhere better, preventing friction on the skin surface.

SKELETAL TRACTION

1. Treat all entry sites as surgical wounds. a. Cleanse entry site according to institutional policy or guidelines. This should be done at least once per shift. b. Assess the entry site every shift for indications of infection or slippage.	1. Reduces the chance of infection along the pin or screw tract. a. Policies vary. Cleansing the pin site prevents infection, promotes comfort by preventing skin from adhering to pin. b. Notify health care provider if either of these conditions exists.
2. Protect the exposed ends of skeletal traction pins.	2. Protects the health care provider as well as the child from injury.

SPECIFIC TRACTION TYPES: BRYANT'S *(SEE ACCOMPANYING FIGURE)*

Indications
1. To reduce fractures of the femur in children younger than age 2 or weighing less than 30 lb (14 kg).
2. Also used to stabilize the hip joint when casting is not indicated.
3. Preoperatively to attempt reduction of a congenitally dislocated hip in the same age group.

Mechanism of Action
Involves the bilateral vertical extension of the child's legs. The child's weight serves as the countertraction. Skin traction is applied to both limbs to minimize potential trauma and maintain stability and alignment of child.

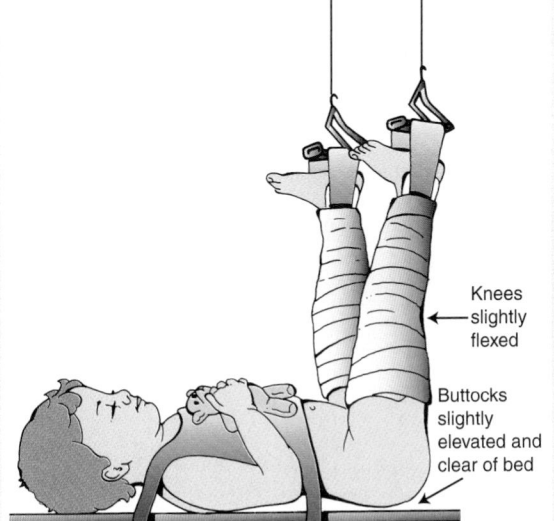

Knees slightly flexed

Buttocks slightly elevated and clear of bed

Bryant's traction.

continued

PROCEDURE GUIDELINES 54-2   **CARE OF A CHILD IN TRACTION** *CONTINUED*

Nursing Action	Rationale

1. Maintain appropriate position:
  a. The legs are extended at right angles to the body.
  b. The hips are elevated slightly from the bed.
  c. The buttocks are elevated slightly from the bed.
  d. The heels and ankles are free from pressure.
2. Check condition and position of elastic bandages every shift. Rewrap as indicated and permitted by the health care provider.
	1. Proper positioning is needed to achieve desired results.
	
	  c. This ensures proper traction pull.
	  d. Prevents skin breakdown.
	2. Elastic bandages can cause compression and compromise circulation. In addition, force across skin surfaces needs to be constant and free from constriction to prevent skin breakdown and ensure adequate traction force.

RUSSEL'S TRACTION *(SEE ACCOMPANYING FIGURE)*

Indications
1. To reduce fractures of the femur or hip.
2. Treatment of specific types of knee injuries or contractures.

Mechanism of Action
Traction force is applied to the limb through application of skin traction. This can be accomplished with traction tapes or a traction boot in older individuals.

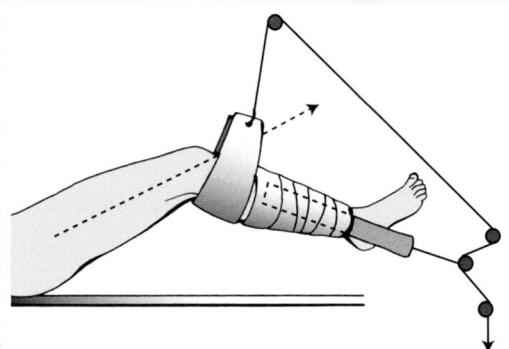

Russel's traction.

1. Application of elastic bandages:
  a. Wrap bandages from ankle to thigh on patients younger than 2 years of age.
  b. Older patients should have bandages wrapped from ankle to the knee.
2. Place foot support against both feet.
3. Keep the heel free from the bed.
 	
4. Carefully assess the popliteal space for signs of pressure from the knee sling.
5. Assess the neurovascular status of limb at least every 2 hours.
6. Make certain that the footplate or spreader block is wide enough.
	1. Proper application of the tapes prevents neurovascular compromise and ensures proper and adequate pull on the extremity.
	
	2. This prevents footdrop.
	3. Prevents pressure sores and ensures continuous traction pull.
	4. Prevents pressure sores, or neurovascular compression.
	5. Early detection can prevent injury to patient.
	
	6. Prevents pressure sores and circulatory compromise.

PROCEDURE GUIDELINES 54-2   *CONTINUED*

Nursing Action	**Rationale**

90-DEGREE–90-DEGREE TRACTION (90–90) *(SEE ACCOMPANYING FIGURE)*

Indications

To reduce fractures of the femur when skin traction is inadequate.

Mechanism of Action

Traction force is applied through skeletal traction pin placed through the distal femur. A short leg cast or foam boot may be used to help suspend the lower leg. Traction force is only applied to femur through pin. Only enough weight should be used to hold lower limb suspended.

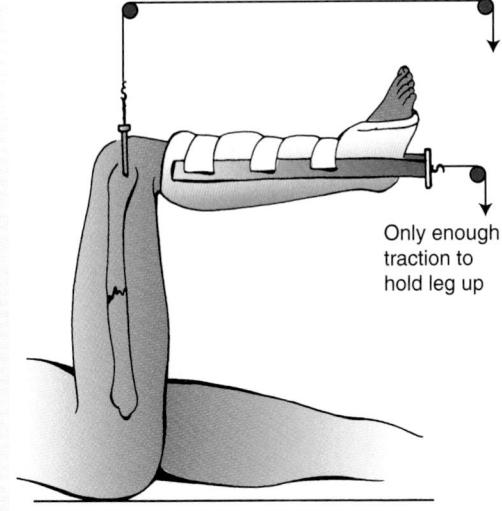

Only enough traction to hold leg up

90–90 traction.

BUCK'S EXTENSION

Indications

Used to correct or prevent knee and hip contractures, to rest the limb, to prevent spasm of injured muscles or joints, or to temporarily immobilize a fractured limb.

Mechanism of Action

The traction force is delivered through a traction boot or skin traction in a straight line.

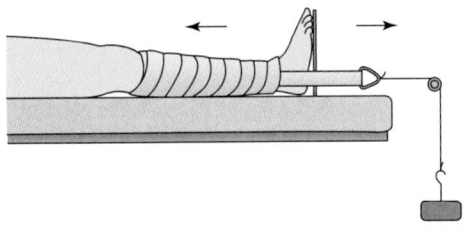

Buck's extension.

BALANCED SUSPENSION WITH THOMAS SPLINT AND PEARSON ATTACHMENT

Indications

Used in older children and adolescents for fractured femurs, to rest an injured lower extremity or joint.

Mechanism of Action

Thomas splint suspends the thigh; Pearson attachment applied to the splint allows knee flexion and supports the leg below the knee.

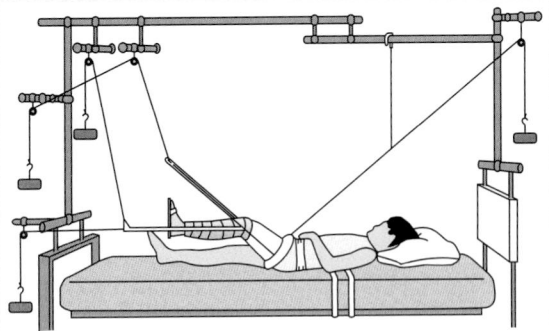

Balanced suspension.

continued

PROCEDURE GUIDELINES 54-2   **CARE OF A CHILD IN TRACTION** *CONTINUED*

Nursing Action	Rationale

DUNLOP'S TRACTION (OVERHEAD 90–90) *(SEE ACCOMPANYING FIGURE)*

Indications

Used to treat fractures of the humerus and injuries in or around the shoulder girdle.

Mechanism of Action

Traction force is applied usually through skin traction on the upper arm only. Occasionally, skeletal traction through an olecranon screw or pin in the distal humerus may be indicated. The lower arm is held in balanced suspension only. The elbow is maintained at 90 degrees of flexion or slightly more.

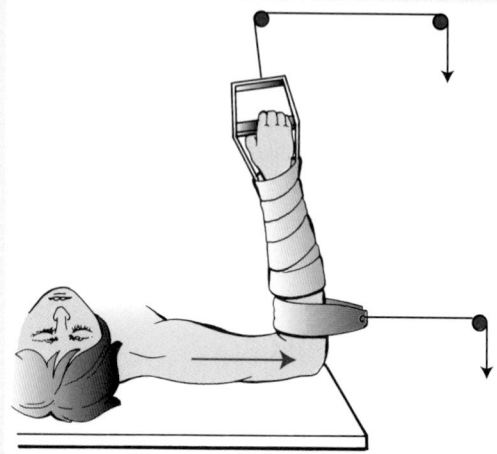

Dunlop's traction.

1. Be certain that the traction tapes are properly adhered and wrapped.
2. Assess the neurovascular status of the extremity every 2 hours.

1. Prevents damage to the skin and ensures proper pull.

2. Elastic bandages can cause circulatory or neurologic compromise. Early detection can prevent patient harm.

CERVICAL TRACTION *(SEE ACCOMPANYING FIGURE)*

Indications

Used for stabilization of spinal fractures or injuries, muscle spasms, muscle contractures.

Mechanism of Action

Traction force applied through a head halter (skin traction) or directly to the skull by means of Crutchfield tongs or halo apparatus.

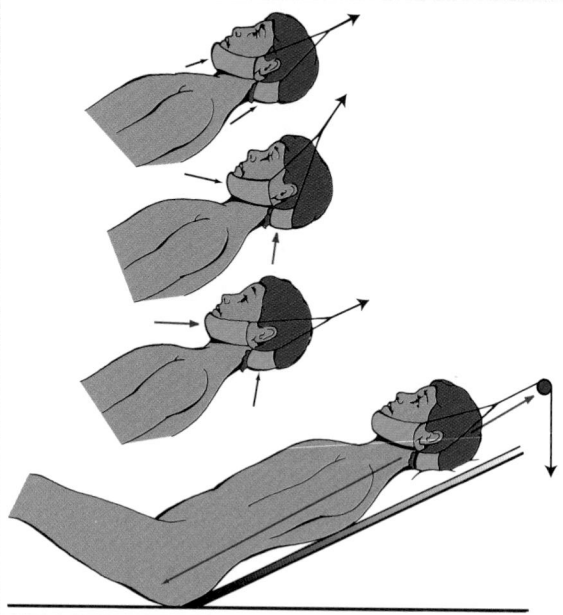

Cervical traction.

PROCEDURE GUIDELINES 54-2   *CONTINUED*

Nursing Action	Rationale
1. Head halter must be assessed for proper positioning. It should not place pressure on ears, skin, or throat.	1. Prevents pressure sores.
2. Maintain flat bed position.	2. Proper spinal alignment is critical to prevent further injury.
3. Keep the child in proper position and alignment.	
4. Crutchfield tongs or halo pin sites should be treated as skeletal traction sites.	4. Prevents infection.
5. If permissible, place the child on a Stryker frame or specially equipped bed.	5. Allows the child to be repositioned without disrupting spinal alignment.

HALO-FEMORAL

Indications

Used to correct severe spinal curvatures either before surgery or after a spinal release before final correction.

Mechanism of Action

A halo is affixed to the skull. A traction pin is placed in each distal femur. Traction force is applied upward to the halo and downward to the femurs, pulling the spine into alignment.

Nursing Action	Rationale
1. General traction considerations must be followed.	
2. Assess the child carefully every 2 hours for any increased complaints of pain, respiratory difficulty, or nerve injury.	2. Complaints should not be ignored, because alteration in any of these can indicate neurologic or spinal injury. Notification of health care provider is vital to prevent further harm.
3. Be alert for symptoms of injury to cranial nerves: a. Lateral gaze paralysis b. Difficulty in swallowing c. Difficulty in coughing d. Voice changes e. Tongue weakness	3. Common cranial nerve injuries: a. Abducens nerve palsy (most common injury) b. Vagus nerve c. Vagus nerve d. Glossopharyngeal nerve e. Hypoglossal nerve
4. Be alert for symptoms of injury to spinal cord: a. Weakness, numbness in legs b. Loss of bladder function c. Upturning or downturning of toes d. Clonus of ankles or knees	4. These complaints may indicate lower spinal nerve root or cauda equina damage and should be reported promptly.
5. Be alert for symptoms of brachial plexus injuries: a. Difficulty in moving hand, shoulder, or arm b. Numbness or weakness in hand	5. These complaints or findings may indicate damage to upper extremity and should be reported promptly.
6. Assess all pin sites for loosening every shift.	6. Loose pins can cause harm to the child as well as prevent proper traction pull.
7. Keep the torque wrench for the halo pins at the bedside at all times.	7. The halo or pins may have to be removed or adjusted in an emergency or to ensure proper tension on the pins.

SELECTED REFERENCES

Adams, J., & Hamblen, D. (1999). *Outline of fractures including joint injuries.* London: Churchill Livingstone.

Adkins, L. (1997). Cast changes: Synthetic versus plaster. *Pediatric Nursing, 23,* 422–427.

Albers, H. W., Hresko, M. T., Carlson, J., & Hall, J. E. (2000). Comparison of single and dual-rod techniques for posterior spinal instrumentation in the treatment of adolescent idiopathic scoliosis. *Spine, 25*(15), 1944–1949.

Alexander, M., & Kuo, K. (1997). Musculoskeletal assessment of the newborn. *Orthopaedic Nursing, 16,* 21–33.

Beaty, J. (1999). *Orthopaedic knowledge update home study syllabus.* Rosemont, IL: Academy of Orthopaedic Surgeons.

Benchot, R. (1996). The adolescent with slipped capital femoral epiphysis. *Journal of Pediatric Nursing, 11,* 175–182.

Benson, M., Fixsen, J., Macnicol, M., & Bleck, E. (1994). *Children's orthopaedics and fractures.* London: Churchill Livingstone.

Blakemore, L. C., Coopeman, D. R., Thompson, G. H., Wathey, C., & Ballock, R. T. (2000). Compartment syndrome in ipsilateral humerus and forearm fractures in children. *Clinical Orthopaedics, 376,* 32–38.

Buckley, S. (1997). Current trends in the treatment of femoral shaft fractures in children and adolescents. *Clinical Orthopaedics and Related Research, 338,* 60–73.

Carpenito, L. (1999). *Handbook of nursing diagnosis* (8th ed.). Philadelphia: Lippincott Williams & Wilkins.

DeBaun, B. (1998). Prevention of infection in the orthopedic surgery patient. *Nursing Clinics of North America, 33,* 671–684.

de Sanctis, N., & Rondinella, F. (2000). Prognostic evaluation of Legg-Calvé-Perthes disease by MRI. Part II: Pathomorphogenesis and new classification. *Journal of Pediatric Orthopedics, 20*(4), 463–470.

England, S., & Sundberg, S. (1996). Management of common pediatric fractures. *Pediatric Clinics of North America, 43,* 991–1012.

Fernbach, S. (1998). Common orthopedic problems of the newborn. *Nursing Clinics of North America, 33,* 583–594.

Gallegos, S., & Michalec, D. (1996). Neurologic assessment of the orthopaedic patient. *Orthopaedic Nursing, 15,* 23–29.

Gordon, J. E., Kelly-Hahn, J., Carpenter, C. J., & Schoenecker, P. L. (2000). Pin site care during external fixation in children: Results of a nihilistic approach. *Journal of Pediatric Orthopedics, 20*(2), 163–165.

Hammond, W., Kay, R., & Skaggs, D. (1998). Supracondylar humerus fractures in children. *AORN Journal, 68,* 186–200.

Hanger, C., & Brncick, N. (1998). Fat embolism syndrome: A complication of orthopaedic trauma. *Orthopaedic Nursing, 17,* 41–58.

Hayes, M. (1995). Traction at home for infants with developmental dysplasis of the hip. *Orthopaedic Nursing, 14,* 33–40.

Houston, M. (1996). Care of the school-aged child in 90/90 traction. *Orthopaedic Nursing, 15,* 57–64.

Houston, R., & Valentine, W. (1998). Complementary and alternative therapies in perinatal populations: A selected review of the current literature. *Journal of Perinatal and Neonatal Nursing, 12,* 1–15.

Hughes, B., Sponseller, P., & Thompson, J. (1995). Pediatric femur fractures: Effects of spica cast treatment on family and community. *Journal of Pediatric Orthopaedics, 15,* 457–460.

Huurman, W., & Ginsburg, G. (1997). Musculoskeletal injury in children. *Pediatrics in Review, 18,* 429–440.

Infante, A. F. Jr., Albert, M. C., Jennings, W. B., & Lehner, J. T. (2000). Immediate hip spica casting for femur fractures in pediatric patients. A review of 175 patients. *Clinical Orthopaedics, 376,* 106–112.

Islam, O., Soboleski, D., Symons, S., Davidson, L. K., Ashworth, M. A., & Babyn, P. (2000). Development and duration of radiographic signs of bone healing in children. *American Journal of Roentgenology, 175*(1), 75–78.

Kadiyala, R., & Waters, P. (1998). Upper extremity pediatric compartment syndromes. *Hand Clinics, 14,* 467–475.

Lamontagne, L., Hepworth, J., Byington, K., & Chang, C. (1997). Child and parent emotional responses during hospitalization for orthopaedic surgery. *American Journal of Maternal Child Nursing, 22,* 299–303.

McCann, S., & Gruen, G. (1997). Fracture blisters: A review of the literature. *Orthopaedic Nursing, 16,* 17–24.

Nichol, D. (1995). Understanding the principles of traction. *Nursing Standard, 9,* 25–28.

Pallija, G., Mondozzi, M., & Webb, A. (1999). Skin care of the pediatric patient. *Journal of Pediatric Nursing, 14,* 80–87.

Paton, R., Srinivasan, M., Shah, B., & Hollis, S. (1999). Ultrasound screening for hips at risk in developmental dysplasia. *Journal of Bone and Joint Surgery, 81B,* 255–258.

Patterson, M. (1998). Child abuse: Assessment and intervention. *Orthopaedic Nursing, 17,* 49–56.

Pizzutillo, P. (1997). *Pediatric orthopaedics in primary practice.* New York: McGraw-Hill.

Prior, M., & Miles, S. (1999). Casting: Part two. *Nursing Standard, 13,* 42–49.

Redfield, R., & Hayes, T. (1998). Orthopaedic infections. *Critical Care Nursing Quarterly, 21,* 24–35.

Rheiner, J., Erickson Megel, M., Hiatt, M., Halbach, R., Cyronek, & Quinn, J. (1998). Nurses' assessments and management of pain in children having orthopedic surgery. *Issues in Comprehensive Pediatric Nursing, 21,* 1–18.

Salter, R. (1999). *Textbook of disorders and injuries of the musculoskeletal system.* Baltimore: Williams & Wilkins.

Shanker, V. S., Hashemi-Nejad, A., Catteral, A., & Jackson, A. (2000). Slipped capital femoral epiphysis: Is the displacement always posterior? *Journal of Pediatric Orthopedics British, 9*(2), 119–121.

Siberry, G. K., & Iannone, R. (Eds.) (2000). *The Harriet Lane handbook* (15th ed.). St Louis: Mosby.

Skaggs, D., & Tolo, V. (1996). Legg-Calvé-Perthes disease. *Journal of the American Academy of Orthopaedic Surgeons, 4,* 9–16.

Staheli, L. (1992). *Fundamentals of pediatric orthopedics.* New York: Raven Press.

Stevens, B., Stockwell, M., Browne, G., Dent, P., Gafni, A., Martin, R., & Anderson, M. (1995). Evaluation of a home-based traction program for children with congenital dislocated hip and Legg-Perthes disease. *Canadian Journal of Nursing Research, 27,* 133–150.

Styrcula, L. (1994). Traction basics: Part IV—traction for lower extremities. *Orthopaedic Nursing, 13,* 59–68.

Veldhuizen, A. G., Wever, D. J., & Webb, P. J. (2000). The aetiology of idiopathic scoliosis: Biomechanical and neuromuscular factors. *European Spine Journal, 9*(3), 178–184.

Waagner, D. C. (2000). Musculoskeletal infections in adolescents. *Adolescent Medicine, 11*(2), 375–400.

Wall, E. J. (2000). Practical primary pediatric orthopedics. *Nursing Clinics of North America, 35*(1), 95–113.

Wenger, D., & Rang, M. (1993). *The art and practice of children's orthopaedics.* New York: Raven Press.

Wong, D. (1996). *Wong and Whaley's clinical manual of pediatric nursing.* St. Louis: Mosby.

Wong, D. (1997). *Whaley and Wong's essentials of pediatric nursing.* St. Louis: Mosby.

Pediatric Integumentary Disorders

BURNS

■ Management of Burns in Children

Burns are a frequent form of childhood injury. They may be caused by heat, electrical energy, or chemicals. The effects of burns are not limited to the burn area. Very serious burns may include:

1. Second-degree burn of 10% or more of the body surface
2. Burns of face, hands, feet, perineum, or joint surfaces
3. Electrical burns
4. Burns in the presence of other injuries
5. Any burn that cannot be cared for adequately at home

Epidemiology

1. Burns are the second leading cause of accidental deaths in childhood, with the highest incidence of burns occurring in children younger than 5 years of age.
2. Children at high risk are of lower socioeconomic status and of single parents. However, any child, supervised or unsupervised, is at risk for a burn injury.
3. Scalds are the leading cause of injury in children, followed by flame burns.
4. Burns from hot liquid are most common in children younger than age 3 years.
   a. Child left unsupervised in tub turns on hot water tap.
   b. Tap water temperature above 125°F (at 130°F it takes only 30 seconds to produce a full-thickness injury in adult skin—less time in the very young).
   c. Child placed in tub of hot water that has not been tested.
   d. Spilling of hot liquid such as coffee or tea on child. Spilling occurs especially when pot handles stick out on top of stove, when hot liquids and foods are removed from microwave oven, and when child grabs or pulls items from surfaces.
   e. Ingestion and aspiration of hot foods and liquids from microwave oven, as well as scald burns to skin and palate from hot formula.
5. Burns from open flames:
   a. House fires.
   b. Child climbing on stove, resulting in ignited clothing.
   c. Children playing with lighters, especially 3- to 10-year-olds.
   d. Playing or working with gasoline.
      (i) Automobile accidents with subsequent fire
      (ii) Juvenile fire setters
6. Electrical burns are most common in toddlers and adolescents and may be caused by:
   a. Child playing with electrical outlets or appliances.
   b. Child playing with extension cords; children often bite through the cord.
   c. Child playing on railroad tracks; climbing trees and touching high-tension wires; lightning.
7. Other causes:
   a. Caustic acid or alkali burns of mouth and esophagus
   b. Chemical burns of the skin—child playing with gasoline that comes in contact with skin (often gasoline ignites)
   c. Burns inflicted on the child as a result of neglect or abuse (an estimated 30% of all burns brought to a hospital; immersion and contact burns most common)
   d. Smoke inhalation and inhalation from products of combustion of synthetics, that is, plastics, rayons; may yield cyanide, formaldehyde
   e. Radiation burns—sunburn most common, may be secondary to cancer radiation therapy
   f. Contact burns from touching hot surfaces, such as radiators or wood-burning stoves
   g. Fireworks burns, often as a result of misuse and lack of adult supervision; may be combined with explosive hand injuries

> **NURSING ALERT**
>
> With combined injury, the trauma takes precedence over the burn.

Pathophysiology and Etiology
See Burns in Adults, page 1045.

Clinical Manifestations
Characteristics of Burn Wounds
1. See page 1050 for characteristics of first-, second-, and third-degree burns.
2. Electrical burns:
   a. Especially of the mouth in child younger than age 2 years; may chew or suck on live wire.
   b. Are progressive and may take up to 3 weeks to fully manifest the full extent of injury

Symptoms of Shock
Symptoms of shock appear soon after the burn.
1. Rapid pulse, low blood pressure
2. Subnormal temperature
3. Pallor, cyanosis, prostration
4. Failure to recognize familiar people
5. Poor muscle tone; may become flaccid

Symptoms of Toxemia
Symptoms may develop 1 to 2 days after burn.
1. Prostration, fever, rapid pulse

> **NURSING ALERT**
>
> The fever of toxemia is not to be confused with expected "burn fever," which may be as high as 103°F (39.5°C) because of the hypermetabolic state.

2. Glucosuria, decreased urinary output
3. Vomiting, edema
4. These symptoms may progress to coma or death.

Upper Respiratory Tract Injury
Causes inflammation or edema of the glottis, vocal cords, and upper trachea and is characterized by symptoms of upper airway obstruction.
1. Dyspnea, tachypnea, hoarseness
2. Stridor, substernal and intercostal retractions, nasal flaring
3. Restlessness, drooling, cough

> **NURSING ALERT**
>
> Hoarseness, drooling, and stridor are leading indicators for immediate intubation.

Smoke Inhalation
May cause no initial symptoms other than mild bronchial obstruction during the initial phase after the burn. Within 6 to 48 hours, the child may develop sudden onset of the following conditions:

1. Bronchiolitis
2. Pulmonary edema (adult respiratory distress syndrome)
3. Severe airway obstruction
4. Delayed damage: up to 7 days after the burn injury

Diagnostic Evaluation
Calculation of the Burn Area
1. "Rule of Nines" (used in assessment of extent of burns in adults) has not proved to be exact when applied to young children; it may be acceptable to use in child older than 10 years of age. It is not recommended for hospital use; the Lund and Browder chart is recommended. Total body surface area (TBSA) is based on age, thus compensating for changes in percentages resulting from growth (Figure 55-1).
   a. During infancy and early childhood, the relative surface area of different parts of the body varies with age.
   b. The younger the child, the greater the proportion of the surface area is constituted by the head and the lesser the proportion of the surface area is constituted by the legs.
2. A rough estimate can be obtained by using the child's hand, which is equal to 1%.

Categorization of Severity of Burn
1. Total area injured, depth of injury, location of injury
2. Age of child
3. Condition of patient (ie, level of consciousness)
4. Medical history (ie, chronic disease)
5. Additional injuries

Schematic Classification of Burn Severity
1. Minor burn—10% TBSA; first- and second-degree burn
2. Moderate burn:
   a. Ten percent to 20% TBSA; second-degree burn
   b. Two percent to 5% TBSA; third-degree burn not involving eyes, ears, face, genitals, hands, or feet or circumferential burns
3. Major burn:
   a. Twenty percent TBSA; second-degree burn.
   b. All third-degree burns greater than 10%; depending on age of child, 5% is sometimes used
   c. All burns involving hands, face, eyes, ears, feet, and/or genitals
   d. All electrical burns
   e. Complicated burn injuries involving fracture or other major trauma
   f. All poor-risk patients (ie, head injury, cancer, lung disease, diabetes)

Treatment
Fluid Resuscitation: Intravenous Fluid Replacement
Note: Controversy exists regarding fluid resuscitation solution and amount.
1. Fluid loss from transcapillary leakage is greatest during the first 12 hours after injury and diminishes to almost zero 12 to 24 hours after injury. Fluid loss after 48 hours is due to vaporization of water from wound.

Area of Body	Relative percentage of body surface (varies by age)					Estimated percentage of body area with:	
	0-1 years	1-4 years	5-9 years	10-15 years	Adult	2nd degree burns	3rd and 4th degree burns
Head	19	17	13	10	7		
Neck	2	2	2	2	2		
Anterior Trunk	13	13	13	13	13		
Posterior Trunk	13	13	13	13	13		
Right buttock	2	2	2	2	2		
Left buttock	2	2	2	2	2		
Genitalia	1	1	1	1	1		
Right upper arm	4	4	4	4	4		
Left upper arm	4	4	4	4	4		
Right lower arm	3	3	3	3	3		
Left lower arm	3	3	3	3	3		
Right hand	2	2	2	2	2		
Left hand	2	2	2	2	2		
Right thigh	5	6	8	8	9		
Left thigh	5	6	8	8	9		
Right lower leg	5	5	5	6	7		
Left lower leg	5	5	5	6	7		
Right foot	3	3	3	3	3		
Left foot	3	3	3	3	3		

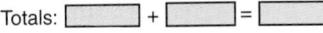

Totals: [＿＿] + [＿＿] = [＿＿]

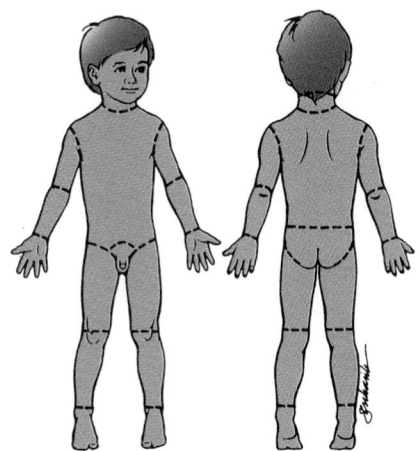

FIGURE 55-1 The Lund and Browder chart is used to determine the extent of burns in children because it is based on age, thus compensating for changes based on growth.

2. Replacement usually consists of Ringer's Lactate solution, an isotonic electrolyte solution.
3. The Parkland formula is commonly used to determine the fluid needed for resuscitation for burns greater than 15% to 20% TBSA (see page 1050). In children, it is recommended that maintenance fluid requirements also be given with the Parkland formula. It is administered in the same manner.
    a. One half of the requirements are given during the first 8 hours.
    b. The remainder is given over the next 24 hours.
    c. Ringer's Lactate may be used.
    d. In children, the second day's crystalloid consists of the maintenance requirements, and 5% D/0.45 or 0.25 saline is used.

Burn Treatment

1. Burns may be treated by the open or closed method or by a combination technique.
2. Children appear to be more mobile when burn injury is covered, because they experience less pain.

3. Hydrotherapy is treatment of choice for cleansing of wounds. Isotonic saline rather than water may be needed for large wounds and small children.
4. Gaining popularity is the use of a shower to facilitate the loosening and removal of sloughing tissue, eschar, exudate, and topical medications. The shower—water about 32°C (90°F)—flows over the child; debridement is then done.
5. See page 1051 for wound cleansing and debridement, hydrotherapy, topical antimicrobials, surgical management, and burn wound grafting.

Complications

Depend on severity of burn injury; commonly occur, especially with severe burn injury.

Acute
1. Infection; burn wound sepsis, pneumonia, urinary tract infection, phlebitis, toxic shock syndrome
2. Curling's (stress) ulcer, gastrointestinal hemorrhage; rarely seen now that histamine 2 (H_2) blockers are commonly used prophylactically, especially in burns greater than 20% TBSA
3. Acute gastric dilation, paralytic ileus; occurs especially in child younger than 2 years of age with greater than 20% injury and develops early in postburn period, lasting 2 to 3 days
4. Renal failure
5. Respiratory failure; severe inhalation injury is the insult most likely to cause death
6. Postburn seizures
7. Hypertension
8. Central nervous system dysfunction
9. Vascular ischemia
10. Anemia and malnutrition; may resolve once burn area is covered
11. Fecal impaction
12. Depression secondary to hospitalization and changing body image

Long-Term
1. Growth and development delays secondary to malnutrition
2. Scarring, disfigurement, and contractures
3. Psychological trauma

Nursing Assessment
1. Initially, perform emergency assessment of the burn patient to determine priorities of care.
   a. Airway, breathing, and circulation: airway may be compromised with inhalation injury
   b. Extent of burn injury
   c. Additional injuries
2. Obtain a history of the injury; for example, ask if the child was involved in an automobile accident or dropped from a window for rescue to help establish if additional injuries may exist.

3. Obtain a complete medical history, including childhood diseases, immunizations (especially tetanus status), current medications, allergies, recent infections.
4. Subsequently, focus assessment on fluid volume balance, condition of the burn wounds, and signs of infection (burn wound, pulmonary, urinary).
5. Assess level of comfort and emotional status; provide reassurance while performing assessment and determining priorities.

Nursing Diagnoses
- Decreased Cardiac Output related to fluid loss and hypermetabolic state
- Risk for Infection related to altered skin integrity, decreased circulation, and immobility
- Impaired Gas Exchange related to inhalation injury, pain, and immobility
- Risk for Injury related to paralytic ileus and stress
- Altered Nutrition: Less Than Body Requirements related to hypermetabolic state and poor appetite
- Impaired Physical Mobility related to dressings, pain, and contractures
- Pain related to burn wound and associated treatments
- Body Image Disturbance related to pain, scarring, and disfigurement
- Fear and Anxiety related to pain, treatments, procedures, and hospitalization
- Altered Parenting related to crisis situation, prolonged hospitalization, and disfigurement

Nursing Interventions
Supporting Cardiac Output
1. Be alert to the symptoms of shock that occur very shortly after a severe burn—tachycardia, hypothermia, hypotension, pallor, prostration, shallow respirations, anuria.
2. Monitor the administration of intravenous fluid, because major burns are followed by a reduction in blood volume due to outflow of plasma into the tissues.
3. Maintain and record intake and output to provide an accurate measure of volume.
   a. Record time and amount of all fluids given.
   b. Measure accurately urinary output every hour and report diminished output as ordered (usually, 0.5 mL/kg/hour is considered minimally acceptable urinary output).
   c. Check specific gravity to determine urine concentration or dilution.
4. With severe burn injuries, insert an indwelling catheter.
5. Weigh daily to help evaluate fluid balance.
6. Monitor sensorium, pulse, pulse pressure, capillary filling, and blood gases.
7. Provide a rich oxygen environment to combat hypoxia, as necessary.
8. Monitor electrolyte and hematocrit results as a guide to fluid replacement.

9. Maintain a warm, humidified ambient environment (especially with burns of 20% TBSA) to maintain body temperature and decrease fluid needs.

Preventing Infection

1. Provide scrupulous skin care to prevent infection and promote healing.

NURSING ALERT

Even with scrupulous skin care, the burn wound is fully colonized in 3 to 5 days. A warm, moist environment sets up an excellent medium for bacterial growth, especially of *Pseudomonas*.

---

2. Prevent child from scratching by administering antipruritics and applying protective devices to hands.
3. Obtain serial cultures as ordered.
4. Observe burn wounds with each dressing change: assess drainage for color, odor, and amount; necrosis; increase in pain; and surrounding erythema, warmth, swelling, and tenderness, which may indicate infection.
5. Administer topical antimicrobials and systemic antibiotics as ordered.
6. Observe for signs of toxemia, such as fever, prostration, tachycardia, vomiting, and oliguria, and report immediately.
7. Be alert for the development of pneumonia or urinary tract infection related to immobility and invasive procedures. Encourage coughing, turning, deep breathing, ambulation, and early discontinuation of indwelling catheter to minimize the complications.
8. Administer tetanus prophylaxis based on immunization history.
   a. If primary series complete (or at least three doses of tetanus toxoid obtained) and last injection within past 5 years, it is not necessary.
   b. If at least three doses obtained and last injection greater than 5 years, give tetanus toxoid.
   c. If two or fewer doses obtained, give tetanus immunoglobulin and tetanus toxoid.
9. Obtain urine, sputum, and blood cultures for two or more consecutive temperatures of 103°F (39.5°C) or a single temperature of 104°F (40°C).

Optimizing Gas Exchange

1. Be alert for and report symptoms of respiratory distress—dyspnea, stridor, tachypnea, restlessness, cyanosis, coughing, increasing hoarseness, drooling.
2. Administer supplemental humidified oxygen.
3. Monitor arterial blood gases.
4. Evaluate the carboxyhemoglobin on arterial blood gases (due to inhalation of carbon monoxide, a product of combustion) and be prepared to support ventilation if signs of hypoxemia and respiratory failure develop.
5. Assist with pulmonary function and bronchoscopy as indicated.
6. Have intubation supplies immediately available. If unable to intubate the child, then tracheostomy may be necessary. If unable to extubate in 14 to 21 days, then may be converted to tracheostomy for continuous pulmonary management.

Relieving Gastric Dilation and Preventing Stress Ulcer

1. Be alert for the development of gastric distention, especially with burns greater than 20% TBSA, associated injury, or tachypnea.
2. Maintain nothing-by-mouth status if distention or decreased bowel sounds develop.
3. Insert nasogastric tube as indicated to prevent vomiting, aspiration, and paralytic ileus.
4. Monitor the return of bowel sounds after nasogastric extubation and before reinstituting oral feeding.
5. Administer H_2 blockers, such as cimetidine (Tagamet), to prevent Curling's ulcer development.

Ensuring Adequate Nutrition for Healing and Growth Needs

1. Be aware that hypernutrition is important because of the extreme hypermetabolism related to large burn injuries.
   a. Twice the predicted basal metabolic rate in calories, based on ideal weight, may be necessary. Caloric recommendation is 1,800 kcal/m² body surface for maintenance, plus 2,000 kcal/m² of burned surface area.
   b. Hypermetabolic state generally subsides when the majority of the wounds are grafted or healed.
   c. High caloric intake to support hypermetabolic state; protein synthesis; calories should come from carbohydrates.
   d. High-protein intake to replace protein lost by exudation; support synthesis of immunoglobulins and structural protein; prevent negative nitrogen balance.
   e. Vitamin and mineral supplement needed, particularly vitamins B and C, iron, and zinc.
2. Maintain ambient temperature at 28°C to 32°C (90°F) to minimize metabolic expenditure by maintaining core temperature.
3. Minimize anorexia to increase caloric intake.
   a. Offer small amounts of food, perhaps four to five feedings rather than three per day.
   b. Give choice of foods; determine favorites.
   c. Provide high-calorie, high-protein oral or nasogastric supplementation as necessary.
   d. Make meals a pleasant time, unassociated with treatments or unpleasant interruptions.
4. Monitor dietary compliance with dietary goals and adjust as needed.
5. Administer total parenteral nutrition if necessary.
6. Administer serum albumin or fresh frozen plasma to combat hypoalbuminemia when burn area exceeds 20% TBSA.
7. Monitor nutritional status through weight gain, wound healing, serum transferrin, and serum albumin.

Preserving Mobility

1. Ensure that physical and occupational therapy are begun early to facilitate rehabilitation.

2. Encourage range-of-motion exercises, ambulation, and positioning to minimize joint and skin complications.
3. Position joint in opposite direction of expected contracture.
4. Apply splints to aid joint positioning and decrease skin contractures and hypertrophy.
5. Apply pressure garments to aid circulation, protect newly healed skin, and prevent and treat hypertrophic scar formation by promoting dermal collagen fiber growth in parallel direction. Encourage use of pressure garments for as long as 12 to 18 months after injury, until the healed skin has matured.
6. Medicate for pain before therapy or exercise to minimize discomfort.
7. Use play opportunities to help the child accept the therapy program (eg, tricycle riding may be used as form of exercise).

Controlling Pain

1. Assess for signs of pain, such as irritability, crying, increased blood pressure, tachycardia, decreased mobility, and inability to sleep.
2. Administer analgesics and/or sedatives to relieve pain.
   a. Analgesia may include, but is not limited to, acetaminophen (Tylenol), acetaminophen with codeine (Tylenol #2 or #3), meperidine (Demerol), morphine, fentanyl (IV or oral), hydroxyzine (Vistaril), and ibuprofen (Motrin).
   b. In severe burns, analgesia should be given intravenously because of lack of absorption of intramuscular injections during the emergency phase.
3. Use an alternating water or sand bed to relieve pressure and provide comfort.
4. Maintain warmth and prevent chilling.
5. Provide diversional activities appropriate for age to distract from focus on pain.
6. Teach simple relaxation techniques, such as relaxation breathing and guided imagery.
7. Recognize that fear may exacerbate discomfort; provide reassurance and empathy.

Preventing Negative Body Image

1. Encourage the child to talk about the way he or she feels and looks.
   a. The child may feel guilty and think that the burn is punishment for some wrong deed.
   b. Small children may be fearful of the appearance of bandages, scars, or pressure garments; offer reassurance.
   c. Encourage the use of play with dolls or puppets, role playing, or picture drawing to help the child express feelings and fears.
2. Treat child with warmth and affection and encourage parents to continually point out their love even though child has a bad burn.
3. Support child in viewing self in mirror when ready and encourage presence of family members.
4. Encourage early contact with other children.

5. Suggest psychiatric consultation for:
   a. Refusing to eat
   b. Resisting all nursing procedures
   c. Resisting socialization
6. Advise parents that separation from the hospital environment, caregivers, and other patients can produce excessive anxiety. Short-time home passes (overnight, weekend) are helpful before final discharge.
7. If the child is school age, help prepare for school reentry; contact teacher or discuss with parents the need to prepare peers for what to expect.
8. Discuss issues of social reentry, such as responding to questions and stares from strangers and perceived rejection by friends.
   a. Refer to a support group and/or have a child who has recovered from burns visit child.
   b. Refer to a burn camp—often this may be the first opportunity for the child to wear a swimsuit after the injury.
9. Initiate family consultation with plastic surgeon about future scar revision.
10. Encourage older child to experiment with clothing and consult with a burn cosmetic specialist to enhance appearance and body image.

Reducing Fear and Anxiety

1. Explain procedures, surgeries, and treatments to the child according to age and level of understanding.
2. Allow the child to express fears through puppets, dolls, water play, clay, and drawings.
3. Expect regression due to the physical pain and psychological trauma the child is going through.
4. Encourage parents to stay with a young child as much as possible.
5. Try to involve child in group play and unit activities.
6. Encourage involvement with treatment plan and self-care activities.

Promoting Effective Parenting

1. Be alert to signs that parents may react to the situation with depression and/or stress syndromes, and encourage counseling for them to promote a healthier family.
2. Encourage parents to assess the effects on siblings at home; they may have needs that are unrecognized or neglected as a result of this crisis.
3. Attempt to have parents become actively involved in the child's care when they are ready to do so.
   a. Advise parents that their visits and involvement can have a positive effect on the child's survival and recovery.
   b. If the parents are unable to visit, telephone calls and family photographs are helpful.
4. Give the parents the opportunity to discuss their feelings.
   a. Parents frequently express guilt regarding their lack of supervision when the accident occurred.
   b. Frequently, burn injury is associated with actual or perceived parental neglect. Remember that this type of injury is sudden and acute, placing the family in a state of crisis.

5. Keep the parents informed of the child's progress.
   a. Begin initial teaching at admission with supportive words and limited technical information.
   b. Education and orientation to the facility and the burn injury will decrease some anxiety and begin to build rapport on which future support can be based.
   c. Encourage meetings with other parents who have coped with trauma.

Community and Home Care Considerations

1. Make routine home visits to perform, teach, and supervise burn wound care.
2. Inspect for signs of infection at every visit.
3. Assess coping ability of child and family to care for child and provide psychological support and counseling referrals as needed.
4. Ensure that parents are able to:
   a. Discuss and demonstrate treatments, procedures, and dressing changes
   b. Obtain equipment necessary to perform treatment at home
   c. Understand reason for and side effects of medications as well as dietary requirements
   d. Follow up at appropriate intervals with the designated health care provider
5. Encourage the use of smoke alarms on every floor in the home, a fire extinguisher, and an emergency fire escape plan.

Family Education and Health Maintenance

1. Teach that special skin care is necessary after burn injury.
   a. Avoid exposure to sunlight; use sunscreen of sun protective factor 24 or higher and apply frequently.
   b. Use pressure garments to prevent hypertrophic scar and keloid formation—worn 23 of 24 hours for effectiveness, over a time period of 1 to $1\frac{1}{2}$ years.
   c. Use lotions and creams to prevent skin from drying, cracking, and itching.
   d. Burn area has decreased sensation to touch, heat, and pressure; take precautions to prevent injury to area.
2. Advise that adjustment after burn is often prolonged and painful. Encourage ongoing family and individual psychological support.
3. Encourage continued physical therapy to prevent contractures and preserve function.
4. Initiate home health, financial assistance, and other referrals as necessary.
5. Teach parents and children the prevention of burn injury as well as other safety measures (see p. 1278).
6. Teach first-aid emergency care for burn injury (ie, cool burned area with cool water, remove clothing, seek medical assistance).
7. Teach children how to stop, drop, and roll if their clothes catch on fire and how to crawl to safety if a fire occurs in the house.

Outcome-Based Evaluation

- Absence of shock: stabilization of vital signs, normal serum and electrolyte values
- Absence of infection: normal laboratory values, clean wound, and normal temperature
- No respiratory distress: stable vital signs, respiratory status, and arterial blood gases
- No gastrointestinal complications: normal bowel sounds and ability to tolerate oral feeding
- Adequate nutritional status: weight gain and wound healing
- Improved mobility: involvement in play and other activities
- Minimal discomfort: stable vital signs, verbalization, and involvement in play
- Positive body image: verbalization, socialization, and ability to look in mirror
- Relief of fear: able to play, participates in care
- Effective parenting: involvement in child's care, accurate discussion of child's progress and treatment plan

DERMATOLOGIC DISORDERS

Atopic Dermatitis (Infantile and Childhood Eczema)

Atopic dermatitis, the most common cause of eczema in childhood, is a characteristic inflammatory response of the skin. The major features include pruritus, a typical morphology and distribution, a chronic or chronically relapsing nature, and a personal or family history of atopy (asthma, hay fever, and atopic dermatitis). There is a tendency toward dry skin and a lower threshold to itching.

Atopic dermatitis affects 10% to 15% of the childhood population. It usually starts after 2 months of age. By age 5, 90% of the patients who will develop atopic dermatitis have already manifested the disease. It may stop after an indefinite period of time, or it may progress from infancy to adulthood with little or no relief. It is rare for adults to develop atopic dermatitis without a history of eczema in childhood.

Pathophysiology and Etiology

1. Atopic dermatitis involves immunologic abnormalities, such as elevated immunoglobulin E levels and increased rates of sensitization to common contact allergens and to intradermal skin tests. Although the exact cause is unknown, there is a constitutional predisposition to develop pruritus. In general, the skin of patients with atopic dermatitis is different from that of healthy patients in the following respects:
   a. Increased tendency toward dryness
   b. Lowered threshold for pruritus from minor irritants, such as soap, wool, perspiration, cold weather, and heat

c. Tendency toward lichenification (leathery thickening of skin) and production of a rash when the skin is rubbed or scratched

2. The etiology is unknown but has familial tendencies. Almost 75% of patients with this form of eczema have a family history of atopic dermatitis, hay fever, or asthma. One-third to one-half of children with eczema will develop hay fever or asthma themselves.

Clinical Manifestations
Age and Distribution of Lesions
Atopic dermatitis is divided into three phases based on the age of the patient and the distribution of the lesions. These are referred to as the infant, childhood, and adult phases.

1. Infant (2 months to 2 years):
   a. The onset is between 2 and 6 months of age. Half of affected infants have spontaneous resolution by age 2 or 3.
   b. Characterized by intense itching, erythema, papules, vesicles, oozing, and crusting (Figure 55-2).
   c. The rash usually begins on the cheeks, forehead, or scalp and then extends to the trunk or extremities in scattered, often symmetric patches. The perioral, perinasal, and diaper areas are usually spared (Figure 55-3).
2. Childhood (4 to 10 years):
   a. Affected persons in this age group are less likely to have exudative and crusted lesions. Eruptions are characteristically more dry and papular and often occur as circumscribed scaly patches. There is a greater tendency toward chronicity and lichenification.
   b. The typical areas of involvement are the face, including the perioral and perinasal areas, neck, antecubital and popliteal fossae, wrists, and ankles.
3. Adult (puberty to old age):
   a. Predominant areas of involvement include the flexor folds, face, neck, upper arms, back, dorsa of the hands and feet, fingers, and toes.

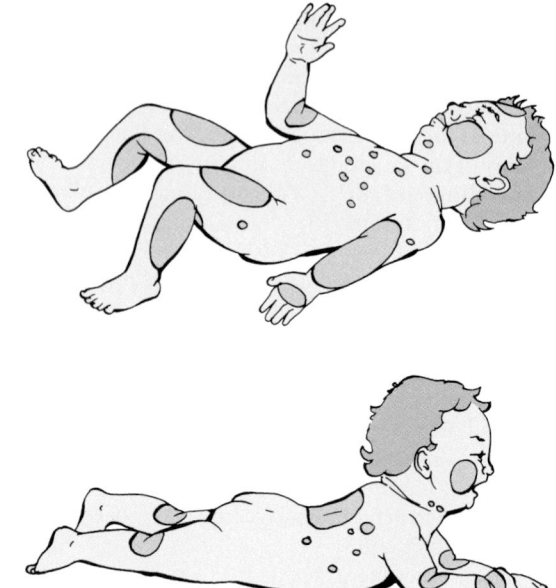

FIGURE 55-3 Infant atopic dermatitis occurs primarily on the face, but may develop on symmetric areas of the body. Diaper areas are usually clear.

b. The eruption appears as thick, dry lesions, confluent papules, and large lichenified plaques. Weeping, crusting, and exudation can occur, but they are usually the result of superimposed external irritation or infection.

Clinical Appearance
Atopic dermatitis is also divided into three stages based on the clinical appearance of the lesions. The acute, subacute, and chronic stages can occur in infants, children, and adults.

1. Acute (Figure 55-4A)—moderate to intense erythema, vesicles, a wet surface, and severe itching.

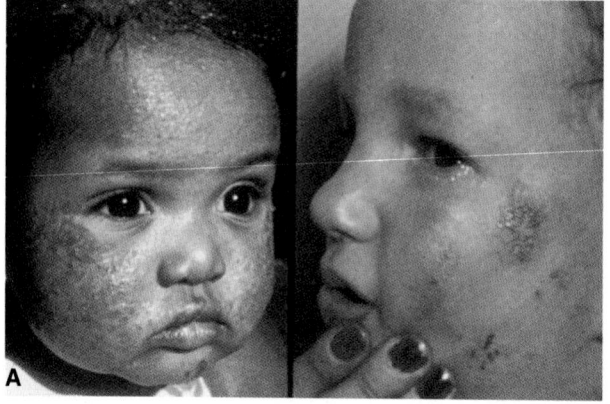
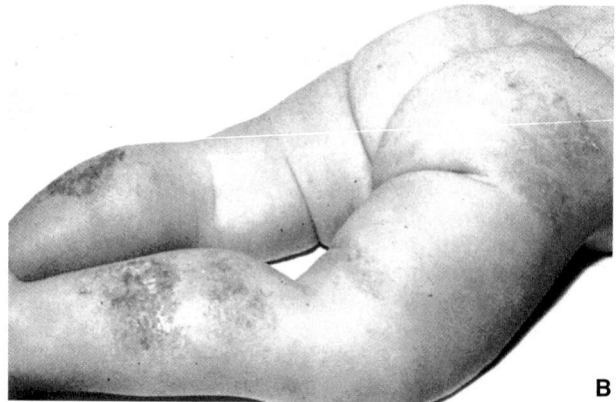

FIGURE 55-2 Infantile atopic dermatitis of the head (**A**) and of the limbs (**B**). (Courtesy of Schering.)

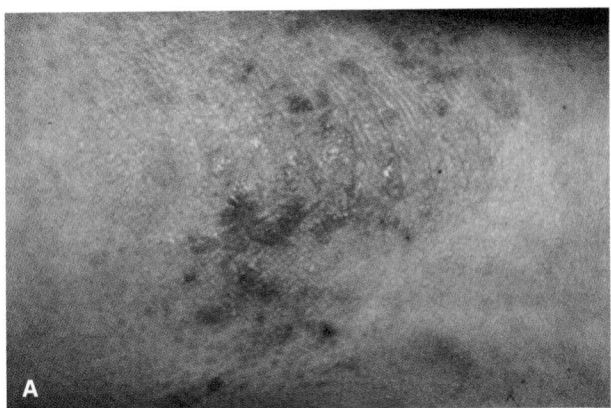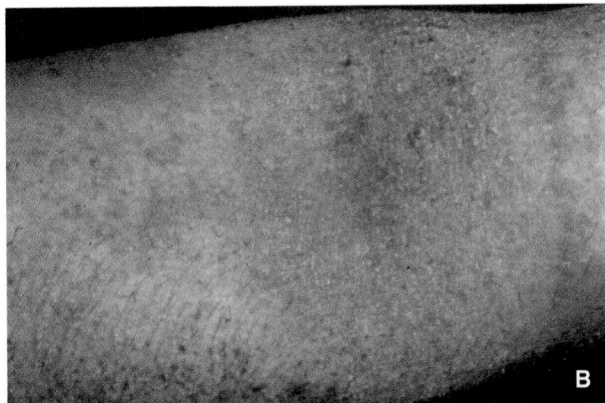

FIGURE 55-4 (**A**) Acute atopic dermatitis. (**B**) Chronic atopic dermatitis. (Courtesy of Schering.)

2. Subacute:
   a. Erythema and scaling are present in various patterns with indistinct borders. The redness may be faint or intense. The surface is dry. There are varying degrees of pruritus.
   b. The subacute stage may be an initial stage or may follow an acute inflammation or exacerbation of a chronic stage. Irritation, allergy, or infection can convert a subacute process into an acute one.
3. Chronic (Figure 55-4B)—the inflamed area thickens and the surface skin markings become more prominent. Thick plaques with deep parallel skin markings are called lichenified. Lichenification is the hallmark of chronic eczema. The surface of the skin is dry and the border of the lesion well defined. There is moderate to intense itching.

Diagnostic Evaluation

Atopic dermatitis is usually a clinical diagnosis based on the evaluation of the aggregate of signs, symptoms, stigmata, course, and associated familial findings. The major features include pruritus, a characteristic morphology and typical distribution for the age of the patient, a chronic or chronically relapsing nature, and a personal or family history of atopic disease. When the diagnosis is in doubt, a skin biopsy may be performed.

Treatment
Acute
1. Open wet dressings for 1 to 3 days
2. Avoidance of any known allergen
3. Topical corticosteroids
   a. Topical corticortcosteroids are ranked into seven groups according to potency. Group 1 contains the most potent topical steroids and group 7 the least potent ones. The concentration listed on the medication does not correlate with its potency or safety, but is merely a statement of its specific chemical formulation.
   b. Very potent (Group 1) topical corticosteroids are avoided in children younger than 12 years of age because of greater skin absorption.

 DRUG ALERT

Topical corticosteroids of adequate strength should be used 2 to 4 times a day for a specific length of time, such as 7 to 21 days, in order to achieve control and avoid side effects. Long-term use of topical corticosteroids can cause striae, cutaneous atrophy, telangiectasia, acne, growth retardation, adrenal suppression, Cushing's syndrome, and cataracts.

4. Oral medications to relieve itching—hydroxyzine hydrochloride (Atarax), diphenhydramine hydrochloride (Benadryl), or promethazine hydrochloride (Phenergan). Diphenhydramine and promethazine cause more sedation than hydroxyzine hydrochloride. Mild sedation may be desirable.
5. Management of secondary infection, if present, with oral antibiotics
6. Initiation of a hypoallergenic diet to eliminate any responsible food for infants and young children with severe, recalcitrant atopic dermatitis

Subacute and Chronic
1. Prevention of dry skin:
   a. Diminish the frequency and duration of bathing.
   b. Use mild soap or hydrophilic lotion.
   c. Lubricate the skin with emollients.
   d. Add tar preparations to the bath water.
   e. Maintain environmental humidity above 40% in winter months.
2. Same measures as the acute stage with exception of wet dressings.

Nursing Assessment
1. Take a nursing history focusing on clinical manifestations:
   a. Onset and duration of rash
   b. Location, course, and distribution of lesions

c. Change in morphology of lesions
d. Local and systemic symptoms
e. Exposure to possible allergens
f. Previous episodes of rashes
g. Personal history of allergies, asthma, or hay fever
h. Family history of eczema, allergies, or hay fever
i. Medications, treatments tried, and their effect
2. Perform a physical assessment.
   a. Examine the entire skin in an orderly fashion with specific attention to the type of lesion (ie, macule, papule, vesicle, etc.), its appearance (shape, border, color, texture, and surface), and its distribution (areas of the body involved).
   b. Note any associated symptoms, such as scratching, fever, or drainage.
3. Document findings:
   a. Describe skin findings using dermatologic terminology.
   b. Draw pictures to facilitate communication.

Nursing Diagnoses

- Impaired Skin Integrity or high risk for impairment, related to skin pathology and scratching
- Sensory/Perceptual Alterations (Tactile), related to skin pathology
- Risk for Infection related to increased bacterial colonization of skin and possible break in defensive barrier

Nursing Interventions

The nurse may perform the following interventions or teach the patient or family to do the following:

Improving Skin Integrity

1. Reduce inflammation during the acute stage with the topical application of open wet dressings.
   a. Use a soft, lightweight cloth, such as a handkerchief, a thin diaper, or strips of bed sheeting. Do not use gauze (adheres to skin), washcloths, or towels (too heavy).
   b. Open wet dressings should be clean. In certain situations, they should be sterile to prevent contamination.
   c. Solutions should be lukewarm or at body temperature to soothe the skin and prevent chilling.
   d. Compresses should be moderately wet, not dripping, and removed after 20 minutes, unless otherwise directed. They should be reapplied three to four times a day.
   e. After the compress, a topical corticosteroid may be applied to further reduce itching and inflammation.
   f. Observe the skin for changes in response to therapy.
2. Prevent dry skin during the subacute and chronic stages.
   a. Decrease the frequency and duration of bathing. Long, hot tub baths are to be avoided.
   b. Avoid hot water and harsh soaps. Patients should bathe in lukewarm water using mild soap (Dove, Neutrogena); avoid bubble baths; rinse well and pat skin dry with towel.

c. If bath water stings, add 1 cup of table salt.
d. Apply unscented emollients (eg, Eucerin, Keri, Lubriderm) within 3 minutes of bathing, when the skin is slightly moist. Creams and ointments are more effective than lotions because they are better at preventing evaporation of water from the skin. Bathing will dry and damage the skin unless an emollient is applied immediately after exiting the bath.
e. Some patients may benefit from soaking in a tar bath for 15 to 20 minutes daily, preferably in the evening. Add to bath water as directed. Tar preparations can stain the skin and clothing and may cause sunlight sensitivity.
f. For patients with extremely dry skin, cleanse with a hydrophilic lotion (eg, Cetaphil). Apply without water until light foam occurs. Remove by wiping with soft cotton cloth or cleansing tissue.
g. Keep environmental humidity above 40% in winter months. Use a humidifier.
h. Observe the skin for changes in response to therapy.

NURSING ALERT

 Apply unscented emollients to the skin within 3 minutes of bathing when the skin has been patted dry but is still moist to maintain a high level of hydration to the epidermis.

Controlling Pruritus

1. Apply topical corticosteroids.
   a. Apply a thin layer of topical corticosteroids to the affected skin two to four times a day as directed. Use only for the duration prescribed.
   b. Observe for possible side effects from long-term use of topical corticosteroids (ie, striae, cutaneous atrophy, telangiectasia, acne, and growth retardation).
   c. Note any scratching and intervene as necessary.
2. Administer oral antipruritic medications.
   a. Give medications exactly as prescribed.
   b. Note the degree of sedation and presence of scratching.
3. Teach the caretaker or family of infants and small children a hypoallergenic diet when indicated.
   a. Write any known allergens on care plan and chart. Inform the dietitian of the child's food allergies.
   b. Avoid substances that have a high potential for sensitization, such as cow's milk, eggs, tomatoes, citrus fruits, chocolate, wheat products, spiced food, fish, nuts, and peanut butter.
   c. A minimal diet is prescribed. The trial diet may be composed of milk substitute, rice cereal, two fruits, two vegetables, beef, a multivitamin, and no eggs.
   d. A new food is added to the diet every 3 to 5 days, during which time the response to the food is observed.
   e. An allergic response occurring during this 3- to 5-day period indicates sensitivity to that food. The food is then eliminated from the diet. If no response is apparent, the food is added to the child's diet.

(text continues on page 1607)

TABLE 55-1 Common Pediatric Skin Problems

Disorder/Organism	Clinical Manifestations	Treatment/Prevention	Nursing/Patient Care Considerations

Impetigo
1. Bacterial infectious disease affecting the superficial layers of the skin and characterized by the formation of vesicles, crusts, or bullae.
2. Etiology and incidence
  a. Caused by *Staphylococcus aureus* and *Streptococcus pyogenes*.
  b. Occurs most frequently when personal hygiene is poor.
  c. Is common in children under 10 years of age.
  d. Spread by close contact—easily conveyed from person to person via hands, nasal discharge, shared towels, toys, etc.; plastic wading pools in summer—when water is not replaced and no disinfectant is used. Is highly contagious.
  e. Any abrasion of skin may serve as portal of entry.
3. Diagnosis
  a. Is usually clinical.
  b. Rarely, a culture of lesion's exudate is indicated to confirm the diagnosis.
	1. Incubation period is 1 to 10 days.
	2. Lesion first appears as pink-red macules that quickly change to vesicles that, in turn, rupture, develop crusts, and leave temporary superficial erythematous area.
	  a. *Bullous* (newborn and older child)—large, thin-roofed blisters break to form thin, light-brown crusts. Lesions may occur anywhere on the body but are more common on the face, axillae, and groin.
	  b. *Crusted* (preschool-age—seen more often in summer on exposed body parts)—lesions appear with thick, yellow crusts; skin around crusts is red and weeping with satellite lesions.
	3. Regional lymphadenopathy is common with secondary infection of insect bites, eczema, poison ivy, and scabies.
	4. Autoinoculation is major cause of spreading.
	5. Pruritus may occur.
		Based on etiology and type of infection.
		1. Gently wash affected area with soap and water three times a day. Crusts and debris can be removed from the affected area by gentle soaking or wet compresses. Use tap water, normal saline or 1:20 Burrow's solution.
		3. Apply topical antibacterial medication such as Bacitracin or mupirocin ointment (Bactroban).
		4. Systemic antibiotics (cephalosporins, erythromycin, or dicloxacillin) if widespread or recurrent.
		5. Prevention—close contact with other children should be avoided until 24 hours after treatment is initiated.
			1. Assess the child's skin condition and document the location and appearance of lesions. Note any new lesions.
			2. Initiate and teach measures to prevent the spread of infection.
			  a. Engage in frequent handwashing. Use separate towels.
			  b. Daily bathing with soap and water. Regular laundering for contaminated bed linens, towels, and clothing.
			  c. Observe drainage/secretion precautions for 24 hours after the start of therapy.
			  d. Isolate the child from direct contact with other children (school or day care) until 24 hours after treatment has started.
			  e. Trim fingernails and toenails. Apply small amount of Bacitracin or mupirocin ointment under the fingernails to prevent the spread of infection.
			  f. Engage the child in diversional activities to discourage scratching.
			3. Be aware that the patient with streptococcal impetigo has an increased risk for acute glomerulonephritis.

Ringworm of the Scalp (tinea capitis)
1. A fungal infection of the scalp and hair follicles.
2. Etiology and incidence
  a. Most ringworm of the scalp is caused by *Trichophyton tonsurans*. *Micosporum canis* and *Micosporum audovinii* are also causative agents.
  b. Is seen primarily in children before puberty (usually ages 3–10 years).
  c. The infection may be spread through child-to-child contact as well as through the common use of towels, pillows, combs, brushes, and hats. Cats and dogs may be the source of the infection.
	1. The lesions appear on the scalp as one or several round patches of inflammation and hair breakage or loss (alopecia).
	2. Pruritus usually occurs in the involved area.
	3. A kerion, an acute inflammation that produces edema, pustules, and granulomatous swelling, may occur.
		1. Microsized griseofulvin (Grifulvin V)—an antifungal antibiotic that is administered orally, 15–20 mg/kg/day (maximum 1 g) in a single dose with a high-fat food for 4–12 weeks. Some children may require higher doses or microsized griseofulvin 20–25 mg/kg/day or ultramicrosized griseofulvin 5–10 mg/kg/day (maximum 750 mg).
		2. Topical antifungal medicines are not effective. Selenium sulfide lotion 2.5% (Selsun Rx+) used twice weekly decreases fungal shedding and may curb infection.
		3. Treatment should be continued for 2 weeks after clinical resolution.
			1. Assess the scalp for characteristic lesions.
			2. Administer or teach patient/family to administer medications as prescribed.
			  a. Be aware of side effects, such as headache, heartburn, nausea, epigastric discomfort, diarrhea, urticaria, photosensitivity, and possible granulocytopenia caused by griseofulvin. Griseofulvin is absorbed more efficiently with a fatty meal. Children can be given the medicine once a day with ice cream or peanut butter.
			3. Teach the child and family methods to prevent further episodes.
			  a. Teach general hygiene measures—regular shampooing and bathing.
			  b. Advise them to avoid sharing hats, combs, brushes, pillows, etc.

(continued)

TABLE 55-1 Common Pediatric Skin Problems (Continued)

Disorder/Organism	Clinical Manifestations	Treatment/Prevention	Nursing/Patient Care Considerations
3. Diagnosis a. Hair or skin scrapings for microscopic evaluation or fungal culture, obtained by rubbing a swab or toothbrush over the affected area. b. Wood's lamp evaluation causes *Microsporum* infections to fluoresce. Since most tinea capitis is now caused by *Trichophyton* infection, this test is no longer that useful.			c. Routine cleaning of heavily contaminated articles such as pillowcases, sheets, towels, hats, bike helmets, combs, brushes, etc. d. All family members and close contacts should be screened for tinea infections. The child's school should be notified to facilitate the screening of classmates. 4. Hair loss is usually temporary, except in some cases with a kerion, when the hair follicles may have been destroyed. 5. Child may attend school once treatment has been initiated. Hats are not necessary.
Pediculosis 1. The infestation of human beings by lice. 2. Etiology a. Three types of lice affect human beings. • Pediculosis capitis (the head louse)—commonly infests school-aged children • Pediculosis corporis (the body louse)—rare in U.S. • Phthirus pubis (the pubic or crab louse)—common in sexually active adolescents or adults—can be found on pubic hair, chest hair, axillary hair, eyebrows, eyelashes, and beards. b. Each type of louse generally remains in the area designated by its name, but it may occasionally be seen in other areas of the body. c. Lice are transmitted by personal contact with people harboring them or through contact with articles that temporarily harbor them (clothing or bed linen). d. There is no evidence that the lice themselves transmit disease. 3. Diagnosis a. Identification of lice or their eggs with the naked eye is possible.	1. Itching in the area affected is the primary symptom of pediculosis. Scratch marks may be evident in these areas. However, not all affected persons itch. 2. Other signs of infestation are pillows or clothing that look unusually dirty. 3. Infested scalp areas may become secondarily infected from scratching. 4. Crusts, lice, nits, eggs, and dirt may combine to cause a foul odor and matted hair. 5. Body lice may produce minute red lesions.	1. *Pediculosis capitis* and *Phthirus pubis* may be treated with over-the-counter agents such as permethrin (NIX) or natural pyrethrin-based products (A-200, RID, R&C shampoo, or Pronto). Lindane 1% (Rx) is indicated for second-line therapy only. Natural pyrethrin-based products and lindane may be reapplied 7–10 days later. Lindane should be avoided in children less than 2 years of age, persons with known seizures, and pregnant or lactating women. 2. For infestation of eyelashes by crab lice, petroleum jelly applied twice daily for 8–10 days is effective. 3. Pediculicides are not necessary for the treatment of Pediculosis corporis. Washing infested clothing and linens, where the lice harbor, in hot water and machine drying (on hot cycle) is adequate. 4. Because pediculicides kill lice shortly after application, the detection of living lice on scalp inspection 24 hours or more after treatment suggests incorrect use, reinfection, or resistance. Immediate retreatment with a different pediculicide followed by a second	1. Administer or teach administration of antiparasitic as directed. Natural pyrethrin-based products work best on dry hair. Permethrin is a cream rinse applied after regular shampooing. 2. Although both pyrethrins and permethrin are quite safe, limit exposure to the skin by rinsing the hair in a sink rather than the shower and use cool water to minimize absorption from vasodilation. 3. Use of a fine-toothed comb aids in the mechanical removal of nits. Soaking the hair in white vinegar and water can facilitate the removal of nits with combing. 4. Inspect the scalp (or have the family inspect the scalp) 24 to 48 hours after treatment to see what lice remain. The presence of large lice may mean that the treatment was ineffective or that the lice are resistant. 5. Provide appropriate teaching for the family to prevent recurrences. a. Wash clothing, bed linens, and towels in hot water and machine dry (on hot cycle). Temperature above 53.5°C (128.3°F) for 5 minutes will kill lice and eggs. Dry cleaning or simply storing contaminated articles in a well-sealed plastic bag for 10 days is also effective. b. Caution against sharing the same hairbrush or comb. Do not wear one another's hats or headgear. Disinfect combs and brushes by soaking in hot water for 10 minutes or washing with a pediculocide shampoo.

b. In active infection, nits and eggs are close to the skin–hair junction and are difficult to remove from the hair.

application 7 days later is recommended.

5. Studies regarding the efficacy of suffocation of lice by the application of occlusive agents such as petroleum jelly, olive oil, or mayonnaise have not been done.

c. Environmental insecticide sprays are not helpful. Vacuuming is a safe alternative.
d. Household, other close contacts, and classmates of the child with head lice should be screened for parasites and treated if affected. Prophylactic treatment of head lice is unnecessary and may increase resistance. Notify the child's school or day care center so classmates can be screened.
f. Children should be allowed back to school or day care the morning after their first treatment.
g. Prophylactic treatment of all sexual contacts of adolescents and adults with pubic lice is warranted because of the high co-infection rate.

Scabies

1. A disease of the skin produced by the burrowing action of a parasite mite in the epidermis, resulting in irritation and the formation of burrows, vesicles, or pustules.
2. Etiology
   a. The mite, *Sarcoptes scabiei*, is the cause of this disorder.
   b. Scabies occurs in persons of all socioeconomic levels, regardless of personal hygiene standards.
   c. Scabies is transmitted by direct skin contact with infected persons or by indirect contact through soiled bed linen, clothing, etc.
3. Diagnosis
   Identification of a mite, ova, or feces from skin scrapings.

1. Itching, particularly at night, is the primary symptom. The onset of itching is usually insidious.
2. Secondary skin infection is common and may confuse the diagnosis.
3. Systemic manifestations are absent, unless they result from the secondary infection.
4. The burrow, a gray or white, tortuous, threadlike line, is seen most commonly in older children and adults between the fingers, in the wrists, in the axillary and buttock folds, along the belt-line, on the male genitalia, on the female breasts, and on the knees, elbows, and ankles.
5. In infants and small children, the lesions may occur on any part of the body and are usually widespread. Vesicles on the palms and soles are characteristic.
6. Incubation period in children without previous exposure is 4–6 weeks.

1. Application of a scabicide to the skin:
   a. The drug of choice is 5% permethrin (Elimite). Alternative drugs are lindane 1% and crotaminton (Eurax). Permethrin should be removed by bathing after 8–14 hours, lindane after 8–12 hours, and crotaminton after 48 hours.
   b. Lindane can cause neurotoxicity from absorption through the skin. It should be avoided in children less than 2 years of age, persons with known seizures, pregnant and lactating women, and persons with extensive dermatitis.
   c. Infected children and adults should apply the scabicidal lotion or cream on the entire body from the neck down. The entire head, neck, and body of infants and young children should be treated. It is not necessary to bathe prior to treatment.

1. Persons caring for affected children should wear gloves.
2. Contagion is unlikely 24 hours after treatment. Children may return to school or day care.
3. Teach the patient and family to launder all clothing, bed linens, and towels used by the patient during the 4 days prior to therapy with hot water and hot drying cycle to kill mites. Clothing that cannot be laundered can be stored in a plastic bag for 1 week. Further environmental disinfection is rarely necessary.
4. Itching may continue 2–3 weeks after successful therapy due to a hypersensitivity reaction to the mites. The use of oral antihistamines and topical corticosteroids can help relieve symptoms.
5. All household and close contacts should be treated prophylactically and at the same time to prevent reinfection. Caretakers with prolonged skin-to-skin contact with infected patients may also benefit from prophylactic treatment. Manifestations of scabies can occur as late as 2 months after exposure.

Oral Candidiasis (Thrush)

1. Oral candidiasis is a mycotic stomatitis characterized by the appearance of white plaques on the oral mucous membranes, the gums, and the tongue. Chronic mucocutaneous candidiasis may be associated with endocrine diseases or immunodeficiency disorders.
2. Etiology
   a. Caused by *Candida albicans*.

1. The infant develops small plaques on the oral mucous membranes, tongue, or gums. These plaques look like curds of milk but cannot be wiped out of the mouth.
2. Most infants with thrush appear to have little pain or discomfort, unless the case is severe and there is erosion and ulceration of the mucosa.

1. Oral administration of nystatin (Mycostatin) in suspension 3–4 times daily is the treatment of choice. Apply ½ dose to each side of the mouth after feeding.
2. Retain in mouth as long as possible before swallowing. Allow the child to swallow any medication to treat any lesions along the gastrointestinal tract.

1. Recognize the appearance of thrush.
2. Be aware of the infant or child who is particularly susceptible to the development of this condition, especially normal newborns under 6 months of age, low-birth-weight infants, immunocompromised or debilitated hosts, and persons on prolonged, broad-spectrum antibiotics.
3. Teach parents to inspect mouth before every feeding for presence of thrush and report the appearance of thrush.

(continued)

TABLE 55-1 Common Pediatric Skin Problems (Continued)

Disorder/Organism	Clinical Manifestations	Treatment/Prevention	Nursing/Patient Care Considerations
b. Maternal vulvovaginitis is the primary source of neonatal thrush. Evaluate for endocrine diseases or immunodeficiency disorders if thrush occurs after 6 months of life or is chronic.	3. The mouth may be dry. 4. Occasionally, the infant may appear to have some difficulty in swallowing or eat less vigorously. 5. Enteric infection is frequently associated with oral thrush.	3. Clotrimazole troches can be used in children older than 3 years of age. 4. Amphotericin B (Fungizone), clotrimazole (Lotrimin), ketoconazole (Nizoral), and newer antifungal agents are used for candidiasis resistant to nystatin. Not all of these drugs are approved for use in infants and children.	
Diaper Dermatitis 1. Candidal diaper dermatitis is a rash characterized by bright red, sharply circumscribed but moist patches with pustular satellite lesions. 2. Etiology a. Caused by *Candida albicans*, which is plentiful in humans and the environment. b. Most frequently seen in infants and toddlers wearing diapers.	1. Buttock rash consisting of erythematous maculopapular eruption with perianal distribution. 2. Generally causes discomfort, especially with wetting and cleanings. Lesions last approximately 2 weeks, desquamate, and resolve without scarring.	1. Keep the affected area clean and dry. 2. Topical application of nystatin (Mycostatin) or miconazole nitrate (Monistat) cream or ointment after gentle cleaning of the affected area. 3. Nystatin may be given orally if rash is persistent. 4. Burow's solution compresses for severe inflammation or vesiculation.	1. Recognize and teach the parents to recognize the appearance of candidal diaper dermatitis and report to health care provider. 2. Allow the infant to go without a diaper for short periods to leave area open to air. 3. Teach parents the general principles of preventing diaper dermatitis. a. Change diaper as soon as possible after wetting or soiling. Prolonged contact of feces with the skin promotes the development of candidal diaper dermatitis. Check diaper frequently. Disposable diapers are useful. b. Wash entire diaper area with warm water thoroughly and dry area before applying clean diaper. Commercial wiping agents may cause burning. c. Use a second hot rinse when washing diapers to neutralize ammonia produced when infant urinates; use vinegar, Borax, or Diaparene in wash. d. Avoid powder and oil, which tend to clog pores and cake on skin, retaining bacteria. e. Avoid occlusive plastic coverings, and tightly pinned or double diapers, all of which tend to increase production and retention of body heat and moisture.

f. Another food substance is then added, and the child is observed for the following 3- to 5-day period. This method is followed until the food allergen is determined.

Preventing Infection

1. Assess and/or treat secondary infection:
   a. Observe the skin for signs of bacterial infection (discharge, oozing, crusts). Report positive findings.
   b. Administer antibiotics as prescribed.
   c. Loosen exudate and crusts with water or wet dressings, unless otherwise specified.
   d. Note changes in the skin in response to therapy.

Family Education and Health Education

1. Teach the patient or family to avoid potential precipitants, including:
   a. Exposure to excessive heat and cold, windy weather, and rapidly changing temperatures.
   b. Contact with wool and occlusive synthetic fabrics, which promote sweating and pruritus. Soft, light-weight cotton fabrics are the preferred wearing apparel.
   c. Participation in strenuous athletic activities that promote sweating. Activities should be modified according to the needs of the child. Swimming is permitted if the child showers afterward and applies a lubricant and/or other topical medications.
   d. Use of irritating soaps, perfumes, detergents, and chemicals.
   e. Stress-stressful situations should be avoided when possible.
   f. Any foods that are associated with skin reactions.
2. Ensure that family knows when to follow up for routine appointments, worsening of condition, and signs of secondary infection.

3. Stress the importance of regular health maintenance examinations, immunizations, and preventive practices.

Outcome-Based Evaluation

- Skin intact with minimal erythema and lichenification
- Verbalizes less itching; less scratching observed
- No signs of secondary infection

Other Dermatologic Disorders

See Table 55-1.

SELECTED REFERENCES

Boiko, S. (2000). Making rash decisions in the diaper area. *Pediatric Annals, 29*(1), 50–56.

Chesney, P. J. & Burgess, I. F. (1998). Lice: Resistance and treatment. *Contemporary Pediatrics, 15*(11), 180–192.

Committee of Infectious Diseases (2000). *Red book 2000: Report of the Committee of Infectious Diseases.* (25th ed.). Elk Grove Village, IL: American Academy of Pediatrics.

Committee of Infectious Diseases (1997). *1997 red book: Report of the Committee of Infectious Diseases* (24th ed.). Elk Grove Village, IL: American Academy of Pediatrics.

Eichenfield, L. F. & Friedlander, S. F. (1998). Coping with chronic dermatitis. *Contemporary Pediatrics, 15*(10), 53–80.

Habif, T. P. (1996). *Clinical dermatology: A color guide to diagnosis and therapy* (3rd ed.). St. Louis: Mosby.

Hall, J.C. (2000). *Sauer's manual of skin diseases.* Philadelphia: Lippincott Williams & Wilkins.

Knoell, K. A. & Greer, K. E. (1999). Atopic dermatitis. *Pediatrics in Review, 20*(2), 46–51.

McEvoy, M. (2000). Pediatric impetigo. *Advance for Nurse Practitioners, 8*(2), 69–71.

Pillitteri, A. (1999). *Maternal and child health nursing* (3rd ed.). Philadelphia: Lippincott Williams & Wilkins.

Resnick, S. (1998). Principles of topical therapy. *Pediatric Annals, 27*(3), 177–184.

Siberry, G. K. & Iannone, R. (Eds.) (2000). *The Harriet Lane handbook* (15th ed.). St. Louis: Mosby.

Stein, D. H. (1998). Tineas—superficial dermatophyte infections. *Pediatrics in Review, 19*(11), 368–372.

Suarez, S. & Friedlander, S. (1998). Antifungal therapy in children: An update. *Pediatric Annals, 27*(3), 177–184.

INTRODUCTION

The spectrum of developmental disabilities is a group of interrelated chronic neurologic handicaps. It includes cerebral palsy, mental retardation, pervasive developmental disorder, autism, learning disabilities, communication disorders, anxiety disorders, and attention deficit disorders. These conditions are suspected or noticed at varying stages during childhood. Some conditions, like Down syndrome, can be recognized prenatally or at birth; other conditions, such as cerebral palsy or autism, may not present themselves until the child fails to meet normal developmental milestones. This phenomenon makes the nurse's role in developmental disabilities crucial. The pediatric nurse who understands that the development of the child occurs in an orderly, predictable manner and who is knowledgeable of what the milestones should be may be the first person to recognize the deviation and raise the suspicion to the parent or pediatrician. Since there are many confusing and overlapping characteristics for many of these conditions, it is of the utmost importance for the health care provider and family to use experienced and knowledgeable developmental specialists to arrive at an accurate diagnosis and arrange an appropriate care plan.

When a known condition exists, the nurse should be aware of the health issues associated with the condition and the resources available to promote the optimal growth and development of the child within the family.

This chapter will provide some cursory information about some of the more common conditions. It is also important to keep in mind that there are differences in the severity of all of the developmental disabilities as well as overlapping conditions.

> ### NURSING ALERT
>
> **Normal child development is very predictable and sequential. The nurse who is knowledgeable about normal development may be the first person to raise the question that a developmental disability exists.**

Signs of Developmental Delay
Criteria for Referral
Communication and Feeding
1. Feeding difficulties—inability to coordinate suck-swallowing to sustain normal weight gain
2. No social smile by 4 months
3. No babbling (Mamma, Dada) by 9 months
4. No Mamma, Dada (specific) by 14 months
5. No name of object (1 word) by 14 months
6. At least 10 words by 18 months (not just repeating)
7. Combines words (eg, me outside, more milk) and uses pronouns by 24 months

> ### NURSING ALERT
>
> **Always rule out vision and hearing impairment when a delay is present.**

Motor Delay
1. Not rolling by 6 months
2. Not sitting by 9 months
3. Not walking by 15 months
4. Not stair-climbing by 2 years

See Chapter 40 for normal pediatric growth and development.

Care of the Child With a Developmental Disability

Nursing Assessment

1. Review the child's record to determine prior existing health problems that may cause or affect the developmental disability. Always rule out a vision or hearing impairment.
2. Assess the family's understanding of the diagnosis and its ramifications. The parents' experiences, cultural biases, cognitive ability, stage of grief, and physical condition affect their ability to assimilate information provided. It will be necessary to repeat the information. (For example, a woman who has just given birth to a child with Down syndrome will not be able to retain much information until her body returns to a state of homeostasis.)
3. Determine the developmental age of the child. The pediatric nurse should be familiar with normal development milestones (Chapter 40, p. 1223), noting the areas of strengths and weaknesses of the child in each area of development, for example, the communication skills are at a 12-month level and the gross motor skills are at a 36-month level. Children who are found to be functioning at one-half or less of their chronologic age have a moderate to severe developmental problem.
4. Administer the Clinical Adaptive Test-Clinical Linguistic Auditory Milestone Scales (CAT-CLAMS). It is a reliable tool that nurses can be trained to use to assess cognitive and communicative development in children at the 1- to 36-month developmental level. It has been found to be more sensitive than the Denver Developmental Screening Scale, because language development is the best early predictor of cognitive abilities (Table 56-1).
5. Assess the functional level of the child. The WeeFIM is a tool used to track functional independence in children. It uses the following categories to describe function: completely dependent, needs some physical assistance, is physically able to perform the task but needs verbal cues and coaching, and completely independent. Functional areas to assess include:
   a. Feeding
   b. Grooming and bathing
   c. Dressing
   d. Mobility
   e. Problem solving
   f. Communication
6. Assess parents' perception of the child's development level and the appropriateness of parental expectations. Use questions such as, "What age child does your child act like?" or "In the area of communication, how does your child's ability compare with other children the same age?"
7. Assess parent–child interaction. Observe and explore bonding and attachment, ability to set appropriate limits, management of behavioral problems, and methods of discipline.
8. Assess the need for additional resources, such as financial aid, transportation, and counseling, for long-term support of child and family.

Nursing Diagnoses

- Impaired Adjustment related to birth/diagnosis of developmentally disabled child
- Altered Parenting related to multiple needs of child and difficult bonding
- Ineffective Infant Feeding Pattern related to protruding tongue, poor muscle tone, and weak sucking
- Altered Growth and Development related to disability
- Social Isolation related to developmental differences from other children
- Risk for Injury related to developmental age

Nursing Interventions

Promoting Adjustment

1. Allow the parents access to the baby at all possible times to promote bonding when parents appear ready.
2. Focus on the positive aspects of the baby and serve as a role model for handling and stimulating.
3. Be cognizant of the grieving process (loss of the "normal child") that families experience when a diagnosis is made, and be aware that spouses can be at different stages.
4. Accept all questions and reactions nonjudgmentally, offering verbal and written explanations.
5. Provide the family a quiet place to discuss their questions with each other and someone knowledgeable about the condition (primary care provider, clinical nurse specialist) to support them in grieving.
6. Offer the family the option to take advantage of counseling. A social worker or psychologist can assist families to deal with immediate reactions. Many parents benefit from continuous or periodic support of counseling professionals.

> **NURSING ALERT**
>
> Children with developmental disabilities and chronic illness are at greater risk of experiencing divorce, child abuse, and neglect than the general population.

Strengthening the Role of Parents

1. Help the family to realize what strengths they have in caring for their child. The role of the parents is critical; a nurturing, loving environment gives the child the best chance at maximizing potential. Individuals who grow up at home have markedly higher adaptive abilities and increased life spans compared with children raised in institutions.
2. Enlist the help of family and siblings who can offer valuable support to the parents and child and assist with stimulation activities. Including siblings in the care can help them feel needed and involved, thus strengthening the family.

TABLE 56-1 The CAT (Clinical Adaptive Test) and CLAMS (Clinical Linguistic Auditory Milestone Scales)

Clinical Linguistic Auditory Milestone Scales (CLAMS)				Clinical Adaptive Test (CAT)	
	Yes	No	Age(mos)		Yes	No
1 month Alerts to sound (0.5).	—	—	—	**1 month** Visually fixates momentarily upon red ring (0.5).	—	—
Soothes when picked up (0.5).	—	—	—	Lifts chin off table in prone (0.5).	—	—
2 months Social smile (1.0).	—	—	—	**2 months** Visually follows ring in circle (0.5). Lifts chest off table prone (0.5).	— —	— —
3 months Cooing (1.0).	—	—	—	**3 months** Visually follows ring horizontally and vertically (0.5). Supports on forearms in prone (0.3). Visual threat (0.3).	— — —	— — —
4 months Orients to voice (0.5). Laughs aloud (0.5).	— —	— —	— —	**4 months** Unfisted (0.3). Manipulates fingers (0.3). Supports on wrists in prone (0.3).	— — —	— — —
5 months Orients toward bell laterally (0.3). Ah-goo (0.3). Razzing (0.3).	— — —	— — —	— — —	**5 months** Pulls down rings (0.3). Transfers (0.3). Regards pellet (0.3).	— — —	— — —
6 months Babbling (1.0).	—	—	—	**6 months** Obtains cube (0.3). Lifts cup (0.3). Radial rake (0.3).	— — —	— — —
7 months Orients toward bell (1.0), upwardly indirectly (90°).	—	—	—	**7 months** Attempts pellet (0.3). Pulls out peg (0.3). Inspects ring (0.3).	— — —	— — —
8 months Says "Dada" inappropriately (0.5). Says "Mama" inappropriately (0.5).	— —	— —	— —	**8 months** Pulls ring by string (0.3). Secures pellet (0.3). Inspects bell (0.3).	— — —	— — —
9 months Orients toward bell upward directly (180°) (0.5). Gesture language (0.5).	— —	— —	— —	**9 months** 30-finger scissor grasp (0.3). Rings bell (0.3). Over the edge for toy (0.3).	— — —	— — —
10 months Understands "no" (0.3). Uses "dada" appropriately (0.3). Uses "mama" appropriately (0.3).	— — —	— — —	— — —	**10 months** Combines cube-cup (0.3). Uncovers bell (0.3). Fingers pegboard (0.3).	— — —	— — —
11 months 1 word (other than "mama" & "dada") (1.0).	—	—	—	**11 months** Mature overhand pincer movement (0.5). Solves cube under cup (0.5).	— —	— —
12 months 1-step command with gesture (0.5). 2-word vocabulary (0.5).	— —	— —	— —	**12 months** Releases 1 cube in cup (0.5). Crayon mark (0.5).	— —	— —
14 months 3-word vocabulary (1.0). Immature jargoning (1.0).	— —	— —	— —	**14 months** Solves glass frustration (0.6). Out-in with peg (0.6). Solves pellet-bottle with demonstration (0.6).	— — —	— — —

(continued)

TABLE 56-1 The CAT and CLAMS (Continued)

Clinical Linguistic Auditory Milestone Scales (CLAMS)				Clinical Adaptive Test (CAT)	
	Yes	No	Age(mos)	Yes	No
16 months Four- to six-word vocabulary (1.0). One-step command without gesture (1.0).	___	___	___		
16 months Solves pellet-bottle spontaneously (0.6). Round block in formboard (0.6). Scribbles in imitation (0.6).				___ ___ ___	___ ___ ___
18 months Mature jargoning (0.5). 7-to-10-word vocabulary (0.5) Body parts (0.5). Points to one picture (0.5).	___ ___ ___ ___	___ ___ ___ ___	___ ___ ___ ___		
18 months 10 cubes in cup (0.5). Solves round hole in formboard reversed (0.5). Spontaneous scribbling with crayon (0.5). Pegboard completed spontaneously (0.5).				___ ___ ___ ___	___ ___ ___ ___
21 months 20-word vocabulary (1.0). 2-word phrases (1.0). Points to two pictures (1.0).	___ ___ ___	___ ___ ___	___ ___ ___		
21 months Obtains object with stick (1.0). Solves square in formboard (1.0). Tower of 3 cubes (1.0).				___ ___ ___	___ ___ ___
24 months 50-word vocabulary (1.0). 2-step command (1.0). Pronouns (I, you, me) inappropriately (1.0).	___ ___ ___	___ ___ ___	___ ___ ___		
24 months Attempts to fold paper (0.7). Horizontal 4-cube train. Imitates stroke with pencil (0.7). Completes formboard (0.7).				___ ___ ___ ___	___ ___ ___ ___
30 months Uses pronouns appropriately (1.5). Concept of one (1.5). Points to 7 pictures (1.5). 2 digits forward (1.5).	___ ___ ___ ___	___ ___ ___ ___	___ ___ ___ ___		
30 months Horizontal-vertical stroke with pencil (1.5). Formboard reversed (1.5). Folds paper with definite crease (1.5). Train with chimney (1.5).				___ ___ ___ ___	___ ___ ___ ___
36 months 250-word vocabulary (1.5). 3-word sentence (1.5) 3-digits forward (1.5). Follows 2 prepositional commands (1.5).	___ ___ ___ ___	___ ___ ___ ___	___ ___ ___ ___		
36 months 3-cube bridge (1.5). Draws circle (1.5). Names 1 color (1.5). Draw-a-person with head plus 1 other body part (1.5).				___ ___ ___ ___	___ ___ ___ ___

Reliability of informant _____
  (0 = unreliable;
  1 = reliable).					

3. If sibling issues arise, suggest counseling.
4. Identify resources available to the family, such as parent support groups, early intervention programs, specialty clinics, pediatrician/primary health care provider, financial support programs, and advocacy groups for individuals with developmental disabilities.
5. For those parents concerned with their ability to care for the child, explore with them their options of adoption or institutionalization in a nonjudgmental manner.

Establishing Effective Feeding Techniques

1. Be aware of the poor neurologic development of children with Down syndrome and of infants with other developmental disabilities and how this interferes with sucking and swallowing.
2. Demonstrate proper feeding positioning, with head elevated, and encourage the parents to always hold the infant during feedings with head elevated and supported in arms.
3. Try different nipples and bottles to determine which is easiest for infant to use without leakage or danger of aspiration.
4. Allow adequate time for feeding, and increase frequency of feedings if infant tires easily.
5. Offer support and guidance for breast-feeding.
6. If feeding remains difficult, consider referral to a speech therapist, who is knowledgeable in the area and may be beneficial.

Promoting Optimum Growth and Development

1. Help the parents to understand the concept of developmental age, and identify the functional level of the child.
2. Determine whether there is consistency between the developmental age of the child and degree of independence. Cognitive and physical limitations may interfere with emerging independence; however, parents may "baby" or overindulge a child who has a disability.

3. Work with parents to set reasonable expectations and to break tasks down into simple, achievable steps. Care should be taken not to address too many areas at one time so as not to overwhelm the family.
4. Use appropriate behavior modification techniques, such as extinction, time-out, and reward, to achieve cooperation and success.
5. Demonstrate and encourage play with the child at the appropriate level to provide stimulation, and work toward achieving developmental milestones.
6. Refer parents to the Early Intervention Program administered by their county so that they can take advantage of the educational and support services available for infants from birth to 3 years of age.
7. If condition is identified after the age of 3 years, refer parents for help through the Pupil Personnel Department of the school system in which they reside.

Providing Meaningful Social Interaction

1. Make parents aware that recreational and leisure-time experiences are valuable in building social skills and self-esteem.
2. Offer suggestions that will be enjoyable and developmentally appropriate for child. In general, individuals with developmental delays do better in small groups. Interaction with both developmentally delayed and non-developmentally delayed peers is desirable. The Special Olympics is one example of an adaptive program. Local programs are available in many areas. Social outings, such as sight-seeing, camping, dances, and dating opportunities, are also important for older children.
3. Praise child for participation in activities, regardless of whether the child succeeds or fails.

Maintaining Safety

1. When handling the infant, provide adequate support with a firm grasp, because infant may be very floppy due to poor muscle tone.
2. Position the infant so that if vomiting should occur, aspiration will be prevented.
   a. Prop infant with a diaper roll so that position will be maintained.
   b. Change position frequently, because the infant is not usually very active.
   c. Continuously check environment for safety needs for this child.

NURSING ALERT

Teach caregivers to base safety needs on the developmental, not the chronologic, age of the child.

3. Advise the parents to:
   a. Maintain constant surveillance of the child when cooking or exposing child to other potential hazards that child may be able to get into but not understand.
   b. Help child to read words such as "danger" and "stop."
   c. Teach child how to call and ask for help.
   d. Teach child to say no to strangers.

e. Provide sex education in a way the child can understand.

Family Education and Health Maintenance

1. Remind the parents to recognize the child's routine health care needs and maintain regular follow-up with a primary care provider.
   a. Immunizations
   b. Regular dental checkups
   c. Visual and hearing examinations
2. Teach parents to provide a therapeutic home environment.
   a. Maintain regular sleeping, eating, working, and playing routines.
   b. Ensure adequate nutrition.
   c. Divide tasks and expectations into small, manageable parts. Give only one or two instructions at a time.
   d. Set firm but reasonable limits on behavior and carry through with consistent discipline.
   e. Avoid situations that cause excessive excitement, stimulation, or fatigue.
   f. Provide energy outlet through physical activity, vocal outlet, and outdoor play.
   g. Channel need for movement into safe, appropriate activities.
3. Discuss preparation for independent living.
   a. Help the parents identify areas of home responsibilities that may be delegated to the retarded child.
   b. Teach habits that are essential to later vocational life, such as getting to places on time, cooperating, focusing on the task at hand, and establishing acceptable interpersonal relationships.
   c. Help the child to develop a set of attitudes and behaviors that will increase motivation.
   d. Refer for vocational assistance to ARC (formerly Association of Retarded Citizens) or other rehabilitative agencies.
4. Refer for genetic consultation for information about genetics of the disorder, risk in subsequent pregnancies (parents) or risk to offspring (patient), or risk to other relatives as it is warranted by the diagnosis.
5. Encourage compliance with the multidimensional treatment plan, and make sure parents know whom to contact when problems arise. Encourage parents to develop a system (such as notebook with calendar) to keep track of all agencies, subspecialists, and professionals who will be involved with their child. It should include names, addresses, phone numbers, appointment dates, health providers' orders, and insurance information.

Outcome-Based Evaluation

- Parents holding infant frequently and seeking information from health care provider
- Parents and siblings feeding and assisting with care of infant
- Infant feeding for 15 to 20 minutes every 1 to 2 hours; taking 50 to 100 mL

- Parents describe developmental level of child and realistic goals for attainment of next milestones
- Parents seeking information about Special Olympics
- Child describes concept of stranger and appropriate response if approached

DEVELOPMENTAL DISABILITIES

Cognitive Developmental Delay

Cognitive developmental delay, also known as *mental retardation,* refers to the most severe, general lack of cognitive and problem-solving skills. The American Association on Mental Deficiency defines mental retardation as a significant subaverage general intellectual functioning existing concurrently with deficits in adaptive behaviors and manifested during the developmental period. There are many causes and a wide range of impairments. Three percent of the U.S. population— 6.6 million people—are considered mentally retarded. Of every 1,000 babies born, 30 will be classified as mentally retarded before they reach the age of 18.

Pathophysiology and Etiology
1. No identifiable organic or biologic cause can be found for 50% of children.
2. Identifiable causes include:
   a. Genetic causes, such as Down syndrome and fragile X syndrome, and inborn errors of metabolism, such as phenylketonuria (PKU)
   b. Congenital anomalies, including brain malformations, hydrocephalus, and microcephaly
   c. Intrauterine influences, such as congenital infections, drug exposure, and teratogens
   d. Perinatal trauma—birth anoxia, intracranial hemorrhage
   e. Postnatal trauma—head injuries from falls, motor vehicle accidents
   f. Postnatal infections (meningitis, sepsis)
   g. Environmental exposure to toxins, such as lead; environmental deprivation; and neglect
3. The malfunctioning brain is poorly understood in most cases, but physiologic alterations identified in some cases include:
   a. Congenital brain malformations, brain tissue damage, or underdevelopment of the brain as shown by abnormal results of computed tomography (CT) scan or magnetic resonance imaging (MRI)
   b. Biochemical or errors of metabolism, in which an absence of an enzyme or hormone produces abnormal brain function or formation, as in PKU or hypothyroidism
4. Intelligence quotient (IQ) is 75 or below; classification has been recently changed to mild and severe and includes both cognitive and functional ability.
   a. The more severe types of mental retardation tend to be diagnosed in early infancy, especially when they coexist with an identifiable syndrome or congenital anomalies.
   b. Milder forms of mental retardation tend to be diagnosed in preschool years, when language and behavioral concerns call attention to slower development.
5. Limitations in adaptive ability occur in communication, self-care, home living, social skills, community use, self-direction, health and safety, functional academics, leisure, and work.

Clinical Manifestations
Developmental delays (failure to achieve age-appropriate skills) are evident to some degree in almost all areas.
Infancy
1. "Poor feeder"—a weak or uncoordinated suck results in poor breast- or bottle-feeding, leading to poor weight gain
2. Delayed or decreased visual alertness and curiosity with poor visual tracking of face or objects
3. Decreased or lack of auditory response
4. Decreased spontaneous activity
5. Delayed head and trunk control

> **NURSING ALERT**
>
> Although 75% of individuals with mental retardation have no physical signs, they often achieve motor milestones at a slower rate.

6. Floppy (hypotonia) or spastic muscle tone
Toddler
1. Delayed independent sitting, crawling, pull to stand, and independent ambulation.
2. Delayed communication—failure to develop receptive and expressive language milestones. Almost half of children with mental retardation are identified after the age of 3 years, when speech delays manifest themselves.
3. Failure of the child to make progress or show interest in the area of independence in self-feeding, dressing, and toilet training may reflect cognitive impairment.
4. Short attention span and distractibility.
5. Behavioral disturbances.
6. Clumsiness.

Diagnostic Evaluation
Federal Law (PL 94-142—Education for All Handicapped Children and PL 101-476— Individuals with Disabilities Education Act [IDEA]) ensures that each child with a delay or suspected of having a delay has a multidisciplinary evaluation by a team. Part C of PL 105-17 called for the creation of statewide, coordinated, multidisciplinary, interagency programs for the provision of early intervention. Each state has its own definitions and organizational framework to provide these services. No single test can diagnose mental retardation. The multidisciplinary evaluation should be individually tailored to the child.

1. Rule out sensory deficits by assessment of vision and hearing.
2. Medical evaluation should include developmental history, sequential developmental assessments, family history, and physical examination. The positive findings determine the direction of the individual evaluation.
   a. Unusual appearance (dysmorphic features) warrants genetic workup.
   b. History consistent with loss of developmental milestones and positive family history warrants workup for presence of an inborn error of metabolism (diagnosed by blood and urine analysis) or lead poisoning.
   c. Children with macrocephaly, microcephaly, or neurologic abnormalities may require a CT scan or MRI.
   d. Electroencephalogram is necessary for children with seizures.
3. Psychological testing (appropriate tests selected by a child psychologist):
   a. The Bayley Scales are used to assess fine motor, gross motor, and language skills and visual problem solving in infants of developmental age of 2 months to 3 years (this test is weighted on nonlanguage items).
   b. The McCarthy Scale offers a "general cognitive index" that is roughly equivalent to an IQ score.
   c. The Stanford-Binet Intelligence Scale is used to test children with mental abilities of 2 years and older.
   d. The Wechsler Preschool and Primary Scale of Intelligence (WPPSI) (1991) measures mental age of 3 to 7 years.
   e. The Wechsler Intelligence Scale for Children (WISC) III (1991) tests children whose functional age is above a 6-year level.
   f. The Vineland Scale tests social-adaptive abilities—self-help skills, self-control, interaction with others, cooperation; the Adaptive Behavior Scale is similar to Vineland but also measures adjustment.

Complications and Associated Findings

1. Seizures
2. Cerebral palsy
3. Sensory deficits
4. Communication disorders (speech and language)
5. Neurodegenerative disorders
6. Psychiatric illness
7. Specific learning disabilities
8. Emotional problems

Management

1. An interdisciplinary team evaluation by a developmental pediatrician, clinical psychologist, and counselor is usually the initial step in the management of mental retardation. This type of evaluation can be obtained through a state or private diagnostic and evaluation center, public school, or university-affiliated program.

2. If a treatable cause is identified, such as an inborn error of metabolism, a therapeutic diet can be instituted. Hypothyroidism can be treated with thyroid hormone.
3. Associated medical problems, such as seizures, poor nutrition, sensory deficits, or dental problems, must be treated to allow the child to maximize his or her potential.
4. A family assessment is essential to address:
   a. Financial stressors—financial aid may be available through Social Security Income, Medicaid, or state and local programs to help families with children with mental retardation
   b. Family coping abilities
   c. Support for siblings
   d. Respite services
   e. Support groups
   f. Recreational programs, for example, Special Olympics, summer camps
   g. Identification of other affected or at-risk persons
5. The initial evaluation often leads to recommendations for more targeted evaluations, such as physical therapy, occupational therapy, and social work assessment.

■ Down Syndrome

Down syndrome, or *trisomy 21,* is the most common identifiable cause of mental retardation and a condition associated with a variety of congenital anomalies. Each child with Down syndrome has a unique set of genes besides the effects of the extra genes on the 21st chromosome, and he or she will need individualized evaluation. The most common life experience of a child with Down syndrome is to live with the family, participate in infant stimulation and preschool programs, and attend school while receiving some support for special education. Adults with Down syndrome can function in supported employment programs and live in small groups. Their life expectancy depends on the presence of medical complications; when there are no complications, life expectancy is slightly shorter than average. Down syndrome is one of the most widely known syndromes associated with mental retardation.

Pathophysiology and Etiology

See Chapter 4, page 33.

Clinical Manifestations and Associated Problems

1. Characteristic facies—brachycephaly; oblique palpebral fissures; epicanthal folds; flat nasal bridge; protruding tongue; small, low-set ears; simean crease of palms (Figure 56-1)
2. Congenital heart defects
3. Mental retardation
4. Hypotonia
5. Growth retardation
6. Scaly, dry skin

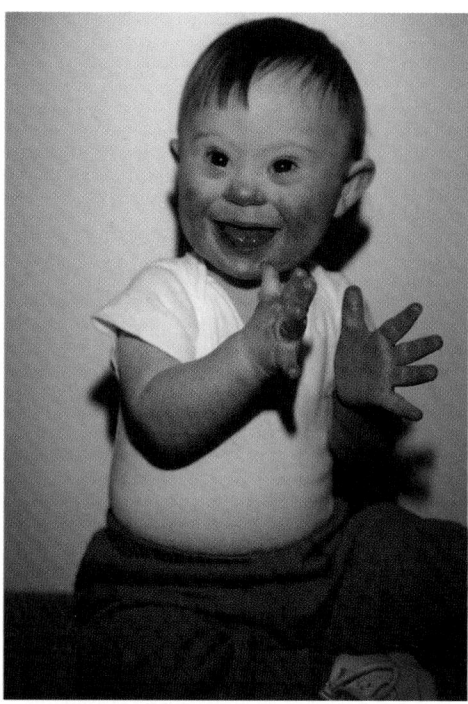

FIGURE 56-1 One-year-old with Down syndrome, recently diagnosed with hypothyroidism.

7. Table 56-2 provides a comprehensive list of potential problems that occur with Down syndrome. Some are identified at birth; others arise and cause difficulties later in the life cycle. Percentages are listed that represent occurrence within the Down syndrome population.

Diagnosis and Management

1. See Cognitive Developmental Delay for general approach to assessment.
2. See Table 56-2 for specific medical issues related to Down syndrome, such as thyroid, cardiac, etc.
3. Alternative therapies—nutritional and supplemental vitamin therapy for Down syndrome remains controversial, and its effects have not been medically proved.

◼ Fragile X Syndrome

Fragile X syndrome is the second most common identifiable cause of mental retardation, as well as the most common inherited cause. Diagnosis is often not made until mid-childhood or later. Chromosome analysis reveals that the long arm of the X chromosome is constricted and appears fragile, but this cannot be detected in all cases; thus, DNA analysis is preferred for diagnosis. This anomaly is seen more commonly in males; however, females can be symptomatic or may display very mild symptoms.

Pathophysiology and Etiology
See Chapter 4, page 33.

TABLE 56-2 Down Syndrome		
Potential Problems	**Evaluation**	**Management**
Congenital heart malformations (ie, AV canal, VSD, PDA, and tetralogy of Fallot) (40%)	Observe for color changes, pulse, and respiratory rate at rest and with stress. Assess tolerance of feeding for early tiring or frequent interruptions in feeding. Echocardiogram usually done during newborn period on all infants with DS.	Early identification and treatment can prevent congestive heart failure and decompensation or poor growth. Medical or surgical correction is possible to repair the defect.
Congenital gastrointestinal malformations (12%): Pyloric stenosis Duodenal atresia, tracheoesophageal fistula	Observe for coughing or vomiting, especially with feeding: bile-stained vomitus suggests lower tract abnormalities; partially digested contents suggest upper tract problem. Observe bowel movements and for distention of abdomen. Radiographic studies are done.	Spillage of material from esophagus into the trachea can cause aspiration and pneumonia. Surgical intervention occurs in early newborn period.
Hypothyroidism (10–20%)	Monitor for weight gain, hair loss, lethargy, short stature, voice changes, and depression (can develop at any time over life cycle). Newborn screening includes T_3, TSH, T_4 biannually.	Thyroid hormone replacement.
Visual defects: Refractive errors (70%) Strabismus (50%) Nystagmus (35%) Cataracts (3%)	Use Teller activity as a visual screen tool for those who cannot cooperate with Snellen chart. Positive findings in first year of life warrant immediate referral to ophthalmologist. All individuals should be seen by an ophthalmologist at 1 year of age, and vision screening should continue throughout life.	Undetected visual deficits can cause failure to achieve developmental milestones and cause permanent loss of vision.

(continued)

TABLE 56-2 Down Syndrome (Continued)

Potential Problems	Evaluation	Management

Hearing defects (60–90%):
   Mild–moderate conductive hearing loss
   Enlarged adenoids
   Sleep apnea
	Assess for curiosity and response to sounds of varying quality. Auditory brain stem response assesses hearing in infants. Sound field testing for children over 1 year of age.
	Tympanometry to assess middle ear function.
		Narrow ear canals and subtle immune deficiencies can cause chronic middle ear infections. Enlarged adenoids can cause upper airway obstruction especially during sleep.
		Treatment can range from antibiotics for simple otitis media to myringotomy tubes, adenoidectomy, or hearing loss.

Hypotonia of infants (100%)	Observe for floppiness, poor head control, poor oral motor function. Infant should be placed on abdomen periodically while being observed and monitored for potential for suffocation.	Physical, occupational, and speech therapy. Adaptive equipment gives extra support to head and neck when handling newborn. Always keep head elevated for at least 1 hour after meals. Change position regularly.
Atlanto-occipital and atlanto-axial subluxation (dislocation of the upper spine due to joint laxity) (15%)	Assess for head tilt; increasing clumsiness, limping, or refusal to walk; weakness of arms. X-ray of spine at age 2 years and then every 5 years during childhood. Precise measurements are taken to document alignment of the skull and vertebrae. Shifting of the two causes compression and neurologic damage.	If present, participation in contact sports and gymnastics is contraindicated. In severe cases, surgery to fuse the vertebrae and occiput and stabilize spinal column.
Gait abnormalities (15%)	Monitor for onset of limp, leg length discrepancy. Hip x-rays can document dislocation or subluxation.	Physical therapy and sometimes orthopedic surgery are necessary.
Failure to thrive	Monitor growth on Down syndrome growth chart. Monitor feedings for length of feeding, feeding schedule, loss of feeding by vomiting or poor seal on nipple. Monitor type of formula and caloric content.	Nutritionist can advise on formula adjustments. Therapists can help with positioning types of nipples used to counteract effects of weak sucking reflex and large, protruding tongue.
Short stature (100%)	Plot growth on Down syndrome growth chart. Monitor stages of puberty. Delayed puberty may warrant further investigation.	Use of human growth hormone may be considered; this is still controversial.
Obesity (50%)	Monitor thyroid hormone levels. Serial monitoring of weight. Monitor for amount of exercise, caloric intake.	Overindulgence by adults or use of food in behavior management increases risk of overeating. Lack of social involvement lead to decreased activity. Behavior modification is necessary.
Malocclusions (60–100%)	Assess for malocclusions, periodontal disease, delayed eruption of teeth. Regular dental checkups begin at age 2.	Encourage good oral hygiene with proper teeth brushing.
Mental retardation with varying degrees from mild to moderate (100%)	Routine developmental assessment using standardized tools of measurement.	Special education and training.
Alzheimer's disease after the age of 40 years (15–30%)	Assess for decreased cognitive function and loss of memory. MRI or CT scan shows areas of plaque.	Increased supervision is needed.
Seizures (6%)	Onset of seizures is seen primarily during adolescence and middle age.	Neurologic evaluation and appropriate antiseizure medications.

Other problems:
   Communication Disorders
   Alopecia 10%
   Leukemia 1%		

VSD: ventricular septal defect; AV: atrioventricular; DS: Down syndrome; T_3: triiodothyronine; TSH: thyroid stimulating hormone; T_4:levothyroxine; MRI: magnetic resonance imaging; CT: computed tomography.

Clinical Manifestations and Associated Problems

1. Mild to moderate mental retardation
2. Elongated face, prominent ears, macrocephaly, high-arched palate
3. Macroorchidism after puberty
4. Autistic-like communication disorders
5. Attention deficit, hyperactivity
6. Self-stimulating and self-injurious behaviors
7. Associated problems, including mitral valve prolapse, seizures, hypotonia, and feeding problems

Diagnosis and Management

1. See Cognitive Developmental Delay for general approach to management.
2. See Table 56-3 for specific medical issues related to Fragile X syndrome.

■ Turner Syndrome

Turner syndrome is a genetic disorder found in females. There is an absence of a normal second sex chromosome. The incidence of this syndrome is approximately 1 in 2500 female live births. Genetic analysis reveals a 45, X chromosome constitution. There are often mosaic variations seen with Turner syndrome.

Pathophysiology and Etiology

See Chapter 4, page 33.

Clinical Manifestations and Associated Problems

1. The most prevalent characteristics of Turner syndrome include:
   a. Short stature, webbed neck, low posterior hairline, edema of the hands and feet (Figure 56-2)
   b. Congenital cardiac defects
   c. Broad chest with inverted or underdeveloped nipples
   d. Immature reproductive organs, primary amennorrhea
   e. Learning disabilities
2. Associated problems include:
   a. Coarctation of the aorta, idiopathic hypertension
   b. Hearing loss—conductive or sensorineural
   c. Obesity, glucose intolerance
   d. Feeding problems
   e. Renal anomalies

TABLE 56-3 Fragile X Syndrome

Potential Problems	Evaluation	Management
Hypotonia of infancy	Assess ability to control head and assume upright posture. Assess feeding for efficient suck and coordination of suck/swallow.	Physical therapy, stimulation program, feeding adaptations.
Seizures (20% of cases)	Assess for muscle tremors, deviation of eyes to one side, rhythmic jerking of the body, and loss of consciousness.	Referral to neurologist for diagnosis and anticonvulsants to treat seizures.
Mitral valve prolapse (80% of males)	Assess dyspnea, cyanosis, murmur. Echocardiogram to evaluate valve function.	Antibiotics for prophylaxis before invasive procedures to prevent endocarditis. Treatment of congestive heart failure; surgical repair may be necessary.
Self-stimulating behavior	Rule out any source of pain (ie, otitis media, tooth pain) that may be causing behavior. Rule out sensory deficits.	Behavior management techniques: Focus on replacing undesirable behaviors with purposeful, meaningful substitutes, with emphasis on positive reinforcement and extinguishing negative reinforcement.
Hyperactivity attention deficits	Assess activity of attention span within the context of the developmental age of the child.	Behavior management and special educational techniques.
Discipline problems	Assess social skills.	Boys tend to do best in self-contained classrooms for children with similar degrees of mental retardation.
Communication disorders	Assess language development (often weakest area of development).	Speech–language therapy can be beneficial.
Poor auditory memory; auditory reception	Assess how child lets needs be known: cries, gestures, single words, and/or sentences.	Speech therapy, behavior modification.
Cognitive dysfunction: Short-term memory deficits Poor problem-solving skills Functional limitations in self-care	Assess for appropriateness of educational placement and child's reaction to situation.	Specialized training and education, assisted living.

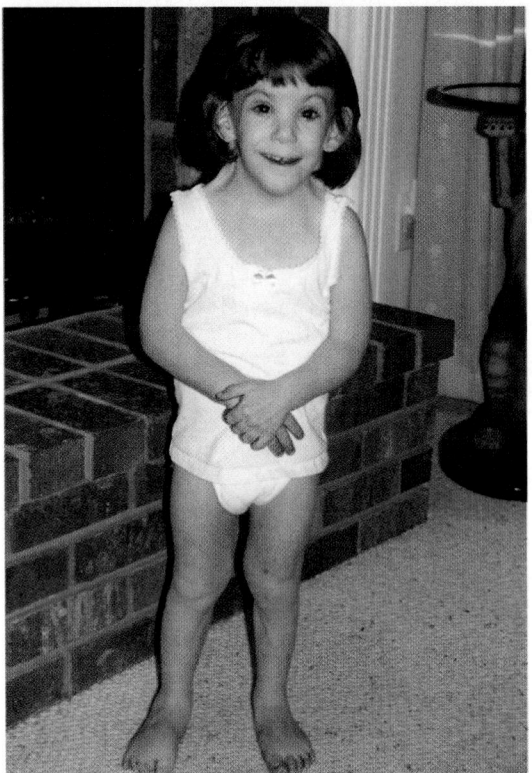

FIGURE 56-2 Three-year-old with Turner syndrome. Note the webbed neck.

Diagnosis and Management
1. See Cognitive Developmental Delay for general approach to assessment.
2. See Table 56-4 for specific medical issues related to Turner syndrome.
3. Diagnosis may occur prenatally through an amniocentesis, with genetic testing, or any time after birth. A preliminary diagnosis may be made based on physical characteristics. This should then be confirmed by genetic testing. A diagnosis may not be made until there is a failure to begin menstruation.

PERVASIVE DEVELOPMENTAL DISORDERS

Pervasive developmental disorders is a term applied to neurologic disorders affecting communicative, social interactive skills as well as characteristic behaviors. The disorders under this heading include autism, Rett's disorder, childhood disintegrative disorder, and Asperger's disorder, as well as a category labeled Pervasive Developmental Disorder Not Otherwise Specified (PDDNOS).

Autism

The diagnosis of autism is based on the display of at least six out of twelve symptoms in three categories. These categories include impairments in social interactions; communication impairments; and display of characteristic behaviors, interests, or activities typically seen with autism. Autism is a lifelong disorder. Most people with autism function with an IQ ranging from 35 to 50. Autism is seen in approximately 2 to 5 per 1000 live births. It is four to five times more prevalent in males than females.

Pathophysiology and Etiology
1. Very little is known about the etiology. No genetic implications have been identified at this time.
2. Studies have shown that the measles, mumps and rubella vaccine does *not* cause autism. Thimerisol, a preservative found in many vaccines, does *not* cause autism.
3. Prior to diagnosis, parents may be initially concerned about their infant's interactions and reactions to various stimuli. Typically, these interactions and reactions will improve to an individualized extent as the child grows and develops.

Diagnosis and Management
1. See Cognitive Developmental Delay, diagnosis and treatment, for general approach to assessment.
2. Alternative treatments: nutrition and vitamin therapy approaches are being investigated but no definitive research is conclusive at this time.

Rett's Disorder

Rett's disorder presents in females with manifestations following "normal" development through the first 5 months of life. This normal period is followed by a loss of previously attained motor skills and coordination. There are also severe delays with expressive and receptive language development as well as psychomotor delays. These regressive symptoms begin before 4 years of age, most commonly appearing in the first or second year. A clinical characteristic correlated with Rett's disorder is a decelerated rate of head growth between 5 and 48 months of life.

Pathophysiology and Etiology
There is very little information regarding the etiology and incidence of Rett's disorder. The incidence of the disorder is rare.

Diagnosis and Management
1. The prognosis of Rett's disorder is very limited. Some small increases in development and interactions may be achieved in late childhood and early adolescence; however, the disorder is lifelong.
2. See Cognitive Developmental Delay for general approach to assessment.

TABLE 56-4 Turner's Syndrome

Potential Problems	Evaluation	Management
Congenital heart malformations: increased incidence of left-sided cardiac anomalies, aortic valve anomalies, coarctation of the aorta	Observe for color changes, pulse, and respiratory rate at rest and with stress. Monitor BP. Assess tolerance of feeding for early tiring or frequent interruptions in feeding. An EKG should be done in the newborn period. A yearly echocardiogram or MRI should be done.	Early identification and treatment can prevent secondary problems. If needed, prophylactic antibiotic for subacute bacterial endocarditis. Referral to a cardiologist.
Renal and renovascular anomalies: horseshoe kidney, duplicated renal pelvis, vascular anomalies	Renal sonogram should be done to rule out anomalies. Routine urinalysis and culture to screen for UTI, glycosuria.	Referral to a nephrologist if a renal anomaly is present. Monitor for the development of DM.
Edema in the hands and feet	Edema may persist for months or may recur; if recurrence, monitor for renal or cardiac causes.	
Dysmorphic features: webbed neck, face, ears	Parents may elect plastic surgery to minimize the visual defects.	Enhances the socialization of Turner syndrome girls in school. May need additional support or therapy.
Nutrition: failure to thrive in the infant period and obesity in childhood	Infants may have inefficient sucking and swallowing reflexes. Monitor growth utilizing a Turner syndrome growth chart.	Nutrition counseling and encouragement of exercise to maintain appropriate weight.
Hearing loss	Hearing loss may be conductive or sensorineural. Routine screening should be performed.	Otitis media should be treated aggressively to minimize the potential hearing loss.
Short stature and failure to develop secondary sex characteristics		Endocrine therapy may be indicated for growth and development. Hormonal therapy may enhance the development of secondary sex characteristics.
Infertility	Ovaries are streaks of connective tissue.	Infertility is generally expected in Turner syndrome. Infertility techniques may be able to assist with childbearing.
Hypothyroidism	Periodic laboratory testing.	Thyroid hormone replacement therapy.
Behavioral problems, learning disabilities		Behavioral management.
Strabismus	If detected, referral to an ophthalmologist is recommended.	Patching or surgical repair
Cognitive function	Average to slightly below-average intelligence. Problem areas include spatial perception and math functions.	Special education

Disintegrative Disorder

Childhood disintegrative disorder follows a period of normal development, as is also seen in Rett's disorder. This normal developmental period lasts at least 2 years and up to 10 years of age. The most common age of onset is between 3 and 4 years of age. The child begins to experience a significant loss of previously acquired skills. Areas that may be affected include expressive/receptive language, social skills or adaptive behavior, bowel and bladder control, and motor skills. The loss of these skills generally reaches a point at which they do not disintegrate further; at this point, some limited improvements may be seen.

Pathophysiology and Etiology
Etiology is unknown. Childhood disintegrative disorder appears to be more common in males. The incidence of this disorder is rare.

Diagnosis and Management
See Cognitive Developmental Delay for general approach to assessment.

Asperger's Disorder

Asperger's disorder is characterized by an impairment of social skills. These interactions include verbal social and nonverbal communication. Often there is a lack of peer relationships that are appropriate for the developmental level. These children will not seek spontaneous interpersonal interactions. Characteristically, they are of average to above-average intelligence and have developed normal language skills in terms of vocabulary and grammar. There are no significant delays in the areas of cognitive development, development of age-appropriate self-help skills, adaptive behavior, and curiosity about the environment. There are common behaviors associated with Asperger's disorder, including a limited range of interest, strict adherence to routines and rituals, and repetitive motor movements or sequences.

Asperger's disorder is one of several developmental disabilities associated with normal intelligence, such as learning disabilities and attention disorders. Academic and functional underachievement in the preschool and school-age child with normal intelligence is the common picture. Proper diagnosis, utilizing a cooperative team effort from several individuals, is imperative to develop an individualized treatment plan.

Pathophysiology and Etiology
The etiology is unknown. Asperger's disorder is often not diagnosed until school age. One study showed the prevalence of Asperger's disorder to be approximately 3 per 1000 children. The male to female ratio is 4:1.

Diagnosis and Management
1. Complete medical review, family history, and physical examination, including vision and hearing assessment and neurologic evaluation to rule out other disorders
2. Psychological testing to determine the exact nature of cognitive and perceptual dysfunctions
3. Behavioral and social assessment
4. Assessment of academic performance
5. MRI and other testing to determine underlying neurologic abnormality
6. Occupational and physical therapy, speech and language evaluations as necessary
7. School evaluation—school psychologists will obtain IQ testing, achievement testing. The teacher's input is also essential. The focus of a school evaluation is to determine eligibility for services. Most school systems will provide services only when moderate to severe problems exist. It may be necessary for the family to provide remediation for problems considered to be mild outside of the educational setting.

■ Pervasive Developmental Disorder Not Otherwise Specified (PDDNOS)
This category is used when the characteristics of a pervasive developmental disorder are present but do not fit in any of the categories as described above or meet the criteria for schizophrenia or avoidant personality disorders.

ATTENTION DISORDERS AND LEARNING DISABILITIES

Attention disorders and learning disabilities are separate but overlapping problems and may need specific approaches based on the nature of the disability. The term "learning disabilities" (LD) is defined by the Interagency Committee of Learning Disabilities (1987) as a "heterogeneous group of disorders manifested by significant difficulties in the acquisition of listening, speaking, reading, writing, reasoning, or mathematical abilities, or of social skills."

An estimated 5% to 10% of children (ranging up to 30%) have attention deficit hyperactivity disorder (ADHD); LD is reportedly present in 12.6% of children by the end of the second grade. Males are diagnosed twice as frequently as females (girls may go undiagnosed because they are less likely to exhibit disruptive behaviors).

Pathophysiology and Etiology
1. Multiple hypotheses exist because the exact causes are unknown. May be genetic.
   a. A family trait—other members of the family often have similar difficulties.
   b. Characteristic of inborn errors of metabolism.
   c. Sex chromosome abnormalities often exhibit these traits.
2. Not shown to be associated with a history of birth trauma or brain damage.
3. Exposure to prenatal and postnatal factors that might adversely affect brain development and function—lead, alcohol, cocaine, central nervous system infections, low birth weight, and prematurity.
4. May coexist with other handicapping conditions, such as spina bifida, cerebral palsy, or seizure disorders.
5. May have biomedical, emotional, social, and environmental components.
6. Attention deficit hyperactivity disorder is an alteration in the response-inhibition mechanisms of the brain controlled by the frontal cortex and reticular activating system; alteration in neurotransmitter.
7. Learning disabilities—authorities are investigating abnormalities in the parietal lobe of the brain and in the central visual pathways located in the occipital lobe.
8. Although emotional and environmental factors play a role, serotonin deficiency may serve as a physiologic basis for these disorders.

■ Attention Disorders
Attention disorders (ADs) are characterized by a cluster of symptoms, including developmentally inappropriate short attention span, impulsivity, and distractibility. Three subtypes of attention disorders are the hyperactive-impulsive type, the inattentive type, and combined. It is a diagnosis of exclusion; other disorders associated with these symptoms must be ruled out before a diagnosis of AD can be

made. Hearing and visual impairments, seizures, mental retardation, learning disabilities, side effects of medications, lead poisoning, and psychiatric disorders are just a few that need to be ruled out.

Learning disabilities and ADHD often occur together.

Clinical Manifestations and Diagnostic Evaluation
Diagnostic Criteria for Attention Deficit Hyperactivity Disorder

The child must experience a disturbance for at least 6 months and exhibit 8 of the following 14 symptoms.

1. Does the child often fidget with hands or feet or squirm in seat?
2. Does the child have difficulty remaining seated when required to do so?
3. Is the child easily distracted by extraneous stimuli?
4. Does the child have difficulty awaiting his or her turn in games or group situations?
5. Does the child often blurt out answers to questions before they have been completed?
6. Does the child often have difficulty following instructions from others?
7. Does the child have difficulty sustaining attention in tasks or play activities?
8. Does the child often shift from one uncompleted activity to another?
9. Does the child have difficulty playing quietly?
10. Does the child often talk excessively?
11. Does the child often interrupt or intrude on others?
12. Does the child often not seem to listen to what is being said to him or her?
13. Does the child often lose things necessary for tasks or activities at school or at home?
14. Does the child often engage in physically dangerous activities without considering possible consequences? (American Psychiatric Association, 1994)

Symptoms

Vary slightly based on the age of the child.
1. Toddlers: constant movement, described as "into everything"; may have focused attention in highly motivated situations.
2. School age: fidgety, easily distracted, does not finish tasks, loses things; school achievement is below child's potential.
3. Attention disorders may be diagnosed as late as college or adulthood.

Management
Multidisciplinary Approach

A multidisciplinary approach, including environmental and behavioral approaches, is the treatment of choice.
Pharmacologic Treatment

1. Central nervous system stimulants work for 70% to 75% of ADHD children (reserved for children older than 7 years of age).

a. Effective in decreasing motor activities and increasing attention span and concentration, thereby allowing child to be more available to learn.
b. Medications used: methylphenidate (Ritalin), dextroamphetamine (Dexadrine), dextroamphetamine and amphetamine (Adderall), pemoline (Cylert) and clonidine (Catapres).
2. Side effects of stimulants:
a. Insomnia may result from increased dosage or if administered too late in the day.
b. Anorexia and temporary growth retardation.
c. Increased pulse and respiratory rates, nervousness, nausea, and stomachache.
d. Liver dysfunction (pemoline): periodic liver function tests are required.
e. Altered effects of many antiseizure drugs and tricyclic antidepressants.
f. Do not cause euphoric effect or addiction in children.

Nursing Responsibilities and Family Education

1. Administer before breakfast and lunch (sustained-release forms do not require a lunch dose).
2. Work with school system to ensure that lunch dose is given.
3. Consider "drug holidays" during vacations and on weekends to monitor effectiveness and the need for change; this is especially recommended at the start of each academic school year.
4. Stimulant medications are not usually given to children younger than 6 years of age.
5. The child is usually started on a small dose, which is gradually increased until the desired response is achieved.
6. Evaluate the child's response to medication by direct observation and consultation with others, such as parent and teachers.

◆ **DRUG ALERT**

Stimulant medications for attention disorders should be used in conjunction with a comprehensive therapeutic regimen and not as the sole method of treatment. Stimulant medications require monitoring and feedback from parents and teachers who directly observe the effects.

■ Learning Disability

Difficulties with academic achievement fall under a broad category of learning problems. The cause or influencing factors can be biomedical, developmental, behavioral, emotional, social, environmental, and family issues. The problem may be in the area of reading, math, written expression, motor skills, and communication disorders. Attention deficit, anxiety, and behavioral disorders must be ruled out.

Clinical Manifestations

1. Symptoms of LD:
   a. School achievement significantly lower than potential
   b. Perceptual-motor impairments
   c. Emotional lability
   d. Speech and language disorders
   e. Coordination deficits
2. There can be a wide range of cognitive ability from mild retardation to above-average intelligence.

Areas of Learning Disabilities

Auditory Perception

Auditory perception is characterized by difficulty distinguishing between similar sounds or words. This includes not being able to process the sounds into words that have a meaning at a rapid enough rate to be able to follow conversations.

1. Visual perception: visual perception difficulties involve problems interpreting what is seen. This may include problems recognizing shapes and positions of letters or words. Depth perception may pose a problem to some children with visual perception disorders.
2. Integrative processing: integrative processing disabilities encompass, to varying degrees, the inability to sequence events or facts; comprehend abstract ideas or implied meanings; and organize information that has been learned and apply it to what has been previously acquired.
3. Memory: the third stage of processing information involves memory. Disabilities generally affect the short-term memory, which stores information that has just been perceived for a brief period before it is either discarded or stored in the long-term memory.
4. Expressive language: characteristics of expressive language disorders are dependent upon the age of the child and the severity of the disorder. This disorder affects the child's verbal communication. Language skills in terms of vocabulary, grammatical content, fluency, and language formulation can be affected.
5. Motor: motor disabilities can affect either gross motor or fine motor muscle groups. A disability affecting the gross motor development can cause children to be "clumsy." These children have a tendency to fall or bump into things and have difficulty running and playing sports. Fine motor disabilities affect the muscles for detailed tasks such as writing, cutting with scissors, painting, etc.

Management and Special Teaching Strategies

1. For visual perceptual deficit—present material verbally; use hands-on experience; tape-record teaching sessions.
2. For auditory perceptual deficit—provide materials in written form; use pictures; provide tactile learning.
3. For integrative deficit—use multisensory approaches; print directions while you verbalize them; use calendars and lists to organize tasks and activities.
4. For motor/expressive deficits—break down skills and projects into their multiple component parts; verbally describe the component parts; provide extra time to perform; allow child to type work rather than using cursive writing.
5. For highly distractible child—provide a structured environment; have child sit in front of class; place child away from doors or windows; decrease clutter on desk.

NURSING ALERT

 Historically, preschool and kindergarten screening tools have not been accurate in predicting LD; newer tests of language and memory appear to be better predictors.

CHILDHOOD PSYCHIATRIC DISORDERS

Psychiatric disorders such as depression and anxiety may masquerade as, or complicate the course of, developmental disabilities.

■ Depression

It is estimated that 1% of preschoolers, 2% of school-aged children, and 5% of adolescents in the U. S. have depression. Symptoms typically include somatic complaints, drop in school performance, apathy, loss of interest, social withdrawal, increased irritability, tearfulness, sleep and appetite changes, and suicidal ideation or behavior. A family history is a risk factor for depression in children. Any disturbance in mood that exists with functional impairment should be considered a psychiatric disorder until proved otherwise.

■ Anxiety Disorder

Exaggerated fears and overall "nervousness" interfering with the child's ability to function at chronologic level.

Other psychiatric disorders that are seen in childhood and adolescence include bipolar disorder, Tourette syndrome, obsessive-compulsive disorder, post-traumatic stress disorder, eating disorders, substance abuse, and schizophrenia. See Chapter 57 for general information.

RESOURCES AND SUPPORT GROUPS

Agencies that may provide information, support, and additional resources include the following:
ARC (formerly Association for Retarded Citizens of the United States)
1010 Wayne Avenue, Suite 650
Silver Spring, MD 20910
301-565-3842
http://thearc.org

Joseph P. Kennedy, Jr., Foundation
1325 G Street, Suite 500
Washington, D.C. 20005-4709
(202)393-1250

National Down Syndrome Congress (publishes Down
Syndrome News, booklets, bibliographies)
7000 Peachtree-Dunwoody Rd. N.E.
Lake Ridge 400 Office Park
Bldg. 5, Suite 100
Atlanta, GA 30328
1-800-232-NDSC
www.ndscenter.org

National Down Syndrome Society
666 Broadway
New York, NY 10012
1-800-221-4602

Parents of Down's Syndrome Children
Local groups listed in phone book or community services
directory.

National Fragile X Foundation
P.O. Box 190488
San Francisco, California 94119
1-800-688-8765
http://nfxf.org

National Information Center for Children and Youth
with Disabilities (NICHCY)
PO Box 1492
Washington, D.C. 20013
www.nichcy.org
1-800-695-0285

Learning Disability Association of America
4156 Library Road
Pittsburgh, PA 15234
(412) 341-1515
www.ldanatl.org

Children and Adults with Attention Deficit Disorders
(CHADD)
8181 Professional Place, Suite 201
Landover, MD 20785
800-233-4050
www.chadd.org

Council for Learning Disabilities
PO Box 40303
Overland Park, KS 66204
(913)492-8755
http://cldinternational.org

SELECTED REFERENCES

American Academy of Child and Adolescent Psychiatry (1999). Practice parameters for the assessment and treatment of children, adolescents, and adults with autism and other pervasive developmental disorders. *Journal of the American Academy of Child and Adolescent Psychiatry, 38*(12), 32S–54S.

American Academy of Pediatrics (1999). The pediatrician's role in development and implementation of an individual education plan (IEP) and/or an individual family service plan (IFSP). *Pediatrics, 104*(1), 124–127.

American Psychiatric Association (1994). *Diagnostic and statistical manual of mental disorders* (4th ed.). Washington, D.C.: American Psychiatric Association.

Batshaw, M., & Perret, Y. (1992). *Children with disabilities: A medical primer* (3rd ed.). Baltimore: Paul Brooks Publishing.

Briskin, H., & Liptak, G. S. (1995). Helping families with children with developmental disabilities. *Pediatric Annals, 24*(5), 262–266.

Capute, A. J., & Accardo, P. J. (1980). *Developmental disabilities in infancy and childhood.* Baltimore: Paul Brooks Publishing.

Castiglia, P. (1997). Attention deficit/hyperactivity disorder. *Journal of Pediatric Health Care, 11*(3), 130–133.

Centers for Disease Control and Prevention, Division of Child Development, Disability, and Health (1999). **www.cdc.gov/nech/programs/cddh/**

Committee on Genetics (1995) Health supervision for children with Turner syndrome. *Pediatrics, 96*(6), 1166–1173.

Epps, S., & Kroeker, R. (1995). Effects of child age and level of developmental delay on family practice physicians' diagnostic impressions. *Mental Retardation, 33*(1), 35–41.

Giangreco, C., Steele, M., Aston, C., Cummins, J., & Wenger, S. (1996). A simplified six-item checklist for screening for fragile X syndrome in the pediatric population. *Journal of Pediatrics, 129*(4), 611–614.

Kutcher, S. (1997). *Child and adolescent psychopharmacology.* Philadelphia: W. B. Saunders.

Levine, M., Carey, W., & Crocker, A. (1999). *Developmental-behavioral pediatrics* (3rd ed.). Philadelphia: W. B. Saunders.

MacDonald, D. (1998). Meeting special learning needs. *RN, 61*(4), 33–34.

McKusick, V. A. (1994). *Mendelian inheritance in man* (11th ed.). Baltimore: Johns Hopkins University Press.

Msall, M. E., Digaudio, K., Duffy, L. C., LaForest, S., & Granger, C. V. (1994). WeeFimm: Normative sample of an instrument for tracking functional dependence in children. *Clinical Pediatrics, 33*(7), 431–438.

National Information Center for Children and Youth with Disabilities (1999). **www.nichcy.org.**

Sanez, R. (1999) Primary care of infants and young children with Down syndrome. *American Family Physician, 59*(2), 381–390.

Sangare, J. (2000). ADHD: Making the appropriate pediatric assessment. *Lippincott's Primary Care Practice, 4*(2), 193–206.

Seideman, R., & Kleine, P. (1995). A theory of transformed parenting: Parenting a child with developmental delay/mental retardation. *Nursing Research, 44*(1), 38–44.

Volkmar, F., Klin, A., Schultz, R. Rubin, E., & Bronen, R. (2000). Asperger's disorder. *American Journal of Psychiatry, 157*(2), 262–267.

Zametkin, A., & Ernst, M. (1999). Current concepts: Problems in the management of attention-deficit-hyperactivity disorder [review article]. *New England Journal of Medicine, 340*(1), 40–46.

PART

5

Psychiatric Nursing

Problems of
Mental Health

ANXIETY-RELATED DISORDERS

■ Anxiety and Dissociative Disorders

The anxiety disorders are the most common of all psychiatric disorders. An individual with one of these disorders experiences physiologic, cognitive, and behavioral symptoms of anxiety. The physiologic manifestations are related to the "fight/flight" response and result in cardiovascular, respiratory, neuromuscular, and gastrointestinal stimulation. The cognitive symptoms include subjective feelings of apprehension, uneasiness, uncertainty, or dread. Behavioral manifestations include irritability, restlessness, pacing, crying and sighing, and complaints of tension and nervousness. The common theme among the anxiety disorders is that the individual experiences a level of anxiety that interferes with functioning in personal, occupational, and social areas.

The dissociative disorders are characterized by an alteration in conscious awareness, which includes forgetfulness, memory loss for past stressful events, feeling disconnected from daily events, or development of distinctly different personalities in one individual.

Classification

Anxiety-related disorders, as defined by the *Diagnostic and Statistical Manual of Mental Disorders,* 4th edition (DSM-IV), include the following:

Anxiety Disorders

1. Panic disorder without agoraphobia
2. Panic disorder with agoraphobia
3. Agoraphobia without history of panic disorder
4. Specific phobia
5. Social phobia
6. Obsessive-compulsive disorder
7. Post-traumatic stress disorder
8. Acute stress disorder
9. Generalized anxiety disorder
10. Anxiety disorder due to a general medical condition
11. Substance-induced anxiety disorder
12. Anxiety disorder not otherwise specified

Dissociative Disorders

1. Dissociative amnesia
2. Dissociative fugue
3. Dissociative identity disorder
4. Depersonalization disorder
5. Dissociative disorder not otherwise specified

Pathophysiology and Etiology

The underlying etiology of anxiety disorders, as well as any of the psychiatric disorders, is complex, having multiple factors that interact. Therefore, it is essential to examine the following factors: (1) biochemical, (2) genetic, (3) psychosocial, and (4) sociocultural.

Biochemical Factors

1. The limbic system, which is called the emotional brain, regulates emotional responses. Anxiety disorders are associated with abnormalities within this system (including the frontal cortex, hypothalamus, amygdala, hippocampus, brain stem, and the autonomic nervous system).
2. Neurotransmitters (NT) and their specific receptor sites function to transmit inhibiting or stimulating messages across the synapses between nerve cells in the brain. Abnormalities in the neurotransmitters or the receptor sites have been associated with multiple psychiatric disorders, including anxiety disorders.
3. Gamma-aminobutryic acid (GABA) is an inhibitory NT that normally acts to decrease anxiety responses. An inadequate amount is associated with increased anxiety.
4. Norepinephrine is a stimulating NT, which is released as part of the fight/flight response and is associated with the cardiovascular and respiratory effects of anxiety. Serotonin is an NT that regulates multiple responses, including sleep and alertness and sensations of hunger and satiation. Serotonin abnormalities may also contribute to the symptoms of anxiety disorders.

5. Panic disorders may be related to the reception of a false signal from the brain that there is a shortage of oxygen or an increase in carbon dioxide (suffocation alarm theory). Persons who have panic attacks have also been reported to have higher levels of norepinephrine.

6. Suppression of cortisol through administration of dexamethasone has been associated with post-traumatic stress disorder, suggesting heightened glucocorticoid feedback sensitivity.

7. Positron emission tomography (PET) and computed tomography (CT) have shown abnormalities in glucose metabolism in the frontal and pre-frontal cortex and the basal ganglia of the brains of individuals with panic disorder. PET scans have also demonstrated increased blood flow and cerebral metabolism in the basal ganglia and frontal cortex of individuals with obsessive-compulsive disorder.

8. Obsessive-compulsive disorder (OCD) has been associated with increased serotonin responsiveness as well as striatum dysfunction. The striatum controls voluntary movement, and it is hypothesized that individuals with OCD may be doing repetitive rituals to "self-medicate" for serotonin deficiencies.

9. Dissociative symptoms have been related to shrinkage of the hippocampus. Studies of physically, sexually, and psychologically abused children found increased EEG abnormalities in the frontal and temporal lobes.

Genetic Factors

1. First-degree relatives of individuals with panic disorder have a four to seven times greater chance of developing this disorder. Twin studies demonstrate a higher concordance rate for monozygotic than dizygotic twins.

2. Approximately 20% of first-degree relatives of persons with agoraphobia also have agoraphobia.

3. Approximately 3% to 7% of persons with OCD have first-degree relatives with the same disorder.

4. Approximately 25% of first-degree relatives with generalized anxiety disorder are also affected by generalized anxiety disorder.

5. Dissociative disorders have not been identified as being genetically transmitted.

Psychosocial Factors

1. Psychodynamic theory describes unconscious conflicts having early childhood origin and resulting from repressed wishes and drives. These conflicts cause guilt and shame, which lead to anxiety and associated symptoms.

2. Interpersonal theory implicates early relationships, which directly affect development of self-concept and self-esteem. Individuals with poor self-concept and decreased self-esteem have increased susceptibility to anxiety-related disorders.

3. Behavioral theory describes anxiety and associated symptoms as a conditioned response to internal and external stressors.

4. Cognitive theory describes faulty thinking patterns that lead to an individual's misperceiving events affecting self, the future, and the world. These faulty thinking patterns contribute to the subjective experience of anxiety.

5. Dissociative disorders are generally associated with traumatic events. An individual responds to severe trauma (especially in early childhood) by "splitting off" or dissociating the self from the memory of the trauma. Severe physical, sexual, and psychological abuse in early childhood is associated with dissociative identity disorder.

Sociocultural Factors

1. Anxiety disorders and ritualistic behaviors are commonly seen in high-technology societies.

2. There is a higher incidence of anxiety disorders in urban communities than in rural communities.

3. Women are diagnosed more often with anxiety disorders except with OCD, which affects men and women equally. It is thought that this may represent a sociocultural rather than a genetic factor.

Clinical Manifestations
See Box 57-1.

Diagnostic Evaluation

1. Measurement tools for anxiety:
   a. Hamilton Anxiety Scale
   b. Graphic Anxiety Scales (GASs)

2. Measurement tools for obsessive-compulsive disorders:
   a. Yale-Brown Obsessive-Compulsive Scale
   b. Florida Obsessive-Compulsive Inventory (FOCI)

3. Sodium lactate infusion or carbon dioxide inhalation will likely produce a panic attack in a person with panic disorder.

4. Increased arousal may be measured through studies of autonomic functioning (ie, heart rate, electromyography, sweat gland activity) in a person with post-traumatic stress disorder.

5. Dexamethasone suppression test (DST) may be used to demonstrate heightened glucocorticoid feedback in individuals with post-traumatic stress disorder.

6. Measurement tools for dissociation:
   a. Dissociation Impulsivity Scale (DIS)
   b. Dissociative Experiences Scale (DES)
   c. Dissociative Disorders Interview Schedule (DDIS)

Management

1. A variety of levels and sites of care can be provided: psychiatric inpatient, outpatient, or home care. Most care is provided on an outpatient basis. Site of care is based on a number of factors, including degree of disability of affected individual, community services available, and insurance and managed care considerations. Generally the recommended treatment is a combination of medication and psychotherapy, along with education of individual and family.

2. Psychoeducational strategies:
   a. Relaxation techniques
   b. Progressive muscle relaxation
   c. Guided imagery or visualization exercises

BOX 57-1   Diagnostic Criteria for Anxiety Disorders

Anxiety Disorders

Acute Stress Disorder

1. Person has been exposed to a traumatic event either witnessed or experienced.
2. Develops three or more of these dissociative symptoms:
   - Subjective sense of numbing
   - Absence of emotional responsiveness
   - Feeling dazed
   - Derealization
   - Depersonalization
   - Dissociative amnesia
3. Duration of 2 days to 4 weeks.

Generalized Anxiety Disorder

1. Persists for at least 6 months.
2. Symptoms present from three of the four categories:
   - Motor tension (eg, trembling, restlessness, inability to relax, and fatigue).
   - Autonomic hyperactivity (eg, sweating, palpitations, cold clammy hands, urinary frequency, lump in throat, pallor or flushing, increased pulse, and rapid respirations).
   - Apprehensiveness (eg, worry, dread, fear, rumination, insomnia, and inability to concentrate).
   - Hypervigilance (eg, feeling edgy, scanning the environment, and distractibility).

Obsessive-Compulsive Disorder

1. Preoccupation with persistent intrusive thoughts (obsessions), repeated performance of rituals designed to prevent some event (compulsions), or both.
2. Anxiety occurs if obsessions or compulsions are resisted and from feeling powerless to resist the thoughts or rituals.

Panic Disorder

1. Recurrent unexpected anxiety attacks.
2. Sudden onset with intense apprehension and dread.
3. At least four of the following symptoms:
   - Dyspnea
   - Chest discomfort
   - Dizziness
   - Hot or cold flashes
   - Tingling of hands or feet
   - Feelings of unreality
   - Palpitations
   - Syncope
   - Diaphoresis
   - Trembling
   - Fear of losing control, going crazy, or dying

Post-traumatic Stress Disorder

1. After experiencing a psychologically traumatic event outside the range of usual experience (eg, rape, combat, bombings, kidnapping), the person reexperiences the event through recurrent dreams and flashbacks.
2. Emotional numbness, detachment, and estrangement may be used to defend against anxiety.

3. May experience sleep disturbance, hypervigilance, guilt about surviving, poor concentration, and avoidance of activities that trigger memory of the event.

Phobias

1. Irrational fear of an object or situation that persists, although the person may recognize it as unreasonable.
2. Types include:
   Agoraphobia: Fear of being alone in open or public places where escape might be difficult; may not leave home.
   Social phobia: Fear of situations in which one might be seen and embarrassed or criticized; fear of eating in public, public speaking, or performing.
   Specific phobia: Fear of a single object, activity, or situation (eg, snakes, closed spaces, and flying).
3. Anxiety is severe if the object, situation, or activity cannot be avoided.

Substance-Induced Anxiety Disorder

1. Prominent anxiety, panic attacks, or obsessions or compulsions predominate.
2. Symptoms developed within 1 month of substance intoxication or withdrawal.
3. Medication use is related to disturbance.
4. The disturbance doesn't occur exclusively during the course of delirium.
5. Significant distress or impairment in social and occupational functioning results.

Dissociative Disorders

Depersonalization Disorder

1. Persistent or recurrent experience of feeling detached from and outside one's mental processes or body.
2. Reality testing remains intact.
3. The experience causes significant impairment in social or occupational functioning or causes marked distress.
4. Does not occur exclusively during course of another mental disorder.

Dissociative Amnesia

1. One of more episodes of inability to recall important information—usually of a traumatic or stressful nature.
2. Other psychological (eg, multiple personality disorder) and physical (eg, substance-induced) disorders are ruled out.

Dissociative Fugue

1. Sudden, unexpected travel away from home or one's place of work with inability to remember past.
2. Confusion about personal identity or assumption of new identity.

Dissociative Identity Disorder

1. Presence of two or more distinct identities, each with its own patterns of relating, perceiving, and thinking.
2. At least two of these identities take control of the person's behavior.
3. Inability to recall important personal information too extensive to be explained by ordinary forgetfulness.
4. Other causes ruled out.

(Adapted from American Psychiatric Association [1994]. *Diagnostic and statistical manual of mental disorders* [4th ed.]. Washington, D.C.: APA.)

d. Stress management

e. Assertiveness training

3. Psychotherapy:

a. Psychodynamic: assists persons in understanding their experiences by identifying unconscious conflicts and developing effective coping behaviors.

b. Behavioral: focuses on the individual problematic behavior and works to modify or extinguish the behavior. One form of behavioral therapy effective in management of phobic disorders is systematic desensitization.

c. Cognitive: assists client to question faulty thought patterns (reframing) and examine alternatives. In post-traumatic stress disorder and dissociative disorders, the client is assisted to view self as a survivor rather than a victim.

d. Hypnotherapy can be used as part of therapy for those suffering dissociative disorders.

e. Support group therapy has been useful in providing a supportive and psychoeducational approach for clients with anxiety or dissociative disorders.

4. Somatic therapies:

a. Biofeedback: relaxation through biofeedback is achieved when a person learns to control physiologic mechanisms that are not ordinarily within his or her awareness. Awareness and control are accomplished by monitoring body processes, including muscle tone, heart rate, and brain waves.

b. Psychopharmacologic: medications used to treat anxiety-related disorders are those that will increase GABA (benzodiazapines), regulate serotonin levels (antidepressants), or reduce physiologic effects of anxiety by causing peripheral beta-adrenergic blockade (beta blockers).

c. Narcotherapy: sodium amobarbital or intravenous sodium thiopental may assist the therapist in gaining access to a patient's repressed memories and buried conflicts. In a person experiencing dissociative amnesia or dissociative fugue, the therapist may explore dissociated events. If the person is diagnosed with dissociative identity disorder, this type of interview may facilitate the access of other personalities.

Complications

1. Undiagnosed medical reasons for anxiety could lead to physical deterioration and a delay in obtaining appropriate medical care. It is important to screen for any co-existing medical illness.

2. If panic and phobic disorders are left untreated, these disorders can lead to increasing social withdrawal and isolation, which may severely impair the person's social and work life.

3. Untreated OCD can lead to aggressive behavior toward self or others as well as depression. It can also lead to injuries from compulsive behavior, such as skin breakdown from repeated handwashing.

4. Undiagnosed or untreated post-traumatic stress disorder or acute stress disorder can lead to substance abuse or dependence, aggressive/violent behavior, and possibly suicide.

5. If a person with a dissociative disorder goes untreated, he or she may develop aggressive behavior toward self or others. Such behaviors may include assaults, depression, post-traumatic stress disorder, psychoactive substance abuse disorder, rape, self-mutilation, and suicide attempts.

Nursing Assessment

1. Assess psychological, cognitive, and behavioral symptoms.

a. Defense mechanisms used and/or coping measures used

b. Mood

c. Suicide potential

d. Thought content and process

e. Severity of subjective experience of anxiety

f. Understanding of specific disorder

2. Explore social functioning.

a. Ability to function in social and work situations

b. Impact of symptoms on the patient's relationships, especially family relationships

c. Diversional and recreational behavior

d. Identification of stressors related to self-concept, role performance, life values, social status, and support systems

e. Benefits (primary and secondary gains) and risks of the presenting symptoms

Nursing Diagnoses

• Anxiety related to unexpected panic attacks or related to re-experiencing traumatic events

• Altered Thought Processes related to severe anxiety

• Social Isolation related to avoidance behavior or related to embarrassment and shame associated with symptoms

• Altered Role Performance related to inability to function in usual social and occupational situations secondary to anxiety-related symptoms

• Personal Identity Disturbance related to a traumatic event

• Risk for Injury related to compulsive behaviors

Nursing Interventions

Reducing Symptoms of Anxiety

1. Help patient identify anxiety-producing situations and plan for such events.

2. Assist patient to develop assertiveness and communication skills.

3. Practice stress-reduction techniques with patient.

4. Teach patient to monitor for objective and subjective manifestations of anxiety.

a. Tachycardia, tachypnea

b. Signs and symptoms associated with autonomic stimulation—perspiration, difficulty concentrating, insomnia

5. Encourage patient to verbalize feelings of anxiety.
6. Administer prescribed anxiolytics to decrease anxiety level.

 DRUG ALERT

Benzodiazepines are associated with tolerance and dependence and are appropriate for short-term use. Withdrawal symptoms may occur when drug is abruptly discontinued. Gradual dosage reduction is necessary. Overdose or taking benzodiazepines with alcohol or other CNS depressants can cause respiratory depression requiring emergency intervention.

Improving Concentration
1. Use short, simple sentences when communicating with patient.
2. Maintain a calm, serene manner.
3. Use adjuncts to verbal communication, such as visual aids and role playing, to stimulate memory and retention of information.
4. Teach relaxation techniques to diminish distress that interferes with concentration ability.

Increasing Social Interaction
1. Encourage discussion of reasons for and feelings about social isolation.
2. Help patient identify specific causes/situations that produce anxiety that inhibits social interaction.
3. Recommend participation in programs directed at specific conflict areas or skill deficiencies. Such programs may focus on assertiveness skills, body awareness, managing multiple role responsibilities, and stress management.

Encouraging Independence
1. Identify secondary benefits, such as decreased responsibility and increased dependency, that inhibit patient's move to independence.
2. Provide experiences in which patient can be successful.
3. Explore alternative methods of meeting dependency needs.
4. Explore beliefs that support a helpless or dependent mode of behavior.
5. Teach and role-play assertive behaviors in specific situations.
6. Assist patient to improve skills based on performance.
7. Encourage family members to avoid fostering dependency.

Strengthening Identity
1. Develop an honest, nonjudgmental relationship with the patient.
2. Try to establish communication between patient's alters.
3. Do not overwhelm patient with information or memories.
4. Assist patient to incorporate dissociated material into conscious memory by encouraging the sharing of painful, repressed memories.
5. Teach patient containment techniques to assist in coping with the painful memories becoming conscious.

Reducing Harm From Behavior
1. Encourage limit setting on ritualistic behavior as part of established treatment plan.
2. Assist patient in listing all of objects and places that trigger anxiety as part of exposure-response prevention program.
3. Use cognitive strategies, such as reframing, to assist patient in placing thoughts and feelings in a different perspective.
4. Participate as member of treatment team in establishing program for systematic desensitization.
5. Intervene as needed and obtain emergency assistance when patient is in immediate danger.

Community and Home Care Considerations
1. Patients with anxiety-related disorders generally are treated in an outpatient setting. Many of these patients may not see a mental health professional but will be treated by their family health care provider, utilizing pharmacologic therapy. Nurses who encounter patients taking medications for anxiety should assess effectiveness and patient knowledge base regarding safe use of these drugs. Patients should be encouraged to utilize anxiety-reduction techniques.
2. Since anxiety disorders will affect family functioning, the nurse should provide support for the family, including teaching family members about the disorder and any treatment measures.
3. Patients may elect to utilize alternative/complementary therapies in order to obtain relief from symptoms. Advise patients not to use any nutritional supplement or "natural" remedy, such as St. John's Wort or kava kava, without discussing it with his or her health care provider; many drug interactions exist (see Appendix IV).

Patient Education and Health Maintenance
1. Teach patient and family members about anxiety.
   a. Define anxiety and differentiate it from fear.
   b. Explain causes of anxiety.
   c. Identity events that can trigger anxiety.
   d. Identify the relevant signs and symptoms of anxiety.
2. Describe the medication regimen, including significant action, side effects, dosage considerations, and any food or drug interactions.
3. Identify, describe, and practice deep-muscle relaxation techniques, relaxation breathing, imagery, and other relaxation therapies (see pp. 27–29).
4. Teach family to give positive reinforcement for use of healthy behaviors.
5. Teach family not to assume responsibilities or roles normally assigned to the patient.
6. Teach family to give attention to the patient, not to the patient's symptoms.
7. Teach alternative ways to perform activities of daily living (ADLs) if physical disability inhibits function and performance.

8. For additional information and support, refer to such agencies as Anxiety Disorders Association of America, 11900 Park Lawn Drive, Suite 100, Rockville, MD 20852, 301-231-9350; *www.adaa.org.*

A number of web sites provide support for individuals and family members. Some examples include Agoraphobic Building Independent Lives: *bhtp:/tgopbi.com/community/ groups/abilpbfl/index.html; HealthyPlace.com* (for sufferers from anxiety disorders); and for panic/anxiety disorders, *http://panicdisorder.about.com/index.htm.*

Outcome-Based Evaluation

- Identifies stressors and demonstrates normal heart rate, respirations, sleep pattern, and subjective feelings of anxiety
- Demonstrates improved concentration and thought processes through improved ability to focus, think, and problem solve
- Reports increased participation in family- and community-related events
- Reports going to work, keeping appointments
- Uses coping strategies for situations that are anxiety provoking.
- No injuries

■ Somatoform Disorders

Somatoform disorders are characterized by complaints of physical symptoms that cannot be explained by known physical mechanisms. These disorders have in common the belief that physical symptoms are real despite any evidence to the contrary. The affected individual experiences changes or loss in physical function. The physical symptoms are not under the individual's voluntary control. Significant impairment occurs in social or occupational functioning.

Classification

1. Somatization disorder
2. Undifferentiated somatoform disorder
3. Conversion disorder
4. Pain disorder
5. Hypochondriasis
6. Body dysmorphic disorder
7. Somatoform disorder not otherwise specified

Pathophysiology and Etiology

The underlying etiology of somatoform disorders is difficult to define. The following factors may interact in the individual with these disorders.

Biochemical Factors

1. An individual with a somatoform disorder may experience high levels of physiologic arousal (increased awareness of somatic sensations).
2. The phenomenon of alexithymia, or deficient communication between brain hemispheres, may result in difficulty expressing emotions directly, and therefore distress may be expressed as physical symptoms.

3. The concept of somatosensory amplification, in which there is the tendency to experience somatic sensation as intense, noxious, and disturbing, may be related to the development of somatoform disorders.

Genetic Factors

1. Somatization disorder has been found to have a 10% to 20% frequency in first-degree female biologic relatives of women with this disorder.
2. Twin studies have validated some increased risk in conversion disorder in monozygotic twins.
3. The genetic basis for other somataform disorders is not well established.

Psychosocial Factors

1. Psychodynamic theory: the psychological source of ego conflict is denied and finds expression through displacement of anxiety onto physical symptoms. Both primary gain (anxiety relief) and secondary gains (increased dependence and relief from normal responsibilities) are common to these disorders.
2. Behavioral theory: the child learns from parent to express anxiety through somatization; secondary gains reinforce symptoms.
3. Cognitive theory: the individual has cognitive distortions in which benign symptoms are magnified and interpreted as serious disease.
4. Family theory: a family system that is undifferentiated may utilize dysfunction in one person as a means to handle anxiety.

Sociocultural factors

1. Incidence of somatoform disorders is highest in rural populations and in low socioeconomic groups.
2. Somatic symptoms are more common in cultures that view direct expression of emotions as unacceptable.
3. Women may experience certain chronic pain conditions more frequently than men (this may have more of a cultural than a genetic basis).

Clinical Manifestations

See Box 57-2.

Diagnostic Evaluation

1. Individuals with somatoform disorders will present in the medical rather than the psychiatric setting because of their belief that the problems are medical.
2. The individual should receive a thorough medical evaluation (if possible, avoiding repeating tests that have already had negative results).
3. The diagnosis of somatoform disorder will be made after a thorough medical evaluation in which no organic basis for the symptoms is validated.

Management

1. Level and setting of care to be provided is determined. In general, the individual will be treated on an outpatient basis, unless underlying mood disorder is present leading to risk for self-harm.

BOX 57-2 Diagnostic Criteria for Somatoform Disorders

Body Dysmorphic Disorder

1. Preoccupation with some imagined defect in appearance in a normal-appearing person (if the defect is present, concern is excessive).
2. Preoccupation causes significant impairment in social or occupational functioning or causes marked distress.

Conversion Disorder

1. Development of a symptom or deficit suggesting:
   - Neurologic disorder (blindness, deafness, loss of touch, or pain sensation)
   - Involuntary motor function (aphonia, impaired coordination, paralysis, seizures, etc.)
2. Not due to malingering or factitious disorder and not culturally sanctioned.
3. Causes impairment in social or occupational functioning, causes marked distress, or requires medical attention.

Hypochondriasis

1. Preoccupation with fears of having or the idea that one has a serious disease.
2. Preoccupation persists despite appropriate medical tests and assurances to the contrary.
3. Other disorders are ruled out, eg, somatic delusional disorders.
4. Preoccupation causes significant impairment in social or occupational functioning or causes marked distress.

Pain Disorder

1. Pain in one or more anatomic sites is a major part of the clinical picture.

2. Causes significant impairment in occupational or social functioning or causes marked distress.
3. Psychological factors are thought to cause onset, severity, or exacerbation.
4. If a medical condition is present, it plays a minor role in accounting for pain.

Somatization Disorder

1. History of many physical complaints before age 30, occurring over a period of years, resulting in change of lifestyle.
2. Complaints must include all of the following:
   - History of pain in at least four different sites or functions.
   - History of at least two GI symptoms other than pain.
   - History of at least one sexual or reproductive symptom.
   - History of at least one symptom defined as or suggesting a neurologic disorder.

Undifferentiated Somatoform Disorder

1. One or more physical complaints:
   - Fatigue
   - Loss of appetite
   - Gastrointestinal symptoms
   - Urinary symptoms
2. No physiologic explanation after an investigation.
3. Symptoms cause clinically significant distress or impairment in social or occupational areas of functioning.
4. Duration of the disturbance is at least 6 months.

(Adapted from American Psychiatric Association [1994]. *Diagnostic and statistical manual of mental disorders* [4th ed.]. Washington, D.C.: APA.)

---

2. Referral to psychiatric treatment is generally rejected by the individual with a somatoform disorder; therefore, the goal of management is to maintain a long-term relationship with a specific health care provider to prevent the patient from seeking multiple providers with multiple recommendations for testing, treatments, and medications.
3. Psychotherapy:
   a. Psychodynamic: assist the individual to express conflicts and emotions verbally rather than displacing them onto physical symptoms.
   b. Behavioral: establish a program whereby adaptive behavior is reinforced and illness behaviors do not receive secondary gains.
   c. Cognitive: restructure belief system that perpetuates illness-related behaviors.
   d. Family therapy: assist family members to define appropriate boundaries and support client in increasing self-responsibility.
4. Somatic therapies: somatoform disorders are usually not treated with psychopharmacologic agents because these patients are susceptible to dependency on medications used.

5. Mood disorders, especially depression, are a common co-morbid problem in individuals with somatoform disorders. Antidepressants may be used to treat the mood disorder.

Complications

1. The patient with a known history of a somatoform disorder may also have a co-existing medical condition that may go undiagnosed. Careful screening is essential to rule out medical problems.
2. Increased risk of suicide and substance abuse/dependence disorders is possible in the patient with an untreated somatoform disorder.

Nursing Assessment

Assess Physical Complaints

1. Current and past history as well as duration of problems
2. Diagnostic testing completed
3. Number of health care providers consulted
4. Types and amounts of medications as well as whether self medicating (over the counter) or prescribed

Assess Psychological Processes

1. Perception of illness and current stressors
2. Self-concept and body image

3. Secondary gains from physical symptoms
4. Mood
5. Suicide potential

Explore Social Functioning

Refer to section on Anxiety Disorders for assessment data.

Nursing Diagnoses

- Anxiety related to multiple physical symptoms and belief that serious disease exists
- Ineffective Individual Coping related to preoccupation with physical symptoms

    Other nursing diagnoses and nursing interventions under Anxiety Disorders may apply.

Nursing Interventions

Encouraging Recognition of Anxiety

1. Discuss current life stressors in the areas of social, occupational, and family functioning.
2. Assist patient to identify anxiety-producing situations and plan coping strategies.
3. Avoid focus on physical symptoms (after appropiate screening to rule out physical origin).
4. Maintain focus on feelings and emotional responses rather than on somatic symptoms.

Improving Coping

1. Teach and reinforce problem-solving approach to stressors.
2. Practice use of stress-reduction techniques with patient.
3. Encourage use of support groups.
4. Set limits on manipulative behaviors in a matter-of-fact manner.
5. Decrease reinforcement of secondary gains for physical symptoms.
6. Help patient identify and use positive means to meet emotional needs.

Community and Home Care Considerations

1. Encourage patient to cooperate with referrals for psychiatric or psychotherapy treatments.
2. Teach patient and family importance of remaining with one health care provider to ensure continuity of care.
3. Nurses who encounter patients with somatoform disorders in the community should maintain a matter-of-fact attitude in order to help decrease emphasis on dramatic symptoms.

Patient Education and Health Maintenance

1. Teach patient and family about the relationship between stressors, anxiety, and physical symptoms.
2. Family should expect person to function despite physical symptoms; doing things for him or her and making decisions will increase dependent behaviors.
3. Family therapy may be helpful in order to clarify roles, communication, and expectations.

Outcome-Based Evaluation

- Verbalizes anxiety about specific problems rather than expressing anxiety with physical symptoms

- Uses stress-management techniques and follows health-promoting lifestyle

MOOD DISTURBANCES

▨ Depressive Disorders

Depressive disorders are considered mood disorders. A mood is a sustained emotion that, when extreme, colors the person's view of the world. The mood disorders are characterized by disturbances in feelings, thinking, and behavior. These disorders may occur on a continuum ranging from severe depression to severe mania (hyperactivity). A depressive illness is painful and can be psychophysiologically debilitating. Depression is much more than just sadness; it affects the way one feels about the future and can alter basic attitudes about the self. A depressed person can become so despairing that he or she expresses hopelessness. When moods become severe or prolonged or interfere with a person's interpersonal or occupational functioning, this may signal a mood disorder.

Pathophysiology and Etiology

The exact causes for depressive disorders have not been established. These disorders are thought to result from complex interactions among a variety of factors.

Biochemical Factors

1. Biogenic amine theory proposes that there is a norepinephrine and serotonin deficiency in individuals with a depressive disorder. Changes in quantity and sensitivity of receptor sites for these neurotransmitters may also be important.
2. Kindling theory describes a process whereby external environmental stressors activate internal physiologic stress responses, which trigger the first depressive episode. Subsequent episodes can occur with less stress in response to the electrophysiologic sensitivity that was established in the brain from the initial episode.
3. Neuroendocrine dysfunction:
    a. Hypothalamic-pituitary-adrenal (HPA axis) dysfunction may be present in some individuals. Abnormalities include increased cortisol levels, resistance of cortisol to suppression by dexamethasone, and blunted adrenocorticotropin hormone response to corticotropin-releasing factor.
    b. Subclinical hypothyroidism has been associated with depression, especially in women.
    c. Dysfunction of circadian rhythms have been theorized to be related to depression. Abnormal sleep EEGs have been demonstrated in many individuals. Increased early morning awakening is common, as are multiple nighttime awakenings.

Genetic Factors

1. Risk of developing a mood disorder is 1.5 to 3 times greater in individuals with a first-degree relative with a mood disorder.
2. Twin studies reveal a higher rate of concordance in monozygotic twins than in dizygotic twins.

3. Research is ongoing related to the investigation of defective genes on chromosome 4 as well as on chromosomes 11, 18, and 21 that may be related to depression.

Medication Factors

1. Many medications have the side effect of depression, including hormones, cardiovascular drugs, psychotropic medications, and anti-inflammatory and anti-ulcer drugs.
2. Clinically significant depressive symptoms are detected in approximately 12% to 36% of individuals with a nonpsychiatric general medical condition.

Psychosocial Factors

1. Psychodynamic theory describes the occurrence of a significant loss (object loss) that is associated with anger and aggression, which is turned inward and leads to negative feelings about self. The negative feelings about the self, including shame and guilt, then lead to depression.
2. Life events and environmental stress, such as loss of a family member through death, divorce, or separation; lack of social support; and significant health problems, have all been associated with the onset of depression.
3. Cognitive theory describes faulty thought patterns, including negative distortions of life experiences, that produce negative self-evaluation, pessimistic thinking, and hopelessness.
4. Learned helplessness theory posits that a person who internalizes the belief that an unwanted event is his or her own fault and that nothing can be done to avoid or change it is prone to developing depression.

Clinical Manifestations

See Box 57-3.

Diagnostic Evaluation

1. Rating scales of depression—to determine presence and severity of the problem:
   a. Zung Self-Rating Scale
   b. Raskin Severity of Depression Scale
   c. Hamilton Depression Scale
   d. Beck Depression Inventory
2. Laboratory studies:
   a. Thyroid function tests and thyrotropin-releasing hormone stimulation test—to detect underlying hypothyroidism, which may cause depression.
   b. Dexamethasone suppression test—to evaluate depression that may be responsive to antidepressant or electroconvulsive therapy (ECT).
   c. Twenty-four hour urinary 3-methoxy-4-hydroxyphenylglycol (MHPG)—may show slightly lower level in unipolar depression than in bipolar depression.
3. Polysomography—an increase in the overall amount of REM sleep and shortened REM latency period in patients with major depression.
4. Additional diagnostic tests to evaluate physical conditions, such as computed tomography (CT) scan or magnetic resonance imaging (MRI), complete blood count (CBC), chemistry panel, rapid plasma reagin (RPR), human immunodeficiency virus (HIV) test, electroencephalogram (EEG), vitamin B_{12} and folate levels, and toxicology studies.

Management

1. Patients may receive treatment in acute inpatient psychiatric hospitals or in the community in an outpatient

---

BOX 57-3 Characteristics of Depressive Disorders

Major Depressive Disorder

1. Occurs over a 2-week period.
2. Represents a change in previous functions.
3. Impairs social and occupational functioning.
4. Five or more of the following occur nearly every day for most waking hours:
   - Depressed mood
   - Anhedonia (inability to experience pleasure)
   - Significant weight loss or gain (more than 5% of body weight per month)
   - Insomnia or hypersomnia
   - Increased or decreased motor activity
   - Anergy (fatigue or loss of energy)
   - Feelings of worthlessness or inappropriate guilt (may be delusional)
   - Decreased concentration or indecisiveness
   - Recurrent thought of death or suicidal ideation (with or without plan)

Specifiers

1. Severity
2. Psychotic features
3. Remission—chronic

4. Seasonal affective disorder related to either winter or summer
5. Catatonic features
6. Melancholic features
7. Atypical features
8. Postpartum onset

Dysthymic Disorder

1. Occurs over a 2-year period (1 year for children and adolescents), presence of depressed mood
2. Still able to function in social and occupational spheres
3. Presence of some of the following:
   - Decreased or increased appetite
   - Insomnia or hypersomnia
   - Anergy or chronic fatigue
   - Anhedonia
   - Decreased self-esteem
   - Poor concentration or difficulty making decisions
   - Perceived inability to cope with routine responsibilities
   - Feelings of hopelessness or despair
   - Pessimistic about the future, brooding over the past, or feeling sorry for self
   - Recurrent thoughts of death or suicide

(Adapted from American Psychiatric Association [1994]. *Diagnostic and statistical manual of mental disorders* [4th ed.]. Washington, D.C.: APA.)

program. Decision about treatment setting is made according to the severity of the patient's illness, with primary concern being the risk of self-harm (suicide) as well as the presence of symptoms that are severely disabling.

2. Inpatient treatment is directed toward medication management and supportive psychotherapy using milieu management.

3. Somatic therapies:
   a. Psychopharmacologic: medications used to treat depression are those that will increase serotonin and/or norepinephrine (Table 57-1).
   b. Electroconvulsive therapy may be used to treat severe depression that is unresponsive to antidepressant medications.

TABLE 57-1 Pharmacology of Antidepressant Medications

Medication: Class/Generic/Trade Name	Therapeutic Dosage Range (mg/day) in Adults	Adverse Reactions
Tricyclic Agents		
Amitriptyline (Elavil, Endep)	75–300 mg	For all tricyclic and tetracyclic agents:
Clomipramine (Anafranil)	75–300 mg	Possibility of enduring a manic episode in bipolar patients.
Desipramine (Norpramin, Pertofrane)	75–300 mg	Anticholinergic effects. Dry mouth, constipation, blurred vision, urinary retention.
Doxepin (Adapin, Sinequan)	75–300 mg	Sedative effects.
Imipramine (Tofranil, Tofranil-PM, Janimine, SK-pramine)	75–300 mg	Autonomic effects: orthostatic hypotension, sweating, palpitations, and increased blood pressure.
Nortriptyline (Aventyl, Pamelor)	40–200 mg	Cardiac effects: tachycardia, T-wave flattening, prolonged QT interval.
Protriptyline (Vivactil)	20–60 mg	Twitch, extrapyramidal movement effects.
Trimipramine (Surmontil)	75–300 mg	
Tetracyclic Agent		
Mirtazapine (Remeron)	15–45 mg	Somnolence, increased appetite, weight gain, dry mouth, constipation.
Bicyclic Agent		
Venlafaxine (Effexor)	375 mg	Nervousness, weight loss, dizziness, hypertension.
Selective Serotonin Reuptake Inhibitors (SSRIs)		
Fluoxetine (Prozac)	10–40 mg	Delayed orgasm, headache, nervousness, insomnia, anxiety, tremor, dizziness, nausea, diarrhea, anorexia, dry mouth.
Paroxetine (Paxil)	20–50 mg	Nausea, dry mouth, headache, somnolence, insomnia, diarrhea, constipation, tremor.
Sertraline (Zoloft)	50–150 mg	Insomnia, diarrhea, nausea, weight loss.
Fluvoxamine (Luvox)	50–300 mg	Nausea, vomiting, drowsiness, anorexia, constipation, tremor, insomnia.
Monoamine Oxidase Inhibitors (MAOIs)		
Isocarboxazid (Marplan)	30–50 mg	For all MAOIs:
Phenelzine (Nardil)	45–90 mg	Orthostatic hypotension, weight gain, edema, insomnia, sexual dysfunction, myoclonus, muscle pains, paresthesias, anticholinergic effects.
Tranylcypromine (Parnate)	20–60 mg	
Pargyline (Eutonyl)	150 mg	
Selegiline (Eldepryl, Deprenyl)	10 mg	Food and beverages containing tyramine in combination with MAOIs as well as combining sympathetic drugs with an MAOI can cause hypertensive crisis.
Dibenzoxazepine Agent		
Amoxapine (Asendin)	100–600 mg	Dizziness, postural hypotension, reflex tachycardia, extrapyramidal movement disorders.
Unicyclic Agent		
Bupropion (Wellbutrin)	225–450 mg	Dry mouth, constipation, headache, insomnia, restlessness, agitation, menstrual irregularities, increased seizure risk.
Triazolopyridine Agent		
Trazodone (Desyrel)	150–600 mg	Sedation, orthostatic hypotension, dizziness, headache, nausea, priapism.
Phenylipiperazine Agent		
Nefazodone (Serzone)	200–600 mg	Postural hypotension, anxiety, nervous tremor, agitation.

c. Ultraviolet light therapy may be recommended for depression that occurs during fall and winter months (seasonal affective disorder).

4. The patient may select complementary/alternative treatments. The use of herbal supplements, especially St. John's wort, is a popular alternative for antidepressant medications (see Appendix IV).

 DRUG ALERT

Antidepressant therapy requires 2 to 4 weeks before beneficial effects occur. Patients cannot combine two different antidepressant drugs because of additive serotonergic effects leading to serotonin syndrome. Hypertensive crisis can occur if patients take an MAOI antidepressant in combination with a sympathomimetic drug or eat foods high in tryamine.

5. Psychotherapy
   a. Psychodynamic therapy assists the patient to become aware of unconscious anger directed toward object loss and "work through" these feelings to alleviate depression.
   b. Cognitive therapy is the recommended psychotherapeutic approach for depression. This approach includes identifying and challenging the accuracy of the patient's negative thought patterns and encouraging behaviors designed to counteract depressive symptoms.
   c. Family therapy assists the patient and family members to increase level of differentiation and therefore function in a more self-responsible manner.

Complications

1. An undiagnosed medical condition causing depressive symptoms could lead to physical deterioration and/or delay in obtaining appropriate treatment.
2. Untreated depressive illness can lead to suicide.
3. Use of alcohol or drugs to "feel better" or numb dysphoric feelings.

Nursing Assessment

1. Assess posture and affect for:
   a. Poor/slumped posture
   b. Appearance of being older than stated age
   c. Facial expression of sadness, dejection
   d. Episodes of weeping
   e. Anhedonia—inability to experience pleasure
2. Assess thought processes.
   a. Identify the presence of suicidal thoughts
   b. Poor judgment, indecisiveness
   c. Impaired problem solving, poor concentration
   d. Negative thoughts
3. Explore feelings for:
   a. Anger and irritability
   b. Anxiety, guilt
   c. Worthlessness
   d. Helplessness, hopelessness

4. Assess physical behavior for:
   a. Psychomotor agitation or retardation
   b. Vegetative signs of depression
      (i) Change in eating patterns
      (ii) Change in sleeping patterns
      (iii) Change in elimination patterns
      (iv) Change in level of interest in sex
5. Assess for evidence of "masked depression."
   a. Hypochondriasis
   b. Psychosomatic disorders
   c. Compulsive gambling
   d. Compulsive overwork
   e. Accident proneness
   f. Eating disorders
   g. Addictive illnesses

Nursing Diagnoses

- Hopelessness related to depressive thoughts
- Risk for Injury related to hopelessness and impaired problem solving
- Self-Care Deficit related to lack of motivation and poor concentration
- Sleep Pattern Disturbance related to insomnia

Other nursing diagnoses that may apply include:
- Dysfunctional Grieving related to unresolved feelings from significant loss
- Social Isolation related to lack of interest or energy to interact with others
- Ineffective Family Coping: Compromised related to impact of symptoms of depression in one member

Nursing Interventions
Strengthening Coping and Sense of Hope

1. Initiate interaction with the patient at a regularly scheduled time.
2. Be clear and honest about your own feelings related to the patient's behavior.
3. Encourage verbal expression of feelings.
4. Validate feelings that are appropriate to the situation.
5. Explore with the patient what is producing and maintaining the feeling of depression.
6. Encourage the patient to identify events that cause unpleasant emotional responses.
7. Assess significant losses the patient has experienced.
8. Identify cultural and social factors that may contribute to how the patient copes with loss and feelings.
9. Assess the patient's support network.

Maintaining Safety

1. Assess current suicide risk.
2. Implement appropriate level of observation based on a focused suicide assessment (eg, constant observation or 15-minute checks).
3. Explain observation precautions to the patient.
4. Remove harmful objects from the patient's possession, and assess environmental safety of the patient's room and unit.
5. Encourage the patient to negotiate a no-self-harm/no-suicide agreement with the staff.

6. Monitor need to revise level of observation.

7. Provide additional structure by keeping the patient involved in therapeutic and psychorehabilitative activities.

Encouraging Participation in Activities of Daily Living

1. Collaborate with occupational and physical therapists to determine patient's functional capacity to accomplish ADLs.

2. If patient is unable to accomplish ADLs independently, provide hygiene activities in collaboration with patient.

3. Acknowledge and reinforce the patient's efforts to maintain appearance; do not rush the patient when self-care is slow.

4. Reinforce what the patient can do rather than what he or she cannot do without assistance.

5. Remain with the patient during mealtime to determine the level of need for assistance or cueing in the ability to eat.

Facilitating Sleep

1. Determine the patient's past and current sleep patterns and sleep hygiene.

2. Ask what strategies the patient has already used to improve sleep, and elicit which ones have been successful.

3. Consider decreasing the amount of daytime sleep by encouraging participation in an activity.

4. Discuss alternative methods for facilitating sleep:
   a. Avoid caffeine.
   b. Avoid emotionally charged or upsetting discussions before bedtime.
   c. Avoid exercise $\frac{1}{2}$ to 1 hour before bed.
   d. Increase physical activity within functional limits.
   e. Use relaxation techniques.
   f. Try a warm bath or warm milk.

5. Administer medications at bedtime that cause sleepiness; avoid administering those at night that cause insomnia.

Community and Home Care Considerations

1. Mood disorders tend to be chronic, with acute episodes that may require inpatient treatment. The patient in the home or community setting will require ongoing monitoring regarding the use of medications as well as support and education in terms of the disorder.

2. Community health care providers, including nurses, must be aware of the need for primary and secondary prevention programs directed at education as well as early case finding and prompt treatment.

Patient Education and Health Maintenance

1. Instruct patient and family members about symptoms of depression.

2. Instruct patient and family members about purpose of antidepressant medication, effects, side effects and their management, and how to recognize early signs and symptoms of relapse.

3. Instruct patient and family members about the effect of a depressive disorder on the family system.

4. Provide patient and family members with written material on coping with depression.

5. Provide patient and family members with information about appropriate community-based programs and support groups. Contact the National Foundation for Depressive Illness, P.O. Box 2257, New York, NY 10016, 800-248-4344.

Outcome-Based Evaluation

- Reports improvement in mood and increased interest in daily living
- Remains safe from self-harm
- Accomplishes activities of daily living in an independent manner
- Obtains a minimum of 5 hours of uninterrupted sleep

■ Bipolar Disorders

The bipolar disorders, also considered mood disorders, include the occurrence of depressive episodes and one or more elated mood episodes. An elated mood can include a range of affect, from normal mood to hypomania to mania. In the most intense presentation, the person with bipolar disorder experiences altered thought processes, which can produce bizarre delusions.

Pathophysiology and Etiology
Genetic Basis

1. Twin studies reveal a concordance rate of 65% in monozygotic twins for bipolar disorder.

2. Risk for developing bipolar disorder is increased 4% to 24% in first-degree relatives of people with bipolar disorder.

3. Current research indicates that defective genes located within chromosomes 18 and 21 may be related to bipolar disorder.

Biochemical Factors

1. Patients with bipolar disorders may have lower plasma norepinephrine, urinary MHPG, and platelet serotonin uptake and higher red blood cell/plasma lithium rates than do unipolar populations.

2. Pathology of the limbic system, basal ganglia, and hypothalamus is proposed to contribute to the development of mood disorders.

Psychosocial Factors

1. Psychosocial stressors appear to have an important role early in the illness, in concert with the electrical kindling and behavioral sensitization models.

2. Mania and hypomania have been viewed by psychoanalytic theorists as a defense against depression.

Clinical Manifestations
See Box 57-4.

Diagnostic Evaluation

1. Rating scale assessment tools:
   a. Mania Rating Scale
   b. Mini-mental Status Examination

BOX 57-4 Characteristics of Bipolar Disorders

Bipolar I Disorder

1. Presence of only one manic episode.
2. No past major depressive episodes.
3. The manic episode is not accounted for by schizoaffective disorder.
4. Manic episode is not superimposed on schizophrenia, schizophreniform disorder, delusional disorder, or psychotic disorder.

Specifiers

- Mixed symptoms
- Severity/psychotic
- Remission specifiers
- Catatonic features
- Postpartum onset

Bipolar II Disorder

1. Presence/history of one or more major depressive episodes.
2. Presence/history of at least one hypomanic episode.
3. There has not been a manic or mixed episode.
4. The symptoms cause clinically significant distress or impairment in social or occupational functioning.

Specifiers

- Hypomanic
- Depressed

Cyclothymic Disorder

- Over a period of 2 years, there are numerous periods without hypomanic symptoms and numerous periods with depressive symptoms that don't meet criteria for a major depressive episode.
- During the 2-year period, the client has not been without these symptoms for more than 2 months at a time.
- No major depressive episode, manic episode, or mixed episode during the first 2 years of the disturbance.
- Symptoms are not due to physiologic aspects.
- Symptoms cause clinically significant distress or impairment in all aspects of functioning.

(Adapted from American Psychiatric Association [1994]. *Diagnostic and statistical manual of mental disorders* [4th ed.]. Washington, D.C.: APA.)

2. There appear to be no laboratory features that distinguish major depressive episodes found in major depressive disorder from those in bipolar I or bipolar II disorder.
3. Complete psychophysiologic examination.
4. Complete assessment to rule out medical conditions.

Management

1. Patients may receive treatment in acute inpatient psychiatric hospitals or in the community in an outpatient program. Decision about treatment setting is made according to severity of patient's illness, including degree of mania and/or depression as well as risk of self-harm or harm to others.

2. Inpatient treatment is directed toward medication management as well as supportive psychotherapy in order to alleviate the acute manic symptoms.
3. Pharmacologic treatment for acute mania consists of the following:
   a. Lithium carbonate (Lithobid)
   b. Anticonvulsants for mood-stabilizing properties, such as gabapentin (Neurontin) and valproate (Depakene)
   c. Neuroleptic agents such as risperidone (Risperdal) utilized for acute psychotic thinking
   d. Benzodiazepines such as clonazepam (Klonopin) or lorazepam (Ativan) used for acute agitation

◆ DRUG ALERT

Patients taking lithium can develop toxicity related to elevated levels in the blood; therefore, lithium blood levels must be monitored periodically. Initial therapy requires daily monitoring until safe, therapeutic level is attained; weekly and then monthly monitoring is then recommended. Lithium toxicity is related to decreased serum sodium levels and inadequate hydration. Therefore, patients taking lithium must have normal sodium intake and at least 2 to 3 L of water daily.

4. Psychotherapy is used as described above in the section related to depression.
5. Psychiatric home care nursing to facilitate compliance with medications and therapeutic interventions.
6. Community-based support group participation.

Complications

1. Untreated bipolar disorder can lead to physical exhaustion.
2. Poor judgment can lead to financial problems.
3. Alcohol and drug abuse problems can develop and cause disruption in the family.
4. Concurrent medical conditions may be exacerbated.

Nursing Assessment

1. Assess mood for stability; range of affect, from elation to irritability to severe agitation; laughing, joking, and talking continuously; uninhibited familiarity with interviewer.
2. Assess behavior for constant activity, starting many projects but finishing few, mild to severe hyperactivity, spending large sums of money, increased appetite, indiscriminate sex, minimal to no sleeping, outlandish or bizarre dress, poor concentration.
3. Assess thought processes for flight of ideas; pressured speech, often with content that is sexually explicit; clang associations (sound of word, rather than its meaning, directs subsequent associations); delusions; hallucinations.

Nursing Diagnoses

- Altered Thought Processes related to biologic changes as demonstrated by agitation, hyperactivity, and inability to concentrate

- Sleep Pattern Disturbance related to hyperactivity and perceived lack of need for sleep
- Altered Family Processes related to role changes, economic strain, and lack of knowledge about the patient's illness
- Altered Nutrition: Less Than Body Requirements related to hyperactivity

Nursing Interventions
Improving Thought Processes and Decreasing Sensory Overload
1. Assess patient's degree of distorted thinking.
2. Redirect the patient when you are unable to follow his or her thought processes.
3. Use brief explanations.
4. Remain consistent in approach and expectations.
5. Frequently reality-orient the patient; speak in a clear, simple manner.
6. Provide the patient with a relaxing area with decreased environmental stimulation.
7. Assist the patient with a gradual and progressive integration into the social environment while observing for behavioral changes that indicate readiness for participation in further activities.

Improving Sleep Pattern
1. Establish a distraction-free environment at bedtime.
2. Help the patient avoid the intake of caffeine and nicotine.
3. Administer prescribed medications as ordered, and monitor the patient's response.

Improving the Effect of Bipolar Illness on Family
1. Assess the family's external support network, and encourage participation in family therapy and support groups.
2. Assess communication and boundaries within the family.
3. Observe and assess interaction patterns within the family, and discuss their influence on the patient and his or her family functioning.
4. Provide the patient and family with information regarding bipolar disorder and the treatment plan, prognosis, and aftercare plan.

Ensuring Adequate Nutrition
1. Maintain accurate documentation of food and fluid intake.
2. Offer small, frequent meals of high-calorie foods. Include food that the patient likes and that can be eaten "on the move."
3. Serve the patient meals in a low-stimulus environment.
4. Monitor the patient's serum electrolyte and albumin levels and weigh every other day.
5. Monitor vital signs.

Patient Education and Health Maintenance
1. Instruct patient and family about bipolar illness, including symptoms of relapse.
2. Instruct patient and family members about psychopharmacologic treatment, including its purpose, effects, side effects, and management.

3. Advise patient and family members about community-based support groups or health care agencies that are relevant to his or her care.

Outcome-Based Evaluation
- Improved thought processes demonstrated by clear sentences with no evidence of flight of ideas and completion of simple tasks
- Sleeping for 5 hours at night
- Family members verbalize realistic, goal-directed thinking related to the patient's abilities, recovery, and control of condition
- No weight loss noted

THOUGHT DISTURBANCES (PSYCHOTIC DISORDERS)

Schizophrenia, Schizophreniform, and Delusional Disorders

The disorders included in this section have defining features of psychotic symptoms. Psychotic symptoms are produced by a loss of ego boundaries and/or a gross impairment in reality testing, which includes prominent hallucinations and delusions, disorganized speech, and grossly disorganized or catatonic behavior. Schizophrenia can be classified as positive or negative type, although most patients have a mixture of these symptoms. The positive symptoms include hallucinations, delusions, loose associations, and bizarre or disorganized behavior. The negative symptoms include restricted emotion (flat affect), anhedonia, avolition, alogia, and social withdrawal.

Pathophysiology and Etiology
The exact causation of these disorders remains unclear. The current consensus is that they result from complex interactions among a variety of factors.

Schizophrenia, Schizophreniform Disorder
1. Genetic factors:
   a. Studies of monozygotic twins reveal a 50% concordance rate with a 15% rate with dizygotic twins.
   b. If one parent is affected with schizophrenia, a 12% rate is demonstrated in the children, while having two parents with the disorder increases the risk to 35% to 39%.
   c. Research is focused on genes on chromosomes 6, 13, 18, and 22 as related to the development of schizophrenia.
2. Biochemical and structural brain factors:
   a. Dopamine hypothesis—hyperactivity in the dopaminergic system, possibly due to receptor neurons that are functionally hyperactive.
   b. Norepinephrine, serotonin, glutamate, and GABA may also have a role in modulating the symptoms of schizophrenia.

c. Endogenous dysfunction of N-methyl-D-aspartate receptor-mediated neurotransmission could lead to the development of schizophrenia.

d. Neuroanatomic studies—cerebral ventricular enlargement; sulcal enlargement; cerebellar atrophy; decreased cranial, cerebral, and frontal size; abnormalities in basal ganglia; structural abnormalities at the cellular level, particularly in the limbic and periventricular regions.

e. Functional and metabolic studies—regional cerebral blood flow studies demonstrated hypofrontality: schizophrenic patients were unable to increase blood flow to their frontal lobes during a task thought to increase frontal lobe functions; positron-emission tomography (PET) studies also consistently found evidence for a relative hypofrontality.

f. Electrophysiologic studies-EEG findings in schizophrenic patients demonstrated decreased alpha and increased delta activity; changes in evoked potentials and amplitude reduction may occur in responses reflecting selective attention and stimulus evaluation. P300 response (reduced amplitude to unexpected stimuli using auditory and visual parameters) is the most pronounced and is prolonged. This defect leads to information or sensory overload and an inability to "screen out" irrelevant stimuli.

g. Research evidence supports speculation that schizophrenia is a neurodevelopmental disorder that may result from brain injury occurring early in life and interfering with normal developmental events.

3. Psychosocial factors:

a. Psychodynamic theory proposes that the essential feature of schizophrenia is a defect in interpersonal relationships due to a withdrawal of the libido into the self.

b. Interpersonal theory proposes that the lack of a warm, nurturing relationship in the early years of life contributes to the lack of self-identity, reality misperception, and relationship withdrawal that is apparent in the disorder.

c. Family theory related to the role of the family in the development of schizophrenia has not been validated by research. An area of family functioning that has been implicated is increased relapse rates in families characterized by high expressed emotion (HEE). This characteristic is described as emotional overinvolvement along with hostile and critical feedback.

Delusional Disorder

1. Little has been established about the etiology of delusional disorder.
2. There is no demonstrated genetic linkage.
3. It is possible that psychosocial stressors have a role in the etiology of delusional disorder in some persons. This is illustrated in some of the rarer conditions, such as shared psychotic disorder.

Clinical Manifestations
See Boxes 57-5 and 57-6.

Diagnostic Evaluation

1. Clinical diagnosis is developed on historical information and thorough mental status examination.
2. No laboratory findings have been identified that are diagnostic of schizophrenia.
3. Routine battery of laboratory tests may be useful in ruling out possible organic etiologies, including CBC, urinalysis, liver function tests, thyroid function tests, RPR, HIV test, serum ceruloplasmin (rules out Wilson's disease), PET scan, CT, and MRI.
4. Rating scale assessment:
   a. Scale for the Assessment of Negative Symptoms
   b. Scale for the Assessment of Positive Symptoms

Management
Schizophrenia and Schizophreniform Disorder

1. Patients may receive treatment in inpatient settings or in community-based outpatient programs or psychiatric home care. The level of care is dependent of the severity of the symptoms and the risk of harm to self and others.
2. These disorders generally require long-term treatment; therefore, a case management approach is important in order to coordinate multiple services.
3. Pharmacologic therapy with either the typical or atypical neuroleptics (antipsychotics) is the mainstay of treatment. The typical neuroleptics have multiple side effects that require careful management (Table 57-2). The atypical neuroleptics have less adverse effects and may also be more effective in decreasing the negative symptoms of schizophrenia. The common atypical neuroleptics include clozapine (Clozaril), olanzapine (Zyprexa), and risperidone (Risperdal). The reader is directed to a pharmacology source for details regarding the typical and atypical neuroleptics.
4. Psychosocial treatments
5. Supportive therapy that is reality oriented and pragmatic
6. Family therapy
7. Psychoeducational individual, group, and family support
8. Support groups in the community
9. Community-based partial hospitalization programs
10. Psychiatric home care nursing
11. Vocational and social skills education

Delusional Disorder

1. Neuroleptic agents have demonstrated some success in reducing the intensity of the delusion.
2. Individual psychotherapy.
3. Hospitalization for comprehensive assessment for diagnostic purposes or if suicidal or homicidal.

BOX 57-5 **Characteristics of Schizophrenia, Schizophreniform, and Schizoaffective Disorders**

Schizophrenia Subtypes

Paranoid
1. Dominant—hallucinations and delusions.
2. No disorganized speech, disorganized behavior, or disorganized affect present.

Disorganized
1. Dominant—disorganized speech and disorganized behavior.
2. Delusions and hallucinations if present are not prominent or fragmented.

Residual
1. No longer has positive symptoms, eg, delusions, hallucinations, or disorganized speech or behaviors.
2. However, persistence of some symptoms is noted, eg,
   - Marked social isolation or withdrawal
   - Marked impairment in role function (wage earner, student, or homemaker)
   - Markedly peculiar behavior
   - Marked impairment in personal hygiene
   - Marked lack of initiative, interest, or energy
   - Blunted or inappropriate affect

Catatonic
1. Motor immobility (waxy flexibility)
2. Excessive purposeless motor activity (agitation)
3. Extreme negativism or mutism
4. Peculiar voluntary movement
   - Posturing
   - Stereotyped movements
   - Prominent mannerisms
   - Prominent grimaces
5. Echolalia or echopraxia

Undifferentiated
1. Has positive symptoms (does have hallucinations, delusions, and bizarre behaviors)
2. No one clinical presentation dominates, eg,
   - Paranoid
   - Disorganized
   - Catatonic

Schizophreniform Disorder
1. Two or more of the following symptoms:
   (1) Delusions
   (2) Hallucinations
   (3) Disorganized speech
   (4) Grossly disorganized or catatonic behavior
       - Affective flattening
       - Alogia (inability to speak)
       - Avolition (inability to make a decision)
2. Schizoaffective and mood disorders, chemical dependence, or a causative general medical condition is ruled out.
3. Lasts at least 1 month but less than 6 months.

Schizoaffective Disorder
1. An uninterrupted period of illness where there was either a major depressive, manic, or mixed episode.
2. Concurrent positive and negative symptoms of schizophrenia.
3. Disturbance not due to direct physiologic effects of a chemical or general medical condition.

(Adapted from American Psychiatric Association [1994]. *Diagnostic and statistical manual of mental disorders* [4th ed.]. Washington, D.C.: APA.)

Complications

1. If left undiagnosed, untreated, or ineffectively treated, schizophrenia can lead to profound inability to function and contribute to the problem of homelessness in our society.
2. Neglect of other medical conditions; therefore, complications due to untreated medical illness are common.
3. Depression and suicide.
4. Chemical use, abuse, or dependency.

Nursing Assessment

Assess for positive symptoms of schizophrenia. These symptoms reflect aberrant mental activity and are usually present early in the first phase of the schizophrenic illness.

Alterations in Thinking

1. Delusion: false, fixed belief that is not amenable to change by reasoning. The most frequent elicited delusions include:
   a. Ideas of reference
   b. Delusions of grandeur
   c. Delusions of jealousy
   d. Delusions of persecution
   e. Somatic delusions
2. Loose associations: the thought process becomes illogical and confused.
3. Neologisms: made-up words that have a special meaning to the delusional person.
4. Concrete thinking: an overemphasis on small or specific details and an impaired ability to abstract.
5. Echolalia: pathologic repeating of another's words.
6. Clang associations: the meaningless rhyming of a word in a forceful way.
7. Word salad: a mixture of words that is meaningless to the listener.

Alterations in Perceiving

1. Hallucinations: sensory perceptions that have no external stimulus. The most common are auditory, visual, gustatory, olfactory, and tactile.
2. Loss of ego boundaries: lack a sense of their body and how they relate to the environment.

BOX 57-6 Characteristics of Psychotic Disorders (Not Schizophrenic)

Delusional Disorder
1. Nonbizarre delusions of at least 1 month's duration.
2. No positive/negative symptoms of schizophrenia present.
3. Tactile/olfactory hallucinations may be present and are related to the delusional theme.
4. Functioning is not markedly impaired and behavior is not obviously bizarre or odd.
5. Only brief mood episodes, if any.
6. Not due to direct physiologic effects of a chemical or a general medical condition.

Psychotic Disorder Due to a General Medical Disorder
1. Prominent hallucinations or delusions.
2. Evidence from the history, physical examination, or lab studies that the disorder is due to physiologic consequences of a general medical condition.
3. Disturbance does not occur exclusively during the course of delirium.

Brief Psychotic Disorder
1. Presence of 1 or more of these symptoms:
   • Delusions
   • Disorganized speech
   • Grossly disorganized or catatonic behavior
   • Hallucinations
2. Duration of the disturbance is at least 1 day and less than 1 month.
3. Eventual return to premorbid level of functioning.

Specifiers:
• With marked stressors
• Without marked stressors
• With postpartum onset

Shared Psychotic Disorder
1. Delusion develops in an individual who has an already established delusion in the context of a close relationship.
2. Delusion is similar in content to the other person's.
3. Disturbance doesn't meet criteria for other psychotic disorders.

Substance-Induced Psychotic Disorder
1. Prominant hallucinations or delusions.
2. There is evidence from the history or physical assessment of the following:
   • Symptoms developed during or within 1 month of substance intoxication/withdrawal.
   • Medication use is related to the disturbance.
3. Disturbance does not occur exclusively during the course of a delirium.

Specifiers
• Specific substance
• Onset during intoxication
• Onset during withdrawal

(Adapted from American Psychiatric Association [1994]. *Diagnostic and statistical manual of mental disorders* [4th ed.]. Washington, D.C.: APA.)

---

a. Depersonalization is a nonspecific feeling or sense that a person has lost his or her identity or is unreal.
b. Derealization is the false perception by a person that the environment has changed.

Alterations in Behavioral Responses
1. Bizarre behavioral patterns:
   a. Motor agitation/restlessness
   b. Automatic obedience/robot-like movement
   c. Negativism
   d. Stereotyped behaviors
   e. Stupor
   f. Waxy flexibility
2. Agitated or impulsive behavior:
   a. Assess for negative symptoms of schizophrenia that reflect a deficiency of mental functioning.
      (i) Alogia—inability to speak
      (ii) Anergia—inability to react
      (iii) Anhedonia—inability to experience pleasure
      (iv) Avolition—inability to choose or decide
      (v) Poor social functioning
      (vi) Poverty of speech
      (vii) Social withdrawal
      (vii) Thought blocking
   b. Assess for associated symptoms of schizophrenia.

(i) Chemical use/abuse/dependence
(ii) Depression
(iii) Fantasy
(iv) Violent or aggressive behavior
(v) Water intoxication
(vi) Withdrawal

Nursing Diagnoses
• Altered Thought Processes related to perceptual and cognitive distortions, as demonstrated by suspiciousness, defensive behavior, and disruptions in thought
• Social Isolation related to an inability to trust
• Risk for Activity Intolerance related to adverse reactions to psychopharmacologic medications
• Ineffective Individual Coping related to misinterpretation of environment and impaired communication ability
• Risk for Violence: Self-directed or directed at others, related to delusional thinking and hallucinatory experiences

Nursing Interventions
Strengthening Differentiation
Between Delusions and Reality
1. Provide the patient with honest and consistent feedback in a nonthreatening manner.

TABLE 57-2 Management of Adverse Effects of Neuroleptic Medications

Symptom	Management
Orthostatic (Postural) Hypotension	Assess for orthostatic blood pressure changes and dizziness and teach the patient: • When rising from bed or chair, get up slowly. • Sit at side of bed for a few minutes, dangling legs. • Do ankle pumps before standing. • Once standing, move slowly. • Don't twist or turn quickly. • Use assistive devices, hand rails, canes, walkers when necessary for functional deficits. • Don't drive or operate machinery when dizzy.
Peripheral Anticholinergic Effects: dry mouth and nose, blurred vision, constipation, urinary retention	Dry mouth: • Brush teeth after each meal with a fluoridated toothpaste. • Rinse mouth frequently. • Limit caffeinated or alcoholic drinks, because they can be dehydrating. • Stop smoking due to the irritation of oral mucosa. • Suck on sugarless candy or gum; avoid sugared candy to decrease the risk of fungal infections and dental caries. • Avoid dry or spicy foods. • Drink fluids between meals unless you are on a specific fluid restriction. • Avoid acidic beverages due to potential irritation. • Use dressing, juices, or sauces (if allowed) to moisten food. Constipation: • Drink fluids (within prescribed limits set by health care provider). • Eat roughage: fruits, vegetables (raw leafy types) to increase bulk and help soften stool. • Eat dried fruits, such as prunes or dates, for laxative effect. • Maintain activity level within functional limits. • Consult with health care provider to determine appropriate use of over-the-counter laxatives (Metamucil, Citrucel) and/or prescribed stool softeners. Urinary retention: • Void at regular intervals • Ensure privacy.
Extrapyramidal Side Effects: Short Term	
Akathisia—restless legs, jitters, nervous energy, motor agitation	• Reassure patient. • Differentiate between agitation and akathisia. • Consider reducing dosage. • Consider switching patient to another class of antipsychotic.
Akinesia—weakness (hypotonia), fatigue, painful muscles, anergy (lack of energy), absence of movement	• Assess functional ability. • Dose reduction or cessation should improve movement if problems are due to akinesia versus psychotic symptoms.
Dystonias, dyskinesias—grimacing, torticollis, intermittent spasms, opisthotonos, oculogyric crises, head-neck stiffness, myoclonic twitches, laryngeal-pharyngeal dystonia	• Consider prophylaxis with anticholinergic medications. • Treat with IM/IV anticholinergics, as prescribed.
Parkinsonian effects—muscle stiffness, cog wheel rigidity, shuffling gait, stooped posture, drooling	• Treat with anticholinergics, as prescribed. • Stop the antipsychotic, as directed.
Long-Term Effects of Neuroleptics	
Tardive dyskinesia—a delayed effect of neuroleptic agents usually occurring after 6 months of treatment involving abnormal, involuntary, irregular, choreoathetoid movements of the muscles of the head, limbs, and trunk.	• Complete regular objective rating/assessment of the movement disorder. • Reduce/stop neuroleptic as directed. • Consider clozapine or respiridol. • Comprehensive medical psychiatric assessment necessary with close monitoring of movement disorder.

IM: intramuscular; IV: intravenous.

2. Avoid challenging the content of the patient's behaviors.
3. Focus interactions on the patient's behaviors.
4. Administer medications as prescribed while monitoring and documenting the patient's response to the medication regimen.
5. Use simple and clear language when speaking with the patient.
6. Explain all procedures, tests, and activities to the patient before starting them, and provide written or video material for learning purposes.

Promoting Socialization

1. Encourage the patient to talk about feelings in the context of a trusting, supportive relationship.
2. Allow patient time to reveal delusions to you without engaging in a power struggle over the content or the reality of the delusions.
3. Use a supportive, empathic approach to focus on the patient's feelings about troubling events and/or conflicts.
4. Provide opportunities for socialization and encourage participation in group activities.
5. Be aware of the patient's personal space and use touch judiciously.
6. Assist the patient to identify behaviors that alienate significant others and family members.

Improving Activity Tolerance

1. Assess the patient's response to prescribed antipsychotic medication.
2. Collaborate with the patient and occupational and physical therapy specialists to assess the patient's ability to perform ADLs.
3. Collaborate with the patient to establish a daily, achievable routine within physical limitations.
4. Teach strategies to manage side effects of antipsychotics that affect the patient's functional status, including the following:
   a. Change positions slowly.
   b. Gradually increase physical activities.
   c. Limit overdoing it in hot, sunny weather.
   d. Use sun precautions.
   e. Use caution in activities if extrapyramidal symptoms develop.

Improving Coping With Thoughts and Feelings

1. Encourage patient to express feelings.
2. Focus on patient's feelings and behavior.
3. Provide honest perceptions of reality and feedback about symptoms and behaviors.
4. Encourage the patient to explore adaptive behaviors that increase his or her abilities and success in socializing and accomplishing ADLs.
5. Decrease environmental stimuli.

Ensuring Safety

1. Monitor the patient for behaviors that indicate increased anxiety.
2. Collaborate with the patient to identify anxious behaviors as well as the causes.
3. Tell the patient that you will help him or her maintain control.
4. Establish consistent limits on the patient's behaviors and clearly communicate these limits to him or her, family members, and health care providers.
5. Secure all potential weapons and articles that could be used to inflict an injury from the patient's room and the unit environment.
6. To prepare for possible continued escalation, form a psychiatric emergency assist team and designate a leader to facilitate an effective and safe aggression-management process.

7. Determine the need for external control, including seclusion and/or restraints. Communicate the decision to the patient and put plan into action.
8. Frequently monitor the patient within the guidelines of the institution's policy on restrictive devices and assess the patient's level of agitation.
9. When the patient's level of agitation begins to decrease and self-control is regained, establish a behavioral agreement that identifies specific behaviors that indicate self-control against a reescalation of agitation.

Community and Home Care Considerations

1. Patients with these disorders may be in supportive housing, such as transitional living halfway houses, foster homes, and board and care homes. Supervision and medication management are important areas of concern for the nurse working in the community.
2. Psychosocial rehabilitation approach may be used in the community setting, where skills necessary for independent living are taught. The patient who has been symptomatic since early adulthood may not have learned these skills. The nurse working in the community setting may work as a member of the treatment team using this approach.

Patient Education and Health Maintenance

1. Instruct the patient and family members in disease process and how to recognize and cope with relapse symptoms.
2. Instruct the patient and family members about the uses, actions, and side effects of any prescribed medications.
3. Instruct the patient and family about community resources, support groups, and possible use of psychiatric home care nursing.
4. For additional information and support, refer to such agencies as National Alliance for Research on Schizophrenia and Depression (NARSAD), 60 Cutter Mill Road, Suite 404, Great Neck, NY 11021, 516-829-0091; *www.narsad.org*.

Outcome-Based Evaluation

- Exhibits improved reality orientation, concentration, and attention span as demonstrated through speech and behavior
- Communicates with family and staff in a clear manner without evidence of loose, dissociated thinking
- Independently maintains personal hygiene
- Participates in activities of daily living with minimal or no direction
- Remains free from harm or violent acts

COGNITIVE IMPAIRMENT DISTURBANCES

◼ Delirium, Dementia, and Amnesic Disorder

Cognitive impairment disturbances encompass specific disorders that produce either temporary or permanent neuronal damage, resulting in psychological or behavioral dysfunction. Cognitive impairment disorders described in the DSM-IV include delirium, dementia, and amnesic disorder.

Delirium is an acute disturbance of consciousness and a change in cognition that develops over a brief time period. Dementia is a chronic disturbance involving multiple cognitive deficits, including memory impairment. Amnesic disorder is characterized by memory impairment in the absence of other significant cognitive impairments.

Pathophysiology and Etiology
Delirium

Can be caused by numerous pathophysiologic conditions. Some of the major possibilities include:

1. CNS pathology: head trauma, hypertensive cerebral changes, seizures, tumors
2. Endocrinopathies: thyroidism, parathyroidism
3. Hypoxemia
4. Hypothermia/hyperthermia
5. Intoxication/abstinence and withdrawal states
6. Metals/toxins/drugs
7. Metabolic: diabetic acidosis, hypoglycemia, acid-base imbalances
8. Hepatic encephalopathy
9. Thiamine deficiency
10. Postoperative states
11. Psychosocial stressors: relocation stress, sensory deprivation/overload, sleep deprivation, immobilization

Primary Dementia

Primary dementias are degenerative disorders that are progressive, irreversible, and not due to any other condition. Specific disorders are dementia of Alzheimer's type (DAT) and vascular dementia (formerly multi-infarct dementia). Dementia of Alzheimer's type demonstrates progression of symptoms from the initial stage, which is characterized by mild cognitive deficits in the area of short-term memory and accomplishment of goal-directed activity, to the final stage in which profound impairment occurs in the areas of cognition and self-care abilities. Research is ongoing; however, DAT is believed to have multiple causative factors. (Also see p. 186 for Alzheimer's disease.)

1. Genetic factors:
   a. Familial Alzheimer's disease (F.A.D.) is associated with abnormal genes on chromosomes 1, 14, and 21.
   b. A specific cholesterol-bearing protein, apolipoprotein E4 (Apo E4), is found on chromosome 19 twice as often in people with DAT as in the general population.
2. Biochemical and brain structural factors:
   a. The neurotransmitter acetylcholine has been implicated in terms of relative deficit and/or receptor abnormalities as related to Alzheimer's disease.
   b. Findings from autopsy reveal presence of brain changes, that is, the presence of amyloid plaques and neurofibrillary tangles associated with nerve cell destruction.
   c. Additional areas of investigation include:
      (i) Slow viral infection
      (ii) Autoimmune processes
      (iii) Head trauma

Secondary Dementias

Occur as a result of another pathologic process.

1. Infection-related dementias:
   a. Acquired immunodeficiency syndrome
   b. Chronic meningitis
   c. Jakob-Creutzfeldt disease
   d. Progressive multifocal leukoencephalopathy
   e. Postencephalitic dementia syndrome
   f. Syphilis
   g. Subacute sclerosing panencephalitis
   h. Tuberculosis
2. Subcortical degenerative disorders:
   a. Huntington's disease
   b. Parkinson's disease
   c. Wilson's disease
   d. Thalamic dementia
3. Hydrocephalic dementias
4. Vascular dementias
5. Traumatic conditions, such as post-traumatic encephalopathy and subdural hematoma
6. Neoplastic dementias:
   a. Glioma
   b. Meningioma
   c. Meningeal carcinomatosis
   d. Metastatic deposits
7. Inflammatory conditions, such as sarcoidosis, systemic lupus erythematosus, and temporal arteritis
8. Toxic conditions, such as alcohol-related syndrome and iatrogenic dementias (anticonvulsants, anticholinergics, antihypertensives, psychotropic agents)
9. Metabolic disorders:
   a. Anemias
   b. Deficiency states (minerals and vitamins)
   c. Cardiac/pulmonary failure
   d. Hepatic encephalopathy
   e. Porphyria
   f. Uremia

Amnesic Disorder

1. Post-traumatic amnesia: head trauma is the most common cause of amnesia
2. Poststroke amnesia: damage to the fornix or hippocampus
3. Neoplasms
4. Anoxic states
5. Herpes simplex encephalitis
6. Hypoglycemic states
7. Epileptic seizures
8. ECT
9. Substance-induced

Clinical Manifestations
See Table 57-3.

Diagnostic Evaluation
A wide variety of diagnostic tests may be done to determine cause. A comprehensive neuropsychiatric evaluation must be completed to make an accurate diagnosis.

TABLE 57-3 Clinical Manifestations: Cognitive Impairment Disorders

Disorder	DSM-IV Diagnoses	Defining Characteristics
Delirium (severe impairment in functioning)	• Delirium due to a general medical condition • Substance-induced delirium • Delirium due to multiple etiologies	• Fluctuating levels of awareness • Clouding of consciousness (confused and disoriented) • Perceptual disturbances (illusions and hallucinations) • Memory, especially recent memory, is disturbed • Alteration in sleep–wake cycle • EEG changes • Abrupt onset may last about 1 week • Reversible when underlying cause has been treated
Dementia (severe impairment in functioning)	• Dementia of the Alzheimer's type • Vascular dementia • Dementia due to a general medical condition • Substance-induced persisting dementia • Dementia due to multiple etiologies	• Slow, insidious onset • Impaired long- and short-term memory • Deterioration of cognitive abilities—judgment, abstract thinking • Often irreversible if untreatable • Personality changes • No or slow EEG changes
Amnesic syndrome (moderate to severe impairment in functioning)	• Amnestic disorder due to a general medical condition • Substance-induced persisting amnestic disorder	• Impairment in short- and long-term memory • Inability to learn new material • Remote memory better than that of recent events • Confabulation • Apathy, lack of initiative • Emotionally bland

DSM-IV: *Diagnostic and statistical manual of mental disorders, 4th Edition,* EEG: electroencephalogram.
(Adapted from American Psychiatric Association [1994]. *Diagnostic and statistical manual of mental disorders* [4th ed.]. Washington, D.C.: APA.)

1. Basic laboratory examination, including CBC with differential, chemistry panel (including blood urea nitrogen, creatine, and ammonia), arterial blood gases, chest x-ray, toxicology screen (comprehensive), thyroid function tests, and serologic tests for syphilis.
2. Additional tests may include CT, MRI, additional blood chemistries (heavy metals, thiamine, folate, antinuclear antibody [ANA], and urinary porphobilinogen), lumbar puncture, PET/single photon emission computer tomography (SPECT) scans
3. Complete mental status examination
4. Comprehensive physical examination

Management
Delirium
1. Treatment generally occurs in acute hospital-based setting where the goal is diagnosis to identify specific reversible causes of the delirium so that treatment is focused on ameliorating the causative factor(s).
2. Pharmacologic therapy is dependent on underlying cause(s). Additional medications may be used that are directed toward the decrease of the acute symptoms of delirium. These include:
   a. Benzodiazepines such as lorazepam (Ativan) for abstinence withdrawal states
   b. Neuroleptics such as risperidone (Risperdal) and haloperidol (Haldol) for agitation
   c. Combined administration of haloperidol and lorazepam for agitated and psychotic symptomatology
3. Environmental management:
   a. Safe, structured environment
   b. Orientation facilitated by accurate clocks and calendars
4. Family teaching regarding the nature of the disorder.
5. Family participation in the treatment plan in order to assist in the management of behavior.

Dementia
1. Treatment is generally community focused; the goal of treatment is to maintain the quality of life as long as possible despite the progressive nature of the disease. Effective treatment is based on:
   a. Diagnosis of primary illness and concurrent psychiatric disorders
   b. Assessment of auditory and visual impairment
   c. Measurement of the degree, nature, and progression of cognitive deficits
   d. Assessment of functional capacity and ability for self-care
   e. Family and social system assessment
2. Environmental strategies in order to assist in maintaining the safety and functional abilities of the patient as long as possible.
3. Pharmacologic therapy used for the person with DAT is directed toward the use of anticholinesterase medications to slow the progression of the disorder by increasing the relative amount of acetylcholine. The medication donepezil (Aricept) is utilized. Other medications may be used for behavioral control and symptom reduction.
   a. Agitation management: neuroleptic agents
   b. Psychosis: neuroleptic agents
   c. Depression: antidepressants, ECT

4. Hypertension management in vascular dementia is important in decreasing the severity of symptoms.
5. Family education is a treatment strategy because statistics indicate that family caregivers provide care for patients with DAT in 7 out of 10 cases. The family and the treatment team collaborate in the delivery of care.

Complications

1. Without accurate diagnosis and treatment, secondary dementias may become permanent.
2. Falls with serious orthopedic or cerebral injuries.
3. Self-inflicted injuries.
4. Aggression or violence toward self, others, or property.
5. Wandering events, in which the person can get lost and potentially suffer exposure, hypothermia, and even death.
6. Serious depression is demonstrated in caregivers who receive inadequate support.

Nursing Assessment

See Table 57-4.
1. Assess the onset and characteristics of symptoms (determine type and stage of disorder).
2. Establish cognitive status using standard measurement tools.
3. Determine self-care abilities.
4. Assess threats to physical safety (eg, wandering, poor reality testing).
5. Assess affect and emotional responsiveness.
6. Assess ability and level of support available to caregiver(s).

Nursing Diagnoses

• Impaired Communication related to cerebral impairment as demonstrated by altered memory, judgment, and word finding
• Self-Care Deficit related to cognitive impairment as demonstrated by inattention and inability to complete ADLs

• Risk for Injury related to cognitive impairment and wandering behavior
• Impaired Social Interaction related to cognitive impairment
• Risk for Violence: Self-directed or directed toward others due to suspicion and inability to recognize people or places

Nursing diagnoses may also include:
• Altered Family Processes related to impact of cognitive deficits on traditional roles and functioning
• Caregiver Role Strain related to lack of adequate support and level of care necessary for the patient with a cognitive impairment disorder

Nursing Interventions
Improving Communication

1. Speak slowly and use short, simple words and phrases.
2. Consistently identify yourself, and address the person by name at each meeting.
3. Focus on one piece of information at a time. Review what has been discussed with patient.
4. If patient has vision or hearing disturbances, have him or her wear prescription eyeglasses and/or a hearing device.
5. Keep environment well lit.
6. Use clocks, calendars, and familiar personal effects in the patient's view.
7. If patient becomes verbally aggressive, identify and acknowledge how he or she is feeling.
8. If patient becomes aggressive, shift the topic to a safer, more familiar one.
9. If patient becomes delusional, acknowledge his or her feelings and reinforce reality. Do not attempt to challenge the content of the delusion.

Promoting Independence in Self-Care

1. Assess and monitor the patient's ability to perform ADLs.
2. Encourage decision making regarding ADLs as much as possible.
3. Label clothes with patient's name, address, and telephone number.

TABLE 57-4 Nursing Assessment for Delirium, Dementia and Amnesic Disorder			
	Delirium	**Dementia**	**Amnestic Disorder**
Onset	Acute	Slow, insidious	Sudden
Course	Usually brief	Progresses over years	Transient or chronic
Mood	Fearfulness, anxiety, irritability	Mood labile, personality traits accentuated	Apathy, agitation, emotional blandness, shallow range of affective expression
Perception	Auditory, visual, tactile hallucinations; illusions	Hallucinations not a prominent feature	No hallucinatory experiences
Memory	Short-term memory impaired	Short-term memory damage followed by long-term memory damage	Impaired ability to learn new information; unable to recall previously learned information or past events
Communication	Slurred speech; confabulation	Normal—early stage: progressive aphasia and confabulation	Confabulation

4. Use clothing with elastic and Velcro for fastenings rather than buttons or zippers, which may be too difficult for the patient to manipulate.
5. Monitor food and fluid intake.
6. Weigh the patient weekly.
7. Provide food that patient can eat while moving.
8. Sit with the patient during meals and assist by cueing.
9. Initiate a bowel and bladder program early in the disease process to maintain continence and prevent constipation or urinary retention.

Ensuring Safety

1. Discuss restriction of driving when recommended.
2. Assess home for safety: remove throw rugs, label rooms, and keep the house well lit.
3. Assess community for safety.
4. Alert neighbors about the patient's wandering behavior.
5. Alert police and have current pictures taken.
6. Provide patient with a Medic-Alert bracelet.
7. Install complex safety locks on doors to outside or basement.
8. Install safety bars in bathroom.
9. Closely observe patient if he or she is smoking.
10. Encourage physical activity during the daytime.
11. Give the patient a card with simple instructions (address and phone number) in case he or she is lost.
12. Use night lights.
13. Install alarm/sensor devices on doors.

Improving Socialization

1. Provide magazines with pictures as reading and language abilities diminish.
2. Encourage participation in simple, familiar group activities, such as singing, reminiscing, and painting.
3. Encourage participation in simple activities that promote the exercise of large muscle groups.

Preventing Violence and Aggression

1. Respond calmly and do not raise your voice.
2. Remove objects that might be used to harm self or others.
3. Identify stressors that increase agitation.
4. Distract patient when an upsetting situation develops.

Community and Home Care Considerations

1. Multidisciplinary team approach is important, along with collaboration among professionals in nursing, medicine, psychiatry, nutrition, social work, pharmacy, and rehabilitative specialties.
2. Nurses involved in community care need to utilize case finding approach as well as provide long-term support for family members involved in caregiving.
3. Adult day care and respite care may be utilized in order to provide the level of care needed by the patient as well as allow the family to continue to maintain normal functioning.

Patient Education and Health Maintenance

1. Instruct the family about the process of the disorder, whether delirium, dementia, or amnesic disorder.
2. Instruct the family about safety measures, environmental supports, and effective interventions for common symptoms in order to provide care in the home.
3. Instruct about and refer family members to community-based groups (adult day care centers, senior assessment centers, home care, respite care, and family support groups).
4. For additional information and support, refer to Alzheimer's Association, 919 North Michigan Avenue, Suite 1000, Chicago, IL 60611-1676, 800-272-3900; or National Institutes of Health, National Institute on Aging, Alzheimer's Disease Education and Referral Center, 1-800-438-4380; *www.alzheimer.org.*

Outcome-Based Evaluation

- Demonstrates decreased anxiety and increased feelings of security in supportive environment
- Maintains maximum degree of orientation and self-care within level of ability
- Safety precautions and close surveillance maintained
- Increased interaction with staff and family members
- Decreased occurrence of acting-out behaviors

SELECTED REFERENCES

American Psychiatric Association (1994). *Diagnostic and statistical manual of mental disorders* (4th ed.). Washington, D. C.: American Psychiatric Association.

Baier, M. & Murrau, R.L. (1999). A descriptive study of insight into illness reported by persons with schizophrenia. *Journal of Psychosocial Nursing and Mental Health Services, 37*(1), 14–21.

Bonnel, W.B. (1996). Not gone and not forgotten: A spouse's experience of late stage Alzheimer's disease. *Journal of Psychosocial Nursing and Mental Health Services, 34*(8), 23–27.

Brown, A. & Lempa, M. (1996). Update on potential causes and new treatments for anxiety disorders. *NARSAD Research Newsletter,* Spring/Summer, 13–18.

Cattell, R.B. & Scheier, I.H. (1963). *IPAT anxiety scale questionnaire manual.* Champaign, IL: Institute for Personality and Ability Testing.

Deglin, J.W. & Hazard Vallerand, A. (1997). *Davis's drug guide for nurses* (5th ed.). Philadelphia: F.A. Davis.

Dossey, B. & Dossey, L. (1998). Attending to holistic care." *American Journal of Nursing, 98*(8), 35–38.

Evans, B. (1999). Complimentary therapies and HIV infection. *American Journal of Nursing, 99*(2), 42–45.

Folstein, M.F. (1975). Mini-mental state: A practical method for grading the cognitive state of patients for the clinician. *Journal of Psychiatric Research, 12,* 189.

Fontaine, K.L. & Fletcher, J.S. (1999). *Psychiatric mental health nursing.* Albany, NY: Delmar.

Frisch, N.C. & Frisch, L.E. (1998). *Psychiatric mental health nursing.* Albany, NY: Delmar.

Glod, C.A. (1998). *Contemporary psychiatric-mental health nursing: The brain-body connection.* Philadelphia: F.A. Davis.

Greenwald, J. (1998). Herbal healing. *Time, 98*(11), 60–69.

Hobbs, H., Wilson, J.H., & Archie, S. (1999). The alumni program: Redefining continuity of care in psychiatry. *Journal of Psychosocial Nursing and Mental Health Services, 37*(1), 23–29.

Huber, J., et al. (1997). *Contempory psychiatric nursing* (5th ed). St. Louis: Mosby.

Isaacs, A. (1998). Depression and your patient. *American Journal of Nursing, 98*(7), 26–31.

Jones, J.E. (1994). Chronic anxiety and the adrenocortical response, and differentiation. *Family Systems: Journal of Natural Systems Thinking in Psychiatry and the Sciences, 94*(1), 24–28.

Keltner, N. (1997). Catastrophic consequences secondary to psychotropic drugs, Part I. *Journal of Psychosocial Nursing and Mental Health Services, 35*(7), 41–45.

Keltner, N., Schweike, L., & Bostrom, C. (1999). *Psychiatric nursing* (3rd ed.). St. Louis: Mosby.

Kerr, M. (1997). A systems model for disease. In Sagar, R. R. (Ed.), *Bowen theory and practice*. Washington, D.C.: Georgetown Family Center.

Mohr, W.K. (1998). Updating what we know about adolescent depression. *Journal of Psychosocial Nursing and Mental Health Services, 36*(9), 12–19.

Newman, C.F. (1999). Cognitive therapy with depressed and suicidal adolescents. *Healing Magazine, 4*(1), 24–27.

Nugent, E. (1998). Try to remember: Reminiscence as a nursing intervention. *Journal of Psychosocial Nursing and Mental Health Services, 33*(11), 7–11.

Vallone, D.C. (1997). Antidepressants and anxiolytics. *RN, 60*(7), 27–33.

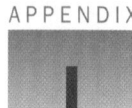
Diagnostic Studies and Interpretation

TEST VALUE STUDIED

Reference Ranges—Hematology
Reference Ranges—Serum, Plasma, and Whole Blood Chemistries
Reference Ranges—Immunodiagnostic Tests
Reference Ranges—Urine Chemistry
Reference Ranges—Cerebrospinal Fluid (CSF)
Miscellaneous Values

SELECTED ABBREVIATIONS USED IN REFERENCE RANGES

■ Conventional Units

kg = kilogram
gm = gram
mg = milligram
μg = microgram
μμg = micromicrogram
ng = nanogram
pg = picogram
dL = 100 milliliters
mL = milliliter

mm^3 = cubic millimeter
fL = femtoliter
mM = millimole
nM = nanomole
mOsm = milliosmole
mm = millimeter
μm = micron or micrometer
mm Hg = millimeters of mercury
U = unit
mU = milliunit
μU = microunit
mEq = milliequivalent
IU = International Unit
mIU = milliInternational Unit

■ SI Units

g = gram
L = liter
d = day
h = hour
mol = mole
mmol = millimole
μmol = micromole
nmol = nanomole
pmol = picomole

TABLE I-1 Reference Ranges—Hematology*

Determination	Reference Range		Clinical Significance
	Conventional Units	*SI Units*	
A₂ hemoglobin	1.5%–3.5% of total hemoglobin	Mass fraction: 0.015–0.035 of total hemoglobin	Increased in certain types of thalassemia
Bleeding time	1–9 min	1–9 min	Prolonged in thrombocytopenia, defective platelet function, and aspirin therapy
Factor V assay (proaccelerin factor)	60%–140%		
Factor VIII assay (anti-hemophiliac factor)	50%–200%		Deficient in classical hemophilia
Factor IX assay (plasma thromboplastin component)	75%–125%		Deficient in Christmas disease (pseudohemophilia)
Factor X (Stuart factor)	60%–140%		Deficient in Stuart clotting defect
Fibrinogen	200–400 mg/dL	2–4 g/dL	Increased in pregnancy, infections accompanied by leukocytosis, nephrosis. Decreased in severe liver disease, abruptio placentae
Fibrin split (degradation) products	Less than 10 mg/L	Less than 10 mg/L	Increased in disseminated intravascular coagulation
Fibrinolysins (whole blood clot lysis time)	No lysis in 24 h		Increased activity associated with massive hemorrhage, extensive surgery, transfusion reactions
Partial thromboplastin time (activated)	20–45 sec		Prolonged in deficiency of fibrinogen, factors II, V, VIII, IX, X, XI, and XII, and in heparin therapy
Prothrombin consumption	Over 20 sec		Impaired in deficiency of factors VIII, IX, and X
Prothrombin time	9.5–12 sec		Prolonged by deficiency of factors I, II, V, VII, and X, far malabsorption, severe liver disease, coumarin anticoagulant therapy.
INR	1.0		INR used to standardize the prothrombin time and anticoagulation therapy
	2–3 for therapy in atrial fibrillation, deep vein thrombosis, and pulmonary embolism 2.5–3.5 for therapy in prosthetic heart valves		
Erythrocyte count	Males: 4,600,000–6,200,000/cu mm	4.6–6.2 × 10¹²/L	Increased in severe diarrhea and dehydration, polycythemia, acute poisoning, pulmonary fibrosis
	Females: 4,200,000–5,400,000/cu mm	4.2–5.4 × 10¹²/L	Decreased in all anemias in leukemia, and after hemorrhage, when blood volume has been restored
Erythrocyte indices			
Mean corpuscular volume (MCV)	80–94 (cu μ)	80–94 fL	Increased in macrocytic anemias; decreased in microcytic anemia
Mean corpuscular hemoglobin (MCH)	27–32 μμg/cell	27–32 pg	Increased in macrocytic anemias; decreased in microcytic anemia
Mean corpuscular hemoglobin concentration (MCHC)	33%–38%	Concentration fraction: 0.33–0.38	Decreased in severe hypochromic anemia
Reticulocytes	0.5%–1.5% of red cells	Number fraction: 0.005–0.015	Increased with any condition stimulating increase in bone marrow activity (ie, infection, blood loss [acute and chronically following iron therapy in iron deficiency anemia], polycythemia rubra vera). Decreased with any condition depressing bone marrow activity, acute leukemia, late stage of severe anemias
Erythrocyte sedimentation rate (ESR)—Westergren method	Males under 50 yr: <15 mm/h	<15 mm/h	Increased in tissue destruction, whether inflammatory or degenerative; during menstruation and pregnancy; and in acute febrile diseases
	Males over 50 yr: <20 mm/h	<20 mm/h	
	Females under 50 yr: <20 mm/h	<20 mm/h	
	Females over 50 yr: <30 mm/h	<30 mm/h	

(continued)

TABLE I-1 Reference Ranges—Hematology* (Continued)

Determination	Reference Range		Clinical Significance
	Conventional Units	*SI Units*	
Erythrocyte sedimentation ratio—Zeta centrifuge	41%–54%	Fraction: 0.41–0.54	Significance similar to ESR
Hematocrit	Males: 42%–50%	Volume fraction: 0.42–0.5	Decreased in severe anemias, anemia of pregnancy, acute massive blood loss
	Females: 40%–48%	Volume fraction: 0.4–0.48	Increased in erythrocytosis of any cause, and in dehydration or hemo-concentration associated with shock
Hemoglobin	Males: 13–18 gm/dL	2.02–2.79 mmol/L	Decreased in various anemias, pregnancy, severe or prolonged hemorrhage, and with excessive fluid intake
	Females: 12–16 gm/dL	1.86–2.48 mmol/L	Increased in polycythemia, chronic obstructive pulmonary disease, failure of oxygenation because of congestive heart failure, and normally in people living at high altitudes
Hemoglobin F	Less than 2% of total hemoglobin	Mass fraction: <0.02	Increased in infants and children, and in thalassemia and many anemias
Leukocyte alkaline phosphatase	Score of 40–100		Increased in polycythemia vera, myelofibrosis, and infections. Decreased in chronic granulocytic leukemia, paroxysmal nocturnal hemoglobinuria, hypoplastic marrow, and viral infections, particularly infectious mononucleosis
Leukocyte count	Total: 5,000–10,000/cu mm	5–10 × 10⁹/L	Elevated in acute infectious diseases, predominantly in the neutrophilic fraction with bacterial diseases, and in the lymphocytic and monocytic fractions in viral diseases
Neutrophils	60%–70%	Number fraction: 0.6–0.7	
Eosinophils	1%–4%	Number fraction: 0.01–0.04	Elevated in acute leukemia, following menstruation, and following surgery or trauma
Basophils	0%–0.5%	Number fraction: 0.00–0.05	Depressed in aplastic anemia, agranulocytosis, and by toxic chemotherapeutic agents used in treating malignancy
Lymphocytes	20%–30%	Number fraction: 0.2–0.3	
Monocytes	2%–6%	Number fraction: 0.02–0.06	Eosinophils elevated in collagen disease, allergy, intestinal parasitosis
Platelet count	100,000–400,000/cu mm	0.1–0.4 × 10¹²/L	Increased in malignancy, myeloproliferative disease, rheumatoid arthritis, and postoperatively; about 50% of patients with unexpected increase of platelet count will be found to have a malignancy Decreased in thrombocytopenic purpura, acute leukemia, aplastic anemia, and during cancer chemotherapy.

* Laboratory values may vary according to the techniques used in different laboratories.

TABLE I-2 Reference Ranges—Serum, Plasma, and Whole Blood Chemistries

Determination	Normal Adult Reference Range		Clinical Significance	
	Conventional Units	SI Units	Increased	Decreased
Acetoacetate	0.2–1.0 mg/dL	19.6–98 µmol/L	Diabetic acidosis Fasting	
Acetone	0.3–2.0 mg/dL	51.6–344.0/µmol/L	Diabetic ketoacidosis Toxemia of pregnancy Carbohydrate-free diet High-fat diet	
Acid, total phosphatase	0–11 UL	0–11 UL	Carcinoma of prostate Advanced Paget's disease Hyperparathyroidism Gaucher's disease	
Acid, phosphatase, prostatic—RLA	0–10 ng/mL Borderline: 2.5–3.3 IU/L	0–10 µg/L	Carcinoma of prostate	
Alkaline phosphatase	Adults: 30–150 mU/mL	30–150 µ/L	Conditions reflecting increased osteoblastic activity of bone Rickets Hyperparathyroidism Hepatic disease Bone disease	
Alkaline phosphatase, thermostable fraction	Thermostable fraction >35%: hepatic disease and combined disease with predominant hepatic component Thermostable fraction between 25% and 35%: combined hepatic and skeletal disease Thermostable fraction <25%: skeletal disease with increased osteoblastic activity			
Adrenocorticotropic hormone (ACTH) (plasma)—RIA*	Less than 50 pg/mL	Less than 50 mg/L	Pituitary-dependent Cushing's syndrome Ectopic ACTH syndrome Primary adrenal atrophy	Adrenocortical tumor Adrenal insufficiency secondary to hypopituitarism
Aldolase	3–8 Sibley-Lehninger U/dL at 37°C	22–59 mU/L at 37°C	Hepatic necrosis Granulocytic leukemia Myocardial infarction Skeletal muscle disease	
Aldosterone (plasma)—RIA	Supine: 3–10 ng/dL Upright: 5–30 ng/dL Adrenal vein 200–800 ng/dL	0.08–0.30 nmol/L 0.14–0.90 nmol/L 5.54–22.16 nmol/L	Primary aldosteronism Secondary aldosteronism	Addison's disease
Alpha-1-antitrypsin	200–400 mg/dL	2–4 g/L		Certain forms of chronic lung and liver disease in young adults
Alpha-1-fetoprotein	None detected		Hepatocarcinoma Metastatic carcinoma of liver Germinal cell carcinoma of the testicle or ovary Fetal neural tube defects—elevation in maternal serum	
Alpha-hydroxybutyric dehydrogenase	Up to 140 U/mL	Up to 140 U/L	Myocardial infarction Granulocytic leukemia Hemolytic anemias Muscular dystrophy	
Ammonia (plasma)	40–80 ug/dL (enzymatic method); varies considerably with method	22.2–44.3/µmol/L	Severe liver disease Hepatic decompensation	

(continued)

TABLE I-2 Reference Ranges—Serum, Plasma, and Whole Blood Chemistries (Continued)

| Determination | Normal Adult Reference Range | | Clinical Significance | |
	Conventional Units	SI Units	Increased	Decreased
Amylase	60–160 Somogyi U/dL	111–296U/L	Acute pancreatitis Mumps Duodenal ulcer Carcinoma of head of pancreas Prolonged elevation with pseudocyst of pancreas Increased by drugs that constrict pancreatic duct sphincters: morphine, codeine, cholinergics	Chronic pancreatitis Pancreatic fibrosis and atrophy Cirrhosis of liver Pregnancy (2nd and 3rd trimesters)
Arsenic	6–20 µg/dL; if 50 µg/dL, suspect toxicity	0.78–2.6 µmol/L	Intentional or unintentional poisoning Excessive occupational exposure	
Ascorbic acid (vitamin C)	0.4–1.5 mg/dL	23–85 µmol/L	Large doses of ascorbic acid as a prophylactic against the common cold	
ALT (alanine aminotransferase), formerly SGPT	10–40 U/mL	5–20 U/L	Same conditions as AST (SGOT), but increase is more marked in liver disease than AST (SGOT)	
AST (aspartate aminotransferase), formerly SGOT	7–40 U/mL	4–20 U/L	Myocardial infarction Skeletal muscle disease Liver disease	
Bilirubin	Total: 0.1–1.2 mg/dL Direct: 0.1–0.2 mg/dL Indirect: 0.1–1 mg/dL	1.7–20.5/µmol/L 1.7–3.4/µmol/L 1.7–17.1 µmol/L	Hemolytic anemia (indirect) Biliary obstruction and disease Hepatocellular damage (hepatitis) Pernicious anemia Hemolytic disease of newborn	
Blood gases Oxygen, arterial (whole blood): Partial pressure (PaO$_2$)	95–100 mm Hg	12.64–13.30kPa	Polycythemia	Anemia Cardiac or pulmonary disease
Saturation (SaO$_2$)	94%–100%	Volume fraction: 0.94–1	Anhydremia	Cardiac decompensation Chronic obstructive lung disease
Carbon dioxide, arterial (whole blood) partial pressure (PaCO$_2$)	35–45 mm Hg	4.66–5.99 kPa	Respiratory acidosis Metabolic alkalosis	Respiratory alkalosis Metabolic acidosis
pH (whole blood, arterial)	7.35–7.45	7.35–7.45	Vomiting Hyperventilation Fever Intestinal obstruction	Uremia Diabetic acidosis Hemorrhage Nephritis
Calcitonin	Basal: nondetectable 400 pg/mL	400 ng/L	Medullary carcinoma of the thyroid Some nonthyroid tumors Zollinger-Ellison syndrome	
Calcium	8.5–10.5 mg/dL	2.125–2.625 mmol/L	Tumor or hyperplasia of parathyroid Hypervitaminosis D Multiple myeloma Nephritis with uremia Malignant tumors Sarcoidosis Hyperthyroidism Skeletal immobilization Excess calcium intake:milk alkali syndrome	Hypoparathyroidism Diarrhea Celiac disease Vitamin D deficiency Acute pancreatitis Nephrosis After parathyroidectomy

TABLE I-2 Reference Ranges—Serum, Plasma, and Whole Blood Chemistries (Continued)

Determination	Normal Adult Reference Range		Clinical Significance	
	Conventional Units	*SI Units*	*Increased*	*Decreased*
CO_2, venous	Adults 24–32 mEq/L Infants: 18–24 mEq/L	24–32 mmol/L 18–24 mmol/L	Tetany Respiratory disease Intestinal obstruction Vomiting	Acidosis Nephritis Eclampsia Diarrhea Anesthesia
Catecholamines (plasma)—RIA	Epinephrine random: up to 90 pg/mL Norepinephrine, random 100 550 pg/mL Dopamine, random up to 130 pg/mL	Up to 490 pmol/L 590–3240 pmol/L Up to 850 pmol/L	Pheochromocytoma	
Ceruloplasmin	30–80 mg/dL	300–800 mg/L		Wilson's disease (hepatolenticular degeneration)
Chloride	95–105 mEq/L	95–105 mmol/L	Nephrosis Nephritis Urinary obstruction Cardiac decompensation Anemia	Diabetes Diarrhea Vomiting Pneumonia Heavy metal poisoning Cushing's syndrome Intestinal obstruction Febrile conditions
Cholesterol	150–200 mg/dL	3.9–5.2 mmol/L	Lipemia Obstructive jaundice Diabetes Hypothyroidism	Pernicious anemia Hemolytic anemia Hyperthyroidism Severe infection Terminal states of debilitating disease
Cholesterol esters	60%–70% of total	Fraction of total cholesterol 0.6–0.7		The esterified fraction decreases in liver diseases
Cholinesterase	Serum: 0.6–1.6 delta pH Red cells—0.6–1 delta pH	0.6–1.6 U 0.6–1 U	Nephrosis Exercise	Nerve gas intoxication (greater effect on red cell activity) Insecticide poisoning
Chorionic gonadotropin, beta subunit	0–5 IU/L	0–5 IU/L	Pregnancy Hydatidiform mole Choriocarcinoma	Threatened abortion Ectopic pregnancy
Complement, human C_3	70–150 mg/dL	880–2520 mg/L	Some inflammatory diseases, acute myocardial infarction, cancer	Acute glomerulonephritis Disseminated lupus erythematosus with renal involvement
Complement C4	16–45 mg/dL	140–510 mg/L	Some inflammatory diseases, acute myocardial infarction, cancer	Often decreased in immunologic disease, especially with active systemic lupus erythematosus Hereditary angioneurotic edema
Complement, total (hemolytic)	90%–94% complement	25–70 U/mL	Some inflammatory diseases	Acute glomerulonephritis Epidemic meningitis Subacute bacterial endocarditis
Copper	70–165 µg/dL	11–25.9 µmol/L	Cirrhosis of liver Pregnancy	Wilson's disease
Cortisol-RIA	8 AM: 7–25/µg/dL 4 PM: 2–9 µg/dL	193–690 nmol/L 55–248 nmol/L	Stress: infectious disease, surgery, burns, etc. Pregnancy Cushing's syndrome Pancreatitis Eclampsia	Addison's disease Anterior pituitary hypofunction

(continued)

TABLE I-2 Reference Ranges—Serum, Plasma, and Whole Blood Chemistries (Continued)

Determination	Normal Adult Reference Range		Clinical Significance	
	Conventional Units	SI Units	Increased	Decreased
C-peptide reactivity	1.5–10 ng/mL	1.5–10 µg/L	Insulinoma	Diabetes
Creatine	0.2–0.8 mg/mL	15.3–61 µmol/L	Pregnancy Skeletal muscle necrosis or atrophy Starvation Hyperthyroidism	
Creatine phosphokinase (CPK)	Males: 50–325 mU/mL Females: 50–250 mU/mL	50–325 U/L 50–250 U/L	Myocardial infarction Skeletal muscle diseases Intramuscular injections Crush syndrome Hypothyroidism Alcohol withdrawal delirium Alcoholic myopathy Cerebrovascular disease	

Creatine phosphoki-nase isoenzymes	MM band present
	  (skeletal muscle)–
	  MB band absent
	  (heart muscle)
			MB band increased in myo-cardial infarction, ischemia	

Creatinine	0.7–1.4 mg/dL	62–124 µmol/L	Nephritis Chronic renal disease	
Creatinine clearance	100–150 mL of blood cleared of creatinine per min	1.67–2.5 mL/s		Kidney diseases
Cryoglobulins, qualitative	Negative		Multiple myeloma Chronic lymphocytic leukemia Lymphosarcoma Systemic lupus erythematosus Rheumatoid arthritis Infective subacute endocarditis Some malignancies Scleroderma	
11-Deoxycortisol	1/µg/dL	<0.029 µmol/L	Hypertensive form of virilizing adrenal hyperplasia due to an 11-β-hydroxylase defect	
Dibucaine number	Normal: 70%–85% inhibition Heterozygote: 50%–65% inhibition Homozygote: 16%–25% inhibition			Important in detecting carriers of abnormal cholinesterase activity who are susceptible to succinylcholine anesthetic shock
Dihydrotestosterone	Males: 50–210 ng/dL Females: none detectable	1.72–7.22 nmol/L		Testicular feminization syndrome

Estradiol—RIA	Females:
	Follicular: 10–90 pg/mL
	Midcycle: 100–500 pg/mL
	Luteal: 50–240 pg/mL
	Follicular phase:
	  2–20 ng/dL
	Midcycle: 12–40 ng/dL
	Luteal phase:
	  10–30 ng/dL
	Postmenopausal:
	  1–5 ng/dL
	Males: 0.5–5 ng/dL
		37–370 pmol/L
		367–1835 pmol/L
		184–881 pmol/L
			Pregnancy	Depressed or failure to peak—ovarian failure

TABLE I-2 Reference Ranges—Serum, Plasma, and Whole Blood Chemistries (Continued)

Determination	Normal Adult Reference Range		Clinical Significance	
	Conventional Units	**SI Units**	**Increased**	**Decreased**
Estriol—RIA	Nonpregnant females: <0.5 ng/mL	<1.75 nmol/L	Pregnancy	Depressed or failure to peak—ovarian failure
	Pregnant females:			
	1st trimester: up to 1 ng/mL	Up to 3.5 nmol/L		
	2nd trimester: 0.8–7 ng/mL	2.8–24.3 nmol/L		
	3rd trimester: 5–25 ng/mL	17.4–86.8 nmol/L		
Estrogens, total—RIA	Females: cycle days:		Pregnancy	Fetal distress
	Day 1–10: 61–394 pg/mL	61–394 ng/L	Measured on a daily basis, can be used to evaluate response of hypogonadotrophic, hypoestrogenic women to human menopausal or pituitary gonadotropin	Ovarian failure
	Day 11–20: 122–437 pg/mL	122–437 ng/L		
	Day 21–30: 156–350 pg/mL	156–350 ng/L		
	Males: 40–115 pg/mL	40–115 ng/L		
Estrone—RIA	Females:			Depressed or failure to peak—ovarian failure
	Day 1–10: 4.3–18 ng/dL	15.9–66.6 pmol/L		
	Day 11–20: 7.5–19.6 ng/dL	27.8–72.5 pmol/L		
	Day 21–30: 13–20 ng/dL	48.1–74 pmol/L		
	Males: 2.5–7.5 ng/dL	9.3–27.8 pmol/L		
Ferritin—RIA	Males: 29–438 ng/mL	29–438 µg/L	Nephritis	Iron deficiency
	Females: 9–219 ng/mL	9–219 µg/L	Hemochromatosis	
			Certain neoplastic diseases	
			Acute myelogenous leukemia	
			Multiple myeloma	
Folic acid—RIA	2.5–20 ng/mL	6–46 nmol/L		Megaloblastic anemias of infancy and pregnancy
				Inadequate diet
				Liver disease
				Malabsorption syndrome
				Severe hemolytic anemia
Follicle stimulating hormone (FSH)—RIA	Males: 2–10 mIU/mL		Menopause and primary ovarian failure	Pituitary failure
	Females:	5–20 IU/L		
	Follicular phase: 5–20 mIU/mL			
	Peak of middle cycle: 12–30 mIU/mL	12–30 IU/L		
	Luteinic phase: 5–15 mIU/mL	5–15 IU/L		
	Menopausal females: 40–200 mIU/mL	40–200 IU/L		
Galactose	<5 mg/dL	<0.28 mmol/L		Galactosemia
Gamma glutamyl transpeptidase	Males: <45 IU/L	45 U/L	Hepatobiliary disease	
	Females: <30 IU/L	30 U/L	Drug toxicity	
			Myocardial infarction	
			Renal infarction	
			Zollinger-Ellison syndrome	
Gastrin—RIA	Fasting: 50–155 pg/mL	50–155 ng/L	Peptic ulceration of the duodenum	
			Pernicious anemia	
	Postprandial: 80–170 pg/mL	80–170 ng/L		

(continued)

TABLE I-2 Reference Ranges—Serum, Plasma, and Whole Blood Chemistries (Continued)

| Determination | Normal Adult Reference Range | | Clinical Significance | |
	Conventional Units	SI Units	Increased	Decreased
Glucose	Fasting: 60–110 mg/dL	3.3–6.05 mmol/L	Diabetes Nephritis	Hyperinsulinism Hypothyroidism
	Postprandial (2 h): 65–140 mg/dL	3.58–7.7 mmol/L	Hyperthyroidism Early hyperpituitarism Cerebral lesions Infections Pregnancy Uremia	Late hyperpituitarism Pernicious vomiting Addison's disease Extensive hepatic damage
Glucose tolerance (oral)	Features of a normal response:		Two-hour value >200 mg/dL (11.1 mmol/L) is diagnostic for diabetes	Decreased 2 and 3 hour values may occur with hypoglycemia
	1. Normal fasting between 60– 110 mg/dL	3.3–6.05 mmol/L		
	2. No sugar in urine			
	3. Upper limits of normal:			
	Fasting = 125	6.88 mmol/L		
	1 hour = 190	10.45 mmol/L		
	2 hours = 140	7.70 mmol/L		
	3 hours = 125	6.88 mmol/L		
Glucose-6-phosphate dehydrogenase (red cells)	Screening: Decolorization in 20–100 min			Drug-induced hemolytic anemia Hemolytic disease of newborn
	Quantitative: 1.86–2.5 IU/mL RBC	1860–2500 U/L		
Glycoprotein (alpha-1-acid)	40–110 mg/dL	400–1100 mg/L	Neoplasm Tuberculosis Diabetes complicated by de- generative vascular disease Pregnancy Rheumatoid arthritis Rheumatic fever Infectious liver disease Lupus erythematosus	
Growth hormone—RIA	< 10 ng/mL	<10 mg/L	Acromegaly	Failure to stimulate with arginine or insulin— hypopituitarism Hemolytic anemia
Haptoglobin	50–250 mg/dL	0.5–2.5 g/L	Pregnancy Estrogen therapy Chronic infections Various inflammatory conditions	Hemolytic blood trans- fusion reaction
Hemoglobin (plasma)	0.5–5 mg/dL	5–50 mg/L	Transfusion reactions Paroxysmal nocturnal hemoglobinuria Intravascular hemolysis	
Glycohemoglobin (GHB, hemoglobin A_{1c}, hemoblobin A1)	Nondiabetics & diabet- ics with good control: 4.4%–6.4%		Suboptimal glucose control	Anemia, pregnancy, chronic renal failure
Hexosaminidase, total	Controls: 333–375 nM/ mL/h	333–375 μmol/ L/h	Sandhoff's disease	Tay-Sachs disease and heterozygotes
Hexosaminidase A	Controls: 49%–68% of total	Fraction of total: 0.49–0.68		
	Heterozygotes: 26%–45% of total	0.26–0.45		
	Tay-Sachs disease: 0%–4% of total	0–0.04		
	Diabetics: 39%–59% of total	0.39–0.59		

TABLE I-2 Reference Ranges—Serum, Plasma, and Whole Blood Chemistries (Continued)

Determination	Normal Adult Reference Range		Clinical Significance	
	Conventional Units	SI Units	Increased	Decreased
High-density lipoprotein cholesterol (HDL cholesterol)	Males: 35–70 mg/dL Females: 35–85 mg/dL	0.91–1.81 mmol/L 0.91–220 mmol/L		HDL cholesterol is lower in patients with increased risk for coronary heart disease
	Males: 0.4–4 ng/mL	1.2–12 nmol/L	Congenital adrenal hyperplasia	
	Females: 0.1–3.3 ng/mL	0.3–10 nmol/L	Pregnancy	
Homocysteine		4–17 µmol/L	Folic acid deficiency Increased risk for vascular disease Homocystinuria	
17 Hydroxy-progesterone—RIA				
Immunoglobulin A	Children: 0.1–0.5 ng/mL	0.3–1.5 nmol/L	Some cases of adrenal or ovarian adenomas	Ataxia telangiectasis Agammaglobulinemia
	Adults: 50–300 mg/dL (in children the normals are lower and vary with age)	0.5–3 g/L	Gamma A myeloma Wiskott-Aldrich syndrome Autoimmune disease Hepatic cirrhosis	Hypogammaglobulinemia, transient Dysgammaglobulinemia Protein-losing enteropathies
Immunoglobulin D	0–30 mg/dL	0–300 mg/L	IgD multiple myeloma Some patients with chronic infectious diseases	
Immunoglobulin E	20–740 ng/mL	20–740 µg/L	Allergic patients and those with parasitic infections	
Immunoglobulin G	Adults: 565–1765 mg/dL	6.35–14 g/L	IgG myeloma Following hyperimmunization Autoimmune disease states Chronic infections	Congenital and acquired hypogammaglobulinemia IgA myelomas, Waldenstrom's (IgM) macroglobulinemia Some malabsorption syndromes Extensive protein loss
Immunoglobulin M	Adults: 55–375 mg/dL	0.4–2.8 g/L	Waldenström's macroglobulinemia Parasitic infections Hepatitis	Agammaglobulinemias Some IgG and IgA myelomas Chronic lymphatic leukemia
Insulin—RIA	5–25 µU/mL	0.2–1 µg/L	Insulinoma Acromegaly	Diabetes mellitus
Iron	50–160/µg/dL	9–29 µmol/L	Pernicious anemia Aplastic anemia Hemolytic anemia Hepatitis Hemochromatosis	Iron deficiency anemia
Iron-binding capacity	IBC: 150–235 µg/dL TIBC: 230–410 µg/dL % Saturation: 20–50	26.9–42.1 µmol/L 41–73 µmol/L Fraction of total iron-binding capacity: 0.2–0.5	Iron deficiency anemia Acute and chronic blood loss Hepatitis	Chronic infectious diseases Cirrhosis
Isocitric dehydrogenase	50–180 U	0.83–3 UIL	Hepatitis, cirrhosis Obstructive jaundice Metastatic carcinoma of the liver Megaloblastic anemia	
Lactic acid (whole blood)	Venous: 5–20 mg/dL Arterial: 3–7 mg/dL	0.6–2.2 mmol/L 0.3–0.8 mmol/L	Increased muscular activity Congestive heart failure Hemorrhage Shock Lactic acidosis	

(continued)

TABLE I-2 Reference Ranges—Serum, Plasma, and Whole Blood Chemistries (Continued)

| Determination | Normal Adult Reference Range | | Clinical Significance | |
	Conventional Units	SI Units	Increased	Decreased
Lactic dehydrogenase (LDH)	100–225 mU/mL	100–225 U/L	Some febrile infections May be increased in severe liver disease Untreated pernicious anemia Myocardial infarction Pulmonary infarction Liver disease	
Lactic dehydrogenase isoenzymes				
Total lactic dehydrogenase	100–225 mU/mL	100–225 U/L Fraction of total LDH:	LDH-1 and LDH-2 are increased in myocardial infarction, megaloblastic anemia, and hemolytic anemia	
LDH-1	20%–35%	0.2–0.35		
LDH-2	25%–40%	0.25–0.4	LDH-4 and LDH-5 are increased in pulmonary infarction, congestive heart failure, and liver disease	
LDH-3	20%–30%	0.2–0.3		
LDH-4	0–20%	0–0.2		
LDH-5	0–25%	0–0.25		
Lead (whole blood)	Up to 40 µg/dL	Up to 2 µmol/L	Lead poisoning	
Leucine aminopeptidase	80–200 U/mL	19.2–48 U/L	Liver or bilary tract diseases Pancreatic disease Metastatic carcinoma of liver and pancreas Biliary obstruction	
Lipase	0.2–1.5 U/mL	55–417 U/L	Acute and chronic pancreatitis Biliary obstruction Cirrhosis Hepatitis Peptic ulcer	
Lipids, total	400–1000 mg/dL	4–10 g/L	Hypothyroidism Diabetes Nephrosis Glomerulonephritis Hyperlipoproteinemias	Hyperthyroidism
Low-density lipoprotein cholesterol (LDL cholesterol)	mg/dL desirable levels: <160 if no coronary artery disease (CAD) and <2 risk factors <130 if no CAD and 2 or more risk factors <100 if CAD present		LDL cholesterol is higher in patients with increased risk for coronary heart disease	

Luteinizing hormone—RIA	Males: 4.9–15 MIU/mL
	Females:
	  Follicular phase: 2–3 MIU/mL
	  Ovulatory peak: 40–200 MIU/mL
	  Luteal phase: 0–20 MIU/mL
	  Postmenopausal: 35–120 mIU/mL
		4.9–15 mg/L
		
		0.5–6.9 mg/L
		
		9.2–46 mg/L
		
		0–5 mg/L
		
		8–27.5 mg/L
			Pituitary tumor
			Ovarian failure
				Depressed or failure to peak—pituitary failure

Lysozyme (muramidase)	2.8–8 µg/mL	2.8–8 mg	Certain types of leukemia (acute monocytic leukemia) Inflammatory states and infections	Acute lymphocytic leukemia
Magnesium	1.3–2.4 mEq/L	0.7–1.2 mmol/L	Excess ingestion of magnesium-containing antacids	Chronic alcoholism Severe renal disease Diarrhea Defective growth
Manganese	0.04–1.4 µg/dL	72.9–255 nmol/L		
Mercury	Up to 10 µg/dL	Up to 0.5/µmol/L	Mercury poisoning	
Myoglobin—RIA	Up to 85 ng/mL	Up to 85 µg/mL	Myocardial infarction Muscle necrosis	

TABLE I-2 Reference Ranges—Serum, Plasma, and Whole Blood Chemistries (Continued)

| Determination | Normal Adult Reference Range | | Clinical Significance | |
	Conventional Units	SI Units	Increased	Decreased
5' Nucleotidase	3.2–11.6 IU/L	3.2–11.6 U/L	Hepatobiliary disease	
Osmolality	280–300 mOsm/kg	280–300 mmol/L	Diabetes insipidus	Inappropriate secretion
			Osmotic diuresis	of ADH
				Addison's disease
Parathyroid hormone	160–350 pg/mL	160–350 ng/L	Hyperparathyroidism	Chronic renal failure
				Hypoparathyroidism
Phenylalanine	1.2–3.5 mg/dL	0.07–0.21 mmol/L	Phenylketonuria	
	1st week			
	0.7–3.5 mg/dL	0.04–0.21 mmol/L		
	thereafter			
Phosphohexose	20–90 IU/L	20–90 U/L	Malignancy	
isomerase			Disease of heart, liver, and	
			skeletal muscles	
Phospholipids	125–300 mg/dL	1.25–3 g/L	Diabetes	
			Nephritis	
Phosphorus, inorganic	2.5–4.5 mg/dL	0.8–1.45 mmol/L	Chronic nephritis	Hyperparathyroidism
			Hypoparathyroidism	Vitamin D deficiency
Potassium	3.8–5 mEq/L	3.8–5 mmol/L	Renal failure	GI losses
			Acidosis	Diuretic administration
			Cell lysis	
			Tissue breakdown or	
			hemolysis	
Progesterone—RIA	Follicular phase: up to	2.5 nmol/L	Useful in evaluation of men-	
	0.8 ng/mL		strual disorders and infertil-	
	Luteal phase:	31.8–63.6 nmol/L	ity and in the evaluation of	
	10–20 ng/mL		placental function during	
	End of cycle: <1 ng/mL	<3 nmol/L	pregnancies complicated by	
	Pregnant: up to 50	Up to 160 nmol/L	toxemia, diabetes mellitus,	
	ng/mL in 20th week		or threatened miscarriage	
Prolactin—RIA	6–24 ng/mL	6–24 µg/L	Pregnancy	
			Functional or structural dis-	
			orders of the hypothalamus	
			Pituitary stalk section	
			Pituitary tumors	
Prostate-specific antigen	<4 ng/mL		Prostatic cancer, benign	
			prostatic hyperplasia,	
			prostatitis	
Protein, total	6–8 gm/dL	60–80 g/L	Hemoconcentration	Malnutrition
Albumin	3.5–5 gm/dL	35–50 g/L	Shock	Hemorrhage
Globulin	1.5–3 gm/dL	15–30 g/L	Multiple myeloma	Loss of plasma from
			(globulin fraction)	burns
			Chronic infections	Proteinuria
			(globulin function)	
			Liver disease (globulin)	
Protein				
Electrophoresis		35–50 g/L		
(cellulose acetate)		24 g/L		
Albumin	3.5–5 gm/dL	6–10 g/L		
Alpha-1 globulin	0.1–0.4 gm/dL	1–4 g/L		
Alpha-2 globulin	0.4–1.2 gm/dL	4–12 g/L		
Beta globulin	0.6–1.2 gm/dL	5–11 g/L		
Gamma globulin	0.5–1.6 gm/dL	5–16 g/L		
Protoporphyrin erythro-	15–100 µg/dL	0.27–1.80 µmol/L	Lead toxicity	
cyte (whole blood)			Erythropoietic porphyria	
Pyridoxine	3.6–18 ng/mL			A wide spectrum of clini-
				cal conditions, such as
				mental depression, pe-
				ripheral neuropathy,
				anemia, neonatal sei-
				zures, and reactions to
				certain drug therapies

(continued)

TABLE I-2 Reference Ranges—Serum, Plasma, and Whole Blood Chemistries (Continued)

| Determination | Normal Adult Reference Range | | Clinical Significance | |
	Conventional Units	SI Units	Increased	Decreased
Pyruvic acid (whole blood)	0.3–0.7 mg/dL	34–80 μmol/L	Diabetes Severe thiamine deficiency Acute phase of some infections, possibly secondary to increased glycogenolysis and glycolysis	

Renin (plasma)—RIA	Normal diet:
	  Supine:
	  0.3–1.9 ng/mL/h
	  Upright:
	  0.6–3.6 ng/mL/h
	
	Low salt diet:
	  Supine:
	  0.9–4.5 ng/mL/h
	  Upright:
	  4.1–9.1 ng/mL/h
		0.08–0.52 ng/L/S
		
		0.16–1.00 μg/L/S
		
		0.25–1.25 μg/L/S
		
		1.13–2.53 μg/L/S
			Renovascular hypertension
			Malignant hypertension
			Untreated Addison's disease
			Primary salt-losing nephropathy
			Low-salt diet
			Diuretic therapy
			
			Hemorrhage
				Frank primary aldosteronism
				Increased salt intake
				Salt-retaining steroid therapy
				Antidiuretic hormone therapy
				Blood transfusion

Sodium	135–145 mEq/L	135–145 mmol/L	Hemoconcentration Nephritis Pyloric obstruction	Alkali deficit Addison's disease Myxedema
Sulfate (inorganic)	0.5–1.5 mg/dL	0.05–0.15 mmol/L	Nephritis Nitrogen retention	
Testosterone—RIA	Females: 25–100 ng/dL Males: 300–800 ng/dL	0.9–3.5 nmol/L 10.5–28 nmol/L	Females: Polycystic ovary Virilizing tumors	Males Orchidectomy for neoplastic disease of the prostate or breast Estrogen therapy Klinefelter's syndrome Hypopituitarism Hypogonadism Hepatic cirrhosis
T_3 (triiodothyronine) uptake	25%–35%	Relative uptake fraction: 0.25–0.35	Hyperthyroidism Thyroxine-binding globulin (TBG) deficiency Androgens and anabolic steroids	Hypothyroidism Pregnancy TBG excess Estrogens and antiovulatory drugs
T_3 total circulating—RIA	75–200 ng/dL	1.15–3.1 nmol/L	Pregnancy Hyperthyroidism	Hypothyroidism
T_4 (thyroxine)—RIA	4.5–11.5 μg/dL	58.5–150 nmol/L	Hyperthyroidism Thyroiditis Elevated thyroxine-binding proteins caused by oral contraceptives Pregnancy	Primary and pituitary hypothyroidism Idiopathic involvement Cases of diminished thyroxine-binding proteins caused by androgenic and anabolic steroids Hypoproteinemia Nephrotic syndrome
T_4, free	1–2.2 ng/dL	13–30 pmol/L	Euthyroid patients with normal free thyroxine levels may have abnormal T3 and T4 levels caused by drug preparations	
Thyroid-stimulating hormone (TSH)—RIA		0.3–5 m/IU/L	Hypothyroidism	Hyperthyroidism
Thyroid-binding globulin	10–26 μg/dL	100–260/μg/L	Hypothyroidism Pregnancy Estrogen therapy Oral contraceptives Genetic and idiopathic liver disease	Use of androgens and anabolic steroids Nephrotic syndrome Marked hypoproteinemia

TABLE I-2 Reference Ranges—Serum, Plasma, and Whole Blood Chemistries (Continued)

Determination	Normal Adult Reference Range		Clinical Significance	
	Conventional Units	SI Units	Increased	Decreased
Transferrin	230–320 mg/dL	2.3–3.2 g/L	Pregnancy Iron deficiency anemia due to hemorrhaging Acute hepatitis Polycythemia Oral contraceptives Primary and secondary hyperlipidemias	Pernicious anemia in relapse Thalassemic and sickle cell anemia Chromatosis Neoplastic and hepatic diseases
Triglycerides	10–150 mg/dL	0.10–1.65 nmol/L		Tryptophan-specific malabsorption syndrome
Troponin T and I	Negative	Negative	Myocardial infarction	
Tryptophan	1.4–3 mg/dL	68.6–147 nmol/L	Tyrosinosis	
Tyrosine	0.5–4 mg/dL	27.6–220.8 mmol/L		
Urea nitrogen (BUN)	10–20 mg/dL	3.6–7.2 mmol/L	Acute glomerulonephritis Obstructive uropathy Mercury poisoning Nephrotic syndrome	Severe hepatic failure Pregnancy
Uric acid	2.5–8 mg/dL	0.15–0 mmol/L	Gouty arthritis Acute leukemia Lymphomas treated by chemotherapy Toxemia of pregnancy	Defective tubular reabsorption
Viscosity	1.4–1.8 relative to water at 37°C (98.6°F)		Patients with marked increases of the gamma globulins	
Vitamin A	50–220 Hg/dL	1.75–7.7 µmol/L	Hypervitaminosis A	Vitamin A deficiency Celiac disease Sprue Obstructive jaundice Giardiasis Parenchymal hepatic disease
Vitamin B, (thiamine)	1.6–4 µg/dL	47.4–135.7 nmol/L		Anorexia Beriberi Polyneuropathy Cardiomyopathies
Vitamin B6 (pyridoxal phosphate)	3.6–18 ng/mL	14.6–72.8 nmol/L		Chronic alcoholism Malnutrition Uremia Neonatal seizures Malabsorption, such as celiac syndrome
Vitamin B12—RIA	130–785 pg/mL	100–580 pmol/L	Hepatic cell damage and in association with the myeloproliferative disorders (the highest levels are encountered in myeloid leukemia)	Strict vegetarianism Alcoholism Pernicious anemia Total or partial gastrectomy Ileal resection Sprue and celiac disease Fish tapeworm infestation
Vitamin E	0.5–2 mg/dL	11.6–46.4 µmol/L		Vitamin E deficiency
Xylose absorption test	2 hr, 30–50 mg/dL	2–3.35 mmol/L		Malabsorption syndrome
Zinc	55–150/µg/dL	7.65–22.95 µmol/L	Coronary artery disease Arteriosclerosis Industrial exposure	Metastatic liver disease Tuberculosis Sprue

* By radioimmunoassay.

TABLE I-3   Reference Ranges—Immunodiagnostic Tests

Determination	Normal Value	Clinical Significance
Acetylcholine receptor binding antibody	Negative or <0.03 nmol/L	Considered to be diagnostic for myasthenia gravis in patients with symptoms.
Anti-ds-DNA antibody	<70 U by enzyme-linked immuno-sorbent assay (ELISA) <1:20 by indirect fluorescence	Valuable in supporting diagnosis or monitoring disease activity and prognosis of systemic lupus erythematosus (SLE).
Antiglomerular basement membrane antibody	Negative or less than 10 U	Primarily used in the differential diagnosis of glomerular nephritis induced by antiglomerular basement membrane antibodies from other types of glomerular nephritis.
Anti-insulin antibody	<3% binding of labeled beef and pork insulin by patient's serum; or <9 mIU/L	Helpful in determining the best therapeutic agent in diabetics and the cause of allergic manifestations. Also used to identify insulin resistance.
Antimitochondrial antibody and anti-smooth muscle antibody	<1:5 and <1:20, respectively	Increased in cirrhosis, autoimmune disease, thyroiditis, pernicious anemia.
Antinuclear antibody	Negative, <1:20	Increased in SLE, chronic hepatitis, scleroderma, leukemia, and mononucleosis.
Anti-parietal cell antibody	Negative, <1:20	Helpful in diagnosing chronic gastric disease and differentiating autoimmune pernicious anemia from other megaloblastic anemias.
Antiribonucleoprotein antibody	Negative	Helpful in differential diagnosis of systemic rheumatic disease.
Antiscleroderma antibody	Negative	Highly diagnostic for scleroderma.
Anti-Smith antibody	Negative	Highly diagnostic of SLE.
Anti-SS-A/anti-SS-B antibody	Negative	SS-A antibodies are found in Sjögren's syndrome alone or associated with lupus. SS-B antibodies are associated with primary Sjögren's syndrome.
Antithyroglobulin and anti-microsomal antibodies	<1:100 titer by gelatin or hemaglutination	Presence and concentration is important in evaluation and treatment of various thyroid disorders, such as Hashimoto's thyroiditis and Graves' disease. May indicate previous autoimmune disorders.
CA 15-3 tumor marker	<22 IU/ml	Increased in metastatic breast cancer.
CA 19-9 tumor marker	<37 IU/ml	Increased in pancreatic, hepatobiliary, gastric, and colorectal cancer, gallstones.
CA 125	0–35 IU/ml	Increased in colon, upper gastrointestinal (GI), ovarian, and other gynecologic cancers: pregnancy, peritonitis.
Carcinoembryonic antigen (CEA)—RLK	0–2.5 11g/L (nonsmoker) 0–5/µg/L (smoker)	The repeatedly high incidence of this antigen in cancers of the colon, rectum, pancreas, and stomach suggests that CEA levels may be useful in the therapeutic monitoring of these conditions, but it is not a screening test
Cold agglutinins	<1:16	Increased in mycoplasma pneumonia, viral illness, mononucleosis, multiple myeloma, scleroderma.
C-reactive protein	<0.8 mg/dL	Increase indicates active inflammation.
Cytomegalovirus antibodies (CMV IgG)	Negative: <0.9 units/mL	Positive >1.0 unit/mL if exposed to CMV at anytime. Acute and convalescent specimens can help identify acute infection.
Cytomegalovirus antibodies (CMV IgM)	Negative: <0.79 Equivocal: 0.80–1.20	Positive >1.20 usually indicates acute infection. Repeat specimen in 1–2 weeks for equivocal result.
Epstein-Barr virus serology (viral capsid antigen IgG and IgM, early antigen IgG, and nuclear antigen IgG)	Negative is <1:20 or <20 for each individual test	Differentiation of acute from chronic or old infection by interpretation of table below.

EBV Interpretation

	VCA-IgG	VCA-IgM	EA-IgG	EBV-NA
Susceptible	−	−	−	−
Acute infection	+	+	±	−
Convalescent phase	+	±	±	+
Chronic or reactivated	+	−	+	±
Old infection	±	−	−	+

Antibody present: +
Antibody absent: −
VCA, viral capsid antigen; EA, early antigen; EBV-NA, Epstein Barr virus-nuclear antigen

TABLE I-3 Reference Ranges—Immunodiagnostic Tests (Continued)

Determination	Normal Value	Clinical Significance
Hepatitis A virus antibodies, IgM (HAV-Ab/IgM)	Negative	Positive in acute-stage hepatitis A; develops early in disease.
Hepatitis A virus antibodies, IgG (HAV-Ab/IgG)	Negative	Positive if previous exposure and immunity to hepatitis A.
Hepatitis B surface antigen (HBsAg)	Negative	Positive in acute-stage hepatitis B.
Hepatitis B surface antibody (HBsAb)	Negative	Positive if previous exposure and immunity to hepatitis B.
Hepatitis C virus antibodies	Negative	Positive in exposure to hepatitis C virus; may indicate acute, chronic, or cleared infection.
Hepatitis C virus RNA	Negative	Positive in hepatitis C infection, can be quantitative
Infectious mononucleosis tests (monospot, monotest, heterophile antigen test, Epstein-Barr virus (EBV), antiviral capsid antigen IgM and IgG)	Negative, <1:80	Positive monospot and monotest are presumptive, positive EBV IgM and IgG indicate acute and recent or past infection, respectively.
Lyme disease titer	Negative, <1:256 by indirect fluorescent antibody method <0.8 by ELISA	Positive results help diagnose Lyme disease. False positive may occur with high rheumatoid factor titers or syphilis. Positive ELISA confirmed by Western blot test.
Pyroglobulin test	Negative	These abnormal proteins may be associated with myeloma, lymphoma, polycythemia vera, and SLE.
Rheumatoid factor	Negative or less than 60 IU/mL	Elevated in rheumatoid arthritis, lupus endocarditis, tuberculosis, syphilis, sarcoidosis, cancer.
T and B cell lymphocyte surface markers T-helper/T-suppressor ratio	T and B cell lymphocyte surface markers: Percent T cells (CD2) 60–88% Percent helper cells (CD4) 34–67% Percent suppressor cells (CD8) 10–42% Percent B cells (CD19) 3–21% Absolute counts: Lymphocytes 0.66–4.60 thou/mL T cells 644–2201 cells/mL Helper cells 493–1191 cells/mL Suppressor T cells 182–785 cells/mL B cells 92–392 cells/mL Lymphocyte ratio: T_H/T_S ratio > 1	Done to evaluate immune system by identifying the specific cells involved in the immune response. Valuable in diagnosis of lymphocytic leukemia, lymphoma, and immunodeficiency diseases including acquired immunodeficiency syndrome, and in the assessment of patient response to chemotherapy and radiation.

TABLE I-4 Reference Ranges—Urine Chemistry

Determination	Normal Adult Reference Range		Clinical Significance	
	Conventional Units	SI Units	Increased	Decreased
Acetone and acetoacetate	Zero		Uncontrolled diabetes Starvation	
Aldosterone	With normal salt diet: Normal: 4–20 µg/24 h Renovascular: 10–40 µg/24 h Tumor: 20–100 µg/24 h	11.1–55.5 nmol/24h 27.7–111 nmol/24 h 55.4–277 nmol/24 h	Primary aldosteronism (adrenocortical tumor) Secondary aldosteronism Salt depletion Potassium loading ACTH in large doses Cardiac failure Cirrhosis with ascites formation Nephrosis Pregnancy	
Alpha amino nitrogen	50–200 mg/24 h	3.6–14.3 nmol/24 h	Leukemia Phenylketonuria Other metabolic diseases	
Amylase	35–260 units excreted per h	6.5–48.1 U/h	Acute pancreatitis	
Arylsulfatase A	>2.4 U/mL			
Bence-Jones protein	None detected		Myeloma	Metachromatic leuko-dystrophy
Calcium	<150 mg/24 h	<3.75 mmol/24 h	Hyperparathyroidism Vitamin D intoxication Fanconi's syndrome	Hypoparathyroidism Vitamin D deficiency
Catecholamines	Total: 0–275 µg/24 h Epinephrine; 10%–40% Norepinephrine: 60%–90%	0–275 µg/24 h Fraction total: 0.10–8.4 Fraction total: 0.60–0.90	Pheochromocytoma Neuroblastoma	
Chorionic gonadotro-phin, qualitative (pregnancy test)	Negative		Pregnancy Chorionepithelioma Hydatidiform mole	
Copper	20–70 µg/24 h	0.32–1.12 µmol/24 h	Wilson's diseases Cirrhosis Nephrosis	
Coproporphyrin	50–300 µg/24 h	0.075–0.45 µmol/24 h	Poliomyelitis Lead poisoning Porphyria	
Cortisol, free	20–90 Hg/24 h	55.2–248.4 mmol/d	Cushing's syndrome	
Creatinine	0–200 mg/24 h	0–1.52 mmol/24 h	Muscular dystrophy Fever Carcinoma of liver Pregnancy Hyperthyroidism Myositis	
Creatine	0.8–2 gm/24 h	7–17.6 mmol/24 h	Typhoid fever Salmonella infections Tetanus	Muscular atrophy Anemia Advanced degeneration of kidneys Leukemia
Creatinine clearance	100–150 mL of blood cleared of creatinine per mm	1.67–2.5 mL/s		Measures glomerular filtration rate Renal diseases
Cystine and cysteine	10–100 mg/24 h	0.08–0.83 mmol/24 h	Cystinuria	
Delta aminolevulimic acid	0–0.54 mg/dL	0–40/µmol/L	Lead poisoning Porphyria hepatica Hepatitis Hepatic carcinoma	
11-Desoxycortisol	20–100 µg/24 h	0.6–2.9/µmol/d	Hypertensive form of virilizing adrenal hyper-plasia due to an 11-beta hydroxylase defect	

TABLE I-4 Reference Ranges—Urine Chemistry (Continued)

Determination	Normal Adult Reference Range		Clinical Significance	
	Conventional Units	SI Units	Increased	Decreased
Estriol (placental)				Decreased values occur with fetal distress of many conditions, including preeclampsia, placental insufficiency, and poorly controlled diabetes mellitus
	Weeks of pregnancy	μm/24 h	mmol/24 h		
	12	<1	<3.5		
	16	2–7	7–24.5		
	20	4–9	14–32		
	24	6–13	21–45.5		
	28	8–22	28–77		
	32	12–43	42–150		
	36	14–45	49–158		
	40	19–46	66.5–160		
Estrogens, total (fluorometric)	Females: Onset of menstruation: 4–25 μg/24 h	4–25 μg/24 h	Hyperestrogenism due to gonadal or adrenal neoplasm	Primary or secondary amenorrhea
	Ovulation peak: 28 μg/24 h	28 μg/24 h		
	Luteal peak: 22–105 μg/24 h	22–105 μg/24 h		
	Menopausal: 1.4–19.6 μg/24 h	1.4–19.6 μg/24 h		
	Males: 5–18 μg/24 h	5–18 μg/24 h		
Etiocholanolone	Males: 1.9–6 mg/24 h	6.5–20.6 μmol/24 h	Adrenogenital syndrome	
	Females: 0.5–4 mg/24 h	1.7–13.8 μmol/24 h	Idiopathic hirsutism	
Follicle-stimulating hormone—RIA	Females: Follicular: 5–20 IU/24 h	5–20 IU/d	Menopause and primary ovarian failure	Pituitary failure
	Luteal: 5–15 IU/24 h	5–15 IU/d		
	Midcycle: 15–60 IU/24 h	15–60 IU/d		
	Menopausal: 50–100 IU/24 h	50–100 IU/d		
	Males: 5–25 IU/24 h	5–25 IU/d		
Glucose	Negative		Diabetes mellitus Pituitary disorders Increased ICP Lesion in floor of 4th ventricle	
Hemoglobin and myoglobin	Negative		Extensive burns Transfusion of incompatible blood Myoglobin increased in severe crushing injuries to muscles	
Homogentistic add, qualitative	Negative		Alkaptonuria Ochronosis	
Homovanillic acid	Up to 15 mg/24 h	Up to 82 μmol/d	Neuroblastoma	
17-hydroxycortico-steroids	2–10 mg/24 h	5.5–27.5 μmol/d	Cushing's disease	Addison's disease Anterior pituitary hypofunction
5-Hydroxyindoleascetic add, qualitative	Negative		Malignant carcinoid tumors	
Hydroxyproline	15–43 mg/24 h	0.11–0.33 μmol/d	Paget disease Fibrous dysplasia Osteomalacia Neoplastic bone diseases Hyperparathyroidism	

(continued)

TABLE I-4 Reference Ranges—Urine Chemistry (Continued)

Determination	Normal Adult Reference Range		Clinical Significance	
	Conventional Units	*SI Units*	*Increased*	*Decreased*
17-ketosteroids, total	Males: 10–22 mg/24 h Females: 6–16 mg/24 h	35–76 µmol/d 21–55 µmol/d	Interstitial cell tumor of testes Simple hirsutism, occasionally Adrenal hyperplasia Cushing's syndrome Adrenal cancer, virilism Adrenoblastoma	Thyrotoxicosis Female hypogonadism Diabetes mellitus Hypertension Debilitating disease of mild to moderate severity Eunuchoidism Addison's disease Panhypopituitarism Myxedema Nephrosis
Lead Luteinizing hormone	Up to 150 µg/24 h Males: 5–18 IU/24 h Females: Follicular phase: 2–25 IU/24 h Ovulatory peak: 30–95 IU/24 h Luteal phase: 2–20 IU/24 h Postmenopausal: 40–110 IU/24 h	Up to 60 µmol/24 h 2–25 IU/d 30–95 IU/d 2–20 IU/d 40–110 IU/d	Lead poisoning Pituitary tumor Ovarian failure	 Depressed or failure to peak—pituitary failure
Metanephines, total	Less than 1.3 mg/24 h	Less than 6.5 µmol/d	Pheochromocytoma, a few patients with pheochromocytoma may have elevated urinary metanephines but normal catecholamines and vanillylmandelic acid (VMA)	
Osmolality	Males: 390–1090 mM/kg Females: 300–1090 mM/kg	390–1090 mmol/kg 300–1090 mmol/kg	Useful in the study of electrolyte and water balance	
Oxalate	Up to 40 mg/24 h	Up to 456/µmol/d	Primary hyperoxaluria	
Phenylpyruvic acid qualitative	Negative		Phenylketonuria	
Phosphorus, inorganic	0.8–1.3 gm/24 h	26–24 mmol/24 h	Hypoparathyroidism Vitamin D intoxication Paget's disease Metastatic neoplasm to bone	Hypoparathyroidism Vitamin D deficiency
Porphobilinogen, qualitative	Negative		Chronic lead poisoning Acute porphyria Liver disease	
Porphobilinogen quantitative	0–1 mg/24 h	0–4.4 µmol/24 h	Acute porphyria Liver disease	
Porphyrins, qualitative	Negative		See porphyrins, quantitative	
Porphyrins, quantitative (coproporphyrin and uroporphyrin)	Coproporphyrin: 50–160 µg/24 h Uroporphyrin: up to 50 µ/24 h	0.075–0.24 µmol/24h Up to 0.06 µmol/24 h	Porphyria Lead poisoning (only coproporphyrin increased)	
Potassium	40–65 mEq/24 h	40–65 mmol/24 h	Hemolysis Chronic renal failure Acidosis Cushing's disease	Diarrhea Adrenocortical insufficiency

TABLE I-4   Reference Ranges—Urine Chemistry (Continued)

| Determination | Normal Adult Reference Range | | Clinical Significance | |
	Conventional Units	SI Units	Increased	Decreased
Pregnanediol	Females:		Corpus luteum cysts	Placental dysfunction
	Proliferative phase: 0.5–1.5 mg/24 h	1.6–4.8 µmol/24 h	When placental tissue remains in the uterus following parturition	Threatened abortion Intrauterine death
	Luteal phase: 2–7 mg/24 h	6–22 µmol/24 h	Some cases of adreno- cortical tumors	
	Menopause: 0.2–1 mg/24 h	0.6–3.1 µmol/24 h		
	Pregnancy:			
	Weeks of gestation mg/24 h	µmol/24 h		
	10–12 5–15	15.6–47		
	12–18 5–25	15.6–78.0		
	18–24 15–33	47.0–103.0		
	24–28 20–42	62.4–131.0		
	28–32 27–47	84.2–146.6		
	Males: 0.1–2 mg/24 h	0.3–6.2 µmol/24 h		
Pregnanetriol	0.4–2.4 mg/24 h	1.2–7.1 µmol/24 h	Congenital adrenal androgenic hyperplasia	
Protein	Up to 100 mg/24 h	Up to 100 mg/24 h	Nephritis Cardiac failure Mercury poisoning Bence-Jones protein in multiple myeloma Febrile states Hematuria	
Sodium	130–200 mEq/24 h	130–200 mmol/24 h	Useful in detecting gross changes in water and salt balance	
Titratable acidity	20–40 mEq/24 h	20–40 mmol/24 h	Metabolic acidosis	Metabolic alkalosis
Urea nitrogen	9–16 gm/24 h	0.32–0.57 mol/L	Excessive protein catabolism	Impaired kidney function
Uric add	250–750 mg/24 h	1.48–4.43 mmol/24 h	Gout	Nephritis
Urobilinogen	Random urine: <0.25 mg/dL	<0.42 mol/24 h	Liver and biliary tract disease	Complete or nearly complete biliary obstruction
	24-hour urine: up to 4 mg/24 h	Up to 6.76 µmol/24 h	Hemolytic anemias	Diarrhea Renal insufficiency
Uroporphyrins	Up to 50 µg/24 h	Up to 0.06 µmol/24 h	Porphyria	
Vanillylmandelic acid (VMA)	0.7–6.8 mg/24 h	3.5–34.3 µmol/24 h	Pheochromocytoma Neuroblastoma Ingestion of coffee, tea, aspirin, bananas, and several different drugs	
Xylose absorption test (5-hour)	16%–33% of ingested xylose	Fraction absorbed: 0.16–0.33		Malabsorption syndromes
Zinc	0.15–1.2 mg/24 h	2.3–18.4 µmol/24 h		

TABLE I-5   Reference Ranges—Cerebrospinal Fluid (CSF)

| Determination | Normal Adult Reference Range | | Clinical Significance | |
	Conventional Units	SI Units	Increased	Decreased
Albumin	15–30 mg/dL	150–300 mg/L	Certain neurologic disorders Lesion in the choroid plexus or blockage of the flow of CSF Damage to the blood central nervous system (CNS) barrier	
Cell count	0–5 mononuclear cells per cu mm	0–5 × 10⁶/L	Bacterial meningitis Neurosyphilis Anterior poliomyelitis Encephalitis lethargica	
Chloride	100–130 mEq/L	100–300 mmol/L	Uremia	Acute generalized meningitis Tuberculous meningitis
Glucose	50–75 mg/dL	2.75–4.13 mmol/L	Diabetes mellitus Diabetic coma Epidemic encephalitis Uremia	Acute meningitides Tuberculous meningitis Insulin shock
Glutamine	6–15 mg/dL	0.41–1 mmol/L	Hepatic encephalopathies, including Reye's syndrome Hepatic coma Cirrhosis	
IgG	0–6.6 mg/dL	0–66 mg/L	Damage to the blood CNS barrier Multiple sclerosis Neurosyphilis Subacute sclerosing panencephalitis Chronic phases of CNS infections	
Lactic acid	<24 mg/dL	<2.7 mmol/L	Bacterial meningitis Hypocapnia Hydrocephalus Brain abscesses Cerebral ischemia	
Lactic dehydrogenase	¹⁄₁₀ that of serum	Activity fraction: 0.1 of serum	CNS disease	
Protein: Lumbar Cisternal Ventricular	 15–45 mg/dL 15–25 mg/dL 5–15 mg/dL	 150–450 mg/L 150–250 mg/L 50–150 mg/L	Acute meningitides Tubercular meningitis Neurosyphilis Poliomyelitis Guillain-Barré syndrome	
Protein electrophoresis (cellulose acetate) Prealbumin Albumin Alpha, globulin Alpha2 globulin Beta globulin Gamma globulin	% of total: 3–7 56–74 2–6.5 3–12 8–18.5 4–14	Fraction: 0.03–0.07 0.56–0.74 0.02–0.065 0.03–0.12 0.08–0.185 0.04–0.14	An increase in the level of albumin alone can be the result of a lesion in the choroid plexus or a blockage of the flow of CSF. An elevated gamma globulin value with a normal albumin level has been reported in multiple sclerosis, neurosyphilis, subacute sclerosing panencephalitis, and the chronic phase of CNS infections. If the blood-CNS barrier has been damaged severely during the course of these diseases, the CSF albumin level may also be elevated.	

TABLE I-6 Miscellaneous Values

Determinations	Normal Value	Clinical Significance	
		Conventional Units	*SI Units*
Acetaminophen	Zero	Therapeutic level = 10–20 μg/mL	10–20 mg/L
Aminophylline (theophylline)	Zero	Therapeutic level = 10–20/μg/mL	10–20 mg/L
Bromide	Zero	Therapeutic level = 5–50 mg/dL	50–500 mg/L
Carbamazepine	Zero	Therapeutic level = 8–12 μg/mL	34–51 μmol/L
Carbon monoxide	0%–2%	Symptoms with >20% saturation	
Chlordiazepoxide	Zero	Therapeutic level = 1–3 μg/mL	1–3 mg/L
Diazepam	Zero	Therapeutic level = 0.5–2.5 μg/dL	5–25 μg/L
Digitoxin	Zero	Therapeutic level = 5–30 ng/mL	5–30 μg/L
Digoxin	Zero	Therapeutic level = 0.5–2 ng/mL	0.5–2/μg/L
Ethanol	0%–0.01%	Legal intoxication level = 0.10% or above 0.3%–0.4% = marked intoxication 0.4%–0.5% = alcoholic stupor	
Gentamicin	Zero	Therapeutic level = 4–10 μg/mL	4–10 mg/L
Lithium	Zero	Therapeutic level = 0.6–1.2 mEq/L	0.6–1.2 mmol/L
Methanol	Zero	May be fatal in concentration as low as 10 mg/dL	100 mg/L
Phenobarbital	Zero	Therapeutic level = 15–40 μg/mL	10–20 mg/L
Phenytoin	Zero	Therapeutic level = 10–20 μg/mL	10–20 mg/L
Primidone	Zero	Therapeutic level = 5–12 μg/mL	5–12 mg/L
Quinidine	Zero	Therapeutic level = 0.2–0.5 mg/dL	2–5 mg/L
Salicylate	Zero	Therapeutic level = 2–25 mg/dL Toxic level = >30 mg/dL	20–250 mg/L 300 mg/L
Vancomycin	Zero	Therapeutic peak 18.0–26.0 μg/mL Therapeutic trough 5.0–10.0 μg/mL	
Amitriptyline	Zero	Therapeutic level 120–250 mg/mL	433–903 nmol/L
Doxepin	Zero	Therapeutic level 30–150 ng/mL	107–537 nmol/L
Imipramine	Zero	Therapeutic level 125–250 ng/mL	446–893 nmol/L
Lidocaine	Zero	Therapeutic level 1.5–6.0 μg/mL	6.4–25.6 μmol/L
Methotrexate	Zero	Toxic (48 hr. after high dose) 454 mg/mL	1000 mmol/L
Propranolol	Zero	Therapeutic level 50–100 ng/mL	193–386 nmol/L
Valproic acid	Zero	Therapeutic level 50–100 g/mg	347–693 mmol/L

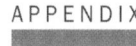

APPENDIX

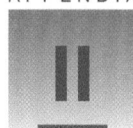

Conversion Tables

Metric Units and Symbols

Quantity	Unit	Symbol	Equivalent
Length	millimeter	mm	1000 mm = 1 m
	centimeter	cm	100 cm = 1 m
	decimeter	dm	10 dm = 1 m
	meter	m	1000 m = 1 km
Volume	cubic centimeter	cc or cm³	1000 cc = 1 cm³ or liter
	milliliter	ml	1000 mL = 1 liter
	cu decimeter	dm³	1000 dm³ = 1 m³
	liter	L	1000 L = 1 m³
Mass	microgram	μg	1000 μg = 1 mg
	milligram	mg	1000 mg = 1 g
	gram	g	1000 g = 1 kg
	kilogram	kg	1000 kg = 1 metric ton (t)

To convert from pounds to kilograms, divide by 2.2.
To convert from kilograms to pounds, multiply by 2.2.

Celsius (Centigrade) and Fahrenheit Temperatures

Celsius (Centigrade) 0°	Fahrenheit 32°
36.0	96.8
36.5	97.7
37.0	98.6
37.5	99.5
38.0	100.4
38.5	101.3
39.0	102.2
39.5	103.1
40.0	104.0
40.5	104.9
41.0	105.8
41.5	106.7
42.0	107.6

To convert degrees F. to degrees C: Subtract 32, then multiply by ⅝.
To convert degrees C. to degrees F: Multiply by ⅝, then add 32.

Table of Metric and Apothecaries' Systems
(Approved *approximate* dose equivalents are enclosed in parentheses. Use exact equivalents in calculations.)

Metric	Apothecaries	Metric	Apothecaries
1 milligram (mg)	¹⁄₆₄ grain	3.888 cubic centimeters or grams	1 dram (4 cc or grams)
64.79 milligrams	1 grain (65 mg)	31.103 cubic centimeters or grams	1 ounce (30 cc or grams)
1 gram	15.43 grains (15 grains)	473.167 cubic centimeters	1 pint (500 cc)
1 cubic centimeter (cc)*	16 minims		

*Note: A cubic centimeter (cc.) is the approximate equivalent of a milliliter (ml.). The terms are used interchangeably in general medicine.

NOMOGRAM FOR ESTIMATING SURFACE AREA OF INFANTS AND YOUNG CHILDREN

HEIGHT		SURFACE AREA	WEIGHT	
feet	centimeters	in square meters	pounds	kilograms

HEIGHT		SURFACE AREA	WEIGHT	
			65	30
			60	
			55	25
		.8	50	
3′	95	.7	45	20
34″	90		40	
32″	85	.6	35	15
30″	80			
28″	75	.5	30	
26″	70			
2′	65	.4	25	10
22″	60		20	
20″	55	.3		
18″	50		15	
16″	45			5
14″	40	.2	10	4
1′	35			3
10″	30			
9″	25		5	2
8″		.1	4	
	20		3	1

To determine the surface area of the patient, draw a straight line between the point representing the patient's height on the left vertical scale to the point representing the patient's weight on the right vertical scale. The point at which this line intersects the middle vertical scale represents the surface area in square meters. (Courtesy of Abbott Laboratories.)

NOMOGRAM FOR ESTIMATING SURFACE AREA OF OLDER CHILDREN AND ADULTS

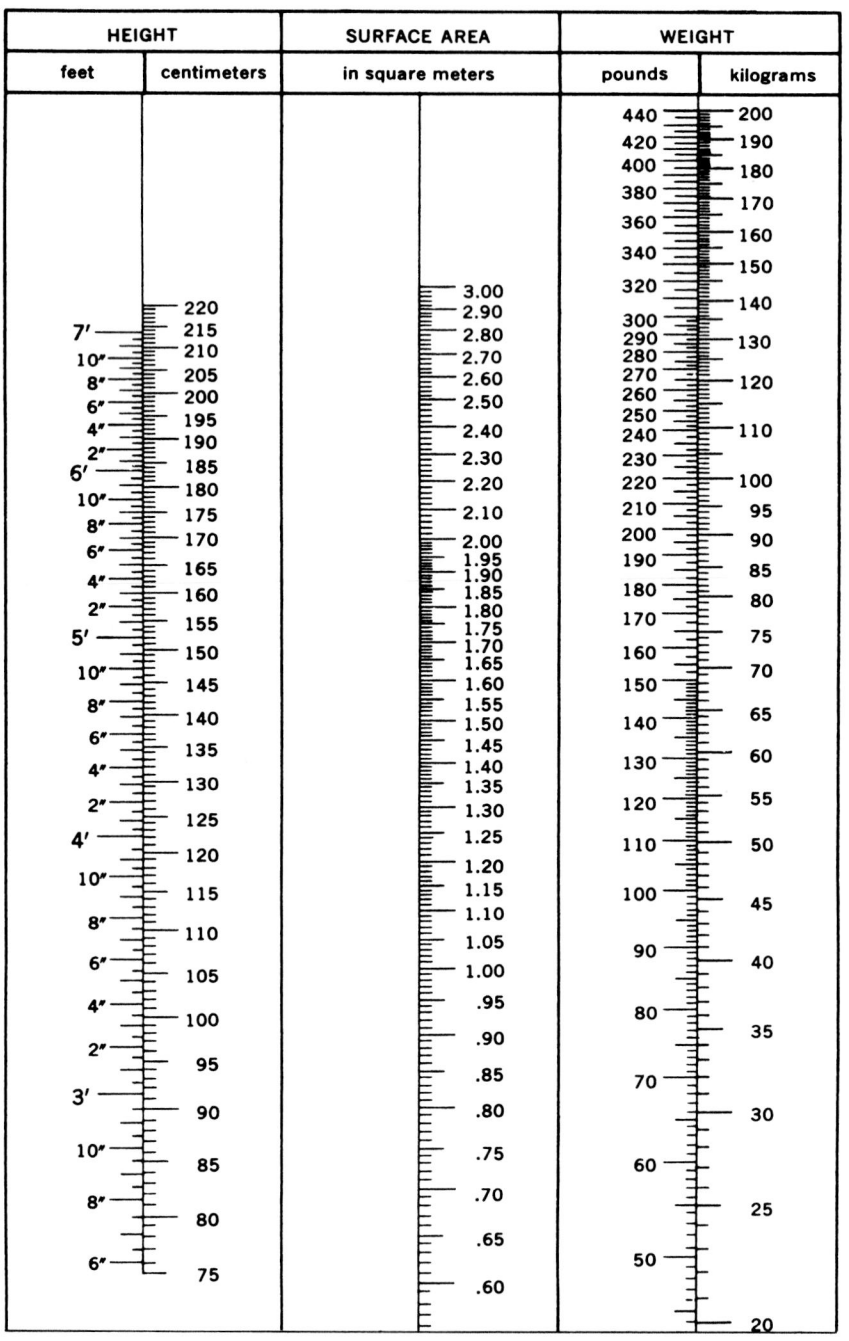

See Nomogram for Estimating Surface Area of Infants and Young Children for instructions on use. (Courtesy of Abbott Laboratories.)

Pediatric Laboratory Values

BLOOD CHEMISTRIES

These values are compiled from a review of current published literature; however, normal values vary with the analytic method used. If any doubt exists, consult your laboratory for its analytical method and normal range of values.

Determination	Conventional Units	SI Units	Determination	Conventional Units	SI Units
Acid phosphatase			Aspartate amino-transferase (AST)		
Newborn	7.4–19.4 U/ml	7.4–19.4 U/ml	Newborn/infant	25–65 U/L	25–65 U/L
2–13 yr	6.4–15.2 U/ml	6.4–15.2 U/ml	Child/adult	0–35 U/L	0–35 U/L
Adult	M: 0.5–11 U/ml	0.5–11.0 U/ml	Bicarbonate		
	F: 0.2–9.5 U/ml	0.2–9.5 U/ml	Premature	18–26 mEq/L	18–26 mmol/L
Alanine aminotrans-ferase (ALT)			Infant	20–25 mEq/L	20–25 mmol/L
			>2 yr	22–26 mEq/L	22–26 mmol/L
Infants	<54 U/L	<54 U/L	Bilirubin (total)		
Children/adults	1–30 U/L	1–30 U/L	Cord	<2 mg/dl	<34 µmol/L
Aldolase			24 h		
Adult	<8 U/L	<8 U/L	Preterm	≤8 mg/dl	≤137 µmol/L
Children	<16 U/L	<16 U/L	Term	≤ 6 mg/dl	≤103 µmol/L
Newborn	<32 U/L	<32 U/L	48 h		
Alkaline phosphatase			Preterm	<12 mg/dl	<205 µmol/L
Infant	150–420 U/L	150–420 U/L	Term	≤ 8 mg/dl	≤137 µmol/L
2–10 yr	100–320 U/L	100–320 U/L	3–5 days		
11–18 yr			Preterm	≤16 mg/dl	≤274 µmol/L
Male	100–390 U/L	50–390 U/L	Term	≤12 mg/dl	≤205 µmol/L
Female	100–320 U/L	100–320 U/L	1 mo-Adult	≤ 2 mg/dl	≤34 µmol/L
Adult	30–120 U/L	30–100 U/L	Conjugated	≤ 0.4 mg/dl	≤9 µmol/L
Alpha-1-antitrypsin	93–224 mg/dl		Calcium (total)		
Alpha-fetoprotein	<30 ng/dl	<0.1 g/L	Premature <1 week	6–10 mg/dl	1.5–2.5 mmol/L
	<30 mcg/L		Full-term <1 week	7–12 mg/dl	1.75–3 mmol/L
Ammonia nitrogen	Newborn:		Child	8–10.5 mg/dl	2–2.6 mmol/L
(venous sample:	90–150 µg/dl	64–107 µmol/L	Adult	8.5–10.5 mg/dl	2.1–2.6 mmol/L
heparinized speci-	>1 month:		Calcium (ionized)	4.4–5.4 mg/dl	0.1–1.35 mmol/L
men in ice water	29–70 µg/dl	21–50 µmol/L	Carbon dioxide		
and analyzed within			(CO_2 content)		
30 min)			Cord blood	14–22 mmol/L	14–22 mmol/L
All ages	0–50 µg/dl	0–35 µmol/L	Child	20–24 mmol/L	20–24 mmol/L
Amylase			Adult	24–30 mmol/L	24–30 mmol/L
Newborn	0–44 U/L	5–65 U/L			*(continued)*
> 1 yr	0–88 U/L	25–125 U/L			
Arsenic	<3 µg/dl	<0.4 mmol/L			

Determination	Conventional Units	SI Units
Carbon monoxide (carboxyhemoglobin)		
Nonsmoker	<2% of total hemoglobin	
Smoker	<10% of total hemoglobin	
Lethal	>60% of total hemoglobin	
Carotenoids (carotenes)		
Infant	20–70 µg/dl	0.37–1.30 µmol/L
Child	40–130 µg/dl	0.74–2.42 µmol/L
Adult	50–250 µg/dl	0.95–4.69 µmol/L
Ceruloplasmin	23–58 mg/dl	210–530 µmol/L
Chloride	99–111 mEq/L	99–111 mmol/L
Cholesterol	See Lipids	
Copper		
0–6 mo	20–70 µg/dl	3.1–11 µmol/L
6 mo–6 yr	90–190 µg/dl	14–30 µmol/L
6–17 yr	80–160 µg/dl	12.6–25 µmol/L
Adult	80–155 µg/dl	12.6–24.4 µmol/L
Creatine Kinase (Creatine Phosphokinase)		

	Upper 95th Percentile (U/L)	
Age	Males	Females
1 d	600	500
2–10 d	440	440
<1 yr	170	170
1–7 yr	109	100
7–9 yr	103	85
9–11 yr	109	88
11–13 yr	108	85
13–15 yr	129	85
15–17 yr	247	74
17–19 yr	190	68

Creatinine (serum)

	Upper Limits, mg/dl (µmol/L)	
Age (yr)	Males	Females
1	0.6 (53)	0.5 (44)
2–3	0.7 (62)	0.6 (53)
4–7	0.8 (71)	0.7 (62)
8–10	0.9 (80)	0.8 (71)
11–12	1.0 (88)	0.9 (80)
13–17	1.2 (106)	1.1 (97)
18–20	1.3 (115)	1.1 (97)
Adult	1.2 (106)	1.4 (124)

Determination	Conventional Units	SI Units
Ferritin		
Children	7–140 ng/ml	7–140 µg/L
Fibrin degradation products		
Titer	1:50 = positive	
Fibrinogen	200–400 mg/dl	2–4 g/L

Determination	Conventional Units	SI Units
Folic acid (folate)	3–17.5 ng/L	4–20 nmol/L
Galactose		
Newborn	0–20 mg/dl	0–1.11 mmol/L
Thereafter	<5 mg/dl	<0.28 mmol/L
Gammaglutamyl transferase (GGT)		
Cord	19–270 U/L	19–270 U/L
Premature	56–233 U/L	56–233 U/L
0–3 wk	0–130 U/L	0–130 U/L
3 wk–3 mo	4–120 U/L	4–120 U/L
>3 mo		
M	5–65 U/L	5–65 U/L
F	5–35 U/L	5–35 U/L
1–15 yr	0–23 U/L	0–23 U/L
Gastrin	<100 pg/ml	<100 ng/L
Glucose (serum)		
Premature	45–100 mg/dl	1.1–3.6 mmol/L
Full term	45–120 mg/dl	1.1–6.4 mmol/L
1 wk–16 yr	60–105 mg/dl	3.3–5.8 nmol/L
>16 yr	70–115 mg/dl	3.9–6.4 nmol/L
Haptoglobin*	400–1800 mg/L	0.4–1.8 g/L
Iron		

	Iron		Iron Binding Capacity		% Saturation
	(µg/dl)	(µmol/L)	(µg/dl)	(µmol/L)	(µg/dl)
Newborn	100–250	18–45	59–175	10.6–31.3	65%
4–10 mo	40–100	7–18	250–400	45–72	25%
3–10 yr	50–120	9–22	250–400	45–72	30%
Adult	50–170	9–30	250–400	45–72	35%

Determination	Conventional Units	SI Units
Ketones		
Qualitative	Negative	
Quantitative	up to 3 mg%	5–30 mg/L
Lactate		
Capillary blood		
Newborn	≤27 mg/dl	<3.0 mmol/L
Child	5–20 mg/dl	0.56–2.25 mmol/L
Venous	5–20 mg/dl	0.5–2.2 mmol/L
Arterial	5–14 mg/dl	0.5–1.6 mmol/L
Lactate dehydrogenase (37°C)		
Newborn	160–1500 U/L	160–1500 U/L
Infant	150–360 U/L	150–360 U/L
Child	150–300 U/L	150–300 U/L
Adult	100–250 U/L	100–250 U/L
Lactate dehydrogenase isoenzymes (% total)		
LD$_1$ Heart		24–34%
LD$_2$ Heart, erythrocytes		35–45%
LD$_3$ Muscle		15–25%
LD$_4$ Liver, trace muscle		4–10%
LD$_5$ Liver, muscle		1–9%
Lipase	4–24 U/dl	20–180 U/L
Lipids		

(continued)

Determination	Conventional Units	SI Units	Determination	Conventional Units	SI Units
Cholesterol (mg/dl)			Pyruvate	0.3–0.9 mg/dl	0.03–0.10 mmol/L
Desirable: <170			Sodium		
Borderline: 170–199			Premature	130–140 mEq/L	130–140 mmol/L
High: ≥200			Older	135–148 mEq/L	135–148 mmol/L
HDL: >45 mg/dl			Transaminase (SGOT)	*See Aspartate Aminotransferase (AST)*	
LDL: (mg/dl)			Transaminase (SGPT)	*See Alanine Aminotransferase (AT)*	
Desirable: <110			Troponin	0.03–0.15 ng/ml	
Borderline: 110–129			Urea nitrogen	7–22 mg/dl	2.5–7.9 mmol/L
High: ≥130			Uric acid		
Magnesium	1.3–2 mEq/L	0.65–1 mmol/L	0–2 yr	2.0–6.4 mg/dl	0.14–0.38 mmol/L
Manganese (blood)			2–12 yr	2.4–5.9 mg/dl	0.14–0.35 mmol/L
Newborn	2.4–9.6 µg/dl	2.44–1.75 µmol/L	12–14 yr	2.4–6.4 mg/dl	0.14–0.38 mmol/L
2–18 yr	0.8–2.1 µg/dl	0.15–0.38 µmol/L	14–adult		
Methemoglobin	1.3% of total Hb		M	3.5–7.2 mg/dl	2–0.43 mmol/L
5′ Nucleotidase	2.2–15 U/L	2.2–15 U/L	F	2.4–6.4 mg/dl	0.14–0.38 mmol/L
Osmolality	285–295 mOsm/kg	270–285 mOsm/L plasma	Vitamin A (retinol)		
			0–1 yr	20–90 µg/dl	0.7–3.14 µmol/L
Phenylalanine			1–5 yr	30–100 µg/dl	1.05–3.50 µmol/L
Premature	2.0–7.5 mg/dl	0.12–0.45 mmol/L	5–16 yr	60–100 µg/dl	2.09–3.50 µmol/L
Newborn	<1.2–3.4 mg/dl	0.07–0.21 mmol/L	Adult	20–80 µg/dl	0.70–2.79 µmol/L
Child	<3 mg/dl	<0.18 mmol/L	Vitamin B$_1$ (thiamine)	5.3–7.9 µg/dl	0.16–0.23 µmol/L
Phosphorus			Vitamin B$_2$ (riboflavin)	3.7–13.7 µg/dl	98–363 mmol/L
Newborn	4.2–9.0 mg/dl	1.36–2.91 mmol/L	Vitamin B$_{12}$ (cobalamin)	130–785 pg/ml	96–579 pmol/L
1 yr	3.8–6.2 mg/dl	1.23–2.0 mmol/L	Vitamin C	0.2–2 mg/dl	11.4–113.6 µmol/L
2–5 yr	3.5–6.8 mg/dl	1.13–2.2 mmol/L	(ascorbic acid)		
Adult	3.0–4.5 mg/dl	0.97–1.45 mmol/L	Vitamin D		
Porcelain	0.52–1.94 mg/dl	0.32–9.93	(1.25 dihydroxy)		
			Newborn	21 ± 2 pg/ml	50 ± 4.8 nmol/L
Potassium			Child	43 ± 3 pg/ml	103 ± 7.2 nmol/L
<10 days of age	4–6 mEq/L	4–6 mmol/L	Adult	29 ± 2 pg/ml	69.6 ± 4.8 nmol/L
>10 days of age	3.5–5 mEq/L	3.5–5 mmol/L	Vitamin E	5–20 µg/dl	8.4–23 µmol/L
Prolactin			Zinc	70–150 µg/dl	10.7–23 µmol/L
Newborn	<200 ng/ml	<200 µg/L			
Adult	<20 ng/ml	<20 µg/L			
Proteins Average (Range) in g/dl					

*Detectable in only 10%–20% of newborns.
(Adapted from Siberry, G. K. & Iannone, R. [Eds.] [2000]. *The Harriet Lane handbook* [15th ed.]. St. Louis: Mosby.)

Age	Total	Albumin	Globulin	Gamma Globulin
Premature	5.5 (4.0–7.0)	3.7 (2.5–4.5)	1.8 (1.2–2.0)	0.7 (0.5–0.9)
FT newborn	6.4 (5.0–7.1)	3.4 (2.5–5.0)	3.1 (1.2–4.0)	0.8 (0.7–0.9)
1-mo	6.6 (4.7–7.4)	3.8 (3.0–4.2)	2.5 (1.0–3.3)	0.3 (0.1–0.5)
3–12 mo	6.8 (5.0–7.5)	3.9 (2.7–5.0)	2.6 (2.0–3.8)	0.6 (0.4–1.2)
1–15 yr	7.4 (6.5–8.6)	4.0 (3.2–5.0)	3.1 (2.0–4.0)	0.9 (0.6–1.2)

Normal Values—Hematology

Age	Hgb (gm %) Mean (−2SD)	HCT (%) Mean (−2SD)	MCV (fl.) Mean (−2SD)	MCHC (gm/% RBC) Mean (−2SD)	Retic (%)	WBC/mm³ × 100 Mean (−2SD)	Plts (10³/mm³) Mean (±2SD)
26–30 wk gestation*	13.4 (11)	41.5 (34.9)	118.2 (106.7)	37.9 (30.6)	—	4.4 (2.7)	254 (180–327)
28 wk	14.5	45	120	31	(5–10)	—	275
32 wk	15.0	47	118	32	(3–10)	—	290
Term† (cord)	16.5 (13.5)	51 (42)	108 (98)	33 (30)	(3–7)	18.1 (9–30)‡	290
1–3 days	18.5 (14.5)	56 (45)	108 (95)	33 (29)	(1.8–4.6)	18.9 (9.4–34)	192
2 wk	16.6 (13.4)	53 (41)	105 (88)	31.4 (28.1)		11.4 (5–20)	252
1 mo	13.9 (10.7)	44 (33)	101 (91)	31.8 (28.1)	(0.1–1.7)	10.8 (5–19.5)	
2 mo	11.2 (9.4)	35 (28)	95 (84)	31.8 (28.3)			
6 mo	12.6 (11.1)	36 (31)	76 (68)	35 (32.7)	(0.7–2.3)	11.9 (6–17.5)	
6 mo—2 yr	12 (10.5)	36 (33)	78 (70)	33 (30)		10.6 (6–17)	(150–350)
2–6 yr	12.5 (11.5)	37 (34)	81 (75)	34 (31)	(0.5–1.0)	8.5 (5–15.5)	(150–350)
6–12 yr	13.5 (11.5)	40 (35)	86 (77)	34 (31)	(0.5–1.0)	8.1 (4.5–13.5)	(150–350)
12–18 yr							
Male	14.5 (13)	43 (36)	88 (78)	34 (31)	(0.5–1.0)	7.8 (4.5–13.5)	(150–350)
Female	14 (12)	41 (37)	90 (78)	34 (31)	(0.5–1.0)	7.8 (4.5–13.5)	(150–350)

* Values are from fetal samplings.
† Under 1 month, capillary Hgb exceeds venous: 1 h–3.6 gm difference; 5 days–2.2 gm difference; 3 wks–1.1 gm difference.
‡ Mean (95% confidence limits).
(Adapted from Siberry, G. K. & Iannone, R. [Eds.] [2000]. *The Harriet Lane handbook* [15th ed.]. St. Louis: Mosby.)

Normal Serologic Reference Values

Determination	Value
Antinuclear antibody	<1:80
Anti-streptolysin O titer*	
Preschool	<1:85
School ages and adults	<1:170
Older adults	<1:85
Anti-hyaluronidase	<1:256
C-reactive Protein	Negative
C₁ Esterase inhibitor	17.4–24 mg/dl
C₃	
1–6 mo	53–175 mg/dl
7–12 mo	75–180 mg/dl
1–5 yr	77–166 mg/dl
6–10 yr	88–199 mg/dl
Adult	83–177 mg/dl
C₄	
1–6 mo	7–42 mg/dl
7–12 mo	9.5–39 mg/dl
1–5 yr	9–40 mg/dl
6–10 yr	12–40 mg/dl
Adult	15–45 mg/dl
C_H50	75–160 U/ml
Rheumatoid factor	<20 negative
	20–40 suggestive
	≥80 positive
Rheumaton titer (modified Waaler-Rose slide test)	Negative ≥10 may be significant
Total B cells	5%–20% of lymphocytes
Total T cells	50%–80% of lymphocytes
T helper cells	34%–56% of lymphocytes
T suppressor cells	18%–32% of lymphocytes
Helper/suppressor ratio	1.1–2.5

* Significant if rising titer can be demonstrated at weekly intervals.
(Adapted from Siberry, G. K. & Iannone, R. [Eds.] [2000]. *The Harriet Lane handbook* [15th ed.]. St. Louis: Mosby.)

Cerebrospinal Fluid Values

Determination	Value
Cell Count	
Preterm mean	9.0 (0–25.4 WBC/mm³) (57% PMNs)
Term mean	8.2 (0.–22.4 WBC/mm³) (61% PMNs)
> 1 mo	0–7 (0% PMNs)
Glucose	
Preterm	24–63 mg/dl (mean 50)
Term	34–119 mg/dl (mean 52)
Child	40–80 mg/dl
CSF Glucose/ Blood Glucose (%)	
Preterm	55–105
Term	44–128
Child	50%
Lactic acid dehydrogenase	20 U/ml (range 5–30 U/ml)
Myelin basic protein	<4 ng/ml
Pressure (initial lumbar puncture)	
Newborn	80–110 (<110) mm H₂O
Infant	<200 (lateral recumbent position)
Child	mm H₂O
Respiratory movements	5–10 mm H₂O
Protein	
Preterm	65–150 mg/dl (mean 115)
Term	20–170 mg/dl (mean 90)
Children	
Ventricular	5–15 mg/dl
Cisternal	5–25 mg/dl
Lumbar	5–40 mg/dl

(Adapted from Siberry, G. K. & Iannone, R. [Eds.] [2000]. *The Harriet Lane handbook* [15th ed.]. St. Louis: Mosby.)

Sample Conversions of Pounds and Ounces to Grams*

Pounds	Ounces															
	0	1	2	3	4	5	6	7	8	9	10	11	12	13	14	15
0	—	28	57	85	113	142	170	198	227	255	283	312	340	369	397	425
1	454	482	510	539	567	595	624	652	680	709	737	765	794	822	850	879
2	907	936	964	992	1021	1049	1077	1106	1134	1162	1191	1219	1247	1276	1304	1332
3	1361	1389	1417	1446	1474	1503	1531	1559	1588	1616	1644	1673	1701	1729	1758	1786
4	1814	1843	1871	1899	1928	1956	1984	2013	2041	2070	2098	2126	2155	2183	2211	2240
5	2268	2296	2325	2353	2381	2410	2438	2466	2495	2532	2551	2580	2608	2637	2665	2693
6	2722	2750	2778	2807	2835	2863	2892	2920	2948	2977	3005	3033	3062	3090	3118	3147

*1 ounce = approximately 30 grams.
(From Avery, GB. [1994]. *Neonatology* [4th ed.]. Philadelphia: J.B. Lippincott.)

Herbal Preparations Used As Health Remedies

Sales of herbal and dietary supplements have skyrocketed over the past decade. Sales have gone from less than $50 million dollars in 1991 to close to $4 billion dollars in 1998. With the passage of the Dietary Supplement Health Education Act of 1994, the burden of proof for these supplements shifted from the manufacturers to prove that a supplement is safe and effective before it can be marketed, to the FDA to prove that a supplement is unsafe before it can be removed from the market. As a result, herbs are more widely available than ever before, and more patients use them.

Patients' use of herbal supplements is not without its dangers. Legislation has not clearly established good manufacturing practices for herbal supplements. As a result, there are no gold standards for potency or prevention of contamination of supplements. As information is more widely shared between countries, such as that contained in the highly visible German Commission E monographs, tightened regulation may occur. Some companies have come forward with standardized extracts, which are often the herbal preparations that are used in controlled studies and give a kind of "fingerprint" of identification to a specific herb. Other companies guarantee potency and purity and freely share their quality control standards with consumers and health professionals. However, not all companies use these standards. As a result, patients can suffer unexpected adverse effects if they are not checking their companies carefully.

Furthermore, clinical data on many herbs are scarce, making predictions for interactions with medications difficult or impossible. Patients often do not tell their providers that they are taking herbs in addition to their medications.

Patients should be encouraged to tell their health care providers about any alternative forms of therapy they are using. Any advice on herbal supplements should be given as objectively as possible to encourage these disclosures.

The herbs and dietary supplements listed in this table are among the most popular on the market. Many of these also have the most clinical data on use. However, designations of efficacy or safety should not be taken as permission to give these medications therapeutically. None of these herbs has undergone long-term, large-scale, randomized, double-blinded trials. None are recognized as safe or effective by the FDA. Most human trials performed with these herbs have been small (fewer than 100—200 subjects). Safety assumes appropriate, short-term use with no contraindications. If herbs are used at all in patients, it should occur only after more conventional therapies have been exhausted, under the supervision of a physician, and with special attention to the adverse effects that could occur with treatment.

In 1983 the FDA proposed a list of unsafe herbs that should not be used in foods, beverages, or drugs. The list was withdrawn but is still widely used. It includes the following: arnica (*Arnica montana*), belladonna/deadly nightshade (*Atropa belladonna*), bittersweet (*Solanum dulcamara*), bloodroot (*Sanguinara canadensis*), calamus (*Acorus calamus*), heliotrope (*Heliotropium eropaeum*), henbane (*Hyoscyamus niger*), Irish broom (*Cytisus scoparius*), jalap root (*Exagonium purga, Ipomoea nutt, Exagonium jalapa*), jimson weed (*Datura stramonium*), lily of the valley (*Convallaria majalis*), lobelia (*Lobelia inflata*), mandrake (*Mandragora officinarum, Podophyllum peltatum*), mistletoe (*Phoradendron flavescens, Vis-*

cum flavescens, Phoradendron juniperinum, Viscum album), morning glory (*Ipomoea purpurea*), periwinkle (*Vinca major, Vinca minor*), poison hemlock (*Conium maculatum*), spindle-tree (*Euonymus europaeus*), tonka bean (*Dipteryx odorata, Coumarouna odorata, Dipteryx oppositifolia, Coumarouna oppositifolia*), wahoo bark (*Euonymus atropurpureus*), white snakeroot (*Eupatorium rugosum, E. ogeratoides, L. urticaefoli*), wormwood (*Artemsia absinthium*), and yohimbe (*Corynanthe yohimbi*). Horse chestnut (*Aesculus hippocastanum*) and St. John's Wort (*Hypericum perforatum*) are also listed; however, side effect incidence has been low in clinical trials when specific extracts were used. Other unsafe herbs include betel nut (*Areca catechu*), chaparral (*Larrea tridenta. L. divaricata, L. mexicana*), coltsfoot (*Tussilago farfara*), comfrey (*Symphytum officinale*), germander (*Teucrium scorodonia*), and pennyroyal (*Hedeoma pulegoides, Mentha pulegium*).

Additional information for health care professionals and clients can be obtained from:

National Institutes of Health/Office of Dietary Supplements at *http://dietary-supplements.info.nih.gov*

FDA Center for Food Safety and Applied Nutrition at *http://vm.cfscan.fda.gov/dms.supplmnt.html*

REFERENCES

Blumenthal, M., Busse, W.R., Goldberg, A., Gruenwald, J., Hall, T., et al. (1998). *The complete Commission E monographs*. Austin, TX: American Botanical Council.

Brevoort, P. (1998). The booming U.S. botanical market: A new overview. *HerbalGram, 44*, 33–46.

Brinker, F. (1998). *Herb contraindications and drug interactions* (2nd ed.). Sandy, OR: Eclectic Medical Publications.

Cauffield, J.S. & Forbes, H.J.M. (1999). Dietary supplements used in the treatment of depression, anxiety, and sleep disorders. *Lippincott's Primary Care Practice, 3*, 290–304.

Da Camara, C.C & Dowless, G.V. (1998). Glucosamine for osteoarthritis. *Annals of Pharmacotherapy, 32*, 580–587.

Der Marderosian, A. (1999). *The review of natural products*. Philadelphia: Facts and Comparisons.

FDA's List of Unsafe Herbs at *http://www.herbsnmore.com/herbs unsafelist.html*. (accessed 12/17/99)

Foster, S. & Tyler, V.E. (1999). *Tyler's honest herbal* (4th ed.). New York: The Haworth Herbal Press.

Leung, A.Y. & Foster, S. (1996). *Encyclopedia of common natural ingredients used in food, drugs, and cosmetics*. New York: John Wiley & Sons.

Newall, C.A., Anderson, L.A. & Phillipson, J.D. (1996). *Herbal medicines: A guide for health-care professionals*. London: The Pharmaceutical Press.

Schulz, V., Hansel, R., & Tyler, V.E. (1998) *Rational phytotherapy*. New York: Springer-Verlag.

Taffe, A.M. & Cauffield, J.S. (1998). "Natural" hormone replacement therapy and dietary supplements used in the treatment of menopausal symptoms. *Lippincott's Primary Care Practice, 3*, 292–304.

Herbal Supplement	Popular Uses	Usual Dose Range	Possible Side Effects	Safety in Pregnancy and Lactation	Possible Medication Interactions	Possible Efficacy / Type of Study	Probable Safety
Cardiovascular and Circulatory							
CoEnzyme Q10, ubiquinone	Heart problems	100–600 mg daily.	None known	Unknown	None known	+, in vitro and human studies	+
Garlic (*Allium sativa*)	Hyperlipidemia, antiplatelet, hypertension, anti-infective, digestive disorders	3.6–5.4 mg allicin/day (enteric-coated, freeze-dried)	Heartburn, flatulence, increased bleeding risk (with >5 cloves garlic/day), possible allergies	Contraindicated	Antiplatelet agents (aspirin, clopidogrel), anticoagulants, including warfarin	+, human studies	+
Green tea (*Camellia sinensis*)	To prevent heart disease, cancer, lower cholesterol, as an antioxidant, an antimicrobial	3–9 cups/day	Possible increased risk for esophageal cancer due to tannin content, not conclusive; asthma	Contraindicated	May prevent absorption of concomitantly administered medications; separate by several hours	+ in vitro ?, human studies	+
Hawthorn (*Crataegus* sp.)	Mild heart failure (NYHA Stage I or II)	0.3–1.0 g dried fruit, 0.5–1.0 mL 1:1 liquid extract or 1–2 mL 1:5 in 45% alcohol tid (standardized to procyanidin or flavinoid content)	Nausea, fatigue, sweating, hand rashes	Contraindicated	Digoxin	?, human studies	+, human studies
Gastrointestinal							
Aloe (*Aloe barbadensis*)	Juice or latex: laxative	20–30 mg hydroxyanthrecene derivatives/day as aloin	Cramps, electrolyte depletion with long-term use	Contraindicated	Digoxin, diuretics, other stimulant laxatives	+, human studies	?
	Gel: wound healing	Apply to affected area as needed	None			+, animal studies	+
Chammomile (*Matricaria recutita*)	Gastrointestinal disorders, inflammation of mucous membranes and skin, sedative, anti-inflammatory, anti-infective	2–8 g dried flowers or 1–4 mL 1:1 in 45% alcohol tid	Allergic reactions, #	Contraindicated	None known	?, human studies	+
Flaxseed (*Linium usitatissimum*)	Constipation, irritable bowel syndrome, diverticulitis, estrogenic effects, hyperlipidemia	15–45 g milled seed; contains alpha-linoleic acid	None known Intestinal obstruction, dehydration: contraindicated	Contraindicated	May decrease absorption of concomitantly administered medications	+, human studies	+
Ginger (*Zingiber officinale*)	Nausea, motion sickness, dyspepsia	0.25–1.0 dried ginger root daily	Gallstones: contraindicated	Unknown	Antiplatelet agents (aspirin, clopidogrel), anticoagulants, including warfarin	+, human studies	+
Licorice (*Glycyrrhiza glabra*)	Coughs, colds, gastric ulcers, liver disease	5–15 g root, approximately 200–600 mg glycyrrhizin	Renal insufficiency, high blood pressure, hypokalemia, heart disease, liver disease, diabetes	Contraindicated	Digoxin, diuretics, corticosteroids, insulin, amoliride, spironolactone, stimulant laxatives	+, human studies	?

Herb	Uses	Dosage	Side effects/Adverse reactions	Pregnancy	Drug interactions	Efficacy	Rating
Milk thistle (*Silybum marianum*)	Dyspepsia, supportive treatment of liver disease, protection from chemical and hepatitis-induced liver damage	12–15 g herb (200–400 mg silymarin as silibinin)	Mild transient gastrointestinal effects Allergic reactions, #	Unknown	None known	+, human studies	+
Endocrine							
Bilberry (*Vaccinium myrtillus*)	Diarrhea, improving visual acuity, diabetes	20–60 g dried berry	None known	Unknown	None known	?, human studies	?
Bitter melon (*Momordica charantia*)	Diabetes	15 g aqueous extract, 50 mL extract	None reported in humans; seeds are toxic, may cause liver damage (animal data)	Contraindicated	May potentiate the effects of sulfonylureas, insulin, other antidiabetic agents	+, animal studies +, human studies	? to +
Dehydroepiandrosterone (DHEA)	Multiple uses, including anti-aging agent, in the place of estrogen replacement therapy, memory loss	25–50 mg po qd	High blood pressure, glucose intolerance, increased risk for breast and prostate cancer	Contraindicated	None known	? to +, human studies	? to (–), human studies
Vascular							
Gingko biloba	Decreased circulation (cerebral, intermittent claudication)	40 mg tid (as Egb-761 or LI 1370; 24% flavinoids and 6% terpenes)	Occasional stomach or intestinal upset, headaches, allergy	Unknown	Antiplatelet agents (aspirin, clopidogrel), anticoagulants, including warfarin	+, human studies	+
Grapeseed extract (*Vitis vinifera*)	Vascular insufficiency	50 mg daily	None reported	Unknown	None reported	+, human studies	+
Horse chestnut (*Aesculus hippocastanum*)	Vascular insufficiency	30–150 mg aesculin/day	Gastrointestinal symptoms Bleeding disorders: contraindicated	Unknown	Antiplatelet agents (aspirin, clopidogrel), anticoagulants, including warfarin	+, human studies	+
Musculoskeletal/Pain							
Indian frankincense tree (*Boswellia serrata*)	Pain reliever, anti-inflammatory, particularly for arthritis	350 mg tid	None reported	Unknown	None reported	?, human studies	+
Devil's claw (*Harpagophytum procumbens*)	To alleviate pain, particularly arthritis and back pain	0.1–0.25 g tid, up to 6 g/day dried root or 50 mg harpagoside	None known	Unknown; may be contraindicated	None reported	?, human studies	? to +
Glucosamine	Arthritis	1500 mg/day	Gastrointestinal side effects	Contraindicated	None known	+	+
Immune System							
Cat's claw, Una de gato (*Uncaria guianensis, U. tomentosa*)	Immunostimulant anti-cancer agent, anti-inflammatory for arthritis, inflammatory bowel disease, etc.	1–5 g powdered bark or one cup of tea 2–3 times daily	None reported	Unknown	None reported	+, in vitro ?, human studies	?
Echinacea (*Echinacea purpura, E. angustiflora, E. pallida*)	Immune-stimulant, colds, upper respiratory tract, externally for wound healing	6–9 mL freshly pressed plant juice; hydroalcoholic extract, maximum of 6–8 weeks*	Allergic reactions, # Autommune diseases (eg, rheumatoid arthritis, lupus), progressive systemic disease (eg, multiple sclerosis), HIV: contraindicated	Unknown	None reported	+, human studies	+, human studies

(continued)

Herbal Supplement	Popular Uses	Usual Dose Range	Possible Side Effects	Safety in Pregnancy and Lactation	Possible Medication Interactions	Possible Efficacy / Type of Study	Probable Safety
Goldenseal (*Hydrastis canadensis*)	Anti-infective, digestive disorders, to mask a positive drug screen	Endangered species, banned from international trade.	None reported Contraindicated in ear infection with purulent discharge	Contraindicated	None reported	?, no effect on drug screens.	+
Korean ginseng (*Panax ginseng*)	"Adaptogen" (increases the body's ability to resist stress and resist disease)	1–2 g ginseng or 200–600 mg standardized extract (4–7% ginsenosides)*	Insomnia, diarrhea, skin eruptions	Contraindicated	Monoamine oxidase inhibitors, caffeine, warfarin, insulin (speculative, AS)	?	+
Siberian ginseng, eluthero, ciwujia (*Elutherococcus senticosus*)	"Adaptogen," particularly to improve athletic performance	2–3 g root/day*	None known BP >180/90 mm Hg; possibly contraindicated	Contraindicated	Barbiturates (speculative, AS), monomycin, kanamycin, insulin (speculative, AS)	?	+
Genitourinary							
Cranberry (*Vaccinium macrocarpon*)	Urinary tract infections, particularly in women	5–20 mL cranberry cocktail/day	None reported	Unknown	None known	+, in vitro, ? human studies	+
Uva Ursi (*Arctostaphylos uva ursi*)	Urinary tract inflammatory disorders, diuretic	1.5–4.0 g (100–210 mg hydroquinone) as a tea qid (no longer than 1 week)	Nausea, vomiting Renal disease: contraindicated	Contraindicated	None known	+, animal studies	?
Saw palmetto (*Serenoa repens*)	Benign prostatic hypertrophy	1–2 s berry or 320 mg lipophilic extract (90% v/v hexane or ethanol) daily	Occasional gastrointestinal side effects	Contraindicated	None known	+, human studies, superior to finasteride, comparable to alpha blocker	+
Gynecologic Conditions							
Black cohosh (*Cimicifuga racemosa*)	Menopausal symptoms, premenstrual syndrome, painful menstruation	Alcohol extract (40–60% v/v) equivalent to 40 mg herb	Occasional gastrointestinal discomfort	Contraindicated	None known	?	?
Chaste berry (*Vitex agnus castus*)	Premenstrual syndrome, irregularities of the menstrual cycle	Aqueous-alcohol extract (50–70% v/v) equivalent to 30–40 mg berry	Occasional pruritus, urticaria	Contraindicated	May interfere with birth-control pills, may antagonize dopamine antagonists (eg, antipsychotics)	? to +, human studies	+
Dong quai (*Angelica sinensis*)	Menopausal symptoms, premenstrual syndrome, painful menstruation	1000–3390 mg/day dried root	Photosensitivity, particularly with high doses	Contraindicated	None known	?	–

Herb	Uses	Dose/Comments	Adverse effects	Pregnancy	Drug interactions		
Evening primrose oil (black currant or borage oil, cisgamma linoleic acid-GLA)	Premenstrual syndrome, rheumatoid arthritis, other autoimmune diseases, multiple sclerosis	Dose dependent on reason for taking; most common range is 2–3 g/day of an 8% GLA preparation	Gastrointestinal symptoms Borage oil may cause liver damage, avoid None reported for other forms of GLA	Unknown	None known	?	?
Soy/phytoestrogens (isoflavones)	As a substitute for estrogen replacement therapy	165 mg isoflavones (45 mg soy flour)	Headaches, oily skin	Do not exceed amounts found in foods	None known	?	?
Neurologic							
Feverfew (*Tanacetum parthenium*)	Migraine headaches	2.5 fresh leaves or 50 mg freeze-dried leaves daily	Mouth ulcers, gastrointestinal symptoms, # Allergic reactions	Contraindicated	None known	+, HS	+, HS
Guarana (*Paullinia cupana*)	Stimulant, weight loss	Contains 2.5–5% caffeine	Nervousness, insomnia, rapid or irregular heart beat, heartburn	Contraindicated	Monoamine oxidase inhibitors, ephedrine, adenosine, beta-blockers, phenyl-propanolamine, lithium, theophylline, and fluoroquinolones	?	?
Ma huang (*Ephedra* sp.)	Stimulant, weight loss, asthma	Contains ephedrine, which is a controlled substance in the United States; the status of ma huang is undetermined	Increases blood pressure and heart rate, palpitations, nervousness, headaches, insomnia and dizziness Contraindicated in heart disease, high blood pressure, diabetes, hyperthyroidism, history of substance abuse	Contraindicated	Theophylline, caffeine, monoamine oxidases, reserpine, amitriptyline	(+) for asthma, ? to (–) for other uses	? to (–)
Psychiatric							
Kava kava (*Piper methysticum*)	Anxiety	Clinical trials (WS 1490): 90–110 mg dried extract (70 mg kava-pyrones) daily	Yellow discoloration of skin, hair and nails, rare allergic reactions Depression: contraindicated	Contraindicated	Benzodiazepines (one case report of coma), alcohol, barbiturates	+, human studies	+
Hops	Insomnia, anxiety, restlessness	Single dose: 0.5 g hops (as a tea)	None known	Unknown	Barbiturates (speculative, AS)	+, animal studies	?
Melatonin	Insomnia, jet lag	Jet lag: 5–10 mg/day Insomnia: dose undefined	Headache, may worsen depression	Unknown	None known	+, small human studies	?
Passion flower (*Passiflora incarnata*)	Insomnia	?	None reported	Unknown	Barbiturates (speculative, AS)	+, animal studies	+

(continued)

Herbal Supplement	Popular Uses	Usual Dose Range	Possible Side Effects	Safety in Pregnancy and Lactation	Possible Medication Interactions	Possible Efficacy	Probable Safety
						Type of Study	
St. John's Wort (*Hypericum perforatum*)	Depression	Clinical trials (extract LI 160): 900–1800 mg/day	Photosensitivity, headache, nausea, vomiting, restless, dizziness, sedation, gastric symptoms	Contraindicated	Possible monoamine oxidase activity; avoid tyramine in diet, caffeine, decongestants, caffeine, SSRIs, amphetamines	+, human studies, = to 150 mg imipramine	+
Valerian (*Valeriana officinalis*)	Insomnia	2–3 g herb (as tea), up to several times daily, 1–2 mL tincture up to several times daily, 450–900 mg extract at bedtime	Cases of hepatotoxicity reported, may have been secondary to substitution with *Teucrium* species	Unknown	Barbiturates, benzodiazepines (speculative, in vitro, AS)	+, but human study results mixed	+

Key: (+) = possibly effective or safe; ? = inconclusive; (–) = ineffective or unsafe; * = prone to adulteration with other plants; # = individuals allergic to ragweed, chrysanthemums, marigolds, daisies, and other members of the *Asteraceae/Compositae* plant family may also be allergic to this plant. AS = animal studies; HS = human studies.

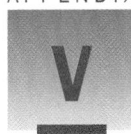
Sources of Further Information

Alzheimer's Association
919 North Michigan Avenue, Suite 1100
Chicago, IL 60611
800-272-3900
www.alz.org

American Academy of Allergy, Asthma, and Immunology
611 E. Wells Street
Milwaukee, WI 53202
414-272-6071
www.aaai.org

American Association of Kidney Patients
100 South Ashley Drive, Suite 200
Tampa, FL 33602
800-749-AAKP
www.aakp.org

American Academy of Medical Acupuncture
5820 Wilshire Blvd.
Los Angeles, CA 90036
323-937-5514
www.medicalacupuncture.org

American Brain Tumor Association
2720 River Road
Des Plaines, IL 60018
800-886-2282
www.abta.org

American Cancer Society (ACS)
19 West 56th Street
New York, NY 10019
212-586-8700, 800-ACS-2345
www.cancer.org

American College of Allergy, Asthma, and Immunology
800-842-7777
www.allergy.mcg.edu

American Council for the Blind
1155 15th Street, N.W., Suite 1004
Washington, DC 20005
202-467-5081
www.acb.org

American Diabetes Association
1660 Duke Street
Alexandria, VA 22314
800-676-4065
www.diabetes.org

American Dietetic Association
216 West Jackson Boulevard
Chicago, IL 60606-6995
800-366-1655

American Foundation for the Blind
11 Penn Plaza, Suite 300
New York, NY 10001
212-502-7600
www.afb.org

American Heart Association
772 Greenville Avenue
Dallas, TX 75231
214-373-6300
www.americanheart.org

American Latex Allergy Association
800-972-5378

American Lung Association
1740 Broadway
New York, NY 10019
212-315-8700
www.lungusa.org

American Pseudo-Obstruction and Hirschsprung's Disease Society
158 Pleasant Street
North Andover, MA 01845
978-685-4477
www.tiac.net/users/aphs

American Psychology and Medical Hypnosis Association
http://APMHA.com

American Social Health Association Herpes Hotline
PO Box 13827
Research Triangle Park, NC 27709
919-361-8488

American Speech Hearing Association
10801 Rockville Pike
Rockville, MD 20852
301-897-5700
800-638-TALK
www.asha.org

American Thyroid Association
www.thyroid.org

Amyotrophic Lateral Sclerosis Association
1021 Ventura Boulevard, Suite 321
Woodland Hills, CA 91364
800-782-4747
www.alsa.org

Anxiety Disorders Association of America
11900 Park Lawn Drive, Suite 100
Rockville, MD 20852
301-231-9350
www.adaa.org

Aplastic Anemia Foundation of America
P.O. Box 613
Annapolis, MD 21404
800-747-2820
www.aamds.org

ARC (formerly Association for Retarded Citizens)
1010 Wayne Avenue, Suite 650
Silver Spring, MD 20910
301-565-3842
http://thearc.org

Arthritis Foundation
1330 West Peachtree Street
Atlanta, GA 30309
404-872-7100
www.arthritis.org

Association of Bladder Exstrophy Children (ABC)
P.O. Box 1472
Wake Forest, NC 27588
919-554-3088
www.bladderexstrophy.com

Brain Injury Association
105 N. Alfred Street
Alexandria, VA 22314
703-236-6000

Candlelighters
3910 Warner Street
Kensington, MD 20895
800-366-2223
www.candlelighters.org

Canadian Celiac Association
www.celiac.ca

Celiac Disease Foundation
www.celiac.org

Celiac Sprue Association
P.O. Box 31700
Omaha, NE 68131
402-558-0600
www.csaceliacs.org

Centers for Disease Control and Prevention
404-639-3534
www.cdc.gov

Centers for Disease Control and Prevention National STD Hotline
800-227-8922

Children and Adults with Attention Deficit Disorders (CHADD)
8181 Professional Place, Suite 201
Landover, MD 20785
800-233-4050
www.chadd.org

Children's Heart Society—Canada
www.childrensheart.org

Choice in Dying
475 Riverside Drive, Room 1852
New York, NY 10115
800-989-9455
www.choices.org

Cleft Palate Foundation
104 South Estes Drive, Suite 204
Chapel Hill, NC 27514
800-242-5338
www.cleftline.org

Congenital Heart Disease Information and Resources
www.tchin.org

Congenital Heart Disease Resource Page
www.csun.edu

Cooley's Anemia Foundation
129-09 26th Avenue, Room 203
Flushing, NY 11354
718-321-2873
www.thalassemia.org

Corporate Angel Network
Westchester County Airport, 1 Loop Road
White Plains, NY 10604
914-328-1313
www.corpangelnetwork.org

Council for Learning Disabilities
P.O. Box 40303
Overland Park, KS 66204
913-492-8755
http://cldinternational.org

Crohn's & Colitis Foundation of America, Inc.
386 Park Avenue South
New York, NY 10016
212-685-3440
www.ccfa.org

Cushing's Support and Research Foundation
www.world.std.com/~csrf

Cystic Fibrosis Foundation
6931 Arlington Road
Bethesda, MD 20814
800-FIGHT CF
www.cff.org

Directory of Genetic Support Groups
http://members.aol.com/dnacutter/all.htm#B

Down Syndrome Parent Network
3226 Fallow Drive
Allentown, PA 18104
800-HELP309
www.dspn.org

Endometriosis Association
8585 North 76th Place
Milwaukee, WI 53223
800-992-3636

Epilepsy Foundation of America
4351 Garden City Drive
Landover, MD 20785
800-332-1000
www.epilepsyfoundation.org

Esophageal Atresia/Tracheoesophageal Fistula (EA/TEF)
    Family and Support Connection
111 West Jackson Blvd., Suite 1145
Chicago, IL 60604
3312-987-9085

Food Allergy Network
800-929-4040
www.foodallergy.org

Guillain-Barré Syndrome Foundation International
PO Box 262
Wynnewood, PA 19096
610-667-0131
www.webmast.com

Hemophilia Association
104 East 40th Street, Suite 506
New York, NY 10016
212-682-5510

Hydrocephalus Association
870 Market Street, Suite 705
San Francisco, CA 94102
415-732-7040
www.hydroassoc.org

Joseph P. Kennedy, Jr. Foundation
1325 G. Street, Suite 500
Washington, DC 20005
202-393-1250

Juvenile Diabetes Foundation International
120 Wall Street
New York, NY 10005
800-JDF-CURE
www.jdf.org

Juvenile Rheumatoid Arthritis (JRA) World
http://jraworld.arthritisinsight.com

Learning Disability Association of America
4156 Library Road
Pittsburgh, PA 15234
412-341-1515
www.ldanatl.org

Leukemia and Lymphoma Society
600 Third Avenue
New York, NY 10016
212-573-8484 or 800-955-4572
www.leukemia-lymphoma.org

Lupus Foundation
1300 Piccard Drive, Suite 200
Rockville, MD 20850-4303
800-558-0120
www.lupus.org

March of Dimes Birth Defects Foundation
1275 Mamaroneck Avenue
White Plains, NY 10605
914-428-7100
www.modimes.org

Medic Alert Foundation
2323 Colorado
Tarlock, CA 95381

Muscular Dystrophy Association
3300 East Sunrise Drive
Tucson, AZ 85718
520-529-2000
www.mdausa.org

Myasthenia Gravis Foundation, Inc.
61 Gramercy Park North, Room 605
New York, NY 10010
212-533-7005
email: *mgfgny@aol.com*

National Adrenal Diseases Foundation
www.medhelp.org/www/nadf.htm

National Alliance for Research on Schizophrenia and Depression
60 Cutter Mill Road, Suite 404
Great Neck, NY 11021
516-829-0091
www.narsad.org

National Cancer Institute
800-4-CANCER

National Clearinghouse on Child Abuse and Neglect
P.O. Box 1182
Washington, DC 20013-1182
800-FYI, 3366
www.calib.com/nccanch

National Coalition of Cancer Survivorship
1010 Wayne Ave., Suite 707
Silver Spring, MD 20910
888-937-6227
www.cansearch.org

National Down Syndrome Congress
7000 Peachtree-Dunwoody Road, N.E.
Lake Ridge 400 Office Park, Bldg. 5, Suite 100
Atlanta, GA 30328
800-232-NDSC
www.ndscenter.org

National Down Syndrome Society
666 Broadway
New York, NY 10012
212-460-9330
www.ndss.org

National Foundation for Depressive Illness
P.O. Box 2257
New York, NY 10116
800-248-4344

National Fragile X Foundation
P.O. Box 190488
San Francisco, CA 94119
800-688-8765
http://nfxf.org

National Herpes Hotline
919-361-8488

National Information Center for Children and Youth With Disabilities (NICHCY)
P.O. Box 1492
Washington, DC 20013
800-695-0285
www.nichcy.org

National Institute of Allergy and Infectious Diseases
NIAID Office of Communications
Bldg. 31, Room 7A-50
31 Center Drive MSC 2520
Bethesda, MD 20892-2520
301-496-5717
www.niaid.nih.gov

National Institute of Diabetes, Gastrointestinal and Kidney Diseases
3 Information Way
Bethesda, MD 20892
301-654-4415
www.niddk.nih.gov

National Institutes of Health, Institute on Aging Alzheimer Disease Education and Referral Center
800-438-4380
www.alzheimer.org

National Kidney Foundation
30 East 33rd Street
New York, NY 10016
212-889-2210
www.kidney.org

National Marrow Donor Program
www.marrow.org

National Multiple Sclerosis Society
733 Third Avenue
New York, NY 10017
212-986-3240
www.nmss.org

National Organization of Mothers of Twins Clubs, Inc.
12404 Princess Jeanne NE
Albuquerque, NM 87112-4640
877-540-2200

National Organization for Rare Disorders, Inc.
P.O. Box 8923
New Fairfield, CT 06812
203-746-6518
www.nord-rdb.com

National Osteoporosis Foundation
800-223-9994
www.nof.org

National Parkinson's Foundation
www.parkinson.org

National Prevention Information Network (information
   on STDs, TB, and AIDS)
1-800-458-5231

National Stroke Association
9709 East Easter Lane
Englewood, CO 80102
303-649-9299
www.stroke.org

Pituitary Tumor Network Association
www.pituitary.com

PMS Access (postmenstrual syndrome)
P.O. Box 9326
Madison, WI 53715
800-222-4767

Prevent Blindness America
500 East Remington Road
Schaumburg, IL 60173
800-331-2020
www.preventblindness.org

Prevent Child Abuse America
332 South Michigan Avenue, Suite 1600
Chicago, IL 60604
800-55NCPCA

Sickle Cell Disease Foundation
5110 West Goldleaf Circle, #150
Los Angeles, CA 90056
323-299-3600
www.scdfc.org

Spina Bifida Association of America
4590 MacArthur Boulevard, N.W., Suite 250
Washington, DC 20007
800-621-3141
www.sbaa.org

Sudden Infant Death Syndrome Foundation
1314 Bedford Avenue, Suite 210
Baltimore, MD 21208
800-638-7437
www.sidsalliance.org

Sudden Infant Death: Information
   and Counseling Program
520 First Avenue, Room 419
New York, NY 10016
212-686-8854

Take Pounds Off Safely (TOPS)
P.O. Box 070360
4575 South Fifth Street
Milwaukee, WI 53207
414-482-4620
www.tops.org

United Cerebral Palsy Association
1660 L. Street, N.W., Suite 700
Washington, DC 20036
800-872-5827
www.ucp.org

United Ostomy Association
19772 MacArthur Blvd., Suite 200
Irvine, CA 92612-2405
800-826-0826
www.uoa.org

United Scleroderma Foundation
89 Newbury Street, Suite 201
Danvers, MA 01923
800-722-HOPE
www.scleroderma.org

US TOO International (prostate cancer support)
930 North York Road, Suite 50
Hinsdale, IL 60521
800-808-7866
www.ustoo.com

Subject Index

Note: Pages in *italics* indicate illustrations; those followed by t indicate tables; and those followed by p indicate procedures.

Art Credit List

The following pieces of art were borrowed from Lippincott Williams & Wilkins sources:

Chapter 5

Figure 5-1: Weber, J. and Kelly, J. (1998). *Health assessment in nursing.* Philadelphia: Lippincott Williams & Wilkins. Photograph by Barbara Proud.

Figure 5-2: Craven, R. and Hirnle, C., (2000). *Fundamentals of nursing: Human health and function,* 3rd edition. Philadelphia: Lippincott Williams & Wilkins.

Figure 5-3: Bickley, L. (1999). *Bates' guide to physical examination and history taking,* 7th edition. Philadelphia: Lippincott Williams & Wilkins

Figure 5-5: Craven, R. and Hirnle, C., (2000). *Fundamentals of nursing: Human health and function,* 3rd edition. Philadelphia: Lippincott Williams & Wilkins.

Figure 5-6: Smeltzer, S. and Bare, B. (2000). *Brunner and Suddarth's textbook of medical-surgical nursing,* 9th edition. Philadelphia: Lippincott Williams & Wilkins.

Figure 5-7: Smeltzer, S and Bare, B. (2000). *Brunner and Suddarth's textbook of medical-surgical nursing,* 9th edition. Philadelphia: Lippincott Williams & Wilkins.

Figure 5-8: Weber, J. and Kelly, J. (1998). *Health assessment in nursing.* Philadelphia: Lippincott Williams & Wilkins. Photograph by Barbara Proud.

Figure 5-9: Weber, J. and Kelly, J. (1998). *Health assessment in nursing.* Philadelphia: Lippincott Williams & Wilkins.

Figure 5-10: Weber, J. and Kelly, J. (1998). *Health assessment in nursing.* Philadelphia: Lippincott Williams & Wilkins. Photograph by Barbara Proud.

Figure 5-11: Craven, R. and Hirnle, C., (2000). *Fundamentals of nursing: Human health and function,* 3rd edition. Philadelphia: Lippincott Williams & Wilkins.

Figure 5-12: Weber, J. and Kelly, J. (1998). *Health assessment in nursing.* Philadelphia: Lippincott Williams & Wilkins. Photograph by Barbara Proud.

Figure 5-14: Weber, J. and Kelly, J. (1998). *Health assessment in nursing.* Philadelphia: Lippincott Williams & Wilkins. Photograph by Barbara Proud.

Figure 5-15: Weber, J. and Kelly, J. (1998). *Health assessment in nursing.* Philadelphia: Lippincott Williams & Wilkins. Photograph by Barbara Proud.

Figure 5-19: Bickley, L. (1999). *Bates' guide to physical examination and history taking,* 7th edition. Philadelphia: Lippincott Williams & Wilkins

Figure 5-20: Bickley, L. (1999). *Bates' guide to physical examination and history taking,* 7th edition. Philadelphia: Lippincott Williams & Wilkins

Figure 5-28: Bickley, L. (1999). *Bates' guide to physical examination and history taking,* 7th edition. Philadelphia: Lippincott Williams & Wilkins

Figure 5-29: Smeltzer, S. and Bare, B. (2000). *Brunner and Suddarth's textbook of medical-surgical nursing,* 9th edition. Philadelphia: Lippincott Williams & Wilkins.

Figure 5-32: Bickley, L. (1999). *Bates' guide to physical examination and history taking,* 7th edition. Philadelphia: Lippincott Williams & Wilkins

Figure 5-33: Weber, J. and Kelly, J. (1998). *Health assessment in nursing.* Philadelphia: Lippincott Williams & Wilkins. Photograph by Barbara Proud.

Figure 5-34: Weber, J. and Kelly, J. (1998). *Health assessment in nursing.* Philadelphia: Lippincott Williams & Wilkins. Photograph by Barbara Proud.

Figure 5-35: Weber, J. and Kelly, J. (1998). *Health assessment in nursing.* Philadelphia: Lippincott Williams & Wilkins. Photograph by Barbara Proud.

Figure 5-36: Bickley, L. (1999). *Bates' guide to physical examination and history taking,* 7th edition. Philadelphia: Lippincott Williams & Wilkins

Figure 5-38: Bickley, L. (1999). *Bates' guide to physical examination and history taking,* 7th edition. Philadelphia: Lippincott Williams & Wilkins

Figure 5-39: Bickley, L. (1999). *Bates' guide to physical examination and history taking,* 7th edition. Philadelphia: Lippincott Williams & Wilkins

Figure 5-40: Bickley, L. (1999). *Bates' guide to physical examination and history taking,* 7th edition. Philadelphia: Lippincott Williams & Wilkins

Figure 5-41: Craven, R. and Hirnle, C., (2000). *Fundamentals of nursing: Human health and function,* 3rd edition. Philadelphia: Lippincott Williams & Wilkins.

Figure 5-45: Weber, J. and Kelly, J. (1998). *Health assessment in nursing.* Philadelphia: Lippincott Williams & Wilkins. Photograph by Barbara Proud.

Figure 5-46: Weber, J. and Kelly, J. (1998). *Health assessment in nursing.* Philadelphia: Lippincott Williams & Wilkins. Photograph by Barbara Proud.

Figure 5-47: Weber, J. and Kelly, J. (1998). *Health assessment in nursing.* Philadelphia: Lippincott Williams & Wilkins. Photograph by Barbara Proud.

Figure 5-48: Weber, J. and Kelly, J. (1998). *Health assessment in nursing.* Philadelphia: Lippincott Williams & Wilkins. Photograph by Barbara Proud.

Figure 5-49: Weber, J. and Kelly, J. (1998). *Health assessment in nursing.* Philadelphia: Lippincott Williams & Wilkins. Photograph by Barbara Proud.

Chapter 6

Figure 6-2: Smeltzer, S. and Bare, B. (2000). *Brunner and Suddarth's textbook of medical-surgical nursing,* 9th edition. Philadelphia: Lippincott Williams & Wilkins.

Chapter 7

Figure 7-4: Smeltzer, S. and Bare, B. (2000). *Brunner and Suddarth's textbook of medical-surgical nursing,* 9th edition. Philadelphia: Lippincott Williams & Wilkins.

Chapter 9

Figure 9-2: Smeltzer, S. and Bare, B. (2000). *Brunner and Suddarth's textbook of medical-surgical nursing,* 9th edition. Philadelphia: Lippincott Williams & Wilkins.

All photos in Box 9-5: Weber, J. and Kelly, J. (1998). *Health assessment in nursing.* Philadelphia: Lippincott Williams & Wilkins. Photographs by Barbara Proud.

Chapter 10

Figure 10-2A: Craven, R. and Hirnle, C., (2000). *Fundamentals of nursing: Human health and function,* 3rd edition. Philadelphia: Lippincott Williams & Wilkins.

Figure 10-4: Smeltzer, S. and Bare, B. (2000). *Brunner and Suddarth's textbook of medical-surgical nursing,* 9th edition. Philadelphia: Lippincott Williams & Wilkins.

Chapter 12

In Procedure Guidelines 12-3: Smeltzer, S. and Bare, B. (2000). *Brunner and Suddarth's textbook of medical-surgical nursing,* 9th edition. Philadelphia: Lippincott Williams & Wilkins.

In Procedure Guidelines 12-5: Smeltzer, S. and Bare, B. (2000). *Brunner and Suddarth's textbook of medical-surgical nursing,* 9th edition. Philadelphia: Lippincott Williams & Wilkins.

Chapter 13

Figure 13-2: Smeltzer, S. and Bare, B. (2000). *Brunner and Suddarth's textbook of medical-surgical nursing,* 9th edition. Philadelphia: Lippincott Williams & Wilkins.

Chapter 14

Figure 14-6: Smeltzer, S. and Bare, B. (2000). *Brunner and Suddarth's textbook of medical-surgical nursing,* 9th edition. Philadelphia: Lippincott Williams & Wilkins.

Chapter 15

Figure 15-5: Smeltzer, S. and Bare, B. (2000). *Brunner and Suddarth's textbook of medical-surgical nursing,* 9th edition. Philadelphia: Lippincott Williams & Wilkins.

Chapter 16

Figure 16-2: Smeltzer, S. and Bare, B. (2000). *Brunner and Suddarth's textbook of medical-surgical nursing,* 9th edition. Philadelphia: Lippincott Williams & Wilkins.

In Procedure Guidelines 16-1: Smeltzer, S. and Bare, B. (2000). *Brunner and Suddarth's textbook of medical-surgical nursing,* 9th edition. Philadelphia: Lippincott Williams & Wilkins.

In Procedure Guidelines 16-4: Bickley, L. (1999). *Bates' guide to physical examination and history taking,* 7th edition. Philadelphia: Lippincott Williams & Wilkins

Chapter 17

Figure 17-1: Smeltzer, S. and Bare, B. (2000). *Brunner and Suddarth's textbook of medical-surgical nursing,* 9th edition. Philadelphia: Lippincott Williams & Wilkins.

Figure 17-3: Bickley, L. (1999). *Bates' guide to physical examination and history taking,* 7th edition. Philadelphia: Lippincott Williams & Wilkins

Figure 17-6: Smeltzer, S. and Bare, B. (2000). *Brunner and Suddarth's textbook of medical-surgical nursing,* 9th edition. Philadelphia: Lippincott Williams & Wilkins.

Chapter 18

Figure 18-7: Smeltzer, S. and Bare, B. (2000). *Brunner and Suddarth's textbook of medical-surgical nursing,* 9th edition. Philadelphia: Lippincott Williams & Wilkins.

Figure 18-8: Smeltzer, S. and Bare, B. (2000). *Brunner and Suddarth's textbook of medical-surgical nursing,* 9th edition. Philadelphia: Lippincott Williams & Wilkins.

In Procedure Guidelines 18-1: Smeltzer, S. and Bare, B. (2000). *Brunner and Suddarth's textbook of medical-surgical nursing,* 9th edition. Philadelphia: Lippincott Williams & Wilkins.

Chapter 19

In Procedure Guidelines 19-2: Smeltzer, S. and Bare, B. (2000). *Brunner and Suddarth's textbook of medical-surgical nursing,* 9th edition. Philadelphia: Lippincott Williams & Wilkins.

Chapter 21

Figure 21-1: Porth, C. (1998). *Pathophysiology: Concepts of altered health states,* 5th ed. Philadelphia: Lippincott-Raven Publishers.

Chapter 21 (cont.)

Figure 21-2: Smeltzer, S. and Bare, B. (2000). *Brunner and Suddarth's textbook of medical-surgical nursing,* 9th edition. Philadelphia: Lippincott Williams & Wilkins.

Figure 21-3: Smeltzer, S. and Bare, B. (2000). *Brunner and Suddarth's textbook of medical-surgical nursing,* 9th edition. Philadelphia: Lippincott Williams & Wilkins.

Figure 21-4: Porth, C. (1998). *Pathophysiology: Concepts of altered health states,* 5th ed. Philadelphia: Lippincott-Raven Publishers.

Figure 21-5: Smeltzer, S. and Bare, B. (2000). *Brunner and Suddarth's textbook of medical-surgical nursing,* 9th edition. Philadelphia: Lippincott Williams & Wilkins.

Figure 21-6: Smeltzer, S. and Bare, B. (2000). *Brunner and Suddarth's textbook of medical-surgical nursing,* 9th edition. Philadelphia: Lippincott Williams & Wilkins.

Chapter 22

Figure 22-2: Smeltzer, S. and Bare, B. (2000). *Brunner and Suddarth's textbook of medical-surgical nursing,* 9th edition. Philadelphia: Lippincott Williams & Wilkins.

Figure 22-4: Smeltzer, S. and Bare, B. (2000). *Brunner and Suddarth's textbook of medical-surgical nursing,* 9th edition. Philadelphia: Lippincott Williams & Wilkins.

Figure 22-5: Reeder, S., Martin, L., and Koniak-Griffin, D., (1997). *Maternity nursing: Family, newborn, and women's health care,* 18th edition. Philadelphia: Lippincott-Raven Publishers.

In Procedure Guidelines 22-1: Smeltzer, S. and Bare, B. (2000). *Brunner and Suddarth's textbook of medical-surgical nursing,* 9th edition. Philadelphia: Lippincott Williams & Wilkins.

Chapter 24

Figure 24-3: Smeltzer, S. and Bare, B. (2000). *Brunner and Suddarth's textbook of medical-surgical nursing,* 9th edition. Philadelphia: Lippincott Williams & Wilkins.

Chapter 25

In Procedure Guidelines 25-2: Smeltzer, S. and Bare, B. (2000). *Brunner and Suddarth's textbook of medical-surgical nursing,* 9th edition. Philadelphia: Lippincott Williams & Wilkins.

Chapter 32

Figure 32-1: Smeltzer, S. and Bare, B. (2000). *Brunner and Suddarth's textbook of medical-surgical nursing*, 9th edition. Philadelphia: Lippincott Williams & Wilkins. Photo by Barbara Proud.

Figure 32-2: Smeltzer, S. and Bare, B. (2000). *Brunner and Suddarth's textbook of medical-surgical nursing*, 9th edition. Philadelphia: Lippincott Williams & Wilkins.

Figure 32-5: Smeltzer, S. and Bare, B. (2000). *Brunner and Suddarth's textbook of medical-surgical nursing*, 9th edition. Philadelphia: Lippincott Williams & Wilkins.

Figure 32-6: Smeltzer, S. and Bare, B. (2000). *Brunner and Suddarth's textbook of medical-surgical nursing*, 9th edition. Philadelphia: Lippincott Williams & Wilkins.

Figure 32-7: Smeltzer, S. and Bare, B. (2000). *Brunner and Suddarth's textbook of medical-surgical nursing*, 9th edition. Philadelphia: Lippincott Williams & Wilkins.

Figure 32-8: Smeltzer, S. and Bare, B. (2000). *Brunner and Suddarth's textbook of medical-surgical nursing*, 9th edition. Philadelphia: Lippincott Williams & Wilkins.

Figure 32-9: Smeltzer, S. and Bare, B. (2000). *Brunner and Suddarth's textbook of medical-surgical nursing*, 9th edition. Philadelphia: Lippincott Williams & Wilkins.

Figure 32-10: Smeltzer, S. and Bare, B. (2000). *Brunner and Suddarth's textbook of medical-surgical nursing*, 9th edition. Philadelphia: Lippincott Williams & Wilkins.

Figure 32-11: Smeltzer, S. and Bare, B. (2000). *Brunner and Suddarth's textbook of medical-surgical nursing*, 9th edition. Philadelphia: Lippincott Williams & Wilkins.

Figure 32-12: Smeltzer, S. and Bare, B. (2000). *Brunner and Suddarth's textbook of medical-surgical nursing*, 9th edition. Philadelphia: Lippincott Williams & Wilkins.

Chapter 33

Figure 33-1: Smeltzer, S. and Bare, B. (2000). *Brunner and Suddarth's textbook of medical-surgical nursing*, 9th edition. Philadelphia: Lippincott Williams & Wilkins.

Figure 33-3: Smeltzer, S. and Bare, B. (2000). *Brunner and Suddarth's textbook of medical-surgical nursing*, 9th edition. Philadelphia: Lippincott Williams & Wilkins.

Figure 33-4: Smeltzer, S. and Bare, B. (2000). *Brunner and Suddarth's textbook of medical-surgical nursing*, 9th edition. Philadelphia: Lippincott Williams & Wilkins.

Figure 33-5, A&B: Smeltzer, S. and Bare, B. (2000). *Brunner and Suddarth's textbook of medical-surgical nursing*, 9th edition. Philadelphia: Lippincott Williams & Wilkins.

Figure 33-5C: Porth, C. (1998). *Pathophysiology: Concepts of altered health states*, 5th ed. Philadelphia: Lippincott-Raven Publishers.

Chapter 35

Figure 35-1: Smeltzer, S. and Bare, B. (2000). *Brunner and Suddarth's textbook of medical-surgical nursing*, 9th edition. Philadelphia: Lippincott Williams & Wilkins.

In Procedure Guidelines 35-5: Smeltzer, S. and Bare, B. (2000). *Brunner and Suddarth's textbook of medical-surgical nursing*, 9th edition. Philadelphia: Lippincott Williams & Wilkins.

Chapter 36

Figure 36-6: Pillitteri, A. (1999). *Maternal and child health nursing: Care of the childbearing and childrearing family*, 3rd edition. Philadelphia: Lippincott-Raven.

Figure 36-7: Pillitteri, A. (1999). *Maternal and child health nursing: Care of the childbearing and childrearing family*, 3rd edition. Philadelphia: Lippincott-Raven.

Figure 36-9: Pillitteri, A. (1999). *Maternal and child health nursing: Care of the childbearing and childrearing family*, 3rd edition. Philadelphia: Lippincott-Raven.

Chapter 37

Figure 37-4: Pillitteri, A. (1999). *Maternal and child health nursing: care of the childbearing and childrearing family*, 3rd edition. Philadelphia: Lippincott-Raven.

Figure 37-6: Pillitteri, A. (1999). *Maternal and child health nursing: Care of the childbearing and childrearing family*, 3rd edition. Philadelphia: Lippincott-Raven.

Figure 37-11: Pillitteri, A. (1999). *Maternal and child health nursing: Care of the childbearing and childrearing family*, 3rd edition. Philadelphia: Lippincott-Raven.

Chapter 38

Figure 38-1: Reeder, S., Martin, L., and Koniak-Griffin, D., (1997). *Maternity nursing: family newborn, and women's health care*, 18th edition. Philadelphia: Lippincott-Raven Publishers.

Figure 38-2: Reeder, S., Martin, L., and Koniak-Griffin, D., (1997). *Maternity nursing: family, newborn, and women's health care*, 18th edition. Philadelphia: Lippincott-Raven Publishers.

Figure 38-4: Reeder, S., Martin, L., and Koniak-Griffin, D., (1997). *Maternity nursing: family, newborn, and women's health care*, 18th edition. Philadelphia: Lippincott-Raven Publishers.

Figure 38-5: Pillitteri, A. (1999). *Maternal and child health nursing: Care of the childbearing and childrearing family*, 3rd edition. Philadelphia: Lippincott-Raven.

Chapter 39

Figure 39-1: Pillitteri, A. (1999). *Maternal and child health nursing: Care of the childbearing and childrearing family*, 3rd edition. Philadelphia: Lippincott-Raven.

Figure 39-2: Pillitteri, A. (1999). *Maternal and child health nursing: Care of the childbearing and childrearing family*, 3rd edition. Philadelphia: Lippincott-Raven.

Figure 39-3: Pillitteri, A. (1999). *Maternal and child health nursing: Care of the childbearing and childrearing family*, 3rd edition. Philadelphia: Lippincott-Raven.

Figure 39-4: Pillitteri, A. (1999). *Maternal and child health nursing: Care of the childbearing and childrearing family*, 3rd edition. Philadelphia: Lippincott-Raven.

Figure 39-5: Reeder, S., Martin, L., and Koniak-Griffin, D., (1997). *Maternity nursing: Family newborn, and women's health care*, 18th edition. Philadelphia: Lippincott-Raven Publishers.

Figure 39-6: Pillitteri, A. (1999). *Maternal and child health nursing: Care of the childbearing and childrearing family*, 3rd edition. Philadelphia: Lippincott-Raven.

Figure 39-7: Pillitteri, A. (1999). *Maternal and child health nursing: Care of the childbearing and childrearing family*, 3rd edition. Philadelphia: Lippincott-Raven.

In Procedure Guidelines 39-1: Pillitteri, A. (1999). *Maternal and child health nursing: Care of the childbearing and childrearing family*, 3rd edition. Philadelphia: Lippincott-Raven.

Chapter 41

Figure 41-1: Pillitteri, A. (1999). *Maternal and child health nursing: Care of the childbearing and childrearing family,* 3rd edition. Philadelphia: Lippincott-Raven.

Chapter 42

Figure 42-3: Pillitteri, A. (1999). *Maternal and child health nursing: Care of the childbearing and childrearing family,* 3rd edition. Philadelphia: Lippincott-Raven.

Chapter 43

Photo in Procedure Guidelines 43-1: Pillitteri, A. (1999). *Maternal and child health nursing: Care of the childbearing and childrearing family,* 3rd edition. Philadelphia: Lippincott-Raven. Photograph by Barbara Proud.

In Procedure Guidelines 43-2: Pillitteri, A. (1999). *Maternal and child health nursing: Care of the childbearing and childrearing family,* 3rd edition. Philadelphia: Lippincott-Raven.

Chapter 44

Figure 44-2: Pillitteri, A. (1999). *Maternal and child health nursing: Care of the*

childbearing and childrearing family, 3rd edition. Philadelphia: Lippincott-Raven.

Photo in Procedure Guidelines 44-2: Pillitteri, A. (1999). *Maternal and child health nursing: Care of the childbearing and childrearing family,* 3rd edition. Philadelphia: Lippincott-Raven. Photograph by Caroline Brown.

Chapter 46

Figure 46-1: Pillitteri, A. (1999). *Maternal and child health nursing: Care of the childbearing and childrearing family,* 3rd edition. Philadelphia: Lippincott-Raven.

Figure 46-2: Pillitteri, A. (1999). *Maternal and child health nursing: Care of the childbearing and childrearing family,* 3rd edition. Philadelphia: Lippincott-Raven.

Figure 46-3: Pillitteri, A. (1999). *Maternal and child health nursing: Care of the childbearing and childrearing family,* 3rd edition. Philadelphia: Lippincott-Raven.

Chapter 47

Figure 47-1: Pillitteri, A. (1999). *Maternal and child health nursing: Care of the*

childbearing and childrearing family, 3rd edition. Philadelphia: Lippincott-Raven.

Chapter 49

Figure 49-1: Pillitteri, A. (1999). *Maternal and child health nursing: Care of the childbearing and childrearing family,* 3rd edition. Philadelphia: Lippincott-Raven.

Chapter 54

Figure 54-5: Pillitteri, A. (1999). *Maternal and child health nursing: Care of the childbearing and* childrearing family, 3rd edition. Philadelphia: Lippincott-Raven.

Buck's Traction in Procedure Guidelines 54-2: Pillitteri, A. (1999). *Maternal and child health nursing: Care of the childbearing and childrearing family,* 3rd edition. Philadelphia: Lippincott-Raven.

Balanced Suspension in Procedure Guidelines 54-2: Pillitteri, A. (1999). *Maternal and child health nursing: Care of the childbearing and childrearing family,* 3rd edition. Philadelphia: Lippincott-Raven.